OPTUM™

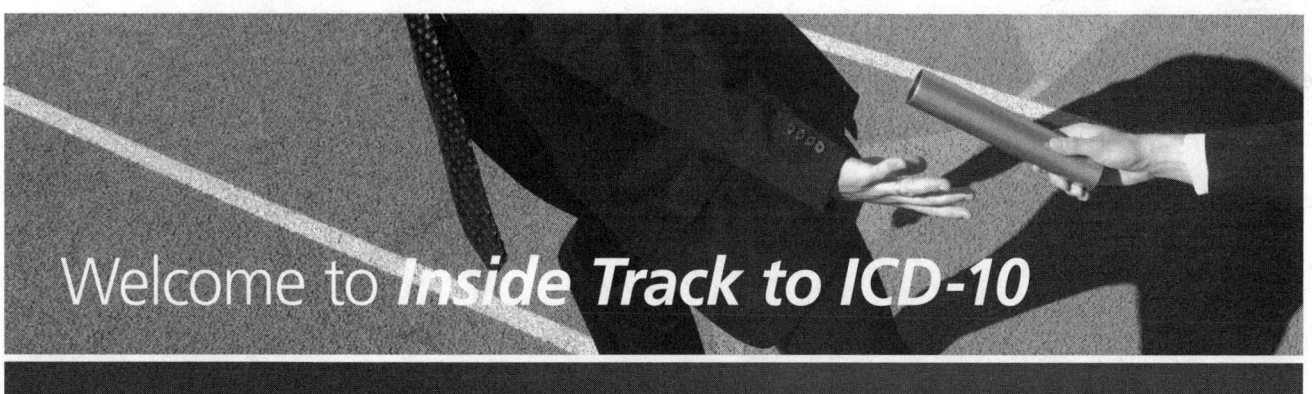

Welcome to *Inside Track to ICD-10*

Be sure to opt in to
Inside Track to ICD-10
(and pass this
great benefit along).

VISIT

OptumCoding.com/InsideTrack
to sign up today or scan the QR
code below with your smartphone.

Optum *Inside Track to ICD-10*, your new ICD-10 source.

Stay informed with *Inside Track to ICD-10*. Gain exclusive access to ICD-10-CM/PCS training and transition information via email when you purchase an ICD-9-CM, ICD-10-CM or ICD-10-PCS code book or sign up at OptumCoding.com/InsideTrack.

- ICD-10-CM/PCS updates and news
- Monthly eNewsletter
- Exclusive offers

Key features and benefits

For no additional cost, become a member of *Inside Track to ICD-10*, and share this benefit with your colleagues. Gain access to the latest tools and updates, conveniently delivered to your inbox to meet your organization's diagnosis coding needs.

- Stay on top of changing health care, code sets, and regulations with *Inside Track to ICD-10*
- Take advantage of the opportunity to participate in customer surveys and forums to help improve Optum diagnosis coding products
- Learn the latest ICD-10-CM/PCS news, transition updates and tips
- Link right to our online resources through *Inside Track to ICD-10* communications
- Learn about new tools available to help with your ICD-10 transition

Order your coding resources and earn rewards at **OptumCoding.com**

Get so much more when you shop at OptumCoding.com

- Find the products you need quickly and easily with our powerful search engine.
- View all available formats and edition years on the same page with consolidated product pages.

- Browse our eCatalog online.
- Chat live with a customer service representative; ask questions about the site or the checkout process.

- Visit Coding Central for expert resources, including articles, *Inside Track to ICD-10,* and coding scenarios to test your knowledge.

Register on OptumCoding.com for a customized website experience:

- View special website promotions/discounts.
- Get product recommendations based on your order history.
- Research your order history.
- Check on shipment status and tracking.
- View invoices and payment history.
- Pay outstanding invoices online.
- Manage your address book.
- Ship orders to multiple locations.
- Renew your order with a single click.

- Compile a wish list of the products you want and purchase when you're ready.

Rewards program

- Register for an account and you are automatically enrolled in our eRewards program! Receive a $50 coupon for every $500 you spend on OptumCoding.com.* When logged in, the eRewards meter keeps track of purchases toward your next reward.

REGISTER NOW: **Visit:** OptumCoding.com/Register   **Call:** 800.464.3649, option 1

RENEW TODAY

SAVE UP TO 25%

when you renew your coding essentials.

Buy 1–2 items, save 15%
Buy 3–5 items, save 20%
Buy 6+ items, save 25%

ITEM #	TITLE INDICATE THE ITEMS YOU WISH TO PURCHASE	QUANTITY	PRICE PER PRODUCT	TOTAL

	Subtotal	
(AK, DE, HI, MT, NH & OR are exempt)	Sales Tax	
1 item $10.95 • 2–4 items $12.95 • 5+ CALL	Shipping & Handling	
	TOTAL AMOUNT ENCLOSED	

Save up to 25% when you renew.

Visit **www.optumcoding.com**
and enter your promo code.

Call **1.800.464.3649, option 1,**
and mention the promo code.

Fax this order form with
purchase order to **801.982.4033.**
*Optum no longer accepts
credit cards by fax.*

Mail this order form with payment and/or purchase order to:
Optum, PO Box 88050, Chicago, IL 60680-9920.
Optum no longer accepts credit cards by mail.

Name

Address

Customer Number   Contact Number

○ CHECK ENCLOSED (PAYABLE TO OPTUM)

○ BILL ME   ○ P.O.#

(   )
Telephone
(   )
Fax

E-mail

Optum respects your right to privacy. We will not sell or rent your email address or fax number to anyone outside Optum and its
business partners. If you would like to remove your name from Optum promotions, please call 1.800.464.3649, option 1.

PROMO CODE
FOBA14C

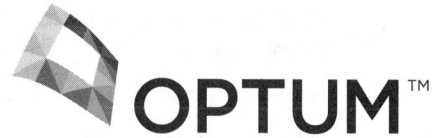

Dear Optum Customer:

Enclosed is the 2014 draft of the International Classification of Diseases, 10th Revision, Clinical Modification (ICD-10-CM) as written by the World Health Organization (WHO) and National Center for Healthcare Statistics (NCHS). These codes will replace the current ICD-9-CM system for medical documentation and reimbursement. Our new ICD-10-CM code book will help you get a head start with training programs and system conversion.

The Department of Health and Human Services (HHS) published the final rule regarding the adoption of both ICD-10-CM and ICD-10-PCS in the January 16, 2009, *Federal Register* (45 CFR part 162 [CMS—0013—FJ]). The initial compliance date for implementation of ICD-10-CM and ICD-10-PCS as a replacement for ICD-9-CM was October 1, 2013. On April 17, 2012, the department of Health and Human Services (HHS) released a notice to postpone the date by which certain health care entities have to comply with International Classification of Diseases, 10th Revision diagnosis and procedure codes (ICD-10). The compliance date for implementation of ICD-10-CM and ICD-10-PCS as a replacement for ICD-9-CM is October 1, 2014.

The ICD-9-CM Coordination and Maintenance Committee implemented a partial code set freeze of the ICD-10-CM codes prior to the initial implementation date of October 1, 2013. As a result, on October 1, 2013, there were only limited code updates to the ICD-10-CM code sets to capture new technologies and diseases as required by section 503(a) of Pub. L. 108-173. With the one-year delay in the compliance and implementation date, the same limited code set freeze will be in effect for October 1, 2014.

Corrections and minor revisions were made to the draft code set for 2014. The complete and official 2014 addenda to ICD-10-CM are available on the government website. Log on http://www.cdc.gov/nchs/icd/icd10cm.htm#10update.

Features and benefits include:

- **Exclusive Optum Edge Color Coding and Icons:**
    - **Optum Exclusive — Xtension 7th Alert Symbol.** This symbol (designed and used exclusively by Optum) alerts the coder to a new ICD-10-CM convention — the use of a "placeholder X"
    - **Optum Exclusive — Key Word.** Green font is used to differentiate key words that appear in similar code descriptions in a given category
    - **Optum Exclusive feature** — Exclusive *following* references and Check Additional Character symbol in the indexes. The *following* references (designed and used exclusively by Optum) help coders locate those alphanumeric codes that are out of sequence in the tabular section .
    - **Optum Exclusive feature** — Exclusive shaded guides in the index help users easily follow the indent levels for the subterms under a main term.
    - check character icons to alert coders to required 4th, 5th, 6th, and 7th characters
    - manifestation color coding to ensure appropriate etiology/manifestation code sequencing with no manifestation code sequenced as a first-listed or principal diagnosis
    - color-coded instructional notes that appear in red font
    - icons, footnotes, and color-coding for identification of Medicare Code Edits (MCEs) (v29) related to age and sex edits, wrong procedure performed, etc.
    - color-coding for identification of "other" and "unspecified" diagnosis codes to assure the most specific code is assigned
- **Illustrations.** Normal anatomy illustrations focusing on the terminology found in ICD-10-CM.
- **Official Preface (2014):** Official preface provided by National Center for Health Statistics (NCHS) as guidance concerning this pre-release draft of ICD-10-CM.
- **Guidelines and Conventions (2014):** The Draft ICD-10-CM Official Guidelines for Coding and Reporting for Acute Short-term and Long-term Hospital Inpatient and Physician Office and Other Outpatient Encounters has been included to assist you with appropriate and consistent code assignment.
- **Index (2014):** Official alphabetic index to the tabular sections.

- **Complete set of ICD-10-CM codes (2014):** All 21 chapters — Infectious and Parasitic Diseases through Injuries, including External Causes and Reasons for Visit.

- **Neoplasm Table (2014):** The Neoplasm Table assists in the indexing and classification of neoplasms within ICD-10-CM.

- **Table of Drugs and Chemicals (2014):** This is a classification of drugs and other chemical substances to assist in the coding of poisoning, overdose states, underdosing, and external causes of adverse effects.

The codes in ICD-10-CM are not currently valid for coding and reporting of medical services for reimbursement purposes. However, the United States began using ICD-10 in 1999 to classify mortality data from death certificates to ensure the international comparability of health statistics.

Thank you for choosing to be an Optum customer. If you have any questions about your *ICD-10-CM Draft 2014* or about any Optum publication, please call our customer service department toll free at (800) 464-3649.

Although this draft of ICD-10-CM is available, the codes in ICD-10-CM are not currently valid for any purpose or use. Updates to this draft are anticipated prior to implementation of ICD-10-CM.

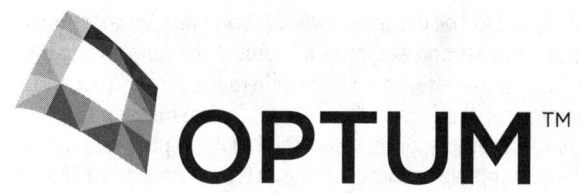

ICD-10-CM

The Complete Official Draft Code Set

2014

Publisher's Notice

The *ICD-10-CM The Complete Official Draft Code Set* is designed to be an accurate and authoritative source regarding coding and every reasonable effort has been made to ensure accuracy and completeness of the content. However, Optum makes no guarantee, warranty, or representation that this publication is accurate, complete or without errors. It is understood that Optum is not rendering any legal or other professional services or advice in this publication and that Optum bears no liability for any results or consequences that may arise from the use of this book.

Our Commitment to Accuracy

Optum is committed to producing accurate and reliable materials.

To report corrections, please visit www.optumcoding.com/accuracy or email accuracy@optum.com. You can also reach customer service by calling 1.800.464.3649, option 1.

Acknowledgments

Anita C. Hart, RHIA, CCS, CCS-P *Product Manager*
Karen Schmidt, BSN, *Technical Director*
Stacy Perry, *Manager, Desktop Publishing*
Lisa Singley, *Project Manager*
Brigid T. Caffrey, BA, BS, CCS, *Clinical/Technical Editor*
Tracy Betzler, *Senior Desktop Publishing Specialist*
Hope M. Dunn, *Senior Desktop Publishing Specialist*
Katie Russell, *Desktop Publishing Specialist*
Kate Holden, *Editor*

Anita Hart, RHIA,CCS, CCS-P

Product Manager, Optum

Ms. Hart's experience includes 15 years conducting and publishing research in clinical medicine and human genetics for Yale University, Massachusetts General Hospital, and Massachusetts Institute of Technology. Her research conclusions have been published in several peer-reviewed journals. In addition, Ms. Hart has supervised medical records management, health information management, coding and reimbursement, and workers' compensation issues as the office manager for a physical therapy rehabilitation clinic. Ms. Hart is an expert in physician and facility coding, reimbursement systems, and compliance issues. She is also the author of several OptumInsight publications and has served as subject matter advisor on numerous other publications for hospital and physician practices. Ms. Hart is the ICD-9-CM and ICD-10-CM/PCS subject matter expert for OptumInsight, has served as product manager for that product line for 15 years, and has presented at numerous national conferences. Ms. Hart is a member of the American Academy of Professional Coders (AAPC) and is a fully credentialed active member of the American Health Information Management Association (AHIMA). Ms. Hart is a current AHIMA Approved ICD-10-CM/PCS Trainer and leads the training initiatives within OptumInsight Coding Solutions business unit.

Contents

Preface

ICD-10-CM Official Preface

This 2014 update of the International Classification of Diseases, 10th revision, Clinical Modification (ICD-10-CM) is being published by the United States government in recognition of its responsibility to promulgate this classification throughout the United States for morbidity coding. The International Statistical Classification of Diseases and Related Health Problems, 10th Revision (ICD-10), published by the World Health Organization (WHO), is the foundation of ICD-10-CM. ICD-10 continues to be the classification used in cause-of-death coding in the United States. The ICD-10-CM is comparable with the ICD-10. The WHO Collaborating Center for the Family of International Classifications in North America, housed at the National Center for Health Statistics (NCHS), has responsibility for the implementation of ICD and other WHO-FIC classifications and serves as a liaison with the WHO, fulfilling international obligations for comparable classifications and the national health data needs of the United States. The historical background of ICD and ICD-10 can be found in the Introduction to the International Classification of Diseases and Related Health Problems (ICD-10), 2008, World Health Organization, Geneva, Switzerland.

ICD-10-CM is the United States' clinical modification of the World Health Organization's ICD-10. The term clinical is used to emphasize the modification's intent: to serve as a useful tool in the area of classification of morbidity data for indexing of medical records, medical care review, and ambulatory and other medical care programs, as well as for basic health statistics. To describe the clinical picture of the patient the codes must be more precise than those needed only for statistical groupings and trend analysis.

Characteristics of ICD-10-CM

ICD-10-CM far exceeds its predecessors in the number of concepts and codes provided. The disease classification has been expanded to include health-related conditions and to provide greater specificity at the sixth and seventh character level. The sixth and seventh characters are not optional and are intended for use in recording the information documented in the clinical record.

Introduction

History and Future of ICD-10-CM

The ICD-10-CM classification system was developed by the National Center for Health Statistics (NCHS) as a clinical modification to the ICD-10 system developed by the World Health Organization (WHO), primarily as a unique system for use in the United States for morbidity and mortality reporting. Although ICD-10-CM has not yet been implemented for use in the United States, ICD-10 has been adopted for use in the coding and classification of mortality data from death certificates. ICD-10 replaced ICD-9 for this purpose as of January 1, 1999. Upon legislative approval, ICD-10-CM is planned as the replacement for ICD-9-CM, volumes 1 and 2.

ICD-10 is the copyrighted product of the World Health Organization (WHO), which has authorized the development of a clinical modification (CM) of ICD-10 for use in the United States. However, all modifications to the ICD-10 must conform to WHO conventions for ICD. The development of ICD-10-CM included comprehensive evaluation by a Technical Advisory Panel and extensive consultation with physician groups, clinical coders, and other industry experts.

The ICD-10-CM draft and crosswalk between ICD-9-CM and ICD-10-CM have been made available on the CMS website for public comment. The initial public comment period extended from December 1997 through February 1998. A field test for ICD-10-CM was conducted in the summer of 2003 jointly by The American Hospital Association (AHA) and the American Health Information Management Association (AHIMA). Public comments and suggestions were reviewed and additional modifications to ICD-10-CM were made. Revisions were made to ICD-10-CM based on the established update process for ICD-9-CM (the ICD-9-CM Coordination and Maintenance Committee) and the World Health Organization's ICD-10 (the Update and Revision Committee).

These revisions to ICD-10-CM have included:

- information relevant to ambulatory and managed care encounters
- expanded injury codes
- creation of combination diagnosis/symptom codes to reduce the number of codes needed to fully describe a condition
- the addition of sixth and seventh character classifications
- incorporation of common 4th and 5th character classifications
- classifications specific to laterality
- classification refinement for increased data granularity

This new structure allows for further expansion than was possible with the ICD-9-CM classification system.

This new 2014 draft update release is available for public viewing. ICD-10-CM codes are not currently valid for any purpose or use other than the reporting of mortality data for death certificates.

The Department of Health and Human Services (HHS) published the final rule regarding the adoption of both ICD-10-CM and ICD-10-PCS in the January 16, 2009 *Federal Register* (45 CFR part 162 [CMS—0013—F]). The initial compliance date for implementation of ICD-10-CM and ICD-10-PCS as a replacement for ICD-9-CM was set at October 1, 2013. On April 17, 2012 the Department of Health and Human Services (HHS) released a notice to postpone the date by which certain health care entities have to comply with International Classification of Diseases, 10th Revision diagnosis and procedure codes (ICD-10). The compliance date for implementation of ICD-10-CM and ICD-10-PCS as a replacement for ICD-9-CM is October 1, 2014.

ICD-10-CM: The Complete Official Draft Code Set

ICD-10-CM: The Complete Official Draft Code Set 2014 edition includes many of the enhancements described below in direct response to requests from our subscribers. Users will find many of the conventions, icons, color bars, and other enhancements familiar since many of these features are similar to the hallmark color coding and symbols of our ICD-9-CM code books.

As you review the content, you will find the following:

- Optum Exclusive feature — Check XTension Alert symbol, indicating the need for one or more "filler" x character assignments in the 5th and/or 6th character position, in order to appropriately assign a required character in the 7th character position
- Optum Exclusive feature — Key word differentiation by the use of a green font that highlights the differentiating terms in similar code descriptions in a given category
- Optum Exclusive color coding, symbols, and footnotes that alert coders to coding and reimbursement issues, including the majority of the Medicare code edits
- Optum Exclusive feature — Exclusive *following* references and Check Additional Character symbol in the indexes. The *following* references (designed and used exclusively by Optum) help coders locate those alphanumeric codes that are out of sequence in the tabular section .
- Optum Exclusive feature — Exclusive shaded guides in the index help users easily follow the indent levels for the subterms under a main term.
- Illustrations featuring anatomy and terminology included in the ICD-10-CM classification system
- The complete ICD-10-CM official guidelines for coding and reporting, published by the U.S. Department of Health and Human Services and approved by the cooperating parties (American Health Information Management Association, National Center for Health Statistics, Centers for Medicare and Medicaid Services, American Hospital Association)
- All the official ICD-10-CM codes, indexes, notes, footnotes, and symbols
- Icons and definitions to differentiate between the two types of Excludes notes
- Check fourth-, fifth-, sixth-, and seventh- character symbols identify codes that require the addition of a fourth, fifth, sixth, or seventh character for code specificity and validity
- Color coding and symbol legend at the bottom of each page

Please review "How to Use *ICD-10-CM: The Complete Official Draft Code Set*" in this section to learn about the features that will help you assign and report correct codes, ensuring appropriate reimbursement.

How to Use the ICD-10-CM (Draft 2014)

This draft of the International Classification of Diseases, 10th Revision, Clinical Modification (ICD-10-CM) is being published by the United States Government in recognition of its responsibility to promulgate this classification throughout the United States for morbidity coding. This code book represents an adaptation of ICD-10 which was created specifically for use in the United States. Future revisions to ICD-10-CM will be made based on the established update process for ICD-9-CM (the ICD-9-CM Coordination and Maintenance Committee) and the World Health Organization's ICD-10 (the Update and Revision Committee). ICD-10-CM has been approved for implementation on October 1, 2014.

Steps to Correct Coding

1. Before beginning to use this code book, review section 1.A., "Conventions," and section 1.B., "General Coding Guidelines of the ICD-10-CM Draft Official Guidelines for Coding and Reporting 2014."

2. Look up the main term in the Alphabetic Index and scan the subterm entries as appropriate. Review continued lines and additional subterms that may appear in the next column or on the next page.

3. Note all parenthetical terms (nonessential modifiers) that help in code selection but do not affect code assignment. Shaded vertical guidelines in the Index are provided to help determine the indentation level for each subterm in relation to the main terms.

4. Pay close attention to the following instructions in the Index:

   - "see," "see also," and "see category" cross-references

   - "with"/"without" notes

   - "omit code" notes

   - "due to" subterms

   - other instructions found in note boxes, such as "code by site"

   - *Following* references and Check Additional Character symbol in the indexes. The *following* references (designed and used exclusively by Optum) help coders locate those alphanumeric codes that are out of sequence in the tabular section.

5. Do not code from the Alphabetic Index without verifying the accuracy of the code in the Tabular List. Locate the code in the alphanumerically arranged Tabular List.

6. To determine the appropriateness of the code selection and proper coding, read all instructional material:

   - "includes" and both types of "excludes" notes

   - "use additional code" and "code first underlying disease" instructions

   - "code also"

   - fourth-, fifth-, and sixth-character requirements and seventh-character extension requirements

   - age and sex symbols

7. Consult the official Draft ICD-10-CM guidelines, which govern the use of specific codes. These guidelines provide both general and chapter-specific coding guidance.

8. Confirm and assign the correct code.

Organization

This book is organized in the following manner:

Introduction

The introductory material in this book includes the ICD-10-CM Official Preface, the history and future of ICD-10-CM as well as an overview of the classification system.

Draft Official ICD-10-CM Conventions and Guidelines

This section provides an explanation of the conventions and guidelines regulating the appropriate assignment and reporting of ICD-10-CM codes. This coding guidance is presented by the National Center for Health Statistics (NCHS), a governmental agency of the Centers for Disease Control and Prevention (CDC), within the United States Department of Health and Human Services (DHHS).

Alphabetic Index to Diseases

The Alphabetic Index to Diseases is arranged in alphabetic order by disease — by specific illness, injury, eponym, abbreviation, or other descriptive diagnostic term. The Index also lists diagnostic terms for other reasons for encounters with health care professionals.

Neoplasm Table

The Neoplasm Table provides the proper code based upon histology of the neoplasm and site.

Table of Drugs and Chemicals

The Table of Drugs and Chemicals is also included within the Alphabetic Index.

The Table of Drugs and Chemicals lists the drug and the specific codes that identify the drug and the intent. No additional external cause of injury and poisoning code is assigned in ICD-10-CM.

Index to External Causes

The Alphabetic Index to External Causes of injuries is arranged in alphabetic order by main term indicating the event.

Tabular List of Diseases

ICD-10-CM codes and descriptors are arranged numerically within the Tabular List of Diseases within 21 separate chapters according to body system or nature of injury and disease. Classifications which were previously considered supplemental to ICD-9-CM (e.g., V codes and E codes) are incorporated into the Tabular Listing of ICD-10-CM as individual chapters. Chapters 20 External Causes of Morbidity and 21 Factors Influencing Health Status and Contact with Health Services include chapter-specific guidelines.

Illustrations

This section includes illustrations of normal anatomy with ICD-10-CM specific terminology.

Use of Official Sources

The *ICD-10-CM: The Complete Official Draft Code Set* contains the official U.S. Department of Health and Human Services, Tenth Revision, Clinical Modification, ICD-10-CM codes, effective for the current year.

The color-coding, footnotes and symbols, which identify coding and reimbursement issues, are derived from official federal government sources, including the Medicare Code Edits (MCE), version 30.0.

ICD-10-CM Draft Official Conventions

The ICD-10-CM conventions are general rules for the use of the classification system, independent of the guidelines. These conventions are incorporated within the Index and Tabular List as instructional notes and are applicable regardless of the health care setting.

Format

ICD-10-CM is divided into two main parts: the Index, an alphabetical list of terms and their corresponding code, and the Tabular List, a sequential, alphanumeric list of codes divided into chapters based on body system or condition. The Index contains the Index to Diseases and Injuries (main index) and the Index to External Causes of Injury. Also included in the main Index is the Neoplasm Table and a Table of Drugs and Chemicals.

The Tabular List contains categories, subcategories, and valid codes. ICD-10-CM is an alphanumeric classification system. The first character of a three-character category is a letter. The second and third characters may be numbers or alpha characters. A three-character category without further subclassification is equivalent to a valid three-character code. Subcategories are either four or five characters. Subcategory characters include either letters or numbers. Codes may be four, five, or six characters in length, in which each level of subdivision after a category is a subcategory. The final level of subdivision is a valid code. The final character in a code may be either a letter or a number.

The ICD-10-CM uses the letter "X" as a place-holder. A placeholder "X" is used as a fifth character place-holder at certain six-character codes to allow for future expansion, without disturbing the sixth-character structure. For instance, an initial encounter for accidental poisoning by penicillin is coded to T36.0X1A. The "X" in the fifth character position is a place-holder, or filler character.

Similarly, certain categories have applicable seventh-character extensions. In these cases, the seventh-character extension is required for all codes within the category, or as otherwise instructed in the Tabular List notations. Seventh-character extensions must always be the last character in the data field. If a code is not a full six characters in length, a dummy place-holder "X" must be used to fill in the empty characters when a seventh character extension is required.

Punctuation

[ ]   In the Tabular List, brackets are used to enclose synonyms, alternative wording, or explanatory phrases. In the Index, brackets are used to identify manifestation codes.

( )   Parentheses are used in both the Index and Tabular List to enclose nonessential modifiers; supplementary words that may be present or absent in the statement of a disease or procedure without affecting the code number to which it is assigned.

:   Colons are used in the Tabular List after an incomplete term that needs one or more of the modifiers following the colon to make it assignable to a given category.

Abbreviations

NEC

The abbreviation NEC, "Not elsewhere classifiable" represents "other specified" in the ICD-10-CM. An index entry that states NEC directs the coder to an "other specified" code in the Tabular List. Codes titled "Other" or "Other specified" in the Tabular List (usually a code with a fourth or sixth character 8 and fifth character 9) are for use when the information in the medical record provides detail for which a specific code does not exist.

NOS

The abbreviation NOS, "Not otherwise specified," in the Tabular List may be interpreted as "unspecified." Codes in the Tabular List with "Unspecified" in the title (usually a code with a fourth or sixth character 9 and fifth character 0) are for use when the information in the medical record is insufficient to assign a more specific code.

Typeface

Boldface

Boldface type is used for main term entries in the Alphabetic Index, and all codes and descriptions in the Tabular List.

Italicized

Italicized type is used for all exclusion notes and to identify manifestation codes, those codes that should not be reported as first-listed (principal) diagnoses.

General Notes

The following conventions and notes appear only in the Tabular List of Diseases:

Includes Notes

The word "Includes" appears immediately under certain categories to further define, clarify, or give examples of the content of a code category.

Inclusion Terms

Lists of inclusion terms are included under certain codes. These terms indicate some of the conditions for which that code number may be used. Inclusion terms may be synonyms with the code title, or, in the case of "other specified" codes, the terms may also provide a list of various conditions included within a classification code. The inclusion terms are not exhaustive. The Index may provide additional terms that may also be assigned to a given code.

Excludes Notes

ICD-10-CM has two types of excludes notes. Each note has a different definition for use. However, they are similar in that they both indicate that codes excluded from each other are independent of each other.

Excludes1

An excludes1 note is a "pure" excludes. It means "NOT CODED HERE!" An excludes1 note indicates mutually exclusive codes; two conditions that cannot be reported together. For example, a congenital form of a disease may not be reported with the acquired form of the same condition. The code excluded should never be reported with the applicable codes listed above the excludes notation.

Excludes2

An excludes2 note means "NOT INCLUDED HERE." An excludes2 note indicates that although the excluded condition is not part of the condition it is excluded from, a patient may have both conditions at the same time. Therefore, when an excludes2 note appears under a code, it may be acceptable to use both the code and the excluded code together if supported by the medical documentation.

Default Codes

In the index, the default code is the code listed next to the main term. The default code represents the condition most commonly associated with the main term. This code may be assigned when documentation does not facilitate reporting a more specific code. Alternately, it may provide an unspecified code for the condition.

Syndromes

Follow the Alphabetic Index guidance when coding syndromes. In the absence of index guidance, assign codes for the documented manifestations of the syndrome.

And

When the term "and" is used in a narrative statement it may be interpreted as "and/or."

With/Without

When "with" and "without" are the two options for the final character of a set of codes, the default is always "without." For five-character codes, a "Ø" as the fifth-position character represents "without", and "1" represents "with." For six-character codes, the sixth-position character "1" represents "with" and "9" represents "without."

Instructional Notes Used in the Tabular List

In the tabular section, the following instructional notes appear in red type for emphasis:

Code First/Use additional code:

These instructional notes are in red type and provide sequencing instruction. They may appear independently of each other or to designate certain etiology/manifestation paired codes. These instructions signal the coder that an additional code should be reported to provide a more complete picture of that diagnosis.

In etiology/manifestation coding, ICD-10-CM requires the underlying condition to be sequenced first, followed by the manifestation. In these situations, codes with "In diseases classified elsewhere" in the code description are never permitted as a first-listed or principal diagnosis code and must be sequenced following the underlying condition code.

Code Also:

A code also note alerts the coder that more than one code may be required to fully describe the condition. Code sequencing is discretionary. Factors that may determine sequencing include severity and reason for the encounter. These coding notes appear in red type.

Additional Conventions

Color-coding and symbols are included to alert the coder to important reimbursement issues affected by the diagnosis code assignment. Some codes may carry more than one color and/or symbol. For a quick reference to the color codes and their meanings, refer to the color/symbol legend located at the bottom of each page in the Tabular Listing.

Additional Characters Required

✓4ᵗʰ This symbol indicates that the code requires a fourth character.

✓5ᵗʰ This symbol indicates that the code requires a fifth character.

✓6ᵗʰ This symbol indicates that the code requires a sixth character.

✓7ᵗʰ This symbol indicates that the code requires a seventh character.

✓x7ᵗʰ This symbol indicates that the code requires a seventh character following the placeholder X. Codes with fewer than six characters that require a seventh character must contain placeholder X to fill the missing

Boldface

Note

The term "Note" appears enclosed within a red icon and precedes the instructional information. These notes function as an alert, to highlight coding instruction within the text.

Key Word

Green font is used throughout the Tabular List of Diseases to differentiate the key words that appear in similar code descriptions in a given category or subcategory.

For example, refer to the list of codes below from category C7A:

C7A.020   Malignant carcinoid tumor of the **appendix**

C7A.021   Malignant carcinoid tumor of the **cecum**

C7A.022   Malignant carcinoid tumor of the **ascending colon**

C7A.023   Malignant carcinoid tumor of the **transverse colon**

C7A.024   Malignant carcinoid tumor of the **descending colon**

C7A.025   Malignant carcinoid tumor of the **sigmoid colon**

C7A.029   Malignant carcinoid tumor of the large intestine, unspecified portion

The portion of the code description that appears in bold font above appears in green font in the Tabular List, to assist the coder in quickly identifying the key terms and in identifying the correct code. This convention is especially useful when the codes describe laterality, such as the following codes from category H40.22:

H40.221   Chronic angle-closure glaucoma, **right** eye

H40.222   Chronic angle-closure glaucoma, **left** eye

H40.223   Chronic angle-closure glaucoma, **bilateral**

H40.229   Chronic angle-closure glaucoma, unspecified eye

The key word convention is only used in those categories in which there are multiple codes with very similar descriptions with only a few words that differentiate them.

Color Coding

Medicare administrative contractors and many payers use Medicare code edits to check the coding accuracy on claims. The coding edit information in this manual is effective from October 1, 2013, to September 30, 2014, reflect those edits used for physician office encounters. This ICD-10 version of the Medicare Code Editor (MCE) is version 30.0. However, the MCE is not intended to be used to process claims since the ICD-10 code set will not be mandated for use until the implementation of ICD-10 beginning on October 1, 2014.

Manifestation Code

These codes appear in italic type, with a blue color bar over the title. A manifestation code cannot be reported as a first-listed or principal diagnosis. By definition, a manifestation code represents a demonstration of some aspect of an underlying disease, which is separately classifiable. In the Alphabetic Index, these codes are listed as the secondary code in brackets. The underlying disease code is listed first.

Age and Sex Edit Symbols

The age edits below address MCE edit 4 and are used to detect inconsistencies between the patient's age and diagnosis. The following edit symbols appear in the Tabular List of Diseases to the right of the code description.

Newborn Age: 0   N
These diagnoses are intended for newborns and neonates and the patient's age must be 0 years.

Pediatric Age: 0-17   P
These diagnoses are intended for children and the patient's age must between 0 and 17 years.

Maternity Age: 12-55   M
These diagnoses are intended for childbearing patients between the age of 12 and 55 years.

Adult Age: 15-124   A
These diagnoses are intended for the patients between the age of 15 and 124 years.

The sex symbols below address MCE edit 3 and are used to detect inconsistencies between the patient's sex and diagnosis. These symbols appear in the Tabular List to the right of the code description.

♂   **Male diagnosis or procedure only**
This symbol appears to the right of the code description. This reference appears in the disease and procedure Tabular List.

♀   **Female diagnosis or procedure only**
This symbol appears to the right of the code description. This reference appears in the disease and procedure Tabular List.

Wrong Procedure Performed Edit

The Wrong Surgery Edit was created to identify cases in which wrong surgeries occurred. Any claim with a code from the Y65.51-Y65.53 will be denied and returned to the provider. A surgical or other invasive procedure is considered to be a wrong procedure if:

- The procedure was performed on the wrong site

- The procedure was performed on the wrong patient, or

- The incorrect procedure was performed on a patient.

Other Notations in the Tabular

Other Specified Code

These codes will appear with a gray color bar over the code description. Use these codes when the documentation indicates a specified diagnosis, but the ICD-10-CM system does not have a specific code that describes the condition. These codes may be stated as "Other" or "Not elsewhere classified (NEC)."

Unspecified Code

These codes will have a yellow color bar over the code description. Use these codes when neither the diagnostic statement nor the documentation provides enough information to assign a more specific diagnosis code. These codes may be stated as "Unspecified" or "Not otherwise specified (NOS)." Note: Do not assign these codes when a more specific diagnosis has been determined.

PDx Symbol

This symbol identifies a Z code that generally is for use as a first-listed (or primary) diagnosis only but may be used as an additional diagnosis if the patient has more than one encounter on the same day or there is more than one reason for the encounter.

The instructions for Z code use contained in the ICD-10-CM official coding guidelines only identify those Z codes that can only be used as a PDx. All other Z codes may either be SDx or PDx, depending upon circumstances of the encounter, by meeting the definition of first-listed or principal diagnosis, and by following any specific Z code guidelines in section I.C.21 a-c. The responsibility of those assigning the Z codes as PDx is to make sure the circumstances of the encounter meet the definition of first-listed or principal diagnosis, follow all coding instructions, and follow the Z code specific guidelines. Optum does not include any SDx edit since there is no official source for it and the Z code use is determined by circumstances of the encounter.

Note: Please note that the symbols indicating the Z code "principal or first-listed only" designation and the Z codes that may be principal or first-listed diagnoses included in the official coding guidelines [Section

1.C.18.e] are consistent with reporting guidelines for health care encounters *excluding acute care inpatient admissions.* These Z codes edits are often in conflict with the inpatient prospective payment system (IPPS) edits. For example, code Z34.90 Encounter for supervision of normal pregnancy, unspecified, unspecified trimester, may be an appropriate primary reason for an outpatient encounter. However, supervision for a normal pregnancy is not an acceptable principal diagnosis or reason for an inpatient admission and will have an unacceptable principal diagnosis edit under inpatient prospective payment system (IPPS).

Other Notations in the Alphabetic Indexes

▽ Subterms under main terms may continue to next column or page. This warning statement is a reminder to always check for additional subterms and information that may continue onto the next page or column before making a final selection.

Following References

The index includes *following* references to assist in locating "out-of-sequence" codes in the Tabular List. "Out-of-sequence" codes contain an alphabetic character (letter) in the third or fourth character position. These codes are placed according to the classification rules — the placement of the codes according to condition — not according to alphabetic or numeric sequencing rules.

Example:

Carcinoma (malignant) (*see also,* Neoplasm, by site, malignant)
   neuroendocrine (*see also* Tumor, neuroendocrine)
      high grade, any site C7A.1 (*following* C75)
      poorly differentiated, any site C7A.1 (*following* C75)

In the tabular rubric, C7A is included after rubric C75 and before C76.

Gout, chronic (*see also* Gout, gouty) M1A.9
   drug-induced M1A.20 (*following* M08)
      ankle M1A.27-(*following* M08)
      elbow M1A.22-(*following* M08)

In the tabular rubric, MIA is included after rubric M08 and before M10.

ICD-10-CM Draft Official Guidelines for Coding and Reporting 2014

Narrative changes appear in **bold** text.

Items underlined have been moved within the guidelines since the 2013 version.

Italics are used to indicate revisions to heading changes.

The Centers for Medicare and Medicaid Services (CMS) and the National Center for Health Statistics (NCHS), two departments within the U.S. Federal Government's Department of Health and Human Services (DHHS) provide the following guidelines for coding and reporting using the International Classification of Diseases, 10th Revision, Clinical Modification (ICD-10-CM). These guidelines should be used as a companion document to the official version of the ICD-10-CM as published on the NCHS website. The ICD-10-CM is a morbidity classification published by the United States for classifying diagnoses and reason for visits in all health care settings. The ICD-10-CM is based on the ICD-10, the statistical classification of disease published by the World Health Organization (WHO).

These guidelines have been approved by the four organizations that make up the Cooperating Parties for the ICD-10-CM: the American Hospital Association (AHA), the American Health Information Management Association (AHIMA), CMS, and NCHS.

These guidelines are a set of rules that have been developed to accompany and complement the official conventions and instructions provided within the ICD-10-CM itself. The instructions and conventions of the classification take precedence over guidelines. These guidelines are based on the coding and sequencing instructions in the Tabular List and Alphabetic Index of ICD-10-CM, but provide additional instruction. Adherence to these guidelines when assigning ICD-10-CM diagnosis codes is required under the Health Insurance Portability and Accountability Act (HIPAA). The diagnosis codes (Tabular List and Alphabetic Index) have been adopted under HIPAA for all healthcare settings. A joint effort between the healthcare provider and the coder is essential to achieve complete and accurate documentation, code assignment, and reporting of diagnoses and procedures. These guidelines have been developed to assist both the healthcare provider and the coder in identifying those diagnoses and procedures that are to be reported. The importance of consistent, complete documentation in the medical record cannot be overemphasized. Without such documentation accurate coding cannot be achieved. The entire record should be reviewed to determine the specific reason for the encounter and the conditions treated.

The term encounter is used for all settings, including hospital admissions. In the context of these guidelines, the term provider is used throughout the guidelines to mean physician or any qualified health care practitioner who is legally accountable for establishing the patient's diagnosis. Only this set of guidelines, approved by the Cooperating Parties, is official.

The guidelines are organized into sections. Section I includes the structure and conventions of the classification and general guidelines that apply to the entire classification, and chapter-specific guidelines that correspond to the chapters as they are arranged in the classification. Section II includes guidelines for selection of principal diagnosis for non-outpatient settings. Section III includes guidelines for reporting additional diagnoses in non-outpatient settings. Section IV is for outpatient coding and reporting. It is necessary to review all sections of the guidelines to fully understand all of the rules and instructions needed to code properly.

Section I. Conventions, general coding guidelines and chapter specific guidelines

The conventions, general guidelines and chapter-specific guidelines are applicable to all health care settings unless otherwise indicated. The conventions and instructions of the classification take precedence over guidelines.

A. Conventions for the ICD-10-CM

The conventions for the ICD-10-CM are the general rules for use of the classification independent of the guidelines. These conventions are incorporated within the Alphabetic Index and Tabular List of the ICD-10-CM as instructional notes.

1. **The Alphabetic Index and Tabular List**
    The ICD-10-CM is divided into the Alphabetic Index, an alphabetical list of terms and their corresponding code, and the Tabular List, a structured chronological list of codes divided into chapters based on body system or condition. The Alphabetic Index consists of the following parts: the Index of Diseases and Injury, the Index of External Causes of Injury, the Table of Neoplasms and the Table of Drugs and Chemicals.

    See Section I.C2. General guidelines

    See Section I.C.19. Adverse effects, poisoning, underdosing and toxic effects

2. **Format and Structure**
    The ICD-10-CM Tabular List contains categories, subcategories and codes. Characters for categories, subcategories and codes may be either a letter or a number. All categories are 3 characters. A three-character category that has no further subdivision is equivalent to a code. Subcategories are either 4 or 5 characters. Codes may be 3, 4, 5, 6 or 7 characters. That is, each level of subdivision after a category is a subcategory. The final level of subdivision is a code. Codes that have applicable 7th characters are still referred to as codes, not subcategories. A code that has an applicable 7th character is considered invalid without the 7th character.

    The ICD-10-CM uses an indented format for ease in reference.

3. **Use of codes for reporting purposes**
    For reporting purposes only codes are permissible, not categories or subcategories, and any applicable 7th character is required.

4. **Placeholder character**
    The ICD-10-CM utilizes a placeholder character "X". The "X" is used as a placeholder at certain codes to allow for future expansion. An example of this is at the poisoning, adverse effect and underdosing codes, categories T36-T50.

    Where a placeholder exists, the X must be used in order for the code to be considered a valid code.

5. **7th Characters**
    Certain ICD-10-CM categories have applicable 7th characters. The applicable 7th character is required for all codes within the category, or as the notes in the Tabular List instruct. The 7th character must always be the 7th character in the data field. If a code that requires a 7th character is not 6 characters, a placeholder X must be used to fill in the empty characters.

6. **Abbreviations**
    a. **Alphabetic Index abbreviations**
        NEC   "Not elsewhere classifiable"
                This abbreviation in the Alphabetic Index represents "other specified". When a specific code is not available for a condition, the Alphabetic Index directs the coder to the "other specified" code in the Tabular List.
        NOS   "Not otherwise specified"
                This abbreviation is the equivalent of unspecified.
    b. **Tabular List abbreviations**
        NEC   "Not elsewhere classifiable"
                This abbreviation in the Tabular List represents "other specified". When a specific code is not available for a condition the Tabular List includes an NEC entry under a code to identify the code as the "other specified" code.
        NOS   "Not otherwise specified"
                This abbreviation is the equivalent of unspecified.

7. **Punctuation**
    [ ]   Brackets are used in the Tabular List to enclose synonyms, alternative wording or explanatory phrases. Brackets are used in the Alphabetic Index to identify manifestation codes.
    ( )   Parentheses are used in both the Alphabetic Index and Tabular List to enclose supplementary words that may be present or absent in the statement of a disease or procedure without affecting the code number to which it is assigned. The terms within the parentheses are referred to as nonessential modifiers. **The nonessential modifiers in the Alphabetic Index to Diseases apply to subterms following a main term except when a nonessential modifier and a subentry are mutually exclusive, the subentry takes precedence. For example, in the ICD-10-CM Alphabetic Index under the main term Enteritis, "acute" is a nonessential modifier and "chronic" is a subentry. In this case, the nonessential modifier "acute" does not apply to the subentry "chronic".**
    :   Colons are used in the Tabular List after an incomplete term which needs one or more of the modifiers following the colon to make it assignable to a given category.

8. **Use of "and"**
    See Section I.A.14. Use of the term "And"

9. **Other and Unspecified codes**
    a. **"Other" codes**
        Codes titled "other" or "other specified" are for use when the information in the medical record provides detail for which a specific code does not exist. Alphabetic Index entries with NEC in the line designate "other" codes in the Tabular List. These Alphabetic Index entries represent specific disease entities for which no specific code exists so the term is included within an "other" code.
    b. **"Unspecified" codes**
        Codes titled "unspecified" are for use when the information in the medical record is insufficient to assign a more specific code. For those categories for which an unspecified code is not provided, the "other specified" code may represent both other and unspecified.

        See Section I.B.18 Use of Signs/Symptom/Unspecified Codes

10. **Includes Notes**
    This note appears immediately under a three character code title to further define, or give examples of, the content of the category.

11. **Inclusion Terms**
    List of terms is included under some codes. These terms are the conditions for which that code is to be used. The terms may be synonyms of the code title, or, in the case of "other specified" codes, the terms are a list of the various conditions assigned to that code. The inclusion terms are not necessarily exhaustive. Additional terms found only in the Alphabetic Index may also be assigned to a code.

12. **Excludes Notes**
    The ICD-10-CM has two types of excludes notes. Each type of note has a different definition for use but they are all similar in that they indicate that codes excluded from each other are independent of each other.
    a. **Excludes1**
        A type 1 Excludes note is a pure excludes note. It means "NOT CODED HERE!" An Excludes1 note indicates that the code excluded should never be used at the same time as the code above the Excludes1 note. An Excludes1 is used when two conditions cannot occur together, such as a congenital form versus an acquired form of the same condition.
    b. **Excludes2**
        A type 2 Excludes note represents "Not included here". An excludes2 note indicates that the condition excluded is not part of the condition represented by the code, but a patient may have both conditions at the same time. When an Excludes2 note appears under a code, it is acceptable to use both the code and the excluded code together, when appropriate.

13. **Etiology/manifestation convention ("code first", "use additional code" and "in diseases classified elsewhere" notes)**
    Certain conditions have both an underlying etiology and multiple body system manifestations due to the underlying etiology. For such conditions, the ICD-10-CM has a coding convention that requires the underlying condition be sequenced first followed by the manifestation.

Wherever such a combination exists, there is a "use additional code" note at the etiology code, and a "code first" note at the manifestation code. These instructional notes indicate the proper sequencing order of the codes, etiology followed by manifestation.

In most cases the manifestation codes will have in the code title, "in diseases classified elsewhere." Codes with this title are a component of the etiology/ manifestation convention. The code title indicates that it is a manifestation code. "In diseases classified elsewhere" codes are never permitted to be used as first-listed or principal diagnosis codes. They must be used in conjunction with an underlying condition code and they must be listed following the underlying condition. See category F02, Dementia in other diseases classified elsewhere, for an example of this convention.

There are manifestation codes that do not have "in diseases classified elsewhere" in the title. For such codes, there is a "use additional code" note at the etiology code and a "code first" note at the manifestation code and the rules for sequencing apply.

In addition to the notes in the Tabular List, these conditions also have a specific Alphabetic Index entry structure. In the Alphabetic Index both conditions are listed together with the etiology code first followed by the manifestation codes in brackets. The code in brackets is always to be sequenced second.

An example of the etiology/manifestation convention is dementia in Parkinson's disease. In the Alphabetic Index, code G20 is listed first, followed by code F02.80 or F02.81 in brackets. Code G20 represents the underlying etiology, Parkinson's disease, and must be sequenced first, whereas codes F02.80 and F02.81 represent the manifestation of dementia in diseases classified elsewhere, with or without behavioral disturbance.

"Code first" and "Use additional code" notes are also used as sequencing rules in the classification for certain codes that are not part of an etiology/ manifestation combination.

See Section I.B.7. Multiple coding for a single condition.

14. "And"
The word "and" should be interpreted to mean either "and" or "or" when it appears in a title.

For example, cases of "tuberculosis of bones", "tuberculosis of joints" and "tuberculosis of bones and joints" are classified to subcategory A18.0, Tuberculosis of bones and joints.

15. "With"
The word "with" should be interpreted to mean "associated with" or "due to" when it appears in a code title, the Alphabetic Index, or an instructional note in the Tabular List.

The word "with" in the Alphabetic Index is sequenced immediately following the main term, not in alphabetical order.

16. "See" and "See Also"
The "see" instruction following a main term in the Alphabetic Index indicates that another term should be referenced. It is necessary to go to the main term referenced with the "see" note to locate the correct code.

A "see also" instruction following a main term in the Alphabetic Index instructs that there is another main term that may also be referenced that may provide additional Alphabetic Index entries that may be useful. It is not necessary to follow the "see also" note when the original main term provides the necessary code.

17. "Code also note"
A "code also" note instructs that two codes may be required to fully describe a condition, but this note does not provide sequencing direction.

18. Default codes
A code listed next to a main term in the ICD-10-CM Alphabetic Index is referred to as a default code. The default code represents that condition that is most commonly associated with the main term, or is the unspecified code for the condition. If a condition is documented in a medical record (for example, appendicitis) without any additional information, such as acute or chronic, the default code should be assigned.

B. General Coding Guidelines

1. Locating a code in the ICD-10-CM
To select a code in the classification that corresponds to a diagnosis or reason for visit documented in a medical record, first locate the term in the Alphabetic Index, and then verify the code in the Tabular List. Read and be guided by instructional notations that appear in both the Alphabetic Index and the Tabular List.

It is essential to use both the Alphabetic Index and Tabular List when locating and assigning a code. The Alphabetic Index does not always provide the full code. Selection of the full code, including laterality and any applicable 7th character can only be done in the Tabular List. A dash (-) at the end of an Alphabetic Index entry indicates that additional characters are required. Even if a dash is not included at the Alphabetic Index entry, it is necessary to refer to the Tabular List to verify that no 7th character is required.

2. Level of Detail in Coding
Diagnosis codes are to be used and reported at their highest number of characters available.

ICD-10-CM diagnosis codes are composed of codes with 3, 4, 5, 6 or 7 characters. Codes with three characters are included in ICD-10-CM as the heading of a category of codes that may be further subdivided by the use of fourth and/or fifth characters and/or sixth characters, which provide greater detail.

A three-character code is to be used only if it is not further subdivided. A code is invalid if it has not been coded to the full number of characters required for that code, including the 7th character, if applicable.

3. Code or codes from A00.0 through T88.9, Z00-Z99.8
The appropriate code or codes from A00.0 through T88.9, Z00-Z99.8 must be used to identify diagnoses, symptoms, conditions, problems, complaints or other reason(s) for the encounter/visit.

4. Signs and symptoms
Codes that describe symptoms and signs, as opposed to diagnoses, are acceptable for reporting purposes when a related definitive diagnosis has not been established (confirmed) by the provider. Chapter 18 of ICD-10-CM, Symptoms, Signs, and Abnormal Clinical and Laboratory Findings, Not Elsewhere Classified (codes R00.0 - R99) contains many, but not all codes for symptoms.

See Section I.B.18 Use of Signs/Symptom/Unspecified Codes

5. Conditions that are an integral part of a disease process
Signs and symptoms that are associated routinely with a disease process should not be assigned as additional codes, unless otherwise instructed by the classification.

6. Conditions that are not an integral part of a disease process
Additional signs and symptoms that may not be associated routinely with a disease process should be coded when present.

7. Multiple coding for a single condition
In addition to the etiology/manifestation convention that requires two codes to fully describe a single condition that affects multiple body systems, there are other single conditions that also require more than one code. "Use additional code" notes are found in the Tabular List at codes that are not part of an etiology/manifestation pair where a secondary code is useful to fully describe a condition. The sequencing rule is the same as the etiology/manifestation pair, "use additional code" indicates that a secondary code should be added.

For example, for bacterial infections that are not included in chapter 1, a secondary code from category B95, Streptococcus, Staphylococcus, and Enterococcus, as the cause of diseases classified elsewhere, or B96, Other bacterial agents as the cause of diseases classified elsewhere, may be required to identify the bacterial organism causing the infection. A "use additional code" note will normally be found at the infectious disease code, indicating a need for the organism code to be added as a secondary code.

"Code first" notes are also under certain codes that are not specifically manifestation codes but may be due to an underlying cause. When there is a "code first" note and an underlying condition is present, the underlying condition should be sequenced first.

"Code, if applicable, any causal condition first", notes indicate that this code may be assigned as a principal diagnosis when the causal condition is unknown or not applicable. If a causal condition is known, then the code for that condition should be sequenced as the principal or first-listed diagnosis.

Multiple codes may be needed for sequela, complication codes and obstetric codes to more fully describe a condition. See the specific guidelines for these conditions for further instruction.

8. Acute and Chronic Conditions
If the same condition is described as both acute (subacute) and chronic, and separate subentries exist in the Alphabetic Index at the same indentation level, code both and sequence the acute (subacute) code first.

9. Combination Code
A combination code is a single code used to classify:

Two diagnoses, or

A diagnosis with an associated secondary process (manifestation)

A diagnosis with an associated complication

Combination codes are identified by referring to subterm entries in the Alphabetic Index and by reading the inclusion and exclusion notes in the Tabular List.

Assign only the combination code when that code fully identifies the diagnostic conditions involved or when the Alphabetic Index so directs. Multiple coding should not be used when the classification provides a combination code that clearly identifies all of the elements documented in the diagnosis. When the combination code lacks necessary specificity in describing the manifestation or complication, an additional code should be used as a secondary code.

10. Sequela (Late Effects)
A sequela is the residual effect (condition produced) after the acute phase of an illness or injury has terminated. There is no time limit on when a sequela code can be used. The residual may be apparent early, such as in cerebral infarction, or it may occur months or years later, such as that due to a previous injury. Coding of sequela generally requires two codes sequenced in the following order: The condition or nature of the sequela is sequenced first. The sequela code is sequenced second.

An exception to the above guidelines are those instances where the code for the sequela is followed by a manifestation code identified in the Tabular List and title, or the sequela code has been expanded (at the fourth, fifth or sixth character levels) to include the manifestation(s). The code for the acute phase of an illness or injury that led to the sequela is never used with a code for the late effect.

See Section I.C.9. Sequelae of cerebrovascular disease

See Section I.C.15. Sequelae of complication of pregnancy, childbirth and the puerperium

See Section I.C.19. Application of 7th characters for Chapter 19

11. Impending or Threatened Condition
Code any condition described at the time of discharge as "impending" or "threatened" as follows:

If it did occur, code as confirmed diagnosis.

If it did not occur, reference the Alphabetic Index to determine if the condition has a subentry term for "impending" or "threatened" and also reference main term entries for "Impending" and for "Threatened."

If the subterms are listed, assign the given code.

If the subterms are not listed, code the existing underlying condition(s) and not the condition described as impending or threatened.

12. Reporting Same Diagnosis Code more than Once
Each unique ICD-10-CM diagnosis code may be reported only once for an encounter. This applies to bilateral conditions when there are no distinct codes identifying laterality or two different conditions classified to the same ICD-10-CM diagnosis code.

13. Laterality
Some ICD-10-CM codes indicate laterality, specifying whether the condition occurs on the left, right or is bilateral. If no bilateral code is provided and the condition is bilateral, assign separate codes for both the left and right side. If the side is not identified in the medical record, assign the code for the unspecified side.

14. Documentation for BMI and Pressure Ulcer Stages
For the Body Mass Index (BMI), depth of non-pressure chronic ulcers and pressure ulcer stage codes, code assignment may be based on medical record documentation from clinicians who are not the patient's provider (i.e., physician or other qualified healthcare practitioner legally accountable for establishing the patient's diagnosis), since this information is typically documented by other clinicians involved in the care of the patient (e.g., a dietitian often documents the BMI and nurses often documents the pressure ulcer stages). However, the associated diagnosis (such as overweight, obesity, or pressure ulcer) must be documented by the patient's provider. If there is conflicting medical record documentation, either from the same clinician or different clinicians, the patient's attending provider should be queried for clarification.

The BMI codes should only be reported as secondary diagnoses. As with all other secondary diagnosis codes, the BMI codes should only be assigned when they meet the definition of a reportable additional diagnosis (see Section III, Reporting Additional Diagnoses).

15. Syndromes
Follow the Alphabetic Index guidance when coding syndromes. In the absence of Alphabetic Index guidance, assign codes for the documented manifestations of the syndrome.

Additional codes for manifestations that are not an integral part of the disease process may also be assigned when the condition does not have a unique code.

16. Documentation of Complications of Care
Code assignment is based on the provider's documentation of the relationship between the condition and the care or procedure. The guideline extends to any complications of care, regardless of the chapter the code is located in. It is important to note that not all conditions that occur during or following medical care or surgery are classified as complications. There must be a cause-and-effect relationship between the care provided and the condition, and an indication in the documentation that it is a complication. Query the provider for clarification, if the complication is not clearly documented.

17. Borderline Diagnosis
If the provider documents a "borderline" diagnosis at the time of discharge, the diagnosis is coded as confirmed, unless the classification provides a specific entry (e.g., borderline diabetes). If a borderline condition has a specific index entry in ICD-10-CM, it should be coded as such. Since borderline conditions are not uncertain diagnoses, no distinction is made between the care setting (inpatient versus outpatient). Whenever the documentation is unclear regarding a borderline condition, coders are encouraged to query for clarification.

18. Use of Sign/Symptom/Unspecified Codes
Sign/symptom and "unspecified" codes have acceptable, even necessary, uses. While specific diagnosis codes should be reported when they are supported by the available medical record documentation and clinical knowledge of the patient's health condition, there are instances when signs/symptoms or unspecified codes are the best choices for accurately reflecting the healthcare encounter. Each healthcare encounter should be coded to the level of certainty known for that encounter.

If a definitive diagnosis has not been established by the end of the encounter, it is appropriate to report codes for sign(s) and/or symptom(s) in lieu of a definitive diagnosis. When sufficient clinical information isn't known or available about a particular health condition to assign a more specific code, it is acceptable to report the appropriate "unspecified" code (e.g., a diagnosis of pneumonia has been determined, but not the specific type). Unspecified codes should be reported when they are the codes that most accurately reflects what is known about the patient's condition at the time of that particular encounter. It would be inappropriate to select a specific code that is not supported by the medical record documentation or conduct medically unnecessary diagnostic testing in order to determine a more specific code.

C. Chapter-Specific Coding Guidelines
In addition to general coding guidelines, there are guidelines for specific diagnoses and/or conditions in the classification. Unless otherwise indicated, these guidelines apply to all health care settings. Please refer to Section II for guidelines on the selection of principal diagnosis.

1. **Chapter 1: Certain Infectious and Parasitic Diseases (A00-B99)**
   a. **Human immunodeficiency virus (HIV) infections**
      1) **Code only confirmed cases**

         Code only confirmed cases of HIV infection/illness. This is an exception to the hospital inpatient guideline Section II, H.

         In this context, "confirmation" does not require documentation of positive serology or culture for HIV; the provider's diagnostic statement that the patient is HIV positive, or has an HIV-related illness is sufficient.

      2) **Selection and sequencing of HIV codes**
         (a) **Patient admitted for HIV-related condition**

            If a patient is admitted for an HIV-related condition, the principal diagnosis should be B20, Human immunodeficiency virus [HIV] disease followed by additional diagnosis codes for all reported HIV-related conditions.

         (b) **Patient with HIV disease admitted for unrelated condition**

            If a patient with HIV disease is admitted for an unrelated condition (such as a traumatic injury), the code for the unrelated condition (e.g., the nature of injury code) should be the principal diagnosis. Other diagnoses would be B20 followed by additional diagnosis codes for all reported HIV-related conditions.

         (c) **Whether the patient is newly diagnosed**

            Whether the patient is newly diagnosed or has had previous admissions/encounters for HIV conditions is irrelevant to the sequencing decision.

         (d) **Asymptomatic human immunodeficiency virus**

            Z21, Asymptomatic human immunodeficiency virus [HIV] infection status, is to be applied when the patient without any documentation of symptoms is listed as being "HIV positive," "known HIV," "HIV test positive," or similar terminology. Do not use this code if the term "AIDS" is used or if the patient is treated for any HIV-related illness or is described as having any condition(s) resulting from his/her HIV positive status; use B20 in these cases.

         (e) **Patients with inconclusive HIV serology**

            Patients with inconclusive HIV serology, but no definitive diagnosis or manifestations of the illness, may be assigned code R75, Inconclusive laboratory evidence of human immunodeficiency virus [HIV].

         (f) **Previously diagnosed HIV-related illness**

            Patients with any known prior diagnosis of an HIV-related illness should be coded to B20. Once a patient has developed an HIV-related illness, the patient should always be assigned code B20 on every subsequent admission/encounter. Patients previously diagnosed with any HIV illness (B20) should never be assigned to R75 or Z21, Asymptomatic human immunodeficiency virus [HIV] infection status.

         (g) **HIV infection in pregnancy, childbirth and the puerperium**

            During pregnancy, childbirth or the puerperium, a patient admitted (or presenting for a health care encounter) because of an HIV-related illness should receive a principal diagnosis code of O98.7-, Human immunodeficiency [HIV] disease complicating pregnancy, childbirth and the puerperium, followed by B20 and the code(s) for the HIV-related illness(es). Codes from Chapter 15 always take sequencing priority.

            Patients with asymptomatic HIV infection status admitted (or presenting for a health care encounter) during pregnancy, childbirth, or the puerperium should receive codes of O98.7- and Z21.

         (h) **Encounters for testing for HIV**

            If a patient is being seen to determine his/her HIV status, use code Z11.4, Encounter for screening for human immunodeficiency virus [HIV]. Use additional codes for any associated high risk behavior.

            If a patient with signs or symptoms is being seen for HIV testing, code the signs and symptoms. An additional counseling code Z71.7, Human immunodeficiency virus [HIV] counseling, may be used if counseling is provided during the encounter for the test.

            When a patient returns to be informed of his/her HIV test results and the test result is negative, use code Z71.7, Human immunodeficiency virus [HIV] counseling.

            If the results are positive, see previous guidelines and assign codes as appropriate.

   b. **Infectious agents as the cause of diseases classified to other chapters**

      Certain infections are classified in chapters other than Chapter 1 and no organism is identified as part of the infection code. In these instances, it is necessary to use an additional code from Chapter 1 to identify the organism. A code from category B95, Streptococcus, Staphylococcus, and Enterococcus as the cause of diseases classified to other chapters, B96, Other bacterial agents as the cause of diseases classified to other chapters, or B97, Viral agents as the cause of diseases classified to other chapters, is to be used as an additional code to identify the organism. An instructional note will be found at the infection code advising that an additional organism code is required.

   c. **Infections resistant to antibiotics**

      Many bacterial infections are resistant to current antibiotics. It is necessary to identify all infections documented as antibiotic resistant. Assign a code from category Z16, Resistance to antimicrobial drugs, following the infection code only if the infection code does not identify drug resistance.

   d. **Sepsis, severe sepsis, and septic shock**
      1) **Coding of sepsis and severe sepsis**
         (a) **Sepsis**

            For a diagnosis of sepsis, assign the appropriate code for the underlying systemic infection. If the type of infection or causal organism is not further specified, assign code A41.9, Sepsis, unspecified organism.

            A code from subcategory R65.2, Severe sepsis, should not be assigned unless severe sepsis or an associated acute organ dysfunction is documented.

            (i) Negative or inconclusive blood cultures and sepsis
               Negative or inconclusive blood cultures do not preclude a diagnosis of sepsis in patients with clinical evidence of the condition, however, the provider should be queried.

            (ii) Urosepsis
               The term urosepsis is a nonspecific term. It is not to be considered synonymous with sepsis. It has no default code in the Alphabetic Index. Should a provider use this term, he/she must be queried for clarification.

            (iii) Sepsis with organ dysfunction
               If a patient has sepsis and associated acute organ dysfunction or multiple organ dysfunction (MOD), follow the instructions for coding severe sepsis.

            (iv) Acute organ dysfunction that is not clearly associated with the sepsis
               If a patient has sepsis and an acute organ dysfunction, but the medical record documentation indicates that the acute organ dysfunction is related to a medical condition other than the sepsis, do not assign a code from subcategory R65.2, Severe sepsis. An acute organ dysfunction must be associated with the sepsis in order to assign the severe sepsis code. If the documentation is not clear as to whether an acute organ dysfunction is related to the sepsis or another medical condition, query the provider.

         (b) **Severe sepsis**

            The coding of severe sepsis requires a minimum of 2 codes: first a code for the underlying systemic infection, followed by a code from subcategory R65.2, Severe sepsis. If the causal organism is not documented, assign code A41.9, Sepsis, unspecified organism, for the infection. Additional code(s) for the associated acute organ dysfunction are also required.

Due to the complex nature of severe sepsis, some cases may require querying the provider prior to assignment of the codes.

2) Septic shock

(a) Septic shock generally refers to circulatory failure associated with severe sepsis, and therefore, it represents a type of acute organ dysfunction. For all cases of septic shock, the code for the underlying systemic infection should be sequenced first, followed by code R65.21, Severe sepsis with septic shock. Any additional codes for the other acute organ dysfunctions should also be assigned.

For cases of septic shock, the code for the systemic infection should be sequenced first, followed by code R65.21, Severe sepsis with septic shock or code T81.12, Postprocedural septic shock. Any additional codes for the other acute organ dysfunctions should also be assigned. As noted in the sequencing instructions in the Tabular List, the code for septic shock cannot be assigned as a principal diagnosis.

3) Sequencing of severe sepsis

If severe sepsis is present on admission, and meets the definition of principal diagnosis, the underlying systemic infection should be assigned as principal diagnosis followed by the appropriate code from subcategory R65.2 as required by the sequencing rules in the Tabular List. A code from subcategory R65.2 can never be assigned as a principal diagnosis.

When severe sepsis develops during an encounter (it was not present on admission) the underlying systemic infection and the appropriate code from subcategory R65.2 should be assigned as secondary diagnoses.

Severe sepsis may be present on admission but the diagnosis may not be confirmed until sometime after admission. If the documentation is not clear whether severe sepsis was present on admission, the provider should be queried.

4) Sepsis and severe sepsis with a localized infection

If the reason for admission is both sepsis or severe sepsis and a localized infection, such as pneumonia or cellulitis, a code(s) for the underlying systemic infection should be assigned first and the code for the localized infection should be assigned as a secondary diagnosis. If the patient has severe sepsis, a code from subcategory R65.2 should also be assigned as a secondary diagnosis. If the patient is admitted with a localized infection, such as pneumonia, and sepsis/severe sepsis doesn't develop until after admission, the localized infection should be assigned first, followed by the appropriate sepsis/severe sepsis codes.

5) Sepsis due to a postprocedural infection

(a) **Documentation of causal relationship**

As with all postprocedural complications, code assignment is based on the provider's documentation of the relationship between the infection and the procedure.

(b) **Sepsis due to a postprocedural infection**

For such cases, the postprocedural infection code, such as, T80.2, Infections following infusion, transfusion, and therapeutic injection, T81.4, Infection following a procedure, T88.0, Infection following immunization, or O86.0, Infection of obstetric surgical wound, should be coded first, followed by the code for the specific infection. If the patient has severe sepsis the appropriate code from subcategory R65.2 should also be assigned with the additional code(s) for any acute organ dysfunction.

(c) **Postprocedural infection and postprocedural septic shock**

In cases where a postprocedural infection has occurred and has resulted in severe sepsis and postprocedural septic shock, the code for the precipitating complication such as code T81.4, Infection following a procedure, or O86.0, Infection of obstetrical surgical wound should be coded first followed by code R65.21, Severe sepsis with septic shock and a code for the systemic infection.

6) Sepsis and severe sepsis associated with a noninfectious process (condition)

In some cases a noninfectious process (condition), such as trauma, may lead to an infection which can result in sepsis or severe sepsis. If sepsis or severe sepsis is documented as associated with a noninfectious condition, such as a burn or serious injury, and this condition meets the definition for principal diagnosis, the code for the noninfectious condition should be sequenced first, followed by the code for the resulting infection. If severe sepsis, is present a code from subcategory R65.2 should also be assigned with any associated organ dysfunction(s) codes. It is not necessary to assign a code from subcategory R65.1, Systemic inflammatory response syndrome (SIRS) of non-infectious origin, for these cases.

If the infection meets the definition of principal diagnosis it should be sequenced before the non-infectious condition. When both the associated non-infectious condition and the infection meet the definition of principal diagnosis either may be assigned as principal diagnosis.

Only one code from category R65, Symptoms and signs specifically associated with systemic inflammation and infection, should be assigned. Therefore, when a non-infectious condition leads to an infection resulting in severe sepsis, assign the appropriate code from subcategory R65.2, Severe sepsis. Do not additionally assign a code from subcategory R65.1, Systemic inflammatory response syndrome (SIRS) of non-infectious origin.

See Section I.C.18. SIRS due to non-infectious process

7) Sepsis and septic shock complicating abortion, pregnancy, childbirth, and the puerperium

See Section I.C.15. Sepsis and septic shock complicating abortion, pregnancy, childbirth and the puerperium

8) Newborn sepsis

See Section I.C.16. f. Bacterial sepsis of Newborn

e. Methicillin resistant *Staphylococcus aureus* (MRSA) conditions

1) Selection and sequencing of MRSA codes

(a) **Combination codes for MRSA infection**

When a patient is diagnosed with an infection that is due to methicillin resistant *Staphylococcus aureus* (MRSA), and that infection has a combination code that includes the causal organism (e.g., sepsis, pneumonia) assign the appropriate combination code for the condition (e.g., code A41.02, Sepsis due to Methicillin resistant *Staphylococcus aureus* or code J15.212, Pneumonia due to Methicillin resistant *Staphylococcus aureus*). Do not assign code B95.62, Methicillin resistant *Staphylococcus aureus* infection as the cause of diseases classified elsewhere, as an additional code because the combination code includes the type of infection and the MRSA organism. Do not assign a code from subcategory Z16.11, Resistance to penicillins, as an additional diagnosis.

See Section C.1. for instructions on coding and sequencing of sepsis and severe sepsis.

(b) **Other codes for MRSA infection**

When there is documentation of a current infection (e.g., wound infection, stitch abscess, urinary tract infection) due to MRSA, and that infection does not have a combination code that includes the causal organism, assign the appropriate code to identify the condition along with code B95.62, Methicillin resistant *Staphylococcus aureus* infection as the cause of diseases classified elsewhere for the MRSA infection. Do not assign a code from subcategory Z16.11, Resistance to penicillins.

(c) **Methicillin susceptible *Staphylococcus aureus* (MSSA) and MRSA colonization**

The condition or state of being colonized or carrying MSSA or MRSA is called colonization or carriage, while an individual person is described as being colonized or being a carrier. Colonization means that MSSA or MSRA is present on or in the body without necessarily causing illness. A positive MRSA colonization test might be documented by the provider as "MRSA screen positive" or "MRSA nasal swab positive".

Assign code Z22.322, Carrier or suspected carrier of Methicillin resistant *Staphylococcus aureus*, for patients documented as having MRSA colonization. Assign code Z22.321, Carrier or suspected carrier of Methicillin susceptible *Staphylococcus aureus*, for patient documented as having MSSA colonization. Colonization is not necessarily indicative of a disease process or as the cause of a specific condition the patient may have unless documented as such by the provider.

(d) MRSA colonization and infection

If a patient is documented as having both MRSA colonization and infection during a hospital admission, code Z22.322, Carrier or suspected carrier of Methicillin resistant *Staphylococcus aureus*, and a code for the MRSA infection may both be assigned.

2. **Chapter 2: Neoplasms (C00-D49)**

General guidelines

Chapter 2 of the ICD-10-CM contains the codes for most benign and all malignant neoplasms. Certain benign neoplasms, such as prostatic adenomas, may be found in the specific body system chapters. To properly code a neoplasm it is necessary to determine from the record if the neoplasm is benign, in-situ, malignant, or of uncertain histologic behavior. If malignant, any secondary (metastatic) sites should also be determined.

Primary malignant neoplasms overlapping site boundaries

A primary malignant neoplasm that overlaps two or more contiguous (next to each other) sites should be classified to the subcategory/code .8 ('overlapping lesion'), unless the combination is specifically indexed elsewhere. For multiple neoplasms of the same site that are not contiguous such as tumors in different quadrants of the same breast, codes for each site should be assigned.

Malignant neoplasm of ectopic tissue

Malignant neoplasms of ectopic tissue are to be coded to the site of origin mentioned, e.g., ectopic pancreatic malignant neoplasms involving the stomach are coded to pancreas, unspecified (C25.9).

The neoplasm table in the Alphabetic Index should be referenced first. However, if the histological term is documented, that term should be referenced first, rather than going immediately to the Neoplasm Table, in order to determine which column in the Neoplasm Table is appropriate. For example, if the documentation indicates "adenoma," refer to the term in the Alphabetic Index to review the entries under this term and the instructional note to "see also neoplasm, by site, benign." The table provides the proper code based on the type of neoplasm and the site. It is important to select the proper column in the table that corresponds to the type of neoplasm. The Tabular List should then be referenced to verify that the correct code has been selected from the table and that a more specific site code does not exist.

See Section I.C.21. Factors influencing health status and contact with health services, Status, for information regarding Z15.0, codes for genetic susceptibility to cancer.

a. **Treatment directed at the malignancy**

If the treatment is directed at the malignancy, designate the malignancy as the principal diagnosis.

The only exception to this guideline is if a patient admission/encounter is solely for the administration of chemotherapy, immunotherapy or radiation therapy, assign the appropriate Z51.- code as the first-listed or principal diagnosis, and the diagnosis or problem for which the service is being performed as a secondary diagnosis.

b. **Treatment of secondary site**

When a patient is admitted because of a primary neoplasm with metastasis and treatment is directed toward the secondary site only, the secondary neoplasm is designated as the principal diagnosis even though the primary malignancy is still present.

c. **Coding and sequencing of complications**

Coding and sequencing of complications associated with the malignancies or with the therapy thereof are subject to the following guidelines:

1) **Anemia associated with malignancy**

When admission/encounter is for management of an anemia associated with the malignancy, and the treatment is only for anemia, the appropriate code for the malignancy is sequenced as the principal or first-listed diagnosis followed by the appropriate code for the anemia (such as code D63.0, Anemia in neoplastic disease).

2) **Anemia associated with chemotherapy, immunotherapy and radiation therapy**

When the admission/encounter is for management of an anemia associated with an adverse effect of the administration of chemotherapy or immunotherapy and the only treatment is for the anemia, the anemia code is sequenced first followed by the appropriate codes for the neoplasm and the adverse effect (T45.1X5, Adverse effect of antineoplastic and immunosuppressive drugs).

When the admission/encounter is for management of an anemia associated with an adverse effect of radiotherapy, the anemia code should be sequenced first, followed by the appropriate neoplasm code and code Y84.2, Radiological procedure and radiotherapy as the cause of abnormal reaction of the patient, or of later complication, without mention of misadventure at the time of the procedure.

3) **Management of dehydration due to the malignancy**

When the admission/encounter is for management of dehydration due to the malignancy and only the dehydration is being treated (intravenous rehydration), the dehydration is sequenced first, followed by the code(s) for the malignancy.

4) **Treatment of a complication resulting from a surgical procedure**

When the admission/encounter is for treatment of a complication resulting from a surgical procedure, designate the complication as the principal or first-listed diagnosis if treatment is directed at resolving the complication.

d. **Primary malignancy previously excised**

When a primary malignancy has been previously excised or eradicated from its site and there is no further treatment directed to that site and there is no evidence of any existing primary malignancy, a code from category Z85, Personal history of malignant neoplasm, should be used to indicate the former site of the malignancy. Any mention of extension, invasion, or metastasis to another site is coded as a secondary malignant neoplasm to that site. The secondary site may be the principal or first-listed with the Z85 code used as a secondary code.

e. **Admissions/Encounters involving chemotherapy, immunotherapy and radiation therapy**

1) **Episode of care involves surgical removal of neoplasm**

When an episode of care involves the surgical removal of a neoplasm, primary or secondary site, followed by adjunct chemotherapy or radiation treatment during the same episode of care, the code for the neoplasm should be assigned as principal or first-listed diagnosis.

2) **Patient admission/encounter solely for administration of chemotherapy, immunotherapy and radiation therapy**

If a patient admission/encounter is solely for the administration of chemotherapy, immunotherapy or radiation therapy assign code Z51.0, Encounter for antineoplastic radiation therapy, or Z51.11, Encounter for antineoplastic chemotherapy, or Z51.12, Encounter for antineoplastic immunotherapy as the first-listed or principal diagnosis. If a patient receives more than one of these therapies during the same admission more than one of these codes may be assigned, in any sequence.

The malignancy for which the therapy is being administered should be assigned as a secondary diagnosis.

3) **Patient admitted for radiation therapy, chemotherapy or immunotherapy and develops complications**

When a patient is admitted for the purpose of radiotherapy, immunotherapy or chemotherapy and develops complications such as uncontrolled nausea and vomiting or dehydration, the principal or first-listed diagnosis is Z51.0, Encounter for antineoplastic radiation therapy, or Z51.11, Encounter for antineoplastic chemotherapy, or Z51.12, Encounter for antineoplastic immunotherapy followed by any codes for the complications.

f. Admission/encounter to determine extent of malignancy

When the reason for admission/encounter is to determine the extent of the malignancy, or for a procedure such as paracentesis or thoracentesis, the primary malignancy or appropriate metastatic site is designated as the principal or first-listed diagnosis, even though chemotherapy or radiotherapy is administered.

g. Symptoms, signs, and abnormal findings listed in Chapter 18 associated with neoplasms

Symptoms, signs, and ill-defined conditions listed in Chapter 18 characteristic of, or associated with, an existing primary or secondary site malignancy cannot be used to replace the malignancy as principal or first-listed diagnosis, regardless of the number of admissions or encounters for treatment and care of the neoplasm.

See section I.C.21. Factors influencing health status and contact with health services, Encounter for prophylactic organ removal.

h. Admission/encounter for pain control/management

See Section I.C.6. for information on coding admission/encounter for pain control/management.

i. Malignancy in two or more noncontiguous sites

A patient may have more than one malignant tumor in the same organ. These tumors may represent different primaries or metastatic disease, depending on the site. Should the documentation be unclear, the provider should be queried as to the status of each tumor so that the correct codes can be assigned.

j. Disseminated malignant neoplasm, unspecified

Code C80.0, Disseminated malignant neoplasm, unspecified, is for use only in those cases where the patient has advanced metastatic disease and no known primary or secondary sites are specified. It should not be used in place of assigning codes for the primary site and all known secondary sites.

k. Malignant neoplasm without specification of site

Code C80.1, Malignant (primary) neoplasm, unspecified, equates to Cancer, unspecified. This code should only be used when no determination can be made as to the primary site of a malignancy. This code should rarely be used in the inpatient setting.

l. Sequencing of neoplasm codes

1) **Encounter for treatment of primary malignancy**

If the reason for the encounter is for treatment of a primary malignancy, assign the malignancy as the principal/first-listed diagnosis. The primary site is to be sequenced first, followed by any metastatic sites.

2) **Encounter for treatment of secondary malignancy**

When an encounter is for a primary malignancy with metastasis and treatment is directed toward the metastatic (secondary) site(s) only, the metastatic site(s) is designated as the principal/first-listed diagnosis. The primary malignancy is coded as an additional code.

3) **Malignant neoplasm in a pregnant patient**

When a pregnant woman has a malignant neoplasm, a code from subcategory O9A.1-, Malignant neoplasm complicating pregnancy, childbirth, and the puerperium, should be sequenced first, followed by the appropriate code from Chapter 2 to indicate the type of neoplasm.

4) **Encounter for complication associated with a neoplasm**

When an encounter is for management of a complication associated with a neoplasm, such as dehydration, and the treatment is only for the complication, the complication is coded first, followed by the appropriate code(s) for the neoplasm.

The exception to this guideline is anemia. When the admission/encounter is for management of an anemia associated with the malignancy, and the treatment is only for anemia, the appropriate code for the malignancy is sequenced as the principal or first-listed diagnosis followed by code D63.0, Anemia in neoplastic disease.

5) **Complication from surgical procedure for treatment of a neoplasm**

When an encounter is for treatment of a complication resulting from a surgical procedure performed for the treatment of the neoplasm, designate the complication as the principal/first-listed diagnosis. See guideline regarding the coding of a current malignancy versus personal history to determine if the code for the neoplasm should also be assigned.

6) **Pathologic fracture due to a neoplasm**

When an encounter is for a pathological fracture due to a neoplasm, and the focus of treatment is the fracture, a code from subcategory M84.5, Pathological fracture in neoplastic disease, should be sequenced first, followed by the code for the neoplasm.

If the focus of treatment is the neoplasm with an associated pathological fracture, the neoplasm code should be sequenced first, followed by a code from M84.5 for the pathological fracture.

m. Current malignancy versus personal history of malignancy

When a primary malignancy has been excised but further treatment, such as an additional surgery for the malignancy, radiation therapy or chemotherapy is directed to that site, the primary malignancy code should be used until treatment is completed.

When a primary malignancy has been previously excised or eradicated from its site, there is no further treatment (of the malignancy) directed to that site, and there is no evidence of any existing primary malignancy, a code from category Z85, Personal history of malignant neoplasm, should be used to indicate the former site of the malignancy.

See Section I.C.21. Factors influencing health status and contact with health services, History (of)

n. Leukemia, multiple myeloma, and malignant plasma cell neoplasms in remission versus personal history

The categories for leukemia, and category C90, Multiple myeloma and malignant plasma cell neoplasms, have codes indicating whether or not the leukemia has achieved remission. There are also codes Z85.6, Personal history of leukemia, and Z85.79, Personal history of other malignant neoplasms of lymphoid, hematopoietic and related tissues. If the documentation is unclear, as to whether the leukemia has achieved remission, the provider should be queried.

See Section I.C.21. Factors influencing health status and contact with health services, History (of)

o. Aftercare following surgery for neoplasm

See Section I.C.21. Factors influencing health status and contact with health services, Aftercare

p. Follow-up care for completed treatment of a malignancy

See Section I.C.21. Factors influencing health status and contact with health services, Follow-up

q. Prophylactic organ removal for prevention of malignancy

See Section I.C. 21, Factors influencing health status and contact with health services, Prophylactic organ removal

r. Malignant neoplasm associated with transplanted organ

A malignant neoplasm of a transplanted organ should be coded as a transplant complication. Assign first the appropriate code from category T86.-, Complications of transplanted organs and tissue, followed by code C80.2, Malignant neoplasm associated with transplanted organ. Use an additional code for the specific malignancy.

3. **Chapter 3: Disease of the Blood and Blood-forming Organs and Certain Disorders Involving the Immune Mechanism (D50-D89)**

Reserved for future guideline expansion

4. **Chapter 4: Endocrine, Nutritional, and Metabolic Diseases (E00-E89)**

a. **Diabetes mellitus**

The diabetes mellitus codes are combination codes that include the type of diabetes mellitus, the body system affected, and the complications affecting that body system. As many codes within a particular category as are necessary to describe all of the complications of the disease may be used. They should be sequenced based on the reason for a particular encounter. Assign as many codes from categories E08 – E13 as needed to identify all of the associated conditions that the patient has.

1) Type of diabetes
The age of a patient is not the sole determining factor, though most type 1 diabetics develop the condition before reaching puberty. For this reason type 1 diabetes mellitus is also referred to as juvenile diabetes.

2) Type of diabetes mellitus not documented
If the type of diabetes mellitus is not documented in the medical record the default is E11.-, Type 2 diabetes mellitus.

3) Diabetes mellitus and the use of insulin
If the documentation in a medical record does not indicate the type of diabetes but does indicate that the patient uses insulin, code E11, Type 2 diabetes mellitus, should be assigned. Code Z79.4, Long-term (current) use of insulin, should also be assigned to indicate that the patient uses insulin. Code Z79.4 should not be assigned if insulin is given temporarily to bring a type 2 patient's blood sugar under control during an encounter.

4) Diabetes mellitus in pregnancy and gestational diabetes
See Section I.C.15. Diabetes mellitus in pregnancy.

See Section I.C.15. Gestational (pregnancy induced) diabetes

5) Complications due to insulin pump malfunction
(a) Underdose of insulin due to insulin pump failure
An underdose of insulin due to an insulin pump failure should be assigned to a code from subcategory T85.6, Mechanical complication of other specified internal and external prosthetic devices, implants and grafts, that specifies the type of pump malfunction, as the principal or first-listed code, followed by code T38.3x6-, Underdosing of insulin and oral hypoglycemic [antidiabetic] drugs. Additional codes for the type of diabetes mellitus and any associated complications due to the underdosing should also be assigned.

(b) Overdose of insulin due to insulin pump failure
The principal or first-listed code for an encounter due to an insulin pump malfunction resulting in an overdose of insulin, should also be T85.6-, Mechanical complication of other specified internal and external prosthetic devices, implants and grafts, followed by code T38.3X1-, Poisoning by insulin and oral hypoglycemic [antidiabetic] drugs, accidental (unintentional).

6) Secondary diabetes mellitus
Codes under categories E08, Diabetes mellitus due to underlying condition, E09, Drug or chemical induced diabetes mellitus, and E13, Other specified diabetes mellitus, identify complications/manifestations associated with secondary diabetes mellitus. Secondary diabetes is always caused by another condition or event (e.g., cystic fibrosis, malignant neoplasm of pancreas, pancreatectomy, adverse effect of drug, or poisoning).

(a) Secondary diabetes mellitus and the use of insulin
For patients who routinely use insulin, code Z79.4, Long-term (current) use of insulin, should also be assigned. Code Z79.4 should not be assigned if insulin is given temporarily to bring a patient's blood sugar under control during an encounter.

(b) Assigning and sequencing secondary diabetes codes and its causes
The sequencing of the secondary diabetes codes in relationship to codes for the cause of the diabetes is based on the Tabular List instructions for categories E08, E09 and E13.

(i) Secondary diabetes mellitus due to pancreatectomy
For postpancreatectomy diabetes mellitus (lack of insulin due to the surgical removal of all or part of the pancreas), assign code E89.1, Postprocedural hypoinsulinemia. Assign a code from category E13 and

a code from subcategory Z90.41-, Acquired absence of pancreas, as additional codes.

(ii) Secondary diabetes due to drugs
Secondary diabetes may be caused by an adverse effect of correctly administered medications, poisoning or sequela of poisoning.
See section I.C.19.e for coding of adverse effects and poisoning, and section I.C.20 for external cause code reporting.

5. Chapter 5: Mental, Behavioral and Neurodevelopmental Disorders (F01 – F99)
a. Pain disorders related to psychological factors
Assign code F45.41, for pain that is exclusively related to psychological disorders. As indicated by the Excludes 1 note under category G89, a code from category G89 should not be assigned with code F45.41

Code F45.42, Pain disorders with related psychological factors, should be used with a code from category G89, Pain, not elsewhere classified, if there is documentation of a psychological component for a patient with acute or chronic pain.
See Section I.C.6. Pain

b. Mental and behavioral disorders due to psychoactive substance use
1) In remission
Selection of codes for "in remission" for categories F10-F19, Mental and behavioral disorders due to psychoactive substance use (categories F10-F19 with -.21) requires the provider's clinical judgment. The appropriate codes for "in remission" are assigned only on the basis of provider documentation (as defined in the Official Guidelines for Coding and Reporting).

2) Psychoactive substance use, abuse and dependence
When the provider documentation refers to use, abuse and dependence of the same substance (e.g. alcohol, opioid, cannabis, etc.), only one code should be assigned to identify the pattern of use based on the following hierarchy:

- If both use and abuse are documented, assign only the code for abuse
- If both abuse and dependence are documented, assign only the code for dependence
- If use, abuse and dependence are all documented, assign only the code for dependence
- If both use and dependence are documented, assign only the code for dependence.

3) Psychoactive substance use
As with all other diagnoses, the codes for psychoactive substance use (F10.9-, F11.9-, F12.9-, F13.9-, F14.9-, F15.9-, F16.9-) should only be assigned based on provider documentation and when they meet the definition of a reportable diagnosis (see Section III, Reporting Additional Diagnoses). The codes are to be used only when the psychoactive substance use is associated with a mental or behavioral disorder, and such a relationship is documented by the provider.

6. Chapter 6: Diseases of Nervous System (G00-G99)
a. Dominant/nondominant side
Codes from category G81, Hemiplegia and hemiparesis, and subcategories, G83.1, Monoplegia of lower limb, G83.2, Monoplegia of upper limb, and G83.3, Monoplegia, unspecified, identify whether the dominant or nondominant side is affected. Should the affected side be documented, but not specified as dominant or nondominant, and the classification system does not indicate a default, code selection is as follows:

- For ambidextrous patients, the default should be dominant.
- If the left side is affected, the default is non-dominant.
- If the right side is affected, the default is dominant.

b. Pain - Category G89
1) General coding information
Codes in category G89, Pain, not elsewhere classified, may be used in conjunction with codes from other categories and

chapters to provide more detail about acute or chronic pain and neoplasm-related pain, unless otherwise indicated below.

If the pain is not specified as acute or chronic, post-thoracotomy, postprocedural, or neoplasm-related, do not assign codes from category G89.

A code from category G89 should not be assigned if the underlying (definitive) diagnosis is known, unless the reason for the encounter is pain control/ management and not management of the underlying condition.

When an admission or encounter is for a procedure aimed at treating the underlying condition (e.g., spinal fusion, kyphoplasty), a code for the underlying condition (e.g., vertebral fracture, spinal stenosis) should be assigned as the principal diagnosis. No code from category G89 should be assigned.

(a) Category G89 codes as principal or first-listed diagnosis
Category G89 codes are acceptable as principal diagnosis or the first-listed code:

- When pain control or pain management is the reason for the admission/encounter (e.g., a patient with displaced intervertebral disc, nerve impingement and severe back pain presents for injection of steroid into the spinal canal). The underlying cause of the pain should be reported as an additional diagnosis, if known.

- When a patient is admitted for the insertion of a neurostimulator for pain control, assign the appropriate pain code as the principal or first-listed diagnosis. When an admission or encounter is for a procedure aimed at treating the underlying condition and a neurostimulator is inserted for pain control during the same admission/encounter, a code for the underlying condition should be assigned as the principal diagnosis and the appropriate pain code should be assigned as a secondary diagnosis.

(b) Use of category G89 codes in conjunction with site specific pain codes
(i) Assigning category G89 and site-specific pain codes
Codes from category G89 may be used in conjunction with codes that identify the site of pain (including codes from chapter 18) if the category G89 code provides additional information. For example, if the code describes the site of the pain, but does not fully describe whether the pain is acute or chronic, then both codes should be assigned.

(ii) Sequencing of category G89 codes with site-specific pain codes
The sequencing of category G89 codes with site-specific pain codes (including chapter 18 codes), is dependent on the circumstances of the encounter/admission as follows:

- If the encounter is for pain control or pain management, assign the code from category G89 followed by the code identifying the specific site of pain (e.g., encounter for pain management for acute neck pain from trauma is assigned code G89.11, Acute pain due to trauma, followed by code M54.2, Cervicalgia, to identify the site of pain).

- If the encounter is for any other reason except pain control or pain management, and a related definitive diagnosis has not been established (confirmed) by the provider, assign the code for the specific site of pain first, followed by the appropriate code from category G89.

2) Pain due to devices, implants and grafts
See Section I.C.19. Pain due to medical devices

3) Postoperative pain
The provider's documentation should be used to guide the coding of postoperative pain, as well as *Section III. Reporting*

Additional Diagnoses and Section IV. Diagnostic Coding and Reporting in the Outpatient Setting.

The default for post-thoracotomy and other postoperative pain not specified as acute or chronic is the code for the acute form.

Routine or expected postoperative pain immediately after surgery should not be coded.

(a) Postoperative pain not associated with specific postoperative complication
Postoperative pain not associated with a specific postoperative complication is assigned to the appropriate postoperative pain code in category G89.

(b) Postoperative pain associated with specific postoperative complication
Postoperative pain associated with a specific postoperative complication (such as painful wire sutures) is assigned to the appropriate code(s) found in Chapter 19, Injury, poisoning, and certain other consequences of external causes. If appropriate, use additional code(s) from category G89 to identify acute or chronic pain (G89.18 or G89.28).

4) Chronic pain
Chronic pain is classified to subcategory G89.2. There is no time frame defining when pain becomes chronic pain. The provider's documentation should be used to guide use of these codes.

5) Neoplasm related pain
Code G89.3 is assigned to pain documented as being related, associated or due to cancer, primary or secondary malignancy, or tumor. This code is assigned regardless of whether the pain is acute or chronic.

This code may be assigned as the principal or first-listed code when the stated reason for the admission/encounter is documented as pain control/pain management. The underlying neoplasm should be reported as an additional diagnosis.

When the reason for the admission/encounter is management of the neoplasm and the pain associated with the neoplasm is also documented, code G89.3 may be assigned as an additional diagnosis. It is not necessary to assign an additional code for the site of the pain.

See Section I.C.2 for instructions on the sequencing of neoplasms for all other stated reasons for the admission/encounter (except for pain control/pain management).

6) Chronic pain syndrome
Central pain syndrome (G89.0) and chronic pain syndrome (G89.4) are different than the term "chronic pain," and therefore codes should only be used when the provider has specifically documented this condition.

See Section I.C.5. Pain disorders related to psychological factors

7. Chapter 7: Diseases of Eye and Adnexa (H00-H59)
a. Glaucoma
1) Assigning glaucoma codes
Assign as many codes from category H40, Glaucoma, as needed to identify the type of glaucoma, the affected eye, and the glaucoma stage.

2) Bilateral glaucoma with same type and stage
When a patient has bilateral glaucoma and both eyes are documented as being the same type and stage, and there is a code for bilateral glaucoma, report only the code for the type of glaucoma, bilateral, with the seventh character for the stage.

When a patient has bilateral glaucoma and both eyes are documented as being the same type and stage, and the classification does not provide a code for bilateral glaucoma (i.e. subcategories H40.10, H40.11 and H40.20) report only one code for the type of glaucoma with the appropriate seventh character for the stage.

3) Bilateral glaucoma stage with different types or stages
When a patient has bilateral glaucoma and each eye is documented as having a different type or stage, and the classification distinguishes laterality, assign the appropriate code for each eye rather than the code for bilateral glaucoma.

When a patient has bilateral glaucoma and each eye is documented as having a different type, and the classification does not distinguish laterality (i.e. subcategories H40.10, H40.11 and H40.20), assign one code for each type of glaucoma with the appropriate seventh character for the stage.

When a patient has bilateral glaucoma and each eye is documented as having the same type, but different stage, and the classification does not distinguish laterality (i.e. subcategories H40.10, H40.11 and H40.20), assign a code for the type of glaucoma for each eye with the seventh character for the specific glaucoma stage documented for each eye.

4) Patient admitted with glaucoma and stage evolves during the admission

If a patient is admitted with glaucoma and the stage progresses during the admission, assign the code for highest stage documented.

5) Indeterminate stage glaucoma

Assignment of the seventh character "4" for "indeterminate stage" should be based on the clinical documentation. The seventh character "4" is used for glaucomas whose stage cannot be clinically determined. This seventh character should not be confused with the seventh character "0", unspecified, which should be assigned when there is no documentation regarding the stage of the glaucoma.

8. Chapter 8: Diseases of Ear and Mastoid Process (H60-H95)
Reserved for future guideline expansion

9. Chapter 9: Diseases of Circulatory System (I00-I99)

a. Hypertension

1) Hypertension with heart disease

Heart conditions classified to I50.- or I51.4-I51.9, are assigned to, a code from category I11, Hypertensive heart disease, when a causal relationship is stated (due to hypertension) or implied (hypertensive). Use an additional code from category I50, Heart failure, to identify the type of heart failure in those patients with heart failure.

The same heart conditions (I50.-, I51.4-I51.9) with hypertension, but without a stated causal relationship, are coded separately. Sequence according to the circumstances of the admission/encounter.

2) Hypertensive chronic kidney disease

Assign codes from category I12, Hypertensive chronic kidney disease, when both hypertension and a condition classifiable to category N18, Chronic kidney disease (CKD), are present. Unlike hypertension with heart disease, ICD-10-CM presumes a cause-and-effect relationship and classifies chronic kidney disease with hypertension as hypertensive chronic kidney disease.

The appropriate code from category N18 should be used as a secondary code with a code from category I12 to identify the stage of chronic kidney disease.

See Section I.C.14. Chronic kidney disease.

If a patient has hypertensive chronic kidney disease and acute renal failure, an additional code for the acute renal failure is required.

3) Hypertensive heart and chronic kidney disease

Assign codes from combination category I13, Hypertensive heart and chronic kidney disease, when both hypertensive kidney disease and hypertensive heart disease are stated in the diagnosis. Assume a relationship between the hypertension and the chronic kidney disease, whether or not the condition is so designated. If heart failure is present, assign an additional code from category I50 to identify the type of heart failure.

The appropriate code from category N18, Chronic kidney disease, should be used as a secondary code with a code from category I13 to identify the stage of chronic kidney disease.

See Section I.C.14. Chronic kidney disease.

The codes in category I13, Hypertensive heart and chronic kidney disease, are combination codes that include hypertension, heart disease and chronic kidney disease. The Includes note at I13 specifies that the conditions included at I11 and I12 are included together in I13. If a patient has hypertension, heart disease and chronic kidney disease then a

code from I13 should be used, not individual codes for hypertension, heart disease and chronic kidney disease, or codes from I11 or I12.

For patients with both acute renal failure and chronic kidney disease an additional code for acute renal failure is required.

4) Hypertensive cerebrovascular disease

For hypertensive cerebrovascular disease, first assign the appropriate code from categories I60-I69, followed by the appropriate hypertension code.

5) Hypertensive retinopathy

Subcategory H35.0, Background retinopathy and retinal vascular changes, should be used with a code from category I10 – I15, Hypertensive disease to include the systemic hypertension. The sequencing is based on the reason for the encounter.

6) Hypertension, secondary

Secondary hypertension is due to an underlying condition. Two codes are required: one to identify the underlying etiology and one from category I15 to identify the hypertension. Sequencing of codes is determined by the reason for admission/encounter.

7) Hypertension, transient

Assign code R03.0, Elevated blood pressure reading without diagnosis of hypertension, unless patient has an established diagnosis of hypertension. Assign code O13.-, Gestational [pregnancy-induced] hypertension without significant proteinuria, or O14.-, Pre-eclampsia, for transient hypertension of pregnancy.

8) Hypertension, controlled

This diagnostic statement usually refers to an existing state of hypertension under control by therapy. Assign the appropriate code from categories I10-I15, Hypertensive diseases.

9) Hypertension, uncontrolled

Uncontrolled hypertension may refer to untreated hypertension or hypertension not responding to current therapeutic regimen. In either case, assign the appropriate code from categories I10-I15, Hypertensive diseases.

b. Atherosclerotic coronary artery disease and angina

ICD-10-CM has combination codes for atherosclerotic heart disease with angina pectoris. The subcategories for these codes are I25.11, Atherosclerotic heart disease of native coronary artery with angina pectoris and I25.7, Atherosclerosis of coronary artery bypass graft(s) and coronary artery of transplanted heart with angina pectoris.

When using one of these combination codes it is not necessary to use an additional code for angina pectoris. A causal relationship can be assumed in a patient with both atherosclerosis and angina pectoris, unless the documentation indicates the angina is due to something other than the atherosclerosis.

If a patient with coronary artery disease is admitted due to an acute myocardial infarction (AMI), the AMI should be sequenced before the coronary artery disease.

See Section I.C.9. Acute myocardial infarction (AMI)

c. Intraoperative and postprocedural cerebrovascular accident

Medical record documentation should clearly specify the cause-and-effect relationship between the medical intervention and the cerebrovascular accident in order to assign a code for intraoperative or postprocedural cerebrovascular accident.

Proper code assignment depends on whether it was an infarction or hemorrhage and whether it occurred intraoperatively or postoperatively. If it was a cerebral hemorrhage, code assignment depends on the type of procedure performed.

d. Sequelae of cerebrovascular disease

1) Category I69, sequelae of cerebrovascular disease

Category I69 is used to indicate conditions classifiable to categories I60-I67 as the causes of sequela (neurologic deficits), themselves classified elsewhere. These "late effects" include neurologic deficits that persist after initial onset of conditions classifiable to categories I60-I67. The neurologic deficits caused by cerebrovascular disease may be present from the onset or may arise at any time after the onset of the condition classifiable to categories I60-I67.

Codes from category I69, Sequelae of cerebrovascular disease, that specify hemiplegia, hemiparesis and monoplegia identify whether the dominant or nondominant side is affected. Should the affected side be documented, but not specified as dominant or nondominant, and the classification system does not indicate a default, code selection is as follows:

- For ambidextrous patients, the default should be dominant.
- If the left side is affected, the default is non-dominant.
- If the right side is affected, the default is dominant.

2) Codes from category I69 with codes from I60-I67
Codes from category I69 may be assigned on a health care record with codes from I60-I67, if the patient has a current cerebrovascular disease and deficits from an old cerebrovascular disease.

3) Codes from category I69 and Personal history of transient ischemic attack (TIA) and cerebral infarction (Z86.73)
Codes from category I69 should not be assigned if the patient does not have neurologic deficits.

See Section I.C.21. 4. History (of) for use of personal history codes

e. Acute myocardial infarction (AMI)

1) ST elevation myocardial infarction (STEMI) and non ST elevation myocardial infarction (NSTEMI)
The ICD-10-CM codes for acute myocardial infarction (AMI) identify the site, such as anterolateral wall or true posterior wall. Subcategories I21.0-I21.2 and code I21.3 are used for ST elevation myocardial infarction (STEMI). Code I21.4, Non-ST elevation (NSTEMI) myocardial infarction, is used for non ST elevation myocardial infarction (NSTEMI) and nontransmural MIs.

If NSTEMI evolves to STEMI, assign the STEMI code. If STEMI converts to NSTEMI due to thrombolytic therapy, it is still coded as STEMI.

For encounters occurring while the myocardial infarction is equal to, or less than, four weeks old, including transfers to another acute setting or a postacute setting, and the patient requires continued care for the myocardial infarction, codes from category I21 may continue to be reported. For encounters after the 4 week time frame and the patient is still receiving care related to the myocardial infarction, the appropriate aftercare code should be assigned, rather than a code from category I21. For old or healed myocardial infarctions not requiring further care, code I25.2, Old myocardial infarction, may be assigned.

2) Acute myocardial infarction, unspecified
Code I21.3, ST elevation (STEMI) myocardial infarction of unspecified site, is the default for the unspecified term acute myocardial infarction. If only STEMI or transmural MI without the site is documented, query the provider as to the site, or assign code I21.3.

3) AMI documented as nontransmural or subendocardial but site provided
If an AMI is documented as nontransmural or subendocardial, but the site is provided, it is still coded as a subendocardial AMI.

See Section I.C.21.3 for information on coding status post administration of tPA in a different facility within the last 24 hrs.

4) Subsequent acute myocardial infarction
A code from category I22, Subsequent ST elevation (STEMI) and non ST elevation (NSTEMI) myocardial infarction, is to be used when a patient who has suffered an AMI has a new AMI within the 4 week time frame of the initial AMI. A code from category I22 must be used in conjunction with a code from category I21. The sequencing of the I22 and I21 codes depends on the circumstances of the encounter.

10. Chapter 10: Diseases of the Respiratory System (J00-J99)

a. Chronic Obstructive Pulmonary Disease [COPD] and Asthma

1) Acute exacerbation of chronic obstructive bronchitis and asthma
The codes in categories J44 and J45 distinguish between uncomplicated cases and those in acute exacerbation. An acute exacerbation is a worsening or a decompensation of a chronic condition. An acute exacerbation is not equivalent to an infection superimposed on a chronic condition, though an exacerbation may be triggered by an infection.

b. Acute Respiratory Failure

1) Acute respiratory failure as principal diagnosis
A code from subcategory J96.0, Acute respiratory failure, or subcategory J96.2, Acute and chronic respiratory failure, may be assigned as a principal diagnosis when it is the condition established after study to be chiefly responsible for occasioning the admission to the hospital, and the selection is supported by the Alphabetic Index and Tabular List. However, chapter-specific coding guidelines (such as obstetrics, poisoning, HIV, newborn) that provide sequencing direction take precedence.

2) Acute respiratory failure as secondary diagnosis
Respiratory failure may be listed as a secondary diagnosis if it occurs after admission, or if it is present on admission, but does not meet the definition of principal diagnosis.

3) Sequencing of acute respiratory failure and another acute condition
When a patient is admitted with respiratory failure and another acute condition, (e.g., myocardial infarction, cerebrovascular accident, aspiration pneumonia), the principal diagnosis will not be the same in every situation. This applies whether the other acute condition is a respiratory or nonrespiratory condition. Selection of the principal diagnosis will be dependent on the circumstances of admission. If both the respiratory failure and the other acute condition are equally responsible for occasioning the admission to the hospital, and there are no chapter-specific sequencing rules, the guideline regarding two or more diagnoses that equally meet the definition for principal diagnosis (Section II, C.) may be applied in these situations.

If the documentation is not clear as to whether acute respiratory failure and another condition are equally responsible for occasioning the admission, query the provider for clarification.

c. Influenza due to certain identified influenza viruses
Code only confirmed cases of influenza due to certain identified influenza viruses (category J09), and due to other identified influenza virus (category J10). This is an exception to the hospital inpatient guideline Section II, H. (Uncertain Diagnosis).

In this context, "confirmation" does not require documentation of positive laboratory testing specific for avian or other novel influenza A or other identified influenza virus. However, coding should be based on the provider's diagnostic statement that the patient has avian influenza, or other novel influenza A, for category J09, or has another particular identified strain of influenza, such as H1N1 or H3N2, but not identified as novel or variant, for category J10.

If the provider records "suspected" or "possible" or "probable" avian influenza, or novel influenza, or other identified influenza, then the appropriate influenza code from category J11, Influenza due to unidentified influenza virus, should be assigned. A code from category J09, Influenza due to certain identified influenza viruses, should not be assigned nor should a code from category J10, Influenza due to other identified influenza virus.

d. Ventilator associated pneumonia

1) Documentation of ventilator associated pneumonia
As with all procedural or postprocedural complications, code assignment is based on the provider's documentation of the relationship between the condition and the procedure.

Code J95.851, Ventilator associated pneumonia, should be assigned only when the provider has documented ventilator associated pneumonia (VAP). An additional code to identify the organism (e.g., Pseudomonas aeruginosa, code B96.5) should also be assigned. Do not assign an additional code from categories J12-J18 to identify the type of pneumonia.

Code J95.851 should not be assigned for cases where the patient has pneumonia and is on a mechanical ventilator and the provider has not specifically stated that the pneumonia is ventilator-associated pneumonia. If the documentation is unclear as to whether the patient has a pneumonia that is a complication attributable to the mechanical ventilator, query the provider.

2) Ventilator associated pneumonia develops after admission

A patient may be admitted with one type of pneumonia (e.g., code J13, Pneumonia due to Streptococcus pneu- monia) and subsequently develop VAP. In this instance, the principal diagnosis would be the appro- priate code from categories J12-J18 for the pneumonia diagnosed at the time of admission. Code J95.851, Ventilator assoc- iated pneumonia, would be assigned as an additional diagnosis when the provider has also documented the presence of ventilator associated pneumonia.

11. Chapter 11: Diseases of the Digestive System (KØØ-K95)

Reserved for future guideline expansion

12. Chapter 12: Diseases of the Skin and Subcutaneous Tissue (LØØ-L99)

a. Pressure ulcer stage codes

1) Pressure ulcer stages

Codes from category L89, Pressure ulcer, are combination codes that identify the site of the pressure ulcer as well as the stage of the ulcer.

The ICD-1Ø-CM classifies pressure ulcer stages based on severity, which is designated by stages 1-4, unspecified stage and unstageable.

Assign as many codes from category L89 as needed to identify all the pressure ulcers the patient has, if applicable.

2) Unstageable pressure ulcers

Assignment of the code for unstageable pressure ulcer (L89.--Ø) should be based on the clinical documentation. These codes are used for pressure ulcers whose stage cannot be clinically determined (e.g., the ulcer is covered by eschar or has been treated with a skin or muscle graft) and pressure ulcers that are documented as deep tissue injury but not documented as due to trauma. This code should not be confused with the codes for unspecified stage (L89.--9). When there is no documentation regarding the stage of the pressure ulcer, assign the appropriate code for unspecified stage (L89.--9).

3) Documented pressure ulcer stage

Assignment of the pressure ulcer stage code should be guided by clinical documentation of the stage or documentation of the terms found in the Alphabetic Index. For clinical terms describing the stage that are not found in the Alphabetic Index, and there is no documentation of the stage, the provider should be queried.

4) Patients admitted with pressure ulcers documented as healed

No code is assigned if the documentation states that the pressure ulcer is completely healed.

5) Patients admitted with pressure ulcers documented as healing

Pressure ulcers described as healing should be assigned the appropriate pressure ulcer stage code based on the documentation in the medical record. If the documentation does not provide information about the stage of the healing pressure ulcer, assign the appropriate code for unspecified stage.

If the documentation is unclear as to whether the patient has a current (new) pressure ulcer or if the patient is being treated for a healing pressure ulcer, query the provider.

6) Patient admitted with pressure ulcer evolving into another stage during the admission

If a patient is admitted with a pressure ulcer at one stage and it progresses to a higher stage, assign the code for the highest stage reported for that site.

13. Chapter 13: Diseases of the Musculoskeletal System and Connective Tissue (MØØ-M99)

a. Site and laterality

Most of the codes within Chapter 13 have site and laterality designations. The site represents the bone, joint or the muscle involved. For some conditions where more than one bone, joint or muscle is usually involved, such as osteoarthritis, there is a "multiple

sites" code available. For categories where no multiple site code is provided and more than one bone, joint or muscle is involved, multiple codes should be used to indicate the different sites involved.

1) Bone versus joint

For certain conditions, the bone may be affected at the upper or lower end, (e.g., avascular necrosis of bone, M87, Osteoporosis, M8Ø, M81). Though the portion of the bone affected may be at the joint, the site designation will be the bone, not the joint.

b. Acute traumatic versus chronic or recurrent musculoskeletal conditions

Many musculoskeletal conditions are a result of previous injury or trauma to a site, or are recurrent conditions. Bone, joint or muscle conditions that are the result of a healed injury are usually found in chapter 13. Recurrent bone, joint or muscle conditions are also usually found in chapter 13. Any current, acute injury should be coded to the appropriate injury code from chapter 19. Chronic or recurrent conditions should generally be coded with a code from chapter 13. If it is difficult to determine from the documentation in the record which code is best to describe a condition, query the provider.

c. Coding of Pathologic Fractures

7th character A is for use as long as the patient is receiving active treatment for the fracture. Examples of active treatment are: surgical treatment, emergency department encounter, evaluation and treatment by a new physician. 7th character, D is to be used for encounters after the patient has completed active treatment. The other 7th characters, listed under each subcategory in the Tabular List, are to be used for subsequent encounters for treatment of problems associated with the healing, such as malunions, nonunions, and sequelae.

Care for complications of surgical treatment for fracture repairs during the healing or recovery phase should be coded with the appropriate complication codes.

See Section I.C.19. Coding of traumatic fractures.

d. Osteoporosis

Osteoporosis is a systemic condition, meaning that all bones of the musculoskeletal system are affected. Therefore, site is not a component of the codes under category M81, Osteoporosis without current pathological fracture. The site codes under category M8Ø, Osteoporosis with current pathological fracture, identify the site of the fracture, not the osteoporosis.

1) Osteoporosis without pathological fracture

Category M81, Osteoporosis without current pathological fracture, is for use for patients with osteoporosis who do not currently have a pathologic fracture due to the osteoporosis, even if they have had a fracture in the past. For patients with a history of osteoporosis fractures, status code Z87.31Ø, Personal history of (healed) osteoporosis fracture, should follow the code from M81.

2) Osteoporosis with current pathological fracture

Category M8Ø, Osteoporosis with current pathological fracture, is for patients who have a current pathologic fracture at the time of an encounter. The codes under M8Ø identify the site of the fracture. A code from category M8Ø, not a traumatic fracture code, should be used for any patient with known osteoporosis who suffers a fracture, even if the patient had a minor fall or trauma, if that fall or trauma would not usually break a normal, healthy bone.

14. Chapter 14: Diseases of Genitourinary System (NØØ-N99)

a. Chronic kidney disease

1) Stages of chronic kidney disease (CKD)

The ICD-1Ø-CM classifies CKD based on severity. The severity of CKD is designated by stages 1-5. Stage 2, code N18.2, equates to mild CKD; stage 3, code N18.3, equates to moderate CKD; and stage 4, code N18.4, equates to severe CKD. Code N18.6, End stage renal disease (ESRD), is assigned when the provider has documented end-stage-renal disease (ESRD).

If both a stage of CKD and ESRD are documented, assign code N18.6 only.

2) Chronic kidney disease and kidney transplant status

Patients who have undergone kidney transplant may still have some form of chronic kidney disease (CKD) because the kidney transplant may not fully restore kidney function. Therefore, the presence of CKD alone does not constitute a transplant complication. Assign the appropriate N18 code for the patient's stage of CKD and code Z94.0, Kidney transplant status. If a transplant complication such as failure or rejection or other transplant complication is documented, see section I.C.19.g for information on coding complications of a kidney transplant. If the documentation is unclear as to whether the patient has a complication of the transplant, query the provider.

3) Chronic kidney disease with other conditions

Patients with CKD may also suffer from other serious conditions, most commonly diabetes mellitus and hypertension. The sequencing of the CKD code in relationship to codes for other contributing conditions is based on the conventions in the Tabular List.

See I.C.9. Hypertensive chronic kidney disease.

See I.C.19. Chronic kidney disease and kidney transplant complications.

15. Chapter 15: Pregnancy, Childbirth, and the Puerperium (O00-O9A)

a. General Rules for Obstetric Cases

1) Codes from chapter 15 and sequencing priority

Obstetric cases require codes from chapter 15, codes in the range O00-O9A, Pregnancy, Childbirth, and the Puerperium. Chapter 15 codes have sequencing priority over codes from other chapters. Additional codes from other chapters may be used in conjunction with chapter 15 codes to further specify conditions. Should the provider document that the pregnancy is incidental to the encounter, then code Z33.1, Pregnant state, incidental, should be used in place of any chapter 15 codes. It is the provider's responsibility to state that the condition being treated is not affecting the pregnancy.

2) Chapter 15 codes used only on the maternal record

Chapter 15 codes are to be used only on the maternal record, never on the record of the newborn.

3) Final character for trimester

The majority of codes in Chapter 15 have a final character indicating the trimester of pregnancy. The timeframes for the trimesters are indicated at the beginning of the chapter. If trimester is not a component of a code it is because the condition always occurs in a specific trimester, or the concept of trimester of pregnancy is not applicable. Certain codes have characters for only certain trimesters because the condition does not occur in all trimesters, but it may occur in more than just one.

Assignment of the final character for trimester should be based on the provider's documentation of the trimester (or number of weeks) for the current admission/encounter. This applies to the assignment of trimester for pre-existing conditions as well as those that develop during or are due to the pregnancy. The provider's documentation of the number of weeks may be used to assign the appropriate code identifying the trimester.

Whenever delivery occurs during the current admission, and there is an "in childbirth" option for the obstetric complication being coded, the "in childbirth" code should be assigned.

4) Selection of trimester for inpatient admissions that encompass more than one trimesters

In instances when a patient is admitted to a hospital for complications of pregnancy during one trimester and remains in the hospital into a subsequent trimester, the trimester character for the antepartum complication code should be assigned on the basis of the trimester when the complication developed, not the trimester of the discharge. If the condition developed prior to the current admission/encounter or represents a pre-existing condition, the trimester character for the trimester at the time of the admission/encounter should be assigned.

5) Unspecified trimester

Each category that includes codes for trimester has a code for "unspecified trimester." The "unspecified trimester" code should rarely be used, such as when the documentation in the record is insufficient to determine the trimester and it is not possible to obtain clarification.

6) 7th character for fetus identification

Where applicable, a 7th character is to be assigned for certain categories (O31, O32, O33.3 - O33.6, O35, O36, O40, O41, O60.1, O60.2, O64, and O69) to identify the fetus for which the complication code applies.

Assign 7th character "0":

- For single gestations

- When the documentation in the record is insufficient to determine the fetus affected and it is not possible to obtain clarification.

- When it is not possible to clinically determine which fetus is affected.

b. Selection of OB principal or first-listed diagnosis

1) Routine outpatient prenatal visits

For routine outpatient prenatal visits when no complications are present, a code from category Z34, Encounter for supervision of normal pregnancy, should be used as the first-listed diagnosis. These codes should not be used in conjunction with chapter 15 codes.

2) Prenatal outpatient visits for high-risk patients

For routine prenatal outpatient visits for patients with high-risk pregnancies, a code from category O09, Supervision of high-risk pregnancy, should be used as the first-listed diagnosis. Secondary chapter 15 codes may be used in conjunction with these codes if appropriate.

3) Episodes when no delivery occurs

In episodes when no delivery occurs, the principal diagnosis should correspond to the principal complication of the pregnancy which necessitated the encounter. Should more than one complication exist, all of which are treated or monitored, any of the complications codes may be sequenced first.

4) When a delivery occurs

When a delivery occurs, the principal diagnosis should correspond to the main circumstances or complication of the delivery. In cases of cesarean delivery, the selection of the principal diagnosis should be the condition established after study that was responsible for the patient's admission. If the patient was admitted with a condition that resulted in the performance of a cesarean procedure, that condition should be selected as the principal diagnosis. If the reason for the admission/encounter was unrelated to the condition resulting in the cesarean delivery, the condition related to the reason for the admission/encounter should be selected as the principal diagnosis.

5) Outcome of delivery

A code from category Z37, Outcome of delivery, should be included on every maternal record when a delivery has occurred. These codes are not to be used on subsequent records or on the newborn record.

c. Pre-existing conditions versus conditions due to the pregnancy

Certain categories in Chapter 15 distinguish between conditions of the mother that existed prior to pregnancy (pre-existing) and those that are a direct result of pregnancy. When assigning codes from Chapter 15, it is important to assess if a condition was pre-existing prior to pregnancy or developed during or due to the pregnancy in order to assign the correct code.

Categories that do not distinguish between pre-existing and pregnancy-related conditions may be used for either. It is acceptable to use codes specifically for the puerperium with codes complicating pregnancy and childbirth if a condition arises postpartum during the delivery encounter.

d. **Pre-existing hypertension in pregnancy**

Category O10, Pre-existing hypertension complicating pregnancy, childbirth and the puerperium, includes codes for hypertensive heart and hypertensive chronic kidney disease. When assigning one of the O10 codes that includes hypertensive heart disease or hypertensive chronic kidney disease, it is necessary to add a secondary code from the appropriate hypertension category to specify the type of heart failure or chronic kidney disease.

See Section I.C.9. Hypertension.

e. **Fetal conditions affecting the management of the mother**

1) **Codes from categories O35 and O36**

Codes from categories O35, Maternal care for known or suspected fetal abnormality and damage, and O36, Maternal care for other fetal problems, are assigned only when the fetal condition is actually responsible for modifying the management of the mother, i.e., by requiring diagnostic studies, additional observation, special care, or termination of pregnancy. The fact that the fetal condition exists does not justify assigning a code from this series to the mother's record.

2) **In utero surgery**

In cases when surgery is performed on the fetus, a diagnosis code from category O35, Maternal care for known or suspected fetal abnormality and damage, should be assigned identifying the fetal condition. Assign the appropriate procedure code for the procedure performed.

No code from Chapter 16, the perinatal codes, should be used on the mother's record to identify fetal conditions. Surgery performed in utero on a fetus is still to be coded as an obstetric encounter.

f. **HIV Infection in pregnancy, childbirth and the puerperium**

During pregnancy, childbirth or the puerperium, a patient admitted because of an HIV-related illness should receive a principal diagnosis from subcategory O98.7-, Human immunodeficiency [HIV] disease complicating pregnancy, childbirth and the puerperium, followed by the code(s) for the HIV-related illness(es).

Patients with asymptomatic HIV infection status admitted during pregnancy, childbirth, or the puerperium should receive codes of O98.7- and Z21, Asymptomatic human immunodeficiency virus [HIV] infection status.

g. **Diabetes mellitus in pregnancy**

Diabetes mellitus is a significant complicating factor in pregnancy. Pregnant women who are diabetic should be assigned a code from category O24, Diabetes mellitus in pregnancy, childbirth, and the puerperium, first, followed by the appropriate diabetes code(s) (E08-E13) from Chapter 4.

h. **Long term use of insulin**

Code Z79.4, Long-term (current) use of insulin, should also be assigned if the diabetes mellitus is being treated with insulin.

i. **Gestational (pregnancy induced) diabetes**

Gestational (pregnancy induced) diabetes can occur during the second and third trimester of pregnancy in women who were not diabetic prior to pregnancy. Gestational diabetes can cause complications in the pregnancy similar to those of pre-existing diabetes mellitus. It also puts the woman at greater risk of developing diabetes after the pregnancy. Codes for gestational diabetes are in subcategory O24.4, Gestational diabetes mellitus. No other code from category O24, Diabetes mellitus in pregnancy, childbirth, and the puerperium, should be used with a code from O24.4.

The codes under subcategory O24.4 include diet controlled and insulin controlled. If a patient with gestational diabetes is treated with both diet and insulin, only the code for insulin-controlled is required.

Code Z79.4, Long-term (current) use of insulin, should not be assigned with codes from subcategory O24.4.

An abnormal glucose tolerance in pregnancy is assigned a code from subcategory O99.81, Abnormal glucose complicating pregnancy, childbirth, and the puerperium.

j. **Sepsis and septic shock complicating abortion, pregnancy, childbirth and the puerperium**

When assigning a chapter 15 code for sepsis complicating abortion, pregnancy, childbirth, and the puerperium, a code for the specific type of infection should be assigned as an additional diagnosis. If severe sepsis is present, a code from subcategory R65.2, Severe sepsis, and code(s) for associated organ dysfunction(s) should also be assigned as additional diagnoses.

k. **Puerperal sepsis**

Code O85, Puerperal sepsis, should be assigned with a secondary code to identify the causal organism (e.g., for a bacterial infection, assign a code from category B95-B96, Bacterial infections in conditions classified elsewhere). A code from category A40, Streptococcal sepsis, or A41, Other sepsis, should not be used for puerperal sepsis. If applicable, use additional codes to identify severe sepsis (R65.2-) and any associated acute organ dysfunction.

l. **Alcohol and tobacco use during pregnancy, childbirth and the puerperium**

1) **Alcohol use during pregnancy, childbirth and the puerperium**

Codes under subcategory O99.31, Alcohol use complicating pregnancy, childbirth, and the puerperium, should be assigned for any pregnancy case when a mother uses alcohol during the pregnancy or postpartum. A secondary code from category F10, Alcohol related disorders, should also be assigned to identify manifestations of the alcohol use.

2) **Tobacco use during pregnancy, childbirth and the puerperium**

Codes under subcategory O99.33, Smoking (tobacco) complicating pregnancy, childbirth, and the puerperium, should be assigned for any pregnancy case when a mother uses any type of tobacco product during the pregnancy or postpartum. A secondary code from category F17, Nicotine dependence, or code Z72.0, Tobacco use, should also be assigned to identify the type of nicotine dependence.

m. **Poisoning, toxic effects, adverse effects and underdosing in a pregnant patient**

A code from subcategory O9A.2, Injury, poisoning and certain other consequences of external causes complicating pregnancy, childbirth, and the puerperium, should be sequenced first, followed by the appropriate injury, poisoning, toxic effect, adverse effect or underdosing code, and then the additional code(s) that specifies the condition caused by the poisoning, toxic effect, adverse effect or underdosing.

See Section I.C.19. Adverse effects, poisoning, underdosing and toxic effects.

n. **Normal delivery, code O80**

1) **Encounter for full term uncomplicated delivery**

Code O80 should be assigned when a woman is admitted for a full-term normal delivery and delivers a single, healthy infant without any complications antepartum, during the delivery, or postpartum during the delivery episode. Code O80 is always a principal diagnosis. It is not to be used if any other code from chapter 15 is needed to describe a current complication of the antenatal, delivery, or perinatal period. Additional codes from other chapters may be used with code O80 if they are not related to or are in any way complicating the pregnancy.

2) **Uncomplicated delivery with resolved antepartum complication**

Code O80 may be used if the patient had a complication at some point during the pregnancy, but the complication is not present at the time of the admission for delivery.

3) **Outcome of delivery for O80**

Z37.0, Single live birth, is the only outcome of delivery code appropriate for use with O80.

o. **The peripartum and postpartum periods**

1) **Peripartum and postpartum periods**

The postpartum period begins immediately after delivery and continues for six weeks following delivery. The peripartum period is defined as the last month of pregnancy to five months postpartum.

2) Peripartum and postpartum complication

A postpartum complication is any complication occurring within the six-week period.

3) Pregnancy-related complications after 6 week period

Chapter 15 codes may also be used to describe pregnancy-related complications after the peripartum or postpartum period if the provider documents that a condition is pregnancy related.

4) Admission for routine postpartum care following delivery outside hospital

When the mother delivers outside the hospital prior to admission and is admitted for routine postpartum care and no complications are noted, code Z39.0, Encounter for care and examination of mother immediately after delivery, should be assigned as the principal diagnosis.

5) Pregnancy associated cardiomyopathy

Pregnancy associated cardiomyopathy, code O90.3, is unique in that it may be diagnosed in the third trimester of pregnancy but may continue to progress months after delivery. For this reason, it is referred to as peripartum cardiomyopathy. Code O90.3 is only for use when the cardiomyopathy develops as a result of pregnancy in a woman who did not have pre-existing heart disease.

p. Code O94, Sequelae of complication of pregnancy, childbirth, and the puerperium

1) Code O94

Code O94, Sequelae of complication of pregnancy, childbirth, and the puerperium, is for use in those cases when an initial complication of a pregnancy develops a sequelae requiring care or treatment at a future date.

2) After the initial postpartum period

This code may be used at any time after the initial postpartum period.

3) Sequencing of code O94

This code, like all late effect codes, is to be sequenced following the code describing the sequelae of the complication.

q. Termination of Pregnancy and Spontaneous Abortions

1) Abortion with liveborn fetus

When an attempted termination of pregnancy results in a liveborn fetus, assign code Z33.2, Encounter for elective termination of pregnancy and a code from category Z37, Outcome of Delivery.

2) Retained products of conception following an abortion

Subsequent encounters for retained products of conception following a spontaneous abortion or elective termination of pregnancy are assigned the appropriate code from category O03, Spontaneous abortion, or codes O07.4, Failed attempted termination of pregnancy without complication and Z33.2, Encounter for elective termination of pregnancy. This advice is appropriate even when the patient was discharged previously with a discharge diagnosis of complete abortion.

3) Complications leading to abortion

Codes from Chapter 15 may be used as additional codes to identify any documented complications of the pregnancy in conjunction with codes in categories in O07 and O08.

r. Abuse in a pregnant patient

For suspected or confirmed cases of abuse of a pregnant patient, a code(s) from subcategories O9A.3, Physical abuse complicating pregnancy, childbirth, and the puerperium, O9A.4, Sexual abuse complicating pregnancy, childbirth, and the puerperium, and O9A.5, Psychological abuse complicating pregnancy, childbirth, and the puerperium, should be sequenced first, followed by the appropriate codes (if applicable) to identify any associated current injury due to physical abuse, sexual abuse, and the perpetrator of abuse.

See Section I.C.19.f. Adult and child abuse, neglect and other maltreatment.

16. Chapter 16: Certain Conditions Origination in the Perinatal Period (P00-P96)

For coding and reporting purposes the perinatal period is defined as before birth through the 28th day following birth. The following guidelines are provided for reporting purposes

a. General Perinatal Rules

1) Use of Chapter 16 codes

Codes in this chapter are <u>never</u> for use on the maternal record. Codes from Chapter 15, the obstetric chapter, are never permitted on the newborn record. Chapter 16 codes may be used throughout the life of the patient if the condition is still present.

2) Principal diagnosis for birth record

When coding the birth episode in a newborn record, assign a code from category Z38, Liveborn infants according to place of birth and type of delivery, as the principal diagnosis. A code from category Z38 is assigned only once, to a newborn at the time of birth. If a newborn is transferred to another institution, a code from category Z38 should not be used at the receiving hospital.

A code from category Z38 is used only on the newborn record, not on the mother's record.

3) Use of codes from other chapters with codes from Chapter 16

Codes from other chapters may be used with codes from chapter 16 if the codes from the other chapters provide more specific detail. Codes for signs and symptoms may be assigned when a definitive diagnosis has not been established. If the reason for the encounter is a perinatal condition, the code from chapter 16 should be sequenced first.

4) Use of Chapter 16 codes after the perinatal period

Should a condition originate in the perinatal period, and continue throughout the life of the patient, the perinatal code should continue to be used regardless of the patient's age.

5) Birth process or community acquired conditions

If a newborn has a condition that may be either due to the birth process or community acquired and the documentation does not indicate which it is, the default is due to the birth process and the code from Chapter 16 should be used. If the condition is community-acquired, a code from Chapter 16 should not be assigned.

6) Code all clinically significant conditions

All clinically significant conditions noted on routine newborn examination should be coded. A condition is clinically significant if it requires:

- clinical evaluation; or
- therapeutic treatment; or
- diagnostic procedures; or
- extended length of hospital stay; or
- increased nursing care and/or monitoring; or
- has implications for future health care needs

Note: The perinatal guidelines listed above are the same as the general coding guidelines for "additional diagnoses", except for the final point regarding implications for future health care needs. Codes should be assigned for conditions that have been specified by the provider as having implications for future health care needs.

b. Observation and evaluation of newborns for suspected conditions not found
Reserved for future expansion

c. Coding Additional Perinatal Diagnoses

1) Assigning codes for conditions that require treatment

Assign codes for conditions that require treatment or further investigation, prolong the length of stay, or require resource utilization.

2) Codes for conditions specified as having implications for future health care needs

Assign codes for conditions that have been specified by the provider as having implications for future health care needs.

Note: This guideline should not be used for adult patients.

d. **Prematurity and fetal growth retardation**

Providers utilize different criteria in determining prematurity. A code for prematurity should not be assigned unless it is documented. Assignment of codes in categories P05, Disorders of newborn related to slow fetal growth and fetal malnutrition, and P07, Disorders of newborn related to short gestation and low birth weight, not elsewhere classified, should be based on the recorded birth weight and estimated gestational age. Codes from category P05 should not be assigned with codes from category P07.

When both birth weight and gestational age are available, two codes from category P07 should be assigned, with the code for birth weight sequenced before the code for gestational age.

A code from P05 and codes from P07.2 and P07.3 may be used to specify weeks of gestation as documented by the provider in the record.

e. **Low birth weight and immaturity status**

Codes from category P07, Disorders of newborn related to short gestation and low birth weight, not elsewhere classified, are for use for a child or adult who was premature or had a low birth weight as a newborn and this is affecting the patient's current health status.

See Section I.C.21. Factors influencing health status and contact with health services, Status.

f. **Bacterial sepsis of newborn**

Category P36, Bacterial sepsis of newborn, includes congenital sepsis. If a perinate is documented as having sepsis without documentation of congenital or community acquired, the default is congenital and a code from category P36 should be assigned. If the P36 code includes the causal organism, an additional code from category B95, Streptococcus, Staphylococcus, and Enterococcus as the cause of diseases classified elsewhere, or B96, Other bacterial agents as the cause of diseases classified elsewhere, should not be assigned. If the P36 code does not include the causal organism, assign an additional code from category B96. If applicable, use additional codes to identify severe sepsis (R65.2-) and any associated acute organ dysfunction.

g. **Stillbirth**

Code P95, Stillbirth, is only for use in institutions that maintain separate records for stillbirths. No other code should be used with P95. Code P95 should not be used on the mother's record.

17. **Chapter 17: Congenital Malformations, Deformations, and Chromosomal Abnormalities (Q00-Q99)**

Assign an appropriate code(s) from categories Q00-Q99, Congenital malformations, deformations, and chromosomal abnormalities when a malformation/deformation or chromosomal abnormality is documented. A malformation/deformation/or chromosomal abnormality may be the principal/first-listed diagnosis on a record or a secondary diagnosis.

When a malformation/deformation/or chromosomal abnormality does not have a unique code assignment, assign additional code(s) for any manifestations that may be present.

When the code assignment specifically identifies the malformation/deformation/or chromosomal abnormality, manifestations that are an inherent component of the anomaly should not be coded separately. Additional codes should be assigned for manifestations that are not an inherent component.

Codes from Chapter 17 may be used throughout the life of the patient. If a congenital malformation or deformity has been corrected, a personal history code should be used to identify the history of the malformation or deformity. Although present at birth, malformation/deformation/or chromosomal abnormality may not be identified until later in life. Whenever the condition is diagnosed by the physician, it is appropriate to assign a code from codes Q00-Q99.

For the birth admission, the appropriate code from category Z38, Liveborn infants, according to place of birth and type of delivery, should be sequenced as the principal diagnosis, followed by any congenital anomaly codes, Q00- Q99.

18. **Chapter 18: Symptoms, Signs, and Abnormal Clinical and Laboratory Findings, Not Elsewhere Classified (R00-R99)**

Chapter 18 includes symptoms, signs, abnormal results of clinical or other investigative procedures, and ill-defined conditions regarding which no diagnosis classifiable elsewhere is recorded. Signs and symptoms that point to a specific diagnosis have been assigned to a category in other chapters of the classification.

a. **Use of symptom codes**

Codes that describe symptoms and signs are acceptable for reporting purposes when a related definitive diagnosis has not been established (confirmed) by the provider.

b. **Use of a symptom code with a definitive diagnosis code**

Codes for signs and symptoms may be reported in addition to a related definitive diagnosis when the sign or symptom is not routinely associated with that diagnosis, such as the various signs and symptoms associated with complex syndromes. The definitive diagnosis code should be sequenced before the symptom code.

Signs or symptoms that are associated routinely with a disease process should not be assigned as additional codes, unless otherwise instructed by the classification.

c. **Combination codes that include symptoms**

ICD-10-CM contains a number of combination codes that identify both the definitive diagnosis and common symptoms of that diagnosis. When using one of these combination codes, an additional code should not be assigned for the symptom.

d. **Repeated falls**

Code R29.6, Repeated falls, is for use for encounters when a patient has recently fallen and the reason for the fall is being investigated.

Code Z91.81, History of falling, is for use when a patient has fallen in the past and is at risk for future falls. When appropriate, both codes R29.6 and Z91.81 may be assigned together.

e. **Coma scale**

The coma scale codes (R40.2-) can be used in conjunction with traumatic brain injury codes, acute cerebrovascular disease or sequelae of cerebrovascular disease codes. These codes are primarily for use by trauma registries, but they may be used in any setting where this information is collected. The coma scale codes should be sequenced after the diagnosis code(s).

These codes, one from each subcategory, are needed to complete the scale. The 7th character indicates when the scale was recorded. The 7th character should match for all three codes.

At a minimum, report the initial score documented on presentation at your facility. This may be a score from the emergency medicine technician (EMT) or in the emergency department. If desired, a facility may choose to capture multiple Glasgow coma scale scores.

Assign code R40.24, Glasgow coma scale, total score, when only the total score is documented in the medical record and not the individual score(s).

f. **Functional quadriplegia**

Functional quadriplegia (code R53.2) is the lack of ability to use one's limbs or to ambulate due to extreme debility. It is not associated with neurologic deficit or injury, and code R53.2 should not be used for cases of neurologic quadriplegia. It should only be assigned if functional quadriplegia is specifically documented in the medical record.

g. **SIRS due to non-infectious process**

The systemic inflammatory response syndrome (SIRS) can develop as a result of certain non-infectious disease processes, such as trauma, malignant neoplasm, or pancreatitis. When SIRS is documented with a noninfectious condition, and no subsequent infection is documented, the code for the underlying condition, such as an injury, should be assigned, followed by code R65.10, Systemic inflammatory response syndrome (SIRS) of non-infectious origin without acute organ dysfunction, or code R65.11, Systemic inflammatory response syndrome (SIRS) of non-infectious origin with acute organ dysfunction. If an associated acute organ dysfunction is documented, the appropriate code(s) for the specific type of organ dysfunction(s) should be assigned in addition to code R65.11. If acute organ dysfunction is documented, but it cannot be determined if the acute organ dysfunction is associated with SIRS or due to another condition (e.g., directly due to the trauma), the provider should be queried.

h. **Death NOS**

Code R99, Ill-defined and unknown cause of mortality, is only for use in the very limited circumstance when a patient who has already died is brought into an emergency department or other healthcare facility and is pronounced dead upon arrival. It does not represent the discharge disposition of death.

19. Chapter 19: Injury, Poisoning, and Certain Other Consequences of External Causes (S00-T88)

a. Application of 7th Characters in Chapter 19

Most categories in chapter 19 have a 7th character requirement for each applicable code. Most categories in this chapter have three 7th character values (with the exception of fractures): A, initial encounter, D, subsequent encounter and S, sequela. Categories for traumatic fractures have additional 7th character values.

7th character "A", initial encounter is used while the patient is receiving active treatment for the condition. Examples of active treatment are: surgical treatment, emergency department encounter, and evaluation and treatment by a new physician.

7th character "D" subsequent encounter is used for encounters after the patient has received active treatment of the condition and is receiving routine care for the condition during the healing or recovery phase. Examples of subsequent care are: cast change or removal, removal of external or internal fixation device, medication adjustment, other aftercare and follow up visits following treatment of the injury or condition.

The aftercare Z codes should not be used for aftercare for conditions such as injuries or poisonings, where 7th characters are provided to identify subsequent care. For example, for aftercare of an injury, assign the acute injury code with the 7th character "D" (subsequent encounter).

7th character "S", sequela, is for use for complications or conditions that arise as a direct result of a condition, such as scar formation after a burn. The scars are sequelae of the burn. When using 7th character "S", it is necessary to use both the injury code that precipitated the sequela and the code for the sequela itself. The "S" is added only to the injury code, not the sequela code. The 7th character "S" identifies the injury responsible for the sequela. The specific type of sequela (e.g. scar) is sequenced first, followed by the injury code.

b. Coding of injuries

When coding injuries, assign separate codes for each injury unless a combination code is provided, in which case the combination code is assigned. Code T07, Unspecified multiple injuries should not be assigned in the inpatient setting unless information for a more specific code is not available. Traumatic injury codes (S00-T14.9) are not to be used for normal, healing surgical wounds or to identify complications of surgical wounds.

The code for the most serious injury, as determined by the provider and the focus of treatment, is sequenced first.

1) Superficial injuries

Superficial injuries such as abrasions or contusions are not coded when associated with more severe injuries of the same site.

2) Primary injury with damage to nerves/blood vessels

When a primary injury results in minor damage to peripheral nerves or blood vessels, the primary injury is sequenced first with additional code(s) for injuries to nerves and spinal cord (such as category S04), and/or injury to blood vessels (such as category S15). When the primary injury is to the blood vessels or nerves, that injury should be sequenced first.

c. Coding of traumatic fractures

The principles of multiple coding of injuries should be followed in coding fractures. Fractures of specified sites are coded individually by site in accordance with both the provisions within categories S02, S12, S22, S32, S42, S49, S52, S59, S62, S72, S79, S82, S89, S92 and the level of detail furnished by medical record content.

A fracture not indicated as open or closed should be coded to closed. A fracture not indicated whether displaced or not displaced should be coded to displaced.

More specific guidelines are as follows:

1) Initial vs. subsequent encounter for fractures

Traumatic fractures are coded using the appropriate 7th character extension for initial encounter (A, B, C) while the patient is receiving active treatment for the fracture. Examples of active treatment are: surgical treatment, emergency

department encounter, and evaluation and treatment by a new physician. The appropriate 7th character for initial encounter should also be assigned for a patient who delayed seeking treatment for the fracture or nonunion.

Fractures are coded using the appropriate 7th character extension for subsequent care for encounters after the patient has completed active treatment of the fracture and is receiving routine care for the fracture during the healing or recovery phase. Examples of fracture aftercare are: cast change or removal, removal of external or internal fixation device, medication adjustment, and follow-up visits following fracture treatment.

Care for complications of surgical treatment for fracture repairs during the healing or recovery phase should be coded with the appropriate complication codes.

Care of complications of fractures, such as malunion and nonunion, should be reported with the appropriate 7th character extensions for subsequent care with nonunion (K, M, N,) or subsequent care with malunion (P, Q, R).

A code from category M80, not a traumatic fracture code, should be used for any patient with known osteoporosis who suffers a fracture, even if the patient had a minor fall or trauma, if that fall or trauma would not usually break a normal, healthy bone.

See Section I.C.13. Osteoporosis.

The aftercare Z codes should not be used for aftercare for traumatic fractures. For aftercare of a traumatic fracture, assign the acute fracture code with the appropriate 7th character.

2) Multiple fractures sequencing

Multiple fractures are sequenced in accordance with the severity of the fracture.

d. Coding of burns and corrosions

The ICD-10-CM makes a distinction between burns and corrosions. The burn codes are for thermal burns, except sunburns, that come from a heat source, such as a fire or hot appliance. The burn codes are also for burns resulting from electricity and radiation. Corrosions are burns due to chemicals. The guidelines are the same for burns and corrosions.

Current burns (T20-T25) are classified by depth, extent and by agent (X code). Burns are classified by depth as first degree (erythema), second degree (blistering), and third degree (full-thickness involvement). Burns of the eye and internal organs (T26-T28) are classified by site, but not by degree.

1) Sequencing of burn and related condition codes

Sequence first the code that reflects the highest degree of burn when more than one burn is present.

a. When the reason for the admission or encounter is for treatment of external multiple burns, sequence first the code that reflects the burn of the highest degree.

b. When a patient has both internal and external burns, the circumstances of admission govern the selection of the principal diagnosis or first-listed diagnosis.

c. When a patient is admitted for burn injuries and other related conditions such as smoke inhalation and/or respiratory failure, the circumstances of admission govern the selection of the principal or first-listed diagnosis.

2) Burns of the same local site

Classify burns of the same local site (three-character category level, T20-T28) but of different degrees to the subcategory identifying the highest degree recorded in the diagnosis.

3) Non-healing burns

Non-healing burns are coded as acute burns.

Necrosis of burned skin should be coded as a non-healed burn.

4) Infected burn

For any documented infected burn site, use an additional code for the infection.

5) Assign separate codes for each burn site

When coding burns, assign separate codes for each burn site. Category T30, Burn and corrosion, body region unspecified is extremely vague and should rarely be used.

6) **Burns and corrosions classified according to extent of body surface involved**

Assign codes from category T31, Burns classified according to extent of body surface involved, or T32, Corrosions classified according to extent of body surface involved, when the site of the burn is not specified or when there is a need for additional data. It is advisable to use category T31 as additional coding when needed to provide data for evaluating burn mortality, such as that needed by burn units. It is also advisable to use category T31 as an additional code for reporting purposes when there is mention of a third-degree burn involving 20 percent or more of the body surface.

Categories T31 and T32 are based on the classic "rule of nines" in estimating body surface involved: head and neck are assigned nine percent, each arm nine percent, each leg 18 percent, the anterior trunk 18 percent, posterior trunk 18 percent, and genitalia one percent. Providers may change these percentage assignments where necessary to accommodate infants and children who have proportionately larger heads than adults, and patients who have large buttocks, thighs, or abdomen that involve burns.

7) **Encounters for treatment of sequela of burns**

Encounters for the treatment of the late effects of burns or corrosions (i.e., scars or joint contractures) should be coded with a burn or corrosion code with the 7th character "S" for sequela.

8) **Sequelae with a late effect code and current burn**

When appropriate, both a code for a current burn or corrosion with 7th character "A" or "D" and a burn or corrosion code with 7th character "S" may be assigned on the same record (when both a current burn and sequelae of an old burn exist). Burns and corrosions do not heal at the same rate and a current healing wound may still exist with sequela of a healed burn or corrosion.

9) **Use of an external cause code with burns and corrosions**

An external cause code should be used with burns and corrosions to identify the source and intent of the burn, as well as the place where it occurred.

e. **Adverse effects, poisoning, underdosing and toxic effects**

Codes in categories T36-T65 are combination codes that include the substance that was taken as well as the intent. No additional external cause code is required for poisonings, toxic effects, adverse effects and underdosing codes.

1) **Do not code directly from the Table of Drugs**

Do not code directly from the Table of Drugs and Chemicals. Always refer back to the Tabular List.

2) **Use as many codes as necessary to describe**

Use as many codes as necessary to describe completely all drugs, medicinal or biological substances.

3) **If the same code would describe the causative agent**

If the same code would describe the causative agent for more than one adverse reaction, poisoning, toxic effect or underdosing, assign the code only once.

4) **If two or more drugs, medicinal or biological substances**

If two or more drugs, medicinal or biological substances are reported, code each individually unless a combination code is listed in the Table of Drugs and Chemicals.

5) **The occurrence of drug toxicity is classified in ICD-10-CM as follows:**

(a) **Adverse effect**

When coding an adverse effect of a drug that has been correctly prescribed and properly administered, assign the appropriate code for the nature of the adverse effect followed by the appropriate code for the adverse effect of the drug (T36-T50). The code for the drug should have a 5th or 6th character "5" (for example T36.0X5-) Examples of the nature of an adverse effect are tachycardia, delirium, gastrointestinal hemorrhaging, vomiting, hypokalemia, hepatitis, renal failure, or respiratory failure.

(b) **Poisoning**

When coding a poisoning or reaction to the improper use of a medication (e.g., overdose, wrong substance given or taken in error, wrong route of administration), first assign the appropriate code from categories T36-T50. The poisoning codes have an associated intent as their 5th or 6th character (accidental, intentional self-harm, assault and undetermined. Use additional code(s) for all manifestations of poisonings.

If there is also a diagnosis of abuse or dependence of the substance, the abuse or dependence is assigned as an additional code.

Examples of poisoning include:

(i) Error was made in drug prescription

Errors made in drug prescription or in the administration of the drug by provider, nurse, patient, or other person.

(ii) Overdose of a drug intentionally taken

If an overdose of a drug was intentionally taken or administered and resulted in drug toxicity, it would be coded as a poisoning.

(iii) Nonprescribed drug taken with correctly prescribed and properly administered drug

If a nonprescribed drug or medicinal agent was taken in combination with a correctly prescribed and properly administered drug, any drug toxicity or other reaction resulting from the interaction of the two drugs would be classified as a poisoning.

(iv) Interaction of drug(s) and alcohol

When a reaction results from the interaction of a drug(s) and alcohol, this would be classified as poisoning.

See Section I.C.4. if poisoning is the result of insulin pump malfunctions.

(c) **Underdosing**

Underdosing refers to taking less of a medication than is prescribed by a provider or a manufacturer's instruction. For underdosing, assign the code from categories T36-T50 (fifth or sixth character "6").

Codes for underdosing should never be assigned as principal or first-listed codes. If a patient has a relapse or exacerbation of the medical condition for which the drug is prescribed because of the reduction in dose, then the medical condition itself should be coded.

Noncompliance (Z91.12-, Z91.13-) or complication of care (Y63.61, Y63.8-Y63.9) codes are to be used with an underdosing code to indicate intent, if known.

(d) **Toxic effects**

When a harmful substance is ingested or comes in contact with a person, this is classified as a toxic effect. The toxic effect codes are in categories T51-T65.

Toxic effect codes have an associated intent: accidental, intentional self-harm, assault and undetermined.

f. **Adult and child abuse, neglect and other maltreatment**

Sequence first the appropriate code from categories T74.- (Adult and child abuse, neglect and other maltreatment, confirmed) or T76.- (Adult and child abuse, neglect and other maltreatment, suspected) for abuse, neglect and other maltreatment, followed by any accompanying mental health and injury code(s).

If the documentation in the medical record states abuse or neglect it is coded as confirmed (T74.-). It is coded as suspected if it is documented as suspected (T76.-).

For cases of confirmed abuse or neglect an external cause code from the assault section (X92-Y08) should be added to identify the cause of any physical injuries. A perpetrator code (Y07) should be added when the perpetrator of the abuse is known. For suspected cases of abuse or neglect, do not report external cause or perpetrator code.

If a suspected case of abuse, neglect or mistreatment is ruled out during an encounter code Z04.71, Encounter for examination and observation following alleged physical adult abuse, ruled out, or code Z04.72, Encounter for examination and observation following alleged child physical abuse, ruled out, should be used, not a code from T76.

If a suspected case of alleged rape or sexual abuse is ruled out during an encounter code Z04.41, Encounter for examination and observation following alleged physical adult abuse, ruled out, or code Z04.42, Encounter for examination and observation following alleged rape or sexual abuse, ruled out, should be used, not a code from T76.

See Section I.C.15. Abuse in a pregnant patient.

g. Complications of care

1) General guidelines for complications of care

(a) Documentation of complications of care
See Section I.B.16. for information on documentation of complications of care.

2) Pain due to medical devices
Pain associated with devices, implants or grafts left in a surgical site (for example painful hip prosthesis) is assigned to the appropriate code(s) found in Chapter 19, Injury, poisoning, and certain other consequences of external causes. Specific codes for pain due to medical devices are found in the T code section of the ICD-10-CM. Use additional code(s) from category G89 to identify acute or chronic pain due to presence of the device, implant or graft (G89.18 or G89.28).

3) Transplant complications

(a) Transplant complications other than kidney
Codes under category T86, Complications of transplanted organs and tissues, are for use for both complications and rejection of transplanted organs. A transplant complication code is only assigned if the complication affects the function of the transplanted organ. Two codes are required to fully describe a transplant complication: the appropriate code from category T86 and a secondary code that identifies the complication.

Pre-existing conditions or conditions that develop after the transplant are not coded as complications unless they affect the function of the transplanted organs.

See I.C.21. for transplant organ removal status

See I.C.2. for malignant neoplasm associated with transplanted organ.

(b) Kidney transplant complications
Patients who have undergone kidney transplant may still have some form of chronic kidney disease (CKD) because the kidney transplant may not fully restore kidney function. Code T86.1- should be assigned for documented complications of a kidney transplant, such as transplant failure or rejection or other transplant complication. Code T86.1- should not be assigned for post kidney transplant patients who have chronic kidney (CKD) unless a transplant complication such as transplant failure or rejection is documented. If the documentation is unclear as to whether the patient has a complication of the transplant, query the provider.

Conditions that affect the function of the transplanted kidney, other than CKD, should be assigned a code from subcategory T86.1, Complications of transplanted organ, Kidney, and a secondary code that identifies the complication.

For patients with CKD following a kidney transplant, but who do not have a complication such as failure or rejection, *see section I.C.14. Chronic kidney disease and kidney transplant status.*

4) Complication codes that include the external cause
As with certain other T codes, some of the complications of care codes have the external cause included in the code. The code includes the nature of the complication as well as the type of procedure that caused the complication. No external cause code indicating the type of procedure is necessary for these codes.

5) Complications of care codes within the body system chapters
Intraoperative and postprocedural complication codes are found within the body system chapters with codes specific to the organs and structures of that body system. These codes should be sequenced first, followed by a code(s) for the specific complication, if applicable.

20. Chapter 20: External Causes of Morbidity (V01-Y99)
Introduction: These guidelines are provided for the reporting of external causes of morbidity codes in order that there will be standardization in the process. These codes are secondary codes for use in any health care setting.

External cause codes are intended to provide data for injury research and evaluation of injury prevention strategies. These codes capture how the injury or health condition happened (cause), the intent (unintentional or accidental; or intentional, such as suicide or assault), the place where the event occurred the activity of the patient at the time of the event, and the person's status (e.g., civilian, military).

There is no national requirement for mandatory ICD-10-CM external cause code reporting. Unless a provider is subject to a state-based external cause code reporting mandate or these codes are required by a particular payer, reporting of ICD-10-CM codes in Chapter 20, External Causes of Morbidity, is not required. In the absence of a mandatory reporting requirement, providers are encouraged to voluntarily report external cause codes, as they provide valuable data for injury research and evaluation of injury prevention strategies.

a. General external cause coding guidelines

1) Used with any code in the range of A00.0-T88.9, Z00-Z99
An external cause code may be used with any code in the range of A00.0-T88.9, Z00-Z99, classification that is a health condition due to an external cause. Though they are most applicable to injuries, they are also valid for use with such things as infections or diseases due to an external source, and other health conditions, such as a heart attack that occurs during strenuous physical activity.

2) External cause code used for length of treatment
Assign the external cause code, with the appropriate 7th character (initial encounter, subsequent encounter or sequela) for each encounter for which the injury or condition is being treated.

3) Use the full range of external cause codes
Use the full range of external cause codes to completely describe the cause, the intent, the place of occurrence, and if applicable, the activity of the patient at the time of the event, and the patient's status, for all injuries, and other health conditions due to an external cause.

4) Assign as many external cause codes as necessary
Assign as many external cause codes as necessary to fully explain each cause. If only one external code can be recorded, assign the code most related to the principal diagnosis.

5) The selection of the appropriate external cause code
The selection of the appropriate external cause code is guided by the Alphabetic Index of External Causes and by Inclusion and Exclusion notes in the Tabular List.

6) External cause code can never be a principal diagnosis
An external cause code can never be a principal (first-listed) diagnosis.

7) Combination external cause codes
Certain of the external cause codes are combination codes that identify sequential events that result in an injury, such as a fall which results in striking against an object. The injury may be due to either event or both. The combination external cause code used should correspond to the sequence of events regardless of which caused the most serious injury.

8) No external cause code needed in certain circumstances
No external cause code from Chapter 20 is needed if the external cause and intent are included in a code from another chapter (e.g. T36.0x1- Poisoning by penicillins, accidental (unintentional)).

b. **Place of occurrence guideline**

Codes from category Y92, Place of occurrence of the external cause, are secondary codes for use after other external cause codes to identify the location of the patient at the time of injury or other condition.

A place of occurrence code is used only once, at the initial encounter for treatment. No 7th characters are used for Y92. Only one code from Y92 should be recorded on a medical record. A place of occurrence code should be used in conjunction with an activity code, Y93.

Do not use place of occurrence code Y92.9 if the place is not stated or is not applicable.

c. **Activity code**

Assign a code from category Y93, Activity code, to describe the activity of the patient at the time the injury or other health condition occurred.

An activity code is used only once, at the initial encounter for treatment. Only one code from Y93 should be recorded on a medical record. An activity code should be used in conjunction with a place of occurrence code, Y92.

The activity codes are not applicable to poisonings, adverse effects, misadventures or sequela.

Do not assign Y93.9, Unspecified activity, if the activity is not stated.

A code from category Y93 is appropriate for use with external cause and intent codes if identifying the activity provides additional information about the event.

d. **Place of occurrence, activity, and status codes used with other external cause code**

When applicable, place of occurrence, activity, and external cause status codes are sequenced after the main external cause code(s). Regardless of the number of external cause codes assigned, there should be only one place of occurrence code, one activity code, and one external cause status code assigned to an encounter.

e. **If the reporting format limits the number of external cause codes**

If the reporting format limits the number of external cause codes that can be used in reporting clinical data, report the code for the cause/intent most related to the principal diagnosis. If the format permits capture of additional external cause codes, the cause/intent, including medical misadventures, of the additional events should be reported rather than the codes for place, activity, or external status.

f. **Multiple external cause coding guidelines**

More than one external cause code is required to fully describe the external cause of an illness or injury. The assignment of external cause codes should be sequenced in the following priority:

If two or more events cause separate injuries, an external cause code should be assigned for each cause. The first-listed external cause code will be selected in the following order:

External codes for child and adult abuse take priority over all other external cause codes.

See Section I.C.19., Child and Adult abuse guidelines.

External cause codes for terrorism events take priority over all other external cause codes except child and adult abuse.

External cause codes for cataclysmic events take priority over all other external cause codes except child and adult abuse and terrorism.

External cause codes for transport accidents take priority over all other external cause codes except cataclysmic events, child and adult abuse and terrorism.

Activity and external cause status codes are assigned following all causal (intent) external cause codes.

The first-listed external cause code should correspond to the cause of the most serious diagnosis due to an assault, accident, or self-harm, following the order of hierarchy listed above.

g. **Child and adult abuse guideline**

Adult and child abuse, neglect and maltreatment are classified as assault. Any of the assault codes may be used to indicate the external cause of any injury resulting from the confirmed abuse.

For confirmed cases of abuse, neglect and maltreatment, when the perpetrator is known, a code from Y07, Perpetrator of maltreatment and neglect, should accompany any other assault codes.

See Section I.C.19. Adult and child abuse, neglect and other maltreatment

h. **Unknown or undetermined intent guideline**

If the intent (accident, self-harm, assault) of the cause of an injury or other condition is unknown or unspecified, code the intent as accidental intent. All transport accident categories assume accidental intent.

1) **Use of undetermined intent**

External cause codes for events of undetermined intent are only for use if the documentation in the record specifies that the intent cannot be determined.

i. **Sequelae (Late Effects) of external cause guidelines**

1) **Sequelae external cause codes**

Sequela are reported using the external cause code with the 7th character extension "S" for sequela. These codes should be used with any report of a late effect or sequela resulting from a previous injury.

2) **Sequela external cause code with a related current injury**

A sequela external cause code should never be used with a related current nature of injury code.

3) **Use of sequela external cause codes for subsequent visits**

Use a late effect external cause code for subsequent visits when a late effect of the initial injury is being treated. Do not use a late effect external cause code for subsequent visits for follow-up care (e.g., to assess healing, to receive rehabilitative therapy) of the injury when no late effect of the injury has been documented.

j. **Terrorism guidelines**

1) **Cause of injury identified by the Federal Government (FBI) as terrorism**

When the cause of an injury is identified by the Federal Government (FBI) as terrorism, the first-listed external cause code should be a code from category Y38, Terrorism. The definition of terrorism employed by the FBI is found at the inclusion note at the beginning of category Y38. Use additional code for place of occurrence (Y92.-). More than one Y38 code may be assigned if the injury is the result of more than one mechanism of terrorism.

2) **Cause of an injury is suspected to be the result of terrorism**

When the cause of an injury is suspected to be the result of terrorism a code from category Y38 should not be assigned. Suspected cases should be classified as assault.

3) **Code Y38.9, terrorism, secondary effects**

Assign code Y38.9, Terrorism, secondary effects, for conditions occurring subsequent to the terrorist event. This code should not be assigned for conditions that are due to the initial terrorist act.

It is acceptable to assign code Y38.9 with another code from Y38 if there is an injury due to the initial terrorist event and an injury that is a subsequent result of the terrorist event.

k. **External cause status**

A code from category Y99, External cause status, should be assigned whenever any other external cause code is assigned for an encounter, including an Activity code, except for the events noted below. Assign a code from category Y99, External cause status, to indicate the work status of the person at the time the event occurred. The status code indicates whether the event occurred during military activity, whether a non-military person was at work, whether an individual including a student or volunteer was involved in a non-work activity at the time of the causal event.

A code from Y99, External cause status, should be assigned, when applicable, with other external cause codes, such as transport accidents and falls. The external cause status codes are not applicable to poisonings, adverse effects, misadventures or late effects.

Do not assign a code from category Y99 if no other external cause codes (cause, activity) are applicable for the encounter.

An external cause status code is used only once, at the initial encounter for treatment. Only one code from Y99 should be recorded on a medical record.

Do not assign code Y99.9, Unspecified external cause status, if the status is not stated.

21. Chapter 21: Factors Influencing Health Status and Contact with Health Services (Z00-Z99)

Note: The chapter specific guidelines provide additional information about the use of Z codes for specified encounters.

a. Use of Z codes in any healthcare setting

Z codes are for use in any healthcare setting. Z codes may be used as either a first-listed (principal diagnosis code in the inpatient setting) or secondary code, depending on the circumstances of the encounter. Certain Z codes may only be used as first-listed or principal diagnosis.

b. Z Codes indicate a reason for an encounter

Z codes are not procedure codes. A corresponding procedure code must accompany a Z code to describe any procedure performed.

c. Categories of Z codes

1) Contact/exposure

Category Z20 indicates contact with, and suspected exposure to, communicable diseases. These codes are for patients who do not show any sign or symptom of a disease but are suspected to have been exposed to it by close personal contact with an infected individual or are in an area where a disease is epidemic.

Category Z77, indicates contact with and suspected exposures hazardous to health.

Contact/exposure codes may be used as a first-listed code to explain an encounter for testing, or, more commonly, as a secondary code to identify a potential risk.

2) Inoculations and vaccinations

Code Z23 is for encounters for inoculations and vaccinations. It indicates that a patient is being seen to receive a prophylactic inoculation against a disease. Procedure codes are required to identify the actual administration of the injection and the type(s) of immunizations given. Code Z23 may be used as a secondary code if the inoculation is given as a routine part of preventive health care, such as a well-baby visit.

3) Status

Status codes indicate that a patient is either a carrier of a disease or has the sequelae or residual of a past disease or condition. This includes such things as the presence of prosthetic or mechanical devices resulting from past treatment. A status code is informative, because the status may affect the course of treatment and its outcome. A status code is distinct from a history code. The history code indicates that the patient no longer has the condition.

A status code should not be used with a diagnosis code from one of the body system chapters, if the diagnosis code includes the information provided by the status code. For example, code Z94.1, Heart transplant status, should not be used with a code from subcategory T86.2, Complications of heart transplant. The status code does not provide additional information. The complication code indicates that the patient is a heart transplant patient.

For encounters for weaning from a mechanical ventilator, assign a code from subcategory J96.1, Chronic respiratory failure, followed by code Z99.11, Dependence on respirator [ventilator] status.

The status Z codes/categories are:

Z14   Genetic carrier

Genetic carrier status indicates that a person carries a gene, associated with a particular disease, which may be passed on to offspring who may develop that disease. The person does not have the disease and is not at risk of developing the disease.

Z15   Genetic susceptibility to disease

Genetic susceptibility indicates that a person has a gene that increases the risk of that person developing the disease.

Codes from category Z15 should not be used as principal or first-listed codes. If the patient has the condition to which he/she is susceptible, and that condition is the reason for the encounter, the code for the current condition should be sequenced first. If the patient is being seen for follow-up after completed treatment for this condition, and the condition no longer exists, a follow-up code should be sequenced first, followed by the appropriate personal history and genetic susceptibility codes. If the purpose of the encounter is genetic counseling associated with procreative management, code Z31.5, Encounter for genetic counseling, should be assigned as the first-listed code, followed by a code from category Z15. Additional codes should be assigned for any applicable family or personal history.

Z16   Resistance to antimicrobial drugs

This code indicates that a patient has a condition that is resistant to antimicrobial drug treatment. Sequence the infection code first.

Z17   Estrogen receptor status

Z18   Retained foreign body fragments

Z21   Asymptomatic HIV infection status

This code indicates that a patient has tested positive for HIV but has manifested no signs or symptoms of the disease.

Z22   Carrier of infectious disease

Carrier status indicates that a person harbors the specific organisms of a disease without manifest symptoms and is capable of transmitting the infection.

Z28.3 Underimmunization status

Z33.1 Pregnant state, incidental

This code is a secondary code only for use when the pregnancy is in no way complicating the reason for visit. Otherwise, a code from the obstetric chapter is required.

Z66   Do not resuscitate

This code may be used when it is documented by the provider that a patient is on do not resuscitate status at any time during the stay.

Z67   Blood type

Z68   Body mass index (BMI)

Z74.01 Bed confinement status

Z76.82 Awaiting organ transplant status

Z78   Other specified health status

Code Z78.1, Physical restraint status, may be used when it is documented by the provider that a patient has been put in restraints during the current encounter. Please note that this code should not be reported when it is documented by the provider that a patient is temporarily restrained during a procedure.

Z79   Long-term (current) drug therapy

Codes from this category indicate a patient's continuous use of a prescribed drug (including such things as aspirin therapy) for the long-term treatment of a condition or for prophylactic use. It is not for use for patients who have addictions to drugs. This subcategory is not for use of medications for detoxification or maintenance programs to prevent withdrawal symptoms in patients with drug dependence (e.g., methadone maintenance for opiate dependence). Assign the appropriate code for the drug dependence instead.

Assign a code from Z79 if the patient is receiving a medication for an extended period as a prophylactic measure (such as for the prevention of deep vein thrombosis) or as treatment of a chronic condition (such as arthritis) or a disease requiring a lengthy course of treatment (such as cancer). Do not assign a code from category Z79 for medication being administered for a brief period of time to treat an acute illness or injury (such as a course of antibiotics to treat acute bronchitis).

Z88　Allergy status to drugs, medicaments and biological substances

　　　Except: Z88.9, Allergy status to unspecified drugs, medicaments and biological substances status

Z89　Acquired absence of limb

Z9Ø　Acquired absence of organs, not elsewhere classified

Z91.Ø-　Allergy status, other than to drugs and biological substances

Z92.82　Status post administration of tPA (rtPA) in a different facility within the last 24 hours prior to admission to a current facility

　　　Assign code Z92.82, Status post administration of tPA (rtPA) in a different facility within the last 24 hours prior to admission to current facility, as a secondary diagnosis when a patient is received by transfer into a facility and documentation indicates they were administered tissue plasminogen activator (tPA) within the last 24 hours prior to admission to the current facility.

　　　This guideline applies even if the patient is still receiving the tPA at the time they are received into the current facility.

　　　The appropriate code for the condition for which the tPA was administered (such as cerebrovascular disease or myocardial infarction) should be assigned first.

　　　Code Z92.82 is only applicable to the receiving facility record and not to the transferring facility record.

Z93　Artificial opening status

Z94　Transplanted organ and tissue status

Z95　Presence of cardiac and vascular implants and grafts

Z96　Presence of other functional implants

Z97　Presence of other devices

Z98　Other postprocedural states

　　　Assign code Z98.85, Transplanted organ removal status, to indicate that a transplanted organ has been previously removed. This code should not be assigned for the encounter in which the transplanted organ is removed. The complication necessitating removal of the transplant organ should be assigned for that encounter.

　　　See section I.C19.g.3. for information on the coding of organ transplant complications.

Z99　Dependence on enabling machines and devices, not elsewhere classified

　　　Note: Categories Z89-Z9Ø and Z93-Z99 are for use only if there are no complications or malfunctions of the organ or tissue replaced, the amputation site or the equipment on which the patient is dependent.

4)　**History (of)**

There are two types of history Z codes, personal and family. Personal history codes explain a patient's past medical condition that no longer exists and is not receiving any treatment, but that has the potential for recurrence, and therefore may require continued monitoring.

Family history codes are for use when a patient has a family member(s) who has had a particular disease that causes the patient to be at higher risk of also contracting the disease.

Personal history codes may be used in conjunction with follow-up codes and family history codes may be used in conjunction with screening codes to explain the need for a test or procedure. History codes are also acceptable on any medical record regardless of the reason for visit. A history of an illness, even if no longer present, is important information that may alter the type of treatment ordered.

The history Z code categories are:

Z8Ø　Family history of primary malignant neoplasm

Z81　Family history of mental and behavioral disorders

Z82　Family history of certain disabilities and chronic diseases (leading to disablement)

Z83　Family history of other specific disorders

Z84　Family history of other conditions

Z85　Personal history of malignant neoplasm

Z86　Personal history of certain other diseases

Z87　Personal history of other diseases and conditions

Z91.4-　Personal history of psychological trauma, not elsewhere classified

Z91.5　Personal history of self-harm

Z91.8-　Other specified personal risk factors, not elsewhere classified

　　　Exception: Z91.83, Wandering in diseases classified elsewhere

Z92　Personal history of medical treatment

　　　Except: Z92.Ø, Personal history of contraception

　　　Except: Z92.82, Status post administration of tPA (rtPA) in a different facility within the last 24 hours prior to admission to a current facility

5)　**Screening**

Screening is the testing for disease or disease precursors in seemingly well individuals so that early detection and treatment can be provided for those who test positive for the disease (e.g., screening mammogram).

The testing of a person to rule out or confirm a suspected diagnosis because the patient has some sign or symptom is a diagnostic examination, not a screening. In these cases, the sign or symptom is used to explain the reason for the test.

A screening code may be a first-listed code if the reason for the visit is specifically the screening exam. It may also be used as an additional code if the screening is done during an office visit for other health problems. A screening code is not necessary if the screening is inherent to a routine examination, such as a pap smear done during a routine pelvic examination.

Should a condition be discovered during the screening then the code for the condition may be assigned as an additional diagnosis.

The Z code indicates that a screening exam is planned. A procedure code is required to confirm that the screening was performed.

The screening Z codes/categories:

Z11　Encounter for screening for infectious and parasitic diseases

Z12　Encounter for screening for malignant neoplasms

Z13　Encounter for screening for other diseases and disorders

　　　Except: Z13.9, Encounter for screening, unspecified

Z36　Encounter for antenatal screening for mother

6)　**Observation**

There are two observation Z code categories. They are for use in very limited circumstances when a person is being observed for a suspected condition that is ruled out. The observation codes are not for use if an injury or illness or any signs or symptoms related to the suspected condition are present. In such cases the diagnosis/symptom code is used with the corresponding external cause code.

The observation codes are to be used as principal diagnosis only. Additional codes may be used in addition to the observation code but only if they are unrelated to the suspected condition being observed.

Codes from subcategory ZØ3.7, Encounter for suspected maternal and fetal conditions ruled out, may either be used as a first-listed or as an additional code assignment depending on the case. They are for use in very limited circumstances on a maternal record when an encounter is for a suspected maternal or fetal condition that is ruled out during that encounter (for example, a maternal or fetal condition may be suspected due to an abnormal test result). These codes should not be used when the condition is confirmed. In those cases, the confirmed condition should be coded. In addition, these codes are not for use if an illness or any signs or symptoms related to the suspected condition or problem are present. In such cases the diagnosis/symptom code is used.

Additional codes may be used in addition to the code from subcategory Z03.7, but only if they are unrelated to the suspected condition being evaluated.

Codes from subcategory Z03.7 may not be used for encounters for antenatal screening of mother. *See Section I.C.21.c.5, Screening.*

For encounters for suspected fetal condition that are inconclusive following testing and evaluation, assign the appropriate code from category O35, O36, O40 or O41.

The observation Z code categories:

Z03   Encounter for medical observation for suspected diseases and conditions ruled out

Z04   Encounter for examination and observation for other reasons
       Except: Z04.9, Encounter for examination and observation for unspecified reason

7) Aftercare

Aftercare visit codes cover situations when the initial treatment of a disease has been performed and the patient requires continued care during the healing or recovery phase, or for the long-term consequences of the disease. The aftercare Z code should not be used if treatment is directed at a current, acute disease. The diagnosis code is to be used in these cases. Exceptions to this rule are codes Z51.0, Encounter for antineoplastic radiation therapy, and codes from subcategory Z51.1, Encounter for antineoplastic chemotherapy and immunotherapy. These codes are to be first-listed, followed by the diagnosis code when a patient's encounter is solely to receive radiation therapy, chemotherapy, or immunotherapy for the treatment of a neoplasm. If the reason for the encounter is more than one type of antineoplastic therapy, code Z51.0 and a code from subcategory Z51.1 may be assigned together, in which case one of these codes would be reported as a secondary diagnosis.

The aftercare Z codes should also not be used for aftercare for injuries. For aftercare of an injury, assign the acute injury code with the appropriate 7th character (for subsequent encounter).

The aftercare codes are generally first-listed to explain the specific reason for the encounter. An aftercare code may be used as an additional code when some type of aftercare is provided in addition to the reason for admission and no diagnosis code is applicable. An example of this would be the closure of a colostomy during an encounter for treatment of another condition.

Aftercare codes should be used in conjunction with other aftercare codes or diagnosis codes to provide better detail on the specifics of an aftercare encounter visit, unless otherwise directed by the classification. Should a patient receive multiple types of antineoplastic therapy during the same encounter, code Z51.0, Encounter for antineoplastic radiation therapy, and codes from subcategory Z51.1, Encounter for antineoplastic chemotherapy and immunotherapy, may be used together on a record. The sequencing of multiple aftercare codes depends on the circumstances of the encounter.

Certain aftercare Z code categories need a secondary diagnosis code to describe the resolving condition or sequelae. For others, the condition is included in the code title.

Additional Z code aftercare category terms include fitting and adjustment, and attention to artificial openings.

Status Z codes may be used with aftercare Z codes to indicate the nature of the aftercare. For example code Z95.1, Presence of aortocoronary bypass graft, may be used with code Z48.812, Encounter for surgical aftercare following surgery on the circulatory system, to indicate the surgery for which the aftercare is being performed. A status code should not be used when the aftercare code indicates the type of status, such as using Z43.0, Encounter for attention to tracheostomy, with Z93.0, Tracheostomy status.

The aftercare Z category/codes:

Z42   Encounter for plastic and reconstructive surgery following medical procedure or healed injury

Z43   Encounter for attention to artificial openings

Z44   Encounter for fitting and adjustment of external prosthetic device

Z45   Encounter for adjustment and management of implanted device

Z46   Encounter for fitting and adjustment of other devices

Z47   Orthopedic aftercare

Z48   Encounter for other postprocedural aftercare

Z49   Encounter for care involving renal dialysis

Z51   Encounter for other aftercare

8) Follow-up

The follow-up codes are used to explain continuing surveillance following completed treatment of a disease, condition, or injury. They imply that the condition has been fully treated and no longer exists. They should not be confused with aftercare codes, or injury codes with a 7th character for subsequent encounter, that explain ongoing care of a healing condition or its sequelae. Follow-up codes may be used in conjunction with history codes to provide the full picture of the healed condition and its treatment. The follow-up code is sequenced first, followed by the history code.

A follow-up code may be used to explain multiple visits. Should a condition be found to have recurred on the follow-up visit, then the diagnosis code for the condition should be assigned in place of the follow-up code.

The follow-up Z code categories:

Z08   Encounter for follow-up examination after completed treatment for malignant neoplasm

Z09   Encounter for follow-up examination after completed treatment for conditions other than malignant neoplasm

Z39   Encounter for maternal postpartum care and examination

9) Donor

Codes in category Z52, Donors of organs and tissues, are used for living individuals who are donating blood or other body tissue. These codes are only for individuals donating for others, not for self-donations. They are not used to identify cadaveric donations.

10) Counseling

Counseling Z codes are used when a patient or family member receives assistance in the aftermath of an illness or injury, or when support is required in coping with family or social problems. They are not used in conjunction with a diagnosis code when the counseling component of care is considered integral to standard treatment.

The counseling Z codes/categories:

Z30.0- Encounter for general counseling and advice on contraception

Z31.5   Encounter for genetic counseling

Z31.6- Encounter for general counseling and advice on procreation

Z32.2   Encounter for childbirth instruction

Z32.3   Encounter for childcare instruction

Z69   Encounter for mental health services for victim and perpetrator of abuse

Z70   Counseling related to sexual attitude, behavior and orientation

Z71   Persons encountering health services for other counseling and medical advice, not elsewhere classified

Z76.81 Expectant mother prebirth pediatrician visit

11) Encounters for obstetrical and reproductive services
See Section I.C.15. Pregnancy, Childbirth, and the Puerperium, for further instruction on the use of these codes.

Z codes for pregnancy are for use in those circumstances when none of the problems or complications included in the codes from the Obstetrics chapter exist (a routine prenatal visit or postpartum care). Codes in category Z34, Encounter for supervision of normal pregnancy, are always first-listed and are not to be used with any other code from the OB chapter. Codes in category Z3A, Weeks of gestation, may be assigned to provide additional information about the pregnancy.

The outcome of delivery, category Z37, should be included on all maternal delivery records. It is always a secondary code.

Codes in category Z3A, Weeks of gestation, may be assigned to provide additional information about the pregnancy. **The date of the admission should be used to determine weeks of gestation for inpatient admissions that encompass more than one gestational week.**

Z codes for family planning (contraceptive) or procreative management and counseling should be included on an obstetric record either during the pregnancy or the postpartum stage, if applicable.

Z codes/categories for obstetrical and reproductive services:

Z30   Encounter for contraceptive management
Z31   Encounter for procreative management
Z32.2 Encounter for childbirth instruction
Z32.3 Encounter for childcare instruction
Z33   Pregnant state
Z34   Encounter for supervision of normal pregnancy
Z36   Encounter for antenatal screening of mother
Z3A   Weeks of gestation
Z37   Outcome of delivery
Z39   Encounter for maternal postpartum care and examination
Z76.81 Expectant mother prebirth pediatrician visit

12) Newborns and Infants

See Section I.C.16. Newborn (Perinatal) Guidelines, for further instruction on the use of these codes.

Newborn Z codes/categories:

Z76.1 Encounter for health supervision and care of foundling
Z00.1- Encounter for routine child health examination
Z38   Liveborn infants according to place of birth and type of delivery

13) Routine and administrative examinations

The Z codes allow for the description of encounters for routine examinations, such as, a general check-up, or, examinations for administrative purposes, such as, a pre-employment physical. The codes are not to be used if the examination is for diagnosis of a suspected condition or for treatment purposes. In such cases the diagnosis code is used. During a routine exam, should a diagnosis or condition be discovered, it should be coded as an additional code. Pre-existing and chronic conditions and history codes may also be included as additional codes as long as the examination is for administrative purposes and not focused on any particular condition.

Some of the codes for routine health examinations distinguish between "with" and "without" abnormal findings. Code assignment depends on the information that is known at the time the encounter is being coded. For example, if no abnormal findings were found during the examination, but the encounter is being coded before test results are back, it is acceptable to assign the code for "without abnormal findings." When assigning a code for "with abnormal findings," additional code(s) should be assigned to identify the specific abnormal finding(s).

Pre-operative examination and pre-procedural laboratory examination Z codes are for use only in those situations when a patient is being cleared for a procedure or surgery and no treatment is given.

The Z codes/categories for routine and administrative examinations:

Z00   Encounter for general examination without complaint, suspected or reported diagnosis
Z01   Encounter for other special examination without complaint, suspected or reported diagnosis
Z02   Encounter for administrative examination
       Except: Z02.9, Encounter for administrative examinations, unspecified

Z32.0- Encounter for pregnancy test

14) Miscellaneous Z codes

The miscellaneous Z codes capture a number of other health care encounters that do not fall into one of the other categories. Certain of these codes identify the reason for the encounter; others are for use as additional codes that provide useful information on circumstances that may affect a patient's care and treatment.

Prophylactic Organ Removal
For encounters specifically for prophylactic removal of an organ (such as prophylactic removal of breasts due to a genetic susceptibility to cancer or a family history of cancer), the principal or first-listed code should be a code from category Z40, Encounter for prophylactic surgery, followed by the appropriate codes to identify the associated risk factor (such as genetic susceptibility or family history).

If the patient has a malignancy of one site and is having prophylactic removal at another site to prevent either a new primary malignancy or metastatic disease, a code for the malignancy should also be assigned in addition to a code from subcategory Z40.0, Encounter for prophylactic surgery for risk factors related to malignant neoplasms. A Z40.0 code should not be assigned if the patient is having organ removal for treatment of a malignancy, such as the removal of the testes for the treatment of prostate cancer.

Miscellaneous Z codes/categories:

Z28   Immunization not carried out
       Except: Z28.3, Underimmunization status
Z40   Encounter for prophylactic surgery
Z41   Encounter for procedures for purposes other than remedying health state
       Except: Z41.9, Encounter for procedure for purposes other than remedying health state, unspecified
Z53   Persons encountering health services for specific procedures and treatment, not carried out
Z55   Problems related to education and literacy
Z56   Problems related to employment and unemployment
Z57   Occupational exposure to risk factors
Z58   Problems related to physical environment
Z59   Problems related to housing and economic circumstances
Z60   Problems related to social environment
Z62   Problems related to upbringing
Z63   Other problems related to primary support group, including family circumstances
Z64   Problems related to certain psychosocial circumstances
Z65   Problems related to other psychosocial circumstances
Z72   Problems related to lifestyle
Z73   Problems related to life management difficulty
Z74   Problems related to care provider dependency
       Except: Z74.01, Bed confinement status
Z75   Problems related to medical facilities and other health care
Z76.0 Encounter for issue of repeat prescription
Z76.3 Healthy person accompanying sick person
Z76.4 Other boarder to healthcare facility
Z76.5 Malingerer [conscious simulation]
Z91.1- Patient's noncompliance with medical treatment and regimen
Z91.83 Wandering in diseases classified elsewhere
Z91.89 Other specified personal risk factors, not elsewhere classified

15) Nonspecific Z codes

Certain Z codes are so non-specific, or potentially redundant with other codes in the classification, that there can be little justification for their use in the inpatient setting. Their use in the outpatient setting should be limited to those instances when there is no further documentation to permit more precise coding. Otherwise, any sign or symptom or any other reason for visit that is captured in another code should be used.

Nonspecific Z codes/categories:

Z02.9   Encounter for administrative examinations, unspecified

Z04.9   Encounter for examination and observation for unspecified reason

Z13.9   Encounter for screening, unspecified

Z41.9   Encounter for procedure for purposes other than remedying health state, unspecified

Z52.9   Donor of unspecified organ or tissue

Z86.59   Personal history of other mental and behavioral disorders

Z88.9   Allergy status to unspecified drugs, medicaments and biological substances status

Z92.0   Personal history of contraception

16) **Z codes that may only be principal/first-listed diagnosis**

The following Z codes/categories may only be reported as the principal/first-listed diagnosis, except when there are multiple encounters on the same day and the medical records for the encounters are combined:

Z00   Encounter for general examination without complaint, suspected or reported diagnosis

Z01   Encounter for other special examination without complaint, suspected or reported diagnosis

Z02   Encounter for administrative examination

Z03   Encounter for medical observation for suspected diseases and conditions ruled out

Z04   Encounter for examination and observation for other reasons

Z31.81   Encounter for male factor infertility in female patient

Z31.82   Encounter for Rh incompatibility status

Z31.83   Encounter for assisted reproductive fertility procedure cycle

Z31.84   Encounter for fertility preservation procedure

Z33.2   Encounter for elective termination of pregnancy

Z34   Encounter for supervision of normal pregnancy

Z38   Liveborn infants according to place of birth and type of delivery

Z39   Encounter for maternal postpartum care and examination

Z42   Encounter for plastic and reconstructive surgery following medical procedure or healed injury

Z51.0   Encounter for antineoplastic radiation therapy

Z51.1-   Encounter for antineoplastic chemotherapy and immunotherapy

Z52   Donors of organs and tissues
         Except: Z52.9, Donor of unspecified organ or tissue

Z76.1   Encounter for health supervision and care of foundling

Z76.2   Encounter for health supervision and care of other healthy infant and child

Z99.12   Encounter for respirator [ventilator] dependence during power failure

Section II. Selection of Principal Diagnosis

The circumstances of inpatient admission always govern the selection of principal diagnosis. The principal diagnosis is defined in the Uniform Hospital Discharge Data Set (UHDDS) as "that condition established after study to be chiefly responsible for occasioning the admission of the patient to the hospital for care."

The UHDDS definitions are used by hospitals to report inpatient data elements in a standardized manner. These data elements and their definitions can be found in the July 31, 1985, Federal Register (Vol. 50, No, 147), pp. 31038-40.

Since that time the application of the UHDDS definitions has been expanded to include all non-outpatient settings (acute care, short term, long term care and psychiatric hospitals; home health agencies; rehab facilities; nursing homes, etc).

In determining principal diagnosis the coding conventions in the ICD-10-CM, the Tabular List and Alphabetic Index take precedence over these official coding guidelines.

(See Section I.A., Conventions for the ICD-10-CM)

The importance of consistent, complete documentation in the medical record cannot be overemphasized. Without such documentation the application of all coding guidelines is a difficult, if not impossible, task.

A. Codes for symptoms, signs, and ill-defined conditions

Codes for symptoms, signs, and ill-defined conditions from Chapter 18 are not to be used as principal diagnosis when a related definitive diagnosis has been established.

B. Two or more interrelated conditions, each potentially meeting the definition for principal diagnosis

When there are two or more interrelated conditions (such as diseases in the same ICD-10-CM chapter or manifestations characteristically associated with a certain disease) potentially meeting the definition of principal diagnosis, either condition may be sequenced first, unless the circumstances of the admission, the therapy provided, the Tabular List, or the Alphabetic Index indicate otherwise.

C. Two or more diagnoses that equally meet the definition for principal diagnosis

In the unusual instance when two or more diagnoses equally meet the criteria for principal diagnosis as determined by the circumstances of admission, diagnostic workup and/or therapy provided, and the Alphabetic Index, Tabular List, or another coding guidelines does not provide sequencing direction, any one of the diagnoses may be sequenced first.

D. Two or more comparative or contrasting conditions

In those rare instances when two or more contrasting or comparative diagnoses are documented as "either/or" (or similar terminology), they are coded as if the diagnoses were confirmed and the diagnoses are sequenced according to the circumstances of the admission. If no further determination can be made as to which diagnosis should be principal, either diagnosis may be sequenced first.

E. A symptom(s) followed by contrasting/comparative diagnoses

When a symptom(s) is followed by contrasting/comparative diagnoses, the symptom code is sequenced first. **However, if the symptom code is integral to the conditions listed, no code for the symptom is reported.** All the contrasting/comparative diagnoses should be coded as additional diagnoses.

F. Original treatment plan not carried out

Sequence as the principal diagnosis the condition, which after study occasioned the admission to the hospital, even though treatment may not have been carried out due to unforeseen circumstances.

G. Complications of surgery and other medical care

When the admission is for treatment of a complication resulting from surgery or other medical care, the complication code is sequenced as the principal diagnosis. If the complication is classified to the T80-T88 series and the code lacks the necessary specificity in describing the complication, an additional code for the specific complication should be assigned.

H. Uncertain diagnosis

If the diagnosis documented at the time of discharge is qualified as "probable", "suspected", "likely", "questionable", "possible", or "still to be ruled out", or other similar terms indicating uncertainty, code the condition as if it existed or was established. The bases for these guidelines are the diagnostic workup, arrangements for further workup or observation, and initial therapeutic approach that correspond most closely with the established diagnosis.

Note: This guideline is applicable only to inpatient admissions to short-term, acute, long-term care and psychiatric hospitals.

I. Admission from observation unit

1. **Admission Following Medical Observation**
   When a patient is admitted to an observation unit for a medical condition, which either worsens or does not improve, and is subsequently admitted as an inpatient of the same hospital for this same medical condition, the principal diagnosis would be the medical condition which led to the hospital admission.

2. **Admission Following Post-Operative Observation**
   When a patient is admitted to an observation unit to monitor a condition (or complication) that develops following outpatient surgery, and then is subsequently admitted as an inpatient of the same hospital, hospitals should apply the Uniform Hospital Discharge Data Set (UHDDS) definition of principal diagnosis as "that condition established after study to be chiefly responsible for occasioning the admission of the patient to the hospital for care."

J. Admission from outpatient surgery

When a patient receives surgery in the hospital's outpatient surgery department and is subsequently admitted for continuing inpatient care at the same hospital, the following guidelines should be followed in selecting the principal diagnosis for the inpatient admission:

- If the reason for the inpatient admission is a complication, assign the complication as the principal diagnosis.
- If no complication, or other condition, is documented as the reason for the inpatient admission, assign the reason for the outpatient surgery as the principal diagnosis.
- If the reason for the inpatient admission is another condition unrelated to the surgery, assign the unrelated condition as the principal diagnosis.

K. Admissions/Encounters for Rehabilitation

When the purpose for the admission/encounter is rehabilitation, sequence first the code for the condition for which the service is being performed. For example, for an admission/encounter for rehabilitation for right-sided dominant hemiplegia following a cerebrovascular infarction, report code I69.351, Hemiplegia and hemiparesis following cerebral infarction affecting right dominant side, as the first-listed or principal diagnosis.

If the condition for which the rehabilitation service is no longer present, report the appropriate aftercare code as the first-listed or principal diagnosis. For example, if a patient with severe degenerative osteoarthritis of the hip, underwent hip replacement and the current encounter/admission is for rehabilitation, report code Z47.1, Aftercare following joint replacement surgery, as the first-listed or principal diagnosis.

See Section I.C.21.c.7, Factors influencing health states and contact with health services, Aftercare.

Section III. Reporting Additional Diagnoses

GENERAL RULES FOR OTHER (ADDITIONAL) DIAGNOSES

For reporting purposes the definition for "other diagnoses" is interpreted as additional conditions that affect patient care in terms of requiring:

- clinical evaluation; or
- therapeutic treatment; or
- diagnostic procedures; or
- extended length of hospital stay; or
- increased nursing care and/or monitoring.

The UHDDS item #11-b defines Other Diagnoses as "all conditions that coexist at the time of admission, that develop subsequently, or that affect the treatment received and/or the length of stay. Diagnoses that relate to an earlier episode which have no bearing on the current hospital stay are to be excluded." UHDDS definitions apply to inpatients in acute care, short-term, long term care and psychiatric hospital setting. The UHDDS definitions are used by acute care short-term hospitals to report inpatient data elements in a standardized manner. These data elements and their definitions can be found in the July 31, 1985, Federal Register (Vol. 50, No, 147), pp. 31038-40.

Since that time the application of the UHDDS definitions has been expanded to include all non-outpatient settings (acute care, short term, long term care and psychiatric hospitals; home health agencies; rehab facilities; nursing homes, etc.).

The following guidelines are to be applied in designating "other diagnoses" when neither the Alphabetic Index nor the Tabular List in ICD-10-CM provide direction. The listing of the diagnoses in the patient record is the responsibility of the attending provider.

A. Previous conditions
If the provider has included a diagnosis in the final diagnostic statement, such as the discharge summary or the face sheet, it should ordinarily be coded. Some providers include in the diagnostic statement resolved conditions or diagnoses and status-post procedures from previous admission that have no bearing on the current stay. Such conditions are not to be reported and are coded only if required by hospital policy.

However, history codes (categories Z80-Z87) may be used as secondary codes if the historical condition or family history has an impact on current care or influences treatment.

B. Abnormal findings
Abnormal findings (laboratory, x-ray, pathologic, and other diagnostic results) are not coded and reported unless the provider indicates their clinical significance. If the findings are outside the normal range and the attending provider has ordered other tests to evaluate the condition or prescribed treatment, it is appropriate to ask the provider whether the abnormal finding should be added.

Please note: This differs from the coding practices in the outpatient setting for coding encounters for diagnostic tests that have been interpreted by a provider.

C. Uncertain Diagnosis
If the diagnosis documented at the time of discharge is qualified as "probable", "suspected", "likely", "questionable", "possible", or "still to be ruled out" or other similar terms indicating uncertainty, code the condition as if it existed or was established. The bases for these guidelines are the diagnostic workup, arrangements for further workup or observation, and initial therapeutic approach that correspond most closely with the established diagnosis.

Note: This guideline is applicable only to inpatient admissions to short-term, acute, long-term care and psychiatric hospitals.

Section IV. Diagnostic Coding and Reporting Guidelines for Outpatient Services

These coding guidelines for outpatient diagnoses have been approved for use by hospitals/ providers in coding and reporting hospital-based outpatient services and provider-based office visits.

Information about the use of certain abbreviations, punctuation, symbols, and other conventions used in the ICD-10-CM Tabular List (code numbers and titles), can be found in Section IA of these guidelines, under "Conventions Used in the Tabular List." **Section I.B. contains general guidelines that apply to the entire classification. Section I.C. contains chapter-specific guidelines that correspond to the chapters as they are arranged in the classification.** Information about the correct sequence to use in finding a code is also described in Section I.

The terms encounter and visit are often used interchangeably in describing outpatient service contacts and, therefore, appear together in these guidelines without distinguishing one from the other.

Though the conventions and general guidelines apply to all settings, coding guidelines for outpatient and provider reporting of diagnoses will vary in a number of instances from those for inpatient diagnoses, recognizing that:

The Uniform Hospital Discharge Data Set (UHDDS) definition of principal diagnosis applies only to inpatients in acute, short-term, long-term care and psychiatric hospitals.

Coding guidelines for inconclusive diagnoses (probable, suspected, rule out, etc.) were developed for inpatient reporting and do not apply to outpatients.

A. Selection of first-listed condition
In the outpatient setting, the term first-listed diagnosis is used in lieu of principal diagnosis.

In determining the first-listed diagnosis the coding conventions of ICD-10-CM, as well as the general and disease specific guidelines take precedence over the outpatient guidelines.

Diagnoses often are not established at the time of the initial encounter/visit. It may take two or more visits before the diagnosis is confirmed.

The most critical rule involves beginning the search for the correct code assignment through the Alphabetic Index. Never begin searching initially in the Tabular List as this will lead to coding errors.

1. Outpatient surgery

When a patient presents for outpatient surgery (same day surgery), code the reason for the surgery as the first-listed diagnosis (reason for the encounter), even if the surgery is not performed due to a contraindication.

2. Observation stay

When a patient is admitted for observation for a medical condition, assign a code for the medical condition as the first-listed diagnosis.

When a patient presents for outpatient surgery and develops complications requiring admission to observation, code the reason for the surgery as the first reported diagnosis (reason for the encounter), followed by codes for the complications as secondary diagnoses.

B. Codes from A00.0 through T88.9, Z00-Z99

The appropriate code(s) from A00.0 through T88.9, Z00-Z99 must be used to identify diagnoses, symptoms, conditions, problems, complaints, or other reason(s) for the encounter/visit.

C. Accurate reporting of ICD-10-CM diagnosis codes

For accurate reporting of ICD-10-CM diagnosis codes, the documentation should describe the patient's condition, using terminology which includes specific diagnoses as well as symptoms, problems, or reasons for the encounter. There are ICD-10-CM codes to describe all of these.

D. Codes that describe symptoms and signs

Codes that describe symptoms and signs, as opposed to diagnoses, are acceptable for reporting purposes when a diagnosis has not been established (confirmed) by the provider. Chapter 18 of ICD-10-CM, Symptoms, Signs, and Abnormal Clinical and Laboratory Findings Not Elsewhere Classified (codes R00-R99) contain many, but not all codes for symptoms.

E. Encounters for circumstances other than a disease or injury

ICD-10-CM provides codes to deal with encounters for circumstances other than a disease or injury. The Factors Influencing Health Status and Contact with Health Services codes (Z00-Z99) are provided to deal with occasions when circumstances other than a disease or injury are recorded as diagnosis or problems.

See Section I.C.21. Factors influencing health status and contact with health services.

F. Level of Detail in Coding

1. ICD-10-CM codes with 3, 4, 5, 6 or 7 characters

ICD-10-CM is composed of codes with 3, 4, 5, 6 or 7 characters. Codes with three characters are included in ICD-10-CM as the heading of a category of codes that may be further subdivided by the use of fourth, fifth, sixth or seventh characters to provide greater specificity.

2. Use of full number of characters required for a code

A three-character code is to be used only if it is not further subdivided. A code is invalid if it has not been coded to the full number of characters required for that code, including the 7th character extension, if applicable.

G. ICD-10-CM code for the diagnosis, condition, problem, or other reason for encounter/visit

List first the ICD-10-CM code for the diagnosis, condition, problem, or other reason for encounter/visit shown in the medical record to be chiefly responsible for the services provided. List additional codes that describe any coexisting conditions. In some cases the first-listed diagnosis may be a symptom when a diagnosis has not been established (confirmed) by the physician.

H. Uncertain diagnosis

Do not code diagnoses documented as "probable," "suspected," "questionable," "rule out," or "working diagnosis" or other similar terms indicating uncertainty. Rather, code the condition(s) to the highest degree of certainty for that encounter/visit, such as symptoms, signs, abnormal test results, or other reason for the visit.

Please note: This differs from the coding practices used by short-term, acute care, long-term care and psychiatric hospitals.

I. Chronic diseases

Chronic diseases treated on an ongoing basis may be coded and reported as many times as the patient receives treatment and care for the condition(s)

J. Code all documented conditions that coexist

Code all documented conditions that coexist at the time of the encounter/visit, and require or affect patient care treatment or management. Do not code conditions that were previously treated and no longer exist. However, history codes (categories Z80-Z87) may be used as secondary codes if the historical condition or family history has an impact on current care or influences treatment.

K. Patients receiving diagnostic services only

For patients receiving diagnostic services only during an encounter/visit, sequence first the diagnosis, condition, problem, or other reason for encounter/visit shown in the medical record to be chiefly responsible for the outpatient services provided during the encounter/visit. Codes for other diagnoses (e.g., chronic conditions) may be sequenced as additional diagnoses.

For encounters for routine laboratory/radiology testing in the absence of any signs, symptoms, or associated diagnosis, assign Z01.89, Encounter for other specified special examinations. If routine testing is performed during the same encounter as a test to evaluate a sign, symptom, or diagnosis, it is appropriate to assign both the Z code and the code describing the reason for the non-routine test.

For outpatient encounters for diagnostic tests that have been interpreted by a physician, and the final report is available at the time of coding, code any confirmed or definitive diagnosis(es) documented in the interpretation. Do not code related signs and symptoms as additional diagnoses.

Please note: This differs from the coding practice in the hospital inpatient setting regarding abnormal findings on test results.

L. Patients receiving therapeutic services only

For patients receiving therapeutic services only during an encounter/visit, sequence first the diagnosis, condition, problem, or other reason for encounter/visit shown in the medical record to be chiefly responsible for the outpatient services provided during the encounter/visit. Codes for other diagnoses (e.g., chronic conditions) may be sequenced as additional diagnoses.

The only exception to this rule is that when the primary reason for the admission/encounter is chemotherapy or radiation therapy, the appropriate Z code for the service is listed first, and the diagnosis or problem for which the service is being performed listed second.

M. Patients receiving preoperative evaluations only

For patients receiving preoperative evaluations only, sequence first a code from subcategory Z01.81, Encounter for pre-procedural examinations, to describe the pre-op consultations. Assign a code for the condition to describe the reason for the surgery as an additional diagnosis. Code also any findings related to the pre-op evaluation.

N. Ambulatory surgery

For ambulatory surgery, code the diagnosis for which the surgery was performed. If the postoperative diagnosis is known to be different from the preoperative diagnosis at the time the diagnosis is confirmed, select the postoperative diagnosis for coding, since it is the most definitive.

O. Routine outpatient prenatal visits

See Section I.C.15. Routine outpatient prenatal visits.

P. Encounters for general medical examinations with abnormal findings

The subcategories for encounters for general medical examinations, Z00.0-, provide codes for with and without abnormal findings. Should a general medical examination result in an abnormal finding, the code for general medical examination with abnormal finding should be assigned as the first-listed diagnosis. A secondary code for the abnormal finding should also be coded.

Q. Encounters for routine health screenings

See Section I.C.21. Factors influencing health status and contact with health services, Screening

Appendix I. Present on Admission Reporting Guidelines

Introduction

These guidelines are to be used as a supplement to the *ICD-10-CM Official Guidelines for Coding and Reporting* to facilitate the assignment of the Present on Admission (POA) indicator for each diagnosis and external cause of injury code reported on claim forms (UB-04 and 837 Institutional).

These guidelines are not intended to replace any guidelines in the main body of the *ICD-10-CM Official Guidelines for Coding and Reporting*. The POA guidelines are not intended to provide guidance on when a condition should be coded, but rather, how to apply the POA indicator to the final set of diagnosis codes that have been assigned in accordance with Sections I, II, and III of the official coding guidelines. Subsequent to the assignment of the ICD-10-CM codes, the POA indicator should then be assigned to those conditions that have been coded.

As stated in the Introduction to the *ICD-10-CM Official Guidelines for Coding and Reporting*, a joint effort between the healthcare provider and the coder is essential to achieve complete and accurate documentation, code assignment, and reporting of diagnoses and procedures. The importance of consistent, complete documentation in the medical record cannot be overemphasized. Medical record documentation from any provider involved in the care and treatment of the patient may be used to support the determination of whether a condition was present on admission or not. In the context of the official coding guidelines, the term "provider" means a physician or any qualified healthcare practitioner who is legally accountable for establishing the patient's diagnosis.

These guidelines are not a substitute for the provider's clinical judgment as to the determination of whether a condition was/was not present on admission. The provider should be queried regarding issues related to the linking of signs/symptoms, timing of test results, and the timing of findings.

General Reporting Requirements

All claims involving inpatient admissions to general acute care hospitals or other facilities that are subject to a law or regulation mandating collection of present on admission information.

Present on admission is defined as present at the time the order for inpatient admission occurs -- conditions that develop during an outpatient encounter, including emergency department, observation, or outpatient surgery, are considered as present on admission.

POA indicator is assigned to principal and secondary diagnoses (as defined in Section II of the Official Guidelines for Coding and Reporting) and the external cause of injury codes.

Issues related to inconsistent, missing, conflicting or unclear documentation must still be resolved by the provider.

If a condition would not be coded and reported based on UHDDS definitions and current official coding guidelines, then the POA indicator would not be reported.

Reporting Options

- Y – Yes
- N – No
- U – Unknown
- W – Clinically undetermined
- Unreported/Not used (or "1" for Medicare usage) – (Exempt from POA reporting)

Reporting Definitions

- Y – present at the time of inpatient admission
- N – not present at the time of inpatient admission
- U – documentation is insufficient to determine if condition is present on admission
- W – provider is unable to clinically determine whether condition was present on admission or not

Timeframe for POA Identification and Documentation

There is no required timeframe as to when a provider (per the definition of "provider" used in these guidelines) must identify or document a condition to be present on admission. In some clinical situations, it may not be possible for a provider to make a definitive diagnosis (or a

condition may not be recognized or reported by the patient) for a period of time after admission. In some cases it may be several days before the provider arrives at a definitive diagnosis. This does not mean that the condition was not present on admission. Determination of whether the condition was present on admission or not will be based on the applicable POA guideline as identified in this document, or on the provider's best clinical judgment.

If at the time of code assignment the documentation is unclear as to whether a condition was present on admission or not, it is appropriate to query the provider for clarification.

Assigning the POA Indicator

Condition is on the "Exempt from Reporting" list

Leave the "present on admission" field blank if the condition is on the list of ICD-10-CM codes for which this field is not applicable. This is the only circumstance in which the field may be left blank.

POA Explicitly Documented

Assign "Y" for any condition the provider explicitly documents as being present on admission.

Assign "N" for any condition the provider explicitly documents as not present at the time of admission.

Conditions diagnosed prior to inpatient admission

Assign "Y" for conditions that were diagnosed prior to admission (example: hypertension, diabetes mellitus, asthma).

Conditions diagnosed during the admission but clearly present before admission

Assign "Y" for conditions diagnosed during the admission that were clearly present but not diagnosed until after admission occurred.

Diagnoses subsequently confirmed after admission are considered present on admission if at the time of admission they are documented as suspected, possible, rule out, differential diagnosis, or constitute an underlying cause of a symptom that is present at the time of admission.

Condition develops during outpatient encounter prior to inpatient admission

Assign "Y" for any condition that develops during an outpatient encounter prior to a written order for inpatient admission.

Documentation does not indicate whether condition was present on admission

Assign "U" when the medical record documentation is unclear as to whether the condition was present on admission. "U" should not be routinely assigned and used only in very limited circumstances. Coders are encouraged to query the providers when the documentation is unclear.

Documentation states that it cannot be determined whether the condition was or was not present on admission

Assign "W" when the medical record documentation indicates that it cannot be clinically determined whether or not the condition was present on admission.

Chronic condition with acute exacerbation during the admission

If a single code identifies both the chronic condition and the acute exacerbation, see POA guidelines pertaining to combination codes.

If a single code only identifies the chronic condition and not the acute exacerbation (e.g., acute exacerbation of chronic leukemia), assign "Y."

Conditions documented as possible, probable, suspected, or rule out at the time of discharge

If the final diagnosis contains a possible, probable, suspected, or rule out diagnosis, and this diagnosis was based on signs, symptoms or clinical findings suspected at the time of inpatient admission, assign "Y."

If the final diagnosis contains a possible, probable, suspected, or rule out diagnosis, and this diagnosis was based on signs, symptoms or clinical findings that were not present on admission, assign "N".

Conditions documented as impending or threatened at the time of discharge

If the final diagnosis contains an impending or threatened diagnosis, and this diagnosis is based on symptoms or clinical findings that were present on admission, assign "Y".

If the final diagnosis contains an impending or threatened diagnosis, and this diagnosis is based on symptoms or clinical findings that were not present on admission, assign "N".

Acute and Chronic Conditions

Assign "Y" for acute conditions that are present at time of admission and N for acute conditions that are not present at time of admission.

Assign "Y" for chronic conditions, even though the condition may not be diagnosed until after admission.

If a single code identifies both an acute and chronic condition, see the POA guidelines for combination codes.

Combination Codes

Assign "N" if any part of the combination code was not present on admission (e.g., COPD with acute exacerbation and the exacerbation was not present on admission; gastric ulcer that does not start bleeding until after admission; asthma patient develops status asthmaticus after admission).

Assign "Y" if all parts of the combination code were present on admission (e.g., patient with acute prostatitis admitted with hematuria).

If the final diagnosis includes comparative or contrasting diagnoses, and both were present, or suspected, at the time of admission, assign "Y".

For infection codes that include the causal organism, assign "Y" if the infection (or signs of the infection) was present on admission, even though the culture results may not be known until after admission (e.g., patient is admitted with pneumonia and the provider documents pseudomonas as the causal organism a few days later).

Same Diagnosis Code for Two or More Conditions

When the same ICD-10-CM diagnosis code applies to two or more conditions during the same encounter (e.g. two separate conditions classified to the same ICD-10-CM diagnosis code):

> Assign "Y" if all conditions represented by the single ICD-10-CM code were present on admission (e.g. bilateral unspecified age-related cataracts).

> Assign "N" if any of the conditions represented by the single ICD-10-CM code was not present on admission (e.g. traumatic secondary and recurrent hemorrhage and seroma is assigned to a single code T79.2, but only one of the conditions was present on admission).

Obstetrical conditions

Whether or not the patient delivers during the current hospitalization does not affect assignment of the POA indicator. The determining factor for POA assignment is whether the pregnancy complication or obstetrical condition described by the code was present at the time of admission or not.

If the pregnancy complication or obstetrical condition was present on admission (e.g., patient admitted in preterm labor), assign "Y".

If the pregnancy complication or obstetrical condition was not present on admission (e.g., 2nd degree laceration during delivery, postpartum hemorrhage that occurred during current hospitalization, fetal distress develops after admission), assign "N".

If the obstetrical code includes more than one diagnosis and any of the diagnoses identified by the code were not present on admission assign "N". (e.g., Category O11, Pre-existing hypertension with pre-eclampsia).

Perinatal conditions

Newborns are not considered to be admitted until after birth. Therefore, any condition present at birth or that developed in utero is considered present at admission and should be assigned "Y". This includes conditions that occur during delivery (e.g., injury during delivery, meconium aspiration, exposure to streptococcus B in the vaginal canal).

Congenital conditions and anomalies

Assign "Y" for congenital conditions and anomalies except for categories Q00-Q99, Congenital anomalies, which are on the exempt list. Congenital conditions are always considered present on admission.

External cause of injury codes

Assign "Y" for any external cause code representing an external cause of morbidity that occurred prior to inpatient admission (e.g., patient fell out of bed at home, patient fell out of bed in emergency room prior to admission).

Assign "N" for any external cause code representing an external cause of morbidity that occurred during inpatient hospitalization (e.g., patient fell out of hospital bed during hospital stay, patient experienced an adverse reaction to a medication administered after inpatient admission).

Categories and Codes Exempt from Diagnosis Present on Admission Requirement

Note: "Diagnosis present on admission" for these code categories are exempt because they represent circumstances regarding the healthcare encounter or factors influencing health status that do not represent a current disease or injury or are always present on admission.

B90–B94	Sequelae of infectious and parasitic diseases
E64	Sequelae of malnutrition and other nutritional deficiences
I25.2	Old myocardial infarction
I69	Sequelae of cerebrovascular disease
O09	Supervision of high risk pregnancy
O66.5	Attempted application of vacuum extractor and forceps
O80	Encounter for full-term uncomplicated delivery
O94	Sequelae of complication of pregnancy, childbirth, and the puerperium
P00	Newborn (suspected to be) affected by maternal conditions that may be unrelated to present pregnancy
Q00 – Q99	Congenital malformations, deformations and chromosomal abnormalities
S00-T88.9	Injury, poisoning and certain other consequences of external causes with 7th character representing subsequent encounter or sequela
V00- V09	Pedestrian injured in transport accident
	Except: V00.81-, Accident with wheelchair (powered)
	V00.83-, Accident with motorized mobility scooter
V10-V19	Pedal cycle rider injured in transport accident
V20-V29	Motorcycle rider injured in transport accident
V30-V39	Occupant of three-wheeled motor vehicle injured in transport accident
V40-V49	Car occupant injured in transport accident
V50-V59	Occupant of pick-up truck or van injured in transport accident
V60-V69	Occupant of heavy transport vehicle injured in transport accident
V70-V79	Bus occupant injured in transport accident
V80-V89	Other land transport accidents
V90-V94	Water transport accidents
V95-V97	Air and space transport accidents
V98-V99	Other and unspecified transport accidents
W03	Other fall on same level due to collision with another person
W09	Fall on and from playground equipment
W14	Fall from tree
W15	Fall from cliff
W17.0	Fall into well
W17.1	Fall into storm drain or manhole
W18.01	Striking against sports equipment with subsequent fall
W20.8	Other cause of strike by thrown, projected or falling object
W21	Striking against or struck by sports equipment
W30	Contact with agricultural machinery
W31	Contact with other and unspecified machinery
W32-W34	Accidental handgun discharge and malfunction
W35- W40	Exposure to inanimate mechanical forces
W52	Crushed, pushed or stepped on by crowd or human stampede
W56	Contact with nonvenomous marine animal
W58	Contact with crocodile or alligator

W61	Contact with birds (domestic) (wild)	
W62	Contact with nonvenomous amphibians	
W89	Exposure to man-made visible and ultraviolet light	
X02	Exposure to controlled fire in building or structure	
X03	Exposure to controlled fire, not in building or structure	
X04	Exposure to ignition of highly flammable material	
X52	Prolonged stay in weightless environment	
X71	Intentional self-harm by drowning and submersion	
	Except: X71.0-, Intentional self-harm by drowning and submersion while in bath tub	
X72	Intentional self-harm by handgun discharge	
X73	Intentional self-harm by rifle, shotgun and larger firearm discharge	
X74	Intentional self-harm by other and unspecified firearm and gun discharge	
X75	Intentional self-harm by explosive material	
X76	Intentional self-harm by smoke, fire and flames	
X77	Intentional self-harm by steam, hot vapors and hot objects	
X81	Intentional self-harm by jumping or lying in front of moving object	
X82	Intentional self-harm by crashing of motor vehicle	
X83	Intentional self-harm by other specified means	
X71-X83	Intentional self-harm	
Y03	**Assault by crashing of motor vehicle**	
Y07	**Perpetrator of assault, maltreatment and neglect**	
Y08.8	**Assault by strike by sports equipment**	
Y21	Drowning and submersion, undetermined intent	
Y22	Handgun discharge, undetermined intent	
Y23	Rifle, shotgun and larger firearm discharge, undetermined intent	
Y24	Other and unspecified firearm discharge, undetermined intent	
Y30	Falling, jumping or pushed from a high place, undetermined intent	
Y32	**Assault by crashing of motor vehicle, undetermined intent**	
Y35	Legal intervention	
Y36	Operations of war	
Y37	Military operations	
Y38	Terrorism	
Y92	Place of occurrence of the external cause	
Y93	Activity code	
Y99	External cause status	
Z00	Encounter for general examination without complaint, suspected or reported diagnosis	
Z01	Encounter for other special examination without complaint, suspected or reported diagnosis	
Z02	Encounter for administrative examination	
Z03	Encounter for medical observation for suspected diseases and conditions ruled out	
Z08	Encounter for follow-up examination following completed treatment for malignant neoplasm	
Z09	Encounter for follow-up examination after completed treatment for conditions other than malignant neoplasm	
Z11	Encounter for screening for infectious and parasitic diseases	
Z11.8	Encounter for screening for other infectious and parasitic diseases	
Z12	Encounter for screening for malignant neoplasms	
Z13	Encounter for screening for other diseases and disorders	
Z13.4	Encounter for screening for certain developmental disorders in childhood	
Z13.5	Encounter for screening for eye and ear disorders	
Z13.6	Encounter for screening for cardiovascular disorders	
Z13.83	Encounter for screening for respiratory disorder NEC	
Z13.89	Encounter for screening for other disorder	
Z14	Genetic carrier	
Z15	Genetic susceptibility to disease	
Z17	Estrogen receptor status	
Z18	Retained foreign body fragments	

Z22	Carrier of infectious disease
Z23	Encounter for immunization
Z28	Immunization not carried out and underimmunization status
Z28.3	Underimmunization status
Z30	Encounter for contraceptive management
Z31	Encounter for procreative management
Z34	Encounter for supervision of normal pregnancy
Z36	Encounter for antenatal screening of mother
Z37	Outcome of delivery
Z38	Liveborn infants according to place of birth and type of delivery
Z39	Encounter for maternal postpartum care and examination
Z41	Encounter for procedures for purposes other than remedying health state
Z42	Encounter for plastic and reconstructive surgery following medical procedure or healed injury
Z43	Encounter for attention to artificial openings
Z44	Encounter for fitting and adjustment of external prosthetic device
Z45	Encounter for adjustment and management of implanted device
Z46	Encounter for fitting and adjustment of other devices
Z47.8	Encounter for other orthopedic aftercare
Z49	Encounter for care involving renal dialysis
Z51	Encounter for other aftercare
Z51.5	Encounter for palliative care
Z51.8	Encounter for other specified aftercare
Z52	Donors of organs and tissues
Z59	Problems related to housing and economic circumstances
Z63	Other problems related to primary support groupincluding family circumstances
Z65	Problems related to other psychosocial circumstances
Z65.8	Other specified problems related to psychosocial circumstances
Z67.1-Z67.9	Blood type
Z68	Body mass index (BMI)
Z72	Problems related to lifestyle
Z74.01	Bed confinement status
Z76	Persons encountering health services in other circumstances
Z77.110-Z77.128	Environmental pollution and hazards in the physical environment
Z78	Other specified health status
Z79	Long term (current) drug therapy
Z80	Family history of primary malignant neoplasm
Z81	Family history of mental and behavioral disorders
Z82	Family history of certain disabilities and chronic diseases (leading to disablement)
Z83	Family history of other specific disorders
Z84	Family history of other conditions
Z85	Personal history of primary malignant neoplasm
Z86	Personal history of certain other diseases
Z87	Personal history of other diseases and conditions
Z87.828	Personal history of other (healed) physical injury and trauma
Z87.891	Personal history of nicotine dependence
Z88	Allergy status to drugs, medicaments and biological substances
Z89	Acquired absence of limb
Z90.710	Acquired absence of both cervix and uterus
Z91.0	Allergy status, other than to drugs and biological substances
Z91.4	Personal history of psychological trauma, not elsewhere classified
Z91.5	Personal history of self-harm
Z91.8	Other specified risk factors, not elsewhere classified
Z92	Personal history of medical treatment
Z93	Artificial opening status
Z94	Transplanted organ and tissue status
Z95	Presence of cardiac and vascular implants and grafts
Z97	Presence of other devices
Z98	Other postprocedural states
Z99	Dependence on enabling machines and devices, not elsewhere classified

ICD-10-CM Index to Diseases and Injuries

A

Aarskog's syndrome Q87.1
Abandonment — *see* Maltreatment
Abasia (-astasia) (hysterical) F44.4
Abderhalden-Kaufmann-Lignac syndrome (cystinosis) E72.04
Abdomen, abdominal (*see also* condition)
  acute R10.0
  angina K55.1
  muscle deficiency syndrome Q79.4
Abdominalgia — *see* Pain, abdominal
Abduction contracture, hip or other joint — *see* Contraction, joint
Aberrant (congenital) (*see also* Malposition, congenital)
  adrenal gland Q89.1
  artery (peripheral) Q27.8
    basilar NEC Q28.1
    cerebral Q28.3
    coronary Q24.5
    digestive system Q27.8
    eye Q15.8
    lower limb Q27.8
    precerebral Q28.1
    pulmonary Q25.79
    renal Q27.2
    retina Q14.1
    specified site NEC Q27.8
    subclavian Q27.8
    upper limb Q27.8
    vertebral Q28.1
  breast Q83.8
  endocrine gland NEC Q89.2
  hepatic duct Q44.5
  pancreas Q45.3
  parathyroid gland Q89.2
  pituitary gland Q89.2
  sebaceous glands, mucous membrane, mouth, congenital Q38.6
  spleen Q89.09
  subclavian artery Q27.8
  thymus (gland) Q89.2
  thyroid gland Q89.2
  vein (peripheral) NEC Q27.8
    cerebral Q28.3
    digestive system Q27.8
    lower limb Q27.8
    precerebral Q28.1
    specified site NEC Q27.8
    upper limb Q27.8
Aberration
  distantial — *see* Disturbance, visual
  mental F99
Abetalipoproteinemia E78.6
Abiotrophy R68.89
Ablatio, ablation
  retinae — *see* Detachment, retina
Ablepharia, ablepharon Q10.3
Abnormal, abnormality, abnormalities (*see also* Anomaly)
  acid-base balance (mixed) E87.4
  albumin R77.0
  alphafetoprotein R77.2
  alveolar ridge K08.9
  anatomical relationship Q89.9
  apertures, congenital, diaphragm Q79.1
  auditory perception H93.29- ☑
    diplacusis — *see* Diplacusis
    hyperacusis — *see* Hyperacusis
    recruitment — *see* Recruitment, auditory
    threshold shift — *see* Shift, auditory threshold
  autosomes Q99.9
    fragile site Q95.5
  basal metabolic rate R94.8
  biosynthesis, testicular androgen E29.1
  bleeding time R79.1
  blood level (of)
    cobalt R79.0
    copper R79.0
    iron R79.0
    lithium R78.89

Abnormal, abnormality, abnormalities — *continued*
  blood level — *continued*
    magnesium R79.0
    mineral NEC R79.0
    zinc R79.0
  blood pressure
    elevated R03.0
    low reading (nonspecific) R03.1
  blood sugar R73.09
  blood-gas level R79.81
  bowel sounds R19.15
    absent R19.11
    hyperactive R19.12
  brain scan R94.02
  breathing R06.9
  caloric test R94.138
  cerebrospinal fluid R83.9
    cytology R83.6
    drug level R83.2
    enzyme level R83.0
    hormones R83.1
    immunology R83.4
    microbiology R83.5
    nonmedicinal level R83.3
    specified type NEC R83.8
  chemistry, blood R79.9
    C-reactive protein R79.82
    drugs — *see* Findings, abnormal, in blood
    gas level R79.81
    minerals R79.0
    pancytopenia D61.818
    PTT R79.1
    specified NEC R79.89
    toxins — *see* Findings, abnormal, in blood
  chest sounds (friction) (rales) R09.89
  chromosome, chromosomal Q99.9
    with more than three X chromosomes, female Q97.1
    analysis result R89.8
      bronchial washings R84.8
      cerebrospinal fluid R83.8
      cervix uteri NEC R87.89
      nasal secretions R84.8
      nipple discharge R89.8
      peritoneal fluid R85.89
      pleural fluid R84.8
      prostatic secretions R86.8
      saliva R85.89
      seminal fluid R86.8
      sputum R84.8
      synovial fluid R89.8
      throat scrapings R84.8
      vagina R87.89
      vulva R87.89
      wound secretions R89.8
    dicentric replacement Q93.2
    ring replacement Q93.2
    sex Q99.8
      female phenotype Q97.9
        specified NEC Q97.8
      male phenotype Q98.9
        specified NEC Q98.8
      structural male Q98.6
    specified NEC Q99.8
  clinical findings NEC R68.89
  coagulation D68.9
    newborn, transient P61.6
    profile R79.1
    time R79.1
  communication — *see* Fistula
  conjunctiva, vascular H11.41- ☑
  coronary artery Q24.5
  cortisol-binding globulin E27.8
  course, eustachian tube Q17.8
  creatinine clearance R94.4
  cytology
    anus R85.619
      atypical squamous cells cannot exclude high grade squamous intraepithelial lesion (ASC-H) R85.611
      atypical squamous cells of undetermined significance (ASC-US) R85.610

Abnormal, abnormality, abnormalities — *continued*
  cytology — *continued*
    anus — *continued*
      cytologic evidence of malignancy R85.614
      high grade squamous intraepithelial lesion (HGSIL) R85.613
      human papillomavirus (HPV) DNA test
        high risk positive R85.81
        low risk positve R85.82
      inadequate smear R85.615
      low grade squamous intraepithelial lesion (LGSIL) R85.612
      satisfactory anal smear but lacking transformation zone R85.616
      specified NEC R85.618
      unsatisfactory smear R85.615
    female genital organs — *see* Abnormal, Papanicolaou (smear)
  dark adaptation curve H53.61
  dentofacial NEC — *see* Anomaly, dentofacial
  development, developmental Q89.9
    central nervous system Q07.9
  diagnostic imaging
    abdomen, abdominal region NEC R93.5
    biliary tract R93.2
    breast R92.8
    central nervous system NEC R90.89
    cerebrovascular NEC R90.89
    coronary circulation R93.1
    digestive tract NEC R93.3
    gastrointestinal (tract) R93.3
    genitourinary organs R93.8
    head R93.0
    heart R93.1
    intrathoracic organ NEC R93.8
    limbs R93.6
    liver R93.2
    lung (field) R91.8
    musculoskeletal system NEC R93.7
    retroperitoneum R93.5
    site specified NEC R93.8
    skin and subcutaneous tissue R93.8
    skull R93.0
    urinary organs R93.4
  direction, teeth, fully erupted M26.30
  ear ossicles, acquired NEC H74.39- ☑
    ankylosis — *see* Ankylosis, ear ossicles
    discontinuity — *see* Discontinuity, ossicles, ear
    partial loss — *see* Loss, ossicles, ear (partial)
  Ebstein Q22.5
  echocardiogram R93.1
  echoencephalogram R90.81
  echogram — *see* Abnormal, diagnostic imaging
  electro-oculogram [EOG] R94.110
  electrocardiogram [ECG] [EKG] R94.31
  electroencephalogram [EEG] R94.01
  electrolyte — *see* Imbalance, electrolyte
  electromyogram [EMG] R94.131
  electrophysiological intracardiac studies R94.39
  electroretinogram [ERG] R94.111
  erythrocytes
    congenital, with perinatal jaundice D58.9
  feces (color) (contents) (mucus) R19.5
  finding — *see* Findings, abnormal, without diagnosis
  fluid
    amniotic — *see* Abnormal, specimen, specified
    cerebrospinal — *see* Abnormal, cerebrospinal fluid
    peritoneal — *see* Abnormal, specimen, digestive organs
    pleural — *see* Abnormal, specimen, respiratory organs
    synovial — *see* Abnormal, specimen, specified
    thorax (bronchial washings) (pleural fluid) — *see* Abnormal, specimen, respiratory organs
    vaginal — *see* Abnormal, specimen, female genital organs
  form
    teeth K00.2
    uterus — *see* Anomaly, uterus
  function studies
    auditory R94.120
    bladder R94.8

Abnormal, abnormality, abnormalities — *continued*

function studies — *continued*
brain R94.09
cardiovascular R94.30
ear R94.128
endocrine NEC R94.7
eye NEC R94.118
kidney R94.4
liver R94.5
nervous system
central NEC R94.09
peripheral NEC R94.138
pancreas R94.8
placenta R94.8
pulmonary R94.2
special senses NEC R94.128
spleen R94.8
thyroid R94.6
vestibular R94.121
gait — *see* Gait
hysterical F44.4
gastrin secretion E16.4
globulin R77.1
cortisol-binding E27.8
thyroid-binding E07.89
glomerular, minor (*see also* N00-N07 with fourth character .0) N05.0
glucagon secretion E16.3
glucose tolerance (test) (non-fasting) R73.09
gravitational (G) forces or states (effect of) T75.81 ☑
hair (color) (shaft) L67.9
specified NEC L67.8
hard tissue formation in pulp (dental) K04.3
head movement R25.0
heart
rate R00.9
specified NEC R00.8
shadow R93.1
sounds NEC R01.2
hemoglobin (disease) (*see also* Disease, hemoglobin) D58.2
trait — *see* Trait, hemoglobin, abnormal
histology NEC R89.7
immunological findings R89.4
in serum R76.9
specified NEC R76.8
increase in appetite R63.2
involuntary movement — *see* Abnormal, movement, involuntary
jaw closure M26.51
karyotype R89.8
kidney function test R94.4
knee jerk R29.2
leukocyte (cell) (differential) NEC D72.9
liver
loss of
height R29.890
weight R63.4
mammogram NEC R92.8
calcification (calculus) R92.1
microcalcification R92.0
Mantoux test R76.11
movement (disorder) (*see also* Disorder, movement)
head R25.0
involuntary R25.9
fasciculation R25.3
of head R25.0
spasm R25.2
specified type NEC R25.8
tremor R25.1
myoglobin (Aberdeen) (Annapolis) R89.7
neonatal screening P09
oculomotor study R94.113
palmar creases Q82.8
Papanicolaou (smear)
anus R85.619
atypical squamous cells cannot exclude high grade squamous intraepithelial lesion (ASC-H) R85.611
atypical squamous cells of undetermined significance (ASC-US) R85.610
cytologic evidence of malignancy R85.614
high grade squamous intraepithelial lesion (HGSIL) R85.613
human papillomavirus (HPV) DNA test
high risk positive R85.81
low risk postive R85.82

Abnormal, abnormality, abnormalities — *continued*

Papanicolaou — *continued*
anus — *continued*
inadequate smear R85.615
low grade squamous intraepithelial lesion (LGSIL) R85.612
satisfactory anal smear but lacking transformation zone R85.616
specified NEC R85.618
unsatisfactory smear R85.615
bronchial washings R84.6
cerebrospinal fluid R83.6
cervix R87.619
atypical squamous cells cannot exclude high grade squamous intraepithelial lesion (ASC-H) R87.611
atypical squamous cells of undetermined significance (ASC-US) R87.610
cytologic evidence of malignancy R87.614
high grade squamous intraepithelial lesion (HGSIL) R87.613
inadequate smear R87.615
low grade squamous intraepithelial lesion (LGSIL) R87.612
non-atypical endometrial cells R87.618
satisfactory cervical smear but lacking transformation zone R87.616
specified NEC R87.618
thin preparaton R87.619
unsatisfactory smear R87.615
nasal secretions R84.6
nipple discharge R89.6
peritoneal fluid R85.69
pleural fluid R84.6
prostatic secretions R86.6
saliva R85.69
seminal fluid R86.6
sites NEC R89.6
sputum R84.6
synovial fluid R89.6
throat scrapings R84.6
vagina R87.629
atypical squamous cells cannot exclude high grade squamous intraepithelial lesion (ASC-H) R87.621
atypical squamous cells of undetermined significance (ASC-US) R87.620
cytologic evidence of malignancy R87.624
high grade squamous intraepithelial lesion (HGSIL) R87.623
inadequate smear R87.625
low grade squamous intraepithelial lesion (LGSIL) R87.622
specified NEC R87.628
thin preparation R87.629
unsatisfactory smear R87.625
vulva R87.69
wound secretions R89.6
partial thromboplastin time (PTT) R79.1
pelvis (bony) — *see* Deformity, pelvis
percussion, chest (tympany) R09.89
periods (grossly) — *see* Menstruation
phonocardiogram R94.39
plasma
protein R77.9
specified NEC R77.8
viscosity R70.1
pleural (folds) Q34.0
posture R29.3
product of conception O02.9
specified type NEC O02.89
prothrombin time (PT) R79.1
pulmonary
artery, congenital Q25.79
function, newborn P28.89
test results R94.2
pulsations in neck R00.2
pupillary H21.56- ☑
function (reaction) (reflex) — *see* Anomaly, pupil, function
radiological examination — *see* Abnormal, diagnostic imaging
red blood cell(s) (morphology) (volume) R71.8
reflex — *see* Reflex
renal function test R94.4
response to nerve stimulation R94.130

Abnormal, abnormality, abnormalities — *continued*

retinal correspondence H53.31
retinal function study R94.111
rhythm, heart (*see also* Arrhythmia)
saliva — *see* Abnormal, specimen, digestive organs
scan
kidney R94.4
liver R93.2
thyroid R94.6
secretion
gastrin E16.4
glucagon E16.3
semen, seminal fluid — *see* Abnormal, specimen, male genital organs
serum level (of)
acid phosphatase R74.8
alkaline phosphatase R74.8
amylase R74.8
enzymes R74.9
specified NEC R74.8
lipase R74.8
triacylglycerol lipase R74.8
shape
gravid uterus — *see* Anomaly, uterus
sinus venosus Q21.1
size, tooth, teeth K00.2
spacing, tooth, teeth, fully erupted M26.30
specimen
digestive organs (peritoneal fluid) (saliva) R85.9
cytology R85.69
drug level R85.2
enzyme level R85.0
histology R85.7
hormones R85.1
immunology R85.4
microbiology R85.5
nonmedicinal level R85.3
specified type NEC R85.89
female genital organs (secretions) (smears) R87.9
cytology R87.69
cervix R87.619
human papillomavirus (HPV) DNA test
high risk positive R87.810
low risk positive R87.820
inadequate (unsatisfactory) smear R87.615
non-atypical endometrial cells R87.618
specified NEC R87.618
vagina R87.629
human papillomavirus (HPV) DNA test
high risk positive R87.811
low risk positive R87.821
inadequate (unsatisfactory) smear R87.625
vulva R87.69
drug level R87.2
enzyme level R87.0
histological R87.7
hormones R87.1
immunology R87.4
microbiology R87.5
nonmedicinal level R87.3
specified type NEC R87.89
male genital organs (prostatic secretions) (semen) R86.9
cytology R86.6
drug level R86.2
enzyme level R86.0
histological R86.7
hormones R86.1
immunology R86.4
microbiology R86.5
nonmedicinal level R86.3
specified type NEC R86.8
nipple discharge — *see* Abnormal, specimen, specified
respiratory organs (bronchial washings) (nasal secretions) (pleural fluid) (sputum) R84.9
cytology R84.6
drug level R84.2
enzyme level R84.0
histology R84.7
hormones R84.1
immunology R84.4
microbiology R84.5
nonmedicinal level R84.3
specified type NEC R84.8

☑ **Additional Character Required — Refer to the Tabular List for Character Selection**   ⬇ **Subterms under main terms may continue to next column or page**

Abnormal, abnormality, abnormalities —
  continued
  specimen — *continued*
    specified organ, system and tissue NOS R89.9
      cytology R89.6
      drug level R89.2
      enzyme level R89.0
      histology R89.7
      hormones R89.1
      immunology R89.4
      microbiology R89.5
      nonmedicinal level R89.3
      specified type NEC R89.8
    synovial fluid — *see* Abnormal, specimen, specified
    thorax (bronchial washings) (pleural fluids) — *see*
      Abnormal, specimen, respiratory organs
    vagina (secretion) (smear) R87.629
    vulva (secretion) (smear) R87.69
    wound secretion — *see* Abnormal, specimen,
      specified
  spermatozoa — *see* Abnormal, specimen, male genital
    organs
  sputum (amount) (color) (odor) R09.3
  stool (color) (contents) (mucus) R19.5
    bloody K92.1
    guaiac positive R19.5
  synchondrosis Q78.8
  thermography (*see also* Abnormal, diagnostic imaging)
    R93.8
  thyroid-binding globulin E07.89
  tooth, teeth (form) (size) K00.2
  toxicology (findings) R78.9
  transport protein E88.09
  tumor marker NEC R97.8
  ultrasound results — *see* Abnormal, diagnostic imag-
    ing
  umbilical cord complicating delivery O69.9 ☑
  urination NEC R39.19
  urine (constituents) R82.90
    bile R82.2
    cytological examination R82.8
    drugs R82.5
    fat R82.0
    glucose R81
    heavy metals R82.6
    hemoglobin R82.3
    histological examination R82.8
    ketones R82.4
    microbiological examination (culture) R82.7
    myoglobin R82.1
    positive culture R82.7
    protein — *see* Proteinuria
    specified substance NEC R82.99
      chromoabnormality NEC R82.91
    substances nonmedical R82.6
  uterine hemorrhage — *see* Hemorrhage, uterus
  vectorcardiogram R94.39
  visually evoked potential (VEP) R94.112
  white blood cells D72.9
    specified NEC D72.89
  X-ray examination — *see* Abnormal, diagnostic
    imaging

Abnormity (any organ or part) — *see* Anomaly
Abocclusion M26.29
  hemolytic disease (newborn) P55.1
  incompatibility reaction ABO — *see* Complication(s),
    transfusion, incompatibility reaction, ABO
Abolition, language R48.8
Aborter, habitual or recurrent — *see* Loss (of), pregnancy, recurrent
Abortion (complete) (spontaneous) O03.9
  with
    retained products of conception — *see* Abortion,
      incomplete
  attempted (elective) (failed) O07.4
    complicated by O07.30
      afibrinogenemia O07.1
      cardiac arrest O07.36
      chemical damage of pelvic organ(s) O07.34
      circulatory collapse O07.31
      cystitis O07.38
      defibrination syndrome O07.1
      electrolyte imbalance O07.33
      embolism (air) (amniotic fluid) (blood clot) (fat)
        (pulmonary) (septic) (soap) O07.2
      endometritis O07.0
      genital tract and pelvic infection O07.0
      hemolysis O07.1

Abortion — *continued*
  attempted — *continued*
    complicated by — *continued*
      hemorrhage (delayed) (excessive) O07.1
      infection
        genital tract or pelvic O07.0
        urinary tract tract O07.38
      intravascular coagulation O07.1
      laceration of pelvic organ(s) O07.34
      metabolic disorder O07.33
      oliguria O07.32
      oophoritis O07.0
      parametritis O07.0
      pelvic peritonitis O07.0
      perforation of pelvic organ(s) O07.34
      renal failure or shutdown O07.32
      salpingitis or salpingo-oophoritis O07.0
      sepsis O07.37
      shock O07.31
      specified condition NEC O07.39
      tubular necrosis (renal) O07.32
      uremia O07.32
      urinary tract infection O07.38
      venous complication NEC O07.35
        embolism (air) (amniotic fluid) (blood clot)
          (fat) (pulmonary) (septic) (soap) O07.2
  complicated (by) (following) O03.80
    afibrinogenemia O03.6
    cardiac arrest O03.86
    chemical damage of pelvic organ(s) O03.84
    circulatory collapse O03.81
    cystitis O03.88
    defibrination syndrome O03.6
    electrolyte imbalance O03.83
    embolism (air) (amniotic fluid) (blood clot) (fat)
      (pulmonary) (septic) (soap) O03.7
    endometritis O03.5
    genital tract and pelvic infection O03.5
    hemolysis O03.6
    hemorrhage (delayed) (excessive) O03.6
    infection
      genital tract or pelvic O03.5
      urinary tract O03.88
    intravascular coagulation O03.6
    laceration of pelvic organ(s) O03.84
    metabolic disorder O03.83
    oliguria O03.82
    oophoritis O03.5
    parametritis O03.5
    pelvic peritonitis O03.5
    perforation of pelvic organ(s) O03.84
    renal failure or shutdown O03.82
    salpingitis or salpingo-oophoritis O03.5
    sepsis O03.87
    shock O03.81
    specified condition NEC O03.89
    tubular necrosis (renal) O03.82
    uremia O03.82
    urinary tract infection O03.88
    venous complication NEC O03.85
      embolism (air) (amniotic fluid) (blood clot) (fat)
        (pulmonary) (septic) (soap) O03.7
  failed — *see* Abortion, attempted
  habitual or recurrent N96
    with current abortion — *see* categories O03-O06
    without current pregnancy N96
    care in current pregnancy O26.2- ☑
  incomplete (spontaneous) O03.4
    complicated (by) (following) O03.30
      afibrinogenemia O03.1
      cardiac arrest O03.36
      chemical damage of pelvic organ(s) O03.34
      circulatory collapse O03.31
      cystitis O03.38
      defibrination syndrome O03.1
      electrolyte imbalance O03.33
      embolism (air) (amniotic fluid) (blood clot) (fat)
        (pulmonary) (septic) (soap) O03.2
      endometritis O03.0
      genital tract and pelvic infection O03.0
      hemolysis O03.1
      hemorrhage (delayed) (excessive) O03.1
      infection
        genital tract or pelvic O03.0
        urinary tract O03.38
      intravascular coagulation O03.1
      laceration of pelvic organ(s) O03.34
      metabolic disorder O03.33

Abortion — *continued*
  incomplete — *continued*
    complicated — *continued*
      oliguria O03.32
      oophoritis O03.0
      parametritis O03.0
      pelvic peritonitis O03.0
      perforation of pelvic organ(s) O03.34
      renal failure or shutdown O03.32
      salpingitis or salpingo-oophoritis O03.0
      sepsis O03.37
      shock O03.31
      specified condition NEC O03.39
      tubular necrosis (renal) O03.32
      uremia O03.32
      urinary infection O03.38
      venous complication NEC O03.35
        embolism (air) (amniotic fluid) (blood clot)
          (fat) (pulmonary) (septic) (soap) O03.2
  induced (encounter for) Z33.2
    complicated by O04.80
      afibrinogenemia O04.6
      cardiac arrest O04.86
      chemical damage of pelvic organ(s) O04.84
      circulatory collapse O04.81
      cystitis O04.88
      defibrination syndrome O04.6
      electrolyte imbalance O04.83
      embolism (air) (amniotic fluid) (blood clot) (fat)
        (pulmonary) (septic) (soap) O04.7
      endometritis O04.5
      genital tract and pelvic infection O04.5
      hemolysis O04.6
      hemorrhage (delayed) (excessive) O04.6
      infection
        genital tract or pelvic O04.5
        urinary tract O04.88
      intravascular coagulation O04.6
      laceration of pelvic organ(s) O04.84
      metabolic disorder O04.83
      oliguria O04.82
      oophoritis O04.5
      parametritis O04.5
      pelvic peritonitis O04.5
      perforation of pelvic organ(s) O04.84
      renal failure or shutdown O04.82
      salpingitis or salpingo-oophoritis O04.5
      sepsis O04.87
      shock O04.81
      specified condition NEC O04.89
      tubular necrosis (renal) O04.82
      uremia O04.82
      urinary tract infection O04.88
      venous complication NEC O04.85
        embolism (air) (amniotic fluid) (blood clot)
          (fat) (pulmonary) (septic) (soap) O04.7
  missed O02.1
  spontaneous — *see* Abortion (complete) (sponta-
    neous)
    threatened O20.0
  threatened (spontaneous) O20.0
  tubal O00.1
Abortus fever A23.1
Aboulomania F60.7
Abrami's disease D59.8
Abramov-Fiedler myocarditis (acute isolated myocarditis) I40.1
Abrasion T14.8
  abdomen, abdominal (wall) S30.811 ☑
  alveolar process S00.512 ☑
  ankle S90.51- ☑
  antecubital space — *see* Abrasion, elbow
  anus S30.817 ☑
  arm (upper) S40.81- ☑
  auditory canal — *see* Abrasion, ear
  auricle — *see* Abrasion, ear
  axilla — *see* Abrasion, arm
  back, lower S30.810 ☑
  breast S20.11- ☑
  brow S00.81 ☑
  buttock S30.810 ☑
  calf — *see* Abrasion, leg
  canthus — *see* Abrasion, eyelid
  cheek S00.81 ☑
    internal S00.512 ☑
  chest wall — *see* Abrasion, thorax
  chin S00.81 ☑
  clitoris S30.814 ☑

Abrasion — *continued*
- cornea S05.0- ☑
- costal region — *see* Abrasion, thorax
- dental K03.1
- digit(s)
  - foot — *see* Abrasion, toe
  - hand — *see* Abrasion, finger
- ear S00.41- ☑
- elbow S50.31- ☑
- epididymis S30.813 ☑
- epigastric region S30.811 ☑
- epiglottis S10.11 ☑
- esophagus (thoracic) S27.818 ☑
  - cervical S10.11 ☑
- eyebrow — *see* Abrasion, eyelid
- eyelid S00.21- ☑
- face S00.81 ☑
- finger(s) S60.41- ☑
  - index S60.41- ☑
  - little S60.41- ☑
  - middle S60.41- ☑
  - ring S60.41- ☑
- flank S30.811 ☑
- foot (except toe(s) alone) S90.81- ☑
  - toe — *see* Abrasion, toe
- forearm S50.81- ☑
  - elbow only — *see* Abrasion, elbow
- forehead S00.81 ☑
- genital organs, external
  - female S30.816 ☑
  - male S30.815 ☑
- groin S30.811 ☑
- gum S00.512 ☑
- hand S60.51- ☑
- head S00.91 ☑
  - ear — *see* Abrasion, ear
  - eyelid — *see* Abrasion, eyelid
  - lip S00.511 ☑
  - nose S00.31 ☑
  - oral cavity S00.512 ☑
  - scalp S00.01 ☑
  - specified site NEC S00.81 ☑
- heel — *see* Abrasion, foot
- hip S70.21- ☑
- inguinal region S30.811 ☑
- interscapular region S20.419 ☑
- jaw S00.81 ☑
- knee S80.21- ☑
- labium (majus) (minus) S30.814 ☑
- larynx S10.11 ☑
- leg (lower) S80.81- ☑
  - knee — *see* Abrasion, knee
  - upper — *see* Abrasion, thigh
- lip S00.511 ☑
- lower back S30.810 ☑
- lumbar region S30.810 ☑
- malar region S00.81 ☑
- mammary — *see* Abrasion, breast
- mastoid region S00.81 ☑
- mouth S00.512 ☑
- nail
  - finger — *see* Abrasion, finger
  - toe — *see* Abrasion, toe
- nape S10.81 ☑
- nasal S00.31 ☑
- neck S10.91 ☑
  - specified site NEC S10.81 ☑
  - throat S10.11 ☑
- nose S00.31 ☑
- occipital region S00.01 ☑
- oral cavity S00.512 ☑
- orbital region — *see* Abrasion, eyelid
- palate S00.512 ☑
- palm — *see* Abrasion, hand
- parietal region S00.01 ☑
- pelvis S30.810 ☑
- penis S30.812 ☑
- perineum
  - female S30.814 ☑
  - male S30.810 ☑
- periocular area — *see* Abrasion, eyelid
- phalanges
  - finger — *see* Abrasion, finger
  - toe — *see* Abrasion, toe
- pharynx S10.11 ☑
- pinna — *see* Abrasion, ear

Abrasion — *continued*
- popliteal space — *see* Abrasion, knee
- prepuce S30.812 ☑
- pubic region S30.810 ☑
- pudendum
  - female S30.816 ☑
  - male S30.815 ☑
- sacral region S30.810 ☑
- scalp S00.01 ☑
- scapular region — *see* Abrasion, shoulder
- scrotum S30.813 ☑
- shin — *see* Abrasion, leg
- shoulder S40.21- ☑
- skin NEC T14.8
- sternal region S20.319 ☑
- submaxillary region S00.81 ☑
- submental region S00.81 ☑
- subungual
  - finger(s) — *see* Abrasion, finger
  - toe(s) — *see* Abrasion, toe
- supraclavicular fossa S10.81 ☑
- supraorbital S00.81 ☑
- temple S00.81 ☑
- temporal region S00.81 ☑
- testis S30.813 ☑
- thigh S70.31- ☑
- thorax, thoracic (wall) S20.91 ☑
  - back S20.41- ☑
  - front S20.31- ☑
- throat S10.11 ☑
- thumb S60.31- ☑
- toe(s) (lesser) S90.416 ☑
  - great S90.41- ☑
- tongue S00.512 ☑
- tooth, teeth (dentifrice) (habitual) (hard tissues) (occupational) (ritual) (traditional) K03.1
- trachea S10.11 ☑
- tunica vaginalis S30.813 ☑
- tympanum, tympanic membrane — *see* Abrasion, ear
- uvula S00.512 ☑
- vagina S30.814 ☑
- vocal cords S10.11 ☑
- vulva S30.814 ☑
- wrist S60.81- ☑

Abrism — *see* Poisoning, food, noxious, plant

Abruptio placentae O45.9- ☑
- with
  - afibrinogenemia O45.01- ☑
  - coagulation defect O45.00- ☑
    - specified NEC O45.09- ☑
  - disseminated intravascular coagulation O45.02- ☑
  - hypofibrinogenemia O45.01- ☑
- specified NEC O45.8- ☑

Abruption, placenta — *see* Abruptio placentae

Abscess (connective tissue) (embolic) (fistulous) (infective) (metastatic) (multiple) (pernicious) (pyogenic) (septic) L02.91
- with
  - diverticular disease (intestine) K57.80
    - with bleeding K57.81
    - large intestine K57.20
      - with
        - bleeding K57.21
        - small intestine K57.40
          - with bleeding K57.41
    - small intestine K57.00
      - with
        - bleeding K57.01
        - large intestine K57.40
          - with bleeding K57.41
  - lymphangitis — *code by* site under Abscess
- abdomen, abdominal
  - cavity K65.1
  - wall L02.211
- abdominopelvic K65.1
- accessory sinus — *see* Sinusitis
- adrenal (capsule) (gland) E27.8
- alveolar K04.7
  - with sinus K04.6
- ambic A06.4
  - brain (and liver or lung abscess) A06.6
  - genitourinary tract A06.82
  - liver (without mention of brain or lung abscess) A06.4
  - lung (and liver) (without mention of brain abscess) A06.5
  - specified site NEC A06.89

Abscess — *continued*
- amebic — *continued*
  - spleen A06.89
- anerobic A48.0
- ankle — *see* Abscess, lower limb
- anorectal K61.2
- antecubital space — *see* Abscess, upper limb
- antrum (chronic) (Highmore) — *see* Sinusitis, maxillary
- anus K61.0
- apical (tooth) K04.7
  - with sinus (alveolar) K04.6
- appendix K35.3
- areola (acute) (chronic) (nonpuerperal) N61
  - puerperal, postpartum or gestational — *see* Infection, nipple
- arm (any part) — *see* Abscess, upper limb
- artery (wall) I77.89
- atheromatous I77.2
- auricle, ear — *see* Abscess, ear, external
- axilla (region) L02.41- ☑
  - lymph gland or node L04.2
- back (any part, except buttock) L02.212
- Bartholin's gland N75.1
  - with
    - abortion — *see* Abortion, by type complicated by, sepsis
    - ectopic or molar pregnancy O08.0
    - following ectopic or molar pregnancy O08.0
- Bezold's — *see* Mastoiditis, acute
- bilharziasis B65.1
- bladder (wall) — *see* Cystitis, specified type NEC
- bone (subperiosteal) (*see also* Osteomyelitis, specified type NEC)
  - accessory sinus (chronic) — *see* Sinusitis
  - chronic or old — *see* Osteomyelitis, chronic
  - jaw (lower) (upper) M27.2
  - mastoid — *see* Mastoiditis, acute, subperiosteal
  - petrous — *see* Petrositis
  - spinal (tuberculous) A18.01
    - nontuberculous — *see* Osteomyelitis, vertebra
- bowel K63.0
- brain (any part) (cystic) (otogenic) G06.0
  - amebic (with abscess of any other site) A06.6
  - gonococcal A54.82
  - pheomycotic (chromomycotic) B43.1
  - tuberculous A17.81
- breast (acute) (chronic) (nonpuerperal) N61
  - newborn P39.0
  - puerperal, postpartum, gestational — *see* Mastitis, obstetric, purulent
- broad ligament N73.2
  - acute N73.0
  - chronic N73.1
- Brodie's (localized) (chronic) M86.8X- ☑
- bronchi J98.09
- buccal cavity K12.2
- bulbourethral gland N34.0
- bursa M71.00
  - ankle M71.07- ☑
  - elbow M71.02- ☑
  - foot M71.07- ☑
  - hand M71.04- ☑
  - hip M71.05- ☑
  - knee M71.06- ☑
  - multiple sites M71.09
  - pharyngeal J39.1
  - shoulder M71.01- ☑
  - specified site NEC M71.08
  - wrist M71.03- ☑
- buttock L02.31
- canthus — *see* Blepharoconjunctivitis
- cartilage — *see* Disorder, cartilage, specified type NEC
- cecum K35.3
- cerebellum, cerebellar G06.0
  - sequelae G09
- cerebral (embolic) G06.0
  - sequelae G09
- cervical (meaning neck) L02.11
  - lymph gland or node L04.0
- cervix (stump) (uteri) — *see* Cervicitis
- cheek (external) L02.01
  - inner K12.2
- chest J86.9
  - with fistula J86.0
  - wall L02.213
- chin L02.01
- choroid — *see* Inflammation, chorioretinal

Abscess — *continued*
  circumtonsillar J36
  cold (lung) (tuberculous) (*see also* Tuberculosis, abscess, lung)
    articular — *see* Tuberculosis, joint
  colon (wall) K63.0
  colostomy K94.02
  conjunctiva — *see* Conjunctivitis, acute
  cornea H16.31- ☑
  corpus
    cavernosum N48.21
    luteum — *see* Oophoritis
  Cowper's gland N34.0
  cranium G06.0
  cul-de-sac (Douglas') (posterior) — *see* Peritonitis, pelvic, female
  cutaneous — *see* Abscess, by site
  dental K04.7
    with sinus (alveolar) K04.6
  dentoalveolar K04.7
    with sinus K04.6
  diaphragm, diaphragmatic K65.1
  Douglas' cul-de-sac or pouch — *see* Peritonitis, pelvic, female
  Dubois A50.59
  ear (middle) (*see also* Otitis, media, suppurative)
    acute — *see* Otitis, media, suppurative, acute
    external H60.0- ☑
  entamebic — *see* Abscess, amebic
  enterostomy K94.12
  epididymis N45.4
  epidural G06.2
    brain G06.0
    spinal cord G06.1
  epiglottis J38.7
  epiploon, epiploic K65.1
  erysipelatous — *see* Erysipelas
  esophagus K20.8
  ethmoid (bone) (chronic) (sinus) J32.2
  external auditory canal — *see* Abscess, ear, external
  extradural G06.2
    brain G06.0
      sequelae G09
    spinal cord G06.1
  extraperitoneal K68.19
  eye — *see* Endophthalmitis, purulent
  eyelid H00.03- ☑
  face (any part, except ear, eye and nose) L02.01
  fallopian tube — *see* Salpingitis
  fascia M72.8
  fauces J39.1
  fecal K63.0
  femoral (region) — *see* Abscess, lower limb
  filaria, filarial — *see* Infestation, filarial
  finger (any) (*see also* Abscess, hand)
    nail — *see* Cellulitis, finger
  foot L02.61- ☑
  forehead L02.01
  frontal sinus (chronic) J32.1
  gallbladder K81.0
  genital organ or tract
    female (external) N76.4
    male N49.9
      multiple sites N49.8
      specified NEC N49.8
  gestational mammary O91.11- ☑
  gestational subareolar O91.11- ☑
  gingival K05.21
  gland, glandular (lymph) (acute) — *see* Lymphadenitis, acute
  gluteal (region) L02.31
  gonorrheal — *see* Gonococcus
  groin L02.214
  gum K05.21
  hand L02.51- ☑
  head NEC L02.811
    face (any part, except ear, eye and nose) L02.01
  heart — *see* Carditis
  heel — *see* Abscess, foot
  helminthic — *see* Infestation, helminth
  hepatic (cholangitic) (hematogenic) (lymphogenic) (pylephlebitic) K75.0
    amebic A06.4
  hip (region) — *see* Abscess, lower limb
  ileocecal K35.3
  ileostomy (bud) K94.12
  iliac (region) L02.214

Abscess — *continued*
  iliac — *continued*
    fossa K35.3
  infraclavicular (fossa) — *see* Abscess, upper limb
  inguinal (region) L02.214
    lymph gland or node L04.1
  intestine, intestinal NEC K63.0
    rectal K61.1
  intra-abdominal (*see also* Abscess, peritoneum) K65.1
    postoperative T81.4 ☑
      retroperitoneal K68.11
  intracranial G06.0
  intramammary — *see* Abscess, breast
  intraorbital — *see* Abscess, orbit
  intraperitoneal K65.1
  intrasphincteric (anus) K61.4
  intraspinal G06.1
  intratonsillar J36
  ischiorectal (fossa) K61.3
  jaw (bone) (lower) (upper) M27.2
  joint — *see* Arthritis, pyogenic or pyemic
    spine (tuberculous) A18.01
      nontuberculous — *see* Spondylopathy, infective
  kidney N15.1
    with calculus N20.0
      with hydronephrosis N13.6
    puerperal (postpartum) O86.21
  knee (*see also* Abscess, lower limb)
    joint M00.9
  labium (majus) (minus) N76.4
  lacrimal
    caruncle — *see* Inflammation, lacrimal, passages, acute
    gland — *see* Dacryoadenitis
    passages (duct) (sac) — *see* Inflammation, lacrimal, passages, acute
  lacunar N34.0
  larynx J38.7
  lateral (alveolar) K04.7
    with sinus K04.6
  leg (any part) — *see* Abscess, lower limb
  lens H27.8
  lingual K14.0
    tonsil J36
  lip K13.0
  Littre's gland N34.0
  liver (cholangitic) (hematogenic) (lymphogenic) (pylephlebitic) (pyogenic) K75.0
    amebic (due to Entamoeba histolytica) (dysenteric) (tropical) A06.4
      with
        brain abscess (and liver or lung abscess) A06.6
        lung abscess A06.5
  loin (region) L02.211
  lower limb L02.41- ☑
  lumbar (tuberculous) A18.01
    nontuberculous L02.212
  lung (miliary) (putrid) J85.2
    with pneumonia J85.1
      due to specified organism (see Pneumonia, in (due to))
    amebic (with liver abscess) A06.5
      with
        brain abscess A06.6
        pneumonia A06.5
  lymph, lymphatic, gland or node (acute) (*see also* Lymphadenitis, acute)
    mesentery I88.0
  malar M27.2
  mammary gland — *see* Abscess, breast
  marginal, anus K61.0
  mastoid — *see* Mastoiditis, acute
  maxilla, maxillary M27.2
    molar (tooth) K04.7
      with sinus K04.6
    premolar K04.7
    sinus (chronic) J32.0
  mediastinum J85.3
  meibomian gland — *see* Hordeolum
  meninges G06.2
  mesentery, mesenteric K65.1
  mesosalpinx — *see* Salpingitis
  mons pubis L02.215
  mouth (floor) K12.2
  muscle — *see* Myositis, infective
  myocardium I40.0

Abscess — *continued*
  nabothian (follicle) — *see* Cervicitis
  nasal J32.9
  nasopharyngeal J39.1
  navel L02.216
    newborn P38.9
      with mild hemorrhage P38.1
      without hemorrhage P38.9
  neck (region) L02.11
    lymph gland or node L04.0
  nephritic — *see* Abscess, kidney
  nipple N61
    associated with
      lactation — *see* Pregnancy, complicated by, pregnancy — *see* Pregnancy, complicated by
  nose (external) (fossa) (septum) J34.0
    sinus (chronic) — *see* Sinusitis
  omentum K65.1
  operative wound T81.4 ☑
  orbit, orbital — *see* Cellulitis, orbit
  otogenic G06.0
  ovary, ovarian (corpus luteum) — *see* Oophoritis
  oviduct — *see* Oophoritis
  palate (soft) K12.2
    hard M27.2
  palmar (space) — *see* Abscess, hand
  pancreas (duct) — *see* Pancreatitis, acute
  parafrenal N48.21
  parametric, parametrium N73.2
    acute N73.0
    chronic N73.1
  paranephric N15.1
  parapancreatic — *see* Pancreatitis, acute
  parapharyngeal J39.0
  pararectal K61.1
  parasinus — *see* Sinusitis
  parauterine (*see also* Disease, pelvis, inflammatory) N73.2
  paravaginal — *see* Vaginitis
  parietal region (scalp) L02.811
  parodontal K05.21
  parotid (duct) (gland) K11.3
    region K12.2
  pectoral (region) L02.213
  pelvis, pelvic
    female — *see* Disease, pelvis, inflammatory
    male, peritoneal K65.1
  penis N48.21
    gonococcal (accessory gland) (periurethral) A54.1
  perianal K61.0
  periapical K04.7
    with sinus (alveolar) K04.6
  periappendicular K35.3
  pericardial I30.1
  pericecal K35.3
  pericemental K05.21
  pericholecystic — *see* Cholecystitis, acute
  pericoronal K05.21
  peridental K05.21
  perimetric (*see also* Disease, pelvis, inflammatory) N73.2
  perinephric, perinephritic — *see* Abscess, kidney
  perineum, perineal (superficial) L02.215
    urethra N34.0
  periodontal (parietal) K05.21
    apical K04.7
  periosteum, periosteal (*see also* Osteomyelitis, specified type NEC)
    with osteomyelitis (*see also* Osteomyelitis, specified type NEC)
      acute — *see* Osteomyelitis, acute
      chronic — *see* Osteomyelitis, chronic
  peripharyngeal J39.0
  peripleuritic J86.9
    with fistula J86.0
  periprostatic N41.2
  perirectal K61.1
  perirenal (tissue) — *see* Abscess, kidney
  perisinuous (nose) — *see* Sinusitis
  peritoneum, peritoneal (perforated) (ruptured) K65.1
    with appendicitis K35.3
    pelvic
      female — *see* Peritonitis, pelvic, female
      male K65.1
    postoperative T81.4 ☑
    puerperal, postpartum, childbirth O85
    tuberculous A18.31
  peritonsillar J36

Abscess — *continued*
- perityphlic K35.3
- periureteral N28.89
- periurethral N34.0
  - gonococcal (accessory gland) (periurethral) A54.1
- periuterine (*see also* Disease, pelvis, inflammatory) N73.2
- perivesical — *see* Cystitis, specified type NEC
- petrous bone — *see* Petrositis
- phagedenic NOS L02.91
  - chancroid A57
- pharynx, pharyngeal (lateral) J39.1
- pilonidal L05.01
- pituitary (gland) E23.6
- pleura J86.9
  - with fistula J86.0
- popliteal — *see* Abscess, lower limb
- post-typhoid A01.09
- postcecal K35.3
- postlaryngeal J38.7
- postnasal J34.0
- postoperative (any site) T81.4 ☑
  - retroperitoneal K68.11
- postpharyngeal J39.0
- posttonsillar J36
- pouch of Douglas — *see* Peritonitis, pelvic, female
- premammary — *see* Abscess, breast
- prepatellar — *see* Abscess, lower limb
- prostate N41.2
  - gonococcal (acute) (chronic) A54.22
- psoas muscle K68.12
- puerperal — *code by* site under Puerperal, abscess
- pulmonary — *see* Abscess, lung
- pulp, pulpal (dental) K04.0
- rectovaginal septum K63.0
- rectovesical — *see* Cystitis, specified type NEC
- rectum K61.1
- renal — *see* Abscess, kidney
- retina — *see* Inflammation, chorioretinal
- retrobulbar — *see* Abscess, orbit
- retrocecal K65.1
- retrolaryngeal J38.7
- retromammary — *see* Abscess, breast
- retroperitoneal NEC K68.19
  - postprocedural K68.11
- retropharyngeal J39.0
- retrouterine — *see* Peritonitis, pelvic, female
- retrovesical — *see* Cystitis, specified type NEC
- root, tooth K04.7
  - with sinus (alveolar) K04.6
- round ligament (*see also* Disease, pelvis, inflammatory) N73.2
- rupture (spontaneous) NOS L02.91
- sacrum (tuberculous) A18.01
  - nontuberculous M46.28
- salivary (duct) (gland) K11.3
- scalp (any part) L02.811
- scapular — *see* Osteomyelitis, specified type NEC
- sclera — *see* Scleritis
- scrofulous (tuberculous) A18.2
- scrotum N49.2
- seminal vesicle N49.0
- septal, dental K04.7
  - with sinus (alveolar) K04.6
- serous — *see* Periostitis
- shoulder (region) — *see* Abscess, upper limb
- sigmoid K63.0
- sinus (accessory) (chronic) (nasal) (*see also* Sinusitis)
  - intracranial venous (any) G06.0
- Skene's duct or gland N34.0
- skin — *see* Abscess, by site
- specified site NEC L02.818
- spermatic cord N49.1
- sphenoidal (sinus) (chronic) J32.3
- spinal cord (any part) (staphylococcal) G06.1
  - tuberculous A17.81
- spine (column) (tuberculous) A18.01
  - epidural G06.1
  - nontuberculous — *see* Osteomyelitis, vertebra
- spleen D73.3
  - amebic A06.89
- stitch T81.4 ☑
- subarachnoid G06.2
  - brain G06.0
  - spinal cord G06.1
- subareolar — *see* Abscess, breast
- subcecal K35.3
- subcutaneous (*see also* Abscess, by site)

Abscess — *continued*
- subcutaneous (*see also* Abscess, by site) — *continued*
  - pheomycotic (chromomycotic) B43.2
- subdiaphragmatic K65.1
- subdural G06.2
  - brain G06.0
    - sequelae G09
  - spinal cord G06.1
- subgaleal L02.811
- subhepatic K65.1
- sublingual K12.2
  - gland K11.3
- submammary — *see* Abscess, breast
- submandibular (region) (space) (triangle) K12.2
  - gland K11.3
- submaxillary (region) L02.01
  - gland K11.3
- submental L02.01
  - gland K11.3
- subperiosteal — *see* Osteomyelitis, specified type NEC
- subphrenic K65.1
  - postoperative T81.4 ☑
- suburethral N34.0
- sudoriparous L75.8
- supraclavicular (fossa) — *see* Abscess, upper limb
- suprapelvic, acute N73.0
- suprarenal (capsule) (gland) E27.8
- sweat gland L74.8
- tear duct — *see* Inflammation, lacrimal, passages, acute
- temple L02.01
- temporal region L02.01
- temporosphenoidal G06.0
- tendon (sheath) M65.00
  - ankle M65.07- ☑
  - foot M65.07- ☑
  - forearm M65.03- ☑
  - hand M65.04- ☑
  - lower leg M65.06- ☑
  - pelvic region M65.05- ☑
  - shoulder region M65.01- ☑
  - specified site NEC M65.08
  - thigh M65.05- ☑
  - upper arm M65.02- ☑
- testis N45.4
- thigh — *see* Abscess, lower limb
- thorax J86.9
  - with fistula J86.0
- throat J39.1
- thumb (*see also* Abscess, hand)
  - nail — *see* Cellulitis, finger
- thymus (gland) E32.1
- thyroid (gland) E06.0
- toe (any) (*see also* Abscess, foot)
  - nail — *see* Cellulitis, toe
- tongue (staphylococcal) K14.0
- tonsil(s) (lingual) J36
- tonsillopharyngeal J36
- tooth, teeth (root) K04.7
  - with sinus (alveolar) K04.6
  - supporting structures NEC K05.21
- trachea J39.8
- trunk L02.219
  - abdominal wall L02.211
  - back L02.212
  - chest wall L02.213
  - groin L02.214
  - perineum L02.215
  - umbilicus L02.216
- tubal — *see* Salpingitis
- tuberculous — *see* Tuberculosis, abscess
- tubo-ovarian — *see* Salpingo-oophoritis
- tunica vaginalis N49.1
- umbilicus L02.216
- upper
  - limb L02.41- ☑
  - respiratory J39.8
- urethral (gland) N34.0
- urinary N34.0
- uterus, uterine (wall) (*see also* Endometritis)
  - ligament (*see also* Disease, pelvis, inflammatory) N73.2
  - neck — *see* Cervicitis
- uvula K12.2
- vagina (wall) — *see* Vaginitis
- vaginorectal — *see* Vaginitis

Abscess — *continued*
- vas deferens N49.1
- vermiform appendix K35.3
- vertebra (column) (tuberculous) A18.01
  - nontuberculous — *see* Osteomyelitis, vertebra
- vesical — *see* Cystitis, specified type NEC
- vesico-uterine pouch — *see* Peritonitis, pelvic, female
- vitreous (humor) — *see* Endophthalmitis, purulent
- vocal cord J38.3
- von Bezold's — *see* Mastoiditis, acute
- vulva N76.4
- vulvovaginal gland N75.1
- web space — *see* Abscess, hand
- wound T81.4 ☑
- wrist — *see* Abscess, upper limb

Absence (of) (organ or part) (complete or partial)
- adrenal (gland) (congenital) Q89.1
  - acquired E89.6
- albumin in blood E88.09
- alimentary tract (congenital) Q45.8
  - upper Q40.8
- alveolar process (acquired) — *see* Anomaly, alveolar
- ankle (acquired) Z89.44- ☑
- anus (congenital) Q42.3
  - with fistula Q42.2
- aorta (congenital) Q25.4
- appendix, congenital Q42.8
- arm (acquired) Z89.20- ☑
  - above elbow Z89.22- ☑
    - congenital (with hand present) — *see* Agenesis, arm, with hand present
      - and hand — *see* Agenesis, forearm, and hand
  - below elbow Z89.21- ☑
    - congenital (with hand present) — *see* Agenesis, arm, with hand present
      - and hand — *see* Agenesis, forearm, and hand
  - congenital — *see* Defect, reduction, upper limb
  - shoulder (following explantation of shoulder joint prosthesis) (joint) (with or without presence of antibiotic-impregnated cement spacer) Z89.23- ☑
    - congenital (with hand present) — *see* Agenesis, arm, with hand present
- artery (congenital) (peripheral) Q27.8
  - brain Q28.3
  - coronary Q24.5
  - pulmonary Q25.79
  - specified NEC Q27.8
  - umbilical Q27.0
- atrial septum (congenital) Q21.1
- auditory canal (congenital) (external) Q16.1
- auricle (ear), congenital Q16.0
- bile, biliary duct, congenital Q44.5
- bladder (acquired) Z90.6
  - congenital Q64.5
- bowel sounds R19.11
- brain Q00.0
  - part of Q04.3
- breast(s) (and nipple(s)) (acquired) Z90.1- ☑
  - congenital Q83.8
- broad ligament Q50.6
- bronchus (congenital) Q32.4
- canaliculus lacrimalis, congenital Q10.4
- cerebellum (vermis) Q04.3
- cervix (acquired) (with uterus) Z90.710
  - with remaining uterus Z90.712
  - congenital Q51.5
- chin, congenital Q18.8
- cilia (congenital) Q10.3
  - acquired — *see* Madarosis
- clitoris (congenital) Q52.6
- coccyx, congenital Q76.49
- cold sense R20.8
- congenital
  - lumen — *see* Atresia
  - organ or site NEC — *see* Agenesis
  - septum — *see* Imperfect, closure
- corpus callosum Q04.0
- cricoid cartilage, congenital Q31.8
- diaphragm (with hernia), congenital Q79.1
- digestive organ(s) or tract, congenital Q45.8
  - acquired NEC Z90.49
  - upper Q40.8
- ductus arteriosus Q28.8
- duodenum (acquired) Z90.49
  - congenital Q41.0

Absence — *continued*
- ear, congenital Q16.9
  - acquired H93.8- ☑
  - auricle Q16.0
  - external Q16.0
  - inner Q16.5
  - lobe, lobule Q17.8
  - middle, except ossicles Q16.4
    - ossicles Q16.3
  - ossicles Q16.3
- ejaculatory duct (congenital) Q55.4
- endocrine gland (congenital) NEC Q89.2
  - acquired E89.89
- epididymis (congenital) Q55.4
  - acquired Z90.79
- epiglottis, congenital Q31.8
- esophagus (congenital) Q39.8
  - acquired (partial) Z90.49
- eustachian tube (congenital) Q16.2
- extremity (acquired) Z89.9
  - congenital Q73.0
  - knee (following explanation of knee joint prosthesis) (joint) (with or without presence of antibiotic-impregnated cement spacer) Z89.52- ☑
  - lower (above knee) Z89.619
    - below knee Z89.51- ☑
  - upper — *see* Absence, arm
- eye (acquired) Z90.01
  - congenital Q11.1
  - muscle (congenital) Q10.3
- eyeball (acquired) Z90.01
- eyelid (fold) (congenital) Q10.3
  - acquired Z90.01
- face, specified part NEC Q18.8
- fallopian tube(s) (acquired) Z90.79
  - congenital Q50.6
- family member (causing problem in home) NEC (*see also* Disruption, family) Z63.32
- femur, congenital — *see* Defect, reduction, lower limb, longitudinal, femur
- fibrinogen (congenital) D68.2
  - acquired D65
- finger(s) (acquired) Z89.02- ☑
  - congenital — *see* Agenesis, hand
- foot (acquired) Z89.43- ☑
  - congenital — *see* Agenesis, foot
- forearm (acquired) — *see* Absence, arm, below elbow
- gallbladder (acquired) Z90.49
  - congenital Q44.0
- gamma globulin in blood D80.1
  - hereditary D80.0
- genital organs
  - acquired (female) (male) Z90.79
  - female, congenital Q52.8
    - external Q52.71
    - internal NEC Q52.8
  - male, congenital Q55.8
- genitourinary organs, congenital NEC
  - female Q52.8
  - male Q55.8
- globe (acquired) Z90.01
  - congenital Q11.1
- glottis, congenital Q31.8
- hand and wrist (acquired) Z89.11- ☑
  - congenital — *see* Agenesis, hand
- head, part (acquired) NEC Z90.09
- heat sense R20.8
- hip (following explanation of hip joint prosthesis) (joint) (with or without presence of antibiotic-impregnated cement spacer) Z89.62- ☑
- hymen (congenital) Q52.4
- ileum (acquired) Z90.49
  - congenital Q41.2
- immunoglobulin, isolated NEC D80.3
  - IgA D80.2
  - IgG D80.3
  - IgM D80.4
- incus (acquired) — *see* Loss, ossicles, ear
  - congenital Q16.3
- inner ear, congenital Q16.5
- intestine (acquired) (small) Z90.49
  - congenital Q41.9
    - specified NEC Q41.8
  - large Z90.49
    - congenital Q42.9
      - specified NEC Q42.8
- iris, congenital Q13.1

Absence — *continued*
- jejunum (acquired) Z90.49
  - congenital Q41.1
- joint
  - acquired
    - hip (following explanation of hip joint prosthesis) (with or without presence of antibiotic-impregnated cement spacer) Z89.62- ☑
    - knee (following explanation of knee joint prosthesis) (with or without presence of antibiotic-impregnated cement spacer) Z89.52- ☑
    - shoulder (following explanation of shoulder joint prosthesis) (with or without presence of antibiotic-impregnated cement spacer) Z89.23- ☑
  - congenital NEC Q74.8
- kidney(s) (acquired) Z90.5
  - congenital Q60.2
    - bilateral Q60.1
    - unilateral Q60.0
- knee (following explanation of knee joint prosthesis) (joint) (with or without presence of antibiotic-impregnated cement spacer) Z89.52- ☑
- labyrinth, membranous Q16.5
- larynx (congenital) Q31.8
  - acquired Z90.02
- leg (acquired) (above knee) Z89.61- ☑
  - below knee (acquired) Z89.51- ☑
  - congenital — *see* Defect, reduction, lower limb
- lens (acquired) (*see also* Aphakia)
  - congenital Q12.3
  - post cataract extraction Z98.4- ☑
- limb (acquired) — *see* Absence, extremity
- lip Q38.6
- liver (congenital) Q44.7
- lung (fissure) (lobe) (bilateral) (unilateral) (congenital) Q33.3
  - acquired (any part) Z90.2
- menstruation — *see* Amenorrhea
- muscle (congenital) (pectoral) Q79.8
  - ocular Q10.3
- neck, part Q18.8
- neutrophil — *see* Agranulocytosis
- nipple(s) (with breast(s)) (acquired) Z90.1- ☑
  - congenital Q83.2
- nose (congenital) Q30.1
  - acquired Z90.09
- organ
  - of Corti, congenital Q16.5
  - or site, congenital NEC Q89.8
    - acquired NEC Z90.89
- osseous meatus (ear) Q16.4
- ovary (acquired)
  - bilateral Z90.722
  - congenital
    - bilateral Q50.02
    - unilateral Q50.01
  - unilateral Z90.721
- oviduct (acquired)
  - bilateral Z90.722
  - congenital Q50.6
  - unilateral Z90.721
- pancreas (congenital) Q45.0
  - acquired Z90.410
    - complete Z90.410
    - partial Z90.411
    - total Z90.410
- parathyroid gland (acquired) E89.2
  - congenital Q89.2
- patella, congenital Q74.1
- penis (congenital) Q55.5
  - acquired Z90.79
- pericardium (congenital) Q24.8
- pituitary gland (congenital) Q89.2
  - acquired E89.3
- prostate (acquired) Z90.79
  - congenital Q55.4
- pulmonary valve Q22.0
- punctum lacrimale (congenital) Q10.4
- radius, congenital — *see* Defect, reduction, upper limb, longitudinal, radius
- rectum (congenital) Q42.1
  - with fistula Q42.0
  - acquired Z90.49
- respiratory organ NOS Q34.9
- rib (acquired) Z90.89

Absence — *continued*
- rib — *continued*
  - congenital Q76.6
- sacrum, congenital Q76.49
- salivary gland(s), congenital Q38.4
- scrotum, congenital Q55.29
- seminal vesicles (congenital) Q55.4
  - acquired Z90.79
- septum
  - atrial (congenital) Q21.1
  - between aorta and pulmonary artery Q21.4
  - ventricular (congenital) Q20.4
- sex chromosome
  - female phenotype Q97.8
  - male phenotype Q98.8
- skull bone (congenital) Q75.8
  - with
    - anencephaly Q00.0
    - encephalocele — *see* Encephalocele
    - hydrocephalus Q03.9
      - with spina bifida — *see* Spina bifida, by site, with hydrocephalus
    - microcephaly Q02
- spermatic cord, congenital Q55.4
- spine, congenital Q76.49
- spleen (congenital) Q89.01
  - acquired Z90.81
- sternum, congenital Q76.7
- stomach (acquired) (partial) Z90.3
  - congenital Q40.2
- superior vena cava, congenital Q26.8
- teeth, tooth (congenital) K00.0
  - acquired (complete) K08.109
    - class I K08.101
    - class II K08.102
    - class III K08.103
    - class IV K08.104
    - due to
      - caries K08.139
        - class I K08.131
        - class II K08.132
        - class III K08.133
        - class IV K08.134
      - periodontal disease K08.129
        - class I K08.121
        - class II K08.122
        - class III K08.123
        - class IV K08.124
      - specified NEC K08.199
        - class I K08.191
        - class II K08.192
        - class III K08.193
        - class IV K08.194
      - trauma K08.119
        - class I K08.111
        - class II K08.112
        - class III K08.113
        - class IV K08.114
    - partial K08.409
      - class I K08.401
      - class II K08.402
      - class III K08.403
      - class IV K08.404
      - due to
        - caries K08.439
          - class I K08.431
          - class II K08.432
          - class III K08.433
          - class IV K08.434
        - periodontal disease K08.429
          - class I K08.421
          - class II K08.422
          - class III K08.423
          - class IV K08.424
        - specified NEC K08.499
          - class I K08.491
          - class II K08.492
          - class III K08.493
          - class IV K08.494
        - trauma K08.419
          - class I K08.411
          - class II K08.412
          - class III K08.413
          - class IV K08.414
- tendon (congenital) Q79.8
- testis (congenital) Q55.0
  - acquired Z90.79
- thumb (acquired) Z89.01- ☑

Absence — *continued*
  thumb — *continued*
    congenital — *see* Agenesis, hand
  thymus gland Q89.2
  thyroid (gland) (acquired) E89.0
    cartilage, congenital Q31.8
    congenital E03.1
  toe(s) (acquired) Z89.42- ☑
    with foot — *see* Absence, foot and ankle
    congenital — *see* Agenesis, foot
    great Z89.41- ☑
  tongue, congenital Q38.3
  trachea (cartilage), congenital Q32.1
  transverse aortic arch, congenital Q25.4
  tricuspid valve Q22.4
  umbilical artery, congenital Q27.0
  upper arm and forearm with hand present, congenital
       — *see* Agenesis, arm, with hand present
  ureter (congenital) Q62.4
    acquired Z90.6
  urethra, congenital Q64.5
  uterus (acquired) Z90.710
    with cervix Z90.710
    with remaining cervical stump Z90.711
    congenital Q51.0
  uvula, congenital Q38.5
  vagina, congenital Q52.0
  vas deferens (congenital) Q55.4
    acquired Z90.79
  vein (peripheral) congenital NEC Q27.8
    cerebral Q28.3
    digestive system Q27.8
    great Q26.8
    lower limb Q27.8
    portal Q26.5
    precerebral Q28.1
    specified site NEC Q27.8
    upper limb Q27.8
  vena cava (inferior) (superior), congenital Q26.8
  ventricular septum Q20.4
  vertebra, congenital Q76.49
  vulva, congenital Q52.71
  wrist (acquired) Z89.12- ☑
Absorbent system disease I87.8
Absorption
  carbohydrate, disturbance K90.4
  chemical — *see* Table of Drugs and Chemicals
    through placenta (newborn) P04.9
      environmental substance P04.6
      nutritional substance P04.5
      obstetric anesthetic or analgesic drug P04.0
  drug NEC — *see* Table of Drugs and Chemicals
    addictive
      through placenta (newborn) P04.49
        cocaine P04.41
    medicinal
      through placenta (newborn) P04.1
    through placenta (newborn) P04.1
      obstetric anesthetic or analgesic drug P04.0
  fat, disturbance K90.4
  pancreatic K90.3
  noxious substance — *see* Table of Drugs and Chemicals
  protein, disturbance K90.4
  starch, disturbance K90.4
  toxic substance — *see* Table of Drugs and Chemicals
  uremic — *see* Uremia
Abstinence symptoms, syndrome
  alcohol F10.239
    with delirium F10.231
  cocaine F14.23
  neonatal P96.1
  nicotine — *see* Dependence, drug, nicotine, with, withdrawal
  opioid F11.93
    with dependence F11.23
  psychoactive NEC F19.939
    with
      delirium F19.931
      dependence F19.239
        with
          delirium F19.231
          perceptual disturbance F19.232
          uncomplicated F19.230
        perceptual disturbance F19.932
        uncomplicated F19.930
  sedative F13.939

Abstinence symptoms, syndrome — *continued*
  sedative — *continued*
    with
      delirium F13.931
      dependence F13.239
        with
          delirium F13.231
          perceptual disturbance F13.232
          uncomplicated F13.230
        perceptual disturbance F13.932
        uncomplicated F13.930
  stimulant NEC F15.93
    with dependence F15.23
Abulia R68.89
Abulomania F60.7
Abuse
  adult — *see* Maltreatment, adult
    as reason for
      couple seeking advice (including offender)
         Z63.0
  alcohol (non-dependent) F10.10
    with
      anxiety disorder F10.180
      intoxication F10.129
        with delirium F10.121
        uncomplicated F10.120
      mood disorder F10.14
      other specified disorder F10.188
      psychosis F10.159
        delusions F10.150
        hallucinations F10.151
      sexual dysfunction F10.181
      sleep disorder F10.182
      unspecified disorder F10.19
    counseling and surveillance Z71.41
  amphetamine (or related substance) — *see* Abuse,
       drug, stimulant NEC
  analgesics (non-prescribed) (over the counter) F55.8
  antacids F55.0
  antidepressants — *see* Abuse, drug, psychoactive NEC
  anxiolytic — *see* Abuse, drug, sedative
  barbiturates — *see* Abuse, drug, sedative
  caffeine — *see* Abuse, drug, stimulant NEC
  cannabis, cannabinoids — *see* Abuse, drug, cannabis
  child — *see* Maltreatment, child
  cocaine — *see* Abuse, drug, cocaine
  drug NEC (non-dependent) F19.10
    with sleep disorder F19.182
    amphetamine type — *see* Abuse, drug, stimulant
       NEC
    analgesics (non-prescribed) (over the counter)
       F55.8
    antacids F55.0
    antidepressants — *see* Abuse, drug, psychoactive
       NEC
    anxiolytics — *see* Abuse, drug, sedative
    barbiturates — *see* Abuse, drug, sedative
    caffeine — *see* Abuse, drug, stimulant NEC
    cannabis F12.10
      with
        anxiety disorder F12.180
        intoxication F12.129
          with
            delirium F12.121
            perceptual disturbance F12.122
          uncomplicated F12.120
        other specified disorder F12.188
        psychosis F12.159
          delusions F12.150
          hallucinations F12.151
        unspecified disorder F12.19
    cocaine F14.10
      with
        anxiety disorder F14.180
        intoxication F14.129
          with
            delirium F14.121
            perceptual disturbance F14.122
          uncomplicated F14.120
        mood disorder F14.14
        other specified disorder F14.188
        psychosis F14.159
          delusions F14.150
          hallucinations F14.151
        sexual dysfunction F14.181
        sleep disorder F14.182
        unspecified disorder F14.19
    counseling and surveillance Z71.51

Abuse — *continued*
  drug — *continued*
    hallucinogen F16.10
      with
        anxiety disorder F16.180
        flashbacks F16.183
        intoxication F16.129
          with
            delirium F16.121
            perceptual disturbance F16.122
          uncomplicated F16.120
        mood disorder F16.14
        other specified disorder F16.188
        perception disorder, persisting F16.183
        psychosis F16.159
          delusions F16.150
          hallucinations F16.151
        unspecified disorder F16.19
    hashish — *see* Abuse, drug, cannabis
    herbal or folk remedies F55.1
    hormones F55.3
    hypnotics — *see* Abuse, drug, sedative
    inhalant F18.10
      with
        anxiety disorder F18.180
        dementia, persisting F18.17
        intoxication F18.129
          with delirium F18.121
          uncomplicated F18.120
        mood disorder F18.14
        other specified disorder F18.188
        psychosis F18.159
          delusions F18.150
          hallucinations F18.151
        unspecified disorder F18.19
    laxatives F55.2
    LSD — *see* Abuse, drug, hallucinogen
    marihuana — *see* Abuse, drug, cannabis
    morphine type (opioids) — *see* Abuse, drug, opioid
    opioid F11.10
      with
        intoxication F11.129
          with
            delirium F11.121
            perceptual disturbance F11.122
          uncomplicated F11.120
        mood disorder F11.14
        other specified disorder F11.188
        psychosis F11.159
          delusions F11.150
          hallucinations F11.151
        sexual dysfunction F11.181
        sleep disorder F11.182
        unspecified disorder F11.19
    PCP (phencyclidine) (or related substance) — *see*
       Abuse, drug, hallucinogen
    psychoactive NEC F19.10
      with
        amnestic disorder F19.16
        anxiety disorder F19.180
        dementia F19.17
        intoxication F19.129
          with
            delirium F19.121
            perceptual disturbance F19.122
          uncomplicated F19.120
        mood disorder F19.14
        other specified disorder F19.188
        psychosis F19.159
          delusions F19.150
          hallucinations F19.151
        sexual dysfunction F19.181
        sleep disorder F19.182
        unspecified disorder F19.19
    sedative, hypnotic or anxiolytic F13.10
      with
        anxiety disorder F13.180
        intoxication F13.129
          with delirium F13.121
          uncomplicated F13.120
        mood disorder F13.14
        other specified disorder F13.188
        psychosis F13.159
          delusions F13.150
          hallucinations F13.151
        sexual dysfunction F13.181
        sleep disorder F13.182
        unspecified disorder F13.19

Abuse — *continued*
  drug — *continued*
    solvent — *see* Abuse, drug, inhalant
    steroids F55.3
    stimulant NEC F15.10
      with
        anxiety disorder F15.180
        intoxication F15.129
          with
            delirium F15.121
            perceptual disturbance F15.122
          uncomplicated F15.120
        mood disorder F15.14
        other specified disorder F15.188
        psychosis F15.159
          delusions F15.150
          hallucinations F15.151
        sexual dysfunction F15.181
        sleep disorder F15.182
        unspecified disorder F15.19
    tranquilizers — *see* Abuse, drug, sedative
    vitamins F55.4
  hallucinogens — *see* Abuse, drug, hallucinogen
  hashish — *see* Abuse, drug, cannabis
  herbal or folk remedies F55.1
  hormones F55.3
  hypnotic — *see* Abuse, drug, sedative
  inhalant — *see* Abuse, drug, inhalant
  laxatives F55.2
  LSD — *see* Abuse, drug, hallucinogen
  marihuana — *see* Abuse, drug, cannabis
  morphine type (opioids) — *see* Abuse, drug, opioid
  non-psychoactive substance NEC F55.8
    antacids F55.0
    folk remedies F55.1
    herbal remedies F55.1
    hormones F55.3
    laxatives F55.2
    steroids F55.3
    vitamins F55.4
  opioids — *see* Abuse, drug, opioid
  PCP (phencyclidine) (or related substance) — *see* Abuse, drug, hallucinogen
  physical (adult) (child) — *see* Maltreatment
  psychoactive substance — *see* Abuse, drug, psychoactive NEC
  psychological (adult) (child) — *see* Maltreatment
  sedative — *see* Abuse, drug, sedative
  sexual — *see* Maltreatment
  solvent — *see* Abuse, drug, inhalant
  steroids F55.3
  vitamins F55.4
Acalculia R48.8
  developmental F81.2
Acanthamebiasis (with) B60.10
  conjunctiva B60.12
  keratoconjunctivitis B60.13
  meningoencephalitis B60.11
  other specified B60.19
Acanthocephaliasis B83.8
Acanthocheilonemiasis B74.4
Acanthocytosis E78.6
Acantholysis L11.9
Acanthosis (acquired) (nigricans) L83
  benign Q82.8
  congenital Q82.8
  seborrheic L82.1
    inflamed L82.0
  tongue K14.3
Acapnia E87.3
Acarbia E87.2
Acardia, acardius Q89.8
Acardiacus amorphus Q89.8
Acardiotrophia I51.4
Acariasis B88.0
  scabies B86
Acarodermatitis (urticarioides) B88.0
Acarophobia F40.218
Acatalasemia, acatalasia E80.3
Acathisia (drug induced) G25.71
Accelerated atrioventricular conduction I45.6
Accentuation of personality traits (type A) Z73.1
Accessory (congenital)
  adrenal gland Q89.1
  anus Q43.4
  appendix Q43.4
  atrioventricular conduction I45.6

Accessory — *continued*
  auditory ossicles Q16.3
  auricle (ear) Q17.0
  biliary duct or passage Q44.5
  bladder Q64.79
  blood vessels NEC Q27.9
    coronary Q24.5
  bone NEC Q79.8
  breast tissue, axilla Q83.1
  carpal bones Q74.0
  cecum Q43.4
  chromosome(s) NEC (nonsex) Q92.9
    with complex rearrangements NEC Q92.5
      seen only at prometaphase Q92.8
    13 — *see* Trisomy, 13
    18 — *see* Trisomy, 18
    21 — *see* Trisomy, 21
    partial Q92.9
    sex
      female phenotype Q97.8
  coronary artery Q24.5
  cusp(s), heart valve NEC Q24.8
    pulmonary Q22.3
  cystic duct Q44.5
  digit(s) Q69.9
  ear (auricle) (lobe) Q17.0
  endocrine gland NEC Q89.2
  eye muscle Q10.3
  eyelid Q10.3
  face bone(s) Q75.8
  fallopian tube (fimbria) (ostium) Q50.6
  finger(s) Q69.0
  foreskin N47.8
  frontonasal process Q75.8
  gallbladder Q44.1
  genital organ(s)
    female Q52.8
      external Q52.79
      internal NEC Q52.8
    male Q55.8
  genitourinary organs NEC Q89.8
    female Q52.8
    male Q55.8
  hallux Q69.2
  heart Q24.8
    valve NEC Q24.8
      pulmonary Q22.3
  hepatic ducts Q44.5
  hymen Q52.4
  intestine (large) (small) Q43.4
  kidney Q63.0
  lacrimal canal Q10.6
  leaflet, heart valve NEC Q24.8
  ligament, broad Q50.6
  liver Q44.7
    duct Q44.5
  lobule (ear) Q17.0
  lung (lobe) Q33.1
  muscle Q79.8
  navicular of carpus Q74.0
  nervous system, part NEC Q07.8
  nipple Q83.3
  nose Q30.8
  organ or site not listed — *see* Anomaly, by site
  ovary Q50.31
  oviduct Q50.6
  pancreas Q45.3
  parathyroid gland Q89.2
  parotid gland (and duct) Q38.4
  pituitary gland Q89.2
  preauricular appendage Q17.0
  prepuce N47.8
  renal arteries (multiple) Q27.2
  rib Q76.6
    cervical Q76.5
  roots (teeth) K00.2
  salivary gland Q38.4
  sesamoid bones Q74.8
    foot Q74.2
    hand Q74.0
  skin tags Q82.8
  spleen Q89.09
  sternum Q76.7
  submaxillary gland Q38.4
  tarsal bones Q74.2
  teeth, tooth K00.1
  tendon Q79.8
  thumb Q69.1

Accessory — *continued*
  thymus gland Q89.2
  thyroid gland Q89.2
  toes Q69.2
  tongue Q38.3
  tooth, teeth K00.1
  tragus Q17.0
  ureter Q62.5
  urethra Q64.79
  urinary organ or tract NEC Q64.8
  uterus Q51.2
  vagina Q52.10
  valve, heart NEC Q24.8
    pulmonary Q22.3
  vertebra Q76.49
  vocal cords Q31.8
  vulva Q52.79
Accident
  birth — *see* Birth, injury
  cardiac — *see* Infarct, myocardium
  cerebral I63.9
  cerebrovascular (embolic) (ischemic) (thrombotic) I63.9
    aborted I63.9
    hemorrhagic — *see* Hemorrhage, intracranial, intracerebral
    old (without sequelae) Z86.73
      with sequelae (of) — *see* Sequelae, infarction, cerebral
  coronary — *see* Infarct, myocardium
  craniovascular I63.9
  vascular, brain I63.9
Accidental — *see* condition
Accommodation (disorder) (*see also* condition)
  hysterical paralysis of F44.89
  insufficiency of H52.4
  paresis — *see* Paresis, of accommodation
  spasm — *see* Spasm, of accommodation
Accouchement — *see* Delivery
Accreta placenta O43.21- ☑
Accretio cordis (nonrheumatic) I31.0
Accretions, tooth, teeth K03.6
Acculturation difficulty Z60.3
Accumulation secretion, prostate N42.89
Acephalia, acephalism, acephalus, acephaly Q00.0
Acephalobrachia monster Q89.8
Acephalochirus monster Q89.8
Acephalogaster Q89.8
Acephalostomus monster Q89.8
Acephalothorax Q89.8
Acerophobia F40.298
Acetonemia R79.89
  in Type 1 diabetes E10.10
    with coma E10.11
Acetonuria R82.4
Achalasia (cardia) (esophagus) K22.0
  congenital Q39.5
  pylorus Q40.0
  sphincteral NEC K59.8
Ache(s) — *see* Pain
Acheilia Q38.6
Achillobursitis — *see* Tendinitis, Achilles
Achillodynia — *see* Tendinitis, Achilles
Achlorhydria, achlorhydric (neurogenic) K31.83
  anemia D50.8
  diarrhea K31.83
  psychogenic F45.8
  secondary to vagotomy K91.1
Achluophobia F40.228
Acholia K82.8
Acholuric jaundice (familial) (splenomegalic) (*see also* Spherocytosis)
  acquired D59.8
Achondrogenesis Q77.0
Achondroplasia (osteosclerosis congenita) Q77.4
Achroma, cutis L80
Achromat (ism), achromatopsia (acquired) (congenital) H53.51
Achromia, congenital — *see* Albinism
Achromia parasitica B36.0
Achylia gastrica K31.89
  psychogenic F45.8
Acid
  burn — *see* Corrosion
  deficiency
    amide nicotinic E52
    ascorbic E54
    folic E53.8

Acid — *continued*
  deficiency — *continued*
    nicotinic E52
    pantothenic E53.8
  intoxication E87.2
  peptic disease K30
  phosphatase deficiency E83.39
  stomach K30
    psychogenic F45.8
Acidemia E87.2
  argininosuccinic E72.22
  isovaleric E71.110
  metabolic (newborn) P19.9
    first noted before onset of labor P19.0
    first noted during labor P19.1
    noted at birth P19.2
  methylmalonic E71.120
  pipecolic E72.3
  propionic E71.121
Acidity, gastric (high) K30
  psychogenic F45.8
Acidocytopenia — *see* Agranulocytosis
Acidocytosis D72.1
Acidopenia — *see* Agranulocytosis
Acidosis (lactic) (respiratory) E87.2
  in Type 1 diabetes E10.10
    with coma E10.11
  kidney, tubular N25.89
  lactic E87.2
  metabolic NEC E87.2
    with respiratory acidosis E87.4
    late, of newborn P74.0
  mixed metabolic and respiratory, newborn P84
  newborn P84
  renal (hyperchloremic) (tubular) N25.89
  respiratory E87.2
    complicated by
      metabolic
        acidosis E87.4
        alkalosis E87.4
Aciduria
  argininosuccinic E72.22
  glutaric (type I) E72.3
    type II E71.313
    type III E71.5- ☑
  orotic (congenital) (hereditary) (pyrimidine deficiency) E79.8
    anemia D53.0
Acladiosis (skin) B36.0
Aclasis, diaphyseal Q78.6
Acleistocardia Q21.1
Aclusion — *see* Anomaly, dentofacial, malocclusion
Acne L70.9
  artificialis L70.8
  atrophica L70.2
  cachecticorum (Hebra) L70.8
  conglobata L70.1
  cystic L70.0
  decalvans L66.2
  excoriée des jeunes filles L70.5
  frontalis L70.2
  indurata L70.0
  infantile L70.4
  keloid L73.0
  lupoid L70.2
  necrotic, necrotica (miliaris) L70.2
  neonatal L70.4
  nodular L70.0
  occupational L70.8
  picker's L70.5
  pustular L70.0
  rodens L70.2
  rosacea L71.9
  specified NEC L70.8
  tropica L70.3
  varioliformis L70.2
  vulgaris L70.0
Acnitis (primary) A18.4
Acosta's disease T70.29 ☑
Acoustic — *see* condition
Acousticophobia F40.298
Acquired (*see also* condition)
  immunodeficiency syndrome (AIDS) B20
Acrania Q00.0
Acroangiodermatitis I78.9
Acroasphyxia, chronic I73.89
Acrobystitis N47.7
Acrocephalopolysyndactyly Q87.0

Acrocephalosyndactyly Q87.0
Acrocephaly Q75.0
Acrochondrohyperplasia — *see* Syndrome, Marfan's
Acrocyanosis I73.8 ☑
  newborn P28.2
    meaning transient blue hands and feet — *omit code*
Acrodermatitis L30.8
  atrophicans (chronica) L90.4
  continua (Hallopeau) L40.2
  enteropathica (hereditary) E83.2
  Hallopeau's L40.2
  infantile papular L44.4
  perstans L40.2
  pustulosa continua L40.2
  recalcitrant pustular L40.2
Acrodynia — *see* Poisoning, mercury
Acromegaly, acromegalia E22.0
Acromelalgia I73.81
Acromicria, acromikria Q79.8
Acronyx L60.0
Acropachy, thyroid — *see* Thyrotoxicosis
Acroparesthesia (simple) (vasomotor) I73.89
Acropathy, thyroid — *see* Thyrotoxicosis
Acrophobia F40.241
Acroposthitis N47.7
Acroscleriasis, acroscleroderma, acrosclerosis — *see* Sclerosis, systemic
Acrosphacelus I96
Acrospiroma, eccrine — *see* Neoplasm, skin, benign
Acrostealgia — *see* Osteochondropathy
Acrotrophodynia — *see* Immersion
ACTH ectopic syndrome E24.3
Actinic — *see* condition
Actinobacillosis, actinobacillus A28.8
  mallei A24.0
  muris A25.1
Actinomyces israelii (infection) — *see* Actinomycosis
Actinomycetoma (foot) B47.1
Actinomycosis, actinomycotic A42.9
  with pneumonia A42.0
  abdominal A42.1
  cervicofacial A42.2
  cutaneous A42.89
  gastrointestinal A42.1
  pulmonary A42.0
  sepsis A42.7
  specified site NEC A42.89
Actinoneuritis G62.82
Action, heart
  disorder I49.9
  irregular I49.9
    psychogenic F45.8
Activated protein C resistance D68.51
Active — *see* condition
Acute (*see also* condition)
  abdomen R10.0
  gallbladder — *see* Cholecystitis, acute
Acyanotic heart disease (congenital) Q24.9
Acystia Q64.5
Adair-Dighton syndrome (brittle bones and blue sclera, deafness) Q78.0
Adamantinoblastoma — *see* Ameloblastoma
Adamantinoma (*see also* Cyst, calcifying odontogenic)
  long bones C40.90
    lower limb C40.2- ☑
    upper limb C40.0- ☑
  malignant C41.1
    jaw (bone) (lower) C41.1
      upper C41.0
  tibial C40.2- ☑
Adamantoblastoma — *see* Ameloblastoma
Adams-Stokes (-Morgagni) disease or syndrome I45.9
Adaption reaction — *see* Disorder, adjustment
Addiction (*see also* Dependence) F19.20
  alcohol, alcoholic (ethyl) (methyl) (wood) (without remission) F10.20
    with remission F10.21
  drug — *see* Dependence, drug
  ethyl alcohol (without remission) F10.20
    with remission F10.21
  heroin — *see* Dependence, drug, opioid
  methyl alcohol (without remission) F10.20
    with remission F10.21
  methylated spirit (without remission) F10.20
    with remission F10.21

Addiction — *continued*
  morphine (-like substances) — *see* Dependence, drug, opioid
  nicotine — *see* Dependence, drug, nicotine
  opium and opioids — *see* Dependence, drug, opioid
  tobacco — *see* Dependence, drug, nicotine
Addison-Biermer anemia (pernicious) D51.0
Addison-Schilder complex E71.528
Addisonian crisis E27.2
Addison's
  anemia (pernicious) D51.0
  disease (bronze) or syndrome E27.1
    tuberculous A18.7
  keloid L94.0
Additional (*see also* Accessory)
  chromosome(s) Q99.8
    21 — *see* Trisomy, 21
    sex — *see* Abnormal, chromosome, sex
Adduction contracture, hip or other joint — *see* Contraction, joint
Adenitis (*see also* Lymphadenitis)
  acute, unspecified site L04.9
  axillary I88.9
    acute L04.2
    chronic or subacute I88.1
  Bartholin's gland N75.8
  bulbourethral gland — *see* Urethritis
  cervical I88.9
    acute L04.0
    chronic or subacute I88.1
  chancroid (Hemophilus ducreyi) A57
  chronic, unspecified site I88.1
  Cowper's gland — *see* Urethritis
  due to Pasteurella multocida (p. septica) A28.0
  epidemic, acute B27.09
  gangrenous L04.9
  gonorrheal NEC A54.89
  groin I88.9
    acute L04.1
    chronic or subacute I88.1
  infectious (acute) (epidemic) B27.09
  inguinal I88.9
    acute L04.1
    chronic or subacute I88.1
  lymph gland or node, except mesenteric I88.9
    acute — *see* Lymphadenitis, acute
    chronic or subacute I88.1
  mesenteric (acute) (chronic) (nonspecific) (subacute) I88.0
  parotid gland (suppurative) — *see* Sialoadenitis
  salivary gland (any) (suppurative) — *see* Sialoadenitis
  scrofulous (tuberculous) A18.2
  Skene's duct or gland — *see* Urethritis
  strumous, tuberculous A18.2
  subacute, unspecified site I88.1
  sublingual gland (suppurative) — *see* Sialoadenitis
  submandibular gland (suppurative) — *see* Sialoadenitis
  submaxillary gland (suppurative) — *see* Sialoadenitis
  tuberculous — *see* Tuberculosis, lymph gland
  urethral gland — *see* Urethritis
  Wharton's duct (suppurative) — *see* Sialoadenitis
Adenoacanthoma — *see* Neoplasm, malignant, by site
Adenoameloblastoma — *see* Cyst, calcifying odontogenic
Adenocarcinoid (tumor) — *see* Neoplasm, malignant, by site
Adenocarcinoma (*see also* Neoplasm, malignant, by site)
  acidophil
    specified site — *see* Neoplasm, malignant, by site
    unspecified site C75.1
  adrenal cortical C74.0- ☑
  alveolar — *see* Neoplasm, lung, malignant
  apocrine
    breast — *see* Neoplasm, breast, malignant
    in situ
      breast D05.8- ☑
      specified site NEC — *see* Neoplasm, skin, in situ
      unspecified site D04.9
    specified site NEC — *see* Neoplasm, skin, malignant
    unspecified site C44.99
  basal cell
    specified site — *see* Neoplasm, skin, malignant
    unspecified site C08.9
  basophil
    specified site — *see* Neoplasm, malignant, by site

Adenocarcinoma — *continued*
  basophil — *continued*
    unspecified site C75.1
  bile duct type C22.1
    liver C22.1
    specified site NEC — *see* Neoplasm, malignant, by site
    unspecified site C22.1
  bronchiolar — *see* Neoplasm, lung, malignant
  bronchioloalveolar — *see* Neoplasm, lung, malignant
  ceruminous C44.29- ☑
  cervix, in situ (*see also* Carcinoma, cervix uteri, in situ) D06.9
  chromophobe
    specified site — *see* Neoplasm, malignant, by site
    unspecified site C75.1
  diffuse type
    specified site — *see* Neoplasm, malignant, by site
    unspecified site C16.9
  duct
    infiltrating
      with Paget's disease — *see* Neoplasm, breast, malignant
      specified site — *see* Neoplasm, malignant, by site
      unspecified site (female) C50.91- ☑
        male C50.92- ☑
    specified site — *see* Neoplasm, malignant, by site
    unspecified site
      female C56.9
      male C61
  eosinophil
    specified site — *see* Neoplasm, malignant, by site
    unspecified site C75.1
  follicular
    with papillary C73
    moderately differentiated C73
    specified site — *see* Neoplasm, malignant, by site
    trabecular C73
    unspecified site C73
    well differentiated C73
  Hurthle cell C73
  in
    adenomatous
      polyposis coli C18.9
  infiltrating duct
    with Paget's disease — *see* Neoplasm, breast, malignant
    specified site — *see* Neoplasm, by site, malignant
    unspecified site (female) C50.91- ☑
      male C50.92- ☑
  inflammatory
    specified site — *see* Neoplasm, by site, malignant
    unspecified site (female) C50.91- ☑
      male C50.92- ☑
  intestinal type
    specified site — *see* Neoplasm, by site, malignant
    unspecified site C16.9
  intracystic papillary
  intraductal
    breast D05.1- ☑
    noninfiltrating
      breast D05.1- ☑
      papillary
        with invasion
          specified site — *see* Neoplasm, by site, malignant
          unspecified site (female) C50.91- ☑
            male C50.92- ☑
        breast D05.1- ☑
        specified site NEC — *see* Neoplasm, in situ, by site
        unspecified site D05.1- ☑
      specified site NEC — *see* Neoplasm, in situ, by site
      unspecified site D05.1- ☑
    papillary
      with invasion
        specified site — *see* Neoplasm, malignant, by site
        unspecified site (female) C50.91- ☑
          male C50.92- ☑
      breast D05.1- ☑
      specified site — *see* Neoplasm, in situ, by site
      unspecified site D05.1- ☑
    specified site NEC — *see* Neoplasm, in situ, by site
    unspecified site D05.1- ☑

Adenocarcinoma — *continued*
  islet cell
    with exocrine, mixed
      specified site — *see* Neoplasm, malignant, by site
      unspecified site C25.9
    pancreas C25.4
    specified site NEC — *see* Neoplasm, malignant, by site
    unspecified site C25.4
  lobular
    in situ
      breast D05.0- ☑
      specified site NEC — *see* Neoplasm, in situ, by site
      unspecified site D05.0- ☑
    specified site — *see* Neoplasm, malignant, by site
    unspecified site (female) C50.91- ☑
      male C50.92- ☑
  mucoid (*see also* Neoplasm, malignant, by site)
    cell
      specified site — *see* Neoplasm, malignant, by site
      unspecified site C75.1
  nonencapsulated sclerosing C73
  papillary
    with follicular C73
    follicular variant C73
    intraductal (noninfiltrating)
      with invasion
        specified site — *see* Neoplasm, malignant, by site
        unspecified site (female) C50.91- ☑
          male C50.92- ☑
      breast D05.1- ☑
      specified site NEC — *see* Neoplasm, in situ, by site
      unspecified site D05.1- ☑
    serous
      specified site — *see* Neoplasm, malignant, by site
      unspecified site C56.9
  papillocystic
    specified site — *see* Neoplasm, malignant, by site
    unspecified site C56.9
  pseudomucinous
    specified site — *see* Neoplasm, malignant, by site
    unspecified site C56.9
  renal cell C64- ☑
  sebaceous — *see* Neoplasm, skin, malignant
  serous (*see also* Neoplasm, malignant, by site)
    papillary
      specified site — *see* Neoplasm, malignant, by site
      unspecified site C56.9
  sweat gland — *see* Neoplasm, skin, malignant
  water-clear cell C75.0

Adenocarcinoma-in-situ (*see also* Neoplasm, in situ, by site)
  breast D05.9- ☑

Adenofibroma
  clear cell — *see* Neoplasm, benign, by site
  endometrioid D27.9
    borderline malignancy D39.10
    malignant C56- ☑
  mucinous
    specified site — *see* Neoplasm, benign, by site
    unspecified site D27.9
  papillary
    specified site — *see* Neoplasm, benign, by site
    unspecified site D27.9
  prostate — *see* Enlargement, enlarged, prostate
  serous
    specified site — *see* Neoplasm, benign, by site
    unspecified site D27.9
  specified site — *see* Neoplasm, benign, by site
  unspecified site D27.9

Adenofibrosis
  breast — *see* Fibroadenosis, breast
  endometrioid N80.0

Adenoiditis (chronic) J35.02
  with tonsillitis J35.03
  acute J03.90
    recurrent J03.91
    specified organism NEC J03.80
      recurrent J03.81
    staphylococcal J03.80

Adenoiditis — *continued*
  acute — *continued*
    staphylococcal — *continued*
      recurrent J03.81
    streptococcal J03.00
      recurrent J03.01
Adenoids — *see* condition
Adenolipoma — *see* Neoplasm, benign, by site
Adenolipomatosis, Launois-Bensaude E88.89
Adenolymphoma
  specified site — *see* Neoplasm, benign, by site
  unspecified site D11.9
Adenoma (*see also* Neoplasm, benign, by site)
  acidophil
    specified site — *see* Neoplasm, benign, by site
    unspecified site D35.2
  acidophil-basophil, mixed
    specified site — *see* Neoplasm, benign, by site
    unspecified site D35.2
  adrenal (cortical) D35.00
    clear cell D35.00
    compact cell D35.00
    glomerulosa cell D35.00
    heavily pigmented variant D35.00
    mixed cell D35.00
  alpha-cell
    pancreas D13.7
    specified site — *see* Neoplasm, benign, by site
    unspecified site D13.7
  alveolar D14.30
  apocrine
    breast D24- ☑
    specified site NEC — *see* Neoplasm, skin, benign, by site
    unspecified site D23.9
  basal cell D11.9
  basophil
    specified site — *see* Neoplasm, benign, by site
    unspecified site D35.2
  basophil-acidophil, mixed
    specified site — *see* Neoplasm, benign, by site
    unspecified site D35.2
  beta-cell
    pancreas D13.7
    specified site NEC — *see* Neoplasm, benign, by site
    unspecified site D13.7
  bile duct D13.4
    common D13.5
    extrahepatic D13.5
    intrahepatic D13.4
    specified site NEC — *see* Neoplasm, benign, by site
    unspecified site D13.4
  black D35.00
  bronchial D38.1
    cylindroid type — *see* Neoplasm, lung, malignant
  ceruminous D23.2- ☑
  chief cell D35.1
  chromophobe
    specified site — *see* Neoplasm, benign, by site
    unspecified site D35.2
  colloid
    specified site — *see* Neoplasm, benign, by site
    unspecified site D34
  duct
  eccrine, papillary — *see* Neoplasm, skin, benign
  endocrine, multiple
    single specified site — *see* Neoplasm, uncertain behavior, by site
    two or more specified sites D44- ☑
    unspecified site D44.9
  endometrioid (*see also* Neoplasm, benign)
    borderline malignancy — *see* Neoplasm, uncertain behavior, by site
  eosinophil
    specified site — *see* Neoplasm, benign, by site
    unspecified site D35.2
  fetal
    specified site — *see* Neoplasm, benign, by site
    unspecified site D34
  follicular
    specified site NEC — *see* Neoplasm, benign, by site
    unspecified site D34
  hepatocellular D13.4
  Hurthle cell D34
  islet cell
    pancreas D13.7
    specified site NEC — *see* Neoplasm, benign, by site
    unspecified site D13.7

Adenoma — *continued*
  liver cell D13.4
  macrofollicular
    specified site — *see* Neoplasm, benign, by site
    unspecified site D34
  malignant, malignum — *see* Neoplasm, malignant, by site
  microcystic
    pancreas D13.7
    specified site NEC — *see* Neoplasm, benign, by site
    unspecified site D13.7
  microfollicular
    specified site — *see* Neoplasm, benign, by site
    unspecified site D34
  mucoid cell
    specified site — *see* Neoplasm, benign, by site
    unspecified site D35.2
  multiple endocrine
    single specified site — *see* Neoplasm, uncertain behavior, by site
    two or more specified sites D44- ☑
    unspecified site D44.9
  nipple D24- ☑
  papillary (*see also* Neoplasm, benign, by site)
    eccrine — *see* Neoplasm, skin, benign, by site
  Pick's tubular
    specified site — *see* Neoplasm, benign, by site
    unspecified site
      female D27.9
      male D29.20
  pleomorphic
    carcinoma in — *see* Neoplasm, salivary gland, malignant
      specified site — *see* Neoplasm, malignant, by site
      unspecified site C08.9
  polypoid (*see also* Neoplasm, benign)
    adenocarcinoma in — *see* Neoplasm, malignant, by site
    adenocarcinoma in situ — *see* Neoplasm, in situ, by site
  prostate — *see* Neoplasm, benign, prostate
  rete cell D29.20
  sebaceous — *see* Neoplasm, skin, benign
  Sertoli cell
    specified site — *see* Neoplasm, benign, by site
    unspecified site
      female D27.9
      male D29.20
  skin appendage — *see* Neoplasm, skin, benign
  sudoriferous gland — *see* Neoplasm, skin, benign
  sweat gland — *see* Neoplasm, skin, benign
  testicular
    specified site — *see* Neoplasm, benign, by site
    unspecified site
      female D27.9
      male D29.20
  tubular (*see also* Neoplasm, benign, by site)
    adenocarcinoma in — *see* Neoplasm, malignant, by site
    adenocarcinoma in situ — *see* Neoplasm, in situ, by site
    Pick's
      specified site — *see* Neoplasm, benign, by site
      unspecified site
        female D27.9
        male D29.20
  tubulovillous (*see also* Neoplasm, benign, by site)
    adenocarcinoma in — *see* Neoplasm, malignant, by site
    adenocarcinoma in situ — *see* Neoplasm, in situ, by site
  villous — *see* Neoplasm, uncertain behavior, by site
    adenocarcinoma in — *see* Neoplasm, malignant, by site
    adenocarcinoma in situ — *see* Neoplasm, in situ, by site
  water-clear cell D35.1
Adenomatosis
  endocrine (multiple) E31.20
    single specified site — *see* Neoplasm, uncertain behavior, by site
  erosive of nipple D24- ☑
  pluriendocrine — *see* Adenomatosis, endocrine
  pulmonary D38.1
    malignant — *see* Neoplasm, lung, malignant
    specified site — *see* Neoplasm, benign, by site

Adenomatosis — *continued*
  unspecified site D12.6
Adenomatous
  goiter (nontoxic) E04.9
    with hyperthyroidism — *see* Hyperthyroidism, with, goiter, nodular
    toxic — *see* Hyperthyroidism, with, goiter, nodular
Adenomyoma (*see also* Neoplasm, benign, by site)
  prostate — *see* Enlarged, prostate
Adenomyometritis N80.0
Adenomyosis N80.0
Adenopathy (lymph gland) R59.9
  generalized R59.1
  inguinal R59.0
  localized R59.0
  mediastinal R59.0
  mesentery R59.0
  syphilitic (secondary) A51.49
  tracheobronchial R59.0
    tuberculous A15.4
      primary (progressive) A15.7
  tuberculous (*see also* Tuberculosis, lymph gland)
    tracheobronchial A15.4
      primary (progressive) A15.7
Adenosalpingitis — *see* Salpingitis
Adenosarcoma — *see* Neoplasm, malignant, by site
Adenosclerosis I88.8
Adenosis (sclerosing) breast — *see* Fibroadenosis, breast
Adenovirus, as cause of disease classified elsewhere B97.0
Adentia (complete) (partial) — *see* Absence, teeth
Adherent (*see also* Adhesions)
  labia (minora) N90.89
  pericardium (nonrheumatic) I31.0
    rheumatic I09.2
  placenta (with hemorrhage) O72.0
    without hemorrhage O73.0
  prepuce, newborn N47.0
  scar (skin) L90.5
  tendon in scar L90.5
Adhesions, adhesive (postinfective) K66.0
  with intestinal obstruction K56.5
  abdominal (wall) — *see* Adhesions, peritoneum
  appendix K38.8
  bile duct (common) (hepatic) K83.8
  bladder (sphincter) N32.89
  bowel — *see* Adhesions, peritoneum
  cardiac I31.0
    rheumatic I09.2
  cecum — *see* Adhesions, peritoneum
  cervicovaginal N88.1
    congenital Q52.8
    postpartal O90.89
      old N88.1
  cervix N88.1
  ciliary body NEC — *see* Adhesions, iris
  clitoris N90.89
  colon — *see* Adhesions, peritoneum
  common duct K83.8
  congenital (*see also* Anomaly, by site)
    fingers — *see* Syndactylism, complex, fingers
    omental, anomalous Q43.3
    peritoneal Q43.3
    tongue (to gum or roof of mouth) Q38.3
  conjunctiva (acquired) H11.21- ☑
    congenital Q15.8
  cystic duct K82.8
  diaphragm — *see* Adhesions, peritoneum
  due to foreign body — *see* Foreign body
  duodenum — *see* Adhesions, peritoneum
  ear
    middle H74.1- ☑
  epididymis N50.8
  epidural — *see* Adhesions, meninges
  epiglottis J38.7
  eyelid H02.59
  female pelvis N73.6
  gallbladder K82.8
  globe H44.89
  heart I31.0
    rheumatic I09.2
  ileocecal (coil) — *see* Adhesions, peritoneum
  ileum — *see* Adhesions, peritoneum
  intestine (*see also* Adhesions, peritoneum)
    with obstruction K56.5
  intra-abdominal — *see* Adhesions, peritoneum
  iris H21.50- ☑

Adhesions, adhesive — *continued*
  iris — *continued*
    anterior H21.51- ☑
    goniosynechiae H21.52- ☑
    posterior H21.54- ☑
    to corneal graft T85.89 ☑
  joint — *see* Ankylosis
    knee M23.8X ☑
    temporomandibular M26.61
  labium (majus) (minus), congenital Q52.5
  liver — *see* Adhesions, peritoneum
  lung J98.4
  mediastinum J98.5
  meninges (cerebral) (spinal) G96.12
    congenital Q07.8
    tuberculous (cerebral) (spinal) A17.0
  mesenteric — *see* Adhesions, peritoneum
  nasal (septum) (to turbinates) J34.89
  ocular muscle — *see* Strabismus, mechanical
  omentum — *see* Adhesions, peritoneum
  ovary N73.6
    congenital (to cecum, kidney or omentum) Q50.39
  paraovarian N73.6
  pelvic (peritoneal)
    female N73.6
      postprocedural N99.4
    male — *see* Adhesions, peritoneum
    postpartal (old) N73.6
    tuberculous A18.17
  penis to scrotum (congenital) Q55.8
  periappendiceal (*see also* Adhesions, peritoneum)
  pericardium (nonrheumatic) I31.0
    focal I31.8
    rheumatic I09.2
    tuberculous A18.84
  pericholecystic K82.8
  perigastric — *see* Adhesions, peritoneum
  periovarian N73.6
  periprostatic N42.89
  perirectal — *see* Adhesions, peritoneum
  perirenal N28.89
  peritoneum, peritoneal (postinfective) (postprocedural) K66.0
    with obstruction (intestinal) K56.5
    congenital Q43.3
    pelvic, female N73.6
      postprocedural N99.4
    postpartal, pelvic N73.6
    to uterus N73.6
  peritubal N73.6
  periureteral N28.89
  periuterine N73.6
  perivesical N32.89
  perivesicular (seminal vesicle) N50.8
  pleura, pleuritic J94.8
    tuberculous NEC A15.6
  pleuropericardial J94.8
  postoperative (gastrointestinal tract) K66.0
    with obstruction K91.3
    due to foreign body accidentally left in wound — *see* Foreign body, accidentally left during a procedure
    pelvic peritoneal N99.4
    urethra — *see* Stricture, urethra, postprocedural
    vagina N99.2
  postpartal, old (vulva or perineum) N90.89
  preputial, prepuce N47.5
  pulmonary J98.4
  pylorus — *see* Adhesions, peritoneum
  sciatic nerve — *see* Lesion, nerve, sciatic
  seminal vesicle N50.8
  shoulder (joint) — *see* Capsulitis, adhesive
  sigmoid flexure — *see* Adhesions, peritoneum
  spermatic cord (acquired) N50.8
    congenital Q55.4
  spinal canal G96.12
  stomach — *see* Adhesions, peritoneum
  subscapular — *see* Capsulitis, adhesive
  temporomandibular M26.61
  tendinitis (*see also* Tenosynovitis, specified type NEC)
    shoulder — *see* Capsulitis, adhesive
  testis N44.8
  tongue, congenital (to gum or roof of mouth) Q38.3
    acquired K14.8
  trachea J39.8
  tubo-ovarian N73.6
  tunica vaginalis N44.8
  uterus N73.6

☑ **Additional Character Required — Refer to the Tabular List for Character Selection**   ▽ **Subterms under main terms may continue to next column or page**

Adhesions, adhesive — *continued*
  uterus — *continued*
    internal N85.6
    to abdominal wall N73.6
  vagina (chronic) N89.5
    postoperative N99.2
  vitreomacular H43.82- ☑
  vitreous H43.89
  vulva N90.89
Adiaspiromycosis B48.8
Adie (-Holmes) **pupil or syndrome** — *see* Anomaly,
    pupil, function, tonic pupil
Adiponecrosis neonatorum P83.8
Adiposis (*see also* Obesity)
  cerebralis E23.6
  dolorosa E88.2
Adiposity (*see also* Obesity)
  heart — *see* Degeneration, myocardial
  localized E65
Adiposogenital dystrophy E23.6
Adjustment
  disorder — *see* Disorder, adjustment
  implanted device — *see* Encounter (for), adjustment
    (of)
  prosthesis, external — *see* Fitting
  reaction — *see* Disorder, adjustment
Administration of tPA (rtPA) in a different facility within
    the last 24 hours prior to admission to current facil-
    ity Z92.82
Admission (for) (*see also* Encounter (for))
  adjustment (of)
    artificial
      arm Z44.00- ☑
        complete Z44.01- ☑
        partial Z44.02- ☑
      eye Z44.2 ☑
      leg Z44.10- ☑
        complete Z44.11- ☑
        partial Z44.12- ☑
    brain neuropacemaker Z46.2
      implanted Z45.42
    breast
      implant Z45.81 ☑
      prosthesis (external) Z44.3 ☑
    colostomy belt Z46.89
    contact lenses Z46.0
    cystostomy device Z46.6
    dental prosthesis Z46.3
    device NEC
      abdominal Z46.89
      implanted Z45.89
        cardiac Z45.09
          defibrillator (with synchronous cardiace
            pacemaker) Z45.02
          pacemaker Z45.018
            pulse generator Z45.010
        hearing device Z45.328
          bone conduction Z45.320
          cochlear Z45.321
        infusion pump Z45.1
        nervous system Z45.49
          CSF drainage Z45.41
          hearing device — *see* Admission, adjust-
            ment, device, implanted, hearing
            device
          neuropacemaker Z45.42
          visual substitution Z45.31
        specified NEC Z45.89
        vascular access Z45.2
        visual substitution Z45.31
      nervous system Z46.2
        implanted — *see* Admission, adjustment,
          device, implanted, nervous system
      orthodontic Z46.4
      prosthetic Z44.9
        arm — *see* Admission, adjustment, artificial,
          arm
        breast Z44.3 ☑
        dental Z46.3
        eye Z44.2 ☑
        leg — *see* Admission, adjustment, artificial,
          leg
        specified type NEC Z44.8
    substitution
      auditory Z46.2

Admission — *continued*
  adjustment — *continued*
    device — *continued*
      substitution — *continued*
        auditory — *continued*
          implanted — *see* Admission, adjust-
            ment, device, implanted, hearing
            device
        nervous system Z46.2
          implanted — *see* Admission, adjust-
            ment, device, implanted, nervous
            system
        visual Z46.2
          implanted Z45.31
    urinary Z46.6
    hearing aid Z46.1
      implanted — *see* Admission, adjustment, de-
        vice, implanted, hearing device
    ileostomy device Z46.89
    intestinal appliance or device NEC Z46.89
    neuropacemaker (brain) (peripheral nerve) (spinal
      cord) Z46.2
      implanted Z45.42
    orthodontic device Z46.4
    orthopedic (brace) (cast) (device) (shoes) Z46.89
    pacemaker
      cardiac Z45.018
        pulse generator Z45.010
      nervous system Z46.2
        implanted Z45.42
    portacath (port-a-cath) Z45.2
    prosthesis Z44.9
      arm — *see* Admission, adjustment, artificial,
        arm
      breast Z44.3 ☑
      dental Z46.3
      eye Z44.2 ☑
      leg — *see* Admission, adjustment, artificial, leg
      specified NEC Z44.8
    spectacles Z46.0
  aftercare (*see also* Aftercare) Z51.89
    postpartum
      immediately after delivery Z39.0
      routine follow-up Z39.2
    radiation therapy (antineoplastic) Z51.0
  attention to artificial opening (of) Z43.9
    artificial vagina Z43.7
    colostomy Z43.3
    cystostomy Z43.5
    enterostomy Z43.4
    gastrostomy Z43.1
    ileostomy Z43.2
    jejunostomy Z43.4
    nephrostomy Z43.6
    specified site NEC Z43.8
      intestinal tract Z43.4
      urinary tract Z43.6
    tracheostomy Z43.0
    ureterostomy Z43.6
    urethrostomy Z43.6
  breast augmentation or reduction Z41.1
  breast reconstruction following mastectomy Z42.1
  change of
    dressing (nonsurgical) Z48.00
    neuropacemaker device (brain) (peripheral nerve)
      (spinal cord) Z46.2
      implanted Z45.42
    surgical dressing Z48.01
  circumcision, ritual or routine (in absence of diagnosis)
    Z41.2
  clinical research investigation (control) (normal com-
    parison) (participant) Z00.6
  contraceptive management Z30.9
  cosmetic surgery NEC Z41.1
  counseling (*see also* Counseling)
    dietary Z71.3
    HIV Z71.7
    human immunodeficiency virus Z71.7
    nonattending third party Z71.0
    procreative management NEC Z31.69
  delivery, full-term, uncomplicated O80
    cesarean, without indication O82
  dietary surveillance and counseling Z71.3
  ear piercing Z41.3
  examination at health care facility (adult) (*see also*
    Examination) Z00.00
    with abnormal findings Z00.01

Admission — *continued*
  examination at health care facility (*see also* Examina-
    tion) — *continued*
    clinical research investigation (control) (normal
      comparison) (participant) Z00.6
    dental Z01.20
      with abnormal findings Z01.21
    donor (potential) Z00.5
    ear Z01.10
      with abnormal findings NEC Z01.118
    eye Z01.00
      with abnormal findings Z01.01
    general, specified reason NEC Z00.8
    hearing Z01.10
      with abnormal findings NEC Z01.118
    postpartum checkup Z39.2
    psychiatric (general) Z00.8
      requested by authority Z04.6
    vision Z01.00
      with abnormal findings Z01.01
  fitting (of)
    artificial
      arm — *see* Admission, adjustment, artificial,
        arm
      eye Z44.2 ☑
      leg — *see* Admission, adjustment, artificial, leg
    brain neuropacemaker Z46.2
      implanted Z45.42
    breast prosthesis (external) Z44.3 ☑
    colostomy belt Z46.89
    contact lenses Z46.0
    cystostomy device Z46.6
    dental prosthesis Z46.3
    dentures Z46.3
    device NEC
      abdominal Z46.89
      nervous system Z46.2
        implanted — *see* Admission, adjustment,
          device, implanted, nervous system
      orthodontic Z46.4
      prosthetic Z44.9
        breast Z44.3 ☑
        dental Z46.3
        eye Z44.2 ☑
      substitution
        auditory Z46.2
          implanted — *see* Admission, adjust-
            ment, device, implanted, hearing
            device
        nervous system Z46.2
          implanted — *see* Admission, adjust-
            ment, device, implanted, nervous
            system
        visual Z46.2
          implanted Z45.31
    hearing aid Z46.1
    ileostomy device Z46.89
    intestinal appliance or device NEC Z46.89
    neuropacemaker (brain) (peripheral nerve) (spinal
      cord) Z46.2
      implanted Z45.42
    orthodontic device Z46.4
    orthopedic device (brace) (cast) (shoes) Z46.89
    prosthesis Z44.9
      arm — *see* Admission, adjustment, artificial,
        arm
      breast Z44.3 ☑
      dental Z46.3
      eye Z44.2 ☑
      leg — *see* Admission, adjustment, artificial, leg
      specified type NEC Z44.8
    spectacles Z46.0
  follow-up examination Z09
  intrauterine device management Z30.431
    initial prescription Z30.014
  mental health evaluation Z00.8
    requested by authority Z04.6
  observation — *see* Observation
  Papanicolaou smear, cervix Z12.4
    for suspected malignant neoplasm Z12.4
  plastic and reconstructive surgery following medical
    procedure or healed injury NEC Z42.8
  plastic surgery, cosmetic NEC Z41.1
  postpartum observation
    immediately after delivery Z39.0
    routine follow-up Z39.2
  poststerilization (for restoration) Z31.0
    aftercare Z31.42

Admission — *continued*
  procreative management Z31.9
  prophylactic (measure)
    organ removal Z40.00
      breast Z40.01
      ovary Z40.02
      specified organ NEC Z40.09
      testes Z40.09
    vaccination Z23
  psychiatric examination (general) Z00.8
    requested by authority Z04.6
  radiation therapy (antineoplastic) Z51.0
  reconstructive surgery following medical procedure or healed injury NEC Z42.8
  removal of
    cystostomy catheter Z43.5
    drains Z48.03
    dressing (nonsurgical) Z48.00
    intrauterine contraceptive device Z30.432
    neuropacemaker (brain) (peripheral nerve) (spinal cord) Z46.2
      implanted Z45.42
    staples Z48.02
    surgical dressing Z48.01
    sutures Z48.02
    ureteral stent Z46.6
  respirator [ventilator] use during power failure Z99.12
  restoration of organ continuity (poststerilization) Z31.0
    aftercare Z31.42
  sensitivity test (*see also* Test, skin)
    allergy NEC Z01.82
    Mantoux Z11.1
  tuboplasty following previous sterilization Z31.0
    aftercare Z31.42
  vasoplasty following previous sterilization Z31.0
    aftercare Z31.42
  vision examination Z01.00
    with abnormal findings Z01.01
  waiting period for admission to other facility Z75.1
Adnexitis (suppurative) — *see* Salpingo-oophoritis
Adolescent X-linked adrenoleukodystrophy E71.521
Adrenal (gland) — *see* condition
Adrenalism, tuberculous A18.7
Adrenalitis, adrenitis E27.8
  autoimmune E27.1
  meningococcal, hemorrhagic A39.1
Adrenarche, premature E27.0
Adrenocortical syndrome — *see* Cushing's, syndrome
Adrenogenital syndrome E25.9
  acquired E25.8
  congenital E25.0
  salt loss E25.0
Adrenogenitalism, congenital E25.0
Adrenoleukodystrophy E71.529
  neonatal E71.511
  X-linked E71.529
    Addison only phenotype E71.528
    Addison-Schilder E71.528
    adolescent E71.521
    adrenomyeloneuropathy E71.522
    childhood cerebral E71.520
    other specified E71.528
Adrenomyeloneuropathy E71.522
Adventitious bursa — *see* Bursopathy, specified type NEC
Adverse effect — *see* Table of Drugs and Chemicals, categories T36-T50, with 6th character 5
Advice — *see* Counseling
Adynamia (episodica) (hereditary) (periodic) G72.3
Aeration lung imperfect, newborn — *see* Atelectasis
Aero-otitis media T70.0 ☑
Aerobullosis T70.3 ☑
Aerocele — *see* Embolism, air
Aerodermectasia
  subcutaneous (traumatic) T79.7 ☑
Aerodontalgia T70.29 ☑
Aeroembolism T70.3 ☑
Aerogenes capsulatus infection A48.0
Aerophagy, aerophagia (psychogenic) F45.8
Aerophobia F40.228
Aerosinusitis T70.1 ☑
Aerotitis T70.0 ☑
Affection — *see* Disease
Afibrinogenemia (*see also* Defect, coagulation) D68.8
  acquired D65
  congenital D68.2
  following ectopic or molar pregnancy O08.1

Afibrinogenemia — *continued*
  in abortion — *see* Abortion, by type, complicated by, afibrinogenemia
  puerperal O72.3
African
  sleeping sickness B56.9
  tick fever A68.1
  trypanosomiasis B56.9
    gambian B56.0
    rhodesian B56.1
After-cataract — *see* Cataract, secondary
Aftercare (*see also* Care) Z51.89
  following surgery (for) (on)
    amputation Z47.81
    attention to
      drains Z48.03
      dressings (nonsurgical) Z48.00
        surgical Z48.01
      sutures Z48.02
    circulatory system Z48.812
    delayed (planned) wound closure Z48.1
    digestive system Z48.815
    explantation of joint prosthesis (staged procedure)
      hip Z47.32
      knee Z47.33
      shoulder Z47.31
    genitourinary system Z48.816
    joint replacement Z47.1
    neoplasm Z48.3
    nervous system Z48.811
    oral cavity Z48.814
    organ transplant
      bone marrow Z48.290
      heart Z48.21
      heart-lung Z48.280
      kidney Z48.22
      liver Z48.23
      lung Z48.24
      multiple organs NEC Z48.288
      specified NEC Z48.298
    orthopedic NEC Z47.89
    planned wound closure Z48.1
    removal of internal fixation device Z47.2
    respiratory system Z48.813
    scoliosis Z47.82
    sense organs Z48.810
    skin and subcutaneous tissue Z48.817
    specified body system
      circulatory Z48.812
      digestive Z48.815
      genitourinary Z48.816
      nervous Z48.811
      oral cavity Z48.814
      respiratory Z48.813
      sense organs Z48.810
      skin and subcutaneous tissue Z48.817
      teeth Z48.814
    specified NEC Z48.89
    spinal Z48.89
    teeth Z48.814
  fracture — *code to* fracture with seventh character D
  involving
    removal of
      drains Z48.03
      dressings (nonsurgical) Z48.00
      staples Z48.02
      surgical dressings Z48.01
      sutures Z48.02
  neuropacemaker (brain) (peripheral nerve) (spinal cord) Z46.2
    implanted Z45.42
  orthopedic NEC Z47.89
  postprocedural — *see* Aftercare, following surgery
Agalactia (primary) O92.3
  elective, secondary or therapeutic O92.5
Agammaglobulinemia (acquired (secondary)) (nonfamilial) D80.1
  with
    immunoglobulin-bearing B-lymphocytes D80.1
    lymphopenia D81.9
  autosomal recessive (Swiss type) D80.0
  Bruton's X-linked D80.0
  common variable (CVAgamma) D80.1
  congenital sex-linked D80.0
  hereditary D80.0
  lymphopenic D81.9
  Swiss type (autosomal recessive) D80.0

Agammaglobulinemia — *continued*
  X-linked (with growth hormone deficiency)(Bruton) D80.0
Aganglionosis (bowel) (colon) Q43.1
Age (old) — *see* Senility
Agenesis
  adrenal (gland) Q89.1
  alimentary tract (complete) (partial) NEC Q45.8
    upper Q40.8
  anus, anal (canal) Q42.3
    with fistula Q42.2
  aorta Q25.4
  appendix Q42.8
  arm (complete) Q71.0- ☑
    with hand present Q71.1- ☑
  artery (peripheral) Q27.9
    brain Q28.3
    coronary Q24.5
    pulmonary Q25.79
    specified NEC Q27.8
    umbilical Q27.0
  auditory (canal) (external) Q16.1
  auricle (ear) Q16.0
  bile duct or passage Q44.5
  bladder Q64.5
  bone Q79.9
  brain Q00.0
    part of Q04.3
  breast (with nipple present) Q83.8
    with absent nipple Q83.0
  bronchus Q32.4
  canaliculus lacrimalis Q10.4
  carpus — *see* Agenesis, hand
  cartilage Q79.9
  cecum Q42.8
  cerebellum Q04.3
  cervix Q51.5
  chin Q18.8
  cilia Q10.3
  circulatory system, part NOS Q28.9
  clavicle Q74.0
  clitoris Q52.6
  coccyx Q76.49
  colon Q42.9
    specified NEC Q42.8
  corpus callosum Q04.0
  cricoid cartilage Q31.8
  diaphragm (with hernia) Q79.1
  digestive organ(s) or tract (complete) (partial) NEC Q45.8
    upper Q40.8
  ductus arteriosus Q28.8
  duodenum Q41.0
  ear Q16.9
    auricle Q16.0
    lobe Q17.8
  ejaculatory duct Q55.4
  endocrine (gland) NEC Q89.2
  epiglottis Q31.8
  esophagus Q39.8
  eustachian tube Q16.2
  eye Q11.1
    adnexa Q15.8
  eyelid (fold) Q10.3
  face
    bones NEC Q75.8
    specified part NEC Q18.8
  fallopian tube Q50.6
  femur — *see* Defect, reduction, lower limb, longitudinal, femur
  fibula — *see* Defect, reduction, lower limb, longitudinal, fibula
  finger (complete) (partial) — *see* Agenesis, hand
  foot (and toes) (complete) (partial) Q72.3- ☑
  forearm (with hand present) — *see* Agenesis, arm, with hand present
    and hand Q71.2- ☑
  gallbladder Q44.0
  gastric Q40.2
  genitalia, genital (organ(s))
    female Q52.8
      external Q52.71
      internal NEC Q52.8
    male Q55.8
  glottis Q31.8
  hair Q84.0
  hand (and fingers) (complete) (partial) Q71.3- ☑
  heart Q24.8

Agenesis — continued
  heart — continued
    valve NEC Q24.8
      pulmonary Q22.0
  hepatic Q44.7
  humerus — see Defect, reduction, upper limb
  hymen Q52.4
  ileum Q41.2
  incus Q16.3
  intestine (small) Q41.9
    large Q42.9
      specified NEC Q42.8
  iris (dilator fibers) Q13.1
  jaw M26.09
  jejunum Q41.1
  kidney(s) (partial) Q60.2
    bilateral Q60.1
    unilateral Q60.0
  labium (majus) (minus) Q52.71
  labyrinth, membranous Q16.5
  lacrimal apparatus Q10.4
  larynx Q31.8
  leg (complete) Q72.0- ☑
    with foot present Q72.1- ☑
    lower leg (with foot present) — see Agenesis, leg,
      with foot present
      and foot Q72.2- ☑
  lens Q12.3
  limb (complete) Q73.0
    lower — see Agenesis, leg
    upper — see Agenesis, arm
  lip Q38.0
  liver Q44.7
  lung (fissure) (lobe) (bilateral) (unilateral) Q33.3
  mandible, maxilla M26.09
  metacarpus — see Agenesis, hand
  metatarsus — see Agenesis, foot
  muscle Q79.8
    eyelid Q10.3
    ocular Q15.8
  musculoskeletal system NEC Q79.8
  nail(s) Q84.3
  neck, part Q18.8
  nerve Q07.8
  nervous system, part NEC Q07.8
  nipple Q83.2
  nose Q30.1
  nuclear Q07.8
  organ
    of Corti Q16.5
    or site not listed — see Anomaly, by site
  osseous meatus (ear) Q16.1
  ovary
    bilateral Q50.02
    unilateral Q50.01
  oviduct Q50.6
  pancreas Q45.0
  parathyroid (gland) Q89.2
  parotid gland(s) Q38.4
  patella Q74.1
  pelvic girdle (complete) (partial) Q74.2
  penis Q55.5
  pericardium Q24.8
  pituitary (gland) Q89.2
  prostate Q55.4
  punctum lacrimale Q10.4
  radioulnar — see Defect, reduction, upper limb
  radius — see Defect, reduction, upper limb, longitudinal, radius
  rectum Q42.1
    with fistula Q42.0
  renal Q60.2
    bilateral Q60.1
    unilateral Q60.0
  respiratory organ NEC Q34.8
  rib Q76.6
  roof of orbit Q75.8
  round ligament Q52.8
  sacrum Q76.49
  salivary gland Q38.4
  scapula Q74.0
  scrotum Q55.29
  seminal vesicles Q55.4
  septum
    atrial Q21.1
    between aorta and pulmonary artery Q21.4
    ventricular Q20.4
  shoulder girdle (complete) (partial) Q74.0

Agenesis — continued
  skull (bone) Q75.8
    with
      anencephaly Q00.0
      encephalocele — see Encephalocele
      hydrocephalus Q03.9
        with spina bifida — see Spina bifida, by site, with hydrocephalus
      microcephaly Q02
  spermatic cord Q55.4
  spinal cord Q06.0
  spine Q76.49
  spleen Q89.01
  sternum Q76.7
  stomach Q40.2
  submaxillary gland(s) (congenital) Q38.4
  tarsus — see Agenesis, foot
  tendon Q79.8
  testicle Q55.0
  thymus (gland) Q89.2
  thyroid (gland) E03.1
    cartilage Q31.8
  tibia — see Defect, reduction, lower limb, longitudinal, tibia
  tibiofibular — see Defect, reduction, lower limb, specified type NEC
  toe (and foot) (complete) (partial) — see Agenesis, foot
  tongue Q38.3
  trachea (cartilage) Q32.1
  ulna — see Defect, reduction, upper limb, longitudinal, ulna
  upper limb — see Agenesis, arm
  ureter Q62.4
  urethra Q64.5
  urinary tract NEC Q64.8
  uterus Q51.0
  uvula Q38.5
  vagina Q52.0
  vas deferens Q55.4
  vein(s) (peripheral) Q27.9
    brain Q28.3
    great NEC Q26.8
    portal Q26.5
  vena cava (inferior) (superior) Q26.8
  vermis of cerebellum Q04.3
  vertebra Q76.49
  vulva Q52.71
Ageusia R43.2
Agitated — see condition
Agitation R45.1
Aglossia (congenital) Q38.3
Aglossia-adactylia syndrome Q87.0
Aglycogenosis E74.00
Agnosia (body image) (other senses) (tactile) R48.1
  developmental F88
  verbal R48.1
    auditory R48.1
      developmental F80.2
    developmental F80.2
  visual (object) R48.3
Agoraphobia F40.00
  with panic disorder F40.01
  without panic disorder F40.02
Agrammatism R48.8
Agranulocytopenia — see Agranulocytosis
Agranulocytosis (chronic) (cyclical) (genetic) (infantile) (periodic) (pernicious) (see also Neutropenia) D70.9
  congenital D70.0
  cytoreductive cancer chemotherapy sequela D71.1
  drug-induced D70.2
    due to cytoreductive cancer chemotherapy D71.1
  due to infection D70.3
  secondary D70.4
    drug-induced D70.2
      due to cytoreductive cancer chemotherapy D71.1
Agraphia (absolute) R48.8
  with alexia R48.0
  developmental F81.81
Ague (dumb) — see Malaria
Agyria Q04.3
Ahumada-del Castillo syndrome E23.0
Aichomophobia F40.298
AIDS (related complex) B20
Ailment heart — see Disease, heart
Ailurophobia F40.218
Ainhum (disease) L94.6

AIPHI (acute idiopathic pulmonary hemorrhage in infants (over 28 days old)) R04.81
Air
  anterior mediastinum J98.2
  compressed, disease T70.3 ☑
  conditioner lung or pneumonitis J67.7
  embolism (artery) (cerebral) (any site) T79.0 ☑
    with ectopic or molar pregnancy O08.2
    due to implanted device NEC — see Complications, by site and type, specified NEC
    following
      abortion — see Abortion by type, complicated by, embolism
      ectopic or molar pregnancy O08.2
      infusion, therapeutic injection or transfusion T80.0 ☑
    in pregnancy, childbirth or puerperium — see Embolism, obstetric
    traumatic T79.0 ☑
  hunger, psychogenic F45.8
  rarefied, effects of — see Effect, adverse, high altitude
  sickness T75.3 ☑
Airplane sickness T75.3 ☑
Akathisia (drug-induced) (treatment-induced) G25.71
  neuroleptic induced (acute) G25.71
Akinesia R29.898
Akinetic mutism R41.89
Akureyri's disease G93.3
Alactasia, congenital E73.0
Alagille's syndrome Q44.7
Alastrim B03
Albers-Schönberg syndrome Q78.2
Albert's syndrome — see Tendinitis, Achilles
Albinism, albino E70.30
  with hematologic abnormality E70.339
    Chédiak-Higashi syndrome E70.330
    Hermansky-Pudlak syndrome E70.331
    other specified E70.338
  I E70.320
  II E70.321
  ocular E70.319
    autosomal recessive E70.311
    other specified E70.318
    X-linked E70.310
  oculocutaneous E70.329
    other specified E70.328
    tyrosinase (ty) negative E70.320
    tyrosinase (ty) positive E70.321
  other specified E70.39
Albinismus E70.30
Albright (-McCune)(-Sternberg) syndrome Q78.1
Albuminous — see condition
Albuminuria, albuminuric (acute) (chronic) (subacute) (see also Proteinuria) R80.9
  complicating pregnancy — see Proteinuria, gestational
    with
      gestational hypertension — see Pre-eclampsia
      pre-existing hypertension — see Hypertension, complicating pregnancy, pre-existing, with, pre-eclampsia
  gestational — see Proteinuria, gestational
    with
      gestational hypertension — see Pre-eclampsia
      pre-existing hypertension — see Hypertension, complicating pregnancy, pre-existing, with, pre-eclampsia
  orthostatic R80.2
  postural R80.2
  pre-eclamptic — see Pre-eclampsia
  scarlatinal A38.8
Albuminurophobia F40.298
Alcaptonuria E70.29
Alcohol, alcoholic, alcohol-induced
  addiction (without remission) F10.20
    with remission F10.21
  amnestic disorder, persisting F10.96
    with dependence F10.26
  brain syndrome, chronic F10.97
    with dependence F10.27
  cardiopathy I42.6
  counseling and surveillance Z71.41
    family member Z71.42
  delirium (acute) (tremens) (withdrawal) F10.231
    with intoxication F10.921
    in
      abuse F10.121
      dependence F10.221

Alcohol, alcoholic, alcohol-induced — continued
  dementia F10.97
    with dependence F10.27
  deterioration F10.97
    with dependence F10.27
  hallucinosis (acute) F10.951
    in
      abuse F10.151
      dependence F10.251
  insanity F10.959
  intoxication (acute) (without dependence) F10.129
    with
      delirium F10.121
      dependence F10.229
        with delirium F10.221
        uncomplicated F10.220
      uncomplicated F10.120
  jealousy F10.988
  Korsakoff's, Korsakov's, Korsakow's F10.26
  liver K70.9
    acute — see Disease, liver, alcoholic, hepatitis
  mania (acute) (chronic) F10.959
  paranoia, paranoid (type) psychosis F10.950
  pellagra E52
  poisoning, accidental (acute) NEC — see Table of Drugs
    and Chemicals, alcohol, poisoning
  psychosis — see Psychosis, alcoholic
  withdrawal (without convulsions) F10.239
    with delirium F10.231
Alcoholism (chronic) (without remission) F10.20
  with
    psychosis — see Psychosis, alcoholic
    remission F10.21
  Korsakov's F10.96
    with dependence F10.26
Alder (-Reilly) **anomaly or syndrome** (leukocyte granulation) D72.0
Aldosteronism E26.9
  familial (type I) E26.02
  glucocorticoid-remediable E26.02
  primary (due to) (bilateral) adrenal hyperplasia E26.09
  primary NEC E26.09
  secondary E26.1
  specified NEC E26.89
Aldosteronoma D44.10
Aldrich (-Wiskott) **syndrome** (eczema-thrombocytopenia) D82.0
Alektorophobia F40.218
Aleppo boil B55.1
Aleukemic — see condition
Aleukia
  congenital D70.0
  hemorrhagica D61.9
    congenital D61.09
  splenica D73.1
Alexia R48.0
  developmental F81.0
  secondary to organic lesion R48.0
Algoneurodystrophy M89.00
  ankle M89.07- ☑
  foot M89.07- ☑
  forearm M89.03- ☑
  hand M89.04- ☑
  lower leg M89.06- ☑
  multiple sites M89.0- ☑
  shoulder M89.01- ☑
  specified site NEC M89.08
  thigh M89.05- ☑
  upper arm M89.02- ☑
Algophobia F40.298
Alienation, mental — see Psychosis
Alkalemia E87.3
Alkalosis E87.3
  metabolic E87.3
    with respiratory acidosis E87.4
  respiratory E87.3
Alkaptonuria E70.29
Allen-Masters syndrome N83.8
Allergy, allergic (reaction) (to) T78.40 ☑
  air-borne substance NEC (rhinitis) J30.89
  alveolitis (extrinsic) J67.9
    due to
      Aspergillus clavatus J67.4
      Cryptostroma corticale J67.6
      organisms (fungal, thermophilic actinomycete)
        growing in ventilation (air conditioning)
        systems J67.7

Allergy, allergic — continued
  alveolitis — continued
    specified type NEC J67.8
  anaphylactic reaction or shock T78.2 ☑
  angioneurotic edema T78.3 ☑
  animal (dander) (epidermal) (hair) (rhinitis) J30.81
  bee sting (anaphylactic shock) — see Toxicity, venom,
    arthropod, bee
  biological — see Allergy, drug
  colitis K52.2
  dander (animal) (rhinitis) J30.81
  dandruff (rhinitis) J30.81
  dental restorative material (existing) K08.55
  dermatitis — see Dermatitis, contact, allergic
  diathesis — see History, allergy
  drug, medicament & biological (any) (external) (internal) T78.40 ☑
    correct substance properly administered — see
      Table of Drugs and Chemicals, by drug, adverse effect
    wrong substance given or taken NEC (by accident)
      — see Table of Drugs and Chemicals, by
      drug, poisoning
  due to pollen J30.1
  dust (house) (stock) (rhinitis) J30.89
    with asthma — see Asthma, allergic extrinsic
  eczema — see Dermatitis, contact, allergic
  epidermal (animal) (rhinitis) J30.81
  feathers (rhinitis) J30.89
  food (any) (ingested) NEC T78.1 ☑
    anaphylactic shock — see Shock, anaphylactic, due
      to food
    dermatitis — see Dermatitis, due to, food
    dietary counseling and surveillance Z71.3
    in contact with skin L23.6
    rhinitis J30.5
    status (without reaction) Z91.018
      eggs Z91.012
      milk products Z91.011
      peanuts Z91.010
      seafood Z91.013
      specified NEC Z91.018
  gastrointestinal K52.2
  grain J30.1
  grass (hay fever) (pollen) J30.1
    asthma — see Asthma, allergic extrinsic
  hair (animal) (rhinitis) J30.81
  history (of) — see History, allergy
  horse serum — see Allergy, serum
  inhalant (rhinitis) J30.89
    pollen J30.1
  kapok (rhinitis) J30.89
  medicine — see Allergy, drug
  milk protein K52.2
  nasal, seasonal due to pollen J30.1
  pneumonia J82
  pollen (any) (hay fever) J30.1
    asthma — see Asthma, allergic extrinsic
  primrose J30.1
  primula J30.1
  purpura D69.0
  ragweed (hay fever) (pollen) J30.1
    asthma — see Asthma, allergic extrinsic
  rose (pollen) J30.1
  seasonal NEC J30.2
  Senecio jacobae (pollen) J30.1
  serum (see also Reaction, serum) T80.69 ☑
    anaphylactic shock T80.59 ☑
  shock (anaphylactic) T78.2 ☑
    due to
      administration of blood and blood products
        T80.51 ☑
      adverse effect of correct medicinal substance
        properly administered T88.6 ☑
      immunization T80.52 ☑
      serum NEC T80.59 ☑
      vaccination T80.52 ☑
  specific NEC T78.49 ☑
  tree (any) (hay fever) (pollen) J30.1
    asthma — see Asthma, allergic extrinsic
  upper respiratory J30.9
  urticaria L50.0
  vaccine — see Allergy, serum
  wheat — see Allergy, food
Allescheriasis B48.2
Alligator skin disease Q80.9
Allocheiria, allochiria R20.8

Almeida's disease — see Paracoccidioidomycosis
Alopecia (hereditaria) (seborrheica) L65.9
  androgenic L64.9
    drug-induced L64.0
    specified NEC L64.8
  areata L63.9
    ophiasis L63.2
    specified NEC L63.8
    totalis L63.0
    universalis L63.1
  cicatricial L66.9
    specified NEC L66.8
  circumscripta L63.9
  congenital, congenitalis Q84.0
  due to cytotoxic drugs NEC L65.8
  mucinosa L65.2
  postinfective NEC L65.8
  postpartum L65.0
  premature L64.8
  specific (syphilitic) A51.32
  specified NEC L65.8
  syphilitic (secondary) A51.32
  totalis (capitis) L63.0
  universalis (entire body) L63.1
  X-ray L58.1
Alpers' disease G31.81
Alpine sickness T70.29 ☑
Alport syndrome Q87.81
ALTE (apparent life threatening event) **in newborn and
    infant** R68.13
Alteration (of), **Altered**
  awareness, transient R40.4
  mental status R41.82
  pattern of family relationships affecting child Z62.898
  sensation
    following
      cerebrovascular disease I69.998
        cerebral infarction I69.398
        intracerebral hemorrhage I69.198
        nontraumatic intracranial hemorrhage NEC
          I69.298
        specified disease NEC I69.898
        subarachnoid hemorrhage I69.098
Alternating — see condition
Altitude, high (effects) — see Effect, adverse, high altitude
Aluminosis (of lung) J63.0
Alveolitis
  allergic (extrinsic) — see Pneumonitis, hypersensitivity
  due to
    Aspergillus clavatus J67.4
    Cryptostroma corticale J67.6
  fibrosing (cryptogenic) (idiopathic) J84.112
  jaw M27.3
  sicca dolorosa M27.3
Alveolus, alveolar — see condition
Alymphocytosis D72.810
  thymic (with immunodeficiency) D82.1
Alymphoplasia, thymic D82.1
Alzheimer's disease or sclerosis — see Disease,
    Alzheimer's
Amastia (with nipple present) Q83.8
  with absent nipple Q83.0
Amathophobia F40.228
Amaurosis (acquired) (congenital) (see also Blindness)
  fugax G45.3
  hysterical F44.6
  Leber's congenital H35.50
  uremic — see Uremia
Amaurotic idiocy (infantile) (juvenile) (late) E75.4
Amaxophobia F40.248
Ambiguous genitalia Q56.4
Amblyopia (congenital) (ex anopsia) (partial) (suppression) H53.00- ☑
  anisometropic — see Amblyopia, refractive
  deprivation H53.01- ☑
  hysterical F44.6
  nocturnal (see also Blindness, night)
    vitamin A deficiency E50.5
  refractive H53.02- ☑
  strabismic H53.03- ☑
  tobacco H53.8
  toxic NEC H53.8
  uremic — see Uremia
Ameba, amebic (histolytica) (see also Amebiasis)
  abscess (liver) A06.4
Amebiasis A06.9

Amebiasis — *continued*
　with abscess — *see* Abscess, amebic
　acute A06.0
　chronic (intestine) A06.1
　　with abscess — *see* Abscess, amebic
　cutaneous A06.7
　cutis A06.7
　cystitis A06.81
　genitourinary tract NEC A06.82
　hepatic — *see* Abscess, liver, amebic
　intestine A06.0
　nondysenteric colitis A06.2
　skin A06.7
　specified site NEC A06.89
Ameboma (of intestine) A06.3
Amelia Q73.0
　lower limb — *see* Agenesis, leg
　upper limb — *see* Agenesis, arm
Ameloblastoma (*see also* Cyst, calcifying odontogenic)
　long bones C40.9- ☑
　　lower limb C40.2- ☑
　　upper limb C40.0- ☑
　malignant C41.1
　　jaw (bone) (lower) C41.1
　　　upper C41.0
　tibial C40.2- ☑
Amelogenesis imperfecta K00.5
　nonhereditaria (segmentalis) K00.4
Amenorrhea N91.2
　hyperhormonal E28.8
　primary N91.0
　secondary N91.1
Amentia — *see* Disability, intellectual
　Meynert's (nonalcoholic) F04
American
　leishmaniasis B55.2
　mountain tick fever A93.2
Ametropia — *see* Disorder, refraction
Amianthosis J61
Amimia R48.8
Amino-acid disorder E72.9
　anemia D53.0
Aminoacidopathy E72.9
Aminoaciduria E72.9
Amnesia R41.3
　anterograde R41.1
　auditory R48.8
　dissociative F44.0
　hysterical F44.0
　postictal in epilepsy — *see* Epilepsy
　psychogenic F44.0
　retrograde R41.2
　transient global G45.4
Amnes(t)ic syndrome (post-traumatic) F04
　induced by
　　alcohol F10.96
　　　with dependence F10.26
　　psychoactive NEC F19.96
　　　with
　　　　abuse F19.16
　　　　dependence F19.26
　　sedative F13.96
　　　with dependence F13.26
Amnion, amniotic — *see* condition
Amnionitis — *see* Pregnancy, complicated by
Amok F68.8
Amoral traits F60.89
Ampulla
　lower esophagus K22.8
　phrenic K22.8
Amputation (*see also* Absence, by site, acquired)
　neuroma (postoperative) (traumatic) — *see* Complications, amputation stump, neuroma
　stump (surgical)
　　abnormal, painful, or with complication (late) — *see* Complications, amputation stump
　　healed or old NOS Z89.9
　traumatic (complete) (partial)
　　arm (upper) (complete) S48.91- ☑
　　　at
　　　　elbow S58.01- ☑
　　　　　partial S58.02- ☑
　　　　shoulder joint (complete) S48.01- ☑
　　　　　partial S48.02- ☑
　　　　between
　　　　　elbow and wrist (complete) S58.11- ☑
　　　　　　partial S58.12- ☑

Amputation — *continued*
　traumatic — *continued*
　　arm — *continued*
　　　between — *continued*
　　　　shoulder and elbow (complete) S48.11- ☑
　　　　　partial S48.12- ☑
　　　partial S48.92- ☑
　　breast (complete) S28.21- ☑
　　　partial S28.22- ☑
　　clitoris (complete) S38.211 ☑
　　　partial S38.212 ☑
　　ear (complete) S08.11- ☑
　　　partial S08.12- ☑
　　finger (complete) (metacarpophalangeal)
　　　　S68.11- ☑
　　　index S68.11- ☑
　　　little S68.11- ☑
　　　middle S68.11- ☑
　　　partial S68.12- ☑
　　　　index S68.12- ☑
　　　　little S68.12- ☑
　　　　middle S68.12- ☑
　　　　ring S68.12- ☑
　　　ring S68.11- ☑
　　　thumb — *see* Amputation, traumatic, thumb
　　　transphalangeal (complete) S68.61- ☑
　　　　index S68.61- ☑
　　　　little S68.61- ☑
　　　　middle S68.61- ☑
　　　　partial S68.62- ☑
　　　　　index S68.62- ☑
　　　　　little S68.62- ☑
　　　　　middle S68.62- ☑
　　　　　ring S68.62- ☑
　　　　ring S68.61- ☑
　　foot (complete) S98.91- ☑
　　　at ankle level S98.01- ☑
　　　　partial S98.02- ☑
　　　midfoot S98.31- ☑
　　　　partial S98.32- ☑
　　　partial S98.92- ☑
　　forearm (complete) S58.91- ☑
　　　at elbow level (complete) S58.01- ☑
　　　　partial S58.02- ☑
　　　between elbow and wrist (complete) S58.11- ☑
　　　　partial S58.12- ☑
　　　partial S58.92- ☑
　　genital organ(s) (external)
　　　female (complete) S38.211 ☑
　　　　partial S38.212 ☑
　　　male
　　　　penis (complete) S38.221 ☑
　　　　　partial S38.222 ☑
　　　　scrotum (complete) S38.231 ☑
　　　　　partial S38.232 ☑
　　　　testes (complete) S38.231 ☑
　　　　　partial S38.232 ☑
　　hand (complete) (wrist level) S68.41- ☑
　　　finger(s) alone — *see* Amputation, traumatic, finger
　　　partial S68.42- ☑
　　　thumb alone — *see* Amputation, traumatic, thumb
　　　transmetacarpal (complete) S68.71- ☑
　　　　partial S68.72- ☑
　　head
　　　ear — *see* Amputation, traumatic, ear
　　　nose (partial) S08.812 ☑
　　　　complete S08.811 ☑
　　　part S08.89 ☑
　　　scalp S08.0 ☑
　　hip (and thigh) (complete) S78.91- ☑
　　　at hip joint (complete) S78.01- ☑
　　　　partial S78.02- ☑
　　　between hip and knee (complete) S78.11- ☑
　　　　partial S78.12- ☑
　　　partial S78.92- ☑
　　labium (majus) (minus) (complete) S38.21- ☑
　　　partial S38.21- ☑
　　leg (lower) S88.91- ☑
　　　at knee level S88.01- ☑
　　　　partial S88.02- ☑
　　　between knee and ankle S88.11- ☑
　　　　partial S88.12- ☑
　　　partial S88.92- ☑
　　nose (partial) S08.812 ☑

Amputation — *continued*
　traumatic — *continued*
　　nose — *continued*
　　　complete S08.811 ☑
　　　penis (complete) S38.221 ☑
　　　　partial S38.222 ☑
　　　scrotum (complete) S38.231 ☑
　　　　partial S38.232 ☑
　　　shoulder — *see* Amputation, traumatic, arm
　　　　at shoulder joint — *see* Amputation, traumatic, arm, at shoulder joint
　　　testes (complete) S38.231 ☑
　　　　partial S38.232 ☑
　　　thigh — *see* Amputation, traumatic, hip
　　　thorax, part of S28.1 ☑
　　　　breast — *see* Amputation, traumatic, breast
　　　thumb (complete) (metacarpophalangeal)
　　　　　S68.01- ☑
　　　　partial S68.02- ☑
　　　　transphalangeal (complete) S68.51- ☑
　　　　　partial S68.52- ☑
　　　toe (lesser) S98.13- ☑
　　　　great S98.11- ☑
　　　　　partial S98.12- ☑
　　　　more than one S98.21- ☑
　　　　　partial S98.22- ☑
　　　　partial S98.14- ☑
　　　vulva (complete) S38.211 ☑
　　　　partial S38.212 ☑
Amputee (bilateral) (old) Z89.9
Amsterdam dwarfism Q87.1
Amusia R48.8
　developmental F80.89
Amyelencephalus, amyelencephaly Q00.0
Amyelia Q06.0
Amygdalitis — *see* Tonsillitis
Amygdalolith J35.8
Amyloid heart (disease) E85.4 [I43]
Amyloidosis (generalized) (primary) E85.9
　with lung involvement E85.4 [J99]
　familial E85.2
　genetic E85.2
　heart E85.4 [I43]
　hemodialysis-associated E85.3
　liver E85.4 [K77]
　localized E85.4
　neuropathic heredofamilial E85.1
　non-neuropathic heredofamilial E85.0
　organ limited E85.4
　Portuguese E85.1
　pulmonary E85.4 [J99]
　secondary systemic E85.3
　skin (lichen) (macular) E85.4 [L99]
　specified NEC E85.8
　subglottic E85.4 [J99]
Amylopectinosis (brancher enzyme deficiency) E74.03
Amylophagia — *see* Pica
Amyoplasia congenita Q79.8
Amyotonia M62.89
　congenita G70.2
Amyotrophia, amyotrophy, amyotrophic G71.8
　congenita Q79.8
　diabetic — *see* Diabetes, amyotrophy
　lateral sclerosis G12.21
　neuralgic G54.5
　spinal progressive G12.21
Anacidity, gastric K31.83
　psychogenic F45.8
Anaerosis of newborn P28.89
Analbuminemia E88.09
Analgesia — *see* Anesthesia
Analphalipoproteinemia E78.6
Anaphylactic
　purpura D69.0
　shock or reaction — *see* Shock, anaphylactic
Anaphylactoid shock or reaction — *see* Shock, anaphylactic
Anaphylactoid syndrome of pregnancy O88.01- ☑
Anaphylaxis — *see* Shock, anaphylactic
Anaplasia cervix (*see also* Dysplasia, cervix) N87.9
Anaplasmosis, human A77.49
Anarthria R47.1
Anasarca R60.1
　cardiac — *see* Failure, heart, congestive
　lung J18.2
　newborn P83.2
　nutritional E43

Anasarca — *continued*
pulmonary J18.2
renal N04.9
Anastomosis
aneurysmal — *see* Aneurysm
arteriovenous ruptured brain I60.8
intestinal K63.89
complicated NEC K91.89
involving urinary tract N99.89
retinal and choroidal vessels (congenital) Q14.8
Anatomical narrow angle H40.03- ☑
Ancylostoma, ancylostomiasis (braziliense) (caninum) (ceylanicum) (duodenale) B76.0
Necator americanus B76.1
Andersen's disease (glycogen storage) E74.09
Anderson-Fabry disease E75.21
Andes disease T70.29 ☑
Andrews' disease (bacterid) L08.89
Androblastoma
benign
specified site — *see* Neoplasm, benign, by site
unspecified site
female D27.9
male D29.20
malignant
specified site — *see* Neoplasm, malignant, by site
unspecified site
female C56.9
male C62.90
specified site — *see* Neoplasm, uncertain behavior, by site
tubular
with lipid storage
specified site — *see* Neoplasm, benign, by site
unspecified site
female D27.9
male D29.20
specified site — *see* Neoplasm, benign, by site
unspecified site
female D27.9
male D29.20
unspecified site
female D39.10
male D40.10
Androgen insensitivity syndrome (*see also* Syndrome, androgen insensitivity) E34.50
Androgen resistance syndrome (*see also* Syndrome, androgen insensitivity) E34.50
Android pelvis Q74.2
with disproportion (fetopelvic) O33.3 ☑
causing obstructed labor O65.3
Androphobia F40.290
Anectasis, pulmonary (newborn) — *see* Atelectasis
Anemia (essential) (general) (hemoglobin deficiency) (infantile) (primary) (profound) D64.9
with (due to) (in)
disorder of
anaerobic glycolysis D55.2
pentose phosphate pathway D55.1
koilonychia D50.9
achlorhydric D50.8
achrestic D53.1
Addison (-Biermer) (pernicious) D51.0
agranulocytic — *see* Agranulocytosis
amino-acid-deficiency D53.0
aplastic D61.9
congenital D61.09
drug-induced D61.1
due to
drugs D61.1
external agents NEC D61.2
infection D61.2
radiation D61.2
idiopathic D61.3
red cell (pure) D60.9
chronic D60.0
congenital D61.01
specified type NEC D60.8
transient D60.1
specified type NEC D61.89
toxic D61.2
aregenerative
congenital D61.09
asiderotic D50.9
atypical (primary) D64.9
Baghdad spring D55.0
Balantidium coli A07.0
Biermer's (pernicious) D51.0

Anemia — *continued*
blood loss (chronic) D50.0
acute D62
bothriocephalus B70.0 [D63.8]
brickmaker's B76.9 [D63.8]
cerebral I67.89
childhood D58.9
chlorotic D50.8
chronic
blood loss D50.0
hemolytic D58.9
idiopathic D59.9
simple D53.9
chronica congenita aregenerativa D61.09
combined system disease NEC D51.0 [G32.0]
due to dietary vitamin B12 deficiency D51.3 [G32.0]
complicating pregnancy, childbirth or puerperium — *see* Pregnancy, complicated by (management affected by), anemia
congenital P61.4
aplastic D61.09
due to isoimmunization NOS P55.9
dyserythropoietic, dyshematopoietic D64.4
following fetal blood loss P61.3
Heinz body D58.2
hereditary hemolytic NOS D58.9
pernicious D51.0
spherocytic D58.0
Cooley's (erythroblastic) D56.1
cytogenic D51.0
deficiency D53.9
6-PGD D55.1
2, 3 diphosphoglycurate mutase D55.2
2, 3 PG D55.2
6 phosphogluconate dehydrogenase D55.1
amino-acid D53.0
combined B12 and folate D53.1
enzyme D55.9
drug-induced (hemolytic) D59.2
glucose-6-phosphate dehydrogenase (G6PD) D55.0
glycolytic D55.2
nucleotide metabolism D55.3
related to hexose monophosphate (HMP) shunt pathway NEC D55.1
specified type NEC D55.8
erythrocytic glutathione D55.1
folate D52.9
dietary D52.0
drug-induced D52.1
folic acid D52.9
dietary D52.0
drug-induced D52.1
G SH D55.1
G6PD D55.0
GGS-R D55.1
glucose-6-phosphate dehydrogenase D55.0
glutathione reductase D55.1
glyceraldehyde phosphate dehydrogenase D55.2
hexokinase D55.2
iron D50.9
secondary to blood loss (chronic) D50.0
nutritional D53.9
with
poor iron absorption D50.8
specified deficiency NEC D53.8
phosphofructo-aldolase D55.2
phosphoglycerate kinase D55.2
PK D55.2
protein D53.0
pyruvate kinase D55.2
transcobalamin II D51.2
triose-phosphate isomerase D55.2
vitamin B12 NOS D51.9
dietary D51.3
due to
intrinsic factor deficiency D51.0
selective vitamin B12 malabsorption with proteinuria D51.1
pernicious D51.0
specified type NEC D51.8
Diamond-Blackfan (congenital hypoplastic) D61.01
dibothriocephalus B70.0 [D63.8]
dimorphic D53.1
diphasic D53.1
Diphyllobothrium (Dibothriocephalus) B70.0 [D63.8]
due to (in) (with)
antineoplastic chemotherapy D64.81

Anemia — *continued*
due to — *continued*
blood loss (chronic) D50.0
acute D62
chemotherapy, antineoplastic D64.81
chronic disease classified elsewhere NEC D63.8
chronic kidney disease D63.1
deficiency
amino-acid D53.0
copper D53.8
folate (folic acid) D52.9
dietary D52.0
drug-induced D52.1
molybdenum D53.8
protein D53.0
zinc D53.8
dietary vitamin B12 deficiency D51.3
disorder of
glutathione metabolism D55.1
nucleotide metabolism D55.3
drug — *see* Anemia, by type (*see also* Table of Drugs and Chemicals)
end stage renal disease D63.1
enzyme disorder D55.9
fetal blood loss P61.3
fish tapeworm (D.latum) infestation B70.0 [D63.8]
hemorrhage (chronic) D50.0
acute D62
impaired absorption D50.9
loss of blood (chronic) D50.0
acute D62
myxedema E03.9 [D63.8]
Necator americanus B76.1 [D63.8]
prematurity P61.2
selective vitamin B12 malabsorption with proteinuria D51.1
transcobalamin II deficiency D51.2
Dyke-Young type (secondary) (symptomatic) D59.1
dyserythropoietic (congenital) D64.4
dyshematopoietic (congenital) D64.4
Egyptian B76.9 [D63.8]
elliptocytosis — *see* Elliptocytosis
enzyme-deficiency, drug-induced D59.2
epidemic (*see also* Ancylostomiasis) B76.9 [D63.8]
erythroblastic
familial D56.1
newborn (*see also* Disease, hemolytic) P55.9
of childhood D56.1
erythrocytic glutathione deficiency D55.1
erythropoietin-resistant anemia (EPO resistant anemia) D63.1
Faber's (achlorhydric anemia) D50.9
factitious (self-induced blood letting) D50.0
familial erythroblastic D56.1
Fanconi's (congenital pancytopenia) D61.09
favism D55.0
fish tapeworm (D. latum) infestation B70.0 [D63.8]
folate (folic acid) deficiency D52.9
glucose-6-phosphate dehydrogenase (G6PD) deficiency D55.0
glutathione-reductase deficiency D55.1
goat's milk D52.0
granulocytic — *see* Agranulocytosis
Heinz body, congenital D58.2
hemolytic D58.9
acquired D59.9
with hemoglobinuria NEC D59.6
autoimmune NEC D59.1
infectious D59.4
specified type NEC D59.8
toxic D59.4
acute D59.9
due to enzyme deficiency specified type NEC D55.8
Lederer's D59.1
autoimmune D59.1
drug-induced D59.0
chronic D58.9
idiopathic D59.9
cold type (secondary) (symptomatic) D59.1
congenital (spherocytic) — *see* Spherocytosis
due to
cardiac conditions D59.4
drugs (nonautoimmune) D59.2
autoimmune D59.0
enzyme disorder D55.9
drug-induced D59.2

☑ **Additional Character Required** — **Refer to the Tabular List for Character Selection** ▽ Subterms under main terms may continue to next column or page

Anemia — continued
  hemolytic — continued
    due to — continued
      presence of shunt or other internal prosthetic device D59.4
    familial D58.9
    hereditary D58.9
      due to enzyme disorder D55.9
        specified type NEC D55.8
      specified type NEC D58.8
    idiopathic (chronic) D59.9
    mechanical D59.4
    microangiopathic D59.4
    nonautoimmune D59.4
      drug-induced D59.2
    nonspherocytic
      congenital or hereditary NEC D55.8
        glucose-6-phosphate dehydrogenase deficiency D55.0
        pyruvate kinase deficiency D55.2
        type
          I D55.1
          II D55.2
      type
        I D55.1
        II D55.2
    secondary D59.4
      autoimmune D59.1
    specified (hereditary) type NEC D58.8
    Stransky-Regala type (see also Hemoglobinopathy) D58.8
    symptomatic D59.4
      autoimmune D59.1
    toxic D59.4
    warm type (secondary) (symptomatic) D59.1
  hemorrhagic (chronic) D50.0
    acute D62
  Herrick's D57.1
  hexokinase deficiency D55.2
  hookworm B76.9 [D63.8]
  hypochromic (idiopathic) (microcytic) (normoblastic) D50.9
    due to blood loss (chronic) D50.0
      acute D62
    familial sex-linked D64.0
    pyridoxine-responsive D64.3
    sideroblastic, sex-linked D64.0
  hypoplasia, red blood cells D61.9
    congenital or familial D61.01
  hypoplastic (idiopathic) D61.9
    congenital or familial (of childhood) D61.01
  hypoproliferative (refractive) D61.9
  idiopathic D64.9
    aplastic D61.3
    hemolytic, chronic D59.9
  in (due to) (with)
    chronic kidney disease D63.1
    end stage renal disease D63.1
    failure, kidney (renal) D63.1
    neoplastic disease (see also Neoplasm) D63.0
  intertropical (see also Ancylostomiasis) D63.8
  iron deficiency D50.9
    secondary to blood loss (chronic) D50.0
      acute D62
    specified type NEC D50.8
  Joseph-Diamond-Blackfan (congenital hypoplastic) D61.01
  Lederer's (hemolytic) D59.1
  leukoerythroblastic D61.82
  macrocytic D53.9
    nutritional D52.0
    tropical D52.8
  malarial (see also Malaria) B54 [D63.8]
  malignant (progressive) D51.0
  malnutrition D53.9
  marsh (see also Malaria) B54 [D63.8]
  Mediterranean (with other hemoglobinopathy) D56.9
  megaloblastic D53.1
    combined B12 and folate deficiency D53.1
    hereditary D51.1
    nutritional D52.0
    orotic aciduria D53.0
    refractory D53.1
    specified type NEC D53.1
  megalocytic D53.1
  microcytic (hypochromic) D50.9
    due to blood loss (chronic) D50.0
      acute D62

Anemia — continued
  microcytic — continued
    familial D56.8
  microdrepanocytosis D57.40
  microelliptopoikilocytic (Rietti-Greppi- Micheli) D56.9
  miner's B76.9 [D63.8]
  myelodysplastic D46.9
  myelofibrosis D75.81
  myelogenous D64.89
  myelopathic D64.89
  myelophthisic D61.82
  myeloproliferative D47.Z9 (following D47.4)
  newborn P61.4
    due to
      ABO (antibodies, isoimmunization, maternal/fetal incompatibility) P55.1
      Rh (antibodies, isoimmunization, maternal/fetal incompatibility) P55.0
    following fetal blood loss P61.3
    posthemorrhagic (fetal) P61.3
  nonspherocytic hemolytic — see Anemia, hemolytic, nonspherocytic
  normocytic (infectional) D64.9
    due to blood loss (chronic) D50.0
      acute D62
    myelophthisic D61.82
  nutritional (deficiency) D53.9
    with
      poor iron absorption D50.8
      specified deficiency NEC D53.8
    megaloblastic D52.0
  of prematurity P61.2
  orotaciduric (congenital) (hereditary) D53.0
  osteosclerotic D64.89
  ovalocytosis (hereditary) — see Elliptocytosis
  paludal (see also Malaria) B54 [D63.8]
  pernicious (congenital) (malignant) (progressive) D51.0
  pleochromic D64.89
    of sprue D52.8
  posthemorrhagic (chronic) D50.0
    acute D62
    newborn P61.3
  postoperative (postprocedural)
    due to (acute) blood loss D62
      chronic blood loss D50.0
    specified NEC D64.9
  postpartum O90.81
  pressure D64.89
  progressive D64.9
    malignant D51.0
    pernicious D51.0
  protein-deficiency D53.0
  pseudoleukemica infantum D64.89
  pure red cell D60.9
    congenital D61.01
  pyridoxine-responsive D64.3
  pyruvate kinase deficiency D55.2
  refractory D46.4
    with
      excess of blasts D46.20
        1 (RAEB 1) D46.21
        2 (RAEB 2) D46.22
        in transformation (RAEB T) — see Leukemia, acute myeloblastic
      hemochromatosis D46.1
      sideroblasts (ring) (RARS) D46.1
    without ring sideroblasts, so stated D46.0
    without sideroblasts without excess of blasts D46.0
    megaloblastic D53.1
    sideroblastic D46.1
    sideropenic D50.9
  Rietti-Greppi-Micheli D56.9
  scorbutic D53.2
  secondary to
    blood loss (chronic) D50.0
      acute D62
    hemorrhage (chronic) D50.0
      acute D62
  semiplastic D61.89
  sickle-cell — see Disease, sickle-cell
  sideroblastic D64.3
    hereditary D64.0
    hypochromic, sex-linked D64.0
    pyridoxine-responsive NEC D64.3
    refractory D46.1
    secondary (due to)
      disease D64.1
      drugs and toxins D64.2

Anemia — continued
  sideroblastic — continued
    specified type NEC D64.3
  sideropenic (refractory) D50.9
    due to blood loss (chronic) D50.0
      acute D62
  simple chronic D53.9
  specified type NEC D64.89
  spherocytic (hereditary) — see Spherocytosis
  splenic D64.89
  splenomegalic D64.89
  stomatocytosis D58.8
  syphilitic (acquired) (late) A52.79 [D63.8]
  target cell D64.89
  thalassemia D56.9
  thrombocytopenic — see Thrombocytopenia
  toxic D61.2
  tropical B76.9 [D63.8]
    macrocytic D52.8
  tuberculous A18.89 [D63.8]
  vegan D51.3
  vitamin
    B6-responsive D64.3
    B12 deficiency (dietary) pernicious D51.0
  von Jaksch's D64.89
  Witts' (achlorhydric anemia) D50.8
Anemophobia F40.228
Anencephalus, anencephaly Q00.0
Anergasia — see Psychosis, organic
Anesthesia, anesthetic R20.0
  complication or reaction NEC (see also Complications, anesthesia) T88.59 ☑
    due to
      correct substance properly administered — see Table of Drugs and Chemicals, by drug, adverse effect
      overdose or wrong substance given — see Table of Drugs and Chemicals, by drug, poisoning
  cornea H18.81- ☑
  dissociative F44.6
  functional (hysterical) F44.6
  hyperesthetic, thalamic G89.0
  hysterical F44.6
  local skin lesion R20.0
  sexual (psychogenic) F52.1
  shock (due to) T88.2 ☑
  skin R20.0
  testicular N50.9
Anetoderma (maculosum) (of) L90.8
  Jadassohn-Pellizzari L90.2
  Schweninger-Buzzi L90.1
Aneurin deficiency E51.9
Aneurysm (anastomotic) (artery) (cirsoid) (diffuse) (false) (fusiform) (multiple) (saccular) I72.9
  abdominal (aorta) I71.4
    ruptured I71.3
    syphilitic A52.01
  aorta, aortic (nonsyphilitic) I71.9
    abdominal I71.4
      ruptured I71.3
    arch I71.2
      ruptured I71.1
    arteriosclerotic I71.9
      ruptured I71.8
    ascending I71.2
      ruptured I71.1
    congenital Q25.4
    descending I71.9
      abdominal I71.4
        ruptured I71.3
      ruptured I71.8
      thoracic I71.2
        ruptured I71.1
    ruptured I71.8
    sinus, congenital Q25.4
    syphilitic A52.01
    thoracic I71.2
      ruptured I71.1
    thoracoabdominal I71.6
      ruptured I71.5
    thorax, thoracic (arch) I71.2
      ruptured I71.1
    transverse I71.2
      ruptured I71.1
    valve (heart) (see also Endocarditis, aortic) I35.8
  arteriosclerotic I72.9
    cerebral I67.1

Aneurysm — *continued*
  arteriosclerotic — *continued*
    cerebral — *continued*
      ruptured — *see* Hemorrhage, intracranial, subarachnoid
  arteriovenous (congenital) (*see also* Malformation, arteriovenous)
    acquired I77.0
      brain I67.1
      coronary I25.41
      pulmonary I28.0
    brain Q28.2
      ruptured I60.8
    peripheral — *see* Malformation, arteriovenous, peripheral
    precerebral vessels Q28.0
    specified site NEC (*see also* Malformation, arteriovenous)
      acquired I77.0
  basal — *see* Aneurysm, brain
  berry (congenital) (nonruptured) I67.1
    ruptured I60.7
  brain I67.1
    arteriosclerotic I67.1
      ruptured — *see* Hemorrhage, intracranial, subarachnoid
    arteriovenous (congenital) (nonruptured) Q28.2
      acquired I67.1
        ruptured I60.8
      ruptured I60.8
    berry (congenital) (nonruptured) I67.1
      ruptured (*see also* Hemorrhage, intracranial, subarachnoid) I60.7
    congenital Q28.3
      ruptured I60.7
    meninges I67.1
      ruptured I60.8
    miliary (congenital) (nonruptured) I67.1
      ruptured (*see also* Hemorrhage, intracranial, subarachnoid) I60.7
    mycotic I33.0
    ruptured — *see* Hemorrhage, intracranial, subarachnoid
    syphilitic (hemorrhage) A52.05
  cardiac (false) (*see also* Aneurysm, heart) I25.3
  carotid artery (common) (external) I72.0
    internal (intracranial) I67.1
      extracranial portion I72.0
      ruptured into brain I60.0- ☑
    syphilitic A52.09
      intracranial A52.05
  cavernous sinus I67.1
    arteriovenous (congenital) (nonruptured) Q28.3
      ruptured I60.8
  celiac I72.8
  central nervous system, syphilitic A52.05
  cerebral — *see* Aneurysm, brain
  chest — *see* Aneurysm, thorax
  circle of Willis I67.1
    congenital Q28.3
      ruptured I60.6
    ruptured I60.6
  common iliac artery I72.3
  congenital (peripheral) Q27.8
    brain Q28.3
      ruptured I60.7
    coronary Q24.5
    digestive system Q27.8
    lower limb Q27.8
    pulmonary Q25.79
    retina Q14.1
    specified site NEC Q27.8
    upper limb Q27.8
  conjunctiva — *see* Abnormality, conjunctiva, vascular
  conus arteriosus — *see* Aneurysm, heart
  coronary (arteriosclerotic) (artery) I25.41
    arteriovenous, congenital Q24.5
    congenital Q24.5
    ruptured — *see* Infarct, myocardium
    syphilitic A52.06
    vein I25.89
  cylindroid (aorta) I71.9
    ruptured I71.8
    syphilitic A52.01
  ductus arteriosus Q25.0
  endocardial, infective (any valve) I33.0
  femoral (artery) (ruptured) I72.4
  gastroduodenal I72.8

Aneurysm — *continued*
  gastroepiploic I72.8
  heart (wall) (chronic or with a stated duration of over 4 weeks) I25.3
    valve — *see* Endocarditis
  hepatic I72.8
  iliac (common) (artery) (ruptured) I72.3
  infective I72.9
    endocardial (any valve) I33.0
  innominate (nonsyphilitic) I72.8
    syphilitic A52.09
  interauricular septum — *see* Aneurysm, heart
  interventricular septum — *see* Aneurysm, heart
  intrathoracic (nonsyphilitic) I71.2
    ruptured I71.1
    syphilitic A52.09
  lower limb I72.4
  lung (pulmonary artery) I28.1
  mediastinal (nonsyphilitic) I72.8
    syphilitic A52.09
  miliary (congenital) I67.1
    ruptured — *see* Hemorrhage, intracerebral, subarachnoid, intracranial
  mitral (heart) (valve) I34.8
  mural — *see* Aneurysm, heart
  mycotic I72.9
    endocardial (any valve) I33.0
    ruptured, brain — *see* Hemorrhage, intracerebral, subarachnoid
  myocardium — *see* Aneurysm, heart
  neck I72.0
  pancreaticoduodenal I72.8
  patent ductus arteriosus Q25.0
  peripheral NEC I72.8
    congenital Q27.8
      digestive system Q27.8
      lower limb Q27.8
      specified site NEC Q27.8
      upper limb Q27.8
  popliteal (artery) (ruptured) I72.4
  precerebral, congenital (nonruptured) Q28.1
  pulmonary I28.1
    arteriovenous Q25.72
      acquired I28.0
    syphilitic A52.09
    valve (heart) — *see* Endocarditis, pulmonary
  racemose (peripheral) I72.9
    congenital — *see* Aneurysm, congenital
  radial I72.1
  Rasmussen NEC A15.0
  renal (artery) I72.2
  retina (*see also* Disorder, retina, microaneurysms)
    congenital Q14.1
    diabetic — *see* Diabetes, microaneurysms, retinal
  sinus of Valsalva Q25.4
  specified NEC I72.8
  spinal (cord) I72.8
    syphilitic (hemorrhage) A52.09
  splenic I72.8
  subclavian (artery) (ruptured) I72.8
    syphilitic A52.09
  superior mesenteric I72.8
  syphilitic (aorta) A52.01
    central nervous system A52.05
    congenital (late) A50.54 [I79.0]
    spine, spinal A52.09
  thoracoabdominal (aorta) I71.6
    ruptured I71.5
    syphilitic A52.01
  thorax, thoracic (aorta) (arch) (nonsyphilitic) I71.2
    ruptured I71.1
    syphilitic A52.01
  traumatic (complication) (early), specified site — *see* Injury, blood vessel
  tricuspid (heart) (valve) I07.8
  ulnar I72.1
  upper limb (ruptured) I72.1
  valve, valvular — *see* Endocarditis
  venous (*see also* Varix) I86.8
    congenital Q27.8
      digestive system Q27.8
      lower limb Q27.8
      specified site NEC Q27.8
      upper limb Q27.8
  ventricle — *see* Aneurysm, heart
  visceral NEC I72.8

Angelman syndrome Q93.5

Anger R45.4

Angiectasis, angiectopia I99.8
Angiitis I77.6
  allergic granulomatous M30.1
  hypersensitivity M31.0
  necrotizing M31.9
    specified NEC M31.8
  nervous system, granulomatous I67.7
Angina (attack) (cardiac) (chest) (heart) (pectoris) (syndrome) (vasomotor) I20.9
  with
    atherosclerotic heart disease — *see* Arteriosclerosis, coronary (artery),
    documented spasm I20.1
  abdominal K55.1
  accelerated — *see* Angina, unstable
  agranulocytic — *see* Agranulocytosis
  angiospastic — *see* Angina, with documented spasm
  aphthous B08.5
  crescendo — *see* Angina, unstable
  croupous J05.0
  cruris I73.9
  de novo effort — *see* Angina, unstable
  diphtheritic, membranous A36.0
  equivalent I20.8
  exudative, chronic J37.0
  following acute myocardial infarction I23.7
  gangrenous diphtheritic A36.0
  intestinal K55.1
  Ludovici K12.2
  Ludwig's K12.2
  malignant diphtheritic A36.0
  membranous J05.0
    diphtheritic A36.0
    Vincent's A69.1
  mesenteric K55.1
  monocytic — *see* Mononucleosis, infectious
  of effort — *see* Angina, specified NEC
  phlegmonous J36
    diphtheritic A36.0
  post-infarctional I23.7
  pre-infarctional — *see* Angina, unstable
  Prinzmetal — *see* Angina, with documented spasm
  progressive — *see* Angina, unstable
  pseudomembranous A69.1
  pultaceous, diphtheritic A36.0
  spasm-induced — *see* Angina, with documented spasm
  specified NEC I20.8
  stable I20.9
  stenocardia — *see* Angina, specified NEC
  stridulous, diphtheritic A36.2
  tonsil J36
  trachealis J05.0
  unstable I20.0
  variant — *see* Angina, with documented spasm
  Vincent's A69.1
  worsening effort — *see* Angina, unstable
Angioblastoma — *see* Neoplasm, connective tissue, uncertain behavior
Angiocholecystitis — *see* Cholecystitis, acute
Angiocholitis (*see also* Cholecystitis, acute) K83.0
Angiodysgenesis spinalis G95.19
Angiodysplasia (cecum) (colon) K55.20
  with bleeding K55.21
  duodenum (and stomach) K31.819
    with bleeding K31.811
  stomach (and duodenum) K31.819
    with bleeding K31.811
Angioedema (allergic) (any site) (with urticaria) T78.3 ☑
  hereditary D84.1
Angioendothelioma — *see* Neoplasm, uncertain behavior, by site
  benign D18.00
    intra-abdominal D18.03
    intracranial D18.02
    skin D18.01
    specified site NEC D18.09
  bone — *see* Neoplasm, bone, malignant
  Ewing's — *see* Neoplasm, bone, malignant
Angioendotheliomatosis C85.8- ☑
Angiofibroma (*see also* Neoplasm, benign, by site)
  juvenile
    specified site — *see* Neoplasm, benign, by site
    unspecified site D10.6
Angiohemophilia (A) (B) D68.0
Angioid streaks (choroid) (macula) (retina) H35.33
Angiokeratoma — *see* Neoplasm, skin, benign

Angiokeratoma — *continued*
  corporis diffusum E75.21
Angioleiomyoma — *see* Neoplasm, connective tissue, benign
Angiolipoma (*see also* Lipoma)
  infiltrating — *see* Lipoma
Angioma (*see also* Hemangioma, by site)
  capillary I78.1
  hemorrhagicum hereditaria I78.0
  intra-abdominal D18.03
  intracranial D18.02
  malignant — *see* Neoplasm, connective tissue, malignant
  plexiform D18.00
    intra-abdominal D18.03
    intracranial D18.02
    skin D18.01
    specified site NEC D18.09
  senile I78.1
  serpiginosum L81.7
  skin D18.01
  specified site NEC D18.09
  spider I78.1
  stellate I78.1
  venous Q28.3
Angiomatosis Q82.8
  bacillary A79.89
  encephalotrigeminal Q85.8
  hemorrhagic familial I78.0
  hereditary familial I78.0
  liver K76.4
Angiomyolipoma — *see* Lipoma
Angiomyoliposarcoma — *see* Neoplasm, connective tissue, malignant
Angiomyoma — *see* Neoplasm, connective tissue, benign
Angiomyosarcoma — *see* Neoplasm, connective tissue, malignant
Angiomyxoma — *see* Neoplasm, connective tissue, uncertain behavior
Angioneurosis F45.8
Angioneurotic edema (allergic) (any site) (with urticaria) T78.3 ☑
  hereditary D84.1
Angiopathia, angiopathy I99.9
  cerebral I67.9
    amyloid E85.4 [I68.0]
  diabetic (peripheral) — *see* Diabetes, angiopathy
  peripheral I73.9
    diabetic — *see* Diabetes, angiopathy
    specified type NEC I73.89
  retinae syphilitica A52.05
  retinalis (juvenilis)
    diabetic — *see* Diabetes, retinopathy
    proliferative — *see* Retinopathy, proliferative
Angiosarcoma (*see also* Neoplasm, connective tissue, malignant)
  liver C22.3
Angiosclerosis — *see* Arteriosclerosis
Angiospasm (peripheral) (traumatic) (vessel) I73.9
  brachial plexus G54.0
  cerebral G45.9
  cervical plexus G54.2
  nerve
    arm — *see* Mononeuropathy, upper limb
      axillary G54.0
      median — *see* Lesion, nerve, median
      ulnar — *see* Lesion, nerve, ulnar
    axillary G54.0
    leg — *see* Mononeuropathy, lower limb
    median — *see* Lesion, nerve, median
    plantar — *see* Lesion, nerve, plantar
    ulnar — *see* Lesion, nerve, ulnar
Angiospastic disease or edema I73.9
Angiostrongyliasis
  due to
    Parastrongylus
      cantonensis B83.2
      costaricensis B81.3
    intestinal B81.3
Anguillulosis — *see* Strongyloidiasis
Angulation
  cecum — *see* Obstruction, intestine
  coccyx (acquired) (*see also* subcategory) M43.8 ☑
    congenital NEC Q76.49
  femur (acquired) (*see also* Deformity, limb, specified type NEC, thigh)

Angulation — *continued*
  femur (*see also* Deformity, limb, specified type, thigh) — *continued*
    congenital Q74.2
  intestine (large) (small) — *see* Obstruction, intestine
  sacrum (acquired) (*see also* subcategory) M43.8 ☑
    congenital NEC Q76.49
  sigmoid (flexure) — *see* Obstruction, intestine
  spine — *see* Dorsopathy, deforming, specified NEC
  tibia (acquired) (*see also* Deformity, limb, specified type NEC, lower leg)
    congenital Q74.2
  ureter N13.5
    with infection N13.6
  wrist (acquired) (*see also* Deformity, limb, specified type NEC, forearm)
    congenital Q74.0
Angulus infectiosus (lips) K13.0
Anhedonia R45.84
Anhidrosis L74.4
Anhydration, anhydremia E86.0
  with
    hypernatremia E87.0
    hyponatremia E87.1
Anhydremia E86.0
  with
    hypernatremia E87.0
    hyponatremia E87.1
Anidrosis L74.4
Aniridia (congenital) Q13.1
Anisakiasis (infection) (infestation) B81.0
Anisakis larvae infestation B81.0
Aniseikonia H52.32
Anisocoria (pupil) H57.02
  congenital Q13.2
Anisocytosis R71.8
Anisometropia (congenital) H52.31
Ankle — *see* condition
Ankyloblepharon (eyelid) (acquired) (*see also* Blepharophimosis)
  filiforme (adnatum) (congenital) Q10.3
  total Q10.3
Ankyloglossia Q38.1
Ankylosis (fibrous) (osseous) (joint) M24.60
  ankle M24.67- ☑
  arthrodesis status Z98.1
  cricoarytenoid (cartilage) (joint) (larynx) J38.7
  dental K03.5
  ear ossicles H74.31- ☑
  elbow M24.62- ☑
  foot M24.67- ☑
  hand M24.64- ☑
  hip M24.65- ☑
  incostapedial joint (infectional) — *see* Ankylosis, ear ossicles
  jaw (temporomandibular) M26.61
  knee M24.66- ☑
  lumbosacral (joint) M43.27
  postoperative (status) Z98.1
  produced by surgical fusion, status Z98.1
  sacro-iliac (joint) M43.28
  shoulder M24.61- ☑
  spine (joint) (*see also* Fusion, spine)
    spondylitic — *see* Spondylitis, ankylosing
  surgical Z98.1
  temporomandibular M26.61
  tooth, teeth (hard tissues) K03.5
  wrist M24.63- ☑
Ankylostoma — *see* Ancylostoma
Ankylostomiasis — *see* Ancylostomiasis
Ankylurethria — *see* Stricture, urethra
Annular (*see also* condition)
  detachment, cervix N88.8
  organ or site, congenital NEC — *see* Distortion
  pancreas (congenital) Q45.1
Anodontia (complete) (partial) (vera) K00.0
  acquired K08.10 ☑
Anomaly, anomalous (congenital) (unspecified type) Q89.9
  abdominal wall NEC Q79.59
  acoustic nerve Q07.8
  adrenal (gland) Q89.1
  Alder (-Reilly) (leukocyte granulation) D72.0
  alimentary tract Q45.9
    upper Q40.9
  alveolar M26.70
    hyperplasia M26.79

Anomaly, anomalous — *continued*
  alveolar — *continued*
    hyperplasia — *continued*
      mandibular M26.72
      maxillary M26.71
    hypoplasia M26.79
      mandibular M26.74
      maxillary M26.73
    ridge (process) M26.79
    specified NEC M26.79
  ankle (joint) Q74.2
  anus Q43.9
  aorta (arch) NEC Q25.4
    coarctation (preductal) (postductal) Q25.1
  aortic cusp or valve Q23.9
  appendix Q43.8
  apple peel syndrome Q41.1
  aqueduct of Sylvius Q03.0
    with spina bifida — *see* Spina bifida, with hydrocephalus
  arm Q74.0
  arteriovenous NEC
    coronary Q24.5
    gastrointestinal Q27.33
      acquired — *see* Angiodysplasia
  artery (peripheral) Q27.9
    basilar NEC Q28.1
    cerebral Q28.3
    coronary Q24.5
    digestive system Q27.8
    eye Q15.8
    great Q25.9
      specified NEC Q25.8
    lower limb Q27.8
    peripheral Q27.9
      specified NEC Q27.8
    pulmonary NEC Q25.79
    renal Q27.2
    retina Q14.1
    specified site NEC Q27.8
    subclavian Q27.8
    umbilical Q27.0
    upper limb Q27.8
    vertebral NEC Q28.1
  aryteno-epiglottic folds Q31.8
  atrial
    bands or folds Q20.8
    septa Q21.1
  atrioventricular
    excitation I45.6
    septum Q21.0
  auditory canal Q17.8
  auricle
    ear Q17.8
      causing impairment of hearing Q16.9
    heart Q20.8
  Axenfeld's Q15.0
  back Q89.9
  band
    atrial Q20.8
    heart Q24.8
    ventricular Q24.8
  Bartholin's duct Q38.4
  biliary duct or passage Q44.5
  bladder Q64.70
    absence Q64.5
    diverticulum Q64.6
    exstrophy Q64.10
      cloacal Q64.12
      extroversion Q64.19
      specified type NEC Q64.19
      supravesical fissure Q64.11
    neck obstruction Q64.31
    specified type NEC Q64.79
  bone Q79.9
    arm Q74.0
    face Q75.9
    leg Q74.2
    pelvic girdle Q74.2
    shoulder girdle Q74.0
    skull Q75.9
      with
        anencephaly Q00.0
        encephalocele — *see* Encephalocele
        hydrocephalus Q03.9
          with spina bifida — *see* Spina bifida, by site, with hydrocephalus
        microcephaly Q02

Anomaly, anomalous — *continued*
jejunum Q43.8
joint Q74.9
    specified NEC Q74.8
Jordan's D72.0
kidney(s) (calyx) (pelvis) Q63.9
    artery Q27.2
    specified NEC Q63.8
Klippel-Feil (brevicollis) Q76.1
knee Q74.1
labium (majus) (minus) Q52.70
labyrinth, membranous Q16.5
lacrimal apparatus or duct Q10.6
larynx, laryngeal (muscle) Q31.9
    web (bed) Q31.0
lens Q12.9
leukocytes, genetic D72.0
    granulation (constitutional) D72.0
lid (fold) Q10.3
ligament Q79.9
    broad Q50.6
    round Q52.8
limb Q74.9
    lower NEC Q74.2
        reduction deformity — *see* Defect, reduction,
            lower limb
    upper Q74.0
lip Q38.0
liver Q44.7
    duct Q44.5
lower limb NEC Q74.2
lumbosacral (joint) (region) Q76.49
    kyphosis — *see* Kyphosis, congenital
    lordosis — *see* Lordosis, congenital
lung (fissure) (lobe) Q33.9
mandible — *see* Anomaly, dentofacial
maxilla — *see* Anomaly, dentofacial
May (-Hegglin) D72.0
meatus urinarius NEC Q64.79
meningeal bands or folds Q07.9
    constriction of Q07.8
        spinal Q06.9
meninges Q07.9
    cerebral Q04.8
    spinal Q06.9
meningocele Q05.9
mesentery Q45.9
metacarpus Q74.0
metatarsus NEC Q74.2
middle ear Q16.4
    ossicles Q16.3
mitral (leaflets) (valve) Q23.9
    insufficiency Q23.3
    specified NEC Q23.8
    stenosis Q23.2
mouth Q38.6
Müllerian (*see also* Anomaly, by site)
    uterus NEC Q51.818
multiple NEC Q89.7
muscle Q79.9
    eyelid Q10.3
musculoskeletal system, except limbs Q79.9
myocardium Q24.8
nail Q84.6
narrowness, eyelid Q10.3
nasal sinus (wall) Q30.8
neck (any part) Q18.9
nerve Q07.9
    acoustic Q07.8
    optic Q07.8
nervous system (central) Q07.9
nipple Q83.9
nose, nasal (bones) (cartilage) (septum) (sinus) Q30.9
    specified NEC Q30.8
ocular muscle Q15.8
omphalomesenteric duct Q43.0
opening, pulmonary veins Q26.4
optic
    disc Q14.2
    nerve Q07.8
opticociliary vessels Q13.2
orbit (eye) Q10.7
organ Q89.9
    of Corti Q16.5
origin
    artery
        innominate Q25.8
        pulmonary Q25.79

Anomaly, anomalous — *continued*
origin — *continued*
    artery — *continued*
        renal Q27.2
        subclavian Q25.8
osseous meatus (ear) Q16.1
ovary Q50.39
oviduct Q50.6
palate (hard) (soft) NEC Q38.5
pancreas or pancreatic duct Q45.3
papillary muscles Q24.8
parathyroid gland Q89.2
paraurethral ducts Q64.79
parotid (gland) Q38.4
patella Q74.1
Pelger-Huët (hereditary hyposegmentation) D72.0
pelvic girdle NEC Q74.2
pelvis (bony) NEC Q74.2
    rachitic E64.3
penis (glans) Q55.69
pericardium Q24.8
peripheral vascular system Q27.9
Peter's Q13.4
pharynx Q38.8
pigmentation L81.9
    congenital Q82.8
pituitary (gland) Q89.2
pleural (folds) Q34.0
portal vein Q26.5
    connection Q26.5
position, tooth, teeth, fully erupted M26.30
    specified NEC M26.39
precerebral vessel Q28.1
prepuce Q55.69
prostate Q55.4
pulmonary Q33.9
    artery NEC Q25.79
    valve Q22.3
        atresia Q22.0
        insufficiency Q22.2
        specified type NEC Q22.3
        stenosis Q22.1
            infundibular Q24.3
            subvalvular Q24.3
    venous connection Q26.4
        partial Q26.3
        total Q26.2
pupil Q13.2
    function H57.00
        anisocoria H57.02
        Argyll Robertson pupil H57.01
        miosis H57.03
        mydriasis H57.04
        specified type NEC H57.09
        tonic pupil H57.05- ☑
pylorus Q40.3
radius Q74.0
rectum Q43.9
reduction (extremity) (limb)
    femur (longitudinal) — *see* Defect, reduction,
        lower limb, longitudinal, femur
    fibula (longitudinal) — *see* Defect, reduction, lower
        limb, longitudinal, fibula
    lower limb — *see* Defect, reduction, lower limb
    radius (longitudinal) — *see* Defect, reduction, up-
        per limb, longitudinal, radius
    tibia (longitudinal) — *see* Defect, reduction, lower
        limb, longitudinal, tibia
    ulna (longitudinal) — *see* Defect, reduction, upper
        limb, longitudinal, ulna
    upper limb — *see* Defect, reduction, upper limb
refraction — *see* Disorder, refraction
renal Q63.9
    artery Q27.2
    pelvis Q63.9
        specified NEC Q63.8
respiratory system Q34.9
    specified NEC Q34.8
retina Q14.1
rib Q76.6
    cervical Q76.5
Rieger's Q13.81
rotation — *see* Malrotation
    hip or thigh Q65.89
round ligament Q52.8
sacroiliac (joint) NEC Q74.2
sacrum NEC Q76.49
    kyphosis — *see* Kyphosis, congenital

Anomaly, anomalous — *continued*
sacrum — *continued*
    lordosis — *see* Lordosis, congenital
saddle nose, syphilitic A50.57
salivary duct or gland Q38.4
scapula Q74.0
scrotum — *see* Malformation, testis and scrotum
sebaceous gland Q82.9
seminal vesicles Q55.4
sense organs NEC Q07.8
sex chromosomes NEC (*see also* Anomaly, chromo-
    somes)
    female phenotype Q97.8
    male phenotype Q98.9
shoulder (girdle) (joint) Q74.0
sigmoid (flexure) Q43.9
simian crease Q82.8
sinus of Valsalva Q25.4
skeleton generalized Q78.9
skin (appendage) Q82.9
skull Q75.9
    with
        anencephaly Q00.0
        encephalocele — *see* Encephalocele
        hydrocephalus Q03.9
            with spina bifida — *see* Spina bifida, by site,
                with hydrocephalus
        microcephaly Q02
specified organ or site NEC Q89.8
spermatic cord Q55.4
spine, spinal NEC Q76.49
    column NEC Q76.49
        kyphosis — *see* Kyphosis, congenital
        lordosis — *see* Lordosis, congenital
    cord Q06.9
    nerve root Q07.8
spleen Q89.09
    agenesis Q89.01
stenonian duct Q38.4
sternum NEC Q76.7
stomach Q40.3
submaxillary gland Q38.4
tarsus NEC Q74.2
tendon Q79.9
testis — *see* Malformation, testis and scrotum
thigh NEC Q74.2
thorax (wall) Q67.8
    bony Q76.9
throat Q38.8
thumb Q74.0
thymus gland Q89.2
thyroid (gland) Q89.2
    cartilage Q31.8
tibia NEC Q74.2
    saber A50.56
toe Q74.2
tongue Q38.3
tooth, teeth K00.9
    eruption K00.6
    position, fully erupted M26.30
    spacing, fully erupted M26.30
trachea (cartilage) Q32.1
tragus Q17.9
tricuspid (leaflet) (valve) Q22.9
    atresia or stenosis Q22.4
    Ebstein's Q22.5
Uhl's (hypoplasia of myocardium, right ventricle) Q24.8
ulna Q74.0
umbilical artery Q27.0
union
    cricoid cartilage and thyroid cartilage Q31.8
    thyroid cartilage and hyoid bone Q31.8
    trachea with larynx Q31.8
upper limb Q74.0
urachus Q64.4
ureter Q62.8
    obstructive NEC Q62.39
        cecoureterocele Q62.32
        orthotopic ureterocele Q62.31
urethra Q64.70
    absence Q64.5
    double Q64.74
    fistula to rectum Q64.73
    obstructive Q64.39
        stricture Q64.32
    prolapse Q64.71
    specified type NEC Q64.79
urinary tract Q64.9

Anomaly, anomalous — *continued*
uterus Q51.9
with only one functioning horn Q51.4
uvula Q38.5
vagina Q52.4
valleculae Q31.8
valve (heart) NEC Q24.8
coronary sinus Q24.5
inferior vena cava Q24.8
pulmonary Q22.3
sinus coronario Q24.5
venae cavae inferioris Q24.8
vas deferens Q55.4
vascular Q27.9
brain Q28.3
ring Q25.4
vein(s) (peripheral) Q27.9
brain Q28.3
cerebral Q28.3
coronary Q24.5
developmental Q28.3
great Q26.9
specified NEC Q26.8
vena cava (inferior) (superior) Q26.9
venous — *see* Anomaly, vein(s)
venous return Q26.8
ventricular
bands or folds Q24.8
septa Q21.0
vertebra Q76.49
kyphosis — *see* Kyphosis, congenital
lordosis — *see* Lordosis, congenital
vesicourethral orifice Q64.79
vessel(s) Q27.9
optic papilla Q14.2
precerebral Q28.1
vitelline duct Q43.0
vitreous body or humor Q14.0
vulva Q52.70
wrist (joint) Q74.0
Anomia R48.8
Anonychia (congenital) Q84.3
acquired L60.8
Anophthalmos, anophthalmus (congenital) (globe) Q11.1
acquired Z90.01
Anopia, anopsia H53.46- ☑
quadrant H53.46- ☑
Anorchia, anorchism, anorchidism Q55.0
Anorexia R63.0
hysterical F44.89
nervosa F50.00
atypical F50.9
binge-eating type F50.2
with purging F50.02
restricting type F50.01
Anorgasmy, psychogenic (female) F52.31
male F52.32
Anosmia R43.0
hysterical F44.6
postinfectional J39.8
Anosognosia R41.89
Anosteoplasia Q78.9
Anovulatory cycle N97.0
Anoxemia R09.02
newborn P84
Anoxia (pathological) R09.02
altitude T70.29 ☑
cerebral G93.1
complicating
anesthesia (general) (local) or other sedation T88.59 ☑
in labor and delivery O74.3
in pregnancy O29.21- ☑
postpartum, puerperal O89.2
delivery (cesarean) (instrumental) O75.4
during a procedure G97.81
newborn P84
resulting from a procedure G97.82
due to
drowning T75.1 ☑
high altitude T70.29 ☑
heart — *see* Insufficiency, coronary
intrauterine P84
myocardial — *see* Insufficiency, coronary
newborn P84
spinal cord G95.11

Anoxia — *continued*
systemic (by suffocation) (low content in atmosphere) — *see* Asphyxia, traumatic
Anteflexion — *see* Anteversion
Antenatal
care (normal pregnancy) Z34.90
screening (encounter for) of mother Z36
Antepartum — *see* condition
Anterior — *see* condition
Antero-occlusion M26.220
Anteversion
cervix — *see* Anteversion, uterus
femur (neck), congenital Q65.89
uterus, uterine (cervix) (postinfectional) (postpartal, old) N85.4
congenital Q51.818
in pregnancy or childbirth — *see* Pregnancy, complicated by
Anthophobia F40.228
Anthracosilicosis J60
Anthracosis (lung) (occupational) J60
lingua K14.3
Anthrax A22.9
with pneumonia A22.1
cerebral A22.8
colitis A22.2
cutaneous A22.0
gastrointestinal A22.2
inhalation A22.1
intestinal A22.2
meningitis A22.8
pulmonary A22.1
respiratory A22.1
sepsis A22.7
specified manifestation NEC A22.8
Anthropoid pelvis Q74.2
with disproportion (fetopelvic) O33.0
Anthropophobia F40.10
generalized F40.11
Antibodies, maternal (blood group) — *see* Isoimmunization, affecting management of pregnancy
anti-D — *see* Isoimmunization, affecting management of pregnancy, Rh
newborn P55.0
Antibody
anticardiolipin R76.0
with
hemorrhagic disorder D68.312
hypercoagulable state D68.61
antiphosphatidylglycerol R76.0
with
hemorrhagic disorder D68.312
hypercoagulable state D68.61
antiphosphatidylinositol R76.0
with
hemorrhagic disorder D68.312
hypercoagulable state D68.61
antiphosphatidylserine R76.0
with
hemorrhagic disorder D68.312
hypercoagulable state D68.61
antiphospholipid R76.0
with
hemorrhagic disorder D68.312
hypercoagulable state D68.61
Anticardiolipin syndrome D68.61
Anticoagulant, circulating (intrinsic) (*see also* Disorder, hemorrhagic) D68.318
drug-induced (extrinsic) (*see also* Disorder, hemorrhagic) D68.32
Antidiuretic hormone syndrome E22.2
Antimonial cholera — *see* Poisoning, antimony
Antiphospholipid
antibody
with hemorrhagic disorder D68.312
syndrome D68.61
Antisocial personality F60.2
Antithrombinemia — *see* Circulating anticoagulants
Antithromboplastinemia D68.318
Antithromboplastinogenemia D68.318
Antitoxin complication or reaction — *see* Complications, vaccination
Antlophobia F40.228
Antritis J32.0
maxilla J32.0
acute J01.00
recurrent J01.01
stomach K29.60

Antritis — *continued*
stomach — *continued*
with bleeding K29.61
Antrum, antral — *see* condition
Anuria R34
calculous (impacted) (recurrent) (*see also* Calculus, urinary) N20.9
following
abortion — *see* Abortion by type complicated by, renal failure
ectopic or molar pregnancy O08.4
newborn P96.0
postprocedural N99.0
postrenal N13.8
traumatic (following crushing) T79.5 ☑
Anus, anal — *see* condition
Anusitis K62.89
Anxiety F41.9
depression F41.8
episodic paroxysmal F41.0
generalized F41.1
hysteria F41.8
neurosis F41.1
panic type F41.0
reaction F41.1
separation, abnormal (of childhood) F93.0
specified NEC F41.8
state F41.1
Aorta, aortic — *see* condition
Aortectasia — *see* Ectasia, aorta
with aneurysm — *see* Aneurysm, aorta
Aortitis (nonsyphilitic) (calcific) I77.6
arteriosclerotic I70.0
Doehle-Heller A52.02
luetic A52.02
rheumatic — *see* Endocarditis, acute, rheumatic
specific (syphilitic) A52.02
syphilitic A52.02
congenital A50.54 [I79.1]
Apathetic thyroid storm — *see* Thyrotoxicosis
Apathy R45.3
Apeirophobia F40.228
Apepsia K30
psychogenic F45.8
Aperistalsis, esophagus K22.0
Apertognathia M26.29
Apert's syndrome Q87.0
Aphagia R13.0
psychogenic F50.9
Aphakia (acquired) (postoperative) H27.0- ☑
congenital Q12.3
Aphasia (amnestic) (global) (nominal) (semantic) (syntactic) R47.01
acquired, with epilepsy (Landau-Kleffner syndrome) — *see* Epilepsy, specified NEC
auditory (developmental) F80.2
developmental (receptive type) F80.2
expressive type F80.1
Wernicke's F80.2
following
cerebrovascular disease I69.920
cerebral infarction I69.320
intracerebral hemorrhage I69.120
nontraumatic intracranial hemorrhage NEC I69.220
specified disease NEC I69.820
subarachnoid hemorrhage I69.020
primary progressive G31.01 [F02.80]
with behavioral disturbance G31.01 [F02.81]
progressive isolated G31.01 [F02.80]
with behavioral disturbance G31.01 [F02.81]
sensory F80.2
syphilis, tertiary A52.19
Wernicke's (developmental) F80.2
Aphonia (organic) R49.1
hysterical F44.4
psychogenic F44.4
Aphthae, aphthous (*see also* condition)
Bednar's K12.0
cachectic K14.0
epizootic B08.8
fever B08.8
oral (recurrent) K12.0
stomatitis (major) (minor) K12.0
thrush B37.0
ulcer (oral) (recurrent) K12.0
genital organ(s) NEC
female N76.6

Aphthae, aphthous — *continued*
  ulcer — *continued*
    genital organ(s) — *continued*
      male N50.8
      larynx J38.7
Apical — *see* condition
Apiphobia F40.218
Aplasia (*see also* Agenesis)
  abdominal muscle syndrome Q79.4
  alveolar process (acquired) — *see* Anomaly, alveolar
    congenital Q38.6
  aorta (congenital) Q25.4
  axialis extracorticalis (congenita) E75.29
  bone marrow (myeloid) D61.9
    congenital D61.01
  brain Q00.0
    part of Q04.3
  bronchus Q32.4
  cementum K00.4
  cerebellum Q04.3
  cervix (congenital) Q51.5
  congenital pure red cell D61.01
  corpus callosum Q04.0
  cutis congenita Q84.8
  erythrocyte congenital D61.01
  extracortical axial E75.29
  eye Q11.1
  fovea centralis (congenital) Q14.1
  gallbladder, congenital Q44.0
  iris Q13.1
  labyrinth, membranous Q16.5
  limb (congenital) Q73.8
    lower — *see* Defect, reduction, lower limb
    upper — *see* Agenesis, arm
  lung, congenital (bilateral) (unilateral) Q33.3
  pancreas Q45.0
  parathyroid-thymic D82.1
  Pelizaeus-Merzbacher E75.29
  penis Q55.5
  prostate Q55.4
  red cell (with thymoma) D60.9
    acquired D60.9
      due to drugs D60.9
    adult D60.9
    chronic D60.0
    congenital D61.01
    constitutional D61.01
    due to drugs D60.9
    hereditary D61.01
    of infants D61.01
    primary D61.01
    pure D61.01
      due to drugs D60.9
    specified type NEC D60.8
    transient D60.1
  round ligament Q52.8
  skin Q84.8
  spermatic cord Q55.4
  spleen Q89.01
  testicle Q55.0
  thymic, with immunodeficiency D82.1
  thyroid (congenital) (with myxedema) E03.1
  uterus Q51.0
  ventral horn cell Q06.1
Apnea, apneic (of) (spells) R06.81
  newborn NEC P28.4
    obstructive P28.4
    sleep (central) (obstructive) (primary) P28.3
  prematurity P28.4
  sleep G47.30
    central (primary) G47.31
      in conditions classified elsewhere G47.37
    obstructive (adult) (pediatric) G47.33
    primary central G47.31
    specified NEC G47.39
Apneumatosis, newborn P28.0
Apocrine metaplasia (breast) — *see* Dysplasia, mammary, specified type NEC
Apophysitis (bone) (*see also* Osteochondropathy)
  calcaneus M92.8
  juvenile M92.9
Apoplectiform convulsions (cerebral ischemia) I67.82
Apoplexia, apoplexy, apoplectic
  adrenal A39.1
  heart (auricle) (ventricle) — *see* Infarct, myocardium
  heat T67.0 ☑
  hemorrhagic (stroke) — *see* Hemorrhage, intracranial

Apoplexia, apoplexy, apoplectic — *continued*
  meninges, hemorrhagic — *see* Hemorrhage, intracranial, subarachnoid
  uremic N18.9 [I68.8]
Appearance
  bizarre R46.1
  specified NEC R46.89
  very low level of personal hygiene R46.0
Appendage
  epididymal (organ of Morgagni) Q55.4
  intestine (epiploic) Q43.8
  preauricular Q17.0
  testicular (organ of Morgagni) Q55.29
Appendicitis (pneumococcal) (retrocecal) K37
  with
    perforation or rupture K35.2
    peritoneal abscess K35.3
    peritonitis NEC K35.3
      generalized (with perforation or rupture) K35.2
      localized (with perforation or rupture) K35.3
  acute (catarrhal) (fulminating) (gangrenous) (obstructive) (retrocecal) (suppurative) K35.80
    with
      peritoneal abscess K35.3
      peritonitis NEC K35.3
        generalized (with perforation or rupture) K35.2
        localized (with perforation or rupture) K35.3
    specified NEC K35.89
  amebic A06.89
  chronic (recurrent) K36
  exacerbation — *see* Appendicitis, acute
  gangrenous — *see* Appendicitis, acute
  healed (obliterative) K36
  interval K36
  neurogenic K36
  obstructive K36
  recurrent K36
  relapsing K36
  subacute (adhesive) K36
  subsiding K36
  suppurative — *see* Appendicitis, acute
  tuberculous A18.32
Appendicopathia oxyurica B80
Appendix, appendicular (*see also* condition)
  epididymis Q55.4
  Morgagni
    female Q50.5
    male (epididymal) Q55.4
      testicular Q55.29
  testis Q55.29
Appetite
  depraved — *see* Pica
  excessive R63.2
  lack or loss (*see also* Anorexia) R63.0
    nonorganic origin F50.8
    psychogenic F50.8
  perverted (hysterical) — *see* Pica
Apple peel syndrome Q41.1
Apprehension state F41.1
Apprehensiveness, abnormal F41.9
Approximal wear K03.0
Apraxia (classic) (ideational) (ideokinetic) (ideomotor) (motor) (verbal) R48.2
  following
    cerebrovascular disease I69.990
      cerebral infarction I69.390
      intracerebral hemorrhage I69.190
      nontraumatic intracranial hemorrhage NEC I69.290
      specified disease NEC I69.890
      subarachnoid hemorrhage I69.090
  oculomotor, congenital H51.8
Aptyalism K11.7
Apudoma — *see* Neoplasm, uncertain behavior, by site
Aqueous misdirection H40.83- ☑
Arabicum elephantiasis — *see* Infestation, filarial
Arachnitis — *see* Meningitis
Arachnodactyly — *see* Syndrome, Marfan's
Arachnoiditis (acute) (adhesive) (basal) (brain) (cerebrospinal) — *see* Meningitis
Arachnophobia F40.210
Arboencephalitis, Australian A83.4
Arborization block (heart) I45.5
ARC (AIDS-related complex) B20
Arc-welder's lung J63.4
Arches — *see* condition

Arcuate uterus Q51.810
Arcuatus uterus Q51.810
Arcus (cornea) senilis — *see* Degeneration, cornea, senile
Areflexia R29.2
Areola — *see* condition
Argentaffinoma (*see also* Neoplasm, uncertain behavior, by site)
  malignant — *see* Neoplasm, malignant, by site
  syndrome E34.0
Argininemia E72.21
Arginosuccinic aciduria E72.22
Argyll Robertson phenomenon, pupil or syndrome (syphilitic) A52.19
  atypical H57.09
  nonsyphilitic H57.09
Argyria, argyriasis
  conjunctival H11.13- ☑
  from drug or medicament — *see* Table of Drugs and Chemicals, by substance
Argyrosis, conjunctival H11.13- ☑
Arhinencephaly Q04.1
Ariboflavinosis E53.0
Arm — *see* condition
Arnold-Chiari disease, obstruction or syndrome (type II) Q07.00
  with
    hydrocephalus Q07.02
      with spina bifida Q07.03
    spina bifida Q07.01
      with hydrocephalus Q07.03
  type III — *see* Encephalocele
  type IV Q04.8
Aromatic amino-acid metabolism disorder E70.9
  specified NEC E70.8
Arousals, confusional G47.51
Arrest, arrested
  cardiac I46.9
    complicating
      abortion — *see* Abortion, by type, complicated by, cardiac arrest
      anesthesia (general) (local) or other sedation — *see* Table of Drugs and Chemicals, by drug
        in labor and delivery O74.2
        in pregnancy O29.11- ☑
          postpartum, puerperal O89.1
        delivery (cesarean) (instrumental) O75.4
    due to
      cardiac condition I46.2
      specified condition NEC I46.8
    intraoperative I97.71- ☑
    newborn P29.81
    postprocedural I97.12- ☑
      obstetric procedure O75.4
  cardiorespiratory — *see* Arrest, cardiac
  circulatory — *see* Arrest, cardiac
  deep transverse O64.0 ☑
  development or growth
    bone — *see* Disorder, bone, development or growth
    child R62.50
    tracheal rings Q32.1
  epiphyseal
    complete
      femur M89.15- ☑
      humerus M89.12- ☑
      tibia M89.16- ☑
      ulna M89.13- ☑
      forearm M89.13- ☑
        specified NEC M89.13- ☑
        ulna — *see* Arrest, epiphyseal, by type, ulna
      lower leg M89.16- ☑
        specified NEC M89.168
        tibia — *see* Arrest, epiphyseal, by type, tibia
    partial
      femur M89.15- ☑
      humerus M89.12- ☑
      tibia M89.16- ☑
      ulna M89.13- ☑
    specified NEC M89.18
  granulopoiesis — *see* Agranulocytosis
  growth plate — *see* Arrest, epiphyseal
  heart — *see* Arrest, cardiac
  legal, anxiety concerning Z65.3
  physeal — *see* Arrest, epiphyseal
  respiratory R09.2
    newborn P28.81

Arrest, arrested — *continued*
  sinus I45.5
  spermatogenesis (complete) — *see* Azoospermia
    incomplete — *see* Oligospermia
  transverse (deep) O64.0 ☑
Arrhenoblastoma
  benign
    specified site — *see* Neoplasm, benign, by site
    unspecified site
      female D27.9
      male D29.20
  malignant
    specified site — *see* Neoplasm, malignant, by site
    unspecified site
      female C56.9
      male C62.90
  specified site — *see* Neoplasm, uncertain behavior, by site
  unspecified site
    female D39.10
    male D40.10
Arrhythmia (auricle) (cardiac) (juvenile) (nodal) (reflex) (sinus) (supraventricular) (transitory) (ventricle) I49.9
  block I45.9
  extrasystolic I49.49
  newborn
    bradycardia P29.12
    occurring before birth P03.819
      before onset of labor P03.810
      during labor P03.811
    tachycardia P29.11
  psychogenic F45.8
  specified NEC I49.8
  vagal R55
  ventricular re-entry I47.0
Arrillaga-Ayerza syndrome (pulmonary sclerosis with pulmonary hypertension) I27.0
Arsenical pigmentation L81.8
  from drug or medicament — *see* Table of Drugs and Chemicals
Arsenism — *see* Poisoning, arsenic
Arterial — *see* condition
Arteriofibrosis — *see* Arteriosclerosis
Arteriolar sclerosis — *see* Arteriosclerosis
Arteriolith — *see* Arteriosclerosis
Arteriolitis I77.6
  necrotizing, kidney I77.5
  renal — *see* Hypertension, kidney
Arteriolosclerosis — *see* Arteriosclerosis
Arterionephrosclerosis — *see* Hypertension, kidney
Arteriopathy I77.9
Arteriosclerosis, arteriosclerotic (diffuse) (obliterans) (of) (senile) (with calcification) I70.90
  aorta I70.0
  arteries of extremities — *see* Arteriosclerosis, extremities
  brain I67.2
  bypass graft
    coronary — *see* Arteriosclerosis, coronary, bypass graft
    extremities — *see* Arteriosclerosis, extremities, bypass graft
  cardiac — *see* Disease, heart, ischemic, atherosclerotic
  cardiopathy — *see* Disease, heart, ischemic, atherosclerotic
  cardiorenal — *see* Hypertension, cardiorenal
  cardiovascular — *see* Disease, heart, ischemic, atherosclerotic
  carotid (*see also* Occlusion, artery, carotid) I65.2- ☑
  central nervous system I67.2
  cerebral I67.2
  cerebrovascular I67.2
  coronary (artery) I25.10
    bypass graft I25.810
      with
        angina pectoris I25.709
          with documented spasm I25.701
          specified type NEC I25.708
          unstable I25.700
        ischemic chest pain I25.709
      autologous artery I25.810
        with
          angina pectoris I25.729
            with documented spasm I25.721
            specified type I25.728
            unstable I25.720
          ischemic chest pain I25.729
      autologous vein I25.810

Arteriosclerosis, arteriosclerotic — *continued*
  coronary — *continued*
    bypass graft — *continued*
      autologous vein — *continued*
        with
          angina pectoris I25.719
            with documented spasm I25.711
            specified type I25.718
            unstable I25.710
          ischemic chest pain I25.719
      nonautologous biological I25.810
        with
          angina pectoris I25.739
            with documented spasm I25.731
            specified type I25.738
            unstable I25.730
          ischemic chest pain I25.739
      specified type NEC I25.810
        with
          angina pectoris I25.799
            with documented spasm I25.791
            specified type I25.798
            unstable I25.790
          ischemic chest pain I25.799
    due to
      calcified coronary lesion (severely) I25.84
      lipid rich plaque I25.83
    native vessel
      with
        angina pectoris I25.119
          with documented spasm I25.111
          specified type NEC I25.118
          unstable I25.110
        ischemic chest pain I25.119
    transplanted heart I25.811
      bypass graft I25.812
        with
          angina pectoris I25.769
            with documented spasm I25.761
            specified type I25.768
            unstable I25.760
          ischemic chest pain I25.769
      native coronary artery I25.811
        with
          angina pectoris I25.759
            with documented spasm I25.751
            specified type I25.758
            unstable I25.750
          ischemic chest pain I25.759
  extremities (native arteries) I70.209
    bypass graft I70.309
      autologous vein graft I70.409
        leg I70.409
          with
            gangrene (and intermittent claudication, rest pain and ulcer) I70.469
            intermittent claudication I70.419
            rest pain (and intermittent claudication) I70.429
          bilateral I70.403
            with
              gangrene (and intermittent claudication, rest pain and ulcer) I70.463
              intermittent claudication I70.463
              rest pain (and intermittent claudication) I70.423
            specified type NEC I70.493
          left I70.402
            with
              gangrene (and intermittent claudication, rest pain and ulcer) I70.462
              intermittent claudication I70.412
              rest pain (and intermittent claudication) I70.422
              ulceration (and intermittent claudication and rest pain) I70.449
                ankle I70.443
                calf I70.442
                foot site NEC I70.445
                heel I70.444
                lower leg NEC I70.448
                midfoot I70.444
                thigh I70.441
              specified type NEC I70.492

Arteriosclerosis, arteriosclerotic — *continued*
  extremities — *continued*
    bypass graft — *continued*
      autologous vein graft — *continued*
        leg — *continued*
          right I70.401
            with
              gangrene (and intermittent claudication, rest pain and ulcer) I70.461
              intermittent claudication I70.411
              rest pain (and intermittent claudication) I70.421
              ulceration (and intermittent claudication and rest pain) I70.439
                ankle I70.433
                calf I70.432
                foot site NEC I70.435
                heel I70.434
                lower leg NEC I70.438
                midfoot I70.434
                thigh I70.431
              specified type NEC I70.491
          specified type NEC I70.499
        specified NEC I70.408
          with
            gangrene (and intermittent claudication, rest pain and ulcer) I70.468
            intermittent claudication I70.418
            rest pain (and intermittent claudication) I70.428
            ulceration (and intermittent claudication and rest pain) I70.45
          specified type NEC I70.498
      leg I70.309
        with
          gangrene (and intermittent claudication, rest pain and ulcer) I70.369
          intermittent claudication I70.319
          rest pain (and intermittent claudication) I70.329
        bilateral I70.303
          with
            gangrene (and intermittent claudication, rest pain and ulcer) I70.363
            intermittent claudication I70.313
            rest pain (and intermittent claudication) I70.323
          specified type NEC I70.393
        left I70.302
          with
            gangrene (and intermittent claudication, rest pain and ulcer) I70.362
            intermittent claudication I70.312
            rest pain (and intermittent claudication) I70.322
            ulceration (and intermittent claudication and rest pain) I70.349
              ankle I70.343
              calf I70.342
              foot site NEC I70.345
              heel I70.344
              lower leg NEC I70.348
              midfoot I70.344
              thigh I70.341
            specified type NEC I70.392
        right I70.301
          with
            gangrene (and intermittent claudication, rest pain and ulcer) I70.361
            intermittent claudication I70.311
            rest pain (and intermittent claudication) I70.321
            ulceration (and intermittent claudication and rest pain) I70.339
              ankle I70.333
              calf I70.332
              foot site NEC I70.335
              heel I70.334
              lower leg NEC I70.338
              midfoot I70.334
              thigh I70.331
            specified type NEC I70.391

Arteriosclerosis, arteriosclerotic — *continued*
  extremities — *continued*
    bypass graft — *continued*
      leg — *continued*
        specified type NEC I70.399
      nonautologous biological graft I70.509
        leg I70.509
          with
            gangrene (and intermittent claudication, rest pain and ulcer) I70.569
            intermittent claudication I70.519
            rest pain (and intermittent claudication) I70.529
        bilateral I70.503
          with
            gangrene (and intermittent claudication, rest pain and ulcer) I70.563
            intermittent claudication I70.513
            rest pain (and intermittent claudication) I70.523
          specified type NEC I70.593
        left I70.502
          with
            gangrene (and intermittent claudication, rest pain and ulcer) I70.562
            intermittent claudication I70.512
            rest pain (and intermittent claudication) I70.522
            ulceration (and intermittent claudication and rest pain) I70.549
              ankle I70.543
              calf I70.542
              foot site NEC I70.545
              heel I70.544
              lower leg NEC I70.548
              midfoot I70.544
              thigh I70.541
          specified type NEC I70.592
        right I70.501
          with
            gangrene (and intermittent claudication, rest pain and ulcer) I70.561
            intermittent claudication I70.511
            rest pain (and intermittent claudication) I70.521
            ulceration (and intermittent claudication and rest pain) I70.539
              ankle I70.533
              calf I70.532
              foot site NEC I70.535
              heel I70.534
              lower leg NEC I70.538
              midfoot I70.534
              thigh I70.531
          specified type NEC I70.591
        specified type NEC I70.599
        specified NEC I70.508
          with
            gangrene (and intermittent claudication, rest pain and ulcer) I70.568
            intermittent claudication I70.518
            rest pain (and intermittent claudication) I70.528
            ulceration (and intermittent claudication and rest pain) I70.55
          specified type NEC I70.598
      nonbiological graft I70.609
        leg I70.609
          with
            gangrene (and intermittent claudication, rest pain and ulcer) I70.669
            intermittent claudication I70.619
            rest pain (and intermittent claudication) I70.629
        bilateral I70.603
          with
            gangrene (and intermittent claudication, rest pain and ulcer) I70.663
            intermittent claudication I70.613

Arteriosclerosis, arteriosclerotic — *continued*
  extremities — *continued*
    bypass graft — *continued*
      nonbiological graft — *continued*
        leg — *continued*
          bilateral — *continued*
            with — *continued*
              rest pain (and intermittent claudication) I70.623
           specified type NEC I70.693
          left I70.602
            with
              gangrene (and intermittent claudication, rest pain and ulcer) I70.662
              intermittent claudication I70.612
              rest pain (and intermittent claudication) I70.622
              ulceration (and intermittent claudication and rest pain) I70.649
                ankle I70.643
                calf I70.642
                foot site NEC I70.645
                heel I70.644
                lower leg NEC I70.648
                midfoot I70.644
                thigh I70.641
           specified type NEC I70.692
          right I70.601
            with
              gangrene (and intermittent claudication, rest pain and ulcer) I70.661
              intermittent claudication I70.611
              rest pain (and intermittent claudication) I70.621
              ulceration (and intermittent claudication and rest pain) I70.639
                ankle I70.633
                calf I70.632
                foot site NEC I70.635
                heel I70.634
                lower leg NEC I70.638
                midfoot I70.634
                thigh I70.631
           specified type NEC I70.691
         specified type NEC I70.699
        specified NEC I70.608
          with
            gangrene (and intermittent claudication, rest pain and ulcer) I70.668
            intermittent claudication I70.618
            rest pain (and intermittent claudication) I70.628
            ulceration (and intermittent claudication and rest pain) I70.65
          specified type NEC I70.698
      specified graft NEC I70.709
        leg I70.709
          with
            gangrene (and intermittent claudication, rest pain and ulcer) I70.769
            intermittent claudication I70.719
            rest pain (and intermittent claudication) I70.729
        bilateral I70.703
          with
            gangrene (and intermittent claudication, rest pain and ulcer) I70.763
            intermittent claudication I70.713
            rest pain (and intermittent claudication) I70.723
          specified type NEC I70.793
        left I70.702
          with
            gangrene (and intermittent claudication, rest pain and ulcer) I70.762
            intermittent claudication I70.712
            rest pain (and intermittent claudication) I70.722

Arteriosclerosis, arteriosclerotic — *continued*
  extremities — *continued*
    bypass graft — *continued*
      specified graft — *continued*
        leg — *continued*
          left — *continued*
            with — *continued*
              ulceration (and intermittent claudication and rest pain) I70.749
                ankle I70.743
                calf I70.742
                foot site NEC I70.745
                heel I70.744
                lower leg NEC I70.748
                midfoot I70.744
                thigh I70.741
           specified type NEC I70.792
         right I70.701
          with
            gangrene (and intermittent claudication, rest pain and ulcer) I70.761
            intermittent claudication I70.711
            rest pain (and intermittent claudication) I70.721
            ulceration (and intermittent claudication and rest pain) I70.739
              ankle I70.733
              calf I70.732
              foot site NEC I70.735
              heel I70.734
              lower leg NEC I70.738
              midfoot I70.734
              thigh I70.731
          specified type NEC I70.791
        specified type NEC I70.799
        specified NEC I70.708
          with
            gangrene (and intermittent claudication, rest pain and ulcer) I70.768
            intermittent claudication I70.718
            rest pain (and intermittent claudication) I70.728
            ulceration (and intermittent claudication and rest pain) I70.75
          specified type NEC I70.798
      specified NEC I70.308
        with
          gangrene (and intermittent claudication, rest pain and ulcer) I70.368
          intermittent claudication I70.318
          rest pain (and intermittent claudication) I70.328
          ulceration (and intermittent claudication and rest pain) I70.35
          specifiec type NEC I70.398
    leg I70.209
      with
        gangrene (and intermittent claudication, rest pain and ulcer) I70.269
        intermittent claudication I70.219
        rest pain (and intermittent claudication) I70.229
      bilateral I70.203
        with
         gangrene (and intermittent claudication, rest pain and ulcer) I70.263
         intermittent claudication I70.213
         rest pain (and intermittent claudication) I70.223
        specified type NEC I70.293
      left I70.202
        with
         gangrene (and intermittent claudication, rest pain and ulcer) I70.262
         intermittent claudication I70.212
         rest pain (and intermittent claudication) I70.222
         ulceration (and intermittent claudication and rest pain) I70.249
          ankle I70.243
          calf I70.242
          foot site NEC I70.245
          heel I70.244
          lower leg NEC I70.248

Arteriosclerosis, arteriosclerotic — *continued*
- extremities — *continued*
  - leg — *continued*
    - left — *continued*
      - with — *continued*
        - ulceration — *continued*
          - midfoot I70.244
          - thigh I70.241
      - specified type NEC I70.292
    - right I70.201
      - with
        - gangrene (and intermittent claudication, rest pain and ulcer) I70.261
        - intermittent claudication I70.211
        - rest pain (and intermittent claudication) I70.221
        - ulceration (and intermittent claudication and rest pain) I70.239
          - ankle I70.233
          - calf I70.232
          - foot site NEC I70.235
          - heel I70.234
          - lower leg NEC I70.238
          - midfoot I70.234
          - thigh I70.231
      - specified type NEC I70.291
    - specified type NEC I70.299
  - specified site NEC I70.208
    - with
      - gangrene (and intermittent claudication, rest pain and ulcer) I70.268
      - intermittent claudication I70.218
      - rest pain (and intermittent claudication) I70.228
      - ulceration (and intermittent claudication and rest pain) I70.25
    - specified type NEC I70.298
- generalized I70.91
- heart (disease) — *see* Arteriosclerosis, coronary (artery),
- kidney — *see* Hypertension, kidney
- medial — *see* Arteriosclerosis, extremities
- mesenteric (artery) K55.1
- Mönckeberg's — *see* Arteriosclerosis, extremities
- myocarditis I51.4
- peripheral (of extremities) — *see* Arteriosclerosis, extremities
- pulmonary (idiopathic) I27.0
- renal (arterioles) (*see also* Hypertension, kidney)
  - artery I70.1
- retina (vascular) I70.8 [H35.0-] ☑
- specified artery NEC I70.8
- spinal (cord) G95.19
- vertebral (artery) I67.2

Arteriospasm I73.9
Arteriovenous — *see* condition
Arteritis I77.6
- allergic M31.0
- aorta (nonsyphilitic) I77.6
  - syphilitic A52.02
- aortic arch M31.4
- brachiocephalic M31.4
- brain I67.7
  - syphilitic A52.04
- cerebral I67.7
  - in systemic lupus erythematosus M32.19
  - listerial A32.89
  - syphilitic A52.04
  - tuberculous A18.89
- coronary (artery) I25.89
  - rheumatic I01.8
    - chronic I09.89
  - syphilitic A52.06
- cranial (left) (right), giant cell M31.6
- deformans — *see* Arteriosclerosis
- giant cell NEC M31.6
  - with polymyalgia rheumatica M31.5
- necrosing or necrotizing M31.9
  - specified NEC M31.8
- nodosa M30.0
- obliterans — *see* Arteriosclerosis
- pulmonary I28.8
- rheumatic — *see* Fever, rheumatic
- senile — *see* Arteriosclerosis
- suppurative I77.2
- syphilitic (general) A52.09
  - brain A52.04
  - coronary A52.06

Arteritis — *continued*
- syphilitic — *continued*
  - spinal A52.09
- temporal, giant cell M31.6
- young female aortic arch syndrome M31.4

Artery, arterial (*see also* condition)
- abscess I77.89
- single umbilical Q27.0

Arthralgia (allergic) (*see also* Pain, joint)
- in caisson disease T70.3 ☑
- temporomandibular M26.62

Arthritis, arthritic (acute) (chronic) (nonpyogenic) (subacute) M19.90
- allergic — *see* Arthritis, specified form NEC
- ankylosing (crippling) (spine) (*see also* Spondylitis, ankylosing)
  - sites other than spine — *see* Arthritis, specified form NEC
- atrophic — *see* Osteoarthritis
  - spine — *see* Spondylitis, ankylosing
- back — *see* Spondylopathy, inflammatory
- blennorrhagic (gonococcal) A54.42
- Charcot's — *see* Arthropathy, neuropathic
  - diabetic — *see* Diabetes, arthropathy, neuropathic
  - syringomyelic G95.0
- chylous (filarial) (*see also* category M01) B74.9
- climacteric (any site) NEC — *see* Arthritis, specified form NEC
- crystal (-induced) — *see* Arthritis, in, crystals
- deformans — *see* Osteoarthritis
- degenerative — *see* Osteoarthritis
- due to or associated with
  - acromegaly E22.0
  - brucellosis — *see* Brucellosis
  - caisson disease T70.3 ☑
  - diabetes — *see* Diabetes, arthropathy
  - dracontiasis (*see also* category M01) B72
  - enteritis NEC
    - regional — *see* Enteritis, regional
  - erysipelas (*see also* category M01) A46
  - erythema
    - epidemic A25.1
    - nodosum L52
  - filariasis NOS B74.9
  - glanders A24.0
  - helminthiasis (*see also* category M01) B83.9
  - hemophilia D66 [M36.2]
  - Henoch- (Schönlein) purpura D69.0 [M36.4]
  - human parvovirus (*see also* category M01) B97.6
  - infectious disease NEC M01 ☑
  - leprosy (*see also* category M01) (*see also* Leprosy) A30.9
  - Lyme disease A69.23
  - mycobacteria (*see also* category M01) A31.8
  - parasitic disease NEC (*see also* category M01) B89
  - paratyphoid fever (*see also* category M01) (*see also* Fever, paratyphoid) A01.4
  - rat bite fever (*see also* category M01) A25.1
  - regional enteritis — *see* Enteritis, regional
  - respiratory disorder NOS J98.9
  - serum sickness (*see also* Reaction, serum) T80.69 ☑
  - syringomyelia G95.0
  - typhoid fever A01.04
- epidemic erythema A25.1
- febrile — *see* Fever, rheumatic
- gonococcal A54.42
- gouty (acute) — *see* Gout, idiopathic
- in (due to)
  - acromegaly (*see also* subcategory M14.8-) E22.0
  - amyloidosis (*see also* subcategory M14.8-) E85.4
  - bacterial disease (*see also* subcategory M01) A49.9
  - Behçet's syndrome M35.2
  - caisson disease (*see also* subcategory M14.8-) T70.3 ☑
  - coliform bacilli (Escherichia coli) — *see* Arthritis, in, pyogenic organism NEC
  - crystals M11.9
    - dicalcium phosphate — *see* Arthritis, in, crystals, specified type NEC
    - hydroxyapatite M11.0- ☑
    - pyrophosphate — *see* Arthritis, in, crystals, specified type NEC
    - specified type NEC M11.80
      - ankle M11.87- ☑
      - elbow M11.82- ☑
      - foot joint M11.87- ☑
      - hand joint M11.84- ☑

Arthritis, arthritic — *continued*
- in — *continued*
  - crystals — *continued*
    - specified type — *continued*
      - hip M11.85- ☑
      - knee M11.86- ☑
      - multiple sites M11.8- ☑
      - shoulder M11.81- ☑
      - vertebrae M11.88
      - wrist M11.83- ☑
  - dermatoarthritis, lipoid E78.81
  - dracontiasis (dracunculiasis) (*see also* category M01) B72
  - endocrine disorder NEC (*see also* subcategory M14.8-) E34.9
  - enteritis, infectious NEC (*see also* category M01) A09
    - specified organism NEC (*see also* category M01) A08.8
  - erythema
    - multiforme (*see also* subcategory M14.8-) L51.9
    - nodosum (*see also* subcategory M14.8-) L52
  - gout — *see* Gout, idiopathic
  - helminthiasis NEC (*see also* category M01) B83.9
  - hemochromatosis (*see also* subcategory M14.8-) E83.118
  - hemoglobinopathy NEC D58.2 [M36.3]
  - hemophilia NEC D66 [M36.2]
  - Hemophilus influenzae M00.8- ☑ [B96.3]
  - Henoch (-Schönlein) purpura D69.0 [M36.4]
  - hyperparathyroidism NEC (*see also* subcategory M14.8-) E21.3
  - hypersensitivity reaction NEC T78.49 ☑ [M36.4]
  - hypogammaglobulinemia (*see also* subcategory M14.8-) D80.1
  - hypothyroidism NEC (*see also* subcategory M14.8-) E03.9
  - infection — *see* Arthritis, pyogenic or pyemic
    - spine — *see* Spondylopathy, infective
  - infectious disease NEC M01 ☑
  - leprosy (*see also* category M01) A30.9
  - leukemia NEC C95.9- ☑ [M36.1]
  - lipoid dermatoarthritis E78.81
  - Lyme disease A69.23
  - Mediterranean fever, familial (*see also* subcategory M14.8-) E85.0
  - Meningococcus A39.83
  - metabolic disorder NEC (*see also* subcategory M14.8-) E88.9
  - multiple myelomatosis C90.0- ☑ [M36.1]
  - mumps B26.85
  - mycosis NEC (*see also* category M01) B49
  - myelomatosis (multiple) C90.0- ☑ [M36.1]
  - neurological disorder NEC G98.0
  - ochronosis (*see also* subcategory M14.8-) E70.29
  - O'nyong-nyong (*see also* category M01) A92.1
  - parasitic disease NEC (*see also* category M01) B89
  - paratyphoid fever (*see also* category M01) A01.4
  - Pseudomonas — *see* Arthritis, pyogenic, bacterial NEC
  - psoriasis L40.50
  - pyogenic organism NEC — *see* Arthritis, pyogenic, bacterial NEC
  - Reiter's disease — *see* Reiter's disease
  - respiratory disorder NEC (*see also* subcategory M14.8-) J98.9
  - reticulosis, malignant (*see also* subcategory M14.8-) C86.0
  - rubella B06.82
  - Salmonella (arizonae) (cholerae-suis) (enteritidis) (typhimurium) A02.23
  - sarcoidosis D86.86
  - specified bacteria NEC — *see* Arthritis, pyogenic, bacterial NEC
  - sporotrichosis B42.82
  - syringomyelia G95.0
  - thalassemia NEC D56.9 [M36.3]
  - tuberculosis — *see* Tuberculosis, arthritis
  - typhoid fever A01.04
  - urethritis, Reiter's — *see* Reiter's disease
  - viral disease NEC (*see also* category M01) B34.9
- infectious or infective (*see also* Arthritis, pyogenic or pyemic)
  - spine — *see* Spondylopathy, infective
- juvenile M08.90
  - with systemic onset — *see* Still's disease
  - ankle M08.97- ☑

Arthritis, arthritic — *continued*
- juvenile — *continued*
  - elbow M08.92- ☑
  - foot joint M08.97- ☑
  - hand joint M08.94- ☑
  - hip M08.95- ☑
  - knee M08.96- ☑
  - multiple site M08.99
  - pauciarticular M08.40
    - ankle M08.47- ☑
    - elbow M08.42- ☑
    - foot joint M08.47- ☑
    - hand joint M08.44- ☑
    - hip M08.45- ☑
    - knee M08.46- ☑
    - shoulder M08.41- ☑
    - vertebrae M08.48
    - wrist M08.43- ☑
  - psoriatic L40.54
  - rheumatoid — *see* Arthritis, rheumatoid, juvenile
  - shoulder M08.91- ☑
  - specified type NEC M08.80
    - ankle M08.87- ☑
    - elbow M08.82- ☑
    - foot joint M08.87- ☑
    - hand joint M08.84- ☑
    - hip M08.85- ☑
    - knee M08.86- ☑
    - multiple site M08.89
    - shoulder M08.81- ☑
    - specified joint NEC M08.88
    - vertebrae M08.88
    - wrist M08.83- ☑
  - wrist M08.93- ☑
- meaning osteoarthritis — *see* Osteoarthritis
- meningococcal A39.83
- menopausal (any site) NEC — *see* Arthritis, specified form NEC
- mutilans (psoriatic) L40.52
- mycotic NEC (*see also* category M01) B49
- neuropathic (Charcot) — *see* Arthropathy, neuropathic
  - diabetic — *see* Diabetes, arthropathy, neuropathic
  - nonsyphilitic NEC G98.0
  - syringomyelic G95.0
- ochronotic (*see also* subcategory M14.8-) E70.29
- palindromic (any site) — *see* Rheumatism, palindromic
- pneumococcal M00.10
  - ankle M00.17- ☑
  - elbow M00.12- ☑
  - foot joint — *see* Arthritis, pneumococcal, ankle
  - hand joint M00.14- ☑
  - hip M00.15- ☑
  - knee M00.16- ☑
  - multiple site M00.19
  - shoulder M00.11- ☑
  - vertebra M00.18
  - wrist M00.13- ☑
- postdysenteric — *see* Arthropathy, postdysenteric
- postmeningococcal A39.84
- postrheumatic, chronic — *see* Arthropathy, postrheumatic, chronic
- primary progressive (*see also* Arthritis, specified form NEC)
  - spine — *see* Spondylitis, ankylosing
- psoriatic L40.50
- purulent (any site except spine) — *see* Arthritis, pyogenic or pyemic
  - spine — *see* Spondylopathy, infective
- pyogenic or pyemic (any site except spine) M00.9
  - bacterial NEC M00.80
    - ankle M00.87- ☑
    - elbow M00.82- ☑
    - foot joint — *see* Arthritis, pyogenic, bacterial NEC, ankle
    - hand joint M00.84- ☑
    - hip M00.85- ☑
    - knee M00.86- ☑
    - multiple site M00.89
    - shoulder M00.81- ☑
    - vertebra M00.88
    - wrist M00.83- ☑
  - pneumococcal — *see* Arthritis, pneumococcal
  - spine — *see* Spondylopathy, infective
  - staphylococcal — *see* Arthritis, staphylococcal
  - streptococcal — *see* Arthritis, streptococcal NEC
    - pneumococcal — *see* Arthritis, pneumococcal

Arthritis, arthritic — *continued*
- reactive — *see* Reiter's disease
- rheumatic (*see also* Arthritis, rheumatoid)
  - acute or subacute — *see* Fever, rheumatic
- rheumatoid M06.9
  - with
    - carditis — *see* Rheumatoid, carditis
    - endocarditis — *see* Rheumatoid, carditis
    - heart involvement NEC — *see* Rheumatoid, carditis
    - lung involvement — *see* Rheumatoid, lung
    - myocarditis — *see* Rheumatoid, carditis
    - myopathy — *see* Rheumatoid, myopathy
    - pericarditis — *see* Rheumatoid, carditis
    - polyneuropathy — *see* Rheumatoid, polyneuropathy
    - rheumatoid factor — *see* Arthritis, rheumatoid, seropositive
    - splenoadenomegaly and leukopenia — *see* Felty's syndrome
    - vasculitis — *see* Rheumatoid, vasculitis
    - visceral involvement NEC — *see* Rheumatoid, arthritis, with involvement of organs NEC
  - juvenile (with or without rheumatoid factor) M08.00
    - ankle M08.07- ☑
    - elbow M08.02- ☑
    - foot joint M08.07- ☑
    - hand joint M08.04- ☑
    - hip M08.05- ☑
    - knee M08.06- ☑
    - multiple site M08.09
    - shoulder M08.01- ☑
    - vertebra M08.08
    - wrist M08.03- ☑
  - seronegative M06.00
    - ankle M06.07- ☑
    - elbow M06.02- ☑
    - foot joint M06.07- ☑
    - hand joint M06.04- ☑
    - hip M06.05- ☑
    - knee M06.06- ☑
    - multiple site M06.09
    - shoulder M06.01- ☑
    - vertebra M06.08
    - wrist M06.03- ☑
  - seropositive M05.9
    - without organ involvement M05.70
      - ankle M05.77- ☑
      - elbow M05.72- ☑
      - foot joint M05.77- ☑
      - hand joint M05.74- ☑
      - hip M05.75- ☑
      - knee M05.76- ☑
      - multiple sites M05.79
      - shoulder M05.71- ☑
      - vertebra — *see* Spondylitis, ankylosing
      - wrist M05.73- ☑
    - specified NEC M05.80
      - ankle M05.87- ☑
      - elbow M05.82- ☑
      - foot joint M05.87- ☑
      - hand joint M05.84- ☑
      - hip M05.85- ☑
      - knee M05.86- ☑
      - multiple sites M05.89
      - shoulder M05.81- ☑
      - vertebra — *see* Spondylitis, ankylosing
      - wrist M05.83- ☑
    - specified type NEC M06.80
      - ankle M06.87- ☑
      - elbow M06.82- ☑
      - foot joint M06.87- ☑
      - hand joint M06.84- ☑
      - hip M06.85- ☑
      - knee M06.86- ☑
      - multiple site M06.89
      - shoulder M06.81- ☑
      - vertebra M06.88
      - wrist M06.83- ☑
  - spine — *see* Spondylitis, ankylosing
- rubella B06.82
- scorbutic (*see also* subcategory M14.8-) E54
- senile or senescent — *see* Osteoarthritis
- septic (any site except spine) — *see* Arthritis, pyogenic or pyemic

Arthritis, arthritic — *continued*
- septic — *see* Arthritis, pyogenic or pyemic — *continued*
  - spine — *see* Spondylopathy, infective
- serum (nontherapeutic) (therapeutic) — *see* Arthropathy, postimmunization
- specified form NEC M13.80
  - ankle M13.87- ☑
  - elbow M13.82- ☑
  - foot joint M13.87- ☑
  - hand joint M13.84- ☑
  - hip M13.85- ☑
  - knee M13.86- ☑
  - multiple site M13.89
  - shoulder M13.81- ☑
  - specified joint NEC M13.88
  - wrist M13.83- ☑
- spine (*see also* Spondylopathy, inflammatory)
  - infectious or infective NEC — *see* Spondylopathy, infective
  - Marie-Strümpell — *see* Spondylitis, ankylosing
  - pyogenic — *see* Spondylopathy, infective
  - rheumatoid — *see* Spondylitis, ankylosing
  - traumatic (old) — *see* Spondylopathy, traumatic
  - tuberculous A18.01
- staphylococcal M00.00
  - ankle M00.07- ☑
  - elbow M00.02- ☑
  - foot joint — *see* Arthritis, staphylococcal, ankle
  - hand joint M00.04- ☑
  - hip M00.05- ☑
  - knee M00.06- ☑
  - multiple site M00.09
  - shoulder M00.01- ☑
  - vertebra M00.08
  - wrist M00.03- ☑
- streptococcal NEC M00.20
  - ankle M00.27- ☑
  - elbow M00.22- ☑
  - foot joint — *see* Arthritis, streptococcal, ankle
  - hand joint M00.24- ☑
  - hip M00.25- ☑
  - knee M00.26- ☑
  - multiple site M00.29
  - shoulder M00.21- ☑
  - vertebra M00.28
  - wrist M00.23- ☑
- suppurative — *see* Arthritis, pyogenic or pyemic
- syphilitic (late) A52.16
  - congenital A50.55 [M12.80]
- syphilitica deformans (Charcot) A52.16
- temporomandibular M26.69
- toxic of menopause (any site) — *see* Arthritis, specified form NEC
- transient — *see* Arthropathy, specified form NEC
- traumatic (chronic) — *see* Arthropathy, traumatic
- tuberculous A18.02
  - spine A18.01
- uratic — *see* Gout, idiopathic
- urethritica (Reiter's) — *see* Reiter's disease
- vertebral — *see* Spondylopathy, inflammatory
- villous (any site) — *see* Arthropathy, specified form NEC

Arthrocele — *see* Effusion, joint
Arthrodesis status Z98.1
Arthrodynia (*see also* Pain, joint)
Arthrodysplasia Q74.9
Arthrofibrosis, joint — *see* Ankylosis
Arthrogryposis (congenital) Q68.8
- multiplex congenita Q74.3
Arthrokatadysis M24.7
Arthropathy (*see also* Arthritis) M12.9
- Charcot's — *see* Arthropathy, neuropathic
  - diabetic — *see* Diabetes, arthropathy, neuropathic
  - syringomyelic G95.0
- cricoarytenoid J38.7
- crystal (-induced) — *see* Arthritis, in, crystals
- diabetic NEC — *see* Diabetes, arthropathy
- distal interphalangeal, psoriatic L40.51
- enteropathic M07.60
  - ankle M07.67- ☑
  - elbow M07.62- ☑
  - foot joint M07.67- ☑
  - hand joint M07.64- ☑
  - hip M07.65- ☑
  - knee M07.66- ☑

Arthropathy — *continued*
  enteropathic — *continued*
    multiple site M07.69
    shoulder M07.61- ☑
    vertebra M07.68
    wrist M07.63- ☑
  following intestinal bypass M02.00
    ankle M02.07- ☑
    elbow M02.02- ☑
    foot joint M02.07- ☑
    hand joint M02.04- ☑
    hip M02.05- ☑
    knee M02.06- ☑
    multiple site M02.09
    shoulder M02.01- ☑
    vertebra M02.08
    wrist M02.03- ☑
  gouty (*see also* Gout, idiopathic)
    in (due to)
      Lesch-Nyhan syndrome E79.1 [M14.8-] ☑
      sickle-cell disorders D57- ☑ [M14.8-] ☑
  hemophilic NEC D66 [M36.2]
    in (due to)
      hyperparathyroidism NEC E21.3 [M14.8-] ☑
      metabolic disease NOS E88.9 [M14.8-] ☑
  in (due to)
    acromegaly E22.0 [M14.8-] ☑
    amyloidosis E85.4 [M14.8-] ☑
    blood disorder NOS D75.9 [M36.3]
    diabetes — *see* Diabetes, arthropathy
    endocrine disease NOS E34.9 [M14.8-] ☑
    erythema
      multiforme L51.9 [M14.8-] ☑
      nodosum L52 [M14.8-] ☑
    hemochromatosis E83.118 [M14.8-] ☑
    hemoglobinopathy NEC D58.2 [M36.3]
    hemophilia NEC D66 [M36.2]
    Henoch-Schönlein purpura D69.0 [M36.4]
    hyperthyroidism E05.90 [M14.8-] ☑
    hypothyroidism E03.9 [M14.8-] ☑
    infective endocarditis I33.0 [M12.80]
    leukemia NEC C95.9- ☑ [M36.1]
    malignant histiocytosis C96.A [M36.1]
    metabolic disease NOS E88.9 [M14.8-] ☑
    multiple myeloma C90.0- ☑ [M36.1]
    neoplastic disease NOS (*see also* Neoplasm)
      D49.9 [M36.1]
    nutritional deficiency (*see also* subcategory
      M14.8-) E63.9
    psoriasis NOS L40.50
    sarcoidosis D86.86
    syphilis (late) A52.77
      congenital A50.55 [M12.80]
    thyrotoxicosis (*see also* subcategory M14.8-) E05.90
    ulcerative colitis K51.90 [M07.60]
    viral hepatitis (postinfectious) NEC B19.9 [M12.80]
    Whipple's disease (*see also* subcategory M14.8-)
      K90.81
  Jaccoud — *see* Arthropathy, postrheumatic, chronic
  juvenile — *see* Arthritis, juvenile
    psoriatic L40.54
    mutilans (psoriatic) L40.52
  neuropathic (Charcot) M14.60
    ankle M14.67- ☑
    diabetic — *see* Diabetes, arthropathy, neuropathic
    elbow M14.62- ☑
    foot joint M14.67- ☑
    hand joint M14.64- ☑
    hip M14.65- ☑
    knee M14.66- ☑
    multiple site M14.69
    nonsyphilitic NEC G98.0
    shoulder M14.61- ☑
    syringomyelic G95.0
    vertebra M14.68
    wrist M14.63- ☑
  osteopulmonary — *see* Osteoarthropathy, hyper-
    trophic, specified NEC
  postdysenteric M02.10
    ankle M02.17- ☑
    elbow M02.12- ☑
    foot joint M02.17- ☑
    hand joint M02.14- ☑
    hip M02.15- ☑
    knee M02.16- ☑
    multiple site M02.19
    shoulder M02.11- ☑

Arthropathy — *continued*
  postdysenteric — *continued*
    vertebra M02.18
    wrist M02.13- ☑
  postimmunization M02.20
    ankle M02.27- ☑
    elbow M02.22- ☑
    foot joint M02.27- ☑
    hand joint M02.24- ☑
    hip M02.25- ☑
    knee M02.26- ☑
    multiple site M02.29
    shoulder M02.21- ☑
    vertebra M02.28
    wrist M02.23- ☑
  postinfectious NEC B99 ☑ [M12.80]
    in (due to)
      enteritis due to Yersinia enterocolitica
        A04.6 [M12.80]
      syphilis A52.77
      viral hepatitis NEC B19.9 [M12.80]
  postrheumatic, chronic (Jaccoud) M12.00
    ankle M12.07- ☑
    elbow M12.02- ☑
    foot joint M12.07- ☑
    hand joint M12.04- ☑
    hip M12.05- ☑
    knee M12.06- ☑
    multiple site M12.09
    shoulder M12.01- ☑
    specified joint NEC M12.08
    vertebrae M12.08
    wrist M12.03- ☑
  psoriatic NEC L40.59
    interphalangeal, distal L40.51
  reactive M02.9
    in (due to)
      infective endocarditis I33.0 [M02.9]
    specified type NEC M02.80
      ankle M02.87- ☑
      elbow M02.82- ☑
      foot joint M02.87- ☑
      hand joint M02.84- ☑
      hip M02.85- ☑
      knee M02.86- ☑
      multiple site M02.89
      shoulder M02.81- ☑
      vertebra M02.88
      wrist M02.83- ☑
  specified form NEC M12.80
    ankle M12.87- ☑
    elbow M12.82- ☑
    foot joint M12.87- ☑
    hand joint M12.84- ☑
    hip M12.85- ☑
    knee M12.86- ☑
    multiple site M12.89
    shoulder M12.81- ☑
    specified joint NEC M12.88
    vertebrae M12.88
    wrist M12.83- ☑
  syringomyelic G95.0
  tabes dorsalis A52.16
  tabetic A52.16
  transient — *see* Arthropathy, specified form NEC
  traumatic M12.50
    ankle M12.57- ☑
    elbow M12.52- ☑
    foot joint M12.57- ☑
    hand joint M12.54- ☑
    hip M12.55- ☑
    knee M12.56- ☑
    multiple site M12.59
    shoulder M12.51- ☑
    specified joint NEC M12.58
    vertebrae M12.58
    wrist M12.53- ☑
Arthropyosis — *see* Arthritis, pyogenic or pyemic
Arthrosis (deformans) (degenerative) (localized) (*see also*
  Osteoarthritis) M19.90
  spine — *see* Spondylosis
Arthus' phenomenon or reaction T78.41 ☑
  due to
    drug — *see* Table of Drugs and Chemicals, by drug
Articular — *see* condition
Articulation, reverse (teeth) M26.24

Artificial
  insemination complication — *see* Complications, arti-
    ficial, fertilization
  opening status (functioning) (without complication)
    Z93.9
    anus (colostomy) Z93.3
    colostomy Z93.3
    cystostomy Z93.50
      appendico-vesicostomy Z93.52
      cutaneous Z93.51
      specified NEC Z93.59
    enterostomy Z93.4
    gastrostomy Z93.1
    ileostomy Z93.2
    intestinal tract NEC Z93.4
    jejunostomy Z93.4
    nephrostomy Z93.6
    specified site NEC Z93.8
    tracheostomy Z93.0
    ureterostomy Z93.6
    urethrostomy Z93.6
    urinary tract NEC Z93.6
    vagina Z93.8
    vagina status Z93.8
Arytenoid — *see* condition
Asbestosis (occupational) J61
ASC-H (atypical squamous cells cannot exclude high
    grade squamous intraepithelial lesion on cytologic
    smear)
  anus R85.611
  cervix R87.611
  vagina R87.621
ASC-US (atypical squamous cells of undetermined signif-
    icance on cytologic smear)
  anus R85.610
  cervix R87.610
  vagina R87.620
Ascariasis B77.9
  with
    complications NEC B77.89
    intestinal complications B77.0
    pneumonia, pneumonitis B77.81
Ascaridosis, ascaridiasis — *see* Ascariasis
Ascaris (infection) (infestation) (lumbricoides) — *see*
    Ascariasis
Ascending — *see* condition
Aschoff's bodies — *see* Myocarditis, rheumatic
Ascites (abdominal) R18.8
  cardiac I50.9
  chylous (nonfilarial) I89.8
    filarial — *see* Infestation, filarial
  due to
    cirrhosis, alcoholic K70.31
    hepatitis
      alcoholic K70.11
      chronic active K71.51
    S. japonicum B65.2
  heart I50.9
  malignant R18.0
  pseudochylous R18.8
  syphilitic A52.74
  tuberculous A18.31
Aseptic — *see* condition
Asherman's syndrome N85.6
Asialia K11.7
Asiatic cholera — *see* Cholera
Asimultagnosia (simultanagnosia) R48.3
Askin's tumor — *see* Neoplasm, connective tissue, ma-
    lignant
Asocial personality F60.2
Asomatognosia R41.4
Aspartylglucosaminuria E77.1
Asperger's disease or syndrome F84.5
Aspergilloma — *see* Aspergillosis
Aspergillosis (with pneumonia) B44.9
  bronchopulmonary, allergic B44.81
  disseminated B44.7
  generalized B44.7
  pulmonary NEC B44.1
    allergic B44.81
    invasive B44.0
  specified NEC B44.89
  tonsillar B44.2
Aspergillus (flavus) (fumigatus) (infection) (terreus) —
    see Aspergillosis
Aspermatogenesis — *see* Azoospermia
Aspermia (testis) — *see* Azoospermia
Asphyxia, asphyxiation (by) R09.01

☑ **Additional Character Required — Refer to the Tabular List for Character Selection**   ▽ **Subterms under main terms may continue to next column or page**

Asphyxia, asphyxiation — *continued*
  antenatal P84
  birth P84
  bunny bag — *see* Asphyxia, due to, mechanical threat to breathing, trapped in bed clothes
  crushing S28.0 ☑
  drowning T75.1 ☑
  gas, fumes, or vapor — *see* Table of Drugs and Chemicals
  inhalation — *see* Inhalation
  intrauterine P84
  local I73.00
    with gangrene I73.01
  mucus (*see also* Foreign body, respiratory tract, causing asphyxia)
  newborn P84
  pathological R09.01
  postnatal P84
    mechanical — *see* Asphyxia, due to, mechanical threat to breathing
  prenatal P84
  reticularis R23.1
  strangulation — *see* Asphyxia, due to, mechanical threat to breathing
  submersion T75.1 ☑
  traumatic T71.9 ☑
    due to
      crushed chest S28.0 ☑
      foreign body (in) — *see* Foreign body, respiratory tract, causing asphyxia
      low oxygen content of ambient air T71.20 ☑
        due to
          being trapped in
            low oxygen environment T71.29 ☑
              in car trunk T71.221 ☑
                circumstances undetermined T71.224 ☑
                done with intent to harm by
                  another person T71.223 ☑
                  self T71.222 ☑
              in refrigerator T71.231 ☑
                circumstances undetermined T71.234 ☑
                done with intent to harm by
                  another person T71.233 ☑
                  self T71.232 ☑
      cave-in T71.21 ☑
      mechanical threat to breathing (accidental) T71.191 ☑
        circumstances undetermined T71.194 ☑
        done with intent to harm by
          another person T71.193 ☑
          self T71.192 ☑
        hanging T71.161 ☑
          circumstances undetermined T71.164 ☑
          done with intent to harm by
            another person T71.163 ☑
            self T71.162 ☑
        plastic bag T71.121 ☑
          circumstances undetermined T71.124 ☑
          done with intent to harm by
            another person T71.123 ☑
            self T71.122 ☑
        smothering
          in furniture T71.151 ☑
            circumstances undetermined T71.154 ☑
            done with intent to harm by
              another person T71.153 ☑
              self T71.152 ☑
          under
            another person's body T71.141 ☑
              circumstances undetermined T71.144 ☑
              done with intent to harm T71.143 ☑
            pillow T71.111 ☑
              circumstances undetermined T71.114 ☑
              done with intent to harm by
                another person T71.113 ☑
                self T71.112 ☑
          trapped in bed clothes T71.131 ☑
            circumstances undetermined T71.134 ☑
            done with intent to harm by
              another person T71.133 ☑
              self T71.132 ☑

Asphyxia, asphyxiation — *continued*
  vomiting, vomitus — *see* Foreign body, respiratory tract, causing asphyxia
Aspiration
  amniotic (clear) fluid (newborn) P24.10
    with
      pneumonia (pneumonitis) P24.11
      respiratory symptoms P24.11
  blood
    newborn (without respiratory symptoms) P24.20
      with
        pneumonia (pneumonitis) P24.21
        respiratory symptoms P24.21
      specified age NEC — *see* Foreign body, respiratory tract
  bronchitis J69.0
  food or foreign body (with asphyxiation) — *see* Asphyxia, food
  liquor (amnii) (newborn) P24.10
    with
      pneumonia (pneumonitis) P24.11
      respiratory symptoms P24.11
  meconium (newborn) (without respiratory symptoms) P24.00
    with
      pneumonia (pneumonitis) P24.01
      respiratory symptoms P24.01
  milk (newborn) (without respiratory symptoms) P24.30
    with
      pneumonia (pneumonitis) P24.31
      respiratory symptoms P24.31
    specified age NEC — *see* Foreign body, respiratory tract
  mucus (*see also* Foreign body, by site, causing asphyxia)
    newborn P24.10
      with
        pneumonia (pneumonitis) P24.11
        respiratory symptoms P24.11
  neonatal P24.9
    specific NEC (without respiratory symptoms) P24.80
      with
        pneumonia (pneumonitis) P24.81
        respiratory symptoms P24.81
  newborn P24.9
    specific NEC (without respiratory symptoms) P24.80
      with
        pneumonia (pneumonitis) P24.81
        respiratory symptoms P24.81
  pneumonia J69.0
  pneumonitis J69.0
  syndrome of newborn — *see* Aspiration, by substance, with pneumonia
  vernix caseosa (newborn) P24.80
    with
      pneumonia (pneumonitis) P24.81
      respiratory symptoms P24.81
  vomitus (*see also* Foreign body, respiratory tract)
    newborn (without respiratory symptoms) P24.30
      with
        pneumonia (pneumonitis) P24.31
        respiratory symptoms P24.31
Asplenia (congenital) Q89.01
  postsurgical Z90.81
Assam fever B55.0
Assault, sexual — *see* Maltreatment
Assmann's focus NEC A15.0
Astasia (-abasia) (hysterical) F44.4
Asteatosis cutis L85.3
Astereognosia, astereognosis R48.1
Asterixis R27.8
  in liver disease K71.3
Asteroid hyalitis — *see* Deposit, crystalline
Asthenia, asthenic R53.1
  cardiac (*see also* Failure, heart) I50.9
    psychogenic F45.8
  cardiovascular (*see also* Failure, heart) I50.9
    psychogenic F45.8
  heart (*see also* Failure, heart) I50.9
    psychogenic F45.8
  hysterical F44.4
  myocardial (*see also* Failure, heart) I50.9
    psychogenic F45.8
  nervous F48.8
  neurocirculatory F45.8
  neurotic F48.8
  psychogenic F48.8
  psychoneurotic F48.8

Asthenia, asthenic — *continued*
  psychophysiologic F48.8
  reaction (psychophysiologic) F48.8
  senile R54
Asthenopia (*see also* Discomfort, visual)
  hysterical F44.6
  psychogenic F44.6
Asthenospermia — *see* Abnormal, specimen, male genital organs
Asthma, asthmatic (bronchial) (catarrh) (spasmodic) J45.909
  with
    chronic obstructive bronchitis J44.9
      with
        acute lower respiratory infection J44.0
        exacerbation (acute) J44.1
    chronic obstructive pulmonary disease J44.9
      with
        acute lower respiratory infection J44.0
        exacerbation (acute) J44.1
    exacerbation (acute) J45.901
    hay fever — *see* Asthma, allergic extrinsic
    rhinitis, allergic — *see* Asthma, allergic extrinsic
    status asthmaticus J45.902
  allergic extrinsic J45.909
    with
      exacerbation (acute) J45.901
      status asthmaticus J45.902
  atopic — *see* Asthma, allergic extrinsic
  cardiac — *see* Failure, ventricular, left
  cardiobronchial I50.1
  childhood J45.909
    with
      exacerbation (acute) J45.901
      status asthmaticus J45.902
  chronic obstructive J44.9
    with
      acute lower respiratory infection J44.0
      exacerbation (acute) J44.1
  collier's J60
  cough variant J45.991
  detergent J69.8
  due to
    detergent J69.8
    inhalation of fumes J68.3
  eosinophilic J82
  extrinsic, allergic — *see* Asthma, allergic extrinsic
  grinder's J62.8
  hay — *see* Asthma, allergic extrinsic
  heart I50.1
  idiosyncratic — *see* Asthma, nonallergic
  intermittent (mild) J45.20
    with
      exacerbation (acute) J45.21
      status asthmaticus J45.22
  intrinsic, nonallergic — *see* Asthma, nonallergic
  Kopp's E32.8
  late-onset J45.909
    with
      exacerbation (acute) J45.901
      status asthmaticus J45.902
  mild intermittent J45.20
    with
      exacerbation (acute) J45.21
      status asthmaticus J45.22
  mild persistent J45.30
    with
      exacerbation (acute) J45.31
      status asthmaticus J45.32
  Millar's (laryngismus stridulus) J38.5
  miner's J60
  mixed J45.909
    with
      exacerbation (acute) J45.901
      status asthmaticus J45.902
  moderate persistent J45.40
    with
      exacerbation (acute) J45.41
      status asthmaticus J45.42
  nervous — *see* Asthma, nonallergic
  nonallergic (intrinsic) J45.909
    with
      exacerbation (acute) J45.901
      status asthmaticus J45.902
  persistent
    mild J45.30
      with
        exacerbation (acute) J45.31

Asthma, asthmatic — *continued*
 persistent — *continued*
  mild — *continued*
   with — *continued*
    status asthmaticus J45.32
  moderate J45.40
   with
    exacerbation (acute) J45.41
    status asthmaticus J45.42
   severe J45.50
    with
     exacerbation (acute) J45.51
     status asthmaticus J45.52
 platinum J45.998
 pneumoconiotic NEC J64
 potter's J62.8
 predominantly allergic J45.909
 psychogenic F54
 pulmonary eosinophilic J82
 red cedar J67.8
 Rostan's I50.1
 sandblaster's J62.8
 sequoiosis J67.8
 severe persistent J45.50
  with
   exacerbation (acute) J45.51
   status asthmaticus J45.52
 specified NEC J45.998
 stonemason's J62.8
 thymic E32.8
 tuberculous — *see* Tuberculosis, pulmonary
 Wichmann's (laryngismus stridulus) J38.5
 wood J67.8
Astigmatism (compound) (congenital) H52.20- ☑
 irregular H52.21- ☑
 regular H52.22- ☑
Astraphobia F40.220
Astroblastoma
 specified site — *see* Neoplasm, malignant, by site
 unspecified site C71.9
Astrocytoma (cystic)
 anaplastic
  specified site — *see* Neoplasm, malignant, by site
  unspecified site C71.9
 fibrillary
  specified site — *see* Neoplasm, malignant, by site
  unspecified site C71.9
 fibrous
  specified site — *see* Neoplasm, malignant, by site
  unspecified site C71.9
 gemistocytic
  specified site — *see* Neoplasm, malignant, by site
  unspecified site C71.9
 juvenile
  specified site — *see* Neoplasm, malignant, by site
  unspecified site C71.9
 pilocytic
  specified site — *see* Neoplasm, malignant, by site
  unspecified site C71.9
 piloid
  specified site — *see* Neoplasm, malignant, by site
  unspecified site C71.9
 protoplasmic
  specified site — *see* Neoplasm, malignant, by site
  unspecified site C71.9
 specified site NEC — *see* Neoplasm, malignant, by site
 subependymal D43.2
  giant cell
   specified site — *see* Neoplasm, uncertain behavior, by site
   unspecified site D43.2
  specified site — *see* Neoplasm, uncertain behavior, by site
  unspecified site D43.2
 unspecified site C71.9
Astroglioma
 specified site — *see* Neoplasm, malignant, by site
 unspecified site C71.9
Asymbolia R48.8
Asymmetry (*see also* Distortion)
 between native and reconstructed breast N65.1
 face Q67.0
 jaw (lower) — *see* Anomaly, dentofacial, jaw-cranial
  base relationship, asymmetry
Asynergia, asynergy R27.8
 ventricular I51.89
Asystole (heart) — *see* Arrest, cardiac

At risk
 for falling Z91.81
Ataxia, ataxy, ataxic R27.0
 acute R27.8
 brain (hereditary) G11.9
 cerebellar (hereditary) G11.9
  with defective DNA repair G11.3
  alcoholic G31.2
  early-onset G11.1
  in
   alcoholism G31.2
   myxedema E03.9 [G13.2]
   neoplastic disease (*see also* Neoplasm)
    D49.9 [G13.1]
   specified disease NEC G32.81
  late-onset (Marie's) G11.2
 cerebral (hereditary) G11.9
 congenital nonprogressive G11.0
 family, familial — *see* Ataxia, hereditary
 following
  cerebrovascular disease I69.993
   cerebral infarction I69.393
   intracerebral hemorrhage I69.193
   nontraumatic intracranial hemorrhage NEC
    I69.293
   specified disease NEC I69.893
   subarachnoid hemorrhage I69.093
 Friedreich's (heredofamilial) (cerebellar) (spinal) G11.1
 gait R26.0
  hysterical F44.4
 general R27.8
 gluten M35.9 [G32.81]
  with celiac disease K90.0 [G32.81]
 hereditary G11.9
  with neuropathy G60.2
  cerebellar — *see* Ataxia, cerebellar
  spastic G11.4
  specified NEC G11.8
  spinal (Friedreich's) G11.1
 heredofamilial — *see* Ataxia, hereditary
 Hunt's G11.1
 hysterical F44.4
 locomotor (progressive) (syphilitic) (partial) (spastic)
  A52.11
  diabetic — *see* Diabetes, ataxia
 Marie's (cerebellar) (heredofamilial) (late- onset) G11.2
 nonorganic origin F44.4
 nonprogressive, congenital G11.0
 psychogenic F44.4
 Roussy-Lévy G60.0
 Sanger-Brown's (hereditary) G11.2
 spastic hereditary G11.4
 spinal
  hereditary (Friedreich's) G11.1
  progressive (syphilitic) A52.11
 spinocerebellar, X-linked recessive G11.1
 telangiectasia (Louis-Bar) G11.3
Ataxia-telangiectasia (Louis-Bar) G11.3
Atelectasis (massive) (partial) (pressure) (pulmonary)
  J98.11
 newborn P28.10
  due to resorption P28.11
  partial P28.19
  primary P28.0
  secondary P28.19
 primary (newborn) P28.0
 tuberculous — *see* Tuberculosis, pulmonary
Atelocardia Q24.9
Atelomyelia Q06.1
Atheroembolism
 of
  extremities
   lower I75.02- ☑
   upper I75.01- ☑
  kidney I75.81
  specified NEC I75.89
Atheroma, atheromatous (*see also* Arteriosclerosis)
  I70.90
 aorta, aortic I70.0
  valve (*see also* Endocarditis, aortic) I35.8
 aorto-iliac I70.0
 artery — *see* Arteriosclerosis
 basilar (artery) I67.2
 carotid (artery) (common) (internal) I67.2
 cerebral (arteries) I67.2
 coronary (artery) I25.10
  with angina pectoris — *see* Arteriosclerosis, coronary (artery),

Atheroma, atheromatous — *continued*
 degeneration — *see* Arteriosclerosis
 heart, cardiac — *see* Disease, heart, ischemic,
  atherosclerotic
 mitral (valve) I34.8
 myocardium, myocardial — *see* Disease, heart, ischemic, atherosclerotic
 pulmonary valve (heart) (*see also* Endocarditis, pulmonary) I37.8
 tricuspid (heart) (valve) I36.8
 valve, valvular — *see* Endocarditis
 vertebral (artery) I67.2
Atheromatosis — *see* Arteriosclerosis
Atherosclerosis (*see also* Arteriosclerosis)
 coronary
  artery I25.10
   with angina pectoris — *see* Arteriosclerosis,
    coronary (artery),
   due to
    calcified coronary lesion (severely) I25.84
    lipid rich plaque I25.83
  transplanted heart I25.811
   bypass graft I25.812
    with angina pectoris — *see* Arteriosclerosis,
     coronary (artery),
   native coronary artery I25.811
    with angina pectoris — *see* Arteriosclerosis,
     coronary (artery),
Athetosis (acquired) R25.8
 bilateral (congenital) G80.3
 congenital (bilateral) (double) G80.3
 double (congenital) G80.3
 unilateral R25.8
Athlete's
 foot B35.3
 heart I51.7
Athrepsia E41
Athyrea (acquired) (*see also* Hypothyroidism)
 congenital E03.1
Atonia, atony, atonic
 bladder (sphincter) (neurogenic) N31.2
 capillary I78.8
 cecum K59.8
  psychogenic F45.8
 colon — *see* Atony, intestine
 congenital P94.2
 esophagus K22.8
 intestine K59.8
  psychogenic F45.8
 stomach K31.89
  neurotic or psychogenic F45.8
 uterus (during labor) O62.2
  with hemorrhage (postpartum) O72.1
  postpartum (with hemorrhage) O72.1
   without hemorrhage O75.89
Atopy — *see* History, allergy
Atransferrinemia, congenital E88.09
Atresia, atretic
 alimentary organ or tract NEC Q45.8
  upper Q40.8
 ani, anus, anal (canal) Q42.3
  with fistula Q42.2
 aorta (arch) (ring) Q25.2
 aortic (orifice) (valve) Q23.0
  arch Q25.2
  congenital with hypoplasia of ascending aorta and
   defective development of left ventricle (with
   mitral stenosis) Q23.4
  in hypoplastic left heart syndrome Q23.4
 aqueduct of Sylvius Q03.0
  with spina bifida — *see* Spina bifida, with hydrocephalus
 artery NEC Q27.8
  cerebral Q28.3
  coronary Q24.5
  digestive system Q27.8
  eye Q15.8
  lower limb Q27.8
  pulmonary Q25.5
  specified site NEC Q27.8
  umbilical Q27.0
  upper limb Q27.8
 auditory canal (external) Q16.1
 bile duct (common) (congenital) (hepatic) Q44.2
  acquired — *see* Obstruction, bile duct
 bladder (neck) Q64.39
  obstruction Q64.31
 bronchus Q32.4

Atresia, atretic — continued
cecum Q42.8
cervix (acquired) N88.2
congenital Q51.828
in pregnancy or childbirth — see Anomaly, cervix, in pregnancy or childbirth
causing obstructed labor O65.5
choana Q30.0
colon Q42.9
specified NEC Q42.8
common duct Q44.2
cricoid cartilage Q31.8
cystic duct Q44.2
acquired K82.8
with obstruction K82.0
digestive organs NEC Q45.8
duodenum Q41.0
ear canal Q16.1
ejaculatory duct Q55.4
epiglottis Q31.8
esophagus Q39.0
with tracheoesophageal fistula Q39.1
eustachian tube Q17.8
fallopian tube (congenital) Q50.6
acquired N97.1
follicular cyst N83.0
foramen of
Luschka Q03.1
with spina bifida — see Spina bifida, with hydrocephalus
Magendie Q03.1
with spina bifida — see Spina bifida, with hydrocephalus
gallbladder Q44.1
genital organ
external
female Q52.79
male Q55.8
internal
female Q52.8
male Q55.8
glottis Q31.8
gullet Q39.0
with tracheoesophageal fistula Q39.1
heart valve NEC Q24.8
pulmonary Q22.0
tricuspid Q22.4
hymen Q52.3
acquired (postinfective) N89.6
ileum Q41.2
intestine (small) Q41.9
large Q42.9
specified NEC Q42.8
iris, filtration angle Q15.0
jejunum Q41.1
lacrimal apparatus Q10.4
larynx Q31.8
meatus urinarius Q64.33
mitral valve Q23.2
in hypoplastic left heart syndrome Q23.4
nares (anterior) (posterior) Q30.0
nasopharynx Q34.8
nose, nostril Q30.0
acquired J34.89
organ or site NEC Q89.8
osseous meatus (ear) Q16.1
oviduct (congenital) Q50.6
acquired N97.1
parotid duct Q38.4
acquired K11.8
pulmonary (artery) Q25.5
valve Q22.0
pulmonic Q22.0
pupil Q13.2
rectum Q42.1
with fistula Q42.0
salivary duct Q38.4
acquired K11.8
sublingual duct Q38.4
acquired K11.8
submandibular duct Q38.4
acquired K11.8
submaxillary duct Q38.4
acquired K11.8
thyroid cartilage Q31.8
trachea Q32.1
tricuspid valve Q22.4
ureter Q62.10

Atresia, atretic — continued
ureter — continued
pelvic junction Q62.11
vesical orifice Q62.12
ureteropelvic junction Q62.11
ureterovesical orifice Q62.12
urethra (valvular) Q64.39
stricture Q64.32
urinary tract NEC Q64.8
uterus Q51.818
acquired N85.8
vagina (congenital) Q52.4
acquired (postinfectional) (senile) N89.5
vas deferens Q55.3
vascular NEC Q27.8
cerebral Q28.3
digestive system Q27.8
lower limb Q27.8
specified site NEC Q27.8
upper limb Q27.8
vein NEC Q27.8
digestive system Q27.8
great Q26.8
lower limb Q27.8
portal Q26.5
pulmonary Q26.3
specified site NEC Q27.8
upper limb Q27.8
vena cava (inferior) (superior) Q26.8
vesicourethral orifice Q64.31
vulva Q52.79
acquired N90.5
Atrichia, atrichosis — see Alopecia
Atrophia (see also Atrophy)
cutis senilis L90.8
due to radiation L57.8
gyrata of choroid and retina H31.23
senilis R54
dermatological L90.8
due to radiation (nonionizing) (solar) L57.8
unguium L60.3
congenita Q84.6
Atrophie blanche (en plaque) (de Milian) L95.0
Atrophoderma, atrophodermia (of) L90.9
diffusum (idiopathic) L90.4
maculatum L90.8
et striatum L90.8
due to syphilis A52.79
syphilitic A51.39
neuriticum L90.8
Pasini and Pierini L90.3
pigmentosum Q82.1
reticulatum symmetricum faciei L66.4
senile L90.8
due to radiation (nonionizing) (solar) L57.8
vermiculata (cheeks) L66.4
Atrophy, atrophic (of)
adrenal (capsule) (gland) E27.49
primary (autoimmune) E27.1
alveolar process or ridge (edentulous) K08.20
anal sphincter (disuse) N81.84
appendix K38.8
arteriosclerotic — see Arteriosclerosis
bile duct (common) (hepatic) K83.8
bladder N32.89
neurogenic N31.8
blanche (en plaque) (of Milian) L95.0
bone (senile) NEC (see also Disorder, bone, specified type NEC)
due to
tabes dorsalis (neurogenic) A52.11
brain (cortex) (progressive) G31.9
frontotemporal circumscribed G31.01 [F02.80]
with behavioral disturbance G31.01 [F02.81]
senile NEC G31.1
breast N64.2
obstetric — see Disorder, breast, specified type NEC
buccal cavity K13.79
cardiac — see Degeneration, myocardial
cartilage (infectional) (joint) — see Disorder, cartilage, specified NEC
cerebellar — see Atrophy, brain
cerebral — see Atrophy, brain
cervix (mucosa) (senile) (uteri) N88.8
menopausal N95.8
Charcot-Marie-Tooth G60.0
choroid (central) (macular) (myopic) (retina) H31.10- ☑

Atrophy, atrophic — continued
choroid — continued
diffuse secondary H31.12- ☑
gyrate H31.23
senile H31.11- ☑
ciliary body — see Atrophy, iris
conjunctiva (senile) H11.89
corpus cavernosum N48.89
cortical — see Atrophy, brain
cystic duct K82.8
Déjérine-Thomas G23.8
disuse NEC — see Atrophy, muscle
Duchenne-Aran G12.21
ear H93.8- ☑
edentulous alveolar ridge K08.20
endometrium (senile) N85.8
cervix N88.8
enteric K63.89
epididymis N50.8
eyeball — see Disorder, globe, degenerated condition, atrophy
eyelid (senile) — see Disorder, eyelid, degenerative
facial (skin) L90.9
fallopian tube (senile) N83.32
with ovary N83.33
fascioscapulohumeral (Landouzy- Déjérine) G71.0
fatty, thymus (gland) E32.8
gallbladder K82.8
gastric K29.40
with bleeding K29.41
gastrointestinal K63.89
glandular I89.8
globe H44.52- ☑
gum K06.0
hair L67.8
heart (brown) — see Degeneration, myocardial
hemifacial Q67.4
Romberg G51.8
infantile E41
paralysis, acute — see Poliomyelitis, paralytic
intestine K63.89
iris (essential) (progressive) H21.26- ☑
specified NEC H21.29
kidney (senile) (terminal) (see also Sclerosis, renal) N26.1
congenital or infantile Q60.5
bilateral Q60.4
unilateral Q60.3
hydronephrotic — see Hydronephrosis
lacrimal gland (primary) H04.14- ☑
secondary H04.15- ☑
Landouzy-Déjérine G71.0
laryngitis, infective J37.0
larynx J38.7
Leber's optic (hereditary) H47.22
lip K13.0
liver (yellow) K72.90
with coma K72.91
acute, subacute K72.00
with coma K72.01
chronic K72.10
with coma K72.11
lung (senile) J98.4
macular (dermatological) L90.8
syphilitic, skin A51.39
striated A52.79
mandible (edentulous) K08.20
minimal K08.21
moderate K08.22
severe K08.23
maxilla K08.20
minimal K08.24
moderate K08.25
severe K08.26
muscle, muscular (diffuse) (general) (idiopathic) (primary) M62.50
ankle M62.57- ☑
Duchenne-Aran G12.21
foot M62.57- ☑
forearm M62.53- ☑
hand M62.54- ☑
infantile spinal G12.0
lower leg M62.56- ☑
multiple sites M62.59
myelopathic — see Atrophy, muscle, spinal
myotonic G71.11
neuritic G58.9
neuropathic (peroneal) (progressive) G60.0

Atrophy, atrophic — *continued*
  muscle, muscular — *continued*
    pelvic (disuse) N81.84
    peroneal G60.0
    progressive (bulbar) G12.21
      adult G12.1
      infantile (spinal) G12.0
      spinal G12.9
        adult G12.1
        infantile G12.0
    pseudohypertrophic G71.0
    shoulder region M62.51- ☑
    specified site NEC M62.58
    spinal G12.9
      adult form G12.1
      Aran-Duchenne G12.21
      childhood form, type II G12.1
      distal G12.1
      hereditary NEC G12.1
      infantile, type I (Werdnig-Hoffmann) G12.0
      juvenile form, type III (Kugelberg- Welander) G12.1
      progressive G12.21
      scapuloperoneal form G12.1
      specified NEC G12.8
    syphilitic A52.78
    thigh M62.55- ☑
    upper arm M62.52- ☑
  myocardium — *see* Degeneration, myocardial
  myometrium (senile) N85.8
    cervix N88.8
  myopathic NEC — *see* Atrophy, muscle
  myotonia G71.11
  nail L60.3
  nasopharynx J31.1
  nerve (*see also* Disorder, nerve)
    abducens — *see* Strabismus, paralytic, sixth nerve
    accessory G52.8
    acoustic or auditory H93.3 ☑
    cranial G52.9
      eighth (auditory) H93.3 ☑
      eleventh (accessory) G52.8
      fifth (trigeminal) G50.8
      first (olfactory) G52.0
      fourth (trochlear) — *see* Strabismus, paralytic, fourth nerve
      second (optic) H47.20
      sixth (abducens) — *see* Strabismus, paralytic, sixth nerve
      tenth (pneumogastric) (vagus) G52.2
      third (oculomotor) — *see* Strabismus, paralytic, third nerve
      twelfth (hypoglossal) G52.3
    hypoglossal G52.3
    oculomotor — *see* Strabismus, paralytic, third nerve
    olfactory G52.0
    optic (papillomacular bundle)
      syphilitic (late) A52.15
        congenital A50.44
    pneumogastric G52.2
    trigeminal G50.8
    trochlear — *see* Strabismus, paralytic, fourth nerve
    vagus (pneumogastric) G52.2
  neurogenic, bone, tabetic A52.11
  nutritional E41
  old age R54
  olivopontocerebellar G23.8
  optic (nerve) H47.20
    glaucomatous H47.23- ☑
    hereditary H47.22
    primary H47.21- ☑
    specified type NEC H47.29- ☑
    syphilitic (late) A52.15
      congenital A50.44
  orbit H05.31- ☑
  ovary (senile) N83.31
    with fallopian tube N83.33
  oviduct (senile) — *see* Atrophy, fallopian tube
  palsy, diffuse (progressive) G12.22
  pancreas (duct) (senile) K86.8
  parotid gland K11.0
  pelvic muscle N81.84
  penis N48.89
  pharynx J39.2
  pluriglandular E31.8
    autoimmune E31.0
  polyarthritis M15.9

Atrophy, atrophic — *continued*
  prostate N42.89
  pseudohypertrophic (muscle) G71.0
  renal (*see also* Sclerosis, renal) N26.1
  retina, retinal (postinfectional) H35.89
  rhinitis J31.0
  salivary gland K11.0
  scar L90.5
  sclerosis, lobar (of brain) G31.09 [F02.80]
    with behavioral disturbance G31.09 [F02.81]
  scrotum N50.8
  seminal vesicle N50.8
  senile R54
    due to radiation (nonionizing) (solar) L57.8
  skin (patches) (spots) L90.9
    degenerative (senile) L90.8
    due to radiation (nonionizing) (solar) L57.8
    senile L90.8
  spermatic cord N50.8
  spinal (acute) (cord) G95.89
    muscular — *see* Atrophy, muscle, spinal
    paralysis G12.20
      acute — *see* Poliomyelitis, paralytic
      meaning progressive muscular atrophy G12.21
  spine (column) — *see* Spondylopathy, specified NEC
  spleen (senile) D73.0
  stomach K29.40
    with bleeding K29.41
  striate (skin) L90.6
    syphilitic A52.79
  subcutaneous L90.9
  sublingual gland K11.0
  submandibular gland K11.0
  submaxillary gland K11.0
  Sudeck's — *see* Algoneurodystrophy
  suprarenal (capsule) (gland) E27.49
    primary E27.1
  systemic affecting central nervous system in
      myxedema E03.9 [G13.2]
      neoplastic disease (*see also* Neoplasm) D49.9 [G13.1]
      specified disease NEC G13.8
  tarso-orbital fascia, congenital Q10.3
  testis N50.0
  thenar, partial — *see* Syndrome, carpal tunnel
  thymus (fatty) E32.8
  thyroid (gland) (acquired) E03.4
    with cretinism E03.1
    congenital (with myxedema) E03.1
  tongue (senile) K14.8
    papillae K14.4
  trachea J39.8
  tunica vaginalis N50.8
  turbinate J34.89
  tympanic membrane (nonflaccid) H73.82- ☑
    flaccid H73.81- ☑
  upper respiratory tract J39.8
  uterus, uterine (senile) N85.8
    cervix N88.8
    due to radiation (intended effect) N85.8
      adverse effect or misadventure N99.89
  vagina (senile) N95.2
  vas deferens N50.8
  vascular I99.8
  vertebra (senile) — *see* Spondylopathy, specified NEC
  vulva (senile) N90.5
  Werdnig-Hoffmann G12.0
  yellow — *see* Failure, hepatic
Attack, attacks
  with alteration of consciousness (with automatisms) — *see* Epilepsy, localization-related, symptomatic, with complex partial seizures
  without alteration of consciousness — *see* Epilepsy, localization-related, symptomatic, with simple partial seizures
  Adams-Stokes I45.9
  akinetic — *see* Epilepsy, generalized, specified NEC
  angina — *see* Angina
  atonic — *see* Epilepsy, generalized, specified NEC
  benign shuddering G25.83
  cataleptic — *see* Catalepsy
  coronary — *see* Infarct, myocardium
  cyanotic, newborn P28.2
  drop NEC R55
  epileptic — *see* Epilepsy
  heart — *see* infarct, myocardium
  hysterical F44.9

Attack, attacks — *continued*
  jacksonian — *see* Epilepsy, localization-related, symptomatic, with simple partial seizures
  myocardium, myocardial — *see* Infarct, myocardium
  myoclonic — *see* Epilepsy, generalized, specified NEC
  panic F41.0
  psychomotor — *see* Epilepsy, localization-related, symptomatic, with complex partial seizures
  salaam — *see* Epilepsy, spasms
  schizophreniform, brief F23
  shuddering, benign G25.83
  Stokes-Adams I45.9
  syncope R55
  transient ischemic (TIA) G45.9
    specified NEC G45.8
  unconsciousness R55
    hysterical F44.89
  vasomotor R55
  vasovagal (paroxysmal) (idiopathic) R55
Attention (to)
  artificial
    opening (of) Z43.9
      digestive tract NEC Z43.4
        colon Z43.3
        ilium Z43.2
        stomach Z43.1
      specified NEC Z43.8
      trachea Z43.0
      urinary tract NEC Z43.6
        cystostomy Z43.5
        nephrostomy Z43.6
        ureterostomy Z43.6
        urethrostomy Z43.6
      vagina Z43.7
  colostomy Z43.3
  cystostomy Z43.5
  deficit disorder or syndrome F98.8
    with hyperactivity — *see* Disorder, attention-deficit hyperactivity
  gastrostomy Z43.1
  ileostomy Z43.2
  jejunostomy Z43.4
  nephrostomy Z43.6
  surgical dressings Z48.01
  sutures Z48.02
  tracheostomy Z43.0
  ureterostomy Z43.6
  urethrostomy Z43.6
Attrition
  gum K06.0
  tooth, teeth (excessive) (hard tissues) K03.0
Atypical, atypism (*see also* condition)
  cells (on cytolgocial smear) (endocervical) (endometri-al) (glandular)
    cervix R87.619
    vagina R87.629
  cervical N87.9
  endometrium N85.9
    hyperplasia N85.00
  parenting situation Z62.9
Auditory — *see* condition
Aujeszky's disease B33.8
Aurantiasis, cutis E67.1
Auricle, auricular (*see also* condition)
  cervical Q18.2
Auriculotemporal syndrome G50.8
Austin Flint murmur (aortic insufficiency) I35.1
Australian
  Q fever A78
  X disease A83.4
Autism, autistic (childhood) (infantile) F84.0
  atypical F84.9
Autodigestion R68.89
Autoerythrocyte sensitization (syndrome) D69.2
Autographism L50.3
Autoimmune
  disease (systemic) M35.9
  inhibitors to clotting factors D68.311
  lymphoproliferative syndrome [ALPS] D89.82
  thyroiditis E06.3
Autointoxication R68.89
Automatism G93.89
  with temporal sclerosis G93.81
  epileptic — *see* Epilepsy, localization-related, symptomatic, with complex partial seizures
  paroxysmal, idiopathic — *see* Epilepsy, localization-related, symptomatic, with complex partial seizures

B

Autonomic, autonomous
  bladder (neurogenic) N31.2
  hysteria seizure F44.5
Autosensitivity, erythrocyte D69.2
Autosensitization, cutaneous L30.2
Autosome — *see* condition by chromosome involved
Autotopagnosia R48.1
Autotoxemia R68.89
Autumn — *see* condition
Avellis' syndrome G46.8
Aversion
  oral R63.3
    newborn P92.-☑
    nonorganic origin F98.2 ☑
  sexual F52.1
Aviator's
  disease or sickness — *see* Effect, adverse, high altitude
  ear T70.0 ☑
Avitaminosis (multiple) (*see also* Deficiency, vitamin) E56.9
  B E53.9
    with
      beriberi E51.11
      pellagra E52
  B2 E53.0
  B6 E53.1
  B12 E53.8
  D E55.9
    with rickets E55.0
  G E53.0
  K E56.1
  nicotinic acid E52
AVNRT (atrioventricular nodal re-entrant tachycardia) I47.1
AVRT (atrioventricular nodal re-entrant tachycardia) I47.1
Avulsion (traumatic)
  blood vessel — *see* Injury, blood vessel
  bone — *see* Fracture, by site
  cartilage (*see also* Dislocation, by site)
    symphyseal (inner), complicating delivery O71.6
  external site other than limb — *see* Wound, open, by site
  eye S05.7- ☑
  head (intracranial)
    external site NEC S08.89 ☑
    scalp S08.0 ☑
  internal organ or site — *see* Injury, by site
  joint (*see also* Dislocation, by site)
    capsule — *see* Sprain, by site
  kidney S37.06- ☑
  ligament — *see* Sprain, by site
  limb (*see also* Amputation, traumatic, by site)
    skin and subcutaneous tissue — *see* Wound, open, by site
  muscle — *see* Injury, muscle
  nerve (root) — *see* Injury, nerve
  scalp S08.0 ☑
  skin and subcutaneous tissue — *see* Wound, open, by site
  spleen S36.032 ☑
  symphyseal cartilage (inner), complicating delivery O71.6
  tendon — *see* Injury, muscle
  tooth S03.2 ☑
Awareness of heart beat R00.2
Axenfeld's
  anomaly or syndrome Q15.0
  degeneration (calcareous) Q13.4
Axilla, axillary (*see also* condition)
  breast Q83.1
Axonotmesis — *see* Injury, nerve
Ayerza's disease or syndrome (pulmonary artery sclerosis with pulmonary hypertension) I27.0
Azoospermia (organic) N46.01
  due to
    drug therapy N46.021
    efferent duct obstruction N46.023
    infection N46.022
    radiation N46.024
    specified cause NEC N46.029
    systemic disease N46.025
Azotemia R79.89
  meaning uremia N19
Aztec ear Q17.3
Azygos
  continuation inferior vena cava Q26.8
  lobe (lung) Q33.1

Baastrup's disease — *see* Kissing spine
Babesiosis B60.0
Babington's disease (familial hemorrhagic telangiectasia) I78.0
Babinski's syndrome A52.79
Baby
  crying constantly R68.11
  floppy (syndrome) P94.2
Bacillary — *see* condition
Bacilluria N39.0
Bacillus (*see also* Infection, bacillus)
  abortus infection A23.1
  anthracis infection A22.9
  coli infection (*see also* Escherichia coli) B96.20
  Flexner's A03.1
  mallei infection A24.0
  Shiga's A03.0
  suipestifer infection — *see* Infection, salmonella
Back — *see* condition
Backache (postural) M54.9
  sacroiliac M53.3
  specified NEC M54.89
Backflow — *see* Reflux
Backward reading (dyslexia) F81.0
Bacteremia R78.81
  with sepsis — *see* Sepsis
Bactericholia — *see* Cholecystitis, acute
Bacterid, bacteride (pustular) L40.3
Bacterium, bacteria, bacterial
  agent NEC, as cause of disease classified elsewhere B96.89
  in blood — *see* Bacteremia
  in urine — *see* Bacteriuria
Bacteriuria, bacteruria N39.0
  asymptomatic N39.0
Bacteroides
  fragilis, as cause of disease classified elsewhere B96.6
Bad
  heart — *see* Disease, heart
  trip
    due to drug abuse — *see* Abuse, drug, hallucinogen
    due to drug dependence — *see* Dependence, drug, hallucinogen
Baelz's disease (cheilitis glandularis apostematosa) K13.0
Baerensprung's disease (eczema marginatum) B35.6
Bagasse disease or pneumonitis J67.1
Bagassosis J67.1
Baker's cyst — *see* Cyst, Baker's
Bakwin-Krida syndrome (craniometaphyseal dysplasia) Q78.5
Balancing side interference M26.56
Balanitis (circinata) (erosiva) (gangrenosa) (phagedenic) (vulgaris) N48.1
  amebic A06.82
  candidal B37.42
  due to Haemophilus ducreyi A57
  gonococcal (acute) (chronic) A54.09
  xerotica obliterans N48.0
Balanoposthitis N47.6
  gonococcal (acute) (chronic) A54.09
  ulcerative (specific) A63.8
Balanorrhagia — *see* Balanitis
Balantidiasis, balantidiosis A07.0
Bald tongue K14.4
Baldness (*see also* Alopecia)
  male-pattern — *see* Alopecia, androgenic
Balkan grippe A78
Balloon disease — *see* Effect, adverse, high altitude
Balo's disease (concentric sclerosis) G37.5
Bamberger-Marie disease — *see* Osteoarthropathy, hypertrophic, specified type NEC
Bancroft's filariasis B74.0
Band(s)
  adhesive — *see* Adhesions, peritoneum
  anomalous or congenital (*see also* Anomaly, by site)
    heart (atrial) (ventricular) Q24.8
    intestine Q43.3
    omentum Q43.3
  cervix N88.1
  constricting, congenital Q79.8
  gallbladder (congenital) Q44.1
  intestinal (adhesive) — *see* Adhesions, peritoneum

Band(s) — *continued*
  obstructive
    intestine K56.5
    peritoneum K56.5
  periappendiceal, congenital Q43.3
  peritoneal (adhesive) — *see* Adhesions, peritoneum
    uterus N73.6
      internal N85.6
    vagina N89.5
Bandemia D72.825
Bandl's ring (contraction), complicating delivery O62.4
Bangkok hemorrhagic fever A91
Bang's disease (brucella abortus) A23.1
Bankruptcy, anxiety concerning Z59.8
Bannister's disease T78.3 ☑
  hereditary D84.1
Banti's disease or syndrome (with cirrhosis) (with portal hypertension) K76.6
Bar, median, prostate — *see* Enlargement, enlarged, prostate
Barcoo disease or rot — *see* Ulcer, skin
Barlow's disease E54
Barodontalgia T70.29 ☑
Baron Münchausen syndrome — *see* Disorder, factitious
Barosinusitis T70.1 ☑
Barotitis T70.0 ☑
Barotrauma T70.29 ☑
  odontalgia T70.29 ☑
  otitic T70.0 ☑
  sinus T70.1 ☑
Barraquer (-Simons) **disease or syndrome** (progressive lipodystrophy) E88.1
Barré-Guillain disease or syndrome G61.0
Barré-Liéou syndrome (posterior cervical sympathetic) M53.0
Barrel chest M95.4
Barrett's
  disease — *see* Barrett's, esophagus
  esophagus K22.70
    with dysplasia K22.719
      high grade K22.711
      low grade K22.710
    without dysplasia K22.70
  syndrome — *see* Barrett's, esophagus
  ulcer K22.10
    with bleeding K22.11
    without bleeding K22.10
Bársony (-Polgár) (-Teschendorf) **syndrome** (corkscrew esophagus) K22.4
Barth syndrome E78.71
Bartholinitis (suppurating) N75.8
  gonococcal (acute) (chronic) (with abscess) A54.1
Bartonellosis A44.9
  cutaneous A44.1
  mucocutaneous A44.1
  specified NEC A44.8
  systemic A44.0
Barton's fracture S52.56- ☑
Bartter's syndrome E26.81
Basal — *see* condition
Basan's (hidrotic) ectodermal dysplasia Q82.4
Baseball finger — *see* Dislocation, finger
Basedow's disease (exophthalmic goiter) — *see* Hyperthyroidism, with, goiter
Basic — *see* condition
Basilar — *see* condition
Bason's (hidrotic) ectodermal dysplasia Q82.4
Basopenia — *see* Agranulocytosis
Basophilia D72.824
Basophilism (cortico-adrenal) (Cushing's) (pituitary) E24.0
Bassen-Kornzweig disease or syndrome E78.6
Bat ear Q17.5
Bateman's
  disease B08.1
  purpura (senile) D69.2
Bathing cramp T75.1 ☑
Bathophobia F40.248
Batten (-Mayou) **disease** E75.4
  retina E75.4 [H36]
Batten-Steinert syndrome G71.11
Battered — *see* Maltreatment
Battey Mycobacterium infection A31.0
Battle exhaustion F43.0
Battledore placenta O43.19- ☑

Baumgarten-Cruveilhier cirrhosis, disease or syndrome K74.69
Bauxite fibrosis (of lung) J63.1
Bayle's disease (general paresis) A52.17
Bazin's disease (primary) (tuberculous) A18.4
Beach ear — see Swimmer's, ear
Beaded hair (congenital) Q84.1
Béal conjunctivitis or syndrome B30.2
Beard's disease (neurasthenia) F48.8
Beat(s)
  atrial, premature I49.1
  ectopic I49.49
  elbow — see Bursitis, elbow
  escaped, heart I49.49
  hand — see Bursitis, hand
  knee — see Bursitis, knee
  premature I49.40
    atrial I49.1
    auricular I49.1
    supraventricular I49.1
Beau's
  disease or syndrome — see Degeneration, myocardial
  lines (transverse furrows on fingernails) L60.4
Bechterev's syndrome — see Spondylitis, ankylosing
Becker's
  cardiomyopathy I42.8
  disease
    idiopathic mural endomyocardial disease I42.3
    myotonia congenita, recessive form G71.12
  dystrophy G71.0
  pigmented hairy nevus D22.5
Beck's syndrome (anterior spinal artery occlusion) I65.8
Beckwith-Wiedemann syndrome Q87.3
Bed confinement status Z74.01
Bed sore — see Ulcer, pressure, by site
Bedbug bite(s) — see Bite(s), by site, superficial, insect
Bedclothes, asphyxiation or suffocation by — see Asphyxia, traumatic, due to, mechanical, trapped
Bednar's
  aphthae K12.0
  tumor — see Neoplasm, malignant, by site
Bedridden Z74.01
Bedsore — see Ulcer, pressure, by site
Bedwetting — see Enuresis
Bee sting (with allergic or anaphylactic shock) — see Toxicity, venom, arthropod, bee
Beer drinker's heart (disease) I42.6
Begbie's disease (exophthalmic goiter) — see Hyperthyroidism, with, goiter
Behavior
  antisocial
    adult Z72.811
    child or adolescent Z72.810
  disorder, disturbance — see Disorder, conduct
  disruptive — see Disorder, conduct
  drug seeking Z72.89
  inexplicable R46.2
  marked evasiveness R46.5
  obsessive-compulsive R46.81
  overactivity R46.3
  poor responsiveness R46.4
  self-damaging (life-style) Z72.89
  sleep-incompatible Z72.821
  slowness R46.4
  specified NEC R46.89
  strange (and inexplicable) R46.2
  suspiciousness R46.5
  type A pattern Z73.1
  undue concern or preoccupation with stressful events R46.6
  verbosity and circumstantial detail obscuring reason for contact R46.7
Behçet's disease or syndrome M35.2
Behr's disease — see Degeneration, macula
Beigel's disease or morbus (white piedra) B36.2
Bejel A65
Bekhterev's syndrome — see Spondylitis, ankylosing
Belching — see Eructation
Bell's
  mania F30.8
  palsy, paralysis G51.0
    infant or newborn P11.3
  spasm G51.3
Bence Jones albuminuria or proteinuria NEC R80.3
Bends T70.3 ☑
Benedikt's paralysis or syndrome G46.3
Benign (see also condition)

Benign — continued
  prostatic hyperplasia — see Hyperplasia, prostate
Bennett's fracture (displaced) S62.21- ☑
Benson's disease — see Deposit, crystalline
Bent
  back (hysterical) F44.4
  nose M95.0
    congenital Q67.4
Bereavement (uncomplicated) Z63.4
Bergeron's disease (hysterical chorea) F44.4
Berger's disease — see Nephropathy, IgA
Beriberi (dry) E51.11
  heart (disease) E51.12
  polyneuropathy E51.11
  wet E51.12
    involving circulatory system E51.11
Berlin's disease or edema (traumatic) S05.8X- ☑
Berlock (berloque) **dermatitis** L56.2
Bernard-Horner syndrome G90.2
Bernard-Soulier disease or thrombopathia D69.1
Bernhardt (-Roth) **disease** — see Mononeuropathy, lower limb, meralgia paresthetica
Bernheim's syndrome — see Failure, heart, congestive
Bertielliasis B71.8
Berylliosis (lung) J63.2
Besnier-Boeck (-Schaumann) **disease** — see Sarcoidosis
Besnier's
  lupus pernio D86.3
  prurigo L20.0
Bestiality F65.89
Best's disease H35.50
Beta-mercaptolactate-cysteine disulfiduria E72.09
Betalipoproteinemia, broad or floating E78.2
Betting and gambling Z72.6
  pathological (compulsive) F63.0
Bezoar T18.9 ☑
  intestine T18.3 ☑
  stomach T18.2 ☑
Bezold's abscess — see Mastoiditis, acute
Bianchi's syndrome R48.8
Bicornate or bicornis uterus Q51.3
  in pregnancy or childbirth O34.59- ☑
    causing obstructed labor O65.5
Bicuspid aortic valve Q23.1
Biedl-Bardet syndrome Q87.89
Bielschowsky (-Jansky) **disease** E75.4
Biermer's (pernicious) anemia or disease D51.0
Biett's disease L93.0
Bifid (congenital)
  apex, heart Q24.8
  clitoris Q52.6
  kidney Q63.8
  nose Q30.2
  patella Q74.1
  scrotum Q55.29
  toe NEC Q74.2
  tongue Q38.3
  ureter Q62.8
  uterus Q51.3
  uvula Q35.7
Biforis uterus (suprasimplex) Q51.3
Bifurcation (congenital)
  gallbladder Q44.1
  kidney pelvis Q63.8
  renal pelvis Q63.8
  rib Q76.6
  tongue, congenital Q38.3
  trachea Q32.1
  ureter Q62.8
  urethra Q64.74
  vertebra Q76.49
Big spleen syndrome D73.1
Bigeminal pulse R00.8
Bilateral — see condition
Bile
  duct — see condition
  pigments in urine R82.2
Bilharziasis (see also Schistosomiasis)
  chyluria B65.0
  cutaneous B65.3
  galacturia B65.0
  hematochyluria B65.0
  intestinal B65.1
  lipemia B65.9
  lipuria B65.0
  oriental B65.2
  piarhemia B65.9

Bilharziasis — continued
  pulmonary NOS B65.9 [J99]
    pneumonia B65.9 [J17]
  tropical hematuria B65.0
  vesical B65.0
Biliary — see condition
Bilirubin metabolism disorder E80.7
  specified NEC E80.6
Bilirubinemia, familial nonhemolytic E80.4
Bilirubinuria R82.2
Biliuria R82.2
Bilocular stomach K31.2
Binswanger's disease I67.3
Biparta, bipartite
  carpal scaphoid Q74.0
  patella Q74.1
  vagina Q52.10
Bird
  face Q75.8
  fancier's disease or lung J67.2
Birt-Hogg-Dube syndrome Q87.89
Birth
  complications in mother — see Delivery, complicated
  compression during NOS P15.9
  defect — see Anomaly
  immature (less than 37 completed weeks) — see Preterm, newborn
    extremely (less than 28 completed weeks) — see Immaturity, extreme
  inattention, at or after — see Maltreatment, child, neglect
  injury NOS P15.9
    basal ganglia P11.1
    brachial plexus NEC P14.3
    brain (compression) (pressure) P11.2
    central nervous system NOS P11.9
    cerebellum P11.1
    cerebral hemorrhage P10.1
    external genitalia P15.5
    eye P15.3
    face P15.4
    fracture
      bone P13.9
        specified NEC P13.8
      clavicle P13.4
      femur P13.2
      humerus P13.3
      long bone, except femur P13.3
      radius and ulna P13.3
      skull P13.0
      spine P11.5
      tibia and fibula P13.3
    intracranial P11.2
      laceration or hemorrhage P10.9
        specified NEC P10.8
    intraventricular hemorrhage P10.2
    laceration
      brain P10.1
      by scalpel P15.8
      peripheral nerve P14.9
    liver P15.0
    meninges
      brain P11.1
      spinal cord P11.5
    nerve
      brachial plexus P14.3
      cranial NEC (except facial) P11.4
      facial P11.3
      peripheral P14.9
      phrenic (paralysis) P14.2
    paralysis
      facial nerve P11.3
      spinal P11.5
    penis P15.5
    rupture
      spinal cord P11.5
    scalp P12.9
    scalpel wound P15.8
    scrotum P15.5
    skull NEC P13.1
      fracture P13.0
    specified type NEC P15.8
    spinal cord P11.5
    spine P11.5
    spleen P15.1
    sternomastoid (hematoma) P15.2
    subarachnoid hemorrhage P10.3
    subcutaneous fat necrosis P15.6

Birth — *continued*
  injury — *continued*
    subdural hemorrhage P10.0
    tentorial tear P10.4
    testes P15.5
    vulva P15.5
  lack of care, at or after — *see* Maltreatment, child, neglect
  neglect, at or after — *see* Maltreatment, child, neglect
  palsy or paralysis, newborn, NOS (birth injury) P14.9
  premature (infant) — *see* Preterm, newborn
  shock, newborn P96.89
  trauma — *see* Birth, injury
  weight
    4000 grams to 4499 grams P08.1
    4500 grams or more P08.0
    low (2499 grams or less) — *see* Low, birthweight
      extremely (999 grams or less) — *see* Low, birthweight, extreme
Birthmark Q82.5
Bisalbuminemia E88.09
Biskra's button B55.1
Bite(s) (animal) (human)
  abdomen, abdominal
    wall S31.159 ☑
      with penetration into peritoneal cavity S31.659 ☑
      epigastric region S31.152 ☑
        with penetration into peritoneal cavity S31.652 ☑
      left
        lower quadrant S31.154 ☑
          with penetration into peritoneal cavity S31.654 ☑
        upper quadrant S31.151 ☑
          with penetration into peritoneal cavity S31.651 ☑
      periumbilic region S31.155 ☑
        with penetration into peritoneal cavity S31.655 ☑
      right
        lower quadrant S31.153 ☑
          with penetration into peritoneal cavity S31.653 ☑
        upper quadrant S31.150 ☑
          with penetration into peritoneal cavity S31.650 ☑
      superficial NEC S30.871 ☑
        insect S30.861 ☑
  alveolar (process) — *see* Bite, oral cavity
  amphibian (venomous) — *see* Venom, bite, amphibian
  animal (*see also* Bite, by site)
    venomous — *see* Venom
  ankle S91.05- ☑
    superficial NEC S90.57- ☑
      insect S90.56- ☑
  antecubital space — *see* Bite, elbow
  anus S31.835 ☑
    superficial NEC S30.877 ☑
      insect S30.867 ☑
  arm (upper) S41.15- ☑
    lower — *see* Bite, forearm
    superficial NEC S40.87- ☑
      insect S40.86- ☑
  arthropod NEC — *see* Venom, bite, arthropod
  auditory canal (external) (meatus) — *see* Bite, ear
  auricle, ear — *see* Bite, ear
  axilla — *see* Bite, arm
  back (*see also* Bite, thorax, back)
    lower S31.050 ☑
      with penetration into retroperitoneal space S31.051 ☑
      superficial NEC S30.870 ☑
        insect S30.860 ☑
  bedbug — *see* Bite(s), by site, superficial, insect
  breast S21.05- ☑
    superficial NEC S20.17- ☑
      insect S20.16- ☑
  brow — *see* Bite, head, specified site NEC
  buttock S31.805 ☑
    left S31.825 ☑
    right S31.815 ☑
    superficial NEC S30.870 ☑
      insect S30.860 ☑
  calf — *see* Bite, leg
  canaliculus lacrimalis — *see* Bite, eyelid

Bite(s) — *continued*
  canthus, eye — *see* Bite, eyelid
  centipede — *see* Toxicity, venom, arthropod, centipede
  cheek (external) S01.45- ☑
    internal — *see* Bite, oral cavity
    superficial NEC S00.87 ☑
      insect S00.86 ☑
  chest wall — *see* Bite, thorax
  chigger B88.0
  chin — *see* Bite, head, specified site NEC
  clitoris — *see* Bite, vulva
  costal region — *see* Bite, thorax
  digit(s)
    hand — *see* Bite, finger
    toe — *see* Bite, toe
  ear (canal) (external) S01.35- ☑
    superficial NEC S00.47- ☑
      insect S00.46- ☑
  elbow S51.05- ☑
    superficial NEC S50.37- ☑
      insect S50.36- ☑
  epididymis — *see* Bite, testis
  epigastric region — *see* Bite, abdomen
  epiglottis — *see* Bite, neck, specified site NEC
  esophagus, cervical S11.25 ☑
    superficial NEC S10.17 ☑
      insect S10.16 ☑
  eyebrow — *see* Bite, eyelid
  eyelid S01.15- ☑
    superficial NEC S00.27- ☑
      insect S00.26- ☑
  face NEC — *see* Bite, head, specified site NEC
  finger(s) S61.259 ☑
    with
      damage to nail S61.359 ☑
    index S61.258 ☑
      with
        damage to nail S61.358 ☑
      left S61.251 ☑
        with
          damage to nail S61.351 ☑
      right S61.250 ☑
        with
          damage to nail S61.350 ☑
      superficial NEC S60.478 ☑
        insect S60.46- ☑
    little S61.25- ☑
      with
        damage to nail S61.35- ☑
      superficial NEC S60.47- ☑
        insect S60.46- ☑
    middle S61.25- ☑
      with
        damage to nail S61.35- ☑
      superficial NEC S60.47- ☑
        insect S60.46- ☑
    ring S61.25- ☑
      with
        damage to nail S61.35- ☑
      superficial NEC S60.47- ☑
        insect S60.46- ☑
    superficial NEC S60.479 ☑
      insect S60.469 ☑
    thumb — *see* Bite, thumb
  flank — *see* Bite, abdomen, wall
  flea — *see* Bite, by site, superficial, insect
  foot (except toe(s) alone) S91.35- ☑
    superficial NEC S90.87- ☑
      insect S90.86- ☑
    toe — *see* Bite, toe
  forearm S51.85- ☑
    elbow only — *see* Bite, elbow
    superficial NEC S50.87- ☑
      insect S50.86- ☑
  forehead — *see* Bite, head, specified site NEC
  genital organs, external
    female S31.552 ☑
      superficial NEC S30.876 ☑
        insect S30.866 ☑
      vagina and vulva — *see* Bite, vulva
    male S31.551 ☑
      penis — *see* Bite, penis
      scrotum — *see* Bite, scrotum
      superficial NEC S30.875 ☑
        insect S30.865 ☑

Bite(s) — *continued*
  genital organs, external — *continued*
    male — *continued*
      testes — *see* Bite, testis
  groin — *see* Bite, abdomen, wall
  gum — *see* Bite, oral cavity
  hand S61.45- ☑
    finger — *see* Bite, finger
    superficial NEC S60.57- ☑
      insect S60.56- ☑
    thumb — *see* Bite, thumb
  head S01.95 ☑
    cheek — *see* Bite, cheek
    ear — *see* Bite, ear
    eyelid — *see* Bite, eyelid
    lip — *see* Bite, lip
    nose — *see* Bite, nose
    oral cavity — *see* Bite, oral cavity
    scalp — *see* Bite, scalp
    specified site NEC S01.85 ☑
      superficial NEC S00.87 ☑
        insect S00.86 ☑
    superficial NEC S00.97 ☑
      insect S00.96 ☑
    temporomandibular area — *see* Bite, cheek
  heel — *see* Bite, foot
  hip S71.05- ☑
    superficial NEC S70.27- ☑
      insect S70.26- ☑
  hymen S31.45 ☑
  hypochondrium — *see* Bite, abdomen, wall
  hypogastric region — *see* Bite, abdomen, wall
  inguinal region — *see* Bite, abdomen, wall
  insect — *see* Bite, by site, superficial, insect
  instep — *see* Bite, foot
  interscapular region — *see* Bite, thorax, back
  jaw — *see* Bite, head, specified site NEC
  knee S81.05- ☑
    superficial NEC S80.27- ☑
      insect S80.26- ☑
  labium (majus) (minus) — *see* Bite, vulva
  lacrimal duct — *see* Bite, eyelid
  larynx S11.015 ☑
    superficial NEC S10.17 ☑
      insect S10.16 ☑
  leg (lower) S81.85- ☑
    ankle — *see* Bite, ankle
    foot — *see* Bite, foot
    knee — *see* Bite, knee
    superficial NEC S80.87- ☑
      insect S80.86- ☑
    toe — *see* Bite, toe
    upper — *see* Bite, thigh
  lip S01.551 ☑
    superficial NEC S00.571 ☑
      insect S00.561 ☑
  lizard (venomous) — *see* Venom, bite, reptile
  loin — *see* Bite, abdomen, wall
  lower back — *see* Bite, back, lower
  lumbar region — *see* Bite, back, lower
  malar region — *see* Bite, head, specified site NEC
  mammary — *see* Bite, breast
  marine animals (venomous) — *see* Toxicity, venom, marine animal
  mastoid region — *see* Bite, head, specified site NEC
  mouth — *see* Bite, oral cavity
  nail
    finger — *see* Bite, finger
    toe — *see* Bite, toe
  nape — *see* Bite, neck, specified site NEC
  nasal (septum) (sinus) — *see* Bite, nose
  nasopharynx — *see* Bite, head, specified site NEC
  neck S11.95 ☑
    involving
      cervical esophagus — *see* Bite, esophagus, cervical
      larynx — *see* Bite, larynx
      pharynx — *see* Bite, pharynx
      thyroid gland S11.15 ☑
      trachea — *see* Bite, trachea
    specified site NEC S11.85 ☑
      superficial NEC S10.87 ☑
        insect S10.86 ☑
    superficial NEC S10.97 ☑
      insect S10.96 ☑
    throat S11.85 ☑

Bite(s) — *continued*
  neck — *continued*
    throat — *continued*
      superficial NEC S10.17 ☑
        insect S10.16 ☑
  nose (septum) (sinus) S01.25 ☑
    superficial NEC S00.37 ☑
      insect S00.36 ☑
  occipital region — *see* Bite, scalp
  oral cavity S01.552 ☑
    superficial NEC S00.572 ☑
      insect S00.562 ☑
  orbital region — *see* Bite, eyelid
  palate — *see* Bite, oral cavity
  palm — *see* Bite, hand
  parietal region — *see* Bite, scalp
  pelvis S31.050 ☑
    with penetration into retroperitoneal space
      S31.051 ☑
    superficial NEC S30.870 ☑
      insect S30.860 ☑
  penis S31.25 ☑
    superficial NEC S30.872 ☑
      insect S30.862 ☑
  perineum
    female — *see* Bite, vulva
    male — *see* Bite, pelvis
  periocular area (with or without lacrimal passages) —
    see Bite, eyelid
  phalanges
    finger — *see* Bite, finger
    toe — *see* Bite, toe
  pharynx S11.25 ☑
    superficial NEC S10.17 ☑
      insect S10.16 ☑
  pinna — *see* Bite, ear
  poisonous — *see* Venom
  popliteal space — *see* Bite, knee
  prepuce — *see* Bite, penis
  pubic region — *see* Bite, abdomen, wall
  rectovaginal septum — *see* Bite, vulva
  red bug B88.0
  reptile NEC (*see also* Venom, bite, reptile)
    nonvenomous — *see* Bite, by site
    snake — *see* Venom, bite, snake
  sacral region — *see* Bite, back, lower
  sacroiliac region — *see* Bite, back, lower
  salivary gland — *see* Bite, oral cavity
  scalp S01.05 ☑
    superficial NEC S00.07 ☑
      insect S00.06 ☑
  scapular region — *see* Bite, shoulder
  scrotum S31.35 ☑
    superficial NEC S30.873 ☑
      insect S30.863 ☑
  sea-snake (venomous) — *see* Toxicity, venom, snake,
    sea snake
  shin — *see* Bite, leg
  shoulder S41.05- ☑
    superficial NEC S40.27- ☑
      insect S40.26- ☑
  snake (*see also* Venom, bite, snake)
    nonvenomous — *see* Bite, by site
  spermatic cord — *see* Bite, testis
  spider (venomous) — *see* Toxicity, venom, spider
    nonvenomous — *see* Bite, by site, superficial, insect
  sternal region — *see* Bite, thorax, front
  submaxillary region — *see* Bite, head, specified site
    NEC
  submental region — *see* Bite, head, specified site NEC
  subungual
    finger(s) — *see* Bite, finger
    toe — *see* Bite, toe
  superficial — *see* Bite, by site, superficial
  supraclavicular fossa S11.85 ☑
  supraorbital — *see* Bite, head, specified site NEC
  temple, temporal region — *see* Bite, head, specified
    site NEC
  temporomandibular area — *see* Bite, cheek
  testis S31.35 ☑
    superficial NEC S30.873 ☑
      insect S30.863 ☑
  thigh S71.15- ☑
    superficial NEC S70.37- ☑
      insect S70.36- ☑
  thorax, thoracic (wall) S21.95 ☑

Bite(s) — *continued*
  thorax, thoracic — *continued*
    back S21.25- ☑
      with penetration into thoracic cavity S21.45- ☑
    breast — *see* Bite, breast
    front S21.15- ☑
      with penetration into thoracic cavity S21.35- ☑
    superficial NEC S20.97 ☑
      back S20.47- ☑
      front S20.37- ☑
      insect S20.96 ☑
        back S20.46- ☑
        front S20.36- ☑
  throat — *see* Bite, neck, throat
  thumb S61.05- ☑
    with
      damage to nail S61.15- ☑
    superficial NEC S60.37- ☑
      insect S60.36- ☑
  thyroid S11.15 ☑
    superficial NEC S10.87 ☑
      insect S10.86 ☑
  toe(s) S91.15- ☑
    with
      damage to nail S91.25- ☑
    great S91.15- ☑
      with
        damage to nail S91.25- ☑
    lesser S91.15- ☑
      with
        damage to nail S91.25- ☑
    superficial NEC S90.47- ☑
      great S90.47- ☑
      insect S90.46- ☑
        great S90.46- ☑
  tongue S01.552 ☑
  trachea S11.025 ☑
    superficial NEC S10.17 ☑
      insect S10.16 ☑
  tunica vaginalis — *see* Bite, testis
  tympanum, tympanic membrane — *see* Bite, ear
  umbilical region S31.155 ☑
  uvula — *see* Bite, oral cavity
  vagina — *see* Bite, vulva
  venomous — *see* Venom
  vocal cords S11.035 ☑
    superficial NEC S10.17 ☑
      insect S10.16 ☑
  vulva S31.45 ☑
    superficial NEC S30.874 ☑
      insect S30.864 ☑
  wrist S61.55- ☑
    superficial NEC S60.87- ☑
      insect S60.86- ☑
Biting, cheek or lip K13.1
Biventricular failure (heart) I50.9
Björck (-Thorson) **syndrome** (malignant carcinoid) E34.0
Black
  death A20.9
  eye S00.1- ☑
  hairy tongue K14.3
  heel (foot) S90.3- ☑
  lung (disease) J60
  palm (hand) S60.22- ☑
Blackfan-Diamond anemia or syndrome (congenital
  hypoplastic anemia) D61.01
Blackhead L70.0
Blackout R55
Bladder — *see* condition
Blast (air) (hydraulic) (immersion) (underwater)
  blindness S05.8X- ☑
  injury
    abdomen or thorax — *see* Injury, by site
    ear (acoustic nerve trauma) — *see* Injury, nerve,
      acoustic, specified type NEC
    syndrome NEC T70.8 ☑
Blastoma — *see* Neoplasm, malignant, by site
  pulmonary — *see* Neoplasm, lung, malignant
Blastomycosis, blastomycotic B40.9
  Brazilian — *see* Paracoccidioidomycosis
  cutaneous B40.3
  disseminated B40.7
  European — *see* Cryptococcosis
  generalized B40.7
  keloidal B48.0
  North American B40.9

Blastomycosis, blastomycotic — *continued*
  primary pulmonary B40.0
  pulmonary B40.2
    acute B40.0
    chronic B40.1
  skin B40.3
  South American — *see* Paracoccidioidomycosis
  specified NEC B40.89
Bleb(s) R23.8
  emphysematous (lung) (solitary) J43.9
  endophthalmitis H59.43
  filtering (vitreous), after glaucoma surgery Z98.83
  inflamed (infected), postprocedural H59.40
    stage 1 H59.41
    stage 2 H59.42
    stage 3 H59.43
  lung (ruptured) J43.9
    congenital — *see* Atelectasis
    newborn P25.8
  subpleural (emphysematous) J43.9
Blebitis, postprocedural H59.40
  stage 1 H59.41
  stage 2 H59.42
  stage 3 H59.43
Bleeder (familial) (hereditary) — *see* Hemophilia
Bleeding (*see also* Hemorrhage)
  anal K62.5
  anovulatory N97.0
  atonic, following delivery O72.1
  capillary I78.8
    puerperal O72.2
  contact (postcoital) N93.0
  due to uterine subinvolution N85.3
  ear — *see* Otorrhagia
  excessive, associated with menopausal onset N92.4
  familial — *see* Defect, coagulation
  following intercourse N93.0
  gastrointestinal K92.2
  hemorrhoids — *see* Hemorrhoids
  intermenstrual (regular) N92.3
    irregular N92.1
  intraoperative — *see* Complication, intraoperative,
    hemorrhage
  irregular N92.6
  menopausal N92.4
  newborn, intraventricular — *see* Newborn, affected
    by, hemorrhage, intraventricular
  nipple N64.59
  nose R04.0
  ovulation N92.3
  postclimacteric N95.0
  postcoital N93.0
  postmenopausal N95.0
  postoperative — *see* Complication, postprocedural,
    hemorrhage
  preclimacteric N92.4
  puberty (excessive, with onset of menstrual periods)
    N92.2
  rectum, rectal K62.5
    newborn P54.2
  tendencies — *see* Defect, coagulation
  throat R04.1
  tooth socket (post-extraction) K91.840
  umbilical stump P51.9
  uterus, uterine NEC N93.9
    climacteric N92.4
    dysfunctional of functional N93.8
    menopausal N92.4
    preclimacteric or premenopausal N92.4
    unrelated to menstrual cycle N93.9
  vagina, vaginal (abnormal) N93.9
    dysfunctional or functional N93.8
    newborn P54.6
  vicarious N94.89
Blennorrhagia, blennorrhagic — *see* Gonorrhea
Blennorrhea (acute) (chronic) (*see also* Gonorrhea)
  inclusion (neonatal) (newborn) P39.1
  lower genitourinary tract (gonococcal) A54.00
  neonatorum (gonococcal ophthalmia) A54.31
Blepharelosis — *see* Entropion
Blepharitis (angularis) (ciliaris) (eyelid) (marginal)
  (nonulcerative) H01.009
  herpes zoster B02.39
  left H01.006
    lower H01.005
    upper H01.004
  right H01.003
    lower H01.002

☑ Additional Character Required — Refer to the Tabular List for Character Selection   ▽ Subterms under main terms may continue to next column or page

Blepharitis — continued
  right — continued
    upper H01.001
  squamous H01.029
    left H01.026
      lower H01.025
      upper H01.024
    right H01.023
      lower H01.022
      upper H01.021
  ulcerative H01.019
    left H01.016
      lower H01.015
      upper H01.014
    right H01.013
      lower H01.012
      upper H01.011
Blepharochalasis H02.30
  congenital Q10.0
  left H02.36
    lower H02.35
    upper H02.34
  right H02.33
    lower H02.32
    upper H02.31
Blepharoclonus H02.59
Blepharoconjunctivitis H10.50- ☑
  angular H10.52- ☑
  contact H10.53- ☑
  ligneous H10.51- ☑
Blepharophimosis (eyelid) H02.529
  congenital Q10.3
  left H02.526
    lower H02.525
    upper H02.524
  right H02.523
    lower H02.522
    upper H02.521
Blepharoptosis H02.40- ☑
  congenital Q10.0
  mechanical H02.41- ☑
  myogenic H02.42- ☑
  neurogenic H02.43- ☑
  paralytic H02.43- ☑
Blepharopyorrhea, gonococcal A54.39
Blepharospasm G24.5
  drug induced G24.01
Blighted ovum O02.0
Blind (see also Blindness)
  bronchus (congenital) Q32.4
  loop syndrome K90.2
    congenital Q43.8
  sac, fallopian tube (congenital) Q50.6
  spot, enlarged — see Defect, visual field, localized, scotoma, blind spot area
  tract or tube, congenital NEC — see Atresia, by site
Blindness (acquired) (congenital) (both eyes) H54.0
  blast S05.8X- ☑
  color — see Deficiency, color vision
  concussion S05.8X- ☑
  cortical H47.619
    left brain H47.612
    right brain H47.611
  day H53.11
  due to injury (current episode) S05.9- ☑
    sequelae — code to injury with seventh character S
  eclipse (total) — see Retinopathy, solar
  emotional (hysterical) F44.6
  face H53.16
  hysterical F44.6
  legal (both eyes) (USA definition) H54.8
  mind R48.8
  night H53.60
    abnormal dark adaptation curve H53.61
    acquired H53.62
    congenital H53.63
    specified type NEC H53.69
    vitamin A deficiency E50.5
  one eye (other eye normal) H54.40
    left (normal vision on right) H54.42
      low vision on right H54.12
    low vision, other eye H54.10
    right (normal vision on left) H54.41
      low vision on left H54.11
  psychic R48.8
  river B73.01
  snow — see Photokeratitis

Blindness — continued
  sun, solar — see Retinopathy, solar
  transient — see Disturbance, vision, subjective, loss, transient
  traumatic (current episode) S05.9- ☑
  word (developmental) F81.0
    acquired R48.0
    secondary to organic lesion R48.0
Blister (nonthermal)
  abdominal wall S30.821 ☑
  alveolar process S00.522 ☑
  ankle S90.52- ☑
  antecubital space — see Blister, elbow
  anus S30.827 ☑
  arm (upper) S40.82- ☑
  auditory canal — see Blister, ear
  auricle — see Blister, ear
  axilla — see Blister, arm
  back, lower S30.820 ☑
  beetle dermatitis L24.89
  breast S20.12- ☑
  brow S00.82 ☑
  calf — see Blister, leg
  canthus — see Blister, eyelid
  cheek S00.82 ☑
    internal S00.522 ☑
  chest wall — see Blister, thorax
  chin S00.82 ☑
  costal region — see Blister, thorax
  digit(s)
    foot — see Blister, toe
    hand — see Blister, finger
  due to burn — see Burn, by site, second degree
  ear S00.42- ☑
  elbow S50.32- ☑
  epiglottis S10.12 ☑
  esophagus, cervical S10.12 ☑
  eyebrow — see Blister, eyelid
  eyelid S00.22- ☑
  face S00.82 ☑
  fever B00.1
  finger(s) S60.429 ☑
    index S60.42- ☑
    little S60.42- ☑
    middle S60.42- ☑
    ring S60.42- ☑
  foot (except toe(s) alone) S90.82- ☑
    toe — see Blister, toe
  forearm S50.82- ☑
    elbow only — see Blister, elbow
  forehead S00.82 ☑
  fracture — omit code
  genital organ
    female S30.826 ☑
    male S30.825 ☑
  gum S00.522 ☑
  hand S60.52- ☑
  head S00.92 ☑
    ear — see Blister, ear
    eyelid — see Blister, eyelid
    lip S00.521 ☑
    nose S00.32 ☑
    oral cavity S00.522 ☑
    scalp S00.02 ☑
    specified site NEC S00.82 ☑
  heel — see Blister, foot
  hip S70.22- ☑
  interscapular region S20.429 ☑
  jaw S00.82 ☑
  knee S80.22- ☑
  larynx S10.12 ☑
  leg (lower) S80.82- ☑
    knee — see Blister, knee
    upper — see Blister, thigh
  lip S00.521 ☑
  malar region S00.82 ☑
  mammary — see Blister, breast
  mastoid region S00.82 ☑
  mouth S00.522 ☑
  multiple, skin, nontraumatic R23.8
  nail
    finger — see Blister, finger
    toe — see Blister, toe
  nasal S00.32 ☑
  neck S10.92 ☑
    specified site NEC S10.82 ☑

Blister — continued
  neck — continued
    throat S10.12 ☑
  nose S00.32 ☑
  occipital region S00.02 ☑
  oral cavity S00.522 ☑
  orbital region — see Blister, eyelid
  palate S00.522 ☑
  palm — see Blister, hand
  parietal region S00.02 ☑
  pelvis S30.820 ☑
  penis S30.822 ☑
  periocular area — see Blister, eyelid
  phalanges
    finger — see Blister, finger
    toe — see Blister, toe
  pharynx S10.12 ☑
  pinna — see Blister, ear
  popliteal space — see Blister, knee
  scalp S00.02 ☑
  scapular region — see Blister, shoulder
  scrotum S30.823 ☑
  shin — see Blister, leg
  shoulder S40.22- ☑
  sternal region S20.329 ☑
  submaxillary region S00.82 ☑
  submental region S00.82 ☑
  subungual
    finger(s) — see Blister, finger
    toe(s) — see Blister, toe
  supraclavicular fossa S10.82 ☑
  supraorbital S00.82 ☑
  temple S00.82 ☑
  temporal region S00.82 ☑
  testis S30.823 ☑
  thermal — see Burn, second degree, by site
  thigh S70.32- ☑
  thorax, thoracic (wall) S20.92 ☑
    back S20.42- ☑
    front S20.32- ☑
  throat S10.12 ☑
  thumb S60.32- ☑
  toe(s) S90.42- ☑
    great S90.42- ☑
  tongue S00.522 ☑
  trachea S10.12 ☑
  tympanum, tympanic membrane — see Blister, ear
  upper arm — see Blister, arm (upper)
  uvula S00.522 ☑
  vagina S30.824 ☑
  vocal cords S10.12 ☑
  vulva S30.824 ☑
  wrist S60.82- ☑
Bloating R14.0
Bloch-Sulzberger disease or syndrome Q82.3
Block, blocked
  alveolocapillary J84.10
  arborization (heart) I45.5
  arrhythmic I45.9
  atrioventricular (incomplete) (partial) I44.30
    with atrioventricular dissociation I44.2
    complete I44.2
      congenital Q24.6
    congenital Q24.6
    first degree I44.0
    second degree (types I and II) I44.1
    specified NEC I44.39
    third degree I44.2
    types I and II I44.1
  auriculoventricular — see Block, atrioventricular
  bifascicular (cardiac) I45.2
  bundle-branch (complete) (false) (incomplete) I45.4
    bilateral I45.2
    left I44.7
      with right bundle branch block I45.2
      hemiblock I44.60
        anterior I44.4
        posterior I44.5
      incomplete I44.7
        with right bundle branch block I45.2
    right I45.10
      with
        left bundle branch block I45.2
        left fascicular block I45.2
      specified NEC I45.19
    Wilson's type I45.19
  cardiac I45.9

Block, blocked — *continued*
- conduction I45.9
  - complete I44.2
- fascicular (left) I44.60
  - anterior I44.4
  - posterior I44.5
  - right I45.0
  - specified NEC I44.69
- foramen Magendie (acquired) G91.1
  - congenital Q03.1
    - with spina bifida — *see* Spina bifida, by site, with hydrocephalus
- heart I45.9
  - bundle branch I45.4
    - bilateral I45.2
  - complete (atrioventricular) I44.2
  - congenital Q24.6
  - first degree (atrioventricular) I44.0
  - second degree (atrioventricular) I44.1
  - specified type NEC I45.5
  - third degree (atrioventricular) I44.2
- hepatic vein I82.0
- intraventricular (nonspecific) I45.4
  - bundle branch
    - bilateral I45.2
- kidney N28.9
  - postcystoscopic or postprocedural N99.0
- Mobitz (types I and II) I44.1
- myocardial — *see* Block, heart
- nodal I45.5
- organ or site, congenital NEC — *see* Atresia, by site
- portal (vein) I81
- second degree (types I and II) I44.1
- sinoatrial I45.5
- sinoauricular I45.5
- third degree I44.2
- trifascicular I45.3
- tubal N97.1
- vein NOS I82.90
- Wenckebach (types I and II) I44.1

Blockage — *see* Obstruction
Blocq's disease F44.4
Blood
- constituents, abnormal R78.9
- disease D75.9
- donor — *see* Donor, blood
- dyscrasia D75.9
  - with
    - abortion — *see* Abortion, by type, complicated by, hemorrhage
    - ectopic pregnancy O08.1
    - molar pregnancy O08.1
  - following ectopic or molar pregnancy O08.1
  - newborn P61.9
  - puerperal, postpartum O72.3
- flukes NEC — *see* Schistosomiasis
- in
  - feces K92.1
    - occult R19.5
  - urine — *see* Hematuria
- mole O02.0
- occult in feces R19.5
- pressure
  - decreased, due to shock following injury T79.4 ☑
  - examination only Z01.30
  - fluctuating I99.8
  - high — *see* Hypertension
    - borderline R03.0
    - incidental reading, without diagnosis of hypertension R03.0
  - low (*see also* Hypotension)
    - incidental reading, without diagnosis of hypotension R03.1
- spitting — *see* Hemoptysis
- staining cornea — *see* Pigmentation, cornea, stromal
- transfusion
  - reaction or complication — *see* Complications, transfusion
- type
  - A (Rh positive) Z67.10
    - Rh negative Z67.11
  - AB (Rh positive) Z67.30
    - Rh negative Z67.31
  - B (Rh positive) Z67.20
    - Rh negative Z67.21
  - O (Rh positive) Z67.40
    - Rh negative Z67.41
  - Rh (positive) Z67.90

Blood — *continued*
- type — *continued*
  - Rh — *continued*
    - negative Z67.91
- vessel rupture — *see* Hemorrhage
- vomiting — *see* Hematemesis
Blood-forming organs, disease D75.9
Bloodgood's disease — *see* Mastopathy, cystic
Bloom (-Machacek)(-Torre) **syndrome** Q82.8
Blount's disease or osteochondrosis — *see* Osteochondrosis, juvenile, tibia
Blue
- baby Q24.9
- diaper syndrome E72.09
- dome cyst (breast) — *see* Cyst, breast
- dot cataract Q12.0
- nevus D22.9
- sclera Q13.5
  - with fragility of bone and deafness Q78.0
- toe syndrome I75.02- ☑
Blueness — *see* Cyanosis
Blues, postpartal O90.6
- baby O90.6
Blurring, visual H53.8
Blushing (abnormal) (excessive) R23.2
BMI — *see* Body, mass index
Boarder, hospital NEC Z76.4
- accompanying sick person Z76.3
- healthy infant or child Z76.2
  - foundling Z76.1
Bockhart's impetigo L01.02
Bodechtel-Guttman disease (subacute sclerosing panencephalitis) A81.1
Boder-Sedgwick syndrome (ataxia-telangiectasia) G11.3
Body, bodies
- Aschoff's — *see* Myocarditis, rheumatic
- asteroid, vitreous — *see* Deposit, crystalline
- cytoid (retina) — *see* Occlusion, artery, retina
- drusen (degenerative) (macula) (retinal) (*see also* Degeneration, macula, drusen)
  - optic disc — *see* Drusen, optic disc
- foreign — *see* Foreign body
- loose
  - joint, except knee — *see* Loose, body, joint
    - knee M23.4- ☑
  - sheath, tendon — *see* Disorder, tendon, specified type NEC
- mass index (BMI)
  - adult
    - 19 or less Z68.1
    - 20.0-20.9 Z68.20
    - 21.0-21.9 Z68.21
    - 22.0-22.9 Z68.22
    - 23.0-23.9 Z68.23
    - 24.0-24.9 Z68.24
    - 25.0-25.9 Z68.25
    - 26.0-26.9 Z68.26
    - 27.0-27.9 Z68.27
    - 28.0-28.9 Z68.28
    - 29.0-29.9 Z68.29
    - 30.0-30.9 Z68.30
    - 31.0-31.9 Z68.31
    - 32.0-32.9 Z68.32
    - 33.0-33.9 Z68.33
    - 34.0-34.9 Z68.34
    - 35.0-35.9 Z68.35
    - 36.0-36.9 Z68.36
    - 37.0-37.9 Z68.37
    - 38.0-38.9 Z68.38
    - 39.0-39.9 Z68.39
    - 40.0-44.9 Z68.41
    - 45.0-49.9 Z68.42
    - 50.0-59.9 Z68.43
    - 60.0-69.9 Z68.44
    - 70 and over Z68.45
  - pediatric
    - 5th percentile to less than 85th percentile for age Z68.52
    - 85th percentile to less than 95th percentile for age Z68.53
    - less than fifth percentile for age Z68.51
    - greater than or equal to ninety-fifth percentile for age Z68.54
- Mooser's A75.2
- rice (*see also* Loose, body, joint)
  - knee M23.4- ☑
- rocking F98.4

Boeck's
- disease or sarcoid — *see* Sarcoidosis
- lupoid (miliary) D86.3
Boerhaave's syndrome (spontaneous esophageal rupture) K22.3
Boggy
- cervix N88.8
- uterus N85.8
Boil (*see also* Furuncle, by site)
- Aleppo B55.1
- Baghdad B55.1
- Delhi B55.1
- lacrimal
  - gland — *see* Dacryoadenitis
  - passages (duct) (sac) — *see* Inflammation, lacrimal, passages, acute
- Natal B55.1
- orbit, orbital — *see* Abscess, orbit
- tropical B55.1
Bold hives — *see* Urticaria
Bombé, iris — *see* Membrane, pupillary
Bone — *see* condition
Bonnevie-Ullrich syndrome Q87.1
Bonnier's syndrome H81.8 ☑
Bonvale dam fever T73.3 ☑
Bony block of joint — *see* Ankylosis
BOOP (bronchiolitis obliterans organized pneumonia) J84.89
Borderline
- diabetes mellitus R73.09
- hypertension R03.0
- osteopenia M85.8- ☑
- pelvis, with obstruction during labor O65.1
- personality F60.3
Borna disease A83.9
Bornholm disease B33.0
Boston exanthem A88.0
Botalli, ductus (patent) (persistent) Q25.0
Bothriocephalus latus infestation B70.0
Botulism (foodborne intoxication) A05.1
- infant A48.51
- non-foodborne A48.52
- wound A48.52
Bouba — *see* Yaws
Bouchard's nodes (with arthropathy) M15.2
Bouffée délirante F23
Bouillaud's disease or syndrome (rheumatic heart disease) I01.9
Bourneville's disease Q85.1
Boutonniere deformity (finger) — *see* Deformity, finger, boutonniere
Bouveret (-Hoffmann) **syndrome** (paroxysmal tachycardia) I47.9
Bovine heart — *see* Hypertrophy, cardiac
Bowel — *see* condition
Bowen's
- dermatosis (precancerous) — *see* Neoplasm, skin, in situ
- disease — *see* Neoplasm, skin, in situ
- epithelioma — *see* Neoplasm, skin, in situ
- type
  - epidermoid carcinoma-in-situ — *see* Neoplasm, skin, in situ
  - intraepidermal squamous cell carcinoma — *see* Neoplasm, skin, in situ
Bowing
- femur (*see also* Deformity, limb, specified type NEC, thigh)
  - congenital Q68.3
- fibula (*see also* Deformity, limb, specified type NEC, lower leg)
  - congenital Q68.4
- forearm — *see* Deformity, limb, specified type NEC, forearm
- leg(s), long bones, congenital Q68.5
- radius — *see* Deformity, limb, specified type NEC, forearm
- tibia (*see also* Deformity, limb, specified type NEC, lower leg)
  - congenital Q68.4
Bowleg(s) (acquired) M21.16- ☑
- congenital Q68.5
- rachitic E64.3
Boyd's dysentery A03.2
Brachial — *see* condition
Brachycardia R00.1
Brachycephaly Q75.0

Bradley's disease A08.19
Bradyarrhythmia, cardiac I49.8
Bradycardia (sinoatrial) (sinus) (vagal) R00.1
  neonatal P29.12
  reflex G90.09
  tachycardia syndrome I49.5
Bradykinesia R25.8
Bradypnea R06.89
Bradytachycardia I49.5
Brailsford's disease or osteochondrosis — see Osteo-
  chondrosis, juvenile, radius
Brain (see also condition)
  death G93.82
  syndrome — see Syndrome, brain
Branched-chain amino-acid disorder E71.2
Branchial — see condition
  cartilage, congenital Q18.2
Branchiogenic remnant (in neck) Q18.0
Brandt's syndrome (acrodermatitis enteropathica) E83.2
Brash (water) R12
Bravais-jacksonian epilepsy — see Epilepsy, localiza-
  tion-related, symptomatic, with simple partial
  seizures
Braxton Hicks contractions — see False, labor
Brazilian leishmaniasis B55.2
BRBPR K62.5
Break, retina (without detachment) H33.30- ☑
  with retinal detachment — see Detachment, retina
  horseshoe tear H33.31- ☑
  multiple H33.33- ☑
  round hole H33.32- ☑
Breakdown
  device, graft or implant (see also Complications, by
    site and type, mechanical) T85.618 ☑
    arterial graft NEC — see Complication, cardiovas-
      cular device, mechanical, vascular
    breast (implant) T85.41 ☑
    catheter NEC T85.618 ☑
      cystostomy T83.010 ☑
      dialysis (renal) T82.41 ☑
        intraperitoneal T85.611 ☑
      infusion NEC T82.514 ☑
        spinal (epidural) (subdural) T85.610 ☑
      urinary (indwelling) T83.018 ☑
    electronic (electrode) (pulse generator) (stimulator)
      bone T84.310 ☑
      cardiac T82.119 ☑
        electrode T82.110 ☑
        pulse generator T82.111 ☑
        specified type NEC T82.118 ☑
      nervous system — see Complication, prosthetic
        device, mechanical, electronic nervous
        system stimulator
      urinary — see Complication, genitourinary,
        device, urinary, mechanical
    fixation, internal (orthopedic) NEC — see Compli-
      cation, fixation device, mechanical
    gastrointestinal — see Complications, prosthetic
      device, mechanical, gastrointestinal device
    genital NEC T83.418 ☑
      intrauterine contraceptive device T83.31 ☑
      penile prosthesis T83.410 ☑
    heart NEC — see Complication, cardiovascular de-
      vice, mechanical
    joint prosthesis — see Complications..., joint prosthe-
      sis, internal, mechanical, by site
    ocular NEC — see Complications, prosthetic device,
      mechanical, ocular device
    orthopedic NEC — see Complication, orthopedic,
      device, mechanical
    specified NEC T85.618 ☑
    sutures, permanent T85.612 ☑
      used in bone repair — see Complications, fixa-
        tion device, internal (orthopedic), me-
        chanical
    urinary NEC (see also Complication, genitourinary,
      device, urinary, mechanical)
      graft T83.21 ☑
    vascular NEC — see Complication, cardiovascular
      device, mechanical
    ventricular intracranial shunt T85.01 ☑
  nervous F48.8
  perineum O90.1
  respirator J95.850
    specified NEC J95.859
  ventilator J95.850

Breakdown — continued
  ventilator — continued
    specified NEC J95.859
Breast (see also condition)
  buds E30.1
    in newborn P96.89
  dense R92.2
  nodule N63
Breath
  foul R19.6
  holder, child R06.89
  holding spell R06.89
  shortness R06.02
Breathing
  labored — see Hyperventilation
  mouth R06.5
    causing malocclusion M26.5 ☑
  periodic R06.3
    high altitude G47.32
Breathlessness R06.81
Breda's disease — see Yaws
Breech presentation (mother) O32.1 ☑
  causing obstructed labor O64.1 ☑
  footling O32.8 ☑
    causing obstructed labor O64.8 ☑
  incomplete O32.8 ☑
    causing obstructed labor O64.8 ☑
Breisky's disease N90.4
Brennemann's syndrome I88.0
Brenner
  tumor (benign) D27.9
    borderline malignancy D39.1- ☑
    malignant C56 ☑
    proliferating D39.1- ☑
Bretonneau's disease or angina A36.0
Breus' mole O02.0
Brevicollis Q76.49
Brickmakers' anemia B76.9 [D63.8]
Bridge, myocardial Q24.5
Bright red blood per rectum (BRBPR) K62.5
Bright's disease (see also Nephritis)
  arteriosclerotic — see Hypertension, kidney
Brill (-Zinsser) **disease** (recrudescent typhus) A75.1
  flea-borne A75.2
  louse-borne A75.1
Brill-Symmers' disease C82.90
Brion-Kayser disease — see Fever, parathyroid
Briquet's disorder or syndrome F45.0
Brissaud's
  infantilism or dwarfism E23.0
  motor-verbal tic F95.2
Brittle
  bones disease Q78.0
  nails L60.3
    congenital Q84.6
Broad (see also condition)
  beta disease E78.2
  ligament laceration syndrome N83.8
Broad- or floating-betalipoproteinemia E78.2
Brock's syndrome (atelectasis due to enlarged lymph
  nodes) J98.19
Brocq-Duhring disease (dermatitis herpetiformis) L13.0
Brodie's abscess or disease M86.8X- ☑
Broken
  arches (see also Deformity, limb, flat foot)
  arm (meaning upper limb) — see Fracture, arm
  back — see Fracture, vertebra
  bone — see Fracture
  implant or internal device — see Complications, by
    site and type, mechanical
  leg (meaning lower limb) — see Fracture, leg
  nose S02.2 ☑
  tooth, teeth — see Fracture, tooth
Bromhidrosis, bromidrosis L75.0
Bromidism, bromism G92
  chronic (dependence) F13.20
  due to
    correct substance properly administered — see
      Table of Drugs and Chemicals, by drug, ad-
      verse effect
    overdose or wrong substance given or taken —
      see Table of Drugs and Chemicals, by drug,
      poisoning
Bromidrosiphobia F40.298
Bronchi, bronchial — see condition
Bronchiectasis (cylindrical) (diffuse) (fusiform) (localized)
  (saccular) J47.9

Bronchiectasis — continued
  with
    acute
      bronchitis J47.0
      lower respiratory infection J47.0
    exacerbation (acute) J47.1
  congenital Q33.4
  tuberculous NEC — see Tuberculosis, pulmonary
Bronchiolectasis — see Bronchiectasis
Bronchiolitis (acute) (infective) (subacute) J21.9
  with
    bronchospasm or obstruction J21.9
    influenza, flu or grippe — see Influenza, with, res-
      piratory manifestations NEC
  chemical (chronic) J68.4
    acute J68.0
  chronic (fibrosing) (obliterative) J44.9
  due to
    external agent — see Bronchitis, acute, due to
    human metapneumovirus J21.1
    respiratory syncytial virus J21.0
    specified organism NEC J21.8
  fibrosa obliterans J44.9
  influenzal — see Influenza, with, respiratory manifes-
    tations NEC
  obliterans J42
    with organizing pneumonia (BOOP) J84.89
  obliterative (chronic) (subacute) J44.9
    due to chemicals, gases, fumes or vapors (inhala-
      tion) J68.4
    due to fumes or vapors J68.4
  respiratory, interstitial lung disease J84.115
Bronchitis (diffuse) (fibrinous) (hypostatic) (infective)
  (membranous) J40
  with
    influenza, flu or grippe — see Influenza, with, res-
      piratory manifestations NEC
    obstruction (airway) (lung) J44.9
    tracheitis (15 years of age and above) J40
      acute or subacute J20.9
      chronic J42
      under 15 years of age J20.9
  acute or subacute (with bronchospasm or obstruction)
    J20.9
    with
      bronchiectasis J47.0
      chronic obstructive pulmonary disease J44.0
    chemical (due to gases, fumes or vapors) J68.0
    due to
      fumes or vapors J68.0
      Haemophilus influenzae J20.1
      Mycoplasma pneumoniae J20.0
      radiation J70.0
      specified organism NEC J20.8
      Streptococcus J20.2
      virus
        coxsackie J20.3
        echovirus J20.7
        parainfluenzae J20.4
        respiratory syncytial J20.5
        rhinovirus J20.6
        viral NEC J20.8
  allergic (acute) J45.909
    with
      exacerbation (acute) J45.901
      status asthmaticus J45.902
  arachidic T17.528 ☑
  aspiration (due to fumes or vapors) J68.0
  asthmatic J45.9 ☑
    chronic J44.9
      with
        acute lower respiratory infection J44.0
        exacerbation (acute) J44.1
  capillary — see Pneumonia, broncho
  caseous (tuberculous) A15.5
  Castellani's A69.8
  catarrhal (15 years of age and above) J40
    acute — see Bronchitis, acute
    chronic J41.0
    under 15 years of age J20.9
  chemical (acute) (subacute) J68.0
    chronic J68.4
    due to fumes or vapors J68.0
      chronic J68.4
  chronic J42
    with
      airways obstruction J44.9
      tracheitis (chronic) J42

Bronchitis — continued
  chronic — continued
    asthmatic (obstructive) J44.9
    catarrhal J41.0
    chemical (due to fumes or vapors) J68.4
    due to
      chemicals, gases, fumes or vapors (inhalation) J68.4
      radiation J70.1
      tobacco smoking J41.0
    emphysematous J44.9
    mucopurulent J41.1
    non-obstructive J41.0
    obliterans J44.9
    obstructive J44.9
    purulent J41.1
    simple J41.0
  croupous — see Bronchitis, acute
  due to gases, fumes or vapors (chemical) J68.0
  emphysematous (obstructive) J44.9
  exudative — see Bronchitis, acute
  fetid J41.1
  grippal — see Influenza, with, respiratory manifestations NEC
  in those under l5 years age — see Bronchitis, acute
    chronic — see Bronchitis, chronic
  influenzal — see Influenza, with, respiratory manifestations NEC
  mixed simple and mucopurulent J41.8
  moulder's J62.8
  mucopurulent (chronic) (recurrent) J41.1
    acute or subacute J20.9
    simple (mixed) J41.8
  obliterans (chronic) J44.9
  obstructive (chronic) (diffuse) J44.9
  pituitous J41.1
  pneumococcal, acute or subacute J20.2
  pseudomembranous, acute or subacute — see Bronchitis, acute
  purulent (chronic) (recurrent) J41.1
    acute or subacute — see Bronchitis, acute
  putrid J41.1
  senile (chronic) J42
  simple and mucopurulent (mixed) J41.8
  smokers' J41.0
  spirochetal NEC A69.8
  subacute — see Bronchitis, acute
  suppurative (chronic) J41.1
    acute or subacute — see Bronchitis, acute
  tuberculous A15.5
  under 15 years of age — see Bronchitis, acute
    chronic — see Bronchitis, chronic
  viral NEC, acute or subacute (see also Bronchitis, acute) J20.8
Bronchoalveolitis J18.0
Bronchoaspergillosis B44.1
Bronchocele meaning goiter E04.0
Broncholithiasis J98.09
  tuberculous NEC A15.5
Bronchomalacia J98.09
  congenital Q32.2
Bronchomycosis NOS B49 [J99]
  candidal B37.1
Bronchopleuropneumonia — see Pneumonia, broncho
Bronchopneumonia — see Pneumonia, broncho
Bronchopneumonitis — see Pneumonia, broncho
Bronchopulmonary — see condition
Bronchopulmonitis — see Pneumonia, broncho
Bronchorrhagia (see Hemoptysis)
Bronchorrhea J98.09
  acute J20.9
  chronic (infective) (purulent) J42
Bronchospasm (acute) J98.01
  with
    bronchiolitis, acute J21.9
    bronchitis, acute (conditions in J20) — see Bronchitis, acute
  due to external agent — see condition, respiratory, acute, due to
  exercise induced J45.990
Bronchospirochetosis A69.8
  Castellani A69.8
Bronchostenosis J98.09
Bronchus — see condition
Brontophobia F40.220
Bronze baby syndrome P83.8
Brooke's tumor — see Neoplasm, skin, benign

Brown enamel of teeth (hereditary) K00.5
Brown-Séquard disease, paralysis or syndrome G83.81
Brown's sheath syndrome H50.61- ✓
Bruce sepsis A23.0
Brucellosis (infection) A23.9
  abortus A23.1
  canis A23.3
  dermatitis A23.9
  melitensis A23.0
  mixed A23.8
  sepsis A23.9
    melitensis A23.0
    specified NEC A23.8
  suis A23.2
Bruck-de Lange disease Q87.1
Bruck's disease — see Deformity, limb
Brugsch's syndrome Q82.8
Bruise (skin surface intact) (see also Contusion)
  with
    open wound — see Wound, open
  internal organ — see Injury, by site
  newborn P54.5
  scalp, due to birth injury, newborn P12.3
  umbilical cord O69.5 ✓
Bruit (arterial) R09.89
  cardiac R01.1
Brush burn — see Abrasion, by site
Bruton's X-linked agammaglobulinemia D80.0
Bruxism
  psychogenic F45.8
  sleep related G47.63
Bubbly lung syndrome P27.0
Bubo I88.8
  blennorrhagic (gonococcal) A54.89
  chancroidal A57
  climatic A55
  due to Haemophilus ducreyi A57
  gonococcal A54.89
  indolent (nonspecific) I88.8
  inguinal (nonspecific) I88.8
    chancroidal A57
    climatic A55
    due to H. ducreyi A57
    infective I88.8
  scrofulous (tuberculous) A18.2
  soft chancre A57
  suppurating — see Lymphadenitis, acute
  syphilitic (primary) A51.0
    congenital A50.07
  tropical A55
  virulent (chancroidal) A57
Bubonic plague A20.0
Bubonocele — see Hernia, inguinal
Buccal — see condition
Buchanan's disease or osteochondrosis M91.0
Buchem's syndrome (hyperostosis corticalis) M85.2
Bucket-handle fracture or tear (semilunar cartilage) — see Tear, meniscus
Budd-Chiari syndrome (hepatic vein thrombosis) I82.0
Budgerigar fancier's disease or lung J67.2
Buds
  breast E30.1
    in newborn P96.89
Buerger's disease (thromboangiitis obliterans) I73.1
Bulbar — see condition
Bulbus cordis (left ventricle) (persistent) Q21.8
Bulimia (nervosa) F50.2
  atypical F50.9
  normal weight F50.9
Bulky
  stools R19.5
  uterus N85.2
Bulla (e) R23.8
  lung (emphysematous) (solitary) J43.9
    newborn P25.8
Bullet wound (see also Wound, open)
  fracture — code as Fracture, by site
  internal organ — see Injury, by site
Bundle
  branch block (complete) (false) (incomplete) — see Block, bundle-branch
  of His — see condition
Bunion — see Deformity, toe, hallux valgus
Buphthalmia, buphthalmos (congenital) Q15.0
Burdwan fever B55.0
Bürger-Grütz disease or syndrome E78.3

Buried
  penis (congenital) Q55.64
    acquired N48.83
  roots K08.3
Burke's syndrome K86.8
Burkitt
  cell leukemia C91.0- ✓
  lymphoma (malignant) C83.7- ✓
    small noncleaved, diffuse C83.7- ✓
    spleen C83.77
    undifferentiated C83.7- ✓
  tumor C83.7- ✓
  type
    acute lymphoblastic leukemia C91.0- ✓
    undifferentiated C83.7- ✓
Burn (electricity) (flame) (hot gas, liquid or hot object) (radiation) (steam) (thermal) T30.0
  abdomen, abdominal (muscle) (wall) T21.02 ✓
    first degree T21.12 ✓
    second degree T21.22 ✓
    third degree T21.32 ✓
  above elbow T22.039 ✓
    first degree T22.139 ✓
    left T22.032 ✓
      first degree T22.132 ✓
      second degree T22.232 ✓
      third degree T22.332 ✓
    right T22.031 ✓
      first degree T22.131 ✓
      second degree T22.231 ✓
      third degree T22.331 ✓
    second degree T22.239 ✓
    third degree T22.339 ✓
  acid (caustic) (external) (internal) — see Corrosion, by site
  alimentary tract NEC T28.2 ✓
    esophagus T28.1 ✓
    mouth T28.0 ✓
    pharynx T28.0 ✓
  alkaline (caustic) (external) (internal) — see Corrosion, by site
  ankle T25.019 ✓
    first degree T25.119 ✓
    left T25.012 ✓
      first degree T25.112 ✓
      second degree T25.212 ✓
      third degree T25.312 ✓
    multiple with foot — see Burn, lower, limb, multiple, ankle and foot
    right T25.011 ✓
      first degree T25.111 ✓
      second degree T25.211 ✓
      third degree T25.311 ✓
    second degree T25.219 ✓
    third degree T25.319 ✓
  anus — see Burn, buttock
  arm (lower) (upper) — see Burn, upper, limb
  axilla T22.049 ✓
    first degree T22.149 ✓
    left T22.042 ✓
      first degree T22.142 ✓
      second degree T22.242 ✓
      third degree T22.342 ✓
    right T22.041 ✓
      first degree T22.141 ✓
      second degree T22.241 ✓
      third degree T22.341 ✓
    second degree T22.249 ✓
    third degree T22.349 ✓
  back (lower) T21.04 ✓
    first degree T21.14 ✓
    second degree T21.24 ✓
    third degree T21.34 ✓
    upper T21.03 ✓
      first degree T21.13 ✓
      second degree T21.23 ✓
      third degree T21.33 ✓
  blisters — code as Burn, second degree, by site
  breast(s) — see Burn, chest wall
  buttock(s) T21.05 ✓
    first degree T21.15 ✓
    second degree T21.25 ✓
    third degree T21.35 ✓
  calf T24.039 ✓
    first degree T24.139 ✓
    left T24.032 ✓

Burn — continued
  calf — continued
    left — continued
      first degree T24.132 ☑
      second degree T24.232 ☑
      third degree T24.332 ☑
    right T24.031 ☑
      first degree T24.131 ☑
      second degree T24.231 ☑
      third degree T24.331 ☑
    second degree T24.239 ☑
    third degree T24.339 ☑
  canthus (eye) — see Burn, eyelid
  caustic acid or alkaline — see Corrosion, by site
  cervix T28.3 ☑
  cheek T20.06 ☑
    first degree T20.16 ☑
    second degree T20.26 ☑
    third degree T20.36 ☑
  chemical (acids) (alkalines) (caustics) (external) (internal) — see Corrosion, by site
  chest wall T21.01 ☑
    first degree T21.11 ☑
    second degree T21.21 ☑
    third degree T21.31 ☑
  chin T20.03 ☑
    first degree T20.13 ☑
    second degree T20.23 ☑
    third degree T20.33 ☑
  colon T28.2 ☑
  conjunctiva (and cornea) — see Burn, cornea
  cornea (and conjunctiva) T26.1- ☑
    chemical — see Corrosion, cornea
  corrosion (external) (internal) — see Corrosion, by site
  deep necrosis of underlying tissue — code as Burn, third degree, by site
  dorsum of hand T23.069 ☑
    first degree T23.169 ☑
    left T23.062 ☑
      first degree T23.162 ☑
      second degree T23.262 ☑
      third degree T23.362 ☑
    right T23.061 ☑
      first degree T23.161 ☑
      second degree T23.261 ☑
      third degree T23.361 ☑
    second degree T23.269 ☑
    third degree T23.369 ☑
  due to ingested chemical agent — see Corrosion, by site
  ear (auricle) (external) (canal) T20.01 ☑
    first degree T20.11 ☑
    second degree T20.21 ☑
    third degree T20.31 ☑
  elbow T22.029 ☑
    first degree T22.129 ☑
    left T22.022 ☑
      first degree T22.122 ☑
      second degree T22.222 ☑
      third degree T22.322 ☑
    right T22.021 ☑
      first degree T22.121 ☑
      second degree T22.221 ☑
      third degree T22.321 ☑
    second degree T22.229 ☑
    third degree T22.329 ☑
  epidermal loss — code as Burn, second degree, by site
  erythema, erythematous — code as Burn, first degree, by site
  esophagus T28.1 ☑
  extent (percentage of body surface)
    less than 10 percent T31.0
    10-19 percent T31.10
      with 0-9 percent third degree burns T31.10
      with 10-19 percent third degree burns T31.11
    20-29 percent T31.20
      with 0-9 percent third degree burns T31.20
      with 10-19 percent third degree burns T31.21
      with 20-29 percent third degree burns T31.22
    30-39 percent T31.30
      with 0-9 percent third degree burns T31.30
      with 10-19 percent third degree burns T31.31
      with 20-29 percent third degree burns T31.32
      with 30-39 percent third degree burns T31.33
    40-49 percent T31.40
      with 0-9 percent third degree burns T31.40

Burn — continued
  extent — continued
    40-49 percent — continued
      with 10-19 percent third degree burns T31.41
      with 20-29 percent third degree burns T31.42
      with 30-39 percent third degree burns T31.43
      with 40-49 percent third degree burns T31.44
    50-59 percent T31.50
      with 0-9 percent third degree burns T31.50
      with 10-19 percent third degree burns T31.51
      with 20-29 percent third degree burns T31.52
      with 30-39 percent third degree burns T31.53
      with 40-49 percent third degree burns T31.54
      with 50-59 percent third degree burns T31.55
    60-69 percent T31.60
      with 0-9 percent third degree burns T31.60
      with 10-19 percent third degree burns T31.61
      with 20-29 percent third degree burns T31.62
      with 30-39 percent third degree burns T31.63
      with 40-49 percent third degree burns T31.64
      with 50-59 percent third degree burns T31.65
      with 60-69 percent third degree burns T31.66
    70-79 percent T31.70
      with 0-9 percent third degree burns T31.70
      with 10-19 percent third degree burns T31.71
      with 20-29 percent third degree burns T31.72
      with 30-39 percent third degree burns T31.73
      with 40-49 percent third degree burns T31.74
      with 50-59 percent third degree burns T31.75
      with 60-69 percent third degree burns T31.76
      with 70-79 percent third degree burns T31.77
    80-89 percent T31.80
      with 0-9 percent third degree burns T31.80
      with 10-19 percent third degree burns T31.81
      with 20-29 percent third degree burns T31.82
      with 30-39 percent third degree burns T31.83
      with 40-49 percent third degree burns T31.84
      with 50-59 percent third degree burns T31.85
      with 60-69 percent third degree burns T31.86
      with 70-79 percent third degree burns T31.87
      with 80-89 percent third degree burns T31.88
    90 percent or more T31.90
      with 0-9 percent third degree burns T31.90
      with 10-19 percent third degree burns T31.91
      with 20-29 percent third degree burns T31.92
      with 30-39 percent third degree burns T31.93
      with 40-49 percent third degree burns T31.94
      with 50-59 percent third degree burns T31.95
      with 60-69 percent third degree burns T31.96
      with 70-79 percent third degree burns T31.97
      with 80-89 percent third degree burns T31.98
      with 90 percent or more third degree burns T31.99
  extremity — see Burn, limb
  eye(s) and adnexa T26.4- ☑
    with resulting rupture and destruction of eyeball T26.2- ☑
    conjunctival sac — see Burn, cornea
    cornea — see Burn, cornea
    lid — see Burn, eyelid
    periocular area — see Burn, eyelid
    specified site NEC T26.3- ☑
  eyeball — see Burn, eye
  eyelid(s) T26.0- ☑
    chemical — see Corrosion, eyelid
  face — see Burn, head
  finger T23.029 ☑
    first degree T23.129 ☑
    left T23.022 ☑
      first degree T23.122 ☑
      second degree T23.222 ☑
      third degree T23.322 ☑
    multiple sites (without thumb) T23.039 ☑
      with thumb T23.049 ☑
        first degree T23.149 ☑
        left T23.042 ☑
          first degree T23.142 ☑
          second degree T23.242 ☑
          third degree T23.342 ☑
        right T23.041 ☑
          first degree T23.141 ☑
          second degree T23.241 ☑
          third degree T23.341 ☑
      second degree T23.249 ☑
      third degree T23.349 ☑
      first degree T23.139 ☑
      left T23.032 ☑

Burn — continued
  finger — continued
    multiple sites — continued
      left — continued
        first degree T23.132 ☑
        second degree T23.232 ☑
        third degree T23.332 ☑
      right T23.031 ☑
        first degree T23.131 ☑
        second degree T23.231 ☑
        third degree T23.331 ☑
      second degree T23.239 ☑
      third degree T23.339 ☑
    right T23.021 ☑
      first degree T23.121 ☑
      second degree T23.221 ☑
      third degree T23.321 ☑
    second degree T23.229 ☑
    third degree T23.329 ☑
  flank — see Burn, abdominal wall
  foot T25.029 ☑
    first degree T25.129 ☑
    left T25.022 ☑
      first degree T25.122 ☑
      second degree T25.222 ☑
      third degree T25.322 ☑
    multiple with ankle — see Burn, lower, limb, multiple, ankle and foot
    right T25.021 ☑
      first degree T25.121 ☑
      second degree T25.221 ☑
      third degree T25.321 ☑
    second degree T25.229 ☑
    third degree T25.329 ☑
  forearm T22.019 ☑
    first degree T22.119 ☑
    left T22.012 ☑
      first degree T22.112 ☑
      second degree T22.212 ☑
      third degree T22.312 ☑
    right T22.011 ☑
      first degree T22.111 ☑
      second degree T22.211 ☑
      third degree T22.311 ☑
    second degree T22.219 ☑
    third degree T22.319 ☑
  forehead T20.06 ☑
    first degree T20.16 ☑
    second degree T20.26 ☑
    third degree T20.36 ☑
  fourth degree — code as Burn, third degree, by site
  friction — see Burn, by site
  from swallowing caustic or corrosive substance NEC — see Corrosion, by site
  full thickness skin loss — code as Burn, third degree, by site
  gastrointestinal tract NEC T28.2 ☑
    from swallowing caustic or corrosive substance T28.7 ☑
  genital organs
    external
      female T21.07 ☑
        first degree T21.17 ☑
        second degree T21.27 ☑
        third degree T21.37 ☑
      male T21.06 ☑
        first degree T21.16 ☑
        second degree T21.26 ☑
        third degree T21.36 ☑
    internal T28.3 ☑
      from caustic or corrosive substance T28.8 ☑
  groin — see Burn, abdominal wall
  hand(s) T23.009 ☑
    back — see Burn, dorsum of hand
    finger — see Burn, finger
    first degree T23.109 ☑
    left T23.002 ☑
      first degree T23.102 ☑
      second degree T23.202 ☑
      third degree T23.302 ☑
    multiple sites with wrist T23.099 ☑
      first degree T23.199 ☑
      left T23.092 ☑
        first degree T23.192 ☑
        second degree T23.292 ☑
        third degree T23.392 ☑

Burn — *continued*

hand(s) — *continued*
  multiple sites with wrist — *continued*
    right T23.091 ☑
      first degree T23.191 ☑
      second degree T23.291 ☑
      third degree T23.391 ☑
    second degree T23.299 ☑
    third degree T23.399 ☑
  palm — *see* Burn, palm
  right T23.001 ☑
    first degree T23.101 ☑
    second degree T23.201 ☑
    third degree T23.301 ☑
  second degree T23.209 ☑
  third degree T23.309 ☑
  thumb — *see* Burn, thumb
head (and face) (and neck) T20.00 ☑
  cheek — *see* Burn, cheek
  chin — *see* Burn, chin
  ear — *see* Burn, ear
  eye(s) only — *see* Burn, eye
  first degree T20.10 ☑
  forehead — *see* Burn, forehead
  lip — *see* Burn, lip
  multiple sites T20.09 ☑
    first degree T20.19 ☑
    second degree T20.29 ☑
    third degree T20.39 ☑
  neck — *see* Burn, neck
  nose — *see* Burn, nose
  scalp — *see* Burn, scalp
  second degree T20.20 ☑
  third degree T20.30 ☑
hip(s) — *see* Burn, lower, limb
inhalation — *see* Burn, respiratory tract
  caustic or corrosive substance (fumes) — *see* Corrosion, respiratory tract
internal organ(s) T28.40 ☑
  alimentary tract T28.2 ☑
    esophagus T28.1 ☑
  eardrum T28.41 ☑
  esophagus T28.1 ☑
  from caustic or corrosive substance (swallowing) NEC — *see* Corrosion, by site
  genitourinary T28.3 ☑
  mouth T28.0 ☑
  pharynx T28.0 ☑
  respiratory tract — *see* Burn, respiratory tract
  specified organ NEC T28.49 ☑
interscapular region — *see* Burn, back, upper
intestine (large) (small) T28.2 ☑
knee T24.029 ☑
  first degree T24.129 ☑
  left T24.022 ☑
    first degree T24.122 ☑
    second degree T24.222 ☑
    third degree T24.322 ☑
  right T24.021 ☑
    first degree T24.121 ☑
    second degree T24.221 ☑
    third degree T24.321 ☑
  second degree T24.229 ☑
  third degree T24.329 ☑
labium (majus) (minus) — *see* Burn, genital organs, external, female
lacrimal apparatus, duct, gland or sac — *see* Burn, eye, specified site NEC
larynx T27.0 ☑
  with lung T27.1 ☑
leg(s) (lower) (upper) — *see* Burn, lower, limb
lightning — *see* Burn, by site
limb(s)
  lower (except ankle or foot alone) — *see* Burn, lower, limb
  upper — *see* Burn, upper limb
lip(s) T20.02 ☑
  first degree T20.12 ☑
  second degree T20.22 ☑
  third degree T20.32 ☑
lower
  back — *see* Burn, back
  limb T24.009 ☑
    ankle — *see* Burn, ankle
    calf — *see* Burn, calf
      first degree T24.109 ☑

Burn — *continued*

lower — *continued*
  limb — *continued*
    foot — *see* Burn, foot
    hip — *see* Burn, thigh
    knee — *see* Burn, knee
    left T24.002 ☑
      first degree T24.102 ☑
      second degree T24.202 ☑
      third degree T24.302 ☑
    multiple sites, except ankle and foot T24.099 ☑
      ankle and foot T25.099 ☑
        first degree T25.199 ☑
        left T25.092 ☑
          first degree T25.192 ☑
          second degree T25.292 ☑
          third degree T25.392 ☑
        right T25.091 ☑
          first degree T25.191 ☑
          second degree T25.291 ☑
          third degree T25.391 ☑
        second degree T25.299 ☑
        third degree T25.399 ☑
      first degree T24.199 ☑
      left T24.092 ☑
        first degree T24.192 ☑
        second degree T24.292 ☑
        third degree T24.392 ☑
      right T24.091 ☑
        first degree T24.191 ☑
        second degree T24.291 ☑
        third degree T24.391 ☑
      second degree T24.299 ☑
      third degree T24.399 ☑
    right T24.001 ☑
      first degree T24.101 ☑
      second degree T24.201 ☑
      third degree T24.301 ☑
    second degree T24.209 ☑
    thigh — *see* Burn, thigh
    third degree T24.309 ☑
    toe — *see* Burn, toe
lung (with larynx and trachea) T27.1 ☑
mouth T28.0 ☑
neck T20.07 ☑
  first degree T20.17 ☑
  second degree T20.27 ☑
  third degree T20.37 ☑
nose (septum) T20.04 ☑
  first degree T20.14 ☑
  second degree T20.24 ☑
  third degree T20.34 ☑
ocular adnexa — *see* Burn, eye
orbit region — *see* Burn, eyelid
palm T23.059 ☑
  first degree T23.159 ☑
  left T23.052 ☑
    first degree T23.152 ☑
    second degree T23.252 ☑
    third degree T23.352 ☑
  right T23.051 ☑
    first degree T23.151 ☑
    second degree T23.251 ☑
    third degree T23.351 ☑
  second degree T23.259 ☑
  third degree T23.359 ☑
partial thickness — *code as* Burn, unspecified degree, by site
pelvis — *see* Burn, trunk
penis — *see* Burn, genital organs, external, male
perineum
  female — *see* Burn, genital organs, external, female
  male — *see* Burn, genital organs, external, male
periocular area — *see* Burn, eyelid
pharynx T28.0 ☑
rectum T28.2 ☑
respiratory tract T27.3 ☑
  larynx — *see* Burn, larynx
  specified part NEC T27.2 ☑
  trachea — *see* Burn, trachea
sac, lacrimal — *see* Burn, eye, specified site NEC
scalp T20.05 ☑
  first degree T20.15 ☑
  second degree T20.25 ☑
  third degree T20.35 ☑

Burn — *continued*

scapular region T22.069 ☑
  first degree T22.169 ☑
  left T22.062 ☑
    first degree T22.162 ☑
    second degree T22.262 ☑
    third degree T22.362 ☑
  right T22.061 ☑
    first degree T22.161 ☑
    second degree T22.261 ☑
    third degree T22.361 ☑
  second degree T22.269 ☑
  third degree T22.369 ☑
sclera — *see* Burn, eye, specified site NEC
scrotum — *see* Burn, genital organs, external, male
shoulder T22.059 ☑
  first degree T22.159 ☑
  left T22.052 ☑
    first degree T22.152 ☑
    second degree T22.252 ☑
    third degree T22.352 ☑
  right T22.051 ☑
    first degree T22.151 ☑
    second degree T22.251 ☑
    third degree T22.351 ☑
  second degree T22.259 ☑
  third degree T22.359 ☑
stomach T28.2 ☑
temple — *see* Burn, head
testis — *see* Burn, genital organs, external, male
thigh T24.019 ☑
  first degree T24.119 ☑
  left T24.012 ☑
    first degree T24.112 ☑
    second degree T24.212 ☑
    third degree T24.312 ☑
  right T24.011 ☑
    first degree T24.111 ☑
    second degree T24.211 ☑
    third degree T24.311 ☑
  second degree T24.219 ☑
  third degree T24.319 ☑
thorax (external) — *see* Burn, trunk
throat (meaning pharynx) T28.0 ☑
thumb(s) T23.019 ☑
  first degree T23.119 ☑
  left T23.012 ☑
    first degree T23.112 ☑
    second degree T23.212 ☑
    third degree T23.312 ☑
  multiple sites with fingers T23.049 ☑
    first degree T23.149 ☑
    left T23.042 ☑
      first degree T23.142 ☑
      second degree T23.242 ☑
      third degree T23.342 ☑
    right T23.041 ☑
      first degree T23.141 ☑
      second degree T23.241 ☑
      third degree T23.341 ☑
    second degree T23.249 ☑
    third degree T23.349 ☑
  right T23.011 ☑
    first degree T23.111 ☑
    second degree T23.211 ☑
    third degree T23.311 ☑
  second degree T23.219 ☑
  third degree T23.319 ☑
toe T25.039 ☑
  first degree T25.139 ☑
  left T25.032 ☑
    first degree T25.132 ☑
    second degree T25.232 ☑
    third degree T25.332 ☑
  right T25.031 ☑
    first degree T25.131 ☑
    second degree T25.231 ☑
    third degree T25.331 ☑
  second degree T25.239 ☑
  third degree T25.339 ☑
tongue T28.0 ☑
tonsil(s) T28.0 ☑
trachea T27.0 ☑
  with lung T27.1 ☑
trunk T21.00 ☑

☑ Additional Character Required — Refer to the Tabular List for Character Selection ▽ Subterms under main terms may continue to next column or page

Burn — *continued*
  trunk — *continued*
    abdominal wall — *see* Burn, abdominal wall
    anus — *see* Burn, buttock
    axilla — *see* Burn, upper limb
    back — *see* Burn, back
    breast — *see* Burn, chest wall
    buttock — *see* Burn, buttock
    chest wall — *see* Burn, chest wall
    first degree T21.10 ☑
    flank — *see* Burn, abdominal wall
    genital
      female — *see* Burn, genital organs, external, female
      male — *see* Burn, genital organs, external, male
    groin — *see* Burn, abdominal wall
    interscapular region — *see* Burn, back, upper
    labia — *see* Burn, genital organs, external, female
    lower back — *see* Burn, back
    penis — *see* Burn, genital organs, external, male
    perineum
      female — *see* Burn, genital organs, external, female
      male — *see* Burn, genital organs, external, male
    scapula region — *see* Burn, scapular region
    scrotum — *see* Burn, genital organs, external, male
    second degree T21.20 ☑
    specified site NEC T21.09 ☑
      first degree T21.19 ☑
      second degree T21.29 ☑
      third degree T21.39 ☑
    testes — *see* Burn, genital organs, external, male
    third degree T21.30 ☑
    upper back — *see* Burn, back, upper
    vulva — *see* Burn, genital organs, external, female
  unspecified site with extent of body surface involved specified
    less than 10 per cent T31.0
    10-19 per cent (0-9 percent third degree) T31.10
      with 10-19 percent third degree T31.11
    20-29 per cent (0-9 percent third degree) T31.20
      with
        10-19 percent third degree T31.21
        20-29 percent third degree T31.22
    30-39 per cent (0-9 percent third degree) T31.30
      with
        10-19 percent third degree T31.31
        20-29 percent third degree T31.32
        30-39 percent third degree T31.33
    40-49 per cent (0-9 percent third degree) T31.40
      with
        10-19 percent third degree T31.41
        20-29 percent third degree T31.42
        30-39 percent third degree T31.43
        40-49 percent third degree T31.44
    50-59 per cent (0-9 percent third degree) T31.50
      with
        10-19 percent third degree T31.51
        20-29 percent third degree T31.52
        30-39 percent third degree T31.53
        40-49 percent third degree T31.54
        50-59 percent third degree T31.55
    60-69 per cent (0-9 percent third degree) T31.60
      with
        10-19 percent third degree T31.61
        20-29 percent third degree T31.62
        30-39 percent third degree T31.63
        40-49 percent third degree T31.64
        50-59 percent third degree T31.65
        60-69 percent third degree T31.66
    70-79 per cent (0-9 percent third degree) T31.70
      with
        10-19 percent third degree T31.71
        20-29 percent third degree T31.72
        30-39 percent third degree T31.73
        40-49 percent third degree T31.74
        50-59 percent third degree T31.75
        60-69 percent third degree T31.76
        70-79 percent third degree T31.77
    80-89 per cent (0-9 percent third degree) T31.80
      with
        10-19 percent third degree T31.81
        20-29 percent third degree T31.82
        30-39 percent third degree T31.83
        40-49 percent third degree T31.84
        50-59 percent third degree T31.85
        60-69 percent third degree T31.86
        70-79 percent third degree T31.87

Burn — *continued*
  unspecified site with extent of body surface involved specified — *continued*
    80-89 per cent — *continued*
      with — *continued*
        80-89 percent third degree T31.88
    90 per cent or more (0-9 percent third degree) T31.90
      with
        10-19 percent third degree T31.91
        20-29 percent third degree T31.92
        30-39 percent third degree T31.93
        40-49 percent third degree T31.94
        50-59 percent third degree T31.95
        60-69 percent third degree T31.96
        70-79 percent third degree T31.97
        80-89 percent third degree T31.98
        90-99 percent third degree T31.99
  upper limb T22.00 ☑
    above elbow — *see* Burn, above elbow
    axilla — *see* Burn, axilla
    elbow — *see* Burn, elbow
    first degree T22.10 ☑
    forearm — *see* Burn, forearm
    hand — *see* Burn, hand
    interscapular region — *see* Burn, back, upper
    multiple sites T22.099 ☑
      first degree T22.199 ☑
      left T22.092 ☑
        first degree T22.192 ☑
        second degree T22.292 ☑
        third degree T22.392 ☑
      right T22.091 ☑
        first degree T22.191 ☑
        second degree T22.291 ☑
        third degree T22.391 ☑
      second degree T22.299 ☑
      third degree T22.399 ☑
    scapular region — *see* Burn, scapular region
    second degree T22.20 ☑
    shoulder — *see* Burn, shoulder
    third degree T22.30 ☑
    wrist — *see* Burn, wrist
  uterus T28.3 ☑
  vagina T28.3 ☑
  vulva — *see* Burn, genital organs, external, female
  wrist T23.079 ☑
    first degree T23.179 ☑
    left T23.072 ☑
      first degree T23.172 ☑
      second degree T23.272 ☑
      third degree T23.372 ☑
    multiple sites with hand T23.099 ☑
      first degree T23.199 ☑
      left T23.092 ☑
        first degree T23.192 ☑
        second degree T23.292 ☑
        third degree T23.392 ☑
      right T23.091 ☑
        first degree T23.191 ☑
        second degree T23.291 ☑
        third degree T23.391 ☑
      second degree T23.299 ☑
      third degree T23.399 ☑
    right T23.071 ☑
      first degree T23.171 ☑
      second degree T23.271 ☑
      third degree T23.371 ☑
    second degree T23.279 ☑
    third degree T23.379 ☑
Burn-out (state) Z73.0
Burnett's syndrome E83.52
Burning
  feet syndrome E53.9
  sensation R20.8
  tongue K14.6
Burns' disease or osteochondrosis — *see* Osteochondrosis, juvenile, ulna
Bursa — *see* condition
Bursitis M71.9
  Achilles — *see* Tendinitis, Achilles
  adhesive — *see* Bursitis, specified NEC
  ankle — *see* Enthesopathy, lower limb, ankle, specified type NEC
  calcaneal — *see* Enthesopathy, foot, specified type NEC

Bursitis — *continued*
  collateral ligament, tibial — *see* Bursitis, tibial collateral
  due to use, overuse, pressure (*see also* Disorder, soft tissue, due to use, specified type NEC)
    specified NEC — *see* Disorder, soft tissue, due to use, specified NEC
  Duplay's M75.0
  elbow NEC M70.3- ☑
    olecranon M70.2- ☑
  finger — *see* Disorder, soft tissue, due to use, specified type NEC, hand
  foot — *see* Enthesopathy, foot, specified type NEC
  gonococcal A54.49
  gouty — *see* Gout, idiopathic
  hand M70.1- ☑
  hip NEC M70.7- ☑
    trochanteric M70.6- ☑
  infective NEC M71.10
    abscess — *see* Abscess, bursa
    ankle M71.17- ☑
    elbow M71.12- ☑
    foot M71.17- ☑
    hand M71.14- ☑
    hip M71.15- ☑
    knee M71.16- ☑
    multiple sites M71.19
    shoulder M71.11- ☑
    specified site NEC M71.18
    wrist M71.13- ☑
  ischial — *see* Bursitis, hip
  knee NEC M70.5- ☑
    prepatellar M70.4- ☑
  occupational NEC (*see also* Disorder, soft tissue, due to, use)
  olecranon — *see* Bursitis, elbow, olecranon
  pharyngeal J39.1
  popliteal — *see* Bursitis, knee
  prepatellar M70.4- ☑
  radiohumeral M77.8
  rheumatoid M06.20
    ankle M06.27- ☑
    elbow M06.22- ☑
    foot joint M06.27- ☑
    hand joint M06.24- ☑
    hip M06.25- ☑
    knee M06.26- ☑
    multiple site M06.29
    shoulder M06.21- ☑
    vertebra M06.28
    wrist M06.23- ☑
  scapulohumeral — *see* Bursitis, shoulder
  semimembranous muscle (knee) — *see* Bursitis, knee
  shoulder M75.5- ☑
    adhesive — *see* Capsulitis, adhesive
  specified NEC M71.50
    ankle M71.57- ☑
    due to use, overuse or pressure — *see* Disorder, soft tissue, due to, use
    elbow M71.52- ☑
    foot M71.57- ☑
    hand M71.54- ☑
    hip M71.55- ☑
    knee M71.56- ☑
    shoulder — *see* Bursitis, shoulder
    specified site NEC M71.58
    tibial collateral M76.4- ☑
    wrist M71.53- ☑
  subacromial — *see* Bursitis, shoulder
  subcoracoid — *see* Bursitis, shoulder
  subdeltoid — *see* Bursitis, shoulder
  syphilitic A52.78
  Thornwaldt, Tornwaldt J39.2
  tibial collateral — *see* Bursitis, tibial collateral
  toe — *see* Enthesopathy, foot, specified type NEC
  trochanteric (area) — *see* Bursitis, hip, trochanteric
  wrist — *see* Bursitis, hand
Bursopathy M71.9
  specified type NEC M71.80
    ankle M71.87- ☑
    elbow M71.82- ☑
    foot M71.87- ☑
    hand M71.84- ☑
    hip M71.85- ☑
    knee M71.86- ☑
    multiple sites M71.89
    shoulder M71.81- ☑

Bursopathy — *continued*
  specified type — *continued*
    specified site NEC M71.88
    wrist M71.83-
Burst stitches or sutures (complication of surgery)
    T81.31 ☑
  external operation wound T81.31 ☑
  internal operation wound T81.32 ☑
Buruli ulcer A31.1
Bury's disease L95.1
Buschke's
  disease B45.3
  scleredema — *see* Sclerosis, systemic
Busse-Buschke disease B45.3
Buttock — *see* condition
Button
  Biskra B55.1
  Delhi B55.1
  oriental B55.1
Buttonhole deformity (finger) — *see* Deformity, finger, boutonniere
Bwamba fever A92.8
Byssinosis J66.0
Bywaters' syndrome T79.5 ☑

C

Cachexia R64
  cancerous R64
  cardiac — *see* Disease, heart
  dehydration E86.0
    with
      hypernatremia E87.0
      hyponatremia E87.1
    due to malnutrition R64
  exophthalmic — *see* Hyperthyroidism
  heart — *see* Disease, heart
  hypophyseal E23.0
  hypopituitary E23.0
  lead — *see* Poisoning, lead
  malignant R64
  marsh — *see* Malaria
  nervous F48.8
  old age R54
  paludal — *see* Malaria
  pituitary E23.0
  renal N28.9
  saturnine — *see* Poisoning, lead
  senile R54
  Simmonds' E23.0
  splenica D73.0
  strumipriva E03.4
  tuberculous NEC — *see* Tuberculosis
Café, au lait spots L81.3
Caffey's syndrome Q78.8
Caisson disease T70.3 ☑
Cake kidney Q63.1
Caked breast (puerperal, postpartum) O92.79
Calabar swelling B74.3
Calcaneal spur — *see* Spur, bone, calcaneal
Calcaneo-apophysitis M92.8
Calcareous — *see* condition
Calcicosis J62.8
Calciferol (vitamin D) deficiency E55.9
  with rickets E55.0
Calcification
  adrenal (capsule) (gland) E27.49
    tuberculous E35 [B90.8]
  aorta I70.0
  artery (annular) — *see* Arteriosclerosis
  auricle (ear) — *see* Disorder, pinna, specified type NEC
  basal ganglia G23.8
  bladder N32.89
    due to Schistosoma hematobium B65.0
  brain (cortex) — *see* Calcification, cerebral
  bronchus J98.09
  bursa M71.40
    ankle M71.47- ☑
    elbow M71.42- ☑
    foot M71.47- ☑
    hand M71.44- ☑
    hip M71.45- ☑
    knee M71.46- ☑
    multiple sites M71.49
    shoulder M75.3- ☑
    specified site NEC M71.48
    wrist M71.43- ☑

Calcification — *continued*
  cardiac — *see* Degeneration, myocardial
  cerebral (cortex) G93.89
    artery I67.2
  cervix (uteri) N88.8
  choroid plexus G93.89
  conjunctiva — *see* Concretion, conjunctiva
  corpora cavernosa (penis) N48.89
  cortex (brain) — *see* Calcification, cerebral
  dental pulp (nodular) K04.2
  dentinal papilla K00.4
  fallopian tube N83.8
  falx cerebri G96.19
  gallbladder K82.8
  general E83.59
  heart (*see also* Degeneration, myocardial)
    valve — *see* Endocarditis
  idiopathic infantile arterial (IIAC) Q28.8
  intervertebral cartilage or disc (postinfective) — *see* Disorder, disc, specified NEC
  intracranial — *see* Calcification, cerebral
  joint — *see* Disorder, joint, specified type NEC
  kidney N28.89
    tuberculous N29 [B90.1]
  larynx (senile) J38.7
  lens — *see* Cataract, specified NEC
  lung (active) (postinfectional) J98.4
    tuberculous B90.9
  lymph gland or node (postinfectional) I89.8
    tuberculous (*see also* Tuberculosis, lymph gland) B90.8
  mammographic R92.1
  massive (paraplegic) — *see* Myositis, ossificans, in, quadriplegia
  medial — *see* Arteriosclerosis, extremities
  meninges (cerebral) (spinal) G96.19
  metastatic E83.59
  Mönckeberg's — *see* Arteriosclerosis, extremities
  muscle M61.9
    due to burns — *see* Myositis, ossificans, in, burns
    paralytic — *see* Myositis, ossificans, in, quadriplegia
    specified type NEC M61.40
      ankle M61.47- ☑
      foot M61.47- ☑
      forearm M61.43- ☑
      hand M61.44- ☑
      lower leg M61.46- ☑
      multiple sites M61.49
      pelvic region M61.45- ☑
      shoulder region M61.41- ☑
      specified site NEC M61.48
      thigh M61.45- ☑
      upper arm M61.42- ☑
  myocardium, myocardial — *see* Degeneration, myocardial
  ovary N83.8
  pancreas K86.8
  penis N48.89
  periarticular — *see* Disorder, joint, specified type NEC
  pericardium (*see also* Pericarditis) I31.1
  pineal gland E34.8
  pleura J94.8
    postinfectional J94.8
    tuberculous NEC B90.9
  pulpal (dental) (nodular) K04.2
  sclera H15.89
  spleen D73.89
  subcutaneous L94.2
  suprarenal (capsule) (gland) E27.49
  tendon (sheath) (*see also* Tenosynovitis, specified type NEC)
    with bursitis, synovitis or tenosynovitis — *see* Tendinitis, calcific
  trachea J39.8
  ureter N28.89
  uterus N85.8
  vitreous — *see* Deposit, crystalline
Calcified — *see* Calcification
Calcinosis (interstitial) (tumoral) (universalis) E83.59
  with Raynaud's phenomenon, esophageal dysfunction, sclerodactyly, telangiectasia (CREST syndrome) M34.1
  circumscripta (skin) L94.2
  cutis L94.2
Calciphylaxis (*see also* Calcification, by site) E83.59
Calcium
  deposits — *see* Calcification, by site

Calcium — *continued*
  metabolism disorder E83.50
  salts or soaps in vitreous — *see* Deposit, crystalline
Calciuria R82.99
Calculi — *see* Calculus
Calculosis, intrahepatic — *see* Calculus, bile duct
Calculus, calculi, calculous
  ampulla of Vater — *see* Calculus, bile duct
  anuria (impacted) (recurrent) (*see also* Calculus, urinary) N20.9
  appendix K38.1
  bile duct (common) (hepatic) K80.50
    with
      calculus of gallbladder — *see* Calculus, gallbladder and bile duct
      cholangitis K80.30
        with
          cholecystitis — *see* Calculus, bile duct, with cholecystitis
          obstruction K80.31
        acute K80.32
          with
            chronic cholangitis K80.36
              with obstruction K80.37
            obstruction K80.33
        chronic K80.34
          with
            acute cholangitis K80.36
              with obstruction K80.37
            obstruction K80.35
      cholecystitis (with cholangitis) K80.40
        with obstruction K80.41
        acute K80.42
          with
            chronic cholecystitis K80.46
              with obstruction K80.47
            obstruction K80.43
        chronic K80.44
          with
            acute cholecystitis K80.46
              with obstruction K80.47
            obstruction K80.45
      obstruction K80.51
  biliary (*see also* Calculus, gallbladder)
    specified NEC K80.80
      with obstruction K80.81
  bilirubin, multiple — *see* Calculus, gallbladder
  bladder (encysted) (impacted) (urinary) (diverticulum) N21.0
  bronchus J98.09
  calyx (kidney) (renal) — *see* Calculus, kidney
  cholesterol (pure) (solitary) — *see* Calculus, gallbladder
  common duct (bile) — *see* Calculus, bile duct
  conjunctiva — *see* Concretion, conjunctiva
  cystic N21.0
    duct — *see* Calculus, gallbladder
  dental (subgingival) (supragingival) K03.6
  diverticulum
    bladder N21.0
    kidney N20.0
  epididymis N50.8
  gallbladder K80.20
    with
      bile duct calculus — *see* Calculus, gallbladder and bile duct
      cholecystitis K80.10
        with obstruction K80.11
        acute K80.00
          with
            chronic cholecystitis K80.12
              with obstruction K80.13
            obstruction K80.01
        chronic K80.10
          with
            acute cholecystitis K80.12
              with obstruction K80.13
            obstruction K80.11
        specified NEC K80.18
          with obstruction K80.19
      obstruction K80.21
  gallbladder and bile duct K80.70
    with
      cholecystitis K80.60
        with obstruction K80.61
        acute K80.62
          with
            chronic cholecystitis K80.66
              with obstruction K80.67

☑ **Additional Character Required** — Refer to the Tabular List for Character Selection   ▼ Subterms under main terms may continue to next column or page

Calculus, calculi, calculous — *continued*
  gallbladder and bile duct — *continued*
    with — *continued*
      cholecystitis — *continued*
        acute — *continued*
          with — *continued*
            obstruction K80.63
        chronic K80.64
          with
            acute cholecystitis K80.66
              with obstruction K80.67
            obstruction K80.65
        obstruction K80.71
  hepatic (duct) — *see* Calculus, bile duct
  ileal conduit N21.8
  intestinal (impaction) (obstruction) K56.49
  kidney (impacted) (multiple) (pelvis) (recurrent) (staghorn) N20.0
    with calculus, ureter N20.2
    congenital Q63.8
  lacrimal passages — *see* Dacryolith
  liver (impacted) — *see* Calculus, bile duct
  lung J98.4
  mammographic R92.1
  nephritic (impacted) (recurrent) — *see* Calculus, kidney
  nose J34.89
  pancreas (duct) K86.8
  parotid duct or gland K11.5
  pelvis, encysted — *see* Calculus, kidney
  prostate N42.0
  pulmonary J98.4
  pyelitis (impacted) (recurrent) N20.0
    with hydronephrosis N13.2
  pyelonephritis (impacted) (recurrent) N20 ☑
    with hydronephrosis N13.2
  renal (impacted) (recurrent) — *see* Calculus, kidney
  salivary (duct) (gland) K11.5
  seminal vesicle N50.8
  staghorn — *see* Calculus, kidney
  Stensen's duct K11.5
  stomach K31.89
  sublingual duct or gland K11.5
    congenital Q38.4
  submandibular duct, gland or region K11.5
  submaxillary duct, gland or region K11.5
  suburethral N21.8
  tonsil J35.8
  tooth, teeth (subgingival) (supragingival) K03.6
  tunica vaginalis N50.8
  ureter (impacted) (recurrent) N20.1
    with calculus, kidney N20.2
      with hydronephrosis N13.2
        with infection N13.6
  urethra (impacted) N21.1
  urinary (duct) (impacted) (passage) (tract) N20.9
    with hydronephrosis N13.2
      with infection N13.6
    in (due to)
    lower N21.9
      specified NEC N21.8
  vagina N89.8
  vesical (impacted) N21.0
  Wharton's duct K11.5
  xanthine E79.8 [N22]
Calicectasis N28.89
Caliectasis N28.89
California
  disease B38.9
  encephalitis A83.5
Caligo cornea — *see* Opacity, cornea, central
Callositas, callosity (infected) L84
Callus (infected) L84
  bone — *see* Osteophyte
  excessive, following fracture — *code as* Sequelae of fracture
Calorie deficiency or malnutrition (*see also* Malnutrition) E46
Calvé-Perthes disease — *see* Legg-Calvé-Perthes disease
Calvé's disease — *see* Osteochondrosis, juvenile, spine
Calvities — *see* Alopecia, androgenic
Cameroon fever — *see* Malaria
Camptocormia (hysterical) F44.4
Camurati-Engelmann syndrome Q78.3
Canal (*see also* condition)
  atrioventricular common Q21.2
Canaliculitis (lacrimal) (acute) (subacute) H04.33- ☑
  Actinomyces A42.89

Canaliculitis — *continued*
  chronic H04.42- ☑
Canavan's disease E75.29
Canceled procedure (surgical) Z53.9
  because of
    contraindication Z53.09
      smoking Z53.01
    left against medical advice (AMA) Z53.21
    patient's decision Z53.20
      for reasons of belief or group pressure Z53.1
      specified reason NEC Z53.29
    specified reason NEC Z53.8
Cancer (*see also* Neoplasm, by site, malignant)
  bile duct type liver C22.1
  blood — *see* Leukemia
  breast (*see also* Neoplasm, breast, malignant) C50.91- ☑
  hepatocellular C22.0
  lung (*see also* Neoplasm, lung, malignant) C34.90
  ovarian (*see also* Neoplasm ovary, malignant) C56.9
  unspecified site (primary) C80.1
Cancer (o)**phobia** F45.29
Cancerous — *see* Neoplasm, malignant, by site
Cancrum oris A69.0
Candidiasis, candidal B37.9
  balanitis B37.42
  bronchitis B37.1
  cheilitis B37.83
  congenital P37.5
  cystitis B37.41
  disseminated B37.7
  endocarditis B37.6
  enteritis B37.82
  esophagitis B37.81
  intertrigo B37.2
  lung B37.1
  meningitis B37.5
  mouth B37.0
  nails B37.2
  neonatal P37.5
  onychia B37.2
  oral B37.0
  osteomyelitis B37.89
  otitis externa B37.84
  paronychia B37.2
  perionyxis B37.2
  pneumonia B37.1
  proctitis B37.82
  pulmonary B37.1
  pyelonephritis B37.49
  sepsis B37.7
  skin B37.2
  specified site NEC B37.89
  stomatitis B37.0
  systemic B37.7
  urethritis B37.41
  urogenital site NEC B37.49
  vagina B37.3
  vulva B37.3
  vulvovaginitis B37.3
Candidid L30.2
Candidosis — *see* Candidiasis
Candiru infection or infestation B88.8
Canities (premature) L67.1
  congenital Q84.2
Canker (mouth) (sore) K12.0
  rash A38.9
Cannabinosis J66.2
Canton fever A75.9
Cantrell's syndrome Q87.89
Capillariasis (intestinal) B81.1
  hepatic B83.8
Capillary — *see* condition
Caplan's syndrome — *see* Rheumatoid, lung
Capsule — *see* condition
Capsulitis (joint) (*see also* Enthesopathy)
  adhesive (shoulder) M75.0- ☑
  hepatic K65.8
  labyrinthine — *see* Otosclerosis, specified NEC
  thyroid E06.9
Caput
  crepitus Q75.8
  medusae I86.8
  succedaneum P12.81
Car sickness T75.3 ☑
Carapata (disease) A68.0
Carate — *see* Pinta

Carbon lung J60
Carbuncle L02.93
  abdominal wall L02.231
  anus K61.0
  auditory canal, external — *see* Abscess, ear, external
  auricle ear — *see* Abscess, ear, external
  axilla L02.43- ☑
  back (any part) L02.232
  breast N61
  buttock L02.33
  cheek (external) L02.03
  chest wall L02.233
  chin L02.03
  corpus cavernosum N48.21
  ear (any part) (external) (middle) — *see* Abscess, ear, external
  external auditory canal — *see* Abscess, ear, external
  eyelid — *see* Abscess, eyelid
  face NEC L02.03
  femoral (region) — *see* Carbuncle, lower limb
  finger — *see* Carbuncle, hand
  flank L02.231
  foot L02.63- ☑
  forehead L02.03
  genital — *see* Abscess, genital
  gluteal (region) L02.33
  groin L02.234
  hand L02.53- ☑
  head NEC L02.831
  heel — *see* Carbuncle, foot
  hip — *see* Carbuncle, lower limb
  kidney — *see* Abscess, kidney
  knee — *see* Carbuncle, lower limb
  labium (majus) (minus) N76.4
  lacrimal
    gland — *see* Dacryoadenitis
    passages (duct) (sac) — *see* Inflammation, lacrimal, passages, acute
  leg — *see* Carbuncle, lower limb
  lower limb L02.43- ☑
  malignant A22.0
  navel L02.236
  neck L02.13
  nose (external) (septum) J34.0
  orbit, orbital — *see* Abscess, orbit
  palmar (space) — *see* Carbuncle, hand
  partes posteriores L02.33
  pectoral region L02.233
  penis N48.21
  perineum L02.235
  pinna — *see* Abscess, ear, external
  popliteal — *see* Carbuncle, lower limb
  scalp L02.831
  seminal vesicle N49.0
  shoulder — *see* Carbuncle, upper limb
  specified site NEC L02.838
  temple (region) L02.03
  thumb — *see* Carbuncle, hand
  toe — *see* Carbuncle, foot
  trunk L02.239
    abdominal wall L02.231
    back L02.232
    chest wall L02.233
    groin L02.234
    perineum L02.235
    umbilicus L02.236
  umbilicus L02.236
  upper limb L02.43- ☑
  urethra N34.0
  vulva N76.4
Carbunculus — *see* Carbuncle
Carcinoid (tumor) — *see* Tumor, carcinoid
Carcinoidosis E34.0
Carcinoma (malignant) (*see also* Neoplasm, by site, malignant)
  acidophil
    specified site — *see* Neoplasm, malignant, by site
    unspecified site C75.1
  acidophil-basophil, mixed
    specified site — *see* Neoplasm, malignant, by site
    unspecified site C75.1
  adnexal (skin) — *see* Neoplasm, skin, malignant
  adrenal cortical C74.0- ☑
  alveolar — *see* Neoplasm, lung, malignant
    cell — *see* Neoplasm, lung, malignant
  ameloblastic C41.1
    upper jaw (bone) C41.0

Carcinoma — continued
  noninfiltrating — continued
    intraductal — continued
      papillary
        breast D05.1- ☑
        specified site NEC — see Neoplasm, in situ, by site
        unspecified site D05.1- ☑
      specified site — see Neoplasm, in situ, by site
      unspecified site D05.1- ☑
      lobular
        breast D05.0- ☑
        specified site NEC — see Neoplasm, in situ, by site
        unspecified site (female) D05.0- ☑
  oat cell
    specified site — see Neoplasm, malignant, by site
    unspecified site C34.90
  odontogenic C41.1
    upper jaw (bone) C41.0
  papillary
    with follicular (mixed) C73
    follicular variant C73
    intraductal (noninfiltrating)
      with invasion
        specified site — see Neoplasm, malignant, by site
        unspecified site (female) C50.91- ☑
          male C50.92- ☑
      breast D05.1- ☑
      specified site NEC — see Neoplasm, in situ, by site
      unspecified site D05.1- ☑
    serous
      specified site — see Neoplasm, malignant, by site
      surface
        specified site — see Neoplasm, malignant, by site
        unspecified site C56.9
      unspecified site C56.9
  papillocystic
    specified site — see Neoplasm, malignant, by site
    unspecified site C56.9
  parafollicular cell
    specified site — see Neoplasm, malignant, by site
    unspecified site C73
  pilomatrix — see Neoplasm, skin, malignant
  pseudomucinous
    specified site — see Neoplasm, malignant, by site
    unspecified site C56.9
  renal cell C64- ☑
  Schmincke — see Neoplasm, nasopharynx, malignant
  Schneiderian
    specified site — see Neoplasm, malignant, by site
    unspecified site C30.0
  sebaceous — see Neoplasm, skin, malignant
  secondary (see also Neoplasm, secondary, by site)
    Merkel cell C7B.1 (following C75)
  secretory, breast — see Neoplasm, breast, malignant
  serous
    papillary
      specified site — see Neoplasm, malignant, by site
      unspecified site C56.9
    surface, papillary
      specified site — see Neoplasm, malignant, by site
      unspecified site C56.9
  Sertoli cell
    specified site — see Neoplasm, malignant, by site
    unspecified site C62.90
      female C56.9
      male C62.90
  skin appendage — see Neoplasm, skin, malignant
  small cell
    fusiform cell
      specified site — see Neoplasm, malignant, by site
      unspecified site C34.90
    intermediate cell
      specified site — see Neoplasm, malignant, by site
      unspecified site C34.90
    large cell
      specified site — see Neoplasm, malignant, by site

Carcinoma — continued
  small cell — continued
    large cell — continued
      unspecified site C34.90
  solid
    with amyloid stroma
      specified site — see Neoplasm, malignant, by site
      unspecified site C73
    microinvasive
      specified site — see Neoplasm, malignant, by site
      unspecified site C53.9
  sweat gland — see Neoplasm, skin, malignant
  theca cell C56.- ☑
  thymic C37
  unspecified site (primary) C80.1
  water-clear cell C75.0
Carcinoma-in-situ (see also Neoplasm, in situ, by site)
  breast NOS D05.9- ☑
    specified type NEC D05.8- ☑
  epidermoid (see also Neoplasm, in situ, by site)
    with questionable stromal invasion
      cervix D06.9
      specified site NEC — see Neoplasm, in situ, by site
      unspecified site D06.9
    Bowen's type — see Neoplasm, skin, in situ
  intraductal
    breast D05.1- ☑
    specified site NEC — see Neoplasm, in situ, by site
    unspecified site D05.1- ☑
  lobular
    with
      infiltrating duct
        breast (female) C50.91- ☑
          male C50.92- ☑
        specified site NEC — see Neoplasm, malignant
        unspecified site (female) C50.91- ☑
          male C50.92- ☑
      intraductal
        breast D05.8- ☑
        specified site NEC — see Neoplasm, in situ, by site
        unspecified site (female) D05.8- ☑
    breast D05.0- ☑
    specified site NEC — see Neoplasm, in situ, by site
    unspecified site D05.0- ☑
  squamous cell (see also Neoplasm, in situ, by site)
    with questionable stromal invasion
      cervix D06.9
      specified site NEC — see Neoplasm, in situ, by site
      unspecified site D06.9
Carcinomaphobia F45.29
Carcinomatosis C80.0
  peritonei C78.6
  unspecified site (primary) (secondary) C80.0
Carcinosarcoma — see Neoplasm, malignant, by site
  embryonal — see Neoplasm, malignant, by site
Cardia, cardial — see condition
Cardiac (see also condition)
  death, sudden — see Arrest, cardiac
  pacemaker
    in situ Z95.0
    management or adjustment Z45.018
  tamponade I31.4
Cardialgia — see Pain, precordial
Cardiectasis — see Hypertrophy, cardiac
Cardiochalasia K21.9
Cardiomalacia I51.5
Cardiomegalia glycogenica diffusa E74.02 [I43]
Cardiomegaly (see also Hypertrophy, cardiac)
  congenital Q24.8
  glycogen E74.02 [I43]
  idiopathic I51.7
Cardiomyoliposis I51.5
Cardiomyopathy (familial) (idiopathic) I42.9
  alcoholic I42.6
  amyloid E85.4 [I43]
  arteriosclerotic — see Disease, heart, ischemic, atherosclerotic
  beriberi E51.12
  cobalt-beer I42.6
  congenital I42.4
  congestive I42.0

Cardiomyopathy — continued
  constrictive NOS I42.5
  dilated I42.0
  due to
    alcohol I42.6
    beriberi E51.12
    cardiac glycogenosis E74.02 [I43]
    drugs I42.7
    external agents NEC I42.7
    Friedreich's ataxia G11.1
    myotonia atrophica G71.11 [I43]
    progressive muscular dystrophy G71.0
  glycogen storage E74.02 [I43]
  hypertensive — see Hypertension, heart
  hypertrophic (nonobstructive) I42.2
    obstructive I42.1
      congenital Q24.8
  in
    Chagas' disease (chronic) B57.2
      acute B57.0
    sarcoidosis D86.85
  ischemic I25.5
  metabolic E88.9 [I43]
    thyrotoxic E05.90 [I43]
      with thyroid storm E05.91 [I43]
  newborn I42.8
    congenital I42.4
  nutritional E63.9 [I43]
    beriberi E51.12
  obscure of Africa I42.8
  peripartum O90.3
  postpartum O90.3
  restrictive NEC I42.5
  rheumatic I09.0
  secondary I42.9
  stress induced I51.81
  takotsubo I51.81
  thyrotoxic E05.90 [I43]
    with thyroid storm E05.91 [I43]
  toxic NEC I42.7
  tuberculous A18.84
  viral B33.24
Cardionephritis — see Hypertension, cardiorenal
Cardionephropathy — see Hypertension, cardiorenal
Cardionephrosis — see Hypertension, cardiorenal
Cardiopathia nigra I27.0
Cardiopathy (see also Disease, heart) I51.9
  idiopathic I42.9
  mucopolysaccharidosis E76.3 [I52]
Cardiopericarditis — see Pericarditis
Cardiophobia F45.29
Cardiorenal — see condition
Cardiorrhexis — see Infarct, myocardium
Cardiosclerosis — see Disease, heart, ischemic, atherosclerotic
Cardiosis — see Disease, heart
Cardiospasm (esophagus) (reflex) (stomach) K22.0
  congenital Q39.5
    with megaesophagus Q39.5
Cardiostenosis — see Disease, heart
Cardiosymphysis I31.0
Cardiovascular — see condition
Carditis (acute) (bacterial) (chronic) (subacute) I51.89
  meningococcal A39.50
  rheumatic — see Disease, heart, rheumatic
  rheumatoid — see Rheumatoid, carditis
  viral B33.20
Care (of) (for) (following)
  child (routine) Z76.2
  family member (handicapped) (sick)
    creating problem for family Z63.6
    provided away from home for holiday relief Z75.5
    unavailable, due to
      absence (person rendering care) (sufferer) Z74.2
      inability (any reason) of person rendering care Z74.2
  foundling Z76.1
  holiday relief Z75.5
  improper — see Maltreatment
  lack of (at or after birth) (infant) — see Maltreatment, child, neglect
  lactating mother Z39.1
  palliative Z51.5
  postpartum
    immediately after delivery Z39.0
    routine follow-up Z39.2
  respite Z75.5

Care — *continued*
  unavailable, due to
    absence of person rendering care Z74.2
    inability (any reason) of person rendering care
      Z74.2
  well-baby Z76.2
Caries
  bone NEC A18.03
  dental K02.9
    arrested (coronal) (root) K02.3
    chewing surface
      limited to enamel K02.51
      penetrating into dentin K02.52
      penetrating into pulp K02.53
    coronal surface
      chewing surface
        limited to enamel K02.51
        penetrating into dentin K02.52
        penetrating into pulp K02.53
      pit and fissure surface
        limited to enamel K02.51
        penetrating into dentin K02.52
        penetrating into pulp K02.53
      smooth surface
        limited to enamel K02.61
        penetrating into dentin K02.62
        penetrating into pulp K02.63
    pit and fissure surface
      limited to enamel K02.51
      penetrating into dentin K02.52
      penetrating into pulp K02.53
    root K02.7
    smooth surface
      limited to enamel K02.61
      penetrating into dentin K02.62
      penetrating into pulp K02.63
  external meatus — *see* Disorder, ear, external, specified type NEC
  hip (tuberculous) A18.02
  initial (tooth)
    chewing surface K02.51
    pit and fissure surface K02.51
    smooth surface K02.61
  knee (tuberculous) A18.02
  labyrinth H83.8 ☑
  limb NEC (tuberculous) A18.03
  mastoid process (chronic) — *see* Mastoiditis, chronic tuberculous A18.03
  middle ear H74.8 ☑
  nose (tuberculous) A18.03
  orbit (tuberculous) A18.03
  ossicles, ear — *see* Abnormal, ear ossicles
  petrous bone — *see* Petrositis
  root (dental) (tooth) K02.7
  sacrum (tuberculous) A18.01
  spine, spinal (column) (tuberculous) A18.01
  syphilitic A52.77
    congenital (early) A50.02 [M90.80]
  tooth, teeth — *see* Caries, dental
  tuberculous A18.03
  vertebra (column) (tuberculous) A18.01
Carious teeth — *see* Caries, dental
Carneous mole O02.0
Carnitine insufficiency E71.40
Carotid body or sinus syndrome G90.01
Carotidynia G90.01
Carotinemia (dietary) E67.1
Carotinosis (cutis) (skin) E67.1
Carpal tunnel syndrome — *see* Syndrome, carpal tunnel
Carpenter's syndrome Q87.0
Carpopedal spasm — *see* Tetany
Carr-Barr-Plunkett syndrome Q97.1
Carrier (suspected) of
  amebiasis Z22.1
  bacterial disease NEC Z22.39
    diphtheria Z22.2
    intestinal infectious NEC Z22.1
      typhoid Z22.0
    meningococcal Z22.31
    sexually transmitted Z22.4
    specified NEC Z22.39
    staphylococcal (Methicillin susceptible) Z22.321
      Methicillin resistant Z22.322
    streptococcal Z22.338
      group B Z22.330
    typhoid Z22.0
  cholera Z22.1
  diphtheria Z22.2

Carrier of — *continued*
  gastrointestinal pathogens NEC Z22.1
  genetic Z14.8
    cystic fibrosis Z14.1
    hemophilia A (asymptomatic) Z14.01
      symptomatic Z14.02
  gonorrhea Z22.4
  HAA (hepatitis Australian-antigen) Z22.59
  HB (c)(s)-AG Z22.51
  hepatitis (viral) Z22.50
    Australia-antigen (HAA) Z22.59
    B surface antigen (HBsAg) Z22.51
      with acute delta- (super)infection B17.0
    C Z22.52
    specified NEC Z22.59
  human T-cell lymphotropic virus type-1 (HTLV-1) infection Z22.6
  infectious organism Z22.9
    specified NEC Z22.8
  meningococci Z22.31
  Salmonella typhosa Z22.0
  serum hepatitis — *see* Carrier, hepatitis
  staphylococci (Methicillin susceptible) Z22.321
    Methicillin resistant Z22.322
  streptococci Z22.338
    group B Z22.330
  syphilis Z22.4
  typhoid Z22.0
  venereal disease NEC Z22.4
Carrion's disease A44.0
Carter's relapsing fever (Asiatic) A68.1
Cartilage — *see* condition
Caruncle (inflamed)
  conjunctiva (acute) — *see* Conjunctivitis, acute
  labium (majus) (minus) N90.89
  lacrimal — *see* Inflammation, lacrimal, passages
  myrtiform N89.8
  urethral (benign) N36.2
Cascade stomach K31.2
Caseation lymphatic gland (tuberculous) A18.2
Cassidy (-Scholte) syndrome (malignant carcinoid) E34.0
Castellani's disease A69.8
Castration, traumatic, male S38.231 ☑
Cat
  cry syndrome Q93.4
  ear Q17.3
  eye syndrome Q92.8
Cat-scratch (*see also* Abrasion)
  disease or fever A28.1
Catabolism, senile R54
Catalepsy (hysterical) F44.2
  schizophrenic F20.2
Cataplexy (idiopathic) — *see* Narcolepsy
Cataract (cortical) (immature) (incipient) H26.9
  with
    neovascularization — *see* Cataract, complicated
  age-related — *see* Cataract, senile
  anterior
    and posterior axial embryonal Q12.0
    pyramidal Q12.0
  associated with
    galactosemia E74.21 [H28]
    myotonic disorders G71.19 [H28]
  blue Q12.0
  central Q12.0
  cerulean Q12.0
  complicated H26.20
    with
      neovascularization H26.21- ☑
      ocular disorder H26.22- ☑
      glaucomatous flecks H26.23- ☑
  congenital Q12.0
  coraliform Q12.0
  coronary Q12.0
  crystalline Q12.0
  diabetic — *see* Diabetes, cataract
  drug-induced H26.3- ☑
  due to
    ocular disorder — *see* Cataract, complicated
    radiation H26.8
  electric H26.8
  extraction status Z98.4- ☑
  glass-blower's H26.8
  heat ray H26.8
  heterochromic — *see* Cataract, complicated
  hypermature — *see* Cataract, senile, morgagnian type

Cataract — *continued*
  in (due to)
    chronic iridocyclitis — *see* Cataract, complicated
    diabetes — *see* Diabetes, cataract
    endocrine disease E34.9 [H28]
    eye disease — *see* Cataract, complicated
    hypoparathyroidism E20.9 [H28]
    malnutrition-dehydration E46 [H28]
    metabolic disease E88.9 [H28]
    myotonic disorders G71.19 [H28]
    nutritional disease E63.9 [H28]
  infantile — *see* Cataract, presenile
  irradiational — *see* Cataract, specified NEC
  juvenile — *see* Cataract, presenile
  malnutrition-dehydration E46 [H28]
  morgagnian — *see* Cataract, senile, morgagnian type
  myotonic G71.19 [H28]
  myxedema E03.9 [H28]
  nuclear
    embryonal Q12.0
    sclerosis — *see* Cataract, senile, nuclear
  presenile H26.00- ☑
    combined forms H26.06- ☑
    cortical H26.01- ☑
    lamellar — *see* Cataract, presenile, cortical
    nuclear H26.03- ☑
    specified NEC H26.09
    subcapsular polar (anterior) H26.04- ☑
      posterior H26.05- ☑
    zonular — *see* Cataract, presenile, cortical
  secondary H26.40
    Soemmering's ring H26.41- ☑
    specified NEC H26.49- ☑
    to eye disease — *see* Cataract, complicated
  senile H25.9
    brunescens — *see* Cataract, senile, nuclear
    combined forms H25.81- ☑
    coronary — *see* Cataract, senile, incipient
    cortical H25.01- ☑
    hypermature — *see* Cataract, senile, morgagnian type
    incipient (mature) (total) H25.09- ☑
      cortical — *see* Cataract, senile, cortical
      subcapsular — *see* Cataract, senile, subcapsular
    morgagnian type (hypermature) H25.2- ☑
    nuclear (sclerosis) H25.1- ☑
    polar subcapsular (anterior) (posterior) — *see* Cataract, senile, incipient
    punctate — *see* Cataract, senile, incipient
    specified NEC H25.89
    subcapsular polar (anterior) H25.03- ☑
      posterior H25.04- ☑
  snowflake — *see* Diabetes, cataract
  specified NEC H26.8
  toxic — *see* Cataract, drug-induced
  traumatic H26.10- ☑
    localized H26.11- ☑
    partially resolved H26.12- ☑
    total H26.13- ☑
  zonular (perinuclear) Q12.0
Cataracta (*see also* Cataract)
  brunescens — *see* Cataract, senile, nuclear
  centralis pulverulenta Q12.0
  cerulea Q12.0
  complicata — *see* Cataract, complicated
  congenita Q12.0
  coralliformis Q12.0
  coronaria Q12.0
  diabetic — *see* Diabetes, cataract
  membranacea
    accreta — *see* Cataract, secondary
    congenita Q12.0
  nigra — *see* Cataract, senile, nuclear
  sunflower — *see* Cataract, complicated
Catarrh, catarrhal (acute) (febrile) (infectious) (inflammation) (*see also* condition) J00
  bronchial — *see* Bronchitis
  chest — *see* Bronchitis
  chronic J31.0
  due to congenital syphilis A50.03
  enteric — *see* Enteritis
  eustachian H68.009
  fauces — *see* Pharyngitis
  gastrointestinal — *see* Enteritis
  gingivitis K05.00
    nonplaque induced K05.01
    plaque induced K05.00

☑ **Additional Character Required** — Refer to the Tabular List for Character Selection   ▽ **Subterms under main terms may continue to next column or page**

Catarrh, catarrhal — *continued*
  hay — *see* Fever, hay
  intestinal — *see* Enteritis
  larynx, chronic J37.0
  liver B15.9
    with hepatic coma B15.0
  lung — *see* Bronchitis
  middle ear, chronic — *see* Otitis, media, nonsuppura-
    tive, chronic, serous
  mouth K12.1
  nasal (chronic) — *see* Rhinitis
  nasobronchial J31.1
  nasopharyngeal (chronic) J31.1
    acute J00
  pulmonary — *see* Bronchitis
  spring (eye) (vernal) — *see* Conjunctivitis, acute, atopic
  summer (hay) — *see* Fever, hay
  throat J31.2
  tubotympanal (*see also* Otitis, media, nonsuppurative)
    chronic — *see* Otitis, media, nonsuppurative,
      chronic, serous
Catatonia (schizophrenic) F20.2
Catatonic
  disorder due to known physiologic condition F06.1
  schizophrenia F20.2
  stupor R40.1
Cauda equina — *see* condition
Cauliflower ear M95.1- ☑
Causalgia (upper limb) G56.4- ☑
  lower limb G57.7- ☑
Cause
  external, general effects T75.89 ☑
Caustic burn — *see* Corrosion, by site
Cavare's disease (familial periodic paralysis) G72.3
Cave-in, injury
  crushing (severe) — *see* Crush
  suffocation — *see* Asphyxia, traumatic, due to low
    oxygen, due to cave-in
Cavernitis (penis) N48.29
Cavernositis N48.29
Cavernous — *see* condition
Cavitation of lung (*see also* Tuberculosis, pulmonary)
  nontuberculous J98.4
Cavities, dental — *see* Caries, dental
Cavity
  lung — *see* Cavitation of lung
  optic papilla Q14.2
  pulmonary — *see* Cavitation of lung
Cavovarus foot, congenital Q66.1
Cavus foot (congenital) Q66.7
  acquired — *see* Deformity, limb, foot, specified NEC
Cazenave's disease L10.2
Cecitis K52.9
  with perforation, peritonitis, or rupture K65.8
Cecum — *see* condition
Celiac
  artery compression syndrome I77.4
  disease K90.0
  infantilism K90.0
Cell(s), **cellular** (*see also* condition)
  in urine R82.99
Cellulitis (diffuse) (phlegmonous) (septic) (suppurative)
    L03.90
  abdominal wall L03.311
  anaerobic A48.0
  ankle — *see* Cellulitis, lower limb
  anus K61.0
  arm — *see* Cellulitis, upper limb
  auricle (ear) — *see* Cellulitis, ear
  axilla L03.11- ☑
  back (any part) L03.312
  broad ligament
    acute N73.0
  buttock L03.317
  cervical (meaning neck) L03.221
  cervix (uteri) — *see* Cervicitis
  cheek (external) L03.211
    internal K12.2
  chest wall L03.313
  chronic L03.90
  clostridial A48.0
  corpus cavernosum N48.22
  digit
    finger — *see* Cellulitis, finger
    toe — *see* Cellulitis, toe
  Douglas' cul-de-sac or pouch
    acute N73.0

Cellulitis — *continued*
  drainage site (following operation) T81.4 ☑
  ear (external) H60.1- ☑
  eosinophilic (granulomatous) L98.3
  erysipelatous — *see* Erysipelas
  external auditory canal — *see* Cellulitis, ear
  eyelid — *see* Abscess, eyelid
  face NEC L03.211
  finger (intrathecal) (periosteal) (subcutaneous) (subcu-
    ticular) L03.01- ☑
  foot — *see* Cellulitis, lower limb
  gangrenous — *see* Gangrene
  genital organ NEC
    female (external) N76.4
    male N49.9
      multiple sites N49.8
      specified NEC N49.8
  gluteal (region) L03.317
  gonococcal A54.89
  groin L03.314
  hand — *see* Cellulitis, upper limb
  head NEC L03.811
    face (any part, except ear, eye and nose) L03.211
  heel — *see* Cellulitis, lower limb
  hip — *see* Cellulitis, lower limb
  jaw (region) L03.211
  knee — *see* Cellulitis, lower limb
  labium (majus) (minus) — *see* Vulvitis
  lacrimal passages — *see* Inflammation, lacrimal, pas-
    sages
  larynx J38.7
  leg — *see* Cellulitis, lower limb
  lip K13.0
  lower limb L03.11- ☑
    toe — *see* Cellulitis, toe
  mouth (floor) K12.2
  multiple sites, so stated L03.90
  nasopharynx J39.1
  navel L03.316
    newborn P38.9
      with mild hemorrhage P38.1
      without hemorrhage P38.9
  neck (region) L03.221
  nose (septum) (external) J34.0
  orbit, orbital H05.01- ☑
  palate (soft) K12.2
  pectoral (region) L03.313
  pelvis, pelvic (chronic)
    female (*see also* Disease, pelvis, inflammatory)
      N73.2
      acute N73.0
    following ectopic or molar pregnancy O08.0
    male K65.0
  penis N48.22
  perineal, perineum L03.315
  perirectal K61.1
  peritonsillar J36
  periurethral N34.0
  periuterine (*see also* Disease, pelvis, inflammatory)
    N73.2
    acute N73.0
  pharynx J39.1
  rectum K61.1
  retroperitoneal K68.9
  round ligament
    acute N73.0
  scalp (any part) L03.811
  scrotum N49.2
  seminal vesicle N49.0
  shoulder — *see* Cellulitis, upper limb
  specified site NEC L03.818
  submandibular (region) (space) (triangle) K12.2
    gland K11.3
  submaxillary (region) K12.2
    gland K11.3
  thigh — *see* Cellulitis, lower limb
  thumb (intrathecal) (periosteal) (subcutaneous) (sub-
    cuticular) — *see* Cellulitis, finger
  toe (intrathecal) (periosteal) (subcutaneous) (subcutic-
    ular) L03.03- ☑
  tonsil J36
  trunk L03.319
    abdominal wall L03.311
    back (any part) L03.312
    buttock L03.317
    chest wall L03.313
    groin L03.314
    perineal, perineum L03.315

Cellulitis — *continued*
  trunk — *continued*
    umbilicus L03.316
  tuberculous (primary) A18.4
  umbilicus L03.316
  upper limb L03.11- ☑
    axilla — *see* Cellulitis, axilla
    finger — *see* Cellulitis, finger
    thumb — *see* Cellulitis, finger
  vaccinal T88.0 ☑
  vocal cord J38.3
  vulva — *see* Vulvitis
  wrist — *see* Cellulitis, upper limb
Cementoblastoma, benign — *see* Cyst, calcifying
  odontogenic
Cementoma — *see* Cyst, calcifying odontogenic
Cementoperiostitis — *see* Periodontitis
Cementosis K03.4
Central auditory processing disorder H93.25
Central pain syndrome G89.0
Cephalematocele, cephal (o)hematocele
  newborn P52.8
    birth injury P10.8
  traumatic — *see* Hematoma, brain
Cephalematoma, cephalhematoma (calcified)
  newborn (birth injury) P12.0
  traumatic — *see* Hematoma, brain
Cephalgia, cephalalgia (*see also* Headache)
  histamine G44.009
    intractable G44.001
    not intractable G44.009
  trigeminal autonomic (TAC) NEC G44.099
    intractable G44.091
    not intractable G44.099
Cephalic — *see* condition
Cephalitis — *see* Encephalitis
Cephalocele — *see* Encephalocele
Cephalomenia N94.89
Cephalopelvic — *see* condition
Cerclage (with cervical incompetence) in pregnancy —
  see Incompetence, cervix, in pregnancy
Cerebellitis — *see* Encephalitis
Cerebellum, cerebellar — *see* condition
Cerebral — *see* condition
Cerebritis — *see* Encephalitis
Cerebro-hepato-renal syndrome Q87.89
Cerebromalacia — *see* Softening, brain
  sequelae of cerebrovascular disease I69.398
Cerebroside lipidosis E75.22
Cerebrospasticity (congenital) G80.1
Cerebrospinal — *see* condition
Cerebrum — *see* condition
Ceroid-lipofuscinosis, neuronal E75.4
Cerumen (accumulation) (impacted) H61.2- ☑
Cervical (*see also* condition)
  auricle Q18.2
  dysplasia in pregnancy — *see* Abnormal, cervix, in
    pregnancy or childbirth
  erosion in pregnancy — *see* Abnormal, cervix, in
    pregnancy or childbirth
  fibrosis in pregnancy — *see* Abnormal, cervix, in
    pregnancy or childbirth
  fusion syndrome Q76.1
  rib Q76.5
  shortening (complicating pregnancy) O26.87- ☑
Cervicalgia M54.2
Cervicitis (acute) (chronic) (nonvenereal) (senile (atrophic)) (subacute) (with ulceration) N72
  with
    abortion — *see* Abortion, by type complicated by
      genital tract and pelvic infection
    ectopic pregnancy O08.0
    molar pregnancy O08.0
  chlamydial A56.09
  gonococcal A54.03
  herpesviral A60.03
  puerperal (postpartum) O86.11
  syphilitic A52.76
  trichomonal A59.09
  tuberculous A18.16
Cervicocolpitis (emphysematosa) (see also Cervicitis)
  N72
Cervix — *see* condition
**Cesarean delivery, previous, affecting management
  of pregnancy** O34.21
Céstan (-Chenais) paralysis or syndrome G46.3
Céstan-Raymond syndrome I65.8

Cestode infestation B71.9
   specified type NEC B71.8
Cestodiasis B71.9
Chabert's disease A22.9
Chacaleh E53.8
Chafing L30.4
Chagas' (-Mazza) disease (chronic) B57.2
   with
      cardiovascular involvement NEC B57.2
      digestive system involvement B57.30
         megacolon B57.32
         megaesophagus B57.31
         other specified B57.39
      megacolon B57.32
      megaesophagus B57.31
      myocarditis B57.2
      nervous system involvement B57.40
         meningitis B57.41
         meningoencephalitis B57.42
         other specified B57.49
      specified organ involvement NEC B57.5
   acute (with) B57.1
      cardiovascular NEC B57.0
      myocarditis B57.0
Chagres fever B50.9
Chairridden Z74.09
Chalasia (cardiac sphincter) K21.9
Chalazion H00.19
   left H00.16
      lower H00.15
      upper H00.14
   right H00.13
      lower H00.12
      upper H00.11
Chalcosis (see also Disorder, globe, degenerative, chalcosis)
   cornea — see Deposit, cornea
   crystalline lens — see Cataract, complicated
   retina H35.89
Chalicosis (pulmonum) J62.8
Chancre (any genital site) (hard) (hunterian) (mixed) (primary) (seronegative) (seropositive) (syphilitic) A51.0
   congenital A50.07
   conjunctiva NEC A51.2
   Ducrey's A57
   extragenital A51.2
   eyelid A51.2
   lip A51.2
   nipple A51.2
   Nisbet's A57
   of
      carate A67.0
      pinta A67.0
      yaws A66.0
   palate, soft A51.2
   phagedenic A57
   simple A57
   soft A57
      bubo A57
      palate A51.2
   urethra A51.0
   yaws A66.0
Chancroid (anus) (genital) (penis) (perineum) (rectum) (urethra) (vulva) A57
Chandler's disease (osteochondritis dissecans, hip) — see Osteochondritis, dissecans, hip
Change(s) (in) (of) (see also Removal)
   arteriosclerotic — see Arteriosclerosis
   bone (see also Disorder, bone)
      diabetic — see Diabetes, bone change
   bowel habit R19.4
   cardiorenal (vascular) — see Hypertension, cardiorenal
   cardiovascular — see Disease, cardiovascular
   circulatory I99.9
   cognitive (mild) (organic) R41.89
   color, tooth, teeth
      during formation K00.8
      posteruptive K03.7
   contraceptive device Z30.433
   corneal membrane H18.30
      Bowman's membrane fold or rupture H18.31- ☑
      Descemet's membrane
         fold H18.32- ☑
         rupture H18.33- ☑
   coronary — see Disease, heart, ischemic
   degenerative, spine or vertebra — see Spondylosis
   dental pulp, regressive K04.2

Change(s) — continued
   dressing (nonsurgical) Z48.00
      surgical Z48.01
   heart — see Disease, heart
   hip joint — see Derangement, joint, hip
   hyperplastic larynx J38.7
   hypertrophic
      nasal sinus J34.89
      turbinate, nasal J34.3
      upper respiratory tract J39.8
   indwelling catheter Z46.6
   inflammatory (see also Inflammation)
      sacroiliac M46.1
   job, anxiety concerning Z56.1
   joint — see Derangement, joint
   life — see Menopause
   mental status R41.82
   minimal (glomerular) (see also N00-N07 with fourth character .0) N05.0
   myocardium, myocardial — see Degeneration, myocardial
   of life — see Menopause
   pacemaker Z45.018
      pulse generator Z45.010
   personality (enduring) F68.8
      due to (secondary to)
         general medical condition F07.0
      secondary (nonspecific) F60.89
   regressive, dental pulp K04.2
   renal — see Disease, renal
   retina H35.9
      myopic H44.2- ☑
   sacroiliac joint M53.3
   senile (see also condition) R54
   sensory R20.8
   skin R23.9
      acute, due to ultraviolet radiation L56.9
         specified NEC L56.8
      chronic, due to nonionizing radiation L57.9
         specified NEC L57.8
      cyanosis R23.0
      flushing R23.2
      pallor R23.1
      petechiae R23.3
      specified change NEC R23.8
      swelling — see Mass, localized
      texture R23.4
   trophic
      arm — see Mononeuropathy, upper limb
      leg — see Mononeuropathy, lower limb
   vascular I99.9
   vasomotor I73.9
   voice R49.9
      psychogenic F44.4
      specified NEC R49.8
Changing sleep-work schedule, affecting sleep G47.26
Changuinola fever A93.8
Chapping skin T69.8 ☑
Charcot-Marie-Tooth disease, paralysis or syndrome G60.0
Charcot's
   arthropathy — see Arthropathy, neuropathic
   cirrhosis K74.3
   disease (tabetic arthropathy) A52.16
   joint (disease) (tabetic) A52.16
      diabetic — see Diabetes, with, arthropathy
      syringomyelic G95.0
   syndrome (intermittent claudication) I73.9
CHARGE association Q89.8
Charley-horse (quadriceps) M62.831
   traumatic (quadriceps) S76.11- ☑
Charlouis' disease — see Yaws
Cheadle's disease E54
Check-up — see Examination
Checking (of)
   cardiac pacemaker (battery) (electrode(s)) Z45.018
      pulse generator Z45.010
   intrauterine contraceptive device Z30.431
Chédiak-Higashi (-Steinbrinck) **syndrome** (congenital gigantism of peroxidase granules) E70.330
Cheek — see condition
Cheese itch B88.0
Cheese-washer's lung J67.8
Cheese-worker's lung J67.8

Cheilitis (acute) (angular) (catarrhal) (chronic) (exfoliative) (gangrenous) (glandular) (infectional) (suppurative) (ulcerative) (vesicular) K13.0
   actinic (due to sun) L56.8
      other than from sun L59.8
   candidal B37.83
Cheilodynia K13.0
Cheiloschisis — see Cleft, lip
Cheilosis (angular) K13.0
   with pellagra E52
   due to
      vitamin B2 (riboflavin) deficiency E53.0
Cheiromegaly M79.89
Cheiropompholyx L30.1
Cheloid — see Keloid
Chemical burn — see Corrosion, by site
Chemodectoma — see Paraganglioma, nonchromaffin
Chemosis, conjunctiva — see Edema, conjunctiva
Chemotherapy (session) (for)
   cancer Z51.11
   neoplasm Z51.11
Cherubism M27.8
Chest — see condition
Cheyne-Stokes breathing (respiration) R06.3
Chiari's
   disease or syndrome (hepatic vein thrombosis) I82.0
   malformation
      type I G93.5
      type II — see Spina bifida
   net Q24.8
Chicago disease B40.9
Chickenpox — see Varicella
Chiclero ulcer or sore B55.1
Chigger (infestation) B88.0
Chignon (disease) B36.8
   newborn (from vacuum extraction) (birth injury) P12.1
Chilaiditi's syndrome (subphrenic displacement, colon) Q43.3
Chilblain(s) (lupus) T69.1 ☑
Child
   custody dispute Z65.3
Childbirth — see Delivery
Childhood
   cerebral X-linked adrenoleukodystrophy E71.520
   period of rapid growth Z00.2
Chill(s) R68.83
   with fever R50.9
   without fever R68.83
   congestive in malarial regions B54
Chilomastigiasis A07.8
Chimera 46,XX/46,XY Q99.0
Chin — see condition
Chinese dysentery A03.9
Chionophobia F40.228
Chitral fever A93.1
Chlamydia, chlamydial A74.9
   cervicitis A56.09
   conjunctivitis A74.0
   cystitis A56.01
   endometritis A56.11
   epididymitis A56.19
   female
      pelvic inflammatory disease A56.11
      pelviperitonitis A56.11
   orchitis A56.19
   peritonitis A74.81
   pharyngitis A56.4
   proctitis A56.3
   psittaci (infection) A70
   salpingitis A56.11
   sexually-transmitted infection NEC A56.8
   specified NEC A74.89
   urethritis A56.01
   vulvovaginitis A56.02
Chlamydiosis — see Chlamydia
Chloasma (skin) (idiopathic) (symptomatic) L81.1
   eyelid H02.719
      hyperthyroid E05.90 [H02.719]
         with thyroid storm E05.91 [H02.719]
      left H02.716
         lower H02.715
         upper H02.714
      right H02.713
         lower H02.712
         upper H02.711
Chloroma C92.3- ☑
Chlorosis D50.9

☑ **Additional Character Required** — Refer to the Tabular List for Character Selection   �假 **Subterms under main terms may continue to next column or page**

Chlorosis — *continued*
Egyptian B76.9 [D63.8]
miner's B76.9 [D63.8]
Chlorotic anemia D50.8
Chocolate cyst (ovary) N80.1
Choked
disc or disk — *see* Papilledema
on food, phlegm, or vomitus NOS — *see* Foreign body, by site
while vomiting NOS — *see* Foreign body, by site
Chokes (resulting from bends) T70.3 —
Choking sensation R09.89
Cholangiectasis K83.8
Cholangiocarcinoma
with hepatocellular carcinoma, combined C22.0
liver C22.1
specified site NEC — *see* Neoplasm, malignant, by site
unspecified site C22.1
Cholangiohepatitis K83.8
due to fluke infestation B66.1
Cholangiohepatoma C22.0
Cholangiolitis (acute) (chronic) (extrahepatic) (gangrenous) (intrahepatic) K83.0
paratyphoidal — *see* Fever, paratyphoid
typhoidal A01.09
Cholangioma D13.4
malignant — *see* Cholangiocarcinoma
Cholangitis (ascending) (primary) (recurrent) (sclerosing) (secondary) (stenosing) (suppurative) K83.0
with calculus, bile duct — *see* Calculus, bile duct, with cholangitis
chronic nonsuppurative destructive K74.3
Cholecystectasia K82.8
Cholecystitis K81.9
with
calculus, stones in
bile duct (common) (hepatic) — *see* Calculus, bile duct, with cholecystitis
cystic duct — *see* Calculus, gallbladder, with cholecystitis
gallbladder — *see* Calculus, gallbladder, with cholecystitis
choledocholithiasis — *see* Calculus, bile duct, with cholecystitis
cholelithiasis — *see* Calculus, gallbladder, with cholecystitis
acute (emphysematous) (gangrenous) (suppurative) K81.0
with
calculus, stones in
cystic duct — *see* Calculus, gallbladder, with cholecystitis, acute
gallbladder — *see* Calculus, gallbladder, with cholecystitis, acute
choledocholithiasis — *see* Calculus, bile duct, with cholecystitis, acute
cholelithiasis — *see* Calculus, gallbladder, with cholecystitis, acute
chronic cholecystitis K81.2
with gallbladder calculus K80.12
with obstruction K80.13
chronic K81.1
with acute cholecystitis K81.2
with gallbladder calculus K80.12
with obstruction K80.13
emphysematous (acute) — *see* Cholecystitis, acute
gangrenous — *see* Cholecystitis, acute
paratyphoidal, current A01.4
suppurative — *see* Cholecystitis, acute
typhoidal A01.09
Cholecystolithiasis — *see* Calculus, gallbladder
Choledochitis (suppurative) K83.0
Choledocholith — *see* Calculus, bile duct
Choledocholithiasis (common duct) (hepatic duct) —
see Calculus, bile duct
cystic — *see* Calculus, gallbladder
typhoidal A01.09
Cholelithiasis (cystic duct) (gallbladder) (impacted) (multiple) — *see* Calculus, gallbladder
bile duct (common) (hepatic) — *see* Calculus, bile duct
hepatic duct — *see* Calculus, bile duct
specified NEC K80.80
with obstruction K80.81
Cholemia (*see also* Jaundice)
familial (simple) (congenital) E80.4
Gilbert's E80.4
Choleperitoneum, choleperitonitis K65.3

Cholera (Asiatic) (epidemic) (malignant) A00.9
antimonial — *see* Poisoning, antimony
classical A00.0
due to Vibrio cholerae 01 A00.9
biovar cholerae A00.0
biovar eltor A00.1
el tor A00.1
el tor A00.1
Cholerine — *see* Cholera
Cholestasis NEC K83.1
with hepatocyte injury K71.0
due to total parenteral nutrition (TPN) K76.89
pure K71.0
Cholesteatoma (ear) (middle) (with reaction) H71.9- ☑
attic H71.0- ☑
external ear (canal) H60.4- ☑
mastoid H71.2- ☑
postmastoidectomy cavity (recurrent) — *see* Complications, postmastoidectomy, recurrent cholesteatoma
recurrent (postmastoidectomy) — *see* Complications, postmastoidectomy, recurrent cholesteatoma
tympanum H71.1- ☑
Cholesteatosis, diffuse H71.3- ☑
Cholesteremia E78.0
Cholesterin in vitreous — *see* Deposit, crystalline
Cholesterol
deposit
retina H35.89
vitreous — *see* Deposit, crystalline
elevated (high) E78.0
with elevated (high) triglycerides E78.2
screening for Z13.220
imbibition of gallbladder K82.4
Cholesterolemia (essential) (familial) (hereditary) (pure) E78.0
Cholesterolosis, cholesterosis (gallbladder) K82.4
cerebrotendinous E75.5
Cholocolic fistula K82.3
Choluria R82.2
Chondritis M94.8X9
aural H61.03- ☑
costal (Tietze's) M94.0
external ear H61.03- ☑
patella, posttraumatic — *see* Chondromalacia, patella
pinna H61.03- ☑
purulent M94.8X- ☑
tuberculous NEC A18.02
intervertebral A18.01
Chondro-osteodysplasia (Morquio-Brailsford type) E76.219
Chondro-osteodystrophy E76.29
Chondro-osteoma — *see* Neoplasm, bone, benign
Chondroblastoma (*see also* Neoplasm, bone, benign)
malignant — *see* Neoplasm, bone, malignant
Chondrocalcinosis M11.20
ankle M11.27- ☑
elbow M11.22- ☑
familial M11.10
ankle M11.17- ☑
elbow M11.12- ☑
foot joint M11.17- ☑
hand joint M11.14- ☑
hip M11.15- ☑
knee M11.16- ☑
multiple site M11.19
shoulder M11.11- ☑
vertebrae M11.18
wrist M11.13- ☑
foot joint M11.27- ☑
hand joint M11.24- ☑
hip M11.25- ☑
knee M11.26- ☑
multiple site M11.29
shoulder M11.21- ☑
specified type NEC M11.20
ankle M11.27- ☑
elbow M11.22- ☑
foot joint M11.27- ☑
hand joint M11.24- ☑
hip M11.25- ☑
knee M11.26- ☑
multiple site M11.29
shoulder M11.21- ☑
vertebrae M11.28
wrist M11.23- ☑
vertebrae M11.28

Chondrocalcinosis — *continued*
wrist M11.23- ☑
Chondrodermatitis nodularis helicis or anthelicis
— *see* Perichondritis, ear
Chondrodysplasia Q78.9
with hemangioma Q78.4
calcificans congenita Q77.3
fetalis Q77.4
metaphyseal (Jansen's) (McKusick's) (Schmid's) Q78.5
punctata Q77.3
Chondrodystrophy, chondrodystrophia (familial) (fetalis) (hypoplastic) Q78.9
calcificans congenita Q77.3
myotonic (congenital) G71.13
punctata Q77.3
Chondroectodermal dysplasia Q77.6
Chondrogenesis imperfecta Q77.4
Chondrolysis M94.35- ☑
Chondroma (*see also* Neoplasm, cartilage, benign)
juxtacortical — *see* Neoplasm, bone, benign
periosteal — *see* Neoplasm, bone, benign
Chondromalacia (systemic) M94.20
acromioclavicular joint M94.21- ☑
ankle M94.27- ☑
elbow M94.22- ☑
foot joint M94.27- ☑
glenohumeral joint M94.21- ☑
hand joint M94.24- ☑
hip M94.25- ☑
knee M94.26- ☑
patella M22.4- ☑
multiple sites M94.29
patella M22.4- ☑
rib M94.28
sacroiliac joint M94.259
shoulder M94.21- ☑
sternoclavicular joint M94.21- ☑
vertebral joint M94.28
wrist M94.23- ☑
Chondromatosis (*see also* Neoplasm, cartilage, uncertain behavior)
internal Q78.4
Chondromyxosarcoma — *see* Neoplasm, cartilage, malignant
Chondropathia tuberosa M94.0
Chondrosarcoma — *see* Neoplasm, cartilage, malignant
juxtacortical — *see* Neoplasm, bone, malignant
mesenchymal — *see* Neoplasm, connective tissue, malignant
myxoid — *see* Neoplasm, cartilage, malignant
Chordee (nonvenereal) N48.89
congenital Q54.4
gonococcal A54.09
Chorditis (fibrinous) (nodosa) (tuberosa) J38.2
Chordoma — *see* Neoplasm, vertebral (column), malignant
Chorea (chronic) (gravis) (posthemiplegic) (senile) (spasmodic) G25.5
with
heart involvement I02.0
active or acute (conditions in I01-) I02.0
rheumatic I02.9
with valvular disorder I02.0
rheumatic heart disease (chronic) (inactive)(quiescent) — *code to* rheumatic heart condition involved
drug-induced G25.4
habit F95.8
hereditary G10
Huntington's G10
hysterical F44.4
minor I02.9
with heart involvement I02.0
progressive G25.5
hereditary G10
rheumatic (chronic) I02.9
with heart involvement I02.0
Sydenham's I02.9
with heart involvement — *see* Chorea, with rheumatic heart disease
nonrheumatic G25.5
Choreoathetosis (paroxysmal) G25.5
Chorioadenoma (destruens) D39.2
Chorioamnionitis O41.12- ☑
Chorioangioma D26.7
Choriocarcinoma — *see* Neoplasm, malignant, by site

Choriocarcinoma — *continued*
  combined with
    embryonal carcinoma — *see* Neoplasm, malignant, by site
    other germ cell elements — *see* Neoplasm, malignant, by site
    teratoma — *see* Neoplasm, malignant, by site
  specified site — *see* Neoplasm, malignant, by site
  unspecified site
    female C58
    male C62.90
Chorioencephalitis (acute) (lymphocytic) (serous) A87.2
Chorioepithelioma — *see* Choriocarcinoma
Choriomeningitis (acute) (lymphocytic) (serous) A87.2
Chorionepithelioma — *see* Choriocarcinoma
Chorioretinitis (*see also* Inflammation, chorioretinal)
  disseminated (*see also* Inflammation, chorioretinal, disseminated)
    in neurosyphilis A52.19
  Egyptian B76.9 [D63.8]
  focal (*see also* Inflammation, chorioretinal, focal)
  histoplasmic B39.9 [H32]
  in (due to)
    histoplasmosis B39.9 [H32]
    syphilis (secondary) A51.43
      late A52.71
    toxoplasmosis (acquired) B58.01
      congenital (active) P37.1 [H32]
    tuberculosis A18.53
  juxtapapillary, juxtapapillaris — *see* Inflammation, chorioretinal, focal, juxtapapillary
  leprous A30.9 [H32]
  miner's B76.9 [D63.8]
  progressive myopia (degeneration) H44.2- ☑
  syphilitic (secondary) A51.43
    congenital (early) A50.01 [H32]
      late A50.32
    late A52.71
  tuberculous A18.53
Chorioretinopathy, central serous H35.71- ☑
Choroid — *see* condition
Choroideremia H31.21
Choroiditis — *see* Chorioretinitis
Choroidopathy — *see* Disorder, choroid
Choroidoretinitis — *see* Chorioretinitis
Choroidoretinopathy, central serous — *see* Chorioretinopathy, central serous
Christian-Weber disease M35.6
Christmas disease D67
Chromaffinoma (*see also* Neoplasm, benign, by site)
  malignant — *see* Neoplasm, malignant, by site
Chromatopsia — *see* Deficiency, color vision
Chromhidrosis, chromidrosis L75.1
Chromoblastomycosis — *see* Chromomycosis
Chromoconversion R82.91
Chromomycosis B43.9
  brain abscess B43.1
  cerebral B43.1
  cutaneous B43.0
  skin B43.0
  specified NEC B43.8
  subcutaneous abscess or cyst B43.2
Chromophytosis B36.0
Chromosome — *see* Anomaly, by chromosome involved
  D (1) — *see* Anomaly, chromosome 13
  E (3) — *see* Anomaly, chromosome 18
  G — *see* Anomaly, chromosome 21
Chromotrichomycosis B36.8
Chronic — *see* condition
  fracture — *see* Fracture, pathological
Churg-Strauss syndrome M30.1
Chyle cyst, mesentery I89.8
Chylocele (nonfilarial) I89.8
  filarial (*see also* Infestation, filarial) B74.9 [N51]
  tunica vaginalis N50.8
    filarial (*see also* Infestation, filarial) B74.9 [N51]
Chylomicronemia (fasting) (with hyperprebetalipoproteinemia) E78.3
Chylopericardium I31.3
  acute I30.9
Chylothorax (nonfilarial) I89.8
  filarial (*see also* Infestation, filarial) B74.9 [J91.8]
Chylous — *see* condition
Chyluria (nonfilarial) R82.0
  due to
    bilharziasis B65.0
    Brugia (malayi) B74.1

Chyluria — *continued*
  due to — *continued*
    Brugia — *continued*
      timori B74.2
    schistosomiasis (bilharziasis) B65.0
    Wuchereria (bancrofti) B74.0
  filarial — *see* Infestation, filarial
Cicatricial (deformity) — *see* Cicatrix
Cicatrix (adherent) (contracted) (painful) (vicious) (*see also* Scar) L90.5
  adenoid (and tonsil) J35.8
  alveolar process M26.79
  anus K62.89
  auricle — *see* Disorder, pinna, specified type NEC
  bile duct (common) (hepatic) K83.8
  bladder N32.89
  bone — *see* Disorder, bone, specified type NEC
  brain G93.89
  cervix (postoperative) (postpartal) N88.1
  common duct K83.8
  cornea H17.9
    tuberculous A18.59
  duodenum (bulb), obstructive K31.5
  esophagus K22.2
  eyelid — *see* Disorder, eyelid function
  hypopharynx J39.2
  lacrimal passages — *see* Obstruction, lacrimal
  larynx J38.7
  lung J98.4
  middle ear H74.8 ☑
  mouth K13.79
  muscle M62.89
    with contracture — *see* Contraction, muscle NEC
  nasopharynx J39.2
  palate (soft) K13.79
  penis N48.89
  pharynx J39.2
  prostate N42.89
  rectum K62.89
  retina — *see* Scar, chorioretinal
  semilunar cartilage — *see* Derangement, meniscus
  seminal vesicle N50.8
  skin L90.5
    infected L08.89
    postinfective L90.5
    tuberculous B90.8
  specified site NEC L90.5
  throat J39.2
  tongue K14.8
  tonsil (and adenoid) J35.8
  trachea J39.8
  tuberculous NEC B90.9
  urethra N36.8
  uterus N85.8
  vagina N89.8
    postoperative N99.2
  vocal cord J38.3
  wrist, constricting (annular) L90.5
CIDP (chronic inflammatory demyelinating polyneuropathy) G61.81
CIN — *see* Neoplasia, intraepithelial, cervix
Cinchonism — *see* Deafness, ototoxic
  correct substance properly administered — *see* Table of Drugs and Chemicals, by drug, adverse effect
  overdose or wrong substance given or taken — *see* Table of Drugs and Chemicals, by drug, poisoning
Circle of Willis — *see* condition
Circular — *see* condition
Circulating anticoagulants (*see also* Disorder, hemorrhagic) D68.318
  due to drugs (*see also* Disorder, hemorrhagic) D68.32
  following childbirth O72.3
Circulation
  collateral, any site I99.8
  defective (lower extremity) I99.8
    congenital Q28.9
  embryonic Q28.9
  failure (peripheral) R57.9
    newborn P29.89
  fetal, persistent P29.3
  heart, incomplete Q28.9
Circulatory system — *see* condition
Circulus senilis (cornea) — *see* Degeneration, cornea, senile
Circumcision (in absence of medical indication) (ritual) (routine) Z41.2
Circumscribed — *see* condition

Circumvallate placenta O43.11- ☑
Cirrhosis, cirrhotic (hepatic) (liver) K74.60
  alcoholic K70.30
    with ascites K70.31
  atrophic — *see* Cirrhosis, liver
  Baumgarten-Cruveilhier K74.69
  biliary (cholangiolitic) (cholangitic) (hypertrophic) (obstructive) (pericholangiolitic) K74.5
    due to
      Clonorchiasis B66.1
      flukes B66.3
    primary K74.3
    secondary K74.4
  cardiac (of liver) K76.1
  Charcot's K74.3
  cholangiolitic, cholangitic, cholostatic (primary) K74.3
  congestive K76.1
  Cruveilhier-Baumgarten K74.69
  cryptogenic (liver) K74.69
  due to
    hepatolenticular degeneration E83.01
    Wilson's disease E83.01
    xanthomatosis E78.2
  fatty K76.0
    alcoholic K70.0
  Hanot's (hypertrophic) K74.3
  hepatic — *see* Cirrhosis, liver
  hypertrophic K74.3
  Indian childhood K74.69
  kidney — *see* Sclerosis, renal
  Laennec's K70.30
    with ascites K70.31
    alcoholic K70.30
      with ascites K70.31
    nonalcoholic K74.69
  liver K74.60
    alcoholic K70.30
      with ascites K70.31
      fatty K70.0
    congenital P78.81
    syphilitic A52.74
  lung (chronic) J84.10
  macronodular K74.69
    alcoholic K70.30
      with ascites K70.31
  micronodular K74.69
    alcoholic K70.30
      with ascites K70.31
  mixed type K74.69
  monolobular K74.3
  nephritis — *see* Sclerosis, renal
  nutritional K74.69
    alcoholic K70.30
      with ascites K70.31
  obstructive — *see* Cirrhosis, biliary
  ovarian N83.8
  pancreas (duct) K86.8
  pigmentary E83.110
  portal K74.69
    alcoholic K70.30
      with ascites K70.31
  postnecrotic K74.69
    alcoholic K70.30
      with ascites K70.31
  pulmonary J84.10
  renal — *see* Sclerosis, renal
  spleen D73.2
  stasis K76.1
  Todd's K74.3
  unilobar K74.3
  xanthomatous (biliary) K74.5
    due to xanthomatosis (familial) (metabolic) (primary) E78.2
Cistern, subarachnoid R93.0
Citrullinemia E72.23
Citrullinuria E72.23
Civatte's disease or poikiloderma L57.3
Clam digger's itch B65.3
Clammy skin R23.1
Clap — *see* Gonorrhea
Clarke-Hadfield syndrome (pancreatic infantilism) K86.8
Clark's paralysis G80.9
Clastothrix L67.8
Claude Bernard-Horner syndrome G90.2
  traumatic — *see* Injury, nerve, cervical sympathetic
Claude's disease or syndrome G46.3
Claudicatio venosa intermittens I87.8

Claudication, intermittent I73.9
 cerebral (artery) G45.9
 spinal cord (arteriosclerotic) G95.19
  syphilitic A52.09
 venous (axillary) I87.8
Claustrophobia F40.240
Clavus (infected) L84
Clawfoot (congenital) Q66.89
 acquired — *see* Deformity, limb, clawfoot
Clawhand (acquired) (*see also* Deformity, limb, clawhand)
 congenital Q68.1
Clawtoe (congenital) Q66.89
 acquired — *see* Deformity, toe, specified NEC
Clay eating — *see* Pica
Cleansing of artificial opening — *see* Attention to, artificial, opening
Cleft (congenital) (*see also* Imperfect, closure)
 alveolar process M26.79
 branchial (cyst) (persistent) Q18.2
 cricoid cartilage, posterior Q31.8
 lip (unilateral) Q36.9
  with cleft palate Q37.9
   hard Q37.1
    with soft Q37.5
   soft Q37.3
    with hard Q37.5
  bilateral Q36.0
   with cleft palate Q37.8
    hard Q37.0
     with soft Q37.4
    soft Q37.2
     with hard Q37.4
  median Q36.1
 nose Q30.2
 palate Q35.9
  with cleft lip (unilateral) Q37.9
   bilateral Q37.8
  hard Q35.1
   with
    cleft lip (unilateral) Q37.1
     bilateral Q37.0
    soft Q35.5
     with cleft lip (unilateral) Q37.5
      bilateral Q37.4
  medial Q35.5
  soft Q35.3
   with
    cleft lip (unilateral) Q37.3
     bilateral Q37.2
    hard Q35.5
     with cleft lip (unilateral) Q37.5
      bilateral Q37.4
 penis Q55.69
 scrotum Q55.29
 thyroid cartilage Q31.8
 uvula Q35.7
Cleidocranial dysostosis Q74.0
Cleptomania F63.2
Clicking hip (newborn) R29.4
Climacteric (female) (*see also* Menopause)
 arthritis (any site) NEC — *see* Arthritis, specified form NEC
 depression (single episode) F32.8
 male (symptoms) (syndrome) NEC N50.8
 paranoid state F22
 polyarthritis NEC — *see* Arthritis, specified form NEC
 symptoms (female) N95.1
Clinical research investigation (clinical trial) (control subject) (normal comparison) (participant) Z00.6
Clitoris — *see* condition
Cloaca (persistent) Q43.7
Clonorchiasis, clonorchis infection (liver) B66.1
Clonus R25.8
Closed bite M26.29
Clostridium (C.) **perfringens, as cause of disease classified elsewhere** B96.7
Closure
 congenital, nose Q30.0
 cranial sutures, premature Q75.0
 defective or imperfect NEC — *see* Imperfect, closure
 fistula, delayed — *see* Fistula
 foramen ovale, imperfect Q21.1
 hymen N89.6
 interauricular septum, defective Q21.1
 interventricular septum, defective Q21.0
 lacrimal duct (*see also* Stenosis, lacrimal, duct)
  congenital Q10.5
 nose (congenital) Q30.0

Closure — *continued*
 nose — *continued*
  acquired M95.0
 of artificial opening — *see* Attention to, artificial, opening
 vagina N89.5
 valve — *see* Endocarditis
 vulva N90.5
Clot (blood) (*see also* Embolism)
 artery (obstruction) (occlusion) — *see* Embolism
 bladder N32.89
 brain (intradural or extradural) — *see* Occlusion, artery, cerebral
 circulation I74.9
 heart (*see also* Infarct, myocardium)
  not resulting in infarction I24.0
 vein — *see* Thrombosis
Clouded state R40.1
 epileptic — *see* Epilepsy, specified NEC
 paroxysmal — *see* Epilepsy, specified NEC
Cloudy antrum, antra J32.0
Clouston's (hidrotic) **ectodermal dysplasia** Q82.4
Clubbed nail pachydermoperiostosis M89.40 [L62]
Clubbing of finger(s) (nails) R68.3
Clubfinger R68.3
 congenital Q68.1
Clubfoot (congenital) Q66.89
 acquired — *see* Deformity, limb, clubfoot
 equinovarus Q66.0
 paralytic — *see* Deformity, limb, clubfoot
Clubhand (congenital) (radial) Q71.4- ☑
 acquired — *see* Deformity, limb, clubhand
Clubnail R68.3
 congenital Q84.6
Clump, kidney Q63.1
Clumsiness, clumsy child syndrome F82
Cluttering F80.81
Clutton's joints A50.51 [M12.80]
Coagulation, intravascular (diffuse) (disseminated)
 (*see also* Defibrination syndrome)
 complicating abortion — *see* Abortion, by type, complicated by, intravascular coagulation
 following ectopic or molar pregnancy O08.1
Coagulopathy (*see also* Defect, coagulation)
 consumption D65
 intravascular D65
  newborn P60
Coalition
 calcaneo-scaphoid Q66.89
 tarsal Q66.89
Coalminer's
 elbow — *see* Bursitis, elbow, olecranon
 lung or pneumoconiosis J60
Coalworker's lung or pneumoconiosis J60
Coarctation
 aorta (preductal) (postductal) Q25.1
 pulmonary artery Q25.71
Coated tongue K14.3
Coats' disease (exudative retinopathy) — *see* Retinopathy, exudative
Cocainism — *see* Dependence, drug, cocaine
Coccidioidomycosis B38.9
 cutaneous B38.3
 disseminated B38.7
 generalized B38.7
 meninges B38.4
 prostate B38.81
 pulmonary B38.2
  acute B38.0
  chronic B38.1
 skin B38.3
 specified NEC B38.89
Coccidioidosis — *see* Coccidioidomycosis
Coccidiosis (intestinal) A07.3
Coccydynia, coccygodynia M53.3
Coccyx — *see* condition
Cochin-China diarrhea K90.1
Cockayne's syndrome Q87.1
Cocked up toe — *see* Deformity, toe, specified NEC
Cock's peculiar tumor L72.3
Codman's tumor — *see* Neoplasm, bone, benign
Coenurosis B71.8
Coffee-worker's lung J67.8
Cogan's syndrome H16.32- ☑
 oculomotor apraxia H51.8
Coitus, painful (female) N94.1
 male N53.12

Coitus, painful — *continued*
 psychogenic F52.6
Cold J00
 with influenza, flu, or grippe — *see* Influenza, with, respiratory manifestations NEC
 agglutinin disease or hemoglobinuria (chronic) D59.1
 bronchial — *see* Bronchitis
 chest — *see* Bronchitis
 common (head) J00
 effects of T69.9 ☑
  specified effect NEC T69.8 ☑
 excessive, effects of T69.9 ☑
  specified effect NEC T69.8 ☑
 exhaustion from T69.8 ☑
 exposure to T69.9 ☑
  specified effect NEC T69.8 ☑
 head J00
 injury syndrome (newborn) P80.0
 on lung — *see* Bronchitis
 rose J30.1
 sensitivity, auto-immune D59.1
 virus J00
Coldsore B00.1
Colibacillosis A49.8
 as the cause of other disease (*see also* Escherichia coli) B96.20
 generalized A41.50
Colic (bilious) (infantile) (intestinal) (recurrent) (spasmodic) R10.83
 abdomen R10.83
  psychogenic F45.8
 appendix, appendicular K38.8
 bile duct — *see* Calculus, bile duct
 biliary — *see* Calculus, bile duct
 common duct — *see* Calculus, bile duct
 cystic duct — *see* Calculus, gallbladder
 Devonshire NEC — *see* Poisoning, lead
 gallbladder — *see* Calculus, gallbladder
 gallstone — *see* Calculus, gallbladder
  gallbladder or cystic duct — *see* Calculus, gallbladder
 hepatic (duct) — *see* Calculus, bile duct
 hysterical F45.8
 kidney N23
 lead NEC — *see* Poisoning, lead
 mucous K58.9
  with diarrhea K58.0
  psychogenic F54
 nephritic N23
 painter's NEC — *see* Poisoning, lead
 pancreas K86.8
 psychogenic F45.8
 renal N23
 saturnine NEC — *see* Poisoning, lead
 ureter N23
 urethral N36.8
  due to calculus N21.1
 uterus NEC N94.89
  menstrual — *see* Dysmenorrhea
 worm NOS B83.9
Colicystitis — *see* Cystitis
Colitis (acute) (catarrhal) (chronic) (noninfective) (hemorrhagic) (*see also* Enteritis) K52.9
 allergic K52.2
 amebic (acute) (*see also* Amebiasis) A06.0
  nondysenteric A06.2
 anthrax A22.2
 bacillary — *see* Infection, Shigella
 balantidial A07.0
 Clostridium difficile A04.7
 coccidial A07.3
 collagenous K52.89
 cystica superficialis K52.89
 dietary counseling and surveillance (for) Z71.3
 dietetic K52.2
 drug-induced K52.1
 due to radiation K52.0
 eosinophilic K52.82
 food hypersensitivity K52.2
 giardial A07.1
 granulomatous — *see* Enteritis, regional, large intestine
 infectious — *see* Enteritis, infectious
 ischemic K55.9
  acute (fulminant) (subacute) K55.0
  chronic K55.1
   due to mesenteric artery insufficiency K55.1

Colitis — continued
- ischemic — continued
  - fulminant (acute) K55.Ø
  - left sided K51.5Ø
    - with
      - abscess K51.514
      - complication K51.519
        - specified NEC K51.518
      - fistula K51.513
      - obstruction K51.512
      - rectal bleeding K51.511
- lymphocytic K52.89
- membranous
  - psychogenic F54
- microscopic (collagenous) (lymphocytic) K52.89
- mucous — see Syndrome, irritable, bowel
  - psychogenic F54
- noninfective K52.9
  - specified NEC K52.89
- polyposa — see Polyp, colon, inflammatory
- protozoal AØ7.9
- pseudomembranous AØ4.7
- pseudomucinous — see Syndrome, irritable, bowel
- regional — see Enteritis, regional, large intestine
- segmental — see Enteritis, regional, large intestine
- septic — see Enteritis, infectious
- spastic K58.9
  - with diarrhea K58.Ø
  - psychogenic F54
- staphylococcal AØ4.8
  - foodborne AØ5.Ø
- subacute ischemic K55.Ø
- thromboulcerative K55.Ø
- toxic NEC K52.1
  - due to Clostridium difficile AØ4.7
- transmural — see Enteritis, regional, large intestine
- trichomonal AØ7.8
- tuberculous (ulcerative) A18.32
- ulcerative (chronic) K51.9Ø
  - with
    - complication K51.919
      - abscess K51.914
      - fistula K51.913
      - obstruction K51.912
      - rectal bleeding K51.911
      - specified complication NEC K51.918
  - enterocolitis — see Enterocolitis, ulcerative
  - ileocolitis — see Ileocolitis, ulcerative
  - mucosal proctocolitis — see Proctocolitis, mucosal
  - proctitis — see Proctitis, ulcerative
  - pseudopolyposis — see Polyp, colon, inflammatory
  - psychogenic F54
  - rectosigmoiditis — see Rectosigmoiditis, ulcerative
  - specified type NEC K51.8Ø
    - with
      - complication K51.819
        - abscess K51.814
        - fistula K51.813
        - obstruction K51.812
        - rectal bleeding K51.811
        - specified complication NEC K51.818

Collagenosis, collagen disease (nonvascular) (vascular) M35.9
- cardiovascular I42.8
- reactive perforating L87.1
- specified NEC M35.8

Collapse R55
- adrenal E27.2
- cardiorespiratory R57.Ø
- cardiovascular R57.Ø
  - newborn P29.89
- circulatory (peripheral) R57.9
  - during or after labor and delivery O75.1
  - following ectopic or molar pregnancy OØ8.3
  - newborn P29.89
- during or
  - after labor and delivery O75.1
  - resulting from a procedure, not elsewhere classified T81.1Ø ☑
- external ear canal — see Stenosis, external ear canal
- general R55
- heart — see Disease, heart
- heat T67.1 ☑
- hysterical F44.89
- labyrinth, membranous (congenital) Q16.5
- lung (massive) (see also Atelectasis) J98.19
  - pressure due to anesthesia (general) (local) or other sedation T88.2 ☑

Collapse — continued
- lung (see also Atelectasis) — continued
  - pressure due to anesthesia or other sedation — continued
    - during labor and delivery O74.1
    - in pregnancy O29.Ø2- ☑
    - postpartum, puerperal O89.Ø9
- myocardial — see Disease, heart
- nervous F48.8
- neurocirculatory F45.8
- nose M95.Ø
- postoperative T81.1Ø ☑
- pulmonary (see also Atelectasis) J98.19
  - newborn — see Atelectasis
- trachea J39.8
- tracheobronchial J98.Ø9
- valvular — see Endocarditis
- vascular (peripheral) R57.9
  - during or after labor and delivery O75.1
  - following ectopic or molar pregnancy OØ8.3
  - newborn P29.89
- vertebra M48.5Ø- ☑
  - cervical region M48.52- ☑
  - cervicothoracic region M48.53- ☑
  - in (due to)
    - metastasis — see Collapse, vertebra, in, specified disease NEC
    - osteoporosis (see also Osteoporosis) M8Ø.88 ☑
      - cervical region M8Ø.88 ☑
      - cervicothoracic region M8Ø.88 ☑
      - lumbar region M8Ø.88 ☑
      - lumbosacral region M8Ø.88 ☑
      - multiple sites M8Ø.88 ☑
      - occipito-atlanto-axial region M8Ø.88 ☑
      - sacrococcygeal region M8Ø.88 ☑
      - thoracic region M8Ø.88 ☑
      - thoracolumbar region M8Ø.88 ☑
    - specified disease NEC M48.5Ø- ☑
      - cervical region M48.52- ☑
      - cervicothoracic region M48.53- ☑
      - lumbar region M48.56- ☑
      - lumbosacral region M48.57- ☑
      - occipito-atlanto-axial region M48.51- ☑
      - sacrococcygeal region M48.58- ☑
      - thoracic region M48.54- ☑
      - thoracolumbar region M48.55- ☑
  - lumbar region M48.56- ☑
  - lumbosacral region M48.57- ☑
  - occipito-atlanto-axial region M48.51- ☑
  - sacrococcygeal region M48.58- ☑
  - thoracic region M48.54- ☑
  - thoracolumbar region M48.55- ☑

Collateral (see also condition)
- circulation (venous) I87.8
- dilation, veins I87.8

Colles' fracture S52.53- ☑
Collet (-Sicard) syndrome G52.7
Collier's asthma or lung J6Ø
Collodion baby Q8Ø.2
Colloid nodule (of thyroid) (cystic) EØ4.1
Coloboma (iris) Q13.Ø
- eyelid Q1Ø.3
- fundus Q14.8
- lens Q12.2
- optic disc (congenital) Q14.2
  - acquired H47.31- ☑
Coloenteritis — see Enteritis
Colon — see condition
Colonization
- MRSA (Methicillin resistant Staphylococcus aureus) Z22.322
- MSSA (Methicillin susceptible Staphylococcus aureus) Z22.321
- status — see Carrier (suspected) of
Coloptosis K63.4
Color blindness — see Deficiency, color vision
Colostomy
- attention to Z43.3
- fitting or adjustment Z46.89
- malfunctioning K94.Ø3
- status Z93.3
Colpitis (acute) — see Vaginitis
Colpocele N81.5
Colpocystitis — see Vaginitis
Colpospasm N94.2
Column, spinal, vertebral — see condition

Coma R4Ø.2Ø
- with
  - motor response (none) R4Ø.231 ☑
    - abnormal R4Ø.233 ☑
    - extension R4Ø.232 ☑
    - flexion withdrawal R4Ø.234 ☑
    - localizes pain R4Ø.235 ☑
    - obeys commands R4Ø.236 ☑
  - opening of eyes (never) R4Ø.211 ☑
    - in response to
      - pain R4Ø.212 ☑
      - sound R4Ø.213 ☑
    - spontaneous R4Ø.214 ☑
  - verbal response (none) R4Ø.221 ☑
    - confused conversation R4Ø.224 ☑
    - inappropriate words R4Ø.223 ☑
    - incomprehensible words R4Ø.222 ☑
    - oriented R4Ø.225 ☑
- eclamptic — see Eclampsia
- epileptic — see Epilepsy
- Glasgow, scale score — see Glasgow coma scale
- hepatic — see Failure, hepatic, by type, with coma
- hyperglycemic (diabetic) — see Diabetes, coma
- hyperosmolar (diabetic) — see Diabetes, coma
- hypoglycemic (diabetic) — see Diabetes, coma, hypoglycemic
  - nondiabetic E15
- in diabetes — see Diabetes, coma
- insulin-induced — see Coma, hypoglycemic
- myxedematous EØ3.5
- newborn P91.5
- persistent vegetative state R4Ø.3
- specified NEC, without documented Glasgow coma scale score, or with partial Glasgow coma scale score reported R4Ø.244
Comatose — see Coma
Combat fatigue F43.Ø
Combined — see condition
Comedo, comedones (giant) L7Ø.Ø
Comedocarcinoma (see also Neoplasm, breast, malignant)
- noninfiltrating
  - breast DØ5.8- ☑
  - specified site — see Neoplasm, in situ, by site
  - unspecified site DØ5.8- ☑
Comedomastitis — see Ectasia, mammary duct
Comminuted fracture — code as Fracture, closed
Common
- arterial trunk Q2Ø.Ø
- atrioventricular canal Q21.2
- atrium Q21.1
- cold (head) JØØ
- truncus (arteriosus) Q2Ø.Ø
- variable immunodeficiency — see Immunodeficiency, common variable
- ventricle Q2Ø.4
Commotio, commotion (current)
- brain — see Injury, intracranial, concussion
- cerebri — see Injury, intracranial, concussion
- retinae SØ5.8X- ☑
- spinal cord — see Injury, spinal cord, by region
- spinalis — see Injury, spinal cord, by region
Communication
- between
  - base of aorta and pulmonary artery Q21.4
  - left ventricle and right atrium Q2Ø.5
  - pericardial sac and pleural sac Q34.8
  - pulmonary artery and pulmonary vein, congenital Q25.72
- congenital between uterus and digestive or urinary tract Q51.7
Compartment syndrome (deep) (posterior) (traumatic) T79.AØ ☑ (following T79.7)
- abdomen T79.A3 ☑ (following T79.7)
- lower extremity (hip, buttock, thigh, leg, foot, toes) T79.A2 ☑ (following T79.7)
- nontraumatic
  - abdomen M79.A3 (following M79.7)
  - lower extremity (hip, buttock, thigh, leg, foot, toes) M79.A2- ☑ (following M79.7)
  - specified site NEC M79.A9 (following M79.7)
  - upper extremity (shoulder, arm, forearm, wrist, hand, fingers) M79.A1- ☑ (following M79.7)
- specified site NEC T79.A9 ☑ (following T79.7)
- upper extremity (shoulder, arm, forearm, wrist, hand, fingers) T79.A1- ☑ (following T79.7)

Compensation
failure — *see* Disease, heart
neurosis, psychoneurosis — *see* Disorder, factitious
Complaint (*see also* Disease)
bowel, functional K59.9
psychogenic F45.8
intestine, functional K59.9
psychogenic F45.8
kidney — *see* Disease, renal
miners' J60
Complete — *see* condition
Complex
Addison-Schilder E71.528
cardiorenal — *see* Hypertension, cardiorenal
Costen's M26.69
disseminated mycobacterium avium- intracellulare (DMAC) A31.2
Eisenmenger's (ventricular septal defect) I27.89
hypersexual F52.8
jumped process, spine — *see* Dislocation, vertebra
primary, tuberculous A15.7
Schilder-Addison E71.528
subluxation (vertebral) M99.19
abdomen M99.19
acromioclavicular M99.17
cervical region M99.11
cervicothoracic M99.11
costochondral M99.18
costovertebral M99.18
head region M99.10
hip M99.15
lower extremity M99.16
lumbar region M99.13
lumbosacral M99.13
occipitocervical M99.10
pelvic region M99.15
pubic M99.15
rib cage M99.18
sacral region M99.14
sacrococcygeal M99.14
sacroiliac M99.14
specified NEC M99.19
sternochondral M99.18
sternoclavicular M99.17
thoracic region M99.12
thoracolumbar M99.12
upper extremity M99.17
Taussig-Bing (transposition, aorta and overriding pulmonary artery) Q20.1
Complication(s) (from) (of)
accidental puncture or laceration during a procedure (of) — *see* Complications, intraoperative (intraprocedural), puncture or laceration
amputation stump (surgical) (late) NEC T87.9
dehiscence T87.81
infection or inflammation T87.40
lower limb T87.4- ☑
upper limb T87.4- ☑
necrosis T87.50
lower limb T87.5- ☑
upper limb T87.5- ☑
neuroma T87.30
lower limb T87.3- ☑
upper limb T87.3- ☑
specified type NEC T87.89
anastomosis (and bypass) (*see also* Complications, prosthetic device or implant)
intestinal (internal) NEC K91.89
involving urinary tract N99.89
urinary tract (involving intestinal tract) N99.89
vascular — *see* Complications, cardiovascular device or implant
anesthesia, anesthetic (*see also* Anesthesia, complication) T88.59 ☑
brain, postpartum, puerperal O89.2
cardiac
in
labor and delivery O74.2
pregnancy O29.19- ☑
postpartum, puerperal O89.1
central nervous system
in
labor and delivery O74.3
pregnancy O29.29- ☑
postpartum, puerperal O89.2
difficult or failed intubation T88.4 ☑
in pregnancy O29.6- ☑

Complication(s) — *continued*
anesthesia, anesthetic (*see also* Anesthesia, complication) — *continued*
failed sedation (conscious) (moderate) during procedure T88.52 ☑
hyperthermia, malignant T88.3 ☑
hypothermia T88.51 ☑
intubation failure T88.4 ☑
malignant hyperthermia T88.3 ☑
pulmonary
in
labor and delivery O74.1
pregnancy NEC O29.09- ☑
postpartum, puerperal O89.09
shock T88.2 ☑
spinal and epidural
in
labor and delivery NEC O74.6
headache O74.5
pregnancy NEC O29.5X- ☑
postpartum, puerperal NEC O89.5
headache O89.4
anti-reflux device — *see* Complications, esophageal anti-reflux device
aortic (bifurcation) graft — *see* Complications, graft, vascular
aortocoronary (bypass) graft — *see* Complications, coronary artery (bypass) graft
aortofemoral (bypass) graft — *see* Complications, extremity artery (bypass) graft
arteriovenous
fistula, surgically created T82.9 ☑
embolism T82.818 ☑
fibrosis T82.828 ☑
hemorrhage T82.838 ☑
infection or inflammation T82.7 ☑
mechanical
breakdown T82.510 ☑
displacement T82.520 ☑
leakage T82.530 ☑
malposition T82.520 ☑
obstruction T82.590 ☑
perforation T82.590 ☑
protrusion T82.590 ☑
pain T82.848 ☑
specified type NEC T82.898 ☑
stenosis T82.858 ☑
thrombosis T82.868 ☑
shunt, surgically created T82.9 ☑
embolism T82.818 ☑
fibrosis T82.828 ☑
hemorrhage T82.838 ☑
infection or inflammation T82.7 ☑
mechanical
breakdown T82.511 ☑
displacement T82.521 ☑
leakage T82.531 ☑
malposition T82.521 ☑
obstruction T82.591 ☑
perforation T82.591 ☑
protrusion T82.591 ☑
pain T82.848 ☑
specified type NEC T82.898 ☑
stenosis T82.858 ☑
thrombosis T82.868 ☑
arthroplasty — *see* Complications, joint prosthesis
artificial
fertilization or insemination N98.9
attempted introduction (of)
embryo in embryo transfer N98.3
ovum following in vitro fertilization N98.2
hyperstimulation of ovaries N98.1
infection N98.0
specified NEC N98.8
heart T82.9 ☑
embolism T82.817 ☑
fibrosis T82.827 ☑
hemorrhage T82.837 ☑
infection or inflammation T82.7 ☑
mechanical
breakdown T82.512 ☑
displacement T82.522 ☑
leakage T82.532 ☑
malposition T82.522 ☑
obstruction T82.592 ☑
perforation T82.592 ☑

Complication(s) — *continued*
artificial — *continued*
heart — *continued*
mechanical — *continued*
protrusion T82.592 ☑
pain T82.847 ☑
specified type NEC T82.897 ☑
stenosis T82.857 ☑
thrombosis T82.867 ☑
opening
cecostomy — *see* Complications, colostomy
colostomy — *see* Complications, colostomy
cystostomy — *see* Complications, cystostomy
enterostomy — *see* Complications, enterostomy
gastrostomy — *see* Complications, gastrostomy
ileostomy — *see* Complications, enterostomy
jejunostomy — *see* Complications, enterostomy
nephrostomy — *see* Complications, stoma, urinary tract
tracheostomy — *see* Complications, tracheostomy
ureterostomy — *see* Complications, stoma, urinary tract
urethrostomy — *see* Complications, stoma, urinary tract
balloon implant or device
gastrointestinal T85.9 ☑
embolism T85.81 ☑
fibrosis T85.82 ☑
hemorrhage T85.83 ☑
infection and inflammation T85.79 ☑
pain T85.84 ☑
specified type NEC T85.89 ☑
stenosis T85.85 ☑
thrombosis T85.86 ☑
vascular (counterpulsation) T82.9 ☑
embolism T82.818 ☑
fibrosis T82.828 ☑
hemorrhage T82.838 ☑
infection or inflammation T82.7 ☑
mechanical
breakdown T82.513 ☑
displacement T82.523 ☑
leakage T82.533 ☑
malposition T82.523 ☑
obstruction T82.593 ☑
perforation T82.593 ☑
protrusion T82.593 ☑
pain T82.848 ☑
specified type NEC T82.898 ☑
stenosis T82.858 ☑
thrombosis T82.868 ☑
bariatric procedure
gastric band procedure K95.09
infection K95.01
specified procedure NEC K95.89
infection K95.81
bile duct implant (prosthetic) T85.9 ☑
embolism T85.81 ☑
fibrosis T85.82 ☑
hemorrhage T85.83 ☑
infection and inflammation T85.79 ☑
mechanical
breakdown T85.510 ☑
displacement T85.520 ☑
malfunction T85.510 ☑
malposition T85.520 ☑
obstruction T85.590 ☑
perforation T85.590 ☑
protrusion T85.590 ☑
specified NEC T85.590 ☑
pain T85.84 ☑
specified type NEC T85.89 ☑
stenosis T85.85 ☑
thrombosis T85.86 ☑
bladder device (auxiliary) — *see* Complications, genitourinary, device or implant, urinary system
bleeding (postoperative) — *see* Complication, postoperative, hemorrhage
intraoperative — *see* Complication, intraoperative, hemorrhage
blood vessel graft — *see* Complications, graft, vascular
bone
device NEC T84.9 ☑
embolism T84.81 ☑

Complication(s) — *continued*
bone — *continued*
  device — *continued*
    fibrosis T84.82 ☑
    hemorrhage T84.83 ☑
    infection or inflammation T84.7 ☑
    mechanical
      breakdown T84.318 ☑
      displacement T84.328 ☑
      malposition T84.328 ☑
      obstruction T84.398 ☑
      perforation T84.398 ☑
      protrusion T84.398 ☑
    pain T84.84 ☑
    specified type NEC T84.89 ☑
    stenosis T84.85 ☑
    thrombosis T84.86 ☑
  graft — *see* Complications, graft, bone
  growth stimulator (electrode) — *see* Complications, electronic stimulator device, bone
  marrow transplant — *see* Complications, transplant, bone, marrow
brain neurostimulator (electrode) — *see* Complications, electronic stimulator device, brain
breast implant (prosthetic) T85.9 ☑
  capsular contracture T85.44 ☑
  embolism T85.81 ☑
  fibrosis T85.82 ☑
  hemorrhage T85.83 ☑
  infection and inflammation T85.79 ☑
  mechanical
    breakdown T85.41 ☑
    displacement T85.42 ☑
    leakage T85.43 ☑
    malposition T85.42 ☑
    obstruction T85.49 ☑
    perforation T85.49 ☑
    protrusion T85.49 ☑
    specified NEC T85.49 ☑
  pain T85.84 ☑
  specified type NEC T85.89 ☑
  stenosis T85.85 ☑
  thrombosis T85.86 ☑
bypass (*see also* Complications, prosthetic device or implant)
  aortocoronary — *see* Complications, coronary artery (bypass) graft
  arterial (*see also* Complications, graft, vascular)
    extremity — *see* Complications, extremity artery (bypass) graft
cardiac (*see also* Disease, heart)
  device, implant or graft T82.9 ☑
    embolism T82.817 ☑
    fibrosis T82.827 ☑
    hemorrhage T82.837 ☑
    infection or inflammation T82.7 ☑
      valve prosthesis T82.6 ☑
    mechanical
      breakdown T82.519 ☑
        specified device NEC T82.518 ☑
      displacement T82.529 ☑
        specified device NEC T82.528 ☑
      leakage T82.539 ☑
        specified device NEC T82.538 ☑
      malposition T82.529 ☑
        specified device NEC T82.528 ☑
      obstruction T82.599 ☑
        specified device NEC T82.598 ☑
      perforation T82.599 ☑
        specified device NEC T82.598 ☑
      protrusion T82.599 ☑
        specified device NEC T82.598 ☑
    pain T82.847 ☑
    specified type NEC T82.897 ☑
    stenosis T82.857 ☑
    thrombosis T82.867 ☑
cardiovascular device, graft or implant T82.9 ☑
  aortic graft — *see* Complications, graft, vascular
  arteriovenous
    fistula, artificial — *see* Complication, arteriovenous, fistula, surgically created
    shunt — *see* Complication, arteriovenous, shunt, surgically created
  artificial heart — *see* Complication, artificial, heart
  balloon (counterpulsation) device — *see* Complication, balloon implant, vascular

Complication(s) — *continued*
cardiovascular device, graft or implant — *continued*
  carotid artery graft — *see* Complications, graft, vascular
  coronary bypass graft — *see* Complication, coronary artery (bypass) graft
  dialysis catheter (vascular) — *see* Complication, catheter, dialysis
  electronic T82.9 ☑
    electrode T82.9 ☑
      embolism T82.817 ☑
      fibrosis T82.827 ☑
      hemorrhage T82.837 ☑
      infection T82.7 ☑
      mechanical
        breakdown T82.110 ☑
        displacement T82.120 ☑
        leakage T82.190 ☑
        obstruction T82.190 ☑
        perforation T82.190 ☑
        protrusion T82.190 ☑
        specified type NEC T82.190 ☑
      pain T82.847 ☑
      specified NEC T82.897 ☑
      stenosis T82.857 ☑
      thrombosis T82.867 ☑
    embolism T82.817 ☑
    fibrosis T82.827 ☑
    hemorrhage T82.837 ☑
    infection T82.7 ☑
    mechanical
      breakdown T82.119 ☑
      displacement T82.129 ☑
      leakage T82.199 ☑
      obstruction T82.199 ☑
      perforation T82.199 ☑
      protrusion T82.199 ☑
      specified type NEC T82.199 ☑
    pain T82.847 ☑
    pulse generator T82.9 ☑
      embolism T82.817 ☑
      fibrosis T82.827 ☑
      hemorrhage T82.837 ☑
      infection T82.7 ☑
      mechanical
        breakdown T82.111 ☑
        displacement T82.121 ☑
        leakage T82.191 ☑
        obstruction T82.191 ☑
        perforation T82.191 ☑
        protrusion T82.191 ☑
        specified type NEC T82.191 ☑
      pain T82.847 ☑
      specified NEC T82.897 ☑
      stenosis T82.857 ☑
      thrombosis T82.867 ☑
    specified condition NEC T82.897 ☑
    specified device NEC T82.9 ☑
      embolism T82.817 ☑
      fibrosis T82.827 ☑
      hemorrhage T82.837 ☑
      infection T82.7 ☑
      mechanical
        breakdown T82.118 ☑
        displacement T82.128 ☑
        leakage T82.198 ☑
        obstruction T82.198 ☑
        perforation T82.198 ☑
        protrusion T82.198 ☑
        specified type NEC T82.198 ☑
      pain T82.847 ☑
      specified NEC T82.897 ☑
      stenosis T82.857 ☑
      thrombosis T82.867 ☑
    stenosis T82.857 ☑
    thrombosis T82.867 ☑
  extremity artery graft — *see* Complication, extremity artery (bypass) graft
  femoral artery graft — *see* Complication, extremity artery (bypass) graft
  heart
    transplant — *see* Complication, transplant, heart
    valve — *see* Complication, prosthetic device, heart valve

Complication(s) — *continued*
cardiovascular device, graft or implant — *continued*
  heart — *continued*
    valve — *see* Complication, prosthetic device, heart valve — *continued*
      graft — *see* Complication, heart, valve, graft
    heart-lung transplant — *see* Complication, transplant, heart, with lung
    infection or inflammation T82.7 ☑
    umbrella device — *see* Complication, umbrella device, vascular
    vascular graft (or anastomosis) — *see* Complication, graft, vascular
  carotid artery (bypass) graft — *see* Complications, graft, vascular
  catheter (device) NEC (*see also* Complications, prosthetic device or implant)
    cystostomy T83.9 ☑
      embolism T83.81 ☑
      fibrosis T83.82 ☑
      hemorrhage T83.83 ☑
      infection and inflammation T83.59 ☑
      mechanical
        breakdown T83.010 ☑
        displacement T83.020 ☑
        leakage T83.030 ☑
        malposition T83.020 ☑
        obstruction T83.090 ☑
        perforation T83.090 ☑
        protrusion T83.090 ☑
        specified NEC T83.090 ☑
      pain T83.84 ☑
      specified type NEC T83.89 ☑
      stenosis T83.85 ☑
      thrombosis T83.86 ☑
    dialysis (vascular) T82.9 ☑
      embolism T82.818 ☑
      fibrosis T82.828 ☑
      hemorrhage T82.838 ☑
      infection and inflammation T82.7 ☑
      intraperitoneal — *see* Complications, catheter, intraperitoneal
      mechanical
        breakdown T82.41 ☑
        displacement T82.42 ☑
        leakage T82.43 ☑
        malposition T82.42 ☑
        obstruction T82.49 ☑
        perforation T82.49 ☑
        protrusion T82.49 ☑
      pain T82.848 ☑
      specified type NEC T82.898 ☑
      stenosis T82.858 ☑
      thrombosis T82.868 ☑
  epidural infusion T85.9 ☑
    embolism T85.81 ☑
    fibrosis T85.82 ☑
    hemorrhage T85.83 ☑
    infection and inflammation T85.79 ☑
    mechanical
      breakdown T85.610 ☑
      displacement T85.620 ☑
      leakage T85.630 ☑
      malfunction T85.610 ☑
      malposition T85.620 ☑
      obstruction T85.690 ☑
      perforation T85.690 ☑
      protrusion T85.690 ☑
      specified NEC T85.690 ☑
    pain T85.84 ☑
    specified type NEC T85.89 ☑
    stenosis T85.85 ☑
    thrombosis T85.86 ☑
  intraperitoneal dialysis T85.9 ☑
    embolism T85.81 ☑
    fibrosis T85.82 ☑
    hemorrhage T85.83 ☑
    infection and inflammation T85.71 ☑
    mechanical
      breakdown T85.611 ☑
      displacement T85.621 ☑
      leakage T85.631 ☑
      malfunction T85.611 ☑
      malposition T85.621 ☑
      obstruction T85.691 ☑

Complication(s) — *continued*
- catheter (*see also* Complications, prosthetic device or implant) — *continued*
  - intraperitoneal dialysis — *continued*
    - mechanical — *continued*
      - perforation T85.691 ☑
      - protrusion T85.691 ☑
      - specified NEC T85.691 ☑
    - pain T85.84 ☑
    - specified type NEC T85.89 ☑
    - stenosis T85.85 ☑
    - thrombosis T85.86 ☑
  - intravenous infusion T82.9 ☑
    - embolism T82.818 ☑
    - fibrosis T82.828 ☑
    - hemorrhage T82.838 ☑
    - infection or inflammation T82.7 ☑
    - mechanical
      - breakdown T82.514 ☑
      - displacement T82.524 ☑
      - leakage T82.534 ☑
      - malposition T82.524 ☑
      - obstruction T82.594 ☑
      - perforation T82.594 ☑
      - protrusion T82.594 ☑
    - pain T82.848 ☑
    - specified type NEC T82.898 ☑
    - stenosis T82.858 ☑
    - thrombosis T82.868 ☑
  - subdural infusion T85.9 ☑
    - embolism T85.81 ☑
    - fibrosis T85.82 ☑
    - hemorrhage T85.83 ☑
    - infection and inflammation T85.79 ☑
    - mechanical
      - breakdown T85.610 ☑
      - displacement T85.620 ☑
      - leakage T85.630 ☑
      - malfunction T85.610 ☑
      - malposition T85.620 ☑
      - obstruction T85.690 ☑
      - perforation T85.690 ☑
      - protrusion T85.690 ☑
      - specified NEC T85.690 ☑
    - pain T85.84 ☑
    - specified type NEC T85.89 ☑
    - stenosis T85.85 ☑
    - thrombosis T85.86 ☑
  - urethral, indwelling T83.9 ☑
    - displacement T83.028 ☑
    - embolism T83.81 ☑
    - fibrosis T83.82 ☑
    - hemorrhage T83.83 ☑
    - infection and inflammation T83.51 ☑
    - leakage T83.038 ☑
    - malposition T83.028 ☑
    - mechanical
      - breakdown T83.018 ☑
    - obstruction (mechanical) T83.098 ☑
    - pain T83.84 ☑
    - perforation T83.098 ☑
    - protrusion T83.098 ☑
    - specified type NEC T83.098 ☑
    - stenosis T83.85 ☑
    - thrombosis T83.86 ☑
  - urinary (indwelling) — *see* Complications, catheter, urethral, indwelling
- cecostomy (stoma) — *see* Complications, colostomy
- cesarean delivery wound NEC O90.89
  - disruption O90.0
  - hematoma O90.2
  - infection (following delivery) O86.0
- chemotherapy (antineoplastic) NEC T88.7 ☑
- chin implant (prosthetic) — *see* Complication, prosthetic device or implant, specified NEC
- circulatory system I99.8
  - intraoperative I97.88
  - postprocedural I97.89
    - following cardiac surgery I97.19- ☑
      - postcardiotomy syndrome I97.0
    - hypertension I97.3
    - lymphedema after mastectomy I97.2
    - postcardiotomy syndrome I97.0
    - specified NEC I97.89
- colostomy (stoma) K94.00
  - hemorrhage K94.01

Complication(s) — *continued*
- colostomy — *continued*
  - infection K94.02
  - malfunction K94.03
  - mechanical K94.03
  - specified complication NEC K94.09
- contraceptive device, intrauterine — *see* Complications, intrauterine, contraceptive device
- cord (umbilical) — *see* Complications, umbilical cord
- corneal graft — *see* Complications, graft, cornea
- coronary artery (bypass) graft T82.9
  - atherosclerosis — *see* Arteriosclerosis, coronary (artery),
  - embolism T82.818 ☑
  - fibrosis T82.828 ☑
  - hemorrhage T82.838 ☑
  - infection and inflammation T82.7 ☑
  - mechanical
    - breakdown T82.211 ☑
    - displacement T82.212 ☑
    - leakage T82.213 ☑
    - malposition T82.212 ☑
    - obstruction T82.218 ☑
    - perforation T82.218 ☑
    - protrusion T82.218 ☑
    - specified NEC T82.218 ☑
  - pain T82.848 ☑
  - specified type NEC T82.897 ☑
  - stenosis T82.858 ☑
  - thrombosis T82.868 ☑
- counterpulsation device (balloon), intra- aortic — *see* Complications, balloon implant, vascular
- cystostomy (stoma) N99.518
  - catheter — *see* Complications, catheter, cystostomy
  - hemorrhage N99.510
  - infection N99.511
  - malfunction N99.512
  - specified type NEC N99.518
- delivery (*see also* Complications, obstetric) O75.9
  - procedure (instrumental) (manual) (surgical) O75.4
  - specified NEC O75.89
- dialysis (peritoneal) (renal) (*see also* Complications, infusion)
  - catheter (vascular) — *see* Complication, catheter, dialysis
    - peritoneal, intraperitoneal — *see* Complications, catheter, intraperitoneal
- dorsal column (spinal) neurostimulator — *see* Complications, electronic stimulator device, spinal cord
- drug NEC T88.7 ☑
- ear procedure (*see also* Disorder, ear)
  - intraoperative H95.88-
    - hematoma — *see* Complications, intraoperative, hemorrhage (hematoma) (of), ear
    - hemorrhage — *see* Complications, intraoperative, hemorrhage (hematoma) (of), ear
    - laceration — *see* Complications, intraoperative, puncture or laceration..., ear
    - specified NEC H95.88-
  - postoperative H95.89-
    - external ear canal stenosis H95.81- ☑
    - hematoma — *see* Complications, postprocedural, hemorrhage (hematoma) (of), ear
    - hemorrhage — *see* Complications, postprocedural, hemorrhage (hematoma) (of), ear
    - postmastoidectomy — *see* Complications, postmastoidectomy
    - specified NEC H95.89-
- ectopic pregnancy O08.9
  - damage to pelvic organs O08.6
  - embolism O08.2
  - genital infection O08.0
  - hemorrhage (delayed) (excessive) O08.1
  - metabolic disorder O08.5
  - renal failure O08.4
  - shock O08.3
  - specified type NEC O08.0
  - venous complication NEC O08.7
- electronic stimulator device
  - bladder (urinary) — *see* Complications, electronic stimulator device, urinary
  - bone T84.9 ☑
    - breakdown T84.310 ☑
    - displacement T84.320 ☑
    - embolism T84.81 ☑
    - fibrosis T84.82 ☑

Complication(s) — *continued*
- electronic stimulator device — *continued*
  - bone — *continued*
    - hemorrhage T84.83 ☑
    - infection or inflammation T84.7 ☑
    - malfunction T84.310 ☑
    - malposition T84.320 ☑
    - mechanical NEC T84.390 ☑
    - obstruction T84.390 ☑
    - pain T84.84 ☑
    - perforation T84.390 ☑
    - protrusion T84.390 ☑
    - specified type NEC T84.89 ☑
    - stenosis T84.85 ☑
    - thrombosis T84.86 ☑
  - brain T85.9 ☑
    - embolism T85.81 ☑
    - fibrosis T85.82 ☑
    - hemorrhage T85.83 ☑
    - infection and inflammation T85.79 ☑
    - mechanical
      - breakdown T85.110 ☑
      - displacement T85.120 ☑
      - leakage T85.190 ☑
      - malposition T85.120 ☑
      - obstruction T85.190 ☑
      - perforation T85.190 ☑
      - protrusion T85.190 ☑
      - specified NEC T85.190 ☑
    - pain T85.84 ☑
    - specified type NEC T85.89 ☑
    - stenosis T85.85 ☑
    - thrombosis T85.86 ☑
  - cardiac (defibrillator) (pacemaker) — *see* Complications, cardiovascular device or implant, electronic
  - muscle T84.9 ☑
    - breakdown T84.418 ☑
    - displacement T84.428 ☑
    - embolism T84.81 ☑
    - fibrosis T84.82 ☑
    - hemorrhage T84.83 ☑
    - infection or inflammation T84.7 ☑
    - mechanical NEC T84.498 ☑
    - pain T84.84 ☑
    - specified type NEC T84.89 ☑
    - stenosis T84.85 ☑
    - thrombosis T84.86 ☑
  - nervous system T85.9 ☑
    - brain — *see* Complications, electronic stimulator device, brain
    - embolism T85.81 ☑
    - fibrosis T85.82 ☑
    - hemorrhage T85.83 ☑
    - infection and inflammation T85.79 ☑
    - mechanical
      - breakdown T85.118 ☑
      - displacement T85.128 ☑
      - leakage T85.199 ☑
      - malposition T85.128 ☑
      - obstruction T85.199 ☑
      - perforation T85.199 ☑
      - protrusion T85.199 ☑
      - specified NEC T85.199 ☑
    - pain T85.84 ☑
    - peripheral nerve — *see* Complications, electronic stimulator device, peripheral nerve
    - specified type NEC T85.89 ☑
    - spinal cord — *see* Complications, electronic stimulator device, spinal cord
    - stenosis T85.85 ☑
    - thrombosis T85.86 ☑
  - peripheral nerve T85.9 ☑
    - embolism T85.81 ☑
    - fibrosis T85.82 ☑
    - hemorrhage T85.83 ☑
    - infection and inflammation T85.79 ☑
    - mechanical
      - breakdown T85.111 ☑
      - displacement T85.121 ☑
      - leakage T85.191 ☑
      - malposition T85.121 ☑
      - obstruction T85.191 ☑
      - perforation T85.191 ☑
      - protrusion T85.191 ☑
      - specified NEC T85.191 ☑

Complication(s) — *continued*
electronic stimulator device — *continued*
  peripheral nerve — *continued*
    pain T85.84 ☑
    specified type NEC T85.89 ☑
    stenosis T85.85 ☑
    thrombosis T85.86 ☑
  spinal cord T85.9 ☑
    embolism T85.81 ☑
    fibrosis T85.82 ☑
    hemorrhage T85.83 ☑
    infection and inflammation T85.79 ☑
    mechanical
      breakdown T85.112 ☑
      displacement T85.122 ☑
      leakage T85.192 ☑
      malposition T85.122 ☑
      obstruction T85.192 ☑
      perforation T85.192 ☑
      protrusion T85.192 ☑
      specified NEC T85.192 ☑
    pain T85.84 ☑
    specified type NEC T85.89 ☑
    stenosis T85.85 ☑
    thrombosis T85.86 ☑
  urinary T83.9 ☑
    embolism T83.81 ☑
    fibrosis T83.82 ☑
    hemorrhage T83.83 ☑
    infection and inflammation T83.59 ☑
    mechanical
      breakdown T83.110 ☑
      displacement T83.120 ☑
      malposition T83.120 ☑
      perforation T83.190 ☑
      protrusion T83.190 ☑
      specified NEC T83.190 ☑
    pain T83.84 ☑
    specified type NEC T83.89 ☑
    stenosis T83.85 ☑
    thrombosis T83.86 ☑
electroshock therapy T88.9 ☑
  specified NEC T88.8 ☑
endocrine E34.9
  postprocedural
    adrenal hypofunction E89.6
    hypoinsulinemia E89.1
    hypoparathyroidism E89.2
    hypopituitarism E89.3
    hypothyroidism E89.0
    ovarian failure E89.40
      asymptomatic E89.40
      symptomatic E89.41
    specified NEC E89.89
    testicular hypofunction E89.5
endodontic treatment NEC M27.59
enterostomy (stoma) K94.10
  hemorrhage K94.11
  infection K94.12
  malfunction K94.13
  mechanical K94.13
  specified complication NEC K94.19
episiotomy, disruption O90.1
esophageal anti-reflux device T85.9 ☑
  embolism T85.81 ☑
  fibrosis T85.82 ☑
  hemorrhage T85.83 ☑
  infection and inflammation T85.79 ☑
  mechanical
    breakdown T85.511 ☑
    displacement T85.521 ☑
    malfunction T85.511 ☑
    malposition T85.521 ☑
    obstruction T85.591 ☑
    perforation T85.591 ☑
    protrusion T85.591 ☑
    specified NEC T85.591 ☑
  pain T85.84 ☑
  specified type NEC T85.89 ☑
  stenosis T85.85 ☑
  thrombosis T85.86 ☑
esophagostomy K94.30
  hemorrhage K94.31
  infection K94.32
  malfunction K94.33
  mechanical K94.33

Complication(s) — *continued*
esophagostomy — *continued*
  specified complication NEC K94.39
extracorporeal circulation T80.90 ☑
extremity artery (bypass) graft T82.9 ☑
  arteriosclerosis — *see* Arteriosclerosis, extremities, bypass graft
  embolism T82.818 ☑
  fibrosis T82.828 ☑
  hemorrhage T82.838 ☑
  infection and inflammation T82.7 ☑
  mechanical
    breakdown T82.318 ☑
      femoral artery T82.312 ☑
    displacement T82.328 ☑
      femoral artery T82.322 ☑
    leakage T82.338 ☑
      femoral artery T82.332 ☑
    malposition T82.328 ☑
      femoral artery T82.322 ☑
    obstruction T82.398 ☑
      femoral artery T82.392 ☑
    perforation T82.398 ☑
      femoral artery T82.392 ☑
    protrusion T82.398 ☑
      femoral artery T82.392 ☑
  pain T82.848 ☑
  specified type NEC T82.898 ☑
  stenosis T82.858 ☑
  thrombosis T82.868 ☑
eye H57.9
  corneal graft — *see* Complications, graft, cornea
  implant (prosthetic) T85.9 ☑
    embolism T85.81 ☑
    fibrosis T85.82 ☑
    hemorrhage T85.83 ☑
    infection and inflammation T85.79 ☑
    mechanical
      breakdown T85.318 ☑
      displacement T85.328 ☑
      leakage T85.398 ☑
      malposition T85.328 ☑
      obstruction T85.398 ☑
      perforation T85.398 ☑
      protrusion T85.398 ☑
      specified NEC T85.398 ☑
    pain T85.84 ☑
    specified type NEC T85.89 ☑
    stenosis T85.85 ☑
    thrombosis T85.86 ☑
  intraocular lens — *see* Complications, intraocular lens
  orbital prosthesis — *see* Complications, orbital prosthesis
female genital N94.9
  device, implant or graft NEC — *see* Complications, genitourinary, device or implant, genital tract
femoral artery (bypass) graft — *see* Complication, extremity artery (bypass) graft
fixation device, internal (orthopedic) T84.9 ☑
  infection and inflammation T84.60 ☑
    arm T84.61- ☑
      humerus T84.61- ☑
      radius T84.61- ☑
      ulna T84.61- ☑
    leg T84.629 ☑
      femur T84.62- ☑
      fibula T84.62- ☑
      tibia T84.62- ☑
    specified site NEC T84.89 ☑
    spine T84.63 ☑
  mechanical
    breakdown
      limb T84.119 ☑
        carpal T84.210 ☑
        femur T84.11- ☑
        fibula T84.11- ☑
        humerus T84.11- ☑
        metacarpal T84.210 ☑
        metatarsal T84.213 ☑
        phalanx
          foot T84.213 ☑
          hand T84.210 ☑
        radius T84.11- ☑
        tarsal T84.213 ☑
        tibia T84.11- ☑

Complication(s) — *continued*
fixation device, internal — *continued*
  mechanical — *continued*
    breakdown — *continued*
      limb — *continued*
        ulna T84.11- ☑
        specified bone NEC T84.218 ☑
        spine T84.216 ☑
    displacement
      limb T84.129 ☑
        carpal T84.220 ☑
        femur T84.12- ☑
        fibula T84.12- ☑
        humerus T84.12- ☑
        metacarpal T84.220 ☑
        metatarsal T84.223 ☑
        phalanx
          foot T84.223 ☑
          hand T84.220 ☑
        radius T84.12- ☑
        tarsal T84.223 ☑
        tibia T84.12- ☑
        ulna T84.12- ☑
        specified bone NEC T84.228 ☑
        spine T84.226 ☑
    malposition — *see* Complications, fixation device, internal, mechanical, displacement
    obstruction — *see* Complications, fixation device, internal, mechanical, specified type NEC
    perforation — *see* Complications, fixation device, internal, mechanical, specified type NEC
    protrusion — *see* Complications, fixation device, internal, mechanical, specified type NEC
    specified type NEC
      limb T84.199 ☑
        carpal T84.290 ☑
        femur T84.19- ☑
        fibula T84.19- ☑
        humerus T84.19- ☑
        metacarpal T84.290 ☑
        metatarsal T84.293 ☑
        phalanx
          foot T84.293 ☑
          hand T84.290 ☑
        radius T84.19- ☑
        tarsal T84.293 ☑
        tibia T84.19- ☑
        ulna T84.19- ☑
        specified bone NEC T84.298 ☑
        vertebra T84.296 ☑
  specified type NEC T84.89 ☑
    embolism T84.81 ☑
    fibrosis T84.82 ☑
    hemorrhage T84.83 ☑
    pain T84.84 ☑
    specified complication NEC T84.89 ☑
    stenosis T84.85 ☑
    thrombosis T84.86 ☑
following
  acute myocardial infarction NEC I23.8
  aneurysm (false) (of cardiac wall) (of heart wall) (ruptured) I23.3
  angina I23.7
  atrial
    septal defect I23.1
    thrombosis I23.6
  cardiac wall rupture I23.3
  chordae tendinae rupture I23.4
  defect
    septal
      atrial (heart) I23.1
      ventricular (heart) I23.2
  hemopericardium I23.0
  papillary muscle rupture I23.5
  rupture
    cardiac wall I23.3
      with hemopericardium I23.0
    chordae tendineae I23.4
    papillary muscle I23.5
  specified NEC I23.8
  thrombosis
    atrium I23.6
    auricular appendage I23.6
    ventricle (heart) I23.6

☑ **Additional Character Required — Refer to the Tabular List for Character Selection**   ▽ **Subterms under main terms may continue to next column or page**

Complication(s) — *continued*
  following — *continued*
    acute myocardial infarction — *continued*
      ventricular
        septal defect I23.2
        thrombosis I23.6
    ectopic or molar pregnancy O08.9
      cardiac arrest O08.81
      sepsis O08.82
      specified type NEC O08.89
      urinary tract infection O08.83
    termination of pregnancy — *see* Abortion
  gastrointestinal K92.9
    bile duct prosthesis — *see* Complications, bile duct
      implant
    esophageal anti-reflux device — *see* Complications,
      esophageal anti-reflux device
    postoperative
      colostomy — *see* Complications, colostomy
      dumping syndrome K91.1
      enterostomy — *see* Complications, enterosto-
        my
      gastrostomy — *see* Complications, gastrostomy
      malabsorption NEC K91.2
      obstruction K91.3
      postcholecystectomy syndrome K91.5
      specified NEC K91.89
      vomiting after GI surgery K91.0
    prosthetic device or implant
      bile duct prosthesis — *see* Complications, bile
        duct implant
      esophageal anti-reflux device — *see* Complica-
        tions, esophageal anti-reflux device
      specified type NEC
        embolism T85.81 ☑
        fibrosis T85.82 ☑
        hemorrhage T85.83 ☑
        mechanical
          breakdown T85.518 ☑
          displacement T85.528 ☑
          malfunction T85.518 ☑
          malposition T85.528 ☑
          obstruction T85.598 ☑
          perforation T85.598 ☑
          protrusion T85.598 ☑
          specified NEC T85.598 ☑
        pain T85.84 ☑
        specified complication NEC T85.89 ☑
        stenosis T85.85 ☑
        thrombosis T85.86 ☑
  gastrostomy (stoma) K94.20
    hemorrhage K94.21
    infection K94.22
    malfunction K94.23
    mechanical K94.23
    specified complication NEC K94.29
  genitourinary
    device or implant T83.9 ☑
      genital tract T83.9 ☑
        infection or inflammation T83.6 ☑
        intrauterine contraceptive device — *see*
          Complications, intrauterine, contra-
          ceptive device
        mechanical — *see* Complications, by device,
          mechanical
        mesh — *see* Complications, mesh
        penile prosthesis — *see* Complications,
          prosthetic device, penile
        specified type NEC T83.89 ☑
          embolism T83.81 ☑
          fibrosis T83.82 ☑
          hemorrhage T83.83 ☑
          pain T83.84 ☑
          specified complication NEC T83.89 ☑
          stenosis T83.85 ☑
          thrombosis T83.86 ☑
        vaginal mesh — *see* Complications, mesh
      urinary system T83.9 ☑
        cystostomy catheter — *see* Complication,
          catheter, cystostomy
        electronic stimulator — *see* Complications,
          electronic stimulator device, urinary
        indwelling urethral catheter — *see* Compli-
          cations, catheter, urethral, indwelling
        infection or inflammation T83.59 ☑
          indwelling urinary catheter T83.51 ☑

Complication(s) — *continued*
  genitourinary — *continued*
    device or implant — *continued*
      urinary system — *continued*
        kidney transplant — *see* Complication,
          transplant, kidney
        organ graft — *see* Complication, graft, uri-
          nary organ
        specified type NEC T83.89 ☑
          embolism T83.81 ☑
          fibrosis T83.82 ☑
          hemorrhage T83.83 ☑
          mechanical T83.198 ☑
            breakdown T83.118 ☑
            displacement T83.128 ☑
            malfunction T83.118 ☑
            malposition T83.128 ☑
            obstruction T83.198 ☑
            perforation T83.198 ☑
            protrusion T83.198 ☑
            specified NEC T83.198 ☑
          pain T83.84 ☑
          specified complication NEC T83.89 ☑
          stenosis T83.85 ☑
          thrombosis T83.86 ☑
        sphincter implant — *see* Complications,
          implant, urinary sphincter
    postprocedural
      pelvic peritoneal adhesions N99.4
      renal failure N99.0
      specified NEC N99.89
      stoma — *see* Complications, stoma, urinary
        tract
      urethral stricture — *see* Stricture, urethra,
        postprocedural
      vaginal
        adhesions N99.2
        vault prolapse N99.3
  graft (bypass) (patch) (*see also* Complications, prosthet-
    ic device or implant)
    aorta — *see* Complications, graft, vascular
    arterial — *see* Complication, graft, vascular
    bone T86.839
      failure T86.831
      infection T86.832
      mechanical T84.318 ☑
        breakdown T84.318 ☑
        displacement T84.328 ☑
        protrusion T84.398 ☑
        specified type NEC T84.398 ☑
      rejection T86.830
      specified type NEC T86.838
    carotid artery — *see* Complications, graft, vascular
    cornea T86.849
      failure T86.841
      infection T86.842
      mechanical T85.398 ☑
        breakdown T85.318 ☑
        displacement T85.328 ☑
        protrusion T85.398 ☑
        specified type NEC T85.398 ☑
      rejection T86.840
      retroprosthetic membrane T85.398 ☑
      specified type NEC T86.848
    femoral artery (bypass) — *see* Complication, ex-
      tremity artery (bypass) graft
    genital organ or tract — *see* Complications, geni-
      tourinary, device or implant, genital tract
    muscle T84.9 ☑
      breakdown T84.410 ☑
      displacement T84.420 ☑
      embolism T84.81 ☑
      fibrosis T84.82 ☑
      hemorrhage T84.83 ☑
      infection and inflammation T84.7 ☑
      mechanical NEC T84.490 ☑
      pain T84.84 ☑
      specified type NEC T84.89 ☑
      stenosis T84.85 ☑
      thrombosis T84.86 ☑
    nerve — *see* Complication, prosthetic device or
      implant, specified NEC
    skin — *see* Complications, prosthetic device or
      implant, skin graft
    tendon T84.9 ☑
      breakdown T84.410 ☑

Complication(s) — *continued*
  graft (*see also* Complications, prosthetic device or im-
    plant) — *continued*
    tendon — *continued*
      displacement T84.420 ☑
      embolism T84.81 ☑
      fibrosis T84.82 ☑
      hemorrhage T84.83 ☑
      infection and inflammation T84.7 ☑
      mechanical NEC T84.490 ☑
      pain T84.84 ☑
      specified type NEC T84.89 ☑
      stenosis T84.85 ☑
      thrombosis T84.86 ☑
    urinary organ T83.9 ☑
      embolism T83.81 ☑
      fibrosis T83.82 ☑
      hemorrhage T83.83 ☑
      infection and inflammation T83.59 ☑
        indwelling urinary catheter T83.51 ☑
      mechanical
        breakdown T83.21 ☑
        displacement T83.22 ☑
        leakage T83.23 ☑
        malposition T83.22 ☑
        obstruction T83.29 ☑
        perforation T83.29 ☑
        protrusion T83.29 ☑
        specified NEC T83.29 ☑
      pain T83.84 ☑
      specified type NEC T83.89 ☑
      stenosis T83.85 ☑
      thrombosis T83.86 ☑
    vascular T82.9 ☑
      embolism T82.818 ☑
      femoral artery — *see* Complication, extremity
        artery (bypass) graft
      fibrosis T82.828 ☑
      hemorrhage T82.838 ☑
      mechanical
        breakdown T82.319 ☑
          aorta (bifurcation) T82.310 ☑
          carotid artery T82.311 ☑
          specified vessel NEC T82.318 ☑
        displacement T82.329 ☑
          aorta (bifurcation) T82.320 ☑
          carotid artery T82.321 ☑
          specified vessel NEC T82.328 ☑
        leakage T82.339 ☑
          aorta (bifurcation) T82.330 ☑
          carotid artery T82.331 ☑
          specified vessel NEC T82.338 ☑
        malposition T82.329 ☑
          aorta (bifurcation) T82.320 ☑
          carotid artery T82.321 ☑
          specified vessel NEC T82.328 ☑
        obstruction T82.399 ☑
          aorta (bifurcation) T82.390 ☑
          carotid artery T82.391 ☑
          specified vessel NEC T82.398 ☑
        perforation T82.399 ☑
          aorta (bifurcation) T82.390 ☑
          carotid artery T82.391 ☑
          specified vessel NEC T82.398 ☑
        protrusion T82.399 ☑
          aorta (bifurcation) T82.390 ☑
          carotid artery T82.391 ☑
          specified vessel NEC T82.398 ☑
      pain T82.848 ☑
      specified complication NEC T82.898 ☑
      stenosis T82.858 ☑
      thrombosis T82.868 ☑
  heart I51.9
    assist device
      infection and inflammation T82.7 ☑
    following acute myocardial infarction — *see*
      Complications, following, acute myocardial
      infarction
    postoperative — *see* Complications, circulatory
      system
    transplant — *see* Complication, transplant, heart
      and lung(s) — *see* Complications, transplant,
      heart, with lung
    valve
      graft (biological) T82.9 ☑
        embolism T82.817 ☑

Complication(s) — *continued*
  heart — *continued*
    valve — *continued*
      graft — *continued*
        fibrosis T82.827 ☑
        hemorrhage T82.837 ☑
        infection and inflammation T82.7 ☑
        mechanical T82.228 ☑
          breakdown T82.221 ☑
          displacement T82.222 ☑
          leakage T82.223 ☑
          malposition T82.222 ☑
          obstruction T82.228 ☑
          perforation T82.228 ☑
          protrusion T82.228 ☑
        pain T82.847 ☑
        specified type NEC T82.897 ☑
        stenosis T82.857 ☑
        thrombosis T82.867 ☑
      prosthesis T82.9 ☑
        embolism T82.817 ☑
        fibrosis T82.827 ☑
        hemorrhage T82.837 ☑
        infection or inflammation T82.6 ☑
        mechanical T82.09 ☑
          breakdown T82.01 ☑
          displacement T82.02 ☑
          leakage T82.03 ☑
          malposition T82.02 ☑
          obstruction T82.09 ☑
          perforation T82.09 ☑
          protrusion T82.09 ☑
        pain T82.847 ☑
        specified type NEC T82.897 ☑
          mechanical T82.09 ☑
        stenosis T82.857 ☑
        thrombosis T82.867 ☑
  hematoma
    intraoperative — *see* Complication, intraoperative, hemorrhage
    postprocedural — *see* Complication, postprocedural, hemorrhage
  hemodialysis — *see* Complications, dialysis
  hemorrhage
    intraoperative — *see* Complication, intraoperative, hemorrhage
    postprocedural — *see* Complication, postprocedural, hemorrhage
  ileostomy (stoma) — *see* Complications, enterostomy
  immunization (procedure) — *see* Complications, vaccination
  implant (*see also* Complications, by site and type)
    urinary sphincter T83.9 ☑
      embolism T83.81 ☑
      fibrosis T83.82 ☑
      hemorrhage T83.83 ☑
      infection and inflammation T83.59 ☑
      mechanical
        breakdown T83.111 ☑
        displacement T83.121 ☑
        leakage T83.191 ☑
        malposition T83.121 ☑
        obstruction T83.191 ☑
        perforation T83.191 ☑
        protrusion T83.191 ☑
        specified NEC T83.191 ☑
      pain T83.84 ☑
      specified type NEC T83.89 ☑
      stenosis T83.85 ☑
      thrombosis T83.86 ☑
  infusion (procedure) T80.90 ☑
    air embolism T80.0 ☑
    blood — *see* Complications, transfusion
    catheter — *see* Complications, catheter
    infection T80.29 ☑
    pump — *see* Complications, cardiovascular, device or implant
    sepsis T80.29 ☑
    serum reaction (*see also* Reaction, serum) T80.69 ☑
      anaphylactic shock (*see also* Shock, anaphylactic) T80.59 ☑
    specified type NEC T80.89 ☑
  inhalation therapy NEC T81.81 ☑
  injection (procedure) T80.90 ☑
    drug reaction — *see* Reaction, drug
    infection T80.29 ☑

Complication(s) — *continued*
  injection — *continued*
    sepsis T80.29 ☑
    serum (prophylactic) (therapeutic) — *see* Complications, vaccination
    specified type NEC T80.89 ☑
    vaccine (any) — *see* Complications, vaccination
  inoculation (any) — *see* Complications, vaccination
  insulin pump
    infection and inflammation T85.72 ☑
    mechanical
      breakdown T85.614 ☑
      displacement T85.624 ☑
      leakage T85.633 ☑
      malposition T85.624 ☑
      obstruction T85.694 ☑
      perforation T85.694 ☑
      protrusion T85.694 ☑
      specified NEC T85.694 ☑
  intestinal pouch NEC K91.858
  intraocular lens (prosthetic) T85.9 ☑
    embolism T85.81 ☑
    fibrosis T85.82 ☑
    hemorrhage T85.83 ☑
    infection and inflammation T85.79 ☑
    mechanical
      breakdown T85.21 ☑
      displacement T85.22 ☑
      malposition T85.22 ☑
      obstruction T85.29 ☑
      perforation T85.29 ☑
      protrusion T85.29 ☑
      specified NEC T85.29 ☑
    pain T85.84 ☑
    specified type NEC T85.89 ☑
    stenosis T85.85 ☑
    thrombosis T85.86 ☑
  intraoperative (intraprocedural)
    cardiac arrest
      during cardiac surgery I97.710
      during other surgery I97.711
    cardiac functional disturbance NEC
      during cardiac surgery I97.790
      during other surgery I97.791
    hemorrhage (hematoma) (of)
      circulatory system organ or structure
        during cardiac bypass I97.411
        during cardiac catheterization I97.410
        during other circulatory system procedure I97.418
        during other procedure I97.42
      digestive system organ
        during procedure on digestive system K91.61
        during procedure on other organ K91.62
      ear
        during procedure on ear and mastoid process H95.21
        during procedure on other organ H95.22
      endocrine system organ or structure
        during procedure on endocrine system organ or structure E36.01
        during procedure on other organ E36.02
      eye and adnexa
        during ophthalmic procedure H59.11- ☑
        during other procedure H59.12- ☑
      genitourinary organ or structure
        during procedure on genitourinary organ or structure N99.61
        during procedure on other organ N99.62
      mastoid process
        during procedure on ear and mastoid process H95.21
        during procedure on other organ H95.22
      musculoskeletal structure
        during musculoskeletal surgery M96.810
        during non-orthopedic surgery M96.811
        during orthopedic surgery M96.810
      nervous system
        during a nervous system procedure G97.31
        during other procedure G97.32
      respiratory system
        during other procedure J95.62
        during procedure on respiratory system organ or structure J95.61
      skin and subcutaneous tissue
        during a dermatologic procedure L76.01

Complication(s) — *continued*
  intraoperative — *continued*
    hemorrhage — *continued*
      skin and subcutaneous tissue — *continued*
        during a procedure on other organ L76.02
      spleen
        during a procedure on other organ D78.02
        during a procedure on the spleen D78.01
    puncture or laceration (accidental) (unintentional) (of)
      brain
        during a nervous system procedure G97.48
        during other procedure G97.49
      circulatory system organ or structure
        during circulatory system procedure I97.51
        during other procedure I97.52
      digestive system
        during procedure on digestive system K91.71
        during procedure on other organ K91.72
      ear
        during procedure on ear and mastoid process H95.31
        during procedure on other organ H95.32
      endocrine system organ or structure
        during procedure on endocrine system organ or structure E36.11
        during procedure on other organ E36.12
      eye and adnexa
        during ophthalmic procedure H59.21- ☑
        during other procedure H59.22- ☑
      genitourinary organ or structure
        during procedure on genitourinary organ or structure N99.71
        during procedure on other organ N99.72
      mastoid process
        during procedure on ear and mastoid process H95.31
        during procedure on other organ H95.32
      musculoskeletal structure
        during musculoskeletal surgery M96.820
        during non-orthopedic surgery M96.821
        during orthopedic surgery M96.820
      nervous system
        during a nervous system procedure G97.48
        during other procedure G97.49
      respiratory system
        during other procedure J95.72
        during procedure on respiratory system organ or structure J95.71
      skin and subcutaneous tissue
        during a dermatologic procedure L76.11
        during a procedure on other organ L76.12
      spleen
        during a procedure on other organ D78.12
        during a procedure on the spleen D78.11
    specified NEC
      circulatory system I97.88
      digestive system K91.81
      ear H95.88
      endocrine system E36.8
      eye and adnexa H59.88
      genitourinary system N99.81
      mastoid process H95.88
      musculoskeletal structure M96.89
      nervous system G97.81
      respiratory system J95.88
      skin and subcutaneous tissue L76.81
      spleen D78.81
  intraperitoneal catheter (dialysis) (infusion) — *see* Complications, catheter, intraperitoneal
  intrauterine
    contraceptive device
      embolism T83.81 ☑
      fibrosis T83.82 ☑
      hemorrhage T83.83 ☑
      infection and inflammation T83.6 ☑
      mechanical
        breakdown T83.31 ☑
        displacement T83.32 ☑
        malposition T83.32 ☑
        obstruction T83.39 ☑
        perforation T83.39 ☑
        protrusion T83.39 ☑
        specified NEC T83.39 ☑
      pain T83.84 ☑
      specified type NEC T83.89 ☑
      stenosis T83.85 ☑

Complication(s) — *continued*
- intrauterine — *continued*
  - contraceptive device — *continued*
    - thrombosis T83.86 ☑
    - procedure (fetal), to newborn P96.5
  - jejunostomy (stoma) — *see* Complications, enterostomy
- joint prosthesis, internal T84.9 ☑
  - breakage (fracture) T84.01- ☑
  - dislocation T84.02- ☑
  - fracture T84.01- ☑
  - infection or inflammation T84.50 ☑
    - hip T84.5- ☑
    - knee T84.5- ☑
    - specified joint NEC T84.59 ☑
  - instability T84.02- ☑
  - malposition — *see* Complications, joint prosthesis, mechanical, displacement
  - mechanical
    - breakage, broken T84.01- ☑
    - dislocation T84.02- ☑
    - fracture T84.01- ☑
    - instability T84.02- ☑
    - leakage — *see* Complications, joint prosthesis, mechanical, specified NEC
    - loosening T84.039 ☑
      - hip T84.03- ☑
      - knee T84.03- ☑
      - specified joint NEC T84.038 ☑
    - obstruction — *see* Complications, joint prosthesis, mechanical, specified NEC
    - perforation — *see* Complications, joint prosthesis, mechanical, specified NEC
    - periprosthetic
      - fracture T84.049 ☑
        - hip T84.04- ☑
        - knee T84.04- ☑
        - other specified joint T84.048 ☑
      - osteolysis T84.059 ☑
        - hip T84.05- ☑
        - knee T84.05- ☑
        - other specified joint T84.058 ☑
    - protrusion — *see* Complications, joint prosthesis, mechanical, specified NEC
    - specified complication NEC T84.099 ☑
      - hip T84.09- ☑
      - knee T84.09- ☑
      - other specified joint T84.098 ☑
    - subluxation T84.02- ☑
    - wear of articular bearing surface T84.069 ☑
      - hip T84.06- ☑
      - knee T84.06- ☑
      - other specified joint T84.068 ☑
  - specified joint NEC T84.89 ☑
  - embolism T84.81 ☑
  - fibrosis T84.82 ☑
  - hemorrhage T84.83 ☑
  - pain T84.84 ☑
  - specified complication NEC T84.89 ☑
  - stenosis T84.85 ☑
  - thrombosis T84.86 ☑
  - subluxation T84.02- ☑
- kidney transplant — *see* Complications, transplant, kidney
- labor O75.9
  - specified NEC O75.89
- liver transplant (immune or nonimmune) — *see* Complications, transplant, liver
- lumbar puncture G97.1
  - cerebrospinal fluid leak G97.0
  - headache or reaction G97.1
- lung transplant — *see* Complications, transplant, lung and heart — *see* Complications, transplant, lung, with heart
- male genital N50.9
  - device, implant or graft — *see* Complications, genitourinary, device or implant, genital tract
  - postprocedural or postoperative — *see* Complications, genitourinary, postprocedural
    - specified NEC N99.89
- mastoid (process) procedure
  - intraoperative H95.88-
    - hematoma — *see* Complications, intraoperative, hemorrhage (hematoma) (of), mastoid process

Complication(s) — *continued*
- mastoid procedure — *continued*
  - intraoperative — *continued*
    - hemorrhage — *see* Complications, intraoperative, hemorrhage (hematoma) (of), mastoid process
    - laceration — *see* Complications, intraoperative, puncture or laceration, mastoid process
    - specified NEC H95.88-
  - postmastoidectomy — *see* Complications, postmastoidectomy
  - postoperative H95.89-
    - external ear canal stenosis H95.81 ☑
    - hematoma — *see* Complications, postprocedural, hemorrhage (hematoma) (of), mastoid process
    - hemorrhage — *see* Complications, postprocedural, hemorrhage (hematoma) (of), mastoid process
    - postmastoidectomy — *see* Complications, postmastoidectomy
    - specified NEC H95.89-
- mastoidectomy cavity — *see* Complications, postmastoidectomy
- mechanical — *see* Complications, by site and type, mechanical
- medical procedures (*see also* Complication(s), intraoperative) T88.9 ☑
- metabolic E88.9
  - postoperative E89.89
    - specified NEC E89.89
- molar pregnancy NOS O08.9
  - damage to pelvic organs O08.6
  - embolism O08.2
  - genital infection O08.0
  - hemorrhage (delayed) (excessive) O08.1
  - metabolic disorder O08.5
  - renal failure O08.4
  - shock O08.3
  - specified type NEC O08.0
  - venous complication NEC O08.7
- musculoskeletal system (*see also* Complication, intraoperative (intraprocedural), by site)
  - device, implant or graft NEC — *see* Complications, orthopedic, device or implant
  - internal fixation (nail) (plate) (rod) — *see* Complications, fixation device, internal
  - joint prosthesis — *see* Complications, joint prosthesis
  - post radiation M96.89
    - kyphosis M96.3
    - scoliosis M96.5
    - specified complication NEC M96.89
  - postoperative (postprocedural) M96.89
    - with osteoporosis — *see* Osteoporosis
    - fracture following insertion of device — *see* Fracture, following insertion of orthopedic implant, joint prosthesis or bone plate
    - joint instability after prosthesis removal M96.89
    - lordosis M96.4
    - postlaminectomy syndrome NEC M96.1
      - kyphosis M96.3
    - pseudarthrosis M96.0
    - specified complication NEC M96.89
- nephrostomy (stoma) — *see* Complications, stoma, urinary tract, external NEC
- nervous system G98.8
  - central G96.9
  - device, implant or graft (*see also* Complication, prosthetic device or implant, specified NEC)
    - electronic stimulator (electrode(s)) — *see* Complications, electronic stimulator device
    - ventricular shunt — *see* Complications, ventricular shunt
  - electronic stimulator (electrode(s)) — *see* Complications, electronic stimulator device
  - postprocedural G97.82
    - intracranial hypotension G97.2
    - specified NEC G97.82
    - spinal fluid leak G97.0
- newborn, due to intrauterine (fetal) procedure P96.5
- nonabsorbable (permanent) sutures — *see* Complication, sutures, permanent
- obstetric O75.9
  - procedure (instrumental) (manual) (surgical)
    - specified NEC O75.4
  - specified NEC O75.89

Complication(s) — *continued*
- obstetric — *continued*
  - surgical wound NEC O90.89
    - hematoma O90.2
    - infection O86.0
  - ocular lens implant — *see* Complications, intraocular lens
- ophthalmologic
  - postprocedural bleb — *see* Blebitis
- orbital prosthesis T85.9 ☑
  - embolism T85.81 ☑
  - fibrosis T85.82 ☑
  - hemorrhage T85.83 ☑
  - infection and inflammation T85.79 ☑
  - mechanical
    - breakdown T85.31- ☑
    - displacement T85.32- ☑
    - malposition T85.32- ☑
    - obstruction T85.39- ☑
    - perforation T85.39- ☑
    - protrusion T85.39- ☑
    - specified NEC T85.39- ☑
  - pain T85.84 ☑
  - specified type NEC T85.89 ☑
  - stenosis T85.85 ☑
  - thrombosis T85.86 ☑
- organ or tissue transplant (partial) (total) — *see* Complications, transplant
- orthopedic (*see also* Disorder, soft tissue)
  - device or implant T84.9 ☑
    - bone
      - device or implant — *see* Complication, bone, device NEC
      - graft — *see* Complication, graft, bone
    - breakdown T84.418 ☑
    - displacement T84.428 ☑
    - electronic bone stimulator — *see* Complications, electronic stimulator device, bone
    - embolism T84.81 ☑
    - fibrosis T84.82 ☑
    - fixation device — *see* Complication, fixation device, internal
    - hemorrhage T84.83 ☑
    - infection or inflammation T84.7 ☑
    - joint prosthesis — *see* Complication, joint prosthesis, internal
    - malfunction T84.418 ☑
    - malposition T84.428 ☑
    - mechanical NEC T84.498 ☑
    - muscle graft — *see* Complications, graft, muscle
    - obstruction T84.498 ☑
    - pain T84.84 ☑
    - perforation T84.498 ☑
    - protrusion T84.498 ☑
    - specified complication NEC T84.89 ☑
    - stenosis T84.85 ☑
    - tendon graft — *see* Complications, graft, tendon
    - thrombosis T84.86 ☑
  - fracture (following insertion of device) — *see* Fracture, following insertion of orthopedic implant, joint prosthesis or bone plate
  - postprocedural M96.89
    - fracture — *see* Fracture, following insertion of orthopedic implant, joint prosthesis or bone plate
    - postlaminectomy syndrome NEC M96.1
      - kyphosis M96.3
      - lordosis M96.4
    - postradiation
      - kyphosis M96.2
      - scoliosis M96.5
    - pseudarthrosis post-fusion M96.0
    - specified type NEC M96.89
  - pacemaker (cardiac) — *see* Complications, cardiovascular device or implant, electronic
  - pancreas transplant — *see* Complications, transplant, pancreas
  - penile prosthesis (implant) — *see* Complications, prosthetic device, penile
  - perfusion NEC T80.90 ☑
  - perineal repair (obstetrical) NEC O90.89
    - disruption O90.1
    - hematoma O90.2
    - infection (following delivery) O86.0
  - phototherapy T88.9 ☑
    - specified NEC T88.8 ☑

Complication(s) — *continued*
- postmastoidectomy NEC H95.19- ☑
  - cyst, mucosal H95.13- ☑
  - granulation H95.12- ☑
  - inflammation, chronic H95.11- ☑
  - recurrent cholesteatoma H95.0- ☑
- postoperative — *see* Complications, postprocedural
  - circulatory — *see* Complications, circulatory system
  - ear — *see* Complications, ear
  - endocrine — *see* Complications, endocrine
  - eye — *see* Complications, eye
  - lumbar puncture G97.1
    - cerebrospinal fluid leak G97.0
  - nervous system (central) (peripheral) — *see* Complications, nervous system
  - respiratory system — *see* Complications, respiratory system
- postprocedural (*see also* Complications, surgical procedure)
  - cardiac arrest
    - following cardiac surgery I97.120
    - following other surgery I97.121
  - cardiac functional disturbance NEC
    - following cardiac surgery I97.190
    - following other surgery I97.191
  - cardiac insufficiency
    - following cardiac surgery I97.110
    - following other surgery I97.111
  - chorioretinal scars following retinal surgery H59.81- ☑
  - following cataract surgery
    - cataract (lens) fragments H59.02- ☑
    - cystoid macular edema H59.03- ☑
    - specified NEC H59.09- ☑
    - vitreous (touch) syndrome H59.01- ☑
  - heart failure
    - following cardiac surgery I97.130
    - following other surgery I97.131
  - hemorrhage (hematoma) (of)
    - circulatory system organ or structure
      - following a cardiac bypass I97.611
      - following a cardiac catheterization I97.610
      - following other circulatory system procedure I97.618
      - following other procedure I97.62
    - digestive system
      - following procedure on digestive system K91.840
      - following procedure on other organ K91.841
    - ear
      - following other procedure H95.42
      - following procedure on ear and mastoid process H95.41
    - endocrine system
      - following endocrine system procedure E89.810
      - following other procedure E89.811
    - eye and adnexa
      - following ophthalmic procedure H59.31- ☑
      - following other procedure H59.32- ☑
    - genitourinary organ or structure
      - following procedure on genitourinary organ or structure N99.820
      - following procedure on other organ N99.821
    - mastoid process
      - following other procedure H95.42
      - following procedure on ear and mastoid process H95.41
    - musculoskeletal structure
      - following musculoskeletal surgery M96.830
      - following non-orthopedic surgery M96.831
      - following orthopedic surgery M96.830
    - nervous system
      - following a nervous system procedure G97.51
      - following other procedure G97.52
    - respiratory system
      - following a respiratory system procedure J95.830
      - following other procedure J95.831
    - skin and subcutaneous tissue
      - following a dermatologic procedure L76.21
      - following a procedure on other organ L76.22
    - spleen
      - following procedure on other organ D78.22
      - following procedure on the spleen D78.21

Complication(s) — *continued*
- postprocedural (*see also* Complications, surgical procedure) — *continued*
  - specified NEC
    - circulatory system I97.89
    - digestive K91.89
    - ear H95.89
    - endocrine E89.89
    - eye and adnexa H59.89
    - genitourinary N99.89
    - mastoid process H95.89
    - metabolic E89.89
    - musculoskeletal structure M96.89
    - nervous system G97.82
    - respiratory system J95.89
    - skin and subcutaneous tissue L76.82
    - spleen D78.89
- pregnancy NEC — *see* Pregnancy, complicated by
- prosthetic device or implant T85.9 ☑
  - bile duct — *see* Complications, bile duct implant
  - breast — *see* Complications, breast implant
  - cardiac and vascular NEC — *see* Complications, cardiovascular device or implant
  - corneal transplant — *see* Complications, graft, cornea
  - electronic nervous system stimulator — *see* Complications, electronic stimulator device
  - epidural infusion catheter — *see* Complications, catheter, epidural
  - esophageal anti-reflux device — *see* Complications, esophageal anti-reflux device
  - genital organ or tract — *see* Complications, genitourinary, device or implant, genital tract
  - heart valve — *see* Complications, heart, valve, prosthesis
  - infection or inflammation T85.79 ☑
    - intestine transplant T86.892
    - liver transplant T86.43
    - lung transplant T86.812
    - pancreas transplant T86.892
    - skin graft T86.822
  - intraocular lens — *see* Complications, intraocular lens
  - intraperitoneal (dialysis) catheter — *see* Complications, catheter, intraperitoneal
  - joint — *see* Complications, joint prosthesis, internal
  - mechanical NEC T85.698 ☑
    - dialysis catheter (vascular) (*see also* Complication, catheter, dialysis, mechanical)
      - peritoneal — *see* Complication, catheter, intraperitoneal, mechanical
    - gastrointestinal device T85.598 ☑
    - ocular device T85.398 ☑
    - subdural (infusion) catheter T85.690 ☑
    - suture, permanent T85.692 ☑
      - that for bone repair — *see* Complications, fixation device, internal (orthopedic), mechanical
    - ventricular shunt
      - breakdown T85.01 ☑
      - displacement T85.02 ☑
      - leakage T85.03 ☑
      - malposition T85.02 ☑
      - obstruction T85.09 ☑
      - perforation T85.09 ☑
      - protrusion T85.09 ☑
      - specified NEC T85.09 ☑
  - mesh
    - erosion (to surrounding organ or tissue) T83.718 ☑
      - vaginal (into pelvic floor muscles) T83.711 ☑
    - exposure (into surrounding organ or tissue) T83.728 ☑
      - vaginal (into vagina) (through vaginal wall) T83.721 ☑
  - orbital — *see* Complications, orbital prosthesis
  - penile T83.9 ☑
    - embolism T83.81 ☑
    - fibrosis T83.82 ☑
    - hemorrhage T83.83 ☑
    - infection and inflammation T83.6 ☑
    - mechanical
      - breakdown T83.410 ☑
      - displacement T83.420 ☑
      - leakage T83.490 ☑
      - malposition T83.420 ☑

Complication(s) — *continued*
- prosthetic device or implant — *continued*
  - penile — *continued*
    - mechanical — *continued*
      - obstruction T83.490 ☑
      - perforation T83.490 ☑
      - protrusion T83.490 ☑
      - specified NEC T83.490 ☑
    - pain T83.84 ☑
    - specified type NEC T83.89 ☑
    - stenosis T83.85 ☑
    - thrombosis T83.86 ☑
  - prosthetic materials NEC
    - erosion (to surrounding organ or tissue) T83.718 ☑
      - vaginal (into pelvic floor muscles) T83.711 ☑
    - exposure (into surrounding organ or tissue) T83.728 ☑
      - vaginal (into vagina) (through vaginal wall) T83.721 ☑
  - skin graft T86.829
    - artificial skin or decellularized allodermis
      - embolism T85.81 ☑
      - fibrosis T85.82 ☑
      - hemorrhage T85.83 ☑
      - infection and inflammation T85.79 ☑
      - mechanical
        - breakdown T85.613 ☑
        - displacement T85.623 ☑
        - malfunction T85.613 ☑
        - malposition T85.623 ☑
        - obstruction T85.693 ☑
        - perforation T85.693 ☑
        - protrusion T85.693 ☑
        - specified NEC T85.693 ☑
      - pain T85.84 ☑
      - specified type NEC T85.89 ☑
      - stenosis T85.85 ☑
      - thrombosis T85.86 ☑
    - failure T86.821
    - infection T86.822
    - rejection T86.820
    - specified NEC T86.828
  - specified NEC T85.9 ☑
    - embolism T85.81 ☑
    - fibrosis T85.82 ☑
    - hemorrhage T85.83 ☑
    - infection and inflammation T85.79 ☑
    - mechanical
      - breakdown T85.618 ☑
      - displacement T85.628 ☑
      - leakage T85.638 ☑
      - malfunction T85.618 ☑
      - malposition T85.628 ☑
      - obstruction T85.698 ☑
      - perforation T85.698 ☑
      - protrusion T85.698 ☑
      - specified NEC T85.698 ☑
    - pain T85.84 ☑
    - specified type NEC T85.89 ☑
    - stenosis T85.85 ☑
    - thrombosis T85.86 ☑
  - subdural infusion catheter — *see* Complications, catheter, subdural
  - sutures — *see* Complications, sutures
  - urinary organ or tract NEC — *see* Complications, genitourinary, device or implant, urinary system
  - vascular — *see* Complications, cardiovascular device or implant
  - ventricular shunt — *see* Complications, ventricular shunt (device)
- puerperium — *see* Puerperal
- puncture, spinal G97.1
  - cerebrospinal fluid leak G97.0
  - headache or reaction G97.1
- pyelogram N99.89
- radiation
  - kyphosis M96.2
  - scoliosis M96.5
- reattached
  - extremity (infection) (rejection)
    - lower T87.1X- ☑
    - upper T87.0X- ☑
  - specified body part NEC T87.2

Complication(s) — *continued*
  reconstructed breast
    asymmetry between native and reconstructed
      breast N65.1
    deformity N65.0
    disproportion between native and reconstructed
      breast N65.1
    excess tissue N65.0
    misshappen N65.0
  reimplant NEC (*see also* Complications, prosthetic de-
      vice or implant)
    limb (infection) (rejection) — *see* Complications,
      reattached, extremity
    organ (partial) (total) — *see* Complications, trans-
      plant
    prosthetic device NEC — *see* Complications, pros-
      thetic device
  renal N28.9
    allograft — *see* Complications, transplant, kidney
    dialysis — *see* Complications, dialysis
  respirator
    mechanical J95.850
      specified NEC J95.859
  respiratory system J98.9
    device, implant or graft — *see* Complication,
      prosthetic device or implant, specified NEC
    lung transplant — *see* Complications, prosthetic
      device or implant, lung transplant
    postoperative J95.89
      air leak J95.812
      Mendelson's syndrome (chemical pneumonitis)
        J95.4
      pneumothorax J95.811
      pulmonary insufficiency (acute) (after nontho-
        racic surgery) J95.2
        chronic J95.3
        following thoracic surgery J95.1
      respiratory failure (acute) J95.821
        acute and chronic J95.822
      specified NEC J95.89
      subglottic stenosis J95.5
      tracheostomy complication — *see* Complica-
        tions, tracheostomy
    therapy T81.89 ☑
  sedation during labor and delivery O74.9
    cardiac O74.2
    central nervous system O74.3
    pulmonary NEC O74.1
  shunt (*see also* Complications, prosthetic device or
      implant)
    arteriovenous — *see* Complications, arteriovenous,
      shunt
    ventricular (communicating) — *see* Complications,
      ventricular shunt
  skin
    graft T86.829
      failure T86.821
      infection T86.822
      rejection T86.820
      specified type NEC T86.828
  spinal
    anesthesia — *see* Complications, anesthesia, spinal
    catheter (epidural) (subdural) — *see* Complications,
      catheter
    puncture or tap G97.1
      cerebrospinal fluid leak G97.0
      headache or reaction G97.1
  stent
    bile duct — *see* Complications, bile duct prosthesis
    urinary T83.9 ☑
      embolism T83.81 ☑
      fibrosis T83.82 ☑
      hemorrhage T83.83 ☑
      infection and inflammation T83.59 ☑
      mechanical
        breakdown T83.112 ☑
        displacement T83.122 ☑
        leakage T83.192 ☑
        malposition T83.122 ☑
        obstruction T83.192 ☑
        perforation T83.192 ☑
        protrusion T83.192 ☑
        specified NEC T83.192 ☑
      pain T83.84 ☑
      specified type NEC T83.89 ☑
      stenosis T83.85 ☑
      thrombosis T83.86 ☑

Complication(s) — *continued*
  stoma
    digestive tract
      colostomy — *see* Complications, colostomy
      enterostomy — *see* Complications, enterosto-
        my
      esophagostomy — *see* Complications,
        esophagostomy
      gastrostomy — *see* Complications, gastrostomy
    urinary tract N99.538
      cystostomy — *see* Complications, cystostomy
      external NOS N99.528
        hemorrhage N99.520
        infection N99.521
        malfunction N99.522
        specified type NEC N99.528
      hemorrhage N99.530
      infection N99.531
      malfunction N99.532
      specified type NEC N99.538
  stomach banding — *see* Complication(s), bariatric
      procedure
  stomach stapling — *see* Complication(s), bariatric
      procedure
  surgical material, nonabsorbable — *see* Complication,
      suture, permanent
  surgical procedure (on) T81.9 ☑
    amputation stump (late) — *see* Complications,
      amputation stump
    cardiac — *see* Complications, circulatory system
    cholesteatoma, recurrent — *see* Complications,
      postmastoidectomy, recurrent
      cholesteatoma
    circulatory (early) — *see* Complications, circulatory
      system
    digestive system — *see* Complications, gastroin-
      testinal
    dumping syndrome (postgastrectomy) K91.1
    ear — *see* Complications, ear
    elephantiasis or lymphedema I97.89
      postmastectomy I97.2
    emphysema (surgical) T81.82 ☑
    endocrine — *see* Complications, endocrine
    eye — *see* Complications, eye
    fistula (persistent postoperative) T81.83 ☑
    foreign body inadvertently left in wound (sponge)
      (suture) (swab) — *see* Foreign body, acciden-
      tally left during a procedure
    gastrointestinal — *see* Complications, gastrointesti-
      nal
    genitourinary NEC N99.89
    hematoma
      intraoperative — *see* Complication, intraopera-
        tive, hemorrhage
      postprocedural — *see* Complication, postpro-
        cedural, hemorrhage
    hemorrhage
      intraoperative — *see* Complication, intraopera-
        tive, hemorrhage
      postprocedural — *see* Complication, postpro-
        cedural, hemorrhage
    hepatic failure K91.82
    hyperglycemia (postpancreatectomy) E89.1
    hypoinsulinemia (postpancreatectomy) E89.1
    hypoparathyroidism (postparathyroidectomy)
      E89.2
    hypopituitarism (posthypophysectomy) E89.3
    hypothyroidism (post-thyroidectomy) E89.0
    intestinal obstruction K91.3
    intracranial hypotension following ventricular
      shunting (ventriculostomy) G97.2
    lymphedema I97.89
      postmastectomy I97.2
    malabsorption (postsurgical) NEC K91.2
      osteoporosis — *see* Osteoporosis, postsurgical
        malabsorption
    mastoidectomy cavity NEC — *see* Complications,
      postmastoidectomy
    metabolic E89.89
      specified NEC E89.89
    musculoskeletal — *see* Complications, muscu-
      loskeletal system
    nervous system (central) (peripheral) — *see* Com-
      plications, nervous system
    ovarian failure E89.40
      asymptomatic E89.40
      symptomatic E89.41

Complication(s) — *continued*
  surgical procedure — *continued*
    peripheral vascular — *see* Complications, surgical
      procedure, vascular
    postcardiotomy syndrome I97.0
    postcholecystectomy syndrome K91.5
    postcommissurotomy syndrome I97.0
    postgastrectomy dumping syndrome K91.1
    postlaminectomy syndrome NEC M96.1
      kyphosis M96.3
    postmastectomy lymphedema syndrome I97.2
    postmastoidectomy cholesteatoma — *see* Compli-
      cations, postmastoidectomy, recurrent
      cholesteatoma
    postvagotomy syndrome K91.1
    postvalvulotomy syndrome I97.0
    pulmonary insufficiency (acute) J95.2
      chronic J95.3
      following thoracic surgery J95.1
    reattached body part — *see* Complications, reat-
      tached
    respiratory — *see* Complications, respiratory sys-
      tem
    shock (hypovolemic) T81.19 ☑
    spleen (postoperative) D78.89
      intraoperative D78.81
    stitch abscess T81.4 ☑
    subglottic stenosis (postsurgical) J95.5
    testicular hypofunction E89.5
    transplant — *see* Complications, organ or tissue
      transplant
    urinary NEC N99.89
    vaginal vault prolapse (posthysterectomy) N99.3
    vascular (peripheral)
      artery T81.719 ☑
        mesenteric T81.710 ☑
        renal T81.711 ☑
        specified NEC T81.718 ☑
      vein T81.72 ☑
    wound infection T81.4 ☑
  suture, permanent (wire) NEC T85.9 ☑
    with repair of bone — *see* Complications, fixation
      device, internal
    embolism T85.81 ☑
    fibrosis T85.82 ☑
    hemorrhage T85.83 ☑
    infection and inflammation T85.79 ☑
    mechanical
      breakdown T85.612 ☑
      displacement T85.622 ☑
      malfunction T85.612 ☑
      malposition T85.622 ☑
      obstruction T85.692 ☑
      perforation T85.692 ☑
      protrusion T85.692 ☑
      specified NEC T85.692 ☑
    pain T85.84 ☑
    specified type NEC T85.89 ☑
    stenosis T85.85 ☑
    thrombosis T85.86 ☑
  tracheostomy J95.00
    granuloma J95.09
    hemorrhage J95.01
    infection J95.02
    malfunction J95.03
    mechanical J95.03
    obstruction J95.03
    specified type NEC J95.09
    tracheo-esophageal fistula J95.04
  transfusion (blood) (lymphocytes) (plasma) T80.92 ☑
    air emblism T80.0 ☑
    circulatory overload E87.71
    febrile nonhemolytic transfusion reaction R50.84
    hemochromatosis E83.111
    hemolysis T80.89 ☑
    hemolytic reaction (antigen unspecified)
      T80.919 ☑
    incompatibility reaction (antigen unspecified)
      T80.919 ☑
      ABO T80.30 ☑
        delayed serologic (DSTR) T80.39 ☑
        hemolytic transfusion reaction (HTR) (un-
          specified time after transfusion)
          T80.319 ☑
          acute (AHTR) (less than 24 hours after
            transfusion) T80.310 ☑

Complication(s) — *continued*
  transfusion — *continued*
    incompatibility reaction — *continued*
      ABO — *continued*
        hemolytic transfusion reaction — *continued*
          delayed (DHTR) (24 hours or more after transfusion) T80.311 ☑
          specified NEC T80.39 ☑
        acute (antigen unspecified) T80.910 ☑
        delayed (antigen unspecified) T80.911 ☑
        delayed serologic (DSTR) T80.89 ☑
        non-ABO (minor antigens (Duffy) (Kell) (Kidd) (Lewis) (M) (N) (P) (S)) T80.A0 ☑ (*following* T80.4)
        delayed serologic (DSTR) T80.A9 ☑ (*following* T80.4)
        hemolytic transfusion reaction (HTR) (unspecified time after transfusion) T80.A19 ☑ (*following* T80.4)
        acute (AHTR) (less than 24 hours after transfusion) T80.A10 ☑ (*following* T80.4)
        delayed (DHTR) (24 hours or more after transfusion) T80.A11 ☑ (*following* T80.4)
        specified NEC T80.A9 ☑ (*following* T80.4)
        Rh (antigens (C) (c) (D) (E) (e)) (factor) T80.40 ☑
        delayed serologic (DSTR) T80.49 ☑
        hemolytic transfusion reaction (HTR) (unspecified time after transfusion) T80.419 ☑
        acute (AHTR) (less than 24 hours after transfusion) T80.410 ☑
        delayed (DHTR) (24 hours or more after transfusion) T80.411 ☑
        specified NEC T80.49 ☑
    infection T80.29 ☑
    reaction NEC T80.89 ☑
    sepsis T80.29 ☑
    shock T80.89 ☑
  transplant T86.90
    bone T86.839
      failure T86.831
      infection T86.832
      rejection T86.830
      specified type NEC T86.838
    bone marrow T86.00
      failure T86.02
      infection T86.03
      rejection T86.01
      specified type NEC T86.09
    cornea T86.849
      failure T86.841
      infection T86.842
      rejection T86.840
      specified type NEC T86.848
    failure T86.92
    heart T86.20
      with lung T86.30
        cardiac allograft vasculopathy T86.290
        failure T86.32
        infection T86.33
        rejection T86.31
        specified type NEC T86.39
      failure T86.22
      infection T86.23
      rejection T86.21
      specified type NEC T86.298
    infection T86.93
    intestine T86.859
      failure T86.851
      infection T86.852
      rejection T86.850
      specified type NEC T86.858
    kidney T86.10
      failure T86.12
      infection T86.13
      rejection T86.11
      specified type NEC T86.19
    liver T86.40
      failure T86.42
      infection T86.43
      rejection T86.41
      specified type NEC T86.49
    lung T86.819
      with heart T86.30
        failure T86.32

Complication(s) — *continued*
  transplant — *continued*
    lung — *continued*
      with heart — *continued*
        infection T86.33
        rejection T86.31
        specified type NEC T86.39
      failure T86.811
      infection T86.812
      rejection T86.810
      specified type NEC T86.818
    malignant neoplasm C80.2
    pancreas T86.899
      failure T86.891
      infection T86.892
      rejection T86.890
      specified type NEC T86.898
    peripheral blood stem cells T86.5
    post-transplant lymphoproliferative disorder (PTLD) D47.Z1 (*following* D47.4)
    rejection T86.91
    skin T86.829
      failure T86.821
      infection T86.822
      rejection T86.820
      specified type NEC T86.828
    specified
      tissue T86.899
        failure T86.891
        infection T86.892
        rejection T86.890
        specified type NEC T86.898
      type NEC T86.99
    stem cell (from peripheral blood) (from umbilical cord) T86.5
    umbilical cord stem cells T86.5
  trauma (early) T79.9
    specified NEC T79.8 ☑
  ultrasound therapy NEC T88.9 ☑
  umbilical cord NEC
    complicating delivery O69.9 ☑
    specified NEC O69.89 ☑
  umbrella device, vascular T82.9 ☑
    embolism T82.818 ☑
    fibrosis T82.828 ☑
    hemorrhage T82.838 ☑
    infection or inflammation T82.7 ☑
    mechanical
      breakdown T82.515 ☑
      displacement T82.525 ☑
      leakage T82.535 ☑
      malposition T82.525 ☑
      obstruction T82.595 ☑
      perforation T82.595 ☑
      protrusion T82.595 ☑
    pain T82.848 ☑
    specified type NEC T82.898 ☑
    stenosis T82.858 ☑
    thrombosis T82.868 ☑
  urethral catheter — *see* Complications, catheter, urethral, indwelling
  vaccination T88.1 ☑
    anaphylaxis NEC T80.52 ☑
    arthropathy — *see* Arthropathy, postimmunization
    cellulitis T88.0 ☑
    encephalitis or encephalomyelitis G04.02
    infection (general) (local) NEC T88.0 ☑
    meningitis G03.8
    myelitis G04.89
    protein sickness T80.62 ☑
    rash T88.1 ☑
    reaction (allergic) T88.1 ☑
      serum T80.62 ☑
    sepsis T88.0 ☑
    serum intoxication, sickness, rash, or other serum reaction NEC T80.62 ☑
    anaphylactic shock T80.52 ☑
    shock (allergic) (anaphylactic) T80.52 ☑
    vaccinia (generalized) (localized) T88.1 ☑
  vas deferens device or implant — *see* Complications, genitourinary, device or implant, genital tract
  vascular I99.9
    device or implant T82.9 ☑
      embolism T82.818 ☑
      fibrosis T82.828 ☑
      hemorrhage T82.838 ☑
      infection or inflammation T82.7 ☑

Complication(s) — *continued*
  vascular — *continued*
    device or implant — *continued*
      mechanical
        breakdown T82.519 ☑
          specified device NEC T82.518 ☑
        displacement T82.529 ☑
          specified device NEC T82.528 ☑
        leakage T82.539 ☑
          specified device NEC T82.538 ☑
        malposition T82.529 ☑
          specified device NEC T82.528 ☑
        obstruction T82.599 ☑
          specified device NEC T82.598 ☑
        perforation T82.599 ☑
          specified device NEC T82.598 ☑
        protrusion T82.599 ☑
          specified device NEC T82.598 ☑
      pain T82.848 ☑
      specified type NEC T82.898 ☑
      stenosis T82.858 ☑
      thrombosis T82.868 ☑
    dialysis catheter — *see* Complication, catheter, dialysis
    following infusion, therapeutic injection or transfusion T80.1 ☑
    graft T82.9
      embolism T82.818 ☑
      fibrosis T82.828 ☑
      hemorrhage T82.838 ☑
      mechanical
        breakdown T82.319 ☑
          aorta (bifurcation) T82.310 ☑
          carotid artery T82.311 ☑
          specified vessel NEC T82.318 ☑
        displacement T82.329 ☑
          aorta (bifurcation) T82.320 ☑
          carotid artery T82.321 ☑
          specified vessel NEC T82.328 ☑
        leakage T82.339 ☑
          aorta (bifurcation) T82.330 ☑
          carotid artery T82.331 ☑
          specified vessel NEC T82.338 ☑
        malposition T82.329 ☑
          aorta (bifurcation) T82.320 ☑
          carotid artery T82.321 ☑
          specified vessel NEC T82.328 ☑
        obstruction T82.399 ☑
          aorta (bifurcation) T82.390 ☑
          carotid artery T82.391 ☑
          specified vessel NEC T82.398 ☑
        perforation T82.399 ☑
          aorta (bifurcation) T82.390 ☑
          carotid artery T82.391 ☑
          specified vessel NEC T82.398 ☑
        protrusion T82.399 ☑
          aorta (bifurcation) T82.390 ☑
          carotid artery T82.391 ☑
          specified vessel NEC T82.398 ☑
      pain T82.848 ☑
      specified complication NEC T82.898 ☑
      stenosis T82.858 ☑
      thrombosis T82.868 ☑
    postoperative — *see* Complications, postoperative, circulatory
  vena cava device (filter) (sieve) (umbrella) — *see* Complications, umbrella device, vascular
  ventilation therapy NEC T81.81 ☑
  ventilator
    mechanical J95.850
      specified NEC J95.859
  ventricular (communicating) shunt (device) T85.9 ☑
    embolism T85.81 ☑
    fibrosis T85.82 ☑
    hemorrhage T85.83 ☑
    infection and inflammation T85.79 ☑
    mechanical
      breakdown T85.01 ☑
      displacement T85.02 ☑
      leakage T85.03 ☑
      malposition T85.02 ☑
      obstruction T85.09 ☑
      perforation T85.09 ☑
      protrusion T85.09 ☑
      specified NEC T85.09 ☑
    pain T85.84 ☑

☑ Additional Character Required — Refer to the Tabular List for Character Selection   ▽ Subterms under main terms may continue to next column or page

Complication(s) — continued
  ventricular shunt — continued
    specified type NEC T85.89 ☑
    stenosis T85.85 ☑
    thrombosis T85.86 ☑
  wire suture, permanent (implanted) — see Complications, suture, permanent
Compressed air disease T70.3 ☑
Compression
  with injury — code by Nature of injury
  artery I77.1
    celiac, syndrome I77.4
  brachial plexus G54.0
  brain (stem) G93.5
    due to
      contusion (diffuse) — see Injury, intracranial, diffuse
        focal — see Injury, intracranial, focal
      injury NEC — see Injury, intracranial, diffuse
      traumatic — see Injury, intracranial, diffuse
  bronchus J98.09
  cauda equina G83.4
  celiac (artery) (axis) I77.4
  cerebral — see Compression, brain
  cervical plexus G54.2
  cord
    spinal — see Compression, spinal
    umbilical — see Compression, umbilical cord
  cranial nerve G52.9
    eighth H93.3 ☑
    eleventh G52.8
    fifth G50.8
    first G52.0
    fourth — see Strabismus, paralytic, fourth nerve
    ninth G52.1
    second — see Disorder, nerve, optic
    seventh G52.8
    sixth — see Strabismus, paralytic, sixth nerve
    tenth G52.2
    third — see Strabismus, paralytic, third nerve
    twelfth G52.3
  diver's squeeze T70.3 ☑
  during birth (newborn) P15.9
  esophagus K22.2
  eustachian tube — see Obstruction, eustachian tube, cartilaginous
  facies Q67.1
  fracture — see Fracture
  heart — see Disease, heart
  intestine — see Obstruction, intestine
  laryngeal nerve, recurrent G52.2
    with paralysis of vocal cords and larynx J38.00
      bilateral J38.02
      unilateral J38.01
  lumbosacral plexus G54.1
  lung J98.4
  lymphatic vessel I89.0
  medulla — see Compression, brain
  nerve (see also Disorder, nerve) G58.9
    arm NEC — see Mononeuropathy, upper limb
    axillary G54.0
    cranial — see Compression, cranial nerve
    leg NEC — see Mononeuropathy, lower limb
    median (in carpal tunnel) — see Syndrome, carpal tunnel
    optic — see Disorder, nerve, optic
    plantar — see Lesion, nerve, plantar
    posterior tibial (in tarsal tunnel) — see Syndrome, tarsal tunnel
    root or plexus NOS (in) G54.9
      intervertebral disc disorder NEC — see Disorder, disc, with, radiculopathy
      with myelopathy — see Disorder, disc, with, myelopathy
      neoplastic disease (see also Neoplasm) D49.9 [G55]
      spondylosis — see Spondylosis, with radiculopathy
    sciatic (acute) — see Lesion, nerve, sciatic
    sympathetic G90.8
    traumatic — see Injury, nerve
    ulnar — see Lesion, nerve, ulnar
    upper extremity NEC — see Mononeuropathy, upper limb
  spinal (cord) G95.20
    by displacement of intervertebral disc NEC (see also Disorder, disc, with, myelopathy)

Compression — continued
  spinal — continued
    nerve root NOS G54.9
      due to displacement of intervertebral disc NEC — see Disorder, disc, with, radiculopathy
      with myelopathy — see Disorder, disc, with, myelopathy
      specified NEC G95.29
    spondylogenic (cervical) (lumbar, lumbosacral) (thoracic) — see Spondylosis, with myelopathy NEC
    anterior — see Syndrome, anterior, spinal artery, compression
    traumatic — see Injury, spinal cord, by region
  subcostal nerve (syndrome) — see Mononeuropathy, upper limb, specified NEC
  sympathetic nerve NEC G90.8
  syndrome T79.5 ☑
  trachea J39.8
  ulnar nerve (by scar tissue) — see Lesion, nerve, ulnar
  umbilical cord
    complicating delivery O69.2 ☑
      cord around neck O69.1 ☑
      prolapse O69.0 ☑
      specified NEC O69.2 ☑
  ureter N13.5
  vein I87.1
  vena cava (inferior) (superior) I87.1
Compulsion, compulsive
  gambling F63.0
  neurosis F42
  personality F60.5
  states F42
  swearing F42
    in Gilles de la Tourette's syndrome F95.2
  tics and spasms F95.9
Concato's disease (pericardial polyserositis) A19.9
  nontubercular I31.1
  pleural — see Pleurisy, with effusion
Concavity chest wall M95.4
Concealed penis Q55.69
Concern (normal) **about sick person in family** Z63.6
Concrescence (teeth) K00.2
Concretio cordis I31.1
  rheumatic I09.2
Concretion (see also Calculus)
  appendicular K38.1
  canaliculus — see Dacryolith
  clitoris N90.89
  conjunctiva H11.12-
  eyelid — see Disorder, eyelid, specified type NEC
  lacrimal passages — see Dacryolith
  prepuce (male) N47.8
  salivary gland (any) K11.5
  seminal vesicle N50.8
  tonsil J35.8
Concussion (brain) (cerebral) (current) S06.0X- ☑
  blast (air) (hydraulic) (immersion) (underwater)
    abdomen or thorax — see Injury, blast, by site
    ear with acoustic nerve injury — see Injury, nerve, acoustic, specified type NEC
  cauda equina S34.3 ☑
  conus medullaris S34.02 ☑
  ocular S05.8X- ☑
  spinal (cord)
    cervical S14.0 ☑
    lumbar S34.01 ☑
    sacral S34.02 ☑
    thoracic S24.0 ☑
  syndrome F07.81
Condition — see Disease
Conditions arising in the perinatal period — see Newborn, affected by
Conduct disorder — see Disorder, conduct
Condyloma A63.0
  acuminatum A63.0
  gonorrheal A54.09
  latum A51.31
  syphilitic A51.31
    congenital A50.07
  venereal, syphilitic A51.31
Conflagration (see also Burn)
  asphyxia (by inhalation of gases, fumes or vapors) (see also Table of Drugs and Chemicals) T59.9- ☑
Conflict (with) (see also Discord)
  family Z73.9
  marital Z63.0

Conflict — continued
  marital — continued
    involving divorce or estrangement Z63.5
  parent-child Z62.820
    parent-adopted child Z62.821
    parent-biological child Z62.820
    parent-foster child Z62.822
  social role NEC Z73.5
Confluent — see condition
Confusion, confused R41.0
  epileptic F05
  mental state (psychogenic) F44.89
  psychogenic F44.89
  reactive (from emotional stress, psychological trauma) F44.89
Confusional arousals G47.51
Congelation T69.9 ☑
Congenital (see also condition)
  aortic septum Q25.4
  intrinsic factor deficiency D51.0
  malformation — see Anomaly
Congestion, congestive
  bladder N32.89
  bowel K63.89
  brain G93.89
  breast N64.59
  bronchial J98.09
  catarrhal J31.0
  chest R09.89
  chill, malarial — see Malaria
  circulatory NEC I99.8
  duodenum K31.89
  eye — see Hyperemia, conjunctiva
  facial, due to birth injury P15.4
  general R68.89
  glottis J37.0
  heart — see Failure, heart, congestive
  hepatic K76.1
  hypostatic (lung) — see Edema, lung
  intestine K63.89
  kidney N28.89
  labyrinth H83.8 ☑
  larynx J37.0
  liver K76.1
  lung R09.89
    active or acute — see Pneumonia
  malaria, malarial — see Malaria
  nasal R09.81
  nose R09.81
  orbit, orbital (see also Exophthalmos)
    inflammatory (chronic) — see Inflammation, orbit
  ovary N83.8
  pancreas K86.8
  pelvic, female N94.89
  pleural J94.8
  prostate (active) N42.1
  pulmonary — see Congestion, lung
  renal N28.89
  retina H35.81
  seminal vesicle N50.1
  spinal cord G95.19
  spleen (chronic) D73.2
  stomach K31.89
  trachea — see Tracheitis
  urethra N36.8
  uterus N85.8
    with subinvolution N85.3
  venous (passive) I87.8
  viscera R68.89
Congestive — see Congestion
Conical
  cervix (hypertrophic elongation) N88.4
  cornea — see Keratoconus
  teeth K00.2
Conjoined twins Q89.4
Conjugal maladjustment Z63.0
  involving divorce or estrangement Z63.5
Conjunctiva — see condition
Conjunctivitis (staphylococcal) (streptococcal) NOS H10.9
  Acanthamoeba B60.12
  acute H10.3- ☑
    atopic H10.1- ☑
    chemical (see also Corrosion, cornea) H10.21- ☑
    mucopurulent H10.02- ☑
      follicular H10.01- ☑
    pseudomembranous H10.22- ☑

Conjunctivitis — *continued*
acute — *continued*
serous except viral H10.23- ☑
viral — *see* Conjunctivitis, viral
toxic H10.21- ☑
adenoviral (acute) (follicular) B30.1
allergic (acute) — *see* Conjunctivitis, acute, atopic
chronic H10.45
vernal H10.44
anaphylactic — *see* Conjunctivitis, acute, atopic
Apollo B30.3
atopic (acute) — *see* Conjunctivitis, acute, atopic
Béal's B30.2
blennorrhagic (gonococcal) (neonatorum) A54.31
chemical (acute) (*see also* Corrosion, cornea)
H10.21- ☑
chlamydial A74.0
due to trachoma A71.1
neonatal P39.1
chronic (nodosa) (petrificans) (phlyctenular) H10.40- ☑
allergic H10.45
vernal H10.44
follicular H10.43- ☑
giant papillary H10.41- ☑
simple H10.42- ☑
vernal H10.44
coxsackievirus 24 B30.3
diphtheritic A36.86
due to
dust — *see* Conjunctivitis, acute, atopic
filariasis B74.9
mucocutaneous leishmaniasis B55.2
enterovirus type 70 (hemorrhagic) B30.3
epidemic (viral) B30.9
hemorrhagic B30.3
gonococcal (neonatorum) A54.31
granular (trachomatous) A71.1
sequelae (late effect) B94.0
hemorrhagic (acute) (epidemic) B30.3
herpes zoster B02.31
in (due to)
Acanthamoeba B60.12
adenovirus (acute) (follicular) B30.1
Chlamydia A74.0
coxsackievirus 24 B30.3
diphtheria A36.86
enterovirus type 70 (hemorrhagic) B30.3
filariasis B74.9
gonococci A54.31
herpes (simplex) virus B00.53
zoster B02.31
infectious disease NEC B99 ☑
meningococci A39.89
mucocutaneous leishmaniasis B55.2
rosacea L71.9
syphilis (late) A52.71
zoster B02.31
inclusion A74.0
infantile P39.1
gonococcal A54.31
Koch-Weeks' — *see* Conjunctivitis, acute, mucopurulent
light — *see* Conjunctivitis, acute, atopic
ligneous — *see* Blepharoconjunctivitis, ligneous
meningococcal A39.89
mucopurulent — *see* Conjunctivitis, acute, mucopurulent
neonatal P39.1
gonococcal A54.31
Newcastle B30.8
of Béal B30.2
parasitic
filariasis B74.9
mucocutaneous leishmaniasis B55.2
Parinaud's H10.89
petrificans H10.89
rosacea L71.9
specified NEC H10.89
swimming-pool B30.1
trachomatous A71.1
acute A71.0
sequelae (late effect) B94.0
traumatic NEC H10.89
tuberculous A18.59
tularemic A21.1
tularensis A21.1
viral B30.9

Conjunctivitis — *continued*
viral — *continued*
due to
adenovirus B30.1
enterovirus B30.3
specified NEC B30.8
Conjunctivochalasis H11.82- ☑
Connective tissue — *see* condition
Conn's syndrome E26.01
Consanguinity Z84.3
counseling Z71.89
Conscious simulation (of illness) Z76.5
Consecutive — *see* condition
Consolidation lung (base) — *see* Pneumonia, lobar
Constipation (atonic) (neurogenic) (simple) (spastic) K59.00
drug-induced — *see* Table of Drugs and Chemicals
outlet dysfunction K59.02
psychogenic F45.8
slow transit K59.01
specified NEC K59.09
Constitutional (*see also* condition)
substandard F60.7
Constitutionally substandard F60.7
Constriction (*see also* Stricture)
auditory canal — *see* Stenosis, external ear canal
bronchial J98.09
duodenum K31.5
esophagus K22.2
external
abdomen, abdominal (wall) S30.841 ☑
alveolar process S00.542 ☑
ankle S90.54- ☑
antecubital space — *see* Constriction, external, forearm
arm (upper) S40.84- ☑
auricle — *see* Constriction, external, ear
axilla — *see* Constriction, external, arm
back, lower S30.840 ☑
breast S20.14- ☑
brow S00.84 ☑
buttock S30.840 ☑
calf — *see* Constriction, external, leg
canthus — *see* Constriction, external, eyelid
cheek S00.84 ☑
internal S00.542 ☑
chest wall — *see* Constriction, external, thorax
chin S00.84 ☑
clitoris S30.844 ☑
costal region — *see* Constriction, external, thorax
digit(s)
foot — *see* Constriction, external, toe
hand — *see* Constriction, external, finger
ear S00.44- ☑
elbow S50.34- ☑
epididymis S30.843 ☑
epigastric region S30.841 ☑
esophagus, cervical S10.14 ☑
eyebrow — *see* Constriction, external, eyelid
eyelid S00.24- ☑
face S00.84 ☑
finger(s) S60.44- ☑
index S60.44- ☑
little S60.44- ☑
middle S60.44- ☑
ring S60.44- ☑
flank S30.841 ☑
foot (except toe(s) alone) S90.84- ☑
toe — *see* Constriction, external, toe
forearm S50.84- ☑
elbow only — *see* Constriction, external, elbow
forehead S00.84 ☑
genital organs, external
female S30.846 ☑
male S30.845 ☑
groin S30.841 ☑
gum S00.542 ☑
hand S60.54- ☑
head S00.94 ☑
ear — *see* Constriction, external, ear
eyelid — *see* Constriction, external, eyelid
lip S00.541 ☑
nose S00.34 ☑
oral cavity S00.542 ☑
scalp S00.04 ☑

Constriction — *continued*
external — *continued*
head — *continued*
specified site NEC S00.84 ☑
heel — *see* Constriction, external, foot
hip S70.24- ☑
inguinal region S30.841 ☑
interscapular region S20.449 ☑
jaw S00.84 ☑
knee S80.24- ☑
labium (majus) (minus) S30.844 ☑
larynx S10.14 ☑
leg (lower) S80.84- ☑
knee — *see* Constriction, external, knee
upper — *see* Constriction, external, thigh
lip S00.541 ☑
lower back S30.840 ☑
lumbar region S30.840 ☑
malar region S00.84 ☑
mammary — *see* Constriction, external, breast
mastoid region S00.84 ☑
mouth S00.542 ☑
nail
finger — *see* Constriction, external, finger
toe — *see* Constriction, external, toe
nasal S00.34 ☑
neck S10.94 ☑
specified site NEC S10.84 ☑
throat S10.14 ☑
nose S00.34 ☑
occipital region S00.04 ☑
oral cavity S00.542 ☑
orbital region — *see* Constriction, external, eyelid
palate S00.542 ☑
palm — *see* Constriction, external, hand
parietal region S00.04 ☑
pelvis S30.840 ☑
penis S30.842 ☑
perineum
female S30.844 ☑
male S30.840 ☑
periocular area — *see* Constriction, external, eyelid
phalanges
finger — *see* Constriction, external, finger
toe — *see* Constriction, external, toe
pharynx S10.14 ☑
pinna — *see* Constriction, external, ear
popliteal space — *see* Constriction, external, knee
prepuce S30.842 ☑
pubic region S30.840 ☑
pudendum
female S30.846 ☑
male S30.845 ☑
sacral region S30.840 ☑
scalp S00.04 ☑
scapular region — *see* Constriction, external, shoulder
scrotum S30.843 ☑
shin — *see* Constriction, external, leg
shoulder S40.24- ☑
sternal region S20.349 ☑
submaxillary region S00.84 ☑
submental region S00.84 ☑
subungual
finger(s) — *see* Constriction, external, finger
toe(s) — *see* Constriction, external, toe
supraclavicular fossa S10.84 ☑
supraorbital S00.84 ☑
temple S00.84 ☑
temporal region S00.84 ☑
testis S30.843 ☑
thigh S70.34- ☑
thorax, thoracic (wall) S20.94 ☑
back S20.44- ☑
front S20.34- ☑
throat S10.14 ☑
thumb S60.34- ☑
toe(s) (lesser) S90.44- ☑
great S90.44- ☑
tongue S00.542 ☑
trachea S10.14 ☑
tunica vaginalis S30.843 ☑
uvula S00.542 ☑
vagina S30.844 ☑
vulva S30.844 ☑
wrist S60.84- ☑

Constriction — *continued*
  gallbladder — *see* Obstruction, gallbladder
  intestine — *see* Obstruction, intestine
  larynx J38.6
    congenital Q31.8
      specified NEC Q31.8
      subglottic Q31.1
  organ or site, congenital NEC — *see* Atresia, by site
  prepuce (acquired) (congenital) N47.1
  pylorus (adult hypertrophic) K31.1
    congenital or infantile Q40.0
      newborn Q40.0
  ring dystocia (uterus) O62.4
  spastic (*see also* Spasm)
    ureter N13.5
  ureter N13.5
    with infection N13.6
  urethra — *see* Stricture, urethra
  visual field (peripheral) (functional) — *see* Defect, visual field
Constrictive — *see* condition
Consultation
  without complaint or sickness Z71.9
    feared complaint unfounded Z71.1
    specified reason NEC Z71.89
  medical — *see* Counseling, medical
  religious Z71.81
  specified reason NEC Z71.89
  spiritual Z71.81
Consumption — *see* Tuberculosis
Contact (with) (*see also* Exposure (to))
  acariasis Z20.7
  AIDS virus Z20.6
  air pollution Z77.110
  algae and algae toxins Z77.121
  algae bloom Z77.121
  anthrax Z20.810
  aromatic amines Z77.020
  aromatic (hazardous) compounds NEC Z77.028
  aromatic dyes NOS Z77.028
  arsenic Z77.010
  asbestos Z77.090
  bacterial disease NEC Z20.818
  benzene Z77.021
  blue-green algae bloom Z77.121
  body fluids (potentially hazardous) Z77.21
  brown tide Z77.121
  chemicals (chiefly nonmedicinal) (hazardous) NEC Z77.098
  cholera Z20.09
  chromium compounds Z77.018
  communicable disease Z20.9
    bacterial NEC Z20.818
    specified NEC Z20.89
    viral NEC Z20.828
  cyanobacteria bloom Z77.121
  dyes Z77.098
  Escherichia coli (E. coli) Z20.01
  fiberglass — *see* Table of Drugs and Chemicals, fiberglass
  German measles Z20.4
  gonorrhea Z20.2
  hazardous metals NEC Z77.018
  hazardous substances NEC Z77.29
  hazards in the physical environment NEC Z77.128
  hazards to health NEC Z77.9
  HIV Z20.6
  HTLV-III/LAV Z20.6
  human immunodeficiency virus (HIV) Z20.6
  infection Z20.9
    specified NEC Z20.89
  infestation (parasitic) NEC Z20.7
  intestinal infectious disease NEC Z20.09
    Escherichia coli (E. coli) Z20.01
  lead Z77.011
  meningococcus Z20.811
  mold (toxic) Z77.120
  nickel dust Z77.018
  noise Z77.122
  parasitic disease Z20.7
  pediculosis Z20.7
  pfiesteria piscicida Z77.121
  poliomyelitis Z20.89
  pollution
    air Z77.110
    environmental NEC Z77.118
    soil Z77.112
    water Z77.111

Contact — *continued*
  polycyclic aromatic hydrocarbons Z77.028
  rabies Z20.3
  radiation, naturally occurring NEC Z77.123
  radon Z77.123
  red tide (Florida) Z77.121
  rubella Z20.4
  sexually-transmitted disease Z20.2
  smallpox (laboratory) Z20.89
  syphilis Z20.2
  tuberculosis Z20.1
  uranium Z77.012
  varicella Z20.820
  venereal disease Z20.2
  viral disease NEC Z20.828
  viral hepatitis Z20.5
  water pollution Z77.111
Contamination, food — *see* Intoxication, foodborne
Contraception, contraceptive
  advice Z30.09
  counseling Z30.09
  device (intrauterine) (in situ) Z97.5
    causing menorrhagia T83.83 ☑
    checking Z30.431
    complications — *see* Complications, intrauterine, contraceptive device
    in place Z97.5
    initial prescription Z30.014
    reinsertion Z30.433
    removal Z30.432
    replacement Z30.433
  emergency (postcoital) Z30.012
  initial prescription Z30.019
    injectable Z30.013
    intrauterine device Z30.014
    pills Z30.011
    postcoital (emergency) Z30.012
    specified type NEC Z30.018
    subdermal implantable Z30.019
  maintenance Z30.40
    examination Z30.8
    injectable Z30.42
    intrauterine device Z30.431
    pills Z30.41
    specified type NEC Z30.49
    subdermal implantable Z30.49
  management Z30.9
    specified NEC Z30.8
  postcoital (emergency) Z30.012
  prescription Z30.019
    repeat Z30.40
  sterilization Z30.2
  surveillance (drug) — *see* Contraception, maintenance
Contraction(s), contracture, contracted
  Achilles tendon (*see also* Short, tendon, Achilles)
    congenital Q66.89
  amputation stump (surgical) (flexion) (late) (next proximal joint) T87.89
  anus K59.8
  bile duct (common) (hepatic) K83.8
  bladder N32.89
    neck or sphincter N32.0
  bowel, cecum, colon or intestine, any part — *see* Obstruction, intestine
  Braxton Hicks — *see* False, labor
  breast implant, capsular T85.44 ☑
  bronchial J98.09
  burn (old) — *see* Cicatrix
  cervix — *see* Stricture, cervix
  cicatricial — *see* Cicatrix
  conjunctiva, trachomatous, active A71.1
    sequelae (late effect) B94.0
  Dupuytren's M72.0
  eyelid — *see* Disorder, eyelid function
  fascia (lata) (postural) M72.8
    Dupuytren's M72.0
    palmar M72.0
    plantar M72.2
  finger NEC (*see also* Deformity, finger)
    congenital Q68.1
    joint — *see* Contraction, joint, hand
  flaccid — *see* Contraction, paralytic
  gallbladder K82.0
  heart valve — *see* Endocarditis
  hip — *see* Contraction, joint, hip
  hourglass
    bladder N32.89
      congenital Q64.79

Contraction(s), contracture, contracted — *continued*
  hourglass — *continued*
    gallbladder K82.0
      congenital Q44.1
    stomach K31.89
      congenital Q40.2
      psychogenic F45.8
    uterus (complicating delivery) O62.4
  hysterical F44.4
  internal os — *see* Stricture, cervix
  joint (abduction) (acquired) (adduction) (flexion) (rotation) M24.50
    ankle M24.57- ☑
    congenital NEC Q68.8
      hip Q65.89
    elbow M24.52- ☑
    foot joint M24.57- ☑
    hand joint M24.54- ☑
    hip M24.55- ☑
      congenital Q65.89
    hysterical F44.4
    knee M24.56- ☑
    shoulder M24.51- ☑
    wrist M24.53- ☑
  kidney (granular) (secondary) N26.9
    congenital Q63.8
    hydronephritic — *see* Hydronephrosis
    Page N26.2
    pyelonephritic — *see* Pyelitis, chronic
    tuberculous A18.11
  ligament (*see also* Disorder, ligament)
    congenital Q79.8
  muscle (postinfective) (postural) NEC M62.40
    with contracture of joint — *see* Contraction, joint
    ankle M62.47- ☑
    congenital Q79.8
      sternocleidomastoid Q68.0
    extraocular — *see* Strabismus
    eye (extrinsic) — *see* Strabismus
    foot M62.47- ☑
    forearm M62.43- ☑
    hand M62.44- ☑
    hysterical F44.4
    ischemic (Volkmann's) T79.6 ☑
    lower leg M62.46- ☑
    multiple sites M62.49
    pelvic region M62.45- ☑
    posttraumatic — *see* Strabismus, paralytic
    psychogenic F45.8
      conversion reaction F44.4
    shoulder region M62.41- ☑
    specified site NEC M62.48
    thigh M62.45- ☑
    upper arm M62.42- ☑
  neck — *see* Torticollis
  ocular muscle — *see* Strabismus
  organ or site, congenital NEC — *see* Atresia, by site
  outlet (pelvis) — *see* Contraction, pelvis
  palmar fascia M72.0
  paralytic
    joint — *see* Contraction, joint
    muscle (*see also* Contraction, muscle NEC)
      ocular — *see* Strabismus, paralytic
  pelvis (acquired) (general) M95.5
    with disproportion (fetopelvic) O33.1
      causing obstructed labor O65.1
    inlet O33.2
    mid-cavity O33.3 ☑
    outlet O33.3 ☑
  plantar fascia M72.2
  premature
    atrium I49.1
    auriculoventricular I49.49
    heart I49.49
    junctional I49.2
    supraventricular I49.1
    ventricular I49.3
  prostate N42.89
  pylorus NEC (*see also* Pylorospasm)
    psychogenic F45.8
  rectum, rectal (sphincter) K59.8
  ring (Bandl's) (complicating delivery) O62.4
  scar — *see* Cicatrix
  spine — *see* Dorsopathy, deforming
  sternocleidomastoid (muscle), congenital Q68.0
  stomach K31.89
    hourglass K31.89

Contraction(s), contracture, contracted — *continued*
  stomach — *continued*
    hourglass — *continued*
      congenital Q40.2
      psychogenic F45.8
    psychogenic F45.8
  tendon (sheath) M62.40
    with contracture of joint — *see* Contraction, joint
    Achilles — *see* Short, tendon, Achilles
    ankle M62.47-
      Achilles — *see* Short, tendon, Achilles
    foot M62.47-
    forearm M62.43-
    hand M62.44-
    lower leg M62.46-
    multiple sites M62.49
    neck M62.48
    pelvic region M62.45-
    shoulder region M62.41-
    specified site NEC M62.48
    thigh M62.45-
    thorax M62.48
    trunk M62.48
    upper arm M62.42-
  toe — *see* Deformity, toe, specified NEC
  ureterovesical orifice (postinfectional) N13.5
    with infection N13.6
  urethra (*see also* Stricture, urethra)
    orifice N32.0
  uterus N85.8
    abnormal NEC O62.9
    clonic (complicating delivery) O62.4
    dyscoordinate (complicating delivery) O62.4
    hourglass (complicating delivery) O62.4
    hypertonic O62.4
    hypotonic NEC O62.2
    inadequate
      primary O62.0
      secondary O62.1
    incoordinate (complicating delivery) O62.4
    poor O62.2
    tetanic (complicating delivery) O62.4
  vagina (outlet) N89.5
  vesical N32.89
    neck or urethral orifice N32.0
  visual field — *see* Defect, visual field, generalized
  Volkmann's (ischemic) T79.6
Contusion (skin surface intact) T14.8
  abdomen, abdominal (muscle) (wall) S30.1
  adnexa, eye NEC S05.8X-
  adrenal gland S37.812
  alveolar process S00.532
  ankle S90.0-
  antecubital space — *see* Contusion, forearm
  anus S30.3
  arm (upper) S40.02-
    lower (with elbow) — *see* Contusion, forearm
  auditory canal — *see* Contusion, ear
  auricle — *see* Contusion, ear
  axilla — *see* Contusion, arm, upper
  back (*see also* Contusion, thorax, back)
    lower S30.0
  bile duct S36.13
  bladder S37.22
  bone NEC T14.8
  brain (diffuse) — *see* Injury, intracranial, diffuse
    focal — *see* Injury, intracranial, focal
  brainstem S06.38-
  breast S20.0-
  broad ligament S37.892
  brow S00.83
  buttock S30.0
  canthus, eye S00.1-
  cauda equina S34.3
  cerebellar, traumatic S06.37-
  cerebral S06.33-
    left side S06.32-
    right side S06.31-
  cheek S00.83
    internal S00.532
  chest (wall) — *see* Contusion, thorax
  chin S00.83
  clitoris S30.23
  colon — *see* Injury, intestine, large, contusion
  common bile duct S36.13
  conjunctiva S05.1-

Contusion — *continued*
  conjunctiva — *continued*
    with foreign body (in conjunctival sac) — *see* Foreign body, conjunctival sac
  conus medullaris (spine) S34.139
  cornea — *see* Contusion, eyeball
    with foreign body — *see* Foreign body, cornea
  corpus cavernosum S30.21
  cortex (brain) (cerebral) — *see* Injury, intracranial, diffuse
    focal — *see* Injury, intracranial, focal
  costal region — *see* Contusion, thorax
  cystic duct S36.13
  diaphragm S27.802
  duodenum S36.420
  ear S00.43-
  elbow S50.0-
    with forearm — *see* Contusion, forearm
  epididymis S30.22
  epigastric region S30.1
  epiglottis S10.0
  esophagus (thoracic) S27.812
    cervical S10.0
  eyeball S05.1-
  eyebrow S00.1-
  eyelid (and periocular area) S00.1-
  face NEC S00.83
  fallopian tube S37.529
    bilateral S37.522
    unilateral S37.521
  femoral triangle S30.1
  finger(s) S60.00
    with damage to nail (matrix) S60.10
    index S60.02-
      with damage to nail S60.12-
    little S60.05-
      with damage to nail S60.15-
    middle S60.03-
      with damage to nail S60.13-
    ring S60.04-
      with damage to nail S60.14-
    thumb — *see* Contusion, thumb
  flank S30.1
  foot (except toe(s) alone) S90.3-
    toe — *see* Contusion, toe
  forearm S50.1-
    elbow only — *see* Contusion, elbow
  forehead S00.83
  gallbladder S36.122
  genital organs, external
    female S30.202
    male S30.201
  globe (eye) — *see* Contusion, eyeball
  groin S30.1
  gum S00.532
  hand S60.22-
    finger(s) — *see* Contusion, finger
    wrist — *see* Contusion, wrist
  head S00.93
    ear — *see* Contusion, ear
    eyelid — *see* Contusion, eyelid
    lip S00.531
    nose S00.33
    oral cavity S00.532
    scalp S00.03
    specified part NEC S00.83
  heel — *see* Contusion, foot
  hepatic duct S36.13
  hip S70.0-
  ileum S36.428
  iliac region S30.1
  inguinal region S30.1
  interscapular region S20.229
  intra-abdominal organ S36.92
    colon — *see* Injury, intestine, large, contusion
    liver S36.112
    pancreas — *see* Contusion, pancreas
    rectum S36.62
    small intestine — *see* Injury, intestine, small, contusion
    specified organ NEC S36.892
    spleen — *see* Contusion, spleen
    stomach S36.32
  iris (eye) — *see* Contusion, eyeball
  jaw S00.83
  jejunum S36.428

Contusion — *continued*
  kidney S37.01-
    major (greater than 2 cm) S37.02-
    minor (less than 2 cm) S37.01-
  knee S80.0-
  labium (majus) (minus) S30.23
  lacrimal apparatus, gland or sac S05.8X-
  larynx S10.0
  leg (lower) S80.1-
    knee — *see* Contusion, knee
  lens — *see* Contusion, eyeball
  lip S00.531
  liver S36.112
  lower back S30.0
  lumbar region S30.0
  lung S27.329
    bilateral S27.322
    unilateral S27.321
  malar region S00.83
  mastoid region S00.83
  membrane, brain — *see* Injury, intracranial, diffuse
    focal — *see* Injury, intracranial, focal
  mesentery S36.892
  mesosalpinx S37.892
  mouth S00.532
  muscle — *see* Contusion, by site
  nail
    finger — *see* Contusion, finger, with damage to nail
    toe — *see* Contusion, toe, with damage to nail
  nasal S00.33
  neck S10.93
    specified site NEC S10.83
    throat S10.0
  nerve — *see* Injury, nerve
  newborn P54.5
  nose S00.33
  occipital
    lobe (brain) — *see* Injury, intracranial, diffuse
      focal — *see* Injury, intracranial, focal
    region (scalp) S00.03
  orbit (region) (tissues) S05.1-
  ovary S37.429
    bilateral S37.422
    unilateral S37.421
  palate S00.532
  pancreas S36.229
    body S36.221
    head S36.220
    tail S36.222
  parietal
    lobe (brain) — *see* Injury, intracranial, diffuse
      focal — *see* Injury, intracranial, focal
    region (scalp) S00.03
  pelvic organ S37.92
    adrenal gland S37.812
    bladder S37.22
    fallopian tube — *see* Contusion, fallopian tube
    kidney — *see* Contusion, kidney
    ovary — *see* Contusion, ovary
    prostate S37.822
    specified organ NEC S37.892
    ureter S37.12
    urethra S37.32
    uterus S37.62
  pelvis S30.0
  penis S30.21
  perineum
    female S30.23
    male S30.0
  periocular area S00.1-
  peritoneum S36.81
  periurethral tissue — *see* Contusion, urethra
  pharynx S10.0
  pinna — *see* Contusion, ear
  popliteal space — *see* Contusion, knee
  prepuce S30.21
  prostate S37.822
  pubic region S30.1
  pudendum
    female S30.202
    male S30.201
  quadriceps femoris — *see* Contusion, thigh
  rectum S36.62
  retroperitoneum S36.892
  round ligament S37.892

☑ **Additional Character Required** — **Refer to the Tabular List for Character Selection**   ▽ **Subterms under main terms may continue to next column or page**

Contusion — *continued*
  sacral region S30.0 ☑
  scalp S00.03 ☑
    due to birth injury P12.3
  scapular region — *see* Contusion, shoulder
  sclera — *see* Contusion, eyeball
  scrotum S30.22 ☑
  seminal vesicle S37.892 ☑
  shoulder S40.01- ☑
  skin NEC T14.8
  small intestine — *see* Injury, intestine, small, contusion
  spermatic cord S30.22 ☑
  spinal cord — *see* Injury, spinal cord, by region
    cauda equina S34.3 ☑
    conus medullaris S34.139 ☑
  spleen S36.029 ☑
    major S36.021 ☑
    minor S36.020 ☑
  sternal region S20.219 ☑
  stomach S36.32 ☑
  subconjunctival S05.1- ☑
  subcutaneous NEC T14.8
  submaxillary region S00.83 ☑
  submental region S00.83 ☑
  subperiosteal NEC T14.8
  subungual
    finger — *see* Contusion, finger, with damage to nail
    toe — *see* Contusion, toe, with damage to nail
  supraclavicular fossa S10.83 ☑
  supraorbital S00.83 ☑
  suprarenal gland S37.812 ☑
  temple (region) S00.83 ☑
  temporal
    lobe (brain) — *see* Injury, intracranial, diffuse
      focal — *see* Injury, intracranial, focal
    region S00.83 ☑
  testis S30.22 ☑
  thigh S70.1- ☑
  thorax (wall) S20.20 ☑
    back S20.22- ☑
    front S20.21- ☑
  throat S10.0 ☑
  thumb S60.01- ☑
    with damage to nail S60.11- ☑
  toe(s) (lesser) S90.12- ☑
    with damage to nail S90.22- ☑
    great S90.11- ☑
      with damage to nail S90.21- ☑
      specified type NEC S90.221 ☑
  tongue S00.532 ☑
  trachea (cervical) S10.0 ☑
    thoracic S27.52 ☑
  tunica vaginalis S30.22 ☑
  tympanum, tympanic membrane — *see* Contusion, ear
  ureter S37.12 ☑
  urethra S37.32 ☑
  urinary organ NEC S37.892 ☑
  uterus S37.62 ☑
  uvula S00.532 ☑
  vagina S30.23 ☑
  vas deferens S37.892 ☑
  vesical S37.22 ☑
  vocal cord(s) S10.0 ☑
  vulva S30.23 ☑
  wrist S60.21- ☑
Conus (congenital) (any type) Q14.8
  cornea — *see* Keratoconus
  medullaris syndrome G95.81
Conversion hysteria, neurosis or reaction F44.9
Converter, tuberculosis (test reaction) R76.11
Conviction (legal), **anxiety concerning** Z65.0
  with imprisonment Z65.1
Convulsions (idiopathic) (*see also* Seizure(s)) R56.9
  apoplectiform (cerebral ischemia) I67.82
  benign neonatal (familial) — *see* Epilepsy, generalized, idiopathic
  dissociative F44.5
  epileptic — *see* Epilepsy
  epileptiform, epileptoid — *see* Seizure, epileptiform
  ether (anesthetic) — *see* Table of Drugs and Chemicals, by drug
  febrile R56.00
    with status epilepticus G40.901
    complex R56.01

Convulsions — *continued*
  febrile — *continued*
    complex — *continued*
      with status epilepticus G40.901
    simple R56.00
  hysterical F44.5
  infantile P90
    epilepsy — *see* Epilepsy
  jacksonian — *see* Epilepsy, localization-related, symptomatic, with simple partial seizures
  myoclonic G25.3
  neonatal, benign (familial) — *see* Epilepsy, generalized, idiopathic
  newborn P90
  obstetrical (nephritic) (uremic) — *see* Eclampsia
  paretic A52.17
  post traumatic R56.1
  psychomotor — *see* Epilepsy, localization-related, symptomatic, with complex partial seizures
  recurrent R56.9
  reflex R25.8
  scarlatinal A38.8
  tetanus, tetanic — *see* Tetanus
  thymic E32.8
Convulsive (*see also* Convulsions)
Cooley's anemia D56.1
Coolie itch B76.9
Cooper's
  disease — *see* Mastopathy, cystic
  hernia — *see* Hernia, abdomen, specified site NEC
Copra itch B88.0
Coprophagy F50.8
Coprophobia F40.298
Coproporphyria, hereditary E80.29
Cor
  biloculare Q20.8
  bovis, bovinum — *see* Hypertrophy, cardiac
  pulmonale (chronic) I27.81
    acute I26.09
  triatriatum, triatrium Q24.2
  triloculare Q20.8
    biatrium Q20.4
    biventriculare Q21.1
Corbus' disease (gangrenous balanitis) N48.1
Cord (*see also* condition)
  around neck (tightly) (with compression) complicating delivery O69.1 ☑
  bladder G95.89
    tabetic A52.19
Cordis ectopia Q24.8
Corditis (spermatic) N49.1
Corectopia Q13.2
Cori's disease (glycogen storage) E74.03
Corkhandler's disease or lung J67.3
Corkscrew esophagus K22.4
Corkworker's disease or lung J67.3
Corn (infected) L84
Cornea (*see also* condition)
  donor Z52.5
  plana Q13.4
Cornelia de Lange syndrome Q87.1
Cornu cutaneum L85.8
Cornual gestation or pregnancy O00.8
Coronary (artery) — *see* condition
Coronavirus, as cause of disease classified elsewhere B97.29
  SARS-associated B97.21
Corpora (*see also* condition)
  amylacea, prostate N42.89
  cavernosa — *see* condition
Corpulence — *see* Obesity
Corpus — *see* condition
Corrected transposition Q20.5
Corrosion (injury) (acid) (caustic) (chemical) (lime) (external) (internal) T30.4
  abdomen, abdominal (muscle) (wall) T21.42 ☑
    first degree T21.52 ☑
    second degree T21.62 ☑
    third degree T21.72 ☑
  above elbow T22.439 ☑
    first degree T22.539 ☑
    left T22.432 ☑
      first degree T22.532 ☑
      second degree T22.632 ☑
      third degree T22.732 ☑
    right T22.431 ☑
      first degree T22.531 ☑

Corrosion — *continued*
  above elbow — *continued*
    right — *continued*
      second degree T22.631 ☑
      third degree T22.731 ☑
    second degree T22.639 ☑
    third degree T22.739 ☑
  alimentary tract NEC T28.7 ☑
  ankle T25.419 ☑
    first degree T25.519 ☑
    left T25.412 ☑
      first degree T25.512 ☑
      second degree T25.612 ☑
      third degree T25.712 ☑
    multiple with foot — *see* Corrosion, lower, limb, multiple, ankle and foot
    right T25.411 ☑
      first degree T25.511 ☑
      second degree T25.611 ☑
      third degree T25.711 ☑
    second degree T25.619 ☑
    third degree T25.719 ☑
  anus — *see* Corrosion, buttock
  arm(s) (meaning upper limb(s)) — *see* Corrosion, upper limb
  axilla T22.449 ☑
    first degree T22.549 ☑
    left T22.442 ☑
      first degree T22.542 ☑
      second degree T22.642 ☑
      third degree T22.742 ☑
    right T22.441 ☑
      first degree T22.541 ☑
      second degree T22.641 ☑
      third degree T22.741 ☑
    second degree T22.649 ☑
    third degree T22.749 ☑
  back (lower) T21.44 ☑
    first degree T21.54 ☑
    second degree T21.64 ☑
    third degree T21.74 ☑
    upper T21.43 ☑
      first degree T21.53 ☑
      second degree T21.63 ☑
      third degree T21.73 ☑
  blisters — *code as* Corrosion, second degree, by site
  breast(s) — *see* Corrosion, chest wall
  buttock(s) T21.45 ☑
    first degree T21.55 ☑
    second degree T21.65 ☑
    third degree T21.75 ☑
  calf T24.439 ☑
    first degree T24.539 ☑
    left T24.432 ☑
      first degree T24.532 ☑
      second degree T24.632 ☑
      third degree T24.732 ☑
    right T24.431 ☑
      first degree T24.531 ☑
      second degree T24.631 ☑
      third degree T24.731 ☑
    second degree T24.639 ☑
    third degree T24.739 ☑
  canthus (eye) — *see* Corrosion, eyelid
  cervix T28.8 ☑
  cheek T20.46 ☑
    first degree T20.56 ☑
    second degree T20.66 ☑
    third degree T20.76 ☑
  chest wall T21.41 ☑
    first degree T21.51 ☑
    second degree T21.61 ☑
    third degree T21.71 ☑
  chin T20.43 ☑
    first degree T20.53 ☑
    second degree T20.63 ☑
    third degree T20.73 ☑
  colon T28.7 ☑
  conjunctiva (and cornea) — *see* Corrosion, cornea
  cornea (and conjunctiva) T26.6- ☑
  deep necrosis of underlying tissue — *code as* Corrosion, third degree, by site
  dorsum of hand T23.469 ☑
    first degree T23.569 ☑
    left T23.462 ☑

Corrosion — *continued*
  interscapular region — *see* Corrosion, back, upper
  intestine (large) (small) T28.7 ☑
  knee T24.429 ☑
    first degree T24.529 ☑
    left T24.422 ☑
      first degree T24.522 ☑
      second degree T24.622 ☑
      third degree T24.722 ☑
    right T24.421 ☑
      first degree T24.521 ☑
      second degree T24.621 ☑
      third degree T24.721 ☑
    second degree T24.629 ☑
    third degree T24.729 ☑
  labium (majus) (minus) — *see* Corrosion, genital organs, external, female
  lacrimal apparatus, duct, gland or sac — *see* Corrosion, eye, specified site NEC
  larynx T27.4 ☑
    with lung T27.5 ☑
  leg(s) (meaning lower limb(s)) — *see* Corrosion, lower limb
  limb(s)
    lower — *see* Corrosion, lower, limb
    upper — *see* Corrosion, upper limb
  lip(s) T20.42 ☑
    first degree T20.52 ☑
    second degree T20.62 ☑
    third degree T20.72 ☑
  lower
    back — *see* Corrosion, back
    limb T24.409 ☑
      ankle — *see* Corrosion, ankle
      calf — *see* Corrosion, calf
      first degree T24.509 ☑
      foot — *see* Corrosion, foot
      knee — *see* Corrosion, knee
      left T24.402 ☑
        first degree T24.502 ☑
        second degree T24.602 ☑
        third degree T24.702 ☑
      multiple sites, except ankle and foot T24.499 ☑
        ankle and foot T25.499 ☑
          first degree T25.599 ☑
          left T25.492 ☑
            first degree T25.592 ☑
            second degree T25.692 ☑
            third degree T25.792 ☑
          right T25.491 ☑
            first degree T25.591 ☑
            second degree T25.691 ☑
            third degree T25.791 ☑
          second degree T25.699 ☑
          third degree T25.799 ☑
        first degree T24.599 ☑
        left T24.492 ☑
          first degree T24.592 ☑
          second degree T24.692 ☑
          third degree T24.792 ☑
        right T24.491 ☑
          first degree T24.591 ☑
          second degree T24.691 ☑
          third degree T24.791 ☑
        second degree T24.699 ☑
        third degree T24.799 ☑
      right T24.401 ☑
        first degree T24.501 ☑
        second degree T24.601 ☑
        third degree T24.701 ☑
      second degree T24.609 ☑
      thigh — *see* Corrosion, thigh
      third degree T24.709 ☑
  lung (with larynx and trachea) T27.5 ☑
  mouth T28.5 ☑
  neck T20.47 ☑
    first degree T20.57 ☑
    second degree T20.67 ☑
    third degree T20.77 ☑
  nose (septum) T20.44 ☑
    first degree T20.54 ☑
    second degree T20.64 ☑
    third degree T20.74 ☑
  ocular adnexa — *see* Corrosion, eye
  orbit region — *see* Corrosion, eyelid

Corrosion — *continued*
  palm T23.459 ☑
    first degree T23.559 ☑
    left T23.452 ☑
      first degree T23.552 ☑
      second degree T23.652 ☑
      third degree T23.752 ☑
    right T23.451 ☑
      first degree T23.551 ☑
      second degree T23.651 ☑
      third degree T23.751 ☑
    second degree T23.659 ☑
    third degree T23.759 ☑
  partial thickness — *code as* Corrosion, unspecified degree, by site
  pelvis — *see* Corrosion, trunk
  penis — *see* Corrosion, genital organs, external, male
  perineum
    female — *see* Corrosion, genital organs, external, female
    male — *see* Corrosion, genital organs, external, male
  periocular area — *see* Corrosion, eyelid
  pharynx T28.5 ☑
  rectum T28.7 ☑
  respiratory tract T27.7 ☑
    larynx — *see* Corrosion, larynx
    specified part NEC T27.6 ☑
    trachea — *see* Corrosion, larynx
  sac, lacrimal — *see* Corrosion, eye, specified site NEC
  scalp T20.45 ☑
    first degree T20.55 ☑
    second degree T20.65 ☑
    third degree T20.75 ☑
  scapular region T22.469 ☑
    first degree T22.569 ☑
    left T22.462 ☑
      first degree T22.562 ☑
      second degree T22.662 ☑
      third degree T22.762 ☑
    right T22.461 ☑
      first degree T22.561 ☑
      second degree T22.661 ☑
      third degree T22.761 ☑
    second degree T22.669 ☑
    third degree T22.769 ☑
  sclera — *see* Corrosion, eye, specified site NEC
  scrotum — *see* Corrosion, genital organs, external, male
  shoulder T22.459 ☑
    first degree T22.559 ☑
    left T22.452 ☑
      first degree T22.552 ☑
      second degree T22.652 ☑
      third degree T22.752 ☑
    right T22.451 ☑
      first degree T22.551 ☑
      second degree T22.651 ☑
      third degree T22.751 ☑
    second degree T22.659 ☑
    third degree T22.759 ☑
  stomach T28.7 ☑
  temple — *see* Corrosion, head
  testis — *see* Corrosion, genital organs, external, male
  thigh T24.419 ☑
    first degree T24.519 ☑
    left T24.412 ☑
      first degree T24.512 ☑
      second degree T24.612 ☑
      third degree T24.712 ☑
    right T24.411 ☑
      first degree T24.511 ☑
      second degree T24.611 ☑
      third degree T24.711 ☑
    second degree T24.619 ☑
    third degree T24.719 ☑
  thorax (external) — *see* Corrosion, trunk
  throat (meaning pharynx) T28.5 ☑
  thumb(s) T23.419 ☑
    first degree T23.519 ☑
    left T23.412 ☑
      first degree T23.512 ☑
      second degree T23.612 ☑
      third degree T23.712 ☑
    multiple sites with fingers T23.449 ☑

Corrosion — *continued*
  thumb(s) — *continued*
    multiple sites with fingers — *continued*
      first degree T23.549 ☑
      left T23.442 ☑
        first degree T23.542 ☑
        second degree T23.642 ☑
        third degree T23.742 ☑
      right T23.441 ☑
        first degree T23.541 ☑
        second degree T23.641 ☑
        third degree T23.741 ☑
      second degree T23.649 ☑
      third degree T23.749 ☑
    right T23.411 ☑
      first degree T23.511 ☑
      second degree T23.611 ☑
      third degree T23.711 ☑
    second degree T23.619 ☑
    third degree T23.719 ☑
  toe T25.439 ☑
    first degree T25.539 ☑
    left T25.432 ☑
      first degree T25.532 ☑
      second degree T25.632 ☑
      third degree T25.732 ☑
    right T25.431 ☑
      first degree T25.531 ☑
      second degree T25.631 ☑
      third degree T25.731 ☑
    second degree T25.639 ☑
    third degree T25.739 ☑
  tongue T28.5 ☑
  tonsil(s) T28.5 ☑
  total body — *see* Corrosion, multiple body regions
  trachea T27.4 ☑
    with lung T27.5 ☑
  trunk T21.40 ☑
    abdominal wall — *see* Corrosion, abdominal wall
    anus — *see* Corrosion, buttock
    axilla — *see* Corrosion, upper limb
    back — *see* Corrosion, back
    breast — *see* Corrosion, chest wall
    buttock — *see* Corrosion, buttock
    chest wall — *see* Corrosion, chest wall
    first degree T21.50 ☑
    flank — *see* Corrosion, abdominal wall
    genital
      female — *see* Corrosion, genital organs, external, female
      male — *see* Corrosion, genital organs, external, male
    groin — *see* Corrosion, abdominal wall
    interscapular region — *see* Corrosion, back, upper
    labia — *see* Corrosion, genital organs, external, female
    lower back — *see* Corrosion, back
    penis — *see* Corrosion, genital organs, external, male
    perineum
      female — *see* Corrosion, genital organs, external, female
      male — *see* Corrosion, genital organs, external, male
    scapular region — *see* Corrosion, upper limb
    scrotum — *see* Corrosion, genital organs, external, male
    second degree T21.60 ☑
    shoulder — *see* Corrosion, upper limb
    specified site NEC T21.49 ☑
      first degree T21.59 ☑
      second degree T21.69 ☑
      third degree T21.79 ☑
    testes — *see* Corrosion, genital organs, external, male
    third degree T21.70 ☑
    upper back — *see* Corrosion, back, upper
    vagina T28.8 ☑
    vulva — *see* Corrosion, genital organs, external, female
  unspecified site with extent of body surface involved specified
    less than 10 per cent T32.0 ☑
    10-19 per cent (0-9 percent third degree) T32.10 ☑
      with 10-19 percent third degree T32.11 ☑
    20-29 per cent (0-9 percent third degree) T32.20 ☑

Corrosion — *continued*
 unspecified site with extent of body surface involved
  specified — *continued*
   20-29 per cent — *continued*
    with
     10-19 percent third degree T32.21
     20-29 percent third degree T32.22
   30-39 per cent (0-9 percent third degree) T32.30
    with
     10-19 percent third degree T32.31
     20-29 percent third degree T32.32
     30-39 percent third degree T32.33
   40-49 per cent (0-9 percent third degree) T32.40
    with
     10-19 percent third degree T32.41
     20-29 percent third degree T32.42
     30-39 percent third degree T32.43
     40-49 percent third degree T32.44
   50-59 per cent (0-9 percent third degree) T32.50
    with
     10-19 percent third degree T32.51
     20-29 percent third degree T32.52
     30-39 percent third degree T32.53
     40-49 percent third degree T32.54
     50-59 percent third degree T32.55
   60-69 per cent (0-9 percent third degree) T32.60
    with
     10-19 percent third degree T32.61
     20-29 percent third degree T32.62
     30-39 percent third degree T32.63
     40-49 percent third degree T32.64
     50-59 percent third degree T32.65
     60-69 percent third degree T32.66
   70-79 per cent (0-9 percent third degree) T32.70
    with
     10-19 percent third degree T32.71
     20-29 percent third degree T32.72
     30-39 percent third degree T32.73
     40-49 percent third degree T32.74
     50-59 percent third degree T32.75
     60-69 percent third degree T32.76
     70-79 percent third degree T32.77
   80-89 per cent (0-9 percent third degree) T32.80
    with
     10-19 percent third degree T32.81
     20-29 percent third degree T32.82
     30-39 percent third degree T32.83
     40-49 percent third degree T32.84
     50-59 percent third degree T32.85
     60-69 percent third degree T32.86
     70-79 percent third degree T32.87
     80-89 percent third degree T32.88
   90 per cent or more (0-9 percent third degree)
    T32.90
    with
     10-19 percent third degree T32.91
     20-29 percent third degree T32.92
     30-39 percent third degree T32.93
     40-49 percent third degree T32.94
     50-59 percent third degree T32.95
     60-69 percent third degree T32.96
     70-79 percent third degree T32.97
     80-89 percent third degree T32.98
     90-99 percent third degree T32.99
 upper limb (axilla) (scapular region) T22.40 ☑
  above elbow — *see* Corrosion, above elbow
  axilla — *see* Corrosion, axilla
  elbow — *see* Corrosion, elbow
  first degree T22.50 ☑
  forearm — *see* Corrosion, forearm
  hand — *see* Corrosion, hand
  interscapular region — *see* Corrosion, back, upper
  multiple sites T22.499 ☑
   first degree T22.599 ☑
   left T22.492 ☑
    first degree T22.592 ☑
    second degree T22.692 ☑
    third degree T22.792 ☑
   right T22.491 ☑
    first degree T22.591 ☑
    second degree T22.691 ☑
    third degree T22.791 ☑
   second degree T22.699 ☑
   third degree T22.799 ☑
  scapular region — *see* Corrosion, scapular region
  second degree T22.60 ☑
  shoulder — *see* Corrosion, shoulder
  third degree T22.70 ☑

Corrosion — *continued*
 upper limb — *continued*
  wrist — *see* Corrosion, hand
 uterus T28.8 ☑
 vagina T28.8 ☑
 vulva — *see* Corrosion, genital organs, external, female
 wrist T23.479 ☑
  first degree T23.579 ☑
  left T23.472 ☑
   first degree T23.572 ☑
   second degree T23.672 ☑
   third degree T23.772 ☑
  multiple sites with hand T23.499 ☑
   first degree T23.599 ☑
   left T23.492 ☑
    first degree T23.592 ☑
    second degree T23.692 ☑
    third degree T23.792 ☑
   right T23.491 ☑
    first degree T23.591 ☑
    second degree T23.691 ☑
    third degree T23.791 ☑
   second degree T23.699 ☑
   third degree T23.799 ☑
  right T23.471 ☑
   first degree T23.571 ☑
   second degree T23.671 ☑
   third degree T23.771 ☑
  second degree T23.679 ☑
  third degree T23.779 ☑
Corrosive burn — *see* Corrosion
Corsican fever — *see* Malaria
Cortical — *see* condition
Cortico-adrenal — *see* condition
Coryza (acute) J00
 with grippe or influenza — *see* Influenza, with, respiratory manifestations NEC
 syphilitic
  congenital (chronic) A50.05
Costen's syndrome or complex M26.69
Costiveness — *see* Constipation
Costochondritis M94.0
Cot death R99
Cotard's syndrome F22
Cotia virus B08.8
Cotton wool spots (retinal) H35.81
Cotungo's disease — *see* Sciatica
Cough (affected) (chronic) (epidemic) (nervous) R05
 with hemorrhage — *see* Hemoptysis
 bronchial R05
  with grippe or influenza — *see* Influenza, with, respiratory manifestations NEC
 functional F45.8
 hysterical F45.8
 laryngeal, spasmodic R05
 psychogenic F45.8
 smokers' J41.0
 tea taster's B49
Counseling (for) Z71.9
 abuse NEC
  perpetrator Z69.82
  victim Z69.81
 alcohol abuser Z71.41
  family Z71.42
 child abuse
  nonparental
   perpetrator Z69.021
   victim Z69.020
  parental
   perpetrator Z69.011
   victim Z69.010
 consanguinity Z71.89
 contraceptive Z30.09
 dietary Z71.3
 drug abuser Z71.51
  family member Z71.52
 family Z71.89
 fertility preservation (prior to cancer therapy) (prior to removal of gonads) Z31.62
 for non-attending third party Z71.0
  related to sexual behavior or orientation Z70.2
 genetic NEC Z31.5
 health (advice) (education) (instruction) — *see* Counseling, medical
 human immunodeficiency virus (HIV) Z71.7
 impotence Z70.1
 insulin pump use Z46.81

Counseling — *continued*
 medical (for) Z71.9
  boarding school resident Z59.3
  consanguinity Z71.89
  feared complaint and no disease found Z71.1
  human immunodeficiency virus (HIV) Z71.7
  institutional resident Z59.3
  on behalf of another Z71.0
   related to sexual behavior or orientation Z70.2
  person living alone Z60.2
  specified reason NEC Z71.89
 natural family planning
  procreative Z31.61
  to avoid pregnancy Z30.02
 perpetrator (of)
  abuse NEC Z69.82
  child abuse
   non-parental Z69.021
   parental Z69.011
  rape NEC Z69.82
  spousal abuse Z69.12
 procreative NEC Z31.69
  fertility preservation (prior to cancer therapy) (prior to removal of gonads) Z31.62
  using natural family planning Z31.61
 promiscuity Z70.1
 rape victim Z69.81
 religious Z71.81
 sex, sexual (related to) Z70.9
  attitude(s) Z70.0
  behavior or orientation Z70.1
  combined concerns Z70.3
  non-responsiveness Z70.1
  on behalf of third party Z70.2
  specified reason NEC Z70.8
 specified reason NEC Z71.89
 spiritual Z71.81
 spousal abuse (perpetrator) Z69.12
  victim Z69.11
 substance abuse Z71.89
  alcohol Z71.41
  drug Z71.51
  tobacco Z71.6
 tobacco use Z71.6
 use (of)
  insulin pump Z46.81
 victim (of)
  abuse Z69.81
  child abuse
   by parent Z69.010
   non-parental Z69.020
  rape NEC Z69.81
Coupled rhythm R00.8
Couvelaire syndrome or uterus (complicating delivery) O45.8X- ☑
Cowperitis — *see* Urethritis
Cowper's gland — *see* condition
Cowpox B08.010
 due to vaccination T88.1 ☑
Coxa
 magna M91.4- ☑
 plana M91.2- ☑
 valga (acquired) (*see also* Deformity, limb, specified type NEC, thigh)
  congenital Q65.81
  sequelae (late effect) of rickets E64.3
 vara (acquired) (*see also* Deformity, limb, specified type NEC, thigh)
  congenital Q65.82
  sequelae (late effect) of rickets E64.3
Coxalgia, coxalgic (nontuberculous) (*see also* Pain, joint, hip)
 tuberculous A18.02
Coxitis — *see* Monoarthritis, hip
Coxsackie (virus) (infection) B34.1
 as cause of disease classified elsewhere B97.11
 carditis B33.20
 central nervous system NEC A88.8
 endocarditis B33.21
 enteritis A08.39
 meningitis (aseptic) A87.0
 myocarditis B33.22
 pericarditis B33.23
 pharyngitis B08.5
 pleurodynia B33.0
 specific disease NEC B33.8
Crabs, meaning pubic lice B85.3
Crack baby P04.41

☑ **Additional Character Required** — Refer to the Tabular List for Character Selection   ▽ **Subterms under main terms may continue to next column or page**

Cracked nipple N64.0
  associated with
    lactation O92.13
    pregnancy O92.11- ☑
    puerperium O92.12
Cracked tooth K03.81
Cradle cap L21.0
Craft neurosis F48.8
Cramp(s) R25.2
  abdominal — *see* Pain, abdominal
  bathing T75.1 ☑
  colic R10.83
    psychogenic F45.8
  due to immersion T75.1 ☑
  fireman T67.2 ☑
  heat T67.2 ☑
  immersion T75.1 ☑
  intestinal — *see* Pain, abdominal
    psychogenic F45.8
  leg, sleep related G47.62
  limb (lower) (upper) NEC R25.2
    sleep related G47.62
  linotypist's F48.8
    organic G25.89
  muscle (limb) (general) R25.2
    due to immersion T75.1 ☑
    psychogenic F45.8
  occupational (hand) F48.8
    organic G25.89
  salt-depletion E87.1
  sleep related, leg G47.62
  stoker's T67.2 ☑
  swimmer's T75.1 ☑
  telegrapher's F48.8
    organic G25.89
  typist's F48.8
    organic G25.89
  uterus N94.89
    menstrual — *see* Dysmenorrhea
  writer's F48.8
    organic G25.89
Cranial — *see* condition
Craniocleidodysostosis Q74.0
Craniofenestria (skull) Q75.8
Craniolacunia (skull) Q75.8
Craniopagus Q89.4
Craniopathy, metabolic M85.2
Craniopharyngeal — *see* condition
Craniopharyngioma D44.4
Craniorachischisis (totalis) Q00.1
Cranioschisis Q75.8
Craniostenosis Q75.0
Craniosynostosis Q75.0
Craniotabes (cause unknown) M83.8
  neonatal P96.3
  rachitic E64.3
  syphilitic A50.56
Cranium — *see* condition
Craw-craw — *see* Onchocerciasis
Creaking joint — *see* Derangement, joint, specified type
    NEC
Creeping
  eruption B76.9
  palsy or paralysis G12.22
Crenated tongue K14.8
Creotoxism A05.9
Crepitus
  caput Q75.8
  joint — *see* Derangement, joint, specified type NEC
Crescent or conus choroid, congenital Q14.3
CREST syndrome M34.1
Cretin, cretinism (congenital) (endemic) (nongoitrous)
    (sporadic) E00.9
  pelvis
    with disproportion (fetopelvic) O33.0
      causing obstructed labor O65.0
  type
    hypothyroid E00.1
    mixed E00.2
    myxedematous E00.1
    neurological E00.0
Creutzfeldt-Jakob disease or syndrome (with demen-
    tia) A81.00
  familial A81.09
  iatrogenic A81.09
  specified NEC A81.09
  sporadic A81.09

Creutzfeldt-Jakob disease or syndrome —
  continued
  variant (vCJD) A81.01
Cri-du-chat syndrome Q93.4
Crib death R99
Cribriform hymen Q52.3
Crigler-Najjar disease or syndrome E80.5
Crime, victim of Z65.4
Crimean hemorrhagic fever A98.0
Criminalism F60.2
Crisis
  abdomen R10.0
  acute reaction F43.0
  addisonian E27.2
  adrenal (cortical) E27.2
  celiac K90.0
  Dietl's N13.8
  emotional (*see also* Disorder, adjustment)
    acute reaction to stress F43.0
    specific to childhood and adolescence F93.8
  glaucomatocyclitic — *see* Glaucoma, secondary, in-
    flammation
  heart — *see* Failure, heart
  nitritoid I95.2
    correct substance properly administered — *see*
      Table of Drugs and Chemicals, by drug, ad-
      verse effect
    overdose or wrong substance given or taken —
      see Table of Drugs and Chemicals, by drug,
      poisoning
  oculogyric H51.8
    psychogenic F45.8
  Pel's (tabetic) A52.11
  psychosexual identity F64.2
  renal N28.0
  sickle-cell D57.00
    with
      acute chest syndrome D57.01
      splenic sequestration D57.02
  state (acute reaction) F43.0
  tabetic A52.11
  thyroid — *see* Thyrotoxicosis with thyroid storm
  thyrotoxic — *see* Thyrotoxicosis with thyroid storm
Crocq's disease (acrocyanosis) I73.89
Crohn's disease — *see* Enteritis, regional
Crooked septum, nasal J34.2
Cross syndrome E70.328
Cross-eye — *see* Strabismus, convergent concomitant
Crossbite (anterior) (posterior) M26.24
Croup, croupous (catarrhal) (infectious) (inflammatory)
    (nondiphtheritic) J05.0
  bronchial J20.9
  diphtheritic A36.2
  false J38.5
  spasmodic J38.5
    diphtheritic A36.2
  stridulous J38.5
    diphtheritic A36.2
Crouzon's disease Q75.1
Crowding, tooth, teeth, fully erupted M26.31
CRST syndrome M34.1
Cruchet's disease A85.8
Cruelty in children (*see also* Disorder, conduct)
Crural ulcer — *see* Ulcer, lower limb
Crush, crushed, crushing T14.8
  abdomen S38.1 ☑
  ankle S97.0- ☑
  arm (upper) (and shoulder) S47.- ☑
  axilla — *see* Crush, arm
  back, lower S38.1 ☑
  buttock S38.1 ☑
  cheek S07.0 ☑
  chest S28.0 ☑
  cranium S07.1 ☑
  ear S07.0 ☑
  elbow S57.0- ☑
  extremity
    lower
      ankle — *see* Crush, ankle
      below knee — *see* Crush, leg
      foot — *see* Crush, foot
      hip — *see* Crush, hip
      knee — *see* Crush, knee
      thigh — *see* Crush, thigh
      toe — *see* Crush, toe
    upper
      below elbow S67.9- ☑

Crush, crushed, crushing — *continued*
  extremity — *continued*
    upper — *continued*
      elbow — *see* Crush, elbow
      finger — *see* Crush, finger
      forearm — *see* Crush, forearm
      hand — *see* Crush, hand
      thumb — *see* Crush, thumb
      upper arm — *see* Crush, arm
      wrist — *see* Crush, wrist
  face S07.0 ☑
  finger(s) S67.1- ☑
    with hand (and wrist) — *see* Crush, hand, specified
      site NEC
    index S67.19- ☑
    little S67.19- ☑
    middle S67.19- ☑
    ring S67.19- ☑
    thumb — *see* Crush, thumb
  foot S97.8- ☑
    toe — *see* Crush, toe
  forearm S57.8- ☑
  genitalia, external
    female S38.002 ☑
      vagina S38.03 ☑
      vulva S38.03 ☑
    male S38.001 ☑
      penis S38.01 ☑
      scrotum S38.02 ☑
      testis S38.02 ☑
  hand (except fingers alone) S67.2- ☑
    with wrist S67.4- ☑
  head S07.9 ☑
    specified NEC S07.8 ☑
  heel — *see* Crush, foot
  hip S77.0- ☑
    with thigh S77.2- ☑
  internal organ (abdomen, chest, or pelvis) NEC T14.8
  knee S87.0- ☑
  labium (majus) (minus) S38.03 ☑
  larynx S17.0 ☑
  leg (lower) S87.8- ☑
    knee — *see* Crush, knee
  lip S07.0 ☑
  lower
    back S38.1 ☑
    leg — *see* Crush, leg
  neck S17.9 ☑
  nerve — *see* Injury, nerve
  nose S07.0 ☑
  pelvis S38.1 ☑
  penis S38.01 ☑
  scalp S07.8 ☑
  scapular region — *see* Crush, arm
  scrotum S38.02 ☑
  severe, unspecified site T14.8
  shoulder (and upper arm) — *see* Crush, arm
  skull S07.1 ☑
  syndrome (complication of trauma) T79.5 ☑
  testis S38.02 ☑
  thigh S77.1- ☑
    with hip S77.2- ☑
  throat S17.8 ☑
  thumb S67.0- ☑
    with hand (and wrist) — *see* Crush, hand, specified
      site NEC
  toe(s) S97.10- ☑
    great S97.11- ☑
    lesser S97.12- ☑
  trachea S17.8 ☑
  vagina S38.03 ☑
  vulva S38.03 ☑
  wrist S67.3- ☑
    with hand S67.4- ☑
Crusta lactea L21.0
Crusts R23.4
Crutch paralysis — *see* Injury, brachial plexus
**Cruveilhier-Baumgarten cirrhosis, disease or syn-
    drome** K74.69
Cruveilhier's atrophy or disease G12.8
Crying (constant) (continuous) (excessive)
  child, adolescent, or adult R45.83
  infant (baby) (newborn) R68.11
Cryofibrinogenemia D89.2
Cryoglobulinemia (essential) (idiopathic) (mixed) (pri-
    mary) (purpura) (secondary) (vasculitis) D89.1

Cryoglobulinemia — *continued*
  with lung involvement D89.1 [J99]
Cryptitis (anal) (rectal) K62.89
Cryptococcosis, cryptococcus (infection) (neoformans) B45.9
  bone B45.3
  cerebral B45.1
  cutaneous B45.2
  disseminated B45.7
  generalized B45.7
  meningitis B45.1
  meningocerebralis B45.1
  osseous B45.3
  pulmonary B45.0
  skin B45.2
  specified NEC B45.8
Cryptopapillitis (anus) K62.89
Cryptophthalmos Q11.2
  syndrome Q87.0
Cryptorchid, cryptorchism, cryptorchidism Q53.9
  bilateral Q53.20
    abdominal Q53.21
    perineal Q53.22
  unilateral Q53.10
    abdominal Q53.11
    perineal Q53.12
Cryptosporidiosis A07.2
  hepatobiliary B88.8
  respiratory B88.8
Cryptostromosis J67.6
Crystalluria R82.99
Cubitus
  congenital Q68.8
  valgus (acquired) M21.0- ☑
    congenital Q68.8
    sequelae (late effect) of rickets E64.3
  varus (acquired) M21.1- ☑
    congenital Q68.8
    sequelae (late effect) of rickets E64.3
Cultural deprivation or shock Z60.3
Curling esophagus K22.4
Curling's ulcer — *see* Ulcer, peptic, acute
Curschmann (-Batten) (-Steinert) **disease or syndrome** G71.11
Curse, Ondine's — *see* Apnea, sleep
Curvature
  organ or site, congenital NEC — *see* Distortion
  penis (lateral) Q55.61
  Pott's (spinal) A18.01
  radius, idiopathic, progressive (congenital) Q74.0
  spine (acquired) (angular) (idiopathic) (incorrect) (postural) — *see* Dorsopathy, deforming
    congenital Q67.5
    due to or associated with
      Charcot-Marie-Tooth disease (*see also* subcategory M49.8) G60.0
      osteitis
        deformans M88.88
        fibrosa cystica (*see also* subcategory M49.8) E21.0
      tuberculosis (Pott's curvature) A18.01
    sequelae (late effect) of rickets E64.3
    tuberculous A18.01
Cushingoid due to steroid therapy E24.2
  correct substance properly administered — *see* Table of Drugs and Chemicals, by drug, adverse effect
  overdose or wrong substance given or taken — *see* Table of Drugs and Chemicals, by drug, poisoning
Cushing's
  syndrome or disease E24.9
    drug-induced E24.2
    iatrogenic E24.2
    pituitary-dependent E24.0
    specified NEC E24.8
  ulcer — *see* Ulcer, peptic, acute
Cusp, Carabelli — *omit code*
Cut (external) (*see also* Laceration)
  muscle — *see* Injury, muscle
Cutaneous (*see also* condition)
  hemorrhage R23.3
  larva migrans B76.9
Cutis (*see also* condition)
  hyperelastica Q82.8
    acquired L57.4
  laxa (hyperelastica) — *see* Dermatolysis
  marmorata R23.8

Cutis — *continued*
  osteosis L94.2
  pendula — *see* Dermatolysis
  rhomboidalis nuchae L57.2
  verticis gyrata Q82.8
    acquired L91.8
Cyanosis R23.0
  due to
    patent foramen botalli Q21.1
    persistent foramen ovale Q21.1
  enterogenous D74.8
  paroxysmal digital — *see* Raynaud's disease
    with gangrene I73.01
  retina, retinal H35.89
Cyanotic heart disease I24.9
  congenital Q24.9
Cycle
  anovulatory N97.0
  menstrual, irregular N92.6
Cyclencephaly Q04.9
Cyclical vomiting (*see also* Vomiting, cyclical) G43.A0 (following G43.7)
  psychogenic F50.8
Cyclitis (*see also* Iridocyclitis) H20.9
  chronic — *see* Iridocyclitis, chronic
  Fuchs' heterochromic H20.81- ☑
  granulomatous — *see* Iridocyclitis, chronic
  lens-induced — *see* Iridocyclitis, lens-induced
  posterior H30.2- ☑
Cycloid personality F34.0
Cyclophoria H50.54
Cyclopia, cyclops Q87.0
Cyclopism Q87.0
Cyclosporiasis A07.4
Cyclothymia F34.0
Cyclothymic personality F34.0
Cyclotropia H50.41- ☑
Cylindroma (*see also* Neoplasm, malignant, by site)
  eccrine dermal — *see* Neoplasm, skin, benign
  skin — *see* Neoplasm, skin, benign
Cylindruria R82.99
Cynanche
  diphtheritic A36.2
  tonsillaris J36
Cynophobia F40.218
Cynorexia R63.2
Cyphosis — *see* Kyphosis
Cyprus fever — *see* Brucellosis
Cyst (colloid) (mucous) (simple) (retention)
  adenoid (infected) J35.8
  adrenal gland E27.8
    congenital Q89.1
  air, lung J98.4
  allantoic Q64.4
  alveolar process (jaw bone) M27.40
  amnion, amniotic O41.8X- ☑
  anterior
    chamber (eye) — *see* Cyst, iris
    nasopalatine K09.1
  antrum J34.1
  anus K62.89
  apical (tooth) (periodontal) K04.8
  appendix K38.8
  arachnoid, brain (acquired) G93.0
    congenital Q04.6
  arytenoid J38.7
  Baker's M71.2- ☑
    ruptured M66.0
    tuberculous A18.02
  Bartholin's gland N75.0
  bile duct (common) (hepatic) K83.5
  bladder (multiple) (trigone) N32.89
  blue dome (breast) — *see* Cyst, breast
  bone (local) NEC M85.60
    aneurysmal M85.50
      ankle M85.57- ☑
      foot M85.57- ☑
      forearm M85.53- ☑
      hand M85.54- ☑
      jaw M27.49
      lower leg M85.56- ☑
      multiple site M85.59
      neck M85.58
      rib M85.58
      shoulder M85.51- ☑
      skull M85.58
      specified site NEC M85.58

Cyst — *continued*
  bone — *continued*
    aneurysmal — *continued*
      thigh M85.55- ☑
      toe M85.57- ☑
      upper arm M85.52- ☑
      vertebra M85.58
    solitary M85.40
      ankle M85.47- ☑
      fibula M85.46- ☑
      foot M85.47- ☑
      hand M85.44- ☑
      humerus M85.42- ☑
      jaw M27.49
      neck M85.48
      pelvis M85.45- ☑
      radius M85.43- ☑
      rib M85.48
      shoulder M85.41- ☑
      skull M85.48
      specified site NEC M85.48
      tibia M85.46- ☑
      toe M85.47- ☑
      ulna M85.43- ☑
      vertebra M85.48
    specified type NEC M85.60
      ankle M85.67- ☑
      foot M85.67- ☑
      forearm M85.63- ☑
      hand M85.64- ☑
      jaw M27.40
        developmental (nonodontogenic) K09.1
        odontogenic K09.0
        latent M27.0
      lower leg M85.66- ☑
      multiple site M85.69
      neck M85.68
      rib M85.68
      shoulder M85.61- ☑
      skull M85.68
      specified site NEC M85.68
      thigh M85.65- ☑
      toe M85.67- ☑
      upper arm M85.62- ☑
      vertebra M85.68
  brain (acquired) G93.0
    congenital Q04.6
    hydatid B67.99 [G94]
    third ventricle (colloid), congenital Q04.6
  branchial (cleft) Q18.0
  branchiogenic Q18.0
  breast (benign) (blue dome) (pedunculated) (solitary) N60.0- ☑
    involution — *see* Dysplasia, mammary, specified type NEC
    sebaceous — *see* Dysplasia, mammary, specified type NEC
  broad ligament (benign) N83.8
  bronchogenic (mediastinal) (sequestration) J98.4
    congenital Q33.0
  buccal K09.8
  bulbourethral gland N36.8
  bursa, bursal NEC M71.30
    with rupture — *see* Rupture, synovium
    ankle M71.37- ☑
    elbow M71.32- ☑
    foot M71.37- ☑
    hand M71.34- ☑
    hip M71.35- ☑
    multiple sites M71.39
    pharyngeal J39.2
    popliteal space — *see* Cyst, Baker's
    shoulder M71.31- ☑
    specified site NEC M71.38
    wrist M71.33- ☑
  calcifying odontogenic D16.5
    upper jaw (bone) (maxilla) D16.4
  canal of Nuck (female) N94.89
    congenital Q52.4
  canthus — *see* Cyst, conjunctiva
  carcinomatous — *see* Neoplasm, malignant, by site
  cauda equina G95.89
  cavum septi pellucidi — *see* Cyst, brain
  celomic (pericardium) Q24.8
  cerebellopontine (angle) — *see* Cyst, brain
  cerebellum — *see* Cyst, brain
  cerebral — *see* Cyst, brain

☑ **Additional Character Required — Refer to the Tabular List for Character Selection**   ▽ **Subterms under main terms may continue to next column or page**

Cyst — *continued*
  cervical lateral Q18.1
  cervix NEC N88.8
    embryonic Q51.6
    nabothian N88.8
  chiasmal optic NEC — *see* Disorder, optic, chiasm
  chocolate (ovary) N80.1
  choledochus, congenital Q44.4
  chorion O41.8X- ☑
  choroid plexus G93.0
  ciliary body — *see* Cyst, iris
  clitoris N90.7
  colon K63.89
  common (bile) duct K83.5
  congenital NEC Q89.8
    adrenal gland Q89.1
    epiglottis Q31.8
    esophagus Q39.8
    fallopian tube Q50.4
    kidney Q61.00
      more than one (multiple) Q61.02
        specified as polycystic Q61.3
          adult type Q61.2
          infantile type NEC Q61.19
            collecting duct dilation Q61.11
      solitary Q61.01
    larynx Q31.8
    liver Q44.6
    lung Q33.0
    mediastinum Q34.1
    ovary Q50.1
    oviduct Q50.4
    periurethral (tissue) Q64.79
    prepuce Q55.69
    salivary gland (any) Q38.4
    sublingual Q38.6
    submaxillary gland Q38.6
    thymus (gland) Q89.2
    tongue Q38.3
    ureterovesical orifice Q62.8
    vulva Q52.79
  conjunctiva H11.44- ☑
  cornea H18.89- ☑
  corpora quadrigemina G93.0
  corpus
    albicans N83.29
    luteum (hemorrhagic) (ruptured) N83.1
  Cowper's gland (benign) (infected) N36.8
  cranial meninges G93.0
  craniobuccal pouch E23.6
  craniopharyngeal pouch E23.6
  cystic duct K82.8
  Cysticercus — *see* Cysticercosis
  Dandy-Walker Q03.1
    with spina bifida — *see* Spina bifida
  dental (root) K04.8
    developmental K09.0
    eruption K09.0
    primordial K09.0
  dentigerous (mandible) (maxilla) K09.0
  dermoid — *see* Neoplasm, benign, by site
    with malignant transformation C56.- ☑
    implantation
      external area or site (skin) NEC L72.0
      iris — *see* Cyst, iris, implantation
      vagina N89.8
      vulva N90.7
    mouth K09.8
    oral soft tissue K09.8
    sacrococcygeal — *see* Cyst, pilonidal
  developmental K09.1
    odontogenic K09.0
    oral region (nonodontogenic) K09.1
    ovary, ovarian Q50.1
  dura (cerebral) G93.0
    spinal G96.19
  ear (external) Q18.1
  echinococcal — *see* Echinococcus
  embryonic
    cervix uteri Q51.6
    fallopian tube Q50.4
    vagina Q51.6
  endometrium, endometrial (uterus) N85.8
    ectopic — *see* Endometriosis
  enterogenous Q43.8
  epidermal, epidermoid (inclusion) (*see also* Cyst, skin)
    L72.0
    mouth K09.8

Cyst — *continued*
  epidermal, epidermoid (*see also* Cyst, skin) — *continued*
    oral soft tissue K09.8
  epididymis N50.3
  epiglottis J38.7
  epiphysis cerebri E34.8
  epithelial (inclusion) L72.0
  epoophoron Q50.5
  eruption K09.0
  esophagus K22.8
  ethmoid sinus J34.1
  external female genital organs NEC N90.7
  eyelid (sebaceous) H02.829
    infected — *see* Hordeolum
    left H02.826
      lower H02.825
      upper H02.824
    right H02.823
      lower H02.822
      upper H02.821
  eye NEC H57.8
    congenital Q15.8
  fallopian tube N83.8
    congenital Q50.4
  fimbrial (twisted) Q50.4
  fissural (oral region) K09.1
  follicle (graafian) (hemorrhagic) N83.0
    nabothian N88.8
  follicular (atretic) (hemorrhagic) (ovarian) N83.0
    dentigerous K09.0
    odontogenic K09.0
    skin L72.9
      specified NEC L72.8
  frontal sinus J34.1
  gallbladder K82.8
  ganglion — *see* Ganglion
  Gartner's duct Q52.4
  gingiva K09.0
  gland of Moll — *see* Cyst, eyelid
  globulomaxillary K09.1
  graafian follicle (hemorrhagic) N83.0
  granulosal lutein (hemorrhagic) N83.1
  hemangiomatous D18.00
    intra-abdominal D18.03
    intracranial D18.02
    skin D18.01
    specified site NEC D18.09
  hydatid (*see also* Echinococcus) B67.90
    brain B67.99 [G94]
    liver (*see also* Cyst, liver, hydatid) B67.8
    lung NEC B67.99 [J99]
    Morgagni
      female Q50.5
      male (epididymal) Q55.4
        testicular Q55.29
    specified site NEC B67.99
  hymen N89.8
    embryonic Q52.4
  hypopharynx J39.2
  hypophysis, hypophyseal (duct) (recurrent) E23.6
    cerebri E23.6
  implantation (dermoid)
    external area or site (skin) NEC L72.0
    iris — *see* Cyst, iris, implantation
    vagina N89.8
    vulva N90.7
  incisive canal K09.1
  inclusion (epidermal) (epithelial) (epidermoid) (squamous) L72.0
    not of skin — *code under* Cyst, by site
  intestine (large) (small) K63.89
  intracranial — *see* Cyst, brain
  intraligamentous (*see also* Disorder, ligament)
    knee — *see* Derangement, knee
  intrasellar E23.6
  iris H21.309
    exudative H21.31- ☑
    idiopathic H21.30- ☑
    implantation H21.32- ☑
    parasitic H21.33- ☑
    pars plana (primary) H21.34- ☑
      exudative H21.35- ☑
  jaw (bone) M27.40
    aneurysmal M27.49
    developmental (odontogenic) K09.0
    fissural K09.1
    hemorrhagic M27.49

Cyst — *continued*
  jaw — *continued*
    traumatic M27.49
  joint NEC — *see* Disorder, joint, specified type NEC
  kidney (acquired) N28.1
    calyceal — *see* Hydronephrosis
    congenital Q61.00
    more than one (multiple) Q61.02
      specified as polycystic Q61.3
        adult type (autosomal dominant) Q61.2
        infantile type (autosomal recessive) NEC
          Q61.19
          collecting duct dilation Q61.11
    pyelogenic — *see* Hydronephrosis
    simple N28.1
    solitary (single) Q61.01
      acquired N28.1
  labium (majus) (minus) N90.7
    sebaceous N90.7
  lacrimal (*see also* Disorder, lacrimal system, specified
    NEC)
    gland H04.13- ☑
    passages or sac — *see* Disorder, lacrimal system,
      specified NEC
  larynx J38.7
  lateral periodontal K09.0
  lens H27.8
    congenital Q12.8
  lip (gland) K13.0
  liver (idiopathic) (simple) K76.89
    congenital Q44.6
    hydatid B67.8
      granulosus B67.0
      multilocularis B67.5
  lung J98.4
    congenital Q33.0
    giant bullous J43.9
  lutein N83.1
  lymphangiomatous D18.1
  lymphoepithelial, oral soft tissue K09.8
  macula — *see* Degeneration, macula, hole
  malignant — *see* Neoplasm, malignant, by site
  mammary gland — *see* Cyst, breast
  mandible M27.40
    dentigerous K09.0
    radicular K04.8
  maxilla M27.40
    dentigerous K09.0
    radicular K04.8
  medial, face and neck Q18.8
  median
    anterior maxillary K09.1
    palatal K09.1
  mediastinum, congenital Q34.1
  meibomian (gland) — *see* Chalazion
    infected — *see* Hordeolum
  membrane, brain G93.0
  meninges (cerebral) G93.0
    spinal G96.19
  meniscus, knee — *see* Derangement, knee, meniscus,
    cystic
  mesentery, mesenteric K66.8
    chyle I89.8
  mesonephric duct
    female Q50.5
    male Q55.4
  milk N64.89
  Morgagni (hydatid)
    female Q50.5
    male (epididymal) Q55.4
      testicular Q55.29
  mouth K09.8
  Müllerian duct Q50.4
    appendix testis Q55.29
    cervix Q51.6
    fallopian tube Q50.4
    female Q50.4
    male Q55.29
    prostatic utricle Q55.4
    vagina (embryonal) Q52.4
  multilocular (ovary) D39.10
    benign — *see* Neoplasm, benign, by site
  myometrium N85.8
  nabothian (follicle) (ruptured) N88.8
  nasoalveolar K09.1
  nasolabial K09.1
  nasopalatine (anterior) (duct) K09.1
  nasopharynx J39.2

Cyst — continued
- neoplastic — see Neoplasm, uncertain behavior, by site
  - benign — see Neoplasm, benign, by site
- nervous system NEC G96.8
- neuroenteric (congenital) Q06.8
- nipple — see Cyst, breast
- nose (turbinates) J34.1
  - sinus J34.1
- odontogenic, developmental K09.0
- omentum (lesser) K66.8
  - congenital Q45.8
- ora serrata — see Cyst, retina, ora serrata
- oral
  - region K09.9
    - developmental (nonodontogenic) K09.1
    - specified NEC K09.8
  - soft tissue K09.9
    - specified NEC K09.8
- orbit H05.81- ☑
- ovary, ovarian (twisted) N83.20
  - adherent N83.20
  - chocolate N80.1
  - corpus
    - albicans N83.29
    - luteum (hemorrhagic) N83.1
  - dermoid D27.9
  - developmental Q50.1
  - due to failure of involution NEC N83.20
  - endometrial N80.1
  - follicular (graafian) (hemorrhagic) N83.0
  - hemorrhagic N83.20
  - in pregnancy or childbirth O34.8- ☑
    - with obstructed labor O65.5
  - multilocular D39.10
  - pseudomucinous D27.9
  - retention N83.29
  - serous N83.29
  - specified NEC N83.29
  - theca lutein (hemorrhagic) N83.1
  - tuberculous A18.18
- oviduct N83.8
- palate (median) (fissural) K09.1
- palatine papilla (jaw) K09.1
- pancreas, pancreatic (hemorrhagic) (true) K86.2
  - congenital Q45.2
  - false K86.3
- paralabral
  - hip M24.85- ☑
  - shoulder S43.43- ☑
- paramesonephric duct Q50.4
  - female Q50.4
  - male Q55.29
- paranephric N28.1
- paraphysis, cerebri, congenital Q04.6
- parasitic B89
- parathyroid (gland) E21.4
- paratubal N83.8
- paraurethral duct N36.8
- paroophoron Q50.5
- parotid gland K11.6
- parovarian Q50.5
- pelvis, female N94.89
  - in pregnancy or childbirth O34.8- ☑
    - causing obstructed labor O65.5
- penis (sebaceous) N48.89
- periapical K04.8
- pericardial (congenital) Q24.8
  - acquired (secondary) I31.8
- pericoronal K09.0
- periodontal K04.8
  - lateral K09.0
- peripelvic (lymphatic) N28.1
- peritoneum K66.8
  - chylous I89.8
- periventricular, acquired, newborn P91.1
- pharynx (wall) J39.2
- pilar L72.11
- pilonidal (infected) (rectum) L05.91
  - with abscess L05.01
  - malignant C44.59- ☑
- pituitary (duct) (gland) E23.6
- placenta O43.19- ☑
- pleura J94.8
- popliteal — see Cyst, Baker's
- porencephalic Q04.6
  - acquired G93.0
- postanal (infected) — see Cyst, pilonidal

Cyst — continued
- postmastoidectomy cavity (mucosal) — see Complications, postmastoidectomy, cyst
- preauricular Q18.1
- prepuce N47.4
  - congenital Q55.69
- primordial (jaw) K09.0
- prostate N42.83
- pseudomucinous (ovary) D27.9
- pupillary, miotic H21.27- ☑
- radicular (residual) K04.8
- radiculodental K04.8
- ranular K11.8
- Rathke's pouch E23.6
- rectum (epithelium) (mucous) K62.89
- renal — see Cyst, kidney
- residual (radicular) K04.8
- retention (ovary) N83.29
  - salivary gland K11.6
- retina H33.19- ☑
  - ora serrata H33.11- ☑
  - parasitic H33.12- ☑
- retroperitoneal K68.9
- sacrococcygeal (dermoid) — see Cyst, pilonidal
- salivary gland or duct (mucous extravasation or retention) K11.6
- Sampson's N80.1
- sclera H15.89
- scrotum L72.9
  - sebaceous L72.3
- sebaceous (duct) (gland) L72.3
  - breast — see Dysplasia, mammary, specified type NEC
  - eyelid — see Cyst, eyelid
  - genital organ NEC
    - female N94.89
    - male N50.8
  - scrotum L72.3
- semilunar cartilage (knee) (multiple) — see Derangement, knee, meniscus, cystic
- seminal vesicle N50.8
- serous (ovary) N83.20
- sinus (accessory) (nasal) J34.1
- Skene's gland N36.8
- skin L72.9
  - breast — see Dysplasia, mammary, specified type NEC
  - epidermal, epidermoid L72.0
  - epithelial L72.0
  - eyelid — see Cyst, eyelid
  - genital organ NEC
    - female N90.7
    - male N50.8
  - inclusion L72.0
  - scrotum L72.9
  - sebaceous L72.3
  - sweat gland or duct L74.8
- solitary
  - bone — see Cyst, bone, solitary
  - jaw M27.40
  - kidney N28.1
- spermatic cord N50.8
- sphenoid sinus J34.1
- spinal meninges G96.19
- spleen NEC D73.4
  - congenital Q89.09
  - hydatid (see also Echinococcus) B67.99 [D77]
- Stafne's M27.0
- subarachnoid intrasellar R93.0
- subcutaneous, pheomycotic (chromomycotic) B43.2
- subdural (cerebral) G93.0
  - spinal cord G96.19
- sublingual gland K11.6
- submandibular gland K11.6
- submaxillary gland K11.6
- suburethral N36.8
- suprarenal gland E27.8
- suprasellar — see Cyst, brain
- sweat gland or duct L74.8
- synovial (see also Cyst, bursa)
  - ruptured — see Rupture, synovium
- tarsal — see Chalazion
- tendon (sheath) — see Disorder, tendon, specified type NEC
- testis N44.2
  - tunica albuginea N44.1
- theca lutein (ovary) N83.1
- Thornwaldt's J39.2

Cyst — continued
- thymus (gland) E32.8
- thyroglossal duct (infected) (persistent) Q89.2
- thyroid (gland) E04.1
- thyrolingual duct (infected) (persistent) Q89.2
- tongue K14.8
- tonsil J35.8
- tooth — see Cyst, dental
- Tornwaldt's J39.2
- trichilemmal (proliferating) L72.12
- trichodermal L72.12
- tubal (fallopian) N83.8
  - inflammatory — see Salpingitis, chronic
- tubo-ovarian N83.8
  - inflammatory N70.13
- tunica
  - albuginea testis N44.1
  - vaginalis N50.8
- turbinate (nose) J34.1
- Tyson's gland N48.89
- urachus, congenital Q64.4
- ureter N28.89
- ureterovesical orifice N28.89
- urethra, urethral (gland) N36.8
- uterine ligament N83.8
- uterus (body) (corpus) (recurrent) N85.8
  - embryonic Q51.818
    - cervix Q51.6
- vagina, vaginal (implantation) (inclusion) (squamous cell) (wall) N89.8
  - embryonic Q52.4
- vallecula, vallecular (epiglottis) J38.7
- vesical (orifice) N32.89
- vitreous body H43.89
- vulva (implantation) (inclusion) N90.7
  - congenital Q52.79
  - sebaceous gland N90.7
- vulvovaginal gland N90.7
- wolffian
  - female Q50.5
  - male Q55.4

Cystadenocarcinoma — see Neoplasm, malignant, by site
- bile duct C22.1
- endometrioid — see Neoplasm, malignant, by site
  - specified site — see Neoplasm, malignant, by site
  - unspecified site
    - female C56.9
    - male C61
- mucinous
  - papillary
    - specified site — see Neoplasm, malignant, by site
    - unspecified site C56.9
  - specified site — see Neoplasm, malignant, by site
  - unspecified site C56.9
- papillary
  - mucinous
    - specified site — see Neoplasm, malignant, by site
    - unspecified site C56.9
  - pseudomucinous
    - specified site — see Neoplasm, malignant, by site
    - unspecified site C56.9
  - serous
    - specified site — see Neoplasm, malignant, by site
    - unspecified site C56.9
  - specified site — see Neoplasm, malignant, by site
  - unspecified site C56.9
- pseudomucinous
  - papillary
    - specified site — see Neoplasm, malignant, by site
    - unspecified site C56.9
  - specified site — see Neoplasm, malignant, by site
  - unspecified site C56.9
- serous
  - papillary
    - specified site — see Neoplasm, malignant, by site
    - unspecified site C56.9
  - specified site — see Neoplasm, malignant, by site
  - unspecified site C56.9

Cystadenofibroma
- clear cell — see Neoplasm, benign, by site
- endometrioid D27.9

Cystadenofibroma — *continued*
  endometrioid — *continued*
    borderline malignancy D39.1- ☑
    malignant C56.- ☑
  mucinous
    specified site — *see* Neoplasm, benign, by site
    unspecified site D27.9
  serous
    specified site — *see* Neoplasm, benign, by site
    unspecified site D27.9
  specified site — *see* Neoplasm, benign, by site
  unspecified site D27.9
Cystadenoma (*see also* Neoplasm, benign, by site)
  bile duct D13.4
  endometrioid — *see* Neoplasm, benign, by site
    borderline malignancy — *see* Neoplasm, uncertain behavior, by site
  malignant — *see* Neoplasm, malignant, by site
  mucinous
    borderline malignancy
      ovary C56.- ☑
      specified site NEC — *see* Neoplasm, uncertain behavior, by site
      unspecified site C56.9
    papillary
      borderline malignancy
        ovary C56.- ☑
        specified site NEC — *see* Neoplasm, uncertain behavior, by site
        unspecified site C56.9
      specified site — *see* Neoplasm, benign, by site
      unspecified site D27.9
    specified site — *see* Neoplasm, benign, by site
    unspecified site D27.9
  papillary
    borderline malignancy
      ovary C56.- ☑
      specified site NEC — *see* Neoplasm, uncertain behavior, by site
      unspecified site C56.9
    lymphomatosum
      specified site — *see* Neoplasm, benign, by site
      unspecified site D11.9
    mucinous
      borderline malignancy
        ovary C56.- ☑
        specified site NEC — *see* Neoplasm, uncertain behavior, by site
        unspecified site C56.9
      specified site — *see* Neoplasm, benign, by site
      unspecified site D27.9
    pseudomucinous
      borderline malignancy
        ovary C56.- ☑
        specified site NEC — *see* Neoplasm, uncertain behavior, by site
        unspecified site C56.9
      specified site — *see* Neoplasm, benign, by site
      unspecified site D27.9
    serous
      borderline malignancy
        ovary C56.- ☑
        specified site NEC — *see* Neoplasm, uncertain behavior, by site
        unspecified site C56.9
      specified site — *see* Neoplasm, benign, by site
      unspecified site D27.9
  pseudomucinous
    borderline malignancy
      ovary C56.- ☑
      specified site NEC — *see* Neoplasm, uncertain behavior, by site
      unspecified site C56.9
    papillary
      borderline malignancy
        ovary C56.- ☑
        specified site NEC — *see* Neoplasm, uncertain behavior, by site
        unspecified site C56.9
      specified site — *see* Neoplasm, benign, by site
      unspecified site D27.9
    specified site — *see* Neoplasm, benign, by site

Cystadenoma — *continued*
  pseudomucinous — *continued*
    unspecified site D27.9
  serous
    borderline malignancy
      ovary C56.- ☑
      specified site NEC — *see* Neoplasm, uncertain behavior, by site
      unspecified site C56.9
    papillary
      borderline malignancy
        ovary C56.- ☑
        specified site NEC — *see* Neoplasm, uncertain behavior, by site
        unspecified site C56.9
      specified site — *see* Neoplasm, benign, by site
      unspecified site D27.9
    specified site — *see* Neoplasm, benign, by site
    unspecified site D27.9
Cystathionine synthase deficiency E72.11
Cystathioninemia E72.19
Cystathioninuria E72.19
Cystic (*see also* condition)
  breast (chronic) — *see* Mastopathy, cystic
  corpora lutea (hemorrhagic) N83.1
  duct — *see* condition
  eyeball (congenital) Q11.0
  fibrosis — *see* Fibrosis, cystic
  kidney (congenital) Q61.9
    adult type Q61.2
    infantile type NEC Q61.19
      collecting duct dilatation Q61.11
    medullary Q61.5
  liver, congenital Q44.6
  lung disease J98.4
    congenital Q33.0
  mastitis, chronic — *see* Mastopathy, cystic
  medullary, kidney Q61.5
  meniscus — *see* Derangement, knee, meniscus, cystic
  ovary N83.20
Cysticercosis, cysticerciasis B69.9
  with
    epileptiform fits B69.0
    myositis B69.81
  brain B69.0
  central nervous system B69.0
  cerebral B69.0
  ocular B69.1
  specified NEC B69.89
Cysticercus cellulose infestation — *see* Cysticercosis
Cystinosis (malignant) E72.04
Cystinuria E72.01
Cystitis (exudative) (hemorrhagic) (septic) (suppurative) N30.90
  with
    fibrosis — *see* Cystitis, chronic, interstitial
    hematuria N30.91
    leukoplakia — *see* Cystitis, chronic, interstitial
    malakoplakia — *see* Cystitis, chronic, interstitial
    metaplasia — *see* Cystitis, chronic, interstitial
    prostatitis N41.3
  acute N30.00
    with hematuria N30.01
    of trigone N30.30
      with hematuria N30.31
  allergic — *see* Cystitis, specified type NEC
  amebic A06.81
  bilharzial B65.9 [N33]
  blennorrhagic (gonococcal) A54.01
  bullous — *see* Cystitis, specified type NEC
  calculous N21.0
  chlamydial A56.01
  chronic N30.20
    with hematuria N30.21
    interstitial N30.10
      with hematuria N30.11
    of trigone N30.30
      with hematuria N30.31
    specified NEC N30.20
      with hematuria N30.21
  cystic (a) — *see* Cystitis, specified type NEC
  diphtheritic A36.85
  echinococcal
    granulosus B67.39

Cystitis — *continued*
  echinococcal — *continued*
    multilocularis B67.69
  emphysematous — *see* Cystitis, specified type NEC
  encysted — *see* Cystitis, specified type NEC
  eosinophilic — *see* Cystitis, specified type NEC
  follicular — *see* Cystitis, of trigone
  gangrenous — *see* Cystitis, specified type NEC
  glandularis — *see* Cystitis, specified type NEC
  gonococcal A54.01
  incrusted — *see* Cystitis, specified type NEC
  interstitial (chronic) — *see* Cystitis, chronic, interstitial
  irradiation N30.40
    with hematuria N30.41
  irritation — *see* Cystitis, specified type NEC
  malignant — *see* Cystitis, specified type NEC
  of trigone N30.30
    with hematuria N30.31
  panmural — *see* Cystitis, chronic, interstitial
  polyposa — *see* Cystitis, specified type NEC
  prostatic N41.3
  puerperal (postpartum) O86.22
  radiation — *see* Cystitis, irradiation
  specified type NEC N30.80
    with hematuria N30.81
  subacute — *see* Cystitis, chronic
  submucous — *see* Cystitis, chronic, interstitial
  syphilitic (late) A52.76
  trichomonal A59.03
  tuberculous A18.12
  ulcerative — *see* Cystitis, chronic, interstitial
Cystocele (-urethrocele)
  female N81.10
    with prolapse of uterus — *see* Prolapse, uterus
    lateral N81.12
    midline N81.11
    paravaginal N81.12
  in pregnancy or childbirth O34.8- ☑
    causing obstructed labor O65.5
  male N32.89
Cystolithiasis N21.0
Cystoma (*see also* Neoplasm, benign, by site)
  endometrial, ovary N80.1
  mucinous
    specified site — *see* Neoplasm, benign, by site
    unspecified site D27.9
  serous
    specified site — *see* Neoplasm, benign, by site
    unspecified site D27.9
  simple (ovary) N83.29
Cystoplegia N31.2
Cystoptosis N32.89
Cystopyelitis — *see* Pyelonephritis
Cystorrhagia N32.89
Cystosarcoma phyllodes D48.6- ☑
  benign D24- ☑
  malignant — *see* Neoplasm, breast, malignant
Cystostomy
  attention to Z43.5
  complication — *see* Complications, cystostomy
  status Z93.50
    appendico-vesicostomy Z93.52
    cutaneous Z93.51
    specified NEC Z93.59
Cystourethritis — *see* Urethritis
Cystourethrocele (*see also* Cystocele)
  female N81.10
    with uterine prolapse — *see* Prolapse, uterus
    lateral N81.12
    midline N81.11
    paravaginal N81.12
  male N32.89
Cytomegalic inclusion disease
  congenital P35.1
Cytomegalovirus infection B25.9
Cytomycosis (reticuloendothelial) B39.4
Cytopenia D75.9
  refractory
    with multilineage dysplasia D46.A (*following* D46.2)
      and ring sideroblasts (RCMD RS) D46.B (*following* D46.2)
Czerny's disease (periodic hydrarthrosis of the knee) — *see* Effusion, joint, knee

D

d-glycericacidemia E72.59
Da Costa's syndrome F45.8
Daae (-Finsen) **disease** (epidemic pleurodynia) B33.0
Dabney's grip B33.0
Dacryoadenitis, dacryadenitis H04.00- ☑
  acute H04.01- ☑
  chronic H04.02- ☑
Dacryocystitis H04.30- ☑
  acute H04.32- ☑
  chronic H04.41- ☑
  neonatal P39.1
  phlegmonous H04.31- ☑
  syphilitic A52.71
    congenital (early) A50.01
  trachomatous, active A71.1
    sequelae (late effect) B94.0
Dacryocystoblenorrhea — see Inflammation, lacrimal, passages, chronic
Dacryocystocele — see Disorder, lacrimal system, changes
Dacryolith, dacryolithiasis H04.51- ☑
Dacryoma — see Disorder, lacrimal system, changes
Dacryopericystitis — see Dacryocystitis
Dacryops H04.11- ☑
Dacryostenosis (see also Stenosis, lacrimal)
  congenital Q10.5
Dactylitis
  bone — see Osteomyelitis
  sickle-cell D57.00
    Hb C D57.219
    Hb SS D57.00
    specified NEC D57.819
  skin L08.9
  syphilitic A52.77
  tuberculous A18.03
Dactylolysis spontanea (ainhum) L94.6
Dactylosymphysis Q70.9
  fingers — see Syndactylism, complex, fingers
  toes — see Syndactylism, complex, toes
Damage
  arteriosclerotic — see Arteriosclerosis
  brain (nontraumatic) G93.9
    anoxic, hypoxic G93.1
      resulting from a procedure G97.82
    child NEC G80.9
    due to birth injury P11.2
  cardiorenal (vascular) — see Hypertension, cardiorenal
  cerebral NEC — see Damage, brain
  coccyx, complicating delivery O71.6
  coronary — see Disease, heart, ischemic
  eye, birth injury P15.3
  liver (nontraumatic) K76.9
    alcoholic K70.9
    due to drugs — see Disease, liver, toxic
    toxic — see Disease, liver, toxic
  medication T88.7 ☑
  pelvic
    joint or ligament, during delivery O71.6
    organ NEC
      during delivery O71.5
      following ectopic or molar pregnancy O08.6
  renal — see Disease, renal
  subendocardium, subendocardial — see Degeneration, myocardial
  vascular I99.9
Dana-Putnam syndrome (subacute combined sclerosis with pernicious anemia) — see Degeneration, combined
Danbolt (-Cross) **syndrome** (acrodermatitis enteropathica) E83.2
Dandruff L21.0
Dandy-Walker syndrome Q03.1
  with spina bifida — see Spina bifida
Danlos' syndrome Q79.6
Darier (-White) **disease** (congenital) Q82.8
  meaning erythema annulare centrifugum L53.1
Darier-Roussy sarcoid D86.3
Darling's disease or histoplasmosis B39.4

Darwin's tubercle Q17.8
Dawson's (inclusion body) **encephalitis** A81.1
De Beurmann (-Gougerot) **disease** B42.1
De la Tourette's syndrome F95.2
De Lange's syndrome Q87.1
De Morgan's spots (senile angiomas) I78.1
De Quervain's
  disease (tendon sheath) M65.4
  syndrome E34.51
  thyroiditis (subacute granulomatous thyroiditis) E06.1
De Toni-Fanconi (-Debré) **syndrome** E72.09
  with cystinosis E72.04
Dead
  fetus, retained (mother) O36.4 ☑
    early pregnancy O02.1
  labyrinth H83.2 ☑
  ovum, retained O02.0
Deaf nonspeaking NEC H91.3
Deafmutism (acquired) (congenital) NEC H91.3
  hysterical F44.6
  syphilitic, congenital (see also subcategory) H94.8 A50.09
Deafness (acquired) (complete) (hereditary) (partial) H91.9-
  with blue sclera and fragility of bone Q78.0
  auditory fatigue — see Deafness, specified type NEC
  aviation T70.0 ☑
    nerve injury — see Injury, nerve, acoustic, specified type NEC
  boilermaker's H83.3 ☑
  central — see Deafness, sensorineural
  conductive H90.2
    and sensorineural, mixed H90.8
      bilateral H90.6
    bilateral H90.0
    unilateral H90.1- ☑
  congenital H90.5
    with blue sclera and fragility of bone Q78.0
  due to toxic agents — see Deafness, ototoxic
  emotional (hysterical) F44.6
  functional (hysterical) F44.6
  high frequency H91.9- ☑
  hysterical F44.6
  low frequency H91.9- ☑
  mental R48.8
  mixed conductive and sensorineural H90.8
    bilateral H90.6
    unilateral H90.7- ☑
  nerve — see Deafness, sensorineural
  neural — see Deafness, sensorineural
  noise-induced (see also subcategory) H83.3 ☑
    nerve injury — see Injury, nerve, acoustic, specified type NEC
  nonspeaking H91.3
  ototoxic H91.0 ☑
  perceptive — see Deafness, sensorineural
  psychogenic (hysterical) F44.6
  sensorineural H90.5
    and conductive, mixed H90.8
      bilateral H90.6
    bilateral H90.3
    unilateral H90.4- ☑
  sensory — see Deafness, sensorineural
  specified type NEC H91.8 ☑
  sudden (idiopathic) H91.2- ☑
  syphilitic A52.15
  transient ischemic H93.01- ☑
  traumatic — see Injury, nerve, acoustic, specified type NEC
  word (developmental) H93.25
Death (cause unknown) (of) (unexplained) (unspecified cause) R99
  brain G93.82
  cardiac (sudden) (with successful resuscitation) — code to underlying disease
    family history of Z82.41
    personal history of Z86.74
  family member (assumed) Z63.4
Debility (chronic) (general) (nervous) R53.81
  congenital or neonatal NOS P96.9
  nervous R53.81
  old age R54

Debility — continued
  senile R54
Débove's disease (splenomegaly) R16.1
Decalcification
  bone — see Osteoporosis
  teeth K03.89
Decapsulation, kidney N28.89
Decay
  dental — see Caries, dental
  senile R54
  tooth, teeth — see Caries, dental
Deciduitis (acute)
  following ectopic or molar pregnancy O08.0
Decline (general) — see Debility
  cognitive, age-associated R41.81
Decompensation
  cardiac (acute) (chronic) — see Disease, heart
  cardiovascular — see Disease, cardiovascular
  heart — see Disease, heart
  hepatic — see Failure, hepatic
  myocardial (acute) (chronic) — see Disease, heart
  respiratory J98.8
Decompression sickness T70.3 ☑
Decrease (d)
  absolute neutrophile count — see Neutropenia
  blood
    platelets — see Thrombocytopenia
    pressure R03.1
      due to shock following
        injury T79.4 ☑
        operation T81.19 ☑
  estrogen E28.39
    postablative E89.40
      asymptomatic E89.40
      symptomatic E89.41
  fragility of erythrocytes D58.8
  function
    lipase (pancreatic) K90.3
    ovary in hypopituitarism E23.0
    parenchyma of pancreas K86.8
    pituitary (gland) (anterior) (lobe) E23.0
      posterior (lobe) E23.0
  functional activity R68.89
  glucose R73.09
  hematocrit R71.0
  hemoglobin R71.0
  leukocytes D72.819
    specified NEC D72.818
  libido R68.82
  lymphocytes D72.810
  platelets D69.6
  respiration, due to shock following injury T79.4 ☑
  sexual desire R68.82
  tear secretion NEC — see Syndrome, dry eye
  tolerance
    fat K90.4
    glucose R73.09
    pancreatic K90.3
    salt and water E87.8
  vision NEC H54.7
  white blood cell count D72.819
    specified NEC D72.818
Decubitus (ulcer) — see Ulcer, pressure, by site
  cervix N86
Deepening acetabulum — see Derangement, joint, specified type NEC, hip
Defect, defective Q89.9
  3-beta-hydroxysteroid dehydrogenase E25.0
  11-hydroxylase E25.0
  21-hydroxylase E25.0
  abdominal wall, congenital Q79.59
  antibody immunodeficiency D80.9
  aorticopulmonary septum Q21.4
  atrial septal (ostium secundum type) Q21.1
    following acute myocardial infarction (current complication) I23.1
    ostium primum type Q21.2
  atrioventricular
    canal Q21.2
    septum Q21.2
  auricular septal Q21.1
  bilirubin excretion NEC E80.6

☑ **Additional Character Required** — Refer to the Tabular List for Character Selection   ⬇ **Subterms under main terms may continue to next column or page**

Defect, defective — *continued*
- biosynthesis, androgen (testicular) E29.1
- bulbar septum Q21.Ø
- catalase E8Ø.3
- cell membrane receptor complex (CR3) D71
- circulation I99.9
  - congenital Q28.9
  - newborn Q28.9
- coagulation (factor) (*see also* Deficiency, factor) D68.9
  - with
    - ectopic pregnancy OØ8.1
    - molar pregnancy OØ8.1
  - acquired D68.4
  - antepartum with hemorrhage — *see* Hemorrhage, antepartum, with coagulation defect
  - due to
    - liver disease D68.4
    - vitamin K deficiency D68.4
  - hereditary NEC D68.2
  - intrapartum O67.Ø
  - newborn, transient P61.6
  - postpartum O72.3
  - specified type NEC D68.8
- complement system D84.1
- conduction (heart) I45.9
  - bone — *see* Deafness, conductive
- congenital, organ or site not listed — *see* Anomaly, by site
- coronary sinus Q21.1
- cushion, endocardial Q21.2
- degradation, glycoprotein E77.1
- dental bridge, crown, fillings — *see* Defect, dental restoration
- dental restoration KØ8.5Ø
  - specified NEC KØ8.59
- dentin (hereditary) KØØ.5
- Descemet's membrane, congenital Q13.89
- developmental (*see also* Anomaly)
  - cauda equina QØ6.3
- diaphragm
  - with elevation, eventration or hernia — *see* Hernia, diaphragm
  - congenital Q79.1
    - with hernia Q79.Ø
    - gross (with hernia) Q79.Ø
- ectodermal, congenital Q82.9
- Eisenmenger's Q21.8
- enzyme
  - catalase E8Ø.3
  - peroxidase E8Ø.3
- esophagus, congenital Q39.9
- extensor retinaculum M62.89
- fibrin polymerization D68.2
- filling
  - bladder R93.4
  - kidney R93.4
  - stomach R93.3
  - ureter R93.4
- Gerbode Q21.Ø
- glycoprotein degradation E77.1
- Hageman (factor) D68.2
- hearing — *see* Deafness
- high grade F7Ø
- interatrial septal Q21.1
- interauricular septal Q21.1
- interventricular septal Q21.Ø
  - with dextroposition of aorta, pulmonary stenosis and hypertrophy of right ventricle Q21.3
  - in tetralogy of Fallot Q21.3
- learning (specific) — *see* Disorder, learning
- lymphocyte function antigen-1 (LFA-1) D84.Ø
- lysosomal enzyme, post-translational modification E77.Ø
- major osseous M89.7Ø
  - ankle M89.77- ☑
  - carpus M89.74- ☑
  - clavicle M89.71- ☑
  - femur M89.75- ☑
  - fibula M89.76- ☑
  - fingers M89.74- ☑
  - foot M89.77- ☑
  - forearm M89.73- ☑
  - hand M89.74- ☑
  - humerus M89.72- ☑
  - lower leg M89.76- ☑
  - metacarpus M89.74- ☑
  - metatarsus M89.77- ☑
  - multiple sites M89.79

Defect, defective — *continued*
- major osseous — *continued*
  - pelvic region M89.75- ☑
  - pelvis M89.75- ☑
  - radius M89.73- ☑
  - scapula M89.71- ☑
  - shoulder region M89.71- ☑
  - specified NEC M89.78
  - tarsus M89.77- ☑
  - thigh M89.75- ☑
  - tibia M89.76- ☑
  - toes M89.77- ☑
  - ulna M89.73- ☑
- mental — *see* Disability, intellectual
- modification, lysosomal enzymes, post-translational E77.Ø
- obstructive, congenital
  - renal pelvis Q62.39
  - ureter Q62.39
    - atresia — *see* Atresia, ureter
    - cecoureterocele Q62.32
    - megaureter Q62.2
    - orthotopic ureterocele Q62.31
- osseous, major M89.7Ø
  - ankle M89.77- ☑
  - carpus M89.74- ☑
  - clavicle M89.71- ☑
  - femur M89.75- ☑
  - fibula M89.76- ☑
  - fingers M89.74- ☑
  - foot M89.77- ☑
  - forearm M89.73- ☑
  - hand M89.74- ☑
  - humerus M89.72- ☑
  - lower leg M89.76- ☑
  - metacarpus M89.74- ☑
  - metatarsus M89.77- ☑
  - multiple sites M89.9
  - pelvic region M89.75- ☑
  - pelvis M89.75- ☑
  - radius M89.73- ☑
  - scapula M89.71- ☑
  - shoulder region M89.71- ☑
  - specified NEC M89.78
  - tarsus M89.77- ☑
  - thigh M89.75- ☑
  - tibia M89.76- ☑
  - toes M89.77- ☑
  - ulna M89.73- ☑
- osteochondral NEC (*see also* Deformity) M95.8-
- ostium
  - primum Q21.2
  - secundum Q21.1
- peroxidase E8Ø.3
- placental blood supply — *see* Insufficiency, placental
- platelets, qualitative D69.1
  - constitutional D68.Ø
- postural NEC, spine — *see* Dorsopathy, deforming
- reduction
  - limb Q73.8
    - lower Q72.9- ☑
      - absence — *see* Agenesis, leg
        - foot — *see* Agenesis, foot
      - longitudinal
        - femur Q72.4- ☑
        - fibula Q72.6- ☑
        - tibia Q72.5- ☑
      - specified type NEC Q72.89- ☑
      - split foot Q72.7- ☑
    - specified type NEC Q73.8
    - upper Q71.9- ☑
      - absence — *see* Agenesis, arm
        - forearm — *see* Agenesis, forearm
        - hand — *see* Agenesis, hand
      - lobster-claw hand Q71.6- ☑
      - longitudinal
        - radius Q71.4- ☑
        - ulna Q71.5- ☑
      - specified type NEC Q71.89- ☑
- renal pelvis Q63.8
  - obstructive Q62.39
- respiratory system, congenital Q34.9
- restoration, dental KØ8.5Ø
  - specified NEC KØ8.59
- retinal nerve bundle fibers H35.89
- septal (heart) NOS Q21.9

Defect, defective — *continued*
- septal — *continued*
  - acquired (atrial) (auricular) (ventricular) (old) I51.Ø
  - atrial Q21.1
    - concurrent with acute myocardial infarction — *see* Infarct, myocardium
    - following acute myocardial infarction (current complication) I23.1
    - ventricular (*see also* Defect, ventricular septal) Q21.Ø
  - sinus venosus Q21.1
- speech R47.9
  - developmental F8Ø.9
  - specified NEC R47.89
- Taussig-Bing (aortic transposition and overriding pulmonary artery) Q2Ø.1
- teeth, wedge KØ3.1
- vascular (local) I99.9
  - congenital Q27.9
- ventricular septal Q21.Ø
  - concurrent with acute myocardial infarction — *see* Infarct, myocardium
  - following acute myocardial infarction (current complication) I23.2
  - in tetralogy of Fallot Q21.3
- vision NEC H54.7
- visual field H53.4Ø
  - bilateral
    - heteronymous H53.47
    - homonymous H53.46- ☑
  - generalized contraction H53.48- ☑
  - localized
    - arcuate H53.43- ☑
    - scotoma (central area) H53.41- ☑
      - blind spot area H53.42- ☑
    - sector H53.43- ☑
    - specified type NEC H53.45- ☑
- voice R49.9
  - specified NEC R49.8
- wedge, tooth, teeth (abrasion) KØ3.1

Deferentitis N49.1
- gonorrheal (acute) (chronic) A54.23

Defibrination (syndrome) D65
- antepartum — *see* Hemorrhage, antepartum, with coagulation defect, disseminated intravascular coagulation
- following ectopic or molar pregnancy OØ8.1
- intrapartum O67.Ø
- newborn P6Ø
- postpartum O72.3

Deficiency, deficient
- 3-beta hydroxysteroid dehydrogenase E25.Ø
- 5-alpha reductase (with male pseudo-hermaphroditism) E29.1
- 11-hydroxylase E25.Ø
- 21-hydroxylase E25.Ø
- abdominal muscle syndrome Q79.4
- AC globulin (congenital) (hereditary) D68.2
  - acquired D68.4
- accelerator globulin (Ac G) (blood) D68.2
- acid phosphatase E83.39
- activating factor (blood) D68.2
- adenosine deaminase (ADA) D81.3
- aldolase (hereditary) E74.19
- alpha-1-antitrypsin E88.Ø1
- amino-acids E72.9
- anemia — *see* Anemia
- aneurin E51.9
- anti-hemophilic
  - factor (A) D66
    - B D67
    - C D68.1
  - globulin (AHG) NEC D66
- antibody with
  - hyperimmunoglobulinemia D8Ø.6
  - near-normal immunoglobins D8Ø.6
- antidiuretic hormone E23.2
- antithrombin (antithrombin III) D68.59
- ascorbic acid E54
- attention (disorder) (syndrome) F98.8
  - with hyperactivity — *see* Disorder, attention-deficit hyperactivity
- autoprothrombin
  - C D68.2
  - I D68.2
  - II D67
- beta-glucuronidase E76.29
- biotin E53.8

Deficiency, deficient — *continued*
- biotin-dependent carboxylase D81.819
- biotinidase D81.810
- brancher enzyme (amylopectinosis) E74.03
- C1 esterase inhibitor (C1-INH) D84.1
- calciferol E55.9
  - with
    - adult osteomalacia M83.8
    - rickets — *see* Rickets
- calcium (dietary) E58
- calorie, severe E43
  - with marasmus E41
    - and kwashiorkor E42
- cardiac — *see* Insufficiency, myocardial
- carnitine E71.40
  - due to
    - hemodialysis E71.43
    - inborn errors of metabolism E71.42
    - Valproic acid therapy E71.43
  - iatrogenic E71.43
  - muscle palmityltransferase E71.314
  - primary E71.41
  - secondary E71.448
- carotene E50.9
- central nervous system G96.8
- ceruloplasmin (Wilson) E83.01
- choline E53.8
- Christmas factor D67
- chromium E61.4
- clotting (blood) (*see also* Deficiency, coagulation factor) D68.9
- clotting factor NEC (hereditary) (*see also* Deficiency, factor) D68.2
- coagulation NOS D68.9
  - with
    - ectopic pregnancy O08.1
    - molar pregnancy O08.1
  - acquired (any) D68.4
  - antepartum hemorrhage — *see* Hemorrhage, antepartum, with coagulation defect
  - clotting factor NEC (*see also* Deficiency, factor) D68.2
  - due to
    - hyperprothrombinemia D68.4
    - liver disease D68.4
    - vitamin K deficiency D68.4
  - newborn, transient P61.6
  - postpartum O72.3
  - specified NEC D68.8
- cognitive F09
- color vision H53.50
  - achromatopsia H53.51
  - acquired H53.52
  - deuteranomaly H53.53
  - protanomaly H53.54
  - specified type NEC H53.59
  - tritanomaly H53.55
- combined glucocorticoid and mineralocorticoid E27.49
- contact factor D68.2
- copper (nutritional) E61.0
- corticoadrenal E27.40
  - primary E27.1
- craniofacial axis Q75.0
- cyanocobalamin E53.8
- debrancher enzyme (limit dextrinosis) E74.03
- dehydrogenase
  - long chain/very long chain acyl CoA E71.310
  - medium chain acyl CoA E71.311
  - short chain acyl CoA E71.312
- diet E63.9
- dihydropyrimidine dehydrogenase (DPD) E88.89
- disaccharidase E73.9
- edema — *see* Malnutrition, severe
- endocrine E34.9
- energy-supply — *see* Malnutrition
- enzymes, circulating NEC E88.09
- ergosterol E55.9
  - with
    - adult osteomalacia M83.8
    - rickets — *see* Rickets
- essential fatty acid (EFA) E63.0
- factor (*see also* Deficiency, coagulation)
  - Hageman D68.2
  - I (congenital) (hereditary) D68.2
  - II (congenital) (hereditary) D68.2
  - IX (congenital) (functional) (hereditary) (with functional defect) D67
  - multiple (congenital) D68.8

Deficiency, deficient — *continued*
- factor (*see also* Deficiency, coagulation) — *continued*
  - multiple — *continued*
    - acquired D68.4
    - V (congenital) (hereditary) D68.2
    - VII (congenital) (hereditary) D68.2
    - VIII (congenital) (functional) (hereditary) (with functional defect) D66
      - with vascular defect D68.0
    - X (congenital) (hereditary) D68.2
    - XI (congenital) (hereditary) D68.1
    - XII (congenital) (hereditary) D68.2
    - XIII (congenital) (hereditary) D68.2
  - femoral, proximal focal (congenital) — *see* Defect, reduction, lower limb, longitudinal, femur
- fibrin-stabilizing factor (congenital) (hereditary) D68.2
  - acquired D68.4
- fibrinase D68.2
- fibrinogen (congenital) (hereditary) D68.2
  - acquired D65
- folate E53.8
- folic acid E53.8
- foreskin N47.3
- fructokinase E74.11
- fructose 1,6-diphosphatase E74.19
- fructose-1-phosphate aldolase E74.19
- galactokinase E74.29
- galactose-1-phosphate uridyl transferase E74.29
- gammaglobulin in blood D80.1
  - hereditary D80.0
- glass factor D68.2
- glucocorticoid E27.49
  - mineralocorticoid E27.49
- glucose-6-phosphatase E74.01
- glucose-6-phosphate dehydrogenase anemia D55.0
- glucuronyl transferase E80.5
- glycogen synthetase E74.09
- gonadotropin (isolated) E23.0
- growth hormone (idiopathic) (isolated) E23.0
- Hageman factor D68.2
- hemoglobin D64.9
- hepatophosphorylase E74.09
- homogentisate 1,2-dioxygenase E70.29
- hormone
  - anterior pituitary (partial) NEC E23.0
    - growth E23.0
  - growth (isolated) E23.0
  - pituitary E23.0
  - testicular E29.1
- hypoxanthine- (guanine)-phosphoribosyltransferase (HG- PRT) (total H-PRT) E79.1
- immunity D84.9
  - cell-mediated D84.8
    - with thrombocytopenia and eczema D82.0
  - combined D81.9
  - humoral D80.9
  - IgA (secretory) D80.2
  - IgG D80.3
  - IgM D80.4
- immuno- — *see* Immunodeficiency
- immunoglobulin, selective
  - A (IgA) D80.2
  - G (IgG) (subclasses) D80.3
  - M (IgM) D80.4
- inositol (B complex) E53.8
- intrinsic
  - factor (congenital) D51.0
  - sphincter N36.42
    - with urethral hypermobility N36.43
- iodine E61.8
  - congenital syndrome — *see* Syndrome, iodine-deficiency, congenital
- iron E61.1
  - anemia D50.9
- kalium E87.6
- kappa-light chain D80.8
- labile factor (congenital) (hereditary) D68.2
  - acquired D68.4
- lacrimal fluid (acquired) (*see also* Syndrome, dry eye)
  - congenital Q10.6
- lactase
  - congenital E73.0
  - secondary E73.1
- Laki-Lorand factor D68.2
- lecithin cholesterol acyltransferase E78.6
- lipocaic K86.8
- lipoprotein (familial) (high density) E78.6

Deficiency, deficient — *continued*
- liver phosphorylase E74.09
- lysosomal alpha-1, 4 glucosidase E74.02
- magnesium E61.2
- major histocompatibility complex
  - class I D81.6
  - class II D81.7
- manganese E61.3
- menadione (vitamin K) E56.1
  - newborn P53
- mental (familial) (hereditary) — *see* Disability, intellectual
- methylenetetrahydrofolate reductase (MTHFR) E72.12
- mineralocorticoid E27.49
  - with glucocorticoid E27.49
- mineral NEC E61.8
- molybdenum (nutritional) E61.5
- moral F60.2
- multiple nutrient elements E61.7
- muscle
  - carnitine (palmityltransferase) E71.314
  - phosphofructokinase E74.09
- myoadenylate deaminase E79.2
- myocardial — *see* Insufficiency, myocardial
- myophosphorylase E74.04
- NADH diaphorase or reductase (congenital) D74.0
- NADH-methemoglobin reductase (congenital) D74.0
- natrium E87.1
- niacin (amide) (-tryptophan) E52
- nicotinamide E52
- nicotinic acid E52
- number of teeth — *see* Anodontia
- nutrient element E61.9
  - multiple E61.7
  - specified NEC E61.8
- nutrition, nutritional E63.9
  - sequelae — *see* Sequelae, nutritional deficiency
  - specified NEC E63.8
- ornithine transcarbamylase E72.4
- ovarian E28.39
- oxygen — *see* Anoxia
- pantothenic acid E53.8
- parathyroid (gland) E20.9
- perineum (female) N81.89
- phenylalanine hydroxylase E70.1
- phosphoenolpyruvate carboxykinase E74.4
- phosphofructokinase E74.19
- phosphomannomutuse E74.8
- phosphomannose isomerase E74.8
- phosphomannosyl mutase E74.8
- phosphorylase kinase, liver E74.09
- pituitary hormone (isolated) E23.0
- plasma thromboplastin
  - antecedent (PTA) D68.1
  - component (PTC) D67
- platelet NEC D69.1
  - constitutional D68.0
- polyglandular E31.8
  - autoimmune E31.0
- potassium (K) E87.6
- prepuce N47.3
- proaccelerin (congenital) (hereditary) D68.2
  - acquired D68.4
- proconvertin factor (congenital) (hereditary) D68.2
  - acquired D68.4
- protein (*see also* Malnutrition) E46
  - anemia D53.0
  - C D68.59
  - S D68.59
- prothrombin (congenital) (hereditary) D68.2
  - acquired D68.4
- Prower factor D68.2
- pseudocholinesterase E88.09
- PTA (plasma thromboplastin antecedent) D68.1
- PTC (plasma thromboplastin component) D67
- purine nucleoside phosphorylase (PNP) D81.5
- pyracin (alpha) (beta) E53.1
- pyridoxal E53.1
- pyridoxamine E53.1
- pyridoxine (derivatives) E53.1
- pyruvate
  - carboxylase E74.4
  - dehydrogenase E74.4
- riboflavin (vitamin B2) E53.0
- salt E87.1
- secretion
  - ovary E28.39
  - salivary gland (any) K11.7

☑ **Additional Character Required** — **Refer to the Tabular List for Character Selection** 🔺 Subterms under main terms may continue to next column or page

Deficiency, deficient — *continued*
  secretion — *continued*
    urine R34
  selenium (dietary) E59
  serum antitrypsin, familial E88.01
  short stature homeobox gene (SHOX)
    with
      dyschondrosteosis Q78.8
      short stature (idiopathic) E34.3
      Turner's syndrome Q96.9
  sodium (Na) E87.1
  SPCA (factor VII) D68.2
  sphincter, intrinsic N36.42
    with urethral hypermobility N36.43
  stable factor (congenital) (hereditary) D68.2
    acquired D68.4
  Stuart-Prower (factor X) D68.2
  sucrase E74.39
  sulfatase E75.29
  sulfite oxidase E72.19
  thiamin, thiaminic (chloride) E51.9
    beriberi (dry) E51.11
      wet E51.12
  thrombokinase D68.2
    newborn P53
  thyroid (gland) — *see* Hypothyroidism
  tocopherol E56.0
  tooth bud K00.0
  transcobalamine II (anemia) D51.2
  vanadium E61.6
  vascular I99.9
  vasopressin E23.2
  viosterol — *see* Deficiency, calciferol
  vitamin (multiple) NOS E56.9
    A E50.9
      with
        Bitot's spot (corneal) E50.1
        follicular keratosis E50.8
        keratomalacia E50.4
        manifestations NEC E50.8
        night blindness E50.5
        scar of cornea, xerophthalmic E50.6
        xeroderma E50.8
        xerophthalmia E50.7
        xerosis
          conjunctival E50.0
            and Bitot's spot E50.1
          cornea E50.2
            and ulceration E50.3
      sequelae E64.1
    B (complex) NOS E53.9
      with
        beriberi (dry) E51.11
          wet E51.12
        pellagra E52
    B1 NOS E51.9
      beriberi (dry) E51.11
        with circulatory system manifestations E51.11
        wet E51.12
    B2 (riboflavin) E53.0
    B6 E53.1
    B12 E53.8
    C E54
      sequelae E64.2
    D E55.9
      with
        adult osteomalacia M83.8
        rickets — *see* Rickets
      25-hydroxylase E83.32
    E E56.0
    folic acid E53.8
    G E53.0
    group B E53.9
      specified NEC E53.8
    H (biotin) E53.8
    K E56.1
      of newborn P53
    nicotinic E52
    P E56.8
    PP (pellagra-preventing) E52
    specified NEC E56.8
    thiamin E51.9
      beriberi — *see* Beriberi
  zinc, dietary E60

Deficit (*see also* Deficiency)
  attention and concentration R41.840
    disorder — *see* Attention, deficit

Deficit — *continued*
  cognitive communication R41.841
  cognitive NEC R41.89
    following
      cerebral infarction I69.31
      cerebrovascular disease I69.91
        specified disease NEC I69.81
      intracerebral hemorrhage I69.11
      nontraumatic intracranial hemorrhage NEC I69.21
      subarachnoid hemorrhage I69.01
  concentration R41.840
  executive function R41.844
  frontal lobe R41.844
  neurologic NEC R29.818
    ischemic
      reversible (RIND) I63.9
        prolonged (PRIND) I63.9
  oxygen R09.02
  prolonged reversible ischemic neurologic (PRIND) I63.9
  psychomotor R41.843
  visuospatial R41.842

Deflection
  radius — *see* Deformity, limb, specified type NEC, forearm
  septum (acquired) (nasal) (nose) J34.2
  spine — *see* Curvature, spine
  turbinate (nose) J34.2

Defluvium
  capillorum — *see* Alopecia
  ciliorum — *see* Madarosis
  unguium L60.8

Deformity Q89.9
  abdomen, congenital Q89.9
  abdominal wall
    acquired M95.8
    congenital Q79.59
  acquired (unspecified site) M95.9
  adrenal gland Q89.1
  alimentary tract, congenital Q45.9
    upper Q40.9
  ankle (joint) (acquired) (*see also* Deformity, limb, lower leg)
    abduction — *see* Contraction, joint, ankle
    congenital Q68.8
    contraction — *see* Contraction, joint, ankle
    specified type NEC — *see* Deformity, limb, foot, specified NEC
  anus (acquired) K62.89
    congenital Q43.9
  aorta (arch) (congenital) Q25.4
    acquired I77.89
  aortic
    arch, acquired I77.89
    cusp or valve (congenital) Q23.8
      acquired (*see also* Endocarditis, aortic) I35.8
  arm (acquired) (upper) (*see also* Deformity, limb, upper arm)
    congenital Q68.8
    forearm — *see* Deformity, limb, forearm
  artery (congenital) (peripheral) NOS Q27.9
    acquired I77.89
    coronary (acquired) I25.9
      congenital Q24.5
    umbilical Q27.0
  atrial septal Q21.1
  auditory canal (external) (congenital) (*see also* Malformation, ear, external)
    acquired — *see* Disorder, ear, external, specified type NEC
  auricle
    ear (congenital) (*see also* Malformation, ear, external)
      acquired — *see* Disorder, pinna, deformity
  back — *see* Dorsopathy, deforming
  bile duct (common) (congenital) (hepatic) Q44.5
    acquired K83.8
  biliary duct or passage (congenital) Q44.5
    acquired K83.8
  bladder (neck) (trigone) (sphincter) (acquired) N32.89
    congenital Q64.79
  bone (acquired) NOS M95.9
    congenital Q79.9
    turbinate M95.0
  brain (congenital) Q04.9
    acquired G93.89
    reduction Q04.3
  breast (acquired) N64.89

Deformity — *continued*
  breast — *continued*
    congenital Q83.9
    reconstructed N65.0
  bronchus (congenital) Q32.4
    acquired NEC J98.09
  bursa, congenital Q79.9
  canaliculi (lacrimalis) (acquired) (*see also* Disorder, lacrimal system, changes)
    congenital Q10.6
  canthus, acquired — *see* Disorder, eyelid, specified type NEC
  capillary (acquired) I78.8
  cardiovascular system, congenital Q28.9
  caruncle, lacrimal (acquired) (*see also* Disorder, lacrimal system, changes)
    congenital Q10.6
  cascade, stomach K31.2
  cecum (congenital) Q43.9
    acquired K63.89
  cerebral, acquired G93.89
    congenital Q04.9
  cervix (uterus) (acquired) NEC N88.8
    congenital Q51.9
  cheek (acquired) M95.2
    congenital Q18.9
  chest (acquired) (wall) M95.4
    congenital Q67.8
    sequelae (late effect) of rickets E64.3
  chin (acquired) M95.2
    congenital Q18.9
  choroid (congenital) Q14.3
    acquired H31.8
    plexus Q07.8
      acquired G96.19
  cicatricial — *see* Cicatrix
  cilia, acquired — *see* Disorder, eyelid, specified type NEC
  clavicle (acquired) M95.8
    congenital Q68.8
  clitoris (congenital) Q52.6
    acquired N90.89
  clubfoot — *see* Clubfoot
  coccyx (acquired) — *see* subcategory M43.8 ☑
  colon (congenital) Q43.9
    acquired K63.89
  concha (ear), congenital (*see also* Malformation, ear, external)
    acquired — *see* Disorder, pinna, deformity
  cornea (acquired) H18.70
    congenital Q13.4
    descemetocele — *see* Descemetocele
    ectasia — *see* Ectasia, cornea
    specified NEC H18.79- ☑
    staphyloma — *see* Staphyloma, cornea
  coronary artery (acquired) I25.9
    congenital Q24.5
  cranium (acquired) — *see* Deformity, skull
  cricoid cartilage (congenital) Q31.8
    acquired J38.7
  cystic duct (congenital) Q44.5
    acquired K82.8
  Dandy-Walker Q03.1
    with spina bifida — *see* Spina bifida
  diaphragm (congenital) Q79.1
    acquired J98.6
  digestive organ NOS Q45.9
  ductus arteriosus Q25.0
  duodenal bulb K31.89
  duodenum (congenital) Q43.9
    acquired K31.89
  dura — *see* Deformity, meninges
  ear (acquired) (*see also* Disorder, pinna, deformity)
    congenital (external) Q17.9
      internal Q16.5
      middle Q16.4
        ossicles Q16.3
      ossicles Q16.3
  ectodermal (congenital) NEC Q84.9
  ejaculatory duct (congenital) Q55.4
    acquired N50.8
  elbow (joint) (acquired) (*see also* Deformity, limb, upper arm)
    congenital Q68.8
    contraction — *see* Contraction, joint, elbow
  endocrine gland NEC Q89.2
  epididymis (congenital) Q55.4
    acquired N50.8

Deformity — *continued*
- epiglottis (congenital) Q31.8
  - acquired J38.7
- esophagus (congenital) Q39.9
  - acquired K22.8
- eustachian tube (congenital) NEC Q17.8
- eye, congenital Q15.9
- eyebrow (congenital) Q18.8
- eyelid (acquired) (*see also* Disorder, eyelid, specified type NEC)
  - congenital Q10.3
- face (acquired) M95.2
  - congenital Q18.9
- fallopian tube, acquired N83.8
- femur (acquired) — *see* Deformity, limb, specified type NEC, thigh
- fetal
  - with fetopelvic disproportion O33.7
  - causing obstructed labor O66.3
- finger (acquired) M20.00- ☑
  - boutonniere M20.02- ☑
  - congenital Q68.1
  - flexion contracture — *see* Contraction, joint, hand
  - mallet finger M20.01- ☑
  - specified NEC M20.09- ☑
  - swan-neck M20.03- ☑
- flexion (joint) (acquired) (*see also* Deformity, limb, flexion) M21.20
  - congenital NOS Q74.9
    - hip Q65.89
- foot (acquired) (*see also* Deformity, limb, lower leg)
  - cavovarus (congenital) Q66.1
  - congenital NOS Q66.9
    - specified type NEC Q66.89
  - specified type NEC — *see* Deformity, limb, foot, specified NEC
  - valgus (congenital) Q66.6
    - acquired — *see* Deformity, valgus, ankle
  - varus (congenital) NEC Q66.3
    - acquired — *see* Deformity, varus, ankle
- forearm (acquired) (*see also* Deformity, limb, forearm)
  - congenital Q68.8
- forehead (acquired) M95.2
  - congenital Q75.8
- frontal bone (acquired) M95.2
  - congenital Q75.8
- gallbladder (congenital) Q44.1
  - acquired K82.8
- gastrointestinal tract (congenital) NOS Q45.9
  - acquired K63.89
- genitalia, genital organ(s) or system NEC
  - female (congenital) Q52.9
    - acquired N94.89
    - external Q52.70
  - male (congenital) Q55.9
    - acquired N50.8
- globe (eye) (congenital) Q15.8
  - acquired H44.89
- gum, acquired NEC K06.8
- hand (acquired) — *see* Deformity, limb, hand
  - congenital Q68.1
- head (acquired) M95.2
  - congenital Q75.8
- heart (congenital) Q24.9
  - septum Q21.9
    - auricular Q21.1
    - ventricular Q21.0
  - valve (congenital) NEC Q24.8
    - acquired — *see* Endocarditis
- heel (acquired) — *see* Deformity, foot
- hepatic duct (congenital) Q44.5
  - acquired K83.8
- hip (joint) (acquired) (*see also* Deformity, limb, thigh)
  - congenital Q65.9
  - due to (previous) juvenile osteochondrosis — *see* Coxa, plana
  - flexion — *see* Contraction, joint, hip
- hourglass — *see* Contraction, hourglass
- humerus (acquired) M21.82- ☑
  - congenital Q74.0
- hypophyseal (congenital) Q89.2
- ileocecal (coil) (valve) (acquired) K63.89
  - congenital Q43.9
- ileum (congenital) Q43.9
  - acquired K63.89
- ilium (acquired) M95.5
  - congenital Q74.2
- integument (congenital) Q84.9

Deformity — *continued*
- intervertebral cartilage or disc (acquired) — *see* Disorder, disc, specified NEC
- intestine (large) (small) (congenital) NOS Q43.9
  - acquired K63.89
- intrinsic minus or plus (hand) — *see* Deformity, limb, specified type NEC, forearm
- iris (acquired) H21.89
  - congenital Q13.2
- ischium (acquired) M95.5
  - congenital Q74.2
- jaw (acquired) (congenital) M26.9
- joint (acquired) NEC M21.90
  - congenital Q68.8
  - elbow M21.92- ☑
  - hand M21.94- ☑
  - hip M21.95- ☑
  - knee M21.96- ☑
  - shoulder M21.92- ☑
  - wrist M21.93- ☑
- kidney(s) (calyx) (pelvis) (congenital) Q63.9
  - acquired N28.89
  - artery (congenital) Q27.2
    - acquired I77.89
- Klippel-Feil (brevicollis) Q76.1
- knee (acquired) NEC (*see also* Deformity, limb, lower leg)
  - congenital Q68.2
- labium (majus) (minus) (congenital) Q52.79
  - acquired N90.89
- lacrimal passages or duct (congenital) NEC Q10.6
  - acquired — *see* Disorder, lacrimal system, changes
- larynx (muscle) (congenital) Q31.8
  - acquired J38.7
  - web (glottic) Q31.0
- leg (upper) (acquired) NEC (*see also* Deformity, limb, thigh)
  - congenital Q68.8
  - lower leg — *see* Deformity, limb, lower leg
- lens (acquired) H27.8
  - congenital Q12.9
- lid (fold) (acquired) (*see also* Disorder, eyelid, specified type NEC)
  - congenital Q10.3
- ligament (acquired) — *see* Disorder, ligament
  - congenital Q79.9
- limb (acquired) M21.90
  - clawfoot M21.53- ☑
  - clawhand M21.51- ☑
  - clubfoot M21.54- ☑
  - clubhand M21.52- ☑
  - congenital, except reduction deformity Q74.9
  - flat foot M21.4- ☑
  - flexion M21.20
    - ankle M21.27- ☑
    - elbow M21.22- ☑
    - finger M21.24- ☑
    - hip M21.25- ☑
    - knee M21.26- ☑
    - shoulder M21.21- ☑
    - toe M21.27- ☑
    - wrist M21.23- ☑
  - foot
    - claw — *see* Deformity, limb, clawfoot
    - club — *see* Deformity, limb, clubfoot
    - drop M21.37- ☑
    - flat — *see* Deformity, limb, flat foot
    - specified NEC M21.6X- ☑
  - forearm M21.93- ☑
  - hand M21.94- ☑
  - lower leg M21.96- ☑
  - specified type NEC M21.80
    - forearm M21.83- ☑
    - lower leg M21.86- ☑
    - thigh M21.85- ☑
    - upper arm M21.82- ☑
  - thigh M21.95- ☑
  - unequal length M21.70
    - short site is
      - femur M21.75- ☑
      - fibula M21.76- ☑
      - humerus M21.72- ☑
      - radius M21.73- ☑
      - tibia M21.76- ☑
      - ulna M21.73- ☑
  - upper arm M21.92- ☑
  - valgus — *see* Deformity, valgus

Deformity — *continued*
- limb — *continued*
  - varus — *see* Deformity, varus
    - wrist drop M21.33- ☑
- lip (acquired) NEC K13.0
  - congenital Q38.0
- liver (congenital) Q44.7
  - acquired K76.89
- lumbosacral (congenital) (joint) (region) Q76.49
  - acquired — *see* subcategory M43.8 ☑
  - kyphosis — *see* Kyphosis, congenital
  - lordosis — *see* Lordosis, congenital
- lung (congenital) Q33.9
  - acquired J98.4
- lymphatic system, congenital Q89.9
- Madelung's (radius) Q74.0
- mandible (acquired) (congenital) M26.9
- maxilla (acquired) (congenital) M26.9
- meninges or membrane (congenital) Q07.9
  - cerebral Q04.8
    - acquired G96.19
  - spinal cord (congenital) G96.19
    - acquired G96.19
- metacarpus (acquired) — *see* Deformity, limb, forearm
  - congenital Q74.0
- metatarsus (acquired) — *see* Deformity, foot
  - congenital Q66.9
- middle ear (congenital) Q16.4
  - ossicles Q16.3
- mitral (leaflets) (valve) I05.8
  - parachute Q23.2
  - stenosis, congenital Q23.2
- mouth (acquired) K13.79
  - congenital Q38.6
- multiple, congenital NEC Q89.7
- muscle (acquired) M62.89
  - congenital Q79.9
    - sternocleidomastoid Q68.0
- musculoskeletal system (acquired) M95.9
  - congenital Q79.9
  - specified NEC M95.8
- nail (acquired) L60.8
  - congenital Q84.6
- nasal — *see* Deformity, nose
- neck (acquired) M95.3
  - congenital Q18.9
    - sternocleidomastoid Q68.0
- nervous system (congenital) Q07.9
- nipple (congenital) Q83.9
  - acquired N64.89
- nose (acquired) (cartilage) M95.0
  - bone (turbinate) M95.0
  - congenital Q30.9
    - bent or squashed Q67.4
  - saddle M95.0
    - syphilitic A50.57
  - septum (acquired) J34.2
    - congenital Q30.8
  - sinus (wall) (congenital) Q30.8
    - acquired M95.0
  - syphilitic (congenital) A50.57
    - late A52.73
- ocular muscle (congenital) Q10.3
  - acquired — *see* Strabismus, mechanical
- opticociliary vessels (congenital) Q13.2
- orbit (eye) (acquired) H05.30
  - atrophy — *see* Atrophy, orbit
  - congenital Q10.7
  - due to
    - bone disease NEC H05.32- ☑
    - trauma or surgery H05.33- ☑
  - enlargement — *see* Enlargement, orbit
  - exostosis — *see* Exostosis, orbit
- organ of Corti (congenital) Q16.5
- ovary (congenital) Q50.39
  - acquired N83.8
- oviduct, acquired N83.8
- palate (congenital) Q38.5
  - acquired M27.8
  - cleft (congenital) — *see* Cleft, palate
- pancreas (congenital) Q45.3
  - acquired K86.8
- parathyroid (gland) Q89.2
- parotid (gland) (congenital) Q38.4
  - acquired K11.8
- patella (acquired) — *see* Disorder, patella, specified NEC
- pelvis, pelvic (acquired) (bony) M95.5

Deformity — *continued*
pelvis, pelvic — *continued*
with disproportion (fetopelvic) O33.0
causing obstructed labor O65.0
congenital Q74.2
rachitic sequelae (late effect) E64.3
penis (glans) (congenital) Q55.69
acquired N48.89
pericardium (congenital) Q24.8
acquired — *see* Pericarditis
pharynx (congenital) Q38.8
acquired J39.2
pinna, acquired (*see also* Disorder, pinna, deformity)
congenital Q17.9
pituitary (congenital) Q89.2
posture — *see* Dorsopathy, deforming
prepuce (congenital) Q55.69
acquired N47.8
prostate (congenital) Q55.4
acquired N42.89
pupil (congenital) Q13.2
acquired — *see* Abnormality, pupillary
pylorus (congenital) Q40.3
acquired K31.89
rachitic (acquired), old or healed E64.3
radius (acquired) (*see also* Deformity, limb, forearm)
congenital Q68.8
rectum (congenital) Q43.9
acquired K62.89
reduction (extremity) (limb), congenital (*see also* condition and site) Q73.8
brain Q04.3
lower — *see* Defect, reduction, lower limb
upper — *see* Defect, reduction, upper limb
renal — *see* Deformity, kidney
respiratory system (congenital) Q34.9
rib (acquired) M95.4
congenital Q76.6
cervical Q76.5
rotation (joint) (acquired) — *see* Deformity, limb, specified site NEC
congenital Q74.9
hip — *see* Deformity, limb, specified type NEC, thigh
congenital Q65.89
sacroiliac joint (congenital) — *see* subcategory Q74.2
acquired — *see* subcategory M43.8 ☑
sacrum (acquired) — *see* subcategory M43.8 ☑
saddle
back — *see* Lordosis
nose M95.0
syphilitic A50.57
salivary gland or duct (congenital) Q38.4
acquired K11.8
scapula (acquired) M95.8
congenital Q68.8
scrotum (congenital) (*see also* Malformation, testis and scrotum)
acquired N50.8
seminal vesicles (congenital) Q55.4
acquired N50.8
septum, nasal (acquired) J34.2
shoulder (joint) (acquired) — *see* Deformity, limb, upper arm
congenital Q74.0
contraction — *see* Contraction, joint, shoulder
sigmoid (flexure) (congenital) Q43.9
acquired K63.89
skin (congenital) Q82.9
skull (acquired) M95.2
congenital Q75.8
with
anencephaly Q00.0
encephalocele — *see* Encephalocele
hydrocephalus Q03.9
with spina bifida — *see* Spina bifida, by site, with hydrocephalus
microcephaly Q02
soft parts, organs or tissues (of pelvis)
in pregnancy or childbirth NEC O34.8- ☑
causing obstructed labor O65.5
spermatic cord (congenital) Q55.4
acquired N50.8
torsion — *see* Torsion, spermatic cord
spinal — *see* Dorsopathy, deforming
column (acquired) — *see* Dorsopathy, deforming
congenital Q67.5
cord (congenital) Q06.9

Deformity — *continued*
spinal — *see* Dorsopathy, deforming — *continued*
cord — *continued*
acquired G95.89
nerve root (congenital) Q07.9
spine (acquired) (i>see also</i> Dorsopathy, deforming)
congenital Q67.5
rachitic E64.3
specified NEC — *see* Dorsopathy, deforming, specified NEC
spleen
acquired D73.89
congenital Q89.09
Sprengel's (congenital) Q74.0
sternocleidomastoid (muscle), congenital Q68.0
sternum (acquired) M95.4
congenital NEC Q76.7
stomach (congenital) Q40.3
acquired K31.89
submandibular gland (congenital) Q38.4
submaxillary gland (congenital) Q38.4
acquired K11.8
talipes — *see* Talipes
testis (congenital) (*see also* Malformation, testis and scrotum)
acquired N44.8
torsion — *see* Torsion, testis
thigh (acquired) (i>see also</i> Deformity, limb, thigh)
congenital NEC Q68.8
thorax (acquired) (wall) M95.4
congenital Q67.8
sequelae of rickets E64.3
thumb (acquired) (*see also* Deformity, finger)
congenital NEC Q68.1
thymus (tissue) (congenital) Q89.2
thyroid (gland) (congenital) Q89.2
cartilage Q31.8
acquired J38.7
tibia (acquired) (*see also* Deformity, limb, specified type NEC, lower leg)
congenital NEC Q68.8
saber (syphilitic) A50.56
toe (acquired) M20.6- ☑
congenital Q66.9
hallux rigidus M20.2- ☑
hallux valgus M20.1- ☑
hallux varus M20.3- ☑
hammer toe M20.4- ☑
specified NEC M20.5X- ☑
tongue (congenital) Q38.3
acquired K14.8
tooth, teeth K00.2
trachea (rings) (congenital) Q32.1
acquired J39.8
transverse aortic arch (congenital) Q25.4
tricuspid (leaflets) (valve) I07.8
atresia or stenosis Q22.4
Ebstein's Q22.5
trunk (acquired) M95.8
congenital Q89.9
ulna (acquired) (*see also* Deformity, limb, forearm)
congenital NEC Q68.8
urachus, congenital Q64.4
ureter (opening) (congenital) Q62.8
acquired N28.89
urethra (congenital) Q64.79
acquired N36.8
urinary tract (congenital) Q64.9
urachus Q64.4
uterus (congenital) Q51.9
acquired N85.8
uvula (congenital) Q38.5
vagina (acquired) N89.8
congenital Q52.4
valgus NEC M21.00
ankle M21.07- ☑
elbow M21.02- ☑
hip M21.05- ☑
knee M21.06- ☑
valve, valvular (congenital) (heart) Q24.8
acquired — *see* Endocarditis
varus NEC M21.10
ankle M21.17- ☑
elbow M21.12- ☑
hip M21.15 ☑
knee M21.16- ☑
tibia — *see* Osteochondrosis, juvenile, tibia

Deformity — *continued*
vas deferens (congenital) Q55.4
acquired N50.8
vein (congenital) Q27.9
great Q26.9
vertebra — *see* Dorsopathy, deforming
vertical talus (congenital) Q66.80
left foot Q66.82
right foot Q66.81
vesicourethral orifice (acquired) N32.89
congenital NEC Q64.79
vessels of optic papilla (congenital) Q14.2
visual field (contraction) — *see* Defect, visual field
vitreous body, acquired H43.89
vulva (congenital) Q52.79
acquired N90.89
wrist (joint) (acquired) (*see also* Deformity, limb, forearm)
congenital Q68.8
contraction — *see* Contraction, joint, wrist

Degeneration, degenerative
adrenal (capsule) (fatty) (gland) (hyaline) (infectional) E27.8
amyloid (*see also* Amyloidosis) E85.9
anterior cornua, spinal cord G12.29
anterior labral S43.49- ☑
aorta, aortic I70.0
fatty I77.89
aortic valve (heart) — *see* Endocarditis, aortic
arteriovascular — *see* Arteriosclerosis
artery, arterial (atheromatous) (calcareous) (*see also* Arteriosclerosis)
cerebral, amyloid E85.4 [I68.0]
medial — *see* Arteriosclerosis, extremities
articular cartilage NEC — *see* Derangement, joint, articular cartilage, by site
atheromatous — *see* Arteriosclerosis
basal nuclei or ganglia G23.9
specified NEC G23.8
bone NEC — *see* Disorder, bone, specified type NEC
brachial plexus G54.0
brain (cortical) (progressive) G31.9
alcoholic G31.2
arteriosclerotic I67.2
childhood G31.9
specified NEC G31.89
cystic G31.89
congenital Q04.6
in
alcoholism G31.2
beriberi E51.2
cerebrovascular disease I67.9
congenital hydrocephalus Q03.9
with spina bifida (*see also* Spina bifida)
Fabry-Anderson disease E75.21
Gaucher's disease E75.22
Hunter's syndrome E76.1
lipidosis
cerebral E75.4
generalized E75.6
mucopolysaccharidosis — *see* Mucopolysaccharidosis
myxedema E03.9 [G32.89]
neoplastic disease (*see also* Neoplasm) [G32.89], D49.6
Niemann-Pick disease E75.249 [G32.89]
sphingolipidosis E75.3 [G32.89]
vitamin B12 deficiency E53.8 [G32.89]
senile NEC G31.1
breast N64.89
Bruch's membrane — *see* Degeneration, choroid
capillaries (fatty) I78.8
amyloid E85.8 [I79.8]
cardiac (*see also* Degeneration, myocardial)
valve, valvular — *see* Endocarditis
cardiorenal — *see* Hypertension, cardiorenal
cardiovascular (*see also* Disease, cardiovascular)
renal — *see* Hypertension, cardiorenal
cerebellar NOS G31.9
alcoholic G31.2
primary (hereditary) (sporadic) G11.9
cerebral — *see* Degeneration, brain
cerebrovascular I67.9
due to hypertension I67.4
cervical plexus G54.2
cervix N88.8
due to radiation (intended effect) N88.8
adverse effect or misadventure N99.89

Degeneration, degenerative — *continued*
 chamber angle H21.21- ☑
 changes, spine or vertebra — *see* Spondylosis
 chorioretinal (*see also* Degeneration, choroid)
  hereditary H31.2Ø
 choroid (colloid) (drusen) H31.1Ø- ☑
  atrophy — *see* Atrophy, choroidal
  hereditary — *see* Dystrophy, choroidal, hereditary
 ciliary body H21.22- ☑
 cochlear — *see* subcategory H83.8 ☑
 combined (spinal cord) (subacute) E53.8 [G32.Ø]
  with anemia (pernicious) D51.Ø [G32.Ø]
   due to dietary vitamin B12 deficiency
       D51.3 [G32.Ø]
  in (due to)
   vitamin B12 deficiency E53.8 [G32.Ø]
       anemia D51.9 [G32.Ø]
 conjunctiva H11.1Ø
  concretions — *see* Concretion, conjunctiva
  deposits — *see* Deposit, conjunctiva
  pigmentations — *see* Pigmentation, conjunctiva
  pinguecula — *see* Pinguecula
  xerosis — *see* Xerosis, conjunctiva
 cornea H18.4Ø
  calcerous H18.43
   band keratopathy H18.42- ☑
  familial, hereditary — *see* Dystrophy, cornea
  hyaline (of old scars) H18.49
  keratomalacia — *see* Keratomalacia
  nodular H18.45- ☑
  peripheral H18.46- ☑
  senile H18.41- ☑
  specified type NEC H18.49
 cortical (cerebellar) (parenchymatous) G31.89
  alcoholic G31.2
  diffuse, due to arteriopathy I67.2
 corticobasal G31.85
 cutis L98.8
  amyloid E85.4 [L99]
 dental pulp KØ4.2
 disc disease — *see* Degeneration, intervertebral disc
   NEC
 dorsolateral (spinal cord) — *see* Degeneration, combined
 extrapyramidal G25.9
 eye, macular (*see also* Degeneration, macula)
  congenital or hereditary — *see* Dystrophy, retina
 facet joints — *see* Spondylosis
 fatty
  liver NEC K76.Ø
   alcoholic K7Ø.Ø
 grey matter (brain) (Alpers') G31.81
 heart (*see also* Degeneration, myocardial)
  amyloid E85.4 [I43]
  atheromatous — *see* Disease, heart, ischemic,
      atherosclerotic
  ischemic — *see* Disease, heart, ischemic
 hepatolenticular (Wilson's) E83.Ø1
 hepatorenal K76.7
 hyaline (diffuse) (generalized)
  localized — *see* Degeneration, by site
 infrapatellar fat pad M79.4
 intervertebral disc NOS
  with
   myelopathy — *see* Disorder, disc, with,
       myelopathy
   radiculitis or radiculopathy — *see* Disorder, disc,
       with, radiculopathy
  cervical, cervicothoracic — *see* Disorder, disc, cer-
      vical, degeneration
   with
    myelopathy — *see* Disorder, disc, cervical,
        with myelopathy
    neuritis, radiculitis or radiculopathy — *see*
        Disorder, disc, cervical, with neuritis
  lumbar region M51.36
   with
    myelopathy M51.Ø6
    neuritis, radiculitis, radiculopathy or sciatica
        M51.16
  lumbosacral region M51.37
   with
    neuritis, radiculitis, radiculopathy or sciatica
        M51.17
  sacrococcygeal region M53.3
  thoracic region M51.34

Degeneration, degenerative — *continued*
 intervertebral disc — *continued*
  thoracic region — *continued*
   with
    myelopathy M51.Ø4
    neuritis, radiculitis, radiculopathy M51.14
  thoracolumbar region M51.35
   with
    myelopathy M51.Ø5
    neuritis, radiculitis, radiculopathy M51.15
 intestine, amyloid E85.4
 iris (pigmentary) H21.23- ☑
 ischemic — *see* Ischemia
 joint disease — *see* Osteoarthritis
 kidney N28.89
  amyloid E85.4 [N29]
  cystic, congenital Q61.9
  fatty N28.89
  polycystic Q61.3
   adult type (autosomal dominant) Q61.2
   infantile type (autosomal recessive) NEC Q61.19
    collecting duct dilatation Q61.11
 Kuhnt-Junius (*see also* Degeneration, macula) H35.32
 lens — *see* Cataract
 lenticular (familial) (progressive) (Wilson's) (with cirrhosis of liver) E83.Ø1
 liver (diffuse) NEC K76.89
  amyloid E85.4 [K77]
  cystic K76.89
   congenital Q44.6
  fatty NEC K76.Ø
   alcoholic K7Ø.Ø
  hypertrophic K76.89
  parenchymatous, acute or subacute K72.ØØ
   with coma K72.Ø1
  pigmentary K76.89
  toxic (acute) K71.9
 lung J98.4
 lymph gland I89.8
  hyaline I89.8
 macula, macular (acquired) (age-related) (senile)
   H35.3Ø
  angioid streaks H35.33
  atrophic age-related H35.31
  congenital or hereditary — *see* Dystrophy, retina
  cystoid H35.35- ☑
  drusen H35.36- ☑
  exudative H35.32
  hole H35.34- ☑
  nonexudative H35.31
  puckering H35.37- ☑
  toxic H35.38- ☑
 membranous labyrinth, congenital (causing impairment of hearing) Q16.5
 meniscus — *see* Derangement, meniscus
 mitral — *see* Insufficiency, mitral
 Mönckeberg's — *see* Arteriosclerosis, extremities
 motor centers, senile G31.1
 multi-system G9Ø.3
 mural — *see* Degeneration, myocardial
 muscle (fatty) (fibrous) (hyaline) (progressive) M62.89
  heart — *see* Degeneration, myocardial
 myelin, central nervous system G37.9
 myocardial, myocardium (fatty) (hyaline) (senile) I51.5
  with rheumatic fever (conditions in IØØ) IØ9.Ø
   active, acute or subacute IØ1.2
    with chorea IØ2.Ø
   inactive or quiescent (with chorea) IØ9.Ø
  hypertensive — *see* Hypertension, heart
  rheumatic — *see* Degeneration, myocardial, with
      rheumatic fever
  syphilitic A52.Ø6
 nasal sinus (mucosa) J32.9
  frontal J32.1
  maxillary J32.Ø
 nerve — *see* Disorder, nerve
 nervous system G31.9
  alcoholic G31.2
  amyloid E85.4 [G99.8]
  autonomic G9Ø.9
  fatty G31.89
  specified NEC G31.89
 nipple N64.89
 olivopontocerebellar (hereditary) (familial) G23.8
 osseous labyrinth — *see* subcategory H83.8 ☑
 ovary N83.8
  cystic N83.2Ø
  microcystic N83.2Ø

Degeneration, degenerative — *continued*
 pallidal pigmentary (progressive) G23.Ø
 pancreas K86.8
  tuberculous A18.83
 penis N48.89
 pigmentary (diffuse) (general)
  localized — *see* Degeneration, by site
  pallidal (progressive) G23.Ø
 pineal gland E34.8
 pituitary (gland) E23.6
 popliteal fat pad M79.4
 posterolateral (spinal cord) — *see* Degeneration,
   combined
 pulmonary valve (heart) I37.8
 pulp (tooth) KØ4.2
 pupillary margin H21.24- ☑
 renal — *see* Degeneration, kidney
 retina H35.9
  hereditary (cerebroretinal) (congenital) (juvenile)
      (macula) (peripheral) (pigmentary) — *see*
      Dystrophy, retina
  Kuhnt-Junius (*see also* Degeneration, macula)
      H35.32
  macula (cystic) (exudative) (hole) (nonexudative)
      (pseudohole) (senile) (toxic) — *see* Degener-
      ation, macula
  peripheral H35.4Ø
   lattice H35.41- ☑
   microcystoid H35.42- ☑
   paving stone H35.43- ☑
   secondary
    pigmentary H35.45- ☑
    vitreoretinal H35.46- ☑
   senile reticular H35.44- ☑
  pigmentary (primary) (*see also* Dystrophy, retina)
   secondary — *see* Degeneration, retina, periph-
      eral, secondary
  posterior pole — *see* Degeneration, macula
 saccule, congenital (causing impairment of hearing)
   Q16.5
 senile R54
  brain G31.1
  cardiac, heart or myocardium — *see* Degeneration,
      myocardial
  motor centers G31.1
  vascular — *see* Arteriosclerosis
 sinus (cystic) (*see also* Sinusitis)
  polypoid J33.1
 skin L98.8
  amyloid E85.4 [L99]
  colloid L98.8
 spinal (cord) G31.89
  amyloid E85.4 [G32.89]
  combined (subacute) — *see* Degeneration, com-
      bined
  dorsolateral — *see* Degeneration, combined
  familial NEC G31.89
  fatty G31.89
  funicular — *see* Degeneration, combined
  posterolateral — *see* Degeneration, combined
  subacute combined — *see* Degeneration, com-
      bined
  tuberculous A17.81
 spleen D73.Ø
  amyloid E85.4 [D77]
 stomach K31.89
 striatonigral G23.2
 suprarenal (capsule) (gland) E27.8
 synovial membrane (pulpy) — *see* Disorder, synovium,
   specified type NEC
 tapetoretinal — *see* Dystrophy, retina
 thymus (gland) E32.8
  fatty E32.8
 thyroid (gland) EØ7.89
 tricuspid (heart) (valve) IØ7.9
 tuberculous NEC — *see* Tuberculosis
 turbinate J34.89
 uterus (cystic) N85.8
 vascular (senile) — *see* Arteriosclerosis
  hypertensive — *see* Hypertension
 vitreoretinal, secondary — *see* Degeneration, retina,
   peripheral, secondary, vitreoretinal
 vitreous (body) H43.81- ☑
 Wallerian — *see* Disorder, nerve
 Wilson's hepatolenticular E83.Ø1
Deglutition
 paralysis R13.Ø

☑ **Additional Character Required — Refer to the Tabular List for Character Selection** ▽ Subterms under main terms may continue to next column or page

Deglutition — *continued*
  paralysis — *continued*
    hysterical F44.4
    pneumonia J69.0
Degos' disease I77.89
Dehiscence (of)
  amputation stump T87.81
  cesarean wound O90.0
  closure of
    cornea T81.31 ☑
    craniotomy T81.32 ☑
    fascia (muscular) (superficial) T81.32 ☑
    internal organ or tissue T81.32 ☑
    laceration (external) (internal) T81.33 ☑
    ligament T81.32 ☑
    mucosa T81.31 ☑
    muscle or muscle flap T81.32 ☑
    ribs or rib cage T81.32 ☑
    skin and subcutaneous tissue (full-thickness) (superficial) T81.31 ☑
    skull T81.32 ☑
    sternum (sternotomy) T81.32 ☑
    tendon T81.32 ☑
    traumatic laceration (external) (internal) T81.33 ☑
  episiotomy O90.1
  operation wound NEC T81.31 ☑
    external operation wound (superficial) T81.31 ☑
    internal operation wound (deep) T81.32 ☑
  perineal wound (postpartum) O90.1
  traumatic injury wound repair T81.33 ☑
  wound T81.30 ☑
    traumatic repair T81.33 ☑
Dehydration E86.0
  hypertonic E87.0
  hypotonic E87.1
  newborn P74.1
Déjérine-Roussy syndrome G89.0
Déjérine-Sottas disease or neuropathy (hypertrophic) G60.0
Déjérine-Thomas atrophy G23.8
Delay, delayed
  any plane in pelvis
    complicating delivery O66.9
  birth or delivery NOS O63.9
  closure, ductus arteriosus (Botalli) P29.3
  coagulation — *see* Defect, coagulation
  conduction (cardiac) (ventricular) I45.9
  delivery, second twin, triplet, etc O63.2
  development R62.50
    global F88
    intellectual (specific) F81.9
    language F80.9
      due to hearing loss F80.4
    learning F81.9
    pervasive F84.9
    physiological R62.50
      specified stage NEC R62.0
    reading F81.0
    sexual E30.0
    speech F80.9
      due to hearing loss F80.4
    spelling F81.81
  gastric emptying K30
  menarche E30.0
  menstruation (cause unknown) N91.0
  milestone R62.0
  passage of meconium (newborn) P76.0
  primary respiration P28.9
  puberty (constitutional) E30.0
  separation of umbilical cord P96.82
  sexual maturation, female E30.0
  sleep phase syndrome G47.21
  union, fracture — *see* Fracture, by site
  vaccination Z28.9
Deletion(s)
  autosome Q93.9
    identified by fluorescence in situ hybridization (FISH) Q93.89
    identified by in situ hybridization (ISH) Q93.89
  chromosome
    with complex rearrangements NEC Q93.7
    part of NEC Q93.5
    seen only at prometaphase Q93.89
    short arm
      22q11.2 Q93.81
      4 Q93.3
      5p Q93.4

Deletion(s) — *continued*
  chromosome — *continued*
    specified NEC Q93.89
    long arm chromosome 18 or 21 Q93.89
      with complex rearrangements NEC Q93.7
    microdeletions NEC Q93.88
Delhi boil or button B55.1
Delinquency (juvenile) (neurotic) F91.8
  group Z72.810
Delinquent immunization status Z28.3
Delirium, delirious (acute or subacute) (not alcohol- or drug-induced) (with dementia) R41.0
  alcoholic (acute) (tremens) (withdrawal) F10.921
    with intoxication F10.921
      in
        abuse F10.121
        dependence F10.221
  due to (secondary to)
    alcohol
      intoxication F10.921
        in
          abuse F10.121
          dependence F10.221
      withdrawal F10.231
    amphetamine intoxication F15.921
      in
        abuse F15.121
        dependence F15.221
    anxiolytic
      intoxication F13.921
        in
          abuse F13.121
          dependence F13.221
      withdrawal F13.231
    cannabis intoxication (acute) F12.921
      in
        abuse F12.121
        dependence F12.221
    cocaine intoxication (acute) F14.921
      in
        abuse F14.121
        dependence F14.221
    general medical condition F05
    hallucinogen intoxication F16.921
      in
        abuse F16.121
        dependence F16.221
    hypnotic
      intoxication F13.921
        in
          abuse F13.121
          dependence F13.221
      withdrawal F13.231
    inhalant intoxication (acute) F18.921
      in
        abuse F18.121
        dependence F18.221
    multiple etiologies F05
    opioid intoxication (acute) F11.921
      in
        abuse F11.121
        dependence F11.221
    phencyclidine intoxication (acute) F16.921
      in
        abuse F16.121
        dependence F16.221
    psychoactive substance NEC intoxication (acute) F19.921
      in
        abuse F19.121
        dependence F19.221
    sedative
      intoxication F13.921
        in
          abuse F13.121
          dependence F13.221
      withdrawal F13.231
    unknown etiology F05
  exhaustion F43.0
  hysterical F44.89
  postprocedural (postoperative) F05
  puerperal F05
  thyroid — *see* Thyrotoxicosis with thyroid storm
  traumatic — *see* Injury, intracranial
  tremens (alcohol-induced) F10.231
    sedative-induced F13.231
Delivery (childbirth) (labor)
  arrested active phase O62.1

Delivery — *continued*
  cesarean (for)
    without indication O82
    abnormal
      pelvis (bony) (deformity) (major) NEC with disproportion (fetopelvic) O33.0
        with obstructed labor O65.0
      presentation or position O32.9 ☑
    abruptio placentae (*see also* Abruptio placentae) O45.9-
    acromion presentation O32.2 ☑
    atony, uterus O62.2
    breech presentation O32.1 ☑
      incomplete O32.8 ☑
    brow presentation O32.3 ☑
    cephalopelvic disproportion O33.9
    cerclage O34.3- ☑
    chin presentation O32.3 ☑
    cicatrix of cervix O34.4- ☑
    contracted pelvis (general)
      inlet O33.2
      outlet O33.3 ☑
    cord presentation or prolapse O69.0 ☑
    cystocele O34.8- ☑
    deformity (acquired) (congenital)
      pelvic organs or tissues NEC O34.8- ☑
      pelvis (bony) NEC O33.0
    disproportion NOS O33.9
    eclampsia — *see* Eclampsia
    face presentation O32.3 ☑
    failed
      forceps O66.5
      induction of labor O61.9
        instrumental O61.1
        mechanical O61.1
        medical O61.0
        specified NEC O61.8
        surgical O61.1
      trial of labor NOS O66.40
        following previous cesarean delivery O66.41
      vacuum extraction O66.5
      ventouse O66.5
    fetal-maternal hemorrhage O43.01- ☑
    hemorrhage (intrapartum) O67.9
      with coagulation defect O67.0
      specified cause NEC O67.8
    high head at term O32.4 ☑
    hydrocephalic fetus O33.6 ☑
    incarceration of uterus O34.51- ☑
    incoordinate uterine action O62.4
    increased size, fetus O33.5 ☑
    inertia, uterus O62.2
      primary O62.0
      secondary O62.1
    lateroversion, uterus O34.59- ☑
    mal lie O32.9 ☑
    malposition
      fetus O32.9 ☑
      pelvic organs or tissues NEC O34.8- ☑
      uterus NEC O34.59- ☑
    malpresentation NOS O32.9 ☑
    oblique presentation O32.2 ☑
    occurring after 37 completed weeks of gestation but before 39 completed weeks gestation due to (spontaneous) onset of labor O75.82
    oversize fetus O33.5 ☑
    pelvic tumor NEC O34.8- ☑
    placenta previa O44.1- ☑
      without hemorrhage O44.0- ☑
    placental insufficiency O36.51- ☑
    planned, occurring after 37 completed weeks of gestation but before 39 completed weeks gestation due to (spontaneous) onset of labor O75.82
    polyp, cervix O34.4- ☑
      causing obstructed labor O65.5
    poor dilatation, cervix O62.0
    pre-eclampsia O14.9- ☑
      mild O14.0- ☑
      moderate O14.0- ☑
      severe
        with hemolysis, elevated liver enzymes and low platelet count (HELLP) O14.2- ☑
    previous
      cesarean delivery O34.21
      surgery (to)
        cervix O34.4- ☑

☑ **Additional Character Required** — Refer to the Tabular List for Character Selection   ▽ **Subterms under main terms may continue to next column or page**

Delivery — *continued*
  complicated — *continued*
    by — *continued*
      malposition, malpresentation
        without obstruction (*see also* Delivery, complicated by, obstruction) O32.9 ☑
          breech O32.1 ☑
          compound O32.6 ☑
          face (brow) (chin) O32.3 ☑
          footling O32.8 ☑
          high head O32.4 ☑
          oblique O32.2 ☑
          specified NEC O32.8 ☑
          transverse O32.2 ☑
          unstable lie O32.0 ☑
      placenta (with hemorrhage) O44.1- ☑
        without hemorrhage O44.0- ☑
      uterus or cervix O65.5
    meconium in amniotic fluid O77.0
    mental disorder NEC O99.344
    metrorrhexis — *see* Delivery, complicated by, rupture, uterus
    nervous system disorder O99.354
    obesity (pre-existing) O99.214
    obesity surgery status O99.844
    obstetric trauma O71.9
      specified NEC O71.89
    obstructed labor
      due to
        breech (complete) (frank) presentation O64.1 ☑
          incomplete O64.8 ☑
        brow presenation O64.3 ☑
        buttock presentation O64.1 ☑
        chin presentation O64.2 ☑
        compound presentation O64.5 ☑
        contracted pelvis O65.1
        deep transverse arrest O64.0 ☑
        deformed pelvis O65.0
        dystocia (fetal) O66.9
          due to
            conjoined twins O66.3
            fetal
              abnormality NEC O66.3
              ascites O66.3
              hydrops O66.3
              meningomyelocele O66.3
              sacral teratoma O66.3
              tumor O66.3
            hydrocephalic fetus O66.3
            shoulder O66.0
        face presentation O64.2 ☑
        fetopelvic disproportion O65.4
        footling presentation O64.8 ☑
        impacted shoulders O66.0
        incomplete rotation of fetal head O64.0 ☑
        large fetus O66.2
        locked twins O66.1
        malposition O64.9 ☑
          specified NEC O64.8 ☑
        malpresentation O64.9 ☑
          specified NEC O64.8 ☑
        multiple fetuses NEC O66.6
        pelvic
          abnormality (maternal) O65.9
          contraction
            inlet O65.2
            mid-cavity O65.3
            organ O65.5
            outlet O65.3
            specified NEC O65.8
          persistent (position)
            occipitoiliac O64.0 ☑
            occipitoposterior O64.0 ☑
            occipitosacral O64.0 ☑
            occipitotransverse O64.0 ☑
        prolapsed arm O64.4 ☑
        shoulder presentation O64.4 ☑
        specified NEC O66.8
    pathological retraction ring, uterus O62.4
    penetration, pregnant uterus by instrument O71.1
    perforation — *see* Delivery, complicated by, laceration

Delivery — *continued*
  complicated — *continued*
    by — *continued*
      placenta, placental
        ablatio (*see also* Abruptio placentae) O45.9- ☑
        abnormality O43.9- ☑
          specified NEC O43.89- ☑
        abruptio (*see also* Abruptio placentae) O45.9- ☑
        accreta O43.21- ☑
        adherent (with hemorrhage) O72.0
          without hemorrhage O73.0
        detachment (premature) (*see also* Abruptio placentae) O45.9- ☑
        disorder O43.9- ☑
          specified NEC O43.89- ☑
        hemorrhage NEC O67.8
        increta O43.22- ☑
        low (implantation) O44.1- ☑
          without hemorrhage O44.0- ☑
        malformation O43.10- ☑
        malposition O44.1- ☑
          without hemorrhage O44.0- ☑
        percreta O43.23- ☑
        previa (central) (lateral) (low) (marginal) (partial) (total) O44.1- ☑
          without hemorrhage O44.0- ☑
        retained (with hemorrhage) O72.0
          without hemorrhage O73.0
        separation (premature) O45.9- ☑
          specified NEC O45.8X- ☑
        vicious insertion O44.1- ☑
      precipitate labor O62.3
      premature rupture, membranes (*see also* Pregnancy, complicated by, premature rupture of membranes) O42.90
      prolapse
        arm or hand O32.2 ☑
        cord (umbilical) O69.0 ☑
        foot or leg O32.8 ☑
        uterus O34.52- ☑
      prolonged labor O63.9
        first stage O63.0
        second stage O63.1
      protozoal disease (maternal) O98.62
      respiratory disease NEC O99.52
      retained membranes or portions of placenta O72.2
        without hemorrhage O73.1
      retarded birth O63.9
      retention of secundines (with hemorrhage) O72.0
        without hemorrhage O73.0
        partial O72.2
          without hemorrhage O73.1
      rupture
        bladder (urinary) O71.5
        cervix O71.3
        pelvic organ NEC O71.5
        urethra O71.5
        uterus (during or after labor) O71.1
          before labor O71.0- ☑
      separation, pubic bone (symphysis pubis) O71.6
      shock O75.1
      shoulder presentation O64.4 ☑
      skin disorder NEC O99.72
      spasm, cervix O62.4
      stenosis or stricture, cervix O65.5
      streptococcus B carrier state O99.824
      subluxation of symphysis (pubis) O26.72
      syphilis (maternal) O98.12
      tear — *see* Delivery, complicated by, laceration
      tetanic uterus O62.4
      trauma (obstetrical) (*see also* Delivery, complicated, by, damage to) O71.9
        non-obstetric O9A.22 (*following* O99)
        periurethral O71.82
        specified NEC O71.89
      tuberculosis (maternal) O98.02
      tumor, pelvic organs or tissues NEC O65.5
      umbilical cord around neck
        with compression O69.1 ☑
        without compression O69.81 ☑
      uterine inertia O62.2
        during latent phase of labor O62.0
        primary O62.0

Delivery — *continued*
  complicated — *continued*
    by — *continued*
      uterine inertia — *continued*
        secondary O62.1
      vasa previa O69.4 ☑
      velamentous insertion of cord O43.12- ☑
    specified complication NEC O75.89
  delayed NOS O63.9
    following rupture of membranes
      artificial O75.5
    second twin, triplet, etc. O63.2
  forceps, low following failed vacuum extraction O66.5
  missed (at or near term) O36.4 ☑
  normal O80
  obstructed — *see* Delivery, complicated by, obstruction
  precipitate O62.3
  preterm (*see also* Pregnancy, complicated by, preterm labor) O60.10 ☑
  spontaneous O80
  term pregnancy NOS O80
  uncomplicated O80
  vaginal, following previous cesarean delivery O34.21
Delusions (paranoid) — *see* Disorder, delusional
Dementia (degenerative (primary)) (old age) (persisting) F03.90
  with
    aggressive behavior F03.91
    behavioral disturbance F03.91
    combative behavior F03.91
    Lewy bodies G31.83 [F02.80]
      with behavioral disturbance G31.83 [F02.81]
    Parkinsonism G31.83 [F02.80]
      with behavioral disturbance G31.83 [F02.81]
    Parkinson's disease G20 [F02.80]
      with behavioral disturbance G20 [F02.81]
    violent behavior F03.91
  alcoholic F10.97
    with dependence F10.27
  Alzheimer's type — *see* Disease, Alzheimer's
  arteriosclerotic — *see* Dementia, vascular
  atypical, Alzheimer's type — *see* Disease, Alzheimer's, specified NEC
  congenital — *see* Disability, intellectual
  frontal (lobe) G31.09 [F02.80]
    with behavioral disturbance G31.09 [F02.81]
  frontotemporal G31.09 [F02.80]
    with behavioral disturbance G31.09 [F02.81]
    specified NEC G31.09 [F02.80]
      with behavioral disturbance G31.09 [F02.81]
  in (due to)
    with behavioral disturbance G31.83 [F02.81]
    alcohol F10.97
      with dependence F10.27
    Alzheimer's disease — *see* Disease, Alzheimer's
    arteriosclerotic brain disease — *see* Dementia, vascular
    cerebral lipidoses E75.- ☑ [F02.80]
      with behavioral disturbance E75.- ☑ [F02.81]
    Creutzfeldt-Jakob disease (*see also* Creutzfeldt-Jakob disease or syndrome (with dementia)) A81.00
    epilepsy G40.- ☑ [F02.80]
      with behavioral disturbance G40.- ☑ [F02.81]
    hepatolenticular degeneration E83.01 [F02.80]
      with behavioral disturbance E83.01 [F02.81]
    human immunodeficiency virus (HIV) disease B20 [F02.80]
      with behavioral disturbance B20 [F02.81]
    Huntington's disease or chorea G10
    hypercalcemia E83.52 [F02.80]
      with behavioral disturbance E83.52 [F02.81]
    hypothyroidism, acquired E03.9 [F02.80]
      with behavioral disturbance E03.9 [F02.81]
      due to iodine deficiency E01.8 [F02.80]
        with behavioral disturbance E01.8 [F02.81]
    inhalants F18.97
      with dependence F18.27
    multiple
      etiologies F03 ☑
      sclerosis G35 [F02.80]
        with behavioral disturbance G35 [F02.81]
    neurosyphilis A52.17 [F02.80]
      with behavioral disturbance A52.17 [F02.81]
      juvenile A50.49 [F02.80]
        with behavioral disturbance A50.49 [F02.81]
    niacin deficiency E52 [F02.80]

Dementia — continued
  in — continued
    niacin deficiency — continued
      with behavioral disturbance E52 [FØ2.81]
    paralysis agitans G2Ø [FØ2.8Ø]
      with behavioral disturbance G2Ø [FØ2.81]
    Parkinson's disease G2Ø [FØ2.8Ø]
    pellagra E52 [FØ2.8Ø]
      with behavioral disturbance E52 [FØ2.81]
    Pick's G31.Ø1 [FØ2.8Ø]
      with behavioral disturbance G31.Ø1 [FØ2.81]
    polyarteritis nodosa M3Ø.Ø [FØ2.8Ø]
      with behavioral disturbance M3Ø.Ø [FØ2.81]
    psychoactive drug F19.97
      with dependence F19.27
      inhalants F18.97
        with dependence F18.27
      sedatives, hypnotics or anxiolytics F13.97
        with dependence F13.27
    sedatives, hypnotics or anxiolytics F13.97
      with dependence F13.27
    systemic lupus erythematosus M32.- ☑ [FØ2.8Ø]
      with behavioral disturbance M32.- ☑ [FØ2.81]
    trypanosomiasis
      African B56.9 [FØ2.8Ø]
        with behavioral disturbance B56.9 [FØ2.81]
    unknown etiology FØ3 ☑
    vitamin B12 deficiency E53.8 [FØ2.8Ø]
      with behavioral disturbance E53.8 [FØ2.81]
    volatile solvents F18.97
      with dependence F18.27
  infantile, infantilis F84.3
  Lewy body G31.83 [FØ2.8Ø]
    with behavioral disturbance G31.83 [FØ2.81]
  multi-infarct — see Dementia, vascular
  paralytica, paralytic (syphilitic) A52.17 [FØ2.8Ø]
    with behavioral disturbance A52.17 [FØ2.81]
    juvenilis A5Ø.45
  paretic A52.17
  praecox — see Schizophrenia
  presenile FØ3 ☑
    Alzheimer's type — see Disease, Alzheimer's, early onset
  primary degenerative FØ3 ☑
  progressive, syphilitic A52.17
  senile FØ3 ☑
    with acute confusional state FØ5
    Alzheimer's type — see Disease, Alzheimer's, late onset
    depressed or paranoid type FØ3 ☑
  vascular (acute onset) (mixed) (multi-infarct) (subcortical) FØ1.5Ø
    with behavioral disturbance FØ1.51
Demineralization, bone — see Osteoporosis
Demodex folliculorum (infestation) B88.Ø
Demophobia F4Ø.248
Demoralization R45.3
Demyelination, demyelinization
  central nervous system G37.9
    specified NEC G37.8
  corpus callosum (central) G37.1
  disseminated, acute G36.9
    specified NEC G36.8
  global G35
  in optic neuritis G36.Ø
Dengue (classical) (fever) A9Ø
  hemorrhagic A91
  sandfly A93.1
Dennie-Marfan syphilitic syndrome A5Ø.45
Dens evaginatus, in dente or invaginatus KØØ.2
Dense breasts R92.2
Density
  increased, bone (disseminated) (generalized) (spotted) — see Disorder, bone, density and structure, specified type NEC
  lung (nodular) J98.4
Dental (see also condition)
  examination ZØ1.2Ø
    with abnormal findings ZØ1.21
  restoration
    aesthetically inadequate or displeasing KØ8.56
    defective KØ8.5Ø
      specified NEC KØ8.59
    failure of marginal integrity KØ8.51
    failure of periodontal anatomical integrity KØ8.54
Dentia praecox KØØ.6
Denticles (pulp) KØ4.2
Dentigerous cyst KØ9.Ø

Dentin
  irregular (in pulp) KØ4.3
  opalescent KØØ.5
  secondary (in pulp) KØ4.3
  sensitive KØ3.89
Dentinogenesis imperfecta KØØ.5
Dentinoma — see Cyst, calcifying odontogenic
Dentition (syndrome) KØØ.7
  delayed KØØ.6
  difficult KØØ.7
  precocious KØØ.6
  premature KØØ.6
  retarded KØØ.6
Dependence (on) (syndrome) F19.2Ø
  with remission F19.21
  alcohol (ethyl) (methyl) (without remission) F1Ø.2Ø
    with
      amnestic disorder, persisting F1Ø.26
      anxiety disorder F1Ø.28Ø
      dementia, persisting F1Ø.27
      intoxication F1Ø.229
        with delirium F1Ø.221
        uncomplicated F1Ø.22Ø
      mood disorder F1Ø.24
      psychotic disorder F1Ø.259
        with
          delusions F1Ø.25Ø
          hallucinations F1Ø.251
      remission F1Ø.21
      sexual dysfunction F1Ø.281
      sleep disorder F1Ø.282
      specified disorder NEC F1Ø.288
      withdrawal F1Ø.239
        with
          delirium F1Ø.231
          perceptual disturbance F1Ø.232
          uncomplicated F1Ø.23Ø
    counseling and surveillance Z71.41
  amobarbital — see Dependence, drug, sedative
  amphetamine(s) (type) — see Dependence, drug, stimulant NEC
  amytal (sodium) — see Dependence, drug, sedative
  analgesic NEC F55.8
  anesthetic (agent) (gas) (general) (local) NEC — see Dependence, drug, psychoactive NEC
  anxiolytic NEC — see Dependence, drug, sedative
  barbital(s) — see Dependence, drug, sedative
  barbiturate(s) (compounds) (drugs classifiable to T42) — see Dependence, drug, sedative
  benzedrine — see Dependence, drug, stimulant NEC
  bhang — see Dependence, drug, cannabis
  bromide(s) NEC — see Dependence, drug, sedative
  caffeine — see Dependence, drug, stimulant NEC
  cannabis (sativa) (indica) (resin) (derivatives) (type) — see Dependence, drug, cannabis
  chloral (betaine) (hydrate) — see Dependence, drug, sedative
  chlordiazepoxide — see Dependence, drug, sedative
  coca (leaf) (derivatives) — see Dependence, drug, cocaine
  cocaine — see Dependence, drug, cocaine
  codeine — see Dependence, drug, opioid
  combinations of drugs F19.2Ø
  D-lysergic acid diethylamide — see Dependence, drug, hallucinogen
  dagga — see Dependence, drug, cannabis
  demerol — see Dependence, drug, opioid
  dexamphetamine — see Dependence, drug, stimulant NEC
  dexedrine — see Dependence, drug, stimulant NEC
  dextro-nor-pseudo-ephedrine — see Dependence, drug, stimulant NEC
  dextromethorphan — see Dependence, drug, opioid
  dextromoramide — see Dependence, drug, opioid
  dextrorphan — see Dependence, drug, opioid
  diazepam — see Dependence, drug, sedative
  dilaudid — see Dependence, drug, opioid
  drug NEC F19.2Ø
    with sleep disorder F19.282
    cannabis F12.2Ø
      with
        anxiety disorder F12.28Ø
        intoxication F12.229
          with
            delirium F12.221
            perceptual disturbance F12.222
          uncomplicated F12.22Ø

Dependence — continued
  drug — continued
    cannabis — continued
      with — continued
        other specified disorder F12.288
        psychosis F12.259
          delusions F12.25Ø
          hallucinations F12.251
        unspecified disorder F12.29
      in remission F12.21
    cocaine F14.2Ø
      with
        anxiety disorder F14.28Ø
        intoxication F14.229
          with
            delirium F14.221
            perceptual disturbance F14.222
          uncomplicated F14.22Ø
        mood disorder F14.24
        other specified disorder F14.288
        psychosis F14.259
          delusions F14.25Ø
          hallucinations F14.251
        sexual dysfunction F14.281
        sleep disorder F14.282
        unspecified disorder F14.29
        withdrawal F14.23
      in remission F14.21
      withdrawal symptoms in newborn P96.1
    counseling and surveillance Z71.51
    hallucinogen F16.2Ø
      with
        anxiety disorder F16.28Ø
        flashbacks F16.283
        intoxication F16.229
          with delirium F16.221
          uncomplicated F16.22Ø
        mood disorder F16.24
        other specified disorder F16.288
        perception disorder, persisting F16.283
        psychosis F16.259
          delusions F16.25Ø
          hallucinations F16.251
        unspecified disorder F16.29
      in remission F16.21
    in remission F19.21
    inhalant F18.2Ø
      with
        anxiety disorder F18.28Ø
        dementia, persisting F18.27
        intoxication F18.229
          with delirium F18.221
          uncomplicated F18.22Ø
        mood disorder F18.24
        other specified disorder F18.288
        psychosis F18.259
          delusions F18.25Ø
          hallucinations F18.251
        unspecified disorder F18.29
      in remission F18.21
    nicotine F17.2ØØ
      with disorder F17.2Ø9
        remission F17.2Ø1
        specified disorder NEC F17.2Ø8
        withdrawal F17.2Ø3
      chewing tobacco F17.22Ø
        with disorder F17.229
          remission F17.221
          specified disorder NEC F17.228
          withdrawal F17.223
      cigarettes F17.21Ø
        with disorder F17.219
          remission F17.211
          specified disorder NEC F17.218
          withdrawal F17.213
      specified product NEC F17.29Ø
        with disorder F17.299
          remission F17.291
          specified disorder NEC F17.298
          withdrawal F17.293
    opioid F11.2Ø
      with
        intoxication F11.229
          with
            delirium F11.221
            perceptual disturbance F11.222
          uncomplicated F11.22Ø
        mood disorder F11.24

☑ **Additional Character Required** — Refer to the Tabular List for Character Selection   ▽ **Subterms under main terms may continue to next column or page**

Dependence — *continued*
  drug — *continued*
    opioid — *continued*
      with — *continued*
        other specified disorder F11.288
        psychosis F11.259
          delusions F11.250
          hallucinations F11.251
        sexual dysfunction F11.281
        sleep disorder F11.282
        unspecified disorder F11.29
        withdrawal F11.23
      in remission F11.21
    psychoactive NEC F19.20
      with
        amnestic disorder F19.26
        anxiety disorder F19.280
        dementia F19.27
        intoxication F19.229
          with
            delirium F19.221
            perceptual disturbance F19.222
          uncomplicated F19.220
        mood disorder F19.24
        other specified disorder F19.288
        psychosis F19.259
          delusions F19.250
          hallucinations F19.251
        sexual dysfunction F19.281
        sleep disorder F19.282
        unspecified disorder F19.29
        withdrawal F19.239
          with
            delirium F19.231
            perceptual disturbance F19.232
          uncomplicated F19.230
    sedative, hypnotic or anxiolytic F13.20
      with
        amnestic disorder F13.26
        anxiety disorder F13.280
        dementia, persisting F13.27
        intoxication F13.229
          with delirium F13.221
          uncomplicated F13.220
        mood disorder F13.24
        other specified disorder F13.288
        psychosis F13.259
          delusions F13.250
          hallucinations F13.251
        sexual dysfunction F13.281
        sleep disorder F13.282
        unspecified disorder F13.29
        withdrawal F13.239
          with
            delirium F13.231
            perceptual disturbance F13.232
          uncomplicated F13.230
      in remission F13.21
    stimulant NEC F15.20
      with
        anxiety disorder F15.280
        intoxication F15.229
          with
            delirium F15.221
            perceptual disturbance F15.222
          uncomplicated F15.220
        mood disorder F15.24
        other specified disorder F15.288
        psychosis F15.259
          delusions F15.250
          hallucinations F15.251
        sexual dysfunction F15.281
        sleep disorder F15.282
        unspecified disorder F15.29
        withdrawal F15.23
      in remission F15.21
  ethyl
    alcohol (without remission) F10.20
      with remission F10.21
    bromide — *see* Dependence, drug, sedative
    carbamate F19.20
    chloride F19.20
    morphine — *see* Dependence, drug, opioid
  ganja — *see* Dependence, drug, cannabis
  glue (airplane) (sniffing) — *see* Dependence, drug,
    inhalant
  glutethimide — *see* Dependence, drug, sedative

Dependence — *continued*
  hallucinogenics — *see* Dependence, drug, hallucinogen
  hashish — *see* Dependence, drug, cannabis
  hemp — *see* Dependence, drug, cannabis
  heroin (salt) (any) — *see* Dependence, drug, opioid
  hypnotic NEC — *see* Dependence, drug, sedative
  Indian hemp — *see* Dependence, drug, cannabis
  inhalants — *see* Dependence, drug, inhalant
  khat — *see* Dependence, drug, stimulant NEC
  laudanum — *see* Dependence, drug, opioid
  LSD (-25) (derivatives) — *see* Dependence, drug, hallucinogen
  luminal — *see* Dependence, drug, sedative
  lysergic acid — *see* Dependence, drug, hallucinogen
  maconha — *see* Dependence, drug, cannabis
  marihuana — *see* Dependence, drug, cannabis
  meprobamate — *see* Dependence, drug, sedative
  mescaline — *see* Dependence, drug, hallucinogen
  methadone — *see* Dependence, drug, opioid
  methamphetamine(s) — *see* Dependence, drug, stimulant NEC
  methaqualone — *see* Dependence, drug, sedative
  methyl
    alcohol (without remission) F10.20
      with remission F10.21
    bromide — *see* Dependence, drug, sedative
    morphine — *see* Dependence, drug, opioid
    phenidate — *see* Dependence, drug, stimulant NEC
    sulfonal — *see* Dependence, drug, sedative
  morphine (sulfate) (sulfite) (type) — *see* Dependence, drug, opioid
  narcotic (drug) NEC — *see* Dependence, drug, opioid
  nembutal — *see* Dependence, drug, sedative
  neraval — *see* Dependence, drug, sedative
  neravan — *see* Dependence, drug, sedative
  neurobarb — *see* Dependence, drug, sedative
  nicotine — *see* Dependence, drug, nicotine
  nitrous oxide F19.20
  nonbarbiturate sedatives and tranquilizers with similar effect — *see* Dependence, drug, sedative
  on
    artificial heart (fully implantable) (mechanical) Z95.812
    aspirator Z99.0
    care provider (because of) Z74.9
      impaired mobility Z74.09
      need for
        assistance with personal care Z74.1
        continuous supervision Z74.3
      no other household member able to render care Z74.2
      specified reason NEC Z74.8
    machine Z99.89
      enabling NEC Z99.89
      specified type NEC Z99.89
    renal dialysis (hemodialysis) (peritoneal) Z99.2
    respirator Z99.11
    ventilator Z99.11
    wheelchair Z99.3
  opiate — *see* Dependence, drug, opioid
  opioids — *see* Dependence, drug, opioid
  opium (alkaloids) (derivatives) (tincture) — *see* Dependence, drug, opioid
  oxygen (long-term) (supplemental) Z99.81
  paraldehyde — *see* Dependence, drug, sedative
  paregoric — *see* Dependence, drug, opioid
  PCP (phencyclidine) (*see also* Abuse, drug, hallucinogen) F16.20
  pentobarbital — *see* Dependence, drug, sedative
  pentobarbitone (sodium) — *see* Dependence, drug, sedative
  pentothal — *see* Dependence, drug, sedative
  peyote — *see* Dependence, drug, hallucinogen
  phencyclidine (PCP) (and related substances) (*see also* Abuse, drug, hallucinogen) F16.20
  phenmetrazine — *see* Dependence, drug, stimulant NEC
  phenobarbital — *see* Dependence, drug, sedative
  polysubstance F19.20
  psilocibin, psilocin, psilocyn, psilocyline — *see* Dependence, drug, hallucinogen
  psychostimulant NEC — *see* Dependence, drug, stimulant NEC
  secobarbital — *see* Dependence, drug, sedative
  seconal — *see* Dependence, drug, sedative

Dependence — *continued*
  sedative NEC — *see* Dependence, drug, sedative
  specified drug NEC — *see* Dependence, drug
  stimulant NEC — *see* Dependence, drug, stimulant NEC
  substance NEC — *see* Dependence, drug
  supplemental oxygen Z99.81
  tobacco — *see* Dependence, drug, nicotine
    counseling and surveillance Z71.6
  tranquilizer NEC — *see* Dependence, drug, sedative
  vitamin B6 E53.1
  volatile solvents — *see* Dependence, drug, inhalant
Dependency
  care-provider Z74.9
  passive F60.7
  reactions (persistent) F60.7
Depersonalization (in neurotic state) (neurotic) (syndrome) F48.1
Depletion
  extracellular fluid E86.9
  plasma E86.1
  potassium E87.6
    nephropathy N25.89
  salt or sodium E87.1
    causing heat exhaustion or prostration T67.4 ☑
    nephropathy N28.9
  volume NOS E86.9
Deployment (current) (military) status Z56.82
  in theater or in support of military war, peacekeeping and humanitarian operations Z56.82
  personal history of Z91.82
    military war, peacekeeping and humanitarian deployment (current or past conflict) Z91.82
  returned from Z91.82
Depolarization, premature I49.40
  atrial I49.1
  junctional I49.2
  specified NEC I49.49
  ventricular I49.3
Deposit
  bone in Boeck's sarcoid D86.89
  calcareous, calcium — *see* Calcification
  cholesterol
    retina H35.89
    vitreous (body) (humor) — *see* Deposit, crystalline
  conjunctiva H11.11- ☑
  cornea H18.00- ☑
    argentous H18.02- ☑
    due to metabolic disorder H18.03- ☑
    Kayser-Fleischer ring H18.04- ☑
    pigmentation — *see* Pigmentation, cornea
  crystalline, vitreous (body) (humor) H43.2- ☑
  hemosiderin in old scars of cornea — *see* Pigmentation, cornea, stromal
  metallic in lens — *see* Cataract, specified NEC
  skin R23.8
  tooth, teeth (betel) (black) (green) (materia alba) (orange) (tobacco) K03.6
  urate, kidney — *see* Calculus, kidney
Depraved appetite — *see* Pica
Depressed
  HDL cholesterol E78.6
Depression (acute) (mental) F32.9
  agitated (single episode) F32.2
  anaclitic — *see* Disorder, adjustment
  anxiety F41.8
    persistent F34.1
  arches (*see also* Deformity, limb, flat foot)
  atypical (single episode) F32.8
  basal metabolic rate R94.8
  bone marrow D75.89
  central nervous system R09.2
  cerebral R29.818
    newborn P91.4
  cerebrovascular I67.9
  chest wall M95.4
  climacteric (single episode) F32.8
  endogenous (without psychotic symptoms) F33.2
    with psychotic symptoms F33.3
  functional activity R68.89
  hysterical F44.89
  involutional (single episode) F32.8
  major F32.9
    with psychotic symptoms F32.3
    recurrent — *see* Disorder, depressive, recurrent
  manic-depressive — *see* Disorder, depressive, recurrent

Depression — *continued*
  masked (single episode) F32.8
  medullary G93.89
  menopausal (single episode) F32.8
  metatarsus — *see* Depression, arches
  monopolar F33.9
  nervous F34.1
  neurotic F34.1
  nose M95.0
  post-psychotic of schizophrenia F32.8
  post-schizophrenic F32.8
  postnatal F53
  postpartum F53
  psychogenic (reactive) (single episode) F32.9
  psychoneurotic F34.1
  psychotic (single episode) F32.3
    recurrent F33.3
  reactive (psychogenic) (single episode) F32.9
    psychotic (single episode) F32.3
  recurrent — *see* Disorder, depressive, recurrent
  respiratory center G93.89
  seasonal — *see* Disorder, depressive, recurrent
  senile F03 ☑
  severe, single episode F32.2
  situational F43.21
  skull Q67.4
  specified NEC (single episode) F32.8
  sternum M95.4
  visual field — *see* Defect, visual field
  vital (recurrent) (without psychotic symptoms) F33.2
    with psychotic symptoms F33.3
      single episode F32.2

Deprivation
  cultural Z60.3
  effects NOS T73.9 ☑
    specified NEC T73.8 ☑
  emotional NEC Z65.8
    affecting infant or child — *see* Maltreatment, child, psychological
  food T73.0 ☑
  protein — *see* Malnutrition
  sleep Z72.820
  social Z60.4
    affecting infant or child — *see* Maltreatment, child, psychological
  specified NEC T73.8 ☑
  vitamins — *see* Deficiency, vitamin
  water T73.1 ☑

Derangement
  ankle (internal) — *see* Derangement, joint, ankle
  cartilage (articular) NEC — *see* Derangement, joint, articular cartilage, by site
    recurrent — *see* Dislocation, recurrent
  cruciate ligament, anterior, current injury — *see* Sprain, knee, cruciate, anterior
  elbow (internal) — *see* Derangement, joint, elbow
  hip (joint) (internal) (old) — *see* Derangement, joint, hip
  joint (internal) M24.9
    ankylosis — *see* Ankylosis
    articular cartilage M24.10
      ankle M24.17- ☑
      elbow M24.12- ☑
      foot M24.17- ☑
      hand M24.14- ☑
      hip M24.15- ☑
      knee NEC M23.9- ☑
      loose body — *see* Loose, body
      shoulder M24.11- ☑
      wrist M24.13- ☑
    contracture — *see* Contraction, joint
    current injury (*see also* Dislocation)
      knee, meniscus or cartilage — *see* Tear, meniscus
    dislocation
      pathological — *see* Dislocation, pathological
      recurrent — *see* Dislocation, recurrent
    knee — *see* Derangement, knee
    ligament — *see* Disorder, ligament
    loose body — *see* Loose, body
    recurrent — *see* Dislocation, recurrent
    specified type NEC M24.80
      ankle M24.87- ☑
      elbow M24.82- ☑
      foot joint M24.87- ☑
      hand joint M24.84- ☑
      hip M24.85- ☑

Derangement — *continued*
  joint — *continued*
    specified type — *continued*
      shoulder M24.81- ☑
      wrist M24.83- ☑
    temporomandibular M26.69
  knee (recurrent) M23.9-
    ligament disruption, spontaneous M23.60- ☑
      anterior cruciate M23.61- ☑
      capsular M23.67- ☑
      instability, chronic M23.5- ☑
      lateral collateral M23.64- ☑
      medial collateral M23.63- ☑
      posterior cruciate M23.62- ☑
    loose body M23.4- ☑
    meniscus M23.30- ☑
      cystic M23.00- ☑
        lateral M23.002
          anterior horn M23.04- ☑
          posterior horn M23.05- ☑
          specified NEC M23.06- ☑
        medial M23.005
          anterior horn M23.01- ☑
          posterior horn M23.02- ☑
          specified NEC M23.03- ☑
      degenerate — *see* Derangement, knee, meniscus, specified NEC
      detached — *see* Derangement, knee, meniscus, specified NEC
      due to old tear or injury M23.20- ☑
        lateral M23.20- ☑
          anterior horn M23.24- ☑
          posterior horn M23.25- ☑
          specified NEC M23.26- ☑
        medial M23.20- ☑
          anterior horn M23.21- ☑
          posterior horn M23.22- ☑
          specified NEC M23.23- ☑
      retained — *see* Derangement, knee, meniscus, specified NEC
      specified NEC M23.30- ☑
        lateral M23.30- ☑
          anterior horn M23.34- ☑
          posterior horn M23.35- ☑
          specified NEC M23.36- ☑
        medial M23.30- ☑
          anterior horn M23.31- ☑
          posterior horn M23.32- ☑
          specified NEC M23.33- ☑
    old M23.8X- ☑
    specified NEC — *see* subcategory M23.8 ☑
  low back NEC — *see* Dorsopathy, specified NEC
  meniscus — *see* Derangement, knee, meniscus
  mental — *see* Psychosis
  patella, specified NEC — *see* Disorder, patella, derangement NEC
  semilunar cartilage (knee) — *see* Derangement, knee, meniscus, specified NEC
  shoulder (internal) — *see* Derangement, joint, shoulder

Dercum's disease E88.2
Derealization (neurotic) F48.1
Dermal — *see* condition
Dermaphytid — *see* Dermatophytosis
Dermatitis (eczematous) L30.9
  ab igne L59.0
  acarine B88.0
  actinic (due to sun) L57.8
    other than from sun L59.8
  allergic — *see* Dermatitis, contact, allergic
  ambustionis, due to burn or scald — *see* Burn
  amebic A06.7
  ammonia L22
  arsenical (ingested) L27.8
  artefacta L98.1
    psychogenic F54
  atopic L20.9
    psychogenic F54
    specified NEC L20.89
  autoimmune progesterone L30.8
  berlock, berloque L56.2
  blastomycotic B40.3
  blister beetle L24.89
  bullous, bullosa L13.9
    mucosynechial, atrophic L12.1
    seasonal L30.8

Dermatitis — *continued*
  bullous, bullosa — *continued*
    specified NEC L13.8
  calorica L59.0
    due to burn or scald — *see* Burn
  caterpillar L24.89
  cercarial B65.3
  combustionis L59.0
    due to burn or scald — *see* Burn
  congelationis T69.1 ☑
  contact (occupational) L25.9
    allergic L23.9
      due to
        adhesives L23.1
        cement L23.5
        chemical products NEC L23.5
        chromium L23.0
        cosmetics L23.2
        dander (cat) (dog) L23.81
        drugs in contact with skin L23.3
        dyes L23.4
        food in contact with skin L23.6
        hair (cat) (dog) L23.81
        insecticide L23.5
        metals L23.0
        nickel L23.0
        plants, non-food L23.7
        plastic L23.5
        rubber L23.5
        specified agent NEC L23.89
    due to
      cement L25.3
      chemical products NEC L25.3
      cosmetics L25.0
      dander (cat) (dog) L23.81
      drugs in contact with skin L25.1
      dyes L25.2
      food in contact with skin L25.4
      hair (cat) (dog) L23.81
      plants, non-food L25.5
      specified agent NEC L25.8
    irritant L24.9
      due to
        cement L25.3
        chemical products NEC L24.5
        cosmetics L24.3
        detergents L24.0
        drugs in contact with skin L24.4
        food in contact with skin L24.6
        oils and greases L24.1
        plants, non-food L24.7
        solvents L24.2
        specified agent NEC L24.89
  contusiformis L52
  diabetic — *see* E08-E13 with .620
  diaper L22
  diphtheritica A36.3
  dry skin L85.3
  due to
    acetone (contact) (irritant) L24.2
    acids (contact) (irritant) L24.5
    adhesive(s) (allergic) (contact) (plaster) L23.1
      irritant L24.5
    alcohol (irritant) (skin contact) (substances in category T51) L24.2
      taken internally L27.8
    alkalis (contact) (irritant) L24.5
    arsenic (ingested) L27.8
    carbon disulfide (contact) (irritant) L24.2
    caustics (contact) (irritant) L24.5
    cement (contact) L25.3
    cereal (ingested) L27.2
    chemical(s) NEC L25.3
      taken internally L27.8
    chlorocompounds L24.2
    chromium (contact) (irritant) L24.81
    coffee (ingested) L27.2
    cold weather L30.8
    cosmetics (contact) L25.0
      allergic L23.2
      irritant L24.3
    cyclohexanes L24.2
    dander (cat) (dog) L23.81
    Demodex species B88.0
    Dermanyssus gallinae B88.0
    detergents (contact) (irritant) L24.0
    dichromate L24.81

☑ **Additional Character Required** — Refer to the Tabular List for Character Selection   ▽ Subterms under main terms may continue to next column or page

Dermatitis — *continued*
  due to — *continued*
    drugs and medicaments (generalized) (internal use) L27.0
      external — *see* Dermatitis, due to, drugs, in contact with skin
      in contact with skin L25.1
        allergic L23.3
        irritant L24.4
      localized skin eruption L27.1
      specified substance — *see* Table of Drugs and Chemicals
    dyes (contact) L25.2
      allergic L23.4
      irritant L24.89
    epidermophytosis — *see* Dermatophytosis
    esters L24.2
    external irritant NEC L24.9
    fish (ingested) L27.2
    flour (ingested) L27.2
    food (ingested) L27.2
      in contact with skin L25.4
    fruit (ingested) L27.2
    furs (allergic) (contact) L23.81
    glues — *see* Dermatitis, due to, adhesives
    glycols L24.2
    greases NEC (contact) (irritant) L24.1
    hair (cat) (dog) L23.81
    hot
      objects and materials — *see* Burn
      weather or places L59.0
    hydrocarbons L24.2
    infrared rays L59.8
    ingestion, ingested substance L27.9
      chemical NEC L27.8
      drugs and medicaments — *see* Dermatitis, due to, drugs
      food L27.2
      specified NEC L27.8
    insecticide in contact with skin L24.5
    internal agent L27.9
      drugs and medicaments (generalized) — *see* Dermatitis, due to, drugs
      food L27.2
    irradiation — *see* Dermatitis, due to, radioactive substance
    ketones L24.2
    lacquer tree (allergic) (contact) L23.7
    light (sun) NEC L57.8
      acute L56.8
      other L59.8
    Liponyssoides sanguineus B88.0
    low temperature L30.8
    meat (ingested) L27.2
    metals, metal salts (contact) (irritant) L24.81
    milk (ingested) L27.2
    nickel (contact) (irritant) L24.81
    nylon (contact) (irritant) L24.5
    oils NEC (contact) (irritant) L24.1
    paint solvent (contact) (irritant) L24.2
    petroleum products (contact) (irritant) (substances in T52.0) L24.2
    plants NEC (contact) L25.5
      allergic L23.7
      irritant L24.7
    plasters (adhesive) (any) (allergic) (contact) L23.1
      irritant L24.5
    plastic (contact) L25.3
    preservatives (contact) — *see* Dermatitis, due to, chemical, in contact with skin
    primrose (allergic) (contact) L23.7
    primula (allergic) (contact) L23.7
    radiation L59.8
      nonionizing (chronic exposure) L57.8
      sun NEC L57.8
        acute L56.8
    radioactive substance L58.9
      acute L58.0
      chronic L58.1
    radium L58.9
      acute L58.0
      chronic L58.1
    ragweed (allergic) (contact) L23.7
    Rhus (allergic) (contact) (diversiloba) (radicans) (toxicodendron) (venenata) (verniciflua) L23.7
    rubber (contact) L24.5
    Senecio jacobaea (allergic) (contact) L23.7

Dermatitis — *continued*
  due to — *continued*
    solvents (contact) (irritant) (substances in category T52) L24.2
    specified agent NEC (contact) L25.8
      allergic L23.89
      irritant L24.89
    sunshine NEC L57.8
      acute L56.8
    tetrachlorethylene (contact) (irritant) L24.2
    toluene (contact) (irritant) L24.2
    turpentine (contact) L24.2
    ultraviolet rays (sun NEC) (chronic exposure) L57.8
      acute L56.8
    vaccine or vaccination L27.0
      specified substance — *see* Table of Drugs and Chemicals
    varicose veins — *see* Varix, leg, with, inflammation
    X-rays L58.9
      acute L58.0
      chronic L58.1
  dyshydrotic L30.1
  dysmenorrheica N94.6
  escharotica — *see* Burn
  exfoliative, exfoliativa (generalized) L26
    neonatorum L00
  eyelid (*see also* Dermatosis, eyelid)
    allergic H01.119
      left H01.116
        lower H01.115
        upper H01.114
      right H01.113
        lower H01.112
        upper H01.111
    contact — *see* Dermatitis, eyelid, allergic
    due to
      Demodex species B88.0
      herpes (zoster) B02.39
        simplex B00.59
    eczematous H01.139
      left H01.136
        lower H01.135
        upper H01.134
      right H01.133
        lower H01.132
        upper H01.131
  facta, factitia, factitial L98.1
    psychogenic F54
  flexural NEC L20.82
  friction L30.4
  fungus B36.9
    specified type NEC B36.8
  gangrenosa, gangrenous infantum L08.0
  harvest mite B88.0
  heat L59.0
  herpesviral, vesicular (ear) (lip) B00.1
  herpetiformis (bullous) (erythematous) (pustular) (vesicular) L13.0
    juvenile L12.2
    senile L12.0
  hiemalis L30.8
  hypostatic, hypostatica — *see* Varix, leg, with, inflammation
  infectious eczematoid L30.3
  infective L30.3
  irritant — *see* Dermatitis, contact, irritant
  Jacquet's (diaper dermatitis) L22
  Leptus B88.0
  lichenified NEC L28.0
  medicamentosa (generalized) (internal use) — *see* Dermatitis, due to drugs
  mite B88.0
  multiformis L13.0
    juvenile L12.2
  napkin L22
  neurotica L13.0
  nummular L30.0
  papillaris capillitii L73.0
  pellagrous E52
  perioral L71.0
  photocontact L56.2
  polymorpha dolorosa L13.0
  pruriginosa L13.0
  pruritic NEC L30.8
  psychogenic F54
  purulent L08.0
  pustular
    contagious B08.02

Dermatitis — *continued*
  pustular — *continued*
    subcorneal L13.1
  pyococcal L08.0
  pyogenica L08.0
  repens L40.2
  Ritter's (exfoliativa) L00
  Schamberg's L81.7
  schistosome B65.3
  seasonal bullous L30.8
  seborrheic L21.9
    infantile L21.1
    specified NEC L21.8
  sensitization NOS L23.9
  septic L08.0
  solare L57.8
  specified NEC L30.8
  stasis I87.2
    with varicose ulcer — *see* Varix, leg, with ulcer, with inflammation
    due to postthrombotic syndrome — *see* Syndrome, postthrombotic
  suppurative L08.0
  traumatic NEC L30.4
  trophoneurotica L13.0
  ultraviolet (sun) (chronic exposure) L57.8
    acute L56.8
  varicose — *see* Varix, leg, with, inflammation
  vegetans L10.1
  verrucosa B43.0
  vesicular, herpesviral B00.1
Dermatoarthritis, lipoid E78.81
Dermatochalasis, eyelid H02.839
  left H02.836
    lower H02.835
    upper H02.834
  right H02.833
    lower H02.832
    upper H02.831
Dermatofibroma (lenticulare) — *see* Neoplasm, skin, benign
  protuberans — *see* Neoplasm, skin, uncertain behavior
Dermatofibrosarcoma (pigmented) (protuberans) — *see* Neoplasm, skin, malignant
Dermatographia L50.3
Dermatolysis (exfoliativa) (congenital) Q82.8
  acquired L57.4
  eyelids — *see* Blepharochalasis
  palpebrarum — *see* Blepharochalasis
  senile L57.4
Dermatomegaly NEC Q82.8
Dermatomucosomyositis M33.10
  with
    myopathy M33.12
    respiratory involvement M33.11
    specified organ involvement NEC M33.19
Dermatomycosis B36.9
  furfuracea B36.0
  specified type NEC B36.8
Dermatomyositis (acute) (chronic) (*see also* Dermatopolymyositis)
  in (due to) neoplastic disease (*see also* Neoplasm) D49.9 [M36.0]
Dermatoneuritis of children — *see* Poisoning, mercury
Dermatophilosis A48.8
Dermatophytid L30.2
Dermatophytide — *see* Dermatophytosis
Dermatophytosis (epidermophyton) (infection) (Microsporum) (tinea) (Trichophyton) B35.9
  beard B35.0
  body B35.4
  capitis B35.0
  corporis B35.4
  deep-seated B35.8
  disseminated B35.8
  foot B35.3
  granulomatous B35.8
  groin B35.6
  hand B35.2
  nail B35.1
  perianal (area) B35.6
  scalp B35.0
  specified NEC B35.8
Dermatopolymyositis M33.90
  with
    myopathy M33.92
    respiratory involvement M33.91
    specified organ involvement NEC M33.99

Dermatopolymyositis — continued
in neoplastic disease (see also Neoplasm)
D49.9 [M36.0]
juvenile M33.00
with
myopathy M33.02
respiratory involvement M33.01
specified organ involvement NEC M33.09
specified NEC M33.10
myopathy M33.12
respiratory involvement M33.11
specified organ involvement NEC M33.19
Dermatopolyneuritis — see Poisoning, mercury
Dermatorrhexis Q79.6
acquired L57.4
Dermatosclerosis (see also Scleroderma)
localized L94.0
Dermatosis L98.9
Andrews' L08.89
Bowen's — see Neoplasm, skin, in situ
bullous L13.9
specified NEC L13.8
exfoliativa L26
eyelid (noninfectious)
dermatitis — see Dermatitis, eyelid
discoid lupus erythematosus — see Lupus, erythematosus, eyelid
xeroderma — see Xeroderma, acquired, eyelid
factitial L98.1
febrile neutrophilic L98.2
gonococcal A54.89
herpetiformis L13.0
juvenile L12.2
linear IgA L13.8
menstrual NEC L98.8
neutrophilic, febrile L98.2
occupational — see Dermatitis, contact
papulosa nigra L82.1
pigmentary L81.9
progressive L81.7
Schamberg's L81.7
psychogenic F54
purpuric, pigmented L81.7
pustular, subcorneal L13.1
transient acantholytic L11.1
Dermographia, dermographism L50.3
Dermoid (cyst) (see also Neoplasm, benign, by site)
with malignant transformation C56- ☑
due to radiation (nonionizing) L57.8
Dermopathy
infiltrative with thyrotoxicosis — see Thyrotoxicosis
nephrogenic fibrosing L90.8
Dermophytosis — see Dermatophytosis
Descemetocele H18.73- ☑
Descemet's membrane — see condition
Descending — see condition
Descensus uteri — see Prolapse, uterus
Desert
rheumatism B38.0
sore — see Ulcer, skin
Desertion (newborn) — see Maltreatment
Desmoid (extra-abdominal) (tumor) — see Neoplasm, connective tissue, uncertain behavior
abdominal D48.1
Despondency F32.9
Desquamation, skin R23.4
Destruction, destructive (see also Damage)
articular facet (see also Derangement, joint, specified type NEC)
knee M23.8X- ☑
vertebra — see Spondylosis
bone (see also Disorder, bone, specified type NEC)
syphilitic A52.77
joint (see also Derangement, joint, specified type NEC)
sacroiliac M53.3
rectal sphincter K62.89
septum (nasal) J34.89
tuberculous NEC — see Tuberculosis
tympanum, tympanic membrane (nontraumatic) — see Disorder, tympanic membrane, specified NEC
vertebral disc — see Degeneration, intervertebral disc
Destructiveness (see also Disorder, conduct)
adjustment reaction — see Disorder, adjustment
Desultory labor O62.2
Detachment
cartilage — see Sprain

Detachment — continued
cervix, annular N88.8
complicating delivery O71.3
choroid (old) (postinfectional) (simple) (spontaneous)
H31.40- ☑
hemorrhagic H31.41- ☑
serous H31.42- ☑
ligament — see Sprain
meniscus (knee) (see also Derangement, knee, meniscus, specified NEC)
current injury — see Tear, meniscus
due to old tear or injury — see Derangement, knee, meniscus, due to old tear
retina (without retinal break) (serous) H33.2- ☑
with retinal:
break H33.00- ☑
giant H33.03- ☑
multiple H33.02- ☑
single H33.01- ☑
dialysis H33.04- ☑
pigment epithelium — see Degeneration, retina, separation of layers, pigment epithelium detachment
rhegmatogenous — see Detachment, retina, with retinal, break
specified NEC H33.8
total H33.05- ☑
traction H33.4- ☑
vitreous (body) H43.81 ☑
Detergent asthma J69.8
Deterioration
epileptic F06.8
general physical R53.81
heart, cardiac — see Degeneration, myocardial
mental — see Psychosis
myocardial, myocardium — see Degeneration, myocardial
senile (simple) R54
Deuteranomaly (anomalous trichromat) H53.53
Deuteranopia (complete) (incomplete) H53.53
Development
abnormal, bone Q79.9
arrested R62.50
bone — see Arrest, development or growth, bone
child R62.50
due to malnutrition E45
defective, congenital (see also Anomaly, by site)
cauda equina Q06.3
left ventricle Q24.8
in hypoplastic left heart syndrome Q23.4
valve Q24.8
pulmonary Q22.3
delayed (see also Delay, development) R62.50
arithmetical skills F81.2
language (skills) (expressive) F80.1
learning skill F81.9
mixed skills F88
motor coordination F82
reading F81.0
specified learning skill NEC F81.89
speech F80.9
spelling F81.81
written expression F81.81
imperfect, congenital (see also Anomaly, by site)
heart Q24.9
lungs Q33.6
incomplete
bronchial tree Q32.4
organ or site not listed — see Hypoplasia, by site
respiratory system Q34.9
sexual, precocious NEC E30.1
tardy, mental (see also Disability, intellectual) F79
Developmental — see condition
testing, child — see Examination, child
Devergie's disease (pityriasis rubra pilaris) L44.0
Deviation (in)
conjugate palsy (eye) (spastic) H51.0
esophagus (acquired) K22.8
eye, skew H51.8
midline (jaw) (teeth) (dental arch) M26.29
specified site NEC — see Malposition
nasal septum J34.2
congenital Q67.4
opening and closing of the mandible M26.53
organ or site, congenital NEC — see Malposition, congenital
septum (nasal) (acquired) J34.2

Deviation — continued
septum — continued
congenital Q67.4
sexual F65.9
bestiality F65.89
erotomania F52.8
exhibitionism F65.2
fetishism, fetishistic F65.0
transvestism F65.1
frotteurism F65.81
masochism F65.51
multiple F65.89
necrophilia F65.89
nymphomania F52.8
pederosis F65.4
pedophilia F65.4
sadism, sadomasochism F65.52
satyriasis F52.8
specified type NEC F65.89
transvestism F64.1
voyeurism F65.3
teeth, midline M26.29
trachea J39.8
ureter, congenital Q62.61
Device
cerebral ventricle (communicating) in situ Z98.2
contraceptive — see Contraceptive, device
drainage, cerebrospinal fluid, in situ Z98.2
Devic's disease G36.0
Devil's
grip B33.0
pinches (purpura simplex) D69.2
Devitalized tooth K04.99
Devonshire colic — see Poisoning, lead
Dextraposition, aorta Q20.3
in tetralogy of Fallot Q21.3
Dextrinosis, limit (debrancher enzyme deficiency)
E74.03
Dextrocardia (true) Q24.0
with
complete transposition of viscera Q89.3
situs inversus Q89.3
Dextrotransposition, aorta Q20.3
Dhat syndrome F48.8
Dhobi itch B35.6
Di George's syndrome D82.1
Di Guglielmo's disease C94.0- ☑
Diabetes, diabetic (mellitus) (sugar) E11.9
with
amyotrophy E11.44
arthropathy NEC E11.618
autonomic (poly)neuropathy E11.43
cataract E11.36
Charcot's joints E11.610
chronic kidney disease E11.22
circulatory complication NEC E11.59
complication E11.8
specified NEC E11.69
dermatitis E11.620
foot ulcer E11.621
gangrene E11.52
gastroparesis E11.43
glomerulonephrosis, intracapillary E11.21
glomerulosclerosis, intercapillary E11.21
hyperglycemia E11.65
hyperosmolarity E11.00
with coma E11.01
hypoglycemia E11.649
with coma E11.641
kidney complications NEC E11.29
Kimmelstiel-Wilson disease E11.21
loss of protective sensation (LOPS) — see Diabetes, by type, with neuropathy
mononeuropathy E11.41
myasthenia E11.44
necrobiosis lipoidica E11.620
nephropathy E11.21
neuralgia E11.42
neurologic complication NEC E11.49
neuropathic arthropathy E11.610
neuropathy E11.40
ophthalmic complication NEC E11.39
oral complication NEC E11.638
periodontal disease E11.630
peripheral angiopathy E11.51
with gangrene E11.52
polyneuropathy E11.42
renal complication NEC E11.29

☑ **Additional Character Required — Refer to the Tabular List for Character Selection**   ▽ **Subterms under main terms may continue to next column or page**

Diabetes, diabetic — *continued*

with — *continued*

renal tubular degeneration E11.29

retinopathy E11.319

with macular edema E11.311

nonproliferative E11.329

with macular edema E11.321

mild E11.329

with macular edema E11.321

moderate E11.339

with macular edema E11.331

severe E11.349

with macular edema E11.341

proliferative E11.359

with macular edema E11.351

skin complication NEC E11.628

skin ulcer NEC E11.622

bronzed E83.110

complicating pregnancy — *see* Pregnancy, complicated by, diabetes

dietary counseling and surveillance Z71.3

due to drug or chemical E09.9

with

amyotrophy E09.44

arthropathy NEC E09.618

autonomic (poly)neuropathy E09.43

cataract E09.36

Charcot's joints E09.610

chronic kidney disease E09.22

circulatory complication NEC E09.59

complication E09.8

specified NEC E09.69

dermatitis E09.620

foot ulcer E09.621

gangrene E09.52

gastroparesis E09.43

glomerulonephrosis, intracapillary E09.21

glomerulosclerosis, intercapillary E09.21

hyperglycemia E09.65

hyperosmolarity E09.00

with coma E09.01

hypoglycemia E09.649

with coma E09.641

ketoacidosis E09.10

with coma E09.11

kidney complications NEC E09.29

Kimmelstiel-Wilson disease E09.21

mononeuropathy E09.41

myasthenia E09.44

necrobiosis lipoidica E09.620

nephropathy E09.21

neuralgia E09.42

neurologic complication NEC E09.49

neuropathic arthropathy E09.610

neuropathy E09.40

ophthalmic complication NEC E09.39

oral complication NEC E09.638

periodontal disease E09.630

peripheral angiopathy E09.51

with gangrene E09.52

polyneuropathy E09.42

renal complication NEC E09.29

renal tubular degeneration E09.29

retinopathy E09.319

with macular edema E09.311

nonproliferative E09.329

with macular edema E09.321

mild E09.329

with macular edema E09.321

moderate E09.339

with macular edema E09.331

severe E09.349

with macular edema E09.341

proliferative E09.359

with macular edema E09.351

skin complication NEC E09.628

skin ulcer NEC E09.622

due to underlying condition E08.9

with

amyotrophy E08.44

arthropathy NEC E08.618

autonomic (poly)neuropathy E08.43

cataract E08.36

Charcot's joints E08.610

chronic kidney disease E08.22

circulatory complication NEC E08.59

complication E08.8

specified NEC E08.69

Diabetes, diabetic — *continued*

due to underlying condition — *continued*

with — *continued*

dermatitis E08.620

foot ulcer E08.621

gangrene E08.52

gastroparesis E08.43

glomerulonephrosis, intracapillary E08.21

glomerulosclerosis, intercapillary E08.21

hyperglycemia E08.65

hyperosmolarity E08.00

with coma E08.01

hypoglycemia E08.649

with coma E08.641

ketoacidosis E08.10

with coma E08.11

kidney complications NEC E08.29

Kimmelstiel-Wilson disease E08.21

mononeuropathy E08.41

myasthenia E08.44

necrobiosis lipoidica E08.620

nephropathy E08.21

neuralgia E08.42

neurologic complication NEC E08.49

neuropathic arthropathy E08.610

neuropathy E08.40

ophthalmic complication NEC E08.39

oral complication NEC E08.638

periodontal disease E08.630

peripheral angiopathy E08.51

with gangrene E08.52

polyneuropathy E08.42

renal complication NEC E08.29

renal tubular degeneration E08.29

retinopathy E08.319

with macular edema E08.311

nonproliferative E08.329

with macular edema E08.321

mild E08.329

with macular edema E08.321

moderate E08.339

with macular edema E08.331

severe E08.349

with macular edema E08.341

proliferative E08.359

with macular edema E08.351

skin complication NEC E08.628

skin ulcer NEC E08.622

gestational (in pregnancy) O24.419

affecting newborn P70.0

diet controlled O24.410

in childbirth O24.429

diet controlled O24.420

insulin (and diet) controlled O24.424

insulin (and diet) controlled O24.414

puerperal O24.439

diet controlled O24.430

insulin (and diet) controlled O24.434

hepatogenous E13.9

inadequately controlled — *code to* Diabetes, by type, with hyperglycemia

insipidus E23.2

nephrogenic N25.1

pituitary E23.2

vasopressin resistant N25.1

insulin dependent — *code to* type of diabetes

juvenile-onset — *see* Diabetes, type 1

ketosis-prone — *see* Diabetes, type 1

latent R73.09

neonatal (transient) P70.2

non-insulin dependent — *code to* type of diabetes

out of control — *code to* Diabetes, by type, with hyperglycemia

phosphate E83.39

poorly controlled — *code to* Diabetes, by type, with hyperglycemia

postpancreatectomy — *see* Diabetes, specified type NEC

postprocedural — *see* Diabetes, specified type NEC

secondary diabetes mellitus NEC — *see* Diabetes, specified type NEC

specified type NEC E13.9

with

amyotrophy E13.44

arthropathy NEC E13.618

autonomic (poly)neuropathy E13.43

cataract E13.36

Charcot's joints E13.610

Diabetes, diabetic — *continued*

specified type — *continued*

with — *continued*

chronic kidney disease E13.22

circulatory complication NEC E13.59

complication E13.8

specified NEC E13.69

dermatitis E13.620

foot ulcer E13.621

gangrene E13.52

gastroparesis E13.43

glomerulonephrosis, intracapillary E13.21

glomerulosclerosis, intercapillary E13.21

hyperglycemia E13.65

hyperosmolarity E13.00

with coma E13.01

hypoglycemia E13.649

with coma E13.641

ketoacidosis E13.10

with coma E13.11

kidney complications NEC E13.29

Kimmelstiel-Wilson disease E13.21

mononeuropathy E13.41

myasthenia E13.44

necrobiosis lipoidica E13.620

nephropathy E13.21

neuralgia E13.42

neurologic complication NEC E13.49

neuropathic arthropathy E13.610

neuropathy E13.40

ophthalmic complication NEC E13.39

oral complication NEC E13.638

periodontal disease E13.630

peripheral angiopathy E13.51

with gangrene E13.52

polyneuropathy E13.42

renal complication NEC E13.29

renal tubular degeneration E13.29

retinopathy E13.319

with macular edema E13.311

nonproliferative E13.329

with macular edema E13.321

mild E13.329

with macular edema E13.321

moderate E13.339

with macular edema E13.331

severe E13.349

with macular edema E13.341

proliferative E13.359

with macular edema E13.351

skin complication NEC E13.628

skin ulcer NEC E13.622

steroid-induced — *see* Diabetes, due to, drug or chemical

type 1 E10.9

with

amyotrophy E10.44

arthropathy NEC E10.618

autonomic (poly)neuropathy E10.43

cataract E10.36

Charcot's joints E10.610

chronic kidney disease E10.22

circulatory complication NEC E10.59

complication E10.8

specified NEC E10.69

dermatitis E10.620

foot ulcer E10.621

gangrene E10.52

gastroparesis E10.43

glomerulonephrosis, intracapillary E10.21

glomerulosclerosis, intercapillary E10.21

hyperglycemia E10.65

hypoglycemia E10.649

with coma E10.641

ketoacidosis E10.10

with coma E10.11

kidney complications NEC E10.29

Kimmelstiel-Wilson disease E10.21

mononeuropathy E10.41

myasthenia E10.44

necrobiosis lipoidica E10.620

nephropathy E10.21

neuralgia E10.42

neurologic complication NEC E10.49

neuropathic arthropathy E10.610

neuropathy E10.40

ophthalmic complication NEC E10.39

oral complication NEC E10.638

Diabetes, diabetic — *continued*
 type 1 — *continued*
  with — *continued*
   periodontal disease E10.630
   peripheral angiopathy E10.51
    with gangrene E10.52
   polyneuropathy E10.42
   renal complication NEC E10.29
   renal tubular degeneration E10.29
   retinopathy E10.319
    with macular edema E10.311
    nonproliferative E10.329
     with macular edema E10.321
     mild E10.329
      with macular edema E10.321
     moderate E10.339
      with macular edema E10.331
     severe E10.349
      with macular edema E10.341
    proliferative E10.359
     with macular edema E10.351
   skin complication NEC E10.628
   skin ulcer NEC E10.622
 type 2 E11.9
  with
   amyotrophy E11.44
   arthropathy NEC E11.618
   autonomic (poly)neuropathy E11.43
   cataract E11.36
   Charcot's joints E11.610
   chronic kidney disease E11.22
   circulatory complication NEC E11.59
   complication E11.8
    specified NEC E11.69
   dermatitis E11.620
   foot ulcer E11.621
   gangrene E11.52
   gastroparesis E11.43
   glomerulonephrosis, intracapillary E11.21
   glomerulosclerosis, intercapillary E11.21
   hyperglycemia E11.65
   hyperosmolarity E11.00
    with coma E11.01
   hypoglycemia E11.649
    with coma E11.641
   kidney complications NEC E11.29
   Kimmelstiel-Wilson disease E11.21
   mononeuropathy E11.41
   myasthenia E11.44
   necrobiosis lipoidica E11.620
   nephropathy E11.21
   neuralgia E11.42
   neurologic complication NEC E11.49
   neuropathic arthropathy E11.610
   neuropathy E11.40
   ophthalmic complication NEC E11.39
   oral complication NEC E11.638
   periodontal disease E11.630
   peripheral angiopathy E11.51
    with gangrene E11.52
   polyneuropathy E11.42
   renal complication NEC E11.29
   renal tubular degeneration E11.29
   retinopathy E11.319
    with macular edema E11.311
    nonproliferative E11.329
     with macular edema E11.321
     mild E11.329
      with macular edema E11.321
     moderate E11.339
      with macular edema E11.331
     severe E11.349
      with macular edema E11.341
    proliferative E11.359
     with macular edema E11.351
   skin complication NEC E11.628
   skin ulcer NEC E11.622
Diacyclothrombopathia D69.1
Diagnosis deferred R69
Dialysis (intermittent) (treatment)
 noncompliance (with) Z91.15
 renal (hemodialysis) (peritoneal), status Z99.2
 retina, retinal — *see* Detachment, retina, with retinal, dialysis
Diamond-Blackfan anemia (congenital hypoplastic) D61.01
Diamond-Gardener syndrome (autoerythrocyte sensitization) D69.2

Diaper rash L22
Diaphoresis (excessive) R61
Diaphragm — *see* condition
Diaphragmalgia R07.1
Diaphragmatitis, diaphragmitis J98.6
Diaphysial aclasis Q78.6
Diaphysitis — *see* Osteomyelitis, specified type NEC
Diarrhea, diarrheal (disease) (infantile) (inflammatory) R19.7
 achlorhydric K31.83
 allergic K52.2
 amebic (*see also* Amebiasis) A06.0
  with abscess — *see* Abscess, amebic
  acute A06.0
  chronic A06.1
  nondysenteric A06.2
 bacillary — *see* Dysentery, bacillary
 balantidial A07.0
 cachectic NEC K52.89
 Chilomastix A07.8
 choleriformis A00.1
 chronic (noninfectious) K52.9
 coccidial A07.3
 Cochin-China K90.1
  strongyloidiasis B78.0
 Dientamoeba A07.8
 dietetic K52.2
 drug-induced K52.1
 due to
  bacteria A04.9
   specified NEC A04.8
  Campylobacter A04.5
  Capillaria philippinensis B81.1
  Clostridium difficile A04.7
  Clostridium perfringens (C) (F) A04.8
  Cryptosporidium A07.2
  drugs K52.1
  Escherichia coli A04.4
   enteroaggregative A04.4
   enterohemorrhagic A04.3
   enteroinvasive A04.2
   enteropathogenic A04.0
   enterotoxigenic A04.1
   specified NEC A04.4
  food hypersensitivity K52.2
  Necator americanus B76.1
  S. japonicum B65.2
  specified organism NEC A08.8
   bacterial A04.8
   viral A08.39
  Staphylococcus A04.8
  Trichuris trichiuria B79
  virus — *see* Enteritis, viral
  Yersinia enterocolitica A04.6
 dysenteric A09
 endemic A09
 epidemic A09
 flagellate A07.9
 Flexner's (ulcerative) A03.1
 functional K59.1
  following gastrointestinal surgery K91.89
  psychogenic F45.8
 Giardia lamblia A07.1
 giardial A07.1
 hill K90.1
 infectious A09
 malarial — *see* Malaria
 mite B88.0
 mycotic NEC B49
 neonatal (noninfectious) P78.3
 nervous F45.8
 neurogenic K59.1
 noninfectious K52.9
 postgastrectomy K91.1
 postvagotomy K91.1
 protozoal A07.9
  specified NEC A07.8
 psychogenic F45.8
 specified
  bacterium NEC A04.8
  virus NEC A08.39
 strongyloidiasis B78.0
 toxic K52.1
 trichomonal A07.8
 tropical K90.1
 tuberculous A18.32
 viral — *see* Enteritis, viral

Diastasis
 cranial bones M84.88
  congenital NEC Q75.8
 joint (traumatic) — *see* Dislocation
 muscle M62.00
  ankle M62.07- ✓
  congenital Q79.8
  foot M62.07- ✓
  forearm M62.03- ✓
  hand M62.04- ✓
  lower leg M62.06- ✓
  pelvic region M62.05- ✓
  shoulder region M62.01- ✓
  specified site NEC M62.08
  thigh M62.05- ✓
  upper arm M62.02- ✓
 recti (abdomen)
  complicating delivery O71.89
  congenital Q79.59
Diastema, tooth, teeth, fully erupted M26.32
Diastematomyelia Q06.2
Diataxia, cerebral G80.4
Diathesis
 allergic — *see* History, allergy
 bleeding (familial) D69.9
 cystine (familial) E72.00
 gouty — *see* Gout
 hemorrhagic (familial) D69.9
  newborn NEC P53
 spasmophilic R29.0
Diaz's disease or osteochondrosis (juvenile) (talus) — *see* Osteochondrosis, juvenile, tarsus
Dibothriocephalus, dibothriocephaliasis (latus) (infection) (infestation) B70.0
 larval B70.1
Dicephalus, dicephaly Q89.4
Dichotomy, teeth K00.2
Dichromat, dichromatopsia (congenital) — *see* Deficiency, color vision
Dichuchwa A65
Dicroceliasis B66.2
Didelphia, didelphys — *see* Double uterus
Didymytis N45.1
 with orchitis N45.3
Dietary
 inadequacy or deficiency E63.9
 surveillance and counseling Z71.3
Dietl's crisis N13.8
Dieulafoy lesion (hemorrhagic)
 duodenum K31.82
 esophagus K22.8
 intestine (colon) K63.81
 stomach K31.82
Difficult, difficulty (in)
 acculturation Z60.3
 feeding R63.3
  newborn P92.9
   breast P92.5
   specified NEC P92.8
  nonorganic (infant or child) F98.29
 intubation, in anesthesia T88.4 ✓
 mechanical, gastroduodenal stoma K91.89
  causing obstruction K91.3
 reading (developmental) F81.0
  secondary to emotional disorders F93.9
 spelling (specific) F81.81
  with reading disorder F81.89
  due to inadequate teaching Z55.8
 swallowing — *see* Dysphagia
 walking R26.2
 work
  conditions NEC Z56.5
  schedule Z56.3
Diffuse — *see* condition
Digestive — *see* condition
Dihydropyrimidine dehydrogenase disease (DPD) E88.89
Diktyoma — *see* Neoplasm, malignant, by site
Dilaceration, tooth K00.4
Dilatation
 anus K59.8
  venule — *see* Hemorrhoids
 aorta (focal) (general) — *see* Ectasia, aorta
  with aneurysm — *see* Aneurysm, aorta
 artery — *see* Aneurysm
 bladder (sphincter) N32.89
  congenital Q64.79

Dilatation — continued
blood vessel I99.8
bronchial J47.9
  with
    exacerbation (acute) J47.1
    lower respiratory infection J47.0
calyx (due to obstruction) — see Hydronephrosis
capillaries I78.8
cardiac (acute) (chronic) (see also Hypertrophy, cardiac)
  congenital Q24.8
    valve NEC Q24.8
      pulmonary Q22.3
  valve — see Endocarditis
cavum septi pellucidi Q06.8
cervix (uteri) (see also Incompetency, cervix)
  incomplete, poor, slow complicating delivery O62.0
colon K59.3
  congenital Q43.1
  psychogenic F45.8
common duct (acquired) K83.8
  congenital Q44.5
cystic duct (acquired) K82.8
  congenital Q44.5
duct, mammary — see Ectasia, mammary duct
duodenum K59.8
esophagus K22.8
  congenital Q39.5
  due to achalasia K22.0
eustachian tube, congenital Q17.8
gallbladder K82.8
gastric — see Dilatation, stomach
heart (acute) (chronic) (see also Hypertrophy, cardiac)
  congenital Q24.8
  valve — see Endocarditis
ileum K59.8
  psychogenic F45.8
jejunum K59.8
  psychogenic F45.8
kidney (calyx) (collecting structures) (cystic)
  (parenchyma) (pelvis) (idiopathic) N28.89
lacrimal passages or duct — see Disorder, lacrimal
  system, changes
lymphatic vessel I89.0
mammary duct — see Ectasia, mammary duct
Meckel's diverticulum (congenital) Q43.0
  malignant — see Table of Neoplasms, small intes-
    tine, malignant
myocardium (acute) (chronic) — see Hypertrophy,
  cardiac
organ or site, congenital NEC — see Distortion
pancreatic duct K86.8
pericardium — see Pericarditis
pharynx J39.2
prostate N42.89
pulmonary
  artery (idiopathic) I28.8
  valve, congenital Q22.3
pupil H57.04
rectum K59.3
saccule, congenital Q16.5
salivary gland (duct) K11.8
sphincter ani K62.89
stomach K31.89
  acute K31.0
  psychogenic F45.8
submaxillary duct K11.8
trachea, congenital Q32.1
ureter (idiopathic) N28.82
  congenital Q62.2
  due to obstruction N13.4
urethra (acquired) N36.8
vasomotor I73.9
vein I86.8
ventricular, ventricle (acute) (chronic) (see also Hypertrophy, cardiac)
  cerebral, congenital Q04.8
venule NEC I86.8
vesical orifice N32.89
Dilated, dilation — see Dilatation
Diminished, diminution
hearing (acuity) — see Deafness
sense or sensation (cold) (heat) (tactile) (vibratory)
  R20.8
vision NEC H54.7
vital capacity R94.2
Diminuta taenia B71.0
Dimitri-Sturge-Weber disease Q85.8

Dimple
parasacral, pilonidal or postanal — see Cyst, pilonidal
Dioctophyme renalis (infection) (infestation) B83.8
Dipetalonemiasis B74.4
Diphallus Q55.69
Diphtheria, diphtheritic (gangrenous) (hemorrhagic)
  A36.9
carrier (suspected) Z22.2
cutaneous A36.3
faucial A36.0
infection of wound A36.3
laryngeal A36.2
myocarditis A36.81
nasal, anterior A36.89
nasopharyngeal A36.1
neurological complication A36.89
pharyngeal A36.0
specified site NEC A36.89
tonsillar A36.0
Diphyllobothriasis (intestine) B70.0
larval B70.1
Diplacusis H93.22- ☑
Diplegia (upper limbs) G83.0
congenital (cerebral) G80.8
facial G51.0
lower limbs G82.20
spastic G80.1
Diplococcus, diplococcal — see condition
Diplopia H53.2
Dipsomania F10.20
  with
    psychosis — see Psychosis, alcoholic
    remission F10.21
Dipylidiasis B71.1
Direction, teeth, abnormal, fully erupted M26.30
Dirofilariasis B74.8
Dirt-eating child F98.3
Disability, disabilities
heart — see Disease, heart
intellectual F79
  with
    autistic features F84.9
  mild (I.Q. 50-69) F70
  moderate (I.Q. 35-49) F71
  profound (I.Q. under 20) F73
  severe (I.Q. 20-34) F72
  specified level NEC F78
knowledge acquisition F81.9
learning F81.9
limiting activities Z73.6
spelling, specific F81.81
Disappearance of family member Z63.4
Disarticulation — see Amputation
meaning traumatic amputation — see Amputation,
  traumatic
Discharge (from)
abnormal finding in — see Abnormal, specimen
breast (female) (male) N64.52
diencephalic autonomic idiopathic — see Epilepsy,
  specified NEC
ear (see also Otorrhea)
  blood — see Otorrhagia
excessive urine R35.8
nipple N64.52
penile R36.9
postnasal R09.82
prison, anxiety concerning Z65.2
urethral R36.9
  without blood R36.0
  hematospermia R36.1
vaginal N89.8
Discitis, diskitis M46.40
cervical region M46.42
cervicothoracic region M46.43
lumbar region M46.46
lumbosacral region M46.47
multiple sites M46.49
occipito-atlanto-axial region M46.41
pyogenic — see Infection, intervertebral disc, pyogenic
sacrococcygeal region M46.48
thoracic region M46.44
thoracolumbar region M46.45
Discoid
meniscus (congenital) Q68.6
semilunar cartilage (congenital) — see Derangement,
  knee, meniscus, specified NEC

Discoloration
nails L60.8
teeth (posteruptive) K03.7
  during formation K00.8
Discomfort
chest R07.89
visual H53.14- ☑
Discontinuity, ossicles, ear H74.2- ☑
Discord (with)
boss Z56.4
classmates Z55.4
counselor Z64.4
employer Z56.4
family Z63.8
fellow employees Z56.4
in-laws Z63.1
landlord Z59.2
lodgers Z59.2
neighbors Z59.2
probation officer Z64.4
social worker Z64.4
teachers Z55.4
workmates Z56.4
Discordant connection
atrioventricular (congenital) Q20.5
ventriculoarterial Q20.3
Discrepancy
centric occlusion maximum intercuspation M26.55
leg length (acquired) — see Deformity, limb, unequal
  length
  congenital — see Defect, reduction, lower limb
uterine size date O26.84- ☑
Discrimination
ethnic Z60.5
political Z60.5
racial Z60.5
religious Z60.5
sex Z60.5
Disease, diseased (see also Syndrome)
absorbent system I87.8
acid-peptic K30
Acosta's T70.29 ☑
Adams-Stokes (-Morgagni) (syncope with heart block)
  I45.9
Addison's anemia (pernicious) D51.0
adenoids (and tonsils) J35.9
adrenal (capsule) (cortex) (gland) (medullary) E27.9
  hyperfunction E27.0
  specified NEC E27.8
ainhum L94.6
airway
  obstructive, chronic J44.9
    due to
      cotton dust J66.0
      specific organic dusts NEC J66.8
  reactive — see Asthma
akamushi (scrub typhus) A75.3
Albers-Schönberg (marble bones) Q78.2
Albert's — see Tendinitis, Achilles
alimentary canal K63.9
alligator-skin Q80.9
  acquired L85.0
alpha heavy chain C88.3
alpine T70.29 ☑
altitude T70.20 ☑
alveolar ridge
  edentulous K06.9
    specified NEC K06.8
alveoli, teeth K08.9
Alzheimer's G30.9 [F02.80]
  with behavioral disturbance G30.9 [F02.81]
  early onset G30.0 [F02.80]
    with behavioral disturbance G30.0 [F02.81]
  late onset G30.1 [F02.80]
    with behavioral disturbance G30.1 [F02.81]
  specified NEC G30.8 [F02.80]
    with behavioral disturbance G30.8 [F02.81]
amyloid — see Amyloidosis
Andersen's (glycogenosis IV) E74.09
Andes T70.29 ☑
Andrews' (bacterid) L08.89
angiospastic I73.9
  cerebral G45.9
  vein I87.8
anterior
  chamber H21.9
  horn cell G12.29

Disease, diseased — *continued*
- antiglomerular basement membrane (anti- GBM) anti-body M31.0
  - tubulo-interstitial nephritis N12
- antral — *see* Sinusitis, maxillary
- anus K62.9
  - specified NEC K62.89
- aorta (nonsyphilitic) I77.9
  - syphilitic NEC A52.02
- aortic (heart) (valve) I35.9
  - rheumatic I06.9
- Apollo B30.3
- aponeuroses — *see* Enthesopathy
- appendix K38.9
  - specified NEC K38.8
- aqueous (chamber) H21.9
- Arnold-Chiari — *see* Arnold-Chiari disease
- arterial I77.9
  - occlusive — *see* Occlusion, by site
    - due to stricture or stenosis I77.1
- arteriocardiorenal — *see* Hypertension, cardiorenal
- arteriolar (generalized) (obliterative) I77.9
- arteriorenal — *see* Hypertension, kidney
- arteriosclerotic (*see also* Arteriosclerosis)
  - cardiovascular — *see* Disease, heart, ischemic, atherosclerotic
  - coronary (artery) — *see* Disease, heart, ischemic, atherosclerotic
  - heart — *see* Disease, heart, ischemic, atherosclerotic
- artery I77.9
  - cerebral I67.9
  - coronary I25.10
    - with angina pectoris — *see* Arteriosclerosis, coronary (artery)
- arthropod-borne NOS (viral) A94
  - specified type NEC A93.8
- atticoantral, chronic H66.20
  - left H66.22
    - with right H66.23
  - right H66.21
    - with left H66.23
- auditory canal — *see* Disorder, ear, external
- auricle, ear NEC — *see* Disorder, pinna
- Australian X A83.4
- autoimmune (systemic) NOS M35.9
  - hemolytic (cold type) (warm type) D59.1
    - drug-induced D59.0
  - thyroid E06.3
- aviator's — *see* Effect, adverse, high altitude
- Ayala's Q78.5
- Ayerza's (pulmonary artery sclerosis with pulmonary hypertension) I27.0
- Babington's (familial hemorrhagic telangiectasia) I78.0
- bacterial A49.9
  - specified NEC A48.8
  - zoonotic A28.9
    - specified type NEC A28.8
- Baelz's (cheilitis glandularis apostematosa) K13.0
- bagasse J67.1
- balloon — *see* Effect, adverse, high altitude
- Bang's (brucella abortus) A23.1
- Bannister's T78.3 ☑
- barometer makers' — *see* Poisoning, mercury
- Barraquer (-Simons') (progressive lipodystrophy) E88.1
- Barrett's — *see* Barrett's, esophagus
- Bartholin's gland N75.9
- basal ganglia G25.9
  - degenerative G23.9
    - specified NEC G23.8
  - specified NEC G25.89
- Basedow's (exophthalmic goiter) — *see* Hyperthyroidism, with, goiter (diffuse)
- Bateman's B08.1
- Batten-Steinert G71.11
- Battey A31.0
- Beard's (neurasthenia) F48.8
- Becker
  - idiopathic mural endomyocardial I42.3
  - myotonia congenita G71.12
- Begbie's (exophthalmic goiter) — *see* Hyperthyroidism, with, goiter (diffuse)
- behavioral, organic F07.9
- Beigel's (white piedra) B36.2
- Benson's — *see* Deposit, crystalline
- Bernard-Soulier (thrombopathy) D69.1
- Bernhardt (-Roth) — *see* Mononeuropathy, lower limb, meralgia paresthetica

Disease, diseased — *continued*
- Biermer's (pernicious anemia) D51.0
- bile duct (common) (hepatic) K83.9
  - with calculus, stones — *see* Calculus, bile duct
  - specified NEC K83.8
- biliary (tract) K83.9
  - specified NEC K83.8
- Billroth's — *see* Spina bifida
- bird fancier's J67.2
- black lung J60
- bladder N32.9
  - in (due to)
    - schistosomiasis (bilharziasis) B65.0 [N33]
  - specified NEC N32.89
- bleeder's D66
- blood D75.9
  - forming organs D75.9
  - vessel I99.9
- Bloodgood's — *see* Mastopathy, cystic
- Bodechtel-Guttmann (subacute sclerosing panencephalitis) A81.1
- bone (*see also* Disorder, bone)
  - aluminum M83.4
  - fibrocystic NEC
    - jaw M27.49
- bone-marrow D75.9
- Borna A83.9
- Bornholm (epidemic pleurodynia) B33.0
- Bouchard's (myopathic dilatation of the stomach) K31.0
- Bouillaud's (rheumatic heart disease) I01.9
- Bourneville (-Brissaud) (tuberous sclerosis) Q85.1
- Bouveret (-Hoffmann) (paroxysmal tachycardia) I47.9
- bowel K63.9
  - functional K59.9
    - psychogenic F45.8
- brain G93.9
  - arterial, artery I67.9
  - arteriosclerotic I67.2
  - congenital Q04.9
  - degenerative — *see* Degeneration, brain
  - inflammatory — *see* Encephalitis
  - organic G93.9
    - arteriosclerotic I67.2
  - parasitic NEC B71.9 [G94]
  - senile NEC G31.1
  - specified NEC G93.89
- breast (*see also* Disorder, breast) N64.9
  - cystic (chronic) — *see* Mastopathy, cystic
  - fibrocystic — *see* Mastopathy, cystic
  - Paget's
    - female, unspecified side C50.91- ☑
    - male, unspecified side C50.92- ☑
  - specified NEC N64.89
- Breda's — *see* Yaws
- Bretonneau's (diphtheritic malignant angina) A36.0
- Bright's — *see* Nephritis
  - arteriosclerotic — *see* Hypertension, kidney
- Brill-Zinsser (recrudescent typhus) A75.1
- Brill's (recrudescent typhus) A75.1
- Brion-Kayser — *see* Fever, paratyphoid
- broad
  - beta E78.2
  - ligament (noninflammatory) N83.9
    - inflammatory — *see* Disease, pelvis, inflammatory
    - specified NEC N83.8
- Brocq-Duhring (dermatitis herpetiformis) L13.0
- Brocq's
  - meaning
    - dermatitis herpetiformis L13.0
    - prurigo L28.2
- bronchopulmonary J98.4
- bronchus NEC J98.09
- bronze Addison's E27.1
  - tuberculous A18.7
- budgerigar fancier's J67.2
- Buerger's (thromboangiitis obliterans) I73.1
- bullous L13.9
  - chronic of childhood L12.2
  - specified NEC L13.8
- Bürger-Grütz (essential familial hyperlipemia) E78.3
- bursa — *see* Bursopathy
- caisson T70.3 ☑
- California — *see* Coccidioidomycosis
- capillaries I78.9
  - specified NEC I78.8
- Carapata A68.0

Disease, diseased — *continued*
- cardiac — *see* Disease, heart
- cardiopulmonary, chronic I27.9
- cardiorenal (hepatic) (hypertensive) (vascular) — *see* Hypertension, cardiorenal
- cardiovascular (atherosclerotic) I25.10
  - with angina pectoris — *see* Arteriosclerosis, coronary (artery),
  - congenital Q28.9
  - hypertensive — *see* Hypertension, heart
  - newborn P29.9
    - specified NEC P29.89
  - renal (hypertensive) — *see* Hypertension, cardiorenal
  - syphilitic (asymptomatic) A52.00
- cartilage — *see* Disorder, cartilage
- Castellani's A69.8
- cat-scratch A28.1
- Cavare's (familial periodic paralysis) G72.3
- cecum K63.9
- celiac (adult) (infantile) K90.0
- cellular tissue L98.9
- central core G71.2
- cerebellar, cerebellum — *see* Disease, brain
- cerebral (*see also* Disease, brain)
  - degenerative — *see* Degeneration, brain
- cerebrospinal G96.9
- cerebrovascular I67.9
  - acute I67.89
    - embolic I63.4- ☑
    - thrombotic I63.3- ☑
  - arteriosclerotic I67.2
  - specified NEC I67.89
- cervix (uteri) (noninflammatory) N88.9
  - inflammatory — *see* Cervicitis
  - specified NEC N88.8
- Chabert's A22.9
- Chandler's (osteochondritis dissecans, hip) — *see* Osteochondritis, dissecans, hip
- Charlouis — *see* Yaws
- Chédiak-Steinbrinck (-Higashi) (congenital gigantism of peroxidase granules) E70.330
- chest J98.6
- Chiari's (hepatic vein thrombosis) I82.0
- Chicago B40.9
- Chignon B36.8
- chigo, chigoe B88.1
- childhood granulomatous D71
- Chinese liver fluke B66.1
- chlamydial A74.9
  - specified NEC A74.89
- cholecystic K82.9
- choroid H31.9
  - specified NEC H31.8
- Christmas D67
- chronic bullous of childhood L12.2
- chylomicron retention E78.3
- ciliary body H21.9
  - specified NEC H21.89
- circulatory (system) NEC I99.8
  - newborn P29.9
  - syphilitic A52.00
    - congenital A50.54
- coagulation factor deficiency (congenital) — *see* Defect, coagulation
- coccidioidal — *see* Coccidioidomycosis
- cold
  - agglutinin or hemoglobinuria D59.1
    - paroxysmal D59.6
  - hemagglutinin (chronic) D59.1
- collagen NOS (nonvascular) (vascular) M35.9
  - specified NEC M35.8
- colon K63.9
  - functional K59.9
    - congenital Q43.2
  - ischemic K55.0
- combined system — *see* Degeneration, combined
- compressed air T70.3 ☑
- Concato's (pericardial polyserositis) A19.9
  - nontubercular I31.1
  - pleural — *see* Pleurisy, with effusion
- conjunctiva H11.9
  - chlamydial A74.0
  - specified NEC H11.89
  - viral B30.9
    - specified NEC B30.8
- connective tissue, systemic (diffuse) M35.9

☑ **Additional Character Required — Refer to the Tabular List for Character Selection**   ▽ Subterms under main terms may continue to next column or page

Disease, diseased — *continued*
  connective tissue, systemic — *continued*
    in (due to)
      hypogammaglobulinemia D80.1 [M36.8]
      ochronosis E70.29 [M36.8]
      specified NEC M35.8
  Conor and Bruch's (boutonneuse fever) A77.1
  Cooper's — *see* Mastopathy, cystic
  Cori's (glycogenosis III) E74.03
  corkhandler's or corkworker's J67.3
  cornea H18.9
    specified NEC H18.89- ☑
  coronary (artery) — *see* Disease, heart, ischemic, atherosclerotic
    congenital Q24.5
    ostial, syphilitic (aortic) (mitral) (pulmonary) A52.03
  corpus cavernosum N48.9
    specified NEC N48.89
  Cotugno's — *see* Sciatica
  coxsackie (virus) NEC B34.1
  cranial nerve NOS G52.9
  Creutzfeldt-Jakob — *see* Creutzfeldt-Jakob disease or syndrome
  Crocq's (acrocyanosis) I73.89
  Crohn's — *see* Enteritis, regional
  Curschmann G71.11
  cystic
    breast (chronic) — *see* Mastopathy, cystic
    kidney, congenital Q61.9
    liver, congenital Q44.6
    lung J98.4
      congenital Q33.0
  cytomegalic inclusion (generalized) B25.9
    with pneumonia B25.0
    congenital P35.1
  cytomegaloviral B25.9
    specified NEC B25.8
  Czerny's (periodic hydrarthrosis of the knee) — *see* Effusion, joint, knee
  Daae (-Finsen) (epidemic pleurodynia) B33.0
  Darling's — *see* Histoplasmosis capsulati
  de Quervain's (tendon sheath) M65.4
    thyroid (subacute granulomatous thyroiditis) E06.1
  Débove's (splenomegaly) R16.1
  deer fly — *see* Tularemia
  Degos' I77.89
  demyelinating, demyelinizating (nervous system) G37.9
    multiple sclerosis G35
    specified NEC G37.8
  dense deposit (*see also* N00-N07 with fourth character .6) N05.6
  deposition, hydroxyapatite — *see* Disease, hydroxyapatite deposition
  Devergie's (pityriasis rubra pilaris) L44.0
  Devic's G36.0
  diaphorase deficiency D74.0
  diaphragm J98.6
  diarrheal, infectious NEC A09
  digestive system K92.9
    specified NEC K92.89
  disc, degenerative — *see* Degeneration, intervertebral disc
  discogenic (*see also* Displacement, intervertebral disc NEC)
    with myelopathy — *see* Disorder, disc, with, myelopathy
  diverticular — *see* Diverticula
  Dubois (thymus) A50.59 [E35]
  Duchenne-Griesinger G71.0
  Duchenne's
    muscular dystrophy G71.0
    pseudohypertrophy, muscles G71.0
  ductless glands E34.9
  Duhring's (dermatitis herpetiformis) L13.0
  duodenum K31.9
    specified NEC K31.89
  Dupré's (meningism) R29.1
  Dupuytren's (muscle contracture) M72.0
  Durand-Nicholas-Favre (climatic bubo) A55
  Duroziez's (congenital mitral stenosis) Q23.2
  ear — *see* Disorder, ear
  Eberth's — *see* Fever, typhoid
  Ebola (virus) A98.4
  Ebstein's heart Q22.5
  Echinococcus — *see* Echinococcus
  echovirus NEC B34.1
  Eddowes' (brittle bones and blue sclera) Q78.0

Disease, diseased — *continued*
  edentulous (alveolar) ridge K06.9
    specified NEC K06.8
  Edsall's T67.2 ☑
  Eichstedt's (pityriasis versicolor) B36.0
  Ellis-van Creveld (chondroectodermal dysplasia) Q77.6
  end stage renal (ESRD) N18.6
    due to hypertension I12.0
  endocrine glands or system NEC E34.9
  endomyocardial (eosinophilic) I42.3
  English (rickets) E55.0
  enteroviral, enterovirus NEC B34.1
    central nervous system NEC A88.8
  epidemic B99.9
    specified NEC B99.8
  epididymis N50.9
  Erb (-Landouzy) G71.0
  Erdheim-Chester (ECD) E88.89
  esophagus K22.9
    functional K22.4
    psychogenic F45.8
    specified NEC K22.8
  Eulenburg's (congenital paramyotonia) G71.19
  eustachian tube — *see* Disorder, eustachian tube
  external
    auditory canal — *see* Disorder, ear, external
    ear — *see* Disorder, ear, external
  extrapyramidal G25.9
    specified NEC G25.89
  eye H57.9
    anterior chamber H21.9
    inflammatory NEC H57.8
    muscle (external) — *see* Strabismus
    specified NEC H57.8
    syphilitic — *see* Oculopathy, syphilitic
  eyeball H44.9
    specified NEC H44.89
  eyelid — *see* Disorder, eyelid
    specified NEC — *see* Disorder, eyelid, specified type NEC
  eyeworm of Africa B74.3
  facial nerve (seventh) G51.9
    newborn (birth injury) P11.3
  Fahr (of brain) G23.8
  Fahr Volhard (of kidney) I12.- ☑
  fallopian tube (noninflammatory) N83.9
    inflammatory — *see* Salpingo-oophoritis
    specified NEC N83.8
  familial periodic paralysis G72.3
  Fanconi's (congenital pancytopenia) D61.09
  fascia NEC (*see also* Disorder, muscle)
    inflammatory — *see* Myositis
    specified NEC M62.89
  Fauchard's (periodontitis) — *see* Periodontitis
  Favre-Durand-Nicolas (climatic bubo) A55
  Fede's K14.0
  Feer's — *see* Poisoning, mercury
  female pelvic inflammatory (*see also* Disease, pelvis, inflammatory) N73.9
    syphilitic (secondary) A51.42
    tuberculous A18.17
  Fernels' (aortic aneurysm) I71.9
  fibrocaseous of lung — *see* Tuberculosis, pulmonary
  fibrocystic — *see* Fibrocystic disease
  Fiedler's (leptospiral jaundice) A27.0
  fifth B08.3
  file-cutter's — *see* Poisoning, lead
  fish-skin Q80.9
    acquired L85.0
  Flajani (-Basedow) (exophthalmic goiter) — *see* Hyperthyroidism, with, goiter (diffuse)
  flax-dresser's J66.1
  fluke — *see* Infestation, fluke
  foot and mouth B08.8
  foot process N04.9
  Forbes' (glycogenosis III) E74.03
  Fordyce-Fox (apocrine miliaria) L75.2
  Fordyce's (ectopic sebaceous glands) (mouth) Q38.6
  Forestier's (rhizomelic pseudopolyarthritis) M35.3
    meaning ankylosing hyperostosis — *see* Hyperostosis, ankylosing
  Fothergill's
    neuralgia — *see* Neuralgia, trigeminal
    scarlatina anginosa A38.9
  Fournier (gangrene) N49.3
    female N76.89
  fourth B08.8
  Fox (-Fordyce) (apocrine miliaria) L75.2

Disease, diseased — *continued*
  Francis' — *see* Tularemia
  Franklin C88.2
  Frei's (climatic bubo) A55
  Friedreich's
    combined systemic or ataxia G11.1
    myoclonia G25.3
  frontal sinus — *see* Sinusitis, frontal
  fungus NEC B49
  Gaisböck's (polycythemia hypertonica) D75.1
  gallbladder K82.9
    calculus — *see* Calculus, gallbladder
    cholecystitis — *see* Cholecystitis
    cholesterolosis K82.4
    fistula — *see* Fistula, gallbladder
    hydrops K82.1
    obstruction — *see* Obstruction, gallbladder
    perforation K82.2
    specified NEC K82.8
  gamma heavy chain C88.2
  Gamna's (siderotic splenomegaly) D73.2
  Gamstorp's (adynamia episodica hereditaria) G72.3
  Gandy-Nanta (siderotic splenomegaly) D73.2
  ganister J62.8
  gastric — *see* Disease, stomach
  gastroesophageal reflux (GERD) K21.9
    with esophagitis K21.0
  gastrointestinal (tract) K92.9
    amyloid E85.4
    functional K59.9
      psychogenic F45.8
    specified NEC K92.89
  Gee (-Herter) (-Heubner) (-Thaysen) (nontropical sprue) K90.0
  genital organs
    female N94.9
    male N50.9
  Gerhardt's (erythromelalgia) I73.81
  Gibert's (pityriasis rosea) L42
  Gierke's (glycogenosis I) E74.01
  Gilles de la Tourette's (motor-verbal tic) F95.2
  gingiva K06.9
    specified NEC K06.8
  gland (lymph) I89.9
  Glanzmann's (hereditary hemorrhagic thrombasthenia) D69.1
  glass-blower's (cataract) — *see* Cataract, specified NEC
    salivary gland hypertrophy K11.1
  Glisson's — *see* Rickets
  globe H44.9
    specified NEC H44.89
  glomerular (*see also* Glomerulonephritis)
    with edema — *see* Nephrosis
    acute — *see* Nephritis, acute
    chronic — *see* Nephritis, chronic
    minimal change N05.0
    rapidly progressive N01.9
  glycogen storage E74.00
    Andersen's E74.09
    Cori's E74.03
    Forbes' E74.03
    generalized E74.00
    glucose-6-phosphatase deficiency E74.01
    heart E74.02 [I43]
    hepatorenal E74.09
    Hers' E74.09
    liver and kidney E74.09
    McArdle's E74.04
    muscle phosphofructokinase E74.09
    myocardium E74.02 [I43]
    Pompe's E74.02
    Tauri's E74.09
    type 0 E74.09
    type I E74.01
    type II E74.02
    type III E74.03
    type IV E74.09
    type V E74.04
    type VI-XI E74.09
    Von Gierke's E74.01
  Goldstein's (familial hemorrhagic telangiectasia) I78.0
  gonococcal NOS A54.9
  graft-versus-host (GVH) D89.813
    acute D89.810
      acute on chronic D89.812
      chronic D89.811
  grainhandler's J67.8
  granulomatous (childhood) (chronic) D71

Disease, diseased — *continued*
  Graves' (exophthalmic goiter) — *see* Hyperthyroidism, with, goiter (diffuse)
  Griesinger's — *see* Ancylostomiasis
  Grisel's M43.6
  Gruby's (tinea tonsurans) B35.0
  Guillain-Barré G61.0
  Guinon's (motor-verbal tic) F95.2
  gum K06.9
  gynecological N94.9
  H (Hartnup's) E72.02
  Haff — *see* Poisoning, mercury
  Hageman (congenital factor XII deficiency) D68.2
  hair (color) (shaft) L67.9
    follicles L73.9
      specified NEC L73.8
  Hamman's (spontaneous mediastinal emphysema) J98.2
  hand, foot and mouth B08.4
  Hansen's — *see* Leprosy
  Hantavirus, with pulmonary manifestations B33.4
    with renal manifestations A98.5
  Harada's H30.81- ☑
  Hartnup (pellagra-cerebellar ataxia-renal aminoaciduria) E72.02
  Hart's (pellagra-cerebellar ataxia-renal aminoaciduria) E72.02
  Hashimoto's (struma lymphomatosa) E06.3
  Hb — *see* Disease, hemoglobin
  heart (organic) I51.9
    with
      pulmonary edema (acute) (*see also* Failure, ventricular, left) I50.1
      rheumatic fever (conditions in I00)
        active I01.9
          with chorea I02.0
          specified NEC I01.8
        inactive or quiescent (with chorea) I09.9
          specified NEC I09.89
    amyloid E85.4 [I43]
    aortic (valve) I35.9
    arteriosclerotic or sclerotic (senile) — *see* Disease, heart, ischemic, atherosclerotic
    artery, arterial — *see* Disease, heart, ischemic, atherosclerotic
    beer drinkers' I42.6
    beriberi (wet) E51.12
    black I27.0
    congenital Q24.9
      cyanotic Q24.9
      specified NEC Q24.8
    coronary — *see* Disease, heart, ischemic
    cryptogenic I51.9
    fibroid — *see* Myocarditis
    functional I51.89
      psychogenic F45.8
    glycogen storage E74.02 [I43]
    gonococcal A54.83
    hypertensive — *see* Hypertension, heart
    hyperthyroid (*see also* Hyperthyroidism) E05.90 [I43]
      with thyroid storm E05.91 [I43]
    ischemic (chronic or with a stated duration of over 4 weeks) I25.9
      atherosclerotic (of) I25.10
        with angina pectoris — *see* Arteriosclerosis, coronary (artery)
        coronary artery bypass graft — *see* Arteriosclerosis, coronary (artery),
      cardiomyopathy I25.5
      diagnosed on ECG or other special investigation, but currently presenting no symptoms I25.6
      silent I25.6
      specified form NEC I25.89
    kyphoscoliotic I27.1
    meningococcal A39.50
      endocarditis A39.51
      myocarditis A39.52
      pericarditis A39.53
    mitral I05.9
      specified NEC I05.8
    muscular — *see* Degeneration, myocardial
    psychogenic (functional) F45.8
    pulmonary (chronic) I27.9
      in schistosomiasis B65.9 [I52]
      specified NEC I27.89

Disease, diseased — *continued*
  heart — *continued*
    rheumatic (chronic) (inactive) (old) (quiescent) (with chorea) I09.9
      active or acute I01.9
        with chorea (acute) (rheumatic) (Sydenham's) I02.0
      specified NEC I09.89
    senile — *see* Myocarditis
    syphilitic A52.06
      aortic A52.03
        aneurysm A52.01
      congenital A50.54 [I52]
    thyrotoxic (*see also* Thyrotoxicosis) E05.90 [I43]
      with thyroid storm E05.91 [I43]
    valve, valvular (obstructive) (regurgitant) (*see also* Endocarditis)
      congenital NEC Q24.8
      pulmonary Q22.3
    vascular — *see* Disease, cardiovascular
  heavy chain NEC C88.2
    alpha C88.3
    gamma C88.2
    mu C88.2
  Hebra's
    pityriasis
      maculata et circinata L42
      rubra pilaris L44.0
    prurigo L28.2
  hematopoietic organs D75.9
  hemoglobin or Hb
    abnormal (mixed) NEC D58.2
      with thalassemia D56.9
    AS genotype D57.3
    Bart's D56.0
    C (Hb-C) D58.2
      with other abnormal hemoglobin NEC D58.2
      elliptocytosis D58.1
      Hb-S D57.2- ☑
      sickle-cell D57.2- ☑
      thalassemia D56.8
    Constant Spring D58.2
    D (Hb-D) D58.2
    E (Hb-E) D58.2
    E-beta thalassemia D56.5
    elliptocytosis D58.1
    H (Hb-H) (thalassemia) D56.0
      with other abnormal hemoglobin NEC D56.9
      Constant Spring D56.0
    I thalassemia D56.9
    M D74.0
    S or SS D57.1
    SC D57.2- ☑
    SD D57.8- ☑
    SE D57.8- ☑
    spherocytosis D58.0
    unstable, hemolytic D58.2
  hemolytic (newborn) P55.9
    autoimmune (cold type) (warm type) D59.1
    drug-induced D59.0
    due to or with
      incompatibility
        ABO (blood group) P55.1
        blood (group) (Duffy) (K(ell)) (Kidd) (Lewis) (M) (S) NEC P55.8
        Rh (blood group) (factor) P55.0
        Rh negative mother P55.0
    specified type NEC P55.8
    unstable hemoglobin D58.2
  hemorrhagic D69.9
    newborn P53
  Henoch (-Schönlein) (purpura nervosa) D69.0
  hepatic — *see* Disease, liver
  hepatolenticular E83.01
  heredodegenerative NEC
    spinal cord G95.89
  herpesviral, disseminated B00.7
  Hers' (glycogenosis VI) E74.09
  Herter (-Gee) (-Heubner) (nontropical sprue) K90.0
  Heubner-Herter (nontropical sprue) K90.0
  high fetal gene or hemoglobin thalassemia D56.9
  Hildenbrand's — *see* Typhus
  hip (joint) M25.9
    congenital Q65.89
    suppurative M00.9
    tuberculous A18.02
  His (-Werner) (trench fever) A79.0
  Hodgson's I71.2

Disease, diseased — *continued*
  Hodgson's — *continued*
    ruptured I71.1
  Holla — *see* Spherocytosis
  hookworm B76.9
    specified NEC B76.8
  host-versus-graft D89.813
    acute D89.810
    acute on chronic D89.812
    chronic D89.811
  human immunodeficiency virus (HIV) B20
  Huntington's G10
  Hutchinson's (cheiropompholyx) — *see* Hutchinson's disease
  hyaline (diffuse) (generalized)
    membrane (lung) (newborn) P22.0
      adult J80
  hydatid — *see* Echinococcus
  hydroxyapatite deposition M11.00
    ankle M11.07- ☑
    elbow M11.02- ☑
    foot joint M11.07- ☑
    hand joint M11.04- ☑
    hip M11.05- ☑
    knee M11.06- ☑
    multiple site M11.09
    shoulder M11.01- ☑
    vertebra M11.08
    wrist M11.03- ☑
  hyperkinetic — *see* Hyperkinesia
  hypertensive — *see* Hypertension
  hypophysis E23.7
  I-cell E77.0
  Iceland G93.3
  immune D89.9
  immunoproliferative (malignant) C88.9
    small intestinal C88.3
    specified NEC C88.8
  inclusion B25.9
    salivary gland B25.9
  infectious, infective B99.9
    congenital P37.9
      specified NEC P37.8
      viral P35.9
        specified type NEC P35.8
    specified NEC B99.8
  inflammatory
    penis N48.29
      abscess N48.21
      cellulitis N48.22
    prepuce N47.7
      balanoposthitis N47.6
    tubo-ovarian — *see* Salpingo-oophoritis
  intervertebral disc (*see also* Disorder, disc)
    with myelopathy — *see* Disorder, disc, with, myelopathy
    cervical, cervicothoracic — *see* Disorder, disc, cervical
      with
        myelopathy — *see* Disorder, disc, cervical, with myelopathy
        neuritis, radiculitis or radiculopathy — *see* Disorder, disc, cervical, with neuritis
        specified NEC — *see* Disorder, disc, cervical, specified type NEC
    lumbar (with)
      myelopathy M51.06
      neuritis, radiculitis, radiculopathy or sciatica M51.16
      specified NEC M51.86
    lumbosacral (with)
      neuritis, radiculitis or radiculopathy or sciatica M51.17
      specified NEC M51.87
    specified NEC — *see* Disorder, disc, specified NEC
    thoracic (with)
      myelopathy M51.04
      neuritis, radiculitis or radiculopathy M51.14
      specified NEC M51.84
    thoracolumbar (with)
      myelopathy M51.05
      neuritis, radiculitis or radiculopathy M51.15
      specified NEC M51.85
  intestine K63.9
    functional K59.9
      psychogenic F45.8
      specified NEC K59.8
    organic K63.9

☑ **Additional Character Required** — **Refer to the Tabular List for Character Selection**   ▽ Subterms under main terms may continue to next column or page

Disease, diseased — *continued*
  intestine — *continued*
    protozoal A07.9
    specified NEC K63.89
  iris H21.9
    specified NEC H21.89
  iron metabolism or storage E83.10
  island (scrub typhus) A75.3
  itai-itai — *see* Poisoning, cadmium
  Jakob-Creutzfeldt — *see* Creutzfeldt-Jakob disease or syndrome
  jaw M27.9
    fibrocystic M27.49
    specified NEC M27.8
  jigger B88.1
  joint (*see also* Disorder, joint)
    Charcot's — *see* Arthropathy, neuropathic (Charcot)
    degenerative — *see* Osteoarthritis
      multiple M15.9
      spine — *see* Spondylosis
    hypertrophic — *see* Osteoarthritis
    sacroiliac M53.3
    specified NEC — *see* Disorder, joint, specified type NEC
    spine NEC — *see* Dorsopathy
    suppurative — *see* Arthritis, pyogenic or pyemic
  Jourdain's (acute gingivitis) K05.00
    nonplaque induced K05.01
    plaque induced K05.00
  Kaschin-Beck (endemic polyarthritis) M12.10
    ankle M12.17- ☑
    elbow M12.12- ☑
    foot joint M12.17- ☑
    hand joint M12.14- ☑
    hip M12.15- ☑
    knee M12.16- ☑
    multiple site M12.19
    shoulder M12.11- ☑
    vertebra M12.18
    wrist M12.13- ☑
  Katayama B65.2
  Kedani (scrub typhus) A75.3
  Keshan E59
  kidney (functional) (pelvis) N28.9
    chronic N18.9
      hypertensive — *see* Hypertension, kidney
      stage 1 N18.1
      stage 2 (mild) N18.2
      stage 3 (moderate) N18.3
      stage 4 (severe) N18.4
      stage 5 N18.5
    complicating pregnancy — *see* Pregnancy, complicated by, renal disease
    cystic (congenital) Q61.9
    fibrocystic (congenital) Q61.8
    hypertensive — *see* Hypertension, kidney
    in (due to)
      schistosomiasis (bilharziasis) B65.9 [N29]
    multicystic Q61.4
    polycystic Q61.3
      adult type Q61.2
      childhood type NEC Q61.19
        collecting duct dilatation Q61.11
  Kimmelstiel (-Wilson) (intercapillary polycystic (congenital) glomerulosclerosis) — *see* E08-E13 with .21
  Kinnier Wilson's (hepatolenticular degeneration) E83.01
  kissing — *see* Mononucleosis, infectious
  Klebs' (*see also* Glomerulonephritis) N05- ☑
  Klippel-Feil (brevicollis) Q76.1
  Köhler-Pellegrini-Stieda (calcification, knee joint) — *see* Bursitis, tibial collateral
  Kok Q89.8
  König's (osteochondritis dissecans) — *see* Osteochondritis, dissecans
  Korsakoff's (nonalcoholic) F04
    alcoholic F10.96
      with dependence F10.26
  Kostmann's (infantile genetic agranulocytosis) D70.0
  kuru A81.81
  Kyasanur Forest A98.2
  labyrinth, ear — *see* Disorder, ear, inner
  lacrimal system — *see* Disorder, lacrimal system
  Lafora's — *see* Epilepsy, generalized, idiopathic
  Lanceraux-Mathieu (leptospiral jaundice) A27.0
  Landry's G61.0

Disease, diseased — *continued*
  Larrey-Weil (leptospiral jaundice) A27.0
  larynx J38.7
  legionnaires' A48.1
    nonpneumonic A48.2
  Lenegre's I44.2
  lens H27.9
    specified NEC H27.8
  Lev's (acquired complete heart block) I44.2
  Lewy body (dementia) G31.83 [F02.80]
    with behavioral disturbance G31.83 [F02.81]
  Lichtheim's (subacute combined sclerosis with pernicious anemia) D51.0
  Lightwood's (renal tubular acidosis) N25.89
  Lignac's (cystinosis) E72.04
  lip K13.0
  lipid-storage E75.6
    specified NEC E75.5
  Lipschütz's N76.6
  liver (chronic) (organic) K76.9
    alcoholic (chronic) K70.9
      acute — *see* Disease, liver, alcoholic, hepatitis
      cirrhosis K70.30
        with ascites K70.31
      failure K70.40
        with coma K70.41
      fatty liver K70.0
      fibrosis K70.2
      hepatitis K70.10
        with ascites K70.11
      sclerosis K70.2
    cystic, congenital Q44.6
    drug-induced (idiosyncratic) (toxic) (predictable) (unpredictable) — *see* Disease, liver, toxic
    end stage K72.90
      due to hepatitis — *see* Hepatitis
    fatty, nonalcoholic (NAFLD) K76.0
      alcoholic K70.0
    fibrocystic (congenital) Q44.6
    fluke
      Chinese B66.1
      oriental B66.1
      sheep B66.3
    glycogen storage E74.09 [K77]
    in (due to)
      schistosomiasis (bilharziasis) B65.9 [K77]
    inflammatory K75.9
      alcoholic K70.1 ☑
      specified NEC K75.89
    polycystic (congenital) Q44.6
    toxic K71.9
      with
        cholestasis K71.0
        cirrhosis (liver) K71.7
        fibrosis (liver) K71.7
        focal nodular hyperplasia K71.8
        hepatic granuloma K71.8
        hepatic necrosis K71.10
          with coma K71.11
        hepatitis NEC K71.6
          acute K71.2
          chronic
            active K71.50
              with ascites K71.51
            lobular K71.4
            persistent K71.3
        lupoid K71.50
          with ascites K71.51
        peliosis hepatis K71.8
        veno-occlusive disease (VOD) of liver K71.8
    veno-occlusive K76.5
  Lobo's (keloid blastomycosis) B48.0
  Lobstein's (brittle bones and blue sclera) Q78.0
  Ludwig's (submaxillary cellulitis) K12.2
  lumbosacral region M53.87
  lung J98.4
    black J60
    congenital Q33.9
    cystic J98.4
      congenital Q33.0
    fibroid (chronic) — *see* Fibrosis, lung
    fluke B66.4
      oriental B66.4
    in
      amyloidosis E85.4 [J99]
      sarcoidosis D86.0
      Sjögren's syndrome M35.02

Disease, diseased — *continued*
  lung — *continued*
    in — *continued*
      systemic
        lupus erythematosus M32.13
        sclerosis M34.81
    interstitial J84.9
      of childhood, specified NEC J84.848
      respiratory bronchiolitis J84.115
      specified NEC J84.89
    obstructive (chronic) J44.9
      with
        acute
          bronchitis J44.0
          exacerbation NEC J44.1
          lower respiratory infection J44.0
        alveolitis, allergic J67.9
        asthma J44.9
        bronchiectasis J47.9
          with
            exacerbation (acute) J47.1
            lower respiratory infection J47.0
        bronchitis J44.9
          with
            exacerbation (acute) J44.1
            lower respiratory infection J44.0
        emphysema J44.9
        hypersensitivity pneumonitis J67.9
      decompensated J44.1
        with
          exacerbation (acute) J44.1
    polycystic J98.4
      congenital Q33.0
    rheumatoid (diffuse) (interstitial) — *see* Rheumatoid, lung
  Lutembacher's (atrial septal defect with mitral stenosis) Q21.1
  Lyme A69.20
  lymphatic (gland) (system) (channel) (vessel) I89.9
  lymphoproliferative D47.9
    specified NEC D47.Z9 (*following* D47.4)
    T-gamma D47.Z9 (*following* D47.4)
    X-linked D82.3
  Magitot's M27.2
  malarial — *see* Malaria
  malignant (*see also* Neoplasm, malignant, by site)
  Manson's B65.1
  maple bark J67.6
  maple-syrup-urine E71.0
  Marburg (virus) A98.3
  Marion's (bladder neck obstruction) N32.0
  Marsh's (exophthalmic goiter) — *see* Hyperthyroidism, with goiter (diffuse)
  mastoid (process) — *see* Disorder, ear, middle
  Mathieu's (leptospiral jaundice) A27.0
  Maxcy's A75.2
  McArdle (-Schmid-Pearson) (glycogenosis V) E74.04
  mediastinum J98.5
  medullary center (idiopathic) (respiratory) G93.89
  Meige's (chronic hereditary edema) Q82.0
  meningococcal — *see* Infection, meningococcal
  mental F99
    organic F09
  mesenchymal M35.9
  mesenteric embolic K55.0
  metabolic, metabolism E88.9
    bilirubin E80.7
  metal-polisher's J62.8
  metastatic (*see also* Neoplasm, secondary, by site) C79.9
  microvascular - code to condition
  microvillus
    atrophy Q43.8
    inclusion (MVD) Q43.8
  middle ear — *see* Disorder, ear, middle
  Mikulicz' (dryness of mouth, absent or decreased lacrimation) K11.8
  Milroy's (chronic hereditary edema) Q82.0
  Minamata — *see* Poisoning, mercury
  minicore G71.2
  Minor's G95.19
  Minot-von Willebrand-Jürgens (angiohemophilia) D68.0
  Minot's (hemorrhagic disease, newborn) P53
  Mitchell's (erythromelalgia) I73.81
  mitral (valve) I05.9
    nonrheumatic I34.9
  mixed connective tissue M35.1

Disease, diseased — continued
- moldy hay J67.0
- Monge's T70.29 ☑
- Morgagni-Adams-Stokes (syncope with heart block) I45.9
- Morgagni's (syndrome) (hyperostosis frontalis interna) M85.2
- Morton's (with metatarsalgia) — *see* Lesion, nerve, plantar
- Morvan's G60.8
- motor neuron (bulbar) (familial) (mixed type) (spinal) G12.20
  - amyotrophic lateral sclerosis G12.21
  - progressive bulbar palsy G12.22
  - specified NEC G12.29
- moyamoya I67.5
- mu heavy chain disease C88.2
- multicore G71.2
- muscle (*see also* Disorder, muscle)
  - inflammatory — *see* Myositis
  - ocular (external) — *see* Strabismus
- musculoskeletal system, soft tissue — *see also* Disorder, soft tissue
  - specified NEC — *see* Disorder, soft tissue, specified type NEC
- mushroom workers' J67.5
- mycotic B49
- myelodysplastic, not classified C94.6
- myeloproliferative, not classified C94.6
  - chronic D47.1
- myocardium, myocardial (*see also* Degeneration, myocardial) I51.5
  - primary (idiopathic) I42.9
- myoneural G70.9
- Naegeli's D69.1
- nails L60.9
  - specified NEC L60.8
- Nairobi (sheep virus) A93.8
- nasal J34.9
- nemaline body G71.2
- nerve — *see* Disorder, nerve
- nervous system G98.8
  - autonomic G90.9
  - central G96.9
    - specified NEC G96.8
  - congenital Q07.9
  - parasympathetic G90.9
  - specified NEC G98.8
  - sympathetic G90.9
  - vegetative G90.9
- neuromuscular system G70.9
- Newcastle B30.8
- Nicolas (-Durand)-Favre (climatic bubo) A55
- nipple N64.9
  - Paget's C50.01- ☑
    - female C50.01- ☑
    - male C50.02- ☑
- Nishimoto (-Takeuchi) I67.5
- nonarthropod-borne NOS (viral) B34.9
  - enterovirus NEC B34.1
- nonautoimmune hemolytic D59.4
  - drug-induced D59.2
- Nonne-Milroy-Meige (chronic hereditary edema) Q82.0
- nose J34.9
- nucleus pulposus — *see* Disorder, disc
- nutritional E63.9
- oast-house-urine E72.19
  - ocular
    - herpesviral B00.50
    - zoster B02.30
- obliterative vascular I77.1
- Ohara's — *see* Tularemia
- Opitz's (congestive splenomegaly) D73.2
- Oppenheim-Urbach (necrobiosis lipoidica diabeticorum) — *see* E08-E13 with .620
- optic nerve NEC — *see* Disorder, nerve, optic
- orbit — *see* Disorder, orbit
- Oriental liver fluke B66.1
- Oriental lung fluke B66.4
- Ormond's N13.5
- Oropouche virus A93.0
- Osler-Rendu (familial hemorrhagic telangiectasia) I78.0
- osteofibrocystic E21.0
- Otto's M24.7
- outer ear — *see* Disorder, ear, external
- ovary (noninflammatory) N83.9
  - cystic N83.20
  - inflammatory — *see* Salpingo-oophoritis

Disease, diseased — continued
- ovary — continued
  - polycystic E28.2
  - specified NEC N83.8
- Owren's (congenital) — *see* Defect, coagulation
- pancreas K86.9
  - cystic K86.2
  - fibrocystic E84.9
  - specified NEC K86.8
- panvalvular I08.9
  - specified NEC I08.8
- parametrium (noninflammatory) N83.9
- parasitic B89
  - cerebral NEC B71.9 [G94]
  - intestinal NOS B82.9
  - mouth B37.0
  - skin NOS B88.9
  - specified type — *see* Infestation
  - tongue B37.0
- parathyroid (gland) E21.5
  - specified NEC E21.4
- Parkinson's G20
- parodontal K05.6
- Parrot's (syphilitic osteochondritis) A50.02
- Parry's (exophthalmic goiter) — *see* Hyperthyroidism, with, goiter (diffuse)
- Parson's (exophthalmic goiter) — *see* Hyperthyroidism, with, goiter (diffuse)
- Paxton's (white piedra) B36.2
- pearl-worker's — *see* Osteomyelitis, specified type NEC
- Pellegrini-Stieda (calcification, knee joint) — *see* Bursitis, tibial collateral
- pelvis, pelvic
  - female NOS N94.9
    - specified NEC N94.89
  - gonococcal (acute) (chronic) A54.24
  - inflammatory (female) N73.9
    - acute N73.0
    - chronic N73.1
    - specified NEC N73.8
    - syphilitic (secondary) A51.42
      - late A52.76
    - tuberculous A18.17
  - organ, female N94.9
  - peritoneum, female NEC N94.89
- penis N48.9
  - inflammatory N48.29
    - abscess N48.21
    - cellulitis N48.22
  - specified NEC N48.89
- periapical tissues NOS K04.90
- periodontal K05.6
  - specified NEC K05.5
- periosteum — *see* Disorder, bone, specified type NEC
- peripheral
  - arterial I73.9
  - autonomic nervous system G90.9
  - nerves — *see* Polyneuropathy
  - vascular NOS I73.9
- peritoneum K66.9
  - pelvic, female NEC N94.89
  - specified NEC K66.8
- persistent mucosal (middle ear) H66.20
  - left H66.22
    - with right H66.23
  - right H66.21
    - with left H66.23
- Petit's — *see* Hernia, abdomen, specified site NEC
- pharynx J39.2
  - specified NEC J39.2
- Phocas' — *see* Mastopathy, cystic
- photochromogenic (acid-fast bacilli) (pulmonary) A31.0
  - nonpulmonary A31.9
- Pick's G31.01 [F02.80]
  - with behavioral disturbance G31.01 [F02.81]
- pigeon fancier's J67.2
- pineal gland E34.8
- pink — *see* Poisoning, mercury
- Pinkus' (lichen nitidus) L44.1
- pinworm B80
- Piry virus A93.8
- pituitary (gland) E23.7
- pituitary-snuff-taker's J67.8
- pleura (cavity) J94.9
  - specified NEC J94.8
- pneumatic drill (hammer) T75.21 ☑

Disease, diseased — continued
- Pollitzer's (hidradenitis suppurativa) L73.2
- polycystic
  - kidney or renal Q61.3
    - adult type Q61.2
    - childhood type NEC Q61.19
      - collecting duct dilatation Q61.11
  - liver or hepatic Q44.6
  - lung or pulmonary J98.4
    - congenital Q33.0
  - ovary, ovaries E28.2
  - spleen Q89.09
- polyethylene T84.05- ☑
- Pompe's (glycogenosis II) E74.02
- Posadas-Wernicke B38.9
- Potain's (pulmonary edema) — *see* Edema, lung
- prepuce N47.8
  - inflammatory N47.7
    - balanoposthitis N47.6
- Pringle's (tuberous sclerosis) Q85.1
- prion, central nervous system A81.9
  - specified NEC A81.89
- prostate N42.9
  - specified NEC N42.89
- protozoal B64
  - acanthamebiasis — *see* Acanthamebiasis
  - African trypanosomiasis — *see* African trypanosomiasis
  - babesiosis B60.0
  - Chagas disease — *see* Chagas disease
  - intestine, intestinal A07.9
  - leishmaniasis — *see* Leishmaniasis
  - malaria — *see* Malaria
  - naegleriasis B60.2
  - pneumocystosis B59
  - specified organism NEC B60.8
  - toxoplasmosis — *see* Toxoplasmosis
- pseudo-Hurler's E77.0
- psychiatric F99
- psychotic — *see* Psychosis
- Puente's (simple glandular cheilitis) K13.0
- puerperal (*see also* Puerperal) O90.89
- pulmonary (*see also* Disease, lung)
  - artery I28.9
  - chronic obstructive J44.9
    - with
      - acute bronchitis J44.0
      - exacerbation (acute) J44.1
      - lower respiratory infection (acute) J44.0
    - decompensated J44.1
      - with
        - exacerbation (acute) J44.1
  - heart I27.9
    - specified NEC I27.89
  - hypertensive (vascular) I27.0
  - valve I37.9
    - rheumatic I09.89
- pulp (dental) NOS K04.90
- pulseless M31.4
- Putnam's (subacute combined sclerosis with pernicious anemia) D51.0
- Pyle (-Cohn) (craniometaphyseal dysplasia) Q78.5
- ragpicker's or ragsorter's A22.1
- Raynaud's — *see* Raynaud's disease
- reactive airway — *see* Asthma
- Reclus' (cystic) — *see* Mastopathy, cystic
- rectum K62.9
  - specified NEC K62.89
- Refsum's (heredopathia atactica polyneuritiformis) G60.1
- renal (functional) (pelvis) (*see also* Disease, kidney) N28.9
  - with
    - edema — *see* Nephrosis
    - glomerular lesion — *see* Glomerulonephritis
      - with edema — *see* Nephrosis
    - interstitial nephritis N12
  - acute N28.9
  - chronic (*see also* Disease, kidney, chronic) N18.9
  - cystic, congenital Q61.9
  - diabetic — *see* E08-E13 with .22
  - end-stage (failure) N18.6
    - due to hypertension I12.0
  - fibrocystic (congenital) Q61.8
  - hypertensive — *see* Hypertension, kidney
  - lupus M32.14
  - phosphate-losing (tubular) N25.0
  - polycystic (congenital) Q61.3

☑ Additional Character Required — Refer to the Tabular List for Character Selection   ▽ Subterms under main terms may continue to next column or page

Disease, diseased — *continued*

renal (*see also* Disease, kidney) — *continued*
   polycystic — *continued*
      adult type Q61.2
      childhood type NEC Q61.19
         collecting duct dilatation Q61.11
      rapidly progressive N06.9
      subacute N01.9
Rendu-Osler-Weber (familial hemorrhagic telangiectasia) I78.0
renovascular (arteriosclerotic) — *see* Hypertension, kidney
respiratory (tract) J98.9
   acute or subacute NOS J06.9
      due to
         chemicals, gases, fumes or vapors (inhalation) J68.3
         external agent J70.9
            specified NEC J70.8
         radiation J70.0
         smoke inhalation J70.5
      noninfectious J39.8
   chronic NOS J98.9
      due to
         chemicals, gases, fumes or vapors J68.4
         external agent J70.9
            specified NEC J70.8
         radiation J70.1
      newborn P27.9
         specified NEC P27.8
   due to
      chemicals, gases, fumes or vapors J68.9
         acute or subacute NEC J68.3
         chronic J68.4
      external agent J70.9
         specified NEC J70.8
      newborn P28.9
         specified type NEC P28.89
   upper J39.9
      acute or subacute J06.9
      noninfectious NEC J39.8
      specified NEC J39.8
      streptococcal J06.9
retina, retinal H35.9
   Batten's or Batten-Mayou E75.4 [H36]
   specified NEC H35.89
rheumatoid — *see* Arthritis, rheumatoid
rickettsial NOS A79.9
   specified type NEC A79.89
Riga (-Fede) (cachectic aphthae) K14.0
Riggs' (compound periodontitis) — *see* Periodontitis
Ritter's L00
Rivalta's (cervicofacial actinomycosis) A42.2
Robles' (onchocerciasis) B73.01
Roger's (congenital interventricular septal defect) Q21.0
Rosenthal's (factor XI deficiency) D68.1
Ross River B33.1
Rossbach's (hyperchlorhydria) K30
Rotes Quérol — *see* Hyperostosis, ankylosing
Roth (-Bernhardt) — *see* Mononeuropathy, lower limb, meralgia paresthetica
Runeberg's (progressive pernicious anemia) D51.0
sacroiliac NEC M53.3
salivary gland or duct K11.9
   inclusion B25.9
   specified NEC K11.8
   virus B25.9
sandworm B76.9
Schimmelbusch's — *see* Mastopathy, cystic
Schmorl's — *see* Schmorl's disease or nodes
Schönlein (-Henoch) (purpura rheumatica) D69.0
Schottmüller's — *see* Fever, paratyphoid
Schultz's (agranulocytosis) — *see* Agranulocytosis
Schwalbe-Ziehen-Oppenheim G24.1
Schwartz-Jampel G71.13
sclera H15.9
   specified NEC H15.89
scrofulous (tuberculous) A18.2
scrotum N50.9
sebaceous glands L73.9
semilunar cartilage, cystic (*see also* Derangement, knee, meniscus, cystic)
seminal vesicle N50.9
serum NEC (*see also* Reaction, serum) T80.69 ☑
sexually transmitted A64
   anogenital
      herpesviral infection — *see* Herpes, anogenital

Disease, diseased — *continued*

sexually transmitted — *continued*
   anogenital — *continued*
      warts A63.0
   chancroid A57
   chlamydial infection — *see* Chlamydia
   gonorrhea — *see* Gonorrhea
   granuloma inguinale A58
   specified organism NEC A63.8
   syphilis — *see* Syphilis
   trichomoniasis — *see* Trichomoniasis
Sézary C84.1- ☑
shimamushi (scrub typhus) A75.3
shipyard B30.0
sickle-cell D57.1
   with crisis (vasoocclusive pain) D57.00
      with
         acute chest syndrome D57.01
         splenic sequestration D57.02
   elliptocytosis D57.8- ☑
   Hb-C D57.20
      with crisis (vasoocclusive pain) D57.219
         with
            acute chest syndrome D57.211
            splenic sequestration D57.212
      without crisis D57.20
   Hb-SD D57.80
      with crisis D57.819
         with
            acute chest syndrome D57.811
            splenic sequestration D57.812
   Hb-SE D57.80
      with crisis D57.819
         with
            acute chest syndrome D57.811
            splenic sequestration D57.812
   specified NEC D57.80
      with crisis D57.819
         with
            acute chest syndrome D57.811
            splenic sequestration D57.812
   spherocytosis D57.80
      with crisis D57.819
         with
            acute chest syndrome D57.811
            splenic sequestration D57.812
   thalassemia D57.40
      with crisis (vasoocclusive pain) D57.419
         with
            acute chest syndrome D57.411
            splenic sequestration D57.412
      without crisis D57.40
silo-filler's J68.8
   bronchitis J68.0
   pneumonitis J68.0
   pulmonary edema J68.1
simian B B00.4
Simons' (progressive lipodystrophy) E88.1
sin nombre virus B33.4
sinus — *see* Sinusitis
Sirkari's B55.0
sixth B08.20
   due to human herpesvirus 6 B08.21
   due to human herpesvirus 7 B08.22
skin L98.9
   due to metabolic disorder NEC E88.9 [L99]
   specified NEC L98.8
slim (HIV) B20
small vessel I73.9
Sneddon-Wilkinson (subcorneal pustular dermatosis) L13.1
South African creeping B88.0
spinal (cord) G95.9
   congenital Q06.9
   specified NEC G95.89
spine (*see also* Spondylopathy)
   joint — *see* Dorsopathy
   tuberculous A18.01
spinocerebellar (hereditary) G11.9
   specified NEC G11.8
spleen D73.9
   amyloid E85.4 [D77]
   organic D73.9
   polycystic Q89.09
   postinfectional D73.89
sponge-diver's — *see* Toxicity, venom, marine animal, sea anemone
Startle Q89.8

Disease, diseased — *continued*

Steinert's G71.11
Sticker's (erythema infectiosum) B08.3
Stieda's (calcification, knee joint) — *see* Bursitis, tibial collateral
Stokes' (exophthalmic goiter) — *see* Hyperthyroidism, with, goiter (diffuse)
Stokes-Adams (syncope with heart block) I45.9
stomach K31.9
   functional, psychogenic F45.8
   specified NEC K31.89
stonemason's J62.8
storage
   glycogen — *see* Disease, glycogen storage
   mucopolysaccharide — *see* Mucopolysaccharidosis
striatopallidal system NEC G25.89
Stuart-Prower (congenital factor X deficiency) D68.2
Stuart's (congenital factor X deficiency) D68.2
subcutaneous tissue — *see* Disease, skin
supporting structures of teeth K08.9
   specified NEC K08.8
suprarenal (capsule) (gland) E27.9
   hyperfunction E27.0
   specified NEC E27.8
sweat glands L74.9
   specified NEC L74.8
Sweeley-Klionsky E75.21
Swift (-Feer) — *see* Poisoning, mercury
swimming-pool granuloma A31.1
Sylvest's (epidemic pleurodynia) B33.0
sympathetic nervous system G90.9
synovium — *see* Disorder, synovium
syphilitic — *see* Syphilis
systemic tissue mast cell C96.2
tanapox (virus) B08.71
Tangier E78.6
Tarral-Besnier (pityriasis rubra pilaris) L44.0
Tauri's E74.09
tear duct — *see* Disorder, lacrimal system
tendon, tendinous (*see also* Disorder, tendon)
   nodular — *see* Trigger finger
terminal vessel I73.9
testis N50.9
thalassemia Hb-S — *see* Disease, sickle-cell, thalassemia
Thaysen-Gee (nontropical sprue) K90.0
Thomsen G71.12
throat J39.2
   septic J02.0
thromboembolic — *see* Embolism
thymus (gland) E32.9
   specified NEC E32.8
thyroid (gland) E07.9
   heart (*see also* Hyperthyroidism) E05.90 [I43]
      with thyroid storm E05.91 [I43]
   specified NEC E07.89
Tietze's M94.0
tongue K14.9
   specified NEC K14.8
tonsils, tonsillar (and adenoids) J35.9
tooth, teeth K08.9
   hard tissues K03.9
      specified NEC K03.89
   pulp NEC K04.99
   specified NEC K08.8
Tourette's F95.2
trachea NEC J39.8
tricuspid I07.9
   nonrheumatic I36.9
triglyceride-storage E75.5
trophoblastic — *see* Mole, hydatidiform
tsutsugamushi A75.3
tube (fallopian) (noninflammatory) N83.9
   inflammatory — *see* Salpingitis
   specified NEC N83.8
tuberculous NEC — *see* Tuberculosis
tubo-ovarian (noninflammatory) N83.9
   inflammatory — *see* Salpingo-oophoritis
   specified NEC N83.8
tubotympanic, chronic — *see* Otitis, media, suppurative, chronic, tubotympanic
tubulo-interstitial N15.9
   specified NEC N15.8
tympanum — *see* Disorder, tympanic membrane
Uhl's Q24.8
Underwood's (sclerema neonatorum) P83.0
Unverricht (-Lundborg) — *see* Epilepsy, generalized, idiopathic

Disease, diseased — *continued*
Urbach-Oppenheim (necrobiosis lipoidica diabeticorum) — *see* E08-E13 with .620
ureter N28.9
    in (due to)
        schistosomiasis (bilharziasis) B65.0 [N29]
urethra N36.9
    specified NEC N36.8
urinary (tract) N39.9
    bladder N32.9
        specified NEC N32.89
    specified NEC N39.8
uterus (noninflammatory) N85.9
    infective — *see* Endometritis
    inflammatory — *see* Endometritis
    specified NEC N85.8
uveal tract (anterior) H21.9
    posterior H31.9
vagabond's B85.1
vagina, vaginal (noninflammatory) N89.9
    inflammatory NEC N76.89
    specified NEC N89.8
valve, valvular I38
    multiple I08.9
        specified NEC I08.8
van Creveld-von Gierke (glycogenosis I) E74.01
vas deferens N50.9
vascular I99.9
    arteriosclerotic — *see* Arteriosclerosis
    ciliary body NEC — *see* Disorder, iris, vascular
    hypertensive — *see* Hypertension
    iris NEC — *see* Disorder, iris, vascular
    obliterative I77.1
        peripheral I73.9
    occlusive I99.8
    peripheral (occlusive) I73.9
        in diabetes mellitus — *see* E08-E13 with .51
vasomotor I73.9
vasospastic I73.9
vein I87.9
venereal (*see also* Disease, sexually transmitted) A64
    chlamydial NEC A56.8
        anus A56.3
        genitourinary NOS A56.2
        pharynx A56.4
        rectum A56.3
    fifth A55
    sixth A55
    specified nature or type NEC A63.8
vertebra, vertebral (*see also* Spondylopathy)
    disc — *see* Disorder, disc
vibration — *see* Vibration, adverse effects
viral, virus (*see also* Disease, by type of virus) B34.9
    arbovirus NOS A94
    arthropod-borne NOS A94
    congenital P35.9
        specified NEC P35.8
    Hanta (with renal manifestations) (Dobrava) (Puumala) (Seoul) A98.5
        with pulmonary manifestations (Andes) (Bayou) (Bermejo) (Black Creek Canal) (Choclo) (Juquitiba) (Laguna negra) (Lechiguanas) (New York) (Oran) (Sin nombre) B33.4
    Hantaan (Korean hemorrhagic fever) A98.5
    human immunodeficiency (HIV) B20
    Kunjin A83.4
    nonarthropod-borne NOS B34.9
    Powassan A84.8
    Rocio (encephalitis) A83.6
    Sin nombre (Hantavirus) (cardio)-pulmonary syndrome) B33.4
    Tahyna B33.8
    vesicular stomatitis A93.8
vitreous H43.9
    specified NEC H43.89
vocal cord J38.3
Volkmann's, acquired T79.6 ☑
von Eulenburg's (congenital paramyotonia) G71.19
von Gierke's (glycogenosis I) E74.01
von Graefe's — *see* Strabismus, paralytic, ophthalmoplegia, progressive
von Willebrand (-Jürgens) (angiohemophilia) D68.0
Vrolik's (osteogenesis imperfecta) Q78.0
vulva (noninflammatory) N90.9
    inflammatory NEC N76.89
    specified NEC N90.89
Wallgren's (obstruction of splenic vein with collateral circulation) I87.8

Disease, diseased — *continued*
Wassilieff's (leptospiral jaundice) A27.0
wasting NEC R64
    due to malnutrition E41
Waterhouse-Friderichsen A39.1
Wegner's (syphilitic osteochondritis) A50.02
Weil's (leptospiral jaundice of lung) A27.0
Weir Mitchell's (erythromelalgia) I73.81
Werdnig-Hoffmann G12.0
Wermer's E31.21
Werner-His (trench fever) A79.0
Werner-Schultz (neutropenic splenomegaly) D73.81
Wernicke-Posadas B38.9
whipworm B79
white blood cells D72.9
    specified NEC D72.89
white matter R90.82
white-spot, meaning lichen sclerosus et atrophicus L90.0
    penis N48.0
    vulva N90.4
Wilkie's K55.1
Wilkinson-Sneddon (subcorneal pustular dermatosis) L13.1
Willis' — *see* Diabetes
Wilson's (hepatolenticular degeneration) E83.01
woolsorter's A22.1
yaba monkey tumor B08.72
yaba pox (virus) B08.72
zoonotic, bacterial A28.9
    specified type NEC A28.8
Disfigurement (due to scar) L90.5
Disgerminoma — *see* Dysgerminoma
DISH (diffuse idiopathic skeletal hyperostosis) — *see* Hyperostosis, ankylosing
Disinsertion, retina — *see* Detachment, retina
Dislocatable hip, congenital Q65.6
Dislocation (articular)
    with fracture — *see* Fracture
    acromioclavicular (joint) S43.10- ☑
        with displacement
            100%-200% S43.12- ☑
            more than 200% S43.13- ☑
        inferior S43.14- ☑
        posterior S43.15- ☑
    ankle S93.0- ☑
    astragalus — *see* Dislocation, ankle
    atlantoaxial S13.121 ☑
    atlantooccipital S13.111 ☑
    atloidooccipital S13.111 ☑
    breast bone S23.29 ☑
    capsule, joint — *code by* site under Dislocation
    carpal (bone) — *see* Dislocation, wrist
    carpometacarpal (joint) NEC S63.05- ☑
        thumb S63.04- ☑
    cartilage (joint) — *code by* site under Dislocation
    cervical spine (vertebra) — *see* Dislocation, vertebra, cervical
    chronic — *see* Dislocation, recurrent
    clavicle — *see* Dislocation, acromioclavicular joint
    coccyx S33.2 ☑
    congenital NEC Q68.8
    coracoid — *see* Dislocation, shoulder
    costal cartilage S23.29 ☑
    costochondral S23.29 ☑
    cricoarytenoid articulation S13.29 ☑
    cricothyroid articulation S13.29 ☑
    dorsal vertebra — *see* Dislocation, vertebra, thoracic
    ear ossicle — *see* Discontinuity, ossicles, ear
    elbow S53.10- ☑
        congenital Q68.8
        pathological — *see* Dislocation, pathological NEC, elbow
        radial head alone — *see* Dislocation, radial head
        recurrent — *see* Dislocation, recurrent, elbow
        traumatic S53.10- ☑
            anterior S53.11- ☑
            lateral S53.14- ☑
            medial S53.13- ☑
            posterior S53.12- ☑
            specified type NEC S53.19- ☑
    eye, nontraumatic — *see* Luxation, globe
    eyeball, nontraumatic — *see* Luxation, globe
    femur
        distal end — *see* Dislocation, knee
        proximal end — *see* Dislocation, hip

Dislocation — *continued*
fibula
    distal end — *see* Dislocation, ankle
    proximal end — *see* Dislocation, knee
finger S63.25- ☑
    index S63.25- ☑
    interphalangeal S63.27- ☑
        distal S63.27- ☑
            index S63.29- ☑
            little S63.29- ☑
            middle S63.29- ☑
            ring S63.29- ☑
        index S63.27- ☑
        little S63.27- ☑
        middle S63.27- ☑
        proximal S63.28- ☑
            index S63.28- ☑
            little S63.28- ☑
            middle S63.28- ☑
            ring S63.28- ☑
        ring S63.27- ☑
    little S63.25- ☑
    metacarpophalangeal S63.26- ☑
        index S63.26- ☑
        little S63.26- ☑
        middle S63.26- ☑
        ring S63.26- ☑
    middle S63.25- ☑
    recurrent — *see* Dislocation, recurrent, finger
    ring S63.25- ☑
    thumb — *see* Dislocation, thumb
foot S93.30- ☑
    recurrent — *see* Dislocation, recurrent, foot
    specified site NEC S93.33- ☑
    tarsal joint S93.31- ☑
    tarsometatarsal joint S93.32- ☑
    toe — *see* Dislocation, toe
fracture — *see* Fracture
glenohumeral (joint) — *see* Dislocation, shoulder
glenoid — *see* Dislocation, shoulder
habitual — *see* Dislocation, recurrent
hip S73.00- ☑
    anterior S73.03- ☑
        obturator S73.02- ☑
    central S73.04- ☑
    congenital (total) Q65.2
        bilateral Q65.1
        partial Q65.5
            bilateral Q65.4
            unilateral Q65.3- ☑
        unilateral Q65.0- ☑
    developmental M24.85- ☑
    pathological — *see* Dislocation, pathological NEC, hip
    posterior S73.01- ☑
    recurrent — *see* Dislocation, recurrent, hip
humerus, proximal end — *see* Dislocation, shoulder
incomplete — *see* Subluxation, by site
incus — *see* Discontinuity, ossicles, ear
infracoracoid — *see* Dislocation, shoulder
innominate (pubic junction) (sacral junction) S33.39 ☑
    acetabulum — *see* Dislocation, hip
interphalangeal (joint(s))
    finger S63.279 ☑
        distal S63.29- ☑
            index S63.29- ☑
            little S63.29- ☑
            middle S63.29- ☑
            ring S63.29- ☑
        index S63.27- ☑
        little S63.27- ☑
        middle S63.27- ☑
        proximal S63.28- ☑
            index S63.28- ☑
            little S63.28- ☑
            middle S63.28- ☑
            ring S63.28- ☑
        ring S63.27- ☑
    foot or toe — *see* Dislocation, toe
    thumb S63.12- ☑
        distal joint S63.14- ☑
        proximal joint S63.13- ☑
jaw (cartilage) (meniscus) S03.0 ☑
joint prosthesis — *see* Complications, joint prosthesis, mechanical, displacement, by site
knee S83.106 ☑

Dislocation — *continued*
knee — *continued*
　cap — *see* Dislocation, patella
　congenital Q68.2
　old M23.8X-
　patella — *see* Dislocation, patella
　pathological — *see* Dislocation, pathological NEC, knee
　proximal tibia
　　anteriorly S83.11- ☑
　　laterally S83.14- ☑
　　medially S83.13- ☑
　　posteriorly S83.12- ☑
　recurrent (*see also* Derangement, knee, specified NEC)
　specified type NEC S83.19- ☑
lacrimal gland H04.16- ☑
lens (complete) H27.10-
　anterior H27.12- ☑
　congenital Q12.1
　ocular implant — *see* Complications, intraocular lens
　partial H27.11- ☑
　posterior H27.13- ☑
　traumatic S05.8X- ☑
ligament — *code by* site under Dislocation
lumbar (vertebra) — *see* Dislocation, vertebra, lumbar
lumbosacral (vertebra) (*see also* Dislocation, vertebra, lumbar)
　congenital Q76.49
mandible S03.0 ☑
meniscus (knee) — *see* Tear, meniscus
　other sites - code by site under Dislocation
metacarpal (bone)
　distal end — *see* Dislocation, finger
　proximal end S63.06- ☑
metacarpophalangeal (joint)
　finger S63.26- ☑
　　index S63.26- ☑
　　little S63.26- ☑
　　middle S63.26- ☑
　　ring S63.26- ☑
　　thumb S63.11- ☑
metatarsal (bone) — *see* Dislocation, foot
metatarsophalangeal (joint(s)) — *see* Dislocation, toe
midcarpal (joint) S63.03- ☑
midtarsal (joint) — *see* Dislocation, foot
neck S13.20 ☑
　specified site NEC S13.29 ☑
　vertebra — *see* Dislocation, vertebra, cervical
nose (septal cartilage) S03.1 ☑
occipitoatloid S13.111 ☑
old — *see* Derangement, joint, specified type NEC
ossicles, ear — *see* Discontinuity, ossicles, ear
partial — *see* Subluxation, by site
patella S83.006 ☑
　congenital Q74.1
　lateral S83.01- ☑
　recurrent (nontraumatic) M22.0- ☑
　　incomplete M22.1- ☑
　specified type NEC S83.09- ☑
pathological NEC M24.30
　ankle M24.37- ☑
　elbow M24.32- ☑
　foot joint M24.37- ☑
　hand joint M24.34- ☑
　hip M24.35- ☑
　knee M24.36- ☑
　lumbosacral joint — *see* subcategory M53.2 ☑
　pelvic region — *see* Dislocation, pathological, hip
　sacroiliac — *see* subcategory M53.2 ☑
　shoulder M24.31- ☑
　wrist M24.33- ☑
pelvis NEC S33.30 ☑
　specified NEC S33.39 ☑
phalanx
　finger or hand — *see* Dislocation, finger
　foot or toe — *see* Dislocation, toe
prosthesis, internal — *see* Complications, prosthetic device, by site, mechanical
radial head S53.006 ☑
　anterior S53.01- ☑
　posterior S53.02- ☑
　specified type NEC S53.09- ☑
radiocarpal (joint) S63.02- ☑
radiohumeral (joint) — *see* Dislocation, radial head

Dislocation — *continued*
radioulnar (joint)
　distal S63.01- ☑
　proximal — *see* Dislocation, elbow
radius
　distal end — *see* Dislocation, wrist
　proximal end — *see* Dislocation, radial head
recurrent M24.40
　ankle M24.47- ☑
　elbow M24.42- ☑
　finger M24.44- ☑
　foot joint M24.47- ☑
　hand joint M24.44- ☑
　hip M24.45- ☑
　knee M24.46- ☑
　　patella — *see* Dislocation, patella, recurrent
　patella — *see* Dislocation, patella, recurrent
　sacroiliac — *see* subcategory M53.2 ☑
　shoulder M24.41- ☑
　toe M24.47- ☑
　vertebra (*see also* subcategory) M43.5 ☑
　　atlantoaxial M43.4
　　　with myelopathy M43.3
　wrist M24.43- ☑
rib (cartilage) S23.29 ☑
sacrococcygeal S33.2 ☑
sacroiliac (joint) (ligament) S33.2 ☑
　congenital Q74.2
　recurrent — *see* subcategory M53.2 ☑
sacrum S33.2 ☑
scaphoid (bone) (hand) (wrist) — *see* Dislocation, wrist
　foot — *see* Dislocation, foot
scapula — *see* Dislocation, shoulder, girdle, scapula
semilunar cartilage, knee — *see* Tear, meniscus
septal cartilage (nose) S03.1 ☑
septum (nasal) (old) J34.2
sesamoid bone — *code by* site under Dislocation
shoulder (blade) (ligament) (joint) (traumatic) S43.006 ☑
　acromioclavicular — *see* Dislocation, acromioclavicular
　chronic — *see* Dislocation, recurrent, shoulder
　congenital Q68.8
　girdle S43.30- ☑
　　scapula S43.31- ☑
　　specified site NEC S43.39- ☑
　humerus S43.00- ☑
　　anterior S43.01- ☑
　　inferior S43.03- ☑
　　posterior S43.02- ☑
　pathological — *see* Dislocation, pathological NEC, shoulder
　recurrent — *see* Dislocation, recurrent, shoulder
　specified type NEC S43.08- ☑
spine
　cervical — *see* Dislocation, vertebra, cervical
　due to birth trauma P11.5
　lumbar — *see* Dislocation, vertebra, lumbar
　thoracic — *see* Dislocation, vertebra, thoracic
spontaneous — *see* Dislocation, pathological
sternoclavicular (joint) S43.206 ☑
　anterior S43.21- ☑
　posterior S43.22- ☑
sternum S23.29 ☑
subglenoid — *see* Dislocation, shoulder
symphysis pubis S33.4 ☑
talus — *see* Dislocation, ankle
tarsal (bone(s)) (joint(s)) — *see* Dislocation, foot
tarsometatarsal (joint(s)) — *see* Dislocation, foot
temporomandibular (joint) S03.0 ☑
thigh, proximal end — *see* Dislocation, hip
thorax S23.20 ☑
　specified site NEC S23.29 ☑
　vertebra — *see* Dislocation, vertebra
thumb S63.10- ☑
　interphalangeal joint — *see* Dislocation, interphalangeal (joint), thumb
　metacarpophalangeal joint — *see* Dislocation, metacarpophalangeal (joint), thumb
thyroid cartilage S13.29 ☑
tibia
　distal end — *see* Dislocation, ankle
　proximal end — *see* Dislocation, knee
tibiofibular (joint)
　distal — *see* Dislocation, ankle

Dislocation — *continued*
tibiofibular — *continued*
　superior — *see* Dislocation, knee
toe(s) S93.106 ☑
　great S93.10- ☑
　　interphalangeal joint S93.11- ☑
　　metatarsophalangeal joint S93.12- ☑
　interphalangeal joint S93.119 ☑
　lesser S93.106 ☑
　　interphalangeal joint S93.11- ☑
　　metatarsophalangeal joint S93.12- ☑
　metatarsophalangeal joint S93.12- ☑
tooth S03.2 ☑
trachea S23.29 ☑
ulna
　distal end S63.07- ☑
　proximal end — *see* Dislocation, elbow
ulnohumeral (joint) — *see* Dislocation, elbow
vertebra (articular process) (body) (traumatic)
　cervical S13.101 ☑
　　atlantoaxial joint S13.121 ☑
　　atlantooccipital joint S13.111 ☑
　　atloidooccipital joint S13.111 ☑
　　joint between
　　　C0 and C1 S13.111 ☑
　　　C1 and C2 S13.121 ☑
　　　C2 and C3 S13.131 ☑
　　　C3 and C4 S13.141 ☑
　　　C4 and C5 S13.151 ☑
　　　C5 and C6 S13.161 ☑
　　　C6 and C7 S13.171 ☑
　　　C7 and T1 S13.181 ☑
　　occipitoatloid joint S13.111 ☑
　congenital Q76.49
　lumbar S33.101 ☑
　　joint between
　　　L1 and L2 S33.111 ☑
　　　L2 and L3 S33.121 ☑
　　　L3 and L4 S33.131 ☑
　　　L4 and L5 S33.141 ☑
　nontraumatic — *see* Displacement, intervertebral disc
　partial — *see* Subluxation, by site
　recurrent NEC — *see* subcategory M43.5 ☑
　thoracic S23.101 ☑
　　joint between
　　　T1 and T2 S23.111 ☑
　　　T2 and T3 S23.121 ☑
　　　T3 and T4 S23.123 ☑
　　　T4 and T5 S23.131 ☑
　　　T5 and T6 S23.133 ☑
　　　T6 and T7 S23.141 ☑
　　　T7 and T8 S23.143 ☑
　　　T8 and T9 S23.151 ☑
　　　T9 and T10 S23.153 ☑
　　　T10 and T11 S23.161 ☑
　　　T11 and T12 S23.163 ☑
　　　T12 and L1 S23.171 ☑
wrist (carpal bone) S63.006 ☑
　carpometacarpal joint — *see* Dislocation, carpometacarpal (joint)
　distal radioulnar joint — *see* Dislocation, radioulnar (joint), distal
　metacarpal bone, proximal — *see* Dislocation, metacarpal (bone), proximal end
　midcarpal — *see* Dislocation, midcarpal (joint)
　radiocarpal joint — *see* Dislocation, radiocarpal (joint)
　recurrent — *see* Dislocation, recurrent, wrist
　specified site NEC S63.09- ☑
　ulna — *see* Dislocation, ulna, distal end
xiphoid cartilage S23.29 ☑
Disorder (of) (*see also* Disease)
acantholytic L11.9
　specified NEC L11.8
acute
　psychotic — *see* Psychosis, acute
　stress F43.0
adjustment (grief) F43.20
　with
　　anxiety F43.22
　　　with depressed mood F43.23
　　conduct disturbance F43.24
　　　with emotional disturbance F43.25
　　depressed mood F43.21
　　　with anxiety F43.23

Disorder — *continued*
 adjustment — *continued*
  with — *continued*
   other specified symptom F43.29
 adrenal (capsule) (gland) (medullary) E27.9
  specified NEC E27.8
 adrenogenital E25.9
  drug-induced E25.8
  iatrogenic E25.8
  idiopathic E25.8
 adult personality (and behavior) F69
  specified NEC F68.8
 affective (mood) — *see* Disorder, mood
 aggressive, unsocialized F91.1
 alcohol-related F10.99
  with
   amnestic disorder, persisting F10.96
   anxiety disorder F10.980
   dementia, persisting F10.97
   intoxication F10.929
    with delirium F10.921
    uncomplicated F10.920
   mood disorder F10.94
   other specified F10.988
   psychotic disorder F10.959
    with
     delusions F10.950
     hallucinations F10.951
   sexual dysfunction F10.981
   sleep disorder F10.982
 allergic — *see* Allergy
 alveolar NEC J84.09
 amino-acid
  cystathioninuria E72.19
  cystinosis E72.04
  cystinuria E72.01
  glycinuria E72.09
  homocystinuria E72.11
  metabolism — *see* Disturbance, metabolism, amino-acid
  specified NEC E72.8
  neonatal, transitory P74.8
  renal transport NEC E72.09
  transport NEC E72.09
 amnesic, amnestic
  alcohol-induced F10.96
   with dependence F10.26
  due to (secondary to) general medical condition F04
  psychoactive NEC-induced F19.96
   with
    abuse F19.16
    dependence F19.26
  sedative, hypnotic or anxiolytic-induced F13.96
   with dependence F13.26
 anaerobic glycolysis with anemia D55.2
 anxiety F41.9
  due to (secondary to)
   alcohol F10.980
   amphetamine F15.980
    in
     abuse F15.180
     dependence F15.280
   anxiolytic F13.980
    in
     abuse F13.180
     dependence F13.280
   caffeine F15.980
    in
     abuse F15.180
     dependence F15.280
   cannabis F12.980
    in
     abuse F12.180
     dependence F12.280
   cocaine F14.980
    in
     abuse F14.180
     dependence F14.180
   general medical condition F06.4
   hallucinogen F16.980
    in
     abuse F16.180
     dependence F16.280
   hypnotic F13.980
    in
     abuse F13.180
     dependence F13.280

Disorder — *continued*
 anxiety — *continued*
  due to — *continued*
   inhalant F18.980
    in
     abuse F18.180
     dependence F18.280
   phencyclidine F16.980
    in
     abuse F16.180
     dependence F16.280
   psychoactive substance NEC F19.980
    in
     abuse F19.180
     dependence F19.280
   sedative F13.980
    in
     abuse F13.180
     dependence F13.280
   volatile solvents F18.980
    in
     abuse F18.180
     dependence F18.280
  generalized F41.1
  mixed
   with depression (mild) F41.8
   specified NEC F41.3
  organic F06.4
  phobic F40.9
   of childhood F40.8
  specified NEC F41.8
 aortic valve — *see* Endocarditis, aortic
 aromatic amino-acid metabolism E70.9
  specified NEC E70.8
 arteriole NEC I77.89
 artery NEC I77.89
 articulation — *see* Disorder, joint
 attachment (childhood)
  disinhibited F94.2
  reactive F94.1
 attention-deficit hyperactivity (adolescent) (adult) (child) F90.9
  combined type F90.2
  hyperactive type F90.1
  inattentive type F90.0
  specified type NEC F90.8
 attention-deficit without hyperactivity (adolescent) (adult) (child) F90.0
 auditory processing (central) H93.25
 autistic F84.0
 autonomic nervous system G90.9
  specified NEC G90.8
 avoidant, child or adolescent F40.10
 balance
  acid-base E87.8
   mixed E87.4
  electrolyte E87.8
  fluid NEC E87.8
 behavioral (disruptive) — *see* Disorder, conduct
 beta-amino-acid metabolism E72.8
 bile acid and cholesterol metabolism E78.70
  Barth syndrome E78.71
  other specified E78.79
  Smith-Lemli-Opitz syndrome E78.72
 bilirubin excretion E80.6
 binocular
  movement H51.9
   convergence
    excess H51.12
    insufficiency H51.11
   internuclear ophthalmoplegia — *see* Ophthalmoplegia, internuclear
   palsy of conjugate gaze H51.0
   specified type NEC H51.8
  vision NEC — *see* Disorder, vision, binocular
 bipolar (I) F31.9
  current episode
   depressed F31.9
    with psychotic features F31.5
    without psychotic features F31.30
     mild F31.31
     moderate F31.32
     severe (without psychotic features) F31.4
      with psychotic features F31.5
   hypomanic F31.0
   manic F31.9
    with psychotic features F31.2
    without psychotic features F31.10

Disorder — *continued*
 bipolar — *continued*
  current episode — *continued*
   manic — *continued*
    without psychotic features — *continued*
     mild F31.11
     moderate F31.12
     severe (without psychotic features) F31.13
      with psychotic features F31.2
   mixed F31.60
    mild F31.61
    moderate F31.62
    severe (without psychotic features) F31.63
     with psychotic features F31.64
    severe depression (without psychotic features) F31.4
     with psychotic features F31.5
  in remission (currently) F31.70
   in full remission
    most recent episode
     depressed F31.76
     hypomanic F31.72
     manic F31.74
     mixed F31.78
   in partial remission
    most recent episode
     depressed F31.75
     hypomanic F31.71
     manic F31.73
     mixed F31.77
  organic F06.30
  single manic episode F30.9
   mild F30.11
   moderate F30.12
   severe (without psychotic symptoms) F30.13
    with psychotic symptoms F30.2
  specified NEC F31.89
 bipolar II F31.81
 bladder N32.9
  functional NEC N31.9
  in schistosomiasis B65.0 [N33]
  specified NEC N32.89
 bleeding D68.9
 blood D75.9
  in congenital early syphilis A50.09 [D77]
 body dysmorphic F45.22
 bone M89.9
  continuity M84.9
   specified type NEC M84.80
    ankle M84.87- ☑
    fibula M84.86- ☑
    foot M84.87- ☑
    hand M84.84- ☑
    humerus M84.82- ☑
    neck M84.88
    pelvis M84.859
    radius M84.83- ☑
    rib M84.88
    shoulder M84.81- ☑
    skull M84.88
    thigh M84.85- ☑
    tibia M84.86- ☑
    ulna M84.83- ☑
    vertebra M84.88
  density and structure M85.9
   cyst (*see also* Cyst, bone, specified type NEC)
    aneurysmal — *see* Cyst, bone, aneurysmal
    solitary — *see* Cyst, bone, solitary
   diffuse idiopathic skeletal hyperostosis — *see* Hyperostosis, ankylosing
   fibrous dysplasia (monostotic) — *see* Dysplasia, fibrous, bone
   fluorosis — *see* Fluorosis, skeletal
   hyperostosis of skull M85.2
   osteitis condensans — *see* Osteitis, condensans
   specified type NEC M85.8- ☑
    ankle M85.87- ☑
    foot M85.87- ☑
    forearm M85.83- ☑
    hand M85.84- ☑
    lower leg M85.86- ☑
    multiple sites M85.89
    neck M85.88
    rib M85.88
    shoulder M85.81- ☑
    skull M85.88
    thigh M85.85- ☑

☑ **Additional Character Required — Refer to the Tabular List for Character Selection**   ▽ **Subterms under main terms may continue to next column or page**

Disorder — *continued*
bone — *continued*
  density and structure — *continued*
    specified type — *continued*
      upper arm M85.82- ☑
      vertebra M85.88
  development and growth NEC M89.20
    carpus M89.24- ☑
    clavicle M89.21- ☑
    femur M89.25- ☑
    fibula M89.26- ☑
    finger M89.24- ☑
    humerus M89.22- ☑
    ilium M89.259
    ischium M89.259
    metacarpus M89.24- ☑
    metatarsus M89.27- ☑
    multiple sites M89.29
    neck M89.28
    radius M89.23- ☑
    rib M89.28
    scapula M89.21- ☑
    skull M89.28
    tarsus M89.27- ☑
    tibia M89.26- ☑
    toe M89.27- ☑
    ulna M89.23- ☑
    vertebra M89.28
    specified type NEC M89.8X- ☑
brachial plexus G54.0
branched-chain amino-acid metabolism E71.2
  specified NEC E71.19
breast N64.9
  agalactia — *see* Agalactia
  associated with
    lactation O92.70
      specified NEC O92.79
    pregnancy O92.20
      specified NEC O92.29
    puerperium O92.20
      specified NEC O92.29
  cracked nipple — *see* Cracked nipple
  galactorrhea — *see* Galactorrhea
  hypogalactia O92.4
  lactation disorder NEC O92.79
  mastitis — *see* Mastitis
  nipple infection — *see* Infection, nipple
  retracted nipple — *see* Retraction, nipple
  specified type NEC N64.89
Briquet's F45.0
bullous, in diseases classified elsewhere L14
cannabis use
  due to drug abuse — *see* Abuse, drug, cannabis
  due to drug dependence — *see* Dependence, drug, cannabis
carbohydrate
  absorption, intestinal NEC E74.39
  metabolism (congenital) E74.9
    specified NEC E74.8
cardiac, functional I51.89
carnitine metabolism E71.40
cartilage M94.9
  articular NEC — *see* Derangement, joint, articular cartilage
  chondrocalcinosis — *see* Chondrocalcinosis
  specified type NEC M94.8X- ☑
    articular — *see* Derangement, joint, articular cartilage
    multiple sites M94.8X0
catatonic
  due to (secondary to) known physiological condition F06.1
  organic F06.1
central auditory processing H93.25
cervical
  region NEC M53.82
  root (nerve) NEC G54.2
character NOS F60.9
childhood disintegrative NEC F84.3
cholesterol and bile acid metabolism E78.70
  Barth syndrome E78.71
  other specified E78.79
  Smith-Lemli-Opitz syndrome E78.72
choroid H31.9
  atrophy — *see* Atrophy, choroid
  degeneration — *see* Degeneration, choroid
  detachment — *see* Detachment, choroid

Disorder — *continued*
choroid — *continued*
  dystrophy — *see* Dystrophy, choroid
  hemorrhage — *see* Hemorrhage, choroid
  rupture — *see* Rupture, choroid
  scar — *see* Scar, chorioretinal
  solar retinopathy — *see* Retinopathy, solar
  specified type NEC H31.8
ciliary body — *see* Disorder, iris
  degeneration — *see* Degeneration, ciliary body
coagulation (factor) (*see also* Defect, coagulation) D68.9
  newborn, transient P61.6
coccyx NEC M53.3
cognitive F09
  due to (secondary to) general medical condition F09
  persisting R41.89
    due to
      alcohol F10.97
        with dependence F10.27
      anxiolytics F13.97
        with dependence F13.27
      hypnotics F13.97
        with dependence F13.27
      sedatives F13.97
        with dependence F13.27
      specified substance NEC F19.97
        with
          abuse F19.17
          dependence F19.27
communication F80.9
conduct (childhood) F91.9
  adjustment reaction — *see* Disorder, adjustment
  adolescent onset type F91.2
  childhood onset type F91.1
  compulsive F63.9
  confined to family context F91.0
  depressive F91.8
  group type F91.2
  hyperkinetic — *see* Disorder, attention-deficit hyperactivity
  oppositional defiance F91.3
  socialized F91.2
  solitary aggressive type F91.1
  specified NEC F91.8
  unsocialized (aggressive) F91.1
conduction, heart I45.9
congenital glycosylation (CDG) E74.8
conjunctiva H11.9
  infection — *see* Conjunctivitis
connective tissue, localized L94.9
  specified NEC L94.8
conversion — *see* Disorder, dissociative
convulsive (secondary) — *see* Convulsions
cornea H18.9
  deformity — *see* Deformity, cornea
  degeneration — *see* Degeneration, cornea
  deposits — *see* Deposit, cornea
  due to contact lens H18.82- ☑
    specified as edema — *see* Edema, cornea
  edema — *see* Edema, cornea
  keratitis — *see* Keratitis
  keratoconjunctivitis — *see* Keratoconjunctivitis
  membrane change — *see* Change, corneal membrane
  neovascularization — *see* Neovascularization, cornea
  scar — *see* Opacity, cornea
  specified type NEC H18.89- ☑
  ulcer — *see* Ulcer, cornea
corpus cavernosum N48.9
cranial nerve — *see* Disorder, nerve, cranial
cyclothymic F34.0
defiant oppositional F91.3
delusional (persistent) (systematized) F22
  induced F24
depersonalization F48.1
depressive F32.9
  major F32.9
    with psychotic symptoms F32.3
    in remission (full) F32.5
      partial F32.4
    recurrent F33.9
    single episode F32.9
      mild F32.0
      moderate F32.1
      severe (without psychotic symptoms) F32.2

Disorder — *continued*
depressive — *continued*
  major — *continued*
    single episode — *continued*
      severe — *continued*
        with psychotic symptoms F32.3
    organic F06.31
    recurrent F33.9
      current episode
        mild F33.0
        moderate F33.1
        severe (without psychotic symptoms) F33.2
          with psychotic symptoms F33.3
      in remission F33.40
        full F33.42
        partial F33.41
      specified NEC F33.8
    single episode — *see* Episode, depressive
developmental F89
  arithmetical skills F81.2
  coordination (motor) F82
  expressive writing F81.81
  language F80.9
    expressive F80.1
    mixed receptive and expressive F80.2
    receptive type F80.2
    specified NEC F80.89
  learning F81.9
    arithmetical F81.2
    reading F81.0
  mixed F88
  motor coordination or function F82
  pervasive F84.9
    specified NEC F84.8
  phonological F80.0
  reading F81.0
  scholastic skills (*see also* Disorder, learning)
    mixed F81.89
  specified NEC F88
  speech F80.9
    articulation F80.0
    specified NEC F80.89
  written expression F81.81
diaphragm J98.6
digestive (system) K92.9
  newborn P78.9
    specified NEC P78.89
  postprocedural — *see* Complication, gastrointestinal
  psychogenic F45.8
disc (intervertebral) M51.9
  with
    myelopathy
      cervical region M50.00
      cervicothoracic region M50.03
      high cervical region M50.01
      lumbar region M51.06
      mid-cervical region M50.02
      sacrococcygeal region M53.3
      thoracic region M51.04
      thoracolumbar region M51.05
    radiculopathy
      cervical region M50.10
      cervicothoracic region M50.13
      high cervical region M50.11
      lumbar region M51.16
      lumbosacral region M51.17
      mid-cervical region M50.12
      sacrococcygeal region M53.3
      thoracic region M51.14
      thoracolumbar region M51.15
  cervical M50.90
    with
      myelopathy M50.00
        C2-C3 M50.01
        C3-C4 M50.01
        C4-C5 M50.02
        C5-C6 M50.02
        C6-C7 M50.02
        C7-T1 M50.03
        cervicothoracic region M50.03
        high cervical region M50.01
        mid-cervical region M50.02
      neuritis, radiculitis or radiculopathy M50.10
        C2-C3 M50.11
        C3-C4 M50.11
        C4-C5 M50.12
        C5-C6 M50.12

Disorder — *continued*
  disc — *continued*
    cervical — *continued*
      with — *continued*
        neuritis, radiculitis or radiculopathy — *continued*
          C6-C7 M50.12
          C7-T1 M50.13
          cervicothoracic region M50.13
          high cervical region M50.11
          mid-cervical region M50.12
        C2-C3 M50.91
        C3-C4 M50.91
        C4-C5 M50.92
        C5-C6 M50.92
        C6-C7 M50.92
        C7-T1 M50.93
        cervicothoracic region M50.93
      degeneration M50.30
        C2-C3 M50.31
        C3-C4 M50.31
        C4-C5 M50.32
        C5-C6 M50.32
        C6-C7 M50.32
        C7-T1 M50.33
        cervicothoracic region M50.33
        high cervical region M50.31
        mid-cervical region M50.32
      displacement M50.20
        C2-C3 M50.21
        C3-C4 M50.21
        C4-C5 M50.22
        C5-C6 M50.22
        C6-C7 M50.22
        C7-T1 M50.23
        cervicothoracic region M50.23
        high cervical region M50.21
        mid-cervical region M50.22
      high cervical region M50.91
      mid-cervical region M50.92
      specified type NEC M50.80
        C2-C3 M50.81
        C3-C4 M50.81
        C4-C5 M50.82
        C5-C6 M50.82
        C6-C7 M50.82
        C7-T1 M50.83
        cervicothoracic region M50.83
        high cervical region M50.81
        mid-cervical region M50.82
    specified NEC
      lumbar region M51.86
      lumbosacral region M51.87
      sacrococcygeal region M53.3
      thoracic region M51.84
      thoracolumbar region M51.85
  disinhibited attachment (childhood) F94.2
  disintegrative, childhood NEC F84.3
  disruptive behavior F98.9
  dissocial personality F60.2
  dissociative F44.9
    affecting
      motor function F44.4
        and sensation F44.7
      sensation F44.6
        and motor function F44.7
    brief reactive F43.0
    due to (secondary to) general medical condition F06.8
    mixed F44.7
    organic F06.8
    other specified NEC F44.89
  double heterozygous sickling — *see* Disease, sickle-cell
  dream anxiety F51.5
  drug induced hemorrhagic D68.32
  drug related F19.99
    abuse — *see* Abuse, drug
    dependence — *see* Dependence, drug
  dysmorphic body F45.1
  dysthymic F34.1
  ear H93.9- ☑
    bleeding — *see* Otorrhagia
    deafness — *see* Deafness
    degenerative H93.09- ☑
    discharge — *see* Otorrhea
    external H61.9- ☑

Disorder — *continued*
  ear — *continued*
    external — *continued*
      auditory canal stenosis — *see* Stenosis, external ear canal
      exostosis — *see* Exostosis, external ear canal
      impacted cerumen — *see* Impaction, cerumen
      otitis — *see* Otitis, externa
      perichondritis — *see* Perichondritis, ear
      pinna — *see* Disorder, pinna
      specified type NEC H61.89- ☑
    inner H83.9- ☑
      vestibular dysfunction — *see* Disorder, vestibular function
    middle H74.9- ☑
      adhesive H74.1- ☑
      ossicle — *see* Abnormal, ear ossicles
      polyp — *see* Polyp, ear (middle)
      specified NEC, in diseases classified elsewhere H75.8- ☑
    postprocedural — *see* Complications, ear, procedure
    specified NEC, in diseases classified elsewhere H94.8- ☑
  eating (adult) (psychogenic) F50.9
    anorexia — *see* Anorexia
    bulimia F50.2
    child F98.29
      pica F98.3
      rumination disorder F98.21
    pica F50.8
      childhood F98.3
  electrolyte (balance) NEC E87.8
    with
      abortion — *see* Abortion by type complicated by specified condition NEC
      ectopic pregnancy O08.5
      molar pregnancy O08.5
    acidosis (metabolic) (respiratory) E87.2
    alkalosis (metabolic) (respiratory) E87.3
  elimination, transepidermal L87.9
    specified NEC L87.8
  emotional (persistent) F34.9
    of childhood F93.9
      specified NEC F93.8
  endocrine E34.9
    postprocedural E89.89
      specified NEC E89.89
  erectile (male) (organic) (*see also* Dysfunction, sexual, male, erectile) N52.9
    nonorganic F52.21
  erythematous — *see* Erythema
  esophagus K22.9
    functional K22.4
    psychogenic F45.8
  eustachian tube H69.9- ☑
    infection — *see* Salpingitis, eustachian
    obstruction — *see* Obstruction, eustachian tube
    patulous — *see* Patulous, eustachian tube
    specified NEC H69.8- ☑
  extrapyramidal G25.9
    in deseases classified elsewhere — *see* category G26
    specified type NEC G25.89
  eye H57.9
    postprocedural — *see* Complication, postprocedural, eye
  eyelid H02.9
    cyst — *see* Cyst, eyelid
    degenerative H02.70
      chloasma — *see* Chloasma, eyelid
      madarosis — *see* Madarosis
      specified type NEC H02.79
      vitiligo — *see* Vitiligo, eyelid
      xanthelasma — *see* Xanthelasma
    dermatochalasis — *see* Dermatochalasis
    edema — *see* Edema, eyelid
    elephantiasis — *see* Elephantiasis, eyelid
    foreign body, retained — *see* Foreign body, retained, eyelid
    function H02.59
      abnormal innervation syndrome — *see* Syndrome, abnormal innervation
      blepharochalasis — *see* Blepharochalasis
      blepharoclonus — *see* Blepharoclonus
      blepharophimosis — *see* Blepharophimosis
      blepharoptosis — *see* Blepharoptosis

Disorder — *continued*
  eyelid — *continued*
    function — *continued*
      lagophthalmos — *see* Lagophthalmos
      lid retraction — *see* Retraction, lid
    hypertrichosis — *see* Hypertrichosis, eyelid
    specified type NEC H02.89
    vascular H02.879
      left H02.876
        lower H02.875
        upper H02.874
      right H02.873
        lower H02.872
        upper H02.871
  factitious F68.10
    with predominantly
      physical symptoms F68.12
        with psychological symptoms F68.13
      psychological symptoms F68.11
        with physical symptoms F68.13
  factor, coagulation — *see* Defect, coagulation
  fatty acid
    metabolism E71.30
      specified NEC E71.39
    oxidation
      LCAD E71.310
      MCAD E71.311
      SCAD E71.312
      specified deficiency NEC E71.318
  feeding (infant or child) (*see also* Disorder, eating) R63.3-
  feigned (with obvious motivation) Z76.5
    without obvious motivation — *see* Disorder, factitious
  female
    hypoactive sexual desire F52.0
    orgasmic F52.31
    sexual arousal F52.22
  fibroblastic M72.9
    specified NEC M72.8
  fluency
    adult onset F98.5
    childhood onset F80.81
    following
      cerebral infarction I69.323
      cerebrovascular disease I69.923
        specified disease NEC I69.823
      intracerebral hemorrhage I69.123
      nontraumatic intracranial hemorrhage NEC I69.223
      subarachnoid hemorrhage I69.023
    in conditions classified elsewhere R47.82
  fluid balance E87.8
  follicular (skin) L73.9
    specified NEC L73.8
  fructose metabolism E74.10
    essential fructosuria E74.11
    fructokinase deficiency E74.11
    fructose-1, 6-diphosphatase deficiency E74.19
    hereditary fructose intolerance E74.12
    other specified E74.19
  functional polymorphonuclear neutrophils D71
  gallbladder, biliary tract and pancreas in diseases classified elsewhere K87
  gamma-glutamyl cycle E72.8
  gastric (functional) K31.9
    motility K30
    psychogenic F45.8
    secretion K30
  gastrointestinal (functional) NOS K92.9
    newborn P78.9
    psychogenic F45.8
  gender-identity or -role F64.9
    childhood F64.2
    effect on relationship F66
    of adolescence or adulthood (nontranssexual) F64.1
    specified NEC F64.8
    uncertainty F66
  genitourinary system
    female N94.9
    male N50.9
    psychogenic F45.8
  globe H44.9
    degenerated condition H44.50
      absolute glaucoma H44.51- ☑
      atrophy H44.52- ☑
      leucocoria H44.53- ☑
    degenerative H44.30

108
☑ Additional Character Required — Refer to the Tabular List for Character Selection
⬙ Subterms under main terms may continue to next column or page

Disorder — *continued*
  globe — *continued*
    degenerative — *continued*
      chalcosis H44.31- ☑
      myopia H44.2- ☑
      siderosis H44.32- ☑
      specified type NEC H44.39- ☑
    endophthalmitis — *see* Endophthalmitis
    foreign body, retained — *see* Foreign body, intraocular, old, retained
    hemophthalmos — *see* Hemophthalmos
    hypotony H44.40
      due to
        ocular fistula H44.42- ☑
        specified disorder NEC H44.43- ☑
      flat anterior chamber H44.41- ☑
      primary H44.44- ☑
    luxation — *see* Luxation, globe
    specified type NEC H44.89
  glomerular (in) N05.9
    amyloidosis E85.4 [N08]
    cryoglobulinemia D89.1 [N08]
    disseminated intravascular coagulation D65 [N08]
    Fabry's disease E75.21 [N08]
    familial lecithin cholesterol acyltransferase deficiency E78.6 [N08]
    Goodpasture's syndrome M31.0
    hemolytic-uremic syndrome D59.3
    Henoch (-Schönlein) purpura D69.0 [N08]
    malariae malaria B52.0
    microscopic polyangiitis M31.7 [N08]
    multiple myeloma C90.0- ☑ [N08]
    mumps B26.83
    schistosomiasis B65.9 [N08]
    sepsis NEC A41.- ☑ [N08]
      streptococcal A40.- ☑ [N08]
    sickle-cell disorders D57.- ☑ [N08]
    strongyloidiasis B78.9 [N08]
    subacute bacterial endocarditis I33.0 [N08]
    syphilis A52.75
    systemic lupus erythematosus M32.14
    thrombotic thrombocytopenic purpura M31.1 [N08]
    Waldenström macroglobulinemia C88.0 [N08]
    Wegener's granulomatosis M31.31
  gluconeogenesis E74.4
  glucosaminoglycan metabolism — *see* Disorder, metabolism, glucosaminoglycan
  glycine metabolism E72.50
    d-glycericacidemia E72.59
    hyperhydroxyprolinemia E72.59
    hyperoxaluria E72.53
    hyperprolinemia E72.59
    non-ketotic hyperglycinemia E72.51
    oxalosis E72.53
    oxaluria E72.53
    sarcosinemia E72.59
    trimethylaminuria E72.52
  glycoprotein metabolism E77.9
    specified NEC E77.8
  habit (and impulse) F63.9
    involving sexual behavior NEC F65.9
    specified NEC F63.89
  heart action I49.9
  hematological D75.9
    newborn (transient) P61.9
      specified NEC P61.8
  hematopoietic organs D75.9
  hemorrhagic NEC D69.9
    drug-induced D68.32
    due to
      extrinsic circulating anticoagulants D68.32
      increase in
        anti-IIa D68.32
        anti-Xa D68.32
      intrinsic
        circulating anticoagulants D68.318
        increase in
          anti-IXa D68.318
          anti-VIIIa D68.318
          anti-XIa D68.318
          antithrombin D68.318
    following childbirth O72.3
  hemostasis — *see* Defect, coagulation
  histidine metabolism E70.40
    histidinemia E70.41
    other specified E70.49

Disorder — *continued*
  hyperkinetic — *see* Disorder, attention-deficit hyperactivity
  hyperleucine-isoleucinemia E71.19
  hypervalinemia E71.19
  hypoactive sexual desire F52.0
  hypochondriacal F45.20
    body dysmorphic F45.22
    neurosis F45.21
    other specified F45.29
  identity
    dissociative F44.81
    of childhood F93.8
  immune mechanism (immunity) D89.9
    specified type NEC D89.89
  impaired renal tubular function N25.9
    specified NEC N25.89
  impulse (control) F63.9
  inflammatory
    pelvic, in diseases classified elsewhere — *see* category N74
    penis N48.29
      abscess N48.21
      cellulitis N48.22
  integument, newborn P83.9
    specified NEC P83.8
  intermittent explosive F63.81
  internal secretion pancreas — *see* Increased, secretion, pancreas, endocrine
  intestine, intestinal
    carbohydrate absorption NEC E74.39
      postoperative K91.2
    functional NEC K59.9
      postoperative K91.89
      psychogenic F45.8
    vascular K55.9
      chronic K55.1
      specified NEC K55.8
  intraoperative (intraprocedural) — *see* Complications, intraoperative
  involuntary emotional expression (IEED) F07.89
  iris H21.9
    adhesions — *see* Adhesions, iris
    atrophy — *see* Atrophy, iris
    chamber angle recession — *see* Recession, chamber angle
    cyst — *see* Cyst, iris
    degeneration — *see* Degeneration, iris
    in diseases classified elsewhere H22
    iridodialysis — *see* Iridodialysis
    iridoschisis — *see* Iridoschisis
    miotic pupillary cyst — *see* Cyst, pupillary
    pupillary
      abnormality — *see* Abnormality, pupillary
      membrane — *see* Membrane, pupillary
    specified type NEC H21.89
    vascular NEC H21.1X- ☑
  iron metabolism E83.10
    specified NEC E83.19
  isovaleric acidemia E71.110
  jaw, developmental M27.0
    temporomandibular — *see* Anomaly, dentofacial, temporomandibular joint
  joint M25.9
    derangement — *see* Derangement, joint
    effusion — *see* Effusion, joint
    fistula — *see* Fistula, joint
    hemarthrosis — *see* Hemarthrosis
    instability — *see* Instability, joint
    osteophyte — *see* Osteophyte
    pain — *see* Pain, joint
    psychogenic F45.8
    specified type NEC M25.80
      ankle M25.87- ☑
      elbow M25.82- ☑
      foot joint M25.87- ☑
      hand joint M25.84- ☑
      hip M25.85- ☑
      knee M25.86- ☑
      shoulder M25.81- ☑
      wrist M25.83- ☑
    stiffness — *see* Stiffness, joint
  ketone metabolism E71.32
  kidney N28.9
    functional (tubular) N25.9
    in
      schistosomiasis B65.9 [N29]

Disorder — *continued*
  kidney — *continued*
    tubular function N25.9
      specified NEC N25.89
  lacrimal system H04.9
    changes H04.69
    fistula — *see* Fistula, lacrimal
    gland H04.19
      atrophy — *see* Atrophy, lacrimal gland
      cyst — *see* Cyst, lacrimal, gland
      dacryops — *see* Dacryops
      dislocation — *see* Dislocation, lacrimal gland
      dry eye syndrome — *see* Syndrome, dry eye
      infection — *see* Dacryoadenitis
    granuloma — *see* Granuloma, lacrimal
    inflammation — *see* Inflammation, lacrimal
    obstruction — *see* Obstruction, lacrimal
    specified NEC H04.89
  lactation NEC O92.79
  language (developmental) F80.9
    expressive F80.1
    mixed receptive and expressive F80.2
    receptive F80.2
  late luteal phase dysphoric N94.89
  learning (specific) F81.9
    acalculia R48.8
    alexia R48.0
    mathematics F81.2
    reading F81.0
    specified NEC F81.89
    spelling F81.81
    written expression F81.81
  lens H27.9
    aphakia — *see* Aphakia
    cataract — *see* Cataract
    dislocation — *see* Dislocation, lens
    specified type NEC H27.8
  ligament M24.20
    ankle M24.27- ☑
    attachment, spine — *see* Enthesopathy, spinal
    elbow M24.22- ☑
    foot joint M24.27- ☑
    hand joint M24.24- ☑
    hip M24.25- ☑
    knee — *see* Derangement, knee, specified NEC
    shoulder M24.21- ☑
    vertebra M24.28
    wrist M24.23- ☑
  ligamentous attachments (*see also* Enthesopathy)
    spine — *see* Enthesopathy, spinal
  lipid
    metabolism, congenital E78.9
    storage E75.6
      specified NEC E75.5
  lipoprotein
    deficiency (familial) E78.6
    metabolism E78.9
      specified NEC E78.89
  liver K76.9
    malarial B54 [K77]
  low back (*see also* Dorsopathy, specified NEC)
  lumbosacral
    plexus G54.1
    root (nerve) NEC G54.4
  lung, interstitial, drug-induced J70.4
    acute J70.2
    chronic J70.3
  lymphoproliferative, post-transplant (PTLD) D47.Z1 (*following* D47.4)
  lysine and hydroxylysine metabolism E72.3
  male
    erectile (organic) (*see also* Dysfunction, sexual, male, erectile) N52.9
      nonorganic F52.21
    hypoactive sexual desire F52.0
    orgasmic F52.32
  manic F30.9
    organic F06.33
  mastoid (*see also* Disorder, ear, middle)
    postprocedural — *see* Complications, ear, procedure
  meniscus — *see* Derangement, knee, meniscus
  menopausal N95.9
    specified NEC N95.8
  menstrual N92.6
    psychogenic F45.8
    specified NEC N92.5
  mental (or behavioral) (nonpsychotic) F99

Disorder — *continued*
  mental — *continued*
    due to (secondary to)
      amphetamine
        due to drug abuse — *see* Abuse, drug, stimulant
        due to drug dependence — *see* Dependence, drug, stimulant
      brain disease, damage and dysfunction F09
      caffeine use
        due to drug abuse — *see* Abuse, drug, stimulant
        due to drug dependence — *see* Dependence, drug, stimulant
      cannabis use
        due to drug abuse — *see* Abuse, drug, cannabis
        due to drug dependence — *see* Dependence, drug, cannabis
      general medical condition F09
      sedative or hypnotic use
        due to drug abuse — *see* Abuse, drug, sedative
        due to drug dependence — *see* Dependence, drug, sedative
      tobacco (nicotine) use — *see* Dependence, drug, nicotine
    following organic brain damage F07.9
      frontal lobe syndrome F07.0
      personality change F07.0
      postconcussional syndrome F07.81
      specified NEC F07.89
    infancy, childhood or adolescence F98.9
    neurotic — *see* Neurosis
    organic or symptomatic F09
    presenile, psychotic F03 ☑
    problem NEC
    psychoneurotic — *see* Neurosis
    psychotic — *see* Psychosis
    puerperal F53
    senile, psychotic NEC F03 ☑
  metabolic, amino acid, transitory, newborn P74.8
  metabolism NOS E88.9
    amino-acid E72.9
      aromatic E70.9
        albinism — *see* Albinism
        histidine E70.40
          histidinemia E70.41
          other specified E70.49
        hyperphenylalaninemia E70.1
          classical phenylketonuria E70.0
        other specified E70.8
        tryptophan E70.5
        tyrosine E70.20
          hypertyrosinemia E70.21
          other specified E70.29
      branched chain E71.2
        3-methylglutaconic aciduria E71.111
        hyperleucine-isoleucinemia E71.19
        hypervalinemia E71.19
        isovaleric acidemia E71.110
        maple syrup urine disease E71.0
        methylmalonic acidemia E71.120
        organic aciduria NEC E71.118
        other specified E71.19
        proprionate NEC E71.128
        proprionic acidemia E71.121
      glycine E72.50
        d-glycericacidemia E72.59
        hyperhydroxyprolinemia E72.59
        hyperoxaluria E72.53
        hyperprolinemia E72.59
        non-ketotic hyperglycinemia E72.51
        other specified E72.59
        sarcosinemia E72.59
        trimethylaminuria E72.52
      hydroxylysine E72.3
      lysine E72.3
      ornithine E72.4
      other specified E72.8
        beta-amino acid E72.8
        gamma-glutamyl cycle E72.8
      straight-chain E72.8
      sulfur-bearing E72.10
        homocystinuria E72.11
        methylenetetrahydrofolate reductase deficiency E72.12
        other specified E72.19

Disorder — *continued*
  metabolism — *continued*
    bile acid and cholesterol metabolism E78.70
    bilirubin E80.7
      specified NEC E80.6
    calcium E83.50
      hypercalcemia E83.52
      hypocalcemia E83.51
      other specified E83.59
    carbohydrate E74.9
      specified NEC E74.8
    cholesterol and bile acid metabolism E78.70
    congenital E88.9
    copper E83.00
      specified type NEC E83.09
      Wilson's disease E83.01
    cystinuria E72.01
    fructose E74.10
    galactose E74.20
    glucosaminoglycan E76.9
      mucopolysaccharidosis — *see* Mucopolysaccharidosis
      specified NEC E76.8
    glutamine E72.8
    glycine E72.50
    glycogen storage (hepatorenal) E74.09
    glycoprotein E77.9
      specified NEC E77.8
    glycosaminoglycan E76.9
      specified NEC E76.8
    in labor and delivery O75.89
    iron E83.10
    isoleucine E71.19
    leucine E71.19
    lipoid E78.9
    lipoprotein E78.9
      specified NEC E78.89
    magnesium E83.40
      hypermagnesemia E83.41
      hypomagnesemia E83.42
      other specified E83.49
    mineral E83.9
      specified NEC E83.89
    mitochondrial E88.40
      MELAS syndrome E88.41
      MERRF syndrome (myoclonic epilepsy associated with ragged-red fibers) E88.42
      other specified E88.49
    ornithine E72.4
    phosphatases E83.30
    phosphorus E83.30
      acid phosphatase deficiency E83.39
      hypophosphatasia E83.39
      hypophosphatemia E83.39
        familial E83.31
      other specified E83.39
      pseudovitamin D deficiency E83.32
    plasma protein NEC E88.09
    porphyrin — *see* Porphyria
    postprocedural E89.89
      specified NEC E89.89
    purine E79.9
      specified NEC E79.8
    pyrimidine E79.9
      specified NEC E79.8
    pyruvate E74.4
    serine E72.8
    sodium E87.8
    specified NEC E88.89
    threonine E72.8
    valine E71.19
    zinc E83.2
  methylmalonic acidemia E71.120
  micturition NEC R39.19
    feeling of incomplete emptying R39.14
    hesitancy R39.11
    poor stream R39.12
    psychogenic F45.8
    split stream R39.13
    straining R39.16
    urgency R39.15
  mitochondrial metabolism E88.40
  mitral (valve) — *see* Endocarditis, mitral
  mixed
    anxiety and depressive F41.8
    of scholastic skills (developmental) F81.89
    receptive expressive language F80.2
  mood F39

Disorder — *continued*
  mood — *continued*
    bipolar — *see* Disorder, bipolar
    depressive — *see* Disorder, depressive
    due to (secondary to)
      alcohol F10.94
      amphetamine F15.94
        in
          abuse F15.14
          dependence F15.24
      anxiolytic F13.94
        in
          abuse F13.14
          dependence F13.24
      cocaine F14.94
        in
          abuse F14.14
          dependence F14.24
      general medical condition F06.30
      hallucinogen F16.94
        in
          abuse F16.14
          dependence F16.24
      hypnotic F13.94
        in
          abuse F13.14
          dependence F13.24
      inhalant F18.94
        in
          abuse F18.14
          dependence F18.24
      opioid F11.94
        in
          abuse F11.14
          dependence F11.24
      phencyclidine (PCP) F16.94
        in
          abuse F16.14
          dependence F16.24
      physiological condition F06.30
        with
          depressive features F06.31
          major depressive-like episode F06.32
          manic features F06.33
          mixed features F06.34
      psychoactive substance NEC F19.94
        in
          abuse F19.14
          dependence F19.24
      sedative F13.94
        in
          abuse F13.14
          dependence F13.24
      volatile solvents F18.94
        in
          abuse F18.14
          dependence F18.24
    manic episode F30.9
      with psychotic symptoms F30.2
      without psychotic symptoms F30.10
        mild F30.11
        moderate F30.12
        severe F30.13
      in remission (full) F30.4
        partial F30.3
      specified type NEC F30.8
    organic F06.30
      right hemisphere F07.89
    persistent F34.9
      cyclothymia F34.0
      dysthymia F34.1
      specified type NEC F34.8
    recurrent F39
    right hemisphere organic F07.89
  movement G25.9
    drug-induced G25.70
      akathisia G25.71
      specified NEC G25.79
    hysterical F44.4
    in diseases classified elsewhere — *see* category G26
    periodic limb G47.61
      sleep related G47.61
    sleep related NEC G47.69
    specified NEC G25.89
    stereotyped F98.4
    treatment-induced G25.9
  multiple personality F44.81

☑ Additional Character Required — Refer to the Tabular List for Character Selection   ▽ Subterms under main terms may continue to next column or page

Disorder — *continued*

muscle M62.9
  attachment, spine — *see* Enthesopathy, spinal
  in trichinellosis — *see* Trichinellosis, with muscle disorder
  psychogenic F45.8
  specified type NEC M62.89
  tone, newborn P94.9
    specified NEC P94.8
muscular
  attachments (*see also* Enthesopathy)
    spine — *see* Enthesopathy, spinal
  urethra N36.44
musculoskeletal system, soft tissue — *see* Disorder, soft tissue
  postprocedural M96.89
  psychogenic F45.8
myoneural G70.9
  due to lead G70.1
  specified NEC G70.89
  toxic G70.1
myotonic NEC G71.19
nail, in diseases classified elsewhere L62
neck region NEC — *see* Dorsopathy, specified NEC
nerve G58.9
  abducent NEC — *see* Strabismus, paralytic, sixth nerve
  accessory G52.8
  acoustic — *see* subcategory H93.3 ☑
  auditory — *see* subcategory H93.3 ☑
  auriculotemporal G50.8
  axillary G54.0
  cerebral — *see* Disorder, nerve, cranial
  cranial G52.9
    eighth — *see* subcategory H93.3 ☑
    eleventh G52.8
    fifth G50.9
    first G52.0
    fourth NEC — *see* Strabismus, paralytic, fourth nerve
    multiple G52.7
    ninth G52.1
    second NEC — *see* Disorder, nerve, optic
    seventh NEC G51.8
    sixth NEC — *see* Strabismus, paralytic, sixth nerve
    specified NEC G52.8
    tenth G52.2
    third NEC — *see* Strabismus, paralytic, third nerve
    twelfth G52.3
  entrapment — *see* Neuropathy, entrapment
  facial G51.9
    specified NEC G51.8
  femoral — *see* Lesion, nerve, femoral
  glossopharyngeal NEC G52.1
  hypoglossal G52.3
  intercostal G58.0
  lateral
    cutaneous of thigh — *see* Mononeuropathy, lower limb, meralgia paresthetica
    popliteal — *see* Lesion, nerve, popliteal
  lower limb — *see* Mononeuropathy, lower limb
  medial popliteal — *see* Lesion, nerve, popliteal, medial
  median NEC — *see* Lesion, nerve, median
  multiple G58.7
  oculomotor NEC — *see* Strabismus, paralytic, third nerve
  olfactory G52.0
  optic NEC H47.09- ☑
    hemorrhage into sheath — *see* Hemorrhage, optic nerve
    ischemic H47.01- ☑
  peroneal — *see* Lesion, nerve, popliteal
  phrenic G58.8
  plantar — *see* Lesion, nerve, plantar
  pneumogastric G52.2
  posterior tibial — *see* Syndrome, tarsal tunnel
  radial — *see* Lesion, nerve, radial
  recurrent laryngeal G52.2
  root G54.9
    cervical G54.2
    lumbosacral G54.1
    specified NEC G54.8
    thoracic G54.3
  sciatic NEC — *see* Lesion, nerve, sciatic

Disorder — *continued*

nerve — *continued*
  specified NEC G58.8
    lower limb — *see* Mononeuropathy, lower limb, specified NEC
    upper limb — *see* Mononeuropathy, upper limb, specified NEC
  sympathetic G90.9
  tibial — *see* Lesion, nerve, popliteal, medial
  trigeminal G50.9
    specified NEC G50.8
  trochlear NEC — *see* Strabismus, paralytic, fourth nerve
  ulnar — *see* Lesion, nerve, ulnar
  upper limb — *see* Mononeuropathy, upper limb
  vagus G52.2
nervous system G98.8
  autonomic (peripheral) G90.9
    specified NEC G90.8
  central G96.9
    specified NEC G96.8
  parasympathetic G90.9
  specified NEC G98.8
  sympathetic G90.9
  vegetative G90.9
neurohypophysis NEC E23.3
neurological NEC R29.818
neuromuscular G70.9
  hereditary NEC G71.9
  specified NEC G70.89
  toxic G70.1
neurotic F48.9
  specified NEC F48.8
neutrophil, polymorphonuclear D71
nicotine use — *see* Dependence, drug, nicotine
nightmare F51.5
nose J34.9
  specified NEC J34.89
obsessive-compulsive F42
odontogenesis NOS K00.9
opioid use
  with
    opioid-induced psychotic disorder F11.959
      with
        delusions F11.950
        hallucinations F11.951
  due to drug abuse — *see* Abuse, drug, opioid
  due to drug dependence — *see* Dependence, drug, opioid
oppositional defiant F91.3
optic
  chiasm H47.49
    due to
      inflammatory disorder H47.41
      neoplasm H47.42
      vascular disorder H47.43
  disc H47.39- ☑
    coloboma — *see* Coloboma, optic disc
    drusen — *see* Drusen, optic disc
    pseudopapilledema — *see* Pseudopapilledema
  radiations — *see* Disorder, visual, pathway
  tracts — *see* Disorder, visual, pathway
orbit H05.9
  cyst — *see* Cyst, orbit
  deformity — *see* Deformity, orbit
  edema — *see* Edema, orbit
  enophthalmos — *see* Enophthalmos
  exophthalmos — *see* Exophthalmos
  hemorrhage — *see* Hemorrhage, orbit
  inflammation — *see* Inflammation, orbit
  myopathy — *see* Myopathy, extraocular muscles
  retained foreign body — *see* Foreign body, orbit, old
  specified type NEC H05.89
organic
  anxiety F06.4
  catatonic F06.1
  delusional F06.2
  dissociative F06.8
  emotionally labile (asthenic) F06.8
  mood (affective) F06.30
  schizophrenia-like F06.2
orgasmic (female) F52.31
  male F52.32
ornithine metabolism E72.4
overanxious F41.1
  of childhood F93.8

Disorder — *continued*

pain
  with related psychological factors F45.42
  exclusively related to psychological factors F45.41
pancreatic internal secretion E16.9
  specified NEC E16.8
panic F41.0
  with agoraphobia F40.01
papulosquamous L44.9
  in diseases classified elsewhere L45
  specified NEC L44.8
paranoid F22
  induced F24
  shared F24
parathyroid (gland) E21.5
  specified NEC E21.4
parietoalveolar NEC J84.09
paroxysmal, mixed R56.9
patella M22.9- ☑
  chondromalacia — *see* Chondromalacia, patella
  derangement NEC M22.3X- ☑
  recurrent
    dislocation — *see* Dislocation, patella, recurrent
    subluxation — *see* Dislocation, patella, recurrent, incomplete
  specified NEC M22.8X- ☑
patellofemoral M22.2X- ☑
pentose phosphate pathway with anemia D55.1
perception, due to hallucinogens F16.983
  in
    abuse F16.183
    dependence F16.283
peripheral nervous system NEC G64
peroxisomal E71.50
  biogenesis
    neonatal adrenoleukodystrophy E71.511
    specified disorder NEC E71.518
    Zellweger syndrome E71.510
  rhizomelic chondrodysplasia punctata E71.540
  specified form NEC E71.548
    group 1 E71.518
    group 2 E71.53
    group 3 E71.542
  X-linked adrenoleukodystrophy E71.529
    adolescent E71.521
    adrenomyeloneuropathy E71.522
    childhood E71.520
    specified form NEC E71.528
  Zellweger-like syndrome E71.541
persistent
  (somatoform) pain F45.41
  affective (mood) F34.9
personality (*see also* Personality) F60.9
  affective F34.0
  aggressive F60.3
  amoral F60.2
  anankastic F60.5
  antisocial F60.2
  anxious F60.6
  asocial F60.2
  asthenic F60.7
  avoidant F60.6
  borderline F60.3
  change (secondary) due to general medical condition F07.0
  compulsive F60.5
  cyclothymic F34.0
  dependent (passive) F60.7
  depressive F34.1
  dissocial F60.2
  emotional instability F60.3
  expansive paranoid F60.0
  explosive F60.3
  following organic brain damage F07.9
  histrionic F60.4
  hyperthymic F34.0
  hypothymic F34.1
  hysterical F60.4
  immature F60.89
  inadequate F60.7
  labile F60.3
  mixed (nonspecific) F60.89
  moral deficiency F60.2
  narcissistic F60.81
  negativistic F60.89
  obsessional F60.5
  obsessive (-compulsive) F60.5
  organic F07.9

Disorder — *continued*
  personality (*see also* Personality) — *continued*
    overconscientious F60.5
    paranoid F60.0
    passive (-dependent) F60.7
    passive-aggressive F60.89
    pathological NEC F60.9
    pseudosocial F60.2
    psychopathic F60.2
    schizoid F60.1
    schizotypal F21
    self-defeating F60.7
    specified NEC F60.89
    type A F60.5
    unstable (emotional) F60.3
  pervasive, developmental F84.9
  phobic anxiety, childhood F40.8
  phosphate-losing tubular N25.0
  pigmentation L81.9
    choroid, congenital Q14.3
    diminished melanin formation L81.6
    iron L81.8
    specified NEC L81.8
  pinna (noninfective) H61.10- ☑
    deformity, acquired H61.11- ☑
    hematoma H61.12- ☑
    perichondritis — *see* Perichondritis, ear
    specified type NEC H61.19- ☑
  pituitary gland E23.7
    iatrogenic (postprocedural) E89.3
    specified NEC E23.6
  platelets D69.1
  plexus G54.9
    specified NEC G54.8
  polymorphonuclear neutrophils D71
  porphyrin metabolism — *see* Porphyria
  post-transplant lymphoproliferative D47.Z1 (*following* D47.4)
  post-traumatic stress (PTSD) F43.10
    acute F43.11
    chronic F43.12
  postconcussional F07.81
  posthallucinogen perception F16.983
    in
      abuse F16.183
      dependence F16.283
  postmenopausal N95.9
    specified NEC N95.8
  postprocedural (postoperative) — *see* Complications, postprocedural
  premenstrual dysphoric (PMDD) N94.3
  prepuce N47.8
  propionic acidemia E71.121
  prostate N42.9
    specified NEC N42.89
  psychogenic NOS (*see also* condition) F45.9
    anxiety F41.8
    appetite F50.9
    asthenic F48.8
    cardiovascular (system) F45.8
    compulsive F42
    cutaneous F54
    depressive F32.9
    digestive (system) F45.8
    dysmenorrheic F45.8
    dyspneic F45.8
    endocrine (system) F54
    eye NEC F45.8
    feeding — *see* Disorder, eating
    functional NEC F45.8
    gastric F45.8
    gastrointestinal (system) F45.8
    genitourinary (system) F45.8
    heart (function) (rhythm) F45.8
    hyperventilatory F45.8
    hypochondriacal — *see* Disorder, hypochondriacal
    intestinal F45.8
    joint F45.8
    learning F81.9
    limb F45.8
    lymphatic (system) F45.8
    menstrual F45.8
    micturition F45.8
    monoplegic NEC F44.4
    motor F44.4
    muscle F45.8
    musculoskeletal F45.8
    neurocirculatory F45.8

Disorder — *continued*
  psychogenic (*see also* condition) — *continued*
    obsessive F42
    occupational F48.8
    organ or part of body NEC F45.8
    paralytic NEC F44.4
    phobic F40.9
    physical NEC F45.8
    rectal F45.8
    respiratory (system) F45.8
    rheumatic F45.8
    sexual (function) F52.9
    skin (allergic) (eczematous) F54
    sleep F51.9
    specified part of body NEC F45.8
    stomach F45.8
  psychological F99
    associated with
      disease classified elsewhere F54
      sexual
        development F66
        relationship F66
        uncertainty about gender identity F66
  psychomotor NEC F44.4
    hysterical F44.4
  psychoneurotic (*see also* Neurosis)
    mixed NEC F48.8
  psychophysiologic — *see* Disorder, somatoform
  psychosexual F65.9
    development F66
    identity of childhood F64.2
  psychosomatic NOS — *see* Disorder, somatoform
    multiple F45.0
    undifferentiated F45.1
  psychotic — *see* Psychosis
    transient (acute) F23
  puberty E30.9
    specified NEC E30.8
  pulmonary (valve) — *see* Endocarditis, pulmonary
  purine metabolism E79.9
  pyrimidine metabolism E79.9
  pyruvate metabolism E74.4
  reactive attachment (childhood) F94.1
  reading R48.0
    developmental (specific) F81.0
  receptive language F80.2
  receptor, hormonal, peripheral (*see also* Syndrome, androgen insensitivity) E34.50
  recurrent brief depressive F33.8
  reflex R29.2
  refraction H52.7
    aniseikonia H52.32
    anisometropia H52.31
    astigmatism — *see* Astigmatism
    hypermetropia — *see* Hypermetropia
    myopia — *see* Myopia
    presbyopia H52.4
    specified NEC H52.6
  relationship F68.8
    due to sexual orientation F66
  REM sleep behavior G47.52
  renal function, impaired (tubular) N25.9
  resonance R49.9
    specified NEC R49.8
  respiratory function, impaired (*see also* Failure, respiration)
    postprocedural — *see* Complication, postoperative, respiratory system
    psychogenic F45.8
  retina H35.9
    angioid streaks H35.33
    changes in vascular appearance H35.01- ☑
    degeneration — *see* Degeneration, retina
    dystrophy (hereditary) — *see* Dystrophy, retina
    edema H35.81
    hemorrhage — *see* Hemorrhage, retina
    ischemia H35.82
    macular degeneration — *see* Degeneration, macula
    microaneurysms H35.04- ☑
    microvascular abnormality NEC H35.09
    neovascularization — *see* Neovascularization, retina
    retinopathy — *see* Retinopathy
    separation of layers H35.70
      central serous chorioretinopathy H35.71- ☑
      pigment epithelium detachment (serous) H35.72- ☑
      hemorrhagic H35.73- ☑

Disorder — *continued*
  retina — *continued*
    specified type NEC H35.89
    telangiectasis — *see* Telangiectasis, retina
    vasculitis — *see* Vasculitis, retina
  retroperitoneal K68.9
  right hemisphere organic affective F07.89
  rumination (infant or child) F98.21
  sacrum, sacrococcygeal NEC M53.3
  schizoaffective F25.9
    bipolar type F25.0
    depressive type F25.1
    manic type F25.0
    mixed type F25.0
    specified NEC F25.8
  schizoid of childhood F84.5
  schizophreniform F20.81
    brief F23
  schizotypal (personality) F21
  secretion, thyrocalcitonin E07.0
  seizure (*see also* Epilepsy) G40.909
    intractable G40.919
      with status epilepticus G40.911
  semantic pragmatic F80.89
    with autism F84.0
  sense of smell R43.1
    psychogenic F45.8
  separation anxiety, of childhood F93.0
  sexual
    arousal, female F52.22
    aversion F52.1
    function, psychogenic F52.9
    maturation F66
    nonorganic F52.9
    preference (*see also* Deviation, sexual) F65.9
      fetishistic transvestism F65.1
    relationship F66
  shyness, of childhood and adolescence F40.10
  sibling rivalry F93.8
  sickle-cell (sickling) (homozygous) — *see* Disease, sickle-cell
    heterozygous D57.3
    specified type NEC D57.8- ☑
    trait D57.3
  sinus (nasal) J34.9
    specified NEC J34.89
  skin L98.9
    atrophic L90.9
      specified NEC L90.8
    granulomatous L92.9
      specified NEC L92.8
    hypertrophic L91.9
      specified NEC L91.8
    infiltrative NEC L98.6
    newborn P83.9
      specified NEC P83.8
    psychogenic (allergic) (eczematous) F54
  sleep G47.9
    breathing-related — *see* Apnea, sleep
    circadian rhythm G47.20
      advance sleep phase type G47.22
      delayed sleep phase type G47.21
      due to
        alcohol
          abuse F10.182
          dependence F10.282
          use F10.982
        amphetamines
          abuse F15.182
          dependence F15.282
          use F15.982
        caffeine
          abuse F15.182
          dependence F15.282
          use F15.982
        cocaine
          abuse F14.182
          dependence F14.282
          use F14.982
        drug NEC
          abuse F19.182
          dependence F19.282
          use F19.982
        opioid
          abuse F11.182
          dependence F11.282
          use F11.982

☑ **Additional Character Required — Refer to the Tabular List for Character Selection** ▽ **Subterms under main terms may continue to next column or page**

Disorder — continued
  sleep — continued
    circadian rhythm — continued
      due to — continued
        psychoactive substance NEC
          abuse F19.182
          dependence F19.282
          use F19.982
        sedative, hypnotic, or anxiolytic
          abuse F13.182
          dependence F13.282
          use F13.982
        stimulant NEC
          abuse F15.182
          dependence F15.282
          use F15.982
      free running type G47.24
      in conditions classified elsewhere G47.27
      irregular sleep wake type G47.23
      jet lag type G47.25
      shift work type G47.26
      specified NEC G47.29
    due to
      alcohol
        abuse F10.182
        dependence F10.282
        use F10.982
      amphetamine
        abuse F15.182
        dependence F15.282
        use F15.982
      anxiolytic
        abuse F13.182
        dependence F13.282
        use F13.982
      caffeine
        abuse F15.182
        dependence F15.282
        use F15.982
      cocaine
        abuse F14.182
        dependence F14.282
        use F14.982
      drug NEC
        abuse F19.182
        dependence F19.282
        use F19.982
      hypnotic
        abuse F13.182
        dependence F13.282
        use F13.982
      opioid
        abuse F11.182
        dependence F11.282
        use F11.982
      psychoactive substance NEC
        abuse F19.182
        dependence F19.282
        use F19.982
      sedative
        abuse F13.182
        dependence F13.282
        use F13.982
      stimulant NEC
        abuse F15.182
        dependence F15.282
        use F15.982
    emotional F51.9
    excessive somnolence — see Hypersomnia
    hypersomnia type — see Hypersomnia
    initiating or maintaining — see Insomnia
    nightmares F51.5
    nonorganic F51.9
      specified NEC F51.8
    parasomnia type G47.50
    specified NEC G47.8
    terrors F51.4
    walking F51.3
  sleep-wake pattern or schedule — see Disorder, sleep, circadian rhythm
  social
    anxiety of childhood F40.10
    functioning in childhood F94.9
      specified NEC F94.8
  soft tissue M79.9
    ankle M79.9
    due to use, overuse and pressure M70.90
      ankle M70.97- ☑

Disorder — continued
  soft tissue — continued
    due to use, overuse and pressure — continued
      bursitis — see Bursitis
      foot M70.97- ☑
      forearm M70.93- ☑
      hand M70.94- ☑
      lower leg M70.96- ☑
      multiple sites M70.99
      pelvic region M70.95- ☑
      shoulder region M70.91- ☑
      specified site NEC M70.98
      specified type NEC M70.80
        ankle M70.87- ☑
        foot M70.87- ☑
        forearm M70.83- ☑
        hand M70.84- ☑
        lower leg M70.86- ☑
        multiple sites M70.89
        pelvic region M70.85- ☑
        shoulder region M70.81- ☑
        specified site NEC M70.88
        thigh M70.85- ☑
        upper arm M70.82- ☑
      thigh M70.95- ☑
      upper arm M70.92- ☑
    foot M79.9
    forearm M79.9
    hand M79.9
    lower leg M79.9
    multiple sites M79.9
    occupational — see Disorder, soft tissue, due to use, overuse and pressure
    pelvic region M79.9
    shoulder region M79.9
    specified type NEC M79.89
    thigh M79.9
    upper arm M79.9
  somatization F45.0
  somatoform F45.9
    pain (persistent) F45.41
    somatization (multiple) (long-lasting) F45.0
    specified NEC F45.8
    undifferentiated F45.1
  somnolence, excessive — see Hypersomnia
  specific
    arithmetical F81.2
    developmental, of motor F82
    reading F81.0
    speech and language F80.9
    spelling F81.81
    written expression F81.81
  speech R47.9
    articulation (functional) (specific) F80.0
    developmental F80.9
    specified NEC R47.89
  spelling (specific) F81.81
  spine (see also Dorsopathy)
    ligamentous or muscular attachments, peripheral — see Enthesopathy, spinal
    specified NEC — see Dorsopathy, specified NEC
  stereotyped, habit or movement F98.4
  stomach (functional) — see Disorder, gastric
  stress F43.9
    post-traumatic F43.10
      acute F43.11
      chronic F43.12
  sulfur-bearing amino-acid metabolism E72.10
  sweat gland (eccrine) L74.9
    apocrine L75.9
      specified NEC L75.8
    specified NEC L74.8
  synovium M67.90
    acromioclavicular M67.91- ☑
    ankle M67.97- ☑
    elbow M67.92- ☑
    foot M67.97- ☑
    forearm M67.93- ☑
    hand M67.94- ☑
    hip M67.95- ☑
    knee M67.96- ☑
    multiple sites M67.99
    rupture — see Rupture, synovium
    shoulder M67.91- ☑
    specified type NEC M67.80
      acromioclavicular M67.81- ☑
      ankle M67.87- ☑

Disorder — continued
  synovium — continued
    specified type — continued
      elbow M67.82- ☑
      foot M67.87- ☑
      hand M67.84- ☑
      hip M67.85- ☑
      knee M67.86- ☑
      multiple sites M67.89
      wrist M67.83- ☑
    synovitis — see Synovitis
    upper arm M67.92- ☑
    wrist M67.93- ☑
  temperature regulation, newborn P81.9
    specified NEC P81.8
  temporomandibular joint — see Anomaly, dentofacial, temporomandibular joint
  tendon M67.90
    acromioclavicular M67.91- ☑
    ankle M67.97- ☑
    contracture — see Contracture, tendon
    elbow M67.92- ☑
    foot M67.97- ☑
    forearm M67.93- ☑
    hand M67.94- ☑
    hip M67.95- ☑
    knee M67.96- ☑
    multiple sites M67.99
    rupture — see Rupture, tendon
    shoulder M67.91- ☑
    specified type NEC M67.80
      acromioclavicular M67.81- ☑
      ankle M67.87- ☑
      elbow M67.82- ☑
      foot M67.87- ☑
      hand M67.84- ☑
      hip M67.85- ☑
      knee M67.86- ☑
      multiple sites M67.89
      trunk M67.88
      wrist M67.83- ☑
    synovitis — see Synovitis
    tendinitis — see Tendinitis
    tenosynovitis — see Tenosynovitis
    trunk M67.98
    upper arm M67.92- ☑
    wrist M67.93- ☑
  thoracic root (nerve) NEC G54.3
  thyrocalcitonin hypersecretion E07.0
  thyroid (gland) E07.9
    function NEC, neonatal, transitory P72.2
    iodine-deficiency related E01.8
    specified NEC E07.89
  tic — see Tic
  tooth K08.9
    development K00.9
      specified NEC K00.8
    eruption K00.6
  Tourette's F95.2
  trance and possession F44.89
  tricuspid (valve) — see Endocarditis, tricuspid
  tryptophan metabolism E70.5
  tubular, phosphate-losing N25.0
  tubulo-interstitial (in)
    brucellosis A23.9 [N16]
    cystinosis E72.04
    diphtheria A36.84
    glycogen storage disease E74.00 [N16]
    leukemia NEC C95.9- ☑ [N16]
    lymphoma NEC C85.9- ☑ [N16]
    mixed cryoglobulinemia D89.1 [N16]
    multiple myeloma C90.0- ☑ [N16]
    Salmonella infection A02.25
    sarcoidosis D86.84
    sepsis A41.9 [N16]
      streptococcal A40.9 [N16]
    systemic lupus erythematosus M32.15
    toxoplasmosis B58.83
    transplant rejection T86.91 [N16]
    Wilson's disease E83.01 [N16]
  tubulo-renal function, impaired N25.9
    specified NEC N25.89
  tympanic membrane H73.9- ☑
    atrophy — see Atrophy, tympanic membrane
    infection — see Myringitis
    perforation — see Perforation, tympanum
    specified NEC H73.89- ☑

Disruption — continued
  ligament(s) (see also Sprain)
    knee
      current injury — see Dislocation, knee
      old (chronic) — see Derangement, knee, insta-
        bility
      spontaneous NEC — see Derangement, knee,
        disruption ligament
    ossicular chain — see Discontinuity, ossicles, ear
  pelvic ring (stable) S32.810 ☑
    unstable S32.811 ☑
  traumatic injury wound repair T81.33 ☑
  wound T81.30 ☑
    episiotomy O90.1
    operation T81.31 ☑
      cesarean O90.0
      external operation wound (superficial)
        T81.31 ☑
      internal operation wound (deep) T81.32 ☑
    perineal (obstetric) O90.1
    traumatic injury repair T81.33 ☑
Dissatisfaction with
  employment Z56.9
  school environment Z55.4
Dissecting — see condition
Dissection
  aorta I71.00
    abdominal I71.02
    thoracic I71.01
    thoracoabdominal I71.03
  artery
    carotid I77.71
    cerebral (nonruptured) I67.0
      ruptured — see Hemorrhage, intracranial,
        subarachnoid
    coronary I25.42
    iliac I77.72
    renal I77.73
    specified NEC I77.79
    vertebral I77.74
  traumatic — see Wound, open, by site
  vascular I99.8
  wound — see Wound, open
Disseminated — see condition
Dissociation
  auriculoventricular or atrioventricular (AV) (any de-
    gree) (isorhythmic) I45.89
    with heart block I44.2
  interference I45.89
Dissociative reaction, state F44.9
Dissolution, vertebra — see Osteoporosis
Distension, distention
  abdomen R14.0
  bladder N32.89
  cecum K63.89
  colon K63.89
  gallbladder K82.8
  intestine K63.89
  kidney N28.89
  liver K76.89
  seminal vesicle N50.8
  stomach K31.89
    acute K31.0
    psychogenic F45.8
  ureter — see Dilatation, ureter
  uterus N85.8
Disto-occlusion (Division I) (Division II) M26.212
Distoma hepaticum infestation B66.3
Distomiasis B66.9
  bile passages B66.3
  hemic B65.9
  hepatic B66.3
    due to Clonorchis sinensis B66.1
  intestinal B66.5
  liver B66.3
    due to Clonorchis sinensis B66.1
  lung B66.4
  pulmonary B66.4
Distomolar (fourth molar) K00.1
Distortion(s) (congenital)
  adrenal (gland) Q89.1
  arm NEC Q68.8
  bile duct or passage Q44.5
  bladder Q64.79
  brain Q04.9
  cervix (uteri) Q51.9
  chest (wall) Q67.8

Distortion(s) — continued
  chest — continued
    bones Q76.8
  clavicle Q74.0
  clitoris Q52.6
  coccyx Q76.49
  common duct Q44.5
  coronary Q24.5
  cystic duct Q44.5
  ear (auricle) (external) Q17.3
    inner Q16.5
    middle Q16.4
      ossicles Q16.3
  endocrine NEC Q89.2
  eustachian tube Q17.8
  eye (adnexa) Q15.8
  face bone(s) NEC Q75.8
  fallopian tube Q50.6
  femur NEC Q68.8
  fibula NEC Q68.8
  finger(s) Q68.1
  foot Q66.9
  genitalia, genital organ(s)
    female Q52.8
      external Q52.79
      internal NEC Q52.8
  gyri Q04.8
  hand bone(s) Q68.1
  heart (auricle) (ventricle) Q24.8
    valve (cusp) Q24.8
  hepatic duct Q44.5
  humerus NEC Q68.8
  hymen Q52.4
  intrafamilial communications Z63.8
  jaw NEC M26.89
  labium (majus) (minus) Q52.79
  leg NEC Q68.8
  lens Q12.8
  liver Q44.7
  lumbar spine Q76.49
    with disproportion O33.8
      causing obstructed labor O65.0
  lumbosacral (joint) (region) Q76.49
    kyphosis — see Kyphosis, congenital
    lordosis — see Lordosis, congenital
  nerve Q07.8
  nose Q30.8
  organ
    of Corti Q16.5
    or site not listed — see Anomaly, by site
  ossicles, ear Q16.3
  oviduct Q50.6
  pancreas Q45.3
  parathyroid (gland) Q89.2
  pituitary (gland) Q89.2
  radius NEC Q68.8
  sacroiliac joint Q74.2
  sacrum Q76.49
  scapula Q74.0
  shoulder girdle Q74.0
  skull bone(s) NEC Q75.8
    with
      anencephalus Q00.0
      encephalocele — see Encephalocele
      hydrocephalus Q03.9
        with spina bifida — see Spina bifida, with
          hydrocephalus
      microcephaly Q02
  spinal cord Q06.8
  spine Q76.49
    kyphosis — see Kyphosis, congenital
    lordosis — see Lordosis, congenital
  spleen Q89.09
  sternum NEC Q76.7
  thorax (wall) Q67.8
    bony Q76.8
  thymus (gland) Q89.2
  thyroid (gland) Q89.2
  tibia NEC Q68.8
  toe(s) Q66.9
  tongue Q38.3
  trachea (cartilage) Q32.1
  ulna NEC Q68.8
  ureter Q62.8
  urethra Q64.79
    causing obstruction Q64.39
  uterus Q51.9
  vagina Q52.4

Distortion(s) — continued
  vertebra Q76.49
    kyphosis — see Kyphosis, congenital
    lordosis — see Lordosis, congenital
  visual (see also Disturbance, vision)
    shape and size H53.15
  vulva Q52.79
  wrist (bones) (joint) Q68.8
Distress
  abdomen — see Pain, abdominal
  acute respiratory (adult) (child) J80
  epigastric R10.13
  fetal P84
    complicating pregnancy — see Stress, fetal
  gastrointestinal (functional) K30
    psychogenic F45.8
  intestinal (functional) NOS K59.9
    psychogenic F45.8
  maternal, during labor and delivery O75.0
  respiratory R06.00
    adult J80
    child J80
    newborn P22.9
      specified NEC P22.8
    orthopnea R06.01
    psychogenic F45.8
    shortness of breath R06.02
    specified type NEC R06.09
Distribution vessel, atypical Q27.9
  coronary artery Q24.5
  precerebral Q28.1
Districhiasis L68.8
Disturbance(s) (see also Disease)
  absorption K90.9
    calcium E58
    carbohydrate K90.4
    fat K90.4
      pancreatic K90.3
    protein K90.4
    starch K90.4
    vitamin — see Deficiency, vitamin
  acid-base equilibrium E87.8
    mixed E87.4
  activity and attention (with hyperkinesis) — see Disor-
    der, attention-deficit hyperactivity
  amino acid transport E72.00
  assimilation, food K90.9
  auditory nerve, except deafness — see subcategory
    H93.3 ☑
  behavior — see Disorder, conduct
  blood clotting (mechanism) (see also Defect, coagula-
    tion) D68.9
  cerebral
    nerve — see Disorder, nerve, cranial
    status, newborn P91.9
      specified NEC P91.8
  circulatory I99.9
  conduct (see also Disorder, conduct) F91.9
    adjustment reaction — see Disorder, adjustment
    compulsive F63.9
    disruptive F91.9
    hyperkinetic — see Disorder, attention-deficit hy-
      peractivity
    socialized F91.2
    specified NEC F91.8
    unsocialized F91.1
  coordination R27.8
  cranial nerve — see Disorder, nerve, cranial
  deep sensibility — see Disturbance, sensation
  digestive K30
    psychogenic F45.8
  electrolyte (see also Imbalance, electrolyte)
    newborn, transitory P74.4
      hyperammonemia P74.6
      potassium balance P74.3
      sodium balance P74.2
      specified type NEC P74.4
  emotions specific to childhood and adolescence F93.9
    with
      anxiety and fearfulness NEC F93.8
      elective mutism F94.0
      oppositional disorder F91.3
      sensitivity (withdrawal) F40.10
      shyness F40.10
      social withdrawal F40.10
    involving relationship problems F93.8
    mixed F93.8
    specified NEC F93.8

Disturbance(s) — continued
  endocrine (gland) E34.9
    neonatal, transitory P72.9
      specified NEC P72.8
  equilibrium R42
  fructose metabolism E74.10
  gait — see Gait
    hysterical F44.4
    psychogenic F44.4
  gastrointestinal (functional) K30
    psychogenic F45.8
  habit, child F98.9
  hearing, except deafness and tinnitus — see Abnormal,
      auditory perception
  heart, functional (conditions in I44-I50)
    due to presence of (cardiac) prosthesis I97.19- ☑
    postoperative I97.89
      cardiac surgery I97.19- ☑
  hormones E34.9
  innervation uterus (parasympathetic) (sympathetic)
      N85.8
  keratinization NEC
    gingiva K05.10
      nonplaque induced K05.11
      plaque induced K05.10
    lip K13.0
    oral (mucosa) (soft tissue) K13.29
    tongue K13.29
  learning (specific) — see Disorder, learning
  memory — see Amnesia
    mild, following organic brain damage F06.8
  mental F99
    associated with diseases classified elsewhere F54
  metabolism E88.9
    with
      abortion — see Abortion, by type with other
          specified complication
      ectopic pregnancy O08.5
      molar pregnancy O08.5
    amino-acid E72.9
      aromatic E70.9
      branched-chain E71.2
      straight-chain E72.8
      sulfur-bearing E72.10
    ammonia E72.20
    arginine E72.21
    arginosuccinic acid E72.22
    carbohydrate E74.9
    cholesterol E78.9
    citrulline E72.23
    cystathionine E72.19
    general E88.9
    glutamine E72.8
    histidine E70.40
    homocystine E72.19
    hydroxylysine E72.3
    in labor or delivery O75.89
    iron E83.10
    lipoid E78.9
    lysine E72.3
    methionine E72.19
    neonatal, transitory P74.9
      calcium and magnesium P71.9
        specified type NEC P71.8
      carbohydrate metabolism P70.9
        specified type NEC P70.8
      specified NEC P74.8
    ornithine E72.4
    phosphate E83.39
    sodium NEC E87.8
    threonine E72.8
    tryptophan E70.5
    tyrosine E70.20
    urea cycle E72.20
  motor R29.2
  nervous, functional R45.0
  neuromuscular mechanism (eye), due to syphilis
      A52.15
  nutritional E63.9
    nail L60.3
  ocular motion H51.9
    psychogenic F45.8
  oculogyric H51.8
    psychogenic F45.8
  oculomotor H51.9
    psychogenic F45.8
  olfactory nerve R43.1
  optic nerve NEC — see Disorder, nerve, optic

Disturbance(s) — continued
  oral epithelium, including tongue NEC K13.29
  perceptual due to
    alcohol withdrawal F10.232
    amphetamine intoxication F15.922
      in
        abuse F15.122
        dependence F15.222
    anxiolytic withdrawal F13.232
    cannabis intoxication (acute) F12.922
      in
        abuse F12.122
        dependence F12.222
    cocaine intoxication (acute) F14.922
      in
        abuse F14.122
        dependence F14.222
    hypnotic withdrawal F13.232
    opioid intoxication (acute) F11.922
      in
        abuse F11.122
        dependence F11.222
    phencyclidine intoxication (acute) F19.922
      in
        abuse F19.122
        dependence F19.222
    sedative withdrawal F13.232
  personality (pattern) (trait) (see also Disorder, person-
      ality) F60.9
    following organic brain damage F07.9
  polyglandular E31.9
    specified NEC E31.8
  potassium balance, newborn P74.3
  psychogenic F45.9
  psychomotor F44.4
  psychophysical visual H53.16
  pupillary — see Anomaly, pupil, function
  reflex R29.2
  rhythm, heart I49.9
  salivary secretion K11.7
  sensation (cold) (heat) (localization) (tactile discrimi-
      nation) (texture) (vibratory) NEC R20.9
    hysterical F44.6
    skin R20.9
      anesthesia R20.0
      hyperesthesia R20.3
      hypoesthesia R20.1
      paresthesia R20.2
      specified type NEC R20.8
    smell R43.9
      and taste (mixed) R43.8
      anosmia R43.0
      parosmia R43.1
      specified NEC R43.8
    taste R43.9
      and smell (mixed) R43.8
      parageusia R43.2
      specified NEC R43.8
  sensory — see Disturbance, sensation
  situational (transient) (see also Disorder, adjustment)
    acute F43.0
  sleep G47.9
    nonorganic origin F51.9
  smell — see Disturbance, sensation, smell
  sociopathic F60.2
  sodium balance, newborn P74.2
  speech R47.9
    developmental F80.9
    specified NEC R47.89
  stomach (functional) K31.9
  sympathetic (nerve) G90.9
  taste — see Disturbance, sensation, taste
  temperature
    regulation, newborn P81.9
      specified NEC P81.8
    sense R20.8
      hysterical F44.6
  tooth
    eruption K00.6
    formation K00.4
    structure, hereditary NEC K00.5
  touch — see Disturbance, sensation
  vascular I99.9
    arteriosclerotic — see Arteriosclerosis
  vasomotor I73.9
  vasospastic I73.9
  vision, visual H53.9

Disturbance(s) — continued
  vision, visual — continued
    following
      cerebral infarction I69.398
      cerebrovascular disease I69.998
        specified NEC I69.898
      intracerebral hemorrhage I69.198
      nontraumatic intracranial hemorrhage NEC
          I69.298
      specified disease NEC I69.898
      subarachnoid hemorrhage I69.098
    psychophysical H53.16
    specified NEC H53.8
    subjective H53.10
      day blindness H53.11
      discomfort H53.14- ☑
      distortions of shape and size H53.15
      loss
        sudden H53.13- ☑
        transient H53.12- ☑
      specified type NEC H53.19
  voice R49.9
    psychogenic F44.4
    specified NEC R49.8
Diuresis R35.8
Diver's palsy, paralysis or squeeze T70.3 ☑
Diverticulitis (acute) K57.92
  bladder — see Cystitis
  ileum — see Diverticulitis, intestine, small
  intestine K57.92
    with
      abscess, perforation or peritonitis K57.80
        with bleeding K57.81
      bleeding K57.93
    congenital Q43.8
    large K57.32
      with
        abscess, perforation or peritonitis K57.20
          with bleeding K57.21
        bleeding K57.33
        small intestine K57.52
          with
            with bleeding K57.41
            abscess, perforation or peritonitis
                K57.40
            bleeding K57.53
    small K57.12
      with
        abscess, perforation or peritonitis K57.00
          with bleeding K57.01
        bleeding K57.13
        large intestine K57.52
          with
            with bleeding K57.41
            abscess, perforation or peritonitis
                K57.40
            bleeding K57.53
Diverticulosis K57.90
  with bleeding K57.91
  large intestine K57.30
    with
      bleeding K57.31
      small intestine K57.50
        with bleeding K57.51
  small intestine K57.10
    with
      bleeding K57.11
      large intestine K57.50
        with bleeding K57.51
Diverticulum, diverticula (multiple) K57.90
  appendix (noninflammatory) K38.2
  bladder (sphincter) N32.3
    congenital Q64.6
  bronchus (congenital) Q32.4
    acquired J98.09
  calyx, calyceal (kidney) N28.89
  cardia (stomach) K31.4
  cecum — see Diverticulosis, intestine, large
    congenital Q43.8
  colon — see Diverticulosis, intestine, large
    congenital Q43.8
  duodenum — see Diverticulosis, intestine, small
    congenital Q43.8
  epiphrenic (esophagus) K22.5
  esophagus (congenital) Q39.6
    acquired (epiphrenic) (pulsion) (traction) K22.5
  eustachian tube — see Disorder, eustachian tube,
      specified NEC

Index

Duchenne's — Dysfunction

Duchenne's
  disease or syndrome
    motor neuron disease G12.22
    muscular dystrophy G71.0
  locomotor ataxia (syphilitic) A52.11
  paralysis
    birth injury P14.0
    due to or associated with
      motor neuron disease G12.22
      muscular dystrophy G71.0
Ducrey's chancre A57
Duct, ductus — see condition
Duhring's disease (dermatitis herpetiformis) L13.0
Dullness, cardiac (decreased) (increased) R01.2
Dumb ague — see Malaria
Dumbness — see Aphasia
Dumdum fever B55.0
Dumping syndrome (postgastrectomy) K91.1
Duodenitis (nonspecific) (peptic) K29.80
  with bleeding K29.81
Duodenocholangitis — see Cholangitis
Duodenum, duodenal — see condition
Duplay's bursitis or periarthritis — see Tendinitis,
    calcific, shoulder
Duplication, duplex (see also Accessory)
  alimentary tract Q45.8
  anus Q43.4
  appendix (and cecum) Q43.4
  biliary duct (any) Q44.5
  bladder Q64.79
  cecum (and appendix) Q43.4
  cervix Q51.820 ✓
  chromosome NEC
    with complex rearrangements NEC Q92.5
    seen only at prometaphase Q92.8
  cystic duct Q44.5
  digestive organs Q45.8
  esophagus Q39.8
  frontonasal process Q75.8
  intestine (large) (small) Q43.4
  kidney Q63.0
  liver Q44.7
  pancreas Q45.3
  penis Q55.69
  respiratory organs NEC Q34.8
  salivary duct Q38.4
  spinal cord (incomplete) Q06.2
  stomach Q40.2
Dupré's disease (meningism) R29.1
Dupuytren's contraction or disease M72.0
Durand-Nicolas-Favre disease A55
Durotomy (inadvertent) (incidental) G97.41
Duroziez's disease (congenital mitral stenosis) Q23.2
Dutton's relapsing fever (West African) A68.1
Dwarfism E34.3
  achondroplastic Q77.4
  congenital E34.3
  constitutional E34.3
  hypochondroplastic Q77.4
  hypophyseal E23.0
  infantile E34.3
  Laron-type E34.3
  Lorain (-Levi) type E23.0
  metatropic Q77.8
  nephrotic-glycosuric (with hypophosphatemic rickets)
      E72.09
  nutritional E45
  pancreatic K86.8
  pituitary E23.0
  renal N25.0
  thanatophoric Q77.1
Dyke-Young anemia (secondary) (symptomatic) D59.1
Dysacusis — see Abnormal, auditory perception
Dysadrenocortism E27.9
  hyperfunction E27.0
Dysarthria R47.1
  following
    cerebral infarction I69.322
    cerebrovascular disease I69.922
      specified disease NEC I69.822
    intracerebral hemorrhage I69.122
    nontraumatic intracranial hemorrhage NEC I69.222
    subarachnoid hemorrhage I69.022
Dysautonomia (familial) G90.1
Dysbarism T70.3 ✓
Dysbasia R26.2
  angiosclerotica intermittens I73.9
  hysterical F44.4

Dysbasia — continued
  lordotica (progressiva) G24.1
  nonorganic origin F44.4
  psychogenic F44.4
Dysbetalipoproteinemia (familial) E78.2
Dyscalculia R48.8
  developmental F81.2
Dyschezia K59.00
Dyschondroplasia (with hemangiomata) Q78.4
Dyschromia (skin) L81.9
Dyscollagenosis M35.9
Dyscranio-pygo-phalangy Q87.0
Dyscrasia
  blood (with) D75.9
    antepartum hemorrhage — see Hemorrhage, an-
        tepartum, with coagulation defect
    intrapartum hemorrhage O67.0
    newborn P61.9
      specified type NEC P61.8
    puerperal, postpartum O72.3
    polyglandular, pluriglandular E31.9
Dysendocrinism E34.9
Dysentery, dysenteric (catarrhal) (diarrhea) (epidemic)
    (hemorrhagic) (infectious) (sporadic) (tropical) A09
  abscess, liver A06.4
  amebic (see also Amebiasis) A06.0
    with abscess — see Abscess, amebic
    acute A06.0
    chronic A06.1
  arthritis (see also category M01) A09
    bacillary (see also category M01) A03.9
  bacillary A03.9
    arthritis (see also category M01) A03.9
    Boyd A03.2
    Flexner A03.1
    Schmitz (-Stutzer) A03.0
    Shiga (-Kruse) A03.0
    Shigella A03.9
      boydii A03.2
      dysenteriae A03.0
      flexneri A03.1
      group A A03.0
      group B A03.1
      group C A03.2
      group D A03.3
      sonnei A03.3
      specified type NEC A03.8
    Sonne A03.3
    specified type NEC A03.8
  balantidial A07.0
  Balantidium coli A07.0
  Boyd's A03.2
  candidal B37.82
  Chilomastix A07.8
  Chinese A03.9
  coccidial A07.3
  Dientamoeba (fragilis) A07.8
  Embadomonas A07.8
  Entamoeba, entamebic — see Dysentery, amebic
  Flexner-Boyd A03.2
  Flexner's A03.1
  Giardia lamblia A07.1
  Hiss-Russell A03.1
  Lamblia A07.1
  leishmanial B55.0
  malarial — see Malaria
  metazoal B82.0
  monilial B37.82
  protozoal A07.9
  Salmonella A02.0
  schistosomal B65.1
  Schmitz (-Stutzer) A03.0
  Shiga (-Kruse) A03.0
  Shigella NOS — see Dysentery, bacillary
  Sonne A03.3
  strongyloidiasis B78.0
  trichomonal A07.8
  viral (see also Enteritis, viral) A08.4
Dysequilibrium R42
Dysesthesia R20.8
  hysterical F44.6
Dysfibrinogenemia (congenital) D68.2
Dysfunction
  adrenal E27.9
    hyperfunction E27.0
  autonomic
    due to alcohol G31.2
    somatoform F45.8

Dysfunction — continued
  bladder N31.9
    neurogenic NOS — see Dysfunction, bladder,
        neuromuscular
    neuromuscular NOS N31.9
      atonic (motor) (sensory) N31.2
      autonomous N31.2
      flaccid N31.2
      nonreflex N31.2
      reflex N31.1
      specified NEC N31.8
      uninhibited N31.0
  bleeding, uterus N93.8
  cerebral G93.89
  colon K59.9
    psychogenic F45.8
  colostomy K94.03
  cystic duct K82.8
  cystostomy (stoma) — see Complications, cystostomy
  ejaculatory N53.19
    anejaculatory orgasm N53.13
    painful N53.12
    premature F52.4
    retarded N53.11
  endocrine NOS E34.9
  endometrium N85.8
  enterostomy K94.13
  gallbladder K82.8
  gastrostomy (stoma) K94.23
  gland, glandular NOS E34.9
  heart I51.89
  hemoglobin D75.89
  hepatic K76.89
  hypophysis E23.7
  hypothalamic NEC E23.3
  ileostomy (stoma) K94.13
  jejunostomy (stoma) K94.13
  kidney — see Disease, renal
  labyrinthine — see subcategory H83.2 ✓
  left ventricular, following sudden emotional stress
      I51.81
  liver K76.89
  male — see Dysfunction, sexual, male
  orgasmic (female) F52.31
    male F52.32
  ovary E28.9
    specified NEC E28.8
  papillary muscle I51.89
  parathyroid E21.4
  physiological NEC R68.89
    psychogenic F59
  pineal gland E34.8
  pituitary (gland) E23.3
  platelets D69.1
  polyglandular E31.9
    specified NEC E31.8
  psychophysiologic F59
  psychosexual F52.9
    with
      dyspareunia F52.6
      premature ejaculation F52.4
      vaginismus F52.5
  pylorus K31.9
  rectum K59.9
    psychogenic F45.8
  reflex (sympathetic) — see Syndrome, pain, complex
      regional I
  segmental — see Dysfunction, somatic
  senile R54
  sexual (due to) R37
    alcohol F10.981
    amphetamine F15.981
      in
        abuse F15.181
        dependence F15.281
    anxiolytic F13.981
      in
        abuse F13.181
        dependence F13.281
    cocaine F14.981
      in
        abuse F14.181
        dependence F14.281
    excessive sexual drive F52.8
    failure of genital response (male) F52.21
      female F52.22
    female N94.9
      aversion F52.1

Dysfunction — continued
  sexual — continued
    female — continued
      dyspareunia N94.1
        psychogenic F52.6
      frigidity F52.22
      nymphomania F52.8
      orgasmic F52.31
      psychogenic F52.9
        aversion F52.1
        dyspareunia F52.6
        frigidity F52.22
        nymphomania F52.8
        orgasmic F52.31
        vaginismus F52.5
      vaginismus N94.2
        psychogenic F52.5
    hypnotic F13.981
      in
        abuse F13.181
        dependence F13.281
    inhibited orgasm (female) F52.31
      male F52.32
    lack
      of sexual enjoyment F52.1
      or loss of sexual desire F52.0
    male N53.9
      anejaculatory orgasm N53.13
      ejaculatory N53.19
        painful N53.12
        premature F52.4
        retarded N53.11
      erectile N52.9
        drug induced N52.2
        due to
          disease classified elsewhere N52.1
          drug N52.2
        postoperative (postprocedural) N52.39
          following
            prostatectomy N52.34
              radical N52.31
            radical cystectomy N52.32
            urethral surgery N52.33
        psychogenic F52.21
        specified cause NEC N52.8
        vasculogenic
          arterial insufficiency N52.01
            with corporo-venous occlusive N52.03
          corporo-venous occlusive N52.02
            with arterial insufficiency N52.03
      impotence — see Dysfunction, sexual, male, erectile
      psychogenic F52.9
        aversion F52.1
        erectile F52.21
        orgasmic F52.32
        premature ejaculation F52.4
        satyriasis F52.8
        specified type NEC F52.8
      specified type NEC N53.8
    nonorganic F52.9
      specified NEC F52.8
    opioid F11.981
      in
        abuse F11.181
        dependence F11.281
    orgasmic dysfunction (female) F52.31
      male F52.32
    premature ejaculation F52.4
    psychoactive substances NEC F19.981
      in
        abuse F19.181
        dependence F19.281
    psychogenic F52.9
    sedative F13.981
      in
        abuse F13.181
        dependence F13.281
    sexual aversion F52.1
    vaginismus (nonorganic) (psychogenic) F52.5
  sinoatrial node I49.5
  somatic M99.09
    abdomen M99.09
    acromioclavicular M99.07
    cervical region M99.01
    cervicothoracic M99.01
    costochondral M99.08

Dysfunction — continued
  somatic — continued
    costovertebral M99.08
    head region M99.00
    hip M99.05
    lower extremity M99.06
    lumbar region M99.03
    lumbosacral M99.03
    occipitocervical M99.00
    pelvic region M99.05
    pubic M99.05
    rib cage M99.08
    sacral region M99.04
    sacrococcygeal M99.04
    sacroiliac M99.04
    specified NEC M99.09
    sternochondral M99.08
    sternoclavicular M99.07
    thoracic region M99.02
    thoracolumbar M99.02
    upper extremity M99.07
  somatoform autonomic F45.8
  stomach K31.89
    psychogenic F45.8
  suprarenal E27.9
    hyperfunction E27.0
  symbolic R48.9
    specified type NEC R48.8
  temporomandibular (joint) M26.69
    joint-pain syndrome M26.62
  testicular (endocrine) E29.9
    specified NEC E29.8
  thymus E32.9
  thyroid E07.9
  ureterostomy (stoma) — see Complications, stoma, urinary tract
  urethrostomy (stoma) — see Complications, stoma, urinary tract
  uterus, complicating delivery O62.9
    hypertonic O62.4
    hypotonic O62.2
      primary O62.0
      secondary O62.1
  ventricular I51.9
    with congestive heart failure I50.9
    left, reversible, following sudden emotional stress I51.81

Dysgenesis
  gonadal (due to chromosomal anomaly) Q96.9
    pure Q99.1
  renal Q60.5
    bilateral Q60.4
    unilateral Q60.3
  reticular D72.0
  tidal platelet D69.3

Dysgerminoma
  specified site — see Neoplasm, malignant, by site
  unspecified site
    female C56.9
    male C62.90

Dysgeusia R43.2
Dysgraphia R27.8
Dyshidrosis, dysidrosis L30.1
Dyskaryotic cervical smear R87.619
Dyskeratosis L85.8
  cervix — see Dysplasia, cervix
  congenital Q82.8
  uterus NEC N85.8
Dyskinesia G24.9
  biliary (cystic duct or gallbladder) K82.8
  drug induced
    orofacial G24.01
  esophagus K22.4
  hysterical F44.4
  intestinal K59.8
  nonorganic origin F44.4
  orofacial (idiopathic) G24.4
    drug induced G24.01
  psychogenic F44.4
  subacute, drug induced G24.01
  tardive G24.01
    neuroleptic induced G24.01
  trachea J39.8
  tracheobronchial J98.09
Dyslalia (developmental) F80.0
Dyslexia R48.0
  developmental F81.0
Dyslipidemia E78.5

Dyslipidemia — continued
  depressed HDL cholesterol E78.6
  elevated fasting triglycerides E78.1
Dysmaturity (see also Light for dates)
  pulmonary (newborn) (Wilson-Mikity) P27.0
Dysmenorrhea (essential) (exfoliative) N94.6
  congestive (syndrome) N94.6
  primary N94.4
  psychogenic F45.8
  secondary N94.5
Dysmetabolic syndrome X E88.81
Dysmetria R27.8
Dysmorphism (due to)
  alcohol Q86.0
  exogenous cause NEC Q86.8
  hydantoin Q86.1
  warfarin Q86.2
Dysmorphophobia (nondelusional) F45.22
  delusional F22
Dysnomia R47.01
Dysorexia R63.0
  psychogenic F50.8
Dysostosis
  cleidocranial, cleidocranialis Q74.0
  craniofacial Q75.1
  Fairbank's (idiopathic familial generalized osteophytosis) Q78.9
  mandibulofacial (incomplete) Q75.4
  multiplex E76.01
  oculomandibular Q75.5
Dyspareunia (female) N94.1
  male N53.12
  nonorganic F52.6
  psychogenic F52.6
  secondary N94.1
Dyspepsia R10.13
  atonic K30
  functional (allergic) (congenital) (gastrointestinal) (occupational) (reflex) K30
  intestinal K59.8
  nervous F45.8
  neurotic F45.8
  psychogenic F45.8
Dysphagia R13.10
  cervical R13.19
  following
    cerebral infarction I69.391
    cerebrovascular disease I69.991
      specified NEC I69.891
    intracerebral hemorrhage I69.191
    nontraumatic intracranial hemorrhage NEC I69.291
    specified disease NEC I69.891
    subarachnoid hemorrhage I69.091
  functional (hysterical) F45.8
  hysterical F45.8
  nervous (hysterical) F45.8
  neurogenic R13.19
  oral phase R13.11
  oropharyngeal phase R13.12
  pharyneal phase R13.13
  pharyngoesophageal phase R13.14
  psychogenic F45.8
  sideropenic D50.1
  spastica K22.4
  specified NEC R13.19
Dysphagocytosis, congenital D71
Dysphasia R47.02
  developmental
    expressive type F80.1
    receptive type F80.2
  following
    cerebrovascular disease I69.921
      cerebral infarction I69.321
      intracerebral hemorrhage I69.121
      nontraumatic intracranial hemorrhage NEC I69.221
      specified disease NEC I69.821
      subarachnoid hemorrhage I69.021
Dysphonia R49.0
  functional F44.4
  hysterical F44.4
  psychogenic F44.4
  spastica J38.3
Dysphoria, postpartal O90.6
Dyspituitarism E23.3
Dysplasia (see also Anomaly)
  acetabular, congenital Q65.89
  alveolar capillary, with vein misalignment J84.843

Eaton-Lambert syndrome — see Syndrome, Lambert-Eaton
Eberth's disease (typhoid fever) A01.00
Ebola virus disease A98.4
Ebstein's anomaly or syndrome (heart) Q22.5
Eccentro-osteochondrodysplasia E76.29
Ecchondroma — see Neoplasm, bone, benign
Ecchondrosis D48.0
Ecchymosis R58
  conjunctiva — see Hemorrhage, conjunctiva
  eye (traumatic) — see Contusion, eyeball
  eyelid (traumatic) — see Contusion, eyelid
  newborn P54.5
  spontaneous R23.3
  traumatic — see Contusion
Echinococciasis — see Echinococcus
Echinococcosis — see Echinococcus
Echinococcus (infection) B67.90
  granulosus B67.4
    bone B67.2
    liver B67.0
    lung B67.1
    multiple sites B67.32
    specified site NEC B67.39
    thyroid B67.31 [E35]
  liver NOS B67.8
    granulosus B67.0
    multilocularis B67.5
  lung NEC B67.99
    granulosus B67.1
    multilocularis B67.69
  multilocularis B67.7
    liver B67.5
    multiple sites B67.61
    specified site NEC B67.69
  specified site NEC B67.99
    granulosus B67.39
    multilocularis B67.69
  thyroid NEC B67.99
    granulosus B67.31 [E35]
    multilocularis B67.69 [E35]
Echinorhynchiasis B83.8
Echinostomiasis B66.8
Echolalia R48.8
Echovirus, as cause of disease classified elsewhere B97.12
Eclampsia, eclamptic (coma) (convulsions) (delirium) (with hypertension) NEC O15.9
  during labor and delivery O15.1
  postpartum O15.2
  pregnancy O15.0- ☑
  puerperal O15.2
Economic circumstances affecting care Z59.9
Economo's disease A85.8
Ectasia, ectasis
  annuloaortic I35.8
  aorta I77.819
    with aneurysm — see Aneurysm, aorta
    abdominal I77.811
    thoracic I77.810
    thoracoabdominal I77.812
  breast — see Ectasia, mammary duct
  capillary I78.8
  cornea H18.71- ☑
  gastric antral vascular (GAVE) K31.819
    with hemorrhage K31.811
    without hemorrhage K31.819
  mammary duct N60.4- ☑
  salivary gland (duct) K11.8
  sclera — see Sclerectasia
Ecthyma L08.0
  contagiosum B08.02
  gangrenosum L08.0
  infectiosum B08.02
Ectocardia Q24.8
Ectodermal dysplasia (anhidrotic) Q82.4
Ectodermosis erosiva pluriorificialis L51.1
Ectopic, ectopia (congenital)
  abdominal viscera Q45.8
    due to defect in anterior abdominal wall Q79.59
  ACTH syndrome E24.3
  adrenal gland Q89.1
  anus Q43.5
  atrial beats I49.1
  beats I49.49
    atrial I49.1
    ventricular I49.3

Ectopic, ectopia — continued
  bladder Q64.10
  bone and cartilage in lung Q33.5
  brain Q04.8
  breast tissue Q83.8
  cardiac Q24.8
  cerebral Q04.8
  cordis Q24.8
  endometrium — see Endometriosis
  gastric mucosa Q40.2
  gestation — see Pregnancy, by site
  heart Q24.8
  hormone secretion NEC E34.2
  kidney (crossed) (pelvis) Q63.2
  lens, lentis Q12.1
  mole — see Pregnancy, by site
  organ or site NEC — see Malposition, congenital
  pancreas Q45.3
  pregnancy — see Pregnancy, ectopic
  pupil — see Abnormality, pupillary
  renal Q63.2
  sebaceous glands of mouth Q38.6
  spleen Q89.09
  testis Q53.00
    bilateral Q53.02
    unilateral Q53.01
  thyroid Q89.2
  tissue in lung Q33.5
  ureter Q62.63
  ventricular beats I49.3
  vesicae Q64.10
Ectromelia Q73.8
  lower limb — see Defect, reduction, limb, lower, specified type NEC
  upper limb — see Defect, reduction, limb, upper, specified type NEC
Ectropion H02.109
  cervix N86
    with cervicitis N72
  congenital Q10.1
  eyelid (paralytic) H02.109
    cicatricial H02.119
      left H02.116
        lower H02.115
        upper H02.114
      right H02.113
        lower H02.112
        upper H02.111
    congenital Q10.1
    left H02.106
      lower H02.105
      upper H02.104
    mechanical H02.129
      left H02.126
        lower H02.125
        upper H02.124
      right H02.123
        lower H02.122
        upper H02.121
    right H02.103
      lower H02.102
      upper H02.101
    senile H02.139
      left H02.136
        lower H02.135
        upper H02.134
      right H02.133
        lower H02.132
        upper H02.131
    spastic H02.149
      left H02.146
        lower H02.145
        upper H02.144
      right H02.143
        lower H02.142
        upper H02.141
  iris H21.89
  lip (acquired) K13.0
    congenital Q38.0
  urethra N36.8
  uvea H21.89
Eczema (acute) (chronic) (erythematous) (fissum) (rubrum) (squamous) (see also Dermatitis) L30.9
  contact — see Dermatitis, contact
  dyshydrotic L30.1
  external ear — see Otitis, externa, acute, eczematoid
  flexural L20.82
  herpeticum B00.0

Eczema — continued
  hypertrophicum L28.0
  hypostatic — see Varix, leg, with, inflammation
  impetiginous L01.1
  infantile (due to any substance) L20.83
    intertriginous L21.1
    seborrheic L21.1
  intertriginous NEC L30.4
    infantile L21.1
  intrinsic (allergic) L20.84
  lichenified NEC L28.0
  marginatum (hebrae) B35.6
  pustular L30.3
  stasis — see Varix, leg, with, inflammation
  vaccination, vaccinatum T88.1 ☑
  varicose — see Varix, leg, with, inflammation
Eczematid L30.2
Eddowes (-Spurway) **syndrome** Q78.0
Edema, edematous (infectious) (pitting) (toxic) R60.9
  with nephritis — see Nephrosis
  allergic T78.3 ☑
  amputation stump (surgical) (sequelae (late effect)) T87.89
  angioneurotic (allergic) (any site) (with urticaria) T78.3 ☑
    hereditary D84.1
  angiospastic I73.9
  Berlin's (traumatic) S05.8X- ☑
  brain (cytotoxic) (vasogenic) G93.6
    due to birth injury P11.0
    newborn (anoxia or hypoxia) P52.4
      birth injury P11.0
    traumatic — see Injury, intracranial, cerebral edema
  cardiac — see Failure, heart, congestive
  cardiovascular — see Failure, heart, congestive
  cerebral — see Edema, brain
  cerebrospinal — see Edema, brain
  cervix (uteri) (acute) N88.8
    puerperal, postpartum O90.89
  chronic hereditary Q82.0
  circumscribed, acute T78.3 ☑
    hereditary D84.1
  conjunctiva H11.42- ☑
  cornea H18.2- ☑
    idiopathic H18.22- ☑
    secondary H18.23- ☑
      due to contact lens H18.21- ☑
  due to
    lymphatic obstruction I89.0
    salt retention E87.0
  epiglottis — see Edema, glottis
  essential, acute T78.3 ☑
    hereditary D84.1
  extremities, lower — see Edema, legs
  eyelid NEC H02.849
    left H02.846
      lower H02.845
      upper H02.844
    right H02.843
      lower H02.842
      upper H02.841
  familial, hereditary Q82.0
  famine — see Malnutrition, severe
  generalized R60.1
  glottis, glottic, glottidis (obstructive) (passive) J38.4
    allergic T78.3 ☑
      hereditary D84.1
  heart — see Failure, heart, congestive
  heat T67.7 ☑
  hereditary Q82.0
  inanition — see Malnutrition, severe
  intracranial G93.6
  iris H21.89
  joint — see Effusion, joint
  larynx — see Edema, glottis
  legs R60.0
    due to venous obstruction I87.1
    hereditary Q82.0
  localized R60.0
    due to venous obstruction I87.1
  lower limbs — see Edema, legs
  lung J81.1
    with heart condition or failure — see Failure, ventricular, left
    acute J81.0
    chemical (acute) J68.1
      chronic J68.1

Edema, edematous — *continued*
- lung — *continued*
  - chronic J81.1
    - due to
      - chemicals, gases, fumes or vapors (inhalation) J68.1
      - external agent J70.9
        - specified NEC J70.8
      - radiation J70.1
    - due to
      - chemicals, fumes or vapors (inhalation) J68.1
      - external agent J70.9
        - specified NEC J70.8
      - high altitude T70.29 ☑
      - near drowning T75.1 ☑
      - radiation J70.0
    - meaning failure, left ventricle I50.1
  - lymphatic I89.0
    - due to mastectomy I97.2
  - macula H35.81
    - cystoid, following cataract surgery — *see* Complications, postprocedural, following cataract surgery
    - diabetic — *see* Diabetes, by type, with, retinopathy, with macular edema
  - malignant — *see* Gangrene, gas
  - Milroy's Q82.0
  - nasopharynx J39.2
  - newborn P83.30
    - hydrops fetalis — *see* Hydrops, fetalis
    - specified NEC P83.39
  - nutritional (*see also* Malnutrition, severe)
    - with dyspigmentation, skin and hair E40
  - optic disc or nerve — *see* Papilledema
  - orbit H05.22- ☑
  - pancreas K86.8
  - papilla, optic — *see* Papilledema
  - penis N48.89
  - periodic T78.3 ☑
    - hereditary D84.1
  - pharynx J39.2
  - pulmonary — *see* Edema, lung
  - Quincke's T78.3 ☑
    - hereditary D84.1
  - renal — *see* Nephrosis
  - retina H35.81
    - diabetic — *see* Diabetes, by type, with, retinopathy, with macular edema
  - salt E87.0
  - scrotum N50.8
  - seminal vesicle N50.8
  - spermatic cord N50.8
  - spinal (cord) (vascular) (nontraumatic) G95.19
  - starvation — *see* Malnutrition, severe
  - stasis — *see* Hypertension, venous, (chronic)
  - subglottic — *see* Edema, glottis
  - supraglottic — *see* Edema, glottis
  - testis N44.8
  - tunica vaginalis N50.8
  - vas deferens N50.8
  - vulva (acute) N90.89

Edentulism — *see* Absence, teeth, acquired

Edsall's disease T67.2 ☑

Educational handicap Z55.9
- specified NEC Z55.8

Edward's syndrome — *see* Trisomy, 18

Effect(s) (of) (from) — *see* Effect, adverse NEC

Effect, adverse
- abnormal gravitational (G) forces or states T75.81 ☑
- abuse — *see* Maltreatment
- air pressure T70.9 ☑
  - specified NEC T70.8 ☑
- altitude (high) — *see* Effect, adverse, high altitude
- anesthesia (*see also* Anesthesia) T88.59 ☑
  - in labor and delivery O74.9
  - in pregnancy NEC O29.3- ☑
  - local, toxic
    - in labor and delivery O74.4
    - postpartum, puerperal O89.3
  - postpartum, puerperal O89.9
  - specified NEC T88.59 ☑
    - in labor and delivery O74.8
    - postpartum, puerperal O89.8
  - spinal and epidural T88.59 ☑
    - headache T88.59 ☑
      - in labor and delivery O74.5
      - postpartum, puerperal O89.4

Effect, adverse — *continued*
- anesthesia (*see also* Anesthesia) — *continued*
  - spinal and epidural — *continued*
    - specified NEC
      - in labor and delivery O74.6
      - postpartum, puerperal O89.5
- antitoxin — *see* Complications, vaccination
- atmospheric pressure T70.9 ☑
  - due to explosion T70.8 ☑
  - high T70.3 ☑
  - low — *see* Effect, adverse, high altitude
  - specified effect NEC T70.8 ☑
- biological, correct substance properly administered — *see* Effect, adverse, drug
- blood (derivatives) (serum) (transfusion) — *see* Complications, transfusion
- chemical substance — *see* Table of Drugs and Chemicals
- cold (temperature) (weather) T69.9 ☑
  - chilblains T69.1 ☑
  - frostbite — *see* Frostbite
  - specified effect NEC T69.8 ☑
- drugs and medicaments T88.7 ☑
  - specified drug — *see* Table of Drugs and Chemicals, by drug, adverse effect
  - specified effect — *code to* condition
- electric current, electricity (shock) T75.4 ☑
  - burn — *see* Burn
- exertion (excessive) T73.3 ☑
- exposure — *see* Exposure
- external cause NEC T75.89 ☑
- foodstuffs T78.1 ☑
  - allergic reaction — *see* Allergy, food
    - causing anaphylaxis — *see* Shock, anaphylactic, due to food
  - noxious — *see* Poisoning, food, noxious
- gases, fumes, or vapors T59.9- ☑
  - specified agent — *see* Table of Drugs and Chemicals
- glue (airplane) sniffing
  - due to drug abuse — *see* Abuse, drug, inhalant
  - due to drug dependence — *see* Dependence, drug, inhalant
- heat — *see* Heat
- high altitude NEC T70.29 ☑
  - anoxia T70.29 ☑
  - on
    - ears T70.0 ☑
    - sinuses T70.1 ☑
  - polycythemia D75.1
- high pressure fluids T70.4 ☑
- hot weather — *see* Heat
- hunger T73.0 ☑
- immersion, foot — *see* Immersion
- immunization — *see* Complications, vaccination
- immunological agents — *see* Complications, vaccination
- infrared (radiation) (rays) NOS T66 ☑
  - dermatitis or eczema L59.8
- infusion — *see* Complications, infusion
- lack of care of infants — *see* Maltreatment, child
- lightning — *see* Lightning
- medical care T88.9 ☑
  - specified NEC T88.8 ☑
- medicinal substance, correct, properly administered — *see* Effect, adverse, drug
- motion T75.3 ☑
- noise, on inner ear — *see* subcategory H83.3 ☑
- overheated places — *see* Heat
- psychosocial, of work environment Z56.5
- radiation (diagnostic) (infrared) (natural source) (therapeutic) (ultraviolet) (X-ray) NOS T66 ☑
  - dermatitis or eczema — *see* Dermatitis, due to, radiation
  - fibrosis of lung J70.1
  - pneumonitis J70.0
  - pulmonary manifestations
    - acute J70.0
    - chronic J70.1
  - skin L59.9
- radioactive substance NOS
  - dermatitis or eczema — *see* Radiodermatitis
- reduced temperature T69.9 ☑
  - immersion foot or hand — *see* Immersion
  - specified effect NEC T69.8 ☑
- serum NEC (*see also* Reaction, serum) T80.69 ☑

Effect, adverse — *continued*
- specified NEC T78.8 ☑
  - external cause NEC T75.89 ☑
- strangulation — *see* Asphyxia, traumatic
- submersion T75.1 ☑
- thirst T73.1 ☑
- toxic — *see* Toxicity
- transfusion — *see* Complications, transfusion
- ultraviolet (radiation) (rays) NOS T66 ☑
  - burn — *see* Burn
  - dermatitis or eczema — *see* Dermatitis, due to, ultraviolet rays
    - acute L56.8
- vaccine (any) — *see* Complications, vaccination
- vibration — *see* Vibration, adverse effects
- water pressure NEC T70.9 ☑
  - specified NEC T70.8 ☑
- weightlessness T75.82 ☑
- whole blood — *see* Complications, transfusion
- work environment Z56.5

Effects, late — *see* Sequelae

Effluvium
- anagen L65.1
- telogen L65.0

Effort syndrome (psychogenic) F45.8

Effusion
- amniotic fluid — *see* Pregnancy, complicated by, prematue rupture of membranes
- brain (serous) G93.6
- bronchial — *see* Bronchitis
- cerebral G93.6
- cerebrospinal (*see also* Meningitis)
  - vessel G93.6
- chest — *see* Effusion, pleura
- chylous, chyliform (pleura) J94.0
- intracranial G93.6
- joint M25.40
  - ankle M25.47- ☑
  - elbow M25.42- ☑
  - foot joint M25.47- ☑
  - hand joint M25.44- ☑
  - hip M25.45- ☑
  - knee M25.46- ☑
  - shoulder M25.41- ☑
  - specified joint NEC M25.48
  - wrist M25.43- ☑
- malignant pleural J91.0
- meninges — *see* Meningitis
- pericardium, pericardial (noninflammatory) I31.3
  - acute — *see* Pericarditis, acute
- peritoneal (chronic) R18.8
- pleura, pleurisy, pleuritic, pleuropericardial J90
  - chylous, chyliform J94.0
  - due to systemic lupus erythematosis M32.13
  - influenzal — *see* Influenza, with, respiratory manifestations NEC
  - malignant J91.0
  - newborn P28.89
  - tuberculous NEC A15.6
    - primary (progressive) A15.7
- spinal — *see* Meningitis
- thorax, thoracic — *see* Effusion, pleura

Egg shell nails L60.3
- congenital Q84.6

Egyptian splenomegaly B65.1

Ehlers-Danlos syndrome Q79.6

Ehrlichiosis A77.40
- due to
  - E. chafeensis A77.41
  - E. sennetsu A79.81
  - specified organism NEC A77.49

Eichstedt's disease B36.0

Eisenmenger's
- complex or syndrome I27.89
- defect Q21.8

Ejaculation
- painful N53.12
- premature F52.4
- retarded N53.11
- retrograde N53.14
- semen, painful N53.12
  - psychogenic F52.6

Ekbom's syndrome (restless legs) G25.81

Ekman's syndrome (brittle bones and blue sclera) Q78.0

Elastic skin Q82.8
- acquired L57.4

Elastofibroma — see Neoplasm, connective tissue, benign
Elastoma (juvenile) Q82.8
    Miescher's L87.2
Elastomyofibrosis I42.4
Elastosis
    actinic, solar L57.8
    atrophicans (senile) L57.4
    perforans serpiginosa L87.2
    senilis L57.4
Elbow — see condition
Electric current, electricity, effects (concussion) (fatal) (nonfatal) (shock) T75.4 ☑
    burn — see Burn
Electric feet syndrome E53.8
Electrocution T75.4 ☑
    from electroshock gun (taser) T75.4 ☑
Electrolyte imbalance E87.8
    with
        abortion — see Abortion by type, complicated by, electrolyte imbalance
        ectopic pregnancy O08.5
        molar pregnancy O08.5
Elephantiasis (nonfilarial) I89.0
    arabicum — see Infestation, filarial
    bancroftian B74.0
    congenital (any site) (hereditary) Q82.0
    due to
        Brugia (malayi) B74.1
            timori B74.2
        mastectomy I97.2
        Wuchereria (bancrofti) B74.0
    eyelid H02.859
        left H02.856
            lower H02.855
            upper H02.854
        right H02.853
            lower H02.852
            upper H02.851
    filarial, filariensis — see Infestation, filarial
    glandular I89.0
    graecorum A30.9
    lymphangiectatic I89.0
    lymphatic vessel I89.0
        due to mastectomy I97.2
    scrotum (nonfilarial) I89.0
    streptococcal I89.0
    surgical I97.89
        postmastectomy I97.2
    telangiectodes I89.0
    vulva (nonfilarial) N90.89
Elevated, elevation
    antibody titer R76.0
    basal metabolic rate R94.8
    blood pressure (see also Hypertension)
        reading (incidental) (isolated) (nonspecific), no diagnosis of hypertension R03.0
    blood sugar R73.9
    body temperature (of unknown origin) R50.9
    C-reactive protein (CRP) R79.82
    cancer antigen 125 [CA 125] R97.1
    carcinoembryonic antigen [CEA] R97.0
    cholesterol E78.0
        with high triglycerides E78.2
    conjugate, eye H51.0
    diaphragm, congenital Q79.1
    erythrocyte sedimentation rate R70.0
    fasting glucose R73.01
    fasting triglycerides E78.1
    finding on laboratory examination — see Findings, abnormal, inconclusive, without diagnosis, by type of exam
    GFR (glomerular filtration rate) — see Findings, abnormal, inconclusive, without diagnosis, by type of exam
    glucose tolerance (oral) R73.02
    immunoglobulin level R76.8
    indoleacetic acid R82.5
    lactic acid dehydrogenase (LDH) level R74.0
    leukocytes D72.829
    lipoprotein a level E78.8 ☑
    liver function
        study R94.5
        test R79.89
            alkaline phosphatase R74.8
            aminotransferase R74.0
            bilirubin R17
            hepatic enzyme R74.8

Elevated, elevation — continued
    liver function — continued
        test — continued
            lactate dehydrogenase R74.0
    lymphocytes D72.820
    prostate specific antigen [PSA] R97.2
    Rh titer — see Complication(s), transfusion, incompatibility reaction, Rh (factor)
    scapula, congenital Q74.0
    sedimentation rate R70.0
    SGOT R74.0
    SGPT R74.0
    transaminase level R74.0
    triglycerides E78.1
        with high cholesterol E78.2
    tumor associated antigens [TAA] NEC R97.8
    tumor specific antigens [TSA] NEC R97.8
    urine level of
        17-ketosteroids R82.5
        catecholamine R82.5
        indoleacetic acid R82.5
        steroids R82.5
        vanillylmandelic acid (VMA) R82.5
    venous pressure I87.8
    white blood cell count D72.829
        specified NEC D72.828
Elliptocytosis (congenital) (hereditary) D58.1
    Hb C (disease) D58.1
    hemoglobin disease D58.1
    sickle-cell (disease) D57.8- ☑
        trait D57.3
Ellis-van Creveld syndrome (chondroectodermal dysplasia) Q77.6
Ellison-Zollinger syndrome E16.4
Elongated, elongation (congenital) (see also Distortion)
    bone Q79.9
    cervix (uteri) Q51.828
        acquired N88.4
        hypertrophic N88.4
    colon Q43.8
    common bile duct Q44.5
    cystic duct Q44.5
    frenulum, penis Q55.69
    labia minora (acquired) N90.6
    ligamentum patellae Q74.1
    petiolus (epiglottidis) Q31.8
    tooth, teeth K00.2
    uvula Q38.6
Eltor cholera A00.1
Emaciation (due to malnutrition) E41
Embadomoniasis A07.8
Embedded tooth, teeth K01.0
    root only K08.3
Embolic — see condition
Embolism (multiple) (paradoxical) I74.9
    air (any site) (traumatic) T79.0 ☑
        following
            abortion — see Abortion by type complicated by embolism
            ectopic pregnancy O08.2
            infusion, therapeutic injection or transfusion T80.0 ☑
            molar pregnancy O08.2
            procedure NEC
                artery T81.719 ☑
                    mesenteric T81.710 ☑
                    renal T81.711 ☑
                    specified NEC T81.718 ☑
                vein T81.72 ☑
        in pregnancy, childbirth or puerperium — see Embolism, obstetric
    amniotic fluid (pulmonary) (see also Embolism, obstetric)
        following
            abortion — see Abortion by type complicated by embolism
            ectopic pregnancy O08.2
            molar pregnancy O08.2
    aorta, aortic I74.10
        abdominal I74.09
            saddle I74.01
        bifurcation I74.09
        saddle I74.01
        thoracic I74.11
    artery I74.9
        auditory, internal I65.8
        basilar — see Occlusion, artery, basilar

Embolism — continued
    artery — continued
        carotid (common) (internal) — see Occlusion, artery, carotid
        cerebellar (anterior inferior) (posterior inferior) (superior) I66.3
        cerebral — see Occlusion, artery, cerebral
        choroidal (anterior) I66.8
        communicating posterior I66.8
        coronary (see also Infarct, myocardium)
            not resulting in infarction I24.0
        extremity I74.4
            lower I74.3
            upper I74.2
        hypophyseal I66.8
        iliac I74.5
        limb I74.4
            lower I74.3
            upper I74.2
        mesenteric (with gangrene) K55.0
        ophthalmic — see Occlusion, artery, retina
        peripheral I74.4
        pontine I66.8
        precerebral — see Occlusion, artery, precerebral
        pulmonary — see Embolism, pulmonary
        renal N28.0
        retinal — see Occlusion, artery, retina
        septic I76
        specified NEC I74.8
        vertebral — see Occlusion, artery, vertebral
    basilar (artery) I65.1
    blood clot
        following
            abortion — see Abortion by type complicated by embolism
            ectopic or molar pregnancy O08.2
            in pregnancy, childbirth or puerperium — see Embolism, obstetric
    brain (see also Occlusion, artery, cerebral)
        following
            abortion — see Abortion by type complicated by embolism
            ectopic or molar pregnancy O08.2
        puerperal, postpartum, childbirth — see Embolism, obstetric
    capillary I78.8
    cardiac (see also Infarct, myocardium)
        not resulting in infarction I24.0
    carotid (artery) (common) (internal) — see Occlusion, artery, carotid
    cavernous sinus (venous) — see Embolism, intracranial venous sinus
    cerebral — see Occlusion, artery, cerebral
    cholesterol — see Atheroembolism
    coronary (artery or vein) (systemic) — see Occlusion, artery, coronary
    due to device, implant or graft (see also Complications, by site and type, specified NEC)
        arterial graft NEC T82.818 ☑
        breast (implant) T85.81 ☑
        catheter NEC T85.81 ☑
            dialysis (renal) T82.818 ☑
                intraperitoneal T85.81 ☑
            infusion NEC T82.818 ☑
                spinal (epidural) (subdural) T85.81 ☑
            urinary (indwelling) T83.81 ☑
        electronic (electrode) (pulse generator) (stimulator)
            bone T84.81 ☑
            cardiac T82.817 ☑
            nervous system (brain) (peripheral nerve) (spinal) T85.81 ☑
            urinary T83.81 ☑
        fixation, internal (orthopedic) NEC T84.81 ☑
        gastrointestinal (bile duct) (esophagus) T85.81 ☑
        genital NEC T83.81 ☑
        heart (graft) (valve) T82.817 ☑
        joint prosthesis T84.81 ☑
        ocular (corneal graft) (orbital implant) T85.81 ☑
        orthopedic (bone graft) NEC T86.838
        specified NEC T85.81 ☑
        urinary (graft) NEC T83.81 ☑
        vascular NEC T82.818 ☑
        ventricular intracranial shunt T85.81 ☑
    extremities
        lower — see Embolism, vein, lower extremity
            arterial I74.3
        upper I74.2

Embolism — *continued*
- eye H34.9
- fat (cerebral) (pulmonary) (systemic) T79.1 ☑
  - complicating delivery — *see* Embolism, obstetric
  - following
    - abortion — *see* Abortion by type complicated by embolism
    - ectopic or molar pregnancy O08.2
- following
  - abortion — *see* Abortion by type complicated by embolism
  - ectopic or molar pregnancy O08.2
  - infusion, therapeutic injection or transfusion
    - air T80.0 ☑
- heart (fatty) (*see also* Infarct, myocardium)
  - not resulting in infarction I24.0
- hepatic (vein) I82.0
- in pregnancy, childbirth or puerperium — *see* Embolism, obstetric
- intestine (artery) (vein) (with gangrene) K55.0
- intracranial (*see also* Occlusion, artery, cerebral)
  - venous sinus (any) G08
    - nonpyogenic I67.6
- intraspinal venous sinuses or veins G08
  - nonpyogenic G95.19
- kidney (artery) N28.0
- lateral sinus (venous) — *see* Embolism, intracranial, venous sinus
- leg — *see* Embolism, vein, lower extremity
  - arterial I74.3
- longitudinal sinus (venous) — *see* Embolism, intracranial, venous sinus
- lung (massive) — *see* Embolism, pulmonary
- meninges I66.8
- mesenteric (artery) (vein) (with gangrene) K55.0
- obstetric (in) (pulmonary)
  - childbirth O88.82
    - air O88.02
    - amniotic fluid O88.12
    - blood clot O88.22
    - fat O88.82
    - pyemic O88.32
    - septic O88.32
    - specified type NEC O88.82
  - pregnancy O88.81- ☑
    - air O88.01- ☑
    - amniotic fluid O88.11- ☑
    - blood clot O88.21- ☑
    - fat O88.81- ☑
    - pyemic O88.31- ☑
    - septic O88.31- ☑
    - specified type NEC O88.81- ☑
  - puerperal O88.83
    - air O88.03
    - amniotic fluid O88.13
    - blood clot O88.23
    - fat O88.83
    - pyemic O88.33
    - septic O88.33
    - specified type NEC O88.83
- ophthalmic — *see* Occlusion, artery, retina
- penis N48.81
- peripheral artery NOS I74.4
- pituitary E23.6
- popliteal (artery) I74.3
- portal (vein) I81
- postoperative, postrpocedural
  - artery T81.719 ☑
    - mesenteric T81.710 ☑
    - renal T81.711 ☑
    - specified NEC T81.718 ☑
  - vein T81.72 ☑
- precerebral artery — *see* Occlusion, artery, precerebral
- puerperal — *see* Embolism, obstetric
- pulmonary (acute) (artery) (vein) I26.99
  - with acute cor pulmonale I26.09
  - chronic I27.82
  - following
    - abortion — *see* Abortion by type complicated by embolism
    - ectopic or molar pregnancy O08.2
  - healed or old Z86.711
  - in pregnancy, childbirth or puerperium — *see* Embolism, obstetric
  - personal history of Z86.711
  - saddle I26.92
    - with acute cor pulmonale I26.02

Embolism — *continued*
- pulmonary — *continued*
  - septic I26.90
    - with acute cor pulmonale I26.01
- pyemic (multiple) I76
  - following
    - abortion — *see* Abortion by type complicated by embolism
    - ectopic or molar pregnancy O08.2
  - Hemophilus influenzae A41.3
  - pneumococcal A40.3
    - with pneumonia J13
  - puerperal, postpartum, childbirth (any organism) — *see* Embolism, obstetric
  - specified organism NEC A41.89
  - staphylococcal A41.2
  - streptococcal A40.9
- renal (artery) N28.0
  - vein I82.3
- retina, retinal — *see* Occlusion, artery, retina
- saddle
  - abdominal aorta I74.01
  - pulmonary artery I26.92
    - with acute cor pulmonale I26.02
- septic (arterial) I76
  - complicating abortion — *see* Abortion, by type, complicated by, embolism
- sinus — *see* Embolism, intracranial, venous sinus
- soap complicating abortion — *see* Abortion, by type, complicated by, embolism
- spinal cord G95.19
  - pyogenic origin G06.1
- spleen, splenic (artery) I74.8
- upper extremity I74.2
- vein (acute) I82.90
  - antecubital I82.61- ☑
    - chronic I82.71- ☑
  - axillary I82.A1- ☑ (*following* I82.7)
    - chronic I82.A2- ☑ (*following* I82.7)
  - basilic I82.61- ☑
    - chronic I82.71- ☑
  - brachial I82.62- ☑
    - chronic I82.72- ☑
  - brachiocephalic (innominate) I82.290
    - chronic I82.291
  - cephalic I82.61- ☑
    - chronic I82.71- ☑
  - chronic I82.91
  - deep (DVT) I82.40- ☑
    - calf I82.4Z- ☑
      - chronic I82.5Z- ☑
    - lower leg I82.4Z- ☑
      - chronic I82.5Z- ☑
    - thigh I82.4Y- ☑
      - chronic I82.5Y- ☑
    - upper leg I82.4Y ☑
      - chronic I82.5Y- ☑
  - femoral I82.41- ☑
    - chronic I82.51- ☑
  - iliac (iliofemoral) I82.42- ☑
    - chronic I82.52- ☑
  - innominate I82.290
    - chronic I82.291
  - internal jugular I82.C1- ☑ (*following* I82.7)
    - chronic I82.C2- ☑ (*following* I82.7)
  - lower extremity
    - deep I82.40- ☑
      - chronic I82.50- ☑
      - specified NEC I82.49- ☑
        - chronic NEC I82.59- ☑
    - distal
      - deep I82.4Z- ☑
    - proximal
      - deep I82.4Y- ☑
        - chronic I82.5Y- ☑
    - superficial I82.81- ☑
  - popliteal I82.43- ☑
    - chronic I82.53- ☑
  - radial I82.62- ☑
    - chronic I82.72- ☑
  - renal I82.3
  - saphenous (greater) (lesser) I82.81- ☑
  - specified NEC I82.890
    - chronic NEC I82.891
  - subclavian I82.B1- ☑ (*following* I82.7)
    - chronic I82.B2- ☑ (*following* I82.7)
  - thoracic NEC I82.290

Embolism — *continued*
- vein — *continued*
  - thoracic — *continued*
    - chronic I82.291
  - tibial I82.44- ☑
    - chronic I82.54- ☑
  - ulnar I82.62- ☑
    - chronic I82.72- ☑
  - upper extremity I82.60- ☑
    - chronic I82.70- ☑
    - deep I82.62- ☑
      - chronic I82.72- ☑
    - superficial I82.61- ☑
      - chronic I82.71- ☑
  - vena cava
    - inferior (acute) I82.220
      - chronic I82.221
    - superior (acute) I82.210
      - chronic I82.211
  - venous sinus G08
  - vessels of brain — *see* Occlusion, artery, cerebral
Embolus — *see* Embolism
Embryoma (*see also* Neoplasm, uncertain behavior, by site)
- benign — *see* Neoplasm, benign, by site
- kidney C64.- ☑
- liver C22.0
- malignant (*see also* Neoplasm, malignant, by site)
  - kidney C64.- ☑
  - liver C22.0
  - testis C62.9- ☑
    - descended (scrotal) C62.1- ☑
    - undescended C62.0- ☑
- testis C62.9- ☑
  - descended (scrotal) C62.1- ☑
  - undescended C62.0- ☑
Embryonic
- circulation Q28.9
- heart Q28.9
- vas deferens Q55.4
Embryopathia NOS Q89.9
Embryotoxon Q13.4
Emesis — *see* Vomiting
Emotional lability R45.86
Emotionality, pathological F60.3
Emotogenic disease — *see* Disorder, psychogenic
Emphysema (atrophic) (bullous) (chronic) (interlobular) (lung) (obstructive) (pulmonary) (senile) (vesicular) J43.9
- cellular tissue (traumatic) T79.7 ☑
  - surgical T81.82 ☑
- centrilobular J43.2
- compensatory J98.3
- congenital (interstitial) P25.0
- conjunctiva H11.89
- connective tissue (traumatic) T79.7 ☑
  - surgical T81.82 ☑
- due to chemicals, gases, fumes or vapors J68.4
- eyelid(s) — *see* Disorder, eyelid, specified type NEC
  - surgical T81.82 ☑
  - traumatic T79.7 ☑
- interstitial J98.2
  - congenital P25.0
  - perinatal period P25.0
- laminated tissue T79.7 ☑
  - surgical T81.82 ☑
- mediastinal J98.2
  - newborn P25.2
- orbit, orbital — *see* Disorder, orbit, specified type NEC
- panacinar J43.1
- panlobular J43.1
- specified NEC J43.8
- subcutaneous (traumatic) T79.7 ☑
  - nontraumatic J98.2
  - postprocedural T81.82 ☑
  - surgical T81.82 ☑
- surgical T81.82 ☑
- thymus (gland) (congenital) E32.8
- traumatic (subcutaneous) T79.7 ☑
- unilateral J43.0
Empty nest syndrome Z60.0
Empyema (acute) (chest) (double) (pleura) (supradiaphragmatic) (thorax) J86.9
- with fistula J86.0
- accessory sinus (chronic) — *see* Sinusitis
- antrum (chronic) — *see* Sinusitis, maxillary
- brain (any part) — *see* Abscess, brain

Empyema — *continued*
  ethmoidal (chronic) (sinus) — *see* Sinusitis, ethmoidal
  extradural — *see* Abscess, extradural
  frontal (chronic) (sinus) — *see* Sinusitis, frontal
  gallbladder K81.0
  mastoid (process) (acute) — *see* Mastoiditis, acute
  maxilla, maxillary M27.2
    sinus (chronic) — *see* Sinusitis, maxillary
  nasal sinus (chronic) — *see* Sinusitis
  sinus (accessory) (chronic) (nasal) — *see* Sinusitis
  sphenoidal (sinus) (chronic) — *see* Sinusitis, sphenoidal
  subarachnoid — *see* Abscess, extradural
  subdural — *see* Abscess, subdural
  tuberculous A15.6
  ureter — *see* Ureteritis
  ventricular — *see* Abscess, brain
En coup de sabre lesion L94.1
Enamel pearls K00.2
Enameloma K00.2
Enanthema, viral B09
Encephalitis (chronic) (hemorrhagic) (idiopathic) (nonepidemic) (spurious) (subacute) G04.90
  acute (*see also* Encephalitis, viral) A86
    disseminated G04.00
      infectious G04.01
      noninfectious G04.81
      postimmunization (postvaccination) G04.02
      postinfectious G04.01
    inclusion body A85.8
    necrotizing hemorrhagic G04.30
      postimmunization G04.32
      postinfectious G04.31
      specified NEC G04.39
  arboviral, arbovirus NEC A85.2
  arthropod-borne NEC (viral) A85.2
  Australian A83.4
  California (virus) A83.5
  Central European (tick-borne) A84.1
  Czechoslovakian A84.1
  Dawson's (inclusion body) A81.1
  diffuse sclerosing A81.1
  disseminated, acute G04.00
  due to
    cat scratch disease A28.1
    human immunodeficiency virus (HIV) disease B20 [G05.3]
    malaria — *see* Malaria
    rickettsiosis — *see* Rickettsiosis
    smallpox inoculation G04.02
    typhus — *see* Typhus
  Eastern equine A83.2
  endemic (viral) A86
  epidemic NEC (viral) A86
  equine (acute) (infectious) (viral) A83.9
    Eastern A83.2
    Venezuelan A92.2
    Western A83.1
  Far Eastern (tick-borne) A84.0
  following vaccination or other immunization procedure G04.02
  herpes zoster B02.0
  herpesviral B00.4
    due to herpesvirus 6 B10.01
    due to herpesvirus 7 B10.09
    specified NEC B10.09
  Ilheus (virus) A83.8
  in (due to)
    actinomycosis A42.82
    adenovirus A85.1
    African trypanosomiasis B56.9 [G05.3]
    Chagas' disease (chronic) B57.42
    cytomegalovirus B25.8
    enterovirus A85.0
    herpes (simplex) virus B00.4
      due to herpesvirus 6 B10.01
      due to herpesvirus 7 B10.09
      specified NEC B10.09
    infectious disease NEC B99 ☑ [G05.3]
    influenza — *see* Influenza, with, encephalopathy
    listeriosis A32.12
    measles B05.0
    mumps B26.2
    naegleriasis B60.2
    parasitic disease NEC B89 [G05.3]
    poliovirus A80.9 [G05.3]
    rubella B06.01

Encephalitis — *continued*
  in — *continued*
    syphilis
      congenital A50.42
      late A52.14
    systemic lupus erythematosus M32.19
    toxoplasmosis (acquired) B58.2
      congenital P37.1
    tuberculosis A17.82
    zoster B02.0
  inclusion body A81.1
  infectious (acute) (virus) NEC A86
  Japanese (B type) A83.0
  La Crosse A83.5
  lead — *see* Poisoning, lead
  lethargica (acute) (infectious) A85.8
  louping ill A84.8
  lupus erythematosus, systemic M32.19
  lymphatica A87.2
  Mengo A85.8
  meningococcal A39.81
  Murray Valley A83.4
  otitic NEC H66.40 [G05.3]
  parasitic NOS B71.9
  periaxial G37.0
  periaxialis (concentrica) (diffuse) G37.5
  postchickenpox B01.11
  postexanthematous NEC B09
  postimmunization G04.02
  postinfectious NEC G04.01
  postmeasles B05.0
  postvaccinal G04.02
  postvaricella B01.11
  postviral NEC A86
  Powassan A84.8
  Rasmussen G04.81
  Rio Bravo A85.8
  Russian
    autumnal A83.0
    spring-summer (taiga) A84.0
  saturnine — *see* Poisoning, lead
  specified NEC G04.81
  St. Louis A83.3
  subacute sclerosing A81.1
  summer A83.0
  suppurative G04.81
  tick-borne A84.9
  Torula, torular (cryptococcal) B45.1
  toxic NEC G92
  trichinosis B75 [G05.3]
  type
    B A83.0
    C A83.3
  van Bogaert's A81.1
  Venezuelan equine A92.2
  Vienna A85.8
  viral, virus A86
    arthropod-borne NEC A85.2
      mosquito-borne A83.9
        Australian X disease A83.4
        California virus A83.5
        Eastern equine A83.2
        Japanese (B type) A83.0
        Murray Valley A83.4
        specified NEC A83.8
        St. Louis A83.3
        type B A83.0
        type C A83.3
        Western equine A83.1
      tick-borne A84.9
        biundulant A84.1
        central European A84.1
        Czechoslovakian A84.1
        diphasic meningoencephalitis A84.1
        Far Eastern A84.0
        Russian spring-summer (taiga) A84.0
        specified NEC A84.8
      specified type NEC A85.8
  Western equine A83.1
Encephalocele Q01.9
  frontal Q01.0
  nasofrontal Q01.1
  occipital Q01.2
  specified NEC Q01.8
Encephalocystocele — *see* Encephalocele
Encephaloduroarteriomyosynangiosis (EDAMS) I67.5
Encephalomalacia (brain) (cerebellar) (cerebral) — *see* Softening, brain

Encephalomeningitis — *see* Meningoencephalitis
Encephalomeningocele — *see* Encephalocele
Encephalomeningomyelitis — *see* Meningoencephalitis
Encephalomyelitis (*see also* Encephalitis) G04.90
  acute disseminated G04.00
    infectious G04.00
    noninfectious G04.81
    postimmunization G04.02
    postinfectious G04.01
  acute necrotizing hemorrhagic G04.30
    postimmunization G04.32
    postinfectious G04.31
    specified NEC G04.39
  benign myalgic G93.3
  equine A83.9
    Eastern A83.2
    Venezuelan A92.2
    Western A83.1
  in diseases classified elsewhere G05.3
  myalgic, benign G93.3
  postchickenpox B01.11
  postinfectious NEC G04.01
  postmeasles B05.0
  postvaccinal G04.02
  postvaricella B01.11
  rubella B06.01
  specified NEC G04.81
  Venezuelan equine A92.2
Encephalomyelocele — *see* Encephalocele
Encephalomyelomeningitis — *see* Meningoencephalitis
Encephalomyelopathy G96.9
Encephalomyeloradiculitis (acute) G61.0
Encephalomyeloradiculoneuritis (acute) (Guillain-Barré) G61.0
Encephalomyeloradiculopathy G96.9
Encephalopathia hyperbilirubinemica, newborn P57.9
  due to isoimmunization (conditions in P55) P57.0
Encephalopathy (acute) G93.40
  acute necrotizing hemorrhagic G04.30
    postimmunization G04.32
    postinfectious G04.31
    specified NEC G04.39
  alcoholic G31.2
  anoxic — *see* Damage, brain, anoxic
  arteriosclerotic I67.2
  centrolobar progressive (Schilder) G37.0
  congenital Q07.9
  degenerative, in specified disease NEC G32.89
  demyelinating callosal G37.1
  due to
    drugs (*see also* Table of Drugs and Chemicals) G92
  hepatic — *see* Failure, hepatic
  hyperbilirubinemic, newborn P57.9
    due to isoimmunization (conditions in P55) P57.0
  hypertensive I67.4
  hypoglycemic E16.2
  hypoxic — *see* Damage, brain, anoxic
  hypoxic ischemic P91.60
    mild P91.61
    moderate P91.62
    severe P91.63
  in (due to) (with)
    birth injury P11.1
    hyperinsulinism E16.1 [G94]
    influenza — *see* Influenza, with, encephalopathy
    lack of vitamin (*see also* Deficiency, vitamin) E56.9 [G32.89]
    neoplastic disease (*see also* Neoplasm) D49.9 [G13.1]
    serum (*see also* Reaction, serum) T80.69 ☑
    syphilis A52.17
    trauma (postconcussional) F07.81
      current injury — *see* Injury, intracranial
    vaccination G04.02
  lead — *see* Poisoning, lead
  metabolic G93.41
    drug induced G92
    toxic G92
  myoclonic, early, symptomatic — *see* Epilepsy, generalized, specified NEC
  necrotizing, subacute (Leigh) G31.82
  pellagrous E52 [G32.89]
  portosystemic — *see* Failure, hepatic
  postcontusional F07.81
    current injury — *see* Injury, intracranial, diffuse

Encephalopathy — continued
  posthypoglycemic (coma) E16.1 [G94]
  postradiation G93.89
  saturnine — see Poisoning, lead
  septic G93.41
  specified NEC G93.49
  spongioform, subacute (viral) A81.09
  toxic G92
    metabolic G92
  traumatic (postconcussional) F07.81
    current injury — see Injury, intracranial
  vitamin B deficiency NEC E53.9 [G32.89]
    vitamin B1 E51.2
    Wernicke's E51.2
Encephalorrhagia — see Hemorrhage, intracranial, intracerebral
Encephalosis, posttraumatic F07.81
Enchondroma (see also Neoplasm, bone, benign)
Enchondromatosis (cartilaginous) (multiple) Q78.4
Encopresis R15.9
  functional F98.1
  nonorganic origin F98.1
  psychogenic F98.1
Encounter (with health service) (for) Z76.89
  adjustment and management (of)
    breast implant Z45.81 ☑
    implanted device NEC Z45.89
    myringotomy device (stent) (tube) Z45.82
  administrative purpose only Z02.9
    examination for
      adoption Z02.82
      armed forces Z02.3
      disability determination Z02.71
      driving license Z02.4
      employment Z02.1
      insurance Z02.6
      medical certificate NEC Z02.79
      paternity testing Z02.81
      residential institution admission Z02.2
      school admission Z02.0
      sports Z02.5
      specified reason NEC Z02.89
  aftercare — see Aftercare
  antenatal screening Z36
  assisted reproductive fertility procedure cycle Z31.83
  blood typing Z01.83
    Rh typing Z01.83
  breast augmentation or reduction Z41.1
  breast implant exchange (different material) (different size) Z45.81 ☑
  breast reconstruction following mastectomy Z42.1
  check-up — see Examination
  chemotherapy for neoplasm Z51.11
  colonoscopy, screening NEC Z12.11
  counseling — see Counseling
  delivery, full-term, uncomplicated O80
    cesarean, without indication O82
  ear piercing Z41.3
  examination — see Examination
  expectant parent(s) (adoptive) pre-birth pediatrician visit Z76.81
  fertility preservation procedure (prior to cancer therapy) (prior to removal of gonads) Z31.84
  fitting (of) — see Fitting (and adjustment) (of)
  genetic
    counseling Z31.5
    testing — see Test, genetic
  hearing conservation and treatment Z01.12
  immunotherapy for neoplasm Z51.12
  in vitro fertilization cycle Z31.83
  instruction (in)
    child care (postpartal) (prenatal) Z32.3
    childbirth Z32.2
    natural family planning
      procreative Z31.61
      to avoid pregnancy Z30.02
  insulin pump titration Z46.81
  joint prosthesis insertion following prior explantation of joint prosthesis (staged procedure)
    hip Z47.32
    knee Z47.33
    shoulder Z47.31
  laboratory (as part of a general medical examination) Z00.00
    with abnormal findings Z00.01
  mental health services (for)
    abuse NEC
      perpetrator Z69.82

Encounter — continued
  mental health services — continued
    abuse — continued
      victim Z69.81
    child abuse
      nonparental
        perpetrator Z69.021
        victim Z69.020
      parental
        perpetrator Z69.011
        victim Z69.010
    spousal or partner abuse
      perpetrator Z69.12
      victim Z69.11
  observation (for) (ruled out)
    exposure to (suspected)
      anthrax Z03.810
      biological agent NEC Z03.818
  pediatrician visit, by expectant parent(s) (adoptive) Z76.81
  plastic and reconstructive surgery following medical procedure or healed injury NEC Z42.8
  pregnancy
    supervision of — see Pregnancy, supervision of
    test Z32.00
      result negative Z32.02
      result positive Z32.01
  radiation therapy (antineoplastic) Z51.0
  radiological (as part of a general medical examination) Z00.00
    with abnormal findings Z00.01
  reconstructive surgery following medical procedure or healed injury NEC Z42.8
  removal (of) (see also Removal)
    artificial
      arm Z44.00- ☑
        complete Z44.01- ☑
        partial Z44.02- ☑
      eye Z44.2- ☑
      leg Z44.10- ☑
        complete Z44.11- ☑
        partial Z44.12- ☑
    breast implant Z45.81 ☑
      tissue expander (without synchronous insertion of permanent implant) Z45.81 ☑
    device Z46.9
      specified NEC Z46.89
    external
      fixation device — code to fracture with seventh character D
      prosthesis, prosthetic device Z44.9
        breast Z44.3- ☑
        specified NEC Z44.8
    implanted device NEC Z45.89
    insulin pump Z46.81
    internal fixation device Z47.2
    myringotomy device (stent) (tube) Z45.82
    nervous system device NEC Z46.2
      brain neuropacemaker Z46.2
      visual substitution device Z46.2
        implanted Z45.31
    non-vascular catheter Z46.82
    orthodontic device Z46.4
    stent
      ureteral Z46.6
    urinary device Z46.6
  repeat cervical smear to confirm findings of recent normal smear following initial abnormal smear Z01.42
  respirator [ventilator] use during power failure Z99.12
  Rh typing Z01.83
  screening — see Screening
  specified NEC Z76.89
  sterilization Z30.2
  suspected condition, ruled out
    amniotic cavity and membrane Z03.71
    cervical shortening Z03.75
    fetal anomaly Z03.73
    fetal growth Z03.74
    maternal and fetal conditions NEC Z03.79
    oligohydramnios Z03.71
    placental problem Z03.72
    polyhydramnios Z03.71
  suspected exposure (to), ruled out
    anthrax Z03.810
    biological agents NEC Z03.818
  termination of pregnancy, elective Z33.2
  testing — see Test

Encounter — continued
  therapeutic drug level monitoring Z51.81
  titration, insulin pump Z46.81
  to determine fetal viability of pregnancy O36.80 ☑
  training
    insulin pump Z46.81
  X-ray of chest (as part of a general medical examination) Z00.00
    with abnormal findings Z00.01
Encystment — see Cyst
Endarteritis (bacterial, subacute) (infective) I77.6
  brain I67.7
  cerebral or cerebrospinal I67.7
  deformans — see Arteriosclerosis
  embolic — see Embolism
  obliterans (see also Arteriosclerosis)
    pulmonary I28.8
  pulmonary I28.8
  retina — see Vasculitis, retina
  senile — see Arteriosclerosis
  syphilitic A52.09
    brain or cerebral A52.04
    congenital A50.54 [I79.8]
  tuberculous A18.89
Endemic — see condition
Endocarditis (chronic) (marantic) (nonbacterial) (thrombotic) (valvular) I38
  with rheumatic fever (conditions in I00)
    active — see Endocarditis, acute, rheumatic
    inactive or quiescent (with chorea) I09.1
  acute or subacute I33.9
    infective I33.0
    rheumatic (aortic) (mitral) (pulmonary) (tricuspid) I01.1
      with chorea (acute) (rheumatic) (Sydenham's) I02.0
  aortic (heart) (nonrheumatic) (valve) I35.8
    with
      mitral disease I08.0
        with tricuspid (valve) disease I08.3
        active or acute I01.1
          with chorea (acute) (rheumatic) (Sydenham's) I02.0
      rheumatic fever (conditions in I00)
        active — see Endocarditis, acute, rheumatic
        inactive or quiescent (with chorea) I06.9
      tricuspid (valve) disease I08.2
        with mitral (valve) disease I08.3
    acute or subacute I33.9
    arteriosclerotic I35.8
    rheumatic I06.9
      with mitral disease I08.0
        with tricuspid (valve) disease I08.3
        active or acute I01.1
          with chorea (acute) (rheumatic) (Sydenham's) I02.0
      active or acute I01.1
        with chorea (acute) (rheumatic) (Sydenham's) I02.0
      specified NEC I06.8
    specified cause NEC I35.8
    syphilitic A52.03
  arteriosclerotic I38
  atypical verrucous (Libman-Sacks) M32.11
  bacterial (acute) (any valve) (subacute) I33.0
  candidal B37.6
  congenital Q24.8
  constrictive I33.0
  Coxiella burnetii A78 [I39]
  Coxsackie B33.21
  due to
    prosthetic cardiac valve T82.6 ☑
    Q fever A78 [I39]
    Serratia marcescens I33.0
    typhoid (fever) A01.02
  gonococcal A54.83
  infectious or infective (acute) (any valve) (subacute) I33.0
  lenta (acute) (any valve) (subacute) I33.0
  Libman-Sacks M32.11
  listerial A32.82
  Löffler's I42.3
  malignant (acute) (any valve) (subacute) I33.0
  meningococcal A39.51
  mitral (chronic) (double) (fibroid) (heart) (inactive) (valve) (with chorea) I05.9
    with
      aortic (valve) disease I08.0

Endocarditis — *continued*
　mitral — *continued*
　　with — *continued*
　　　aortic disease — *continued*
　　　　with tricuspid (valve) disease I08.3
　　　　active or acute I01.1
　　　　　with chorea (acute) (rheumatic) (Sydenham's) I02.0
　　　　rheumatic fever (conditions in I00)
　　　　　active — *see* Endocarditis, acute, rheumatic
　　　　　inactive or quiescent (with chorea) I05.9
　　　　tricuspid (valve) disease I08.1
　　　　　with aortic (valve) disease I08.3
　　　active or acute I01.1
　　　　with chorea (acute) (rheumatic) (Sydenham's) I02.0
　　　bacterial I33.0
　　　arteriosclerotic I34.8
　　　nonrheumatic I34.8
　　　　acute or subacute I33.9
　　　specified NEC I05.8
　monilial B37.6
　multiple valves I08.9
　　specified disorders I08.8
　mycotic (acute) (any valve) (subacute) I33.0
　pneumococcal (acute) (any valve) (subacute) I33.0
　pulmonary (chronic) (heart) (valve) I37.8
　　with rheumatic fever (conditions in I00)
　　　active — *see* Endocarditis, acute, rheumatic
　　　inactive or quiescent (with chorea) I09.89
　　　　with aortic, mitral or tricuspid disease I08.8
　　acute or subacute I33.9
　　　rheumatic I01.1
　　　　with chorea (acute) (rheumatic) (Sydenham's) I02.0
　　arteriosclerotic I37.8
　　congenital Q22.2
　　rheumatic (chronic) (inactive) (with chorea) I09.89
　　　active or acute I01.1
　　　　with chorea (acute) (rheumatic) (Sydenham's) I02.0
　　syphilitic A52.03
　purulent (acute) (any valve) (subacute) I33.0
　Q fever A78 [I39]
　rheumatic (chronic) (inactive) (with chorea) I09.1
　　active or acute (aortic) (mitral) (pulmonary) (tricuspid) I01.1
　　　with chorea (acute) (rheumatic) (Sydenham's) I02.0
　rheumatoid — *see* Rheumatoid, carditis
　septic (acute) (any valve) (subacute) I33.0
　streptococcal (acute) (any valve) (subacute) I33.0
　subacute — *see* Endocarditis, acute
　suppurative (acute) (any valve) (subacute) I33.0
　syphilitic A52.03
　toxic I33.9
　tricuspid (chronic) (heart) (inactive) (rheumatic) (valve) (with chorea) I07.9
　　with
　　　aortic (valve) disease I08.2
　　　　mitral (valve) disease I08.3
　　　mitral (valve) disease I08.1
　　　　aortic (valve) disease I08.3
　　　rheumatic fever (conditions in I00)
　　　　active — *see* Endocarditis, acute, rheumatic
　　　　inactive or quiescent (with chorea) I07.8
　　active or acute I01.1
　　　with chorea (acute) (rheumatic) (Sydenham's) I02.0
　　arteriosclerotic I36.8
　　nonrheumatic I36.8
　　　acute or subacute I33.9
　　specified cause, except rheumatic I36.8
　tuberculous — *see* Tuberculosis, endocarditis
　typhoid A01.02
　ulcerative (acute) (any valve) (subacute) I33.0
　vegetative (acute) (any valve) (subacute) I33.0
　verrucous (atypical) (nonbacterial) (nonrheumatic) M32.11
Endocardium, endocardial (*see also* condition)
　cushion defect Q21.2
Endocervicitis (*see also* Cervicitis)
　due to intrauterine (contraceptive) device T83.6 ☑
　hyperplastic N72
Endocrine — *see* condition
Endocrinopathy, pluriglandular E31.9
Endodontic
　overfill M27.52

Endodontic — *continued*
　underfill M27.53
Endodontitis K04.0
Endomastoiditis — *see* Mastoiditis
Endometrioma N80.9
Endometriosis N80.9
　appendix N80.5
　bladder N80.8
　bowel N80.5
　broad ligament N80.3
　cervix N80.0
　colon N80.5
　cul-de-sac (Douglas') N80.3
　exocervix N80.0
　fallopian tube N80.2
　female genital organ NEC N80.8
　gallbladder N80.8
　in scar of skin N80.6
　internal N80.0
　intestine N80.5
　lung N80.8
　myometrium N80.0
　ovary N80.1
　parametrium N80.3
　pelvic peritoneum N80.3
　peritoneal (pelvic) N80.3
　rectovaginal septum N80.4
　rectum N80.5
　round ligament N80.3
　skin (scar) N80.6
　specified site NEC N80.8
　stromal D39.0
　umbilicus N80.8
　uterus (internal) N80.0
　vagina N80.4
　vulva N80.8
Endometritis (decidual) (nonspecific) (purulent) (senile) (atrophic) (suppurative) N71.9
　with ectopic pregnancy O08.0
　acute N71.0
　blenorrhagic (gonococcal) (acute) (chronic) A54.24
　cervix, cervical (with erosion or ectropion) (*see also* Cervicitis)
　　hyperplastic N72
　chlamydial A56.11
　chronic N71.1
　following
　　abortion — *see* Abortion by type complicated by genital infection
　　ectopic or molar pregnancy O08.0
　gonococcal, gonorrheal (acute) (chronic) A54.24
　hyperplastic (*see also* Hyperplasia, endometrial) N85.00
　　cervix N72
　puerperal, postpartum, childbirth O86.12
　subacute N71.0
　tuberculous A18.17
Endometrium — *see* condition
Endomyocardiopathy, South African I42.3
Endomyocarditis — *see* Endocarditis
Endomyofibrosis I42.3
Endomyometritis — *see* Endometritis
Endopericarditis — *see* Endocarditis
Endoperineuritis — *see* Disorder, nerve
Endophlebitis — *see* Phlebitis
Endophthalmia — *see* Endophthalmitis, purulent
Endophthalmitis (acute) (infective) (metastatic) (subacute) H44.009
　bleb associated (*see also* Bleb, inflammed (infected), postprocedural H59.4 ☑
　gonorrheal A54.39
　in (due to)
　　cysticercosis B69.1
　　onchocerciasis B73.01
　　toxocariasis B83.0
　panuveitis — *see* Panuveitis
　parasitic H44.12- ☑
　purulent H44.00- ☑
　　panophthalmitis — *see* Panophthalmitis
　　vitreous abscess H44.02- ☑
　specified NEC H44.19
　sympathetic — *see* Uveitis, sympathetic
Endosalpingioma D28.2
Endosalpingiosis N94.89
Endosteitis — *see* Osteomyelitis
Endothelioma, bone — *see* Neoplasm, bone, malignant
Endotheliosis (hemorrhagic infectional) D69.8

Endotoxemia — code to condition
Endotrachelitis — *see* Cervicitis
Engelmann (-Camurati) **syndrome** Q78.3
English disease — *see* Rickets
Engman's disease L30.3
Engorgement
　breast N64.59
　　newborn P83.4
　　puerperal, postpartum O92.79
　lung (passive) — *see* Edema, lung
　pulmonary (passive) — *see* Edema, lung
　stomach K31.89
　venous, retina — *see* Occlusion, retina, vein, engorgement
Enlargement, enlarged (*see also* Hypertrophy)
　adenoids J35.2
　　with tonsils J35.3
　alveolar ridge K08.8
　　congenital — *see* Anomaly, alveolar
　apertures of diaphragm (congenital) Q79.1
　gingival K06.1
　heart, cardiac — *see* Hypertrophy, cardiac
　lacrimal gland, chronic H04.03- ☑
　liver — *see* Hypertrophy, liver
　lymph gland or node R59.9
　　generalized R59.1
　　localized R59.0
　orbit H05.34- ☑
　organ or site, congenital NEC — *see* Anomaly, by site
　parathyroid (gland) E21.0
　pituitary fossa R93.0
　prostate N40.0
　　with lower urinary tract symptoms (LUTS) N40.1
　　without lower urinary tract symptoms (LUTS) N40.0
　sella turcica R93.0
　spleen — *see* Splenomegaly
　thymus (gland) (congenital) E32.0
　thyroid (gland) — *see* Goiter
　tongue K14.8
　tonsils J35.1
　　with adenoids J35.3
　uterus N85.2
Enophthalmos H05.40- ☑
　due to
　　orbital tissue atrophy H05.41- ☑
　　trauma or surgery H05.42- ☑
Enostosis M27.8
Entamebic, entamebiasis — *see* Amebiasis
Entanglement
　umbilical cord(s) O69.2 ☑
　　with compression O69.2 ☑
　　　without compression O69.82 ☑
　　around neck (with compression) O69.1 ☑
　　　without compression O69.81 ☑
　　of twins in monoamniotic sac O69.2 ☑
Enteralgia — *see* Pain, abdominal
Enteric — *see* condition
Enteritis (acute) (diarrheal) (hemorrhagic) (noninfective) (septic) K52.9
　adenovirus A08.2
　aertrycke infection A02.0
　allergic K52.2
　ambic (acute) A06.0
　　with abscess — *see* Abscess, amebic
　　chronic A06.1
　　　with abscess — *see* Abscess, amebic
　　　nondysenteric A06.2
　　nondysenteric A06.2
　astrovirus A08.32
　bacillary NOS A03.9
　bacterial A04.9
　　specified NEC A04.8
　calicivirus A08.31
　candidal B37.82
　Chilomastix A07.8
　choleriformis A00.1
　chronic (noninfective) K52.9
　　ulcerative — *see* Colitis, ulcerative
　cicatrizing (chronic) — *see* Enteritis, regional, small intestine
　Clostridium
　　botulinum (food poisoning) A05.1
　　difficile A04.7
　coccidial A07.3
　coxsackie virus A08.39
　dietetic K52.2
　drug-induced K52.1

Enteritis — continued
due to
astrovirus A08.32
calicivirus A08.31
coxsackie virus A08.39
drugs K52.1
echovirus A08.39
enterovirus NEC A08.39
food hypersensitivity K52.2
infectious organism (bacterial) (viral) — see Enteritis, infectious
torovirus A08.39
Yersinia enterocolitica A04.6
echovirus A08.39
eltor A00.1
enterovirus NEC A08.39
eosinophilic K52.81
epidemic (infectious) A09
fulminant K55.0
gangrenous — see Enteritis, infectious
giardial A07.1
infectious NOS A09
due to
adenovirus A08.2
Aerobacter aerogenes A04.8
Arizona (bacillus) A02.0
bacteria NOS A04.9
specified NEC A04.8
Campylobacter A04.5
Clostridium difficile A04.7
Clostridium perfringens A04.8
Enterobacter aerogenes A04.8
enterovirus A08.39
Escherichia coli A04.4
enteroaggregative A04.4
enterohemorrhagic A04.3
enteroinvasive A04.2
enteropathogenic A04.0
enterotoxigenic A04.1
specified NEC A04.4
specified
bacteria NEC A04.8
virus NEC A08.39
Staphylococcus A04.8
virus NEC A08.4
specified type NEC A08.39
Yersinia enterocolitica A04.6
specified organism NEC A08.8
influenzal — see Influenza, with, digestive manifestations
ischemic K55.9
acute K55.0
chronic K55.1
microsporidial A07.8
mucomembranous, myxomembranous — see Syndrome, irritable bowel
mucous — see Syndrome, irritable bowel
necroticans A05.2
necrotizing of newborn — see Enterocolitis, necrotizing, in newborn
neurogenic — see Syndrome, irritable bowel
newborn necrotizing — see Enterocolitis, necrotizing, in newborn
noninfectious K52.9
norovirus A08.11
parasitic NEC B82.9
paratyphoid (fever) — see Fever, paratyphoid
protozoal A07.9
specified NEC A07.8
radiation K52.0
regional (of) K50.90
with
complication K50.919
abscess K50.914
fistula K50.913
intestinal obstruction K50.912
rectal bleeding K50.911
specified complication NEC K50.918
colon — see Enteritis, regional, large intestine
duodenum — see Enteritis, regional, small intestine
ileum — see Enteritis, regional, small intestine
jejunum — see Enteritis, regional, small intestine
large bowel — see Enteritis, regional, large intestine
large intestine (colon) (rectum) K50.10
with
complication K50.119
abscess K50.114

Enteritis — continued
regional — continued
large intestine — continued
with — continued
complication — continued
fistula K50.113
intestinal obstruction K50.112
rectal bleeding K50.111
small intestine (duodenum) (ileum) (jejunum) involvement K50.80
with
complication K50.819
abscess K50.814
fistula K50.813
intestinal obstruction K50.812
rectal bleeding K50.811
specified complication NEC K50.818
specified complication NEC K50.118
rectum — see Enteritis, regional, large intestine
small intestine (duodenum) (ileum) (jejunum) K50.00
with
complication K50.019
abscess K50.014
fistula K50.013
intestinal obstruction K50.012
large intestine (colon) (rectum) involvement K50.80
with
complication K50.819
abscess K50.814
fistula K50.813
intestinal obstruction K50.812
rectal bleeding K50.811
specified complication NEC K50.818
rectal bleeding K50.011
specified complication NEC K50.018
rotaviral A08.0
Salmonella, salmonellosis (arizonae) (cholerae-suis) (enteritidis) (typhimurium) A02.0
segmental — see Enteritis, regional
septic A09
Shigella — see Infection, Shigella
small round structured NEC A08.19
spasmodic, spastic — see Syndrome, irritable bowel
staphylococcal A04.8
due to food A05.0
torovirus A08.39
toxic NEC K52.1
due to Clostridium difficile A04.7
trichomonal A07.8
tuberculous A18.32
typhosa A01.00
ulcerative (chronic) — see Colitis, ulcerative
viral A08.4
adenovirus A08.2
enterovirus A08.39
Rotavirus A08.0
small round structured NEC A08.19
specified NEC A08.39
virus specified NEC A08.39
Enterobiasis B80
Enterobius vermicularis (infection) (infestation) B80
Enterocele (see also Hernia, abdomen)
pelvic, pelvis (acquired) (congenital) N81.5
vagina, vaginal (acquired) (congenital) NEC N81.5
Enterocolitis (see also Enteritis) K52.9
due to Clostridium difficile A04.7
fulminant ischemic K55.0
granulomatous — see Enteritis, regional
hemorrhagic (acute) K55.0
chronic K55.1
infectious NEC A09
ischemic K55.9
necrotizing
due to Clostridium difficile A04.7
in newborn P77.9
stage 1 (without pneumatosis, without perforation) P77.1
stage 2 (with pneumatosis, without perforation) P77.2
stage 3 (with pneumatosis, with perforation) P77.3
noninfectious K52.9
newborn — see Enterocolitis, necrotizing, in newborn

Enterocolitis — continued
pseudomembranous (newborn) A04.7
radiation K52.0
newborn — see Enterocolitis, necrotizing, in newborn
ulcerative (chronic) — see Pancolitis, ulcerative (chronic)
Enterogastritis — see Enteritis
Enteropathy K63.9
gluten-sensitive K90.0
hemorrhagic, terminal K55.0
protein-losing K90.4
Enteroperitonitis — see Peritonitis
Enteroptosis K63.4
Enterorrhagia K92.2
Enterospasm (see also Syndrome, irritable, bowel)
psychogenic F45.8
Enterostenosis (see also Obstruction, intestine) K56.69
Enterostomy
complication — see Complication, enterostomy
status Z93.4
Enterovirus, as cause of disease classified elsewhere
B97.10
coxsackievirus B97.11
echovirus B97.12
other specified B97.19
Enthesopathy (peripheral) M77.9
Achilles tendinitis — see Tendinitis, Achilles
ankle and tarsus M77.9
specified type NEC — see Enthesopathy, foot, specified type NEC
anterior tibial syndrome M76.81- ☑
calcaneal spur — see Spur, bone, calcaneal
elbow region M77.8
lateral epicondylitis — see Epicondylitis, lateral
medial epicondylitis — see Epicondylitis, medial
foot NEC M77.9
metatarsalgia — see Metatarsalgia
specified type NEC M77.5- ☑
forearm M77.9
gluteal tendinitis — see Tendinitis, gluteal
hand M77.9
hip — see Enthesopathy, lower limb, specified type NEC
iliac crest spur — see Spur, bone, iliac crest
iliotibial band syndrome — see Syndrome, iliotibial band
knee — see Enthesopathy, lower limb, lower leg, specified type NEC
lateral epicondylitis — see Epicondylitis, lateral
lower limb (excluding foot) M76.9
Achilles tendinitis — see Tendinitis, Achilles
anterior tibial syndrome M76.81- ☑
gluteal tendinitis — see Tendinitis, gluteal
iliac crest spur — see Spur, bone, iliac crest
iliotibial band syndrome — see Syndrome, iliotibial band
patellar tendinitis — see Tendinitis, patellar
pelvic region — see Enthesopathy, lower limb, specified type NEC
peroneal tendinitis — see Tendinitis, peroneal
posterior tibial syndrome M76.82- ☑
psoas tendinitis — see Tendinitis, psoas
shoulder M77.9
specified type NEC M76.89- ☑
tibial collateral bursitis — see Bursitis, tibial collateral
medial epicondylitis — see Epicondylitis, medial
metatarsalgia — see Metatarsalgia
multiple sites M77.9
patellar tendinitis — see Tendinitis, patellar
pelvis M77.9
periarthritis of wrist — see Periarthritis, wrist
peroneal tendinitis — see Tendinitis, peroneal
posterior tibial syndrome M76.82- ☑
psoas tendinitis — see Tendinitis, psoas
shoulder region — see Lesion, shoulder
specified site NEC M77.9
specified type NEC M77.8
spinal M46.00
cervical region M46.02
cervicothoracic region M46.03
lumbar region M46.06
lumbosacral region M46.07
multiple sites M46.09
occipito-atlanto-axial region M46.01
sacrococcygeal region M46.08

Epilepsy, epileptic, epilepsia — *continued*
  partialis continua (*see also* Kozhevnikof's epilepsy)
    G40.1- ☑
  peripheral — *see* Epilepsy, specified NEC
  procursiva — *see* Epilepsy, localization-related,
    symptomatic, with simple partial seizures
  progressive (familial) myoclonic — *see* Epilepsy, gen-
    eralized, idiopathic
  reflex — *see* Epilepsy, specified NEC
  related to
    alcohol G40.509
      not intractable G40.509
        with status epilepticus G40.501
        without status epliepticus G40.509
    drugs G40.509
      not intractable G40.509
        with status epilepticus G40.501
        without status epliepticus G40.509
    external causes G40.509
      not intractable G40.509
        with status epilepticus G40.501
        without status epliepticus G40.509
    hormonal changes G40.509
      not intractable G40.509
        with status epilepticus G40.501
        without status epliepticus G40.509
    sleep deprivation G40.509
      not intractable G40.509
        with status epilepticus G40.501
        without status epliepticus G40.509
    stress G40.509
      not intractable G40.509
        with status epilepticus G40.501
        without status epliepticus G40.509
  somatomotor — *see* Epilepsy, localization-related,
    symptomatic, with simple partial seizures
  somatosensory — *see* Epilepsy, localization-related,
    symptomatic, with simple partial seizures
  spasms G40.822
    intractable G40.824
      with status epilepticus G40.823
      without status epilepticus G40.824
    not intractable G40.822
      with status epilepticus G40.821
      without status epilepticus G40.822
  specified NEC G40.802
    intractable G40.804
      with status epilepticus G40.803
      without status epilepticus G40.804
    not intractable G40.802
      with status epilepticus G40.801
      without status epilepticus G40.802
  syndromes
    generalized
      idiopathic G40.309
        intractable G40.319
          with status epilepticus G40.311
          without status epilepticus G40.319
        not intractable G40.309
          with status epilepticus G40.301
          without status epilepticus G40.309
      specified NEC G40.409
        intractable G40.419
          with status epilepticus G40.411
          without status epilepticus G40.419
        not intractable G40.409
          with status epilepticus G40.401
          without status epilepticus G40.409
    localization-related (focal) (partial)
      idiopathic G40.009
        with seizures of localized onset G40.009
          intractable G40.019
            with status epilepticus G40.011
            without status epilepticus G40.019
          not intractable G40.009
            with status epilepticus G40.001
            without status epilepticus G40.009
      symptomatic
        with complex partial seizures G40.209
          intractable G40.219
            with status epilepticus G40.211
            without status epilepticus G40.219
          not intractable G40.209
            with status epilepticus G40.201
            without status epilepticus G40.209
        with simple partial seizures G40.109
          intractable G40.119
            with status epilepticus G40.111

Epilepsy, epileptic, epilepsia — *continued*
  syndromes — *continued*
    localization-related — *continued*
      symptomatic — *continued*
        with simple partial seizures — *continued*
          intractable — *continued*
            without status epilepticus G40.119
          not intractable G40.109
            with status epilepticus G40.101
            without status epilepticus G40.109
      specified NEC G40.802
        intractable G40.804
          with status epilepticus G40.803
          without status epilepticus G40.804
        not intractable G40.802
          with status epilepticus G40.801
          without status epilepticus G40.802
    tonic (-clonic) — *see* Epilepsy, generalized, specified
      NEC
    twilight F05
    uncinate (gyrus) — *see* Epilepsy, localization-related,
      symptomatic, with complex partial seizures
    Unverricht (-Lundborg) (familial myoclonic) — *see*
      Epilepsy, generalized, idiopathic
    visceral — *see* Epilepsy, specified NEC
    visual — *see* Epilepsy, specified NEC
Epiloia Q85.1
Epimenorrhea N92.0
Epipharyngitis — *see* Nasopharyngitis
Epiphora H04.20- ☑
  due to
    excess lacrimation H04.21- ☑
    insufficient drainage H04.22- ☑
Epiphyseal arrest — *see* Arrest, epiphyseal
Epiphyseolysis, epiphysiolysis — *see* Osteochondropa-
  thy
Epiphysitis (*see also* Osteochondropathy)
  juvenile M92.9
  syphilitic (congenital) A50.02
Epiplocele — *see* Hernia, abdomen
Epiploitis — *see* Peritonitis
Epiplosarcomphalocele — *see* Hernia, umbilicus
Episcleritis (suppurative) H15.10- ☑
  in (due to)
    syphilis A52.71
    tuberculosis A18.51
  nodular H15.12- ☑
  periodica fugax H15.11- ☑
    angioneurotic — *see* Edema, angioneurotic
  syphilitic (late) A52.71
  tuberculous A18.51
Episode
  affective, mixed F39
  depersonalization (in neurotic state) F48.1
  depressive F32.9
    major F32.9
      mild F32.0
      moderate F32.1
      severe (without psychotic symptoms) F32.2
        with psychotic symptoms F32.3
      recurrent F33.9
        brief F33.8
      specified NEC F32.8
  hypomanic F30.8
  manic F30.9
    with
      psychotic symptoms F30.2
      remission (full) F30.4
        partial F30.3
    without psychotic symptoms F30.10
      mild F30.11
      moderate F30.12
      severe (without psychotic symptoms) F30.13
        with psychotic symptoms F30.2
    other specified F30.8
    recurrent F31.89
  psychotic F23
    organic F06.8
  schizophrenic (acute) NEC, brief F23
Epispadias (female) (male) Q64.0
Episplenitis D73.89
Epistaxis (multiple) R04.0
  hereditary I78.0
  vicarious menstruation N94.89
Epithelioma (malignant) (*see also* Neoplasm, malignant,
  by site)
  adenoides cysticum — *see* Neoplasm, skin, benign
  basal cell — *see* Neoplasm, skin, malignant

Epithelioma — *continued*
  benign — *see* Neoplasm, benign, by site
  Bowen's — *see* Neoplasm, skin, in situ
  calcifying, of Malherbe — *see* Neoplasm, skin, benign
  external site — *see* Neoplasm, skin, malignant
  intraepidermal, Jadassohn — *see* Neoplasm, skin, be-
    nign
  squamous cell — *see* Neoplasm, malignant, by site
Epitheliomatosis pigmented Q82.1
Epitheliopathy, multifocal placoid pigment
  H30.14- ☑
Epithelium, epithelial — *see* condition
Epituberculosis (with atelectasis) (allergic) A15.7
Eponychia Q84.6
Epstein's
  nephrosis or syndrome — *see* Nephrosis
  pearl K09.8
Epulis (gingiva) (fibrous) (giant cell) K06.8
Equinia A24.0
Equinovarus (congenital) (talipes) Q66.0
  acquired — *see* Deformity, limb, clubfoot
Equivalent
  convulsive (abdominal) — *see* Epilepsy, specified NEC
  epileptic (psychic) — *see* Epilepsy, localization-related,
    symptomatic, with complex partial seizures
Erb (-Duchenne) **paralysis** (birth injury) (newborn) P14.0
Erb-Goldflam disease or syndrome G70.00
  with exacerbation (acute) G70.01
  in crisis G70.01
Erb's
  disease G71.0
  palsy, paralysis (brachial) (birth) (newborn) P14.0
    spinal (spastic) syphilitic A52.17
  pseudohypertrophic muscular dystrophy G71.0
Erdheim's syndrome (acromegalic macrospondylitis)
  E22.0
Erection, painful (persistent) — *see* Priapism
Ergosterol deficiency (vitamin D) E55.9
  with
    adult osteomalacia M83.8
    rickets — *see* Rickets
Ergotism (*see also* Poisoning, food, noxious, plant)
  from ergot used as drug (migraine therapy) — *see*
    Table of Drugs and Chemicals
Erosio interdigitalis blastomycetica B37.2
Erosion
  artery I77.2
    without rupture I77.89
  bone — *see* Disorder, bone, density and structure,
    specified NEC
  bronchus J98.09
  cartilage (joint) — *see* Disorder, cartilage, specified
    type NEC
  cervix (uteri) (acquired) (chronic) (congenital) N86
    with cervicitis N72
  cornea (nontraumatic) — *see* Ulcer, cornea
    recurrent H18.83- ☑
    traumatic — *see* Abrasion, cornea
  dental (idiopathic) (occupational) (due to diet, drugs
    or vomiting) K03.2
  duodenum, postpyloric — *see* Ulcer, duodenum
  esophagus K22.10
    with bleeding K22.11
  gastric — *see* Ulcer, stomach
  gastrojejunal — *see* Ulcer, gastrojejunal
  implanted mesh — *see* Complications, mesh
  intestine K63.3
  lymphatic vessel I89.8
  pylorus, pyloric (ulcer) — *see* Ulcer, stomach
  spine, aneurysmal A52.09
  stomach — *see* Ulcer, stomach
  teeth (idiopathic) (occupational) (due to diet, drugs
    or vomiting) K03.2
  urethra N36.8
  uterus N85.8
Erotomania F52.8
Error
  metabolism, inborn — *see* Disorder, metabolism
  refractive — *see* Disorder, refraction
Eructation R14.2
  nervous or psychogenic F45.8
Eruption
  creeping B76.9
  drug (generalized) (taken internally) L27.0
    fixed L27.1
    in contact with skin — *see* Dermatitis, due to drugs
    localized L27.1

  ☑ **Additional Character Required** — Refer to the Tabular List for Character Selection   🔻 **Subterms under main terms may continue to next column or page**

Eruption — continued
  Hutchinson, summer L56.4
  Kaposi's varicelliform B00.0
  napkin L22
  polymorphous light (sun) L56.4
  recalcitrant pustular L13.8
  ringed R23.8
  skin (nonspecific) R21
    creeping (meaning hookworm) B76.9
    due to inoculation/vaccination (generalized) (see
      also Dermatitis, due to, vaccine) L27.0
        localized L27.1
    erysipeloid A26.0
    feigned L98.1
    Kaposi's varicelliform B00.0
    lichenoid L28.0
    meaning dermatitis — see Dermatitis
    toxic NEC L53.0
  tooth, teeth, abnormal (incomplete) (late) (premature)
    (sequence) K00.6
  vesicular R23.8
Erysipelas (gangrenous) (infantile) (newborn) (phleg-
    monous) (suppurative) A46
  external ear A46 [H62.40]
  puerperal, postpartum O86.89
Erysipeloid A26.9
  cutaneous (Rosenbach's) A26.0
  disseminated A26.8
  sepsis A26.7
  specified NEC A26.8
Erythema, erythematous (infectional) (inflammation)
    L53.9
  ab igne L59.0
  annulare (centrifugum) (rheumaticum) L53.1
  arthriticum epidemicum A25.1
  brucellum — see Brucellosis
  chronic figurate NEC L53.3
  chronicum migrans (Borrelia burgdorferi) A69.20
  diaper L22
  due to
    chemical NEC L53.0
      in contact with skin L24.5
    drug (internal use) — see Dermatitis, due to, drugs
  elevatum diutinum L95.1
  endemic E52
  epidemic, arthritic A25.1
  figuratum perstans L53.3
  gluteal L22
  heat — code by site under Burn, first degree
  ichthyosiforme congenitum bullous Q80.3
  in diseases classified elsewhere L54
  induratum (nontuberculous) L52
    tuberculous A18.4
  infectiosum B08.3
  intertrigo L30.4
  iris L51.9
  marginatum L53.2
    in (due to) acute rheumatic fever I00
  medicamentosum — see Dermatitis, due to, drugs
  migrans A26.0
    chronicum A69.20
    tongue K14.1
  multiforme (major) (minor) L51.9
    bullous, bullosum L51.1
    conjunctiva L51.1
    nonbullous L51.0
    pemphigoides L12.0
    specified NEC L51.8
  napkin L22
  neonatorum P83.8
    toxic P83.1
  nodosum L52
    tuberculous A18.4
  palmar L53.8
  pernio T69.1 ☑
  rash, newborn P83.8
  scarlatiniform (recurrent) (exfoliative) L53.8
  solare L55.0
  specified NEC L53.8
  toxic, toxicum NEC L53.0
    newborn P83.1
  tuberculous (primary) A18.4
Erythematous, erythematosus — see condition
Erythermalgia (primary) I73.81
Erythralgia I73.81
Erythrasma L08.1
Erythredema (polyneuropathy) — see Poisoning, mer-
    cury

Erythremia (acute) C94.0- ☑
  chronic D45
  secondary D75.1
Erythroblastopenia (see also Aplasia, red cell) D60.9
  congenital D61.01
Erythroblastophthisis D61.09
Erythroblastosis (fetalis) (newborn) P55.9
  due to
    ABO (antibodies) (incompatibility) (isoimmuniza-
      tion) P55.1
    Rh (antibodies) (incompatibility) (isoimmunization)
      P55.0
Erythrocyanosis (crurum) I73.89
Erythrocythemia — see Erythremia
Erythrocytosis (megalosplenic) (secondary) D75.1
  familial D75.0
  oval, hereditary — see Elliptocytosis
  secondary D75.1
  stress D75.1
Erythroderma (secondary) (see also Erythema) L53.9
  bullous ichthyosiform, congenital Q80.3
  desquamativum L21.1
  ichthyosiform, congenital (bullous) Q80.3
  neonatorum P83.8
  psoriaticum L40.8
Erythrodysesthesia, palmar plantar (PPE) L27.1
Erythrogenesis imperfecta D61.09
Erythroleukemia C94.0- ☑
Erythromelalgia I73.81
Erythrophagocytosis D75.89
Erythrophobia F40.298
Erythroplakia, oral epithelium, and tongue K13.29
Erythroplasia (Queyrat) D07.4
  specified site — see Neoplasm, skin, in situ
  unspecified site D07.4
Escherichia coli (E. coli), **as cause of disease classified**
    elsewhere B96.20
  non-O157 Shiga toxin-producing (with known O
    group) B96.22
  non-Shiga toxin-producing B96.29
  O157 B96.21
  O157 with confirmation of Shiga toxin when H antigen
    is unknown, or is not H7 B96.21
  O157:H- (nonmotile) with confirmation of Shiga toxin
    B96.21
  O157:H7 with or without confirmation of Shiga toxin-
    production B96.21
    specified NEC B96.22
  Shiga toxin-producing (with unspecified O group)
    (STEC) B96.23
  specified NEC B96.29
Esophagismus K22.4
Esophagitis (acute) (alkaline) (chemical) (chronic) (infec-
    tional) (necrotic) (peptic) (postoperative) K20.9
  candidal B37.81
  due to gastrointestinal reflux disease K21.0
  eosinophilic K20.0
  reflux K21.0
  specified NEC K20.8
  tuberculous A18.83
  ulcerative K22.10
    with bleeding K22.11
Esophagocele K22.5
Esophagomalacia K22.8
Esophagospasm K22.4
Esophagostenosis K22.2
Esophagostomiasis B81.8
Esophagotracheal — see condition
Esophagus — see condition
Esophoria H50.51
  convergence, excess H51.12
  divergence, insufficiency H51.8
Esotropia — see Strabismus, convergent concomitant
Espundia B55.2
Essential — see condition
Esthesioneuroblastoma C30.0
Esthesioneurocytoma C30.0
Esthesioneuroepithelioma C30.0
Esthiomene A55
Estivo-autumnal malaria (fever) B50.9
Estrangement (marital) Z63.5
  parent-child NEC Z62.890
Estriasis — see Myiasis
Ethanolism — see Alcoholism
Etherism — see Dependence, drug, inhalant
Ethmoid, ethmoidal — see condition

Ethmoiditis (chronic) (nonpurulent) (purulent) (see also
    Sinusitis, ethmoidal)
  influenzal — see Influenza, with, respiratory manifes-
    tations NEC
  Woakes' J33.1
Ethylism — see Alcoholism
Eulenburg's disease (congenital paramyotonia) G71.19
Eumycetoma B47.0
Eunuchoidism E29.1
  hypogonadotropic E23.0
European blastomycosis — see Cryptococcosis
Eustachian — see condition
Evaluation (for) (of)
  development state
    adolescent Z00.3
    period of
      delayed growth in childhood Z00.70
        with abnormal findings Z00.71
      rapid growth in childhood Z00.2
    puberty Z00.3
  growth and developmental state (period of rapid
    growth) Z00.2
  delayed growth Z00.70
    with abnormal findings Z00.71
  mental health (status) Z00.8
    requested by authority Z04.6
  period of
    delayed growth in childhood Z00.70
      with abnormal findings Z00.71
    rapid growth in childhood Z00.2
  suspected condition — see Observation
Evans syndrome D69.41
Event, apparent life threatening in newborn and
    infant (ALTE) R68.13
Eventration (see also Hernia, ventral)
  colon into chest — see Hernia, diaphragm
  diaphragm (congenital) Q79.1
Eversion
  bladder N32.89
  cervix (uteri) N86
    with cervicitis N72
  foot NEC (see also Deformity, valgus, ankle)
    congenital Q66.6
  punctum lacrimale (postinfectional) (senile) H04.52- ☑
  ureter (meatus) N28.89
  urethra (meatus) N36.8
  uterus N81.4
Evidence
  cytologic
    of malignancy on anal smear R85.614
    of malignancy on cervical smear R87.614
    of malignancy on vaginal smear R87.624
Evisceration
  birth injury P15.8
  traumatic NEC
    eye — see Enucleated eye
Evulsion — see Avulsion
Ewing's sarcoma or tumor — see Neoplasm, bone,
    malignant
Examination (for) (following) (general) (of) (routine)
    Z00.00-
  with abnormal findings Z00.01
  abuse, physical (alleged), ruled out
    adult Z04.71
    child Z04.72
  adolescent (development state) Z00.3
  alleged rape or sexual assault (victim), ruled out
    adult Z04.41
    child Z04.42
  allergy Z01.82
  annual (adult) (periodic) (physical) Z00.00
    with abnormal findings Z00.01
    gynecological Z01.419
      with abnormal findings Z01.411
  antibody response Z01.84
  blood — see Examination, laboratory
  blood pressure Z01.30
    with abnormal findings Z01.31
  cancer staging — see Neoplasm, malignant, by site
  cervical Papanicolaou smear Z12.4
    as part of routine gynecological examination
      Z01.419
      with abnormal findings Z01.411
  child (over 28 days old) Z00.129
    with abnormal findings Z00.121
    under 28 days old — see Newborn, examination
  clinical research control or normal comparison (con-
    trol) (participant) Z00.6

Examination — *continued*
  contraceptive (drug) maintenance (routine) Z30.8
    device (intrauterine) Z30.431
  dental Z01.20
    with abnormal findings Z01.21
  developmental — *see* Examination, child
  donor (potential) Z00.5
  ear Z01.10
    with abnormal findings NEC Z01.118
  eye Z01.00
    with abnormal findings Z01.01
  follow-up (routine) (following) Z09
    chemotherapy NEC Z09
      malignant neoplasm Z08
    fracture Z09
    malignant neoplasm Z08
    postpartum Z39.2
    psychotherapy Z09
    radiotherapy NEC Z09
      malignant neoplasm Z08
    surgery NEC Z09
      malignant neoplasm Z08
  following
    accident NEC Z04.3
      transport Z04.1
      work Z04.2
    assault, alleged, ruled out
      adult Z04.71
      child Z04.72
    motor vehicle accident Z04.1
    treatment (for) Z09
      combined NEC Z09
        fracture Z09
        malignant neoplasm Z08
      malignant neoplasm Z08
      mental disorder Z09
      specified condition NEC Z09
  gynecological Z01.419
    with abnormal findings Z01.411
    for contraceptive maintenance Z30.8
  health — *see* Examination, medical
  hearing Z01.10
    with abnormal findings NEC Z01.118
    following failed hearing screening Z01.110
  immunity status testing Z01.84
  laboratory (as part of a general medical examination) Z00.00
    with abnormal findings Z00.01
    preprocedural Z01.812
  lactating mother Z39.1
  medical (adult) (for) (of) Z00.00
    with abnormal findings Z00.01
    administrative purpose only Z02.9
      specified NEC Z02.89
    admission to
      armed forces Z02.3
      old age home Z02.2
      prison Z02.89
      residential institution Z02.2
      school Z02.0
        following illness or medical treatment Z02.0
      summer camp Z02.89
    adoption Z02.82
    blood alcohol or drug level Z02.83
    camp (summer) Z02.89
    clinical research, normal subject (control) (participant) Z00.6
    control subject in clinical research (normal comparison) (participant) Z00.6
    donor (potential) Z00.5
    driving license Z02.4
    general (adult) Z00.00
      with abnormal findings Z00.01
    immigration Z02.89
    insurance purposes Z02.6
    marriage Z02.89
    medicolegal reasons NEC Z04.8
    naturalization Z02.89
    participation in sport Z02.5
    paternity testing Z02.81
    population survey Z00.8
    pre-employment Z02.1
    pre-operative — *see* Examination, pre-procedural
    pre-procedural
      cardiovascular Z01.810
      respiratory Z01.811
      specified NEC Z01.818

Examination — *continued*
  medical — *continued*
    preschool children
      for admission to school Z02.0
    prisoners
      for entrance into prison Z02.89
    recruitment for armed forces Z02.3
    specified NEC Z00.8
    sport competition Z02.5
  medicolegal reason NEC Z04.8
  newborn — *see* Newborn, examination
  pelvic (annual) (periodic) Z01.419
    with abnormal findings Z01.411
  period of rapid growth in childhood Z00.2
  periodic (adult) (annual) (routine) Z00.00
    with abnormal findings Z00.01
  physical (adult) (*see also* Examination, medical) Z00.00
    sports Z02.5
  postpartum
    immediately after delivery Z39.0
    routine follow-up Z39.2
  pre-chemotherapy (antineoplastic) Z01.818
  pre-procedural (pre-operative)
    cardiovascular Z01.810
    laboratory Z01.812
    respiratory Z01.811
    specified NEC Z01.818
  prenatal (normal pregnancy) (*see also* Pregnancy, normal) Z34.9- ☑
  prior to chemotherapy (antineoplastic) Z01.818
  psychiatric NEC Z00.8
    follow-up not needing further care Z09
    requested by authority Z04.6
  radiological (as part of a general medical examination) Z00.00
    with abnormal findings Z00.01
  repeat cervical smear to confirm findings of recent normal smear following initial abnormal smear Z01.42
  skin (hypersensitivity) Z01.82
  special (*see also* Examination, by type) Z01.89
    specified type NEC Z01.89
  specified type or reason NEC Z04.8
  teeth Z01.20
    with abnormal findings Z01.21
  urine — *see* Examination, laboratory
  vision Z01.00
    with abnormal findings Z01.01
Exanthem, exanthema (*see also* Rash)
  with enteroviral vesicular stomatitis B08.4
  Boston A88.0
  epidemic with meningitis A88.0 [G02]
  subitum B08.20
    due to human herpesvirus 6 B08.21
    due to human herpesvirus 7 B08.22
  viral, virus B09
    specified type NEC B08.8
Excess, excessive, excessively
  alcohol level in blood R78.0
  androgen (ovarian) E28.1
  attrition, tooth, teeth K03.0
  carotene, carotin (dietary) E67.1
  cold, effects of T69.9 ☑
    specified effect NEC T69.8 ☑
  convergence H51.12
  crying
    in child, adolescent, or adult R45.83
    in infant R68.11
  development, breast N62
  divergence H51.8
  drinking (alcohol) NEC (without dependence) F10.10
    habitual (continual) (without remission) F10.20
  eating R63.2
  estrogen E28.0
  fat (*see also* Obesity)
    in heart — *see* Degeneration, myocardial
    localized E65
  foreskin N47.8
  gas R14.0
  glucagon E16.3
  heat — *see* Heat
  intermaxillary vertical dimension of fully erupted teeth M26.37
  interocclusal distance of fully erupted teeth M26.37
  kalium E87.5
  large
    colon K59.3
      congenital Q43.8

Excess, excessive, excessively — *continued*
  large — *continued*
    infant P08.0
    organ or site, congenital NEC — *see* Anomaly, by site
  long
    organ or site, congenital NEC — *see* Anomaly, by site
  menstruation (with regular cycle) N92.0
    with irregular cycle N92.1
  napping Z72.821
  natrium E87.0
  number of teeth K00.1
  nutrient (dietary) NEC R63.2
  potassium (K) E87.5
  salivation K11.7
  secretion (*see also* Hypersecretion)
    milk O92.6
    sputum R09.3
    sweat R61
  sexual drive F52.8
  short
    organ or site, congenital NEC — *see* Anomaly, by site
    umbilical cord in labor or delivery O69.3 ☑
  skin, eyelid (acquired) — *see* Blepharochalasis
    congenital Q10.3
  sodium (Na) E87.0
  spacing of fully erupted teeth M26.32
  sputum R09.3
  sweating R61
  thirst R63.1
    due to deprivation of water T73.1 ☑
  tuberosity of jaw M26.07
  vitamin
    A (dietary) E67.0
      administered as drug (prolonged intake) — *see* Table of Drugs and Chemicals, vitamins, adverse effect
      overdose or wrong substance given or taken — *see* Table of Drugs and Chemicals, vitamins, poisoning
    D (dietary) E67.3
      administered as drug (prolonged intake) — *see* Table of Drugs and Chemicals, vitamins, adverse effect
      overdose or wrong substance given or taken — *see* Table of Drugs and Chemicals, vitamins, poisoning
  weight
    gain R63.5
    loss R63.4
Excitability, abnormal, under minor stress (personality disorder) F60.3
Excitation
  anomalous atrioventricular I45.6
  psychogenic F30.8
  reactive (from emotional stress, psychological trauma) F30.8
Excitement
  hypomanic F30.8
  manic F30.9
  mental, reactive (from emotional stress, psychological trauma) F30.8
  state, reactive (from emotional stress, psychological trauma) F30.8
Excoriation (traumatic) (*see also* Abrasion)
  neurotic L98.1
Exfoliation
  due to erythematous conditions according to extent of body surface involved L49.0
    less than 10 percent of body surface L49.0
    10-19 percent of body surface L49.1
    20-29 percent of body surface L49.2
    30-39 percent of body surface L49.3
    40-49 percent of body surface L49.4
    50-59 percent of body surface L49.5
    60-69 percent of body surface L49.6
    70-79 percent of body surface L49.7
    80-89 percent of body surface L49.8
    90-99 percent of body surface L49.9
  teeth, due to systemic causes K08.0
Exfoliative — *see* condition
Exhaustion, exhaustive (physical NEC) R53.83
  battle F43.0
  cardiac — *see* Failure, heart
  delirium F43.0

Exhaustion, exhaustive — *continued*
  due to
    cold T69.8 ☑
    excessive exertion T73.3 ☑
    exposure T73.2 ☑
    neurasthenia F48.8
  heart — *see* Failure, heart
  heat (*see also* Heat, exhaustion) T67.5 ☑
    due to
      salt depletion T67.4 ☑
      water depletion T67.3 ☑
  maternal, complicating delivery O75.81
  mental F48.8
  myocardium, myocardial — *see* Failure, heart
  nervous F48.8
  old age R54
  psychogenic F48.8
  psychosis F43.0
  senile R54
  vital NEC Z73.0
Exhibitionism F65.2
Exocervicitis — *see* Cervicitis
Exomphalos Q79.2
  meaning hernia — *see* Hernia, umbilicus
Exophoria H50.52
  convergence, insufficiency H51.11
  divergence, excess H51.8
Exophthalmos H05.2- ☑
  congenital Q15.8
  constant NEC H05.24- ☑
  displacement, globe — *see* Displacement, globe
  due to thyrotoxicosis (hyperthyroidism) — *see* Hyper-
    thyroidism, with, goiter (diffuse)
  dysthyroid — *see* Hyperthyroidism, with, goiter (dif-
    fuse)
  goiter — *see* Hyperthyroidism, with, goiter (diffuse)
  intermittent NEC H05.25- ☑
  malignant — *see* Hyperthyroidism, with, goiter (dif-
    fuse)
  orbital
    edema — *see* Edema, orbit
    hemorrhage — *see* Hemorrhage, orbit
  pulsating NEC H05.26- ☑
  thyrotoxic, thyrotropic — *see* Hyperthyroidism, with,
    goiter (diffuse)
Exostosis (*see also* Disorder, bone)
  cartilaginous — *see* Neoplasm, bone, benign
  congenital (multiple) Q78.6
  external ear canal H61.81- ☑
  gonococcal A54.49
  jaw (bone) M27.8
  multiple, congenital Q78.6
  orbit H05.35- ☑
  osteocartilaginous — *see* Neoplasm, bone, benign
  syphilitic A52.77
Exotropia — *see* Strabismus, divergent concomitant
Explanation of
  investigation finding Z71.2
  medication Z71.89
Exposure (to) (*see also* Contact, with) T75.89 ☑
  acariasis Z20.7
  AIDS virus Z20.6
  air pollution Z77.110
  algae and algae toxins Z77.121
  algae bloom Z77.121
  anthrax Z20.810
  aromatic amines Z77.020
  aromatic (hazardous) compounds NEC Z77.028
  aromatic dyes NOS Z77.028
  arsenic Z77.010
  asbestos Z77.090
  bacterial disease NEC Z20.818
  benzene Z77.021
  blue-green algae bloom Z77.121
  body fluids (potentially hazardous) Z77.21
  brown tide Z77.121
  chemicals (chiefly nonmedicinal) (hazardous) NEC
    Z77.098
  cholera Z20.09
  chromium compounds Z77.018
  cold, effects of T69.9 ☑
    specified effect NEC T69.8 ☑
  communicable disease Z20.9
    bacterial NEC Z20.818
    specified NEC Z20.89
    viral NEC Z20.828
  cyanobacteria bloom Z77.121

Exposure — *continued*
  disaster Z65.5
  discrimination Z60.5
  dyes Z77.098
  effects of T73.9 ☑
  environmental tobacco smoke (acute) (chronic) Z77.22
  Escherichia coli (E. coli) Z20.01
  exhaustion due to T73.2 ☑
  fiberglass — *see* Table of Drugs and Chemicals, fiber-
    glass
  German measles Z20.4
  gonorrhea Z20.2
  hazardous metals NEC Z77.018
  hazardous substances NEC Z77.29
  hazards in the physical environment NEC Z77.128
  hazards to health NEC Z77.9
  human immunodeficiency virus (HIV) Z20.6
  human T-lymphotropic virus type-1 (HTLV-1) Z20.89
  implanted
    mesh — *see* Complications, mesh
    prosthetic materials NEC — *see* Complications,
      prosthetic materials NEC
  infestation (parasitic) NEC Z20.7
  intestinal infectious disease NEC Z20.09
    Escherichia coli (E. coli) Z20.01
  lead Z77.011
  meningococcus Z20.811
  mold (toxic) Z77.120
  nickel dust Z77.018
  noise Z77.122
  occupational
    air contaminants NEC Z57.39
    dust Z57.2
    environmental tobacco smoke Z57.31
    extreme temperature Z57.6
    noise Z57.0
    radiation Z57.1
    risk factors Z57.9
      specified NEC Z57.8
    toxic agents (gases) (liquids) (solids) (vapors) in
      agriculture Z57.4
    toxic agents (gases) (liquids) (solids) (vapors) in
      industry NEC Z57.5
    vibration Z57.7
  parasitic disease NEC Z20.7
  pediculosis Z20.7
  persecution Z60.5
  pfiesteria piscicida Z77.121
  poliomyelitis Z20.89
  pollution
    air Z77.110
    environmental NEC Z77.118
    soil Z77.112
    water Z77.111
  polycyclic aromatic hydrocarbons Z77.028
  prenatal (drugs) (toxic chemicals) — *see* Newborn,
    affected by (suspected to be), noxious sub-
    stances transmitted via placenta or breast milk
  rabies Z20.3
  radiation, naturally occurring NEC Z77.123
  radon Z77.123
  red tide (Florida) Z77.121
  rubella Z20.4
  second hand tobacco smoke (acute) (chronic) Z77.22
    in the perinatal period P96.81
  sexually-transmitted disease Z20.2
  smallpox (laboratory) Z20.89
  syphilis Z20.2
  terrorism Z65.4
  torture Z65.4
  tuberculosis Z20.1
  uranium Z77.012
  varicella Z20.820
  venereal disease Z20.2
  viral disease NEC Z20.828
  war Z65.5
  water pollution Z77.111
Exsanguination — *see* Hemorrhage
Exstrophy
  abdominal contents Q45.8
  bladder Q64.10
    cloacal Q64.12
    specified type NEC Q64.19
    supravesical fissure Q64.11
Extensive — *see* condition
Extra (*see also* Accessory)
  marker chromosomes (normal individual) Q92.61
    in abnormal individual Q92.62

Extra — *continued*
  rib Q76.6
    cervical Q76.5
Extrasystoles (supraventricular) I49.49
  atrial I49.1
  auricular I49.1
  junctional I49.2
  ventricular I49.3
Extrauterine gestation or pregnancy — *see* Pregnancy, by site
Extravasation
  blood R58
  chyle into mesentery I89.8
  pelvicalyceal N13.8
  pyelosinus N13.8
  urine (from ureter) R39.0
  vesicant agent
    antineoplastic chemotherapy T80.810 ☑
    other agent NEC T80.818 ☑
Extremity — *see* condition, limb
Extrophy — *see* Exstrophy
Extroversion
  bladder Q64.19
  uterus N81.4
    complicating delivery O71.2
    postpartal (old) N81.4
Extruded tooth (teeth) M26.34
Extrusion
  breast implant (prosthetic) T85.42 ☑
  eye implant (globe) (ball) T85.328 ☑
  intervertebral disc — *see* Displacement, intervertebral
    disc
  ocular lens implant (prosthetic) — *see* Complications,
    intraocular lens
  vitreous — *see* Prolapse, vitreous
Exudate
  pleural — *see* Effusion, pleura
  retina H35.89
Exudative — *see* condition
Eye, eyeball, eyelid — *see* condition
Eyestrain — *see* Disturbance, vision, subjective
Eyeworm disease of Africa B74.3

F

Faber's syndrome (achlorhydric anemia) D50.9
Fabry (-Anderson) **disease** E75.21
Faciocephalalgia, autonomic (*see also* Neuropathy,
  peripheral, autonomic) G90.09
Factor(s)
  psychic, associated with diseases classified elsewhere
    F54
  psychological
    affecting physical conditions F54
    or behavioral
      affecting general medical condition F54
      associated with disorders or diseases classified
      elsewhere F54
Fahr disease (of brain) G23.8
Fahr Volhard disease (of kidney) I12.- ☑
Failure, failed
  abortion — *see* Abortion, attempted
  aortic (valve) I35.8
    rheumatic I06.8
  attempted abortion — *see* Abortion, attempted
  biventricular I50.9
  bone marrow — *see* Anemia, aplastic
  cardiac — *see* Failure, heart
  cardiorenal (chronic) I50.9
    hypertensive I13.2
  cardiorespiratory (*see also* Failure, heart) R09.2
  cardiovascular (chronic) — *see* Failure, heart
  cerebrovascular I67.9
  cervical dilatation in labor O62.0
  circulation, circulatory (peripheral) R57.9
    newborn P29.89
  compensation — *see* Disease, heart
  compliance with medical treatment or regimen — *see*
    Noncompliance
  congestive — *see* Failure, heart, congestive
  dental implant (endosseous) M27.69
    due to
      failure of dental prosthesis M27.63
      lack of attached gingiva M27.62
      occlusal trauma (poor prosthetic design)
        M27.62
      parafunctional habits M27.62

☑ **Additional Character Required — Refer to the Tabular List for Character Selection**   ▽ **Subterms under main terms may continue to next column or page**

Falling, falls — *continued*
  any organ or part — *see* Prolapse
Fallopian
  insufflation Z31.41
  tube — *see* condition
Fallot's
  pentalogy Q21.8
  tetrad or tetralogy Q21.3
  triad or trilogy Q22.3
False (*see also* condition)
  croup J38.5
  joint — *see* Nonunion, fracture
  labor (pains) O47.9
    at or after 37 completed weeks of gestation O47.1
    before 37 completed weeks of gestation O47.0- ☑
  passage, urethra (prostatic) N36.5
  pregnancy F45.8
Family, familial (*see also* condition)
  disruption Z63.8
    involving divorce or separation Z63.5
  Li-Fraumeni (syndrome) Z15.01
  planning advice Z30.09
  problem Z63.9
    specified NEC Z63.8
  retinoblastoma C69.2- ☑
Famine (effects of) T73.0 ☑
  edema — *see* Malnutrition, severe
Fanconi (-de Toni)(-Debré) **syndrome** E72.09
  with cystinosis E72.04
Fanconi's anemia (congenital pancytopenia) D61.09
Farber's disease or syndrome E75.29
Farcy A24.0
Farmer's
  lung J67.0
  skin L57.8
Farsightedness — *see* Hypermetropia
Fascia — *see* condition
Fasciculation R25.3
Fasciitis M72.9
  diffuse (eosinophilic) M35.4
  infective M72.8
    necrotizing M72.6
  necrotizing M72.6
  nodular M72.4
  perirenal (with ureteral obstruction) N13.5
    with infection N13.6
  plantar M72.2
  specified NEC M72.8
  traumatic (old) M72.8
    current — *code by* site under Sprain
Fascioliasis B66.3
Fasciolopsis, fasciolopsiasis (intestinal) B66.5
Fascioscapulohumeral myopathy G71.0
Fast pulse R00.0
Fat
  embolism — *see* Embolism, fat
  excessive (*see also* Obesity)
    in heart — *see* Degeneration, myocardial
  in stool R19.5
  localized (pad) E65
    heart — *see* Degeneration, myocardial
    knee M79.4
    retropatellar M79.4
  necrosis
    breast N64.1
    mesentery K65.4
    omentum K65.4
  pad E65
    knee M79.4
Fatigue R53.83
  auditory deafness — *see* Deafness
  chronic R53.82
  combat F43.0
  general R53.83
    psychogenic F48.8
  heat (transient) T67.6 ☑
  muscle M62.89
  myocardium — *see* Failure, heart
  neoplasm-related R53.0
  nervous, neurosis F48.8
  operational F48.8
  psychogenic (general) F48.8
  senile R54
  voice R49.8
Fatness — *see* Obesity
Fatty (*see also* condition)
  apron E65

Fatty — *continued*
  degeneration — *see* Degeneration, fatty
  heart (enlarged) — *see* Degeneration, myocardial
  liver NEC K76.0
    alcoholic K70.0
    nonalcoholic K76.0
  necrosis — *see* Degeneration, fatty
Fauces — *see* condition
Fauchard's disease (periodontitis) — *see* Periodontitis
Faucitis J02.9
Favism (anemia) D55.0
Favus — *see* Dermatophytosis
Fazio-Londe disease or syndrome G12.1
Fear complex or reaction F40.9
Fear of — *see* Phobia
Feared complaint unfounded Z71.1
Febris, febrile (*see also* Fever)
  flava (*see also* Fever, yellow) A95.9
  melitensis A23.0
  pestis — *see* Plague
  recurrens — *see* Fever, relapsing
  rubra A38.9
Fecal
  incontinence R15.9
  smearing R15.1
  soiling R15.1
  urgency R15.2
Fecalith (impaction) K56.41
  appendix K38.1
  congenital P76.8
Fede's disease K14.0
Feeble rapid pulse due to shock following injury
  T79.4 ☑
Feeble-minded F70
Feeding
  difficulties R63.3
  problem R63.3
    newborn P92.9
      specified NEC P92.8
    nonorganic (adult) — *see* Disorder, eating
Feeling (of)
  foreign body in throat R09.89
Feer's disease — *see* Poisoning, mercury
Feet — *see* condition
Feigned illness Z76.5
Feil-Klippel syndrome (brevicollis) Q76.1
Feinmesser's (hidrotic) **ectodermal dysplasia** Q82.4
Felon (*see also* Cellulitis, digit)
  with lymphangitis — *see* Lymphangitis, acute, digit
Felty's syndrome M05.00
  ankle M05.07- ☑
  elbow M05.02- ☑
  foot joint M05.07- ☑
  hand joint M05.04- ☑
  hip M05.05- ☑
  knee M05.06- ☑
  multiple site M05.09
  shoulder M05.01- ☑
  vertebra — *see* Spondylitis, ankylosing
  wrist M05.03- ☑
Female genital cutting status — *see* Female genital
    mutilation status (FGM)
Female genital mutilation status (FGM) N90.810
  specified NEC N90.818
  type I (clitorectomy status) N90.811
  type II (clitorectomy with excision of labia minora sta-
    tus) N90.812
  type III (infibulation status) N90.813
  type IV N90.818
Femur, femoral — *see* condition
Fenestration, fenestrated (*see also* Imperfect, closure)
  aortico-pulmonary Q21.4
  cusps, heart valve NEC Q24.8
    pulmonary Q22.3
  pulmonic cusps Q22.3
Fernell's disease (aortic aneurysm) I71.9
Fertile eunuch syndrome E23.0
Fetid
  breath R19.6
  sweat L75.0
Fetishism F65.0
  transvestic F65.1
Fetus, fetal (*see also* condition)
  alcohol syndrome (dysmorphic) Q86.0
  compressus O31.0- ☑
  hydantoin syndrome Q86.1

Fetus, fetal — *continued*
  lung tissue P28.0
  papyraceous O31.0- ☑
Fever (inanition) (of unknown origin) (persistent) (with
    chills) (with rigor) R50.9
  abortus A23.1
  Aden (dengue) A90
  African tick-borne A68.1
  American
    mountain (tick) A93.2
    spotted A77.0
  aphthous B08.8
  arbovirus, arboviral A94
    hemorrhagic A94
    specified NEC A93.8
  Argentinian hemorrhagic A96.0
  Assam B55.0
  Australian Q A78
  Bangkok hemorrhagic A91
  Barmah forest A92.8
  Bartonella A44.0
  bilious, hemoglobinuric B50.8
  blackwater B50.8
  blister B00.1
  Bolivian hemorrhagic A96.1
  Bonvale dam T73.3 ☑
  boutonneuse A77.1
  brain — *see* Encephalitis
  Brazilian purpuric A48.4
  breakbone A90
  Bullis A77.0
  Bunyamwera A92.8
  Burdwan B55.0
  Bwamba A92.8
  Cameroon — *see* Malaria
  Canton A75.9
  cat-scratch A28.1
  catarrhal (acute) J00
    chronic J31.0
  Central Asian hemorrhagic A98.0
  cerebral — *see* Encephalitis
  cerebrospinal meningococcal A39.0
  Chagres B50.9
  Chandipura A92.8
  Changuinola A93.1
  Charcot's (biliary) (hepatic) (intermittent) — *see* Calcu-
    lus, bile duct
  Chikungunya (viral) (hemorrhagic) A92.0
  Chitral A93.1
  Colombo — *see* Fever, paratyphoid
  Colorado tick (virus) A93.2
  congestive (remittent) — *see* Malaria
  Congo virus A98.0
  continued malarial B50.9
  Corsican — *see* Malaria
  Crimean-Congo hemorrhagic A98.0
  Cyprus — *see* Brucellosis
  dandy A90
  deer fly — *see* Tularemia
  dengue (virus) A90
    hemorrhagic A91
    sandfly A93.1
  desert B38.0
  drug induced R50.2
  due to
    conditions classified elsewhere R50.81
    heat T67.0 ☑
  enteric A01.00
  enteroviral exanthematous (Boston exanthem) A88.0
  ephemeral (of unknown origin) R50.9
  epidemic hemorrhagic A98.5
  erysipelatous — *see* Erysipelas
  estivo-autumnal (malarial) B50.9
  famine A75.0
  five day A79.0
  following delivery O86.4
  Fort Bragg A27.89
  gastroenteric A01.00
  gastromalarial — *see* Malaria
  Gibraltar — *see* Brucellosis
  glandular — *see* Mononucleosis, infectious
  Guama (viral) A92.8
  Haverhill A25.1
  hay (allergic) J30.1
    with asthma (bronchial) J45.909
      with
        exacerbation (acute) J45.901
        status asthmaticus J45.902

Index

Fever — Fever

Fever — *continued*
hay — *continued*
   due to
      allergen other than pollen J30.89
      pollen, any plant or tree J30.1
heat (effects) T67.0 ☑
hematuric, bilious B50.8
hemoglobinuric (malarial) (bilious) B50.8
hemorrhagic (arthropod-borne) NOS A94
   with renal syndrome A98.5
   arenaviral A96.9
      specified NEC A96.8
   Argentinian A96.0
   Bangkok A91
   Bolivian A96.1
   Central Asian A98.0
   Chikungunya A92.0
   Crimean-Congo A98.0
   dengue (virus) A91
   epidemic A98.5
   Junin (virus) A96.0
   Korean A98.5
   Kyasanur forest A98.2
   Machupo (virus) A96.1
   mite-borne A93.8
   mosquito-borne A92.8
   Omsk A98.1
   Philippine A91
   Russian A98.5
   Singapore A91
   Southeast Asia A91
   Thailand A91
   tick-borne NEC A93.8
   viral A99
      specified NEC A98.8
hepatic — *see* Cholecystitis
herpetic — *see* Herpes
icterohemorrhagic A27.0
Indiana A93.8
infective B99.9
   specified NEC B99.8
intermittent (bilious) (*see also* Malaria)
   of unknown origin R50.9
   pernicious B50.9
iodide R50.2
Japanese river A75.3
jungle (*see also* Malaria)
   yellow A95.0
Junin (virus) hemorrhagic A96.0
Katayama B65.2
kedani A75.3
Kenya (tick) A77.1
Kew Garden A79.1
Korean hemorrhagic A98.5
Lassa A96.2
Lone Star A77.0
Machupo (virus) hemorrhagic A96.1
malaria, malarial — *see* Malaria
Malta A23.9
Marseilles A77.1
marsh — *see* Malaria
Mayaro (viral) A92.8
Mediterranean (*see also* Brucellosis) A23.9
   familial E85.0
   tick A77.1
meningeal — *see* Meningitis
Meuse A79.0
Mexican A75.2
mianeh A68.1
miasmatic — *see* Malaria
mosquito-borne (viral) A92.9
   hemorrhagic A92.8
mountain (*see also* Brucellosis)
   meaning Rocky Mountain spotted fever A77.0
   tick (American) (Colorado) (viral) A93.2
Mucambo (viral) A92.8
mud A27.9
Neapolitan — *see* Brucellosis
neutropenic D70.9
newborn P81.9
   environmental P81.0
Nine-Mile A78
non-exanthematous tick A93.2
North Asian tick-borne A77.2
Omsk hemorrhagic A98.1
O'nyong-nyong (viral) A92.1
Oropouche (viral) A93.0
Oroya A44.0

paludal — *see* Malaria
Panama (malarial) B50.9
Pappataci A93.1
paratyphoid A01.4
   A A01.1
   B A01.2
   C A01.3
parrot A70
periodic (Mediterranean) E85.0
persistent (of unknown origin) R50.9
petechial A39.0
pharyngoconjunctival B30.2
Philippine hemorrhagic A91
phlebotomus A93.1
Piry (virus) A93.8
Pixuna (viral) A92.8
Plasmodium ovale B53.0
polioviral (nonparalytic) A80.4
Pontiac A48.2
postimmunization R50.83
postoperative R50.82
   due to infection T81.4 ☑
posttransfusion R50.84
postvaccination R50.83
presenting with conditions classified elsewhere R50.81
pretibial A27.89
puerperal O86.4
Q A78
quadrilateral A78
quartan (malaria) B52.9
Queensland (coastal) (tick) A77.3
quintan A79.0
rabbit — *see* Tularemia
rat-bite A25.9
   due to
      Spirillum A25.0
      Streptobacillus moniliformis A25.1
recurrent — *see* Fever, relapsing
relapsing (Borrelia) A68.9
   Carter's (Asiatic) A68.1
   Dutton's (West African) A68.1
   Koch's A68.9
   louse-borne A68.0
   Novy's
      louse-borne A68.0
      tick-borne A68.1
   Obermeyer's (European) A68.0
   tick-borne A68.1
remittent (bilious) (congestive) (gastric) — *see* Malaria
rheumatic (active) (acute) (chronic) (subacute) I00
   with central nervous system involvement I02.9
   active with heart involvement — *see* category
      I01 ☑
   inactive or quiescent with
      cardiac hypertrophy I09.89
      carditis I09.9
      endocarditis I09.1
         aortic (valve) I06.9
            with mitral (valve) disease I08.0
         mitral (valve) I05.9
            with aortic (valve) disease I08.0
         pulmonary (valve) I09.89
         tricuspid (valve) I07.8
      heart disease NEC I09.89
      heart failure (congestive) (conditions in I50.9)
         I09.81
      left ventricular failure (conditions in I50.1)
         I09.81
      myocarditis, myocardial degeneration (conditions in I51.4) I09.0
      pancarditis I09.9
      pericarditis I09.2
Rift Valley (viral) A92.4
Rocky Mountain spotted A77.0
rose J30.1
Ross River B33.1
Russian hemorrhagic A98.5
San Joaquin (Valley) B38.0
sandfly A93.1
Sao Paulo A77.0
scarlet A38.9
seven day (leptospirosis) (autumnal) (Japanese) A27.89
   dengue A90
shin-bone A79.0
Singapore hemorrhagic A91
solar A90
Songo A98.5

sore B00.1
South African tick-bite A68.1
Southeast Asia hemorrhagic A91
spinal — *see* Meningitis
spirillary A25.0
splenic — *see* Anthrax
spotted A77.9
   American A77.0
   Brazilian A77.0
   cerebrospinal meningitis A39.0
   Colombian A77.0
   due to Rickettsia
      australis A77.3
      conorii A77.1
      rickettsii A77.0
      sibirica A77.2
      specified type NEC A77.8
   Ehrlichiosis A77.40
      due to
         E. chafeensis A77.41
         specified organism NEC A77.49
   Rocky Mountain A77.0
steroid R50.2
streptobacillary A25.1
subtertian B50.9
Sumatran mite A75.3
sun A90
swamp A27.9
swine A02.8
sylvatic, yellow A95.0
Tahyna B33.8
tertian — *see* Malaria, tertian
Thailand hemorrhagic A91
thermic T67.0 ☑
three-day A93.1
tick
   American mountain A93.2
   Colorado A93.2
   Kemerovo A93.8
   Mediterranean A77.1
   mountain A93.2
   nonexanthematous A93.2
   Quaranfil A93.8
tick-bite NEC A93.8
tick-borne (hemorrhagic) NEC A93.8
trench A79.0
tsutsugamushi A75.3
typhogastric A01.00
typhoid (abortive) (hemorrhagic) (intermittent) (malignant) A01.00
   complicated by
      arthritis A01.04
      heart involvement A01.02
      meningitis A01.01
      osteomyelitis A01.05
      pneumonia A01.03
      specified NEC A01.09
typhomalarial — *see* Malaria
typhus — *see* Typhus (fever)
undulant — *see* Brucellosis
unknown origin R50.9
uveoparotid D86.89
valley B38.0
Venezuelan equine A92.2
vesicular stomatitis A93.8
viral hemorrhagic — *see* Fever, hemorrhagic, by type of virus
Volhynian A79.0
Wesselsbron (viral) A92.8
West
   African B50.8
   Nile (viral) A92.30
      with
         complications NEC A92.39
         cranial nerve disorders A92.32
         encephalitis A92.31
         encephalomyelitis A92.31
         neurologic manifestation NEC A92.32
         optic neuritis A92.32
         polyradiculitis A92.32
Whitmore's — *see* Melioidosis
Wolhynian A79.0
worm B83.9
yellow A95.9
   jungle A95.0
   sylvatic A95.0
   urban A95.1

Fever — *continued*
  Zika (viral) A92.8
Fibrillation
  atrial or auricular (established) I48.91
    chronic I48.2
    paroxysmal I48.0
    permanent I48.2
    persistent I48.1
  cardiac I49.8
  heart I49.8
  muscular M62.89
  ventricular I49.01
Fibrin
  ball or bodies, pleural (sac) J94.1
  chamber, anterior (eye) (gelatinous exudate) — *see* Iridocyclitis, acute
Fibrinogenolysis — *see* Fibrinolysis
Fibrinogenopenia D68.8
  acquired D65
  congenital D68.2
Fibrinolysis (hemorrhagic) (acquired) D65
  antepartum hemorrhage — *see* Hemorrhage, antepartum, with coagulation defect
  following
    abortion — *see* Abortion by type complicated by hemorrhage
    ectopic or molar pregnancy O08.1
  intrapartum O67.0
  newborn, transient P60
  postpartum O72.3
Fibrinopenia (hereditary) D68.2
  acquired D68.4
Fibrinopurulent — *see* condition
Fibrinous — *see* condition
Fibro-odontoma, ameloblastic — *see* Cyst, calcifying odontogenic
Fibro-osteoma — *see* Neoplasm, bone, benign
Fibroadenoma
  cellular intracanalicular D24- ☑
  giant D24- ☑
  intracanalicular
    cellular D24- ☑
    giant D24- ☑
    specified site — *see* Neoplasm, benign, by site
    unspecified site D24- ☑
  juvenile D24- ☑
  pericanalicular
    specified site — *see* Neoplasm, benign, by site
    unspecified site D24- ☑
  phyllodes D24- ☑
  prostate D29.1
  specified site NEC — *see* Neoplasm, benign, by site
  unspecified site D24- ☑
Fibroadenosis, breast (chronic) (cystic) (diffuse) (periodic) (segmental) N60.2- ☑
Fibroangioma (*see also* Neoplasm, benign, by site)
  juvenile
    specified site — *see* Neoplasm, benign, by site
    unspecified site D10.6
Fibrochondrosarcoma — *see* Neoplasm, cartilage, malignant
Fibrocystic
  disease (*see also* Fibrosis, cystic)
    breast — *see* Mastopathy, cystic
    jaw M27.49
    kidney (congenital) Q61.8
    liver Q44.6
    pancreas E84.9
  kidney (congenital) Q61.8
Fibrodysplasia ossificans progressiva — *see* Myositis, ossificans, progressiva
Fibroelastosis (cordis) (endocardial) (endomyocardial) I42.4
Fibroid (tumor) (*see also* Neoplasm, connective tissue, benign)
  disease, lung (chronic) — *see* Fibrosis, lung
  heart (disease) — *see* Myocarditis
  in pregnancy or childbirth O34.1- ☑
    causing obstructed labor O65.5
  induration, lung (chronic) — *see* Fibrosis, lung
  lung — *see* Fibrosis, lung
  pneumonia (chronic) — *see* Fibrosis, lung
  uterus D25.9
Fibrolipoma — *see* Lipoma
Fibroliposarcoma — *see* Neoplasm, connective tissue, malignant
Fibroma (*see also* Neoplasm, connective tissue, benign)

Fibroma — *continued*
  ameloblastic — *see* Cyst, calcifying odontogenic
  bone (nonossifying) — *see* Disorder, bone, specified type NEC
    ossifying — *see* Neoplasm, bone, benign
  cementifying — *see* Neoplasm, bone, benign
  chondromyxoid — *see* Neoplasm, bone, benign
  desmoplastic — *see* Neoplasm, connective tissue, uncertain behavior
  durum — *see* Neoplasm, connective tissue, benign
  fascial — *see* Neoplasm, connective tissue, benign
  invasive — *see* Neoplasm, connective tissue, uncertain behavior
  molle — *see* Lipoma
  myxoid — *see* Neoplasm, connective tissue, benign
  nasopharynx, nasopharyngeal (juvenile) D10.6
  nonosteogenic (nonossifying) — *see* Dysplasia, fibrous
  odontogenic (central) — *see* Cyst, calcifying odontogenic
  ossifying — *see* Neoplasm, bone, benign
  periosteal — *see* Neoplasm, bone, benign
  soft — *see* Lipoma
Fibromatosis M72.9
  abdominal — *see* Neoplasm, connective tissue, uncertain behavior
  aggressive — *see* Neoplasm, connective tissue, uncertain behavior
  congenital generalized — *see* Neoplasm, connective tissue, uncertain behavior
  Dupuytren's M72.0
  gingival K06.1
  palmar (fascial) M72.0
  plantar (fascial) M72.2
  pseudosarcomatous (proliferative) (subcutaneous) M72.4
  retroperitoneal D48.3
  specified NEC M72.8
Fibromyalgia M79.7
Fibromyoma (*see also* Neoplasm, connective tissue, benign)
  uterus (corpus) (*see also* Leiomyoma, uterus)
    in pregnancy or childbirth — *see* Fibroid, in pregnancy or childbirth
      causing obstructed labor O65.5
Fibromyositis M79.7
Fibromyxolipoma D17.9
Fibromyxoma — *see* Neoplasm, connective tissue, benign
Fibromyxosarcoma — *see* Neoplasm, connective tissue, malignant
Fibroplasia, retrolental H35.17- ☑
Fibropurulent — *see* condition
Fibrosarcoma (*see also* Neoplasm, connective tissue, malignant)
  ameloblastic C41.1
    upper jaw (bone) C41.0
  congenital — *see* Neoplasm, connective tissue, malignant
  fascial — *see* Neoplasm, connective tissue, malignant
  infantile — *see* Neoplasm, connective tissue, malignant
  odontogenic C41.1
    upper jaw (bone) C41.0
  periosteal — *see* Neoplasm, bone, malignant
Fibrosclerosis
  breast N60.3- ☑
  multifocal M35.5
  penis (corpora cavernosa) N48.6
Fibrosis, fibrotic
  adrenal (gland) E27.8
  amnion O41.8X- ☑
  anal papillae K62.89
  arteriocapillary — *see* Arteriosclerosis
  bladder N32.89
    interstitial — *see* Cystitis, chronic, interstitial
    localized submucosal — *see* Cystitis, chronic, interstitial
    panmural — *see* Cystitis, chronic, interstitial
  breast — *see* Fibrosclerosis, breast
  capillary (*see also* Arteriosclerosis) I70.90
    lung (chronic) — *see* Fibrosis, lung
  cardiac — *see* Myocarditis
  cervix N88.8
  chorion O41.8X- ☑
  corpus cavernosum (sclerosing) N48.6
  cystic (of pancreas) E84.9

Fibrosis, fibrotic — *continued*
  cystic — *continued*
    with
      distal intestinal obstruction syndrome E84.19
      fecal impaction E84.19
      intestinal manifestations NEC E84.19
      pulmonary manifestations E84.0
      specified manifestations NEC E84.8
  due to device, implant or graft (*see also* Complications, by site and type, specified NEC) T85.82 ☑
    arterial graft NEC T82.828 ☑
    breast (implant) T85.82 ☑
    catheter NEC T85.82 ☑
      dialysis (renal) T82.828 ☑
        intraperitoneal T85.82 ☑
      infusion NEC T82.828 ☑
        spinal (epidural) (subdural) T85.82 ☑
      urinary (indwelling) T83.82 ☑
    electronic (electrode) (pulse generator) (stimulator)
      bone T84.82 ☑
      cardiac T82.827 ☑
      nervous system (brain) (peripheral nerve) (spinal) T85.82 ☑
      urinary T83.82 ☑
    fixation, internal (orthopedic) NEC T84.82 ☑
    gastrointestinal (bile duct) (esophagus) T85.82 ☑
    genital NEC T83.82 ☑
    heart NEC T82.827 ☑
    joint prosthesis T84.82 ☑
    ocular (corneal graft) (orbital implant) NEC T85.82 ☑
    orthopedic NEC T84.82 ☑
    specified NEC T85.82 ☑
    urinary NEC T83.82 ☑
    vascular NEC T82.828 ☑
    ventricular intracranial shunt T85.82 ☑
  ejaculatory duct N50.8
  endocardium — *see* Endocarditis
  endomyocardial (tropical) I42.3
  epididymis N50.8
  eye muscle — *see* Strabismus, mechanical
  heart — *see* Myocarditis
  hepatic — *see* Fibrosis, liver
  hepatolienal (portal hypertension) K76.6
  hepatosplenic (portal hypertension) K76.6
  infrapatellar fat pad M79.4
  intrascrotal N50.8
  kidney N26.9
  liver K74.0
    with sclerosis K74.2
    alcoholic K70.2
  lung (atrophic) (chronic) (confluent) (massive) (perialveolar) (peribronchial) J84.10
    with
      anthracosilicosis J60
      anthracosis J60
      asbestosis J61
      bagassosis J67.1
      bauxite J63.1
      berylliosis J63.2
      byssinosis J66.0
      calcicosis J62.8
      chalicosis J62.8
      dust reticulation J64
      farmer's lung J67.0
      ganister disease J62.8
      graphite J63.3
      pneumoconiosis NOS J64
      siderosis J63.4
      silicosis J62.8
    capillary J84.10
    congenital P27.8
    diffuse (idiopathic) J84.10
      chemicals, gases, fumes or vapors (inhalation) J68.4
      interstitial J84.10
        acute J84.114
      talc J62.0
    following radiation J70.1
    idiopathic J84.112
    postinflammatory J84.10
    silicotic J62.8
    tuberculous — *see* Tuberculosis, pulmonary
  lymphatic gland I89.8
  median bar — *see* Hyperplasia, prostate
  mediastinum (idiopathic) J98.5
  meninges G96.19

Fibrosis, fibrotic — *continued*
　myocardium, myocardial — *see* Myocarditis
　ovary N83.8
　oviduct N83.8
　pancreas K86.8
　penis NEC N48.6
　pericardium I31.0
　perineum, in pregnancy or childbirth O34.7- ☑
　　causing obstructed labor O65.5
　pleura J94.1
　popliteal fat pad M79.4
　prostate (chronic) — *see* Hyperplasia, prostate
　pulmonary (*see also* Fibrosis, lung) J84.10
　　congenital P27.8
　　idiopathic J84.112
　rectal sphincter K62.89
　retroperitoneal, idiopathic (with ureteral obstruction) N13.5
　　with infection N13.6
　sclerosing mesenteric (idiopathic) K65.4
　scrotum N50.8
　seminal vesicle N50.8
　senile R54
　skin L90.5
　spermatic cord N50.8
　spleen D73.89
　　in schistosomiasis (bilharziasis) B65.9 [D77]
　subepidermal nodular — *see* Neoplasm, skin, benign
　submucous (oral) (tongue) K13.5
　testis N44.8
　　chronic, due to syphilis A52.76
　thymus (gland) E32.8
　tongue, submucous K13.5
　tunica vaginalis N50.8
　uterus (non-neoplastic) N85.8
　vagina N89.8
　valve, heart — *see* Endocarditis
　vas deferens N50.8
　vein I87.8
Fibrositis (periarticular) M79.7
　nodular, chronic (Jaccoud's) (rheumatoid) — *see* Arthropathy, postrheumatic, chronic
Fibrothorax J94.1
Fibrotic — *see* Fibrosis
Fibrous — *see* condition
Fibroxanthoma (*see also* Neoplasm, connective tissue, benign)
　atypical — *see* Neoplasm, connective tissue, uncertain behavior
　malignant — *see* Neoplasm, connective tissue, malignant
Fibroxanthosarcoma — *see* Neoplasm, connective tissue, malignant
Fiedler's
　disease (icterohemorrhagic leptospirosis) A27.0
　myocarditis (acute) I40.1
Fifth disease B08.3
　venereal A55
Filaria, filarial, filariasis — *see* Infestation, filarial
Filatov's disease — *see* Mononucleosis, infectious
File-cutter's disease — *see* Poisoning, lead
Filling defect
　biliary tract R93.2
　bladder R93.4
　duodenum R93.3
　gallbladder R93.2
　gastrointestinal tract R93.3
　intestine R93.3
　kidney R93.4
　stomach R93.3
　ureter R93.4
Fimbrial cyst Q50.4
Financial problem affecting care NOS Z59.9
　bankruptcy Z59.8
　foreclosure on loan Z59.8
Findings, abnormal, inconclusive, without diagnosis
　(*see also* Abnormal)
　17-ketosteroids, elevated R82.5
　acetonuria R82.4
　alcohol in blood R78.0
　anisocytosis R71.8
　antenatal screening of mother O28.9
　　biochemical O28.1
　　chromosomal O28.5
　　cytological O28.2
　　genetic O28.5
　　hematological O28.0
　　radiological O28.4

Findings, abnormal, inconclusive, without diagnosis — *continued*
　antenatal screening of mother — *continued*
　　specified NEC O28.8
　　ultrasonic O28.3
　antibody titer, elevated R76.0
　anticardiolipin antibody R76.0
　antiphosphatidylglycerol antibody R76.0
　antiphosphatidylinositol antibody R76.0
　antiphosphatidylserine antibody R76.0
　antiphospholipid antibody R76.0
　bacteriuria N39.0
　bicarbonate E87.8
　bile in urine R82.2
　blood sugar R73.09
　　high R73.9
　　low (transient) E16.2
　body fluid or substance, specified NEC R88.8
　casts, urine R82.99
　catecholamines R82.5
　cells, urine R82.99
　chloride E87.8
　cholesterol E78.9
　　high R78.0
　　　with high triglycerides E78.2
　chyluria R82.0
　cloudy
　　dialysis effluent R88.0
　　urine R82.90
　creatinine clearance R94.4
　crystals, urine R82.99
　culture
　　blood R78.81
　　positive — *see* Positive, culture
　echocardiogram R93.1
　electrolyte level, urinary R82.99
　function study NEC R94.8
　　bladder R94.8
　　endocrine NEC R94.7
　　　thyroid R94.6
　　kidney R94.4
　　liver R94.5
　　pancreas R94.8
　　placenta R94.8
　　pulmonary R94.2
　　spleen R94.8
　gallbladder, nonvisualization R93.2
　glucose (tolerance test) (non-fasting) R73.09
　glycosuria R81
　heart
　　shadow R93.1
　　sounds R01.2
　hematinuria R82.3
　hematocrit drop (precipitous) R71.0
　hemoglobinuria R82.3
　human papillomavirus (HPV) DNA test positive
　　cervix
　　　high risk R87.810
　　　low risk R87.820
　　vagina
　　　high risk R87.811
　　　low risk R87.821
　in blood (of substance not normally found in blood) R78.9
　　addictive drug NEC R78.4
　　alcohol (excessive level) R78.0
　　cocaine R78.2
　　hallucinogen R78.3
　　heavy metals (abnormal level) R78.79
　　lead R78.71
　　lithium (abnormal level) R78.89
　　opiate drug R78.1
　　psychotropic drug R78.5
　　specified substance NEC R78.89
　　steroid agent R78.6
　indoleacetic acid, elevated R82.5
　ketonuria R82.4
　lactic acid dehydrogenase (LDH) R74.0
　liver function test R79.89
　mammogram NEC R92.8
　　calcification (calculus) R92.1
　　inconclusive result (due to dense breasts) R92.2
　　microcalcification R92.0
　mediastinal shift R93.8
　melanin, urine R82.99
　myoglobinuria R82.1
　neonatal screening P09
　nonvisualization of gallbladder R93.2

Findings, abnormal, inconclusive, without diagnosis — *continued*
　odor of urine NOS R82.90
　Papanicolaou cervix R87.619
　　non-atypical endometrial cells R87.618
　pneumoencephalogram R93.0
　poikilocytosis R71.8
　potassium (deficiency) E87.6
　　excess E87.5
　PPD R76.11
　radiologic (X-ray) R93.8
　　abdomen R93.5
　　biliary tract R93.2
　　breast R92.8
　　gastrointestinal tract R93.3
　　genitourinary organs R93.8
　　head R93.0
　　inconclusive due to excess body fat of patient R93.9
　　intrathoracic organs NEC R93.1
　　placenta R93.8
　　retroperitoneum R93.5
　　skin R93.8
　　skull R93.0
　　subcutaneous tissue R93.8
　red blood cell (count) (morphology) (sickling) (volume) R71.8
　scan NEC R94.8
　　bladder R94.8
　　bone R94.8
　　kidney R94.4
　　liver R93.2
　　lung R94.2
　　pancreas R94.8
　　placental R94.8
　　spleen R94.8
　　thyroid R94.6
　sedimentation rate, elevated R70.0
　SGOT R74.0
　SGPT R74.0
　sodium (deficiency) E87.1
　　excess E87.0
　specified body fluid NEC R88.8
　stress test R94.39
　thyroid (function) (metabolic rate) (scan) (uptake) R94.6
　transaminase (level) R74.0
　triglycerides E78.9
　　high E78.1
　　　with high cholesterol E78.2
　tuberculin skin test (without active tuberculosis) R76.11
　urine R82.90
　　acetone R82.4
　　bacteria N39.0
　　bile R82.2
　　casts or cells R82.99
　　chyle R82.0
　　culture positive R82.7
　　glucose R81
　　hemoglobin R82.3
　　ketone R82.4
　　sugar R81
　vanillylmandelic acid (VMA), elevated R82.5
　vectorcardiogram (VCG) R94.39
　ventriculogram R93.0
　white blood cell (count) (differential) (morphology) D72.9
　xerography R92.8
Finger — *see* condition
Fire, Saint Anthony's — *see* Erysipelas
Fire-setting
　pathological (compulsive) F63.1
Fish hook stomach K31.89
Fishmeal-worker's lung J67.8
Fissure, fissured
　anus, anal K60.2
　　acute K60.0
　　chronic K60.1
　　congenital Q43.8
　ear, lobule, congenital Q17.8
　epiglottis (congenital) Q31.8
　larynx J38.7
　　congenital Q31.8
　lip K13.0
　　congenital — *see* Cleft, lip
　nipple N64.0
　　associated with
　　　lactation O92.13

Fissure, fissured — continued
  nipple — continued
    associated with — continued
      pregnancy O92.11- ☑
      puerperium O92.12
  nose Q30.2
  palate (congenital) — see Cleft, palate
  skin R23.4
  spine (congenital) (see also Spina bifida)
    with hydrocephalus — see Spina bifida, by site,
      with hydrocephalus
  tongue (acquired) K14.5
    congenital Q38.3
Fistula (cutaneous) L98.8
  abdomen (wall) K63.2
    bladder N32.2
    intestine NEC K63.2
    ureter N28.89
    uterus N82.5
  abdominorectal K63.2
  abdominosigmoidal K63.2
  abdominothoracic J86.0
  abdominouterine N82.5
    congenital Q51.7
  abdominovesical N32.2
  accessory sinuses — see Sinusitis
  actinomycotic — see Actinomycosis
  alveolar antrum — see Sinusitis, maxillary
  alveolar process K04.6
  anorectal K60.5
  antrobuccal — see Sinusitis, maxillary
  antrum — see Sinusitis, maxillary
  anus, anal (recurrent) (infectional) K60.3
    congenital Q43.6
      with absence, atresia and stenosis Q42.2
    tuberculous A18.32
  aorta-duodenal I77.2
  appendix, appendicular K38.3
  arteriovenous (acquired) (nonruptured) I77.0
    brain I67.1
      congenital Q28.2
        ruptured I60.8
      ruptured I60.8
    cerebral — see Fistula, arteriovenous, brain
    congenital (peripheral) (see also Malformation, ar-
      teriovenous)
      brain Q28.2
        ruptured I60.8
      coronary Q24.5
      pulmonary Q25.72
    coronary I25.41
      congenital Q24.5
    pulmonary I28.0
      congenital Q25.72
    surgically created (for dialysis) Z99.2
      complication — see Complication, arteriove-
        nous, fistula, surgically created
    traumatic — see Injury, blood vessel
  artery I77.2
  aural (mastoid) — see Mastoiditis, chronic
  auricle (see also Disorder, pinna, specified type NEC)
    congenital Q18.1
  Bartholin's gland N82.8
  bile duct (common) (hepatic) K83.3
    with calculus, stones — see Calculus, bile duct
  biliary (tract) — see Fistula, bile duct
  bladder (sphincter) NEC (see also Fistula, vesico-) N32.2
    into seminal vesicle N32.2
  bone (see also Disorder, bone, specified type NEC)
    with osteomyelitis, chronic — see Osteomyelitis,
      chronic, with draining sinus
  brain G93.89
    arteriovenous (acquired) I67.1
      congenital Q28.2
  branchial (cleft) Q18.0
  branchiogenous Q18.0
  breast N61
    puerperal, postpartum or gestational, due to mas-
      titis (purulent) — see Mastitis, obstetric, pu-
      rulent
  bronchial J86.0
  bronchocutaneous, bronchomediastinal, bronchopleu-
    ral, bronchopleuromediastinal (infective) J86.0
    tuberculous NEC A15.5
  bronchoesophageal J86.0
    congenital Q39.2
      with atresia of esophagus Q39.1
  bronchovisceral J86.0

Fistula — continued
  buccal cavity (infective) K12.2
  cecosigmoidal K63.2
  cecum K63.2
  cerebrospinal (fluid) G96.0
  cervical, lateral Q18.1
  cervicoaural Q18.1
  cervicosigmoidal N82.4
  cervicovesical N82.1
  cervix N82.8
  chest (wall) J86.0
  cholecystenteric — see Fistula, gallbladder
  cholecystocolic — see Fistula, gallbladder
  cholecystocolonic — see Fistula, gallbladder
  cholecystoduodenal — see Fistula, gallbladder
  cholecystogastric — see Fistula, gallbladder
  cholecystointestinal — see Fistula, gallbladder
  choledochoduodenal — see Fistula, bile duct
  cholocolic K82.3
  coccyx — see Sinus, pilonidal
  colon K63.2
  colostomy K94.09
  common duct — see Fistula, bile duct
  congenital, site not listed — see Anomaly, by site
  coronary, arteriovenous I25.41
    congenital Q24.5
  costal region J86.0
  cul-de-sac, Douglas' N82.8
  cystic duct (see also Fistula, gallbladder)
    congenital Q44.5
  dental K04.6
  diaphragm J86.0
  duodenum K31.6
  ear (external) (canal) — see Disorder, ear, external,
    specified type NEC
  enterocolic K63.2
  enterocutaneous K63.2
  enterouterine N82.4
    congenital Q51.7
  enterovaginal N82.4
    congenital Q52.2
    large intestine N82.3
    small intestine N82.2
  enterovesical N32.1
  epididymis N50.8
    tuberculous A18.15
  esophagobronchial J86.0
    congenital Q39.2
      with atresia of esophagus Q39.1
  esophagocutaneous K22.8
  esophagopleural-cutaneous J86.0
  esophagotracheal J86.0
    congenital Q39.2
      with atresia of esophagus Q39.1
  esophagus K22.8
    congenital Q39.2
      with atresia of esophagus Q39.1
  ethmoid — see Sinusitis, ethmoidal
  eyeball (cornea) (sclera) — see Disorder, globe, hy-
    potony
  eyelid H01.8
  fallopian tube, external N82.5
  fecal K63.2
    congenital Q43.6
  from periapical abscess K04.6
  frontal sinus — see Sinusitis, frontal
  gallbladder K82.3
    with calculus, cholelithiasis, stones — see Calculus,
      gallbladder
  gastric K31.6
  gastrocolic K31.6
    congenital Q40.2
    tuberculous A18.32
  gastroenterocolic K31.6
  gastroesophageal K31.6
  gastrojejunal K31.6
  gastrojejunocolic K31.6
  genital tract (female) N82.9
    specified NEC N82.8
    to intestine NEC N82.4
    to skin N82.5
  hepatic artery-portal vein, congenital Q26.6
  hepatopleural J86.0
  hepatopulmonary J86.0
  ileorectal or ileosigmoidal K63.2
  ileovaginal N82.2
  ileovesical N32.1
  ileum K63.2

Fistula — continued
  in ano K60.3
    tuberculous A18.32
  inner ear (labyrinth) — see subcategory H83.1 ☑
  intestine NEC K63.2
  intestinocolonic (abdominal) K63.2
  intestinoureteral N28.89
  intestinouterine N82.4
  intestinovaginal N82.4
    large intestine N82.3
    small intestine N82.2
  intestinovesical N32.1
  ischiorectal (fossa) K61.3
  jejunum K63.2
  joint M25.10
    ankle M25.17- ☑
    elbow M25.12- ☑
    foot joint M25.17- ☑
    hand joint M25.14- ☑
    hip M25.15- ☑
    knee M25.16- ☑
    shoulder M25.11- ☑
    specified joint NEC M25.18
    tuberculous — see Tuberculosis, joint
    vertebrae M25.18
    wrist M25.13- ☑
  kidney N28.89
  labium (majus) (minus) N82.8
  labyrinth — see subcategory H83.1 ☑
  lacrimal (gland) (sac) H04.61- ☑
  lacrimonasal duct — see Fistula, lacrimal
  laryngotracheal, congenital Q34.8
  larynx J38.7
  lip K13.0
    congenital Q38.0
  lumbar, tuberculous A18.01
  lung J86.0
  lymphatic I89.8
  mammary (gland) N61
  mastoid (process) (region) — see Mastoiditis, chronic
  maxillary J32.0
  medial, face and neck Q18.8
  mediastinal J86.0
  mediastinobronchial J86.0
  mediastinocutaneous J86.0
  middle ear — see subcategory H74.8 ☑
  mouth K12.2
  nasal J34.89
    sinus — see Sinusitis
  nasopharynx J39.2
  nipple N64.0
  nose J34.89
  oral (cutaneous) K12.2
    maxillary J32.0
    nasal (with cleft palate) — see Cleft, palate
  orbit, orbital — see Disorder, orbit, specified type NEC
  oroantral J32.0
  oviduct, external N82.5
  palate (hard) M27.8
  pancreatic K86.8
  pancreaticoduodenal K86.8
  parotid (gland) K11.4
    region K12.2
  penis N48.89
  perianal K60.3
  pericardium (pleura) (sac) — see Pericarditis
  pericecal K63.2
  perineorectal K60.4
  perineosigmoidal K63.2
  perineum, perineal (with urethral involvement) NEC
    N36.0
    tuberculous A18.13
    ureter N28.89
  perirectal K60.4
    tuberculous A18.32
  peritoneum K65.9
  pharyngoesophageal J39.2
  pharynx J39.2
    branchial cleft (congenital) Q18.0
  pilonidal (infected) (rectum) — see Sinus, pilonidal
  pleura, pleural, pleurocutaneous, pleuroperitoneal
    J86.0
    tuberculous NEC A15.6
  pleuropericardial I31.8
  portal vein-hepatic artery, congenital Q26.6
  postauricular H70.81- ☑
  postoperative, persistent T81.83 ☑
    specified site — see Fistula, by site

Fistula — *continued*
preauricular (congenital) Q18.1
prostate N42.89
pulmonary J86.0
arteriovenous I28.0
congenital Q25.72
tuberculous — *see* Tuberculosis, pulmonary
pulmonoperitoneal J86.0
rectolabial N82.4
rectosigmoid (intercommunicating) K63.2
rectoureteral N28.89
rectourethral N36.0
congenital Q64.73
rectouterine N82.4
congenital Q51.7
rectovaginal N82.3
congenital Q52.2
tuberculous A18.18
rectovesical N32.1
congenital Q64.79
rectovesicovaginal N82.3
rectovulval N82.4
congenital Q52.79
rectum (to skin) K60.4
congenital Q43.6
with absence, atresia and stenosis Q42.0
tuberculous A18.32
renal N28.89
retroauricular — *see* Fistula, postauricular
salivary duct or gland (any) K11.4
congenital Q38.4
scrotum (urinary) N50.8
tuberculous A18.15
semicircular canals — *see* subcategory H83.1 ☑
sigmoid K63.2
to bladder N32.1
sinus — *see* Sinusitis
skin L98.8
to genital tract (female) N82.5
splenocolic D73.89
stercoral K63.2
stomach K31.6
sublingual gland K11.4
submandibular gland K11.4
submaxillary (gland) K11.4
region K12.2
thoracic J86.0
duct I89.8
thoracoabdominal J86.0
thoracogastric J86.0
thoracointestinal J86.0
thorax J86.0
thyroglossal duct Q89.2
thyroid E07.89
trachea, congenital (external) (internal) Q32.1
tracheoesophageal J86.0
congenital Q39.2
with atresia of esophagus Q39.1
following tracheostomy J95.04
traumatic arteriovenous — *see* Injury, blood vessel, by site
tuberculous — *code by* site under Tuberculosis
typhoid A01.09
umbilicourinary Q64.8
urachus, congenital Q64.4
ureter (persistent) N28.89
ureteroabdominal N28.89
ureterorectal N28.89
ureterosigmoido-abdominal N28.89
ureterovaginal N82.1
ureterovesical N32.2
urethra N36.0
congenital Q64.79
tuberculous A18.13
urethroperineal N36.0
urethroperineovesical N32.2
urethrorectal N36.0
congenital Q64.73
urethroscrotal N50.8
urethrovaginal N82.1
urethrovesical N32.2
urinary (tract) (persistent) (recurrent) N36.0
uteroabdominal N82.5
congenital Q51.7
uteroenteric, uterointestinal N82.4
congenital Q51.7
uterorectal N82.4
congenital Q51.7

Fistula — *continued*
uteroureteric N82.1
uterourethral Q51.7
uterovaginal N82.8
uterovesical N82.1
congenital Q51.7
uterus N82.8
vagina (postpartal) (wall) N82.8
vaginocutaneous (postpartal) N82.5
vaginointestinal NEC N82.4
large intestine N82.3
small intestine N82.2
vaginoperineal N82.5
vasocutaneous, congenital Q55.7
vesical NEC N32.2
vesicoabdominal N32.2
vesicocervicovaginal N82.1
vesicocolic N32.1
vesicocutaneous N32.2
vesicoenteric N32.1
vesicointestinal N32.1
vesicometrorectal N82.4
vesicoperineal N32.2
vesicorectal N32.1
congenital Q64.79
vesicosigmoidal N32.1
vesicosigmoidovaginal N82.3
vesicoureteral N32.2
vesicoureterovaginal N82.1
vesicourethral N32.2
vesicourethrorectal N32.1
vesicouterine N82.1
congenital Q51.7
vesicovaginal N82.0
vulvorectal N82.4
congenital Q52.79
Fit R56.9
epileptic — *see* Epilepsy
fainting R55
hysterical F44.5
newborn P90
Fitting (and adjustment) (of)
artificial
arm — *see* Admission, adjustment, artificial, arm
breast Z44.3 ☑
eye Z44.2 ☑
leg — *see* Admission, adjustment, artificial, leg
automatic implantable cardiac defibrillator (with synchronous cardiac pacemaker) Z45.02
brain neuropacemaker Z46.2
implanted Z45.42
cardiac defibrillator — *see* Fitting (and adjustment) (of), automatic implantable cardiac defibrillator
catheter, non-vascular Z46.82
colostomy belt Z46.89
contact lenses Z46.0
cystostomy device Z46.6
defibrillator, cardiac — *see* Fitting (and adjustment) (of), automatic implantable cardiac defibrillator
dentures Z46.3
device NOS Z46.9
abdominal Z46.89
gastrointestinal NEC Z46.59
implanted NEC Z45.89
nervous system Z46.2
implanted — *see* Admission, adjustment, device, implanted, nervous system
orthodontic Z46.4
orthoptic Z46.0
orthotic Z46.89
prosthetic (external) Z44.9
breast Z44.3 ☑
dental Z46.3
eye Z44.2 ☑
specified NEC Z44.8
specified NEC Z46.89
substitution
auditory Z46.2
implanted — *see* Admission, adjustment, device, implanted, hearing device
nervous system Z46.2
implanted — *see* Admission, adjustment, device, implanted, nervous system
visual Z46.2
implanted Z45.31
urinary Z46.6
gastric lap band Z46.51
gastrointestinal appliance NEC Z46.59

Fitting — *continued*
glasses (reading) Z46.0
hearing aid Z46.1
ileostomy device Z46.89
insulin pump Z46.81
intestinal appliance NEC Z46.89
myringotomy device (stent) (tube) Z45.82
neuropacemaker Z46.2
implanted Z45.42
non-vascular catheter Z46.82
orthodontic device Z46.4
orthopedic device (brace) (cast) (corset) (shoes) Z46.89
pacemaker (cardiac) Z45.018
nervous system (brain) (peripheral nerve) (spinal cord) Z46.2
implanted Z45.42
pulse generator Z45.010
portacath (port-a-cath) Z45.2
prosthesis (external) Z44.9
arm — *see* Admission, adjustment, artificial, arm
breast Z44.3 ☑
dental Z46.3
eye Z44.2 ☑
leg — *see* Admission, adjustment, artificial, leg
specified NEC Z44.8
spectacles Z46.0
wheelchair Z46.89
Fitzhugh-Curtis syndrome
due to
Chlamydia trachomatis A74.81
Neisseria gonorrhorea (gonococcal peritonitis) A54.85
Fitz's syndrome (acute hemorrhagic pancreatitis) K85.8
Fixation
joint — *see* Ankylosis
larynx J38.7
stapes — *see* Ankylosis, ear ossicles
deafness — *see* Deafness, conductive
uterus (acquired) — *see* Malposition, uterus
vocal cord J38.3
Flabby ridge K06.8
Flaccid (*see also* condition)
palate, congenital Q38.5
Flail
chest S22.5 ☑
newborn (birth injury) P13.8
joint (paralytic) M25.20
ankle M25.27- ☑
elbow M25.22- ☑
foot joint M25.27- ☑
hand joint M25.24- ☑
hip M25.25- ☑
knee M25.26- ☑
shoulder M25.21- ☑
specified joint NEC M25.28
wrist M25.23- ☑
Flajani's disease — *see* Hyperthyroidism, with, goiter (diffuse)
Flap, liver K71.3
Flashbacks (residual to hallucinogen use) F16.283
Flat
chamber (eye) — *see* Disorder, globe, hypotony, flat anterior chamber
chest, congenital Q67.8
foot (acquired) (fixed type) (painful) (postural) (*see also* Deformity, limb, flat foot)
congenital (rigid) (spastic (everted)) Q66.5- ☑
rachitic sequelae (late effect) E64.3
organ or site, congenital NEC — *see* Anomaly, by site
pelvis M95.5
with disproportion (fetopelvic) O33.0
causing obstructed labor O65.0
congenital Q74.2
Flatau-Schilder disease G37.0
Flatback syndrome M40.30
lumbar region M40.36
lumbosacral region M40.37
thoracolumbar region M40.35
Flattening
head, femur M89.8X5
hip — *see* Coxa, plana
lip (congenital) Q18.8
nose (congenital) Q67.4
acquired M95.0
Flatulence R14.3
psychogenic F45.8
Flatus R14.3

Flatus — *continued*
  vaginalis N89.8
Flax-dresser's disease J66.1
Flea bite — *see* Injury, bite, by site, superficial, insect
Flecks, glaucomatous (subcapsular) — *see* Cataract, complicated
Fleischer (-Kayser) **ring** (cornea) H18.04- ☑
Fleshy mole O02.0
Flexibilitas cerea — *see* Catalepsy
Flexion
  amputation stump (surgical) T87.89
  cervix — *see* Malposition, uterus
  contracture, joint — *see* Contraction, joint
  deformity, joint (*see also* Deformity, limb, flexion) M21.20
    hip, congenital Q65.89
  uterus (*see also* Malposition, uterus)
    lateral — *see* Lateroversion, uterus
Flexner-Boyd dysentery A03.2
Flexner's dysentery A03.1
Flexure — *see* Flexion
Flint murmur (aortic insufficiency) I35.1
Floater, vitreous — *see* Opacity, vitreous
Floating
  cartilage (joint) (*see also* Loose, body, joint)
    knee — *see* Derangement, knee, loose body
  gallbladder, congenital Q44.1
  kidney N28.89
    congenital Q63.8
  spleen D73.89
Flooding N92.0
Floor — *see* condition
Floppy
  baby syndrome (nonspecific) P94.2
  iris syndrome (intraoperative) (IFIS) H21.81
  nonrheumatic mitral valve syndrome I34.1
Flu (*see also* Influenza)
  avian (*see also* Influenza, due to, identified novel influenza A virus) J09.X2
  bird (*see also* Influenza, due to, identified novel influenza A virus) J09.X2
  intestinal NEC A08.4
  swine (viruses that normally cause infections in pigs) (*see also* Influenza, due to, identified novel influenza A virus) J09.X2
Fluctuating blood pressure I99.8
Fluid
  abdomen R18.8
  chest J94.8
  heart — *see* Failure, heart, congestive
  joint — *see* Effusion, joint
  loss (acute) E86.9
    with
      hypernatremia E87.0
      hyponatremia E87.1
  lung — *see* Edema, lung
  overload E87.70
    specified NEC E87.79
  peritoneal cavity R18.8
  pleural cavity J94.8
  retention R60.9
Flukes NEC (*see also* Infestation, fluke)
  blood NEC — *see* Schistosomiasis
  liver B66.3
Fluor (vaginalis) N89.8
  trichomonal or due to Trichomonas (vaginalis) A59.00
Fluorosis
  dental K00.3
  skeletal M85.10
    ankle M85.17- ☑
    foot M85.17- ☑
    forearm M85.13- ☑
    hand M85.14- ☑
    lower leg M85.16- ☑
    multiple site M85.19
    neck M85.18
    rib M85.18
    shoulder M85.11- ☑
    skull M85.18
    specified site NEC M85.18
    thigh M85.15- ☑
    toe M85.17- ☑
    upper arm M85.12- ☑
    vertebra M85.18
Flush syndrome E34.0
Flushing R23.2
  menopausal N95.1

Flutter
  atrial or auricular I48.92
    atypical I48.4
    type I I48.3
    type II I48.4
    typical I48.3
  heart I49.8
    atrial or auricular I48.92
      atypical I48.4
      type I I48.3
      type II I48.4
      typical I48.3
    ventricular I49.02
  ventricular I49.02
FNHTR (febrile nonhemolytic transfusion reaction) R50.84
Fochier's abscess — *code by* site under Abscess
Focus, Assmann's — *see* Tuberculosis, pulmonary
Fogo selvagem L10.3
Foix-Alajouanine syndrome G95.19
Fold, folds (anomalous) (*see also* Anomaly, by site)
  Descemet's membrane — *see* Change, corneal membrane, Descemet's, fold
  epicanthic Q10.3
  heart Q24.8
Folie à deux F24
Follicle
  cervix (nabothian) (ruptured) N88.8
  graafian, ruptured, with hemorrhage N83.0
  nabothian N88.8
Follicular — *see* condition
Folliculitis (superficial) L73.9
  abscedens et suffodiens L66.3
  cyst N83.0
  decalvans L66.2
  deep — *see* Furuncle, by site
  gonococcal (acute) (chronic) A54.01
  keloid, keloidalis L73.0
  pustular L01.02
  ulerythematosa reticulata L66.4
Folliculome lipidique
  specified site — *see* Neoplasm, benign, by site
  unspecified site
    female D27.9
    male D29.20
Følling's disease E70.0
Follow-up — *see* Examination, follow-up
Fong's syndrome (hereditary osteo-onychodysplasia) Q78.5
Food
  allergy L27.2
  asphyxia (from aspiration or inhalation) — *see* Foreign body, by site
  choked on — *see* Foreign body, by site
  deprivation T73.0
    specified kind of food NEC E63.8
  intoxication — *see* Poisoning, food
  lack of T73.0 ☑
  poisoning — *see* Poisoning, food
  rejection NEC — *see* Disorder, eating
  strangulation or suffocation — *see* Foreign body, by site
  toxemia — *see* Poisoning, food
Foot — *see* condition
Foramen ovale (nonclosure) (patent) (persistent) Q21.1
Forbes' glycogen storage disease E74.03
Fordyce-Fox disease L75.2
Fordyce's disease (mouth) Q38.6
Forearm — *see* condition
Foreign body
  with
    laceration — *see* Laceration, by site, with foreign body
    puncture wound — *see* Puncture, by site, with foreign body
  accidentally left following a procedure T81.509 ☑
    aspiration T81.506 ☑
      resulting in
        adhesions T81.516 ☑
        obstruction T81.526 ☑
        perforation T81.536 ☑
        specified complication NEC T81.596 ☑
    cardiac catheterization T81.505 ☑
      resulting in
        acute reaction T81.60 ☑
          aseptic peritonitis T81.61 ☑
          specified NEC T81.69 ☑
        adhesions T81.515 ☑

Foreign body — *continued*
  accidentally left following a procedure — *continued*
    cardiac catheterization — *continued*
      resulting in — *continued*
        obstruction T81.525 ☑
        perforation T81.535 ☑
        specified complication NEC T81.595 ☑
    causing
      acute reaction T81.60 ☑
        aseptic peritonitis T81.61 ☑
        specified complication NEC T81.69 ☑
      adhesions T81.519 ☑
      aseptic peritonitis T81.61 ☑
      obstruction T81.529 ☑
      perforation T81.539 ☑
      specified complication NEC T81.599 ☑
    endoscopy T81.504 ☑
      resulting in
        adhesions T81.514 ☑
        obstruction T81.524 ☑
        perforation T81.534 ☑
        specified complication NEC T81.594 ☑
    immunization T81.503 ☑
      resulting in
        adhesions T81.513 ☑
        obstruction T81.523 ☑
        perforation T81.533 ☑
        specified complication NEC T81.593 ☑
    infusion T81.501 ☑
      resulting in
        adhesions T81.511 ☑
        obstruction T81.521 ☑
        perforation T81.531 ☑
        specified complication NEC T81.591 ☑
    injection T81.503 ☑
      resulting in
        adhesions T81.513 ☑
        obstruction T81.523 ☑
        perforation T81.533 ☑
        specified complication NEC T81.593 ☑
    kidney dialysis T81.502 ☑
      resulting in
        adhesions T81.512 ☑
        obstruction T81.522 ☑
        perforation T81.532 ☑
        specified complication NEC T81.592 ☑
    packing removal T81.507 ☑
      resulting in
        acute reaction T81.60 ☑
          aseptic peritonitis T81.61 ☑
          specified NEC T81.69 ☑
        adhesions T81.517 ☑
        obstruction T81.527 ☑
        perforation T81.537 ☑
        specified complication NEC T81.597 ☑
    puncture T81.506 ☑
      resulting in
        adhesions T81.516 ☑
        obstruction T81.526 ☑
        perforation T81.536 ☑
        specified complication NEC T81.596 ☑
    specified procedure NEC T81.508 ☑
      resulting in
        acute reaction T81.60 ☑
          aseptic peritonitis T81.61 ☑
          specified NEC T81.69 ☑
        adhesions T81.518 ☑
        obstruction T81.528 ☑
        perforation T81.538 ☑
        specified complication NEC T81.598 ☑
    surgical operation T81.500 ☑
      resulting in
        acute reaction T81.60 ☑
          aseptic peritonitis T81.61 ☑
          specified NEC T81.69 ☑
        adhesions T81.510 ☑
        obstruction T81.520 ☑
        perforation T81.530 ☑
        specified complication NEC T81.590 ☑
    transfusion T81.501 ☑
      resulting in
        adhesions T81.511 ☑
        obstruction T81.521 ☑
        perforation T81.531 ☑
        specified complication NEC T81.591 ☑

Foreign body — continued

- alimentary tract T18.9 ☑
  - anus T18.5 ☑
  - colon T18.4 ☑
  - esophagus — see Foreign body, esophagus
  - mouth T18.0 ☑
  - multiple sites T18.8 ☑
  - rectosigmoid (junction) T18.5 ☑
  - rectum T18.5 ☑
  - small intestine T18.3 ☑
  - specified site NEC T18.8 ☑
  - stomach T18.2 ☑
- anterior chamber (eye) S05.5- ☑
- auditory canal — see Foreign body, entering through orifice, ear
- bronchus T17.508 ☑
  - causing
    - asphyxiation T17.500 ☑
      - food (bone) (seed) T17.520 ☑
      - gastric contents (vomitus) T17.510 ☑
      - specified type NEC T17.590 ☑
    - injury NEC T17.508 ☑
      - food (bone) (seed) T17.528 ☑
      - gastric contents (vomitus) T17.518 ☑
      - specified type NEC T17.598 ☑
- canthus — see Foreign body, conjunctival sac
- ciliary body (eye) S05.5- ☑
- conjunctival sac T15.1- ☑
- cornea T15.0- ☑
- entering through orifice
  - accessory sinus T17.0 ☑
  - alimentary canal T18.9 ☑
    - multiple parts T18.8 ☑
    - specified part NEC T18.8 ☑
  - alveolar process T18.0 ☑
  - antrum (Highmore's) T17.0 ☑
  - anus T18.5 ☑
  - appendix T18.4 ☑
  - auditory canal — see Foreign body, entering through orifice, ear
  - auricle — see Foreign body, entering through orifice, ear
  - bladder T19.1 ☑
  - bronchioles — see Foreign body, respiratory tract, specified site NEC
  - bronchus (main) — see Foreign body, bronchus
  - buccal cavity T18.0 ☑
  - canthus (inner) — see Foreign body, conjunctival sac
  - cecum T18.4 ☑
  - cervix (canal) (uteri) T19.3 ☑
  - colon T18.4 ☑
  - conjunctival sac — see Foreign body, conjunctival sac
  - cornea — see Foreign body, cornea
  - digestive organ or tract NOS T18.9 ☑
    - multiple parts T18.8 ☑
    - specified part NEC T18.8 ☑
  - duodenum T18.3 ☑
  - ear (external) T16.- ☑
  - esophagus — see Foreign body, esophagus
  - eye (external) NOS T15.9- ☑
    - conjunctival sac — see Foreign body, conjunctival sac
    - cornea — see Foreign body, cornea
    - specified part NEC T15.8- ☑
  - eyeball (see also Foreign body, entering through orifice, eye, specified part NEC)
    - with penetrating wound — see Puncture, eyeball
  - eyelid (see also Foreign body, conjunctival sac) with
    - laceration — see Laceration, eyelid, with foreign body
    - puncture — see Puncture, eyelid, with foreign body
    - superficial injury — see Foreign body, superficial, eyelid
  - gastrointestinal tract T18.9 ☑
    - multiple parts T18.8 ☑
    - specified part NEC T18.8 ☑
  - genitourinary tract T19.9 ☑
    - multiple parts T19.8 ☑
    - specified part NEC T19.8 ☑
  - globe — see Foreign body, entering through orifice, eyeball

Foreign body — continued

- entering through orifice — continued
  - gum T18.0 ☑
  - Highmore's antrum T17.0 ☑
  - hypopharynx — see Foreign body, pharynx
  - ileum T18.3 ☑
  - intestine (small) T18.3 ☑
    - large T18.4 ☑
  - lacrimal apparatus (punctum) — see Foreign body, entering through orifice, eye, specified part NEC
  - large intestine T18.4 ☑
  - larynx — see Foreign body, larynx
  - lung — see Foreign body, respiratory tract, specified site NEC
  - maxillary sinus T17.0 ☑
  - mouth T18.0 ☑
  - nasal sinus T17.0 ☑
  - nasopharynx — see Foreign body, pharynx
  - nose (passage) T17.1 ☑
  - nostril T17.1 ☑
  - oral cavity T18.0 ☑
  - palate T18.0 ☑
  - penis T19.4 ☑
  - pharynx — see Foreign body, pharynx
  - piriform sinus — see Foreign body, pharynx
  - rectosigmoid (junction) T18.5 ☑
  - rectum T18.5 ☑
  - respiratory tract — see Foreign body, respiratory tract
  - sinus (accessory) (frontal) (maxillary) (nasal) T17.0 ☑
    - piriform — see Foreign body, pharynx
  - small intestine T18.3 ☑
  - stomach T18.2 ☑
  - suffocation by — see Foreign body, by site
  - tear ducts or glands — see Foreign body, entering through orifice, eye, specified part NEC
  - throat — see Foreign body, pharynx
  - tongue T18.0 ☑
  - tonsil, tonsillar (fossa) — see Foreign body, pharynx
  - trachea — see Foreign body, trachea
  - ureter T19.8 ☑
  - urethra T19.0 ☑
  - uterus (any part) T19.3 ☑
  - vagina T19.2 ☑
  - vulva T19.2 ☑
- esophagus T18.108 ☑
  - causing
    - injury NEC T18.108 ☑
      - food (bone) (seed) T18.128 ☑
      - gastric contents (vomitus) T18.118 ☑
      - specified type NEC T18.198 ☑
    - tracheal compression T18.100 ☑
      - food (bone) (seed) T18.120 ☑
      - gastric contents (vomitus) T18.110 ☑
      - specified type NEC T18.190 ☑
- felling of, in throat R09.89
- fragment — see Retained, foreign body fragments (type of)
- genitourinary tract T19.9 ☑
  - bladder T19.1 ☑
  - multiple parts T19.8 ☑
  - penis T19.4 ☑
  - specified site NEC T19.8 ☑
  - urethra T19.0 ☑
  - uterus T19.3 ☑
    - IUD Z97.5
  - vagina T19.2 ☑
    - contraceptive device Z97.5
  - vulva T19.2 ☑
- granuloma (old) (soft tissue) (see also Granuloma, foreign body)
  - skin L92.3
- in
  - laceration — see Laceration, by site, with foreign body
  - puncture wound — see Puncture, by site, with foreign body
  - soft tissue (residual) M79.5
- inadvertently left in operation wound — see Foreign body, accidentally left during a procedure
- ingestion, ingested NOS T18.9 ☑
- inhalation or inspiration — see Foreign body, by site

Foreign body — continued

- internal organ, not entering through a natural orifice — code as specific injury with foreign body
- intraocular S05.5- ☑
  - old, retained (nonmagnetic) H44.70- ☑
    - anterior chamber H44.71- ☑
    - ciliary body H44.72- ☑
    - iris H44.72- ☑
    - lens H44.73- ☑
    - magnetic H44.60- ☑
      - anterior chamber H44.61- ☑
      - ciliary body H44.62- ☑
      - iris H44.62- ☑
      - lens H44.63- ☑
      - posterior wall H44.64- ☑
      - specified site NEC H44.69- ☑
      - vitreous body H44.65- ☑
    - posterior wall H44.74- ☑
    - specified site NEC H44.79- ☑
    - vitreous body H44.75- ☑
  - iris — see Foreign body, intraocular
- lacrimal punctum — see Foreign body, entering through orifice, eye, specified part NEC
- larynx T17.308 ☑
  - causing
    - asphyxiation T17.300 ☑
      - food (bone) (seed) T17.320 ☑
      - gastric contents (vomitus) T17.310 ☑
      - specified type NEC T17.390 ☑
    - injury NEC T17.308 ☑
      - food (bone) (seed) T17.328 ☑
      - gastric contents (vomitus) T17.318 ☑
      - specified type NEC T17.398 ☑
- lens — see Foreign body, intraocular
- ocular muscle S05.4- ☑
  - old, retained — see Foreign body, orbit, old
- old or residual
  - soft tissue (residual) M79.5
- operation wound, left accidentally — see Foreign body, accidentally left during a procedure
- orbit S05.4- ☑
  - old, retained H05.5- ☑
- pharynx T17.208 ☑
  - causing
    - asphyxiation T17.200 ☑
      - food (bone) (seed) T17.220 ☑
      - gastric contents (vomitus) T17.210 ☑
      - specified type NEC T17.290 ☑
    - injury NEC T17.208 ☑
      - food (bone) (seed) T17.228 ☑
      - gastric contents (vomitus) T17.218 ☑
      - specified type NEC T17.298 ☑
- respiratory tract T17.908 ☑
  - bronchioles — see Foreign body, respiratory tract, specified site NEC
  - bronchus — see Foreign body, bronchus
  - causing
    - asphyxiation T17.900 ☑
      - food (bone) (seed) T17.920 ☑
      - gastric contents (vomitus) T17.910 ☑
      - specified type NEC T17.990 ☑
    - injury NEC T17.908 ☑
      - food (bone) (seed) T17.928 ☑
      - gastric contents (vomitus) T17.918 ☑
      - specified type NEC T17.998 ☑
  - larynx — see Foreign body, larynx
  - lung — see Foreign body, respiratory tract, specified site NEC
  - multiple parts — see Foreign body, respiratory tract, specified site NEC
  - nasal sinus T17.0 ☑
  - nasopharynx — see Foreign body, pharynx
  - nose T17.1 ☑
  - nostril T17.1 ☑
  - pharynx — see Foreign body, pharynx
  - specified site NEC T17.808 ☑
    - causing
      - asphyxiation T17.800 ☑
        - food (bone) (seed) T17.820 ☑
        - gastric contents (vomitus) T17.810 ☑
        - specified type NEC T17.890 ☑
      - injury NEC T17.808 ☑
        - food (bone) (seed) T17.828 ☑
        - gastric contents (vomitus) T17.818 ☑
        - specified type NEC T17.898 ☑
  - throat — see Foreign body, pharynx

Foreign body — *continued*
  respiratory tract — *continued*
    trachea — *see* Foreign body, trachea
  retained (old) (nonmagnetic) (in)
    anterior chamber (eye) — *see* Foreign body, intraocular, old, retained, anterior chamber
      magnetic — *see* Foreign body, intraocular, old, retained, magnetic, anterior chamber
    ciliary body — *see* Foreign body, intraocular, old, retained, ciliary body
      magnetic — *see* Foreign body, intraocular, old, retained, magnetic, ciliary body
    eyelid H02.819
      left H02.816
        lower H02.815
        upper H02.814
      right H02.813
        lower H02.812
        upper H02.811
    fragments — *see* Retained, foreign body fragments (type of)
    globe — *see* Foreign body, intraocular, old, retained
      magnetic — *see* Foreign body, intraocular, old, retained, magnetic
    intraocular — *see* Foreign body, intraocular, old, retained
      magnetic — *see* Foreign body, intraocular, old, retained, magnetic
    iris — *see* Foreign body, intraocular, old, retained, iris
      magnetic — *see* Foreign body, intraocular, old, retained, magnetic, iris
    lens — *see* Foreign body, intraocular, old, retained, lens
      magnetic — *see* Foreign body, intraocular, old, retained, magnetic, lens
    muscle — *see* Foreign body, retained, soft tissue
    orbit — *see* Foreign body, orbit, old
    posterior wall of globe — *see* Foreign body, intraocular, old, retained, posterior wall
      magnetic — *see* Foreign body, intraocular, old, retained, magnetic, posterior wall
    retrobulbar — *see* Foreign body, orbit, old, retrobulbar
    soft tissue M79.5
    vitreous — *see* Foreign body, intraocular, old, retained, vitreous body
      magnetic — *see* Foreign body, intraocular, old, retained, magnetic, vitreous body
  retina S05.5- ☑
  superficial, without open wound
    abdomen, abdominal (wall) S30.851 ☑
    alveolar process S00.552 ☑
    ankle S90.55- ☑
    antecubital space — *see* Foreign body, superficial, forearm
    anus S30.857 ☑
    arm (upper) S40.85- ☑
    auditory canal — *see* Foreign body, superficial, ear
    auricle — *see* Foreign body, superficial, ear
    axilla — *see* Foreign body, superficial, arm
    back, lower S30.850 ☑
    breast S20.15- ☑
    brow S00.85 ☑
    buttock S30.850 ☑
    calf — *see* Foreign body, superficial, leg
    canthus — *see* Foreign body, superficial, eyelid
    cheek S00.85 ☑
      internal S00.552 ☑
    chest wall — *see* Foreign body, superficial, thorax
    chin S00.85 ☑
    clitoris S30.854 ☑
    costal region — *see* Foreign body, superficial, thorax
    digit(s)
      foot — *see* Foreign body, superficial, toe
      hand — *see* Foreign body, superficial, finger
    ear S00.45- ☑
    elbow S50.35- ☑
    epididymis S30.853 ☑
    epigastric region S30.851 ☑
    epiglottis S10.15 ☑
    esophagus, cervical S10.15 ☑
    eyebrow — *see* Foreign body, superficial, eyelid
    eyelid S00.25- ☑
    face S00.85 ☑

Foreign body — *continued*
  superficial, without open wound — *continued*
    finger(s) S60.459 ☑
      index S60.45- ☑
      little S60.45- ☑
      middle S60.45- ☑
      ring S60.45- ☑
    flank S30.851 ☑
    foot (except toe(s) alone) S90.85- ☑
      toe — *see* Foreign body, superficial, toe
    forearm S50.85- ☑
      elbow only — *see* Foreign body, superficial, elbow
    forehead S00.85 ☑
    genital organs, external
      female S30.856 ☑
      male S30.855 ☑
    groin S30.851 ☑
    gum S00.552 ☑
    hand S60.55- ☑
    head S00.95 ☑
      ear — *see* Foreign body, superficial, ear
      eyelid — *see* Foreign body, superficial, eyelid
      lip S00.551 ☑
      nose S00.35 ☑
      oral cavity S00.552 ☑
      scalp S00.05 ☑
      specified site NEC S00.85 ☑
    heel — *see* Foreign body, superficial, foot
    hip S70.25- ☑
    inguinal region S30.851 ☑
    interscapular region S20.459 ☑
    jaw S00.85 ☑
    knee S80.25- ☑
    labium (majus) (minus) S30.854 ☑
    larynx S10.15 ☑
    leg (lower) S80.85- ☑
      knee — *see* Foreign body, superficial, knee
      upper — *see* Foreign body, superficial, thigh
    lip S00.551 ☑
    lower back S30.850 ☑
    lumbar region S30.850 ☑
    malar region S00.85 ☑
    mammary — *see* Foreign body, superficial, breast
    mastoid region S00.85 ☑
    mouth S00.552 ☑
    nail
      finger — *see* Foreign body, superficial, finger
      toe — *see* Foreign body, superficial, toe
    nape S10.85 ☑
    nasal S00.35 ☑
    neck S10.95 ☑
      specified site NEC S10.85 ☑
      throat S10.15 ☑
    nose S00.35 ☑
    occipital region S00.05 ☑
    oral cavity S00.552 ☑
    orbital region — *see* Foreign body, superficial, eyelid
    palate S00.552 ☑
    palm — *see* Foreign body, superficial, hand
    parietal region S00.05 ☑
    pelvis S30.850 ☑
    penis S30.852 ☑
    perineum
      female S30.854 ☑
      male S30.850 ☑
    periocular area — *see* Foreign body, superficial, eyelid
    phalanges
      finger — *see* Foreign body, superficial, finger
      toe — *see* Foreign body, superficial, toe
    pharynx S10.15 ☑
    pinna — *see* Foreign body, superficial, ear
    popliteal space — *see* Foreign body, superficial, knee
    prepuce S30.852 ☑
    pubic region S30.850 ☑
    pudendum
      female S30.856 ☑
      male S30.855 ☑
    sacral region S30.850 ☑
    scalp S00.05 ☑
    scapular region — *see* Foreign body, superficial, shoulder
    scrotum S30.853 ☑

Foreign body — *continued*
  superficial, without open wound — *continued*
    shin — *see* Foreign body, superficial, leg
    shoulder S40.25- ☑
    sternal region S20.359 ☑
    submaxillary region S00.85 ☑
    submental region S00.85 ☑
    subungual
      finger(s) — *see* Foreign body, superficial, finger
      toe(s) — *see* Foreign body, superficial, toe
    supraclavicular fossa S10.85 ☑
    supraorbital S00.85 ☑
    temple S00.85 ☑
    temporal region S00.85 ☑
    testis S30.853 ☑
    thigh S70.35- ☑
    thorax, thoracic (wall) S20.95 ☑
      back S20.45- ☑
      front S20.35- ☑
    throat S10.15 ☑
    thumb S60.35- ☑
    toe(s) (lesser) S90.456 ☑
      great S90.45- ☑
    tongue S00.552 ☑
    trachea S10.15 ☑
    tunica vaginalis S30.853 ☑
    tympanum, tympanic membrane — *see* Foreign body, superficial, ear
    uvula S00.552 ☑
    vagina S30.854 ☑
    vocal cords S10.15 ☑
    vulva S30.854 ☑
    wrist S60.85- ☑
  swallowed T18.9 ☑
  trachea T17.408 ☑
    causing
      asphyxiation T17.400 ☑
        food (bone) (seed) T17.420 ☑
        gastric contents (vomitus) T17.410 ☑
        specified type NEC T17.490 ☑
      injury NEC T17.408 ☑
        food (bone) (seed) T17.428 ☑
        gastric contents (vomitus) T17.418 ☑
        specified type NEC T17.498 ☑
  type of fragment — *see* Retained, foreign body fragments (type of)
  vitreous (humor) S05.5- ☑
Forestier's disease (rhizomelic pseudopolyarthritis) M35.3
  meaning ankylosing hyperostosis — *see* Hyperostosis, ankylosing
Formation
  hyalin in cornea — *see* Degeneration, cornea
  sequestrum in bone (due to infection) — *see* Osteomyelitis, chronic
  valve
    colon, congenital Q43.8
    ureter (congenital) Q62.39
Formication R20.2
Fort Bragg fever A27.89
Fossa (*see also* condition)
  pyriform — *see* condition
Foster-Kennedy syndrome H47.14- ☑
Fothergill's
  disease (trigeminal neuralgia) (*see also* Neuralgia, trigeminal)
  scarlatina anginosa A38.9
Foul breath R19.6
Foundling Z76.1
Fournier disease or gangrene N49.3
  female N76.89
Fourth
  cranial nerve — *see* condition
  molar K00.1
Foville's (peduncular) **disease or syndrome** G46.3
Fox (-Fordyce) disease (apocrine miliaria) L75.2
Fracture, burst — *see* Fracture, traumatic, by site
Fracture, chronic — *see* Fracture, pathological
Fracture, insufficiency — *see* Fracture, pathologic, by site
Fracture, pathological (pathologic) (*see also* Fracture, traumatic) M84.40 ☑
  ankle M84.47- ☑
  carpus M84.44- ☑
  clavicle M84.41- ☑
  dental implant M27.63

Fracture, pathological — *continued*
dental restorative material K08.539
  with loss of material K08.531
  without loss of material K08.530
due to
  neoplastic disease NEC (*see also* Neoplasm)
    M84.50 ☑
    ankle M84.57- ☑
    carpus M84.54- ☑
    clavicle M84.51- ☑
    femur M84.55- ☑
    fibula M84.56- ☑
    finger M84.54- ☑
    hip M84.559 ☑
    humerus M84.52- ☑
    ilium M84.550 ☑
    ischium M84.550 ☑
    metacarpus M84.54- ☑
    metatarsus M84.57- ☑
    neck M84.58 ☑
    pelvis M84.550 ☑
    radius M84.53- ☑
    rib M84.58 ☑
    scapula M84.51- ☑
    skull M84.58 ☑
    specified site NEC M84.58 ☑
    tarsus M84.57- ☑
    tibia M84.56- ☑
    toe M84.57- ☑
    ulna M84.53- ☑
    vertebra M84.58 ☑
  osteoporosis M80.80 ☑
    disuse — *see* Osteoporosis, specified type NEC,
      with pathological fracture
    drug-induced — *see* Osteoporosis, drug in-
      duced, with pathological fracture
    idiopathic — *see* Osteoporosis, specified type
      NEC, with pathological fracture
    postmenopausal — *see* Osteoporosis, post-
      menopausal, with pathological fracture
    postoophorectomy — *see* Osteoporosis, pos-
      toophorectomy, with pathological frac-
      ture
    postsurgical malabsorption — *see* Osteoporo-
      sis, specified type NEC, with pathological
      fracture
    specified cause NEC — *see* Osteoporosis, spec-
      ified type NEC, with pathological fracture
  specified disease NEC M84.60 ☑
    ankle M84.67- ☑
    carpus M84.64- ☑
    clavicle M84.61- ☑
    femur M84.65- ☑
    fibula M84.66- ☑
    finger M84.64- ☑
    hip M84.65- ☑
    humerus M84.62- ☑
    ilium M84.650 ☑
    ischium M84.650 ☑
    metacarpus M84.64- ☑
    metatarsus M84.67- ☑
    neck M84.68 ☑
    radius M84.63- ☑
    rib M84.68 ☑
    scapula M84.61- ☑
    skull M84.68 ☑
    tarsus M84.67- ☑
    tibia M84.66- ☑
    toe M84.67- ☑
    ulna M84.63- ☑
    vertebra M84.68 ☑
  femur M84.45- ☑
  fibula M84.46- ☑
  finger M84.44- ☑
  hip M84.459 ☑
  humerus M84.42- ☑
  ilium M84.454 ☑
  ischium M84.454 ☑
  joint prosthesis — *see* Complications, joint prosthesis,
    mechanical, breakdown, by site
    periprosthetic — *see* Complications, joint prosthe-
      sis, mechanical, periprosthesis, fracture, by
      site
  metacarpus M84.44- ☑
  metatarsus M84.47- ☑
  neck M84.48 ☑

Fracture, pathological — *continued*
  pelvis M84.454 ☑
  radius M84.43- ☑
  restorative material (dental) K08.539
    with loss of material K08.531
    without loss of material K08.530
  rib M84.48 ☑
  scapula M84.41- ☑
  skull M84.48 ☑
  tarsus M84.47- ☑
  tibia M84.46- ☑
  toe M84.47- ☑
  ulna M84.43- ☑
  vertebra M84.48 ☑
Fracture, traumatic (abduction) (adduction) (separation)
    (*see also* Fracture, pathological) T14.8
  acetabulum S32.40- ☑
    column
      anterior (displaced) (iliopubic) S32.43- ☑
        nondisplaced S32.436 ☑
      posterior (displaced) (ilioischial) S32.443 ☑
        nondisplaced S32.44- ☑
    dome (displaced) S32.48- ☑
      nondisplaced S32.48 ☑
    specified NEC S32.49- ☑
    transverse (displaced) S32.45- ☑
      with associated posterior wall fracture (dis-
        placed) S32.46- ☑
        nondisplaced S32.46- ☑
      nondisplaced S32.45- ☑
    wall
      anterior (displaced) S32.41- ☑
        nondisplaced S32.41- ☑
      medial (displaced) S32.47- ☑
        nondisplaced S32.47- ☑
      posterior (displaced) S32.42- ☑
        with associated transverse fracture (dis-
          placed) S32.46- ☑
          nondisplaced S32.46- ☑
        nondisplaced S32.42- ☑
  acromion — *see* Fracture, scapula, acromial process
  ankle S82.899 ☑
    bimalleolar (displaced) S82.84- ☑
      nondisplaced S82.84- ☑
    lateral malleolus only (displaced) S82.6- ☑
      nondisplaced S82.6- ☑
    medial malleolus (displaced) S82.5- ☑
      associated with Maisonneuve's fracture — *see*
        Fracture, Maisonneuve's
      nondisplaced S82.5- ☑
    talus — *see* Fracture, tarsal, talus
    trimalleolar (displaced) S82.85- ☑
      nondisplaced S82.85- ☑
  arm (upper) (*see also* Fracture, humerus, shaft)
    humerus — *see* Fracture, humerus
    radius — *see* Fracture, radius
    ulna — *see* Fracture, ulna
  astragalus — *see* Fracture, tarsal, talus
  atlas — *see* Fracture, neck, cervical vertebra, first
  axis — *see* Fracture, neck, cervical vertebra, second
  back — *see* Fracture, vertebra
  Barton's — *see* Barton's fracture
  base of skull — *see* Fracture, skull, base
  basicervical (basal) (femoral) S72.0 ☑
  Bennett's — *see* Bennett's fracture
  bimalleolar — *see* Fracture, ankle, bimalleolar
  blow-out S02.3 ☑
  bone NEC T14.8
    birth injury P13.9
    following insertion of orthopedic implant, joint
      prosthesis or bone plate — *see* Fracture,
      following insertion of orthopedic implant,
      joint prosthesis or bone plate
    in (due to) neoplastic disease NEC — *see* Fracture,
      pathological, due to, neoplastic disease
    pathological (cause unknown) — *see* Fracture,
      pathological
  breast bone — *see* Fracture, sternum
  bucket handle (semilunar cartilage) — *see* Tear,
    meniscus
  burst — *see* Fracture, traumatic, by site
  calcaneus — *see* Fracture, tarsal, calcaneus
  carpal bone(s) S62.10- ☑
    capitate (displaced) S62.13- ☑
      nondisplaced S62.13- ☑
    cuneiform — *see* Fracture, carpal bone, triquetrum

Fracture, traumatic — *continued*
  carpal bone(s) — *continued*
    hamate (body) (displaced) S62.143 ☑
      hook process (displaced) S62.15- ☑
        nondisplaced S62.15- ☑
      nondisplaced S62.14- ☑
    larger multangular — *see* Fracture, carpal bones,
      trapezium
    lunate (displaced) S62.12- ☑
      nondisplaced S62.12- ☑
    navicular S62.00- ☑
      distal pole (displaced) S62.01- ☑
        nondisplaced S62.01- ☑
      middle third (displaced) S62.02- ☑
        nondisplaced S62.02- ☑
      proximal third (displaced) S62.03- ☑
        nondisplaced S62.03- ☑
      volar tuberosity — *see* Fracture, carpal bones,
        navicular, distal pole
    os magnum — *see* Fracture, carpal bones, capitate
    pisiform (displaced) S62.16- ☑
      nondisplaced S62.16- ☑
    semilunar — *see* Fracture, carpal bones, lunate
    smaller multangular — *see* Fracture, carpal bones,
      trapezoid
    trapezium (displaced) S62.17- ☑
      nondisplaced S62.17- ☑
    trapezoid (displaced) S62.18- ☑
      nondisplaced S62.18- ☑
    triquetrum (displaced) S62.11- ☑
      nondisplaced S62.11- ☑
    unciform — *see* Fracture, carpal bones, hamate
  cervical — *see* Fracture, vertebra, cervical
  clavicle S42.00- ☑
    acromial end (displaced) S42.03- ☑
      nondisplaced S42.03- ☑
    birth injury P13.4
    lateral end — *see* Fracture, clavicle, acromial end
    shaft (displaced) S42.02- ☑
      nondisplaced S42.02- ☑
    sternal end (anterior) (displaced) S42.01- ☑
      nondisplaced S42.01- ☑
      posterior S42.01- ☑
  coccyx S32.2 ☑
  collapsed — *see* Collapse, vertebra
  collar bone — *see* Fracture, clavicle
  Colles' — *see* Colles' fracture
  compression, not due to trauma — *see* Collapse, ver-
    tebra
  coronoid process — *see* Fracture, ulna, upper end,
    coronoid process
  corpus cavernosum penis S39.840 ☑
  costochondral cartilage S23.41 ☑
  costochondral, costosternal junction — *see* Fracture,
    rib
  cranium — *see* Fracture, skull
  cricoid cartilage S12.8 ☑
  cuboid (ankle) — *see* Fracture, tarsal, cuboid
  cuneiform
    foot — *see* Fracture, tarsal, cuneiform
    wrist — *see* Fracture, carpal, triquetrum
  delayed union — *see* Delay, union, fracture
  dental restorative material K08.539
    with loss of material K08.531
    without loss of material K08.530
  due to
    birth injury — *see* Birth, injury, fracture
    osteoporosis — *see* Osteoporosis, with fracture
  Dupuytren's — *see* Fracture, ankle, lateral malleolus
  elbow S42.40- ☑
  ethmoid (bone) (sinus) — *see* Fracture, skull, base
  face bone S02.92 ☑
  fatigue (*see also* Fracture, stress)
    vertebra M48.40 ☑
      cervical region M48.42 ☑
      cervicothoracic region M48.43 ☑
      lumbar region M48.46 ☑
      lumbosacral region M48.47 ☑
      occipito-atlanto-axial region M48.41 ☑
      sacrococcygeal region M48.48 ☑
      thoracic region M48.44 ☑
      thoracolumbar region M48.45 ☑
  femur, femoral S72.9- ☑
    basicervical (basal) S72.0 ☑
    birth injury P13.2
    capital epiphyseal S79.01- ☑

Fracture, traumatic — *continued*
  femur, femoral — *continued*
    condyles, epicondyles — *see* Fracture, femur, lower end
    distal end — *see* Fracture, femur, lower end
    epiphysis
      head — *see* Fracture, femur, upper end, epiphysis
      lower — *see* Fracture, femur, lower end, epiphysis
      upper — *see* Fracture, femur, upper end, epiphysis
    following insertion of implant, prosthesis or plate M96.66- ☑
    head — *see* Fracture, femur, upper end, head
    intertrochanteric — *see* Fracture, femur, trochanteric
    intratrochanteric — *see* Fracture, femur, trochanteric
    lower end S72.40- ☑
      condyle (displaced) S72.41- ☑
        lateral (displaced) S72.42- ☑
          nondisplaced S72.42- ☑
        medial (displaced) S72.43- ☑
          nondisplaced S72.43- ☑
        nondisplaced S72.41- ☑
      epiphysis (displaced) S72.44- ☑
        nondisplaced S72.44- ☑
      physeal S79.10- ☑
        Salter-Harris
          Type I S79.11- ☑
          Type II S79.12- ☑
          Type III S79.13- ☑
          Type IV S79.14- ☑
        specified NEC S79.19- ☑
      specified NEC S72.49- ☑
      supracondylar (displaced) S72.45- ☑
        with intracondylar extension (displaced) S72.46- ☑
          nondisplaced S72.46- ☑
        nondisplaced S72.45- ☑
      torus S72.47- ☑
    neck — *see* Fracture, femur, upper end, neck
    pertrochanteric — *see* Fracture, femur, trochanteric
    shaft (lower third) (middle third) (upper third) S72.30- ☑
      comminuted (displaced) S72.35- ☑
        nondisplaced S72.35- ☑
      oblique (displaced) S72.33- ☑
        nondisplaced S72.33- ☑
      segmental (displaced) S72.36- ☑
        nondisplaced S72.36- ☑
      specified NEC S72.39- ☑
      spiral (displaced) S72.34- ☑
        nondisplaced S72.34- ☑
      transverse (displaced) S72.32- ☑
        nondisplaced S72.32- ☑
    specified site NEC — *see* subcategory S72.8 ☑
    subcapital (displaced) S72.01- ☑
    subtrochanteric (region) (section) (displaced) S72.2- ☑
      nondisplaced S72.2- ☑
    transcervical — *see* Fracture, femur, upper end, neck
    transtrochanteric — *see* Fracture, femur, trochanteric
    trochanteric S72.10- ☑
      apophyseal (displaced) S72.14- ☑
        nondisplaced S72.14- ☑
      greater trochanter (displaced) S72.11- ☑
        nondisplaced S72.11- ☑
      intertrochanteric (displaced) S72.13- ☑
        nondisplaced S72.13- ☑
      lesser trochanter (displaced) S72.12- ☑
        nondisplaced S72.12- ☑
    upper end S72.00- ☑
      apophyseal (displaced) S72.13- ☑
        nondisplaced S72.13- ☑
      cervicotrochanteric — *see* Fracture, femur, upper end, neck, base
      epiphysis (displaced) S72.02- ☑
        nondisplaced S72.02- ☑
      head S72.05- ☑
        articular (displaced) S72.06- ☑
          nondisplaced S72.06- ☑

Fracture, traumatic — *continued*
  femur, femoral — *continued*
    upper end — *continued*
      head — *continued*
        specified NEC S72.09- ☑
      intertrochanteric (displaced) S72.14- ☑
        nondisplaced S72.14- ☑
      intracapsular S72.01- ☑
      midcervical (displaced) S72.03- ☑
        nondisplaced S72.03- ☑
      neck S72.00- ☑
        base (displaced) S72.04- ☑
          nondisplaced S72.04- ☑
        specified NEC S72.09- ☑
      pertrochanteric — *see* Fracture, femur, upper end, trochanteric
      physeal S79.00- ☑
        Salter-Harris type I S79.01- ☑
        specified NEC S79.09- ☑
      subcapital (displaced) S72.01- ☑
      subtrochanteric (displaced) S72.2- ☑
        nondisplaced S72.2- ☑
      transcervical — *see* Fracture, femur, upper end, midcervical
      trochanteric S72.10- ☑
        greater (displaced) S72.11- ☑
          nondisplaced S72.11- ☑
        lesser (displaced) S72.12- ☑
          nondisplaced S72.12- ☑
  fibula (shaft) (styloid) S82.40- ☑
    comminuted (displaced) S82.45- ☑
      nondisplaced S82.45- ☑
    following insertion of implant, prosthesis or plate M96.67- ☑
    involving ankle or malleolus — *see* Fracture, fibula, lateral malleolus
    lateral malleolus (displaced) S82.6- ☑
      nondisplaced S82.6- ☑
    lower end
      physeal S89.30- ☑
        Salter-Harris
          Type I S89.31- ☑
          Type II S89.32- ☑
        specified NEC S89.39- ☑
      specified NEC S82.83- ☑
      torus S82.82- ☑
    oblique (displaced) S82.43- ☑
      nondisplaced S82.43- ☑
    segmental (displaced) S82.46- ☑
      nondisplaced S82.46- ☑
    specified NEC S82.49- ☑
    spiral (displaced) S82.44- ☑
      nondisplaced S82.44- ☑
    transverse (displaced) S82.42- ☑
      nondisplaced S82.42- ☑
    upper end
      physeal S89.20- ☑
        Salter-Harris
          Type I S89.21- ☑
          Type II S89.22- ☑
        specified NEC S89.29- ☑
      specified NEC S82.83- ☑
      torus S82.81- ☑
  finger (except thumb) S62.60- ☑
    distal phalanx (displaced) S62.63- ☑
      nondisplaced S62.66- ☑
    index S62.60- ☑
      distal phalanx (displaced) S62.63- ☑
        nondisplaced S62.66- ☑
      medial phalanx (displaced) S62.62- ☑
        nondisplaced S62.65- ☑
      proximal phalanx (displaced) S62.61- ☑
        nondisplaced S62.64- ☑
    little S62.60- ☑
      distal phalanx (displaced) S62.63- ☑
        nondisplaced S62.66- ☑
      medial phalanx (displaced) S62.62- ☑
        nondisplaced S62.65- ☑
      proximal phalanx (displaced) S62.61- ☑
        nondisplaced S62.64- ☑
    medial phalanx (displaced) S62.62- ☑
      nondisplaced S62.65- ☑
    middle S62.60- ☑
      distal phalanx (displaced) S62.63- ☑
        nondisplaced S62.66- ☑
      medial phalanx (displaced) S62.62- ☑

Fracture, traumatic — *continued*
  finger — *continued*
    middle — *continued*
      medial phalanx — *continued*
        nondisplaced S62.65- ☑
      proximal phalanx (displaced) S62.61- ☑
        nondisplaced S62.64- ☑
    proximal phalanx (displaced) S62.61- ☑
      nondisplaced S62.64- ☑
    ring S62.60- ☑
      distal phalanx (displaced) S62.63- ☑
        nondisplaced S62.66- ☑
      medial phalanx (displaced) S62.62- ☑
        nondisplaced S62.65- ☑
      proximal phalanx (displaced) S62.61- ☑
        nondisplaced S62.64- ☑
    thumb — *see* Fracture, thumb
  following insertion (intraoperative) (postoperative) of orthopedic implant, joint prosthesis or bone plate M96.69
    femur M96.66- ☑
    fibula M96.67- ☑
    humerus M96.62- ☑
    pelvis M96.65
    radius M96.63- ☑
    specified bone NEC M96.69
    tibia M96.67- ☑
    ulna M96.63- ☑
  foot S92.90- ☑
    astragalus — *see* Fracture, tarsal, talus
    calcaneus — *see* Fracture, tarsal, calcaneus
    cuboid — *see* Fracture, tarsal, cuboid
    cuneiform — *see* Fracture, tarsal, cuneiform
    metatarsal — *see* Fracture, metatarsal
    navicular — *see* Fracture, tarsal, navicular
    talus — *see* Fracture, tarsal, talus
    tarsal — *see* Fracture, tarsal
    toe — *see* Fracture, toe
  forearm S52.9- ☑
    radius — *see* Fracture, radius
    ulna — *see* Fracture, ulna
  fossa (anterior) (middle) (posterior) S02.19 ☑
  frontal (bone) (skull) S02.0 ☑
    sinus S02.19 ☑
  glenoid (cavity) (scapula) — *see* Fracture, scapula, glenoid cavity
  greenstick — *see* Fracture, by site
  hallux — *see* Fracture, toe, great
  hand S62.9- ☑
    carpal — *see* Fracture, carpal bone
    finger (except thumb) — *see* Fracture, finger
    metacarpal — *see* Fracture, metacarpal
    navicular (scaphoid) (hand) — *see* Fracture, carpal bone, navicular
    thumb — *see* Fracture, thumb
  healed or old
    with complications — *code by* Nature of the complication
  heel bone — *see* Fracture, tarsal, calcaneus
  Hill-Sachs S42.29- ☑
  hip — *see* Fracture, femur, neck
  humerus S42.30- ☑
    anatomical neck — *see* Fracture, humerus, upper end
    articular process — *see* Fracture, humerus, lower end
    capitellum — *see* Fracture, humerus, lower end, condyle, lateral
    distal end — *see* Fracture, humerus, lower end
    epiphysis
      lower — *see* Fracture, humerus, lower end, physeal
      upper — *see* Fracture, humerus, upper end, physeal
    external condyle — *see* Fracture, humerus, lower end, condyle, lateral
    following insertion of implant, prosthesis or plate M96.62- ☑
    great tuberosity — *see* Fracture, humerus, upper end, greater tuberosity
    intercondylar — *see* Fracture, humerus, lower end
    internal epicondyle — *see* Fracture, humerus, lower end, epicondyle, medial
    lesser tuberosity — *see* Fracture, humerus, upper end, lesser tuberosity
    lower end S42.40- ☑

Fracture, traumatic — *continued*
  humerus — *continued*
    lower end — *continued*
      condyle
        lateral (displaced) S42.45- ☑
          nondisplaced S42.45- ☑
        medial (displaced) S42.46- ☑
          nondisplaced S42.46- ☑
      epicondyle
        lateral (displaced) S42.43- ☑
          nondisplaced S42.43- ☑
        medial (displaced) S42.44- ☑
          incarcerated S42.44- ☑
          nondisplaced S42.44- ☑
      physeal S49.10- ☑
        Salter-Harris
          Type I S49.11- ☑
          Type II S49.12- ☑
          Type III S49.13- ☑
          Type IV S49.14- ☑
          specified NEC S49.19- ☑
      specified NEC (displaced) S42.49- ☑
        nondisplaced S42.49- ☑
      supracondylar (simple) (displaced) S42.41- ☑
        comminuted (displaced) S42.42- ☑
          nondisplaced S42.42- ☑
        nondisplaced S42.41- ☑
      torus S42.48- ☑
      transcondylar (displaced) S42.47- ☑
        nondisplaced S42.47- ☑
    proximal end — *see* Fracture, humerus, upper end
    shaft S42.30- ☑
      comminuted (displaced) S42.35- ☑
        nondisplaced S42.35- ☑
      greenstick S42.31- ☑
      oblique (displaced) S42.33- ☑
        nondisplaced S42.33- ☑
      segmental (displaced) S42.36- ☑
        nondisplaced S42.36- ☑
      specified NEC S42.39- ☑
      spiral (displaced) S42.34- ☑
        nondisplaced S42.34- ☑
      transverse (displaced) S42.32- ☑
        nondisplaced S42.32- ☑
    supracondylar — *see* Fracture, humerus, lower end
    surgical neck — *see* Fracture, humerus, upper end, surgical neck
    trochlea — *see* Fracture, humerus, lower end, condyle, medial
    tuberosity — *see* Fracture, humerus, upper end
    upper end S42.20- ☑
      anatomical neck — *see* Fracture, humerus, upper end, specified NEC
      articular head — *see* Fracture, humerus, upper end, specified NEC
      epiphysis — *see* Fracture, humerus, upper end, physeal
      greater tuberosity (displaced) S42.25- ☑
        nondisplaced S42.25- ☑
      lesser tuberosity (displaced) S42.26- ☑
        nondisplaced S42.26- ☑
      physeal S49.00- ☑
        Salter-Harris
          Type I S49.01- ☑
          Type II S49.02- ☑
          Type III S49.03- ☑
          Type IV S49.04- ☑
          specified NEC S49.09- ☑
      specified NEC (displaced) S42.29- ☑
        nondisplaced S42.29- ☑
      surgical neck (displaced) S42.21- ☑
        four-part S42.24- ☑
        nondisplaced S42.21- ☑
        three-part S42.23- ☑
        two-part (displaced) S42.22- ☑
          nondisplaced S42.22- ☑
      torus S42.27- ☑
      transepiphyseal — *see* Fracture, humerus, upper end, physeal
  hyoid bone S12.8- ☑
  ilium S32.30- ☑
    with disruption of pelvic ring — *see* Disruption, pelvic ring
    avulsion (displaced) S32.31- ☑
      nondisplaced S32.31- ☑
    specified NEC S32.39- ☑

Fracture, traumatic — *continued*
  impaction, impacted — *code as* Fracture, by site
  innominate bone — *see* Fracture, ilium
  instep — *see* Fracture, foot
  ischium S32.60- ☑
    with disruption of pelvic ring — *see* Disruption, pelvic ring
    avulsion (displaced) S32.61- ☑
      nondisplaced S32.61- ☑
    specified NEC S32.69- ☑
  jaw (bone) (lower) — *see* Fracture, mandible
    upper — *see* Fracture, maxilla
  joint prosthesis — *see* Complications, joint prosthesis, mechanical, breakdown, by site
    periprosthetic — *see* Complications, joint prosthesis, mechanical, periprosthesis, fracture, by site
  knee cap — *see* Fracture, patella
  larynx S12.8 ☑
  late effects — *see* Sequelae, fracture
  leg (lower) S82.9- ☑
    ankle — *see* Fracture, ankle
    femur — *see* Fracture, femur
    fibula — *see* Fracture, fibula
    malleolus — *see* Fracture, ankle
    patella — *see* Fracture, patella
    specified site NEC S82.89- ☑
    tibia — *see* Fracture, tibia
  lumbar spine — *see* Fracture, vertebra, lumbar
  lumbosacral spine S32.9 ☑
  Maisonneuve's (displaced) S82.86- ☑
    nondisplaced S82.86- ☑
  malar bone (*see also* Fracture, maxilla) S02.400 ☑
  malleolus — *see* Fracture, ankle
  malunion — *see* Fracture, by site
  mandible (lower jaw (bone)) S02.609 ☑
    alveolus S02.67 ☑
    angle (of jaw) S02.65 ☑
    body, unspecified S02.600 ☑
    condylar process S02.61 ☑
    coronoid process S02.63 ☑
    ramus, unspecified S02.64 ☑
    specified site NEC S02.69 ☑
    subcondylar process S02.62 ☑
    symphysis S02.66 ☑
  manubrium (sterni) S22.21 ☑
    dissociation from sternum S22.23 ☑
  march — *see* Fracture, traumatic, stress, by site
  maxilla, maxillary (bone) (sinus) (superior) (upper jaw) S02.401 ☑
    alveolus S02.42 ☑
    inferior — *see* Fracture, mandible
    LeFort I S02.411 ☑
    LeFort II S02.412 ☑
    LeFort III S02.413 ☑
  metacarpal S62.309 ☑
    base (displaced) S62.319 ☑
      nondisplaced S62.349 ☑
    fifth S62.30- ☑
      base (displaced) S62.31- ☑
        nondisplaced S62.34- ☑
      neck (displaced) S62.33- ☑
        nondisplaced S62.36- ☑
      shaft (displaced) S62.32- ☑
        nondisplaced S62.35- ☑
      specified NEC S62.398 ☑
    first S62.20- ☑
      base NEC (displaced) S62.23- ☑
        nondisplaced S62.23- ☑
      Bennett's — *see* Bennett's fracture
      neck (displaced) S62.25- ☑
        nondisplaced S62.25- ☑
      shaft (displaced) S62.24- ☑
        nondisplaced S62.24- ☑
      specified NEC S62.29- ☑
    fourth S62.30- ☑
      base (displaced) S62.31- ☑
        nondisplaced S62.34- ☑
      neck (displaced) S62.33- ☑
        nondisplaced S62.36- ☑
      shaft (displaced) S62.32- ☑
        nondisplaced S62.35- ☑
      specified NEC S62.39- ☑
    neck (displaced) S62.33- ☑
      nondisplaced S62.36- ☑
    Rolando's — *see* Rolando's fracture

Fracture, traumatic — *continued*
  metacarpal — *continued*
    second S62.30- ☑
      base (displaced) S62.31- ☑
        nondisplaced S62.34- ☑
      neck (displaced) S62.33- ☑
        nondisplaced S62.36- ☑
      shaft (displaced) S62.32- ☑
        nondisplaced S62.35- ☑
      specified NEC S62.39- ☑
    shaft (displaced) S62.32- ☑
      nondisplaced S62.35- ☑
    specified NEC S62.399 ☑
    third S62.30- ☑
      base (displaced) S62.31- ☑
        nondisplaced S62.34- ☑
      neck (displaced) S62.33- ☑
        nondisplaced S62.36- ☑
      shaft (displaced) S62.32- ☑
        nondisplaced S62.35- ☑
      specified NEC S62.39- ☑
  metastatic — *see* Fracture, pathological, due to, neoplastic disease (*see also* Neoplasm)
  metatarsal bone S92.30- ☑
    fifth (displaced) S92.35- ☑
      nondisplaced S92.35- ☑
    first (displaced) S92.31- ☑
      nondisplaced S92.31- ☑
    fourth (displaced) S92.34- ☑
      nondisplaced S92.34- ☑
    second (displaced) S92.32- ☑
      nondisplaced S92.32- ☑
    third (displaced) S92.33- ☑
      nondisplaced S92.33- ☑
  Monteggia's — *see* Monteggia's fracture
  multiple
    hand (and wrist) NEC — *see* Fracture, by site
    ribs — *see* Fracture, rib, multiple
  nasal (bone(s)) S02.2 ☑
  navicular (scaphoid) (foot) (*see also* Fracture, tarsal, navicular)
    hand — *see* Fracture, carpal, navicular
  neck S12.9 ☑
    cervical vertebra S12.9 ☑
      fifth (displaced) S12.400 ☑
        nondisplaced S12.401 ☑
        specified type NEC (displaced) S12.490 ☑
          nondisplaced S12.491 ☑
      first (displaced) S12.000 ☑
        burst (stable) S12.01 ☑
          unstable S12.02 ☑
        lateral mass (displaced) S12.040 ☑
          nondisplaced S12.041 ☑
        nondisplaced S12.001 ☑
        posterior arch (displaced) S12.030 ☑
          nondisplaced S12.031 ☑
        specified type NEC (displaced) S12.090 ☑
          nondisplaced S12.091 ☑
      fourth (displaced) S12.300 ☑
        nondisplaced S12.301 ☑
        specified type NEC (displaced) S12.390 ☑
          nondisplaced S12.391 ☑
      second (displaced) S12.100 ☑
        dens (anterior) (displaced) (type II) S12.110 ☑
          nondisplaced S12.112 ☑
          posterior S12.111 ☑
          specified type NEC (displaced) S12.120 ☑
            nondisplaced S12.121 ☑
        nondisplaced S12.101 ☑
        specified type NEC (displaced) S12.190 ☑
          nondisplaced S12.191 ☑
      seventh (displaced) S12.600 ☑
        nondisplaced S12.601 ☑
        specified type NEC (displaced) S12.690 ☑
          displaced S12.691 ☑
      sixth (displaced) S12.500 ☑
        nondisplaced S12.501 ☑
        specified type NEC (displaced) S12.590 ☑
          displaced S12.591 ☑
      third (displaced) S12.200 ☑
        nondisplaced S12.201 ☑
        specified type NEC (displaced) S12.290 ☑
          displaced S12.291 ☑

Fracture, traumatic — *continued*
  neck — *continued*
    hyoid bone S12.8 ☑
    larynx S12.8 ☑
    specified site NEC S12.8 ☑
    thyroid cartilage S12.8 ☑
    trachea S12.8 ☑
  neoplastic NEC — *see* Fracture, pathological, due to, neoplastic disease
  neural arch — *see* Fracture, vertebra
  newborn — *see* Birth, injury, fracture
  nontraumatic — *see* Fracture, pathological
  nonunion — *see* Nonunion, fracture
  nose, nasal (bone) (septum) S02.2 ☑
  occiput — *see* Fracture, skull, base, occiput
  odontoid process — *see* Fracture, neck, cervical vertebra, second
  olecranon (process) (ulna) — *see* Fracture, ulna, upper end, olecranon process
  orbit, orbital (bone) (region) S02.8 ☑
    floor (blow-out) S02.3 ☑
    roof S02.19 ☑
  os
    calcis — *see* Fracture, tarsal, calcaneus
    magnum — *see* Fracture, carpal, capitate
    pubis — *see* Fracture, pubis
  palate S02.8 ☑
  parietal bone (skull) S02.0 ☑
  patella S82.00- ☑
    comminuted (displaced) S82.04- ☑
      nondisplaced S82.04- ☑
    longitudinal (displaced) S82.02- ☑
      nondisplaced S82.02- ☑
    osteochondral (displaced) S82.01- ☑
      nondisplaced S82.01- ☑
    specified NEC S82.09- ☑
    transverse (displaced) S82.03- ☑
      nondisplaced S82.03- ☑
  pedicle (of vertebral arch) — *see* Fracture, vertebra
  pelvis, pelvic (bone) S32.9 ☑
    acetabulum — *see* Fracture, acetabulum
    circle — *see* Disruption, pelvic ring
    following insertion of implant, prosthesis or plate M96.65
    ilium — *see* Fracture, ilium
    ischium — *see* Fracture, ischium
    multiple
      with disruption of pelvic ring (circle) — *see* Disruption, pelvic ring
      without disruption of pelvic ring (circle) S32.82 ☑
    pubis — *see* Fracture, pubis
    sacrum — *see* Fracture, sacrum
    specified site NEC S32.89 ☑
  phalanx
    foot — *see* Fracture, toe
    hand — *see* Fracture, finger
  pisiform — *see* Fracture, carpal, pisiform
  pond — *see* Fracture, skull
  prosthetic device, internal — *see* Complications, prosthetic device, by site, mechanical
  pubis S32.50- ☑
    with disruption of pelvic ring — *see* Disruption, pelvic ring
    specified site NEC S32.59- ☑
    superior rim S32.51- ☑
  radius S52.9- ☑
    distal end — *see* Fracture, radius, lower end
    following insertion of implant, prosthesis or plate M96.63- ☑
    head — *see* Fracture, radius, upper end, head
    lower end S52.50- ☑
      Barton's — *see* Barton's fracture
      Colles' — *see* Colles' fracture
      extraarticular NEC S52.55- ☑
      intraarticular NEC S52.57- ☑
      physeal S59.20- ☑
        Salter-Harris
          Type I S59.21- ☑
          Type II S59.22- ☑
          Type III S59.23- ☑
          Type IV S59.24- ☑
        specified NEC S59.29- ☑
      Smith's — *see* Smith's fracture
      specified NEC S52.59- ☑
      styloid process (displaced) S52.51- ☑

Fracture, traumatic — *continued*
  radius — *continued*
    lower end — *continued*
      styloid process — *continued*
        nondisplaced S52.51- ☑
      torus S52.52- ☑
    neck — *see* Fracture, radius, upper end
    proximal end — *see* Fracture, radius, upper end
    shaft S52.30- ☑
      bent bone S52.38- ☑
      comminuted (displaced) S52.35- ☑
        nondisplaced S52.35- ☑
      Galeazzi's — *see* Galeazzi's fracture
      greenstick S52.31- ☑
      oblique (displaced) S52.33- ☑
        nondisplaced S52.33- ☑
      segmental (displaced) S52.36- ☑
        nondisplaced S52.36- ☑
      specified NEC S52.39- ☑
      spiral (displaced) S52.34- ☑
        nondisplaced S52.34- ☑
      transverse (displaced) S52.32- ☑
        nondisplaced S52.32- ☑
    upper end S52.10- ☑
      head (displaced) S52.12- ☑
        nondisplaced S52.12- ☑
      neck (displaced) S52.13- ☑
        nondisplaced S52.13- ☑
      physeal S59.10- ☑
        Salter-Harris
          Type I S59.11- ☑
          Type II S59.12- ☑
          Type III S59.13- ☑
          Type IV S59.14- ☑
        specified NEC S59.19- ☑
      specified NEC S52.18- ☑
      torus S52.11- ☑
  ramus
    inferior or superior, pubis — *see* Fracture, pubis
    mandible — *see* Fracture, mandible
  restorative material (dental) K08.539
    with loss of material K08.531
    without loss of material K08.530
  rib S22.3- ☑
    with flail chest — *see* Flail, chest
    multiple S22.4- ☑
      with flail chest — *see* Flail, chest
  root, tooth — *see* Fracture, tooth
  sacrum S32.10 ☑
    specified NEC S32.19 ☑
    Type
      1 S32.14 ☑
      2 S32.15 ☑
      3 S32.16 ☑
      4 S32.17 ☑
    Zone
      I S32.119 ☑
        displaced (minimally) S32.111 ☑
          severely S32.112 ☑
        nondisplaced S32.110 ☑
      II S32.129 ☑
        displaced (minimally) S32.121 ☑
          severely S32.122 ☑
        nondisplaced S32.120 ☑
      III S32.139 ☑
        displaced (minimally) S32.131 ☑
          severely S32.132 ☑
        nondisplaced S32.130 ☑
  scaphoid (hand) (*see also* Fracture, carpal, navicular)
    foot — *see* Fracture, tarsal, navicular
  scapula S42.10- ☑
    acromial process (displaced) S42.12- ☑
      nondisplaced S42.12- ☑
    body (displaced) S42.11- ☑
      nondisplaced S42.11- ☑
    coracoid process (displaced) S42.13- ☑
      nondisplaced S42.13- ☑
    glenoid cavity (displaced) S42.14- ☑
      nondisplaced S42.14- ☑
    neck (displaced) S42.15- ☑
      nondisplaced S42.15- ☑
    specified NEC S42.19- ☑
  semilunar bone, wrist — *see* Fracture, carpal, lunate
  sequelae — *see* Sequelae, fracture
  sesamoid bone
    hand — *see* Fracture, carpal

Fracture, traumatic — *continued*
  sesamoid bone — *continued*
    other — *code by* site under Fracture
  shepherd's — *see* Fracture, tarsal, talus
  shoulder (girdle) S42.9- ☑
    blade — *see* Fracture, scapula
  sinus (ethmoid) (frontal) S02.19 ☑
  skull S02.91 ☑
    base S02.10 ☑
      occiput S02.119 ☑
        condyle S02.113 ☑
          type I S02.110 ☑
          type II S02.111 ☑
          type III S02.112 ☑
        specified NEC S02.118 ☑
      specified NEC S02.19 ☑
    birth injury P13.0
    frontal bone S02.0 ☑
    parietal bone S02.0 ☑
    specified site NEC S02.8 ☑
    temporal bone S02.19 ☑
    vault S02.0 ☑
  Smith's — *see* Smith's fracture
  sphenoid (bone) (sinus) S02.19 ☑
  spine — *see* Fracture, vertebra
  spinous process — *see* Fracture, vertebra
  spontaneous (cause unknown) — *see* Fracture, pathological
  stave (of thumb) — *see* Fracture, metacarpal, first
  sternum S22.20 ☑
    with flail chest — *see* Flail, chest
    body S22.22 ☑
    manubrium S22.21 ☑
    xiphoid (process) S22.24 ☑
  stress M84.30 ☑
    ankle M84.37- ☑
    carpus M84.34- ☑
    clavicle M84.31- ☑
    femoral neck M84.359 ☑
    femur M84.35- ☑
    fibula M84.36- ☑
    finger M84.34- ☑
    hip M84.359 ☑
    humerus M84.32- ☑
    ilium M84.350 ☑
    ischium M84.350 ☑
    metacarpus M84.34- ☑
    metatarsus M84.37- ☑
    neck — *see* Fracture, fatigue, vertebra
    pelvis M84.350 ☑
    radius M84.33- ☑
    rib M84.38 ☑
    scapula M84.31- ☑
    skull M84.38 ☑
    tarsus M84.37- ☑
    tibia M84.36- ☑
    toe M84.37- ☑
    ulna M84.33- ☑
    vertebra — *see* Fracture, fatigue, vertebra
  supracondylar, elbow — *see* Fracture, humerus, lower end, supracondylar
  symphysis pubis — *see* Fracture, pubis
  talus (ankle bone) — *see* Fracture, tarsal, talus
  tarsal bone(s) S92.20- ☑
    astragalus — *see* Fracture, tarsal, talus
    calcaneus S92.00- ☑
      anterior process (displaced) S92.02- ☑
        nondisplaced S92.02- ☑
      body (displaced) S92.01- ☑
        nondisplaced S92.01- ☑
      extraarticular NEC (displaced) S92.05- ☑
        nondisplaced S92.05- ☑
      intraarticular (displaced) S92.06- ☑
        nondisplaced S92.06- ☑
      tuberosity (displaced) S92.04- ☑
        avulsion (displaced) S92.03- ☑
          nondisplaced S92.03- ☑
        nondisplaced S92.04- ☑
    cuboid (displaced) S92.21- ☑
      nondisplaced S92.21- ☑
    cuneiform
      intermediate (displaced) S92.23- ☑
        nondisplaced S92.23- ☑
      lateral (displaced) S92.22- ☑
        nondisplaced S92.22- ☑
      medial (displaced) S92.24- ☑

Fracture, traumatic — *continued*
  tarsal bone(s) — *continued*
    cuneiform — *continued*
      medial — *continued*
        nondisplaced S92.24- ☑
      navicular (displaced) S92.25- ☑
        nondisplaced S92.25- ☑
      scaphoid — *see* Fracture, tarsal, navicular
    talus S92.10- ☑
      avulsion (displaced) S92.15- ☑
        nondisplaced S92.15- ☑
      body (displaced) S92.12- ☑
        nondisplaced S92.12- ☑
      dome (displaced) S92.14- ☑
        nondisplaced S92.14- ☑
      head (displaced) S92.12- ☑
        nondisplaced S92.12- ☑
      lateral process (displaced) S92.14- ☑
        nondisplaced S92.14- ☑
      neck (displaced) S92.11- ☑
        nondisplaced S92.11- ☑
      posterior process (displaced) S92.13- ☑
        nondisplaced S92.13- ☑
      specified NEC S92.19- ☑
  temporal bone (styloid) S02.19 ☑
  thorax (bony) S22.9 ☑
    with flail chest — *see* Flail, chest
    rib S22.3- ☑
      multiple S22.4- ☑
        with flail chest — *see* Flail, chest
    sternum S22.20 ☑
      body S22.22 ☑
      manubrium S22.21 ☑
      xiphoid process S22.24 ☑
    vertebra (displaced) S22.009 ☑
      burst (stable) S22.001 ☑
        unstable S22.002 ☑
      eighth S22.069 ☑
        burst (stable) S22.061 ☑
          unstable S22.062 ☑
        specified type NEC S22.068 ☑
        wedge compression S22.060 ☑
      eleventh S22.089 ☑
        burst (stable) S22.081 ☑
          unstable S22.082 ☑
        specified type NEC S22.088 ☑
        wedge compression S22.080 ☑
      fifth S22.059 ☑
        burst (stable) S22.051 ☑
          unstable S22.052 ☑
        specified type NEC S22.058 ☑
        wedge compression S22.050 ☑
      first S22.019 ☑
        burst (stable) S22.011 ☑
          unstable S22.012 ☑
        specified type NEC S22.018 ☑
        wedge compression S22.010 ☑
      fourth S22.049 ☑
        burst (stable) S22.041 ☑
          unstable S22.042 ☑
        specified type NEC S22.048 ☑
        wedge compression S22.040 ☑
      ninth S22.079 ☑
        burst (stable) S22.071 ☑
          unstable S22.072 ☑
        specified type NEC S22.078 ☑
        wedge compression S22.070 ☑
      nondisplaced S22.001 ☑
      second S22.029 ☑
        burst (stable) S22.021 ☑
          unstable S22.022 ☑
        specified type NEC S22.028 ☑
        wedge compression S22.020 ☑
      seventh S22.069 ☑
        burst (stable) S22.061 ☑
          unstable S22.062 ☑
        specified type NEC S22.068 ☑
        wedge compression S22.060 ☑
      sixth S22.059 ☑
        burst (stable) S22.051 ☑
          unstable S22.052 ☑
        specified type NEC S22.058 ☑
        wedge compression S22.050 ☑
      specified type NEC S22.008 ☑
      tenth S22.079 ☑

Fracture, traumatic — *continued*
  thorax — *continued*
    vertebra — *continued*
      tenth — *continued*
        burst (stable) S22.071 ☑
          unstable S22.072 ☑
        specified type NEC S22.078 ☑
        wedge compression S22.070 ☑
      third S22.039 ☑
        burst (stable) S22.031 ☑
          unstable S22.032 ☑
        specified type NEC S22.038 ☑
        wedge compression S22.030 ☑
      twelfth S22.089 ☑
        burst (stable) S22.081 ☑
          unstable S22.082 ☑
        specified type NEC S22.088 ☑
        wedge compression S22.080 ☑
      wedge compression S22.000 ☑
  thumb S62.50- ☑
    distal phalanx (displaced) S62.52- ☑
      nondisplaced S62.52- ☑
    proximal phalanx (displaced) S62.51- ☑
      nondisplaced S62.51- ☑
  thyroid cartilage S12.8 ☑
  tibia (shaft) S82.20- ☑
    comminuted (displaced) S82.25- ☑
      nondisplaced S82.25- ☑
    condyles — *see* Fracture, tibia, upper end
    distal end — *see* Fracture, tibia, lower end
    epiphysis
      lower — *see* Fracture, tibia, lower end
      upper — *see* Fracture, tibia, upper end
    following insertion of implant, prosthesis or plate M96.67- ☑
    head (involving knee joint) — *see* Fracture, tibia, upper end
    intercondyloid eminence — *see* Fracture, tibia, upper end
    involving ankle or malleolus — *see* Fracture, ankle, medial malleolus
    lower end S82.30- ☑
      physeal S89.10- ☑
        Salter-Harris
          Type I S89.11- ☑
          Type II S89.12- ☑
          Type III S89.13- ☑
          Type IV S89.14- ☑
        specified NEC S89.19- ☑
      pilon (displaced) S82.87- ☑
        nondisplaced S82.87- ☑
      specified NEC S82.39- ☑
      torus S82.31- ☑
    malleolus — *see* Fracture, ankle, medial malleolus
    oblique (displaced) S82.23- ☑
      nondisplaced S82.23- ☑
    pilon — *see* Fracture, tibia, lower end, pilon
    proximal end — *see* Fracture, tibia, upper end
    segmental (displaced) S82.26- ☑
      nondisplaced S82.26- ☑
    specified NEC S82.29- ☑
    spine — *see* Fracture, upper end, spine
    spiral (displaced) S82.24- ☑
      nondisplaced S82.24- ☑
    transverse (displaced) S82.22- ☑
      nondisplaced S82.22- ☑
    tuberosity — *see* Fracture, tibia, upper end, tuberosity
    upper end S82.10- ☑
      bicondylar (displaced) S82.14- ☑
        nondisplaced S82.14- ☑
      lateral condyle (displaced) S82.12- ☑
        nondisplaced S82.12- ☑
      medial condyle (displaced) S82.13- ☑
        nondisplaced S82.13- ☑
      physeal S89.00- ☑
        Salter-Harris
          Type I S89.01- ☑
          Type II S89.02- ☑
          Type III S89.03- ☑
          Type IV S89.04- ☑
        specified NEC S89.09- ☑
      plateau — *see* Fracture, tibia, upper end, bicondylar
      specified NEC S82.19- ☑
      spine (displaced) S82.11- ☑

Fracture, traumatic — *continued*
  tibia — *continued*
    upper end — *continued*
      spine — *continued*
        nondisplaced S82.11- ☑
        torus S82.16- ☑
      tuberosity (displaced) S82.15- ☑
        nondisplaced S82.15- ☑
  toe S92.91- ☑
    great (displaced) S92.40- ☑
      distal phalanx (displaced) S92.42- ☑
        nondisplaced S92.42- ☑
      nondisplaced S92.40- ☑
      proximal phalanx (displaced) S92.41- ☑
        nondisplaced S92.41- ☑
      specified NEC S92.49- ☑
    lesser (displaced) S92.50- ☑
      distal phalanx (displaced) S92.53- ☑
        nondisplaced S92.53- ☑
      medial phalanx (displaced) S92.52- ☑
        nondisplaced S92.52- ☑
      nondisplaced S92.50- ☑
      proximal phalanx (displaced) S92.51- ☑
        nondisplaced S92.51- ☑
      specified NEC S92.59- ☑
  tooth (root) S02.5
  trachea (cartilage) S12.8 ☑
  transverse process — *see* Fracture, vertebra
  trapezium or trapezoid bone — *see* Fracture, carpal
  trimalleolar — *see* Fracture, ankle, trimalleolar
  triquetrum (cuneiform of carpus) — *see* Fracture, carpal, triquetrum
  trochanter — *see* Fracture, femur, trochanteric
  tuberosity (external) — *code by* site under Fracture
  ulna (shaft) S52.20- ☑
    bent bone S52.28- ☑
    coronoid process — *see* Fracture, ulna, upper end, coronoid process
    distal end — *see* Fracture, ulna, lower end
    following insertion of implant, prosthesis or plate M96.63- ☑
    head S52.00- ☑
    lower end S52.60- ☑
      physeal S59.00- ☑
        Salter-Harris
          Type I S59.01- ☑
          Type II S59.02- ☑
          Type III S59.03- ☑
          Type IV S59.04- ☑
        specified NEC S59.09- ☑
      specified NEC S52.69- ☑
      styloid process (displaced) S52.61- ☑
        nondisplaced S52.61- ☑
      torus S52.62- ☑
    proximal end — *see* Fracture, ulna, upper end
    shaft S52.20- ☑
      comminuted (displaced) S52.25- ☑
        nondisplaced S52.25- ☑
      greenstick S52.21- ☑
      Monteggia's — *see* Monteggia's fracture
      oblique (displaced) S52.23- ☑
        nondisplaced S52.23- ☑
      segmental (displaced) S52.26- ☑
        nondisplaced S52.26- ☑
      specified NEC S52.29- ☑
      spiral (displaced) S52.24- ☑
        nondisplaced S52.24- ☑
      transverse (displaced) S52.22- ☑
        nondisplaced S52.22- ☑
    upper end S52.00- ☑
      coronoid process (displaced) S52.04- ☑
        nondisplaced S52.04- ☑
      olecranon process (displaced) S52.02- ☑
        with intraarticular extension S52.03- ☑
        nondisplaced S52.02- ☑
          with intraarticular extension S52.03- ☑
      specified NEC S52.09- ☑
      torus S52.01- ☑
  unciform — *see* Fracture, carpal, hamate
  vault of skull S02.0 ☑
  vertebra, vertebral (arch) (body) (column) (neural arch) (pedicle) (spinous process) (transverse process)
    atlas — *see* Fracture, neck, cervical vertebra, first
    axis — *see* Fracture, neck, cervical vertebra, second
    cervical (teardrop) S12.9 ☑

☑ **Additional Character Required** — Refer to the Tabular List for Character Selection   ▽ **Subterms under main terms may continue to next column or page**

Fracture, traumatic — *continued*
  vertebra, vertebral — *continued*
    cervical — *continued*
      axis — *see* Fracture, neck, cervical vertebra, second
      first (atlas) — *see* Fracture, neck, cervical vertebra, first
      second (axis) — *see* Fracture, neck, cervical vertebra, second
      chronic M84.48 ☑
    coccyx S32.2 ☑
    dorsal — *see* Fracture, thorax, vertebra
    lumbar S32.009 ☑
      burst (stable) S32.001 ☑
        unstable S32.002 ☑
      fifth S32.059 ☑
        burst (stable) S32.051 ☑
          unstable S32.052 ☑
        specified type NEC S32.058 ☑
        wedge compression S32.050 ☑
      first S32.019 ☑
        burst (stable) S32.011 ☑
          unstable S32.012 ☑
        specified type NEC S32.018 ☑
        wedge compression S32.010 ☑
      fourth S32.049 ☑
        burst (stable) S32.041 ☑
          unstable S32.042 ☑
        specified type NEC S32.048 ☑
        wedge compression S32.040 ☑
      second S32.029 ☑
        burst (stable) S32.021 ☑
          unstable S32.022 ☑
        specified type NEC S32.028 ☑
        wedge compression S32.020 ☑
      specified type NEC S32.008 ☑
      third S32.039 ☑
        burst (stable) S32.031 ☑
          unstable S32.032 ☑
        specified type NEC S32.038 ☑
        wedge compression S32.030 ☑
      wedge compression S32.000 ☑
    metastatic — *see* Collapse, vertebra, in, specified disease NEC (*see also* Neoplasm)
    newborn (birth injury) P11.5
    sacrum S32.10 ☑
      specified NEC S32.19 ☑
      Type
        1 S32.14 ☑
        2 S32.15 ☑
        3 S32.16 ☑
        4 S32.17 ☑
      Zone
        I S32.119 ☑
          displaced (minimally) S32.111 ☑
            severely S32.112 ☑
          nondisplaced S32.110 ☑
        II S32.129 ☑
          displaced (minimally) S32.121 ☑
            severely S32.122 ☑
          nondisplaced S32.120 ☑
        III S32.139 ☑
          displaced (minimally) S32.131 ☑
            severely S32.132 ☑
          nondisplaced S32.130 ☑
    thoracic — *see* Fracture, thorax, vertebra
  vertex S02.0 ☑
  vomer (bone) S02.2 ☑
  wrist S62.10- ☑
    carpal — *see* Fracture, carpal bone
    navicular (scaphoid) (hand) — *see* Fracture, carpal, navicular
  xiphisternum, xiphoid (process) S22.24 ☑
  zygoma S02.402 ☑
Fragile, fragility
  autosomal site Q95.5
  bone, congenital (with blue sclera) Q78.0
  capillary (hereditary) D69.8
  hair L67.8
  nails L60.3
  non-sex chromosome site Q95.5
  X chromosome Q99.2
Fragilitas
  crinium L67.8
  ossium (with blue sclerae) (hereditary) Q78.0
  unguium L60.3

Fragilitas — *continued*
  unguium — *continued*
    congenital Q84.6
Fragments, cataract (lens), **following cataract surgery** H59.02-
  retained foreign body — *see* Retained, foreign body fragments (type of)
Frailty (frail) R54
  mental R41.81
Frambesia, frambesial (tropica) (*see also* Yaws)
  initial lesion or ulcer A66.0
  primary A66.0
Frambeside
  gummatous A66.4
  of early yaws A66.2
Frambesioma A66.1
Franceschetti-Klein (-Wildervanck) **disease or syndrome** Q75.4
Francis' disease — *see* Tularemia
Franklin disease C88.2
Frank's essential thrombocytopenia D69.3
Fraser's syndrome Q87.0
Freckle(s) L81.2
  malignant melanoma in — *see* Melanoma
  melanotic (Hutchinson's) — *see* Melanoma, in situ
  retinal D49.81
Frederickson's hyperlipoproteinemia, type
  I and V E78.3
  IIA E78.0
  IIB and III E78.2
  IV E78.1
Freeman Sheldon syndrome Q87.0
Freezing (*see also* Effect, adverse, cold) T69.9 ☑
Freiberg's disease (infraction of metatarsal head or osteochondrosis) — *see* Osteochondrosis, juvenile, metatarsus
Frei's disease A55
Fremitus, friction, cardiac R01.2
Frenum, frenulum
  external os Q51.828
  tongue (shortening) (congenital) Q38.1
Frequency micturition (nocturnal) R35.0
  psychogenic F45.8
Frey's syndrome
  auriculotemporal G50.8
  hyperhidrosis L74.52
Friction
  burn — *see* Burn, by site
  fremitus, cardiac R01.2
  precordial R01.2
  sounds, chest R09.89
Friderichsen-Waterhouse syndrome or disease A39.1
Friedländer's B (bacillus) **NEC** (*see also* condition) A49.8
Friedreich's
  ataxia G11.1
  combined systemic disease G11.1
  facial hemihypertrophy Q67.4
  sclerosis (cerebellum) (spinal cord) G11.1
Frigidity F52.22
Fröhlich's syndrome E23.6
Frontal (*see also* condition)
  lobe syndrome F07.0
Frostbite (superficial) T33.90 ☑
  with
    partial thickness skin loss — *see* Frostbite (superficial), by site
    tissue necrosis T34.90 ☑
  abdominal wall T33.3 ☑
    with tissue necrosis T34.3 ☑
  ankle T33.81- ☑
    with tissue necrosis T34.81- ☑
  arm T33.4- ☑
    with tissue necrosis T34.4- ☑
    finger(s) — *see* Frostbite, finger
    hand — *see* Frostbite, hand
    wrist — *see* Frostbite, wrist
  ear T33.01- ☑
    with tissue necrosis T34.01- ☑
  face T33.09 ☑
    with tissue necrosis T34.09 ☑
  finger T33.53- ☑
    with tissue necrosis T34.53- ☑
  foot T33.82- ☑
    with tissue necrosis T34.82- ☑
  hand T33.52- ☑
    with tissue necrosis T34.52- ☑
  head T33.09 ☑

Frostbite — *continued*
  head — *continued*
    with tissue necrosis T34.09 ☑
    ear — *see* Frostbite, ear
    nose — *see* Frostbite, nose
  hip (and thigh) T33.6- ☑
    with tissue necrosis T34.6- ☑
  knee T33.7- ☑
    with tissue necrosis T34.7- ☑
  leg T33.9- ☑
    with tissue necrosis T34.9- ☑
    ankle — *see* Frostbite, ankle
    foot — *see* Frostbite, foot
    knee — *see* Frostbite, knee
    lower T33.7- ☑
      with tissue necrosis T34.7- ☑
    thigh — *see* Frostbite, hip
    toe — *see* Frostbite, toe
  limb
    lower T33.99 ☑
      with tissue necrosis T34.99 ☑
    upper — *see* Frostbite, arm
  neck T33.1 ☑
    with tissue necrosis T34.1 ☑
  nose T33.02 ☑
    with tissue necrosis T34.02 ☑
  pelvis T33.3 ☑
    with tissue necrosis T34.3 ☑
  specified site NEC T33.99 ☑
    with tissue necrosis T34.99 ☑
  thigh — *see* Frostbite, hip
  thorax T33.2 ☑
    with tissue necrosis T34.2 ☑
  toes T33.83- ☑
    with tissue necrosis T34.83- ☑
  trunk T33.99 ☑
    with tissue necrosis T34.99 ☑
  wrist T33.51- ☑
    with tissue necrosis T34.51- ☑
Frotteurism F65.81
Frozen (*see also* Effect, adverse, cold) T69.9 ☑
  pelvis (female) N94.89
    male K66.8
  shoulder — *see* Capsulitis, adhesive
Fructokinase deficiency E74.11
Fructose 1,6 diphosphatase deficiency E74.19
Fructosemia (benign) (essential) E74.12
Fructosuria (benign) (essential) E74.11
Fuchs'
  black spot (myopic) H44.2- ☑
  dystrophy (corneal endothelium) H18.51
  heterochromic cyclitis — *see* Cyclitis, Fuchs' heterochromic
Fucosidosis E77.1
Fugue R68.89
  dissociative F44.1
  hysterical (dissociative) F44.1
  postictal in epilepsy — *see* Epilepsy
  reaction to exceptional stress (transient) F43.0
Fulminant, fulminating — *see* condition
Functional (*see also* condition)
  bleeding (uterus) N93.8
Functioning, intellectual, borderline R41.83
Fundus — *see* condition
Fungemia NOS B49
Fungus, fungous
  cerebral G93.89
  disease NOS B49
  infection — *see* Infection, fungus
Funiculitis (acute) (chronic) (endemic) N49.1
  gonococcal (acute) (chronic) A54.23
  tuberculous A18.15
Funnel
  breast (acquired) M95.4
    congenital Q67.6
    sequelae (late effect) of rickets E64.3
  chest (acquired) M95.4
    congenital Q67.6
    sequelae (late effect) of rickets E64.3
  pelvis (acquired) M95.5
    with disproportion (fetopelvic) O33.3 ☑
      causing obstructed labor O65.3
    congenital Q74.2
FUO (fever of unknown origin) R50.9
Furfur L21.0
  microsporon B36.0

Furrier's lung J67.8
Furrowed K14.5
  nail(s) (transverse) L60.4
    congenital Q84.6
  tongue K14.5
    congenital Q38.3
Furuncle L02.92
  abdominal wall L02.221
  ankle — *see* Furuncle, lower limb
  antecubital space — *see* Furuncle, upper limb
  anus K61.0
  arm — *see* Furuncle, upper limb
  auditory canal, external — *see* Abscess, ear, external
  auricle (ear) — *see* Abscess, ear, external
  axilla (region) L02.42- ☑
  back (any part) L02.222
  breast N61
  buttock L02.32
  cheek (external) L02.02
  chest wall L02.223
  chin L02.02
  corpus cavernosum N48.21
  ear, external — *see* Abscess, ear, external
  external auditory canal — *see* Abscess, ear, external
  eyelid — *see* Abscess, eyelid
  face L02.02
  femoral (region) — *see* Furuncle, lower limb
  finger — *see* Furuncle, hand
  flank L02.221
  foot L02.62- ☑
  forehead L02.02
  gluteal (region) L02.32
  groin L02.224
  hand L02.52- ☑
  head L02.821
    face L02.02
  hip — *see* Furuncle, lower limb
  kidney — *see* Abscess, kidney
  knee — *see* Furuncle, lower limb
  labium (majus) (minus) N76.4
  lacrimal
    gland — *see* Dacryoadenitis
    passages (duct) (sac) — *see* Inflammation, lacrimal, passages, acute
  leg (any part) — *see* Furuncle, lower limb
  lower limb L02.42- ☑
  malignant A22.0
  mouth K12.2
  navel L02.226

Furuncle — *continued*
  neck L02.12
  nose J34.0
  orbit, orbital — *see* Abscess, orbit
  palmar (space) — *see* Furuncle, hand
  partes posteriores L02.32
  pectoral region L02.223
  penis N48.21
  perineum L02.225
  pinna — *see* Abscess, ear, external
  popliteal — *see* Furuncle, lower limb
  prepatellar — *see* Furuncle, lower limb
  scalp L02.821
  seminal vesicle N49.0
  shoulder — *see* Furuncle, upper limb
  specified site NEC L02.828
  submandibular K12.2
  temple (region) L02.02
  thumb — *see* Furuncle, hand
  toe — *see* Furuncle, foot
  trunk L02.229
    abdominal wall L02.221
    back L02.222
    chest wall L02.223
    groin L02.224
    perineum L02.225
    umbilicus L02.226
  umbilicus L02.226
  upper limb L02.42- ☑
  vulva N76.4
Furunculosis — *see* Furuncle
Fused — *see* Fusion, fused
Fusion, fused (congenital)
  astragaloscaphoid Q74.2
  atria Q21.1
  auditory canal Q16.1
  auricles, heart Q21.1
  binocular with defective stereopsis H53.32
  bone Q79.8
  cervical spine M43.22
  choanal Q30.0
  commissure, mitral valve Q23.2
  cusps, heart valve NEC Q24.8
    mitral Q23.2
    pulmonary Q22.1
    tricuspid Q22.4
  ear ossicles Q16.3
  fingers Q70.0 ☑
  hymen Q52.3

Fusion, fused — *continued*
  joint (acquired) (*see also* Ankylosis)
    congenital Q74.8
  kidneys (incomplete) Q63.1
  labium (majus) (minus) Q52.5
  larynx and trachea Q34.8
  limb, congenital Q74.8
    lower Q74.2
    upper Q74.0
  lobes, lung Q33.8
  lumbosacral (acquired) M43.27
    arthrodesis status Z98.1
    congenital Q76.49
    postprocedural status Z98.1
  nares, nose, nasal, nostril(s) Q30.0
  organ or site not listed — *see* Anomaly, by site
  ossicles Q79.9
    auditory Q16.3
  pulmonic cusps Q22.1
  ribs Q76.6
  sacroiliac (joint) (acquired) M43.28
    arthrodesis status Z98.1
    congenital Q74.2
    postprocedural status Z98.1
  spine (acquired) NEC M43.20
    arthrodesis status Z98.1
    cervical region M43.22
    cervicothoracic region M43.23
    congenital Q76.49
    lumbar M43.26
    lumbosacral region M43.27
    occipito-atlanto-axial region M43.21
    postoperative status Z98.1
    sacrococcygeal region M43.28
    thoracic region M43.24
    thoracolumbar region M43.25
  sublingual duct with submaxillary duct at opening in mouth Q38.4
  testes Q55.1
  toes Q70.2- ☑
  tooth, teeth K00.2
  trachea and esophagus Q39.8
  twins Q89.4
  vagina Q52.4
  ventricles, heart Q21.0
  vertebra (arch) — *see* Fusion, spine
  vulva Q52.5
Fusospirillosis (mouth) (tongue) (tonsil) A69.1
Fussy baby R68.12

G

Gain in weight (abnormal) (excessive) (*see also* Weight, gain)
Gaisböck's disease (polycythemia hypertonica) D75.1
Gait abnormality R26.9
  ataxic R26.0
  falling R29.6
  hysterical (ataxic) (staggering) F44.4
  paralytic R26.1
  spastic R26.1
  specified type NEC R26.89
  staggering R26.0
  unsteadiness R26.81
  walking difficulty NEC R26.2
Galactocele (breast) N64.89
  puerperal, postpartum O92.79
Galactokinase deficiency E74.29
Galactophoritis N61
  gestational, puerperal, postpartum O91.2- ☑
Galactorrhea O92.6
  not associated with childbirth N64.3
Galactosemia (classic) (congenital) E74.21
Galactosuria E74.29
Galacturia R82.0
  schistosomiasis (bilharziasis) B65.0
Galeazzi's fracture S52.37- ☑
Galen's vein — *see* condition
Gall duct — *see* condition
Gallbladder (*see also* condition)
  acute K81.0
Gallop rhythm R00.8
Gallstone (colic) (cystic duct) (gallbladder) (impacted) (multiple) (*see also* Calculus, gallbladder)
  with
    cholecystitis — *see* Calculus, gallbladder, with cholecystitis
  bile duct (common) (hepatic) — *see* Calculus, bile duct
  causing intestinal obstruction K56.3
  specified NEC K80.80
    with obstruction K80.81
Gambling Z72.6
  pathological (compulsive) F63.0
Gammopathy (of undetermined significance [MGUS]) D47.2
  associated with lymphoplasmacytic dyscrasia D47.2
  monoclonal D47.2
  polyclonal D89.0
Gamna's disease (siderotic splenomegaly) D73.1
Gamophobia F40.298
Gampsodactylia (congenital) Q66.7
Gamstorp's disease (adynamia episodica hereditaria) G72.3
Gandy-Nanta disease (siderotic splenomegaly) D73.1
Gang
  membership offenses Z72.810
Gangliocytoma D36.10
Ganglioglioma — *see* Neoplasm, uncertain behavior, by site
Ganglion (compound) (diffuse) (joint) (tendon (sheath)) M67.40
  ankle M67.47- ☑
  foot M67.47- ☑
  forearm M67.43- ☑
  hand M67.44- ☑
  lower leg M67.46- ☑
  multiple sites M67.49
  of yaws (early) (late) A66.6
  pelvic region M67.45- ☑
  periosteal — *see* Periostitis
  shoulder region M67.41- ☑
  specified site NEC M67.48
  thigh region M67.45- ☑
  tuberculous A18.09
  upper arm M67.42- ☑
  wrist M67.43- ☑
Ganglioneuroblastoma — *see* Neoplasm, nerve, malignant
Ganglioneuroma D36.10

Ganglioneuroma — *continued*
  malignant — *see* Neoplasm, nerve, malignant
Ganglioneuromatosis D36.10
Ganglionitis
  fifth nerve — *see* Neuralgia, trigeminal
  gasserian (postherpetic) (postzoster) B02.21
  geniculate G51.1
    newborn (birth injury) P11.3
    postherpetic, postzoster B02.21
  herpes zoster B02.21
  postherpetic geniculate B02.21
Gangliosidosis E75.10
  GM1 E75.19
  GM2 E75.00
    other specified E75.09
    Sandhoff disease E75.01
    Tay-Sachs disease E75.02
  GM3 E75.19
  mucolipidosis IV E75.11
Gangosa A66.5
Gangrene, gangrenous (connective tissue) (dropsical) (dry) (moist) (skin) (ulcer) (*see also* Necrosis) I96
  with diabetes (mellitus) — *see* Diabetes, gangrene
  abdomen (wall) I96
  alveolar M27.3
  appendix K35.80
    with
      perforation or rupture K35.2
      peritoneal abscess K35.3
      peritonitis NEC K35.3
        generalized (with perforation or rupture) K35.2
        localized (with perforation or rupture) K35.3
  arteriosclerotic (general) (senile) — *see* Arteriosclerosis, extremities, with, gangrene
  auricle I96
  Bacillus welchii A48.0
  bladder (infectious) — *see* Cystitis, specified type NEC
  bowel, cecum, or colon — *see* Gangrene, intestine
  Clostridium perfringens or welchii A48.0
  cornea H18.89- ☑
  corpora cavernosa N48.29
    noninfective N48.89
  cutaneous, spreading I96
  decubital — *see* Ulcer, pressure, by site
  diabetic (any site) — *see* Diabetes, gangrene
  emphysematous — *see* Gangrene, gas
  epidemic — *see* Poisoning, food, noxious, plant
  epididymis (infectional) N45.1
  erysipelas — *see* Erysipelas
  extremity (lower) (upper) I96
  Fournier N49.3
    female N76.89
  fusospirochetal A69.0
  gallbladder — *see* Cholecystitis, acute
  gas (bacillus) A48.0
    following
      abortion — *see* Abortion by type complicated by infection
      ectopic or molar pregnancy O08.0
  glossitis K14.0
  hernia — *see* Hernia, by site, with gangrene
  intestine, intestinal (hemorrhagic) (massive) K55.0
    with
      mesenteric embolism K55.0
      obstruction — *see* Obstruction, intestine
  laryngitis J04.0
  limb (lower) (upper) I96
  lung J85.0
    spirochetal A69.8
  lymphangitis I89.1
  Meleney's (synergistic) — *see* Ulcer, skin
  mesentery K55.0
    with
      embolism K55.0
      intestinal obstruction — *see* Obstruction, intestine
  mouth A69.0
  ovary — *see* Oophoritis
  pancreas K85.9
  penis N48.29
    noninfective N48.89

Gangrene, gangrenous — *continued*
  perineum I96
  pharynx (*see also* Pharyngitis)
    Vincent's A69.1
  presenile I73.1
  progressive synergistic — *see* Ulcer, skin
  pulmonary J85.0
  pulpal (dental) K04.1
  quinsy J36
  Raynaud's (symmetric gangrene) I73.01
  retropharyngeal J39.2
  scrotum N49.3
    noninfective N50.8
  senile (atherosclerotic) — *see* Arteriosclerosis, extremities, with, gangrene
  spermatic cord N49.1
    noninfective N50.8
  spine I96
  spirochetal NEC A69.8
  spreading cutaneous I96
  stomatitis A69.0
  symmetrical I73.01
  testis (infectional) N45.2
    noninfective N44.8
  throat (*see also* Pharyngitis)
    diphtheritic A36.0
    Vincent's A69.1
  thyroid (gland) E07.89
  tooth (pulp) K04.1
  tuberculous NEC — *see* Tuberculosis
  tunica vaginalis N49.1
    noninfective N50.8
  umbilicus I96
  uterus — *see* Endometritis
  uvulitis K12.2
  vas deferens N49.1
    noninfective N50.8
  vulva N76.89
Ganister disease J62.8
Ganser's syndrome (hysterical) F44.89
Gardner-Diamond syndrome (autoerythrocyte sensitization) D69.2
Gargoylism E76.01
Garré's disease, osteitis (sclerosing), osteomyelitis — *see* Osteomyelitis, specified type NEC
Garrod's pad, knuckle M72.1
Gartner's duct
  cyst Q52.4
  persistent Q50.6
Gas R14.3
  asphyxiation, inhalation, poisoning, suffocation NEC — *see* Table of Drugs and Chemicals
  excessive R14.0
  gangrene A48.0
    following
      abortion — *see* Abortion by type complicated by infection
      ectopic or molar pregnancy O08.0
  on stomach R14.0
  pains R14.1
Gastralgia (*see also* Pain, abdominal)
Gastrectasis K31.0
  psychogenic F45.8
Gastric — *see* condition
Gastrinoma
  malignant
    pancreas C25.4
      specified site NEC — *see* Neoplasm, malignant, by site
      unspecified site C25.4
  specified site — *see* Neoplasm, uncertain behavior
  unspecified site D37.9
Gastritis (simple) K29.70
  with bleeding K29.71
  acute (erosive) K29.00
    with bleeding K29.01
  alcoholic K29.20
    with bleeding K29.21
  allergic K29.60
    with bleeding K29.61
  atrophic (chronic) K29.40
    with bleeding K29.41

Index

Gastritis — Glaucoma

Gastritis — *continued*
  chronic (antral) (fundal) K29.5Ø
    with bleeding K29.51
    atrophic K29.4Ø
      with bleeding K29.41
    superficial K29.3Ø
      with bleeding K29.31
  dietary counseling and surveillance Z71.3
  due to diet deficiency E63.9
  eosinophilic K52.81
  giant hypertrophic K29.6Ø
    with bleeding K29.61
  granulomatous K29.6Ø
    with bleeding K29.61
  hypertrophic (mucosa) K29.6Ø
    with bleeding K29.61
  nervous F54
  spastic K29.6Ø
    with bleeding K29.61
  specified NEC K29.6Ø
    with bleeding K29.61
  superficial chronic K29.3Ø
    with bleeding K29.31
  tuberculous A18.83
  viral NEC AØ8.4
Gastrocarcinoma — *see* Neoplasm, malignant, stomach
Gastrocolic — *see* condition
Gastrodisciasis, gastrodiscoidiasis B66.8
Gastroduodenitis K29.9Ø
  with bleeding K29.91
  virus, viral AØ8.4
    specified type NEC AØ8.39
Gastrodynia — *see* Pain, abdominal
Gastroenteritis (acute) (chronic) (noninfectious) (*see also* Enteritis) K52.9
  allergic K52.2
  dietetic K52.2
  drug-induced K52.1
  due to
    Cryptosporidium AØ7.2
    drugs K52.1
    food poisoning — *see* Intoxication, foodborne
    radiation K52.Ø
  eosinophilic K52.81
  epidemic (infectious) AØ9
  food hypersensitivity K52.2
  infectious — *see* Enteritis, infectious
  influenzal — *see* Influenza, with gastroenteritis
  noninfectious K52.9
    specified NEC K52.89
  rotaviral AØ8.Ø
  Salmonella AØ2.Ø
  toxic K52.1
  viral NEC AØ8.4
    acute infectious AØ8.39
      type Norwalk AØ8.11
    infantile (acute) AØ8.39
    Norwalk agent AØ8.11
    rotaviral AØ8.Ø
    severe of infants AØ8.39
    specified type NEC AØ8.39
Gastroenteropathy (*see also* Gastroenteritis) K52.9
  acute, due to Norovirus AØ8.11
  acute, due to Norwalk agent AØ8.11
  infectious AØ9
Gastroenteroptosis K63.4
Gastroesophageal laceration- hemorrhage syndrome K22.6
Gastrointestinal — *see* condition
Gastrojejunal — *see* condition
Gastrojejunitis (*see also* Enteritis) K52.9
Gastrojejunocolic — *see* condition
Gastroliths K31.89
Gastromalacia K31.89
Gastroparalysis K31.84
  diabetic — *see* Diabetes, gastroparalysis
Gastroparesis K31.84
  diabetic — *see* Diabetes, by type, with gastroparesis
Gastropathy K31.9
  congestive portal K31.89
  erythematous K29.7Ø
  exudative K9Ø.89
  portal hypertensive K31.89
Gastroptosis K31.89
Gastrorrhagia K92.2
  psychogenic F45.8
Gastroschisis (congenital) Q79.3
Gastrospasm (neurogenic) (reflex) K31.89

Gastrospasm — *continued*
  neurotic F45.8
  psychogenic F45.8
Gastrostaxis — *see* Gastritis, with bleeding
Gastrostenosis K31.89
Gastrostomy
  attention to Z43.1
  status Z93.1
Gastrosuccorrhea (continuous) (intermittent) K31.89
  neurotic F45.8
  psychogenic F45.8
Gatophobia F4Ø.218
Gaucher's disease or splenomegaly (adult) (infantile) E75.22
Gee (-Herter)(-Thaysen) **disease** (nontropical sprue) K9Ø.Ø
Gélineau's syndrome G47.419
  with cataplexy G47.411
Gemistocytoma
  specified site — *see* Neoplasm, malignant, by site
  unspecified site C71.9
Gemination, tooth, teeth KØØ.2
General, generalized — *see* condition
Genetic
  carrier (status)
    cystic fibrosis Z14.1
    hemophilia A (asymptomatic) Z14.Ø1
      symptomatic Z14.Ø2
    specified NEC Z14.8
  susceptibility to disease NEC Z15.89
    malignant neoplasm Z15.Ø9
      breast Z15.Ø1
      endometrium Z15.Ø4
      ovary Z15.Ø2
      prostate Z15.Ø3
      specified NEC Z15.Ø9
    multiple endocrine neoplasia Z15.81
Genital — *see* condition
Genito-anorectal syndrome A55
Genitourinary system — *see* condition
Genu
  congenital Q74.1
  extrorsum (acquired) (*see also* Deformity, varus, knee)
    congenital Q74.1
    sequelae (late effect) of rickets E64.3
  introrsum (acquired) (*see also* Deformity, valgus, knee)
    congenital Q74.1
    sequelae (late effect) of rickets E64.3
  rachitic (old) E64.3
  recurvatum (acquired) (*see also* Deformity, limb, specified type NEC, lower leg)
    congenital Q68.2
    sequelae (late effect) of rickets E64.3
  valgum (acquired) (knock-knee) M21.Ø6- ☑
    congenital Q74.1
    sequelae (late effect) of rickets E64.3
  varum (acquired) (bowleg) M21.16- ☑
    congenital Q74.1
    sequelae (late effect) of rickets E64.3
Geographic tongue K14.1
Geophagia — *see* Pica
Geotrichosis B48.3
  stomatitis B48.3
Gephyrophobia F4Ø.242
Gerbode defect Q21.Ø
GERD (gastroesophageal reflux disease) K21.9
Gerhardt's
  disease (erythromelalgia) I73.81
  syndrome (vocal cord paralysis) J38.ØØ
    bilateral J38.Ø2
    unilateral J38.Ø1
German measles (*see also* Rubella)
  exposure to Z2Ø.4
Germinoblastoma (diffuse) C85.9- ☑
  follicular C82.9- ☑
Germinoma — *see* Neoplasm, malignant, by site
Gerontoxon — *see* Degeneration, cornea, senile
Gerstmann-Sträussler-Scheinker syndrome (GSS) A81.82
Gerstmann's syndrome R48.8
  developmental F81.2
Gestation (period) (*see also* Pregnancy)
  ectopic — *see* Pregnancy, by site
  multiple O3Ø.9- ☑
    greater than quadruplets — *see* Pregnancy, multiple (gestation), specified NEC
    specified NEC — *see* Pregnancy, multiple (gestation), specified NEC

Gestational
  mammary abscess O91.11- ☑
  purulent mastitis O91.11- ☑
  subareolar abscess O91.11- ☑
Ghon tubercle, primary infection A15.7
Ghost
  teeth KØØ.4
  vessels (cornea) H16.41- ☑
Ghoul hand A66.3
Gianotti-Crosti disease L44.4
Giant
  cell
    epulis KØ6.8
    peripheral granuloma KØ6.8
  esophagus, congenital Q39.5
  kidney, congenital Q63.3
  urticaria T78.3 ☑
    hereditary D84.1
Giardiasis AØ7.1
Gibert's disease or pityriasis L42
Giddiness R42
  hysterical F44.89
  psychogenic F45.8
Gierke's disease (glycogenosis I) E74.Ø1
Gigantism (cerebral) (hypophyseal) (pituitary) E22.Ø
  constitutional E34.4
Gilbert's disease or syndrome E8Ø.4
Gilchrist's disease B4Ø.9
Gilford-Hutchinson disease E34.8
Gilles de la Tourette's disease or syndrome (motor-verbal tic) F95.2
Gingivitis KØ5.1Ø
  acute (catarrhal) KØ5.ØØ
    necrotizing A69.1
    nonplaque induced KØ5.Ø1
    plaque induced KØ5.ØØ
  chronic (desquamative) (hyperplastic) (simple marginal) (ulcerative) KØ5.1Ø
    nonplaque induced KØ5.11
    plaque induced KØ5.1Ø
  expulsiva — *see* Periodontitis
  necrotizing ulcerative (acute) A69.1
  pellagrous E52
    acute necrotizing A69.1
  Vincent's A69.1
Gingivoglossitis K14.Ø
Gingivopericementitis — *see* Periodontitis
Gingivosis — *see* Gingivitis, chronic
Gingivostomatitis KØ5.1Ø
  herpesviral BØØ.2
  necrotizing ulcerative (acute) A69.1
Gland, glandular — *see* condition
Glanders A24.Ø
Glanzmann (-Naegeli) **disease or thrombasthenia** D69.1
Glasgow coma scale
  total score
    3-8 R4Ø.243
    9-12 R4Ø.242
    13-15 R4Ø.241
Glass-blower's disease (cataract) — *see* Cataract, specified NEC
Glaucoma H4Ø.9
  with
    increased episcleral venous pressure H4Ø.81- ☑
    pseudoexfoliation of lens — *see* Glaucoma, open angle, primary, capsular
  absolute H44.51- ☑
  angle-closure (primary) H4Ø.2Ø- ☑
    acute (attack) (crisis) H4Ø.21- ☑
    chronic H4Ø.22- ☑
    intermittent H4Ø.23- ☑
    residual stage H4Ø.24- ☑
  borderline H4Ø.ØØ- ☑
  capsular (with pseudoexfoliation of lens) — *see* Glaucoma, open angle, primary, capsular
  childhood Q15.Ø
  closed angle — *see* Glaucoma, angle-closure
  congenital Q15.Ø
  corticosteroid-induced — *see* Glaucoma, secondary, drugs
  hypersecretion H4Ø.82- ☑
  in (due to)
    amyloidosis E85.4 [H42]
    aniridia Q13.1 [H42]
    concussion of globe — *see* Glaucoma, secondary, trauma

Glaucoma — continued
in — continued
dislocation of lens — see Glaucoma, secondary
disorder of lens NEC — see Glaucoma, secondary
drugs — see Glaucoma, secondary, drugs
endocrine disease NOS E34.9 [H42]
eye
inflammation — see Glaucoma, secondary, inflammation
trauma — see Glaucoma, secondary, trauma
hypermature cataract — see Glaucoma, secondary
iridocyclitis — see Glaucoma, secondary, inflammation
lens disorder — see Glaucoma, secondary
Lowe's syndrome E72.03 [H42]
metabolic disease NOS E88.9 [H42]
ocular disorders NEC — see Glaucoma, secondary
onchocerciasis B73.02
pupillary block — see Glaucoma, secondary
retinal vein occlusion — see Glaucoma, secondary
Rieger's anomaly Q13.81 [H42]
rubeosis of iris — see Glaucoma, secondary
tumor of globe — see Glaucoma, secondary
infantile Q15.0
low tension — see Glaucoma, open angle, primary, low-tension
malignant H40.83- ☑
narrow angle — see Glaucoma, angle-closure
newborn Q15.0
noncongestive (chronic) — see Glaucoma, open angle
nonobstructive — see Glaucoma, open angle
obstructive (see also Glaucoma, angle-closure)
due to lens changes — see Glaucoma, secondary
open angle H40.10- ☑
primary H40.11- ☑
capsular (with pseudoexfoliation of lens) H40.14- ☑
low-tension H40.12- ☑
pigmentary H40.13- ☑
residual stage H40.15- ☑
phacolytic — see Glaucoma, secondary
pigmentary — see Glaucoma, open angle, primary, pigmentary
postinfectious — see Glaucoma, secondary, inflammation
secondary (to) H40.5- ☑
drugs H40.6- ☑
inflammation H40.4- ☑
trauma H40.3- ☑
simple (chronic) H40.11 ☑
simplex H40.11 ☑
specified type NEC H40.89
suspect H40.00- ☑
syphilitic A52.71
traumatic (see also Glaucoma, secondary, trauma)
newborn (birth injury) P15.3
tuberculous A18.59
Glaucomatous flecks (subcapsular) — see Cataract, complicated
Glazed tongue K14.4
Gleet (gonococcal) A54.01
Glénard's disease K63.4
Glioblastoma (multiforme)
with sarcomatous component
specified site — see Neoplasm, malignant, by site
unspecified site C71.9
giant cell
specified site — see Neoplasm, malignant, by site
unspecified site C71.9
specified site — see Neoplasm, malignant, by site
unspecified site C71.9
Glioma (malignant)
astrocytic
specified site — see Neoplasm, malignant, by site
unspecified site C71.9
mixed
specified site — see Neoplasm, malignant, by site
unspecified site C71.9
nose Q30.8
specified site NEC — see Neoplasm, malignant, by site
subependymal D43.2
specified site — see Neoplasm, uncertain behavior, by site
unspecified site D43.2
unspecified site C71.9
Gliomatosis cerebri C71.0

Glioneuroma — see Neoplasm, uncertain behavior, by site
Gliosarcoma
specified site — see Neoplasm, malignant, by site
unspecified site C71.9
Gliosis (cerebral) G93.89
spinal G95.89
Glisson's disease — see Rickets
Globinuria R82.3
Globus (hystericus) F45.8
Glomangioma D18.00
intra-abdominal D18.03
intracranial D18.02
skin D18.01
specified site NEC D18.09
Glomangiomyoma D18.00
intra-abdominal D18.03
intracranial D18.02
skin D18.01
specified site NEC D18.09
Glomangiosarcoma — see Neoplasm, connective tissue, malignant
Glomerular
disease in syphilis A52.75
nephritis — see Glomerulonephritis
Glomerulitis — see Glomerulonephritis
Glomerulonephritis (see also Nephritis) N05.9
with
edema — see Nephrosis
minimal change N05.0
minor glomerular abnormality N05.0
acute N00.9
chronic N03.9
crescentic (diffuse) NEC (see also N00-N07 with fourth character .7) N05.7
dense deposit (see also N00-N07 with fourth character .6) N05.6
diffuse
crescentic (see also N00-N07 with fourth character .7) N05.7
endocapillary proliferative (see also N00-N07 with fourth character .4) N05.4
membranous (see also N00-N07 with fourth character .2) N05.2
mesangial proliferative (see also N00-N07 with fourth character .3) N05.3
mesangiocapillary (see also N00-N07 with fourth character .5) N05.5
sclerosing N05.8
endocapillary proliferative (diffuse) NEC (see also N00-N07 with fourth character .4) N05.4
extracapillary NEC (see also N00-N07 with fourth character .7) N05.7
focal (and segmental) (see also N00-N07 with fourth character .1) N05.1
hypocomplementemic — see Glomerulonephritis, membranoproliferative
IgA — see Nephropathy, IgA
immune complex (circulating) NEC N05.8
in (due to)
amyloidosis E85.4 [N08]
bilharziasis B65.9 [N08]
cryoglobulinemia D89.1 [N08]
defibrination syndrome D65 [N08]
diabetes mellitus — see Diabetes, glomerulosclerosis
disseminated intravascular coagulation D65 [N08]
Fabry (-Anderson) disease E75.21 [N08]
Goodpasture's syndrome M31.0
hemolytic-uremic syndrome D59.3
Henoch (-Schönlein) purpura D69.0 [N08]
lecithin cholesterol acyltransferase deficiency E78.6 [N08]
microscopic polyangiitis M31.7 [N08]
multiple myeloma C90.0- ☑ [N08]
Plasmodium malariae B52.0
schistosomiasis B65.9 [N08]
sepsis A41.9 [N08]
streptococcal A40- ☑ [N08]
sickle-cell disorders D57.- ☑ [N08]
strongyloidiasis B78.9 [N08]
subacute bacterial endocarditis I33.0 [N08]
syphilis (late) congenital A50.59 [N08]
systemic lupus erythematosus M32.14
thrombotic thrombocytopenic purpura M31.1 [N08]
typhoid fever A01.09
Waldenström macroglobulinemia C88.0 [N08]

Glomerulonephritis — continued
in — continued
Wegener's granulomatosis M31.31
latent or quiescent N03.9
lobular, lobulonodular — see Glomerulonephritis, membranoproliferative
membranoproliferative (diffuse)(type 1 or 3) (see also N00-N07 with fourth character .5) N05.5
dense deposit (type 2) NEC (see also N00-N07 with fourth character .6) N05.6
membranous (diffuse) NEC (see also N00-N07 with fourth character .2) N05.2
mesangial
IgA/IgG — see Nephropathy, IgA
proliferative (diffuse) NEC (see also N00-N07 with fourth character .3) N05.3
mesangiocapillary (diffuse) NEC (see also N00-N07 with fourth character .5) N05.5
necrotic, necrotizing NEC (see also N00- N07 with fourth character .8) N05.8
nodular — see Glomerulonephritis, membranoproliferative
poststreptococcal NEC N05.9
acute N00.9
chronic N03.9
rapidly progressive N01.9
proliferative NEC (see also N00-N07 with fourth character .8) N05.8
diffuse (lupus) M32.14
rapidly progressive N01.9
sclerosing, diffuse N05.8
specified pathology NEC (see also N00- N07 with fourth character .8) N05.8
subacute N01.9
Glomerulopathy — see Glomerulonephritis
Glomerulosclerosis (see also Sclerosis, renal)
intercapillary (nodular) (with diabetes) — see Diabetes, glomerulosclerosis
intracapillary — see Diabetes, glomerulosclerosis
Glossagra K14.6
Glossalgia K14.6
Glossitis (chronic superficial) (gangrenous) (Moeller's) K14.0
areata exfoliativa K14.1
atrophic K14.4
benign migratory K14.1
cortical superficial, sclerotic K14.0
Hunter's D51.0
interstitial, sclerous K14.0
median rhomboid K14.2
pellagrous E52
superficial, chronic K14.0
Glossocele K14.8
Glossodynia K14.6
exfoliativa K14.4
Glossoncus K14.8
Glossopathy K14.9
Glossophytia K14.3
Glossoplegia K14.8
Glossoptosis K14.8
Glossopyrosis K14.6
Glossotrichia K14.3
Glossy skin L90.8
Glottis — see condition
Glottitis (see also Laryngitis) J04.0
Glucagonoma
pancreas
benign D13.7
malignant C25.4
uncertain behavior D37.8
specified site NEC
benign — see Neoplasm, benign, by site
malignant — see Neoplasm, malignant, by site
uncertain behavior — see Neoplasm, uncertain behavior, by site
unspecified site
benign D13.7
malignant C25.4
uncertain behavior D37.8
Glucoglycinuria E72.51
Glucose-galactose malabsorption E74.39
Glue
ear — see Otitis, media, nonsuppurative, chronic, mucoid
sniffing (airplane) — see Abuse, drug, inhalant
dependence — see Dependence, drug, inhalant
Glutaric aciduria E72.3

Glycinemia E72.51
Glycinuria (renal) (with ketosis) E72.09
Glycogen
  infiltration — *see* Disease, glycogen storage
  storage disease — *see* Disease, glycogen storage
Glycogenosis (diffuse) (generalized) (*see also* Disease, glycogen storage)
  cardiac E74.02 [I43]
  diabetic, secondary — *see* Diabetes, glycogenosis, secondary
  pulmonary interstitial J84.842
Glycopenia E16.2
Glycosuria R81
  renal E74.8
Gnathostoma spinigerum (infection) (infestation), **gnathostomiasis** (wandering swelling) B83.1
Goiter (plunging) (substernal) E04.9
  with
    hyperthyroidism (recurrent) — *see* Hyperthyroidism, with, goiter
    thyrotoxicosis — *see* Hyperthyroidism, with, goiter
  adenomatous — *see* Goiter, nodular
  cancerous C73
  congenital (nontoxic) E03.0
    diffuse E03.0
    parenchymatous E03.0
    transitory, with normal functioning P72.0
  cystic E04.2
    due to iodine-deficiency E01.1
  due to
    enzyme defect in synthesis of thyroid hormone E07.1
    iodine-deficiency (endemic) E01.2
  dyshormonogenetic (familial) E07.1
  endemic (iodine-deficiency) E01.2
    diffuse E01.0
    multinodular E01.1
  exophthalmic — *see* Hyperthyroidism, with, goiter
  iodine-deficiency (endemic) E01.2
    diffuse E01.0
    multinodular E01.1
    nodular E01.1
  lingual Q89.2
  lymphadenoid E06.3
  malignant C73
  multinodular (cystic) (nontoxic) E04.2
    toxic or with hyperthyroidism E05.20
      with thyroid storm E05.21
  neonatal NEC P72.0
  nodular (nontoxic) (due to) E04.9
    with
      hyperthyroidism E05.20
        with thyroid storm E05.21
      thyrotoxicosis E05.20
        with thyroid storm E05.21
    endemic E01.1
    iodine-deficiency E01.1
    sporadic E04.9
    toxic E05.20
      with thyroid storm E05.21
  nontoxic E04.9
    diffuse (colloid) E04.0
    multinodular E04.2
    simple E04.0
    specified NEC E04.8
    uninodular E04.1
  simple E04.0
  toxic — *see* Hyperthyroidism, with, goiter
  uninodular (nontoxic) E04.1
    toxic or with hyperthyroidism E05.10
      with thyroid storm E05.11
Goiter-deafness syndrome E07.1
Goldberg syndrome Q89.8
Goldberg-Maxwell syndrome E34.51
Goldblatt's hypertension or kidney I70.1
Goldenhar (-Gorlin) **syndrome** Q87.0
Goldflam-Erb disease or syndrome G70.00
  with exacerbation (acute) G70.01
  in crisis G70.01
Goldscheider's disease Q81.8
Goldstein's disease (familial hemorrhagic telangiectasia) I78.0
Golfer's elbow — *see* Epicondylitis, medial
Gonadoblastoma
  specified site — *see* Neoplasm, uncertain behavior, by site
  unspecified site
    female D39.10

Gonadoblastoma — *continued*
  unspecified site — *continued*
    male D40.10
Gonecystitis — *see* Vesiculitis
Gongylonemiasis B83.8
Goniosynechiae — *see* Adhesions, iris, goniosynechiae
Gonococcemia A54.86
Gonococcus, gonococcal (disease) (infection) (*see also* condition) A54.9
  anus A54.6
  bursa, bursitis A54.49
  conjunctiva, conjunctivitis (neonatorum) A54.31
  endocardium A54.83
  eye A54.30
    conjunctivitis A54.31
    iridocyclitis A54.32
    keratitis A54.33
    newborn A54.31
    other specified A54.39
  fallopian tubes (acute) (chronic) A54.24
  genitourinary (organ) (system) (tract) (acute)
    lower A54.00
      with abscess (accessory gland) (periurethral) A54.1
    upper (*see also* condition) A54.29
  heart A54.83
  iridocyclitis A54.32
  joint A54.42
  lymphatic (gland) (node) A54.89
  meninges, meningitis A54.81
  musculoskeletal A54.40
    arthritis A54.42
    osteomyelitis A54.43
    other specified A54.49
    spondylopathy A54.41
  pelviperitonitis A54.24
  pelvis (acute) (chronic) A54.24
  pharynx A54.5
  proctitis A54.6
  pyosalpinx (acute) (chronic) A54.24
  rectum A54.6
  skin A54.89
  specified site NEC A54.89
  tendon sheath A54.49
  throat A54.5
  urethra (acute) (chronic) A54.01
    with abscess (accessory gland) (periurethral) A54.1
  vulva (acute) (chronic) A54.02
Gonocytoma
  specified site — *see* Neoplasm, uncertain behavior, by site
  unspecified site
    female D39.10
    male D40.10
Gonorrhea (acute) (chronic) A54.9
  Bartholin's gland (acute) (chronic) (purulent) A54.02
    with abscess (accessory gland) (periurethral) A54.1
  bladder A54.01
  cervix A54.03
  conjunctiva, conjunctivitis (neonatorum) A54.31
  contact Z20.2
  Cowper's gland (with abscess) A54.1
  exposure to Z20.2
  fallopian tube (acute) (chronic) A54.24
  kidney (acute) (chronic) A54.21
  lower genitourinary tract A54.00
    with abscess (accessory gland) (periurethral) A54.1
  ovary (acute) (chronic) A54.24
  pelvis (acute) (chronic) A54.24
    female pelvic inflammatory disease A54.24
  penis A54.09
  prostate (acute) (chronic) A54.22
  seminal vesicle (acute) (chronic) A54.23
  specified site not listed (*see also* Gonococcus) A54.89
  spermatic cord (acute) (chronic) A54.23
  urethra A54.01
    with abscess (accessory gland) (periurethral) A54.1
  vagina A54.02
  vas deferens (acute) (chronic) A54.23
  vulva A54.02
Goodall's disease A08.19
Goodpasture's syndrome M31.0
Gopalan's syndrome (burning feet) E53.0
Gorlin-Chaudry-Moss syndrome Q87.0
Gottron's papules L94.4
Gougerot-Blum syndrome (pigmented purpuric lichenoid dermatitis) L81.7

Gougerot-Carteaud disease or syndrome (confluent reticulate papillomatosis) L83
Gougerot's syndrome (trisymptomatic) L81.7
Gouley's syndrome (constrictive pericarditis) I31.1
Goundou A66.6
Gout, chronic (*see also* Gout, gouty) M1A.9 ☑ (*following* M08)
  drug-induced M1A.20 ☑ (*following* M08)
    ankle M1A.27- ☑ (*following* M08)
    elbow M1A.22- ☑ (*following* M08)
    foot joint M1A.27- ☑ (*following* M08)
    hand joint M1A.24- ☑ (*following* M08)
    hip M1A.25- ☑ (*following* M08)
    knee M1A.26- ☑ (*following* M08)
    multiple site M1A.29- ☑ (*following* M08)
    shoulder M1A.21- ☑ (*following* M08)
    vertebrae M1A.28 ☑ (*following* M08)
    wrist M1A.23- ☑ (*following* M08)
  idiopathic M1A.00 ☑ (*following* M08)
    ankle M1A.07- ☑ (*following* M08)
    elbow M1A.02- ☑ (*following* M08)
    foot joint M1A.07- ☑ (*following* M08)
    hand joint M1A.04- ☑ (*following* M08)
    hip M1A.05- ☑ (*following* M08)
    knee M1A.06- ☑ (*following* M08)
    multiple site M1A.09 ☑ (*following* M08)
    shoulder M1A.01- ☑ (*following* M08)
    vertebrae M1A.08 ☑ (*following* M08)
    wrist M1A.03- ☑ (*following* M08)
  in (due to) renal impairment M1A.30 ☑ (*following* M08)
    ankle M1A.37- ☑ (*following* M08)
    elbow M1A.32- ☑ (*following* M08)
    foot joint M1A.37- ☑ (*following* M08)
    hand joint M1A.34- ☑ (*following* M08)
    hip M1A.35- ☑ (*following* M08)
    knee M1A.36- ☑ (*following* M08)
    multiple site M1A.39 ☑ (*following* M08)
    shoulder M1A.31- ☑ (*following* M08)
    vertebrae M1A.38 ☑ (*following* M08)
    wrist M1A.33- ☑ (*following* M08)
  lead-induced M1A.10 ☑ (*following* M08)
    ankle M1A.17- ☑ (*following* M08)
    elbow M1A.12- ☑ (*following* M08)
    foot joint M1A.17- ☑ (*following* M08)
    hand joint M1A.14- ☑ (*following* M08)
    hip M1A.15- ☑ (*following* M08)
    knee M1A.16- ☑ (*following* M08)
    multiple site M1A.19 ☑ (*following* M08)
    shoulder M1A.11- ☑ (*following* M08)
    vertebrae M1A.18 ☑ (*following* M08)
    wrist M1A.13- ☑ (*following* M08)
  primary — *see* Gout, chronic, idiopathic
  saturnine — *see* Gout, chronic, lead-induced
  secondary NEC M1A.40 ☑ (*following* M08)
    ankle M1A.47- ☑ (*following* M08)
    elbow M1A.42- ☑ (*following* M08)
    foot joint M1A.47- ☑ (*following* M08)
    hand joint M1A.44- ☑ (*following* M08)
    hip M1A.45- ☑ (*following* M08)
    knee M1A.46- ☑ (*following* M08)
    multiple site M1A.49 ☑ (*following* M08)
    shoulder M1A.41- ☑ (*following* M08)
    vertebrae M1A.48 ☑ (*following* M08)
    wrist M1A.43- ☑ (*following* M08)
  syphilitic (*see also* subcategory M14.8-) A52.77
  tophi M1A.9 ☑ (*following* M08)
Gout, gouty (acute) (attack) (flare) (*see also* Gout, chronic) M10.9
  drug-induced M10.20
    ankle M10.27- ☑
    elbow M10.22- ☑
    foot joint M10.27- ☑
    hand joint M10.24- ☑
    hip M10.25- ☑
    knee M10.26- ☑
    multiple site M10.29
    shoulder M10.21- ☑
    vertebrae M10.28
    wrist M10.23- ☑
  idiopathic M10.00
    ankle M10.07- ☑
    elbow M10.02- ☑
    foot joint M10.07- ☑
    hand joint M10.04- ☑
    hip M10.05- ☑

154

☑ **Additional Character Required — Refer to the Tabular List for Character Selection**   ▽ **Subterms under main terms may continue to next column or page**

Gout, gouty — *continued*
  idiopathic — *continued*
    knee M10.06- ☑
    multiple site M10.09
    shoulder M10.01- ☑
    vertebrae M10.08
    wrist M10.03- ☑
  in (due to) renal impairment M10.30
    ankle M10.37- ☑
    elbow M10.32- ☑
    foot joint M10.37- ☑
    hand joint M10.34- ☑
    hip M10.35- ☑
    knee M10.36- ☑
    multiple site M10.39
    shoulder M10.31- ☑
    vertebrae M10.38
    wrist M10.33- ☑
  lead-induced M10.10
    ankle M10.17- ☑
    elbow M10.12- ☑
    foot joint M10.17- ☑
    hand joint M10.14- ☑
    hip M10.15- ☑
    knee M10.16- ☑
    multiple site M10.19
    shoulder M10.11- ☑
    vertebrae M10.18
    wrist M10.13- ☑
  primary — *see* Gout, idiopathic
  saturnine — *see* Gout, lead-induced
  secondary NEC M10.40
    ankle M10.47- ☑
    elbow M10.42- ☑
    foot joint M10.47- ☑
    hand joint M10.44- ☑
    hip M10.45- ☑
    knee M10.46- ☑
    multiple site M10.49
    shoulder M10.41- ☑
    vertebrae M10.48
    wrist M10.43- ☑
  syphilitic (*see also* subcategory M14.8-) A52.77
  tophi — *see* Gout, chronic
Gower's
  muscular dystrophy G71.0
  syndrome (vasovagal attack) R55
Gradenigo's syndrome — *see* Otitis, media, suppurative, acute
Graefe's disease — *see* Strabismus, paralytic, ophthalmoplegia, progressive
Graft-versus-host disease D89.813
  acute D89.810
  acute on chronic D89.812
  chronic D89.811
Grain mite (itch) B88.0
Grainhandler's disease or lung J67.8
Grand mal — *see* Epilepsy, generalized, specified NEC
Grand multipara status only (not pregnant) Z64.1
  pregnant — *see* Pregnancy, complicated by, grand multiparity
Granite worker's lung J62.8
Granular (*see also* condition)
  inflammation, pharynx J31.2
  kidney (contracting) — *see* Sclerosis, renal
  liver K74.69
Granulation tissue (abnormal) (excessive) L92.9
  postmastoidectomy cavity — *see* Complications, postmastoidectomy, granulation
Granulocytopenia (primary) (malignant) — *see* Agranulocytosis
Granuloma L92.9
  abdomen K66.8
    from residual foreign body L92.3
    pyogenicum L98.0
  actinic L57.5
  annulare (perforating) L92.0
  apical K04.5
  aural — *see* Otitis, externa, specified NEC
  beryllium (skin) L92.3
  bone
    eosinophilic C96.6
    from residual foreign body — *see* Osteomyelitis, specified type NEC
    lung C96.6
  brain (any site) G06.0
    schistosomiasis B65.9 [G07]

Granuloma — *continued*
  canaliculus lacrimalis — *see* Granuloma, lacrimal
  candidal (cutaneous) B37.2
  cerebral (any site) G06.0
  coccidioidal (primary) (progressive) B38.7
    lung B38.1
    meninges B38.4
  colon K63.89
  conjunctiva H11.22- ☑
  dental K04.5
  ear, middle — *see* Cholesteatoma
  eosinophilic C96.6
    bone C96.6
    lung C96.6
    oral mucosa K13.4
    skin L92.2
  eyelid H01.8
  facial (e) L92.2
  foreign body (in soft tissue) NEC M60.20
    ankle M60.27- ☑
    foot M60.27- ☑
    forearm M60.23- ☑
    hand M60.24- ☑
    in operation wound — *see* Foreign body, accidentally left during a procedure
    lower leg M60.26- ☑
    pelvic region M60.25- ☑
    shoulder region M60.21- ☑
    skin L92.3
    specified site NEC M60.28
    subcutaneous tissue L92.3
    thigh M60.25- ☑
    upper arm M60.22- ☑
  gangraenescens M31.2
  genito-inguinale A58
  giant cell (central) (reparative) (jaw) M27.1
    gingiva (peripheral) K06.8
  gland (lymph) I88.8
  hepatic NEC K75.3
    in (due to)
      berylliosis J63.2 [K77]
      sarcoidosis D86.89
  Hodgkin C81.9 ☑
  ileum K63.89
  infectious B99.9
    specified NEC B99.8
  inguinale (Donovan) (venereal) A58
  intestine NEC K63.89
  intracranial (any site) G06.0
  intraspinal (any part) G06.1
  iridocyclitis — *see* Iridocyclitis, chronic
  jaw (bone) (central) M27.1
    reparative giant cell M27.1
  kidney (*see also* Infection, kidney) N15.8
  lacrimal H04.81- ☑
  larynx J38.7
  lethal midline (faciale(e)) M31.2
  liver NEC — *see* Granuloma, hepatic
  lung (infectious) (*see also* Fibrosis, lung)
    coccidioidal B38.1
    eosinophilic C96.6
  Majocchi's B35.8
  malignant (facial(e)) M31.2
  mandible (central) M27.1
  midline (lethal) M31.2
  monilial (cutaneous) B37.2
  nasal sinus — *see* Sinusitis
  operation wound T81.89 ☑
    foreign body — *see* Foreign body, accidentally left during a procedure
    stitch T81.89 ☑
    talc — *see* Foreign body, accidentally left during a procedure
  oral mucosa K13.4
  orbit, orbital H05.11- ☑
  paracoccidioidal B41.8
  penis, venereal A58
  periapical K04.5
  peritoneum K66.8
    due to ova of helminths NOS (*see also* Helminthiasis) B83.9 [K67]
  postmastoidectomy cavity — *see* Complications, postmastoidectomy, recurrent cholesteatoma
  prostate N42.89
  pudendi (ulcerating) A58
  pulp, internal (tooth) K03.3
  pyogenic, pyogenicum (of) (skin) L98.0
    gingiva K06.8

Granuloma — *continued*
  pyogenic, pyogenicum — *continued*
    maxillary alveolar ridge K04.5
    oral mucosa K13.4
  rectum K62.89
  reticulohistiocytic D76.3
  rubrum nasi L74.8
  Schistosoma — *see* Schistosomiasis
  septic (skin) L98.0
  silica (skin) L92.3
  sinus (accessory) (infective) (nasal) — *see* Sinusitis
  skin L92.9
    from residual foreign body L92.3
    pyogenicum L98.0
  spine
    syphilitic (epidural) A52.19
    tuberculous A18.01
  stitch (postoperative) T81.89 ☑
  suppurative (skin) L98.0
  swimming pool A31.1
  talc (*see also* Granuloma, foreign body)
    in operation wound — *see* Foreign body, accidentally left during a procedure
  telangiectaticum (skin) L98.0
  tracheostomy J95.09
  trichophyticum B35.8
  tropicum A66.4
  umbilicus L92.9
  urethra N36.8
  uveitis — *see* Iridocyclitis, chronic
  vagina A58
  venereum A58
  vocal cord J38.3
Granulomatosis L92.9
  lymphoid C83.8- ☑
  miliary (listerial) A32.89
  necrotizing, respiratory M31.30
  progressive septic D71
  specified NEC L92.8
  Wegener's M31.30
    with renal involvement M31.31
Granulomatous tissue (abnormal) (excessive) L92.9
Granulosis rubra nasi L74.8
Graphite fibrosis (of lung) J63.3
Graphospasm F48.8
  organic G25.89
Grating scapula M89.8X1
Gravel (urinary) — *see* Calculus, urinary
Graves' disease — *see* Hyperthyroidism, with, goiter
Gravis — *see* condition
Grawitz tumor C64.- ☑
Gray syndrome (newborn) P93.0
Grayness, hair (premature) L67.1
  congenital Q84.2
Green sickness D50.8
Greenfield's disease
  meaning
    concentric sclerosis (encephalitis periaxialis concentrica) G37.5
    metachromatic leukodystrophy E75.25
Greenstick fracture — *code as* Fracture, by site
Grey syndrome (newborn) P93.0
Grief F43.21
  prolonged F43.29
  reaction (*see also* Disorder, adjustment) F43.20
Griesinger's disease B76.9
Grinder's lung or pneumoconiosis J62.8
Grinding, teeth
  psychogenic F45.8
  sleep related G47.63
Grip
  Dabney's B33.0
  devil's B33.0
Grippe, grippal (*see also* Influenza)
  Balkan A78
  summer, of Italy A93.1
Grisel's disease M43.6
Groin — *see* condition
Grooved tongue K14.5
Ground itch B76.9
Grover's disease or syndrome L11.1
Growing pains, children R29.898
Growth (fungoid) (neoplastic) (new) (*see also* Neoplasm)
  adenoid (vegetative) J35.8
  benign — *see* Neoplasm, benign, by site
  malignant — *see* Neoplasm, malignant, by site
  rapid, childhood Z00.2

Index

Growth — Headache

Growth — *continued*
  secondary — *see* Neoplasm, secondary, by site
Gruby's disease B35.0
Gubler-Millard paralysis or syndrome G46.3
Guerin-Stern syndrome Q74.3
Guidance, insufficient anterior (occlusal) M26.54
Guillain-Barré disease or syndrome G61.0
  sequelae G65.0
Guinea worms (infection) (infestation) B72
Guinon's disease (motor-verbal tic) F95.2
Gull's disease E03.4
Gum — *see* condition
Gumboil K04.7
  with sinus K04.6
Gumma (syphilitic) A52.79
  artery A52.09
    cerebral A52.04
  bone A52.77
    of yaws (late) A66.6
  brain A52.19
  cauda equina A52.19
  central nervous system A52.3
  ciliary body A52.71
  congenital A50.59
  eyelid A52.71
  heart A52.06
  intracranial A52.19
  iris A52.71
  kidney A52.75
  larynx A52.73
  leptomeninges A52.19
  liver A52.74
  meninges A52.19
  myocardium A52.06
  nasopharynx A52.73
  neurosyphilitic A52.3
  nose A52.73
  orbit A52.71
  palate (soft) A52.79
  penis A52.76
  pericardium A52.06
  pharynx A52.73
  pituitary A52.79
  scrofulous (tuberculous) A18.4
  skin A52.79
  specified site NEC A52.79
  spinal cord A52.19
  tongue A52.79
  tonsil A52.73
  trachea A52.73
  tuberculous A18.4
  ulcerative due to yaws A66.4
  ureter A52.75
  yaws A66.4
    bone A66.6
Gunn's syndrome Q07.8
Gunshot wound (*see also* Wound, open)
  fracture — *code as* Fracture, by site
  internal organs — *see* Injury, by site
Gynandrism Q56.0
Gynandroblastoma
  specified site — *see* Neoplasm, uncertain behavior,
    by site
  unspecified site
    female D39.10
    male D40.10
Gynecological examination (periodic) (routine) Z01.419
  with abnormal findings Z01.411
Gynecomastia N62
Gynephobia F40.291
Gyrate scalp Q82.8

H

H (Hartnup's) **disease** E72.02
Haas' disease or osteochondrosis (juvenile) (head of
  humerus) — *see* Osteochondrosis, juvenile,
  humerus
Habit, habituation
  bad sleep Z72.821
  chorea F95.8
  disturbance, child F98.9
  drug — *see* Dependence, drug
  irregular sleep Z72.821
  laxative F55.2
  spasm — *see* Tic
  tic — *see* Tic

Haemophilus (H.) **influenzae, as cause of disease
classified elsewhere** B96.3
Haff disease — *see* Poisoning, mercury
Hageman's factor defect, deficiency or disease D68.2
Haglund's disease or osteochondrosis (juvenile) (os
  tibiale externum) — *see* Osteochondrosis, juvenile,
  tarsus
Hailey-Hailey disease Q82.8
Hair (*see also* condition)
  plucking F63.3
    in stereotyped movement disorder F98.4
  tourniquet syndrome (*see also* Constriction, external,
    by site)
    finger S60.44- ☑
    penis S30.842 ☑
    thumb S60.34- ☑
    toe S90.44- ☑
Hair-pulling, pathological (compulsive) F63.3
Hairball in stomach T18.2 ☑
Hairy black tongue K14.3
Half vertebra Q76.49
Halitosis R19.6
Hallerman-Streiff syndrome Q87.0
Hallervorden-Spatz disease G23.0
Hallopeau's acrodermatitis or disease L40.2
Hallucination R44.3
  auditory R44.0
  gustatory R44.2
  olfactory R44.2
  specified NEC R44.2
  tactile R44.2
  visual R44.1
Hallucinosis (chronic) F28
  alcoholic (acute) F10.951
    in
      abuse F10.151
      dependence F10.251
  drug-induced F19.951
    cannabis F12.951
    cocaine F14.951
    hallucinogen F16.151
    in
      abuse F19.151
        cannabis F12.151
        cocaine F14.151
        hallucinogen F16.151
        inhalant F18.151
        opioid F11.151
        sedative, anxiolytic or hypnotic F13.151
        stimulant NEC F15.151
      dependence F19.251
        cannabis F12.251
        cocaine F14.251
        hallucinogen F16.251
        inhalant F18.251
        opioid F11.251
        sedative, anxiolytic or hypnotic F13.251
        stimulant NEC F15.251
    inhalant F18.951
    opioid F11.951
    sedative, anxiolytic or hypnotic F13.951
    stimulant NEC F15.951
  organic F06.0
Hallux
  deformity (acquired) NEC M20.5X- ☑
  limitus M20.5X- ☑
  malleus (acquired) NEC M20.3- ☑
  rigidus (acquired) M20.2- ☑
    congenital Q74.2
    sequelae (late effect) of rickets E64.3
  valgus (acquired) M20.1- ☑
    congenital Q66.6
  varus (acquired) M20.3- ☑
    congenital Q66.3
Halo, visual H53.19
Hamartoma, hamartoblastoma Q85.9
  epithelial (gingival), odontogenic, central or peripheral
    — *see* Cyst, calcifying odontogenic
Hamartosis Q85.9
Hamman-Rich syndrome J84.114
Hammer toe (acquired) NEC (*see also* Deformity, toe,
  hammer toe)
  congenital Q66.89
  sequelae (late effect) of rickets E64.3
Hand — *see* condition
Hand-foot syndrome L27.1
Hand-Schüller-Christian disease or syndrome C96.5

Handicap, handicapped
  educational Z55.9
  specified NEC Z55.8
Hanging (asphyxia) (strangulation) (suffocation) — *see*
  Asphyxia, traumatic, due to mechanical threat
Hangnail (*see also* Cellulitis, digit)
  with lymphangitis — *see* Lymphangitis, acute, digit
Hangover (alcohol) F10.129
Hanhart's syndrome Q87.0
Hanot-Chauffard (-Troisier) **syndrome** E83.19
Hanot's cirrhosis or disease K74.3
Hansen's disease — *see* Leprosy
Hantaan virus disease (Korean hemorrhagic fever) A98.5
Hantavirus disease (with renal manifestations) (Dobra-
  va) (Puumala) (Seoul) A98.5
  with pulmonary manifestations (Andes) (Bayou)
    (Bermejo) (Black Creek Canal) (Choclo) (Juquiti-
    ba) (Laguna negra) (Lechiguanas) (New York)
    (Oran) (Sin nombre) B33.4
Happy puppet syndrome Q93.5
Harada's disease or syndrome H30.81- ☑
Hardening
  artery — *see* Arteriosclerosis
  brain G93.89
Harelip (complete) (incomplete) — *see* Cleft, lip
Harlequin (newborn) Q80.4
Harley's disease D59.6
Harmful use (of)
  alcohol F10.10
  anxiolytics — *see* Abuse, drug, sedative
  cannabinoids — *see* Abuse, drug, cannabis
  cocaine — *see* Abuse, drug, cocaine
  drug — *see* Abuse, drug
  hallucinogens — *see* Abuse, drug, hallucinogen
  hypnotics — *see* Abuse, drug, sedative
  opioids — *see* Abuse, drug, opioid
  PCP (phencyclidine) — *see* Abuse, drug, hallucinogen
  sedatives — *see* Abuse, drug, sedative
  stimulants NEC — *see* Abuse, drug, stimulant
Harris' lines — *see* Arrest, epiphyseal
Hartnup's disease E72.02
Harvester's lung J67.0
Harvesting ovum for in vitro fertilization Z31.83
Hashimoto's disease or thyroiditis E06.3
Hashitoxicosis (transient) E06.3
Hassal-Henle bodies or warts (cornea) H18.49
Haut mal — *see* Epilepsy, generalized, specified NEC
Haverhill fever A25.1
Hay fever (*see also* Fever, hay) J30.1
Hayem-Widal syndrome D59.8
Haygarth's nodes M15.8
Haymaker's lung J67.0
Hb (abnormal)
  Bart's disease D56.0
  disease — *see* Disease, hemoglobin
  trait — *see* Trait
Head — *see* condition
Headache R51
  allergic NEC G44.89
  associated with sexual activity G44.82
  chronic daily R51
  cluster G44.009
    chronic G44.029
      intractable G44.021
      not intractable G44.029
    episodic G44.019
      intractable G44.011
      not intractable G44.019
    intractable G44.001
    not intractable G44.009
  cough (primary) G44.83
  daily chronic R51
  drug-induced NEC G44.40
    intractable G44.41
    not intractable G44.40
  exertional (primary) G44.84
  histamine G44.009
    intractable G44.001
    not intractable G44.009
  hypnic G44.81
  lumbar puncture G97.1
  medication overuse G44.40
    intractable G44.41
    not intractable G44.40
  menstrual — *see* Migraine, menstrual
  migraine (type) (*see also* Migraine) G43.909
  nasal septum R51

Headache — *continued*
　neuralgiform, short lasting unilateral, with conjunctival injection and tearing (SUNCT) G44.059
　　intractable G44.051
　　not intractable G44.059
　new daily persistent (NDPH) G44.52
　orgasmic G44.82
　periodic syndromes in adults and children G43.C0 (*following* G43.7)
　　with refractory migraine G43.C1 (*following* G43.7)
　　without refractory migraine G43.C0 (*following* G43.7)
　　intractable G43.C1 (*following* G43.7)
　　not intractable G43.C0 (*following* G43.7)
　post-traumatic G44.309
　　acute G44.319
　　　intractable G44.311
　　　not intractable G44.319
　　chronic G44.329
　　　intractable G44.321
　　　not intractable G44.329
　　intractable G44.301
　　not intractable G44.309
　postspinal puncture G97.1
　pre-menstrual — *see* Migraine, menstrual
　preorgasmic G44.82
　primary
　　cough G44.83
　　exertional G44.84
　　stabbing G44.85
　　thunderclap G44.53
　rebound G44.40
　　intractable G44.41
　　not intractable G44.40
　short lasting unilateral neuralgiform, with conjunctival injection and tearing (SUNCT) G44.059
　　intractable G44.051
　　not intractable G44.059
　specified syndrome NEC G44.89
　spinal and epidural anesthesia - induced T88.59 ☑
　　in labor and delivery O74.5
　　in pregnancy O29.4- ☑
　　postpartum, puerperal O89.4
　spinal fluid loss (from puncture) G97.1
　stabbing (primary) G44.85
　tension (-type) G44.209
　　chronic G44.229
　　　intractable G44.221
　　　not intractable G44.229
　　episodic G44.219
　　　intractable G44.211
　　　not intractable G44.219
　　intractable G44.201
　　not intractable G44.209
　thunderclap (primary) G44.53
　vascular NEC G44.1
Healthy
　infant
　　accompanying sick mother Z76.3
　　receiving care Z76.2
　person accompanying sick person Z76.3
Hearing examination Z01.10
　with abnormal findings NEC Z01.118
　following failed hearing screening Z01.110
　for hearing conservation and treatment Z01.12
Heart — *see* condition
Heart beat
　abnormality R00.9
　　specified NEC R00.8
　awareness R00.2
　rapid R00.0
　slow R00.1
Heartburn R12
　psychogenic F45.8
Heat (effects) T67.9 ☑
　apoplexy T67.0 ☑
　burn (*see also* Burn) L55.9
　collapse T67.1 ☑
　cramps T67.2 ☑
　dermatitis or eczema L59.0
　edema T67.7 ☑
　erythema — *code by site under* Burn, first degree
　excessive T67.9 ☑
　　specified effect NEC T67.8 ☑
　exhaustion T67.5 ☑
　　anhydrotic T67.3 ☑
　　due to
　　　salt (and water) depletion T67.4 ☑

Heat — *continued*
　exhaustion — *continued*
　　due to — *continued*
　　　water depletion T67.3 ☑
　　　　with salt depletion T67.4 ☑
　fatigue (transient) T67.6 ☑
　fever T67.0 ☑
　hyperpyrexia T67.0 ☑
　prickly L74.0
　prostration — *see* Heat, exhaustion
　pyrexia T67.0 ☑
　rash L74.0
　specified effect NEC T67.8 ☑
　stroke T67.0 ☑
　sunburn — *see* Sunburn
　syncope T67.1 ☑
Heavy-for-dates NEC (infant) (4000g to 4499g) P08.1
　exceptionally (4500g or more) P08.0
Hebephrenia, hebephrenic (schizophrenia) F20.1
Heberden's disease or nodes (with arthropathy) M15.1
Hebra's
　pityriasis L26
　prurigo L28.2
Heel — *see* condition
Heerfordt's disease D86.89
Hegglin's anomaly or syndrome D72.0
Heilmeyer-Schoner disease D45
Heine-Medin disease A80.9
Heinz body anemia, congenital D58.2
Heliophobia F40.228
Heller's disease or syndrome F84.3
HELLP syndrome (hemolysis, elevated liver enzymes and low platelet count) O14.2- ☑
Helminthiasis (*see also* Infestation, helminth)
　Ancylostoma B76.0
　intestinal B82.0
　　mixed types (types classifiable to more than one of the titles B65.0-B81.3 and B81.8) B81.4
　　specified type NEC B81.8
　mixed types (intestinal) (types classifiable to more than one of the titles B65.0-B81.3 and B81.8) B81.4
　Necator (americanus) B76.1
　specified type NEC B83.8
Heloma L84
Hemangioblastoma — *see* Neoplasm, connective tissue, uncertain behavior
　malignant — *see* Neoplasm, connective tissue, malignant
Hemangioendothelioma (*see also* Neoplasm, uncertain behavior, by site)
　benign D18.00
　　intra-abdominal D18.03
　　intracranial D18.02
　　skin D18.01
　　specified site NEC D18.09
　bone (diffuse) — *see* Neoplasm, bone, malignant
　epithelioid (*see also* Neoplasm, uncertain behavior, by site)
　　malignant — *see* Neoplasm, malignant, by site
　malignant — *see* Neoplasm, connective tissue, malignant
Hemangiofibroma — *see* Neoplasm, benign, by site
Hemangiolipoma — *see* Lipoma
Hemangioma D18.00
　arteriovenous D18.00
　　intra-abdominal D18.03
　　intracranial D18.02
　　skin D18.01
　　specified site NEC D18.09
　capillary D18.00
　　intra-abdominal D18.03
　　intracranial D18.02
　　skin D18.01
　　specified site NEC D18.09
　cavernous D18.00
　　intra-abdominal D18.03
　　intracranial D18.02
　　skin D18.01
　　specified site NEC D18.09
　epithelioid D18.00
　　intra-abdominal D18.03
　　intracranial D18.02
　　skin D18.01
　　specified site NEC D18.09
　histiocytoid D18.00
　　intra-abdominal D18.03

Hemangioma — *continued*
　histiocytoid — *continued*
　　intracranial D18.02
　　skin D18.01
　　specified site NEC D18.09
　infantile D18.00
　　intra-abdominal D18.03
　　intracranial D18.02
　　skin D18.01
　　specified site NEC D18.09
　intra-abdominal D18.03
　intracranial D18.02
　intramuscular D18.00
　　intra-abdominal D18.03
　　intracranial D18.02
　　skin D18.01
　　specified site NEC D18.09
　juvenile D18.00
　malignant — *see* Neoplasm, connective tissue, malignant
　plexiform D18.00
　　intra-abdominal D18.03
　　intracranial D18.02
　　skin D18.01
　　specified site NEC D18.09
　racemose D18.00
　　intra-abdominal D18.03
　　intracranial D18.02
　　skin D18.01
　　specified site NEC D18.09
　sclerosing — *see* Neoplasm, skin, benign
　simplex D18.00
　　intra-abdominal D18.03
　　intracranial D18.02
　　skin D18.01
　　specified site NEC D18.09
　skin D18.01
　specified site NEC D18.09
　venous D18.00
　　intra-abdominal D18.03
　　intracranial D18.02
　　skin D18.01
　　specified site NEC D18.09
　verrucous keratotic D18.00
　　intra-abdominal D18.03
　　intracranial D18.02
　　skin D18.01
　　specified site NEC D18.09
Hemangiomatosis (systemic) I78.8
　involving single site — *see* Hemangioma
Hemangiopericytoma (*see also* Neoplasm, connective tissue, uncertain behavior)
　benign — *see* Neoplasm, connective tissue, benign
　malignant — *see* Neoplasm, connective tissue, malignant
Hemangiosarcoma — *see* Neoplasm, connective tissue, malignant
Hemarthrosis (nontraumatic) M25.00
　ankle M25.07- ☑
　elbow M25.02- ☑
　foot joint M25.07- ☑
　hand joint M25.04- ☑
　hip M25.05- ☑
　in hemophilic arthropathy — *see* Arthropathy, hemophilic
　knee M25.06- ☑
　shoulder M25.01- ☑
　specified joint NEC M25.08
　traumatic — *see* Sprain, by site
　vertebrae M25.08
　wrist M25.03- ☑
Hematemesis K92.0
　with ulcer — *code by site under* Ulcer, with hemorrhage K27.4
　newborn, neonatal P54.0
　　due to swallowed maternal blood P78.2
Hematidrosis L74.8
Hematinuria (*see also* Hemoglobinuria)
　malarial B50.8
Hematobilia K83.8
Hematocele
　female NEC N94.89
　　with ectopic pregnancy O00.9
　　ovary N83.8
　male N50.1
Hematochezia (*see also* Melena) K92.1
Hematochyluria (*see also* Infestation, filarial)
　schistosomiasis (bilharziasis) B65.0

Hematocolpos (with hematometra or hematosalpinx) N89.7
Hematocornea — *see* Pigmentation, cornea, stromal
Hematogenous — *see* condition
Hematoma (traumatic) (skin surface intact) (*see also* Contusion)
  with
    injury of internal organs — *see* Injury, by site
    open wound — *see* Wound, open
  amputation stump (surgical) (late) T87.89
  aorta, dissecting I71.00
    abdominal I71.02
    thoracic I71.01
    thoracoabdominal I71.03
  aortic intramural — *see* Dissection, aorta
  arterial (complicating trauma) — *see* Injury, blood vessel, by site
  auricle — *see* Contusion, ear
    nontraumatic — *see* Disorder, pinna, hematoma
  birth injury NEC P15.8
  brain (traumatic)
    with
      cerebral laceration or contusion (diffuse) — *see* Injury, intracranial, diffuse
      focal — *see* Injury, intracranial, focal
    cerebellar, traumatic S06.37- ☑
    intracerebral, traumatic — *see* Injury, intracranial, intracerebral hemorrhage
    newborn NEC P52.4
      birth injury P10.1
    nontraumatic — *see* Hemorrhage, intracranial
    subarachnoid, arachnoid, traumatic — *see* Injury, intracranial, subarachnoid hemorrhage
    subdural, traumatic — *see* Injury, intracranial, subdural hemorrhage
  breast (nontraumatic) N64.89
  broad ligament (nontraumatic) N83.7
    traumatic S37.892 ☑
  cerebellar, traumatic S06.37- ☑
  cerebral — *see* Hematoma, brain
  cerebrum S06.36- ☑
    left S06.35- ☑
    right S06.34- ☑
  cesarean delivery wound O90.2
  complicating delivery (perineal) (pelvic) (vagina) (vulva) O71.7
  corpus cavernosum (nontraumatic) N48.89
  epididymis (nontraumatic) N50.1
  epidural (traumatic) — *see* Injury, intracranial, epidural hemorrhage
    spinal — *see* Injury, spinal cord, by region
  episiotomy O90.2
  face, birth injury P15.4
  genital organ NEC (nontraumatic)
    female (nonobstetric) N94.89
      traumatic S30.202 ☑
    male N50.1
      traumatic S30.201 ☑
  internal organs — *see* Injury, by site
  intracerebral, traumatic — *see* Injury, intracranial, intracerebral hemorrhage
  intraoperative — *see* Complications, intraoperative, hemorrhage
  labia (nontraumatic) (nonobstetric) N90.89
  liver (subcapsular) (nontraumatic) K76.89
    birth injury P15.0
  mediastinum — *see* Injury, intrathoracic
  mesosalpinx (nontraumatic) N83.7
    traumatic S37.898 ☑
  muscle — code by site under Contusion
  nontraumatic
    muscle M79.81
    soft tissue M79.81
  obstetrical surgical wound O90.2
  orbit, orbital (nontraumatic) (*see also* Hemorrhage, orbit)
    traumatic — *see* Contusion, orbit
  pelvis (female) (nontraumatic) (nonobstetric) N94.89
    obstetric O71.7
    traumatic — *see* Injury, by site
  penis (nontraumatic) N48.89
    birth injury P15.5
  perianal (nontraumatic) K64.5
  perineal S30.23 ☑
    complicating delivery O71.7
  perirenal — *see* Injury, kidney
  pinna — *see* Contusion, ear

Hematoma — *continued*
  pinna — *see* Contusion, ear — *continued*
    nontraumatic — *see* Disorder, pinna, hematoma
  placenta O43.89- ☑
  postoperative (postprocedural) — *see* Complication, postprocedural, hemorrhage
  retroperitoneal (nontraumatic) K66.1
    traumatic S36.892 ☑
  scrotum, superficial S30.22 ☑
    birth injury P15.5
  seminal vesicle (nontraumatic) N50.1
    traumatic S37.892 ☑
  spermatic cord (traumatic) S37.892 ☑
    nontraumatic N50.1
  spinal (cord) (meninges) (*see also* Injury, spinal cord, by region)
    newborn (birth injury) P11.5
  spleen D73.5
    intraoperative — *see* Complications, intraoperative, hemorrhage, spleen
    postprocedural (postoperative) — *see* Complications, postprocedural, hemorrhage, spleen
  sternocleidomastoid, birth injury P15.2
  sternomastoid, birth injury P15.2
  subarachnoid (traumatic) — *see* Injury, intracranial, subarachnoid hemorrhage
    newborn (nontraumatic) P52.5
      due to birth injury P10.3
    nontraumatic — *see* Hemorrhage, intracranial, subarachnoid
  subdural (traumatic) — *see* Injury, intracranial, subdural hemorrhage
    newborn (localized) P52.8
      birth injury P10.0
    nontraumatic — *see* Hemorrhage, intracranial, subdural
  superficial, newborn P54.5
  testis (nontraumatic) N50.1
    birth injury P15.5
  tunica vaginalis (nontraumatic) N50.1
  umbilical cord, complicating delivery O69.5 ☑
  uterine ligament (broad) (nontraumatic) N83.7
    traumatic S37.892 ☑
  vagina (ruptured) (nontraumatic) N89.8
    complicating delivery O71.7
  vas deferens (nontraumatic) N50.1
    traumatic S37.892 ☑
  vitreous — *see* Hemorrhage, vitreous
  vulva (nontraumatic) (nonobstetric) N90.89
    complicating delivery O71.7
    newborn (birth injury) P15.5
Hematometra N85.7
  with hematocolpos N89.7
Hematomyelia (central) G95.19
  newborn (birth injury) P11.5
  traumatic T14.8
Hematomyelitis G04.90
Hematoperitoneum — *see* Hemoperitoneum
Hematophobia F40.230
Hematopneumothorax (see Hemothorax)
Hematopoiesis, cyclic D70.4
Hematoporphyria — *see* Porphyria
Hematorachis, hematorrhachis G95.19
  newborn (birth injury) P11.5
Hematosalpinx N83.6
  with
    hematocolpos N89.7
    hematometra N85.7
      with hematocolpos N89.7
  infectional — *see* Salpingitis
Hematospermia R36.1
Hematothorax (see Hemothorax)
Hematuria R31.9
  benign (familial) (of childhood) (*see also* Hematuria, idiopathic)
    essential microscopic R31.1
  due to sulphonamide, sulfonamide — *see* Table of Drugs and Chemicals, by drug
  endemic (*see also* Schistosomiasis) B65.0
  gross R31.0
  idiopathic N02.9
    with glomerular lesion
      crescentic (diffuse) glomerulonephritis N02.7
      dense deposit disease N02.6
      endocapillary proliferative glomerulonephritis N02.4

Hematuria — *continued*
  idiopathic — *continued*
    with glomerular lesion — *continued*
      focal and segmental hyalinosis or sclerosis N02.1
      membranoproliferative (diffuse) N02.5
      membranous (diffuse) N02.2
      mesangial proliferative (diffuse) N02.3
      mesangiocapillary (diffuse) N02.5
      minor abnormality N02.0
      proliferative NEC N02.8
      specified pathology NEC N02.8
  intermittent — *see* Hematuria, idiopathic
  malarial B50.8
  microscopic NEC R31.2
    benign essential R31.1
  paroxysmal (*see also* Hematuria, idiopathic)
    nocturnal D59.5
  persistent — *see* Hematuria, idiopathic
  recurrent — *see* Hematuria, idiopathic
  tropical (*see also* Schistosomiasis) B65.0
  tuberculous A18.13
Hemeralopia (day blindness) H53.11
  vitamin A deficiency E50.5
Hemi-akinesia R41.4
Hemi-inattention R41.4
Hemianalgesia R20.0
Hemianencephaly Q00.0
Hemianesthesia R20.0
Hemianopia, hemianopsia (heteronymous) H53.47
  homonymous H53.46- ☑
  syphilitic A52.71
Hemiathetosis R25.8
Hemiatrophy R68.89
  cerebellar G31.9
  face, facial, progressive (Romberg) G51.8
  tongue K14.8
Hemiballism (us) G25.5
Hemicardia Q24.8
Hemicephalus, hemicephaly Q00.0
Hemichorea G25.5
Hemicolitis, left — *see* Colitis, left sided
Hemicrania
  congenital malformation Q00.0
  continua G44.51
  meaning migraine (*see also* Migraine) G43.909
  paroxysmal G44.039
    chronic G44.049
      intractable G44.041
      not intractable G44.049
    episodic G44.039
      intractable G44.031
      not intractable G44.039
    intractable G44.031
    not intractable G44.039
Hemidystrophy — *see* Hemiatrophy
Hemiectromelia Q73.8
Hemihypalgesia R20.8
Hemihypesthesia R20.1
Hemimelia Q73.8
  lower limb — *see* Defect, reduction, lower limb, specified type NEC
  upper limb — *see* Defect, reduction, upper limb, specified type NEC
Hemiparalysis — *see* Hemiplegia
Hemiparesis — *see* Hemiplegia
Hemiparesthesia R20.2
Hemiparkinsonism G20
Hemiplegia G81.9- ☑
  alternans facialis G83.89
  ascending NEC G81.90
    spinal G95.89
  congenital (cerebral) G80.8
    spastic G80.2
  embolic (current episode) I63.4- ☑
  flaccid G81.0- ☑
  following
    cerebrovascular disease I69.959
      cerebral infarction I69.35- ☑
      intracerebral hemorrhage I69.15- ☑
      nontraumatic intracranial hemorrhage NEC I69.25- ☑
      specified disease NEC I69.85- ☑
      stroke NOS I69.35- ☑
      subarachnoid hemorrhage I69.05- ☑
  hysterical F44.4
  newborn NEC P91.8

Hemiplegia — *continued*
  newborn — *continued*
    birth injury P11.9
  spastic G81.1- ☑
    congenital G80.2
  thrombotic (current episode) I63.3 ☑
Hemisection, spinal cord — *see* Injury, spinal cord, by region
Hemispasm (facial) R25.2
Hemisporosis B48.8
Hemitremor R25.1
Hemivertebra Q76.49
  failure of segmentation with scoliosis Q76.3
  fusion with scoliosis Q76.3
Hemochromatosis E83.119
  with refractory anemia D46.1
  due to repeated red blood cell transfusion E83.111
  hereditary (primary) E83.110
  primary E83.110
  specified NEC E83.118
Hemoglobin (*see also* condition)
  abnormal (disease) — *see* Disease, hemoglobin
  AS genotype D57.3
  Constant Spring D58.2
  E-beta thalassemia D56.5
  fetal, hereditary persistence (HPFH) D56.4
  H Constant Spring D56.0
  low NOS D64.9
  S (Hb S), heterozygous D57.3
Hemoglobinemia D59.9
  due to blood transfusion T80.89 ☑
  paroxysmal D59.6
    nocturnal D59.5
Hemoglobinopathy (mixed) D58.2
  with thalassemia D56.8
  sickle-cell D57.1
    with thalassemia D57.40
      with crisis (vasoocclusive pain) D57.419
        with
          acute chest syndrome D57.411
          splenic sequestration D57.412
      without crisis D57.40
Hemoglobinuria R82.3
  with anemia, hemolytic, acquired (chronic) NEC D59.6
  cold (agglutinin) (paroxysmal) (with Raynaud's syndrome) D59.6
  due to exertion or hemolysis NEC D59.6
  intermittent D59.6
  malarial B50.8
  march D59.6
  nocturnal (paroxysmal) D59.5
  paroxysmal (cold) D59.6
    nocturnal D59.5
Hemolymphangioma D18.1
Hemolysis
  intravascular
    with
      abortion — *see* Abortion, by type, complicated by, hemorrhage
      ectopic or molar pregnancy O08.1
      hemorrhage
        antepartum — *see* Hemorrhage, antepartum, with coagulation defect
        intrapartum (*see also* Hemorrhage, complicating, delivery) O67.0
    postpartum O72.3
  neonatal (excessive) P58.9
    specified NEC P58.8
Hemolytic — *see* condition
Hemopericardium I31.2
  following acute myocardial infarction (current complication) I23.0
  newborn P54.8
  traumatic — *see* Injury, heart, with hemopericardium
Hemoperitoneum K66.1
  infectional K65.9
  traumatic S36.899 ☑
    with open wound — *see* Wound, open, with penetration into peritoneal cavity
Hemophilia (classical) (familial) (hereditary) D66
  A D66
  acquired D68.311
  autoimmune D68.311
  B D67
  C D68.1
  calcipriva (*see also* Defect, coagulation) D68.4
  nonfamilial (*see also* Defect, coagulation) D68.4
  secondary D68.311

Hemophilia — *continued*
  vascular D68.0
Hemophthalmos H44.81- ☑
Hemopneumothorax (*see also* Hemothorax)
  traumatic S27.2 ☑
Hemoptysis R04.2
  newborn P26.9
  tuberculous — *see* Tuberculosis, pulmonary
Hemorrhage, hemorrhagic (concealed) R58
  abdomen R58
  accidental antepartum — *see* Hemorrhage, antepartum
  acute idiopathic pulmonary, in infants R04.81
  adenoid J35.8
  adrenal (capsule) (gland) E27.49
    medulla E27.8
    newborn P54.4
  after delivery — *see* Hemorrhage, postpartum
  alveolar
    lung, newborn P26.8
    process K08.8
  alveolus K08.8
  amputation stump (surgical) T87.89
  anemia (chronic) D50.0
    acute D62
  antepartum (with) O46.90
    with coagulation defect O46.00- ☑
      afibrinogenemia O46.01- ☑
      disseminated intravascular coagulation O46.02- ☑
      hypofibrinogenemia O46.01- ☑
      specified defect NEC O46.09- ☑
    before 20 weeks gestation O20.9
      specified type NEC O20.8
      threatened abortion O20.0
    due to
      abruptio placenta (*see also* Abruptio placentae) O45.9- ☑
      leiomyoma, uterus — *see* Hemorrhage, antepartum, specified cause NEC
      placenta previa O44.1- ☑
    specified cause NEC — *see* subcategory O46.8X- ☑
  anus (sphincter) K62.5
  apoplexy (stroke) — *see* Hemorrhage, intracranial, intracerebral
  arachnoid — *see* Hemorrhage, intracranial, subarachnoid
  artery R58
    brain — *see* Hemorrhage, intracranial, intracerebral
  basilar (ganglion) I61.0
  bladder N32.89
  bowel K92.2
    newborn P54.3
  brain (miliary) (nontraumatic) — *see* Hemorrhage, intracranial, intracerebral
    due to
      birth injury P10.1
      syphilis A52.05
    epidural or extradural (traumatic) — *see* Injury, intracranial, epidural hemorrhage
    newborn P52.4
      birth injury P10.1
    subarachnoid — *see* Hemorrhage, intracranial, subarachnoid
    subdural — *see* Hemorrhage, intracranial, subdural
  brainstem (nontraumatic) I61.3
    traumatic S06.38- ☑
  breast N64.59
  bronchial tube — *see* Hemorrhage, lung
  bronchopulmonary — *see* Hemorrhage, lung
  bronchus — *see* Hemorrhage, lung
  bulbar I61.5
  capillary I78.8
    primary D69.8
  cecum K92.2
  cerebellar, cerebellum (nontraumatic) I61.4
    newborn P52.6
    traumatic S06.37- ☑
  cerebral, cerebrum (*see also* Hemorrhage, intracranial, intracerebral)
    lobe I61.1
    newborn (anoxic) P52.4
      birth injury P10.1
  cerebromeningeal I61.8
  cerebrospinal — *see* Hemorrhage, intracranial, intracerebral
  cervix (uteri) (stump) NEC N88.8

Hemorrhage, hemorrhagic — *continued*
  chamber, anterior (eye) — *see* Hyphema
  childbirth — *see* Hemorrhage, complicating, delivery
  choroid H31.30- ☑
    expulsive H31.31- ☑
  ciliary body — *see* Hyphema
  cochlea — *see* subcategory H83.8 ☑
  colon K92.2
  complicating
    abortion — *see* Abortion, by type, complicated by, hemorrhage
    delivery O67.9
      associated with coagulation defect (afibrinogenemia) (DIC) (hyperfibrinolysis) O67.0
      specified cause NEC O67.8
    surgical procedure — *see* Hemorrhage, intraoperative
  conjunctiva H11.3- ☑
    newborn P54.8
  cord, newborn (stump) P51.9
  corpus luteum (ruptured) cyst N83.1
  cortical (brain) I61.1
  cranial — *see* Hemorrhage, intracranial
  cutaneous R23.3
    due to autosensitivity, erythrocyte D69.2
    newborn P54.5
  delayed
    following ectopic or molar pregnancy O08.1
    postpartum O72.2
  diathesis (familial) D69.9
  disease D69.9
    newborn P53
    specified type NEC D69.8
  due to or associated with
    afibrinogenemia or other coagulation defect (conditions in categories D65- D69)
      antepartum — *see* Hemorrhage, antepartum, with coagulation defect
      intrapartum O67.0
  dental implant M27.61
  device, implant or graft (*see also* Complications, by site and type, specified NEC) T85.83 ☑
    arterial graft NEC T82.838 ☑
    breast T85.83 ☑
    catheter NEC T85.83 ☑
      dialysis (renal) T82.838 ☑
        intraperitoneal T85.83 ☑
      infusion NEC T82.838 ☑
        spinal (epidural) (subdural) T85.83 ☑
      urinary (indwelling) T83.83 ☑
    electronic (electrode) (pulse generator) (stimulator)
      bone T84.83 ☑
      cardiac T82.837 ☑
      nervous system (brain) (peripheral nerve) (spinal) T85.83 ☑
      urinary T83.83 ☑
    fixation, internal (orthopedic) NEC T84.83 ☑
    gastrointestinal (bile duct) (esophagus) T85.83 ☑
    genital NEC T83.83 ☑
    heart NEC T82.837 ☑
    joint prosthesis T84.83 ☑
    ocular (corneal graft) (orbital implant) NEC T85.83 ☑
    orthopedic NEC T84.83 ☑
      bone graft T86.838
    specified NEC T85.83 ☑
    urinary NEC T83.83 ☑
    vascular NEC T82.838 ☑
    ventricular intracranial shunt T85.83 ☑
  duodenum, duodenal K92.2
    ulcer — *see* Ulcer, duodenum, with hemorrhage
  dura mater — *see* Hemorrhage, intracranial, subdural
  endotracheal — *see* Hemorrhage, lung
  epicranial subaponeurotic (massive), birth injury P12.2
  epidural (traumatic) (*see also* Injury, intracranial, epidural hemorrhage)
    nontraumatic I62.1
  esophagus K22.8
    varix I85.01
      secondary I85.11
  excessive, following ectopic gestation (subsequent episode) O08.1
  extradural (traumatic) — *see* Injury, intracranial, epidural hemorrhage
    birth injury P10.8

Hemorrhage, hemorrhagic — *continued*
extradural — *see* Injury, intracranial, epidural hemorrhage — *continued*
newborn (anoxic) (nontraumatic) P52.8
nontraumatic I62.1
eye NEC H57.8
fundus — *see* Hemorrhage, retina
lid — *see* Disorder, eyelid, specified type NEC
fallopian tube N83.6
fibrinogenolysis — *see* Fibrinolysis
fibrinolytic (acquired) — *see* Fibrinolysis
from
ear (nontraumatic) — *see* Otorrhagia
tracheostomy stoma J95.01
fundus, eye — *see* Hemorrhage, retina
funis — *see* Hemorrhage, umbilicus, cord
gastric — *see* Hemorrhage, stomach
gastroenteric K92.2
newborn P54.3
gastrointestinal (tract) K92.2
newborn P54.3
genital organ, male N50.1
genitourinary (tract) NOS R31.9
gingiva K06.8
globe (eye) — *see* Hemophthalmos
graafian follicle cyst (ruptured) N83.0
gum K06.8
heart I51.89
hypopharyngeal (throat) R04.1
intermenstrual (regular) N92.3
irregular N92.1
internal (organs) NEC R58
capsule I61.0
ear — *see* subcategory H83.8 ☑
newborn P54.8
intestine K92.2
newborn P54.3
intra-abdominal R58
intra-alveolar (lung), newborn P26.8
intracerebral (nontraumatic) — *see* Hemorrhage, intracranial, intracerebral
intracranial (nontraumatic) I62.9
birth injury P10.9
epidural, nontraumatic I62.1
extradural, nontraumatic I62.1
intracerebral (nontraumatic) (in) I61.9
brain stem I61.3
cerebellum I61.4
hemisphere I61.2
cortical (superficial) I61.1
subcortical (deep) I61.0
intraoperative
during a nervous system procedure G97.31
during other procedure G97.32
intraventricular I61.5
multiple localized I61.6
newborn P52.4
birth injury P10.1
postprocedural
following a nervous system procedure
G97.51
following other procedure G97.52
specified NEC I61.8
superficial I61.1
traumatic (diffuse) — *see* Injury, intracranial,
diffuse
focal — *see* Injury, intracranial, focal
newborn P52.9
specified NEC P52.8
subarachnoid (nontraumatic) (from) I60.9
intracranial (cerebral) artery I60.7
anterior communicating I60.2- ☑
basilar I60.4
carotid siphon and bifurcation I60.0- ☑
communicating I60.7
anterior I60.2- ☑
posterior I60.3- ☑
middle cerebral I60.1- ☑
posterior communicating I60.3- ☑
specified artery NEC I60.6
vertebral I60.5- ☑
newborn P52.5
birth injury P10.3
specified NEC I60.8
traumatic S06.6X- ☑
subdural (nontraumatic) I62.00
acute I62.01
birth injury P10.0

Hemorrhage, hemorrhagic — *continued*
intracranial — *continued*
subdural — *continued*
chronic I62.03
newborn (anoxic) (hypoxic) P52.8
birth injury P10.0
spinal G95.19
subacute I62.02
traumatic — *see* Injury, intracranial, subdural
hemorrhage
traumatic — *see* Injury, intracranial, focal brain injury
intramedullary NEC G95.19
intraocular — *see* Hemophthalmos
intraoperative, intraprocedural — *see* Complication,
hemorrhage (hematoma), intraoperative (intraprocedural), by site
intrapartum — *see* Hemorrhage, complicating, delivery
intrapelvic
female N94.89
male K66.1
intraperitoneal K66.1
intrapontine I61.3
intraprocedural — *see* Complication, hemorrhage
(hematoma), intraoperative (intraprocedural),
by site
intrauterine N85.7
complicating delivery (*see also* Hemorrhage, complicating, delivery) O67.9
postpartum — *see* Hemorrhage, postpartum
intraventricular I61.5
newborn (nontraumatic) (*see also* Newborn, affected by, hemorrhage) P52.3
due to birth injury P10.2
grade
1 P52.0
2 P52.1
3 P52.21
4 P52.22
intravesical N32.89
iris (postinfectional) (postinflammatory) (toxic) — *see*
Hyphema
joint (nontraumatic) — *see* Hemarthrosis
kidney N28.89
knee (joint) (nontraumatic) — *see* Hemarthrosis, knee
labyrinth — *see* subcategory H83.8 ☑
lenticular striate artery I61.0
ligature, vessel — *see* Hemorrhage, postoperative
liver K76.89
lung R04.89
newborn P26.9
massive P26.1
specified NEC P26.8
tuberculous — *see* Tuberculosis, pulmonary
massive umbilical, newborn P51.0
mediastinum — *see* Hemorrhage, lung
medulla I61.3
membrane (brain) I60.8
spinal cord — *see* Hemorrhage, spinal cord
meninges, meningeal (brain) (middle) I60.8
spinal cord — *see* Hemorrhage, spinal cord
mesentery K66.1
metritis — *see* Endometritis
mouth K13.79
mucous membrane NEC R58
newborn P54.8
muscle M62.89
nail (subungual) L60.8
nasal turbinate R04.0
newborn P54.8
navel, newborn P51.9
newborn P54.9
specified NEC P54.8
nipple N64.59
nose R04.0
newborn P54.8
omentum K66.1
optic nerve (sheath) H47.02- ☑
orbit, orbital H05.23- ☑
ovary NEC N83.8
oviduct N83.6
pancreas K86.8
parathyroid (gland) (spontaneous) E21.4
parturition — *see* Hemorrhage, complicating, delivery
penis N48.89
pericardium, pericarditis I31.2
peritoneum, peritoneal K66.1

Hemorrhage, hemorrhagic — *continued*
peritonsillar tissue J35.8
due to infection J36
petechial R23.3
due to autosensitivity, erythrocyte D69.2
pituitary (gland) E23.6
pleura — *see* Hemorrhage, lung
polioencephalitis, superior E51.2
polymyositis — *see* Polymyositis
pons, pontine I61.3
posterior fossa (nontraumatic) I61.8
newborn P52.6
postmenopausal N95.0
postnasal R04.0
postoperative — *see* Complications, postprocedural,
hemorrhage, by site
postpartum NEC (following delivery of placenta) O72.1
delayed or secondary O72.2
retained placenta O72.0
third stage O72.0
pregnancy — *see* Hemorrhage, antepartum
preretinal — *see* Hemorrhage, retina
prostate N42.1
puerperal — *see* Hemorrhage, postpartum
delayed or secondary O72.2
pulmonary R04.89
newborn P26.9
massive P26.1
specified NEC P26.8
tuberculous — *see* Tuberculosis, pulmonary
purpura (primary) D69.3
rectum (sphincter) K62.5
newborn P54.2
recurring, following initial hemorrhage at time of injury
T79.2 ☑
renal N28.89
respiratory passage or tract R04.9
specified NEC R04.89
retina, retinal (vessels) H35.6- ☑
diabetic — *see* Diabetes, retinal, hemorrhage
retroperitoneal R58
scalp R58
scrotum N50.1
secondary (nontraumatic) R58
following initial hemorrhage at time of injury
T79.2 ☑
seminal vesicle N50.1
skin R23.3
newborn P54.5
slipped umbilical ligature P51.8
spermatic cord N50.1
spinal (cord) G95.19
newborn (birth injury) P11.5
spleen D73.5
intraoperative — *see* Complications, intraoperative,
hemorrhage, spleen
postprocedural — *see* Complications, postprocedural, hemorrhage, spleen
stomach K92.2
newborn P54.3
ulcer — *see* Ulcer, stomach, with hemorrhage
subarachnoid (nontraumatic) — *see* Hemorrhage, intracranial, subarachnoid
subconjunctival (*see also* Hemorrhage, conjunctiva)
birth injury P15.3
subcortical (brain) I61.0
subcutaneous R23.3
subdiaphragmatic R58
subdural (acute) (nontraumatic) — *see* Hemorrhage,
intracranial, subdural
subependymal
newborn P52.0
with intraventricular extension P52.1
and intracerebral extension P52.22
subgaleal P12.1
subhyaloid — *see* Hemorrhage, retina
subperiosteal — *see* Disorder, bone, specified type
NEC
subretinal — *see* Hemorrhage, retina
subtentorial — *see* Hemorrhage, intracranial, subdural
subungual L60.8
suprarenal (capsule) (gland) E27.49
newborn P54.4
tentorium (traumatic) NEC — *see* Hemorrhage, brain
newborn (birth injury) P10.4
testis N50.1
third stage (postpartum) O72.0
thorax — *see* Hemorrhage, lung

☑ **Additional Character Required — Refer to the Tabular List for Character Selection**

▽ **Subterms under main terms may continue to next column or page**

Hemorrhage, hemorrhagic — *continued*
  throat R04.1
  thymus (gland) E32.8
  thyroid (cyst) (gland) E07.89
  tongue K14.8
  tonsil J35.8
  trachea — *see* Hemorrhage, lung
  tracheobronchial R04.89
    newborn P26.0
  traumatic — *code to* specific injury
    cerebellar — *see* Hemorrhage, brain
    intracranial — *see* Hemorrhage, brain
    recurring or secondary (following initial hemor-
      rhage at time of injury) T79.2 ☑
  tuberculous NEC (*see also* Tuberculosis, pulmonary)
    A15.0
  tunica vaginalis N50.1
  ulcer — *code by* site under Ulcer, with hemorrhage
    K27.4
  umbilicus, umbilical
    cord
      after birth, newborn P51.9
      complicating delivery O69.5 ☑
    newborn P51.9
      massive P51.0
      slipped ligature P51.8
    stump P51.9
  urethra (idiopathic) N36.8
  uterus, uterine (abnormal) N93.9
    climacteric N92.4
    complicating delivery — *see* Hemorrhage, compli-
      cating, delivery
    dysfunctional or functional N93.8
    intermenstrual (regular) N92.3
      irregular N92.1
    postmenopausal N95.0
    postpartum — *see* Hemorrhage, postpartum
    preclimacteric or premenopausal N92.4
    prepubertal N93.8
    pubertal N92.2
  vagina (abnormal) N93.9
    newborn P54.6
  vas deferens N50.1
  vasa previa O69.4 ☑
  ventricular I61.5
  vesical N32.89
  viscera NEC R58
    newborn P54.8
  vitreous (humor) (intraocular) H43.1- ☑
  vulva N90.89
Hemorrhoids (bleeding) (without mention of degree)
    K64.9
  1st degree (grade/stage I) (without prolapse outside
    of anal canal) K64.0
  2nd degree (grade/stage II) (that prolapse with
    straining but retract spontaneously) K64.1
  3rd degree (grade/stage III) (that prolapse with
    straining and require manual replacement back
    inside anal canal) K64.2
  4th degree (grade/stage IV) (with prolapsed tissue that
    cannot be manually replaced) K64.3
  complicating
    pregnancy O22.4 ☑
    puerperium O87.2
  external K64.4
    with
      thrombosis K64.5
  internal (without mention of degree) K64.8
  prolapsed K64.8
  skin tags
    anus K64.4
    residual K64.4
  specified NEC K64.8
  strangulated (*see also* Hemorrhoids, by degree) K64.8
  thrombosed (*see also* Hemorrhoids, by degree) K64.5
  ulcerated (*see also* Hemorrhoids, by degree) K64.8
Hemosalpinx N83.6
  with
    hematocolpos N89.7
    hematometra N85.7
      with hematocolpos N89.7
Hemosiderosis (dietary) E83.19
  pulmonary, idiopathic E83.1- ☑ [J84.03]
  transfusion T80.89 ☑
Hemothorax (bacterial) (nontuberculous) J94.2
  newborn P54.8
  traumatic S27.1 ☑
    with pneumothorax S27.2 ☑

Hemothorax — *continued*
  tuberculous NEC A15.6
Henoch (-Schönlein) **disease or syndrome** (purpura)
    D69.0
Henpue, henpuye A66.6
Hepar lobatum (syphilitic) A52.74
Hepatalgia K76.89
Hepatitis K75.9
  acute B17.9
    with coma K72.01
    with hepatic failure — *see* Failure, hepatic
    alcoholic — *see* Hepatitis, alcoholic
    infectious B15.9
      with hepatic coma B15.0
    viral B17.9
  alcoholic (acute) (chronic) K70.10
    with ascites K70.11
  amebic — *see* Abscess, liver, amebic
  anicteric, (viral) — *see* Hepatitis, viral
  antigen-associated (HAA) — *see* Hepatitis, B
  Australia-antigen (positive) — *see* Hepatitis, B
  autoimmune K75.4
  B B19.10
    with hepatic coma B19.11
    acute B16.9
      with
        delta-agent (coinfection) (without hepatic
          coma) B16.1
          with hepatic coma B16.0
        hepatic coma (without delta-agent coinfec-
          tion) B16.2
    chronic B18.1
      with delta-agent B18.0
  bacterial NEC K75.89
  C (viral) B19.20
    with hepatic coma B19.21
    acute B17.10
      with hepatic coma B17.11
    chronic B18.2
  catarrhal (acute) B15.9
    with hepatic coma B15.0
  cholangiolitic K75.89
  cholestatic K75.89
  chronic K73.9
    active NEC K73.2
    lobular NEC K73.1
    persistent NEC K73.0
    specified NEC K73.8
  cytomegaloviral B25.1
  due to ethanol (acute) (chronic) — *see* Hepatitis, alco-
    holic
  epidemic B15.9
    with hepatic coma B15.0
  fulminant NEC (viral) — *see* Hepatitis, viral
  granulomatous NEC K75.3
  herpesviral B00.81
  history of
    B Z86.19
    C Z86.19
  homologous serum — *see* Hepatitis, viral, type B
  in (due to)
    mumps B26.81
    toxoplasmosis (acquired) B58.1
      congenital (active) P37.1 [K77]
  infectious, infective (acute) (chronic) (subacute) B15.9
    with hepatic coma B15.0
  inoculation — *see* Hepatitis, viral, type B
  interstitial (chronic) K74.69
  lupoid NEC K75.4
  malignant NEC (with hepatic failure) K72.90
    with coma K72.91
  neonatal (idiopathic) (toxic) P59.29
  neonatal giant cell P59.29
  newborn P59.29
  post-transfusion — *see* Hepatitis, viral, type B
  postimmunization — *see* Hepatitis, viral, type B
  reactive, nonspecific K75.2
  serum — *see* Hepatitis, viral, type B
  specified type NEC
    with hepatic failure — *see* Failure, hepatic
  syphilitic (late) A52.74
    congenital (early) A50.08 [K77]
      late A50.59 [K77]
    secondary A51.45
  toxic (*see also* Disease, liver, toxic) K71.6
  tuberculous A18.83
  viral, virus B19.9
    with hepatic coma B19.0

Hepatitis — *continued*
  viral, virus — *continued*
    acute B17.9
    chronic B18.9
      specified NEC B18.8
      type
        B B18.1
          with delta-agent B18.0
        C B18.2
    congenital P35.3
    coxsackie B33.8 [K77]
    cytomegalic inclusion B25.1
    in remission, any type — *code to* Hepatitis, chronic,
      by type
    non-A, non-B B17.8
    specified type NEC (with or without coma) B17.8
      type
        A B15.9
          with hepatic coma B15.0
        B B19.10
          with hepatic coma B19.11
          acute B16.9
            with
              delta-agent (coinfection) (without
                hepatic coma) B16.1
                with hepatic coma B16.0
              hepatic coma (without delta-agent
                coinfection) B16.2
          chronic B18.1
            with delta-agent B18.0
        C B19.20
          with hepatic coma B19.21
          acute B17.10
            with hepatic coma B17.11
          chronic B18.2
        E B17.2
    non-A, non-B B17.8
Hepatization lung (acute) — *see* Pneumonia, lobar
Hepatoblastoma C22.2
Hepatocarcinoma C22.0
Hepatocholangiocarcinoma C22.0
Hepatocholangioma, benign D13.4
Hepatocholangitis K75.89
Hepatolenticular degeneration E83.01
Hepatoma (malignant) C22.0
  benign D13.4
  embryonal C22.0
Hepatomegaly (*see also* Hypertrophy, liver)
  with splenomegaly R16.2
  congenital Q44.7
  in mononucleosis
    gammaherpesviral B27.09
    infectious specified NEC B27.89
Hepatoptosis K76.89
Hepatorenal syndrome following labor and delivery
    O90.4
Hepatosis K76.89
Hepatosplenomegaly R16.2
  hyperlipemic (Bürger-Grütz type) E78.3 [K77]
Hereditary — *see* condition
Heredodegeneration, macular — *see* Dystrophy, retina
Heredopathia atactica polyneuritiformis G60.1
Heredosyphilis — *see* Syphilis, congenital
Herlitz' syndrome Q81.1
Hermansky-Pudlak syndrome E70.331
Hermaphrodite, hermaphroditism (true) Q56.0
  46,XX with streak gonads Q99.1
  46,XX/46,XY Q99.0
  46,XY with streak gonads Q99.1
  chimera 46,XX/46,XY Q99.0
Hernia, hernial (acquired) (recurrent) K46.9
  with
    gangrene — *see* Hernia, by site, with, gangrene
    incarceration — *see* Hernia, by site, with, obstruc-
      tion
    irreducible — *see* Hernia, by site, with, obstruction
    obstruction — *see* Hernia, by site, with, obstruction
    strangulation — *see* Hernia, by site, with, obstruc-
      tion
  abdomen, abdominal K46.9
    with
      gangrene (and obstruction) K46.1
      obstruction K46.0
    femoral — *see* Hernia, femoral
    incisional — *see* Hernia, incisional
    inguinal — *see* Hernia, inguinal
    specified site NEC K45.8

Hernia, hernial — *continued*
  abdomen, abdominal — *continued*
    specified site — *continued*
      with
        gangrene (and obstruction) K45.1
        obstruction K45.0
      umbilical — *see* Hernia, umbilical
      wall — *see* Hernia, ventral
  appendix — *see* Hernia, abdomen
  bladder (mucosa) (sphincter)
    congenital (female) (male) Q79.51
    female — *see* Cystocele
    male N32.89
  brain, congenital — *see* Encephalocele
  cartilage, vertebra — *see* Displacement, intervertebral disc
  cerebral, congenital (*see also* Encephalocele)
    endaural Q01.8
  ciliary body (traumatic) S05.2- ☑
  colon — *see* Hernia, abdomen
  Cooper's — *see* Hernia, abdomen, specified site NEC
  crural — *see* Hernia, femoral
  diaphragm, diaphragmatic K44.9
    with
      gangrene (and obstruction) K44.1
      obstruction K44.0
    congenital Q79.0
  direct (inguinal) — *see* Hernia, inguinal
  diverticulum, intestine — *see* Hernia, abdomen
  double (inguinal) — *see* Hernia, inguinal, bilateral
  due to adhesions (with obstruction) K56.5
  epigastric (*see also* Hernia, ventral) K43.9
  esophageal hiatus — *see* Hernia, hiatal
  external (inguinal) — *see* Hernia, inguinal
  fallopian tube N83.4
  fascia M62.89
  femoral K41.90
    with
      gangrene (and obstruction) K41.40
        not specified as recurrent K41.40
        recurrent K41.41
      obstruction K41.30
        not specified as recurrent K41.30
        recurrent K41.31
    bilateral K41.20
      with
        gangrene (and obstruction) K41.10
          not specified as recurrent K41.10
          recurrent K41.11
        obstruction K41.00
          not specified as recurrent K41.00
          recurrent K41.01
      not specified as recurrent K41.20
      recurrent K41.21
    not specified as recurrent K41.90
    recurrent K41.91
    unilateral K41.90
      with
        gangrene (and obstruction) K41.40
          not specified as recurrent K41.40
          recurrent K41.41
        obstruction K41.30
          not specified as recurrent K41.30
          recurrent K41.31
      not specified as recurrent K41.90
      recurrent K41.91
  foramen magnum G93.5
    congenital Q01.8
  funicular (umbilical) (*see also* Hernia, umbilicus)
    spermatic (cord) — *see* Hernia, inguinal
  gastrointestinal tract — *see* Hernia, abdomen
  Hesselbach's — *see* Hernia, femoral, specified site NEC
  hiatal (esophageal) (sliding) K44.9
    with
      gangrene (and obstruction) K44.1
      obstruction K44.0
    congenital Q40.1
  hypogastric — *see* Hernia, ventral
  incarcerated (*see also* Hernia, by site, with obstruction)
    with gangrene — *see* Hernia, by site, with gangrene
  incisional K43.2
    with
      gangrene (and obstruction) K43.1
      obstruction K43.0
  indirect (inguinal) — *see* Hernia, inguinal
  inguinal (direct) (external) (funicular) (indirect) (internal) (oblique) (scrotal) (sliding) K40.90

Hernia, hernial — *continued*
  inguinal — *continued*
    with
      gangrene (and obstruction) K40.40
        not specified as recurrent K40.40
        recurrent K40.41
      obstruction K40.30
        not specified as recurrent K40.30
        recurrent K40.31
    bilateral K40.20
      with
        gangrene (and obstruction) K40.10
          not specified as recurrent K40.10
          recurrent K40.11
        obstruction K40.00
          not specified as recurrent K40.00
          recurrent K40.01
      not specified as recurrent K40.20
      recurrent K40.21
    not specified as recurrent K40.90
    recurrent K40.91
    unilateral K40.90
      with
        gangrene (and obstruction) K40.40
          not specified as recurrent K40.40
          recurrent K40.41
        obstruction K40.30
          not specified as recurrent K40.30
          recurrent K40.31
      not specified as recurrent K40.90
      recurrent K40.91
  internal (*see also* Hernia, abdomen)
    inguinal — *see* Hernia, inguinal
  interstitial — *see* Hernia, abdomen
  intervertebral cartilage or disc — *see* Displacement, intervertebral disc
  intestine, intestinal — *see* Hernia, by site
  intra-abdominal — *see* Hernia, abdomen
  iris (traumatic) S05.2- ☑
  irreducible (*see also* Hernia, by site, with obstruction)
    with gangrene — *see* Hernia, by site, with gangrene
  ischiatic — *see* Hernia, abdomen, specified site NEC
  ischiorectal — *see* Hernia, abdomen, specified site NEC
  lens (traumatic) S05.2- ☑
  linea (alba) (semilunaris) — *see* Hernia, ventral
  Littre's — *see* Hernia, abdomen
  lumbar — *see* Hernia, abdomen, specified site NEC
  lung (subcutaneous) J98.4
  mediastinum J98.5
  mesenteric (internal) — *see* Hernia, abdomen
  midline — *see* Hernia, ventral
  muscle (sheath) M62.89
  nucleus pulposus — *see* Displacement, intervertebral disc
  oblique (inguinal) — *see* Hernia, inguinal
  obstructive (*see also* Hernia, by site, with obstruction)
    with gangrene — *see* Hernia, by site, with gangrene
  obturator — *see* Hernia, abdomen, specified site NEC
  omental — *see* Hernia, abdomen
  ovary N83.4
  oviduct N83.4
  paraesophageal (*see also* Hernia, diaphragm)
    congenital Q40.1
  parastomal K43.5
    with
      gangrene (and obstruction) K43.4
      obstruction K43.3
  paraumbilical — *see* Hernia, umbilicus
  perineal — *see* Hernia, abdomen, specified site NEC
  Petit's — *see* Hernia, abdomen, specified site NEC
  postoperative — *see* Hernia, incisional
  pregnant uterus — *see* Abnormal, uterus in pregnancy or childbirth
  prevesical N32.89
  properitoneal — *see* Hernia, abdomen, specified site NEC
  pudendal — *see* Hernia, abdomen, specified site NEC
  rectovaginal N81.6
  retroperitoneal — *see* Hernia, abdomen, specified site NEC
  Richter's — *see* Hernia, abdomen, with obstruction
  Rieux's, Riex's — *see* Hernia, abdomen, specified site NEC

Hernia, hernial — *continued*
  sac condition (adhesion) (dropsy) (inflammation) (laceration) (suppuration) — *code by site under* Hernia
  sciatic — *see* Hernia, abdomen, specified site NEC
  scrotum, scrotal — *see* Hernia, inguinal
  sliding (inguinal) (*see also* Hernia, inguinal)
    hiatus — *see* Hernia, hiatal
  spigelian — *see* Hernia, ventral
  spinal — *see* Spina bifida
  strangulated (*see also* Hernia, by site, with obstruction)
    with gangrene — *see* Hernia, by site, with gangrene
  subxiphoid — *see* Hernia, ventral
  supra-umbilicus — *see* Hernia, ventral
  tendon — *see* Disorder, tendon, specified type NEC
  Treitz's (fossa) — *see* Hernia, abdomen, specified site NEC
  tunica vaginalis Q55.29
  umbilicus, umbilical K42.9
    with
      gangrene (and obstruction) K42.1
      obstruction K42.0
  ureter N28.89
  urethra, congenital Q64.79
  urinary meatus, congenital Q64.79
  uterus N81.4
    pregnant — *see* Abnormal, uterus in pregnancy or childbirth
  vaginal (anterior) (wall) — *see* Cystocele
  Velpeau's — *see* Hernia, femoral
  ventral K43.9
    with
      gangrene (and obstruction) K43.7
      obstruction K43.6
    incisional K43.2
      with
        gangrene (and obstruction) K43.1
        obstruction K43.0
    recurrent — *see* Hernia, incisional
    specified NEC K43.9
      with
        gangrene (and obstruction) K43.7
        obstruction K43.6
  vesical
    congenital (female) (male) Q79.51
    female — *see* Cystocele
    male N32.89
  vitreous (into wound) S05.2- ☑
    into anterior chamber — *see* Prolapse, vitreous
Herniation (*see also* Hernia)
  brain (stem) G93.5
  cerebral G93.5
  mediastinum J98.5
  nucleus pulposus — *see* Displacement, intervertebral disc
Herpangina B08.5
Herpes, herpesvirus, herpetic B00.9
  anogenital A60.9
    perianal skin A60.1
    rectum A60.1
    urogenital tract A60.00
      cervix A60.03
      male genital organ NEC A60.02
      penis A60.01
      specified site NEC A60.09
      vagina A60.04
      vulva A60.04
  blepharitis (zoster) B02.39
    simplex B00.59
  circinatus B35.4
    bullosus L12.0
  conjunctivitis (simplex) B00.53
    zoster B02.31
  cornea B02.33
  encephalitis B00.4
    due to herpesvirus 6 B10.01
    due to herpesvirus 7 B10.09
    specified NEC B10.09
  eye (zoster) B02.30
    simplex B00.50
  eyelid (zoster) B02.39
    simplex B00.59
  facialis B00.1
  febrilis B00.1
  geniculate ganglionitis B02.21
  genital, genitalis A60.00
    female A60.09

Herpes, herpesvirus, herpetic — continued
genital, genitalis — continued
male A60.02
gestational, gestationis O26.4- ☑
gingivostomatitis B00.2
human B00.9
1 — see Herpes, simplex
2 — see Herpes, simplex
3 — see Varicella
4 — see Mononucleosis, Epstein-Barr (virus)
5 — see Disease, cytomegalic inclusion (generalized)
6
encephalitis B10.01
specified NEC B10.81
7
encephalitis B10.09
specified NEC B10.82
8 B10.89
infection NEC B10.89
Kaposi's sarcoma associated B10.89
iridocyclitis (simplex) B00.51
zoster B02.32
iris (vesicular erythema multiforme) L51.9
iritis (simplex) B00.51
Kaposi's sarcoma associated B10.89
keratitis (simplex) (dendritic) (disciform) (interstitial) B00.52
zoster (interstitial) B02.33
keratoconjunctivitis (simplex) B00.52
zoster B02.33
labialis B00.1
lip B00.1
meningitis (simplex) B00.3
zoster B02.1
ophthalmicus (zoster) NEC B02.30
simplex B00.50
penis A60.01
perianal skin A60.1
pharyngitis, pharyngotonsillitis B00.2
rectum A60.1
scrotum A60.02
sepsis B00.7
simplex B00.9
complicated NEC B00.89
congenital P35.2
conjunctivitis B00.53
external ear B00.1
eyelid B00.59
hepatitis B00.81
keratitis (interstitial) B00.52
myleitis B00.82
specified complication NEC B00.89
visceral B00.89
stomatitis B00.2
tonsurans B35.0
visceral B00.89
vulva A60.04
whitlow B00.89
zoster (see also condition) B02.9
auricularis B02.21
complicated NEC B02.8
conjunctivitis B02.31
disseminated B02.7
encephalitis B02.0
eye (lid) B02.39
geniculate ganglionitis B02.21
keratitis (interstitial) B02.33
meningitis B02.1
myelitis B02.24
neuritis, neuralgia B02.29
ophthalmicus NEC B02.30
oticus B02.21
polyneuropathy B02.23
specified complication NEC B02.8
trigeminal neuralgia B02.22
Herpesvirus (human) — see Herpes
Herpetophobia F40.218
Herrick's anemia — see Disease, sickle-cell
Hers' disease E74.09
Herter-Gee syndrome K90.0
Herxheimer's reaction R68.89
Hesitancy
of micturition R39.11
urinary R39.11
Hesselbach's hernia — see Hernia, femoral, specified site NEC
Heterochromia (congenital) Q13.2

Heterochromia — continued
cataract — see Cataract, complicated
cyclitis (Fuchs) — see Cyclitis, Fuchs' heterochromic
hair L67.1
iritis — see Cyclitis, Fuchs' heterochromic
retained metallic foreign body (nonmagnetic) — see Foreign body, intraocular, old, retained
magnetic — see Foreign body, intraocular, old, retained, magnetic
uveitis — see Cyclitis, Fuchs' heterochromic
Heterophoria — see Strabismus, heterophoria
Heterophyes, heterophyiasis (small intestine) B66.8
Heterotopia, heterotopic (see also Malposition, congenital)
cerebralis Q04.8
Heterotropia — see Strabismus
Heubner-Herter disease K90.0
Hexadactylism Q69.9
HGSIL (cytology finding) (high grade squamous intraepithelial lesion on cytologic smear) (Pap smear finding)
anus R85.613
cervix R87.613
biopsy (histology) finding — code to CIN II or CIN III
vagina R87.623
biopsy (histology) finding — code to VAIN II or VAIN III
Hibernoma — see Lipoma
Hiccup, hiccough R06.6
epidemic B33.0
psychogenic F45.8
Hidden penis (congenital) Q55.64
acquired N48.83
Hidradenitis (axillaris) (suppurative) L73.2
Hidradenoma (nodular) (see also Neoplasm, skin, benign)
clear cell — see Neoplasm, skin, benign
papillary — see Neoplasm, skin, benign
Hidrocystoma — see Neoplasm, skin, benign
High
altitude effects T70.20 ☑
anoxia T70.29 ☑
on
ears T70.0 ☑
sinuses T70.1 ☑
polycythemia D75.1
arch
foot Q66.7
palate, congenital Q38.5
arterial tension — see Hypertension
basal metabolic rate R94.8
blood pressure (see also Hypertension)
borderline R03.0
reading (incidental) (isolated) (nonspecific), without diagnosis of hypertension R03.0
cholesterol E78.0
with high triglycerides E78.2
diaphragm (congenital) Q79.1
expressed emotional level within family Z63.8
head at term O32.4 ☑
palate, congenital Q38.5
risk
infant NEC Z76.2
sexual behavior (heterosexual) Z72.51
bisexual Z72.53
homosexual Z72.52
temperature (of unknown origin) R50.9
thoracic rib Q76.6
triglycerides E78.1
with high cholesterol E78.2
Hildenbrand's disease A75.0
Hilum — see condition
Hip — see condition
Hippel's disease Q85.8
Hippophobia F40.218
Hippus H57.09
Hirschsprung's disease or megacolon Q43.1
Hirsutism, hirsuties L68.0
Hirudiniasis
external B88.3
internal B83.4
His-Werner disease A79.0
Hiss-Russell dysentery A03.1
Histidinemia, histidinuria E70.41
Histiocytoma (see also Neoplasm, skin, benign)
fibrous (see also Neoplasm, skin, benign)

Histiocytoma — continued
fibrous (see also Neoplasm, skin, benign) — continued
atypical — see Neoplasm, connective tissue, uncertain behavior
malignant — see Neoplasm, connective tissue, malignant
Histiocytosis D76.3
acute differentiated progressive C96.0
Langerhans' cell NEC C96.6
multifocal X
multisystemic (disseminated) C96.0
unisystemic C96.5
pulmonary, adult (adult PLCH) J84.82
unifocal (X) C96.6
lipid, lipoid D76.3
essential E75.29
malignant C96.A (following C96.6)
mononuclear phagocytes NEC D76.1
Langerhans' cells C96.6
non-Langerhans cell D76.3
polyostotic sclerosing D76.3
sinus, with massive lymphadenopathy D76.3
syndrome NEC D76.3
X NEC C96.6
acute (progressive) C96.0
chronic C96.6
multifocal C96.5
multisystemic C96.0
unifocal C96.6
Histoplasmosis B39.9
with pneumonia NEC B39.2
African B39.5
American — see Histoplasmosis, capsulati
capsulati B39.4
disseminated B39.3
generalized B39.3
pulmonary B39.2
acute B39.0
chronic B39.1
Darling's B39.4
duboisii B39.5
lung NEC B39.2
History
family (of) (see also History, personal (of))
alcohol abuse Z81.1
allergy NEC Z84.89
anemia Z83.2
arthritis Z82.61
asthma Z82.5
blindness Z82.1
cardiac death (sudden) Z82.41
carrier of genetic disease Z84.81
chromosomal anomaly Z82.79
chronic
disabling disease NEC Z82.8
lower respiratory disease Z82.5
colonic polyps Z83.71
congenital malformations and deformations Z82.79
polycystic kidney Z82.71
consanguinity Z84.3
deafness Z82.2
diabetes mellitus Z83.3
disability NEC Z82.8
disease or disorder (of)
allergic NEC Z84.89
behavioral NEC Z81.8
blood and blood-forming organs Z83.2
cardiovascular NEC Z82.49
chronic disabling NEC Z82.8
digestive Z83.79
ear NEC Z83.52
endocrine NEC Z83.49
eye NEC Z83.518
glaucoma Z83.511
genitourinary NEC Z84.2
glaucoma Z83.511
hematological Z83.2
immune mechanism Z83.2
infectious NEC Z83.1
ischemic heart Z82.49
kidney Z84.1
mental NEC Z81.8
metabolic Z83.49
musculoskeletal NEC Z82.69
neurological NEC Z82.0
nutritional Z83.49
parasitic NEC Z83.1

History — *continued*
- family (*see also* History, personal) — *continued*
  - disease or disorder — *continued*
    - psychiatric NEC Z81.8
    - respiratory NEC Z83.6
    - skin and subcutaneous tissue NEC Z84.0
    - specified NEC Z84.89
  - drug abuse NEC Z81.3
  - epilepsy Z82.0
  - genetic disease carrier Z84.81
  - glaucoma Z83.511
  - hearing loss Z82.2
  - human immunodeficiency virus (HIV) infection Z83.0
  - Huntington's chorea Z82.0
  - intellectual disability Z81.0
  - leukemia Z80.6
  - malignant neoplasm (of) NOS Z80.9
    - bladder Z80.52
    - breast Z80.3
    - bronchus Z80.1
    - digestive organ Z80.0
    - gastrointestinal tract Z80.0
    - genital organ Z80.49
      - ovary Z80.41
      - prostate Z80.42
      - specified organ NEC Z80.49
      - testis Z80.43
    - hematopoietic NEC Z80.7
    - intrathoracic organ NEC Z80.2
    - kidney Z80.51
    - lung Z80.1
    - lymphatic NEC Z80.7
    - ovary Z80.41
    - prostate Z80.42
    - respiratory organ NEC Z80.2
    - specified site NEC Z80.8
    - testis Z80.43
    - trachea Z80.1
    - urinary organ or tract Z80.59
      - bladder Z80.52
      - kidney Z80.51
  - mental
    - disorder NEC Z81.8
  - multiple endocrine neoplasia (MEN) syndrome Z83.41
  - osteoporosis Z82.62
  - polycystic kidney Z82.71
  - polyps (colon) Z83.71
  - psychiatric disorder Z81.8
  - psychoactive substance abuse NEC Z81.3
  - respiratory condition NEC Z83.6
    - asthma and other lower respiratory conditions Z82.5
  - self-harmful behavior Z81.8
  - skin condition Z84.0
  - specified condition NEC Z84.89
  - stroke (cerebrovascular) Z82.3
  - substance abuse NEC Z81.4
    - alcohol Z81.1
    - drug NEC Z81.3
    - psychoactive NEC Z81.3
    - tobacco Z81.2
  - sudden cardiac death Z82.41
  - tobacco abuse Z81.2
  - violence, violent behavior Z81.8
  - visual loss Z82.1
- personal (of) (*see also* History, family (of))
  - abuse
    - adult Z91.419
      - physical and sexual Z91.410
      - psychological Z91.411
    - childhood Z62.819
      - physical Z62.810
      - psychological Z62.811
      - sexual Z62.810
  - alcohol dependence F10.21
  - allergy (to) Z88.9
    - analgesic agent NEC Z88.6
    - anesthetic Z88.4
    - anti-infective agent NEC Z88.3
    - antibiotic agent NEC Z88.1
    - contrast media Z91.041
    - drugs, medicaments and biological substances Z88.9
      - specified NEC Z88.8
    - food Z91.018
      - additives Z91.02

History — *continued*
- personal (*see also* History, family) — *continued*
  - allergy — *continued*
    - food — *continued*
      - eggs Z91.012
      - milk products Z91.011
      - peanuts Z91.010
      - seafood Z91.013
      - specified food NEC Z91.018
    - insect Z91.038
      - bee Z91.030
    - latex Z91.040
    - medicinal agents Z88.9
      - specified NEC Z88.8
    - narcotic agent NEC Z88.5
    - nonmedicinal agents Z91.048
    - penicillin Z88.0
    - serum Z88.7
    - specified NEC Z91.09
    - sulfonamides Z88.2
    - vaccine Z88.7
  - anaphylactic shock Z87.892
  - anaphylaxis Z87.892
  - behavioral disorders Z86.59
  - benign carcinoid tumor Z86.012
  - benign neoplasm Z86.018
    - brain Z86.011
    - carcinoid Z86.012
    - colonic polyps Z86.010
  - brain injury (traumatic) Z87.820
  - breast implant removal Z98.86
  - calculi, renal Z87.442
  - cancer — *see* History, personal (of), malignant neoplasm (of)
  - cardiac arrest (death), successfully resuscitated Z86.74
  - cerebral infarction without residual deficit Z86.73
  - cervical dysplasia Z87.410
  - chemotherapy for neoplastic condition Z92.21
  - childhood abuse — *see* History, personal (of), abuse
  - cleft lip (corrected) Z87.730
  - cleft palate (corrected) Z87.730
  - collapsed vertebra (healed) Z87.311
    - due to osteoporosis Z87.310
  - combat and operational stress reaction Z86.51
  - congenital malformation (corrected) Z87.798
    - circulatory system (corrected) Z87.74
    - digestive system (corrected) NEC Z87.738
    - ear (corrected) Z87.720
    - eye (corrected) Z87.721
    - face and neck (corrected) Z87.790
    - genitourinary system (corrected) NEC Z87.718
    - heart (corrected) Z87.74
    - integument (corrected) Z87.76
    - limb(s) (corrected) Z87.76
    - musculoskeletal system (corrected) Z87.76
    - neck (corrected) Z87.790
    - nervous system (corrected) NEC Z87.728
    - respiratory system (corrected) Z87.75
    - sense organs (corrected) NEC Z87.728
    - specified NEC Z87.798
  - contraception Z92.0
  - deployment (military) Z91.82
  - diabetic foot ulcer Z86.31
  - disease or disorder (of) Z87.898
    - anaphylaxis Z87.892
    - blood and blood-forming organs Z86.2
    - circulatory system Z86.79
      - specified condition NEC Z86.79
    - connective tissue Z87.39
    - digestive system Z87.19
      - colonic polyp Z86.010
      - peptic ulcer disease Z87.11
      - specified condition NEC Z87.19
    - ear Z86.69
    - endocrine Z86.39
      - diabetic foot ulcer Z86.31
      - gestational diabetes Z86.32
      - specified type NEC Z86.39
    - eye Z86.69
    - genital (track) system NEC
      - female Z87.42
      - male Z87.438
    - hematological Z86.2
    - Hodgkin Z85.71
    - immune mechanism Z86.2
    - infectious Z86.19

History — *continued*
- personal (*see also* History, family) — *continued*
  - disease or disorder — *continued*
    - infectious — *continued*
      - malaria Z86.13
      - Methicillin resistant Staphylococcus aureus (MRSA) Z86.14
      - poliomyelitis Z86.12
      - specified NEC Z86.19
      - tuberculosis Z86.11
    - mental NEC Z86.59
    - metabolic Z86.39
      - diabetic foot ulcer Z86.31
      - gestational diabetes Z86.32
      - specified type NEC Z86.39
    - musculoskeletal NEC Z87.39
    - nervous system Z86.69
    - nutritional Z86.39
    - parasitic Z86.19
    - respiratory system NEC Z87.09
    - sense organs Z86.69
    - skin Z87.2
    - specified site or type NEC Z87.898
    - subcutaneous tissue Z87.2
    - trophoblastic Z87.59
    - urinary system NEC Z87.448
  - drug dependence — *see* Dependence, drug, by type, in remission
  - drug therapy
    - antineoplastic chemotherapy Z92.21
    - estrogen Z92.23
    - immunosupression Z92.25
    - inhaled steroids Z92.240
    - monoclonal drug Z92.22
    - specified NEC Z92.29
    - steroid Z92.241
    - systemic steroids Z92.241
  - dysplasia
    - cervical Z87.410
    - prostatic Z87.430
    - vaginal Z87.411
    - vulvar Z87.412
  - embolism (venous) Z86.718
    - pulmonary Z86.711
  - encephalitis Z86.61
  - estrogen therapy Z92.23
  - extracorporeal membrane oxygenation (ECMO) Z92.81
  - failed conscious sedation Z92.83
  - failed moderate sedation Z92.83
  - fall, falling Z91.81
  - fracture (healed)
    - fatigue Z87.312
    - fragility Z87.310
    - osteoporosis Z87.310
    - pathological NEC Z87.311
    - stress Z87.312
    - traumatic Z87.81
  - gestational diabetes Z86.32
  - hepatitis
    - B Z86.19
    - C Z86.19
  - Hodgkin disease Z85.71
  - hyperthermia, malignant Z88.4
  - hypospadias (corrected) Z87.710
  - hysterectomy Z90.710
  - immunosupression therapy Z92.25
  - in situ neoplasm
    - breast Z86.000
    - cervix uteri Z86.001
    - specified NEC Z86.008
  - in utero procedure during pregnancy Z98.870
  - in utero procedure while a fetus Z98.871
  - infection NEC Z86.19
    - central nervous system Z86.61
    - Methicillin resistant Staphylococcus aureus (MRSA) Z86.14
    - urinary (recurrent) (tract) Z87.440
  - injury NEC Z87.828
  - irradiation Z92.3
  - kidney stones Z87.442
  - leukemia Z85.6
  - lymphoma (non-Hodgkin) Z85.72
  - malignant melanoma (skin) Z85.820
  - malignant neoplasm (of) Z85.9
    - accessory sinuses Z85.22
    - anus NEC Z85.048
      - carcinoid Z85.040

   ☑ **Additional Character Required — Refer to the Tabular List for Character Selection**   ▽ **Subterms under main terms may continue to next column or page**

History — continued
  personal (see also History, family) — continued
    malignant neoplasm — continued
      bladder Z85.51
      bone Z85.830
      brain Z85.841
      breast Z85.3
      bronchus NEC Z85.118
        carcinoid Z85.110
      carcinoid — see History, personal (of), malignant neoplasm, by site, carcinioid
      cervix Z85.41
      colon NEC Z85.038
        carcinoid Z85.030
      digestive organ Z85.00
        specified NEC Z85.09
      endocrine gland NEC Z85.858
      epididymis Z85.48
      esophagus Z85.01
      eye Z85.840
      gastrointestinal tract — see History, malignant neoplasm, digestive organ
      genital organ
        female Z85.40
          specified NEC Z85.44
        male Z85.45
          specified NEC Z85.49
      hematopoietic NEC Z85.79
      intrathoracic organ Z85.20
      kidney NEC Z85.528
        carcinoid Z85.520
      large intestine NEC Z85.038
        carcinoid Z85.030
      larynx Z85.21
      liver Z85.05
      lung NEC Z85.118
        carcinoid Z85.110
      mediastinum Z85.29
      Merkel cell Z85.821
      Methicillin resistant Staphylococcus aureus (MRSA) Z86.14
      middle ear Z85.22
      nasal cavities Z85.22
      nervous system NEC Z85.848
      oral cavity Z85.819
        specified site NEC Z85.818
      ovary Z85.43
      pancreas Z85.07
      pelvis Z85.53
      pharynx Z85.819
        specified site NEC Z85.818
      pleura Z85.29
      prostate Z85.46
      rectosigmoid junction NEC Z85.048
        carcinoid Z85.040
      rectum NEC Z85.048
        carcinoid Z85.040
      respiratory organ Z85.20
      sinuses, accessory Z85.22
      skin NEC Z85.828
        melanoma Z85.820
        Merkel cell Z85.821
      small intestine NEC Z85.068
        carcinoid Z85.060
      soft tissue Z85.831
      specified site NEC Z85.89
      stomach NEC Z85.028
        carcinoid Z85.020
      testis Z85.47
      thymus NEC Z85.238
        carcinoid Z85.230
      thyroid Z85.850
      tongue Z85.810
      trachea Z85.12
      urinary organ or tract Z85.50
        specified NEC Z85.59
      uterus Z85.42
    maltreatment Z91.89
    medical treatment NEC Z92.89
    melanoma (malignant) (skin) Z85.820
    meningitis Z86.61
    mental disorder Z86.59
    Merkel cell carcinoma (skin) Z85.821
    Methicillin resistant Staphylococcus aureus (MRSA) Z86.14
    military deployment Z91.82
    military war, peacekeeping and humanitarian deployment (current or past conflict) Z91.82

History — continued
  personal (see also History, family) — continued
    myocardial infarction (old) I25.2
    neglect (in)
      adult Z91.412
      childhood Z62.812
    neoplasm
      benign Z86.018
        brain Z86.011
        colon polyp Z86.010
      in situ
        breast Z86.000
        cervix uteri Z86.001
        specified NEC Z86.008
      malignant — see History of, malignant neoplasm
      uncertain behavior Z86.03
    nephrotic syndrome Z87.441
    nicotine dependence Z87.891
    noncompliance with medical treatment or regimen — see Noncompliance
    nutritional deficiency Z86.39
    obstetric complications Z87.59
      childbirth Z87.59
      pre-term labor Z87.51
      pregnancy Z87.59
      puerperium Z87.59
    osteoporosis fractures Z87.31 ☑
    parasuicide (attempt) Z91.5
    physical trauma NEC Z87.828
      self-harm or suicide attempt Z91.5
    pneumonia (recurrent) Z87.01
    poisoning NEC Z91.89
      self-harm or suicide attempt Z91.5
    poor personal hygiene Z91.89
    preterm labor Z87.51
    procedure during pregnancy Z98.870
    procedure while a fetus Z98.871
    prolonged reversible ischemic neurologic deficit (PRIND) Z86.73
    prostatic dysplasia Z87.430
    psychological
      abuse
        adult Z91.411
        child Z62.811
      trauma, specified NEC Z91.49
    radiation therapy Z92.3
    removal
      implant
        breast Z98.86
    renal calculi Z87.442
    respiratory condition NEC Z87.09
    retained foreign body fully removed Z87.821
    risk factors NEC Z91.89
    self-harm Z91.5
    self-poisoning attempt Z91.5
    sex reassignment Z87.890
    sleep-wake cycle problem Z72.821
    specified NEC Z87.898
    steroid therapy (systemic) Z92.241
      inhaled Z92.240
    stroke without residual deficits Z86.73
    substance abuse NEC F10-F19 with fifth character 1
    sudden cardiac arrest Z86.74
    sudden cardiac death successfully resuscitated Z86.74
    suicide attempt Z91.5
    surgery NEC Z98.89
      sex reassignment Z87.890
      transplant — see Transplant
    thrombophlebitis Z86.72
    thrombosis (venous) Z86.718
      pulmonary Z86.711
    tobacco dependence Z87.891
    transient ischemic attack (TIA) without residual deficits Z86.73
    trauma (physical) NEC Z87.828
      psychological NEC Z91.49
      self-harm Z91.5
    traumatic brain injury Z87.820
    unhealthy sleep-wake cycle Z72.821
    urinary calculi Z87.442
    urinary (recurrent) (tract) infection(s) Z87.440
    vaginal dysplasia Z87.411
    venous thrombosis or embolism Z86.718
      pulmonary Z86.711
    vulvar dysplasia Z87.412

HIV (see also Human, immunodeficiency virus) B20
  laboratory evidence (nonconclusive) R75
  nonconclusive test (in infants) R75
  positive, seropositive Z21
Hives (bold) — see Urticaria
Hoarseness R49.0
Hobo Z59.0
Hodgkin disease — see Lymphoma, Hodgkin
Hodgson's disease I71.2
  ruptured I71.1
Hoffa-Kastert disease E88.89
Hoffa's disease E88.89
Hoffmann-Bouveret syndrome I47.9
Hoffmann's syndrome E03.9 [G73.7]
Hole (round)
  macula H35.34- ☑
  retina (without detachment) — see Break, retina, round hole
    with detachment — see Detachment, retina, with retinal, break
Holiday relief care Z75.5
Hollenhorst's plaque — see Occlusion, artery, retina
Hollow foot (congenital) Q66.7
  acquired — see Deformity, limb, foot, specified NEC
Holoprosencephaly Q04.2
Holt-Oram syndrome Q87.2
Homelessness Z59.0
Homesickness — see Disorder, adjustment
Homocystinemia, homocystinuria E72.11
Homogentisate 1,2-dioxygenase deficiency E70.29
Homologous serum hepatitis (prophylactic) (therapeutic) — see Hepatitis, viral, type B
Honeycomb lung J98.4
  congenital Q33.0
Hooded
  clitoris Q52.6
  penis Q55.69
Hookworm (anemia) (disease) (infection) (infestation) B76.9
  specified NEC B76.8
Hordeolum (eyelid) (externum) (recurrent) H00.019
  internum H00.029
    left H00.026
      lower H00.025
      upper H00.024
    right H00.023
      lower H00.022
      upper H00.021
  left H00.016
    lower H00.015
    upper H00.014
  right H00.013
    lower H00.012
    upper H00.011
Horn
  cutaneous L85.8
  nail L60.2
    congenital Q84.6
Horner (-Claude Bernard) **syndrome** G90.2
  traumatic — see Injury, nerve, cervical sympathetic
Horseshoe kidney (congenital) Q63.1
Horton's headache or neuralgia G44.099
  intractable G44.091
  not intractable G44.099
Hospital hopper syndrome — see Disorder, factitious
Hospitalism in children — see Disorder, adjustment
Hostility R45.5
  towards child Z62.3
Hot flashes
  menopausal N95.1
Hourglass (contracture) (see also Contraction, hourglass)
  stomach K31.89
    congenital Q40.2
    stricture K31.2
Household, housing circumstance affecting care Z59.9
  specified NEC Z59.8
Housemaid's knee — see Bursitis, prepatellar
Hudson (-Ståhli) **line** (cornea) — see Pigmentation, cornea, anterior
Human
  bite (open wound) (see also Bite)
    intact skin surface — see Bite, superficial
  herpesvirus — see Herpes
  immunodeficiency virus (HIV) disease (infection) B20
    asymptomatic status Z21
    contact Z20.6

Human — *continued*
  immunodeficiency virus disease — *continued*
    counseling Z71.7
    dementia B20 [F02.80]
      with behavioral disturbance B20 [F02.81]
    exposure to Z20.6
    laboratory evidence R75
    type-2 (HIV 2) as cause of disease classified elsewhere B97.35
  papillomavirus (HPV)
    DNA test positive
      high risk
        cervix R87.810
        vagina R87.811
      low risk
        cervix R87.820
        vagina R87.821
    screening for Z11.51
  T-cell lymphotropic virus
    type-1 (HTLV-I) infection B33.3
      as cause of disease classified elsewhere B97.33
      carrier Z22.6
    type-2 (HTLV-II) as cause of disease classified elsewhere B97.34
Humidifier lung or pneumonitis J67.7
Humiliation (experience) **in childhood** Z62.898
Humpback (acquired) — *see* Kyphosis
Hunchback (acquired) — *see* Kyphosis
Hunger T73.0 ☑
  air, psychogenic F45.8
Hungry bone syndrome E83.81
Hunner's ulcer — *see* Cystitis, chronic, interstitial
Hunter's
  glossitis D51.0
  syndrome E76.1
Huntington's disease or chorea G10
  with dementia G10 [F02.80]
    with behavioral disturbance G10 [F02.81]
Hunt's
  disease or syndrome (herpetic geniculate ganglionitis) B02.21
    dyssynergia cerebellaris myoclonica G11.1
  neuralgia B02.21
Hurler (-Scheie) **disease or syndrome** E76.02
Hurst's disease G36.1
Hurthle cell
  adenocarcinoma C73
  adenoma D34
  carcinoma C73
  tumor D34
Hutchinson-Boeck disease or syndrome — *see* Sarcoidosis
Hutchinson-Gilford disease or syndrome E34.8
Hutchinson's
  disease, meaning
    angioma serpiginosum L81.7
    pompholyx (cheiropompholyx) L30.1
    prurigo estivalis L56.4
    summer eruption or summer prurigo L56.4
  melanotic freckle — *see* Melanoma, in situ
    malignant melanoma in — *see* Melanoma
  teeth or incisors (congenital syphilis) A50.52
  triad (congenital syphilis) A50.53
Hyalin plaque, sclera, senile H15.89
Hyaline membrane (disease) (lung) (pulmonary) (newborn) P22.0
Hyalinosis
  cutis (et mucosae) E78.89
  focal and segmental (glomerular) (*see also* N00-N07 with fourth character .1) N05.1
Hyalitis, hyalosis, asteroid (*see also* Deposit, crystalline)
  syphilitic (late) A52.71
Hydatid
  cyst or tumor — *see* Echinococcus
  mole — *see* Hydatidiform mole
  Morgagni
    female Q50.5
    male (epididymal) Q55.4
      testicular Q55.29
Hydatidiform mole (benign) (complicating pregnancy) (delivered) (undelivered) O01.9
  classical O01.0
  complete O01.0
  incomplete O01.1
  invasive D39.2
  malignant D39.2
  partial O01.1
Hydatidosis — *see* Echinococcus

Hydradenitis (axillaris) (suppurative) L73.2
Hydradenoma — *see* Hidradenoma
Hydramnios O40.- ☑
Hydrancephaly, hydranencephaly Q04.3
  with spina bifida — *see* Spina bifida, with hydrocephalus
Hydrargyrism NEC — *see* Poisoning, mercury
Hydrarthrosis (*see also* Effusion, joint)
  gonococcal A54.42
  intermittent M12.40
    ankle M12.47- ☑
    elbow M12.42- ☑
    foot joint M12.47- ☑
    hand joint M12.44- ☑
    hip M12.45- ☑
    knee M12.46- ☑
    multiple site M12.49
    shoulder M12.41- ☑
    specified joint NEC M12.48
    wrist M12.43- ☑
  of yaws (early) (late) (*see also* subcategory M14.8-) A66.6
  syphilitic (late) A52.77
    congenital A50.55 [M12.80]
Hydremia D64.89
Hydrencephalocele (congenital) — *see* Encephalocele
Hydrencephalomeningocele (congenital) — *see* Encephalocele
Hydroa R23.8
  aestivale L56.4
  vacciniforme L56.4
Hydroadenitis (axillaris) (suppurative) L73.2
Hydrocalycosis — *see* Hydronephrosis
Hydrocele (spermatic cord) (testis) (tunica vaginalis) N43.3
  canal of Nuck N94.89
  communicating N43.2
    congenital P83.5
  congenital P83.5
  encysted N43.0
  female NEC N94.89
  infected N43.1
  newborn P83.5
  round ligament N94.89
  specified NEC N43.2
  spinalis — *see* Spina bifida
  vulva N90.89
Hydrocephalus (acquired) (external) (internal) (malignant) (recurrent) G91.9
  aqueduct Sylvius stricture Q03.0
  causing disproportion O33.6 ☑
    with obstructed labor O66.3
  communicating G91.0
  congenital (external) (internal) Q03.9
    with spina bifida Q05.4
      cervical Q05.0
      dorsal Q05.1
      lumbar Q05.2
      lumbosacral Q05.2
      sacral Q05.3
      thoracic Q05.1
      thoracolumbar Q05.1
    specified NEC Q03.8
  due to toxoplasmosis (congenital) P37.1
  foramen Magendie block (acquired) G91.1
    congenital (*see also* Hydrocephalus, congenital) Q03.1
  in (due to)
    infectious disease NEC B89 [G91.4]
    neoplastic disease NEC (*see also* Neoplasm) G91.4
    parasitic disease B89 [G91.4]
  newborn Q03.9
    with spina bifida — *see* Spina bifida, with hydrocephalus
  noncommunicating G91.1
  normal pressure G91.2
    secondary G91.0
  obstructive G91.1
  otitic G93.2
  post-traumatic NEC G91.3
  secondary G91.4
    post-traumatic G91.3
  specified NEC G91.8
  syphilitic, congenital A50.49
Hydrocolpos (congenital) N89.8
Hydrocystoma — *see* Neoplasm, skin, benign
Hydroencephalocele (congenital) — *see* Encephalocele

Hydroencephalomeningocele (congenital) — *see* Encephalocele
Hydrohematopneumothorax — *see* Hemothorax
Hydromeningitis — *see* Meningitis
Hydromeningocele (spinal) (*see also* Spina bifida)
  cranial — *see* Encephalocele
Hydrometra N85.8
Hydrometrocolpos N89.8
Hydromicrocephaly Q02
Hydromphalos (since birth) Q45.8
Hydromyelia Q06.4
Hydromyelocele — *see* Spina bifida
Hydronephrosis (atrophic) (early) (functionless) (intermittent) (primary) (secondary) NEC N13.30
  with
    infection N13.6
    obstruction (by) (of)
      renal calculus N13.2
        with infection N13.6
      ureteral NEC N13.1
        with infection N13.6
        calculus N13.2
          with infection N13.6
      ureteropelvic junction (congenital) Q62.0
        with infection N13.6
      ureteral stricture NEC N13.1
        with infection N13.6
  congenital Q62.0
  specified type NEC N13.39
  tuberculous A18.11
Hydropericarditis — *see* Pericarditis
Hydropericardium — *see* Pericarditis
Hydroperitoneum R18.8
Hydrophobia — *see* Rabies
Hydrophthalmos Q15.0
Hydropneumohemothorax — *see* Hemothorax
Hydropneumopericarditis — *see* Pericarditis
Hydropneumopericardium — *see* Pericarditis
Hydropneumothorax J94.8
  traumatic — *see* Injury, intrathoracic, lung
  tuberculous NEC A15.6
Hydrops R60.9
  abdominis R18.8
  articulorum intermittens — *see* Hydrarthrosis, intermittent
  cardiac — *see* Failure, heart, congestive
  causing obstructed labor (mother) O66.3
  endolymphatic H81.0- ☑
  fetal — *see* Pregnancy, complicated by, hydrops, fetalis
  fetalis P83.2
    due to
      ABO isoimmunization P56.0
      alpha thalassemia D56.0
      hemolytic disease P56.90
        specified NEC P56.99
      isoimmunization (ABO) (Rh) P56.0
      other specified nonhemolytic disease NEC P83.2
      Rh incompatibility P56.0
    during pregnancy — *see* Pregnancy, complicated by, hydrops, fetalis
  gallbladder K82.1
  joint — *see* Effusion, joint
  labyrinth H81.0- ☑
  newborn (idiopathic) P83.2
    due to
      ABO isoimmunization P56.0
      alpha thalassemia D56.0
      hemolytic disease P56.90
        specified NEC P56.99
      isoimmunization (ABO) (Rh) P56.0
      Rh incompatibility P56.0
  nutritional — *see* Malnutrition, severe
  pericardium — *see* Pericarditis
  pleura — *see* Hydrothorax
  spermatic cord — *see* Hydrocele
Hydropyonephrosis N13.6
Hydrorachis Q06.4
Hydrorrhea (nasal) J34.89
  pregnancy — *see* Rupture, membranes, premature
Hydrosadenitis (axillaris) (suppurative) L73.2
Hydrosalpinx (fallopian tube) (follicularis) N70.11
Hydrothorax (double) (pleura) J94.8
  chylous (nonfilarial) I89.8
    filarial (*see also* Infestation, filarial) B74.9 [J91.8]
  traumatic — *see* Injury, intrathoracic
  tuberculous NEC (non primary) A15.6
Hydroureter (*see also* Hydronephrosis) N13.4

☑ Additional Character Required — Refer to the Tabular List for Character Selection   ▽ Subterms under main terms may continue to next column or page

Hypermenorrhea N92.0
Hypermethioninemia E72.19
Hypermetropia (congenital) H52.0- ☑
Hypermobility, hypermotility
  cecum — see Syndrome, irritable bowel
  coccyx — see subcategory M53.2 ☑
  colon — see Syndrome, irritable bowel
    psychogenic F45.8
  ileum K58.9
  intestine (see also Syndrome, irritable bowel) K58.9
    psychogenic F45.8
  meniscus (knee) — see Derangement, knee, meniscus
  scapula — see Instability, joint, shoulder
  stomach K31.89
    psychogenic F45.8
  syndrome M35.7
  urethra N36.41
    with intrinsic sphincter deficiency N36.43
Hypernasality R49.21
Hypernatremia E87.0
Hypernephroma C64.- ☑
Hyperopia — see Hypermetropia
Hyperorexia nervosa F50.2
Hyperornithinemia E72.4
Hyperosmia R43.1
Hyperosmolality E87.0
Hyperostosis (monomelic) (see also Disorder, bone, density and structure, specified NEC)
  ankylosing (spine) M48.10
    cervical region M48.12
    cervicothoracic region M48.13
    lumbar region M48.16
    lumbosacral region M48.17
    multiple sites M48.19
    occipito-atlanto-axial region M48.11
    sacrococcygeal region M48.18
    thoracic region M48.14
    thoracolumbar region M48.15
  cortical (skull) M85.2
    infantile M89.8X- ☑
  frontal, internal of skull M85.2
  interna frontalis M85.2
  skeletal, diffuse idiopathic — see Hyperostosis, ankylosing
  skull M85.2
    congenital Q75.8
  vertebral, ankylosing — see Hyperostosis, ankylosing
Hyperovarism E28.8
Hyperoxaluria (primary) E72.53
Hyperparathyroidism E21.3
  primary E21.0
  secondary (renal) N25.81
    non-renal E21.1
  specified NEC E21.2
  tertiary E21.2
Hyperpathia R20.8
Hyperperistalsis R19.2
  psychogenic F45.8
Hyperpermeability, capillary I78.8
Hyperphagia R63.2
Hyperphenylalaninemia NEC E70.1
Hyperphoria (alternating) H50.53
Hyperphosphatemia E83.39
Hyperpiesis, hyperpiesia — see Hypertension
Hyperpigmentation (see also Pigmentation)
  melanin NEC L81.4
  postinflammatory L81.0
Hyperpinealism E34.8
Hyperpituitarism E22.9
Hyperplasia, hyperplastic
  adenoids J35.2
  adrenal (capsule) (cortex) (gland) E27.8
    with
      sexual precocity (male) E25.9
        congenital E25.0
      virilism, adrenal E25.9
        congenital E25.0
      virilization (female) E25.9
        congenital E25.0
    congenital E25.0
    salt-losing E25.0
  adrenomedullary E27.5
  angiolymphoid, eosinophilia (ALHE) D18.01
  appendix (lymphoid) K38.0
  artery, fibromuscular I77.3
  bone (see also Hypertrophy, bone)
    marrow D75.89

Hyperplasia, hyperplastic — continued
  breast (see also Hypertrophy, breast)
    ductal (atypical) N60.9- ☑
  C-cell, thyroid E07.0
  cementation (tooth) (teeth) K03.4
  cervical gland R59.0
  cervix (uteri) (basal cell) (endometrium) (polypoid) (see also Dysplasia, cervix)
    congenital Q51.828
  clitoris, congenital Q52.6
  denture K06.2
  endocervicitis N72
  endometrium, endometrial (adenomatous) (benign) (cystic) (glandular) (glandular-cystic) (polypoid) N85.00
    with atypia N85.02
    cervix — see Dysplasia, cervix
    complex (without atypia) N85.01
    simple (without atypia) N85.01
  epithelial L85.9
    focal, oral, including tongue K13.29
    nipple N62
    skin L85.9
    tongue K13.29
    vaginal wall N89.3
  erythroid D75.89
  fibromuscular of artery (carotid) (renal) I77.3
  genital
    female NEC N94.89
    male N50.8
  gingiva K06.1
  glandularis cystica uteri (interstitialis) (see also Hyperplasia, endometrial) N85.00
  gum K06.1
  hymen, congenital Q52.4
  irritative, edentulous (alveolar) K06.2
  jaw M26.09
    alveolar M26.79
    lower M26.03
      alveolar M26.72
    upper M26.01
      alveolar M26.71
  kidney (congenital) Q63.3
  labia N90.6
    epithelial N90.3
  liver (congenital) Q44.7
    nodular, focal K76.89
  lymph gland or node R59.9
  mandible, mandibular M26.03
    alveolar M26.72
    unilateral condylar M27.8
  maxilla, maxillary M26.01
    alveolar M26.71
  myometrium, myometrial N85.2
  neuroendocrine cell, of infancy J84.841
  nose
    lymphoid J34.89
    polypoid J33.9
  oral mucosa (irritative) K13.6
  organ or site, congenital NEC — see Anomaly, by site
  ovary N83.8
  palate, papillary (irritative) K13.6
  pancreatic islet cells E16.9
    alpha E16.8
      with excess
        gastrin E16.4
        glucagon E16.3
    beta E16.1
  parathyroid (gland) E21.0
  pharynx (lymphoid) J39.2
  prostate (adenofibromatous) (nodular) N40.0
    with lower urinary tract symptoms (LUTS) N40.1
    without lower urinary tract symptoms (LUTS) N40.0
  renal artery I77.89
  reticulo-endothelial (cell) D75.89
  salivary gland (any) K11.1
  Schimmelbusch's — see Mastopathy, cystic
  suprarenal capsule (gland) E27.8
  thymus (gland) (persistent) E32.0
  thyroid (gland) — see Goiter
  tonsils (faucial) (infective) (lingual) (lymphoid) J35.1
    with adenoids J35.3
  unilateral condylar M27.8
  uterus, uterine N85.2
    endometrium (glandular) (see also Hyperplasia, endometrial) N85.00
  vulva N90.6
    epithelial N90.3

Hyperpnea — see Hyperventilation
Hyperpotassemia E87.5
Hyperprebetalipoproteinemia (familial) E78.1
Hyperprolactinemia E22.1
Hyperprolinemia (type I) (type II) E72.59
Hyperproteinemia E88.09
Hyperprothrombinemia, causing coagulation factor deficiency D68.4
Hyperpyrexia R50.9
  heat (effects) T67.0 ☑
  malignant, due to anesthetic T88.3 ☑
  rheumatic — see Fever, rheumatic
  unknown origin R50.9
Hypersalivation K11.7
Hypersecretion
  ACTH (not associated with Cushing's syndrome) E27.0
    pituitary E24.0
  adrenaline E27.5
  adrenomedullary E27.5
  androgen (testicular) E29.0
    ovarian (drug-induced) (iatrogenic) E28.1
  calcitonin E07.0
  catecholamine E27.5
  corticoadrenal E24.9
  cortisol E24.9
  epinephrine E27.5
  estrogen E28.0
  gastric K31.89
    psychogenic F45.8
  gastrin E16.4
  glucagon E16.3
  hormone(s)
    ACTH (not associated with Cushing's syndrome) E27.0
      pituitary E24.0
    antidiuretic E22.2
    growth E22.0
    intestinal NEC E34.1
    ovarian androgen E28.1
    pituitary E22.9
    testicular E29.0
    thyroid stimulating E05.80
      with thyroid storm E05.81
  insulin — see Hyperinsulinism
  lacrimal glands — see Epiphora
  medulloadrenal E27.5
  milk O92.6
  ovarian androgens E28.1
  salivary gland (any) K11.7
  thyrocalcitonin E07.0
  upper respiratory J39.8
Hypersegmentation, leukocytic, hereditary D72.0
Hypersensitive, hypersensitiveness, hypersensitivity (see also Allergy)
  carotid sinus G90.01
  colon — see Irritable, colon
  drug T88.7 ☑
  gastrointestinal K52.2
    psychogenic F45.8
  labyrinth — see subcategory H83.2 ☑
  pain R20.8
  pneumonitis — see Pneumonitis, allergic
  reaction T78.40 ☑
    upper respiratory tract NEC J39.3
Hypersomnia (organic) G47.10
  due to
    alcohol
      abuse F10.182
      dependence F10.282
      use F10.982
    amphetamines
      abuse F15.182
      dependence F15.282
      use F15.982
    caffeine
      abuse F15.182
      dependence F15.282
      use F15.982
    cocaine
      abuse F14.182
      dependence F14.282
      use F14.982
    drug NEC
      abuse F19.182
      dependence F19.282
      use F19.982
    medical condition G47.14
    mental disorder F51.13

Hypersomnia — *continued*
  due to — *continued*
    opioid
      abuse F11.182
      dependence F11.282
      use F11.982
    psychoactive substance NEC
      abuse F19.182
      dependence F19.282
      use F19.982
    sedative, hypnotic, or anxiolytic
      abuse F13.182
      dependence F13.282
      use F13.982
    stimulant NEC
      abuse F15.182
      dependence F15.282
      use F15.982
  idiopathic G47.11
    with long sleep time G47.11
    without long sleep time G47.12
  menstrual related G47.13
  nonorganic origin F51.11
    specified NEC F51.19
  not due to a substance or known physiological condi-
    tion F51.11
    specified NEC F51.19
  primary F51.11
  recurrent G47.13
  specified NEC G47.19
Hypersplenia, hypersplenism D73.1
Hyperstimulation, ovaries (associated with induced
  ovulation) N98.1
Hypersusceptibility — *see* Allergy
Hypertelorism (ocular) (orbital) Q75.2
Hypertension, hypertensive (accelerated) (benign)
  (essential) (idiopathic) (malignant) (systemic) I10
  with
    heart involvement (conditions in I51.4 - I51.9 due
      to hypertension) — *see* Hypertension, heart
    kidney involvement — *see* Hypertension, kidney
  benign, intracranial G93.2
  borderline R03.0
  cardiorenal (disease) I13.10
    with heart failure I13.0
      with stage 1 through stage 4 chronic kidney
        disease I13.0
      with stage 5 or end stage renal disease I13.2
    without heart failure I13.10
      with stage 1 through stage 4 chronic kidney
        disease I13.10
      with stage 5 or end stage renal disease I13.11
  cardiovascular
    disease (arteriosclerotic) (sclerotic) — *see* Hyper-
      tension, heart
    renal (disease) — *see* Hypertension, cardiorenal
  chronic venous — *see* Hypertension, venous (chronic)
  complicating
    childbirth (labor) O10.92
      with
        heart disease O10.12
          with renal disease O10.32
        renal disease O10.22
          with heart disease O10.32
      essential O10.02
      secondary O10.42
    pregnancy O16.- ☑
      with edema (*see also* Pre-eclampsia) O14.9- ☑
      gestational (pregnancy induced) (transient)
        (without proteinuria) O13.- ☑
      with proteinuria O14.9- ☑
        mild pre-eclampsia O14.0- ☑
        moderate pre-eclampsia O14.0- ☑
        severe pre-eclampsia O14.1- ☑
          with hemolysis, elevated liver en-
            zymes and low platelet count
            (HELLP) O14.2- ☑
    pre-existing O10.91- ☑
      with
        heart disease O10.11- ☑
          with renal disease O10.31- ☑
        pre-eclampsia O11.- ☑
        renal disease O10.21- ☑
          with heart disease O10.31- ☑
      essential O10.01- ☑
      secondary O10.41- ☑
    puerperium, pre-existing O10.93

Hypertension, hypertensive — *continued*
  complicating — *continued*
    puerperium, pre-existing — *continued*
      with
        heart disease O10.13
          with renal disease O10.33
        renal disease O10.23
          with heart disease O10.33
      essential O10.03
      pregnancy-induced O13.9
      secondary O10.43
  due to
    endocrine disorders I15.2
    pheochromocytoma I15.2
    renal disorders NEC I15.1
      arterial I15.0
    renovascular disorders I15.0
    specified disease NEC I15.8
  encephalopathy I67.4
  gestational (without significant proteinuria) (pregnan-
    cy-induced) (transient) O13.- ☑
    with significant proteinuria — *see* Pre-eclampsia
  Goldblatt's I70.1
  heart (disease) (conditions in I51.4-I51.9 due to hyper-
    tension) I11.9
    with
      heart failure (congestive) I11.0
      kidney disease (chronic) — *see* Hypertension,
        cardiorenal
  intracranial (benign) G93.2
  kidney I12.9
    with
      heart disease — *see* Hypertension, cardiorenal
      stage 1 through stage 4 chronic kidney disease
        I12.9
      stage 5 chronic kidney disease (CKD) or end
        stage renal disease (ESRD) I12.0
  lesser circulation I27.0
  newborn P29.2
    pulmonary (persistent) P29.3
  ocular H40.05- ☑
  pancreatic duct — *code to* underlying condition
    with chronic pancreatitis K86.1
  portal (due to chronic liver disease) (idiopathic) K76.6
    gastropathy K31.89
    in (due to) schistosomiasis (bilharziasis) B65.9 [K77]
  postoperative I97.3
  psychogenic F45.8
  pulmonary (artery) (secondary) NEC I27.2
    with
      cor pulmonale (chronic) I27.2
        acute I26.09
      right heart ventricular strain/failure I27.2
        acute I26.09
    of newborn (persistent) P29.3
    primary (idiopathic) I27.0
  renal — *see* Hypertension, kidney
  renovascular I15.0
  secondary NEC I15.9
    due to
      endocrine disorders I15.2
      pheochromocytoma I15.2
      renal disorders NEC I15.1
        arterial I15.0
      renovascular disorders I15.0
      specified NEC I15.8
  venous (chronic)
    due to
      deep vein thrombosis — *see* Syndrome, post-
        thrombotic
    idiopathic I87.309
      with
        inflammation I87.32- ☑
          with ulcer I87.33- ☑
        specified complication NEC I87.39- ☑
        ulcer I87.31- ☑
          with inflammation I87.33- ☑
      asymptomatic I87.30- ☑
Hypertensive urgency — *see* Hypertension
Hyperthecosis ovary E28.8
Hyperthermia (of unknown origin) (*see also* Hyperpyrex-
  ia)
  malignant, due to anesthesia T88.3 ☑
  newborn P81.9
    environmental P81.0
Hyperthyroid (recurrent) — *see* Hyperthyroidism
Hyperthyroidism (latent) (pre-adult) (recurrent) E05.90

Hyperthyroidism — *continued*
  with
    goiter (diffuse) E05.00
      with thyroid storm E05.01
      nodular (multinodular) E05.20
        with thyroid storm E05.21
        uninodular E05.10
          with thyroid storm E05.11
    storm E05.91
  due to ectopic thyroid tissue E05.30
    with thyroid storm E05.31
  neonatal, transitory P72.1
  specified NEC E05.80
    with thyroid storm E05.81
Hypertony, hypertonia, hypertonicity
  bladder N31.8
  congenital P94.1
  stomach K31.89
    psychogenic F45.8
  uterus, uterine (contractions) (complicating delivery)
    O62.4
Hypertrichosis L68.9
  congenital Q84.2
  eyelid H02.869
    left H02.866
      lower H02.865
      upper H02.864
    right H02.863
      lower H02.862
      upper H02.861
  lanuginosa Q84.2
    acquired L68.1
  localized L68.2
  specified NEC L68.8
Hypertriglyceridemia, essential E78.1
Hypertrophy, hypertrophic
  adenofibromatous, prostate — *see* Enlargement, en-
    larged, prostate
  adenoids (infective) J35.2
    with tonsils J35.3
  adrenal cortex E27.8
  alveolar process or ridge — *see* Anomaly, alveolar
  anal papillae K62.89
  artery I77.89
    congenital NEC Q27.8
      digestive system Q27.8
      lower limb Q27.8
      specified site NEC Q27.8
      upper limb Q27.8
  auricular — *see* Hypertrophy, cardiac
  Bartholin's gland N75.8
  bile duct (common) (hepatic) K83.8
  bladder (sphincter) (trigone) N32.89
  bone M89.30
    carpus M89.34- ☑
    clavicle M89.31- ☑
    femur M89.35- ☑
    fibula M89.36- ☑
    finger M89.34- ☑
    humerus M89.32- ☑
    ilium M89.359
    ischium M89.359
    metacarpus M89.34- ☑
    metatarsus M89.37- ☑
    multiple sites M89.39
    neck M89.38
    radius M89.33- ☑
    rib M89.38
    scapula M89.31- ☑
    skull M89.38
    tarsus M89.37- ☑
    tibia M89.36- ☑
    toe M89.37- ☑
    ulna M89.33- ☑
    vertebra M89.38
  brain G93.89
  breast N62
    cystic — *see* Mastopathy, cystic
    newborn P83.4
    pubertal, massive N62
    puerperal, postpartum — *see* Disorder, breast,
      specified type NEC
    senile (parenchymatous) N62
  cardiac (chronic) (idiopathic) I51.7
    with rheumatic fever (conditions in I00)
      active I01.8
      inactive or quiescent (with chorea) I09.89
    congenital NEC Q24.8

Hypertrophy, hypertrophic — *continued*
  cardiac — *continued*
    fatty — *see* Degeneration, myocardial
    hypertensive — *see* Hypertension, heart
    rheumatic (with chorea) I09.89
      active or acute I01.8
        with chorea I02.0
    valve — *see* Endocarditis
  cartilage — *see* Disorder, cartilage, specified type NEC
  cecum — *see* Megacolon
  cervix (uteri) N88.8
    congenital Q51.828
    elongation N88.4
  clitoris (cirrhotic) N90.89
    congenital Q52.6
  colon (*see also* Megacolon)
    congenital Q43.2
  conjunctiva, lymphoid H11.89
  corpora cavernosa N48.89
  cystic duct K82.8
  duodenum K31.89
  endometrium (glandular) (*see also* Hyperplasia, endometrial) N85.00
    cervix N88.8
  epididymis N50.8
  esophageal hiatus (congenital) Q79.1
    with hernia — *see* Hernia, hiatal
  eyelid — *see* Disorder, eyelid, specified type NEC
  fat pad E65
    knee (infrapatellar) (popliteal) (prepatellar) (retropatellar) M79.4
  foot (congenital) Q74.2
  frenulum, frenum (tongue) K14.8
    lip K13.0
  gallbladder K82.8
  gastric mucosa K29.60
    with bleeding K29.61
  gland, glandular R59.9
    generalized R59.1
    localized R59.0
  gum (mucous membrane) K06.1
  heart (idiopathic) (*see also* Hypertrophy, cardiac)
    valve (*see also* Endocarditis) I38
  hemifacial Q67.4
  hepatic — *see* Hypertrophy, liver
  hiatus (esophageal) Q79.1
  hilus gland R59.0
  hymen, congenital Q52.4
  ileum K63.89
  intestine NEC K63.89
  jejunum K63.89
  kidney (compensatory) N28.81
    congenital Q63.3
  labium (majus) (minus) N90.6
  ligament — *see* Disorder, ligament
  lingual tonsil (infective) J35.1
    with adenoids J35.3
  lip K13.0
    congenital Q18.6
  liver R16.0
    acute K76.89
    cirrhotic — *see* Cirrhosis, liver
    congenital Q44.7
    fatty — *see* Fatty, liver
  lymph, lymphatic gland R59.9
    generalized R59.1
    localized R59.0
    tuberculous — *see* Tuberculosis, lymph gland
  mammary gland — *see* Hypertrophy, breast
  Meckel's diverticulum (congenital) Q43.0
    malignant — *see* Table of Neoplasms, small intestine, malignant
  median bar — *see* Hyperplasia, prostate
  meibomian gland — *see* Chalazion
  meniscus, knee, congenital Q74.1
  metatarsal head — *see* Hypertrophy, bone, metatarsus
  metatarsus — *see* Hypertrophy, bone, metatarsus
  mucous membrane
    alveolar ridge K06.2
    gum K06.1
    nose (turbinate) J34.3
  muscle M62.89
  muscular coat, artery I77.89
  myocardium (*see also* Hypertrophy, cardiac)
    idiopathic I42.2
  myometrium N85.2
  nail L60.2
    congenital Q84.5

Hypertrophy, hypertrophic — *continued*
  nasal J34.89
    alae J34.89
    bone J34.89
    cartilage J34.89
    mucous membrane (septum) J34.3
    sinus J34.89
    turbinate J34.3
  nasopharynx, lymphoid (infectional) (tissue) (wall) J35.2
  nipple N62
  organ or site, congenital NEC — *see* Anomaly, by site
  ovary N83.8
  palate (hard) M27.8
    soft K13.79
  pancreas, congenital Q45.3
  parathyroid (gland) E21.0
  parotid gland K11.1
  penis N48.89
  pharyngeal tonsil J35.2
  pharynx J39.2
    lymphoid (infectional) (tissue) (wall) J35.2
  pituitary (anterior) (fossa) (gland) E23.6
  prepuce (congenital) N47.8
    female N90.89
  prostate — *see* Enlargement, enlarged, prostate
    congenital Q55.4
  pseudomuscular G71.0
  pylorus (adult) (muscle) (sphincter) K31.1
    congenital or infantile Q40.0
  rectal, rectum (sphincter) K62.89
  rhinitis (turbinate) J31.0
  salivary gland (any) K11.1
    congenital Q38.4
  scaphoid (tarsal) — *see* Hypertrophy, bone, tarsus
  scar L91.0
  scrotum N50.8
  seminal vesicle N50.8
  sigmoid — *see* Megacolon
  skin L91.9
    specified NEC L91.8
  spermatic cord N50.8
  spleen — *see* Splenomegaly
  spondylitis — *see* Spondylosis
  stomach K31.89
  sublingual gland K11.1
  submandibular gland K11.1
  suprarenal cortex (gland) E27.8
  synovial NEC M67.20
    acromioclavicular M67.21- ☑
    ankle M67.27- ☑
    elbow M67.22- ☑
    foot M67.27- ☑
    hand M67.24- ☑
    hip M67.25- ☑
    knee M67.26- ☑
    multiple sites M67.29
    specified site NEC M67.28
    wrist M67.23- ☑
  tendon — *see* Disorder, tendon, specified type NEC
  testis N44.8
    congenital Q55.29
  thymic, thymus (gland) (congenital) E32.0
  thyroid (gland) — *see* Goiter
  toe (congenital) Q74.2
    acquired (*see also* Deformity, toe, specified NEC)
  tongue K14.8
    congenital Q38.2
    papillae (foliate) K14.3
  tonsils (faucial) (infective) (lingual) (lymphoid) J35.1
    with adenoids J35.3
  tunica vaginalis N50.8
  ureter N28.89
  urethra N36.8
  uterus N85.2
    neck (with elongation) N88.4
    puerperal O90.89
  uvula K13.79
  vagina N89.8
  vas deferens N50.8
  vein I87.8
  ventricle, ventricular (heart) (*see also* Hypertrophy, cardiac)
    congenital Q24.8
    in tetralogy of Fallot Q21.3
  verumontanum N36.8
  vocal cord J38.3
  vulva N90.6

Hypertrophy, hypertrophic — *continued*
  vulva — *continued*
    stasis (nonfilarial) N90.6
Hypertropia H50.2- ☑
Hypertyrosinemia E70.21
Hyperuricemia (asymptomatic) E79.0
Hypervalinemia E71.19
Hyperventilation (tetany) R06.4
  hysterical F45.8
  psychogenic F45.8
  syndrome F45.8
Hypervitaminosis (dietary) NEC E67.8
  A E67.0
    administered as drug (prolonged intake) — *see* Table of Drugs and Chemicals, vitamins, adverse effect
    overdose or wrong substance given or taken — *see* Table of Drugs and Chemicals, vitamins, poisoning
  B6 E67.2
  D E67.3
    administered as drug (prolonged intake) — *see* Table of Drugs and Chemicals, vitamins, adverse effect
    overdose or wrong substance given or taken — *see* Table of Drugs and Chemicals, vitamins, poisoning
  K E67.8
    administered as drug (prolonged intake) — *see* Table of Drugs and Chemicals, vitamins, adverse effect
    overdose or wrong substance given or taken — *see* Table of Drugs and Chemicals, vitamins, poisoning
Hypervolemia E87.70
  specified NEC E87.79
Hypesthesia R20.1
  cornea — *see* Anesthesia, cornea
Hyphema H21.0- ☑
  traumatic S05.1- ☑
Hypo-osmolality E87.1
Hypo-ovarianism, hypo-ovarism E28.39
Hypoacidity, gastric K31.89
  psychogenic F45.8
Hypoadrenalism, hypoadrenia E27.40
  primary E27.1
  tuberculous A18.7
Hypoadrenocorticism E27.40
  pituitary E23.0
  primary E27.1
Hypoalbuminemia E88.09
Hypoaldosteronism E27.40
Hypoalphalipoproteinemia E78.6
Hypobarism T70.29 ☑
Hypobaropathy T70.29 ☑
Hypobetalipoproteinemia (familial) E78.6
Hypocalcemia E83.51
  dietary E58
  neonatal P71.1
    due to cow's milk P71.0
  phosphate-loading (newborn) P71.1
Hypochloremia E87.8
Hypochlorhydria K31.89
  neurotic F45.8
  psychogenic F45.8
Hypochondria, hypochondriac, hypochondriasis (reaction) F45.21
  sleep F51.03
Hypochondrogenesis Q77.0
Hypochondroplasia Q77.4
Hypochromasia, blood cells D50.8
Hypodontia — *see* Anodontia
Hypoeosinophilia D72.89
Hypoesthesia R20.1
Hypofibrinogenemia D68.8
  acquired D65
  congenital (hereditary) D68.2
Hypofunction
  adrenocortical E27.40
    drug-induced E27.3
    postprocedural E89.6
    primary E27.1
  adrenomedullary, postprocedural E89.6
  cerebral R29.818
  corticoadrenal NEC E27.40
  intestinal K59.8
  labyrinth — *see* subcategory H83.2 ☑

Hypofunction — *continued*
　ovary E28.39
　pituitary (gland) (anterior) E23.0
　testicular E29.1
　　postprocedural (postsurgical) (postirradiation) (iatrogenic) E89.5
Hypogalactia O92.4
Hypogammaglobulinemia (*see also* Agammaglobulinemia) D80.1
　hereditary D80.0
　nonfamilial D80.1
　transient, of infancy D80.7
Hypogenitalism (congenital) — *see* Hypogonadism
Hypoglossia Q38.3
Hypoglycemia (spontaneous) E16.2
　coma E15
　　diabetic — *see* Diabetes, coma
　diabetic — *see* Diabetes, hypoglycemia
　dietary counseling and surveillance Z71.3
　drug-induced E16.0
　　with coma (nondiabetic) E15
　due to insulin E16.0
　　with coma (nondiabetic) E15
　　therapeutic misadventure — *see* subcategory T38.3 ☑
　functional, nonhyperinsulinemic E16.1
　iatrogenic E16.0
　　with coma (nondiabetic) E15
　in infant of diabetic mother P70.1
　　gestational diabetes P70.0
　infantile E16.1
　leucine-induced E71.19
　neonatal (transitory) P70.4
　　iatrogenic P70.3
　reactive (not drug-induced) E16.1
　transitory neonatal P70.4
Hypogonadism
　female E28.39
　hypogonadotropic E23.0
　male E29.1
　ovarian (primary) E28.39
　pituitary E23.0
　testicular (primary) E29.1
Hypohidrosis, hypoidrosis L74.4
Hypoinsulinemia, postprocedural E89.1
Hypokalemia E87.6
Hypoleukocytosis — *see* Agranulocytosis
Hypolipoproteinemia (alpha) (beta) E78.6
Hypomagnesemia E83.42
　neonatal P71.2
Hypomania, hypomanic reaction F30.8
Hypomenorrhea — *see* Oligomenorrhea
Hypometabolism R63.8
Hypomotility
　gastrointestinal (tract) K31.89
　　psychogenic F45.8
　intestine K59.8
　　psychogenic F45.8
　stomach K31.89
　　psychogenic F45.8
Hyponasality R49.22
Hyponatremia E87.1
Hypoparathyroidism E20.9
　familial E20.8
　idiopathic E20.0
　neonatal, transitory P71.4
　postprocedural E89.2
　specified NEC E20.8
Hypoperfusion (in)
　newborn P96.89
Hypopharyngitis — *see* Laryngopharyngitis
Hypophoria H50.53
Hypophosphatemia, hypophosphatasia (acquired) (congenital) (renal) E83.39
　familial E83.31
Hypophyseal, hypophysis (*see also* condition)
　dwarfism E23.0
　gigantism E22.0 ☑
Hypopiesis — *see* Hypotension
Hypopinealism E34.8
Hypopituitarism (juvenile) E23.0
　drug-induced E23.1
　due to
　　hypophysectomy E89.3
　　radiotherapy E89.3
　iatrogenic NEC E23.1
　postirradiation E89.3

Hypopituitarism — *continued*
　postpartum E23.0
　postprocedural E89.3
Hypoplasia, hypoplastic
　adrenal (gland), congenital Q89.1
　alimentary tract, congenital Q45.8
　　upper Q40.8
　anus, anal (canal) Q42.3
　　with fistula Q42.2
　aorta, aortic Q25.4
　　ascending, in hypoplastic left heart syndrome Q23.4
　　valve Q23.1
　　　in hypoplastic left heart syndrome Q23.4
　areola, congenital Q83.8
　arm (congenital) — *see* Defect, reduction, upper limb
　artery (peripheral) Q27.8
　　brain (congenital) Q28.3
　　coronary Q24.5
　　digestive system Q27.8
　　lower limb Q27.8
　　pulmonary Q25.79
　　　functional, unilateral J43.0
　　retinal (congenital) Q14.1
　　specified site NEC Q27.8
　　umbilical Q27.8
　　upper limb Q27.8
　auditory canal Q17.8
　　causing impairment of hearing Q16.9
　biliary duct or passage Q44.5
　bone NOS Q79.9
　　face Q75.8
　　marrow D61.9
　　　megakaryocytic D69.49
　　skull — *see* Hypoplasia, skull
　brain Q02
　　gyri Q04.3
　　part of Q04.3
　breast (areola) N64.82
　bronchus Q32.4
　cardiac Q24.8
　carpus — *see* Defect, reduction, upper limb, specified type NEC
　cartilage hair Q78.5
　cecum Q42.8
　cementum K00.4
　cephalic Q02
　cerebellum Q04.3
　cervix (uteri), congenital Q51.821
　clavicle (congenital) Q74.0
　coccyx Q76.49
　colon Q42.9
　　specified NEC Q42.8
　corpus callosum Q04.0
　cricoid cartilage Q31.2
　digestive organ(s) or tract NEC Q45.8
　　upper (congenital) Q40.8
　ear (auricle) (lobe) Q17.2
　　middle Q16.4
　enamel of teeth (neonatal) (postnatal) (prenatal) K00.4
　endocrine (gland) NEC Q89.2
　endometrium N85.8
　epididymis (congenital) Q55.4
　epiglottis Q31.2
　erythroid, congenital D61.01
　esophagus (congenital) Q39.8
　eustachian tube Q17.8
　eye Q11.2
　eyelid (congenital) Q10.3
　face Q18.8
　　bone(s) Q75.8
　femur (congenital) — *see* Defect, reduction, lower limb, specified type NEC
　fibula (congenital) — *see* Defect, reduction, lower limb, specified type NEC
　finger (congenital) — *see* Defect, reduction, upper limb, specified type NEC
　focal dermal Q82.8
　foot — *see* Defect, reduction, lower limb, specified type NEC
　gallbladder Q44.0
　genitalia, genital organ(s)
　　female, congenital Q52.8
　　　external Q52.79
　　　internal NEC Q52.8
　　in adiposogenital dystrophy E23.6
　glottis Q31.2
　hair Q84.2

Hypoplasia, hypoplastic — *continued*
　hand (congenital) — *see* Defect, reduction, upper limb, specified type NEC
　heart Q24.8
　humerus (congenital) — *see* Defect, reduction, upper limb, specified type NEC
　intestine (small) Q41.9
　　large Q42.9
　　specified NEC Q42.8
　jaw M26.09
　　alveolar M26.79
　　lower M26.04
　　　alveolar M26.74
　　upper M26.02
　　　alveolar M26.73
　kidney(s) Q60.5
　　bilateral Q60.4
　　unilateral Q60.3
　labium (majus) (minus), congenital Q52.79
　larynx Q31.2
　left heart syndrome Q23.4
　leg (congenital) — *see* Defect, reduction, lower limb
　limb Q73.8
　　lower (congenital) — *see* Defect, reduction, lower limb
　　upper (congenital) — *see* Defect, reduction, upper limb
　liver Q44.7
　lung (lobe) (not associated with short gestation) Q33.6
　　associated with immaturity, low birth weight, prematurity, or short gestation P28.0
　mammary (areola), congenital Q83.8
　mandible, mandibular M26.04
　　alveolar M26.74
　　unilateral condylar M27.8
　maxillary M26.02
　　alveolar M26.73
　medullary D61.9
　megakaryocytic D69.49
　metacarpus — *see* Defect, reduction, upper limb, specified type NEC
　metatarsus — *see* Defect, reduction, lower limb, specified type NEC
　muscle Q79.8
　nail(s) Q84.6
　nose, nasal Q30.1
　optic nerve H47.03- ☑
　osseous meatus (ear) Q17.8
　ovary, congenital Q50.39
　pancreas Q45.0
　parathyroid (gland) Q89.2
　parotid gland Q38.4
　patella Q74.1
　pelvis, pelvic girdle Q74.2
　penis (congenital) Q55.62
　peripheral vascular system Q27.8
　　digestive system Q27.8
　　lower limb Q27.8
　　specified site NEC Q27.8
　　upper limb Q27.8
　pituitary (gland) (congenital) Q89.2
　pulmonary (not associated with short gestation) Q33.6
　　artery, functional J43.0
　　associated with short gestation P28.0
　radioulnar — *see* Defect, reduction, upper limb, specified type NEC
　radius — *see* Defect, reduction, upper limb
　rectum Q42.1
　　with fistula Q42.0
　respiratory system NEC Q34.8
　rib Q76.6
　right heart syndrome Q22.6
　sacrum Q76.49
　scapula Q74.0
　scrotum Q55.1
　shoulder girdle Q74.0
　skin Q82.8
　skull (bone) Q75.8
　　with
　　　anencephaly Q00.0
　　　encephalocele — *see* Encephalocele
　　　hydrocephalus Q03.9
　　　　with spina bifida — *see* Spina bifida, by site, with hydrocephalus
　　　microcephaly Q02
　spinal (cord) (ventral horn cell) Q06.1
　spine Q76.49
　sternum Q76.7

Hypoplasia, hypoplastic — *continued*
  tarsus — *see* Defect, reduction, lower limb, specified
    type NEC
  testis Q55.1
  thymic, with immunodeficiency D82.1
  thymus (gland) Q89.2
    with immunodeficiency D82.1
  thyroid (gland) E03.1
    cartilage Q31.2
  tibiofibular (congenital) — *see* Defect, reduction,
    lower limb, specified type NEC
  toe — *see* Defect, reduction, lower limb, specified type
    NEC
  tongue Q38.3
  Turner's K00.4
  ulna (congenital) — *see* Defect, reduction, upper limb
  umbilical artery Q27.0
  unilateral condylar M27.8
  ureter Q62.8
  uterus, congenital Q51.811
  vagina Q52.4
  vascular NEC peripheral Q27.8
    brain Q28.3
    digestive system Q27.8
    lower limb Q27.8
    specified site NEC Q27.8
    upper limb Q27.8
  vein(s) (peripheral) Q27.8
    brain Q28.3
    digestive system Q27.8
    great Q26.8
    lower limb Q27.8
    specified site NEC Q27.8
    upper limb Q27.8
  vena cava (inferior) (superior) Q26.8
  vertebra Q76.49
  vulva, congenital Q52.79
  zonule (ciliary) Q12.8
Hypopotassemia E87.6
Hypoproconvertinemia, congenital (hereditary) D68.2
Hypoproteinemia E77.8
Hypoprothrombinemia (congenital) (hereditary) (idiopathic) D68.2
  acquired D68.4
  newborn, transient P61.6
Hypoptyalism K11.7
Hypopyon (eye) (anterior chamber) — *see* Iridocyclitis,
  acute, hypopyon
Hypopyrexia R68.0
Hyporeflexia R29.2
Hyposecretion
  ACTH E23.0
  antidiuretic hormone E23.2
  ovary E28.39
  salivary gland (any) K11.7
  vasopressin E23.2
Hyposegmentation, leukocytic, hereditary D72.0
Hyposiderinemia D50.9
Hypospadias Q54.9
  balanic Q54.0
  coronal Q54.0
  glandular Q54.0
  penile Q54.1
  penoscrotal Q54.2
  perineal Q54.3
  specified NEC Q54.8
Hypospermatogenesis — *see* Oligospermia
Hyposplenism D73.0
Hypostasis pulmonary, passive — *see* Edema, lung
Hypostatic — *see* condition
Hyposthenuria N28.89
Hypotension (arterial) (constitutional) I95.9
  chronic I95.89
  drug-induced I95.2
  due to (of) hemodialysis I95.3
  iatrogenic I95.89
  idiopathic (permanent) I95.0
  intra-dialytic I95.3
  intracranial, following ventricular shunting (ventricu-
    lostomy) G97.2
  maternal, syndrome (following labor and delivery)
    O26.5- ☑
  neurogenic, orthostatic G90.3
  orthostatic (chronic) I95.1
    due to drugs I95.2
    neurogenic G90.3
  postoperative I95.81
  postural I95.1

Hypotension — *continued*
  specified NEC I95.89
Hypothermia (accidental) T68 ☑
  due to anesthesia, anesthetic T88.51 ☑
  low environmental temperature T68 ☑
  neonatal P80.9
    environmental (mild) NEC P80.8
    mild P80.8
    severe (chronic) (cold injury syndrome) P80.0
    specified NEC P80.8
  not associated with low environmental temperature
    R68.0
Hypothyroidism (acquired) E03.9
  congenital (without goiter) E03.1
    with goiter (diffuse) E03.0
  due to
    exogenous substance NEC E03.2
    iodine-deficiency, acquired E01.8
      subclinical E02
    irradiation therapy E89.0
    medicament NEC E03.2
    P-aminosalicylic acid (PAS) E03.2
    phenylbutazone E03.2
    resorcinol E03.2
    sulfonamide E03.2
    surgery E89.0
    thiourea group drugs E03.2
  iatrogenic NEC E03.2
  iodine-deficiency (acquired) E01.8
    congenital — *see* Syndrome, iodine- deficiency,
      congenital
    subclinical E02
  neonatal, transitory P72.2
  postinfectious E03.3
  postirradiation E89.0
  postprocedural E89.0
  postsurgical E89.0
  specified NEC E03.8
  subclinical, iodine-deficiency related E02
Hypotonia, hypotonicity, hypotony
  bladder N31.2
  congenital (benign) P94.2
  eye — *see* Disorder, globe, hypotony
Hypotrichosis — *see* Alopecia
Hypotropia H50.2- ☑
Hypoventilation R06.89
  congenital central alveolar G47.35
  sleep related
    idiopathic nonobstructive alveolar G47.34
    in conditions classified elsewhere G47.36
Hypovitaminosis — *see* Deficiency, vitamin
Hypovolemia E86.1
  surgical shock T81.19 ☑
  traumatic (shock) T79.4 ☑
Hypoxemia R09.02
  newborn P84
  sleep related, in conditions classified elsewhere G47.36
Hypoxia (see also Anoxia) R09.02
  cerebral, during a procedure NEC G97.81
    postprocedural NEC G97.82
  intrauterine P84
  myocardial — *see* Insufficiency, coronary
  newborn P84
  sleep-related G47.34
Hypsarrhythmia — *see* Epilepsy, generalized, specified
  NEC
Hysteralgia, pregnant uterus O26.89- ☑
Hysteria, hysterical (conversion) (dissociative state)
  F44.9
  anxiety F41.8
  convulsions F44.5
  psychosis, acute F44.9
Hysteroepilepsy F44.5

I

Ichthyoparasitism due to Vandellia cirrhosa B88.8
Ichthyosis (congenital) Q80.9
  acquired L85.0
  fetalis Q80.4
  hystrix Q80.8
  lamellar Q80.2
  lingual K13.29
  palmaris and plantaris Q82.8
  simplex Q80.0
  vera Q80.8
  vulgaris Q80.0

Ichthyosis — *continued*
  X-linked Q80.1
Ichthyotoxism — *see* Poisoning, fish
  bacterial — *see* Intoxication, foodborne
Icteroanemia, hemolytic (acquired) D59.9
  congenital — *see* Spherocytosis
Icterus (see also Jaundice)
  conjunctiva R17
  gravis, newborn P55.0
  hematogenous (acquired) D59.9
  hemolytic (acquired) D59.9
    congenital — *see* Spherocytosis
  hemorrhagic (acute) (leptospiral) (spirochetal) A27.0
    newborn P53
  infectious B15.9
    with hepatic coma B15.0
    leptospiral A27.0
    spirochetal A27.0
  neonatorum — *see* Jaundice, newborn
  newborn P59.9
  spirochetal A27.0
Ictus solaris, solis T67.0 ☑
Id reaction (due to bacteria) L30.2
Ideation
  homicidal R45.850
  suicidal R45.851
Identity disorder (child) F64.9
  gender role F64.2
  psychosexual F64.2
Idioglossia F80.0
Idiopathic — *see* condition
Idiot, idiocy (congenital) F73
  amaurotic (Bielschowsky(-Jansky)) (family) (infantile
    (late)) (juvenile (late)) (Vogt-Spielmeyer) E75.4
  microcephalic Q02
IgE asthma J45.909
IIAC (idiopathic infantile arterial calcification) Q28.8
Ileitis (chronic) (noninfectious) (see also Enteritis) K52.9
  backwash — *see* Pancolitis, ulcerative (chronic)
  infectious A09
  regional (ulcerative) — *see* Enteritis, regional, small
    intestine
  segmental — *see* Enteritis, regional
  terminal (ulcerative) — *see* Enteritis, regional, small
    intestine
Ileocolitis (see also Enteritis) K52.9
  infectious A09
  regional — *see* Enteritis, regional
Ileostomy
  attention to Z43.2
  malfunctioning K94.13
  status Z93.2
    with complication — *see* Complications, enteros-
      tomy
Ileotyphus — *see* Typhoid
Ileum — *see* condition
Ileus (bowel) (colon) (inhibitory) (intestine) K56.7
  adynamic K56.0
  due to gallstone (in intestine) K56.3
  duodenal (chronic) K31.5
  gallstone K56.3
  mechanical NEC K56.69
  meconium P76.0
    in cystic fibrosis E84.11
    meaning meconium plug (without cystic fibrosis)
      P76.0
  myxedema K59.8
  neurogenic K56.0
    Hirschsprung's disease or megacolon Q43.1
  newborn
    due to meconium P76.0
      in cystic fibrosis E84.11
      meaning meconium plug (without cystic fibro-
        sis) P76.0
    transitory P76.1
  obstructive K56.69
  paralytic K56.0
Iliac — *see* condition
Iliotibial band syndrome M76.3- ☑
Illiteracy Z55.0
Illness (see also Disease) R69
  manic-depressive — *see* Disorder, bipolar
Imbalance R26.89
  autonomic G90.8
  constituents of food intake E63.1
  electrolyte E87.8

☑ Additional Character Required — Refer to the Tabular List for Character Selection   ▽ Subterms under main terms may continue to next column or page

Imbalance — continued
  electrolyte — continued
    with
      abortion — see Abortion by type, complicated by, electrolyte imbalance
      molar pregnancy O08.5
    due to hyperemesis gravidarum O21.1
    following ectopic or molar pregnancy O08.5
    neonatal, transitory NEC P74.4
      potassium P74.3
      sodium P74.2
  endocrine E34.9
  eye muscle NOS H50.9
  hormone E34.9
  hysterical F44.4
  labyrinth — see subcategory H83.2 ☑
  posture R29.3
  protein-energy — see Malnutrition
  sympathetic G90.8
Imbecile, imbecility (I.Q. 35-49) F71
Imbedding, intrauterine device T83.39 ☑
Imbibition, cholesterol (gallbladder) K82.4
Imbrication, teeth,, fully erupted M26.30
Imerslund (-Gräsbeck) **syndrome** D51.1
Immature (see also Immaturity)
  birth (less than 37 completed weeks) — see Preterm, newborn
    extremely (less than 28 completed weeks) — see Immaturity, extreme
  personality F60.89
Immaturity (less than 37 completed weeks) (see also Preterm, newborn)
  extreme of newborn (less than 28 completed weeks of gestation) (less than 196 completed days of gestation) (unspecified weeks of gestation) P07.20
    gestational age
      less than 23 completed weeks P07.21
      23 completed weeks (23 weeks, 0 days through 23 weeks, 6 days) P07.22
      24 completed weeks (24 weeks, 0 days through 24 weeks, 6 days) P07.23
      25 completed weeks (25 weeks, 0 days through 25 weeks, 6 days) P07.24
      26 completed weeks (26 weeks, 0 days through 26 weeks, 6 days) P07.25
      27 completed weeks (27 weeks, 0 days through 27 weeks, 6 days) P07.26
  fetus or infant light-for-dates — see Light-for-dates
  lung, newborn P28.0
  organ or site NEC — see Hypoplasia
  pulmonary, newborn P28.0
  reaction F60.89
  sexual (female) (male), after puberty E30.0
Immersion T75.1 ☑
  foot T69.02- ☑
  hand T69.01- ☑
Immobile, immobility
  complete, due to severe physical disability or frailty R53.2
  intestine K59.8
  syndrome (paraplegic) M62.3
Immune reconstitution (inflammatory) syndrome [IRIS] D89.3
Immunization (see also Vaccination)
  ABO — see Incompatibility, ABO
    in newborn P55.1
  complication — see Complications, vaccination
  encounter for Z23
  not done (not carried out) Z28.9
    because (of)
      acute illness of patient Z28.01
      allergy to vaccine (or component) Z28.04
      caregiver refusal Z28.82
      chronic illness of patient Z28.02
      contraindication NEC Z28.09
      group pressure Z28.1
      guardian refusal Z28.82
      immune compromised state of patient Z28.03
      parent refusal Z28.82
      patient had disease being vaccinated against Z28.81
      patient refusal Z28.21
      patient's belief Z28.1
      religious beliefs of patient Z28.1
      specified reason NEC Z28.89
        of patient Z28.29
      unspecified patient reason Z28.20

Immunization — continued
  Rh factor
    affecting management of pregnancy NEC O36.09- ☑
      anti-D antibody O36.01- ☑
    from transfusion — see Complication(s), transfusion, incompatibility reaction, Rh (factor)
Immunocytoma C83.0- ☑
Immunodeficiency D84.9
  with
    adenosine-deaminase deficiency D81.3
    antibody defects D80.9
      specified type NEC D80.8
    hyperimmunoglobulinemia D80.6
    increased immunoglobulin M (IgM) D80.5
    major defect D82.9
      specified type NEC D82.8
    partial albinism D82.8
    short-limbed stature D82.2
    thrombocytopenia and eczema D82.0
  antibody with
    hyperimmunoglobulinemia D80.6
    near-normal immunoglobulins D80.6
  autosomal recessive, Swiss type D80.0
  combined D81.9
    biotin-dependent carboxylase D81.819
      biotinidase D81.810
      holocarboxylase synthetase D81.818
      specified type NEC D81.818
    severe (SCID) D81.9
      with
        low or normal B-cell numbers D81.2
        low T- and B-cell numbers D81.1
        reticular dysgenesis D81.0
    specified type NEC D81.89
  common variable D83.9
    with
      abnormalities of B-cell numbers and function D83.0
      autoantibodies to B- or T-cells D83.2
      immunoregulatory T-cell disorders D83.1
    specified type NEC D83.8
  following hereditary defective response to Epstein-Barr virus (EBV) D82.3
  selective, immunoglobulin
    A (IgA) D80.2
    G (IgG) (subclasses) D80.3
    M (IgM) D80.4
  severe combined (SCID) D81.9
  specified type NEC D84.8
  X-linked, with increased IgM D80.5
Immunotherapy (encounter for)
  antineoplastic Z51.12
Impaction, impacted
  bowel, colon, rectum (see also Impaction, fecal) K56.49
    by gallstone K56.3
  calculus — see Calculus
  cerumen (ear) (external) H61.2- ☑
  cuspid — see Impaction, tooth
  dental (same or adjacent tooth) K01.1
  fecal, feces K56.41
  fracture — see Fracture, by site
  gallbladder — see Calculus, gallbladder
  gallstone(s) — see Calculus, gallbladder
    bile duct (common) (hepatic) — see Calculus, bile duct
    cystic duct — see Calculus, gallbladder
    in intestine, with obstruction (any part) K56.3
  intestine (calculous) NEC (see also Impaction, fecal) K56.49
    gallstone, with ileus K56.3
  intrauterine device (IUD) T83.39 ☑
  molar — see Impaction, tooth
  shoulder, causing obstructed labor O66.0
  tooth, teeth K01.1
  turbinate J34.89
Impaired, impairment (function)
  auditory discrimination — see Abnormal, auditory perception
  cognitive, mild, so stated G31.84
  dual sensory Z73.82
  fasting glucose R73.01
  glucose tolerance (oral) R73.02
  hearing — see Deafness
  heart — see Disease, heart
  kidney N28.9
    disorder resulting from N25.9
      specified NEC N25.89

Impaired, impairment — continued
  liver K72.90
    with coma K72.91
  mastication K08.8
  mild cognitive, so stated G31.84
  mobility
    ear ossicles — see Ankylosis, ear ossicles
    requiring care provider Z74.09
  myocardium, myocardial — see Insufficiency, myocardial
  rectal sphincter R19.8
  renal (acute) (chronic) N28.9
    disorder resulting from N25.9
      specified NEC N25.89
  vision NEC H54.7
    both eyes H54.3
Impediment, speech R47.9
  psychogenic (childhood) F98.8
  slurring R47.81
  specified NEC R47.89
Impending
  coronary syndrome I20.0
  delirium tremens F10.239
  myocardial infarction I20.0
Imperception auditory (acquired) (see also Deafness)
  congenital H93.25
Imperfect
  aeration, lung (newborn) NEC — see Atelectasis
  closure (congenital)
    alimentary tract NEC Q45.8
      lower Q43.8
      upper Q40.8
    atrioventricular ostium Q21.2
    atrium (secundum) Q21.1
    branchial cleft or sinus Q18.0
    choroid Q14.3
    cricoid cartilage Q31.8
    cusps, heart valve NEC Q24.8
      pulmonary Q22.3
    ductus
      arteriosus Q25.0
      Botalli Q25.0
    ear drum (causing impairment of hearing) Q16.4
    esophagus with communication to bronchus or trachea Q39.1
    eyelid Q10.3
    foramen
      botalli Q21.1
      ovale Q21.1
    genitalia, genital organ(s) or system
      female Q52.8
        external Q52.79
        internal NEC Q52.8
      male Q55.8
    glottis Q31.8
    interatrial ostium or septum Q21.1
    interauricular ostium or septum Q21.1
    interventricular ostium or septum Q21.0
    larynx Q31.8
    lip — see Cleft, lip
    nasal septum Q30.3
    nose Q30.2
    omphalomesenteric duct Q43.0
    optic nerve entry Q14.2
    organ or site not listed — see Anomaly, by site
    ostium
      interatrial Q21.1
      interauricular Q21.1
      interventricular Q21.0
    palate — see Cleft, palate
    preauricular sinus Q18.1
    retina Q14.1
    roof of orbit Q75.8
    sclera Q13.5
    septum
      aorticopulmonary Q21.4
      atrial (secundum) Q21.1
      between aorta and pulmonary artery Q21.4
      heart Q21.9
      interatrial (secundum) Q21.1
      interauricular (secundum) Q21.1
      interventricular Q21.0
        in tetralogy of Fallot Q21.3
      nasal Q30.3
      ventricular Q21.0
        with pulmonary stenosis or atresia, dextra-position of aorta, and hypertrophy of right ventricle Q21.3

Imperfect — *continued*
  closure — *continued*
    septum — *continued*
      ventricular — *continued*
        in tetralogy of Fallot Q21.3
    skull Q75.0
      with
        anencephaly Q00.0
        encephalocele — *see* Encephalocele
        hydrocephalus Q03.9
          with spina bifida — *see* Spina bifida, by
            site, with hydrocephalus
        microcephaly Q02
    spine (with meningocele) — *see* Spina bifida
    trachea Q32.1
    tympanic membrane (causing impairment of
      hearing) Q16.4
    uterus Q51.818
    vitelline duct Q43.0
  erection — *see* Dysfunction, sexual, male, erectile
  fusion — *see* Imperfect, closure
  inflation, lung (newborn) — *see* Atelectasis
  posture R29.3
  rotation, intestine Q43.3
  septum, ventricular Q21.0
Imperfectly descended testis — *see* Cryptorchid
Imperforate (congenital) (*see also* Atresia)
  anus Q42.3
    with fistula Q42.2
  cervix (uteri) Q51.828
  esophagus Q39.0
    with tracheoesophageal fistula Q39.1
  hymen Q52.3
  jejunum Q41.1
  pharynx Q38.8
  rectum Q42.1
    with fistula Q42.0
  urethra Q64.39
  vagina Q52.4
Impervious (congenital) (*see also* Atresia)
  anus Q42.3
    with fistula Q42.2
  bile duct Q44.2
  esophagus Q39.0
    with tracheoesophageal fistula Q39.1
  intestine (small) Q41.9
    large Q42.9
      specified NEC Q42.8
  rectum Q42.1
    with fistula Q42.0
  ureter — *see* Atresia, ureter
  urethra Q64.39
Impetiginization of dermatoses L01.1
Impetigo (any organism) (any site) (circinate) (contagiosa) (simplex) (vulgaris) L01.00
  Bockhart's L01.02
  bullous, bullosa L01.03
  external ear L01.00 [H62.40]
  follicularis L01.02
  furfuracea L30.5
  herpetiformis L40.1
    nonobstetrical L40.1
  neonatorum L01.03
  nonbullous L01.01
  specified type NEC L01.09
  ulcerative L01.09
Impingement (on teeth)
  soft tissue
    anterior M26.81
    posterior M26.82
Implant, endometrial N80.9
Implantation
  anomalous — *see* Anomaly, by site
    ureter Q62.63
  cyst
    external area or site (skin) NEC L72.0
    iris — *see* Cyst, iris, implantation
    vagina N89.8
    vulva N90.7
  dermoid (cyst) — *see* Implantation, cyst
Impotence (sexual) N52.9
  counseling Z70.1
  organic origin (*see also* Dysfunction, sexual, male,
    erectile) N52.9
  psychogenic F52.21
Impression, basilar Q75.8
Imprisonment, anxiety concerning Z65.1
Improper care (child) (newborn) — *see* Maltreatment

Improperly tied umbilical cord (causing hemorrhage)
  P51.8
Impulsiveness (impulsive) R45.87
Inability to swallow — *see* Aphagia
Inaccessible, inaccessibility
  health care NEC Z75.3
    due to
      waiting period Z75.2
        for admission to facility elsewhere Z75.1
  other helping agencies Z75.4
Inactive — *see* condition
Inadequate, inadequacy
  aesthetics of dental restoration K08.56
  biologic, constitutional, functional, or social F60.7
  development
    child R62.50
    genitalia
      after puberty NEC E30.0
      congenital
        female Q52.8
          external Q52.79
          internal Q52.8
        male Q55.8
    lungs Q33.6
      associated with short gestation P28.0
    organ or site not listed — *see* Anomaly, by site
  diet (causing nutritional deficiency) E63.9
  eating habits Z72.4
  environment, household Z59.1
  family support Z63.8
  food (supply) NEC Z59.4
    hunger effects T73.0 ☑
  functional F60.7
  household care, due to
    family member
      handicapped or ill Z74.2
      on vacation Z75.5
      temporarily away from home Z74.2
    technical defects in home Z59.1
    temporary absence from home of person rendering
      care Z74.2
  housing (heating) (space) Z59.1
  income (financial) Z59.6
  intrafamilial communication Z63.8
  material resources Z59.9
  mental — *see* Disability, intellectual
  parental supervision or control of child Z62.0
  personality F60.7
  pulmonary
    function R06.89
      newborn P28.5
    ventilation, newborn P28.5
  sample of cytologic smear
    anus R85.615
    cervix R87.615
    vagina R87.625
  social F60.7
    insurance Z59.7
    skills NEC Z73.4
  supervision of child by parent Z62.0
  teaching affecting education Z55.8
  welfare support Z59.7
Inanition R64
  with edema — *see* Malnutrition, severe
  due to
    deprivation of food T73.0 ☑
    malnutrition — *see* Malnutrition
  fever R50.9
Inappropriate
  change in quantitative human chorionic gonadotropin
    (hCG) in early pregnancy O02.81
  diet or eating habits Z72.4
  level of quantitative human chorionic gonadotropin
    (hCG) for gestational age in early pregnancy
    O02.81
  secretion
    antidiuretic hormone (ADH) (excessive) E22.2
      deficiency E23.2
    pituitary (posterior) E22.2
Inattention at or after birth — *see* Neglect
Incarceration, incarcerated
  enterocele K46.0
    gangrenous K46.1
  epiplocele K46.0
    gangrenous K46.1
  exophthalmos K42.0
    gangrenous K42.1
  hernia (*see also* Hernia, by site, with obstruction)

Incarceration, incarcerated — *continued*
  hernia (*see also* Hernia, by site, with obstruction) —
    continued
    with gangrene — *see* Hernia, by site, with gan-
      grene
  iris, in wound — *see* Injury, eye, laceration, with pro-
    lapse
  lens, in wound — *see* Injury, eye, laceration, with
    prolapse
  omphalocele K42.0
  prison, anxiety concerning Z65.1
  rupture — *see* Hernia, by site
  sarcoepiplocele K46.0
    gangrenous K46.1
  sarcoepiplomphalocele K42.0
    with gangrene K42.1
  uterus N85.8
    gravid O34.51- ☑
      causing obstructed labor O65.5
Incised wound
  external — *see* Laceration
  internal organs — *see* Injury, by site
Incision, incisional
  hernia K43.2
    with
      gangrene (and obstruction) K43.1
      obstruction K43.0
  surgical, complication — *see* Complications, surgical
    procedure
  traumatic
    external — *see* Laceration
    internal organs — *see* Injury, by site
Inclusion
  azurophilic leukocytic D72.0
  blennorrhea (neonatal) (newborn) P39.1
  gallbladder in liver (congenital) Q44.1
Incompatibility
  ABO
    affecting management of pregnancy O36.11- ☑
      anti-A sensitization O36.11- ☑
      anti-B sensitization O36.19- ☑
      specified NEC O36.19- ☑
    infusion or transfusion reaction — *see* Complica-
      tion(s), transfusion, incompatibility reaction,
      ABO
    newborn P55.1
  blood (group) (Duffy) (K(ell)) (Kidd) (Lewis) (M) (S) NEC
    affecting management of pregnancy O36.11- ☑
      anti-A sensitization O36.11- ☑
      anti-B sensitization O36.19- ☑
    infusion or transfusion reaction T80.89 ☑
    newborn P55.8
  divorce or estrangement Z63.5
  Rh (blood group) (factor) Z31.82
    affecting management of pregnancy NEC
      O36.09- ☑
      anti-D antibody O36.01- ☑
    infusion or transfusion reaction — *see* Complica-
      tion(s), transfusion, incompatibility reaction,
      Rh (factor)
    newborn P55.0
  rhesus — *see* Incompatibility, Rh
Incompetency, incompetent, incompetence
  annular
    aortic (valve) — *see* Insufficiency, aortic
    mitral (valve) I34.0
    pulmonary valve (heart) I37.1
  aortic (valve) — *see* Insufficiency, aortic
  cardiac valve — *see* Endocarditis
  cervix, cervical (os) N88.3
    in pregnancy O34.3- ☑
  chronotropic I45.89
    with
      autonomic dysfunction G90.8
      ischemic heart disease I25.89
      left ventricular dysfunction I51.89
      sinus node dysfunction I49.8
  esophagogastric (junction) (sphincter) K22.0
  mitral (valve) — *see* Insufficiency, mitral
  pelvic fundus N81.89
  pubocervical tissue N81.82
  pulmonary valve (heart) I37.1
    congenital Q22.3
  rectovaginal tissue N81.83
  tricuspid (annular) (valve) — *see* Insufficiency, tricuspid
  valvular — *see* Endocarditis
    congenital Q24.8

174

☑ **Additional Character Required** — Refer to the Tabular List for Character Selection   ▽ **Subterms under main terms may continue to next column or page**

Incompetency, incompetent, incompetence — *continued*
 vein, venous (saphenous) (varicose) — *see* Varix, leg
Incomplete (*see also* condition)
 bladder, emptying R33.9
 defecation R15.0
 expansion lungs (newborn) NEC — *see* Atelectasis
 rotation, intestine Q43.3
Inconclusive
 diagnostic imaging due to excess body fat of patient R93.9
 findings on diagnostic imaging of breast NEC R92.8
 mammogram (due to dense breasts) R92.2
Incontinence R32
 anal sphincter R15.9
 feces R15.9
  nonorganic origin F98.1
 overflow N39.490
 psychogenic F45.8
 rectal R15.9
 reflex N39.498
 stress (female) (male) N39.3
  and urge N39.46
 urethral sphincter R32
 urge N39.41
  and stress (female) (male) N39.46
 urine (urinary) R32
  continuous N39.45
  due to cognitive impairment, or severe physical disability or immobility R39.81
  functional R39.81
  mixed (stress and urge) N39.46
  nocturnal N39.44
  nonorganic origin F98.0
  overflow N39.490
  post dribbling N39.43
  reflex N39.498
  specified NEC N39.498
  stress (female) (male) N39.3
   and urge N39.46
  total N39.498
  unaware N39.42
  urge N39.41
   and stress (female) (male) N39.46
Incontinentia pigmenti Q82.3
Incoordinate, incoordination
 esophageal-pharyngeal (newborn) — *see* Dysphagia
 muscular R27.8
 uterus (action) (contractions) (complicating delivery) O62.4
Increase, increased
 abnormal, in development R63.8
 androgens (ovarian) E28.1
 anticoagulants (antithrombin) (anti-VIIIa) (anti-IXa) (anti-Xa) (anti-XIa) — *see* Circulating anticoagulants
 cold sense R20.8
 estrogen E28.0
 function
  adrenal
   cortex — *see* Cushing's, syndrome
   medulla E27.5
  pituitary (gland) (anterior) (lobe) E22.9
   posterior E22.2
 heat sense R20.8
 intracranial pressure (benign) G93.2
 permeability, capillaries I78.8
 pressure, intracranial G93.2
 secretion
  gastrin E16.4
  glucagon E16.3
  pancreas, endocrine E16.9
   growth hormone-releasing hormone E16.8
   pancreatic polypeptide E16.8
   somatostatin E16.8
   vasoactive-intestinal polypeptide E16.8
 sphericity, lens Q12.4
 splenic activity D73.1
 venous pressure I87.8
  portal K76.6
Increta placenta O43.22- ☑
Incrustation, cornea, foreign body (lead)(zinc) — *see* Foreign body, cornea
Incyclophoria H50.54
Incyclotropia — *see* Cyclotropia
Indeterminate sex Q56.4
India rubber skin Q82.8
Indigestion (acid) (bilious) (functional) K30

Indigestion — *continued*
 catarrhal K31.89
 due to decomposed food NOS A05.9
 nervous F45.8
 psychogenic F45.8
Indirect — *see* condition
Induratio penis plastica N48.6
Induration, indurated
 brain G93.89
 breast (fibrous) N64.51
  puerperal, postpartum O92.29
 broad ligament N83.8
 chancre
  anus A51.1
  congenital A50.07
  extragenital NEC A51.2
 corpora cavernosa (penis) (plastic) N48.6
 liver (chronic) K76.89
 lung (black) (chronic) (fibroid) (*see also* Fibrosis, lung) J84.10
  essential brown J84.03
 penile (plastic) N48.6
 phlebitic — *see* Phlebitis
 skin R23.4
Inebriety (without dependence) — *see* Alcohol, intoxication
Inefficiency, kidney N28.9
Inelasticity, skin R23.4
Inequality, leg (length) (acquired) (*see also* Deformity, limb, unequal length)
 congenital — *see* Defect, reduction, lower limb
 lower leg — *see* Deformity, limb, unequal length
Inertia
 bladder (neurogenic) N31.2
 stomach K31.89
  psychogenic F45.8
 uterus, uterine during labor O62.2
  during latent phase of labor O62.0
  primary O62.0
  secondary O62.1
 vesical (neurogenic) N31.2
Infancy, infantile, infantilism (*see also* condition)
 celiac K90.0
 genitalia, genitals (after puberty) E30.0
 Herter's (nontropical sprue) K90.0
 intestinal K90.0
 Lorain E23.0
 pancreatic K86.8
 pelvis M95.5
  with disproportion (fetopelvic) O33.1
   causing obstructed labor O65.1
 pituitary E23.0
 renal N25.0
 uterus — *see* Infantile, genitalia
Infant(s) (*see also* Infancy)
 excessive crying R68.11
 irritable child R68.12
 lack of care — *see* Neglect
 liveborn (singleton) Z38.2
  born in hospital Z38.00
   by cesarean Z38.01
  born outside hospital Z38.1
  multiple NEC Z38.8
   born in hospital Z38.68
    by cesarean Z38.69
   born outside hospital Z38.7
  quadruplet Z38.8
   born in hospital Z38.63
    by cesarean Z38.64
   born outside hospital Z38.7
  quintuplet Z38.8
   born in hospital Z38.65
    by cesarean Z38.66
   born outside hospital Z38.7
  triplet Z38.8
   born in hospital Z38.61
    by cesarean Z38.62
   born outside hospital Z38.7
  twin Z38.5
   born in hospital Z38.30
    by cesarean Z38.31
   born outside hospital Z38.4
 of diabetic mother (syndrome of) P70.1
  gestational diabetes P70.0
Infantile (*see also* condition)
 genitalia, genitals E30.0
 os, uterine E30.0
 penis E30.0

Infantile — *continued*
 testis E29.1
 uterus E30.0
Infantilism — *see* Infancy
Infarct, infarction
 adrenal (capsule) (gland) E27.49
 appendices epiploicae K55.0
 bowel K55.0
 brain (stem) — *see* Infarct, cerebral
 breast N64.89
 brewer's (kidney) N28.0
 cardiac — *see* Infarct, myocardium
 cerebellar — *see* Infarct, cerebral
 cerebral (*see also* Occlusion, artery cerebral or precerebral, with infarction) I63.9
  aborted I63.9
  cortical I63.9
  due to
   cerebral venous thrombosis, nonpyogenic I63.6
   embolism
    cerebral arteries I63.4- ☑
    precerebral arteries I63.1- ☑
   occlusion NEC
    cerebral arteries I63.5- ☑
    precerebral arteries I63.2- ☑
   stenosis NEC
    cerebral arteries I63.5- ☑
    precerebral arteries I63.2- ☑
   thrombosis
    cerebral artery I63.3- ☑
    precerebral artery I63.0- ☑
  intraoperative
   during cardiac surgery I97.810
   during other surgery I97.811
  postprocedural
   following cardiac surgery I97.820
   following other surgery I97.821
  specified NEC I63.8
 colon (acute) (agnogenic) (embolic) (hemorrhagic) (nonocclusive) (nonthrombotic) (occlusive) (segmental) (thrombotic) (with gangrene) K55.0
 coronary artery — *see* Infarct, myocardium
 embolic — *see* Embolism
 fallopian tube N83.8
 gallbladder K82.8
 heart — *see* Infarct, myocardium
 hepatic K76.3
 hypophysis (anterior lobe) E23.6
 impending (myocardium) I20.0
 intestine (acute) (agnogenic) (embolic) (hemorrhagic) (nonocclusive) (nonthrombotic) (occlusive) (thrombotic) (with gangrene) K55.0
 kidney N28.0
 liver K76.3
 lung (embolic) (thrombotic) — *see* Embolism, pulmonary
 lymph node I89.8
 mesentery, mesenteric (embolic) (thrombotic) (with gangrene) K55.0
 muscle (ischemic) M62.20
  ankle M62.27- ☑
  foot M62.27- ☑
  forearm M62.23- ☑
  hand M62.24- ☑
  lower leg M62.26- ☑
  pelvic region M62.25- ☑
  shoulder region M62.21- ☑
  specified site NEC M62.28
  thigh M62.25- ☑
  upper arm M62.22- ☑
 myocardium, myocardial (acute) (with stated duration of 4 weeks or less) I21.3
  diagnosed on ECG, but presenting no symptoms I25.2
  healed or old I25.2
  intraoperative
   during cardiac surgery I97.790
   during other surgery I97.791
  non-Q wave I21.4
  non-ST elevation (NSTEMI) I21.4
   subsequent I22.2
  nontransmural I21.4
  past (diagnosed on ECG or other investigation, but currently presenting no symptoms) I25.2
  postprocedural
   following cardiac surgery I97.190
   following other surgery I97.191
  Q wave (see also, Infarct, myocardium, by site) I21.3

Infarct, infarction — *continued*
  myocardium, myocardial — *continued*
    ST elevation (STEMI) I21.3
      anterior (anteroapical) (anterolateral) (anteroseptal) (Q wave) (wall) I21.09
        subsequent I22.0
      inferior (diaphragmatic) (inferolateral) (inferoposterior) (wall) NEC I21.19
        subsequent I22.1
      inferoposterior transmural (Q wave) I21.11
      involving
        coronary artery of anterior wall NEC I21.09
        coronary artery of inferior wall NEC I21.19
        diagonal coronary artery I21.02
        left anterior descending coronary artery I21.02
        left circumflex coronary artery I21.21
        left main coronary artery I21.01
        oblique marginal coronary artery I21.21
        right coronary artery I21.11
      lateral (apical-lateral) (basal-lateral) (high) I21.29
        subsequent I22.8
      posterior (posterobasal) (posterolateral) (posteroseptal) (true) I21.29
        subsequent I22.8
      septal I21.29
        subsequent I22.8
      specified NEC I21.29
        subsequent I22.8
      subsequent I22.9
    subsequent (recurrent) (reinfarction) I22.9
      anterior (anteroapical) (anterolateral) (anteroseptal) (wall) I22.0
      diaphragmatic (wall) I22.1
      inferior (diaphragmatic) (inferolateral) (inferoposterior) (wall) I22.1
      lateral (apical-lateral) (basal-lateral) (high) I22.8
      non-ST elevation (NSTEMI) I22.2
      posterior (posterobasal) (posterolateral) (posteroseptal) (true) I22.8
      septal I22.8
      specified NEC I22.8
      ST elevation I22.9
        anterior (anteroapical) (anterolateral) (anteroseptal) (wall) I22.0
        inferior (diaphragmatic) (inferolateral) (inferoposterior) (wall) I22.1
        specified NEC I22.8
      subendocardial I22.2
      transmural I22.9
        anterior (anteroapical) (anterolateral) (anteroseptal) (wall) I22.0
        diaphragmatic (wall) I22.1
        inferior (diaphragmatic) (inferolateral) (inferoposterior) (wall) I22.1
        lateral (apical-lateral) (basal-lateral) (high) I22.8
        posterior (posterobasal) (posterolateral) (posteroseptal) (true) I22.8
        specified NEC I22.8
    syphilitic A52.06
    transmural I21.3
      anterior (anteroapical) (anterolateral) (anteroseptal) (Q wave) (wall) NEC I21.09
      inferior (diaphragmatic) (inferolateral) (inferoposterior) (Q wave) (wall) NEC I21.19
      inferoposterior (Q wave) I21.11
      lateral (apical-lateral) (basal-lateral) (high) NEC I21.29
      posterior (posterobasal) (posterolateral) (posteroseptal) (true) NEC I21.29
      septal NEC I21.29
      specified NEC I21.29
    nontransmural I21.4
  omentum K55.0
  ovary N83.8
  pancreas K86.8
  papillary muscle — *see* Infarct, myocardium
  parathyroid gland E21.4
  pituitary (gland) E23.6
  placenta O43.81- ☑
  prostate N42.89
  pulmonary (artery) (vein) (hemorrhagic) — *see* Embolism, pulmonary
  renal (embolic) (thrombotic) N28.0
  retina, retinal (artery) — *see* Occlusion, artery, retina
  spinal (cord) (acute) (embolic) (nonembolic) G95.11

Infarct, infarction — *continued*
  spleen D73.5
    embolic or thrombotic I74.8
  subendocardial (acute) (nontransmural) I21.4
  suprarenal (capsule) (gland) E27.49
  testis N50.1
  thrombotic (*see also* Thrombosis)
    artery, arterial — *see* Embolism
  thyroid (gland) E07.89
  ventricle (heart) — *see* Infarct, myocardium
Infecting — *see* condition
Infection, infected, infective (opportunistic) B99.9
  with
    drug resistant organism — *see* Resistance (to), drug (*see also* specific organism)
    lymphangitis — *see* Lymphangitis
    organ dysfunction (acute) R65.20
      with septic shock R65.21
  abscess (skin) — *code by* site under Abscess
  Absidia — *see* Mucormycosis
  Acanthamoeba — *see* Acanthamebiasis
  Acanthocheilonema (perstans) (streptocerca) B74.4
  accessory sinus (chronic) — *see* Sinusitis
  achorion — *see* Dermatophytosis
  Acremonium falciforme B47.0
  acromioclavicular M00.9
  Actinobacillus (actinomycetem-comitans) A28.8
    mallei A24.0
    muris A25.1
  Actinomadura B47.1
  Actinomyces (israelii) (*see also* Actinomycosis) A42.9
  Actinomycetales — *see* Actinomycosis
  actinomycotic NOS — *see* Actinomycosis
  adenoid (and tonsil) J03.90
    chronic J35.02
  adenovirus NEC
    as cause of disease classified elsewhere B97.0
    unspecified nature or site B34.0
  aerogenes capsulatus A48.0
  aertrycke — *see* Infection, salmonella
  alimentary canal NOS — *see* Enteritis, infectious
  Allescheria boydii B48.2
  Alternaria B48.8
  alveolus, alveolar (process) K04.7
  Ameba, amebic (histolytica) — *see* Amebiasis
  amniotic fluid, sac or cavity O41.10- ☑
    chorioamnionitis O41.12- ☑
    placentitis O41.14- ☑
  amputation stump (surgical) — *see* Complication, amputation stump, infection
  Ancylostoma (duodenalis) B76.0
  Anisakiasis, Anisakis larvae B81.0
  anthrax — *see* Anthrax
  antrum (chronic) — *see* Sinusitis, maxillary
  anus, anal (papillae) (sphincter) K62.89
  arbovirus (arbor virus) A94
    specified type NEC A93.8
  artificial insemination N98.0
  Ascaris lumbricoides — *see* Ascariasis
  Ascomycetes B47.0
  Aspergillus (flavus) (fumigatus) (terreus) — *see* Aspergillosis
  atypical
    acid-fast (bacilli) — *see* Mycobacterium, atypical
    mycobacteria — *see* Mycobacterium, atypical
    virus A81.9
      specified type NEC A81.89
  auditory meatus (external) — *see* Otitis, externa, infective
  auricle (ear) — *see* Otitis, externa, infective
  axillary gland (lymph) L04.2
  Bacillus A49.9
    abortus A23.1
    anthracis — *see* Anthrax
    Ducrey's (any location) A57
    Flexner's A03.1
    Friedländer's NEC A49.8
    gas (gangrene) A48.0
    mallei A24.0
    melitensis A23.0
    paratyphoid, paratyphosus A01.4
      A A01.1
      B A01.2
      C A01.3
    Shiga (-Kruse) A03.0
    suipestifer — *see* Infection, salmonella
    swimming pool A31.1

Infection, infected, infective — *continued*
  Bacillus — *continued*
    typhosa A01.00
    welchii — *see* Gangrene, gas
  bacterial NOS A49.9
    as cause of disease classified elsewhere B96.89
      Bacteroides fragilis [B. fragilis] B96.6
      Clostridium perfringens [C. perfringens] B96.7
      Enterobacter sakazakii B96.89
      Enterococcus B95.2
      Escherichia coli [E. coli] (*see also* Escherichia coli) B96.20
      Helicobacter pylori [H.pylori] B96.81
      Hemophilus influenzae [H. influenzae] B96.3
      Klebsiella pneumoniae [K. pneumoniae] B96.1
      Mycoplasma pneumoniae [M. pneumoniae] B96.0
      Proteus (mirabilis) (morganii) B96.4
      Pseudomonas (aeruginosa) (mallei) (pseudomallei) B96.5
      Staphylococcus B95.8
        aureus (methicillin susceptible) (MSSA) B95.61
          methicillin resistant (MRSA) B95.62
        specified NEC B95.7
      Streptococcus B95.5
        group A B95.0
        group B B95.1
        pneumoniae B95.3
        specified NEC B95.4
      Vibrio vulnificus B96.82
    specified NEC A48.8
  Bacterium
    paratyphosum A01.4
      A A01.1
      B A01.2
      C A01.3
    typhosum A01.00
  Bacteroides NEC A49.8
    fragilis, as cause of disease classified elsewhere B96.6
  Balantidium coli A07.0
  Bartholin's gland N75.8
  Basidiobolus B46.8
  bile duct (common) (hepatic) — *see* Cholangitis
  bladder — *see* Cystitis
  Blastomyces, blastomycotic (*see also* Blastomycosis)
    brasiliensis — *see* Paracoccidioidomycosis
    dermatitidis — *see* Blastomycosis
    European — *see* Cryptococcosis
    Loboi B48.0
    North American B40.9
    South American — *see* Paracoccidioidomycosis
  bleb, postprocedure — *see* Blebitis
  bone — *see* Osteomyelitis
  Bordetella — *see* Whooping cough
  Borrelia bergdorfi A69.20
  brain (*see also* Encephalitis) G04.90
    membranes — *see* Meningitis
    septic G06.0
      meninges — *see* Meningitis, bacterial
  branchial cyst Q18.0
  breast — *see* Mastitis
  bronchus — *see* Bronchitis
  Brucella A23.9
    abortus A23.1
    canis A23.3
    melitensis A23.0
    mixed A23.8
    specified NEC A23.8
    suis A23.2
  Brugia (malayi) B74.1
    timori B74.2
  bursa — *see* Bursitis, infective
  buttocks (skin) L08.9
  Campylobacter, intestinal A04.5
    as cause of disease classified elsewhere B96.81
  Candida (albicans) (tropicalis) — *see* Candidiasis
  candiru B88.8
  Capillaria (intestinal) B81.1
    hepatica B83.8
    philippinensis B81.1
  cartilage — *see* Disorder, cartilage, specified type NEC
  cat liver fluke B66.0
  catheter-related bloodstream (CRBSI) T80.211 ☑
  cellulitis — *code by* site under Cellulitis
  central line-associated T80.219 ☑
    bloodstream (CLABSI) T80.211 ☑

☑ **Additional Character Required** — Refer to the Tabular List for Character Selection   ▽ **Subterms under main terms may continue to next column or page**

Infection, infected, infective — *continued*
- central line-associated — *continued*
  - specified NEC T80.218 ☑
- Cephalosporium falciforme B47.0
- cerebrospinal — *see* Meningitis
- cervical gland (lymph) L04.0
- cervix — *see* Cervicitis
- cesarean delivery wound (puerperal) O86.0
- cestodes — *see* Infestation, cestodes
- chest J22
- Chilomastix (intestinal) A07.8
- Chlamydia, chlamydial A74.9
  - anus A56.3
  - genitourinary tract A56.2
    - lower A56.00
    - specified NEC A56.19
  - lymphogranuloma A55
  - pharynx A56.4
  - psittaci A70
  - rectum A56.3
  - sexually transmitted NEC A56.8
- cholera — *see* Cholera
- Cladosporium
  - bantianum (brain abscess) B43.1
  - carrionii B43.0
  - castellanii B36.1
  - trichoides (brain abscess) B43.1
  - werneckii B36.1
- Clonorchis (sinensis) (liver) B66.1
- Clostridium NEC
  - bifermentans A48.0
  - botulinum (food poisoning) A05.1
    - infant A48.51
    - wound A48.52
  - difficile
    - as cause of disease classified elsewhere B96.89
    - foodborne (disease) A04.7
    - gas gangrene A48.0
    - necrotizing enterocolitis A04.7
    - sepsis A41.4
  - gas-forming NEC A48.0
  - histolyticum A48.0
  - novyi, causing gas gangrene A48.0
  - oedematiens A48.0
  - perfringens
    - as cause of disease classified elsewhere B96.7
    - due to food A05.2
    - foodborne (disease) A05.2
    - gas gangrene A48.0
    - sepsis A41.4
  - septicum, causing gas gangrene A48.0
  - sordellii, causing gas gangrene A48.0
  - welchii
    - as cause of disease classified elsewhere B96.7
    - foodborne (disease) A05.2
    - gas gangrene A48.0
    - necrotizing enteritis A05.2
    - sepsis A41.4
- Coccidioides (immitis) — *see* Coccidioidomycosis
- colon — *see* Enteritis, infectious
- colostomy K94.02
- common duct — *see* Cholangitis
- congenital P39.9
  - Candida (albicans) P37.5
  - cytomegalovirus P35.1
  - hepatitis, viral P35.3
  - herpes simplex P35.2
  - infectious or parasitic disease P37.9
    - specified NEC P37.8
  - listeriosis (disseminated) P37.2
  - malaria NEC P37.4
    - falciparum P37.3
  - Plasmodium falciparum P37.3
  - poliomyelitis P35.8
  - rubella P35.0
  - skin P39.4
  - toxoplasmosis (acute) (subacute) (chronic) P37.1
  - tuberculosis P37.0
  - urinary (tract) P39.3
  - vaccinia P35.8
  - virus P35.9
    - specified type NEC P35.8
- Conidiobolus B46.8
- coronavirus NEC B34.2
  - as cause of disease classified elsewhere B97.29
  - severe acute respiratory syndrome (SARS associated) B97.21
- corpus luteum — *see* Salpingo-oophoritis

Infection, infected, infective — *continued*
- Corynebacterium diphtheriae — *see* Diphtheria
- cotia virus B08.8
- Coxiella burnetii A78
- coxsackie — *see* Coxsackie
- Cryptococcus neoformans — *see* Cryptococcosis
- Cryptosporidium A07.2
- Cunninghamella — *see* Mucormycosis
- cyst — *see* Cyst
- cystic duct (*see also* Cholecystitis) K81.9
- Cysticercus cellulosae — *see* Cysticercosis
- cytomegalovirus, cytomegaloviral B25.9
  - congenital P35.1
  - maternal, maternal care for (suspected) damage to fetus O35.3 ☑
  - mononucleosis B27.10
    - with
      - complication NEC B27.19
      - meningitis B27.12
      - polyneuropathy B27.11
- delta-agent (acute), in hepatitis B carrier B17.0
- dental (pulpal origin) K04.7
- Deuteromycetes B47.0
- Dicrocoelium dendriticum B66.2
- Dipetalonema (perstans) (streptocerca) B74.4
- diphtherial — *see* Diphtheria
- Diphyllobothrium (adult) (latum) (pacificum) B70.0
  - larval B70.1
- Diplogonoporus (grandis) B71.8
- Dipylidium caninum B67.4
- Dirofilaria B74.8
- Dracunculus medinensis B72
- Drechslera (hawaiiensis) B43.8
- Ducrey Haemophilus (any location) A57
- due to or resulting from
  - artificial insemination N98.0
  - central venous catheter T80.219 ☑
    - bloodstream T80.211 ☑
    - exit or insertion site T80.212 ☑
    - localized T80.212 ☑
    - port or reservoir T80.212 ☑
    - specified NEC T80.218 ☑
    - tunnel T80.212 ☑
  - device, implant or graft (*see also* Complications, by site and type, infection or inflammation) T85.79 ☑
    - arterial graft NEC T82.7 ☑
    - breast (implant) T85.79 ☑
    - catheter NEC T85.79 ☑
      - dialysis (renal) T82.7 ☑
        - intraperitoneal T85.71 ☑
      - infusion NEC T82.7 ☑
        - spinal (epidural) (subdural) T85.79 ☑
      - urinary (indwelling) T83.51 ☑
    - electronic (electrode) (pulse generator) (stimulator)
      - bone T84.7 ☑
      - cardiac T82.7 ☑
      - nervous system (brain) (peripheral nerve) (spinal) T85.79 ☑
      - urinary T83.59 ☑
    - fixation, internal (orthopedic) NEC — *see* Complication, fixation device, infection
    - gastrointestinal (bile duct) (esophagus) T85.79 ☑
    - genital NEC T83.6 ☑
    - heart NEC T82.7 ☑
      - valve (prosthesis) T82.6 ☑
        - graft T82.7 ☑
    - joint prosthesis — *see* Complication, joint prosthesis, infection
    - ocular (corneal graft) (orbital implant) NEC T85.79 ☑
    - orthopedic NEC T84.7 ☑
    - specified NEC T85.79 ☑
    - urinary NEC T83.59 ☑
    - vascular NEC T82.7 ☑
    - ventricular intracranial shunt T85.79 ☑
  - Hickman catheter T80.219 ☑
    - bloodstream T80.211 ☑
    - localized T80.212 ☑
    - specified NEC T80.218 ☑
  - immunization or vaccination T88.0 ☑
  - infusion, injection or transfusion NEC T80.29 ☑
  - injury NEC — *code by* site under Wound, open
  - peripherally inserted central catheter (PICC) T80.219 ☑

Infection, infected, infective — *continued*
- due to or resulting from — *continued*
  - peripherally inserted central catheter — *continued*
    - bloodstream T80.211 ☑
    - localized T80.212 ☑
    - specified NEC T80.218 ☑
  - portacath (port-a-cath) T80.219 ☑
    - bloodstream T80.211 ☑
    - localized T80.212 ☑
    - specified NEC T80.218 ☑
  - surgery T81.4 ☑
  - triple lumen catheter T80.219 ☑
    - bloodstream T80.211 ☑
    - localized T80.212 ☑
    - specified NEC T80.218 ☑
  - umbilical venous catheter T80.219 ☑
    - bloodstream T80.211 ☑
    - localized T80.212 ☑
    - specified NEC T80.218 ☑
- during labor NEC O75.3
- ear (middle) (*see also* Otitis media)
  - external — *see* Otitis, externa, infective
  - inner — *see* subcategory H83.0 ☑
- Eberthella typhosa A01.00
- Echinococcus — *see* Echinococcus
- echovirus
  - as cause of disease classified elsewhere B97.12
  - unspecified nature or site B34.1
- endocardium I33.0
- endocervix — *see* Cervicitis
- Entamoeba — *see* Amebiasis
- enteric — *see* Enteritis, infectious
- Enterobacter sakazakii B96.89
- Enterobius vermicularis B80
- enterostomy K94.12
- enterovirus B34.1
  - as cause of disease classified elsewhere B97.10
    - coxsackievirus B97.11
    - echovirus B97.12
    - specified NEC B97.19
- Entomophthora B46.8
- Epidermophyton — *see* Dermatophytosis
- epididymis — *see* Epididymitis
- episiotomy (puerperal) O86.0
- Erysipelothrix (insidiosa) (rhusiopathiae) — *see* Erysipeloid
- erythema infectiosum B08.3
- Escherichia (E.) coli NEC A49.8
  - as cause of disease classified elsewhere (*see also* Escherichia coli) B96.20
  - congenital P39.8
    - sepsis P36.4
  - generalized A41.51
  - intestinal — *see* Enteritis, infectious, due to, Escherichia coli
- ethmoidal (chronic) (sinus) — *see* Sinusitis, ethmoidal
- eustachian tube (ear) — *see* Salpingitis, eustachian
- external auditory canal (meatus) NEC — *see* Otitis, externa, infective
- eye (purulent) — *see* Endophthalmitis, purulent
- eyelid — *see* Inflammation, eyelid
- fallopian tube — *see* Salpingo-oophoritis
- Fasciola (gigantica) (hepatica) (indica) B66.3
- Fasciolopsis (buski) B66.5
- filarial — *see* Infestation, filarial
- finger (skin) L08.9
  - nail L03.01- ☑
    - fungus B35.1
- fish tapeworm B70.0
  - larval B70.1
- flagellate, intestinal A07.9
- fluke — *see* Infestation, fluke
- focal
  - teeth (pulpal origin) K04.7
  - tonsils J35.01
- Fonsecaea (compactum) (pedrosoi) B43.0
- food — *see* Intoxication, foodborne
- foot (skin) L08.9
  - dermatophytic fungus B35.3
- Francisella tularensis — *see* Tularemia
- frontal (sinus) (chronic) — *see* Sinusitis, frontal
- fungus NOS B49
  - beard B35.0
  - dermatophytic — *see* Dermatophytosis
  - foot B35.3
  - groin B35.6

Infection, infected, infective — *continued*
  fungus — *continued*
    hand B35.2
    nail B35.1
    pathogenic to compromised host only B48.8
    perianal (area) B35.6
    scalp B35.0
    skin B36.9
      foot B35.3
      hand B35.2
      toenails B35.1
  Fusarium B48.8
  gallbladder — *see* Cholecystitis
  gas bacillus — *see* Gangrene, gas
  gastrointestinal — *see* Enteritis, infectious
  generalized NEC — *see* Sepsis
  genital organ or tract
    female — *see* Disease, pelvis, inflammatory
    male N49.9
      multiple sites N49.8
      specified NEC N49.8
  Ghon tubercle, primary A15.7
  Giardia lamblia A07.1
  gingiva (chronic) K05.10
    acute K05.00
      nonplaque induced K05.01
      plaque induced K05.00
    nonplaque induced K05.11
    plaque induced K05.10
  glanders A24.0
  glenosporopsis B48.0
  Gnathostoma (spinigerum) B83.1
  Gongylonema B83.8
  gonococcal — *see* Gonococcus
  gram-negative bacilli NOS A49.9
  guinea worm B72
  gum (chronic) K05.10
    acute K05.00
      nonplaque induced K05.01
      plaque induced K05.00
    nonplaque induced K05.11
    plaque induced K05.10
  Haemophilus — *see* Infection, Hemophilus
  heart — *see* Carditis
  Helicobacter pylori A04.8
    as cause of disease classified elsewhere B96.81
  helminths B83.9
    intestinal B82.0
      mixed (types classifiable to more than one of
        the titles B65.0–B81.3 and B81.8) B81.4
      specified type NEC B81.8
    specified type NEC B83.8
  Hemophilus
    aegyptius, systemic A48.4
    ducrey (any location) A57
    generalized A41.3
    influenzae NEC A49.2
      as cause of disease classified elsewhere B96.3
  herpes (simplex) (*see also* Herpes)
    congenital P35.2
    disseminated B00.7
    zoster B02.9
  herpesvirus, herpesviral — *see* Herpes
  Heterophyes (heterophyes) B66.8
  hip (joint) NEC M00.9
    due to internal joint prosthesis
      left T84.52 ☑
      right T84.51 ☑
    skin NEC L08.9
  Histoplasma — *see* Histoplasmosis
    American B39.4
    capsulatum B39.4
  hookworm B76.9
  human
    papilloma virus A63.0
    T-cell lymphotropic virus type-1 (HTLV-1) B33.3
  hydrocele N43.0
  Hymenolepis B71.0
  hypopharynx — *see* Pharyngitis
  inguinal (lymph) glands L04.1
    due to soft chancre A57
  intervertebral disc, pyogenic M46.30
    cervical region M46.32
    cervicothoracic region M46.33
    lumbar region M46.36
    lumbosacral region M46.37
    multiple sites M46.39
    occipito-atlanto-axial region M46.31

Infection, infected, infective — *continued*
  intervertebral disc, pyogenic — *continued*
    sacrococcygeal region M46.38
    thoracic region M46.34
    thoracolumbar region M46.35
  intestine, intestinal — *see* Enteritis, infectious
    specified NEC A08.8
  intra-amniotic affecting newborn NEC P39.2
  Isospora belli or hominis A07.3
  Japanese B encephalitis A83.0
  jaw (bone) (lower) (upper) M27.2
  joint NEC M00.9
    due to internal joint prosthesis T84.50 ☑
  kidney (cortex) (hematogenous) N15.9
    with calculus N20.0
      with hydronephrosis N13.6
    following ectopic gestation O08.83
    pelvis and ureter (cystic) N28.85
    puerperal (postpartum) O86.21
    specified NEC N15.8
  Klebsiella (K.) pneumoniae NEC A49.8
    as cause of disease classified elsewhere B96.1
  knee (joint) NEC M00.9
    due to internal joint prosthesis
      left T84.54 ☑
      right T84.53 ☑
    joint M00.9
    skin L08.9
  Koch's — *see* Tuberculosis
  labia (majora) (minora) (acute) — *see* Vulvitis
  lacrimal
    gland — *see* Dacryoadenitis
    passages (duct) (sac) — *see* Inflammation, lacrimal,
      passages
  lancet fluke B66.2
  larynx NEC J38.7
  leg (skin) NOS L08.9
  Legionella pneumophila A48.1
    nonpneumonic A48.2
  Leishmania (*see also* Leishmaniasis)
    aethiopica B55.1
    braziliensis B55.2
    chagasi B55.0
    donovani B55.0
    infantum B55.0
    major B55.1
    mexicana B55.1
    tropica B55.1
  lentivirus, as cause of disease classified elsewhere
    B97.31
  Leptosphaeria senegalensis B47.0
  Leptospira interrogans A27.9
    autumnalis A27.89
    canicola A27.89
    hebdomadis A27.89
    icterohaemorrhagiae A27.0
    pomona A27.89
    specified type NEC A27.89
  leptospirochetal NEC — *see* Leptospirosis
  Listeria monocytogenes (*see also* Listeriosis)
    congenital P37.2
  Loa loa B74.3
    with conjunctival infestation B74.3
    eyelid B74.3
  Loboa loboi B48.0
  local, skin (staphylococcal) (streptococcal) L08.9
    abscess — *code by* site under Abscess
    cellulitis — *code by* site under Cellulitis
    specified NEC L08.89
    ulcer — *see* Ulcer, skin
  Loefflerella mallei A24.0
  lung (*see also* Pneumonia) J18.9
    atypical Mycobacterium A31.0
    spirochetal A69.8
    tuberculous — *see* Tuberculosis, pulmonary
    virus — *see* Pneumonia, viral
  lymph gland (*see also* Lymphadenitis, acute)
    mesenteric I88.0
  lymphoid tissue, base of tongue or posterior pharynx,
    NEC (chronic) J35.03
  Madurella (grisea) (mycetomii) B47.0
  major
    following ectopic or molar pregnancy O08.0
    puerperal, postpartum, childbirth O85
  Malassezia furfur B36.0
  Malleomyces
    mallei A24.0
    pseudomallei (whitmori) — *see* Melioidosis

Infection, infected, infective — *continued*
  mammary gland N61
  Mansonella (ozzardi) (perstans) (streptocerca) B74.4
  mastoid — *see* Mastoiditis
  maxilla, maxillary M27.2
    sinus (chronic) — *see* Sinusitis, maxillary
  mediastinum J98.5
  Medina (worm) B72
  meibomian cyst or gland — *see* Hordeolum
  meninges — *see* Meningitis, bacterial
  meningococcal (*see also* condition) A39.9
    adrenals A39.1
    brain A39.81
    cerebrospinal A39.0
    conjunctiva A39.89
    endocardium A39.51
    heart A39.50
      endocardium A39.51
      myocardium A39.52
      pericardium A39.53
    joint A39.83
    meninges A39.0
    meningococcemia A39.4
      acute A39.2
      chronic A39.3
    myocardium A39.52
    pericardium A39.53
    retrobulbar neuritis A39.82
    specified site NEC A39.89
  mesenteric lymph nodes or glands NEC I88.0
  Metagonimus B66.8
  metatarsophalangeal M00.9
  methicillin
    resistant Staphylococcus aureus (MRSA) A49.02
    susceptible Staphylococcus aureus (MSSA) A49.01
  Microsporum, microsporic — *see* Dermatophytosis
  mixed flora (bacterial) NEC A49.8
  Monilia — *see* Candidiasis
  Monosporium apiospermum B48.2
  mouth, parasitic B37.0
  Mucor — *see* Mucormycosis
  muscle NEC — *see* Myositis, infective
  mycelium NOS B49
  mycetoma B47.9
    actinomycotic NEC B47.1
    mycotic NEC B47.0
  Mycobacterium, mycobacterial — *see* Mycobacterium
  Mycoplasma NEC A49.3
    pneumoniae, as cause of disease classified else-
      where B96.0
  mycotic NOS B49
    pathogenic to compromised host only B48.8
    skin NOS B36.9
  myocardium NEC I40.0
  nail (chronic)
    with lymphangitis — *see* Lymphangitis, acute,
      digit
    finger L03.01- ☑
      fungus B35.1
    ingrowing L60.0
    toe L03.03- ☑
      fungus B35.1
  nasal sinus (chronic) — *see* Sinusitis
  nasopharynx — *see* Nasopharyngitis
  navel L08.82
  Necator americanus B76.1
  Neisseria — *see* Gonococcus
  Neotestudina rosatii B47.0
  newborn P39.9
    intra-amniotic NEC P39.2
    skin P39.4
    specified type NEC P39.8
  nipple N61
    associated with
      lactation O91.03
      pregnancy O91.01- ☑
      puerperium O91.02
  Nocardia — *see* Nocardiosis
  obstetrical surgical wound (puerperal) O86.0
  Oesophagostomum (apiostomum) B81.8
  Oestrus ovis — *see* Myiasis
  Oidium albicans B37.9
  Onchocerca (volvulus) — *see* Onchocerciasis
  oncovirus, as cause of disease classified elsewhere
    B97.32
  operation wound T81.4 ☑
  Opisthorchis (felineus) (viverrini) B66.0
  orbit, orbital — *see* Inflammation, orbit

☑ Additional Character Required — Refer to the Tabular List for Character Selection   ▽ Subterms under main terms may continue to next column or page

Infection, infected, infective — *continued*
- orthopoxvirus NEC B08.09
- ovary — *see* Salpingo-oophoritis
- Oxyuris vermicularis B80
- pancreas (acute) K85.9
  - abscess — *see* Pancreatitis, acute
  - specified NEC K85.8
- papillomavirus, as cause of disease classified elsewhere B97.7
- papovavirus NEC B34.4
- Paracoccidioides brasiliensis — *see* Paracoccidioidomycosis
- Paragonimus (westermani) B66.4
- parainfluenza virus B34.8
- parameningococcus NOS A39.9
- parapoxvirus B08.60
  - specified NEC B08.69
- parasitic B89
- Parastrongylus
  - cantonensis B83.2
  - costaricensis B81.3
  - paratyphoid A01.4
    - Type A A01.1
    - Type B A01.2
    - Type C A01.3
- paraurethral ducts N34.2
- parotid gland — *see* Sialoadenitis
- parvovirus NEC B34.3
  - as cause of disease classified elsewhere B97.6
- Pasteurella NEC A28.0
  - multocida A28.0
  - pestis — *see* Plague
  - pseudotuberculosis A28.0
  - septica (cat bite) (dog bite) A28.0
  - tularensis — *see* Tularemia
- pelvic, female — *see* Disease, pelvis, inflammatory
- Penicillium (marneffei) B48.4
- penis (glans) (retention) NEC N48.29
- periapical K04.5
- peridental, periodontal K05.20
  - generalized K05.22
  - localized K05.21
- perinatal period P39.9
  - specified type NEC P39.8
- perineal repair (puerperal) O86.0
- periorbital — *see* Inflammation, orbit
- perirectal K62.89
- perirenal — *see* Infection, kidney
- peritoneal — *see* Peritonitis
- periureteral N28.89
- Petriellidium boydii B48.2
- pharynx (*see also* Pharyngitis)
  - coxsackievirus B08.5
  - posterior, lymphoid (chronic) J35.03
- Phialophora
  - gougerotii (subcutaneous abscess or cyst) B43.2
  - jeanselmei (subcutaneous abscess or cyst) B43.2
  - verrucosa (skin) B43.0
- Piedraia hortae B36.3
- pinta A67.9
  - intermediate A67.1
  - late A67.2
  - mixed A67.3
  - primary A67.0
- pinworm B80
- pityrosporum furfur B36.0
- pleuro-pneumonia-like organism (PPLO) NEC A49.3
  - as cause of disease classified elsewhere B96.0
- pneumococcus, pneumococcal NEC A49.1
  - as cause of disease classified elsewhere B95.3
  - generalized (purulent) A40.3
    - with pneumonia J13
- Pneumocystis carinii (pneumonia) B59
- Pneumocystis jiroveci (pneumonia) B59
- port or reservoir T80.212 ☑
- postoperative T81.4 ☑
- postoperative wound T81.4 ☑
- postprocedural T81.4 ☑
- postvaccinal T88.0 ☑
- prepuce NEC N47.7
  - with penile inflammation N47.6
- prion — *see* Disease, prion, central nervous system
- prostate (capsule) — *see* Prostatitis
- Proteus (mirabilis) (morganii) (vulgaris) NEC A49.8
  - as cause of disease classified elsewhere B96.4
- protozoal NEC B64
  - intestinal A07.9
    - specified NEC A07.8

Infection, infected, infective — *continued*
- protozoal — *continued*
  - specified NEC B60.8
- Pseudoallescheria boydii B48.2
- Pseudomonas NEC A49.8
  - as cause of disease classified elsewhere B96.5
  - mallei A24.0
  - pneumonia J15.1
  - pseudomallei — *see* Melioidosis
- puerperal O86.4
  - genitourinary tract NEC O86.89
  - major or generalized O85
  - minor O86.4
  - specified NEC O86.89
- pulmonary — *see* Infection, lung
- purulent — *see* Abscess
- Pyrenochaeta romeroi B47.0
- Q fever A78
- rectum (sphincter) K62.89
- renal (*see also* Infection, kidney)
  - pelvis and ureter (cystic) N28.85
- reovirus, as cause of disease classified elsewhere B97.5
- respiratory (tract) NEC J98.8
  - acute J22
  - chronic J98.8
  - influenzal (upper) (acute) — *see* Influenza, with, respiratory manifestations NEC
  - lower (acute) J22
    - chronic — *see* Bronchitis, chronic
  - rhinovirus J00
  - syncytial virus, as cause of disease classified elsewhere B97.4
  - upper (acute) NOS J06.9
    - chronic J39.8
    - streptococcal J06.9
    - viral NOS J06.9
- resulting from
  - presence of internal prosthesis, implant, graft — *see* Complications, by site and type, infection
- retortamoniasis A07.8
- retroperitoneal NEC K68.9
- retrovirus B33.3
  - as cause of disease classified elsewhere B97.30
    - human
      - immunodeficiency, type 2 (HIV 2) B97.35
      - T-cell lymphotropic
        - type I (HTLV-I) B97.33
        - type II (HTLV-II) B97.34
    - lentivirus B97.31
    - oncovirus B97.32
    - specified NEC B97.39
- Rhinosporidium (seeberi) B48.1
- rhinovirus
  - as cause of disease classified elsewhere B97.89
  - unspecified nature or site B34.8
- Rhizopus — *see* Mucormycosis
- rickettsial NOS A79.9
- roundworm (large) NEC B82.0
  - Ascariasis (*see also* Ascariasis) B77.9
- rubella — *see* Rubella
- Saccharomyces — *see* Candidiasis
- salivary duct or gland (any) — *see* Sialoadenitis
- Salmonella (aertrycke) (arizonae) (callinarum) (cholerae-suis) (enteritidis) (suipestifer) (typhimurium) A02.9
  - with
    - (gastro)enteritis A02.0
    - sepsis A02.1
    - specified manifestation NEC A02.8
  - due to food (poisoning) A02.9
  - hirschfeldii A01.3
  - localized A02.20
    - arthritis A02.23
    - meningitis A02.21
    - osteomyelitis A02.24
    - pneumonia A02.22
    - pyelonephritis A02.25
    - specified NEC A02.29
  - paratyphi A01.4
    - A A01.1
    - B A01.2
    - C A01.3
  - schottmuelleri A01.2
  - typhi, typhosa — *see* Typhoid
- Sarcocystis A07.8
- scabies B86
- Schistosoma — *see* Infestation, Schistosoma
- scrotum (acute) NEC N49.2

Infection, infected, infective — *continued*
- seminal vesicle — *see* Vesiculitis
- septic
  - localized, skin — *see* Abscess
- sheep liver fluke B66.3
- Shigella A03.9
  - boydii A03.2
  - dysenteriae A03.0
  - flexneri A03.1
  - group
    - A A03.0
    - B A03.1
    - C A03.2
    - D A03.3
  - Schmitz (-Stutzer) A03.0
  - schmitzii A03.0
  - shigae A03.0
  - sonnei A03.3
  - specified NEC A03.8
- shoulder (joint) NEC M00.9
  - due to internal joint prosthesis T84.59 ☑
  - skin NEC L08.9
- sinus (accessory) (chronic) (nasal) (*see also* Sinusitis)
  - pilonidal — *see* Sinus, pilonidal
  - skin NEC L08.89
- Skene's duct or gland — *see* Urethritis
- skin (local) (staphylococcal) (streptococcal) L08.9
  - abscess — *code by* site under Abscess
  - cellulitis — *code by* site under Cellulitis
  - due to fungus B36.9
    - specified type NEC B36.8
  - mycotic B36.9
    - specified type NEC B36.8
  - newborn P39.4
  - ulcer — *see* Ulcer, skin
- slow virus A81.9
  - specified NEC A81.89
- Sparganum (mansoni) (proliferum) (baxteri) B70.1
- specific (*see also* Syphilis)
  - to perinatal period — *see* Infection, congenital
- specified NEC B99.8
- spermatic cord NEC N49.1
- sphenoidal (sinus) — *see* Sinusitis, sphenoidal
- spinal cord NOS (*see also* Myelitis) G04.91
  - abscess G06.1
  - meninges — *see* Meningitis
  - streptococcal G04.89
- Spirillum A25.0
- spirochetal NOS A69.9
  - lung A69.8
  - specified NEC A69.8
- Spirometra larvae B70.1
- spleen D73.89
- Sporotrichum, Sporothrix (schenckii) — *see* Sporotrichosis
- staphylococcal, unspecified site
  - as cause of disease classified elsewhere B95.8
    - aureus (methicillin susceptible) (MSSA) B95.61
      - methicillin resistant (MRSA) B95.62
    - specified NEC B95.7
  - aureus (methicillin susceptible) (MSSA) A49.01
    - methicillin resistant (MRSA) A49.02
  - food poisoning A05.0
  - generalized (purulent) A41.2
  - pneumonia — *see* Pneumonia, staphylococcal
- Stellantchasmus falcatus B66.8
- streptobacillus moniliformis A25.1
- streptococcal NEC A49.1
  - as cause of disease classified elsewhere B95.5
  - B genitourinary complicating
    - childbirth O98.82
    - pregnancy O98.81- ☑
    - puerperium O98.83
  - congenital
    - sepsis P36.10
      - group B P36.0
      - specified NEC P36.19
  - generalized (purulent) A40.9
- Streptomyces B47.1
- Strongyloides (stercoralis) — *see* Strongyloidiasis
- stump (amputation) (surgical) — *see* Complication, amputation stump, infection
- subcutaneous tissue, local L08.9
- suipestifer — *see* Infection, salmonella
- swimming pool bacillus A31.1
- Taenia — *see* Infestation, Taenia
- Taeniarhynchus saginatus B68.1
- tapeworm — *see* Infestation, tapeworm

Infection, infected, infective — *continued*
tendon (sheath) — *see* Tenosynovitis, infective NEC
Ternidens diminutus B81.8
testis — *see* Orchitis
threadworm B80
throat — *see* Pharyngitis
thyroglossal duct K14.8
toe (skin) L08.9
  cellulitis L03.03- ☑
    fungus B35.1
  nail L03.03- ☑
    fungus B35.1
tongue NEC K14.0
  parasitic B37.0
tonsil (and adenoid) (faucial) (lingual) (pharyngeal) —
  see Tonsillitis
tooth, teeth K04.7
  periapical K04.7
  peridental, periodontal K05.20
    generalized K05.22
    localized K05.21
  pulp K04.0
  socket M27.3
TORCH — *see* Infection, congenital
  without active infection P00.2
Torula histolytica — *see* Cryptococcosis
Toxocara (canis) (cati) (felis) B83.0
Toxoplasma gondii — *see* Toxoplasma
trachea, chronic J42
trematode NEC — *see* Infestation, fluke
trench fever A79.0
Treponema pallidum — *see* Syphilis
Trichinella (spiralis) B75
Trichomonas A59.9
  cervix A59.09
  intestine A07.8
  prostate A59.02
  specified site NEC A59.8
  urethra A59.03
  urogenitalis A59.00
  vagina A59.01
  vulva A59.01
Trichophyton, trichophytic — *see* Dermatophytosis
Trichosporon (beigelii) cutaneum B36.2
Trichostrongylus B81.2
Trichuris (trichiura) B79
Trombicula (irritans) B88.0
Trypanosoma
  brucei
    gambiense B56.0
    rhodesiense B56.1
  cruzi — *see* Chagas' disease
tubal — *see* Salpingo-oophoritis
tuberculous NEC — *see* Tuberculosis
tubo-ovarian — *see* Salpingo-oophoritis
tunica vaginalis N49.1
tunnel T80.212 ☑
tympanic membrane NEC — *see* Myringitis
typhoid (abortive) (ambulant) (bacillus) — *see* Typhoid
typhus A75.9
  flea-borne A75.2
  mite-borne A75.3
  recrudescent A75.1
  tick-borne A77.9
    African A77.1
    North Asian A77.2
umbilicus L08.82
ureter N28.86
urethra — *see* Urethritis
urinary (tract) N39.0
  bladder — *see* Cystitis
  complicating
    pregnancy O23.4- ☑
      specified type NEC O23.3- ☑
  kidney — *see* Infection, kidney
  newborn P39.3
  puerperal (postpartum) O86.20
  tuberculous A18.13
  urethra — *see* Urethritis
uterus, uterine — *see* Endometritis
vaccination T88.0 ☑
vaccinia not from vaccination B08.011
vagina (acute) — *see* Vaginitis
varicella B01.9
varicose veins — *see* Varix
vas deferens NEC N49.1
vesical — *see* Cystitis

Infection, infected, infective — *continued*
Vibrio
  cholerae A00.0
    El Tor A00.1
  parahaemolyticus (food poisoning) A05.3
  vulnificus
    as cause of disease classified elsewhere B96.82
    foodborne intoxication A05.5
Vincent's (gum) (mouth) (tonsil) A69.1
virus, viral NOS B34.9
  adenovirus
    as cause of disease classified elsewhere B97.0
    unspecified nature or site B34.0
  arborvirus, arbovirus arthropod-borne A94
  as cause of disease classified elsewhere B97.89
    adenovirus B97.0
    coronavirus B97.29
      SARS-associated B97.21
    coxsackievirus B97.11
    echovirus B97.12
    enterovirus B97.10
      coxsackievirus B97.11
      echovirus B97.12
      specified NEC B97.19
    human
      immunodeficiency, type 2 (HIV 2) B97.35
      metapneumovirus B97.81
      T-cell lymphotropic,
        type I (HTLV-I) B97.33
        type II (HTLV-II) B97.34
    papillomavirus B97.7
    parvovirus B97.6
    reovirus B97.5
    respiratory syncytial B97.4
    retrovirus B97.30
      human
        immunodeficiency, type 2 (HIV 2) B97.35
        T-cell lymphotropic,
          type I (HTLV-I) B97.33
          type II (HTLV-II) B97.34
      lentivirus B97.31
      oncovirus B97.32
      specified NEC B97.39
    specified NEC B97.89
  central nervous system A89
    atypical A81.9
      specified NEC A81.89
    enterovirus NEC A88.8
      meningitis A87.0
    slow virus A81.9
      specified NEC A81.89
    specified NEC A88.8
  chest J98.8
  cotia B08.8
  coxsackie (*see also* Infection, coxsackie) B34.1
    as cause of disease classified elsewhere B97.11
  ECHO
    as cause of disease classified elsewhere B97.12
    unspecified nature or site B34.1
  encephalitis, tick-borne A84.9
  enterovirus, as cause of disease classified elsewhere
    B97.10
    coxsackievirus B97.11
    echovirus B97.12
    specified NEC B97.19
  exanthem NOS B09
  human metapneumovirus as cause of disease
    classified elsewhere B97.81
  human papilloma as cause of disease classified
    elsewhere B97.7
  intestine — *see* Enteritis, viral
  respiratory syncytial
    as cause of disease classified elsewhere B97.4
    bronchopneumonia J12.1
    common cold syndrome J00
    nasopharyngitis (acute) J00
  rhinovirus
    as cause of disease classified elsewhere B97.89
    unspecified nature or site B34.8
  slow A81.9
    specified NEC A81.89
  specified type NEC B33.8
    as cause of disease classified elsewhere B97.89
    unspecified nature or site B34.8
  unspecified nature or site B34.9
  West Nile — *see* Virus, West Nile
vulva (acute) — *see* Vulvitis
West Nile — *see* Virus, West Nile

Infection, infected, infective — *continued*
whipworm B79
worms B83.9
  specified type NEC B83.8
Wuchereria (bancrofti) B74.0
  malayi B74.1
yatapoxvirus B08.70
  specified NEC B08.79
yeast (*see also* Candidiasis) B37.9
yellow fever — *see* Fever, yellow
Yersinia
  enterocolitica (intestinal) A04.6
  pestis — *see* Plague
  pseudotuberculosis A28.2
Zeis' gland — *see* Hordeolum
zoonotic bacterial NOS A28.9
Zopfia senegalensis B47.0
Infective, infectious — *see* condition
Infertility
female N97.9
  age-related N97.8
  associated with
    anovulation N97.0
    cervical (mucus) disease or anomaly N88.3
    congenital anomaly
      cervix N88.3
      fallopian tube N97.1
      uterus N97.2
      vagina N97.8
    dysmucorrhea N88.3
    fallopian tube disease or anomaly N97.1
    pituitary-hypothalamic origin E23.0
    specified origin NEC N97.8
    Stein-Leventhal syndrome E28.2
    uterine disease or anomaly N97.2
    vaginal disease or anomaly N97.8
  due to
    cervical anomaly N88.3
    fallopian tube anomaly N97.1
    ovarian failure E28.39
    Stein-Leventhal syndrome E28.2
    uterine anomaly N97.2
    vaginal anomaly N97.8
  nonimplantation N97.2
  origin
    cervical N88.3
    tubal (block) (occlusion) (stenosis) N97.1
    uterine N97.2
    vaginal N97.8
male N46.9
  azoospermia N46.01
    extratesticular cause N46.029
      drug therapy N46.021
      efferent duct obstruction N46.023
      infection N46.022
      radiation N46.024
      specified cause NEC N46.029
      systemic disease N46.025
  oligospermia N46.11
    extratesticular cause N46.129
      drug therapy N46.121
      efferent duct obstruction N46.123
      infection N46.122
      radiation N46.124
      specified cause NEC N46.129
      systemic disease N46.125
  specified type NEC N46.8
Infestation B88.9
Acanthocheilonema (perstans) (streptocerca) B74.4
Acariasis B88.0
  demodex folliculorum B88.0
  sarcoptes scabiei B86
  trombiculae B88.0
Agamofilaria streptocerca B74.4
Ancylostoma, ankylostoma (braziliense) (caninum)
  (ceylanicum) (duodenale) B76.0
  americanum B76.1
  new world B76.1
Anisakis larvae, anisakiasis B81.0
arthropod NEC B88.2
Ascaris lumbricoides — *see* Ascariasis
Balantidium coli A07.0
beef tapeworm B68.1
Bothriocephalus (latus) B70.0
  larval B70.1
broad tapeworm B70.0
  larval B70.1
Brugia (malayi) B74.1

☑ Additional Character Required — Refer to the Tabular List for Character Selection   ▽ Subterms under main terms may continue to next column or page

Infestation — *continued*
- Brugia — *continued*
  - timori B74.2
- candiru B88.8
- Capillaria
  - hepatica B83.8
  - philippinensis B81.1
- cat liver fluke B66.0
- cestodes B71.9
  - diphyllobothrium — *see* Infestation, diphyllobothrium
  - dipylidiasis B71.1
  - hymenolepiasis B71.0
  - specified type NEC B71.8
- chigger B88.0
- chigo, chigoe B88.1
- Clonorchis (sinensis) (liver) B66.1
- coccidial A07.3
- crab-lice B85.3
- Cysticercus cellulosae — *see* Cysticercosis
- Demodex (folliculorum) B88.0
- Dermanyssus gallinae B88.0
- Dermatobia (hominis) — *see* Myiasis
- Dibothriocephalus (latus) B70.0
  - larval B70.1
- Dicrocoelium dendriticum B66.2
- Diphyllobothrium (adult) (latum) (intestinal) (pacificum) B70.0
  - larval B70.1
- Diplogonoporus (grandis) B71.8
- Dipylidium caninum B67.4
- Distoma hepaticum B66.3
- dog tapeworm B67.4
- Dracunculus medinensis B72
- dragon worm B72
- dwarf tapeworm B71.0
- Echinococcus — *see* Echinococcus
- Echinostomum ilocanum B66.8
- Entamoeba (histolytica) — *see* Infection, Ameba
- Enterobius vermicularis B80
- eyelid
  - in (due to)
    - leishmaniasis B55.1
    - loiasis B74.3
    - onchocerciasis B73.09
    - phthiriasis B85.3
    - parasitic NOS B89
- eyeworm B74.3
- Fasciola (gigantica) (hepatica) (indica) B66.3
- Fasciolopsis (buski) (intestine) B66.5
- filarial B74.9
  - bancroftian B74.0
  - conjunctiva B74.9
  - due to
    - Acanthocheilonema (perstans) (streptocerca) B74.4
    - Brugia (malayi) B74.1
      - timori B74.2
    - Dracunculus medinensis B72
    - guinea worm B72
    - loa loa B74.3
    - Mansonella (ozzardi) (perstans) (streptocerca) B74.4
    - Onchocerca volvulus B73.00
      - eye B73.00
      - eyelid B73.09
    - Wuchereria (bancrofti) B74.0
  - Malayan B74.1
  - ozzardi B74.4
  - specified type NEC B74.8
- fish tapeworm B70.0
  - larval B70.1
- fluke B66.9
  - blood NOS — *see* Schistosomiasis
  - cat liver B66.0
  - intestinal B66.5
  - lancet B66.2
  - liver (sheep) B66.3
    - cat B66.0
    - Chinese B66.1
    - due to clonorchiasis B66.1
    - oriental B66.1
  - lung (oriental) B66.4
  - sheep liver B66.3
  - specified type NEC B66.8
- fly larvae — *see* Myiasis
- Gasterophilus (intestinalis) — *see* Myiasis
- Gastrodiscoides hominis B66.8

Infestation — *continued*
- Giardia lamblia A07.1
- Gnathostoma (spinigerum) B83.1
- Gongylonema B83.8
- guinea worm B72
- helminth B83.9
  - angiostrongyliasis B83.2
    - intestinal B81.3
  - gnathostomiasis B83.1
  - hirudiniasis, internal B83.4
  - intestinal B82.0
    - angiostrongyliasis B81.3
    - anisakiasis B81.0
    - ascariasis — *see* Ascariasis
    - capillariasis B81.1
    - cysticercosis — *see* Cysticercosis
    - diphyllobothriasis — *see* Infestation, diphyllobothriasis
    - dracunculiasis B72
    - echinococcus — *see* Echinococcosis
    - enterobiasis B80
    - filariasis — *see* Infestation, filarial
    - fluke — *see* Infestation, fluke
    - hookworm — *see* Infestation, hookworm
    - mixed (types classifiable to more than one of the titles B65.0-B81.3 and B81.8) B81.4
    - onchocerciasis — *see* Onchocerciasis
    - schistosomiasis — *see* Infestation, schistosoma
    - specified
      - cestode NEC — *see* Infestation, cestode
      - type NEC B81.8
    - strongyloidiasis — *see* Strongyloidiasis
    - taenia — *see* Infestation, taenia
    - trichinellosis B75
    - trichostrongyliasis B81.2
    - trichuriasis B79
  - specified type NEC B83.8
  - syngamiasis B83.3
  - visceral larva migrans B83.0
- Heterophyes (heterophyes) B66.8
- hookworm B76.9
  - ancylostomiasis B76.0
  - necatoriasis B76.1
  - specified type NEC B76.8
- Hymenolepis (diminuta) (nana) B71.0
- intestinal NEC B82.9
- leeches (aquatic) (land) — *see* Hirudiniasis
- Leishmania — *see* Leishmaniasis
- lice, louse — *see* Infestation, Pediculus
- Linguatula B88.8
- Liponyssoides sanguineus B88.0
- Loa loa B74.3
  - conjunctiva B74.3
  - eyelid B74.3
- louse — *see* Infestation, Pediculus
- maggots — *see* Myiasis
- Mansonella (ozzardi) (perstans) (streptocerca) B74.4
- Medina (worm) B72
- Metagonimus (yokogawai) B66.8
- microfilaria streptocerca — *see* Onchocerciasis
  - eye B73.00
  - eyelid B73.09
- mites B88.9
  - scabic B86
- Monilia (albicans) — *see* Candidiasis
- mouth B37.0
- Necator americanus B76.1
- nematode NEC (intestinal) B82.0
  - Ancylostoma B76.0
  - conjunctiva NEC B83.9
  - Enterobius vermicularis B80
  - Gnathostoma spinigerum B83.1
  - physaloptera B80
  - specified NEC B81.8
  - trichostrongylus B81.2
  - trichuris (trichuria) B79
- Oesophagostomum (apiostomum) B81.8
- Oestrus ovis (*see also* Myiasis) B87.9
- Onchocerca (volvulus) — *see* Onchocerciasis
- Opisthorchis (felineus) (viverrini) B66.0
- orbit, parasitic NOS B89
- Oxyuris vermicularis B80
- Paragonimus (westermani) B66.4
- parasite, parasitic B89
  - eyelid B89
  - intestinal NOS B82.9
  - mouth B37.0
  - skin B88.9

Infestation — *continued*
- parasite, parasitic — *continued*
  - tongue B37.0
- Parastrongylus
  - cantonensis B83.2
  - costaricensis B81.3
- Pediculus B85.2
  - body B85.1
  - capitis (humanus) (any site) B85.0
  - corporis (humanus) (any site) B85.1
  - head B85.0
  - mixed (classifiable to more than one of the titles B85.0 - B85.3) B85.4
  - pubis (any site) B85.3
- Pentastoma B88.8
- Phthirus (pubis) (any site) B85.3
  - with any infestation classifiable to B85.0 - B85.2 B85.4
- pinworm B80
- pork tapeworm (adult) B68.0
- protozoal NEC B64
  - intestinal A07.9
    - specified NEC A07.8
  - specified NEC B60.8
- pubic, louse B85.3
- rat tapeworm B71.0
- red bug B88.0
- roundworm (large) NEC B82.0
  - Ascariasis (*see also* Ascariasis) B77.9
- sandflea B88.1
- Sarcoptes scabiei B86
- scabies B86
- Schistosoma B65.9
  - bovis B65.8
  - cercariae B65.3
  - haematobium B65.0
  - intercalatum B65.8
  - japonicum B65.2
  - mansoni B65.1
  - mattheei B65.8
  - mekongi B65.8
  - specified type NEC B65.8
  - spindale B65.8
- screw worms — *see* Myiasis
- skin NOS B88.9
- Sparganum (mansoni) (proliferum) (baxteri) B70.1
  - larval B70.1
- specified type NEC B88.8
- Spirometra larvae B70.1
- Stellantchasmus falcatus B66.8
- Strongyloides stercoralis — *see* Strongyloidiasis
- Taenia B68.9
  - diminuta B71.0
  - echinococcus — *see* Echinococcus
  - mediocanellata B68.1
  - nana B71.0
  - saginata B68.1
  - solium (intestinal form) B68.0
    - larval form — *see* Cysticercosis
- Taeniarhynchus saginatus B68.1
- tapeworm B71.9
  - beef B68.1
  - broad B70.0
    - larval B70.1
  - dog B67.4
  - dwarf B71.0
  - fish B70.0
    - larval B70.1
  - pork B68.0
  - rat B71.0
- Ternidens diminutus B81.8
- Tetranychus molestissimus B88.0
- threadworm B80
- tongue B37.0
- Toxocara (canis) (cati) (felis) B83.0
- trematode(s) NEC — *see* Infestation, fluke
- Trichinella (spiralis) B75
- Trichocephalus B79
- Trichomonas — *see* Trichomoniasis
- Trichostrongylus B81.2
- Trichuris (trichiura) B79
- Trombicula (irritans) B88.0
- Tunga penetrans B88.1
- Uncinaria americana B76.1
- Vandellia cirrhosa B88.8
- whipworm B79
- worms B83.9
  - intestinal B82.0

Infestation — *continued*
  Wuchereria (bancrofti) B74.Ø
Infiltrate, infiltration
  amyloid (generalized) (localized) — *see* Amyloidosis
  calcareous NEC R89.7
    localized — *see* Degeneration, by site
  calcium salt R89.7
  cardiac
    fatty — *see* Degeneration, myocardial
    glycogenic E74.Ø2 [I43]
  corneal — *see* Edema, cornea
  eyelid — *see* Inflammation, eyelid
  glycogen, glycogenic — *see* Disease, glycogen storage
  heart, cardiac
    fatty — *see* Degeneration, myocardial
    glycogenic E74.Ø2 [I43]
  inflammatory in vitreous H43.89
  kidney N28.89
  leukemic — *see* Leukemia
  liver K76.89
    fatty — *see* Fatty, liver NEC
    glycogen (*see also* Disease, glycogen storage)
      E74.Ø3 [K77]
  lung R91.8
    eosinophilic J82
  lymphatic (*see also* Leukemia, lymphatic) C91.9- ☑
    gland I88.9
  muscle, fatty M62.89
  myocardium, myocardial
    fatty — *see* Degeneration, myocardial
    glycogenic E74.Ø2 [I43]
  on chest x-ray R91.8
  pulmonary R91.8
    with eosinophilia J82
  skin (lymphocytic) L98.6
  thymus (gland) (fatty) E32.8
  urine R39.Ø
  vesicant agent
    antineoplastic chemotherapy T8Ø.81Ø ☑
    other agent NEC T8Ø.818 ☑
  vitreous body H43.89
Infirmity R68.89
  senile R54
Inflammation, inflamed, inflammatory (with exudation)
  abducent (nerve) — *see* Strabismus, paralytic, sixth nerve
  accessory sinus (chronic) — *see* Sinusitis
  adrenal (gland) E27.8
  alveoli, teeth M27.3
    scorbutic E54
  anal canal, anus K62.89
  antrum (chronic) — *see* Sinusitis, maxillary
  appendix — *see* Appendicitis
  arachnoid — *see* Meningitis
  areola N61
    puerperal, postpartum or gestational — *see* Infection, nipple
  areolar tissue NOS LØ8.9
  artery — *see* Arteritis
  auditory meatus (external) — *see* Otitis, externa
  Bartholin's gland N75.8
  bile duct (common) (hepatic) or passage — *see* Cholangitis
  bladder — *see* Cystitis
  bone — *see* Osteomyelitis
  brain (*see also* Encephalitis)
    membrane — *see* Meningitis
  breast N61
    puerperal, postpartum, gestational — *see* Mastitis, obstetric
  broad ligament — *see* Disease, pelvis, inflammatory
  bronchi — *see* Bronchitis
  catarrhal JØØ
  cecum — *see* Appendicitis
  cerebral (*see also* Encephalitis)
    membrane — *see* Meningitis
  cerebrospinal
    meningococcal A39.Ø
  cervix (uteri) — *see* Cervicitis
  chest J98.8
  chorioretinal H3Ø.9- ☑
    cyclitis — *see* Cyclitis
    disseminated H3Ø.1Ø- ☑
      generalized H3Ø.13- ☑
      peripheral H3Ø.12- ☑
      posterior pole H3Ø.11- ☑

Inflammation, inflamed, inflammatory — *continued*
  chorioretinal — *continued*
    epitheliopathy — *see* Epitheliopathy
    focal H3Ø.ØØ- ☑
      juxtapapillary H3Ø.Ø1- ☑
      macular H3Ø.Ø4- ☑
      paramacular — *see* Inflammation, chorioretinal, focal, macular
      peripheral H3Ø.Ø3- ☑
      posterior pole H3Ø.Ø2- ☑
    specified type NEC H3Ø.89- ☑
  choroid — *see* Inflammation, chorioretinal
  chronic, postmastoidectomy cavity — *see* Complications, postmastoidectomy, inflammation
  colon — *see* Enteritis
  connective tissue (diffuse) NEC — *see* Disorder, soft tissue, specified type NEC
  cornea — *see* Keratitis
  corpora cavernosa N48.29
  cranial nerve — *see* Disorder, nerve, cranial
  Douglas' cul-de-sac or pouch (chronic) N73.Ø
  due to device, implant or graft (*see also* Complications, by site and type, infection or inflammation)
    arterial graft T82.7 ☑
    breast (implant) T85.79 ☑
    catheter T85.79 ☑
      dialysis (renal) T82.7 ☑
        intraperitoneal T85.71 ☑
      infusion T82.7 ☑
        spinal (epidural) (subdural) T85.79 ☑
      urinary (indwelling) T83.51 ☑
    electronic (electrode) (pulse generator) (stimulator)
      bone T84.7 ☑
      cardiac T82.7 ☑
      nervous system (brain) (peripheral nerve) (spinal) T85.79 ☑
      urinary T83.59 ☑
    fixation, internal (orthopedic) NEC — *see* Complication, fixation device, infection
    gastrointestinal (bile duct) (esophagus) T85.79 ☑
    genital NEC T83.6 ☑
    heart NEC T82.7 ☑
      valve (prosthesis) T82.6 ☑
        graft T82.7 ☑
    joint prosthesis — *see* Complication, joint prosthesis, infection
    ocular (corneal graft) (orbital implant) NEC T85.79 ☑
    orthopedic NEC T84.7 ☑
    specified NEC T85.79 ☑
    urinary NEC T83.59 ☑
    vascular NEC T82.7 ☑
    ventricular intracranial shunt T85.79 ☑
  duodenum K29.8Ø
    with bleeding K29.81
  dura mater — *see* Meningitis
  ear (middle) (*see also* Otitis, media)
    external — *see* Otitis, externa
    inner — *see* subcategory H83.Ø ☑
  epididymis — *see* Epididymitis
  esophagus K2Ø.9
  ethmoidal (sinus) (chronic) — *see* Sinusitis, ethmoidal
  eustachian tube (catarrhal) — *see* Salpingitis, eustachian
  eyelid HØ1.9
    abscess — *see* Abscess, eyelid
    blepharitis — *see* Blepharitis
    chalazion — *see* Chalazion
    dermatosis (noninfectious) — *see* Dermatosis, eyelid
    hordeolum — *see* Hordeolum
    specified NEC HØ1.8
  fallopian tube — *see* Salpingo-oophoritis
  fascia — *see* Myositis
  follicular, pharynx J31.2
  frontal (sinus) (chronic) — *see* Sinusitis, frontal
  gallbladder — *see* Cholecystitis
  gastric — *see* Gastritis
  gastrointestinal — *see* Enteritis
  genital organ (internal) (diffuse)
    female — *see* Disease, pelvis, inflammatory
    male N49.9
      multiple sites N49.8
      specified NEC N49.8
  gland (lymph) — *see* Lymphadenitis

Inflammation, inflamed, inflammatory — *continued*
  glottis — *see* Laryngitis
  granular, pharynx J31.2
  gum KØ5.1Ø
    nonplaque induced KØ5.11
    plaque induced KØ5.1Ø
  heart — *see* Carditis
  hepatic duct — *see* Cholangitis
  ileoanal (internal) pouch K91.85Ø
  ileum (*see also* Enteritis)
    regional or terminal — *see* Enteritis, regional
  intestinal pouch K91.85Ø
  intestine (any part) — *see* Enteritis
  jaw (acute) (bone) (chronic) (lower) (suppurative) (upper) M27.2
  joint NEC — *see* Arthritis
    sacroiliac M46.1
  kidney — *see* Nephritis
  knee (joint) M13.169
    tuberculous A18.Ø2
  labium (majus) (minus) — *see* Vulvitis
  lacrimal
    gland — *see* Dacryoadenitis
    passages (duct) (sac) (*see also* Dacryocystitis)
      canaliculitis — *see* Canaliculitis, lacrimal
  larynx — *see* Laryngitis
  leg NOS LØ8.9
  lip K13.Ø
  liver (capsule) (*see also* Hepatitis)
    chronic K73.9
    suppurative K75.Ø
  lung (acute) (*see also* Pneumonia)
    chronic J98.4
  lymph gland or node — *see* Lymphadenitis
  lymphatic vessel — *see* Lymphangitis
  maxilla, maxillary M27.2
    sinus (chronic) — *see* Sinusitis, maxillary
  membranes of brain or spinal cord — *see* Meningitis
  meninges — *see* Meningitis
  mouth K12.1
  muscle — *see* Myositis
  myocardium — *see* Myocarditis
  nasal sinus (chronic) — *see* Sinusitis
  nasopharynx — *see* Nasopharyngitis
  navel LØ8.82
  nerve NEC — *see* Neuralgia
  nipple N61
    puerperal, postpartum or gestational — *see* Infection, nipple
  nose — *see* Rhinitis
  oculomotor (nerve) — *see* Strabismus, paralytic, third nerve
  optic nerve — *see* Neuritis, optic
  orbit (chronic) HØ5.1Ø
    acute HØ5.ØØ
      abscess — *see* Abscess, orbit
      cellulitis — *see* Cellulitis, orbit
      osteomyelitis — *see* Osteomyelitis, orbit
      periostitis — *see* Periostitis, orbital
      tenonitis — *see* Tenonitis, eye
    granuloma — *see* Granuloma, orbit
    myositis — *see* Myositis, orbital
  ovary — *see* Salpingo-oophoritis
  oviduct — *see* Salpingo-oophoritis
  pancreas (acute) — *see* Pancreatitis
  parametrium N73.Ø
  parotid region LØ8.9
  pelvis, female — *see* Disease, pelvis, inflammatory
  penis (corpora cavernosa) N48.29
  perianal K62.89
  pericardium — *see* Pericarditis
  perineum (female) (male) LØ8.9
  perirectal K62.89
  peritoneum — *see* Peritonitis
  periuterine — *see* Disease, pelvis, inflammatory
  perivesical — *see* Cystitis
  petrous bone (acute) (chronic) — *see* Petrositis
  pharynx (acute) — *see* Pharyngitis
  pia mater — *see* Meningitis
  pleura — *see* Pleurisy
  polyp, colon (*see also* Polyp, colon, inflammatory) K51.4Ø
  prostate (*see also* Prostatitis)
    specified type NEC N41.8
  rectosigmoid — *see* Rectosigmoiditis
  rectum (*see also* Proctitis) K62.89

Inflammation, inflamed, inflammatory — *continued*
  respiratory, upper (*see also* Infection, respiratory, upper) J06.9
    acute, due to radiation J70.0
    chronic, due to external agent — *see* condition, respiratory, chronic, due to
    due to
      chemicals, gases, fumes or vapors (inhalation) J68.2
      radiation J70.1
  retina — *see* Chorioretinitis
  retrocecal — *see* Appendicitis
  retroperitoneal — *see* Peritonitis
  salivary duct or gland (any) (suppurative) — *see* Sialoadenitis
  scorbutic, alveoli, teeth E54
  scrotum N49.2
  seminal vesicle — *see* Vesiculitis
  sigmoid — *see* Enteritis
  sinus — *see* Sinusitis
  Skene's duct or gland — *see* Urethritis
  skin L08.9
  spermatic cord N49.1
  sphenoidal (sinus) — *see* Sinusitis, sphenoidal
  spinal
    cord — *see* Encephalitis
    membrane — *see* Meningitis
    nerve — *see* Disorder, nerve
  spine — *see* Spondylopathy, inflammatory
  spleen (capsule) D73.89
  stomach — *see* Gastritis
  subcutaneous tissue L08.9
  suprarenal (gland) E27.8
  synovial — *see* Tenosynovitis
  tendon (sheath) NEC — *see* Tenosynovitis
  testis — *see* Orchitis
  throat (acute) — *see* Pharyngitis
  thymus (gland) E32.8
  thyroid (gland) — *see* Thyroiditis
  tongue K14.0
  tonsil — *see* Tonsillitis
  trachea — *see* Tracheitis
  trochlear (nerve) — *see* Strabismus, paralytic, fourth nerve
  tubal — *see* Salpingo-oophoritis
  tuberculous NEC — *see* Tuberculosis
  tubo-ovarian — *see* Salpingo-oophoritis
  tunica vaginalis N49.1
  tympanic membrane — *see* Tympanitis
  umbilicus, umbilical L08.82
  uterine ligament — *see* Disease, pelvis, inflammatory
  uterus (catarrhal) — *see* Endometritis
  uveal tract (anterior) NOS (*see also* Iridocyclitis)
    posterior — *see* Chorioretinitis
  vagina — *see* Vaginitis
  vas deferens N49.1
  vein (*see also* Phlebitis)
    intracranial or intraspinal (septic) G08
    thrombotic I80.9
      leg — *see* Phlebitis, leg
      lower extremity — *see* Phlebitis, leg
  vocal cord J38.3
  vulva — *see* Vulvitis
  Wharton's duct or gland (suppurative) — *see* Sialoadenitis
Inflation, lung, imperfect (newborn) — *see* Atelectasis
Influenza (bronchial) (epidemic) (respiratory (upper)) (unidentified influenza virus) J11.1
  with
    digestive manifestations J11.2
    encephalopathy J11.81
    enteritis J11.2
    gastroenteritis J11.2
    gastrointestinal manifestations J11.2
    laryngitis J11.1
    myocarditis J11.82
    otitis media J11.83
    pharyngitis J11.1
    pneumonia J11.00
      specified type J11.08
    respiratory manifestations NEC J11.1
    specified manifestation NEC J11.89
  A/H5N1 (*see also* Influenza, due to, identified novel influenza A virus) J09.X2
  avian (*see also* Influenza, due to, identified novel influenza A virus) J09.X2

Influenza — *continued*
  bird (*see also* Influenza, due to, identified novel influenza A virus) J09.X2
  due to
    avian (*see also* Influenza, due to, identified novel influenza A virus) J09.X2
    identified influenza virus NEC J10.1
      with
        digestive manifestations J10.2
        encephalopathy J10.81
        enteritis J10.2
        gastroenteritis J10.2
        gastrointestinal manifestations J10.2
        laryngitis J10.1
        myocarditis J10.82
        otitis media J10.83
        pharyngitis J10.1
        pneumonia (unspecified type) J10.00
          with same identified influenza virus J10.01
          specified type NEC J10.08
        respiratory manifestations NEC J10.1
        specified manifestation NEC J10.89
    identified novel influenza A virus J09.X2
      with
        digestive manifestations J09.X3
        encephalopathy J09.X9
        enteritis J09.X3
        gastroenteritis J09.X3
        gastrointestinal manifestations J09.X3
        laryngitis J09.X2
        myocarditis J09.X9
        otitis media J09.X9
        pharyngitis J09.X2
        pneumonia J09.X1
        respiratory manifestations NEC J09.X2
        specified manifestation NEC J09.X9
        upper respiratory symptoms J09.X2
    novel (2009) H1N1 influenza (*see also* Influenza, due to, identified influenza virus NEC) J10.1
    novel influenza A/H1N1 (*see also* Influenza, due to, identified influenza virus NEC) J10.1
    of other animal origin, not bird or swine (*see also* Influenza, due to, identified novel influenza A virus) J09.X2
    swine (viruses that normally cause infections in pigs) (*see also* Influenza, due to, identified novel influenza A virus) J09.X2
Influenza-like disease — *see* Influenza
Influenzal — *see* Influenza
Infraction, Freiberg's (metatarsal head) — *see* Osteochondrosis, juvenile, metatarsus
Infraeruption of tooth (teeth) M26.34
Infusion complication, misadventure, or reaction — *see* Complications, infusion
Ingestion
  chemical — *see* Table of Drugs and Chemicals, by substance, poisoning
  drug or medicament
    correct substance properly administered — *see* Table of Drugs and Chemicals, by drug, adverse effect
    overdose or wrong substance given or taken — *see* Table of Drugs and Chemicals, by drug, poisoning
  foreign body — *see* Foreign body, alimentary tract
  tularemia A21.3
Ingrowing
  hair (beard) L73.1
  nail (finger) (toe) L60.0
Inguinal (*see also* condition)
  testicle Q53.9
    bilateral Q53.21
    unilateral Q53.11
Inhalation
  anthrax A22.1
  flame T27.3 ☑
  food or foreign body — *see* Foreign body, by site
  gases, fumes, or vapors NEC T59.9- ☑
    specified agent — *see* Table of Drugs and Chemicals, by substance
  liquid or vomitus — *see* Asphyxia
  meconium (newborn) P24.00
    with
      with respiratory symptoms P24.01
      pneumonia (pneumonitis) P24.01
  mucus — *see* Asphyxia, mucus

Inhalation — *continued*
  oil or gasoline (causing suffocation) — *see* Foreign body, by site
  smoke J70.5
    due to chemicals, gases, fumes and vapors J68.9
  steam — *see* Toxicity, vapors
  stomach contents or secretions — *see* Foreign body, by site
    due to anesthesia (general) (local) or other sedation T88.59 ☑
      in labor and delivery O74.0
      in pregnancy O29.01- ☑
      postpartum, puerperal O89.01
Inhibition, orgasm
  female F52.31
  male F52.32
Inhibitor, systemic lupus erythematosus (presence of) D68.62
Iniencephalus, iniencephaly Q00.2
Injection, traumatic jet (air) (industrial) (water) (paint or dye) T70.4
Injury (*see also* specified injury type) T14.90
  abdomen, abdominal S39.91 ☑
    blood vessel — *see* Injury, blood vessel, abdomen
    cavity — *see* Injury, intra-abdominal
    contusion S30.1 ☑
    internal — *see* Injury, intra-abdominal
    intra-abdominal organ — *see* Injury, intra-abdominal
    nerve — *see* Injury, nerve, abdomen
    open — *see* Wound, open, abdomen
    specified NEC S39.81 ☑
    superficial — *see* Injury, superficial, abdomen
  Achilles tendon S86.00- ☑
    laceration S86.02- ☑
    specified type NEC S86.09- ☑
    strain S86.01- ☑
  acoustic, resulting in deafness — *see* Injury, nerve, acoustic
  adrenal (gland) S37.819 ☑
    contusion S37.812 ☑
    laceration S37.813 ☑
    specified type NEC S37.818 ☑
  alveolar (process) S09.93 ☑
  ankle S99.91- ☑
    contusion — *see* Contusion, ankle
    dislocation — *see* Dislocation, ankle
    fracture — *see* Fracture, ankle
    nerve — *see* Injury, nerve, ankle
    open — *see* Wound, open, ankle
    specified type NEC S99.81- ☑
    sprain — *see* Sprain, ankle
    superficial — *see* Injury, superficial, ankle
  anterior chamber, eye — *see* Injury, eye, specified site NEC
  anus — *see* Injury, abdomen
  aorta (thoracic) S25.00 ☑
    abdominal S35.00 ☑
      laceration (minor) (superficial) S35.01 ☑
        major S35.02 ☑
      specified type NEC S35.09 ☑
    laceration (minor) (superficial) S25.01 ☑
      major S25.02 ☑
    specified type NEC S25.09 ☑
  arm (upper) S49.9- ☑
    blood vessel — *see* Injury, blood vessel, arm
    contusion — *see* Contusion, arm, upper
    fracture — *see* Fracture, humerus
    lower — *see* Injury, forearm
    muscle — *see* Injury, muscle, shoulder
    nerve — *see* Injury, nerve, arm
    open — *see* Wound, open, arm
    specified type NEC S49.8- ☑
    superficial — *see* Injury, superficial, arm
  artery (complicating trauma) (*see also* Injury, blood vessel, by site)
    cerebral or meningeal — *see* Injury, intracranial
  auditory canal (external) (meatus) S09.91 ☑
  auricle, auris, ear S09.91 ☑
  axilla — *see* Injury, shoulder
  back — *see* Injury, back, lower
  bile duct S36.13 ☑
  birth (*see also* Birth, injury) P15.9
  bladder (sphincter) S37.20 ☑
    at delivery O71.5
    contusion S37.22 ☑

Index

Injury — Injury

Injury — continued
  bladder — continued
    laceration S37.23 ☑
    obstetrical trauma O71.5
    specified type NEC S37.29 ☑
  blast (air) (hydraulic) (immersion) (underwater) NEC T14.8
    acoustic nerve trauma — see Injury, nerve, acoustic
    bladder — see Injury, bladder
    brain — see Concussion
    colon — see Injury, intestine, large
    ear (primary) S09.31- ☑
      secondary S09.39- ☑
    generalized T70.8 ☑
    lung — see Injury, intrathoracic, lung
    multiple body organs T70.8 ☑
    peritoneum S36.81 ☑
    rectum S36.61 ☑
    retroperitoneum S36.898 ☑
    small intestine S36.419 ☑
      duodenum S36.410 ☑
      specified site NEC S36.418 ☑
    specified
      intra-abdominal organ NEC S36.898 ☑
      pelvic organ NEC S37.899 ☑
  blood vessel NEC T14.8
    abdomen S35.9 ☑
      aorta — see Injury, aorta, abdominal
      celiac artery — see Injury, blood vessel, celiac artery
      iliac vessel — see Injury, blood vessel, iliac
      laceration S35.91 ☑
      mesenteric vessel — see Injury, mesenteric
      portal vein — see Injury, blood vessel, portal vein
      renal vessel — see Injury, blood vessel, renal
      specified vessel NEC S35.8X- ☑
      splenic vessel — see Injury, blood vessel, splenic
      vena cava — see Injury, vena cava, inferior
    ankle — see Injury, blood vessel, foot
    aorta (abdominal) (thoracic) — see Injury, aorta
    arm (upper) NEC S45.90- ☑
      forearm — see Injury, blood vessel, forearm
      laceration S45.91- ☑
      specified
        site NEC S45.80- ☑
          laceration S45.81- ☑
          specified type NEC S45.89- ☑
        type NEC S45.99- ☑
      superficial vein S45.30- ☑
        laceration S45.31- ☑
        specified type NEC S45.39- ☑
    axillary
      artery S45.00- ☑
        laceration S45.01- ☑
        specified type NEC S45.09- ☑
      vein S45.20- ☑
        laceration S45.21- ☑
        specified type NEC S45.29- ☑
    azygos vein — see Injury, blood vessel, thoracic, specified site NEC
    brachial
      artery S45.10- ☑
        laceration S45.11- ☑
        specified type NEC S45.19- ☑
      vein S45.20- ☑
        laceration S45.219 ☑
        specified type NEC S45.29- ☑
    carotid artery (common) (external) (internal, extracranial) S15.00- ☑
      internal, intracranial S06.8- ☑
      laceration (minor) (superficial) S15.01- ☑
        major S15.02- ☑
      specified type NEC S15.09- ☑
    celiac artery S35.219
      branch S35.299 ☑
        laceration (minor) (superficial) S35.291 ☑
          major S35.292 ☑
        specified NEC S35.298 ☑
      laceration (minor) (superficial) S35.211 ☑
        major S35.212 ☑
      specified type NEC S35.218 ☑
    cerebral — see Injury, intracranial
    deep plantar — see Injury, blood vessel, plantar artery

Injury — continued
  blood vessel — continued
    digital (hand) — see Injury, blood vessel, finger
    dorsal
      artery (foot) S95.00- ☑
        laceration S95.01- ☑
        specified type NEC S95.09- ☑
      vein (foot) S95.20- ☑
        laceration S95.21- ☑
        specified type NEC S95.29- ☑
    due to accidental laceration during procedure — see Laceration, accidental complicating surgery
    extremity — see Injury, blood vessel, limb
    femoral
      artery (common) (superficial) S75.00- ☑
        laceration (minor) (superficial) S75.01- ☑
          major S75.02- ☑
        specified type NEC S75.09- ☑
      vein (hip level) (thigh level) S75.10- ☑
        laceration (minor) (superficial) S75.11- ☑
          major S75.12- ☑
        specified type NEC S75.19- ☑
    finger S65.50- ☑
      index S65.50- ☑
        laceration S65.51- ☑
        specified type NEC S65.59- ☑
      laceration S65.51- ☑
      little S65.50- ☑
        laceration S65.51- ☑
        specified type NEC S65.59- ☑
      middle S65.50- ☑
        laceration S65.51- ☑
        specified type NEC S65.59- ☑
      specified type NEC S65.59- ☑
      thumb — see Injury, blood vessel, thumb
    foot S95.90- ☑
      dorsal
        artery — see Injury, blood vessel, dorsal, artery
        vein — see Injury, blood vessel, dorsal, vein
      laceration S95.91- ☑
      plantar artery — see Injury, blood vessel, plantar artery
      specified
        site NEC S95.80- ☑
          laceration S95.81- ☑
          specified type NEC S95.89- ☑
        specified type NEC S95.99- ☑
    forearm S55.90- ☑
      laceration S55.91- ☑
      radial artery — see Injury, blood vessel, radial artery
      specified
        site NEC S55.80- ☑
          laceration S55.81- ☑
          specified type NEC S55.89- ☑
        type NEC S55.99- ☑
      ulnar artery — see Injury, blood vessel, ulnar artery
      vein S55.20- ☑
        laceration S55.21- ☑
        specified type NEC S55.29- ☑
    gastric
      artery — see Injury, mesenteric, artery, branch
      vein — see Injury, blood vessel, abdomen
    gastroduodenal artery — see Injury, mesenteric, artery, branch
    greater saphenous vein (lower leg level) S85.30- ☑
      hip (and thigh) level S75.20- ☑
        laceration (minor) (superficial) S75.21- ☑
          major S75.22- ☑
        specified type NEC S75.29- ☑
      laceration S85.31- ☑
      specified type NEC S85.39- ☑
    hand (level) S65.90- ☑
      finger — see Injury, blood vessel, finger
      laceration S65.91- ☑
      palmar arch — see Injury, blood vessel, palmar arch
      radial artery — see Injury, blood vessel, radial artery, hand
      specified
        site NEC S65.80- ☑
          laceration S65.81- ☑
          specified type NEC S65.89-

Injury — continued
  blood vessel — continued
    hand — continued
      specified — continued
        type NEC S65.99- ☑
      thumb — see Injury, blood vessel, thumb
      ulnar artery — see Injury, blood vessel, ulnar artery, hand
    head S09.0 ☑
      intracranial — see Injury, intracranial
      multiple S09.0 ☑
    hepatic
      artery — see Injury, mesenteric, artery
      vein — see Injury, vena cava, inferior
    hip S75.90- ☑
      femoral artery — see Injury, blood vessel, femoral, artery
      femoral vein — see Injury, blood vessel, femoral, vein
      greater saphenous vein — see Injury, blood vessel, greater saphenous, hip level
      laceration S75.91- ☑
      specified
        site NEC S75.80- ☑
          laceration S75.81- ☑
          specified type NEC S75.89- ☑
        type NEC S75.99- ☑
    hypogastric (artery) (vein) — see Injury, blood vessel, iliac
    iliac S35.5- ☑
      artery S35.51- ☑
      specified vessel NEC S35.5- ☑
      uterine vessel — see Injury, blood vessel, uterine
      vein S35.51- ☑
    innominate — see Injury, blood vessel, thoracic, innominate
    intercostal (artery) (vein) — see Injury, blood vessel, thoracic, intercostal
    jugular vein (external) S15.20- ☑
      internal S15.30- ☑
        laceration (minor) (superficial) S15.31- ☑
          major S15.32- ☑
        specified type NEC S15.39- ☑
      laceration (minor) (superficial) S15.21- ☑
        major S15.22- ☑
      specified type NEC S15.29- ☑
    leg (level) (lower) S85.90- ☑
      greater saphenous — see Injury, blood vessel, greater saphenous
      laceration S85.91- ☑
      lesser saphenous — see Injury, blood vessel, lesser saphenous
      peroneal artery — see Injury, blood vessel, peroneal artery
      popliteal
        artery — see Injury, blood vessel, popliteal, artery
        vein — see Injury, blood vessel, popliteal, vein
      specified
        site NEC S85.80- ☑
          laceration S85.81- ☑
          specified type NEC S85.89- ☑
        type NEC S85.99- ☑
      thigh — see Injury, blood vessel, hip
      tibial artery — see Injury, blood vessel, tibial artery
    lesser saphenous vein (lower leg level) S85.40- ☑
      laceration S85.41- ☑
      specified type NEC S85.49- ☑
    limb
      lower — see Injury, blood vessel, leg
      upper — see Injury, blood vessel, arm
    lower back — see Injury, blood vessel, abdomen
      specified NEC — see Injury, blood vessel, abdomen, specified, site NEC
    mammary (artery) (vein) — see Injury, blood vessel, thoracic, specified site NEC
    mesenteric (inferior) (superior)
      artery — see Injury, mesenteric, artery
      vein — see Injury, blood vessel, mesenteric, vein
    neck S15.9 ☑
      specified site NEC S15.8 ☑
    ovarian (artery) (vein) — see subcategory S35.8 ☑

☑ **Additional Character Required — Refer to the Tabular List for Character Selection**   ▽ **Subterms under main terms may continue to next column or page**

Injury — continued
  blood vessel — continued
    palmar arch (superficial) S65.20- ☑
      deep S65.30- ☑
        laceration S65.31- ☑
        specified type NEC S65.39- ☑
      laceration S65.21- ☑
      specified type NEC S65.29- ☑
    pelvis — see Injury, blood vessel, abdomen
      specified NEC — see Injury, blood vessel, abdomen, specified, site NEC
    peroneal artery S85.20- ☑
      laceration S85.21- ☑
      specified type NEC S85.29- ☑
    plantar artery (deep) (foot) S95.10- ☑
      laceration S95.11- ☑
      specified type NEC S95.19- ☑
    popliteal
      artery S85.00- ☑
        laceration S85.01- ☑
        specified type NEC S85.09- ☑
      vein S85.50- ☑
        laceration S85.51- ☑
        specified type NEC S85.59- ☑
    portal vein S35.319 ☑
      laceration S35.311 ☑
      specified type NEC S35.318 ☑
    precerebral — see Injury, blood vessel, neck
    pulmonary (artery) (vein) — see Injury, blood vessel, thoracic, pulmonary
    radial artery (forearm level) S55.10- ☑
      hand and wrist (level) S65.10- ☑
        laceration S65.11- ☑
        specified type NEC S65.19- ☑
      laceration S55.11- ☑
      specified type NEC S55.19- ☑
    renal
      artery S35.40- ☑
        laceration S35.41- ☑
        specified NEC S35.49- ☑
      vein S35.40- ☑
        laceration S35.41- ☑
        specified NEC S35.49- ☑
    saphenous vein (greater) (lower leg level) — see Injury, blood vessel, greater saphenous
      hip and thigh level — see Injury, blood vessel, greater saphenous, hip level
      lesser — see Injury, blood vessel, lesser saphenous
    shoulder
      specified NEC — see Injury, blood vessel, arm, specified site NEC
      superficial vein — see Injury, blood vessel, arm, superficial vein
    specified NEC T14.8
    splenic
      artery — see Injury, blood vessel, celiac artery, branch
      vein S35.329 ☑
        laceration S35.321 ☑
        specified NEC S35.328 ☑
    subclavian — see Injury, blood vessel, thoracic, innominate
    thigh — see Injury, blood vessel, hip
    thoracic S25.90 ☑
      aorta S25.00 ☑
        laceration (minor) (superficial) S25.01 ☑
          major S25.02 ☑
        specified type NEC S25.09 ☑
      azygos vein — see Injury, blood vessel, thoracic, specified, site NEC
      innominate
        artery S25.10- ☑
          laceration (minor) (superficial) S25.11- ☑
            major S25.12- ☑
          specified type NEC S25.19- ☑
        vein S25.30- ☑
          laceration (minor) (superficial) S25.31- ☑
            major S25.32- ☑
          specified type NEC S25.39- ☑
      intercostal S25.50- ☑
        laceration S25.51- ☑
        specified type NEC S25.59- ☑
      laceration S25.91 ☑

Injury — continued
  blood vessel — continued
    thoracic — continued
      mammary vessel — see Injury, blood vessel, thoracic, specified, site NEC
      pulmonary S25.40- ☑
        laceration (minor) (superficial) S25.41- ☑
          major S25.42- ☑
        specified type NEC S25.49- ☑
      specified
        site NEC S25.80- ☑
          laceration S25.81 ☑
          specified type NEC S25.89 ☑
        type NEC S25.99 ☑
      subclavian — see Injury, blood vessel, thoracic, innominate
      vena cava (superior) S25.20 ☑
        laceration (minor) (superficial) S25.21 ☑
          major S25.22 ☑
        specified type NEC S25.29 ☑
    thumb S65.40- ☑
      laceration S65.41- ☑
      specified type NEC S65.49- ☑
    tibial artery S85.10- ☑
      anterior S85.13- ☑
        laceration S85.14- ☑
        specified injury NEC S85.15- ☑
      laceration S85.11- ☑
      posterior S85.16- ☑
        laceration S85.17- ☑
        specified injury NEC S85.18- ☑
      specified injury NEC S85.12- ☑
    ulnar artery (forearm level) S55.00- ☑
      hand and wrist (level) S65.00- ☑
        laceration S65.01- ☑
        specified type NEC S65.09- ☑
      laceration S55.01- ☑
      specified type NEC S55.09- ☑
    upper arm (level) — see Injury, blood vessel, arm
      superficial vein — see Injury, blood vessel, arm, superficial vein
    uterine S35.5- ☑
      artery S35.53- ☑
      vein S35.53- ☑
    vena cava — see Injury, vena cava
    vertebral artery S15.10- ☑
      laceration (minor) (superficial) S15.11- ☑
        major S15.12- ☑
      specified type NEC S15.19- ☑
    wrist (level) — see Injury, blood vessel, hand
  brachial plexus S14.3 ☑
    newborn P14.3
  brain (traumatic) S06.9- ☑
    diffuse (axonal) S06.2X- ☑
    focal S06.30- ☑
    traumatic — see category S06 ☑
  brainstem S06.38- ☑
  breast NOS S29.9
  broad ligament — see Injury, pelvic organ, specified site NEC
  bronchus, bronchi — see Injury, intrathoracic, bronchus
  brow S09.90 ☑
  buttock S39.92 ☑
  canthus, eye S05.90 ☑
  cardiac plexus — see Injury, nerve, thorax, sympathetic
  cauda equina S34.3 ☑
  cavernous sinus — see Injury, intracranial
  cecum — see Injury, colon
  celiac ganglion or plexus — see Injury, nerve, lumbosacral, sympathetic
  cerebellum — see Injury, intracranial
  cerebral — see Injury, intracranial
  cervix (uteri) — see Injury, uterus
  cheek (wall) S09.93 ☑
  chest — see Injury, thorax
  childbirth (newborn) (see also Birth, injury)
    maternal NEC O71.9
  chin S09.93 ☑
  choroid (eye) — see Injury, eye, specified site NEC
  clitoris S39.94 ☑
  coccyx (see also Injury, back, lower)
    complicating delivery O71.6
  colon — see Injury, intestine, large
  common bile duct — see Injury, liver
  conjunctiva (superficial) — see Injury, eye, conjunctiva

Injury — continued
  conus medullaris — see Injury, spinal, sacral
  cord
    spermatic (pelvic region) S37.898 ☑
      scrotal region S39.848 ☑
    spinal — see Injury, spinal cord, by region
  cornea — see Injury, eye, specified site NEC
    abrasion — see Injury, eye, cornea, abrasion
  cortex (cerebral) (see also Injury, intracranial)
    visual — see Injury, nerve, optic
  costal region NEC S29.9 ☑
  costochondral NEC S29.9 ☑
  cranial
    cavity — see Injury, intracranial
    nerve — see Injury, nerve, cranial
  crushing — see Crush
  cutaneous sensory nerve
  cystic duct — see Injury, liver
  deep tissue — see Contusion, by site
    meaning pressure ulcer — see Ulcer, pressure, unstageable, by site
  delivery (newborn) P15.9
    maternal NEC O71.9
  Descemet's membrane — see Injury, eyeball, penetrating
  diaphragm — see Injury, intrathoracic, diaphragm
  duodenum — see Injury, intestine, small, duodenum
  ear (auricle) (external) (canal) S09.91 ☑
    abrasion — see Abrasion, ear
    bite — see Bite, ear
    blister — see Blister, ear
    bruise — see Contusion, ear
    contusion — see Contusion, ear
    external constriction — see Constriction, external, ear
    hematoma — see Hematoma, ear
    inner — see Injury, ear, middle
    laceration — see Laceration, ear
    middle S09.30- ☑
      blast — see Injury, blast, ear
      specified NEC S09.39- ☑
    puncture — see Puncture, ear
    superficial — see Injury, superficial, ear
  eighth cranial nerve (acoustic or auditory) — see Injury, nerve, acoustic
  elbow S59.90- ☑
    contusion — see Contusion, elbow
    dislocation — see Dislocation, elbow
    fracture — see Fracture, ulna, upper end
    open — see Wound, open, elbow
    specified NEC S59.80- ☑
    sprain — see Sprain, elbow
    superficial — see Injury, superficial, elbow
  eleventh cranial nerve (accessory) — see Injury, nerve, accessory
  epididymis S39.94 ☑
  epigastric region S39.91 ☑
  epiglottis NEC S19.89 ☑
  esophageal plexus — see Injury, nerve, thorax, sympathetic
  esophagus (thoracic part) (see also Injury, intrathoracic, esophagus)
    cervical NEC S19.85 ☑
  eustachian tube S09.30 ☑
  eye S05.9- ☑
    avulsion S05.7- ☑
    ball — see Injury, eyeball
    conjunctiva S05.0- ☑
    cornea
      abrasion S05.0- ☑
      laceration S05.3- ☑
        with prolapse S05.2- ☑
    lacrimal apparatus S05.8X- ☑
    orbit penetration S05.4- ☑
    specified site NEC S05.8X- ☑
  eyeball S05.8X- ☑
    contusion S05.1- ☑
    penetrating S05.6- ☑
      with
        foreign body S05.5- ☑
        prolapse or loss of intraocular tissue S05.2- ☑
        without prolapse or loss of intraocular tissue S05.3- ☑
    specified type NEC S05.8- ☑
  eyebrow S09.93 ☑

Injury — continued
eyelid S09.93 ☑
  abrasion — see Abrasion, eyelid
  contusion — see Contusion, eyelid
  open — see Wound, open, eyelid
face S09.93 ☑
fallopian tube S37.509 ☑
  bilateral S37.502 ☑
    blast injury S37.512 ☑
    contusion S37.522 ☑
    laceration S37.532 ☑
    specified type NEC S37.592 ☑
  blast injury (primary) S37.519 ☑
    bilateral S37.512 ☑
    secondary — see Injury, fallopian tube, specified type NEC
    unilateral S37.511 ☑
  contusion S37.529 ☑
    bilateral S37.522 ☑
    unilateral S37.521 ☑
  laceration S37.539 ☑
    bilateral S37.532 ☑
    unilateral S37.531 ☑
  specified type NEC S37.599 ☑
    bilateral S37.592 ☑
    unilateral S37.591 ☑
  unilateral S37.501 ☑
    blast injury S37.511 ☑
    contusion S37.521 ☑
    laceration S37.531 ☑
    specified type NEC S37.591 ☑
fascia — see Injury, muscle
fifth cranial nerve (trigeminal) — see Injury, nerve, trigeminal
finger (nail) S69.9- ☑
  blood vessel — see Injury, blood vessel, finger
  contusion — see Contusion, finger
  dislocation — see Dislocation, finger
  fracture — see Fracture, finger
  muscle — see Injury, muscle, finger
  nerve — see Injury, nerve, digital, finger
  open — see Wound, open, finger
  specified NEC S69.8- ☑
  sprain — see Sprain, finger
  superficial — see Injury, superficial, finger
first cranial nerve (olfactory) — see Injury, nerve, olfactory
flank — see Injury, abdomen
foot S99.92- ☑
  blood vessel — see Injury, blood vessel, foot
  contusion — see Contusion, foot
  dislocation — see Dislocation, foot
  fracture — see Fracture, foot
  muscle — see Injury, muscle, foot
  open — see Wound, open, foot
  specified type NEC S99.82- ☑
  sprain — see Sprain, foot
  superficial — see Injury, superficial, foot
forceps NOS P15.9
forearm S59.91- ☑
  blood vessel — see Injury, blood vessel, forearm
  contusion — see Contusion, forearm
  fracture — see Fracture, forearm
  muscle — see Injury, muscle, forearm
  nerve — see Injury, nerve, forearm
  open — see Wound, open, forearm
  specified NEC S59.81- ☑
  superficial — see Injury, superficial, forearm
forehead S09.90 ☑
fourth cranial nerve (trochlear) — see Injury, nerve, trochlear
gallbladder S36.129 ☑
  contusion S36.122 ☑
  laceration S36.123 ☑
  specified NEC S36.128 ☑
ganglion
  celiac, coeliac — see Injury, nerve, lumbosacral, sympathetic
  gasserian — see Injury, nerve, trigeminal
  stellate — see Injury, nerve, thorax, sympathetic
  thoracic sympathetic — see Injury, nerve, thorax, sympathetic
gasserian ganglion — see Injury, nerve, trigeminal
gastric artery — see Injury, blood vessel, celiac artery, branch

Injury — continued
gastroduodenal artery — see Injury, blood vessel, celiac artery, branch
gastrointestinal tract — see Injury, intra-abdominal
  with open wound into abdominal cavity — see Wound, open, with penetration into peritoneal cavity
  colon — see Injury, intestine, large
  rectum — see Injury, intestine, large, rectum
    with open wound into abdominal cavity S36.61
  small intestine — see Injury, intestine, small
  specified site NEC — see Injury, intra-abdominal, specified, site NEC
  stomach — see Injury, stomach
genital organ(s)
  external S39.94 ☑
    specified NEC S39.848 ☑
  internal S37.90 ☑
    fallopian tube — see Injury, fallopian tube
    ovary — see Injury, ovary
    prostate — see Injury, prostate
    seminal vesicle — see Injury, pelvis, organ, specified site NEC
    uterus — see Injury, uterus
    vas deferens — see Injury, pelvis, organ, specified site NEC
  obstetrical trauma O71.9
gland
  lacrimal laceration — see Injury, eye, specified site NEC
  salivary S09.90 ☑
  thyroid NEC S19.84 ☑
globe (eye) S05.90 ☑
  specified NEC S05.8X- ☑
groin — see Injury, abdomen
gum S09.90 ☑
hand S69.9- ☑
  blood vessel — see Injury, blood vessel, hand
  contusion — see Contusion, hand
  fracture — see Fracture, hand
  muscle — see Injury, muscle, hand
  nerve — see Injury, nerve, hand
  open — see Wound, open, hand
  specified NEC S69.8- ☑
  sprain — see Sprain, hand
  superficial — see Injury, superficial, hand
head S09.90 ☑
  with loss of consciousness S06.9- ☑
  specified NEC S09.8 ☑
heart S26.90 ☑
  with hemopericardium S26.00 ☑
    contusion S26.01 ☑
    laceration (mild) S26.020 ☑
      major S26.022 ☑
      moderate S26.021 ☑
    specified type NEC S26.09 ☑
  without hemopericardium S26.10 ☑
    contusion S26.11 ☑
    laceration S26.12 ☑
    specified type NEC S26.19 ☑
  contusion S26.91 ☑
  laceration S26.92 ☑
  specified type NEC S26.99 ☑
heel — see Injury, foot
hepatic
  artery — see Injury, blood vessel, celiac artery, branch
  duct — see Injury, liver
  vein — see Injury, vena cava, inferior
hip S79.91- ☑
  blood vessel — see Injury, blood vessel, hip
  contusion — see Contusion, hip
  dislocation — see Dislocation, hip
  fracture — see Fracture, femur, neck
  muscle — see Injury, muscle, hip
  nerve — see Injury, nerve, hip
  open — see Wound, open, hip
  specified NEC S79.81- ☑
  sprain — see Sprain, hip
  superficial — see Injury, superficial, hip
hymen S39.94 ☑
hypogastric
  blood vessel — see Injury, blood vessel, iliac
  plexus — see Injury, nerve, lumbosacral, sympathetic

Injury — continued
ileum — see Injury, intestine, small
iliac region S39.91 ☑
instrumental (during surgery) — see Laceration, accidental complicating surgery
  birth injury — see Birth, injury
  nonsurgical — see Injury, by site
  obstetrical O71.9
    bladder O71.5
    cervix O71.3
    high vaginal O71.4
    perineal NOS O70.9
    urethra O71.5
    uterus O71.5
      with rupture or perforation O71.1
internal T14.8
  aorta — see Injury, aorta
  bladder (sphincter) — see Injury, bladder
    with
      ectopic or molar pregnancy O08.6
      following ectopic or molar pregnancy O08.6
      obstetrical trauma O71.5
  bronchus, bronchi — see Injury, intrathoracic, bronchus
  cecum — see Injury, intestine, large
  cervix (uteri) (see also Injury, uterus)
    with ectopic or molar pregnancy O08.6
    following ectopic or molar pregnancy O08.6
    obstetrical trauma O71.3
  chest — see Injury, intrathoracic
  gastrointestinal tract — see Injury, intra-abdominal
  heart — see Injury, heart
  intestine NEC — see Injury, intestine
  intrauterine — see Injury, uterus
  mesentery — see Injury, intra-abdominal, specified, site NEC
  pelvis, pelvic (organ) S37.90 ☑
    following ectopic or molar pregnancy (subsequent episode) O08.6
    obstetrical trauma NEC O71.5
      rupture or perforation O71.1
    specified NEC S39.83 ☑
  rectum — see Injury, intestine, large, rectum
  stomach — see Injury, stomach
  ureter — see Injury, ureter
  urethra (sphincter) following ectopic or molar pregnancy O08.6
  uterus — see Injury, uterus
interscapular area — see Injury, thorax
intestine
  large S36.509 ☑
    ascending (right) S36.500 ☑
      blast injury (primary) S36.510 ☑
        secondary S36.590 ☑
      contusion S36.520 ☑
      laceration S36.530 ☑
      specified type NEC S36.590 ☑
    blast injury (primary) S36.519 ☑
      ascending (right) S36.510 ☑
      descending (left) S36.512 ☑
      rectum S36.61 ☑
      sigmoid S36.513 ☑
      specified site NEC S36.518 ☑
      transverse S36.511 ☑
    contusion S36.529 ☑
      ascending (right) S36.520 ☑
      descending (left) S36.522 ☑
      rectum S36.62 ☑
      sigmoid S36.523 ☑
      specified site NEC S36.528 ☑
      transverse S36.521 ☑
    descending (left) S36.502 ☑
      blast injury (primary) S36.512 ☑
        secondary S36.592 ☑
      contusion S36.522 ☑
      laceration S36.532 ☑
      specified type NEC S36.592 ☑
    laceration S36.539 ☑
      ascending (right) S36.530 ☑
      descending (left) S36.532 ☑
      rectum S36.63 ☑
      sigmoid S36.533 ☑
      specified site NEC S36.538 ☑
      transverse S36.531 ☑
    rectum S36.60 ☑
      blast injury (primary) S36.61 ☑

Injury — *continued*
  intestine — *continued*
    large — *continued*
      rectum — *continued*
        blast injury — *continued*
          secondary S36.69 ☑
        contusion S36.62 ☑
        laceration S36.63 ☑
        specified type NEC S36.69 ☑
      sigmoid S36.503 ☑
        blast injury (primary) S36.513 ☑
          secondary S36.593 ☑
        contusion S36.523 ☑
        laceration S36.533 ☑
        specified type NEC S36.593 ☑
      specified
        site NEC S36.508 ☑
          blast injury (primary) S36.518 ☑
            secondary S36.598 ☑
          contusion S36.528 ☑
          laceration S36.538 ☑
          specified type NEC S36.598 ☑
        type NEC S36.599 ☑
          ascending (right) S36.590 ☑
          descending (left) S36.592 ☑
          rectum S36.69 ☑
          sigmoid S36.593 ☑
          specified site NEC S36.598 ☑
          transverse S36.591 ☑
      transverse S36.501 ☑
        blast injury (primary) S36.511 ☑
          secondary S36.591 ☑
        contusion S36.521 ☑
        laceration S36.531 ☑
        specified type NEC S36.591 ☑
    small S36.409 ☑
      blast injury (primary) S36.419 ☑
        duodenum S36.410 ☑
        secondary S36.499 ☑
          duodenum S36.490 ☑
          specified site NEC S36.498 ☑
        specified site NEC S36.418 ☑
      contusion S36.429 ☑
        duodenum S36.420 ☑
        specified site NEC S36.428 ☑
      duodenum S36.400 ☑
        blast injury (primary) S36.410 ☑
          secondary S36.490 ☑
        contusion S36.420 ☑
        laceration S36.430 ☑
        specified NEC S36.490 ☑
      laceration S36.439 ☑
        duodenum S36.430 ☑
        specified site NEC S36.438 ☑
      specified
        site NEC S36.408 ☑
        type NEC S36.499 ☑
          duodenum S36.490 ☑
          specified site NEC S36.498 ☑
  intra-abdominal S36.90 ☑
    adrenal gland — *see* Injury, adrenal gland
    bladder — *see* Injury, bladder
    colon — *see* Injury, intestine, large
    contusion S36.92 ☑
    fallopian tube — *see* Injury, fallopian tube
    gallbladder — *see* Injury, gallbladder
    intestine — *see* Injury, intestine
    kidney — *see* Injury, kidney
    laceration S36.93 ☑
    liver — *see* Injury, liver
    ovary — *see* Injury, ovary
    pancreas — *see* Injury, pancreas
    pelvic NOS S37.90 ☑
    peritoneum — *see* Injury, intra-abdominal, specified, site NEC
    prostate — *see* Injury, prostate
    rectum — *see* Injury, intestine, large, rectum
    retroperitoneum — *see* Injury, intra-abdominal, specified, site NEC
    seminal vesicle — *see* Injury, pelvis, organ, specified site NEC
    small intestine — *see* Injury, intestine, small
    specified
      pelvic S37.90 ☑
        specified
          site NEC S37.899 ☑

Injury — *continued*
  intra-abdominal — *continued*
    specified — *continued*
      pelvic — *continued*
        specified — *continued*
          site — *continued*
            specified type NEC S37.898 ☑
          type NEC S37.99 ☑
        site NEC S36.899 ☑
          contusion S36.892 ☑
          laceration S36.893 ☑
          specified type NEC S36.898 ☑
        type NEC S36.99 ☑
      spleen — *see* Injury, spleen
      stomach — *see* Injury, stomach
      ureter — *see* Injury, ureter
      urethra — *see* Injury, urethra
      uterus — *see* Injury, uterus
      vas deferens — *see* Injury, pelvis, organ, specified site NEC
  intracranial (traumatic) S06.9- ☑
    cerebellar hemorrhage, traumatic — *see* Injury, intracranial, focal
    cerebral edema, traumatic S06.1X- ☑
      diffuse S06.1X- ☑
      focal S06.1X- ☑
    diffuse (axonal) S06.2X- ☑
    epidural hemorrhage (traumatic) S06.4X- ☑
    focal brain injury S06.30- ☑
      contusion — *see* Contusion, cerebral
      laceration — *see* Laceration, cerebral
      intracerebral hemorrhage, traumatic S06.36- ☑
        left side S06.35- ☑
        right side S06.34- ☑
    subarachnoid hemorrhage, traumatic S06.6X- ☑
    subdural hemorrhage, traumatic S06.5X- ☑
  intraocular — *see* Injury, eyeball, penetrating
  intrathoracic S27.9 ☑
    bronchus S27.409 ☑
      bilateral S27.402 ☑
      blast injury (primary) S27.419 ☑
        bilateral S27.412 ☑
        secondary — *see* Injury, intrathoracic, bronchus, specified type NEC
        unilateral S27.411 ☑
      contusion S27.429 ☑
        bilateral S27.422 ☑
        unilateral S27.421 ☑
      laceration S27.439 ☑
        bilateral S27.432 ☑
        unilateral S27.431 ☑
      specified type NEC S27.499 ☑
        bilateral S27.492 ☑
        unilateral S27.491 ☑
      unilateral S27.401 ☑
    diaphragm S27.809 ☑
      contusion S27.802 ☑
      laceration S27.803 ☑
      specified type NEC S27.808 ☑
    esophagus (thoracic) S27.819 ☑
      contusion S27.812 ☑
      laceration S27.813 ☑
      specified type NEC S27.818 ☑
    heart — *see* Injury, heart
    hemopneumothorax S27.2 ☑
    hemothorax S27.1 ☑
    lung S27.309 ☑
      aspiration J69.0
      bilateral S27.302 ☑
      blast injury (primary) S27.319 ☑
        bilateral S27.312 ☑
        secondary — *see* Injury, intrathoracic, lung, specified type NEC
        unilateral S27.311 ☑
      contusion S27.329 ☑
        bilateral S27.322 ☑
        unilateral S27.321 ☑
      laceration S27.339 ☑
        bilateral S27.332 ☑
        unilateral S27.331 ☑
      specified type NEC S27.399 ☑
        bilateral S27.392 ☑
        unilateral S27.391 ☑
      unilateral S27.301 ☑
    pleura S27.60 ☑
      laceration S27.63 ☑

Injury — *continued*
  intrathoracic — *continued*
    pleura — *continued*
      specified type NEC S27.69 ☑
      pneumothorax S27.0 ☑
    specified organ NEC S27.899 ☑
      contusion S27.892 ☑
      laceration S27.893 ☑
      specified type NEC S27.898 ☑
    thoracic duct — *see* Injury, intrathoracic, specified organ NEC
    thymus gland — *see* Injury, intrathoracic, specified organ NEC
    trachea, thoracic S27.50 ☑
      blast (primary) S27.51 ☑
      contusion S27.52 ☑
      laceration S27.53 ☑
      specified type NEC S27.59 ☑
  iris — *see* Injury, eye, specified site NEC
    penetrating — *see* Injury, eyeball, penetrating
  jaw S09.93 ☑
  jejunum — *see* Injury, intestine, small
  joint NOS T14.8
    old or residual — *see* Disorder, joint, specified type NEC
  kidney S37.00- ☑
    acute (nontraumatic) N17.9
    contusion — *see* Contusion, kidney
    laceration — *see* Laceration, kidney
    specified NEC S37.09- ☑
  knee S89.9- ☑
    contusion — *see* Contusion, knee
    dislocation — *see* Dislocation, knee
    meniscus (lateral) (medial) — *see* Sprain, knee, specified site NEC
      old injury or tear — *see* Derangement, knee, meniscus, due to old injury
    open — *see* Wound, open, knee
    specified NEC S89.8- ☑
    sprain — *see* Sprain, knee
    superficial — *see* Injury, superficial, knee
  labium (majus) (minus) S39.94 ☑
  labyrinth, ear S09.30- ☑
  lacrimal apparatus, duct, gland, or sac — *see* Injury, eye, specified site NEC
  larynx NEC S19.81 ☑
  leg (lower) S89.9- ☑
    blood vessel — *see* Injury, blood vessel, leg
    contusion — *see* Contusion, leg
    fracture — *see* Fracture, leg
    muscle — *see* Injury, muscle, leg
    nerve — *see* Injury, nerve, leg
    open — *see* Wound, open, leg
    specified NEC S89.8- ☑
    superficial — *see* Injury, superficial, leg
  lens, eye — *see* Injury, eye, specified site NEC
    penetrating — *see* Injury, eyeball, penetrating
  limb NEC T14.8
  lip S09.93 ☑
  liver S36.119 ☑
    contusion S36.112 ☑
    laceration S36.113 ☑
      major (stellate) S36.116 ☑
      minor S36.114 ☑
      moderate S36.115 ☑
    specified NEC S36.118 ☑
  lower back S39.92 ☑
    specified NEC S39.82 ☑
  lumbar, lumbosacral (region) S39.92 ☑
    plexus — *see* Injury, lumbosacral plexus
  lumbosacral plexus S34.4 ☑
  lung (*see also* Injury, intrathoracic, lung)
    aspiration J69.0
    transfusion-related (TRALI) J95.84
  lymphatic thoracic duct — *see* Injury, intrathoracic, specified organ NEC
  malar region S09.93 ☑
  mastoid region S09.90 ☑
  maxilla S09.93 ☑
  mediastinum — *see* Injury, intrathoracic, specified organ NEC
  membrane, brain — *see* Injury, intracranial
  meningeal artery — *see* Injury, intracranial, subdural hemorrhage
  meninges (cerebral) — *see* Injury, intracranial

Injury — *continued*
  mesenteric
    artery
      branch S35.299 ☑
        laceration (minor) (superficial) S35.291 ☑
          major S35.292 ☑
        specified NEC S35.298 ☑
      inferior S35.239 ☑
        laceration (minor) (superficial) S35.231 ☑
          major S35.232 ☑
        specified NEC S35.238 ☑
      superior S35.229 ☑
        laceration (minor) (superficial) S35.221 ☑
          major S35.222 ☑
        specified NEC S35.228 ☑
    plexus (inferior) (superior) — *see* Injury, nerve, lumbosacral, sympathetic
    vein
      inferior S35.349 ☑
        laceration S35.341 ☑
        specified NEC S35.348 ☑
      superior S35.339 ☑
        laceration S35.331 ☑
        specified NEC S35.338 ☑
  mesentery — *see* Injury, intra-abdominal, specified site NEC
  mesosalpinx — *see* Injury, pelvic organ, specified site NEC
  middle ear S09.30- ☑
  midthoracic region NOS S29.9 ☑
  mouth S09.93 ☑
  multiple NOS T07
  muscle (and fascia) (and tendon)
    abdomen S39.001 ☑
      laceration S39.021 ☑
      specified type NEC S39.091 ☑
      strain S39.011 ☑
    abductor
      thumb, forearm level — *see* Injury, muscle, thumb, abductor
    adductor
      thigh S76.20- ☑
        laceration S76.22- ☑
        specified type NEC S76.29- ☑
        strain S76.21- ☑
    ankle — *see* Injury, muscle, foot
    anterior muscle group, at leg level (lower) S86.20- ☑
      laceration S86.22- ☑
      specified type NEC S86.29- ☑
      strain S86.21- ☑
    arm (upper) — *see* Injury, muscle, shoulder
    biceps (parts NEC) S46.20- ☑
      laceration S46.22- ☑
      long head S46.10- ☑
        laceration S46.12- ☑
        specified type NEC S46.19- ☑
        strain S46.11- ☑
      specified type NEC S46.29- ☑
      strain S46.21- ☑
    extensor
      finger(s) (other than thumb) — *see* Injury, muscle, finger by site, extensor
      forearm level, specified NEC — *see* Injury, muscle, forearm, extensor
      thumb — *see* Injury, muscle, thumb, extensor
      toe (large) (ankle level) (foot level) — *see* Injury, muscle, toe, extensor
    finger
      extensor (forearm level) S56.40- ☑
        hand level S66.309 ☑
          laceration S66.329 ☑
          specified type NEC S66.399 ☑
          strain S66.319 ☑
        laceration S56.429 ☑
        specified type NEC S56.499 ☑
        strain S56.419 ☑
      flexor (forearm level) S56.10- ☑
        hand level S66.109 ☑
          laceration S66.129 ☑
          specified type NEC S66.199 ☑
          strain S66.119 ☑
        laceration S56.129 ☑
        specified type NEC S56.199 ☑
        strain S56.119 ☑

Injury — *continued*
  muscle — *continued*
    finger — *continued*
      index
        extensor (forearm level)
          hand level S66.308 ☑
            laceration S66.32- ☑
            specified type NEC S66.39- ☑
            strain S66.31- ☑
          specified type NEC S56.492- ☑
        flexor (forearm level)
          hand level S66.108 ☑
            laceration S66.12- ☑
            specified type NEC S66.19- ☑
            strain S66.11- ☑
          specified type NEC S56.19- ☑
          strain S56.11- ☑
        intrinsic S66.50- ☑
          laceration S66.52- ☑
          specified type NEC S66.59- ☑
          strain S66.51- ☑
      intrinsic S66.509 ☑
        laceration S66.529 ☑
        specified type NEC S66.599 ☑
        strain S66.519 ☑
      little
        extensor (forearm level)
          hand level S66.30- ☑
            laceration S66.32- ☑
            specified type NEC S66.39- ☑
            strain S66.31- ☑
          laceration S56.42- ☑
          specified type NEC S56.49- ☑
          strain S56.41- ☑
        flexor (forearm level)
          hand level S66.10- ☑
            laceration S66.12- ☑
            specified type NEC S66.19- ☑
            strain S66.11- ☑
          laceration S56.12- ☑
          specified type NEC S56.19- ☑
          strain S56.11- ☑
        intrinsic S66.50- ☑
          laceration S66.52- ☑
          specified type NEC S66.59- ☑
          strain S66.51- ☑
      middle
        extensor (forearm level)
          hand level S66.30- ☑
            laceration S66.32- ☑
            specified type NEC S66.39- ☑
            strain S66.31- ☑
          laceration S56.42- ☑
          specified type NEC S56.49- ☑
          strain S56.41- ☑
        flexor (forearm level)
          hand level S66.10- ☑
            laceration S66.12- ☑
            specified type NEC S66.19- ☑
            strain S66.11- ☑
          laceration S56.12- ☑
          specified type NEC S56.19- ☑
          strain S56.11- ☑
        intrinsic S66.50- ☑
          laceration S66.52- ☑
          specified type NEC S66.59- ☑
          strain S66.51- ☑
      ring
        extensor (forearm level)
          hand level S66.30- ☑
            laceration S66.32- ☑
            specified type NEC S66.39- ☑
            strain S66.31- ☑
          laceration S56.42- ☑
          specified type NEC S56.49- ☑
          strain S56.41- ☑
        flexor (forearm level)
          hand level S66.10- ☑
            laceration S66.12- ☑
            specified type NEC S66.19- ☑
            strain S66.11- ☑
          laceration S56.12- ☑
          specified type NEC S56.19- ☑
          strain S56.11- ☑
        intrinsic S66.50- ☑
          laceration S66.52-

Injury — *continued*
  muscle — *continued*
    finger — *continued*
      ring — *continued*
        intrinsic — *continued*
          specified type NEC S66.59- ☑
          strain S66.51- ☑
    flexor
      finger(s) (other than thumb) — *see* Injury, muscle, finger
      forearm level, specified NEC — *see* Injury, muscle, forearm, flexor
      thumb — *see* Injury, muscle, thumb, flexor
      toe (long) (ankle level) (foot level) — *see* Injury, muscle, toe, flexor
    foot S96.90- ☑
      intrinsic S96.20- ☑
        laceration S96.22- ☑
        specified type NEC S96.29- ☑
        strain S96.21- ☑
      laceration S96.92- ☑
      long extensor, toe — *see* Injury, muscle, toe, extensor
      long flexor, toe — *see* Injury, muscle, toe, flexor
      specified
        site NEC S96.80- ☑
          laceration S96.82- ☑
          specified type NEC S96.89- ☑
          strain S96.81- ☑
          type S96.99- ☑
      strain S96.91- ☑
    forearm (level) S56.90- ☑
      extensor S56.50- ☑
        laceration S56.52- ☑
        specified type NEC S56.59- ☑
        strain S56.51- ☑
      flexor S56.20- ☑
        laceration S56.22- ☑
        specified type NEC S56.29- ☑
        strain S56.21- ☑
      laceration S56.92- ☑
      specified S56.99- ☑
        site NEC S56.80- ☑
          laceration S56.82- ☑
          strain S56.81- ☑
          type NEC S56.89- ☑
      strain S56.91- ☑
    hand (level) S66.90- ☑
      laceration S66.92- ☑
      specified
        site NEC S66.80- ☑
          laceration S66.82- ☑
          specified type NEC S66.89- ☑
          strain S66.81- ☑
          type NEC S66.99- ☑
      strain S66.91- ☑
    head S09.10 ☑
      laceration S09.12 ☑
      specified type NEC S09.19 ☑
      strain S09.11 ☑
    hip NEC S76.00- ☑
      laceration S76.02- ☑
      specified type NEC S76.09- ☑
      strain S76.01- ☑
    intrinsic
      ankle and foot level — *see* Injury, muscle, foot, intrinsic
      finger (other than thumb) — *see* Injury, muscle, finger by site, intrinsic
      foot (level) — *see* Injury, muscle, foot, intrinsic
      thumb — *see* Injury, muscle, thumb, intrinsic
    leg (level) (lower) S86.90- ☑
      Achilles tendon — *see* Injury, Achilles tendon
      anterior muscle group — *see* Injury, muscle, anterior muscle group
      laceration S86.92- ☑
      peroneal muscle group — *see* Injury, muscle, peroneal muscle group
      posterior muscle group — *see* Injury, muscle, posterior muscle group, leg level
      specified
        site NEC S86.80- ☑
          laceration S86.82- ☑
          specified type NEC S86.89- ☑
          strain S86.81- ☑
          type NEC S86.99- ☑

188

☑ Additional Character Required — Refer to the Tabular List for Character Selection   ▽ Subterms under main terms may continue to next column or page

Injury — *continued*
  muscle — *continued*
    leg — *continued*
      strain S86.91- ☑
    long
      extensor toe, at ankle and foot level — *see* Injury, muscle, toe, extensor
      flexor, toe, at ankle and foot level — *see* Injury, muscle, toe, flexor
      head, biceps — *see* Injury, muscle, biceps, long head
    lower back S39.002 ☑
      laceration S39.022 ☑
      specified type NEC S39.092 ☑
      strain S39.012 ☑
    neck (level) S16.9 ☑
      laceration S16.2 ☑
      specified type NEC S16.8 ☑
      strain S16.1 ☑
    pelvis S39.003 ☑
      laceration S39.023 ☑
      specified type NEC S39.093 ☑
      strain S39.013 ☑
    peroneal muscle group, at leg level (lower) S86.30- ☑
      laceration S86.32- ☑
      specified type NEC S86.39- ☑
      strain S86.31- ☑
    posterior muscle (group)
      leg level (lower) S86.10- ☑
        laceration S86.12- ☑
        specified type NEC S86.19- ☑
        strain S86.11- ☑
      thigh level S76.30- ☑
        laceration S76.32- ☑
        specified type NEC S76.39- ☑
        strain S76.31- ☑
    quadriceps (thigh) S76.10- ☑
      laceration S76.12- ☑
      specified type NEC S76.19- ☑
      strain S76.11- ☑
    shoulder S46.90- ☑
      laceration S46.92- ☑
      rotator cuff — *see* Injury, rotator cuff
      specified site S46.80- ☑
        laceration S46.82- ☑
        specified type NEC S46.89- ☑
        strain S46.81- ☑
      specified type NEC S46.99- ☑
      strain S46.91- ☑
    thigh NEC (level) S76.90- ☑
      adductor — *see* Injury, muscle, adductor, thigh
      laceration S76.92- ☑
      posterior muscle (group) — *see* Injury, muscle, posterior muscle, thigh level
      quadriceps — *see* Injury, muscle, quadriceps
      specified
        site NEC S76.80- ☑
          laceration S76.82- ☑
          specified type NEC S76.89- ☑
          strain S76.81- ☑
        type NEC S76.99- ☑
      strain S76.91- ☑
    thorax (level) S29.009 ☑
      back wall S29.002 ☑
      front wall S29.001 ☑
      laceration S29.029 ☑
        back wall S29.022 ☑
        front wall S29.021 ☑
      specified type NEC S29.099 ☑
        back wall S29.092 ☑
        front wall S29.091 ☑
      strain S29.019 ☑
        back wall S29.012 ☑
        front wall S29.011 ☑
    thumb
      abductor (forearm level) S56.30- ☑
        laceration S56.32- ☑
        specified type NEC S56.39- ☑
        strain S56.31- ☑
      extensor (forearm level) S56.30- ☑
        hand level S66.20- ☑
          laceration S66.22- ☑
          specified type NEC S66.29- ☑
          strain S66.21- ☑
        laceration S56.32- ☑

Injury — *continued*
  muscle — *continued*
    thumb — *continued*
      extensor — *continued*
        specified type NEC S56.39- ☑
        strain S56.31- ☑
      flexor (forearm level) S56.00- ☑
        hand level S66.00- ☑
          laceration S66.02- ☑
          specified type NEC S66.09- ☑
          strain S66.01- ☑
        laceration S56.02- ☑
        specified type NEC S56.09- ☑
        strain S56.01- ☑
        wrist level — *see* Injury, muscle, thumb, flexor, hand level
      intrinsic S66.40- ☑
        laceration S66.42- ☑
        specified type NEC S66.49- ☑
        strain S66.41- ☑
    toe (*see also* Injury, muscle, foot)
      extensor, long S96.10- ☑
        laceration S96.12- ☑
        specified type NEC S96.19- ☑
        strain S96.11- ☑
      flexor, long S96.00- ☑
        laceration S96.02- ☑
        specified type NEC S96.09- ☑
        strain S96.01- ☑
    triceps S46.30- ☑
      laceration S46.32- ☑
      specified type NEC S46.39- ☑
      strain S46.31- ☑
    wrist (and hand) level — *see* Injury, muscle, hand
  musculocutaneous nerve — *see* Injury, nerve, musculocutaneous
  myocardium — *see* Injury, heart
  nape — *see* Injury, neck
  nasal (septum) (sinus) S09.92 ☑
  nasopharynx S09.92 ☑
  neck S19.9 ☑
    specified NEC S19.80 ☑
      specified site NEC S19.89 ☑
  nerve NEC T14.8
    abdomen S34.9 ☑
      peripheral S34.6 ☑
      specified site NEC S34.8 ☑
    abducens S04.4- ☑
      contusion S04.4- ☑
      laceration S04.4- ☑
      specified type NEC S04.4- ☑
    abducent — *see* Injury, nerve, abducens
    accessory S04.7- ☑
      contusion S04.7- ☑
      laceration S04.7- ☑
      specified type NEC S04.7- ☑
    acoustic S04.6- ☑
      contusion S04.6- ☑
      laceration S04.6- ☑
      specified type NEC S04.6- ☑
    ankle S94.9- ☑
      cutaneous sensory S94.3- ☑
      specified site NEC — *see* subcategory S94.8 ☑
    anterior crural, femoral — *see* Injury, nerve, femoral
    arm (upper) S44.9- ☑
      axillary — *see* Injury, nerve, axillary
      cutaneous — *see* Injury, nerve, cutaneous, arm
      median — *see* Injury, nerve, median, upper arm
      musculocutaneous — *see* Injury, nerve, musculocutaneous
      radial — *see* Injury, nerve, radial, upper arm
      specified site NEC — *see* subcategory S44.8 ☑
      ulnar — *see* Injury, nerve, ulnar, arm
    auditory — *see* Injury, nerve, acoustic
    axillary S44.3- ☑
    brachial plexus — *see* Injury, brachial plexus
    cervical sympathetic S14.5 ☑
    cranial S04.9 ☑
      contusion S04.9 ☑
      eighth (acoustic or auditory) — *see* Injury, nerve, acoustic
      eleventh (accessory) — *see* Injury, nerve, accessory
      fifth (trigeminal) — *see* Injury, nerve, trigeminal
      first (olfactory) — *see* Injury, nerve, olfactory
      fourth (trochlear) — *see* Injury, nerve, trochlear

Injury — *continued*
  nerve — *continued*
    cranial — *continued*
      laceration S04.9 ☑
      ninth (glossopharyngeal) — *see* Injury, nerve, glossopharyngeal
      second (optic) — *see* Injury, nerve, optic
      seventh (facial) — *see* Injury, nerve, facial
      sixth (abducent) — *see* Injury, nerve, abducens
      specified
        nerve NEC S04.89- ☑
          contusion S04.89- ☑
          laceration S04.89- ☑
          specified type NEC S04.89- ☑
        type NEC S04.9 ☑
      tenth (pneumogastric or vagus) — *see* Injury, nerve, vagus
      third (oculomotor) — *see* Injury, nerve, oculomotor
      twelfth (hypoglossal) — *see* Injury, nerve, hypoglossal
    cutaneous sensory
      ankle (level) S94.3- ☑
      arm (upper) (level) S44.5- ☑
      foot (level) — *see* Injury, nerve, cutaneous sensory, ankle
      forearm (level) S54.3- ☑
      hip (level) S74.2- ☑
      leg (lower level) S84.2- ☑
      shoulder (level) — *see* Injury, nerve, cutaneous sensory, arm
      thigh (level) — *see* Injury, nerve, cutaneous sensory, hip
    deep peroneal — *see* Injury, nerve, peroneal, foot
    digital
      finger S64.4- ☑
        index S64.49- ☑
        little S64.49- ☑
        middle S64.49- ☑
        ring S64.49- ☑
      thumb S64.3- ☑
      toe — *see* Injury, nerve, ankle, specified site NEC
    eighth cranial (acoustic or auditory) — *see* Injury, nerve, acoustic
    eleventh cranial (accessory) — *see* Injury, nerve, accessory
    facial S04.5- ☑
      contusion S04.5- ☑
      laceration S04.5- ☑
      newborn P11.3
      specified type NEC S04.5- ☑
    femoral (hip level) (thigh level) S74.1- ☑
    fifth cranial (trigeminal) — *see* Injury, nerve, trigeminal
    finger (digital) — *see* Injury, nerve, digital, finger
    first cranial (olfactory) — *see* Injury, nerve, olfactory
    foot S94.9- ☑
      cutaneous sensory S94.3- ☑
      deep peroneal S94.2- ☑
      lateral plantar S94.0- ☑
      medial plantar S94.1- ☑
      specified site NEC — *see* subcategory S94.8 ☑
    forearm (level) S54.9- ☑
      cutaneous sensory — *see* Injury, nerve, cutaneous sensory, forearm
      median — *see* Injury, nerve, median
      radial — *see* Injury, nerve, radial
      specified site NEC — *see* subcategory S54.8 ☑
      ulnar — *see* Injury, nerve, ulnar
    fourth cranial (trochlear) — *see* Injury, nerve, trochlear
    glossopharyngeal S04.89- ☑
      specified type NEC S04.89- ☑
    hand S64.9- ☑
      median — *see* Injury, nerve, median, hand
      radial — *see* Injury, nerve, radial, hand
      specified NEC — *see* subcategory S64.8 ☑
      ulnar — *see* Injury, nerve, ulnar, hand
    hip (level) S74.9- ☑
      cutaneous sensory — *see* Injury, nerve, cutaneous sensory, hip
      femoral — *see* Injury, nerve, femoral
      sciatic — *see* Injury, nerve, sciatic
      specified site NEC — *see* subcategory S74.8 ☑
    hypoglossal S04.89- ☑

Injury — *continued*
  nerve — *continued*
    hypoglossal — *continued*
      specified type NEC S04.89- ☑
    lateral plantar S94.0- ☑
    leg (lower) S84.9- ☑
      cutaneous sensory — *see* Injury, nerve, cutaneous sensory, leg
      peroneal — *see* Injury, nerve, peroneal
      specified site NEC — *see* subcategory S84.8 ☑
      tibial — *see* Injury, nerve, tibial
      upper — *see* Injury, nerve, thigh
    lower
      back — *see* Injury, nerve, abdomen, specified site NEC
        peripheral — *see* Injury, nerve, abdomen, peripheral
      limb — *see* Injury, nerve, leg
    lumbar plexus — *see* Injury, nerve, lumbosacral, sympathetic
    lumbar spinal — *see* Injury, nerve, spinal, lumbar
    lumbosacral
      plexus — *see* Injury, nerve, lumbosacral, sympathetic
      sympathetic S34.5 ☑
    medial plantar S94.1- ☑
    median (forearm level) S54.1- ☑
      hand (level) S64.1- ☑
      upper arm (level) S44.1- ☑
      wrist (level) — *see* Injury, nerve, median, hand
    musculocutaneous S44.4- ☑
    musculospiral (upper arm level) — *see* Injury, nerve, radial, upper arm
    neck S14.9 ☑
      peripheral S14.4 ☑
      specified site NEC S14.8 ☑
      sympathetic S14.5 ☑
    ninth cranial (glossopharyngeal) — *see* Injury, nerve, glossopharyngeal
    oculomotor S04.1- ☑
      contusion S04.1- ☑
      laceration S04.1- ☑
      specified type NEC S04.1- ☑
    olfactory S04.81- ☑
      specified type NEC S04.81- ☑
    optic S04.01- ☑
      contusion S04.01- ☑
      laceration S04.01- ☑
      specified type NEC S04.01- ☑
    pelvic girdle — *see* Injury, nerve, hip
    pelvis — *see* Injury, nerve, abdomen, specified site NEC
      peripheral — *see* Injury, nerve, abdomen, peripheral
    peripheral NEC T14.8
      abdomen — *see* Injury, nerve, abdomen, peripheral
      lower back — *see* Injury, nerve, abdomen, peripheral
      neck — *see* Injury, nerve, neck, peripheral
      pelvis — *see* Injury, nerve, abdomen, peripheral
      specified NEC T14.8
    peroneal (lower leg level) S84.1- ☑
      foot S94.2- ☑
    plexus
      brachial — *see* Injury, brachial plexus
      celiac, coeliac — *see* Injury, nerve, lumbosacral, sympathetic
      mesenteric, inferior — *see* Injury, nerve, lumbosacral, sympathetic
      sacral — *see* Injury, lumbosacral plexus
      spinal
        brachial — *see* Injury, brachial plexus
        lumbosacral — *see* Injury, lumbosacral plexus
    pneumogastric — *see* Injury, nerve, vagus
    radial (forearm level) S54.2- ☑
      hand (level) S64.2- ☑
      upper arm (level) S44.2- ☑
      wrist (level) — *see* Injury, nerve, radial, hand
    root — *see* Injury, nerve, spinal, root
    sacral plexus — *see* Injury, lumbosacral plexus
    sacral spinal — *see* Injury, nerve, spinal, sacral
    sciatic (hip level) (thigh level) S74.0- ☑
    second cranial (optic) — *see* Injury, nerve, optic
    seventh cranial (facial) — *see* Injury, nerve, facial

Injury — *continued*
  nerve — *continued*
    shoulder — *see* Injury, nerve, arm
    sixth cranial (abducent) — *see* Injury, nerve, abducens
    spinal
      plexus — *see* Injury, nerve, plexus, spinal
      root
        cervical S14.2 ☑
        dorsal S24.2 ☑
        lumbar S34.21 ☑
        sacral S34.22 ☑
        thoracic — *see* Injury, nerve, spinal, root, dorsal
    splanchnic — *see* Injury, nerve, lumbosacral, sympathetic
    sympathetic NEC — *see* Injury, nerve, lumbosacral, sympathetic
      cervical — *see* Injury, nerve, cervical sympathetic
    tenth cranial (pneumogastric or vagus) — *see* Injury, nerve, vagus
    thigh (level) — *see* Injury, nerve, hip
      cutaneous sensory — *see* Injury, nerve, cutaneous sensory, hip
      femoral — *see* Injury, nerve, femoral
      sciatic — *see* Injury, nerve, sciatic
      specified NEC — *see* Injury, nerve, hip
    third cranial (oculomotor) — *see* Injury, nerve, oculomotor
    thorax S24.9 ☑
      peripheral S24.3 ☑
      specified site NEC S24.8 ☑
      sympathetic S24.4 ☑
    thumb, digital — *see* Injury, nerve, digital, thumb
    tibial (lower leg level) (posterior) S84.0- ☑
    toe — *see* Injury, nerve, ankle
    trigeminal S04.3- ☑
      contusion S04.3- ☑
      laceration S04.3- ☑
      specified type NEC S04.3- ☑
    trochlear S04.2- ☑
      contusion S04.2- ☑
      laceration S04.2- ☑
      specified type NEC S04.2- ☑
    twelfth cranial (hypoglossal) — *see* Injury, nerve, hypoglossal
    ulnar (forearm level) S54.0- ☑
      arm (upper) (level) S44.0- ☑
      hand (level) S64.0- ☑
      wrist (level) — *see* Injury, nerve, ulnar, hand
    vagus S04.89- ☑
      specified type NEC S04.89- ☑
    wrist (level) — *see* Injury, nerve, hand
  ninth cranial nerve (glossopharyngeal) — *see* Injury, nerve, glossopharyngeal
  nose (septum) S09.92 ☑
  obstetrical O71.9
    specified NEC O71.89
  occipital (region) (scalp) S09.90 ☑
    lobe — *see* Injury, intracranial
  optic chiasm S04.02 ☑
  optic radiation S04.03- ☑
  optic tract and pathways S04.03- ☑
  orbit, orbital (region) — *see* Injury, eye
    penetrating (with foreign body) — *see* Injury, eye, orbit, penetrating
    specified NEC — *see* Injury, eye, specified site NEC
  ovary, ovarian S37.409 ☑
    bilateral S37.402 ☑
      contusion S37.422 ☑
      laceration S37.432 ☑
      specified type NEC S37.492 ☑
    blood vessel — *see* Injury, blood vessel, ovarian
    contusion S37.429 ☑
      bilateral S37.422 ☑
      unilateral S37.421 ☑
    laceration S37.439 ☑
      bilateral S37.432 ☑
      unilateral S37.431 ☑
    specified type NEC S37.499 ☑
      bilateral S37.492 ☑
      unilateral S37.491 ☑
    unilateral S37.401 ☑
      contusion S37.421 ☑
      laceration S37.431 ☑

Injury — *continued*
  ovary, ovarian — *continued*
    unilateral — *continued*
      specified type NEC S37.491 ☑
  palate (hard) (soft) S09.93 ☑
  pancreas S36.209 ☑
    body S36.201 ☑
      contusion S36.221 ☑
      laceration S36.231 ☑
        major S36.261 ☑
        minor S36.241 ☑
        moderate S36.251 ☑
      specified type NEC S36.291 ☑
    contusion S36.229 ☑
    head S36.200 ☑
      contusion S36.220 ☑
      laceration S36.230 ☑
        major S36.260 ☑
        minor S36.240 ☑
        moderate S36.250 ☑
      specified type NEC S36.290 ☑
    laceration S36.239 ☑
      major S36.269 ☑
      minor S36.249 ☑
      moderate S36.259 ☑
    specified type NEC S36.299 ☑
    tail S36.202 ☑
      contusion S36.222 ☑
      laceration S36.232 ☑
        major S36.262 ☑
        minor S36.242 ☑
        moderate S36.252 ☑
      specified type NEC S36.292 ☑
  parietal (region) (scalp) S09.90 ☑
    lobe — *see* Injury, intracranial
  patellar ligament (tendon) S76.10- ☑
    laceration S76.12- ☑
    specified NEC S76.19- ☑
    strain S76.11- ☑
  pelvis, pelvic (floor) S39.93 ☑
    complicating delivery O70.1
    joint or ligament, complicating delivery O71.6
    organ S37.90 ☑
      with ectopic or molar pregnancy O08.6
      complication of abortion — *see* Abortion
      contusion S37.92 ☑
      following ectopic or molar pregnancy O08.6
      laceration S37.93 ☑
      obstetrical trauma NEC O71.5
      specified
        site NEC S37.899 ☑
          contusion S37.892 ☑
          laceration S37.893 ☑
          specified type NEC S37.898 ☑
        type NEC S37.99 ☑
    specified NEC S39.83 ☑
  penis S39.94 ☑
  perineum S39.94 ☑
  peritoneum S36.81 ☑
    laceration S36.893 ☑
  periurethral tissue — *see* Injury, urethra
    complicating delivery O71.82
  phalanges
    foot — *see* Injury, foot
    hand — *see* Injury, hand
  pharynx NEC S19.85 ☑
  pleura — *see* Injury, intrathoracic, pleura
  plexus
    brachial — *see* Injury, brachial plexus
    cardiac — *see* Injury, nerve, thorax, sympathetic
    celiac, coeliac — *see* Injury, nerve, lumbosacral, sympathetic
    esophageal — *see* Injury, nerve, thorax, sympathetic
    hypogastric — *see* Injury, nerve, lumbosacral, sympathetic
    lumbar, lumbosacral — *see* Injury, lumbosacral plexus
    mesenteric — *see* Injury, nerve, lumbosacral, sympathetic
    pulmonary — *see* Injury, nerve, thorax, sympathetic
  postcardiac surgery (syndrome) I97.0
  prepuce S39.94 ☑
  prostate S37.829 ☑
    contusion S37.822 ☑

☑ Additional Character Required — Refer to the Tabular List for Character Selection   ▽ Subterms under main terms may continue to next column or page

Injury — *continued*
 prostate — *continued*
  laceration S37.823 ☑
  specified type NEC S37.828 ☑
 pubic region S39.94 ☑
 pudendum S39.94 ☑
 pulmonary plexus — *see* Injury, nerve, thorax, sympathetic
 rectovaginal septum NEC S39.83 ☑
 rectum — *see* Injury, intestine, large, rectum
 retina — *see* Injury, eye, specified site NEC
  penetrating — *see* Injury, eyeball, penetrating
 retroperitoneal — *see* Injury, intra-abdominal, specified site NEC
 rotator cuff (muscle(s)) (tendon(s)) S46.00- ☑
  laceration S46.02- ☑
  specified type NEC S46.09- ☑
  strain S46.01- ☑
 round ligament — *see* Injury, pelvic organ, specified site NEC
 sacral plexus — *see* Injury, lumbosacral plexus
 salivary duct or gland S09.93 ☑
 scalp S09.90 ☑
  newborn (birth injury) P12.9
   due to monitoring (electrode) (sampling incision) P12.4
   specified NEC P12.89
    caput succedaneum P12.81
 scapular region — *see* Injury, shoulder
 sclera — *see* Injury, eye, specified site NEC
  penetrating — *see* Injury, eyeball, penetrating
 scrotum S39.94 ☑
 second cranial nerve (optic) — *see* Injury, nerve, optic
 seminal vesicle — *see* Injury, pelvic organ, specified site NEC
 seventh cranial nerve (facial) — *see* Injury, nerve, facial
 shoulder S49.9- ☑
  blood vessel — *see* Injury, blood vessel, arm
  contusion — *see* Contusion, shoulder
  dislocation — *see* Dislocation, shoulder
  fracture — *see* Fracture, shoulder
  muscle — *see* Injury, muscle, shoulder
  nerve — *see* Injury, nerve, shoulder
  open — *see* Wound, open, shoulder
  specified type NEC S49.8- ☑
  sprain — *see* Sprain, shoulder girdle
  superficial — *see* Injury, superficial, shoulder
 sinus
  cavernous — *see* Injury, intracranial
  nasal S09.92 ☑
 sixth cranial nerve (abducent) — *see* Injury, nerve, abducens
 skeleton, birth injury P13.9
  specified part NEC P13.8
 skin NEC T14.8
  surface intact — *see* Injury, superficial
 skull NEC S09.90 ☑
 specified NEC T14.8
 spermatic cord (pelvic region) S37.898 ☑
  scrotal region S39.848 ☑
 spinal (cord)
  cervical (neck) S14.109 ☑
   anterior cord syndrome S14.139 ☑
    C1 level S14.131 ☑
    C2 level S14.132 ☑
    C3 level S14.133 ☑
    C4 level S14.134 ☑
    C5 level S14.135 ☑
    C6 level S14.136 ☑
    C7 level S14.137 ☑
    C8 level S14.138 ☑
   Brown-Séquard syndrome S14.149 ☑
    C1 level S14.141 ☑
    C2 level S14.142 ☑
    C3 level S14.143 ☑
    C4 level S14.144 ☑
    C5 level S14.145 ☑
    C6 level S14.146 ☑
    C7 level S14.147 ☑
    C8 level S14.148 ☑
   C1 level S14.101 ☑
   C2 level S14.102 ☑
   C3 level S14.103 ☑
   C4 level S14.104 ☑
   C5 level S14.105 ☑
   C6 level S14.106 ☑

Injury — *continued*
 spinal — *continued*
  cervical — *continued*
   C7 level S14.107 ☑
   C8 level S14.108 ☑
   central cord syndrome S14.129 ☑
    C1 level S14.121 ☑
    C2 level S14.122 ☑
    C3 level S14.123 ☑
    C4 level S14.124 ☑
    C5 level S14.125 ☑
    C6 level S14.126 ☑
    C7 level S14.127 ☑
    C8 level S14.128 ☑
   complete lesion S14.119 ☑
    C1 level S14.111 ☑
    C2 level S14.112 ☑
    C3 level S14.113 ☑
    C4 level S14.114 ☑
    C5 level S14.115 ☑
    C6 level S14.116 ☑
    C7 level S14.117 ☑
    C8 level S14.118 ☑
   concussion S14.0 ☑
   edema S14.0 ☑
   incomplete lesion specified NEC S14.159 ☑
    C1 level S14.151 ☑
    C2 level S14.152 ☑
    C3 level S14.153 ☑
    C4 level S14.154 ☑
    C5 level S14.155 ☑
    C6 level S14.156 ☑
    C7 level S14.157 ☑
    C8 level S14.158 ☑
   posterior cord syndrome S14.159 ☑
    C1 level S14.151 ☑
    C2 level S14.152 ☑
    C3 level S14.153 ☑
    C4 level S14.154 ☑
    C5 level S14.155 ☑
    C6 level S14.156 ☑
    C7 level S14.157 ☑
    C8 level S14.158 ☑
  dorsal — *see* Injury, spinal, thoracic
  lumbar S34.109 ☑
   complete lesion S34.119 ☑
    L1 level S34.111 ☑
    L2 level S34.112 ☑
    L3 level S34.113 ☑
    L4 level S34.114 ☑
    L5 level S34.115 ☑
   concussion S34.01 ☑
   edema S34.01 ☑
   incomplete lesion S34.129 ☑
    L1 level S34.121 ☑
    L2 level S34.122 ☑
    L3 level S34.123 ☑
    L4 level S34.124 ☑
    L5 level S34.125 ☑
   L1 level S34.101 ☑
   L2 level S34.102 ☑
   L3 level S34.103 ☑
   L4 level S34.104 ☑
   L5 level S34.105 ☑
  nerve root NEC
   cervical — *see* Injury, nerve, spinal, root, cervical
   dorsal — *see* Injury, nerve, spinal, root, dorsal
   lumbar S34.21 ☑
   sacral S34.22 ☑
   thoracic — *see* Injury, nerve, spinal, root, dorsal
  plexus
   brachial — *see* Injury, brachial plexus
   lumbosacral — *see* Injury, lumbosacral plexus
  sacral S34.139 ☑
   complete lesion S34.131 ☑
   incomplete lesion S34.132 ☑
  thoracic S24.109 ☑
   anterior cord syndrome S24.139 ☑
    T1 level S24.131 ☑
    T2-T6 level S24.132 ☑
    T7-T10 level S24.133 ☑
    T11-T12 level S24.134 ☑
   Brown-Séquard syndrome S24.149 ☑
    T1 level S24.141 ☑

Injury — *continued*
 spinal — *continued*
  thoracic — *continued*
   Brown-Séquard syndrome — *continued*
    T2-T6 level S24.142 ☑
    T7-T10 level S24.143 ☑
    T11-T12 level S24.144 ☑
   complete lesion S24.119 ☑
    T1 level S24.111 ☑
    T2-T6 level S24.112 ☑
    T7-T10 level S24.113 ☑
    T11-T12 level S24.114 ☑
   concussion S24.0 ☑
   edema S24.0 ☑
   incomplete lesion specified NEC S24.159 ☑
    T1 level S24.151 ☑
    T2-T6 level S24.152 ☑
    T7-T10 level S24.153 ☑
    T11-T12 level S24.154 ☑
   posterior cord syndrome S24.159 ☑
    T1 level S24.151 ☑
    T2-T6 level S24.152 ☑
    T7-T10 level S24.153 ☑
    T11-T12 level S24.154 ☑
   T1 level S24.101 ☑
   T2-T6 level S24.102 ☑
   T7-T10 level S24.103 ☑
   T11-T12 level S24.104 ☑
 splanchnic nerve — *see* Injury, nerve, lumbosacral, sympathetic
 spleen S36.00 ☑
  contusion S36.029 ☑
   major S36.021 ☑
   minor S36.020 ☑
  laceration S36.039 ☑
   major (massive) (stellate) S36.032 ☑
   moderate S36.031 ☑
   superficial (capsular) (minor) S36.030 ☑
  specified type NEC S36.09 ☑
 splenic artery — *see* Injury, blood vessel, celiac artery, branch
 stellate ganglion — *see* Injury, nerve, thorax, sympathetic
 sternal region S29.9 ☑
 stomach S36.30 ☑
  contusion S36.32 ☑
  laceration S36.33 ☑
  specified type NEC S36.39 ☑
 subconjunctival — *see* Injury, eye, conjunctiva
 subcutaneous NEC T14.8
 submaxillary region S09.93 ☑
 submental region S09.93 ☑
 subungual
  fingers — *see* Injury, hand
  toes — *see* Injury, foot
 superficial NEC T14.8
  abdomen, abdominal (wall) S30.92 ☑
   abrasion S30.811 ☑
    bite S30.871 ☑
     insect S30.861 ☑
    contusion S30.1 ☑
    external constriction S30.841 ☑
    foreign body S30.851 ☑
  abrasion — *see* Abrasion, by site
  adnexa, eye NEC — *see* Injury, eye, specified site NEC
  alveolar process — *see* Injury, superficial, oral cavity
  ankle S90.91- ☑
   abrasion — *see* Abrasion, ankle
   bite — *see* Bite, ankle
   blister — *see* Blister, ankle
   contusion — *see* Contusion, ankle
   external constriction — *see* Constriction, external, ankle
   foreign body — *see* Foreign body, superficial, ankle
  anus S30.98 ☑
  arm (upper) S40.92- ☑
   abrasion — *see* Abrasion, arm
   bite — *see* Bite, superficial, arm
   blister — *see* Blister, arm (upper)
   contusion — *see* Contusion, arm
   external constriction — *see* Constriction, external, arm

Injury — *continued*
  superficial — *continued*
    arm — *continued*
      foreign body — *see* Foreign body, superficial, arm
      auditory canal (external) (meatus) — *see* Injury, superficial, ear
      auricle — *see* Injury, superficial, ear
      axilla — *see* Injury, superficial, arm
      back (*see also* Injury, superficial, thorax, back)
        lower S30.91 ☑
          abrasion S30.810 ☑
          contusion S30.0 ☑
          external constriction S30.840 ☑
          superficial
            bite NEC S30.870 ☑
            insect S30.860 ☑
            foreign body S30.850 ☑
      bite NEC — *see* Bite, superficial NEC, by site
      blister — *see* Blister, by site
      breast S20.10- ☑
        abrasion — *see* Abrasion, breast
        bite — *see* Bite, superficial, breast
        contusion — *see* Contusion, breast
        external constriction — *see* Constriction, external, breast
        foreign body — *see* Foreign body, superficial, breast
      brow — *see* Injury, superficial, head, specified NEC
      buttock S30.91 ☑
      calf — *see* Injury, superficial, leg
      canthus, eye — *see* Injury, superficial, periocular area
      cheek (external) — *see* Injury, superficial, head, specified NEC
        internal — *see* Injury, superficial, oral cavity
      chest wall — *see* Injury, superficial, thorax
      chin — *see* Injury, superficial, head NEC
      clitoris S30.95 ☑
      conjunctiva — *see* Injury, eye, conjunctiva
        with foreign body (in conjunctival sac) — *see* Foreign body, conjunctival sac
      contusion — *see* Contusion, by site
      costal region — *see* Injury, superficial, thorax
      digit(s)
        hand — *see* Injury, superficial, finger
      ear (auricle) (canal) (external) S00.40- ☑
        abrasion — *see* Abrasion, ear
        bite — *see* Bite, superficial, ear
        contusion — *see* Contusion, ear
        external constriction — *see* Constriction, external, ear
        foreign body — *see* Foreign body, superficial, ear
      elbow S50.90- ☑
        abrasion — *see* Abrasion, elbow
        bite — *see* Bite, superficial, elbow
        blister — *see* Blister, elbow
        contusion — *see* Contusion, elbow
        external constriction — *see* Constriction, external, elbow
        foreign body — *see* Foreign body, superficial, elbow
      epididymis S30.94 ☑
      epigastric region S30.92 ☑
      epiglottis — *see* Injury, superficial, throat
      esophagus
        cervical — *see* Injury, superficial, throat
      external constriction — *see* Constriction, external, by site
      extremity NEC T14.8
      eyeball NEC — *see* Injury, eye, specified site NEC
      eyebrow — *see* Injury, superficial, periocular area
      eyelid S00.20- ☑
        abrasion — *see* Abrasion, eyelid
        bite — *see* Bite, superficial, eyelid
        contusion — *see* Contusion, eyelid
        external constriction — *see* Constriction, external, eyelid
        foreign body — *see* Foreign body, superficial, eyelid
      face NEC — *see* Injury, superficial, head, specified NEC
      finger(s) S60.949 ☑
        abrasion — *see* Abrasion, finger
        bite — *see* Bite, superficial, finger

Injury — *continued*
  superficial — *continued*
    finger(s) — *continued*
      blister — *see* Blister, finger
      contusion — *see* Contusion, finger
      external constriction — *see* Constriction, external, finger
      foreign body — *see* Foreign body, superficial, finger
      index S60.94- ☑
      insect bite — *see* Bite, by site, superficial, insect
      little S60.94- ☑
      middle S60.94- ☑
      ring S60.94- ☑
    flank S30.92 ☑
    foot S90.92- ☑
      abrasion — *see* Abrasion, foot
      bite — *see* Bite, foot
      blister — *see* Blister, foot
      contusion — *see* Contusion, foot
      external constriction — *see* Constriction, external, foot
      foreign body — *see* Foreign body, superficial, foot
    forearm S50.91- ☑
      abrasion — *see* Abrasion, forearm
      bite — *see* Bite, forearm, superficial
      blister — *see* Blister, forearm
      contusion — *see* Contusion, forearm
      elbow only — *see* Injury, superficial, elbow
      external constriction — *see* Constriction, external, forearm
      foreign body — *see* Foreign body, superficial, forearm
    forehead — *see* Injury, superficial, head NEC
    foreign body — *see* Foreign body, superficial
    genital organs, external
      female S30.97 ☑
      male S30.96 ☑
    globe (eye) — *see* Injury, eye, specified site NEC
    groin S30.92 ☑
    gum — *see* Injury, superficial, oral cavity
    hand S60.92- ☑
      abrasion — *see* Abrasion, hand
      bite — *see* Bite, superficial, hand
      contusion — *see* Contusion, hand
      external constriction — *see* Constriction, external, hand
      foreign body — *see* Foreign body, superficial, hand
    head S00.90 ☑
      ear — *see* Injury, superficial, ear
      eyelid — *see* Injury, superficial, eyelid
      nose S00.30 ☑
      oral cavity S00.502 ☑
      scalp S00.00 ☑
      specified site NEC S00.80 ☑
    heel — *see* Injury, superficial, foot
    hip S70.91- ☑
      abrasion — *see* Abrasion, hip
      bite — *see* Bite, superficial, hip
      blister — *see* Blister, hip
      contusion — *see* Contusion, hip
      external constriction — *see* Constriction, external, hip
      foreign body — *see* Foreign body, superficial, hip
    iliac region — *see* Injury, superficial, abdomen
    inguinal region — *see* Injury, superficial, abdomen
    insect bite — *see* Bite, by site, superficial, insect
    interscapular region — *see* Injury, superficial, thorax, back
    jaw — *see* Injury, superficial, head, specified NEC
    knee S80.91- ☑
      abrasion — *see* Abrasion, knee
      bite — *see* Bite, superficial, knee
      blister — *see* Blister, knee
      contusion — *see* Contusion, knee
      external constriction — *see* Constriction, external, knee
      foreign body — *see* Foreign body, superficial, knee
    labium (majus) (minus) S30.95 ☑
    lacrimal (apparatus) (gland) (sac) — *see* Injury, eye, specified site NEC
    larynx — *see* Injury, superficial, throat

Injury — *continued*
  superficial — *continued*
    leg (lower) S80.92- ☑
      abrasion — *see* Abrasion, leg
      bite — *see* Bite, superficial, leg
      contusion — *see* Contusion, leg
      external constriction — *see* Constriction, external, leg
      foreign body — *see* Foreign body, superficial, leg
      knee — *see* Injury, superficial, knee
    limb NEC T14.8
    lip S00.501 ☑
    lower back S30.91 ☑
    lumbar region S30.91 ☑
    malar region — *see* Injury, superficial, head, specified NEC
    mammary — *see* Injury, superficial, breast
    mastoid region — *see* Injury, superficial, head, specified NEC
    mouth — *see* Injury, superficial, oral cavity
    muscle NEC T14.8
    nail NEC T14.8
      finger — *see* Injury, superficial, finger
      toe — *see* Injury, superficial, toe
    nasal (septum) — *see* Injury, superficial, nose
    neck S10.90 ☑
      specified site NEC S10.80 ☑
    nose (septum) S00.30 ☑
    occipital region — *see* Injury, superficial, scalp
    oral cavity S00.502 ☑
    orbital region — *see* Injury, superficial, periocular area
    palate — *see* Injury, superficial, oral cavity
    palm — *see* Injury, superficial, hand
    parietal region — *see* Injury, superficial, scalp
    pelvis S30.91 ☑
      girdle — *see* Injury, superficial, hip
    penis S30.93 ☑
    perineum
      female S30.95 ☑
      male S30.91 ☑
    periocular area S00.20- ☑
      abrasion — *see* Abrasion, eyelid
      bite — *see* Bite, superficial, eyelid
      contusion — *see* Contusion, eyelid
      external constriction — *see* Constriction, external, eyelid
      foreign body — *see* Foreign body, superficial, eyelid
    phalanges
      finger — *see* Injury, superficial, finger
      toe — *see* Injury, superficial, toe
    pharynx — *see* Injury, superficial, throat
    pinna — *see* Injury, superficial, ear
    popliteal space — *see* Injury, superficial, knee
    prepuce S30.93 ☑
    pubic region S30.91 ☑
    pudendum
      female S30.97 ☑
      male S30.96 ☑
    sacral region S30.91 ☑
    scalp S00.00 ☑
    scapular region — *see* Injury, superficial, shoulder
    sclera — *see* Injury, eye, specified site NEC
    scrotum S30.94 ☑
    shin — *see* Injury, superficial, leg
    shoulder S40.91- ☑
      abrasion — *see* Abrasion, shoulder
      bite — *see* Bite, superficial, shoulder
      blister — *see* Blister, shoulder
      contusion — *see* Contusion, shoulder
      external constriction — *see* Constriction, external, shoulder
      foreign body — *see* Foreign body, superficial, shoulder
    skin NEC T14.8
    sternal region — *see* Injury, superficial, thorax, front
    subconjunctival — *see* Injury, eye, specified site NEC
    subcutaneous NEC T14.8
    submaxillary region — *see* Injury, superficial, head, specified NEC
    submental region — *see* Injury, superficial, head, specified NEC

☑ **Additional Character Required** — Refer to the Tabular List for Character Selection   ▽ **Subterms under main terms may continue to next column or page**

Injury — *continued*
  superficial — *continued*
    subungual
      finger(s) — *see* Injury, superficial, finger
      toe(s) — *see* Injury, superficial, toe
    supraclavicular fossa — *see* Injury, superficial, neck
    supraorbital — *see* Injury, superficial, head, specified NEC
    temple — *see* Injury, superficial, head, specified NEC
    temporal region — *see* Injury, superficial, head, specified NEC
    testis S30.94 ☑
    thigh S70.92- ☑
      abrasion — *see* Abrasion, thigh
      bite — *see* Bite, superficial, thigh
      blister — *see* Blister, thigh
      contusion — *see* Contusion, thigh
      external constriction — *see* Constriction, external, thigh
      foreign body — *see* Foreign body, superficial, thigh
    thorax, thoracic (wall) S20.90 ☑
      abrasion — *see* Abrasion, thorax
      back S20.40- ☑
      bite — *see* Bite, thorax, superficial
      blister — *see* Blister, thorax
      contusion — *see* Contusion, thorax
      external constriction — *see* Constriction, external, thorax
      foreign body — *see* Foreign body, superficial, thorax
      front S20.30- ☑
    throat S10.10 ☑
      abrasion S10.11 ☑
      bite S10.17 ☑
        insect S10.16 ☑
      blister S10.12 ☑
      contusion S10.0 ☑
      external constriction S10.14 ☑
      foreign body S10.15 ☑
    thumb S60.93- ☑
      abrasion — *see* Abrasion, thumb
      bite — *see* Bite, superficial, thumb
      blister — *see* Blister, thumb
      contusion — *see* Contusion, thumb
      external constriction — *see* Constriction, external, thumb
      foreign body — *see* Foreign body, superficial, thumb
      insect bite — *see* Bite, by site, superficial, insect
      specified type NEC S60.39 ☑
    toe(s) S90.93- ☑
      abrasion — *see* Abrasion, toe
      bite — *see* Bite, toe
      blister — *see* Blister, toe
      contusion — *see* Contusion, toe
      external constriction — *see* Constriction, external, toe
      foreign body — *see* Foreign body, superficial, toe
      great S90.93- ☑
    tongue — *see* Injury, superficial, oral cavity
    tooth, teeth — *see* Injury, superficial, oral cavity
    trachea S10.10 ☑
    tunica vaginalis S30.94 ☑
    tympanum, tympanic membrane — *see* Injury, superficial, ear
    uvula — *see* Injury, superficial, oral cavity
    vagina S30.95 ☑
    vocal cords — *see* Injury, superficial, throat
    vulva S30.95 ☑
    wrist S60.91- ☑
  supraclavicular region — *see* Injury, neck
  supraorbital S09.93 ☑
  suprarenal gland (multiple) — *see* Injury, adrenal
  surgical complication (external or internal site) — *see* Laceration, accidental complicating surgery
  temple S09.90 ☑
  temporal region S09.90 ☑
  tendon (*see also* Injury, muscle, by site)
    abdomen — *see* Injury, muscle, abdomen
    Achilles — *see* Injury, Achilles tendon
    lower back — *see* Injury, muscle, lower back
    pelvic organs — *see* Injury, muscle, pelvis

Injury — *continued*
  tenth cranial nerve (pneumogastric or vagus) — *see* Injury, nerve, vagus
  testis S39.94 ☑
  thigh S79.92- ☑
    blood vessel — *see* Injury, blood vessel, hip
    contusion — *see* Contusion, thigh
    fracture — *see* Fracture, femur
    muscle — *see* Injury, muscle, thigh
    nerve — *see* Injury, nerve, thigh
    open — *see* Wound, open, thigh
    specified NEC S79.82- ☑
    superficial — *see* Injury, superficial, thigh
  third cranial nerve (oculomotor) — *see* Injury, nerve, oculomotor
  thorax, thoracic S29.9 ☑
    blood vessel — *see* Injury, blood vessel, thorax
    cavity — *see* Injury, intrathoracic
    dislocation — *see* Dislocation, thorax
    external (wall) S29.9 ☑
      contusion — *see* Contusion, thorax
      nerve — *see* Injury, nerve, thorax
      open — *see* Wound, open, thorax
      specified NEC S29.8 ☑
      sprain — *see* Sprain, thorax
      superficial — *see* Injury, superficial, thorax
    fracture — *see* Fracture, thorax
    internal — *see* Injury, intrathoracic
    intrathoracic organ — *see* Injury, intrathoracic
    sympathetic ganglion — *see* Injury, nerve, thorax, sympathetic
  throat (*see also* Injury, neck) S19.9 ☑
  thumb S69.9- ☑
    blood vessel — *see* Injury, blood vessel, thumb
    contusion — *see* Contusion, thumb
    dislocation — *see* Dislocation, thumb
    fracture — *see* Fracture, thumb
    muscle — *see* Injury, muscle, thumb
    nerve — *see* Injury, nerve, digital, thumb
    open — *see* Wound, open, thumb
    specified NEC S69.8- ☑
    sprain — *see* Sprain, thumb
    superficial — *see* Injury, superficial, thumb
  thymus (gland) — *see* Injury, intrathoracic, specified organ NEC
  thyroid (gland) NEC S19.84 ☑
  toe S99.92- ☑
    contusion — *see* Contusion, toe
    dislocation — *see* Dislocation, toe
    fracture — *see* Fracture, toe
    muscle — *see* Injury, muscle, toe
    open — *see* Wound, open, toe
    specified type NEC S99.82- ☑
    sprain — *see* Sprain, toe
    superficial — *see* Injury, superficial, toe
  tongue S09.93 ☑
  tonsil S09.93 ☑
  tooth S09.93 ☑
  trachea (cervical) NEC S19.82 ☑
    thoracic — *see* Injury, intrathoracic, trachea, thoracic
  transfusion-related acute lung (TRALI) J95.84
  tunica vaginalis S39.94 ☑
  twelfth cranial nerve (hypoglossal) — *see* Injury, nerve, hypoglossal
  ureter S37.10 ☑
    contusion S37.12 ☑
    laceration S37.13 ☑
    specified type NEC S37.19 ☑
  urethra (sphincter) S37.30 ☑
    at delivery O71.5
    contusion S37.32 ☑
    laceration S37.33 ☑
    specified type NEC S37.39 ☑
  urinary organ S37.90 ☑
    contusion S37.92 ☑
    laceration S37.93 ☑
    specified
      site NEC S37.899 ☑
        contusion S37.892 ☑
        laceration S37.893 ☑
        specified type NEC S37.898 ☑
      type NEC S37.99 ☑
  uterus, uterine S37.60 ☑
    with ectopic or molar pregnancy O08.6
    blood vessel — *see* Injury, blood vessel, iliac

Injury — *continued*
  uterus, uterine — *continued*
    contusion S37.62 ☑
    laceration S37.63 ☑
      cervix at delivery O71.3
    rupture associated with obstetrics — *see* Rupture, uterus
    specified type NEC S37.69 ☑
  uvula S09.93 ☑
  vagina S39.93 ☑
    abrasion S30.814 ☑
    bite S31.45 ☑
      insect S30.864 ☑
      superficial NEC S30.874 ☑
    contusion S30.23 ☑
    crush S38.03 ☑
    during delivery — *see* Laceration, vagina, during delivery
    external constriction S30.844 ☑
    insect bite S30.864 ☑
    laceration S31.41 ☑
      with foreign body S31.42 ☑
    open wound S31.40 ☑
    puncture S31.43 ☑
      with foreign body S31.44 ☑
    superficial S30.95 ☑
      foreign body S30.854 ☑
  vas deferens — *see* Injury, pelvic organ, specified site NEC
  vascular NEC T14.8
  vein — *see* Injury, blood vessel
  vena cava (superior) S25.20 ☑
    inferior S35.10 ☑
      laceration (minor) (superficial) S35.11 ☑
        major S35.12 ☑
      specified type NEC S35.19 ☑
    laceration (minor) (superficial) S25.21 ☑
      major S25.22 ☑
    specified type NEC S25.29 ☑
  vesical (sphincter) — *see* Injury, bladder
  visual cortex S04.04- ☑
  vitreous (humor) S05.90 ☑
    specified NEC S05.8X- ☑
  vocal cord NEC S19.83 ☑
  vulva S39.94 ☑
    abrasion S30.814 ☑
    bite S31.45 ☑
      insect S30.864 ☑
      superficial NEC S30.874 ☑
    contusion S30.23 ☑
    crush S38.03 ☑
    during delivery — *see* Laceration, perineum, female, during delivery
    external constriction S30.844 ☑
    insect bite S30.864 ☑
    laceration S31.41 ☑
      with foreign body S31.42 ☑
    open wound S31.40 ☑
    puncture S31.43 ☑
      with foreign body S31.44 ☑
    superficial S30.95 ☑
      foreign body S30.854 ☑
  whiplash (cervical spine) S13.4 ☑
  wrist S69.9- ☑
    blood vessel — *see* Injury, blood vessel, hand
    contusion — *see* Contusion, wrist
    dislocation — *see* Dislocation, wrist
    fracture — *see* Fracture, wrist
    muscle — *see* Injury, muscle, hand
    nerve — *see* Injury, nerve, hand
    open — *see* Wound, open, wrist
    specified NEC S69.8- ☑
    sprain — *see* Sprain, wrist
    superficial — *see* Injury, superficial, wrist
Inoculation (*see also* Vaccination)
  complication or reaction — *see* Complications, vaccination
Insanity, insane (*see also* Psychosis)
  adolescent — *see* Schizophrenia
  confusional F28
    acute or subacute F05
  delusional F22
  senile F03 ☑
Insect
  bite — *see* Bite, by site, superficial, insect

Insect — continued
  venomous, poisoning NEC (by) — see Venom, arthropod
Insensitivity
  adrenocorticotropin hormone (ACTH) E27.49
  androgen E34.50
    complete E34.51
    partial E34.52
Insertion
  cord (umbilical) lateral or velamentous O43.12- ☑
  intrauterine contraceptive device (encounter for) — see Intrauterine contraceptive device
Insolation (sunstroke) T67.0 ☑
Insomnia (organic) G47.00
  without objective findings F51.02
  adjustment F51.02
  adjustment disorder F51.02
  behavioral, of childhood Z73.819
    combined type Z73.812
    limit setting type Z73.811
    sleep-onset association type Z73.810
  childhood Z73.819
  chronic F51.04
    somatized tension F51.04
  conditioned F51.04
  due to
    alcohol
      abuse F10.182
      dependence F10.282
      use F10.982
    amphetamines
      abuse F15.182
      dependence F15.282
      use F15.982
    anxiety disorder F51.05
    caffeine
      abuse F15.182
      dependence F15.282
      use F15.982
    cocaine
      abuse F14.182
      dependence F14.282
      use F14.982
    depression F51.05
    drug NEC
      abuse F19.182
      dependence F19.282
      use F19.982
    medical condition G47.01
    mental disorder NEC F51.05
    opioid
      abuse F11.182
      dependence F11.282
      use F11.982
    psychoactive substance NEC
      abuse F19.182
      dependence F19.182
      use F19.982
    sedative, hypnotic, or anxiolytic
      abuse F13.182
      dependence F13.282
      use F13.982
    stimulant NEC
      abuse F15.182
      dependence F15.282
      use F15.982
  fatal familial (FFI) A81.83
  idiopathic F51.01
  learned F51.3
  nonorganic origin F51.01
  not due to a substance or known physiological condition F51.01
    specified NEC F51.09
  paradoxical F51.03
  primary F51.01
  psychiatric F51.05
  psychophysiologic F51.04
  related to psychopathology F51.05
  short-term F51.02
  specified NEC G47.09
  stress-related F51.02
  transient F51.02
Inspiration
  food or foreign body — see Foreign body, by site
  mucus — see Asphyxia, mucus
Inspissated bile syndrome (newborn) P59.1
Instability
  emotional (excessive) F60.3

Instability — continued
  joint (post-traumatic) M25.30
    ankle M25.37- ☑
    due to old ligament injury — see Disorder, ligament
    elbow M25.32- ☑
    flail — see Flail, joint
    foot M25.37- ☑
    hand M25.34- ☑
    hip M25.35- ☑
    knee M25.36- ☑
    lumbosacral — see subcategory M53.2 ☑
    prosthesis — see Complications, joint prosthesis, mechanical, displacement, by site
    sacroiliac — see subcategory M53.2 ☑
    secondary to
      old ligament injury — see Disorder, ligament
      removal of joint prosthesis M96.89
    shoulder (region) M25.31- ☑
    spine — see subcategory M53.2 ☑
    wrist M25.33- ☑
  knee (chronic) M23.5- ☑
  lumbosacral — see subcategory M53.2 ☑
  nervous F48.8
  personality (emotional) F60.3
  spine — see Instability, joint, spine
  vasomotor R55
Institutional syndrome (childhood) F94.2
Institutionalization, affecting child Z62.22
  disinhibited attachment F94.2
Insufficiency, insufficient
  accommodation, old age H52.4
  adrenal (gland) E27.40
    primary E27.1
  adrenocortical E27.40
    drug-induced E27.3
    iatrogenic E27.3
    primary E27.1
  anterior (occlusal) guidance M26.54
  anus K62.89
  aortic (valve) I35.1
    with
      mitral (valve) disease I08.0
        with tricuspid (valve) disease I08.3
      stenosis I35.2
      tricuspid (valve) disease I08.2
        with mitral (valve) disease I08.3
    congenital Q23.1
    rheumatic I06.1
      with
        mitral (valve) disease I08.0
          with tricuspid (valve) disease I08.3
        stenosis I06.2
          with mitral (valve) disease I08.0
            with tricuspid (valve) disease I08.3
        tricuspid (valve) disease I08.2
          with mitral (valve) disease I08.3
    specified cause NEC I35.1
    syphilitic A52.03
  arterial I77.1
    basilar G45.0
    carotid (hemispheric) G45.1
    cerebral I67.81
    coronary (acute or subacute) I24.8
    mesenteric K55.1
    peripheral I73.9
    precerebral (multiple) (bilateral) G45.2
    vertebral G45.0
  arteriovenous I99.8
  biliary K83.8
  cardiac (see also Insufficiency, myocardial)
    due to presence of (cardiac) prosthesis I97.11- ☑
    postprocedural I97.11- ☑
  cardiorenal, hypertensive I13.2
  cardiovascular — see Disease, cardiovascular
  cerebrovascular (acute) I67.81
    with transient focal neurological signs and symptoms G45.8
  circulatory NEC I99.8
    newborn P29.89
  convergence H51.11
  coronary (acute or subacute) I24.8
    chronic or with a stated duration of over 4 weeks I25.89
  corticoadrenal E27.40
    primary E27.1
  dietary E63.9
  divergence H51.8

Insufficiency, insufficient — continued
  food T73.0 ☑
  gastroesophageal K22.8
  gonadal
    ovary E28.39
    testis E29.1
  heart (see also Insufficiency, myocardial)
    newborn P29.0
    valve — see Endocarditis
  hepatic — see Failure, hepatic
  idiopathic autonomic G90.09
  interocclusal distance of fully erupted teeth (ridge) M26.36
  kidney N28.9
    acute N28.9
    chronic N18.9
  lacrimal (secretion) H04.12- ☑
    passages — see Stenosis, lacrimal
  liver — see Failure, hepatic
  lung — see Insufficiency, pulmonary
  mental (congenital) — see Disability, intellectual
  mesenteric K55.1
  mitral (valve) I34.0
    with
      aortic valve disease I08.0
        with tricuspid (valve) disease I08.3
      obstruction or stenosis I05.2
        with aortic valve disease I08.0
      tricuspid (valve) disease I08.1
        with aortic (valve) disease I08.3
    congenital Q23.3
    rheumatic I05.1
      with
        aortic valve disease I08.0
          with tricuspid (valve) disease I08.3
        obstruction or stenosis I05.2
          with aortic valve disease I08.0
            with tricuspid (valve) disease I08.3
        tricuspid (valve) disease I08.1
          with aortic (valve) disease I08.3
      active or acute I01.1
        with chorea, rheumatic (Sydenham's) I02.0
    specified cause, except rheumatic I34.0
  muscle (see also Disease, muscle)
    heart — see Insufficiency, myocardial
  ocular NEC H50.9
  myocardial, myocardium (with arteriosclerosis) I50.9
    with
      rheumatic fever (conditions in I00) I09.0
        active, acute or subacute I01.2
          with chorea I02.0
        inactive or quiescent (with chorea) I09.0
    congenital Q24.8
    hypertensive — see Hypertension, heart
    newborn P29.0
    rheumatic I09.0
      active, acute, or subacute I01.2
    syphilitic A52.06
  nourishment T73.0 ☑
  pancreatic K86.8
  parathyroid (gland) E20.9
  peripheral vascular (arterial) I73.9
  pituitary E23.0
  placental (mother) O36.51- ☑
  platelets D69.6
  prenatal care affecting management of pregnancy O09.3- ☑
  progressive pluriglandular E31.0
  pulmonary J98.4
    acute, following surgery (nonthoracic) J95.2
      thoracic J95.1
    chronic, following surgery J95.3
    following
      shock J98.4
      trauma J98.4
    newborn P28.5
    valve I37.1
      with stenosis I37.2
      congenital Q22.2
      rheumatic I09.89
        with aortic, mitral or tricuspid (valve) disease I08.8
  pyloric K31.89
  renal (acute) N28.9
    chronic N18.9
  respiratory R06.89
    newborn P28.5
  rotation — see Malrotation

Insufficiency, insufficient — *continued*
  sleep syndrome F51.12
  social insurance Z59.7
  suprarenal E27.40
    primary E27.1
  tarso-orbital fascia, congenital Q10.3
  testis E29.1
  thyroid (gland) (acquired) E03.9
    congenital E03.1
  tricuspid (valve) (rheumatic) I07.1
    with
      aortic (valve) disease I08.2
        with mitral (valve) disease I08.3
      mitral (valve) disease I08.1
        with aortic (valve) disease I08.3
      obstruction or stenosis I07.2
        with aortic (valve) disease I08.2
          with mitral (valve) disease I08.3
    congenital Q22.8
    nonrheumatic I36.1
      with stenosis I36.2
  urethral sphincter R32
  valve, valvular (heart) — *see* Endocarditis
    congenital Q24.8
  vascular I99.8
    intestine K55.9
      acute K55.0
      mesenteric K55.1
    peripheral I73.9
    renal — *see* Hypertension, kidney
  velopharyngeal
    acquired K13.79
    congenital Q38.8
  venous (chronic) (peripheral) I87.2
  ventricular — *see* Insufficiency, myocardial
  welfare support Z59.7
Insufflation, fallopian Z31.41
Insular — *see* condition
Insulinoma
  pancreas
    benign D13.7
    malignant C25.4
    uncertain behavior D37.8
  specified site
    benign — *see* Neoplasm, by site, benign
    malignant — *see* Neoplasm, by site, malignant
    uncertain behavior — *see* Neoplasm, by site, uncertain behavior
  unspecified site
    benign D13.7
    malignant C25.4
    uncertain behavior D37.8
Insuloma — *see* Insulinoma
Interference
  balancing side M26.56
  non-working side M26.56
Intermenstrual — *see* condition
Intermittent — *see* condition
Internal — *see* condition
Interrogation
  cardiac defibrillator (automatic) (implantable) Z45.02
  cardiac pacemaker Z45.018
  cardiac (event) (loop) recorder Z45.09
  infusion pump (implanted) (intrathecal) Z45.1
  neurostimulator Z46.2
Interruption
  bundle of His I44.30
  phase-shift, sleep cycle — *see* Disorder, sleep, circadian rhythm
  sleep phase-shift, or 24 hour sleep-wake cycle — *see* Disorder, sleep, circadian rhythm
Interstitial — *see* condition
Intertrigo L30.4
  labialis K13.0
Intervertebral disc — *see* condition
Intestine, intestinal — *see* condition
Intolerance
  carbohydrate K90.4
  disaccharide, hereditary E73.0
  fat NEC K90.4
    pancreatic K90.3
  food K90.4
    dietary counseling and surveillance Z71.3
  fructose E74.10
    hereditary E74.12
  glucose (-galactose) E74.39
  gluten K90.0
  lactose E73.9

Intolerance — *continued*
  lactose — *continued*
    specified NEC E73.8
  lysine E72.3
  milk NEC K90.4
    lactose E73.9
  protein K90.4
  starch NEC K90.4
  sucrose (-isomaltose) E74.31
Intoxicated NEC (without dependence) — *see* Alcohol, intoxication
Intoxication
  acid E87.2
  alcoholic (acute) (without dependence) — *see* Alcohol, intoxication
  alimentary canal K52.1
  amphetamine (without dependence) — *see* Abuse, drug, stimulant, with intoxication
    with dependence — *see* Dependence, drug, stimulant, with intoxication
  anxiolytic (acute) (without dependence) — *see* Abuse, drug, sedative, with intoxication
    with dependence — *see* Dependence, drug, sedative, with intoxication
  caffeine (acute) (without dependence) — *see* Abuse, drug, stimulant, with intoxication
    with dependence — *see* Dependence, drug, stimulant, with intoxication
  cannabinoids (acute) (without dependence) — *see* Abuse, drug, cannabis, with intoxication
    with dependence — *see* Dependence, drug, cannabis, with intoxication
  chemical — *see* Table of Drugs and Chemicals
    via placenta or breast milk — *see* - Absorption, chemical, through placenta
  cocaine (acute) (without dependence) — *see* Abuse, drug, cocaine, with intoxication
    with dependence — *see* Dependence, drug, cocaine, with intoxication
  drug
    acute (without dependence) — *see* Abuse, drug, by type with intoxication
      with dependence — *see* Dependence, drug, by type with intoxication
    addictive
      via placenta or breast milk — *see* Absorption, drug, addictive, through placenta
    newborn P93.8
      gray baby syndrome P93.0
    overdose or wrong substance given or taken — *see* Table of Drugs and Chemicals, by drug, poisoning
  enteric K52.1
  foodborne A05.9
    bacterial A05.9
    classical (Clostridium botulinum) A05.1
    due to
      Bacillus cereus A05.4
      bacterium A05.9
        specified NEC A05.8
      Clostridium
        botulinum A05.1
        perfringens A05.2
        welchii A05.2
      Salmonella A02.9
        with
          (gastro)enteritis A02.0
          localized infection(s) A02.20
            arthritis A02.23
            meningitis A02.21
            osteomyelitis A02.24
            pneumonia A02.22
            pyelonephritis A02.25
            specified NEC A02.29
          sepsis A02.1
          specified manifestation NEC A02.8
      Staphylococcus A05.0
      Vibrio
        parahaemolyticus A05.3
        vulnificus A05.5
    enterotoxin, staphylococcal A05.0
    noxious — *see* Poisoning, food, noxious
  gastrointestinal K52.1
  hallucinogenic (without dependence) — *see* Abuse, drug, hallucinogen, with intoxication
    with dependence — *see* Dependence, drug, hallucinogen, with intoxication

Intoxication — *continued*
  hypnotic (acute) (without dependence) — *see* Abuse, drug, sedative, with intoxication
    with dependence — *see* Dependence, drug, sedative, with intoxication
  inhalant (acute) (without dependence) — *see* Abuse, drug, inhalant, with intoxication
    with dependence — *see* Dependence, drug, inhalant, with intoxication
  meaning
    inebriation — *see* category F10 ☑
    poisoning — *see* Table of Drugs and Chemicals
  methyl alcohol (acute) (without dependence) — *see* Alcohol, intoxication
  opioid (acute) (without dependence) — *see* Abuse, drug, opioid, with intoxication
    with dependence — *see* Dependence, drug, opioid, with intoxication
  pathologic NEC (without dependence) — *see* Alcohol, intoxication
  phencyclidine (without dependence) — *see* Abuse, drug, psychoactive NEC, with intoxication
    with dependence — *see* Dependence, drug, psychoactive NEC, with intoxication
  potassium (K) E87.5
  psychoactive substance NEC (without dependence) — *see* Abuse, drug, psychoactive NEC, with intoxication
    with dependence — *see* Dependence, drug, psychoactive NEC, with intoxication
  sedative (acute) (without dependence) — *see* Abuse, drug, sedative, with intoxication
    with dependence — *see* Dependence, drug, sedative, with intoxication
  serum (*see also* Reaction, serum) T80.69 ☑
  uremic — *see* Uremia
  volatile solvents (acute) (without dependence) — *see* Abuse, drug, inhalant, with intoxication
    with dependence — *see* Dependence, drug, inhalant, with intoxication
  water E87.79
Intracranial — *see* condition
Intrahepatic gallbladder Q44.1
Intraligamentous — *see* condition
Intrathoracic (*see also* condition)
  kidney Q63.2
Intrauterine contraceptive device
  checking Z30.431
  in situ Z97.5
  insertion Z30.430
    immediately following removal Z30.433
  management Z30.431
  reinsertion Z30.433
  removal Z30.432
  replacement Z30.433
  retention in pregnancy O26.3- ☑
Intraventricular — *see* condition
Intrinsic deformity — *see* Deformity
Intubation, difficult or failed T88.4 ☑
Intumescence, lens (eye) (cataract) — *see* Cataract
Intussusception (bowel) (colon) (enteric) (ileocecal) (ileocolic) (intestine) (rectum) K56.1
  appendix K38.8
  congenital Q43.8
  ureter (with obstruction) N13.5
Invagination (bowel, colon, intestine or rectum) K56.1
Inversion
  albumin-globulin (A-G) ratio E88.09
  bladder N32.89
  cecum — *see* Intussusception
  cervix N88.8
  chromosome in normal individual Q95.1
  circadian rhythm — *see* Disorder, sleep, circadian rhythm
  nipple N64.59
    congenital Q83.8
    gestational — *see* Retraction, nipple
    puerperal, postpartum — *see* Retraction, nipple
  nyctohemeral rhythm — *see* Disorder, sleep, circadian rhythm
  optic papilla Q14.2
  organ or site, congenital NEC — *see* Anomaly, by site
  sleep rhythm — *see* Disorder, sleep, circadian rhythm
  testis (congenital) Q55.29
  uterus (chronic) (postinfectional) (postpartal, old) N85.5
    postpartum O71.2

Inversion — *continued*
  vagina (posthysterectomy) N99.3
  ventricular Q20.5
Investigation (*see also* Examination) Z04.9
  clinical research subject (control) (normal comparison) (participant) Z00.6
Involuntary movement, abnormal R25.9
Involution, involutional (*see also* condition)
  breast, cystic — *see* Dysplasia, mammary, specified type NEC
  depression (single episode) F32.8
    recurrent episode F33.9
  melancholia (recurrent episode) (single episode) F32.8
  ovary, senile — *see* Atrophy, ovary
  thymus failure E32.8
I.Q.
  under 20 F73
  20-34 F72
  35-49 F71
  50-69 F70
IRDS (type I) P22.0
  type II P22.1
Irideremia Q13.1
Iridis rubeosis — *see* Disorder, iris, vascular
Iridochoroiditis (panuveitis) — *see* Panuveitis
Iridocyclitis H20.9-
  acute H20.0- ☑
    hypopyon H20.05- ☑
    primary H20.01- ☑
    recurrent H20.02- ☑
    secondary (noninfectious) H20.04- ☑
      infectious H20.03- ☑
  chronic H20.1- ☑
  due to allergy — *see* Iridocyclitis, acute, secondary
  endogenous — *see* Iridocyclitis, acute, primary
  Fuchs' — *see* Cyclitis, Fuchs' heterochromic
  gonococcal A54.32
  granulomatous — *see* Iridocyclitis, chronic
  herpes, herpetic (simplex) B00.51
    zoster B02.32
  hypopyon — *see* Iridocyclitis, acute, hypopyon
  in (due to)
    ankylosing spondylitis M45.9
    gonococcal infection A54.32
    herpes (simplex) virus B00.51
      zoster B02.32
    infectious disease NOS B99 ☑
    parasitic disease NOS B89 [H22]
    sarcoidosis D86.83
    syphilis A51.43
    tuberculosis A18.54
    zoster B02.32
  lens-induced H20.2- ☑
  nongranulomatous — *see* Iridocyclitis, acute
  recurrent — *see* Iridocyclitis, acute, recurrent
  rheumatic — *see* Iridocyclitis, chronic
  subacute — *see* Iridocyclitis, acute
  sympathetic — *see* Uveitis, sympathetic
  syphilitic (secondary) A51.43
  tuberculous (chronic) A18.54
  Vogt-Koyanagi H20.82- ☑
Iridocyclochoroiditis (panuveitis) — *see* Panuveitis
Iridodialysis H21.53- ☑
Iridodonesis H21.89
Iridoplegia (complete) (partial) (reflex) H57.09
Iridoschisis H21.25- ☑
Iris (*see also* condition)
  bombé — *see* Membrane, pupillary
Iritis (*see also* Iridocyclitis)
  chronic — *see* Iridocyclitis, chronic
  diabetic — *see* E08-E13 with .39
  due to
    herpes simplex B00.51
    leprosy A30.9 [H22]
  gonococcal A54.32
  gouty M10.9
  granulomatous — *see* Iridocyclitis, chronic
  lens induced — *see* Iridocyclitis, lens-induced
  papulosa (syphilitic) A52.71
  rheumatic — *see* Iridocyclitis, chronic
  syphilitic (secondary) A51.43
    congenital (early) A50.01
    late A52.71
  tuberculous A18.54
Iron — *see* condition
Iron-miner's lung J63.4
Irradiated enamel (tooth, teeth) K03.89

Irradiation effects, adverse T66 ☑
Irreducible, irreducibility — *see* condition
Irregular, irregularity
  action, heart I49.9
  alveolar process K08.8
  bleeding N92.6
  breathing R06.89
  contour of cornea (acquired) — *see* Deformity, cornea
    congenital Q13.4
  contour, reconstructed breast N65.0
  dentin (in pulp) K04.3
  eye movements H55.89
    nystagmus — *see* Nystagmus
    saccadic H55.81
  labor O62.2
  menstruation (cause unknown) N92.6
  periods N92.6
  prostate N42.9
  pupil — *see* Abnormality, pupillary
  reconstructed breast N65.0
  respiratory R06.89
  septum (nasal) J34.2
  shape, organ or site, congenital NEC — *see* Distortion
  sleep-wake pattern (rhythm) G47.23
Irritable, irritability R45.4
  bladder N32.89
  bowel (syndrome) K58.9
    with diarrhea K58.0
    psychogenic F45.8
  bronchial — *see* Bronchitis
  cerebral, in newborn P91.3
  colon K58.9
    with diarrhea K58.0
    psychogenic F45.8
  duodenum K59.8
  heart (psychogenic) F45.8
  hip — *see* Derangement, joint, specified type NEC, hip
  ileum K59.8
  infant R68.12
  jejunum K59.8
  rectum K59.8
  stomach K31.89
    psychogenic F45.8
  sympathetic G90.8
  urethra N36.8
Irritation
  anus K62.89
  axillary nerve G54.0
  bladder N32.89
  brachial plexus G54.0
  bronchial — *see* Bronchitis
  cervical plexus G54.2
  cervix — *see* Cervicitis
  choroid, sympathetic — *see* Endophthalmitis
  cranial nerve — *see* Disorder, nerve, cranial
  gastric K31.89
    psychogenic F45.8
  globe, sympathetic — *see* Uveitis, sympathetic
  labyrinth — *see* subcategory H83.2 ☑
  lumbosacral plexus G54.1
  meninges (traumatic) — *see* Injury, intracranial
    nontraumatic — *see* Meningismus
  nerve — *see* Disorder, nerve
  nervous R45.0
  penis N48.89
  perineum NEC L29.3
  peripheral autonomic nervous system G90.8
  peritoneum — *see* Peritonitis
  pharynx J39.2
  plantar nerve — *see* Lesion, nerve, plantar
  spinal (cord) (traumatic) (*see also* Injury, spinal cord, by region)
    nerve G58.9
      root NEC — *see* Radiculopathy
    nontraumatic — *see* Myelopathy
  stomach K31.89
    psychogenic F45.8
  sympathetic nerve NEC G90.8
  ulnar nerve — *see* Lesion, nerve, ulnar
  vagina N89.8
Ischemia, ischemic I99.8
  bowel (transient)
    acute K55.0
    chronic K55.1
    due to mesenteric artery insufficiency K55.1
  brain — *see* Ischemia, cerebral
  cardiac (see Disease, heart, ischemic)
  cardiomyopathy I25.5

Ischemia, ischemic — *continued*
  cerebral (chronic) (generalized) I67.82
    arteriosclerotic I67.2
    intermittent G45.9
    newborn P91.0
    recurrent focal G45.8
    transient G45.9
  colon chronic (due to mesenteric artery insufficiency) K55.1
  coronary — *see* Disease, heart, ischemic
  demand (coronary) (*see also* Angina) I24.8
  heart (chronic or with a stated duration of over 4 weeks) I25.9
    acute or with a stated duration of 4 weeks or less I24.9
    subacute I24.9
  infarction, muscle — *see* Infarct, muscle
  intestine (large) (small) (transient) K55.9
    acute K55.0
    chronic K55.1
    due to mesenteric artery insufficiency K55.1
  kidney N28.0
  mesenteric, acute K55.0
  muscle, traumatic T79.6 ☑
  myocardium, myocardial (chronic or with a stated duration of over 4 weeks) I25.9
    acute, without myocardial infarction I24.0
    silent (asymptomatic) I25.6
    transient of newborn P29.4
  renal N28.0
  retina, retinal — *see* Occlusion, artery, retina
  small bowel
    acute K55.0
    chronic K55.1
    due to mesenteric artery insufficiency K55.1
  spinal cord G95.11
  subendocardial — *see* Insufficiency, coronary
  supply (coronary) (*see also* Angina) I25.9
    due to vasospasm I20.1
Ischial spine — *see* condition
Ischialgia — *see* Sciatica
Ischiopagus Q89.4
Ischium, ischial — *see* condition
Ischuria R34
Iselin's disease or osteochondrosis — *see* Osteochondrosis, juvenile, metatarsus
Islands of
  parotid tissue in
    lymph nodes Q38.6
    neck structures Q38.6
  submaxillary glands in
    fascia Q38.6
    lymph nodes Q38.6
    neck muscles Q38.6
Islet cell tumor, pancreas D13.7
Isoimmunization NEC (*see also* Incompatibility)
  affecting management of pregnancy (ABO) (with hydrops fetalis) O36.11- ☑
    anti-A sensitization O36.11- ☑
    anti-B sensitization O36.19- ☑
    anti-c sensitization O36.09- ☑
    anti-C sensitization O36.09- ☑
    anti-E sensitization O36.09- ☑
    anti-e sensitization O36.09- ☑
    Rh NEC O36.09- ☑
      anti-D antibody O36.01- ☑
    specified NEC O36.19- ☑
  newborn P55.9
    with
      hydrops fetalis P56.0
      kernicterus P57.0
    ABO (blood groups) P55.1
    Rhesus (Rh) factor P55.0
    specified type NEC P55.8
Isolation, isolated
  dwelling Z59.8
  family Z63.79
  social Z60.4
Isoleucinosis E71.19
Isomerism atrial appendages (with asplenia or polysplenia) Q20.6
Isosporiasis, isosporosis A07.3
Isovaleric acidemia E71.110
Issue of
  medical certificate Z02.79
    for disability determination Z02.71

Issue of — *continued*
   repeat prescription (appliance) (glasses) (medicinal
    substance, medicament, medicine) Z76.0
     contraception — *see* Contraception
Itch, itching (*see also* Pruritus)
   baker's L23.6
   barber's B35.0
   bricklayer's L24.5
   cheese B88.0
   clam digger's B65.3
   coolie B76.9
   copra B88.0
   dew B76.9
   dhobi B35.6
   filarial — *see* Infestation, filarial
   grain B88.0
   grocer's B88.0
   ground B76.9
   harvest B88.0
   jock B35.6
   Malabar B35.5
    beard B35.0
    foot B35.3
    scalp B35.0
   meaning scabies B86
   Norwegian B86
   perianal L29.0
   poultrymen's B88.0
   sarcoptic B86
   scabies B86
   scrub B88.0
   straw B88.0
   swimmer's B65.3
   water B76.9
   winter L29.8
Ivemark's syndrome (asplenia with congenital heart
   disease) Q89.01
Ivory bones Q78.2
Ixodiasis NEC B88.8

J

Jaccoud's syndrome — *see* Arthropathy, postrheumatic,
   chronic
Jackson's
   membrane Q43.3
   paralysis or syndrome G83.89
   veil Q43.3
Jacquet's dermatitis (diaper dermatitis) L22
Jadassohn-Pellizari's disease or anetoderma L90.2
Jadassohn's
   blue nevus — *see* Nevus
   intraepidermal epithelioma — *see* Neoplasm, skin,
    benign
Jaffe-Lichtenstein (-Uehlinger) **syndrome** — *see* Dys-
   plasia, fibrous, bone NEC
Jakob-Creutzfeldt disease or syndrome — *see*
   Creutzfeldt-Jakob disease or syndrome
Jaksch-Luzet disease D64.89
Jamaican
   neuropathy G92
   paraplegic tropical ataxic-spastic syndrome G92
Janet's disease F48.8
Janiceps Q89.4
Jansky-Bielschowsky amaurotic idiocy E75.4
Japanese
   B-type encephalitis A83.0
   river fever A75.3
Jaundice (yellow) R17
   acholuric (familial) (splenomegalic) (*see also* Sphero-
    cytosis)
    acquired D59.8
   breast-milk (inhibitor) P59.3
   catarrhal (acute) B15.9
    with hepatic coma B15.0
   cholestatic (benign) R17
   due to or associated with
    delayed conjugation P59.8
     associated with (due to) preterm delivery P59.0
    preterm delivery P59.0
   epidemic (catarrhal) B15.9
    with hepatic coma B15.0
    leptospiral A27.0
    spirochetal A27.0
   familial nonhemolytic (congenital) (Gilbert) E80.4
    Crigler-Najjar E80.5
   febrile (acute) B15.9
    with hepatic coma B15.0

Jaundice — *continued*
   febrile — *continued*
    leptospiral A27.0
    spirochetal A27.0
   hematogenous D59.9
   hemolytic (acquired) D59.9
    congenital — *see* Spherocytosis
   hemorrhagic (acute) (leptospiral) (spirochetal) A27.0
   infectious (acute) (subacute) B15.9
    with hepatic coma B15.0
    leptospiral A27.0
    spirochetal A27.0
   leptospiral (hemorrhagic) A27.0
   malignant (without coma) K72.90
    with coma K72.91
   neonatal — *see* Jaundice, newborn
   newborn P59.9
    due to or associated with
     ABO
      antibodies P55.1
      incompatibility, maternal/fetal P55.1
      isoimmunization P55.1
     absence or deficiency of enzyme system for
      bilirubin conjugation (congenital) P59.8
     bleeding P58.1
     breast milk inhibitors to conjugation P59.3
      associated with preterm delivery P59.0
     bruising P58.0
     Crigler-Najjar syndrome E80.5
     delayed conjugation P59.8
      associated with preterm delivery P59.0
     drugs or toxins
      given to newborn P58.42
      transmitted from mother P58.41
     excessive hemolysis P58.9
      due to
       bleeding P58.1
       bruising P58.0
       drugs or toxins
        given to newborn P58.42
        transmitted from mother P58.41
       infection P58.2
       polycythemia P58.3
       swallowed maternal blood P58.5
      specified type NEC P58.8
     galactosemia E74.21
     Gilbert syndrome E80.4
     hemolytic disease P55.9
      ABO isoimmunization P55.1
      Rh isoimmunization P55.0
      specified NEC P55.8
     hepatocellular damage P59.20
      specified NEC P59.29
     hereditary hemolytic anemia P58.8
     hypothyroidism, congenital E03.1
     incompatibility, maternal/fetal NOS P55.9
     infection P58.2
     inspissated bile syndrome P59.1
     isoimmunization NOS P55.9
     mucoviscidosis E84.9
     polycythemia P58.3
     preterm delivery P59.0
     Rh
      antibodies P55.0
      incompatibility, maternal/fetal P55.0
      isoimmunization P55.0
     specified cause NEC P59.8
     swallowed maternal blood P58.5
    spherocytosis (congenital) D58.0
   nonhemolytic congenital familial (Gilbert) E80.4
   nuclear, newborn (*see also* Kernicterus of newborn)
    P57.9
   obstructive (*see also* Obstruction, bile duct) K83.1
   post-immunization — *see* Hepatitis, viral, type, B
   post-transfusion — *see* Hepatitis, viral, type, B
   regurgitation (*see also* Obstruction, bile duct) K83.1
   serum (homologous) (prophylactic) (therapeutic) —
    see Hepatitis, viral, type, B
   spirochetal (hemorrhagic) A27.0
   symptomatic R17
    newborn P59.9
Jaw — *see* condition
Jaw-winking phenomenon or syndrome Q07.8
Jealousy
   alcoholic F10.988
   childhood F93.8
   sibling F93.8
Jejunitis — *see* Enteritis

Jejunostomy status Z93.4
Jejunum, jejunal — *see* condition
Jensen's disease — *see* Inflammation, chorioretinal, fo-
   cal, juxtapapillary
Jerks, myoclonic G25.3
Jervell-Lange-Nielsen syndrome I45.81
Jeune's disease Q77.2
Jigger disease B88.1
Job's syndrome (chronic granulomatous disease) D71
Joint (*see also* condition)
   mice — *see* Loose, body, joint
    knee M23.4- ☑
Jordan's anomaly or syndrome D72.0
Joseph-Diamond-Blackfan anemia (congenital hy-
   poplastic) D61.01
Jungle yellow fever A95.0
Jüngling's disease — *see* Sarcoidosis
Juvenile — *see* condition

K

Kahler's disease C90.0- ☑
Kakke E51.11
Kala-azar B55.0
Kallmann's syndrome E23.0
Kanner's syndrome (autism) — *see* Psychosis, childhood
Kaposi's
   dermatosis (xeroderma pigmentosum) Q82.1
   lichen ruber L44.0
    acuminatus L44.0
   sarcoma
    colon C46.4
    connective tissue C46.1
    gastrointestinal organ C46.4
    lung C46.5- ☑
    lymph node (multiple) C46.3
    palate (hard) (soft) C46.2
    rectum C46.4
    skin (multiple sites) C46.0
    specified site NEC C46.7
    stomach C46.4
    unspecified site C46.9
   varicelliform eruption B00.0
    vaccinia T88.1 ☑
Kartagener's syndrome or triad (sinusitis, bronchiectasis, situs inversus) Q89.3
Karyotype
   with abnormality except iso (Xq) Q96.2
   45,X Q96.0
   46,X
    iso (Xq) Q96.1
   46,XX Q98.3
    with streak gonads Q50.32
    hermaphrodite (true) Q99.1
    male Q98.3
   46,XY
    with streak gonads Q56.1
    female Q97.3
    hermaphrodite (true) Q99.1
   47,XXX Q97.0
   47,XXY Q98.0
   47,XYY Q98.5
Kaschin-Beck disease — *see* Disease, Kaschin-Beck
Katayama's disease or fever B65.2
Kawasaki's syndrome M30.3
Kayser-Fleischer ring (cornea) (pseudosclerosis)
   H18.04- ☑
Kaznelson's syndrome (congenital hypoplastic anemia)
   D61.01
Kearns-Sayre syndrome H49.81- ☑
Kedani fever A75.3
Kelis L91.0
Kelly (-Patterson) **syndrome** (sideropenic dysphagia)
   D50.1
Keloid, cheloid L91.0
   acne L73.0
   Addison's L94.0
   cornea — *see* Opacity, cornea
   Hawkin's L91.0
   scar L91.0
Keloma L91.0
Kenya fever A77.1
Keratectasia (*see also* Ectasia, cornea)
   congenital Q13.4
Keratinization of alveolar ridge mucosa
   excessive K13.23
   minimal K13.22

Keratinized residual ridge mucosa
- excessive K13.23
- minimal K13.22

Keratitis (nodular) (nonulcerative) (simple) (zonular) H16.9
- with ulceration (central) (marginal) (perforated) (ring) — see Ulcer, cornea
- actinic — see Photokeratitis
- arborescens (herpes simplex) B00.52
- areolar H16.11- ☑
- bullosa H16.8
- deep H16.309
  - specified type NEC H16.399
- dendritic (a) (herpes simplex) B00.52
- disciform (is) (herpes simplex) B00.52
  - varicella B01.81
- filamentary H16.12- ☑
- gonococcal (congenital or prenatal) A54.33
- herpes, herpetic (simplex) B00.52
  - zoster B02.33
- in (due to)
  - acanthamebiasis B60.13
  - adenovirus B30.0
  - exanthema (see also Exanthem) B09
  - herpes (simplex) virus B00.52
  - measles B05.81
  - syphilis A50.31
  - tuberculosis A18.52
  - zoster B02.33
- interstitial (nonsyphilitic) H16.30- ☑
  - diffuse H16.32- ☑
  - herpes, herpetic (simplex) B00.52
    - zoster B02.33
  - sclerosing H16.33- ☑
  - specified type NEC H16.39- ☑
  - syphilitic (congenital) (late) A50.31
  - tuberculous A18.52
- macular H16.11- ☑
- nummular H16.11- ☑
- oyster shuckers' H16.8
- parenchymatous — see Keratitis, interstitial
- petrificans H16.8
- postmeasles B05.81
- punctata
  - leprosa A30.9 [H16.14-] ☑
  - syphilitic (profunda) A50.31
- punctate H16.14- ☑
- purulent H16.8
- rosacea L71.8
- sclerosing H16.33- ☑
- specified type NEC H16.8
- stellate H16.11- ☑
- striate H16.11- ☑
- superficial H16.10- ☑
  - with conjunctivitis — see Keratoconjunctivitis
  - due to light — see Photokeratitis
- suppurative H16.8
- syphilitic (congenital) (prenatal) A50.31
- trachomatous A71.1
  - sequelae B94.0
- tuberculous A18.52
- vesicular H16.8
- xerotic (see also Keratomalacia) H16.8
  - vitamin A deficiency E50.4

Kerato-uveitis — see Iridocyclitis
Keratoacanthoma L85.8
Keratocele — see Descemetocele
Keratoconjunctivitis H16.20- ☑
- Acanthamoeba B60.13
- adenoviral B30.0
- epidemic B30.0
- exposure H16.21- ☑
- herpes (simplex) B00.52
  - zoster B02.33
- in exanthema (see also Exanthem) B09
- infectious B30.0
- lagophthalmic — see Keratoconjunctivitis, specified type NEC
- neurotrophic H16.23- ☑
- phlyctenular H16.25- ☑
- postmeasles B05.81
- shipyard B30.0
- sicca (Sjogren's) M35.0- ☑
  - not Sjogren's H16.22- ☑
- specified type NEC H16.29- ☑
- tuberculous (phlyctenular) A18.52
- vernal H16.26- ☑

Keratoconus H18.60- ☑
- congenital Q13.4
- stable H18.61- ☑
- unstable H18.62- ☑

Keratocyst (dental) (odontogenic) — see Cyst, calcifying odontogenic
Keratoderma, keratodermia (congenital) (palmaris et plantaris) (symmetrical) Q82.8
- acquired L85.1
  - in diseases classified elsewhere L86
- climactericum L85.1
- gonococcal A54.89
- gonorrheal A54.89
- punctata L85.2
- Reiter's — see Reiter's disease

Keratodermatocele — see Descemetocele
Keratoglobus H18.79 ☑
- congenital Q15.8
  - with glaucoma Q15.0

Keratohemia — see Pigmentation, cornea, stromal
Keratoiritis (see also Iridocyclitis)
- syphilitic A50.39
- tuberculous A18.54

Keratoma L57.0
- palmaris and plantaris hereditarium Q82.8
- senile L57.0

Keratomalacia H18.44- ☑
- vitamin A deficiency E50.4

Keratomegaly Q13.4
Keratomycosis B49
- nigrans, nigricans (palmaris) B36.1

Keratopathy H18.9
- band H18.42- ☑
- bullous (aphakic), following cataract surgery H59.01- ☑
- bullous H18.1- ☑

Keratoscleritis, tuberculous A18.52
Keratosis L57.0
- actinic L57.0
- arsenical L85.8
- congenital, specified NEC Q80.8
- female genital NEC N94.89
- follicularis Q82.8
  - acquired L11.0
  - congenita Q82.8
  - et parafollicularis in cutem penetrans L87.0
  - spinulosa (decalvans) Q82.8
  - vitamin A deficiency E50.8
- gonococcal A54.89
- male genital (external) N50.8
- nigricans L83
- obturans, external ear (canal) — see Cholesteatoma, external ear
- palmaris et plantaris (inherited) (symmetrical) Q82.8
  - acquired L85.1
- penile N48.89
- pharynx J39.2
- pilaris, acquired L85.8
- punctata (palmaris et plantaris) L85.2
- scrotal N50.8
- seborrheic L82.1
  - inflamed L82.0
- senile L57.0
- solar L57.0
- tonsillaris J35.8
- vagina N89.4
- vegetans Q82.8
- vitamin A deficiency E50.8
- vocal cord J38.3

Kerion (celsi) B35.0
Kernicterus of newborn (not due to isoimmunization) P57.9
- due to isoimmunization (conditions in P55.0-P55.9) P57.0
- specified type NEC P57.8

Kerunoparalysis T75.09 ☑
Keshan disease E59
Ketoacidosis E87.2
- diabetic — see Diabetes, by type, with ketoacidosis

Ketonuria R82.4
Ketosis NEC E88.89
- diabetic — see Diabetes, by type, with with ketoacidosis

Kew Garden fever A79.1
Kidney — see condition
Kienböck's disease (see also Osteochondrosis, juvenile, hand, carpal lunate)

Kienböck's disease — continued
- adult M93.1

Kimmelstiel (-Wilson) **disease** — see Diabetes, Kimmelstiel (-Wilson) disease
Kink, kinking
- artery I77.1
- hair (acquired) L67.8
- ileum or intestine — see Obstruction, intestine
- Lane's — see Obstruction, intestine
- organ or site, congenital NEC — see Anomaly, by site
- ureter (pelvic junction) N13.5
  - with
    - hydronephrosis N13.1
      - with infection N13.6
    - pyelonephritis (chronic) N11.1
  - congenital Q62.39
- vein(s) I87.8
  - caval I87.1
  - peripheral I87.1

Kinnier Wilson's disease (hepatolenticular degeneration) E83.01
Kissing spine M48.20
- cervical region M48.22
- cervicothoracic region M48.23
- lumbar region M48.26
- lumbosacral region M48.27
- occipito-atlanto-axial region M48.21
- thoracic region M48.24
- thoracolumbar region M48.25

Klatskin's tumor C22.1
Klauder's disease A26.8
Klebs' disease (see also Glomerulonephritis) N05- ☑
Klebsiella (K.) pneumoniae, as cause of disease classified elsewhere B96.1
Klein (e)-Levin syndrome G47.13
Kleptomania F63.2
Klinefelter's syndrome Q98.4
- karyotype 47,XXY Q98.0
- male with more than two X chromosomes Q98.1

Klippel-Feil deficiency, disease, or syndrome (brevicollis) Q76.1
Klippel-Trenaunay (-Weber) **syndrome** Q87.2
Klippel's disease I67.2
Klumpke (-Déjerine) **palsy, paralysis** (birth) (newborn) P14.1
Knee — see condition
Knock knee (acquired) M21.06- ☑
- congenital Q74.1

Knot(s)
- intestinal, syndrome (volvulus) K56.2
- surfer S89.8- ☑
- umbilical cord (true) O69.2 ☑

Knotting (of)
- hair L67.8
- intestine K56.2

Knuckle pad (Garrod's) M72.1
Koch-Weeks' conjunctivitis — see Conjunctivitis, acute, mucopurulent
Koch's
- infection — see Tuberculosis
- relapsing fever A68.9

Köebner's syndrome Q81.8
Köenig's disease (osteochondritis dissecans) — see Osteochondritis, dissecans
Köhler-Pellegrini-Steida disease or syndrome (calcification, knee joint) — see Bursitis, tibial collateral
Köhler's disease
- patellar — see Osteochondrosis, juvenile, patella
- tarsal navicular — see Osteochondrosis, juvenile, tarsus

Koilonychia L60.3
- congenital Q84.6

Kojevnikov's, epilepsy — see Kozhevnikof's epilepsy
Koplik's spots B05.9
Kopp's asthma E32.8
Korsakoff's (Wernicke) **disease, psychosis or syndrome** (alcoholic) F10.96
- with dependence F10.26
- drug-induced
  - due to drug abuse — see Abuse, drug, by type, with amnestic disorder
  - due to drug dependence — see Dependence, drug, by type, with amnestic disorder
- nonalcoholic F04

Korsakov's disease, psychosis or syndrome — see Korsakoff's disease
Korsakow's disease, psychosis or syndrome — see Korsakoff's disease

☑ Additional Character Required — Refer to the Tabular List for Character Selection ▽ Subterms under main terms may continue to next column or page

Kostmann's disease or syndrome (infantile genetic agranulocytosis) — *see* Agranulocytosis
Kozhevnikof's epilepsy G40.109
    intractable G40.119
        with status epilepticus G40.111
        without status epilepticus G40.119
    not intractable G40.109
        with status epilepticus G40.101
        without status epilepticus G40.109
Krabbe's
    disease E75.23
    syndrome, congenital muscle hypoplasia Q79.8
Kraepelin-Morel disease — *see* Schizophrenia
Kraft-Weber-Dimitri disease Q85.8
Kraurosis
    ani K62.89
    penis N48.0
    vagina N89.8
    vulva N90.4
Kreotoxism A05.9
Krukenberg's
    spindle — *see* Pigmentation, cornea, posterior
    tumor C79.6- ☑
Kufs' disease E75.4
Kugelberg-Welander disease G12.1
Kuhnt-Junius degeneration (*see also* Degeneration, macula) H35.32
Kümmell's disease or spondylitis — *see* Spondylopathy, traumatic
Kupffer cell sarcoma C22.3
Kuru A81.81
Kussmaul's
    disease M30.0
    respiration E87.2
        in diabetic acidosis — *see* Diabetes, by type, with ketoacidosis
Kwashiorkor E40
    marasmic, marasmus type E42
Kyasanur Forest disease A98.2
Kyphoscoliosis, kyphoscoliotic (acquired) (*see also* Scoliosis) M41.9
    congenital Q67.5
    heart (disease) I27.1
    sequelae of rickets E64.3
    tuberculous A18.01
Kyphosis, kyphotic (acquired) M40.209
    cervical region M40.202
    cervicothoracic region M40.203
    congenital Q76.419
        cervical region Q76.412
        cervicothoracic region Q76.413
        occipito-atlanto-axial region Q76.411
        thoracic region Q76.414
        thoracolumbar region Q76.415
    Morquio-Brailsford type (spinal) (*see also* subcategory M49.8) E76.219
    postlaminectomy M96.3
    postradiation therapy M96.2
    postural (adolescent) M40.00
        cervicothoracic region M40.03
        thoracic region M40.04
        thoracolumbar region M40.05
    secondary NEC M40.10
        cervical region M40.12
        cervicothoracic region M40.13
        thoracic region M40.14
        thoracolumbar region M40.15
    sequelae of rickets E64.3
    specified type NEC M40.299
        cervical region M40.292
        cervicothoracic region M40.293
        thoracic region M40.294
        thoracolumbar region M40.295
    syphilitic, congenital A50.56
    thoracic region M40.204
    thoracolumbar region M40.205
    tuberculous A18.01
Kyrle disease L87.0

L

L-shaped kidney Q63.8
Labia, labium — *see* condition
Labile
    blood pressure R09.89
    vasomotor system I73.9
Labioglossal paralysis G12.29

Labium leporinum — *see* Cleft, lip
Labor — *see* Delivery
Labored breathing — *see* Hyperventilation
Labyrinthitis (circumscribed) (destructive) (diffuse) (inner ear) (latent) (purulent) (suppurative) (*see also* subcategory) H83.0 ☑
    syphilitic A52.79
Laceration
    with abortion — *see* Abortion, by type, complicated by laceration of pelvic organs
    abdomen, abdominal
        wall S31.119 ☑
            with
                foreign body S31.129 ☑
                penetration into peritoneal cavity S31.619 ☑
                    with foreign body S31.629 ☑
            epigastric region S31.112 ☑
                with
                    foreign body S31.122 ☑
                    penetration into peritoneal cavity S31.612 ☑
                        with foreign body S31.622 ☑
            left
                lower quadrant S31.114 ☑
                  with
                    foreign body S31.124 ☑
                    penetration into peritoneal cavity S31.614 ☑
                        with foreign body S31.624 ☑
                upper quadrant S31.111 ☑
                  with
                    foreign body S31.121 ☑
                    penetration into peritoneal cavity S31.611 ☑
                        with foreign body S31.621 ☑
            periumbilic region S31.115 ☑
                with
                    foreign body S31.125 ☑
                    penetration into peritoneal cavity S31.615 ☑
                      with foreign body S31.625 ☑
            right
                lower quadrant S31.113 ☑
                  with
                    foreign body S31.123 ☑
                    penetration into peritoneal cavity S31.613 ☑
                        with foreign body S31.623 ☑
                upper quadrant S31.110 ☑
                  with
                    foreign body S31.120 ☑
                    penetration into peritoneal cavity S31.610 ☑
                        with foreign body S31.620 ☑
    accidental, complicating surgery — *see* Complications, surgical, accidental puncture or laceration
    Achilles tendon S86.02- ☑
    adrenal gland S37.813 ☑
    alveolar (process) — *see* Laceration, oral cavity
    ankle S91.01- ☑
        with
            foreign body S91.02- ☑
    antecubital space — *see* Laceration, elbow
    anus (sphincter) S31.831 ☑
        with
            ectopic or molar pregnancy O08.6
            foreign body S31.832 ☑
        complicating delivery — *see* Delivery, complicated, by, laceration, anus (sphincter)
        following ectopic or molar pregnancy O08.6
        nontraumatic, nonpuerperal — *see* Fissure, anus
    arm (upper) S41.11- ☑
        with foreign body S41.12- ☑
        lower — *see* Laceration, forearm
    auditory canal (external) (meatus) — *see* Laceration, ear
    auricle, ear — *see* Laceration, ear
    axilla — *see* Laceration, arm
    back (*see also* Laceration, thorax, back)
        lower S31.010 ☑
            with
                foreign body S31.020 ☑
                    with penetration into retroperitoneal space S31.021 ☑

Laceration — *continued*
    back (*see also* Laceration, thorax, back) — *continued*
        lower — *continued*
            with — *continued*
                penetration into retroperitoneal space S31.011 ☑
    bile duct S36.13 ☑
    bladder S37.23 ☑
        with ectopic or molar pregnancy O08.6
        following ectopic or molar pregnancy O08.6
        obstetrical trauma O71.5
    blood vessel — *see* Injury, blood vessel
    bowel (*see also* Laceration, intestine)
        with ectopic or molar pregnancy O08.6
        complicating abortion — *see* Abortion, by type, complicated by, specified condition NEC
        following ectopic or molar pregnancy O08.6
        obstetrical trauma O71.5
    brain (any part) (cortex) (diffuse) (membrane) (*see also* Injury, intracranial, diffuse)
        during birth P10.8
            with hemorrhage P10.1
        focal — *see* Injury, intracranial, focal brain injury
    brainstem S06.38- ☑
    breast S21.01- ☑
        with foreign body S21.02- ☑
    broad ligament S37.893 ☑
        with ectopic or molar pregnancy O08.6
        following ectopic or molar pregnancy O08.6
        laceration syndrome N83.8
        obstetrical trauma O71.6
        syndrome (laceration) N83.8
    buttock S31.801 ☑
        with foreign body S31.802 ☑
        left S31.821 ☑
            with foreign body S31.822 ☑
        right S31.811 ☑
            with foreign body S31.812 ☑
    calf — *see* Laceration, leg
    canaliculus lacrimalis — *see* Laceration, eyelid
    canthus, eye — *see* Laceration, eyelid
    capsule, joint — *see* Sprain
    causing eversion of cervix uteri (old) N86
    central (perineal), complicating delivery O70.9
    cerebellum, traumatic S06.37- ☑
    cerebral S06.33- ☑
        during birth P10.8
            with hemorrhage P10.1
        left side S06.32- ☑
        right side S06.31- ☑
    cervix (uteri)
        with ectopic or molar pregnancy O08.6
        following ectopic or molar pregnancy O08.6
        nonpuerperal, nontraumatic N88.1
        obstetrical trauma (current) O71.3
        old (postpartal) N88.1
        traumatic S37.63 ☑
    cheek (external) S01.41- ☑
        with foreign body S01.42- ☑
        internal — *see* Laceration, oral cavity
    chest wall — *see* Laceration, thorax
    chin — *see* Laceration, head, specified site NEC
    chordae tendinae NEC I51.1
        concurrent with acute myocardial infarction — *see* Infarct, myocardium
        following acute myocardial infarction (current complication) I23.4
    clitoris — *see* Laceration, vulva
    colon — *see* Laceration, intestine, large, colon
    common bile duct S36.13 ☑
    cortex (cerebral) — *see* Injury, intracranial, diffuse
    costal region — *see* Laceration, thorax
    cystic duct S36.13 ☑
    diaphragm S27.803 ☑
    digit(s)
        foot — *see* Laceration, toe
        hand — *see* Laceration, finger
    duodenum S36.430 ☑
    ear (canal) (external) S01.31- ☑
        with foreign body S01.32- ☑
        drum S09.2- ☑
    elbow S51.01- ☑
        with
            foreign body S51.02- ☑
    epididymis — *see* Laceration, testis

Laceration — *continued*
epigastric region — *see* Laceration, abdomen, wall, epigastric region
esophagus K22.8
  traumatic
    cervical S11.21 ☑
      with foreign body S11.22 ☑
    thoracic S27.813 ☑
eye (ball) S05.3- ☑
  with prolapse or loss of intraocular tissue S05.2- ☑
  penetrating S05.6- ☑
eyebrow — *see* Laceration, eyelid
eyelid S01.11- ☑
  with foreign body S01.12- ☑
face NEC — *see* Laceration, head, specified site NEC
fallopian tube S37.539 ☑
  bilateral S37.532 ☑
  unilateral S37.531 ☑
finger(s) S61.219 ☑
  with
    damage to nail S61.319 ☑
      with
        foreign body S61.329 ☑
    foreign body S61.229 ☑
  index S61.218 ☑
    with
      damage to nail S61.318 ☑
        with
          foreign body S61.328 ☑
      foreign body S61.228 ☑
    left S61.211 ☑
      with
        damage to nail S61.311 ☑
          with
            foreign body S61.321 ☑
        foreign body S61.221 ☑
    right S61.210 ☑
      with
        damage to nail S61.310 ☑
          with
            foreign body S61.320 ☑
        foreign body S61.220 ☑
  little S61.218 ☑
    with
      damage to nail S61.318 ☑
        with
          foreign body S61.328 ☑
      foreign body S61.228 ☑
    left S61.217 ☑
      with
        damage to nail S61.317 ☑
          with
            foreign body S61.327 ☑
        foreign body S61.227 ☑
    right S61.216 ☑
      with
        damage to nail S61.316 ☑
          with
            foreign body S61.326 ☑
        foreign body S61.226 ☑
  middle S61.218 ☑
    with
      damage to nail S61.318 ☑
        with
          foreign body S61.328 ☑
      foreign body S61.228 ☑
    left S61.213 ☑
      with
        damage to nail S61.313 ☑
          with
            foreign body S61.323 ☑
        foreign body S61.223 ☑
    right S61.212 ☑
      with
        damage to nail S61.312 ☑
          with
            foreign body S61.322 ☑
        foreign body S61.222 ☑
  ring S61.218 ☑
    with
      damage to nail S61.318 ☑
        with
          foreign body S61.328 ☑
      foreign body S61.228 ☑
    left S61.215 ☑

Laceration — *continued*
finger(s) — *continued*
  ring — *continued*
    left — *continued*
      with
        damage to nail S61.315 ☑
          with
            foreign body S61.325 ☑
        foreign body S61.225 ☑
    right S61.214 ☑
      with
        damage to nail S61.314 ☑
          with
            foreign body S61.324 ☑
        foreign body S61.224 ☑
flank S31.119 ☑
  with foreign body S31.129 ☑
foot (except toe(s) alone) S91.319 ☑
  with foreign body S91.329 ☑
  left S91.312 ☑
    with foreign body S91.322 ☑
  right S91.311 ☑
    with foreign body S91.321 ☑
  toe — *see* Laceration, toe
forearm S51.819 ☑
  with
    foreign body S51.829 ☑
  elbow only — *see* Laceration, elbow
  left S51.812 ☑
    with
      foreign body S51.822 ☑
  right S51.811 ☑
    with
      foreign body S51.821 ☑
forehead S01.81 ☑
  with foreign body S01.82 ☑
fourchette O70.0
  with ectopic or molar pregnancy O08.6
  complicating delivery O70.0
  following ectopic or molar pregnancy O08.6
gallbladder S36.123 ☑
genital organs, external
  female S31.512 ☑
    with foreign body S31.522 ☑
    vagina — *see* Laceration, vagina
    vulva — *see* Laceration, vulva
  male S31.511 ☑
    with foreign body S31.521 ☑
    penis — *see* Laceration, penis
    scrotum — *see* Laceration, scrotum
    testis — *see* Laceration, testis
groin — *see* Laceration, abdomen, wall
gum — *see* Laceration, oral cavity
hand S61.419 ☑
  with
    foreign body S61.429 ☑
  finger — *see* Laceration, finger
  left S61.412 ☑
    with
      foreign body S61.422 ☑
  right S61.411 ☑
    with
      foreign body S61.421 ☑
  thumb — *see* Laceration, thumb
head S01.91 ☑
  with foreign body S01.92 ☑
  cheek — *see* Laceration, cheek
  ear — *see* Laceration, ear
  eyelid — *see* Laceration, eyelid
  lip — *see* Laceration, lip
  nose — *see* Laceration, nose
  oral cavity — *see* Laceration, oral cavity
  scalp S01.01 ☑
    with foreign body S01.02 ☑
  specified site NEC S01.81 ☑
    with foreign body S01.82 ☑
  temporomandibular area — *see* Laceration, cheek
heart — *see* Injury, heart, laceration
heel — *see* Laceration, foot
hepatic duct S36.13 ☑
hip S71.019 ☑
  with foreign body S71.029 ☑
  left S71.012 ☑
    with foreign body S71.022 ☑
  right S71.011 ☑
    with foreign body S71.021 ☑

Laceration — *continued*
hymen — *see* Laceration, vagina
hypochondrium — *see* Laceration, abdomen, wall
hypogastric region — *see* Laceration, abdomen, wall
ileum S36.438 ☑
inguinal region — *see* Laceration, abdomen, wall
instep — *see* Laceration, foot
internal organ — *see* Injury, by site
interscapular region — *see* Laceration, thorax, back
intestine
  large
    colon S36.539 ☑
      ascending S36.530 ☑
      descending S36.532 ☑
      sigmoid S36.533 ☑
      specified site NEC S36.538 ☑
    rectum S36.63 ☑
      transverse S36.531 ☑
  small S36.439 ☑
    duodenum S36.430 ☑
    specified site NEC S36.438 ☑
intra-abdominal organ S36.93 ☑
  intestine — *see* Laceration, intestine
  liver — *see* Laceration, liver
  pancreas — *see* Laceration, pancreas
  peritoneum S36.81 ☑
  specified site NEC S36.893 ☑
  spleen — *see* Laceration, spleen
  stomach — *see* Laceration, stomach
intracranial NEC (*see also* Injury, intracranial, diffuse)
  birth injury P10.9
jaw — *see* Laceration, head, specified site NEC
jejunum S36.438 ☑
joint capsule — *see* Sprain, by site
kidney S37.03- ☑
  major (greater than 3 cm) (massive) (stellate) S37.06- ☑
  minor (less than 1 cm) S37.04- ☑
  moderate (1 to 3 cm) S37.05- ☑
    multiple S37.06- ☑
knee S81.01- ☑
  with foreign body S81.02- ☑
labium (majus) (minus) — *see* Laceration, vulva
lacrimal duct — *see* Laceration, eyelid
large intestine — *see* Laceration, intestine, large
larynx S11.011 ☑
  with foreign body S11.012 ☑
leg (lower) S81.819 ☑
  with foreign body S81.829 ☑
  foot — *see* Laceration, foot
  knee — *see* Laceration, knee
  left S81.812 ☑
    with foreign body S81.822 ☑
  right S81.811 ☑
    with foreign body S81.821 ☑
  upper — *see* Laceration, thigh
ligament — *see* Sprain
lip S01.511 ☑
  with foreign body S01.521 ☑
liver S36.113 ☑
  major (stellate) S36.116 ☑
  minor S36.114 ☑
  moderate S36.115 ☑
loin — *see* Laceration, abdomen, wall
lower back — *see* Laceration, back, lower
lumbar region — *see* Laceration, back, lower
lung S27.339 ☑
  bilateral S27.332 ☑
  unilateral S27.331 ☑
malar region — *see* Laceration, head, specified site NEC
mammary — *see* Laceration, breast
mastoid region — *see* Laceration, head, specified site NEC
meninges — *see* Injury, intracranial, diffuse
meniscus — *see* Tear, meniscus
mesentery S36.893 ☑
mesosalpinx S37.893 ☑
mouth — *see* Laceration, oral cavity
muscle — *see* Injury, muscle, by site, laceration
nail
  finger — *see* Laceration, finger, with damage to nail
  toe — *see* Laceration, toe, with damage to nail
nasal (septum) (sinus) — *see* Laceration, nose

☑ Additional Character Required — Refer to the Tabular List for Character Selection   ▽ Subterms under main terms may continue to next column or page

Laceration — *continued*
- nasopharynx — *see* Laceration, head, specified site NEC
- neck S11.91 ☑
  - with foreign body S11.92 ☑
  - involving
    - cervical esophagus S11.21 ☑
      - with foreign body S11.22 ☑
    - larynx — *see* Laceration, larynx
    - pharynx — *see* Laceration, pharynx
    - thyroid gland — *see* Laceration, thyroid gland
    - trachea — *see* Laceration, trachea
  - specified site NEC S11.81 ☑
    - with foreign body S11.82 ☑
- nerve — *see* Injury, nerve
- nose (septum) (sinus) S01.21 ☑
  - with foreign body S01.22 ☑
- ocular NOS S05.3-
  - adnexa NOS S01.11-
- oral cavity S01.512 ☑
  - with foreign body S01.522 ☑
- orbit (eye) — *see* Wound, open, ocular, orbit
- ovary S37.439 ☑
  - bilateral S37.432 ☑
  - unilateral S37.431 ☑
- palate — *see* Laceration, oral cavity
- palm — *see* Laceration, hand
- pancreas S36.239 ☑
- pelvic S31.010 ☑
  - with
    - foreign body S31.020 ☑
      - penetration into retroperitoneal cavity S31.021 ☑
    - penetration into retroperitoneal cavity S31.011 ☑
  - floor (*see also* Laceration, back, lower)
    - with ectopic or molar pregnancy O08.6
    - complicating delivery O70.1
    - following ectopic or molar pregnancy O08.6
    - old (postpartal) N81.89
  - organ S37.93 ☑
- penis S31.21 ☑
  - with foreign body S31.22 ☑
- perineum
  - female S31.41 ☑
    - with
      - ectopic or molar pregnancy O08.6
      - foreign body S31.42 ☑
    - during delivery O70.9
      - first degree O70.0
      - fourth degree O70.3
      - second degree O70.1
      - third degree O70.2
    - old (postpartal) N81.89
    - postpartal N81.89
    - secondary (postpartal) O90.1
  - male S31.119 ☑
    - with foreign body S31.129 ☑
- periocular area (with or without lacrimal passages) — *see* Laceration, eyelid
- peritoneum S36.893 ☑
- periumbilic region — *see* Laceration, abdomen, wall, periumbilic
- periurethral tissue — *see* Laceration, urethra
- phalanges
  - finger — *see* Laceration, finger
  - toe — *see* Laceration, toe
- pharynx S11.21 ☑
  - with foreign body S11.22 ☑
- pinna — *see* Laceration, ear
- popliteal space — *see* Laceration, knee
- prepuce — *see* Laceration, penis
- prostate S37.823 ☑
- pubic region S31.119 ☑
  - with foreign body S31.129 ☑
- pudendum — *see* Laceration, genital organs, external
- rectovaginal septum — *see* Laceration, vagina
- rectum S36.63 ☑
- retroperitoneum S36.893 ☑
- round ligament S37.893 ☑
- sacral region — *see* Laceration, back, lower
- sacroiliac region — *see* Laceration, back, lower
- salivary gland — *see* Laceration, oral cavity
- scalp S01.01 ☑
  - with foreign body S01.02 ☑
- scapular region — *see* Laceration, shoulder

Laceration — *continued*
- scrotum S31.31 ☑
  - with foreign body S31.32 ☑
- seminal vesicle S37.893 ☑
- shin — *see* Laceration, leg
- shoulder S41.019 ☑
  - with foreign body S41.029 ☑
  - left S41.012 ☑
    - with foreign body S41.022 ☑
  - right S41.011 ☑
    - with foreign body S41.021 ☑
- small intestine — *see* Laceration, intestine, small
- spermatic cord — *see* Laceration, testis
- spinal cord (meninges) (*see also* Injury, spinal cord, by region)
  - due to injury at birth P11.5
  - newborn (birth injury) P11.5
- spleen S36.039 ☑
  - major (massive) (stellate) S36.032 ☑
  - moderate S36.031 ☑
  - superficial (minor) S36.030 ☑
- sternal region — *see* Laceration, thorax, front
- stomach S36.33 ☑
- submaxillary region — *see* Laceration, head, specified site NEC
- submental region — *see* Laceration, head, specified site NEC
- subungual
  - finger(s) — *see* Laceration, finger, with damage to nail
  - toe(s) — *see* Laceration, toe, with damage to nail
- suprarenal gland — *see* Laceration, adrenal gland
- temple, temporal region — *see* Laceration, head, specified site NEC
- temporomandibular area — *see* Laceration, cheek
- tendon — *see* Injury, muscle, by site, laceration
  - Achilles S86.02- ☑
- tentorium cerebelli — *see* Injury, intracranial, diffuse
- testis S31.31 ☑
  - with foreign body S31.32 ☑
- thigh S71.11- ☑
  - with foreign body S71.12- ☑
- thorax, thoracic (wall) S21.91 ☑
  - with foreign body S21.92 ☑
    - back S21.22- ☑
      - with penetration into thoracic cavity S21.42- ☑
    - front S21.12- ☑
      - with penetration into thoracic cavity S21.32- ☑
  - back S21.21- ☑
    - with
      - foreign body S21.22- ☑
        - with penetration into thoracic cavity S21.42- ☑
      - penetration into thoracic cavity S21.41- ☑
  - breast — *see* Laceration, breast
  - front S21.11- ☑
    - with
      - foreign body S21.12- ☑
        - with penetration into thoracic cavity S21.32- ☑
      - penetration into thoracic cavity S21.31- ☑
- thumb S61.019 ☑
  - with
    - damage to nail S61.119 ☑
      - with foreign body S61.129 ☑
    - foreign body S61.029 ☑
  - left S61.012 ☑
    - with
      - damage to nail S61.112 ☑
        - with foreign body S61.122 ☑
      - foreign body S61.022 ☑
  - right S61.011 ☑
    - with
      - damage to nail S61.111 ☑
        - with foreign body S61.121 ☑
      - foreign body S61.021 ☑
- thyroid gland S11.11 ☑
  - with foreign body S11.12 ☑
- toe(s) S91.119 ☑
  - with
    - damage to nail S91.219 ☑

Laceration — *continued*
- toe(s) — *continued*
  - with — *continued*
    - damage to nail — *continued*
      - with
        - foreign body S91.229 ☑
      - foreign body S91.129 ☑
    - great S91.113 ☑
      - with
        - damage to nail S91.213 ☑
          - with foreign body S91.223 ☑
        - foreign body S91.123 ☑
      - left S91.112 ☑
        - with
          - damage to nail S91.212 ☑
            - with foreign body S91.222 ☑
          - foreign body S91.122 ☑
      - right S91.111 ☑
        - with
          - damage to nail S91.211 ☑
            - with foreign body S91.221 ☑
          - foreign body S91.121 ☑
    - lesser S91.116 ☑
      - with
        - damage to nail S91.216 ☑
          - with foreign body S91.226 ☑
        - foreign body S91.126 ☑
      - left S91.115 ☑
        - with
          - damage to nail S91.215 ☑
            - with foreign body S91.225 ☑
          - foreign body S91.125 ☑
      - right S91.114 ☑
        - with
          - damage to nail S91.214 ☑
            - with foreign body S91.224 ☑
          - foreign body S91.124 ☑
- tongue — *see* Laceration, oral cavity
- trachea S11.021 ☑
  - with foreign body S11.022 ☑
- tunica vaginalis — *see* Laceration, testis
- tympanum, tympanic membrane — *see* Laceration, ear, drum
- umbilical region S31.115 ☑
  - with foreign body S31.125 ☑
- ureter S37.13 ☑
- urethra S37.33 ☑
  - with or following ectopic or molar pregnancy O08.6
  - obstetrical trauma O71.5
- urinary organ NEC S37.893 ☑
- uterus S37.63 ☑
  - with ectopic or molar pregnancy O08.6
  - following ectopic or molar pregnancy O08.6
  - nonpuerperal, nontraumatic N85.8
  - obstetrical trauma NEC O71.81
  - old (postpartal) N85.8
- uvula — *see* Laceration, oral cavity
- vagina S31.41 ☑
  - with
    - ectopic or molar pregnancy O08.6
    - foreign body S31.42 ☑
  - during delivery O71.4
    - with perineal laceration — *see* Laceration, perineum, female, during delivery
  - following ectopic or molar pregnancy O08.6
  - nonpuerperal, nontraumatic N89.8
  - old (postpartal) N89.8
- vas deferens S37.893 ☑
- vesical — *see* Laceration, bladder
- vocal cords S11.031 ☑
  - with foreign body S11.032 ☑
- vulva S31.41 ☑
  - with
    - ectopic or molar pregnancy O08.6
    - foreign body S31.42 ☑
  - complicating delivery O70.0
  - following ectopic or molar pregnancy O08.6
  - nonpuerperal, nontraumatic N90.89
  - old (postpartal) N90.89
- wrist S61.519 ☑

Laceration — *continued*
wrist — *continued*
with
foreign body S61.529 ☑
left S61.512 ☑
with
foreign body S61.522 ☑
right S61.511 ☑
with
foreign body S61.521 ☑
Lack of
achievement in school Z55.3
adequate
food Z59.4
intermaxillary vertical dimension of fully erupted teeth M26.36
sleep Z72.820
appetite (see Anorexia) R63.0
awareness R41.9
care
in home Z74.2
of infant (at or after birth) T76.02 ☑
confirmed T74.02 ☑
cognitive functions R41.9
coordination R27.9
ataxia R27.0
specified type NEC R27.8
development (physiological) R62.50
failure to thrive (child over 28 days old) R62.51
adult R62.7
newborn P92.6
short stature R62.52
specified type NEC R62.59
energy R53.83
financial resources Z59.6
food T73.0 ☑
growth R62.52
heating Z59.1
housing (permanent) (temporary) Z59.0
adequate Z59.1
learning experiences in childhood Z62.898
leisure time (affecting life-style) Z73.2
material resources Z59.9
memory (*see also* Amnesia)
mild, following organic brain damage F06.8
ovulation N97.0
parental supervision or control of child Z62.0
person able to render necessary care Z74.2
physical exercise Z72.3
play experience in childhood Z62.898
posterior occlusal support M26.57
relaxation (affecting life-style) Z73.2
sexual
desire F52.0
enjoyment F52.1
shelter Z59.0
sleep (adequate) Z72.820
supervision of child by parent Z62.0
support, posterior occlusal M26.57
water T73.1 ☑
Lacrimal — *see* condition
Lacrimation, abnormal — *see* Epiphora
Lacrimonasal duct — *see* condition
Lactation, lactating (breast) (puerperal, postpartum)
associated
cracked nipple O92.13
retracted nipple O92.03
defective O92.4
disorder NEC O92.79
excessive O92.6
failed (complete) O92.3
partial O92.4
mastitis NEC — *see* Mastitis, obstetric
mother (care and/or examination) Z39.1
nonpuerperal N64.3
Lacticemia, excessive E87.2
Lacunar skull Q75.8
Laennec's cirrhosis K74.69
alcoholic K70.30
with ascites K70.31
Lafora's disease — *see* Epilepsy, generalized, idiopathic
Lag, lid (nervous) — *see* Retraction, lid
Lagophthalmos (eyelid) (nervous) H02.209
cicatricial H02.219
left H02.216
lower H02.215
upper H02.214
right H02.213

Lagophthalmos — *continued*
cicatricial — *continued*
right — *continued*
lower H02.212
upper H02.211
keratoconjunctivitis — *see* Keratoconjunctivitis
left H02.206
lower H02.205
upper H02.204
mechanical H02.229
left H02.226
lower H02.225
upper H02.224
right H02.223
lower H02.222
upper H02.221
paralytic H02.239
left H02.236
lower H02.235
upper H02.234
right H02.233
lower H02.232
upper H02.231
right H02.203
lower H02.202
upper H02.201
Laki-Lorand factor deficiency — *see* Defect, coagulation, specified type NEC
Lalling F80.0
Lambert-Eaton syndrome — *see* Syndrome, Lambert-Eaton
Lambliasis, lambliosis A07.1
Landau-Kleffner syndrome — *see* Epilepsy, specified NEC
Landouzy-Déjérine dystrophy or facioscapulohumeral atrophy G71.0
Landouzy's disease (icterohemorrhagic leptospirosis) A27.0
Landry-Guillain-Barré, syndrome or paralysis G61.0
Landry's disease or paralysis G61.0
Lane's
band Q43.3
kink — *see* Obstruction, intestine
syndrome K90.2
Langdon Down syndrome — *see* Trisomy, 21
Lapsed immunization schedule status Z28.3
Large
baby (regardless of gestational age) (4000g to 4499g) P08.1
ear, congenital Q17.1
physiological cup Q14.2
stature R68.89
Large-for-dates NEC (infant) (4000g to 4499g) P08.1
affecting management of pregnancy O36.6- ☑
exceptionally (4500g or more) P08.0
Larsen-Johansson disease orosteochondrosis — *see* Osteochondrosis, juvenile, patella
Larsen's syndrome (flattened facies and multiple congenital dislocations) Q74.8
Larva migrans
cutaneous B76.9
Ancylostoma B76.0
visceral B83.0
Laryngeal — *see* condition
Laryngismus (stridulus) J38.5
congenital P28.89
diphtheritic A36.2
Laryngitis (acute) (edematous) (fibrinous) (infective) (infiltrative) (malignant) (membranous) (phlegmonous) (pneumococcal) (pseudomembranous) (septic) (subglottic) (suppurative) (ulcerative) J04.0
with
influenza, flu, or grippe — *see* Influenza, with, laryngitis
tracheitis (acute) — *see* Laryngotracheitis
atrophic J37.0
catarrhal J37.0
chronic J37.0
with tracheitis (chronic) J37.1
diphtheritic A36.2
due to external agent — *see* Inflammation, respiratory, upper, due to
H. influenzae J04.0
Hemophilus influenzae J04.0
hypertrophic J37.0
influenzal — *see* Influenza, with, respiratory manifestations NEC
obstructive J05.0

Laryngitis — *continued*
sicca J37.0
spasmodic J05.0
acute J04.0
streptococcal J04.0
stridulous J05.0
syphilitic (late) A52.73
congenital A50.59 [J99]
early A50.03 [J99]
tuberculous A15.5
Vincent's A69.1
Laryngocele (congenital) (ventricular) Q31.3
Laryngofissure J38.7
congenital Q31.8
Laryngomalacia (congenital) Q31.5
Laryngopharyngitis (acute) J06.0
chronic J37.0
due to external agent — *see* Inflammation, respiratory, upper, due to
Laryngoplegia J38.00
bilateral J38.02
unilateral J38.01
Laryngoptosis J38.7
Laryngospasm J38.5
Laryngostenosis J38.6
Laryngotracheitis (acute) (Infectional) (infective) (viral) J04.2
atrophic J37.1
catarrhal J37.1
chronic J37.1
diphtheritic A36.2
due to external agent — *see* Inflammation, respiratory, upper, due to
Hemophilus influenzae J04.2
hypertrophic J37.1
influenzal — *see* Influenza, with, respiratory manifestations NEC
pachydermic J38.7
sicca J37.1
spasmodic J38.5
acute J05.0
streptococcal J04.2
stridulous J38.5
syphilitic (late) A52.73
congenital A50.59 [J99]
early A50.03 [J99]
tuberculous A15.5
Vincent's A69.1
Laryngotracheobronchitis — *see* Bronchitis
Larynx, laryngeal — *see* condition
Lassa fever A96.2
Lassitude — *see* Weakness
Late
talker R62.0
walker R62.0
Late effect(s) — *see* Sequelae
Latent — *see* condition
Laterocession — *see* Lateroversion
Lateroflexion — *see* Lateroversion
Lateroversion
cervix — *see* Lateroversion, uterus
uterus, uterine (cervix) (postinfectional) (postpartal, old) N85.4
congenital Q51.818
in pregnancy or childbirth O34.59- ☑
Lathyrism — *see* Poisoning, food, noxious, plant
Launois' syndrome (pituitary gigantism) E22.0
Launois-Bensaude adenolipomatosis E88.89
Laurence-Moon (-Bardet)-**Biedl syndrome** Q87.89
Lax, laxity (see also Relaxation)
ligament (ous) (*see also* Disorder, ligament)
familial M35.7
knee — *see* Derangement, knee
skin (acquired) L57.4
congenital Q82.8
Laxative habit F55.2
Lazy leukocyte syndrome D70.8
Lead miner's lung J63.6
Leak, leakage
air NEC J93.82
postprocedural J95.812
amniotic fluid — *see* Rupture, membranes, premature
blood (microscopic), fetal, into maternal circulation
affecting management of pregnancy — *see* Pregnancy, complicated by
cerebrospinal fluid G96.0
from spinal (lumbar) puncture G97.0

Leak, leakage — *continued*
  device, implant or graft (*see also* Complications, by site and type, mechanical)
    arterial graft NEC — *see* Complication, cardiovascular device, mechanical, vascular
    breast (implant) T85.43 ☑
    catheter NEC T85.638 ☑
      dialysis (renal) T82.43 ☑
        intraperitoneal T85.631 ☑
      infusion NEC T82.534 ☑
        spinal (epidural) (subdural) T85.630 ☑
      urinary, indwelling T83.038 ☑
        cystostomy T83.030 ☑
    gastrointestinal — *see* Complications, prosthetic device, mechanical, gastrointestinal device
    genital NEC T83.498 ☑
      penile prosthesis T83.490 ☑
    heart NEC — *see* Complication, cardiovascular device, mechanical
    joint prosthesis — *see* Complications, joint prosthesis, mechanical, specified NEC, by site
    ocular NEC — *see* Complications, prosthetic device, mechanical, ocular device
    orthopedic NEC — *see* Complication, orthopedic, device, mechanical
    persistent air J93.82
    specified NEC T85.638 ☑
    urinary NEC (*see also* Complication, genitourinary, device, urinary, mechanical)
      graft T83.23 ☑
    vascular NEC — *see* Complication, cardiovascular device, mechanical
    ventricular intracranial shunt T85.03 ☑
  urine — *see* Incontinence
Leaky heart — *see* Endocarditis
Learning defect (specific) F81.9
Leather bottle stomach C16.9
Leber's
  congenital amaurosis H35.50
  optic atrophy (hereditary) H47.22
Lederer's anemia D59.1
Leeches (external) — *see* Hirudiniasis
Leg — *see* condition
Legg (-Calvé)-**Perthes disease, syndrome or osteochondrosis** M91.1- ☑
Legionellosis A48.1
  nonpneumonic A48.2
Legionnaires'
  disease A48.1
    nonpneumonic A48.2
  pneumonia A48.1
Leigh's disease G31.82
Leiner's disease L21.1
Leiofibromyoma — *see* Leiomyoma
Leiomyoblastoma — *see* Neoplasm, connective tissue, benign
Leiomyofibroma (*see also* Neoplasm, connective tissue, benign)
  uterus (cervix) (corpus) D25.9
Leiomyoma (*see also* Neoplasm, connective tissue, benign)
  bizarre — *see* Neoplasm, connective tissue, benign
  cellular — *see* Neoplasm, connective tissue, benign
  epithelioid — *see* Neoplasm, connective tissue, benign
  uterus (cervix) (corpus) D25.9
    intramural D25.1
    submucous D25.0
    subserosal D25.2
  vascular — *see* Neoplasm, connective tissue, benign
Leiomyoma, leiomyomatosis (intravascular) — *see* Neoplasm, connective tissue, uncertain behavior
Leiomyosarcoma (*see also* Neoplasm, connective tissue, malignant)
  epithelioid — *see* Neoplasm, connective tissue, malignant
  myxoid — *see* Neoplasm, connective tissue, malignant
Leishmaniasis B55.9
  American (mucocutaneous) B55.2
    cutaneous B55.1
  Asian Desert B55.1
  Brazilian B55.2
  cutaneous (any type) B55.1
  dermal (*see also* Leishmaniasis, cutaneous)
    post-kala-azar B55.0
  eyelid B55.1
  infantile B55.0
  Mediterranean B55.0

Leishmaniasis — *continued*
  mucocutaneous (American) (New World) B55.2
  naso-oral B55.2
  nasopharyngeal B55.2
  old world B55.1
  tegumentaria diffusa B55.1
  visceral B55.0
Leishmanoid, dermal (*see also* Leishmaniasis, cutaneous)
  post-kala-azar B55.0
Lenegre's disease I44.2
Lengthening, leg — *see* Deformity, limb, unequal length
Lennert's lymphoma — *see* Lymphoma, Lennert's
Lennox-Gastaut syndrome G40.812
  intractable G40.814
    with status epilepticus G40.813
    without status epilepticus G40.814
  not intractable G40.812
    with status epilepticus G40.811
    without status epilepticus G40.812
Lens — *see* condition
Lenticonus (anterior) (posterior) (congenital) Q12.8
Lenticular degeneration, progressive E83.01
Lentiglobus (posterior) (congenital) Q12.8
Lentigo (congenital) L81.4
  maligna (*see also* Melanoma, in situ)
    melanoma — *see* Melanoma
Lentivirus, as cause of disease classified elsewhere B97.31
Leontiasis
  ossium M85.2
  syphilitic (late) A52.78
    congenital A50.59
Lepothrix A48.8
Lepra — *see* Leprosy
Leprechaunism E34.8
Leprosy A30.- ☑
  with muscle disorder A30.9 [M63.80]
    ankle A30.9 [M63.87-] ☑
    foot A30.9 [M63.87-] ☑
    forearm A30.9 [M63.83-] ☑
    hand A30.9 [M63.84-] ☑
    lower leg A30.9 [M63.86-] ☑
    multiple sites A30.9 [M63.89]
    pelvic region A30.9 [M63.85-] ☑
    shoulder region A30.9 [M63.81-] ☑
    specified site NEC A30.9 [M63.88]
    thigh A30.9 [M63.85-] ☑
    upper arm A30.9 [M63.82-] ☑
  anesthetic A30.9
  BB A30.3
  BL A30.4
  borderline (infiltrated) (neuritic) A30.3
    lepromatous A30.4
    tuberculoid A30.2
  BT A30.2
  dimorphous (infiltrated) (neuritic) A30.3
  I A30.0
  indeterminate (macular) (neuritic) A30.0
  lepromatous (diffuse) (infiltrated) (macular) (neuritic) (nodular) A30.5
  LL A30.5
  macular (early) (neuritic) (simple) A30.9
  maculoanesthetic A30.9
  mixed A30.3
  neural A30.9
  nodular A30.5
  primary neuritic A30.3
  specified type NEC A30.8
  TT A30.1
  tuberculoid (major) (minor) A30.1
Leptocytosis, hereditary D56.9
Leptomeningitis (chronic) (circumscribed) (hemorrhagic) (nonsuppurative) — *see* Meningitis
Leptomeningopathy G96.19
Leptospiral — *see* condition
Leptospirochetal — *see* condition
Leptospirosis A27.9
  canicola A27.89
  due to Leptospira interrogans serovar icterohaemorrhagiae A27.0
  icterohemorrhagica A27.0
  pomona A27.89
  Weil's disease A27.0
Leptus dermatitis B88.0
Leri-Weill syndrome Q77.8
Leriche's syndrome (aortic bifurcation occlusion) I74.09

Leri's pleonosteosis Q78.8
Lermoyez' syndrome — *see* Vertigo, peripheral NEC
Lesch-Nyhan syndrome E79.1
Leser-Trélat disease L82.1
  inflamed L82.0
Lesion(s) (nontraumatic)
  abducens nerve — *see* Strabismus, paralytic, sixth nerve
  alveolar process K08.9
  angiocentric immunoproliferative D47.Z9 (*following* D47.4)
  anorectal K62.9
  aortic (valve) I35.9
  auditory nerve — *see* subcategory H93.3 ☑
  basal ganglion G25.9
  bile duct — *see* Disease, bile duct
  biomechanical M99.9
    specified type NEC M99.89
      abdomen M99.89
      acromioclavicular M99.87
      cervical region M99.81
      cervicothoracic M99.81
      costochondral M99.88
      costovertebral M99.88
      head region M99.80
      hip M99.85
      lower extremity M99.86
      lumbar region M99.83
      lumbosacral M99.83
      occipitocervical M99.80
      pelvic region M99.85
      pubic M99.85
      rib cage M99.88
      sacral region M99.84
      sacrococcygeal M99.84
      sacroiliac M99.84
      specified NEC M99.89
      sternochondral M99.88
      sternoclavicular M99.87
      thoracic region M99.82
      thoracolumbar M99.82
      upper extremity M99.87
  bladder N32.9
  bone — *see* Disorder, bone
  brachial plexus G54.0
  brain G93.9
    congenital Q04.9
    vascular I67.9
      degenerative I67.9
      hypertensive I67.4
  buccal cavity K13.79
  calcified — *see* Calcification
  canthus — *see* Disorder, eyelid
  carate — *see* Pinta, lesions
  cardia K22.9
  cardiac (*see also* Disease, heart) I51.9
    congenital Q24.9
    valvular — *see* Endocarditis
  cauda equina G83.4
  cecum K63.9
  cerebral — *see* Lesion, brain
  cerebrovascular I67.9
    degenerative I67.9
    hypertensive I67.4
  cervical (nerve) root NEC G54.2
  chiasmal — *see* Disorder, optic, chiasm
  chorda tympani G51.8
  coin, lung R91.1
  colon K63.9
  congenital — *see* Anomaly, by site
  conjunctiva H11.9
  conus medullaris — *see* Injury, conus medullaris
  coronary artery — *see* Ischemia, heart
  cranial nerve G52.9
    eighth — *see* Disorder, ear
    eleventh G52.9
    fifth G50.9
    first G52.0
    fourth — *see* Strabismus, paralytic, fourth nerve
    seventh G51.9
    sixth — *see* Strabismus, paralytic, sixth nerve
    tenth G52.2
    twelfth G52.3
  cystic — *see* Cyst
  degenerative — *see* Degeneration
  duodenum K31.9
  edentulous (alveolar) ridge, associated with trauma, due to traumatic occlusion K06.2

Lesion(s) — *continued*
en coup de sabre L94.1
eyelid — *see* Disorder, eyelid
gasserian ganglion G50.8
gastric K31.9
gastroduodenal K31.9
gastrointestinal K63.9
gingiva, associated with trauma K06.2
glomerular
   focal and segmental (*see also* N00-N07 with fourth
      character .1) N05.1
   minimal change (*see also* N00-N07 with fourth
      character .0) N05.0
heart (organic) — *see* Disease, heart
hyperchromic, due to pinta (carate) A67.1
hyperkeratotic — *see* Hyperkeratosis
hypothalamic E23.7
ileocecal K63.9
ileum K63.9
iliohypogastric nerve G57.8- ☑
inflammatory — *see* Inflammation
intestine K63.9
intracerebral — *see* Lesion, brain
intrachiasmal (optic) — *see* Disorder, optic, chiasm
intracranial, space-occupying R90.0
joint — *see* Disorder, joint
   sacroiliac (old) M53.3
keratotic — *see* Keratosis
kidney — *see* Disease, renal
laryngeal nerve (recurrent) G52.2
lip K13.0
liver K76.9
lumbosacral
   plexus G54.1
   root (nerve) NEC G54.4
lung (coin) R91.1
maxillary sinus J32.0
mitral I05.9
Morel-Lavallée — *see* Hematoma, by site
motor cortex NEC G93.89
mouth K13.79
nerve G58.9
   femoral G57.2- ☑
   median G56.1- ☑
      carpal tunnel syndrome — *see* Syndrome,
        carpal tunnel
   plantar G57.6- ☑
   popliteal (lateral) G57.3- ☑
      medial G57.4- ☑
   radial G56.3- ☑
   sciatic G57.0- ☑
   spinal — *see* Injury, nerve, spinal
   ulnar G56.2- ☑
nervous system, congenital Q07.9
nonallopathic — *see* Lesion, biomechanical
nose (internal) J34.89
obstructive — *see* Obstruction
obturator nerve G57.8- ☑
oral mucosa K13.70
organ or site NEC — *see* Disease, by site
osteolytic — *see* Osteolysis
peptic K27.9
periodontal, due to traumatic occlusion K05.5
pharynx J39.2
pigment, pigmented (skin) L81.9
pinta — *see* Pinta, lesions
polypoid — *see* Polyp
prechiasmal (optic) — *see* Disorder, optic, chiasm
primary (*see also* Syphilis, primary) A51.0
   carate A67.0
   pinta A67.0
   yaws A66.0
pulmonary J98.4
   valve I37.9
pylorus K31.9
rectosigmoid K63.9
retina, retinal H35.9
sacroiliac (joint) (old) M53.3
salivary gland K11.9
   benign lymphoepithelial K11.8
saphenous nerve G57.8- ☑
sciatic nerve G57.0- ☑
secondary — *see* Syphilis, secondary
shoulder (region) M75.9- ☑
   specified NEC M75.8- ☑
sigmoid K63.9
sinus (accessory) (nasal) J34.89

Lesion(s) — *continued*
skin L98.9
   suppurative L08.0
SLAP S43.43- ☑
spinal cord G95.9
   congenital Q06.9
spleen D73.89
stomach K31.9
superior glenoid labrum S43.43- ☑
syphilitic — *see* Syphilis
tertiary — *see* Syphilis, tertiary
thoracic root (nerve) NEC G54.3
tonsillar fossa J35.9
tooth, teeth K08.9
   white spot
      chewing surface K02.51
      pit and fissure surface K02.51
      smooth surface K02.61
traumatic — *see* specific type of injury by site
tricuspid (valve) I07.9
   nonrheumatic I36.9
trigeminal nerve G50.9
ulcerated or ulcerative — *see* Ulcer, skin
uterus N85.9
vagus nerve G52.2
valvular — *see* Endocarditis
vascular I99.9
   affecting central nervous system I67.9
   following trauma NEC T14.8
   umbilical cord, complicating delivery O69.5 ☑
warty — *see* Verruca
white spot (tooth)
   chewing surface K02.51
   pit and fissure surface K02.51
   smooth surface K02.61
Lethargic — *see* condition
Lethargy R53.83
Letterer-Siwe's disease C96.0
Leukemia, leukemic C95.9- ☑
acute basophilic C94.8- ☑
acute bilineal C95.0- ☑
acute erythroid C94.0- ☑
acute lymphoblastic C91.0- ☑
acute megakaryoblastic C94.2- ☑
acute megakaryocytic C94.2- ☑
acute mixed lineage C95.0- ☑
acute monoblastic (monoblastic/monocytic) C93.0- ☑
acute monocytic (monoblastic/monocytic) C93.0- ☑
acute myeloblastic (minimal differentiation) (with
   maturation) C92.0- ☑
acute myeloid
   with
      11q23-abnormality C92.6- ☑
      dysplasia of remaining hematopoesis and/or
        myelodysplastic disease in its history
        C92.A- ☑ (*following* C92.6)
      multilineage dysplasia C92.A- ☑ (*following*
        C92.6)
      variation of MLL-gene C92.6- ☑
   M6 (a)(b) C94.0- ☑
   M7 C94.2- ☑
acute myelomonocytic C92.5- ☑
acute promyelocytic C92.4- ☑
adult T-cell (HTLV-1-associated) (acute variant)
   (chronic variant) (lymphomatoid variant)
   (smouldering variant) C91.5- ☑
aggressive NK-cell C94.8- ☑
AML (1/ETO) (M0) (M1) (M2) (without a FAB classification) C92.0- ☑
AML M3 C92.4- ☑
AML M4 (Eo with inv(16) or t(16;16)) C92.5- ☑
AML M5 C93.0- ☑
AML M5a C93.0- ☑
AML M5b C93.0- ☑
AML Me with t (15;17) and variants C92.4- ☑
atypical chronic myeloid, BCR/ABL-negative C92.2- ☑
biphenotypic acute C95.0- ☑
blast cell C95.0- ☑
Burkitt-type, mature B-cell C91.A- ☑ (*following* C91.6)
chronic lymphocytic, of B-cell type C91.1- ☑
chronic monocytic C93.1- ☑
chronic myelogenous (Philadelphia chromosome (Ph1)
   positive) (t(9;22)) (q34;q11) (with crisis of blast
   cells) C92.1- ☑
chronic myeloid, BCR/ABL-positive C92.1- ☑
   atypical, BCR/ABL-negative C92.2- ☑
chronic myelomonocytic C93.1- ☑

chronic neutrophilic D47.1
CMML (-1) (-2) (with eosinophilia) C93.1- ☑
granulocytic (*see also* Category C92) C92.9- ☑
hairy cell C91.4- ☑
juvenile myelomonocytic C93.3- ☑
lymphoid C91.9- ☑
   specified NEC C91.Z- ☑ (*following* C91.6)
mast cell C94.3- ☑
mature B-cell, Burkitt-type C91.A- ☑ (*following* C91.6)
monocytic (subacute) C93.9- ☑
   specified NEC C93.Z- ☑ (*following* C93.3)
myelogenous (*see also* Category C92) C92.9- ☑
myeloid C92.9- ☑
   specified NEC C92.Z- ☑ (*following* C92.6)
plasma cell C90.1- ☑
plasmacytic C90.1- ☑
prolymphocytic
   of B-cell type C91.3- ☑
   of T-cell type C91.6- ☑
specified NEC C94.8- ☑
stem cell, of unclear lineage C95.0- ☑
subacute lymphocytic C91.9- ☑
T-cell large granular lymphocytic C91.Z- ☑ (*following*
   C91.6)
unspecified cell type C95.9- ☑
   acute C95.0- ☑
   chronic C95.1- ☑
Leukemoid reaction (*see also* Reaction, leukemoid)
   D72.823
Leukoaraiosis (hypertensive) I67.81
Leukoariosis — *see* Leukoaraiosis
Leukocoria — *see* Disorder, globe, degenerated condition, leucocoria
Leukocytopenia D72.819
Leukocytosis D72.829
   eosinophilic D72.1
Leukoderma, leukodermia NEC L81.5
   syphilitic A51.39
      late A52.79
Leukodystrophy E75.29
Leukoedema, oral epithelium K13.29
Leukoencephalitis G04.81
   acute (subacute) hemorrhagic G36.1
      postimmunization or postvaccinal G04.02
   postinfectious G04.01
   subacute sclerosing A81.1
   van Bogaert's (sclerosing) A81.1
Leukoencephalopathy (*see also* Encephalopathy)
   G93.49
   Binswanger's I67.3
   heroin vapor G92
   metachromatic E75.25
   multifocal (progressive) A81.2
   postimmunization and postvaccinal G04.02
   progressive multifocal A81.2
   reversible, posterior G93.6
   van Bogaert's (sclerosing) A81.1
   vascular, progressive I67.3
Leukoerythroblastosis D75.9
Leukokeratosis (*see also* Leukoplakia)
   mouth K13.21
   nicotina palati K13.24
   oral mucosa K13.21
   tongue K13.21
   vocal cord J38.3
Leukokraurosis vulva (e) N90.4
Leukoma (cornea) (*see also* Opacity, cornea)
   adherent H17.0- ☑
   interfering with central vision — *see* Opacity, cornea,
      central
Leukomalacia, cerebral, newborn P91.2
   periventricular P91.2
Leukomelanopathy, hereditary D72.0
Leukonychia (punctata) (striata) L60.8
   congenital Q84.4
Leukopathia unguium L60.8
   congenital Q84.4
Leukopenia D72.819
   basophilic D72.818
   chemotherapy (cancer) induced D70.1
   congenital D70.0
   cyclic D70.0
   drug induced NEC D70.2
      due to cytoreductive cancer chemotherapy D70.1
   eosinophilic D72.818
   familial D70.0

Leukopenia — *continued*
  infantile genetic D70.0
  malignant D70.9
  periodic D70.0
  transitory neonatal P61.5
Leukopenic — *see* condition
Leukoplakia
  anus K62.89
  bladder (postinfectional) N32.89
  buccal K13.21
  cervix (uteri) N88.0
  esophagus K22.8
  gingiva K13.21
  hairy (oral mucosa) (tongue) K13.3
  kidney (pelvis) N28.89
  larynx J38.7
  lip K13.21
  mouth K13.21
  oral epithelium, including tongue (mucosa) K13.21
  palate K13.21
  pelvis (kidney) N28.89
  penis (infectional) N48.0
  rectum K62.89
  syphilitic (late) A52.79
  tongue K13.21
  ureter (postinfectional) N28.89
  urethra (postinfectional) N36.8
  uterus N85.8
  vagina N89.4
  vocal cord J38.3
  vulva N90.4
Leukorrhea N89.8
  due to Trichomonas (vaginalis) A59.00
  trichomonal A59.00
Leukosarcoma C85.9- ☑
Levocardia (isolated) Q24.1
  with situs inversus Q89.3
Levotransposition Q20.5
Lev's disease or syndrome (acquired complete heart block) I44.2
Levulosuria — *see* Fructosuria
Levurid L30.2
Lewy body (ies) (dementia) (disease) G31.83
Leyden-Moebius dystrophy G71.0
Leydig cell
  carcinoma
    specified site — *see* Neoplasm, malignant, by site
    unspecified site
      female C56.9-
      male C62.9- ☑
  tumor
    benign
      specified site — *see* Neoplasm, benign, by site
      unspecified site
        female D27.- ☑
        male D29.2- ☑
    malignant
      specified site — *see* Neoplasm, malignant, by site
      unspecified site
        female C56.- ☑
        male C62.9- ☑
    specified site — *see* Neoplasm, uncertain behavior, by site
    unspecified site
      female D39.1- ☑
      male D40.1- ☑
Leydig-Sertoli cell tumor
  specified site — *see* Neoplasm, benign, by site
  unspecified site
    female D27.- ☑
    male D29.2- ☑
LGSIL (Low grade squamous intraepithelial lesion on cytologic smear of)
  anus R85.612
  cervix R87.612
  vagina R87.622
Liar, pathologic F60.2
Libido
  decreased R68.82
Libman-Sacks disease M32.11
Lice (infestation) B85.2
  body (Pediculus corporis) B85.1
  crab B85.3
  head (Pediculus capitis) B85.0
  mixed (classifiable to more than one of the titles B85.0-B85.3) B85.4

Lice — *continued*
  pubic (Phthirus pubis) B85.3
Lichen L28.0
  albus L90.0
    penis N48.0
    vulva N90.4
  amyloidosis E85.4 [L99]
  atrophicus L90.0
    penis N48.0
    vulva N90.4
  congenital Q82.8
  myxedematosus L98.5
  nitidus L44.1
  pilaris Q82.8
    acquired L85.8
  planopilaris L66.1
  planus (chronicus) L43.9
    annularis L43.8
    bullous L43.1
    follicular L66.1
    hypertrophic L43.0
    moniliformis L44.3
    of Wilson L43.9
    specified NEC L43.8
    subacute (active) L43.3
    tropicus L43.3
  ruber
    acuminatus L44.0
    moniliformis L44.3
    planus L43.9
  sclerosus (et atrophicus) L90.0
    penis N48.0
    vulva N90.4
  scrofulosus (primary) (tuberculous) A18.4
  simplex (chronicus) (circumscriptus) L28.0
  striatus L44.2
  urticatus L28.2
Lichenification L28.0
Lichenoides tuberculosis (primary) A18.4
Lichtheim's disease or syndrome — *see* Degeneration, combined
Lien migrans D73.89
Ligament — *see* condition
Light
  for gestational age — *see* Light for dates
  headedness R42
Light-for-dates (infant) P05.00
  with weight of
    500-749 grams P05.02
    750-999 grams P05.03
    1000-1249 grams P05.04
    1250-1499 grams P05.05
    1500-1749 grams P05.06
    1750-1999 grams P05.07
    2000-2499 grams P05.08
    499 grams or less P05.01
  affecting management of pregnancy O36.59- ☑
  and small-for-dates — *see* Small for dates
Lightning (effects) (stroke) (struck by) T75.00 ☑
  burn — *see* Burn
  foot E53.8
  shock T75.01 ☑
  specified effect NEC T75.09 ☑
Lightwood-Albright syndrome N25.89
Lightwood's disease or syndrome (renal tubular acidosis) N25.89
Lignac (-de Toni) (-Fanconi) (-Debré) **disease or syndrome** E72.09
  with cystinosis E72.04
Ligneous thyroiditis E06.5
Likoff's syndrome I20.8
Limb — *see* condition
Limbic epilepsy personality syndrome F07.0
Limitation, limited
  activities due to disability Z73.6
  cardiac reserve — *see* Disease, heart
  eye muscle duction, traumatic — *see* Strabismus, mechanical
  mandibular range of motion M26.52
Lindau (-von Hippel) **disease** Q85.8
Line(s)
  Beau's L60.4
  Harris' — *see* Arrest, epiphyseal
  Hudson's (cornea) — *see* Pigmentation, cornea, anterior
  Stähli's (cornea) — *see* Pigmentation, cornea, anterior
Linea corneae senilis — *see* Change, cornea, senile

Lingua
  geographica K14.1
  nigra (villosa) K14.3
  plicata K14.5
  tylosis K13.29
Lingual — *see* condition
Linguatulosis B88.8
Linitis (gastric) **plastica** C16.9
Lip — *see* condition
Lipedema — *see* Edema
Lipemia (*see also* Hyperlipidemia)
  retina, retinalis E78.3
Lipidosis E75.6
  cerebral (infantile) (juvenile) (late) E75.4
  cerebroretinal E75.4
  cerebroside E75.22
  cholesterol (cerebral) E75.5
  glycolipid E75.21
  hepatosplenomegalic E78.3
  sphingomyelin — *see* Niemann-Pick disease or syndrome
  sulfatide E75.29
Lipoadenoma — *see* Neoplasm, benign, by site
Lipoblastoma — *see* Lipoma
Lipoblastomatosis — *see* Lipoma
Lipochondrodystrophy E76.01
Lipochrome histiocytosis (familial) D71
Lipodermatosclerosis — *see* Varix, leg, with, inflammation
  ulcerated — *see* Varix, leg, with, ulcer, with inflammation by site
Lipodystrophia progressiva E88.1
Lipodystrophy (progressive) E88.1
  insulin E88.1
  intestinal K90.81
  mesenteric K65.4
Lipofibroma — *see* Lipoma
Lipofuscinosis, neuronal (with ceroidosis) E75.4
Lipogranuloma, sclerosing L92.8
Lipogranulomatosis E78.89
Lipoid (*see also* condition)
  histiocytosis D76.3
    essential E75.29
  nephrosis N04.9
  proteinosis of Urbach E78.89
Lipoidemia — *see* Hyperlipidemia
Lipoidosis — *see* Lipidosis
Lipoma D17.9
  fetal D17.9
    fat cell D17.9
  infiltrating D17.9
  intramuscular D17.9
  pleomorphic D17.9
  site classification
    arms (skin) (subcutaneous) D17.2- ☑
    connective tissue D17.30
      intra-abdominal D17.5
      intrathoracic D17.4
      peritoneum D17.79
      retroperitoneum D17.79
      specified site NEC D17.39
      spermatic cord D17.6
    face (skin) (subcutaneous) D17.0
    genitourinary organ NEC D17.72
    head (skin) (subcutaneous) D17.0
    intra-abdominal D17.5
    intrathoracic D17.4
    kidney D17.71
    legs (skin) (subcutaneous) D17.2- ☑
    neck (skin) (subcutaneous) D17.0
    peritoneum D17.79
    retroperitoneum D17.79
    skin D17.30
      specified site NEC D17.39
    specified site NEC D17.79
    spermatic cord D17.6
    subcutaneous D17.30
      specified site NEC D17.39
    trunk (skin) (subcutaneous) D17.1
    unspecified D17.9
  spindle cell D17.9
Lipomatosis E88.2
  dolorosa (Dercum) E88.2
  fetal — *see* Lipoma
  Launois-Bensaude E88.89
Lipomyoma — *see* Lipoma
Lipomyxoma — *see* Lipoma

Lipomyxosarcoma — *see* Neoplasm, connective tissue, malignant
Lipoprotein metabolism disorder E78.9
Lipoproteinemia E78.5
  broad-beta E78.2
  floating-beta E78.2
  hyper-pre-beta E78.1
Liposarcoma (*see also* Neoplasm, connective tissue, malignant)
  dedifferentiated — *see* Neoplasm, connective tissue, malignant
  differentiated type — *see* Neoplasm, connective tissue, malignant
  embryonal — *see* Neoplasm, connective tissue, malignant
  mixed type — *see* Neoplasm, connective tissue, malignant
  myxoid — *see* Neoplasm, connective tissue, malignant
  pleomorphic — *see* Neoplasm, connective tissue, malignant
  round cell — *see* Neoplasm, connective tissue, malignant
  well differentiated type — *see* Neoplasm, connective tissue, malignant
Liposynovitis prepatellaris E88.89
Lipping, cervix N86
Lipschütz disease or ulcer N76.6
Lipuria R82.0
  schistosomiasis (bilharziasis) B65.0
Lisping F80.0
Lissauer's paralysis A52.17
Lissencephalia, lissencephaly Q04.3
Listeriosis, listerellosis A32.9
  congenital (disseminated) P37.2
  cutaneous A32.0
  neonatal, newborn (disseminated) P37.2
  oculoglandular A32.81
  specified NEC A32.89
Lithemia E79.0
Lithiasis — *see* Calculus
Lithosis J62.8
Lithuria R82.99
Litigation, anxiety concerning Z65.3
Little leaguer's elbow — *see* Epicondylitis, medial
Little's disease G80.9
Littre's
  gland — *see* condition
  hernia — *see* Hernia, abdomen
Littritis — *see* Urethritis
Livedo (annularis) (racemosa) (reticularis) R23.1
Liver — *see* condition
Living alone (problems with) Z60.2
  with handicapped person Z74.2
Lloyd's syndrome — *see* Adenomatosis, endocrine
Loa loa, loaiasis, loasis B74.3
Lobar — *see* condition
Lobomycosis B48.0
Lobo's disease B48.0
Lobotomy syndrome F07.0
Lobster-claw hand Q71.6- ☑
Lobulation (congenital) (*see also* Anomaly, by site)
  kidney, Q63.1
  liver, abnormal Q44.7
  spleen Q89.09
Lobule, lobular — *see* condition
Local, localized — *see* condition
Locked twins causing obstructed labor O66.1
Locked-in state G83.5
Locking
  joint — *see* Derangement, joint, specified type NEC
    knee — *see* Derangement, knee
Lockjaw — *see* Tetanus
Löffler's
  endocarditis I42.3
  eosinophilia J82
  pneumonia J82
  syndrome (eosinophilic pneumonitis) J82
Loiasis (with conjunctival infestation) (eyelid) B74.3
Lone Star fever A77.0
Long
  labor O63.9
    first stage O63.0
    second stage O63.1
  QT syndrome I45.81
Long-term (current) (prophylactic) **drug therapy** (use of)

Long-term (current) (prophylactic) **drug therapy** — *continued*
  agents affecting estrogen receptors and estrogen levels NEC Z79.818
  anastrozole (Arimidex) Z79.811
  anti-inflammatory, non-steroidal (NSAID) Z79.1
  antibiotics Z79.2
    short-term use — *omit code*
  anticoagulants Z79.01
  antiplatelet Z79.02
  antithrombotics Z79.02
  aromatase inhibitors Z79.811
  aspirin Z79.82
  birth control pill or patch Z79.3
  bisphosphonates Z79.83
  contraceptive, oral Z79.3
  drug, specified NEC Z79.899
  estrogen receptor downregulators Z79.818
  Evista Z79.810
  exemestane (Aromasin) Z79.811
  Fareston Z79.810
  fulvestrant (Faslodex) Z79.818
  gonadotropin-releasing hormone (GnRH) agonist Z79.818
  goserelin acetate (Zoladex) Z79.818
  hormone replacement (postmenopausal) Z79.890
  insulin Z79.4
  letrozole (Femara) Z79.811
  leuprolide acetate (leuprorelin) (Lupron) Z79.818
  megestrol acetate (Megace) Z79.818
  methadone for pain management Z79.891
  Nolvadex Z79.810
  non-steroidal anti-inflammatories (NSAID) Z79.1
  opiate analgesic Z79.891
  oral contraceptive Z79.3
  raloxifene (Evista) Z79.810
  selective estrogen receptor modulators (SERMs) Z79.810
  steroids
    inhaled Z79.51
    systemic Z79.52
  tamoxifen (Nolvadex) Z79.810
  toremifene (Fareston) Z79.810
Longitudinal stripes or grooves, nails L60.8
  congenital Q84.6
Loop
  intestine — *see* Volvulus
  vascular on papilla (optic) Q14.2
Loose (*see also* condition)
  body
    joint M24.00
      ankle M24.07- ☑
      elbow M24.02- ☑
      hand M24.04- ☑
      hip M24.05- ☑
      knee M23.4- ☑
      shoulder (region) M24.01- ☑
      specified site NEC M24.08
      toe M24.07- ☑
      vertebra M24.08
      wrist M24.03- ☑
    knee M23.4- ☑
    sheath, tendon — *see* Disorder, tendon, specified type NEC
  cartilage — *see* Loose, body, joint
  tooth, teeth K08.8
Loosening
  aseptic
    joint prosthesis — *see* Complications, joint prosthesis, mechanical, loosening, by site
  epiphysis — *see* Osteochondropathy
  mechanical
    joint prosthesis — *see* Complications, joint prosthesis, mechanical, loosening, by site
Looser-Milkman (-Debray) **syndrome** M83.8
Lop ear (deformity) Q17.3
Lorain (-Levi) **short stature syndrome** E23.0
Lordosis M40.50
  acquired — *see* Lordosis, specified type NEC
  congenital Q76.429
    lumbar region Q76.426
    lumbosacral region Q76.427
    sacral region Q76.428
    sacrococcygeal region Q76.428
    thoracolumbar region Q76.425
  lumbar region M40.56
  lumbosacral region M40.57
  postsurgical M96.4

Lordosis — *continued*
  postural — *see* Lordosis, specified type NEC
  rachitic (late effect) (sequelae) E64.3
  sequelae of rickets E64.3
  specified type NEC M40.40
    lumbar region M40.46
    lumbosacral region M40.47
    thoracolumbar region M40.45
  thoracolumbar region M40.55
  tuberculous A18.01
Loss (of)
  appetite (*see* Anorexia) R63.0
    hysterical F50.8
    nonorganic origin F50.8
    psychogenic F50.8
  blood — *see* Hemorrhage
  consciousness, transient R55
    traumatic — *see* Injury, intracranial
  control, sphincter, rectum R15.9
    nonorganic origin F98.1
  elasticity, skin R23.4
  family (member) in childhood Z62.898
  fluid (acute) E86.9
    with
      hypernatremia E87.0
      hyponatremia E87.1
  function of labyrinth — *see* subcategory H83.2 ☑
  hair, nonscarring — *see* Alopecia
  hearing (*see also* Deafness)
    central NOS H90.5
    neural NOS H90.5
    perceptive NOS H90.5
    sensorineural NOS H90.5
    sensory NOS H90.5
  height R29.890
  limb or member, traumatic, current — *see* Amputation, traumatic
  love relationship in childhood Z62.898
  memory (*see also* Amnesia)
    mild, following organic brain damage F06.8
  mind — *see* Psychosis
  occlusal vertical dimension of fully erupted teeth M26.37
  organ or part — *see* Absence, by site, acquired
  ossicles, ear (partial) H74.32- ☑
  parent in childhood Z63.4
  pregnancy, recurrent N96
    without current pregnancy N96
    care in current pregnancy O26.2- ☑
  recurrent pregnancy — *see* Loss, pregnancy, recurrent
  self-esteem, in childhood Z62.898
  sense of
    smell — *see* Disturbance, sensation, smell
    taste — *see* Disturbance, sensation, taste
    touch R20.8
  sensory R44.9
    dissociative F44.6
  sexual desire F52.0
  sight (acquired) (complete) (congenital) — *see* Blindness
  substance of
    bone — *see* Disorder, bone, density and structure, specified NEC
    cartilage — *see* Disorder, cartilage, specified type NEC
    auricle (ear) — *see* Disorder, pinna, specified type NEC
    vitreous (humor) H15.89
  tooth, teeth — *see* Absence, teeth, acquired
  vision, visual H54.7
    both eyes H54.3
    one eye H54.60
      left (normal vision on right) H54.62
      right (normal vision on left) H54.61
    specified as blindness — *see* Blindness
    subjective
      sudden H53.13- ☑
      transient H53.12- ☑
  vitreous — *see* Prolapse, vitreous
  voice — *see* Aphonia
  weight (abnormal) (cause unknown) R63.4
Louis-Bar syndrome (ataxia-telangiectasia) G11.3
Louping ill (encephalitis) A84.8
Louse, lousiness — *see* Lice
Low
  achiever, school Z55.3
  back syndrome M54.5

Low — *continued*
  basal metabolic rate R94.8
  birthweight (2499 grams or less) P07.10
    with weight of
      1000-1249 grams P07.14
      1250-1499 grams P07.15
      1500-1749 grams P07.16
      1750-1999 grams P07.17
      2000-2499 grams P07.18
    extreme (999 grams or less) P07.00
      with weight of
        500-749 grams P07.02
        750-999 grams P07.03
        499 grams or less P07.01
    for gestational age — *see* Light for dates
  blood pressure (*see also* Hypotension)
    reading (incidental) (isolated) (nonspecific) R03.1
  cardiac reserve — *see* Disease, heart
  function (*see also* Hypofunction)
    kidney N28.9
  hematocrit D64.9
  hemoglobin D64.9
  income Z59.6
  level of literacy Z55.0
  lying
    kidney N28.89
    organ or site, congenital — *see* Malposition, congenital
  output syndrome (cardiac) — *see* Failure, heart
  platelets (blood) — *see* Thrombocytopenia
  reserve, kidney N28.89
  salt syndrome E87.1
  self esteem R45.81
  set ears Q17.4
  vision H54.2
    one eye (other eye normal) H54.50
      left (normal vision on right) H54.52
      other eye blind — *see* Blindness
      right (normal vision on left) H54.51
Low-density-lipoprotein-type (LDL) **hyperlipoproteinemia** E78.0
Lowe's syndrome E72.03
Lown-Ganong-Levine syndrome I45.6
LSD reaction (acute) (without dependence) F16.90
  with dependence F16.20
Ludwig's angina or disease K12.2
Lues (venerea), **luetic** — *see* Syphilis
Luetscher's syndrome (dehydration) E86.0
Lumbago, lumbalgia M54.5
  with sciatica M54.4- ☑
    due to intervertebral disc disorder M51.17
  due to displacement, intervertebral disc M51.27
    with sciatica M51.17
Lumbar — *see* condition
Lumbarization, vertebra, congenital Q76.49
Lumbermen's itch B88.0
Lump — *see* Mass
Lunacy — *see* Psychosis
Lung — *see* condition
Lupoid (miliary) **of Boeck** D86.3
Lupus
  anticoagulant D68.62
    with
      hemorrhagic disorder D68.312
      hypercoagulable state D68.62
      finding without diagnosis R76.0
  discoid (local) L93.0
  erythematosus (discoid) (local) L93.0
    disseminated — *see* Lupus, erythematosus, systemic
    eyelid H01.129
      left H01.126
        lower H01.125
        upper H01.124
      right H01.123
        lower H01.122
        upper H01.121
    profundus L93.2
    specified NEC L93.2
    subacute cutaneous L93.1
    systemic M32.9
      with organ or system involvement M32.10
        endocarditis M32.11
        lung M32.13
        pericarditis M32.12
        renal (glomerular) M32.14
          tubulo-interstitial M32.15
        specified organ or system NEC M32.19

Lupus — *continued*
  erythematosus — *continued*
    systemic — *continued*
      drug-induced M32.0
      inhibitor (presence of) D68.62
        with
          hemorrhagic disorder D68.312
          hypercoagulable state D68.62
          finding without diagnosis R76.0
      specified NEC M32.8
  exedens A18.4
  hydralazine M32.0
    correct substance properly administered — *see* Table of Drugs and Chemicals, by drug, adverse effect
    overdose or wrong substance given or taken — *see* Table of Drugs and Chemicals, by drug, poisoning
  nephritis (chronic) M32.14
  nontuberculous, not disseminated L93.0
  panniculitis L93.2
  pernio (Besnier) D86.3
  systemic — *see* Lupus, erythematosus, systemic
  tuberculous A18.4
    eyelid A18.4
  vulgaris A18.4
    eyelid A18.4
Luteinoma D27.- ☑
Lutembacher's disease or syndrome (atrial septal defect with mitral stenosis) Q21.1
Luteoma D27.- ☑
Lutz (-Splendore-de Almeida) **disease** — *see* Paracoccidioidomycosis
Luxation (*see also* Dislocation)
  eyeball (nontraumatic) — *see* Luxation, globe
    birth injury P15.3
  globe, nontraumatic H44.82- ☑
  lacrimal gland — *see* Dislocation, lacrimal gland
  lens (old) (partial) (spontaneous)
    congenital Q12.1
      syphilitic A50.39
Lycanthropy F22
Lyell's syndrome L51.2
  due to drug L51.2
    correct substance properly administered — *see* Table of Drugs and Chemicals, by drug, adverse effect
    overdose or wrong substance given or taken — *see* Table of Drugs and Chemicals, by drug, poisoning
Lyme disease A69.20
Lymph
  gland or node — *see* condition
  scrotum — *see* Infestation, filarial
Lymphadenitis I88.9
  with ectopic or molar pregnancy O08.0
  acute L04.9
    axilla L04.2
    face L04.0
    head L04.0
    hip L04.3
    limb
      lower L04.3
      upper L04.2
    neck L04.0
    shoulder L04.2
    specified site NEC L04.8
    trunk L04.1
  anthracosis (occupational) J60
  any site, except mesenteric I88.9
    chronic I88.1
    subacute I88.1
  breast
    gestational — *see* Mastitis, obstetric
    puerperal, postpartum (nonpurulent) O91.22
  chancroidal (congenital) A57
  chronic I88.1
    mesenteric I88.0
  due to
    Brugia (malayi) B74.1
      timori B74.2
    chlamydial lymphogranuloma A55
    diphtheria (toxin) A36.89
    lymphogranuloma venereum A55
    Wuchereria bancrofti B74.0
  following ectopic or molar pregnancy O08.0
  gonorrheal A54.89
  infective — *see* Lymphadenitis, acute

Lymphadenitis — *continued*
  mesenteric (acute) (chronic) (nonspecific) (subacute) I88.0
    due to Salmonella typhi A01.09
    tuberculous A18.39
  mycobacterial A31.8
  purulent — *see* Lymphadenitis, acute
  pyogenic — *see* Lymphadenitis, acute
  regional, nonbacterial I88.8
  septic — *see* Lymphadenitis, acute
  subacute, unspecified site I88.1
  suppurative — *see* Lymphadenitis, acute
  syphilitic (early) (secondary) A51.49
    late A52.79
  tuberculous — *see* Tuberculosis, lymph gland
  venereal (chlamydial) A55
Lymphadenoid goiter E06.3
Lymphadenopathy (generalized) R59.1
  angioimmunoblastic, with dysproteinemia (AILD) C86.5
  due to toxoplasmosis (acquired) B58.89
    congenital (acute) (subacute) (chronic) P37.1
  localized R59.0
  syphilitic (early) (secondary) A51.49
Lymphadenosis R59.1
Lymphangiectasis I89.0
  conjunctiva H11.89
  postinfectional I89.0
  scrotum I89.0
Lymphangiectatic elephantiasis, nonfilarial I89.0
Lymphangioendothelioma D18.1
  malignant — *see* Neoplasm, connective tissue, malignant
Lymphangioleiomyomatosis J84.81
Lymphangioma D18.1
  capillary D18.1
  cavernous D18.1
  cystic D18.1
  malignant — *see* Neoplasm, connective tissue, malignant
Lymphangiomyoma D18.1
Lymphangiomyomatosis J84.81
Lymphangiosarcoma — *see* Neoplasm, connective tissue, malignant
Lymphangitis I89.1
  with
    abscess — *code by* site under Abscess
    cellulitis — *code by* site under Cellulitis
    ectopic or molar pregnancy O08.0
  acute L03.91
    abdominal wall L03.321
    ankle — *see* Lymphangitis, acute, lower limb
    arm — *see* Lymphangitis, acute, upper limb
    auricle (ear) — *see* Lymphangitis, acute, ear
    axilla L03.12- ☑
    back (any part) L03.322
    buttock L03.327
    cervical (meaning neck) L03.222
    cheek (external) L03.212
    chest wall L03.323
    digit
      finger — *see* Lymphangitis, acute, finger
      toe — *see* Lymphangitis, acute, toe
    ear (external) H60.1- ☑
    external auditory canal — *see* Lymphangitis, acute, ear
    eyelid — *see* Abscess, eyelid
    face NEC L03.212
    finger (intrathecal) (periosteal) (subcutaneous) (subcuticular) L03.02- ☑
    foot — *see* Lymphangitis, acute, lower limb
    gluteal (region) L03.327
    groin L03.324
    hand — *see* Lymphangitis, acute, upper limb
    head NEC L03.891
      face (any part, except ear, eye and nose) L03.212
    heel — *see* Lymphangitis, acute, lower limb
    hip — *see* Lymphangitis, acute, lower limb
    jaw (region) L03.212
    knee — *see* Lymphangitis, acute, lower limb
    leg — *see* Lymphangitis, acute, lower limb
    lower limb L03.12- ☑
      toe — *see* Lymphangitis, acute, toe
    navel L03.326
    neck (region) L03.222
    orbit, orbital — *see* Cellulitis, orbit

Lymphangitis — continued
  acute — continued
    pectoral (region) LØ3.323
    perineal, perineum LØ3.325
    scalp (any part) LØ3.891
    shoulder — see Lymphangitis, acute, upper limb
    specified site NEC LØ3.898
    thigh — see Lymphangitis, acute, lower limb
    thumb (intrathecal) (periosteal) (subcutaneous) (subcuticular) — see Lymphangitis, acute, finger
    toe (intrathecal) (periosteal) (subcutaneous) (subcuticular) LØ3.Ø4- ☑
    trunk LØ3.329
      abdominal wall LØ3.321
      back (any part) LØ3.322
      buttock LØ3.327
      chest wall LØ3.323
      groin LØ3.324
      perineal, perineum LØ3.325
      umbilicus LØ3.326
    upper limb LØ3.12- ☑
      axilla — see Lymphangitis, acute, axilla
      finger — see Lymphangitis, acute, finger
      thumb — see Lymphangitis, acute, finger
      wrist — see Lymphangitis, acute, upper limb
  breast
    gestational — see Mastitis, obstetric
  chancroidal A57
  chronic (any site) I89.1
  due to
    Brugia (malayi) B74.1
      timori B74.2
    Wuchereria bancrofti B74.Ø
  following ectopic or molar pregnancy OØ8.89
  penis
    acute N48.29
    gonococcal (acute) (chronic) A54.Ø9
  puerperal, postpartum, childbirth O86.89
  strumous, tuberculous A18.2
  subacute (any site) I89.1
  tuberculous — see Tuberculosis, lymph gland
Lymphatic (vessel) — see condition
Lymphatism E32.8
Lymphectasia I89.Ø
Lymphedema (acquired) (see also Elephantiasis)
  congenital Q82.Ø
  hereditary (chronic) (idiopathic) Q82.Ø
  postmastectomy I97.2
  praecox I89.Ø
  secondary I89.Ø
  surgical NEC I97.89
    postmastectomy (syndrome) I97.2
Lymphoblastic — see condition
Lymphoblastoma (diffuse) — see Lymphoma, lymphoblastic (diffuse)
  giant follicular — see Lymphoma, lymphoblastic (diffuse)
  macrofollicular — see Lymphoma, lymphoblastic (diffuse)
Lymphocele I89.8
Lymphocytic
  chorioencephalitis (acute) (serous) A87.2
  choriomeningitis (acute) (serous) A87.2
  meningoencephalitis A87.2
Lymphocytoma, benign cutis L98.8
Lymphocytopenia D72.81Ø
Lymphocytosis (symptomatic) D72.82Ø
  infectious (acute) B33.8
Lymphoepithelioma — see Neoplasm, malignant, by site
Lymphogranuloma (malignant) (see also Lymphoma, Hodgkin)
  chlamydial A55
  inguinale A55
  venereum (any site) (chlamydial) (with stricture of rectum) A55
Lymphogranulomatosis (malignant) (see also Lymphoma, Hodgkin)
  benign (Boeck's sarcoid) (Schaumann's) D86.1
Lymphohistiocytosis, hemophagocytic (familial) D76.1
Lymphoid — see condition
Lymphoma (of) (malignant) C85.9Ø
  adult T-cell (HTLV-1-associated) (acute variant) (chronic variant) (lymphomatoid variant) (smouldering variant) C91.5- ☑

Lymphoma — continued
  anaplastic large cell
    ALK-negative C84.7- ☑
    ALK-positive C84.6- ☑
    CD3Ø-positive C84.6- ☑
    primary cutaneous C86.6
  angioimmunoblastic T-cell C86.5
  B-cell C85.1- ☑
  B-precursor C83.5- ☑
  BALT C88.4
  blastic NK-cell C86.4
  bronchial-associated lymphoid tissue [BALT-lymphoma] C88.4
  Burkitt (atypical) C83.7- ☑
  Burkitt-like C83.7- ☑
  centrocytic C83.1- ☑
  cutaneous follicle center C82.6- ☑
  cutaneous T-cell C84.A- ☑ (following C84.7)
  diffuse follicle center C82.5- ☑
  diffuse large cell C83.3- ☑
    anaplastic C83.3- ☑
    B-cell C83.3- ☑
    CD3Ø-positive C83.3- ☑
    centroblastic C83.3- ☑
    immunoblastic C83.3- ☑
    plasmablastic C83.3- ☑
    subtype not specified C83.3- ☑
    T-cell rich C83.3- ☑
  enteropathy-type (associated) (intestinal) T-cell C86.2
  extranodal marginal zone B-cell lymphoma of mucosa-associated lymphoid tissue [MALT-lymphoma] C88.4
  extranodal NK/T-cell, nasal type C86.Ø
  follicular C82.9- ☑
    grade
      I C82.Ø- ☑
      II C82.1- ☑
      III C82.2- ☑
      IIIa C82.3- ☑
      IIIb C82.4- ☑
    specified NEC C82.8- ☑
  hepatosplenic T-cell (alpha-beta) (gamma-delta) C86.1
  histiocytic C85.9- ☑
    true C96.A (following C96.6)
  Hodgkin C81.9 ☑
    classical C81.7- ☑
      lymphocyte depleted C81.3- ☑
      lymphocyte-rich C81.4- ☑
      mixed cellularity C81.2- ☑
      nodular sclerosis C81.1- ☑
      specified NEC C81.7- ☑
    lymphocyte depleted classical C81.3- ☑
    lymphocyte-rich classical C81.4- ☑
    mixed cellularity classical C81.2- ☑
    nodular
      lymphocyte predominant C81.Ø- ☑
      sclerosis classical C81.1- ☑
  intravascular large B-cell C83.8- ☑
  Lennert's C84.4- ☑
  lymphoblastic (diffuse) C83.5- ☑
  lymphoblastic B-cell C83.5- ☑
  lymphoblastic T-cell C83.5- ☑
  lymphoepithelioid C84.4- ☑
  lymphoplasmacytic C83.Ø- ☑
    with IgM-production C88.Ø
  MALT C88.4
  mantle cell C83.1- ☑
  mature T-cell NEC C84.4- ☑
  mature T/NK-cell C84.4- ☑
    specified NEC C84.Z- ☑ (following C84.7)
  mediastinal (thymic) large B-cell C85.2- ☑
  Mediterranean C88.3
  mucosa-associated lymphoid tissue [MALT-lymphoma] C88.4
  NK/T cell C84.9- ☑
  nodal marginal zone C83.Ø- ☑
  non-follicular (diffuse) C83.9- ☑
    specified NEC C83.8- ☑
  non-Hodgkin (see also Lymphoma, by type) C85.9- ☑
    specified NEC C85.8- ☑
  non-leukemic variant of B-CLL C83.Ø- ☑
  peripheral T-cell, not classified C84.4- ☑
  primary cutaneous
    anaplastic large cell C86.6
    CD3Ø-positive large T-cell C86.6
  primary effusion B-cell C83.8- ☑

Lymphoma — continued
  SALT C88.4
  skin-associated lymphoid tissue [SALT-lymphoma] C88.4
  small cell B-cell C83.Ø- ☑
  splenic marginal zone C83.Ø- ☑
  subcutaneous panniculitis-like T-cell C86.3
  T-precursor C83.5- ☑
  true histiocytic C96.A (following C96.6)
Lymphomatosis — see Lymphoma
Lymphopathia venereum, veneris A55
Lymphopenia D72.81Ø
Lymphoplasmacytic leukemia — see Leukemia, chronic lymphocytic, B-cell type
Lymphoproliferation, X-linked disease D82.3
Lymphoreticulosis, benign (of inoculation) A28.1
Lymphorrhea I89.8
Lymphosarcoma (diffuse) (see also Lymphoma) C85.9- ☑
Lymphostasis I89.8
Lypemania — see Melancholia
Lysine and hydroxylysine metabolism disorder E72.3
Lyssa — see Rabies

M

Macacus ear Q17.3
Maceration, wet feet, tropical (syndrome) T69.Ø2- ☑
MacLeod's syndrome J43.Ø
Macrocephalia, macrocephaly Q75.3
Macrocheilia, macrochilia (congenital) Q18.6
Macrocolon (see also Megacolon) Q43.1
Macrocornea Q15.8
  with glaucoma Q15.Ø
Macrocytic — see condition
Macrocytosis D75.89
Macrodactylia, macrodactylism (fingers) (thumbs) Q74.Ø
  toes Q74.2
Macrodontia KØØ.2
Macrogenia M26.Ø5
Macrogenitosomia (adrenal) (male) (praecox) E25.9
  congenital E25.Ø
Macroglobulinemia (idiopathic) (primary) C88.Ø
  monoclonal (essential) D47.2
  Waldenström C88.Ø
Macroglossia (congenital) Q38.2
  acquired K14.8
Macrognathia, macrognathism (congenital) (mandibular) (maxillary) M26.Ø9
Macrogyria (congenital) QØ4.8
Macrohydrocephalus — see Hydrocephalus
Macromastia — see Hypertrophy, breast
Macrophthalmos Q11.3
  in congenital glaucoma Q15.Ø
Macropsia H53.15
Macrosigmoid K59.3
  congenital Q43.2
Macrospondylitis , acromegalic E22.Ø
Macrostomia (congenital) Q18.4
Macrotia (external ear) (congenital) Q17.1
Macula
  cornea, corneal — see Opacity, cornea
  degeneration (atrophic) (exudative) (senile) (see also Degeneration, macula)
    hereditary — see Dystrophy, retina
Maculae ceruleae B85.1
Maculopathy, toxic — see Degeneration, macula, toxic
Madarosis (eyelid) HØ2.729
  left HØ2.726
    lower HØ2.725
    upper HØ2.724
  right HØ2.723
    lower HØ2.722
    upper HØ2.721
Madelung's
  deformity (radius) Q74.Ø
  disease
    radial deformity Q74.Ø
    symmetrical lipomas, neck E88.89
Madness — see Psychosis
Madura
  foot B47.9
    actinomycotic B47.1
    mycotic B47.Ø
Maduromycosis B47.Ø
Maffucci's syndrome Q78.4

Magnesium metabolism disorder — *see* Disorder, metabolism, magnesium
Main en griffe (acquired) (*see also* Deformity, limb, clawhand)
  congenital Q74.0
Maintenance (encounter for)
  antineoplastic chemotherapy Z51.11
  antineoplastic radiation therapy Z51.0
  methadone F11.20
Majocchi's
  disease L81.7
  granuloma B35.8
Major — *see* condition
Mal de los pintos — *see* Pinta
Mal de mer T75.3 ☑
Malabar itch (any site) B35.5
Malabsorption K90.9
  calcium K90.89
  carbohydrate K90.4
  disaccharide E73.9
  fat K90.4
  galactose E74.20
  glucose (-galactose) E74.39
  intestinal K90.9
    specified NEC K90.89
  isomaltose E74.31
  lactose E73.9
  methionine E72.19
  monosaccharide E74.39
  postgastrectomy K91.2
  postsurgical K91.2
  protein K90.4
  starch K90.4
  sucrose E74.39
  syndrome K90.9
    postsurgical K91.2
Malacia, bone (adult) M83.9
  juvenile — *see* Rickets
Malacoplakia
  bladder N32.89
  pelvis (kidney) N28.89
  ureter N28.89
  urethra N36.8
Malacosteon, juvenile — *see* Rickets
Maladaptation — *see* Maladjustment
Maladie de Roger Q21.0
Maladjustment
  conjugal Z63.0
    involving divorce or estrangement Z63.5
  educational Z55.4
  family Z63.9
  marital Z63.0
    involving divorce or estrangement Z63.5
  occupational NEC Z56.89
  simple, adult — *see* Disorder, adjustment
  situational — *see* Disorder, adjustment
  social Z60.9
    due to
      acculturation difficulty Z60.3
      discrimination and persecution (perceived) Z60.5
      exclusion and isolation Z60.4
      life-cycle (phase of life) transition Z60.0
      rejection Z60.4
      specified reason NEC Z60.8
Malaise R53.81
Malakoplakia — *see* Malacoplakia
Malaria, malarial (fever) B54
  with
    blackwater fever B50.8
      hemoglobinuric (bilious) B50.8
    hemoglobinuria B50.8
  accidentally induced (therapeutically) — *code by* type under Malaria
  algid B50.9
  cerebral B50.0 [G94]
  clinically diagnosed (without parasitological confirmation) B54
  congenital NEC P37.4
    falciparum P37.3
  congestion, congestive B54
  continued (fever) B50.9
  estivo-autumnal B50.9
  falciparum B50.9
    with complications NEC B50.8
      cerebral B50.0 [G94]
    severe B50.8
  hemorrhagic B54

Malaria, malarial — *continued*
  malariae B52.9
    with
      complications NEC B52.8
      glomerular disorder B52.0
  malignant (tertian) — *see* Malaria, falciparum
  mixed infections — *code to* first listed type in B50-B53
  ovale B53.0
  parasitologically confirmed NEC B53.8
  pernicious, acute — *see* Malaria, falciparum
  Plasmodium (P.)
    falciparum NEC — *see* Malaria, falciparum
    malariae NEC B52.9
      with Plasmodium
        falciparum (and or vivax) — *see* Malaria, falciparum
        vivax (*see also* Malaria, vivax)
          and falciparum — *see* Malaria, falciparum
    ovale B53.0
      with Plasmodium malariae (*see also* Malaria, malariae)
        and vivax (*see also* Malaria, vivax)
          and falciparum — *see* Malaria, falciparum
    simian B53.1
      with Plasmodium malariae (*see also* Malaria, malariae)
        and vivax (*see also* Malaria, vivax)
          and falciparum — *see* Malaria, falciparum
    vivax NEC B51.9
      with Plasmodium falciparum — *see* Malaria, falciparum
  quartan — *see* Malaria, malariae
  quotidian — *see* Malaria, falciparum
  recurrent B54
  remittent B54
  specified type NEC (parasitologically confirmed) B53.8
  spleen B54
  subtertian (fever) — *see* Malaria, falciparum
  tertian (benign) (*see also* Malaria, vivax)
    malignant B50.9
  tropical B50.9
  typhoid B54
  vivax B51.9
    with
      complications NEC B51.8
      ruptured spleen B51.0
Malassez's disease (cystic) N50.8
Malassimilation K90.9
Maldescent, testis Q53.9
  bilateral Q53.20
    abdominal Q53.21
    perineal Q53.22
  unilateral Q53.10
    abdominal Q53.11
    perineal Q53.12
Maldevelopment (*see also* Anomaly)
  brain Q07.9
  colon Q43.9
  hip Q74.2
    congenital dislocation Q65.2
      bilateral Q65.1
      unilateral Q65.0- ☑
  mastoid process Q75.8
  middle ear Q16.4
    except ossicles Q16.4
    ossicles Q16.3
  ossicles Q16.3
  spine Q76.49
  toe Q74.2
Male type pelvis Q74.2
  with disproportion (fetopelvic) O33.3 ☑
    causing obstructed labor O65.3
Malformation (congenital) (*see also* Anomaly)
  adrenal gland Q89.1
  affecting multiple systems with skeletal changes NEC Q87.5
  alimentary tract Q45.9
    specified type NEC Q45.8
    upper Q40.9
      specified type NEC Q40.8
  aorta Q25.9
    atresia Q25.2
    coarctation (preductal) (postductal) Q25.1
    patent ductus arteriosus Q25.0
    specified type NEC Q25.4

Malformation — *continued*
  aorta — *continued*
    stenosis (supravalvular) Q25.3
  aortic valve Q23.9
    specified NEC Q23.8
  arteriovenous, aneurysmatic (congenital) Q27.30
    brain Q28.2
    cerebral Q28.2
    peripheral Q27.30
      digestive system Q27.33
      lower limb Q27.32
      other specified site Q27.39
      renal vessel Q27.34
      upper limb Q27.31
    precerebral vessels (nonruptured) Q28.0
  auricle
    ear (congenital) Q17.3
      acquired H61.119
        left H61.112
          with right H61.113
        right H61.111
          with left H61.113
  bile duct Q44.5
  bladder Q64.79
    aplasia Q64.5
    diverticulum Q64.6
    exstrophy — *see* Exstrophy, bladder
    neck obstruction Q64.31
  bone Q79.9
    face Q75.9
      specified type NEC Q75.8
    skull Q75.9
      specified type NEC Q75.8
  brain (multiple) Q04.9
    arteriovenous Q28.2
    specified type NEC Q04.8
  branchial cleft Q18.2
  breast Q83.9
    specified type NEC Q83.8
  broad ligament Q50.6
  bronchus Q32.4
  bursa Q79.9
  cardiac
    chambers Q20.9
      specified type NEC Q20.8
    septum Q21.9
      specified type NEC Q21.8
  cerebral Q04.9
    vessels Q28.3
  cervix uteri Q51.9
    specified type NEC Q51.828
  Chiari
    Type I G93.5
    Type II Q07.01
  choroid (congenital) Q14.3
    plexus Q07.8
  circulatory system Q28.9
  cochlea Q16.5
  cornea Q13.4
  coronary vessels Q24.5
  corpus callosum (congenital) Q04.0
  diaphragm Q79.1
  digestive system NEC, specified type NEC Q45.8
  dura Q07.9
    brain Q04.9
    spinal Q06.9
  ear Q17.9
    causing impairment of hearing Q16.9
    external Q17.9
      accessory auricle Q17.0
      causing impairment of hearing Q16.9
        absence of
          auditory canal Q16.1
          auricle Q16.0
      macrotia Q17.1
      microtia Q17.2
      misplacement Q17.4
      misshapen NEC Q17.3
      prominence Q17.5
      specified type NEC Q17.8
    inner Q16.5
    middle Q16.4
      absence of eustachian tube Q16.2
      ossicles (fusion) Q16.3
    ossicles Q16.3
    specified type NEC Q17.8
  epididymis Q55.4
  esophagus Q39.9

Malformation — *continued*
  esophagus — *continued*
    specified type NEC Q39.8
  eye Q15.9
    lid Q10.3
    specified NEC Q15.8
  fallopian tube Q50.6
  genital organ — *see* Anomaly, genitalia
  great
    artery Q25.9
      aorta — *see* Malformation, aorta
      pulmonary artery — *see* Malformation, pulmonary, artery
      specified type NEC Q25.8
    vein Q26.9
      anomalous
        portal venous connection Q26.5
        pulmonary venous connection Q26.4
          partial Q26.3
          total Q26.2
        persistent left superior vena cava Q26.1
        portal vein-hepatic artery fistula Q26.6
        specified type NEC Q26.8
        vena cava stenosis, congenital Q26.0
  gum Q38.6
  hair Q84.2
  heart Q24.9
    specified type NEC Q24.8
  integument Q84.9
    specified type NEC Q84.8
  internal ear Q16.5
  intestine Q43.9
    specified type NEC Q43.8
  iris Q13.2
  joint Q74.9
    ankle Q74.2
    lumbosacral Q76.49
    sacroiliac Q74.2
    specified type NEC Q74.8
  kidney Q63.9
    accessory Q63.0
    giant Q63.3
    horseshoe Q63.1
    hydronephrosis Q62.0
    malposition Q63.2
    specified type NEC Q63.8
  lacrimal apparatus Q10.6
  lingual Q38.3
  lip Q38.0
  liver Q44.7
  lung Q33.9
  meninges or membrane (congenital) Q07.9
    cerebral Q04.8
    spinal (cord) Q06.9
  middle ear Q16.4
    ossicles Q16.3
  mitral valve Q23.9
    specified NEC Q23.8
  Mondini's (congenital) (malformation, cochlea) Q16.5
  mouth (congenital) Q38.6
  multiple types NEC Q89.7
  musculoskeletal system Q79.9
  myocardium Q24.8
  nail Q84.6
  nervous system (central) Q07.9
  nose Q30.9
    specified type NEC Q30.8
  optic disc Q14.2
  orbit Q10.7
  ovary Q50.39
  palate Q38.5
  parathyroid gland Q89.2
  pelvic organs or tissues NEC
    in pregnancy or childbirth O34.8- ☑
      causing obstructed labor O65.5
  penis Q55.69
    aplasia Q55.5
    curvature (lateral) Q55.61
    hypoplasia Q55.62
  pericardium Q24.8
  peripheral vascular system Q27.9
    specified type NEC Q27.8
  pharynx Q38.8
  precerebral vessels Q28.1
  prostate Q55.4
  pulmonary
    arteriovenous Q25.72
    artery Q25.9

Malformation — *continued*
  pulmonary — *continued*
    artery — *continued*
      atresia Q25.5
      specified type NEC Q25.79
      stenosis Q25.6
    valve Q22.3
  renal artery Q27.2
  respiratory system Q34.9
  retina Q14.1
  scrotum — *see* Malformation, testis and scrotum
  seminal vesicles Q55.4
  sense organs NEC Q07.9
  skin Q82.9
  specified NEC Q89.8
  spinal
    cord Q06.9
    nerve root Q07.8
  spine Q76.49
    kyphosis — *see* Kyphosis, congenital
    lordosis — *see* Lordosis, congenital
  spleen Q89.09
  stomach Q40.3
    specified type NEC Q40.2
  teeth, tooth K00.9
  tendon Q79.9
  testis and scrotum Q55.20
    aplasia Q55.0
    hypoplasia Q55.1
    polyorchism Q55.21
    retractile testis Q55.22
    scrotal transposition Q55.23
    specified NEC Q55.29
  thorax, bony Q76.9
  throat Q38.8
  thyroid gland Q89.2
  tongue (congenital) Q38.3
    hypertrophy Q38.2
    tie Q38.1
  trachea Q32.1
  tricuspid valve Q22.9
    specified type NEC Q22.8
  umbilical cord NEC (complicating delivery) O69.89 ☑
  umbilicus Q89.9
  ureter Q62.8
    agenesis Q62.4
    duplication Q62.5
    malposition — *see* Malposition, congenital, ureter
    obstructive defect — *see* Defect, obstructive, ureter
    vesico-uretero-renal reflux Q62.7
  urethra Q64.79
    aplasia Q64.5
    duplication Q64.74
    posterior valves Q64.2
    prolapse Q64.71
    stricture Q64.32
  urinary system Q64.9
  uterus Q51.9
    specified type NEC Q51.818
  vagina Q52.4
  vas deferens Q55.4
    atresia Q55.3
  vascular system, peripheral Q27.9
  venous — *see* Anomaly, vein(s)
  vulva Q52.70
Malfunction (*see also* Dysfunction)
  cardiac electronic device T82.119 ☑
    electrode T82.110 ☑
    pulse generator T82.111 ☑
    specified type NEC T82.118 ☑
  catheter device NEC T85.618 ☑
    cystostomy T83.010 ☑
    dialysis (renal) (vascular) T82.41 ☑
      intraperitoneal T85.611 ☑
    infusion NEC T82.514 ☑
      spinal (epidural) (subdural) T85.610 ☑
    urinary, indwelling T83.018 ☑
  colostomy K94.03
    valve K94.03
  cystostomy (stoma) N99.512
    catheter T83.010 ☑
  enteric stoma K94.13
  enterostomy K94.13
  esophagostomy K94.33
  gastroenteric K31.89
  gastrostomy K94.23
  ileostomy K94.13
    valve K94.13

Malfunction — *continued*
  jejunostomy K94.13
  pacemaker — *see* Malfunction, cardiac electronic device
  prosthetic device, internal — *see* Complications, prosthetic device, by site, mechanical
  tracheostomy J95.03
  urinary device NEC — *see* Complication, genitourinary, device, urinary, mechanical
  valve
    colostomy K94.03
    heart T82.09 ☑
    ileostomy K94.13
  vascular graft or shunt NEC — *see* Complication, cardiovascular device, mechanical, vascular
  ventricular (communicating shunt) T85.01 ☑
Malherbe's tumor — *see* Neoplasm, skin, benign
Malibu disease L98.8-
Malignancy (*see also* Neoplasm, malignant, by site)
  unspecified site (primary) C80.1
Malignant — *see* condition
Malingerer, malingering Z76.5
Mallet finger (acquired) — *see* Deformity, finger, mallet finger
  congenital Q74.0
  sequelae of rickets E64.3
Malleus A24.0
Mallory-Weiss syndrome K22.6
Mallory's bodies R89.7
Malnutrition E46
  degree
    first E44.1
    mild (protein) E44.1
    moderate (protein) E44.0
    second E44.0
    severe (protein-energy) E43
      intermediate form E42
        with
          kwashiorkor (and marasmus) E42
          marasmus E41
    third E43
  following gastrointestinal surgery K91.2
  intrauterine
    light-for-dates — *see* Light for dates
    small-for-dates — *see* Small for dates
  lack of care, or neglect (child) (infant) T76.02 ☑
    confirmed T74.02 ☑
  malignant E40
  protein E46
    calorie E46
      mild E44.1
      moderate E44.0
      severe E43
        intermediate form E42
          with
            kwashiorkor (and marasmus) E42
            marasmus E41
    energy E46
      mild E44.1
      moderate E44.0
      severe E43
        intermediate form E42
          with
            kwashiorkor (and marasmus) E42
            marasmus E41
  severe (protein-energy) E43
    with
      kwashiorkor (and marasmus) E42
      marasmus E41
Malocclusion (teeth) M26.4
  Angle's M26.219
    class I M26.211
    class II M26.212
    class III M26.213
  due to
    abnormal swallowing M26.59
    mouth breathing M26.59
    tongue, lip or finger habits M26.59
  temporomandibular (joint) M26.69
Malposition
  cervix — *see* Malposition, uterus
  congenital
    adrenal (gland) Q89.1
    alimentary tract Q45.8
      lower Q43.89
      upper Q40.8
    aorta Q25.4
    appendix Q43.8

☑ **Additional Character Required** — Refer to the Tabular List for Character Selection   ▽ Subterms under main terms may continue to next column or page

Malposition — continued
  congenital — continued
    arterial trunk Q20.0
    artery (peripheral) Q27.8
      coronary Q24.5
      digestive system Q27.8
      lower limb Q27.8
      pulmonary Q25.79
      specified site NEC Q27.8
      upper limb Q27.8
    auditory canal Q17.8
      causing impairment of hearing Q16.9
    auricle (ear) Q17.4
      causing impairment of hearing Q16.9
      cervical Q18.2
    biliary duct or passage Q44.5
    bladder (mucosa) — see Exstrophy, bladder
    brachial plexus Q07.8
    brain tissue Q04.8
    breast Q83.8
    bronchus Q32.4
    cecum Q43.8
    clavicle Q74.0
    colon Q43.8
    digestive organ or tract NEC Q45.8
      lower Q43.8
      upper Q40.8
    ear (auricle) (external) Q17.4
      ossicles Q16.3
    endocrine (gland) NEC Q89.2
    epiglottis Q31.8
    eustachian tube Q17.8
    eye Q15.8
    facial features Q18.8
    fallopian tube Q50.6
    finger(s) Q68.1
      supernumerary Q69.0
    foot Q66.9
    gallbladder Q44.1
    gastrointestinal tract Q45.8
    genitalia, genital organ(s) or tract
      female Q52.8
        external Q52.79
        internal NEC Q52.8
      male Q55.8
    glottis Q31.8
    hand Q68.1
    heart Q24.8
      dextrocardia Q24.0
        with complete transposition of viscera Q89.3
    hepatic duct Q44.5
    hip (joint) Q65.89
    intestine (large) (small) Q43.8
      with anomalous adhesions, fixation or malrotation Q43.3
    joint NEC Q68.8
    kidney Q63.2
    larynx Q31.8
    limb Q68.8
      lower Q68.8
      upper Q68.8
    liver Q44.7
    lung (lobe) Q33.8
    nail(s) Q84.6
    nerve Q07.8
    nervous system NEC Q07.8
    nose, nasal (septum) Q30.8
    organ or site not listed — see Anomaly, by site
    ovary Q50.39
    pancreas Q45.3
    parathyroid (gland) Q89.2
    patella Q74.1
    peripheral vascular system Q27.8
    pituitary (gland) Q89.2
    respiratory organ or system NEC Q34.8
    rib (cage) Q76.6
      supernumerary in cervical region Q76.5
    scapula Q74.0
    shoulder Q74.0
    spinal cord Q06.8
    spleen Q89.09
    sternum NEC Q76.7
    stomach Q40.2
    symphysis pubis Q74.2
    thymus (gland) Q89.2
    thyroid (gland) (tissue) Q89.2
      cartilage Q31.8
    toe(s) Q66.9

Malposition — continued
  congenital — continued
    toe(s) — continued
      supernumerary Q69.2
    tongue Q38.3
    trachea Q32.1
    ureter Q62.60
      deviation Q62.61
      displacement Q62.62
      ectopia Q62.63
      specified type NEC Q62.69
    uterus Q51.818
    vein(s) (peripheral) Q27.8
      great Q26.8
    vena cava (inferior) (superior) Q26.8
  device, implant or graft (see also Complications, by site and type, mechanical) T85.628 ☑
    arterial graft NEC — see Complication, cardiovascular device, mechanical, vascular
    breast (implant) T85.42 ☑
    catheter NEC T85.628 ☑
      cystostomy T83.020 ☑
      dialysis (renal) T82.42 ☑
        intraperitoneal T85.621 ☑
      infusion NEC T82.524 ☑
        spinal (epidural) (subdural) T85.620 ☑
      urinary, indwelling T83.028 ☑
    electronic (electrode) (pulse generator) (stimulator)
      bone T84.320 ☑
      cardiac T82.129 ☑
        electrode T82.120 ☑
        pulse generator T82.121 ☑
        specified type NEC T82.128 ☑
      nervous system — see Complication, prosthetic device, mechanical, electronic nervous system stimulator
      urinary — see Complication, genitourinary, device, urinary, mechanical
    fixation, internal (orthopedic) NEC — see Complication, fixation device, mechanical
    gastrointestinal — see Complications, prosthetic device, mechanical, gastrointestinal device
    genital NEC T83.428 ☑
      intrauterine contraceptive device T83.32 ☑
      penile prosthesis T83.420 ☑
    heart NEC — see Complication, cardiovascular device, mechanical
    joint prosthesis — see Complication, joint prosthesis, mechanical
    ocular NEC — see Complications, prosthetic device, mechanical, ocular device
    orthopedic NEC — see Complication, orthopedic, device, mechanical
    specified NEC T85.628 ☑
    urinary NEC (see also Complication, genitourinary, device, urinary, mechanical)
      graft T83.22 ☑
    vascular NEC — see Complication, cardiovascular device, mechanical
    ventricular intracranial shunt T85.02 ☑
  fetus — see Pregnancy, complicated by (management affected by), presentation, fetal
  gallbladder K82.8
  gastrointestinal tract, congenital Q45.8
  heart, congenital NEC Q24.8
  joint prosthesis — see Complications, joint prosthesis, mechanical, displacement, by site
  stomach K31.89
    congenital Q40.2
  tooth, teeth, fully erupted M26.30
  uterus (acute) (acquired) (adherent) (asymptomatic) (postinfectional) (postpartal, old) N85.4
    anteflexion or anteversion N85.4
    congenital Q51.818
    flexion N85.4
      lateral — see Lateroversion, uterus
    inversion N85.5
    lateral (flexion) (version) — see Lateroversion, uterus
      in pregnancy or childbirth — see subcategory O34.5 ☑
    retroflexion or retroversion — see Retroversion, uterus
Malposture R29.3
Malrotation
  cecum Q43.3
  colon Q43.3

Malrotation — continued
  intestine Q43.3
  kidney Q63.2
Malta fever — see Brucellosis
Maltreatment
  adult
    abandonment
      confirmed T74.01 ☑
      suspected T76.01 ☑
    confirmed T74.91 ☑
    history of Z91.419
    neglect
      confirmed T74.01 ☑
      suspected T76.01 ☑
    physical abuse
      confirmed T74.11 ☑
      suspected T76.11 ☑
    psychological abuse
      confirmed T74.31 ☑
      history of Z91.411
      suspected T76.31 ☑
    sexual abuse
      confirmed T74.21 ☑
      suspected T76.21 ☑
    suspected T76.91 ☑
  child
    abandonment
      confirmed T74.02 ☑
      suspected T76.02 ☑
    confirmed T74.92 ☑
    history of — see History, personal (of), abuse
    neglect
      confirmed T74.02 ☑
      history of — see History, personal (of), abuse
      suspected T76.02 ☑
    physical abuse
      confirmed T74.12 ☑
      history of — see History, personal (of), abuse
      suspected T76.12 ☑
    psychological abuse
      confirmed T74.32 ☑
      history of — see History, personal (of), abuse
      suspected T76.32 ☑
    sexual abuse
      confirmed T74.22 ☑
      history of — see History, personal (of), abuse
      suspected T76.22 ☑
    suspected T76.92 ☑
  personal history of Z91.89
Maltworker's lung J67.4
Malunion, fracture — see Fracture, by site
Mammillitis N61
  puerperal, postpartum O91.02
Mammitis — see Mastitis
Mammogram (examination) Z12.39
  routine Z12.31
Mammoplasia N62
Management (of)
  bone conduction hearing device (implanted) Z45.320
  cardiac pacemaker NEC Z45.018
  cerebrospinal fluid drainage device Z45.41
  cochlear device (implanted) Z45.321
  contraceptive Z30.9
    specified NEC Z30.8
  implanted device Z45.9
    specified NEC Z45.89
  infusion pump Z45.1
  procreative Z31.9
    male factor infertility in female Z31.81
    specified NEC Z31.89
  prosthesis (external) (see also Fitting) Z44.9
    implanted Z45.9
      specified NEC Z45.89
  renal dialysis catheter Z49.01
  vascular access device Z45.2
Mangled — see specified injury by site
Mania (monopolar) (see also Disorder, mood, manic episode)
  with psychotic symptoms F30.2
  without psychotic symptoms F30.10
    mild F30.11
    moderate F30.12
    severe F30.13
  Bell's F30.8
  chronic (recurrent) F31.89
  hysterical F44.89
  puerperal F30.8

Mania — *continued*
 recurrent F31.89
Manic-depressive insanity, psychosis, or syndrome — *see* Disorder, bipolar
Mannosidosis E77.1
Mansonelliasis, mansonellosis B74.4
Manson's
 disease B65.1
 schistosomiasis B65.1
Manual — *see* condition
Maple-bark-stripper's lung (disease) J67.6
Maple-syrup-urine disease E71.0
Marable's syndrome (celiac artery compression) I77.4
Marasmus E41
 due to malnutrition E41
 intestinal E41
 nutritional E41
 senile R54
 tuberculous NEC — *see* Tuberculosis
Marble
 bones Q78.2
 skin R23.8
Marburg virus disease A98.3
March
 fracture — *see* Fracture, traumatic, stress, by site
 hemoglobinuria D59.6
Marchesani (-Weill) **syndrome** Q87.0
Marchiafava (-Bignami) **syndrome or disease** G37.1
Marchiafava-Micheli syndrome D59.5
Marcus Gunn's syndrome Q07.8
Marfan's syndrome — *see* Syndrome, Marfan's
Marie-Bamberger disease — *see* Osteoarthropathy, hypertrophic, specified NEC
Marie-Charcot-Tooth neuropathic muscular atrophy G60.0
Marie-Strümpell arthritis, disease or spondylitis — *see* Spondylitis, ankylosing
Marie's
 cerebellar ataxia (late-onset) G11.2
 disease or syndrome (acromegaly) E22.0
Marion's disease (bladder neck obstruction) N32.0
Marital conflict Z63.0
Mark
 port wine Q82.5
 raspberry Q82.5
 strawberry Q82.5
 stretch L90.6
 tattoo L81.8
Marker heterochromatin — *see* Extra, marker chromosomes
Maroteaux-Lamy syndrome (mild) (severe) E76.29
Marrow (bone)
 arrest D61.9
 poor function D75.89
Marseilles fever A77.1
Marsh fever — *see* Malaria
Marshall's (hidrotic) **ectodermal dysplasia** Q82.4
Marsh's disease (exophthalmic goiter) E05.00
 with storm E05.01
Masculinization (female) **with adrenal hyperplasia** E25.9
 congenital E25.0
Masculinovoblastoma D27.- ☑
Masochism (sexual) F65.51
Mason's lung J62.8
Mass
 abdominal R19.00
  epigastric R19.06
  generalized R19.07
  left lower quadrant R19.04
  left upper quadrant R19.02
  periumbilic R19.05
  right lower quadrant R19.03
  right upper quadrant R19.01
  specified site NEC R19.09
 breast N63
 chest R22.2
 cystic — *see* Cyst
 ear H93.8- ☑
 head R22.0
 intra-abdominal (diffuse) (generalized) — *see* Mass, abdominal
 kidney N28.89
 liver R16.0
 localized (skin) R22.9
  chest R22.2
  head R22.0

Mass — *continued*
 localized — *continued*
  limb
   lower R22.4- ☑
   upper R22.3- ☑
  neck R22.1
  trunk R22.2
 lung R91.8
 malignant — *see* Neoplasm, malignant, by site
 neck R22.1
 pelvic (diffuse) (generalized) — *see* Mass, abdominal
 specified organ NEC — *see* Disease, by site
 splenic R16.1
 substernal thyroid — *see* Goiter
 superficial (localized) R22.9
 umbilical (diffuse) (generalized) R19.09
Massive — *see* condition
Mast cell
 disease, systemic tissue D47.0
 leukemia C94.3- ☑
 sarcoma C96.2
 tumor D47.0
  malignant C96.2
Mastalgia N64.4
Masters-Allen syndrome N83.8
Mastitis (acute) (diffuse) (nonpuerperal) (subacute) N61
 chronic (cystic) — *see* Mastopathy, cystic
 cystic (Schimmelbusch's type) — *see* Mastopathy, cystic
 fibrocystic — *see* Mastopathy, cystic
 infective N61
  newborn P39.0
 interstitial, gestational or puerperal — *see* Mastitis, obstetric
 neonatal (noninfective) P83.4
  infective P39.0
 obstetric (interstitial) (nonpurulent)
  associated with
   lactation O91.23
   pregnancy O91.21- ☑
   puerperium O91.22
  purulent
   associated with
    lactation O91.13
    pregnancy O91.11- ☑
    puerperium O91.12
 periductal — *see* Ectasia, mammary duct
 phlegmonous — *see* Mastopathy, cystic
 plasma cell — *see* Ectasia, mammary duct
Mastocytoma D47.0
 malignant C96.2
Mastocytosis Q82.2
 aggressive systemic C96.2
 indolent systemic D47.0
 malignant C96.2
 systemic, associated with clonal hematopoetic non-mast-cell disease (SM-AHNMD) D47.0
Mastodynia N64.4
Mastoid — *see* condition
Mastoidalgia — *see* subcategory H92.0 ☑
Mastoiditis (coalescent) (hemorrhagic) (suppurative) H70.9- ☑
 acute, subacute H70.00- ☑
  complicated NEC H70.09- ☑
  subperiosteal H70.01- ☑
 chronic (necrotic) (recurrent) H70.1- ☑
 in (due to)
  infectious disease NEC B99 ☑ [H75.0-] ☑
  parasitic disease NEC B89 [H75.0-] ☑
  tuberculosis A18.03
 petrositis — *see* Petrositis
 postauricular fistula — *see* Fistula, postauricular
 specified NEC H70.89- ☑
 tuberculous A18.03
Mastopathy, mastopathia N64.9
 chronica cystica — *see* Mastopathy, cystic
 cystic (chronic) (diffuse) N60.1- ☑
  with epithelial proliferation N60.3- ☑
 diffuse cystic — *see* Mastopathy, cystic
 estrogenic, oestrogenica N64.89
 ovarian origin N64.89
Mastoplasia, mastoplastia N62
Masturbation (excessive) F98.8
Maternal care (for) — *see* Pregnancy (complicated by) (management affected by)
Matheiu's disease (leptospiral jaundice) A27.0

Mauclaire's disease or osteochondrosis — *see* Osteochondrosis, juvenile, hand, metacarpal
Maxcy's disease A75.2
Maxilla, maxillary — *see* condition
May (-Hegglin) **anomaly or syndrome** D72.0
McArdle (-Schmid)(-Pearson) **disease** (glycogen storage) E74.04
McCune-Albright syndrome Q78.1
McQuarrie's syndrome (idiopathic familial hypoglycemia) E16.2
Meadow's syndrome Q86.1
Measles (black) (hemorrhagic) (suppressed) B05.9
 with
  complications NEC B05.89
  encephalitis B05.0
  intestinal complications B05.4
  keratitis (keratoconjunctivitis) B05.81
  meningitis B05.1
  otitis media B05.3
  pneumonia B05.2
 French — *see* Rubella
 German — *see* Rubella
 Liberty — *see* Rubella
Meat-wrappers' asthma J68.9
Meatitis, urethral — *see* Urethritis
Meatus, meatal — *see* condition
Meckel-Gruber syndrome Q61.9
Meckel's diverticulitis, diverticulum (displaced) (hypertrophic) Q43.0
 malignant — *see* Table of Neoplasms, small intestine, malignant
Meconium
 ileus, newborn P76.0
  in cystic fibrosis E84.11
  meaning meconium plug (without cystic fibrosis) P76.0
 obstruction, newborn P76.0
  due to fecaliths P76.0
  in mucoviscidosis E84.11
 peritonitis P78.0
 plug syndrome (newborn) NEC P76.0
Median (*see also* condition)
 arcuate ligament syndrome I77.4
 bar (prostate) (vesical orifice) — *see* Hyperplasia, prostate
 rhomboid glossitis K14.2
Mediastinal shift R93.8
Mediastinitis (acute) (chronic) J98.5
 syphilitic A52.73
 tuberculous A15.8
Mediastinopericarditis (*see also* Pericarditis)
 acute I30.9
 adhesive I31.0
 chronic I31.8
  rheumatic I09.2
Mediastinum, mediastinal — *see* condition
Medicine poisoning — *see* Table of Drugs and Chemicals, by drug, poisoning
Mediterranean
 fever — *see* Brucellosis
  familial E85.0
  tick A77.1
 kala-azar B55.0
 leishmaniasis B55.0
 tick fever A77.1
Medulla — *see* condition
Medullary cystic kidney Q61.5
Medullated fibers
 optic (nerve) Q14.8
 retina Q14.1
Medulloblastoma
 desmoplastic C71.6
 specified site — *see* Neoplasm, malignant, by site
 unspecified site C71.6
Medulloepithelioma (*see also* Neoplasm, malignant, by site)
 teratoid — *see* Neoplasm, malignant, by site
Medullomyoblastoma
 specified site — *see* Neoplasm, malignant, by site
 unspecified site C71.6
Meekeren-Ehlers-Danlos syndrome Q79.6
Megacolon (acquired) (functional) (not Hirschsprung's disease) (in) K59.3
 Chagas' disease B57.32
 congenital, congenitum (aganglionic) Q43.1
 Hirschsprung's (disease) Q43.1
 toxic NEC K59.3

Megacolon — *continued*
   toxic — *continued*
      due to Clostridium difficile A04.7
Megaesophagus (functional) K22.0
   congenital Q39.5
   in (due to) Chagas' disease B57.31
Megalencephaly Q04.5
Megalerythema (epidemic) B08.3
Megaloappendix Q43.8
Megalocephalus, megalocephaly NEC Q75.3
Megalocornea Q15.8
   with glaucoma Q15.0
Megalocytic anemia D53.1
Megalodactylia (fingers) (thumbs) (congenital) Q74.0
   toes Q74.2
Megaloduodenum Q43.8
Megaloesophagus (functional) K22.0
   congenital Q39.5
Megalogastria (acquired) K31.89
   congenital Q40.2
Megalophthalmos Q11.3
Megalopsia H53.15
Megalosplenia — *see* Splenomegaly
Megaloureter N28.82
   congenital Q62.2
Megarectum K62.89
Megasigmoid K59.3
   congenital Q43.2
Megaureter N28.82
   congenital Q62.2
Megavitamin-B6 syndrome E67.2
Megrim — *see* Migraine
Meibomian
   cyst, infected — *see* Hordeolum
   gland — *see* condition
   sty, stye — *see* Hordeolum
Meibomitis — *see* Hordeolum
Meige-Milroy disease (chronic hereditary edema) Q82.0
Meige's syndrome Q82.0
Melalgia, nutritional E53.8
Melancholia F32.9
   climacteric (single episode) F32.8
      recurrent episode F33.9
   hypochondriac F45.29
   intermittent (single episode) F32.8
      recurrent episode F33.9
   involutional (single episode) F32.8
      recurrent episode F33.9
   menopausal (single episode) F32.8
      recurrent episode F33.9
   puerperal F32.8
   reactive (emotional stress or trauma) F32.3
   recurrent F33.9
   senile F03 ☑
   stuporous (single episode) F32.8
      recurrent episode F33.9
Melanemia R79.89
Melanoameloblastoma — *see* Neoplasm, bone, benign
Melanoblastoma — *see* Melanoma
Melanocarcinoma — *see* Melanoma
Melanocytoma, eyeball D31.4- ☑
Melanocytosis, neurocutaneous Q82.8
Melanoderma, melanodermia L81.4
Melanodontia, infantile K03.89
Melanodontoclasia K03.89
Melanoepithelioma — *see* Melanoma
Melanoma (malignant) C43.9
   acral lentiginous, malignant — *see* Melanoma, skin, by site
   amelanotic — *see* Melanoma, skin, by site
   balloon cell — *see* Melanoma, skin, by site
   benign — *see* Nevus
   desmoplastic, malignant — *see* Melanoma, skin, by site
   epithelioid cell — *see* Melanoma, skin, by site
      with spindle cell, mixed — *see* Melanoma, skin, by site
   in
      giant pigmented nevus — *see* Melanoma, skin, by site
      Hutchinson's melanotic freckle — *see* Melanoma, skin, by site
      junctional nevus — *see* Melanoma, skin, by site
      precancerous melanosis — *see* Melanoma, skin, by site
   in situ D03.9
      abdominal wall D03.59

Melanoma — *continued*
   in situ — *continued*
      ala nasi D03.39
      ankle D03.7- ☑
      anus, anal (margin) (skin) D03.51
      arm D03.6- ☑
      auditory canal D03.2- ☑
      auricle (ear) D03.2- ☑
      auricular canal (external) D03.2- ☑
      axilla, axillary fold D03.59
      back D03.59
      breast D03.52
      brow D03.39
      buttock D03.59
      canthus (eye) D03.1- ☑
      cheek (external) D03.39
      chest wall D03.59
      chin D03.39
      choroid D03.8
      conjunctiva D03.8
      ear (external) D03.2- ☑
      external meatus (ear) D03.2- ☑
      eye D03.8
      eyebrow D03.39
      eyelid (lower) (upper) D03.1- ☑
      face D03.30
         specified NEC D03.39
      female genital organ (external) NEC D03.8
      finger D03.6- ☑
      flank D03.59
      foot D03.7- ☑
      forearm D03.6- ☑
      forehead D03.39
      foreskin D03.8
      gluteal region D03.59
      groin D03.59
      hand D03.6- ☑
      heel D03.7- ☑
      helix D03.2- ☑
      hip D03.7- ☑
      interscapular region D03.59
      iris D03.8
      jaw D03.39
      knee D03.7- ☑
      labium (majus) (minus) D03.8
      lacrimal gland D03.8
      leg D03.7- ☑
      lip (lower) (upper) D03.0
      lower limb NEC D03.7- ☑
      male genital organ (external) NEC D03.8
      nail D03.9
         finger D03.6- ☑
         toe D03.7- ☑
      neck D03.4
      nose (external) D03.39
      orbit D03.8
      penis D03.8
      perianal skin D03.51
      perineum D03.51
      pinna D03.2- ☑
      popliteal fossa or space D03.7- ☑
      prepuce D03.8
      pudendum D03.8
      retina D03.8
      retrobulbar D03.8
      scalp D03.4
      scrotum D03.8
      shoulder D03.6- ☑
      specified site NEC D03.8
      submammary fold D03.52
      temple D03.39
      thigh D03.7- ☑
      toe D03.7- ☑
      trunk NEC D03.59
      umbilicus D03.59
      upper limb NEC D03.6- ☑
      vulva D03.8
   juvenile — *see* Nevus
   malignant, of soft parts except skin — *see* Neoplasm, connective tissue, malignant
   metastatic
      breast C79.81
      genital organ C79.82
      specified site NEC C79.89
   neurotropic, malignant — *see* Melanoma, skin, by site
   nodular — *see* Melanoma, skin, by site
   regressing, malignant — *see* Melanoma, skin, by site

Melanoma — *continued*
   skin C43.9
      abdominal wall C43.59
      ala nasi C43.31
      ankle C43.7- ☑
      anus, anal (skin) C43.51
      arm C43.6- ☑
      auditory canal (external) C43.2- ☑
      auricle (ear) C43.2- ☑
      auricular canal (external) C43.2- ☑
      axilla, axillary fold C43.59
      back C43.59
      breast (female) (male) C43.52
      brow C43.39
      buttock C43.59
      canthus (eye) C43.1- ☑
      cheek (external) C43.39
      chest wall C43.59
      chin C43.39
      ear (external) C43.2- ☑
      elbow C43.6- ☑
      external meatus (ear) C43.2- ☑
      eyebrow C43.39
      eyelid (lower) (upper) C43.1- ☑
      face C43.30
         specified NEC C43.39
      female genital organ (external) NEC C51.9
      finger C43.6- ☑
      flank C43.59
      foot C43.7- ☑
      forearm C43.6- ☑
      forehead C43.39
      foreskin C60.0
      glabella C43.39
      gluteal region C43.59
      groin C43.59
      hand C43.6- ☑
      heel C43.7- ☑
      helix C43.2- ☑
      hip C43.7- ☑
      interscapular region C43.59
      jaw (external) C43.39
      knee C43.7- ☑
      labium C51.9
         majus C51.0
         minus C51.1
      leg C43.7- ☑
      lip (lower) (upper) C43.0
      lower limb NEC C43.7- ☑
      male genital organ (external) NEC C63.9
      nail
         finger C43.6- ☑
         toe C43.7- ☑
      nasolabial groove C43.39
      nates C43.59
      neck C43.4
      nose (external) C43.31
      overlapping site C43.8
      palpebra C43.1- ☑
      penis C60.9
      perianal skin C43.51
      perineum C43.51
      pinna C43.2- ☑
      popliteal fossa or space C43.7- ☑
      prepuce C60.0
      pudendum C51.9
      scalp C43.4
      scrotum C63.2
      shoulder C43.6- ☑
      skin NEC C43.9
      submammary fold C43.52
      temple C43.39
      thigh C43.7- ☑
      toe C43.7- ☑
      trunk NEC C43.59
      umbilicus C43.59
      upper limb NEC C43.6- ☑
      vulva C51.9
         overlapping sites C51.8
   spindle cell
      with epithelioid, mixed — *see* Melanoma, skin, by site
      type A C69.4- ☑
      type B C69.4- ☑
   superficial spreading — *see* Melanoma, skin, by site
Melanosarcoma (*see also* Melanoma)
   epithelioid cell — *see* Melanoma

Melanosis L81.4
  addisonian E27.1
    tuberculous A18.7
  adrenal E27.1
  colon K63.89
  conjunctiva — *see* Pigmentation, conjunctiva
    congenital Q13.89
  cornea (presenile) (senile) (*see also* Pigmentation, cornea)
    congenital Q13.4
  eye NEC H57.8
    congenital Q15.8
  lenticularis progressiva Q82.1
  liver K76.89
  precancerous (*see also* Melanoma, in situ)
    malignant melanoma in — *see* Melanoma
  Riehl's L81.4
  sclera H15.89
    congenital Q13.89
  suprarenal E27.1
  tar L81.4
  toxic L81.4
Melanuria R82.99
MELAS syndrome E88.41
Melasma L81.1
  adrenal (gland) E27.1
  suprarenal (gland) E27.1
Melena K92.1
  with ulcer — *code by* site under Ulcer, with hemorrhage K27.4
  due to swallowed maternal blood P78.2
  newborn, neonatal P54.1
    due to swallowed maternal blood P78.2
Meleney's
  gangrene (cutaneous) — *see* Ulcer, skin
  ulcer (chronic undermining) — *see* Ulcer, skin
Melioidosis A24.9
  acute A24.1
  chronic A24.2
  fulminating A24.1
  pneumonia A24.1
  pulmonary (chronic) A24.2
    acute A24.1
    subacute A24.2
  sepsis A24.1
  specified NEC A24.3
  subacute A24.2
Melitensis, febris A23.0
Melkersson (-Rosenthal) **syndrome** G51.2
Mellitus, diabetes — *see* Diabetes
Melorheostosis (bone) — *see* Disorder, bone, density and structure, specified NEC
Meloschisis Q18.4
Melotia Q17.4
Membrana
  capsularis lentis posterior Q13.89
  epipapillaris Q14.2
Membranacea placenta O43.19- ☑
Membranaceous uterus N85.8
Membrane(s), membranous (*see also* condition)
  cyclitic — *see* Membrane, pupillary
  folds, congenital — *see* Web
  Jackson's Q43.3
  over face of newborn P28.9
  premature rupture — *see* Rupture, membranes, premature
  pupillary H21.4- ☑
    persistent Q13.89
  retained (with hemorrhage) (complicating delivery) O72.2
    without hemorrhage O73.1
  secondary cataract — *see* Cataract, secondary
  unruptured (causing asphyxia) — *see* Asphyxia, newborn
  vitreous — *see* Opacity, vitreous, membranes and strands
Membranitis — *see* Chorioamnionitis
Memory disturbance, lack or loss (*see also* Amnesia)
  mild, following organic brain damage F06.8
Menadione deficiency E56.1
Menarche
  delayed E30.0
  precocious E30.1
Mendacity, pathologic F60.2
Mendelson's syndrome (due to anesthesia) J95.4
  in labor and delivery O74.0
  in pregnancy O29.01- ☑

Mendelson's syndrome — *continued*
  obstetric O74.0
  postpartum, puerperal O89.01
Ménétrier's disease or syndrome K29.60
  with bleeding K29.61
Ménière's disease, syndrome or vertigo H81.0- ☑
Meninges, meningeal — *see* condition
Meningioma (*see also* Neoplasm, meninges, benign)
  angioblastic — *see* Neoplasm, meninges, benign
  angiomatous — *see* Neoplasm, meninges, benign
  endotheliomatous — *see* Neoplasm, meninges, benign
  fibroblastic — *see* Neoplasm, meninges, benign
  fibrous — *see* Neoplasm, meninges, benign
  hemangioblastic — *see* Neoplasm, meninges, benign
  hemangiopericytic — *see* Neoplasm, meninges, benign
  malignant — *see* Neoplasm, meninges, malignant
  meningiothelial — *see* Neoplasm, meninges, benign
  meningotheliomatous — *see* Neoplasm, meninges, benign
  mixed — *see* Neoplasm, meninges, benign
  multiple — *see* Neoplasm, meninges, uncertain behavior
  papillary — *see* Neoplasm, meninges, uncertain behavior
  psammomatous — *see* Neoplasm, meninges, benign
  syncytial — *see* Neoplasm, meninges, benign
  transitional — *see* Neoplasm, meninges, benign
Meningiomatosis (diffuse) — *see* Neoplasm, meninges, uncertain behavior
Meningism — *see* Meningismus
Meningismus (infectional) (pneumococcal) R29.1
  due to serum or vaccine R29.1
  influenzal — *see* Influenza, with, manifestations NEC
Meningitis (basal) (basic) (brain) (cerebral) (cervical) (congestive) (diffuse) (hemorrhagic) (infantile) (membranous) (metastatic) (nonspecific) (pontine) (progressive) (simple) (spinal) (subacute) (sympathetic) (toxic) G03.9
  abacterial G03.0
  actinomycotic A42.81
  adenoviral A87.1
  arbovirus A87.8
  aseptic (acute) G03.0
  bacterial G00.9
    Escherichia coli (E. coli) G00.8
    Friedländer (bacillus) G00.8
    gram-negative G00.9
    H. influenzae G00.0
    Klebsiella G00.8
    pneumococcal G00.1
    specified organism NEC G00.8
    staphylococcal G00.3
    streptococcal (acute) G00.2
  benign recurrent (Mollaret) G03.2
  candidal B37.5
  caseous (tuberculous) A17.0
  cerebrospinal A39.0
  chronic NEC G03.1
  clear cerebrospinal fluid NEC G03.0
  coxsackievirus A87.0
  cryptococcal B45.1
  diplococcal (gram positive) A39.0
  echovirus A87.0
  enteroviral A87.0
  eosinophilic B83.2
  epidemic NEC A39.0
  Escherichia coli (E. coli) G00.8
  fibrinopurulent G00.9
    specified organism NEC G00.8
  Friedländer (bacillus) G00.8
  gonococcal A54.81
  gram-negative cocci G00.9
  gram-positive cocci G00.9
  H. influenzae G00.0
  Haemophilus (influenzae) G00.0
  in (due to)
    adenovirus A87.1
    African trypanosomiasis B56.9 [G02]
    anthrax A22.8
    bacterial disease NEC A48.8 [G01]
    Chagas' disease (chronic) B57.41
    chickenpox B01.0
    coccidioidomycosis B38.4
    Diplococcus pneumoniae G00.1
    enterovirus A87.0
    herpes (simplex) virus B00.3
      zoster B02.1

Meningitis — *continued*
  in — *continued*
    infectious mononucleosis B27.92
    leptospirosis A27.81
    Listeria monocytogenes A32.11
    Lyme disease A69.21
    measles B05.1
    mumps (virus) B26.1
    neurosyphilis (late) A52.13
    parasitic disease NEC B89 [G02]
    poliovirus A80.9 [G02]
    preventive immunization, inoculation or vaccination G03.8
    rubella B06.02
    Salmonella infection A02.21
    specified cause NEC G03.8
    typhoid fever A01.01
    varicella B01.0
    viral disease NEC A87.8
    whooping cough A37.90
    zoster B02.1
  infectious G00.9
  influenzal (H. influenzae) G00.0
  Klebsiella G00.8
  leptospiral (aseptic) A27.81
  lymphocytic (acute) (benign) (serous) A87.2
  meningococcal A39.0
  Mima polymorpha G00.8
  Mollaret (benign recurrent) G03.2
  monilial B37.5
  mycotic NEC B49 [G02]
  Neisseria A39.0
  nonbacterial G03.0
  nonpyogenic NEC G03.0
  ossificans G96.19
  pneumococcal G00.1
  poliovirus A80.9 [G02]
  postmeasles B05.1
  purulent G00.9
    specified organism NEC G00.8
  pyogenic G00.9
    specified organism NEC G00.8
  Salmonella (arizonae) (Cholerae-Suis) (enteritidis) (typhimurium) A02.21
  septic G00.9
    specified organism NEC G00.8
  serosa circumscripta NEC G03.0
  serous NEC G93.2
  specified organism NEC G00.8
  sporotrichosis B42.81
  staphylococcal G00.3
  sterile G03.0
  streptococcal (acute) G00.2
  suppurative G00.9
    specified organism NEC G00.8
  syphilitic (late) (tertiary) A52.13
    acute A51.41
    congenital A50.41
    secondary A51.41
  Torula histolytica (cryptococcal) B45.1
  traumatic (complication of injury) T79.8 ☑
  tuberculous A17.0
  typhoid A01.01
  viral NEC A87.9
  Yersinia pestis A20.3
Meningocele (spinal) (*see also* Spina bifida)
  with hydrocephalus — *see* Spina bifida, by site, with hydrocephalus
  acquired (traumatic) G96.19
  cerebral — *see* Encephalocele
Meningocerebritis — *see* Meningoencephalitis
Meningococcemia A39.4
  acute A39.2
  chronic A39.3
Meningococcus, meningococcal (*see also* condition) A39.9
  adrenalitis, hemorrhagic A39.1
  carrier (suspected) of Z22.31
  meningitis (cerebrospinal) A39.0
Meningoencephalitis (*see also* Encephalitis) G04.90
  acute NEC (*see also* Encephalitis, viral) A86
  bacterial NEC G04.2
  California A83.5
  diphasic A84.1
  eosinophilic B83.2
  epidemic A39.81
  herpesviral, herpetic B00.4
    due to herpesvirus 6 B10.01

Meningoencephalitis — *continued*
  herpesviral, herpetic — *continued*
    due to herpesvirus 7 B10.09
    specified NEC B10.09
  in (due to)
    blastomycosis NEC B40.81
    diseases classified elsewhere G05.3
    free-living amebae B60.2
    H. influenzae G00.0
    Hemophilus influenzae (H .influenzae) G04.2
    herpes B00.4
      due to herpesvirus 6 B10.01
      due to herpesvirus 7 B10.09
      specified NEC B10.09
    Lyme disease A69.22
    mercury — *see* subcategory T56.1 ☑
    mumps B26.2
    Naegleria (amebae) (organisms) (fowleri) B60.2
    Parastrongylus cantonensis B83.2
    toxoplasmosis (acquired) B58.2
      congenital P37.1
  infectious (acute) (viral) A86
  influenzal (H. influenzae) G04.2
  Listeria monocytogenes A32.12
  lymphocytic (serous) A87.2
  mumps B26.2
  parasitic NEC B89 [G05.3]
  pneumococcal G00.1
  primary amebic B60.2
  specific (syphilitic) A52.14
  specified organism NEC G04.81
  staphylococcal G04.2
  streptococcal G04.2
  syphilitic A52.14
  toxic NEC G92
    due to mercury — *see* subcategory T56.1 ☑
  tuberculous A17.82
  virus NEC A86
Meningoencephalocele (*see also* Encephalocele)
  syphilitic A52.19
    congenital A50.49
Meningoencephalomyelitis (*see also* Meningoencephalitis)
  acute NEC (viral) A86
    disseminated G04.00
      postimmunization or postvaccination G04.02
      postinfectious G04.01
  due to
    actinomycosis A42.82
    Torula B45.1
    Toxoplasma or toxoplasmosis (acquired) B58.2
      congenital P37.1
  postimmunization or postvaccination G04.02
Meningoencephalomyelopathy G96.9
Meningoencephalopathy G96.9
Meningomyelitis (*see also* Meningoencephalitis)
  bacterial NEC G04.2
  blastomycotic NEC B40.81
  cryptococcal B45.1
  in diseases classified elsewhere G05.4
  meningococcal A39.81
  syphilitic A52.14
  tuberculous A17.82
Meningomyelocele (*see also* Spina bifida)
  syphilitic A52.19
Meningomyeloneuritis — *see* Meningoencephalitis
Meningoradiculitis — *see* Meningitis
Meningovascular — *see* condition
Menkes' disease or syndrome E83.09
  meaning maple-syrup-urine disease E71.0
Menometrorrhagia N92.1
Menopause, menopausal (asymptomatic) (state) Z78.0
  arthritis (any site) NEC — *see* Arthritis, specified form NEC
  bleeding N92.4
  depression (single episode) F32.8
    agitated (single episode) F32.2
      recurrent episode F33.9
    psychotic (single episode) F32.8
      recurrent episode F33.9
    recurrent episode F33.9
  melancholia (single episode) F32.8
    recurrent episode F33.9
  paranoid state F22
  premature E28.319
    asymptomatic E28.319
      postirradiation E89.40
      postsurgical E89.40

Menopause, menopausal — *continued*
  premature — *continued*
    symptomatic E28.310
      postirradiation E89.41
      postsurgical E89.41
  psychosis NEC F28
  symptomatic N95.1
  toxic polyarthritis NEC — *see* Arthritis, specified form NEC
Menorrhagia (primary) N92.0
  climacteric N92.4
    menopausal N92.4
  menopausal N92.4
  postclimacteric N95.0
  postmenopausal N95.0
  preclimacteric or premenopausal N92.4
  pubertal (menses retained) N92.2
Menostaxis N92.0
Menses, retention N94.89
Menstrual — *see* Menstruation
Menstruation
  absent — *see* Amenorrhea
  anovulatory N97.0
  cycle, irregular N92.6
  delayed N91.0
  disorder N93.9
    psychogenic F45.8
  during pregnancy O20.8
  excessive (with regular cycle) N92.0
    with irregular cycle N92.1
    at puberty N92.2
  frequent N92.0
  infrequent — *see* Oligomenorrhea
  irregular N92.6
    specified NEC N92.5
  latent N92.5
  membranous N92.5
  painful (*see also* Dysmenorrhea) N94.6
    primary N94.4
    psychogenic F45.8
    secondary N94.5
  passage of clots N92.0
  precocious E30.1
  protracted N92.5
  rare — *see* Oligomenorrhea
  retained N94.89
  retrograde N92.5
  scanty — *see* Oligomenorrhea
  suppression N94.89
  vicarious (nasal) N94.89
Mental (*see also* condition)
  deficiency — *see* Disability, intellectual
  deterioration — *see* Psychosis
  disorder — *see* Disorder, mental
  exhaustion F48.8
  insufficiency (congenital) — *see* Disability, intellectual
  observation without need for further medical care Z03.89
  retardation — *see* Disability, intellectual
  subnormality — *see* Disability, intellectuall
  upset — *see* Disorder, mental
Meralgia paresthetica G57.1- ☑
Mercurial — *see* condition
Mercurialism — *see* subcategory T56.1 ☑
Merkel cell tumor — *see* Carcinoma, Merkel cell
Merocele — *see* Hernia, femoral
Meromelia
  lower limb — *see* Defect, reduction, lower limb
    intercalary
      femur — *see* Defect, reduction, lower limb, specified type NEC
        tibiofibular (complete) (incomplete) — *see* Defect, reduction, lower limb
  upper limb — *see* Defect, reduction, upper limb
    intercalary, humeral, radioulnar — *see* Agenesis, arm, with hand present
MERRF syndrome (myoclonic epilepsy associated with ragged-red fiber) E88.42
Merzbacher-Pelizaeus disease E75.29
Mesaortitis — *see* Aortitis
Mesarteritis — *see* Arteritis
Mesencephalitis — *see* Encephalitis
Mesenchymoma (*see also* Neoplasm, connective tissue, uncertain behavior)
  benign — *see* Neoplasm, connective tissue, benign
  malignant — *see* Neoplasm, connective tissue, malignant

Mesenteritis
  retractile K65.4
  sclerosing K65.4
Mesentery, mesenteric — *see* condition
Mesio-occlusion M26.213
Mesiodens, mesiodentes K00.1
Mesocolon — *see* condition
Mesonephroma (malignant) — *see* Neoplasm, malignant, by site
  benign — *see* Neoplasm, benign, by site
Mesophlebitis — *see* Phlebitis
Mesostromal dysgenesis Q13.89
Mesothelioma (malignant) C45.9
  benign
    mesentery D19.1
    mesocolon D19.1
    omentum D19.1
    peritoneum D19.1
    pleura D19.0
    specified site NEC D19.7
    unspecified site D19.9
  biphasic C45.9
    benign
      mesentery D19.1
      mesocolon D19.1
      omentum D19.1
      peritoneum D19.1
      pleura D19.0
      specified site NEC D19.7
      unspecified site D19.9
  cystic D48.4
  epithelioid C45.9
    benign
      mesentery D19.1
      mesocolon D19.1
      omentum D19.1
      peritoneum D19.1
      pleura D19.0
      specified site NEC D19.7
      unspecified site D19.9
  fibrous C45.9
    benign
      mesentery D19.1
      mesocolon D19.1
      omentum D19.1
      peritoneum D19.1
      pleura D19.0
      specified site NEC D19.7
      unspecified site D19.9
  site classification
    liver C45.7
    lung C45.7
    mediastinum C45.7
    mesentery C45.1
    mesocolon C45.1
    omentum C45.1
    pericardium C45.2
    peritoneum C45.1
    pleura C45.0
      parietal C45.0
    retroperitoneum C45.7
    specified site NEC C45.7
    unspecified site C45.9
Metabolic syndrome E88.81
Metagonimiasis B66.8
Metagonimus infestation (intestine) B66.8
Metal
  pigmentation L81.8
  polisher's disease J62.8
Metamorphopsia H53.15
Metaplasia
  apocrine (breast) — *see* Dysplasia, mammary, specified type NEC
  cervix (squamous) — *see* Dysplasia, cervix
  endometrium (squamous) (uterus) N85.8
  esophagus
  kidney (pelvis) (squamous) N28.89
  myelogenous D73.1
  myeloid (agnogenic) (megakaryocytic) D73.1
  spleen D73.1
  squamous cell, bladder N32.89
Metastasis, metastatic
  abscess — *see* Abscess
  calcification E83.59
  cancer
    from specified site — *see* Neoplasm, malignant, by site

Metastasis, metastatic — *continued*
  cancer — *continued*
    to specified site — *see* Neoplasm, secondary, by site
    deposits (in) — *see* Neoplasm, secondary, by site
    disease (*see also* Neoplasm, secondary, by site) C79.9
    spread (to) — *see* Neoplasm, secondary, by site
Metastrongyliasis B83.8
Metatarsalgia M77.4- ☑
  anterior G57.6- ☑
  Morton's G57.6- ☑
Metatarsus, metatarsal (*see also* condition)
  valgus (abductus), congenital Q66.6
  varus (adductus) (congenital) Q66.2
Methadone use F11.20
Methemoglobinemia D74.9
  acquired (with sulfhemoglobinemia) D74.8
  congenital D74.0
  enzymatic (congenital) D74.0
  Hb M disease D74.0
  hereditary D74.0
  toxic D74.8
Methemoglobinuria — *see* Hemoglobinuria
Methioninemia E72.19
Methylmalonic acidemia E71.120
Metritis (catarrhal) (hemorrhagic) (septic) (suppurative)
    (*see also* Endometritis)
  cervical — *see* Cervicitis
Metropathia hemorrhagica N93.8
Metroperitonitis — *see* Peritonitis, pelvic, female
Metrorrhagia N92.1
  climacteric N92.4
  menopausal N92.4
  postpartum NEC (atonic) (following delivery of placenta) O72.1
    delayed or secondary O72.2
  preclimacteric or premenopausal N92.4
  psychogenic F45.8
Metrorrhexis — *see* Rupture, uterus
Metrosalpingitis N70.91
Metrostaxis N93.8
Metrovaginitis — *see* Endometritis
Meyer-Schwickerath and Weyers syndrome Q87.0
Meynert's amentia (nonalcoholic) F04
  alcoholic F10.96
    with dependence F10.26
Mibelli's disease (porokeratosis) Q82.8
Mice, joint — *see* Loose, body, joint
  knee M23.4- ☑
Micrencephalon, micrencephaly Q02
Microalbuminuria R80.9
Microaneurysm, retinal (*see also* Disorder, retina, microaneurysms)
  diabetic — *see* E08-E13 with .31
Microangiopathy (peripheral) I73.9
  thrombotic M31.1
Microcalcifications, breast R92.0
Microcephalus, microcephalic, microcephaly Q02
  due to toxoplasmosis (congenital) P37.1
Microcheilia Q18.7
Microcolon (congenital) Q43.8
Microcornea (congenital) Q13.4
Microcytic — *see* condition
Microdeletions NEC Q93.88
Microdontia K00.2
Microdrepanocytosis D57.40
  with crisis (vasoocclusive pain) D57.419
    with
      acute chest syndrome D57.411
      splenic sequestration D57.412
Microembolism
  atherothrombotic — *see* Atheroembolism
  retinal — *see* Occlusion, artery, retina
Microencephalon Q02
Microfilaria streptocerca infestation — *see* Onchocerciasis
Microgastria (congenital) Q40.2
Microgenia M26.06
Microgenitalia, congenital
  female Q52.8
  male Q55.8
Microglioma — *see* Lymphoma, non-Hodgkin, specified NEC
Microglossia (congenital) Q38.3
Micrognathia, micrognathism (congenital) (mandibular) (maxillary) M26.09
Microgyria (congenital) Q04.3

Microinfarct of heart — *see* Insufficiency, coronary
Microlentia (congenital) Q12.8
Microlithiasis, alveolar, pulmonary J84.02
Micromastia N64.82
Micromyelia (congenital) Q06.8
Micropenis Q55.62
Microphakia (congenital) Q12.8
Microphthalmos, microphthalmia (congenital) Q11.2
  due to toxoplasmosis P37.1
Micropsia H53.15
Microscopic polyangiitis (polyarteritis) M31.7
Microsporidiosis B60.8
  intestinal A07.8
Microsporon furfur infestation B36.0
Microsporosis (*see also* Dermatophytosis)
  nigra B36.1
Microstomia (congenital) Q18.5
Microtia (congenital) (external ear) Q17.2
Microtropia H50.40
Microvillus inclusion disease (MVD) (MVID) Q43.8
Micturition
  disorder NEC R39.19
    psychogenic F45.8
  frequency R35.0
    psychogenic F45.8
  hesitancy R39.11
  incomplete emptying R39.14
  nocturnal R35.1
  painful R30.9
    dysuria R30.0
    psychogenic F45.8
    tenesmus R30.1
  poor stream R39.12
  split stream R39.13
  straining R39.16
  urgency R39.15
Mid plane — *see* condition
Middle
  ear — *see* condition
  lobe (right) syndrome J98.19
Miescher's elastoma L87.2
Mietens' syndrome Q87.2
Migraine (idiopathic) G43.909
  with aura (acute-onset) (prolonged) (typical) (without headache) G43.109
    with refractory migraine G43.119
      with status migrainosus G43.111
      without status migrainosus G43.119
    without mention of refractory migraine G43.109
      with status migrainosus G43.101
      without status migrainosus G43.109
    intractable G43.119
      with status migrainosus G43.111
      without status migrainosus G43.119
    not intractable G43.109
      with status migrainosus G43.101
      without status migrainosus G43.109
    persistent G43.509
      with cerebral infarction G43.609
        with refractory migraine G43.619
          with status migrainosus G43.611
          without status migrainosus G43.619
        without refractory migraine G43.609
          with status migrainosus G43.601
          without status migrainosus G43.609
        intractable G43.619
          with status migrainosus G43.611
          without status migrainosus G43.619
        not intractable G43.609
          with status migrainosus G43.601
          without status migrainosus G43.609
      without cerebral infarction G43.509
        with refractory migraine G43.519
          with status migrainosus G43.511
          without status migrainosus G43.519
        without refractory migraine G43.509
          with status migrainosus G43.501
          without status migrainosus G43.509
        intractable G43.519
          with status migrainosus G43.511
          without status migrainosus G43.519
        not intractable G43.509
          with status migrainosus G43.501
          without status migrainosus G43.509
  with refractory migraine G43.919
    with status migrainosus G43.911
    without status migrainosus G43.919
  without aura G43.009

Migraine — *continued*
  without aura — *continued*
    with refractory migraine G43.019
      with status migrainosus G43.011
      without status migrainosus G43.019
    without mention of refractory migraine G43.009
      with status migrainosus G43.001
      without status migrainosus G43.009
    chronic G43.709
      with refractory migraine G43.719
        with status migrainosus G43.711
        without status migrainosus G43.719
      without refractory migraine G43.709
        with status migrainosus G43.701
        without status migrainosus G43.709
      intractable
        with status migrainosus G43.711
        without status migrainosus G43.719
      not intractable
        with status migrainosus G43.701
        without status migrainosus G43.709
    intractable
      with status migrainosus G43.011
      without status migrainosus G43.019
    not intractable
      with status migrainosus G43.001
      without status migrainosus G43.009
  without refractory migraine G43.909
    with status migrainosus G43.901
    without status migrainosus G43.919
  abdominal G43.D0 (*following* G43.7)
    with refractory migraine G43.D1 (*following* G43.7)
    without refractory migraine G43.D0 (*following* G43.7)
    intractable G43.D1 (*following* G43.7)
    not intractable G43.D0 (*following* G43.7)
  basilar — *see* Migraine, with aura
  classical — *see* Migraine, with aura
  common — *see* Migraine, without aura
  complicated G43.109
  equivalents — *see* Migraine, with aura
  familiar — *see* Migraine, hemiplegic
  hemiplegic G43.409
    with refractory migraine G43.419
      with status migrainosus G43.411
      without status migrainosus G43.419
    without refractory migraine G43.409
      with status migrainosus G43.401
      without status migrainosus G43.409
    intractable G43.419
      with status migrainosus G43.411
      without status migrainosus G43.419
    not intractable G43.409
      with status migrainosus G43.401
      without status migrainosus G43.409
  intractable G43.919
    with status migrainosus G43.911
    without status migrainosus G43.919
  menstrual G43.829
    with refractory migraine G43.839
      with status migrainosus G43.831
      without status migrainosus G43.839
    without refractory migraine G43.829
      with status migrainosus G43.821
      without status migrainosus G43.829
    intractable G43.839
      with status migrainosus G43.831
      without status migrainosus G43.839
    not intractable 4G43.829
      with status migrainosus G43.821
      without status migrainosus G43.829
  menstrually related — *see* Migraine, menstrual
  not intractable G43.909
    with status migrainosus G43.901
    without status migrainosus G43.919
  ophthalmoplegic G43.B0 (*following* G43.7)
    with refractory migraine G43.B1 (*following* G43.7)
    without refractory migraine G43.B0 (*following* G43.7)
    intractable G43.B1 (*following* G43.7)
    not intractable G43.B0 (*following* G43.7)
  persistent aura (with, without) cerebral infarction — *see* Migraine, with aura, persistent
  pre-menstrual — *see* Migraine, menstrual
  preceded or accompanied by transient focal neurological phenomena — *see* Migraine, with aura
  pure menstrual — *see* Migraine, menstrual
  retinal — *see* Migraine, with aura

Index

Migraine — Mononucleosis, infectious

Migraine — *continued*
  specified NEC G43.809
    intractable G43.819
      with status migrainosus G43.811
      without status migrainosus G43.819
    not intractable G43.809
      with status migrainosus G43.801
      without status migrainosus G43.809
  sporadic — *see* Migraine, hemiplegic
  transformed — *see* Migraine, without aura, chronic
  triggered seizures — *see* Migraine, with aura
Migrant, social Z59.0
Migration, anxiety concerning Z60.3
Migratory, migrating (*see also* condition)
  person Z59.0
  testis Q55.29
Mikity-Wilson disease or syndrome P27.0
Mikulicz' disease or syndrome K11.8
Miliaria L74.3
  alba L74.1
  apocrine L75.2
  crystallina L74.1
  profunda L74.2
  rubra L74.0
  tropicalis L74.2
Miliary — *see* condition
Milium L72.0
  colloid L57.8
Milk
  crust L21.0
  excessive secretion O92.6
  poisoning — *see* Poisoning, food, noxious
  retention O92.79
  sickness — *see* Poisoning, food, noxious
  spots I31.0
Milk-alkali disease or syndrome E83.52
Milk-leg (deep vessels) (nonpuerperal) — *see* Embolism, vein, lower extremity
  complicating pregnancy O22.3- ☑
  puerperal, postpartum, childbirth O87.1
Milkman's disease or syndrome M83.8
Milky urine — *see* Chyluria
Millard-Gubler (-Foville) **paralysis or syndrome** G46.3
Millar's asthma J38.5
Miller Fisher syndrome G61.0
Mills' disease — *see* Hemiplegia
Millstone maker's pneumoconiosis J62.8
Milroy's disease (chronic hereditary edema) Q82.0
Minamata disease T26.1- ☑
Miners' asthma or lung J60
Minkowski-Chauffard syndrome — *see* Spherocytosis
Minor — *see* condition
Minor's disease (hematomyelia) G95.19
Minot-von Willebrand-Jurgens disease or syndrome (angiohemophilia) D68.0
Minot's disease (hemorrhagic disease), newborn P53
Minus (and plus) **hand** (intrinsic) — *see* Deformity, limb, specified type NEC, forearm
Miosis (pupil) H57.03
Mirizzi's syndrome (hepatic duct stenosis) K83.1
Mirror writing F81.0
Misadventure (of) (prophylactic) (therapeutic) (*see also* Complications) T88.9 ☑
  administration of insulin (by accident) — *see* subcategory T38.3 ☑
  infusion — *see* Complications, infusion
  local applications (of fomentations, plasters, etc.) T88.9 ☑
    burn or scald — *see* Burn
    specified NEC T88.8 ☑
  medical care (early) (late) T88.9 ☑
    adverse effect of drugs or chemicals — *see* Table of Drugs and Chemicals
    burn or scald — *see* Burn
    specified NEC T88.8 ☑
  specified NEC T88.8 ☑
  surgical procedure (early) (late) — *see* Complications, surgical procedure
  transfusion — *see* Complications, transfusion
  vaccination or other immunological procedure — *see* Complications, vaccination
Miscarriage O03.9
Misdirection, aqueous H40.83- ☑
Misperception, sleep state F51.02
Misplaced, misplacement
  ear Q17.4
  kidney (acquired) N28.89

Misplaced, misplacement — *continued*
  kidney — *continued*
    congenital Q63.2
  organ or site, congenital NEC — *see* Malposition, congenital
Missed
  abortion O02.1
  delivery O36.4 ☑
Missing — *see* Absence
Misuse of drugs F19.99
Mitchell's disease (erythromelalgia) I73.81
Mite(s) (infestation) B88.9
  diarrhea B88.0
  grain (itch) B88.0
  hair follicle (itch) B88.0
  in sputum B88.0
Mitral — *see* condition
Mittelschmerz N94.0
Mixed — *see* condition
MNGIE (Mitochondrial Neurogastrointestinal Encephalopathy) **syndrome** E88.49
Mobile, mobility
  cecum Q43.3
  excessive — *see* Hypermobility
  gallbladder, congenital Q44.1
  kidney N28.89
  organ or site, congenital NEC — *see* Malposition, congenital
Mobitz heart block (atrioventricular) I44.1
Moebius, Möbius
  disease (ophthalmoplegic migraine) — *see* Migraine, ophthalmoplegic
  syndrome Q87.0
    congenital oculofacial paralysis (with other anomalies) Q87.0
    ophthalmoplegic migraine — *see* Migraine, ophthalmoplegic
Moeller's glossitis K14.0
Mohr's syndrome (Types I and II) Q87.0
Mola destruens D39.2
Molar pregnancy O02.0
Molarization of premolars K00.2
Molding, head (during birth) — *omit code*
Mole (pigmented) (*see also* Nevus)
  blood O02.0
  Breus' O02.0
  cancerous — *see* Melanoma
  carneous O02.0
  destructive D39.2
  fleshy O02.0
  hydatid, hydatidiform (benign) (complicating pregnancy) (delivered) (undelivered) O01.9
    classical O01.0
    complete O01.0
    incomplete O01.1
    invasive D39.2
    malignant D39.2
    partial O01.1
  intrauterine O02.0
  invasive (hydatidiform) D39.2
  malignant
    meaning
      malignant hydatidiform mole D39.2
      melanoma — *see* Melanoma
  nonhydatidiform O02.0
  nonpigmented — *see* Nevus
  pregnancy NEC O02.0
  skin — *see* Nevus
  tubal O00.1
  vesicular — *see* Mole, hydatidiform
Molimen, molimina (menstrual) N94.3
Molluscum contagiosum (epitheliale) B08.1
Mönckeberg's arteriosclerosis, disease, or sclerosis — *see* Arteriosclerosis, extremities
Mondini's malformation (cochlea) Q16.5
Mondor's disease I80.8
Monge's disease T70.29 ☑
Monilethrix (congenital) Q84.1
Moniliasis (*see also* Candidiasis) B37.9
  neonatal P37.5
Monitoring (encounter for)
  therapeutic drug level Z51.81
Monkey malaria B53.1
Monkeypox B04
Monoarthritis M13.10
  ankle M13.17- ☑
  elbow M13.12- ☑

Monoarthritis — *continued*
  foot joint M13.17- ☑
  hand joint M13.14- ☑
  hip M13.15- ☑
  knee M13.16- ☑
  shoulder M13.11- ☑
  wrist M13.13- ☑
Monoblastic — *see* condition
Monochromat (ism), monochromatopsia (acquired) (congenital) H53.51
Monocytic — *see* condition
Monocytopenia D72.818
Monocytosis (symptomatic) D72.821
Monomania — *see* Psychosis
Mononeuritis G58.9
  cranial nerve — *see* Disorder, nerve, cranial
  femoral nerve G57.2- ☑
  lateral
    cutaneous nerve of thigh G57.1- ☑
    popliteal nerve G57.3- ☑
  lower limb G57.9- ☑
    specified nerve NEC G57.8- ☑
  medial popliteal nerve G57.4- ☑
  median nerve G56.1- ☑
  multiplex G58.7
  plantar nerve G57.6- ☑
  posterior tibial nerve G57.5- ☑
  radial nerve G56.3- ☑
  sciatic nerve G57.0- ☑
  specified NEC G58.8
  tibial nerve G57.4- ☑
  ulnar nerve G56.2- ☑
  upper limb G56.9- ☑
    specified nerve NEC G56.8- ☑
  vestibular — *see* subcategory H93.3 ☑
Mononeuropathy G58.9
  carpal tunnel syndrome — *see* Syndrome, carpal tunnel
  diabetic NEC — *see* E08-E13 with .41
  femoral nerve — *see* Lesion, nerve, femoral
  ilioinguinal nerve G57.8- ☑
  in diseases classified elsewhere — *see* category G59
  intercostal G58.0
  lower limb G57.9- ☑
    causalgia — *see* Causalgia, lower limb
    femoral nerve — *see* Lesion, nerve, femoral
    meralgia paresthetica G57.1- ☑
    plantar nerve — *see* Lesion, nerve, plantar
    popliteal nerve — *see* Lesion, nerve, popliteal
    sciatic nerve — *see* Lesion, nerve, sciatic
    specified NEC G57.8- ☑
    tarsal tunnel syndrome — *see* Syndrome, tarsal tunnel
  median nerve — *see* Lesion, nerve, median
  multiplex G58.7
  obturator nerve G57.8- ☑
  popliteal nerve — *see* Lesion, nerve, popliteal
  radial nerve — *see* Lesion, nerve, radial
  saphenous nerve G57.8- ☑
  specified NEC G58.8
  tarsal tunnel syndrome — *see* Syndrome, tarsal tunnel
  tuberculous A17.83
  ulnar nerve — *see* Lesion, nerve, ulnar
  upper limb G56.9- ☑
    carpal tunnel syndrome — *see* Syndrome, carpal tunnel
    causalgia — *see* Causalgia
    median nerve — *see* Lesion, nerve, median
    radial nerve — *see* Lesion, nerve, radial
    specified site NEC G56.8- ☑
    ulnar nerve — *see* Lesion, nerve, ulnar
Mononucleosis, infectious B27.90
  with
    complication NEC B27.99
    meningitis B27.92
    polyneuropathy B27.91
  cytomegaloviral B27.10
    with
      complication NEC B27.19
      meningitis B27.12
      polyneuropathy B27.11
  Epstein-Barr (virus) B27.00
    with
      complication NEC B27.09
      meningitis B27.02
      polyneuropathy B27.01

Mononucleosis, infectious — continued
  gammaherpesviral B27.00
    with
      complication NEC B27.09
      meningitis B27.02
      polyneuropathy B27.01
    specified NEC B27.80
      with
        complication NEC B27.89
        meningitis B27.82
        polyneuropathy B27.81
Monoplegia G83.3- ☑
  congenital (cerebral) G80.8
    spastic G80.1
  embolic (current episode) I63.4 ☑
  following
    cerebrovascular disease
      cerebral infarction
        lower limb I69.34- ☑
        upper limb I69.33- ☑
      intracerebral hemorrhage
        lower limb I69.14- ☑
        upper limb I69.13- ☑
      lower limb I69.94- ☑
      nontraumatic intracranial hemorrhage NEC
        lower limb I69.24- ☑
        upper limb I69.23- ☑
      specified disease NEC
        lower limb I69.84- ☑
        upper limb I69.83- ☑
      stroke NOS
        lower limb I69.34- ☑
        upper limb I69.33- ☑
      subarachnoid hemorrhage
        lower limb I69.04- ☑
        upper limb I69.03- ☑
      upper limb I69.93- ☑
  hysterical (transient) F44.4
  lower limb G83.1- ☑
  psychogenic (conversion reaction) F44.4
  thrombotic (current episode) I63.3 ☑
  transient R29.818
  upper limb G83.2- ☑
Monorchism, monorchidism Q55.0
Monosomy (see also Deletion, chromosome) Q93.9
  specified NEC Q93.89
  whole chromosome
    meiotic nondisjunction Q93.0
    mitotic nondisjunction Q93.1
    mosaicism Q93.1
  X Q96.9
Monster, monstrosity (single) Q89.7
  acephalic Q00.0
  twin Q89.4
Monteggia's fracture (-dislocation) S52.27- ☑
Mooren's ulcer (cornea) — see Ulcer, cornea, Mooren's
Moore's syndrome — see Epilepsy, specified NEC
Mooser-Neill reaction A75.2
Mooser's bodies A75.2
Morbidity not stated or unknown R69
Morbilli — see Measles
Morbus (see also Disease)
  angelicus, anglorum E55.0
  Beigel B36.2
  caducus — see Epilepsy
  celiacus K90.0
  comitialis — see Epilepsy
  cordis (see also Disease, heart) I51.9
    valvulorum — see Endocarditis
  coxae senilis M16.9
    tuberculous A18.02
  hemorrhagicus neonatorum P53
  maculosus neonatorum P54.5
Morel (-Stewart)(-Morgagni) **syndrome** M85.2
Morel-Kraepelin disease — see Schizophrenia
Morel-Moore syndrome M85.2
Morgagni-Stewart-Morel syndrome M85.2
Morgagni-Stokes-Adams syndrome I45.9
Morgagni-Turner (-Albright) **syndrome** Q96.9
Morgagni's
  cyst, organ, hydatid, or appendage
    female Q50.5
    male (epididymal) Q55.4
      testicular Q55.29
  syndrome M85.2
Moria F07.0
Moron (I.Q. 50-69) F70

Morphea L94.0
Morphinism (without remission) F11.20
  with remission F11.21
Morphinomania (without remission) F11.20
  with remission F11.21
Morquio (-Ullrich)(-Brailsford) **disease or syndrome** —
  see Mucopolysaccharidosis
Mortification (dry) (moist) — see Gangrene
Morton's metatarsalgia (neuralgia)(neuroma) (syn-
  drome) G57.6- ☑
Morvan's disease or syndrome G60.8
Mosaicism, mosaic (autosomal) (chromosomal)
  45,X/46,XX Q96.3
  45,X/other cell lines NEC with abnormal sex chromo-
    some Q96.4
  sex chromosome
    female Q97.8
    lines with various numbers of X chromosomes
      Q97.2
    male Q98.7
  XY Q96.3
Moschowitz' disease M31.1
Mother yaw A66.0
Motion sickness (from travel, any vehicle) (from round-
  abouts or swings) T75.3 ☑
Mottled, mottling, teeth (enamel) (endemic) (nonen-
  demic) K00.3
Mounier-Kuhn syndrome Q32.4
  with bronchiectasis J47.9
    exacerbation (acute) J47.1
    lower respiratory infection J47.0
  acquired J98.09
    with bronchiectasis J47.9
      with
        exacerbation (acute) J47.1
        lower respiratory infection J47.0
Mountain
  sickness T70.29 ☑
    with polycythemia , acquired (acute) D75.1
  tick fever A93.2
Mouse, joint — see Loose, body, joint
  knee M23.4- ☑
Mouth — see condition
Movable
  coccyx — see subcategory M53.2 ☑
  kidney N28.89
    congenital Q63.8
  spleen D73.89
Movements, dystonic R25.8
Moyamoya disease I67.5
MRSA (Methicillin resistant Staphylococcus aureus)
  infection A49.02
    as the cause of diseases classified elsewhere B95.62
  sepsis A41.02
MSSA (Methicillin susceptible Staphylococcus aureus)
  infection A49.01
    as the cause of diseases classified elsewhere B95.61
  sepsis A41.01
Mucha-Habermann disease L41.0
Mucinosis (cutaneous) (focal) (papular) (skin) L98.5
  oral K13.79
Mucocele
  appendix K38.8
  buccal cavity K13.79
  gallbladder K82.1
  lacrimal sac, chronic H04.43- ☑
  nasal sinus J34.1
  nose J34.1
  salivary gland (any) K11.6
  sinus (accessory) (nasal) J34.1
  turbinate (bone) (middle) (nasal) J34.1
  uterus N85.8
Mucolipidosis
  I E77.1
  II, III E77.0
  IV E75.11
Mucopolysaccharidosis E76.3
  beta-gluduronidase deficiency E76.29
  cardiopathy E76.3 [I52]
  Hunter's syndrome E76.1
  Hurler-Scheie syndrome E76.02
  Hurler's syndrome E76.01
  Maroteaux-Lamy syndrome E76.29
  Morquio syndrome E76.219
    A E76.210
    B E76.211
    classic E76.210

Mucopolysaccharidosis — continued
  Sanfilippo syndrome E76.22
  Scheie's syndrome E76.03
  specified NEC E76.29
  type
    I
      Hurler-Scheie syndrome E76.02
      Hurler's syndrome E76.01
      Scheie's syndrome E76.03
    II E76.1
    III E76.22
    IV E76.219
    IVA E76.210
    IVB E76.211
    VI E76.29
    VII E76.29
Mucormycosis B46.5
  cutaneous B46.3
  disseminated B46.4
  gastrointestinal B46.2
  generalized B46.4
  pulmonary B46.0
  rhinocerebral B46.1
  skin B46.3
  subcutaneous B46.3
Mucositis (ulcerative) K12.30
  due to drugs NEC K12.32
  gastrointestinal K92.81
  mouth (oral) (oropharyngeal) K12.30
    due to antineoplastic therapy K12.31
    due to drugs NEC K12.32
    due to radiation K12.33
    specified NEC K12.39
    viral K12.39
  nasal J34.81
  oral cavity — see Mucositis, mouth
  oral soft tissues — see Mucositis, mouth
  vagina and vulva N76.81
Mucositis necroticans agranulocytica — see Agranulocytosis
Mucous (see also condition)
  patches (syphilitic) A51.39
    congenital A50.07
Mucoviscidosis E84.9
  with meconium obstruction E84.11
Mucus
  asphyxia or suffocation — see Asphyxia, mucus
  in stool R19.5
  plug — see Asphyxia, mucus
Muguet B37.0
Mulberry molars (congenital syphilis) A50.52
Müllerian mixed tumor
  specified site — see Neoplasm, malignant, by site
  unspecified site C54.9
Multicystic kidney (development) Q61.4
Multiparity (grand) Z64.1
  affecting management of pregnancy, labor and deliv-
    ery (supervision only) O09.4- ☑
  requiring contraceptive management — see Contra-
    ception
Multipartita placenta O43.19- ☑
Multiple, multiplex (see also condition)
  digits (congenital) Q69.9
  endocrine neoplasia — see Neoplasia, endocrine,
    multiple (MEN)
  personality F44.81
Mumps B26.9
  arthritis B26.85
  complication NEC B26.89
  encephalitis B26.2
  hepatitis B26.81
  meningitis (aseptic) B26.1
  meningoencephalitis B26.2
  myocarditis B26.82
  oophoritis B26.89
  orchitis B26.0
  pancreatitis B26.3
  polyneuropathy B26.84
Mumu (see also Infestation, filarial) B74.9 [N51]
Münchhausen's syndrome — see Disorder, factitious
Münchmeyer's syndrome — see Myositis, ossificans,
  progressiva
Mural — see condition
Murmur (cardiac) (heart) (organic) R01.1
  abdominal R19.15
  aortic (valve) — see Endocarditis, aortic
  benign R01.0
  diastolic — see Endocarditis

Murmur — *continued*
Flint I35.1
functional R01.0
Graham Steell I37.1
innocent R01.0
mitral (valve) — *see* Insufficiency, mitral
nonorganic R01.0
presystolic, mitral — *see* Insufficiency, mitral
pulmonic (valve) I37.8
systolic (valvular) — *see* Endocarditis
tricuspid (valve) I07.9
valvular — *see* Endocarditis
Murri's disease (intermittent hemoglobinuria) D59.6
Muscle, muscular (*see also* condition)
carnitine (palmityltransferase) deficiency E71.314
Musculoneuralgia — *see* Neuralgia
Mushroom-workers' (pickers') disease or lung J67.5
Mushrooming hip — *see* Derangement, joint, specified
NEC, hip
Mutation(s)
factor V Leiden D68.51
prothrombin gene D68.52
surfactant, of lung J84.83
Mutism (*see also* Aphasia)
deaf (acquired) (congenital) NEC H91.3
elective (adjustment reaction) (childhood) F94.0
hysterical F44.4
selective (childhood) F94.0
MVD (microvillus inclusion disease) Q43.8
MVID (microvillus inclusion disease) Q43.8
Myalgia M79.1
epidemic (cervical) B33.0
traumatic NEC T14.8
Myasthenia G70.9
congenital G70.2
cordis — *see* Failure, heart
developmental G70.2
gravis G70.00
with exacerbation (acute) G70.01
in crisis G70.01
neonatal, transient P94.0
pseudoparalytica G70.00
with exacerbation (acute) G70.01
in crisis G70.01
stomach, psychogenic F45.8
syndrome
in
diabetes mellitus — *see* E08-E13 with .44
neoplastic disease (*see also* Neoplasm)
D49.9 [G73.3]
pernicious anemia D51.0 [G73.3]
thyrotoxicosis E05.90 [G73.3]
with thyroid storm E05.91 [G73.3]
Myasthenic M62.81
Mycelium infection B49
Mycetismus — *see* Poisoning, food, noxious, mushroom
Mycetoma B47.9
actinomycotic B47.1
bone (mycotic) B47.9 [M90.80]
eumycotic B47.0
foot B47.9
actinomycotic B47.1
mycotic B47.0
madurae NEC B47.9
mycotic B47.0
maduromycotic B47.0
mycotic B47.0
nocardial B47.1
Mycobacteriosis — *see* Mycobacterium
Mycobacterium, mycobacterial (infection) A31.9
anonymous A31.9
atypical A31.9
cutaneous A31.1
pulmonary A31.0
tuberculous — *see* Tuberculosis, pulmonary
specified site NEC A31.8
avium (intracellulare complex) A31.0
balnei A31.1
Battey A31.0
chelonei A31.8
cutaneous A31.1
extrapulmonary systemic A31.8
fortuitum A31.8
intracellulare (Battey bacillus) A31.0
kakaferifu A31.8
kansasii (yellow bacillus) A31.0
kasongo A31.8
leprae (*see also* Leprosy) A30.9

Mycobacterium, mycobacterial — *continued*
luciflavum A31.1
marinum (M. balnei) A31.1
nonspecific — *see* Mycobacterium, atypical
pulmonary (atypical) A31.0
tuberculous — *see* Tuberculosis, pulmonary
scrofulaceum A31.8
simiae A31.8
systemic, extrapulmonary A31.8
szulgai A31.8
terrae A31.8
triviale A31.8
tuberculosis (human, bovine) — *see* Tuberculosis
ulcerans A31.1
xenopi A31.8
Mycoplasma (M.) pneumoniae, as cause of disease classified elsewhere B96.0
Mycosis, mycotic B49
cutaneous NEC B36.9
ear B36.8
fungoides (extranodal) (solid organ) C84.0- ☑
mouth B37.0
nails B35.1
opportunistic B48.8
skin NEC B36.9
specified NEC B48.8
stomatitis B37.0
vagina, vaginitis (candidal) B37.3
Mydriasis (pupil) H57.04
Myelatelia Q06.1
Myelinolysis, pontine, central G37.2
Myelitis (acute) (ascending) (childhood) (chronic) (descending) (diffuse) (disseminated) (idiopathic) (pressure) (progressive) (spinal cord) (subacute) (*see also* Encephalitis) G04.91
herpes simplex B00.82
herpes zoster B02.24
in diseases classified elsewhere G05.4
necrotizing, subacute G37.4
optic neuritis in G36.0
postchickenpox B01.12
postherpetic B02.24
postimmunization G04.89
postinfectious NEC G04.89
postvaccinal G04.89
specified NEC G04.89
syphilitic (transverse) A52.14
toxic G92
transverse (in demyelinating diseases of central nervous system) G37.3
tuberculous A17.82
varicella B01.12
Myelo-osteo-musculodysplasia hereditaria Q79.8
Myeloblastic — *see* condition
Myeloblastoma
granular cell (*see also* Neoplasm, connective tissue)
malignant — *see* Neoplasm, connective tissue, malignant
tongue D10.1
Myelocele — *see* Spina bifida
Myelocystocele — *see* Spina bifida
Myelocytic — *see* condition
Myelodysplasia D46.9
specified NEC D46.Z (*following* D46.4)
spinal cord (congenital) Q06.1
Myelodysplastic syndrome D46.9
with
5q deletion D46.C (*following* D46.2)
isolated del (5q) chromosomal abnormality D46.C (*following* D46.2)
specified NEC D46.Z (*following* D46.4)
Myeloencephalitis — *see* Encephalitis
Myelofibrosis D75.81
with myeloid metaplasia D47.4
acute C94.4- ☑
idiopathic (chronic) D47.4
primary D47.1
secondary D75.81
in myeloproliferative disease D47.4
Myelogenous — *see* condition
Myeloid — *see* condition
Myelokathexis D70.9
Myeloleukodystrophy E75.29
Myelolipoma — *see* Lipoma
Myeloma (multiple) C90.0- ☑
monostotic C90.3 ☑
plasma cell C90.0- ☑

Myeloma — *continued*
plasma cell C90.0- ☑
solitary (*see also* Plasmacytoma, solitary) C90.3- ☑
Myelomalacia G95.89
Myelomatosis C90.0- ☑
Myelomeningitis — *see* Meningoencephalitis
Myelomeningocele (spinal cord) — *see* Spina bifida
Myelopathic
anemia D64.89
muscle atrophy — *see* Atrophy, muscle, spinal
pain syndrome G89.0
Myelopathy (spinal cord) G95.9
drug-induced G95.89
in (due to)
degeneration or displacement, intervertebral disc NEC — *see* Disorder, disc, with, myelopathy
infection — *see* Encephalitis
intervertebral disc disorder (*see also* Disorder, disc, with, myelopathy)
mercury — *see* subcategory T56.1 ☑
neoplastic disease (*see also* Neoplasm) D49.9 [G99.2]
pernicious anemia D51.0 [G99.2]
spondylosis — *see* Spondylosis, with myelopathy NEC
necrotic (subacute) (vascular) G95.19
radiation-induced G95.89
spondylogenic NEC — *see* Spondylosis, with myelopathy NEC
toxic G95.89
transverse, acute G37.3
vascular G95.19
vitamin B12 E53.8 [G32.0]
Myelophthisis D61.82
Myeloradiculitis G04.91
Myeloradiculodysplasia (spinal) Q06.1
Myelosarcoma C92.3- ☑
Myelosclerosis D75.89
with myeloid metaplasia D47.4
disseminated, of nervous system G35
megakaryocytic D47.4
with myeloid metaplasia D47.4
Myelosis
acute C92.0- ☑
aleukemic C92.9- ☑
chronic D47.1
erythremic (acute) C94.0- ☑
megakaryocytic C94.2- ☑
nonleukemic D72.828
subacute C92.9- ☑
Myiasis (cavernosa) B87.9
aural B87.4
creeping B87.0
cutaneous B87.0
dermal B87.0
ear (external) (middle) B87.4
eye B87.2
genitourinary B87.81
intestinal B87.82
laryngeal B87.3
nasopharyngeal B87.3
ocular B87.2
orbit B87.2
skin B87.0
specified site NEC B87.89
traumatic B87.1
wound B87.1
Myoadenoma, prostate — *see* Hyperplasia, prostate
Myoblastoma
granular cell (*see also* Neoplasm, connective tissue, benign)
malignant — *see* Neoplasm, connective tissue, malignant
tongue D10.1
Myocardial — *see* condition
Myocardiopathy (congestive) (constrictive) (familial) (hypertrophic nonobstructive) (idiopathic) (infiltrative) (obstructive) (primary) (restrictive) (sporadic) (*see also* Cardiomyopathy) I42.9
alcoholic I42.6
cobalt-beer I42.6
glycogen storage E74.02 [I43]
hypertrophic obstructive I42.1
in (due to)
beriberi E51.12
cardiac glycogenosis E74.02 [I43]
Friedreich's ataxia G11.1 [I43]

Myocardiopathy — *continued*
in — *continued*
myotonia atrophica G71.11 [I43]
progressive muscular dystrophy G71.0 [I43]
obscure (African) I42.8
secondary I42.9
thyrotoxic E05.90 [I43]
with storm E05.91 [I43]
toxic NEC I42.7
Myocarditis (with arteriosclerosis)(chronic)(fibroid) (interstitial) (old) (progressive) (senile) I51.4
with
rheumatic fever (conditions in I00) I09.0
active — *see* Myocarditis, acute, rheumatic
inactive or quiescent (with chorea) I09.0
active I40.9
rheumatic I01.2
with chorea (acute) (rheumatic) (Sydenham's) I02.0
acute or subacute (interstitial) I40.9
due to
streptococcus (beta-hemolytic) I01.2
idiopathic I40.1
rheumatic I01.2
with chorea (acute) (rheumatic) (Sydenham's) I02.0
specified NEC I40.8
aseptic of newborn B33.22
bacterial (acute) I40.0
Coxsackie (virus) B33.22
diphtheritic A36.81
eosinophilic I40.1
epidemic of newborn (Coxsackie) B33.22
Fiedler's (acute) (isolated) I40.1
giant cell (acute) (subacute) I40.1
gonococcal A54.83
granulomatous (idiopathic) (isolated) (nonspecific) I40.1
hypertensive — *see* Hypertension, heart
idiopathic (granulomatous) I40.1
in (due to)
diphtheria A36.81
epidemic louse-borne typhus A75.0 [I41]
Lyme disease A69.29
sarcoidosis D86.85
scarlet fever A38.1
toxoplasmosis (acquired) B58.81
typhoid A01.02
typhus NEC A75.9 [I41]
infective I40.0
influenzal — *see* Influenza, with, myocarditis
isolated (acute) I40.1
meningococcal A39.52
mumps B26.82
nonrheumatic, active I40.9
parenchymatous I40.9
pneumococcal I40.0
rheumatic (chronic) (inactive) (with chorea) I09.0
active or acute I01.2
with chorea (acute) (rheumatic) (Sydenham's) I02.0
rheumatoid — *see* Rheumatoid, carditis
septic I40.0
staphylococcal I40.0
suppurative I40.0
syphilitic (chronic) A52.06
toxic I40.8
rheumatic — *see* Myocarditis, acute, rheumatic
tuberculous A18.84
typhoid A01.02
valvular — *see* Endocarditis
virus, viral I40.0
of newborn (Coxsackie) B33.22
Myocardium, myocardial — *see* condition
Myocardosis — *see* Cardiomyopathy
Myoclonus, myoclonic, myoclonia (familial) (essential) (multifocal) (simplex) G25.3
drug-induced G25.3
epilepsy (*see also* Epilepsy, generalized, specified NEC) G40.4- ☑
familial (progressive) G25.3
epileptica G40.409
with status epilepticus G40.401
facial G51.3
familial progressive G25.3
Friedreich's G25.3
jerks G25.3
massive G25.3

Myoclonus, myoclonic, myoclonia — *continued*
palatal G25.3
pharyngeal G25.3
Myocytolysis I51.5
Myodiastasis — *see* Diastasis, muscle
Myoendocarditis — *see* Endocarditis
Myoepithelioma — *see* Neoplasm, benign, by site
Myofasciitis (acute) — *see* Myositis
Myofibroma (*see also* Neoplasm, connective tissue, benign)
uterus (cervix) (corpus) — *see* Leiomyoma
Myofibromatosis D48.1
infantile Q89.8
Myofibrosis M62.89
heart — *see* Myocarditis
scapulohumeral — *see* Lesion, shoulder, specified NEC
Myofibrositis M79.7
scapulohumeral — *see* Lesion, shoulder, specified NEC
Myoglobulinuria, myoglobinuria (primary) R82.1
Myokymia, facial G51.4
Myolipoma — *see* Lipoma
Myoma (*see also* Neoplasm, connective tissue, benign)
malignant — *see* Neoplasm, connective tissue, malignant
prostate D29.1
uterus (cervix) (corpus) — *see* Leiomyoma
Myomalacia M62.89
Myometritis — *see* Endometritis
Myometrium — *see* condition
Myonecrosis, clostridial A48.0
Myopathy G72.9
acute
necrotizing G72.81
quadriplegic G72.81
alcoholic G72.1
benign congenital G71.2
central core G71.2
centronuclear G71.2
congenital (benign) G71.2
critical illness G72.81
distal G71.0
drug-induced G72.0
endocrine NEC E34.9 [G73.7]
extraocular muscles H05.82- ☑
facioscapulohumeral G71.0
hereditary G71.9
specified NEC G71.8
immune NEC G72.49
in (due to)
Addison's disease E27.1 [G73.7]
alcohol G72.1
amyloidosis E85.0 [G73.7]
cretinism E00.9 [G73.7]
Cushing's syndrome E24.9 [G73.7]
drugs G72.0
endocrine disease NEC E34.9 [G73.7]
giant cell arteritis M31.6 [G73.7]
glycogen storage disease E74.00 [G73.7]
hyperadrenocorticism E24.9 [G73.7]
hyperparathyroidism NEC E21.3 [G73.7]
hypoparathyroidism E20.9 [G73.7]
hypopituitarism E23.0 [G73.7]
hypothyroidism E03.9 [G73.7]
infectious disease NEC B99 ☑ [G73.7]
lipid storage disease E75.6 [G73.7]
metabolic disease NEC E88.9 [G73.7]
myxedema E03.9 [G73.7]
parasitic disease NEC B89 [G73.7]
polyarteritis nodosa M30.0 [G73.7]
rheumatoid arthritis — *see* Rheumatoid, myopathy
sarcoidosis D86.87
scleroderma M34.82
sicca syndrome M35.03
Sjögren's syndrome M35.03
systemic lupus erythematosus M32.19
thyrotoxicosis (hyperthyroidism) E05.90 [G73.7]
with thyroid storm E05.91 [G73.7]
toxic agent NEC G72.2
inflammatory NEC G72.49
intensive care (ICU) G72.81
limb-girdle G71.0
mitochondrial NEC G71.3
myotubular G71.2
mytonic, proximal (PROMM) G71.11
nemaline G71.2
ocular G71.0
oculopharyngeal G71.0
of critical illness G72.81

Myopathy — *continued*
primary G71.9
specified NEC G71.8
progressive NEC G72.89
proximal myotonic (PROMM) G71.11
rod G71.2
scapulohumeral G71.0
specified NEC G72.89
toxic G72.2
Myopericarditis (*see also* Pericarditis)
chronic rheumatic I09.2
Myopia (axial) (congenital) H52.1- ☑
degenerative (malignant) H44.2- ☑
malignant H44.2- ☑
pernicious H44.2- ☑
progressive high (degenerative) H44.2- ☑
Myosarcoma — *see* Neoplasm, connective tissue, malignant
Myosis (pupil) H57.03
stromal (endolymphatic) D39.0
Myositis M60.9
clostridial A48.0
due to posture — *see* Myositis, specified type NEC
epidemic B33.0
fibrosa or fibrous (chronic), Volkmann's T79.6 ☑
foreign body granuloma — *see* Granuloma, foreign body
in (due to)
bilharziasis B65.9 [M63.8-] ☑
cysticercosis B69.81
leprosy A30.9 [M63.8-] ☑
mycosis B49 [M63.8-] ☑
sarcoidosis D86.87
schistosomiasis B65.9 [M63.8-] ☑
syphilis
late A52.78
secondary A51.49
toxoplasmosis (acquired) B58.82
trichinellosis B75 [M63.8-] ☑
tuberculosis A18.09
inclusion body [IBM] G72.41
infective M60.009
arm M60.002
left M60.001
right M60.000
leg M60.005
left M60.004
right M60.003
lower limb M60.005
ankle M60.07- ☑
foot M60.07- ☑
lower leg M60.06- ☑
thigh M60.05- ☑
toe M60.07- ☑
multiple sites M60.09
specified site NEC M60.08
upper limb M60.002
finger M60.04- ☑
forearm M60.03- ☑
hand M60.04- ☑
shoulder region M60.01- ☑
upper arm M60.02- ☑
interstitial M60.10
ankle M60.17- ☑
foot M60.17- ☑
forearm M60.13- ☑
hand M60.14- ☑
lower leg M60.16- ☑
multiple sites M60.19
shoulder region M60.11- ☑
specified site NEC M60.18
thigh M60.15- ☑
upper arm M60.12- ☑
mycotic B49 [M63.8-] ☑
orbital, chronic H05.12- ☑
ossificans or ossifying (circumscripta) (*see also* Ossification, muscle, specified NEC)
in (due to)
burns M61.30
ankle M61.37- ☑
foot M61.37- ☑
forearm M61.33- ☑
hand M61.34- ☑
lower leg M61.36- ☑
multiple sites M61.39
pelvic region M61.35- ☑
shoulder region M61.31- ☑

Myositis — continued
- ossificans or ossifying (see also Ossification, muscle, specified) — continued
  - in — continued
    - burns — continued
      - specified site NEC M61.38
        - thigh M61.35-
        - upper arm M61.32-
      - quadriplegia or paraplegia M61.20
        - ankle M61.27-
        - foot M61.27-
        - forearm M61.23-
        - hand M61.24-
        - lower leg M61.26-
        - multiple sites M61.29
        - pelvic region M61.25-
        - shoulder region M61.21-
        - specified site NEC M61.28
        - thigh M61.25-
        - upper arm M61.22-
  - progressiva M61.10
    - ankle M61.17-
    - finger M61.14-
    - foot M61.17-
    - forearm M61.13-
    - hand M61.14-
    - lower leg M61.16-
    - multiple sites M61.19
    - pelvic region M61.15-
    - shoulder region M61.11-
    - specified site NEC M61.18
    - thigh M61.15-
    - toe M61.17-
    - upper arm M61.12-
  - traumatica M61.00
    - ankle M61.07-
    - foot M61.07-
    - forearm M61.03-
    - hand M61.04-

Myositis — continued
- ossificans or ossifying (see also Ossification, muscle, specified) — continued
  - traumatica — continued
    - lower leg M61.06-
    - multiple sites M61.09
    - pelvic region M61.05-
    - shoulder region M61.01-
    - specified site NEC M61.08
    - thigh M61.05-
    - upper arm M61.02-
  - purulent — see Myositis, infective
  - specified type NEC M60.80
    - ankle M60.87-
    - foot M60.87-
    - forearm M60.83-
    - hand M60.84-
    - lower leg M60.86-
    - multiple sites M60.89
    - pelvic region M60.85-
    - shoulder region M60.81-
    - specified site NEC M60.88
    - thigh M60.85-
    - upper arm M60.82-
  - suppurative — see Myositis, infective
  - traumatic (old) — see Myositis, specified type NEC

Myospasia impulsiva F95.2
Myotonia (acquisita) (intermittens) M62.89
- atrophica G71.11
- chondrodystrophic G71.13
- congenita (acetazolamide responsive) (dominant) (recessive) G71.12
- drug-induced G71.14
- dystrophica G71.11
- fluctuans G71.19
- levior G71.12
- permanens G71.19
- symptomatic G71.19

Myotonic pupil — see Anomaly, pupil, function, tonic pupil
Myriapodiasis B88.2
Myringitis H73.2-
- with otitis media — see Otitis, media
- acute H73.00-
  - bullous H73.01-
  - specified NEC H73.09-
- bullous — see Myringitis, acute, bullous
- chronic H73.1-
Mysophobia F40.228
Mytilotoxism — see Poisoning, fish
Myxadenitis labialis K13.0
Myxedema (adult) (idiocy) (infantile) (juvenile) (see also Hypothyroidism) E03.9
- circumscribed E05.90
  - with storm E05.91
- coma E03.5
- congenital E00.1
- cutis L98.5
- localized (pretibial) E05.90
  - with storm E05.91
- papular L98.5
Myxochondrosarcoma — see Neoplasm, cartilage, malignant
Myxofibroma — see Neoplasm, connective tissue, benign
- odontogenic — see Cyst, calcifying odontogenic
Myxofibrosarcoma — see Neoplasm, connective tissue, malignant
Myxolipoma D17.9
Myxoliposarcoma — see Neoplasm, connective tissue, malignant
Myxoma (see also Neoplasm, connective tissue, benign)
- nerve sheath — see Neoplasm, nerve, benign
- odontogenic — see Cyst, calcifying odontogenic
Myxosarcoma — see Neoplasm, connective tissue, malignant

N

Naegeli's
  disease Q82.8
  leukemia, monocytic C93.1- ☑
Naegleriasis (with meningoencephalitis) B60.2
Naffziger's syndrome G54.0
Naga sore — *see* Ulcer, skin
Nägele's pelvis M95.5
  with disproportion (fetopelvic) O33.0
    causing obstructed labor O65.0
Nail (*see also* condition)
  biting F98.8
  patella syndrome Q87.2
Nanism, nanosomia — *see* Dwarfism
Nanophyetiasis B66.8
Nanukayami A27.89
Napkin rash L22
Narcolepsy G47.419
  with cataplexy G47.411
  in conditions classified elsewhere G47.429
    with cataplexy G47.421
Narcosis R06.89
Narcotism — *see* Dependence
NARP (Neuropathy, Ataxia and Retinitis pigmentosa) syndrome E88.49
Narrow
  anterior chamber angle H40.03- ☑
  pelvis — *see* Contraction, pelvis
Narrowing (*see also* Stenosis)
  artery I77.1
    auditory, internal I65.8
    basilar — *see* Occlusion, artery, basilar
    carotid — *see* Occlusion, artery, carotid
    cerebellar — *see* Occlusion, artery, cerebellar
    cerebral — *see* Occlusion artery, cerebral
    choroidal — *see* Occlusion, artery, cerebral, specified NEC
    communicating posterior — *see* Occlusion, artery, cerebral, specified NEC
    coronary (*see also* Disease, heart, ischemic, atherosclerotic)
      congenital Q24.5
        syphilitic A50.54 [I52]
      due to syphilis NEC A52.06
    hypophyseal — *see* Occlusion, artery, cerebral, specified NEC
    pontine — *see* Occlusion, artery, cerebral, specified NEC
    precerebral — *see* Occlusion, artery, precerebral
    vertebral — *see* Occlusion, artery, vertebral
  auditory canal (external) — *see* Stenosis, external ear canal
  eustachian tube — *see* Obstruction, eustachian tube
  eyelid — *see* Disorder, eyelid function
  larynx J38.6
  mesenteric artery K55.0
  palate M26.89
  palpebral fissure — *see* Disorder, eyelid function
  ureter N13.5
    with infection N13.6
  urethra — *see* Stricture, urethra
Narrowness, abnormal, eyelid Q10.3
Nasal — *see* condition
Nasolachrymal, nasolacrimal — *see* condition
Nasopharyngeal (*see also* condition)
  pituitary gland Q89.2
  torticollis M43.6
Nasopharyngitis (acute) (infective) (streptococcal) (subacute) J00
  chronic (suppurative) (ulcerative) J31.1
Nasopharynx, nasopharyngeal — *see* condition
Natal tooth, teeth K00.6
Nausea (without vomiting) R11.0
  with vomiting R11.2
  gravidarum — *see* Hyperemesis, gravidarum
  marina T75.3 ☑
  navalis T75.3 ☑
Navel — *see* condition
Neapolitan fever — *see* Brucellosis

Near drowning T75.1 ☑
Near-syncope R55
Nearsightedness — *see* Myopia
Nebula, cornea — *see* Opacity, cornea
Necator americanus infestation B76.1
Necatoriasis B76.1
Neck — *see* condition
Necrobiosis R68.89
  lipoidica NEC L92.1
    with diabetes — *see* E08-E13 with .620
Necrolysis, toxic epidermal L51.2
  due to drug
    correct substance properly administered — *see* Table of Drugs and Chemicals, by drug, adverse effect
    overdose or wrong substance given or taken — *see* Table of Drugs and Chemicals, by drug, poisoning
Necrophilia F65.89
Necrosis, necrotic (ischemic) (*see also* Gangrene)
  adrenal (capsule) (gland) E27.49
  amputation stump (surgical) (late) T87.50
    arm T87.5- ☑
    leg T87.5- ☑
  antrum J32.0
  aorta (hyaline) (*see also* Aneurysm, aorta)
    cystic medial — *see* Dissection, aorta
  artery I77.5
  bladder (aseptic) (sphincter) N32.89
  bone (*see also* Osteonecrosis) M87.9
    aseptic or avascular — *see* Osteonecrosis
      idiopathic M87.00
    ethmoid J32.2
    jaw M27.2
    tuberculous — *see* Tuberculosis, bone
  brain I67.89
  breast (aseptic) (fat) (segmental) N64.1
  bronchus J98.09
  central nervous system NEC I67.89
  cerebellar I67.89
  cerebral I67.89
  colon K55.0
  cornea H18.40
  cortical (acute) (renal) N17.1
  cystic medial (aorta) — *see* Dissection, aorta
  dental pulp K04.1
  esophagus K22.8
  ethmoid (bone) J32.2
  eyelid — *see* Disorder, eyelid, degenerative
  fat, fatty (generalized) (*see also* Disorder, soft tissue, specified type NEC)
    abdominal wall K65.4
    breast (aseptic) (segmental) N64.1
    localized — *see* Degeneration, by site, fatty
    mesentery K65.4
    omentum K65.4
    pancreas K86.8
    peritoneum K65.4
    skin (subcutaneous), newborn P83.0
    subcutaneous, due to birth injury P15.6
  gallbladder — *see* Cholecystitis, acute
  heart — *see* Infarct, myocardium
  hip, aseptic or avascular — *see* Osteonecrosis, by type, femur
  intestine (acute) (hemorrhagic) (massive) K55.0
  jaw M27.2
  kidney (bilateral) N28.0
    acute N17.9
    cortical (acute) (bilateral) N17.1
      with ectopic or molar pregnancy O08.4
    medullary (bilateral) (in acute renal failure) (papillary) N17.2
    papillary (bilateral) (in acute renal failure) N17.2
    tubular N17.0
      with ectopic or molar pregnancy O08.4
      complicating
        abortion — *see* Abortion, by type, complicated by, tubular necrosis
        ectopic or molar pregnancy O08.4
        pregnancy — *see* Pregnancy, complicated by, diseases of, specified type or system NEC

Necrosis, necrotic — *continued*
  kidney — *continued*
    tubular — *continued*
      following ectopic or molar pregnancy O08.4
      traumatic T79.5 ☑
  larynx J38.7
  liver (with hepatic failure) (cell) — *see* Failure, hepatic
    hemorrhagic, central K76.2
  lung J85.0
  lymphatic gland — *see* Lymphadenitis, acute
  mammary gland (fat) (segmental) N64.1
  mastoid (chronic) — *see* Mastoiditis, chronic
  medullary (acute) (renal) N17.2
  mesentery K55.0
    fat K65.4
  mitral valve — *see* Insufficiency, mitral
  myocardium, myocardial — *see* Infarct, myocardium
  nose J34.0
  omentum (with mesenteric infarction) K55.0
    fat K65.4
  orbit, orbital — *see* Osteomyelitis, orbit
  ossicles, ear — *see* Abnormal, ear ossicles
  ovary N70.92
  pancreas (aseptic) (duct) (fat) K86.8
    acute (infective) — *see* Pancreatitis, acute
    infective — *see* Pancreatitis, acute
  papillary (acute) (renal) N17.2
  perineum N90.89
  peritoneum (with mesenteric infarction) K55.0
    fat K65.4
  pharynx J02.9
    in granulocytopenia — *see* Neutropenia
    Vincent's A69.1
  phosphorus — *see* subcategory T54.2 ☑
  pituitary (gland) (postpartum) (Sheehan) E23.0
  pressure — *see* Ulcer, pressure, by site
  pulmonary J85.0
  pulp (dental) K04.1
  radiation — *see* Necrosis, by site
  radium — *see* Necrosis, by site
  renal — *see* Necrosis, kidney
  sclera H15.89
  scrotum N50.8
  skin or subcutaneous tissue NEC I96
  spine, spinal (column) (*see also* Osteonecrosis, by type, vertebra)
    cord G95.19
  spleen D73.5
  stomach K31.89
  stomatitis (ulcerative) A69.0
  subcutaneous fat, newborn P83.8
  subendocardial (acute) I21.4
    chronic I25.89
  suprarenal (capsule) (gland) E27.49
  testis N50.8
  thymus (gland) E32.8
  tonsil J35.8
  trachea J39.8
  tuberculous NEC — *see* Tuberculosis
  tubular (acute) (anoxic) (renal) (toxic) N17.0
    postprocedural N99.0
  vagina N89.8
  vertebra (*see also* Osteonecrosis, by type, vertebra)
    tuberculous A18.01
  vulva N90.89
  X-ray — *see* Necrosis, by site
Necrospermia — *see* Infertility, male
Need (for)
  care provider because (of)
    assistance with personal care Z74.1
    continuous supervision required Z74.3
    impaired mobility Z74.09
    no other household member able to render care Z74.2
    specified reason NEC Z74.8
  immunization — *see* Vaccination
  vaccination — *see* Vaccination
Neglect
  adult
    confirmed T74.01 ☑
    history of Z91.412
    suspected T76.01 ☑

☑ Additional Character Required — Refer to the Tabular List for Character Selection   ▽ Subterms under main terms may continue to next column or page

Nephropathy — *continued*
  hereditary — *continued*
    with — *continued*
      specified morphological changes NEC N07.8
  hypercalcemic N25.89
  hypertensive — *see* Hypertension, kidney
  hypokalemic (vacuolar) N25.89
  IgA N02.8
    with glomerular lesion N02.9
      focal and segmental hyalinosis or sclerosis N02.1
      membranoproliferative (diffuse) N02.5
      membranous (diffuse) N02.2
      mesangial proliferative (diffuse) N02.3
      mesangiocapillary (diffuse) N02.5
      proliferative NEC N02.8
      specified pathology NEC N02.8
  lead N14.3
  membranoproliferative (diffuse) N02.5
  membranous (diffuse) N02.2
  mesangial (IgA/IgG) — *see* Nephropathy, IgA
    proliferative (diffuse) N02.3
  mesangiocapillary (diffuse) N02.5
  obstructive N13.8
  phenacetin N17.2
  phosphate-losing N25.0
  potassium depletion N25.89
  pregnancy-related O26.83- ☑
  proliferative NEC (*see also* N00-N07 with fourth character .8) N05.8
  protein-losing N25.89
  saturnine N14.3
  sickle-cell D57.- ☑ [N08]
  toxic NEC N14.4
    due to
      drugs N14.2
        analgesic N14.0
        specified NEC N14.1
      heavy metals N14.3
  vasomotor N17.0
  water-losing N25.89
Nephroptosis N28.83
Nephropyosis — *see* Abscess, kidney
Nephrorrhagia N28.89
Nephrosclerosis (arteriolar)(arteriosclerotic) (chronic) (hyaline) (*see also* Hypertension, kidney)
  hyperplastic — *see* Hypertension, kidney
  senile N26.9
Nephrosis, nephrotic (Epstein's) (syndrome) (congenital) N04.9
  with
    foot process disease N04.9
    glomerular lesion N04.1
    hypocomplementemic N04.5
  acute N04.9
  anoxic — *see* Nephrosis, tubular
  chemical — *see* Nephrosis, tubular
  cholemic K76.7
  diabetic — *see* E08-E13 with .21
  Finnish type (congenital) Q89.8
  hemoglobin N10
  hemoglobinuric — *see* Nephrosis, tubular
  in
    amyloidosis E85.4 [N08]
    diabetes mellitus — *see* E08-E13 with .21
    epidemic hemorrhagic fever A98.5
    malaria (malariae) B52.0
  ischemic — *see* Nephrosis, tubular
  lipoid N04.9
  lower nephron — *see* Nephrosis, tubular
  malarial (malariae) B52.0
  minimal change N04.0
  myoglobin N10
  necrotizing — *see* Nephrosis, tubular
  osmotic (sucrose) N25.89
  radiation N04.9
  syphilitic (late) A52.75
  toxic — *see* Nephrosis, tubular
  tubular (acute) N17.0
    postprocedural N99.0
    radiation N04.9
Nephrosonephritis, hemorrhagic (endemic) A98.5
Nephrostomy
  attention to Z43.6
  status Z93.6
Nerve (*see also* condition)
  injury — *see* Injury, nerve, by body site
Nerves R45.0

Nervous (*see also* condition) R45.0
  heart F45.8
  stomach F45.8
  tension R45.0
Nervousness R45.0
Nesidioblastoma
  pancreas D13.7
  specified site NEC — *see* Neoplasm, benign, by site
  unspecified site D13.7
Nettleship's syndrome Q82.2
Neumann's disease or syndrome L10.1
Neuralgia, neuralgic (acute) M79.2
  accessory (nerve) G52.8
  acoustic (nerve) — *see* subcategory H93.3 ☑
  auditory (nerve) — *see* subcategory H93.3 ☑
  ciliary G44.009
    intractable G44.001
    not intractable G44.009
  cranial
    nerve (*see also* Disorder, nerve, cranial)
      fifth or trigeminal — *see* Neuralgia, trigeminal
    postherpetic, postzoster B02.29
  ear — *see* subcategory H92.0 ☑
  facialis vera G51.1
  Fothergill's — *see* Neuralgia, trigeminal
  glossopharyngeal (nerve) G52.1
  Horton's G44.099
    intractable G44.091
    not intractable G44.099
  Hunt's B02.21
  hypoglossal (nerve) G52.3
  infraorbital — *see* Neuralgia, trigeminal
  malarial — *see* Malaria
  migrainous G44.009
    intractable G44.001
    not intractable G44.009
  Morton's G57.6- ☑
  nerve, cranial — *see* Disorder, nerve, cranial
  nose G52.0
  occipital M54.81
  olfactory G52.0
  penis N48.9
  perineum R10.2
  postherpetic NEC B02.29
    trigeminal B02.22
  pubic region R10.2
  scrotum R10.2
  Sluder's G44.89
  specified nerve NEC G58.8
  spermatic cord R10.2
  sphenopalatine (ganglion) G90.09
  trifacial — *see* Neuralgia, trigeminal
  trigeminal G50.0
    postherpetic, postzoster B02.22
  vagus (nerve) G52.2
  writer's F48.8
    organic G25.89
Neurapraxia — *see* Injury, nerve
Neurasthenia F48.8
  cardiac F45.8
  gastric F45.8
  heart F45.8
Neurilemmoma (*see also* Neoplasm, nerve, benign)
  acoustic (nerve) D33.3
  malignant (*see also* Neoplasm, nerve, malignant)
    acoustic (nerve) C72.4- ☑
Neurilemmosarcoma — *see* Neoplasm, nerve, malignant
Neurinoma — *see* Neoplasm, nerve, benign
Neurinomatosis — *see* Neoplasm, nerve, uncertain behavior
Neuritis (rheumatoid) M79.2
  abducens (nerve) — *see* Strabismus, paralytic, sixth nerve
  accessory (nerve) G52.8
  acoustic (nerve) (*see also* subcategory) H93.3 ☑
    in (due to)
      infectious disease NEC B99 ☑ [H94.0-] ☑
      parasitic disease NEC B89 [H94.0-] ☑
      syphilitic A52.15
  alcoholic G62.1
    with psychosis — *see* Psychosis, alcoholic
  amyloid, any site E85.4 [G63]
  auditory (nerve) — *see* subcategory H93.3 ☑
  brachial — *see* Radiculopathy
    due to displacement, intervertebral disc — *see* Disorder, disc, cervical, with neuritis

Neuritis — *continued*
  cranial nerve
    due to Lyme disease A69.22
    eighth or acoustic or auditory — *see* subcategory H93.3 ☑
    eleventh or accessory G52.8
    fifth or trigeminal G51.0
    first or olfactory G52.0
    fourth or trochlear — *see* Strabismus, paralytic, fourth nerve
    second or optic — *see* Neuritis, optic
    seventh or facial G51.8
      newborn (birth injury) P11.3
    sixth or abducent — *see* Strabismus, paralytic, sixth nerve
    tenth or vagus G52.2
    third or oculomotor — *see* Strabismus, paralytic, third nerve
    twelfth or hypoglossal G52.3
  Déjérine-Sottas G60.0
  diabetic (mononeuropathy) — *see* E08-E13 with .41
    polyneuropathy — *see* E08-E13 with .42
  due to
    beriberi E51.11
    displacement, prolapse or rupture, intervertebral disc — *see* Disorder, disc, with, radiculopathy
    herniation, nucleus pulposus M51.9 [G55]
  endemic E51.11
  facial G51.8
    newborn (birth injury) P11.3
  general — *see* Polyneuropathy
  geniculate ganglion G51.1
    due to herpes (zoster) B02.21
  gouty M10.00 [G63]
  hypoglossal (nerve) G52.3
  ilioinguinal (nerve) G57.9- ☑
  infectious (multiple) NEC G61.0
  interstitial hypertrophic progressive G60.0
  lumbar M54.16
  lumbosacral M54.17
  multiple (*see also* Polyneuropathy)
    endemic E51.11
    infective, acute G61.0
  multiplex endemica E51.11
  nerve root — *see* Radiculopathy
  oculomotor (nerve) — *see* Strabismus, paralytic, third nerve
  olfactory nerve G52.0
  optic (nerve) (hereditary) (sympathetic) H46.9
    with demyelination G36.0
    in myelitis G36.0
    nutritional H46.2
    papillitis — *see* Papillitis, optic
    retrobulbar H46.1- ☑
    specified type NEC H46.8
    toxic H46.3
  peripheral (nerve) G62.9
    multiple — *see* Polyneuropathy
    single — *see* Mononeuritis
  pneumogastric (nerve) G52.2
  postherpetic, postzoster B02.29
  progressive hypertrophic interstitial G60.0
  retrobulbar (*see also* Neuritis, optic, retrobulbar)
    in (due to)
      late syphilis A52.15
      meningococcal infection A39.82
    meningococcal A39.82
    syphilitic A52.15
  sciatic (nerve) (*see also* Sciatica)
    due to displacement of intervertebral disc — *see* Disorder, disc, with, radiculopathy
  serum (*see also* Reaction, serum) T80.69 ☑
  shoulder-girdle G54.5
  specified nerve NEC G58.8
  spinal (nerve) root — *see* Radiculopathy
  syphilitic A52.15
  thenar (median) G56.1- ☑
  thoracic M54.14
  toxic NEC G62.2
  trochlear (nerve) — *see* Strabismus, paralytic, fourth nerve
  vagus (nerve) G52.2
Neuroastrocytoma — *see* Neoplasm, uncertain behavior, by site
Neuroavitaminosis E56.9 [G99.8]
Neuroblastoma
  olfactory C30.0
  specified site — *see* Neoplasm, malignant, by site

Neuroblastoma — *continued*
  unspecified site C74.90
Neurochorioretinitis — *see* Chorioretinitis
Neurocirculatory asthenia F45.8
Neurocysticercosis B69.0
Neurocytoma — *see* Neoplasm, benign, by site
Neurodermatitis (circumscribed) (circumscripta) (local)
  L28.0
  atopic L20.81
  diffuse (Brocq) L20.81
  disseminated L20.81
Neuroencephalomyelopathy, optic G36.0
Neuroepithelioma (*see also* Neoplasm, malignant, by
  site)
  olfactory C30.0
Neurofibroma (*see also* Neoplasm, nerve, benign)
  melanotic — *see* Neoplasm, nerve, benign
  multiple — *see* Neurofibromatosis
  plexiform — *see* Neoplasm, nerve, benign
Neurofibromatosis (multiple) (nonmalignant) Q85.00
  acoustic Q85.02
  malignant — *see* Neoplasm, nerve, malignant
  specified NEC Q85.09
  type 1 (von Recklinghausen) Q85.01
  type 2 Q85.02
Neurofibrosarcoma — *see* Neoplasm, nerve, malignant
Neurogenic (*see also* condition)
  bladder (*see also* Dysfunction, bladder, neuromuscular)
    N31.9
    cauda equina syndrome G83.4
  bowel NEC K59.2
  heart F45.8
Neuroglioma — *see* Neoplasm, uncertain behavior, by
  site
Neurolabyrinthitis (of Dix and Hallpike) — *see* Neuronitis, vestibular
Neurolathyrism — *see* Poisoning, food, noxious, plant
Neuroleprosy A30.9
Neuroma (*see also* Neoplasm, nerve, benign)
  acoustic (nerve) D33.3
  amputation (stump) (traumatic) (surgical complication)
    (late) T87.3- ☑
    arm T87.3- ☑
    leg T87.3- ☑
  digital (toe) G57.6- ☑
  interdigital (toe) G58.8
    lower limb G57.8- ☑
    upper limb G56.8- ☑
  intermetatarsal G57.8- ☑
  Morton's G57.6- ☑
  nonneoplastic
    arm G56.9- ☑
    leg G57.9- ☑
    lower extremity G57.9- ☑
    upper extremity G56.9- ☑
  optic (nerve) D33.3
  plantar G57.6- ☑
  plexiform — *see* Neoplasm, nerve, benign
  surgical (nonneoplastic)
    arm G56.9- ☑
    leg G57.9- ☑
    lower extremity G57.9- ☑
    upper extremity G56.9- ☑
Neuromyalgia — *see* Neuralgia
Neuromyasthenia (epidemic) (postinfectious) G93.3
Neuromyelitis G36.9
  ascending G61.0
  optica G36.0
Neuromyopathy G70.9
  paraneoplastic D49.9 [G13.0]
Neuromyotonia (Isaacs) G71.19
Neuronevus — *see* Nevus
Neuronitis G58.9
  ascending (acute) G57.2- ☑
  vestibular H81.2- ☑
Neuroparalytic — *see* condition
Neuropathy, neuropathic G62.9
  acute motor G62.81
  alcoholic G62.1
    with psychosis — *see* Psychosis, alcoholic
  arm G56.9- ☑
  autonomic, peripheral — *see* Neuropathy, peripheral,
    autonomic
  axillary G56.9- ☑
  bladder N31.9
    atonic (motor) (sensory) N31.2
    autonomous N31.2

Neuropathy, neuropathic — *continued*
  bladder — *continued*
    flaccid N31.2
    nonreflex N31.2
    reflex N31.1
    uninhibited N31.0
  brachial plexus G54.0
  cervical plexus G54.2
  chronic
    progressive segmentally demyelinating G62.89
    relapsing demyelinating G62.89
  Déjérine-Sottas G60.0
  diabetic — *see* E08-E13 with .40
    mononeuropathy — *see* E08-E13 with .41
    polyneuropathy — *see* E08-E13 with .42
  entrapment G58.9
    iliohypogastric nerve G57.8- ☑
    ilioinguinal nerve G57.8- ☑
    lateral cutaneous nerve of thigh G57.1- ☑
    median nerve G56.0- ☑
    obturator nerve G57.8- ☑
    peroneal nerve G57.3- ☑
    posterior tibial nerve G57.5- ☑
    saphenous nerve G57.8- ☑
    ulnar nerve G56.2- ☑
  facial nerve G51.9
  hereditary G60.9
    motor and sensory (types I-IV) G60.0
    sensory G60.8
    specified NEC G60.8
  hypertrophic G60.0
    Charcot-Marie-Tooth G60.0
    Déjérine-Sottas G60.0
    interstitial progressive G60.0
    of infancy G60.0
    Refsum G60.1
  idiopathic G60.9
    progressive G60.3
    specified NEC G60.8
  in association with hereditary ataxia G60.2
  intercostal G58.0
  ischemic — *see* Disorder, nerve
  Jamaica (ginger) G62.2
  leg NEC G57.9- ☑
  lower extremity G57.9- ☑
  lumbar plexus G54.1
  median nerve G56.1- ☑
  motor and sensory (*see also* Polyneuropathy)
    hereditary (types I-IV) G60.0
  multiple (acute) (chronic) — *see* Polyneuropathy
  optic (nerve) (*see also* Neuritis, optic)
    ischemic H47.01- ☑
  paraneoplastic (sensorial) (Denny Brown) D49.9 [G13.0]
  peripheral (nerve) (*see also* Polyneuropathy) G62.9
    autonomic G90.9
      idiopathic G90.09
      in (due to)
        amyloidosis E85.4 [G99.0]
        diabetes mellitus — *see* E08-E13 with .43
        endocrine disease NEC E34.9 [G99.0]
        gout M10.00 [G99.0]
        hyperthyroidism E05.90 [G99.0]
          with thyroid storm E05.91 [G99.0]
        metabolic disease NEC E88.9 [G99.0]
    idiopathic G60.9
      progressive G60.3
    in (due to)
      antitetanus serum G62.0
      arsenic G62.2
      drugs NEC G62.0
      lead G62.2
      organophosphate compounds G62.2
      toxic agent NEC G62.2
  plantar nerves G57.6- ☑
  progressive
    hypertrophic interstitial G60.0
    inflammatory G62.81
  radicular NEC — *see* Radiculopathy
  sacral plexus G54.1
  sciatic G57.0- ☑
  serum G61.1
  toxic NEC G62.2
  trigeminal sensory G50.8
  ulnar nerve G56.2- ☑
  uremic N18.9 [G63]
  vitamin B12 E53.8 [G63]
    with anemia (pernicious) D51.0 [G63]
      due to dietary deficiency D51.3 [G63]

Neurophthisis (*see also* Disorder, nerve)
  peripheral, diabetic — *see* E08-E13 with .42
Neuroretinitis — *see* Chorioretinitis
Neuroretinopathy, hereditary optic H47.22
Neurosarcoma — *see* Neoplasm, nerve, malignant
Neurosclerosis — *see* Disorder, nerve
Neurosis, neurotic F48.9
  anankastic F42
  anxiety (state) F41.1
    panic type F41.0
  asthenic F48.8
  bladder F45.8
  cardiac (reflex) F45.8
  cardiovascular F45.8
  character F60.9
  colon F45.8
  compensation F68.1 ☑
  compulsive, compulsion F42
  conversion F44.9
  craft F48.8
  cutaneous F45.8
  depersonalization F48.1
  depressive (reaction) (type) F34.1
  environmental F48.8
  excoriation L98.1
  fatigue F48.8
  functional — *see* Disorder, somatoform
  gastric F45.8
  gastrointestinal F45.8
  heart F45.8
  hypochondriacal F45.21
  hysterical F44.9
  incoordination F45.8
    larynx F45.8
    vocal cord F45.8
  intestine F45.8
  larynx (sensory) F45.8
    hysterical F44.4
  mixed NEC F48.8
  musculoskeletal F45.8
  obsessional F42
  obsessive-compulsive F42
  occupational F48.8
  ocular NEC F45.8
  organ — *see* Disorder, somatoform
  pharynx F45.8
  phobic F40.9
  posttraumatic (situational) F43.10
    acute F43.11
    chronic F43.12
  psychasthenic (type) F48.8
  railroad F48.8
  rectum F45.8
  respiratory F45.8
  rumination F45.8
  sexual F65.9
  situational F48.8
  social F40.10
    generalized F40.11
  specified type NEC F48.8
  state F48.9
    with depersonalization episode F48.1
  stomach F45.8
  traumatic F43.10
    acute F43.11
    chronic F43.12
  vasomotor F45.8
  visceral F45.8
  war F48.8
Neurospongioblastosis diffusa Q85.1
Neurosyphilis (arrested) (early) (gumma) (late) (latent)
  (recurrent) (relapse) A52.3
  with ataxia (cerebellar) (locomotor) (spastic) (spinal)
    A52.19
  aneurysm (cerebral) A52.05
  arachnoid (adhesive) A52.13
  arteritis (any artery) (cerebral) A52.04
  asymptomatic A52.2
  congenital A50.40
  dura (mater) A52.13
  general paresis A52.17
  hemorrhagic A52.05
  juvenile (asymptomatic) (meningeal) A50.40
  leptomeninges (aseptic) A52.13
  meningeal, meninges (adhesive) A52.13
  meningitis A52.13
  meningovascular (diffuse) A52.13
  optic atrophy A52.15

Neurosyphilis — *continued*
  parenchymatous (degenerative) A52.19
  paresis, paretic A52.17
    juvenile A50.45
  remission in (sustained) A52.3
  serological (without symptoms) A52.2
  specified nature or site NEC A52.19
  tabes, tabetic (dorsalis) A52.11
    juvenile A50.45
  taboparesis A52.17
    juvenile A50.45
  thrombosis (cerebral) A52.05
  vascular (cerebral) NEC A52.05
Neurothekeoma — *see* Neoplasm, nerve, benign
Neurotic — *see* Neurosis
Neurotoxemia — *see* Toxemia
Neutroclusion M26.211
Neutropenia, neutropenic (chronic) (genetic) (idiopathic) (immune) (infantile) (malignant) (pernicious) (splenic) D70.9
  congenital (primary) D70.0
  cyclic D70.4
  cytoreductive cancer chemotherapy sequela D70.1
  drug-induced D70.2
    due to cytoreductive cancer chemotherapy D70.1
  due to infection D70.3
  fever D70.9
  neonatal, transitory (isoimmune) (maternal transfer) P61.5
  periodic D70.4
  secondary (cyclic) (periodic) (splenic) D70.4
    drug-induced D70.2
      due to cytoreductive cancer chemotherapy D70.1
  toxic D70.8
Neutrophilia, hereditary giant D72.0
Nevocarcinoma — *see* Melanoma
Nevus D22.9
  achromic — *see* Neoplasm, skin, benign
  amelanotic — *see* Neoplasm, skin, benign
  angiomatousD18.00
    intra-abdominal D18.03
    intracranial D18.02
    skin D18.01
    specified site NEC D18.09
  araneus I78.1
  balloon cell — *see* Neoplasm, skin, benign
  bathing trunk D48.5
  blue — *see* Neoplasm, skin, benign
    cellular — *see* Neoplasm, skin, benign
    giant — *see* Neoplasm, skin, benign
    Jadassohn's — *see* Neoplasm, skin, benign
    malignant — *see* Melanoma
  capillary D18.00
    intra-abdominal D18.03
    intracranial D18.02
    skin D18.01
    specified site NEC D18.09
  cavernous D18.00
    intra-abdominal D18.03
    intracranial D18.02
    skin D18.01
    specified site NEC D18.09
  cellular — *see* Neoplasm, skin, benign
    blue — *see* Neoplasm, skin, benign
  choroid D31.3- ☑
  comedonicus Q82.5
  conjunctiva D31.0- ☑
  dermal — *see* Neoplasm, skin, benign
    with epidermal nevus — *see* Neoplasm, skin, benign
  dysplastic — *see* Neoplasm, skin, benign
  eye D31.9- ☑
  flammeus Q82.5
  hemangiomatous D18.00
    intra-abdominal D18.03
    intracranial D18.02
    skin D18.01
    specified site NEC D18.09
  iris D31.4- ☑
  lacrimal gland D31.5- ☑
  lymphatic D18.1
  magnocellular
    specified site — *see* Neoplasm, benign, by site
    unspecified site D31.40
  malignant — *see* Melanoma
  meaning hemangioma D18.00
    intra-abdominal D18.03

Nevus — *continued*
  meaning hemangioma — *continued*
    intracranial D18.02
    skin D18.01
    specified site NEC D18.09
  mouth (mucosa) D10.30
    specified site NEC D10.39
    white sponge Q38.6
  multiplex Q85.1
  non-neoplastic I78.1
  oral mucosa D10.30
    specified site NEC D10.39
    white sponge Q38.6
  orbit D31.6- ☑
  pigmented
    giant (*see also* Neoplasm, skin, uncertain behavior) D48.5
      malignant melanoma in — *see* Melanoma
  portwine Q82.5
  retina D31.2- ☑
  retrobulbar D31.6- ☑
  sanguineous Q82.5
  senile I78.1
  skin D22.9
    abdominal wall D22.5
    ala nasi D22.39
    ankle D22.7- ☑
    anus, anal D22.5
    arm D22.6- ☑
    auditory canal (external) D22.2- ☑
    auricle (ear) D22.2- ☑
    auricular canal (external) D22.2- ☑
    axilla, axillary fold D22.5
    back D22.5
    breast D22.5
    brow D22.39
    buttock D22.5
    canthus (eye) D22.1- ☑
    cheek (external) D22.39
    chest wall D22.5
    chin D22.39
    ear (external) D22.2- ☑
    external meatus (ear) D22.2- ☑
    eyebrow D22.39
    eyelid (lower) (upper) D22.1- ☑
    face D22.30
      specified NEC D22.39
    female genital organ (external) NEC D28.0
    finger D22.6- ☑
    flank D22.5
    foot D22.7- ☑
    forearm D22.6- ☑
    forehead D22.39
    foreskin D29.0
    genital organ (external) NEC
      female D28.0
      male D29.9
    gluteal region D22.5
    groin D22.5
    hand D22.6- ☑
    heel D22.7- ☑
    helix D22.2- ☑
    hip D22.7- ☑
    interscapular region D22.5
    jaw D22.39
    knee D22.7- ☑
    labium (majus) (minus) D28.0
    leg D22.7- ☑
    lip (lower) (upper) D22.0
    lower limb D22.7- ☑
    male genital organ (external) D29.9
    nail D22.9
      finger D22.6- ☑
      toe D22.7- ☑
    nasolabial groove D22.39
    nates D22.5
    neck D22.4
    nose (external) D22.39
    palpebra D22.1- ☑
    penis D29.0
    perianal skin D22.5
    perineum D22.5
    pinna D22.2- ☑
    popliteal fossa or space D22.7- ☑
    prepuce D29.0
    pudendum D28.0
    scalp D22.4

Nevus — *continued*
  skin — *continued*
    scrotum D29.4
    shoulder D22.6- ☑
    submammary fold D22.5
    temple D22.39
    thigh D22.7- ☑
    toe D22.7- ☑
    trunk NEC D22.5
    umbilicus D22.5
    upper limb D22.6- ☑
    vulva D28.0
  specified site NEC — *see* Neoplasm, by site, benign
  spider I78.1
  stellar I78.1
  strawberry Q82.5
  Sutton's — *see* Neoplasm, skin, benign
  unius lateris Q82.5
  Unna's Q82.5
  vascular Q82.5
  verrucous Q82.5
Newborn (infant) (liveborn) (singleton) Z38.2
  abstinence syndrome P96.1
  acne L70.4
  affected by (suspected to be)
    abnormalities of membranes P02.9
      specified NEC P02.8
    abruptio placenta P02.1
    amino-acid metabolic disorder, transitory P74.8
    amniocentesis (while in utero) P00.6
    amnionitis P02.7
    apparent life threatening event (ALTE) R68.13
    bleeding (into)
      cerebral cortex P52.22
      germinal matrix P52.0
      ventricles P52.1
    breech delivery P03.0
    cardiac arrest P29.81
    cardiomyopathy I42.8
      congenital I42.4
    cerebral ischemia P91.0
    Cesarean delivery P03.4
    chemotherapy agents P04.1
    chorioamnionitis P02.7
    cocaine (crack) P04.41
    complications of labor and delivery P03.9
      specified NEC P03.89
    compression of umbilical cord NEC P02.5
    contracted pelvis P03.1
    delivery P03.9
      Cesarean P03.4
      forceps P03.2
      vacuum extractor P03.3
    entanglement (knot) in umbilical cord P02.5
    environmental chemicals P04.6
    fetal (intrauterine)
      growth retardation P05.9
      malnutrition not light or small for gestational age P05.2
    forceps delivery P03.2
    heart rate abnormalities
      bradycardia P29.12
      intrauterine P03.819
        before onset of labor P03.810
        during labor P03.811
      tachycardia P29.11
    hemorrhage (antepartum) P02.1
      cerebellar (nontraumatic) P52.6
      intracerebral (nontraumatic) P52.4
      intracranial (nontraumatic) P52.9
        specified NEC P52.8
      intraventricular (nontraumatic) P52.3
        grade 1 P52.0
        grade 2 P52.1
        grade 3 P52.21
        grade 4 P52.22
      posterior fossa (nontraumatic) P52.6
      subarachnoid (nontraumatic) P52.5
      subependymal P52.0
        with intracerebral extension P52.22
        with intraventricular extension P52.1
          with enlargment of ventricles P52.21
        without intraventricular extension P52.0
    hypoxic ischemic encephalopathy [HIE] P91.60
      mild P91.61
      moderate P91.62
      severe P91.63
    induction of labor P03.89

☑ **Additional Character Required — Refer to the Tabular List for Character Selection**

�E **Subterms under main terms may continue to next column or page**

Index

Newborn — Nodule

Newborn — continued
  affected by — continued
    intestinal perforation P78.0
    intrauterine (fetal) blood loss P50.9
      due to (from)
        cut end of co-twin cord P50.5
        hemorrhage into
          co-twin P50.3
            maternal circulation P50.4
          placenta P50.2
        ruptured cord blood P50.1
        vasa previa P50.0
      specified NEC P50.8
    intrauterine (fetal) hemorrhage P50.9
    intrauterine (in utero) procedure P96.5
    malpresentation (malposition) NEC P03.1
    maternal (complication of) (use of)
      alcohol P04.3
      analgesia (maternal) P04.0
      anesthesia (maternal) P04.0
      blood loss P02.1
      circulatory disease P00.3
      condition P00.9
        specified NEC P00.89
      delivery P03.9
        Cesarean P03.4
        forceps P03.2
        vacuum extractor P03.3
      diabetes mellitus (pre-existing) P70.1
      disorder P00.9
        specified NEC P00.89
      drugs (addictive) (illegal) NEC P04.49
      ectopic pregnancy P01.4
      gestational diabetes P70.0
      hemorrhage P02.1
      hypertensive disorder P00.0
      incompetent cervix P01.0
      infectious disease P00.2
      injury P00.5
      labor and delivery P03.9
      malpresentation before labor P01.7
      maternal death P01.6
      medical procedure P00.7
      medication P04.1
      multiple pregnancy P01.5
      nutritional disorder P00.4
      oligohydramnios P01.2
      parasitic disease P00.2
      periodontal disease P00.81
      placenta previa P02.0
      polyhydramnios P01.3
      precipitate delivery P03.5
      pregnancy P01.9
        specified P01.8
      premature rupture of membranes P01.1
      renal disease P00.1
      respiratory disease P00.3
      surgical procedure P00.6
      urinary tract disease P00.1
      uterine contraction (abnormal) P03.6
    meconium peritonitis P78.0
    medication (legal) (maternal use) (prescribed) P04.1
    membrane abnormalities P02.9
      specified NEC P02.8
    membranitis P02.7
    methamphetamine(s) P04.49
    mixed metabolic and respiratory acidosis P84
    neonatal abstinence syndrome P96.1
    noxious substances transmitted via placenta or
        breast milk P04.9
      specified NEC P04.8
    nutritional supplements P04.5
    placenta previa P02.0
    placental
      abnormality (functional) (morphological)
        P02.20
        specified NEC P02.29
      dysfunction P02.29
      infarction P02.29
      insufficiency P02.29
      separation NEC P02.1
      transfusion syndromes P02.3
    placentitis P02.7
    precipitate delivery P03.5
    prolapsed cord P02.4
    respiratory arrest P28.81
    slow intrauterine growth P05.9
    tobacco P04.2

Newborn — continued
  affected by — continued
    twin to twin transplacental transfusion P02.3
    umbilical cord (tightly) around neck P02.5
    umbilical cord condition P02.60
      short cord P02.69
      specified NEC P02.69
    uterine contractions (abnormal) P03.6
    vasa previa P02.69
      from intrauterine blood loss P50.0
  apnea P28.3
    obstructive P28.4
    primary P28.3
    specified P28.4
  born in hospital Z38.00
    by cesarean Z38.01
  born outside hospital Z38.1
  breast buds P96.89
  breast engorgement P83.4
  check-up — see Newborn, examination
  convulsion P90
  dehydration P74.1
  examination
    8 to 28 days old Z00.111
    under 8 days old Z00.110
  fever P81.9
    environmentally-induced P81.0
  hyperbilirubinemia P59.9
    of prematurity P59.0
  hypernatremia P74.2
  hyponatremia P74.2
  infection P39.9
    candidal P37.5
    specified NEC P39.8
    urinary tract P39.3
  jaundice P59.8
    due to
      breast milk inhibitor P59.3
      hepatocellular damage P59.20
        specified NEC P59.29
      preterm delivery P59.0
    of prematurity P59.0
    specified NEC P59.8
  late metabolic acidosis P74.0
  mastitis P39.0
    infective P39.0
    noninfective P83.4
  multiple born NEC Z38.8
    born in hospital Z38.68
      by cesarean Z38.69
    born outside hospital Z38.7
  omphalitis P38.9
    with mild hemorrhage P38.1
    without hemorrhage P38.9
  post-term P08.21
  prolonged gestation (over 42 completed weeks)
    P08.22
  quadruplet Z38.8
    born in hospital Z38.63
      by cesarean Z38.64
    born outside hospital Z38.7
  quintuplet Z38.8
    born in hospital Z38.65
      by cesarean Z38.66
    born outside hospital Z38.7
  seizure P90
  sepsis (congenital) P36.9
    due to
      anaerobes NEC P36.5
      Escherichia coli P36.4
      Staphylococcus P36.30
        aureus P36.2
        specified NEC P36.39
      Streptococcus P36.10
        group B P36.0
        specified NEC P36.19
    specified NEC P36.8
  triplet Z38.8
    born in hospital Z38.61
      by cesarean Z38.62
    born outside hospital Z38.7
  twin Z38.5
    born in hospital Z38.30
      by cesarean Z38.31
    born outside hospital Z38.4
  vomiting P92.09
    bilious P92.01
  weight check Z00.111

Newcastle conjunctivitis or disease B30.8
Nezelof's syndrome (pure alymphocytosis) D81.4
Niacin (amide) **deficiency** E52
Nicolas (-Durand)-**Favre disease** A55
Nicotine — see Tobacco
Nicotinic acid deficiency E52
Niemann-Pick disease or syndrome E75.249
  specified NEC E75.248
  type
    A E75.240
    B E75.241
    C E75.242
    D E75.243
Night
  blindness — see Blindness, night
  sweats R61
  terrors (child) F51.4
Nightmares (REM sleep type) F51.5
Nipple — see condition
Nisbet's chancre A57
Nishimoto (-Takeuchi) **disease** I67.5
Nitritoid crisis or reaction — see Crisis, nitritoid
Nitrosohemoglobinemia D74.8
Njovera A65
Nocardiosis, nocardiasis A43.9
  cutaneous A43.1
  lung A43.0
  pneumonia A43.0
  pulmonary A43.0
  specified site NEC A43.8
Nocturia R35.1
  psychogenic F45.8
Nocturnal — see condition
Nodal rhythm I49.8
Node(s) (see also Nodule)
  Bouchard's (with arthropathy) M15.2
  Haygarth's M15.8
  Heberden's (with arthropathy) M15.1
  larynx J38.7
  lymph — see condition
  milker's B08.03
  Osler's I33.0
  Schmorl's — see Schmorl's disease
  singer's J38.2
  teacher's J38.2
  tuberculous — see Tuberculosis, lymph gland
  vocal cord J38.2
Nodule(s), **nodular**
  actinomycotic — see Actinomycosis
  breast NEC N63
  colloid (cystic), thyroid E04.1
  cutaneous — see Swelling, localized
  endometrial (stromal) D26.1
  Haygarth's M15.8
  inflammatory — see Inflammation
  juxta-articular
    syphilitic A52.77
    yaws A66.7
  larynx J38.7
  lung, solitary (subsegmental branch of the bronchial
    tree) R91.1
    multiple R91.8
  milker's B08.03
  prostate N40.2
    with lower urinary tract symptoms (LUTS) N40.3
    without lower urinary tract symtpoms (LUTS) N40.2
  pulmonary, solitary (subsegmental branch of the
    bronchial tree) R91.1
  retrocardiac R09.89
  rheumatoid M06.30
    ankle M06.37- ☑
    elbow M06.32- ☑
    foot joint M06.37- ☑
    hand joint M06.34- ☑
    hip M06.35- ☑
    knee M06.36- ☑
    multiple site M06.39
    shoulder M06.31- ☑
    vertebra M06.38
    wrist M06.33- ☑
  scrotum (inflammatory) N49.2
  singer's J38.2
  solitary, lung (subsegmental branch of the bronchial
    tree) R91.1
    multiple R91.8
  subcutaneous — see Swelling, localized
  teacher's J38.2

Nodule(s), nodular — *continued*
  thyroid (cold) (gland) (nontoxic) E04.1
    with thyrotoxicosis E05.20
      with thyroid storm E05.21
    toxic or with hyperthyroidism E05.20
      with thyroid storm E05.21
  vocal cord J38.2
Noma (gangrenous) (hospital) (infective) A69.0
  auricle I96
  mouth A69.0
  pudendi N76.89
  vulvae N76.89
Nomad, nomadism Z59.0
Non-Hodgkin lymphoma NEC — *see* Lymphoma, non-Hodgkin
Non-ketotic hyperglycinemia E72.51
Non-working side interference M26.56
Nonautoimmune hemolytic anemia D59.4
  drug-induced D59.2
Nonclosure (*see also* Imperfect, closure)
  ductus arteriosus (Botallo's) Q25.0
  foramen
    botalli Q21.1
    ovale Q21.1
Noncompliance Z91.19
  with
    dialysis Z91.15
    dietary regimen Z91.11
    medical treatment Z91.19
    medication regimen NEC Z91.14
      underdosing (*see also* Table of Drugs and Chemicals, categories T36-T50, with final character 6) Z91.14
        intentional NEC Z91.128
          due to financial hardship of patient Z91.120
        unintentional NEC Z91.138
          due to patient's age related debility Z91.130
    renal dialysis Z91.15
Nondescent (congenital) (*see also* Malposition, congenital)
  cecum Q43.3
  colon Q43.3
  testicle Q53.9
    bilateral Q53.20
      abdominal Q53.21
      perineal Q53.22
    unilateral Q53.10
      abdominal Q53.11
      perineal Q53.12
Nondevelopment
  brain Q02
    part of Q04.3
  heart Q24.8
  organ or site, congenital NEC — *see* Hypoplasia
Nonengagement
  head NEC O32.4
    in labor, causing obstructed labor O64.8 ☑
Nonexanthematous tick fever A93.2
Nonexpansion, lung (newborn) P28.0
Nonfunctioning
  cystic duct (*see also* Disease, gallbladder) K82.8
  gallbladder (*see also* Disease, gallbladder) K82.8
  kidney N28.9
  labyrinth — *see* subcategory H83.2 ☑
Nonimplantation, ovum N97.2
Noninsufflation, fallopian tube N97.1
Nonne-Milroy syndrome Q82.0
Nonovulation N97.0
Nonpatent fallopian tube N97.1
Nonpneumatization, lung NEC P28.0
Nonrotation — *see* Malrotation
Nonsecretion, urine — *see* Anuria
Nonunion
  fracture — *see* Fracture, by site
  organ or site, congenital NEC — *see* Imperfect, closure
  symphysis pubis, congenital Q74.2
Nonvisualization, gallbladder R93.2
Nonvital, nonvitalized tooth K04.99
Noonan's syndrome Q87.1
Normocytic anemia (infectional) due to blood loss (chronic) D50.0
  acute D62
Norrie's disease (congenital) Q15.8
North American blastomycosis B40.9
Norwegian itch B86

Nose, nasal — *see* condition
Nose-picking F98.8
Nosebleed R04.0
Nosomania F45.21
Nosophobia F45.22
Nostalgia F43.20
Notch of iris Q13.2
Notching nose, congenital (tip) Q30.2
Nothnagel's
  syndrome — *see* Strabismus, paralytic, third nerve
  vasomotor acroparesthesia I73.89
Novy's relapsing fever A68.9
  louse-borne A68.0
  tick-borne A68.1
Noxious
  foodstuffs, poisoning by — *see* Poisoning, food, noxious, plant
  substances transmitted through placenta or breast milk P04.9
Nucleus pulposus — *see* condition
Numbness R20.0
Nuns' knee — *see* Bursitis, prepatellar
Nursemaid's elbow S53.03- ☑
Nutcracker esophagus K22.4
Nutmeg liver K76.1
Nutrient element deficiency E61.9
  specified NEC E61.8
Nutrition deficient or insufficient (*see also* Malnutrition) E46
  due to
    insufficient food T73.0 ☑
    lack of
      care (child) T76.02 ☑
        adult T76.01 ☑
      food T73.0 ☑
Nutritional stunting E45
Nyctalopia (night blindness) — *see* Blindness, night
Nycturia R35.1
  psychogenic F45.8
Nymphomania F52.8
Nystagmus H55.00
  benign paroxysmal — *see* Vertigo, benign paroxysmal
  central positional H81.4- ☑
  congenital H55.01
  dissociated H55.04
  latent H55.02
  miners' H55.09
  positional
    benign paroxysmal H81.4- ☑
    central H81.4- ☑
  specified form NEC H55.09
  visual deprivation H55.03

O

Obermeyer's relapsing fever (European) A68.0
Obesity E66.9
  with alveolar hyperventilation E66.2
  adrenal E27.8
  complicating
    childbirth O99.214
    pregnancy O99.21- ☑
    puerperium O99.215
  constitutional E66.8
  dietary counseling and surveillance Z71.3
  drug-induced E66.1
  due to
    drug E66.1
    excess calories E66.09
      morbid E66.01
      severe E66.01
  endocrine E66.8
  endogenous E66.8
  familial E66.8
  glandular E66.8
  hypothyroid — *see* Hypothyroidism
  morbid E66.01
    with alveolar hypoventilation E66.2
    due to excess calories E66.01
  nutritional E66.09
  pituitary E23.6
  severe E66.01
  specified type NEC E66.8
Oblique — *see* condition
Obliteration
  appendix (lumen) K38.8
  artery I77.1

Obliteration — *continued*
  bile duct (noncalculous) K83.1
  common duct (noncalculous) K83.1
  cystic duct — *see* Obstruction, gallbladder
  disease, arteriol I77.1
  endometrium N85.8
  eye, anterior chamber — *see* Disorder, globe, hypotony
  fallopian tube N97.1
  lymphatic vessel I89.0
    due to mastectomy I97.2
  organ or site, congenital NEC — *see* Atresia, by site
  ureter N13.5
    with infection N13.6
  urethra — *see* Stricture, urethra
  vein I87.8
  vestibule (oral) K08.8
Observation (following) (for) (without need for further medical care) Z04.9
  accident NEC Z04.3
    at work Z04.2
    transport Z04.1
  adverse effect of drug Z03.6
  alleged rape or sexual assault (victim), ruled out
    adult Z04.41
    child Z04.42
  criminal assault Z04.8
  development state
    adolescent Z00.3
    period of rapid growth in childhood Z00.2
    puberty Z00.3
  disease, specified NEC Z03.89
  following work accident Z04.2
  growth and development state — *see* Observation, development state
  injuries (accidental) NEC (*see also* Observation, accident)
  newborn (for suspected condition, ruled out) — *see* Newborn, affected by (suspected to be), maternal (complication of) (use of)
  postpartum
    immediately after delivery Z39.0
    routine follow-up Z39.2
  pregnancy (normal) (without complication) Z34.9- ☑
    high risk O09.9- ☑
  suicide attempt, alleged NEC Z03.89
    self-poisoning Z03.6
  suspected, ruled out (*see also* Suspected condition, ruled out)
    abuse, physical
      adult Z04.71
      child Z04.72
    accident at work Z04.2
    adult battering victim Z04.71
    child battering victim Z04.72
    condition NEC Z03.89
      newborn — *see* Newborn, affected by (suspected to be), maternal (complication of) (use of)
    drug poisoning or adverse effect Z03.6
    exposure (to)
      anthrax Z03.810
      biological agent NEC Z03.818
    inflicted injury NEC Z04.8
    suicide attempt, alleged Z03.89
      self-poisoning Z03.6
    toxic effects from ingested substance (drug) (poison) Z03.6
  toxic effects from ingested substance (drug) (poison) Z03.6
Obsession, obsessional state F42
Obsessive-compulsive neurosis or reaction F42
Obstetric embolism, septic — *see* Embolism, obstetric, septic
Obstetrical trauma (complicating delivery) O71.9
  with or following ectopic or molar pregnancy O08.6
  specified type NEC O71.89
Obstipation — *see* Constipation
Obstruction, obstructed, obstructive
  airway J98.8
    with
      allergic alveolitis J67.9
      asthma J45.909
        with
          exacerbation (acute) J45.901
          status asthmaticus J45.902
      bronchiectasis J47.9

Obstruction, obstructed, obstructive — *continued*
airway — *continued*
   with — *continued*
      bronchiectasis — *continued*
         with
            exacerbation (acute) J47.1
            lower respiratory infection J47.0
         bronchitis (chronic) J44.9
         emphysema J43.9
      chronic J44.9
         with
            allergic alveolitis — *see* Pneumonitis, hyper-
               sensitivity
            bronchiectasis J47.9
               with
                  exacerbation (acute) J47.1
                  lower respiratory infection J47.0
      due to
         foreign body — *see* Foreign body, by site,
            causing asphyxia
         inhalation of fumes or vapors J68.9
         laryngospasm J38.5
   ampulla of Vater K83.1
   aortic (heart) (valve) — *see* Stenosis, aortic
   aortoiliac I74.09
   aqueduct of Sylvius G91.1
      congenital Q03.0
         with spina bifida — *see* Spina bifida, by site,
            with hydrocephalus
   Arnold-Chiari — *see* Arnold-Chiari disease
   artery (*see also* Embolism, artery) I74.9
      basilar (complete) (partial) — *see* Occlusion, artery,
         basilar
      carotid (complete) (partial) — *see* Occlusion, artery,
         carotid
      cerebellar — *see* Occlusion, artery, cerebellar
      cerebral (anterior) (middle) (posterior) — *see* Oc-
         clusion, artery, cerebral
      precerebral — *see* Occlusion, artery, precerebral
      renal N28.0
      retinal NEC — *see* Occlusion, artery, retina
      vertebral (complete) (partial) — *see* Occlusion,
         artery, vertebral
   band (intestinal) K56.69
   bile duct or passage (common) (hepatic) (noncalcu-
      lous) K83.1
      with calculus K80.51
      congenital (causing jaundice) Q44.3
   biliary (duct) (tract) K83.1
      gallbladder K82.0
   bladder-neck (acquired) N32.0
      congenital Q64.31
      due to hyperplasia (hypertrophy) of prostate —
         see Hyperplasia, prostate
   bowel — *see* Obstruction, intestine
   bronchus J98.09
   canal, ear — *see* Stenosis, external ear canal
   cardia K22.2
   caval veins (inferior) (superior) I87.1
   cecum — *see* Obstruction, intestine
   circulatory I99.8
   colon — *see* Obstruction, intestine
   common duct (noncalculous) K83.1
   coronary (artery) — *see* Occlusion, coronary
   cystic duct (*see also* Obstruction, gallbladder)
      with calculus K80.21
   device, implant or graft (*see also* Complications, by
      site and type, mechanical) T85.698 ☑
      arterial graft NEC — *see* Complication, cardiovas-
         cular device, mechanical, vascular
      catheter NEC T85.628 ☑
         cystostomy T83.090 ☑
         dialysis (renal) T82.49 ☑
            intraperitoneal T85.691 ☑
         infusion NEC T82.594 ☑
            spinal (epidural) (subdural) T85.690 ☑
         urinary, indwelling T83.098 ☑
      due to infection T85.79 ☑
      gastrointestinal — *see* Complications, prosthetic
         device, mechanical, gastrointestinal device
      genital NEC T83.498 ☑
         intrauterine contraceptive device T83.39 ☑
         penile prosthesis T83.490 ☑
      heart NEC — *see* Complication, cardiovascular de-
         vice, mechanical
      joint prosthesis — *see* Complications, joint prosthe-
         sis, mechanical, specified NEC, by site

Obstruction, obstructed, obstructive — *continued*
device, implant or graft (*see also* Complications, by site
   and type, mechanical) — *continued*
   orthopedic NEC — *see* Complication, orthopedic,
      device, mechanical
   specified NEC T85.628 ☑
   urinary NEC (*see also* Complication, genitourinary,
      device, urinary, mechanical)
      graft T83.29 ☑
   vascular NEC — *see* Complication, cardiovascular
      device, mechanical
   ventricular intracranial shunt T85.09 ☑
due to foreign body accidentally left in operative
   wound T81.529 ☑
duodenum K31.5
ejaculatory duct N50.8
esophagus K22.2
eustachian tube (complete) (partial) H68.10- ☑
   cartilagenous (extrinsic) H68.13- ☑
      intrinsic H68.12- ☑
   osseous H68.11- ☑
fallopian tube (bilateral) N97.1
fecal K56.41
   with hernia — *see* Hernia, by site, with obstruction
foramen of Monro (congenital) Q03.8
   with spina bifida — *see* Spina bifida, by site, with
      hydrocephalus
foreign body — *see* Foreign body
gallbladder K82.0
   with calculus, stones K80.21
   congenital Q44.1
gastric outlet K31.1
gastrointestinal — *see* Obstruction, intestine
hepatic K76.89
   duct (noncalculous) K83.1
ileum — *see* Obstruction, intestine
iliofemoral (artery) I74.5
intestine K56.60
   with
      adhesions (intestinal) (peritoneal) K56.5
   adynamic K56.0
   by gallstone K56.3
   congenital (small) Q41.9
      large Q42.9
         specified part NEC Q42.8
   neurogenic K56.0
      Hirschsprung's disease or megacolon Q43.1
   newborn P76.9
      due to
         fecaliths P76.8
         inspissated milk P76.2
         meconium (plug) P76.0
            in mucoviscidosis E84.11
      specified NEC P76.8
   postoperative K91.3
   reflex K56.0
   specified NEC K56.69
   volvulus K56.2
intracardiac ball valve prosthesis T82.09 ☑
jejunum — *see* Obstruction, intestine
joint prosthesis — *see* Complications, joint prosthesis,
   mechanical, specified NEC, by site
kidney (calices) N28.89
labor — *see* Delivery
lacrimal (passages) (duct)
   by
      dacryolith — *see* Dacryolith
      stenosis — *see* Stenosis, lacrimal
   congenital Q10.5
   neonatal H04.53- ☑
lacrimonasal duct — *see* Obstruction, lacrimal
lacteal, with steatorrhea K90.2
laryngitis — *see* Laryngitis
larynx NEC J38.6
   congenital Q31.8
lung J98.4
   disease, chronic J44.9
lymphatic I89.0
meconium (plug)
   newborn P76.0
      due to fecaliths P76.0
         in mucoviscidosis E84.11
mitral — *see* Stenosis, mitral
nasal J34.89
nasolacrimal duct (*see also* Obstruction, lacrimal)
   congenital Q10.5
nasopharynx J39.2
nose J34.89

Obstruction, obstructed, obstructive — *continued*
organ or site, congenital NEC — *see* Atresia, by site
pancreatic duct K86.8
parotid duct or gland K11.8
pelviureteral junction N13.5
   congenital Q62.39
pharynx J39.2
portal (circulation) (vein) I81
prostate (*see also* Hyperplasia, prostate)
   valve (urinary) N32.0
pulmonary valve (heart) I37.0
pyelonephritis (chronic) N11.1
pylorus
   adult K31.1
   congenital or infantile Q40.0
rectosigmoid — *see* Obstruction, intestine
rectum K62.4
renal N28.89
   outflow N13.8
   pelvis, congenital Q62.39
respiratory J98.8
   chronic J44.9
retinal (vessels) H34.9
salivary duct (any) K11.8
   with calculus K11.5
sigmoid — *see* Obstruction, intestine
sinus (accessory) (nasal) J34.89
Stensen's duct K11.8
stomach NEC K31.89
   acute K31.0
   congenital Q40.2
   due to pylorospasm K31.3
submandibular duct K11.8
submaxillary gland K11.8
   with calculus K11.5
thoracic duct I89.0
thrombotic — *see* Thrombosis
trachea J39.8
tracheostomy airway J95.03
tricuspid (valve) — *see* Stenosis, tricuspid
upper respiratory, congenital Q34.8
ureter (functional) (pelvic junction) NEC N13.5
   with
      hydronephrosis N13.1
         with infection N13.6
      pyelonephritis (chronic) N11.1
   congenital Q62.39
   due to calculus — *see* Calculus, ureter
urethra NEC N36.8
   congenital Q64.39
urinary (moderate) N13.9
   due to hyperplasia (hypertrophy) of prostate —
      see Hyperplasia, prostate
   organ or tract (lower) N13.9
   prostatic valve N32.0
   specified NEC N13.8
uropathy N13.9
uterus N85.8
vagina N89.5
valvular — *see* Endocarditis
vein, venous I87.1
   caval (inferior) (superior) I87.1
   thrombotic — *see* Thrombosis
vena cava (inferior) (superior) I87.1
vesical NEC N32.0
vesicourethral orifice N32.0
   congenital Q64.31
vessel NEC I99.8
Obturator — *see* condition
Occlusal wear, teeth K03.0
Occlusio pupillae — *see* Membrane, pupillary
Occlusion, occluded
anus K62.4
   congenital Q42.3
      with fistula Q42.2
aortoiliac (chronic) I74.09
aqueduct of Sylvius G91.1
   congenital Q03.0
      with spina bifida — *see* Spina bifida, by site,
         with hydrocephalus
artery (*see also* Embolism, artery) I74.9
   auditory, internal I65.8
   basilar I65.1
      with
         infarction I63.22
            due to
               embolism I63.12
               thrombosis I63.02

Occlusion, occluded — *continued*
  artery (*see also* Embolism, artery) — *continued*
    brain or cerebral I66.9
      with infarction (due to) I63.5 ☑
        embolism I63.4 ☑
        thrombosis I63.3 ☑
    carotid I65.2- ☑
      with
        infarction I63.23- ☑
          due to
            embolism I63.13- ☑
            thrombosis I63.03- ☑
    cerebellar (anterior inferior) (posterior inferior) (superior) I66.3
      with infarction I63.54- ☑
        due to
          embolism I63.44- ☑
          thrombosis I63.34- ☑
    cerebral I66.9
      with infarction I63.50
        due to
          embolism I63.40
            specified NEC I63.49
          thrombosis I63.30
            specified NEC I63.39
      anterior I66.1- ☑
        with infarction I63.52- ☑
          due to
            embolism I63.42- ☑
            thrombosis I63.32- ☑
      middle I66.0- ☑
        with infarction I63.51- ☑
          due to
            embolism I63.41- ☑
            thrombosis I63.31- ☑
      posterior I66.2- ☑
        with infarction I63.53- ☑
          due to
            embolism I63.43- ☑
            thrombosis I63.33- ☑
      specified NEC I66.8
        with infarction I63.59
          due to
            embolism I63.4 ☑
            thrombosis I63.3 ☑
    choroidal (anterior) — *see* Occlusion, artery, precerebral, specified NEC
    communicating posterior — *see* Occlusion, artery, cerebral, specified NEC
    complete
      coronary I25.82
      extremities I70.92
    coronary (acute) (thrombotic) (without myocardial infarction) I24.0
      with myocardial infarction — *see* Infarction, myocardium
      chronic total I25.82
      complete I25.82
      healed or old I25.2
      total (chronic) I25.82
    hypophyseal — *see* Occlusion, artery, precerebral, specified NEC
    iliac I74.5
    lower extremities due to stenosis or stricture I77.1
    mesenteric (embolic) (thrombotic) K55.0
    perforating — *see* Occlusion, artery, cerebral, specified NEC
    peripheral I77.9
      thrombotic or embolic I74.4
    pontine — *see* Occlusion, artery, cerebral, specified NEC
    precerebral I65.9
      with infarction I63.20
        due to
          embolism I63.10
            specified NEC I63.19
          thrombosis I63.00
            specified NEC I63.09
        specified NEC I63.29
      basilar — *see* Occlusion, artery, basilar
      carotid — *see* Occlusion, artery, carotid
      puerperal O88.23
      specified NEC I65.8
        with infarction I63.29
          due to
            embolism I63.19
            thrombosis I63.00

Occlusion, occluded — *continued*
  artery (*see also* Embolism, artery) — *continued*
    precerebral — *continued*
      vertebral — *see* Occlusion, artery, vertebral
    renal N28.0
    retinal
      branch H34.23- ☑
      central H34.1- ☑
      partial H34.21- ☑
      transient H34.0- ☑
    spinal — *see* Occlusion, artery, precerebral, vertebral
    total (chronic)
      coronary I25.82
      extremities I70.92
    vertebral I65.0- ☑
      with
        infarction I63.21- ☑
          due to
            embolism I63.11- ☑
            thrombosis I63.01- ☑
  basilar artery — *see* Occlusion, artery, basilar
  bile duct (common) (hepatic) (noncalculous) K83.1
  bowel — *see* Obstruction, intestine
  carotid (artery) (common) (internal) — *see* Occlusion, artery, carotid
  centric (of teeth) M26.59
    maximum intercuspation discrepancy M26.55
  cerebellar (artery) — *see* Occlusion, artery, cerebellar
  cerebral (artery) — *see* Occlusion, artery, cerebral
  cerebrovascular (*see also* Occlusion, artery, cerebral)
    with infarction I63.5 ☑
  cervical canal — *see* Stricture, cervix
  cervix (uteri) — *see* Stricture, cervix
  choanal Q30.0
  choroidal (artery) — *see* Occlusion, artery, precerebral, specified NEC
  colon — *see* Obstruction, intestine
  communicating posterior artery — *see* Occlusion, artery, precerebral, specified NEC
  coronary (artery) (vein) (thrombotic) (*see also* Infarct, myocardium)
    chronic total I25.82
    healed or old I25.2
    not resulting in infarction I24.0
    total (chronic) I25.82
  cystic duct — *see* Obstruction, gallbladder
  embolic — *see* Embolism
  fallopian tube N97.1
    congenital Q50.6
  gallbladder (*see also* Obstruction, gallbladder)
    congenital (causing jaundice) Q44.1
  gingiva, traumatic K06.2
  hymen N89.6
    congenital Q52.3
  hypophyseal (artery) — *see* Occlusion, artery, precerebral, specified NEC
  iliac artery I74.5
  intestine — *see* Obstruction, intestine
  lacrimal passages — *see* Obstruction, lacrimal
  lung J98.4
  lymph or lymphatic channel I89.0
  mammary duct N64.89
  mesenteric artery (embolic) (thrombotic) K55.0
  nose J34.89
    congenital Q30.0
  organ or site, congenital NEC — *see* Atresia, by site
  oviduct N97.1
    congenital Q50.6
  peripheral arteries
    due to stricture or stenosis I77.1
    upper extremity I74.2
  pontine (artery) — *see* Occlusion, artery, precerebral, specified NEC
  posterior lingual, of mandibular teeth M26.29
  precerebral artery — *see* Occlusion, artery, precerebral
  punctum lacrimale — *see* Obstruction, lacrimal
  pupil — *see* Membrane, pupillary
  pylorus, adult (*see also* Stricture, pylorus) K31.1
  renal artery N28.0
  retina, retinal
    artery — *see* Occlusion, artery, retinal
    vein (central) H34.81- ☑
      engorgement H34.82- ☑
      tributary H34.83- ☑
    vessels H34.9

Occlusion, occluded — *continued*
  spinal artery — *see* Occlusion, artery, precerebral, vertebral
  teeth (mandibular) (posterior lingual) M26.29
  thoracic duct I89.0
  thrombotic — *see* Thrombosis, artery
  traumatic
    edentulous (alveolar) ridge K06.2
    gingiva K06.2
    periodontal K05.5
  tubal N97.1
  ureter (complete) (partial) N13.5
    congenital Q62.10
  ureteropelvic junction N13.5
    congenital Q62.11
  ureterovesical orifice N13.5
    congenital Q62.12
  urethra — *see* Stricture, urethra
  uterus N85.8
  vagina N89.5
  vascular NEC I99.8
  vein — *see* Thrombosis
    retinal — *see* Occlusion, retinal, vein
  vena cava (inferior) (superior) — *see* Embolism, vena cava
  ventricle (brain) NEC G91.1
  vertebral (artery) — *see* Occlusion, artery, vertebral
  vessel (blood) I99.8
  vulva N90.5

Occult
  blood in feces (stools) R19.5

Occupational
  problems NEC Z56.89

Ochlophobia — *see* Agoraphobia

Ochronosis (endogenous) E70.29

Ocular muscle — *see* condition

Oculogyric crisis or disturbance H51.8
  psychogenic F45.8

Oculomotor syndrome H51.9

Oculopathy
  syphilitic NEC A52.71
    congenital
      early A50.01
      late A50.30
    early (secondary) A51.43
    late A52.71

Oddi's sphincter spasm K83.4

Odontalgia K08.8

Odontoameloblastoma — *see* Cyst, calcifying odontogenic

Odontoclasia K03.89

Odontodysplasia, regional K00.4

Odontogenesis imperfecta K00.5

Odontoma (ameloblastic) (complex) (compound) (fibroameloblastic) — *see* Cyst, calcifying odontogenic

Odontomyelitis (closed) (open) K04.0

Odontorrhagia K08.8

Odontosarcoma, ameloblastic C41.1
  upper jaw (bone) C41.0

Oestriasis — *see* Myiasis

Oguchi's disease H53.63

Ohara's disease — *see* Tularemia

Oidiomycosis — *see* Candidiasis

Oidium albicans infection — *see* Candidiasis

Old age (without mention of debility) R54
  dementia F03 ☑

Old (previous) **myocardial infarction** I25.2

Olfactory — *see* condition

Oligemia — *see* Anemia

Oligoastrocytoma
  specified site — *see* Neoplasm, malignant, by site
  unspecified site C71.9

Oligocythemia D64.9

Oligodendroblastoma
  specified site — *see* Neoplasm, malignant
  unspecified site C71.9

Oligodendroglioma
  anaplastic type
    specified site — *see* Neoplasm, malignant, by site
    unspecified site C71.9
  specified site — *see* Neoplasm, malignant, by site
  unspecified site C71.9

Oligodontia — *see* Anodontia

Oligoencephalon Q02

Oligohidrosis L74.4

Oligohydramnios O41.0- ☑

Oligohydrosis L74.4

Ossification — continued
  myocardium, myocardial — see Degeneration, myocardial
  penis N48.89
  periarticular — see Disorder, joint, specified type NEC
  pinna — see Disorder, pinna, specified type NEC
  rider's bone — see Ossification, muscle, specified NEC
  sclera H15.89
  subperiosteal, post-traumatic M89.8X- ☑
  tendon — see Disorder, tendon, specified type NEC
  trachea J39.8
  tympanic membrane — see Disorder, tympanic
    membrane, specified NEC
  vitreous (humor) — see Deposit, crystalline
Osteitis (see also Osteomyelitis)
  alveolar M27.3
  condensans M85.30
    ankle M85.37- ☑
    foot M85.37- ☑
    forearm M85.33- ☑
    hand M85.34- ☑
    lower leg M85.36- ☑
    multiple site M85.39
    neck M85.38
    rib M85.38
    shoulder M85.31- ☑
    skull M85.38
    specified site NEC M85.38
    thigh M85.35- ☑
    toe M85.37- ☑
    upper arm M85.32- ☑
    vertebra M85.38
  deformans M88.9
    in (due to)
      malignant neoplasm of bone C41.9 [M90.60]
      neoplastic disease (see also Neoplasm)
        D49.9 [M90.60]
        carpus D49.9 [M90.64-] ☑
        clavicle D49.9 [M90.61-] ☑
        femur D49.9 [M90.65-] ☑
        fibula D49.9 [M90.66-] ☑
        finger D49.9 [M90.64-] ☑
        humerus D49.9 [M90.62-] ☑
        ilium D49.9 [M90.65-] ☑
        ischium D49.9 [M90.65-] ☑
        metacarpus D49.9 [M90.64-] ☑
        metatarsus D49.9 [M90.67-] ☑
        multiple sites D49.9 [M90.69]
        neck D49.9 [M90.68]
        radius D49.9 [M90.63-] ☑
        rib D49.9 [M90.68]
        scapula D49.9 [M90.61-] ☑
        skull D49.9 [M90.68]
        tarsus D49.9 [M90.67-] ☑
        tibia D49.9 [M90.66-] ☑
        toe D49.9 [M90.67-] ☑
        ulna D49.9 [M90.63-] ☑
        vertebra D49.9 [M90.68]
    skull M88.0
    specified NEC — see Paget's disease, bone, by site
    vertebra M88.1
  due to yaws A66.6
  fibrosa NEC — see Cyst, bone, by site
    circumscripta — see Dysplasia, fibrous, bone NEC
    cystica (generalisata) E21.0
      disseminata Q78.1
      osteoplastica E21.0
    fragilitans Q78.0
  Garr's (sclerosing) — see Osteomyelitis, specified type NEC
  jaw (acute) (chronic) (lower) (suppurative) (upper) M27.2
  parathyroid E21.0
  petrous bone (acute) (chronic) — see Petrositis
  sclerotic, nonsuppurative — see Osteomyelitis, specified type NEC
  tuberculosa A18.09
    cystica D86.89
    multiplex cystoides D86.89
Osteo-onycho-arthro-dysplasia Q79.8
Osteo-onychodysplasia, hereditary Q79.8
Osteoarthritis M19.90
  ankle M19.07- ☑
  elbow M19.02- ☑
  foot joint M19.07- ☑
  generalized M15.9
    erosive M15.4

Osteoarthritis — continued
  generalized — continued
    primary M15.0
    specified NEC M15.8
  hand joint M19.04- ☑
    first carpometacarpal joint M18.9-
  hip M16.1- ☑
    bilateral M16.0
    due to hip dysplasia (unilateral) M16.3- ☑
      bilateral M16.2
  interphalangeal
    distal (Heberden) M15.1
    proximal (Bouchard) M15.2
  knee M17.9-
    bilateral M17.0
  post-traumatic NEC M19.92
    ankle M19.17- ☑
    elbow M19.12- ☑
    foot joint M19.17- ☑
    hand joint M19.14- ☑
      first carpometacarpal joint M18.3- ☑
        bilateral M18.2
    hip M16.5- ☑
      bilateral M16.4
    knee M17.3- ☑
      bilateral M17.2
    shoulder M19.11- ☑
    wrist M19.13- ☑
  primary M19.91
    ankle M19.07- ☑
    elbow M19.02- ☑
    foot joint M19.07- ☑
    hand joint M19.04- ☑
      first carpometacarpal joint M18.1- ☑
        bilateral M18.0
    hip M16.1- ☑
      bilateral M16.0
    knee M17.1- ☑
      bilateral M17.0
    shoulder M19.01- ☑
    spine — see Spondylosis
    wrist M19.03- ☑
  secondary M19.93
    ankle M19.27- ☑
    elbow M19.22- ☑
    foot joint M19.27- ☑
    hand joint M19.24- ☑
      first carpometacarpal joint M18.5- ☑
        bilateral M18.4
    hip M16.7
      bilateral M16.6
    knee M17.5
      bilateral M17.4
    multiple M15.3
    shoulder M19.21- ☑
    spine — see Spondylosis
    wrist M19.23- ☑
  shoulder M19.01- ☑
  spine — see Spondylosis
  wrist M19.03- ☑
Osteoarthropathy (hypertrophic) M19.90
  ankle — see Osteoarthritis, primary, ankle
  elbow — see Osteoarthritis, primary, elbow
  foot joint — see Osteoarthritis, primary, foot
  hand joint — see Osteoarthritis, primary, hand joint
  knee joint — see Osteoarthritis, primary, knee
  multiple site — see Osteoarthritis, primary, multiple joint
  pulmonary (see also Osteoarthropathy, specified type NEC)
    hypertrophic — see Osteoarthropathy, hypertrophic, specified type NEC
  secondary — see Osteoarthropathy, specified type NEC
  secondary hypertrophic — see Osteoarthropathy, specified type NEC
  shoulder — see Osteoarthritis, primary, shoulder
  specified joint NEC — see Osteoarthritis, primary, specified joint NEC
  specified type NEC M89.40
    carpus M89.44- ☑
    clavicle M89.41- ☑
    femur M89.45- ☑
    fibula M89.46- ☑
    finger M89.44- ☑
    humerus M89.42- ☑
    ilium M89.459

Osteoarthropathy — continued
  specified type — continued
    ischium M89.459
    metacarpus M89.44- ☑
    metatarsus M89.47- ☑
    multiple sites M89.49
    neck M89.48
    radius M89.43- ☑
    rib M89.48
    scapula M89.41- ☑
    skull M89.48
    tarsus M89.47- ☑
    tibia M89.46- ☑
    toe M89.47- ☑
    ulna M89.43- ☑
    vertebra M89.48
  spine — see Spondylosis
  wrist — see Osteoarthritis, primary, wrist
Osteoarthrosis (degenerative) (hypertrophic) (joint) (see also Osteoarthritis)
  deformans alkaptonurica E70.29 [M36.8]
  erosive M15.4
  generalized M15.9
    primary M15.0
  polyarticular M15.9
  spine — see Spondylosis
Osteoblastoma — see Neoplasm, bone, benign
  aggressive — see Neoplasm, bone, uncertain behavior
Osteochondritis (see also Osteochondropathy, by site)
  Brailsford's — see Osteochondrosis, juvenile, radius
  dissecans M93.20
    ankle M93.27- ☑
    elbow M93.22- ☑
    foot M93.27- ☑
    hand M93.24- ☑
    hip M93.25- ☑
    knee M93.26- ☑
    multiple sites M93.29
    shoulder joint M93.21- ☑
    specified site NEC M93.28
    wrist M93.23- ☑
  juvenile M92.9
    patellar — see Osteochondrosis, juvenile, patella
  syphilitic (congenital) (early) A50.02 [M90.80]
    ankle A50.02 [M90.87-] ☑
    elbow A50.02 [M90.82-] ☑
    foot A50.02 [M90.87-] ☑
    forearm A50.02 [M90.83-] ☑
    hand A50.02 [M90.84-] ☑
    hip A50.02 [M90.85-] ☑
    knee A50.02 [M90.86-] ☑
    multiple sites A50.02 [M90.89]
    shoulder joint A50.02 [M90.81-] ☑
    specified site NEC A50.02 [M90.88]
Osteochondroarthrosis deformans endemica — see Disease, Kaschin-Beck
Osteochondrodysplasia Q78.9
  with defects of growth of tubular bones and spine Q77.9
  specified NEC Q77.8
  specified NEC Q78.8
Osteochondrodystrophy E78.9
Osteochondrolysis — see Osteochondritis, dissecans
Osteochondroma — see Neoplasm, bone, benign
Osteochondromatosis D48.0
  syndrome Q78.4
Osteochondromyxosarcoma — see Neoplasm, bone, malignant
Osteochondropathy M93.90
  ankle M93.97- ☑
  elbow M93.92- ☑
  foot M93.97- ☑
  hand M93.94- ☑
  hip M93.95- ☑
  Kienböck's disease of adults M93.1
  knee M93.96- ☑
  multiple joints M93.99
  osteochondritis dissecans — see Osteochondritis, dissecans
  osteochondrosis — see Osteochondrosis
  shoulder region M93.91- ☑
  slipped upper femoral epiphysis — see Slipped, epiphysis, upper femoral
  specified joint NEC M93.98
  specified type NEC M93.80
    ankle M93.87- ☑
    elbow M93.82- ☑

Osteochondropathy — *continued*
　specified type — *continued*
　　foot M93.87- ☑
　　hand M93.84- ☑
　　hip M93.85- ☑
　　knee M93.86- ☑
　　multiple joints M93.89
　　shoulder region M93.81- ☑
　　specified joint NEC M93.88
　　wrist M93.83- ☑
　syphilitic, congenital
　　early A50.02 [M90.80]
　　late A50.56 [M90.80]
　wrist M93.93- ☑
Osteochondrosarcoma — *see* Neoplasm, bone, malignant
Osteochondrosis (*see also* Osteochondropathy, by site)
　acetabulum (juvenile) M91.0
　adult — *see* Osteochondropathy, specified type NEC, by site
　astragalus (juvenile) — *see* Osteochondrosis, juvenile, tarsus
　Blount's — *see* Osteochondrosis, juvenile, tibia
　Buchanan's M91.0
　Burns' — *see* Osteochondrosis, juvenile, ulna
　calcaneus (juvenile) — *see* Osteochondrosis, juvenile, tarsus
　capitular epiphysis (femur) (juvenile) — *see* Legg-Calvé-Perthes disease
　carpal (juvenile) (lunate) (scaphoid) — *see* Osteochondrosis, juvenile, hand, carpal lunate
　　adult M93.1
　coxae juvenilis — *see* Legg-Calvé-Perthes disease
　deformans juvenilis, coxae — *see* Legg-Calvé-Perthes disease
　Diaz's — *see* Osteochondrosis, juvenile, tarsus
　dissecans (knee) (shoulder) — *see* Osteochondritis, dissecans
　femoral capital epiphysis (juvenile) — *see* Legg-Calvé-Perthes disease
　femur (head), juvenile — *see* Legg-Calvé-Perthes disease
　fibula (juvenile) — *see* Osteochondrosis, juvenile, fibula
　foot NEC (juvenile) M92.8
　Freiberg's — *see* Osteochondrosis, juvenile, metatarsus
　Haas' (juvenile) — *see* Osteochondrosis, juvenile, humerus
　Haglund's — *see* Osteochondrosis, juvenile, tarsus
　hip (juvenile) — *see* Legg-Calvé-Perthes disease
　humerus (capitulum) (head) (juvenile) — *see* Osteochondrosis, juvenile, humerus
　ilium, iliac crest (juvenile) M91.0
　ischiopubic synchondrosis M91.0
　Iselin's — *see* Osteochondrosis, juvenile, metatarsus
　juvenile, juvenilis M92.9
　　after congenital dislocation of hip reduction — *see* Osteochondrosis, juvenile, hip, specified NEC
　　arm — *see* Osteochondrosis, juvenile, upper limb NEC
　　capitular epiphysis (femur) — *see* Legg-Calvé-Perthes disease
　　clavicle, sternal epiphysis — *see* Osteochondrosis, juvenile, upper limb NEC
　　coxae — *see* Legg-Calvé-Perthes disease
　　deformans M92.9
　　fibula M92.5- ☑
　　foot NEC M92.8
　　hand M92.20- ☑
　　　carpal lunate M92.21- ☑
　　　metacarpal head M92.22- ☑
　　　specified site NEC M92.29- ☑
　　head of femur — *see* Legg-Calvé-Perthes disease
　　hip and pelvis M91.9- ☑
　　　coxa plana — *see* Coxa, plana
　　　femoral head — *see* Legg-Calvé-Perthes disease
　　　pelvis M91.0
　　　pseudocoxalgia — *see* Pseudocoxalgia
　　　specified NEC M91.8- ☑
　　humerus M92.0- ☑
　　limb
　　　lower NEC M92.8
　　　upper NEC — *see* Osteochondrosis, juvenile, upper limb NEC
　　medial cuneiform bone — *see* Osteochondrosis, juvenile, tarsus
　　metatarsus M92.7- ☑

Osteochondrosis — *continued*
　juvenile, juvenilis — *continued*
　　patella M92.4- ☑
　　radius M92.1- ☑
　　specified site NEC M92.8
　　spine M42.00
　　　cervical region M42.02
　　　cervicothoracic region M42.03
　　　lumbar region M42.06
　　　lumbosacral region M42.07
　　　multiple sites M42.09
　　　occipito-atlanto-axial region M42.01
　　　sacrococcygeal region M42.08
　　　thoracic region M42.04
　　　thoracolumbar region M42.05
　　tarsus M92.6- ☑
　　tibia M92.5- ☑
　　ulna M92.1- ☑
　　upper limb NEC M92.3- ☑
　　vertebra (body) (epiphyseal plates) (Calvé's) (Scheuermann's) — *see* Osteochondrosis, juvenile, spine
　Kienböck's — *see* Osteochondrosis, juvenile, hand, carpal lunate
　　adult M93.1
　Köhler's
　　patellar — *see* Osteochondrosis, juvenile, patella
　　tarsal navicular — *see* Osteochondrosis, juvenile, tarsus
　Legg-Perthes (-Calvé)(-Waldenström) — *see* Legg-Calvé-Perthes disease
　limb
　　lower NEC (juvenile) M92.8
　　upper NEC (juvenile) — *see* Osteochondrosis, juvenile, upper limb NEC
　lunate bone (carpal) (juvenile) (*see also* Osteochondrosis, juvenile, hand, carpal lunate)
　　adult M93.1
　Mauclaire's — *see* Osteochondrosis, juvenile, hand, metacarpal
　metacarpal (head) (juvenile) — *see* Osteochondrosis, juvenile, hand, metacarpal
　metatarsus (fifth) (head) (juvenile) (second) — *see* Osteochondrosis, juvenile, metatarsus
　navicular (juvenile) — *see* Osteochondrosis, juvenile, tarsus
　os
　　calcis (juvenile) — *see* Osteochondrosis, juvenile, tarsus
　　tibiale externum (juvenile) — *see* Osteochondrosis, juvenile, tarsus
　Osgood-Schlatter — *see* Osteochondrosis, juvenile, tibia
　Panner's — *see* Osteochondrosis, juvenile, humerus
　patellar center (juvenile) (primary) (secondary) — *see* Osteochondrosis, juvenile, patella
　pelvis (juvenile) M91.0
　Pierson's M91.0
　radius (head) (juvenile) — *see* Osteochondrosis, juvenile, radius
　Scheuermann's — *see* Osteochondrosis, juvenile, spine
　Sever's — *see* Osteochondrosis, juvenile, tarsus
　Sinding-Larsen — *see* Osteochondrosis, juvenile, patella
　spine M42.9
　　adult M42.10
　　　cervical region M42.12
　　　cervicothoracic region M42.13
　　　lumbar region M42.16
　　　lumbosacral region M42.17
　　　multiple sites M42.19
　　　occipito-atlanto-axial region M42.11
　　　sacrococcygeal region M42.18
　　　thoracic region M42.14
　　　thoracolumbar region M42.15
　　juvenile — *see* Osteochondrosis, juvenile, spine
　symphysis pubis (juvenile) M91.0
　syphilitic (congenital) A50.02
　talus (juvenile) — *see* Osteochondrosis, juvenile, tarsus
　tarsus (navicular) (juvenile) — *see* Osteochondrosis, juvenile, tarsus
　tibia (proximal) (tubercle) (juvenile) — *see* Osteochondrosis, juvenile, tibia
　tuberculous — *see* Tuberculosis, bone
　ulna (lower) (juvenile) — *see* Osteochondrosis, juvenile, ulna
　van Neck's M91.0

Osteochondrosis — *continued*
　vertebral — *see* Osteochondrosis, spine
Osteoclastoma D48.0
　malignant — *see* Neoplasm, bone, malignant
Osteodynia — *see* Disorder, bone, specified type NEC
Osteodystrophy Q78.9
　azotemic N25.0
　congenital Q78.9
　parathyroid, secondary E21.1
　renal N25.0
Osteofibroma — *see* Neoplasm, bone, benign
Osteofibrosarcoma — *see* Neoplasm, bone, malignant
Osteogenesis imperfecta Q78.0
Osteogenic — *see* condition
Osteolysis M89.50
　carpus M89.54- ☑
　clavicle M89.51- ☑
　femur M89.55- ☑
　fibula M89.56- ☑
　finger M89.54- ☑
　humerus M89.52- ☑
　ilium M89.559
　ischium M89.559
　joint prosthesis (periprosthetic) — *see* Complications, joint prosthesis, mechanical, periprosthetic, osteolysis, by site
　metacarpus M89.54- ☑
　metatarsus M89.57- ☑
　multiple sites M89.59
　neck M89.58
　periprosthetic — *see* Complications, joint prosthesis, mechanical, periprosthetic, osteolysis, by site
　radius M89.53- ☑
　rib M89.58
　scapula M89.51- ☑
　skull M89.58
　tarsus M89.57- ☑
　tibia M89.56- ☑
　toe M89.57- ☑
　ulna M89.53- ☑
　vertebra M89.58
Osteoma (*see also* Neoplasm, bone, benign)
　osteoid (*see also* Neoplasm, bone, benign)
　　giant — *see* Neoplasm, bone, benign
Osteomalacia M83.9
　adult M83.9
　　drug-induced NEC M83.5
　　due to
　　　malabsorption (postsurgical) M83.2
　　　malnutrition M83.3
　　specified NEC M83.8
　aluminium-induced M83.4
　infantile — *see* Rickets
　juvenile — *see* Rickets
　oncogenic E83.89
　pelvis M83.8
　puerperal M83.0
　senile M83.1
　vitamin-D-resistant in adults E83.31 [M90.8-] ☑
　　carpus E83.31 [M90.84-] ☑
　　clavicle E83.31 [M90.81-] ☑
　　femur E83.31 [M90.85-] ☑
　　fibula E83.31 [M90.86-] ☑
　　finger E83.31 [M90.84-] ☑
　　humerus E83.31 [M90.82-] ☑
　　ilium E83.31 [M90.859]
　　ischium E83.31 [M90.859]
　　metacarpus E83.31 [M90.84-] ☑
　　metatarsus E83.31 [M90.87-] ☑
　　multiple sites E83.31 [M90.89]
　　neck E83.31 [M90.88]
　　radius E83.31 [M90.83-] ☑
　　rib E83.31 [M90.88]
　　scapula E83.31 [M90.819]
　　skull E83.31 [M90.88]
　　tarsus E83.31 [M90.879]
　　tibia E83.31 [M90.869]
　　toe E83.31 [M90.879]
　　ulna E83.31 [M90.839]
　　vertebra E83.31 [M90.88]
Osteomyelitis (general) (infective) (localized) (neonatal) (purulent) (septic) (staphylococcal) (streptococcal) (suppurative) (with periostitis) M86.9
　acute M86.10
　　carpus M86.14- ☑
　　clavicle M86.11- ☑
　　femur M86.15- ☑

Osteomyelitis — *continued*
  acute — *continued*
    fibula M86.16- ☑
    finger M86.14- ☑
    hematogenous M86.00
      carpus M86.04- ☑
      clavicle M86.01- ☑
      femur M86.05- ☑
      fibula M86.06- ☑
      finger M86.04- ☑
      humerus M86.02- ☑
      ilium M86.059
      ischium M86.059
      mandible M27.2
      metacarpus M86.04- ☑
      metatarsus M86.07- ☑
      multiple sites M86.09
      neck M86.08
      orbit H05.02- ☑
      petrous bone — *see* Petrositis
      radius M86.03- ☑
      rib M86.08
      scapula M86.01- ☑
      skull M86.08
      tarsus M86.07- ☑
      tibia M86.06- ☑
      toe M86.07- ☑
      ulna M86.03- ☑
      vertebra — *see* Osteomyelitis, vertebra
    humerus M86.12- ☑
    ilium M86.159
    ischium M86.159
    mandible M27.2
    metacarpus M86.14- ☑
    metatarsus M86.17- ☑
    multiple sites M86.19
    neck M86.18
    orbit H05.02- ☑
    petrous bone — *see* Petrositis
    radius M86.13- ☑
    rib M86.18
    scapula M86.11- ☑
    skull M86.18
    tarsus M86.17- ☑
    tibia M86.16- ☑
    toe M86.17- ☑
    ulna M86.13- ☑
    vertebra — *see* Osteomyelitis, vertebra
  chronic (or old) M86.60
    with draining sinus M86.40
      carpus M86.44- ☑
      clavicle M86.41- ☑
      femur M86.45- ☑
      fibula M86.46- ☑
      finger M86.44- ☑
      humerus M86.42- ☑
      ilium M86.459
      ischium M86.459
      mandible M27.2
      metacarpus M86.44- ☑
      metatarsus M86.47- ☑
      multiple sites M86.49
      neck M86.48
      orbit H05.02- ☑
      petrous bone — *see* Petrositis
      radius M86.43- ☑
      rib M86.48
      scapula M86.41- ☑
      skull M86.48
      tarsus M86.47- ☑
      tibia M86.46- ☑
      toe M86.47- ☑
      ulna M86.43- ☑
      vertebra — *see* Osteomyelitis, vertebra
    carpus M86.64- ☑
    clavicle M86.61- ☑
    femur M86.65- ☑
    fibula M86.66- ☑
    finger M86.64- ☑
    hematogenous NEC M86.50
      carpus M86.54- ☑
      clavicle M86.51- ☑
      femur M86.55- ☑
      fibula M86.56- ☑
      finger M86.54- ☑
      humerus M86.52- ☑

Osteomyelitis — *continued*
  chronic — *continued*
    hematogenous — *continued*
      ilium M86.559
      ischium M86.559
      mandible M27.2
      metacarpus M86.54- ☑
      metatarsus M86.57- ☑
      multifocal M86.30
        carpus M86.34- ☑
        clavicle M86.31- ☑
        femur M86.35- ☑
        fibula M86.36- ☑
        finger M86.34- ☑
        humerus M86.32- ☑
        ilium M86.359
        ischium M86.359
        metacarpus M86.34- ☑
        metatarsus M86.37- ☑
        multiple sites M86.39
        neck M86.38
        radius M86.33- ☑
        rib M86.38
        scapula M86.31- ☑
        skull M86.38
        tarsus M86.37- ☑
        tibia M86.36- ☑
        toe M86.37- ☑
        ulna M86.33- ☑
        vertebra — *see* Osteomyelitis, vertebra
      multiple sites M86.59
      neck M86.58
      orbit H05.02- ☑
      petrous bone — *see* Petrositis
      radius M86.53- ☑
      rib M86.58
      scapula M86.51- ☑
      skull M86.58
      tarsus M86.57- ☑
      tibia M86.56- ☑
      toe M86.57- ☑
      ulna M86.53- ☑
      vertebra — *see* Osteomyelitis, vertebra
    humerus M86.62- ☑
    ilium M86.659
    ischium M86.659
    mandible M27.2
    metacarpus M86.64- ☑
    metatarsus M86.67- ☑
    multifocal — *see* Osteomyelitis, chronic, hematogenous, multifocal
    multiple sites M86.69
    neck M86.68
    orbit H05.02- ☑
    petrous bone — *see* Petrositis
    radius M86.63- ☑
    rib M86.68
    scapula M86.61- ☑
    skull M86.68
    tarsus M86.67- ☑
    tibia M86.66- ☑
    toe M86.67- ☑
    ulna M86.63- ☑
    vertebra — *see* Osteomyelitis, vertebra
  echinococcal B67.2
  Garr's — *see* Osteomyelitis, specified type NEC
  jaw (acute) (chronic) (lower) (neonatal) (suppurative) (upper) M27.2
  nonsuppurating — *see* Osteomyelitis, specified type NEC
  orbit H05.02- ☑
  petrous bone — *see* Petrositis
  Salmonella (arizonae) (cholerae-suis) (enteritidis) (typhimurium) A02.24
  sclerosing, nonsuppurative — *see* Osteomyelitis, specified type NEC
  specified type NEC (*see also* subcategory) M86.8X- ☑
    mandible M27.2
    orbit H05.02- ☑
    petrous bone — *see* Petrositis
    vertebra — *see* Osteomyelitis, vertebra
  subacute M86.20
    carpus M86.24- ☑
    clavicle M86.21- ☑
    femur M86.25- ☑
    fibula M86.26- ☑

Osteomyelitis — *continued*
  subacute — *continued*
    finger M86.24- ☑
    humerus M86.22- ☑
    mandible M27.2
    metacarpus M86.24- ☑
    metatarsus M86.27- ☑
    multiple sites M86.29
    neck M86.28
    orbit H05.02- ☑
    petrous bone — *see* Petrositis
    radius M86.23- ☑
    rib M86.28
    scapula M86.21- ☑
    skull M86.28
    tarsus M86.27- ☑
    tibia M86.26- ☑
    toe M86.27- ☑
    ulna M86.23- ☑
    vertebra — *see* Osteomyelitis, vertebra
  syphilitic A52.77
    congenital (early) A50.02 [M90.80]
  tuberculous — *see* Tuberculosis, bone
  typhoid A01.05
  vertebra M46.20
    cervical region M46.22
    cervicothoracic region M46.23
    lumbar region M46.26
    lumbosacral region M46.27
    occipito-atlanto-axial region M46.21
    sacrococcygeal region M46.28
    thoracic region M46.24
    thoracolumbar region M46.25
Osteomyelofibrosis D75.89
Osteomyelosclerosis D75.89
Osteonecrosis M87.9
  due to
    drugs — *see* Osteonecrosis, secondary, due to, drugs
    trauma — *see* Osteonecrosis, secondary, due to, trauma
  idiopathic aseptic M87.00
    ankle M87.07- ☑
    carpus M87.03- ☑
    clavicle M87.01- ☑
    femur M87.05- ☑
    fibula M87.06- ☑
    finger M87.04- ☑
    humerus M87.02- ☑
    ilium M87.050
    ischium M87.050
    metacarpus M87.04- ☑
    metatarsus M87.07- ☑
    multiple sites M87.09
    neck M87.08
    pelvis M87.050
    radius M87.03- ☑
    rib M87.08
    scapula M87.01- ☑
    skull M87.08
    tarsus M87.07- ☑
    tibia M87.06- ☑
    toe M87.07- ☑
    ulna M87.03- ☑
    vertebra M87.08
  secondary NEC M87.30
    carpus M87.33- ☑
    clavicle M87.31- ☑
    due to
      drugs M87.10
        carpus M87.13- ☑
        clavicle M87.11- ☑
        femur M87.15- ☑
        fibula M87.16- ☑
        finger M87.14- ☑
        humerus M87.12- ☑
        ilium M87.159
        ischium M87.159
        jaw M87.180
        metacarpus M87.14- ☑
        metatarsus M87.17- ☑
        multiple sites M87.19
        neck M87.18
        radius M87.13- ☑
        rib M87.18
        scapula M87.11- ☑
        skull M87.18 ☑

Index

Osteomyelitis — Osteonecrosis

Osteonecrosis — *continued*
  secondary — *continued*
    due to — *continued*
      drugs — *continued*
        tarsus M87.17- ☑
        tibia M87.16- ☑
        toe M87.17- ☑
        ulna M87.13- ☑
        vertebra M87.18 ☑
      hemoglobinopathy NEC D58.2 [M90.50]
        carpus D58.2 [M90.54-] ☑
        clavicle D58.2 [M90.51-] ☑
        femur D58.2 [M90.55-] ☑
        fibula D58.2 [M90.56-] ☑
        finger D58.2 [M90.54-] ☑
        humerus D58.2 [M90.52-] ☑
        ilium D58.2 [M90.55-] ☑
        ischium D58.2 [M90.55-] ☑
        metacarpus D58.2 [M90.54-] ☑
        metatarsus D58.2 [M90.57-] ☑
        multiple sites D58.2 [M90.58]
        neck D58.2 [M90.58]
        radius D58.2 [M90.53-] ☑
        rib D58.2 [M90.58]
        scapula D58.2 [M90.51-] ☑
        skull D58.2 [M90.58]
        tarsus D58.2 [M90.57-] ☑
        tibia D58.2 [M90.56-] ☑
        toe D58.2 [M90.57-] ☑
        ulna D58.2 [M90.53-] ☑
        vertebra D58.2 [M90.58]
    trauma (previous) M87.20
      carpus M87.23- ☑
      clavicle M87.21- ☑
      femur M87.25- ☑
      fibula M87.26- ☑
      finger M87.24- ☑
      humerus M87.22- ☑
      ilium M87.25- ☑
      ischium M87.25- ☑
      metacarpus M87.24- ☑
      metatarsus M87.27- ☑
      multiple sites M87.29
      neck M87.28
      radius M87.23- ☑
      rib M87.28
      scapula M87.21- ☑
      skull M87.28
      tarsus M87.27- ☑
      tibia M87.26- ☑
      toe M87.27- ☑
      ulna M87.23- ☑
      vertebra M87.28
    femur M87.35- ☑
    fibula M87.36- ☑
    finger M87.34- ☑
    humerus M87.32- ☑
    ilium M87.350
    in
      caisson disease T70.3 ☑ [M90.50]
        carpus T70.3 ☑ [M90.54-] ☑
        clavicle T70.3 ☑ [M90.51-] ☑
        femur T70.3 ☑ [M90.55-] ☑
        fibula T70.3 ☑ [M90.56-] ☑
        finger T70.3 ☑ [M90.54-] ☑
        humerus T70.3 ☑ [M90.52-] ☑
        ilium T70.3 ☑ [M90.55-] ☑
        ischium T70.3 ☑ [M90.55-] ☑
        metacarpus T70.3 ☑ [M90.54-] ☑
        metatarsus T70.3 ☑ [M90.57-] ☑
        multiple sites T70.3 ☑ [M90.59]
        neck T70.3 ☑ [M90.58]
        radius T70.3 ☑ [M90.53-] ☑
        rib T70.3 ☑ [M90.58]
        scapula T70.3 ☑ [M90.51-] ☑
        skull T70.3 ☑ [M90.58]
        tarsus T70.3 ☑ [M90.57-] ☑
        tibia T70.3 ☑ [M90.56-] ☑
        toe T70.3 ☑ [M90.57-] ☑
        ulna T70.3 ☑ [M90.53-] ☑
        vertebra T70.3 ☑ [M90.58]
    ischium M87.350
    metacarpus M87.34- ☑
    metatarsus M87.37- ☑
    multiple site M87.39
    neck M87.38

Osteonecrosis — *continued*
  secondary — *continued*
    radius M87.33- ☑
    rib M87.38
    scapula M87.319
    skull M87.38
    tarsus M87.379
    tibia M87.366
    toe M87.379
    ulna M87.33- ☑
    vertebra M87.38
  specified type NEC M87.80
    carpus M87.83- ☑
    clavicle M87.81- ☑
    femur M87.85- ☑
    fibula M87.86- ☑
    finger M87.84- ☑
    humerus M87.82- ☑
    ilium M87.85- ☑
    ischium M87.85- ☑
    metacarpus M87.84- ☑
    metatarsus M87.87- ☑
    multiple sites M87.89
    neck M87.88
    radius M87.83- ☑
    rib M87.88-
    scapula M87.81- ☑
    skull M87.88
    tarsus M87.87- ☑
    tibia M87.86- ☑
    toe M87.87- ☑
    ulna M87.83- ☑
    vertebra M87.88

Osteopathia condensans disseminata Q78.8
Osteopathy (*see also* Osteomyelitis, Osteonecrosis, Osteoporosis)
  after poliomyelitis M89.60
    carpus M89.64- ☑
    clavicle M89.61- ☑
    femur M89.65- ☑
    fibula M89.66- ☑
    finger M89.64- ☑
    humerus M89.62- ☑
    ilium M89.659
    ischium M89.659
    metacarpus M89.64- ☑
    metatarsus M89.67- ☑
    multiple sites M89.69
    neck M89.68
    radius M89.63- ☑
    rib M89.68
    scapula M89.61- ☑
    skull M89.68
    tarsus M89.67- ☑
    tibia M89.66- ☑
    toe M89.67- ☑
    ulna M89.63- ☑
    vertebra M89.68
  in (due to)
    renal osteodystrophy N25.0
    specified diseases classified elsewhere — *see* subcategory M90.8
Osteopenia M85.8-
  borderline M85.8- ☑
Osteoperiostitis — *see* Osteomyelitis, specified type NEC
Osteopetrosis (familial) Q78.2
Osteophyte M25.70
  ankle M25.77- ☑
  elbow M25.72- ☑
  foot joint M25.77- ☑
  hand joint M25.74- ☑
  hip M25.75- ☑
  knee M25.76- ☑
  shoulder M25.71- ☑
  spine M25.78
  vertebrae M25.78
  wrist M25.73- ☑
Osteopoikilosis Q78.8
Osteoporosis (female) (male) M81.0
  with current pathological fracture M80.00 ☑
  age-related M81.0
    with current pathologic fracture M80.00 ☑
      carpus M80.04- ☑
      clavicle M80.01- ☑
      fibula M80.06- ☑

Osteoporosis — *continued*
  age-related — *continued*
    with current pathologic fracture — *continued*
      finger M80.04- ☑
      humerus M80.02- ☑
      ilium M80.05- ☑
      ischium M80.05- ☑
      metacarpus M80.04- ☑
      metatarsus M80.07- ☑
      pelvis M80.05- ☑
      radius M80.03- ☑
      scapula M80.01- ☑
      tarsus M80.07- ☑
      tibia M80.06- ☑
      toe M80.07- ☑
      ulna M80.03- ☑
      vertebra M80.08 ☑
  disuse M81.8
    with current pathological fracture M80.80 ☑
      carpus M80.84- ☑
      clavicle M80.81- ☑
      fibula M80.86- ☑
      finger M80.84- ☑
      humerus M80.82- ☑
      ilium M80.85- ☑
      ischium M80.85- ☑
      metacarpus M80.84- ☑
      metatarsus M80.87- ☑
      pelvis M80.85- ☑
      radius M80.83- ☑
      scapula M80.81- ☑
      tarsus M80.87- ☑
      tibia M80.86- ☑
      toe M80.87- ☑
      ulna M80.83- ☑
      vertebra M80.88 ☑
  drug-induced — *see* Osteoporosis, specified type NEC
  idiopathic — *see* Osteoporosis, specified type NEC
  involutional — *see* Osteoporosis, age-related
  Lequesne M81.6
  localized M81.6
  post-traumatic — *see* Osteoporosis, specified type NEC
  postmenopausal M81.0
    with pathological fracture M80.00 ☑
      carpus M80.04- ☑
      clavicle M80.01- ☑
      fibula M80.06- ☑
      finger M80.04- ☑
      humerus M80.02- ☑
      ilium M80.05- ☑
      ischium M80.05- ☑
      metacarpus M80.04- ☑
      metatarsus M80.07- ☑
      pelvis M80.05- ☑
      radius M80.03- ☑
      scapula M80.01- ☑
      tarsus M80.07- ☑
      tibia M80.06- ☑
      toe M80.07- ☑
      ulna M80.03- ☑
      vertebra M80.08 ☑
  postoophorectomy — *see* Osteoporosis, specified type NEC
  postsurgical malabsorption — *see* Osteoporosis, specified type NEC
  senile — *see* Osteoporosis, age-related
  specified type NEC M81.8
    with pathological fracture M80.80 ☑
      carpus M80.84- ☑
      clavicle M80.81- ☑
      fibula M80.86- ☑
      finger M80.84- ☑
      humerus M80.82- ☑
      ilium M80.85- ☑
      ischium M80.85- ☑
      metacarpus M80.84- ☑
      metatarsus M80.87- ☑
      pelvis M80.85- ☑
      radius M80.83- ☑
      scapula M80.81- ☑
      tarsus M80.87- ☑
      tibia M80.86- ☑
      toe M80.87- ☑
      ulna M80.83- ☑
      vertebra M80.88 ☑

Osteopsathyrosis (idiopathica) Q78.Ø
Osteoradionecrosis, jaw (acute) (chronic) (lower) (suppurative) (upper) M27.2
Osteosarcoma (any form) — see Neoplasm, bone, malignant
Osteosclerosis Q78.2
  acquired M85.8- ☑
  congenita Q77.4
  fragilitas (generalisata) Q78.2
  myelofibrosis D75.81
Osteosclerotic anemia D64.89
Osteosis
  cutis L94.2
  renal fibrocystic N25.Ø
Österreicher-Turner syndrome Q87.2
Ostium
  atrioventriculare commune Q21.2
  primum (arteriosum) (defect) (persistent) Q21.2
  secundum (arteriosum) (defect) (patent) (persistent) Q21.1
Ostrum-Furst syndrome Q75.8
Otalgia H92.Ø ☑
Otitis (acute) H66.9Ø
  with effusion (see also Otitis, media, nonsuppurative)
    purulent — see Otitis, media, suppurative
  adhesive — see subcategory H74.1
  chronic (see also Otitis, media, chronic)
    with effusion (see also Otitis, media, nonsuppurative, chronic)
  externa H6Ø.9- ☑
    abscess — see Abscess, ear, external
    acute (noninfective) H6Ø.5Ø- ☑
      actinic H6Ø.51- ☑
      chemical H6Ø.52- ☑
      contact H6Ø.53- ☑
      eczematoid H6Ø.54- ☑
      infective — see Otitis, externa, infective
      reactive H6Ø.55- ☑
      specified NEC H6Ø.59- ☑
    cellulitis — see Cellulitis, ear
    chronic H6Ø.6- ☑
    diffuse — see Otitis, externa, infective, diffuse
    hemorrhagic — see Otitis, externa, infective, hemorrhagic
    in (due to)
      aspergillosis B44.89
      candidiasis B37.84
      erysipelas A46 [H62.4Ø]
      herpes (simplex) virus infection BØØ.1
        zoster BØ2.8
      impetigo LØ1.ØØ [H62.4Ø]
      infectious disease NEC B99 [H62.4-] ☑
      mycosis NEC B36.9 [H62.4Ø]
      parasitic disease NEC B89 [H62.4Ø]
      viral disease NEC B34.9 [H62.4Ø]
      zoster BØ2.8
    infective NEC H6Ø.39- ☑
      abscess — see Abscess, ear, external
      cellulitis — see Cellulitis, ear
      diffuse H6Ø.31- ☑
      hemorrhagic H6Ø.32- ☑
      swimmer's ear — see Swimmer's, ear
    malignant H6Ø.2- ☑
    mycotic B36.9 [H62.4Ø]
    necrotizing — see Otitis, externa, malignant
    Pseudomonas aeruginosa — see Otitis, externa, malignant
    reactive — see Otitis, externa, acute, reactive
    specified NEC — see subcategory H6Ø.8 ☑
    tropical B36.8
  insidiosa — see Otosclerosis
  interna H83.Ø ☑
  media (hemorrhagic) (staphylococcal) (streptococcal) H66.9- ☑
    with effusion (nonpurulent) — see Otitis, media, nonsuppurative
    acute, subacute H66.9Ø
      allergic — see Otitis, media, nonsuppurative, acute, allergic
      exudative — see Otitis, media, nonsuppurative, acute
      mucoid — see Otitis, media, nonsuppurative, acute
      necrotizing (see also Otitis, media, suppurative, acute)
        in
          measles BØ5.3

Otitis — continued
  media — continued
    acute, subacute — continued
      necrotizing (see also Otitis, media, suppurative, acute) — continued
        in — continued
          scarlet fever A38.Ø
      nonsuppurative NEC — see Otitis, media, nonsuppurative, acute
      purulent — see Otitis, media, suppurative, acute
      sanguinous — see Otitis, media, suppurative, acute
      secretory — see Otitis, media, nonsuppurative, acute, serous
      seromucinous — see Otitis, media, nonsuppurative, acute
      serous — see Otitis, media, nonsuppurative, acute, serous
      suppurative — see Otitis, media, suppurative, acute
    allergic — see Otitis, media, nonsuppurative
    catarrhal — see Otitis, media, nonsuppurative
    chronic H66.9Ø
      with effusion (nonpurulent) — see Otitis, media, nonsuppurative, chronic
      allergic — see Otitis, media, nonsuppurative, chronic, allergic
      benign suppurative — see Otitis, media, suppurative, chronic, tubotympanic
      catarrhal — see Otitis, media, nonsuppurative, chronic, serous
      exudative — see Otitis, media, nonsuppurative, chronic
      mucinous — see Otitis, media, nonsuppurative, chronic, mucoid
      mucoid — see Otitis, media, nonsuppurative, chronic, mucoid
      nonsuppurative NEC — see Otitis, media, nonsuppurative, chronic
      purulent — see Otitis, media, suppurative, chronic
      secretory — see Otitis, media, nonsuppurative, chronic, mucoid
      seromucinous — see Otitis, media, nonsuppurative, chronic
      serous — see Otitis, media, nonsuppurative, chronic, serous
      suppurative — see Otitis, media, suppurative, chronic
      transudative — see Otitis, media, nonsuppurative, chronic, mucoid
    exudative — see Otitis, media, nonsuppurative
    in (due to) (with)
      influenza — see Influenza, with, otitis media
      measles BØ5.3
      scarlet fever A38.Ø
      tuberculosis A18.6
      viral disease NEC B34.- ☑ [H67.-] ☑
    mucoid — see Otitis, media, nonsuppurative
    nonsuppurative H65.9- ☑
      acute or subacute NEC H65.19- ☑
        allergic H65.11- ☑
          recurrent H65.11- ☑
        recurrent H65.19- ☑
        secretory — see Otitis, media, nonsuppurative, serous
        serous H65.Ø- ☑
          recurrent H65.Ø- ☑
      chronic H65.49- ☑
        allergic H65.41- ☑
        mucoid H65.3- ☑
        serous H65.2- ☑
    postmeasles BØ5.3
    purulent — see Otitis, media, suppurative
    secretory — see Otitis, media, nonsuppurative
    seromucinous — see Otitis, media, nonsuppurative
    serous — see Otitis, media, nonsuppurative
    suppurative H66.4- ☑
      acute H66.ØØ- ☑
        with rupture of ear drum H66.Ø1- ☑
        recurrent H66.ØØ- ☑
          with rupture of ear drum H66.Ø1- ☑
      chronic (see also subcategory) H66.3 ☑
        atticoantral H66.2- ☑
        benign — see Otitis, media, suppurative, chronic, tubotympanic

Otitis — continued
  media — continued
    suppurative — continued
      chronic (see also subcategory) — continued
        tubotympanic H66.1- ☑
    transudative — see Otitis, media, nonsuppurative
    tuberculous A18.6
Otocephaly Q18.2
Otolith syndrome — see subcategory H81.8 ☑
Otomycosis (diffuse) **NEC** B36.9 [H62.4Ø]
  in
    aspergillosis B44.89
    candidiasis B37.84
    moniliasis B37.84
Otoporosis — see Otosclerosis
Otorrhagia (nontraumatic) H92.2- ☑
  traumatic — code by Type of injury
Otorrhea H92.1- ☑
  cerebrospinal G96.Ø
Otosclerosis (general) H8Ø.9- ☑
  cochlear (endosteal) H8Ø.2- ☑
  involving
    otic capsule — see Otosclerosis, cochlear
    oval window
      nonobliterative H8Ø.Ø- ☑
      obliterative H8Ø.1- ☑
    round window — see Otosclerosis, cochlear
  nonobliterative — see Otosclerosis, involving, oval window, nonobliterative
  obliterative — see Otosclerosis, involving, oval window, obliterative
  specified NEC H8Ø.8- ☑
Otospongiosis — see Otosclerosis
Otto's disease or pelvis M24.7
Outcome of delivery Z37.9
  multiple births Z37.9
    all liveborn Z37.5Ø
      quadruplets Z37.52
      quintuplets Z37.53
      sextuplets Z37.54
      specified number NEC Z37.59
      triplets Z37.51
    all stillborn Z37.7
    some liveborn Z37.6Ø
      quadruplets Z37.62
      quintuplets Z37.63
      sextuplets Z37.64
      specified number NEC Z37.69
      triplets Z37.61
  single NEC Z37.9
    liveborn Z37.Ø
    stillborn Z37.1
  twins NEC Z37.9
    both liveborn Z37.2
    both stillborn Z37.4
    one liveborn, one stillborn Z37.3
Outlet — see condition
Ovalocytosis (congenital) (hereditary) — see Elliptocytosis
Ovarian — see Condition
Ovariocele N83.4
Ovaritis (cystic) — see Oophoritis
Ovary, ovarian (see also condition)
  resistant syndrome E28.39
  vein syndrome N13.8
Overactive (see also Hyperfunction)
  adrenal cortex NEC E27.Ø
  bladder N32.81
  hypothalamus E23.3
  thyroid — see Hyperthyroidism
Overactivity R46.3
  child — see Disorder, attention-deficit hyperactivity
Overbite (deep) (excessive) (horizontal) (vertical) M26.29
Overbreathing — see Hyperventilation
Overconscientious personality F6Ø.5
Overdevelopment — see Hypertrophy
Overdistension — see Distension
Overdose, overdosage (drug) — see Table of Drugs and Chemicals, by drug, poisoning
Overeating R63.2
  nonorganic origin F5Ø.8
  psychogenic F5Ø.8
Overexertion (effects) (exhaustion) T73.3 ☑
Overexposure (effects) T73.9 ☑
  exhaustion T73.2 ☑
Overfeeding — see Overeating
  newborn P92.4

Overfill, endodontic M27.52
Overgrowth, bone — see Hypertrophy, bone
Overhanging of dental restorative material (unrepairable) K08.52
Overheated (places) (effects) — see Heat
Overjet (excessive horizontal) M26.23
Overlaid, overlying (suffocation) — see Asphyxia, traumatic, due to mechanical threat
Overlap, excessive horizontal (teeth) M26.23
Overlapping toe (acquired) (see also Deformity, toe, specified NEC)
  congenital (fifth toe) Q66.89
Overload
  circulatory, due to transfusion (blood) (blood components) (TACO) E87.71
  fluid E87.70
    due to transfusion (blood) (blood components) E87.71
    specified NEC E87.79
  iron, due to repeated red blood cell transfusions E83.111
  potassium (K) E87.5
  sodium (Na) E87.0
Overnutrition — see Hyperalimentation
Overproduction (see also Hypersecretion)
  ACTH E27.0
  catecholamine E27.5
  growth hormone E22.0
Overprotection, child by parent Z62.1
Overriding
  aorta Q25.4
  finger (acquired) — see Deformity, finger
    congenital Q68.1
  toe (acquired) (see also Deformity, toe, specified NEC)
    congenital Q66.89
Overstrained R53.83
  heart — see Hypertrophy, cardiac
Overuse, muscle NEC M70.8- ☑
Overweight E66.3
Overworked R53.83
Oviduct — see condition
Ovotestis Q56.0
Ovulation (cycle)
  failure or lack of N97.0
  pain N94.0
Ovum — see condition
Owren's disease or syndrome (parahemophilia) D68.2
Ox heart — see Hypertrophy, cardiac
Oxalosis E72.53
Oxaluria E72.53
Oxycephaly, oxycephalic Q75.0
  syphilitic, congenital A50.02
Oxyuriasis B80
Oxyuris vermicularis (infestation) B80
Ozena J31.0

P

Pachyderma, pachydermia L85.9
  larynx (verrucosa) J38.7
Pachydermatocele (congenital) Q82.8
Pachydermoperiostosis (see also Osteoarthropathy, hypertrophic, specified type NEC)
  clubbed nail M89.40 [L62]
Pachygyria Q04.3
Pachymeningitis (adhesive) (basal) (brain) (cervical) (chronic)(circumscribed) (external) (fibrous) (hemorrhagic) (hypertrophic) (internal) (purulent) (spinal) (suppurative) — see Meningitis
Pachyonychia (congenital) Q84.5
Pacinian tumor — see Neoplasm, skin, benign
Pad, knuckle or Garrod's M72.1
Paget-Schroetter syndrome I82.890
Paget's disease
  with infiltrating duct carcinoma — see Neoplasm, breast, malignant
  bone M88.9
    carpus M88.84- ☑
    clavicle M88.81- ☑
    femur M88.85- ☑
    fibula M88.86- ☑
    finger M88.84- ☑
    humerus M88.82- ☑
    ilium M88.85-
    in neoplastic disease — see Osteitis, deformans, in neoplastic disease
    ischium M88.85- ☑

Paget's disease — continued
  bone — continued
    metacarpus M88.84- ☑
    metatarsus M88.87- ☑
    multiple sites M88.89
    neck M88.88
    radius M88.83- ☑
    rib M88.88
    scapula M88.81- ☑
    skull M88.0
    tarsus M88.87- ☑
    tibia M88.86- ☑
    toe M88.87- ☑
    ulna M88.83- ☑
    vertebra M88.88
  breast (female) C50.01- ☑
    male C50.02- ☑
  extramammary (see also Neoplasm, skin, malignant)
    anus C21.0
      margin C44.590
      skin C44.590
  intraductal carcinoma — see Neoplasm, breast, malignant
  malignant — see Neoplasm, skin, malignant
    breast (female) C50.01- ☑
      male C50.02- ☑
    unspecified site (female) C50.01- ☑
      male C50.02- ☑
  mammary — see Paget's disease, breast
  nipple — see Paget's disease, breast
  osteitis deformans — see Paget's disease, bone
Pain(s) (see also Painful) R52
  abdominal R10.9
    colic R10.83
    generalized R10.84
      with acute abdomen R10.0
    lower R10.30
      left quadrant R10.32
      pelvic or perineal R10.2
      periumbilical R10.33
      right quadrant R10.31
    rebound — see Tenderness, abdominal, rebound
    severe with abdominal rigidity R10.0
    tenderness — see Tenderness, abdominal
    upper R10.10
      epigastric R10.13
      left quadrant R10.12
      right quadrant R10.11
  acute R52
    due to trauma G89.11
    neoplasm related G89.3
    post-thoracotomy G89.12
    postprocedural NEC G89.18
    specified by site — code to Pain, by site
  adnexa (uteri) R10.2
  anginoid — see Pain, precordial
  anus K62.89
  arm — see Pain, limb, upper
  axillary (axilla) M79.62- ☑
  back (postural) M54.9
  bladder R39.89
    associated with micturition — see Micturition, painful
  bone — see Disorder, bone, specified type NEC
  breast N64.4
  broad ligament R10.2
  cancer associated (acute) (chronic) G89.3
  cecum — see Pain, abdominal
  cervicobrachial M53.1
  chest (central) R07.9
    anterior wall R07.89
    atypical R07.89
    ischemic I20.9
    musculoskeletal R07.89
    non-cardiac R07.89
    on breathing R07.1
    pleurodynia R07.81
    precordial R07.2
    wall (anterior) R07.89
  chronic G89.29
    associated with significant psychosocial dysfunction G89.4
    due to trauma G89.21
    neoplasm related G89.3
    post-thoracotomy G89.22
    postoperative NEC G89.28
    postprocedural NEC G89.28

Pain(s) — continued
  chronic — continued
    specified NEC G89.29
  coccyx M53.3
  colon — see Pain, abdominal
  coronary — see Angina
  costochondral R07.1
  diaphragm R07.1
  due to cancer G89.3
  due to device, implant or graft (see also Complications, by site and type, specified NEC) T85.84 ☑
    arterial graft NEC T82.848 ☑
    breast (implant) T85.84 ☑
    catheter NEC T85.84 ☑
      dialysis (renal) T82.848 ☑
        intraperitoneal T85.84 ☑
      infusion NEC T82.848 ☑
        spinal (epidural) (subdural) T85.84 ☑
      urinary (indwelling) T83.84 ☑
    electronic (electrode) (pulse generator) (stimulator)
      bone T84.84 ☑
      cardiac T82.847 ☑
      nervous system (brain) (peripheral nerve) (spinal) T85.84 ☑
      urinary T83.84 ☑
    fixation, internal (orthopedic) NEC T84.84 ☑
    gastrointestinal (bile duct) (esophagus) T85.84 ☑
    genital NEC T83.84 ☑
    heart NEC T82.847 ☑
    infusion NEC T85.84 ☑
    joint prosthesis T84.84 ☑
    ocular (corneal graft) (orbital implant) NEC T85.84 ☑
    orthopedic NEC T84.84 ☑
    specified NEC T85.84 ☑
    urinary NEC T83.84 ☑
    vascular NEC T82.848 ☑
    ventricular intracranial shunt T85.84 ☑
  due to malignancy (primary) (secondary) G89.3
  ear — see subcategory H92.0 ☑
  epigastric, epigastrium R10.13
  eye — see Pain, ocular
  face, facial R51
    atypical G50.1
  female genital organs NEC N94.89
  finger — see Pain, limb, upper
  flank — see Pain, abdominal
  foot — see Pain, limb, lower
  gallbladder K82.9
  gas (intestinal) R14.1
  gastric — see Pain, abdominal
  generalized NOS R52
  genital organ
    female N94.89
    male N50.8
  groin — see Pain, abdominal, lower
  hand — see Pain, limb, upper
  head — see Headache
  heart — see Pain, precordial
  infra-orbital — see Neuralgia, trigeminal
  intercostal R07.82
  intermenstrual N94.0
  jaw R68.84
  joint M25.50
    ankle M25.57- ☑
    elbow M25.52- ☑
    finger M79.64- ☑
    foot M79.67- ☑
    hand M79.64- ☑
    hip M25.55- ☑
    knee M25.56- ☑
    shoulder M25.51- ☑
    toe M79.67- ☑
    wrist M25.53- ☑
  kidney N23
  laryngeal R07.0
  leg — see Pain, limb, lower
  limb M79.609
    lower M79.60- ☑
      foot M79.67- ☑
      lower leg M79.66- ☑
      thigh M79.65- ☑
      toe M79.67- ☑
    upper M79.60- ☑
      axilla M79.62- ☑
      finger M79.64- ☑

Pain(s) — *continued*
  limb — *continued*
    upper — *continued*
      forearm M79.63- ☑
      hand M79.64- ☑
      upper arm M79.62- ☑
  loin M54.5
  low back M54.5
  lumbar region M54.5
  mandibular R68.84
  mastoid — *see* subcategory H92.0 ☑
  maxilla R68.84
  menstrual (*see also* Dysmenorrhea) N94.6
  metacarpophalangeal (joint) — *see* Pain, joint, hand
  metatarsophalangeal (joint) — *see* Pain, joint, foot
  mouth K13.79
  muscle — *see* Myalgia
  musculoskeletal (*see also* Pain, by site) M79.1
  myofascial M79.1
  nasal J34.89
  nasopharynx J39.2
  neck NEC M54.2
  nerve NEC — *see* Neuralgia
  neuromuscular — *see* Neuralgia
  nose J34.89
  ocular H57.1- ☑
  ophthalmic — *see* Pain, ocular
  orbital region — *see* Pain, ocular
  ovary N94.89
  over heart — *see* Pain, precordial
  ovulation N94.0
  pelvic (female) R10.2
  penis N48.89
  pericardial — *see* Pain, precordial
  perineal, perineum R10.2
  pharynx J39.2
  pleura, pleural, pleuritic R07.81
  post-thoracotomy G89.12
  postoperative NOS G89.18
  postprocedural NOS G89.18
  precordial (region) R07.2
  premenstrual N94.3
  psychogenic (persistent) (any site) F45.41
  radicular (spinal) — *see* Radiculopathy
  rectum K62.89
  respiration R07.1
  retrosternal R07.2
  rheumatoid, muscular — *see* Myalgia
  rib R07.81
  root (spinal) — *see* Radiculopathy
  round ligament (stretch) R10.2
  sacroiliac M53.3
  sciatic — *see* Sciatica
  scrotum N50.8
  seminal vesicle N50.8
  shoulder M25.51- ☑
  spermatic cord N50.8
  spinal root — *see* Radiculopathy
  spine M54.9
    cervical M54.2
    low back M54.5
      with sciatica M54.4- ☑
    thoracic M54.6
  stomach — *see* Pain, abdominal
  substernal R07.2
  temporomandibular (joint) M26.62
  testis N50.8
  thoracic spine M54.6
    with radicular and visceral pain M54.14
  throat R07.0
  tibia — *see* Pain, limb, lower
  toe — *see* Pain, limb, lower
  tongue K14.6
  tooth K08.8
  trigeminal — *see* Neuralgia, trigeminal
  tumor associated G89.3
  ureter N23
  urinary (organ) (system) N23
  uterus NEC N94.89
  vagina R10.2
  vertebrogenic (syndrome) M54.89
  vesical R39.89
    associated with micturition — *see* Micturition, painful
  vulva R10.2
Painful (*see also* Pain)
  coitus
    female N94.1

Painful — *continued*
  coitus — *continued*
    male N53.12
    psychogenic F52.6
  ejaculation (semen) N53.12
    psychogenic F52.6
  erection — *see* Priapism
  feet syndrome E53.8
  joint replacement (hip) (knee) T84.84 ☑
  menstruation — *see* Dysmenorrhea
    psychogenic F45.8
  micturition — *see* Micturition, painful
  respiration R07.1
  scar NEC L90.5
  wire sutures T81.89 ☑
Painter's colic — *see* subcategory T56.0 ☑
Palate — *see* condition
Palatoplegia K13.79
Palatoschisis — *see* Cleft, palate
Palilalia R48.8
Palliative care Z51.5
Pallor R23.1
  optic disc, temporal — *see* Atrophy, optic
Palmar (*see also* condition)
  fascia — *see* condition
Palpable
  cecum K63.89
  kidney N28.89
  ovary N83.8
  prostate N42.9
  spleen — *see* Splenomegaly
Palpitations (heart) R00.2
  psychogenic F45.8
Palsy (*see also* Paralysis) G83.9
  atrophic diffuse (progressive) G12.22
  Bell's (*see also* Palsy, facial)
    newborn P11.3
  brachial plexus NEC G54.0
    newborn (birth injury) P14.3
  brain — *see* Palsy, cerebral
  bulbar (progressive) (chronic) G12.22
    of childhood (Fazio-Londe) G12.1
    pseudo NEC G12.29
    supranuclear (progressive) G23.1
  cerebral (congenital) G80.9
    ataxic G80.4
    athetoid G80.3
    choreathetoid G80.3
    diplegic G80.8
      spastic G80.1
    dyskinetic G80.3
      athetoid G80.3
      choreathetoid G80.3
      distonic G80.3
    dystonic G80.3
    hemiplegic G80.8
      spastic G80.2
    mixed G80.8
    monoplegic G80.8
      spastic G80.1
    paraplegic G80.8
      spastic G80.1
    quadriplegic G80.8
      spastic G80.0
    spastic G80.1
      diplegic G80.1
      hemiplegic G80.2
      monoplegic G80.1
      quadriplegic G80.0
      specified NEC G80.1
      tetrapelgic G80.0
    specified NEC G80.8
    syphilitic A52.12
      congenital A50.49
    tetraplegic G80.8
      spastic G80.0
  cranial nerve (*see also* Disorder, nerve, cranial)
    multiple G52.7
      in
        infectious disease B99 ☑ [G53]
        neoplastic disease (*see also* Neoplasm) D49.9 [G53]
        parasitic disease B89 [G53]
        sarcoidosis D86.82
  creeping G12.22
  diver's T70.3 ☑
  Erb's P14.0
  facial G51.0

Palsy — *continued*
  facial — *continued*
    newborn (birth injury) P11.3
  glossopharyngeal G52.1
  Klumpke (-Déjérine) P14.1
  lead — *see* subcategory T56.0 ☑
  median nerve (tardy) G56.1- ☑
  nerve G58.9
    specified NEC G58.8
  peroneal nerve (acute) (tardy) G57.3- ☑
  progressive supranuclear G23.1
  pseudobulbar NEC G12.29
  radial nerve (acute) G56.3- ☑
  seventh nerve (*see also* Palsy, facial)
    newborn P11.3
  shaking — *see* Parkinsonism
  spastic (cerebral) (spinal) G80.1
  ulnar nerve (tardy) G56.2- ☑
  wasting G12.29
Paludism — *see* Malaria
Panangiitis M30.0
Panaris, panaritium (*see also* Cellulitis, digit)
  with lymphangitis — *see* Lymphangitis, acute, digit
Panarteritis nodosa M30.0
  brain or cerebral I67.7
Pancake heart R93.1
  with cor pulmonale (chronic) I27.81
Pancarditis (acute) (chronic) I51.89
  rheumatic I09.89
    active or acute I01.8
Pancoast's syndrome or tumor C34.1- ☑
Pancolitis, ulcerative (chronic) K51.00
  with
    abscess K51.014
    complication K51.019
    fistula K51.013
    obstruction K51.012
    rectal bleeding K51.011
    specified complication NEC K51.018
Pancreas, pancreatic — *see* condition
Pancreatitis (annular) (apopleptic) (calcareous) (edematous) (hemorrhagic) (malignant) (recurrent) (subacute) (suppurative) K85.9
  acute K85.9
    alcohol induced K85.2
    biliary K85.1
    drug induced K85.3
    gallstone K85.1
    idiopathic K85.0
    specified NEC K85.8
  chronic (infectious) K86.1
    alcohol-induced K86.0
    recurrent K86.1
    relapsing K86.1
  cystic (chronic) K86.1
  cytomegaloviral B25.2
  fibrous (chronic) K86.1
  gallstone K85.1
  gangrenous K85.8
  interstitial (chronic) K86.1
    acute K85.8
  mumps B26.3
  recurrent (chronic) K86.1
  relapsing, chronic K86.1
  syphilitic A52.74
Pancreatoblastoma — *see* Neoplasm, pancreas, malignant
Pancreolithiasis K86.8
Pancytolysis D75.89
Pancytopenia (acquired) D61.818
  with
    malformations D61.09
    myelodysplastic syndrome — *see* Syndrome, myelodysplastic
  antineoplastic chemotherapy induced D61.810
  congenital D61.09
  drug-induced NEC D61.811
Panencephalitis, subacute, sclerosing A81.1
Panhematopenia D61.9
  congenital D61.09
  constitutional D61.09
  splenic, primary D73.1
Panhemocytopenia D61.9
  congenital D61.09
  constitutional D61.09
Panhypogonadism E29.1
Panhypopituitarism E23.0
  prepubertal E23.0

Panic (attack) (state) F41.0
  reaction to exceptional stress (transient) F43.0
Panmyelopathy, familial, constitutional D61.09
Panmyelophthisis D61.82
  congenital D61.09
Panmyelosis (acute) (with myelofibrosis) C94.4- ☑
Panner's disease — see Osteochondrosis, juvenile,
  humerus
Panneuritis endemica E51.11
Panniculitis (nodular) (nonsuppurative) M79.3
  back M54.00
    cervical region M54.02
    cervicothoracic region M54.03
    lumbar region M54.06
    lumbosacral region M54.07
    multiple sites M54.09
    occipito-atlanto-axial region M54.01
    sacrococcygeal region M54.08
    thoracic region M54.04
    thoracolumbar region M54.05
  lupus L93.2
  mesenteric K65.4
  neck M54.02
    cervicothoracic region M54.03
    occipito-atlanto-axial region M54.01
  relapsing M35.6
Panniculus adiposus (abdominal) E65
Pannus (allergic) (cornea) (degenerativus) (keratic)
  H16.42-
  abdominal (symptomatic) E65
  trachomatosus, trachomatous (active) A71.1
Panophthalmitis H44.01- ☑
Pansinusitis (chronic) (hyperplastic) (nonpurulent) (purulent) J32.4
  acute J01.40
    recurrent J01.41
  tuberculous A15.8
Panuveitis (sympathetic) H44.11- ☑
Panvalvular disease I08.9
  specified NEC I08.8
Papanicolaou smear, cervix Z12.4
  as part of routine gynecological examination Z01.419
    with abnormal findings Z01.411
  for suspected neoplasm Z12.4
  nonspecific abnormal finding R87.619
  routine Z01.419
    with abnormal findings Z01.411
Papilledema (choked disc) H47.10
  associated with
    decreased ocular pressure H47.12
    increased intracranial pressure H47.11
    retinal disorder H47.13
  Foster-Kennedy syndrome H47.14- ☑
Papillitis H46.00
  anus K62.89
  chronic lingual K14.4
  necrotizing, kidney N17.2
  optic H46.0- ☑
  rectum K62.89
  renal, necrotizing N17.2
  tongue K14.0
Papilloma (see also Neoplasm, benign, by site)
  acuminatum (female) (male) (anogenital) A63.0
  benign pinta (primary) A67.0
  bladder (urinary) (transitional cell) D41.4
  choroid plexus (lateral ventricle) (third ventricle) D33.0
    anaplastic C71.5
    fourth ventricle D33.1
    malignant C71.5
  renal pelvis (transitional cell) D41.1- ☑
    benign D30.1- ☑
  Schneiderian
    specified site — see Neoplasm, benign, by site
    unspecified site D14.0
  serous surface
    borderline malignancy
      specified site — see Neoplasm, uncertain be-
        havior, by site
      unspecified site D39.10
    specified site — see Neoplasm, benign, by site
    unspecified site D27.9
  transitional (cell)
    bladder (urinary) D41.4
    inverted type — see Neoplasm, uncertain behavior,
      by site
    renal pelvis D41.1- ☑
    ureter D41.2- ☑

Papilloma — continued
  ureter (transitional cell) D41.2- ☑
    benign D30.2- ☑
  urothelial — see Neoplasm, uncertain behavior, by
    site
  villous — see Neoplasm, uncertain behavior, by site
    adenocarcinoma in — see Neoplasm, malignant,
      by site
    in situ — see Neoplasm, in situ
  yaws, plantar or palmar A66.1
Papillomata, multiple, of yaws A66.1
Papillomatosis (see also Neoplasm, benign, by site)
  confluent and reticulated L83
  cystic, breast — see Mastopathy, cystic
  ductal, breast — see Mastopathy, cystic
  intraductal (diffuse) — see Neoplasm, benign, by site
  subareolar duct D24- ☑
Papillomavirus, as cause of disease classified else-
  where B97.7
Papillon-Léage and Psaume syndrome Q87.0
Papule(s) R23.8
  carate (primary) A67.0
  fibrous, of nose D22.39
  Gottron's L94.4
  pinta (primary) A67.0
Papulosis
  lymphomatoid C86.6
  malignant I77.89
Papyraceous fetus O31.0- ☑
Para-albuminemia E88.09
Paracephalus Q89.7
Parachute mitral valve Q23.2
Paracoccidioidomycosis B41.9
  disseminated B41.7
  generalized B41.7
  mucocutaneous-lymphangitic B41.8
  pulmonary B41.0
  specified NEC B41.8
  visceral B41.8
Paradentosis K05.4
Paraffinoma T88.8 ☑
Paraganglioma D44.7
  adrenal D35.0- ☑
    malignant C74.1- ☑
  aortic body D44.7
    malignant C75.5
  carotid body D44.6
    malignant C75.4
  chromaffin (see also Neoplasm, benign, by site)
    malignant — see Neoplasm, malignant, by site
  extra-adrenal D44.7
    malignant C75.5
      specified site — see Neoplasm, malignant, by
        site
      unspecified site C75.5
    specified site — see Neoplasm, uncertain behavior,
      by site
    unspecified site D44.7
  gangliocytic D13.2
    specified site — see Neoplasm, benign, by site
    unspecified site D13.2
  glomus jugulare D44.7
    malignant C75.5
  jugular D44.7
  malignant C75.5
    specified site — see Neoplasm, malignant, by site
    unspecified site C75.5
  nonchromaffin D44.7
    malignant C75.5
      specified site — see Neoplasm, malignant, by
        site
      unspecified site C75.5
    specified site — see Neoplasm, uncertain behavior,
      by site
    unspecified site D44.7
  parasympathetic D44.7
    specified site — see Neoplasm, uncertain behavior,
      by site
    unspecified site D44.7
  specified site — see Neoplasm, uncertain behavior,
    by site
  sympathetic D44.7
    specified site — see Neoplasm, uncertain behavior,
      by site
    unspecified site D44.7
  unspecified site D44.7
Parageusia R43.2

Parageusia — continued
  psychogenic F45.8
Paragonimiasis B66.4
Paragranuloma, Hodgkin — see Lymphoma, Hodgkin,
  classical, specified NEC
Parahemophilia (see also Defect, coagulation) D68.2
Parakeratosis R23.4
  variegata L41.0
Paralysis, paralytic (complete) (incomplete) G83.9
  with
    syphilis A52.17
  abducens, abducent (nerve) — see Strabismus, para-
    lytic, sixth nerve
  abductor, lower extremity G57.9- ☑
  accessory nerve G52.8
  accommodation (see also Paresis, of accommodation)
    hysterical F44.89
  acoustic nerve (except Deafness) H93.3 ☑
  agitans (see also Parkinsonism) G20
    arteriosclerotic G21.4
  alternating (oculomotor) G83.89
  amyotrophic G12.21
  ankle G57.9- ☑
  anus (sphincter) K62.89
  arm — see Monoplegia, upper limb
  ascending (spinal), acute G61.0
  association G12.29
  asthenic bulbar G70.00
    with exacerbation (acute) G70.01
    in crisis G70.01
  ataxic (hereditary) G11.9
    general (syphilitic) A52.17
  atrophic G58.9
    infantile, acute — see Poliomyelitis, paralytic
    progressive G12.22
    spinal (acute) — see Poliomyelitis, paralytic
  axillary G54.0
  Babinski-Nageotte's G83.89
  Bell's G51.0
    newborn P11.3
  Benedikt's G46.3
  birth injury P14.9
    spinal cord P11.5
  bladder (neurogenic) (sphincter) N31.2
  bowel, colon or intestine K56.0
  brachial plexus G54.0
    birth injury P14.3
    newborn (birth injury) P14.3
  brain G83.9
    diplegia G83.0
    triplegia G83.89
  bronchial J98.09
  Brown-Séquard G83.81
  bulbar (chronic) (progressive) G12.22
    infantile — see Poliomyelitis, paralytic
    poliomyelitic — see Poliomyelitis, paralytic
    pseudo G12.29
  bulbospinal G70.00
    with exacerbation (acute) G70.01
    in crisis G70.01
  cardiac (see also Failure, heart) I50.9
  cerebrocerebellar, diplegic G80.1
  cervical
    plexus G54.2
    sympathetic G90.09
  Céstan-Chenais G46.3
  Charcot-Marie-Tooth type G60.0
  Clark's G80.9
  colon K56.0
  compressed air T70.3 ☑
  compression
    arm G56.9- ☑
    leg G57.9- ☑
    lower extremity G57.9- ☑
    upper extremity G56.9- ☑
  congenital (cerebral) — see Palsy, cerebral
  conjugate movement (gaze) (of eye) H51.0
    cortical (nuclear) (supranuclear) H51.0
  cordis — see Failure, heart
  cranial or cerebral nerve G52.9
  creeping G12.22
  crossed leg G83.89
  crutch — see Injury, brachial plexus
  deglutition R13.0
    hysterical F44.4
  dementia A52.17
  descending (spinal) NEC G12.29
  diaphragm (flaccid) J98.6

Paralysis, paralytic — *continued*
diaphragm — *continued*
    due to accidental dissection of phrenic nerve during procedure — *see* Puncture, accidental complicating surgery
digestive organs NEC K59.8
diplegic — *see* Diplegia
divergence (nuclear) H51.8
diver's T70.3 ☑
Duchenne's
    birth injury P14.0
    due to or associated with
        motor neuron disease G12.22
        muscular dystrophy G71.0
due to intracranial or spinal birth injury — *see* Palsy, cerebral
embolic (current episode) I63.4 ☑
Erb (-Duchenne) (birth) (newborn) P14.0
Erb's syphilitic spastic spinal A52.17
esophagus K22.8
eye muscle (extrinsic) H49.9
    intrinsic (*see also* Paresis, of accommodation)
facial (nerve) G51.0
    birth injury P11.3
    congenital P11.3
    following operation NEC — *see* Puncture, accidental complicating surgery
    newborn (birth injury) P11.3
familial (recurrent) (periodic) G72.3
    spastic G11.4
fauces J39.2
finger G56.9- ☑
gait R26.1
gastric nerve (nondiabetic) G52.2
gaze, conjugate H51.0
general (progressive) (syphilitic) A52.17
    juvenile A50.45
glottis J38.00
    bilateral J38.02
    unilateral J38.01
gluteal G54.1
Gubler (-Millard) G46.3
hand — *see* Monoplegia, upper limb
heart — *see* Arrest, cardiac
hemiplegic — *see* Hemiplegia
hyperkalemic periodic (familial) G72.3
hypoglossal (nerve) G52.3
hypokalemic periodic G72.3
hysterical F44.4
ileus K56.0
infantile (*see also* Poliomyelitis, paralytic) A80.30
    bulbar — *see* Poliomyelitis, paralytic
    cerebral — *see* Palsy, cerebral
    spastic — *see* Palsy, cerebral, spastic
infective — *see* Poliomyelitis, paralytic
inferior nuclear G83.9
internuclear — *see* Ophthalmoplegia, internuclear
intestine K56.0
iris H57.09
    due to diphtheria (toxin) A36.89
ischemic, Volkmann's (complicating trauma) T79.6 ☑
Jackson's G83.89
jake — *see* Poisoning, food, noxious, plant
Jamaica ginger (jake) G62.2
juvenile general A50.45
Klumpke (-Déjérine) (birth) (newborn) P14.1
labioglossal (laryngeal) (pharyngeal) G12.29
Landry's G61.0
laryngeal nerve (recurrent) (superior) (unilateral) J38.00
    bilateral J38.02
    unilateral J38.01
larynx J38.00
    bilateral J38.02
    due to diphtheria (toxin) A36.2
    unilateral J38.01
lateral G12.21
lead T56.0 ☑
left side — *see* Hemiplegia
leg G83.1- ☑
    both — *see* Paraplegia
    crossed G83.89
    hysterical F44.4
    psychogenic F44.4
    transient or transitory R29.818
        traumatic NEC — *see* Injury, nerve, leg
levator palpebrae superioris — *see* Blepharoptosis, paralytic
limb — *see* Monoplegia

Paralysis, paralytic — *continued*
lip K13.0
    Lissauer's A52.17
lower limb — *see* Monoplegia, lower limb
    both — *see* Paraplegia
lung J98.4
median nerve G56.1- ☑
medullary (tegmental) G83.89
mesencephalic NEC G83.89
    tegmental G83.89
middle alternating G83.89
Millard-Gubler-Foville G46.3
monoplegic — *see* Monoplegia
motor G83.9
muscle, muscular NEC G72.89
    due to nerve lesion G58.9
    eye (extrinsic) H49.9
        intrinsic — *see* Paresis, of accommodation
        oblique — *see* Strabismus, paralytic, fourth nerve
    iris sphincter H21.9
    ischemic (Volkmann's) (complicating trauma) T79.6 ☑
    progressive G12.21
    pseudohypertrophic G71.0
musculocutaneous nerve G56.9- ☑
musculospiral G56.9- ☑
nerve (*see also* Disorder, nerve)
    abducent — *see* Strabismus, paralytic, sixth nerve
    accessory G52.8
    auditory (except Deafness) H93.3 ☑
    birth injury P14.9
    cranial or cerebral G52.9
    facial G51.0
        birth injury P11.3
        congenital P11.3
        newborn (birth injury) P11.3
    fourth or trochlear — *see* Strabismus, paralytic, fourth nerve
    newborn (birth injury) P14.9
    oculomotor — *see* Strabismus, paralytic, third nerve
    phrenic (birth injury) P14.2
    radial G56.3- ☑
    seventh or facial G51.0
        newborn (birth injury) P11.3
    sixth or abducent — *see* Strabismus, paralytic, sixth nerve
    syphilitic A52.15
    third or oculomotor — *see* Strabismus, paralytic, third nerve
    trigeminal G50.9
    trochlear — *see* Strabismus, paralytic, fourth nerve
    ulnar G56.2- ☑
normokalemic periodic G72.3
ocular H49.9
    alternating G83.89
oculofacial, congenital (Moebius) Q87.0
oculomotor (external bilateral) (nerve) — *see* Strabismus, paralytic, third nerve
palate (soft) K13.79
paratrigeminal G50.9
periodic (familial) (hyperkalemic) (hypokalemic) (myotonic) (normokalemic) (potassium sensitive) (secondary) G72.3
peripheral autonomic nervous system — *see* Neuropathy, peripheral, autonomic
peroneal (nerve) G57.3- ☑
pharynx J39.2
phrenic nerve G56.8- ☑
plantar nerve(s) G57.6- ☑
pneumogastric nerve G52.2
poliomyelitis (current) — *see* Poliomyelitis, paralytic
popliteal nerve G57.3- ☑
postepileptic transitory G83.84
progressive (atrophic) (bulbar) (spinal) G12.22
    general A52.17
    infantile acute — *see* Poliomyelitis, paralytic
    supranuclear G23.1
pseudobulbar G12.29
pseudohypertrophic (muscle) G71.0
psychogenic F44.4
quadriceps G57.9- ☑
quadriplegic — *see* Tetraplegia
radial nerve G56.3- ☑
rectus muscle (eye) H49.9
recurrent isolated sleep G47.53

Paralysis, paralytic — *continued*
respiratory (muscle) (system) (tract) R06.81
    center NEC G93.89
    congenital P28.89
    newborn P28.89
right side — *see* Hemiplegia
saturnine T56.0 ☑
sciatic nerve G57.0- ☑
senile G83.9
shaking — *see* Parkinsonism
shoulder G56.9- ☑
sleep, recurrent isolated G47.53
spastic G83.9
    cerebral — *see* Palsy, cerebral, spastic
    congenital (cerebral) — *see* Palsy, cerebral, spastic
    familial G11.4
    hereditary G11.4
    quadriplegic G80.0
    syphilitic (spinal) A52.17
sphincter, bladder — *see* Paralysis, bladder
spinal (cord) G83.9
    accessory nerve G52.8
    acute — *see* Poliomyelitis, paralytic
    ascending acute G61.0
    atrophic (acute) (*see also* Poliomyelitis, paralytic)
        spastic, syphilitic A52.17
    congenital NEC — *see* Palsy, cerebral
    hereditary G95.89
    infantile — *see* Poliomyelitis, paralytic
    progressive G12.21
    sequelae NEC G83.89
sternomastoid G52.8
stomach K31.84
    diabetic — *see* Diabetes, by type, with gastroparesis
    nerve G52.2
        diabetic — *see* Diabetes, by type, with gastroparesis
stroke — *see* Infarct, brain
subcapsularis G56.8- ☑
supranuclear (progressive) G23.1
sympathetic G90.8
    cervical G90.09
    nervous system — *see* Neuropathy, peripheral, autonomic
syndrome G83.9
    specified NEC G83.89
syphilitic spastic spinal (Erb's) A52.17
thigh G57.9- ☑
throat J39.2
    diphtheritic A36.0
    muscle J39.2
thrombotic (current episode) I63.3 ☑
thumb G56.9- ☑
tick — *see* Toxicity, venom, arthropod, specified NEC
Todd's (postepileptic transitory paralysis) G83.84
toe G57.6- ☑
tongue K14.8
transient R29.5
    arm or leg NEC R29.818
    traumatic NEC — *see* Injury, nerve
trapezius G52.8
traumatic, transient NEC — *see* Injury, nerve
trembling — *see* Parkinsonism
triceps brachii G56.9- ☑
trigeminal nerve G50.9
trochlear (nerve) — *see* Strabismus, paralytic, fourth nerve
ulnar nerve G56.2- ☑
upper limb — *see* Monoplegia, upper limb
uremic N18.9 [G99.8]
uveoparotitic D86.89
uvula K13.79
    postdiphtheritic A36.0
vagus nerve G52.2
vasomotor NEC G90.8
velum palati K13.79
vesical — *see* Paralysis, bladder
vestibular nerve (except Vertigo) H93.3 ☑
vocal cords J38.00
    bilateral J38.02
    unilateral J38.01
Volkmann's (complicating trauma) T79.6 ☑
wasting G12.29
Weber's G46.3
wrist G56.9- ☑
Paramedial urethrovesical orifice Q64.79

Paramenia N92.6
Parametritis (*see also* Disease, pelvis, inflammatory)
  N73.2
  acute N73.0
  complicating abortion — *see* Abortion, by type, complicated by, parametritis
Parametrium, parametric — *see* condition
Paramnesia — *see* Amnesia
Paramolar K00.1
Paramyloidosis E85.8
Paramyoclonus multiplex G25.3
Paramyotonia (congenita) G71.19
Parangi — *see* Yaws
Paranoia (querulans) F22
  senile F03 ☑
Paranoid
  dementia (senile) F03 ☑
    praecox — *see* Schizophrenia
  personality F60.0
  psychosis (climacteric) (involutional) (menopausal)
    F22
    psychogenic (acute) F23
    senile F03 ☑
  reaction (acute) F23
    chronic F22
  schizophrenia F20.0
  state (climacteric) (involutional) (menopausal) (simple)
    F22
    senile F03 ☑
  tendencies F60.0
  traits F60.0
  trends F60.0
  type, psychopathic personality F60.0
Paraparesis — *see* Paraplegia
Paraphasia R47.02
Paraphilia F65.9
Paraphimosis (congenital) N47.2
  chancroidal A57
Paraphrenia, paraphrenic (late) F22
  schizophrenia F20.0
Paraplegia (lower) G82.20
  ataxic — *see* Degeneration, combined, spinal cord
  complete G82.21
  congenital (cerebral) G80.8
    spastic G80.1
  familial spastic G11.4
  functional (hysterical) F44.4
  hereditary, spastic G11.4
  hysterical F44.4
  incomplete G82.22
  Pott's A18.01
  psychogenic F44.4
  spastic
    Erb's spinal, syphilitic A52.17
    hereditary G11.4
    tropical G04.1
  syphilitic (spastic) A52.17
  tropical spastic G04.1
Parapoxvirus B08.60
  specified NEC B08.69
Paraproteinemia D89.2
  benign (familial) D89.2
  monoclonal D47.2
  secondary to malignant disease D47.2
Parapsoriasis L41.9
  en plaques L41.4
  guttata L41.1
  large plaque L41.4
  retiform, retiformis L41.5
  small plaque L41.3
  specified NEC L41.8
  varioliformis (acuta) L41.0
Parasitic (*see also* condition)
  disease NEC B89
  stomatitis B37.0
  sycosis (beard) (scalp) B35.0
  twin Q89.4
Parasitism B89
  intestinal B82.9
  skin B88.9
  specified — *see* Infestation
Parasitophobia F40.218
Parasomnia G47.50
  due to
    alcohol
      abuse F10.182
      dependence F10.282

Parasomnia — *continued*
  due to — *continued*
    alcohol — *continued*
      use F10.982
    amphetamines
      abuse F15.182
      dependence F15.282
      use F15.982
    caffeine
      abuse F15.182
      dependence F15.282
      use F15.982
    cocaine
      abuse F14.182
      dependence F14.282
      use F14.982
    drug NEC
      abuse F19.182
      dependence F19.282
      use F19.982
    opioid
      abuse F11.182
      dependence F11.282
      use F11.982
    psychoactive substance NEC
      abuse F19.182
      dependence F19.282
      use F19.982
    sedative, hypnotic, or anxiolytic
      abuse F13.182
      dependence F13.282
      use F13.982
    stimulant NEC
      abuse F15.182
      dependence F15.282
      use F15.982
  in conditions classified elsewhere G47.54
  nonorganic origin F51.8
  organic G47.50
  specified NEC G47.59
Paraspadias Q54.9
Paraspasmus facialis G51.8
Parasuicide (attempt)
  history of (personal) Z91.5
    in family Z81.8
Parathyroid gland — *see* condition
Parathyroid tetany E20.9
Paratrachoma A74.0
Paratyphilitis — *see* Appendicitis
Paratyphoid (fever) — *see* Fever, paratyphoid
Paratyphus — *see* Fever, paratyphoid
Paraurethral duct Q64.79
  nonorganic origin F51.5
Paraurethritis (*see also* Urethritis)
  gonococcal (acute) (chronic) (with abscess) A54.1
Paravaccinia NEC B08.04
Paravaginitis — *see* Vaginitis
Parencephalitis (*see also* Encephalitis)
  sequelae G09
Parent-child conflict — *see* Conflict, parent-child
  estrangement NEC Z62.890
Paresis (*see also* Paralysis)
  accommodation — *see* Paresis, of accommodation
  Bernhardt's G57.1- ☑
  bladder (sphincter) (*see also* Paralysis, bladder)
    tabetic A52.17
  bowel, colon or intestine K56.0
  extrinsic muscle, eye H49.9
  general (progressive) (syphilitic) A52.17
    juvenile A50.45
  heart — *see* Failure, heart
  insane (syphilitic) A52.17
  juvenile (general) A50.45
  of accommodation H52.52- ☑
  peripheral progressive (idiopathic) G60.3
  pseudohypertrophic G71.0
  senile G83.9
  syphilitic (general) A52.17
    congenital A50.45
  vesical NEC N31.2
Paresthesia (*see also* Disturbance, sensation)
  Bernhardt G57.1- ☑
Paretic — *see* condition
Parinaud's
  conjunctivitis H10.89
  oculoglandular syndrome H10.89
  ophthalmoplegia H49.88- ☑
Parkinsonism (idiopathic) (primary) G20

Parkinsonism — *continued*
  with neurogenic orthostatic hypotension (symptomatic) G90.3
  arteriosclerotic G21.4
  dementia G31.83 [F02.80]
    with behavioral disturbance G31.83 [F02.81]
  due to
    drugs NEC G21.19
      neuroleptic G21.11
  neuroleptic induced G21.11
  postencephalitic G21.3
  secondary G21.9
    due to
      arteriosclerosis G21.4
      drugs NEC G21.19
        neuroleptic G21.11
      encephalitis G21.3
      external agents NEC G21.2
      syphilis A52.19
    specified NEC G21.8
  syphilitic A52.19
  treatment-induced NEC G21.19
  vascular G21.4
Parkinson's disease, syndrome or tremor — *see* Parkinsonism
Parodontitis — *see* Periodontitis
Parodontosis K05.4
Paronychia (*see also* Cellulitis, digit)
  with lymphangitis — *see* Lymphangitis, acute, digit
  candidal (chronic) B37.2
  tuberculous (primary) A18.4
Parorexia (psychogenic) F50.8
Parosmia R43.1
  psychogenic F45.8
Parotid gland — *see* condition
Parotitis, parotiditis (allergic)(nonspecific toxic) (purulent) (septic) (suppurative) (*see also* Sialoadenitis)
  epidemic — *see* Mumps
  infectious — *see* Mumps
  postoperative K91.89
  surgical K91.89
Parrot fever A70
Parrot's disease (early congenital syphilitic pseudoparalysis) A50.02
Parry-Romberg syndrome G51.8
Parry's disease or syndrome E05.00
  with thyroid storm E05.01
Pars planitis — *see* Cyclitis
Parsonage (-Aldren)-**Turner syndrome** G54.5
Parson's disease (exophthalmic goiter) E05.00
  with thyroid storm E05.01
Particolored infant Q82.8
Parturition — *see* Delivery
Parulis K04.7
  with sinus K04.6
Parvovirus, as cause of disease classified elsewhere B97.6
Pasini and Pierini's atrophoderma L90.3
Passage
  false, urethra N36.5
  meconium (newborn) during delivery P03.82
  of sounds or bougies — *see* Attention to, artificial, opening
Passive — *see* condition
  smoking Z77.22
Pasteurella septica A28.0
Pasteurellosis — *see* Infection, Pasteurella
PAT (paroxysmal atrial tachycardia) I47.1
Patau's syndrome — *see* Trisomy, 13
Patches
  mucous (syphilitic) A51.39
    congenital A50.07
  smokers' (mouth) K13.24
Patellar — *see* condition
Patent (*see also* Imperfect, closure)
  canal of Nuck Q52.4
  cervix N88.3
  ductus arteriosus or Botallo's Q25.0
  foramen
    botalli Q21.1
    ovale Q21.1
  interauricular septum Q21.1
  interventricular septum Q21.0
  omphalomesenteric duct Q43.0
  os (uteri) — *see* Patent, cervix
  ostium secundum Q21.1
  urachus Q64.4

Patent — *continued*
vitelline duct Q43.Ø
Paterson (-Brown)(-Kelly) **syndrome or web** D50.1
Pathologic, pathological (*see also* condition)
asphyxia RØ9.Ø1
fire-setting F63.1
gambling F63.Ø
ovum OØ2.Ø
resorption, tooth KØ3.3
stealing F63.2
Pathology (of) — *see* Disease
periradicular, associated with previous endodontic treatment NEC M27.59
Pattern, sleep-wake, irregular G47.23
Patulous (*see also* Imperfect, closure (congenital))
alimentary tract Q45.8
lower Q43.8
upper Q4Ø.8
eustachian tube H69.Ø- ☑
Pause, sinoatrial I49.5
Paxton's disease B36.2
Pearl(s)
enamel KØØ.2
Epstein's KØ9.8
Pearl-worker's disease — *see* Osteomyelitis, specified type NEC
Pectenosis K62.4
Pectoral — *see* condition
Pectus
carinatum (congenital) Q67.7
acquired M95.4
rachitic sequelae (late effect) E64.3
excavatum (congenital) Q67.6
acquired M95.4
rachitic sequelae (late effect) E64.3
recurvatum (congenital) Q67.6
Pedatrophia E41
Pederosis F65.4
Pediculosis (infestation) B85.2
capitis (head-louse) (any site) B85.Ø
corporis (body-louse) (any site) B85.1
eyelid B85.Ø
mixed (classifiable to more than one of the titles B85.Ø-B85.3) B85.4
pubis (pubic louse) (any site) B85.3
vestimenti B85.1
vulvae B85.3
Pediculus (infestation) — *see* Pediculosis
Pedophilia F65.4
Peg-shaped teeth KØØ.2
Pelade — *see* Alopecia, areata
Pelger-Huët anomaly or syndrome D72.Ø
Peliosis (rheumatica) D69.Ø
hepatis K76.4
with toxic liver disease K71.8
Pelizaeus-Merzbacher disease E75.29
Pellagra (alcoholic) (with polyneuropathy) E52
Pellagra-cerebellar-ataxia-renal aminoaciduria syndrome E72.Ø2
Pellegrini (-Stieda) **disease or syndrome** — *see* Bursitis, tibial collateral
Pellizzi's syndrome E34.8
Pel's crisis A52.11
Pelvic (*see also* condition)
examination (periodic) (routine) ZØ1.419
with abnormal findings ZØ1.411
kidney, congenital Q63.2
Pelviolithiasis — *see* Calculus, kidney
Pelviperitonitis (*see also* Peritonitis, pelvic)
gonococcal A54.24
puerperal O85
Pelvis — *see* condition or type
Pemphigoid L12.9
benign, mucous membrane L12.1
bullous L12.Ø
cicatricial L12.1
juvenile L12.2
ocular L12.1
specified NEC L12.8
Pemphigus L1Ø.9
benign familial (chronic) Q82.8
Brazilian L1Ø.3
circinatus L13.Ø
conjunctiva L12.1
drug-induced L1Ø.5
erythematosus L1Ø.4
foliaceus L1Ø.2

Pemphigus — *continued*
gangrenous — *see* Gangrene
neonatorum LØ1.Ø3
ocular L12.1
paraneoplastic L1Ø.81
specified NEC L1Ø.89
syphilitic (congenital) A5Ø.Ø6
vegetans L1Ø.1
vulgaris L1Ø.Ø
wildfire L1Ø.3
Pendred's syndrome EØ7.1
Pendulous
abdomen, in pregnancy — *see* Pregnancy, complicated by, abnormal, pelvic organs or tissues NEC
breast N64.89
Penetrating wound (*see also* Puncture)
with internal injury — *see* Injury, by site
eyeball — *see* Puncture, eyeball
orbit (with or without foreign body) — *see* Puncture, orbit
uterus by instrument with or following ectopic or molar pregnancy OØ8.6
Penicillosis B48.4
Penis — *see* condition
Penitis N48.29
Pentalogy of Fallot Q21.8
Pentasomy X syndrome Q97.1
Pentosuria (essential) E74.8
Percreta placenta - O43.23 ☑
Peregrinating patient — *see* Disorder, factitious
Perforation, perforated (nontraumatic) (of)
accidental during procedure (blood vessel) (nerve) (organ) — *see* Complication, accidental puncture or laceration
antrum — *see* Sinusitis, maxillary
appendix K35.2
atrial septum, multiple Q21.1
attic, ear — *see* Perforation, tympanum, attic
bile duct (common) (hepatic) K83.2
cystic K82.2
bladder (urinary)
with or following ectopic or molar pregnancy OØ8.6
obstetrical trauma O71.5
traumatic S37.29 ☑
at delivery O71.5
bowel K63.1
with or following ectopic or molar pregnancy OØ8.6
newborn P78.Ø
obstetrical trauma O71.5
traumatic — *see* Laceration, intestine
broad ligament N83.8
with or following ectopic or molar pregnancy OØ8.6
obstetrical trauma O71.6
by
device, implant or graft (*see also* Complications, by site and type, mechanical) T85.628 ☑
arterial graft NEC — *see* Complication, cardiovascular device, mechanical, vascular
breast (implant) T85.49 ☑
catheter NEC T85.698 ☑
cystostomy T83.Ø90 ☑
dialysis (renal) T82.49 ☑
intraperitoneal T85.691 ☑
infusion NEC T82.594 ☑
spinal (epidural) (subdural) T85.69Ø ☑
electronic (electrode) (pulse generator) (stimulator)
bone T84.39Ø ☑
cardiac T82.199 ☑
electrode T82.19Ø ☑
pulse generator T82.191 ☑
specified type NEC T82.198 ☑
nervous system — *see* Complication, prosthetic device, mechanical, electronic nervous system stimulator
urinary — *see* Complication, genitourinary, device, urinary, mechanical
fixation, internal (orthopedic) NEC — *see* Complication, fixation device, mechanical
gastrointestinal — *see* Complications, prosthetic device, mechanical, gastrointestinal device
genital NEC T83.498 ☑
intrauterine contraceptive device T83.39 ☑
penile prosthesis T83.49Ø ☑
heart NEC — *see* Complication, cardiovascular device, mechanical

Perforation, perforated — *continued*
by — *continued*
device, implant or graft (*see also* Complications, by site and type, mechanical) — *continued*
joint prosthesis — *see* Complications, joint prosthesis, mechanical, specified NEC, by site
ocular NEC — *see* Complications, prosthetic device, mechanical, ocular device
orthopedic NEC — *see* Complication, orthopedic, device, mechanical
specified NEC T85.628 ☑
urinary, indwelling T83.Ø98 ☑
urinary NEC (*see also* Complication, genitourinary, device, urinary, mechanical)
graft T83.29 ☑
vascular NEC — *see* Complication, cardiovascular device, mechanical
ventricular intracranial shunt T85.Ø9 ☑
foreign body left accidentally in operative wound T81.539 ☑
instrument (any) during a procedure, accidental — *see* Puncture, accidental complicating surgery
cecum K35.2
cervix (uteri) N88.8
with or following ectopic or molar pregnancy OØ8.6
obstetrical trauma O71.3
colon K63.1
newborn P78.Ø
obstetrical trauma O71.5
traumatic — *see* Laceration, intestine, large
common duct (bile) K83.2
cornea (due to ulceration) — *see* Ulcer, cornea, perforated
cystic duct K82.2
diverticulum (intestine) K57.8Ø
with bleeding K57.81
large intestine K57.2Ø
with
bleeding K57.21
small intestine K57.4Ø
with bleeding K57.41
small intestine K57.ØØ
with
bleeding K57.Ø1
large intestine K57.4Ø
with bleeding K57.41
ear drum — *see* Perforation, tympanum
esophagus K22.3
ethmoidal sinus — *see* Sinusitis, ethmoidal
frontal sinus — *see* Sinusitis, frontal
gallbladder K82.2
heart valve — *see* Endocarditis
ileum K63.1
newborn P78.Ø
obstetrical trauma O71.5
traumatic — *see* Laceration, intestine, small
instrumental, surgical (accidental) (blood vessel) (nerve) (organ) — *see* Puncture, accidental complicating surgery
intestine NEC K63.1
with ectopic or molar pregnancy OØ8.6
newborn P78.Ø
obstetrical trauma O71.5
traumatic — *see* Laceration, intestine
ulcerative NEC K63.1
newborn P78.Ø
jejunum, jejunal K63.1
obstetrical trauma O71.5
traumatic — *see* Laceration, intestine, small
ulcer — *see* Ulcer, gastrojejunal, with perforation
joint prosthesis — *see* Complications, joint prosthesis, mechanical, specified NEC, by site
mastoid (antrum) (cell) — *see* Disorder, mastoid, specified NEC
maxillary sinus — *see* Sinusitis, maxillary
membrana tympani — *see* Perforation, tympanum
nasal
septum J34.89
congenital Q3Ø.3
syphilitic A52.73
sinus J34.89
congenital Q3Ø.8
due to sinusitis — *see* Sinusitis
palate (*see also* Cleft, palate) Q35.9
syphilitic A52.79

☑ Additional Character Required — Refer to the Tabular List for Character Selection   ▽ Subterms under main terms may continue to next column or page

Perforation, perforated — *continued*
  palatine vault (*see also* Cleft, palate, hard) Q35.1
    syphilitic A52.79
      congenital A50.59
  pars flaccida (ear drum) — *see* Perforation, tympanum, attic
  pelvic
    floor S31.030 ☑
      with
        ectopic or molar pregnancy O08.6
        penetration into retroperitoneal space S31.031
        retained foreign body S31.040 ☑
          with penetration into retroperitoneal space S31.041 ☑
      following ectopic or molar pregnancy O08.6
      obstetrical trauma O70.1
    organ S37.99 ☑
      adrenal gland S37.818 ☑
      bladder — *see* Perforation, bladder
      fallopian tube S37.599 ☑
        bilateral S37.592 ☑
        unilateral S37.591 ☑
      kidney S37.09- ☑
        obstetrical trauma O71.5
      ovary S37.499 ☑
        bilateral S37.492 ☑
        unilateral S37.491 ☑
      prostate S37.828 ☑
      specified organ NEC S37.898 ☑
      ureter — *see* Perforation, ureter
      urethra — *see* Perforation, urethra
      uterus — *see* Perforation, uterus
  perineum — *see* Laceration, perineum
  pharynx J39.2
  rectum K63.1
    newborn P78.0
    obstetrical trauma O71.5
    traumatic S36.63 ☑
  root canal space due to endodontic treatment M27.51
  sigmoid K63.1
    newborn P78.0
    obstetrical trauma O71.5
    traumatic S36.533 ☑
  sinus (accessory) (chronic) (nasal) J34.89
  sphenoidal sinus — *see* Sinusitis, sphenoidal
  surgical (accidental) (by instrument) (blood vessel) (nerve) (organ) — *see* Puncture, accidental complicating surgery
  traumatic
    external — *see* Puncture
    eye — *see* Puncture, eyeball
    internal organ — *see* Injury, by site
  tympanum, tympanic (membrane) (persistent post-traumatic) (postinflammatory) H72.9- ☑
    attic H72.1- ☑
      multiple — *see* Perforation, tympanum, multiple
      total — *see* Perforation, tympanum, total
    central H72.0- ☑
      multiple — *see* Perforation, tympanum, multiple
      total — *see* Perforation, tympanum, total
    marginal NEC — *see* subcategory H72.2 ☑
    multiple H72.81- ☑
    pars flaccida — *see* Perforation, tympanum, attic
    total H72.82- ☑
    traumatic, current episode S09.2- ☑
  typhoid, gastrointestinal — *see* Typhoid
  ulcer — *see* Ulcer, by site, with perforation
  ureter N28.89
    traumatic S37.19 ☑
  urethra N36.8
    with ectopic or molar pregnancy O08.6
    following ectopic or molar pregnancy O08.6
    obstetrical trauma O71.5
    traumatic S37.39 ☑
      at delivery O71.5
  uterus
    with ectopic or molar pregnancy O08.6
    by intrauterine contraceptive device T83.39 ☑
    following ectopic or molar pregnancy O08.6
    obstetrical trauma O71.1
    traumatic S37.69 ☑
      obstetric O71.1
  uvula K13.79
    syphilitic A52.79

Perforation, perforated — *continued*
  vagina O71.4
    obstetrical trauma O71.4
    other trauma — *see* Puncture, vagina
Periadenitis mucosa necrotica recurrens K12.0
Periappendicitis (acute) — *see* Appendicitis
Periarteritis nodosa (disseminated) (infectious) (necrotizing) M30.0
Periarthritis (joint) (*see also* Enthesopathy)
  Duplay's M75.0- ☑
  gonococcal A54.42
  humeroscapularis — *see* Capsulitis, adhesive
  scapulohumeral — *see* Capsulitis, adhesive
  shoulder — *see* Capsulitis, adhesive
  wrist M77.2- ☑
Periarthrosis (angioneural) — *see* Enthesopathy
Pericapsulitis, adhesive (shoulder) — *see* Capsulitis, adhesive
Pericarditis (with decompensation) (with effusion) I31.9
  with rheumatic fever (conditions in I00)
    active — *see* Pericarditis, rheumatic
    inactive or quiescent I09.2
  acute (hemorrhagic) (nonrheumatic) (Sicca) I30.9
    with chorea (acute) (rheumatic) (Sydenham's) I02.0
    benign I30.8
    nonspecific I30.0
    rheumatic I01.0
      with chorea (acute) (Sydenham's) I02.0
  adhesive or adherent (chronic) (external) (internal) I31.0
    acute — *see* Pericarditis, acute
    rheumatic I09.2
  bacterial (acute) (subacute) (with serous or seropurulent effusion) I30.1
  calcareous I31.1
  cholesterol (chronic) I31.8
    acute I30.9
  chronic (nonrheumatic) I31.9
    rheumatic I09.2
  constrictive (chronic) I31.1
  coxsackie B33.23
  fibrinocaseous (tuberculous) A18.84
  fibrinopurulent I30.1
  fibrinous I30.8
  fibrous I31.0
  gonococcal A54.83
  idiopathic I30.0
  in systemic lupus erythematosus M32.12
  infective I30.1
  meningococcal A39.53
  neoplastic (chronic) I31.8
    acute I30.9
  obliterans, obliterating I31.0
  plastic I31.0
  pneumococcal I30.1
  postinfarction I24.1
  purulent I30.1
  rheumatic (active) (acute) (with effusion) (with pneumonia) I01.0
    with chorea (acute) (rheumatic) (Sydenham's) I02.0
    chronic or inactive (with chorea) I09.2
  rheumatoid — *see* Rheumatoid, carditis
  septic I30.1
  serofibrinous I30.8
  staphylococcal I30.1
  streptococcal I30.1
  suppurative I30.1
  syphilitic A52.06
  tuberculous A18.84
  uremic N18.9 [I32]
  viral I30.1
Pericardium, pericardial — *see* condition
Pericellulitis — *see* Cellulitis
Pericementitis (chronic) (suppurative) (*see also* Periodontitis)
  acute K05.20
    generalized K05.22
    localized K05.21
Perichondritis
  auricle — *see* Perichondritis, ear
  bronchus J98.09
  ear (external) H61.00- ☑
    acute H61.01- ☑
    chronic H61.02- ☑
  external auditory canal — *see* Perichondritis, ear
  larynx J38.7
    syphilitic A52.73
    typhoid A01.09

Perichondritis — *continued*
  nose J34.89
  pinna — *see* Perichondritis, ear
  trachea J39.8
Periclasia K05.4
Pericoronitis — *see* Periodontitis
Pericystitis N30.90
  with hematuria N30.91
Peridiverticulitis (intestine) K57.92
  cecum — *see* Diverticulitis, intestine, large
  colon — *see* Diverticulitis, intestine, large
  duodenum — *see* Diverticulitis, intestine, small
  intestine — *see* Diverticulitis, intestine
  jejunum — *see* Diverticulitis, intestine, small
  rectosigmoid — *see* Diverticulitis, intestine, large
  rectum — *see* Diverticulitis, intestine, large
  sigmoid — *see* Diverticulitis, intestine, large
Periendocarditis — *see* Endocarditis
Periepididymitis N45.1
Perifolliculitis L01.02
  abscedens, caput, scalp L66.3
  capitis, abscedens (et suffodiens) L66.3
  superficial pustular L01.02
Perihepatitis K65.8
Perilabyrinthitis (acute) — *see* subcategory H83.0 ☑
Perimeningitis — *see* Meningitis
Perimetritis — *see* Endometritis
Perimetrosalpingitis — *see* Salpingo-oophoritis
Perineocele N81.81
Perinephric, perinephritic — *see* condition
Perinephritis (*see also* Infection, kidney)
  purulent — *see* Abscess, kidney
Perineum, perineal — *see* condition
Perineuritis NEC — *see* Neuralgia
Periodic — *see* condition
Periodontitis (chronic) (complex) (compound) (local) (simplex) K05.30
  acute K05.20
    generalized K05.22
    localized K05.21
  apical K04.5
    acute (pulpal origin) K04.4
  generalized K05.32
  localized K05.31
Periodontoclasia K05.4
Periodontosis (juvenile) K05.4
Periods (*see also* Menstruation)
  heavy N92.0
  irregular N92.6
  shortened intervals (irregular) N92.1
Perionychia (*see also* Cellulitis, digit)
  with lymphangitis — *see* Lymphangitis, acute, digit
Perioophoritis — *see* Salpingo-oophoritis
Periorchitis N45.2
Periosteum, periosteal — *see* condition
Periostitis (albuminosa) (circumscribed) (diffuse) (infective) (monomelic) (*see also* Osteomyelitis)
  alveolar M27.3
  alveolodental M27.3
  dental M27.3
  gonorrheal A54.43
  jaw (lower) (upper) M27.2
  orbit H05.03- ☑
  syphilitic A52.77
    congenital (early) A50.02 [M90.80]
    secondary A51.46
  tuberculous — *see* Tuberculosis, bone
  yaws (hypertrophic) (early) (late) A66.6 [M90.80]
Periostosis (hyperplastic) (*see also* Disorder, bone, specified type NEC)
  with osteomyelitis — *see* Osteomyelitis, specified type NEC
Peripartum
  cardiomyopathy O90.3
Periphlebitis — *see* Phlebitis
Periproctitis K62.89
Periprostatitis — *see* Prostatitis
Perirectal — *see* condition
Perirenal — *see* condition
Perisalpingitis — *see* Salpingo-oophoritis
Perisplenitis (infectional) D73.89
Peristalsis, visible or reversed R19.2
Peritendinitis — *see* Enthesopathy
Peritoneum, peritoneal — *see* condition
Peritonitis (adhesive) (bacterial) (fibrinous) (hemorrhagic) (idiopathic) (localized) (perforative) (primary) (with adhesions) (with effusion) K65.9

Index

Peritonitis — Perversion, perverted

Peritonitis — *continued*
with or following
  abscess K65.1
  appendicitis K35.2
    with perforation or rupture K35.2
    generalized K35.2
    localized K35.3
  diverticular disease (intestine) K57.80
    with bleeding K57.81
    ectopic or molar pregnancy O08.0
    large intestine K57.20
      with
        bleeding K57.21
        small intestine K57.40
          with bleeding K57.41
    small intestine K57.00
      with
        bleeding K57.01
        large intestine K57.40
          with bleeding K57.41
acute (generalized) K65.0
aseptic T81.61 ☑
bile, biliary K65.3
chemical T81.61 ☑
chlamydial A74.81
chronic proliferative K65.8
complicating abortion — *see* Abortion, by type, complicated by, pelvic peritonitis
congenital P78.1
diaphragmatic K65.0
diffuse K65.0
diphtheritic A36.89
disseminated K65.0
due to
  bile K65.3
  foreign
    body or object accidentally left during a procedure (instrument) (sponge) (swab) T81.599 ☑
    substance accidentally left during a procedure (chemical) (powder) (talc) T81.61 ☑
  talc T81.61 ☑
  urine K65.8
eosinophilic K65.8
  acute K65.0
fibrocaseous (tuberculous) A18.31
fibropurulent K65.0
following ectopic or molar pregnancy O08.0
general (ized) K65.0
gonococcal A54.85
meconium (newborn) P78.0
neonatal P78.1
  meconium P78.0
pancreatic K65.0
paroxysmal, familial E85.0
  benign E85.0
pelvic
  female N73.5
    acute N73.3
    chronic N73.4
      with adhesions N73.6
  male K65.0
periodic, familial E85.0
proliferative, chronic K65.8
puerperal, postpartum, childbirth O85
purulent K65.0
septic K65.0
specified NEC K65.8
spontaneous bacterial K65.2
subdiaphragmatic K65.0
subphrenic K65.0
suppurative K65.0
syphilitic A52.74
  congenital (early) A50.08 [K67]
talc T81.61 ☑
tuberculous A18.31
urine K65.8
Peritonsillar — *see* condition
Peritonsillitis J36
Perityphlitis K37
Periureteritis N28.89
Periurethral — *see* condition
Periurethritis (gangrenous) — *see* Urethritis
Periuterine — *see* condition
Perivaginitis — *see* Vaginitis
Perivasculitis, retinal H35.06- ☑
Perivasitis (chronic) N49.1
Perivesiculitis (seminal) — *see* Vesiculitis

Perlèche NEC K13.0
due to
  candidiasis B37.83
  moniliasis B37.83
  riboflavin deficiency E53.0
  vitamin B2 (riboflavin) deficiency E53.0
Pernicious — *see* condition
Pernio, perniosis T69.1 ☑
Perpetrator (of abuse) — *see* Index to External Causes of Injury, Perpetrator
Persecution
delusion F22
social Z60.5
Perseveration (tonic) R48.8
Persistence, persistent (congenital)
anal membrane Q42.3
  with fistula Q42.2
arteria stapedia Q16.3
atrioventricular canal Q21.2
branchial cleft Q18.0
bulbus cordis in left ventricle Q21.8
canal of Cloquet Q14.0
capsule (opaque) Q12.8
cilioretinal artery or vein Q14.8
cloaca Q43.7
communication — *see* Fistula, congenital
convolutions
  aortic arch Q25.4
  fallopian tube Q50.6
  oviduct Q50.6
  uterine tube Q50.6
double aortic arch Q25.4
ductus arteriosus (Botalli) Q25.0
fetal
  circulation P29.3
  form of cervix (uteri) Q51.828
  hemoglobin, hereditary (HPFH) D56.4
foramen
  Botalli Q21.1
  ovale Q21.1
Gartner's duct Q52.4
hemoglobin, fetal (hereditary) (HPFH) D56.4
hyaloid
  artery (generally incomplete) Q14.0
  system Q14.8
hymen, in pregnancy or childbirth — *see* Pregnancy, complicated by, abnormal, vulva
lanugo Q84.2
left
  posterior cardinal vein Q26.8
  root with right arch of aorta Q25.4
  superior vena cava Q26.1
Meckel's diverticulum Q43.0
  malignant — *see* Table of Neoplasms, small intestine, malignant
mucosal disease (middle ear) — *see* Otitis, media, suppurative, chronic, tubotympanic
nail(s), anomalous Q84.6
omphalomesenteric duct Q43.0
organ or site not listed — *see* Anomaly, by site
ostium
  atrioventriculare commune Q21.2
  primum Q21.2
  secundum Q21.1
ovarian rests in fallopian tube Q50.6
pancreatic tissue in intestinal tract Q43.8
primary (deciduous)
  teeth K00.6
  vitreous hyperplasia Q14.0
pupillary membrane Q13.89
rhesus (Rh) titer — *see* Complication(s), transfusion, incompatibility reaction, Rh (factor)
right aortic arch Q25.4
sinus
  urogenitalis
    female Q52.8
    male Q55.8
  venosus with imperfect incorporation in right auricle Q26.8
thymus (gland) (hyperplasia) E32.0
thyroglossal duct Q89.2
thyrolingual duct Q89.2
truncus arteriosus or communis Q20.0
tunica vasculosa lentis Q12.2
umbilical sinus Q64.4
urachus Q64.4
vitelline duct Q43.0

Person (with)
admitted for clinical research, as a control subject (normal comparison) (participant) Z00.6
awaiting admission to adequate facility elsewhere Z75.1
concern (normal) about sick person in family Z63.6
consulting on behalf of another Z71.0
feigning illness Z76.5
living (in)
  without
    adequate housing (heating) (space) Z59.1
    housing (permanent) (temporary) Z59.0
    person able to render necessary care Z74.2
    shelter Z59.0
  alone Z60.2
  boarding school Z59.3
  residential institution Z59.3
on waiting list Z75.1
sick or handicapped in family Z63.6
Personality (disorder) F60.9
accentuation of traits (type A pattern) Z73.1
affective F34.0
aggressive F60.3
amoral F60.2
anacastic, anankastic F60.5
antisocial F60.2
anxious F60.6
asocial F60.2
asthenic F60.7
avoidant F60.6
borderline F60.3
change due to organic condition (enduring) F07.0
compulsive F60.5
cycloid F34.0
cyclothymic F34.0
dependent F60.7
depressive F34.1
dissocial F60.2
dual F44.81
eccentric F60.89
emotionally unstable F60.3
expansive paranoid F60.0
explosive F60.3
fanatic F60.0
haltose type F60.89
histrionic F60.4
hyperthymic F34.0
hypothymic F34.1
hysterical F60.4
immature F60.89
inadequate F60.7
labile (emotional) F60.3
mixed (nonspecific) F60.81
morally defective F60.2
multiple F44.81
narcissistic F60.81
obsessional F60.5
obsessive (-compulsive) F60.5
organic F07.0
overconscientious F60.5
paranoid F60.0
passive (-dependent) F60.7
passive-aggressive F60.89
pathologic F60.9
pattern defect or disturbance F60.9
pseudopsychopathic (organic) F07.0
pseudoretarded (organic) F07.0
psychoinfantile F60.4
psychoneurotic NEC F60.89
psychopathic F60.2
querulant F60.0
sadistic F60.89
schizoid F60.1
self-defeating F60.7
sensitive paranoid F60.0
sociopathic (amoral) (antisocial) (asocial) (dissocial) F60.2
specified NEC F60.89
type A Z73.1
unstable (emotional) F60.3
Perthes' disease — *see* Legg-Calvé-Perthes disease
Pertussis (*see also* Whooping cough) A37.90
Perversion, perverted
appetite F50.8
  psychogenic F50.8
function
  pituitary gland E23.2
    posterior lobe E22.2

Perversion, perverted — *continued*
  sense of smell and taste R43.8
    psychogenic F45.8
  sexual — *see* Deviation, sexual
Pervious, congenital (*see also* Imperfect, closure)
  ductus arteriosus Q25.0
Pes (congenital) (*see also* Talipes)
  acquired (*see also* Deformity, limb, foot, specified NEC)
    planus — *see* Deformity, limb, flat foot
  adductus Q66.89
  cavus Q66.7
  deformity NEC, acquired — *see* Deformity, limb, foot, specified NEC
  planus (acquired) (any degree) (*see also* Deformity, limb, flat foot)
    rachitic sequelae (late effect) E64.3
  valgus Q66.6
Pest, pestis — *see* Plague
Petechia, petechiae R23.3
  newborn P54.5
Petechial typhus A75.9
Peter's anomaly Q13.4
Petit mal seizure — *see* Epilepsy, generalized, specified NEC
Petit's hernia — *see* Hernia, abdomen, specified site NEC
Petrellidosis B48.2
Petrositis H70.20- ☑
  acute H70.21- ☑
  chronic H70.22- ☑
Peutz-Jeghers disease or syndrome Q85.8
Peyronie's disease N48.6
Pfeiffer's disease — *see* Mononucleosis, infectious
Phagedena (dry) (moist) (sloughing) (*see also* Gangrene)
  geometric L88
  penis N48.29
  tropical — *see* Ulcer, skin
  vulva N76.6
Phagedenic — *see* condition
Phakoma H35.89
Phakomatosis (*see also* specific eponymous syndromes) Q85.9
  Bourneville's Q85.1
  specified NEC Q85.8
Phantom limb syndrome (without pain) G54.7
  with pain G54.6
Pharyngeal pouch syndrome D82.1
Pharyngitis (acute) (catarrhal)(gangrenous) (infective) (malignant) (membranous) (phlegmonous) (pseudomembranous) (simple) (subacute) (suppurative) (ulcerative) (viral) J02.9
  with influenza, flu, or grippe — *see* Influenza, with, pharyngitis
  aphthous B08.5
  atrophic J31.2
  chlamydial A56.4
  chronic (atrophic) (granular) (hypertrophic) J31.2
  coxsackievirus B08.5
  diphtheritic A36.0
  enteroviral vesicular B08.5
  follicular (chronic) J31.2
  fusospirochetal A69.1
  gonococcal A54.5
  granular (chronic) J31.2
  herpesviral B00.2
  hypertrophic J31.2
  infectional, chronic J31.2
  influenzal — *see* Influenza, with, respiratory manifestations NEC
  lymphonodular, acute (enteroviral) B08.8
  pneumococcal J02.8
  purulent J02.9
  putrid J02.9
  septic J02.0
  sicca J31.2
  specified organism NEC J02.8
  staphylococcal J02.8
  streptococcal J02.0
  syphilitic, congenital (early) A50.03
  tuberculous A15.8
  vesicular, enteroviral B08.5
  viral NEC J02.8
Pharyngoconjunctivitis, viral B30.2
Pharyngolaryngitis (acute) J06.0
  chronic J37.0
Pharyngoplegia J39.2
Pharyngotonsillitis, herpesviral B00.2

Pharyngotracheitis, chronic J42
Pharynx, pharyngeal — *see* condition
Phenomenon
  Arthus' — *see* Arthus' phenomenon
  jaw-winking Q07.8
  lupus erythematosus (LE) cell M32.9
  Raynaud's (secondary) I73.00
    with gangrene I73.01
  vasomotor R55
  vasospastic I73.9
  vasovagal R55
  Wenckebach's I44.1
Phenylketonuria E70.1
  classical E70.0
  maternal E70.1
Pheochromoblastoma
  specified site — *see* Neoplasm, malignant, by site
  unspecified site C74.10
Pheochromocytoma
  malignant
    specified site — *see* Neoplasm, malignant, by site
    unspecified site C74.10
  specified site — *see* Neoplasm, benign, by site
  unspecified site D35.00
Pheohyphomycosis — *see* Chromomycosis
Pheomycosis — *see* Chromomycosis
Phimosis (congenital) (due to infection) N47.1
  chancroidal A57
Phlebectasia (*see also* Varix)
  congenital Q27.4
Phlebitis (infective) (pyemic) (septic) (suppurative) I80.9
  antepartum — *see* Thrombophlebitis, antepartum
  blue — *see* Phlebitis, leg, deep
  breast, superficial I80.8
  cavernous (venous) sinus — *see* Phlebitis, intracranial (venous) sinus
  cerebral (venous) sinus — *see* Phlebitis, intracranial (venous) sinus
  chest wall, superficial I80.8
  cranial (venous) sinus — *see* Phlebitis, intracranial (venous) sinus
  deep (vessels) — *see* Phlebitis, leg, deep
  due to implanted device — *see* Complications, by site and type, specified NEC
  during or resulting from a procedure T81.72 ☑
  femoral vein (superficial) I80.1- ☑
  femoropopliteal vein I80.0- ☑
  gestational — *see* Phlebopathy, gestational
  hepatic veins I80.8
  iliofemoral — *see* Phlebitis, femoral vein
  intracranial (venous) sinus (any) G08
    nonpyogenic I67.6
  intraspinal venous sinuses and veins G08
    nonpyogenic G95.19
  lateral (venous) sinus — *see* Phlebitis, intracranial (venous) sinus
  leg I80.3
    antepartum — *see* Thrombophlebitis, antepartum
    deep (vessels) NEC I80.20- ☑
      iliac I80.21- ☑
      popliteal vein I80.22- ☑
      specified vessel NEC I80.29- ☑
      tibial vein I80.23- ☑
    femoral vein (superficial) I80.1- ☑
    superficial (vessels) I80.0- ☑
  longitudinal sinus — *see* Phlebitis, intracranial (venous) sinus
  lower limb — *see* Phlebitis, leg
  migrans, migrating (superficial) I82.1
  pelvic
    with ectopic or molar pregnancy O08.0
    following ectopic or molar pregnancy O08.0
    puerperal, postpartum O87.1
  popliteal vein — *see* Phlebitis, leg, deep, popliteal
  portal (vein) K75.1
  postoperative T81.72 ☑
  pregnancy — *see* Thrombophlebitis, antepartum
  puerperal, postpartum, childbirth O87.0
    deep O87.1
    pelvic O87.1
    superficial O87.0
  retina — *see* Vasculitis, retina
  saphenous (accessory) (great) (long) (small) — *see* Phlebitis, leg, superficial
  sinus (meninges) — *see* Phlebitis, intracranial (venous) sinus
  specified site NEC I80.8

Phlebitis — *continued*
  syphilitic A52.09
  tibial vein — *see* Phlebitis, leg, deep, tibial
  ulcerative I80.9
    leg — *see* Phlebitis, leg
  umbilicus I80.8
  uterus (septic) — *see* Endometritis
  varicose (leg) (lower limb) — *see* Varix, leg, with, inflammation
Phlebofibrosis I87.8
Phleboliths I87.8
Phlebopathy,
  gestational O22.9- ☑
  puerperal O87.9
Phlebosclerosis I87.8
Phlebothrombosis (*see also* Thrombosis)
  antepartum — *see* Thrombophlebitis, antepartum
  pregnancy — *see* Thrombophlebitis, antepartum
  puerperal — *see* Thrombophlebitis, puerperal
Phlebotomus fever A93.1
Phlegmasia
  alba dolens O87.1
    nonpuerperal — *see* Phlebitis, femoral vein
  cerulea dolens — *see* Phlebitis, leg, deep
Phlegmon — *see* Abscess
Phlegmonous — *see* condition
Phlyctenulosis (allergic) (keratoconjunctivitis) (nontuberculous) (*see also* Keratoconjunctivitis)
  cornea — *see* Keratoconjunctivitis
  tuberculous A18.52
Phobia, phobic F40.9
  animal F40.218
    spiders F40.210
  examination F40.298
  reaction F40.9
  simple F40.298
  social F40.10
    generalized F40.11
  specific (isolated) F40.298
    animal F40.218
      spiders F40.210
    blood F40.230
    injection F40.231
    injury F40.233
    men F40.290
    natural environment F40.228
      thunderstorms F40.220
    situational F40.248
      bridges F40.242
      closed in spaces F40.240
      flying F40.243
      heights F40.241
    specified focus NEC F40.298
    transfusion F40.231
    women F40.291
  specified NEC F40.8
    medical care NEC F40.232
  state F40.9
Phocas' disease — *see* Mastopathy, cystic
Phocomelia Q73.1
  lower limb — *see* Agenesis, leg, with foot present
  upper limb — *see* Agenesis, arm, with hand present
Phoria H50.50
Phosphate-losing tubular disorder N25.0
Phosphatemia E83.39
Phosphaturia E83.39
Photodermatitis (sun) L56.8
  chronic L57.8
  due to drug L56.8
  light other than sun L59.8
Photokeratitis H16.13- ☑
Photophobia H53.14- ☑
Photophthalmia — *see* Photokeratitis
Photopsia H53.19
Photoretinitis — *see* Retinopathy, solar
Photosensitivity, photosensitization (sun) skin L56.8
  light other than sun L59.8
Phrenitis — *see* Encephalitis
Phrynoderma (vitamin A deficiency) E50.8
Phthiriasis (pubis) B85.3
  with any infestation classifiable to B85.0-B85.2 B85.4
Phthirus infestation — *see* Phthiriasis
Phthisis (*see also* Tuberculosis)
  bulbi (infectional) — *see* Disorder, globe, degenerated condition, atrophy
  eyeball (due to infection) — *see* Disorder, globe, degenerated condition, atrophy

Phycomycosis — see Zygomycosis
Physalopteriasis B81.8
Physical restraint status Z78.1
Phytobezoar T18.9 ☑
  intestine T18.3 ☑
  stomach T18.2 ☑
Pian — see Yaws
Pianoma A66.1
Pica F50.8
  in adults F50.8
  infant or child F98.3
Pick-Niemann disease — see Niemann-Pick disease or syndrome
Picking, nose F98.8
Pick's
  cerebral atrophy G31.01 [F02.80]
    with behavioral disturbance G31.01 [F02.81]
  disease or syndrome (brain) G31.01 [F02.80]
    with behavioral disturbance G31.01 [F02.81]
Pickwickian syndrome E66.2
Piebaldism E70.39
Piedra (beard) (scalp) B36.8
  black B36.3
  white B36.2
Pierre Robin deformity or syndrome Q87.0
Pierson's disease or osteochondrosis M91.0
Pig-bel A05.2
Pigeon
  breast or chest (acquired) M95.4
    congenital Q67.7
      rachitic sequelae (late effect) E64.3
  breeder's disease or lung J67.2
  fancier's disease or lung J67.2
  toe — see Deformity, toe, specified NEC
Pigmentation (abnormal) (anomaly) L81.9
  conjunctiva H11.13- ☑
  cornea (anterior) H18.01- ☑
    posterior H18.05- ☑
    stromal H18.06- ☑
  diminished melanin formation NEC L81.6
  iron L81.8
  lids, congenital Q82.8
  limbus corneae — see Pigmentation, cornea
  metals L81.8
  optic papilla, congenital Q14.2
  retina, congenital (grouped) (nevoid) Q14.1
  scrotum, congenital Q82.8
  tattoo L81.8
Piles (see also Hemorrhoids) K64.9
Pili
  annulati or torti (congenital) Q84.1
  incarnati L73.1
Pill roller hand (intrinsic) — see Parkinsonism
Pilomatrixoma — see Neoplasm, skin, benign
  malignant — see Neoplasm, skin, malignant
Pilonidal — see condition
Pimple R23.8
Pinched nerve — see Neuropathy, entrapment
Pindborg tumor — see Cyst, calcifying odontogenic
Pineal body or gland — see condition
Pinealoblastoma C75.3
Pinealoma D44.5
  malignant C75.3
Pineoblastoma C75.3
Pineocytoma D44.5
Pinguecula H11.15- ☑
Pingueculitis H10.81- ☑
Pinhole meatus (see also Stricture, urethra) N35.9
Pink
  disease — see subcategory T56.1 ☑
  eye — see Conjunctivitis, acute, mucopurulent
Pinkus' disease (lichen nitidus) L44.1
Pinpoint
  meatus — see Stricture, urethra
  os (uteri) — see Stricture, cervix
Pins and needles R20.2
Pinta A67.9
  cardiovascular lesions A67.2
  chancre (primary) A67.0
  erythematous plaques A67.1
  hyperchromic lesions A67.1
  hyperkeratosis A67.1
  lesions A67.9
    cardiovascular A67.2
    hyperchromic A67.1
    intermediate A67.1
    late A67.2

Pinta — continued
  lesions — continued
    mixed A67.3
    primary A67.0
    skin (achromic) (cicatricial) (dyschromic) A67.2
      hyperchromic A67.1
      mixed (achromic and hyperchromic) A67.3
  papule (primary) A67.0
  skin lesions (achromic) (cicatricial) (dyschromic) A67.2
    hyperchromic A67.1
    mixed (achromic and hyperchromic) A67.3
  vitiligo A67.2
Pintids A67.1
Pinworm (disease) (infection) (infestation) B80
Piroplasmosis B60.0
Pistol wound — see Gunshot wound
Pitchers' elbow — see Derangement, joint, specified type NEC, elbow
Pithecoid pelvis Q74.2
  with disproportion (fetopelvic) O33.0
    causing obstructed labor O65.0
Pithiatism F48.8
Pitted — see Pitting
Pitting (see also Edema) R60.9
  lip R60.0
  nail L60.8
  teeth K00.4
Pituitary gland — see condition
Pituitary-snuff-taker's disease J67.8
Pityriasis (capitis) L21.0
  alba L30.5
  circinata (et maculata) L42
  furfuracea L21.0
  Hebra's L26
  lichenoides L41.0
    chronica L41.1
    et varioliformis (acuta) L41.0
  maculata (et circinata) L30.5
  nigra B36.1
  pilaris, Hebra's L44.0
  rosea L42
  rotunda L44.8
  rubra (Hebra) pilaris L44.0
  simplex L30.5
  specified type NEC L30.5
  streptogenes L30.5
  versicolor (scrotal) B36.0
Placenta, placental — see Pregnancy, complicated by (care of) (management affected by), specified condition
Placentitis O41.14- ☑
Plagiocephaly Q67.3
Plague A20.9
  abortive A20.8
  ambulatory A20.8
  asymptomatic A20.8
  bubonic A20.0
  cellulocutaneous A20.1
  cutaneobubonic A20.1
  lymphatic gland A20.0
  meningitis A20.3
  pharyngeal A20.8
  pneumonic (primary) (secondary) A20.2
  pulmonary, pulmonic A20.2
  septicemic A20.7
  tonsillar A20.8
    septicemic A20.7
Planning, family
  contraception Z30.9
  procreation Z31.69
Plaque(s)
  artery, arterial — see Arteriosclerosis
  calcareous — see Calcification
  coronary, lipid rich I25.83
  epicardial I31.8
  erythematous, of pinta A67.1
  Hollenhorst's — see Occlusion, artery, retina
  lipid rich, coronary I25.83
  pleural (without asbestos) J92.9
    with asbestos J92.0
  tongue K13.29
Plasmacytoma C90.3- ☑
  extramedullary C90.2- ☑
  medullary C90.0- ☑
  solitary C90.3- ☑
Plasmacytopenia D72.818
Plasmacytosis D72.822
Plaster ulcer — see Ulcer, pressure, by site

Plateau iris syndrome (post-iridectomy) (postprocedural) (without glaucoma) H21.82
  with glaucoma H40.22- ☑
Platybasia Q75.8
Platyonychia (congenital) Q84.6
  acquired L60.8
Platypelloid pelvis M95.5
  with disproportion (fetopelvic) O33.0
    causing obstructed labor O65.0
  congenital Q74.2
Platyspondylisis Q76.49
Plaut (-Vincent) **disease** (see also Vincent's) A69.1
Plethora R23.2
  newborn P61.1
Pleura, pleural — see condition
Pleuralgia R07.81
Pleurisy (acute) (adhesive) (chronic) (costal) (diaphragmatic) (double) (dry) (fibrinous) (fibrous) (interlobar) (latent) (plastic) (primary) (residual) (sicca) (sterile) (subacute) (unresolved) R09.1
  with
    adherent pleura J86.0
    effusion J90
      chylous, chyliform J94.0
      tuberculous (non primary) A15.6
        primary (progressive) A15.7
      tuberculosis — see Pleurisy, tuberculous (non primary)
  encysted — see Pleurisy, with effusion
  exudative — see Pleurisy, with effusion
  fibrinopurulent, fibropurulent — see Pyothorax
  hemorrhagic — see Hemothorax
  pneumococcal J90
  purulent — see Pyothorax
  septic — see Pyothorax
  serofibrinous — see Pleurisy, with effusion
  seropurulent — see Pyothorax
  serous — see Pleurisy, with effusion
  staphylococcal J86.9
  streptococcal J90
  suppurative — see Pyothorax
  traumatic (post) (current) — see Injury, intrathoracic, pleura
  tuberculous (with effusion) (non primary) A15.6
    primary (progressive) A15.7
Pleuritis sicca — see Pleurisy
Pleuro-pneumonia-like-organism (PPLO), as cause of disease classified elsewhere B96.0
Pleurobronchopneumonia — see Pneumonia, broncho-
Pleurodynia R07.81
  epidemic B33.0
  viral B33.0
Pleuropericarditis (see also Pericarditis)
  acute I30.9
Pleuropneumonia (acute) (bilateral) (double) (septic) (see also Pneumonia) J18.8
  chronic — see Fibrosis, lung
Pleurorrhea — see Pleurisy, with effusion
Plexitis, brachial G54.0
Plica
  polonica B85.0
  syndrome, knee M67.5- ☑
  tonsil J35.8
Plicated tongue K14.5
Plug
  bronchus NEC J98.09
  meconium (newborn) NEC syndrome P76.0
  mucus — see Asphyxia, mucus
Plumbism — see subcategory T56.0 ☑
Plummer-Vinson syndrome D50.1
Plummer's disease E05.20
  with thyroid storm E05.21
Pluricarential syndrome of infancy E40
Plus (and minus) **hand** (intrinsic) — see Deformity, limb, specified type NEC, forearm
Pneumathemia — see Air, embolism
Pneumatic hammer (drill) syndrome T75.21 ☑
Pneumatocele (lung) J98.4
  intracranial G93.89
  tension J44.9
Pneumatosis
  cystoides intestinalis K63.89
  intestinalis K63.89
  peritonei K66.8
Pneumaturia R39.89
Pneumoblastoma — see Neoplasm, lung, malignant
Pneumocephalus G93.89

☑ **Additional Character Required** — Refer to the Tabular List for Character Selection   ▽ Subterms under main terms may continue to next column or page

Pneumococcemia A40.3
Pneumococcus, pneumococcal — *see* condition
Pneumoconiosis (due to) (inhalation of) J64
  with tuberculosis (any type in A15) J65
  aluminum J63.0
  asbestos J61
  bagasse, bagassosis J67.1
  bauxite J63.1
  beryllium J63.2
  coal miners' (simple) J60
  coalworkers' (simple) J60
  collier's J60
  cotton dust J66.0
  diatomite (diatomaceous earth) J62.8
  dust
    inorganic NEC J63.6
    lime J62.8
    marble J62.8
    organic NEC J66.8
  fumes or vapors (from silo) J68.9
  graphite J63.3
  grinder's J62.8
  kaolin J62.8
  mica J62.8
  millstone maker's J62.8
  mineral fibers NEC J61
  miner's J60
  moldy hay J67.0
  potter's J62.8
  rheumatoid — *see* Rheumatoid, lung
  sandblaster's J62.8
  silica, silicate NEC J62.8
    with carbon J60
  stonemason's J62.8
  talc (dust) J62.0
Pneumocystis carinii pneumonia B59
Pneumocystis jiroveci (pneumonia) B59
Pneumocystosis (with pneumonia) B59
Pneumohemopericardium I31.2
Pneumohemothorax J94.2
  traumatic S27.2 ☑
Pneumohydropericardium — *see* Pericarditis
Pneumohydrothorax — *see* Hydrothorax
Pneumomediastinum J98.2
  congenital or perinatal P25.2
Pneumomycosis B49 [J99]
Pneumonia (acute) (double) (migratory) (purulent)
  (septic) (unresolved) J18.9
  with
    influenza — *see* Influenza, with, pneumonia
    lung abscess J85.1
      due to specified organism — *see* Pneumonia,
        in (due to)
  adenoviral J12.0
  adynamic J18.2
  alba A50.04
  allergic (eosinophilic) J82
  alveolar — *see* Pneumonia, lobar
  anaerobes J15.8
  anthrax A22.1
  apex, apical — *see* Pneumonia, lobar
  Ascaris B77.81
  aspiration J69.0
    due to
      aspiration of microorganisms
        bacterial J15.9
        viral J12.9
      food (regurgitated) J69.0
      gastric secretions J69.0
      milk (regurgitated) J69.0
      oils, essences J69.1
      solids, liquids NEC J69.8
      vomitus J69.0
    newborn P24.81
      amniotic fluid (clear) P24.11
      blood P24.21
      food (regurgitated) P24.31
      liquor (amnii) P24.11
      meconium P24.01
      milk P24.31
      mucus P24.11
      specified NEC P24.81
      stomach contents P24.31
    postprocedural J95.4
  atypical NEC J18.9
  bacillus J15.9
    specified NEC J15.8
  bacterial J15.9

Pneumonia — *continued*
  bacterial — *continued*
    specified NEC J15.8
  Bacteroides (fragilis) (oralis) (melaninogenicus) J15.8
  basal, basic, basilar — *see* Pneumonia, by type
  bronchiolitis obliterans organized (BOOP) J84.89
  broncho-, bronchial (confluent) (croupous) (diffuse)
    (disseminated) (hemorrhagic) (involving lobes)
    (lobar) (terminal) J18.0
    allergic (eosinophilic) J82
    aspiration — *see* Pneumonia, aspiration
    bacterial J15.9
      specified NEC J15.8
    chronic — *see* Fibrosis, lung
    diplococcal J13
    Eaton's agent J15.7
    Escherichia coli (E. coli) J15.5
    Friedländer's bacillus J15.0
    Hemophilus influenzae J14
    hypostatic J18.2
    inhalation (*see also* Pneumonia, aspiration)
      due to fumes or vapors (chemical) J68.0
      of oils or essences J69.1
    Klebsiella (pneumoniae) J15.0
    lipid, lipoid J69.1
      endogenous J84.89
    Mycoplasma (pneumoniae) J15.7
    pleuro-pneumonia-like-organisms (PPLO) J15.7
    pneumococcal J13
    Proteus J15.6
    Pseudomonas J15.1
    Serratia marcescens J15.6
    specified organism NEC J16.8
    staphylococcal — *see* Pneumonia, staphylococcal
    streptococcal NEC J15.4
      group B J15.3
      pneumoniae J13
    viral, virus — *see* Pneumonia, viral
  Butyrivibrio (fibriosolvens) J15.8
  Candida B37.1
  caseous — *see* Tuberculosis, pulmonary
  catarrhal — *see* Pneumonia, broncho
  chlamydial J16.0
    congenital P23.1
  cholesterol J84.89
  cirrhotic (chronic) — *see* Fibrosis, lung
  Clostridium (haemolyticum) (novyi) J15.8
  confluent — *see* Pneumonia, broncho
  congenital (infective) P23.9
    due to
      bacterium NEC P23.6
      Chlamydia P23.1
      Escherichia coli P23.4
      Haemophilus influenzae P23.6
      infective organism NEC P23.8
      Klebsiella pneumoniae P23.6
      Mycoplasma P23.6
      Pseudomonas P23.5
      Staphylococcus P23.2
      Streptococcus (except group B) P23.6
        group B P23.3
      viral agent P23.0
    specified NEC P23.8
  croupous — *see* Pneumonia, lobar
  cryptogenic organizing J84.116
  cytomegalic inclusion B25.0
  cytomegaloviral B25.0
  deglutition — *see* Pneumonia, aspiration
  desquamative interstitial J84.117
  diffuse — *see* Pneumonia, broncho
  diplococcal, diplococcus (broncho-) (lobar) J13
  disseminated (focal) — *see* Pneumonia, broncho
  Eaton's agent J15.7
  embolic, embolism — *see* Embolism, pulmonary
  Enterobacter J15.6
  eosinophilic J82
  Escherichia coli (E. coli) J15.5
  Eubacterium J15.8
  fibrinous — *see* Pneumonia, lobar
  fibroid, fibrous (chronic) — *see* Fibrosis, lung
  Friedländer's bacillus J15.0
  Fusobacterium (nucleatum) J15.8
  gangrenous J85.0
  giant cell (measles) B05.2
  gonococcal A54.84
  gram-negative bacteria NEC J15.6
    anaerobic J15.8
  Hemophilus influenzae (broncho) (lobar) J14

Pneumonia — *continued*
  human metapneumovirus J12.3
  hypostatic (broncho) (lobar) J18.2
  in (due to)
    actinomycosis A42.0
    adenovirus J12.0
    anthrax A22.1
    ascariasis B77.81
    aspergillosis B44.9
    Bacillus anthracis A22.1
    Bacterium anitratum J15.6
    candidiasis B37.1
    chickenpox B01.2
    Chlamydia J16.0
      neonatal P23.1
    coccidioidomycosis B38.2
      acute B38.0
      chronic B38.1
    cytomegalovirus disease B25.0
    Diplococcus (pneumoniae) J13
    Eaton's agent J15.7
    Enterobacter J15.6
    Escherichia coli (E. coli) J15.5
    Friedländer's bacillus J15.0
    fumes and vapors (chemical) (inhalation) J68.0
    gonorrhea A54.84
    Hemophilus influenzae (H. influenzae) J14
    Herellea J15.6
    histoplasmosis B39.2
      acute B39.0
      chronic B39.1
    human metapneumovirus J12.3
    Klebsiella (pneumoniae) J15.0
    measles B05.2
    Mycoplasma (pneumoniae) J15.7
    nocardiosis, nocardiasis A43.0
    ornithosis A70
    parainfluenza virus J12.2
    pleuro-pneumonia-like-organism (PPLO) J15.7
    pneumococcus J13
    pneumocystosis (Pneumocystis carinii) (Pneumo-
      cystis jiroveci) B59
    Proteus J15.6
    Pseudomonas NEC J15.1
      pseudomallei A24.1
    psittacosis A70
    Q fever A78
    respiratory syncytial virus J12.1
    rheumatic fever I00 [J17]
    rubella B06.81
    Salmonella (infection) A02.22
      typhi A01.03
    schistosomiasis B65.9 [J17]
    Serratia marcescens J15.6
    specified
      bacterium NEC J15.8
      organism NEC J16.8
    spirochetal NEC A69.8
    Staphylococcus J15.20
      aureus (methicillin susceptible) (MSSA) J15.211
        methicillin resistant (MRSA) J15.212
      specified NEC J15.29
    Streptococcus J15.4
      group B J15.3
      pneumoniae J13
      specified NEC J15.4
    toxoplasmosis B58.3
    tularemia A21.2
    typhoid (fever) A01.03
    varicella B01.2
    virus — *see* Pneumonia, viral
    whooping cough A37.91
      due to
        Bordetella parapertussis A37.11
        Bordetella pertussis A37.01
        specified NEC A37.81
    Yersinia pestis A20.2
  inhalation of food or vomit — *see* Pneumonia, aspira-
    tion
  interstitial J84.9
    chronic J84.111
    desquamative J84.117
    due to
      collagen vascular disease J84.17
      known underlying cause J84.17
    idiopathic NOS J84.111
    in disease classified elsewhere J84.17

Index

Pneumonia — Poisoning

Pneumonia — *continued*
  interstitial — *continued*
    lymphocytic (due to collagen vascular disease) (in diseases classified elsewhere) J84.17
    lymphoid J84.2
    non-specific J84.89
      due to
        collagen vascular disease J84.17
        known underlying cause J84.17
      idiopathic J84.113
      in diseases classified elsewhere J84.17
    plasma cell B59
    pseudomonas J15.1
    usual J84.112
      due to collagen vascular disease J84.17
      idiopathic J84.112
      in diseases classified elsewhere J84.17
  Klebsiella (pneumoniae) J15.0
  lipid, lipoid (exogenous) J69.1
    endogenous J84.89
  lobar (disseminated) (double) (interstitial) J18.1
    bacterial J15.9
      specified NEC J15.8
    chronic — *see* Fibrosis, lung
    Escherichia coli (E. coli) J15.5
    Friedländer's bacillus J15.0
    Hemophilus influenzae J14
    hypostatic J18.2
    Klebsiella (pneumoniae) J15.0
    pneumococcal J13
    Proteus J15.6
    Pseudomonas J15.1
    specified organism NEC J16.8
    staphylococcal — *see* Pneumonia, staphylococcal
    streptococcal NEC J15.4
    Streptococcus pneumoniae J13
    viral, virus — *see* Pneumonia, viral
  lobular — *see* Pneumonia, broncho
  Löffler's J82
  lymphoid interstitial J84.2
  massive — *see* Pneumonia, lobar
  meconium P24.01
  MSSA (methicillin susceptible Staphylococcus aureus) J15.211
  multilobar — *see* Pneumonia, by type
  Mycoplasma (pneumoniae) J15.7
  necrotic J85.0
  neonatal P23.9
    aspiration — *see* Aspiration, by substance, with pneumonia
  nitrogen dioxide J68.9
  organizing J84.89
    due to
      collagen vascular disease J84.17
      known underlying cause J84.17
      in diseases classified elsewhere J84.17
  orthostatic J18.2
  parainfluenza virus J12.2
  parenchymatous — *see* Fibrosis, lung
  passive J18.2
  patchy — *see* Pneumonia, broncho
  Peptococcus J15.8
  Peptostreptococcus J15.8
  plasma cell (of infants) B59
  pleuro-pneumonia-like organism (PPLO) J15.7
  pleurolobar — *see* Pneumonia, lobar
  pneumococcal (broncho) (lobar) J13
  Pneumocystis (carinii) (jiroveci) B59
  postinfectional NEC B99 ☑ [J17]
  postmeasles B05.2
  Proteus J15.6
  Pseudomonas J15.1
  psittacosis A70
  radiation J70.0
  respiratory syncytial virus J12.1
  resulting from a procedure J95.89
  rheumatic I00 [J17]
  Salmonella (arizonae) (cholerae-suis) (enteritidis) (typhimurium) A02.22
    typhi A01.03
    typhoid fever A01.03
  SARS-associated coronavirus J12.81
  segmented, segmental — *see* Pneumonia, broncho-
  Serratia marcescens J15.6
  specified NEC J18.8
    bacterium NEC J15.8
    organism NEC J16.8
    virus NEC J12.89

Pneumonia — *continued*
  spirochetal NEC A69.8
  staphylococcal (broncho) (lobar) J15.20
    aureus (methicillin susceptible) (MSSA) J15.211
      methicillin resistant (MRSA) J15.212
    specified NEC J15.29
  static, stasis J18.2
  streptococcal NEC (broncho) (lobar) J15.4
    group
      A J15.4
      B J15.3
      specified NEC J15.4
  Streptococcus pneumoniae J13
  syphilitic, congenital (early) A50.04
  traumatic (complication) (early) (secondary) T79.8 ☑
  tuberculous (any) — *see* Tuberculosis, pulmonary
  tularemic A21.2
  varicella B01.2
  Veillonella J15.8
  ventilator associated J95.851
  viral, virus (broncho) (interstitial) (lobar) J12.9
    adenoviral J12.0
    congenital P23.0
    human metapneumovirus J12.3
    parainfluenza J12.2
    respiratory syncytial J12.1
    SARS-associated coronavirus J12.81
    specified NEC J12.89
  white (congenital) A50.04
Pneumonic — *see* condition
Pneumonitis (acute) (primary) (*see also* Pneumonia)
  air-conditioner J67.7
  allergic (due to) J67.9
    organic dust NEC J67.8
    red cedar dust J67.8
    sequoiosis J67.8
    wood dust J67.8
  aspiration J69.0
    due to
      anesthesia J95.4
        during
          labor and delivery O74.0
          pregnancy O29.01- ☑
          puerperium O89.01
      fumes or gases J68.0
    obstetric O74.0
  chemical (due to gases, fumes or vapors) (inhalation) J68.0
    due to anesthesia J95.4
  cholesterol J84.89
  chronic — *see* Fibrosis, lung
  congenital rubella P35.0
  crack (cocaine) J68.0
  due to
    beryllium J68.0
    cadmium J68.0
    crack (cocaine) J68.0
    detergent J69.8
    fluorocarbon-polymer J68.0
    food, vomit (aspiration) J69.0
    fumes or vapors J68.0
    gases, fumes or vapors (inhalation) J68.0
    inhalation
      blood J69.8
      essences J69.1
      food (regurgitated), milk, vomit J69.0
      oils, essences J69.1
      saliva J69.0
      solids, liquids NEC J69.8
    manganese J68.0
    nitrogen dioxide J68.0
    oils, essences J69.1
    solids, liquids NEC J69.8
    toxoplasmosis (acquired) B58.3
      congenital P37.1
    vanadium J68.0
    ventilator J95.851
  eosinophilic J82
  hypersensitivity J67.9
    air conditioner lung J67.7
    bagassosis J67.1
    bird fancier's lung J67.2
    farmer's lung J67.0
    maltworker's lung J67.4
    maple bark-stripper's lung J67.6
    mushroom worker's lung J67.5
    specified organic dust NEC J67.8
    suberosis J67.3

Pneumonitis — *continued*
  interstitial (chronic) J84.89
    acute J84.114
    lymphoid J84.2
    non-specific J84.89
      idiopathic J84.113
  lymphoid, interstitial J84.2
  meconium P24.01
  postanesthetic J95.4
    correct substance properly administered — *see* Table of Drugs and Chemicals, by drug, adverse effect
    in labor and delivery O74.0
    in pregnancy O29.01- ☑
    obstetric O74.0
    overdose or wrong substance given or taken (by accident) — *see* Table of Drugs and Chemicals, by drug, poisoning
    postpartum, puerperal O89.01
  postoperative J95.4
    obstetric O74.0
  radiation J70.0
  rubella, congenital P35.0
  ventilation (air-conditioning) J67.7
  ventilator associated J95.851
  wood-dust J67.8
Pneumonoconiosis — *see* Pneumoconiosis
Pneumoparotid K11.8
Pneumopathy NEC J98.4
  alveolar J84.09
  due to organic dust NEC J66.8
  parietoalveolar J84.09
Pneumopericarditis (*see also* Pericarditis)
  acute I30.9
Pneumopericardium (*see also* Pericarditis)
  congenital P25.3
  newborn P25.3
  traumatic (post) — *see* Injury, heart
Pneumophagia (psychogenic) F45.8
Pneumopleurisy, pneumopleuritis (*see also* Pneumonia) J18.8
Pneumopyopericardium I30.1
Pneumopyothorax — *see* Pyopneumothorax
  with fistula J86.0
Pneumorrhagia (*see also* Hemorrhage, lung)
  tuberculous — *see* Tuberculosis, pulmonary
Pneumothorax NOS J93.9
  acute J93.83
  chronic J93.81
  congenital P25.1
  perinatal period P25.1
  postprocedural J95.811
  specified NEC J93.83
  spontaneous NOS J93.83
    newborn P25.1
    primary J93.11
    secondary J93.12
    tension J93.0
  tense valvular, infectional J93.0
  tension (spontaneous) J93.0
  traumatic S27.0 ☑
    with hemothorax S27.2 ☑
  tuberculous — *see* Tuberculosis, pulmonary
Podagra (*see also* Gout) M10.9
Podencephalus Q01.9
Poikilocytosis R71.8
Poikiloderma L81.6
  Civatte's L57.3
  congenital Q82.8
  vasculare atrophicans L94.5
Poikilodermatomyositis M33.10
  with
    myopathy M33.12
    respiratory involvement M33.11
    specified organ involvement NEC M33.19
Pointed ear (congenital) Q17.3
Poison ivy, oak, sumac or other plant dermatitis (allergic) (contact) L23.7
Poisoning (acute) (*see also* Table of Drugs and Chemicals)
  algae and toxins T65.82- ☑
  Bacillus B (aertrycke) (cholerae (suis)) (paratyphosus) (suipestifer) A02.9
    botulinus A05.1
  bacterial toxins A05.9
  berries, noxious — *see* Poisoning, food, noxious, berries
  botulism A05.1
  ciguatera fish T61.0- ☑

Poisoning — *continued*
  Clostridium botulinum A05.1
  death-cap (Amanita phalloides) (Amanita verna) — *see* Poisoning, food, noxious, mushrooms
  drug — *see* Table of Drugs and Chemicals, by drug, poisoning
  epidemic, fish (noxious) — *see* Poisoning, seafood
    bacterial A05.9
  fava bean D55.0
  fish (noxious) T61.9- ☑
    bacterial — *see* Intoxication, foodborne, by agent
    ciguatera fish — *see* Poisoning, ciguatera fish
    scombroid fish — *see* Poisoning, scombroid fish
    specified type NEC T61.77- ☑
  food (acute) (diseased) (infected) (noxious) NEC T62.9- ☑
    bacterial — *see* Intoxication, foodborne, by agent
    due to
      Bacillus (aertrycke) (choleraesuis) (paratyphosus) (suipestifer) A02.9
        botulinus A05.1
      Clostridium (perfringens) (Welchii) A05.2
      salmonella (aertrycke) (callinarum) (choleraesuis) (enteritidis) (paratyphi) (suipestifer) A02.9
        with
          gastroenteritis A02.0
          sepsis A02.1
      staphylococcus A05.0
      Vibrio
        parahaemolyticus A05.3
        vulnificus A05.5
    noxious or naturally toxic T62.9- ☑
      berries — *see* subcategory T62.1 ☑
      fish — *see* Poisoning, seafood
      mushrooms — *see* subcategory T62.0X ☑
      plants NEC — *see* subcategory T62.2X ☑
      seafood — *see* Poisoning, seafood
      specified NEC — *see* subcategory T62.8X ☑
  ichthyotoxism — *see* Poisoning, seafood
  kreotoxism, food A05.9
  latex T65.81- ☑
  lead T56.0- ☑
  mushroom — *see* Poisoning, food, noxious, mushroom
  mussels (*see also* Poisoning, shellfish)
    bacterial — *see* Intoxication, foodborne, by agent
  nicotine (tobacco) T65.2- ☑
  noxious foodstuffs — *see* Poisoning, food, noxious
  plants, noxious — *see* Poisoning, food, noxious, plants NEC
  ptomaine — *see* Poisoning, food
  radiation J70.0
  Salmonella (arizonae) (cholerae-suis) (enteritidis) (typhimurium) A02.9
  scombroid fish T61.1- ☑
  seafood (noxious) T61.9- ☑
    bacterial — *see* Intoxication, foodborne, by agent
    fish — *see* Poisoning, fish
    shellfish — *see* Poisoning, shellfish
    specified NEC — *see* subcategory T61.8X ☑
  shellfish (amnesic) (azaspiracid) (diarrheic) (neurotoxic) (noxious) (paralytic) T61.78- ☑
    bacterial — *see* Intoxication, foodborne, by agent
    ciguatera mollusk — *see* Poisoning, ciguatera fish
  specified substance NEC T65.891 ☑
  Staphylococcus, food A05.0
  tobacco (nicotine) T65.2- ☑
  water E87.79
Poker spine — *see* Spondylitis, ankylosing
Poland syndrome Q79.8
Polioencephalitis (acute) (bulbar) A80.9
  inferior G12.22
  influenzal — *see* Influenza, with, encephalopathy
  superior hemorrhagic (acute) (Wernicke's) E51.2
  Wernicke's E51.2
Polioencephalomyelitis (acute) (anterior) A80.9
  with beriberi E51.2
Polioencephalopathy, superior hemorrhagic E51.2
  with
    beriberi E51.11
    pellagra E52
Poliomeningoencephalitis — *see* Meningoencephalitis
Poliomyelitis (acute) (anterior) (epidemic) A80.9
  with paralysis (bulbar) — *see* Poliomyelitis, paralytic
  abortive A80.4
  ascending (progressive) — *see* Poliomyelitis, paralytic
  bulbar (paralytic) — *see* Poliomyelitis, paralytic

Poliomyelitis — *continued*
  congenital P35.8
  nonepidemic A80.9
  nonparalytic A80.4
  paralytic A80.30
    specified NEC A80.39
    vaccine-associated A80.0
    wild virus
      imported A80.1
      indigenous A80.2
  spinal, acute A80.9
Poliosis (eyebrow) (eyelashes) L67.1
  circumscripta, acquired L67.1
Pollakiuria R35.0
  psychogenic F45.8
Pollinosis J30.1
Pollitzer's disease L73.2
Polyadenitis (*see also* Lymphadenitis)
  malignant A20.0
Polyalgia M79.89
Polyangiitis M30.0
  microscopic M31.7
  overlap syndrome M30.8
Polyarteritis
  microscopic M31.7
  nodosa M30.0
    with lung involvement M30.1
    juvenile M30.2
    related condition NEC M30.8
Polyarthralgia — *see* Pain, joint
Polyarthritis, polyarthropathy (*see also* Arthritis) M13.0
  due to or associated with other specified conditions — *see* Arthritis
  epidemic (Australian) (with exanthema) B33.1
  infective — *see* Arthritis, pyogenic or pyemic
  inflammatory M06.4
  juvenile (chronic) (seronegative) M08.3
  migratory — *see* Fever, rheumatic
  rheumatic, acute — *see* Fever, rheumatic
Polyarthrosis M15.9
  post-traumatic M15.3
  primary M15.0
  specified NEC M15.8
Polycarential syndrome of infancy E40
Polychondritis (atrophic) (chronic) (*see also* Disorder, cartilage, specified type NEC)
  relapsing M94.1
Polycoria Q13.2
Polycystic (disease)
  degeneration, kidney Q61.3
    autosomal dominant (adult type) Q61.2
    autosomal recessive (infantile type) NEC Q61.19
  kidney Q61.3
    autosomal
      dominant Q61.2
      recessive NEC Q61.19
    autosomal dominant (adult type) Q61.2
    autosomal recessive (childhood type) NEC Q61.19
    infantile type NEC Q61.19
  liver Q44.6
  lung J98.4
    congenital Q33.0
  ovary, ovaries E28.2
  spleen Q89.09
Polycythemia (secondary) D75.1
  acquired D75.1
  benign (familial) D75.0
  due to
    donor twin P61.1
    erythropoietin D75.1
    fall in plasma volume D75.1
    high altitude D75.1
    maternal-fetal transfusion P61.1
    stress D75.1
  emotional D75.1
  erythropoietin D75.1
  familial (benign) D75.0
  Gaisböck's (hypertonica) D75.1
  high altitude D75.1
  hypertonica D75.1
  hypoxemic D75.1
  neonatorum P61.1
  nephrogenous D75.1
  relative D75.1
  secondary D75.1
  spurious D75.1
  stress D75.1
  vera D45

Polycytosis cryptogenica D75.1
Polydactylism, polydactyly Q69.9
  toes Q69.2
Polydipsia R63.1
Polydystrophy, pseudo-Hurler E77.0
Polyembryoma — *see* Neoplasm, malignant, by site
Polyglandular
  deficiency E31.0
  dyscrasia E31.9
  dysfunction E31.9
  syndrome E31.8
Polyhydramnios O40.- ☑
Polymastia Q83.1
Polymenorrhea N92.0
Polymyalgia M35.3
  arteritica, giant cell M31.5
  rheumatica M35.3
    with giant cell arteritis M31.5
Polymyositis (acute) (chronic) (hemorrhagic) M33.20
  with
    myopathy M33.22
    respiratory involvement M33.21
    skin involvement — *see* Dermatopolymyositis
    specified organ involvement NEC M33.29
  ossificans (generalisata) (progressiva) — *see* Myositis, ossificans, progressiva
Polyneuritis, polyneuritic (*see also* Polyneuropathy)
  acute (post-)infective G61.0
  alcoholic G62.1
  cranialis G52.7
  demyelinating, chronic inflammatory (CIDP) G61.81
  diabetic — *see* Diabetes, polyneuropathy
  diphtheritic A36.83
  due to lack of vitamin NEC E56.9 [G63]
  endemic E51.11
  erythredema — *see* subcategory T56.1 ☑
  febrile, acute G61.0
  hereditary ataxic G60.1
  idiopathic, acute G61.0
  infective (acute) G61.0
  inflammatory, chronic demyelinating (CIDP) G61.81
  nutritional E63.9 [G63]
  postinfective (acute) G61.0
  specified NEC G62.89
Polyneuropathy (peripheral) G62.9
  alcoholic G62.1
  amyloid (Portuguese) E85.1 [G63]
  arsenical G62.2
  critical illness G62.81
  demyelinating, chronic inflammatory (CIDP) G61.81
  diabetic — *see* Diabetes, polyneuropathy
  drug-induced G62.0
  hereditary G60.9
    specified NEC G60.8
  idiopathic G60.9
    progressive G60.3
  in (due to)
    alcohol G62.1
      sequelae G65.2
    amyloidosis, familial (Portuguese) E85.1 [G63]
    antitetanus serum G61.1
    arsenic G62.2
      sequelae G65.2
    avitaminosis NEC E56.9 [G63]
    beriberi E51.11
    collagen vascular disease NEC M35.9 [G63]
    deficiency (of)
      B (-complex) vitamins E53.9 [G63]
      vitamin B6 E53.1 [G63]
    diabetes — *see* Diabetes, polyneuropathy
    diphtheria A36.83
    drug or medicament G62.0
      correct substance properly administered — *see* Table of Drugs and Chemicals, by drug, adverse effect
      overdose or wrong substance given or taken — *see* Table of Drugs and Chemicals, by drug, poisoning
    endocrine disease NEC E34.9 [G63]
    herpes zoster B02.23
    hypoglycemia E16.2 [G63]
    infectious
      disease NEC B99 ☑ [G63]
      mononucleosis B27.91
    lack of vitamin NEC E56.9 [G63]
    lead G62.2
      sequelae G65.2
    leprosy A30.9 [G63]

Polyneuropathy — continued
  in — continued
   Lyme disease A69.22
   metabolic disease NEC E88.9 [G63]
   microscopic polyangiitis M31.7 [G63]
   mumps B26.84
   neoplastic disease (see also Neoplasm) D49.9 [G63]
   nutritional deficiency NEC E63.9 [G63]
   organophosphate compounds G62.2
    sequelae G65.2
   parasitic disease NEC B89 [G63]
   pellagra E52 [G63]
   polyarteritis nodosa M30.0
   porphyria E80.20 [G63]
   radiation G62.82
   rheumatoid arthritis — see Rheumatoid, polyneu-
    ropathy
   sarcoidosis D86.89
   serum G61.1
   syphilis (late) A52.15
    congenital A50.43
   systemic
    connective tissue disorder M35.9 [G63]
    lupus erythematosus M32.19
   toxic agent NEC G62.2
    sequelae G65.2
   triorthocresyl phosphate G62.2
    sequelae G65.2
   tuberculosis A17.89
   uremia N18.9 [G63]
   vitamin B12 deficiency E53.8 [G63]
    with anemia (pernicious) D51.0 [G63]
     due to dietary deficiency D51.3 [G63]
   zoster B02.23
  inflammatory G61.9
   chronic demyelinating (CIDP) G61.81
   sequelae G65.1
   specified NEC G61.89
  lead G62.2
   sequelae G65.2
  nutritional NEC E63.9 [G63]
  postherpetic (zoster) B02.23
  progressive G60.3
  radiation-induced G62.82
  sensory (hereditary) (idiopathic) G60.8
  specified NEC G62.89
  syphilitic (late) A52.15
   congenital A50.43
Polyopia H53.8
Polyorchism, polyorchidism Q55.21
Polyosteoarthritis (see also Osteoarthritis, generalized)
  M15.9
  post-traumatic M15.3
  specified NEC M15.8
Polyostotic fibrous dysplasia Q78.1
Polyotia Q17.0
Polyp, polypus
  accessory sinus J33.8
  adenocarcinoma in — see Neoplasm, malignant, by
   site
  adenocarcinoma in situ in — see Neoplasm, in situ, by
   site
  adenoid tissue J33.0
  adenomatous (see also Neoplasm, benign, by site)
   adenocarcinoma in — see Neoplasm, malignant,
    by site
   adenocarcinoma in situ in — see Neoplasm, in situ,
    by site
   carcinoma in — see Neoplasm, malignant, by site
   carcinoma in situ in — see Neoplasm, in situ, by
    site
   multiple — see Neoplasm, benign
    adenocarcinoma in — see Neoplasm, malig-
     nant, by site
    adenocarcinoma in situ in — see Neoplasm, in
     situ, by site
  antrum J33.8
  anus, anal (canal) K62.0
  Bartholin's gland N84.3
  bladder D41.4
  carcinoma in — see Neoplasm, malignant, by site
  carcinoma in situ in — see Neoplasm, in situ, by site
  cecum D12.0
  cervix (uteri) N84.1
   in pregnancy or childbirth — see Pregnancy,
    complicated by, abnormal, cervix
   mucous N84.1
   nonneoplastic N84.1

Polyp, polypus — continued
  choanal J33.0
  cholesterol K82.4
  clitoris N84.3
  colon K63.5
   adenomatous D12.6
   ascending D12.2
   cecum D12.0
   descending D12.4
   inflammatory K51.40
    with
     abscess K51.414
     complication K51.419
      specified NEC K51.418
     fistula K51.413
     intestinal obstruction K51.412
     rectal bleeding K51.411
   sigmoid D12.5
   transverse D12.3
  corpus uteri N84.0
  dental K04.0
  duodenum K31.7
  ear (middle) H74.4- ☑
  endometrium N84.0
  ethmoidal (sinus) J33.8
  fallopian tube N84.8
  female genital tract N84.9
   specified NEC N84.8
  frontal (sinus) J33.8
  gallbladder K82.4
  gingiva, gum K06.8
  labia, labium (majus) (minus) N84.3
  larynx (mucous) J38.1
   adenomatous D14.1
  malignant — see Neoplasm, malignant, by site
  maxillary (sinus) J33.8
  middle ear — see Polyp, ear (middle)
  myometrium N84.0
  nares
   anterior J33.9
   posterior J33.0
  nasal (mucous) J33.9
   cavity J33.0
   septum J33.0
  nasopharyngeal J33.0
  nose (mucous) J33.9
  oviduct N84.8
  pharynx J39.2
  placenta O90.89
  prostate — see Enlargement, enlarged, prostate
  pudenda, pudendum N84.3
  pulpal (dental) K04.0
  rectum (nonadenomatous) K62.1
   adenomatous — see Polyp, adenomatous
  septum (nasal) J33.0
  sinus (accessory) (ethmoidal) (frontal) (maxillary)
   (sphenoidal) J33.8
  sphenoidal (sinus) J33.8
  stomach K31.7
   adenomatous D13.1
  tube, fallopian N84.8
  turbinate, mucous membrane J33.8
  umbilical, newborn P83.6
  ureter N28.89
  urethra N36.2
  uterus (body) (corpus) (mucous) N84.0
   cervix N84.1
   in pregnancy or childbirth — see Pregnancy,
    complicated by, tumor, uterus
  vagina N84.2
  vocal cord (mucous) J38.1
  vulva N84.3
Polyphagia R63.2
Polyploidy Q92.7
Polypoid — see condition
Polyposis (see also Polyp)
  coli (adenomatous) D12.6
   adenocarcinoma in C18.9
   adenocarcinoma in situ in — see Neoplasm, in situ,
    by site
   carcinoma in C18.9
  colon (adenomatous) D12.6
  familial D12.6
   adenocarcinoma in situ in — see Neoplasm, in situ,
    by site
  intestinal (adenomatous) D12.6
  malignant lymphomatous C83.1- ☑

Polyposis — continued
  multiple, adenomatous (see also Neoplasm, benign)
   D36.9
Polyradiculitis — see Polyneuropathy
Polyradiculoneuropathy (acute) (postinfective) (seg-
  mentally demyelinating) G61.0
Polyserositis
  due to pericarditis I31.1
  pericardial I31.1
  periodic, familial E85.0
  tuberculous A19.9
   acute A19.1
   chronic A19.8
Polysplenia syndrome Q89.09
Polysyndactyly (see also Syndactylism, syndactyly) Q70.4
Polytrichia L68.3
Polyunguia Q84.6
Polyuria R35.8
  nocturnal R35.1
  psychogenic F45.8
Pompe's disease (glycogen storage) E74.02
Pompholyx L30.1
Poncet's disease (tuberculous rheumatism) A18.09
Pond fracture — see Fracture, skull
Ponos B55.0
Pons, pontine — see condition
Poor
  aesthetic of existing restoration of tooth K08.56
  contractions, labor O62.2
  gingival margin to tooth restoration K08.51
  personal hygiene R46.0
  prenatal care, affecting management of pregnancy
   — see Pregnancy, complicated by, insufficient,
   prenatal care
  sucking reflex (newborn) R29.2
  urinary stream R39.12
  vision NEC H54.7
Poradenitis, nostras inguinalis or venerea A55
Porencephaly (congenital) (developmental) (true) Q04.6
  acquired G93.0
  nondevelopmental G93.0
  traumatic (post) F07.89
Porocephaliasis B88.8
Porokeratosis Q82.8
Poroma, eccrine — see Neoplasm, skin, benign
Porphyria (South African) E80.20
  acquired E80.20
  acute intermittent (hepatic) (Swedish) E80.21
  cutanea tarda (hereditary) (symptomatic) E80.1
  due to drugs E80.20
   correct substance properly administered — see
    Table of Drugs and Chemicals, by drug, ad-
    verse effect
   overdose or wrong substance given or taken —
    see Table of Drugs and Chemicals, by drug,
    poisoning
  erythropoietic (congenital) (hereditary) E80.0
  hepatocutaneous type E80.1
  secondary E80.20
  toxic NEC E80.20
  variegata E80.20
Porphyrinuria — see Porphyria
Porphyruria — see Porphyria
Port wine nevus, mark, or stain Q82.5
Portal — see condition
Posadas-Wernicke disease B38.9
Positive
  culture (nonspecific)
   blood R78.81
   bronchial washings R84.5
   cerebrospinal fluid R83.5
   cervix uteri R87.5
   nasal secretions R84.5
   nipple discharge R89.5
   nose R84.5
    staphylococcus (Methicillin susceptible) Z22.321
     Methicillin resistant Z22.322
   peritoneal fluid R85.5
   pleural fluid R84.5
   prostatic secretions R86.5
   saliva R85.5
   seminal fluid R86.5
   sputum R84.5
   synovial fluid R89.5
   throat scrapings R84.5
   urine R82.7
   vagina R87.5
   vulva R87.5

Positive — *continued*
  culture — *continued*
    wound secretions R89.5
  PPD (skin test) R76.11
  serology for syphilis A53.0
    with signs or symptoms — *code as* Syphilis, by site
      and stage
    false R76.8
  skin test, tuberculin (without active tuberculosis)
    R76.11
  test, human immunodeficiency virus (HIV) R75
  VDRL A53.0
    with signs or symptoms — *code by* site and stage
      under Syphilis A53.9
  Wassermann reaction A53.0
Post-dates (40-42 weeks) (pregnancy) (mother) O48.0
  more than 42 weeks gestation O48.1
Post-term (40-42 weeks) (pregnancy) (mother) O48.0
  infant P08.21
  more than 42 weeks gestation (mother) O48.1
Post-traumatic brain syndrome, nonpsychotic F07.81
Post-typhoid abscess A01.09
Postcardiotomy syndrome I97.0
Postcaval ureter Q62.62
Postcholecystectomy syndrome K91.5
Postclimacteric bleeding N95.0
Postcommissurotomy syndrome I97.0
Postconcussional syndrome F07.81
Postcontusional syndrome F07.81
Postcricoid region — *see* condition
Postencephalitic syndrome F07.89
Posterior — *see* condition
Posterolateral sclerosis (spinal cord) — *see* Degeneration, combined
Postexanthematous — *see* condition
Postfebrile — *see* condition
Postgastrectomy dumping syndrome K91.1
Posthemiplegic chorea — *see* Monoplegia
Posthemorrhagic anemia (chronic) D50.0
  acute D62
  newborn P61.3
Postherpetic neuralgia (zoster) B02.29
  trigeminal B02.22
Posthitis N47.7
Postimmunization complication or reaction — *see* Complications, vaccination
Postinfectious — *see* condition
Postlaminectomy syndrome NEC M96.1
Postleukotomy syndrome F07.0
Postmastectomy lymphedema (syndrome) I97.2
Postmaturity, postmature (over 42 weeks)
  maternal (over 42 weeks gestation) O48.1
  newborn P08.22
Postmeasles complication NEC (*see also* condition)
  B05.89
Postmenopausal
  endometrium (atrophic) N95.8
    suppurative (*see also* Endometritis) N71.9
  osteoporosis — *see* Osteoporosis, postmenopausal
Postnasal drip R09.82
  due to
    allergic rhinitis — *see* Rhinitis, allergic
    common cold J00
    gastroesophageal reflux — *see* Reflux, gastroesophageal
    nasopharyngitis — *see* Nasopharyngitis
    other known condition — *code to* condition
    sinusitis — *see* Sinusitis
Postnatal — *see* condition
Postoperative (postprocedural) — *see* Complication, postprocedural
  pneumothorax, therapeutic Z98.3
  state NEC Z98.89
Postpancreatectomy hyperglycemia E89.1
Postpartum — *see* Puerperal
Postphlebitic syndrome — *see* Syndrome, postthrombotic
Postpolio (myelitic) **syndrome** G14
Postpoliomyelitic (*see also* condition)
  osteopathy — *see* Osteopathy, after poliomyelitis
Postprocedural (*see also* Postoperative)
  hypoinsulinemia E89.1
Postschizophrenic depression F32.8
Postsurgery status (*see also* Status (post))
  pneumothorax, therapeutic Z98.3
Postures, hysterical F44.2

Postvaccinal reaction or complication — *see* Complications, vaccination
Postvalvulotomy syndrome I97.0
Potain's
  disease (pulmonary edema) — *see* Edema, lung
  syndrome (gastrectasis with dyspepsia) K31.0
Potter's
  asthma J62.8
  facies Q60.6
  lung J62.8
  syndrome (with renal agenesis) Q60.6
Pott's
  curvature (spinal) A18.01
  disease or paraplegia A18.01
  spinal curvature A18.01
  tumor, puffy — *see* Osteomyelitis, specified type NEC
Pouch
  bronchus Q32.4
  Douglas' — *see* condition
  esophagus, esophageal, congenital Q39.6
    acquired K22.5
  gastric K31.4
  Hartmann's K82.8
  pharynx, pharyngeal (congenital) Q38.7
Pouchitis K91.850
Poultrymen's itch B88.0
Poverty NEC Z59.6
  extreme Z59.5
Poxvirus NEC B08.8
Prader-Willi syndrome Q87.1
Pre-eclampsia O14.9- ☑
  with pre-existing hypertension — *see* Hypertension, complicating pregnancy, pre-existing, with, pre-eclampsia
  mild O14.0- ☑
  moderate O14.0- ☑
  severe O14.1- ☑
    with hemolysis, elevated liver enzymes and low platelet count (HELLP) O14.2- ☑
Pre-eruptive color change, teeth, tooth K00.8
Pre-excitation atrioventricular conduction I45.6
Pre-kwashiorkor — *see* Malnutrition, severe
Pre-syncope R55
Preauricular appendage or tag Q17.0
Prebetalipoproteinemia (acquired) (essential) (familial) (hereditary) (primary) (secondary) E78.1
  with chylomicronemia E78.3
Precipitate labor or delivery O62.3
Preclimacteric bleeding (menorrhagia) N92.4
Precocious
  adrenarche E30.1
  menarche E30.1
  menstruation E30.1
  pubarche E30.1
  puberty E30.1
    central E22.8
  sexual development NEC E30.1
  thelarche E30.8
Precocity, sexual (constitutional) (cryptogenic) (female) (idiopathic) (male) E30.1
  with adrenal hyperplasia E25.9
    congenital E25.0
Precordial pain R07.2
Predeciduous teeth K00.2
Prediabetes, prediabetic R73.09
  complicating
    pregnancy — *see* Pregnancy, complicated by, diseases of, specified type or system NEC
    puerperium O99.89
Predislocation status of hip at birth Q65.6
Preglaucoma H40.00- ☑
Pregnancy (single) (uterine) (*see also* Delivery and Puerperal)

> *Note: The Tabular must be reviewed for assignment of appropriate seventh character for multiple gestation codes in Chapter 15*

> *Note: The Tabular must be reviewed for assignment of the appropriate character indicating the trimester of the pregnancy*

  abdominal (ectopic) O00.0
    with viable fetus O36.7- ☑
  ampullar O00.1
  biochemical O02.81
  broad ligament O00.8
  cervical O00.8

Pregnancy — *continued*
  chemical O02.81
  complicated by (care of) (management affected by)
    abnormal, abnormality
      cervix O34.4- ☑
        causing obstructed labor O65.5
      cord (umbilical) O69.9
      findings on antenatal screening of mother O28.9
        biochemical O28.1
        chromosomal O28.5
        cytological O28.2
        genetic O28.5
        hematological O28.0
        radiological O28.4
        specified NEC O28.8
        ultrasonic O28.3
      glucose (tolerance) NEC O99.810
      pelvic organs O34.9- ☑
        specified NEC O34.8- ☑
          causing obstructed labor O65.5
      pelvis (bony) (major) NEC O33.0
      perineum O34.7- ☑
      position
        placenta O44.1- ☑
          without hemorrhage O44.0- ☑
        uterus O34.59- ☑
      uterus O34.59- ☑
        causing obstructed labor O65.5
        congenital O34.0- ☑
      vagina O34.6- ☑
        causing obstructed labor O65.5
      vulva O34.7- ☑
        causing obstructed labor O65.5
    abruptio placentae — *see* Abruptio placentae
    abscess or cellulitis
      bladder O23.1- ☑
      breast O91.11- ☑
      genital organ or tract O23.9- ☑
    abuse
      physical O9A.31 ☑ (*following* O99)
      psychological O9A.51 ☑ (*following* O99)
      sexual O9A.41 ☑ (*following* O99)
    adverse effect anesthesia O29.9- ☑
      aspiration pneumonitis O29.01- ☑
      cardiac arrest O29.11- ☑
      cardiac complication NEC O29.19- ☑
      cardiac failure O29.12- ☑
      central nervous system complication NEC O29.29- ☑
      cerebral anoxia O29.21- ☑
      failed or difficult intubation O29.6- ☑
      inhalation of stomach contents or secretions NOS O29.01- ☑
      local, toxic reaction O29.3X- ☑
      Mendelson's syndrome O29.01- ☑
      pressure collapse of lung O29.02- ☑
      pulmonary complications NEC O29.09- ☑
      specified NEC O29.8X- ☑
      spinal and epidural type NEC O29.5X- ☑
        induced headache O29.4- ☑
    albuminuria O12.1- ☑
    alcohol use O99.31- ☑
    amnionitis O41.12- ☑
    anaphylactoid syndrome of pregnancy O88.01- ☑
    anemia (conditions in D50-D64) (pre-existing) O99.01- ☑
      complicating the puerperium O99.03
    antepartum hemorrhage O46.9- ☑
      with coagulation defect — *see* Hemorrhage, antepartum, with coagulation defect
      specified NEC O46.8X- ☑
    appendicitis O99.61- ☑
    atrophy (yellow) (acute) liver (subacute) O26.61- ☑
    bariatric surgery status O99.84- ☑
    bicornis or bicornuate uterus O34.59- ☑
    biliary tract problems O26.61- ☑
    breech presentation O32.1 ☑
    cardiovascular diseases (conditions in I00-I09, I20-I52, I70-I99) O99.41- ☑
    cerebrovascular disorders (conditions in I60-I69) O99.41- ☑
    cervical shortening O26.87- ☑
    cervicitis O23.51- ☑
    chloasma (gravidarum) O26.89- ☑
    cholecystitis O99.61- ☑

Pregnancy — continued
  complicated by — continued
    cholestasis (intrahepatic) O26.61- ☑
    chorioamnionitis O41.12- ☑
    circulatory system disorder (conditions in I00-I09, I20-I99, O99.41-)
    compound presentation O32.6 ☑
    conjoined twins O30.02- ☑
    connective system disorders (conditions in M00-M99) O99.89
    contracted pelvis (general) O33.1
      inlet O33.2
      outlet O33.3 ☑
    convulsions (eclamptic) (uremic) (see also Eclampsia) O15.9
    cracked nipple O92.11- ☑
    cystitis O23.1- ☑
    cystocele O34.8- ☑
    death of fetus (near term) O36.4 ☑
      early pregnancy O02.1
      of one fetus or more in multiple gestation O31.2- ☑
    deciduitis O41.14- ☑
    decreased fetal movement O36.81- ☑
    dental problems O99.61- ☑
    diabetes (mellitus) O24.91- ☑
      gestational (pregnancy induced) — see Diabetes, gestational
      pre-existing O24.31- ☑
        specified NEC O24.81- ☑
        type 1 O24.01- ☑
        type 2 O24.11- ☑
    digestive system disorders (conditions in K00-K93) O99.61- ☑
    diseases of — see Pregnancy, complicated by, specified body system disease
      biliary tract O26.61- ☑
      blood NEC (conditions in D65-D77) O99.11- ☑
      liver O26.61- ☑
      specified NEC O99.89
    disorders of — see Pregnancy, complicated by, specified body system disorder
      amniotic fluid and membranes O41.9- ☑
        specified NEC O41.8X- ☑
      biliary tract O26.61- ☑
      ear and mastoid process (conditions in H60-H95) O99.89
      eye and adnexa (conditions in H00-H59) O99.89
      liver O26.61- ☑
      skin (conditions in L00-L99) O99.71- ☑
      specified NEC O99.89
    displacement, uterus NEC O34.59- ☑
      causing obstructed labor O65.5
    disproportion (due to) O33.9
      fetal deformities NEC O33.7
      generally contracted pelvis O33.1
      hydrocephalic fetus O33.6 ☑
      inlet contraction of pelvis O33.2
      mixed maternal and fetal origin O33.4 ☑
      specified NEC O33.8
    double uterus O34.59- ☑
      causing obstructed labor O65.5
    drug use (conditions in F11-F19) O99.32- ☑
    eclampsia, eclamptic (coma) (convulsions) (delirium) (nephritis) (uremia) (see also Eclampsia) O15.- ☑
    ectopic pregnancy — see Pregnancy, ectopic
    edema O12.0- ☑
      with
        gestational hypertension, mild (see also Pre-eclampsia) O14.0- ☑
        proteinuria O12.2- ☑
    effusion, amniotic fluid — see Pregnancy, complicated by, premature rupture of membranes
    elderly
      multigravida O09.52- ☑
      primigravida O09.51- ☑
    embolism (see also Embolism, obstetric, pregnancy) O88.- ☑
    endocrine diseases NEC O99.28- ☑
    endometritis O86.12
    excessive weight gain O26.0- ☑
    exhaustion O26.81- ☑
      during labor and delivery O75.81
    face presentation O32.3
    failed induction of labor O61.9
      instrumental O61.1

Pregnancy — continued
  complicated by — continued
    failed induction of labor — continued
      mechanical O61.1
      medical O61.0
      specified NEC O61.8
      surgical O61.1
    failed or difficult intubation for anesthesia O29.6- ☑
    false labor (pains) O47.9
      at or after 37 completed weeks of pregnancy O47.1
      before 37 completed weeks of pregnancy O47.0- ☑
    fatigue O26.81- ☑
      during labor and delivery O75.81
    fatty metamorphosis of liver O26.61- ☑
    female genital mutilation O34.8- ☑ [N90.81-] ☑
    fetal (maternal care for)
      abnormality or damage O35.9 ☑
        acid-base balance O68
        specified type NEC O35.8 ☑
      acidemia O68
      acidosis O68
      alkalosis O68
      anemia and thrombocytopenia O36.82- ☑
      anencephaly O35.0
      chromosomal abnormality (conditions in Q90-Q99) O35.1
      conjoined twins O30.02- ☑
      damage from
        amniocentesis O35.7 ☑
        biopsy procedures O35.7 ☑
        drug addiction O35.5 ☑
        hematological investigation O35.7 ☑
        intrauterine contraceptive device O35.7 ☑
        maternal
          alcohol addiction O35.4 ☑
          cytomegalovirus infection O35.3 ☑
          disease NEC O35.8 ☑
          drug addiction O35.5 ☑
          listeriosis O35.8 ☑
          rubella O35.3 ☑
          toxoplasmosis O35.8 ☑
          viral infection O35.3 ☑
        medical procedure NEC O35.7 ☑
        radiation O35.6 ☑
      death (near term) O36.4 ☑
        early pregnancy O02.1
      decreased movement O36.81- ☑
      disproportion due to deformity (fetal) O33.7
      excessive growth (large for dates) O36.6- ☑
      growth retardation O36.59- ☑
        light for dates O36.59- ☑
        small for dates O36.59- ☑
      heart rate irregularity (bradycardia) (decelerations) (tachycardia) O76
      hereditary disease O35.2 ☑
      hydrocephalus O35.0 ☑
      intrauterine death O36.4 ☑
      poor growth O36.59- ☑
        light for dates O36.59- ☑
        small for dates O36.59- ☑
      problem O36.9- ☑
        specified NEC O36.89- ☑
      reduction (elective) O31.3- ☑
      selective termination O31.3- ☑
      spina bifida O35.0 ☑
      thrombocytopenia O36.82- ☑
    fibroid (tumor) (uterus) O34.1- ☑
    fissure of nipple O92.11- ☑
    gallstones O99.61- ☑
    gastric banding status O99.84- ☑
    gastric bypass status O99.84- ☑
    genital herpes (asymptomatic) (history of) (inactive) O98.51- ☑
    genital tract infection O23.9- ☑
    glomerular diseases (conditions in N00-N07) O26.83- ☑
      with hypertension, pre-existing — see Hypertension, complicating, pregnancy, pre-existing, with, renal disease
    gonorrhea O98.21- ☑
    grand multiparity O09.4 ☑
    habitual aborter — see Pregnancy, complicated by, recurrent pregnancy loss

Pregnancy — continued
  complicated by — continued
    HELLP syndrome (hemolysis, elevated liver enzymes and low platelet count) O14.2- ☑
    hemorrhage
      antepartum — see Hemorrhage, antepartum
      before 20 completed weeks gestation O20.9
        specified NEC O20.8
      due to premature separation, placenta (see also Abruptio placentae) O45.9- ☑
      early O20.9
        specified NEC O20.8
      threatened abortion O20.0
    hemorrhoids O22.4- ☑
    hepatitis (viral) O98.41- ☑
    herniation of uterus O34.59- ☑
    high
      head at term O32.4 ☑
      risk — see Supervision (of) (for), high-risk
    history of in utero procedure during previous pregnancy O09.82- ☑
    HIV O98.71- ☑
    human immunodeficiency virus (HIV) disease O98.71- ☑
    hydatidiform mole (see also Mole, hydatidiform) O01.9
    hydramnios O40.- ☑
    hydrocephalic fetus (disproportion) O33.6 ☑
    hydrops
      amnii O40.- ☑
      fetalis O36.2- ☑
        associated with isoimmunization (see also Pregnancy, complicated by, isoimmunization) O36.11- ☑
    hydrorrhea O42.90
    hyperemesis (gravidarum) (mild) (see also Hyperemesis, gravidarum) O21.0
    hypertension — see Hypertension, complicating pregnancy
    hypertensive
      heart and renal disease, pre-existing — see Hypertension, complicating, pregnancy, pre-existing, with, heart disease, with renal disease
      heart disease, pre-existing — see Hypertension, complicating, pregnancy, pre-existing, with, heart disease
      renal disease, pre-existing — see Hypertension, complicating, pregnancy, pre-existing, with, renal disease
    hypotension O26.5- ☑
    immune disorders NEC (conditions in D80-D89) O99.11- ☑
    incarceration, uterus O34.51- ☑
    incompetent cervix O34.3- ☑
    inconclusive fetal viability O36.80 ☑
    infection(s) O98.91- ☑
      amniotic fluid or sac O41.10- ☑
      bladder O23.1- ☑
      carrier state NEC O99.830
        streptococcus B O99.820
      genital organ or tract O23.9- ☑
        specified NEC O23.59- ☑
      genitourinary tract O23.9- ☑
      gonorrhea O98.21- ☑
      hepatitis (viral) O98.41- ☑
      HIV O98.71- ☑
      human immunodeficiency virus (HIV) O98.71- ☑
      kidney O23.0- ☑
      nipple O91.01- ☑
      parasitic disease O98.91- ☑
        specified NEC O98.81- ☑
      protozoal disease O98.61- ☑
      sexually transmitted NEC O98.31- ☑
      specified type NEC O98.81- ☑
      syphilis O98.11- ☑
      tuberculosis O98.01- ☑
      urethra O23.2- ☑
      urinary (tract) O23.4- ☑
        specified NEC O23.3- ☑
      viral disease O98.51- ☑
    injury or poisoning (conditions in S00-T88) O9A.21- ☑ (following O99)
      due to abuse
        physical O9A.31- ☑ (following O99)

☑ Additional Character Required — Refer to the Tabular List for Character Selection   ▽ Subterms under main terms may continue to next column or page

Pregnancy — *continued*
  complicated by — *continued*
    young mother — *continued*
      primigravida O09.61- ☑
  complicated NOS O26.9- ☑
  concealed O09.3- ☑
  continuing following
    elective fetal reduction of one or more fetus
      O31.3- ☑
    intrauterine death of one or more fetus O31.2- ☑
    spontaneous abortion of one or more fetus
      O31.1- ☑
  cornual O00.8
  ectopic (ruptured) O00.9
    abdominal O00.0
      with viable fetus O36.7- ☑
    cervical O00.8
    complicated (by) O08.9
      afibrinogenemia O08.1
      cardiac arrest O08.81
      chemical damage of pelvic organ(s) O08.6
      circulatory collapse O08.3
      defibrination syndrome O08.1
      electrolyte imbalance O08.5
      embolism (amniotic fluid) (blood clot) (pulmonary) (septic) O08.2
      endometritis O08.0
      genital tract and pelvic infection O08.0
      hemorrhage (delayed) (excessive) O08.1
      infection
        genital tract or pelvic O08.0
          kidney O08.83
          urinary tract O08.3
      intravascular coagulation O08.1
      laceration of pelvic organ(s) O08.6
      metabolic disorder O08.5
      oliguria O08.4
      oophoritis O08.0
      parametritis O08.0
      pelvic peritonitis O08.0
      perforation of pelvic organ(s) O08.6
      renal failure or shutdown O08.4
      salpingitis or salpingo-oophoritis O08.0
      sepsis O08.82
      shock O08.83
        septic O08.82
      specified condition NEC O08.89
      tubular necrosis (renal) O08.4
      uremia O08.4
      urinary infection O08.83
      venous complication NEC O08.7
        embolism O08.2
    cornual O00.8
    intraligamentous O00.8
    mural O00.8
    ovarian O00.2
    specified site NEC O00.8
    tubal (ruptured) O00.1
  examination (normal) Z34.9- ☑
    first Z34.0- ☑
    high-risk — *see* Pregnancy, supervision of, high-risk
    specified Z34.8- ☑
  extrauterine — *see* Pregnancy, ectopic
  fallopian O00.1
  false F45.8
  hidden O09.3- ☑
  high-risk — *see* Pregnancy, supervision of, high-risk
  incidental finding Z33.1
  interstitial O00.8
  intraligamentous O00.8
  intramural O00.8
  intraperitoneal O00.0
  isthmian O00.1
  mesometric (mural) O00.8
  molar NEC O02.0
    complicated (by) O08.9
      afibrinogenemia O08.1
      cardiac arrest O08.81
      chemical damage of pelvic organ(s) O08.6
      circulatory collapse O08.3
      defibrination syndrome O08.1
      electrolyte imbalance O08.5
      embolism (amniotic fluid) (blood clot) (pulmonary) (septic) O08.2
      endometritis O08.0
      genital tract and pelvic infection O08.0
      hemorrhage (delayed) (excessive) O08.1

Pregnancy — *continued*
  molar — *continued*
    complicated — *continued*
      infection
        genital tract or pelvic O08.0
          kidney O08.83
          urinary tract O08.83
      intravascular coagulation O08.1
      laceration of pelvic organ(s) O08.6
      metabolic disorder O08.5
      oliguria O08.4
      oophoritis O08.0
      parametritis O08.0
      pelvic peritonitis O08.0
      perforation of pelvic organ(s) O08.6
      renal failure or shutdown O08.4
      salpingitis or salpingo-oophoritis O08.0
      sepsis O08.82
      shock O08.3
        septic O08.82
      specified condition NEC O08.89
      tubular necrosis (renal) O08.4
      uremia O08.4
      urinary infection O08.83
      venous complication NEC O08.7
        embolism O08.2
    hydatidiform (*see also* Mole, hydatidiform) O01.9
  multiple (gestation) O30.9- ☑
    greater than quadruplets — *see* Pregnancy, multiple (gestation), specified NEC
    specified NEC O30.80- ☑
      with
        two or more monoamniotic fetuses
          O30.82- ☑
        two or more monochorionic fetuses
          O30.81- ☑
      two or more monoamniotic fetuses O30.82- ☑
      two or more monochorionic fetuses O30.81- ☑
      unable to determine number of placenta and
        number of amniotic sacs O30.89- ☑
      unspecified number of placenta and unspecified number of amniotic sacs O30.80- ☑
  mural O00.8
  normal (supervision of) Z34.9- ☑
    first Z34.0- ☑
    high-risk — *see* Pregnancy, supervision of, high-risk
    specified Z34.8- ☑
  ovarian O00.2
  post-term (40 to 42 weeks) O48.0
  postmature (40 to 42 weeks) O48.0
    more than 42 weeks gestation O48.1
  prenatal care only Z34.9- ☑
    first Z34.0- ☑
    high-risk — *see* Pregnancy, supervision of, high-risk
    specified Z34.8- ☑
  prolonged (more than 42 weeks gestation) O48.1
  quadruplet O30.20- ☑
    with
      two or more monoamniotic fetuses O30.22- ☑
      two or more monochorionic fetuses O30.21- ☑
    two or more monoamniotic fetuses O30.22- ☑
    two or more monochorionic fetuses O30.21- ☑
    unable to determine number of placenta and
      number of amniotic sacs O30.29- ☑
    unspecified number of placenta and unspecified
      number of amniotic sacs O30.20- ☑
  quintuplet — *see* Pregnancy, multiple (gestation), specified NEC
  sextuplet — *see* Pregnancy, multiple (gestation), specified NEC
  supervision of
    concealed pregnancy O09.3- ☑
    elderly mother
      multigravida O09.52- ☑
      primigravida O09.51- ☑
    hidden pregnancy O09.3- ☑
    high-risk O09.9- ☑
      due to (history of)
        ectopic pregnancy O09.1- ☑
        elderly — *see* Pregnancy, supervision, elderly mother
        grand multiparity O09.4 ☑
        in utero procedure during previous pregnancy O09.82- ☑
        in vitro fertilization O09.81- ☑

Pregnancy — *continued*
  supervision of — *continued*
    high-risk — *continued*
      due to — *continued*
        infertility O09.0- ☑
        insufficient prenatal care O09.3- ☑
        molar pregnancy O09.1- ☑
        multiple previous pregnancies O09.4- ☑
        older mother — *see* Pregnancy, supervision of, elderly mother
        poor reproductive or obstetric history NEC
          O09.29- ☑
        pre-term labor O09.21- ☑
        previous
          neonatal death O09.29- ☑
        social problems O09.7- ☑
        specified NEC O09.89- ☑
        very young mother — *see* Pregnancy, supervision, young mother
      resulting from in vitro fertilization O09.81- ☑
    normal Z34.9- ☑
      first Z34.0- ☑
      specified NEC Z34.8- ☑
    young mother
      multigravida O09.62- ☑
      primigravida O09.61- ☑
  triplet O30.10- ☑
    with
      two or more monoamniotic fetuses O30.12- ☑
      two or more monochrorionic fetuses O30.11- ☑
    two or more monoamniotic fetuses O30.12- ☑
    two or more monochrorionic fetuses O30.11- ☑
    unable to determine number of placenta and
      number of amniotic sacs O30.19- ☑
    unspecified number of placenta and unspecified
      number of amniotic sacs O30.10- ☑
  tubal (with abortion) (with rupture) O00.1
  twin O30.00- ☑
    conjoined O30.02- ☑
    dichorionic/diamniotic (two placenta, two amniotic
      sacs) O30.04- ☑
    monochorionic/diamniotic (one placenta, two
      amniotic sacs) O30.03- ☑
    monochorionic/monoamniotic (one placenta, one
      amniotic sac) O30.01- ☑
    unable to determine number of placenta and
      number of amniotic sacs O30.09- ☑
    unspecified number of placenta and unspecified
      number of amniotic sacs O30.00- ☑
  unwanted Z64.0
  weeks of gestation
    less than 8 weeks Z3A.01 (*following Z36*)
    10 weeks Z3A.10 (*following Z36*)
    11 weeks Z3A.11 (*following Z36*)
    12 weeks Z3A.12 (*following Z36*)
    13 weeks Z3A.13 (*following Z36*)
    14 weeks Z3A.14 (*following Z36*)
    15 weeks Z3A.15 (*following Z36*)
    16 weeks Z3A.16 (*following Z36*)
    17 weeks Z3A.17 (*following Z36*)
    18 weeks Z3A.18 (*following Z36*)
    19 weeks Z3A.19 (*following Z36*)
    20 weeks Z3A.20 (*following Z36*)
    21 weeks Z3A.21 (*following Z36*)
    22 weeks Z3A.22 (*following Z36*)
    23 weeks Z3A.23 (*following Z36*)
    24 weeks Z3A.24 (*following Z36*)
    25 weeks Z3A.25 (*following Z36*)
    26 weeks Z3A.26 (*following Z36*)
    27 weeks Z3A.27 (*following Z36*)
    28 weeks Z3A.28 (*following Z36*)
    29 weeks Z3A.29 (*following Z36*)
    30 weeks Z3A.30 (*following Z36*)
    31 weeks Z3A.31 (*following Z36*)
    32 weeks Z3A.32 (*following Z36*)
    33 weeks Z3A.33 (*following Z36*)
    34 weeks Z3A.34 (*following Z36*)
    35 weeks Z3A.35 (*following Z36*)
    36 weeks Z3A.36 (*following Z36*)
    37 weeks Z3A.37 (*following Z36*)
    38 weeks Z3A.38 (*following Z36*)
    39 weeks Z3A.39 (*following Z36*)
    40 weeks Z3A.40 (*following Z36*)
    41 weeks Z3A.41 (*following Z36*)
    42 weeks Z3A.42 (*following Z36*)
    8 weeks Z3A.08 (*following Z36*)
    9 weeks Z3A.09 (*following Z36*)

☑ Additional Character Required — Refer to the Tabular List for Character Selection   ▽ Subterms under main terms may continue to next column or page

Pregnancy — continued
weeks of gestation — continued
greater than 42 weeks Z3A.49 (following Z36)
not specified Z3A.00 (following Z36)
Preiser's disease — see Osteonecrosis, secondary, due to, trauma, metacarpus
Preleukemia (syndrome) D46.9
Preluxation, hip, congenital Q65.6
Premature (see also condition)
adrenarche E27.0
aging E34.8
beats I49.40
atrial I49.1
auricular I49.1
supraventricular I49.1
birth NEC — see Preterm, newborn
closure, foramen ovale Q21.8
contraction
atrial I49.1
atrioventricular I49.2
auricular I49.1
auriculoventricular I49.49
heart (extrasystole) I49.49
junctional I49.2
ventricular I49.3
delivery (see also Pregnancy, complicated by, preterm labor) O60.10 ☑
ejaculation F52.4
infant NEC — see Preterm, newborn
light-for-dates — see Light for dates
labor — see Pregnancy, complicated by, preterm labor
lungs P28.0
menopause E28.319
asymptomatic E28.319
symptomatic E28.310
newborn
less than 37 completed weeks — see Preterm, newborn
extreme (less than 28 completed weeks) — see Immaturity, extreme
puberty E30.1
rupture membranes or amnion — see Pregnancy, complicated by, premature rupture of membranes
senility E34.8
thelarche E30.8
ventricular systole I49.3
Prematurity NEC (less than 37 completed weeks) — see Preterm, newborn
extreme (less than 28 completed weeks) — see Immaturity, extreme
Premenstrual
dysphoric disorder (PMDD) N94.3
tension (syndrome) N94.3
Premolarization, cuspids K00.2
Prenatal
care, normal pregnancy — see Pregnancy, normal
screening of mother Z36
teeth K00.6
Preparatory care for subsequent treatment NEC
for dialysis Z49.01
peritoneal Z49.02
Prepartum — see condition
Preponderance, left or right ventricular I51.7
Prepuce — see condition
PRES (posterior reversible encephalopathy syndrome) I67.83
Presbycardia R54
Presbycusis, presbyacusia H91.1- ☑
Presbyesophagus K22.8
Presbyophrenia F03 ☑
Presbyopia H52.4
Prescription of contraceptives (initial) Z30.019
emergency (postcoital) Z30.012
implantable subdermal Z30.019
injectable Z30.013
intrauterine contraceptive device Z30.014
pills Z30.011
postcoital (emergency) Z30.012
repeat Z30.40
implantable subdermal Z30.49
injectable Z30.42
pills Z30.41
specified type NEC Z30.49
specified type NEC Z30.018
Presence (of)
ankle-joint implant (functional) (prosthesis) Z96.66- ☑

Presence — continued
aortocoronary (bypass) graft Z95.1
arterial-venous shunt (dialysis) Z99.2
artificial
eye (globe) Z97.0
heart (fully implantable) (mechanical) Z95.812
valve Z95.2
larynx Z96.3
lens (intraocular) Z96.1
limb (complete) (partial) Z97.1- ☑
arm Z97.1- ☑
bilateral Z97.15
leg Z97.1- ☑
bilateral Z97.16
audiological implant (functional) Z96.29
bladder implant (functional) Z96.0
bone
conduction hearing device Z96.29
implant (functional) NEC Z96.7
joint (prosthesis) — see Presence, joint implant
cardiac
defibrillator (functional) (with synchronous cardiac pacemaker) Z95.810
implant or graft Z95.9
specified type NEC Z95.818
pacemaker Z95.0
cerebrospinal fluid drainage device Z98.2
cochlear implant (functional) Z96.21
contact lens (es) Z97.3
coronary artery graft or prosthesis Z95.5
CSF shunt Z98.2
dental prosthesis device Z97.2
dentures Z97.2
device (external) NEC Z97.8
cardiac NEC Z95.818
heart assist Z95.811
implanted (functional) Z96.9
specified NEC Z96.89
prosthetic Z97.8
ear implant Z96.20
cochlear implant Z96.21
myringotomy tube Z96.22
specified type NEC Z96.29
elbow-joint implant (functional) (prosthesis) Z96.62- ☑
endocrine implant (functional) NEC Z96.49
eustachian tube stent or device (functional) Z96.29
external hearing-aid or device Z97.4
finger-joint implant (functional) (prosthetic) Z96.69- ☑
functional implant Z96.9
specified NEC Z96.89
graft
cardiac NEC Z95.818
vascular NEC Z95.828
hearing-aid or device (external) Z97.4
implant (bone) (cochlear) (functional) Z96.21
heart assist device Z95.811
heart valve implant (functional) Z95.2
prosthetic Z95.2
specified type NEC Z95.4
xenogenic Z95.3
hip-joint implant (functional) (prosthesis) Z96.64- ☑
implanted device (artificial) (functional) (prosthetic) Z96.9
automatic cardiac defibrillator (with synchronous cardiac pacemaker) Z95.810
cardiac pacemaker Z95.0
cochlear Z96.21
dental Z96.5
heart Z95.812
heart valve Z95.2
prosthetic Z95.2
specified NEC Z95.4
xenogenic Z95.3
insulin pump Z96.41
intraocular lens Z96.1
joint Z96.60
ankle Z96.66- ☑
elbow Z96.62- ☑
finger Z96.69- ☑
hip Z96.64- ☑
knee Z96.65- ☑
shoulder Z96.61- ☑
specified NEC Z96.698
wrist Z96.63- ☑
larynx Z96.3
myringotomy tube Z96.22
otological Z96.20

Presence — continued
implanted device — continued
otological — continued
cochlear Z96.21
eustachian stent Z96.29
myringotomy Z96.22
specified NEC Z96.29
stapes Z96.29
skin Z96.81
skull plate Z96.7
specified NEC Z96.89
urogenital Z96.0
insulin pump (functional) Z96.41
intestinal bypass or anastomosis Z98.0
intraocular lens (functional) Z96.1
intrauterine contraceptive device (IUD) Z97.5
intravascular implant (functional) (prosthetic) NEC Z95.9
coronary artery Z95.5
defibrillator (with synchronous cardiac pacemaker) Z95.810
peripheral vessel (with angioplasty) Z95.820
joint implant (prosthetic) (any) Z96.60
ankle — see Presence, ankle joint implant
elbow — see Presence, elbow joint implant
finger — see Presence, finger joint implant
hip — see Presence, hip joint implant
knee — see Presence, knee joint implant
shoulder — see Presence, shoulder joint implant
specified joint NEC Z96.698
wrist — see Presence, wrist joint implant
knee-joint implant (functional) (prosthesis) Z96.65- ☑
laryngeal implant (functional) Z96.3
mandibular implant (dental) Z96.5
myringotomy tube(s) Z96.22
orthopedic-joint implant (prosthetic) (any) — see Presence, joint implant
otological implant (functional) Z96.29
shoulder-joint implant (functional) (prosthesis) Z96.61- ☑
skull-plate implant Z96.7
spectacles Z97.3
stapes implant (functional) Z96.29
systemic lupus erythematosus [SLE] inhibitor D68.62
tendon implant (functional) (graft) Z96.7
tooth root(s) implant Z96.5
ureteral stent Z96.0
urethral stent Z96.0
urogenital implant (functional) Z96.0
vascular implant or device Z95.9
access port device Z95.828
specified type NEC Z95.828
wrist-joint implant (functional) (prosthesis) Z96.63- ☑
Presenile (see also condition)
dementia F03 ☑
premature aging E34.8
Presentation, fetal — see Delivery, complicated by, malposition
Prespondylolisthesis (congenital) Q76.2
Pressure
area, skin — see Ulcer, pressure, by site
brachial plexus G54.0
brain G93.5
injury at birth NEC P11.1
cerebral — see Pressure, brain
chest R07.89
cone, tentorial G93.5
hyposystolic (see also Hypotension)
incidental reading, without diagnosis of hypotension R03.1
increased
intracranial (benign) G93.2
injury at birth P11.0
intraocular H40.05- ☑
lumbosacral plexus G54.1
mediastinum J98.5
necrosis (chronic) — see Ulcer, pressure, by site
parental, inappropriate (excessive) Z62.6
sore (chronic) — see Ulcer, pressure, by site
spinal cord G95.20
ulcer (chronic) — see Ulcer, pressure, by site
venous, increased I87.8
Preterm
delivery (see also Pregnancy, complicated by, preterm labor) O60.10 ☑
labor — see Pregnancy, complicated by, preterm labor
newborn (infant) P07.30

Preterm — *continued*
  newborn — *continued*
    gestational age
      28 completed weeks (28 weeks, Ø days through 28 weeks, 6 days) P07.31
      29 completed weeks (29 weeks, Ø days through 29 weeks, 6 days) P07.32
      3Ø completed weeks (3Ø weeks, Ø days through 3Ø weeks, 6 days) P07.33
      31 completed weeks (31 weeks, Ø days through 31 weeks, 6 days) P07.34
      32 completed weeks (32 weeks, Ø days through 32 weeks, 6 days) P07.35
      33 completed weeks (33 weeks, Ø days through 33 weeks, 6 days) P07.36
      34 completed weeks (34 weeks, Ø days through 34 weeks, 6 days) P07.37
      35 completed weeks (35 weeks, Ø days through 35 weeks, 6 days) P07.38
      36 completed weeks (36 weeks, Ø days through 36 weeks, 6 days) P07.39

Previa
  placenta (low) (marginal) (partial) (total) (with hemorrhage) O44.1- ☑
    without hemorrhage O44.Ø- ☑
  vasa O69.4 ☑

Priapism N48.3Ø
  due to
    disease classified elsewhere N48.32
    drug N48.33
    specified cause NEC N48.39
    trauma N48.31

Prickling sensation (skin) R2Ø.2

Prickly heat L74.Ø

Primary — *see* condition

Primigravida
  elderly, affecting management of pregnancy, labor and delivery (supervision only) — *see* Pregnancy, complicated by, elderly, primigravida
  older, affecting management of pregnancy, labor and delivery (supervision only) — *see* Pregnancy, complicated by, elderly, primigravida
  very young, affecting management of pregnancy, labor and delivery (supervision only) — *see* Pregnancy, complicated by, young mother, primigravida

Primipara
  elderly, affecting management of pregnancy, labor and delivery (supervision only) — *see* Pregnancy, complicated by, elderly, primigravida
  older, affecting management of pregnancy, labor and delivery (supervision only) — *see* Pregnancy, complicated by, elderly, primigravida
  very young, affecting management of pregnancy, labor and delivery (supervision only) — *see* Pregnancy, complicated by, young mother, primigravida

Primus varus (bilateral) Q66.2

PRIND (Prolonged reversible ischemic neurologic deficit) I63.9

Pringle's disease (tuberous sclerosis) Q85.1

Prinzmetal angina I2Ø.1

Prizefighter ear — *see* Cauliflower ear

Problem (with) (related to)
  academic Z55.8
  acculturation Z6Ø.3
  adjustment (to)
    change of job Z56.1
    life-cycle transition Z6Ø.Ø
    pension Z6Ø.Ø
    retirement Z6Ø.Ø
  adopted child Z62.821
  alcoholism in family Z63.72
  atypical parenting situation Z62.9
  bankruptcy Z59.8
  behavioral (adult) F69
    drug seeking Z72.89
  birth of sibling affecting child Z62.898
  care (of)
    provider dependency Z74.9
      specified NEC Z74.8
    sick or handicapped person in family or household Z63.6
  child
    abuse (affecting the child) — *see* Maltreatment, child
    custody or support proceedings Z65.3
    in care of non-parental family member Z62.21
    in foster care Z62.21
    in welfare custody Z62.21

Problem — *continued*
  child — *continued*
    living in orphanage or group home Z62.22
  child-rearing Z62.9
    specified NEC Z62.898
  communication (developmental) F8Ø.9
  conflict or discord (with)
    boss Z56.4
    classmates Z55.4
    counselor Z64.4
    employer Z56.4
    family Z63.9
      specified NEC Z63.8
    probation officer Z64.4
    social worker Z64.4
    teachers Z55.4
    workmates Z56.4
  conviction in legal proceedings Z65.Ø
    with imprisonment Z65.1
  counselor Z64.4
  creditors Z59.8
  digestive K92.9
  drug addict in family Z63.72
  ear — *see* Disorder, ear
  economic Z59.9
    affecting care Z59.9
    specified NEC Z59.8
  education Z55.9
    specified NEC Z55.8
  employment Z56.9
    change of job Z56.1
    discord Z56.4
    environment Z56.5
    sexual harassment Z56.81
    specified NEC Z56.89
    stressful schedule Z56.3
    stress NEC Z56.6
    threat of job loss Z56.2
    unemployment Z56.Ø
  enuresis, child F98.Ø
  eye H57.9
  failed examinations (school) Z55.2
  falling Z91.81
  family (*see also* Disruption, family) Z63.9
    specified NEC Z63.8
  feeding (elderly) (infant) R63.3
    newborn P92.9
      breast P92.5
      overfeeding P92.4
      slow P92.2
      specified NEC P92.8
      underfeeding P92.3
    nonorganic F5Ø.8
  finance Z59.9
    specified NEC Z59.8
  foreclosure on loan Z59.8
  foster child Z62.822
  frightening experience(s) in childhood Z62.898
  genital NEC
    female N94.9
    male N5Ø.9
  health care Z75.9
    specified NEC Z75.8
  hearing — *see* Deafness
  homelessness Z59.Ø
  housing Z59.9
    inadequate Z59.1
    isolated Z59.8
    specified NEC Z59.8
  identity (of childhood) F93.8
  illegitimate pregnancy (unwanted) Z64.Ø
  illiteracy Z55.Ø
  impaired mobility Z74.Ø9
  imprisonment or incarceration Z65.1
  in-law Z63.1
  inadequate teaching affecting education Z55.8
  inappropriate (excessive) parental pressure Z62.6
  influencing health status NEC Z78.9
  institutionalization, affecting child Z62.22
  intrafamilial communication Z63.8
  jealousy, child F93.8
  landlord Z59.2
  language (developmental) F8Ø.9
  learning (developmental) F81.9
  legal Z65.3
    conviction without imprisonment Z65.Ø
    imprisonment Z65.1
    release from prison Z65.2

Problem — *continued*
  life-management Z73.9
    specified NEC Z73.89
  life-style Z72.9
    gambling Z72.6
    high-risk sexual behavior (heterosexual) Z72.51
      bisexual Z72.53
      homosexual Z72.52
    inappropriate eating habits Z72.4
    self-damaging behavior NEC Z72.89
    specified NEC Z72.89
    tobacco use Z72.Ø
  literacy Z55.9
    low level Z55.Ø
    specified NEC Z55.8
  living alone Z6Ø.2
  lodgers Z59.2
  loss of love relationship in childhood Z62.898
  marital Z63.Ø
    involving
      divorce Z63.5
      estrangement Z63.5
      gender identity F66
  mastication KØ8.8
  medical
    care, within family Z63.6
    facilities Z75.9
      specified NEC Z75.8
  mental F48.9
  multiparity Z64.1
  negative life events in childhood Z62.9
    altered pattern of family relationships Z62.898
    frightening experience Z62.898
    loss of
      love relationship Z62.898
      self-esteem Z62.898
    physical abuse (alleged) — *see* Maltreatment, child
    removal from home Z62.29
    specified event NEC Z62.898
  neighbor Z59.2
  neurological NEC R29.818
  new step-parent affecting child Z62.898
  none (feared complaint unfounded) Z71.1
  occupational NEC Z56.89
  parent-child — *see* Conflict, parent-child
  personal hygiene Z91.89
  personality F69
  phase-of-life transition, adjustment Z6Ø.Ø
  presence of sick or disabled person in family or household Z63.79
    needing care Z63.6
  primary support group (family) Z63.9
    specified NEC Z63.8
  probation officer Z64.4
  psychiatric F99
  psychosexual (development) F66
  psychosocial Z65.9
    specified NEC Z65.8
  relationship Z63.9
    childhood F93.8
  release from prison Z65.2
  removal from home affecting child Z62.29
  seeking and accepting known hazardous and harmful
    behavioral or psychological interventions Z65.8
    chemical, nutritional or physical interventions Z65.8
  sexual function (nonorganic) F52.9
  sight H54.7
  sleep disorder, child F51.9
  smell — *see* Disturbance, sensation, smell
  social
    environment Z6Ø.9
      specified NEC Z6Ø.8
    exclusion and rejection Z6Ø.4
    worker Z64.4
  speech R47.9
    developmental F8Ø.9
    specified NEC R47.89
  swallowing — *see* Dysphagia
  taste — *see* Disturbance, sensation, taste
  tic, child F95.Ø
  underachievement in school Z55.3
  unemployment Z56.Ø
    threatened Z56.2
  unwanted pregnancy Z64.Ø
  upbringing Z62.9
    specified NEC Z62.898
  urinary N39.9
  voice production R47.89

☑ **Additional Character Required** — Refer to the Tabular List for Character Selection   Subterms under main terms may continue to next column or page

Problem — *continued*
  work schedule (stressful) Z56.3
Procedure (surgical)
  for purpose other than remedying health state Z41.9
    specified NEC Z41.8
  not done Z53.9
    because of
      administrative reasons Z53.8
      contraindication Z53.09
        smoking Z53.01
      patient's decision Z53.20
        for reasons of belief or group pressure Z53.1
        left against medical advice (AMA) Z53.21
        specified reason NEC Z53.29
      specified reason NEC Z53.8
Procidentia (uteri) N81.3
Proctalgia K62.89
  fugax K59.4
  spasmodic K59.4
Proctitis K62.89
  amebic (acute) A06.0
  chlamydial A56.3
  gonococcal A54.6
  granulomatous — *see* Enteritis, regional, large intestine
  herpetic A60.1
  radiation K62.7
  tuberculous A18.32
  ulcerative (chronic) K51.20
    with
      complication K51.219
        abscess K51.214
        fistula K51.213
        obstruction K51.212
        rectal bleeding K51.211
        specified NEC K51.218
Proctocele
  female (without uterine prolapse) N81.6
    with uterine prolapse N81.2
      complete N81.3
  male K62.3
Proctocolitis, mucosal — *see* Rectosigmoiditis, ulcerative
Proctoptosis K62.3
Proctorrhagia K62.5
Proctosigmoiditis K63.89
  ulcerative (chronic) — *see* Rectosigmoiditis, ulcerative
Proctospasm K59.4
  psychogenic F45.8
Profichet's disease — *see* Disorder, soft tissue, specified type NEC
Progeria E34.8
Prognathism (mandibular) (maxillary) M26.19
Progonoma (melanotic) — *see* Neoplasm, benign, by site
Progressive — *see* condition
Prolactinoma
  specified site — *see* Neoplasm, benign, by site
  unspecified site D35.2
Prolapse, prolapsed
  anus, anal (canal) (sphincter) K62.2
  arm or hand O32.2 ☑
    causing obstructed labor O64.4 ☑
  bladder (mucosa) (sphincter) (acquired)
    congenital Q79.4
    female — *see* Cystocele
    male N32.89
  breast implant (prosthetic) T85.49 ☑
  cecostomy K94.09
  cecum K63.4
  cervix, cervical (hypertrophied) N81.2
    anterior lip, obstructing labor O65.5
    congenital Q51.828
    postpartal, old N81.2
    stump N81.85
  ciliary body (traumatic) — *see* Laceration, eye(ball), with prolapse or loss of interocular tissue
  colon (pedunculated) K63.4
  colostomy K94.09
  disc (intervertebral) — *see* Displacement, intervertebral disc
  eye implant (orbital) T85.398 ☑
    lens (ocular) — *see* Complications, intraocular lens
  fallopian tube N83.4
  gastric (mucosa) K31.89
  genital, female N81.9
    specified NEC N81.89
  globe, nontraumatic — *see* Luxation, globe

Prolapse, prolapsed — *continued*
  ileostomy bud K94.19
  intervertebral disc — *see* Displacement, intervertebral disc
  intestine (small) K63.4
  iris (traumatic) — *see* Laceration, eye(ball), with prolapse or loss of interocular tissue
    nontraumatic H21.89
  kidney N28.83
    congenital Q63.2
  laryngeal muscles or ventricle J38.7
  liver K76.89
  meatus urinarius N36.8
  mitral (valve) I34.1
  ocular lens implant — *see* Complications, intraocular lens
  organ or site, congenital NEC — *see* Malposition, congenital
  ovary N83.4
  pelvic floor, female N81.89
  perineum, female N81.89
  rectum (mucosa) (sphincter) K62.3
    due to trichuris trichuria B79
  spleen D73.89
  stomach K31.89
  umbilical cord
    complicating delivery O69.0 ☑
  urachus, congenital Q64.4
  ureter N28.89
    with obstruction N13.5
      with infection N13.6
  ureterovesical orifice N28.89
  urethra (acquired) (infected) (mucosa) N36.8
    congenital Q64.71
  urinary meatus N36.8
    congenital Q64.72
  uterovaginal N81.4
    complete N81.3
    incomplete N81.2
  uterus (with prolapse of vagina) N81.4
    complete N81.3
    congenital Q51.818
    first degree N81.2
    in pregnancy or childbirth — *see* Pregnancy, complicated by, abnormal, uterus
    incomplete N81.2
    postpartal (old) N81.4
    second degree N81.2
    third degree N81.3
  uveal (traumatic) — *see* Laceration, eye(ball), with prolapse or loss of interocular tissue
  vagina (anterior) (wall) — *see* Cystocele
    with prolapse of uterus N81.4
      complete N81.3
      incomplete N81.2
    posterior wall N81.6
    posthysterectomy N99.3
  vitreous (humor) H43.0- ☑
    in wound — *see* Laceration, eye(ball), with prolapse or loss of interocular tissue
  womb — *see* Prolapse, uterus
Prolapsus, female N81.9
  specified NEC N81.89
Proliferation(s)
  primary cutaneous CD30-positive large T-cell C86.6
Proliferative — *see* condition
Prolonged, prolongation (of)
  bleeding (time) (idiopathic) R79.1
  coagulation (time) R79.1
  gestation (over 42 completed weeks)
    mother O48.1
    newborn P08.22
  interval I44.0
  labor O63.9
    first stage O63.0
    second stage O63.1
  partial thromboplastin time (PTT) R79.1
  pregnancy (more than 42 weeks gestation) O48.1
  prothrombin time R79.1
  QT interval I45.81
  uterine contractions in labor O62.4
Prominence, prominent
  auricle (congenital) (ear) Q17.5
  ischial spine or sacral promontory
    with disproportion (fetopelvic) O33.0
      causing obstructed labor O65.0
  nose (congenital) acquired M95.0
Promiscuity — *see* High, risk, sexual behavior

Pronation
  ankle — *see* Deformity, limb, foot, specified NEC
  foot (*see also* Deformity, limb, foot, specified NEC)
    congenital Q74.2
Prophylactic
  administration of
    antibiotics, long-term Z79.2
      short-term use — *omit code*
    drug (*see also* Long-term (current) drug therapy (use of)) Z79.899
    medication Z79.899
  organ removal (for neoplasia management) Z40.00
    breast Z40.01
    ovary Z40.02
    specified site NEC Z40.09
  surgery Z40.9
    for risk factors related to malignant neoplasm — *see* Prophylactic, organ removal
    specified NEC Z40.8
  vaccination Z23
Propionic acidemia E71.121
Proptosis (ocular) (*see also* Exophthalmos)
  thyroid — *see* Hyperthyroidism, with goiter
Prosecution, anxiety concerning Z65.3
Prosopagnosia R48.3
Prostadynia N42.81
Prostate, prostatic — *see* condition
Prostatism — *see* Hyperplasia, prostate
Prostatitis (congestive) (suppurative) (with cystitis) N41.9
  acute N41.0
  cavitary N41.8
  chronic N41.1
  diverticular N41.8
  due to Trichomonas (vaginalis) A59.02
  fibrous N41.1
  gonococcal (acute) (chronic) A54.22
  granulomatous N41.4
  hypertrophic N41.1
  subacute N41.1
  trichomonal A59.02
  tuberculous A18.14
Prostatocystitis N41.3
Prostatorrhea N42.89
Prostatosis N42.82
Prostration R53.83
  heat (*see also* Heat, exhaustion)
    anhydrotic T67.3 ☑
    due to
      salt (and water) depletion T67.4 ☑
      water depletion T67.3 ☑
  nervous F48.8
  senile R54
Protanomaly (anomalous trichromat) H53.54
Protanopia (complete) (incomplete) H53.54
Protection (against) (from) — *see* Prophylactic
Protein
  deficiency NEC — *see* Malnutrition
  malnutrition — *see* Malnutrition
  sickness (*see also* Reaction, serum) T80.69 ☑
Proteinemia R77.9
Proteinosis
  alveolar (pulmonary) J84.01
  lipid or lipoid (of Urbach) E78.89
Proteinuria R80.9
  Bence Jones R80.3
  complicating pregnancy — *see* Proteinuria, gestational
  gestational O12.1- ☑
    with edema O12.2- ☑
  idiopathic R80.0
  isolated R80.0
    with glomerular lesion N06.9
      dense deposit disease N06.6
      diffuse
        crescentic glomerulonephritis N06.7
        endocapillary proliferative glomerulonephritis N06.4
        mesangiocapillary glomerulonephritis N06.5
      focal and segmental hyalinosis or sclerosis N06.1
      membranous (diffuse) N06.2
      mesangial proliferative (diffuse) N06.3
      minimal change N06.0
      specified pathology NEC N06.8
  orthostatic R80.2
    with glomerular lesion — *see* Proteinuria, isolated, with glomerular lesion
  persistent R80.1

Proteinuria — *continued*
  persistent — *continued*
    with glomerular lesion — *see* Proteinuria, isolated, with glomerular lesion
    postural R80.2
      with glomerular lesion — *see* Proteinuria, isolated, with glomerular lesion
  pre-eclamptic — *see* Pre-eclampsia
  specified type NEC R80.8
Proteolysis, pathologic D65
Proteus (mirabilis) (morganii), **as cause of disease classified elsewhere** B96.4
Prothrombin gene mutation D68.52
Protoporphyria, erythropoietic E80.0
Protozoal (*see also* condition)
  disease B64
    specified NEC B60.8
Protrusion, protrusio
  acetabuli M24.7
  acetabulum (into pelvis) M24.7
  device, implant or graft (*see also* Complications, by site and type, mechanical) T85.698 ☑
    arterial graft NEC — *see* Complication, cardiovascular device, mechanical, vascular
    breast (implant) T85.49 ☑
    catheter NEC T85.698 ☑
      cystostomy T83.090 ☑
      dialysis (renal) T82.49 ☑
        intraperitoneal T85.691 ☑
      infusion NEC T82.594 ☑
        spinal (epidural) (subdural) T85.690 ☑
      urinary, indwelling T83.098 ☑
    electronic (electrode) (pulse generator) (stimulator)
      bone T84.390 ☑
      nervous system — *see* Complication, prosthetic device, mechanical, electronic nervous system stimulator
    fixation, internal (orthopedic) NEC — *see* Complication, fixation device, mechanical
    gastrointestinal — *see* Complications, prosthetic device, mechanical, gastrointestinal device
    genital NEC T83.498 ☑
      intrauterine contraceptive device T83.39 ☑
      penile prosthesis T83.490 ☑
    heart NEC — *see* Complication, cardiovascular device, mechanical
    joint prosthesis — *see* Complications, joint prosthesis, mechanical, specified NEC, by site
    ocular NEC — *see* Complications, prosthetic device, mechanical, ocular device
    orthopedic NEC — *see* Complication, orthopedic, device, mechanical
    specified NEC T85.628 ☑
    urinary NEC (*see also* Complication, genitourinary, device, urinary, mechanical)
      graft T83.29 ☑
    vascular NEC — *see* Complication, cardiovascular device, mechanical
    ventricular intracranial shunt T85.09 ☑
  intervertebral disc — *see* Displacement, intervertebral disc
  joint prosthesis — *see* Complications, joint prosthesis, mechanical, specified NEC, by site
  nucleus pulposus — *see* Displacement, intervertebral disc
Prune belly (syndrome) Q79.4
Prurigo (ferox) (gravis) (Hebrae) (Hebra's) (mitis) (simplex) L28.2
  Besnier's L20.0
  estivalis L56.4
  nodularis L28.1
  psychogenic F45.8
Pruritus, pruritic (essential) L29.9
  ani, anus L29.0
    psychogenic F45.8
  anogenital L29.3
    psychogenic F45.8
  due to onchocerca volvulus B73.1
  gravidarum — *see* Pregnancy, complicated by, specified pregnancy-related condition NEC
  hiemalis L29.8
  neurogenic (any site) F45.8
  perianal L29.0
  psychogenic (any site) F45.8
  scroti, scrotum L29.1
    psychogenic F45.8
  senile, senilis L29.8

Pruritus, pruritic — *continued*
  specified NEC L29.8
    psychogenic F45.8
  Trichomonas A59.9
  vulva, vulvae L29.2
    psychogenic F45.8
Pseudarthrosis, pseudoarthrosis (bone) — *see* Nonunion, fracture
  clavicle, congenital Q74.0
  joint, following fusion or arthrodesis M96.0
Pseudo-Cushing's syndrome, alcohol-induced E24.4
Pseudo-Hurler's polydystrophy E77.0
Pseudo-obstruction intestine (acute) (chronic) (idiopathic) (intermittent secondary) (primary) K59.8
Pseudoaneurysm — *see* Aneurysm
Pseudoangina (pectoris) — *see* Angina
Pseudoangioma I81
Pseudoarteriosus Q28.8
Pseudoarthrosis — *see* Pseudarthrosis
Pseudobulbar affect (PBA) F48.8
Pseudochromhidrosis L67.8
Pseudocirrhosis, liver, pericardial I31.1
Pseudocowpox B08.03
Pseudocoxalgia M91.3- ☑
Pseudocroup J38.5
Pseudocyesis F45.8
Pseudocyst
  lung J98.4
  pancreas K86.3
  retina — *see* Cyst, retina
Pseudoelephantiasis neuroarthritica Q82.0
Pseudoexfoliation, capsule (lens) — *see* Cataract, specified NEC
Pseudofolliculitis barbae L73.1
Pseudoglioma H44.89
Pseudohemophilia (Bernuth's) (hereditary) (type B) D68.0
  Type A D69.8
  vascular D69.8
Pseudohermaphroditism Q56.3
  adrenal E25.8
  female Q56.2
    with adrenocortical disorder E25.8
    without adrenocortical disorder Q56.2
    adrenal, congenital E25.0
  male Q56.1
    with
      5-alpha-reductase deficiency E29.1
      adrenocortical disorder E25.8
      androgen resistance E34.51
      cleft scrotum Q56.1
      feminizing testis E34.51
    without gonadal disorder Q56.1
    adrenal E25.8
Pseudohydrocephalus G93.2
Pseudohypertrophic muscular dystrophy (Erb's) G71.0
Pseudohypertrophy, muscle G71.0
Pseudohypoparathyroidism E20.1
Pseudoinsomnia F51.03
Pseudoleukemia, infantile D64.89
Pseudomembranous — *see* condition
Pseudomeningocele (cerebral) (infective) (post-traumatic) G96.19
  postprocedural (spinal) G97.82
Pseudomenses (newborn) P54.6
Pseudomenstruation (newborn) P54.6
Pseudomonas
  aeruginosa, as cause of disease classified elsewhere B96.5
  mallei infection A24.0
    as cause of disease classified elsewhere B96.5
  pseudomallei, as cause of disease classified elsewhere B96.5
Pseudomyotonia G71.19
Pseudomyxoma peritonei C78.6
Pseudoneuritis, optic (nerve) (disc) (papilla), **congenital** Q14.2
Pseudopapilledema H47.33- ☑
  congenital Q14.2
Pseudoparalysis
  arm or leg R29.818
  atonic, congenital P94.2
Pseudopelade L66.0
Pseudophakia Z96.1
Pseudopolyarthritis, rhizomelic M35.3
Pseudopolycythemia D75.1
Pseudopseudohypoparathyroidism E20.1

Pseudopterygium H11.81- ☑
Pseudoptosis (eyelid) — *see* Blepharochalasis
Pseudopuberty, precocious
  female heterosexual E25.8
  male isosexual E25.8
Pseudorickets (renal) N25.0
Pseudorubella B08.20
Pseudosclerema, newborn P83.8
Pseudosclerosis (brain)
  Jakob's — *see* Creutzfeldt-Jakob disease or syndrome of Westphal (Strümpell) E83.01
  spastic — *see* Creutzfeldt-Jakob disease or syndrome
Pseudotetanus — *see* Convulsions
Pseudotetany R29.0
  hysterical F44.5
Pseudotruncus arteriosus Q25.4
Pseudotuberculosis A28.2
  enterocolitis A04.8
  pasteurella (infection) A28.0
Pseudotumor
  cerebri G93.2
  orbital H05.11 ☑
Pseudoxanthoma elasticum Q82.8
Psilosis (sprue) (tropical) K90.1
  nontropical K90.0
Psittacosis A70
Psoitis M60.88
Psoriasis L40.9
  arthropathic L40.50
    arthritis mutilans L40.52
    distal interphalangeal L40.51
    juvenile L40.54
    other specified L40.59
    spondylitis L40.53
  buccal K13.29
  flexural L40.8
  guttate L40.4
  mouth K13.29
  nummular L40.0
  plaque L40.0
  psychogenic F54
  pustular (generalized) L40.1
    palmaris et plantaris L40.3
  specified NEC L40.8
  vulgaris L40.0
Psychasthenia F48.8
Psychiatric disorder or problem F99
Psychogenic (*see also* condition)
  factors associated with physical conditions F54
Psychological and behavioral factors affecting medical condition F59
Psychoneurosis, psychoneurotic (*see also* Neurosis)
  anxiety (state) F41.1
  depersonalization F48.1
  hypochondriacal F45.21
  hysteria F44.9
  neurasthenic F48.8
  personality NEC F60.89
Psychopathy, psychopathic
  affectionless F94.2
  autistic F84.5
  constitution, post-traumatic F07.81
  personality — *see* Disorder, personality
  sexual — *see* Deviation, sexual
  state F60.2
Psychosexual identity disorder of childhood F64.2
Psychosis, psychotic F29
  acute (transient) F23
    hysterical F44.9
  affective — *see* Disorder, mood
  alcoholic F10.959
    with
      abuse F10.159
      anxiety disorder F10.980
        with
          abuse F10.180
          dependence F10.280
      delirium tremens F10.231
      delusions F10.950
        with
          abuse F10.150
          dependence F10.250
      dementia F10.97
        with dependence F10.27
      dependence F10.259
      hallucinosis F10.951

☑ **Additional Character Required** — Refer to the Tabular List for Character Selection

▼ **Subterms under main terms may continue to next column or page**

Psychosis, psychotic — *continued*
  alcoholic — *continued*
    with — *continued*
      hallucinosis — *continued*
        with
          abuse F10.151
          dependence F10.251
      mood disorder F10.94
        with
          abuse F10.14
          dependence F10.24
      paranoia F10.950
        with
          abuse F10.150
          dependence F10.250
      persisting amnesia F10.96
        with dependence F10.26
    amnestic confabulatory F10.96
      with dependence F10.26
    delirium tremens F10.231
    Korsakoff's, Korsakov's, Korsakow's F10.26
    paranoid type F10.950
      with
        abuse F10.150
        dependence F10.250
  anergastic — *see* Psychosis, organic
  arteriosclerotic (simple type) (uncomplicated) F01.50
    with behavioral disturbance F01.51
  childhood F84.0
    atypical F84.8
  climacteric — *see* Psychosis, involutional
  confusional F29
    acute or subacute F05
    reactive F23
  cycloid F23
  depressive — *see* Disorder, depressive
  disintegrative (childhood) F84.3
  drug-induced — *see* F11-F19 with .X59
    paranoid and hallucinatory states — *see* F11-F19
      with .X50 or .X51
  due to or associated with
    addiction, drug — *see* F11-F19 with .X59
    dependence
      alcohol F10.259
      drug — *see* F11-F19 with .X59
    epilepsy F06.8
    Huntington's chorea F06.8
    ischemia, cerebrovascular (generalized) F06.8
    multiple sclerosis F06.8
    physical disease F06.8
    presenile dementia F03 ☑
    senile dementia F03 ☑
    vascular disease (arteriosclerotic) (cerebral) F01.50
      with behavioral disturbance F01.51
  epileptic F06.8
  episode F23
    due to or associated with physical condition F06.8
  exhaustive F43.0
  hallucinatory, chronic F28
  hypomanic F30.8
  hysterical (acute) F44.9
  induced F24
  infantile F84.0
    atypical F84.8
  infective (acute) (subacute) F05
  involutional F28
    depressive — *see* Disorder, depressive
    melancholic — *see* Disorder, depressive
    paranoid (state) F22
  Korsakoff's, Korsakov's, Korsakow's (nonalcoholic) F04
    alcoholic F10.96
      in dependence F10.26
    induced by other psychoactive substance — *see*
      categories F11-F19 with .X5X
  mania, manic (single episode) F30.2
    recurrent type F31.89
  manic-depressive — *see* Disorder, mood
  menopausal — *see* Psychosis, involutional
  mixed schizophrenic and affective F25.8
  multi-infarct (cerebrovascular) F01.50
    with behavioral disturbance F01.51
  nonorganic F29
    specified NEC F28
  organic F09
    due to or associated with
      arteriosclerosis (cerebral) — *see* Psychosis, ar-
        teriosclerotic

Psychosis, psychotic — *continued*
  organic — *continued*
    due to or associated with — *continued*
      cerebrovascular disease, arteriosclerotic — *see*
        Psychosis, arteriosclerotic
      childbirth — *see* Psychosis, puerperal
      Creutzfeldt-Jakob disease or syndrome — *see*
        Creutzfeldt-Jakob disease or syndrome
      dependence, alcohol F10.259
      disease
        alcoholic liver F10.259
        brain, arteriosclerotic — *see* Psychosis, arte-
          riosclerotic
        cerebrovascular F01.50
          with behavioral disturbance F01.51
        Creutzfeldt-Jakob — *see* Creutzfeldt-Jakob
          disease or syndrome
        endocrine or metabolic F06.8
          acute or subacute F05
        liver, alcoholic F10.259
      epilepsy transient (acute) F05
      infection
        brain (intracranial) F06.8
          acute or subacute F05
      intoxication
        alcoholic (acute) F10.259
        drug F11-F19 with .X59
      ischemia, cerebrovascular (generalized) — *see*
        Psychosis, arteriosclerotic
      puerperium — *see* Psychosis, puerperal
      trauma, brain (birth) (from electric current)
        (surgical) F06.8
        acute or subacute F05
    infective F06.8
      acute or subacute F05
    post-traumatic F06.8
      acute or subacute F05
  paranoiac F22
  paranoid (climacteric) (involutional) (menopausal) F22
    psychogenic (acute) F23
    schizophrenic F20.0
    senile F03 ☑
  postpartum F53
  presbyophrenic (type) F03 ☑
  presenile F03 ☑
  psychogenic (paranoid) F23
    depressive F32.3
  puerperal F53
    specified type — *see* Psychosis, by type
  reactive (brief) (transient) (emotional stress) (psycho-
    logical trauma) F23
    depressive F32.3
      recurrent F33.3
    excitative type F30.8
  schizoaffective F25.9
    depressive type F25.1
    manic type F25.0
  schizophrenia, schizophrenic — *see* Schizophrenia
  schizophrenia-like, in epilepsy F06.2
  schizophreniform F20.81
    affective type F25.9
    brief F23
    confusional type F23
    depressive type F25.1
    manic type F25.0
    mixed type F25.0
  senile NEC F03 ☑
    depressed or paranoid type F03 ☑
    simple deterioration F03 ☑
    specified type — *code to* condition
  shared F24
  situational (reactive) F23
  symbiotic (childhood) F84.3
  symptomatic F09
Psychosomatic — *see* Disorder, psychosomatic
Psychosyndrome, organic F07.9
**Psychotic episode due to or associated with physical
  condition** F06.8
Pterygium (eye) H11.00- ☑
  amyloid H11.01- ☑
  central H11.02- ☑
  colli Q18.3
  double H11.03- ☑
  peripheral
    progressive H11.05- ☑
    stationary H11.04- ☑
  recurrent H11.06- ☑

Ptilosis (eyelid) — *see* Madarosis
Ptomaine (poisoning) — *see* Poisoning, food
Ptosis (*see also* Blepharoptosis)
  adiposa (false) — *see* Blepharoptosis
  breast N64.81
  cecum K63.4
  colon K63.4
  congenital (eyelid) Q10.0
    specified site NEC — *see* Anomaly, by site
  eyelid — *see* Blepharoptosis
    congenital Q10.0
  gastric K31.89
  intestine K63.4
  kidney N28.83
  liver K76.89
  renal N28.83
  splanchnic K63.4
  spleen D73.89
  stomach K31.89
  viscera K63.4
PTP D69.51
Ptyalism (periodic) K11.7
  hysterical F45.8
  pregnancy — *see* Pregnancy, complicated by, specified
    pregnancy-related condition NEC
  psychogenic F45.8
Ptyalolithiasis K11.5
Pubarche, precocious E30.1
Pubertas praecox E30.1
Puberty (development state) Z00.3
  bleeding (excessive) N92.2
  delayed E30.0
  precocious (constitutional) (cryptogenic) (idiopathic)
    E30.1
    central E22.8
    due to
      ovarian hyperfunction E28.1
        estrogen E28.0
      testicular hyperfunction E29.0
  premature E30.1
    due to
      adrenal cortical hyperfunction E25.8
      pineal tumor E34.8
      pituitary (anterior) hyperfunction E22.8
Puckering, macula — *see* Degeneration, macula, puckering
Pudenda, pudendum — *see* condition
Puente's disease (simple glandular cheilitis) K13.0
Puerperal, puerperium (complicated by, complications)
  abnormal glucose (tolerance test) O99.815
  abscess
    areola O91.02
      associated with lactation O91.03
    Bartholin's gland O86.19
    breast O91.12
      associated with lactation O91.13
    cervix (uteri) O86.11
    genital organ NEC O86.19
    kidney O86.21
    mammary O91.12
      associated with lactation O91.13
    nipple O91.02
      associated with lactation O91.03
    peritoneum O85
    subareolar O91.12
      associated with lactation O91.13
    urinary tract — *see* Puerperal, infection, urinary
    uterus O86.12
    vagina (wall) O86.13
    vaginorectal O86.13
    vulvovaginal gland O86.13
  adnexitis O86.19
  afibrinogenemia, or other coagulation defect O72.3
  albuminuria (acute) (subacute) — *see* Proteinuria,
    gestational
  alcohol use O99.315
  anemia O90.81
    pre-existing (pre-pregnancy) O99.03
  anesthetic death O89.8
  apoplexy O99.43
  bariatric surgery status O99.845
  blood disorder NEC O99.13
  blood dyscrasia O72.3
  cardiomyopathy O90.3
  cerebrovascular disorder (conditions in I60-I69) O99.43
  cervicitis O86.11
  circulatory system disorder O99.43
  coagulopathy (any) O72.3

Puerperal, puerperium — *continued*
- complications O90.9
  - specified NEC O90.89
- convulsions — *see* Eclampsia
- cystitis O86.22
- cystopyelitis O86.29
- delirium NEC F05
- diabetes O24.93
  - gestational — *see* Puerperal, gestational diabetes
  - pre-existing O24.33
    - specified NEC O24.83
    - type 1 O24.03
    - type 2 O24.13
- digestive system disorder O99.63
- disease O90.9
  - breast NEC O92.29
  - cerebrovascular (acute) O99.43
  - nonobstetric NEC O99.89
  - tubo-ovarian O86.19
  - Valsuani's O99.03
- disorder O90.9
  - biliary tract O26.63
  - lactation O92.70
  - liver O26.63
  - nonobstetric NEC O99.89
- disruption
  - cesarean wound O90.0
  - episiotomy wound O90.1
  - perineal laceration wound O90.1
- drug use O99.325
- eclampsia (with pre-existing hypertension) O15.2
- embolism (pulmonary) (blood clot) — *see* Embolism, obstetric, puerperal
- endocrine, nutritional or metabolic disease NEC O99.285
- endophlebitis — *see* Puerperal, phlebitis
- endotrachelitis O86.11
- failure
  - lactation (complete) O92.3
    - partial O92.4
  - renal, acute O90.4
- fever (of unknown origin) O86.4
  - septic O85
- fissure, nipple O92.12
  - associated with lactation O92.13
- fistula
  - breast (due to mastitis) O91.12
    - associated with lactation O91.13
  - nipple O91.02
    - associated with lactation O91.03
- galactophoritis O91.22
  - associated with lactation O91.23
- galactorrhea O92.6
- gastric banding status O99.845
- gastric bypass status O99.845
- gastrointestinal disease NEC O99.63
- gestational diabetes O24.439
  - diet controlled O24.430
  - insulin (and diet) controlled O24.434
- gonorrhea O98.23
- hematoma, subdural O99.43
- hemiplegia, cerebral O99.355
  - due to cerbrovascular disorder O99.43
- hemorrhage O72.1
  - brain O99.43
  - bulbar O99.43
  - cerebellar O99.43
  - cerebral O99.43
  - cortical O99.43
  - delayed or secondary O72.2
  - extradural O99.43
  - internal capsule O99.43
  - intracranial O99.43
  - intrapontine O99.43
  - meningeal O99.43
  - pontine O99.43
  - retained placenta O72.0
  - subarachnoid O99.43
  - subcortical O99.43
  - subdural O99.43
  - third stage O72.0
  - uterine, delayed O72.2
  - ventricular O99.43
- hemorrhoids O87.2
- hepatorenal syndrome O90.4
- hypertension — *see* Hypertension, complicating, puerperium
- hypertrophy, breast O92.29

Puerperal, puerperium — *continued*
- induration breast (fibrous) O92.29
- infection O86.4
  - cervix O86.11
  - generalized O85
  - genital tract NEC O86.19
    - obstetric surgical wound O86.0
  - kidney (bacillus coli) O86.21
  - maternal O98.93
    - carrier state NEC O99.835
    - gonorrhea O98.23
    - human immunodeficiency virus (HIV) O98.73
    - protozoal O98.63
    - sexually transmitted NEC O98.33
    - specified NEC O98.83
    - streptococcus B carrier state O99.825
    - syphilis O98.13
    - tuberculosis O98.03
    - viral hepatitis O98.43
    - viral NEC O98.53
  - nipple O91.02
    - associated with lactation O91.03
  - peritoneum O85
  - renal O86.21
  - specified NEC O86.89
  - urinary (asymptomatic) (tract) NEC O86.20
    - bladder O86.22
    - kidney O86.21
    - specified site NEC O86.29
    - urethra O86.22
  - vagina O86.13
  - vein — *see* Puerperal, phlebitis
- ischemia, cerebral O99.43
- lymphangitis O86.89
  - breast O91.22
    - associated with lactation O91.23
- malignancy O9A.13 (*following* O99)
- malnutrition O25.3
- mammillitis O91.02
  - associated with lactation O91.03
- mammitis O91.22
  - associated with lactation O91.23
- mania F30.8
- mastitis O91.22
  - associated with lactation O91.23
  - purulent O91.12
    - associated with lactation O91.13
- melancholia — *see* Disorder, depressive
- mental disorder NEC O99.345
- metroperitonitis O85
- metrorrhagia — *see* Hemorrhage, postpartum
- metrosalpingitis O86.19
- metrovaginitis O86.13
- milk leg O87.1
- monoplegia, cerebral O99.43
- mood disturbance O90.6
- necrosis, liver (acute) (subacute) (conditions in subcategory K72.0) O26.63
  - with renal failure O90.4
- nervous system disorder O99.355
- obesity (pre-existing prior to pregnancy) O99.215
- obesity surgery status O99.845
- occlusion, precerebral artery O99.43
- paralysis
  - bladder (sphincter) O90.89
  - cerebral O99.43
- paralytic stroke O99.43
- parametritis O85
- paravaginitis O86.13
- pelviperitonitis O85
- perimetritis O86.12
- perimetrosalpingitis O86.19
- perinephritis O86.21
- periphlebitis — *see* Puerperal phlebitis
- peritoneal infection O85
- peritonitis (pelvic) O85
- perivaginitis O86.13
- phlebitis O87.0
  - deep O87.1
  - pelvic O87.1
  - superficial O87.0
- phlebothrombosis, deep O87.1
- phlegmasia alba dolens O87.1
- placental polyp O90.89
- pneumonia, embolic — *see* Embolism, obstetric, puerperal
- pre-eclampsia — *see* Pre-eclampsia
- psychosis F53

Puerperal, puerperium — *continued*
- pyelitis O86.21
- pyelocystitis O86.29
- pyelonephritis O86.21
- pyelonephrosis O86.21
- pyemia O85
- pyocystitis O86.29
- pyohemia O85
- pyometra O86.12
- pyonephritis O86.21
- pyosalpingitis O86.19
- pyrexia (of unknown origin) O86.4
- renal
  - disease NEC O90.89
  - failure O90.4
- respiratory disease NEC O99.53
- retention
  - decidua — *see* Retention, decidua
  - placenta O72.0
  - secundines — *see* Retention, secundines
- retrated nipple O92.02
- salpingo-ovaritis O86.19
- salpingoperitonitis O85
- secondary perineal tear O90.1
- sepsis (pelvic) O85
- sepsis O85
- septic thrombophlebitis O86.81
- skin disorder NEC O99.73
- specified condition NEC O99.89
- stroke O99.43
- subinvolution (uterus) O90.89
- subluxation of symphysis (pubis) O26.73
- suppuration — *see* Puerperal, abscess
- tetanus A34
- thelitis O91.02
  - associated with lactation O91.03
- thrombocytopenia O72.3
- thrombophlebitis (superficial) O87.0
  - deep O87.1
  - pelvic O87.1
  - septic O86.81
- thrombosis (venous) — *see* Thrombosis, puerperal
- thyroiditis O90.5
- toxemia (eclamptic) (pre-eclamptic) (with convulsions) O15.2
- trauma, non-obstetric O9A.23 (*following* O99)
  - caused by abuse (physical) (suspected) O9A.33 (*following* O99)
    - confirmed O9A.33 (*following* O99)
    - psychological (suspected) O9A.53 (*following* O99)
      - confirmed O9A.53 (*following* O99)
    - sexual (suspected) O9A.43 (*following* O99)
      - confirmed O9A.43 (*following* O99)
- uremia (due to renal failure) O90.4
- urethritis O86.22
- vaginitis O86.13
- varicose veins (legs) O87.4
  - vulva or perineum O87.8
- venous O87.9
- vulvitis O86.19
- vulvovaginitis O86.13
- white leg O87.1

Puerperium — *see* Puerperal

Pulmolithiasis J98.4

Pulmonary — *see* condition

Pulpitis (acute) (anachoretic) (chronic) (hyperplastic) (irreversible) (putrescent) (reversible) (suppurative) (ulcerative) K04.0

Pulpless tooth K04.99

Pulse
- alternating R00.8
- bigeminal R00.8
- fast R00.0
- feeble, rapid due to shock following injury T79.4 ☑
- rapid R00.0
- weak R09.89

Pulsus alternans or trigeminus R00.8

Punch drunk F07.81

Punctum lacrimale occlusion — *see* Obstruction, lacrimal

Puncture
- abdomen, abdominal
  - wall S31.139 ☑
    - with
      - foreign body S31.149 ☑
      - penetration into peritoneal cavity S31.639 ☑

☑ **Additional Character Required** — Refer to the Tabular List for Character Selection   ▽ Subterms under main terms may continue to next column or page

Index

Puncture — Puncture

Puncture — *continued*
- genital organs, external
  - female S31.532 ☑
    - with foreign body S31.542 ☑
    - vagina — *see* Puncture, vagina
    - vulva — *see* Puncture, vulva
  - male S31.531 ☑
    - with foreign body S31.541 ☑
    - penis — *see* Puncture, penis
    - scrotum — *see* Puncture, scrotum
    - testis — *see* Puncture, testis
- groin — *see* Puncture, abdomen, wall
- gum — *see* Puncture, oral cavity
- hand S61.439 ☑
  - with
    - foreign body S61.449 ☑
  - finger — *see* Puncture, finger
  - left S61.432 ☑
    - with
      - foreign body S61.442 ☑
  - right S61.431 ☑
    - with
      - foreign body S61.441 ☑
  - thumb — *see* Puncture, thumb
- head S01.93 ☑
  - with foreign body S01.94 ☑
  - cheek — *see* Puncture, cheek
  - ear — *see* Puncture, ear
  - eyelid — *see* Puncture, eyelid
  - lip — *see* Puncture, oral cavity
  - nose — *see* Puncture, nose
  - oral cavity — *see* Puncture, oral cavity
  - scalp S01.03 ☑
    - with foreign body S01.04 ☑
  - specified site NEC S01.83 ☑
    - with foreign body S01.84 ☑
  - temporomandibular area — *see* Puncture, cheek
- heart S26.99 ☑
  - with hemopericardium S26.09 ☑
  - without hemopericardium S26.19 ☑
- heel — *see* Puncture, foot
- hip S71.039 ☑
  - with foreign body S71.049 ☑
  - left S71.032 ☑
    - with foreign body S71.042 ☑
  - right S71.031 ☑
    - with foreign body S71.041 ☑
- hymen — *see* Puncture, vagina
- hypochondrium — *see* Puncture, abdomen, wall
- hypogastric region — *see* Puncture, abdomen, wall
- inguinal region — *see* Puncture, abdomen, wall
- instep — *see* Puncture, foot
- internal organs — *see* Injury, by site
- interscapular region — *see* Puncture, thorax, back
- intestine
  - large
    - colon S36.599 ☑
      - ascending S36.590 ☑
      - descending S36.592 ☑
      - sigmoid S36.593 ☑
      - specified site NEC S36.598 ☑
      - transverse S36.591 ☑
    - rectum S36.69 ☑
  - small S36.499 ☑
    - duodenum S36.490 ☑
    - specified site NEC S36.498 ☑
- intra-abdominal organ S36.99 ☑
  - gallbladder S36.128 ☑
  - intestine — *see* Puncture, intestine
  - liver S36.118 ☑
  - pancreas — *see* Puncture, pancreas
  - peritoneum S36.81 ☑
  - specified site NEC S36.898 ☑
  - spleen S36.09 ☑
  - stomach S36.39 ☑
- jaw — *see* Puncture, head, specified site NEC
- knee S81.039 ☑
  - with foreign body S81.049 ☑
  - left S81.032 ☑
    - with foreign body S81.042 ☑
  - right S81.031 ☑
    - with foreign body S81.041 ☑
- labium (majus) (minus) — *see* Puncture, vulva
- lacrimal duct — *see* Puncture, eyelid
- larynx S11.013 ☑
  - with foreign body S11.014 ☑

Puncture — *continued*
- leg (lower) S81.839 ☑
  - with foreign body S81.849 ☑
  - foot — *see* Puncture, foot
  - knee — *see* Puncture, knee
  - left S81.832 ☑
    - with foreign body S81.842 ☑
  - right S81.831 ☑
    - with foreign body S81.841 ☑
  - upper — *see* Puncture, thigh
- lip S01.531 ☑
  - with foreign body S01.541 ☑
- loin — *see* Puncture, abdomen, wall
- lower back — *see* Puncture, back, lower
- lumbar region — *see* Puncture, back, lower
- malar region — *see* Puncture, head, specified site NEC
- mammary — *see* Puncture, breast
- mastoid region — *see* Puncture, head, specified site NEC
- mouth — *see* Puncture, oral cavity
- nail
  - finger — *see* Puncture, finger, with damage to nail
  - toe — *see* Puncture, toe, with damage to nail
- nasal (septum) (sinus) — *see* Puncture, nose
- nasopharynx — *see* Puncture, head, specified site NEC
- neck S11.93 ☑
  - with foreign body S11.94 ☑
  - involving
    - cervical esophagus — *see* Puncture, cervical esophagus
    - larynx — *see* Puncture, larynx
    - pharynx — *see* Puncture, pharynx
    - thyroid gland — *see* Puncture, thyroid gland
    - trachea — *see* Puncture, trachea
  - specified site NEC S11.83 ☑
    - with foreign body S11.84 ☑
- nose (septum) (sinus) S01.23 ☑
  - with foreign body S01.24 ☑
- ocular — *see* Puncture, eyeball
- oral cavity S01.532 ☑
  - with foreign body S01.542 ☑
- orbit S05.4- ☑
- palate — *see* Puncture, oral cavity
- palm — *see* Puncture, hand
- pancreas S36.299 ☑
  - body S36.291 ☑
  - head S36.290 ☑
  - tail S36.292 ☑
- pelvis — *see* Puncture, back, lower
- penis S31.23 ☑
  - with foreign body S31.24 ☑
- perineum
  - female S31.43 ☑
    - with foreign body S31.44 ☑
  - male S31.139 ☑
    - with foreign body S31.149 ☑
- periocular area (with or without lacrimal passages) — *see* Puncture, eyelid
- phalanges
  - finger — *see* Puncture, finger
  - toe — *see* Puncture, toe
- pharynx S11.23 ☑
  - with foreign body S11.24 ☑
- pinna — *see* Puncture, ear
- popliteal space — *see* Puncture, knee
- prepuce — *see* Puncture, penis
- pubic region S31.139 ☑
  - with foreign body S31.149 ☑
- pudendum — *see* Puncture, genital organs, external
- rectovaginal septum — *see* Puncture, vagina
- sacral region — *see* Puncture, back, lower
- sacroiliac region — *see* Puncture, back, lower
- salivary gland — *see* Puncture, oral cavity
- scalp S01.03 ☑
  - with foreign body S01.04 ☑
- scapular region — *see* Puncture, shoulder
- scrotum S31.33 ☑
  - with foreign body S31.34 ☑
- shin — *see* Puncture, leg
- shoulder S41.039 ☑
  - with foreign body S41.049 ☑
  - left S41.032 ☑
    - with foreign body S41.042 ☑
  - right S41.031 ☑
    - with foreign body S41.041 ☑
- spermatic cord — *see* Puncture, testis

Puncture — *continued*
- sternal region — *see* Puncture, thorax, front
- submaxillary region — *see* Puncture, head, specified site NEC
- submental region — *see* Puncture, head, specified site NEC
- subungual
  - finger(s) — *see* Puncture, finger, with damage to nail
  - toe — *see* Puncture, toe, with damage to nail
- supraclavicular fossa — *see* Puncture, neck, specified site NEC
- temple, temporal region — *see* Puncture, head, specified site NEC
- temporomandibular area — *see* Puncture, cheek
- testis S31.33 ☑
  - with foreign body S31.34 ☑
- thigh S71.139 ☑
  - with foreign body S71.149 ☑
  - left S71.132 ☑
    - with foreign body S71.142 ☑
  - right S71.131 ☑
    - with foreign body S71.141 ☑
- thorax, thoracic (wall) S21.93 ☑
  - with foreign body S21.94 ☑
  - back S21.23- ☑
    - with
      - foreign body S21.24- ☑
        - with penetration S21.44 ☑
      - penetration S21.43 ☑
  - breast — *see* Puncture, breast
  - front S21.13- ☑
    - with
      - foreign body S21.14- ☑
        - with penetration S21.34 ☑
      - penetration S21.33 ☑
- throat — *see* Puncture, neck
- thumb S61.039 ☑
  - with
    - damage to nail S61.139 ☑
      - with
        - foreign body S61.149 ☑
    - foreign body S61.049 ☑
  - left S61.032 ☑
    - with
      - damage to nail S61.132 ☑
        - with
          - foreign body S61.142 ☑
      - foreign body S61.042 ☑
  - right S61.031 ☑
    - with
      - damage to nail S61.131 ☑
        - with
          - foreign body S61.141 ☑
      - foreign body S61.041 ☑
- thyroid gland S11.13 ☑
  - with foreign body S11.14 ☑
- toe(s) S91.139 ☑
  - with
    - damage to nail S91.239 ☑
      - with
        - foreign body S91.249 ☑
    - foreign body S91.149 ☑
  - great S91.133 ☑
    - with
      - damage to nail S91.233 ☑
        - with
          - foreign body S91.243 ☑
      - foreign body S91.143 ☑
    - left S91.132 ☑
      - with
        - damage to nail S91.232 ☑
          - with
            - foreign body S91.242 ☑
        - foreign body S91.142 ☑
    - right S91.131 ☑
      - with
        - damage to nail S91.231 ☑
          - with
            - foreign body S91.241 ☑
        - foreign body S91.141 ☑
  - lesser S91.136 ☑
    - with
      - damage to nail S91.236 ☑
        - with
          - foreign body S91.246 ☑

Puncture — *continued*
  toe(s) — *continued*
    lesser — *continued*
      with — *continued*
        foreign body S91.146 ☑
      left S91.135 ☑
        with
          damage to nail S91.235 ☑
            with
              foreign body S91.245 ☑
          foreign body S91.145 ☑
      right S91.134 ☑
        with
          damage to nail S91.234 ☑
            with
              foreign body S91.244 ☑
          foreign body S91.144 ☑
  tongue — *see* Puncture, oral cavity
  trachea S11.023 ☑
    with foreign body S11.024 ☑
  tunica vaginalis — *see* Puncture, testis
  tympanum, tympanic membrane S09.2- ☑
  umbilical region S31.135 ☑
    with foreign body S31.145 ☑
  uvula — *see* Puncture, oral cavity
  vagina S31.43 ☑
    with foreign body S31.44 ☑
  vocal cords S11.033 ☑
    with foreign body S11.034 ☑
  vulva S31.43 ☑
    with foreign body S31.44 ☑
  wrist S61.539 ☑
    with
      foreign body S61.549 ☑
    left S61.532 ☑
      with
        foreign body S61.542 ☑
    right S61.531 ☑
      with
        foreign body S61.541 ☑
PUO (pyrexia of unknown origin) R50.9
Pupillary membrane (persistent) Q13.89
Pupillotonia — *see* Anomaly, pupil, function, tonic pupil
Purpura D69.2
  abdominal D69.0
  allergic D69.0
  anaphylactoid D69.0
  annularis telangiectodes L81.7
  arthritic D69.0
  autoerythrocyte sensitization D69.2
  autoimmune D69.0
  bacterial D69.0
  Bateman's (senile) D69.2
  capillary fragility (hereditary) (idiopathic) D69.8
  cryoglobulinemic D89.1
  Devil's pinches D69.2
  fibrinolytic — *see* Fibrinolysis
  fulminans, fulminous D65
  gangrenous D65
  hemorrhagic, hemorrhagica D69.3
    not due to thrombocytopenia D69.0
  Henoch (-Schönlein) (allergic) D69.0
  hypergammaglobulinemic (benign) (Waldenström)
    D89.0
  idiopathic (thrombocytopenic) D69.3
    nonthrombocytopenic D69.0
  immune thrombocytopenic D69.3
  infectious D69.0
  malignant D69.0
  neonatorum P54.5
  nervosa D69.0
  newborn P54.5
  nonthrombocytopenic D69.2
    hemorrhagic D69.0
    idiopathic D69.0
  nonthrombopenic D69.2
  peliosis rheumatica D69.0
  posttransfusion (post-transfusion) (from (fresh) whole
    blood or blood products) D69.51
  primary D69.49
  red cell membrane sensitivity D69.2
  rheumatica D69.0
  Schönlein (-Henoch) (allergic) D69.0
  scorbutic E54 [D77]
  senile D69.2
  simplex D69.2
  symptomatica D69.0

Purpura — *continued*
  telangiectasia annularis L81.7
  thrombocytopenic D69.49
    congenital D69.42
    hemorrhagic D69.3
    hereditary D69.42
    idiopathic D69.3
    immune D69.3
    neonatal, transitory P61.0
    thrombotic M31.1
  thrombohemolytic — *see* Fibrinolysis
  thrombolytic — *see* Fibrinolysis
  thrombopenic D69.49
  thrombotic, thrombocytopenic M31.1
  toxic D69.0
  vascular D69.0
  visceral symptoms D69.0
Purpuric spots R23.3
Purulent — *see* condition
Pus
  in
    stool R19.5
    urine N39.0
  tube (rupture) — *see* Salpingo-oophoritis
Pustular rash L08.0
Pustule (nonmalignant) L08.9
  malignant A22.0
Pustulosis palmaris et plantaris L40.3
Putnam (-Dana) **disease or syndrome** — *see* Degeneration, combined
Putrescent pulp (dental) K04.1
Pyarthritis, pyarthrosis — *see* Arthritis, pyogenic or pyemic
  tuberculous — *see* Tuberculosis, joint
Pyelectasis — *see* Hydronephrosis
Pyelitis (congenital) (uremic) (*see also* Pyelonephritis)
  with
    calculus — *see* category N20 ☑
      with hydronephrosis N13.2
    contracted kidney N11.9
  acute N10
  chronic N11.9
    with calculus — *see* category N20 ☑
      with hydronephrosis N13.2
  cystica N28.84
  puerperal (postpartum) O86.21
  tuberculous A18.11
Pyelocystitis — *see* Pyelonephritis
Pyelonephritis (*see also* Nephritis, tubulo-interstitial)
  with
    calculus — *see* category N20 ☑
      with hydronephrosis N13.2
    contracted kidney N11.9
  acute N10
  calculous — *see* category N20 ☑
    with hydronephrosis N13.2
  chronic N11.9
    with calculus — *see* category N20 ☑
      with hydronephrosis N13.2
    associated with ureteral obstruction or stricture
      N11.1
    nonobstructive N11.8
      with reflux (vesicoureteral) N11.0
    obstructive N11.1
    specified NEC N11.8
  in (due to)
    brucellosis A23.9 [N16]
    cryoglobulinemia (mixed) D89.1 [N16]
    cystinosis E72.04
    diphtheria A36.84
    glycogen storage disease E74.09 [N16]
    leukemia NEC C95.9- ☑ [N16]
    lymphoma NEC C85.90 [N16]
    multiple myeloma C90.0- ☑ [N16]
    obstruction N11.1
    Salmonella infection A02.25
    sarcoidosis D86.84
    sepsis A41.9 [N16]
    Sjögren's disease M35.04
    toxoplasmosis B58.83
    transplant rejection T86.91 [N16]
    Wilson's disease E83.01 [N16]
  nonobstructive N12
    with reflux (vesicoureteral) N11.0
    chronic N11.8
  syphilitic A52.75
Pyelonephrosis (obstructive) N11.1
  chronic N11.9

Pyelophlebitis I80.8
Pyeloureteritis cystica N28.85
Pyemia, pyemic (fever) (infection) (purulent) (*see also* Sepsis)
  joint — *see* Arthritis, pyogenic or pyemic
  liver K75.1
  pneumococcal A40.3
  portal K75.1
  postvaccinal T88.0 ☑
  puerperal, postpartum, childbirth O85
  specified organism NEC A41.89
  tuberculous — *see* Tuberculosis, miliary
Pygopagus Q89.4
Pyknoepilepsy (idiopathic) — *see* Pyknolepsy
Pyknolepsy G40.A09 (*following* G40.3)
  intractable G40.A19 (*following* G40.3)
    with status epilepticus G40.A11 (*following* G40.3)
    without status epilepticus G40.A19 (*following* G40.3)
  not intractable G40.A09 (*following* G40.3)
    with status epilepticus G40.A01 (*following* G40.3)
    without status epilepticus G40.A09 (*following* G40.3)
Pylephlebitis K75.1
Pyle's syndrome Q78.5
Pylethrombophlebitis K75.1
Pylethrombosis K75.1
Pyloritis K29.90
  with bleeding K29.91
Pylorospasm (reflex) **NEC** K31.3
  congenital or infantile Q40.0
  neurotic F45.8
  newborn Q40.0
  psychogenic F45.8
Pylorus, pyloric — *see* condition
Pyo-oophoritis — *see* Salpingo-oophoritis
Pyo-ovarium — *see* Salpingo-oophoritis
Pyoarthrosis — *see* Arthritis, pyogenic or pyemic
Pyocele
  mastoid — *see* Mastoiditis, acute
  sinus (accessory) — *see* Sinusitis
  turbinate (bone) J32.9
  urethra (*see also* Urethritis) N34.0
Pyocolpos — *see* Vaginitis
Pyocystitis N30.80
  with hematuria N30.81
Pyoderma, pyodermia L08.0
  gangrenosum L88
  newborn P39.4
  phagedenic L88
  vegetans L08.81
Pyodermatitis L08.0
  vegetans L08.81
Pyogenic — *see* condition
Pyohydronephrosis N13.6
Pyometra, pyometrium, pyometritis — *see* Endometritis
Pyomyositis (tropical) — *see* Myositis, infective
Pyonephritis N12
Pyonephrosis N13.6
  tuberculous A18.11
Pyopericarditis, pyopericardium I30.1
Pyophlebitis — *see* Phlebitis
Pyopneumopericardium I30.1
Pyopneumothorax (infective) J86.9
  with fistula J86.0
  tuberculous NEC A15.6
Pyosalpinx, pyosalpingitis (*see also* Salpingo-oophoritis)
Pyothorax J86.9
  with fistula J86.0
  tuberculous NEC A15.6
Pyoureter N28.89
  tuberculous A18.11
Pyramidopallidonigral syndrome G20
Pyrexia (of unknown origin) R50.9
  atmospheric T67.0 ☑
  during labor NEC O75.2
  heat T67.0 ☑
  newborn P81.9
    environmentally-induced P81.0
  persistent R50.9
  puerperal O86.4
Pyroglobulinemia NEC E88.09
Pyromania F63.1
Pyrosis R12
Pyuria (bacterial) N39.0

Q

Q fever A78
  with pneumonia A78
Quadricuspid aortic valve Q23.8
Quadrilateral fever A78
Quadriparesis — *see* Quadriplegia
  meaning muscle weakness M62.81
Quadriplegia G82.50
  complete
    C1-C4 level G82.51
    C5-C7 level G82.53
  congenital (cerebral) (spinal) G80.8
    spastic G80.0
  embolic (current episode) I63.4 ☑
  functional R53.2
  incomplete
    C1-C4 level G82.52
    C5-C7 level G82.54
  thrombotic (current episode) I63.3 ☑
  traumatic — *code to* injury with seventh character S
    current episode — *see* Injury, spinal (cord), cervical
Quadruplet, pregnancy — *see* Pregnancy, quadruplet
Quarrelsomeness F60.3
Queensland fever A77.3
Quervain's disease M65.4
  thyroid E06.1
Queyrat's erythroplasia D07.4
  penis D07.4
  specified site — *see* Neoplasm, skin, in situ
  unspecified site D07.4
Quincke's disease or edema T78.3 ☑
  hereditary D84.1
Quinsy (gangrenous) J36
Quintan fever A79.0
Quintuplet, pregnancy — *see* Pregnancy, quintuplet

R

Rabbit fever — *see* Tularemia
Rabies A82.9
  contact Z20.3
  exposure to Z20.3
  inoculation reaction — *see* Complications, vaccination
  sylvatic A82.0
  urban A82.1
Rachischisis — *see* Spina bifida
Rachitic (*see also* condition)
  deformities of spine (late effect) (sequelae) E64.3
  pelvis (late effect) (sequelae) E64.3
    with disproportion (fetopelvic) O33.0
      causing obstructed labor O65.0
Rachitis, rachitism (acute) (tarda) (*see also* Rickets)
  renalis N25.0
  sequelae E64.3
Radial nerve — *see* condition
Radiation
  burn — *see* Burn
  effects NOS T66 ☑
  sickness NOS T66 ☑
  therapy, encounter for Z51.0
Radiculitis (pressure) (vertebrogenic) — *see* Radiculopathy
Radiculomyelitis (*see also* Encephalitis)
  toxic, due to
    Clostridium tetani A35
    Corynebacterium diphtheriae A36.82
Radiculopathy M54.10
  cervical region M54.12
  cervicothoracic region M54.13
  due to
    disc disorder
      C3 M50.11
      C4 M50.11
      C5 M50.12
      C6 M50.12
      C7 M50.12
      C8 M50.13
    displacement of intervertebral disc — *see* Disorder, disc, with, radiculopathy
  leg M54.1- ☑
  lumbar region M54.16
  lumbosacral region M54.17
  occipito-atlanto-axial region M54.11
  postherpetic B02.29
  sacrococcygeal region M54.18

Radiculopathy — *continued*
  syphilitic A52.11
  thoracic region (with visceral pain) M54.14
  thoracolumbar region M54.15
Radiodermal burns (acute, chronic, or occupational) — *see* Burn
Radiodermatitis L58.9
  acute L58.0
  chronic L58.1
Radiotherapy session Z51.0
Rage, meaning rabies — *see* Rabies
Ragpicker's disease A22.1
Ragsorter's disease A22.1
Raillietiniasis B71.8
Railroad neurosis F48.8
Railway spine F48.8
Raised (*see also* Elevated)
  antibody titer R76.0
Rake teeth, tooth M26.39
Rales R09.89
Ramifying renal pelvis Q63.8
Ramsay-Hunt disease or syndrome (*see also* Hunt's disease) B02.21
  meaning dyssynergia cerebellaris myoclonica G11.1
Ranula K11.6
  congenital Q38.4
Rape
  adult
    confirmed T74.21 ☑
    suspected T76.21 ☑
  alleged, observation or examination, ruled out
    adult Z04.41
    child Z04.42
  child
    confirmed T74.22 ☑
    suspected T76.22 ☑
Rapid
  feeble pulse, due to shock, following injury T79.4 ☑
  heart (beat) R00.0
    psychogenic F45.8
  second stage (delivery) O62.3
  time-zone change syndrome — *see* Disorder, sleep, circadian rhythm, psychogenic
Rarefaction, bone — *see* Disorder, bone, density and structure, specified NEC
Rash (toxic) R21
  canker A38.9
  diaper L22
  drug (internal use) L27.0
    contact (*see also* Dermatitis, due to, drugs, external) L25.1
  following immunization T88.1 ☑
  food — *see* Dermatitis, due to, food
  heat L74.0
  napkin (psoriasiform) L22
  nettle — *see* Urticaria
  pustular L08.0
  rose R21
    epidemic B06.9
  scarlet A38.9
  serum (*see also* Reaction, serum) T80.69 ☑
  wandering tongue K14.1
Rasmussen aneurysm — *see* Tuberculosis, pulmonary
Rasmussen encephalitis G04.81
Rat-bite fever A25.9
  due to Streptobacillus moniliformis A25.1
  spirochetal (morsus muris) A25.0
Rathke's pouch tumor D44.3
Raymond (-Céstan) **syndrome** I65.8
Raynaud's disease, phenomenon or syndrome (secondary) I73.00
  with gangrene (symmetric) I73.01
RDS (newborn) (type I) P22.0
  type II P22.1
Reaction (*see also* Disorder)
  adaptation — *see* Disorder, adjustment
  adjustment (anxiety) (conduct disorder) (depressiveness) (distress) — *see* Disorder, adjustment
    with
      mutism, elective (child) (adolescent) F94.0
  adverse
    food (any) (ingested) NEC T78.1 ☑
      anaphylactic — *see* Shock, anaphylactic, due to food
  affective — *see* Disorder, mood
  allergic — *see* Allergy
  anaphylactic — *see* Shock, anaphylactic

Reaction — *continued*
  anaphylactoid — *see* Shock, anaphylactic
  anesthesia — *see* Anesthesia, complication
  antitoxin (prophylactic) (therapeutic) — *see* Complications, vaccination
  anxiety F41.1
  Arthus — *see* Arthus' phenomenon
  asthenic F48.8
  combat and operational stress F43.0
  compulsive F42
  conversion F44.9
  crisis, acute F43.0
  deoxyribonuclease (DNA) (DNase) hypersensitivity D69.2
  depressive (single episode) F32.9
    affective (single episode) F31.4
      recurrent episode F33.9
    neurotic F34.1
    psychoneurotic F34.1
    psychotic F32.3
    recurrent — *see* Disorder, depressive, recurrent
  dissociative F44.9
  drug NEC T88.7 ☑
    addictive — *see* Dependence, drug
      transmitted via placenta or breast milk — *see* Absorption, drug, addictive, through placenta
    allergic — *see* Allergy, drug
    lichenoid L43.2
    newborn P93.8
      gray baby syndrome P93.0
    overdose or poisoning (by accident) — *see* Table of Drugs and Chemicals, by drug, poisoning
    photoallergic L56.1
    phototoxic L56.0
    withdrawal — *see* Dependence, by drug, with, withdrawal
      infant of dependent mother P96.1
      newborn P96.1
    wrong substance given or taken (by accident) — *see* Table of Drugs and Chemicals, by drug, poisoning
  fear F40.9
    child (abnormal) F93.8
  febrile nonhemolytic transfusion (FNHTR) R50.84
  fluid loss, cerebrospinal G97.1
  foreign
    body NEC — *see* Granuloma, foreign body
      in operative wound (inadvertently left) — *see* Foreign body, accidentally left during a procedure
    substance accidentally left during a procedure (chemical) (powder) (talc) T81.60 ☑
      aseptic peritonitis T81.61 ☑
      body or object (instrument) (sponge) (swab) — *see* Foreign body, accidentally left during a procedure
    specified reaction NEC T81.69 ☑
  grief — *see* Disorder, adjustment
  Herxheimer's R68.89
  hyperkinetic — *see* Hyperkinesia
  hypochondriacal F45.20
  hypoglycemic, due to insulin E16.0
    with coma (diabetic) — *see* Diabetes, coma
      nondiabetic E15
    therapeutic misadventure — *see* subcategory T38.3 ☑
  hypomanic F30.8
  hysterical F44.9
  immunization — *see* Complications, vaccination
  incompatibility
    ABO blood group (infusion) (transfusion) — *see* Complication(s), transfusion, incompatibility reaction, ABO
      delayed serologic T80.39 ☑
    minor blood group (Duffy) (E) (K(ell)) (Kidd) (Lewis) (M) (N) (P) (S) T80.89 ☑
    Rh (factor) (infusion) (transfusion) — *see* Complication(s), transfusion, incompatibility reaction, Rh (factor)
  inflammatory — *see* Infection
  infusion — *see* Complications, infusion
  inoculation (immune serum) — *see* Complications, vaccination
  insulin T38.3- ☑
  involutional psychotic — *see* Disorder, depressive
  leukemoid D72.823

☑ Additional Character Required — Refer to the Tabular List for Character Selection   Subterms under main terms may continue to next column or page

Reaction — continued
  leukemoid — continued
    basophilic D72.823
    lymphocytic D72.823
    monocytic D72.823
    myelocytic D72.823
    neutrophilic D72.823
  LSD (acute)
    due to drug abuse — see Abuse, drug, hallucino-
      gen
    due to drug dependence — see Dependence, drug,
      hallucinogen
  lumbar puncture G97.1
  manic-depressive — see Disorder, bipolar
  neurasthenic F48.8
  neurogenic — see Neurosis
  neurotic F48.9
  neurotic-depressive F34.1
  nitritoid — see Crisis, nitritoid
  nonspecific
    to
      cell mediated immunity measurement of gam-
        ma interferon antigen response without
        active tuberculosis R76.12
      QuantiFERON-TB test (QFT) without active tu-
        berculosis R76.12
      tuberculin test (see also Reaction, tuberculin
        skin test) R76.11
  obsessive-compulsive F42
  organic, acute or subacute — see Delirium
  paranoid (acute) F23
    chronic F22
    senile F03 ☑
  passive dependency F60.7
  phobic F40.9
  post-traumatic stress, uncomplicated Z73.3
  psychogenic F99
  psychoneurotic (see also Neurosis)
    compulsive F42
    depersonalization F48.1
    depressive F34.1
    hypochondriacal F45.20
    neurasthenic F48.8
    obsessive F42
  psychophysiologic — see Disorder, somatoform
  psychosomatic — see Disorder, somatoform
  psychotic — see Psychosis
  scarlet fever toxin — see Complications, vaccination
  schizophrenic F23
    acute (brief) (undifferentiated) F23
    latent F21
    undifferentiated (acute) (brief) F23
  serological for syphilis — see Serology for syphilis
  serum T80.69 ☑
    anaphylactic (immediate) (see also Shock, anaphy-
      lactic) T80.59 ☑
    specified reaction NEC
      due to
        administration of blood and blood products
          T80.61 ☑
        immunization T80.62 ☑
        serum specified NEC T80.69 ☑
        vaccination T80.62 ☑
  situational — see Disorder, adjustment
  somatization — see Disorder, somatoform
  spinal puncture G97.1
  stress (severe) F43.9
    acute (agitation) ("daze") (disorientation) (distur-
      bance of consciousness) (flight reaction)
      (fugue) F43.0
    specified NEC F43.8
  surgical procedure — see Complications, surgical
    procedure
  tetanus antitoxin — see Complications, vaccination
  toxic, to local anesthesia T81.89 ☑
    in labor and delivery O74.4
    in pregnancy O29.3X- ☑
    postpartum, puerperal O89.3
  toxin-antitoxin — see Complications, vaccination
  transfusion (blood) (bone marrow) (lymphocytes) (al-
    lergic) — see Complications, transfusion
  tuberculin skin test, abnormal R76.11
  vaccination (any) — see Complications, vaccination
  withdrawing, child or adolescent F93.8
Reactive airway disease — see Asthma
Reactive depression — see Reaction, depressive

Rearrangement
  chromosomal
    balanced (in) Q95.9
      abnormal individual (autosomal) Q95.2
      non-sex (autosomal) chromosomes Q95.2
      sex/non-sex chromosomes Q95.3
      specified NEC Q95.8
Recalcitrant patient — see Noncompliance
Recanalization, thrombus — see Thrombosis
Recession, receding
  chamber angle (eye) H21.55- ☑
  chin M26.09
  gingival (generalized) (localized) (postinfective)
    (postoperative) K06.0
Recklinghausen disease Q85.01
  bones E21.0
Reclus' disease (cystic) — see Mastopathy, cystic
Recrudescent typhus (fever) A75.1
Recruitment, auditory H93.21- ☑
Rectalgia K62.89
Rectitis K62.89
Rectocele
  female (without uterine prolapse) N81.6
    with uterine prolapse N81.4
      incomplete N81.2
  in pregnancy — see Pregnancy, complicated by, ab-
    normal, pelvic organs or tissues NEC
  male K62.3
Rectosigmoid junction — see condition
Rectosigmoiditis K63.89
  ulcerative (chronic) K51.30
    with
      complication K51.319
        abscess K51.314
        fistula K51.313
        obstruction K51.312
        rectal bleeding K51.311
        specified NEC K51.318
Rectourethral — see condition
Rectovaginal — see condition
Rectovesical — see condition
Rectum, rectal — see condition
Recurrent — see condition
  pregnancy loss — see Loss (of), pregnancy, recurrent
Red bugs B88.0
Red tide (see also Table of Drugs and Chemicals)
  T65.82- ☑
Red-cedar lung or pneumonitis J67.8
Reduced
  mobility Z74.09
  ventilatory or vital capacity R94.2
Redundant, redundancy
  anus (congenital) Q43.8
  clitoris N90.89
  colon (congenital) Q43.8
  foreskin (congenital) N47.8
  intestine (congenital) Q43.8
  labia N90.6
  organ or site, congenital NEC — see Accessory
  panniculus (abdominal) E65
  prepuce (congenital) N47.8
  pylorus K31.89
  rectum (congenital) Q43.8
  scrotum N50.8
  sigmoid (congenital) Q43.8
  skin (of face) L57.4
    eyelids — see Blepharochalasis
  stomach K31.89
Reduplication — see Duplication
Reflex R29.2
  hyperactive gag J39.2
  pupillary, abnormal — see Anomaly, pupil, function
  vasoconstriction I73.9
  vasovagal R55
Reflux K21.9
  acid K21.9
  esophageal K21.9
    with esophagitis K21.0
    newborn P78.83
  gastroesophageal K21.9
    with esophagitis K21.0
  mitral — see Insufficiency, mitral
  ureteral — see Reflux, vesicoureteral
  vesicoureteral (with scarring) N13.70
    with
      nephropathy N13.729
        with hydroureter N13.739

Reflux — continued
  vesicoureteral — continued
    with — continued
      nephropathy — continued
        with hydroureter — continued
          bilateral N13.732
          unilateral N13.731
        without hydroureter N13.729
          bilateral N13.722
          unilateral N13.721
          bilateral N13.722
          unilateral N13.721
      pyelonephritis (chronic) N11.0
      without nephropathy N13.71
      congenital Q62.7
Reforming, artificial openings — see Attention to, artificial, opening
Refractive error — see Disorder, refraction
Refsum's disease or syndrome G60.1
Refusal of
  food, psychogenic F50.8
  treatment (because of) Z53.20
    left against medical advice (AMA) Z53.21
    patient's decision NEC Z53.29
    reasons of belief or group pressure Z53.1
Regional — see condition
Regurgitation R11.10
  aortic (valve) — see Insufficiency, aortic
  food (see also Vomiting)
    with reswallowing — see Rumination
    newborn P92.1
  gastric contents — see Vomiting
  heart — see Endocarditis
  mitral (valve) — see Insufficiency, mitral
    congenital Q23.3
  myocardial — see Endocarditis
  pulmonary (valve) (heart) I37.1
    congenital Q22.2
    syphilitic A52.03
  tricuspid — see Insufficiency, tricuspid
  valve, valvular — see Endocarditis
    congenital Q24.8
  vesicoureteral — see Reflux, vesicoureteral
Reichmann's disease or syndrome K31.89
Reifenstein syndrome E34.52
Reinsertion, contraceptive device Z30.433
Reiter's disease, syndrome, or urethritis M02.30
  ankle M02.37- ☑
  elbow M02.32- ☑
  foot joint M02.37- ☑
  hand joint M02.34- ☑
  hip M02.35- ☑
  knee M02.36- ☑
  multiple site M02.39
  shoulder M02.31- ☑
  vertebra M02.38
  wrist M02.33- ☑
Rejection
  food, psychogenic F50.8
  transplant T86.91
    bone T86.830
      marrow T86.01
    cornea T86.840
    heart T86.21
      with lung(s) T86.31
    intestine T86.850
    kidney T86.11
    liver T86.41
    lung(s) T86.810
      with heart T86.31
    organ (immune or nonimmune cause) T86.91
    pancreas T86.890
    skin (allograft) (autograft) T86.820
    specified NEC T86.890
    stem cell (peripheral blood) (umbilical cord) T86.5
Relapsing fever A68.9
  Carter's (Asiatic) A68.1
  Dutton's (West African) A68.1
  Koch's A68.9
  louse-borne (epidemic) A68.0
  Novy's (American) A68.1
  Obermeyers's (European) A68.0
  Spirillum A68.9
  tick-borne (endemic) A68.1
Relationship
  occlusal
    open anterior M26.220

Relationship — *continued*
occlusal — *continued*
open posterior M26.221
Relaxation
anus (sphincter) K62.89
psychogenic F45.8
arch (foot) (*see also* Deformity, limb, flat foot)
back ligaments — *see* Instability, joint, spine
bladder (sphincter) N31.2
cardioesophageal K21.9
cervix — *see* Incompetency, cervix
diaphragm J98.6
joint (capsule) (ligament) (paralytic) — *see* Flail, joint
congenital NEC Q74.8
lumbosacral (joint) — *see* subcategory M53.2 ☑
pelvic floor N81.89
perineum N81.89
posture R29.3
rectum (sphincter) K62.89
sacroiliac (joint) — *see* subcategory M53.2 ☑
scrotum N50.8
urethra (sphincter) N36.44
vesical N31.2
Release from prison, anxiety concerning Z65.2
Remains
canal of Cloquet Q14.0
capsule (opaque) Q14.8
Remittent fever (malarial) B54
Remnant
canal of Cloquet Q14.0
capsule (opaque) Q14.8
cervix, cervical stump (acquired) (postoperative) N88.8
cystic duct, postcholecystectomy K91.5
fingernail L60.8
congenital Q84.6
meniscus, knee — *see* Derangement, knee, meniscus, specified NEC
thyroglossal duct Q89.2
tonsil J35.8
infected (chronic) J35.01
urachus Q64.4
Removal (from) (of)
artificial
arm Z44.00- ☑
complete Z44.01- ☑
partial Z44.02- ☑
eye Z44.2- ☑
leg Z44.10- ☑
complete Z44.11- ☑
partial Z44.12- ☑
breast implant Z45.81 ☑
cardiac pulse generator (battery) (end-of-life) Z45.010
catheter (urinary) (indwelling) Z46.6
from artificial opening — *see* Attention to, artificial, opening
non-vascular Z46.82
vascular NEC Z45.2
device Z46.9
contraceptive Z30.432
implanted NEC Z45.89
specified NEC Z46.89
drains Z48.03
dressing (nonsurgical) Z48.00
surgical Z48.01
external
fixation device — *code to* fracture with seventh character D
prosthesis, prosthetic device Z44.9
breast Z44.3- ☑
specified NEC Z44.8
home in childhood (to foster home or institution) Z62.29
ileostomy Z43.2
insulin pump Z46.81
myringotomy device (stent) (tube) Z45.82
nervous system device NEC Z46.2
brain neuropacemaker Z46.2
visual substitution device Z46.2
implanted Z45.31
non-vascular catheter Z46.82
organ, prophylactic (for neoplasia management) — *see* Prophylactic, organ removal
orthodontic device Z46.4
staples Z48.02
stent
ureteral Z46.6
suture Z48.02
urinary device Z46.6

Removal — *continued*
vascular access device or catheter Z45.2
Ren
arcuatus Q63.1
mobile, mobilis N28.89
congenital Q63.8
unguliformis Q63.1
Renal — *see* condition
Rendu-Osler-Weber disease or syndrome I78.0
Reninoma D41.0- ☑
Renon-Delille syndrome E23.3
Reovirus, as cause of disease classified elsewhere B97.5
Repeated falls NEC R29.6
Replaced chromosome by dicentric ring Q93.2
Replacement by artificial or mechanical device or prosthesis of
bladder Z96.0
blood vessel NEC Z95.828
bone NEC Z96.7
cochlea Z96.21
coronary artery Z95.5
eustachian tube Z96.29
eye globe Z97.0
heart Z95.812
valve Z95.2
prosthetic Z95.2
specified NEC Z95.4
xenogenic Z95.3
intestine Z96.89
joint Z96.60
hip — *see* Presence, hip joint implant
knee — *see* Presence, knee joint implant
specified site NEC Z96.698
larynx Z96.3
lens Z96.1
limb(s) — *see* Presence, artificial, limb
mandible NEC (for tooth root implant(s)) Z96.5
organ NEC Z96.89
peripheral vessel NEC Z95.828
stapes Z96.29
teeth Z97.2
tendon Z96.7
tissue NEC Z96.89
tooth root(s) Z96.5
vessel NEC Z95.828
coronary (artery) Z95.5
Request for expert evidence Z04.8
Reserve, decreased or low
cardiac — *see* Disease, heart
kidney N28.89
Residual (*see also* condition)
ovary syndrome N99.83
state, schizophrenic F20.5
urine R39.19
Resistance, resistant (to)
activated protein C D68.51
complicating pregnancy O26.89 ☑
insulin E88.81
organism(s)
to
drug
aminoglycosides Z16.29
amoxicillin Z16.11
ampicillin Z16.11
antibiotic(s) Z16.20
multiple Z16.24
specified NEC Z16.29
antifungal Z16.32
antimicrobial (single) Z16.30
multiple Z16.35
specified NEC Z16.39
antimycbacterial (single) Z16.341
multiple Z16.342
antiparasitic Z16.31
antiviral Z16.33
beta lactam antibiotics Z16.10
specified NEC Z16.19
cephalosporins Z16.19
extended beta lactamase (ESBL) Z16.12
fluoroquinolones Z16.23
macrolides Z16.29
methicillin — *see* MRSA
multiple drugs (MDRO)
antibiotics Z16.24
penicillins Z16.11
quinine (and related compounds) Z16.31
quinolones Z16.23

Resistance, resistant — *continued*
organism(s) — *continued*
to — *continued*
drug — *continued*
sulfonamides Z16.29
tetracyclines Z16.29
tuberculostatics (single) Z16.341
multiple Z16.342
vancomycin Z16.21
related antibiotics Z16.22
thyroid hormone E07.89
Resorption
dental (roots) K03.3
alveoli M26.79
teeth (external) (internal) (pathological) (roots) K03.3
Respiration
Cheyne-Stokes R06.3
decreased due to shock, following injury T79.4 ☑
disorder of, psychogenic F45.8
insufficient, or poor R06.89
newborn P28.5
painful R07.1
sighing, psychogenic F45.8
Respiratory (*see also* condition)
distress syndrome (newborn) (type I) P22.0
type II P22.1
syncytial virus, as cause of disease classified elsewhere B97.4
Respite care Z75.5
Response (drug)
photoallergic L56.1
phototoxic L56.0
Restless legs (syndrome) G25.81
Restlessness R45.1
Restoration (of)
dental
aesthetically inadequate or displeasing K08.56
defective K08.50
specified NEC K08.59
failure of marginal integrity K08.51
failure of periodontal anatomical intergrity K08.54
organ continuity from previous sterilization (tuboplasty) (vasoplasty) Z31.0
aftercare Z31.42
tooth (existing)
contours biologically incompatible with oral health K08.54
open margins K08.51
overhanging K08.52
poor aesthetic K08.56
poor gingival margins K08.51
unsatisfactory, of tooth K08.50
specified NEC K08.59
Restorative material (dental)
allergy to K08.55
fractured K08.539
with loss of material K08.531
without loss of material K08.530
unrepairable overhanging of K08.52
Restriction of housing space Z59.1
Rests, ovarian, in fallopian tube Q50.6
Restzustand (schizophrenic) F20.5
Retained (*see also* Retention)
cholelithiasis following cholecystectomy K91.86
foreign body fragments (type of) Z18.9
acrylics Z18.2
animal quill(s) or spines Z18.31
cement Z18.83
concrete Z18.83
crystalline Z18.83
depleted isotope Z18.09
depleted uranium Z18.01
diethylhexylphthalates Z18.2
glass Z18.81
isocyanate Z18.2
magnetic metal Z18.11
metal Z18.10
nonmagnectic metal Z18.12
nontherapeutic radioactive Z18.09
organic NEC Z18.39
plastic Z18.2
quill(s) (animal) Z18.31
radioactive (nontherapeutic) NEC Z18.09
specified NEC Z18.89
spine(s) (animal) Z18.31
stone Z18.83
tooth (teeth) Z18.32
wood Z18.33

Retained — *continued*
- fragments (type of) Z18.9
  - acrylics Z18.2
  - animal quill(s) or spines Z18.31
  - cement Z18.83
  - concrete Z18.83
  - crystalline Z18.83
  - depleted isotope Z18.09
  - depleted uranium Z18.01
  - diethylhexylphthalates Z18.2
  - glass Z18.81
  - isocyanate Z18.2
  - magnetic metal Z18.11
  - metal Z18.10
  - nonmagnectic metal Z18.12
  - nontherapeutic radioactive Z18.09
  - organic NEC Z18.39
  - plastic Z18.2
  - quill(s) (animal) Z18.31
  - radioactive (nontherapeutic) NEC Z18.09
  - specified NEC Z18.89
  - spine(s) (animal) Z18.31
  - stone Z18.83
  - tooth (teeth) Z18.32
  - wood Z18.33
- gallstones, following cholecystectomy K91.86

Retardation
- development, developmental, specific — *see* Disorder, developmental
- endochondral bone growth — *see* Disorder, bone, development or growth
- growth R62.50
  - due to malnutrition E45
- mental — *see* Disability, intellectual
- motor function, specific F82
- physical (child) R62.52
  - due to malnutrition E45
- reading (specific) F81.0
- spelling (specific) (without reading disorder) F81.81

Retching — *see* Vomiting

Retention (*see also* Retained)
- bladder — *see* Retention, urine
- carbon dioxide E87.2
- cholelithiasis following cholecystectomy K91.86
- cyst — *see* Cyst
- dead
  - fetus (at or near term) (mother) O36.4 ☑
    - early fetal death O02.1
    - ovum O02.0
- decidua (fragments) (following delivery) (with hemorrhage) O72.2
  - without hemorrhage O73.1
- deciduous tooth K00.6
- dental root K08.3
- fecal — *see* Constipation
- fetus
  - dead O36.4 ☑
    - early O02.1
- fluid R60.9
- foreign body (*see also* Foreign body, retained)
  - current trauma — *code as* Foreign body, by site or type
- gallstones, following cholecystectomy K91.86
- gastric K31.89
- intrauterine contraceptive device, in pregnancy — *see* Pregnancy, complicated by, retention, intrauterine device
- membranes (complicating delivery) (with hemorrhage) O72.2
  - with abortion — *see* Abortion, by type
  - without hemorrhage O73.1
- meniscus — *see* Derangement, meniscus
- menses N94.89
- milk (puerperal, postpartum) O92.79
- nitrogen, extrarenal R39.2
- ovary syndrome N99.83
- placenta (total) (with hemorrhage) O72.0
  - without hemorrhage O73.0
  - portions or fragments (with hemorrhage) O72.2
    - without hemorrhage O73.1
- products of conception
  - early pregnancy (dead fetus) O02.1
  - following
    - delivery (with hemorrhage) O72.2
      - without hemorrhage O73.1
- secundines (following delivery) (with hemorrhage) O72.0
  - without hemorrhage O73.0

Retention — *continued*
- secundines — *continued*
  - complicating puerperium (delayed hemorrhage) O72.2
  - partial O72.2
    - without hemorrhage O73.1
- smegma, clitoris N90.89
- urine R33.9
  - drug-induced R33.0
  - due to hyperplasia (hypertrophy) of prostate — *see* Hyperplasia, prostate
  - organic R33.8
    - drug-induced R33.0
  - psychogenic F45.8
  - specified NEC R33.8
- water (in tissues) — *see* Edema

Reticulation, dust — *see* Pneumoconiosis

Reticulocytosis R70.1

Reticuloendotheliosis
- acute infantile C96.0
- leukemic C91.4- ☑
- malignant C96.9
- nonlipid C96.0

Reticulohistiocytoma (giant-cell) D76.3

Reticuloid, actinic L57.1

Reticulosis (skin)
- acute of infancy C96.0
- hemophagocytic, familial D76.1
- histiocytic medullary C96.9
- lipomelanotic I89.8
- malignant (midline) C86.0
- nonlipid C96.0
- polymorphic C83.8- ☑
- Sézary — *see* Sézary disease

Retina, retinal (*see also* condition)
- dark area D49.81

Retinitis (*see also* Inflammation, chorioretinal)
- albuminurica N18.9 [H32]
- diabetic — *see* Diabetes, retinitis
- disciformis — *see* Degeneration, macula
- focal — *see* Inflammation, chorioretinal, focal
- gravidarum — *see* Pregnancy, complicated by, specified pregnancy-related condition NEC
- juxtapapillaris — *see* Inflammation, chorioretinal, focal, juxtapapillary
- luetic — *see* Retinitis, syphilitic
- pigmentosa H35.52
- proliferans — *see* Disorder, globe, degenerative, specified type NEC
- proliferating — *see* Disorder, globe, degenerative, specified type NEC
- renal N18.9 [H32]
- syphilitic (early) (secondary) A51.43
  - central, recurrent A52.71
  - congenital (early) A50.01 [H32]
  - late A52.71
- tuberculous A18.53

Retinoblastoma C69.2- ☑
- differentiated C69.2- ☑
- undifferentiated C69.2- ☑

Retinochoroiditis (*see also* Inflammation, chorioretinal)
- disseminated — *see* Inflammation, chorioretinal, disseminated
  - syphilitic A52.71
- focal — *see* Inflammation, chorioretinal
- juxtapapillaris — *see* Inflammation, chorioretinal, focal, juxtapapillary

Retinopathy (background) H35.00
- arteriosclerotic I70.8 [H35.0-]
- atherosclerotic I70.8 [H35.0-]
- central serous — *see* Chorioretinopathy, central serous
- Coats H35.02- ☑
- diabetic — *see* Diabetes, retinopathy
- exudative H35.02- ☑
- hypertensive H35.03- ☑
- in (due to)
  - diabetes — *see* Diabetes, retinopathy
  - sickle-cell disorders D57.- ☑ [H36]
- of prematurity H35.10- ☑
  - stage 0 H35.11- ☑
  - stage 1 H35.12- ☑
  - stage 2 H35.13- ☑
  - stage 3 H35.14- ☑
  - stage 4 H35.15- ☑
  - stage 5 H35.16- ☑
- pigmentary, congenital — *see* Dystrophy, retina
- proliferative NEC H35.2- ☑

Retinopathy — *continued*
- proliferative — *continued*
  - diabetic — *see* Diabetes, retinopathy, proliferative
  - sickle-cell D57.- ☑ [H36]
- solar H31.02- ☑

Retinoschisis H33.10- ☑
- congenital Q14.1
- specified type NEC H33.19- ☑

Retortamoniasis A07.8

Retractile testis Q55.22

Retraction
- cervix — *see* Retroversion, uterus
- drum (membrane) — *see* Disorder, tympanic membrane, specified NEC
- finger — *see* Deformity, finger
- lid H02.539
  - left H02.536
    - lower H02.535
    - upper H02.534
  - right H02.533
    - lower H02.532
    - upper H02.531
- lung J98.4
- mediastinum J98.5
- nipple N64.53
  - associated with
    - lactation O92.03
    - pregnancy O92.01- ☑
    - puerperium O92.02
  - congenital Q83.8
- palmar fascia M72.0
- pleura — *see* Pleurisy
- ring, uterus (Bandl's) (pathological) O62.4
- sternum (congenital) Q76.7
  - acquired M95.4
- uterus — *see* Retroversion, uterus
- valve (heart) — *see* Endocarditis

Retrobulbar — *see* condition

Retrocecal — *see* condition

Retrocession — *see* Retroversion

Retrodisplacement — *see* Retroversion

Retroflection, retroflexion — *see* Retroversion

Retrognathia, retrognathism (mandibular) (maxillary) M26.19

Retrograde menstruation N92.5

Retroperineal — *see* condition

Retroperitoneal — *see* condition

Retroperitonitis K68.9

Retropharyngeal — *see* condition

Retroplacental — *see* condition

Retroposition — *see* Retroversion

Retroprosthetic membrane T85.398 ☑

Retrosternal thyroid (congenital) Q89.2

Retroversion, retroverted
- cervix — *see* Retroversion, uterus
- female NEC — *see* Retroversion, uterus
- iris H21.89
- testis (congenital) Q55.29
- uterus (acquired) (acute) (any degree) (asymptomatic) (cervix) (postinfectional) (postpartal, old) N85.4
  - congenital Q51.818
  - in pregnancy O34.53- ☑

Retrovirus, as cause of disease classified elsewhere B97.30
- human
  - immunodeficiency, type 2 (HIV 2) B97.35
  - T-cell lymphotropic
    - type I (HTLV-I) B97.33
    - type II (HTLV-II) B97.34
- lentivirus B97.31
- oncovirus B97.32
- specified NEC B97.39

Retrusion, premaxilla (developmental) M26.09

Rett's disease or syndrome F84.2

Reverse peristalsis R19.2

Reye's syndrome G93.7

Rh (factor)
- hemolytic disease (newborn) P55.0
- incompatibility, immunization or sensitization
  - affecting management of pregnancy NEC O36.09- ☑
    - anti-D antibody O36.01- ☑
  - newborn P55.0
  - transfusion reaction — *see* Complication(s), transfusion, incompatibility reaction, Rh (factor)
- negative mother affecting newborn P55.0

Rh — continued
  titer elevated — see Complication(s), transfusion, incompatibility reaction, Rh (factor)
  transfusion reaction — see Complication(s), transfusion, incompatibility reaction, Rh (factor)
Rhabdomyolysis (idiopathic) NEC M62.82
  traumatic T79.6 ☑
Rhabdomyoma (see also Neoplasm, connective tissue, benign)
  adult — see Neoplasm, connective tissue, benign
  fetal — see Neoplasm, connective tissue, benign
  glycogenic — see Neoplasm, connective tissue, benign
Rhabdomyosarcoma (any type) — see Neoplasm, connective tissue, malignant
Rhabdosarcoma — see Rhabdomyosarcoma
Rhesus (factor) **incompatibility** — see Rh, incompatibility
Rheumatic (acute) (subacute) (chronic)
  adherent pericardium I09.2
  coronary arteritis I01.9
  degeneration, myocardium I09.0
  fever (acute) — see Fever, rheumatic
  heart — see Disease, heart, rheumatic
  myocardial degeneration — see Degeneration, myocardium
  myocarditis (chronic) (inactive) (with chorea) I09.0
    with chorea (acute) (rheumatic) (Sydenham's) I02.0
    active or acute I01.2
  pancarditis, acute I01.8
    with chorea (acute (rheumatic) Sydenham's) I02.0
  pericarditis (active) (acute) (with effusion) (with pneumonia) I01.0
    with chorea (acute) (rheumatic) (Sydenham's) I02.0
    chronic or inactive I09.2
  pneumonia I00 [J17]
  torticollis M43.6
  typhoid fever A01.09
Rheumatism (articular) (neuralgic) (nonarticular) M79.0
  gout — see Arthritis, rheumatoid
  intercostal, meaning Tietze's disease M94.0
  palindromic (any site) M12.30
    ankle M12.37- ☑
    elbow M12.32- ☑
    foot joint M12.37- ☑
    hand joint M12.34- ☑
    hip M12.35- ☑
    knee M12.36- ☑
    multiple site M12.39
    shoulder M12.31- ☑
    specified joint NEC M12.38
    vertebrae M12.38
    wrist M12.33- ☑
  sciatic M54.4- ☑
Rheumatoid (see also condition)
  arthritis (see also Arthritis, rheumatoid)
    with involvement of organs NEC M05.60
      ankle M05.67- ☑
      elbow M05.62- ☑
      foot joint M05.67- ☑
      hand joint M05.64- ☑
      hip M05.65- ☑
      knee M05.66- ☑
      multiple site M05.69
      shoulder M05.61- ☑
      vertebra — see Spondylitis, ankylosing
      wrist M05.63- ☑
    seronegative — see Arthritis, rheumatoid, seronegative
    seropositive — see Arthritis, rheumatoid, seropositive
  carditis M05.30
    ankle M05.37- ☑
    elbow M05.32- ☑
    foot joint M05.37- ☑
    hand joint M05.34- ☑
    hip M05.35- ☑
    knee M05.36- ☑
    multiple site M05.39
    shoulder M05.31- ☑
    vertebra — see Spondylitis, ankylosing
    wrist M05.33- ☑
  endocarditis — see Rheumatoid, carditis
  lung (disease) M05.10
    ankle M05.17- ☑
    elbow M05.12- ☑
    foot joint M05.17- ☑
    hand joint M05.14- ☑

Rheumatoid — continued
  lung — continued
    hip M05.15- ☑
    knee M05.16- ☑
    multiple site M05.19
    shoulder M05.11- ☑
    vertebra — see Spondylitis, ankylosing
    wrist M05.13- ☑
  myocarditis — see Rheumatoid, carditis
  myopathy M05.40
    ankle M05.47- ☑
    elbow M05.42- ☑
    foot joint M05.47- ☑
    hand joint M05.44- ☑
    hip M05.45- ☑
    knee M05.46- ☑
    multiple site M05.49
    shoulder M05.41- ☑
    vertebra — see Spondylitis, ankylosing
    wrist M05.43- ☑
  pericarditis — see Rheumatoid, carditis
  polyarthritis — see Arthritis, rheumatoid
  polyneuropathy M05.50
    ankle M05.57- ☑
    elbow M05.52- ☑
    foot joint M05.57- ☑
    hand joint M05.54- ☑
    hip M05.55- ☑
    knee M05.56- ☑
    multiple site M05.59
    shoulder M05.51- ☑
    vertebra — see Spondylitis, ankylosing
    wrist M05.53- ☑
  vasculitis M05.20
    ankle M05.27- ☑
    elbow M05.22- ☑
    foot joint M05.27- ☑
    hand joint M05.24- ☑
    hip M05.25- ☑
    knee M05.26- ☑
    multiple site M05.29
    shoulder M05.21- ☑
    vertebra — see Spondylitis, ankylosing
    wrist M05.23- ☑
Rhinitis (atrophic) (catarrhal) (chronic) (croupous) (fibrinous) (granulomatous) (hyperplastic) (hypertrophic) (membranous) (obstructive) (purulent) (suppurative) (ulcerative) J31.0
  with
    sore throat — see Nasopharyngitis
  acute J00
  allergic J30.9
    with asthma J45.909
      with
        exacerbation (acute) J45.901
        status asthmaticus J45.902
    due to
      food J30.5
      pollen J30.1
    nonseasonal J30.89
    perennial J30.89
    seasonal NEC J30.2
    specified NEC J30.89
  infective J00
  pneumococcal J00
  syphilitic A52.73
    congenital A50.05 [J99]
  tuberculous A15.8
  vasomotor J30.0
Rhinoantritis (chronic) — see Sinusitis, maxillary
Rhinodacryolith — see Dacryolith
Rhinolith (nasal sinus) J34.89
Rhinomegaly J34.89
Rhinopharyngitis (acute) (subacute) (see also Nasopharyngitis)
  chronic J31.1
  destructive ulcerating A66.5
  mutilans A66.5
Rhinophyma L71.1
Rhinorrhea J34.89
  cerebrospinal (fluid) G96.0
  paroxysmal — see Rhinitis, allergic
  spasmodic — see Rhinitis, allergic
Rhinosalpingitis — see Salpingitis, eustachian
Rhinoscleroma A48.8
Rhinosporidiosis B48.1
Rhinovirus infection NEC B34.8

Rhizomelic chondrodysplasia punctata E71.540
Rhythm
  atrioventricular nodal I49.8
  disorder I49.9
    coronary sinus I49.8
    ectopic I49.8
    nodal I49.8
  escape I49.9
  heart, abnormal I49.9
  idioventricular I44.2
  nodal I49.8
  sleep, inversion G47.2- ☑
    nonorganic origin — see Disorder, sleep, circadian rhythm, psychogenic
Rhytidosis facialis L98.8
Rib (see also condition)
  cervical Q76.5
Riboflavin deficiency E53.0
Rice bodies (see also Loose, body, joint)
  knee M23.4- ☑
Richter syndrome — see Leukemia, chronic lymphocytic, B-cell type
Richter's hernia — see Hernia, abdomen, with obstruction
Ricinism — see Poisoning, food, noxious, plant
Rickets (active) (acute) (adolescent) (chest wall) (congenital) (current) (infantile) (intestinal) E55.0
  adult — see Osteomalacia
  celiac K90.0
  hypophosphatemic with nephrotic-glycosuric dwarfism E72.09
  inactive E64.3
  kidney N25.0
  renal N25.0
  sequelae, any E64.3
  vitamin-D-resistant E83.31 [M90.80]
Rickettsial disease A79.9
  specified type NEC A79.89
Rickettsialpox (Rickettsia akari) A79.1
Rickettsiosis A79.9
  due to
    Ehrlichia sennetsu A79.81
    Rickettsia akari (rickettsialpox) A79.1
  specified type NEC A79.89
  tick-borne A77.9
  vesicular A79.1
Rider's bone — see Ossification, muscle, specified NEC
Ridge, alveolus (see also condition)
  flabby K06.8
Ridged ear, congenital Q17.3
Riedel's
  lobe, liver Q44.7
  struma, thyroiditis or disease E06.5
Rieger's anomaly or syndrome Q13.81
Riehl's melanosis L81.4
Rietti-Greppi-Micheli anemia D56.9
Rieux's hernia — see Hernia, abdomen, specified site NEC
Riga (-Fede) **disease** K14.0
Riggs' disease — see Periodontitis
Right middle lobe syndrome J98.11
Rigid, rigidity (see also condition)
  abdominal R19.30
    with severe abdominal pain R10.0
    epigastric R19.36
    generalized R19.37
    left lower quadrant R19.34
    left upper quadrant R19.32
    periumbilic R19.35
    right lower quadrant R19.33
    right upper quadrant R19.31
  articular, multiple, congenital Q68.8
  cervix (uteri) in pregnancy — see Pregnancy, complicated by, abnormal, cervix
  hymen (acquired) (congenital) N89.6
  nuchal R29.1
  pelvic floor in pregnancy — see Pregnancy, complicated by, abnormal, pelvic organs or tissues NEC
  perineum or vulva in pregnancy — see Pregnancy, complicated by, abnormal, vulva
  spine — see Dorsopathy, specified NEC
  vagina in pregnancy — see Pregnancy, complicated by, abnormal, vagina
Rigors R68.89
  with fever R50.9
Riley-Day syndrome G90.1
RIND (reversible ischemic neurologic deficit) I63.9

☑ **Additional Character Required — Refer to the Tabular List for Character Selection**
    Subterms under main terms may continue to next column or page

Ring(s)
- aorta (vascular) Q25.4
- Bandl's O62.4
- contraction, complicating delivery O62.4
- esophageal, lower (muscular) K22.2
- Fleischer's (cornea) H18.04- ☑
- hymenal, tight (acquired) (congenital) N89.6
- Kayser-Fleischer (cornea) H18.04- ☑
- retraction, uterus, pathological O62.4
- Schatzki's (esophagus) (lower) K22.2
  - congenital Q39.3
- Soemmerring's — *see* Cataract, secondary
- vascular (congenital) Q25.8
  - aorta Q25.4

Ringed hair (congenital) Q84.1

Ringworm B35.9
- beard B35.0
- black dot B35.0
- body B35.4
- Burmese B35.5
- corporeal B35.4
- foot B35.3
- groin B35.6
- hand B35.2
- honeycomb B35.0
- nails B35.1
- perianal (area) B35.6
- scalp B35.0
- specified NEC B35.8
- Tokelau B35.5

Rise, venous pressure I87.8

Risk, suicidal
- meaning personal history of attempted suicide Z91.5
- meaning suicidal ideation — *see* Ideation, suicidal

Ritter's disease L00
Rivalry, sibling Z62.891
Rivalta's disease A42.2
River blindness B73.01
Robert's pelvis Q74.2
- with disproportion (fetopelvic) O33.0
  - causing obstructed labor O65.0
Robin (-Pierre) **syndrome** Q87.0
Robinow-Silvermann-Smith syndrome Q87.1
Robinson's (hidrotic) **ectodermal dysplasia or syndrome** Q82.4
Robles' disease B73.01
Rocky Mountain (spotted) **fever** A77.0
Roetheln — *see* Rubella
Roger's disease Q21.0
Rokitansky-Aschoff sinuses (gallbladder) K82.8
Rolando's fracture (displaced) S62.22- ☑
- nondisplaced S62.22- ☑
Romano-Ward (prolonged QT interval) **syndrome** I45.81
Romberg's disease or syndrome G51.8
Roof, mouth — *see* condition
Rosacea L71.9
- acne L71.9
- keratitis L71.8
- specified NEC L71.8
Rosary, rachitic E55.0
Rose
- cold J30.1
- fever J30.1
- rash R21
  - epidemic B06.9
Rosenbach's erysipeloid A26.0
Rosenthal's disease or syndrome D68.1
Roseola B09
- infantum B08.20
  - due to human herpesvirus 6 B08.21
  - due to human herpesvirus 7 B08.22
Ross River disease or fever B33.1
Rossbach's disease K31.89
- psychogenic F45.8
Rostan's asthma (cardiac) — *see* Failure, ventricular, left
Rotation
- anomalous, incomplete or insufficient, intestine Q43.3
- cecum (congenital) Q43.3
- colon (congenital) Q43.3
- spine, incomplete or insufficient — *see* Dorsopathy, deforming, specified NEC
- tooth, teeth, fully erupted M26.35
- vertebra, incomplete or insufficient — *see* Dorsopathy, deforming, specified NEC
Rotes Quérol disease or syndrome — *see* Hyperostosis, ankylosing

Roth (-Bernhardt) **disease or syndrome** — *see* Meralgia paraesthetica
Rothmund (-Thomson) **syndrome** Q82.8
Rotor's disease or syndrome E80.6
Round
- back (with wedging of vertebrae) — *see* Kyphosis
  - sequelae (late effect) of rickets E64.3
- worms (large) (infestation) NEC B82.0
  - Ascariasis (*see also* Ascariasis) B77.9
Roussy-Lévy syndrome G60.0
Rubella (German measles) B06.9
- complication NEC B06.09
  - neurological B06.00
- congenital P35.0
- contact Z20.4
- exposure to Z20.4
- maternal
  - care for (suspected) damage to fetus O35.3 ☑
    - manifest rubella in infant P35.0
    - suspected damage to fetus affecting management of pregnancy O35.3 ☑
- specified complications NEC B06.89
Rubeola (meaning measles) — *see* Measles
- meaning rubella — *see* Rubella
Rubeosis, iris — *see* Disorder, iris, vascular
Rubinstein-Taybi syndrome Q87.2
Rudimentary (congenital) (*see also* Agenesis)
- arm — *see* Defect, reduction, upper limb
- bone Q79.9
- cervix uteri Q51.828
- eye Q11.2
- lobule of ear Q17.3
- patella Q74.1
- respiratory organs in thoracopagus Q89.4
- tracheal bronchus Q32.4
- uterus Q51.818
  - in male Q56.1
- vagina Q52.0
Ruled out condition — *see* Observation, suspected
Rumination R11.10
- with nausea R11.2
- disorder of infancy F98.21
- neurotic F42
- newborn P92.1
- obsessional F42
- psychogenic F42
Runeberg's disease D51.0
Runny nose R09.89
Rupia (syphilitic) A51.39
- congenital A50.06
- tertiary A52.79
Rupture, ruptured
- abscess (spontaneous) — *code by* site under Abscess
- aneurysm — *see* Aneurysm
- anus (sphincter) — *see* Laceration, anus
- aorta, aortic I71.8
  - abdominal I71.3
  - arch I71.1
  - ascending I71.1
  - descending I71.8
    - abdominal I71.3
    - thoracic I71.1
  - syphilitic A52.01
  - thoracoabdominal I71.5
  - thorax, thoracic I71.1
  - transverse I71.1
  - traumatic — *see* Injury, aorta, laceration, major
  - valve or cusp (*see also* Endocarditis, aortic) I35.8
- appendix (with peritonitis) K35.2
- arteriovenous fistula, brain I60.8
- artery I77.2
  - brain — *see* Hemorrhage, intracranial, intracerebral
  - coronary — *see* Infarct, myocardium
  - heart — *see* Infarct, myocardium
  - pulmonary I28.8
  - traumatic (complication) — *see* Injury, blood vessel
- bile duct (common) (hepatic) K83.2
  - cystic K82.2
- bladder (sphincter) (nontraumatic) (spontaneous) N32.89
  - following ectopic or molar pregnancy O08.6
  - obstetrical trauma O71.5
  - traumatic S37.29 ☑
- blood vessel (*see also* Hemorrhage)
  - brain — *see* Hemorrhage, intracranial, intracerebral
  - heart — *see* Infarct, myocardium

Rupture, ruptured — *continued*
- blood vessel (*see also* Hemorrhage) — *continued*
  - traumatic (complication) — *see* Injury, blood vessel, laceration, major, by site
- bone — *see* Fracture
- bowel (nontraumatic) K63.1
- brain
  - aneurysm (congenital) (*see also* Hemorrhage, intracranial, subarachnoid)
    - syphilitic A52.05
  - hemorrhagic — *see* Hemorrhage, intracranial, intracerebral
- capillaries I78.8
- cardiac (auricle) (ventricle) (wall) I23.3
  - with hemopericardium I23.0
  - infectional I40.9
  - traumatic — *see* Injury, heart
- cartilage (articular) (current) (*see also* Sprain)
  - knee S83.3- ☑
  - semilunar — *see* Tear, meniscus
- cecum (with peritonitis) K65.0
  - with peritoneal abscess K35.3
  - traumatic S36.598 ☑
- celiac artery, traumatic — *see* Injury, blood vessel, celiac artery, laceration, major
- cerebral aneurysm (congenital) (see Hemorrhage, intracranial, subarachnoid)
- cervix (uteri)
  - with ectopic or molar pregnancy O08.6
  - following ectopic or molar pregnancy O08.6
  - obstetrical trauma O71.3
  - traumatic S37.69 ☑
- chordae tendineae NEC I51.1
  - concurrent with acute myocardial infarction — *see* Infarct, myocardium
  - following acute myocardial infarction (current complication) I23.4
- choroid (direct) (indirect) (traumatic) H31.32- ☑
- circle of Willis I60.6
- colon (nontraumatic) K63.1
  - traumatic — *see* Injury, intestine, large
- cornea (traumatic) — *see* Injury, eye, laceration
- coronary (artery) (thrombotic) — *see* Infarct, myocardium
- corpus luteum (infected) (ovary) N83.1
- cyst — *see* Cyst
- cystic duct K82.2
- Descemet's membrane — *see* Change, corneal membrane, Descemet's, rupture
  - traumatic — *see* Injury, eye, laceration
- diaphragm, traumatic — *see* Injury, intrathoracic, diaphragm
- disc — *see* Rupture, intervertebral disc
- diverticulum (intestine) K57.80
  - with bleeding K57.81
    - bladder N32.3
  - large intestine K57.20
    - with
      - bleeding K57.21
      - small intestine K57.40
        - with bleeding K57.41
  - small intestine K57.00
    - with
      - bleeding K57.01
      - large intestine K57.40
        - with bleeding K57.41
- duodenal stump K31.89
- ear drum (nontraumatic) (*see also* Perforation, tympanum)
  - traumatic S09.2- ☑
    - due to blast injury — *see* Injury, blast, ear
- esophagus K22.3
- eye (without prolapse or loss of intraocular tissue) — *see* Injury, eye, laceration
- fallopian tube NEC (nonobstetric) (nontraumatic) N83.8
  - due to pregnancy O00.1
- fontanel P13.1
- gallbladder K82.2
  - traumatic S36.128 ☑
- gastric (*see also* Rupture, stomach)
  - vessel K92.2
- globe (eye) (traumatic) — *see* Injury, eye, laceration
- graafian follicle (hematoma) N83.0
- heart — *see* Rupture, cardiac
- hymen (nontraumatic) (nonintentional) N89.8
- internal organ, traumatic — *see* Injury, by site

Rupture, ruptured — *continued*
  intervertebral disc — *see* Displacement, intervertebral disc
    traumatic — *see* Rupture, traumatic, intervertebral disc
  intestine NEC (nontraumatic) K63.1
    traumatic — *see* Injury, intestine
  iris (*see also* Abnormality, pupillary)
    traumatic — *see* Injury, eye, laceration
  joint capsule, traumatic — *see* Sprain
  kidney (traumatic) S37.06- ☑
    birth injury P15.8
    nontraumatic N28.89
  lacrimal duct (traumatic) — *see* Injury, eye, specified site NEC
  lens (cataract) (traumatic) — *see* Cataract, traumatic
  ligament, traumatic — *see* Rupture, traumatic, ligament, by site
  liver S36.116 ☑
    birth injury P15.0
  lymphatic vessel I89.8
  marginal sinus (placental) (with hemorrhage) — *see* Hemorrhage, antepartum, specified cause NEC
  membrana tympani (nontraumatic) — *see* Perforation, tympanum
  membranes (spontaneous)
    artificial
      delayed delivery following O75.5
    delayed delivery following — *see* Pregnancy, complicated by, premature rupture of membranes
  meningeal artery I60.8
  meniscus (knee) (*see also* Tear, meniscus)
    old — *see* Derangement, meniscus
    site other than knee — *code as* Sprain
  mesenteric artery, traumatic — *see* Injury, mesenteric, artery, laceration, major
  mesentery (nontraumatic) K66.8
    traumatic — *see* Injury, intra-abdominal, specified, site NEC
  mitral (valve) I34.8
  muscle (traumatic) (*see also* Strain)
    diastasis — *see* Diastasis, muscle
    nontraumatic M62.10
      ankle M62.17-
      foot M62.17-
      forearm M62.13-
      hand M62.14-
      lower leg M62.16-
      pelvic region M62.15-
      shoulder region M62.11-
      specified site NEC M62.18
      thigh M62.15-
      upper arm M62.12-
    traumatic — *see* Strain, by site
  musculotendinous junction NEC, nontraumatic — *see* Rupture, tendon, spontaneous
  mycotic aneurysm causing cerebral hemorrhage — *see* Hemorrhage, intracranial, subarachnoid
  myocardium, myocardial — *see* Rupture, cardiac
    traumatic — *see* Injury, heart
  nontraumatic, meaning hernia — *see* Hernia
  obstructed — *see* Hernia, by site, obstructed
  operation wound — *see* Disruption, wound, operation
  ovary, ovarian N83.8
    corpus luteum cyst N83.1
    follicle (graafian) N83.0
  oviduct (nonobstetric) (nontraumatic) N83.8
    due to pregnancy O00.1
  pancreas (nontraumatic) K86.8
    traumatic S36.299 ☑
  papillary muscle NEC I51.2
    following acute myocardial infarction (current complication) I23.5
  pelvic
    floor, complicating delivery O70.1
    organ NEC, obstetrical trauma O71.5
  perineum (nontraumatic) N90.89
    complicating delivery — *see* Delivery, complicated, by, laceration, anus (sphincter)
  postoperative wound — *see* Disruption, wound, operation
  prostate (traumatic) S37.828 ☑
  pulmonary
    artery I28.8
    valve (heart) I37.8
    vein I28.8

Rupture, ruptured — *continued*
  pulmonary — *continued*
    vessel I28.8
  pus tube — *see* Salpingitis
  pyosalpinx — *see* Salpingitis
  rectum (nontraumatic) K63.1
    traumatic S36.69 ☑
  retina, retinal (traumatic) (without detachment) (*see also* Break, retina)
    with detachment — *see* Detachment, retina, with retinal, break
  rotator cuff (nontraumatic) M75.10- ☑
    complete M75.12- ☑
    incomplete M75.11- ☑
  sclera — *see* Injury, eye, laceration
  sigmoid (nontraumatic) K63.1
    traumatic S36.593 ☑
  spinal cord (*see also* Injury, spinal cord, by region)
    due to injury at birth P11.5
    newborn (birth injury) P11.5
  spleen (traumatic) S36.09 ☑
    birth injury P15.1
    congenital (birth injury) P15.1
    due to P. vivax malaria B51.0
    nontraumatic D73.5
    spontaneous D73.5
  splenic vein R58
    traumatic — *see* Injury, blood vessel, splenic vein
  stomach (nontraumatic) (spontaneous) K31.89
    traumatic S36.39 ☑
  supraspinatus (complete) (incomplete) (nontraumatic) — *see* Tear, rotator cuff
  symphysis pubis
    obstetric O71.6
    traumatic S33.4 ☑
  synovium (cyst) M66.10
    ankle M66.17- ☑
    elbow M66.12- ☑
    finger M66.14- ☑
    foot M66.17- ☑
    forearm M66.13- ☑
    hand M66.14- ☑
    pelvic region M66.15- ☑
    shoulder region M66.11- ☑
    specified site NEC M66.18
    thigh M66.15- ☑
    toe M66.17- ☑
    upper arm M66.12- ☑
    wrist M66.13- ☑
  tendon (traumatic) — *see* Strain
    nontraumatic (spontaneous) M66.9
      ankle M66.87- ☑
      extensor M66.20
        ankle M66.27- ☑
        foot M66.27- ☑
        forearm M66.23- ☑
        hand M66.24- ☑
        lower leg M66.26- ☑
        multiple sites M66.29
        pelvic region M66.25- ☑
        shoulder region M66.21- ☑
        specified site NEC M66.28
        thigh M66.25- ☑
        upper arm M66.22- ☑
      flexor M66.30
        ankle M66.37- ☑
        foot M66.37- ☑
        forearm M66.33- ☑
        hand M66.34- ☑
        lower leg M66.36- ☑
        multiple sites M66.39
        pelvic region M66.35- ☑
        shoulder region M66.31- ☑
        specified site NEC M66.38
        thigh M66.35- ☑
        upper arm M66.32- ☑
      foot M66.87- ☑
      forearm M66.83- ☑
      hand M66.84- ☑
      lower leg M66.86- ☑
      multiple sites M66.89
      pelvic region M66.85- ☑
      shoulder region M66.81- ☑
      specified
        site NEC M66.88
        tendon M66.80

Rupture, ruptured — *continued*
  tendon — *see* Strain — *continued*
    nontraumatic — *continued*
      thigh M66.85- ☑
      upper arm M66.82- ☑
  thoracic duct I89.8
  tonsil J35.8
  traumatic
    aorta — *see* Injury, aorta, laceration, major
    diaphragm — *see* Injury, intrathoracic, diaphragm
    external site — *see* Wound, open, by site
    eye — *see* Injury, eye, laceration
    internal organ — *see* Injury, by site
    intervertebral disc
      cervical S13.0 ☑
      lumbar S33.0 ☑
      thoracic S23.0 ☑
    kidney S37.06- ☑
    ligament (*see also* Sprain)
      ankle — *see* Sprain, ankle
      carpus — *see* Rupture, traumatic, ligament, wrist
      collateral (hand) — *see* Rupture, traumatic, ligament, finger, collateral
      finger (metacarpophalangeal) (interphalangeal) S63.40- ☑
        collateral S63.41- ☑
          index S63.41- ☑
          little S63.41- ☑
          middle S63.41- ☑
          ring S63.41- ☑
        index S63.40- ☑
        little S63.40- ☑
        middle S63.40- ☑
        palmar S63.42- ☑
          index S63.42- ☑
          little S63.42- ☑
          middle S63.42- ☑
          ring S63.42- ☑
        ring S63.40- ☑
        specified site NEC S63.499 ☑
          index S63.49- ☑
          little S63.49- ☑
          middle S63.49- ☑
          ring S63.49- ☑
        volar plate S63.43- ☑
          index S63.43- ☑
          little S63.43- ☑
          middle S63.43- ☑
          ring S63.43- ☑
      foot — *see* Sprain, foot
      radial collateral S53.2- ☑
      radiocarpal — *see* Rupture, traumatic, ligament, wrist, radiocarpal
      ulnar collateral S53.3- ☑
      ulnocarpal — *see* Rupture, traumatic, ligament, wrist, ulnocarpal
      wrist S63.30- ☑
        collateral S63.31- ☑
        radiocarpal S63.32- ☑
        specified site NEC S63.39- ☑
        ulnocarpal (palmar) S63.33- ☑
    liver S36.116 ☑
    membrana tympani — *see* Rupture, ear drum, traumatic
    muscle or tendon — *see* Strain
    myocardium — *see* Injury, heart
    pancreas S36.299 ☑
    rectum S36.69 ☑
    sigmoid S36.593 ☑
    spleen S36.09 ☑
    stomach S36.39 ☑
    symphysis pubis S33.4 ☑
    tympanum, tympanic (membrane) — *see* Rupture, ear drum, traumatic
    ureter S37.19 ☑
    uterus S37.69 ☑
    vagina — *see* Injury, vagina
    vena cava — *see* Injury, vena cava, laceration, major
  tricuspid (heart) (valve) I07.8
  tube, tubal (nonobstetric) (nontraumatic) N83.8
    abscess — *see* Salpingitis
    due to pregnancy O00.1

Rupture, ruptured — *continued*
  tympanum, tympanic (membrane) (nontraumatic) (*see also* Perforation, tympanic membrane) H72.9- ☑
    traumatic — *see* Rupture, ear drum, traumatic
  umbilical cord, complicating delivery O69.89 ☑
  ureter (traumatic) S37.19 ☑
    nontraumatic N28.89
  urethra (nontraumatic) N36.8
    with ectopic or molar pregnancy O08.6
    following ectopic or molar pregnancy O08.6
    obstetrical trauma O71.5
    traumatic S37.39 ☑
  uterosacral ligament (nonobstetric) (nontraumatic) N83.8
  uterus (traumatic) S37.69 ☑
    before labor O71.0- ☑
    during or after labor O71.1
    nonpuerperal, nontraumatic N85.8
    pregnant (during labor) O71.1
      before labor O71.0- ☑
  vagina — *see* Injury, vagina
  valve, valvular (heart) — *see* Endocarditis
  varicose vein — *see* Varix
  varix — *see* Varix
  vena cava R58
    traumatic — *see* Injury, vena cava, laceration, major
  vesical (urinary) N32.89
  vessel (blood) R58
    pulmonary I28.8
    traumatic — *see* Injury, blood vessel
  viscus R19.8
  vulva complicating delivery O70.0
Russell-Silver syndrome Q87.1
Russian spring-summer type encephalitis A84.0
Rust's disease (tuberculous cervical spondylitis) A18.01
Ruvalcaba-Myhre-Smith syndrome E71.440
Rytand-Lipsitch syndrome I44.2

S

Saber, sabre shin or tibia (syphilitic) A50.56 [M90.8-] ☑
Sac lacrimal — *see* condition
Saccharomyces infection B37.9
Saccharopinuria E72.3
Saccular — *see* condition
Sacculation
  aorta (nonsyphilitic) — *see* Aneurysm, aorta
  bladder N32.3
  intralaryngeal (congenital) (ventricular) Q31.3
  larynx (congenital) (ventricular) Q31.3
  organ or site, congenital — *see* Distortion
  pregnant uterus — *see* Pregnancy, complicated by, abnormal, uterus
  ureter N28.89
  urethra N36.1
  vesical N32.3
Sachs' amaurotic familial idiocy or disease E75.02
Sachs-Tay disease E75.02
Sacks-Libman disease M32.11
Sacralgia M53.3
Sacralization Q76.49
Sacrodynia M53.3
Sacroiliac joint — *see* condition
Sacroiliitis NEC M46.1
Sacrum — *see* condition
Saddle
  back — *see* Lordosis
  embolus
    abdominal aorta I74.01
    pulmonary artery I26.92
      with acute cor pulmonale I26.02
  injury — *code to* condition
  nose M95.0
    due to syphilis A50.57
Sadism (sexual) F65.52
Sadness, postpartal O90.6
Sadomasochism F65.50
Saemisch's ulcer (cornea) — *see* Ulcer, cornea, central
Sahib disease B55.0
Sailors' skin L57.8
Saint
  Anthony's fire — *see* Erysipelas
  triad — *see* Hernia, diaphragm
  Vitus' dance — *see* Chorea, Sydenham's
Salaam
  attack(s) — *see* Epilepsy, spasms

Salaam — *continued*
  tic R25.8
Salicylism
  abuse F55.8
  overdose or wrong substance given — *see* Table of Drugs and Chemicals, by drug, poisoning
Salivary duct or gland — *see* condition
Salivation, excessive K11.7
Salmonella — *see* Infection, Salmonella
Salmonellosis A02.0
Salpingitis (catarrhal) (fallopian tube) (nodular) (pseudofollicular) (purulent) (septic) N70.91
  with oophoritis N70.93
  acute N70.01
    with oophoritis N70.03
  chlamydial A56.11
  chronic N70.11
    with oophoritis N70.13
  complicating abortion — *see* Abortion, by type, complicated by, salpingitis
  ear — *see* Salpingitis, eustachian
  eustachian (tube) H68.00- ☑
    acute H68.01- ☑
    chronic H68.02- ☑
  follicularis N70.11
    with oophoritis N70.13
  gonococcal (acute) (chronic) A54.24
  interstitial, chronic N70.11
    with oophoritis N70.13
  isthmica nodosa N70.11
    with oophoritis N70.13
  specific (gonococcal) (acute) (chronic) A54.24
  tuberculous (acute) (chronic) A18.17
  venereal (gonococcal) (acute) (chronic) A54.24
Salpingo-oophoritis (catarrhal) (purulent) (ruptured) (septic) (suppurative) N70.93
  acute N70.03
    with ectopic or molar pregnancy O08.0
    following ectopic or molar pregnancy O08.0
    gonococcal A54.24
  chronic N70.13
  following ectopic or molar pregnancy O08.0
  gonococcal (acute) (chronic) A54.24
  puerperal O86.19
  specific (gonococcal) (acute) (chronic) A54.24
  subacute N70.03
  tuberculous (acute) (chronic) A18.17
  venereal (gonococcal) (acute) (chronic) A54.24
Salpingo-ovaritis — *see* Salpingo-oophoritis
Salpingocele N83.4
Salpingoperitonitis — *see* Salpingo-oophoritis
Salzmann's nodular dystrophy — *see* Degeneration, cornea, nodular
Sampson's cyst or tumor N80.1
San Joaquin (Valley) **fever** B38.0
Sandblaster's asthma, lung or pneumoconiosis J62.8
Sander's disease (paranoia) F22
Sandfly fever A93.1
Sandhoff's disease E75.01
Sanfilippo (Type B) (Type C) (Type D) **syndrome** E76.22
Sanger-Brown ataxia G11.2
Sao Paulo fever or typhus A77.0
Saponification, mesenteric K65.8
Sarcocele (benign)
  syphilitic A52.76
    congenital A50.59
Sarcocystosis A07.8
Sarcoepiplocele — *see* Hernia
Sarcoepiplomphalocele Q79.2
Sarcoid (*see also* Sarcoidosis)
  arthropathy D86.86
  Boeck's D86.9
  Darier-Roussy D86.3
  iridocyclitis D86.83
  meningitis D86.81
  myocarditis D86.85
  myositis D86.87
  pyelonephritis D86.84
  Spiegler-Fendt L08.89
Sarcoidosis D86.9
  with
    cranial nerve palsies D86.82
    hepatic granuloma D86.89
    polyarthritis D86.86
    tubulo-interstitial nephropathy D86.84
  combined sites NEC D86.89
  lung D86.0

Sarcoidosis — *continued*
  lung — *continued*
    and lymph nodes D86.2
  lymph nodes D86.1
    and lung D86.2
  meninges D86.81
  skin D86.3
  specified type NEC D86.89
Sarcoma (of) (*see also* Neoplasm, connective tissue, malignant)
  alveolar soft part — *see* Neoplasm, connective tissue, malignant
  ameloblastic C41.1
    upper jaw (bone) C41.0
  botryoid — *see* Neoplasm, connective tissue, malignant
  botryoides — *see* Neoplasm, connective tissue, malignant
  cerebellar C71.6
    circumscribed (arachnoidal) C71.6
  circumscribed (arachnoidal) cerebellar C71.6
  clear cell (*see also* Neoplasm, connective tissue, malignant)
    kidney C64.- ☑
  dendritic cells (accessory cells) C96.4
  embryonal — *see* Neoplasm, connective tissue, malignant
  endometrial (stromal) C54.1
    isthmus C54.0
  epithelioid (cell) — *see* Neoplasm, connective tissue, malignant
  Ewing's — *see* Neoplasm, bone, malignant
  follicular dendritic cell C96.4
  germinoblastic (diffuse) — *see* Lymphoma, diffuse large cell
    follicular — *see* Lymphoma, follicular, specified NEC
  giant cell (except of bone) (*see also* Neoplasm, connective tissue, malignant)
    bone — *see* Neoplasm, bone, malignant
  glomoid — *see* Neoplasm, connective tissue, malignant
  granulocytic C92.3- ☑
  hemangioendothelial — *see* Neoplasm, connective tissue, malignant
  hemorrhagic, multiple — *see* Sarcoma, Kaposi's
  histiocytic C96.A (*following* C96.6)
  Hodgkin — *see* Lymphoma, Hodgkin
  immunoblastic (diffuse) — *see* Lymphoma, diffuse large cell
  interdigitating dendritic cell C96.4
  Kaposi's
    colon C46.4
    connective tissue C46.1
    gastrointestinal organ C46.4
    lung C46.5- ☑
    lymph node(s) C46.3
    palate (hard) (soft) C46.2
    rectum C46.4
    skin C46.0
    specified site NEC C46.7
    stomach C46.4
    unspecified site C46.9
  Kupffer cell C22.3
  Langerhans cell C96.4
  leptomeningeal — *see* Neoplasm, meninges, malignant
  liver NEC C22.4
  lymphangioendothelial — *see* Neoplasm, connective tissue, malignant
  lymphoblastic — *see* Lymphoma, lymphoblastic (diffuse)
  lymphocytic — *see* Lymphoma, small cell B-cell
  mast cell C96.2
  melanotic — *see* Melanoma
  meningeal — *see* Neoplasm, meninges, malignant
  meningothelial — *see* Neoplasm, meninges, malignant
  mesenchymal (*see also* Neoplasm, connective tissue, malignant)
    mixed — *see* Neoplasm, connective tissue, malignant
  mesothelial — *see* Mesothelioma
  monstrocellular
    specified site — *see* Neoplasm, malignant, by site
    unspecified site C71.9
  myeloid C92.3- ☑
  neurogenic — *see* Neoplasm, nerve, malignant

Sarcoma — *continued*
odontogenic C41.1
upper jaw (bone) C41.0
osteoblastic — *see* Neoplasm, bone, malignant
osteogenic (*see also* Neoplasm, bone, malignant)
juxtacortical — *see* Neoplasm, bone, malignant
periosteal — *see* Neoplasm, bone, malignant
periosteal (*see also* Neoplasm, bone, malignant)
osteogenic — *see* Neoplasm, bone, malignant
pleomorphic cell — *see* Neoplasm, connective tissue, malignant
reticulum cell (diffuse) — *see* Lymphoma, diffuse large cell
nodular — *see* Lymphoma, follicular
pleomorphic cell type — *see* Lymphoma, diffuse large cell
rhabdoid — *see* Neoplasm, malignant, by site
round cell — *see* Neoplasm, connective tissue, malignant
small cell — *see* Neoplasm, connective tissue, malignant
soft tissue — *see* Neoplasm, connective tissue, malignant
spindle cell — *see* Neoplasm, connective tissue, malignant
stromal (endometrial) C54.1
isthmus C54.0
synovial (*see also* Neoplasm, connective tissue, malignant)
biphasic — *see* Neoplasm, connective tissue, malignant
epithelioid cell — *see* Neoplasm, connective tissue, malignant
spindle cell — *see* Neoplasm, connective tissue, malignant
Sarcomatosis
meningeal — *see* Neoplasm, meninges, malignant
specified site NEC — *see* Neoplasm, connective tissue, malignant
unspecified site C80.1
Sarcosinemia E72.59
Sarcosporidiosis (intestinal) A07.8
Satiety, early R68.81
Saturnine — *see* condition
Saturnism
overdose or wrong substance given or taken — *see* Table of Drugs and Chemicals, by drug, poisoning
Satyriasis F52.8
Sauriasis — *see* Ichthyosis
SBE (subacute bacterial endocarditis) I33.0
Scabies (any site) B86
Scabs R23.4
Scaglietti-Dagnini syndrome E22.0
Scald — *see* Burn
Scalenus anticus (anterior) **syndrome** G54.0
Scales R23.4
Scaling, skin R23.4
Scalp — *see* condition
Scapegoating affecting child Z62.3
Scaphocephaly Q75.0
Scapulalgia M89.8X1
Scapulohumeral myopathy G71.0
Scar, scarring (*see also* Cicatrix) L90.5
adherent L90.5
atrophic L90.5
cervix
in pregnancy or childbirth — *see* Pregnancy, complicated by, abnormal cervix
cheloid L91.0
chorioretinal H31.00- ☑
posterior pole macula H31.01- ☑
postsurgical H59.81- ☑
solar retinopathy H31.02- ☑
specified type NEC H31.09- ☑
choroid — *see* Scar, chorioretinal
conjunctiva H11.24- ☑
cornea H17.9
xerophthalmic (*see also* Opacity, cornea)
vitamin A deficiency E50.6
duodenum, obstructive K31.5
hypertrophic L91.0
keloid L91.0
labia N90.89
lung (base) J98.4
macula — *see* Scar, chorioretinal, posterior pole
muscle M62.89

Scar, scarring — *continued*
myocardium, myocardial I25.2
painful L90.5
posterior pole (eye) — *see* Scar, chorioretinal, posterior pole
retina — *see* Scar, chorioretinal
trachea J39.8
uterus N85.8
in pregnancy O34.29
vagina N89.8
postoperative N99.2
vulva N90.89
Scarabiasis B88.2
Scarlatina (anginosa) (maligna) (ulcerosa) A38.9
myocarditis (acute) A38.1
old — *see* Myocarditis
otitis media A38.0
Scarlet fever (albuminuria) (angina) A38.9
Schamberg's disease (progressive pigmentary dermatosis) L81.7
Schatzki's ring (acquired) (esophagus) (lower) K22.2
congenital Q39.3
Schaufenster krankheit I20.8
Schaumann's
benign lymphogranulomatosis D86.1
disease or syndrome — *see* Sarcoidosis
Scheie's syndrome E76.03
Schenck's disease B42.1
Scheuermann's disease or osteochondrosis — *see* Osteochondrosis, juvenile, spine
Schilder (-Flatau) **disease** G37.0
Schilling-type monocytic leukemia C93.0- ☑
Schimmelbusch's disease, cystic mastitis, or hyperplasia — *see* Mastopathy, cystic
Schistosoma infestation — *see* Infestation, Schistosoma
Schistosomiasis B65.9
with muscle disorder B65.9 [M63.80]
ankle B65.9 [M63.87-] ☑
foot B65.9 [M63.87-] ☑
forearm B65.9 [M63.83-] ☑
hand B65.9 [M63.84-] ☑
lower leg B65.9 [M63.86-] ☑
multiple sites B65.9 [M63.89]
pelvic region B65.9 [M63.85-] ☑
shoulder region B65.9 [M63.81-] ☑
specified site NEC B65.9 [M63.88]
thigh B65.9 [M63.85-] ☑
upper arm B65.9 [M63.82-] ☑
Asiatic B65.2
bladder B65.0
chestermani B65.8
colon B65.1
cutaneous B65.3
due to
S. haematobium B65.0
S. japonicum B65.2
S. mansoni B65.1
S. mattheii B65.8
Eastern B65.2
genitourinary tract B65.0
intestinal B65.1
lung NEC B65.9 [J99]
pneumonia B65.9 [J17]
Manson's (intestinal) B65.1
oriental B65.2
pulmonary NEC B65.9 [J99]
pneumonia B65.9
Schistosoma
haematobium B65.0
japonicum B65.2
mansoni B65.1
specified type NEC B65.8
urinary B65.0
vesical B65.0
Schizencephaly Q04.6
Schizoaffective psychosis F25.9
Schizodontia K00.2
Schizoid personality F60.1
Schizophrenia, schizophrenic F20.9
acute (brief) (undifferentiated) F23
atypical (form) F20.3
borderline F21
catalepsy F20.2
catatonic (type) (excited) (withdrawn) F20.2
cenesthopathic, cenesthesiopathic F20.89
childhood type F84.5
chronic undifferentiated F20.5

Schizophrenia, schizophrenic — *continued*
cyclic F25.0
disorganized (type) F20.1
flexibilitas cerea F20.2
hebephrenic (type) F20.1
incipient F21
latent F21
negative type F20.5
paranoid (type) F20.0
paraphrenic F20.0
post-psychotic depression F32.8
prepsychotic F21
prodromal F21
pseudoneurotic F21
pseudopsychopathic F21
reaction F23
residual (state) (type) F20.5
restzustand F20.5
schizoaffective (type) — *see* Psychosis, schizoaffective
simple (type) F20.89
simplex F20.89
specified type NEC F20.89
stupor F20.2
syndrome of childhood F84.5
undifferentiated (type) F20.3
chronic F20.5
Schizothymia (persistent) F60.1
Schlatter-Osgood disease or osteochondrosis — *see* Osteochondrosis, juvenile, tibia
Schlatter's tibia — *see* Osteochondrosis, juvenile, tibia
Schmidt's syndrome (polyglandular, autoimmune) E31.0
Schmincke's carcinoma or tumor — *see* Neoplasm, nasopharynx, malignant
Schmitz (-Stutzer) **dysentery** A03.0
Schmorl's disease or nodes
lumbar region M51.46
lumbosacral region M51.47
sacrococcygeal region M53.3
thoracic region M51.44
thoracolumbar region M51.45
Schneiderian
papilloma — *see* Neoplasm, nasopharynx, benign
specified site — *see* Neoplasm, benign, by site
unspecified site D14.0
specified site — *see* Neoplasm, malignant, by site
unspecified site C30.0
Scholte's syndrome (malignant carcinoid) E34.0
Scholz (-Bielchowsky-Henneberg) **disease or syndrome** E75.25
Schönlein (-Henoch) disease or purpura (primary) (rheumatic) D69.0
Schottmuller's disease A01.4
Schroeder's syndrome (endocrine hypertensive) E27.0
Schüller-Christian disease or syndrome C96.5
Schultze's type acroparesthesia, simple I73.89
Schultz's disease or syndrome — *see* Agranulocytosis
Schwalbe-Ziehen-Oppenheim disease G24.1
Schwannoma (*see also* Neoplasm, nerve, benign)
malignant (*see also* Neoplasm, nerve, malignant)
with rhabdomyoblastic differentiation — *see* Neoplasm, nerve, malignant
melanocytic — *see* Neoplasm, nerve, benign
pigmented — *see* Neoplasm, nerve, benign
Schwannomatosis Q85.03
Schwartz (-Jampel) **syndrome** G71.13
Schwartz-Bartter syndrome E22.2
Schweniger-Buzzi anetoderma L90.1
Sciatic — *see* condition
Sciatica (infective)
with lumbago M54.4- ☑
due to intervertebral disc disorder — *see* Disorder, disc, with, radiculopathy
due to displacement of intervertebral disc (with lumbago) — *see* Disorder, disc, with, radiculopathy
wallet M54.3- ☑
Scimitar syndrome Q26.8
Sclera — *see* condition
Sclerectasia H15.84- ☑
Scleredema
adultorum — *see* Sclerosis, systemic
Buschke's — *see* Sclerosis, systemic
newborn P83.0
Sclerema (adiposum) (edematosum) (neonatorum) (newborn) P83.0
adultorum — *see* Sclerosis, systemic
Scleriasis — *see* Scleroderma
Scleritis H15.00- ☑

Scleritis — *continued*
  with corneal involvement H15.04- ☑
    anterior H15.01- ☑
    brawny H15.02- ☑
    in (due to) zoster B02.34
    posterior H15.03- ☑
    specified type NEC H15.09- ☑
  syphilitic A52.71
  tuberculous (nodular) A18.51
Sclerochoroiditis H31.8
Scleroconjunctivitis — *see* Scleritis
Sclerocystic ovary syndrome E28.2
Sclerodactyly, sclerodactylia L94.3
Scleroderma, sclerodermia (acrosclerotic) (diffuse)
    (generalized) (progressive) (pulmonary) (*see also*
    Sclerosis, systemic) M34.9
  circumscribed L94.0
  linear L94.1
  localized L94.0
  newborn P83.8
  systemic M34.9
Sclerokeratitis H16.8
  tuberculous A18.52
Scleroma nasi A48.8
Scleromalacia (perforans) H15.05- ☑
Scleromyxedema L98.5
Sclérose en plaques G35
Sclerosis, sclerotic
  adrenal (gland) E27.8
  Alzheimer's — *see* Disease, Alzheimer's
  amyotrophic (lateral) G12.21
  aorta, aortic I70.0
    valve — *see* Endocarditis, aortic
  artery, arterial, arteriolar, arteriovascular — *see* Arteriosclerosis
  ascending multiple G35
  brain (generalized) (lobular) G37.9
    artery, arterial I67.2
    diffuse G37.0
    disseminated G35
    insular G35
    Krabbe's E75.23
    miliary G35
    multiple G35
    presenile (Alzheimer's) — *see* Disease, Alzheimer's, early onset
    senile (arteriosclerotic) I67.2
    stem, multiple G35
    tuberous Q85.1
  bulbar, multiple G35
  bundle of His I44.39
  cardiac — *see* Disease, heart, ischemic, atherosclerotic
  cardiorenal — *see* Hypertension, cardiorenal
  cardiovascular (*see also* Disease, cardiovascular)
    renal — *see* Hypertension, cardiorenal
  cerebellar — *see* Sclerosis, brain
  cerebral — *see* Sclerosis, brain
  cerebrospinal (disseminated) (multiple) G35
  cerebrovascular I67.2
  choroid — *see* Degeneration, choroid
  combined (spinal cord) (*see also* Degeneration, combined)
      multiple G35
  concentric (Balo) G37.5
  cornea — *see* Opacity, cornea
  coronary (artery) I25.10
    with angina pectoris — *see* Arteriosclerosis, coronary (artery),
  corpus cavernosum
    female N90.89
    male N48.6
  diffuse (brain) (spinal cord) G37.0
  disseminated G35
  dorsal G35
  dorsolateral (spinal cord) — *see* Degeneration, combined
  endometrium N85.5
  extrapyramidal G25.9
  eye, nuclear (senile) — *see* Cataract, senile, nuclear
  focal and segmental (glomerular) (*see also* N00-N07 with fourth character .1) N05.1
  Friedreich's (spinal cord) G11.1
  funicular (spermatic cord) N50.8
  general (vascular) — *see* Arteriosclerosis
  gland (lymphatic) I89.8
  hepatic K74.1
    alcoholic K70.2

Sclerosis, sclerotic — *continued*
  hereditary
    cerebellar G11.9
    spinal (Friedreich's ataxia) G11.1
  hippocampal G93.81
  insular G35
  kidney — *see* Sclerosis, renal
  larynx J38.7
  lateral (amyotrophic) (descending) (primary) (spinal) G12.21
  lens, senile nuclear — *see* Cataract, senile, nuclear
  liver K74.1
    with fibrosis K74.2
      alcoholic K70.2
    alcoholic K70.2
    cardiac K76.1
  lung — *see* Fibrosis, lung
  mastoid — *see* Mastoiditis, chronic
  mesial temporal G93.81
  mitral I05.8
  Mönckeberg's (medial) — *see* Arteriosclerosis, extremities
  multiple (brain stem) (cerebral) (generalized) (spinal cord) G35
  myocardium, myocardial — *see* Disease, heart, ischemic, atherosclerotic
  nuclear (senile), eye — *see* Cataract, senile, nuclear
  ovary N83.8
  pancreas K86.8
  penis N48.6
  peripheral arteries — *see* Arteriosclerosis, extremities
  plaques G35
  pluriglandular E31.8
  polyglandular E31.8
  posterolateral (spinal cord) — *see* Degeneration, combined
  presenile (Alzheimer's) — *see* Disease, Alzheimer's, early onset
  primary, lateral G12.29
  progressive, systemic M34.0
  pulmonary — *see* Fibrosis, lung
    artery I27.0
    valve (heart) — *see* Endocarditis, pulmonary
  renal N26.9
    with
      cystine storage disease E72.09
      hypertensive heart disease (conditions in I11) — *see* Hypertension, cardiorenal
    arteriolar (hyaline) (hyperplastic) — *see* Hypertension, kidney
  retina (senile) (vascular) H35.00
  senile (vascular) — *see* Arteriosclerosis
  spinal (cord) (progressive) G95.89
    ascending G61.0
    combined (*see also* Degeneration, combined)
      multiple G35
      syphilitic A52.11
    disseminated G35
    dorsolateral — *see* Degeneration, combined
    hereditary (Friedreich's) (mixed form) G11.1
    lateral (amyotrophic) G12.21
    multiple G35
    posterior (syphilitic) A52.11
  stomach K31.89
  subendocardial, congenital I42.4
  systemic M34.9
    with
      lung involvement M34.81
      myopathy M34.82
      polyneuropathy M34.83
    drug-induced M34.2
    due to chemicals NEC M34.2
    progressive M34.0
    specified NEC M34.89
  temporal (mesial) G93.81
  tricuspid (heart) (valve) I07.8
  tuberous (brain) Q85.1
  tympanic membrane — *see* Disorder, tympanic membrane, specified NEC
  valve, valvular (heart) — *see* Endocarditis
  vascular — *see* Arteriosclerosis
  vein I87.8
Scoliosis (acquired) (postural) M41.9
  adolescent (idiopathic) — *see* Scoliosis, idiopathic, juvenile
  congenital Q67.5
    due to bony malformation Q76.3
    failure of segmentation (hemivertebra) Q76.3

Scoliosis — *continued*
  congenital — *continued*
    hemivertebra fusion Q76.3
    postural Q67.5
  idiopathic M41.20
    adolescent M41.129
      cervical region M41.122
      cervicothoracic region M41.123
      lumbar region M41.126
      lumbosacral region M41.127
      thoracic region M41.124
      thoracolumbar region M41.125
    cervical region M41.22
    cervicothoracic region M41.23
    infantile M41.00
      cervical region M41.02
      cervicothoracic region M41.03
      lumbar region M41.06
      lumbosacral region M41.07
      sacrococcygeal region M41.08
      thoracic region M41.04
      thoracolumbar region M41.05
    juvenile M41.119
      cervical region M41.112
      cervicothoracic region M41.113
      lumbar region M41.116
      lumbosacral region M41.117
      thoracic region M41.114
      thoracolumbar region M41.115
    lumbar region M41.26
    lumbosacral region M41.27
    thoracic region M41.24
    thoracolumbar region M41.25
  neuromuscular M41.40
    cervical region M41.42
    cervicothoracic region M41.43
    lumbar region M41.46
    lumbosacral region M41.47
    occipito-atlanto-axial region M41.41
    thoracic region M41.44
    thoracolumbar region M41.45
  paralytic — *see* Scoliosis, neuromuscular
  postradiation therapy M96.5
  rachitic (late effect or sequelae) E64.3 [M49.80]
    cervical region E64.3 [M49.82]
    cervicothoracic region E64.3 [M49.83]
    lumbar region E64.3 [M49.86]
    lumbosacral region E64.3 [M49.87]
    multiple sites E64.3 [M49.89]
    occipito-atlanto-axial region E64.3 [M49.81]
    sacrococcygeal region E64.3 [M49.88]
    thoracic region E64.3 [M49.84]
    thoracolumbar region E64.3 [M49.85]
  sciatic M54.4- ☑
  secondary (to) NEC M41.50
    cerebral palsy, Friedreich's ataxia, poliomyelitis, neuromuscular disorders — *see* Scoliosis, neuromuscular
    cervical region M41.52
    cervicothoracic region M41.53
    lumbar region M41.56
    lumbosacral region M41.57
    thoracic region M41.54
    thoracolumbar region M41.55
  specified form NEC M41.80
    cervical region M41.82
    cervicothoracic region M41.83
    lumbar region M41.86
    lumbosacral region M41.87
    thoracic region M41.84
    thoracolumbar region M41.85
  thoracogenic M41.30
    thoracic region M41.34
    thoracolumbar region M41.35
  tuberculous A18.01
Scoliotic pelvis
  with disproportion (fetopelvic) O33.0
    causing obstructed labor O65.0
Scorbutus, scorbutic (*see also* Scurvy)
  anemia D53.2
Scotoma (arcuate) (Bjerrum) (central) (ring) (*see also* Defect, visual field, localized, scotoma)
  scintillating H53.19
Scratch — *see* Abrasion
Scratchy throat R09.89
Screening (for) Z13.9
  alcoholism Z13.89
  anemia Z13.0

▽ Subterms under main terms may continue to next column or page   ☑ Additional Character Required — Refer to the Tabular List for Character Selection

Index

Screening — Seizure(s)

Screening — continued
anomaly, congenital Z13.89
antenatal, of mother Z36
arterial hypertension Z13.6
arthropod-borne viral disease NEC Z11.59
bacteriuria, asymptomatic Z13.89
behavioral disorder Z13.89
brain injury, traumatic Z13.850
bronchitis, chronic Z13.83
brucellosis Z11.2
cardiovascular disorder Z13.6
cataract Z13.5
chlamydial diseases Z11.8
cholera Z11.0
chromosomal abnormalities (nonprocreative) NEC
Z13.79
colonoscopy Z12.11
congenital
dislocation of hip Z13.89
eye disorder Z13.5
malformation or deformation Z13.89
contamination NEC Z13.88
cystic fibrosis Z13.228
dengue fever Z11.59
dental disorder Z13.84
depression Z13.89
developmental handicap Z13.4
in early childhood Z13.4
diabetes mellitus Z13.1
diphtheria Z11.2
disability, intellectual Z13.4
disease or disorder Z13.9
bacterial NEC Z11.2
intestinal infectious Z11.0
respiratory tuberculosis Z11.1
blood or blood-forming organ Z13.0
cardiovascular Z13.6
Chagas' Z11.6
chlamydial Z11.8
dental Z13.89
developmental Z13.4
digestive tract NEC Z13.818
lower GI Z13.811
upper GI Z13.810
ear Z13.5
endocrine Z13.29
eye Z13.5
genitourinary Z13.89
heart Z13.6
human immunodeficiency virus (HIV) infection
Z11.4
immunity Z13.0
infection
intestinal Z11.0
specified NEC Z11.6
infectious Z11.9
mental Z13.89
metabolic Z13.228
neurological Z13.89
nutritional Z13.21
metabolic Z13.228
lipoid disorders Z13.220
protozoal Z11.6
intestinal Z11.0
respiratory Z13.83
rheumatic Z13.828
rickettsial Z11.8
sexually-transmitted NEC Z11.3
human immunodeficiency virus (HIV) Z11.4
sickle-cell (trait) Z13.0
skin Z13.89
specified NEC Z13.89
spirochetal Z11.8
thyroid Z13.29
vascular Z13.6
venereal Z11.3
viral NEC Z11.59
human immunodeficiency virus (HIV) Z11.4
intestinal Z11.0
elevated titer Z13.89
emphysema Z13.83
encephalitis, viral (mosquito- or tick-borne) Z11.59
exposure to contaminants (toxic) Z13.88
fever
dengue Z11.59
hemorrhagic Z11.59
yellow Z11.59
filariasis Z11.6

Screening — continued
galactosemia Z13.228
gastrointestinal condition Z13.818
genetic (nonprocreative) - for procreative management — see Testing, genetic, for procreative
management
disease carrier status (nonprocreative) Z13.71
specified NEC (nonprocreative) Z13.79
genitourinary condition Z13.89
glaucoma Z13.5
gonorrhea Z11.3
gout Z13.89
helminthiasis (intestinal) Z11.6
hematopoietic malignancy Z12.89
hemoglobinopathies NEC Z13.0
hemorrhagic fever Z11.59
Hodgkin disease Z12.89
human immunodeficiency virus (HIV) Z11.4
human papillomavirus Z11.51
hypertension Z13.6
immunity disorders Z13.0
infection
mycotic Z11.8
parasitic Z11.8
ingestion of radioactive substance Z13.88
intellectual disability Z13.4
intestinal
helminthiasis Z11.6
infectious disease Z11.0
leishmaniasis Z11.6
leprosy Z11.2
leptospirosis Z11.8
leukemia Z12.89
lymphoma Z12.89
malaria Z11.6
malnutrition Z13.29
metabolic Z13.228
nutritional Z13.21
measles Z11.59
mental disorder Z13.89
metabolic errors, inborn Z13.228
multiphasic Z13.89
musculoskeletal disorder Z13.828
osteoporosis Z13.820
mycoses Z11.8
myocardial infarction (acute) Z13.6
neoplasm (malignant) (of) Z12.9
bladder Z12.6
blood Z12.89
breast Z12.39
routine mammogram Z12.31
cervix Z12.4
colon Z12.11
genitourinary organs NEC Z12.79
bladder Z12.6
cervix Z12.4
ovary Z12.73
prostate Z12.5
testis Z12.71
vagina Z12.72
hematopoietic system Z12.89
intestinal tract Z12.10
colon Z12.11
rectum Z12.12
small intestine Z12.13
lung Z12.2
lymph (glands) Z12.89
nervous system Z12.82
oral cavity Z12.81
prostate Z12.5
rectum Z12.12
respiratory organs Z12.2
skin Z12.83
small intestine Z12.13
specified site NEC Z12.89
stomach Z12.0
nephropathy Z13.89
nervous system disorders NEC Z13.858
neurological condition Z13.89
osteoporosis Z13.820
parasitic infestation Z11.9
specified NEC Z11.8
phenylketonuria Z13.228
plague Z11.2
poisoning (chemical) (heavy metal) Z13.88
poliomyelitis Z11.59
postnatal, chromosomal abnormalities Z13.89
prenatal, of mother Z36

Screening — continued
protozoal disease Z11.6
intestinal Z11.0
pulmonary tuberculosis Z11.1
radiation exposure Z13.88
respiratory condition Z13.83
respiratory tuberculosis Z11.1
rheumatoid arthritis Z13.828
rubella Z11.59
schistosomiasis Z11.6
sexually-transmitted disease NEC Z11.3
human immunodeficiency virus (HIV) Z11.4
sickle-cell disease or trait Z13.0
skin condition Z13.89
sleeping sickness Z11.6
special Z13.9
specified NEC Z13.89
syphilis Z11.3
tetanus Z11.2
trachoma Z11.8
traumatic brain injury Z13.850
trypanosomiasis Z11.6
tuberculosis, respiratory Z11.1
venereal disease Z11.3
viral encephalitis (mosquito- or tick-borne) Z11.59
whooping cough Z11.2
worms, intestinal Z11.6
yaws Z11.8
yellow fever Z11.59
Scrofula, scrofulosis (tuberculosis of cervical lymph
glands) A18.2
Scrofulide (primary) (tuberculous) A18.4
Scrofuloderma, scrofulodermia (any site) (primary)
A18.4
Scrofulosus lichen (primary) (tuberculous) A18.4
Scrofulous — see condition
Scrotal tongue K14.5
Scrotum — see condition
Scurvy, scorbutic E54
anemia D53.2
gum E54
infantile E54
rickets E55.0 [M90.80]
Sealpox B08.62
Seasickness T75.3 ☑
Seatworm (infection) (infestation) B80
Sebaceous (see also condition)
cyst — see Cyst, sebaceous
Seborrhea, seborrheic L21.9
capillitii R23.8
capitis L21.0
dermatitis L21.9
infantile L21.1
eczema L21.9
infantile L21.1
sicca L21.0
Seckel's syndrome Q87.1
Seclusion, pupil — see Membrane, pupillary
Second hand tobacco smoke exposure (acute)
(chronic) Z77.22
in the perinatal period P96.81
Secondary
dentin (in pulp) K04.3
neoplasm, secondaries — see Table of Neoplasms,
secondary
Secretion
antidiuretic hormone, inappropriate E22.2
catecholamine, by pheochromocytoma E27.5
hormone
antidiuretic, inappropriate (syndrome) E22.2
by
carcinoid tumor E34.0
pheochromocytoma E27.5
ectopic NEC E34.2
urinary
excessive R35.8
suppression R34
Section
nerve, traumatic — see Injury, nerve
Segmentation, incomplete (congenital) (see also Fusion)
bone NEC Q78.8
lumbosacral (joint) (vertebra) Q76.49
Seitelberger's syndrome (infantile neuraxonal dystrophy) G31.89
Seizure(s) (see also Convulsions) R56.9
akinetic — see Epilepsy, generalized, specified NEC
atonic — see Epilepsy, generalized, specified NEC

☑ **Additional Character Required** — Refer to the Tabular List for Character Selection   ▽ **Subterms under main terms may continue to next column or page**

Seizure(s) — *continued*
  autonomic (hysterical) F44.5
  convulsive — *see* Convulsions
  cortical (focal) (motor) — *see* Epilepsy, localization-
    related, symptomatic, with simple partial
    seizures
  disorder (*see also* Epilepsy) G40.909
  due to stroke — *see* Sequelae (of), disease, cerebrovas-
    cular, by type, specified NEC
  epileptic — *see* Epilepsy
  febrile (simple) R56.00
    with status epilepticus G40.901
    complex (atypical) (complicated) R56.01
      with status epilepticus G40.901
  grand mal G40.409
    intractable G40.419
      with status epilepticus G40.411
      without status epilepticus G40.419
    not intractable G40.409
      with status epilepticus G40.401
      without status epilepticus G40.409
  heart — *see* Disease, heart
  hysterical F44.5
  intractable G40.919
    with status epilepticus G40.911
  Jacksonian (focal) (motor type) (sensory type) — *see*
    Epilepsy, localization-related, symptomatic, with
    simple partial seizures
  newborn P90
  nonspecific epileptic
    atonic — *see* Epilepsy, generalized, specified NEC
    clonic — *see* Epilepsy, generalized, specified NEC
    myoclonic — *see* Epilepsy, generalized, specified
      NEC
    tonic — *see* Epilepsy, generalized, specified NEC
    tonic-clonic — *see* Epilepsy, generalized, specified
      NEC
  partial, developing into secondarily generalized
    seizures
    complex — *see* Epilepsy, localization-related,
      symptomatic, with complex partial seizures
    simple — *see* Epilepsy, localization-related, symp-
      tomatic, with simple partial seizures
  petit mal G40.409
    intractable G40.419
      with status epilepticus G40.411
      without status epilepticus G40.419
    not intractable G40.409
      with status epilepticus G40.401
      without status epilepticus G40.409
  post traumatic R56.1
  recurrent G40.909
  specified NEC G40.89
  uncinate — *see* Epilepsy, localization-related, symp-
    tomatic, with complex partial seizures
Selenium deficiency, dietary E59
Self-damaging behavior (life-style) Z72.89
Self-harm (attempted)
  history (personal) Z91.5
    in family Z81.8
Self-mutilation (attempted)
  history (personal) Z91.5
    in family Z81.8
Self-poisoning
  history (personal) Z91.5
    in family Z81.8
  observation following (alleged) attempt Z03.6
Semicoma R40.1
Seminal vesiculitis N49.0
Seminoma C62.9- ☑
  specified site — *see* Neoplasm, malignant, by site
Senear-Usher disease or syndrome L10.4
Senectus R54
Senescence (without mention of psychosis) R54
Senile, senility (*see also* condition) R41.81
  with
    acute confusional state F05
    mental changes NOS F03 ☑
    psychosis NEC — *see* Psychosis, senile
  asthenia R54
  cervix (atrophic) N88.8
  debility R54
  endometrium (atrophic) N85.8
  fallopian tube (atrophic) — *see* Atrophy, fallopian tube
  heart (failure) R54
  ovary (atrophic) — *see* Atrophy, ovary
  premature E34.8

Senile, senility — *continued*
  vagina, vaginitis (atrophic) N95.2
  wart L82.1
Sensation
  burning (skin) R20.8
    tongue K14.6
  loss of R20.8
  prickling (skin) R20.2
  tingling (skin) R20.2
Sense loss
  smell — *see* Disturbance, sensation, smell
  taste — *see* Disturbance, sensation, taste
  touch R20.8
Sensibility disturbance (cortical) (deep) (vibratory)
  R20.9
Sensitive, sensitivity (*see also* Allergy)
  carotid sinus G90.01
  child (excessive) F93.8
  cold, autoimmune D59.1
  dentin K03.89
  latex Z91.040
  methemoglobin D74.8
  tuberculin, without clinical or radiological symptoms
    R76.11
  visual
    glare H53.71
    impaired contrast H53.72
Sensitiver Beziehungswahn F22
Sensitization, auto-erythrocytic D69.2
Separation
  anxiety, abnormal (of childhood) F93.0
  apophysis, traumatic — *code as* Fracture, by site
  choroid — *see* Detachment, choroid
  epiphysis, epiphyseal
    nontraumatic (*see also* Osteochondropathy, speci-
      fied type NEC)
      upper femoral — *see* Slipped, epiphysis, upper
        femoral
    traumatic — *code as* Fracture, by site
  fracture — *see* Fracture
  infundibulum cardiac from right ventricle by a partition
    Q24.3
  joint (traumatic) (current) — *code by* site under Dislo-
    cation
  pubic bone, obstetrical trauma O71.6
  retina, retinal — *see* Detachment, retina
  symphysis pubis, obstetrical trauma O71.6
  tracheal ring, incomplete, congenital Q32.1
Sepsis (generalized) (unspecified organism) A41.9
  with
    organ dysfunction (acute) (multiple) R65.20
      with septic shock R65.21
  actinomycotic A42.7
  adrenal hemorrhage syndrome (meningococcal) A39.1
  anaerobic A41.4
  Bacillus anthracis A22.7
  Brucella (*see also* Brucellosis) A23.9
  candidal B37.7
  cryptogenic A41.9
  due to device, implant or graft T85.79 ☑
    arterial graft NEC T82.7 ☑
    breast (implant) T85.79 ☑
    catheter NEC T85.79 ☑
      dialysis (renal) T82.7 ☑
        intraperitoneal T85.71 ☑
      infusion NEC T82.7 ☑
        spinal (epidural) (subdural) T85.79 ☑
      urinary (indwelling) T83.51 ☑
    ectopic or molar pregnancy O08.82
    electronic (electrode) (pulse generator) (stimulator)
      bone T84.7 ☑
      cardiac T82.7 ☑
      nervous system (brain) (peripheral nerve)
        (spinal) T85.79 ☑
      urinary T83.59 ☑
    fixation, internal (orthopedic) — *see* Complication,
      fixation device, infection
    gastrointestinal (bile duct) (esophagus) T85.79 ☑
    genital T83.6 ☑
    heart NEC T82.7 ☑
      valve (prosthesis) T82.6 ☑
        graft T82.7 ☑
    joint prosthesis — *see* Complication, joint prosthe-
      sis, infection
    ocular (corneal graft) (orbital implant) T85.79 ☑
    orthopedic NEC T84.7 ☑

Sepsis — *continued*
  due to device, implant or graft — *continued*
    orthopedic — *continued*
      fixation device, internal — *see* Complication,
        fixation device, infection
    specified NEC T85.79 ☑
    vascular T82.7 ☑
    ventricular intracranial shunt T85.79 ☑
  during labor O75.3
  Enterococcus A41.81
  Erysipelothrix (rhusiopathiae) (erysipeloid) A26.7
  Escherichia coli (E. coli) A41.5 ☑
  extraintestinal yersiniosis A28.2
  following
    abortion (subsequent episode) O08.0
      current episode — *see* Abortion
    ectopic or molar pregnancy O08.82
    immunization T88.0 ☑
    infusion, therapeutic injection or transfusion NEC
      T80.29 ☑
  gangrenous A41.9
  gonococcal A54.86
  Gram-negative (organism) A41.5 ☑
    anaerobic A41.4
  Haemophilus influenzae A41.3
  herpesviral B00.7
  intra-abdominal K65.1
  intraocular — *see* Endophthalmitis, purulent
  Listeria monocytogenes A32.7
  localized — *code to* specific localized infection
    in operation wound T81.4 ☑
    skin — *see* Abscess
  malleus A24.0
  melioidosis A24.1
  meningeal — *see* Meningitis
  meningococcal A39.4
    acute A39.2
    chronic A39.3
  MSSA (Methicillin susceptible Staphylococcus aureus)
    A41.01
  newborn P36.9
    due to
      anaerobes NEC P36.5
      Escherichia coli P36.4
      Staphylococcus P36.30
        aureus P36.2
        specified NEC P36.39
      Streptococcus P36.10
        group B P36.0
        specified NEC P36.19
    specified NEC P36.8
  Pasteurella multocida A28.0
  pelvic, puerperal, postpartum, childbirth O85
  pneumococcal A40.3
  postprocedural T81.4 ☑
  puerperal, postpartum, childbirth (pelvic) O85
  Salmonella (arizonae) (cholerae-suis) (enteritidis) (ty-
    phimurium) A02.1
  severe R65.20
    with septic shock R65.21
  Shigella (*see also* Dysentery, bacillary) A03.9
  skin, localized — *see* Abscess
  specified organism NEC A41.89
  Staphylococcus, staphylococcal A41.2
    aureus (methicillin susceptible) (MSSA) A41.01
      methicillin resistant (MRSA) A41.02
    coagulase-negative A41.1
    specified NEC A41.1
  Streptococcus, streptococcal A40.9
    agalactiae A40.1
    group
      A A40.0
      B A40.1
      D A41.81
    neonatal P36.10
      group B P36.0
      specified NEC P36.19
    pneumoniae A40.3
    pyogenes A40.0
    specified NEC A40.8
  tracheostomy stoma J95.02
  tularemic A21.7
  umbilical, umbilical cord (newborn) — *see* Sepsis,
    newborn
  Yersinia pestis A20.7
Septate — *see* Septum
Septic — *see* condition
  arm — *see* Cellulitis, upper limb

Index

Septic — Sequelae

Septic — *continued*
  arm — *see* Cellulitis, upper limb — *continued*
    with lymphangitis — *see* Lymphangitis, acute,
      upper limb
  embolus — *see* Embolism
  finger — *see* Cellulitis, digit
    with lymphangitis — *see* Lymphangitis, acute,
      digit
  foot — *see* Cellulitis, lower limb
    with lymphangitis — *see* Lymphangitis, acute,
      lower limb
  gallbladder (acute) K81.0
  hand — *see* Cellulitis, upper limb
    with lymphangitis — *see* Lymphangitis, acute,
      upper limb
  joint — *see* Arthritis, pyogenic or pyemic
  leg — *see* Cellulitis, lower limb
    with lymphangitis — *see* Lymphangitis, acute,
      lower limb
  nail (*see also* Cellulitis, digit)
    with lymphangitis — *see* Lymphangitis, acute,
      digit
  sore (*see also* Abscess)
    throat J02.0
      streptococcal J02.0
  spleen (acute) D73.89
  teeth, tooth (pulpal origin) K04.4
  throat — *see* Pharyngitis
  thrombus — *see* Thrombosis
  toe — *see* Cellulitis, digit
    with lymphangitis — *see* Lymphangitis, acute,
      digit
  tonsils, chronic J35.01
    with adenoiditis J35.03
  uterus — *see* Endometritis
Septicemia A41.9
  meaning sepsis — *see* Sepsis
Septum, septate (congenital) (*see also* Anomaly, by site)
  anal Q42.3
    with fistula Q42.2
  aqueduct of Sylvius Q03.0
    with spina bifida — *see* Spina bifida, by site, with
      hydrocephalus
  uterus (complete) (partial) Q51.2
  vagina Q52.10
    in pregnancy — *see* Pregnancy, complicated by,
      abnormal vagina
      causing obstructed labor O65.5
    longitudinal (with or without obstruction) Q52.12
    transverse Q52.11
Sequelae (of) (*see also* condition)
  abscess, intracranial or intraspinal (conditions in G06)
    G09
  amputation — *code to* injury with seventh character
    S
  burn and corrosion — *code to* injury with seventh
    character S
  calcium deficiency E64.8
  cerebrovascular disease — *see* Sequelae, disease,
    cerebrovascular
  childbirth O94
  contusion — *code to* injury with seventh character S
  corrosion — *see* Sequelae, burn and corrosion
  crushing injury — *code to* injury with seventh charac-
    ter S
  disease
    cerebrovascular I69.90
      alteration of sensation I69.998
      aphasia I69.920
      apraxia I69.990
      ataxia I69.993
      cognitive deficits I69.91
      disturbance of vision I69.998
      dysarthria I69.922
      dysphagia I69.991
      dysphasia I69.921
      facial droop I69.992
      facial weakness I69.992
      fluency disorder I69.923
      hemiplegia I69.95- ☑
      hemorrhage
        intracerebral — *see* Sequelae, hemorrhage,
          intracerebral
        intracranial, nontraumatic NEC — *see* Seque-
          lae, hemorrhage, intracranial, nontrau-
          matic

Sequelae — *continued*
  disease — *continued*
    cerebrovascular — *continued*
      hemorrhage — *continued*
        subarachnoid — *see* Sequelae, hemorrhage,
          subarachnoid
      language deficit I69.928
      monoplegia
        lower limb I69.84- ☑
        upper limb I69.93- ☑
      paralytic syndrome I69.96- ☑
      specified effect NEC I69.998
      specified type NEC I69.80
        alteration of sensation I69.898
        aphasia I69.820
        apraxia I69.890
        ataxia I69.893
        cognitive deficits I69.81
        disturbance of vision I69.898
        dysarthria I69.822
        dysphagia I69.891
        dysphasia I69.821
        facial droop I69.892
        facial weakness I69.892
        fluency disorder I69.823
        hemiplegia I69.85- ☑
        language deficit I69.828
        monoplegia
          lower limb I69.84- ☑
          upper limb I69.83- ☑
        paralytic syndrome I69.86- ☑
        specified effect NEC I69.898
      speech deficit I69.928
        speech deficit I69.828
      stroke NOS — *see* Sequelae, stroke NOS
    dislocation — *code to* injury with seventh character S
    encephalitis or encephalomyelitis (conditions in G04)
      G09
      in infectious disease NEC B94.8
      viral B94.1
    external cause — *code to* injury with seventh character
      S
    foreign body entering natural orifice — *code to* injury
      with seventh character S
    fracture — *code to* injury with seventh character S
    frostbite — *code to* injury with seventh character S
    Hansen's disease B92
    hemorrhage
      intracerebral I69.10
        alteration of sensation I69.198
        aphasia I69.120
        apraxia I69.190
        ataxia I69.193
        cognitive deficits I69.11
        disturbance of vision I69.198
        dysarthria I69.122
        dysphagia I69.191
        dysphasia I69.121
        facial droop I69.192
        facial weakness I69.192
        fluency disorder I69.123
        hemiplegia I69.15- ☑
        language deficit NEC I69.128
        monoplegia
          lower limb I69.14- ☑
          upper limb I69.13- ☑
        paralytic syndrome I69.16- ☑
        specified effect NEC I69.198
        speech deficit NEC I69.128
      intracranial, nontraumatic NEC I69.20
        alteration of sensation I69.298
        aphasia I69.220
        apraxia I69.290
        ataxia I69.293
        cognitive deficits I69.21
        disturbance of vision I69.298
        dysarthria I69.222
        dysphagia I69.291
        dysphasia I69.221
        facial droop I69.292
        facial weakness I69.292
        fluency disorder I69.223
        hemiplegia I69.25- ☑
        language deficit NEC I69.228
        monoplegia
          lower limb I69.24- ☑
          upper limb I69.23- ☑
        paralytic syndrome I69.26- ☑

Sequelae — *continued*
  hemorrhage — *continued*
    intracranial, nontraumatic — *continued*
      specified effect NEC I69.298
      speech deficit NEC I69.228
    subarachnoid I69.00
      alteration of sensation I69.098
      aphasia I69.020
      apraxia I69.090
      ataxia I69.093
      cognitive deficits I69.01
      disturbance of vision I69.098
      dysarthria I69.022
      dysphagia I69.091
      dysphasia I69.021
      facial droop I69.092
      facial weakness I69.092
      fluency disorder I69.023
      hemiplegia I69.05- ☑
      language deficit NEC I69.028
      monoplegia
        lower limb I69.04- ☑
        upper limb I69.03- ☑
      paralytic syndrome I69.06- ☑
      specified effect NEC I69.098
      speech deficit NEC I69.028
  hepatitis, viral B94.2
  hyperalimentation E68
  infarction
    cerebral I69.30
      alteration of sensation I69.398
      aphasia I69.320
      apraxia I69.390
      ataxia I69.393
      cognitive deficits I69.31
      disturbance of vision I69.398
      dysarthria I69.322
      dysphagia I69.391
      dysphasia I69.321
      facial droop I69.392
      facial weakness I69.392
      fluency disorder I69.323
      hemiplegia I69.35- ☑
      language deficit NEC I69.328
      monoplegia
        lower limb I69.34- ☑
        upper limb I69.33- ☑
      paralytic syndrome I69.36- ☑
      specified effect NEC I69.398
      speech deficit NEC I69.328
  infection, pyogenic, intracranial or intraspinal G09
  infectious disease B94.9
    specified NEC B94.8
  injury — *code to* injury with seventh character S
  leprosy B92
  meningitis
    bacterial (conditions in G00) G09
    other or unspecified cause (conditions in G03) G09
  muscle (and tendon) injury — *code to* injury with
    seventh character S
  myelitis — *see* Sequelae, encephalitis
  niacin deficiency E64.8
  nutritional deficiency E64.9
    specified NEC E64.8
  obstetrical condition O94
  parasitic disease B94.9
  phlebitis or thrombophlebitis of intracranial or in-
    traspinal venous sinuses and veins (conditions
    in G08) G09
  poisoning — *code to* poisoning with seventh character
    S
    nonmedicinal substance — *see* Sequelae, toxic ef-
      fect, nonmedicinal substance
  poliomyelitis (acute) B91
  pregnancy O94
  protein-energy malnutrition E64.0
  puerperium O94
  rickets E64.3
  selenium deficiency E64.8
  sprain and strain — *code to* injury with seventh char-
    acter S
  stroke NOS I69.30
    alteration in sensation I69.398
    aphasia I69.320
    apraxia I69.390
    ataxia I69.393
    cognitive deficits I69.31
    disturbance of vision I69.398

Sequelae — *continued*
  stroke — *continued*
    dysarthria I69.322
    dysphagia I69.391
    dysphasia I69.321
    facial droop I69.392
    facial weakness I69.392
    hemiplegia I69.35- ☑
    language deficit NEC I69.328
    monoplegia
      lower limb I69.34- ☑
      upper limb I69.33- ☑
    paralytic syndrome I69.36- ☑
    specified effect NEC I69.398
    speech deficit NEC I69.328
  tendon and muscle injury — *code to* injury with seventh character S
  thiamine deficiency E64.8
  trachoma B94.0
  tuberculosis B90.9
    bones and joints B90.2
    central nervous system B90.0
    genitourinary B90.1
    pulmonary (respiratory) B90.9
    specified organs NEC B90.8
  viral
    encephalitis B94.1
    hepatitis B94.2
  vitamin deficiency NEC E64.8
    A E64.1
    B E64.8
    C E64.2
  wound, open — *code to* injury with seventh character S
Sequestration (*see also* Sequestrum)
  lung, congenital Q33.2
Sequestrum
  bone — *see* Osteomyelitis, chronic
  dental M27.2
  jaw bone M27.2
  orbit — *see* Osteomyelitis, orbit
  sinus (accessory) (nasal) — *see* Sinusitis
Sequoiosis lung or pneumonitis J67.8
Serology for syphilis
  doubtful
    with signs or symptoms — *code by* site and stage under Syphilis
    follow-up of latent syphilis — *see* Syphilis, latent
  negative, with signs or symptoms — *code by* site and stage under Syphilis
  positive A53.0
    with signs or symptoms — *code by* site and stage under Syphilis
  reactivated A53.0
Seroma (*see also* Hematoma)
  traumatic, secondary and recurrent T79.2 ☑
Seropurulent — *see* condition
Serositis, multiple K65.8
  pericardial I31.1
  peritoneal K65.8
Serous — *see* condition
Sertoli cell
  adenoma
    specified site — *see* Neoplasm, benign, by site
    unspecified site
      female D27.9
      male D29.20
  carcinoma
    specified site — *see* Neoplasm, malignant, by site
    unspecified site (male) C62.9- ☑
      female C56.9
  tumor
    with lipid storage
      specified site — *see* Neoplasm, benign, by site
      unspecified site
        female D27.9
        male D29.20
    specified site — *see* Neoplasm, benign, by site
    unspecified site
      female D27.9
      male D29.20
Sertoli-Leydig cell tumor — *see* Neoplasm, benign, by site
  specified site — *see* Neoplasm, benign, by site
  unspecified site
    female D27.9
    male D29.20

Serum
  allergy, allergic reaction (*see also* Reaction, serum) T80.69 ☑
    shock (*see also* Shock, anaphylactic) T80.59 ☑
  arthritis (*see also* Reaction, serum) T80.69 ☑
  complication or reaction NEC (*see also* Reaction, serum) T80.69 ☑
  disease NEC (*see also* Reaction, serum) T80.69 ☑
  hepatitis (*see also* Hepatitis, viral, type B)
    carrier (suspected) of Z22.51
  intoxication (*see also* Reaction, serum) T80.69 ☑
  neuritis (*see also* Reaction, serum) T80.69 ☑
  neuropathy G61.1
  poisoning NEC (*see also* Reaction, serum) T80.69 ☑
  rash NEC (*see also* Reaction, serum) T80.69 ☑
  reaction NEC (*see also* Reaction, serum) T80.69 ☑
  sickness NEC (*see also* Reaction, serum) T80.69 ☑
  urticaria (*see also* Reaction, serum) T80.69 ☑
Sesamoiditis M25.8- ☑
Severe sepsis R65.20
  with septic shock R65.21
Sever's disease or osteochondrosis — *see* Osteochondrosis, juvenile, tarsus
Sex
  chromosome mosaics Q97.8
    lines with various numbers of X chromosomes Q97.2
  education Z70.8
  reassignment surgery status Z87.890
Sextuplet pregnancy — *see* Pregnancy, sextuplet
Sexual
  function, disorder of (psychogenic) F52.9
  immaturity (female) (male) E30.0
  impotence (psychogenic) organic origin NEC — *see* Dysfunction, sexual, male
  precocity (constitutional) (cryptogenic)(female) (idiopathic) (male) E30.1
Sexuality, pathologic — *see* Deviation, sexual
Sézary disease C84.1- ☑
Shadow, lung R91.8
Shaking palsy or paralysis — *see* Parkinsonism
Shallowness, acetabulum — *see* Derangement, joint, specified type NEC, hip
Shaver's disease J63.1
Sheath (tendon) — *see* condition
Sheathing, retinal vessels H35.01- ☑
Shedding
  nail L60.8
  premature, primary (deciduous) teeth K00.6
Sheehan's disease or syndrome E23.0
Shelf, rectal K62.89
Shell teeth K00.5
Shellshock (current) F43.0
  lasting state — *see* Disorder, post-traumatic stress
Shield kidney Q63.1
Shift
  auditory threshold (temporary) H93.24- ☑
  mediastinal R93.8
Shifting sleep-work schedule (affecting sleep) G47.26
Shiga (-Kruse) **dysentery** A03.0
Shiga's bacillus A03.0
Shigella (dysentery) — *see* Dysentery, bacillary
Shigellosis A03.9
  Group A A03.0
  Group B A03.1
  Group C A03.2
  Group D A03.3
Shin splints S86.89- ☑
Shingles — *see* Herpes, zoster
Shipyard disease or eye B30.0
Shirodkar suture, in pregnancy — *see* Pregnancy, complicated by, incompetent cervix
Shock R57.9
  with ectopic or molar pregnancy O08.3
  adrenal (cortical) (Addisonian) E27.2
  adverse food reaction (anaphylactic) — *see* Shock, anaphylactic, due to food
  allergic — *see* Shock, anaphylactic
  anaphylactic T78.2 ☑
    chemical — *see* Table of Drugs and Chemicals
    due to drug or medicinal substance
      correct substance properly administered T88.6 ☑
      overdose or wrong substance given or taken (by accident) — *see* Table of Drugs and Chemicals, by drug, poisoning

Shock — *continued*
  anaphylactic — *continued*
    due to food (nonpoisonous) T78.00 ☑
      additives T78.06 ☑
      dairy products T78.07 ☑
      eggs T78.08 ☑
      fish T78.03 ☑
        shellfish T78.02 ☑
      fruit T78.04 ☑
      milk T78.07 ☑
      nuts T78.05 ☑
        peanuts T78.01 ☑
      peanuts T78.01 ☑
      seeds T78.05 ☑
      specified type NEC T78.09 ☑
      vegetable T78.04 ☑
    following sting(s) — *see* Venom
    immunization T80.52 ☑
    serum T80.59 ☑
      blood and blood products T80.51 ☑
      immunization T80.52 ☑
      specified NEC T80.59 ☑
      vaccination T80.52 ☑
  anaphylactoid — *see* Shock, anaphylactic
  anesthetic
    correct substance properly administered T88.2 ☑
    overdose or wrong substance given or taken — *see* Table of Drugs and Chemicals, by drug, poisoning
    specified anesthetic — *see* Table of Drugs and Chemicals, by drug, poisoning
  cardiogenic R57.0
  chemical substance — *see* Table of Drugs and Chemicals
  complicating ectopic or molar pregnancy O08.3
  culture — *see* Disorder, adjustment
  drug
    due to correct substance properly administered T88.6 ☑
    overdose or wrong substance given or taken (by accident) — *see* Table of Drugs and Chemicals, by drug, poisoning
  during or after labor and delivery O75.1
  electric T75.4 ☑
    (taser) T75.4 ☑
  endotoxic R65.21
    postprocedural (during or resulting from a procedure, not elsewhere classified) T81.12 ☑
  following
    ectopic or molar pregnancy O08.3
    injury (immediate) (delayed) T79.4 ☑
    labor and delivery O75.1
  food (anaphylactic) — *see* Shock, anaphylactic, due to food
  from electroshock gun (taser) T75.4 ☑
  gram-negative R65.21
    postprocedural (during or resulting from a procedure, not elsewhere classified) T81.12 ☑
  hematologic R57.8
  hemorrhagic
    surgery (intraoperative) (postoperative) T81.19 ☑
    trauma T79.4 ☑
  hypovolemic R57.1
    surgical T81.19 ☑
    traumatic T79.4 ☑
  insulin E15
    therapeutic misadventure — *see* subcategory T38.3 ☑
  kidney N17.0
    traumatic (following crushing) T79.5 ☑
  lightning T75.01 ☑
  lung J80
  obstetric O75.1
    with ectopic or molar pregnancy O08.3
    following ectopic or molar pregnancy O08.3
  pleural (surgical) T81.19 ☑
    due to trauma T79.4 ☑
  postprocedural (postoperative) T81.10 ☑
    with ectopic or molar pregnancy O08.3
    cardiogenic T81.11 ☑
    endotoxic T81.12 ☑
    following ectopic or molar pregnancy O08.3
    gram-negative T81.12 ☑
    hypovolemic T81.19 ☑
    septic T81.12 ☑
    specified type NEC T81.19 ☑

Shock — *continued*
- psychic F43.Ø
- septic (due to severe sepsis) R65.21
- specified NEC R57.8
- surgical T81.1Ø ☑
- taser gun (taser) T75.4 ☑
- therapeutic misadventure NEC T81.1Ø ☑
- thyroxin
  - overdose or wrong substance given or taken — *see* Table of Drugs and Chemicals, by drug, poisoning
- toxic, syndrome A48.3
- transfusion — *see* Complications, transfusion
- traumatic (immediate) (delayed) T79.4 ☑

Shoemaker's chest M95.4

Short, shortening, shortness
- arm (acquired) (*see also* Deformity, limb, unequal length)
  - congenital Q71.81- ☑
  - forearm — *see* Deformity, limb, unequal length
- bowel syndrome K91.2
- breath RØ6.Ø2
- cervical (complicating pregnancy) O26.87- ☑
  - non-gravid uterus N88.3
- common bile duct, congenital Q44.5
- cord (umbilical), complicating delivery O69.3 ☑
- cystic duct, congenital Q44.5
- esophagus (congenital) Q39.8
- femur (acquired) — *see* Deformity, limb, unequal length, femur
  - congenital — *see* Defect, reduction, lower limb, longitudinal, femur
- frenum, frenulum, linguae (congenital) Q38.1
- hip (acquired) (*see also* Deformity, limb, unequal length)
  - congenital Q65.89
- leg (acquired) (*see also* Deformity, limb, unequal length)
  - congenital Q72.81- ☑
  - lower leg (*see also* Deformity, limb, unequal length)
- limbed stature, with immunodeficiency D82.2
- lower limb (acquired) (*see also* Deformity, limb, unequal length)
  - congenital Q72.81- ☑
- organ or site, congenital NEC — *see* Distortion
- palate, congenital Q38.5
- radius (acquired) (*see also* Deformity, limb, unequal length)
  - congenital — *see* Defect, reduction, upper limb, longitudinal, radius
- rib syndrome Q77.2
- stature (child) (hereditary) (idiopathic) NEC R62.52
  - constitutional E34.3
  - due to endocrine disorder E34.3
  - Laron-type E34.3
- tendon (*see also* Contraction, tendon)
  - with contracture of joint — *see* Contraction, joint
  - Achilles (acquired) M67.Ø- ☑
    - congenital Q66.89
  - congenital Q79.8
- thigh (acquired) (*see also* Deformity, limb, unequal length, femur)
  - congenital — *see* Defect, reduction, lower limb, longitudinal, femur
- tibialis anterior (tendon) — *see* Contraction, tendon
- umbilical cord
  - complicating delivery O69.3 ☑
- upper limb, congenital — *see* Defect, reduction, upper limb, specified type NEC
- urethra N36.8
- uvula, congenital Q38.5
- vagina (congenital) Q52.4

Shortsightedness — *see* Myopia

Shoshin (acute fulminating beriberi) E51.11

Shoulder — *see* condition

Shovel-shaped incisors KØØ.2

Shower, thromboembolic — *see* Embolism

Shunt
- arterial-venous (dialysis) Z99.2
- arteriovenous, pulmonary (acquired) I28.Ø
  - congenital Q25.72
- cerebral ventricle (communicating) in situ Z98.2
- surgical, prosthetic, with complications — *see* Complications, cardiovascular, device or implant

Shutdown, renal N28.9

Shy-Drager syndrome G9Ø.3

Sialadenitis, sialadenosis (any gland) (chronic) (periodic) (suppurative) — *see* Sialoadenitis

Sialectasia K11.8

Sialidosis E77.1

Sialitis, silitis (any gland) (chronic) (suppurative) — *see* Sialoadenitis

Sialoadenitis (any gland) (periodic) (suppurative) K11.2Ø
- acute K11.21
  - recurrent K11.22
- chronic K11.23

Sialoadenopathy K11.9

Sialoangitis — *see* Sialoadenitis

Sialodochitis (fibrinosa) — *see* Sialoadenitis

Sialodocholithiasis K11.5

Sialolithiasis K11.5

Sialometaplasia, necrotizing K11.8

Sialorrhea (*see also* Ptyalism)
- periodic — *see* Sialoadenitis

Sialosis K11.7

Siamese twin Q89.4

Sibling rivalry Z62.891

Sicard's syndrome G52.7

Sicca syndrome M35.ØØ
- with
  - keratoconjunctivitis M35.Ø1
  - lung involvement M35.Ø2
  - myopathy M35.Ø3
  - renal tubulo-interstitial disorders M35.Ø4
- specified organ involvement NEC M35.Ø9

Sick R69
- or handicapped person in family Z63.79
  - needing care at home Z63.6
- sinus (syndrome) I49.5

Sick-euthyroid syndrome EØ7.81

Sickle-cell
- anemia — *see* Disease, sickle-cell
- trait D57.3

Sicklemia (*see also* Disease, sickle-cell)
- trait D57.3

Sickness
- air (travel) T75.3 ☑
- airplane T75.3 ☑
- alpine T7Ø.29 ☑
- altitude T7Ø.2Ø ☑
- Andes T7Ø.29 ☑
- aviator's T7Ø.29 ☑
- balloon T7Ø.29 ☑
- car T75.3 ☑
- compressed air T7Ø.3 ☑
- decompression T7Ø.3 ☑
- green D5Ø.8
- milk — *see* Poisoning, food, noxious
- motion T75.3 ☑
- mountain T7Ø.29 ☑
  - acute D75.1
- protein (*see also* Reaction, serum) T8Ø.69 ☑
- radiation T66
- roundabout (motion) T75.3 ☑
- sea T75.3 ☑
- serum NEC (*see also* Reaction, serum) T8Ø.69 ☑
- sleeping (African) B56.9
  - by Trypanosoma B56.9
    - brucei
      - gambiense B56.Ø
      - rhodesiense B56.1
    - East African B56.1
    - Gambian B56.Ø
    - Rhodesian B56.1
    - West African B56.Ø
- swing (motion) T75.3 ☑
- train (railway) (travel) T75.3 ☑
- travel (any vehicle) T75.3 ☑

Sideropenia — *see* Anemia, iron deficiency

Siderosilicosis J62.8

Siderosis (lung) J63.4
- eye (globe) — *see* Disorder, globe, degenerative, siderosis

Siemens' syndrome (ectodermal dysplasia) Q82.8

Sighing RØ6.89
- psychogenic F45.8

Sigmoid (*see also* condition)
- flexure — *see* condition
- kidney Q63.1

Sigmoiditis (*see also* Enteritis) K52.9
- infectious AØ9
- noninfectious K52.9

Silfversköld's syndrome Q78.9

Silicosiderosis J62.8

Silicosis, silicotic (simple) (complicated) J62.8
- with tuberculosis J65

Silicotuberculosis J65

Silo-fillers' disease J68.8
- bronchitis J68.Ø
- pneumonitis J68.Ø
- pulmonary edema J68.1

Silver's syndrome Q87.1

Simian malaria B53.1

Simmonds' cachexia or disease E23.Ø

Simons' disease or syndrome (progressive lipodystrophy) E88.1

Simple, simplex — *see* condition

Simulation, conscious (of illness) Z76.5

Simultanagnosia (asimultagnosia) R48.3

Sin Nombre virus disease (Hantavirus) (cardio)-pulmonary syndrome) B33.4

Sinding-Larsen disease or osteochondrosis — *see* Osteochondrosis, juvenile, patella

Singapore hemorrhagic fever A91

Singer's node or nodule J38.2

Single
- atrium Q21.2
- coronary artery Q24.5
- umbilical artery Q27.Ø
- ventricle Q2Ø.4

Singultus RØ6.6
- epidemicus B33.Ø

Sinus (*see also* Fistula)
- abdominal K63.89
- arrest I45.5
- arrhythmia I49.8
- bradycardia RØØ.1
- branchial cleft (internal) (external) Q18.Ø
- coccygeal — *see* Sinus, pilonidal
- dental KØ4.6
- dermal (congenital) QØ6.8
  - with abscess QØ6.8
  - coccygeal, pilonidal — *see* Sinus, coccygeal
- infected, skin NEC LØ8.89
- marginal, ruptured or bleeding — *see* Hemorrhage, antepartum, specified cause NEC
- medial, face and neck Q18.8
- pause I45.5
- pericranii QØ1.9
- pilonidal (infected) (rectum) LØ5.92
  - with abscess LØ5.Ø2
- preauricular Q18.1
- rectovaginal N82.3
- Rokitansky-Aschoff (gallbladder) K82.8
- sacrococcygeal (dermoid) (infected) — *see* Sinus, pilonidal
- tachycardia RØØ.Ø
  - paroxysmal I47.1
- tarsi syndrome M25.57- ☑
- testis N5Ø.8
- tract (postinfective) — *see* Fistula
- urachus Q64.4

Sinusitis (accessory) (chronic) (hyperplastic) (nasal) (nonpurulent) (purulent) J32.9
- acute JØ1.9Ø
  - ethmoidal JØ1.2Ø
    - recurrent JØ1.21
  - frontal JØ1.1Ø
    - recurrent JØ1.11
  - involving more than one sinus, other than pansinusitis JØ1.8Ø
    - recurrent JØ1.81
  - maxillary JØ1.ØØ
    - recurrent JØ1.Ø1
  - pansinusitis JØ1.4Ø
    - recurrent JØ1.41
  - recurrent JØ1.91
  - specified NEC JØ1.8Ø
    - recurrent JØ1.81
  - sphenoidal JØ1.3Ø
    - recurrent JØ1.31
- allergic — *see* Rhinitis, allergic
- due to high altitude T7Ø.1 ☑
- ethmoidal J32.2
  - acute JØ1.2Ø
    - recurrent JØ1.21
- frontal J32.1
  - acute JØ1.1Ø
    - recurrent JØ1.11
- influenzal — *see* Influenza, with, respiratory manifestations NEC

Sinusitis — *continued*
  involving more than one sinus but not pansinusitis
    J32.8
    acute J01.80
      recurrent J01.81
  maxillary J32.0
    acute J01.00
      recurrent J01.01
  sphenoidal J32.3
    acute J01.30
      recurrent J01.31
  tuberculous, any sinus A15.8
Sinusitis-bronchiectasis-situs inversus (syndrome)
  (triad) Q89.3
Sipple's syndrome E31.22
Sirenomelia (syndrome) Q87.2
Siriasis T67.0 ☑
Sirkari's disease B55.0
Siti A65
Situation, psychiatric F99
Situational
  disturbance (transient) — *see* Disorder, adjustment
    acute F43.0
  maladjustment — *see* Disorder, adjustment
  reaction — *see* Disorder, adjustment
    acute F43.0
Situs inversus or transversus (abdominalis) (thoracis)
  Q89.3
Sixth disease B08.20
  due to human herpesvirus 6 B08.21
  due to human herpesvirus 7 B08.22
Sjögren-Larsson syndrome Q87.1
Sjögren's syndrome or disease — *see* Sicca syndrome
Skeletal — *see* condition
Skene's gland — *see* condition
Skenitis — *see* Urethritis
Skerljevo A65
Skevas-Zerfus disease — *see* Toxicity, venom, marine
    animal, sea anemone
Skin (*see also* condition)
  clammy R23.1
  donor — *see* Donor, skin
  hidebound M35.9
Slate-dressers' or slate-miners' lung J62.8
Sleep
  apnea — *see* Apnea, sleep
  deprivation Z72.820
  disorder or disturbance G47.9
    child F51.9
    nonorganic origin F51.9
    specified NEC G47.8
  disturbance G47.9
    nonorganic origin F51.9
  drunkenness F51.9
  rhythm inversion G47.2- ☑
  terrors F51.4
  walking F51.3
    hysterical F44.89
Sleep hygiene
  abuse Z72.821
  inadequate Z72.821
  poor Z72.821
Sleep-wake schedule disorder G47.20
Sleeping sickness — *see* Sickness, sleeping
Sleeplessness — *see* Insomnia
  menopausal N95.1
Slim disease (in HIV infection) B20
Slipped, slipping
  epiphysis (traumatic) (*see also* Osteochondropathy,
      specified type NEC)
    capital femoral (traumatic)
      acute (on chronic) S79.01- ☑
    current traumatic — *code as* Fracture, by site
    upper femoral (nontraumatic) M93.00- ☑
      acute M93.01- ☑
        on chronic M93.03- ☑
      chronic M93.02- ☑
  intervertebral disc — *see* Displacement, intervertebral
      disc
  ligature, umbilical P51.8
  patella — *see* Disorder, patella, derangement NEC
  rib M89.8X8
  sacroiliac joint — *see* subcategory M53.2 ☑
  tendon — *see* Disorder, tendon
  ulnar nerve, nontraumatic — *see* Lesion, nerve, ulnar
  vertebra NEC — *see* Spondylolisthesis
Slocumb's syndrome E27.0

Sloughing (multiple) (phagedena) (skin) (*see also* Gan-
    grene)
  abscess — *see* Abscess
  appendix K38.8
  fascia — *see* Disorder, soft tissue, specified type NEC
  scrotum N50.8
  tendon — *see* Disorder, tendon
  transplanted organ — *see* Rejection, transplant
  ulcer — *see* Ulcer, skin
Slow
  feeding, newborn P92.2
  flow syndrome, coronary I20.8
  heart (beat) R00.1
Slowing, urinary stream R39.19
Sluder's neuralgia (syndrome) G44.89
Slurred, slurring speech R47.81
Small (ness)
  for gestational age — *see* Small for dates
  introitus, vagina N89.6
  kidney (unknown cause) N27.9
    bilateral N27.1
    unilateral N27.0
  ovary (congenital) Q50.39
  pelvis
    with disproportion (fetopelvic) O33.1
      causing obstructed labor O65.1
  uterus N85.8
  white kidney N03.9
Small-and-light-for-dates — *see* Small for dates
Small-for-dates (infant) P05.10
  with weight of
    500-749 grams P05.12
    750-999 grams P05.13
    1000-1249 grams P05.14
    1250-1499 grams P05.15
    1500-1749 grams P05.16
    1750-1999 grams P05.17
    2000-2499 grams P05.18
    499 grams or less P05.11
Smallpox B03
Smearing, fecal R15.1
Smith-Lemli-Opitz syndrome E78.72
Smith's fracture S52.54- ☑
Smoker — *see* Dependence, drug, nicotine
Smoker's
  bronchitis J41.0
  cough J41.0
  palate K13.24
  throat J31.2
  tongue K13.24
Smoking
  passive Z77.22
Smothering spells R06.81
Snaggle teeth, tooth M26.39
Snapping
  finger — *see* Trigger finger
  hip — *see* Derangement, joint, specified type NEC, hip
    involving the iliotibial band M76.3- ☑
  knee — *see* Derangement, knee
    involving the iliotibial band M76.3- ☑
Sneddon-Wilkinson disease or syndrome (sub-corneal
    pustular dermatosis) L13.1
Sneezing (intractable) R06.7
Sniffing
  cocaine
    abuse — *see* Abuse, drug, cocaine
    dependence — *see* Dependence, drug, cocaine
  gasoline
    abuse — *see* Abuse, drug, inhalant
    dependence — *see* Dependence, drug, inhalant
  glue (airplane)
    abuse — *see* Abuse, drug, inhalant
    drug dependence — *see* Dependence, drug, in-
        halant
Sniffles
  newborn P28.89
Snoring R06.83
Snow blindness — *see* Photokeratitis
Snuffles (non-syphilitic) R06.5
  newborn P28.89
  syphilitic (infant) A50.05 [J99]
Social
  exclusion Z60.4
    due to discrimination or persecution (perceived)
        Z60.5
  migrant Z59.0
    acculturation difficulty Z60.3

Social — *continued*
  rejection Z60.4
    due to discrimination or persecution Z60.5
  role conflict NEC Z73.5
  skills inadequacy NEC Z73.4
  transplantation Z60.3
Sodoku A25.0
Soemmerring's ring — *see* Cataract, secondary
Soft (*see also* condition)
  nails L60.3
Softening
  bone — *see* Osteomalacia
  brain (necrotic) (progressive) G93.89
    congenital Q04.8
    embolic I63.4 ☑
    hemorrhagic — *see* Hemorrhage, intracranial, in-
        tracerebral
    occlusive I63.5 ☑
    thrombotic I63.3 ☑
  cartilage M94.2- ☑
    patella M22.4- ☑
  cerebellar — *see* Softening, brain
  cerebral — *see* Softening, brain
  cerebrospinal — *see* Softening, brain
  myocardial, heart — *see* Degeneration, myocardial
  spinal cord G95.89
  stomach K31.89
Soldier's
  heart F45.8
  patches I31.0
Solitary
  cyst, kidney N28.1
  kidney, congenital Q60.0
Solvent abuse — *see* Abuse, drug, inhalant
  dependence — *see* Dependence, drug, inhalant
Somatization reaction, somatic reaction — *see* Disor-
    der, somatoform
Somnambulism F51.3
  hysterical F44.89
Somnolence R40.0
  nonorganic origin F51.11
Sonne dysentery A03.3
Soor B37.0
Sore
  bed — *see* Ulcer, pressure, by site
  chiclero B55.1
  Delhi B55.1
  desert — *see* Ulcer, skin
  eye H57.1- ☑
  Lahore B55.1
  mouth K13.79
    canker K12.0
  muscle M79.1
  Naga — *see* Ulcer, skin
  of skin — *see* Ulcer, skin
  oriental B55.1
  pressure — *see* Ulcer, pressure, by site
  skin L98.9
  soft A57
  throat (acute) (*see also* Pharyngitis)
    with influenza, flu, or grippe — *see* Influenza, with,
        respiratory manifestations NEC
    chronic J31.2
    coxsackie (virus) B08.5
    diphtheritic A36.0
    herpesviral B00.2
    influenzal — *see* Influenza, with, respiratory mani-
        festations NEC
    septic J02.0
    streptococcal (ulcerative) J02.0
    viral NEC J02.8
      coxsackie B08.5
    tropical — *see* Ulcer, skin
    veldt — *see* Ulcer, skin
Soto's syndrome (cerebral gigantism) Q87.3
South African cardiomyopathy syndrome I42.8
Southeast Asian hemorrhagic fever A91
Spacing
  abnormal, tooth, teeth, fully erupted M26.30
  excessive, tooth, fully erupted M26.32
Spade-like hand (congenital) Q68.1
Spading nail L60.8
  congenital Q84.6
Spanish collar N47.1
Sparganosis B70.1
Spasm(s), spastic, spasticity (*see also* condition) R25.2
  accommodation — *see* Spasm, of accommodation

Spasm(s), spastic, spasticity — *continued*
- ampulla of Vater K83.4
- anus, ani (sphincter) (reflex) K59.4
  - psychogenic F45.8
- artery I73.9
  - cerebral G45.9
- Bell's G51.3
- bladder (sphincter, external or internal) N32.89
  - psychogenic F45.8
- bronchus, bronchiole J98.01
- cardia K22.0
- cardiac I20.1
- carpopedal — *see* Tetany
- cerebral (arteries) (vascular) G45.9
- cervix, complicating delivery O62.4
- ciliary body (of accommodation) — *see* Spasm, of accommodation
- colon K58.9
  - with diarrhea K58.0
  - psychogenic F45.8
- common duct K83.8
- compulsive — *see* Tic
- conjugate H51.8
- coronary (artery) I20.1
- diaphragm (reflex) R06.6
  - epidemic B33.0
  - psychogenic F45.8
- duodenum K59.8
- epidemic diaphragmatic (transient) B33.0
- esophagus (diffuse) K22.4
  - psychogenic F45.8
- facial G51.3
- fallopian tube N83.8
- gastrointestinal (tract) K31.89
  - psychogenic F45.8
- glottis J38.5
  - hysterical F44.4
  - psychogenic F45.8
    - conversion reaction F44.4
  - reflex through recurrent laryngeal nerve J38.5
- habit — *see* Tic
- heart I20.1
- hemifacial (clonic) G51.3
- hourglass — *see* Contraction, hourglass
- hysterical F44.4
- infantile — *see* Epilepsy, spasms
- inferior oblique, eye H51.8
- intestinal (*see also* Syndrome, irritable bowel) K58.9
  - psychogenic F45.8
- larynx, laryngeal J38.5
  - hysterical F44.4
  - psychogenic F45.8
    - conversion reaction F44.4
- levator palpebrae superioris — *see* Disorder, eyelid function
- muscle NEC M62.838
  - back M62.830
- nerve, trigeminal G51.0
- nervous F45.8
- nodding F98.4
- occupational F48.8
- oculogyric H51.8
  - psychogenic F45.8
- of accommodation H52.53- ☑
- ophthalmic artery — *see* Occlusion, artery, retina
- perineal, female N94.89
- peroneo-extensor (*see also* Deformity, limb, flat foot)
- pharynx (reflex) J39.2
  - hysterical F45.8
  - psychogenic F45.8
- psychogenic F45.8
- pylorus NEC K31.3
  - adult hypertrophic K31.89
  - congenital or infantile Q40.0
  - psychogenic F45.8
- rectum (sphincter) K59.4
  - psychogenic F45.8
- retinal (artery) — *see* Occlusion, artery, retina
- sigmoid (*see also* Syndrome, irritable bowel) K58.9
  - psychogenic F45.8
- sphincter of Oddi K83.4
- stomach K31.89
  - neurotic F45.8
- throat J39.2
  - hysterical F45.8
  - psychogenic F45.8
- tic F95.9
  - chronic F95.1

Spasm(s), spastic, spasticity — *continued*
- tic — *continued*
  - transient of childhood F95.0
- tongue K14.8
- torsion (progressive) G24.1
- trigeminal nerve — *see* Neuralgia, trigeminal
- ureter N13.5
- urethra (sphincter) N35.9
- uterus N85.8
  - complicating labor O62.4
- vagina N94.2
  - psychogenic F52.5
- vascular I73.9
- vasomotor I73.9
- vein NEC I87.8
- viscera — *see* Pain, abdominal

Spasmodic — *see* condition
Spasmophilia — *see* Tetany
Spasmus nutans F98.4
Spastic, spasticity (*see also* Spasm)
- child (cerebral) (congenital) (paralysis) G80.1

Speaker's throat R49.8
Specific, specified — *see* condition
Speech
- defect, disorder, disturbance, impediment R47.9
  - psychogenic, in childhood and adolescence F98.8
  - slurring R47.81
  - specified NEC R47.89
Spencer's disease A08.19
Spens' syndrome (syncope with heart block) I45.9
Sperm counts (fertility testing) Z31.41
- postvasectomy Z30.8
- reversal Z31.42
Spermatic cord — *see* condition
Spermatocele N43.40
- congenital Q55.4
- multiple N43.42
- single N43.41
Spermatocystitis N49.0
Spermatocytoma C62.9- ☑
- specified site — *see* Neoplasm, malignant, by site
Spermatorrhea N50.8
Sphacelus — *see* Gangrene
Sphenoidal — *see* condition
Sphenoiditis (chronic) — *see* Sinusitis, sphenoidal
Sphenopalatine ganglion neuralgia G90.09
Sphericity, increased, lens (congenital) Q12.4
Spherocytosis (congenital) (familial) (hereditary) D58.0
- hemoglobin disease D58.0
- sickle-cell (disease) D57.8- ☑
Spherophakia Q12.4
Sphincter — *see* condition
Sphincteritis, sphincter of Oddi — *see* Cholangitis
Sphingolipidosis E75.3
- specified NEC E75.29
Sphingomyelinosis E75.3
Spicule tooth K00.2
Spider
- bite — *see* Toxicity, venom, spider
- fingers — *see* Syndrome, Marfan's
- nevus I78.1
- toes — *see* Syndrome, Marfan's
- vascular I78.1
Spiegler-Fendt
- benign lymphocytoma L98.8
- sarcoid L08.89
Spielmeyer-Vogt disease E75.4
Spina bifida (aperta) Q05.9
- with hydrocephalus NEC Q05.4
- cervical Q05.5
  - with hydrocephalus Q05.0
- dorsal Q05.6
  - with hydrocephalus Q05.1
- lumbar Q05.7
  - with hydrocephalus Q05.2
- lumbosacral Q05.7
  - with hydrocephalus Q05.2
- occulta Q76.0
- sacral Q05.8
  - with hydrocephalus Q05.3
- thoracic Q05.6
  - with hydrocephalus Q05.1
- thoracolumbar Q05.6
  - with hydrocephalus Q05.1
Spindle, Krukenberg's — *see* Pigmentation, cornea, posterior
Spine, spinal — *see* condition

Spiradenoma (eccrine) — *see* Neoplasm, skin, benign
Spirillosis A25.0
Spirillum
- minus A25.0
- obermeieri infection A68.0
Spirochetal — *see* condition
Spirochetosis A69.9
- arthritic, arthritica A69.9
- bronchopulmonary A69.8
- icterohemorrhagic A27.0
- lung A69.8
Spirometrosis B70.1
Spitting blood — *see* Hemoptysis
Splanchnoptosis K63.4
Spleen, splenic — *see* condition
Splenectasis — *see* Splenomegaly
Splenitis (interstitial) (malignant) (nonspecific) D73.89
- malarial (*see also* Malaria) B54 [D77]
- tuberculous A18.85
Splenocele D73.89
Splenomegaly, splenomegalia (Bengal) (cryptogenic) (idiopathic) (tropical) R16.1
- with hepatomegaly R16.2
- cirrhotic D73.2
- congenital Q89.09
- congestive, chronic D73.2
- Egyptian B65.1
- Gaucher's E75.22
- malarial (*see also* Malaria) B54 [D77]
- neutropenic D73.81
- Niemann-Pick — *see* Niemann-Pick disease or syndrome
- siderotic D73.2
- syphilitic A52.79
  - congenital (early) A50.08 [D77]
Splenopathy D73.9
Splenoptosis D73.89
Splenosis D73.89
Splinter — *see* Foreign body, superficial, by site
Split, splitting ☑
- foot Q72.7- ☑
- heart sounds R01.2
- lip, congenital — *see* Cleft, lip
- nails L60.3
- urinary stream R39.13
Spondylarthrosis — *see* Spondylosis
Spondylitis (chronic) (*see also* Spondylopathy, inflammatory)
- ankylopoietica — *see* Spondylitis, ankylosing
- ankylosing (chronic) M45.9
  - with lung involvement M45.9 [J99]
  - cervical region M45.2
  - cervicothoracic region M45.3
  - juvenile M08.1
  - lumbar region M45.6
  - lumbosacral region M45.7
  - multiple sites M45.0
  - occipito-atlanto-axial region M45.1
  - sacrococcygeal region M45.8
  - thoracic region M45.4
  - thoracolumbar region M45.5
- atrophic (ligamentous) — *see* Spondylitis, ankylosing
- deformans (chronic) — *see* Spondylosis
- gonococcal A54.41
- gouty M10.08
- in (due to)
  - brucellosis A23.9 [M49.80]
    - cervical region A23.9 [M49.82]
    - cervicothoracic region A23.9 [M49.83]
    - lumbar region A23.9 [M49.86]
    - lumbosacral region A23.9 [M49.87]
    - multiple sites A23.9 [M49.89]
    - occipito-atlanto-axial region A23.9 [M49.81]
    - sacrococcygeal region A23.9 [M49.88]
    - thoracic region A23.9 [M49.84]
    - thoracolumbar region A23.9 [M49.85]
  - enterobacteria (*see also* subcategory M49.8) A04.9
  - tuberculosis A18.01
- infectious NEC — *see* Spondylopathy, infective
- juvenile ankylosing (chronic) M08.1
- Kümmell's — *see* Spondylopathy, traumatic
- Marie-Strümpell — *see* Spondylitis, ankylosing
- muscularis — *see* Spondylopathy, specified NEC
- psoriatic L40.53
- rheumatoid — *see* Spondylitis, ankylosing
- rhizomelica — *see* Spondylitis, ankylosing
- sacroiliac NEC M46.1

Spondylitis — *continued*
  senescent, senile — *see* Spondylosis
  traumatic (chronic) or post-traumatic — *see* Spondylopathy, traumatic
  tuberculous A18.01
  typhosa A01.05
Spondylolisthesis (acquired) (degenerative) M43.10
  with disproportion (fetopelvic) O33.0
    causing obstructed labor O65.0
  cervical region M43.12
  cervicothoracic region M43.13
  congenital Q76.2
  lumbar region M43.16
  lumbosacral region M43.17
  multiple sites M43.19
  occipito-atlanto-axial region M43.11
  sacrococcygeal region M43.18
  thoracic region M43.14
  thoracolumbar region M43.15
  traumatic (old) M43.10
    acute
      fifth cervical (displaced) S12.430 ☑
        nondisplaced S12.431 ☑
        specified type NEC (displaced) S12.450 ☑
          nondisplaced S12.451 ☑
        type III S12.44 ☑
      fourth cervical (displaced) S12.330 ☑
        nondisplaced S12.331 ☑
        specified type NEC (displaced) S12.350 ☑
          nondisplaced S12.351 ☑
        type III S12.34 ☑
      second cervical (displaced) S12.130 ☑
        nondisplaced S12.131 ☑
        specified type NEC (displaced) S12.150 ☑
          nondisplaced S12.151 ☑
        type III S12.14 ☑
      seventh cervical (displaced) S12.630 ☑
        nondisplaced S12.631 ☑
        specified type NEC (displaced) S12.650 ☑
          nondisplaced S12.651 ☑
        type III S12.64 ☑
      sixth cervical (displaced) S12.530 ☑
        nondisplaced S12.531 ☑
        specified type NEC (displaced) S12.550 ☑
          nondisplaced S12.551 ☑
        type III S12.54 ☑
      third cervical (displaced) S12.230 ☑
        nondisplaced S12.231 ☑
        specified type NEC (displaced) S12.250 ☑
          nondisplaced S12.251 ☑
        type III S12.24 ☑
Spondylolysis (acquired) M43.00
  cervical region M43.02
  cervicothoracic region M43.03
  congenital Q76.2
  lumbar region M43.06
  lumbosacral region M43.07
    with disproportion (fetopelvic) O33.0
      causing obstructed labor O65.8
  multiple sites M43.09
  occipito-atlanto-axial region M43.01
  sacrococcygeal region M43.08
  thoracic region M43.04
  thoracolumbar region M43.05
Spondylopathy M48.9
  infective NEC M46.50
    cervical region M46.52
    cervicothoracic region M46.53
    lumbar region M46.56
    lumbosacral region M46.57
    multiple sites M46.59
    occipito-atlanto-axial region M46.51
    sacrococcygeal region M46.58
    thoracic region M46.54
    thoracolumbar region M46.55
  inflammatory M46.90
    cervical region M46.92
    cervicothoracic region M46.93
    lumbar region M46.96
    lumbosacral region M46.97
    multiple sites M46.99
    occipito-atlanto-axial region M46.91
    sacrococcygeal region M46.98
    specified type NEC M46.80
      cervical region M46.82
      cervicothoracic region M46.83
      lumbar region M46.86

Spondylopathy — *continued*
  inflammatory — *continued*
    specified type — *continued*
      lumbosacral region M46.87
      multiple sites M46.89
      occipito-atlanto-axial region M46.81
      sacrococcygeal region M46.88
      thoracic region M46.84
      thoracolumbar region M46.85
    thoracic region M46.94
    thoracolumbar region M46.95
  neuropathic, in
    syringomyelia and syringobulbia G95.0
    tabes dorsalis A52.11
  specified NEC — *see* subcategory M48.8 ☑
  traumatic M48.30
    cervical region M48.32
    cervicothoracic region M48.33
    lumbar region M48.36
    lumbosacral region M48.37
    occipito-atlanto-axial region M48.31
    sacrococcygeal region M48.38
    thoracic region M48.34
    thoracolumbar region M48.35
Spondylosis M47.9
  with
    disproportion (fetopelvic) O33.0
      causing obstructed labor O65.0
    myelopathy NEC M47.10
      cervical region M47.12
      cervicothoracic region M47.13
      lumbar region M47.16
      occipito-atlanto-axial region M47.11
      thoracic region M47.14
      thoracolumbar region M47.15
    radiculopathy M47.20
      cervical region M47.22
      cervicothoracic region M47.23
      lumbar region M47.26
      lumbosacral region M47.27
      occipito-atlanto-axial region M47.21
      sacrococcygeal region M47.28
      thoracic region M47.24
      thoracolumbar region M47.25
  without myelopathy or radiculopathy M47.819
    cervical region M47.812
    cervicothoracic region M47.813
    lumbar region M47.816
    lumbosacral region M47.817
    occipito-atlanto-axial region M47.811
    sacrococcygeal region M47.818
    thoracic region M47.814
    thoracolumbar region M47.815
  specified NEC M47.899
    cervical region M47.892
    cervicothoracic region M47.893
    lumbar region M47.896
    lumbosacral region M47.897
    occipito-atlanto-axial region M47.891
    sacrococcygeal region M47.898
    thoracic region M47.894
    thoracolumbar region M47.895
  traumatic — *see* Spondylopathy, traumatic
Sponge
  inadvertently left in operation wound — *see* Foreign body, accidentally left during a procedure
  kidney (medullary) Q61.5
Sponge-diver's disease — *see* Toxicity, venom, marine animal, sea anemone
Spongioblastoma (any type) — *see* Neoplasm, malignant, by site
  specified site — *see* Neoplasm, malignant, by site
  unspecified site C71.9
Spongioneuroblastoma — *see* Neoplasm, malignant, by site
Spontaneous (*see also* condition)
  fracture (cause unknown) — *see* Fracture, pathological
Spoon nail L60.3
  congenital Q84.6
Sporadic — *see* condition
Sporothrix schenckii infection — *see* Sporotrichosis
Sporotrichosis B42.9
  arthritis B42.82
  disseminated B42.7
  generalized B42.7
  lymphocutaneous (fixed) (progressive) B42.1
  pulmonary B42.0
  specified NEC B42.89

Spots, spotting (in) (of)
  Bitot's (*see also* Pigmentation, conjunctiva)
    in the young child E50.1
    vitamin A deficiency E50.1
  café, au lait L81.3
  Cayenne pepper I78.1
  cotton wool, retina — *see* Occlusion, artery, retina
  de Morgan's (senile angiomas) I78.1
  Fuchs' black (myopic) H44.2- ☑
  intermenstrual (regular) N92.0
    irregular N92.1
  Koplik's B05.9
  liver L81.4
  pregnancy O26.85- ☑
  purpuric R23.3
  ruby I78.1
Spotted fever — *see* Fever, spotted N92.3
Sprain (joint) (ligament)
  acromioclavicular joint or ligament S43.5- ☑
  ankle S93.40- ☑
    calcaneofibular ligament S93.41- ☑
    deltoid ligament S93.42- ☑
    internal collateral ligament — *see* Sprain, ankle, specified ligament NEC
    specified ligament NEC S93.49- ☑
    talofibular ligament — *see* Sprain, ankle, specified ligament NEC
    tibiofibular ligament S93.43- ☑
  anterior longitudinal, cervical S13.4 ☑
  atlas, atlanto-axial, atlanto-occipital S13.4 ☑
  breast bone — *see* Sprain, sternum
  calcaneofibular — *see* Sprain, ankle
  carpal — *see* Sprain, wrist
  carpometacarpal — *see* Sprain, hand, specified site NEC
  cartilage
    costal S23.41 ☑
    semilunar (knee) — *see* Sprain, knee, specified site NEC
      with current tear — *see* Tear, meniscus
    thyroid region S13.5 ☑
    xiphoid — *see* Sprain, sternum
  cervical, cervicodorsal, cervicothoracic S13.4 ☑
  chondrosternal S23.421 ☑
  coracoclavicular S43.8- ☑
  coracohumeral S43.41- ☑
  coronary, knee — *see* Sprain, knee, specified site NEC
  costal cartilage S23.41 ☑
  cricoarytenoid articulation or ligament S13.5 ☑
  cricothyroid articulation S13.5 ☑
  cruciate, knee — *see* Sprain, knee, cruciate
  deltoid, ankle — *see* Sprain, ankle
  dorsal (spine) S23.3 ☑
  elbow S53.40- ☑
    radial collateral ligament S53.43- ☑
    radiohumeral S53.41- ☑
    rupture
      radial collateral ligament — *see* Rupture, traumatic, ligament, radial collateral
      ulnar collateral ligament — *see* Rupture, traumatic, ligament, ulnar collateral
    specified type NEC S53.49- ☑
    ulnar collateral ligament S53.44- ☑
    ulnohumeral S53.42- ☑
  femur, head — *see* Sprain, hip
  fibular collateral, knee — *see* Sprain, knee, collateral
  fibulocalcaneal — *see* Sprain, ankle
  finger(s) S63.61- ☑
    index S63.61- ☑
    interphalangeal (joint) S63.63- ☑
      index S63.63- ☑
      little S63.63- ☑
      middle S63.63- ☑
      ring S63.63- ☑
    little S63.61- ☑
    metacarpophalangeal (joint) S63.65- ☑
    middle S63.61- ☑
    ring S63.61- ☑
    specified site NEC S63.69- ☑
      index S63.69- ☑
      little S63.69- ☑
      middle S63.69- ☑
      ring S63.69- ☑
  foot S93.60- ☑
    specified ligament NEC S93.69- ☑
    tarsal ligament S93.61- ☑

Sprain — *continued*
  foot — *continued*
    tarsometatarsal ligament S93.62- ☑
    toe — *see* Sprain, toe
  hand S63.9- ☑
    finger — *see* Sprain, finger
    specified site NEC — *see* subcategory S63.8 ☑
    thumb — *see* Sprain, thumb
  head S03.9 ☑
  hip S73.10- ☑
    iliofemoral ligament S73.11- ☑
    ischiocapsular (ligament) S73.12- ☑
    specified NEC S73.19- ☑
  iliofemoral — *see* Sprain, hip
  innominate
    acetabulum — *see* Sprain, hip
    sacral junction S33.6 ☑
  internal
    collateral, ankle — *see* Sprain, ankle
    semilunar cartilage — *see* Sprain, knee, specified
      site NEC
  interphalangeal
    finger — *see* Sprain, finger, interphalangeal (joint)
    toe — *see* Sprain, toe, interphalangeal joint
  ischiocapsular — *see* Sprain, hip
  ischiofemoral — *see* Sprain, hip
  jaw (articular disc) (cartilage) (meniscus) S03.4 ☑
    old M26.69
  knee S83.9- ☑
    collateral ligament S83.40- ☑
      lateral (fibular) S83.42- ☑
      medial (tibial) S83.41- ☑
    cruciate ligament S83.50- ☑
      anterior S83.51- ☑
      posterior S83.52- ☑
    lateral (fibular) collateral ligament S83.42- ☑
    medial (tibial) collateral ligament S83.41- ☑
    patellar ligament S76.11- ☑
    specified site NEC S83.8X- ☑
    superior tibiofibular joint (ligament) S83.6- ☑
  lateral collateral, knee — *see* Sprain, knee, collateral
  lumbar (spine) S33.5 ☑
  lumbosacral S33.9 ☑
  mandible (articular disc) S03.4 ☑
    old M26.69
  medial collateral, knee — *see* Sprain, knee, collateral
  meniscus
    jaw S03.4 ☑
      old M26.69
    knee — *see* Sprain, knee, specified site NEC
      with current tear — *see* Tear, meniscus
        old — *see* Derangement, knee, meniscus,
          due to old tear
    mandible S03.4 ☑
      old M26.69
  metacarpal (distal) (proximal) — *see* Sprain, hand,
    specified site NEC
  metacarpophalangeal — *see* Sprain, finger, metacar-
    pophalangeal (joint)
  metatarsophalangeal — *see* Sprain, toe, metatarsopha-
    langeal joint
  midcarpal — *see* Sprain, hand, specified site NEC
  midtarsal — *see* Sprain, foot, specified site NEC
  neck S13.9 ☑
    anterior longitudinal cervical ligament S13.4 ☑
    atlanto-axial joint S13.4 ☑
    atlanto-occipital joint S13.4 ☑
    cervical spine S13.4 ☑
    cricoarytenoid ligament S13.5 ☑
    cricothyroid ligament S13.5 ☑
    specified site NEC S13.8 ☑
    thyroid region (cartilage) S13.5 ☑
  nose S03.8 ☑
  orbicular, hip — *see* Sprain, hip
  patella — *see* Sprain, knee, specified site NEC
  patellar ligament S76.11- ☑
  pelvis NEC S33.8 ☑
  phalanx
    finger — *see* Sprain, finger
    toe — *see* Sprain, toe
  pubofemoral — *see* Sprain, hip
  radiocarpal — *see* Sprain, wrist
  radiohumeral — *see* Sprain, elbow
  radius, collateral — *see* Rupture, traumatic, ligament,
    radial collateral
  rib (cage) S23.41 ☑

Sprain — *continued*
  rotator cuff (capsule) S43.42- ☑
  sacroiliac (region)
    chronic or old — *see* subcategory M53.2 ☑
    joint S33.6 ☑
  scaphoid (hand) — *see* Sprain, hand, specified site
    NEC
  scapula (r) — *see* Sprain, shoulder girdle, specified site
    NEC
  semilunar cartilage (knee) — *see* Sprain, knee, speci-
    fied site NEC
    with current tear — *see* Tear, meniscus
      old — *see* Derangement, knee, meniscus, due
        to old tear
  shoulder joint S43.40- ☑
    acromioclavicular joint (ligament) — *see* Sprain,
      acromioclavicular joint
    blade — *see* Sprain, shoulder, girdle, specified site
      NEC
    coracoclavicular joint (ligament) — *see* Sprain,
      coracoclavicular joint
    coracohumeral ligament — *see* Sprain, coraco-
      humeral joint
    girdle S43.9- ☑
      specified site NEC S43.8- ☑
    rotator cuff — *see* Sprain, rotator cuff
    specified site NEC S43.49- ☑
    sternoclavicular joint (ligament) — *see* Sprain,
      sternoclavicular joint
  spine
    cervical S13.4 ☑
    lumbar S33.5 ☑
    thoracic S23.3 ☑
  sternoclavicular joint S43.6- ☑
  sternum S23.429 ☑
    chondrosternal joint S23.421 ☑
    specified site NEC S23.428 ☑
    sternoclavicular (joint) (ligament) S23.420 ☑
  symphysis
    jaw S03.4 ☑
      old M26.69
    mandibular S03.4 ☑
      old M26.69
  talofibular — *see* Sprain, ankle
  tarsal — *see* Sprain, foot, specified site NEC
  tarsometatarsal — *see* Sprain, foot, specified site NEC
  temporomandibular S03.4 ☑
    old M26.69
  thorax S23.9 ☑
    ribs S23.41 ☑
    specified site NEC S23.8 ☑
    spine S23.3 ☑
    sternum — *see* Sprain, sternum
  thumb S63.60- ☑
    interphalangeal (joint) S63.62- ☑
    metacarpophalangeal (joint) S63.64- ☑
    specified site NEC S63.68- ☑
  thyroid cartilage or region S13.5 ☑
  tibia (proximal end) — *see* Sprain, knee, specified site
    NEC
  tibial collateral, knee — *see* Sprain, knee, collateral
  tibiofibular
    distal — *see* Sprain, ankle
    superior — *see* Sprain, knee, specified site NEC
  toe(s) S93.50- ☑
    great S93.50- ☑
    interphalangeal joint S93.51- ☑
      great S93.51- ☑
      lesser S93.51- ☑
    lesser S93.50- ☑
    metatarsophalangeal joint S93.52- ☑
      great S93.52- ☑
      lesser S93.52- ☑
  ulna, collateral — *see* Rupture, traumatic, ligament,
    ulnar collateral
  ulnohumeral — *see* Sprain, elbow
  wrist S63.50- ☑
    carpal S63.51- ☑
    radiocarpal S63.52- ☑
    specified site NEC S63.59- ☑
  xiphoid cartilage — *see* Sprain, sternum
Sprengel's deformity (congenital) Q74.0
Sprue (tropical) K90.1
  celiac K90.0
  idiopathic K90.0
  meaning thrush B37.0

Sprue — *continued*
  nontropical K90.0
Spur, bone (*see also* Enthesopathy)
  calcaneal M77.3- ☑
  iliac crest M76.2- ☑
  nose (septum) J34.89
Spurway's syndrome Q78.0
Sputum
  abnormal (amount) (color) (odor) (purulent) R09.3
  blood-stained R04.2
  excessive (cause unknown) R09.3
Squamous (*see also* condition)
  epithelium in
    cervical canal (congenital) Q51.828
    uterine mucosa (congenital) Q51.818
Squashed nose M95.0
  congenital Q67.4
Squeeze, diver's T70.3 ☑
Squint (*see also* Strabismus)
  accommodative — *see* Strabismus, convergent con-
    comitant
St. Hubert's disease A82.9
Stab (*see also* Laceration)
  internal organs — *see* Injury, by site
Stafne's cyst or cavity M27.0
Staggering gait R26.0
  hysterical F44.4
Staghorn calculus — *see* Calculus, kidney
Stähli's line (cornea) (pigment) — *see* Pigmentation,
  cornea, anterior
Stain, staining
  meconium (newborn) P96.83
  port wine Q82.5
  tooth, teeth (hard tissues) (extrinsic) K03.6
    due to
      accretions K03.6
      deposits (betel) (black) (green) (materia alba)
        (orange) (soft) (tobacco) K03.6
      metals (copper) (silver) K03.7
      nicotine K03.6
      pulpal bleeding K03.7
      tobacco K03.6
    intrinsic K00.8
Stammering (*see also* Disorder, fluency) F80.81
Standstill
  auricular I45.5
  cardiac — *see* Arrest, cardiac
  sinoatrial I45.5
  ventricular — *see* Arrest, cardiac
Stannosis J63.5
Stanton's disease — *see* Melioidosis
Staphlitis (acute) (catarrhal) (chronic) (gangrenous)
  (membranous) (suppurative) (ulcerative) K12.2
Staphylococcal scalded skin syndrome L00
Staphylococcemia A41.2
Staphylococcus, staphylococcal (*see also* condition)
  as cause of disease classified elsewhere B95.8
    aureus (methicillin susceptible) (MSSA) B95.61
      methicillin resistant (MRSA) B95.62
    specified NEC, as cause of disease classified elsewhere
      B95.7
Staphyloma (sclera)
  cornea H18.72- ☑
  equatorial H15.81- ☑
  localized (anterior) H15.82- ☑
  posticum H15.83- ☑
  ring H15.85- ☑
Stargardt's disease — *see* Dystrophy, retina
Starvation (inanition) (due to lack of food) T73.0 ☑
  edema — *see* Malnutrition, severe
Stasis
  bile (noncalculous) K83.1
  bronchus J98.09
    with infection — *see* Bronchitis
  cardiac — *see* Failure, heart, congestive
  cecum K59.8
  colon K59.8
  dermatitis — *see* Varix, leg, with, inflammation
  duodenal K31.5
  eczema — *see* Varix, leg, with, inflammation
  edema — *see* Hypertension, venous (chronic), idiopath-
    ic
  foot T69.0- ☑
  ileocecal coil K59.8
  ileum K59.8
  intestinal K59.8
  jejunum K59.8

☑ **Additional Character Required — Refer to the Tabular List for Character Selection**   ▽ **Subterms under main terms may continue to next column or page**

Stasis — *continued*
 kidney N19
 liver (cirrhotic) K76.1
 lymphatic I89.8
 pneumonia J18.2
 pulmonary — *see* Edema, lung
 rectal K59.8
 renal N19
  tubular N17.0
 ulcer — *see* Varix, leg, with, ulcer
  without varicose veins I87.2
 urine — *see* Retention, urine
 venous I87.8
State (of)
 affective and paranoid, mixed, organic psychotic F06.8
 agitated R45.1
  acute reaction to stress F43.0
 anxiety (neurotic) F41.1
 apprehension F41.1
 burn-out Z73.0
 climacteric, female Z78.0
  symptomatic N95.1
 compulsive F42
  mixed with obsessional thoughts F42
 confusional (psychogenic) F44.89
  acute (*see also* Delirium)
   with
    arteriosclerotic dementia F01.50
     with behavioral disturbance F01.51
    senility or dementia F05
   alcoholic F10.231
   epileptic F05
  reactive (from emotional stress, psychological
   trauma) F44.89
  subacute — *see* Delirium
 convulsive — *see* Convulsions
 crisis F43.0
 depressive F32.9
  neurotic F34.1
 dissociative F44.9
 emotional shock (stress) R45.7
 hypercoagulation — *see* Hypercoagulable
 locked-in G83.5
 menopausal Z78.0
  symptomatic N95.1
 neurotic F48.9
  with depersonalization F48.1
 obsessional F42
 oneiroid (schizophrenia-like) F23
 organic
  hallucinatory (nonalcoholic) F06.0
  paranoid (-hallucinatory) F06.2
 panic F41.0
 paranoid F22
  climacteric F22
  involutional F22
  menopausal F22
  organic F06.2
  senile F03 ☑
  simple F22
 persistent vegetative R40.3
 phobic F40.9
 postleukotomy F07.0
 pregnant, incidental Z33.1
 psychogenic, twilight F44.89
 psychopathic (constitutional) F60.2
 psychotic, organic (*see also* Psychosis, organic)
  mixed paranoid and affective F06.8
  senile or presenile F03 ☑
  transient NEC F06.8
   with
    depression F06.31
    hallucinations F06.0
 residual schizophrenic F20.5
 restlessness R45.1
 stress (emotional) R45.7
 tension (mental) F48.9
  specified NEC F48.8
 transient organic psychotic NEC F06.8
  depressive type F06.31
  hallucinatory type F06.30
 twilight
  epileptic F05
  psychogenic F44.89
 vegetative, persistent R40.3
 vital exhaustion Z73.0
 withdrawal, — *see* Withdrawal, state
Status (post) (*see also* Presence (of))

Status — *continued*
 absence, epileptic — *see* Epilepsy, by type, with status
  epilepticus
 administration of tPA (rtPA) in a different facility
  within the last 24 hours prior to admission to
  current facility Z92.82
 adrenalectomy (unilateral) (bilateral) E89.6
 anastomosis Z98.0
 anginosus I20.9
 angioplasty (peripheral) Z98.62
  with implant Z95.820
  coronary artery Z98.61
   with implant Z95.5
 aortocoronary bypass Z95.1
 arthrodesis Z98.1
 artificial opening (of) Z93.9
  gastrointestinal tract Z93.4
  specified NEC Z93.8
  urinary tract Z93.6
  vagina Z93.8
 asthmaticus — *see* Asthma, by type, with status asthmaticus
 awaiting organ transplant Z76.82
 bariatric surgery Z98.84
 bed confinement Z74.01
 bleb, filtering (vitreous), after glaucoma surgery Z98.83
 breast implant Z98.82
  removal Z98.86
 cataract extraction Z98.4- ☑
 cholecystectomy Z90.49
 clitoridectomy N90.811
  with excision of labia minora N90.812
 colectomy (complete) (partial) Z90.49
 colonization — *see* Carrier (suspected) of
 colostomy Z93.3
 convulsivus idiopathicus — *see* Epilepsy, by type, with
  status epilepticus
 coronary artery angioplasty — *see* Status, angioplasty,
  coronary artery
 cystectomy (urinary bladder) Z90.6
 cystostomy Z93.50
  appendico-vesicostomy Z93.52
  cutaneous Z93.51
  specified NEC Z93.59
 delinquent immunization Z28.3
 dental Z98.818
  crown Z98.811
  fillings Z98.811
  restoration Z98.811
  sealant Z98.810
  specified NEC Z98.818
 deployment (current) (military) Z56.82
 dialysis (hemodialysis) (peritoneal) Z99.2
 do not resuscitate (DNR) Z66
 donor — *see* Donor
 embedded fragments — *see* Retained, foreign body
  fragments (type of)
 embedded splinter — *see* Retained, foreign body
  fragments (type of)
 enterostomy Z93.4
 epileptic, epilepticus (*see also* Epilepsy, by type, with
  status epilepticus) G40.901
 estrogen receptor
  negative Z17.1
  positive Z17.0
 female genital cutting — *see* Female genital mutilation
  status
 female genital mutilation — *see* Female genital mutilation status
 filtering (vitreous) bleb after glaucoma surgery Z98.83
 gastrectomy (complete) (partial) Z90.3
 gastric banding Z98.84
 gastric bypass for obesity Z98.84
 gastrostomy Z93.1
 human immunodeficiency virus (HIV) infection,
  asymptomatic Z21
 hysterectomy (complete) (total) Z90.710
  partial (with remaining cervial stump) Z90.711
 ileostomy Z93.2
 implant
  breast Z98.82
 infibulation N90.813
 intestinal bypass Z98.0
 jejunostomy Z93.4
 lapsed immunization schedule Z28.3
 laryngectomy Z90.02
 lymphaticus E32.8
 marmoratus G80.3

Status — *continued*
 mastectomy (unilateral) (bilateral) Z90.1- ☑
 military deployment status (current) Z56.82
  in theater or in support of military war, peacekeeping and humanitarian operations Z56.82
 nephrectomy (unilateral) (bilateral) Z90.5
 nephrostomy Z93.6
 obesity surgery Z98.84
 oophorectomy
  bilateral Z90.722
  unilateral Z90.721
 organ replacement
  by artificial or mechanical device or prosthesis of
   artery Z95.828
   bladder Z96.0
   blood vessel Z95.828
   breast Z97.8
   eye globe Z97.0
   heart Z95.812
    valve Z95.2
   intestine Z97.8
   joint Z96.60
    hip — *see* Presence, hip joint implant
    knee — *see* Presence, knee joint implant
    specified site NEC Z96.698
   kidney Z97.8
   larynx Z96.3
   lens Z96.1
   limbs — *see* Presence, artificial, limb
   liver Z97.8
   lung Z97.8
   pancreas Z97.8
  by organ transplant (heterologous)(homologous)
   — *see* Transplant
 pacemaker
  brain Z96.89
  cardiac Z95.0
  specified NEC Z96.89
 pancreatectomy Z90.410
  complete Z90.410
  partial Z90.411
  total Z90.410
 physical restraint Z78.1
 pneumonectomy (complete) (partial) Z90.2
 pneumothorax, therapeutic Z98.3
 postcommotio cerebri F07.81
 postoperative (postprocedural) NEC Z98.89
  breast implant Z98.82
  dental Z98.818
   crown Z98.811
   fillings Z98.811
   restoration Z98.811
   sealant Z98.810
   specified NEC Z98.818
  pneumothorax, therapeutic Z98.3
 postpartum (routine follow-up) Z39.2
  care immediately after delivery Z39.0
 postsurgical (postprocedural) NEC Z98.89
  pneumothorax, therapeutic Z98.3
 pregnancy, incidental Z33.1
 prosthesis coronary angioplasty Z95.5
 pseudophakia Z96.1
 renal dialysis (hemodialysis) (peritoneal) Z99.2
 retained foreign body — *see* Retained, foreign body
  fragments (type of)
 reversed jejunal transposition (for bypass) Z98.0
 salpingo-oophorectomy
  bilateral Z90.722
  unilateral Z90.721
 sex reassignment surgery status Z87.890
 shunt
  arteriovenous (for dialysis) Z99.2
  cerebrospinal fluid Z98.2
  ventricular (communicating) (for drainage) Z98.2
 splenectomy Z90.81
 thymicolymphaticus E32.8
 thymicus E32.8
 thymolymphaticus E32.8
 thyroidectomy (hypothyroidism) E89.0
 tooth (teeth) extraction (*see also* Absence, teeth, acquired) K08.409
 tPA (rtPA) administration in a different facility within
  the last 24 hours prior to admission to current
  facility Z92.82
 tracheostomy Z93.0
 transplant — *see* Transplant
  organ removed Z98.85
 tubal ligation Z98.51

⩔ Subterms under main terms may continue to next column or page ☑ Additional Character Required — Refer to the Tabular List for Character Selection 283

Index

Stasis — Status

Status — continued
underimmunization Z28.3
ureterostomy Z93.6
urethrostomy Z93.6
vagina, artificial Z93.8
vasectomy Z98.52
wheelchair confinement Z99.3
Stealing
child problem F91.8
in company with others Z72.810
pathological (compulsive) F63.2
Steam burn — see Burn
Steatocystoma multiplex L72.2
Steatohepatitis (nonalcoholic) (NASH) K75.81
Steatoma L72.3
eyelid (cystic) — see Dermatosis, eyelid
infected — see Hordeolum
Steatorrhea (chronic) K90.4
with lacteal obstruction K90.2
idiopathic (adult) (infantile) K90.0
pancreatic K90.3
primary K90.0
tropical K90.1
Steatosis E88.89
heart — see Degeneration, myocardial
kidney N28.89
liver NEC K76.0
Steele-Richardson-Olszewski disease or syndrome
G23.1
Stein-Leventhal syndrome E28.2
Steinbrocker's syndrome G90.8
Steinert's disease G71.11
Stein's syndrome E28.2
STEMI (see also Infarct, myocardium, ST elevation) I21.3
Stenocardia I20.8
Stenocephaly Q75.8
Stenosis, stenotic (cicatricial) (see also Stricture)
ampulla of Vater K83.1
anus, anal (canal) (sphincter) K62.4
and rectum K62.4
congenital Q42.3
with fistula Q42.2
aorta (ascending) (supraventricular) (congenital) Q25.3
arteriosclerotic I70.0
calcified I70.0
aortic (valve) I35.0
with insufficiency I35.2
congenital Q23.0
rheumatic I06.0
with
incompetency, insufficiency or regurgitation
I06.2
with mitral (valve) disease I08.0
with tricuspid (valve) disease I08.3
mitral (valve) disease I08.0
with tricuspid (valve) disease I08.3
tricuspid (valve) disease I08.2
with mitral (valve) disease I08.3
specified cause NEC I35.0
syphilitic A52.03
aqueduct of Sylvius (congenital) Q03.0
with spina bifida — see Spina bifida, by site, with
hydrocephalus
acquired G91.1
artery NEC (see also Arteriosclerosis) I77.1
celiac I77.4
cerebral — see Occlusion, artery, cerebral
extremities — see Arteriosclerosis, extremities
precerebral — see Occlusion, artery, precerebral
pulmonary (congenital) Q25.6
acquired I28.8
renal I70.1
bile duct (common) (hepatic) K83.1
congenital Q44.3
bladder-neck (acquired) N32.0
congenital Q64.31
brain G93.89
bronchus J98.09
congenital Q32.3
syphilitic A52.72
cardia (stomach) K22.2
congenital Q39.3
cardiovascular — see Disease, cardiovascular
caudal M48.08
cervix, cervical (canal) N88.2
congenital Q51.828
in pregnancy or childbirth — see Pregnancy,
complicated by, abnormal cervix

Stenosis, stenotic — continued
colon (see also Obstruction, intestine)
congenital Q42.9
specified NEC Q42.8
colostomy K94.03
common (bile) duct K83.1
congenital Q44.3
coronary (artery) — see Disease, heart, ischemic,
atherosclerotic
cystic duct — see Obstruction, gallbladder
due to presence of device, implant or graft (see also
Complications, by site and type, specified NEC)
T85.85 ☑
arterial graft NEC T82.858 ☑
breast (implant) T85.85 ☑
catheter T85.85 ☑
dialysis (renal) T82.858 ☑
intraperitoneal T85.85 ☑
infusion NEC T82.858 ☑
spinal (epidural) (subdural) T85.85 ☑
urinary (indwelling) T83.85 ☑
fixation, internal (orthopedic) NEC T84.85 ☑
gastrointestinal (bile duct) (esophagus) T85.85 ☑
genital NEC T83.85 ☑
heart NEC T82.857 ☑
joint prosthesis T84.85 ☑
ocular (corneal graft) (orbital implant) NEC
T85.85 ☑
orthopedic NEC T84.85 ☑
specified NEC T85.85 ☑
urinary NEC T83.85 ☑
vascular NEC T82.858 ☑
ventricular intracranial shunt T85.85 ☑
duodenum K31.5
congenital Q41.0
ejaculatory duct NEC N50.8
endocervical os — see Stenosis, cervix
enterostomy K94.13
esophagus K22.2
congenital Q39.3
syphilitic A52.79
congenital A50.59 [K23]
eustachian tube — see Obstruction, eustachian tube
external ear canal (acquired) H61.30- ☑
congenital Q16.1
due to
inflammation H61.32- ☑
trauma H61.31- ☑
postprocedural H95.81- ☑
specified cause NEC H61.39- ☑
gallbladder — see Obstruction, gallbladder
glottis J38.6
heart valve (congenital) Q24.8
aortic Q23.0
mitral Q23.2
pulmonary Q22.1
tricuspid Q22.4
hepatic duct K83.1
hymen N89.6
hypertrophic subaortic (idiopathic) I42.1
ileum K56.69
congenital Q41.2
infundibulum cardia Q24.3
intervertebral foramina (see also Lesion, biomechanical, specified NEC)
connective tissue M99.79
abdomen M99.79
cervical region M99.71
cervicothoracic M99.71
head region M99.70
lumbar region M99.73
lumbosacral M99.73
occipitocervical M99.70
sacral region M99.74
sacrococcygeal M99.74
sacroiliac M99.74
specified NEC M99.79
thoracic region M99.72
thoracolumbar M99.72
disc M99.79
abdomen M99.79
cervical region M99.71
cervicothoracic M99.71
head region M99.70
lower extremity M99.76
lumbar region M99.73
lumbosacral M99.73

Stenosis, stenotic — continued
intervertebral foramina (see also Lesion, biomechanical,
specified) — continued
disc — continued
occipitocervical M99.70
pelvic M99.75
rib cage M99.78
sacral region M99.74
sacrococcygeal M99.74
sacroiliac M99.74
specified NEC M99.79
thoracic region M99.72
thoracolumbar M99.72
upper extremity M99.77
osseous M99.69
abdomen M99.69
cervical region M99.61
cervicothoracic M99.61
head region M99.60
lower extremity M99.66
lumbar region M99.63
lumbosacral M99.63
occipitocervical M99.60
pelvic M99.65
rib cage M99.68
sacral region M99.64
sacrococcygeal M99.64
sacroiliac M99.64
specified NEC M99.69
thoracic region M99.62
thoracolumbar M99.62
upper extremity M99.67
subluxation — see Stenosis, intervertebral foramina, osseous
intestine (see also Obstruction, intestine)
congenital (small) Q41.9
large Q42.9
specified NEC Q42.8
specified NEC Q41.8
jejunum K56.69
congenital Q41.1
lacrimal (passage)
canaliculi H04.54- ☑
congenital Q10.5
duct H04.55- ☑
punctum H04.56- ☑
sac H04.57- ☑
lacrimonasal duct — see Stenosis, lacrimal, duct
congenital Q10.5
larynx J38.6
congenital NEC Q31.8
subglottic Q31.1
syphilitic A52.73
congenital A50.59 [J99]
mitral (chronic) (inactive) (valve) I05.0
with
aortic valve disease I08.0
incompetency, insufficiency or regurgitation
I05.2
active or acute I01.1
with rheumatic or Sydenham's chorea I02.0
congenital Q23.2
specified cause, except rheumatic I34.2
syphilitic A52.03
myocardium, myocardial (see also Degeneration, myocardial)
hypertrophic subaortic (idiopathic) I42.1
nares (anterior) (posterior) J34.89
congenital Q30.0
nasal duct (see also Stenosis, lacrimal, duct)
congenital Q10.5
nasolacrimal duct (see also Stenosis, lacrimal, duct)
congenital Q10.5
neural canal (see also Lesion, biomechanical, specified
NEC)
connective tissue M99.49
abdomen M99.49
cervical region M99.41
cervicothoracic M99.41
head region M99.40
lower extremity M99.46
lumbar region M99.43
lumbosacral M99.43
occipitocervical M99.40
pelvic M99.45
rib cage M99.48
sacral region M99.44
sacrococcygeal M99.44

☑ **Additional Character Required — Refer to the Tabular List for Character Selection**   ▽ **Subterms under main terms may continue to next column or page**

Stenosis, stenotic — continued

neural canal (see also Lesion, biomechanical, specified) — continued

connective tissue — continued

sacroiliac M99.44

specified NEC M99.49

thoracic region M99.42

thoracolumbar M99.42

upper extremity M99.47

intervertebral disc M99.59

abdomen M99.59

cervical region M99.51

cervicothoracic M99.51

head region M99.50

lower extremity M99.56

lumbar region M99.53

lumbosacral M99.53

occipitocervical M99.50

pelvic M99.55

rib cage M99.58

sacral region M99.54

sacrococcygeal M99.54

sacroiliac M99.54

specified NEC M99.59

thoracic region M99.52

thoracolumbar M99.52

upper extremity M99.57

osseous M99.39

abdomen M99.39

cervical region M99.31

cervicothoracic M99.31

head region M99.30

lower extremity M99.36

lumbar region M99.33

lumbosacral M99.33

occipitocervical M99.30

pelvic M99.35

rib cage M99.38

sacral region M99.34

sacrococcygeal M99.34

sacroiliac M99.34

specified NEC M99.39

thoracic region M99.32

thoracolumbar M99.32

upper extremity M99.37

subluxation M99.29

cervical region M99.21

cervicothoracic M99.21

head region M99.20

lower extremity M99.26

lumbar region M99.23

lumbosacral M99.23

occipitocervical M99.20

pelvic M99.25

rib cage M99.28

sacral region M99.24

sacrococcygeal M99.24

sacroiliac M99.24

specified NEC M99.29

thoracic region M99.22

thoracolumbar M99.22

upper extremity M99.27

organ or site, congenital NEC — see Atresia, by site

papilla of Vater K83.1

pulmonary (artery) (congenital) Q25.6

with ventricular septal defect, transposition of aorta, and hypertrophy of right ventricle Q21.3

acquired I28.8

in tetralogy of Fallot Q21.3

infundibular Q24.3

subvalvular Q24.3

supravalvular Q25.6

valve I37.0

with insufficiency I37.2

congenital Q22.1

rheumatic I09.89

with aortic, mitral or tricuspid (valve) disease I08.8

vein, acquired I28.8

vessel NEC I28.8

pulmonic (congenital) Q22.1

infundibular Q24.3

subvalvular Q24.3

pylorus (hypertrophic) (acquired) K31.1

adult K31.1

congenital Q40.0

infantile Q40.0

Stenosis, stenotic — continued

rectum (sphincter) — see Stricture, rectum

renal artery I70.1

congenital Q27.1

salivary duct (any) K11.8

sphincter of Oddi K83.1

spinal M48.00

cervical region M48.02

cervicothoracic region M48.03

lumbar region M48.06

lumbosacral region M48.07

occipito-atlanto-axial region M48.01

sacrococcygeal region M48.08

thoracic region M48.04

thoracolumbar region M48.05

stomach, hourglass K31.2

subaortic (congenital) Q24.4

hypertrophic (idiopathic) I42.1

subglottic J38.6

congenital Q31.1

postprocedural J95.5

trachea J39.8

congenital Q32.1

syphilitic A52.73

tuberculous NEC A15.5

tracheostomy J95.03

tricuspid (valve) I07.0

with

aortic (valve) disease I08.2

incompetency, insufficiency or regurgitation I07.2

with aortic (valve) disease I08.2

with mitral (valve) disease I08.3

mitral (valve) disease I08.1

with aortic (valve) disease I08.3

congenital Q22.4

nonrheumatic I36.0

with insufficiency I36.2

tubal N97.1

ureter — see Atresia, ureter

ureteropelvic junction, congenital Q62.11

ureterovesical orifice, congenital Q62.12

urethra (valve) (see also Stricture, urethra)

congenital Q64.32

urinary meatus, congenital Q64.33

vagina N89.5

congenital Q52.4

in pregnancy — see Pregnancy, complicated by, abnormal vagina

causing obstructed labor O65.5

valve (cardiac) (heart) (see also Endocarditis) I38

congenital Q24.8

aortic Q23.0

mitral Q23.2

pulmonary Q22.1

tricuspid Q22.4

vena cava (inferior) (superior) I87.1

congenital Q26.0

vesicourethral orifice Q64.31

vulva N90.5

Stent jail T82.897 ☑

Stercolith (impaction) K56.41

appendix K38.1

Stercoraceous, stercoral ulcer K63.3

anus or rectum K62.6

Stereotypies NEC F98.4

Sterility — see Infertility

Sterilization — see Encounter (for), sterilization

Sternalgia — see Angina

Sternopagus Q89.4

Sternum bifidum Q76.7

Steroid

effects (adverse) (adrenocortical) (iatrogenic)

cushingoid E24.2

correct substance properly administered — see Table of Drugs and Chemicals, by drug, adverse effect

overdose or wrong substance given or taken — see Table of Drugs and Chemicals, by drug, poisoning

diabetes — see subcategory E09 ☑

correct substance properly administered — see Table of Drugs and Chemicals, by drug, adverse effect

overdose or wrong substance given or taken — see Table of Drugs and Chemicals, by drug, poisoning

fever R50.2

Steroid — continued

effects — continued

insufficiency E27.3

correct substance properly administered — see Table of Drugs and Chemicals, by drug, adverse effect

overdose or wrong substance given or taken — see Table of Drugs and Chemicals, by drug, poisoning

responder H40.04- ☑

Stevens-Johnson disease or syndrome L51.1

toxic epidermal necrolysis overlap L51.3

Stewart-Morel syndrome M85.2

Sticker's disease B08.3

Sticky eye — see Conjunctivitis, acute, mucopurulent

Stieda's disease — see Bursitis, tibial collateral

Stiff neck — see Torticollis

Stiff-man syndrome G25.82

Stiffness, joint NEC M25.60

ankle M25.67- ☑

ankylosis — see Ankylosis, joint

contracture — see Contraction, joint

elbow M25.62- ☑

foot M25.67- ☑

hand M25.64- ☑

hip M25.65- ☑

knee M25.66- ☑

shoulder M25.61- ☑

wrist M25.63- ☑

Stigmata congenital syphilis A50.59

Still-Felty syndrome — see Felty's syndrome

Stillbirth P95

Still's disease or syndrome (juvenile) M08.20

adult-onset M06.1

ankle M08.27- ☑

elbow M08.22- ☑

foot joint M08.27- ☑

hand joint M08.24- ☑

hip M08.25- ☑

knee M08.26- ☑

multiple site M08.29

shoulder M08.21- ☑

vertebra M08.28

wrist M08.23- ☑

Stimulation, ovary E28.1

Sting (venomous) (with allergic or anaphylactic shock) — see Table of Drugs and Chemicals, by animal or substance, poisoning

Stippled epiphyses Q78.8

Stitch

abscess T81.4 ☑

burst (in operation wound) — see Disruption, wound, operation

Stokes' disease E05.00

with thyroid storm E05.01

Stokes-Adams disease or syndrome I45.9

Stokvis (-Talma) **disease** D74.8

Stoma malfunction

colostomy K94.03

enterostomy K94.13

gastrostomy K94.23

ileostomy K94.13

tracheostomy J95.03

Stomach — see condition

Stomatitis (denture) (ulcerative) K12.1

angular K13.0

due to dietary or vitamin deficiency E53.0

aphthous K12.0

bovine B08.61

candidal B37.0

catarrhal K12.1

diphtheritic A36.89

due to

dietary deficiency E53.0

thrush B37.0

vitamin deficiency

B group NEC E53.9

B2 (riboflavin) E53.0

epidemic B08.8

epizootic B08.8

follicular K12.1

gangrenous A69.0

Geotrichum B48.3

herpesviral, herpetic B00.2

herpetiformis K12.0

malignant K12.1

membranous acute K12.1

Stomatitis — continued
   monilial B37.0
   mycotic B37.0
   necrotizing ulcerative A69.0
   parasitic B37.0
   septic K12.1
   spirochetal A69.1
   suppurative (acute) K12.2
   ulceromembranous A69.1
   vesicular K12.1
     with exanthem (enteroviral) B08.4
     virus disease A93.8
   Vincent's A69.1
Stomatocytosis D58.8
Stomatomycosis B37.0
Stomatorrhagia K13.79
Stone(s) (see also Calculus)
   bladder (diverticulum) N21.0
   cystine E72.09
   heart syndrome I50.1
   kidney N20.0
   prostate N42.0
   pulpal (dental) K04.2
   renal N20.0
   salivary gland or duct (any) K11.5
   urethra (impacted) N21.1
   urinary (duct) (impacted) (passage) N20.9
     bladder (diverticulum) N21.0
     lower tract N21.9
     specified NEC N21.8
   xanthine E79.8 [N22]
Stonecutter's lung J62.8
Stonemason's asthma, disease, lung or pneumoconiosis J62.8
Stoppage
   heart — see Arrest, cardiac
   urine — see Retention, urine
Storm, thyroid — see Thyrotoxicosis
Strabismus (congenital) (nonparalytic) H50.9
   concomitant H50.40
     convergent — see Strabismus, convergent concomitant
     divergent — see Strabismus, divergent concomitant
   convergent concomitant H50.00
     accommodative component H50.43
     alternating H50.05
       with
         A pattern H50.06
         specified nonconcomitances NEC H50.08
         V pattern H50.07
     monocular H50.01- ☑
       with
         A pattern H50.02- ☑
         specified nonconcomitances NEC H50.04- ☑
         V pattern H50.03- ☑
       intermittent H50.31- ☑
         alternating H50.32
   cyclotropia H50.1- ☑
   divergent concomitant H50.10
     alternating H50.15
       with
         A pattern H50.16
         specified noncomitances NEC H50.18
         V pattern H50.17
     monocular H50.11- ☑
       with
         A pattern H50.12- ☑
         specified noncomitances NEC H50.14- ☑
         V pattern H50.13- ☑
       intermittent H50.33 ☑
         alternating H50.34
   Duane's syndrome H50.81- ☑
   due to adhesions, scars H50.69
   heterophoria H50.50
     alternating H50.55
     cyclophoria H50.54
     esophoria H50.51
     exophoria H50.52
     vertical H50.53
   heterotropia H50.40
     intermittent H50.30
   hypertropia H50.2- ☑
   hypotropia — see Hypertropia
   latent H50.50
   mechanical H50.60
     Brown's sheath syndrome H50.61- ☑

Strabismus — continued
   mechanical — continued
     specified type NEC H50.69
   monofixation syndrome H50.42
   paralytic H49.9
     abducens nerve H49.2- ☑
     fourth nerve H49.1- ☑
     Kearns-Sayre syndrome H49.81- ☑
     ophthalmoplegia (external)
       progressive H49.4- ☑
         with pigmentary retinopathy H49.81- ☑
       total H49.3- ☑
     sixth nerve H49.2- ☑
     specified type NEC H49.88- ☑
     third nerve H49.0- ☑
     trochlear nerve H49.1- ☑
   specified type NEC H50.89
   vertical H50.2- ☑
Strain
   back S39.012 ☑
   cervical S16.1 ☑
   eye NEC — see Disturbance, vision, subjective
   heart — see Disease, heart
   low back S39.012 ☑
   mental NOS Z73.3
     work-related Z56.6
   muscle (tendon) — see Injury, muscle, by site, strain
   neck S16.1 ☑
   physical NOS Z73.3
     work-related Z56.6
   postural (see also Disorder, soft tissue, due to use)
   psychological NEC Z73.3
   tendon — see Injury, muscle, by site, strain
Straining, on urination R39.16
Strand, vitreous — see Opacity, vitreous, membranes and strands
Strangulation, strangulated (see also Asphyxia, traumatic)
   appendix K38.8
   bladder-neck N32.0
   bowel or colon K56.2
   food or foreign body — see Foreign body, by site
   hemorrhoids — see Hemorrhoids, with complication
   hernia (see also Hernia, by site, with obstruction)
     with gangrene — see Hernia, by site, with gangrene
   intestine (large) (small) K56.2
     with hernia (see also Hernia, by site, with obstruction)
       with gangrene — see Hernia, by site, with gangrene
   mesentery K56.2
   mucus — see Asphyxia, mucus
   omentum K56.2
   organ or site, congenital NEC — see Atresia, by site
   ovary — see Torsion, ovary
   penis N48.89
     foreign body T19.4 ☑
   rupture — see Hernia, by site, with obstruction
   stomach due to hernia (see also Hernia, by site, with obstruction)
     with gangrene — see Hernia, by site, with gangrene
   vesicourethral orifice N32.0
Strangury R30.0
Straw itch B88.0
Strawberry
   gallbladder K82.4
   mark Q82.5
   tongue (red) (white) K14.3
Streak(s)
   macula, angioid H35.33
   ovarian Q50.32
Strephosymbolia F81.0
   secondary to organic lesion R48.8
Streptobacillary fever A25.1
Streptobacillosis A25.1
Streptobacillus moniliformis A25.1
Streptococcus, streptococcal (see also condition)
   as cause of disease classified elsewhere B95.5
   group
     A, as cause of disease classified elsewhere B95.0
     B, as cause of disease classified elsewhere B95.1
     D, as cause of disease classified elsewhere B95.2
   pneumoniae, as cause of disease classified elsewhere B95.3

Streptococcus, streptococcal — continued
   specified NEC, as cause of disease classified elsewhere B95.4
Streptomycosis B47.1
Streptotrichosis A48.8
Stress F43.9
   family — see Disruption, family
   fetal P84
     complicating pregnancy O77.9
     due to drug administration O77.1
   mental NEC Z73.3
     work-related Z56.6
   physical NEC Z73.3
     work-related Z56.6
   polycythemia D75.1
   reaction (see also Reaction, stress) F43.9
   work schedule Z56.3
Stretching, nerve — see Injury, nerve
Striae albicantes, atrophicae or distensae (cutis) L90.6
Stricture (see also Stenosis)
   ampulla of Vater K83.1
   anus (sphincter) K62.4
     congenital Q42.3
       with fistula Q42.2
     infantile Q42.3
       with fistula Q42.2
   aorta (ascending) (congenital) Q25.3
     arteriosclerotic I70.0
     calcified I70.0
     supravalvular, congenital Q25.3
   aortic (valve) — see Stenosis, aortic
   aqueduct of Sylvius (congenital) Q03.0
     with spina bifida — see Spina bifida, by site, with hydrocephalus
     acquired G91.1
   artery I77.1
     basilar — see Occlusion, artery, basilar
     carotid — see Occlusion, artery, carotid
     celiac I77.4
     congenital (peripheral) Q27.8
       cerebral Q28.3
       coronary Q24.5
       digestive system Q27.8
       lower limb Q27.8
       retinal Q14.1
       specified site NEC Q27.8
       umbilical Q27.0
       upper limb Q27.8
     coronary — see Disease, heart, ischemic, atherosclerotic
       congenital Q24.5
     precerebral — see Occlusion, artery, precerebral
     pulmonary (congenital) Q25.6
       acquired I28.8
     renal I70.1
     vertebral — see Occlusion, artery, vertebral
   auditory canal (external) (congenital)
     acquired — see Stenosis, external ear canal
   bile duct (common) (hepatic) K83.1
     congenital Q44.3
     postoperative K91.89
   bladder N32.89
     neck N32.0
   bowel — see Obstruction, intestine
   brain G93.89
   bronchus J98.09
     congenital Q32.3
     syphilitic A52.72
   cardia (stomach) K22.2
     congenital Q39.3
   cardiac (see also Disease, heart)
     orifice (stomach) K22.2
   cecum — see Obstruction, intestine
   cervix, cervical (canal) N88.2
     congenital Q51.828
     in pregnancy — see Pregnancy, complicated by, abnormal cervix
       causing obstructed labor O65.5
   colon (see also Obstruction, intestine)
     congenital Q42.9
       specified NEC Q42.8
   colostomy K94.03
   common (bile) duct K83.1
   coronary (artery) — see Disease, heart, ischemic, atherosclerotic
   cystic duct — see Obstruction, gallbladder
   digestive organs NEC, congenital Q45.8
   duodenum K31.5

Stricture — *continued*
  duodenum — *continued*
    congenital Q41.0
  ear canal (external) (congenital) Q16.1
    acquired — *see* Stricture, auditory canal, acquired
  ejaculatory duct N50.8
  enterostomy K94.13
  esophagus K22.2
    congenital Q39.3
    syphilitic A52.79
      congenital A50.59 [K23]
  eustachian tube (*see also* Obstruction, eustachian tube)
    congenital Q17.8
  fallopian tube N97.1
    gonococcal A54.24
    tuberculous A18.17
  gallbladder — *see* Obstruction, gallbladder
  glottis J38.6
  heart (*see also* Disease, heart)
    valve (*see also* Endocarditis) I38
      aortic Q23.0
      mitral Q23.4
      pulmonary Q22.1
      tricuspid Q22.4
  hepatic duct K83.1
  hourglass, of stomach K31.2
  hymen N89.6
  hypopharynx J39.2
  ileum K56.69
    congenital Q41.2
  intestine (*see also* Obstruction, intestine)
    congenital (small) Q41.9
      large Q42.9
        specified NEC Q42.8
      specified NEC Q41.8
    ischemic K55.1
  jejunum K56.69
    congenital Q41.1
  lacrimal passages (*see also* Stenosis, lacrimal)
    congenital Q10.5
  larynx J38.6
    congenital NEC Q31.8
      subglottic Q31.1
    syphilitic A52.73
      congenital A50.59 [J99]
  meatus
    ear (congenital) Q16.1
      acquired — *see* Stricture, auditory canal, acquired
    osseous (ear) (congenital) Q16.1
      acquired — *see* Stricture, auditory canal, acquired
    urinarius (*see also* Stricture, urethra)
      congenital Q64.33
  mitral (valve) — *see* Stenosis, mitral
  myocardium, myocardial I51.5
    hypertrophic subaortic (idiopathic) I42.1
  nares (anterior) (posterior) J34.89
    congenital Q30.0
  nasal duct (*see also* Stenosis, lacrimal, duct)
    congenital Q10.5
  nasolacrimal duct (*see also* Stenosis, lacrimal, duct)
    congenital Q10.5
  nasopharynx J39.2
    syphilitic A52.73
  nose J34.89
    congenital Q30.0
  nostril (anterior) (posterior) J34.89
    congenital Q30.0
    syphilitic A52.73
      congenital A50.59 [J99]
  organ or site, congenital NEC — *see* Atresia, by site
  os uteri — *see* Stricture, cervix
  osseous meatus (ear) (congenital) Q16.1
    acquired — *see* Stricture, auditory canal, acquired
  oviduct — *see* Stricture, fallopian tube
  pelviureteric junction (congenital) Q62.11
  penis, by foreign body T19.4 ☑
  pharynx J39.2
  prostate N42.89
  pulmonary, pulmonic
    artery (congenital) Q25.6
      acquired I28.8
      noncongenital I28.8
    infundibulum (congenital) Q24.3
    valve I37.0
      congenital Q22.1
    vein, acquired I28.8

Stricture — *continued*
  pulmonary, pulmonic — *continued*
    vessel NEC I28.8
  punctum lacrimale (*see also* Stenosis, lacrimal, punctum)
    congenital Q10.5
  pylorus (hypertrophic) K31.1
    adult K31.1
    congenital Q40.0
    infantile Q40.0
  rectosigmoid K56.69
  rectum (sphincter) K62.4
    congenital Q42.1
      with fistula Q42.0
    due to
      chlamydial lymphogranuloma A55
      irradiation K91.89
      lymphogranuloma venereum A55
    gonococcal A54.6
    inflammatory (chlamydial) A55
    syphilitic A52.74
    tuberculous A18.32
  renal artery I70.1
    congenital Q27.1
  salivary duct or gland (any) K11.8
  sigmoid (flexure) — *see* Obstruction, intestine
  spermatic cord N50.8
  stoma (following) (of)
    colostomy K94.03
    enterostomy K94.13
    gastrostomy K94.23
    ileostomy K94.13
    tracheostomy J95.03
  stomach K31.89
    congenital Q40.2
    hourglass K31.2
  subaortic Q24.4
    hypertrophic (acquired) (idiopathic) I42.1
  subglottic J38.6
  syphilitic NEC A52.79
  trachea J39.8
    congenital Q32.1
    syphilitic A52.73
    tuberculous NEC A15.5
  tracheostomy J95.03
  tricuspid (valve) — *see* Stenosis, tricuspid
  tunica vaginalis N50.8
  ureter (postoperative) N13.5
    with
      hydronephrosis N13.1
        with infection N13.6
      pyelonephritis (chronic) N11.1
    congenital — *see* Atresia, ureter
    tuberculous A18.11
  ureteropelvic junction (congenital) Q62.11
  ureterovesical orifice N13.5
    with infection N13.6
  urethra (organic) (spasmodic) N35.9
    associated with schistosomiasis B65.0 [N37]
    congenital Q64.39
      valvular (posterior) Q64.2
    due to
      infection — *see* Stricture, urethra, postinfective
      trauma — *see* Stricture, urethra, post-traumatic
    gonococcal, gonorrheal A54.01
    infective NEC — *see* Stricture, urethra, postinfective
    late effect (sequelae) of injury — *see* Stricture, urethra, post-traumatic
    post-traumatic
      female N35.028
        due to childbirth N35.021
      male N35.014
        anterior urethra N35.013
        bulbous urethra N35.011
        meatal N35.010
        membranous urethra N35.012
    postcatheterization — *see* Stricture, urethra, postprocedural
    postinfective NEC
      female N35.12
      male N35.119
        anterior urethra N35.114
        bulbous urethra N35.112
        meatal N35.111
        membranous urethra N35.113
    postobstetric N35.021
    postoperative — *see* Stricture, urethra, postprocedural

Stricture — *continued*
  urethra — *continued*
    postprocedural
      female N99.12
      male N99.114
        anterior urethra N99.113
        bulbous urethra N99.111
        meatal N99.110
        membranous urethra N99.112
    sequela (late effect) of
      childbirth N35.021
      injury — *see* Stricture, urethra, post-traumatic
    specified cause NEC N35.8
    syphilitic A52.76
    traumatic — *see* Stricture, urethra, post-traumatic
    valvular (posterior), congenital Q64.2
  urinary meatus — *see* Stricture, urethra
  uterus, uterine (synechiae) N85.6
    os (external) (internal) — *see* Stricture, cervix
  vagina (outlet) — *see* Stenosis, vagina
  valve (cardiac) (heart) (*see also* Endocarditis)
    congenital
      aortic Q23.0
      mitral Q23.2
      pulmonary Q22.1
      tricuspid Q22.4
  vas deferens N50.8
    congenital Q55.4
  vein I87.1
  vena cava (inferior) (superior) NEC I87.1
    congenital Q26.0
  vesicourethral orifice N32.0
    congenital Q64.31
  vulva (acquired) N90.5
Stridor R06.1
  congenital (larynx) P28.89
Stridulous — *see* condition
Stroke (apoplectic) (brain) (embolic) (ischemic) (paralytic) (thrombotic) I63.9
  epileptic — *see* Epilepsy
  heat T67.0 ☑
  in evolution I63.9
  intraoperative
    during cardiac surgery I97.810
    during other surgery I97.811
  lightning — *see* Lightning
  meaning
    cerebral hemorrhage — *code to* Hemorrhage, intracranial
    cerebral infarction — *code to* Infarction, cerebral
  postprocedural
    following cardiac surgery I97.820
    following other surgery I97.821
  unspecified (NOS) I63.9
Stromatosis, endometrial D39.0
Strongyloidiasis, strongyloidosis B78.9
  cutaneous B78.1
  disseminated B78.7
  intestinal B78.0
Strophulus pruriginosus L28.2
Struck by lightning — *see* Lightning
Struma (*see also* Goiter)
  Hashimoto E06.3
  lymphomatosa E06.3
  nodosa (simplex) E04.9
    endemic E01.2
      multinodular E01.1
    multinodular E04.2
      iodine-deficiency related E01.1
    toxic or with hyperthyroidism E05.20
      with thyroid storm E05.21
      multinodular E05.20
        with thyroid storm E05.21
      uninodular E05.10
        with thyroid storm E05.11
    toxicosa E05.20
      with thyroid storm E05.21
      multinodular E05.20
        with thyroid storm E05.21
      uninodular E05.10
        with thyroid storm E05.11
    uninodular E04.1
  ovarii D27.- ☑
  Riedel's E06.5
Strumipriva cachexia E03.4
Strümpell-Marie spine — *see* Spondylitis, ankylosing
Strümpell-Westphal pseudosclerosis E83.01
Stuart deficiency disease (factor X) D68.2

Stuart-Prower factor deficiency (factor X) D68.2
Student's elbow — *see* Bursitis, elbow, olecranon
Stump — *see* Amputation
Stunting, nutritional E45
Stupor (catatonic) R40.1
  depressive F32.8
  dissociative F44.2
  manic F30.2
  manic-depressive F31.89
  psychogenic (anergic) F44.2
  reaction to exceptional stress (transient) F43.0
Sturge (-Weber) (-Dimitri) (-Kalischer) **disease or syndrome** Q85.8
Stuttering F80.81
  adult onset F98.5
  childhood onset F80.81
  following cerebrovascular disease — *see* Disorder, fluency. following cerebrovascular disease
  in conditions classified elsewhere R47.82
Sty, stye (external) (internal) (meibomian) (zeisian) — *see* Hordeolum
Subacidity, gastric K31.89
  psychogenic F45.8
Subacute — *see* condition
Subarachnoid — *see* condition
Subcortical — *see* condition
Subcostal syndrome, nerve compression — *see* Mononeuropathy, upper limb, specified site NEC
Subcutaneous, subcuticular — *see* condition
Subdural — *see* condition
Subendocardium — *see* condition
Subependymoma
  specified site — *see* Neoplasm, uncertain behavior, by site
  unspecified site D43.2
Suberosis J67.3
Subglossitis — *see* Glossitis
Subhemophilia D66
Subinvolution
  breast (postlactational) (postpuerperal) N64.89
  puerperal O90.89
  uterus (chronic) (nonpuerperal) N85.3
    puerperal O90.89
Sublingual — *see* condition
Sublinguitis — *see* Sialoadenitis
Subluxatable hip Q65.6
Subluxation (*see also* Dislocation)
  acromioclavicular S43.11- ☑
  ankle S93.0- ☑
  atlantoaxial, recurrent M43.4
    with myelopathy M43.3
  carpometacarpal (joint) NEC S63.05- ☑
    thumb S63.04- ☑
  complex, vertebral — *see* Complex, subluxation
  congenital (*see also* Malposition, congenital)
    hip — *see* Dislocation, hip, congenital, partial
    joint (excluding hip)
      lower limb Q68.8
      shoulder Q68.8
      upper limb Q68.8
  elbow (traumatic) S53.10- ☑
    anterior S53.11- ☑
    lateral S53.14- ☑
    medial S53.13- ☑
    posterior S53.12- ☑
    specified type NEC S53.19- ☑
  finger S63.20- ☑
    index S63.20- ☑
    interphalangeal S63.22- ☑
      distal S63.24- ☑
        index S63.24- ☑
        little S63.24- ☑
        middle S63.24- ☑
        ring S63.24- ☑
      index S63.22- ☑
      little S63.22- ☑
      middle S63.22- ☑
      proximal S63.23- ☑
        index S63.23- ☑
        little S63.23- ☑
        middle S63.23- ☑
        ring S63.23- ☑
      ring S63.22- ☑
    little S63.20- ☑
    metacarpophalangeal S63.21- ☑
      index S63.21- ☑

      little S63.21- ☑
      middle S63.21- ☑
      ring S63.21- ☑
    middle S63.20- ☑
    ring S63.20- ☑
  foot S93.30- ☑
    specified site NEC S93.33- ☑
    tarsal joint S93.31- ☑
    tarsometatarsal joint S93.32- ☑
    toe — *see* Subluxation, toe
  hip S73.00- ☑
    anterior S73.03- ☑
      obturator S73.02- ☑
    central S73.04- ☑
    posterior S73.01- ☑
  interphalangeal (joint)
    finger S63.22- ☑
      distal joint S63.24- ☑
        index S63.24- ☑
        little S63.24- ☑
        middle S63.24- ☑
        ring S63.24- ☑
      index S63.22- ☑
      little S63.22- ☑
      middle S63.22- ☑
      proximal joint S63.23- ☑
        index S63.23- ☑
        little S63.23- ☑
        middle S63.23- ☑
        ring S63.23- ☑
      ring S63.22- ☑
    thumb S63.12- ☑
      distal joint S63.14- ☑
      proximal joint S63.13- ☑
    toe S93.13- ☑
      great S93.13- ☑
      lesser S93.13- ☑
  joint prosthesis — *see* Complications, joint prosthesis, mechanical, displacement, by site
  knee S83.10- ☑
    cap — *see* Subluxation, patella
    patella — *see* Subluxation, patella
    proximal tibia
      anteriorly S83.11- ☑
      laterally S83.14- ☑
      medially S83.13- ☑
      posteriorly S83.12- ☑
      specified type NEC S83.19- ☑
  lens — *see* Dislocation, lens, partial
  ligament, traumatic — *see* Sprain, by site
  metacarpal (bone)
    proximal end S63.06- ☑
  metacarpophalangeal (joint)
    finger S63.21- ☑
      index S63.21- ☑
      little S63.21- ☑
      middle S63.21- ☑
      ring S63.21- ☑
    thumb S63.11- ☑
  metatarsophalangeal joint S93.14- ☑
    great toe S93.14- ☑
    lesser toe S93.14- ☑
  midcarpal (joint) S63.03- ☑
  patella S83.00- ☑
    lateral S83.01- ☑
    recurrent (nontraumatic) — *see* Dislocation, patella, recurrent, incomplete
    specified type NEC S83.09- ☑
  pathological — *see* Dislocation, pathological
  radial head S53.00- ☑
    anterior S53.01- ☑
    nursemaid's elbow S53.03- ☑
    posterior S53.02- ☑
    specified type NEC S53.09- ☑
  radiocarpal (joint) S63.02- ☑
  radioulnar (joint)
    distal S63.01- ☑
    proximal — *see* Subluxation, elbow
  shoulder
    congenital Q68.8
    girdle S43.30- ☑
      scapula S43.31- ☑
      specified site NEC S43.39- ☑

Subluxation — *continued*
  shoulder — *continued*
    traumatic S43.00- ☑
      anterior S43.01- ☑
      inferior S43.03- ☑
      posterior S43.02- ☑
      specified type NEC S43.08- ☑
  sternoclavicular (joint) S43.20- ☑
    anterior S43.21- ☑
    posterior S43.22- ☑
  symphysis (pubis)
  thumb S63.103 ☑
    interphalangeal joint — *see* Subluxation, interphalangeal (joint), thumb
    metacarpophalangeal joint — *see* Subluxation, metacarpophalangeal (joint), thumb
  toe(s) S93.10- ☑
    great S93.10- ☑
      interphalangeal joint S93.13- ☑
      metatarsophalangeal joint S93.14- ☑
    interphalangeal joint S93.13- ☑
    lesser S93.10- ☑
      interphalangeal joint S93.13- ☑
      metatarsophalangeal joint S93.14- ☑
    metatarsophalangeal joint S93.149 ☑
  ulna
    distal end S63.07- ☑
    proximal end — *see* Subluxation, elbow
  ulnohumeral joint — *see* Subluxation, elbow
  vertebral
    recurrent NEC — *see* subcategory M43.5 ☑
    traumatic
      cervical S13.100 ☑
        atlantoaxial joint S13.120 ☑
        atlantooccipital joint S13.110 ☑
        atloidooccipital joint S13.110 ☑
        joint between
          C0 and C1 S13.110 ☑
          C1 and C2 S13.120 ☑
          C2 and C3 S13.130 ☑
          C3 and C4 S13.140 ☑
          C4 and C5 S13.150 ☑
          C5 and C6 S13.160 ☑
          C6 and C7 S13.170 ☑
          C7 and T1 S13.180 ☑
        occipitoatloid joint S13.110 ☑
      lumbar S33.100 ☑
        joint between
          L1 and L2 S33.110 ☑
          L2 and L3 S33.120 ☑
          L3 and L4 S33.130 ☑
          L4 and L5 S33.140 ☑
      thoracic S23.100 ☑
        joint between
          T1 and T2 S23.110 ☑
          T2 and T3 S23.120 ☑
          T3 and T4 S23.122 ☑
          T4 and T5 S23.130 ☑
          T5 and T6 S23.132 ☑
          T6 and T7 S23.140 ☑
          T7 and T8 S23.142 ☑
          T8 and T9 S23.150 ☑
          T9 and T10 S23.152 ☑
          T10 and T11 S23.160 ☑
          T11 and T12 S23.162 ☑
          T12 and L1 S23.170 ☑
  wrist (carpal bone) S63.00- ☑
    carpometacarpal joint — *see* Subluxation, carpometacarpal (joint)
    distal radioulnar joint — *see* Subluxation, radioulnar (joint), distal
    metacarpal bone, proximal — *see* Subluxation, metacarpal (bone), proximal end
    midcarpal — *see* Subluxation, midcarpal (joint)
    radiocarpal joint — *see* Subluxation, radiocarpal (joint)
    recurrent — *see* Dislocation, recurrent, wrist
    specified site NEC S63.09- ☑
    ulna — *see* Subluxation, ulna, distal end
Submaxillary — *see* condition
Submersion (fatal) (nonfatal) T75.1 ☑
Submucous — *see* condition
Subnormal, subnormality
  accommodation (old age) H52.4
  mental — *see* Disability, intellectual
  temperature (accidental) T68 ☑

☑ Additional Character Required — Refer to the Tabular List for Character Selection

▽ Subterms under main terms may continue to next column or page

Subphrenic — *see* condition
Subscapular nerve — *see* condition
Subseptus uterus Q51.2
Subsiding appendicitis K36
Substernal thyroid E04.9
  congenital Q89.2
Substitution disorder F44.9
Subtentorial — *see* condition
Subthyroidism (acquired) (*see also* Hypothyroidism)
  congenital E03.1
Succenturiate placenta O43.19- ☑
Sucking thumb, child (excessive) F98.8
Sudamen, sudamina L74.1
Sudanese kala-azar B55.0
Sudden
  hearing loss — *see* Deafness, sudden
  heart failure — *see* Failure, heart
Sudeck's atrophy, disease, or syndrome — *see* Algo-
  neurodystrophy
Suffocation — *see* Asphyxia, traumatic
Sugar
  blood
    high (transient) R73.9
    low (transient) E16.2
  in urine R81
Suicide, suicidal (attempted) T14.91
  by poisoning — *see* Table of Drugs and Chemicals
  history of (personal) Z91.5
    in family Z81.8
  ideation — *see* Ideation, suicidal
  risk
    meaning personal history of attempted suicide
      Z91.5
    meaning suicidal ideation — *see* Ideation, suicidal
  tendencies
    meaning personal history of attempted suicide
      Z91.5
    meaning suicidal ideation — *see* Ideation, suicidal
  trauma — *see* nature of injury by site
Suipestifer infection — *see* Infection, salmonella
Sulfhemoglobinemia, sulphemoglobinemia (acquired) (with methemoglobinemia) D74.8
Sumatran mite fever A75.3
Summer — *see* condition
Sunburn L55.9
  first degree L55.0
  second degree L55.1
  third degree L55.2
SUNCT (short lasting unilateral neuralgiform headache
  with conjunctival injection and tearing) G44.059
  intractable G44.051
  not intractable G44.059
Sunken acetabulum — *see* Derangement, joint, specified type NEC, hip
Sunstroke T67.0 ☑
Superfecundation — *see* Pregnancy, multiple
Superfetation — *see* Pregnancy, multiple
Superinvolution (uterus) N85.8
Supernumerary (congenital)
  aortic cusps Q23.8
  auditory ossicles Q16.3
  bone Q79.8
  breast Q83.1
  carpal bones Q74.0
  cusps, heart valve NEC Q24.8
    aortic Q23.8
    mitral Q23.2
    pulmonary Q22.3
  digit(s) Q69.9
  ear (lobule) Q17.0
  fallopian tube Q50.6
  finger Q69.0
  hymen Q52.4
  kidney Q63.0
  lacrimonasal duct Q10.6
  lobule (ear) Q17.0
  mitral cusps Q23.2
  muscle Q79.8
  nipple(s) Q83.3
  organ or site not listed — *see* Accessory
  ossicles, auditory Q16.3
  ovary Q50.31
  oviduct Q50.6
  pulmonary, pulmonic cusps Q22.3
  rib Q76.6
    cervical or first (syndrome) Q76.5
  roots (of teeth) K00.2

Supernumerary — *continued*
  spleen Q89.09
  tarsal bones Q74.2
  teeth K00.1
  testis Q55.29
  thumb Q69.1
  toe Q69.2
  uterus Q51.2
  vagina Q52.1 ☑
  vertebra Q76.49
Supervision (of)
  contraceptive — *see* Prescription, contraceptives
  dietary (for) Z71.3
    allergy (food) Z71.3
    colitis Z71.3
    diabetes mellitus Z71.3
    food allergy or intolerance Z71.3
    gastritis Z71.3
    hypercholesterolemia Z71.3
    hypoglycemia Z71.3
    intolerance (food) Z71.3
    obesity Z71.3
    specified NEC Z71.3
  healthy infant or child Z76.2
    foundling Z76.1
  high-risk pregnancy — *see* Pregnancy, complicated
    by, high, risk
  lactation Z39.1
  pregnancy — *see* Pregnancy, supervision of
Supplemental teeth K00.1
Suppression
  binocular vision H53.34
  lactation O92.5
  menstruation N94.89
  ovarian secretion E28.39
  renal N28.9
  urine, urinary secretion R34
Suppuration, suppurative (*see also* condition)
  accessory sinus (chronic) — *see* Sinusitis
  adrenal gland
  antrum (chronic) — *see* Sinusitis, maxillary
  bladder — *see* Cystitis
  brain G06.0
    sequelae G09
  breast N61
    puerperal, postpartum or gestational — *see* Masti-
      tis, obstetric, purulent
  dental periosteum M27.3
  ear (middle) (*see also* Otitis, media)
    external NEC — *see* Otitis, externa, infective
    internal — *see* subcategory H83.0 ☑
  ethmoidal (chronic) (sinus) — *see* Sinusitis, ethmoidal
  fallopian tube — *see* Salpingo-oophoritis
  frontal (chronic) (sinus) — *see* Sinusitis, frontal
  gallbladder (acute) K81.0
  gum K05.20
    generalized K05.22
    localized K05.21
  intracranial G06.0
  joint — *see* Arthritis, pyogenic or pyemic
  labyrinthine — *see* subcategory H83.0 ☑
  lung — *see* Abscess, lung
  mammary gland N61
    puerperal, postpartum O91.12
      associated with lactation O91.13
  maxilla, maxillary M27.2
    sinus (chronic) — *see* Sinusitis, maxillary
  muscle — *see* Myositis, infective
  nasal sinus (chronic) — *see* Sinusitis
  pancreas, acute K85.8
  parotid gland — *see* Sialoadenitis
  pelvis, pelvic
    female — *see* Disease, pelvis, inflammatory
    male K65.0
  pericranial — *see* Osteomyelitis
  salivary duct or gland (any) — *see* Sialoadenitis
  sinus (accessory) (chronic) (nasal) — *see* Sinusitis
  sphenoidal sinus (chronic) — *see* Sinusitis, sphenoidal
  thymus (gland) E32.1
  thyroid (gland) E06.0
  tonsil — *see* Tonsillitis
  uterus — *see* Endometritis
Supraeruption of tooth (teeth) M26.34
Supraglottitis J04.30
  with obstruction J04.31
Suprarenal (gland) — *see* condition
Suprascapular nerve — *see* condition

Suprasellar — *see* condition
Surfer's knots or nodules S89.8- ☑
Surgical
  emphysema T81.82 ☑
  procedures, complication or misadventure — *see*
    Complications, surgical procedures
  shock T81.10 ☑
Surveillance (of) (for) (*see also* Observation)
  alcohol abuse Z71.41
  contraceptive — *see* Prescription, contraceptives
  dietary Z71.3
  drug abuse Z71.51
Susceptibility to disease, genetic Z15.89
  malignant neoplasm Z15.09
    breast Z15.01
    endometrium Z15.04
    ovary Z15.02
    prostate Z15.03
    specified NEC Z15.09
  multiple endocrine neoplasia Z15.81
Suspected condition, ruled out (*see also* Observation,
  suspected)
  amniotic cavity and membrane Z03.71
  cervical shortening Z03.75
  fetal anomaly Z03.73
  fetal growth Z03.74
  maternal and fetal conditions NEC Z03.79
  oligohydramnios Z03.71
  placental problem Z03.72
  polyhydramnios Z03.71
Suspended uterus
  in pregnancy or childbirth — *see* Pregnancy, compli-
    cated by, abnormal uterus
Sutton's nevus D22.9
Suture
  burst (in operation wound) T81.31 ☑
    external operation wound T81.31 ☑
    internal operation wound T81.32 ☑
  inadvertently left in operation wound — *see* Foreign
    body, accidentally left during a procedure
  removal Z48.02
Swab inadvertently left in operation wound — *see*
  Foreign body, accidentally left during a procedure
Swallowed, swallowing
  difficulty — *see* Dysphagia
  foreign body — *see* Foreign body, alimentary tract
Swan-neck deformity (finger) — *see* Deformity, finger,
  swan-neck
Swearing, compulsive F42
  in Gilles de la Tourette's syndrome F95.2
Sweat, sweats
  fetid L75.0
  night R61
Sweating, excessive R61
Sweeley-Klionsky disease E75.21
Sweet's disease or dermatosis L98.2
Swelling (of) R60.9
  abdomen, abdominal (not referable to any particular
    organ) — *see* Mass, abdominal
  ankle — *see* Effusion, joint, ankle
  arm M79.89
    forearm M79.89
  breast N63
  Calabar B74.3
  cervical gland R59.0
  chest, localized R22.2
  ear H93.8- ☑
  extremity (lower) (upper) — *see* Disorder, soft tissue,
    specified type NEC
  finger M79.89
  foot M79.89
  glands R59.9
    generalized R59.1
    localized R59.0
  hand M79.89
  head (localized) R22.0
  inflammatory — *see* Inflammation
  intra-abdominal — *see* Mass, abdominal
  joint — *see* Effusion, joint
  leg M79.89
    lower M79.89
  limb — *see* Disorder, soft tissue, specified type NEC
  localized (skin) R22.9
    chest R22.2
    head R22.0
    limb
      lower — *see* Mass, localized, limb, lower

Swelling — continued
  localized — continued
    limb — continued
      upper — see Mass, localized, limb, upper
    neck R22.1
    trunk R22.2
  neck (localized) R22.1
  pelvic — see Mass, abdominal
  scrotum N50.8
  splenic — see Splenomegaly
  testis N50.8
  toe M79.89
  umbilical R19.09
  wandering, due to Gnathostoma (spinigerum) B83.1
  white — see Tuberculosis, arthritis
Swift (-Feer) disease
  overdose or wrong substance given or taken — see Table of Drugs and Chemicals, by drug, poisoning
Swimmer's
  cramp T75.1 ☑
  ear H60.33- ☑
  itch B65.3
Swimming in the head R42
Swollen — see Swelling
Swyer syndrome Q99.1
Sycosis L73.8
  barbae (not parasitic) L73.8
  contagiosa (mycotic) B35.0
  lupoides L73.8
  mycotic B35.0
  parasitic B35.0
  vulgaris L73.8
Sydenham's chorea — see Chorea, Sydenham's
Sylvatic yellow fever A95.0
Sylvest's disease B33.0
Symblepharon H11.23- ☑
  congenital Q10.3
Symond's syndrome G93.2
Sympathetic — see condition
Sympatheticotonia G90.8
Sympathicoblastoma
  specified site — see Neoplasm, malignant, by site
  unspecified site C74.90
Sympathogonioma — see Sympathicoblastoma
Symphalangy (fingers) (toes) Q70.9
Symptoms NEC R68.89
  breast NEC N64.59
  development NEC R63.8
  factitious, self-induced — see Disorder, factitious
  genital organs, female R10.2
  involving
    abdomen NEC R19.8
    appearance NEC R46.89
    awareness R41.9
      altered mental status R41.82
      amnesia — see Amnesia
      borderline intellectual functioning R41.83
      coma — see Coma
      disorientation R41.0
      neurologic neglect syndrome R41.4
      senile cognitive decline R41.81
      specified symptom NEC R41.89
    behavior NEC R46.89
    cardiovascular system NEC R09.89
    chest NEC R09.89
    circulatory system NEC R09.89
    cognitive functions R41.9
      altered mental status R41.82
      amnesia — see Amnesia
      borderline intellectual functioning R41.83
      coma — see Coma
      disorientation R41.0
      neurologic neglect syndrome R41.4
      senile cognitive decline R41.81
      specified symptom NEC R41.89
    development NEC R62.50
    digestive system NEC R19.8
    emotional state NEC R45.89
      emotional lability R45.86
    food and fluid intake R63.8
    general perceptions and sensations R44.9
      specified NEC R44.8
    musculoskeletal system R29.91
      specified NEC R29.898
    nervous system R29.90
      specified NEC R29.818
    pelvis NEC R19.8

Symptoms — continued
  involving — continued
    respiratory system NEC R09.89
    skin and integument R23.9
    urinary system R39.9
  menopausal N95.1
  metabolism NEC R63.8
  neurotic F48.8
  of infancy R68.19
  pelvis NEC, female R10.2
  skin and integument NEC R23.9
  subcutaneous tissue NEC R23.9
Sympus Q74.2
Syncephalus Q89.4
Synchondrosis
  abnormal (congenital) Q78.8
  ischiopubic M91.0
Synchysis (scintillans) (senile) (vitreous body) H43.89
Syncope (near) (pre-) R55
  anginosa I20.8
  bradycardia R00.1
  cardiac R55
  carotid sinus G90.01
  due to spinal (lumbar) puncture G97.1
  heart R55
  heat T67.1 ☑
  laryngeal R05
  psychogenic F48.8
  tussive R05
  vasoconstriction R55
  vasodepressor R55
  vasomotor R55
  vasovagal R55
Syndactylism, syndactyly Q70.9
  complex (with synostosis)
    fingers Q70.0- ☑
    toes Q70.2- ☑
  simple (without synostosis)
    fingers Q70.1- ☑
    toes Q70.3- ☑
Syndrome (see also Disease)
  48,XXXX Q97.1
  49,XXXXX Q97.1
  5q minus NOS D46.C (following D46.2)
  abdominal
    acute R10.0
    muscle deficiency Q79.4
  abnormal innervation H02.519
    left H02.516
      lower H02.515
      upper H02.514
    right H02.513
      lower H02.512
      upper H02.511
  abstinence, neonatal P96.1
  acid pulmonary aspiration, obstetric O74.0
  acquired immunodeficiency — see Human, immunodeficiency virus (HIV) disease
  acute abdominal R10.0
  acute respiratory distress (adult) (child) J80
  Adair-Dighton Q78.0
  Adams-Stokes (-Morgagni) I45.9
  adiposogenital E23.6
  adrenal
    hemorrhage (meningococcal) A39.1
    meningococcic A39.1
  adrenocortical — see Cushing's, syndrome
  adrenogenital E25.9
    congenital, associated with enzyme deficiency E25.0
  afferent loop NEC K91.89
  Alagille's Q44.7
  alcohol withdrawal (without convulsions) — see Dependence, alcohol, with, withdrawal
  Alder's D72.0
  Aldrich (-Wiskott) D82.0
  alien hand R41.4
  Alport Q87.81
  alveolar hypoventilation E66.2
  alveolocapillary block J84.10
  amnesic, amnestic (confabulatory) (due to) — see Disorder, amnesic
  amyostatic (Wilson's disease) E83.01
  androgen insensitivity E34.50
    complete E34.51
    partial E34.52
  androgen resistance (see also Syndrome, androgen insensitivity) E34.50

Syndrome — continued
  Angelman Q93.5
  anginal — see Angina
  ankyloglossia superior Q38.1
  anterior
    chest wall R07.89
    cord G83.82
    spinal artery G95.19
      compression M47.019
        cervical region M47.012
        cervicothoracic region M47.013
        lumbar region M47.016
        occipito-atlanto-axial region M47.011
        thoracic region M47.014
        thoracolumbar region M47.015
    tibial M76.81- ☑
  antibody deficiency D80.9
    agammaglobulinemic D80.1
      hereditary D80.0
    congenital D80.0
    hypogammaglobulinemic D80.1
      hereditary D80.0
  anticardiolipin (-antibody) D68.61
  antiphospholipid (-antibody) D68.61
  aortic
    arch M31.4
    bifurcation I74.09
  aortomesenteric duodenum occlusion K31.5
  apical ballooning (transient left ventricular) I51.81
  arcuate ligament I77.4
  argentaffin, argintaffinoma E34.0
  Arnold-Chiari — see Arnold-Chiari disease
  Arrillaga-Ayerza I27.0
  Asherman's N85.6
  aspiration, of newborn — see Aspiration, by substance, with pneumonia
    meconium P24.01
  ataxia-telangiectasia G11.3
  auriculotemporal G50.8
  autoerythrocyte sensitization (Gardner-Diamond) D69.2
  autoimmune lymphoproliferative [ALPS] D89.82
  autoimmune polyglandular E31.0
  autosomal — see Abnormal, autosomes
  Avellis' G46.8
  Ayerza (-Arrillaga) I27.0
  Babinski-Nageotte G83.89
  Bakwin-Krida Q79.8
  bare lymphocyte D81.6
  Barré-Guillain G61.0
  Barré-Liéou M53.0
  Barrett's — see Barrett's, esophagus
  Barsony-Polgar K22.4
  Bársony-Teschendorf K22.4
  Barth E78.71
  Bartter's E26.81
  basal cell nevus Q87.89
  Basedow's E05.00
    with thyroid storm E05.01
  basilar artery G45.0
  Batten-Steinert G71.11
  battered
    baby or child — see Maltreatment, child, physical abuse
    spouse — see Maltreatment, adult, physical abuse
  Beals Q87.40
  Beau's I51.5
  Beck's I65.8
  Benedikt's G46.3
  Béquez César (-Steinbrinck-Chédiak-Higashi) E70.330
  Bernhardt-Roth — see Meralgia paresthetica
  Bernheim's I50.9
  big spleen D73.1
  bilateral polycystic ovarian E28.2
  Bing-Horton's — see Horton's headache
  Birt-Hogg-Dube syndrome Q87.89
  Björck (-Thorsen) E34.0
  black
    lung J60
    widow spider bite — see Toxicity, venom, spider, black widow
  Blackfan-Diamond D61.01
  blind loop K90.2
    congenital Q43.8
    postsurgical K91.2
  blue sclera Q78.0
  blue toe I75.02- ☑
  Boder-Sedgewick G11.3

Syndrome — *continued*
  Boerhaave's K22.3
  Borjeson Forssman Lehmann Q89.8
  Bouillaud's I01.9
  Bourneville (-Pringle) Q85.1
  Bouveret (-Hoffman) I47.9
  brachial plexus G54.0
  bradycardia-tachycardia I49.5
  brain (nonpsychotic) F09
    with psychosis, psychotic reaction F09
    acute or subacute — *see* Delirium
    congenital — *see* Disability, intellectual
    organic F09
      post-traumatic (nonpsychotic) F07.81
        psychotic F09
    personality change F07.0
    post-traumatic, nonpsychotic F07.81
    postcontusional F07.81
    psycho-organic F09
    psychotic F06.8
  brain stem stroke G46.3
  Brandt's (acrodermatitis enteropathica) E83.2
  broad ligament laceration N83.8
  Brock's J98.11
  bronze baby P83.8
  Brown-Sequard G83.81
  bubbly lung P27.0
  Buchem's M85.2
  Budd-Chiari I82.0
  bulbar (progressive) G12.22
  Bürger-Grütz E78.3
  Burke's K86.8
  Burnett's (milk-alkali) E83.52
  burning feet E53.9
  Bywaters' T79.5 ☑
  Call-Fleming I67.841
  carbohydrate-deficient glycoprotein (CDGS) E77.8
  carcinogenic thrombophlebitis I82.1
  carcinoid E34.0
  cardiac asthma I50.1
  cardiacos negros I27.0
  cardiofaciocutaneous Q87.89
  cardiopulmonary-obesity E66.2
  cardiorenal — *see* Hypertension, cardiorenal
  cardiorespiratory distress (idiopathic), newborn P22.0
  cardiovascular renal — *see* Hypertension, cardiorenal
  carotid
    artery (hemispheric) (internal) G45.1
      body G90.01
      sinus G90.01
  carpal tunnel G56.0- ☑
  Cassidy (-Scholte) E34.0
  cat cry Q93.4
  cat eye Q92.8
  cauda equina G83.4
  causalgia — *see* Causalgia
  celiac K90.0
    artery compression I77.4
    axis I77.4
  central pain G89.0
  cerebellar
    hereditary G11.9
    stroke G46.4
  cerebellomedullary malformation — *see* Spina bifida
  cerebral
    artery
      anterior G46.1
      middle G46.0
      posterior G46.2
    gigantism E22.0
  cervical (root) M53.1
    disc — *see* Disorder, disc, cervical, with neuritis
    fusion Q76.1
    posterior, sympathicus M53.0
    rib Q76.5
    sympathetic paralysis G90.2
  cervicobrachial (diffuse) M53.1
  cervicocranial M53.0
  cervicodorsal outlet G54.2
  cervicothoracic outlet G54.0
  Céstan (-Raymond) I65.8
  Charcot-Weiss-Baker G90.09
  Charcot's (angina cruris) (intermittent claudication) I73.9
  CHARGE Q89.8
  Chédiak-Higashi (-Steinbrinck) E70.330
  chest wall R07.1
  Chiari's (hepatic vein thrombosis) I82.0

Syndrome — *continued*
  Chilaiditi's Q43.3
  child maltreatment — *see* Maltreatment, child
  chondrocostal junction M94.0
  chondroectodermal dysplasia Q77.6
  chromosome 4 short arm deletion Q93.3
  chromosome 5 short arm deletion Q93.4
  chronic
    pain G89.4
      personality F68.8
  Clarke-Hadfield K86.8
  Clerambault's automatism G93.89
  Clouston's (hidrotic ectodermal dysplasia) Q82.4
  clumsiness, clumsy child F82
  cluster headache G44.009
    intractable G44.001
    not intractable G44.009
  Coffin-Lowry Q89.8
  cold injury (newborn) P80.0
  combined immunity deficiency D81.9
  compartment (deep) (posterior) (traumatic) T79.A0 ☑ (*following* T79.7)
    abdomen T79.A3 ☑ (*following* T79.7)
    lower extremity (hip, buttock, thigh, leg, foot, toes) T79.A2 ☑ (*following* T79.7)
    nontraumatic
      abdomen M79.A3 (*following* M79.7)
      lower extremity (hip, buttock, thigh, leg, foot, toes) M79.A2- ☑ (*following* M79.7)
      specified site NEC M79.A9 (*following* M79.7)
      upper extremity (shoulder, arm, forearm, wrist, hand, fingers) M79.A1- ☑ (*following* M79.7)
    postprocedural — *see* Syndrome, compartment, nontraumatic
    specified site NEC T79.A9 ☑ (*following* T79.7)
    upper extremity (shoulder, arm, forearm, wrist, hand, fingers) T79.A1 ☑ (*following* T79.7)
  complex regional pain — *see* Syndrome, pain, complex regional
  compression T79.5 ☑
    anterior spinal — *see* Syndrome, anterior, spinal artery, compression
    cauda equina G83.4
    celiac artery I77.4
    vertebral artery M47.029
      cervical region M47.022
      occipito-atlanto-axial region M47.021
  concussion F07.81
  congenital
    affecting multiple systems NEC Q87.89
    central alveolar hypoventilation G47.35
    facial diplegia Q87.0
    muscular hypertrophy-cerebral Q87.89
    oculo-auriculovertebral Q87.0
    oculofacial diplegia (Moebius) Q87.0
    rubella (manifest) P35.0
  congestion-fibrosis (pelvic), female N94.89
  congestive dysmenorrhea N94.6
  connective tissue M35.9
    overlap NEC M35.1
  Conn's E26.01
  conus medullaris G95.81
  cord
    anterior G83.82
    posterior G83.83
  coronary
    acute NEC I24.9
    insufficiency or intermediate I20.0
    slow flow I20.8
  Costen's (complex) M26.69
  costochondral junction M94.0
  costoclavicular G54.0
  costovertebral E22.0
  Cowden Q85.8
  craniovertebral M53.0
  Creutzfeldt-Jakob — *see* Creutzfeldt-Jakob disease or syndrome
  cri-du-chat Q93.4
  crib death R99
  cricopharyngeal — *see* Dysphagia
  croup J05.0
  CRPS I — *see* Syndrome, pain, complex regional I
  crush T79.5 ☑
  cryptophthalmos Q87.0
  cubital tunnel — *see* Lesion, nerve, ulnar
  Curschmann (-Batten) (-Steinert) G71.11
  Cushing's E24.9

Syndrome — *continued*
  Cushing's — *continued*
    alcohol-induced E24.4
    drug-induced E24.2
    due to
      alcohol
      drugs E24.2
      ectopic ACTH E24.3
      overproduction of pituitary ACTH E24.0
      overdose or wrong substance given or taken — *see* Table of Drugs and Chemicals, by drug, poisoning
    pituitary-dependent E24.0
    specified type NEC E24.8
  cystic duct stump K91.5
  Dana-Putnam D51.0
  Danbolt (-Cross) (acrodermatitis enteropathica) E83.2
  Dandy-Walker Q03.1
    with spina bifida Q07.01
  Danlos' Q79.8
  De Quervain E34.51
  de Toni-Fanconi (-Debré) E72.09
    with cystinosis E72.04
  defibrination (*see also* Fibrinolysis)
    with
      antepartum hemorrhage — *see* Hemorrhage, antepartum, with coagulation defect
      intrapartum hemorrhage — *see* Hemorrhage, complicating, delivery
    newborn P60
    postpartum O72.3
  Degos' I77.89
  Déjérine-Roussy G89.0
  delayed sleep phase G47.21
  demyelinating G37.9
  dependence — *see* F10-F19 with fourth character .2
  depersonalization (-derealization) F48.1
  di George's D82.1
  diabetes mellitus in newborn infant P70.2
  diabetes mellitus-hypertension-nephrosis — *see* Diabetes, nephrosis
  diabetes-nephrosis — *see* Diabetes, nephrosis
  diabetic amyotrophy — *see* Diabetes, amyotrophy
  Diamond-Blackfan D61.01
  Diamond-Gardener D69.2
  DIC (diffuse or disseminated intravascular coagulopathy) D65
  Dighton's Q78.0
  disequilibrium E87.8
  Döhle body-panmyelopathic D72.0
  dorsolateral medullary G46.4
  double athetosis G80.3
  Down (*see also* Down syndrome) Q90.9
  Dresbach's (elliptocytosis) D58.1
  Dressler's (postmyocardial infarction) I24.1
    postcardiotomy I97.0
  drug withdrawal, infant of dependent mother P96.1
  dry eye H04.12- ☑
  due to abnormality
    chromosomal Q99.9
      sex
        female phenotype Q97.9
        male phenotype Q98.9
        specified NEC Q99.8
  dumping (postgastrectomy) K91.1
    nonsurgical K31.89
  Dupré's (meningism) R29.1
  dysmetabolic X E88.81
  dyspraxia, developmental F82
  Eagle-Barrett Q79.4
  Eaton-Lambert — *see* Syndrome, Lambert-Eaton
  Ebstein's Q22.5
  ectopic ACTH E24.3
  eczema-thrombocytopenia D82.0
  Eddowes' Q78.8
  effort (psychogenic) F45.8
  Ehlers-Danlos Q79.6
  Eisenmenger's I27.89
  Ekman's Q78.0
  electric feet E53.8
  Ellis-van Creveld Q77.6
  empty nest Z60.0
  endocrine-hypertensive E27.0
  entrapment — *see* Neuropathy, entrapment
  eosinophilia-myalgia M35.8
  epileptic (*see also* Epilepsy, by type)
    absence G40.A09 (*following* G40.3)
      intractable G40.A19 (*following* G40.3)

Syndrome — *continued*
  epileptic (*see also* Epilepsy, by type) — *continued*
    absence — *continued*
      intractable — *continued*
        with status epilepticus G40.A11 (*following* G40.3)
        without status epilepticus G40.A19 (*following* G40.3)
      not intractable G40.A09 (*following* G40.3)
        with status epilepticus G40.A01 (*following* G40.3)
        without status epilepticus G40.A09 (*following* G40.3)
  Erdheim-Chester (ECD) E88.89
  Erdheim's E22.0
  erythrocyte fragmentation D59.4
  Evans D69.41
  exhaustion F48.8
  extrapyramidal G25.9
    specified NEC G25.89
  eye retraction — *see* Strabismus
  eyelid-malar-mandible Q87.0
  Faber's D50.9
  facial pain, paroxysmal G50.0
  Fallot's Q21.3
  familial eczema-thrombocytopenia (Wiskott-Aldrich) D82.0
  Fanconi (-de Toni) (-Debré) E72.09
    with cystinosis E72.04
  Fanconi's (anemia) (congenital pancytopenia) D61.09
  fatigue
    chronic R53.82
    psychogenic F48.8
  faulty bowel habit K59.3
  Feil-Klippel (brevicollis) Q76.1
  Felty's — *see* Felty's syndrome
  fertile eunuch E23.0
  fetal
    alcohol (dysmorphic) Q86.0
    hydantoin Q86.1
  Fiedler's I40.1
  first arch Q87.0
  fish odor E72.8
  Fisher's G61.0
  Fitzhugh-Curtis
    due to
      Chlamydia trachomatis A74.81
      Neisseria gonorrhorea (gonococcal peritonitis) A54.85
  Fitz's K85.8
  Flajani (-Basedow) E05.00
    with thyroid storm E05.01
  flatback — *see* Flatback syndrome
  floppy
    baby P94.2
    iris (intraoeprative) (IFIS) H21.81
    mitral valve I34.1
  flush E34.0
  Foix-Alajouanine G95.19
  Fong's Q79.8
  foramen magnum G93.5
  Foster-Kennedy H47.14- ☑
  Foville's (peduncular) G46.3
  fragile X Q99.2
  Franceschetti Q75.4
  Frey's
    auriculotemporal G50.8
    hyperhidrosis L74.52
  Friderichsen-Waterhouse A39.1
  Froin's G95.89
  frontal lobe F07.0
  Fukuhara E88.49
  functional
    bowel K59.9
    prepubertal castrate E29.1
  Gaisböck's D75.1
  ganglion (basal ganglia brain) G25.9
    geniculi G51.1
  Gardner-Diamond D69.2
  gastroesophageal
    junction K22.0
    laceration-hemorrhage K22.6
  gastrojejunal loop obstruction K91.89
  Gee-Herter-Heubner K90.0
  Gelineau's G47.419
    with cataplexy G47.411
  genito-anorectal A55
  Gerstmann-Sträussler-Scheinker (GSS) A81.82

Syndrome — *continued*
  Gianotti-Crosti L44.4
  giant platelet (Bernard-Soulier) D69.1
  Gilles de la Tourette's F95.2
  goiter-deafness E07.1
  Goldberg Q89.8
  Goldberg-Maxwell E34.51
  Good's D83.8
  Gopalan' (burning feet) E53.8
  Gorlin's Q87.89
  Gougerot-Blum L81.7
  Gouley's I31.1
  Gower's R55
  gray or grey (newborn) P93.0
    platelet D69.1
  Gubler-Millard G46.3
  Guillain-Barré (-Strohl) G61.0
  gustatory sweating G50.8
  Hadfield-Clarke K86.8
  hair tourniquet — *see* Constriction, external, by site
  Hamman's J98.19
  hand-foot L27.1
  hand-shoulder G90.8
  hantavirus (cardio)-pulmonary (HPS) (HCPS) B33.4
  happy puppet Q93.5
  Harada's H30.81- ☑
  Hayem-Faber D50.9
  headache NEC G44.89
    complicated NEC G44.59
  Heberden's I20.8
  Hedinger's E34.0
  Hegglin's D72.0
  HELLP (hemolysis, elevated liver enzymes and low platelet count) O14.2- ☑
  hemolytic-uremic D59.3
  hemophagocytic, infection-associated D76.2
  Henoch-Schönlein D69.0
  hepatic flexure K59.8
  hepatopulmonary K76.81
  hepatorenal K76.7
    following delivery O90.4
    postoperative or postprocedural K91.83
    postpartum, puerperal O90.4
  hepatourologic K76.7
  Herter (-Gee) (nontropical sprue) K90.0
  Heubner-Herter K90.0
  Heyd's K76.7
  Hilger's G90.09
  histamine-like (fish poisoning) — *see* Poisoning, fish
  histiocytic D76.3
  histiocytosis NEC D76.3
  HIV infection, acute B20
  Hoffmann-Werdnig G12.0
  Hollander-Simons E88.1
  Hoppe-Goldflam G70.00
    with exacerbation (acute) G70.01
    in crisis G70.01
  Horner's G90.2
  hungry bone E83.81
  hunterian glossitis D51.0
  Hutchinson's triad A50.53
  hyperabduction G54.0
  hyperammonemia-hyperornithinemia-homocitrullinemia E72.4
  hypereosinophilic (idiopathic) D72.1
  hyperimmunoglobulin E (IgE) D82.4
  hyperkalemic E87.5
  hyperkinetic — *see* Hyperkinesia
  hypermobility M35.7
  hypernatremia E87.0
  hyperosmolarity E87.0
  hyperperfusion G97.82
  hypersplenic D73.1
  hypertransfusion, newborn P61.1
  hyperventilation F45.8
  hyperviscosity (of serum)
    polycythemic D75.1
    sclerothymic D58.8
  hypoglycemic (familial) (neonatal) E16.2
  hypokalemic E87.6
  hyponatremic E87.1
  hypopituitarism E23.0
  hypoplastic left-heart Q23.4
  hypopotassemia E87.6
  hyposmolality E87.1
  hypotension, maternal O26.5- ☑
  hypothenar hammer I73.89
  ICF (intravascular coagulation-fibrinolysis) D65

Syndrome — *continued*
  idiopathic
    cardiorespiratory distress, newborn P22.0
    nephrotic (infantile) N04.9
  iliotibial band M76.3- ☑
  immobility, immobilization (paraplegic) M62.3
  immune reconstitution D89.3
  immune reconstitution inflammatory [IRIS] D89.3
  immunity deficiency, combined D81.9
  immunodeficiency
    acquired — *see* Human, immunodeficiency virus (HIV) disease
    combined D81.9
  impending coronary I20.0
  impingement, shoulder M75.4- ☑
  inappropriate secretion of antidiuretic hormone E22.2
  infant
    gestational diabetes P70.0
    of diabetic mother P70.1
  infantilism (pituitary) E23.0
  inferior vena cava I87.1
  inspissated bile (newborn) P59.1
  institutional (childhood) F94.2
  insufficient sleep F51.12
  intermediate coronary (artery) I20.0
  interspinous ligament — *see* Spondylopathy, specified NEC
  intestinal
    carcinoid E34.0
    knot K56.2
  intravascular coagulation-fibrinolysis (ICF) D65
  iodine-deficiency, congenital E00.9
    type
      mixed E00.2
      myxedematous E00.1
      neurological E00.0
  IRDS (idiopathic respiratory distress, newborn) P22.0
  irritable
    bowel K58.9
      with diarrhea K58.0
      psychogenic F45.8
    heart (psychogenic) F45.8
    weakness F48.8
  ischemic bowel (transient) K55.9
    chronic K55.1
    due to mesenteric artery insufficiency K55.1
  IVC (intravascular coagulopathy) D65
  Ivemark's Q89.01
  Jaccoud's — *see* Arthropathy, postrheumatic, chronic
  Jackson's G83.89
  Jakob-Creutzfeldt — *see* Creutzfeldt-Jakob disease or syndrome
  jaw-winking Q07.8
  Jervell-Lange-Nielsen I45.81
  jet lag G47.25
  Job's D71
  Joseph-Diamond-Blackfan D61.01
  jugular foramen G52.7
  Kabuki Q89.8
  Kanner's (autism) F84.0
  Kartagener's Q89.3
  Kelly's D50.1
  Kimmelstiel-Wilson — *see* Diabetes, specified type, with Kimmelstiel-Wilson disease
  Klein (e)-Levine G47.13
  Klippel-Feil (brevicollis) Q76.1
  Köhler-Pellegrini-Steida — *see* Bursitis, tibial collateral
  König's K59.8
  Korsakoff (-Wernicke) (nonalcoholic) F04
    alcoholic F10.26
  Kostmann's D70.0
  Krabbe's congenital muscle hypoplasia Q79.8
  labyrinthine — *see* subcategory H83.2 ☑
  lacunar NEC G46.7
  Lambert-Eaton G70.80
    in
      neoplastic disease G73.1
      specified disease NEC G70.81
  Landau-Kleffner — *see* Epilepsy, specified NEC
  Larsen's Q74.8
  lateral
    cutaneous nerve of thigh G57.1- ☑
    medullary G46.4
  Launois' E22.0
  lazy
    leukocyte D70.8
    posture M62.3
  Lemiere I80.8

☑ **Additional Character Required — Refer to the Tabular List for Character Selection** 　　 ◥◤ **Subterms under main terms may continue to next column or page**

Syndrome — *continued*
- Lennox-Gastaut G40.812
  - intractable G40.814
    - with status epilepticus G40.813
    - without status epilepticus G40.814
  - not intractable G40.812
    - with status epilepticus G40.811
    - without status epilepticus G40.812
- lenticular, progressive E83.01
- Leopold-Levi's E05.90
- Lev's I44.2
- Li-Fraumeni Z15.01
- Lichtheim's D51.0
- Lightwood's N25.89
- Lignac (de Toni) (-Fanconi) (-Debré) E72.09
  - with cystinosis E72.04
- Likoff's I20.8
- limbic epilepsy personality F07.0
- liver-kidney K76.7
- lobotomy F07.0
- Loffler's J82
- long arm 18 or 21 deletion Q93.89
- long QT I45.81
- Louis-Barré G11.3
- low
  - atmospheric pressure T70.29 ☑
  - back M54.5
  - output (cardiac) I50.9
- lower radicular, newborn (birth injury) P14.8
- Luetscher's (dehydration) E86.0
- Lupus anticoagulant D68.62
- Lutembacher's Q21.1
- macrophage activation D76.1
  - due to infection D76.2
- magnesium-deficiency R29.0
- Mal de Debarquement R42
- malabsorption K90.9
  - postsurgical K91.2
- malformation, congenital, due to
  - alcohol Q86.0
  - exogenous cause NEC Q86.8
  - hydantoin Q86.1
  - warfarin Q86.2
- malignant
  - carcinoid E34.0
  - neuroleptic G21.0
- Mallory-Weiss K22.6
- mandibulofacial dysostosis Q75.4
- manic-depressive — *see* Disorder, bipolar, affective
- maple-syrup-urine E71.0
- Marable's I77.4
- Marfan's Q87.40
  - with
    - cardiovascular manifestations Q87.418
      - aortic dilation Q87.410
    - ocular manifestations Q87.42
    - skeletal manifestations Q87.43
- Marie's (acromegaly) E22.0
- maternal hypotension — *see* Syndrome, hypotension, maternal
- May (-Hegglin) D72.0
- McArdle (-Schmidt) (-Pearson) E74.04
- McQuarrie's E16.2
- meconium plug (newborn) P76.0
- median arcuate ligament I77.4
- Meekeren-Ehlers-Danlos Q79.6
- megavitamin-B6 E67.2
- Meige G24.4
- MELAS E88.41
- Mendelson's O74.0
- MERRF (myoclonic epilepsy associated with ragged-red fibers) E88.42
- mesenteric
  - artery (superior) K55.1
  - vascular insufficiency K55.1
- metabolic E88.81
- metastatic carcinoid E34.0
- micrognathia-glossoptosis Q87.0
- midbrain NEC G93.89
- middle lobe (lung) J98.19
- middle radicular G54.0
- migraine (*see also* Migraine) G43.909
- Mikulicz' K11.8
- milk-alkali E83.52
- Millard-Gubler G46.3
- Miller-Dieker Q93.88
- Miller-Fisher G61.0
- Minkowski-Chauffard D58.0

Syndrome — *continued*
- Mirizzi's K83.1
- MNGIE (Mitochondrial Neurogastrointestinal Encephalopathy) E88.49
- Möbius, ophthalmoplegic migraine — *see* Migraine, ophthalmoplegic
- monofixation H50.42
- Morel-Moore M85.2
- Morel-Morgagni M85.2
- Morgagni (-Morel) (-Stewart) M85.2
- Morgagni-Adams-Stokes I45.9
- Mounier-Kuhn Q32.4
  - with bronchiectasis J47.9
    - with
      - exacerbation (acute) J47.1
      - lower respiratory infection J47.0
  - acquired J98.09
    - with bronchiectasis J47.9
      - with
        - exacerbation (acute) J47.1
        - lower respiratory infection J47.0
- mucocutaneous lymph node (acute febrile) (MCLS) M30.3
- multiple endocrine neoplasia (MEN) — *see* Neoplasia, endocrine, multiple (MEN)
- multiple operations — *see* Disorder, factitious
- myasthenic G70.9
  - in
    - diabetes mellitus — *see* Diabetes, amyotrophy
    - endocrine disease NEC E34.9 [G73.3]
    - neoplastic disease (*see also* Neoplasm) D49.9 [G73.3]
    - thyrotoxicosis (hyperthyroidism) E05.90 [G73.3]
      - with thyroid storm E05.91 [G73.3]
- myelodysplastic D46.9
  - with
    - 5q deletion D46.C (*following* D46.2)
    - isolated del (5q) chromosomal abnormality D46.C (*following* D46.2)
    - lesions, low grade D46.20
    - specified NEC D46.Z (*following* D46.4)
- myelopathic pain G89.0
- myeloproliferative (chronic) D47.1
- myofascial pain M79.1
- Naffziger's G54.0
- nail patella Q87.2
- NARP (Neuropathy, Ataxia and Retinitis pigmentosa) E88.49
- neonatal abstinence P96.1
- nephritic (*see also* Nephritis)
  - with edema — *see* Nephrosis
  - acute N00.9
  - chronic N03.9
  - rapidly progressive N01.9
- nephrotic (congenital) (*see also* Nephrosis) N04.9
  - with
    - dense deposit disease N04.6
    - diffuse
      - crescentic glomerulonephritis N04.7
      - endocapillary proliferative glomerulonephritis N04.4
      - membranous glomerulonephritis N04.2
      - mesangial proliferative glomerulonephritis N04.3
      - mesangiocapillary glomerulonephritis N04.5
    - focal and segmental glomerular lesions N04.1
    - minor glomerular abnormality N04.0
    - specified morphological changes NEC N04.8
  - diabetic — *see* Diabetes, nephrosis
- neurologic neglect R41.4
- Nezelof's D81.4
- Nonne-Milroy-Meige Q82.0
- Nothnagel's vasomotor acroparesthesia I73.89
- oculomotor H51.9
- ophthalmoplegia-cerebellar ataxia — *see* Strabismus, paralytic, third nerve
- oral-facial-digital Q87.0
- organic
  - affective F06.30
  - amnesic (not alcohol- or drug-induced) F04
  - brain F09
  - depressive F06.31
  - hallucinosis F06.0
  - personality F07.0
- Ormond's N13.5
- oro-facial-digital Q87.0
- os trigonum Q68.8
- Osler-Weber-Rendu I78.0

Syndrome — *continued*
- osteoporosis-osteomalacia M83.8
- Osterreicher-Turner Q79.8
- oto-palatal-digital Q87.0
- otolith — *see* subcategory H81.8 ☑
- outlet (thoracic) G54.0
- ovary
  - polycystic E28.2
  - resistant E28.39
  - sclerocystic E28.2
- Owren's D68.2
- Paget-Schroetter I82.890
- pain (*see also* Pain)
  - complex regional I G90.50
    - lower limb G90.52- ☑
    - specified site NEC G90.59
    - upper limb G90.51- ☑
  - complex regional II — *see* Causalgia
- painful
  - bruising D69.2
  - feet E53.8
  - prostate N42.81
- paralysis agitans — *see* Parkinsonism
- paralytic G83.9
  - specified NEC G83.89
- Parinaud's H51.0
- parkinsonian — *see* Parkinsonism
- Parkinson's — *see* Parkinsonism
- paroxysmal facial pain G50.0
- Parry's E05.00
  - with thyroid storm E05.01
- Parsonage (-Aldren)-Turner G54.5
- patella clunk M25.86- ☑
- Paterson (-Brown) (-Kelly) D50.1
- pectoral girdle I77.89
- pectoralis minor I77.89
- Pelger-Huet D72.0
- pellagra-cerebellar ataxia-renal aminoaciduria E72.02
- pellagroid E52
- Pellegrini-Stieda — *see* Bursitis, tibial collateral
- pelvic congestion-fibrosis, female N94.89
- penta X Q97.1
- peptic ulcer — *see* Ulcer, peptic
- perabduction I77.89
- periodic headache, in adults and children — *see* Headache, periodic syndromes in adults and children
- periurethral fibrosis N13.5
- phantom limb (without pain) G54.7
  - with pain G54.6
- pharyngeal pouch D82.1
- Pick's (heart) (liver) I31.1
- Pickwickian E66.2
- PIE (pulmonary infiltration with eosinophilia) J82
- pigmentary pallidal degeneration (progressive) G23.0
- pineal E34.8
- pituitary E22.0
- placental transfusion — *see* Pregnancy, complicated by, placental transfusion syndromes
- plantar fascia M72.2
- plateau iris (post-iridectomy) (postprocedural) H21.82
- Plummer-Vinson D50.1
- pluricarential of infancy E40
- plurideficiency E40
- pluriglandular (compensatory) E31.8
  - autoimmune E31.0
- pneumatic hammer T75.21 ☑
- polyangiitis overlap M30.8
- polycarential of infancy E40
- polyglandular E31.8
  - autoimmune E31.0
- polysplenia Q89.09
- pontine NEC G93.89
- popliteal
  - artery entrapment I77.89
  - web Q87.89
- post chemoembolization — *code to* associated conditions
- postcardiac injury
  - postcardiotomy I97.0
  - postmyocardial infarction I24.1
- postcardiotomy I97.0
- postcholecystectomy K91.5
- postcommissurotomy I97.0
- postconcussional F07.81
- postcontusional F07.81
- postencephalitic F07.89

Syndrome — continued
- posterior
  - cervical sympathetic M53.0
  - cord G83.83
  - fossa compression G93.5
  - reversible encephalopathy (PRES) I67.83
- postgastrectomy (dumping) K91.1
- postgastric surgery K91.1
- postinfarction I24.1
- postlaminectomy NEC M96.1
- postleukotomy F07.0
- postmastectomy lymphedema I97.2
- postmyocardial infarction I24.1
- postoperative NEC T81.9 ☑
  - blind loop K90.2
- postpartum panhypopituitary (Sheehan) E23.0
- postpolio (myelitic) G14
- postthrombotic I87.009
  - with
    - inflammation I87.02- ☑
      - with ulcer I87.03- ☑
    - specified complication NEC I87.09- ☑
    - ulcer I87.01- ☑
      - with inflammation I87.03- ☑
  - asymptomatic I87.00- ☑
- postvagotomy K91.1
- postvalvulotomy I97.0
- postviral NEC G93.3
  - fatigue G93.3
- Potain's K31.0
- potassium intoxication E87.5
- precerebral artery (multiple) (bilateral) G45.2
- preinfarction I20.0
- preleukemic D46.9
- premature senility E34.8
- premenstrual dysphoric N94.3
- premenstrual tension N94.3
- Prinzmetal-Massumi R07.1
- prune belly Q79.4
- pseudo -Turner's Q87.1
- pseudocarpal tunnel (sublimis) — see Syndrome, carpal tunnel
- pseudoparalytica G70.00
  - with exacerbation (acute) G70.01
  - in crisis G70.01
- psycho-organic (nonpsychotic severity) F07.9
  - acute or subacute F05
  - depressive type F06.31
  - hallucinatory type F06.0
  - nonpsychotic severity F07.0
  - specified NEC F07.89
- pulmonary
  - arteriosclerosis I27.0
  - dysmaturity (Wilson-Mikity) P27.0
  - hypoperfusion (idiopathic) P22.0
  - renal (hemorrhagic) (Goodpasture's) M31.0
- pure
  - motor lacunar G46.5
  - sensory lacunar G46.6
- Putnam-Dana D51.0
- pyramidopallidonigral G20
- pyriformis — see Lesion, nerve, sciatic
- QT interval prolongation I45.81
- radicular NEC — see Radiculopathy
  - upper limbs, newborn (birth injury) P14.3
- rapid time-zone change G47.25
- Rasmussen G04.81
- Raymond (-Céstan) I65.8
- Raynaud's I73.00
  - with gangrene I73.01
- RDS (respiratory distress syndrome, newborn) P22.0
- reactive airways dysfunction J68.3
- Refsum's G60.1
- Reifenstein E34.52
- renal glomerulohyalinosis-diabetic — see Diabetes, nephrosis
- Rendu-Osler-Weber I78.0
- residual ovary N99.83
- resistant ovary E28.39
- respiratory
  - distress
    - acute J80
      - adult J80
      - child J80
    - newborn (idiopathic) (type I) P22.0
      - type II P22.1
- restless legs G25.81
- retinoblastoma (familial) C69.2 ☑

Syndrome — continued
- retroperitoneal fibrosis N13.5
- retroviral seroconversion (acute) Z21
- Reye's G93.7
- Richter — see Leukemia, chronic lymphocytic, B-cell type
- Ridley's I50.1
- right
  - heart, hypoplastic Q22.6
  - ventricular obstruction — see Failure, heart, congestive
- Romano-Ward (prolonged QT interval) I45.81
- rotator cuff, shoulder (see also Tear, rotator cuff) M75.10- ☑
- Rotes Quérol — see Hyperostosis, ankylosing
- Roth — see Meralgia paresthetica
- rubella (congenital) P35.0
- Ruvalcaba-Myhre-Smith E71.440
- Rytand-Lipsitch I44.2
- salt
  - depletion E87.1
    - due to heat NEC T67.8 ☑
      - causing heat exhaustion or prostration T67.4 ☑
  - low E87.1
- salt-losing N28.89
- Scaglietti-Dagnini E22.0
- scalenus anticus (anterior) G54.0
- scapulocostal — see Mononeuropathy, upper limb, specified site NEC
- scapuloperoneal G71.0
- schizophrenic, of childhood NEC F84.5
- Schnitzler D47.2
- Scholte's E34.0
- Schroeder's E27.0
- Schüller-Christian C96.5
- Schwachman's — see Syndrome, Shwachman's
- Schwartz (-Jampel) G71.13
- Schwartz-Bartter E22.2
- scimitar Q26.8
- sclerocystic ovary E28.2
- Seitelberger's G31.89
- septicemic adrenal hemorrhage A39.1
- seroconversion, retroviral (acute) Z21
- serous meningitis G93.2
- severe acute respiratory (SARS) J12.81
- shaken infant T74.4 ☑
- shock (traumatic) T79.4 ☑
  - kidney N17.0
  - following crush injury T79.5 ☑
  - toxic A48.3
- shock-lung J80
- Shone's — code to specific anomalies
- short
  - bowel K91.2
  - rib Q77.2
- shoulder-hand — see Algoneurodystrophy
- Shwachman's D70.4
- sicca — see Sicca syndrome
- sick
  - cell E87.1
  - sinus I49.5
- sick-euthyroid E07.81
- sideropenic D50.1
- Siemens' ectodermal dysplasia Q82.4
- Silfverskjöld's Q78.9
- Simons' E88.1
- sinus tarsi M25.57- ☑
- sinusitis-bronchiectasis-situs inversus Q89.3
- Sipple's E31.22
- sirenomelia Q87.2
- Slocumb's E27.0
- slow flow, coronary I20.8
- Sluder's G44.89
- Smith-Magenis Q93.88
- Sneddon-Wilkinson L13.1
- Sotos' Q22.0
- South African cardiomyopathy I42.8
- spasmodic
  - upward movement, eyes H51.8
  - winking F95.8
- Spen's I45.9
- splenic
  - agenesis Q89.01
  - flexure K59.8
  - neutropenia D73.81
- Spurway's Q78.0
- staphylococcal scalded skin L00

Syndrome — continued
- Stein-Leventhal E28.2
- Stein's E28.2
- Stevens-Johnson syndrome L51.1
  - toxic epidermal necrolysis overlap L51.3
- Stewart-Morel M85.2
- Stickler Q89.8
- stiff baby Q89.8
- stiff man G25.82
- Still-Felty — see Felty's syndrome
- Stokes (-Adams) I45.9
- stone heart I50.1
- straight back, congenital Q76.49
- subclavian steal G45.8
- subcoracoid-pectoralis minor G54.0
- subcostal nerve compression I77.89
- subphrenic interposition Q43.3
- superior
  - cerebellar artery I63.8
  - mesenteric artery K55.1
  - semi-circular canal dehiscence H83.8X- ☑
  - vena cava I87.1
- supine hypotensive (maternal) — see Syndrome, hypotension, maternal
- suprarenal cortical E27.0
- supraspinatus (see also Tear, rotator cuff) M75.10- ☑
- Susac G93.49
- swallowed blood P78.2
- sweat retention L74.0
- Swyer Q99.1
- Symond's G93.2
- sympathetic
  - cervical paralysis G90.2
  - pelvic, female N94.89
- systemic inflammatory response (SIRS), of non-infectious origin (without organ dysfunction) R65.10
  - with acute organ dysfunction R65.11
- tachycardia-bradycardia I49.5
- takotsubo I51.81
- TAR (thrombocytopenia with absent radius) Q87.2
- tarsal tunnel G57.5- ☑
- teething K00.7
- tegmental G93.89
- telangiectasic-pigmentation-cataract Q82.8
- temporal pyramidal apex — see Otitis, media, suppurative, acute
- temporomandibular joint-pain-dysfunction M26.62
- Terry's H44.2- ☑
- testicular feminization (see also Syndrome, androgen insensitivity) E34.51
- thalamic pain (hyperesthetic) G89.0
- thoracic outlet (compression) G54.0
- Thorson-Björck E34.0
- thrombocytopenia with absent radius (TAR) Q87.2
- thyroid-adrenocortical insufficiency E31.0
- tibial
  - anterior M76.81- ☑
  - posterior M76.82- ☑
- Tietze's M94.0
- time-zone (rapid) G47.25
- Toni-Fanconi E72.09
  - with cystinosis E72.04
- Touraine's Q79.8
- tourniquet — see Constriction, external, by site
- toxic shock A48.3
- transient left ventricular apical ballooning I51.81
- traumatic vasospastic T75.22 ☑
- Treacher Collins Q75.4
- triple X, female Q97.0
- trisomy Q92.9
  - 13 Q91.7
    - meiotic nondisjunction Q91.4
    - mitotic nondisjunction Q91.5
    - mosaicism Q91.5
    - translocation Q91.6
  - 18 Q91.3
    - meiotic nondisjunction Q91.0
    - mitotic nondisjunction Q91.1
    - mosaicism Q91.1
    - translocation Q91.2
  - 20 (q)(p) Q92.8
  - 21 Q90.9
    - meiotic nondisjunction Q90.0
    - mitotic nondisjunction Q90.1
    - mosaicism Q90.1
    - translocation Q90.2
  - 22 Q92.8
- tropical wet feet T69.0- ☑

Syndrome — continued
Trousseau's I82.1
tumor lysis (following antineoplastic chemotherapy) (spontaneous) NEC E88.3
Twiddler's (due to)
automatic implantable defibrillator T82.198 ☑
cardiac pacemaker T82.198 ☑
Unverricht (-Lundborg) — see Epilepsy, generalized, idiopathic
upward gaze H51.8
uremia, chronic (see also Disease, kidney, chronic) N18.9
urethral N34.3
urethro-oculo-articular — see Reiter's disease
urohepatic K76.7
vago-hypoglossal G52.7
van Buchem's M85.2
van der Hoeve's Q78.0
vascular NEC in cerebrovascular disease G46.8
vasoconstriction, reversible cerebrovascular I67.841
vasomotor I73.9
vasospastic (traumatic) T75.22 ☑
vasovagal R55
VATER Q87.2
velo-cardio-facial Q93.81
vena cava (inferior) (superior) (obstruction) I87.1
vertebral
artery G45.0
compression — see Syndrome, anterior, spinal artery, compression
steal G45.0
vertebro-basilar artery G45.0
vertebrogenic (pain) M54.89
vertiginous — see Disorder, vestibular function
Vinson-Plummer D50.1
virus B34.9
visceral larva migrans B83.0
visual disorientation H53.8
vitamin B6 deficiency E53.1
vitreal corneal H59.01- ☑
vitreous (touch) H59.01- ☑
Vogt-Koyanagi H20.82- ☑
Volkmann's T79.6 ☑
von Schroetter's I82.890
von Willebrand (-Jürgen) D68.0
Waldenström-Kjellberg D50.1
Wallenberg's G46.3
water retention E87.79
Waterhouse (-Friderichsen) A39.1
Weber-Gubler G46.3
Weber-Leyden G46.3
Weber's G46.3
Wegener's M31.30
with
kidney involvement M31.31
lung involvement M31.30
with kidney involvement M31.31
Weingarten's (tropical eosinophilia) J82
Weiss-Baker G90.09
Werdnig-Hoffman G12.0
Wermer's E31.21
Werner's E34.8
Wernicke-Korsakoff (nonalcoholic) F04
alcoholic F10.26
Westphal-Strümpell E83.01
West's — see Epilepsy, spasms
wet
feet (maceration) (tropical) T69.0- ☑
lung, newborn P22.1
whiplash S13.4 ☑
whistling face Q87.0
Wilkie's K55.1
Wilkinson-Sneddon L13.1
Willebrand (-Jürgens) D68.0
Wilson's (hepatolenticular degeneration) E83.01
Wiskott-Aldrich D82.0
withdrawal — see Withdrawal, state
drug
infant of dependent mother P96.1
therapeutic use, newborn P96.2
Woakes' (ethmoiditis) J33.1
Wright's (hyperabduction) I77.89
X I20.9
XXXX Q97.1
XXXXX Q97.1
XXXXY Q98.1
XXY Q98.0
yellow nail L60.5

Syndrome — continued
Zahorsky's B08.5
Zellweger syndrome E71.510
Zellweger-like syndrome E71.541
Synechia (anterior) (iris) (posterior) (pupil) (see also Adhesions, iris)
intra-uterine (traumatic) N85.6
Synesthesia R20.8
Syngamiasis, syngamosis B83.3
Synodontia K00.2
Synorchidism, synorchism Q55.1
Synostosis (congenital) Q78.8
astragalo-scaphoid Q74.2
radioulnar Q74.0
Synovial sarcoma — see Neoplasm, connective tissue, malignant
Synovioma (malignant) (see also Neoplasm, connective tissue, malignant)
benign — see Neoplasm, connective tissue, benign
Synoviosarcoma — see Neoplasm, connective tissue, malignant
Synovitis (see also Tenosynovitis)
crepitant
hand M70.0- ☑
wrist M70.03- ☑
gonococcal A54.49
gouty — see Gout, idiopathic
in (due to)
crystals M65.8- ☑
gonorrhea A54.49
syphilis (late) A52.78
use, overuse, pressure — see Disorder, soft tissue, due to use
infective NEC — see Tenosynovitis, infective NEC
specified NEC — see Tenosynovitis, specified type NEC
syphilitic A52.78
congenital (early) A50.02
toxic — see Synovitis, transient
transient M67.3- ☑
ankle M67.37- ☑
elbow M67.32- ☑
foot joint M67.37- ☑
hand joint M67.34- ☑
hip M67.35- ☑
knee M67.36- ☑
multiple site M67.39
pelvic region M67.35- ☑
shoulder M67.31- ☑
specified joint NEC M67.38
wrist M67.33- ☑
traumatic, current — see Sprain
tuberculous — see Tuberculosis, synovitis
villonodular (pigmented) M12.2- ☑
ankle M12.27- ☑
elbow M12.22- ☑
foot joint M12.27- ☑
hand joint M12.24- ☑
hip M12.25- ☑
knee M12.26- ☑
multiple site M12.29
pelvic region M12.25- ☑
shoulder M12.21- ☑
specified joint NEC M12.28
vertebrae M12.28
wrist M12.23- ☑
Syphilid A51.39
congenital A50.06
newborn A50.06
tubercular (late) A52.79
Syphilis, syphilitic (acquired) A53.9
abdomen (late) A52.79
acoustic nerve A52.15
adenopathy (secondary) A51.49
adrenal (gland) (with cortical hypofunction) A52.79
age under 2 years NOS (see also Syphilis, congenital, early)
acquired A51.9
alopecia (secondary) A51.32
anemia (late) A52.79 [D63.8]
aneurysm (aorta) (ruptured) A52.01
central nervous system A52.05
congenital A50.54 [I79.0]
anus (late) A52.74
primary A51.1
secondary A51.39
aorta (arch) (abdominal) (thoracic) A52.02
aneurysm A52.01

Syphilis, syphilitic — continued
aortic (insufficiency) (regurgitation) (stenosis) A52.03
aneurysm A52.01
arachnoid (adhesive) (cerebral) (spinal) A52.13
asymptomatic — see Syphilis, latent
ataxia (locomotor) A52.11
atrophoderma maculatum A51.39
auricular fibrillation A52.06
bladder (late) A52.76
bone A52.77
secondary A51.46
brain A52.17
breast (late) A52.79
bronchus (late) A52.72
bubo (primary) A51.0
bulbar palsy A52.19
bursa (late) A52.78
cardiac decompensation A52.06
cardiovascular A52.00
central nervous system (late) (recurrent) (relapse) (tertiary) A52.3
with
ataxia A52.11
general paralysis A52.17
juvenile A50.45
paresis (general) A52.17
juvenile A50.45
tabes (dorsalis) A52.11
juvenile A50.45
taboparesis A52.17
juvenile A50.45
aneurysm A52.05
congenital A50.40
juvenile A50.40
remission in (sustained) A52.3
serology doubtful, negative, or positive A52.3
specified nature or site NEC A52.19
vascular A52.05
cerebral A52.17
meningovascular A52.13
nerves (multiple palsies) A52.15
sclerosis A52.17
thrombosis A52.05
cerebrospinal (tabetic type) A52.12
cerebrovascular A52.05
cervix (late) A52.76
chancre (multiple) A51.0
extragenital A51.2
Rollet's A51.0
Charcot's joint A52.16
chorioretinitis A51.43
congenital A50.01
late A52.71
prenatal A50.01
choroiditis — see Syphilitic chorioretinitis
choroidoretinitis — see Syphilitic chorioretinitis
ciliary body (secondary) A51.43
late A52.71
colon (late) A52.74
combined spinal sclerosis A52.11
condyloma (latum) A51.31
congenital A50.9
with
paresis (general) A50.45
tabes (dorsalis) A50.45
taboparesis A50.45
early, or less than 2 years after birth NEC A50.2
with manifestations — see Syphilis, congenital, early, symptomatic
latent (without manifestations) A50.1
negative spinal fluid test A50.1
serology positive A50.1
symptomatic A50.09
cutaneous A50.06
mucocutaneous A50.07
oculopathy A50.01
osteochondropathy A50.02
pharyngitis A50.03
pneumonia A50.04
rhinitis A50.05
visceral A50.08
chorioretinitis, choroiditis A50.01 [H32]
interstitial keratitis A50.31
juvenile neurosyphilis A50.45
late, or 2 years or more after birth NEC A50.7
chorioretinitis, choroiditis A50.32
interstitial keratitis A50.31
juvenile neurosyphilis A50.45

Syphilis, syphilitic — *continued*
congenital — *continued*
late, or 2 years or more after birth — *continued*
latent (without manifestations) A50.6
negative spinal fluid test A50.6
serology positive A50.6
symptomatic or with manifestations NEC A50.59
arthropathy A50.55
cardiovascular A50.54
Clutton's joints A50.51
Hutchinson's teeth A50.52
Hutchinson's triad A50.53
osteochondropathy A50.56
saddle nose A50.57
conjugal A53.9
tabes A52.11
conjunctiva (late) A52.71
contact Z20.2
cord bladder A52.19
cornea, late A52.71
coronary (artery) (sclerosis) A52.06
coryza, congenital A50.05
cranial nerve A52.15
multiple palsies A52.15
cutaneous — *see* Syphilis, skin
dacryocystitis (late) A52.71
degeneration, spinal cord A52.12
dementia paralytica A52.17
juvenilis A50.45
destruction of bone A52.77
dilatation, aorta A52.01
due to blood transfusion A53.9
dura mater A52.13
ear A52.79
inner A52.79
nerve (eighth) A52.15
neurorecurrence A52.15
early A51.9
cardiovascular A52.00
central nervous system A52.3
latent (without manifestations) (less than 2 years after infection) A51.5
negative spinal fluid test A51.5
serological relapse after treatment A51.5
serology positive A51.5
relapse (treated, untreated) A51.9
skin A51.39
symptomatic A51.9
extragenital chancre A51.2
primary, except extragenital chancre A51.0
secondary (*see also* Syphilis, secondary) A51.39
relapse (treated, untreated) A51.49
ulcer A51.39
eighth nerve (neuritis) A52.15
endemic A65
endocarditis A52.03
aortic A52.03
pulmonary A52.03
epididymis (late) A52.76
epiglottis (late) A52.73
epiphysitis (congenital) (early) A50.02
episcleritis (late) A52.71
esophagus A52.79
eustachian tube A52.73
exposure to Z20.2
eye A52.71
eyelid (late) (with gumma) A52.71
fallopian tube (late) A52.76
fracture A52.77
gallbladder (late) A52.74
gastric (polyposis) (late) A52.74
general A53.9
paralysis A52.17
juvenile A50.45
genital (primary) A51.0
glaucoma A52.71
gumma NEC A52.79
cardiovascular system A52.00
central nervous system A52.3
congenital A50.59
heart (block) (decompensation) (disease) (failure) A52.06 [I52]
valve NEC A52.03
hemianesthesia A52.19
hemianopsia A52.71
hemiparesis A52.17
hemiplegia A52.17

Syphilis, syphilitic — *continued*
hepatic artery A52.09
hepatis A52.74
hepatomegaly, congenital A50.08
hereditaria tarda — *see* Syphilis, congenital, late
hereditary — *see* Syphilis, congenital
Hutchinson's teeth A50.52
hyalitis A52.71
inactive — *see* Syphilis, latent
infantum — *see* Syphilis, congenital
inherited — *see* Syphilis, congenital
internal ear A52.79
intestine (late) A52.74
iris, iritis (secondary) A51.43
late A52.71
joint (late) A52.77
keratitis (congenital) (interstitial) (late) A50.31
kidney (late) A52.75
lacrimal passages (late) A52.71
larynx (late) A52.73
late A52.9
cardiovascular A52.00
central nervous system A52.3
kidney A52.75
latent or 2 years or more after infection (without manifestations) A52.8
negative spinal fluid test A52.8
serology positive A52.8
paresis A52.17
specified site NEC A52.79
symptomatic or with manifestations A52.79
tabes A52.11
latent A53.0
with signs or symptoms — *code by* site and stage under Syphilis
early, or less than 2 years after infection A51.5
central nervous system A52.2
date of infection unspecified A53.0
follow-up of latent syphilis A53.0
date of infection unspecified A53.0
late, or 2 years or more after infection A52.8
late, or 2 years or more after infection A52.8
positive serology (only finding) A53.0
early, or less than 2 years after infection A51.5
date of infection unspecified A53.0
late, or 2 years or more after infection A52.8
lens (late) A52.71
leukoderma A51.39
late A52.79
lienitis A52.79
lip A51.39
chancre (primary) A51.2
late A52.79
Lissauer's paralysis A52.17
liver A52.74
locomotor ataxia A52.11
lung A52.72
lymph gland (early) (secondary) A51.49
late A52.79
lymphadenitis (secondary) A51.49
macular atrophy of skin A51.39
striated A52.79
mediastinum (late) A52.73
meninges (adhesive) (brain) (spinal cord) A52.13
meningitis A52.13
acute (secondary) A51.41
congenital A50.41
meningoencephalitis A52.14
meningovascular A52.13
congenital A50.41
mesarteritis A52.09
brain A52.04
middle ear A52.77
mitral stenosis A52.03
monoplegia A52.17
mouth (secondary) A51.39
late A52.79
mucocutaneous (secondary) A51.39
late A52.79
mucous
membrane (secondary) A51.39
late A52.79
patches A51.39
congenital A50.07
mulberry molars A50.52
muscle A52.78
myocardium A52.06
nasal sinus (late) A52.73

Syphilis, syphilitic — *continued*
neonatorum — *see* Syphilis, congenital
nephrotic syndrome (secondary) A51.44
nerve palsy (any cranial nerve) A52.15
multiple A52.15
nervous system, central A52.3
neuritis A52.15
acoustic A52.15
neurorecidive of retina A52.19
neuroretinitis A52.19
newborn — *see* Syphilis, congenital
nodular superficial (late) A52.79
nonvenereal A65
nose (late) A52.73
saddle back deformity A50.57
occlusive arterial disease A52.09
oculopathy A52.71
ophthalmic (late) A52.71
optic nerve (atrophy) (neuritis) (papilla) A52.15
orbit (late) A52.71
organic A53.9
osseous (late) A52.77
osteochondritis (congenital) (early) A50.02 [M90.80]
osteoporosis A52.77
ovary (late) A52.76
oviduct (late) A52.76
palate (late) A52.79
pancreas (late) A52.74
paralysis A52.17
general A52.17
juvenile A50.45
paresis (general) A52.17
juvenile A50.45
paresthesia A52.19
Parkinson's disease or syndrome A52.19
paroxysmal tachycardia A52.06
pemphigus (congenital) A50.06
penis (chancre) A51.0
late A52.76
pericardium A52.06
perichondritis, larynx (late) A52.73
periosteum (late) A52.77
congenital (early) A50.02 [M90.80]
early (secondary) A51.46
peripheral nerve A52.79
petrous bone (late) A52.77
pharynx (late) A52.73
secondary A51.39
pituitary (gland) A52.79
pleura (late) A52.73
pneumonia, white A50.04
pontine lesion A52.17
portal vein A52.09
primary A51.0
anal A51.1
and secondary — *see* Syphilis, secondary
central nervous system A52.3
extragenital chancre NEC A51.2
fingers A51.2
genital A51.0
lip A51.2
specified site NEC A51.2
tonsils A51.2
prostate (late) A52.76
ptosis (eyelid) A52.71
pulmonary (late) A52.72
artery A52.09
pyelonephritis (late) A52.75
recently acquired, symptomatic A51.9
rectum (late) A52.74
respiratory tract (late) A52.73
retina, late A52.71
retrobulbar neuritis A52.15
salpingitis A52.76
sclera (late) A52.71
sclerosis
cerebral A52.17
coronary A52.06
multiple A52.11
scotoma (central) A52.71
scrotum (late) A52.76
secondary (and primary) A51.49
adenopathy A51.49
anus A51.39
bone A51.46
chorioretinitis, choroiditis A51.43
hepatitis A51.45
liver A51.45

Syphilis, syphilitic — *continued*
   secondary — *continued*
      lymphadenitis A51.49
      meningitis (acute) A51.41
      mouth A51.39
      mucous membranes A51.39
      periosteum, periostitis A51.46
      pharynx A51.39
      relapse (treated, untreated) A51.49
      skin A51.39
      specified form NEC A51.49
      tonsil A51.39
      ulcer A51.39
      viscera NEC A51.49
      vulva A51.39
   seminal vesicle (late) A52.76
   seronegative with signs or symptoms — *code by* site and stage under Syphilis
   seropositive
      with signs or symptoms — *code by* site and stage under Syphilis
      follow-up of latent syphilis — *see* Syphilis, latent
      only finding — *see* Syphilis, latent
   seventh nerve (paralysis) A52.15
   sinus, sinusitis (late) A52.73
   skeletal system A52.77
   skin (with ulceration) (early) (secondary) A51.39
      late or tertiary A52.79
   small intestine A52.74
   spastic spinal paralysis A52.17
   spermatic cord (late) A52.76
   spinal (cord) A52.12
   spleen A52.79
   splenomegaly A52.79
   spondylitis A52.77
   staphyloma A52.71
   stigmata (congenital) A50.59
   stomach A52.74
   synovium A52.78

Syphilis, syphilitic — *continued*
   tabes dorsalis (late) A52.11
      juvenile A50.45
   tabetic type A52.11
      juvenile A50.45
   taboparesis A52.17
      juvenile A50.45
   tachycardia A52.06
   tendon (late) A52.78
   tertiary A52.9
      with symptoms NEC A52.79
      cardiovascular A52.00
      central nervous system A52.3
      multiple NEC A52.79
      specified site NEC A52.79
   testis A52.76
   thorax A52.73
   throat A52.73
   thymus (gland) (late) A52.79
   thyroid (late) A52.79
   tongue (late) A52.79
   tonsil (lingual) (late) A52.73
      primary A51.2
      secondary A51.39
   trachea (late) A52.73
   tunica vaginalis (late) A52.76
   ulcer (any site) (early) (secondary) A51.39
      late A52.79
      perforating A52.79
         foot A52.11
   urethra (late) A52.76
   urogenital (late) A52.76
   uterus (late) A52.76
   uveal tract (secondary) A51.43
      late A52.71
   uveitis (secondary) A51.43
      late A52.71
   uvula (late) (perforated) A52.79
   vagina A51.0

Syphilis, syphilitic — *continued*
   vagina — *continued*
      late A52.76
   valvulitis NEC A52.03
   vascular A52.00
      brain (cerebral) A52.05
   ventriculi A52.74
   vesicae urinariae (late) A52.76
   viscera (abdominal) (late) A52.74
      secondary A51.49
   vitreous (opacities) (late) A52.71
      hemorrhage A52.71
   vulva A51.0
      late A52.76
      secondary A51.39
Syphiloma A52.79
   cardiovascular system A52.00
   central nervous system A52.3
   circulatory system A52.00
   congenital A50.59
Syphilophobia F45.29
Syringadenoma (*see also* Neoplasm, skin, benign)
   papillary –- *see* Neoplasm, skin, benign
Syringobulbia G95.0
Syringocystadenoma — *see* Neoplasm, skin, benign
   papillary — *see* Neoplasm, skin, benign
Syringoma (*see also* Neoplasm, skin, benign)
   chondroid — *see* Neoplasm, skin, benign
Syringomyelia G95.0
Syringomyelitis — *see* Encephalitis
Syringomyelocele — *see* Spina bifida
Syringopontia G95.0
System, systemic (*see also* condition)
   disease, combined — *see* Degeneration, combined
   inflammatory response syndrome (SIRS) of non-infectious origin (without organ dysfunction) R65.10
      with acute organ dysfunction R65.11
   lupus erythematosus M32.9
      inhibitor present D68.62

T

T-shaped incisors K00.2
Tabacism, tabacosis, tabagism (*see also* Poisoning, tobacco)
  meaning dependence (without remission) F17.200
    with
      disorder F17.299
        remission F17.211
        specified disorder NEC F17.298
        withdrawal F17.203
Tabardillo A75.9
  flea-borne A75.2
  louse-borne A75.0
Tabes, tabetic A52.10
  with
    central nervous system syphilis A52.10
    Charcot's joint A52.16
    cord bladder A52.19
    crisis, viscera (any) A52.19
    paralysis, general A52.17
    paresis (general) A52.17
    perforating ulcer (foot) A52.19
  arthropathy (Charcot) A52.16
  bladder A52.19
  bone A52.11
  cerebrospinal A52.12
  congenital A50.45
  conjugal A52.10
  dorsalis A52.11
    juvenile A50.49
  juvenile A50.49
  latent A52.19
  mesenterica A18.39
  paralysis, insane, general A52.17
  spasmodic A52.17
  syphilis (cerebrospinal) A52.12
Taboparalysis A52.17
Taboparesis (remission) A52.17
  juvenile A50.45
TAC (trigeminal autonomic cephalgia) **NEC** G44.099
  intractable G44.091
  not intractable G44.099
Tache noir S60.22- ☑
Tachyalimentation K91.2
Tachyarrhythmia, tachyrhythmia — *see* Tachycardia
Tachycardia R00.0
  atrial (paroxysmal) I47.1
  auricular I47.1
  AV nodal re-entry (re-entrant) I47.1
  junctional (paroxysmal) I47.1
  newborn P29.11
  nodal (paroxysmal) I47.1
  non-paroxysmal AV nodal I45.89
  paroxysmal (sustained) (nonsustained) I47.9
    with sinus bradycardia I49.5
    atrial (PAT) I47.1
    atrioventricular (AV) (re-entrant) I47.1
      psychogenic F54
    junctional I47.1
      ectopic I47.1
    nodal I47.1
    psychogenic (atrial) (supraventricular) (ventricular) F54
    supraventricular (sustained) I47.1
      psychogenic F54
    ventricular I47.2
      psychogenic F54
  psychogenic F45.8
  sick sinus I49.5
  sinoauricular NOS R00.0
    paroxysmal I47.1
  sinus [sinusal] NOS R00.0
    paroxysmal I47.1
  supraventricular I47.1
  ventricular (paroxysmal) (sustained) I47.2
    psychogenic F54
Tachygastria K31.89
Tachypnea R06.82
  hysterical F45.8
  newborn (idiopathic) (transitory) P22.1
  psychogenic F45.8

Tachypnea — *continued*
  transitory, of newborn P22.1
TACO (transfusion associated circulatory overload) E87.71
Taenia (infection) (infestation) B68.9
  diminuta B71.0
  echinococcal infestation B67.90
  mediocanellata B68.1
  nana B71.0
  saginata B68.1
  solium (intestinal form) B68.0
    larval form — *see* Cysticercosis
Taeniasis (intestine) — *see* Taenia
Tag (hypertrophied skin) (infected) L91.8
  adenoid J35.8
  anus K64.4
  hemorrhoidal K64.4
  hymen N89.8
  perineal N90.89
  preauricular Q17.0
  sentinel K64.4
  skin L91.8
    accessory (congenital) Q82.8
    anus K64.4
    congenital Q82.8
    preauricular Q17.0
  tonsil J35.8
  urethra, urethral N36.8
  vulva N90.89
Tahyna fever B33.8
Takahara's disease E80.3
Takayasu's disease or syndrome M31.4
Talcosis (pulmonary) J62.0
Talipes (congenital) Q66.89
  acquired, planus — *see* Deformity, limb, flat foot
  asymmetric Q66.89
  calcaneovalgus Q66.4
  calcaneovarus Q66.1
  calcaneus Q66.89
  cavus Q66.7
  equinovalgus Q66.6
  equinovarus Q66.0
  equinus Q66.89
  percavus Q66.7
  planovalgus Q66.6
  planus (acquired) (any degree) (*see also* Deformity, limb, flat foot)
    congenital Q66.5- ☑
    due to rickets (sequelae) E64.3
  valgus Q66.6
  varus Q66.3
Tall stature, constitutional E34.4
Talma's disease M62.89
Talon noir S90.3- ☑
  hand S60.22- ☑
  heel S90.3- ☑
  toe S90.1- ☑
Tamponade, heart I31.4
Tanapox (virus disease) B08.71
Tangier disease E78.6
Tantrum, child problem F91.8
Tapeworm (infection) (infestation) — *see* Infestation, tapeworm
Tapia's syndrome G52.7
TAR (thrombocytopenia with absent radius) **syndrome** Q87.2
Tarral-Besnier disease L44.0
Tarsal tunnel syndrome — *see* Syndrome, tarsal tunnel
Tarsalgia — *see* Pain, limb, lower
Tarsitis (eyelid) H01.8
  syphilitic A52.71
  tuberculous A18.4
Tartar (teeth) (dental calculus) K03.6
Tattoo (mark) L81.8
Tauri's disease E74.09
Taurodontism K00.2
Taussig-Bing syndrome Q20.1
Tay-Sachs amaurotic familial idiocy or disease E75.02
Taybi's syndrome Q87.2
TBI (traumatic brain injury) — *see* category S06 ☑
Teacher's node or nodule J38.2
Tear, torn (traumatic) (*see also* Laceration)
  with abortion — *see* Abortion

Tear, torn — *continued*
  annular fibrosis M51.35
  anus, anal (sphincter) S31.831 ☑
    complicating delivery
      with third degree perineal laceration O70.2
        with mucosa O70.3
      without third degree perineal laceration O70.4
    nontraumatic (healed) (old) K62.81
  articular cartilage, old — *see* Derangement, joint, articular cartilage, by site
  bladder
    with ectopic or molar pregnancy O08.6
    following ectopic or molar pregnancy O08.6
    obstetrical O71.5
    traumatic — *see* Injury, bladder
  bowel
    with ectopic or molar pregnancy O08.6
    following ectopic or molar pregnancy O08.6
    obstetrical trauma O71.5
  broad ligament
    with ectopic or molar pregnancy O08.6
    following ectopic or molar pregnancy O08.6
    obstetrical trauma O71.6
  bucket handle (knee) (meniscus) — *see* Tear, meniscus
  capsule, joint — *see* Sprain
  cartilage (*see also* Sprain)
    articular, old — *see* Derangement, joint, articular cartilage, by site
  cervix
    with ectopic or molar pregnancy O08.6
    following ectopic or molar pregnancy O08.6
    obstetrical trauma (current) O71.3
    old N88.1
    traumatic — *see* Injury, uterus
  dural G97.41
    nontraumatic G96.11
  internal organ — *see* Injury, by site
  knee cartilage
    articular (current) S83.3- ☑
    old — *see* Derangement, knee, meniscus, due to old tear
  ligament — *see* Sprain
  meniscus (knee) (current injury) S83.209 ☑
    bucket-handle S83.20- ☑
    lateral
      bucket-handle S83.25- ☑
      complex S83.27- ☑
      peripheral S83.26- ☑
      specified type NEC S83.28- ☑
    medial
      bucket-handle S83.21- ☑
      complex S83.23- ☑
      peripheral S83.22- ☑
      specified type NEC S83.24- ☑
    old — *see* Derangement, knee, meniscus, due to old tear
    site other than knee — *code as* Sprain
    specified type NEC S83.20- ☑
  muscle — *see* Strain
  pelvic
    floor, complicating delivery O70.1
    organ NEC, obstetrical trauma O71.5
      with ectopic or molar pregnancy O08.6
      following ectopic or molar pregnancy O08.6
  perineal, secondary O90.1
  periurethral tissue, obstetrical trauma O71.82
    with ectopic or molar pregnancy O08.6
    following ectopic or molar pregnancy O08.6
  rectovaginal septum — *see* Laceration, vagina
  retina, retinal (without detachment) (horseshoe) (*see also* Break, retina, horseshoe)
    with detachment — *see* Detachment, retina, with retinal, break
  rotator cuff (nontraumatic) M75.10- ☑
    complete M75.12- ☑
    incomplete M75.11- ☑
    traumatic S46.01- ☑
    capsule S43.42- ☑
  semilunar cartilage, knee — *see* Tear, meniscus
  supraspinatus (complete) (incomplete) (nontraumatic) (*see also* Tear, rotator cuff) M75.10- ☑
  tendon — *see* Strain

Tear, torn — *continued*
  tentorial, at birth P10.4
  umbilical cord
    complicating delivery O69.89 ☑
  urethra
    with ectopic or molar pregnancy O08.6
    following ectopic or molar pregnancy O08.6
    obstetrical trauma O71.5
  uterus — *see* Injury, uterus
  vagina — *see* Laceration, vagina
  vessel, from catheter — *see* Puncture, accidental
    complicating surgery
  vulva, complicating delivery O70.0
Tear-stone — *see* Dacryolith
Teeth (*see also* condition)
  grinding
    psychogenic F45.8
    sleep related G47.63
Teething (syndrome) K00.7
Telangiectasia, telangiectasis (verrucous) I78.1
  ataxic (cerebellar) (Louis-Bar) G11.3
  familial I78.0
  hemorrhagic, hereditary (congenital) (senile) I78.0
  hereditary, hemorrhagic (congenital) (senile) I78.0
  juxtafoveal H35.07- ☑
  macular H35.07- ☑
  parafoveal H35.07- ☑
  retinal (idiopathic) (juxtafoveal) (macular) (parafoveal)
    H35.07- ☑
  spider I78.1
Telephone scatologia F65.89
Telescoped bowel or intestine K56.1
  congenital Q43.8
Temperature
  body, high (of unknown origin) R50.9
  cold, trauma from T69.9 ☑
    newborn P80.0
    specified effect NEC T69.8 ☑
Temple — *see* condition
Temporal — *see* condition
Temporomandibular joint pain-dysfunction syn-
    drome M26.62
Temporosphenoidal — *see* condition
Tendency
  bleeding — *see* Defect, coagulation
  suicide
    meaning personal history of attempted suicide
      Z91.5
    meaning suicidal ideation — *see* Ideation, suicidal
  to fall R29.6
Tenderness, abdominal R10.819
  epigastric R10.816
  generalized R10.817
  left lower quadrant R10.814
  left upper quadrant R10.812
  periumbilic R10.815
  rebound R10.829
    epigastric R10.826
    generalized R10.827
    left lower quadrant R10.824
    left upper quadrant R10.822
    periumbilic R10.825
    right lower quadrant R10.823
    right upper quadrant R10.821
  right lower quadrant R10.813
  right upper quadrant R10.811
Tendinitis, tendonitis (*see also* Enthesopathy)
  Achilles M76.6- ☑
  adhesive — *see* Tenosynovitis, specified type NEC
    shoulder — *see* Capsulitis, adhesive
  bicipital M75.2- ☑
  calcific M65.2- ☑
    ankle M65.27- ☑
    foot M65.27- ☑
    forearm M65.23- ☑
    hand M65.24- ☑
    lower leg M65.26- ☑
    multiple sites M65.29
    pelvic region M65.25- ☑
    shoulder M75.3- ☑
    specified site NEC M65.28
    thigh M65.25- ☑
    upper arm M65.22- ☑
  due to use, overuse, pressure (*see also* Disorder, soft
    tissue, due to use)
    specified NEC — *see* Disorder, soft tissue, due to
      use, specified NEC

Tendinitis, tendonitis — *continued*
  gluteal M76.0- ☑
  patellar M76.5- ☑
  peroneal M76.7- ☑
  psoas M76.1- ☑
  tibial (posterior) M76.82- ☑
    anterior M76.81- ☑
  trochanteric — *see* Bursitis, hip, trochanteric
Tendon — *see* condition
Tendosynovitis — *see* Tenosynovitis
Tenesmus (rectal) R19.8
  vesical R30.1
Tennis elbow — *see* Epicondylitis, lateral
Tenonitis (*see also* Tenosynovitis)
  eye (capsule) H05.04- ☑
Tenontosynovitis — *see* Tenosynovitis
Tenontothecitis — *see* Tenosynovitis
Tenophyte — *see* Disorder, synovium, specified type
    NEC
Tenosynovitis (*see also* Synovitis) M65.9
  adhesive — *see* Tenosynovitis, specified type NEC
    shoulder — *see* Capsulitis, adhesive
  bicipital (calcifying) — *see* Tendinitis, bicipital
  gonococcal A54.49
  in (due to)
    crystals M65.8- ☑
    gonorrhea A54.49
    syphilis (late) A52.78
    use, overuse, pressure (*see also* Disorder, soft tissue,
      due to use)
      specified NEC — *see* Disorder, soft tissue, due
        to use, specified NEC
  infective NEC M65.1- ☑
    ankle M65.17- ☑
    foot M65.17- ☑
    forearm M65.13- ☑
    hand M65.14- ☑
    lower leg M65.16- ☑
    multiple sites M65.19
    pelvic region M65.15- ☑
    shoulder region M65.11- ☑
    specified site NEC M65.18
    thigh M65.15- ☑
    upper arm M65.12- ☑
  radial styloid M65.4
  shoulder region M65.81- ☑
    adhesive — *see* Capsulitis, adhesive
  specified type NEC M65.88-
    ankle M65.87- ☑
    foot M65.87- ☑
    forearm M65.83- ☑
    hand M65.84- ☑
    lower leg M65.86- ☑
    multiple sites M65.89
    pelvic region M65.85- ☑
    shoulder region M65.81- ☑
    specified site NEC M65.88
    thigh M65.85- ☑
    upper arm M65.82- ☑
  tuberculous — *see* Tuberculosis, tenosynovitis
Tenovaginitis — *see* Tenosynovitis
Tension
  arterial, high (*see also* Hypertension)
    without diagnosis of hypertension R03.0
  headache G44.209
    intractable G44.201
    not intractable G44.209
  nervous R45.0
  pneumothorax J93.0
  premenstrual N94.3
  state (mental) F48.9
Tentorium — *see* condition
Teratencephalus Q89.8
Teratism Q89.7
Teratoblastoma (malignant) — *see* Neoplasm, malig-
    nant, by site
Teratocarcinoma (*see also* Neoplasm, malignant, by
    site)
  liver C22.7
Teratoma (solid) (*see also* Neoplasm, uncertain behavior,
    by site)
  with embryonal carcinoma, mixed — *see* Neoplasm,
    malignant, by site
  with malignant transformation — *see* Neoplasm, ma-
    lignant, by site
  adult (cystic) — *see* Neoplasm, benign, by site

Teratoma — *continued*
  benign — *see* Neoplasm, benign, by site
  combined with choriocarcinoma — *see* Neoplasm,
    malignant, by site
  cystic (adult) — *see* Neoplasm, benign, by site
  differentiated — *see* Neoplasm, benign, by site
  embryonal (*see also* Neoplasm, malignant, by site)
    liver C22.7
  immature — *see* Neoplasm, malignant, by site
  liver C22.7
    adult, benign, cystic, differentiated type or mature
      D13.4
  malignant (*see also* Neoplasm, malignant, by site)
    anaplastic — *see* Neoplasm, malignant, by site
    intermediate — *see* Neoplasm, malignant, by site
      specified site — *see* Neoplasm, malignant, by
        site
      unspecified site C62.90
    undifferentiated — *see* Neoplasm, malignant, by
      site
  mature — *see* Neoplasm, uncertain behavior, by site
    malignant — *see* Neoplasm, by site, malignant, by
      site
  ovary D27.- ☑
    embryonal, immature or malignant C56- ☑
  solid — *see* Neoplasm, uncertain behavior, by site
  testis C62.9- ☑
    adult, benign, cystic, differentiated type or mature
      D29.2- ☑
    scrotal C62.1- ☑
    undescended C62.0- ☑
Termination
  anomalous (*see also* Malposition, congenital)
    right pulmonary vein Q26.3
  pregnancy, elective Z33.2
Ternidens diminutus infestation B81.8
Ternidensiasis B81.8
Terror(s) night (child) F51.4
Terrorism, victim of Z65.4
Terry's syndrome H44.2- ☑
Tertiary — *see* condition
Test, tests, testing (for)
  adequacy (for dialysis)
    hemodialysis Z49.31
    peritoneal Z49.32
  blood pressure Z01.30
    abnormal reading — *see* Blood, pressure
  blood typing Z01.83
    Rh typing Z01.83
  blood-alcohol Z04.8
    positive — *see* Findings, abnormal, in blood
  blood-drug Z04.8
    positive — *see* Findings, abnormal, in blood
  cardiac pulse generator (battery) Z45.010
  fertility Z31.41
  genetic
    disease carrier status for procreative management
      female Z31.430
      male Z31.440
    male partner of patient with recurrent pregnancy
      loss Z31.441
    procreative management NEC
      female Z31.438
      male Z31.448
  hearing Z01.10
    with abnormal findings NEC Z01.118
  HIV (human immunodeficiency virus)
    nonconclusive (in infants) R75
    positive Z21
    seropositive Z21
  immunity status Z01.84
  intelligence NEC Z01.89
  laboratory (as part of a general medical examination)
      Z00.00
    with abnormal finding Z00.01
    for medicolegal reason NEC Z04.8
  male partner of patient with recurrent pregnancy loss
      Z31.441
  Mantoux (for tuberculosis) Z11.1
    abnormal result R76.11
  pregnancy, positive first pregnancy — *see* Pregnancy,
    normal, first
  procreative Z31.49
    fertility Z31.41
  skin, diagnostic
    allergy Z01.82

Test, tests, testing — *continued*
  skin, diagnostic — *continued*
    allergy — *continued*
      special screening examination — *see* Screening, by name of disease
      Mantoux Z11.1
      tuberculin Z11.1
    specified NEC Z01.89
    tuberculin Z11.1
      abnormal result R76.11
    vision Z01.00
      with abnormal findings Z01.01
    Wassermann Z11.3
      positive — *see* Serology for syphilis, positive
Testicle, testicular, testis (*see also* condition)
  feminization syndrome (*see also* Syndrome, androgen insensitivity) E34.51
  migrans Q55.29
Tetanus, tetanic (cephalic) (convulsions) A35
  with
    abortion A34
    ectopic or molar pregnancy O08.0
    following ectopic or molar pregnancy O08.0
    inoculation reaction (due to serum) — *see* Complications, vaccination
  neonatorum A33
  obstetrical A34
  puerperal, postpartum, childbirth A34
Tetany (due to) R29.0
  alkalosis E87.3
  associated with rickets E55.0
  convulsions R29.0
    hysterical F44.5
  functional (hysterical) F44.5
  hyperkinetic R29.0
    hysterical F44.5
  hyperpnea R06.4
    hysterical F44.5
    psychogenic F45.8
  hyperventilation (*see also* Hyperventilation) R06.4
    hysterical F44.5
  neonatal (without calcium or magnesium deficiency) P71.3
  parathyroid (gland) E20.9
  parathyroprival E89.2
  post- (para)thyroidectomy E89.2
  postoperative E89.2
  pseudotetany R29.0
  psychogenic (conversion reaction) F44.5
Tetralogy of Fallot Q21.3
Tetraplegia (chronic) (*see also* Quadriplegia) G82.50-
Thailand hemorrhagic fever A91
Thalassanemia — *see* Thalassemia
Thalassemia (anemia) (disease) D56.9
  with other hemoglobinopathy D56.8
  alpha (major) (severe) (triple gene defect) D56.0
    minor D56.3
    silent carrier D56.3
    trait D56.3
  beta (severe) D56.1
    homozygous D56.1
    major D56.1
    minor D56.3
    trait D56.3
  delta-beta (homozygous) D56.2
    minor D56.3
    trait D56.3
  dominant D56.8
  hemoglobin
    C D56.8
    E-beta D56.5
  intermedia D56.1
  major D56.1
  minor D56.3
  mixed D56.8
  sickle-cell — *see* Disease, sickle-cell, thalassemia
  specified type NEC D56.8
  trait D56.3
  variants D56.8
Thanatophoric dwarfism or short stature Q77.1
Thaysen-Gee disease (nontropical sprue) K90.0
Thaysen's disease K90.0
Thecoma D27- ☑
  luteinized D27- ☑
  malignant C56- ☑
Thelarche, premature E30.8
Thelaziasis B83.8
Thelitis N61

Thelitis — *continued*
  puerperal, postpartum or gestational — *see* Infection, nipple
Therapeutic — *see* condition
Therapy
  drug, long-term (current) (prophylactic)
    agents affecting estrogen receptors and estrogen levels NEC Z79.818
    anastrozole (Arimidex) Z79.811
    anti-inflammatory Z79.1
    antibiotics Z79.2
      short-term use — *omit code*
    anticoagulants Z79.01
    antiplatelet Z79.02
    antithrombotics Z79.02
    aromatase inhibitors Z79.811
    aspirin Z79.82
    birth control pill or patch Z79.3
    bisphosphonates Z79.83
    contraceptive, oral Z79.3
    drug, specified NEC Z79.899
    estrogen receptor downregulators Z79.818
    Evista Z79.810
    exemestane (Aromasin) Z79.811
    Fareston Z79.810
    fulvestrant (Faslodex) Z79.818
    gonadotropin-releasing hormone (GnRH) agonist Z79.818
    goserelin acetate (Zoladex) Z79.818
    hormone replacement (postmenopausal) Z79.890
    insulin Z79.4
    letrozole (Femara) Z79.811
    leuprolide acetate (leuprorelin) (Lupron) Z79.818
    megestrol acetate (Megace) Z79.818
    methadone
      for pain management Z79.891
      maintenance therapy F11.20
    Nolvadex Z79.810
    opiate analgesic Z79.891
    oral contraceptive Z79.3
    raloxifene (Evista) Z79.810
    selective estrogen receptor modulators (SERMs) Z79.810
    short term — *omit code*
    steroids
      inhaled Z79.51
      systemic Z79.52
    tamoxifen (Nolvadex) Z79.810
    toremifene (Fareston) Z79.810
Thermic — *see* condition
Thermography (abnormal) (*see also* Abnormal, diagnostic imaging) R93.8
  breast R92.8
Thermoplegia T67.0 ☑
Thesaurismosis, glycogen — *see* Disease, glycogen storage
Thiamin deficiency E51.9
  specified NEC E51.8
Thiaminic deficiency with beriberi E51.11
Thibierge-Weissenbach syndrome — *see* Sclerosis, systemic
Thickening
  bone — *see* Hypertrophy, bone
  breast N64.59
  endometrium R93.8
  epidermal L85.9
    specified NEC L85.8
  hymen N89.6
  larynx J38.7
  nail L60.2
    congenital Q84.5
  periosteal — *see* Hypertrophy, bone
  pleura J92.9
    with asbestos J92.0
  skin R23.4
  subepiglottic J38.7
  tongue K14.8
  valve, heart — *see* Endocarditis
Thigh — *see* condition
Thinning vertebra — *see* Spondylopathy, specified NEC
Thirst, excessive R63.1
  due to deprivation of water T73.1 ☑
Thomsen disease G71.12
Thoracic (*see also* condition)
  kidney Q63.2
  outlet syndrome G54.0
Thoracogastroschisis (congenital) Q79.8
Thoracopagus Q89.4

Thorax — *see* condition
Thorn's syndrome N28.89
Thorson-Björck syndrome E34.0
Threadworm (infection) (infestation) B80
Threatened
  abortion O20.0
    with subsequent abortion O03.9
  job loss, anxiety concerning Z56.2
  labor (without delivery) O47.9
    after 37 completed weeks of gestation O47.1
    before 37 completed weeks of gestation O47.0- ☑
  loss of job, anxiety concerning Z56.2
  miscarriage O20.0
  unemployment, anxiety concerning Z56.2
Three-day fever A93.1
Threshers' lung J67.0
Thrix annulata (congenital) Q84.1
Throat — *see* condition
Thrombasthenia (Glanzmann) (hemorrhagic) (hereditary) D69.1
Thromboangiitis I73.1
  obliterans (general) I73.1
    cerebral I67.89
    vessels
      brain I67.89
      spinal cord I67.89
Thromboarteritis — *see* Arteritis
Thromboasthenia (Glanzmann) (hemorrhagic) (hereditary) D69.1
Thrombocytasthenia (Glanzmann) D69.1
Thrombocythemia (essential) (hemorrhagic) (idiopathic) (primary) D47.3
Thrombocytopathy (dystrophic) (granulopenic) D69.1
Thrombocytopenia, thrombocytopenic D69.6
  with absent radius (TAR) Q87.2
  congenital D69.42
  dilutional D69.59
  due to
    (massive) blood transfusion D69.59
    drugs D69.59
    extracorporeal circulation of blood D69.59
    platelet alloimmunization D69.59
  essential D69.3
  heparin induced (HIT) D75.82
  hereditary D69.42
  idiopathic D69.3
  neonatal, transitory P61.0
    due to
      exchange transfusion P61.0
      idiopathic maternal thrombocytopenia P61.0
      isoimmunization P61.0
  primary NEC D69.49
    idiopathic D69.3
  puerperal, postpartum O72.3
  secondary D69.59
  transient neonatal P61.0
Thrombocytosis, essential D47.3
  primary D47.3
Thromboembolism — *see* Embolism
Thrombopathy (Bernard-Soulier) D69.1
  constitutional D68.0
  Willebrand-Jurgens D68.0
Thrombopenia — *see* Thrombocytopenia
Thrombophilia D68.59
  primary NEC D68.59
  secondary NEC D68.69
  specified NEC D68.69
Thrombophlebitis I80.9
  antepartum O22.2- ☑
    deep O22.3- ☑
    superficial O22.2- ☑
  cavernous (venous) sinus G08
    complicating pregnancy O22.5- ☑
    nonpyogenic I67.6
  cerebral (sinus) (vein) G08
    nonpyogenic I67.6
    sequelae G09
  due to implanted device — *see* Complications, by site and type, specified NEC
  during or resulting from a procedure NEC T81.72 ☑
  femoral vein (superficial) I80.1- ☑
  femoropopliteal vein I80.0- ☑
  hepatic (vein) I80.8
  idiopathic, recurrent I82.1
  iliofemoral I80.1- ☑
  intracranial venous sinus (any) G08
    nonpyogenic I67.6

Thrombophlebitis — *continued*
　intracranial venous sinus — *continued*
　　sequelae G09
　intraspinal venous sinuses and veins G08
　　nonpyogenic G95.19
　lateral (venous) sinus G08
　　nonpyogenic I67.6
　leg I80.299
　　superficial I80.0- ☑
　longitudinal (venous) sinus G08
　　nonpyogenic I67.6
　lower extremity I80.299
　migrans, migrating I82.1
　pelvic
　　with ectopic or molar pregnancy O08.0
　　following ectopic or molar pregnancy O08.0
　　puerperal O87.1
　popliteal vein — *see* Phlebitis, leg, deep, popliteal
　portal (vein) K75.1
　postoperative T81.72 ☑
　pregnancy — *see* Thrombophlebitis, antepartum
　puerperal, postpartum, childbirth O87.0
　　deep O87.1
　　pelvic O87.1
　　septic O86.81
　　superficial O87.0
　saphenous (greater) (lesser) I80.0- ☑
　sinus (intracranial) G08
　　nonpyogenic I67.6
　specified site NEC I80.8
　tibial vein I80.23- ☑
Thrombosis, thrombotic (bland) (multiple) (progressive)
　　(silent) (vessel) I82.90
　anal K64.5
　antepartum — *see* Thrombophlebitis, antepartum
　aorta, aortic I74.10
　　abdominal I74.09
　　　saddle I74.01
　　bifurcation I74.09
　　saddle I74.01
　　specified site NEC I74.19
　　terminal I74.09
　　thoracic I74.11
　　valve — *see* Endocarditis, aortic
　apoplexy I63.3 ☑
　artery, arteries (postinfectional) I74.9
　　auditory, internal — *see* Occlusion, artery, precerebral, specified NEC
　　basilar — *see* Occlusion, artery, basilar
　　carotid (common) (internal) — *see* Occlusion, artery, carotid
　　cerebellar (anterior inferior) (posterior inferior) (superior) — *see* Occlusion, artery, cerebellar
　　cerebral — *see* Occlusion, artery, cerebral
　　choroidal (anterior) — *see* Occlusion, artery, cerebral, specified NEC
　　communicating, posterior — *see* Occlusion, artery, cerebral, specified NEC
　　coronary (*see also* Infarct, myocardium)
　　　not resulting in infarction I24.0
　　hepatic I74.8
　　hypophyseal — *see* Occlusion, artery, cerebral, specified NEC
　　iliac I74.5
　　limb I74.4
　　　lower I74.3
　　　upper I74.2
　　meningeal, anterior or posterior — *see* Occlusion, artery, cerebral, specified NEC
　　mesenteric (with gangrene) K55.0
　　ophthalmic — *see* Occlusion, artery, retina
　　pontine — *see* Occlusion, artery, cerebral, specified NEC
　　precerebral — *see* Occlusion, artery, precerebral
　　pulmonary (iatrogenic) — *see* Embolism, pulmonary
　　renal N28.0
　　retinal — *see* Occlusion, artery, retina
　　spinal, anterior or posterior G95.11
　　traumatic NEC T14.8
　　vertebral — *see* Occlusion, artery, vertebral
　atrium, auricular (*see also* Infarct, myocardium)
　　following acute myocardial infarction (current complication) I23.6
　　not resulting in infarction I24.0
　basilar (artery) — *see* Occlusion, artery, basilar
　brain (artery) (stem) (*see also* Occlusion, artery, cerebral)

Thrombosis, thrombotic — *continued*
　brain (*see also* Occlusion, artery, cerebral) — *continued*
　　due to syphilis A52.05
　　puerperal O99.43
　　sinus — *see* Thrombosis, intracranial venous sinus
　capillary I78.8
　cardiac (*see also* Infarct, myocardium)
　　not resulting in infarction I24.0
　　valve — *see* Endocarditis
　carotid (artery) (common) (internal) — *see* Occlusion, artery, carotid
　cavernous (venous) sinus — *see* Thrombosis, intracranial venous sinus
　cerebellar artery (anterior inferior) (posterior inferior) (superior) I66.3
　cerebral (artery) — *see* Occlusion, artery, cerebral
　cerebrovenous sinus (*see also* Thrombosis, intracranial venous sinus)
　　puerperium O87.3
　chronic I82.91
　coronary (artery) (vein) (*see also* Infarct, myocardium)
　　not resulting in infarction I24.0
　corpus cavernosum N48.89
　cortical I66.9
　deep — *see* Embolism, vein, lower extremity
　due to device, implant or graft (*see also* Complications, by site and type, specified NEC) T85.86 ☑
　　arterial graft NEC T82.868 ☑
　　breast (implant) T85.86 ☑
　　catheter NEC T85.86 ☑
　　　dialysis (renal) T82.868 ☑
　　　　intraperitoneal T85.86 ☑
　　　infusion NEC T82.868 ☑
　　　　spinal (epidural) (subdural) T85.86 ☑
　　　urinary (indwelling) T83.86 ☑
　　electronic (electrode) (pulse generator) (stimulator)
　　　bone T84.86 ☑
　　　cardiac T82.867 ☑
　　　nervous system (brain) (peripheral nerve) (spinal) T85.86 ☑
　　　urinary T83.86 ☑
　　fixation, internal (orthopedic) NEC T84.86 ☑
　　gastrointestinal (bile duct) (esophagus) T85.86 ☑
　　genital NEC T83.86 ☑
　　heart T82.867 ☑
　　joint prosthesis T84.86 ☑
　　ocular (corneal graft) (orbital implant) NEC T85.86 ☑
　　orthopedic NEC T84.86 ☑
　　specified NEC T85.86 ☑
　　urinary NEC T83.86 ☑
　　vascular NEC T82.868 ☑
　　ventricular intracranial shunt T85.86 ☑
　during the puerperium — *see* Thrombosis, puerperal
　endocardial (*see also* Infarct, myocardium)
　　not resulting in infarction I24.0
　eye — *see* Occlusion, retina
　genital organ
　　female NEC N94.89
　　　pregnancy — *see* Thrombophlebitis, antepartum
　　male N50.1
　gestational — *see* Phlebopathy, gestational
　heart (chamber) (*see also* Infarct, myocardium)
　　not resulting in infarction I24.0
　hepatic (vein) I82.0
　　artery I74.8
　history (of) Z86.718
　intestine (with gangrene) K55.0
　intracardiac NEC (apical) (atrial) (auricular) (ventricular) (old) I51.3
　intracranial (arterial) I66.9
　　venous sinus (any) G08
　　　nonpyogenic origin I67.6
　　　puerperium O87.3
　intramural (*see also* Infarct, myocardium)
　　not resulting in infarction I24.0
　intraspinal venous sinuses and veins G08
　　nonpyogenic G95.19
　kidney (artery) N28.0
　lateral (venous) sinus — *see* Thrombosis, intracranial venous sinus
　leg — *see* Thrombosis, vein, lower extremity
　　arterial I74.3
　liver (venous) I82.0
　　artery I74.8

Thrombosis, thrombotic — *continued*
　liver — *continued*
　　portal vein I81
　longitudinal (venous) sinus — *see* Thrombosis, intracranial venous sinus
　lower limb — *see* Thrombosis, vein, lower extremity
　lung (iatrogenic) (postoperative) — *see* Embolism, pulmonary
　meninges (brain) (arterial) I66.8
　mesenteric (artery) (with gangrene) K55.0
　　vein (inferior) (superior) I81
　mitral I34.8
　mural (*see also* Infarct, myocardium)
　　due to syphilis A52.06
　　not resulting in infarction I24.0
　omentum (with gangrene) K55.0
　ophthalmic — *see* Occlusion, retina
　pampiniform plexus (male) N50.1
　parietal (*see also* Infarct, myocardium)
　　not resulting in infarction I24.0
　penis, superficial vein N48.81
　perianal venous K64.5
　peripheral arteries I74.4
　　upper I74.2
　personal history (of) Z86.718
　portal I81
　　due to syphilis A52.09
　precerebral artery — *see* Occlusion, artery, precerebral
　puerperal, postpartum O87.0
　　brain (artery) O99.43
　　　venous (sinus) O87.3
　　cardiac O99.43
　　cerebral (artery) O99.43
　　　venous (sinus) O87.3
　　superficial O87.0
　pulmonary (artery) (iatrogenic) (postoperative) (vein) — *see* Embolism, pulmonary
　renal (artery) N28.0
　　vein I82.3
　resulting from presence of device, implant or graft — *see* Complications, by site and type, specified NEC
　retina, retinal — *see* Occlusion, retina
　scrotum N50.1
　seminal vesicle N50.1
　sigmoid (venous) sinus — *see* Thrombosis, intracranial venous sinus
　sinus, intracranial (any) — *see* Thrombosis, intracranial venous sinus
　specified site NEC I82.890
　　chronic I82.891
　spermatic cord N50.1
　spinal cord (arterial) G95.11
　　due to syphilis A52.09
　　pyogenic origin G06.1
　spleen, splenic D73.5
　　artery I74.8
　testis N50.1
　traumatic NEC T14.8
　tricuspid I07.8
　tumor — *see* Neoplasm, unspecified behavior, by site
　tunica vaginalis N50.1
　umbilical cord (vessels), complicating delivery O69.5 ☑
　vas deferens N50.1
　vein (acute) I82.90
　　antecubital I82.61- ☑
　　　chronic I82.71- ☑
　　axillary I82.A1- ☑ (*following* I82.7)
　　　chronic I82.A2- ☑ (*following* I82.7)
　　basilic I82.61- ☑
　　　chronic I82.71- ☑
　　brachial I82.62- ☑
　　　chronic I82.72- ☑
　　brachiocephalic (innominate) I82.290
　　　chronic I82.291
　　cephalic I82.61- ☑
　　　chronic I82.71- ☑
　　cerebral, nonpyogenic I67.6
　　chronic I82.91
　　deep (DVT) I82.40- ☑
　　　calf I82.4Z- ☑
　　　　chronic I82.5Z- ☑
　　　lower leg I82.4Z- ☑
　　　　chronic I82.5Z- ☑
　　　thigh I82.4Y- ☑
　　　　chronic I82.5Y- ☑
　　　upper leg I82.4Y ☑

Todd's
- cirrhosis K74.3
- paralysis (postepileptic) (transitory) G83.84

Toe — *see* condition

Toilet, artificial opening — *see* Attention to, artificial, opening

Tokelau (ringworm) B35.5

Tollwut — *see* Rabies

Tommaselli's disease R31.9
- correct substance properly administered — *see* Table of Drugs and Chemicals, by drug, adverse effect
- overdose or wrong substance given or taken — *see* Table of Drugs and Chemicals, by drug, poisoning

Tongue (*see also* condition)
- tie Q38.1

Toni-Fanconi syndrome (cystinosis) E72.09
- with cystinosis E72.04

Tonic pupil — *see* Anomaly, pupil, function, tonic pupil

Tonsil — *see* condition

Tonsillitis (acute) (catarrhal) (croupous) (follicular) (gangrenous) (infective) (lacunar) (lingual) (malignant) (membranous) (parenchymatous) (phlegmonous) (pseudomembranous) (purulent) (septic) (subacute) (suppurative) (toxic) (ulcerative) (vesicular) (viral) J03.90
- chronic J35.01
  - with adenoiditis J35.03
- diphtheritic A36.0
- hypertrophic J35.01
  - with adenoiditis J35.03
- recurrent J03.91
- specified organism NEC J03.80
  - recurrent J03.81
- staphylococcal J03.80
  - recurrent J03.81
- streptococcal J03.00
  - recurrent J03.01
- tuberculous A15.8
- Vincent's A69.1

Tooth, teeth — *see* condition

Toothache K08.8

Topagnosis R20.8

Tophi — *see* Gout, chronic

TORCH infection — *see* Infection, congenital
- without active infection P00.2

Torn — *see* Tear

Tornwaldt's cyst or disease J39.2

Torsion
- accessory tube — *see* Torsion, fallopian tube
- adnexa (female) — *see* Torsion, fallopian tube
- aorta, acquired I77.1
- appendix epididymis N44.04
- appendix testis N44.03
- bile duct (common) (hepatic) K83.8
  - congenital Q44.5
- bowel, colon or intestine K56.2
- cervix — *see* Malposition, uterus
- cystic duct K82.8
- dystonia — *see* Dystonia, torsion
- epididymis (appendix) N44.04
- fallopian tube N83.52
  - with ovary N83.53
- gallbladder K82.8
  - congenital Q44.1
- hydatid of Morgagni
  - female N83.52
  - male N44.03
- kidney (pedicle) (leading to infarction) N28.0
- Meckel's diverticulum (congenital) Q43.0
  - malignant — *see* Table of Neoplasms, small intestine, malignant
- mesentery K56.2
- omentum K56.2
- organ or site, congenital NEC — *see* Anomaly, by site
- ovary (pedicle) N83.51
  - with fallopian tube N83.53
  - congenital Q50.2
- oviduct — *see* Torsion, fallopian tube
- penis (acquired) N48.82
  - congenital Q55.63
- spasm — *see* Dystonia, torsion
- spermatic cord N44.02
  - extravaginal N44.01
  - intravaginal N44.02
- spleen D73.5
- testis, testicle N44.00
  - appendix N44.03

Torsion — *continued*
- tibia — *see* Deformity, limb, specified type NEC, lower leg
- uterus — *see* Malposition, uterus

Torticollis (intermittent) (spastic) M43.6
- congenital (sternomastoid) Q68.0
- due to birth injury P15.8
- hysterical F44.4
- ocular R29.891
- psychogenic F45.8
  - conversion reaction F44.4
- rheumatic M43.6
- rheumatoid M06.88
- spasmodic G24.3
- traumatic, current S13.4 ☑

Tortipelvis G24.1

Tortuous
- artery I77.1
- organ or site, congenital NEC — *see* Distortion
- retinal vessel, congenital Q14.1
- ureter N13.8
- urethra N36.8
- vein — *see* Varix

Torture, victim of Z65.4

Torula, torular (histolytica) (infection) — *see* Cryptococcosis

Torulosis — *see* Cryptococcosis

Torus (mandibularis) (palatinus) M27.0
- fracture — *see* Fracture, by site, torus

Touraine's syndrome Q79.8

Tourette's syndrome F95.2

Tourniquet syndrome — *see* Constriction, external, by site

Tower skull Q75.0
- with exophthalmos Q87.0

Toxemia R68.89
- bacterial — *see* Sepsis
- burn — *see* Burn
- eclamptic (with pre-existing hypertension) — *see* Eclampsia
- erysipelatous — *see* Erysipelas
- fatigue R68.89
- food — *see* Poisoning, food
- gastrointestinal K52.1
- intestinal K52.1
- kidney — *see* Uremia
- malarial — *see* Malaria
- myocardial — *see* Myocarditis, toxic
- of pregnancy — *see* Pre-eclampsia
- pre-eclamptic — *see* Pre-eclampsia
- small intestine K52.1
- staphylococcal, due to food A05.0
- stasis R68.89
- uremic — *see* Uremia
- urinary — *see* Uremia

Toxemica cerebropathia psychica (nonalcoholic) F04
- alcoholic — *see* Alcohol, amnestic disorder

Toxic (poisoning) (*see also* condition) T65.91 ☑
- effect — *see* Table of Drugs and Chemicals, by substance, poisoning
- shock syndrome A48.3
- thyroid (gland) — *see* Thyrotoxicosis

Toxicemia — *see* Toxemia

Toxicity — *see* Table of Drugs and Chemicals, by substance, poisoning
- fava bean D55.0
- food, noxious — *see* Poisoning, food
- from drug or nonmedicinal substance — *see* Table of Drugs and Chemicals, by drug

Toxicosis (*see also* Toxemia)
- capillary, hemorrhagic D69.0

Toxinfection, gastrointestinal K52.1

Toxocariasis B83.0

Toxoplasma, toxoplasmosis (acquired) B58.9
- with
  - hepatitis B58.1
  - meningoencephalitis B58.2
  - ocular involvement B58.00
  - other organ involvement B58.89
  - pneumonia, pneumonitis B58.3
- congenital (acute) (subacute) (chronic) P37.1
- maternal, manifest toxoplasmosis in infant (acute) (subacute) (chronic) P37.1

tPA (rtPA) **administration in a different facility within the last 24 hours prior to admission to current facility** Z92.82

Trabeculation, bladder N32.89

Trachea — *see* condition

Tracheitis (catarrhal) (infantile) (membranous) (plastic) (septal) (suppurative) (viral) J04.10
- with
  - bronchitis (15 years of age and above) J40
    - acute or subacute — *see* Bronchitis, acute
    - chronic J42
    - tuberculous NEC A15.5
    - under 15 years of age J20.9
  - laryngitis (acute) J04.2
    - chronic J37.1
    - tuberculous NEC A15.5
- acute J04.10
  - with obstruction J04.11
- chronic J42
  - with
    - bronchitis (chronic) J42
    - laryngitis (chronic) J37.1
  - diphtheritic (membranous) A36.89
  - due to external agent — *see* Inflammation, respiratory, upper, due to
  - syphilitic A52.73
  - tuberculous A15.5

Trachelitis (nonvenereal) — *see* Cervicitis

Tracheobronchial — *see* condition

Tracheobronchitis (15 years of age and above) (*see also* Bronchitis)
- due to
  - Bordetella bronchiseptica A37.80
    - with pneumonia A37.81
  - Francisella tularensis A21.8

Tracheobronchomegaly Q32.4
- with bronchiectasis J47.9
  - with
    - exacerbation (acute) J47.1
    - lower respiratory infection J47.0
- acquired J98.09
  - with bronchiectasis J47.9
    - with
      - exacerbation (acute) J47.1
      - lower respiratory infection J47.0

Tracheobronchopneumonitis — *see* Pneumonia, broncho-

Tracheocele (external) (internal) J39.8
- congenital Q32.1

Tracheomalacia J39.8
- congenital Q32.0

Tracheopharyngitis (acute) J06.9
- chronic J42
- due to external agent — *see* Inflammation, respiratory, upper, due to

Tracheostenosis J39.8

Tracheostomy
- complication — *see* Complication, tracheostomy
- status Z93.0
  - attention to Z43.0
  - malfunctioning J95.03

Trachoma, trachomatous A71.9
- active (stage) A71.1
- contraction of conjunctiva A71.1
- dubium A71.0
- healed or sequelae B94.0
- initial (stage) A71.0
- pannus A71.1
- Türck's J37.0

Traction, vitreomacular H43.82- ☑

Train sickness T75.3 ☑

Trait(s)
- Hb-S D57.3
- hemoglobin
  - abnormal NEC D58.2
    - with thalassemia D56.3
  - C — *see* Disease, hemoglobin C
  - S (Hb-S) D57.3
- Lepore D56.3
- personality, accentuated Z73.1
- sickle-cell D57.3
  - with elliptocytosis or spherocytosis D57.3
- type A personality Z73.1

Tramp Z59.0

Trance R41.89
- hysterical F44.89

Transaminasemia R74.0

Transection
- abdomen (partial) S38.3 ☑
- aorta (incomplete) (*see also* Injury, aorta)
  - complete — *see* Injury, aorta, laceration, major

Transection — *continued*
- carotid artery (incomplete) (*see also* Injury, blood vessel, carotid, laceration)
  - complete — *see* Injury, blood vessel, carotid, laceration, major
- celiac artery (incomplete) S35.211 ☑
  - branch (incomplete) S35.291 ☑
    - complete S35.292 ☑
  - complete S35.212 ☑
- innominate
  - artery (incomplete) (*see also* Injury, blood vessel, thoracic, innominate, artery, laceration)
    - complete — *see* Injury, blood vessel, thoracic, innominate, artery, laceration, major
  - vein (incomplete) (*see also* Injury, blood vessel, thoracic, innominate, vein, laceration)
    - complete — *see* Injury, blood vessel, thoracic, innominate, vein, laceration, major
- jugular vein (external) (incomplete) (*see also* Injury, blood vessel, jugular vein, laceration)
  - complete — *see* Injury, blood vessel, jugular vein, laceration, major
  - internal (incomplete) (*see also* Injury, blood vessel, jugular vein, internal, laceration)
    - complete — *see* Injury, blood vessel, jugular vein, internal, laceration, major
- mesenteric artery (incomplete) (*see also* Injury, mesenteric, artery, laceration)
  - complete — *see* Injury, mesenteric artery, laceration, major
- pulmonary vessel (incomplete) (*see also* Injury, blood vessel, thoracic, pulmonary, laceration)
  - complete — *see* Injury, blood vessel, thoracic, pulmonary, laceration, major
- subclavian — *see* Transection, innominate
- vena cava (incomplete) (*see also* Injury, vena cava)
  - complete — *see* Injury, vena cava, laceration, major
- vertebral artery (incomplete) (*see also* Injury, blood vessel, vertebral, laceration)
  - complete — *see* Injury, blood vessel, vertebral, laceration, major

Transfusion
- associated (red blood cell) hemochromatosis E83.111
- blood
  - ABO incompatible — *see* Complication(s), transfusion, incompatibility reaction, ABO
  - minor blood group (Duffy) (E) (K(ell)) (Kidd) (Lewis) (M) (N) (P) (S) T80.89 ☑
  - reaction or complication — *see* Complications, transfusion
- fetomaternal (mother) — *see* Pregnancy, complicated by, placenta, transfusion syndrome
- maternofetal (mother) — *see* Pregnancy, complicated by, placenta, transfusion syndrome
- placental (syndrome) (mother) — *see* Pregnancy, complicated by, placenta, transfusion syndrome
- reaction (adverse) — *see* Complications, transfusion
- related acute lung injury (TRALI) J95.84
- twin-to-twin — *see* Pregnancy, complicated by, placenta, transfusion syndrome, fetus to fetus

Transient (meaning homeless) (*see also* condition) Z59.0

Translocation
- balanced autosomal Q95.9
  - in normal individual Q95.0
- chromosomes NEC Q99.8
  - balanced and insertion in normal individual Q95.0
- Down syndrome Q90.2
- trisomy
  - 13 Q91.6
  - 18 Q91.2
  - 21 Q90.2

Translucency, iris — *see* Degeneration, iris
Transmission of chemical substances through the placenta — *see* Absorption, chemical, through placenta
Transparency, lung, unilateral J43.0
Transplant (ed) (status) Z94.9
- awaiting organ Z76.82
- bone Z94.6
  - marrow Z94.81
- candidate Z76.82
- complication — *see* Complication, transplant
- cornea Z94.7
- heart Z94.1
  - and lung(s) Z94.3
  - valve Z95.2
    - prosthetic Z95.2

Transplant — *continued*
- heart — *continued*
  - valve — *continued*
    - specified NEC Z95.4
    - xenogenic Z95.3
- intestine Z94.82
- kidney Z94.0
- liver Z94.4
- lung(s) Z94.2
  - and heart Z94.3
- organ (failure) (infection) (rejection) Z94.9
  - removal status Z98.85
- pancreas Z94.83
- skin Z94.5
- social Z60.3
- specified organ or tissue NEC Z94.89
- stem cells Z94.84
- tissue Z94.9

Transplants, ovarian, endometrial N80.1
Transposed — *see* Transposition
Transposition (congenital) (*see also* Malposition, congenital)
- abdominal viscera Q89.3
- aorta (dextra) Q20.3
- appendix Q43.8
- colon Q43.8
- corrected Q20.5
- great vessels (complete) (partial) Q20.3
- heart Q24.0
  - with complete transposition of viscera Q89.3
- intestine (large) (small) Q43.8
- reversed jejunal (for bypass) (status) Z98.0
- scrotum Q55.23
- stomach Q40.2
  - with general transposition of viscera Q89.3
- tooth, teeth, fully erupted M26.30
- vessels, great (complete) (partial) Q20.3
- viscera (abdominal) (thoracic) Q89.3

Transsexualism F64.1
Transverse (*see also* condition)
- arrest (deep), in labor O64.0 ☑
- lie (mother) O32.2 ☑
  - causing obstructed labor O64.8 ☑

Transvestism, transvestitism (dual-role) F64.1
- fetishistic F65.1

Trapped placenta (with hemorrhage) O72.0
- without hemorrhage O73.0

Trauma, traumatism (*see also* Injury)
- acoustic — *see* subcategory H83.3 ☑
- birth — *see* Birth, injury
- complicating ectopic or molar pregnancy O08.6
- during delivery O71.9
- following ectopic or molar pregnancy O08.6
- obstetric O71.9
  - specified NEC O71.89

Traumatic (*see also* condition)
- brain injury — *see* category S06 ☑

Treacher Collins syndrome Q75.4
Treitz's hernia — *see* Hernia, abdomen, specified site NEC
Trematode infestation — *see* Infestation, fluke
Trematodiasis — *see* Infestation, fluke
Trembling paralysis — *see* Parkinsonism
Tremor(s) R25.1
- drug induced G25.1
- essential (benign) G25.0
- familial G25.0
- hereditary G25.0
- hysterical F44.4
- intention G25.2
- medication induced postural G25.1
- mercurial — *see* subcategory T56.1 ☑
- Parkinson's — *see* Parkinsonism
- psychogenic (conversion reaction) F44.4
- senilis R54
- specified type NEC G25.2

Trench
- fever A79.0
- foot — *see* Immersion, foot
- mouth A69.1

Treponema pallidum infection — *see* Syphilis
Treponematosis
- due to
  - T. pallidum — *see* Syphilis
  - T. pertenue — *see* Yaws

Triad
- Hutchinson's (congenital syphilis) A50.53

Triad — *continued*
- Kartagener's Q89.3
- Saint's — *see* Hernia, diaphragm

Trichiasis (eyelid) H02.059
- with entropion — *see* Entropion
- left H02.056
  - lower H02.055
  - upper H02.054
- right H02.053
  - lower H02.052
  - upper H02.051

Trichinella spiralis (infection) (infestation) B75
Trichinellosis, trichiniasis, trichinelliasis, trichinosis B75
- with muscle disorder B75 [M63.80]
  - ankle B75 [M63.87-] ☑
  - foot B75 [M63.87-] ☑
  - forearm B75 [M63.83-] ☑
  - hand B75 [M63.84-] ☑
  - lower leg B75 [M63.86-] ☑
  - multiple sites B75 [M63.89]
  - pelvic region B75 [M63.85-] ☑
  - shoulder region B75 [M63.81-] ☑
  - specified site NEC B75 [M63.88]
  - thigh B75 [M63.85-] ☑
  - upper arm B75 [M63.82-] ☑

Trichobezoar T18.9 ☑
- intestine T18.3 ☑
- stomach T18.2 ☑

Trichocephaliasis, trichocephalosis B79
Trichocephalus infestation B79
Trichoclasis L67.8
Trichoepithelioma (*see also* Neoplasm, skin, benign)
- malignant — *see* Neoplasm, skin, malignant

Trichofolliculoma — *see* Neoplasm, skin, benign
Tricholemmoma — *see* Neoplasm, skin, benign
Trichomoniasis A59.9
- bladder A59.03
- cervix A59.09
- intestinal A07.8
- prostate A59.02
- seminal vesicles A59.09
- specified site NEC A59.8
- urethra A59.03
- urogenitalis A59.00
- vagina A59.01
- vulva A59.01

Trichomycosis
- axillaris A48.8
- nodosa, nodularis B36.8

Trichonodosis L67.8
Trichophytid, trichophyton infection — *see* Dermatophytosis
Trichophytobezoar T18.9 ☑
- intestine T18.3 ☑
- stomach T18.2 ☑

Trichophytosis — *see* Dermatophytosis
Trichoptilosis L67.8
Trichorrhexis (nodosa) (invaginata) L67.0
Trichosis axillaris A48.8
Trichosporosis nodosa B36.2
Trichostasis spinulosa (congenital) Q84.1
Trichostrongyliasis, trichostrongylosis (small intestine) B81.2
Trichostrongylus infection B81.2
Trichotillomania F63.3
Trichromat, trichromatopsia, anomalous (congenital) H53.55
Trichuriasis B79
Trichuris trichiura (infection) (infestation) (any site) B79
Tricuspid (valve) — *see* condition
Trifid (*see also* Accessory)
- kidney (pelvis) Q63.8
- tongue Q38.3

Trigeminal neuralgia — *see* Neuralgia, trigeminal
Trigeminy R00.8
Trigger finger (acquired) M65.30
- congenital Q74.0
- index finger M65.32- ☑
- little finger M65.35- ☑
- middle finger M65.33- ☑
- ring finger M65.34- ☑
- thumb M65.31- ☑

Trigonitis (bladder) (chronic) (pseudomembranous) N30.30
- with hematuria N30.31

Trigonocephaly Q75.0

Trilocular heart — see Cor triloculare
Trimethylaminuria E72.52
Tripartite placenta O43.19- ☑
Triphalangeal thumb Q74.0
Triple (see also Accessory)
　kidneys Q63.0
　uteri Q51.818
　X, female Q97.0
Triplegia G83.89
　congenital G80.8
Triplet (newborn) (see also Newborn, triplet)
　complicating pregnancy — see Pregnancy, triplet
Triplication — see Accessory
Triploidy Q92.7
Trismus R25.2
　neonatorum A33
　newborn A33
Trisomy (syndrome) Q92.9
　13 (partial) Q91.7
　　meiotic nondisjunction Q91.4
　　mitotic nondisjunction Q91.5
　　mosaicism Q91.5
　　translocation Q91.6
　18 (partial) Q91.3
　　meiotic nondisjunction Q91.0
　　mitotic nondisjunction Q91.1
　　mosaicism Q91.1
　　translocation Q91.2
　20 Q92.8
　21 (partial) Q90.9
　　meiotic nondisjunction Q90.0
　　mitotic nondisjunction Q90.1
　　mosaicism Q90.1
　　translocation Q90.2
　22 Q92.8
　autosomes Q92.9
　chromosome specified NEC Q92.8
　　partial Q92.2
　　　due to unbalanced translocation Q92.5
　　specified NEC Q92.8
　　whole (nonsex chromosome)
　　　meiotic nondisjunction Q92.0
　　　mitotic nondisjunction Q92.1
　　　mosaicism Q92.1
　due to
　　dicentrics — see Extra, marker chromosomes
　　extra rings — see Extra, marker chromosomes
　　isochromosomes — see Extra, marker chromosomes
　　specified NEC Q92.8
　whole chromosome Q92.9
　　meiotic nondisjunction Q92.0
　　mitotic nondisjunction Q92.1
　　mosaicism Q92.1
　　partial Q92.9
　　specified NEC Q92.8
Tritanomaly, tritanopia H53.55
Trombiculosis, trombiculiasis, trombidiosis B88.0
Trophedema (congenital) (hereditary) Q82.0
Trophoblastic disease (see also Mole, hydatidiform) O01.9
Tropholymphedema Q82.0
Trophoneurosis NEC G96.8
　disseminated M34.9
Tropical — see condition
Trouble (see also Disease)
　heart — see Disease, heart
　kidney — see Disease, renal
　nervous R45.0
　sinus — see Sinusitis
Trousseau's syndrome (thrombophlebitis migrans) I82.1
Truancy, childhood
　from school Z72.810
Truncus
　arteriosus (persistent) Q20.0
　communis Q20.0
Trunk — see condition
Trypanosomiasis
　African B56.9
　　by Trypanosoma brucei
　　　gambiense B56.0
　　　rhodesiense B56.1
　American — see Chagas' disease
　Brazilian — see Chagas' disease
　by Trypanosoma
　　brucei gambiense B56.0
　　brucei rhodesiense B56.1

Trypanosomiasis — continued
　by Trypanosoma — continued
　　cruzi — see Chagas' disease
　　gambiensis, Gambian B56.0
　　rhodesiensis, Rhodesian B56.1
　South American — see Chagas' disease
　where
　　African trypanosomiasis is prevalent B56.9
　　Chagas' disease is prevalent B57.2
Tsutsugamushi (disease) (fever) A75.3
Tube, tubal, tubular — see condition
Tubercle (see also Tuberculosis)
　brain, solitary A17.81
　Darwin's Q17.8
　Ghon, primary infection A15.7
Tuberculid, tuberculide (indurating, subcutaneous) (lichenoid) (miliary) (papulonecrotic) (primary) (skin) A18.4
Tuberculoma (see also Tuberculosis)
　brain A17.81
　meninges (cerebral) (spinal) A17.1
　spinal cord A17.81
Tuberculosis, tubercular, tuberculous (calcification) (calcified) (caseous) (chromogenic acid-fast bacilli) (degeneration) (fibrocaseous) (fistula) (interstitial) (isolated circumscribed lesions) (necrosis) (parenchymatous) (ulcerative) A15.9
　with pneumoconiosis (any condition in J60-J64) J65
　abdomen (lymph gland) A18.39
　abscess (respiratory) A15.9
　　bone A18.03
　　　hip A18.02
　　　knee A18.02
　　　sacrum A18.01
　　　specified site NEC A18.03
　　　spinal A18.01
　　　vertebra A18.01
　　brain A17.81
　　breast A18.89
　　Cowper's gland A18.15
　　dura (mater) (cerebral) (spinal) A17.81
　　epidural (cerebral) (spinal) A17.81
　　female pelvis A18.17
　　frontal sinus A15.8
　　genital organs NEC A18.10
　　genitourinary A18.10
　　gland (lymphatic) — see Tuberculosis, lymph gland
　　hip A18.02
　　intestine A18.32
　　ischiorectal A18.32
　　joint NEC A18.02
　　　hip A18.02
　　　knee A18.02
　　　specified NEC A18.02
　　　vertebral A18.01
　　kidney A18.11
　　knee A18.02
　　latent R76.11
　　lumbar (spine) A18.01
　　lung — see Tuberculosis, pulmonary
　　meninges (cerebral) (spinal) A17.0
　　muscle A18.09
　　perianal (fistula) A18.32
　　perinephritic A18.11
　　perirectal A18.32
　　rectum A18.32
　　retropharyngeal A15.8
　　sacrum A18.01
　　scrofulous A18.2
　　scrotum A18.15
　　skin (primary) A18.4
　　spinal cord A17.81
　　spine or vertebra (column) A18.01
　　subdiaphragmatic A18.31
　　testis A18.15
　　urinary A18.13
　　uterus A18.17
　accessory sinus — see Tuberculosis, sinus
　Addison's disease A18.7
　adenitis — see Tuberculosis, lymph gland
　adenoids A15.8
　adenopathy — see Tuberculosis, lymph gland
　adherent pericardium A18.84
　adnexa (uteri) A18.17
　adrenal (capsule) (gland) A18.7
　alimentary canal A18.32
　anemia A18.89
　ankle (joint) (bone) A18.02

Tuberculosis, tubercular, tuberculous — continued
　anus A18.32
　apex, apical — see Tuberculosis, pulmonary
　appendicitis, appendix A18.32
　arachnoid A17.0
　artery, arteritis A18.89
　　cerebral A18.89
　arthritis (chronic) (synovial) A18.02
　　spine or vertebra (column) A18.01
　articular — see Tuberculosis, joint
　ascites A18.31
　asthma — see Tuberculosis, pulmonary
　axilla, axillary (gland) A18.2
　bladder A18.12
　bone A18.03
　　hip A18.02
　　knee A18.02
　　limb NEC A18.03
　　sacrum A18.01
　　spine or vertebral column A18.01
　bowel (miliary) A18.32
　brain A17.81
　breast A18.89
　broad ligament A18.17
　bronchi, bronchial, bronchus A15.5
　　ectasia, ectasis (bronchiectasis) — see Tuberculosis, pulmonary
　　fistula A15.5
　　　primary (progressive) A15.7
　　gland or node A15.4
　　　primary (progressive) A15.7
　　lymph gland or node A15.4
　　　primary (progressive) A15.7
　bronchiectasis — see Tuberculosis, pulmonary
　bronchitis A15.5
　bronchopleural A15.6
　bronchopneumonia, bronchopneumonic — see Tuberculosis, pulmonary
　bronchorrhagia A15.5
　bronchotracheal A15.5
　bronze disease A18.7
　buccal cavity A18.83
　bulbourethral gland A18.15
　bursa A18.09
　cachexia A15.9
　cardiomyopathy A18.84
　caries — see Tuberculosis, bone
　cartilage A18.02
　　intervertebral A18.01
　catarrhal — see Tuberculosis, respiratory
　cecum A18.32
　cellulitis (primary) A18.4
　cerebellum A17.81
　cerebral, cerebrum A17.81
　cerebrospinal A17.81
　　meninges A17.0
　cervical (lymph gland or node) A18.2
　cervicitis, cervix (uteri) A18.16
　chest — see Tuberculosis, respiratory
　chorioretinitis A18.53
　choroid, choroiditis A18.53
　ciliary body A18.54
　colitis A18.32
　collier's J65
　colliquativa (primary) A18.4
　colon A18.32
　complex, primary A15.7
　congenital P37.0
　conjunctiva A18.59
　connective tissue (systemic) A18.89
　contact Z20.1
　cornea (ulcer) A18.52
　Cowper's gland A18.15
　coxae A18.02
　coxalgia A18.02
　cul-de-sac of Douglas A18.17
　curvature, spine A18.01
　cutis (colliquativa) (primary) A18.4
　cyst, ovary A18.18
　cystitis A18.12
　dactylitis A18.03
　diarrhea A18.32
　diffuse — see Tuberculosis, miliary
　digestive tract A18.32
　disseminated — see Tuberculosis, miliary
　duodenum A18.32
　dura (mater) (cerebral) (spinal) A17.0
　　abscess (cerebral) (spinal) A17.81

Tuberculosis, tubercular, tuberculous — *continued*
- dysentery A18.32
- ear (inner) (middle) A18.6
  - bone A18.03
  - external (primary) A18.4
  - skin (primary) A18.4
- elbow A18.02
- emphysema — *see* Tuberculosis, pulmonary
- empyema A15.6
- encephalitis A17.82
- endarteritis A18.89
- endocarditis A18.84
  - aortic A18.84
  - mitral A18.84
  - pulmonary A18.84
  - tricuspid A18.84
- endocrine glands NEC A18.82
- endometrium A18.17
- enteric, enterica, enteritis A18.32
- enterocolitis A18.32
- epididymis, epididymitis A18.15
- epidural abscess (cerebral) (spinal) A17.81
- epiglottis A15.5
- episcleritis A18.51
- erythema (induratum) (nodosum) (primary) A18.4
- esophagus A18.83
- eustachian tube A18.6
- exposure (to) Z20.1
- exudative — *see* Tuberculosis, pulmonary
- eye A18.50
- eyelid (primary) (lupus) A18.4
- fallopian tube (acute) (chronic) A18.17
- fascia A18.09
- fauces A15.8
- female pelvic inflammatory disease A18.17
- finger A18.03
- first infection A15.7
- gallbladder A18.83
- ganglion A18.09
- gastritis A18.83
- gastrocolic fistula A18.32
- gastroenteritis A18.32
- gastrointestinal tract A18.32
- general, generalized — *see* Tuberculosis, miliary
- genital organs A18.10
- genitourinary A18.10
- genu A18.02
- glandula suprarenalis A18.7
- glandular, general A18.2
- glottis A15.5
- grinder's J65
- gum A18.83
- hand A18.03
- heart A18.84
- hematogenous — *see* Tuberculosis, miliary
- hemoptysis — *see* Tuberculosis, pulmonary
- hemorrhage NEC — *see* Tuberculosis, pulmonary
- hemothorax A15.6
- hepatitis A18.83
- hilar lymph nodes A15.4
  - primary (progressive) A15.7
- hip (joint) (disease) (bone) A18.02
- hydropneumothorax A15.6
- hydrothorax A15.6
- hypoadrenalism A18.7
- hypopharynx A15.8
- ileocecal (hyperplastic) A18.32
- ileocolitis A18.32
- ileum A18.32
- iliac spine (superior) A18.03
- immunological findings only A15.7
- indurativa (primary) A18.4
- infantile A15.7
- infection A15.9
  - without clinical manifestations A15.7
- infraclavicular gland A18.2
- inguinal gland A18.2
- inguinalis A18.2
- intestine (any part) A18.32
- iridocyclitis A18.54
- iris, iritis A18.54
- ischiorectal A18.32
- jaw A18.03
- jejunum A18.32
- joint A18.02
  - vertebral A18.01
- keratitis (interstitial) A18.52
- keratoconjunctivitis A18.52

Tuberculosis, tubercular, tuberculous — *continued*
- kidney A18.11
- knee (joint) A18.02
- kyphosis, kyphoscoliosis A18.01
- laryngitis A15.5
- larynx A15.5
- leptomeninges, leptomeningitis (cerebral) (spinal) A17.0
- lichenoides (primary) A18.4
- linguae A18.83
- lip A18.83
- liver A18.83
- lordosis A18.01
- lung — *see* Tuberculosis, pulmonary
- lupus vulgaris A18.4
- lymph gland or node (peripheral) A18.2
  - abdomen A18.39
  - bronchial A15.4
    - primary (progressive) A15.7
  - cervical A18.2
  - hilar A15.4
    - primary (progressive) A15.7
  - intrathoracic A15.4
    - primary (progressive) A15.7
  - mediastinal A15.4
    - primary (progressive) A15.7
  - mesenteric A18.39
  - retroperitoneal A18.39
  - tracheobronchial A15.4
    - primary (progressive) A15.7
- lymphadenitis — *see* Tuberculosis, lymph gland
- lymphangitis — *see* Tuberculosis, lymph gland
- lymphatic (gland) (vessel) — *see* Tuberculosis, lymph gland
- mammary gland A18.89
- marasmus A15.9
- mastoiditis A18.03
- mediastinal lymph gland or node A15.4
  - primary (progressive) A15.7
- mediastinitis A15.8
  - primary (progressive) A15.7
- mediastinum A15.8
  - primary (progressive) A15.7
- medulla A17.81
- melanosis, Addisonian A18.7
- meninges, meningitis (basilar) (cerebral) (cerebrospinal) (spinal) A17.0
- meningoencephalitis A17.82
- mesentery, mesenteric (gland or node) A18.39
- miliary A19.9
  - acute A19.2
    - multiple sites A19.1
    - single specified site A19.0
  - chronic A19.8
  - specified NEC A19.8
- millstone makers' J65
- miner's J65
- molder's J65
- mouth A18.83
- multiple A19.9
  - acute A19.1
  - chronic A19.8
- muscle A18.09
- myelitis A17.82
- myocardium, myocarditis A18.84
- nasal (passage) (sinus) A15.8
- nasopharynx A15.8
- neck gland A18.2
- nephritis A18.11
- nerve (mononeuropathy) A17.83
- nervous system A17.9
- nose (septum) A15.8
- ocular A18.50
- omentum A18.31
- oophoritis (acute) (chronic) A18.17
- optic (nerve trunk) (papilla) A18.59
- orbit A18.59
- orchitis A18.15
- organ, specified NEC A18.89
- osseous — *see* Tuberculosis, bone
- osteitis — *see* Tuberculosis, bone
- osteomyelitis — *see* Tuberculosis, bone
- otitis media A18.6
- ovary, ovaritis (acute) (chronic) A18.17
- oviduct (acute) (chronic) A18.17
- pachymeningitis A17.0
- palate (soft) A18.83
- pancreas A18.83

Tuberculosis, tubercular, tuberculous — *continued*
- papulonecrotic (a) (primary) A18.4
- parathyroid glands A18.82
- paronychia (primary) A18.4
- parotid gland or region A18.83
- pelvis (bony) A18.03
- penis A18.15
- peribronchitis A15.5
- pericardium, pericarditis A18.84
- perichondritis, larynx A15.5
- periostitis — *see* Tuberculosis, bone
- perirectal fistula A18.32
- peritoneum NEC A18.31
- peritonitis A18.31
- pharynx, pharyngitis A15.8
- phlyctenulosis (keratoconjunctivitis) A18.52
- phthisis NEC — *see* Tuberculosis, pulmonary
- pituitary gland A18.82
- pleura, pleural, pleurisy, pleuritis (fibrinous) (obliterative) (purulent) (simple plastic) (with effusion) A15.6
  - primary (progressive) A15.7
- pneumonia, pneumonic — *see* Tuberculosis, pulmonary
- pneumothorax (spontaneous) (tense valvular) — *see* Tuberculosis, pulmonary
- polyneuropathy A17.89
- polyserositis A19.9
  - acute A19.1
  - chronic A19.8
- potter's J65
- prepuce A18.15
- primary (complex) A15.7
- proctitis A18.32
- prostate, prostatitis A18.14
- pulmonalis — *see* Tuberculosis, pulmonary
- pulmonary (cavitated) (fibrotic) (infiltrative) (nodular) A15.0
  - childhood type or first infection A15.7
  - primary (complex) A15.7
- pyelitis A18.11
- pyelonephritis A18.11
- pyemia — *see* Tuberculosis, miliary
- pyonephrosis A18.11
- pyopneumothorax A15.6
- pyothorax A15.6
- rectum (fistula) (with abscess) A18.32
- reinfection stage — *see* Tuberculosis, pulmonary
- renal A18.11
- renis A18.11
- respiratory A15.9
  - primary A15.7
  - specified site NEC A15.8
- retina, retinitis A18.53
- retroperitoneal (lymph gland or node) A18.39
- rheumatism NEC A18.09
- rhinitis A15.8
- sacroiliac (joint) A18.01
- sacrum A18.01
- salivary gland A18.83
- salpingitis (acute) (chronic) A18.17
- sandblaster's J65
- sclera A18.51
- scoliosis A18.01
- scrofulous A18.2
- scrotum A18.15
- seminal tract or vesicle A18.15
- senile A15.9
- septic — *see* Tuberculosis, miliary
- shoulder (joint) A18.02
  - blade A18.03
- sigmoid A18.32
- sinus (any nasal) A15.8
  - bone A18.03
  - epididymis A18.15
- skeletal NEC A18.03
- skin (any site) (primary) A18.4
- small intestine A18.32
- soft palate A18.83
- spermatic cord A18.15
- spine, spinal (column) A18.01
  - cord A17.81
  - medulla A17.81
  - membrane A17.0
  - meninges A17.0
- spleen, splenitis A18.85
- spondylitis A18.01
- sternoclavicular joint A18.02

☑ **Additional Character Required** — Refer to the Tabular List for Character Selection   ▽ **Subterms under main terms may continue to next column or page**

Tuberculosis, tubercular, tuberculous — *continued*
  stomach A18.83
  stonemason's J65
  subcutaneous tissue (cellular) (primary) A18.4
  subcutis (primary) A18.4
  subdeltoid bursa A18.83
  submaxillary (region) A18.83
  supraclavicular gland A18.2
  suprarenal (capsule) (gland) A18.7
  swelling, joint (*see also* category M01) (*see also* Tuberculosis, joint) A18.02
  symphysis pubis A18.02
  synovitis A18.09
    articular A18.02
    spine or vertebra A18.01
  systemic — *see* Tuberculosis, miliary
  tarsitis A18.4
  tendon (sheath) — *see* Tuberculosis, tenosynovitis
  tenosynovitis A18.09
    spine or vertebra A18.01
  testis A18.15
  throat A15.8
  thymus gland A18.82
  thyroid gland A18.81
  tongue A18.83
  tonsil, tonsillitis A15.8
  trachea, tracheal A15.5
    lymph gland or node A15.4
      primary (progressive) A15.7
  tracheobronchial A15.5
    lymph gland or node A15.4
      primary (progressive) A15.7
  tubal (acute) (chronic) A18.17
  tunica vaginalis A18.15
  ulcer (skin) (primary) A18.4
    bowel or intestine A18.32
    specified NEC — *see* Tuberculosis, by site
  unspecified site A15.9
  ureter A18.11
  urethra, urethral (gland) A18.13
  urinary organ or tract A18.13
  uterus A18.17
  uveal tract A18.54
  uvula A18.83
  vagina A18.18
  vas deferens A18.15
  verruca, verrucosa (cutis) (primary) A18.4
  vertebra (column) A18.01
  vesiculitis A18.15
  vulva A18.18
  wrist (joint) A18.02
Tuberculum
  Carabelli — *see* Excludes Note at K00.2
  occlusal — *see* Excludes Note at K00.2
  paramolare K00.2
Tuberosity, enitre maxillary M26.07
Tuberous sclerosis (brain) Q85.1
Tubo-ovarian — *see* condition
Tuboplasty, after previous sterilization Z31.0
  aftercare Z31.42
Tubotympanitis, catarrhal (chronic) — *see* Otitis, media, nonsuppurative, chronic, serous
Tularemia A21.9
  with
    conjunctivitis A21.1
    pneumonia A21.2
  abdominal A21.3
  bronchopneumonic A21.2
  conjunctivitis A21.1
  cryptogenic A21.3
  enteric A21.3
  gastrointestinal A21.3
  generalized A21.7
  ingestion A21.3
  intestinal A21.3
  oculoglandular A21.1
  ophthalmic A21.1
  pneumonia (any), pneumonic A21.2
  pulmonary A21.2
  sepsis A21.7
  specified NEC A21.8
  typhoidal A21.7
  ulceroglandular A21.0
Tularensis conjunctivitis A21.1
Tumefaction (*see also* Swelling)
  liver — *see* Hypertrophy, liver
Tumor (*see also* Neoplasm, unspecified behavior, by site)

Tumor — *continued*
  acinar cell — *see* Neoplasm, uncertain behavior, by site
  acinic cell — *see* Neoplasm, uncertain behavior, by site
  adenocarcinoid — *see* Neoplasm, malignant, by site
  adenomatoid (*see also* Neoplasm, benign, by site)
    odontogenic — *see* Cyst, calcifying odontogenic
  adnexal (skin) — *see* Neoplasm, skin, benign, by site
  adrenal
    cortical (benign) D35.0- ☑
      malignant C74.0- ☑
    rest — *see* Neoplasm, benign, by site
  alpha-cell
    malignant
      pancreas C25.4
      specified site NEC — *see* Neoplasm, malignant, by site
      unspecified site C25.4
    pancreas D13.7
    specified site NEC — *see* Neoplasm, benign, by site
    unspecified site D13.7
  aneurysmal — *see* Aneurysm
  aortic body D44.7
    malignant C75.5
  Askin's — *see* Neoplasm, connective tissue, malignant
  basal cell (*see also* Neoplasm, skin, uncertain behavior) D48.5
  Bednar — *see* Neoplasm, skin, malignant
  benign (unclassified) — *see* Neoplasm, benign, by site
  beta-cell
    malignant
      pancreas C25.4
      specified site NEC — *see* Neoplasm, malignant, by site
      unspecified site C25.4
    pancreas D13.7
    specified site NEC — *see* Neoplasm, benign, by site
    unspecified site D13.7
  Brenner D27.9
    borderline malignancy D39.1- ☑
    malignant C56- ☑
    proliferating D39.1- ☑
  bronchial alveolar, intravascular D38.1
  Brooke's — *see* Neoplasm, skin, benign
  brown fat — *see* Lipoma
  Burkitt — *see* Lymphoma, Burkitt
  calcifying epithelial odontogenic — *see* Cyst, calcifying odontogenic
  carcinoid
    benign D3A.00 (*following* D36)
      appendix D3A.020 (*following* D36)
      ascending colon D3A.022 (*following* D36)
      bronchus (lung) D3A.090 (*following* D36)
      cecum D3A.021 (*following* D36)
      colon D3A.029 (*following* D36)
      descending colon D3A.024 (*following* D36)
      duodenum D3A.010 (*following* D36)
      foregut NOS D3A.094 (*following* D36)
      hindgut NOS D3A.096 (*following* D36)
      ileum D3A.012 (*following* D36)
      jejunum D3A.011 (*following* D36)
      kidney D3A.093 (*following* D36)
      large intestine D3A.029 (*following* D36)
      lung (bronchus) D3A.090 (*following* D36)
      midgut NOS D3A.095 (*following* D36)
      rectum D3A.026 (*following* D36)
      sigmoid colon D3A.025 (*following* D36)
      small intestine D3A.019 (*following* D36)
      specified NEC D3A.098 (*following* D36)
      stomach D3A.092 (*following* D36)
      thymus D3A.091 (*following* D36)
      transverse colon D3A.023 (*following* D36)
    malignant C7A.00 (*following* C75)
      appendix C7A.020 (*following* C75)
      ascending colon C7A.022 (*following* C75)
      bronchus (lung) C7A.090 (*following* C75)
      cecum C7A.021 (*following* C75)
      colon C7A.029 (*following* C75)
      descending colon C7A.024 (*following* C75)
      duodenum C7A.010 (*following* C75)
      foregut NOS C7A.094 (*following* C75)
      hindgut NOS C7A.096 (*following* C75)
      ileum C7A.012 (*following* C75)
      jejunum C7A.011 (*following* C75)
      kidney C7A.093 (*following* C75)
      large intestine C7A.029 (*following* C75)
      lung (bronchus) C7A.090 (*following* C75)

Tumor — *continued*
  carcinoid — *continued*
    malignant — *continued*
      midgut NOS C7A.095 (*following* C75)
      rectum C7A.026 (*following* C75)
      sigmoid colon C7A.025 (*following* C75)
      small intestine C7A.019 (*following* C75)
      specified NEC C7A.098 (*following* C75)
      stomach C7A.092 (*following* C75)
      thymus C7A.091 (*following* C75)
      transverse colon C7A.023 (*following* C75)
    mesentary metastasis C7B.04 (*following* C75)
    secondary C7B.00 (*following* C75)
      bone C7B.03 (*following* C75)
      distant lymph nodes C7B.01 (*following* C75)
      liver C7B.02 (*following* C75)
      peritoneum C7B.04 (*following* C75)
      specified NEC C7B.09 (*following* C75)
  carotid body D44.6
    malignant C75.4
  cells (*see also* Neoplasm, unspecified behavior, by site)
    benign — *see* Neoplasm, benign, by site
    malignant — *see* Neoplasm, malignant, by site
    uncertain whether benign or malignant — *see* Neoplasm, uncertain behavior, by site
  cervix, in pregnancy or childbirth — *see* Pregnancy, complicated by, tumor, cervix
  chondromatous giant cell — *see* Neoplasm, bone, benign
  chromaffin (*see also* Neoplasm, benign, by site)
    malignant — *see* Neoplasm, malignant, by site
  Cock's peculiar L72.3
  Codman's — *see* Neoplasm, bone, benign
  dentigerous, mixed — *see* Cyst, calcifying odontogenic
  dermoid — *see* Neoplasm, benign, by site
    with malignant transformation C56- ☑
  desmoid (extra-abdominal) (*see also* Neoplasm, connective tissue, uncertain behavior)
    abdominal — *see* Neoplasm, connective tissue, uncertain behavior
  embolus — *see* Neoplasm, secondary, by site
  embryonal (mixed) (*see also* Neoplasm, uncertain behavior, by site)
    liver C22.7
  endodermal sinus
    specified site — *see* Neoplasm, malignant, by site
    unspecified site
      female C56.- ☑
      male C62.90
  epithelial
    benign — *see* Neoplasm, benign, by site
    malignant — *see* Neoplasm, malignant, by site
  Ewing's — *see* Neoplasm, bone, malignant, by site
  fatty — *see* Lipoma
  fibroid — *see* Leiomyoma
  G cell
    malignant
      pancreas C25.4
      specified site NEC — *see* Neoplasm, malignant, by site
      unspecified site C25.4
    specified site — *see* Neoplasm, uncertain behavior, by site
    unspecified site D37.8
  germ cell (*see also* Neoplasm, malignant, by site)
    mixed — *see* Neoplasm, malignant, by site
  ghost cell, odontogenic — *see* Cyst, calcifying odontogenic
  giant cell (*see also* Neoplasm, uncertain behavior, by site)
    bone D48.0
      malignant — *see* Neoplasm, bone, malignant
    chondromatous — *see* Neoplasm, bone, benign
    malignant — *see* Neoplasm, malignant, by site
    soft parts — *see* Neoplasm, connective tissue, uncertain behavior
      malignant — *see* Neoplasm, connective tissue, malignant
  glomus D18.00
    intra-abdominal D18.03
    intracranial D18.02
    jugulare D44.7
      malignant C75.5
    skin D18.01
    specified site NEC D18.09
  gonadal stromal — *see* Neoplasm, uncertain behavior, by site

Tumor — *continued*
  granular cell (*see also* Neoplasm, connective tissue, benign)
    malignant — *see* Neoplasm, connective tissue, malignant
  granulosa cell D39.1- ☑
    juvenile D39.1- ☑
    malignant C56- ☑
  granulosa cell-theca cell D39.1- ☑
    malignant C56- ☑
  Grawitz's C64- ☑
  hemorrhoidal — *see* Hemorrhoids
  hilar cell D27- ☑
  hilus cell D27- ☑
  Hurthle cell (benign) D34
    malignant C73
  hydatid — *see* Echinococcus
  hypernephroid (*see also* Neoplasm, uncertain behavior, by site)
  interstitial cell (*see also* Neoplasm, uncertain behavior, by site)
    benign — *see* Neoplasm, benign, by site
    malignant — *see* Neoplasm, malignant, by site
  intravascular bronchial alveolar D38.1
  islet cell — *see* Neoplasm, benign, by site
    malignant — *see* Neoplasm, malignant, by site
      pancreas C25.4
      specified site NEC — *see* Neoplasm, malignant, by site
      unspecified site C25.4
    pancreas D13.7
    specified site NEC — *see* Neoplasm, benign, by site
    unspecified site D13.7
  juxtaglomerular D41.0- ☑
  Klatskin's C22.1
  Krukenberg's C79.6- ☑
  Leydig cell — *see* Neoplasm, uncertain behavior, by site
    benign — *see* Neoplasm, benign, by site
      specified site — *see* Neoplasm, benign, by site
      unspecified site
        female D27.9
        male D29.20
    malignant — *see* Neoplasm, malignant, by site
      specified site — *see* Neoplasm, malignant, by site
      unspecified site
        female C56.9
        male C62.90
    specified site — *see* Neoplasm, uncertain behavior, by site
    unspecified site
      female D39.10
      male D40.10
  lipid cell, ovary D27- ☑
  lipoid cell, ovary D27- ☑
  malignant (*see also* Neoplasm, malignant, by site) C80.1
    fusiform cell (type) C80.1
    giant cell (type) C80.1
    localized, plasma cell — *see* Plasmacytoma, solitary
    mixed NEC C80.1
    small cell (type) C80.1
    spindle cell (type) C80.1
    unclassified C80.1
  mast cell D47.0
    malignant C96.2
  melanotic, neuroectodermal — *see* Neoplasm, benign, by site
  Merkel cell — *see* Carcinoma, Merkel cell
  mesenchymal
    malignant — *see* Neoplasm, connective tissue, malignant
    mixed — *see* Neoplasm, connective tissue, uncertain behavior
  mesodermal, mixed (*see also* Neoplasm, malignant, by site)
    liver C22.4
  mesonephric (*see also* Neoplasm, uncertain behavior, by site)
    malignant — *see* Neoplasm, malignant, by site
  metastatic
    from specified site — *see* Neoplasm, malignant, by site
    of specified site — *see* Neoplasm, malignant, by site

Tumor — *continued*
  metastatic — *continued*
    to specified site — *see* Neoplasm, secondary, by site
  mixed NEC (*see also* Neoplasm, benign, by site)
    malignant — *see* Neoplasm, malignant, by site
  mucinous of low malignant potential
    specified site — *see* Neoplasm, malignant, by site
    unspecified site C56.9
  mucocarcinoid
    specified site — *see* Neoplasm, malignant, by site
    unspecified site C18.1
  mucoepidermoid — *see* Neoplasm, uncertain behavior, by site
  Müllerian, mixed
    specified site — *see* Neoplasm, malignant, by site
    unspecified site C54.9
  myoepithelial — *see* Neoplasm, benign, by site
  neuroectodermal (peripheral) — *see* Neoplasm, malignant, by site
    primitive
      specified site — *see* Neoplasm, malignant, by site
      unspecified site C71.9
  neuroendocrine D3A.8 (*following* D36)
    malignant poorly differentiated C7A.1 (*following* C75)
    secondary NEC C7B.8 (*following* C75)
    specified NEC C7A.8 (*following* C75)
  neurogenic olfactory C30.0
  nonencapsulated sclerosing C73
  odontogenic (adenomatoid) (benign) (calcifying epithelial) (keratocystic) (squamous) — *see* Cyst, calcifying odontogenic
    malignant C41.1
      upper jaw (bone) C41.0
  ovarian stromal D39.1- ☑
  ovary, in pregnancy — *see* Pregnancy, complicated by
  pacinian — *see* Neoplasm, skin, benign
  Pancoast's — *see* Pancoast's syndrome
  papillary (*see also* Papilloma)
    cystic D37.9
    mucinous of low malignant potential C56- ☑
      specified site — *see* Neoplasm, malignant, by site
      unspecified site C56.9
    serous of low malignant potential
      specified site — *see* Neoplasm, malignant, by site
      unspecified site C56.9
  pelvic, in pregnancy or childbirth — *see* Pregnancy, complicated by
  phantom F45.8
  phyllodes D48.6- ☑
    benign D24- ☑
    malignant — *see* Neoplasm, breast, malignant
  Pindborg — *see* Cyst, calcifying odontogenic
  placental site trophoblastic D39.2
  plasma cell (malignant) (localized) — *see* Plasmacytoma, solitary
  polyvesicular vitelline
    specified site — *see* Neoplasm, malignant, by site
    unspecified site
      female C56.9
      male C62.90
  Pott's puffy — *see* Osteomyelitis, specified NEC
  Rathke's pouch D44.3
  retinal anlage — *see* Neoplasm, benign, by site
  salivary gland type, mixed — *see* Neoplasm, salivary gland, benign
    malignant — *see* Neoplasm, salivary gland, malignant
  Sampson's N80.1
  Schmincke's — *see* Neoplasm, nasopharynx, malignant
  sclerosing stromal D27- ☑
  sebaceous — *see* Cyst, sebaceous
  secondary — *see* Neoplasm, secondary, by site
    carcinoid C7B.00 (*following* C75)
      bone C7B.03 (*following* C75)
      distant lymph nodes C7B.01 (*following* C75)
      liver C7B.02 (*following* C75)
      peritoneum C7B.04 (*following* C75)
      specified NEC C7B.09 (*following* C75)
    neuroendocrine NEC C7B.8 (*following* C75)
  serous of low malignant potential
    specified site — *see* Neoplasm, malignant, by site

Tumor — *continued*
  serous of low malignant potential — *continued*
    unspecified site C56.9
  Sertoli cell — *see* Neoplasm, benign, by site
    with lipid storage
      specified site — *see* Neoplasm, benign, by site
      unspecified site
        female D27.9
        male D29.20
    specified site — *see* Neoplasm, benign, by site
    unspecified site
      female D27.9
      male D29.20
  Sertoli-Leydig cell — *see* Neoplasm, benign, by site
    specified site — *see* Neoplasm, benign, by site
    unspecified site
      female D27.9
      male D29.20
  sex cord (-stromal) — *see* Neoplasm, uncertain behavior, by site
    with annular tubules D39.1- ☑
  skin appendage — *see* Neoplasm, skin, benign
  smooth muscle — *see* Neoplasm, connective tissue, uncertain behavior
  soft tissue
    benign — *see* Neoplasm, connective tissue, benign
    malignant — *see* Neoplasm, connective tissue, malignant
  sternomastoid (congenital) Q68.0
  stromal
    endometrial D39.0
    gastric D48.1
      benign D21.4
      malignant C16.9
      uncertain behavior D48.1
    gastrointestinal
      benign D21.4
      malignant C49.4
      uncertain behavior D48.1
    intestine
      benign D21.4
      malignant C49.4
      uncertain behavior D48.1
    ovarian D39.1- ☑
    stomach
      benign D21.4
      malignant C16.9
      uncertain behavior D48.1
  sweat gland (*see also* Neoplasm, skin, uncertain behavior)
    benign — *see* Neoplasm, skin, benign
    malignant — *see* Neoplasm, skin, malignant
  syphilitic, brain A52.17
  testicular D40.10
  testicular stromal D40.1- ☑
  theca cell D27.- ☑
  theca cell-granulosa cell D39.1- ☑
  Triton, malignant — *see* Neoplasm, nerve, malignant
  trophoblastic, placental site D39.2
  turban D23.4
  uterus (body), in pregnancy or childbirth — *see* Pregnancy, complicated by, tumor, uterus
  vagina, in pregnancy or childbirth — *see* Pregnancy, complicated by
  varicose — *see* Varix
  von Recklinghausen's — *see* Neurofibromatosis
  vulva or perineum, in pregnancy or childbirth — *see* Pregnancy, complicated by
    causing obstructed labor O65.5
  Warthin's — *see* Neoplasm, salivary gland, benign
  Wilms' C64- ☑
  yolk sac — *see* Neoplasm, malignant, by site
    specified site — *see* Neoplasm, malignant, by site
    unspecified site
      female C56.9
      male C62.90

Tumor lysis syndrome (following antineoplastic chemotherapy) (spontaneous) NEC E88.3
Tumorlet — *see* Neoplasm, uncertain behavior, by site
Tungiasis B88.1
Tunica vasculosa lentis Q12.2
Turban tumor D23.4
Türck's trachoma J37.0
Turner-Kieser syndrome Q79.8
Turner-like syndrome Q87.1
Turner-Ullrich syndrome Q96.9

☑ Additional Character Required — Refer to the Tabular List for Character Selection   ▽ Subterms under main terms may continue to next column or page

Turner's
  hypoplasia (tooth) K00.4
  syndrome Q96.9
    specified NEC Q96.8
  tooth K00.4
Tussis convulsiva — see Whooping cough
Twiddler's syndrome (due to)
  automatic implantable defibrillatorT82.198
  cardiac pacemaker T82.198 ☑
Twilight state
  epileptic F05
  psychogenic F44.89
Twin (newborn) (see also Newborn, twin)
  conjoined Q89.4
  pregnancy — see Pregnancy, twin, conjoined
Twinning, teeth K00.2
Twist, twisted
  bowel, colon or intestine K56.2
  hair (congenital) Q84.1
  mesentery K56.2
  omentum K56.2
  organ or site, congenital NEC — see Anomaly, by site
  ovarian pedicle — see Torsion, ovary
Twitching R25.3
Tylosis (acquired) L84
  buccalis K13.29
  linguae K13.29
  palmaris et plantaris (congenital) (inherited) Q82.8
    acquired L85.1
Tympanism R14.0
Tympanites (abdominal) (intestinal) R14.0
Tympanitis — see Myringitis
Tympanosclerosis H74.0 ☑
Tympanum — see condition
Tympany
  abdomen R14.0
  chest R09.89
Type A behavior pattern Z73.1
Typhlitis — see Appendicitis
Typhoenteritis — see Typhoid
Typhoid (abortive) (ambulant) (any site) (clinical) (fever)
      (hemorrhagic) (infection) (intermittent) (malignant)
      (rheumatic) (Widal negative) A01.00
  with pneumonia A01.03
  abdominal A01.09
  arthritis A01.04
  carrier (suspected) of Z22.0
  cholecystitis (current) A01.09
  endocarditis A01.02
  heart involvement A01.02
  inoculation reaction — see Complications, vaccination
  meningitis A01.01
  mesenteric lymph nodes A01.09
  myocarditis A01.02
  osteomyelitis A01.05
  perichondritis, larynx A01.09
  pneumonia A01.03
  specified NEC A01.09
  spine A01.05
  ulcer (perforating) A01.09
Typhomalaria (fever) — see Malaria
Typhomania A01.00
Typhoperitonitis A01.09
Typhus (fever) A75.9
  abdominal, abdominalis — see Typhoid
  African tick A77.1
  amarillic A95.9
  brain A75.9 [G94]
  cerebral A75.9 [G94]
  classical A75.0
  due to Rickettsia
    prowazekii A75.0
      recrudescent A75.1
    tsutsugamushi A75.3
    typhi A75.2
  endemic (flea-borne) A75.2
  epidemic (louse-borne) A75.0
  exanthematicus SAI A75.0
    brillii SAI A75.1
    mexicanus SAI A75.2
    typhus murinus A75.2
  exanthematic NEC A75.0
  flea-borne A75.2
  India tick A77.1
  Kenya (tick) A77.1
  louse-borne A75.0
  Mexican A75.2
  mite-borne A75.3

Typhus — continued
  murine A75.2
  North Asian tick-borne A77.2
  petechial A75.9
  Queensland tick A77.3
  rat A75.2
  recrudescent A75.1
  recurrens — see Fever, relapsing
  Sao Paulo A77.0
  scrub (China) (India) (Malaysia) (New Guinea) A75.3
  shop (of Malaysia) A75.2
  Siberian tick A77.2
  tick-borne A77.9
  tropical (mite-borne) A75.3
Tyrosinemia E70.21
  newborn, transitory P74.5
Tyrosinosis E70.21
Tyrosinuria E70.29

U

Uhl's anomaly or disease Q24.8
Ulcer, ulcerated, ulcerating, ulceration, ulcerative
  alveolar process M27.3
  amebic (intestine) A06.1
    skin A06.7
  anastomotic — see Ulcer, gastrojejunal
  anorectal K62.6
  antral — see Ulcer, stomach
  anus (sphincter) (solitary) K62.6
  aorta — see Aneurysm
  aphthous (oral) (recurrent) K12.0
    genital organ(s)
      female N76.6
      male N50.8
  artery I77.2
  atrophic — see Ulcer, skin
    decubitus — see Ulcer, pressure, by site
  back L98.429
    with
      bone necrosis L98.424
      exposed fat layer L98.422
      muscle necrosis L98.423
      skin breakdown only L98.421
  Barrett's (esophagus) K22.10
    with bleeding K22.11
  bile duct (common) (hepatic) K83.8
  bladder (solitary) (sphincter) NEC N32.89
    bilharzial B65.9 [N33]
    in schistosomiasis (bilharzial) B65.9 [N33]
    submucosal — see Cystitis, interstitial
    tuberculous A18.12
  bleeding K27.4
  bone — see Osteomyelitis, specified type NEC
  bowel — see Ulcer, intestine
  breast N61
  bronchus J98.09
  buccal (cavity) (traumatic) K12.1
  Buruli A31.1
  buttock L98.419
    with
      bone necrosis L98.414
      exposed fat layer L98.412
      muscle necrosis L98.413
      skin breakdown only L98.411
  cancerous — see Neoplasm, malignant, by site
  cardia K22.10
    with bleeding K22.11
  cardioesophageal (peptic) K22.10
    with bleeding K22.11
  cecum — see Ulcer, intestine
  cervix (uteri) (decubitus) (trophic) N86
    with cervicitis N72
  chancroidal A57
  chiclero B55.1
  chronic (cause unknown) — see Ulcer, skin
  Cochin-China B55.1
  colon — see Ulcer, intestine
  conjunctiva H10.89
  cornea H16.00- ☑
    with hypopyon H16.03- ☑
    central H16.01- ☑
    dendritic (herpes simplex) B00.52
    marginal H16.04- ☑
    Mooren's H16.05- ☑
    mycotic H16.06- ☑
    perforated H16.07- ☑

Ulcer, ulcerated, ulcerating, ulceration, ulcerative
  — continued
  cornea — continued
    ring H16.02- ☑
    tuberculous (phlyctenular) A18.52
  corpus cavernosum (chronic) N48.5
  crural — see Ulcer, lower limb
  Curling's — see Ulcer, peptic, acute
  Cushing's — see Ulcer, peptic, acute
  cystic duct K82.8
  cystitis (interstitial) — see Cystitis, interstitial
  decubitus — see Ulcer, pressure, by site
  dendritic, cornea (herpes simplex) B00.52
  diabetes, diabetic — see Diabetes, ulcer
  Dieulafoy's K25.0
  due to
    infection NEC — see Ulcer, skin
    radiation NEC L59.8
    trophic disturbance (any region) — see Ulcer, skin
    X-ray L58.1
  duodenum, duodenal (eroded) (peptic) K26.9
    with
      hemorrhage K26.4
        and perforation K26.6
      perforation K26.5
    acute K26.3
      with
        hemorrhage K26.0
          and perforation K26.2
        perforation K26.1
    chronic K26.7
      with
        hemorrhage K26.4
          and perforation K26.6
        perforation K26.5
  dysenteric A09
  elusive — see Cystitis, interstitial
  endocarditis (acute) (chronic) (subacute) I28.8
  epiglottis J38.7
  esophagus (peptic) K22.10
    with bleeding K22.11
    due to
      aspirin K22.10
        with bleeding K22.11
      gastrointestinal reflux disease K21.0
      ingestion of chemical or medicament K22.10
        with bleeding K22.11
    fungal K22.10
      with bleeding K22.11
    infective K22.10
      with bleeding K22.11
    varicose — see Varix, esophagus
  eyelid (region) H01.8
  fauces J39.2
  Fenwick (-Hunner) (solitary) — see Cystitis, interstitial
  fistulous — see Ulcer, skin
  foot (indolent) (trophic) — see Ulcer, lower limb
  frambesial, initial A66.0
  frenum (tongue) K14.0
  gallbladder or duct K82.8
  gangrenous — see Gangrene
  gastric — see Ulcer, stomach
  gastrocolic — see Ulcer, gastrojejunal
  gastroduodenal — see Ulcer, peptic
  gastroesophageal — see Ulcer, stomach
  gastrointestinal — see Ulcer, gastrojejunal
  gastrojejunal (peptic) K28.9
    with
      hemorrhage K28.4
        and perforation K28.6
      perforation K28.5
    acute K28.3
      with
        hemorrhage K28.0
          and perforation K28.2
        perforation K28.1
    chronic K28.7
      with
        hemorrhage K28.4
          and perforation K28.6
        perforation K28.5
  gastrojejunocolic — see Ulcer, gastrojejunal
  gingiva K06.8
  gingivitis K05.10
    nonplaque induced K05.11
    plaque induced K05.10
  glottis J38.7
  granuloma of pudenda A58

Ulcer, ulcerated, ulcerating, ulceration, ulcerative — *continued*
- gum K06.8
- gumma, due to yaws A66.4
- heel — *see* Ulcer, lower limb
- hemorrhoid (*see also* Hemorrhoids, by degree) K64.8
- Hunner's — *see* Cystitis, interstitial
- hypopharynx J39.2
- hypopyon (chronic) (subacute) — *see* Ulcer, cornea, with hypopyon
- hypostaticum — *see* Ulcer, varicose
- ileum — *see* Ulcer, intestine
- intestine, intestinal K63.3
  - with perforation K63.1
  - amebic A06.1
  - duodenal — *see* Ulcer, duodenum
  - granulocytopenic (with hemorrhage) — *see* Neutropenia
  - marginal — *see* Ulcer, gastrojejunal
  - perforating K63.1
    - newborn P78.0
  - primary, small intestine K63.3
  - rectum K62.6
  - stercoraceous, stercoral K63.3
  - tuberculous A18.32
  - typhoid (fever) — *see* Typhoid
  - varicose I86.8
- jejunum, jejunal — *see* Ulcer, gastrojejunal
- keratitis — *see* Ulcer, cornea
- knee — *see* Ulcer, lower limb
- labium (majus) (minus) N76.6
- laryngitis — *see* Laryngitis
- larynx (aphthous) (contact) J38.7
  - diphtheritic A36.2
- leg — *see* Ulcer, lower limb
- lip K13.0
- Lipschütz's N76.6
- lower limb (atrophic) (chronic) (neurogenic) (perforating) (pyogenic) (trophic) (tropical) L97.909
  - with
    - bone necrosis L97.904
    - exposed fat layer L97.902
    - muscle necrosis L97.903
    - skin breakdown only L97.901
  - ankle L97.309
    - with
      - bone necrosis L97.304
      - exposed fat layer L97.302
      - muscle necrosis L97.303
      - skin breakdown only L97.301
    - left L97.329
      - with
        - bone necrosis L97.324
        - exposed fat layer L97.322
        - muscle necrosis L97.323
        - skin breakdown only L97.321
    - right L97.319
      - with
        - bone necrosis L97.314
        - exposed fat layer L97.312
        - muscle necrosis L97.313
        - skin breakdown only L97.311
  - calf L97.209
    - with
      - bone necrosis L97.204
      - exposed fat layer L97.202
      - muscle necrosis L97.203
      - skin breakdown only L97.201
    - left L97.229
      - with
        - bone necrosis L97.224
        - exposed fat layer L97.222
        - muscle necrosis L97.223
        - skin breakdown only L97.221
    - right L97.219
      - with
        - bone necrosis L97.214
        - exposed fat layer L97.212
        - muscle necrosis L97.213
        - skin breakdown only L97.211
  - decubitus — *see* Ulcer, pressure, by site
  - foot specified NEC L97.509
    - with
      - bone necrosis L97.504
      - exposed fat layer L97.502
      - muscle necrosis L97.503
      - skin breakdown only L97.501
    - left L97.529

Ulcer, ulcerated, ulcerating, ulceration, ulcerative — *continued*
- lower limb — *continued*
  - foot specified — *continued*
    - left — *continued*
      - with
        - bone necrosis L97.524
        - exposed fat layer L97.522
        - muscle necrosis L97.523
        - skin breakdown only L97.521
    - right L97.519
      - with
        - bone necrosis L97.514
        - exposed fat layer L97.512
        - muscle necrosis L97.513
        - skin breakdown only L97.511
  - heel L97.409
    - with
      - bone necrosis L97.404
      - exposed fat layer L97.402
      - muscle necrosis L97.403
      - skin breakdown only L97.401
    - left L97.429
      - with
        - bone necrosis L97.424
        - exposed fat layer L97.422
        - muscle necrosis L97.423
        - skin breakdown only L97.421
    - right L97.419
      - with
        - bone necrosis L97.414
        - exposed fat layer L97.412
        - muscle necrosis L97.413
        - skin breakdown only L97.411
  - left L97.929
    - with
      - bone necrosis L97.924
      - exposed fat layer L97.922
      - muscle necrosis L97.923
      - skin breakdown only L97.921
  - leprous A30.1
  - lower leg NOS L97.909
    - with
      - bone necrosis L97.904
      - exposed fat layer L97.902
      - muscle necrosis L97.903
      - skin breakdown only L97.901
    - left L97.929
      - with
        - bone necrosis L97.924
        - exposed fat layer L97.922
        - muscle necrosis L97.923
        - skin breakdown only L97.921
    - right L97.919
      - with
        - bone necrosis L97.914
        - exposed fat layer L97.912
        - muscle necrosis L97.913
        - skin breakdown only L97.911
    - specified site NEC L97.809
      - with
        - bone necrosis L97.804
        - exposed fat layer L97.802
        - muscle necrosis L97.803
        - skin breakdown only L97.801
      - left L97.829
        - with
          - bone necrosis L97.824
          - exposed fat layer L97.822
          - muscle necrosis L97.823
          - skin breakdown only L97.821
      - right L97.819
        - with
          - bone necrosis L97.814
          - exposed fat layer L97.812
          - muscle necrosis L97.813
          - skin breakdown only L97.811
  - midfoot L97.409
    - with
      - bone necrosis L97.404
      - exposed fat layer L97.402
      - muscle necrosis L97.403
      - skin breakdown only L97.401
    - left L97.429
      - with
        - bone necrosis L97.424
        - exposed fat layer L97.422
        - muscle necrosis L97.423

Ulcer, ulcerated, ulcerating, ulceration, ulcerative — *continued*
- lower limb — *continued*
  - midfoot — *continued*
    - left — *continued*
      - with — *continued*
        - skin breakdown only L97.421
    - right L97.419
      - with
        - bone necrosis L97.414
        - exposed fat layer L97.412
        - muscle necrosis L97.413
        - skin breakdown only L97.411
    - right L97.919
      - with
        - bone necrosis L97.914
        - exposed fat layer L97.912
        - muscle necrosis L97.913
        - skin breakdown only L97.911
    - syphilitic A52.19
    - thigh L97.109
      - with
        - bone necrosis L97.104
        - exposed fat layer L97.102
        - muscle necrosis L97.103
        - skin breakdown only L97.101
      - left L97.129
        - with
          - bone necrosis L97.124
          - exposed fat layer L97.122
          - muscle necrosis L97.123
          - skin breakdown only L97.121
      - right L97.119
        - with
          - bone necrosis L97.114
          - exposed fat layer L97.112
          - muscle necrosis L97.113
          - skin breakdown only L97.111
    - toe L97.509
      - with
        - bone necrosis L97.504
        - exposed fat layer L97.502
        - muscle necrosis L97.503
        - skin breakdown only L97.501
      - left L97.529
        - with
          - bone necrosis L97.524
          - exposed fat layer L97.522
          - muscle necrosis L97.523
          - skin breakdown only L97.521
      - right L97.519
        - with
          - bone necrosis L97.514
          - exposed fat layer L97.512
          - muscle necrosis L97.513
          - skin breakdown only L97.511
    - varicose — *see* Varix, leg, with, ulcer
- luetic — *see* Ulcer, syphilitic
- lung J98.4
  - tuberculous — *see* Tuberculosis, pulmonary
- malignant — *see* Neoplasm, malignant, by site
- marginal NEC — *see* Ulcer, gastrojejunal
- meatus (urinarius) N34.2
- Meckel's diverticulum Q43.0
  - malignant — *see* Table of Neoplasms, small intestine, malignant
- Meleney's (chronic undermining) — *see* Ulcer, skin
- Mooren's (cornea) — *see* Ulcer, cornea, Mooren's
- mycobacterial (skin) A31.1
- nasopharynx J39.2
- neck, uterus N86
- neurogenic NEC — *see* Ulcer, skin
- nose, nasal (passage) (infective) (septum) J34.0
  - skin — *see* Ulcer, skin
  - spirochetal A69.8
  - varicose (bleeding) I86.8
- oral mucosa (traumatic) K12.1
- palate (soft) K12.1
- penis (chronic) N48.5
- peptic (site unspecified) K27.9
  - with
    - hemorrhage K27.4
      - and perforation K27.6
    - perforation K27.5
  - acute K27.3
    - with
      - hemorrhage K27.0
        - and perforation K27.2

☑ **Additional Character Required** — Refer to the Tabular List for Character Selection   ▽ **Subterms under main terms may continue to next column or page**

Ulcer, ulcerated, ulcerating, ulceration, ulcerative
— *continued*
peptic — *continued*
  acute — *continued*
    with — *continued*
      perforation K27.1
  chronic K27.7
    with
      hemorrhage K27.4
        and perforation K27.6
      perforation K27.5
  esophagus K22.10
    with bleeding K22.11
  newborn P78.82
  perforating K27.5
  skin — *see* Ulcer, skin
peritonsillar J35.8
phagedenic (tropical) — *see* Ulcer, skin
pharynx J39.2
phlebitis — *see* Phlebitis
plaster — *see* Ulcer, pressure, by site
popliteal space — *see* Ulcer, lower limb
postpyloric — *see* Ulcer, duodenum
prepuce N47.7
prepyloric — *see* Ulcer, stomach
pressure (pressure area) L89.9- ☑
  ankle L89.5- ☑
  back L89.1- ☑
  buttock L89.3- ☑
  coccyx L89.15- ☑
  contiguous site of back, buttock, hip L89.4- ☑
  elbow L89.0- ☑
  face L89.81- ☑
  head L89.81- ☑
  heel L89.6- ☑
  hip L89.2- ☑
  sacral region (tailbone) L89.15- ☑
  specified site NEC L89.89- ☑
  stage 1 (healing) (pre-ulcer skin changes limited to persistent focal edema)
    ankle L89.5- ☑
    back L89.1- ☑
    buttock L89.3- ☑
    coccyx L89.15- ☑
    contiguous site of back, buttock, hip L89.4- ☑
    elbow L89.0- ☑
    face L89.81- ☑
    head L89.81- ☑
    heel L89.6- ☑
    hip L89.2- ☑
    sacral region (tailbone) L89.15- ☑
    specified site NEC L89.89- ☑
  stage 2 (healing) (abrasion, blister, partial thickness skin loss involving epidermis and/or dermis)
    ankle L89.5- ☑
    back L89.1- ☑
    buttock L89.3- ☑
    coccyx L89.15- ☑
    contiguous site of back, buttock, hip L89.4- ☑
    elbow L89.0- ☑
    face L89.81- ☑
    head L89.81- ☑
    heel L89.6- ☑
    hip L89.2- ☑
    sacral region (tailbone) L89.15- ☑
    specified site NEC L89.89- ☑
  stage 3 (healing) (full thickness skin loss involving damage or necrosis of subcutaneous tissue)
    ankle L89.5- ☑
    back L89.1- ☑
    buttock L89.3- ☑
    coccyx L89.15- ☑
    contiguous site of back, buttock, hip L89.4- ☑
    elbow L89.0- ☑
    face L89.81- ☑
    head L89.81- ☑
    heel L89.6- ☑
    hip L89.2- ☑
    sacral region (tailbone) L89.15- ☑
    specified site NEC L89.89- ☑
  stage 4 (healing) (necrosis of soft tissues through to underlying muscle, tendon, or bone)
    ankle L89.5- ☑
    back L89.1- ☑
    buttock L89.3- ☑
    coccyx L89.15- ☑

Ulcer, ulcerated, ulcerating, ulceration, ulcerative
— *continued*
pressure — *continued*
  stage 4 — *continued*
    contiguous site of back, buttock, hip L89.4- ☑
    elbow L89.0- ☑
    face L89.81- ☑
    head L89.81- ☑
    heel L89.6- ☑
    hip L89.2- ☑
    sacral region (tailbone) L89.15- ☑
    specified site NEC L89.89- ☑
  unspecified stage
    ankle L89.5- ☑
    back L89.1- ☑
    buttock L89.3- ☑
    coccyx L89.15- ☑
    contiguous site of back, buttock, hip L89.4- ☑
    elbow L89.0- ☑
    face L89.81- ☑
    head L89.81- ☑
    heel L89.6- ☑
    hip L89.2- ☑
    sacral region (tailbone) L89.15- ☑
    specified site NEC L89.89- ☑
  unstageable
    ankle L89.5- ☑
    back L89.1- ☑
    buttock L89.3- ☑
    coccyx L89.15- ☑
    contiguous site of back, buttock, hip L89.4- ☑
    elbow L89.0- ☑
    face L89.81- ☑
    head L89.81- ☑
    heel L89.6- ☑
    hip L89.2- ☑
    sacral region (tailbone) L89.15- ☑
    specified site NEC L89.89- ☑
primary of intestine K63.3
  with perforation K63.1
prostate N41.9
pyloric — *see* Ulcer, stomach
rectosigmoid K63.3
  with perforation K63.1
rectum (sphincter) (solitary) K62.6
  stercoraceous, stercoral K62.6
retina — *see* Inflammation, chorioretinal
rodent (*see also* Neoplasm, skin, malignant)
sclera — *see* Scleritis
scrofulous (tuberculous) A18.2
scrotum N50.8
  tuberculous A18.15
  varicose I86.1
seminal vesicle N50.8
sigmoid — *see* Ulcer, intestine
skin (atrophic) (chronic) (neurogenic) (non-healing) (perforating) (pyogenic) (trophic) (tropical) L98.499
  with gangrene — *see* Gangrene
  amebic A06.7
  back — *see* Ulcer, back
  buttock — *see* Ulcer, buttock
  decubitus — *see* Ulcer, pressure
  lower limb — *see* Ulcer, lower limb
  mycobacterial A31.1
  specified site NEC L98.499
    with
      bone necrosis L98.494
      exposed fat layer L98.492
      muscle necrosis L98.493
      skin breakdown only L98.491
  tuberculous (primary) A18.4
  varicose — *see* Ulcer, varicose
sloughing — *see* Ulcer, skin
solitary, anus or rectum (sphincter) K62.6
sore throat J02.9
  streptococcal J02.0
spermatic cord N50.8
spine (tuberculous) A18.01
stasis (venous) — *see* Varix, leg, with, ulcer
  without varicose veins I87.2
stercoraceous, stercoral K63.3
  with perforation K63.1
  anus or rectum K62.6
stoma, stomal — *see* Ulcer, gastrojejunal
stomach (eroded) (peptic) (round) K25.9

Ulcer, ulcerated, ulcerating, ulceration, ulcerative
— *continued*
stomach — *continued*
  with
    hemorrhage K25.4
      and perforation K25.6
    perforation K25.5
  acute K25.3
    with
      hemorrhage K25.0
        and perforation K25.2
      perforation K25.1
  chronic K25.7
    with
      hemorrhage K25.4
        and perforation K25.6
      perforation K25.5
stomal — *see* Ulcer, gastrojejunal
stomatitis K12.1
stress — *see* Ulcer, peptic
strumous (tuberculous) A18.2
submucosal, bladder — *see* Cystitis, interstitial
syphilitic (any site) (early) (secondary) A51.39
  late A52.79
    perforating A52.79
      foot A52.11
testis N50.8
thigh — *see* Ulcer, lower limb
throat J39.2
  diphtheritic A36.0
toe — *see* Ulcer, lower limb
tongue (traumatic) K14.0
tonsil J35.8
  diphtheritic A36.0
trachea J39.8
trophic — *see* Ulcer, skin
tropical — *see* Ulcer, skin
tuberculous — *see* Tuberculosis, ulcer
tunica vaginalis N50.8
turbinate J34.89
typhoid (perforating) — *see* Typhoid
unspecified site — *see* Ulcer, skin
urethra (meatus) — *see* Urethritis
uterus N85.8
  cervix N86
    with cervicitis N72
  neck N86
    with cervicitis N72
vagina N76.5
  in Behçet's disease M35.2 [N77.0]
  pessary N89.8
valve, heart I33.0
varicose (lower limb, any part) (*see also* Varix, leg, with, ulcer)
  broad ligament I86.2
  esophagus — *see* Varix, esophagus
  inflamed or infected — *see* Varix, leg, with ulcer, with inflammation
  nasal septum I86.8
  perineum I86.3
  scrotum I86.1
  specified site NEC I86.8
  sublingual I86.0
  vulva I86.3
vas deferens N50.8
vulva (acute) (infectional) N76.6
  in (due to)
    Behçet's disease M35.2 [N77.0]
    herpesviral (herpes simplex) infection A60.04
    tuberculosis A18.18
vulvobuccal, recurring N76.6
X-ray L58.1
yaws A66.4
Ulcerosa scarlatina A38.8
Ulcus (*see also* Ulcer)
  cutis tuberculosum A18.4
  duodeni — *see* Ulcer, duodenum
  durum (syphilitic) A51.0
    extragenital A51.2
  gastrojejunale — *see* Ulcer, gastrojejunal
  hypostaticum — *see* Ulcer, varicose
  molle (cutis) (skin) A57
  serpens corneae — *see* Ulcer, cornea, central
  ventriculi — *see* Ulcer, stomach
Ulegyria Q04.8
Ulerythema
  ophryogenes, congenital Q84.2
  sycosiforme L73.8

Ullrich (-Bonnevie)(-Turner) **syndrome** Q87.1
Ullrich-Feichtiger syndrome Q87.0
Ulnar — *see* condition
Ulorrhagia, ulorrhea K06.8
Umbilicus, umbilical — *see* condition
Unacceptable
    contours of tooth K08.54
    morphology of tooth K08.54
Unavailability (of)
    bed at medical facility Z75.1
    health service-related agencies Z75.4
    medical facilities (at) Z75.3
        due to
            investigation by social service agency Z75.2
            lack of services at home Z75.0
            remoteness from facility Z75.3
            waiting list Z75.1
        home Z75.0
        outpatient clinic Z75.3
    schooling Z55.1
    social service agencies Z75.4
Uncinaria americana infestation B76.1
Uncinariasis B76.9
Uncongenial work Z56.5
Unconscious (ness) — *see* Coma
Under observation — *see* Observation
Underachievement in school Z55.3
Underdevelopment (*see also* Undeveloped)
    nose Q30.1
    sexual E30.0
Underdosing (*see also* Table of Drugs and Chemicals,
    categories T36-T50, with final character 6) Z91.14
    intentional NEC Z91.128
        due to financial hardship of patient Z91.120
    unintentional NEC Z91.138
        due to patient's age related debility Z91.130
Underfeeding, newborn P92.3
Underfill, endodontic M27.53
Underimmunization status Z28.3
Undernourishment — *see* Malnutrition
Undernutrition — *see* Malnutrition
Underweight R63.6
    for gestational age — *see* Light for dates
Underwood's disease P83.0
Undescended (*see also* Malposition, congenital)
    cecum Q43.3
    colon Q43.3
    testicle — *see* Cryptorchid
Undeveloped, undevelopment (*see also* Hypoplasia)
    brain (congenital) Q02
    cerebral (congenital) Q02
    heart Q24.8
    lung Q33.6
    testis E29.1
    uterus E30.0
Undiagnosed (disease) R69
Undulant fever — *see* Brucellosis
Unemployment, anxiety concerning Z56.0
    threatened Z56.2
Unequal length (acquired) (limb) (*see also* Deformity,
    limb, unequal length)
    leg (*see also* Deformity, limb, unequal length)
        congenital Q72.9- ☑
Unextracted dental root K08.3
Unguis incarnatus L60.0
Unhappiness R45.2
Unicornate uterus Q51.4
Unilateral (*see also* condition)
    development, breast N64.89
    organ or site, congenital NEC — *see* Agenesis, by site
Unilocular heart Q20.8
Union, abnormal (*see also* Fusion)
    larynx and trachea Q34.8
Universal mesentery Q43.3
Unrepairable overhanging of dental restorative
    materials K08.52
Unsatisfactory
    restoration of tooth K08.50
        specified NEC K08.59
    sample of cytologic smear
        anus R85.615
        cervix R87.615
        vagina R87.625
    surroundings Z59.1
        work Z56.5
Unsoundness of mind — *see* Psychosis

Unstable
    back NEC — *see* Instability, joint, spine
    hip (congenital) Q65.6
        acquired — *see* Derangement, joint, specified type
            NEC, hip
    joint — *see* Instability, joint
        secondary to removal of joint prosthesis M96.89
    lie (mother) O32.0 ☑
    lumbosacral joint (congenital)
        acquired — *see* subcategory M53.2 ☑
    sacroiliac — *see* subcategory M53.2 ☑
    spine NEC — *see* Instability, joint, spine
Unsteadiness on feet R26.81
Untruthfulness, child problem F91.8
Unverricht (-Lundborg) **disease or epilepsy** — *see*
    Epilepsy, generalized, idiopathic
Unwanted pregnancy Z64.0
Upbringing, institutional Z62.22
    away from parents NEC Z62.29
    in care of non-parental family member Z62.21
    in foster care Z62.21
    in orphanage or group home Z62.22
    in welfare custody Z62.21
Upper respiratory — *see* condition
Upset
    gastric K30
    gastrointestinal K30
        psychogenic F45.8
    intestinal (large) (small) K59.9
        psychogenic F45.8
    menstruation N93.9
    mental F48.9
    stomach K30
        psychogenic F45.8
Urachus (*see also* condition)
    patent or persistent Q64.4
Urbach-Oppenheim disease (necrobiosis lipoidica dia-
    beticorum) — *see* E08-E13 with .620
Urbach-Wiethe disease E78.89
Urbach's lipoid proteinosis E78.89
Urban yellow fever A95.1
Urea
    blood, high — *see* Uremia
    cycle metabolism disorder — *see* Disorder, urea cycle
        metabolism
Uremia, uremic N19
    with
        ectopic or molar pregnancy O08.4
        polyneuropathy N18.9 [G63]
    chronic (*see also* Disease, kidney, chronic) N18.9
        due to hypertension — *see* Hypertensive, kidney
    complicating
        ectopic or molar pregnancy O08.4
    congenital P96.0
    extrarenal R39.2
    following ectopic or molar pregnancy O08.4
    newborn P96.0
    prerenal R39.2
Ureter, ureteral — *see* condition
Ureteralgia N23
Ureterectasis — *see* Hydroureter
Ureteritis N28.89
    cystica N28.86
    due to calculus N20.1
        with calculus, kidney N20.2
            with hydronephrosis N13.2
    gonococcal (acute) (chronic) A54.21
    nonspecific N28.89
Ureterocele N28.89
    congenital (orthotopic) Q62.31
        ectopic Q62.32
Ureterolith, ureterolithiasis — *see* Calculus, ureter
Ureterostomy
    attention to Z43.6
    status Z93.6
Urethra, urethral — *see* condition
Urethralgia R39.89
Urethritis (anterior) (posterior) N34.2
    calculous N21.1
    candidal B37.41
    chlamydial A56.01
    diplococcal (gonococcal) A54.01
        with abscess (accessory gland) (periurethral) A54.1
    gonococcal A54.01
        with abscess (accessory gland) (periurethral) A54.1
    nongonococcal N34.1
        Reiter's — *see* Reiter's disease

Urethritis — *continued*
    nonspecific N34.1
    nonvenereal N34.1
    postmenopausal N34.2
    puerperal O86.22
    Reiter's — *see* Reiter's disease
    specified NEC N34.2
    trichomonal or due to Trichomonas (vaginalis) A59.03
Urethrocele N81.0
    with
        cystocele — *see* Cystocele
        prolapse of uterus — *see* Prolapse, uterus
Urethrolithiasis (with colic or infection) N21.1
Urethrorectal — *see* condition
Urethrorrhagia N36.8
Urethrorrhea R36.9
Urethrostomy
    attention to Z43.6
    status Z93.6
Urethrotrigonitis — *see* Trigonitis
Urethrovaginal — *see* condition
Urgency
    fecal R15.2
    hypertensive — *see* Hypertension
    urinary N39.41
Urhidrosis, uridrosis L74.8
Uric acid in blood (increased) E79.0
Uricacidemia (asymptomatic) E79.0
Uricemia (asymptomatic) E79.0
Uricosuria R82.99
Urinary — *see* condition
Urination
    frequent R35.0
    painful R30.9
Urine
    blood in — *see* Hematuria
    discharge, excessive R35.8
    enuresis, nonorganic origin F98.0
    extravasation R39.0
    frequency R35.0
    incontinence R32
        nonorganic origin F98.0
    intermittent stream R39.19
    pus in N39.0
    retention or stasis R33.9
        organic R33.8
            drug-induced R33.0
        psychogenic F45.8
    secretion
        deficient R34
        excessive R35.8
        frequency R35.0
    stream
        intermittent R39.19
        slowing R39.19
        splitting R39.13
        weak R39.12
Urinemia — *see* Uremia
Urinoma, urethra N36.8
Uroarthritis, infectious (Reiter's) — *see* Reiter's disease
Urodialysis R34
Urolithiasis — *see* Calculus, urinary
Uronephrosis — *see* Hydronephrosis
Uropathy N39.9
    obstructive N13.9
        specified NEC N13.8
    reflux N13.9
        specified NEC N13.8
    vesicoureteral reflux-associated — *see* Reflux, vesi-
        coureteral
Urosepsis — *code to* condition
Urticaria L50.9
    with angioneurotic edema T78.3 ☑
        hereditary D84.1
    allergic L50.0
    cholinergic L50.5
    chronic L50.8
    cold, familial L50.2
    contact L50.6
    dermatographic L50.3
    due to
        cold or heat L50.2
        drugs L50.0
        food L50.0
        inhalants L50.0
        plants L50.6
        serum (*see also* Reaction, serum) T80.69 ☑

Urticaria — continued
  factitial L50.3
  giant T78.3 ☑
    hereditary D84.1
  gigantea T78.3 ☑
  idiopathic L50.1
  larynx T78.3 ☑
    hereditary D84.1
  neonatorum P83.8
  nonallergic L50.1
  papulosa (Hebra) L28.2
  pigmentosa Q82.2
  recurrent periodic L50.8
  serum (see also Reaction, serum) T80.69 ☑
  solar L56.3
  specified type NEC L50.8
  thermal (cold) (heat) L50.2
  vibratory L50.4
  xanthelasmoidea Q82.2
Use (of)
  alcohol F10.99
    with sleep disorder F10.982
    harmful — see Abuse, alcohol
  amphetamines — see Use, stimulant NEC
  caffeine — see Use, stimulant NEC
  cannabis F12.90
    with
      anxiety disorder F12.980
      intoxication F12.929
        with
          delirium F12.921
          perceptual disturbance F12.922
        uncomplicated F12.920
      other specified disorder F12.988
      psychosis F12.959
        delusions F12.950
        hallucinations F12.951
      unspecified disorder F12.99
  cocaine F14.90
    with
      anxiety disorder F14.980
      intoxication F14.929
        with
          delirium F14.921
          perceptual disturbance F14.922
        uncomplicated F14.920
      other specified disorder F14.988
      psychosis F14.959
        delusions F14.950
        hallucinations F14.951
      sexual dysfunction F14.981
      sleep disorder F14.982
      unspecified disorder F14.99
    harmful — see Abuse, drug, cocaine
  drug(s) NEC F19.90
    with sleep disorder F19.982
    harmful — see Abuse, drug, by type
  hallucinogen NEC F16.90
    with
      anxiety disorder F16.980
      intoxication F16.929
        with
          delirium F16.921
        uncomplicated F16.920
      mood disorder F16.94
      other specified disorder F16.988
      perception disorder (flashbacks) F16.983
      psychosis F16.959
        delusions F16.950
        hallucinations F16.951
      unspecified disorder F16.99
    harmful — see Abuse, drug, hallucinogen NEC
  inhalants F18.90
    with
      anxiety disorder F18.980
      intoxication F18.929
        with delirium F18.921
        uncomplicated F18.920
      mood disorder F18.94
      other specified disorder F18.988
      persisting dementia F18.97
      psychosis F18.959
        delusions F18.950
        hallucinations F18.951
      unspecified disorder F18.99
    harmful — see Abuse, drug, inhalant
  methadone F11.20
  nonprescribed drugs F19.90

Use — continued
  nonprescribed drugs — continued
    harmful — see Abuse, non-psychoactive substance
  opioid F11.90
    with
      disorder F11.99
        mood F11.94
        sleep F11.982
        specified type NEC F11.988
      intoxication F11.929
        with
          delirium F11.921
          perceptual disturbance F11.922
        uncomplicated F11.920
      withdrawal F11.93
    harmful — see Abuse, drug, opioid
  patent medicines F19.90
    harmful — see Abuse, non-psychoactive substance
  psychoactive drug NEC F19.90
    with
      anxiety disorder F19.980
      intoxication F19.929
        with
          delirium F19.921
          perceptual disturbance F19.922
        uncomplicated F19.920
      mood disorder F19.94
      other specified disorder F19.988
      persisting
        amnestic disorder F19.96
        dementia F19.97
      psychosis F19.959
        delusions F19.950
        hallucinations F19.951
      sexual dysfunction F19.981
      sleep disorder F19.982
      unspecified disorder F19.99
      withdrawal F19.939
        with
          delirium F19.931
          perceptual disturbance F19.932
        uncomplicated F19.930
    harmful — see Abuse, drug NEC, psychoactive NEC
  sedative, hypnotic, or anxiolytic F13.90
    with
      anxiety disorder F13.980
      intoxication F13.929
        with
          delirium F13.921
        uncomplicated F13.920
      other specified disorder F13.988
      persisting
        amnestic disorder F13.96
        dementia F13.97
      psychosis F13.959
        delusions F13.950
        hallucinations F13.951
      sexual dysfunction F13.981
      sleep disorder F13.982
      unspecified disorder F13.99
    harmful — see Abuse, drug, sedative, hypnotic, or anxiolytic
  stimulant NEC F15.90
    with
      anxiety disorder F15.980
      intoxication F15.929
        with
          delirium F15.921
          perceptual disturbance F15.922
        uncomplicated F15.920
      mood disorder F15.94
      other specified disorder F15.988
      psychosis F15.959
        delusions F15.950
        hallucinations F15.951
      sexual dysfunction F15.981
      sleep disorder F15.982
      unspecified disorder F15.99
      withdrawal F15.93
    harmful — see Abuse, drug, stimulant NEC
  tobacco Z72.0
    with dependence — see Dependence, drug, nicotine
  volatile solvents (see also Use, inhalant) F18.90
    harmful — see Abuse, drug, inhalant
Usher-Senear disease or syndrome L10.4
Uta B55.1
Uteromegaly N85.2

Uterovaginal — see condition
Uterovesical — see condition
Uveal — see condition
Uveitis (anterior) (see also Iridocyclitis)
  acute — see Iridocyclitis, acute
  chronic — see Iridocyclitis, chronic
  due to toxoplasmosis (acquired) B58.09
    congenital P37.1
  granulomatous — see Iridocyclitis, chronic
  heterochromic — see Cyclitis, Fuchs' heterochromic
  lens-induced — see Iridocyclitis, lens-induced
  posterior — see Chorioretinitis
  sympathetic H44.13- ☑
  syphilitic (secondary) A51.43
    congenital (early) A50.01
    late A52.71
  tuberculous A18.54
Uveoencephalitis — see Inflammation, chorioretinal
Uveokeratitis — see Iridocyclitis
Uveoparotitis D86.89
Uvula — see condition
Uvulitis (acute) (catarrhal) (chronic) (membranous)
    (suppurative) (ulcerative) K12.2

V

Vaccination (prophylactic)
  complication or reaction — see Complications, vaccination
  delayed Z28.9
  encounter for Z23
  not done — see Immunization, not done, because (of)
Vaccinia (generalized) (localized) T88.1 ☑
  without vaccination B08.011
  congenital P35.8
Vacuum, in sinus (accessory) (nasal) J34.89
Vagabond, vagabondage Z59.0
Vagabond's disease B85.1
Vagina, vaginal — see condition
Vaginalitis (tunica) (testis) N49.1
Vaginismus (reflex) N94.2
  functional F52.5
  nonorganic F52.5
  psychogenic F52.5
  secondary N94.2
Vaginitis (acute) (circumscribed) (diffuse) (emphysematous) (nonvenereal) (ulcerative) N76.0
  with ectopic or molar pregnancy O08.0
  ambic A06.82
  atrophic, postmenopausal N95.2
  bacterial N76.0
  blennorrhagic (gonococcal) A54.02
  candidal B37.3
  chlamydial A56.02
  chronic N76.1
  due to Trichomonas (vaginalis) A59.01
  following ectopic or molar pregnancy O08.0
  gonococcal A54.02
    with abscess (accessory gland) (periurethral) A54.1
  granuloma A58
  in (due to)
    candidiasis B37.3
    herpesviral (herpes simplex) infection A60.04
    pinworm infection B80 [N77.1]
  monilial B37.3
  mycotic (candidal) B37.3
  postmenopausal atrophic N95.2
  puerperal (postpartum) O86.13
  senile (atrophic) N95.2
  subacute or chronic N76.1
  syphilitic (early) A51.0
    late A52.76
  trichomonal A59.01
  tuberculous A18.18
Vaginosis — see Vaginitis
Vagotonia G52.2
Vagrancy Z59.0
VAIN — see Neoplasia, intraepithelial, vagina
Vallecula — see condition
Valley fever B38.0
Valsuani's disease — see Anemia, obstetric
Valve, valvular (formation) (see also condition)
  cerebral ventricle (communicating) in situ Z98.2
  cervix, internal os Q51.828
  congenital NEC — see Atresia, by site
  ureter (pelvic junction) (vesical orifice) Q62.39
  urethra (congenital) (posterior) Q64.2

Valvulitis (chronic) — *see* Endocarditis
Valvulopathy — *see* Endocarditis
Van Bogaert-Scherer-Epstein disease or syndrome E75.5
Van Bogaert's leukoencephalopathy (sclerosing) (subacute) A81.1
Van Buchem's syndrome M85.2
Van Creveld-von Gierke disease E74.01
Van der Hoeve (-de Kleyn) **syndrome** Q78.0
Van der Woude's syndrome Q38.0
Van Neck's disease or osteochondrosis M91.0
Vanishing lung J44.9
Vapor asphyxia or suffocation T59.9 ☑
  specified agent — *see* Table of Drugs and Chemicals
Variance, lethal ball, prosthetic heart valve T82.09 ☑
Variants, thalassemic D56.8
Variations in hair color L67.1
Varicella B01.9
  with
    complications NEC B01.89
    encephalitis B01.11
    encephalomyelitis B01.11
    meningitis B01.0
    myelitis B01.12
    pneumonia B01.2
  congenital P35.8
Varices — *see* Varix
Varicocele (scrotum) (thrombosed) I86.1
  ovary I86.2
  perineum I86.3
  spermatic cord (ulcerated) I86.1
Varicose
  aneurysm (ruptured) I77.0
  dermatitis — *see* Varix, leg, with, inflammation
  eczema — *see* Varix, leg, with, inflammation
  phlebitis — *see* Varix, with, inflammation
  tumor — *see* Varix
  ulcer (lower limb, any part) (*see also* Varix, leg, with, ulcer)
    anus (*see also* Hemorrhoids) K64.8
    esophagus — *see* Varix, esophagus
    inflamed or infected — *see* Varix, leg, with ulcer, with inflammation
    nasal septum I86.8
    perineum I86.3
    scrotum I86.1
    specified site NEC I86.8
  vein — *see* Varix
  vessel — *see* Varix, leg
Varicosis, varicosities, varicosity — *see* Varix
Variola (major) (minor) B03
Varioloid B03
Varix (lower limb) (ruptured) I83.90
  with
    edema I83.899
    inflammation I83.10
      with ulcer (venous) I83.209
    pain I83.819
    specified complication NEC I83.899
    stasis dermatitis I83.10
      with ulcer (venous) I83.209
    swelling I83.899
    ulcer I83.009
      with inflammation I83.209
  aneurysmal I77.0
  asymptomatic I83.9- ☑
  bladder I86.2
  broad ligament I86.2
  complicating
    childbirth (lower extremity) O87.4
      anus or rectum O87.2
      genital (vagina, vulva or perineum) O87.8
    pregnancy (lower extremity) O22.0- ☑
      anus or rectum O22.4- ☑
      genital (vagina, vulva or perineum) O22.1- ☑
    puerperium (lower extremity) O87.4
      anus or rectum O87.2
      genital (vagina, vulva, perineum) O87.8
  congenital (any site) Q27.8
  esophagus (idiopathic) (primary) (ulcerated) I85.00
    bleeding I85.01
    congenital Q27.8
    in (due to)
      alcoholic liver disease I85.10
        bleeding I85.11
      cirrhosis of liver I85.10
        bleeding I85.11

Varix — *continued*
  esophagus — *continued*
    in — *continued*
      portal hypertension I85.10
        bleeding I85.11
      schistosomiasis I85.10
        bleeding I85.11
      toxic liver disease I85.10
        bleeding I85.11
    secondary I85.10
      bleeding I85.11
  gastric I86.4
  inflamed or infected I83.10
    ulcerated I83.209
  labia (majora) I86.3
  leg (asymptomatic) I83.90
    with
      edema I83.899
      inflammation I83.10
        with ulcer — *see* Varix, leg, with, ulcer, with inflammation by site
      pain I83.819
      specified complication NEC I83.899
      swelling I83.899
      ulcer I83.009
        with inflammation I83.209
        ankle I83.003
          with inflammation I83.203
        calf I83.002
          with inflammation I83.202
        foot NEC I83.005
          with inflammation I83.205
        heel I83.004
          with inflammation I83.204
        lower leg NEC I83.008
          with inflammation I83.208
        midfoot I83.004
          with inflammation I83.204
        thigh I83.001
          with inflammation I83.201
    bilateral (asymptomatic) I83.93
      with
        edema I83.893
        pain I83.813
        specified complication NEC I83.893
        swelling I83.893
        ulcer I83.009
          with inflammation I83.209
    left (asymptomatic) I83.92
      with
        edema I83.892
        inflammation I83.12
          with ulcer — *see* Varix, leg, with, ulcer, with inflammation by site
        pain I83.812
        specified complication NEC I83.892
        swelling I83.892
        ulcer I83.029
          with inflammation I83.229
          ankle I83.023
            with inflammation I83.223
          calf I83.022
            with inflammation I83.222
          foot NEC I83.025
            with inflammation I83.225
          heel I83.024
            with inflammation I83.224
          lower leg NEC I83.028
            with inflammation I83.228
          midfoot I83.024
            with inflammation I83.224
          thigh I83.021
            with inflammation I83.221
    right (asymptomatic) I83.91
      with
        edema I83.891
        inflammation I83.11
          with ulcer — *see* Varix, leg, with, ulcer, with inflammation by site
        pain I83.811
        specified complication NEC I83.891
        swelling I83.891
        ulcer I83.019
          with inflammation I83.219
          ankle I83.013
            with inflammation I83.213
          calf I83.012
            with inflammation I83.212

Varix — *continued*
  leg — *continued*
    right — *continued*
      with — *continued*
        ulcer — *continued*
          foot NEC I83.015
            with inflammation I83.215
          heel I83.014
            with inflammation I83.214
          lower leg NEC I83.018
            with inflammation I83.218
          midfoot I83.014
            with inflammation I83.214
          thigh I83.011
            with inflammation I83.211
  nasal septum I86.8
  orbit I86.8
    congenital Q27.8
  ovary I86.2
  papillary I78.1
  pelvis I86.2
  perineum I86.3
  pharynx I86.8
  placenta O43.89- ☑
  renal papilla I86.8
  retina H35.09
  scrotum (ulcerated) I86.1
  sigmoid colon I86.8
  specified site NEC I86.8
  spinal (cord) (vessels) I86.8
  spleen, splenic (vein) (with phlebolith) I86.8
  stomach I86.4
  sublingual I86.0
  ulcerated I83.009
    inflamed or infected I83.209
  uterine ligament I86.2
  vagina I86.8
  vocal cord I86.8
  vulva I86.3
Vas deferens — *see* condition
Vas deferentitis N49.1
Vasa previa O69.4 ☑
  hemorrhage from, affecting newborn P50.0
Vascular (*see also* condition)
  loop on optic papilla Q14.2
  spasm I73.9
  spider I78.1
Vascularization, cornea — *see* Neovascularization, cornea
Vasculitis I77.6
  allergic D69.0
  cryoglobulinemic D89.1
  disseminated I77.6
  hypocomplementemic M31.8
  kidney I77.89
  livedoid L95.0
  nodular L95.8
  retina H35.06- ☑
  rheumatic — *see* Fever, rheumatic
  rheumatoid — *see* Rheumatoid, vasculitis
  skin (limited to) L95.9
    specified NEC L95.8
Vasculopathy, necrotizing M31.9
  cardiac allograft T86.290
  specified NEC M31.8
Vasitis (nodosa) N49.1
  tuberculous A18.15
Vasodilation I73.9
Vasomotor — *see* condition
Vasoplasty, after previous sterilization Z31.0
  aftercare Z31.42
Vasospasm (vasoconstriction) I73.9
  cerebral (cerebrovascular) (artery) I67.848
    reversible I67.841
  coronary I20.1
  nerve
    arm — *see* Mononeuropathy, upper limb
    brachial plexus G54.0
    cervical plexus G54.2
    leg — *see* Mononeuropathy, lower limb
  peripheral NOS I73.9
  retina (artery) — *see* Occlusion, artery, retina
Vasospastic — *see* condition
Vasovagal attack (paroxysmal) R55
  psychogenic F45.8
VATER syndrome Q87.2
Vater's ampulla — *see* condition

Vegetation, vegetative
- adenoid (nasal fossa) J35.8
- endocarditis (acute) (any valve) (subacute) I33.0
- heart (mycotic) (valve) I33.0

Veil
- Jackson's Q43.3

Vein, venous — *see* condition
Veldt sore — *see* Ulcer, skin
Velpeau's hernia — *see* Hernia, femoral
Venereal
- bubo A55
- disease A64
- granuloma inguinale A58
- lymphogranuloma (Durand-Nicolas-Favre) A55

Venofibrosis I87.8
Venom, venomous — *see* Table of Drugs and Chemicals, by animal or substance, poisoning
Venous — *see* condition
Ventilator lung, newborn P27.8
Ventral — *see* condition
Ventricle, ventricular (*see also* condition)
- escape I49.3
- inversion Q20.5

Ventriculitis (cerebral) (*see also* Encephalitis) G04.90
Ventriculostomy status Z98.2
Vernet's syndrome G52.7
Verneuil's disease (syphilitic bursitis) A52.78
Verruca (due to HPV) (filiformis) (simplex) (viral) (vulgaris) B07.9
- acuminata A63.0
- necrogenica (primary) (tuberculosa) A18.4
- plana B07.8
- plantaris B07.0
- seborrheica L82.1
  - inflamed L82.0
- senile (seborrheic) L82.1
  - inflamed L82.0
- tuberculosa (primary) A18.4
- venereal A63.0

Verrucosities — *see* Verruca
Verruga peruana, peruviana A44.1
Version
- with extraction
- cervix — *see* Malposition, uterus
- uterus (postinfectional) (postpartal, old) — *see* Malposition, uterus

Vertebra, vertebral — *see* condition
Vertical talus (congenital) Q66.80
- left foot Q66.82
- right foot Q66.81

Vertigo R42
- auditory — *see* Vertigo, aural
- aural H81.31- ☑
- benign paroxysmal (positional) H81.1- ☑
- central (origin) H81.4- ☑
- cerebral H81.4- ☑
- Dix and Hallpike (epidemic) — *see* Neuronitis, vestibular
- due to infrasound T75.23 ☑
- epidemic A88.1
  - Dix and Hallpike — *see* Neuronitis, vestibular
  - Pedersen's — *see* Neuronitis, vestibular
  - vestibular neuronitis — *see* Neuronitis, vestibular
- hysterical F44.89
- infrasound T75.23 ☑
- labyrinthine — *see* subcategory H81.0 ☑
- laryngeal R05
- malignant positional H81.4- ☑
- Ménière's — *see* subcategory H81.0 ☑
- menopausal N95.1
- otogenic — *see* Vertigo, aural
- paroxysmal positional, benign — *see* Vertigo, benign paroxysmal
- Pedersen's (epidemic) — *see* Neuronitis, vestibular
- peripheral NEC H81.39- ☑
- positional
  - benign paroxysmal — *see* Vertigo, benign paroxysmal
  - malignant H81.4- ☑

Very-low-density-lipoprotein-type (VLDL) **hyperlipoproteinemia** E78.1
Vesania — *see* Psychosis
Vesical — *see* condition
Vesicle
- cutaneous R23.8
- seminal — *see* condition
- skin R23.8

Vesicocolic — *see* condition
Vesicoperineal — *see* condition
Vesicorectal — *see* condition
Vesicourethrorectal — *see* condition
Vesicovaginal — *see* condition
Vesicular — *see* condition
Vesiculitis (seminal) N49.0
- amebic A06.82
- gonorrheal (acute) (chronic) A54.23
- trichomonal A59.09
- tuberculous A18.15

Vestibulitis (ear) (*see also* subcategory) H83.0 ☑
- nose (external) J34.89
- vulvar N94.810

Vestibulopathy , acute peripheral (recurrent) — *see* Neuronitis, vestibular
Vestige, vestigial (*see also* Persistence)
- branchial Q18.0
- structures in vitreous Q14.0

Vibration
- adverse effects T75.20 ☑
  - pneumatic hammer syndrome T75.21 ☑
  - specified effect NEC T75.29 ☑
  - vasospastic syndrome T75.22 ☑
  - vertigo from infrasound T75.23 ☑
- exposure (occupational) Z57.7
- vertigo T75.23 ☑

Vibriosis A28.9
Victim (of)
- crime Z65.4
- disaster Z65.5
- terrorism Z65.4
- torture Z65.4
- war Z65.5

Vidal's disease L28.0
Villaret's syndrome G52.7
Villous — *see* condition
VIN — *see* Neoplasia, intraepithelial, vulva
Vincent's infection (angina) (gingivitis) A69.1
- stomatitis NEC A69.1

Vinson-Plummer syndrome D50.1
Violence, physical R45.6
Viosterol deficiency — *see* Deficiency, calciferol
Vipoma — *see* Neoplasm, malignant, by site
Viremia B34.9
Virilism (adrenal) E25.9
- congenital E25.0

Virilization (female) (suprarenal) E25.9
- congenital E25.0
- isosexual E28.2

Virulent bubo A57
Virus, viral (*see also* condition)
- as cause of disease classified elsewhere B97.89
- cytomegalovirus B25.9
- human immunodeficiency (HIV) — *see* Human, immunodeficiency virus (HIV) disease
- infection — *see* Infection, virus
- specified NEC B34.8
- swine influenza (viruses that normally cause infections in pigs) (*see also* Influenza, due to, identified novel influenza A virus) J09.X2
- West Nile (fever) A92.30
  - with
    - complications NEC A92.39
    - cranial nerve disorders A92.32
    - encephalitis A92.31
    - encephalomyelitis A92.31
    - neurologic manifestation NEC A92.32
    - optic neuritis A92.32
    - polyradiculitis A92.32

Viscera, visceral — *see* condition
Visceroptosis K63.4
Visible peristalsis R19.2
Vision, visual
- binocular, suppression H53.34
- blurred, blurring H53.8
  - hysterical F44.6
- defect, defective NEC H54.7
- disorientation (syndrome) H53.8
- disturbance H53.9
  - hysterical F44.6
- double H53.2
- examination Z01.00
  - with abnormal findings Z01.01
- field, limitation (defect) — *see* Defect, visual field
- hallucinations R44.1
- halos H53.19

Vision, visual — *continued*
- loss — *see* Loss, vision
  - sudden — *see* Disturbance, vision, subjective, loss, sudden
- low (both eyes) — *see* Low, vision
- perception, simultaneous without fusion H53.33

Vitality, lack or want of R53.83
- newborn P96.89

Vitamin deficiency — *see* Deficiency, vitamin
Vitelline duct, persistent Q43.0
Vitiligo L80
- eyelid H02.739
  - left H02.736
    - lower H02.735
    - upper H02.734
  - right H02.733
    - lower H02.732
    - upper H02.731
- pinta A67.2
- vulva N90.89

Vitreal corneal syndrome H59.01- ☑
Vitreoretinopathy, proliferative (*see also* Retinopathy, proliferative)
- with retinal detachment — *see* Detachment, retina, traction

Vitreous (*see also* condition)
- touch syndrome — *see* Complication, postprocedural, following cataract surgery

Vocal cord — *see* condition
Vogt-Koyanagi syndrome H20.82- ☑
Vogt-Spielmeyer amaurotic idiocy or disease E75.4
Vogt's disease or syndrome G80.3
Voice
- change R49.9
  - specified NEC R49.8
- loss — *see* Aphonia

Volhynian fever A79.0
Volkmann's ischemic contracture or paralysis (complicating trauma) T79.6 ☑
Volvulus (bowel) (colon) (duodenum) (intestine) K56.2
- with perforation K56.2
- congenital Q43.8
- fallopian tube — *see* Torsion, fallopian tube
- oviduct — *see* Torsion, fallopian tube
- stomach (due to absence of gastrocolic ligament) K31.89

Vomiting R11.10
- with nausea R11.2
- without nausea R11.11
- asphyxia — *see* Foreign body, by site, causing asphyxia, gastric contents
- bilious (cause unknown) R11.14
  - following gastro-intestinal surgery K91.0
  - in newborn P92.01
- blood — *see* Hematemesis
- causing asphyxia, choking, or suffocation — *see* Foreign body, by site
- cyclical G43.A0 (*following* G43.7)
  - with refractory migraine G43.A1 (*following* G43.7)
  - without refractory migraine G43.A0 (*following* G43.7)
  - intractable G43.A1 (*following* G43.7)
  - not intractable G43.A0 (*following* G43.7)
  - psychogenic F50.8
- fecal mater R11.13
- following gastrointestinal surgery K91.0
  - psychogenic F50.8
- functional K31.89
- hysterical F50.8
- nervous F50.8
- neurotic F50.8
- newborn NEC P92.09
  - bilious P92.01
- periodic R11.10
  - psychogenic F50.8
- projectile R11.12
- psychogenic F50.8
- uremic — *see* Uremia

Vomito negro — *see* Fever, yellow
Von Bezold's abscess — *see* Mastoiditis, acute
Von Economo-Cruchet disease A85.8
Von Eulenburg's disease G71.19
Von Gierke's disease E74.01
Von Hippel (-Lindau) **disease or syndrome** Q85.8
Von Jaksch's anemia or disease D64.89
Von Recklinghausen
- disease (neurofibromatosis) Q85.01

Von Recklinghausen — *continued*
  disease — *continued*
    bones E21.0
Von Schroetter's syndrome I82.890
Von Willebrand (-Jurgens)(-Minot) **disease or syndrome** D68.0
Von Zumbusch's disease L40.1
Voyeurism F65.3
Vrolik's disease Q78.0
Vulva — *see* condition
Vulvismus N94.2
Vulvitis (acute) (allergic) (atrophic) (hypertrophic) (intertriginous) (senile) N76.2
  with ectopic or molar pregnancy O08.0
  adhesive, congenital Q52.79
  blennorrhagic (gonococcal) A54.02
  candidal B37.3
  chlamydial A56.02
  due to Haemophilus ducreyi A57
  following ectopic or molar pregnancy O08.0
  gonococcal A54.02
    with abscess (accessory gland) (periurethral) A54.1
  herpesviral A60.04
  leukoplakic N90.4
  monilial B37.3
  puerperal (postpartum) O86.19
  subacute or chronic N76.3
  syphilitic (early) A51.0
    late A52.76
  trichomonal A59.01
  tuberculous A18.18
Vulvodynia N94.819
  specified NEC N94.818
Vulvorectal — *see* condition
Vulvovaginitis (acute) — *see* Vaginitis

W

Waiting list, person on Z75.1
  for organ transplant Z76.82
  undergoing social agency investigation Z75.2
Waldenström
  hypergammaglobulinemia D89.0
  syndrome or macroglobulinemia C88.0
Waldenström-Kjellberg syndrome D50.1
Walking
  difficulty R26.2
    psychogenic F44.4
  sleep F51.3
    hysterical F44.89
Wall, abdominal — *see* condition
Wallenberg's disease or syndrome G46.3
Wallgren's disease I87.8
Wandering
  gallbladder, congenital Q44.1
  in diseases classified elsewhere Z91.83
  kidney, congenital Q63.8
  organ or site, congenital NEC — *see* Malposition, congenital, by site
  pacemaker (heart) I49.8
  spleen D73.89
War neurosis F48.8
Wart (due to HPV) (filiform) (infectious) (viral) B07.9
  anogenital region (venereal) A63.0
  common B07.8
  external genital organs (venereal) A63.0
  flat B07.8
  Hassal-Henle's (of cornea) H18.49
  Peruvian A44.1
  plantar B07.0
  prosector (tuberculous) A18.4
  seborrheic L82.1
    inflamed L82.0
  senile (seborrheic) L82.1
    inflamed L82.0
  tuberculous A18.4
  venereal A63.0
Warthin's tumor — *see* Neoplasm, salivary gland, benign
Wassilieff's disease A27.0
Wasting
  disease R64
    due to malnutrition E41
  extreme (due to malnutrition) E41
  muscle NEC — *see* Atrophy, muscle
Water
  clefts (senile cataract) — *see* Cataract, senile, incipient
  deprivation of T73.1 ☑

Water — *continued*
  intoxication E87.79
  itch B76.9
  lack of T73.1 ☑
  loading E87.70
  on
    brain — *see* Hydrocephalus
    chest J94.8
  poisoning E87.79
Water-losing nephritis N25.89
Waterbrash R12
Waterhouse (-Friderichsen) **syndrome or disease** (meningococcal) A39.1
Watermelon stomach K31.819
  with hemorrhage K31.811
  without hemorrhage K31.819
Watsoniasis B66.8
Wax in ear — *see* Impaction, cerumen
Weak, weakening, weakness (generalized) R53.1
  arches (acquired) (*see also* Deformity, limb, flat foot)
  bladder (sphincter) R32
  facial R29.810
    following
      cerebrovascular disease I69.992
        cerebral infarction I69.392
        intracerebral hemorrhage I69.192
        nontraumatic intracranial hemorrhage NEC I69.292
        specified disease NEC I69.892
        stroke I69.392
        subarachnoid hemorrhage I69.092
  foot (double) — *see* Weak, arches
  heart, cardiac — *see* Failure, heart
  mind F70
  muscle M62.81
  myocardium — *see* Failure, heart
  newborn P96.89
  pelvic fundus N81.89
  pubocervical tissue N81.82
  rectovaginal tissue N81.83
  senile R54
  urinary stream R39.12
  valvular — *see* Endocarditis
Wear, worn (with normal or routine use)
  articular bearing surface of internal joint prosthesis — *see* Complications, joint prosthesis, mechanical, wear of articular bearing surfaces, by site
  device, implant or graft — *see* Complications, by site, mechanical complication
  tooth, teeth (approximal) (hard tissues) (interproximal) (occlusal) K03.0
Weather, weathered
  effects of
    cold T69.9 ☑
      specified effect NEC T69.8 ☑
    hot — *see* Heat
  skin L57.8
Weaver's syndrome Q87.3
Web, webbed (congenital)
  duodenal Q43.8
  esophagus Q39.4
  fingers Q70.1- ☑
  larynx (glottic) (subglottic) Q31.0
  neck (pterygium colli) Q18.3
  Paterson-Kelly D50.1
  popliteal syndrome Q87.89
  toes Q70.3- ☑
Weber-Christian disease M35.6
Weber-Cockayne syndrome (epidermolysis bullosa) Q81.8
Weber-Gubler syndrome G46.3
Weber-Leyden syndrome G46.3
Weber-Osler syndrome I78.0
Weber's paralysis or syndrome G46.3
Wedge-shaped or wedging vertebra — *see* Collapse, vertebra NEC
Wegener's granulomatosis or syndrome M31.30
  with
    kidney involvement M31.31
    lung involvement M31.30
      with kidney involvement M31.31
Wegner's disease A50.02
Weight
  1000-2499 grams at birth (low) — *see* Low, birthweight
  999 grams or less at birth (extremely low) — *see* Low, birthweight, extreme

Weight — *continued*
  gain (abnormal) (excessive) R63.5
    in pregnancy — *see* Pregnancy, complicated by, excessive weight gain
    low — *see* Pregnancy, complicated by, insufficient, weight gain
  loss (abnormal) (cause unknown) R63.4
Weightlessness (effect of) T75.82 ☑
Weil (l)-**Marchesani syndrome** Q87.1
Weil's disease A27.0
Weingarten's syndrome J82
Weir Mitchell's disease I73.81
Weiss-Baker syndrome G90.09
Wells' disease L98.3
Wen — *see* Cyst, sebaceous
Wenckebach's block or phenomenon I44.1
Werdnig-Hoffmann syndrome (muscular atrophy) G12.0
Werlhof's disease D69.3
Wermer's disease or syndrome E31.21
Werner-His disease A79.0
Werner's disease or syndrome E34.8
Wernicke-Korsakoff's syndrome or psychosis (alcoholic) F10.96
  with dependence F10.26
  drug-induced
    due to drug abuse — *see* Abuse, drug, by type, with amnestic disorder
    due to drug dependence — *see* Dependence, drug, by type, with amnestic disorder
  nonalcoholic F04
Wernicke-Posadas disease B38.9
Wernicke's
  developmental aphasia F80.2
  disease or syndrome E51.2
  encephalopathy E51.2
  polioencephalitis, superior E51.2
West African fever B50.8
Westphal-Strümpell syndrome E83.01
West's syndrome — *see* Epilepsy, spasms
Wet
  feet, tropical (maceration) (syndrome) — *see* Immersion, foot
  lung (syndrome), newborn P22.1
Wharton's duct — *see* condition
Wheal — *see* Urticaria
Wheezing R06.2
Whiplash injury S13.4 ☑
Whipple's disease (*see also* subcategory M14.8-) K90.81
Whipworm (disease) (infection) (infestation) B79
Whistling face Q87.0
White (*see also* condition)
  kidney, small N03.9
  leg, puerperal, postpartum, childbirth O87.1
  mouth B37.0
  patches of mouth K13.29
  spot lesions, teeth
    chewing surface K02.51
    pit and fissure surface K02.51
    smooth surface K02.61
Whitehead L70.0
Whitlow (*see also* Cellulitis, digit)
  with lymphangitis — *see* Lymphangitis, acute, digit
  herpesviral B00.89
Whitmore's disease or fever — *see* Melioidosis
Whooping cough A37.90
  with pneumonia A37.91
    due to Bordetella
      bronchiseptica A37.81
      parapertussis A37.11
      pertussis A37.01
    specified organism NEC A37.81
  due to
    Bordetella
      bronchiseptica A37.80
        with pneumonia A37.81
      parapertussis A37.10
        with pneumonia A37.11
      pertussis A37.00
        with pneumonia A37.01
      specified NEC A37.80
        with pneumonia A37.81
Wichman's asthma J38.5
Wide cranial sutures, newborn P96.3
Widening aorta — *see* Ectasia, aorta
  with aneurysm — *see* Aneurysm, aorta
Wilkie's disease or syndrome K55.1

Index

Wound, open — Wound, open

Wound, open — *continued*
  finger(s) — *continued*
    ring — *continued*
      left — *continued*
        with damage to nail S61.305 ☑
      right S61.204 ☑
        with damage to nail S61.304 ☑
  flank — *see* Wound, open, abdomen, wall
  foot (except toe(s) alone) S91.30- ☑
    with amputation — *see* Amputation, traumatic, foot
    bite — *see* Bite, foot
    laceration — *see* Laceration, foot
    puncture — *see* Puncture, foot
    toe — *see* Wound, open, toe
  forearm S51.80- ☑
    with
      amputation — *see* Amputation, traumatic, forearm
    bite — *see* Bite, forearm
    elbow only — *see* Wound, open, elbow
    laceration — *see* Laceration, forearm
    puncture — *see* Puncture, forearm
  forehead — *see* Wound, open, head, specified site NEC
  genital organs, external
    with amputation — *see* Amputation, traumatic, genital organs
    bite — *see* Bite, genital organ
    female S31.502 ☑
      vagina S31.40 ☑
      vulva S31.40 ☑
    laceration — *see* Laceration, genital organ
    male S31.501 ☑
      penis S31.20 ☑
      scrotum S31.30 ☑
      testes S31.30 ☑
    puncture — *see* Puncture, genital organ
  globe (eye) — *see* Wound, open, ocular
  groin — *see* Wound, open, abdomen, wall
  gum — *see* Wound, open, oral cavity
  hand S61.40- ☑
    with
      amputation — *see* Amputation, traumatic, hand
    bite — *see* Bite, hand
    finger(s) — *see* Wound, open, finger
    laceration — *see* Laceration, hand
    puncture — *see* Puncture, hand
    thumb — *see* Wound, open, thumb
  head S01.90 ☑
    bite — *see* Bite, head
    cheek — *see* Wound, open, cheek
    ear — *see* Wound, open, ear
    eyelid — *see* Wound, open, eyelid
    laceration — *see* Laceration, head
    lip — *see* Wound, open, lip
    nose S01.20 ☑
    oral cavity — *see* Wound, open, oral cavity
    puncture — *see* Puncture, head
    scalp — *see* Wound, open, scalp
    specified site NEC S01.80 ☑
    temporomandibular area — *see* Wound, open, cheek
  heel — *see* Wound, open, foot
  hip S71.00- ☑
    with amputation — *see* Amputation, traumatic, hip
    bite — *see* Bite, hip
    laceration — *see* Laceration, hip
    puncture — *see* Puncture, hip
  hymen S31.40 ☑
    bite — *see* Bite, vulva
    laceration — *see* Laceration, vagina
    puncture — *see* Puncture, vagina
  hypochondrium S31.109 ☑
    bite — *see* Bite, hypochondrium
    laceration — *see* Laceration, hypochondrium
    puncture — *see* Puncture, hypochondrium
  hypogastric region S31.109 ☑
    bite — *see* Bite, hypogastric region
    laceration — *see* Laceration, hypogastric region
    puncture — *see* Puncture, hypogastric region
  iliac (region) — *see* Wound, open, inguinal region
  inguinal region S31.109 ☑
    bite — *see* Bite, abdomen, wall, lower quadrant
    laceration — *see* Laceration, inguinal region

Wound, open — *continued*
  inguinal region — *continued*
    puncture — *see* Puncture, inguinal region
  instep — *see* Wound, open, foot
  interscapular region — *see* Wound, open, thorax, back
  intraocular — *see* Wound, open, ocular
  iris — *see* Wound, open, ocular
  jaw — *see* Wound, open, head, specified site NEC
  knee S81.00- ☑
    bite — *see* Bite, knee
    laceration — *see* Laceration, knee
    puncture — *see* Puncture, knee
  labium (majus) (minus) — *see* Wound, open, vulva
  laceration — *see* Laceration, by site
  lacrimal duct — *see* Wound, open, eyelid
  larynx S11.019 ☑
    bite — *see* Bite, larynx
    laceration — *see* Laceration, larynx
    puncture — *see* Puncture, larynx
  left
    lower quadrant S31.104 ☑
      with penetration into peritoneal cavity S31.604 ☑
      bite — *see* Bite, abdomen, wall, left, lower quadrant
      laceration — *see* Laceration, abdomen, wall, left, lower quadrant
      puncture — *see* Puncture, abdomen, wall, left, lower quadrant
    upper quadrant S31.101 ☑
      with penetration into peritoneal cavity S31.601 ☑
      bite — *see* Bite, abdomen, wall, left, upper quadrant
      laceration — *see* Laceration, abdomen, wall, left, upper quadrant
      puncture — *see* Puncture, abdomen, wall, left, upper quadrant
  leg (lower) S81.80- ☑
    with amputation — *see* Amputation, traumatic, leg
    ankle — *see* Wound, open, ankle
    bite — *see* Bite, leg
    foot — *see* Wound, open, foot
    knee — *see* Wound, open, knee
    laceration — *see* Laceration, leg
    puncture — *see* Puncture, leg
    toe — *see* Wound, open, toe
    upper — *see* Wound, open, thigh
  lip S01.501 ☑
    bite — *see* Bite, lip
    laceration — *see* Laceration, lip
    puncture — *see* Puncture, lip
  loin S31.109 ☑
    bite — *see* Bite, abdomen, wall
    laceration — *see* Laceration, loin
    puncture — *see* Puncture, loin
  lower back — *see* Wound, open, back, lower
  lumbar region — *see* Wound, open, back, lower
  malar region — *see* Wound, open, head, specified site NEC
  mammary — *see* Wound, open, breast
  mastoid region — *see* Wound, open, head, specified site NEC
  mouth — *see* Wound, open, oral cavity
  nail
    finger — *see* Wound, open, finger, with damage to nail
    toe — *see* Wound, open, toe, with damage to nail
  nape (neck) — *see* Wound, open, neck
  nasal (septum) (sinus) — *see* Wound, open, nose
  nasopharynx — *see* Wound, open, head, specified site NEC
  neck S11.90 ☑
    bite — *see* Bite, neck
    involving
      cervical esophagus S11.20 ☑
      larynx — *see* Wound, open, larynx
      pharynx S11.20 ☑
      thyroid S11.10 ☑
      trachea (cervical) S11.029 ☑
        bite — *see* Bite, trachea
        laceration S11.021 ☑
          with foreign body S11.022 ☑
        puncture S11.023 ☑
          with foreign body S11.024 ☑

Wound, open — *continued*
  neck — *continued*
    laceration — *see* Laceration, neck
    puncture — *see* Puncture, neck
    specified site NEC S11.80 ☑
      specified type NEC S11.89 ☑
  nose (septum) (sinus) S01.20 ☑
    with amputation — *see* Amputation, traumatic, nose
    bite — *see* Bite, nose
    laceration — *see* Laceration, nose
    puncture — *see* Puncture, nose
  ocular S05.90 ☑
    avulsion (traumatic enucleation) S05.7- ☑
    eyeball S05.6- ☑
      with foreign body S05.5- ☑
    eyelid — *see* Wound, open, eyelid
    laceration and rupture S05.3- ☑
      with prolapse or loss of intraocular tissue S05.2- ☑
    orbit (penetrating) (with or without foreign body) S05.4- ☑
    periocular area — *see* Wound, open, eyelid
    specified NEC S05.8X- ☑
  oral cavity S01.502 ☑
    bite S01.552 ☑
    laceration — *see* Laceration, oral cavity
    puncture — *see* Puncture, oral cavity
  orbit — *see* Wound, open, ocular, orbit
  palate — *see* Wound, open, oral cavity
  palm — *see* Wound, open, hand
  pelvis, pelvic (*see also* Wound, open, back, lower)
    girdle — *see* Wound, open, hip
  penetrating — *see* Puncture, by site
  penis S31.20 ☑
    with amputation — *see* Amputation, traumatic, penis
    bite S31.25 ☑
    laceration — *see* Laceration, penis
    puncture — *see* Puncture, penis
  perineum
    bite — *see* Bite, perineum
    female S31.502 ☑
    laceration — *see* Laceration, perineum
    male S31.501 ☑
    puncture — *see* Puncture, perineum
  periocular area (with or without lacrimal passages) — *see* Wound, open, eyelid
  periumbilic region S31.105 ☑
    with penetration into peritoneal cavity S31.605 ☑
    bite — *see* Bite, abdomen, wall, periumbilic region
    laceration — *see* Laceration, abdomen, wall, periumbilic region
    puncture — *see* Puncture, abdomen, wall, periumbilic region
  phalanges
    finger — *see* Wound, open, finger
    toe — *see* Wound, open, toe
  pharynx S11.20 ☑
  pinna — *see* Wound, open, ear
  popliteal space — *see* Wound, open, knee
  prepuce — *see* Wound, open, penis
  pubic region — *see* Wound, open, back, lower
  pudendum — *see* Wound, open, genital organs, external
  puncture wound — *see* Puncture
  rectovaginal septum — *see* Wound, open, vagina
  right
    lower quadrant S31.103 ☑
      with penetration into peritoneal cavity S31.603 ☑
      bite — *see* Bite, abdomen, wall, right, lower quadrant
      laceration — *see* Laceration, abdomen, wall, right, lower quadrant
      puncture — *see* Puncture, abdomen, wall, right, lower quadrant
    upper quadrant S31.100 ☑
      with penetration into peritoneal cavity S31.600 ☑
      bite — *see* Bite, abdomen, wall, right, upper quadrant
      laceration — *see* Laceration, abdomen, wall, right, upper quadrant
      puncture — *see* Puncture, abdomen, wall, right, upper quadrant

      ☑ **Additional Character Required — Refer to the Tabular List for Character Selection**   ▼ **Subterms under main terms may continue to next column or page**

Wound, open — *continued*
- sacral region — *see* Wound, open, back, lower
- sacroiliac region — *see* Wound, open, back, lower
- salivary gland — *see* Wound, open, oral cavity
- scalp S01.00 ☑
  - bite S01.05 ☑
  - laceration — *see* Laceration, scalp
  - puncture — *see* Puncture, scalp
- scalpel, newborn (birth injury) P15.8
- scapular region — *see* Wound, open, shoulder
- sclera — *see* Wound, open, ocular
- scrotum S31.30 ☑
  - with amputation — *see* Amputation, traumatic, scrotum
  - bite S31.35 ☑
  - laceration — *see* Laceration, scrotum
  - puncture — *see* Puncture, scrotum
- shin — *see* Wound, open, leg
- shoulder S41.00- ☑
  - with amputation — *see* Amputation, traumatic, arm
  - bite — *see* Bite, shoulder
  - laceration — *see* Laceration, shoulder
  - puncture — *see* Puncture, shoulder
- skin NOS T14.8
- spermatic cord — *see* Wound, open, testis
- sternal region — *see* Wound, open, thorax, front wall
- submaxillary region — *see* Wound, open, head, specified site NEC
- submental region — *see* Wound, open, head, specified site NEC
- subungual
  - finger(s) — *see* Wound, open, finger
  - toe(s) — *see* Wound, open, toe
- supraclavicular region — *see* Wound, open, neck, specified site NEC
- temple, temporal region — *see* Wound, open, head, specified site NEC
- temporomandibular area — *see* Wound, open, cheek
- testis S31.30 ☑
  - with amputation — *see* Amputation, traumatic, testes
  - bite S31.35 ☑
  - laceration — *see* Laceration, testis
  - puncture — *see* Puncture, testis
- thigh S71.10- ☑
  - with amputation — *see* Amputation, traumatic, hip
  - bite — *see* Bite, thigh
  - laceration — *see* Laceration, thigh
  - puncture — *see* Puncture, thigh
- thorax, thoracic (wall) S21.90 ☑
  - back S21.20- ☑
    - with penetration S21.40 ☑
  - bite — *see* Bite, thorax
  - breast — *see* Wound, open, breast
  - front S21.10- ☑
    - with penetration S21.30 ☑
  - laceration — *see* Laceration, thorax
  - puncture — *see* Puncture, thorax
- throat — *see* Wound, open, neck
- thumb S61.009 ☑
  - with
    - amputation — *see* Amputation, traumatic, thumb
    - damage to nail S61.109 ☑
  - bite — *see* Bite, thumb
  - laceration — *see* Laceration, thumb
  - left S61.002 ☑
    - with
      - damage to nail S61.102 ☑
  - puncture — *see* Puncture, thumb
  - right S61.001 ☑
    - with
      - damage to nail S61.101 ☑
- thyroid (gland) — *see* Wound, open, neck, thyroid
- toe(s) S91.109 ☑
  - with
    - amputation — *see* Amputation, traumatic, toe
    - damage to nail S91.209 ☑
  - bite — *see* Bite, toe
  - great S91.103 ☑
    - with
      - damage to nail S91.203 ☑
    - left S91.102 ☑

Wound, open — *continued*
- toe(s) — *continued*
  - great — *continued*
    - left — *continued*
      - with
        - damage to nail S91.202 ☑
    - right S91.101 ☑
      - with
        - damage to nail S91.201 ☑
  - laceration — *see* Laceration, toe
  - lesser S91.106 ☑
    - with
      - damage to nail S91.206 ☑
    - left S91.105 ☑
      - with
        - damage to nail S91.205 ☑
    - right S91.104 ☑
      - with
        - damage to nail S91.204 ☑
  - puncture — *see* Puncture, toe
- tongue — *see* Wound, open, oral cavity
- trachea (cervical region) — *see* Wound, open, neck, trachea
- tunica vaginalis — *see* Wound, open, testis
- tympanum, tympanic membrane S09.2- ☑
  - laceration — *see* Laceration, ear, drum
  - puncture — *see* Puncture, tympanum
- umbilical region — *see* Wound, open, abdomen, wall, periumbilic region
- uvula — *see* Wound, open, oral cavity
- vagina S31.40 ☑
  - bite S31.45 ☑
  - laceration — *see* Laceration, vagina
  - puncture — *see* Puncture, vagina
- vitreous (humor) — *see* Wound, open, ocular
- vocal cord S11.039 ☑
  - bite — *see* Bite, vocal cord
  - laceration S11.031 ☑
    - with foreign body S11.032 ☑
  - puncture S11.033 ☑
    - with foreign body S11.034 ☑
- vulva S31.40 ☑
  - with amputation — *see* Amputation, traumatic, vulva
  - bite S31.45 ☑
  - laceration — *see* Laceration, vulva
  - puncture — *see* Puncture, vulva
- wrist S61.50- ☑
  - bite — *see* Bite, wrist
  - laceration — *see* Laceration, wrist
  - puncture — *see* Puncture, wrist

Wound, superficial — *see* Injury (*see also* specified injury type)
Wright's syndrome G54.0
Wrist — *see* condition
Wrong drug (by accident) (given in error) — *see* Table of Drugs and Chemicals, by drug, poisoning
Wry neck — *see* Torticollis
Wuchereria (bancrofti) **infestation** B74.0
Wuchereriasis B74.0
Wuchernde Struma Langhans C73

X

X-ray (of)
- abnormal findings — *see* Abnormal, diagnostic imaging
- breast (mammogram) (routine) Z12.31
- chest
  - routine (as part of a general medical examination) Z00.00
    - with abnormal findings Z00.01
- routine (as part of a general medical examination) Z00.00
  - with abnormal findings Z00.01
Xanthelasma (eyelid) (palpebrarum) H02.60
- left H02.66
  - lower H02.65
  - upper H02.64
- right H02.63
  - lower H02.62
  - upper H02.61
Xanthelasmatosis (essential) E78.2
Xanthinuria, hereditary E79.8
Xanthoastrocytoma
- specified site — *see* Neoplasm, malignant, by site

Xanthoastrocytoma — *continued*
- unspecified site C71.9
Xanthofibroma — *see* Neoplasm, connective tissue, benign
Xanthogranuloma D76.3
Xanthoma(s), xanthomatosis (primary) (familial) (hereditary) E75.5
- with
  - hyperlipoproteinemia
    - Type I E78.3
    - Type III E78.2
    - Type IV E78.1
    - Type V E78.3
- cerebrotendinous E75.5
- cutaneotendinous E75.5
- disseminatum (skin) E78.2
- eruptive E78.2
- hypercholesterinemic E78.0
- hypercholesterolemic E78.0
- hyperlipidemic E78.5
- joint E75.5
- multiple (skin) E78.2
- tendon (sheath) E75.5
- tuberosum E78.2
- tuberous E78.2
- tubo-eruptive E78.2
- verrucous, oral mucosa K13.4
Xanthosis R23.8
Xenophobia F40.10
Xeroderma (*see also* Ichthyosis)
- acquired L85.0
  - eyelid H01.149
    - left H01.146
      - lower H01.145
      - upper H01.144
    - right H01.143
      - lower H01.142
      - upper H01.141
- pigmentosum Q82.1
- vitamin A deficiency E50.8
Xerophthalmia (vitamin A deficiency) E50.7
- unrelated to vitamin A deficiency — *see* Keratoconjunctivitis
Xerosis
- conjunctiva H11.14- ☑
  - with Bitot's spots (*see also* Pigmentation, conjunctiva)
    - vitamin A deficiency E50.1
  - vitamin A deficiency E50.0
- cornea H18.89- ☑
  - with ulceration — *see* Ulcer, cornea
    - vitamin A deficiency E50.3
  - vitamin A deficiency E50.2
- cutis L85.3
- skin L85.3
Xerostomia K11.7
Xiphopagus Q89.4
XO syndrome Q96.9
XXXXY syndrome Q98.1
XXY syndrome Q98.0

Y

Yaba pox (virus disease) B08.72
Yatapoxvirus B08.70
- specified NEC B08.79
Yawning R06.89
- psychogenic F45.8
Yaws A66.9
- cutaneous, less than five years after infection A66.2
- bone lesions A66.6
- butter A66.1
- chancre A66.0
- early (cutaneous) (macular) (maculopapular) (micropapular) (papular) A66.2
  - frambeside A66.2
  - skin lesions NEC A66.2
- eyelid A66.2
- ganglion A66.6
- gangosis, gangosa A66.5
- gumma, gummata A66.4
  - bone A66.6
- gummatous
  - frambeside A66.4
  - osteitis A66.6
  - periostitis A66.6
- hydrarthrosis (*see also* subcategory M14.8-) A66.6
- hyperkeratosis (early) (late) A66.3

Yaws — *continued*
 initial lesions A66.0
 joint lesions (*see also* subcategory M14.8-) A66.6
 juxta-articular nodules A66.7
 late nodular (ulcerated) A66.4
 latent (without clinical manifestations) (with positive
   serology) A66.8
 mother A66.0
 mucosal A66.7
 multiple papillomata A66.1
 nodular, late (ulcerated) A66.4
 osteitis A66.6
 papilloma, plantar or palmar A66.1
 periostitis (hypertrophic) A66.6
 specified NEC A66.7
 ulcers A66.4

Yaws — *continued*
 wet crab A66.1
Yeast infection (*see also* Candidiasis) B37.9
Yellow
 atrophy (liver) — *see* Failure, hepatic
 fever — *see* Fever, yellow
 jack — *see* Fever, yellow
 jaundice — *see* Jaundice
 nail syndrome L60.5
Yersiniosis (*see also* Infection, Yersinia)
 extraintestinal A28.2
 intestinal A04.6

Z

Zahorsky's syndrome (herpangina) B08.5

Zellweger's syndrome Q87.89
Zenker's diverticulum (esophagus) K22.5
Ziehen-Oppenheim disease G24.1
Zieve's syndrome K70.0
Zinc
 deficiency, dietary E60
 metabolism disorder E83.2
Zollinger-Ellison syndrome E16.4
Zona — *see* Herpes, zoster
Zoophobia F40.218
Zoster (herpes) — *see* Herpes, zoster
Zygomycosis B46.9
 specified NEC B46.8
Zymotic — *see* condition

☑ **Additional Character Required — Refer to the Tabular List for Character Selection** ▽ **Subterms under main terms may continue to next column or page**

Note: The list below gives the code number for neoplasms by anatomical site. For each site there are six possible code numbers according to whether the neoplasm in question is malignant, benign, in situ, of uncertain behavior, or of unspecified nature. The description of the neoplasm will often indicate which of the six columns is appropriate; e.g., malignant melanoma of skin, benign fibroadenoma of breast, carcinoma in situ of cervix uteri. Where such descriptors are not present, the remainder of the Index should be consulted where guidance is given to the appropriate column for each morphological (histological) variety listed; e.g., Mesonephroma – see Neoplasm, malignant; Embryoma (see also Neoplasm, uncertain behavior); Disease, Bowen's – see Neoplasm, skin, in situ. However, the guidance in the Index can be overridden if one of the descriptors mentioned above is present; e.g., malignant adenoma of colon is coded to C18.9 and not to D12.6 as the adjective "malignant" overrides the Index entry "Adenoma (see also Neoplasm, benign)." Codes listed with a dash -, following the code have a required 5th character for laterality. The tabular list must be reviewed for the complete code.

	Malignant Primary	Malignant Secondary	Ca in situ	Benign	Uncertain	Unspecified Behavior
Neoplasm, neoplastic	C80.1	C79.9	D09.9	D36.9	D48.9	D49.9
abdomen, abdominal	C76.2	C79.8✓	D09.8	D36.7	D48.7	D49.89
cavity	C76.2	C79.8✓	D09.8	D36.7	D48.7	D49.89
organ	C76.2	C79.8✓	D09.8	D36.7	D48.7	D49.89
viscera	C76.2	C79.8✓	D09.8	D36.7	D48.7	D49.89
wall — *see also* Neoplasm, abdomen, wall, skin	C44.509	C79.2	D04.5	D23.5	D48.5	D49.2
connective tissue	C49.4	C79.8✓	—	D21.4	D48.1	D49.2
skin	C44.509	—	—	—	—	—
basal cell carcinoma	C44.519	—	—	—	—	—
specified type NEC	C44.599	—	—	—	—	—
squamous cell carcinoma	C44.529	—	—	—	—	—
abdominopelvic	C76.8	C79.8✓	—	D36.7	D48.7	D49.89
accessory sinus — *see* Neoplasm, sinus						
acoustic nerve	C72.4✓	C79.49	—	D33.3	D43.3	D49.7
adenoid (pharynx) (tissue)	C11.1	C79.89	D00.08	D10.6	D37.05	D49.0
adipose tissue — *see also* Neoplasm, connective tissue	C49.4	C79.89	—	D21.9	D48.1	D49.2
adnexa (uterine)	C57.4	C79.89	D07.39	D28.7	D39.8	D49.5
adrenal	C74.9✓	C79.7✓	D09.3	D35.0✓	D44.1✓	D49.7
capsule	C74.9✓	C79.7✓	D09.3	D35.0✓	D44.1✓	D49.7
cortex	C74.0✓	C79.7✓	D09.3	D35.0✓	D44.1✓	D49.7
gland	C74.9✓	C79.7✓	D09.3	D35.0✓	D44.1✓	D49.7
medulla	C74.1✓	C79.7✓	D09.3	D35.0✓	D44.1✓	D49.7
ala nasi (external) — *see also* Neoplasm, skin, nose	C44.301	C79.2	D04.39	D23.39	D48.5	D49.2
alimentary canal or tract NEC	C26.9	C78.80	D01.9	D13.9	D37.9	D49.0
alveolar	C03.9	C79.89	D00.03	D10.39	D37.09	D49.0
mucosa	C03.9	C79.89	D00.03	D10.39	D37.09	D49.0
lower	C03.1	C79.89	D00.03	D10.39	D37.09	D49.0
upper	C03.0	C79.89	D00.03	D10.39	D37.09	D49.0
ridge or process	C41.1	C79.51	—	D16.5	D48.0	D49.2
carcinoma	C03.9	C79.8✓	—	—	—	—
lower	C03.1	C79.8✓	—	—	—	—
upper	C03.0	C79.8✓	—	—	—	—
lower	C41.1	C79.51	—	D16.5	D48.0	D49.2
mucosa	C03.9	C79.89	D00.03	D10.39	D37.09	D49.0
lower	C03.1	C79.89	D00.03	D10.39	D37.09	D49.0
upper	C03.0	C79.89	D00.03	D10.39	D37.09	D49.0
upper	C41.0	C79.51	—	D16.4	D48.0	D49.2
sulcus	C06.1	C79.89	D00.02	D10.39	D37.09	D49.0
alveolus	C03.9	C79.89	D00.03	D10.39	D37.09	D49.0
lower	C03.1	C79.89	D00.03	D10.39	D37.09	D49.0
upper	C03.0	C79.89	D00.03	D10.39	D37.09	D49.0
ampulla of Vater	C24.1	C78.89	D01.5	D13.5	D37.6	D49.0
ankle NEC	C76.5✓	C79.89	D04.7✓	D36.7	D48.7	D49.89

	Malignant Primary	Malignant Secondary	Ca in situ	Benign	Uncertain	Unspecified Behavior
Neoplasm, neoplastic — *continued*						
anorectum, anorectal (junction)	C21.8	C78.5	D01.3	D12.9	D37.8	D49.0
antecubital fossa or space	C76.4✓	C79.89	D04.6✓	D36.7	D48.7	D49.89
antrum (Highmore) (maxillary)	C31.0	C78.39	D02.3	D14.0	D38.5	D49.1
pyloric	C16.3	C78.89	D00.2	D13.1	D37.1	D49.0
tympanicum	C30.1	C78.39	D02.3	D14.0	D38.5	D49.1
anus, anal	C21.0	C78.5	D01.3	D12.9	D37.8	D49.0
canal	C21.1	C78.5	D01.3	D12.9	D37.8	D49.0
cloacogenic zone	C21.2	C78.5	D01.3	D12.9	D37.8	D49.0
margin — *see also* Neoplasm, anus, skin	C44.500	C79.2	D04.5	D23.5	D48.5	D49.2
overlapping lesion with rectosigmoid junction or rectum	C21.8	—	—	—	—	—
skin	C44.500	C79.2	D04.5	D23.5	D48.5	D49.2
basal cell carcinoma	C44.510	—	—	—	—	—
specified type NEC	C44.590	—	—	—	—	—
squamous cell carcinoma	C44.520	—	—	—	—	—
sphincter	C21.1	C78.5	D01.3	D12.9	D37.8	D49.0
aorta (thoracic)	C49.3	C79.89	—	D21.3	D48.1	D49.2
abdominal	C49.4	C79.89	—	D21.4	D48.1	D49.2
aortic body	C75.5	C79.89	—	D35.6	D44.7	D49.7
aponeurosis	C49.9	C79.89	—	D21.9	D48.1	D49.2
palmar	C49.1✓	C79.89	—	D21.1✓	D48.1	D49.2
plantar	C49.2✓	C79.89	—	D21.2✓	D48.1	D49.2
appendix	C18.1	C78.5	D01.0	D12.1	D37.3	D49.0
arachnoid	C70.9	C79.49	—	D32.9	D42.9	D49.7
cerebral	C70.0	C79.32	—	D32.0	D42.0	D49.7
spinal	C70.1	C79.49	—	D32.1	D42.1	D49.7
areola	C50.0✓	C79.81	D05✓	D24✓	D48.6✓	D49.3
arm NEC	C76.4✓	C79.89	D04.6✓	D36.7	D48.7	D49.89
artery — *see* Neoplasm, connective tissue						
aryepiglottic fold	C13.1	C79.89	D00.08	D10.7	D37.05	D49.0
hypopharyngeal aspect	C13.1	C79.89	D00.08	D10.7	D37.05	D49.0
laryngeal aspect	C32.1	C78.39	D02.0	D14.1	D38.0	D49.1
marginal zone	C13.1	C79.89	D00.08	D10.7	D37.05	D49.0
arytenoid (cartilage)	C32.3	C78.39	D02.0	D14.1	D38.0	D49.1
fold — *see* Neoplasm, aryepiglottic						
associated with transplanted organ	C80.2	—	—	—	—	—
atlas	C41.2	C79.51	—	D16.6	D48.0	D49.2
atrium, cardiac	C38.0	C79.89	—	D15.1	D48.7	D49.89
auditory						
canal (external) (skin) A81	C44.20✓	C79.2	D04.2✓	D23.2✓	D48.5	D49.2
internal	C30.1	C78.39	D02.3	D14.0	D38.5	D49.1
nerve	C72.4✓	C79.49	—	D33.3	D43.3	D49.7
tube	C30.1	C78.39	D02.3	D14.0	D38.5	D49.1
opening	C11.2	C79.89	D00.08	D10.6	D37.05	D49.0
auricle, ear — *see also* Neoplasm, skin, ear	C44.20✓	C79.2	D04.2✓	D23.2✓	D48.5	D49.2
auricular canal (external) — *see also* Neoplasm, skin, ear	C44.20✓	C79.2	D04.2✓	D23.2✓	D48.5	D49.2
internal	C30.1	C78.39	D02.3	D14.0	D38.5	D49.2
autonomic nerve or nervous system NEC (see Neoplasm, nerve, peripheral)						
axilla, axillary	C76.1	C79.89	D09.8	D36.7	D48.7	D49.89
fold — *see also* Neoplasm, skin, trunk	C44.509	C79.2	D04.5	D23.5	D48.5	D49.2
back NEC	C76.8	C79.89	D04.5	D36.7	D48.7	D49.89

Neoplasm, neoplastic — continued	Malignant Primary	Malignant Secondary	Ca in situ	Benign	Uncertain	Unspecified Behavior
Bartholin's gland	C51.0	C79.82	D07.1	D28.0	D39.8	D49.5
basal ganglia	C71.0	C79.31	—	D33.0	D43.0	D49.6
basis pedunculi	C71.7	C79.31	—	D33.1	D43.1	D49.6
bile or biliary (tract)	C24.9	C78.89	D01.5	D13.5	D37.6	D49.0
canaliculi (biliferi) (intrahepatic)	C22.1	C78.7	D01.5	D13.4	D37.6	D49.0
canals, interlobular	C22.1	C78.89	D01.5	D13.4	D37.6	D49.0
duct or passage (common) (cystic) (extrahepatic)	C24.0	C78.89	D01.5	D13.5	D37.6	D49.0
interlobular	C22.1	C78.89	D01.5	D13.4	D37.6	D49.0
intrahepatic	C22.1	C78.7	D01.5	D13.4	D37.6	D49.0
and extrahepatic	C24.8	C78.89	D01.5	D13.5	D37.6	D49.0
bladder (urinary)	C67.9	C79.11	D09.0	D30.3	D41.4	D49.4
dome	C67.1	C79.11	D09.0	D30.3	D41.4	D49.4
neck	C67.5	C79.11	D09.0	D30.3	D41.4	D49.4
orifice	C67.9	C79.11	D09.0	D30.3	D41.4	D49.4
ureteric	C67.6	C79.11	D09.0	D30.3	D41.4	D49.4
urethral	C67.5	C79.11	D09.0	D30.3	D41.4	D49.4
overlapping lesion	C67.8	—	—	—	—	—
sphincter	C67.8	C79.11	D09.0	D30.3	D41.4	D49.4
trigone	C67.0	C79.11	D09.0	D30.3	D41.4	D49.4
urachus	C67.7	C79.11	D09.0	D30.3	D41.4	D49.4
wall	C67.9	C79.11	D09.0	D30.3	D41.4	D49.4
anterior	C67.3	C79.11	D09.0	D30.3	D41.4	D49.4
lateral	C67.2	C79.11	D09.0	D30.3	D41.4	D49.4
posterior	C67.4	C79.11	D09.0	D30.3	D41.4	D49.4
blood vessel — see Neoplasm, connective tissue						
bone (periosteum)	C41.9	C79.51	—	D16.9	D48.0	D49.2
acetabulum	C41.4	C79.51	—	D16.8-	D48.0	D49.2
ankle	C40.3-☑	C79.51	—	D16.3-☑	—	—
arm NEC	C40.0-☑	C79.51	—	D16.0-☑	—	—
astragalus	C40.3-☑	C79.51	—	D16.3-☑	—	—
atlas	C41.2	C79.51	—	D16.6-	D48.0	D49.2
axis	C41.2	C79.51	—	D16.6-	D48.0	D49.2
back NEC	C41.2	C79.51	—	D16.6-	D48.0	D49.2
calcaneus	C40.3-☑	C79.51	—	D16.3-☑	—	—
calvarium	C41.0	C79.51	—	D16.4-	D48.0	D49.2
carpus (any)	C40.1-☑	C79.51	—	D16.1-☑	—	—
cartilage NEC	C41.9	C79.51	—	D16.9-	D48.0	D49.2
clavicle	C41.3	C79.51	—	D16.7-	D48.0	D49.2
clivus	C41.0	C79.51	—	D16.4-	D48.0	D49.2
coccygeal vertebra	C41.4	C79.51	—	D16.8-	D48.0	D49.2
coccyx	C41.4	C79.51	—	D16.8-	D48.0	D49.2
costal cartilage	C41.3	C79.51	—	D16.7-	D48.0	D49.2
costovertebral joint	C41.3	C79.51	—	D16.7-	D48.0	D49.2
cranial	C41.0	C79.51	—	D16.4-	D48.0	D49.2
cuboid	C40.3-☑	C79.51	—	D16.3-☑	—	—
cuneiform	C41.9	C79.51	—	D16.9-	D48.0	D49.2
elbow	C40.0-☑	C79.51	—	D16.0-☑	—	—
ethmoid (labyrinth)	C41.0	C79.51	—	D16.4-	D48.0	D49.2
face	C41.0	C79.51	—	D16.4-	D48.0	D49.2
femur (any part)	C40.2-☑	C79.51	—	D16.2-☑	—	—
fibula (any part)	C40.2-☑	C79.51	—	D16.2-☑	—	—
finger (any)	C40.1-☑	C79.51	—	D16.1-☑	—	—
foot	C40.3-☑	C79.51	—	D16.3-☑	—	—
forearm	C40.0-☑	C79.51	—	D16.0-☑	—	—
frontal	C41.0	C79.51	—	D16.4-	D48.0	D49.2
hand	C40.1-☑	C79.51	—	D16.1-☑	—	—
heel	C40.3-☑	C79.51	—	D16.3-☑	—	—
hip	C41.4	C79.51	—	D16.8-	D48.0	D49.2
humerus (any part)	C40.0-☑	C79.51	—	D16.0-☑	—	—
hyoid	C41.0	C79.51	—	D16.4-	D48.0	D49.2
ilium	C41.4	C79.51	—	D16.8-	D48.0	D49.2
innominate	C41.4	C79.51	—	D16.8-	D48.0	D49.2
intervertebral cartilage or disc	C41.2	C79.51	—	D16.6-	D48.0	D49.2
ischium	C41.4	C79.51	—	D16.8-	D48.0	D49.2
jaw (lower)	C41.1	C79.51	—	D16.5-	D48.0	D49.2
knee	C40.2-☑	C79.51	—	D16.2-☑	—	—
leg NEC	C40.2-☑	C79.51	—	D16.2-☑	—	—
limb NEC	C40.9-☑	C79.51	—	D16.9-	—	—

Neoplasm, neoplastic — continued	Malignant Primary	Malignant Secondary	Ca in situ	Benign	Uncertain	Unspecified Behavior
bone — continued						
limb — continued						
lower (long bones)	C40.2-☑	C79.51	—	D16.2-☑	—	—
short bones	C40.3-☑	C79.51	—	D16.3-☑	—	—
upper (long bones)	C40.0-☑	C79.51	—	D16.0-☑	—	—
short bones	C40.1-☑	C79.51	—	D16.1-☑	—	—
malar	C41.0	C79.51	—	D16.4-	D48.0	D49.2
mandible	C41.1	C79.51	—	D16.5-	D48.0	D49.2
marrow NEC (any bone)	C96.9	C79.52	—	—	D47.9	D49.89
mastoid	C41.0	C79.51	—	D16.4-	D48.0	D49.2
maxilla, maxillary (superior)	C41.0	C79.51	—	D16.4-	D48.0	D49.2
inferior	C41.1	C79.51	—	D16.5-	D48.0	D49.2
metacarpus (any)	C40.1-☑	C79.51	—	D16.1-☑	—	—
metatarsus (any)	C40.3-☑	C79.51	—	D16.3-☑	—	—
navicular ankle	C40.3-☑	C79.51	—	—	—	—
hand	C40.1-☑	C79.51	—	—	—	—
nose, nasal	C41.0	C79.51	—	D16.4-	D48.0	D49.2
occipital	C41.0	C79.51	—	D16.4-	D48.0	D49.2
orbit	C41.0	C79.51	—	D16.4-	D48.0	D49.2
overlapping sites	C40.8-☑	—	—	—	—	—
parietal	C41.0	C79.51	—	D16.4-	D48.0	D49.2
patella	C40.2-☑	C79.51	—	—	—	—
pelvic	C41.4	C79.51	—	D16.8	D48.0	D49.2
phalanges foot	C40.3-☑	C79.51	—	—	—	—
hand	C40.1-☑	C79.51	—	—	—	—
pubic	C41.4	C79.51	—	D16.8	D48.0	D49.2
radius (any part)	C40.0-☑	C79.51	—	D16.0-☑	—	—
rib	C41.3	C79.51	—	D16.7	D48.0	D49.2
sacral vertebra	C41.4	C79.51	—	D16.8	D48.0	D49.2
sacrum	C41.4	C79.51	—	D16.8	D48.0	D49.2
scaphoid of ankle	C40.3-☑	C79.51	—	—	—	—
of hand	C40.1-☑	C79.51	—	—	—	—
scapula (any part)	C40.0-☑	C79.51	—	D16.0-☑	—	—
sella turcica	C41.0	C79.51	—	D16.4-	D48.0	D49.2
shoulder	C40.0-☑	C79.51	—	D16.0-☑	—	—
skull	C41.0	C79.51	—	D16.4-	D48.0	D49.2
sphenoid	C41.0	C79.51	—	D16.4-	D48.0	D49.2
spine, spinal (column)	C41.2	C79.51	—	D16.6	D48.0	D49.2
coccyx	C41.4	C79.51	—	D16.8	D48.0	D49.2
sacrum	C41.4	C79.51	—	D16.8	D48.0	D49.2
sternum	C41.3	C79.51	—	D16.7	D48.0	D49.2
tarsus (any)	C40.3-☑	C79.51	—	—	—	—
temporal	C41.0	C79.51	—	D16.4-	D48.0	D49.2
thumb	C40.1-☑	C79.51	—	—	—	—
tibia (any part)	C40.2-☑	C79.51	—	—	—	—
toe (any)	C40.3-☑	C79.51	—	—	—	—
trapezium	C40.1-☑	C79.51	—	—	—	—
trapezoid	C40.1-☑	C79.51	—	—	—	—
turbinate	C41.0	C79.51	—	D16.4-	D48.0	D49.2
ulna (any part)	C40.0-☑	C79.51	—	D16.0-☑	—	—
unciform	C40.1-☑	C79.51	—	—	—	—
vertebra (column)	C41.2	C79.51	—	D16.6	D48.0	D49.2
coccyx	C41.4	C79.51	—	D16.8	D48.0	D49.2
sacrum	C41.4	C79.51	—	D16.8	D48.0	D49.2
vomer	C41.0	C79.51	—	D16.4-	D48.0	D49.2
wrist	C40.1-☑	C79.51	—	—	—	—
xiphoid process	C41.3	C79.51	—	D16.7	D48.0	D49.2
zygomatic	C41.0	C79.51	—	D16.4-	D48.0	D49.2
book-leaf (mouth) — ventral surface of tongue and floor of mouth	C06.89	C79.89	D00.00	D10.39	D37.09	D49.0
bowel — see Neoplasm, intestine						
brachial plexus	C47.1☑	C79.89	—	D36.12	D48.2	D49.2
brain NEC	C71.9	C79.31	—	D33.2	D43.2	D49.6
basal ganglia	C71.0	C79.31	—	D33.0	D43.0	D49.6
cerebellopontine angle	C71.6	C79.31	—	D33.1	D43.1	D49.6
cerebellum NOS	C71.6	C79.31	—	D33.1	D43.1	D49.6
cerebrum	C71.0	C79.31	—	D33.0	D43.0	D49.6

☑ Additional Character Required — Refer to the Tabular List for Character Selection   ▽ Subterms under main terms may continue to next column or page

Neoplasm, neoplastic —	Malignant Primary	Malignant Secondary	Ca in situ	Benign	Uncertain	Unspecified Behavior
continued						
brain — *continued*						
choroid plexus	C71.7	C79.31	—	D33.1	D43.1	D49.6
corpus callosum	C71.8	C79.31	—	D33.2	D43.2	D49.6
corpus striatum	C71.0	C79.31	—	D33.0	D43.0	D49.6
cortex (cerebral)	C71.0	C79.31	—	D33.0	D43.0	D49.6
frontal lobe	C71.1	C79.31	—	D33.0	D43.0	D49.6
globus pallidus	C71.0	C79.31	—	D33.0	D43.0	D49.6
hippocampus	C71.2	C79.31	—	D33.0	D43.0	D49.6
hypothalamus	C71.0	C79.31	—	D33.0	D43.0	D49.6
internal capsule	C71.0	C79.31	—	D33.0	D43.0	D49.6
medulla oblongata	C71.7	C79.31	—	D33.1	D43.1	D49.6
meninges	C70.0	C79.32	—	D32.0	D42.0	D49.7
midbrain	C71.7	C79.31	—	D33.1	D43.1	D49.6
occipital lobe	C71.4	C79.31	—	D33.0	D43.0	D49.6
overlapping lesion	C71.8	C79.31	—	—	—	—
parietal lobe	C71.3	C79.31	—	D33.0	D43.0	D49.6
peduncle	C71.7	C79.31	—	D33.1	D43.1	D49.6
pons	C71.7	C79.31	—	D33.1	D43.1	D49.6
stem	C71.7	C79.31	—	D33.1	D43.1	D49.6
tapetum	C71.8	C79.31	—	D33.2	D43.2	D49.6
temporal lobe	C71.2	C79.31	—	D33.0	D43.0	D49.6
thalamus	C71.0	C79.31	—	D33.0	D43.0	D49.6
uncus	C71.2	C79.31	—	D33.0	D43.0	D49.6
ventricle (floor)	C71.5	C79.31	—	D33.0	D43.0	D49.6
fourth	C71.7	C79.31	—	D33.1	D43.1	D49.6
branchial (cleft) (cyst) (vestiges)	C10.4	C79.89	D00.08	D10.5	D37.05	D49.0
breast (connective tissue) (glandular tissue) (soft parts)	C50.9☑	C79.81	D05☑	D24☑	D48.6☑	D49.3
areola	C50.0-☑	C79.81	D05.-☑	D24.-☑	D48.6☑	D49.3
axillary tail	C50.6-☑	C79.81	D05.-☑	D24.-☑	D48.6☑	D49.3
central portion	C50.1-☑	C79.81	D05.-☑	D24.-☑	D48.6☑	D49.3
inner	C50.8-☑	C79.81	D05.-☑	D24.-☑	D48.6☑	D49.3
lower-inner quadrant	C50.3-☑	C79.81	D05.-☑	D24.-☑	D48.6☑	D49.3
lower-outer quadrant	C50.5-☑	C79.81	D05.-☑	D24.-☑	D48.6☑	D49.3
lower	C50.8-☑	C79.81	D05.-☑	D24.-☑	D48.6☑	D49.3
mastectomy site (skin) — *see also* Neoplasm, breast, skin	C44.501	C79.2	—	—	—	—
specified as breast tissue	C50.8-☑	C79.81	—	—	—	—
midline	C50.8-☑	C79.81	D05.-☑	D24.-☑	D48.6☑	D49.3
nipple	C50.0-☑	C79.81	D05.-☑	D24.-☑	D48.6☑	D49.3
outer	C50.8-☑	C79.81	D05.-☑	D24.-☑	D48.6☑	D49.3
overlapping lesion	C50.8-☑	—	—	—	—	—
skin	C44.501	C79.2	D04.5	D23.5	D48.5	D49.2
basal cell carcinoma	C44.511	—	—	—	—	—
specified type NEC	C44.591	—	—	—	—	—
squamous cell carcinoma	C44.521	—	—	—	—	—
tail (axillary)	C50.6-☑	C79.81	D05.-☑	D24.-☑	D48.6-☑	D49.3
upper-inner quadrant	C50.2-☑	C79.81	D05.-☑	D24.-☑	D48.6☑	D49.3
upper-outer quadrant	C50.4-☑	C79.81	D05.-☑	D24.-☑	D48.6☑	D49.3
upper	C50.8-☑	C79.81	D05.-☑	D24.-☑	D48.6☑	D49.3
broad ligament	C57.1☑	C79.82	D07.39	D28.2	D39.8	D49.5
bronchiogenic, bronchogenic (lung)	C34.9☑	C78.0☑	D02.2☑	D14.3☑	D38.1	D49.1
bronchiole	C34.9☑	C78.0☑	D02.2☑	D14.3☑	D38.1	D49.1
bronchus	C34.9☑	C78.0☑	D02.2☑	D14.3☑	D38.1	D49.1
carina	C34.0-☑	C78.0-☑	D02.2-☑	D14.3-☑	D38.1	D49.1
lower lobe of lung	C34.3-☑	C78.0-☑	D02.2-☑	D14.3-☑	D38.1	D49.1
main	C34.0-☑	C78.0-☑	D02.2-☑	D14.3-☑	D38.1	D49.1
middle lobe of lung	C34.2	C78.0-☑	D02.21	D14.31	D38.1	D49.1
overlapping lesion	C34.8-☑	—	—	—	—	—
upper lobe of lung	C34.1-☑	C78.0-☑	D02.2-☑	D14.3-☑	D38.1	D49.1
brow	C44.309	C79.2	D04.39	D23.39	D48.5	D49.2
basal cell carcinoma	C44.319	—	—	—	—	—
specified type NEC	C44.399	—	—	—	—	—

Neoplasm, neoplastic —	Malignant Primary	Malignant Secondary	Ca in situ	Benign	Uncertain	Unspecified Behavior
continued						
brow — *continued*						
squamous cell carcinoma	C44.329	—	—	—	—	—
buccal (cavity)	C06.9	C79.89	D00.00	D10.39	D37.09	D49.0
commissure	C06.0	C79.89	D00.02	D10.39	D37.09	D49.0
groove (lower) (upper)	C06.1	C79.89	D00.02	D10.39	D37.09	D49.0
mucosa	C06.0	C79.89	D00.02	D10.39	D37.09	D49.0
sulcus (lower) (upper)	C06.1	C79.89	D00.02	D10.39	D37.09	D49.0
bulbourethral gland	C68.0	C79.19	D09.19	D30.4	D41.3	D49.5
bursa — *see* Neoplasm, connective tissue						
buttock NEC	C76.3	C79.89	D04.5	D36.7	D48.7	D49.89
calf	C76.5☑	C79.89	D04.7☑	D36.7	D48.7	D49.89
calvarium	C41.0	C79.51	—	D16.4	D48.0	D49.2
calyx, renal	C65☑	C79.0☑	D09.19	D30.1☑	D41.1☑	D49.5
canal						
anal	C21.1	C78.5	D01.3	D12.9	D37.8	D49.0
auditory (external) — *see also* Neoplasm, skin, ear	C44.20-☑	C79.2	D04.2-☑	D23.2-☑	D48.5	D49.2
auricular (external) — *see also* Neoplasm, skin, ear	C44.20-☑	C79.2	D04.2-☑	D23.2-☑	D48.5	D49.2
canaliculi, biliary (biliferi) (intrahepatic)	C22.1	C78.7	D01.5	D13.4	D37.6	D49.0
canthus (eye) (inner) (outer)	C44.10☑	C79.2	D04.1☑	D23.1☑	D48.5	D49.2
basal cell carcinoma	C44.11-☑	—	—	—	—	—
specified type NEC	C44.19-☑	—	—	—	—	—
squamous cell carcinoma	C44.12-☑	—	—	—	—	—
capillary — *see* Neoplasm, connective tissue						
caput coli	C18.0	C78.5	D01.0	D12.0	D37.4	D49.0
carcinoid — *see* Tumor, carcinoid						
cardia (gastric)	C16.0	C78.89	D00.2	D13.1	D37.1	D49.0
cardiac orifice (stomach)	C16.0	C78.89	D00.2	D13.1	D37.1	D49.0
cardio-esophageal junction	C16.0	C78.89	D00.2	D13.1	D37.1	D49.0
cardio-esophagus	C16.0	C78.89	D00.2	D13.1	D37.1	D49.0
carina (bronchus)	C34.0☑	C78.0☑	D02.2☑	D14.3☑	D38.1	D49.1
carotid (artery)	C49.0	C79.89	—	D21.0	D48.1	D49.2
body	C75.4	C79.89	—	D35.5	D44.6	D49.7
carpus (any bone)	C40.1☑	C79.51	—	D16.1☑	—	—
cartilage (articular) (joint) NEC — *see also* Neoplasm, bone	C41.9	C79.51	—	D16.9	D48.0	D49.2
arytenoid	C32.3	C78.39	D02.0	D14.1	D38.0	D49.1
auricular	C49.0	C79.89	—	D21.0	D48.1	D49.2
bronchi	C34.0-☑	C78.39	—	D14.3-☑	D38.1	D49.1
costal	C41.3	C79.51	—	D16.7	D48.0	D49.2
cricoid	C32.3	C78.39	D02.0	D14.1	D38.0	D49.1
cuneiform	C32.3	C78.39	D02.0	D14.1	D38.0	D49.1
ear (external)	C49.0	C79.89	—	D21.0	D48.1	D49.2
ensiform	C41.3	C79.51	—	D16.7	D48.0	D49.2
epiglottis	C32.1	C78.39	D02.0	D14.1	D38.0	D49.1
anterior surface	C10.1	C79.89	D00.08	D10.5	D37.05	D49.0
eyelid	C49.0	C79.89	—	D21.0	D48.1	D49.2
intervertebral	C41.2	C79.51	—	D16.6	D48.0	D49.2
larynx, laryngeal	C32.3	C78.39	D02.0	D14.1	D38.0	D49.1
nose, nasal	C30.0	C78.39	D02.3	D14.0	D38.5	D49.1
pinna	C49.0	C79.89	—	D21.0	D48.1	D49.2
rib	C41.3	C79.51	—	D16.7	D48.0	D49.2
semilunar (knee)	C40.2-☑	C79.51	—	D16.2-☑	D48.0	D49.2
thyroid	C32.3	C78.39	D02.0	D14.1	D38.0	D49.1
trachea	C33	C78.39	D02.1	D14.2	D38.1	D49.1
cauda equina	C72.1	C79.49	—	D33.4	D43.4	D49.7
cavity						
buccal	C06.9	C79.89	D00.00	D10.30	D37.09	D49.0
nasal	C30.0	C78.39	D02.3	D14.0	D38.5	D49.1
oral	C06.9	C79.89	D00.00	D10.30	D37.09	D49.0
peritoneal	C48.2	C78.6	—	D20.1	D48.4	D49.0
tympanic	C30.1	C78.39	D02.3	D14.0	D38.5	D49.1
cecum	C18.0	C78.5	D01.0	D12.0	D37.4	D49.0

Neoplasm, central nervous system — Neoplasm, connective tissue NEC

Neoplasm Table

Neoplasm, neoplastic — continued

	Malignant Primary	Malignant Secondary	Ca in situ	Benign	Uncertain	Unspecified Behavior
central nervous system	C72.9	C79.40	—	—	—	—
cerebellopontine (angle)	C71.6	C79.31	—	D33.1	D43.1	D49.6
cerebellum, cerebellar	C71.6	C79.31	—	D33.1	D43.1	D49.6
cerebrum, cerebral (cortex) (hemisphere) (white matter)	C71.0	C79.31	—	D33.0	D43.0	D49.6
meninges	C70.0	C79.32	—	D32.0	D42.0	D49.7
peduncle	C71.7	C79.31	—	D33.1	D43.1	D49.6
ventricle	C71.5	C79.31	—	D33.0	D43.0	D49.6
fourth	C71.7	C79.31	—	D33.1	D43.1	D49.6
cervical region	C76.0	C79.89	D09.8	D36.7	D48.7	D49.89
cervix (cervical) (uteri) (uterus)	C53.9	C79.82	D06.9	D26.0	D39.0	D49.5
canal	C53.0	C79.82	D06.0	D26.0	D39.0	D49.5
endocervix (canal) (gland)	C53.0	C79.82	D06.0	D26.0	D39.0	D49.5
exocervix	C53.1	C79.82	D06.1	D26.0	D39.0	D49.5
external os	C53.1	C79.82	D06.1	D26.0	D39.0	D49.5
internal os	C53.0	C79.82	D06.0	D26.0	D39.0	D49.5
nabothian gland	C53.0	C79.82	D06.0	D26.0	D39.0	D49.5
overlapping lesion	C53.8	—	—	—	—	—
squamocolumnar junction	C53.8	C79.82	D06.7	D26.0	D39.0	D49.5
stump	C53.8	C79.82	D06.7	D26.0	D39.0	D49.5
cheek	C76.0	C79.89	D09.8	D36.7	D48.7	D49.89
external	C44.309	C79.2	D04.39	D23.39	D48.5	D49.2
basal cell carcinoma	C44.319	—	—	—	—	—
specified type NEC	C44.399	—	—	—	—	—
squamous cell carcinoma	C44.329	—	—	—	—	—
inner aspect	C06.0	C79.89	D00.02	D10.39	D37.09	D49.0
internal	C06.0	C79.89	D00.02	D10.39	D37.09	D49.0
mucosa	C06.0	C79.89	D00.02	D10.39	D37.09	D49.0
chest (wall) NEC	C76.1	C79.89	D09.8	D36.7	D48.7	D49.89
chiasma opticum	C72.3✓	C79.49	—	D33.3	D43.3	D49.7
chin	C44.309	C79.2	D04.39	D23.39	D48.5	D49.2
basal cell carcinoma	C44.319	—	—	—	—	—
specified type NEC	C44.399	—	—	—	—	—
squamous cell carcinoma	C44.329	—	—	—	—	—
choana	C11.3	C79.89	D00.08	D10.6	D37.05	D49.0
cholangiole	C22.1	C78.89	D01.5	D13.4	D37.6	D49.0
choledochal duct	C24.0	C78.89	D01.5	D13.5	D37.6	D49.0
choroid	C69.3✓	C79.49	D09.2✓	D31.3✓	D48.7	D49.81
plexus	C71.5	C79.31	—	D33.0	D43.0	D49.6
ciliary body	C69.4✓	C79.49	D09.2✓	D31.4✓	D48.7	D49.89
clavicle	C41.3	C79.51	—	D16.7	D48.0	D49.2
clitoris	C51.2	C79.82	D07.1	D28.0	D39.8	D49.5
clivus	C41.0	C79.51	—	D16.4	D48.0	D49.2
cloacogenic zone	C21.2	C78.5	D01.3	D12.9	D37.8	D49.0
coccygeal body or glomus	C49.5	C79.89	—	D21.5	D48.1	D49.2
vertebra	C41.4	C79.51	—	D16.8	D48.0	D49.2
coccyx	C41.4	C79.51	—	D16.8	D48.0	D49.2
colon — *see also* Neoplasm, intestine, large	C18.9	C78.5	—	—	—	—
with rectum	C19	C78.5	D01.1	D12.7	D37.5	D49.0
columnella — *see also* Neoplasm, skin, face	C44.390	C79.2	D04.39	D23.39	D48.5	D49.2
column, spinal — *see* Neoplasm, spine						
commissure labial, lip	C00.6	C79.89	D00.01	D10.39	D37.01	D49.0
laryngeal	C32.0	C78.39	D02.0	D14.1	D38.0	D49.1
common (bile) duct	C24.0	C78.89	D01.5	D13.5	D37.6	D49.0
concha — *see also* Neoplasm, skin, ear	C44.20-✓	C79.2	D04.2-✓	D23.2-✓	D48.5	D49.2
nose	C30.0	C78.39	D02.3	D14.0	D38.5	D49.1
conjunctiva	C69.0-✓	C79.49	D09.2-✓	D31.0-✓	D48.7	D49.89

Neoplasm, neoplastic — continued

	Malignant Primary	Malignant Secondary	Ca in situ	Benign	Uncertain	Unspecified Behavior
connective tissue NEC	C49.9	C79.89	—	D21.9	D48.1	D49.2

Note: For neoplasms of connective tissue (blood vessel, bursa, fascia, ligament, muscle, peripheral nerves, sympathetic and parasympathetic nerves and ganglia, synovia, tendon, etc.) or of morphological types that indicate connective tissue, code according to the list under "Neoplasm, connective tissue". For sites that do not appear in this list, code to neoplasm of that site; e.g., fibrosarcoma, pancreas (C25.9)

Note: Morphological types that indicate connective tissue appear in their proper place in the alphabetic index with the instruction "see Neoplasm, connective tissue ...."

	Malignant Primary	Malignant Secondary	Ca in situ	Benign	Uncertain	Unspecified Behavior
abdomen	C49.4	C79.89	—	D21.4	D48.1	D49.2
abdominal wall	C49.4	C79.89	—	D21.4	D48.1	D49.2
ankle	C49.2-✓	C79.89	—	D21.2-✓	D48.1	D49.2
antecubital fossa or space	C49.1-✓	C79.89	—	D21.1-✓	D48.1	D49.2
arm	C49.1-✓	C79.89	—	D21.1-✓	D48.1	D49.2
auricle (ear)	C49.0	C79.89	—	D21.0	D48.1	D49.2
axilla	C49.3	C79.89	—	D21.3	D48.1	D49.2
back	C49.6	C79.89	—	D21.6	D48.1	D49.2
breast — *see* Neoplasm, breast						
buttock	C49.5	C79.89	—	D21.5	D48.1	D49.2
calf	C49.2-✓	C79.89	—	D21.2-✓	D48.1	D49.2
cervical region	C49.0	C79.89	—	D21.0	D48.1	D49.2
cheek	C49.0	C79.89	—	D21.0	D48.1	D49.2
chest (wall)	C49.3	C79.89	—	D21.3	D48.1	D49.2
chin	C49.0	C79.89	—	D21.0	D48.1	D49.2
diaphragm	C49.3	C79.89	—	D21.3	D48.1	D49.2
ear (external)	C49.0	C79.89	—	D21.0	D48.1	D49.2
elbow	C49.1-✓	C79.89	—	D21.1-✓	D48.1	D49.2
extrarectal	C49.5	C79.89	—	D21.5	D48.1	D49.2
extremity	C49.9	C79.89	—	D21.9	D48.1	D49.2
lower	C49.2-✓	C79.89	—	D21.2-✓	D48.1	D49.2
upper	C49.1-✓	C79.89	—	D21.1-✓	D48.1	D49.2
eyelid	C49.0	C79.89	—	D21.0	D48.1	D49.2
face	C49.0	C79.89	—	D21.0	D48.1	D49.2
finger	C49.1-✓	C79.89	—	D21.1-✓	D48.1	D49.2
flank	C49.6	C79.89	—	D21.6	D48.1	D49.2
foot	C49.2-✓	C79.89	—	D21.2-✓	D48.1	D49.2
forearm	C49.1-✓	C79.89	—	D21.1-✓	D48.1	D49.2
forehead	C49.0	C79.89	—	D21.0	D48.1	D49.2
gastric	C49.4	C79.89	—	D21.4	D48.1	D49.2
gastrointestinal	C49.4	C79.89	—	D21.4	D48.1	D49.2
gluteal region	C49.5	C79.89	—	D21.5	D48.1	D49.2
great vessels NEC	C49.3	C79.89	—	D21.3	D48.1	D49.2
groin	C49.5	C79.89	—	D21.5	D48.1	D49.2
hand	C49.1-✓	C79.89	—	D21.1-✓	D48.1	D49.2
head	C49.0	C79.89	—	D21.0	D48.1	D49.2
heel	C49.2-✓	C79.89	—	D21.2-✓	D48.1	D49.2
hip	C49.2-✓	C79.89	—	D21.2-✓	D48.1	D49.2
hypochondrium	C49.4	C79.89	—	D21.4	D48.1	D49.2
iliopsoas muscle	C49.5	C79.89	—	D21.5	D48.1	D49.2
infraclavicular region	C49.3	C79.89	—	D21.3	D48.1	D49.2
inguinal (canal) (region)	C49.5	C79.89	—	D21.5	D48.1	D49.2
intestinal	C49.4	C79.89	—	D21.4	D48.1	D49.2
intrathoracic	C49.3	C79.89	—	D21.3	D48.1	D49.2
ischiorectal fossa	C49.5	C79.89	—	D21.5	D48.1	D49.2
jaw	C03.9	C79.89	D00.03	D10.39	D48.1	D49.0
knee	C49.2-✓	C79.89	—	D21.2-✓	D48.1	D49.2
leg	C49.2-✓	C79.89	—	D21.2-✓	D48.1	D49.2
limb NEC	C49.9	C79.89	—	D21.9	D48.1	D49.2
lower	C49.2-✓	C79.89	—	D21.2-✓	D48.1	D49.2
upper	C49.1-✓	C79.89	—	D21.1-✓	D48.1	D49.2
nates	C49.5	C79.89	—	D21.5	D48.1	D49.2
neck	C49.0	C79.89	—	D21.0	D48.1	D49.2
orbit	C69.6-✓	C79.49	D09.2-✓	D31.6-✓	D48.1	D49.89
overlapping lesion	C49.8	—	—	—	—	—
para-urethral	C49.5	C79.89	—	D21.5	D48.1	D49.2
pararectal	C49.5	C79.89	—	D21.5	D48.1	D49.2
paravaginal	C49.5	C79.89	—	D21.5	D48.1	D49.2
pelvis (floor)	C49.5	C79.89	—	D21.5	D48.1	D49.2
pelvo-abdominal	C49.8	C79.89	—	D21.6	D48.1	D49.2
perineum	C49.5	C79.89	—	D21.5	D48.1	D49.2
perirectal (tissue)	C49.5	C79.89	—	D21.5	D48.1	D49.2

☑ Additional Character Required — Refer to the Tabular List for Character Selection   ▽ Subterms under main terms may continue to next column or page

Neoplasm, neoplastic —	Malignant Primary	Malignant Secondary	Ca in situ	Benign	Uncertain	Unspecified Behavior
continued						
connective tissue —						
continued						
periurethral						
(tissue)	C49.5	C79.89	—	D21.5	D48.1	D49.2
popliteal fossa or						
space	C49.2-☑	C79.89	—	D21.2-☑	D48.1	D49.2
presacral	C49.5	C79.89	—	D21.5	D48.1	D49.2
psoas muscle	C49.4	C79.89	—	D21.4	D48.1	D49.2
pterygoid fossa	C49.0	C79.89	—	D21.0	D48.1	D49.2
rectovaginal septum or						
wall	C49.5	C79.89	—	D21.5	D48.1	D49.2
rectovesical	C49.5	C79.89	—	D21.5	D48.1	D49.2
retroperitoneum	C48.0	C78.6	—	D20.0	D48.3	D49.0
sacrococcygeal						
region	C49.5	C79.89	—	D21.5	D48.1	D49.2
scalp	C49.0	C79.89	—	D21.0	D48.1	D49.2
scapular region	C49.3	C79.89	—	D21.3	D48.1	D49.2
shoulder	C49.1-☑	C79.89	—	D21.1-☑	D48.1	D49.2
skin (dermis) NEC — *see also* Neoplasm, skin,						
by site	C44.90	C79.2	D04.9	D23.9	D48.5	D49.2
stomach	C49.4	C79.89	—	D21.4	D48.1	D49.2
submental	C49.0	C79.89	—	D21.0	D48.1	D49.2
supraclavicular						
region	C49.0	C79.89	—	D21.0	D48.1	D49.2
temple	C49.0	C79.89	—	D21.0	D48.1	D49.2
temporal region	C49.0	C79.89	—	D21.0	D48.1	D49.2
thigh	C49.2-☑	C79.89	—	D21.2-☑	D48.1	D49.2
thoracic (duct)						
(wall)	C49.3	C79.89	—	D21.3	D48.1	D49.2
thorax	C49.3	C79.89	—	D21.3	D48.1	D49.2
thumb	C49.1-☑	C79.89	—	D21.1-☑	D48.1	D49.2
toe	C49.2-☑	C79.89	—	D21.2-☑	D48.1	D49.2
trunk	C49.6	C79.89	—	D21.6	D48.1	D49.2
umbilicus	C49.4	C79.89	—	D21.4	D48.1	D49.2
vesicorectal	C49.5	C79.89	—	D21.5	D48.1	D49.2
wrist	C49.1-☑	C79.89	—	D21.1-☑	D48.1	D49.2
conus medullaris	C72.0	C79.49	—	D33.4	D43.4	D49.7
cord (true) (vocal)	C32.0	C78.39	D02.0	D14.0	D38.0	D49.1
false	C32.1	C78.39	D02.0	D14.1	D38.0	D49.1
spermatic	C63.1-☑	C79.82	D07.69	D29.8	D40.8	D49.5
spinal (cervical)						
(lumbar)						
(thoracic)	C72.0	C79.49	—	D33.4	D43.4	D49.7
cornea (limbus)	C69.1-☑	C79.49	D09.2-☑	D31.1-☑	D48.7	D49.89
corpus						
albicans	C56.-☑	C79.6-☑	D07.39	D27.-☑	D39.1-☑	D49.5
callosum, brain	C71.0	C79.31	—	D33.2	D43.2	D49.6
cavernosum	C60.2	C79.82	D07.4	D29.0	D40.8	D49.5
gastric	C16.2	C78.89	D00.2	D13.1	D37.1	D49.0
overlapping sites	C54.8	—	—	—	—	—
penis	C60.2	C79.82	D07.4	D29.0	D40.8	D49.5
striatum,						
cerebrum	C71.0	C79.31	—	D33.0	D43.0	D49.6
uteri	C54.9	C79.82	D07.0	D26.1	D39.0	D49.5
isthmus	C54.0	C79.82	D07.0	D26.1	D39.0	D49.5
cortex						
adrenal	C74.0-☑	C79.7-☑	D09.3	D35.0-☑	D44.1-☑	D49.7
cerebral	C71.0	C79.31	—	D33.0	D43.0	D49.6
costal cartilage	C41.3	C79.51	—	D16.7	D48.0	D49.2
costovertebral joint	C41.3	C79.51	—	D16.7	D48.0	D49.2
Cowper's gland	C68.0	C79.19	D09.19	D30.4	D41.3	D49.5
cranial (fossa, any)	C71.9	C79.31	—	D33.2	D43.2	D49.6
meninges	C70.0	C79.32	—	D32.0	D42.0	D49.7
nerve	C72.50	C79.49	—	D33.3	D43.3	D49.7
specified NEC	C72.59	C79.49	—	D33.3	D43.3	D49.7
craniobuccal pouch	C75.2	C79.89	D09.3	D35.2	D44.3	D49.7
craniopharyngeal (duct)						
(pouch)	C75.2	C79.89	D09.3	D35.3	D44.4	D49.7
cricoid	C13.0	C79.89	D00.08	D10.7	D37.05	D49.0
cartilage	C32.3	C78.39	D02.0	D14.1	D38.0	D49.1
cricopharynx	C13.0	C79.89	D00.08	D10.7	D37.05	D49.0
crypt of Morgagni	C21.8	C78.5	D01.3	D12.9	D37.8	D49.0
crystalline lens	C69.4-☑	C79.49	D09.2-☑	D31.4-☑	D48.7	D49.89
cul-de-sac						
(Douglas')	C48.1	C78.6	—	D20.1	D48.4	D49.0
cuneiform cartilage	C32.3	C78.39	D02.0	D14.1	D38.0	D49.1
cutaneous — *see* Neoplasm, skin						
cutis — *see* Neoplasm, skin						

Neoplasm, neoplastic —	Malignant Primary	Malignant Secondary	Ca in situ	Benign	Uncertain	Unspecified Behavior
continued						
cystic (bile) duct						
(common)	C24.0	C78.89	D01.5	D13.5	D37.6	D49.0
dermis — *see* Neoplasm, skin						
diaphragm	C49.3	C79.89	—	D21.3	D48.1	D49.2
digestive organs, system, tube, or tract						
NEC	C26.9	C78.89	D01.9	D13.9	D37.9	D49.0
disc, intervertebral	C41.2	C79.51	—	D16.6	D48.0	D49.2
disease, generalized	C80.0	—	—	—	—	—
disseminated	C80.0	—	—	—	—	—
Douglas' cul-de-sac or						
pouch	C48.1	C78.6	—	D20.1	D48.4	D49.0
duodenojejunal						
junction	C17.8	C78.4	D01.49	D13.39	D37.2	D49.0
duodenum	C17.0	C78.4	D01.49	D13.2	D37.2	D49.0
dura (cranial)						
(mater)	C70.9	C79.49	—	D32.9	D42.9	D49.7
cerebral	C70.0	C79.32	—	D32.0	D42.0	D49.7
spinal	C70.1	C79.49	—	D32.1	D42.1	D49.7
ear (external) — *see also* Neoplasm, skin,						
ear	C44.20-☑	C79.2	D04.2-☑	D23.2-☑	D48.5	D49.2
auricle or auris — *see also* Neoplasm, skin,						
ear	C44.20-☑	C79.2	D04.2-☑	D23.2-☑	D48.5	D49.2
canal, external — *see also* Neoplasm, skin,						
ear	C44.20-☑	C79.2	D04.2-☑	D23.2-☑	D48.5	D49.2
cartilage	C49.0	C79.89	—	D21.0	D48.1	D49.2
external meatus — *see also* Neoplasm, skin,						
ear	C44.20-☑	C79.2	D04.2-☑	D23.2-☑	D48.5	D49.2
inner	C30.1	C78.39	D02.3	D14.0	D38.5	D49.1
lobule — *see also* Neoplasm, skin,						
ear	C44.20-☑	C79.2	D04.2-☑	D23.2-☑	D48.5	D49.2
middle	C30.1	C78.39	D02.3	D14.0	D38.5	D49.1
overlapping lesion with accessory						
sinuses	C31.8	—	—	—	—	—
skin	C44.20-☑	C79.2	D04.2-☑	D23.2-☑	D48.5	D49.2
basal cell						
carcinoma	C44.21-☑	—	—	—	—	—
specified type						
NEC	C44.29-☑	—	—	—	—	—
squamous cell						
carcinoma	C44.22-☑	—	—	—	—	—
earlobe	C44.20-☑	C79.2	D04.2-☑	D23.2-☑	D48.5	D49.2
basal cell						
carcinoma	C44.21-☑	—	—	—	—	—
specified type NEC	C44.29-☑	—	—	—	—	—
squamous cell						
carcinoma	C44.22-☑	—	—	—	—	—
ejaculatory duct	C63.7	C79.82	D07.69	D29.8	D40.8	D49.5
elbow NEC	C76.4-☑	C79.89	D04.6-☑	D36.7	D48.7	D49.89
endocardium	C38.0	C79.89	—	D15.1	D48.7	D49.89
endocervix (canal)						
(gland)	C53.0	C79.82	D06.0	D26.0	D39.0	D49.5
endocrine gland						
NEC	C75.9	C79.89	D09.3	D35.9	D44.9	D49.7
pluriglandular	C75.8	C79.89	D09.3	D35.7	D44.9	D49.7
endometrium (gland)						
(stroma)	C54.1	C79.82	D07.0	D26.1	D39.0	D49.5
ensiform cartilage	C41.3	C79.51	—	D16.7	D48.0	D49.2
enteric — *see* Neoplasm, intestine						
ependyma (brain)	C71.5	C79.31	—	D33.0	D43.0	D49.6
fourth ventricle	C71.7	C79.31	—	D33.1	D43.1	D49.6
epicardium	C38.0	C79.89	—	D15.1	D48.7	D49.89
epididymis	C63.0-☑	C79.82	D07.69	D29.3-☑	D40.8	D49.5
epidural	C72.9	C79.49	—	D33.9	D43.9	D49.7
epiglottis	C32.1	C78.39	D02.0	D14.1	D38.0	D49.1
anterior aspect or						
surface	C10.1	C79.89	D00.08	D10.5	D37.05	D49.0
cartilage	C32.3	C78.39	D02.0	D14.1	D38.0	D49.1
free border						
(margin)	C10.1	C79.89	D00.08	D10.5	D37.05	D49.0
junctional region	C10.8	C79.89	D00.08	D10.5	D37.05	D49.0
posterior (laryngeal)						
surface	C32.1	C78.39	D02.0	D14.1	D38.0	D49.1

Neoplasm, neoplastic —
continued

	Malignant Primary	Malignant Secondary	Ca in situ	Benign	Uncertain	Unspecified Behavior
epiglottis — *continued*						
suprahyoid portion	C32.1	C78.39	D02.0	D14.1	D38.0	D49.1
esophagogastric junction	C16.0	C78.89	D00.2	D13.1	D37.1	D49.0
esophagus	C15.9	C78.89	D00.1	D13.0	D37.8	D49.0
abdominal	C15.5	C78.89	D00.1	D13.0	D37.8	D49.0
cervical	C15.3	C78.89	D00.1	D13.0	D37.8	D49.0
distal (third)	C15.5	C78.89	D00.1	D13.0	D37.8	D49.0
lower (third)	C15.5	C78.89	D00.1	D13.0	D37.8	D49.0
middle (third)	C15.4	C78.89	D00.1	D13.0	D37.8	D49.0
overlapping lesion	C15.8	—	—	—	—	—
proximal (third)	C15.3	C78.89	D00.1	D13.0	D37.8	D49.0
thoracic	C15.4	C78.89	D00.1	D13.0	D37.8	D49.0
upper (third)	C15.3	C78.89	D00.1	D13.0	D37.8	D49.0
ethmoid (sinus)	C31.1	C78.39	D02.3	D14.0	D38.5	D49.1
bone or labyrinth	C41.0	C79.51	—	D16.4-	D48.0	D49.2
eustachian tube	C30.1	C78.39	D02.3	D14.0	D38.5	D49.1
exocervix	C53.1	C79.82	D06.1	D26.0	D39.0	D49.5
external						
meatus (ear) — *see also* Neoplasm, skin, ear	C44.20-✓	C79.2	D04.2-✓	D23.2-✓	D48.5	D49.2
os, cervix uteri	C53.1	C79.82	D06.1	D26.0	D39.0	D49.5
extradural	C72.9	C79.49	—	D33.9	D43.9	D49.7
extrahepatic (bile) duct	C24.0	C78.89	D01.5	D13.5	D37.6	D49.0
overlapping lesion with gallbladder	C24.8	—	—	—	—	—
extraocular muscle	C69.6-✓	C79.49	D09.2-✓	D31.6-✓	D48.7	D49.89
extrarectal	C76.3	C79.89	D09.8	D36.7	D48.7	D49.89
extremity	C76.8	C79.89	D04.8	D36.7	D48.7	D49.89
lower	C76.5-✓	C79.89	D04.7-✓	D36.7	D48.7	D49.89
upper	C76.4-✓	C79.89	D04.6-✓	D36.7	D48.7	D49.89
eyeball	C69.9-✓	C79.49	D09.2-✓	D31.9-✓	D48.7	D49.89
eyebrow	C44.309	C79.2	D04.39	D23.39	D48.5	D49.2
basal cell carcinoma	C44.319	—				
specified type NEC	C44.399	—				
squamous cell carcinoma	C44.329	—				
eyelid (lower) (skin) (upper)	C44.10-✓					
basal cell carcinoma	C44.11-✓					
cartilage	C49.0	C79.89		D21.0	D48.1	D49.2
specified type NEC	C44.19-✓					
squamous cell carcinoma	C44.12-✓	—				
eye NEC	C69.9-✓	C79.49	D09.2✓	D31.9✓	D48.7	D49.89
overlapping sites	C69.8-✓					
face NEC	C76.0	C79.89	D04.39	D36.7	D48.7	D49.89
fallopian tube (accessory)	C57.0-✓	C79.82	D07.39	D28.2	D39.8	D49.5
falx (cerebella) (cerebri)	C70.0	C79.32	—	D32.0	D42.0	D49.7
fascia — *see also* Neoplasm, connective tissue						
palmar	C49.1-✓	C79.89	—	D21.1-✓	D48.1	D49.2
plantar	C49.2-✓	C79.89	—	D21.2-✓	D48.1	D49.2
fatty tissue — *see* Neoplasm, connective tissue						
fauces, faucial NEC	C10.9	C79.89	D00.08	D10.5	D37.05	D49.0
pillars	C09.1	C79.89	D00.08	D10.5	D37.05	D49.0
tonsil	C09.9	C79.89	D00.08	D10.4	D37.05	D49.0
femur (any part)	C40.2-✓	—	—	D16.2-✓	—	—
fetal membrane	C58	C79.82	D07.0	D26.7	D39.2	D49.5
fibrous tissue — *see* Neoplasm, connective tissue						
fibula (any part)	C40.2-✓	C79.51	—	D16.2-✓	—	—
filum terminale	C72.0	C79.49	—	D33.4	D43.4	D49.7
finger NEC	C76.4-✓	C79.89	D04.6-✓	D36.7	D48.7	D49.89
flank NEC	C76.8	C79.89	D04.5	D36.7	D48.7	D49.89
follicle, nabothian	C53.0	C79.82	D06.0	D26.0	D39.0	D49.5
foot NEC	C76.5-✓	C79.89	D04.7-✓	D36.7	D48.7	D49.89
forearm NEC	C76.4-✓	C79.89	D04.6-✓	D36.7	D48.7	D49.89
forehead (skin)	C44.309	C79.2	D04.39	D23.39	D48.5	D49.2

Neoplasm, neoplastic —
continued

	Malignant Primary	Malignant Secondary	Ca in situ	Benign	Uncertain	Unspecified Behavior
forehead — *continued*						
basal cell carcinoma	C44.319	—	—	—	—	—
specified type NEC	C44.399	—				
squamous cell carcinoma	C44.329	—				
foreskin	C60.0	C79.82	D07.4	D29.0	D40.8	D49.5
fornix						
pharyngeal	C11.3	C79.89	D00.08	D10.6	D37.05	D49.0
vagina	C52	C79.82	D07.2	D28.1	D39.8	D49.5
fossa (of)						
anterior (cranial)	C71.9	C79.31	—	D33.2	D43.2	D49.6
cranial	C71.9	C79.31	—	D33.2	D43.2	D49.6
ischiorectal	C76.3	C79.89	D09.8	D36.7	D48.7	D49.89
middle (cranial)	C71.9	C79.31	—	D33.2	D43.2	D49.6
piriform	C12	C79.89	D00.08	D10.7	D37.05	D49.0
pituitary	C75.1	C79.89	D09.3	D35.2	D44.3	D49.7
posterior (cranial)	C71.9	C79.31	—	D33.2	D43.2	D49.6
pterygoid	C49.0	C79.89	—	D21.0	D48.1	D49.2
pyriform	C12	C79.89	D00.08	D10.7	D37.05	D49.0
Rosenmuller	C11.2	C79.89	D00.08	D10.6	D37.05	D49.0
tonsillar	C09.0	C79.89	D00.08	D10.5	D37.05	D49.0
fourchette	C51.9	C79.82	D07.1	D28.0	D39.8	D49.5
frenulum						
labii — *see* Neoplasm, lip, internal						
linguae	C02.2	C79.89	D00.07	D10.1	D37.02	D49.0
frontal						
bone	C41.0	C79.51	—	D16.4-	D48.0	D49.2
lobe, brain	C71.1	C79.31	—	D33.0	D43.0	D49.6
pole	C71.1	C79.31	—	D33.0	D43.0	D49.6
sinus	C31.2	C78.39	D02.3	D14.0	D38.5	D49.1
fundus						
stomach	C16.1	C78.89	D00.2	D13.1	D37.1	D49.0
uterus	C54.3	C79.82	D07.0	D26.1	D39.0	D49.5
gallbladder	C23	C78.89	D01.5	D13.5	D37.6	D49.0
overlapping lesion with extrahepatic bile ducts	C24.8	—	—	—	—	—
gall duct (extrahepatic)	C24.0	C78.89	D01.5	D13.5	D37.6	D49.0
intrahepatic	C22.1	C78.7	D01.5	D13.4	D37.6	D49.0
ganglia — *see also* Neoplasm, nerve, peripheral	C47.9	C79.89	—	D36.10	D48.2	D49.2
basal	C71.0	C79.31	—	D33.0	D43.0	D49.6
cranial nerve	C72.50	C79.49	—	D33.3	D43.3	D49.7
Gartner's duct	C52	C79.82	D07.2	D28.1	D39.8	D49.5
gastric — *see* Neoplasm, stomach						
gastrocolic	C26.9	C78.89	D01.9	D13.9	D37.9	D49.0
gastroesophageal junction	C16.0	C78.89	D00.2	D13.1	D37.1	D49.0
gastrointestinal (tract) NEC	C26.9	C78.89	D01.9	D13.9	D37.9	D49.0
generalized	C80.0	—	—	—	—	—
genital organ or tract						
female NEC	C57.9	C79.82	D07.30	D28.9	D39.9	D49.5
overlapping lesion	C57.8	—	—	—	—	—
specified site NEC	C57.7	C79.82	D07.39	D28.7	D39.8	D49.5
male NEC	C63.9	C79.82	D07.60	D29.9	D40.9	D49.5
overlapping lesion	C63.8	—	—	—	—	—
specified site NEC	C63.7	C79.82	D07.69	D29.8	D40.8	D49.5
genitourinary tract						
female	C57.9	C79.82	D07.30	D28.9	D39.9	D49.5
male	C63.9	C79.82	D07.60	D29.9	D40.9	D49.5
gingiva (alveolar) (marginal)	C03.9	C79.89	D00.03	D10.39	D37.09	D49.0
lower	C03.1	C79.89	D00.03	D10.39	D37.09	D49.0
mandibular	C03.1	C79.89	D00.03	D10.39	D37.09	D49.0
maxillary	C03.0	C79.89	D00.03	D10.39	D37.09	D49.0
upper	C03.0	C79.89	D00.03	D10.39	D37.09	D49.0
gland, glandular (lymphatic) (system) — *see also* Neoplasm, lymph gland						
endocrine NEC	C75.9	C79.89	D09.3	D35.9	D44.9	D49.7

✓ Additional Character Required — Refer to the Tabular List for Character Selection   ▽ Subterms under main terms may continue to next column or page

Neoplasm, neoplastic — continued	Malignant Primary	Malignant Secondary	Ca in situ	Benign	Uncertain	Unspecified Behavior
gland, glandular — see also Neoplasm, lymph gland — continued						
salivary — see Neoplasm, salivary gland						
glans penis	C60.1	C79.82	D07.4	D29.0	D40.8	D49.5
globus pallidus	C71.0	C79.31	—	D33.0	D43.0	D49.6
glomus						
coccygeal	C49.5	C79.89	—	D21.5	D48.1	D49.2
jugularis	C75.5	C79.89	—	D35.6	D44.7	D49.7
glosso-epiglottic fold(s)	C10.1	C79.89	D00.08	D10.5	D37.05	D49.0
glossopalatine fold	C09.1	C79.89	D00.08	D10.5	D37.05	D49.0
glossopharyngeal sulcus	C09.0	C79.89	D00.08	D10.5	D37.05	D49.0
glottis	C32.0	C78.39	D02.0	D14.1	D38.0	D49.1
gluteal region	C76.3	C79.89	D04.5	D36.7	D48.7	D49.89
great vessels NEC	C49.3	C79.89	—	D21.3	D48.1	D49.2
groin NEC	C76.3	C79.89	D04.5	D36.7	D48.7	D49.89
gum	C03.9	C79.89	D00.03	D10.39	D37.09	D49.0
lower	C03.1	C79.89	D00.03	D10.39	D37.09	D49.0
upper	C03.0	C79.89	D00.03	D10.39	D37.09	D49.0
hand NEC	C76.4- ☑	C79.89	D04.6- ☑	D36.7	D48.7	D49.89
head NEC	C76.0	C79.89	D04.4	D36.7	D48.7	D49.89
heart	C38.0	C79.89	—	D15.1	D48.7	D49.89
heel NEC	C76.5- ☑	C79.89	D04.7- ☑	D36.7	D48.7	D49.89
helix — see also Neoplasm, skin, ear	C44.20- ☑	C79.2	D04.2- ☑	D23.2- ☑	D48.5	D49.2
hematopoietic, hemopoietic tissue NEC	C96.9	—	—	—	—	—
specified NEC	C96.Z	—	—	—	—	—
hemisphere, cerebral	C71.0	C79.31	—	D33.0	D43.0	D49.6
hemorrhoidal zone	C21.1	C78.5	D01.3	D12.9	D37.8	D49.0
hepatic — see also Index to disease, by histology	C22.9	C78.7	D01.5	D13.4	D37.6	D49.0
duct (bile)	C24.0	C78.89	D01.5	D13.5	D37.6	D49.0
flexure (colon)	C18.3	C78.5	D01.0	D12.3	D37.4	D49.0
primary	C22.8	C78.7	D01.5	D13.4	D37.6	D49.0
hepatobiliary	C24.9	C78.89	D01.5	D13.5	D37.6	D49.0
hepatoblastoma	C22.2	C78.7	D01.5	D13.4	D37.6	D49.0
hepatoma	C22.0	C78.7	D01.5	D13.4	D37.6	D49.0
hilus of lung	C34.0- ☑	C78.0- ☑	D02.2- ☑	D14.3- ☑	D38.1	D49.1
hippocampus, brain	C71.2	C79.31	—	D33.0	D43.0	D49.6
hip NEC	C76.5- ☑	C79.89	D04.7- ☑	D36.7	D48.7	D49.89
humerus (any part)	C40.0- ☑	C79.51	—	D16.0- ☑	—	—
hymen	C52	C79.82	D07.2	D28.1	D39.8	D49.5
hypopharynx, hypopharyngeal NEC	C13.9	C79.89	D00.08	D10.7	D37.05	D49.0
overlapping lesion	C13.8	—	—	—	—	—
postcricoid region	C13.0	C79.89	D00.08	D10.7	D37.05	D49.0
posterior wall	C13.2	C79.89	D00.08	D10.7	D37.05	D49.0
pyriform fossa (sinus)	C12	C79.89	D00.08	D10.7	D37.05	D49.0
hypophysis	C75.1	C79.89	D09.3	D35.2	D44.3	D49.7
hypothalamus	C71.0	C79.31	—	D33.0	D43.0	D49.6
ileocecum, ileocecal (coil) (junction) (valve)	C18.0	C78.5	D01.0	D12.0	D37.4	D49.0
ileum	C17.2	C78.4	D01.49	D13.39	D37.2	D49.0
ilium	C41.4	C79.51	—	D16.8	D48.0	D49.2
immunoproliferative NEC	C88.9	—	—	—	—	—
infraclavicular (region)	C76.1	C79.89	D04.5	D36.7	D48.7	D49.89
inguinal (region)	C76.3	C79.89	D04.5	D36.7	D48.7	D49.89
insula	C71.0	C79.31	—	D33.0	D43.0	D49.6
insular tissue (pancreas)	C25.4	C78.89	D01.7	D13.7	D37.8	D49.0
brain	C71.0	C79.31	—	D33.0	D43.0	D49.6
interarytenoid fold	C13.1	C78.39	D00.08	D10.7	D37.05	D49.0
hypopharyngeal aspect	C13.1	C79.89	D00.08	D10.7	D37.05	D49.0
laryngeal aspect	C32.1	C78.39	D02.0	D14.1	D38.0	D49.1
marginal zone	C13.1	C79.89	D00.08	D10.7	D37.05	D49.0
interdental papillae	C03.9	C79.89	D00.03	D10.39	D37.09	D49.0

Neoplasm, neoplastic — continued	Malignant Primary	Malignant Secondary	Ca in situ	Benign	Uncertain	Unspecified Behavior
interdental papillae — continued						
lower	C03.1	C79.89	D00.03	D10.39	D37.09	D49.0
upper	C03.0	C79.89	D00.03	D10.39	D37.09	D49.0
internal						
capsule	C71.0	C79.31	—	D33.0	D43.0	D49.6
os (cervix)	C53.0	C79.82	D06.0	D26.0	D39.0	D49.5
intervertebral cartilage or disc	C41.2	C79.51	—	D16.6	D48.0	D49.2
intestine, intestinal	C26.0	C78.80	D01.40	D13.9	D37.8	D49.0
large	C18.9	C78.5	D01.0	D12.6	D37.4	D49.0
appendix	C18.1	C78.5	D01.0	D12.1	D37.3	D49.0
caput coli	C18.0	C78.5	D01.0	D12.0	D37.4	D49.0
cecum	C18.0	C78.5	D01.0	D12.0	D37.4	D49.0
colon	C18.9	C78.5	D01.0	D12.6	D37.4	D49.0
and rectum	C19	C78.5	D01.1	D12.7	D37.5	D49.0
ascending	C18.2	C78.5	D01.0	D12.2	D37.4	D49.0
caput	C18.0	C78.5	D01.0	D12.0	D37.4	D49.0
descending	C18.6	C78.5	D01.0	D12.4	D37.4	D49.0
distal	C18.6	C78.5	D01.0	D12.4	D37.4	D49.0
left	C18.6	C78.5	D01.0	D12.4	D37.4	D49.0
overlapping lesion	C18.8	—	—	—	—	—
pelvic	C18.7	C78.5	D01.0	D12.5	D37.4	D49.0
right	C18.2	C78.5	D01.0	D12.2	D37.4	D49.0
sigmoid (flexure)	C18.7	C78.5	D01.0	D12.5	D37.4	D49.0
transverse	C18.4	C78.5	D01.0	D12.3	D37.4	D49.0
hepatic flexure	C18.3	C78.5	D01.0	D12.3	D37.4	D49.0
ileocecum, ileocecal (coil) (valve)	C18.0	C78.5	D01.0	D12.0	D37.4	D49.0
overlapping lesion	C18.8	—	—	—	—	—
sigmoid flexure (lower) (upper)	C18.7	C78.5	D01.0	D12.5	D37.4	D49.0
splenic flexure	C18.5	C78.5	D01.0	D12.3	D37.4	D49.0
small	C17.9	C78.4	D01.40	D13.30	D37.2	D49.0
duodenum	C17.0	C78.4	D01.49	D13.2	D37.2	D49.0
ileum	C17.2	C78.4	D01.49	D13.39	D37.2	D49.0
jejunum	C17.1	C78.4	D01.49	D13.39	D37.2	D49.0
overlapping lesion	C17.8	—	—	—	—	—
tract NEC	C26.0	C78.89	D01.40	D13.9	D37.8	D49.0
intra-abdominal	C76.2	C79.89	D09.8	D36.7	D48.7	D49.89
intracranial NEC	C71.9	C79.31	—	D33.2	D43.2	D49.6
intrahepatic (bile) duct	C22.1	C78.7	D01.5	D13.4	D37.6	D49.0
intraocular	C69.9- ☑	C79.49	D09.2- ☑	D31.9- ☑	D48.7	D49.89
intraorbital	C69.6- ☑	C79.49	D09.2- ☑	D31.6- ☑	D48.7	D49.89
intrasellar	C75.1	C79.89	D09.3	D35.2	D44.3	D49.7
intrathoracic (cavity) (organs)	C76.1	C79.89	D09.8	D15.9	D48.7	D49.89
specified NEC	C76.1	C79.89	D09.8	D15.7	—	—
iris	C69.4- ☑	C79.49	D09.2- ☑	D31.4- ☑	D48.7	D49.89
ischiorectal (fossa)	C76.3	C79.89	D09.8	D36.7	D48.7	D49.89
ischium	C41.4	C79.51	—	D16.8	D48.0	D49.2
island of Reil	C71.0	C79.31	—	D33.0	D43.0	D49.6
islands or islets of Langerhans	C25.4	C78.89	D01.7	D13.7	D37.8	D49.0
isthmus uteri	C54.0	C79.82	D07.0	D26.1	D39.0	D49.5
jaw	C76.0	C79.89	D09.8	D36.7	D48.7	D49.89
bone	C41.1	C79.51	—	D16.5-	D48.0	D49.2
lower	C41.1	C79.51	—	D16.5-	—	—
upper	C41.0	C79.51	—	D16.4-	—	—
carcinoma (any type) (lower) (upper)	C76.0	C79.89	—	—	—	—
skin — see also Neoplasm, skin, face	C44.309	C79.2	D04.39	D23.39	D48.5	D49.2
soft tissues	C03.9	C79.89	D00.03	D10.39	D37.09	D49.0
lower	C03.1	C79.89	D00.03	D10.39	D37.09	D49.0
upper	C03.0	C79.89	D00.03	D10.39	D37.09	D49.0
jejunum	C17.1	C78.4	D01.49	D13.39	D37.2	D49.0
joint NEC — see also Neoplasm, bone	C41.9	C79.51	—	D16.9-	D48.0	D49.2
acromioclavicular	C40.0- ☑	C79.51	—	D16.0- ☑	—	—
bursa or synovial membrane — see						

Neoplasm, neoplastic —	Malignant Primary	Malignant Secondary	Ca in situ	Benign	Uncertain	Unspecified Behavior
continued						
joint — *see also*						
Neoplasm, bone —						
continued						
bursa or synovial						
membrane — *see*						
Neoplasm,						
connective tissue						
— *continued*						
Neoplasm,						
connective tissue						
costovertebral	C41.3	C79.51	—	D16.7	D48.0	D49.2
sternocostal	C41.3	C79.51	—	D16.7	D48.0	D49.2
temporomandibular	C41.1	C79.51	—	D16.5-	D48.0	D49.2
junction						
anorectal	C21.8	C78.5	D01.3	D12.9	D37.8	D49.0
cardioesophageal	C16.0	C78.89	D00.2	D13.1	D37.1	D49.0
esophagogastric	C16.0	C78.89	D00.2	D13.1	D37.1	D49.0
gastroesophageal	C16.0	C78.89	D00.2	D13.1	D37.1	D49.0
hard and soft						
palate	C05.9	C79.89	D00.00	D10.39	D37.09	D49.0
ileocecal	C18.0	C78.5	D01.0	D12.0	D37.4	D49.0
pelvirectal	C19	C78.5	D01.1	D12.7	D37.5	D49.0
pelviureteric	C65.-☑	C79.0-☑	D09.19	D30.1-☑	D41.1-☑	D49.5
rectosigmoid	C19	C78.5	D01.1	D12.7	D37.5	D49.0
squamocolumnar, of						
cervix	C53.8	C79.82	D06.7	D26.0	D39.0	D49.5
Kaposi's sarcoma — *see*						
Kaposi's, sarcoma						
kidney						
(parenchymal)	C64.-☑	C79.0-☑	D09.19	D30.0-☑	D41.0-☑	D49.5
calyx	C65.-☑	C79.0-☑	D09.19	D30.1-☑	D41.1-☑	D49.5
hilus	C65.-☑	C79.0-☑	D09.19	D30.1-☑	D41.1-☑	D49.5
pelvis	C65.-☑	C79.0-☑	D09.19	D30.1-☑	D41.1-☑	D49.5
knee NEC	C76.5-☑	C79.89	D04.7-☑	D36.7	D48.7	D49.89
labia (skin)	C51.9	C79.82	D07.1	D28.0	D39.8	D49.5
majora	C51.0	C79.82	D07.1	D28.0	D39.8	D49.5
minora	C51.1	C79.82	D07.1	D28.0	D39.8	D49.5
labial — *see also*						
Neoplasm, lip	C00.9	C79.89	D00.01	D10.0	D37.01	D49.0
sulcus (lower)						
(upper)	C06.1	C79.89	D00.02	D10.39	D37.09	D49.0
labium (skin)	C51.9	C79.82	D07.1	D28.0	D39.8	D49.5
majus	C51.0	C79.82	D07.1	D28.0	D39.8	D49.5
minus	C51.1	C79.82	D07.1	D28.0	D39.8	D49.5
lacrimal						
canaliculi	C69.5-☑	C79.49	D09.2-☑	D31.5-☑	D48.7	D49.89
duct (nasal)	C69.5-☑	C79.49	D09.2-☑	D31.5-☑	D48.7	D49.89
gland	C69.5-☑	C79.49	D09.2-☑	D31.5-☑	D48.7	D49.89
punctum	C69.5-☑	C79.49	D09.2-☑	D31.5-☑	D48.7	D49.89
sac	C69.5-☑	C79.49	D09.2-☑	D31.5-☑	D48.7	D49.89
Langerhans, islands or						
islets	C25.4	C78.89	D01.7	D13.7	D37.8	D49.0
laryngopharynx	C13.9	C79.89	D00.08	D10.7	D37.05	D49.0
larynx, laryngeal						
NEC	C32.9	C78.39	D02.0	D14.1	D38.0	D49.1
aryepiglottic fold	C32.1	C78.39	D02.0	D14.1	D38.0	D49.1
cartilage (arytenoid)						
(cricoid)						
(cuneiform)						
(thyroid)	C32.3	C78.39	D02.0	D14.1	D38.0	D49.1
commissure (anterior)						
(posterior)	C32.0	C78.39	D02.0	D14.1	D38.0	D49.1
extrinsic NEC	C32.1	C78.39	D02.0	D14.1	D38.0	D49.1
meaning						
hypopharynx	C13.9	C79.89	D00.08	D10.7	D37.05	D49.0
interarytenoid fold	C32.1	C78.39	D02.0	D14.1	D38.0	D49.1
intrinsic	C32.0	C78.39	D02.0	D14.1	D38.0	D49.1
overlapping lesion	C32.8	—	—	—	—	—
ventricular band	C32.1	C78.39	D02.0	D14.1	D38.0	D49.1
leg NEC	C76.5-☑	C79.89	D04.7-☑	D36.7	D48.7	D49.89
lens, crystalline	C69.4-☑	C79.49	D09.2-☑	D31.4-☑	D48.7	D49.89
lid (lower) (upper)	C44.10-☑	C79.2	D04.1-☑	D23.1-☑	D48.5	D49.2
basal cell						
carcinoma	C44.11-☑	—	—	—	—	—
specified type NEC	C44.19-☑	—	—	—	—	—
squamous cell						
carcinoma	C44.12-☑	—	—	—	—	—
ligament — *see also*						
Neoplasm, connective						
tissue						

Neoplasm, neoplastic —	Malignant Primary	Malignant Secondary	Ca in situ	Benign	Uncertain	Unspecified Behavior
continued						
ligament — *see also*						
Neoplasm, connective						
tissue — *continued*						
broad	C57.1☑	C79.82	D07.39	D28.2	D39.8	D49.5
Mackenrodt's	C57.7	C79.82	D07.39	D28.7	D39.8	D49.5
non-uterine — *see*						
Neoplasm,						
connective tissue						
round	C57.2☑	C79.82	—	D28.2	D39.8	D49.5
sacro-uterine	C57.3	C79.82	—	D28.2	D39.8	D49.5
uterine	C57.3	C79.82	—	D28.2	D39.8	D49.5
utero-ovarian	C57.7	C79.82	D07.39	D28.2	D39.8	D49.5
uterosacral	C57.3	C79.82	—	D28.2	D39.8	D49.5
limb	C76.8	C79.89	D04.8	D36.7	D48.7	D49.89
lower	C76.5-☑	C79.89	D04.7-☑	D36.7	D48.7	D49.89
upper	C76.4-☑	C79.89	D04.6-☑	D36.7	D48.7	D49.89
limbus of cornea	C69.1-☑	C79.49	D09.2-☑	D31.1-☑	D48.7	D49.89
lingual NEC — *see also*						
Neoplasm,						
tongue	C02.9	C79.89	D00.07	D10.1	D37.02	D49.0
lingula, lung	C34.1-☑	C78.0-☑	D02.2-☑	D14.3-☑	D38.1	D49.1
lip	C00.9	C79.89	D00.01	D10.0	D37.01	D49.0
buccal aspect — *see*						
Neoplasm, lip,						
internal						
commissure	C00.6	C79.89	D00.01	D10.0	D37.01	D49.0
external	C00.2	C79.89	D00.01	D10.0	D37.01	D49.0
lower	C00.1	C79.89	D00.01	D10.0	D37.01	D49.0
upper	C00.0	C79.89	D00.01	D10.0	D37.01	D49.0
frenulum — *see*						
Neoplasm, lip,						
internal						
inner aspect — *see*						
Neoplasm, lip,						
internal						
internal	C00.5	C79.89	D00.01	D10.0	D37.01	D49.0
lower	C00.4	C79.89	D00.01	D10.0	D37.01	D49.0
upper	C00.3	C79.89	D00.01	D10.0	D37.01	D49.0
lipstick area	C00.2	C79.89	D00.01	D10.0	D37.01	D49.0
lower	C00.1	C79.89	D00.01	D10.0	D37.01	D49.0
upper	C00.0	C79.89	D00.01	D10.0	D37.01	D49.0
lower	C00.1	C79.89	D00.01	D10.0	D37.01	D49.0
internal	C00.4	C79.89	D00.01	D10.0	D37.01	D49.0
mucosa — *see*						
Neoplasm, lip,						
internal						
oral aspect — *see*						
Neoplasm, lip,						
internal						
overlapping lesion	C00.8	—	—	—	—	—
with oral cavity or						
pharynx	C14.8	—	—	—	—	—
skin (commissure)						
(lower)						
(upper)	C44.00	C79.2	D04.0	D23.0	D48.5	D49.2
basal cell						
carcinoma	C44.01	—	—	—	—	—
specified type						
NEC	C44.09	—	—	—	—	—
squamous cell						
carcinoma	C44.02	—	—	—	—	—
upper	C00.0	C79.89	D00.01	D10.0	D37.01	D49.0
internal	C00.3	C79.89	D00.01	D10.0	D37.01	D49.0
vermilion border	C00.2	C79.89	D00.01	D10.0	D37.01	D49.0
lower	C00.1	C79.89	D00.01	D10.0	D37.01	D49.0
upper	C00.0	C79.89	D00.01	D10.0	D37.01	D49.0
lipomatous — *see*						
Lipoma, by site						
liver — *see also* Index to						
disease, by						
histology	C22.9	C78.7	D01.5	D13.4	D37.6	D49.0
primary	C22.8	C78.7	D01.5	D13.4	D37.6	D49.0
lumbosacral plexus	C47.5	C79.89	—	D36.16	D48.2	D49.2
lung	C34.9-☑	C78.0-☑	D02.2-☑	D14.3-☑	D38.1	D49.1
azygos lobe	C34.1-☑	C78.0-☑	D02.2-☑	D14.3-☑	D38.1	D49.1
carina	C34.0-☑	C78.0-☑	D02.2-☑	D14.3-☑	D38.1	D49.1
hilus	C34.0-☑	C78.0-☑	D02.2-☑	D14.3-☑	D38.1	D49.1
lingula	C34.1-☑	C78.0-☑	D02.2-☑	D14.3-☑	D38.1	D49.1
lobe NEC	C34.9-☑	C78.0-☑	D02.2-☑	D14.3-☑	D38.1	D49.1
lower lobe	C34.3-☑	C78.0-☑	D02.2-☑	D14.3-☑	D38.1	D49.1

☑ Additional Character Required — Refer to the Tabular List for Character Selection   ▽ Subterms under main terms may continue to next column or page

Neoplasm, neoplastic —	Malignant Primary	Malignant Secondary	Ca in situ	Benign	Uncertain	Unspecified Behavior
continued						
lung — *continued*						
main bronchus	C34.0-☑	C78.0-☑	D02.2-☑	D14.3-☑	D38.1	D49.1
mesothelioma — *see* Mesothelioma						
middle lobe	C34.2	C78.0-☑	D02.21	D14.31	D38.1	D49.1
overlapping lesion	C34.8-☑	—	—	—	—	—
upper lobe	C34.1-☑	C78.0-☑	D02.2-☑	D14.3-☑	D38.1	D49.1
lymph, lymphatic channel						
NEC	C49.9	C79.89	—	D21.9	D48.1	D49.2
gland (secondary)	—	C77.9	—	D36.0	D48.7	D49.89
abdominal	—	C77.2	—	D36.0	D48.7	D49.89
aortic	—	C77.2	—	D36.0	D48.7	D49.89
arm	—	C77.3	—	D36.0	D48.7	D49.89
auricular (anterior)						
(posterior)	—	C77.0	—	D36.0	D48.7	D49.89
axilla, axillary	—	C77.3	—	D36.0	D48.7	D49.89
brachial	—	C77.3	—	D36.0	D48.7	D49.89
bronchial	—	C77.1	—	D36.0	D48.7	D49.89
bronchopulmonary	—	C77.1	—	D36.0	D48.7	D49.89
celiac	—	C77.2	—	D36.0	D48.7	D49.89
cervical	—	C77.0	—	D36.0	D48.7	D49.89
cervicofacial	—	C77.0	—	D36.0	D48.7	D49.89
Cloquet	—	C77.4	—	D36.0	D48.7	D49.89
colic	—	C77.2	—	D36.0	D48.7	D49.89
common duct	—	C77.2	—	D36.0	D48.7	D49.89
cubital	—	C77.3	—	D36.0	D48.7	D49.89
diaphragmatic	—	C77.1	—	D36.0	D48.7	D49.89
epigastric, inferior	—	C77.1	—	D36.0	D48.7	D49.89
epitrochlear	—	C77.3	—	D36.0	D48.7	D49.89
esophageal	—	C77.1	—	D36.0	D48.7	D49.89
face	—	C77.0	—	D36.0	D48.7	D49.89
femoral	—	C77.4	—	D36.0	D48.7	D49.89
gastric	—	C77.2	—	D36.0	D48.7	D49.89
groin	—	C77.4	—	D36.0	D48.7	D49.89
head	—	C77.0	—	D36.0	D48.7	D49.89
hepatic	—	C77.2	—	D36.0	D48.7	D49.89
hilar						
(pulmonary)	—	C77.1	—	D36.0	D48.7	D49.89
splenic	—	C77.2	—	D36.0	D48.7	D49.89
hypogastric	—	C77.5	—	D36.0	D48.7	D49.89
ileocolic	—	C77.2	—	D36.0	D48.7	D49.89
iliac	—	C77.5	—	D36.0	D48.7	D49.89
infraclavicular	—	C77.3	—	D36.0	D48.7	D49.89
inguina, inguinal	—	C77.4	—	D36.0	D48.7	D49.89
innominate	—	C77.1	—	D36.0	D48.7	D49.89
intercostal	—	C77.1	—	D36.0	D48.7	D49.89
intestinal	—	C77.2	—	D36.0	D48.7	D49.89
intrabdominal	—	C77.2	—	D36.0	D48.7	D49.89
intrapelvic	—	C77.5	—	D36.0	D48.7	D49.89
intrathoracic	—	C77.1	—	D36.0	D48.7	D49.89
jugular	—	C77.0	—	D36.0	D48.7	D49.89
leg	—	C77.4	—	D36.0	D48.7	D49.89
limb						
lower	—	C77.4	—	D36.0	D48.7	D49.89
upper	—	C77.3	—	D36.0	D48.7	D49.89
lower limb	—	C77.4	—	D36.0	D48.7	D49.89
lumbar	—	C77.2	—	D36.0	D48.7	D49.89
mandibular	—	C77.0	—	D36.0	D48.7	D49.89
mediastinal	—	C77.1	—	D36.0	D48.7	D49.89
mesenteric (inferior) (superior)	—	C77.2	—	D36.0	D48.7	D49.89
midcolic	—	C77.2	—	D36.0	D48.7	D49.89
multiple sites in categories C77.0-C77.5	—	C77.8	—	D36.0	D48.7	D49.89
neck	—	C77.0	—	D36.0	D48.7	D49.89
obturator	—	C77.5	—	D36.0	D48.7	D49.89
occipital	—	C77.0	—	D36.0	D48.7	D49.89
pancreatic	—	C77.2	—	D36.0	D48.7	D49.89
para-aortic	—	C77.2	—	D36.0	D48.7	D49.89
paracervical	—	C77.5	—	D36.0	D48.7	D49.89
parametrial	—	C77.5	—	D36.0	D48.7	D49.89
parasternal	—	C77.1	—	D36.0	D48.7	D49.89
parotid	—	C77.0	—	D36.0	D48.7	D49.89
pectoral	—	C77.3	—	D36.0	D48.7	D49.89
pelvic	—	C77.5	—	D36.0	D48.7	D49.89
peri-aortic	—	C77.2	—	D36.0	D48.7	D49.89
peripancreatic	—	C77.2	—	D36.0	D48.7	D49.89
popliteal	—	C77.4	—	D36.0	D48.7	D49.89
porta hepatis	—	C77.2	—	D36.0	D48.7	D49.89

Neoplasm, neoplastic —	Malignant Primary	Malignant Secondary	Ca in situ	Benign	Uncertain	Unspecified Behavior
continued						
lymph, lymphatic channel — *continued*						
gland — *continued*						
portal	—	C77.2	—	D36.0	D48.7	D49.89
preauricular	—	C77.0	—	D36.0	D48.7	D49.89
prelaryngeal	—	C77.0	—	D36.0	D48.7	D49.89
presymphysial	—	C77.5	—	D36.0	D48.7	D49.89
pretracheal	—	C77.0	—	D36.0	D48.7	D49.89
primary (any site) NEC	C96.9	—	—	—	—	—
pulmonary (hiler)	—	C77.1	—	D36.0	D48.7	D49.89
pyloric	—	C77.2	—	D36.0	D48.7	D49.89
retroperitoneal	—	C77.2	—	D36.0	D48.7	D49.89
retropharyngeal	—	C77.0	—	D36.0	D48.7	D49.89
Rosenmuller's	—	C77.4	—	D36.0	D48.7	D49.89
sacral	—	C77.5	—	D36.0	D48.7	D49.89
scalene	—	C77.0	—	D36.0	D48.7	D49.89
site NEC	—	C77.9	—	D36.0	D48.7	D49.89
splenic (hilar)	—	C77.2	—	D36.0	D48.7	D49.89
subclavicular	—	C77.3	—	D36.0	D48.7	D49.89
subinguinal	—	C77.4	—	D36.0	D48.7	D49.89
sublingual	—	C77.0	—	D36.0	D48.7	D49.89
submandibular	—	C77.0	—	D36.0	D48.7	D49.89
submaxillary	—	C77.0	—	D36.0	D48.7	D49.89
submental	—	C77.0	—	D36.0	D48.7	D49.89
subscapular	—	C77.3	—	D36.0	D48.7	D49.89
supraclavicular	—	C77.0	—	D36.0	D48.7	D49.89
thoracic	—	C77.1	—	D36.0	D48.7	D49.89
tibial	—	C77.4	—	D36.0	D48.7	D49.89
tracheal	—	C77.1	—	D36.0	D48.7	D49.89
tracheobronchial	—	C77.1	—	D36.0	D48.7	D49.89
upper limb	—	C77.3	—	D36.0	D48.7	D49.89
Virchow's	—	C77.0	—	D36.0	D48.7	D49.89
node — *see also* Neoplasm, lymph gland						
primary NEC	C96.9	—	—	—	—	—
vessel — *see also* Neoplasm, connective tissue	C49.9	C79.89	—	D21.9	D48.1	D49.2
Mackenrodt's ligament	C57.7	C79.82	D07.39	D28.7	D39.8	D49.5
malar	C41.0	C79.51	—	D16.4-	D48.0	D49.2
region — *see* Neoplasm, cheek						
mammary gland — *see* Neoplasm, breast						
mandible	C41.1	C79.51	—	D16.5-	D48.0	D49.2
alveolar						
mucosa (carcinoma)	C03.1	C79.89	D00.03	D10.39	D37.09	D49.0
ridge or process	C41.1	C79.51	—	D16.5-	D48.0	D49.2
marrow (bone) NEC	C96.9	C79.52	—	—	D47.9	D49.89
mastectomy site (skin) — *see also* Neoplasm, breast, skin	C44.501	C79.2	—	—	—	—
specified as breast tissue	C50.8-☑	C79.81	—	—	—	—
mastoid (air cells) (antrum) (cavity)	C30.1	C78.39	D02.3	D14.0	D38.5	D49.1
bone or process	C41.0	C79.51	—	D16.4-	D48.0	D49.2
maxilla, maxillary (superior)	C41.0	C79.51	—	D16.4-	D48.0	D49.2
alveolar						
mucosa	C03.0	C79.89	D00.03	D10.39	D37.09	D49.0
ridge or process (carcinoma)	C41.0	C79.51	—	D16.4-	D48.0	D49.2
antrum	C31.0	C78.39	D02.3	D14.0	D38.5	D49.1
carcinoma	C03.0	C79.51	—	—	—	—
inferior — *see* Neoplasm, mandible						
sinus	C31.0	C78.39	D02.3	D14.0	D38.5	D49.1
meatus external (ear) — *see also* Neoplasm, skin, ear	C44.20-☑	C79.2	D04.2-☑	D23.2-☑	D48.5	D49.2
Meckel diverticulum, malignant	C17.3	C78.4	D01.49	D13.39	D37.2	D49.0

Neoplasm Table

Neoplasm, mediastinum, mediastinal — Neoplasm, nerve

Neoplasm, neoplastic — continued	Malignant Primary	Malignant Secondary	Ca in situ	Benign	Uncertain	Unspecified Behavior
mediastinum, mediastinal	C38.3	C78.1	—	D15.2	D38.3	D49.89
anterior	C38.1	C78.1	—	D15.2	D38.3	D49.89
posterior	C38.2	C78.1	—	D15.2	D38.3	D49.89
medulla						
adrenal	C74.1-☑	C79.7-☑	D09.3	D35.0-☑	D44.1-☑	D49.7
oblongata	C71.7	C79.31		D33.1	D43.1	D49.6
meibomian gland	C44.10-☑	C79.2	D04.1-☑	D23.1-☑	D48.5	D49.2
basal cell carcinoma	C44.11-☑	—	—	—	—	—
specified type NEC	C44.19-☑	—	—	—	—	—
squamous cell carcinoma	C44.12-☑	—	—	—	—	—
melanoma — see Melanoma						
meninges	C70.9	C79.49	—	D32.9	D42.9	D49.7
brain	C70.0	C79.32	—	D32.0	D42.0	D49.7
cerebral	C70.0	C79.32	—	D32.0	D42.0	D49.7
crainial	C70.0	C79.32	—	D32.0	D42.0	D49.7
intracranial	C70.0	C79.32	—	D32.0	D42.0	D49.7
spinal (cord)	C70.1	C79.49	—	D32.1	D42.1	D49.7
meniscus, knee joint (lateral) (medial)	C40.2-☑	C79.51		D16.2-☑	D48.0	D49.2
Merkel cell — see Carcinoma, Merkel cell						
mesentery, mesenteric	C48.1	C78.6		D20.1	D48.4	D49.0
mesoappendix	C48.1	C78.6		D20.1	D48.4	D49.0
mesocolon	C48.1	C78.6		D20.1	D48.4	D49.0
mesopharynx — see Neoplasm, oropharynx						
mesosalpinx	C57.1☑	C79.82	D07.39	D28.2	D39.8	D49.5
mesothelial tissue — see Mesothelioma						
mesothelioma — see Mesothelioma						
mesovarium	C57.1☑	C79.82	D07.39	D28.2	D39.8	D49.5
metacarpus (any bone)	C40.1-☑	C79.51		D16.1-☑		
metastatic NEC — see also Neoplasm, by site, secondary	—	C79.9	—	—	—	—
metatarsus (any bone)	C40.3-☑	C79.51		D16.3-☑		
midbrain	C71.7	C79.31		D33.1	D43.1	D49.6
milk duct — see Neoplasm, breast						
mons						
pubis	C51.9	C79.82	D07.1	D28.0	D39.8	D49.5
veneris	C51.9	C79.82	D07.1	D28.0	D39.8	D49.5
motor tract	C72.9	C79.49	—	D33.9	D43.9	D49.7
brain	C71.9	C79.31	—	D33.2	D43.2	D49.6
cauda equina	C72.1	C79.49	—	D33.4	D43.4	D49.7
spinal	C72.0	C79.49	—	D33.4	D43.4	D49.7
mouth	C06.9	C79.89	D00.00	D10.30	D37.09	D49.0
book-leaf	C06.89	C79.89	—	—	—	—
floor	C04.9	C79.89	D00.06	D10.2	D37.09	D49.0
anterior portion	C04.0	C79.89	D00.06	D10.2	D37.09	D49.0
lateral portion	C04.1	C79.89	D00.06	D10.2	D37.09	D49.0
overlapping lesion	C04.8	—	—	—	—	—
overlapping NEC	C06.80	—	—	—	—	—
roof	C05.9	C79.89	D00.00	D10.39	D37.09	D49.0
specified part NEC	C06.89	C79.89	D00.00	D10.39	D37.09	D49.0
vestibule	C06.1	C79.89	D00.00	D10.39	D37.09	D49.0
mucosa						
alveolar (ridge or process)	C03.9	C79.89	D00.03	D10.39	D37.09	D49.0
lower	C03.1	C79.89	D00.03	D10.39	D37.09	D49.0
upper	C03.0	C79.89	D00.03	D10.39	D37.09	D49.0
buccal	C06.0	C79.89	D00.02	D10.39	D37.09	D49.0
cheek	C06.0	C79.89	D00.02	D10.39	D37.09	D49.0
lip — see Neoplasm, lip, internal						
nasal	C30.0	C78.39	D02.3	D14.0	D38.5	D49.1
oral	C06.0	C79.89	D00.02	D10.39	D37.09	D49.0
Mullerian duct						
female	C57.7	C79.82	D07.39	D28.7	D39.8	D49.5
male	C63.7	C79.82	D07.69	D29.8	D40.8	D49.5

Neoplasm, neoplastic — continued	Malignant Primary	Malignant Secondary	Ca in situ	Benign	Uncertain	Unspecified Behavior
muscle — see also Neoplasm, connective tissue						
extraocular	C69.6-☑	C79.49	D09.2-☑	D31.6-☑	D48.7	D49.89
myocardium	C38.0	C79.89	—	D15.1	D48.7	D49.89
myometrium	C54.2	C79.82	D07.0	D26.1	D39.0	D49.5
myopericardium	C38.0	C79.89	—	D15.1	D48.7	D49.89
nabothian gland (follicle)	C53.0	C79.82	D06.0	D26.0	D39.0	D49.5
nail — see also Neoplasm, skin, limb	C44.90	C79.2	D04.9	D23.9	D48.5	D49.2
finger — see also Neoplasm, skin, limb, upper	C44.60-☑	C79.2	D04.6-☑	D23.6-☑	D48.5	D49.2
toe — see also Neoplasm, skin, limb, lower	C44.70-☑	C79.2	D04.7-☑	D23.7-☑	D48.5	D49.2
nares, naris (anterior) (posterior)	C30.0	C78.39	D02.3	D14.0	D38.5	D49.1
nasal — see Neoplasm, nose						
nasolabial groove — see also Neoplasm, skin, face	C44.309	C79.2	D04.39	D23.39	D48.5	D49.2
nasolacrimal duct	C69.5-☑	C79.49	D09.2-☑	D31.5-☑	D48.7	D49.89
nasopharynx, nasopharyngeal	C11.9	C79.89	D00.08	D10.6	D37.05	D49.0
floor	C11.3	C79.89	D00.08	D10.6	D37.05	D49.0
overlapping lesion	C11.8	—	—	—	—	—
roof	C11.0	C79.89	D00.08	D10.6	D37.05	D49.0
wall	C11.9	C79.89	D00.08	D10.6	D37.05	D49.0
anterior	C11.3	C79.89	D00.08	D10.6	D37.05	D49.0
lateral	C11.2	C79.89	D00.08	D10.6	D37.05	D49.0
posterior	C11.1	C79.89	D00.08	D10.6	D37.05	D49.0
superior	C11.0	C79.89	D00.08	D10.6	D37.05	D49.0
nates — see also Neoplasm, skin, trunk	C44.509	C79.2	D04.5	D23.5	D48.5	D49.2
neck NEC	C76.0	C79.89	D09.8	D36.7	D48.7	D49.89
skin	C44.40			—	—	—
basal cell carcinoma	C44.41					
specified type NEC	C44.49					
squamous cell carcinoma	C44.42	—				
nerve (ganglion)	C47.9	C79.89	—	D36.10	D48.2	D49.2
abducens	C72.59	C79.49	—	D33.3	D43.3	D49.7
accessory (spinal)	C72.59	C79.49	—	D33.3	D43.3	D49.7
acoustic	C72.4-☑	C79.49	—	D33.3	D43.3	D49.7
auditory	C72.4-☑	C79.49	—	D33.3	D43.3	D49.7
autonomic NEC — see also Neoplasm, nerve, peripheral	C47.9	C79.89	—	D36.10	D48.2	D49.2
brachial	C47.1-☑	C79.89	—	D36.12	D48.2	D49.2
cranial	C72.50	C79.49	—	D33.3	D43.3	D49.7
specified NEC	C72.59	C79.49	—	D33.3	D43.3	D49.7
facial	C72.59	C79.49	—	D33.3	D43.3	D49.7
femoral	C47.2-☑	C79.89	—	D36.13	D48.2	D49.2
ganglion NEC — see also Neoplasm, nerve, peripheral	C47.9	C79.89	—	D36.10	D48.2	D49.2
glossopharyngeal	C72.59	C79.49	—	D33.3	D43.3	D49.7
hypoglossal	C72.59	C79.49	—	D33.3	D43.3	D49.7
intercostal	C47.3	C79.89	—	D36.14	D48.2	D49.2
lumbar	C47.6	C79.89	—	D36.17	D48.2	D49.2
median	C47.1-☑	C79.89	—	D36.12	D48.2	D49.2
obturator	C47.2-☑	C79.89	—	D36.13	D48.2	D49.2
oculomotor	C72.59	C79.49	—	D33.3	D43.3	D49.7
olfactory	C47.2-☑	C79.49	—	D33.3	D43.3	D49.7
optic	C72.3-☑	C79.49	—	D33.3	D43.3	D49.7
parasympathetic NEC	C47.9	C79.89	—	D36.10	D48.2	D49.2
peripheral NEC	C47.9	C79.89	—	D36.10	D48.2	D49.2
abdomen	C47.4	C79.89	—	D36.15	D48.2	D49.2
abdominal wall	C47.4	C79.89	—	D36.15	D48.2	D49.2
ankle	C47.2-☑	C79.89	—	D36.13	D48.2	D49.2

☑ **Additional Character Required** — Refer to the Tabular List for Character Selection   ▽ **Subterms under main terms may continue to next column or page**

Neoplasm, neoplastic —	Malignant Primary	Malignant Secondary	Ca in situ	Benign	Uncertain	Unspecified Behavior
continued						
nerve — *continued*						
peripheral — *continued*						
antecubital fossa or						
space	C47.1-☑	C79.89	—	D36.12	D48.2	D49.2
arm	C47.1-☑	C79.89	—	D36.12	D48.2	D49.2
auricle (ear)	C47.0	C79.89	—	D36.11	D48.2	D49.2
axilla	C47.3	C79.89	—	D36.12	D48.2	D49.2
back	C47.6	C79.89	—	D36.17	D48.2	D49.2
buttock	C47.5	C79.89	—	D36.16	D48.2	D49.2
calf	C47.2-☑	C79.89	—	D36.13	D48.2	D49.2
cervical region	C47.0	C79.89	—	D36.11	D48.2	D49.2
cheek	C47.0	C79.89	—	D36.11	D48.2	D49.2
chest (wall)	C47.3	C79.89	—	D36.14	D48.2	D49.2
chin	C47.0	C79.89	—	D36.11	D48.2	D49.2
ear (external)	C47.0	C79.89	—	D36.11	D48.2	D49.2
elbow	C47.1-☑	C79.89	—	D36.12	D48.2	D49.2
extrarectal	C47.5	C79.89	—	D36.16	D48.2	D49.2
extremity	C47.9	C79.89	—	D36.10	D48.2	D49.2
lower	C47.2-☑	C79.89	—	D36.13	D48.2	D49.2
upper	C47.1-☑	C79.89	—	D36.12	D48.2	D49.2
eyelid	C47.0	C79.89	—	D36.11	D48.2	D49.2
face	C47.0	C79.89	—	D36.11	D48.2	D49.2
finger	C47.1-☑	C79.89	—	D36.12	D48.2	D49.2
flank	C47.6	C79.89	—	D36.17	D48.2	D49.2
foot	C47.2-☑	C79.89	—	D36.13	D48.2	D49.2
forearm	C47.1-☑	C79.89	—	D36.12	D48.2	D49.2
forehead	C47.0	C79.89	—	D36.11	D48.2	D49.2
gluteal region	C47.5	C79.89	—	D36.16	D48.2	D49.2
groin	C47.5	C79.89	—	D36.16	D48.2	D49.2
hand	C47.1-☑	C79.89	—	D36.12	D48.2	D49.2
head	C47.0	C79.89	—	D36.11	D48.2	D49.2
heel	C47.2-☑	C79.89	—	D36.13	D48.2	D49.2
hip	C47.2-☑	C79.89	—	D36.13	D48.2	D49.2
infraclavicular						
region	C47.3	C79.89	—	D36.14	D48.2	D49.2
inguinal (canal)						
(region)	C47.5	C79.89	—	D36.16	D48.2	D49.2
intrathoracic	C47.3	C79.89	—	D36.14	D48.2	D49.2
ischiorectal						
fossa	C47.5	C79.89	—	D36.16	D48.2	D49.2
knee	C47.2-☑	C79.89	—	D36.13	D48.2	D49.2
leg	C47.2-☑	C79.89	—	D36.13	D48.2	D49.2
limb NEC	C47.9	C79.89	—	D36.10	D48.2	D49.2
lower	C47.2-☑	C79.89	—	D36.13	D48.2	D49.2
upper	C47.1-☑	C79.89	—	D36.12	D48.2	D49.2
nates	C47.5	C79.89	—	D36.16	D48.2	D49.2
neck	C47.0	C79.89	—	D36.11	D48.2	D49.2
orbit	C69.6-☑	C79.49	—	D31.6-☑	D48.7	D49.2
pararectal	C47.5	C79.89	—	D36.16	D48.2	D49.2
paraurethral	C47.5	C79.89	—	D36.16	D48.2	D49.2
paravaginal	C47.5	C79.89	—	D36.16	D48.2	D49.2
pelvis (floor)	C47.5	C79.89	—	D36.16	D48.2	D49.2
pelvoabdominal	C47.8	C79.89	—	D36.17	D48.2	D49.2
perineum	C47.5	C79.89	—	D36.16	D48.2	D49.2
perirectal						
(tissue)	C47.5	C79.89	—	D36.16	D48.2	D49.2
periurethral						
(tissue)	C47.5	C79.89	—	D36.16	D48.2	D49.2
popliteal fossa or						
space	C47.2-☑	C79.89	—	D36.13	D48.2	D49.2
presacral	C47.5	C79.89	—	D36.16	D48.2	D49.2
pterygoid fossa	C47.0	C79.89	—	D36.11	D48.2	D49.2
rectovaginal septum						
or wall	C47.5	C79.89	—	D36.16		D49.2
rectovesical	C47.5	C79.89	—	D36.16		D49.2
sacrococcygeal						
region	C47.5	C79.89	—	D36.16	D48.2	D49.2
scalp	C47.0	C79.89	—	D36.11	D48.2	D49.2
scapular region	C47.3	C79.89	—	D36.14	D48.2	D49.2
shoulder	C47.1-☑	C79.89	—	D36.12	D48.2	D49.2
submental	C47.0	C79.89	—	D36.11	D48.2	D49.2
supraclavicular						
region	C47.0	C79.89	—	D36.11	D48.2	D49.2
temple	C47.0	C79.89	—	D36.11	D48.2	D49.2
temporal region	C47.0	C79.89	—	D36.11	D48.2	D49.2
thigh	C47.2-☑	C79.89	—	D36.13	D48.2	D49.2
thoracic (duct)						
(wall)	C47.3	C79.89	—	D36.14	D48.2	D49.2
thorax	C47.3	C79.89	—	D36.14	D48.2	D49.2
thumb	C47.1-☑	C79.89	—	D36.12	D48.2	D49.2

Neoplasm, neoplastic —	Malignant Primary	Malignant Secondary	Ca in situ	Benign	Uncertain	Unspecified Behavior
continued						
nerve — *continued*						
peripheral — *continued*						
toe	C47.2-☑	C79.89	—	D36.13	D48.2	D49.2
trunk	C47.6	C79.89	—	D36.17	D48.2	D49.2
umbilicus	C47.4	C79.89	—	D36.15	D48.2	D49.2
vesicorectal	C47.5	C79.89	—	D36.16	D48.2	D49.2
wrist	C47.1-☑	C79.89	—	D36.12	D48.2	D49.2
radial	C47.1-☑	C79.89	—	D36.12	D48.2	D49.2
sacral	C47.5	C79.89	—	D36.16	D48.2	D49.2
sciatic	C47.2-☑	C79.89	—	D36.13	D48.2	D49.2
spinal NEC	C47.9	C79.89	—	D36.10	D48.2	D49.2
accessory	C72.59	C79.49	—	D33.3	D43.3	D49.7
sympathetic NEC — *see*						
also Neoplasm,						
nerve,						
peripheral	C47.9	C79.89	—	D36.10	D48.2	D49.2
trigeminal	C72.59	C79.49	—	D33.3	D43.3	D49.7
trochlear	C72.59	C79.49	—	D33.3	D43.3	D49.7
ulnar	C47.1-☑	C79.89	—	D36.12	D48.2	D49.2
vagus	C72.59	C79.49	—	D33.3	D43.3	D49.7
nervous system						
(central)	C72.9	C79.40	—	D33.9	D43.9	D49.7
autonomic — *see*						
Neoplasm, nerve,						
peripheral						
parasympathetic — *see*						
Neoplasm, nerve,						
peripheral						
specified site NEC		C79.49	—	D33.7	D43.8	
sympathetic — *see*						
Neoplasm, nerve,						
peripheral						
nevus — *see* Nevus						
nipple	C50.0-☑	C79.81	D05.-☑	D24.-☑	—	—
nose, nasal	C76.0	C79.89	D09.8	D36.7	D48.7	D49.89
ala (external) (nasi) —						
see also Neoplasm,						
nose, skin	C44.301	C79.2	D04.39	D23.39	D48.5	D49.2
bone	C41.0	C79.51	—	D16.4-	D48.0	D49.2
cartilage	C30.0	C78.39	D02.3	D14.0	D38.5	D49.1
cavity	C30.0	C78.39	D02.3	D14.0	D38.5	D49.1
choana	C11.3	C79.89	D00.08	D10.6	D37.05	D49.0
external (skin) — *see*						
also Neoplasm,						
nose, skin	C44.301	C79.2	D04.39	D23.39	D48.5	D49.2
fossa	C30.0	C78.39	D02.3	D14.0	D38.5	D49.1
internal	C30.0	C78.39	D02.3	D14.0	D38.5	D49.1
mucosa	C30.0	C78.39	D02.3	D14.0	D38.5	D49.1
septum	C30.0	C78.39	D02.3	D14.0	D38.5	D49.1
posterior margin	C11.3	C79.89	D00.08	D10.6	D37.05	D49.0
sinus — *see* Neoplasm,						
sinus						
skin	C44.301	C79.2	D04.39	D23.39	D48.5	D49.2
basal cell						
carcinoma	C44.311	—	—	—	—	—
specified type						
NEC	C44.391	—	—	—	—	—
squamous cell						
carcinoma	C44.321	—	—	—	—	—
turbinate						
(mucosa)	C30.0	C78.39	D02.3	D14.0	D38.5	D49.1
bone	C41.0	C79.51	—	D16.4-	D48.0	D49.2
vestibule	C30.0	C78.39	D02.3	D14.0	D38.5	D49.1
nostril	C30.0	C78.39	D02.3	D14.0	D38.5	D49.1
nucleus pulposus	C41.2	C79.51	—	D16.6	D48.0	D49.2
occipital						
bone	C41.0	C79.51	—	D16.4-	D48.0	D49.2
lobe or pole, brain	C71.4	C79.31	—	D33.0	D43.0	D49.6
odontogenic — *see*						
Neoplasm, jaw bone						
olfactory nerve or						
bulb	C72.2-☑	C79.49	—	D33.3	D43.3	D49.7
olive (brain)	C71.7	C79.31	—	D33.1	D43.1	D49.6
omentum	C48.1	C78.6	—	D20.1	D48.4	D49.0
operculum (brain)	C71.0	C79.31	—	D33.0	D43.0	D49.6
optic nerve, chiasm, or						
tract	C72.3-☑	C79.49	—	D33.3	D43.3	D49.7
oral (cavity)	C06.9	C79.89	D00.00	D10.30	D37.09	D49.0
ill-defined	C14.8	C79.89	D00.00	D10.30	D37.09	D49.0
mucosa	C06.9	C79.89	D00.02	D10.39	D37.09	D49.0
orbit	C69.6-☑	C79.49	D09.2-☑	D31.6-☑	D48.7	D49.89

Neoplasm, neoplastic — continued	Malignant Primary	Malignant Secondary	Ca in situ	Benign	Uncertain	Unspecified Behavior
orbit — continued						
autonomic nerve	C69.6-✓	C79.49	—	D31.6-✓	D48.7	D49.2
bone	C41.0	C79.51	—	D48.0	D48.7	D49.2
eye	C69.6-✓	C79.49	D09.2-✓	D31.6-✓	D48.7	D49.89
peripheral nerves	C69.6-✓	C79.49	—	D31.6-✓	D48.7	D49.2
soft parts	C69.6-✓	C79.49	D09.2-✓	D31.6-✓	D48.7	D49.89
organ of Zuckerkandl	C75.5	C79.89	—	D35.6	D44.7	D49.7
oropharynx	C10.9	C79.89	D00.08	D10.5	D37.05	D49.0
branchial cleft (vestige)	C10.4	C79.89	D00.08	D10.5	D37.05	D49.0
junctional region	C10.8	C79.89	D00.08	D10.5	D37.05	D49.0
lateral wall	C10.2	C79.89	D00.08	D10.5	D37.05	D49.0
overlapping lesion	C10.8	—	—	—	—	—
pillars or fauces	C09.1	C79.89	D00.08	D10.5	D37.05	D49.0
posterior wall	C10.3	C79.89	D00.08	D10.5	D37.05	D49.0
vallecula	C10.0	C79.89	D00.08	D10.5	D37.05	D49.0
os						
external	C53.1	C79.82	D06.1	D26.0	D39.0	D49.5
internal	C53.0	C79.82	D06.0	D26.0	D39.0	D49.5
ovary	C56.-✓	C79.6-✓	D07.39	D27.-✓	D39.1-✓	D49.5
oviduct	C57.0-✓	C79.82	D07.39	D28.2	D39.8	D49.5
palate	C05.9	C79.89	D00.00	D10.39	D37.09	D49.0
hard	C05.0	C79.89	D00.05	D10.39	D37.09	D49.89
junction of hard and soft palate	C05.9	C79.89	D00.00	D10.39	D37.09	D49.0
overlapping lesions	C05.8	—	—	—	—	—
soft	C05.1	C79.89	D00.04	D10.39	D37.09	D49.0
nasopharyngeal surface	C11.3	C79.89	D00.08	D10.6	D37.05	D49.0
posterior surface	C11.3	C79.89	D00.08	D10.6	D37.05	D49.0
superior surface	C11.3	C79.89	D00.08	D10.6	D37.05	D49.0
palatoglossal arch	C09.1	C79.89	D00.00	D10.5	D37.09	D49.0
palatopharyngeal arch	C09.1	C79.89	D00.00	D10.5	D37.09	D49.0
pallium	C71.0	C79.31	—	D33.0	D43.0	D49.6
palpebra	C44.10-✓	C79.2	D04.1-✓	D23.1-✓	D48.5	D49.2
basal cell carcinoma	C44.11-✓	—	—	—	—	—
specified type NEC	C44.19-✓	—	—	—	—	—
squamous cell carcinoma	C44.12-✓	—	—	—	—	—
pancreas	C25.9	C78.89	D01.7	D13.6	D37.8	D49.0
body	C25.1	C78.89	D01.7	D13.6	D37.8	D49.0
duct (of Santorini) (of Wirsung)	C25.3	C78.89	D01.7	D13.6	D37.8	D49.0
ectopic tissue	C25.7	C78.89	—	D13.6	D37.8	D49.0
head	C25.0	C78.89	D01.7	D13.6	D37.8	D49.0
islet cells	C25.4	C78.89	D01.7	D13.7	D37.8	D49.0
neck	C25.7	C78.89	D01.7	D13.6	D37.8	D49.0
overlapping lesion	C25.8	—	—	—	—	—
tail	C25.2	C78.89	D01.7	D13.6	D37.8	D49.0
para-aortic body	C75.5	C79.89	—	D35.6	D44.7	D49.7
paraganglion NEC	C75.5	C79.89	—	D35.6	D44.7	D49.7
parametrium	C57.3	C79.82	—	D28.2	D39.8	D49.5
paranephric	C48.0	C78.6	—	D20.0	D48.3	D49.0
pararectal	C76.3	C79.89	—	D36.7	D48.7	D49.89
parasagittal (region)	C76.0	C79.89	D09.8	D36.7	D48.7	D49.89
parasellar	C72.9	C79.49	—	D33.9	D43.8	D49.7
parathyroid (gland)	C75.0	C79.89	D09.3	D35.1	D44.2	D49.7
paraurethral	C76.3	C79.89	—	D36.7	D48.7	D49.89
gland	C68.1	C79.19	D09.19	D30.8	D41.8	D49.5
paravaginal	C76.3	C79.89	—	D36.7	D48.7	D49.89
parenchyma, kidney	C64.-✓	C79.0-✓	D09.19	D30.0-✓	D41.0-✓	D49.5
parietal						
bone	C41.0	C79.51	—	D16.4-	D48.0	D49.2
lobe, brain	C71.3	C79.31	—	D33.0	D43.0	D49.6
paroophoron	C57.1✓	C79.82	D07.39	D28.2	D39.8	D49.5
parotid (duct) (gland)	C07	C79.89	D00.00	D11.0	D37.030	D49.0
parovarium	C57.1✓	C79.82	D07.39	D28.2	D39.8	D49.5
patella	C40.20	C79.51	—	D16.8	D48.0	D49.2
peduncle, cerebral	C71.7	C79.31	—	D33.1	D43.1	D49.6
pelvirectal junction	C19	C78.5	D01.1	D12.7	D37.5	D49.0
pelvis, pelvic	C76.3	C79.89	D09.8	D36.7	D48.7	D49.89
bone	C41.4	C79.51	—	D16.8	D48.0	D49.2
floor	C76.3	C79.89	D09.8	D36.7	D48.7	D49.89
renal	C65.-✓	C79.0-✓	D09.19	D30.1-✓	D41.1-✓	D49.5
viscera	C76.3	C79.89	D09.8	D36.7	D48.7	D49.89

Neoplasm, neoplastic — continued	Malignant Primary	Malignant Secondary	Ca in situ	Benign	Uncertain	Unspecified Behavior
pelvis, pelvic — continued						
wall	C76.3	C79.89	D09.8	D36.7	D48.7	D49.89
pelvo-abdominal	C76.8	C79.89	D09.8	D36.7	D48.7	D49.89
penis	C60.9	C79.82	D07.4	D29.0	D40.8	D49.5
body	C60.2	C79.82	D07.4	D29.0	D40.8	D49.5
corpus (cavernosum)	C60.2	C79.82	D07.4	D29.0	D40.8	D49.5
glans	C60.1	C79.82	D07.4	D29.0	D40.8	D49.5
overlapping sites	C60.8	—	—	—	—	—
skin NEC	C60.9	C79.82	D07.4	D29.0	D40.8	D49.5
periadrenal (tissue)	C48.0	C78.6	—	D20.0	D48.3	D49.0
perianal (skin) — see also Neoplasm, anus, skin	C44.500	C79.2	D04.5	D23.5	D48.5	D49.2
pericardium	C38.0	C79.89	—	D15.1	D48.7	D49.89
perinephric	C48.0	C78.6	—	D20.0	D48.3	D49.0
perineum	C76.3	C79.89	D09.8	D36.7	D48.7	D49.0
periodontal tissue NEC	C03.9	C79.89	D00.03	D10.39	D37.09	D49.0
periosteum — see Neoplasm, bone						
peripancreatic	C48.0	C78.6	—	D20.0	D48.3	D49.0
peripheral nerve NEC	C47.9	C79.89	—	D36.10	D48.2	D49.2
perirectal (tissue)	C76.3	C79.89	—	D36.7	D48.7	D49.89
perirenal (tissue)	C48.0	C78.6	—	D20.0	D48.3	D49.0
peritoneum, peritoneal (cavity)	C48.2	C78.6	—	D20.1	D48.4	D49.0
benign mesothelial tissue — see Mesothelioma, benign						
overlapping lesion with digestive organs	C48.8	—	—	—	—	—
	C26.9	—	—	—	—	—
parietal	C48.1	C78.6	—	D20.1	D48.4	D49.0
pelvic	C48.1	C78.6	—	D20.1	D48.4	D49.0
specified part NEC	C48.1	C78.6	—	D20.1	D48.4	D49.0
peritonsillar (tissue)	C76.0	C79.89	D09.8	D36.7	D48.7	D49.89
periurethral tissue	C76.3	C79.89	—	D36.7	D48.7	D49.89
phalanges						
foot	C40.3-✓	C79.51	—	D16.3-✓	—	—
hand	C40.1-✓	C79.51	—	D16.1-✓	—	—
pharynx, pharyngeal	C14.0	C79.89	D00.08	D10.9	D37.05	D49.0
bursa	C11.1	C79.89	D00.08	D10.6	D37.05	D49.0
fornix	C11.3	C79.89	D00.08	D10.6	D37.05	D49.0
recess	C11.2	C79.89	D00.08	D10.6	D37.05	D49.0
region	C14.0	C79.89	D00.08	D10.9	D37.05	D49.0
tonsil	C11.1	C79.89	D00.08	D10.6	D37.05	D49.0
wall (lateral) (posterior)	C14.0	C79.89	D00.08	D10.9	D37.05	D49.0
pia mater	C70.9	C79.40	—	D32.9	D42.9	D49.7
cerebral	C70.0	C79.32	—	D32.0	D42.0	D49.7
cranial	C70.0	C79.32	—	D32.0	D42.0	D49.7
spinal	C70.1	C79.49	—	D32.1	D42.1	D49.7
pillars of fauces	C09.1	C79.89	D00.08	D10.5	D37.05	D49.0
pineal (body) (gland)	C75.3	C79.89	D09.3	D35.4	D44.5	D49.7
pinna (ear) NEC — see also Neoplasm, skin, ear	C44.20-✓	C79.2	D04.2-✓	D23.2-✓	D48.5	D49.2
piriform fossa or sinus	C12	C79.89	D00.08	D10.7	D37.05	D49.0
pituitary (body) (fossa) (gland) (lobe)	C75.1	C79.89	D09.3	D35.2	D44.3	D49.7
placenta	C58	C79.82	D07.0	D26.7	D39.2	D49.5
pleura, pleural (cavity)	C38.4	C78.2	—	D19.0	D38.2	D49.1
overlapping lesion with heart or mediastinum	C38.8	—	—	—	—	—
parietal	C38.4	C78.2	—	D19.0	D38.2	D49.1
visceral	C38.4	C78.2	—	D19.0	D38.2	D49.1
plexus						
brachial	C47.1-✓	C79.89	—	D36.12	D48.2	D49.2
cervical	C47.0	C79.89	—	D36.11	D48.2	D49.2
choroid	C71.5	C79.31	—	D33.0	D43.0	D49.6
lumbosacral	C47.5	C79.89	—	D36.16	D48.2	D49.2
sacral	C47.5	C79.89	—	D36.16	D48.2	D49.2
pluriendocrine	C75.8	C79.89	D09.3	D35.7	D44.9	D49.7
pole						

✓ **Additional Character Required** — Refer to the Tabular List for Character Selection   ▽ **Subterms under main terms may continue to next column or page**

Neoplasm, neoplastic — continued	Malignant Primary	Malignant Secondary	Ca in situ	Benign	Uncertain	Unspecified Behavior
pole — continued						
frontal	C71.1	C79.31	—	D33.0	D43.0	D49.6
occipital	C71.4	C79.31	—	D33.0	D43.0	D49.6
pons (varolii)	C71.7	C79.31	—	D33.1	D43.1	D49.6
popliteal fossa or space	C76.5-☑	C79.89	D04.7-☑	D36.7	D48.7	D49.89
postcricoid (region)	C13.0	C79.89	D00.08	D10.7	D37.05	D49.0
posterior fossa (cranial)	C71.9	C79.31	—	D33.2	D43.2	D49.6
postnasal space	C11.9	C79.89	D00.08	D10.6	D37.05	D49.0
prepuce	C60.0	C79.82	D07.4	D29.0	D40.8	D49.5
prepylorus	C16.4	C78.89	D00.2	D13.1	D37.1	D49.0
presacral (region)	C76.3	C79.89	—	D36.7	D48.7	D49.89
prostate (gland)	C61	C79.82	D07.5	D29.1	D40.0	D49.5
utricle	C68.0	C79.19	D09.19	D30.4	D41.3	D49.5
pterygoid fossa	C49.0	C79.89	—	D21.0	D48.1	D49.2
pubic bone	C41.4	C79.51	—	D16.8	D48.0	D49.2
pudenda, pudendum (female)	C51.9	C79.82	D07.1	D28.0	D39.8	D49.5
pulmonary — see also Neoplasm, lung	C34.9-☑	C78.0-☑	D02.2-☑	D14.3-☑	D38.1	D49.1
putamen	C71.0	C79.31	—	D33.0	D43.0	D49.6
pyloric						
antrum	C16.3	C78.89	D00.2	D13.1	D37.1	D49.0
canal	C16.4	C78.89	D00.2	D13.1	D37.1	D49.0
pylorus	C16.4	C78.89	D00.2	D13.1	D37.1	D49.0
pyramid (brain)	C71.7	C79.31	—	D33.1	D43.1	D49.6
pyriform fossa or sinus	C12	C79.89	D00.08	D10.7	D37.05	D49.0
radius (any part)	C40.0-☑	C79.51	—	D16.0-☑	—	—
Rathke's pouch	C75.1	C79.89	D09.3	D35.2	D44.3	D49.7
rectosigmoid (junction)	C19	C78.5	D01.1	D12.7	D37.5	D49.0
overlapping lesion with anus or rectum	C21.8	—	—	—	—	—
rectouterine pouch	C48.1	C78.6	—	D20.1	D48.4	D49.0
rectovaginal septum or wall	C76.3	C79.89	D09.8	D36.7	D48.7	D49.89
rectovesical septum	C76.3	C79.89	D09.8	D36.7	D48.7	D49.89
rectum (ampulla)	C20	C78.5	D01.2	D12.8	D37.5	D49.0
and colon	C19	C78.5	D01.1	D12.7	D37.5	D49.0
overlapping lesion with anus or rectosigmoid junction	C21.8	—	—	—	—	—
renal	C64.-☑	C79.0-☑	D09.19	D30.0-☑	D41.0-☑	D49.5
calyx	C65.-☑	C79.0-☑	D09.19	D30.1-☑	D41.1-☑	D49.5
hilus	C65.-☑	C79.0-☑	D09.19	D30.1-☑	D41.1-☑	D49.5
parenchyma	C64.-☑	C79.0-☑	D09.19	D30.0-☑	D41.0-☑	D49.5
pelvis	C65.-☑	C79.0-☑	D09.19	D30.1-☑	D41.1-☑	D49.5
respiratory						
organs or system NEC	C39.9	C78.30	D02.4	D14.4	D38.6	D49.1
tract NEC	C39.9	C78.30	D02.4	D14.4	D38.5	D49.1
upper	C39.0	C78.30	D02.4	D14.4	D38.5	D49.1
retina	C69.2-☑	C79.49	D09.2-☑	D31.2-☑	D48.7	D49.81
retro-orbital	C76.0	C79.89	D09.8	D36.7	D48.7	D49.89
retrobulbar	C69.6-☑	C79.49	—	D31.6-☑	D48.7	D49.89
retrocecal	C48.0	C78.6	—	D20.0	D48.3	D49.0
retromolar (area) (triangle) (trigone)	C06.2	C79.89	D00.00	D10.39	D37.09	D49.0
retroperitoneal (space) (tissue)	C48.0	C78.6	—	D20.0	D48.3	D49.0
retroperitoneum	C48.0	C78.6	—	D20.0	D48.3	D49.0
retropharyngeal	C14.0	C79.89	D00.08	D10.9	D37.05	D49.0
retrovesical (septum)	C76.3	C79.89	D09.8	D36.7	D48.7	D49.89
rhinencephalon	C71.0	C79.31	—	D33.0	D43.0	D49.6
rib	C41.3	C79.51	—	D16.7	D48.0	D49.2
Rosenmuller's fossa	C11.2	C79.89	D00.08	D10.6	D37.05	D49.0
round ligament	C57.2-☑	C79.82	—	D28.2	D39.8	D49.5
sacrococcyx, sacrococcygeal	C41.4	C79.51	—	D16.8	D48.0	D49.2
region	C76.3	C79.89	D09.8	D36.7	D48.7	D49.89
sacrouterine ligament	C57.3	C79.82	—	D28.2	D39.8	D49.5
sacrum, sacral (vertebra)	C41.4	C79.51	—	D16.8	D48.0	D49.2

Neoplasm, neoplastic — continued	Malignant Primary	Malignant Secondary	Ca in situ	Benign	Uncertain	Unspecified Behavior
salivary gland or duct (major)	C08.9	C79.89	D00.00	D11.9	D37.039	D49.0
minor NEC	C06.9	C79.89	D00.00	D10.39	D37.04	D49.0
overlapping lesion	C08.9	—	—	—	—	—
parotid	C07	C79.89	D00.00	D11.0	D37.030	D49.0
pluriglandular	C08.9	C79.89	D00.00	D11.9	D37.039	D49.0
sublingual	C08.1	C79.89	D00.00	D11.7	D37.031	D49.0
submandibular	C08.0	C79.89	D00.00	D11.7	D37.032	D49.0
submaxillary	C08.0	C79.89	D00.00	D11.7	D37.032	D49.0
salpinx (uterine)	C57.0-☑	C79.82	D07.39	D28.2	D39.8	D49.5
Santorini's duct	C25.3	C78.89	D01.7	D13.6	D37.8	D49.0
scalp	C44.40	C79.2	D04.4	D23.4	D48.5	D49.2
basal cell carcinoma	C44.41	—	—	—	—	—
specified type NEC	C44.49	—	—	—	—	—
squamous cell carcinoma	C44.42	—	—	—	—	—
scapula (any part)	C40.0-☑	C79.51	—	D16.0-☑	—	—
scapular region	C76.1	C79.89	D09.8	D36.7	D48.7	D49.89
scar NEC — see also Neoplasm, skin, by site	C44.90	C79.2	D04.9	D23.9	D48.5	D49.2
sciatic nerve	C47.2-☑	C79.89	—	D36.13	D48.2	D49.2
sclera	C69.4-☑	C79.49	D09.2-☑	D31.4-☑	D48.7	D49.89
scrotum (skin)	C63.2	C79.82	D07.61	D29.4	D40.8	D49.5
sebaceous gland — see Neoplasm, skin						
sella turcica	C75.1	C79.89	D09.3	D35.2	D44.3	D49.7
bone	C41.0	C79.51	—	D16.4-	D48.0	D49.2
semilunar cartilage (knee)	C40.2-☑	C79.51	—	D16.2-☑	D48.0	D49.2
seminal vesicle	C63.7	C79.82	D07.69	D29.8	D40.8	D49.5
septum						
nasal	C30.0	C78.39	D02.3	D14.0	D38.5	D49.1
posterior margin	C11.3	C79.89	D00.08	D10.6	D37.05	D49.0
rectovaginal	C76.3	C79.89	D09.8	D36.7	D48.7	D49.89
rectovesical	C76.3	C79.89	D09.8	D36.7	D48.7	D49.89
urethrovaginal	C57.9	C79.82	D07.30	D28.9	D39.9	D49.5
vesicovaginal	C57.9	C79.82	D07.30	D28.9	D39.9	D49.5
shoulder NEC	C76.4-☑	C79.89	D04.6-☑	D36.7	D48.7	D49.89
sigmoid flexure (lower) (upper)	C18.7	C78.5	D01.0	D12.5	D37.4	D49.0
sinus (accessory)	C31.9	C78.39	D02.3	D14.0	D38.5	D49.1
bone (any)	C41.0	C79.51	—	D16.4-	D48.0	D49.2
ethmoidal	C31.1	C78.39	D02.3	D14.0	D38.5	D49.1
frontal	C31.2	C78.39	D02.3	D14.0	D38.5	D49.1
maxillary	C31.0	C78.39	D02.3	D14.0	D38.5	D49.1
nasal, paranasal NEC	C31.9	C78.39	D02.3	D14.0	D38.5	D49.1
overlapping lesion	C31.8	—	—	—	—	—
pyriform	C12	C79.89	D00.08	D10.7	D37.05	D49.0
sphenoid	C31.3	C78.39	D02.3	D14.0	D38.5	D49.1
skeleton, skeletal NEC	C41.9	C79.51	—	D16.9-	D48.0	D49.2
Skene's gland	C68.1	C79.19	D09.19	D30.8	D41.8	D49.5
skin NOS	C44.90	C79.2	D04.9	D23.9	D48.5	D49.2
abdominal wall	C44.509	C79.2	D04.5	D23.5	D48.5	D49.2
basal cell carcinoma	C44.519	—	—	—	—	—
specified type NEC	C44.599	—	—	—	—	—
squamous cell carcinoma	C44.529	—	—	—	—	—
ala nasi — see also Neoplasm, nose, skin	C44.301	C79.2	D04.39	D23.39	D48.5	D49.2
ankle — see also Neoplasm, skin, limb, lower	C44.70-☑	C79.2	D04.7-☑	D23.7-☑	D48.5	D49.2
antecubital space — see also Neoplasm, skin, limb, upper	C44.60-☑	C79.2	D04.6-☑	D23.6-☑	D48.5	D49.2
anus	C44.500	C79.2	D04.5	D23.5	D48.5	D49.2
basal cell carcinoma	C44.510	—	—	—	—	—
specified type NEC	C44.590	—	—	—	—	—
squamous cell carcinoma	C44.520	—	—	—	—	—

Neoplasm, neoplastic — continued

skin — continued

Site	Malignant Primary	Malignant Secondary	Ca in situ	Benign	Uncertain	Unspecified Behavior
arm — see also Neoplasm, skin, limb, upper	C44.60-✓	C79.2	D04.6-✓	D23.6-✓	D48.5	D49.2
auditory canal (external) — see also Neoplasm, skin, ear	C44.20-✓	C79.2	D04.2-✓	D23.2-✓	D48.5	D49.2
auricle (ear) — see also Neoplasm, skin, ear	C44.20-✓	C79.2	D04.2-✓	D23.2-✓	D48.5	D49.2
auricular canal (external) — see also Neoplasm, skin, ear	C44.20-✓	C79.2	D04.2-✓	D23.2-✓	D48.5	D49.2
axilla, axillary fold — see also Neoplasm, skin, trunk	C44.509	C79.2	D04.5	D23.5	D48.5	D49.2
back — see also Neoplasm, skin, trunk	C44.509	C79.2	D04.5	D23.5	D48.5	D49.2
basal cell carcinoma	C44.91	—	—	—	—	—
breast	C44.501	C79.2	D04.5	D23.5	D48.5	D49.2
basal cell carcinoma	C44.511	—	—	—	—	—
specified type NEC	C44.591					
squamous cell carcinoma	C44.521					
brow — see also Neoplasm, skin, face	C44.309	C79.2	D04.39	D23.39	D48.5	D49.2
buttock — see also Neoplasm, skin, trunk	C44.509	C79.2	D04.5	D23.5	D48.5	D49.2
calf — see also Neoplasm, skin, limb, lower	C44.70-✓	C79.2	D04.7-✓	D23.7-✓	D48.5	D49.2
canthus (eye) (inner) (outer)	C44.10-✓	C79.2	D04.1-✓	D23.1-✓	D48.5	D49.2
basal cell carcinoma	C44.11-✓	—	—	—	—	—
specified type NEC	C44.19-✓	—	—	—	—	—
squamous cell carcinoma	C44.12-✓	—	—	—	—	—
cervical region — see also Neoplasm, skin, neck	C44.40	C79.2	D04.4	D23.4	D48.5	D49.2
cheek (external) — see also Neoplasm, skin, face	C44.309	C79.2	D04.39	D23.39	D48.5	D49.2
chest (wall) — see also Neoplasm, skin, trunk	C44.509	C79.2	D04.5	D23.5	D48.5	D49.2
chin — see also Neoplasm, skin, face	C44.309	C79.2	D04.39	D23.39	D48.5	D49.2
clavicular area — see also Neoplasm, skin, trunk	C44.509	C79.2	D04.5	D23.5	D48.5	D49.2
clitoris	C51.2	C79.82	D07.1	D28.0	D39.8	D49.5
columnella — see also Neoplasm, skin, face	C44.309	C79.2	D04.39	D23.39	D48.5	D49.2
concha — see also Neoplasm, skin, ear	C44.20-✓	C79.2	D04.2-✓	D23.2-✓	D48.5	D49.2
ear (external)	C44.20-✓	C79.2	D04.2-✓	D23.2-✓	D48.5	D49.2
basal cell carcinoma	C44.21-✓	—	—	—	—	—
specified type NEC	C44.29-✓	—	—	—	—	—
squamous cell carcinoma	C44.22-✓	—	—	—	—	—
elbow — see also Neoplasm, skin, limb, upper	C44.60-✓	C79.2	D04.6-✓	D23.6-✓	D48.5	D49.2

Neoplasm, neoplastic — continued

skin — continued

Site	Malignant Primary	Malignant Secondary	Ca in situ	Benign	Uncertain	Unspecified Behavior
eyebrow — see also Neoplasm, skin, face	C44.309	C79.2	D04.39	D23.39	D48.5	D49.2
eyelid	C44.10-✓	C79.2	D04.1-✓	D23.1-✓	D48.5	D49.2
basal cell carcinoma	C44.11-✓	—	—	—	—	—
specified type NEC	C44.19-✓	—	—	—	—	—
squamous cell carcinoma	C44.12-✓	—	—	—	—	—
face NOS	C44.300	C79.2	D04.30	D23.30	D48.5	D49.2
basal cell carcinoma	C44.310	—	—	—	—	—
specified type NEC	C44.390	—	—	—	—	—
squamous cell carcinoma	C44.320	—	—	—	—	—
female genital organs (external)	C51.9	C79.82	D07.1	D28.0	D39.8	D49.5
clitoris	C51.2	C79.82	D07.1	D28.0	D39.8	D49.5
labium NEC	C51.9	C79.82	D07.1	D28.0	D39.8	D49.5
majus	C51.0	C79.82	D07.1	D28.0	D39.8	D49.5
minus	C51.1	C79.82	D07.1	D28.0	D39.8	D49.5
pudendum	C51.9	C79.82	D07.1	D28.0	D39.8	D49.5
vulva	C51.9	C79.82	D07.1	D28.0	D39.8	D49.5
finger — see also Neoplasm, skin, limb, upper	C44.60-✓	C79.2	D04.6-✓	D23.6-✓	D48.5	D49.2
flank — see also Neoplasm, skin, trunk	C44.509	C79.2	D04.5	D23.5	D48.5	D49.2
foot — see also Neoplasm, skin, limb, lower	C44.70-✓	C79.2	D04.7-✓	D23.7-✓	D48.5	D49.2
forearm — see also Neoplasm, skin, limb, upper	C44.60-✓	C79.2	D04.6-✓	D23.6-✓	D48.5	D49.2
forehead — see also Neoplasm, skin, face	C44.309	C79.2	D04.39	D23.39	D48.5	D49.2
glabella — see also Neoplasm, skin, face	C44.309	C79.2	D04.39	D23.39	D48.5	D49.2
gluteal region — see also Neoplasm, skin, trunk	C44.509	C79.2	D04.5	D23.5	D48.5	D49.2
groin — see also Neoplasm, skin, trunk	C44.509	C79.2	D04.5	D23.5	D48.5	D49.2
hand — see also Neoplasm, skin, limb, upper	C44.60-✓	C79.2	D04.6-✓	D23.6-✓	D48.5	D49.2
head NEC — see also Neoplasm, skin, scalp	C44.40	C79.2	D04.4	D23.4	D48.5	D49.2
heel — see also Neoplasm, skin, limb, lower	C44.70-✓	C79.2	D04.7-✓	D23.7-✓	D48.5	D49.2
helix — see also Neoplasm, skin, ear	C44.20-✓	C79.2	D04.2-✓	D23.2-✓	D48.5	D49.2
hip — see also Neoplasm, skin, limb, lower	C44.70-✓	C79.2	D04.7-✓	D23.7-✓	D48.5	D49.2
infraclavicular region — see also Neoplasm, skin, trunk	C44.509	C79.2	D04.5	D23.5	D48.5	D49.2
inguinal region — see also Neoplasm, skin, trunk	C44.509	C79.2	D04.5	D23.5	D48.5	D49.2
jaw — see also Neoplasm, skin, face	C44.309	C79.2	D04.39	D23.39	D48.5	D49.2
Kaposi's sarcoma — see Kaposi's, sarcoma, skin						
knee — see also Neoplasm, skin, limb, lower	C44.70-✓	C79.2	D04.7-✓	D23.7-✓	D48.5	D49.2
labia						

✓ Additional Character Required — Refer to the Tabular List for Character Selection   ▽ Subterms under main terms may continue to next column or page

Neoplasm, neoplastic — continued	Malignant Primary	Malignant Secondary	Ca in situ	Benign	Uncertain	Unspecified Behavior
skin — continued						
labia — continued						
majora	C51.0	C79.82	D07.1	D28.0	D39.8	D49.5
minora	C51.1	C79.82	D07.1	D28.0	D39.8	D49.5
leg — see also						
Neoplasm, skin, limb, lower	C44.70-☑	C79.2	D04.7-☑	D23.7-☑	D48.5	D49.2
lid (lower) (upper)	C44.10-☑	C79.2	D04.1-☑	D23.1-☑	D48.5	D49.2
basal cell carcinoma	C44.11-☑	—	—	—	—	—
specified type NEC	C44.19-☑	—	—	—	—	—
squamous cell carcinoma	C44.12-☑	—	—	—	—	—
limb NEC	C44.90	C79.2	D04.9	D23.9	D48.5	D49.2
basal cell carcinoma	C44.91	—	—	—	—	—
lower	C44.70-☑	C79.2	D04.7-☑	D23.7-☑	D48.5	D49.2
basal cell carcinoma	C44.71-☑	—	—	—	—	—
specified type NEC	C44.79-☑	—	—	—	—	—
squamous cell carcinoma	C44.72-☑	—	—	—	—	—
upper	C44.60-☑	C79.2	D04.6-☑	D23.6-☑	D48.5	D49.2
basal cell carcinoma	C44.61-☑	—	—	—	—	—
specified type NEC	C44.69-☑	—	—	—	—	—
squamous cell carcinoma	C44.62-☑	—	—	—	—	—
lip (lower) (upper)	C44.00	C79.2	D04.0	D23.0	D48.5	D49.2
basal cell carcinoma	C44.01	—	—	—	—	—
specified type NEC	C44.09	—	—	—	—	—
squamous cell carcinoma	C44.02	—	—	—	—	—
male genital organs	C63.9	C79.82	D07.60	D29.9	D40.8	D49.5
penis	C60.9	C79.82	D07.4	D29.0	D40.8	D49.5
prepuce	C60.0	C79.82	D07.4	D29.0	D40.8	D49.5
scrotum	C63.2	C79.82	D07.61	D29.4	D40.8	D49.5
mastectomy site (skin) — see also						
Neoplasm, skin, breast	C44.501	C79.2	—	—	—	—
specified as breast tissue	C50.8-☑	C79.81	—	—	—	—
meatus, acoustic (external) — see also Neoplasm, skin, ear	C44.20-☑	C79.2	D04.2-☑	D23.2-☑	D48.5	D49.2
melanotic — see Melanoma						
Merkel cell — see Carcinoma, Merkel cell						
nates — see also Neoplasm, skin, trunk	C44.509	C79.2	D04.5	D23.5	D48.5	D49.2
neck	C44.40	C79.2	D04.4	D23.4	D48.5	D49.2
basal cell carcinoma	C44.41	—	—	—	—	—
specified type NEC	C44.49	—	—	—	—	—
squamous cell carcinoma	C44.42	—	—	—	—	—
nevus — see Nevus, skin						
nose (external) — see also Neoplasm, nose, skin	C44.301	C79.2	D04.39	D23.39	D48.5	D49.2
overlapping lesion	C44.80	—	—	—	—	—
basal cell carcinoma	C44.81	—	—	—	—	—
specified type NEC	C44.89	—	—	—	—	—
squamous cell carcinoma	C44.82	—	—	—	—	—

Neoplasm, neoplastic — continued	Malignant Primary	Malignant Secondary	Ca in situ	Benign	Uncertain	Unspecified Behavior
skin — continued						
palm — see also						
Neoplasm, skin, limb, upper	C44.60-☑	C79.2	D04.6-☑	D23.6-☑	D48.5	D49.2
palpebra	C44.10-☑	C79.2	D04.1-☑	D23.1-☑	D48.5	D49.2
basal cell carcinoma	C44.11-☑	—	—	—	—	—
specified type NEC	C44.19-☑	—	—	—	—	—
squamous cell carcinoma	C44.12-☑	—	—	—	—	—
penis NEC	C60.9	C79.82	D07.4	D29.0	D40.8	D49.5
perianal — see also Neoplasm, skin, anus	C44.500	C79.2	D04.5	D23.5	D48.5	D49.2
perineum — see also Neoplasm, skin, anus	C44.500	C79.2	D04.5	D23.5	D48.5	D49.2
pinna — see also Neoplasm, skin, ear	C44.20-☑	C79.2	D04.2-☑	D23.2-☑	D48.5	D49.2
plantar — see also Neoplasm, skin, limb, lower	C44.70-☑	C79.2	D04.7-☑	D23.7-☑	D48.5	D49.2
popliteal fossa or space — see also Neoplasm, skin, limb, lower	C44.70-☑	C79.2	D04.7-☑	D23.7-☑	D48.5	D49.2
prepuce	C60.0	C79.82	D07.4	D29.0	D40.8	D49.5
pubes — see also Neoplasm, skin, trunk	C44.509	C79.2	D04.5	D23.5	D48.5	D49.2
sacrococcygeal region — see also Neoplasm, skin, trunk	C44.509	C79.2	D04.5	D23.5	D48.5	D49.2
scalp	C44.40	C79.2	D04.4	D23.4	D48.5	D49.2
basal cell carcinoma	C44.41	—	—	—	—	—
specified type NEC	C44.49	—	—	—	—	—
squamous cell carcinoma	C44.42	—	—	—	—	—
scapular region — see also Neoplasm, skin, trunk	C44.509	C79.2	D04.5	D23.5	D48.5	D49.2
scrotum	C63.2	C79.82	D07.61	D29.4	D40.8	D49.5
shoulder — see also Neoplasm, skin, limb, upper	C44.60-☑	C79.2	D04.6-☑	D23.6-☑	D48.5	D49.2
sole (foot) — see also Neoplasm, skin, limb, lower	C44.70-☑	C79.2	D04.7-☑	D23.7-☑	D48.5	D49.2
specified sites NEC	C44.80	C79.2	D04.8	D23.9	D48.5	D49.2
basal cell carcinoma	C44.81	—	—	—	—	—
specified type NEC	C44.89	—	—	—	—	—
squamous cell carcinoma	C44.82	—	—	—	—	—
specified type NEC	C44.99	—	—	—	—	—
squamous cell carcinoma	C44.92	—	—	—	—	—
submammary fold — see also Neoplasm, skin, trunk	C44.509	C79.2	D04.5	D23.5	D48.5	D49.2
supraclavicular region — see also Neoplasm, skin, neck	C44.40	C79.2	D04.4	D23.4	D48.5	D49.2
temple — see also Neoplasm, skin, face	C44.309	C79.2	D04.39	D23.39	D48.5	D49.2
thigh — see also Neoplasm, skin, limb, lower	C44.70-☑	C79.2	D04.7-☑	D23.7-☑	D48.5	D49.2
thoracic wall — see also Neoplasm, skin, trunk	C44.509	C79.2	D04.5	D23.5	D48.5	D49.2

Neoplasm, neoplastic — continued	Malignant Primary	Malignant Secondary	Ca in situ	Benign	Uncertain	Unspecified Behavior
skin — continued						
thumb — see also Neoplasm, skin, limb, upper	C44.60-☑	C79.2	D04.6-☑	D23.6-☑	D48.5	D49.2
toe — see also Neoplasm, skin, limb, lower	C44.70-☑	C79.2	D04.7-☑	D23.7-☑	D48.5	D49.2
tragus — see also Neoplasm, skin, ear	C44.20-☑	C79.2	D04.2-☑	D23.2-☑	D48.5	D49.2
trunk	C44.509	C79.2	D04.5	D23.5	D48.5	D49.2
basal cell carcinoma	C44.519	—	—	—	—	—
specified type NEC	C44.599	—	—	—	—	—
squamous cell carcinoma	C44.529	—	—	—	—	—
umbilicus — see also Neoplasm, skin, trunk	C44.509	C79.2	D04.5	D23.5	D48.5	D49.2
vulva	C51.9	C79.82	D07.1	D28.0	D39.8	D49.5
overlapping lesion	C51.8					
wrist — see also Neoplasm, skin, limb, upper	C44.60-☑	C79.2	D04.6-☑	D23.6-☑	D48.5	D49.2
skull	C41.0	C79.51		D16.4-	D48.0	D49.2
soft parts or tissues — see Neoplasm, connective tissue						
specified site NEC	C76.8	C79.89	D09.8	D36.7	D48.7	D49.89
spermatic cord	C63.1-☑	C79.82	D07.69	D29.8	D40.8	D49.5
sphenoid	C31.3	C78.39	D02.3	D14.0	D38.5	D49.1
bone	C41.0	C79.51	—	D16.4-	D48.0	D49.2
sinus	C31.3	C78.39	D02.3	D14.0	D38.5	D49.1
sphincter						
anal	C21.1	C78.5	D01.3	D12.9	D37.8	D49.0
of Oddi	C24.0	C78.89	D01.5	D13.5	D37.6	D49.0
spine, spinal (column)	C41.2	C79.51	—	D16.6	D48.0	D49.2
bulb	C71.7	C79.31	—	D33.1	D43.1	D49.6
coccyx	C41.4	C79.51	—	D16.8	D48.0	D49.2
cord (cervical) (lumbar) (sacral) (thoracic)	C72.0	C79.49	—	D33.4	D43.4	D49.7
dura mater	C70.1	C79.49	—	D32.1	D42.1	D49.7
lumbosacral	C41.2	C79.51	—	D16.6	D48.0	D49.2
marrow NEC	C96.9	C79.52	—	—	D47.9	D49.89
membrane	C70.1	C79.49	—	D32.1	D42.1	D49.7
meninges	C70.1	C79.49	—	D32.1	D42.1	D49.7
nerve (root)	C47.9	C79.89	—	D36.10	D48.2	D49.2
pia mater	C70.1	C79.49	—	D32.1	D42.1	D49.7
root	C47.9	C79.89	—	D36.10	D48.2	D49.2
sacrum	C41.4	C79.51	—	D16.8	D48.0	D49.2
spleen, splenic NEC	C26.1	C78.89	D01.7	D13.9	D37.8	D49.0
flexure (colon)	C18.5	C78.5	D01.0	D12.3	D37.4	D49.0
stem, brain	C71.7	C79.31	—	D33.1	D43.1	D49.6
Stensen's duct	C07	C79.89	D00.00	D11.0	D37.030	D49.0
sternum	C41.3	C79.51	—	D16.7	D48.0	D49.2
stomach	C16.9	C78.89	D00.2	D13.1	D37.1	D49.0
antrum (pyloric)	C16.3	C78.89	D00.2	D13.1	D37.1	D49.0
body	C16.2	C78.89	D00.2	D13.1	D37.1	D49.0
cardia	C16.0	C78.89	D00.2	D13.1	D37.1	D49.0
cardiac orifice	C16.0	C78.89	D00.2	D13.1	D37.1	D49.0
corpus	C16.2	C78.89	D00.2	D13.1	D37.1	D49.0
fundus	C16.1	C78.89	D00.2	D13.1	D37.1	D49.0
greater curvature NEC	C16.6	C78.89	D00.2	D13.1	D37.1	D49.0
lesser curvature NEC	C16.5	C78.89	D00.2	D13.1	D37.1	D49.0
overlapping lesion	C16.8	—	—	—	—	—
prepylorus	C16.4	C78.89	D00.2	D13.1	D37.1	D49.0
pylorus	C16.4	C78.89	D00.2	D13.1	D37.1	D49.0
wall NEC	C16.9	C78.89	D00.2	D13.1	D37.1	D49.0
anterior NEC	C16.8	C78.89	D00.2	D13.1	D37.1	D49.0
posterior NEC	C16.8	C78.89	D00.2	D13.1	D37.1	D49.0
stroma, endometrial	C54.1	C79.82	D07.0	D26.1	D39.0	D49.5
stump, cervical	C53.8	C79.82	D06.7	D26.0	D39.0	D49.5
subcutaneous (nodule) (tissue) NEC — see						

Neoplasm, neoplastic — continued	Malignant Primary	Malignant Secondary	Ca in situ	Benign	Uncertain	Unspecified Behavior
subcutaneous — see Neoplasm, connective tissue — continued Neoplasm, connective tissue						
subdural	C70.9	C79.32	—	D32.9	D42.9	D49.7
subglottis, subglottic	C32.2	C78.39	D02.0	D14.1	D38.0	D49.1
sublingual	C04.9	C79.89	D00.06	D10.2	D37.09	D49.0
gland or duct	C08.1	C79.89	D00.00	D11.7	D37.031	D49.0
submandibular gland	C08.0	C79.89	D00.00	D11.7	D37.032	D49.0
submaxillary gland or duct	C08.0	C79.89	D00.00	D11.7	D37.032	D49.0
submental	C76.0	C79.89	D09.8	D36.7	D48.7	D49.89
subpleural	C34.9-☑	C78.0-☑	D02.2-☑	D14.3-☑	D38.1	D49.1
substernal	C38.1	C78.1	—	D15.2	D38.3	D49.89
sudoriferous, sudoriparous gland, site unspecified	C44.90	C79.2	D04.9	D23.9	D48.5	D49.2
specified site — see Neoplasm, skin						
supraclavicular region	C76.0	C79.89	D09.8	D36.7	D48.7	D49.89
supraglottis	C32.1	C78.39	D02.0	D14.1	D38.0	D49.1
suprarenal	C74.9-☑	C79.7-☑	D09.3	D35.0-☑	D44.1-☑	D49.7
capsule	C74.9-☑	C79.7-☑	D09.3	D35.0-☑	D44.1-☑	D49.7
cortex	C74.0-☑	C79.7-☑	D09.3	D35.0-☑	D44.1-☑	D49.7
gland	C74.9-☑	C79.7-☑	D09.3	D35.0-☑	D44.1-☑	D49.7
medulla	C74.1-☑	C79.7-☑	D09.3	D35.0-☑	D44.1-☑	D49.7
suprasellar (region)	C71.9	C79.31	—	D33.2	D42.2	D49.6
supratentorial (brain) NEC	C71.0	C79.31	—	D33.0	D43.0	D49.6
sweat gland (apocrine) (eccrine), site unspecified	C44.90	C79.2	D04.9	D23.9	D48.5	D49.2
specified site — see Neoplasm, skin						
sympathetic nerve or nervous system NEC	C47.9	C79.89	—	D36.10	D48.2	D49.2
symphysis pubis	C41.4	C79.51	—	D16.8	D48.0	D49.2
synovial membrane — see Neoplasm, connective tissue						
tapetum, brain	C71.8	C79.31	—	D33.2	D43.2	D49.6
tarsus (any bone)	C40.3-☑	C79.51	—	D16.3-☑	—	—
temple (skin) — see also Neoplasm, skin, face	C44.309	C79.2	D04.39	D23.39	D48.5	D49.2
temporal						
bone	C41.0	C79.51	—	D16.4-	D48.0	D49.2
lobe or pole	C71.2	C79.31	—	D33.0	D43.0	D49.6
region	C76.0	C79.89	D09.8	D36.7	D48.7	D49.89
skin — see also Neoplasm, skin, face	C44.309	C79.2	D04.39	D23.39	D48.5	D49.2
tendon (sheath) — see Neoplasm, connective tissue						
tentorium (cerebelli)	C70.0	C79.32	—	D32.0	D42.0	D49.7
testis, testes	C62.9-☑	C79.82	D07.69	D29.2-☑	D40.1-☑	D49.5
descended	C62.1-☑	C79.82	D07.69	D29.2-☑	D40.1-☑	D49.5
ectopic	C62.0-☑	C79.82	D07.69	D29.2-☑	D40.1-☑	D49.5
retained	C62.0-☑	C79.82	D07.69	D29.2-☑	D40.1-☑	D49.5
scrotal	C62.1-☑	C79.82	D07.69	D29.2-☑	D40.1-☑	D49.5
undescended	C62.0-☑	C79.82	D07.69	D29.2-☑	D40.1-☑	D49.5
unspecified whether descended or undescended	C62.9-☑	C79.82	D07.69	D29.2-☑	D40.1-☑	D49.5
thalamus	C71.0	C79.31	—	D33.0	D43.0	D49.6
thigh NEC	C76.5-☑	C79.89	D04.7-☑	D36.7	D48.7	D49.89
thorax, thoracic (cavity) (organs NEC)	C76.1	C79.89	D09.8	D36.7	D48.7	D49.89
duct	C49.3	C79.89	—	D21.3	D48.1	D49.2
wall NEC	C76.1	C79.89	D09.8	D36.7	D48.7	D49.89
throat	C14.0	C79.89	D00.08	D10.9	D37.05	D49.0
thumb NEC	C76.4-☑	C79.89	D04.6-☑	D36.7	D48.7	D49.89
thymus (gland)	C37	C79.89	D09.3	D15.0	D38.4	D49.89
thyroglossal duct	C73	C79.89	D09.3	D34	D44.0	D49.7

☑ **Additional Character Required** — Refer to the Tabular List for Character Selection   ▽ **Subterms under main terms may continue to next column or page**

Neoplasm, neoplastic —
continued

	Malignant Primary	Malignant Secondary	Ca in situ	Benign	Uncertain	Unspecified Behavior
thyroid (gland)	C73	C79.89	D09.3	D34	D44.0	D49.7
cartilage	C32.3	C78.39	D02.0	D14.1	D38.0	D49.1
tibia (any part)	C40.2-☑	C79.51	—	D16.2-☑	—	D49.2
toe NEC	C76.5-☑	C79.89	D04.7-☑	D36.7	D48.7	D49.89
tongue	C02.9	C79.89	D00.07	D10.1	D37.02	D49.0
anterior (two-thirds)						
NEC	C02.3	C79.89	D00.07	D10.1	D37.02	D49.0
dorsal surface	C02.0	C79.89	D00.07	D10.1	D37.02	D49.0
ventral surface	C02.2	C79.89	D00.07	D10.1	D37.02	D49.0
base (dorsal surface)	C01	C79.89	D00.07	D10.1	D37.02	D49.0
border (lateral)	C02.1	C79.89	D00.07	D10.1	D37.02	D49.0
dorsal surface NEC	C02.0	C79.89	D00.07	D10.1	D37.02	D49.0
fixed part NEC	C01	C79.89	D00.07	D10.1	D37.02	D49.0
foreamen cecum	C02.0	C79.89	D00.07	D10.1	D37.02	D49.0
frenulum linguae	C02.2	C79.89	D00.07	D10.1	D37.02	D49.0
junctional zone	C02.8	C79.89	D00.07	D10.1	D37.02	D49.0
margin (lateral)	C02.1	C79.89	D00.07	D10.1	D37.02	D49.0
midline NEC	C02.0	C79.89	D00.07	D10.1	D37.02	D49.0
mobile part NEC	C02.3	C79.89	D00.07	D10.1	D37.02	D49.0
overlapping lesion	C02.8	—	—	—	—	—
posterior (third)	C01	C79.89	D00.07	D10.1	D37.02	D49.0
root	C01	C79.89	D00.07	D10.1	D37.02	D49.0
surface (dorsal)	C02.0	C79.89	D00.07	D10.1	D37.02	D49.0
base	C01	C79.89	D00.07	D10.1	D37.02	D49.0
ventral	C02.2	C79.89	D00.07	D10.1	D37.02	D49.0
tip	C02.1	C79.89	D00.07	D10.1	D37.02	D49.0
tonsil	C02.4	C79.89	D00.07	D10.1	D37.02	D49.0
tonsil	C09.9	C79.89	D00.08	D10.4	D37.05	D49.0
fauces, faucial	C09.9	C79.89	D00.08	D10.4	D37.05	D49.0
lingual	C02.4	C79.89	D00.07	D10.1	D37.02	D49.0
overlapping sites	C09.8	—	—	—	—	—
palatine	C09.9	C79.89	D00.08	D10.4	D37.05	D49.0
pharyngeal	C11.1	C79.89	D00.08	D10.6	D37.05	D49.0
pillar (anterior) (posterior)	C09.1	C79.89	D00.08	D10.5	D37.05	D49.0
tonsillar fossa	C09.0	C79.89	D00.08	D10.5	D37.05	D49.0
tooth socket NEC	C03.9	C79.89	D00.03	D10.39	D37.09	D49.0
trachea (cartilage) (mucosa)	C33	C78.39	D02.1	D14.2	D38.1	D49.1
overlapping lesion with bronchus or lung	C34.8-☑	—	—	—	—	—
tracheobronchial	C34.8-☑	C78.39	D02.1	D14.2	D38.1	D49.1
overlapping lesion with lung	C34.8-☑	—	—	—	—	—
tragus — *see also* Neoplasm, skin, ear	C44.20-☑	C79.2	D04.2-☑	D23.2-☑	D48.5	D49.2
trunk NEC	C76.8	C79.89	D04.5	D36.7	D48.7	D49.89
tubo-ovarian	C57.8	C79.82	D07.39	D28.7	D39.8	D49.5
tunica vaginalis	C63.7	C79.82	D07.69	D29.8	D40.8	D49.5
turbinate (bone)	C41.0	C79.51	—	D16.4-	D48.0	D49.2
nasal	C30.0	C78.39	D02.3	D14.0	D38.5	D49.1
tympanic cavity	C30.1	C78.39	D02.3	D14.0	D38.5	D49.1
ulna (any part)	C40.0-☑	C79.51	—	D16.0-☑	—	D49.2
umbilicus, umbilical — *see also* Neoplasm, skin, trunk	C44.509	C79.2	D04.5	D23.5	D48.5	D49.2
uncus, brain	C71.2	C79.31	—	D33.0	D43.0	D49.6
unknown site or unspecified	C80.1	C79.9	D09.9	D36.9	D48.9	D49.9
urachus	C67.7	C79.11	D09.0	D30.3	D41.4	D49.4
ureter-bladder (junction)	C67.6	C79.11	D09.0	D30.3	D41.4	D49.4
ureter, ureteral	C66.-☑	C79.19	D09.19	D30.2-☑	D41.2-☑	D49.5
orifice (bladder)	C67.6	C79.11	D09.0	D30.3	D41.4	D49.4
urethra, urethral (gland)	C68.0	C79.19	D09.19	D30.4	D41.3	D49.5
orifice, internal	C67.5	C79.11	D09.0	D30.3	D41.4	D49.4
urethrovaginal (septum)	C57.9	C79.82	D07.30	D28.9	D39.8	D49.5
urinary organ or system	C68.9	C79.10	D09.10	D30.9	D41.9	D49.5
bladder — *see* Neoplasm, bladder						
overlapping lesion	C68.8	—	—	—	—	—
specified sites NEC	C68.8	C79.19	D09.19	D30.8	D41.8	D49.5
utero-ovarian	C57.8	C79.82	D07.39	D28.7	D39.8	D49.5
ligament	C57.1☑	C79.82	D07.39	D28.2	D39.8	D49.5
uterosacral ligament	C57.3	C79.82		D28.2	D39.8	

Neoplasm, neoplastic —
continued

	Malignant Primary	Malignant Secondary	Ca in situ	Benign	Uncertain	Unspecified Behavior
uterus, uteri, uterine	C55	C79.82	D07.0	D26.9	D39.0	D49.5
adnexa NEC	C57.4	C79.82	D07.39	D28.7	D39.8	D49.5
body	C54.9	C79.82	D07.0	D26.1	D39.0	D49.5
cervix	C53.9	C79.82	D06.9	D26.0	D39.0	D49.5
cornu	C54.9	C79.82	D07.0	D26.1	D39.0	D49.5
corpus	C54.9	C79.82	D07.0	D26.1	D39.0	
endocervix (canal) (gland)	C53.0	C79.82	D06.0	D26.0	D39.0	D49.5
endometrium	C54.1	C79.82	D07.0	D26.1	D39.0	D49.5
exocervix	C53.1	C79.82	D06.1	D26.0	D39.0	D49.5
external os	C53.1	C79.82	D06.1	D26.0	D39.0	D49.5
fundus	C54.3	C79.82	D07.0	D26.1	D39.0	D49.5
internal os	C53.0	C79.82	D06.0	D26.0	D39.0	D49.5
isthmus	C54.0	C79.82	D07.0	D26.1	D39.0	D49.5
ligament	C57.3	C79.82		D28.2	D39.8	D49.5
broad	C57.1☑	C79.82	D07.39	D28.2	D39.8	D49.5
round	C57.2☑	C79.82	—	D28.2	D39.8	D49.5
lower segment	C54.0	C79.82	D07.0	D26.1	D39.0	D49.5
myometrium	C54.2	C79.82	D07.0	D26.1	D39.0	D49.5
overlapping sites	C54.8	—	—	—	—	—
squamocolumnar junction	C53.8	C79.82	D06.7	D26.0	D39.0	D49.5
tube	C57.0-☑	C79.82	D07.39	D28.2	D39.8	D49.5
utricle, prostatic	C68.0	C79.19	—	D30.4	D41.3	D49.5
uveal tract	C69.4-☑	C79.49	D09.2-☑	D31.4-☑	D48.7	D49.89
uvula	C05.2	C79.89	D00.04	D10.39	D37.09	D49.0
vagina, vaginal (fornix) (vault) (wall)	C52	C79.82	D07.2	D28.1	D39.8	D49.5
vaginovesical	C57.9	C79.82	D07.30	D28.9	D39.9	D49.5
septum	C57.9	C79.82	D07.30	D28.9	D39.9	D49.5
vallecula (epiglottis)	C10.0	C79.89	D00.08	D10.5	D37.05	D49.0
vascular — *see* Neoplasm, connective tissue						
vas deferens	C63.1-☑	C79.82	D07.69	D29.8	D40.8	D49.5
Vater's ampulla	C24.1	C78.89	D01.5	D13.5	D37.6	D49.0
vein, venous — *see* Neoplasm, connective tissue						
vena cava (abdominal) (inferior)	C49.4	C79.89	—	D21.4	D48.1	D49.2
superior	C49.3	C79.89	—	D21.3	D48.1	D49.2
ventricle (cerebral) (floor) (lateral) (third)	C71.5	C79.31	—	D33.0	D43.0	D49.6
cardiac (left) (right)	C38.0	C79.89	—	D15.1	D48.7	D49.89
fourth	C71.7	C79.31	—	D33.1	D43.1	D49.6
ventricular band of larynx	C32.1	C78.39	D02.0	D14.1	D38.0	D49.1
ventriculus — *see* Neoplasm, stomach						
vermillion border — *see* Neoplasm, lip						
vermis, cerebellum	C71.6	C79.31	—	D33.1	D43.1	D49.6
vertebra (column)	C41.2	C79.51	—	D16.6	D48.0	D49.2
coccyx	C41.4	C79.51	—	D16.8-	D48.0	D49.2
marrow NEC	C96.9	C79.52	—	—	D47.9	D49.89
sacrum	C41.4	C79.51	—	D16.8-	D48.0	D49.2
vesical — *see* Neoplasm, bladder						
vesicle, seminal	C63.7	C79.82	D07.69	D29.8	D40.8	D49.5
vesicocervical tissue	C57.9	C79.82	D07.30	D28.9	D39.9	D49.5
vesicorectal	C76.3	C79.82	D09.8	D36.7	D48.7	D49.89
vesicovaginal	C57.9	C79.82	D07.30	D28.9	D39.9	D49.5
septum	C57.9	C79.82	D07.30	D28.9	D39.8	D49.5
vessel (blood) — *see* Neoplasm, connective tissue						
vestibular gland, greater	C51.0	C79.82	D07.1	D28.0	D39.8	D49.5
vestibule						
mouth	C06.1	C79.89	D00.00	D10.39	D37.09	D49.0
nose	C30.0	C78.39	D02.3	D14.0	D38.5	D49.1
Virchow's gland	C77.0	C77.0	—	D36.0	D48.7	D49.89
viscera NEC	C76.8	C79.89	D09.8	D36.7	D48.7	D49.89
vocal cords (true)	C32.0	C78.39	D02.0	D14.1	D38.0	D49.1
false	C32.1	C78.39	D02.0	D14.1	D38.0	D49.1
vomer	C41.0	C79.51	—	D16.4-	D48.0	D49.2
vulva	C51.9	C79.82	D07.1	D28.0	D39.8	D49.5
vulvovaginal gland	C51.0	C79.82	D07.1	D28.0	D39.8	D49.5
Waldeyer's ring	C14.2	C79.89	D00.08	D10.9	D37.05	D49.0
Wharton's duct	C08.0	C79.89	D00.00	D11.7	D37.032	D49.0

	Malignant Primary	Malignant Secondary	Ca in situ	Benign	Uncertain	Unspecified Behavior
Neoplasm, neoplastic — *continued*						
white matter (central) (cerebral)	C71.Ø	C79.31	—	D33.Ø	D43.Ø	D49.6
windpipe	C33	C78.39	DØ2.1	D14.2	D38.1	D49.1
Wirsung's duct	C25.3	C78.89	DØ1.7	D13.6	D37.8	D49.Ø
wolffian (body) (duct)						
female	C57.7	C79.82	DØ7.39	D28.7	D39.8	D49.5
male	C63.7	C79.82	DØ7.69	D29.8	D40.8	D49.5
womb — *see* Neoplasm, uterus						
wrist NEC	C76.4-☑	C79.89	DØ4.6-☑	D36.7	D48.7	D49.89
xiphoid process	C41.3	C79.51	—	D16.7	D48.Ø	D49.2
Zuckerkandl organ	C75.5	C79.89	—	D35.6	D44.7	D49.7

ICD-1Ø-CM Table of Drugs and Chemicals

Substance	Poisoning, Accidental (unintentional)	Poisoning, Intentional Self-harm	Poisoning, Assault	Poisoning, Undetermined	Adverse Effect	Under-dosing
14-Hydroxydihydromorphinone	T40.2X1	T40.2X2	T40.2X3	T40.2X4	T40.2X5	T40.2X6
1-Propanol	T51.3X1	T51.3X2	T51.3X3	T51.3X4	—	—
2,3,7,8-Tetrachlorodibenzo-p-dioxin	T53.7X1	T53.7X2	T53.7X3	T53.7X4	—	—
2,4,5-T (trichlorophenoxyacetic acid)	T60.1X1	T60.1X2	T60.1X3	T60.1X4	—	—
2,4,5-Trichlorophenoxyacetic acid	T60.3X1	T60.3X2	T60.3X3	T60.3X4	—	—
2,4-D (dichlorophenoxyacetic acid)	T60.3X1	T60.3X2	T60.3X3	T60.3X4	—	—
2,4-Toluene diisocyanate	T65.0X1	T65.0X2	T65.0X3	T65.0X4	—	—
2-Deoxy-5-fluorouridine	T45.1X1	T45.1X2	T45.1X3	T45.1X4	T45.1X5	T45.1X6
2-Ethoxyethanol	T52.3X1	T52.3X2	T52.3X3	T52.3X4	—	—
2-Methoxyethanol	T52.3X1	T52.3X2	T52.3X3	T52.3X4	—	—
2-Propanol	T51.2X1	T51.2X2	T51.2X3	T51.2X4	—	—
4-Aminobutyric acid	T43.8X1	T43.8X2	T43.8X3	T43.8X4	T43.8X5	T43.8X6
4-Aminophenol derivatives	T39.1X1	T39.1X2	T39.1X3	T39.1X4	T39.1X5	T39.1X6
5-Deoxy-5-fluorouridine	T45.1X1	T45.1X2	T45.1X3	T45.1X4	T45.1X5	T45.1X6
5-Methoxypsoralen (5-MOP)	T50.991	T50.992	T50.993	T50.994	T50.995	T50.996
8-Aminoquinoline drugs	T37.2X1	T37.2X2	T37.2X3	T37.2X4	T37.2X5	T37.2X6
8-Methoxypsoralen (8-MOP)	T50.991	T50.992	T50.993	T50.994	T50.995	T50.996
ABOB	T37.5X1	T37.5X2	T37.5X3	T37.5X4	T37.5X5	T37.5X6
Abrine	T62.2X1	T62.2X2	T62.2X3	T62.2X4	—	—
Abrus (seed)	T62.2X1	T62.2X2	T62.2X3	T62.2X4	—	—
Absinthe	T51.0X1	T51.0X2	T51.0X3	T51.0X4	—	—
beverage	T51.0X1	T51.0X2	T51.0X3	T51.0X4	—	—
Acaricide	T60.8X1	T60.8X2	T60.8X3	T60.8X4	—	—
Acebutolol	T44.7X1	T44.7X2	T44.7X3	T44.7X4	T44.7X5	T44.7X6
Acecarbromal	T42.6X1	T42.6X2	T42.6X3	T42.6X4	T42.6X5	T42.6X6
Aceclidine	T44.1X1	T44.1X2	T44.1X3	T44.1X4	T44.1X5	T44.1X6
Acedapsone	T37.0X1	T37.0X2	T37.0X3	T37.0X4	T37.0X5	T37.0X6
Acefylline piperazine	T48.6X1	T48.6X2	T48.6X3	T48.6X4	T48.6X5	T48.6X6
Acemorphan	T40.2X1	T40.2X2	T40.2X3	T40.2X4	T40.2X5	T40.2X6
Acenocoumarin	T45.511	T45.512	T45.513	T45.514	T45.515	T45.516
Acenocoumarol	T45.511	T45.512	T45.513	T45.514	T45.515	T45.516
Acepifylline	T48.6X1	T48.6X2	T48.6X3	T48.6X4	T48.6X5	T48.6X6
Acepromazine	T43.3X1	T43.3X2	T43.3X3	T43.3X4	T43.3X5	T43.3X6
Acesulfamethoxypyridazine	T37.0X1	T37.0X2	T37.0X3	T37.0X4	T37.0X5	T37.0X6
Acetal	T52.8X1	T52.8X2	T52.8X3	T52.8X4	—	—
Acetaldehyde (vapor)	T52.8X1	T52.8X2	T52.8X3	T52.8X4	—	—
liquid	T65.891	T65.892	T65.893	T65.894	—	—
Acetaminophen	T39.1X1	T39.1X2	T39.1X3	T39.1X4	T39.1X5	T39.1X6
Acetaminosalol	T39.1X1	T39.1X2	T39.1X3	T39.1X4	T39.1X5	T39.1X6
Acetanilide	T39.1X1	T39.1X2	T39.1X3	T39.1X4	T39.1X5	T39.1X6
Acetarsol	T37.3X1	T37.3X2	T37.3X3	T37.3X4	T37.3X5	T37.3X6
Acetazolamide	T50.2X1	T50.2X2	T50.2X3	T50.2X4	T50.2X5	T50.2X6
Acetiamine	T45.2X1	T45.2X2	T45.2X3	T45.2X4	T45.2X5	T45.2X6
Acetic						
acid	T54.2X1	T54.2X2	T54.2X3	T54.2X4	—	—
with sodium acetate (ointment)	T49.3X1	T49.3X2	T49.3X3	T49.3X4	T49.3X5	T49.3X6
ester (solvent)(vapor)	T52.8X1	T52.8X2	T52.8X3	T52.8X4	—	—
irrigating solution	T50.3X1	T50.3X2	T50.3X3	T50.3X4	T50.3X5	T50.3X6
medicinal (lotion)	T49.2X1	T49.2X2	T49.2X3	T49.2X4	T49.2X5	T49.2X6
anhydride	T65.891	T65.892	T65.893	T65.894	—	—
ether (vapor)	T52.8X1	T52.8X2	T52.8X3	T52.8X4	—	—
Acetohexamide	T38.3X1	T38.3X2	T38.3X3	T38.3X4	T38.3X5	T38.3X6
Acetohydroxamic acid	T50.991	T50.992	T50.993	T50.994	T50.995	T50.996
Acetomenaphthone	T45.7X1	T45.7X2	T45.7X3	T45.7X4	T45.7X5	T45.7X6
Acetomorphine	T40.1X1	T40.1X2	T40.1X3	T40.1X4	—	—
Acetone (oils)	T52.4X1	T52.4X2	T52.4X3	T52.4X4	—	—
chlorinated	T52.4X1	T52.4X2	T52.4X3	T52.4X4	—	—
vapor	T52.4X1	T52.4X2	T52.4X3	T52.4X4	—	—
Acetonitrile	T52.8X1	T52.8X2	T52.8X3	T52.8X4	—	—
Acetophenazine	T43.3X1	T43.3X2	T43.3X3	T43.3X4	T43.3X5	T43.3X6
Acetophenetedin	T39.1X1	T39.1X2	T39.1X3	T39.1X4	T39.1X5	T39.1X6
Acetophenone	T52.4X1	T52.4X2	T52.4X3	T52.4X4	—	—
Acetorphine	T40.2X1	T40.2X2	T40.2X3	T40.2X4	—	—
Acetosulfone (sodium)	T37.1X1	T37.1X2	T37.1X3	T37.1X4	T37.1X5	T37.1X6
Acetrizoate (sodium)	T50.8X1	T50.8X2	T50.8X3	T50.8X4	T50.8X5	T50.8X6
Acetrizoic acid	T50.8X1	T50.8X2	T50.8X3	T50.8X4	T50.8X5	T50.8X6
Acetyl						
bromide	T53.6X1	T53.6X2	T53.6X3	T53.6X4	—	—
chloride	T53.6X1	T53.6X2	T53.6X3	T53.6X4	—	—
Acetylcarbromal	T42.6X1	T42.6X2	T42.6X3	T42.6X4	T42.6X5	T42.6X6

Substance	Poisoning, Accidental (unintentional)	Poisoning, Intentional Self-harm	Poisoning, Assault	Poisoning, Undetermined	Adverse Effect	Under-dosing
Acetylcholine						
chloride	T44.1X1	T44.1X2	T44.1X3	T44.1X4	T44.1X5	T44.1X6
derivative	T44.1X1	T44.1X2	T44.1X3	T44.1X4	T44.1X5	T44.1X6
Acetylcysteine	T48.4X1	T48.4X2	T48.4X3	T48.4X4	T48.4X5	T48.4X6
Acetyldigitoxin	T46.0X1	T46.0X2	T46.0X3	T46.0X4	T46.0X5	T46.0X6
Acetyldigoxin	T46.0X1	T46.0X2	T46.0X3	T46.0X4	T46.0X5	T46.0X6
Acetyldihydrocodeine	T40.2X1	T40.2X2	T40.2X3	T40.2X4	—	—
Acetyldihydrocodeinone	T40.2X1	T40.2X2	T40.2X3	T40.2X4	—	—
Acetylene (gas)	T59.891	T59.892	T59.893	T59.894	—	—
dichloride	T53.6X1	T53.6X2	T53.6X3	T53.6X4	—	—
incomplete combustion of	T58.11	T58.12	T58.13	T58.14	—	—
industrial	T59.891	T59.892	T59.893	T59.894	—	—
tetrachloride	T53.6X1	T53.6X2	T53.6X3	T53.6X4	—	—
vapor	T53.6X1	T53.6X2	T53.6X3	T53.6X4	—	—
Acetylphenneturide	T42.6X1	T42.6X2	T42.6X3	T42.6X4	T42.6X5	T42.6X6
Acetylphenylhydrazine	T39.8X1	T39.8X2	T39.8X3	T39.8X4	T39.8X5	T39.8X6
Acetylsalicylic acid (salts)	T39.011	T39.012	T39.013	T39.014	T39.015	T39.016
enteric coated	T39.011	T39.012	T39.013	T39.014	T39.015	T39.016
Acetylsulfamethoxypyridazine	T37.0X1	T37.0X2	T37.0X3	T37.0X4	T37.0X5	T37.0X6
Achromycin	T36.4X1	T36.4X2	T36.4X3	T36.4X4	T36.4X5	T36.4X6
ophthalmic preparation	T49.5X1	T49.5X2	T49.5X3	T49.5X4	T49.5X5	T49.5X6
topical NEC	T49.0X1	T49.0X2	T49.0X3	T49.0X4	T49.0X5	T49.0X6
Aciclovir	T37.5X1	T37.5X2	T37.5X3	T37.5X4	T37.5X5	T37.5X6
Acidifying agent NEC	T50.901	T50.902	T50.903	T50.904	T50.905	T50.906
Acid (corrosive) NEC	T54.2X1	T54.2X2	T54.2X3	T54.2X4	—	—
Acipimox	T46.6X1	T46.6X2	T46.6X3	T46.6X4	T46.6X5	T46.6X6
Acitretin	T50.991	T50.992	T50.993	T50.994	T50.995	T50.996
Aclarubicin	T45.1X1	T45.1X2	T45.1X3	T45.1X4	T45.1X5	T45.1X6
Aclatonium napadisilate	T48.1X1	T48.1X2	T48.1X3	T48.1X4	T48.1X5	T48.1X6
Aconite (wild)	T46.991	T46.992	T46.993	T46.994	T46.995	T46.996
Aconitine	T46.991	T46.992	T46.993	T46.994	T46.995	T46.996
Aconitum ferox	T46.991	T46.992	T46.993	T46.994	T46.995	T46.996
Acridine	T65.6X1	T65.6X2	T65.6X3	T65.6X4	—	—
vapor	T59.891	T59.892	T59.893	T59.894	—	—
Acriflavine	T37.91	T37.92	T37.93	T37.94	T37.95	T37.96
Acriflavinium chloride	T49.0X1	T49.0X2	T49.0X3	T49.0X4	T49.0X5	T49.0X6
Acrinol	T49.0X1	T49.0X2	T49.0X3	T49.0X4	T49.0X5	T49.0X6
Acrisorcin	T49.0X1	T49.0X2	T49.0X3	T49.0X4	T49.0X5	T49.0X6
Acrivastine	T45.0X1	T45.0X2	T45.0X3	T45.0X4	T45.0X5	T45.0X6
Acrolein (gas)	T59.891	T59.892	T59.893	T59.894	—	—
liquid	T54.1X1	T54.1X2	T54.1X3	T54.1X4	—	—
Acrylamide	T65.891	T65.892	T65.893	T65.894	—	—
Acrylic resin	T49.3X1	T49.3X2	T49.3X3	T49.3X4	T49.3X5	T49.3X6
Acrylonitrile	T65.891	T65.892	T65.893	T65.894	—	—
Actaea spicata	T62.2X1	T62.2X2	T62.2X3	T62.2X4	—	—
berry	T62.1X1	T62.1X2	T62.1X3	T62.1X4	—	—
Acterol	T37.3X1	T37.3X2	T37.3X3	T37.3X4	T37.3X5	T37.3X6
ACTH	T38.811	T38.812	T38.813	T38.814	T38.815	T38.816
Actinomycin C	T45.1X1	T45.1X2	T45.1X3	T45.1X4	T45.1X5	T45.1X6
Actinomycin D	T45.1X1	T45.1X2	T45.1X3	T45.1X4	T45.1X5	T45.1X6
Activated charcoal — see also Charcoal, medicinal	T47.6X1	T47.6X2	T47.6X3	T47.6X4	T47.6X5	T47.6X6
Acyclovir	T37.5X1	T37.5X2	T37.5X3	T37.5X4	T37.5X5	T37.5X6
Adenine	T45.2X1	T45.2X2	T45.2X3	T45.2X4	T45.2X5	T45.2X6
arabinoside	T37.5X1	T37.5X2	T37.5X3	T37.5X4	T37.5X5	T37.5X6
Adenosine (phosphate)	T46.2X1	T46.2X2	T46.2X3	T46.2X4	T46.2X5	T46.2X6
ADH	T38.891	T38.892	T38.893	T38.894	T38.895	T38.896
Adhesive NEC	T65.891	T65.892	T65.893	T65.894	—	—
Adicillin	T36.0X1	T36.0X2	T36.0X3	T36.0X4	T36.0X5	T36.0X6
Adiphenine	T44.3X1	T44.3X2	T44.3X3	T44.3X4	T44.3X5	T44.3X6
Adipiodone	T50.8X1	T50.8X2	T50.8X3	T50.8X4	T50.8X5	T50.8X6
Adjunct, pharmaceutical	T50.901	T50.902	T50.903	T50.904	T50.905	T50.906
Adrenal (extract, cortex or medulla) (glucocorticoids) (hormones) (mineralocorticoids)	T38.0X1	T38.0X2	T38.0X3	T38.0X4	T38.0X5	T38.0X6
ENT agent	T49.6X1	T49.6X2	T49.6X3	T49.6X4	T49.6X5	T49.6X6
ophthalmic preparation	T49.5X1	T49.5X2	T49.5X3	T49.5X4	T49.5X5	T49.5X6
topical NEC	T49.0X1	T49.0X2	T49.0X3	T49.0X4	T49.0X5	T49.0X6
Adrenalin — see Adrenaline						
Adrenaline	T44.5X1	T44.5X2	T44.5X3	T44.5X4	T44.5X5	T44.5X6
Adrenergic NEC	T44.901	T44.902	T44.903	T44.904	T44.905	T44.906
blocking agent NEC	T44.8X1	T44.8X2	T44.8X3	T44.8X4	T44.8X5	T44.8X6
beta, heart	T44.7X1	T44.7X2	T44.7X3	T44.7X4	T44.7X5	T44.7X6
specified NEC	T44.991	T44.992	T44.993	T44.994	T44.995	T44.996
Adrenochrome						
derivative	T46.991	T46.992	T46.993	T46.994	T46.995	T46.996

Substance	Poisoning, Accidental (unintentional)	Poisoning, Intentional Self-harm	Poisoning, Assault	Poisoning, Undetermined	Adverse Effect	Under-dosing
Adrenochrome — *continued*						
(mono) semicarbazone	T46.991	T46.992	T46.993	T46.994	T46.995	T46.996
Adrenocorticotrophic hormone	T38.811	T38.812	T38.813	T38.814	T38.815	T38.816
Adrenocorticotrophin	T38.811	T38.812	T38.813	T38.814	T38.815	T38.816
Adriamycin	T45.1X1	T45.1X2	T45.1X3	T45.1X4	T45.1X5	T45.1X6
Aerosol spray NEC	T65.91	T65.92	T65.93	T65.94	—	—
Aerosporin	T36.8X1	T36.8X2	T36.8X3	T36.8X4	T36.8X5	T36.8X6
ENT agent	T49.6X1	T49.6X2	T49.6X3	T49.6X4	T49.6X5	T49.6X6
ophthalmic preparation	T49.5X1	T49.5X2	T49.5X3	T49.5X4	T49.5X5	T49.5X6
topical NEC	T49.0X1	T49.0X2	T49.0X3	T49.0X4	T49.0X5	T49.0X6
Aethusa cynapium	T62.2X1	T62.2X2	T62.2X3	T62.2X4		
Afghanistan black	T40.7X1	T40.7X2	T40.7X3	T40.7X4	T40.7X5	T40.7X6
Aflatoxin	T64.01	T64.02	T64.03	T64.04		
Afloqualone	T42.8X1	T42.8X2	T42.8X3	T42.8X4	T42.8X5	T42.8X6
African boxwood	T62.2X1	T62.2X2	T62.2X3	T62.2X4		
Agar	T47.4X1	T47.4X2	T47.4X3	T47.4X4	T47.4X5	T47.4X6
Agonist						
predominantly						
alpha-adrenoreceptor	T44.4X1	T44.4X2	T44.4X3	T44.4X4	T44.4X5	T44.4X6
beta-adrenoreceptor	T44.5X1	T44.5X2	T44.5X3	T44.5X4	T44.5X5	T44.5X6
Agricultural agent NEC	T65.91	T65.92	T65.93	T65.94	—	—
Agrypnal	T42.3X1	T42.3X2	T42.3X3	T42.3X4	T42.3X5	T42.3X6
AHLG	T50.Z11	T50.Z12	T50.Z13	T50.Z14	T50.Z15	T50.Z16
Air contaminant(s), **source/type NOS**	T65.91	T65.92	T65.93	T65.94	—	—
Ajmaline	T46.2X1	T46.2X2	T46.2X3	T46.2X4	T46.2X5	T46.2X6
Akee	T62.1X1	T62.1X2	T62.1X3	T62.1X4		
Akrinol	T49.0X1	T49.0X2	T49.0X3	T49.0X4	T49.0X5	T49.0X6
Akritoin	T37.8X1	T37.8X2	T37.8X3	T37.8X4	T37.8X5	T37.8X6
Alacepril	T46.4X1	T46.4X2	T46.4X3	T46.4X4	T46.4X5	T46.4X6
Alantolactone	T37.4X1	T37.4X2	T37.4X3	T37.4X4	T37.4X5	T37.4X6
Albamycin	T36.8X1	T36.8X2	T36.8X3	T36.8X4	T36.8X5	T36.8X6
Albendazole	T37.4X1	T37.4X2	T37.4X3	T37.4X4	T37.4X5	T37.4X6
Albumin						
bovine	T45.8X1	T45.8X2	T45.8X3	T45.8X4	T45.8X5	T45.8X6
human serum	T45.8X1	T45.8X2	T45.8X3	T45.8X4	T45.8X5	T45.8X6
salt-poor	T45.8X1	T45.8X2	T45.8X3	T45.8X4	T45.8X5	T45.8X6
normal human serum	T45.8X1	T45.8X2	T45.8X3	T45.8X4	T45.8X5	T45.8X6
Albuterol	T48.6X1	T48.6X2	T48.6X3	T48.6X4	T48.6X5	T48.6X6
Albutoin	T42.0X1	T42.0X2	T42.0X3	T42.0X4	T42.0X5	T42.0X6
Alclometasone	T49.0X1	T49.0X2	T49.0X3	T49.0X4	T49.0X5	T49.0X6
Alcohol	T51.91	T51.92	T51.93	T51.94	—	—
absolute	T51.0X1	T51.0X2	T51.0X3	T51.0X4	—	—
beverage	T51.0X1	T51.0X2	T51.0X3	T51.0X4	—	—
allyl	T51.8X1	T51.8X2	T51.8X3	T51.8X4	—	—
amyl	T51.3X1	T51.3X2	T51.3X3	T51.3X4	—	—
antifreeze	T51.1X1	T51.1X2	T51.1X3	T51.1X4	—	—
beverage	T51.0X1	T51.0X2	T51.0X3	T51.0X4	—	—
butyl	T51.3X1	T51.3X2	T51.3X3	T51.3X4	—	—
dehydrated	T51.0X1	T51.0X2	T51.0X3	T51.0X4	—	—
beverage	T51.0X1	T51.0X2	T51.0X3	T51.0X4	—	—
denatured	T51.0X1	T51.0X2	T51.0X3	T51.0X4	—	—
deterrent NEC	T50.6X1	T50.6X2	T50.6X3	T50.6X4	T50.6X5	T50.6X6
diagnostic (gastric function)	T50.8X1	T50.8X2	T50.8X3	T50.8X4	T50.8X5	T50.8X6
ethyl	T51.0X1	T51.0X2	T51.0X3	T51.0X4	—	—
beverage	T51.0X1	T51.0X2	T51.0X3	T51.0X4	—	—
grain	T51.0X1	T51.0X2	T51.0X3	T51.0X4	—	—
beverage	T51.0X1	T51.0X2	T51.0X3	T51.0X4	—	—
industrial	T51.0X1	T51.0X2	T51.0X3	T51.0X4	—	—
isopropyl	T51.2X1	T51.2X2	T51.2X3	T51.2X4	—	—
methyl	T51.1X1	T51.1X2	T51.1X3	T51.1X4	—	—
preparation for consumption	T51.0X1	T51.0X2	T51.0X3	T51.0X4	—	—
propyl	T51.3X1	T51.3X2	T51.3X3	T51.3X4	—	—
secondary	T51.2X1	T51.2X2	T51.2X3	T51.2X4	—	—
radiator	T51.1X1	T51.1X2	T51.1X3	T51.1X4	—	—
rubbing	T51.2X1	T51.2X2	T51.2X3	T51.2X4	—	—
specified type NEC	T51.8X1	T51.8X2	T51.8X3	T51.8X4	—	—
surgical	T51.0X1	T51.0X2	T51.0X3	T51.0X4	—	—
vapor (from any type of Alcohol)	T59.891	T59.892	T59.893	T59.894	—	—
wood	T51.1X1	T51.1X2	T51.1X3	T51.1X4	—	—
Alcuronium (chloride)	T48.1X1	T48.1X2	T48.1X3	T48.1X4	T48.1X5	T48.1X6
Aldactone	T50.0X1	T50.0X2	T50.0X3	T50.0X4	T50.0X5	T50.0X6
Aldesulfone sodium	T37.1X1	T37.1X2	T37.1X3	T37.1X4	T37.1X5	T37.1X6
Aldicarb	T60.0X1	T60.0X2	T60.0X3	T60.0X4		
Aldomet	T46.5X1	T46.5X2	T46.5X3	T46.5X4	T46.5X5	T46.5X6
Aldosterone	T50.0X1	T50.0X2	T50.0X3	T50.0X4	T50.0X5	T50.0X6
Aldrin (dust)	T60.1X1	T60.1X2	T60.1X3	T60.1X4		
Aleve — *see* Naproxen						
Alexitol sodium	T47.1X1	T47.1X2	T47.1X3	T47.1X4	T47.1X5	T47.1X6

Substance	Poisoning, Accidental (unintentional)	Poisoning, Intentional Self-harm	Poisoning, Assault	Poisoning, Undetermined	Adverse Effect	Under-dosing
Alfacalcidol	T45.2X1	T45.2X2	T45.2X3	T45.2X4	T45.2X5	T45.2X6
Alfadolone	T41.1X1	T41.1X2	T41.1X3	T41.1X4	T41.1X5	T41.1X6
Alfaxalone	T41.1X1	T41.1X2	T41.1X3	T41.1X4	T41.1X5	T41.1X6
Alfentanil	T40.4X1	T40.4X2	T40.4X3	T40.4X4	T40.4X5	T40.4X6
Alfuzosin (hydrochloride)	T44.8X1	T44.8X2	T44.8X3	T44.8X4	T44.8X5	T44.8X6
Algae (harmful) (toxin)	T65.821	T65.822	T65.823	T65.824	—	—
Algeldrate	T47.1X1	T47.1X2	T47.1X3	T47.1X4	T47.1X5	T47.1X6
Algin	T47.8X1	T47.8X2	T47.8X3	T47.8X4	T47.8X5	T47.8X6
Alglucerase	T45.3X1	T45.3X2	T45.3X3	T45.3X4	T45.3X5	T45.3X6
Alidase	T45.3X1	T45.3X2	T45.3X3	T45.3X4	T45.3X5	T45.3X6
Alimemazine	T43.3X1	T43.3X2	T43.3X3	T43.3X4	T43.3X5	T43.3X6
Aliphatic thiocyanates	T65.0X1	T65.0X2	T65.0X3	T65.0X4		
Alizapride	T45.0X1	T45.0X2	T45.0X3	T45.0X4	T45.0X5	T45.0X6
Alkali (caustic)	T54.3X1	T54.3X2	T54.3X3	T54.3X4		
Alkaline antiseptic solution (aromatic)	T49.6X1	T49.6X2	T49.6X3	T49.6X4	T49.6X5	T49.6X6
Alkalinizing agents (medicinal)	T50.901	T50.902	T50.903	T50.904	T50.905	T50.906
Alkalizing agent NEC	T50.901	T50.902	T50.903	T50.904	T50.905	T50.906
Alka-seltzer	T39.011	T39.012	T39.013	T39.014	T39.015	T39.016
Alkavervir	T46.5X1	T46.5X2	T46.5X3	T46.5X4	T46.5X5	T46.5X6
Alkonium (bromide)	T49.0X1	T49.0X2	T49.0X3	T49.0X4	T49.0X5	T49.0X6
Alkylating drug NEC	T45.1X1	T45.1X2	T45.1X3	T45.1X4	T45.1X5	T45.1X6
antimyeloproliferative	T45.1X1	T45.1X2	T45.1X3	T45.1X4	T45.1X5	T45.1X6
lymphatic	T45.1X1	T45.1X2	T45.1X3	T45.1X4	T45.1X5	T45.1X6
Alkylisocyanate	T65.0X1	T65.0X2	T65.0X3	T65.0X4		
Allantoin	T49.4X1	T49.4X2	T49.4X3	T49.4X4	T49.4X5	T49.4X6
Allegron	T43.011	T43.012	T43.013	T43.014	T43.015	T43.016
Allethrin	T49.0X1	T49.0X2	T49.0X3	T49.0X4	T49.0X5	T49.0X6
Allobarbital	T42.3X1	T42.3X2	T42.3X3	T42.3X4	T42.3X5	T42.3X6
Allopurinol	T50.4X1	T50.4X2	T50.4X3	T50.4X4	T50.4X5	T50.4X6
Allyl						
alcohol	T51.8X1	T51.8X2	T51.8X3	T51.8X4	—	—
disulfide	T46.6X1	T46.6X2	T46.6X3	T46.6X4	T46.6X5	T46.6X6
Allylestrenol	T38.5X1	T38.5X2	T38.5X3	T38.5X4	T38.5X5	T38.5X6
Allylisopropylacetylurea	T42.6X1	T42.6X2	T42.6X3	T42.6X4	T42.6X5	T42.6X6
Allylisopropylmalonylurea	T42.3X1	T42.3X2	T42.3X3	T42.3X4	T42.3X5	T42.3X6
Allylthiourea	T49.3X1	T49.3X2	T49.3X3	T49.3X4	T49.3X5	T49.3X6
Allyltribromide	T42.6X1	T42.6X2	T42.6X3	T42.6X4	T42.6X5	T42.6X6
Allypropymal	T42.3X1	T42.3X2	T42.3X3	T42.3X4	T42.3X5	T42.3X6
Almagate	T47.1X1	T47.1X2	T47.1X3	T47.1X4	T47.1X5	T47.1X6
Almasilate	T47.1X1	T47.1X2	T47.1X3	T47.1X4	T47.1X5	T47.1X6
Almitrine	T50.7X1	T50.7X2	T50.7X3	T50.7X4	T50.7X5	T50.7X6
Aloes	T47.2X1	T47.2X2	T47.2X3	T47.2X4	T47.2X5	T47.2X6
Aloglutamol	T47.1X1	T47.1X2	T47.1X3	T47.1X4	T47.1X5	T47.1X6
Aloin	T47.2X1	T47.2X2	T47.2X3	T47.2X4	T47.2X5	T47.2X6
Aloxidone	T42.2X1	T42.2X2	T42.2X3	T42.2X4	T42.2X5	T42.2X6
Alpha						
acetyldigoxin	T46.0X1	T46.0X2	T46.0X3	T46.0X4	T46.0X5	T46.0X6
adrenergic blocking drug	T44.6X1	T44.6X2	T44.6X3	T44.6X4	T44.6X5	T44.6X6
amylase	T45.3X1	T45.3X2	T45.3X3	T45.3X4	T45.3X5	T45.3X6
tocoferol (acetate)	T45.2X1	T45.2X2	T45.2X3	T45.2X4	T45.2X5	T45.2X6
tocopherol	T45.2X1	T45.2X2	T45.2X3	T45.2X4	T45.2X5	T45.2X6
Alphadolone	T41.1X1	T41.1X2	T41.1X3	T41.1X4	T41.1X5	T41.1X6
Alphaprodine	T40.4X1	T40.4X2	T40.4X3	T40.4X4	T40.4X5	T40.4X6
Alphaxalone	T41.1X1	T41.1X2	T41.1X3	T41.1X4	T41.1X5	T41.1X6
Alprazolam	T42.4X1	T42.4X2	T42.4X3	T42.4X4	T42.4X5	T42.4X6
Alprenolol	T44.7X1	T44.7X2	T44.7X3	T44.7X4	T44.7X5	T44.7X6
Alprostadil	T46.7X1	T46.7X2	T46.7X3	T46.7X4	T46.7X5	T46.7X6
Alsactide	T38.811	T38.812	T38.813	T38.814	T38.815	T38.816
Alseroxylon	T46.5X1	T46.5X2	T46.5X3	T46.5X4	T46.5X5	T46.5X6
Alteplase	T45.611	T45.612	T45.613	T45.614	T45.615	T45.616
Altizide	T50.2X1	T50.2X2	T50.2X3	T50.2X4	T50.2X5	T50.2X6
Altretamine	T45.1X1	T45.1X2	T45.1X3	T45.1X4	T45.1X5	T45.1X6
Alum (medicinal)	T49.4X1	T49.4X2	T49.4X3	T49.4X4	T49.4X5	T49.4X6
nonmedicinal (ammonium) (potassium)	T56.891	T56.892	T56.893	T56.894		
Aluminium, aluminum						
acetate	T49.2X1	T49.2X2	T49.2X3	T49.2X4	T49.2X5	T49.2X6
solution	T49.0X1	T49.0X2	T49.0X3	T49.0X4	T49.0X5	T49.0X6
aspirin	T39.011	T39.012	T39.013	T39.014	T39.015	T39.016
bis (acetylsalicylate)	T39.011	T39.012	T39.013	T39.014	T39.015	T39.016
carbonate (gel, basic)	T47.1X1	T47.1X2	T47.1X3	T47.1X4	T47.1X5	T47.1X6
chlorhydroxide-complex	T47.1X1	T47.1X2	T47.1X3	T47.1X4	T47.1X5	T47.1X6
chloride	T49.2X1	T49.2X2	T49.2X3	T49.2X4	T49.2X5	T49.2X6
clofibrate	T46.6X1	T46.6X2	T46.6X3	T46.6X4	T46.6X5	T46.6X6
diacetate	T49.2X1	T49.2X2	T49.2X3	T49.2X4	T49.2X5	T49.2X6
glycinate	T47.1X1	T47.1X2	T47.1X3	T47.1X4	T47.1X5	T47.1X6
hydroxide (gel)	T47.1X1	T47.1X2	T47.1X3	T47.1X4	T47.1X5	T47.1X6
hydroxide-magnesium carb. gel	T47.1X1	T47.1X2	T47.1X3	T47.1X4		
magnesium silicate	T47.1X1	T47.1X2	T47.1X3	T47.1X4	T47.1X5	T47.1X6
nicotinate	T46.7X1	T46.7X2	T46.7X3	T46.7X4	T46.7X5	T46.7X6

340

Additional Character May Be Required — Refer to the Tabular List for Character Selection   ▽ Subterms under main terms may continue to next column or page

Substance	Poisoning, Accidental (unintentional)	Poisoning, Intentional Self-harm	Poisoning, Assault	Poisoning, Undetermined	Adverse Effect	Under-dosing
Aluminium, aluminum — *continued*						
ointment (surgical) (topical)	T49.3X1	T49.3X2	T49.3X3	T49.3X4	T49.3X5	T49.3X6
phosphate	T47.1X1	T47.1X2	T47.1X3	T47.1X4	T47.1X5	T47.1X6
salicylate	T39.091	T39.092	T39.093	T39.094	T39.095	T39.096
silicate	T47.1X1	T47.1X2	T47.1X3	T47.1X4	T47.1X5	T47.1X6
sodium silicate	T47.1X1	T47.1X2	T47.1X3	T47.1X4	T47.1X5	T47.1X6
subacetate	T49.2X1	T49.2X2	T49.2X3	T49.2X4	T49.2X5	T49.2X6
sulfate	T49.0X1	T49.0X2	T49.0X3	T49.0X4	T49.0X5	T49.0X6
tannate	T47.6X1	T47.6X2	T47.6X3	T47.6X4	T47.6X5	T47.6X6
topical NEC	T49.3X1	T49.3X2	T49.3X3	T49.3X4	T49.3X5	T49.3X6
Alurate	T42.3X1	T42.3X2	T42.3X3	T42.3X4	T42.3X5	T42.3X6
Alverine	T44.3X1	T44.3X2	T44.3X3	T44.3X4	T44.3X5	T44.3X6
Alvodine	T40.2X1	T40.2X2	T40.2X3	T40.2X4	T40.2X5	T40.2X6
Amanita phalloides	T62.0X1	T62.0X2	T62.0X3	T62.0X4	—	—
Amanitine	T62.0X1	T62.0X2	T62.0X3	T62.0X4	—	—
Amantadine	T42.8X1	T42.8X2	T42.8X3	T42.8X4	T42.8X5	T42.8X6
Ambazone	T49.6X1	T49.6X2	T49.6X3	T49.6X4	T49.6X5	T49.6X6
Ambenonium (chloride)	T44.0X1	T44.0X2	T44.0X3	T44.0X4	T44.0X5	T44.0X6
Ambroxol	T48.4X1	T48.4X2	T48.4X3	T48.4X4	T48.4X5	T48.4X6
Ambuphylline	T48.6X1	T48.6X2	T48.6X3	T48.6X4	T48.6X5	T48.6X6
Ambutonium bromide	T44.3X1	T44.3X2	T44.3X3	T44.3X4	T44.3X5	T44.3X6
Amcinonide	T49.0X1	T49.0X2	T49.0X3	T49.0X4	T49.0X5	T49.0X6
Amdinocilline	T36.0X1	T36.0X2	T36.0X3	T36.0X4	T36.0X5	T36.0X6
Ametazole	T50.8X1	T50.8X2	T50.8X3	T50.8X4	T50.8X5	T50.8X6
Amethocaine	T41.3X1	T41.3X2	T41.3X3	T41.3X4	T41.3X5	T41.3X6
regional	T41.3X1	T41.3X2	T41.3X3	T41.3X4	T41.3X5	T41.3X6
spinal	T41.3X1	T41.3X2	T41.3X3	T41.3X4	T41.3X5	T41.3X6
Amethopterin	T45.1X1	T45.1X2	T45.1X3	T45.1X4	T45.1X5	T45.1X6
Amezinium metilsulfate	T44.991	T44.992	T44.993	T44.994	T44.995	T44.996
Amfebutamone	T43.291	T43.292	T43.293	T43.294	T43.295	T43.296
Amfepramone	T50.5X1	T50.5X2	T50.5X3	T50.5X4	T50.5X5	T50.5X6
Amfetamine	T43.621	T43.622	T43.623	T43.624	T43.625	T43.626
Amfetaminil	T43.621	T43.622	T43.623	T43.624	T43.625	T43.626
Amfomycin	T36.8X1	T36.8X2	T36.8X3	T36.8X4	T36.8X5	T36.8X6
Amidefrine mesilate	T48.5X1	T48.5X2	T48.5X3	T48.5X4	T48.5X5	T48.5X6
Amidone	T40.3X1	T40.3X2	T40.3X3	T40.3X4	T40.3X5	T40.3X6
Amidopyrine	T39.2X1	T39.2X2	T39.2X3	T39.2X4	T39.2X5	T39.2X6
Amidotrizoate	T50.8X1	T50.8X2	T50.8X3	T50.8X4	T50.8X5	T50.8X6
Amiflamine	T43.1X1	T43.1X2	T43.1X3	T43.1X4	T43.1X5	T43.1X6
Amikacin	T36.5X1	T36.5X2	T36.5X3	T36.5X4	T36.5X5	T36.5X6
Amikhelline	T46.3X1	T46.3X2	T46.3X3	T46.3X4	T46.3X5	T46.3X6
Amiloride	T50.2X1	T50.2X2	T50.2X3	T50.2X4	T50.2X5	T50.2X6
Aminacrine	T49.0X1	T49.0X2	T49.0X3	T49.0X4	T49.0X5	T49.0X6
Amineptine	T43.011	T43.012	T43.013	T43.014	T43.015	T43.016
Aminitrozole	T37.3X1	T37.3X2	T37.3X3	T37.3X4	T37.3X5	T37.3X6
Aminoacetic acid (derivatives)	T50.3X1	T50.3X2	T50.3X3	T50.3X4	T50.3X5	T50.3X6
Amino acids	T50.3X1	T50.3X2	T50.3X3	T50.3X4	T50.3X5	T50.3X6
Aminoacridine	T49.0X1	T49.0X2	T49.0X3	T49.0X4	T49.0X5	T49.0X6
Aminobenzoic acid (-p)	T49.3X1	T49.3X2	T49.3X3	T49.3X4	T49.3X5	T49.3X6
Aminocaproic acid	T45.621	T45.622	T45.623	T45.624	T45.625	T45.626
Aminoethylisothiourium	T45.8X1	T45.8X2	T45.8X3	T45.8X4	T45.8X5	T45.8X6
Aminofenazone	T39.2X1	T39.2X2	T39.2X3	T39.2X4	T39.2X5	T39.2X6
Aminoglutethimide	T45.1X1	T45.1X2	T45.1X3	T45.1X4	T45.1X5	T45.1X6
Aminohippuric acid	T50.8X1	T50.8X2	T50.8X3	T50.8X4	T50.8X5	T50.8X6
Aminomethylbenzoic acid	T45.691	T45.692	T45.693	T45.694	T45.695	T45.696
Aminometradine	T50.2X1	T50.2X2	T50.2X3	T50.2X4	T50.2X5	T50.2X6
Aminopentamide	T44.3X1	T44.3X2	T44.3X3	T44.3X4	T44.3X5	T44.3X6
Aminophenazone	T39.2X1	T39.2X2	T39.2X3	T39.2X4	T39.2X5	T39.2X6
Aminophenol	T54.0X1	T54.0X2	T54.0X3	T54.0X4	—	—
Aminophenylpyridone	T43.591	T43.592	T43.593	T43.594	T43.595	T43.596
Aminophylline	T48.6X1	T48.6X2	T48.6X3	T48.6X4	T48.6X5	T48.6X6
Aminopterin sodium	T45.1X1	T45.1X2	T45.1X3	T45.1X4	T45.1X5	T45.1X6
Aminopyrine	T39.2X1	T39.2X2	T39.2X3	T39.2X4	T39.2X5	T39.2X6
Aminorex	T50.5X1	T50.5X2	T50.5X3	T50.5X4	T50.5X5	T50.5X6
Aminosalicylic acid	T37.1X1	T37.1X2	T37.1X3	T37.1X4	T37.1X5	T37.1X6
Aminosalylum	T37.1X1	T37.1X2	T37.1X3	T37.1X4	T37.1X5	T37.1X6
Amiodarone	T46.2X1	T46.2X2	T46.2X3	T46.2X4	T46.2X5	T46.2X6
Amiphenazole	T50.7X1	T50.7X2	T50.7X3	T50.7X4	T50.7X5	T50.7X6
Amiquinsin	T46.5X1	T46.5X2	T46.5X3	T46.5X4	T46.5X5	T46.5X6
Amisometradine	T50.2X1	T50.2X2	T50.2X3	T50.2X4	T50.2X5	T50.2X6
Amisulpride	T43.591	T43.592	T43.593	T43.594	T43.595	T43.596
Amitriptyline	T43.011	T43.012	T43.013	T43.014	T43.015	T43.016
Amitriptylinoxide	T43.011	T43.012	T43.013	T43.014	T43.015	T43.016
Amlexanox	T48.6X1	T48.6X2	T48.6X3	T48.6X4	T48.6X5	T48.6X6
Ammonia (fumes) (gas) (vapor)	T59.891	T59.892	T59.893	T59.894	—	—
aromatic spirit	T48.991	T48.992	T48.993	T48.994	T48.995	T48.996
liquid (household)	T54.3X1	T54.3X2	T54.3X3	T54.3X4	—	—
Ammoniated mercury	T49.0X1	T49.0X2	T49.0X3	T49.0X4	T49.0X5	T49.0X6
Ammonium						
acid tartrate	T49.5X1	T49.5X2	T49.5X3	T49.5X4	T49.5X5	T49.5X6
Ammonium — *continued*						
bromide	T42.6X1	T42.6X2	T42.6X3	T42.6X4	T42.6X5	T42.6X6
carbonate	T54.3X1	T54.3X2	T54.3X3	T54.3X4	—	—
chloride	T50.991	T50.992	T50.993	T50.994	T50.995	T50.996
expectorant	T48.4X1	T48.4X2	T48.4X3	T48.4X4	T48.4X5	T48.4X6
compounds (household) NEC	T54.3X1	T54.3X2	T54.3X3	T54.3X4	—	—
fumes (any usage)	T59.891	T59.892	T59.893	T59.894	—	—
industrial	T54.3X1	T54.3X2	T54.3X3	T54.3X4	—	—
ichthyosulronate	T49.4X1	T49.4X2	T49.4X3	T49.4X4	T49.4X5	T49.4X6
mandelate	T37.91	T37.92	T37.93	T37.94	T37.95	T37.96
sulfamate	T60.3X1	T60.3X2	T60.3X3	T60.3X4	—	—
sulfonate resin	T47.8X1	T47.8X2	T47.8X3	T47.8X4	T47.8X5	T47.8X6
Amobarbital (sodium)	T42.3X1	T42.3X2	T42.3X3	T42.3X4	T42.3X5	T42.3X6
Amodiaquine	T37.2X1	T37.2X2	T37.2X3	T37.2X4	T37.2X5	T37.2X6
Amopyroquin (e)	T37.2X1	T37.2X2	T37.2X3	T37.2X4	T37.2X5	T37.2X6
Amoxapine	T43.011	T43.012	T43.013	T43.014	T43.015	T43.016
Amoxicillin	T36.0X1	T36.0X2	T36.0X3	T36.0X4	T36.0X5	T36.0X6
Amperozide	T43.591	T43.592	T43.593	T43.594	T43.595	T43.596
Amphenidone	T43.591	T43.592	T43.593	T43.594	T43.595	T43.596
Amphetamine NEC	T43.621	T43.622	T43.623	T43.624	T43.625	T43.626
Amphomycin	T36.8X1	T36.8X2	T36.8X3	T36.8X4	T36.8X5	T36.8X6
Amphotalide	T37.4X1	T37.4X2	T37.4X3	T37.4X4	T37.4X5	T37.4X6
Amphotericin B	T36.7X1	T36.7X2	T36.7X3	T36.7X4	T36.7X5	T36.7X6
topical	T49.0X1	T49.0X2	T49.0X3	T49.0X4	T49.0X5	T49.0X6
Ampicillin	T36.0X1	T36.0X2	T36.0X3	T36.0X4	T36.0X5	T36.0X6
Amprotropine	T44.3X1	T44.3X2	T44.3X3	T44.3X4	T44.3X5	T44.3X6
Amsacrine	T45.1X1	T45.1X2	T45.1X3	T45.1X4	T45.1X5	T45.1X6
Amygdaline	T62.2X1	T62.2X2	T62.2X3	T62.2X4	—	—
Amyl						
acetate	T52.8X1	T52.8X2	T52.8X3	T52.8X4	—	—
vapor	T59.891	T59.892	T59.893	T59.894	—	—
alcohol	T51.3X1	T51.3X2	T51.3X3	T51.3X4	—	—
chloride	T53.6X1	T53.6X2	T53.6X3	T53.6X4	—	—
formate	T52.8X1	T52.8X2	T52.8X3	T52.8X4	—	—
nitrite	T46.3X1	T46.3X2	T46.3X3	T46.3X4	T46.3X5	T46.3X6
propionate	T65.891	T65.892	T65.893	T65.894	—	—
Amylase	T47.5X1	T47.5X2	T47.5X3	T47.5X4	T47.5X5	T47.5X6
Amyleine, regional	T41.3X1	T41.3X2	T41.3X3	T41.3X4	T41.3X5	T41.3X6
Amylene						
dichloride	T53.6X1	T53.6X2	T53.6X3	T53.6X4	—	—
hydrate	T51.3X1	T51.3X2	T51.3X3	T51.3X4	—	—
Amylmetacresol	T49.6X1	T49.6X2	T49.6X3	T49.6X4	T49.6X5	T49.6X6
Amylobarbitone	T42.3X1	T42.3X2	T42.3X3	T42.3X4	T42.3X5	T42.3X6
Amylocaine, regional	T41.3X1	T41.3X2	T41.3X3	T41.3X4	T41.3X5	T41.3X6
infiltration (subcutaneous)	T41.3X1	T41.3X2	T41.3X3	T41.3X4	T41.3X5	T41.3X6
nerve block (peripheral) (plexus)	T41.3X1	T41.3X2	T41.3X3	T41.3X4	T41.3X5	T41.3X6
spinal	T41.3X1	T41.3X2	T41.3X3	T41.3X4	T41.3X5	T41.3X6
topical (surface)	T41.3X1	T41.3X2	T41.3X3	T41.3X4	T41.3X5	T41.3X6
Amylopectin	T47.6X1	T47.6X2	T47.6X3	T47.6X4	T47.6X5	T47.6X6
Amytal (sodium)	T42.3X1	T42.3X2	T42.3X3	T42.3X4	T42.3X5	T42.3X6
Anabolic steroid	T38.7X1	T38.7X2	T38.7X3	T38.7X4	T38.7X5	T38.7X6
Analeptic NEC	T50.7X1	T50.7X2	T50.7X3	T50.7X4	T50.7X5	T50.7X6
Analgesic	T39.91	T39.92	T39.93	T39.94	T39.95	T39.96
anti-inflammatory NEC	T39.91	T39.92	T39.93	T39.94	T39.95	T39.96
propionic acid derivative	T39.311	T39.312	T39.313	T39.314	T39.315	T39.316
antirheumatic NEC	T39.4X1	T39.4X2	T39.4X3	T39.4X4	T39.4X5	T39.4X6
aromatic NEC	T39.1X1	T39.1X2	T39.1X3	T39.1X4	T39.1X5	T39.1X6
narcotic NEC	T40.601	T40.602	T40.603	T40.604	T40.605	T40.606
combination	T40.601	T40.602	T40.603	T40.604	T40.605	T40.606
obstetric	T40.601	T40.602	T40.603	T40.604	T40.605	T40.606
non-narcotic NEC	T39.91	T39.92	T39.93	T39.94	T39.95	T39.96
combination	T39.91	T39.92	T39.93	T39.94	T39.95	T39.96
pyrazole	T39.2X1	T39.2X2	T39.2X3	T39.2X4	T39.2X5	T39.2X6
specified NEC	T39.8X1	T39.8X2	T39.8X3	T39.8X4	T39.8X5	T39.8X6
Analgin	T39.2X1	T39.2X2	T39.2X3	T39.2X4	T39.2X5	T39.2X6
Anamirta cocculus	T62.1X1	T62.1X2	T62.1X3	T62.1X4	—	—
Ancillin	T36.0X1	T36.0X2	T36.0X3	T36.0X4	T36.0X5	T36.0X6
Ancrod	T45.691	T45.692	T45.693	T45.694	T45.695	T45.696
Androgen	T38.7X1	T38.7X2	T38.7X3	T38.7X4	T38.7X5	T38.7X6
Androgen-estrogen mixture	T38.7X1	T38.7X2	T38.7X3	T38.7X4	T38.7X5	T38.7X6
Androstalone	T38.7X1	T38.7X2	T38.7X3	T38.7X4	T38.7X5	T38.7X6
Androstanolone	T38.7X1	T38.7X2	T38.7X3	T38.7X4	T38.7X5	T38.7X6
Androsterone	T38.7X1	T38.7X2	T38.7X3	T38.7X4	T38.7X5	T38.7X6
Anemone pulsatilla	T62.2X1	T62.2X2	T62.2X3	T62.2X4	—	—
Anesthesia						
caudal	T41.3X1	T41.3X2	T41.3X3	T41.3X4	T41.3X5	T41.3X6
endotracheal	T41.0X1	T41.0X2	T41.0X3	T41.0X4	T41.0X5	T41.0X6
epidural	T41.3X1	T41.3X2	T41.3X3	T41.3X4	T41.3X5	T41.3X6
inhalation	T41.0X1	T41.0X2	T41.0X3	T41.0X4	T41.0X5	T41.0X6
local	T41.3X1	T41.3X2	T41.3X3	T41.3X4	T41.3X5	T41.3X6

Table of Drugs and Chemicals

Anesthesia — Antifreeze

Substance	Poisoning, Accidental (unintentional)	Poisoning, Intentional Self-harm	Poisoning, Assault	Poisoning, Undetermined	Adverse Effect	Under-dosing
Anesthesia — *continued*						
mucosal	T41.3X1	T41.3X2	T41.3X3	T41.3X4	T41.3X5	T41.3X6
muscle relaxation	T48.1X1	T48.1X2	T48.1X3	T48.1X4	T48.1X5	T48.1X6
nerve blocking	T41.3X1	T41.3X2	T41.3X3	T41.3X4	T41.3X5	T41.3X6
plexus blocking	T41.3X1	T41.3X2	T41.3X3	T41.3X4	T41.3X5	T41.3X6
potentiated	T41.201	T41.202	T41.203	T41.204	T41.205	T41.206
rectal	T41.201	T41.202	T41.203	T41.204	T41.205	T41.206
general	T41.201	T41.202	T41.203	T41.204	T41.205	T41.206
local	T41.3X1	T41.3X2	T41.3X3	T41.3X4	T41.3X5	T41.3X6
regional	T41.3X1	T41.3X2	T41.3X3	T41.3X4	T41.3X5	T41.3X6
surface	T41.3X1	T41.3X2	T41.3X3	T41.3X4	T41.3X5	T41.3X6
Anesthetic NEC — *see also*	T41.41	T41.42	T41.43	T41.44	T41.45	T41.46
Anesthesia						
with muscle relaxant	T41.201	T41.202	T41.203	T41.204	T41.205	T41.206
general	T41.201	T41.202	T41.203	T41.204	T41.205	T41.206
local	T41.3X1	T41.3X2	T41.3X3	T41.3X4	T41.3X5	T41.3X6
gaseous NEC	T41.0X1	T41.0X2	T41.0X3	T41.0X4	T41.0X5	T41.0X6
general NEC	T41.201	T41.202	T41.203	T41.204	T41.205	T41.206
halogenated hydrocarbon derivatives NEC	T41.0X1	T41.0X2	T41.0X3	T41.0X4	T41.0X5	T41.0X6
infiltration NEC	T41.3X1	T41.3X2	T41.3X3	T41.3X4	T41.3X5	T41.3X6
intravenous NEC	T41.1X1	T41.1X2	T41.1X3	T41.1X4	T41.1X5	T41.1X6
local NEC	T41.3X1	T41.3X2	T41.3X3	T41.3X4	T41.3X5	T41.3X6
rectal	T41.201	T41.202	T41.203	T41.204	T41.205	T41.206
general	T41.201	T41.202	T41.203	T41.204	T41.205	T41.206
local	T41.3X1	T41.3X2	T41.3X3	T41.3X4	T41.3X5	T41.3X6
regional NEC	T41.3X1	T41.3X2	T41.3X3	T41.3X4	T41.3X5	T41.3X6
spinal NEC	T41.3X1	T41.3X2	T41.3X3	T41.3X4	T41.3X5	T41.3X6
thiobarbiturate	T41.1X1	T41.1X2	T41.1X3	T41.1X4	T41.1X5	T41.1X6
topical	T41.3X1	T41.3X2	T41.3X3	T41.3X4	T41.3X5	T41.3X6
Aneurine	T45.2X1	T45.2X2	T45.2X3	T45.2X4	T45.2X5	T45.2X6
Angio-Conray	T50.8X1	T50.8X2	T50.8X3	T50.8X4	T50.8X5	T50.8X6
Angiotensin	T44.5X1	T44.5X2	T44.5X3	T44.5X4	T44.5X5	T44.5X6
Angiotensinamide	T44.991	T44.992	T44.993	T44.994	T44.995	T44.996
Anhydrohydroxy-progesterone	T38.5X1	T38.5X2	T38.5X3	T38.5X4	T38.5X5	T38.5X6
Anhydron	T50.2X1	T50.2X2	T50.2X3	T50.2X4	T50.2X5	T50.2X6
Anileridine	T40.4X1	T40.4X2	T40.4X3	T40.4X4	T40.4X5	T40.4X6
Aniline (dye) (liquid)	T65.3X1	T65.3X2	T65.3X3	T65.3X4	—	—
analgesic	T39.1X1	T39.1X2	T39.1X3	T39.1X4	T39.1X5	T39.1X6
derivatives, therapeutic NEC	T39.1X1	T39.1X2	T39.1X3	T39.1X4	T39.1X5	T39.1X6
vapor	T65.3X1	T65.3X2	T65.3X3	T65.3X4	—	—
Aniscoropine	T44.3X1	T44.3X2	T44.3X3	T44.3X4	T44.3X5	T44.3X6
Anise oil	T47.5X1	T47.5X2	T47.5X3	T47.5X4	T47.5X5	T47.5X6
Anisidine	T65.3X1	T65.3X2	T65.3X3	T65.3X4	—	—
Anisindione	T45.511	T45.512	T45.513	T45.514	T45.515	T45.516
Anisotropine methyl-bromide	T44.3X1	T44.3X2	T44.3X3	T44.3X4	T44.3X5	T44.3X6
Anistreplase	T45.611	T45.612	T45.613	T45.614	T45.615	T45.616
Anorexiant (central)	T50.5X1	T50.5X2	T50.5X3	T50.5X4	T50.5X5	T50.5X6
Anorexic agents	T50.5X1	T50.5X2	T50.5X3	T50.5X4	T50.5X5	T50.5X6
Ansamycin	T36.6X1	T36.6X2	T36.6X3	T36.6X4	T36.6X5	T36.6X6
Ant (bite) (sting)	T63.421	T63.422	T63.423	T63.424	—	—
Antabuse	T50.6X1	T50.6X2	T50.6X3	T50.6X4	T50.6X5	T50.6X6
Antacid NEC	T47.1X1	T47.1X2	T47.1X3	T47.1X4	T47.1X5	T47.1X6
Antagonist						
Aldosterone	T50.0X1	T50.0X2	T50.0X3	T50.0X4	T50.0X5	T50.0X6
alpha-adrenoreceptor	T44.6X1	T44.6X2	T44.6X3	T44.6X4	T44.6X5	T44.6X6
anticoagulant	T45.7X1	T45.7X2	T45.7X3	T45.7X4	T45.7X5	T45.7X6
beta-adrenoreceptor	T44.7X1	T44.7X2	T44.7X3	T44.7X4	T44.7X5	T44.7X6
extrapyramidal NEC	T44.3X1	T44.3X2	T44.3X3	T44.3X4	T44.3X5	T44.3X6
folic acid	T45.1X1	T45.1X2	T45.1X3	T45.1X4	T45.1X5	T45.1X6
H2 receptor	T47.0X1	T47.0X2	T47.0X3	T47.0X4	T47.0X5	T47.0X6
heavy metal	T45.8X1	T45.8X2	T45.8X3	T45.8X4	T45.8X5	T45.8X6
narcotic analgesic	T50.7X1	T50.7X2	T50.7X3	T50.7X4	T50.7X5	T50.7X6
opiate	T50.7X1	T50.7X2	T50.7X3	T50.7X4	T50.7X5	T50.7X6
pyrimidine	T45.1X1	T45.1X2	T45.1X3	T45.1X4	T45.1X5	T45.1X6
serotonin	T46.5X1	T46.5X2	T46.5X3	T46.5X4	T46.5X5	T46.5X6
Antazolin (e)	T45.0X1	T45.0X2	T45.0X3	T45.0X4	T45.0X5	T45.0X6
Anterior pituitary hormone NEC	T38.811	T38.812	T38.813	T38.814	T38.815	T38.816
Anthelmintic NEC	T37.4X1	T37.4X2	T37.4X3	T37.4X4	T37.4X5	T37.4X6
Anthiolimine	T37.4X1	T37.4X2	T37.4X3	T37.4X4	T37.4X5	T37.4X6
Anthralin	T49.4X1	T49.4X2	T49.4X3	T49.4X4	T49.4X5	T49.4X6
Anthramycin	T45.1X1	T45.1X2	T45.1X3	T45.1X4	T45.1X5	T45.1X6
Antiadrenergic NEC	T44.8X1	T44.8X2	T44.8X3	T44.8X4	T44.8X5	T44.8X6
Antiallergic NEC	T45.0X1	T45.0X2	T45.0X3	T45.0X4	T45.0X5	T45.0X6
Antiandrogen NEC	T38.6X1	T38.6X2	T38.6X3	T38.6X4	T38.6X5	T38.6X6
Anti-anemic (drug) (preparation)	T45.8X1	T45.8X2	T45.8X3	T45.8X4	T45.8X5	T45.8X6
Antianxiety drug NEC	T43.501	T43.502	T43.503	T43.504	T43.505	T43.506
Antiaris toxicaria	T65.891	T65.892	T65.893	T65.894	—	—
Antiarteriosclerotic drug	T46.6X1	T46.6X2	T46.6X3	T46.6X4	T46.6X5	T46.6X6
Antiasthmatic drug NEC	T48.6X1	T48.6X2	T48.6X3	T48.6X4	T48.6X5	T48.6X6
Antibiotic NEC	T36.91	T36.92	T36.93	T36.94	T36.95	T36.96
aminoglycoside	T36.5X1	T36.5X2	T36.5X3	T36.5X4	T36.5X5	T36.5X6
anticancer	T45.1X1	T45.1X2	T45.1X3	T45.1X4	T45.1X5	T45.1X6
antifungal	T36.7X1	T36.7X2	T36.7X3	T36.7X4	T36.7X5	T36.7X6
antimycobacterial	T36.5X1	T36.5X2	T36.5X3	T36.5X4	T36.5X5	T36.5X6
antineoplastic	T45.1X1	T45.1X2	T45.1X3	T45.1X4	T45.1X5	T45.1X6
b-lactam NEC	T36.1X1	T36.1X2	T36.1X3	T36.1X4	T36.1X5	T36.1X6
cephalosporin (group)	T36.1X1	T36.1X2	T36.1X3	T36.1X4	T36.1X5	T36.1X6
chloramphenicol (group)	T36.2X1	T36.2X2	T36.2X3	T36.2X4	T36.2X5	T36.2X6
ENT	T49.6X1	T49.6X2	T49.6X3	T49.6X4	T49.6X5	T49.6X6
eye	T49.5X1	T49.5X2	T49.5X3	T49.5X4	T49.5X5	T49.5X6
fungicidal (local)	T49.0X1	T49.0X2	T49.0X3	T49.0X4	T49.0X5	T49.0X6
intestinal	T36.8X1	T36.8X2	T36.8X3	T36.8X4	T36.8X5	T36.8X6
local	T49.0X1	T49.0X2	T49.0X3	T49.0X4	T49.0X5	T49.0X6
macrolides	T36.3X1	T36.3X2	T36.3X3	T36.3X4	T36.3X5	T36.3X6
polypeptide	T36.8X1	T36.8X2	T36.8X3	T36.8X4	T36.8X5	T36.8X6
specified NEC	T36.8X1	T36.8X2	T36.8X3	T36.8X4	T36.8X5	T36.8X6
tetracycline (group)	T36.4X1	T36.4X2	T36.4X3	T36.4X4	T36.4X5	T36.4X6
throat	T49.6X1	T49.6X2	T49.6X3	T49.6X4	T49.6X5	T49.6X6
Anticancer agents NEC	T45.1X1	T45.1X2	T45.1X3	T45.1X4	T45.1X5	T45.1X6
Anticholesterolemic drug NEC	T46.6X1	T46.6X2	T46.6X3	T46.6X4	T46.6X5	T46.6X6
Anticholinergic NEC	T44.3X1	T44.3X2	T44.3X3	T44.3X4	T44.3X5	T44.3X6
Anticholinesterase	T44.0X1	T44.0X2	T44.0X3	T44.0X4	T44.0X5	T44.0X6
organophosphorus	T44.0X1	T44.0X2	T44.0X3	T44.0X4	T44.0X5	T44.0X6
insecticide	T60.0X1	T60.0X2	T60.0X3	T60.0X4	—	—
nerve gas	T59.891	T59.892	T59.893	T59.894	—	—
reversible	T44.0X1	T44.0X2	T44.0X3	T44.0X4	T44.0X5	T44.0X6
ophthalmological	T49.5X1	T49.5X2	T49.5X3	T49.5X4	T49.5X5	T49.5X6
Anticoagulant NEC	T45.511	T45.512	T45.513	T45.514	T45.515	T45.516
Antagonist	T45.7X1	T45.7X2	T45.7X3	T45.7X4	T45.7X5	T45.7X6
Anti-common-cold drug NEC	T48.5X1	T48.5X2	T48.5X3	T48.5X4	T48.5X5	T48.5X6
Anticonvulsant	T42.71	T42.72	T42.73	T42.74	T42.75	T42.76
barbiturate	T42.3X1	T42.3X2	T42.3X3	T42.3X4	T42.3X5	T42.3X6
combination (with barbiturate)	T42.3X1	T42.3X2	T42.3X3	T42.3X4	T42.3X5	T42.3X6
hydantoin	T42.0X1	T42.0X2	T42.0X3	T42.0X4	T42.0X5	T42.0X6
hypnotic NEC	T42.6X1	T42.6X2	T42.6X3	T42.6X4	T42.6X5	T42.6X6
oxazolidinedione	T42.2X1	T42.2X2	T42.2X3	T42.2X4	T42.2X5	T42.2X6
pyrimidinedione	T42.6X1	T42.6X2	T42.6X3	T42.6X4	T42.6X5	T42.6X6
specified NEC	T42.6X1	T42.6X2	T42.6X3	T42.6X4	T42.6X5	T42.6X6
succinimide	T42.2X1	T42.2X2	T42.2X3	T42.2X4	T42.2X5	T42.2X6
Antidepressant	T43.201	T43.202	T43.203	T43.204	T43.205	T43.206
monoamine oxidase inhibitor	T43.1X1	T43.1X2	T43.1X3	T43.1X4	T43.1X5	T43.1X6
selective serotonin norepinephrine reuptake inhibitor	T43.211	T43.212	T43.213	T43.214	T43.215	T43.216
selective serotonin reuptake inhibitor	T43.221	T43.222	T43.223	T43.224	T43.225	T43.226
specified NEC	T43.291	T43.292	T43.293	T43.294	T43.295	T43.296
tetracyclic	T43.021	T43.022	T43.023	T43.024	T43.025	T43.026
triazolopyridine	T43.211	T43.212	T43.213	T43.214	T43.215	T43.216
tricyclic	T43.011	T43.012	T43.013	T43.014	T43.015	T43.016
Antidiabetic NEC	T38.3X1	T38.3X2	T38.3X3	T38.3X4	T38.3X5	T38.3X6
biguanide	T38.3X1	T38.3X2	T38.3X3	T38.3X4	T38.3X5	T38.3X6
and sulfonyl combined	T38.3X1	T38.3X2	T38.3X3	T38.3X4	T38.3X5	T38.3X6
combined	T38.3X1	T38.3X2	T38.3X3	T38.3X4	T38.3X5	T38.3X6
sulfonylurea	T38.3X1	T38.3X2	T38.3X3	T38.3X4	T38.3X5	T38.3X6
Antidiarrheal drug NEC	T47.6X1	T47.6X2	T47.6X3	T47.6X4	T47.6X5	T47.6X6
absorbent	T47.6X1	T47.6X2	T47.6X3	T47.6X4	T47.6X5	T47.6X6
Anti-D immunoglobulin (human)	T50.Z11	T50.Z12	T50.Z13	T50.Z14	T50.Z15	T50.Z16
Antidiphtheria serum	T50.Z11	T50.Z12	T50.Z13	T50.Z14	T50.Z15	T50.Z16
Antidiuretic hormone	T38.891	T38.892	T38.893	T38.894	T38.895	T38.896
Antidote NEC	T50.6X1	T50.6X2	T50.6X3	T50.6X4	T50.6X5	T50.6X6
heavy metal	T45.8X1	T45.8X2	T45.8X3	T45.8X4	T45.8X5	T45.8X6
Antidysrhythmic NEC	T46.2X1	T46.2X2	T46.2X3	T46.2X4	T46.2X5	T46.2X6
Antiemetic drug	T45.0X1	T45.0X2	T45.0X3	T45.0X4	T45.0X5	T45.0X6
Antiepilepsy agent	T42.71	T42.72	T42.73	T42.74	T42.75	T42.76
combination	T42.5X1	T42.5X2	T42.5X3	T42.5X4	T42.5X5	T42.5X6
mixed	T42.5X1	T42.5X2	T42.5X3	T42.5X4	T42.5X5	T42.5X6
specified, NEC	T42.6X1	T42.6X2	T42.6X3	T42.6X4	T42.6X5	T42.6X6
Antiestrogen NEC	T38.6X1	T38.6X2	T38.6X3	T38.6X4	T38.6X5	T38.6X6
Antifertility pill	T38.4X1	T38.4X2	T38.4X3	T38.4X4	T38.4X5	T38.4X6
Antifibrinolytic drug	T45.621	T45.622	T45.623	T45.624	T45.625	T45.626
Antifilarial drug	T37.4X1	T37.4X2	T37.4X3	T37.4X4	T37.4X5	T37.4X6
Antiflatulent	T47.5X1	T47.5X2	T47.5X3	T47.5X4	T47.5X5	T47.5X6
Antifreeze	T65.91	T65.92	T65.93	T65.94	—	—
alcohol	T51.1X1	T51.1X2	T51.1X3	T51.1X4	—	—
ethylene glycol	T51.8X1	T51.8X2	T51.8X3	T51.8X4	—	—

Substance	Poisoning, Accidental (unintentional)	Poisoning, Intentional Self-harm	Poisoning, Assault	Poisoning, Undetermined	Adverse Effect	Under-dosing
Antifungal						
antibiotic (systemic)	T36.7X1	T36.7X2	T36.7X3	T36.7X4	T36.7X5	T36.7X6
anti-infective NEC	T37.91	T37.92	T37.93	T37.94	T37.95	T37.96
disinfectant, local	T49.0X1	T49.0X2	T49.0X3	T49.0X4	T49.0X5	T49.0X6
nonmedicinal (spray)	T60.3X1	T60.3X2	T60.3X3	T60.3X4	—	—
topical	T49.0X1	T49.0X2	T49.0X3	T49.0X4	T49.0X5	T49.0X6
Anti-gastric-secretion drug NEC	T47.1X1	T47.1X2	T47.1X3	T47.1X4	T47.1X5	T47.1X6
Antigonadotrophin NEC	T38.6X1	T38.6X2	T38.6X3	T38.6X4	T38.6X5	T38.6X6
Antihallucinogen	T43.501	T43.502	T43.503	T43.504	T43.505	T43.506
Antihelmintics	T37.4X1	T37.4X2	T37.4X3	T37.4X4	T37.4X5	T37.4X6
Antihemophilic						
factor	T45.8X1	T45.8X2	T45.8X3	T45.8X4	T45.8X5	T45.8X6
fraction	T45.8X1	T45.8X2	T45.8X3	T45.8X4	T45.8X5	T45.8X6
globulin concentrate	T45.7X1	T45.7X2	T45.7X3	T45.7X4	T45.7X5	T45.7X6
human plasma	T45.8X1	T45.8X2	T45.8X3	T45.8X4	T45.8X5	T45.8X6
plasma, dried	T45.7X1	T45.7X2	T45.7X3	T45.7X4	T45.7X5	T45.7X6
Antihemorrhoidal preparation	T49.2X1	T49.2X2	T49.2X3	T49.2X4	T49.2X5	T49.2X6
Antiheparin drug	T45.7X1	T45.7X2	T45.7X3	T45.7X4	T45.7X5	T45.7X6
Antihistamine	T45.0X1	T45.0X2	T45.0X3	T45.0X4	T45.0X5	T45.0X6
Antihookworm drug	T37.4X1	T37.4X2	T37.4X3	T37.4X4	T37.4X5	T37.4X6
Anti-human lymphocytic globulin	T50.Z11	T50.Z12	T50.Z13	T50.Z14	T50.Z15	T50.Z16
Antihyperlipidemic drug	T46.6X1	T46.6X2	T46.6X3	T46.6X4	T46.6X5	T46.6X6
Antihypertensive drug NEC	T46.5X1	T46.5X2	T46.5X3	T46.5X4	T46.5X5	T46.5X6
Anti-infective NEC	T37.91	T37.92	T37.93	T37.94	T37.95	T37.96
anthelmintic	T37.4X1	T37.4X2	T37.4X3	T37.4X4	T37.4X5	T37.4X6
antibiotics	T36.91	T36.92	T36.93	T36.94	T36.95	T36.96
specified NEC	T36.8X1	T36.8X2	T36.8X3	T36.8X4	T36.8X5	T36.8X6
antimalarial	T37.2X1	T37.2X2	T37.2X3	T37.2X4	T37.2X5	T37.2X6
antimycobacterial NEC	T37.1X1	T37.1X2	T37.1X3	T37.1X4	T37.1X5	T37.1X6
antibiotics	T36.5X1	T36.5X2	T36.5X3	T36.5X4	T36.5X5	T36.5X6
antiprotozoal NEC	T37.3X1	T37.3X2	T37.3X3	T37.3X4	T37.3X5	T37.3X6
blood	T37.2X1	T37.2X2	T37.2X3	T37.2X4	T37.2X5	T37.2X6
antiviral	T37.5X1	T37.5X2	T37.5X3	T37.5X4	T37.5X5	T37.5X6
arsenical	T37.8X1	T37.8X2	T37.8X3	T37.8X4	T37.8X5	T37.8X6
bismuth, local	T49.0X1	T49.0X2	T49.0X3	T49.0X4	T49.0X5	T49.0X6
ENT	T49.6X1	T49.6X2	T49.6X3	T49.6X4	T49.6X5	T49.6X6
eye NEC	T49.5X1	T49.5X2	T49.5X3	T49.5X4	T49.5X5	T49.5X6
heavy metals NEC	T37.8X1	T37.8X2	T37.8X3	T37.8X4	T37.8X5	T37.8X6
local NEC	T49.0X1	T49.0X2	T49.0X3	T49.0X4	T49.0X5	T49.0X6
specified NEC	T49.0X1	T49.0X2	T49.0X3	T49.0X4	T49.0X5	T49.0X6
mixed	T37.91	T37.92	T37.93	T37.94	T37.95	T37.96
ophthalmic preparation	T49.5X1	T49.5X2	T49.5X3	T49.5X4	T49.5X5	T49.5X6
topical NEC	T49.0X1	T49.0X2	T49.0X3	T49.0X4	T49.0X5	T49.0X6
Anti-inflammatory drug NEC	T39.391	T39.392	T39.393	T39.394	T39.395	T39.396
local	T49.0X1	T49.0X2	T49.0X3	T49.0X4	T49.0X5	T49.0X6
nonsteroidal NEC	T39.391	T39.392	T39.393	T39.394	T39.395	T39.396
propionic acid derivative	T39.311	T39.312	T39.313	T39.314	T39.315	T39.316
specified NEC	T39.391	T39.392	T39.393	T39.394	T39.395	T39.396
Antikaluretic	T50.3X1	T50.3X2	T50.3X3	T50.3X4	T50.3X5	T50.3X6
Antiknock (tetraethyl lead)	T56.0X1	T56.0X2	T56.0X3	T56.0X4	—	—
Antilipemic drug NEC	T46.6X1	T46.6X2	T46.6X3	T46.6X4	T46.6X5	T46.6X6
Antimalarial	T37.2X1	T37.2X2	T37.2X3	T37.2X4	T37.2X5	T37.2X6
prophylactic NEC	T37.2X1	T37.2X2	T37.2X3	T37.2X4	T37.2X5	T37.2X6
pyrimidine derivative	T37.2X1	T37.2X2	T37.2X3	T37.2X4	T37.2X5	T37.2X6
Antimetabolite	T45.1X1	T45.1X2	T45.1X3	T45.1X4	T45.1X5	T45.1X6
Antimitotic agent	T45.1X1	T45.1X2	T45.1X3	T45.1X4	T45.1X5	T45.1X6
Antimony (compounds) (vapor) **NEC**	T56.891	T56.892	T56.893	T56.894	—	—
anti-infectives	T37.8X1	T37.8X2	T37.8X3	T37.8X4	T37.8X5	T37.8X6
dimercaptosuccinate	T37.3X1	T37.3X2	T37.3X3	T37.3X4	T37.3X5	T37.3X6
hydride	T56.891	T56.892	T56.893	T56.894	—	—
pesticide (vapor)	T60.8X1	T60.8X2	T60.8X3	T60.8X4	—	—
potassium (sodium)	T37.8X1	T37.8X2	T37.8X3	T37.8X4	T37.8X5	T37.8X6
tartrate						
sodium	T37.3X1	T37.3X2	T37.3X3	T37.3X4	T37.3X5	T37.3X6
dimercaptosuccinate						
tartrated	T37.8X1	T37.8X2	T37.8X3	T37.8X4	T37.8X5	T37.8X6
Antimuscarinic NEC	T44.3X1	T44.3X2	T44.3X3	T44.3X4	T44.3X5	T44.3X6
Antimycobacterial drug NEC	T37.1X1	T37.1X2	T37.1X3	T37.1X4	T37.1X5	T37.1X6
antibiotics	T36.5X1	T36.5X2	T36.5X3	T36.5X4	T36.5X5	T36.5X6
combination	T37.1X1	T37.1X2	T37.1X3	T37.1X4	T37.1X5	T37.1X6
Antinausea drug	T45.0X1	T45.0X2	T45.0X3	T45.0X4	T45.0X5	T45.0X6
Antinematode drug	T37.4X1	T37.4X2	T37.4X3	T37.4X4	T37.4X5	T37.4X6
Antineoplastic NEC	T45.1X1	T45.1X2	T45.1X3	T45.1X4	T45.1X5	T45.1X6
alkaloidal	T45.1X1	T45.1X2	T45.1X3	T45.1X4	T45.1X5	T45.1X6
antibiotics	T45.1X1	T45.1X2	T45.1X3	T45.1X4	T45.1X5	T45.1X6
combination	T45.1X1	T45.1X2	T45.1X3	T45.1X4	T45.1X5	T45.1X6
estrogen	T38.5X1	T38.5X2	T38.5X3	T38.5X4	T38.5X5	T38.5X6
Antineoplastic — *continued*						
steroid	T38.7X1	T38.7X2	T38.7X3	T38.7X4	T38.7X5	T38.7X6
Antiparasitic drug (systemic)	T37.91	T37.92	T37.93	T37.94	T37.95	T37.96
local	T49.0X1	T49.0X2	T49.0X3	T49.0X4	T49.0X5	T49.0X6
specified NEC	T37.8X1	T37.8X2	T37.8X3	T37.8X4	T37.8X5	T37.8X6
Antiparkinsonism drug NEC	T42.8X1	T42.8X2	T42.8X3	T42.8X4	T42.8X5	T42.8X6
Antiperspirant NEC	T49.2X1	T49.2X2	T49.2X3	T49.2X4	T49.2X5	T49.2X6
Antiphlogistic NEC	T39.4X1	T39.4X2	T39.4X3	T39.4X4	T39.4X5	T39.4X6
Antiplatyhelmintic drug	T37.4X1	T37.4X2	T37.4X3	T37.4X4	T37.4X5	T37.4X6
Antiprotozoal drug NEC	T37.3X1	T37.3X2	T37.3X3	T37.3X4	T37.3X5	T37.3X6
blood	T37.2X1	T37.2X2	T37.2X3	T37.2X4	T37.2X5	T37.2X6
local	T49.0X1	T49.0X2	T49.0X3	T49.0X4	T49.0X5	T49.0X6
Antipruritic drug NEC	T49.1X1	T49.1X2	T49.1X3	T49.1X4	T49.1X5	T49.1X6
Antipsychotic drug	T43.501	T43.502	T43.503	T43.504	T43.505	T43.506
specified NEC	T43.591	T43.592	T43.593	T43.594	T43.595	T43.596
Antipyretic	T39.91	T39.92	T39.93	T39.94	T39.95	T39.96
specified NEC	T39.8X1	T39.8X2	T39.8X3	T39.8X4	T39.8X5	T39.8X6
Antipyrine	T39.2X1	T39.2X2	T39.2X3	T39.2X4	T39.2X5	T39.2X6
Antirabies hyperimmune serum	T50.Z11	T50.Z12	T50.Z13	T50.Z14	T50.Z15	T50.Z16
Antirheumatic NEC	T39.4X1	T39.4X2	T39.4X3	T39.4X4	T39.4X5	T39.4X6
Antirigidity drug NEC	T42.8X1	T42.8X2	T42.8X3	T42.8X4	T42.8X5	T42.8X6
Antischistosomal drug	T37.4X1	T37.4X2	T37.4X3	T37.4X4	T37.4X5	T37.4X6
Antiscorpion sera	T50.Z11	T50.Z12	T50.Z13	T50.Z14	T50.Z15	T50.Z16
Antiseborrheics	T49.4X1	T49.4X2	T49.4X3	T49.4X4	T49.4X5	T49.4X6
Antiseptics (external) (medicinal)	T49.0X1	T49.0X2	T49.0X3	T49.0X4	T49.0X5	T49.0X6
Antistine	T45.0X1	T45.0X2	T45.0X3	T45.0X4	T45.0X5	T45.0X6
Antitapeworm drug	T37.4X1	T37.4X2	T37.4X3	T37.4X4	T37.4X5	T37.4X6
Antitetanus immunoglobulin	T50.Z11	T50.Z12	T50.Z13	T50.Z14	T50.Z15	T50.Z16
Antithyroid drug NEC	T38.2X1	T38.2X2	T38.2X3	T38.2X4	T38.2X5	T38.2X6
Antitoxin	T50.Z11	T50.Z12	T50.Z13	T50.Z14	T50.Z15	T50.Z16
diphtheria	T50.Z11	T50.Z12	T50.Z13	T50.Z14	T50.Z15	T50.Z16
gas gangrene	T50.Z11	T50.Z12	T50.Z13	T50.Z14	T50.Z15	T50.Z16
tetanus	T50.Z11	T50.Z12	T50.Z13	T50.Z14	T50.Z15	T50.Z16
Antitrichomonal drug	T37.3X1	T37.3X2	T37.3X3	T37.3X4	T37.3X5	T37.3X6
Antituberculars	T37.1X1	T37.1X2	T37.1X3	T37.1X4	T37.1X5	T37.1X6
antibiotics	T36.5X1	T36.5X2	T36.5X3	T36.5X4	T36.5X5	T36.5X6
Antitussive NEC	T48.3X1	T48.3X2	T48.3X3	T48.3X4	T48.3X5	T48.3X6
codeine mixture	T40.2X1	T40.2X2	T40.2X3	T40.2X4	T40.2X5	T40.2X6
opiate	T40.2X1	T40.2X2	T40.2X3	T40.2X4	T40.2X5	T40.2X6
Antivaricose drug	T46.8X1	T46.8X2	T46.8X3	T46.8X4	T46.8X5	T46.8X6
Antivenin, antivenom (sera)	T50.Z11	T50.Z12	T50.Z13	T50.Z14	T50.Z15	T50.Z16
crotaline	T50.Z11	T50.Z12	T50.Z13	T50.Z14	T50.Z15	T50.Z16
spider bite	T50.Z11	T50.Z12	T50.Z13	T50.Z14	T50.Z15	T50.Z16
Antivertigo drug	T45.0X1	T45.0X2	T45.0X3	T45.0X4	T45.0X5	T45.0X6
Antiviral drug NEC	T37.5X1	T37.5X2	T37.5X3	T37.5X4	T37.5X5	T37.5X6
eye	T49.5X1	T49.5X2	T49.5X3	T49.5X4	T49.5X5	T49.5X6
Antiwhipworm drug	T37.4X1	T37.4X2	T37.4X3	T37.4X4	T37.4X5	T37.4X6
Ant poison — *see* Insecticide						
Antrol — *see also* by specific chemical substance	T60.91	T60.92	T60.93	T60.94	—	—
fungicide	T60.91	T60.92	T60.93	T60.94	—	—
ANTU (alpha naphthylthiourea)	T60.4X1	T60.4X2	T60.4X3	T60.4X4	—	—
Apalcillin	T36.0X1	T36.0X2	T36.0X3	T36.0X4	T36.0X5	T36.0X6
APC	T48.5X1	T48.5X2	T48.5X3	T48.5X4	T48.5X5	T48.5X6
Aplonidine	T44.4X1	T44.4X2	T44.4X3	T44.4X4	T44.4X5	T44.4X6
Apomorphine	T47.7X1	T47.7X2	T47.7X3	T47.7X4	T47.7X5	T47.7X6
Appetite depressants, central	T50.5X1	T50.5X2	T50.5X3	T50.5X4	T50.5X5	T50.5X6
Apraclonidine (hydrochloride)	T44.4X1	T44.4X2	T44.4X3	T44.4X4	T44.4X5	T44.4X6
Apresoline	T46.5X1	T46.5X2	T46.5X3	T46.5X4	T46.5X5	T46.5X6
Aprindine	T46.2X1	T46.2X2	T46.2X3	T46.2X4	T46.2X5	T46.2X6
Aprobarbital	T42.3X1	T42.3X2	T42.3X3	T42.3X4	T42.3X5	T42.3X6
Apronalide	T42.6X1	T42.6X2	T42.6X3	T42.6X4	T42.6X5	T42.6X6
Aprotinin	T45.621	T45.622	T45.623	T45.624	T45.625	T45.626
Aptocaine	T41.3X1	T41.3X2	T41.3X3	T41.3X4	T41.3X5	T41.3X6
Aqua fortis	T54.2X1	T54.2X2	T54.2X3	T54.2X4	—	—
Ara-A	T37.5X1	T37.5X2	T37.5X3	T37.5X4	T37.5X5	T37.5X6
Ara-C	T45.1X1	T45.1X2	T45.1X3	T45.1X4	T45.1X5	T45.1X6
Arachis oil	T49.3X1	T49.3X2	T49.3X3	T49.3X4	T49.3X5	T49.3X6
cathartic	T47.4X1	T47.4X2	T47.4X3	T47.4X4	T47.4X5	T47.4X6
Aralen	T37.2X1	T37.2X2	T37.2X3	T37.2X4	T37.2X5	T37.2X6
Arecoline	T44.1X1	T44.1X2	T44.1X3	T44.1X4	T44.1X5	T44.1X6
Arginine	T50.991	T50.992	T50.993	T50.994	T50.995	T50.996
glutamate	T50.991	T50.992	T50.993	T50.994	T50.995	T50.996
Argyrol	T49.0X1	T49.0X2	T49.0X3	T49.0X4	T49.0X5	T49.0X6
ENT agent	T49.6X1	T49.6X2	T49.6X3	T49.6X4	T49.6X5	T49.6X6

Table of Drugs and Chemicals

Argyrol — Benzalkonium

Substance	Poisoning, Accidental (unintentional)	Poisoning, Intentional Self-harm	Poisoning, Assault	Poisoning, Undetermined	Adverse Effect	Under-dosing
Argyrol — continued						
ophthalmic preparation	T49.5X1	T49.5X2	T49.5X3	T49.5X4	T49.5X5	T49.5X6
Aristocort	T38.0X1	T38.0X2	T38.0X3	T38.0X4	T38.0X5	T38.0X6
ENT agent	T49.6X1	T49.6X2	T49.6X3	T49.6X4	T49.6X5	T49.6X6
ophthalmic preparation	T49.5X1	T49.5X2	T49.5X3	T49.5X4	T49.5X5	T49.5X6
topical NEC	T49.0X1	T49.0X2	T49.0X3	T49.0X4	T49.0X5	T49.0X6
Aromatics, corrosive	T54.1X1	T54.1X2	T54.1X3	T54.1X4	—	—
disinfectants	T54.1X1	T54.1X2	T54.1X3	T54.1X4	—	—
Arsenate of lead	T57.0X1	T57.0X2	T57.0X3	T57.0X4	—	—
herbicide	T57.0X1	T57.0X2	T57.0X3	T57.0X4	—	—
Arsenic, arsenicals (compounds) (dust) (vapor) **NEC**	T57.0X1	T57.0X2	T57.0X3	T57.0X4	—	—
anti-infectives	T37.8X1	T37.8X2	T37.8X3	T37.8X4	T37.8X5	T37.8X6
pesticide (dust) (fumes)	T57.0X1	T57.0X2	T57.0X3	T57.0X4	—	—
Arsine (gas)	T57.0X1	T57.0X2	T57.0X3	T57.0X4	—	—
Arsphenamine (silver)	T37.8X1	T37.8X2	T37.8X3	T37.8X4	T37.8X5	T37.8X6
Arsthinol	T37.3X1	T37.3X2	T37.3X3	T37.3X4	T37.3X5	T37.3X6
Artane	T44.3X1	T44.3X2	T44.3X3	T44.3X4	T44.3X5	T44.3X6
Arthropod (venomous) **NEC**	T63.481	T63.482	T63.483	T63.484	—	—
Articaine	T41.3X1	T41.3X2	T41.3X3	T41.3X4	T41.3X5	T41.3X6
Asbestos	T57.8X1	T57.8X2	T57.8X3	T57.8X4	—	—
Ascaridole	T37.4X1	T37.4X2	T37.4X3	T37.4X4	T37.4X5	T37.4X6
Ascorbic acid	T45.2X1	T45.2X2	T45.2X3	T45.2X4	T45.2X5	T45.2X6
Asiaticoside	T49.0X1	T49.0X2	T49.0X3	T49.0X4	T49.0X5	T49.0X6
Asparaginase	T45.1X1	T45.1X2	T45.1X3	T45.1X4	T45.1X5	T45.1X6
Aspidium (oleoresin)	T37.4X1	T37.4X2	T37.4X3	T37.4X4	T37.4X5	T37.4X6
Aspirin (aluminum) (soluble)	T39.011	T39.012	T39.013	T39.014	T39.015	T39.016
Aspoxicillin	T36.0X1	T36.0X2	T36.0X3	T36.0X4	T36.0X5	T36.0X6
Astemizole	T45.0X1	T45.0X2	T45.0X3	T45.0X4	T45.0X5	T45.0X6
Astringent (local)	T49.2X1	T49.2X2	T49.2X3	T49.2X4	T49.2X5	T49.2X6
specified NEC	T49.2X1	T49.2X2	T49.2X3	T49.2X4	T49.2X5	T49.2X6
Astromicin	T36.5X1	T36.5X2	T36.5X3	T36.5X4	T36.5X5	T36.5X6
Ataractic drug NEC	T43.501	T43.502	T43.503	T43.504	T43.505	T43.506
Atenolol	T44.7X1	T44.7X2	T44.7X3	T44.7X4	T44.7X5	T44.7X6
Atonia drug, intestinal	T47.4X1	T47.4X2	T47.4X3	T47.4X4	T47.4X5	T47.4X6
Atophan	T50.4X1	T50.4X2	T50.4X3	T50.4X4	T50.4X5	T50.4X6
Atracurium besilate	T48.1X1	T48.1X2	T48.1X3	T48.1X4	T48.1X5	T48.1X6
Atropine	T44.3X1	T44.3X2	T44.3X3	T44.3X4	T44.3X5	T44.3X6
derivative	T44.3X1	T44.3X2	T44.3X3	T44.3X4	T44.3X5	T44.3X6
methonitrate	T44.3X1	T44.3X2	T44.3X3	T44.3X4	T44.3X5	T44.3X6
Attapulgite	T47.6X1	T47.6X2	T47.6X3	T47.6X4	T47.6X5	T47.6X6
Auramine	T65.891	T65.892	T65.893	T65.894	—	—
dye	T65.6X1	T65.6X2	T65.6X3	T65.6X4	—	—
fungicide	T60.3X1	T60.3X2	T60.3X3	T60.3X4	—	—
Auranofin	T39.4X1	T39.4X2	T39.4X3	T39.4X4	T39.4X5	T39.4X6
Aurantiin	T46.991	T46.992	T46.993	T46.994	T46.995	T46.996
Aureomycin	T36.4X1	T36.4X2	T36.4X3	T36.4X4	T36.4X5	T36.4X6
ophthalmic preparation	T49.5X1	T49.5X2	T49.5X3	T49.5X4	T49.5X5	T49.5X6
topical NEC	T49.0X1	T49.0X2	T49.0X3	T49.0X4	T49.0X5	T49.0X6
Aurothioglucose	T39.4X1	T39.4X2	T39.4X3	T39.4X4	T39.4X5	T39.4X6
Aurothioglycanide	T39.4X1	T39.4X2	T39.4X3	T39.4X4	T39.4X5	T39.4X6
Aurothiomalate sodium	T39.4X1	T39.4X2	T39.4X3	T39.4X4	T39.4X5	T39.4X6
Aurotioprol	T39.4X1	T39.4X2	T39.4X3	T39.4X4	T39.4X5	T39.4X6
Automobile fuel	T52.0X1	T52.0X2	T52.0X3	T52.0X4	—	—
Autonomic nervous system agent NEC	T44.901	T44.902	T44.903	T44.904	T44.905	T44.906
Avlosulfon	T37.1X1	T37.1X2	T37.1X3	T37.1X4	T37.1X5	T37.1X6
Avomine	T42.6X1	T42.6X2	T42.6X3	T42.6X4	T42.6X5	T42.6X6
Axerophthol	T45.2X1	T45.2X2	T45.2X3	T45.2X4	T45.2X5	T45.2X6
Azacitidine	T45.1X1	T45.1X2	T45.1X3	T45.1X4	T45.1X5	T45.1X6
Azacyclonol	T43.591	T43.592	T43.593	T43.594	T43.595	T43.596
Azadirachta	T60.2X1	T60.2X2	T60.2X3	T60.2X4	—	—
Azanidazole	T37.3X1	T37.3X2	T37.3X3	T37.3X4	T37.3X5	T37.3X6
Azapetine	T46.7X1	T46.7X2	T46.7X3	T46.7X4	T46.7X5	T46.7X6
Azapropazone	T39.2X1	T39.2X2	T39.2X3	T39.2X4	T39.2X5	T39.2X6
Azaribine	T45.1X1	T45.1X2	T45.1X3	T45.1X4	T45.1X5	T45.1X6
Azaserine	T45.1X1	T45.1X2	T45.1X3	T45.1X4	T45.1X5	T45.1X6
Azatadine	T45.0X1	T45.0X2	T45.0X3	T45.0X4	T45.0X5	T45.0X6
Azatepa	T45.1X1	T45.1X2	T45.1X3	T45.1X4	T45.1X5	T45.1X6
Azathioprine	T45.1X1	T45.1X2	T45.1X3	T45.1X4	T45.1X5	T45.1X6
Azelaic acid	T49.0X1	T49.0X2	T49.0X3	T49.0X4	T49.0X5	T49.0X6
Azelastine	T45.0X1	T45.0X2	T45.0X3	T45.0X4	T45.0X5	T45.0X6
Azidocillin	T36.0X1	T36.0X2	T36.0X3	T36.0X4	T36.0X5	T36.0X6
Azidothymidine	T37.5X1	T37.5X2	T37.5X3	T37.5X4	T37.5X5	T37.5X6
Azinphos (ethyl) (methyl)	T60.0X1	T60.0X2	T60.0X3	T60.0X4	—	—
Aziridine (chelating)	T54.1X1	T54.1X2	T54.1X3	T54.1X4	—	—
Azithromycin	T36.3X1	T36.3X2	T36.3X3	T36.3X4	T36.3X5	T36.3X6
Azlocillin	T36.0X1	T36.0X2	T36.0X3	T36.0X4	T36.0X5	T36.0X6
Azobenzene smoke	T65.3X1	T65.3X2	T65.3X3	T65.3X4	—	—
acaricide	T60.8X1	T60.8X2	T60.8X3	T60.8X4	—	—
Azosulfamide	T37.0X1	T37.0X2	T37.0X3	T37.0X4	T37.0X5	T37.0X6
AZT	T37.5X1	T37.5X2	T37.5X3	T37.5X4	T37.5X5	T37.5X6
Aztreonam	T36.1X1	T36.1X2	T36.1X3	T36.1X4	T36.1X5	T36.1X6
Azulfidine	T37.0X1	T37.0X2	T37.0X3	T37.0X4	T37.0X5	T37.0X6
Azuresin	T50.8X1	T50.8X2	T50.8X3	T50.8X4	T50.8X5	T50.8X6
b-acetyldigoxin	T46.0X1	T46.0X2	T46.0X3	T46.0X4	T46.0X5	T46.0X6
P-Acetamidophenol	T39.1X1	T39.1X2	T39.1X3	T39.1X4	T39.1X5	T39.1X6
Bacampicillin	T36.0X1	T36.0X2	T36.0X3	T36.0X4	T36.0X5	T36.0X6
Bacillus						
lactobacillus	T47.8X1	T47.8X2	T47.8X3	T47.8X4	T47.8X5	T47.8X6
subtilis	T47.6X1	T47.6X2	T47.6X3	T47.6X4	T47.6X5	T47.6X6
Bacimycin	T49.0X1	T49.0X2	T49.0X3	T49.0X4	T49.0X5	T49.0X6
ophthalmic preparation	T49.5X1	T49.5X2	T49.5X3	T49.5X4	T49.5X5	T49.5X6
Bacitracin zinc	T49.0X1	T49.0X2	T49.0X3	T49.0X4	T49.0X5	T49.0X6
with neomycin	T49.0X1	T49.0X2	T49.0X3	T49.0X4	T49.0X5	T49.0X6
ENT agent	T49.6X1	T49.6X2	T49.6X3	T49.6X4	T49.6X5	T49.6X6
ophthalmic preparation	T49.5X1	T49.5X2	T49.5X3	T49.5X4	T49.5X5	T49.5X6
topical NEC	T49.0X1	T49.0X2	T49.0X3	T49.0X4	T49.0X5	T49.0X6
Baclofen	T42.8X1	T42.8X2	T42.8X3	T42.8X4	T42.8X5	T42.8X6
Baking soda	T50.991	T50.992	T50.993	T50.994	T50.995	T50.996
BAL	T45.8X1	T45.8X2	T45.8X3	T45.8X4	T45.8X5	T45.8X6
Bambuterol	T48.6X1	T48.6X2	T48.6X3	T48.6X4	T48.6X5	T48.6X6
Bamethan (sulfate)	T46.7X1	T46.7X2	T46.7X3	T46.7X4	T46.7X5	T46.7X6
Bamifylline	T48.6X1	T48.6X2	T48.6X3	T48.6X4	T48.6X5	T48.6X6
Bamipine	T45.0X1	T45.0X2	T45.0X3	T45.0X4	T45.0X5	T45.0X6
Baneberry — see Actaea spicata						
Banewort — see Belladonna						
Barbenyl	T42.3X1	T42.3X2	T42.3X3	T42.3X4	T42.3X5	T42.3X6
Barbexaclone	T42.6X1	T42.6X2	T42.6X3	T42.6X4	T42.6X5	T42.6X6
Barbital	T42.3X1	T42.3X2	T42.3X3	T42.3X4	T42.3X5	T42.3X6
sodium	T42.3X1	T42.3X2	T42.3X3	T42.3X4	T42.3X5	T42.3X6
Barbitone	T42.3X1	T42.3X2	T42.3X3	T42.3X4	T42.3X5	T42.3X6
Barbiturate NEC	T42.3X1	T42.3X2	T42.3X3	T42.3X4	T42.3X5	T42.3X6
with tranquilizer	T42.3X1	T42.3X2	T42.3X3	T42.3X4	T42.3X5	T42.3X6
anesthetic (intravenous)	T41.1X1	T41.1X2	T41.1X3	T41.1X4	T41.1X5	T41.1X6
Barium (carbonate) (chloride) (sulfite)	T57.8X1	T57.8X2	T57.8X3	T57.8X4	—	—
diagnostic agent	T50.8X1	T50.8X2	T50.8X3	T50.8X4	T50.8X5	T50.8X6
pesticide	T60.4X1	T60.4X2	T60.4X3	T60.4X4	—	—
rodenticide	T60.4X1	T60.4X2	T60.4X3	T60.4X4	—	—
sulfate (medicinal)	T50.8X1	T50.8X2	T50.8X3	T50.8X4	T50.8X5	T50.8X6
Barrier cream	T49.3X1	T49.3X2	T49.3X3	T49.3X4	T49.3X5	T49.3X6
Basic fuchsin	T49.0X1	T49.0X2	T49.0X3	T49.0X4	T49.0X5	T49.0X6
Battery acid or fluid	T54.2X1	T54.2X2	T54.2X3	T54.2X4	—	—
Bay rum	T51.8X1	T51.8X2	T51.8X3	T51.8X4	—	—
b-benzalbutyramide	T46.6X1	T46.6X2	T46.6X3	T46.6X4	T46.6X5	T46.6X6
BCG (vaccine)	T50.A91	T50.A92	T50.A93	T50.A94	T50.A95	T50.A96
BCNU	T45.1X1	T45.1X2	T45.1X3	T45.1X4	T45.1X5	T45.1X6
Bearsfoot	T62.2X1	T62.2X2	T62.2X3	T62.2X4	—	—
Beclamide	T42.6X1	T42.6X2	T42.6X3	T42.6X4	T42.6X5	T42.6X6
Beclomethasone	T44.5X1	T44.5X2	T44.5X3	T44.5X4	T44.5X5	T44.5X6
Bee (sting) (venom)	T63.441	T63.442	T63.443	T63.444	—	—
Befunolol	T49.5X1	T49.5X2	T49.5X3	T49.5X4	T49.5X5	T49.5X6
Bekanamycin	T36.5X1	T36.5X2	T36.5X3	T36.5X4	T36.5X5	T36.5X6
Belladonna — see also Nightshade						
alkaloids	T44.3X1	T44.3X2	T44.3X3	T44.3X4	T44.3X5	T44.3X6
extract	T44.3X1	T44.3X2	T44.3X3	T44.3X4	T44.3X5	T44.3X6
herb	T44.3X1	T44.3X2	T44.3X3	T44.3X4	T44.3X5	T44.3X6
Bemegride	T50.7X1	T50.7X2	T50.7X3	T50.7X4	T50.7X5	T50.7X6
Benactyzine	T44.3X1	T44.3X2	T44.3X3	T44.3X4	T44.3X5	T44.3X6
Benadryl	T45.0X1	T45.0X2	T45.0X3	T45.0X4	T45.0X5	T45.0X6
Benaprizine	T44.3X1	T44.3X2	T44.3X3	T44.3X4	T44.3X5	T44.3X6
Benazepril	T46.4X1	T46.4X2	T46.4X3	T46.4X4	T46.4X5	T46.4X6
Bencyclane	T46.7X1	T46.7X2	T46.7X3	T46.7X4	T46.7X5	T46.7X6
Bendazol	T46.3X1	T46.3X2	T46.3X3	T46.3X4	T46.3X5	T46.3X6
Bendrofluazide	T50.2X1	T50.2X2	T50.2X3	T50.2X4	T50.2X5	T50.2X6
Bendroflumethiazide	T50.2X1	T50.2X2	T50.2X3	T50.2X4	T50.2X5	T50.2X6
Benemid	T50.4X1	T50.4X2	T50.4X3	T50.4X4	T50.4X5	T50.4X6
Benethamine penicillin	T36.0X1	T36.0X2	T36.0X3	T36.0X4	T36.0X5	T36.0X6
Benexate	T47.1X1	T47.1X2	T47.1X3	T47.1X4	T47.1X5	T47.1X6
Benfluorex	T46.6X1	T46.6X2	T46.6X3	T46.6X4	T46.6X5	T46.6X6
Benfotiamine	T45.2X1	T45.2X2	T45.2X3	T45.2X4	T45.2X5	T45.2X6
Benisone	T49.0X1	T49.0X2	T49.0X3	T49.0X4	T49.0X5	T49.0X6
Benomyl	T60.0X1	T60.0X2	T60.0X3	T60.0X4	—	—
Benoquin	T49.8X1	T49.8X2	T49.8X3	T49.8X4	T49.8X5	T49.8X6
Benoxinate	T41.3X1	T41.3X2	T41.3X3	T41.3X4	T41.3X5	T41.3X6
Benperidol	T43.4X1	T43.4X2	T43.4X3	T43.4X4	T43.4X5	T43.4X6
Benproperine	T48.3X1	T48.3X2	T48.3X3	T48.3X4	T48.3X5	T48.3X6
Benserazide	T42.8X1	T42.8X2	T42.8X3	T42.8X4	T42.8X5	T42.8X6
Bentazepam	T42.4X1	T42.4X2	T42.4X3	T42.4X4	T42.4X5	T42.4X6
Bentiromide	T50.8X1	T50.8X2	T50.8X3	T50.8X4	T50.8X5	T50.8X6
Bentonite	T49.3X1	T49.3X2	T49.3X3	T49.3X4	T49.3X5	T49.3X6
Benzalbutyramide	T46.6X1	T46.6X2	T46.6X3	T46.6X4	T46.6X5	T46.6X6
Benzalkonium (chloride)	T49.0X1	T49.0X2	T49.0X3	T49.0X4	T49.0X5	T49.0X6
ophthalmic preparation	T49.5X1	T49.5X2	T49.5X3	T49.5X4	T49.5X5	T49.5X6

Additional Character May Be Required — Refer to the Tabular List for Character Selection
🔺 Subterms under main terms may continue to next column or page

Substance	Poisoning, Accidental (unintentional)	Poisoning, Intentional Self-harm	Poisoning, Assault	Poisoning, Undetermined	Adverse Effect	Under-dosing
Benzamidosalicylate (calcium)	T37.1X1	T37.1X2	T37.1X3	T37.1X4	T37.1X5	T37.1X6
Benzamine	T41.3X1	T41.3X2	T41.3X3	T41.3X4	T41.3X5	T41.3X6
lactate	T49.1X1	T49.1X2	T49.1X3	T49.1X4	T49.1X5	T49.1X6
Benzamphetamine	T50.5X1	T50.5X2	T50.5X3	T50.5X4	T50.5X5	T50.5X6
Benzapril hydrochloride	T46.5X1	T46.5X2	T46.5X3	T46.5X4	T46.5X5	T46.5X6
Benzathine benzylpenicillin	T36.0X1	T36.0X2	T36.0X3	T36.0X4	T36.0X5	T36.0X6
Benzathine penicillin	T36.0X1	T36.0X2	T36.0X3	T36.0X4	T36.0X5	T36.0X6
Benzatropine	T42.8X1	T42.8X2	T42.8X3	T42.8X4	T42.8X5	T42.8X6
Benzbromarone	T50.4X1	T50.4X2	T50.4X3	T50.4X4	T50.4X5	T50.4X6
Benzcarbimine	T45.1X1	T45.1X2	T45.1X3	T45.1X4	T45.1X5	T45.1X6
Benzedrex	T44.991	T44.992	T44.993	T44.994	T44.995	T44.996
Benzedrine (amphetamine)	T43.621	T43.622	T43.623	T43.624	T43.625	T43.626
Benzenamine	T65.3X1	T65.3X2	T65.3X3	T65.3X4	—	—
Benzene	T52.1X1	T52.1X2	T52.1X3	T52.1X4	—	—
homologues (acetyl) (dimethyl) (methyl) (solvent)	T52.2X1	T52.2X2	T52.2X3	T52.2X4	—	—
Benzethonium (chloride)	T49.0X1	T49.0X2	T49.0X3	T49.0X4	T49.0X5	T49.0X6
Benzfetamine	T50.5X1	T50.5X2	T50.5X3	T50.5X4	T50.5X5	T50.5X6
Benzhexol	T44.3X1	T44.3X2	T44.3X3	T44.3X4	T44.3X5	T44.3X6
Benzhydramine (chloride)	T45.0X1	T45.0X2	T45.0X3	T45.0X4	T45.0X5	T45.0X6
Benzidine	T65.891	T65.892	T65.893	T65.894	—	—
Benzilonium bromide	T44.3X1	T44.3X2	T44.3X3	T44.3X4	T44.3X5	T44.3X6
Benzimidazole	T60.3X1	T60.3X2	T60.3X3	T60.3X4	—	—
Benzin (e) — see Ligroin						
Benziodarone	T46.3X1	T46.3X2	T46.3X3	T46.3X4	T46.3X5	T46.3X6
Benznidazole	T37.3X1	T37.3X2	T37.3X3	T37.3X4	T37.3X5	T37.3X6
Benzocaine	T41.3X1	T41.3X2	T41.3X3	T41.3X4	T41.3X5	T41.3X6
Benzodiapin	T42.4X1	T42.4X2	T42.4X3	T42.4X4	T42.4X5	T42.4X6
Benzodiazepine NEC	T42.4X1	T42.4X2	T42.4X3	T42.4X4	T42.4X5	T42.4X6
Benzoic acid	T49.0X1	T49.0X2	T49.0X3	T49.0X4	T49.0X5	T49.0X6
with salicylic acid	T49.0X1	T49.0X2	T49.0X3	T49.0X4	T49.0X5	T49.0X6
Benzoin (tincture)	T48.5X1	T48.5X2	T48.5X3	T48.5X4	T48.5X5	T48.5X6
Benzol (benzene)	T52.1X1	T52.1X2	T52.1X3	T52.1X4	—	—
vapor	T52.0X1	T52.0X2	T52.0X3	T52.0X4	—	—
Benzomorphan	T40.2X1	T40.2X2	T40.2X3	T40.2X4	T40.2X5	T40.2X6
Benzonatate	T48.3X1	T48.3X2	T48.3X3	T48.3X4	T48.3X5	T48.3X6
Benzophenones	T49.3X1	T49.3X2	T49.3X3	T49.3X4	T49.3X5	T49.3X6
Benzopyrone	T46.991	T46.992	T46.993	T46.994	T46.995	T46.996
Benzothiadiazides	T50.2X1	T50.2X2	T50.2X3	T50.2X4	T50.2X5	T50.2X6
Benzoxonium chloride	T49.0X1	T49.0X2	T49.0X3	T49.0X4	T49.0X5	T49.0X6
Benzoylpas calcium	T37.1X1	T37.1X2	T37.1X3	T37.1X4	T37.1X5	T37.1X6
Benzoyl peroxide	T49.0X1	T49.0X2	T49.0X3	T49.0X4	T49.0X5	T49.0X6
Benzperidin	T43.591	T43.592	T43.593	T43.594	T43.595	T43.596
Benzperidol	T43.591	T43.592	T43.593	T43.594	T43.595	T43.596
Benzphetamine	T50.5X1	T50.5X2	T50.5X3	T50.5X4	T50.5X5	T50.5X6
Benzpyrinium bromide	T44.1X1	T44.1X2	T44.1X3	T44.1X4	T44.1X5	T44.1X6
Benzquinamide	T45.0X1	T45.0X2	T45.0X3	T45.0X4	T45.0X5	T45.0X6
Benzthiazide	T50.2X1	T50.2X2	T50.2X3	T50.2X4	T50.2X5	T50.2X6
Benztropine						
anticholinergic	T44.3X1	T44.3X2	T44.3X3	T44.3X4	T44.3X5	T44.3X6
antiparkinson	T42.8X1	T42.8X2	T42.8X3	T42.8X4	T42.8X5	T42.8X6
Benzydamine	T49.0X1	T49.0X2	T49.0X3	T49.0X4	T49.0X5	T49.0X6
Benzyl						
acetate	T52.8X1	T52.8X2	T52.8X3	T52.8X4	—	—
alcohol	T49.0X1	T49.0X2	T49.0X3	T49.0X4	T49.0X5	T49.0X6
benzoate	T49.0X1	T49.0X2	T49.0X3	T49.0X4	T49.0X5	T49.0X6
Benzoic acid	T49.0X1	T49.0X2	T49.0X3	T49.0X4	T49.0X5	T49.0X6
morphine	T40.2X1	T40.2X2	T40.2X3	T40.2X4	—	—
nicotinate	T46.6X1	T46.6X2	T46.6X3	T46.6X4	T46.6X5	T46.6X6
penicillin	T36.0X1	T36.0X2	T36.0X3	T36.0X4	T36.0X5	T36.0X6
Benzylhydrochlorthiazide	T50.2X1	T50.2X2	T50.2X3	T50.2X4	T50.2X5	T50.2X6
Benzylpenicillin	T36.0X1	T36.0X2	T36.0X3	T36.0X4	T36.0X5	T36.0X6
Benzylthiouracil	T38.2X1	T38.2X2	T38.2X3	T38.2X4	T38.2X5	T38.2X6
Bephenium hydroxynaphthoate	T37.4X1	T37.4X2	T37.4X3	T37.4X4	T37.4X5	T37.4X6
Bepridil	T46.1X1	T46.1X2	T46.1X3	T46.1X4	T46.1X5	T46.1X6
Bergamot oil	T65.891	T65.892	T65.893	T65.894	—	—
Bergapten	T50.991	T50.992	T50.993	T50.994	T50.995	T50.996
Berries, poisonous	T62.1X1	T62.1X2	T62.1X3	T62.1X4	—	—
Beryllium (compounds)	T56.7X1	T56.7X2	T56.7X3	T56.7X4	—	—
beta adrenergic blocking agent, heart	T44.7X1	T44.7X2	T44.7X3	T44.7X4	T44.7X5	T44.7X6
Betacarotene	T45.2X1	T45.2X2	T45.2X3	T45.2X4	T45.2X5	T45.2X6
Beta-Chlor	T42.6X1	T42.6X2	T42.6X3	T42.6X4	T42.6X5	T42.6X6
Betahistine	T46.7X1	T46.7X2	T46.7X3	T46.7X4	T46.7X5	T46.7X6
Betaine	T47.5X1	T47.5X2	T47.5X3	T47.5X4	T47.5X5	T47.5X6
Betamethasone	T49.0X1	T49.0X2	T49.0X3	T49.0X4	T49.0X5	T49.0X6
topical	T49.0X1	T49.0X2	T49.0X3	T49.0X4	T49.0X5	T49.0X6
Betamicin	T36.8X1	T36.8X2	T36.8X3	T36.8X4	T36.8X5	T36.8X6
Betanidine	T46.5X1	T46.5X2	T46.5X3	T46.5X4	T46.5X5	T46.5X6
Betaxolol	T44.7X1	T44.7X2	T44.7X3	T44.7X4	T44.7X5	T44.7X6

Substance	Poisoning, Accidental (unintentional)	Poisoning, Intentional Self-harm	Poisoning, Assault	Poisoning, Undetermined	Adverse Effect	Under-dosing
Betazole	T50.8X1	T50.8X2	T50.8X3	T50.8X4	T50.8X5	T50.8X6
Bethanechol	T44.1X1	T44.1X2	T44.1X3	T44.1X4	T44.1X5	T44.1X6
chloride	T44.1X1	T44.1X2	T44.1X3	T44.1X4	T44.1X5	T44.1X6
Bethanidine	T46.5X1	T46.5X2	T46.5X3	T46.5X4	T46.5X5	T46.5X6
Betoxycaine	T41.3X1	T41.3X2	T41.3X3	T41.3X4	T41.3X5	T41.3X6
Betula oil	T49.3X1	T49.3X2	T49.3X3	T49.3X4	T49.3X5	T49.3X6
Bevantolol	T44.7X1	T44.7X2	T44.7X3	T44.7X4	T44.7X5	T44.7X6
Bevonium metilsulfate	T44.3X1	T44.3X2	T44.3X3	T44.3X4	T44.3X5	T44.3X6
Bezafibrate	T46.6X1	T46.6X2	T46.6X3	T46.6X4	T46.6X5	T46.6X6
Bezitramide	T40.4X1	T40.4X2	T40.4X3	T40.4X4	T40.4X5	T40.4X6
BHA	T50.991	T50.992	T50.993	T50.994	T50.995	T50.996
Bhang	T40.7X1	T40.7X2	T40.7X3	T40.7X4	T40.7X5	T40.7X6
BHC (medicinal)	T49.0X1	T49.0X2	T49.0X3	T49.0X4	T49.0X5	T49.0X6
nonmedicinal (vapor)	T53.6X1	T53.6X2	T53.6X3	T53.6X4	—	—
Bialamicol	T37.3X1	T37.3X2	T37.3X3	T37.3X4	T37.3X5	T37.3X6
Bibenzonium bromide	T48.3X1	T48.3X2	T48.3X3	T48.3X4	T48.3X5	T48.3X6
Bibrocathol	T49.5X1	T49.5X2	T49.5X3	T49.5X4	T49.5X5	T49.5X6
Bichloride of mercury — see Mercury, chloride						
Bichromates (calcium) (potassium)(sodium) (crystals)	T57.8X1	T57.8X2	T57.8X3	T57.8X4		
fumes	T56.2X1	T56.2X2	T56.2X3	T56.2X4		
Biclotymol	T49.6X1	T49.6X2	T49.6X3	T49.6X4	T49.6X5	T49.6X6
Bicucculine	T50.7X1	T50.7X2	T50.7X3	T50.7X4	T50.7X5	T50.7X6
Bifemelane	T43.291	T43.292	T43.293	T43.294	T43.295	T43.296
Biguanide derivatives, oral	T38.3X1	T38.3X2	T38.3X3	T38.3X4	T38.3X5	T38.3X6
Bile salts	T47.5X1	T47.5X2	T47.5X3	T47.5X4	T47.5X5	T47.5X6
Biligrafin	T50.8X1	T50.8X2	T50.8X3	T50.8X4	T50.8X5	T50.8X6
Bilopaque	T50.8X1	T50.8X2	T50.8X3	T50.8X4	T50.8X5	T50.8X6
Binifibrate	T46.6X1	T46.6X2	T46.6X3	T46.6X4	T46.6X5	T46.6X6
Binitrobenzol	T65.3X1	T65.3X2	T65.3X3	T65.3X4		
Bioflavonoid(s)	T46.991	T46.992	T46.993	T46.994	T46.995	T46.996
Biological substance NEC	T50.901	T50.902	T50.903	T50.904	T50.905	T50.906
Biotin	T45.2X1	T45.2X2	T45.2X3	T45.2X4	T45.2X5	T45.2X6
Biperiden	T44.3X1	T44.3X2	T44.3X3	T44.3X4	T44.3X5	T44.3X6
Bisacodyl	T47.2X1	T47.2X2	T47.2X3	T47.2X4	T47.2X5	T47.2X6
Bisbentiamine	T45.2X1	T45.2X2	T45.2X3	T45.2X4	T45.2X5	T45.2X6
Bisbutiamine	T45.2X1	T45.2X2	T45.2X3	T45.2X4	T45.2X5	T45.2X6
Bisdequalinium (salts) (diacetate)	T49.6X1	T49.6X2	T49.6X3	T49.6X4	T49.6X5	T49.6X6
Bishydroxycoumarin	T45.511	T45.512	T45.513	T45.514	T45.515	T45.516
Bismarsen	T37.8X1	T37.8X2	T37.8X3	T37.8X4	T37.8X5	T37.8X6
Bismuth salts	T47.6X1	T47.6X2	T47.6X3	T47.6X4	T47.6X5	T47.6X6
aluminate	T47.1X1	T47.1X2	T47.1X3	T47.1X4	T47.1X5	T47.1X6
anti-infectives	T37.8X1	T37.8X2	T37.8X3	T37.8X4	T37.8X5	T37.8X6
formic iodide	T49.0X1	T49.0X2	T49.0X3	T49.0X4	T49.0X5	T49.0X6
glycolylarsenate	T49.0X1	T49.0X2	T49.0X3	T49.0X4	T49.0X5	T49.0X6
nonmedicinal (compounds) NEC	T65.91	T65.92	T65.93	T65.94	—	—
subcarbonate	T47.6X1	T47.6X2	T47.6X3	T47.6X4	T47.6X5	T47.6X6
subsalicylate	T37.8X1	T37.8X2	T37.8X3	T37.8X4	T37.8X5	T37.8X6
sulfarsphenamine	T37.8X1	T37.8X2	T37.8X3	T37.8X4	T37.8X5	T37.8X6
Bisoprolol	T44.7X1	T44.7X2	T44.7X3	T44.7X4	T44.7X5	T44.7X6
Bisoxatin	T47.2X1	T47.2X2	T47.2X3	T47.2X4	T47.2X5	T47.2X6
Bisulepin (hydrochloride)	T45.0X1	T45.0X2	T45.0X3	T45.0X4	T45.0X5	T45.0X6
Bithionol	T37.8X1	T37.8X2	T37.8X3	T37.8X4	T37.8X5	T37.8X6
anthelminthic	T37.4X1	T37.4X2	T37.4X3	T37.4X4	T37.4X5	T37.4X6
Bitolterol	T48.6X1	T48.6X2	T48.6X3	T48.6X4	T48.6X5	T48.6X6
Bitoscanate	T37.4X1	T37.4X2	T37.4X3	T37.4X4	T37.4X5	T37.4X6
Bitter almond oil	T62.8X1	T62.8X2	T62.8X3	T62.8X4		
Bittersweet	T62.2X1	T62.2X2	T62.2X3	T62.2X4		
Black						
flag	T60.91	T60.92	T60.93	T60.94		
henbane	T62.2X1	T62.2X2	T62.2X3	T62.2X4		
leaf (40)	T60.91	T60.92	T60.93	T60.94		
widow spider (bite)	T63.311	T63.312	T63.313	T63.314		
antivenin	T50.Z11	T50.Z12	T50.Z13	T50.Z14	T50.Z15	T50.Z16
Blast furnace gas (carbon monoxide from)	T58.8X1	T58.8X2	T58.8X3	T58.8X4		
Bleach	T54.91	T54.92	T54.93	T54.94		
Bleaching agent (medicinal)	T49.4X1	T49.4X2	T49.4X3	T49.4X4	T49.4X5	T49.4X6
Bleomycin	T45.1X1	T45.1X2	T45.1X3	T45.1X4	T45.1X5	T45.1X6
Blockain	T41.3X1	T41.3X2	T41.3X3	T41.3X4	T41.3X5	T41.3X6
infiltration (subcutaneous)	T41.3X1	T41.3X2	T41.3X3	T41.3X4	T41.3X5	T41.3X6
nerve block (peripheral) (plexus)	T41.3X1	T41.3X2	T41.3X3	T41.3X4	T41.3X5	T41.3X6
topical (surface)	T41.3X1	T41.3X2	T41.3X3	T41.3X4	T41.3X5	T41.3X6
Blockers, calcium channel	T46.1X1	T46.1X2	T46.1X3	T46.1X4	T46.1X5	T46.1X6
Blood (derivatives) (natural) (plasma) (whole)	T45.8X1	T45.8X2	T45.8X3	T45.8X4	T45.8X5	T45.8X6
dried	T45.8X1	T45.8X2	T45.8X3	T45.8X4	T45.8X5	T45.8X6
drug affecting NEC	T45.91	T45.92	T45.93	T45.94	T45.95	T45.96

Table of Drugs and Chemicals

Blood — Butyl

Substance	Poisoning, Accidental (unintentional)	Poisoning, Intentional Self-harm	Poisoning, Assault	Poisoning, Undetermined	Adverse Effect	Under-dosing
Blood — continued						
expander NEC	T45.8X1	T45.8X2	T45.8X3	T45.8X4	T45.8X5	T45.8X6
fraction NEC	T45.8X1	T45.8X2	T45.8X3	T45.8X4	T45.8X5	T45.8X6
substitute (macromolecular)	T45.8X1	T45.8X2	T45.8X3	T45.8X4	T45.8X5	T45.8X6
Blue velvet	T40.2X1	T40.2X2	T40.2X3	T40.2X4	—	—
Bone meal	T62.8X1	T62.8X2	T62.8X3	T62.8X4	—	—
Bonine	T45.0X1	T45.0X2	T45.0X3	T45.0X4	T45.0X5	T45.0X6
Bopindolol	T44.7X1	T44.7X2	T44.7X3	T44.7X4	T44.7X5	T44.7X6
Boracic acid	T49.0X1	T49.0X2	T49.0X3	T49.0X4	T49.0X5	T49.0X6
ENT agent	T49.6X1	T49.6X2	T49.6X3	T49.6X4	T49.6X5	T49.6X6
ophthalmic preparation	T49.5X1	T49.5X2	T49.5X3	T49.5X4	T49.5X5	T49.5X6
Borane complex	T57.8X1	T57.8X2	T57.8X3	T57.8X4	—	—
Borate(s)	T57.8X1	T57.8X2	T57.8X3	T57.8X4	—	—
buffer	T50.991	T50.992	T50.993	T50.994	T50.995	T50.996
cleanser	T54.91	T54.92	T54.93	T54.94	—	—
sodium	T57.8X1	T57.8X2	T57.8X3	T57.8X4	—	—
Borax (cleanser)	T54.91	T54.92	T54.93	T54.94	—	—
Bordeaux mixture	T60.3X1	T60.3X2	T60.3X3	T60.3X4	—	—
Boric acid	T49.0X1	T49.0X2	T49.0X3	T49.0X4	T49.0X5	T49.0X6
ENT agent	T49.6X1	T49.6X2	T49.6X3	T49.6X4	T49.6X5	T49.6X6
ophthalmic preparation	T49.5X1	T49.5X2	T49.5X3	T49.5X4	T49.5X5	T49.5X6
Bornaprine	T44.3X1	T44.3X2	T44.3X3	T44.3X4	T44.3X5	T44.3X6
Boron	T57.8X1	T57.8X2	T57.8X3	T57.8X4	—	—
hydride NEC	T57.8X1	T57.8X2	T57.8X3	T57.8X4	—	—
fumes or gas	T57.8X1	T57.8X2	T57.8X3	T57.8X4	—	—
trifluoride	T59.891	T59.892	T59.893	T59.894	—	—
Botox	T48.291	T48.292	T48.293	T48.294	T48.295	T48.296
Botulinus anti-toxin (type A, B)	T50.Z11	T50.Z12	T50.Z13	T50.Z14	T50.Z15	T50.Z16
Brake fluid vapor	T59.891	T59.892	T59.893	T59.894	—	—
Brallobarbital	T42.3X1	T42.3X2	T42.3X3	T42.3X4	T42.3X5	T42.3X6
Bran (wheat)	T47.4X1	T47.4X2	T47.4X3	T47.4X4	T47.4X5	T47.4X6
Brass (fumes)	T56.891	T56.892	T56.893	T56.894	—	—
Brasso	T52.0X1	T52.0X2	T52.0X3	T52.0X4	—	—
Bretylium tosilate	T46.2X1	T46.2X2	T46.2X3	T46.2X4	T46.2X5	T46.2X6
Brevital (sodium)	T41.1X1	T41.1X2	T41.1X3	T41.1X4	T41.1X5	T41.1X6
Brinase	T45.3X1	T45.3X2	T45.3X3	T45.3X4	T45.3X5	T45.3X6
British antilewisite	T45.8X1	T45.8X2	T45.8X3	T45.8X4	T45.8X5	T45.8X6
Brodifacoum	T60.4X1	T60.4X2	T60.4X3	T60.4X4	—	—
Bromal (hydrate)	T42.6X1	T42.6X2	T42.6X3	T42.6X4	T42.6X5	T42.6X6
Bromazepam	T42.4X1	T42.4X2	T42.4X3	T42.4X4	T42.4X5	T42.4X6
Bromazine	T45.0X1	T45.0X2	T45.0X3	T45.0X4	T45.0X5	T45.0X6
Brombenzylcyanide	T59.3X1	T59.3X2	T59.3X3	T59.3X4	—	—
Bromelains	T45.3X1	T45.3X2	T45.3X3	T45.3X4	T45.3X5	T45.3X6
Bromethalin	T60.4X1	T60.4X2	T60.4X3	T60.4X4	—	—
Bromide salts	T42.6X1	T42.6X2	T42.6X3	T42.6X4	T42.6X5	T42.6X6
Bromindione	T45.511	T45.512	T45.513	T45.514	T45.515	T45.516
Bromine						
compounds (medicinal)	T42.6X1	T42.6X2	T42.6X3	T42.6X4	T42.6X5	T42.6X6
sedative	T42.6X1	T42.6X2	T42.6X3	T42.6X4	T42.6X5	T42.6X6
vapor	T59.891	T59.892	T59.893	T59.894	—	—
Bromisoval	T42.6X1	T42.6X2	T42.6X3	T42.6X4	T42.6X5	T42.6X6
Bromisovalum	T42.6X1	T42.6X2	T42.6X3	T42.6X4	T42.6X5	T42.6X6
Bromobenzylcyanide	T59.3X1	T59.3X2	T59.3X3	T59.3X4	—	—
Bromochlorosalicylani-lide	T49.0X1	T49.0X2	T49.0X3	T49.0X4	T49.0X5	T49.0X6
Bromocriptine	T42.8X1	T42.8X2	T42.8X3	T42.8X4	T42.8X5	T42.8X6
Bromodiphenhydramine	T45.0X1	T45.0X2	T45.0X3	T45.0X4	T45.0X5	T45.0X6
Bromoform	T42.6X1	T42.6X2	T42.6X3	T42.6X4	T42.6X5	T42.6X6
Bromophenol blue reagent	T50.991	T50.992	T50.993	T50.994	T50.995	T50.996
Bromopride	T47.8X1	T47.8X2	T47.8X3	T47.8X4	T47.8X5	T47.8X6
Bromosalicylchloranitide	T49.0X1	T49.0X2	T49.0X3	T49.0X4	T49.0X5	T49.0X6
Bromosalicylhydroxamic acid	T37.1X1	T37.1X2	T37.1X3	T37.1X4	T37.1X5	T37.1X6
Bromo-seltzer	T39.1X1	T39.1X2	T39.1X3	T39.1X4	T39.1X5	T39.1X6
Bromoxynil	T60.3X1	T60.3X2	T60.3X3	T60.3X4	—	—
Bromperidol	T43.4X1	T43.4X2	T43.4X3	T43.4X4	T43.4X5	T43.4X6
Brompheniramine	T45.0X1	T45.0X2	T45.0X3	T45.0X4	T45.0X5	T45.0X6
Bromsulfophthalein	T50.8X1	T50.8X2	T50.8X3	T50.8X4	T50.8X5	T50.8X6
Bromural	T42.6X1	T42.6X2	T42.6X3	T42.6X4	T42.6X5	T42.6X6
Bromvaletone	T42.6X1	T42.6X2	T42.6X3	T42.6X4	T42.6X5	T42.6X6
Bronchodilator NEC	T48.6X1	T48.6X2	T48.6X3	T48.6X4	T48.6X5	T48.6X6
Brotizolam	T42.4X1	T42.4X2	T42.4X3	T42.4X4	T42.4X5	T42.4X6
Brovincamine	T46.7X1	T46.7X2	T46.7X3	T46.7X4	T46.7X5	T46.7X6
Brown recluse spider (bite) (venom)	T63.331	T63.332	T63.333	T63.334	—	—
Brown spider (bite) (venom)	T63.391	T63.392	T63.393	T63.394	—	—
Broxaterol	T48.6X1	T48.6X2	T48.6X3	T48.6X4	T48.6X5	T48.6X6
Broxuridine	T45.1X1	T45.1X2	T45.1X3	T45.1X4	T45.1X5	T45.1X6
Broxyquinoline	T37.8X1	T37.8X2	T37.8X3	T37.8X4	T37.8X5	T37.8X6
Bruceine	T48.291	T48.292	T48.293	T48.294	T48.295	T48.296
Brucia	T62.2X1	T62.2X2	T62.2X3	T62.2X4	—	—
Brucine	T65.1X1	T65.1X2	T65.1X3	T65.1X4	—	—
Brunswick green — *see* Copper						
Bruten — *see* Ibuprofen						
Bryonia	T47.2X1	T47.2X2	T47.2X3	T47.2X4	T47.2X5	T47.2X6
Buclizine	T45.0X1	T45.0X2	T45.0X3	T45.0X4	T45.0X5	T45.0X6
Buclosamide	T49.0X1	T49.0X2	T49.0X3	T49.0X4	T49.0X5	T49.0X6
Budesonide	T44.5X1	T44.5X2	T44.5X3	T44.5X4	T44.5X5	T44.5X6
Budralazine	T46.5X1	T46.5X2	T46.5X3	T46.5X4	T46.5X5	T46.5X6
Bufferin	T39.011	T39.012	T39.013	T39.014	T39.015	T39.016
Buflomedil	T46.7X1	T46.7X2	T46.7X3	T46.7X4	T46.7X5	T46.7X6
Buformin	T38.3X1	T38.3X2	T38.3X3	T38.3X4	T38.3X5	T38.3X6
Bufotenine	T40.991	T40.992	T40.993	T40.994	—	—
Bufrolin	T48.6X1	T48.6X2	T48.6X3	T48.6X4	T48.6X5	T48.6X6
Bufylline	T48.6X1	T48.6X2	T48.6X3	T48.6X4	T48.6X5	T48.6X6
Bulk filler	T50.5X1	T50.5X2	T50.5X3	T50.5X4	T50.5X5	T50.5X6
cathartic	T47.4X1	T47.4X2	T47.4X3	T47.4X4	T47.4X5	T47.4X6
Bumetanide	T50.1X1	T50.1X2	T50.1X3	T50.1X4	T50.1X5	T50.1X6
Bunaftine	T46.2X1	T46.2X2	T46.2X3	T46.2X4	T46.2X5	T46.2X6
Bunamiodyl	T50.8X1	T50.8X2	T50.8X3	T50.8X4	T50.8X5	T50.8X6
Bunazosin	T44.6X1	T44.6X2	T44.6X3	T44.6X4	T44.6X5	T44.6X6
Bunitrolol	T44.7X1	T44.7X2	T44.7X3	T44.7X4	T44.7X5	T44.7X6
Buphenine	T46.7X1	T46.7X2	T46.7X3	T46.7X4	T46.7X5	T46.7X6
Bupivacaine	T41.3X1	T41.3X2	T41.3X3	T41.3X4	T41.3X5	T41.3X6
infiltration (subcutaneous)	T41.3X1	T41.3X2	T41.3X3	T41.3X4	T41.3X5	T41.3X6
nerve block (peripheral) (plexus)	T41.3X1	T41.3X2	T41.3X3	T41.3X4	T41.3X5	T41.3X6
spinal	T41.3X1	T41.3X2	T41.3X3	T41.3X4	T41.3X5	T41.3X6
Bupranolol	T44.7X1	T44.7X2	T44.7X3	T44.7X4	T44.7X5	T44.7X6
Buprenorphine	T40.4X1	T40.4X2	T40.4X3	T40.4X4	T40.4X5	T40.4X6
Bupropion	T43.291	T43.292	T43.293	T43.294	T43.295	T43.296
Burimamide	T47.1X1	T47.1X2	T47.1X3	T47.1X4	T47.1X5	T47.1X6
Buserelin	T38.891	T38.892	T38.893	T38.894	T38.895	T38.896
Buspirone	T43.591	T43.592	T43.593	T43.594	T43.595	T43.596
Busulfan, busulphan	T45.1X1	T45.1X2	T45.1X3	T45.1X4	T45.1X5	T45.1X6
Butabarbital (sodium)	T42.3X1	T42.3X2	T42.3X3	T42.3X4	T42.3X5	T42.3X6
Butabarbitone	T42.3X1	T42.3X2	T42.3X3	T42.3X4	T42.3X5	T42.3X6
Butabarpal	T42.3X1	T42.3X2	T42.3X3	T42.3X4	T42.3X5	T42.3X6
Butacaine	T41.3X1	T41.3X2	T41.3X3	T41.3X4	T41.3X5	T41.3X6
Butalamine	T46.7X1	T46.7X2	T46.7X3	T46.7X4	T46.7X5	T46.7X6
Butalbital	T42.3X1	T42.3X2	T42.3X3	T42.3X4	T42.3X5	T42.3X6
Butallylonal	T42.3X1	T42.3X2	T42.3X3	T42.3X4	T42.3X5	T42.3X6
Butamben	T41.3X1	T41.3X2	T41.3X3	T41.3X4	T41.3X5	T41.3X6
Butamirate	T48.3X1	T48.3X2	T48.3X3	T48.3X4	T48.3X5	T48.3X6
Butane (distributed in mobile container)	T59.891	T59.892	T59.893	T59.894	—	—
distributed through pipes	T59.891	T59.892	T59.893	T59.894	—	—
incomplete combustion	T58.11	T58.12	T58.13	T58.14	—	—
Butanilicaine	T41.3X1	T41.3X2	T41.3X3	T41.3X4	T41.3X5	T41.3X6
Butanol	T51.3X1	T51.3X2	T51.3X3	T51.3X4	—	—
Butanone, 2-butanone	T52.4X1	T52.4X2	T52.4X3	T52.4X4	—	—
Butantrone	T49.4X1	T49.4X2	T49.4X3	T49.4X4	T49.4X5	T49.4X6
Butaperazine	T43.3X1	T43.3X2	T43.3X3	T43.3X4	T43.3X5	T43.3X6
Butazolidin	T39.2X1	T39.2X2	T39.2X3	T39.2X4	T39.2X5	T39.2X6
Butetamate	T48.6X1	T48.6X2	T48.6X3	T48.6X4	T48.6X5	T48.6X6
Butethal	T42.3X1	T42.3X2	T42.3X3	T42.3X4	T42.3X5	T42.3X6
Butethamate	T44.3X1	T44.3X2	T44.3X3	T44.3X4	T44.3X5	T44.3X6
Buthalitone (sodium)	T41.1X1	T41.1X2	T41.1X3	T41.1X4	T41.1X5	T41.1X6
Butisol (sodium)	T42.3X1	T42.3X2	T42.3X3	T42.3X4	T42.3X5	T42.3X6
Butizide	T50.2X1	T50.2X2	T50.2X3	T50.2X4	T50.2X5	T50.2X6
Butobarbital	T42.3X1	T42.3X2	T42.3X3	T42.3X4	T42.3X5	T42.3X6
sodium	T42.3X1	T42.3X2	T42.3X3	T42.3X4	T42.3X5	T42.3X6
Butobarbitone	T42.3X1	T42.3X2	T42.3X3	T42.3X4	T42.3X5	T42.3X6
Butoconazole (nitrate)	T49.0X1	T49.0X2	T49.0X3	T49.0X4	T49.0X5	T49.0X6
Butorphanol	T40.4X1	T40.4X2	T40.4X3	T40.4X4	T40.4X5	T40.4X6
Butriptyline	T43.011	T43.012	T43.013	T43.014	T43.015	T43.016
Butropium bromide	T44.3X1	T44.3X2	T44.3X3	T44.3X4	T44.3X5	T44.3X6
Buttercups	T62.2X1	T62.2X2	T62.2X3	T62.2X4	—	—
Butter of antimony — *see* Antimony						
Butyl						
acetate (secondary)	T52.8X1	T52.8X2	T52.8X3	T52.8X4	—	—
alcohol	T51.3X1	T51.3X2	T51.3X3	T51.3X4	—	—
aminobenzoate	T41.3X1	T41.3X2	T41.3X3	T41.3X4	T41.3X5	T41.3X6
butyrate	T52.8X1	T52.8X2	T52.8X3	T52.8X4	—	—
carbinol	T51.3X1	T51.3X2	T51.3X3	T51.3X4	—	—
carbitol	T52.3X1	T52.3X2	T52.3X3	T52.3X4	—	—
cellosolve	T52.3X1	T52.3X2	T52.3X3	T52.3X4	—	—
chloral (hydrate)	T42.6X1	T42.6X2	T42.6X3	T42.6X4	T42.6X5	T42.6X6
formate	T52.8X1	T52.8X2	T52.8X3	T52.8X4	—	—
lactate	T52.8X1	T52.8X2	T52.8X3	T52.8X4	—	—
propionate	T52.8X1	T52.8X2	T52.8X3	T52.8X4	—	—
scopolamine bromide	T44.3X1	T44.3X2	T44.3X3	T44.3X4	T44.3X5	T44.3X6
thiobarbital sodium	T41.1X1	T41.1X2	T41.1X3	T41.1X4	T41.1X5	T41.1X6

Additional Character May Be Required — Refer to the Tabular List for Character Selection

▽ Subterms under main terms may continue to next column or page

Substance	Poisoning, Accidental (unintentional)	Poisoning, Intentional Self-harm	Poisoning, Assault	Poisoning, Undetermined	Adverse Effect	Underdosing
Butylated hydroxyanisole	T50.991	T50.992	T50.993	T50.994	T50.995	T50.996
Butylchloral hydrate	T42.6X1	T42.6X2	T42.6X3	T42.6X4	T42.6X5	T42.6X6
Butyltoluene	T52.2X1	T52.2X2	T52.2X3	T52.2X4	—	—
Butyn	T41.3X1	T41.3X2	T41.3X3	T41.3X4	T41.3X5	T41.3X6
Butyrophenone (-based tranquilizers)	T43.4X1	T43.4X2	T43.4X3	T43.4X4	T43.4X5	T43.4X6
Cabergoline	T42.8X1	T42.8X2	T42.8X3	T42.8X4	T42.8X5	T42.8X6
Cacodyl, cacodylic acid	T57.0X1	T57.0X2	T57.0X3	T57.0X4	—	—
Cactinomycin	T45.1X1	T45.1X2	T45.1X3	T45.1X4	T45.1X5	T45.1X6
Cade oil	T49.4X1	T49.4X2	T49.4X3	T49.4X4	T49.4X5	T49.4X6
Cadexomer iodine	T49.0X1	T49.0X2	T49.0X3	T49.0X4	T49.0X5	T49.0X6
Cadmium (chloride) (fumes) (oxide)	T56.3X1	T56.3X2	T56.3X3	T56.3X4	—	—
sulfide (medicinal) NEC	T49.4X1	T49.4X2	T49.4X3	T49.4X4	T49.4X5	T49.4X6
Cadralazine	T46.5X1	T46.5X2	T46.5X3	T46.5X4	T46.5X5	T46.5X6
Caffeine	T43.611	T43.612	T43.613	T43.614	T43.615	T43.616
Calabar bean	T62.2X1	T62.2X2	T62.2X3	T62.2X4	—	—
Caladium seguinum	T62.2X1	T62.2X2	T62.2X3	T62.2X4	—	—
Calamine (lotion)	T49.3X1	T49.3X2	T49.3X3	T49.3X4	T49.3X5	T49.3X6
Calcifediol	T45.2X1	T45.2X2	T45.2X3	T45.2X4	T45.2X5	T45.2X6
Calciferol	T45.2X1	T45.2X2	T45.2X3	T45.2X4	T45.2X5	T45.2X6
Calcitonin	T50.991	T50.992	T50.993	T50.994	T50.995	T50.996
Calcitriol	T45.2X1	T45.2X2	T45.2X3	T45.2X4	T45.2X5	T45.2X6
Calcium	T50.3X1	T50.3X2	T50.3X3	T50.3X4	T50.3X5	T50.3X6
actylsalicylate	T39.011	T39.012	T39.013	T39.014	T39.015	T39.016
benzamidosalicylate	T37.1X1	T37.1X2	T37.1X3	T37.1X4	T37.1X5	T37.1X6
bromide	T42.6X1	T42.6X2	T42.6X3	T42.6X4	T42.6X5	T42.6X6
bromolactobionate	T42.6X1	T42.6X2	T42.6X3	T42.6X4	T42.6X5	T42.6X6
carbaspirin	T39.011	T39.012	T39.013	T39.014	T39.015	T39.016
carbimide	T50.6X1	T50.6X2	T50.6X3	T50.6X4	T50.6X5	T50.6X6
carbonate	T47.1X1	T47.1X2	T47.1X3	T47.1X4	T47.1X5	T47.1X6
chloride	T50.991	T50.992	T50.993	T50.994	T50.995	T50.996
anhydrous	T50.991	T50.992	T50.993	T50.994	T50.995	T50.996
cyanide	T57.8X1	T57.8X2	T57.8X3	T57.8X4	—	—
dioctyl sulfosuccinate	T47.4X1	T47.4X2	T47.4X3	T47.4X4	T47.4X5	T47.4X6
disodium edathamil	T45.8X1	T45.8X2	T45.8X3	T45.8X4	T45.8X5	T45.8X6
disodium edetate	T45.8X1	T45.8X2	T45.8X3	T45.8X4	T45.8X5	T45.8X6
dobesilate	T46.991	T46.992	T46.993	T46.994	T46.995	T46.996
EDTA	T45.8X1	T45.8X2	T45.8X3	T45.8X4	T45.8X5	T45.8X6
ferrous citrate	T45.4X1	T45.4X2	T45.4X3	T45.4X4	T45.4X5	T45.4X6
folinate	T45.8X1	T45.8X2	T45.8X3	T45.8X4	T45.8X5	T45.8X6
glubionate	T50.3X1	T50.3X2	T50.3X3	T50.3X4	T50.3X5	T50.3X6
gluconate	T50.3X1	T50.3X2	T50.3X3	T50.3X4	T50.3X5	T50.3X6
gluconogalactogluconate	T50.3X1	T50.3X2	T50.3X3	T50.3X4	T50.3X5	T50.3X6
hydrate, hydroxide	T54.3X1	T54.3X2	T54.3X3	T54.3X4	—	—
hypochlorite	T54.3X1	T54.3X2	T54.3X3	T54.3X4	—	—
iodide	T48.4X1	T48.4X2	T48.4X3	T48.4X4	T48.4X5	T48.4X6
ipodate	T50.8X1	T50.8X2	T50.8X3	T50.8X4	T50.8X5	T50.8X6
lactate	T50.3X1	T50.3X2	T50.3X3	T50.3X4	T50.3X5	T50.3X6
leucovorin	T45.8X1	T45.8X2	T45.8X3	T45.8X4	T45.8X5	T45.8X6
mandelate	T37.91	T37.92	T37.93	T37.94	T37.95	T37.96
oxide	T54.3X1	T54.3X2	T54.3X3	T54.3X4	—	—
pantothenate	T45.2X1	T45.2X2	T45.2X3	T45.2X4	T45.2X5	T45.2X6
phosphate	T50.3X1	T50.3X2	T50.3X3	T50.3X4	T50.3X5	T50.3X6
salicylate	T39.091	T39.092	T39.093	T39.094	T39.095	T39.096
salts	T50.3X1	T50.3X2	T50.3X3	T50.3X4	T50.3X5	T50.3X6
Calculus-dissolving drug	T50.991	T50.992	T50.993	T50.994	T50.995	T50.996
Calomel	T49.0X1	T49.0X2	T49.0X3	T49.0X4	T49.0X5	T49.0X6
Caloric agent	T50.3X1	T50.3X2	T50.3X3	T50.3X4	T50.3X5	T50.3X6
Calusterone	T38.7X1	T38.7X2	T38.7X3	T38.7X4	T38.7X5	T38.7X6
Camazepam	T42.4X1	T42.4X2	T42.4X3	T42.4X4	T42.4X5	T42.4X6
Camomile	T49.0X1	T49.0X2	T49.0X3	T49.0X4	T49.0X5	T49.0X6
Camoquin	T37.2X1	T37.2X2	T37.2X3	T37.2X4	T37.2X5	T37.2X6
Camphor						
insecticide	T60.2X1	T60.2X2	T60.2X3	T60.2X4	—	—
medicinal	T49.8X1	T49.8X2	T49.8X3	T49.8X4	T49.8X5	T49.8X6
Camylofin	T44.3X1	T44.3X2	T44.3X3	T44.3X4	T44.3X5	T44.3X6
Cancer chemotherapy drug regimen	T45.1X1	T45.1X2	T45.1X3	T45.1X4	T45.1X5	T45.1X6
Candeptin	T49.0X1	T49.0X2	T49.0X3	T49.0X4	T49.0X5	T49.0X6
Candicidin	T49.0X1	T49.0X2	T49.0X3	T49.0X4	T49.0X5	T49.0X6
Cannabinol	T40.7X1	T40.7X2	T40.7X3	T40.7X4	T40.7X5	T40.7X6
Cannabis (derivatives)	T40.7X1	T40.7X2	T40.7X3	T40.7X4	T40.7X5	T40.7X6
Canned heat	T51.1X1	T51.1X2	T51.1X3	T51.1X4	—	—
Canrenoic acid	T50.0X1	T50.0X2	T50.0X3	T50.0X4	T50.0X5	T50.0X6
Canrenone	T50.0X1	T50.0X2	T50.0X3	T50.0X4	T50.0X5	T50.0X6
Cantharides, cantharidin, cantharis	T49.8X1	T49.8X2	T49.8X3	T49.8X4	T49.8X5	T49.8X6
Canthaxanthin	T50.991	T50.992	T50.993	T50.994	T50.995	T50.996
Capillary-active drug NEC	T46.901	T46.902	T46.903	T46.904	T46.905	T46.906
Capreomycin	T36.8X1	T36.8X2	T36.8X3	T36.8X4	T36.8X5	T36.8X6
Capsicum	T49.4X1	T49.4X2	T49.4X3	T49.4X4	T49.4X5	T49.4X6
Captafol	T60.3X1	T60.3X2	T60.3X3	T60.3X4	—	—

Substance	Poisoning, Accidental (unintentional)	Poisoning, Intentional Self-harm	Poisoning, Assault	Poisoning, Undetermined	Adverse Effect	Underdosing
Captan	T60.3X1	T60.3X2	T60.3X3	T60.3X4	—	—
Captodiame, captodiamine	T43.591	T43.592	T43.593	T43.594	T43.595	T43.596
Captopril	T46.4X1	T46.4X2	T46.4X3	T46.4X4	T46.4X5	T46.4X6
Caramiphen	T44.3X1	T44.3X2	T44.3X3	T44.3X4	T44.3X5	T44.3X6
Carazolol	T44.7X1	T44.7X2	T44.7X3	T44.7X4	T44.7X5	T44.7X6
Carbachol	T44.1X1	T44.1X2	T44.1X3	T44.1X4	T44.1X5	T44.1X6
Carbacrylamine (resin)	T50.3X1	T50.3X2	T50.3X3	T50.3X4	T50.3X5	T50.3X6
Carbamate (insecticide)	T60.0X1	T60.0X2	T60.0X3	T60.0X4	—	—
Carbamate (sedative)	T42.6X1	T42.6X2	T42.6X3	T42.6X4	T42.6X5	T42.6X6
herbicide	T60.0X1	T60.0X2	T60.0X3	T60.0X4	—	—
insecticide	T60.0X1	T60.0X2	T60.0X3	T60.0X4	—	—
Carbamazepine	T42.1X1	T42.1X2	T42.1X3	T42.1X4	T42.1X5	T42.1X6
Carbamide	T47.3X1	T47.3X2	T47.3X3	T47.3X4	T47.3X5	T47.3X6
peroxide	T49.0X1	T49.0X2	T49.0X3	T49.0X4	T49.0X5	T49.0X6
topical	T49.8X1	T49.8X2	T49.8X3	T49.8X4	T49.8X5	T49.8X6
Carbamylcholine chloride	T44.1X1	T44.1X2	T44.1X3	T44.1X4	T44.1X5	T44.1X6
Carbaril	T60.0X1	T60.0X2	T60.0X3	T60.0X4	—	—
Carbarsone	T37.3X1	T37.3X2	T37.3X3	T37.3X4	T37.3X5	T37.3X6
Carbaryl	T60.0X1	T60.0X2	T60.0X3	T60.0X4	—	—
Carbaspirin	T39.011	T39.012	T39.013	T39.014	T39.015	T39.016
Carbazochrome (salicylate) (sodium sulfonate)	T49.4X1	T49.4X2	T49.4X3	T49.4X4	T49.4X5	T49.4X6
Carbenicillin	T36.0X1	T36.0X2	T36.0X3	T36.0X4	T36.0X5	T36.0X6
Carbenoxolone	T47.1X1	T47.1X2	T47.1X3	T47.1X4	T47.1X5	T47.1X6
Carbetapentane	T48.3X1	T48.3X2	T48.3X3	T48.3X4	T48.3X5	T48.3X6
Carbethyl salicylate	T39.091	T39.092	T39.093	T39.094	T39.095	T39.096
Carbidopa (with levodopa)	T42.8X1	T42.8X2	T42.8X3	T42.8X4	T42.8X5	T42.8X6
Carbimazole	T38.2X1	T38.2X2	T38.2X3	T38.2X4	T38.2X5	T38.2X6
Carbinol	T51.1X1	T51.1X2	T51.1X3	T51.1X4	—	—
Carbinoxamine	T45.0X1	T45.0X2	T45.0X3	T45.0X4	T45.0X5	T45.0X6
Carbiphene	T39.8X1	T39.8X2	T39.8X3	T39.8X4	T39.8X5	T39.8X6
Carbitol	T52.3X1	T52.3X2	T52.3X3	T52.3X4	—	—
Carbocaine	T41.3X1	T41.3X2	T41.3X3	T41.3X4	T41.3X5	T41.3X6
infiltration (subcutaneous)	T41.3X1	T41.3X2	T41.3X3	T41.3X4	T41.3X5	T41.3X6
nerve block (peripheral) (plexus)	T41.3X1	T41.3X2	T41.3X3	T41.3X4	T41.3X5	T41.3X6
topical (surface)	T41.3X1	T41.3X2	T41.3X3	T41.3X4	T41.3X5	T41.3X6
Carbocisteine	T48.4X1	T48.4X2	T48.4X3	T48.4X4	T48.4X5	T48.4X6
Carbocromen	T46.3X1	T46.3X2	T46.3X3	T46.3X4	T46.3X5	T46.3X6
Carbol fuchsin	T49.0X1	T49.0X2	T49.0X3	T49.0X4	T49.0X5	T49.0X6
Carbolic acid — *see also* Phenol	T54.0X1	T54.0X2	T54.0X3	T54.0X4	—	—
Carbolonium (bromide)	T48.1X1	T48.1X2	T48.1X3	T48.1X4	T48.1X5	T48.1X6
Carbo medicinalis	T47.6X1	T47.6X2	T47.6X3	T47.6X4	T47.6X5	T47.6X6
Carbomycin	T36.8X1	T36.8X2	T36.8X3	T36.8X4	T36.8X5	T36.8X6
Carbon						
bisulfide (liquid)	T65.4X1	T65.4X2	T65.4X3	T65.4X4	—	—
vapor	T65.4X1	T65.4X2	T65.4X3	T65.4X4	—	—
dioxide (gas)	T59.7X1	T59.7X2	T59.7X3	T59.7X4	—	—
medicinal	T41.5X1	T41.5X2	T41.5X3	T41.5X4	T41.5X5	T41.5X6
nonmedicinal	T59.7X1	T59.7X2	T59.7X3	T59.7X4	—	—
snow	T49.4X1	T49.4X2	T49.4X3	T49.4X4	T49.4X5	T49.4X6
disulfide (liquid)	T65.4X1	T65.4X2	T65.4X3	T65.4X4	—	—
vapor	T65.4X1	T65.4X2	T65.4X3	T65.4X4	—	—
monoxide (from incomplete combustion)	T58.91	T58.92	T58.93	T58.94	—	—
blast furnace gas	T58.8X1	T58.8X2	T58.8X3	T58.8X4	—	—
butane (distributed in mobile container)	T58.11	T58.12	T58.13	T58.14	—	—
distributed through pipes	T58.11	T58.12	T58.13	T58.14	—	—
charcoal fumes	T58.2X1	T58.2X2	T58.2X3	T58.2X4	—	—
coal	T58.2X1	T58.2X2	T58.2X3	T58.2X4	—	—
coke (in domestic stoves, fireplaces)	T58.2X1	T58.2X2	T58.2X3	T58.2X4	—	—
exhaust gas (motor) not in transit	T58.01	T58.02	T58.03	T58.04	—	—
combustion engine, any not in watercraft	T58.01	T58.02	T58.03	T58.04	—	—
farm tractor, not in transit	T58.01	T58.02	T58.03	T58.04	—	—
gas engine	T58.01	T58.02	T58.03	T58.04	—	—
motor pump	T58.01	T58.02	T58.03	T58.04	—	—
motor vehicle, not in transit	T58.01	T58.02	T58.03	T58.04	—	—
fuel (in domestic use)	T58.2X1	T58.2X2	T58.2X3	T58.2X4	—	—
gas (piped)	T58.11	T58.12	T58.13	T58.14	—	—
in mobile container	T58.11	T58.12	T58.13	T58.14	—	—
piped (natural)	T58.11	T58.12	T58.13	T58.14	—	—
utility	T58.11	T58.12	T58.13	T58.14	—	—
in mobile container	T58.11	T58.12	T58.13	T58.14	—	—
gas (piped)	T58.11	T58.12	T58.13	T58.14	—	—
illuminating gas	T58.11	T58.12	T58.13	T58.14	—	—

Table of Drugs and Chemicals

Carbon — Central nervous system

Substance	Poisoning, Accidental (unintentional)	Poisoning, Intentional Self-harm	Poisoning, Assault	Poisoning, Undetermined	Adverse Effect	Under-dosing
Carbon — *continued*						
monoxide — *continued*						
industrial fuels or gases, any	T58.8X1	T58.8X2	T58.8X3	T58.8X4	—	—
kerosene (in domestic stoves, fireplaces)	T58.2X1	T58.2X2	T58.2X3	T58.2X4	—	—
kiln gas or vapor	T58.8X1	T58.8X2	T58.8X3	T58.8X4	—	—
motor exhaust gas, not in transit	T58.01	T58.02	T58.03	T58.04	—	—
piped gas (manufactured)(natural)	T58.11	T58.12	T58.13	T58.14	—	—
producer gas	T58.8X1	T58.8X2	T58.8X3	T58.8X4	—	—
propane (distributed in mobile container)	T58.11	T58.12	T58.13	T58.14	—	—
distributed through pipes	T58.11	T58.12	T58.13	T58.14	—	—
solid (in domestic stoves, fireplaces)	T58.2X1	T58.2X2	T58.2X3	T58.2X4	—	—
specified source NEC	T58.8X1	T58.8X2	T58.8X3	T58.8X4	—	—
stove gas	T58.11	T58.12	T58.13	T58.14	—	—
piped	T58.11	T58.12	T58.13	T58.14	—	—
utility gas	T58.11	T58.12	T58.13	T58.14	—	—
piped	T58.11	T58.12	T58.13	T58.14	—	—
water gas	T58.11	T58.12	T58.13	T58.14	—	—
wood (in domestic stoves, fireplaces)	T58.2X1	T58.2X2	T58.2X3	T58.2X4	—	—
tetrachloride (vapor) NEC	T53.0X1	T53.0X2	T53.0X3	T53.0X4	—	—
liquid (cleansing agent) NEC	T53.0X1	T53.0X2	T53.0X3	T53.0X4	—	—
solvent	T53.0X1	T53.0X2	T53.0X3	T53.0X4	—	—
Carbonic acid gas	T59.7X1	T59.7X2	T59.7X3	T59.7X4	—	—
anhydrase inhibitor NEC	T50.2X1	T50.2X2	T50.2X3	T50.2X4	T50.2X5	T50.2X6
Carbophenothion	T60.0X1	T60.0X2	T60.0X3	T60.0X4	—	—
Carboplatin	T45.1X1	T45.1X2	T45.1X3	T45.1X4	T45.1X5	T45.1X6
Carboprost	T48.0X1	T48.0X2	T48.0X3	T48.0X4	T48.0X5	T48.0X6
Carboquone	T45.1X1	T45.1X2	T45.1X3	T45.1X4	T45.1X5	T45.1X6
Carbowax	T49.3X1	T49.3X2	T49.3X3	T49.3X4	T49.3X5	T49.3X6
Carboxymethylcellulose	T47.4X1	T47.4X2	T47.4X3	T47.4X4	T47.4X5	T47.4X6
Carbrital	T42.3X1	T42.3X2	T42.3X3	T42.3X4	T42.3X5	T42.3X6
Carbromal	T42.6X1	T42.6X2	T42.6X3	T42.6X4	T42.6X5	T42.6X6
Carbutamide	T38.3X1	T38.3X2	T38.3X3	T38.3X4	T38.3X5	T38.3X6
Carbuterol	T48.6X1	T48.6X2	T48.6X3	T48.6X4	T48.6X5	T48.6X6
Cardiac						
depressants	T46.2X1	T46.2X2	T46.2X3	T46.2X4	T46.2X5	T46.2X6
rhythm regulator	T46.2X1	T46.2X2	T46.2X3	T46.2X4	T46.2X5	T46.2X6
specified NEC	T46.2X1	T46.2X2	T46.2X3	T46.2X4	T46.2X5	T46.2X6
Cardiografin	T50.8X1	T50.8X2	T50.8X3	T50.8X4	T50.8X5	T50.8X6
Cardiogreen	T50.8X1	T50.8X2	T50.8X3	T50.8X4	T50.8X5	T50.8X6
Cardiotonic (glycoside) **NEC**	T46.0X1	T46.0X2	T46.0X3	T46.0X4	T46.0X5	T46.0X6
Cardiovascular drug NEC	T46.901	T46.902	T46.903	T46.904	T46.905	T46.906
Cardrase	T50.2X1	T50.2X2	T50.2X3	T50.2X4	T50.2X5	T50.2X6
Carfecillin	T36.0X1	T36.0X2	T36.0X3	T36.0X4	T36.0X5	T36.0X6
Carfenazine	T43.3X1	T43.3X2	T43.3X3	T43.3X4	T43.3X5	T43.3X6
Carfusin	T49.0X1	T49.0X2	T49.0X3	T49.0X4	T49.0X5	T49.0X6
Carindacillin	T36.0X1	T36.0X2	T36.0X3	T36.0X4	T36.0X5	T36.0X6
Carisoprodol	T42.8X1	T42.8X2	T42.8X3	T42.8X4	T42.8X5	T42.8X6
Carmellose	T47.4X1	T47.4X2	T47.4X3	T47.4X4	T47.4X5	T47.4X6
Carminative	T47.5X1	T47.5X2	T47.5X3	T47.5X4	T47.5X5	T47.5X6
Carmofur	T45.1X1	T45.1X2	T45.1X3	T45.1X4	T45.1X5	T45.1X6
Carmustine	T45.1X1	T45.1X2	T45.1X3	T45.1X4	T45.1X5	T45.1X6
Carotene	T45.2X1	T45.2X2	T45.2X3	T45.2X4	T45.2X5	T45.2X6
Carphenazine	T43.3X1	T43.3X2	T43.3X3	T43.3X4	T43.3X5	T43.3X6
Carpipramine	T42.4X1	T42.4X2	T42.4X3	T42.4X4	T42.4X5	T42.4X6
Carprofen	T39.311	T39.312	T39.313	T39.314	T39.315	T39.316
Carpronium chloride	T44.3X1	T44.3X2	T44.3X3	T44.3X4	T44.3X5	T44.3X6
Carrageenan	T47.8X1	T47.8X2	T47.8X3	T47.8X4	T47.8X5	T47.8X6
Carteolol	T44.7X1	T44.7X2	T44.7X3	T44.7X4	T44.7X5	T44.7X6
Carter's Little Pills	T47.2X1	T47.2X2	T47.2X3	T47.2X4	T47.2X5	T47.2X6
Cascara (sagrada)	T47.2X1	T47.2X2	T47.2X3	T47.2X4	T47.2X5	T47.2X6
Cassava	T62.2X1	T62.2X2	T62.2X3	T62.2X4	—	—
Castellani's paint	T49.0X1	T49.0X2	T49.0X3	T49.0X4	T49.0X5	T49.0X6
Castor						
bean	T62.2X1	T62.2X2	T62.2X3	T62.2X4	—	—
oil	T47.2X1	T47.2X2	T47.2X3	T47.2X4	T47.2X5	T47.2X6
Catalase	T45.3X1	T45.3X2	T45.3X3	T45.3X4	T45.3X5	T45.3X6
Caterpillar (sting)	T63.431	T63.432	T63.433	T63.434	—	—
Catha (edulis) (tea)	T43.691	T43.692	T43.693	T43.694	—	—
Cathartic NEC	T47.4X1	T47.4X2	T47.4X3	T47.4X4	T47.4X5	T47.4X6
anthacene derivative	T47.2X1	T47.2X2	T47.2X3	T47.2X4	T47.2X5	T47.2X6
bulk	T47.4X1	T47.4X2	T47.4X3	T47.4X4	T47.4X5	T47.4X6
contact	T47.2X1	T47.2X2	T47.2X3	T47.2X4	T47.2X5	T47.2X6
emollient NEC	T47.4X1	T47.4X2	T47.4X3	T47.4X4	T47.4X5	T47.4X6
irritant NEC	T47.2X1	T47.2X2	T47.2X3	T47.2X4	T47.2X5	T47.2X6

Substance	Poisoning, Accidental (unintentional)	Poisoning, Intentional Self-harm	Poisoning, Assault	Poisoning, Undetermined	Adverse Effect	Under-dosing
Cathartic — *continued*						
mucilage	T47.4X1	T47.4X2	T47.4X3	T47.4X4	T47.4X5	T47.4X6
saline	T47.3X1	T47.3X2	T47.3X3	T47.3X4	T47.3X5	T47.3X6
vegetable	T47.2X1	T47.2X2	T47.2X3	T47.2X4	T47.2X5	T47.2X6
Cathine	T50.5X1	T50.5X2	T50.5X3	T50.5X4	T50.5X5	T50.5X6
Cathomycin	T36.8X1	T36.8X2	T36.8X3	T36.8X4	T36.8X5	T36.8X6
Cation exchange resin	T50.3X1	T50.3X2	T50.3X3	T50.3X4	T50.3X5	T50.3X6
Caustic(s) NEC	T54.91	T54.92	T54.93	T54.94	—	—
alkali	T54.3X1	T54.3X2	T54.3X3	T54.3X4	—	—
hydroxide	T54.3X1	T54.3X2	T54.3X3	T54.3X4	—	—
potash	T54.3X1	T54.3X2	T54.3X3	T54.3X4	—	—
soda	T54.3X1	T54.3X2	T54.3X3	T54.3X4	—	—
specified NEC	T54.91	T54.92	T54.93	T54.94	—	—
Ceepryn	T49.0X1	T49.0X2	T49.0X3	T49.0X4	T49.0X5	T49.0X6
ENT agent	T49.6X1	T49.6X2	T49.6X3	T49.6X4	T49.6X5	T49.6X6
lozenges	T49.6X1	T49.6X2	T49.6X3	T49.6X4	T49.6X5	T49.6X6
Cefacetrile	T36.1X1	T36.1X2	T36.1X3	T36.1X4	T36.1X5	T36.1X6
Cefaclor	T36.1X1	T36.1X2	T36.1X3	T36.1X4	T36.1X5	T36.1X6
Cefadroxil	T36.1X1	T36.1X2	T36.1X3	T36.1X4	T36.1X5	T36.1X6
Cefalexin	T36.1X1	T36.1X2	T36.1X3	T36.1X4	T36.1X5	T36.1X6
Cefaloglycin	T36.1X1	T36.1X2	T36.1X3	T36.1X4	T36.1X5	T36.1X6
Cefaloridine	T36.1X1	T36.1X2	T36.1X3	T36.1X4	T36.1X5	T36.1X6
Cefalosporins	T36.1X1	T36.1X2	T36.1X3	T36.1X4	T36.1X5	T36.1X6
Cefalotin	T36.1X1	T36.1X2	T36.1X3	T36.1X4	T36.1X5	T36.1X6
Cefamandole	T36.1X1	T36.1X2	T36.1X3	T36.1X4	T36.1X5	T36.1X6
Cefamycin antibiotic	T36.1X1	T36.1X2	T36.1X3	T36.1X4	T36.1X5	T36.1X6
Cefapirin	T36.1X1	T36.1X2	T36.1X3	T36.1X4	T36.1X5	T36.1X6
Cefatrizine	T36.1X1	T36.1X2	T36.1X3	T36.1X4	T36.1X5	T36.1X6
Cefazedone	T36.1X1	T36.1X2	T36.1X3	T36.1X4	T36.1X5	T36.1X6
Cefazolin	T36.1X1	T36.1X2	T36.1X3	T36.1X4	T36.1X5	T36.1X6
Cefbuperazone	T36.1X1	T36.1X2	T36.1X3	T36.1X4	T36.1X5	T36.1X6
Cefetamet	T36.1X1	T36.1X2	T36.1X3	T36.1X4	T36.1X5	T36.1X6
Cefixime	T36.1X1	T36.1X2	T36.1X3	T36.1X4	T36.1X5	T36.1X6
Cefmenoxime	T36.1X1	T36.1X2	T36.1X3	T36.1X4	T36.1X5	T36.1X6
Cefmetazole	T36.1X1	T36.1X2	T36.1X3	T36.1X4	T36.1X5	T36.1X6
Cefminox	T36.1X1	T36.1X2	T36.1X3	T36.1X4	T36.1X5	T36.1X6
Cefonicid	T36.1X1	T36.1X2	T36.1X3	T36.1X4	T36.1X5	T36.1X6
Cefoperazone	T36.1X1	T36.1X2	T36.1X3	T36.1X4	T36.1X5	T36.1X6
Ceforanide	T36.1X1	T36.1X2	T36.1X3	T36.1X4	T36.1X5	T36.1X6
Cefotaxime	T36.1X1	T36.1X2	T36.1X3	T36.1X4	T36.1X5	T36.1X6
Cefotetan	T36.1X1	T36.1X2	T36.1X3	T36.1X4	T36.1X5	T36.1X6
Cefotiam	T36.1X1	T36.1X2	T36.1X3	T36.1X4	T36.1X5	T36.1X6
Cefoxitin	T36.1X1	T36.1X2	T36.1X3	T36.1X4	T36.1X5	T36.1X6
Cefpimizole	T36.1X1	T36.1X2	T36.1X3	T36.1X4	T36.1X5	T36.1X6
Cefpiramide	T36.1X1	T36.1X2	T36.1X3	T36.1X4	T36.1X5	T36.1X6
Cefradine	T36.1X1	T36.1X2	T36.1X3	T36.1X4	T36.1X5	T36.1X6
Cefroxadine	T36.1X1	T36.1X2	T36.1X3	T36.1X4	T36.1X5	T36.1X6
Cefsulodin	T36.1X1	T36.1X2	T36.1X3	T36.1X4	T36.1X5	T36.1X6
Ceftazidime	T36.1X1	T36.1X2	T36.1X3	T36.1X4	T36.1X5	T36.1X6
Cefteram	T36.1X1	T36.1X2	T36.1X3	T36.1X4	T36.1X5	T36.1X6
Ceftezole	T36.1X1	T36.1X2	T36.1X3	T36.1X4	T36.1X5	T36.1X6
Ceftizoxime	T36.1X1	T36.1X2	T36.1X3	T36.1X4	T36.1X5	T36.1X6
Ceftriaxone	T36.1X1	T36.1X2	T36.1X3	T36.1X4	T36.1X5	T36.1X6
Cefuroxime	T36.1X1	T36.1X2	T36.1X3	T36.1X4	T36.1X5	T36.1X6
Cefuzonam	T36.1X1	T36.1X2	T36.1X3	T36.1X4	T36.1X5	T36.1X6
Celestone	T38.0X1	T38.0X2	T38.0X3	T38.0X4	T38.0X5	T38.0X6
topical	T49.0X1	T49.0X2	T49.0X3	T49.0X4	T49.0X5	T49.0X6
Celiprolol	T44.7X1	T44.7X2	T44.7X3	T44.7X4	T44.7X5	T44.7X6
Cellosolve	T52.91	T52.92	T52.93	T52.94	—	—
Cell stimulants and proliferants	T49.8X1	T49.8X2	T49.8X3	T49.8X4	T49.8X5	T49.8X6
Cellulose						
cathartic	T47.4X1	T47.4X2	T47.4X3	T47.4X4	T47.4X5	T47.4X6
hydroxyethyl	T47.4X1	T47.4X2	T47.4X3	T47.4X4	T47.4X5	T47.4X6
nitrates (topical)	T49.3X1	T49.3X2	T49.3X3	T49.3X4	T49.3X5	T49.3X6
oxidized	T49.4X1	T49.4X2	T49.4X3	T49.4X4	T49.4X5	T49.4X6
Centipede (bite)	T63.411	T63.412	T63.413	T63.414	—	—
Central nervous system						
depressants	T42.71	T42.72	T42.73	T42.74	T42.75	T42.76
anesthetic (general) NEC	T41.201	T41.202	T41.203	T41.204	T41.205	T41.206
gases NEC	T41.0X1	T41.0X2	T41.0X3	T41.0X4	T41.0X5	T41.0X6
intravenous	T41.1X1	T41.1X2	T41.1X3	T41.1X4	T41.1X5	T41.1X6
barbiturates	T42.3X1	T42.3X2	T42.3X3	T42.3X4	T42.3X5	T42.3X6
benzodiazepines	T42.4X1	T42.4X2	T42.4X3	T42.4X4	T42.4X5	T42.4X6
bromides	T42.6X1	T42.6X2	T42.6X3	T42.6X4	T42.6X5	T42.6X6
cannabis sativa	T40.7X1	T40.7X2	T40.7X3	T40.7X4	T40.7X5	T40.7X6
chloral hydrate	T42.6X1	T42.6X2	T42.6X3	T42.6X4	T42.6X5	T42.6X6
ethanol	T51.0X1	T51.0X2	T51.0X3	T51.0X4	—	—
hallucinogenics	T40.901	T40.902	T40.903	T40.904	T40.905	T40.906
hypnotics	T42.71	T42.72	T42.73	T42.74	T42.75	T42.76
specified NEC	T42.6X1	T42.6X2	T42.6X3	T42.6X4	T42.6X5	T42.6X6
muscle relaxants	T42.8X1	T42.8X2	T42.8X3	T42.8X4	T42.8X5	T42.8X6
paraldehyde	T42.6X1	T42.6X2	T42.6X3	T42.6X4	T42.6X5	T42.6X6

Additional Character May Be Required — Refer to the Tabular List for Character Selection

Subterms under main terms may continue to next column or page

Substance	Poisoning, Accidental (unintentional)	Poisoning, Intentional Self-harm	Poisoning, Assault	Poisoning, Undetermined	Adverse Effect	Underdosing
Central nervous system — *continued*						
depressants — *continued*						
sedatives;	T42.71	T42.72	T42.73	T42.74	T42.75	T42.76
sedative-hypnotics						
mixed NEC	T42.6X1	T42.6X2	T42.6X3	T42.6X4	T42.6X5	T42.6X6
specified NEC	T42.6X1	T42.6X2	T42.6X3	T42.6X4	T42.6X5	T42.6X6
muscle-tone depressants	T42.8X1	T42.8X2	T42.8X3	T42.8X4	T42.8X5	T42.8X6
stimulants	T43.601	T43.602	T43.603	T43.604	T43.605	T43.606
amphetamines	T43.621	T43.622	T43.623	T43.624	T43.625	T43.626
analeptics	T50.7X1	T50.7X2	T50.7X3	T50.7X4	T50.7X5	T50.7X6
antidepressants	T43.201	T43.202	T43.203	T43.204	T43.205	T43.206
opiate antagonists	T50.7X1	T50.7X2	T50.7X3	T50.7X4	T50.7X5	T50.7X6
specified NEC	T43.691	T43.692	T43.693	T43.694	T43.695	T43.696
Cephalexin	T36.1X1	T36.1X2	T36.1X3	T36.1X4	T36.1X5	T36.1X6
Cephaloglycin	T36.1X1	T36.1X2	T36.1X3	T36.1X4	T36.1X5	T36.1X6
Cephaloridine	T36.1X1	T36.1X2	T36.1X3	T36.1X4	T36.1X5	T36.1X6
Cephalosporins	T36.1X1	T36.1X2	T36.1X3	T36.1X4	T36.1X5	T36.1X6
N (adicillin)	T36.0X1	T36.0X2	T36.0X3	T36.0X4	T36.0X5	T36.0X6
Cephalothin	T36.1X1	T36.1X2	T36.1X3	T36.1X4	T36.1X5	T36.1X6
Cephalotin	T36.1X1	T36.1X2	T36.1X3	T36.1X4	T36.1X5	T36.1X6
Cephradine	T36.1X1	T36.1X2	T36.1X3	T36.1X4	T36.1X5	T36.1X6
Cerbera (odallam)	T62.2X1	T62.2X2	T62.2X3	T62.2X4	—	—
Cerberin	T46.0X1	T46.0X2	T46.0X3	T46.0X4	T46.0X5	T46.0X6
Cerebral stimulants	T43.601	T43.602	T43.603	T43.604	T43.605	T43.606
psychotherapeutic	T43.601	T43.602	T43.603	T43.604	T43.605	T43.606
specified NEC	T43.691	T43.692	T43.693	T43.694	T43.695	T43.696
Cerium oxalate	T45.0X1	T45.0X2	T45.0X3	T45.0X4	T45.0X5	T45.0X6
Cerous oxalate	T45.0X1	T45.0X2	T45.0X3	T45.0X4	T45.0X5	T45.0X6
Ceruletide	T50.8X1	T50.8X2	T50.8X3	T50.8X4	T50.8X5	T50.8X6
Cetalkonium (chloride)	T49.0X1	T49.0X2	T49.0X3	T49.0X4	T49.0X5	T49.0X6
Cethexonium chloride	T49.0X1	T49.0X2	T49.0X3	T49.0X4	T49.0X5	T49.0X6
Cetiedil	T46.7X1	T46.7X2	T46.7X3	T46.7X4	T46.7X5	T46.7X6
Cetirizine	T45.0X1	T45.0X2	T45.0X3	T45.0X4	T45.0X5	T45.0X6
Cetomacrogol	T50.991	T50.992	T50.993	T50.994	T50.995	T50.996
Cetotiamine	T45.2X1	T45.2X2	T45.2X3	T45.2X4	T45.2X5	T45.2X6
Cetoxime	T45.0X1	T45.0X2	T45.0X3	T45.0X4	T45.0X5	T45.0X6
Cetraxate	T47.1X1	T47.1X2	T47.1X3	T47.1X4	T47.1X5	T47.1X6
Cetrimide	T49.0X1	T49.0X2	T49.0X3	T49.0X4	T49.0X5	T49.0X6
Cetrimonium (bromide)	T49.0X1	T49.0X2	T49.0X3	T49.0X4	T49.0X5	T49.0X6
Cetylpyridinium chloride	T49.0X1	T49.0X2	T49.0X3	T49.0X4	T49.0X5	T49.0X6
ENT agent	T49.6X1	T49.6X2	T49.6X3	T49.6X4	T49.6X5	T49.6X6
lozenges	T49.6X1	T49.6X2	T49.6X3	T49.6X4	T49.6X5	T49.6X6
Cevadilla — *see* Sabadilla						
Cevitamic acid	T45.2X1	T45.2X2	T45.2X3	T45.2X4	T45.2X5	T45.2X6
Chalk, precipitated	T47.1X1	T47.1X2	T47.1X3	T47.1X4	T47.1X5	T47.1X6
Chamomile	T49.0X1	T49.0X2	T49.0X3	T49.0X4	T49.0X5	T49.0X6
Ch'an su	T46.0X1	T46.0X2	T46.0X3	T46.0X4	T46.0X5	T46.0X6
Charcoal	T47.6X1	T47.6X2	T47.6X3	T47.6X4	T47.6X5	T47.6X6
activated — *see also* Charcoal, medicinal	T47.6X1	T47.6X2	T47.6X3	T47.6X4	T47.6X5	T47.6X6
fumes (Carbon monoxide)	T58.2X1	T58.2X2	T58.2X3	T58.2X4	—	—
industrial	T58.8X1	T58.8X2	T58.8X3	T58.8X4	—	—
medicinal (activated)	T47.6X1	T47.6X2	T47.6X3	T47.6X4	T47.6X5	T47.6X6
antidiarrheal	T47.6X1	T47.6X2	T47.6X3	T47.6X4	T47.6X5	T47.6X6
poison control	T47.8X1	T47.8X2	T47.8X3	T47.8X4	T47.8X5	T47.8X6
specified use other than for diarrhea	T47.8X1	T47.8X2	T47.8X3	T47.8X4	T47.8X5	T47.8X6
topical	T49.8X1	T49.8X2	T49.8X3	T49.8X4	T49.8X5	T49.8X6
Chaulmosulfone	T37.1X1	T37.1X2	T37.1X3	T37.1X4	T37.1X5	T37.1X6
Chelating agent NEC	T50.6X1	T50.6X2	T50.6X3	T50.6X4	T50.6X5	T50.6X6
Chelidonium majus	T62.2X1	T62.2X2	T62.2X3	T62.2X4	—	—
Chemical substance NEC	T65.91	T65.92	T65.93	T65.94	—	—
Chenodeoxycholic acid	T47.5X1	T47.5X2	T47.5X3	T47.5X4	T47.5X5	T47.5X6
Chenodiol	T47.5X1	T47.5X2	T47.5X3	T47.5X4	T47.5X5	T47.5X6
Chenopodium	T37.4X1	T37.4X2	T37.4X3	T37.4X4	T37.4X5	T37.4X6
Cherry laurel	T62.2X1	T62.2X2	T62.2X3	T62.2X4	—	—
Chinidin (e)	T46.2X1	T46.2X2	T46.2X3	T46.2X4	T46.2X5	T46.2X6
Chiniofon	T37.8X1	T37.8X2	T37.8X3	T37.8X4	T37.8X5	T37.8X6
Chlophedianol	T48.3X1	T48.3X2	T48.3X3	T48.3X4	T48.3X5	T48.3X6
Chloral	T42.6X1	T42.6X2	T42.6X3	T42.6X4	T42.6X5	T42.6X6
derivative	T42.6X1	T42.6X2	T42.6X3	T42.6X4	T42.6X5	T42.6X6
hydrate	T42.6X1	T42.6X2	T42.6X3	T42.6X4	T42.6X5	T42.6X6
Chloralamide	T42.6X1	T42.6X2	T42.6X3	T42.6X4	T42.6X5	T42.6X6
Chloralodol	T42.6X1	T42.6X2	T42.6X3	T42.6X4	T42.6X5	T42.6X6
Chloralose	T60.4X1	T60.4X2	T60.4X3	T60.4X4	—	—
Chlorambucil	T45.1X1	T45.1X2	T45.1X3	T45.1X4	T45.1X5	T45.1X6
Chloramine	T57.8X1	T57.8X2	T57.8X3	T57.8X4	—	—
T	T49.0X1	T49.0X2	T49.0X3	T49.0X4	T49.0X5	T49.0X6
topical	T49.0X1	T49.0X2	T49.0X3	T49.0X4	T49.0X5	T49.0X6
Chloramphenicol	T36.2X1	T36.2X2	T36.2X3	T36.2X4	T36.2X5	T36.2X6
ENT agent	T49.6X1	T49.6X2	T49.6X3	T49.6X4	T49.6X5	T49.6X6
ophthalmic preparation	T49.5X1	T49.5X2	T49.5X3	T49.5X4	T49.5X5	T49.5X6
Chloramphenicol — *continued*						
topical NEC	T49.0X1	T49.0X2	T49.0X3	T49.0X4	T49.0X5	T49.0X6
Chlorate (potassium) (sodium)	T60.3X1	T60.3X2	T60.3X3	T60.3X4	—	—
NEC						
herbicide	T60.3X1	T60.3X2	T60.3X3	T60.3X4	—	—
Chlorazanil	T50.2X1	T50.2X2	T50.2X3	T50.2X4	T50.2X5	T50.2X6
Chlorbenzene, chlorbenzol	T53.7X1	T53.7X2	T53.7X3	T53.7X4	—	—
Chlorbenzoxamine	T44.3X1	T44.3X2	T44.3X3	T44.3X4	T44.3X5	T44.3X6
Chlorbutol	T42.6X1	T42.6X2	T42.6X3	T42.6X4	T42.6X5	T42.6X6
Chlorcyclizine	T45.0X1	T45.0X2	T45.0X3	T45.0X4	T45.0X5	T45.0X6
Chlordan (e) (dust)	T60.1X1	T60.1X2	T60.1X3	T60.1X4	—	—
Chlordantoin	T49.0X1	T49.0X2	T49.0X3	T49.0X4	T49.0X5	T49.0X6
Chlordiazepoxide	T42.4X1	T42.4X2	T42.4X3	T42.4X4	T42.4X5	T42.4X6
Chlordiethyl benzamide	T49.3X1	T49.3X2	T49.3X3	T49.3X4	T49.3X5	T49.3X6
Chloresium	T49.8X1	T49.8X2	T49.8X3	T49.8X4	T49.8X5	T49.8X6
Chlorethiazol	T42.6X1	T42.6X2	T42.6X3	T42.6X4	T42.6X5	T42.6X6
Chlorethyl — *see* Ethyl chloride						
Chloretone	T42.6X1	T42.6X2	T42.6X3	T42.6X4	T42.6X5	T42.6X6
Chlorex	T53.6X1	T53.6X2	T53.6X3	T53.6X4	—	—
insecticide	T60.1X1	T60.1X2	T60.1X3	T60.1X4	—	—
Chlorfenvinphos	T60.0X1	T60.0X2	T60.0X3	T60.0X4	—	—
Chlorhexadol	T42.6X1	T42.6X2	T42.6X3	T42.6X4	T42.6X5	T42.6X6
Chlorhexamide	T45.1X1	T45.1X2	T45.1X3	T45.1X4	T45.1X5	T45.1X6
Chlorhexidine	T49.0X1	T49.0X2	T49.0X3	T49.0X4	T49.0X5	T49.0X6
Chlorhydroxyquinolin	T49.0X1	T49.0X2	T49.0X3	T49.0X4	T49.0X5	T49.0X6
Chlorimipramine	T43.011	T43.012	T43.013	T43.014	T43.015	T43.016
Chlorinated						
camphene	T53.6X1	T53.6X2	T53.6X3	T53.6X4	—	—
diphenyl	T53.7X1	T53.7X2	T53.7X3	T53.7X4	—	—
hydrocarbons NEC	T53.91	T53.92	T53.93	T53.94	—	—
solvents	T53.91	T53.92	T53.93	T53.94	—	—
lime (bleach)	T54.3X1	T54.3X2	T54.3X3	T54.3X4	—	—
and boric acid solution	T49.0X1	T49.0X2	T49.0X3	T49.0X4	T49.0X5	T49.0X6
naphthalene (insecticide)	T60.1X1	T60.1X2	T60.1X3	T60.1X4	—	—
industrial (non-pesticide)	T53.7X1	T53.7X2	T53.7X3	T53.7X4	—	—
pesticide NEC	T60.8X1	T60.8X2	T60.8X3	T60.8X4	—	—
soda — *see also* sodium hypochlorite						
solution	T49.0X1	T49.0X2	T49.0X3	T49.0X4	T49.0X5	T49.0X6
Chlorine (fumes) (gas)	T59.4X1	T59.4X2	T59.4X3	T59.4X4	—	—
bleach	T54.3X1	T54.3X2	T54.3X3	T54.3X4	—	—
compound gas NEC	T59.4X1	T59.4X2	T59.4X3	T59.4X4	—	—
disinfectant	T59.4X1	T59.4X2	T59.4X3	T59.4X4	—	—
releasing agents NEC	T59.4X1	T59.4X2	T59.4X3	T59.4X4	—	—
Chlorisondamine chloride	T46.991	T46.992	T46.993	T46.994	T46.995	T46.996
Chlormadinone	T38.5X1	T38.5X2	T38.5X3	T38.5X4	T38.5X5	T38.5X6
Chlormephos	T60.0X1	T60.0X2	T60.0X3	T60.0X4	—	—
Chlormerodrin	T50.2X1	T50.2X2	T50.2X3	T50.2X4	T50.2X5	T50.2X6
Chlormethiazole	T42.6X1	T42.6X2	T42.6X3	T42.6X4	T42.6X5	T42.6X6
Chlormethine	T45.1X1	T45.1X2	T45.1X3	T45.1X4	T45.1X5	T45.1X6
Chlormethylenecycline	T36.4X1	T36.4X2	T36.4X3	T36.4X4	T36.4X5	T36.4X6
Chlormezanone	T42.6X1	T42.6X2	T42.6X3	T42.6X4	T42.6X5	T42.6X6
Chloroacetic acid	T60.3X1	T60.3X2	T60.3X3	T60.3X4	—	—
Chloroacetone	T59.3X1	T59.3X2	T59.3X3	T59.3X4	—	—
Chloroacetophenone	T59.3X1	T59.3X2	T59.3X3	T59.3X4	—	—
Chloroaniline	T53.7X1	T53.7X2	T53.7X3	T53.7X4	—	—
Chlorobenzene, chlorobenzol	T53.7X1	T53.7X2	T53.7X3	T53.7X4	—	—
Chlorobromomethane (fire extinguisher)	T53.6X1	T53.6X2	T53.6X3	T53.6X4	—	—
Chlorobutanol	T49.0X1	T49.0X2	T49.0X3	T49.0X4	T49.0X5	T49.0X6
Chlorocresol	T49.0X1	T49.0X2	T49.0X3	T49.0X4	T49.0X5	T49.0X6
Chlorodehydromethyl-testosterone	T38.7X1	T38.7X2	T38.7X3	T38.7X4	T38.7X5	T38.7X6
Chlorodinitrobenzene	T53.7X1	T53.7X2	T53.7X3	T53.7X4	—	—
dust or vapor	T53.7X1	T53.7X2	T53.7X3	T53.7X4	—	—
Chlorodiphenyl	T53.7X1	T53.7X2	T53.7X3	T53.7X4	—	—
Chloroethane — *see* Ethyl chloride						
Chloroethylene	T53.6X1	T53.6X2	T53.6X3	T53.6X4	—	—
Chlorofluorocarbons	T53.5X1	T53.5X2	T53.5X3	T53.5X4	—	—
Chloroform (fumes) (vapor)	T53.1X1	T53.1X2	T53.1X3	T53.1X4	—	—
anesthetic	T41.0X1	T41.0X2	T41.0X3	T41.0X4	T41.0X5	T41.0X6
solvent	T53.1X1	T53.1X2	T53.1X3	T53.1X4	—	—
water, concentrated	T41.0X1	T41.0X2	T41.0X3	T41.0X4	T41.0X5	T41.0X6
Chloroguanide	T37.2X1	T37.2X2	T37.2X3	T37.2X4	T37.2X5	T37.2X6
Chloromycetin	T36.2X1	T36.2X2	T36.2X3	T36.2X4	T36.2X5	T36.2X6
ENT agent	T49.6X1	T49.6X2	T49.6X3	T49.6X4	T49.6X5	T49.6X6
ophthalmic preparation	T49.5X1	T49.5X2	T49.5X3	T49.5X4	T49.5X5	T49.5X6
otic solution	T49.6X1	T49.6X2	T49.6X3	T49.6X4	T49.6X5	T49.6X6
topical NEC	T49.0X1	T49.0X2	T49.0X3	T49.0X4	T49.0X5	T49.0X6
Chloronitrobenzene	T53.7X1	T53.7X2	T53.7X3	T53.7X4	—	—
dust or vapor	T53.7X1	T53.7X2	T53.7X3	T53.7X4	—	—

Substance	Poisoning, Accidental (unintentional)	Poisoning, Intentional Self-harm	Poisoning, Assault	Poisoning, Undetermined	Adverse Effect	Under-dosing
Chlorophacinone	T60.4X1	T60.4X2	T60.4X3	T60.4X4	—	—
Chlorophenol	T53.7X1	T53.7X2	T53.7X3	T53.7X4	—	—
Chlorophenothane	T60.1X1	T60.1X2	T60.1X3	T60.1X4	—	—
Chlorophyll	T50.991	T50.992	T50.993	T50.994	T50.995	T50.996
Chloropicrin (fumes)	T53.6X1	T53.6X2	T53.6X3	T53.6X4	—	—
fumigant	T60.8X1	T60.8X2	T60.8X3	T60.8X4	—	—
fungicide	T60.3X1	T60.3X2	T60.3X3	T60.3X4	—	—
pesticide	T60.8X1	T60.8X2	T60.8X3	T60.8X4	—	—
Chloroprocaine	T41.3X1	T41.3X2	T41.3X3	T41.3X4	T41.3X5	T41.3X6
infiltration (subcutaneous)	T41.3X1	T41.3X2	T41.3X3	T41.3X4	T41.3X5	T41.3X6
nerve block (peripheral) (plexus)	T41.3X1	T41.3X2	T41.3X3	T41.3X4	T41.3X5	T41.3X6
spinal	T41.3X1	T41.3X2	T41.3X3	T41.3X4		T41.3X6
Chloroptic	T49.5X1	T49.5X2	T49.5X3	T49.5X4	T49.5X5	T49.5X6
Chloropurine	T45.1X1	T45.1X2	T45.1X3	T45.1X4	T45.1X5	T45.1X6
Chloropyramine	T45.0X1	T45.0X2	T45.0X3	T45.0X4	T45.0X5	T45.0X6
Chloropyrifos	T60.0X1	T60.0X2	T60.0X3	T60.0X4	—	—
Chloropyrilene	T45.0X1	T45.0X2	T45.0X3	T45.0X4	T45.0X5	T45.0X6
Chloroquine	T37.2X1	T37.2X2	T37.2X3	T37.2X4	T37.2X5	T37.2X6
Chlorothalonil	T60.3X1	T60.3X2	T60.3X3	T60.3X4	—	—
Chlorothen	T45.0X1	T45.0X2	T45.0X3	T45.0X4	T45.0X5	T45.0X6
Chlorothiazide	T50.2X1	T50.2X2	T50.2X3	T50.2X4	T50.2X5	T50.2X6
Chlorothymol	T49.4X1	T49.4X2	T49.4X3	T49.4X4	T49.4X5	T49.4X6
Chlorotrianisene	T38.5X1	T38.5X2	T38.5X3	T38.5X4	T38.5X5	T38.5X6
Chlorovinyldichloroarsine, not in war	T57.0X1	T57.0X2	T57.0X3	T57.0X4	—	—
Chloroxine	T49.4X1	T49.4X2	T49.4X3	T49.4X4	T49.4X5	T49.4X6
Chloroxylenol	T49.0X1	T49.0X2	T49.0X3	T49.0X4	T49.0X5	T49.0X6
Chlorphenamine	T45.0X1	T45.0X2	T45.0X3	T45.0X4	T45.0X5	T45.0X6
Chlorphenesin	T42.8X1	T42.8X2	T42.8X3	T42.8X4	T42.8X5	T42.8X6
topical (antifungal)	T49.0X1	T49.0X2	T49.0X3	T49.0X4	T49.0X5	T49.0X6
Chlorpheniramine	T45.0X1	T45.0X2	T45.0X3	T45.0X4	T45.0X5	T45.0X6
Chlorphenoxamine	T45.0X1	T45.0X2	T45.0X3	T45.0X4	T45.0X5	T45.0X6
Chlorphentermine	T50.5X1	T50.5X2	T50.5X3	T50.5X4	T50.5X5	T50.5X6
Chlorprocaine — see Chloroprocaine						
Chlorproguanil	T37.2X1	T37.2X2	T37.2X3	T37.2X4	T37.2X5	T37.2X6
Chlorpromazine	T43.3X1	T43.3X2	T43.3X3	T43.3X4	T43.3X5	T43.3X6
Chlorpropamide	T38.3X1	T38.3X2	T38.3X3	T38.3X4	T38.3X5	T38.3X6
Chlorprothixene	T43.4X1	T43.4X2	T43.4X3	T43.4X4	T43.4X5	T43.4X6
Chlorquinaldol	T49.0X1	T49.0X2	T49.0X3	T49.0X4	T49.0X5	T49.0X6
Chlorquinol	T49.0X1	T49.0X2	T49.0X3	T49.0X4	T49.0X5	T49.0X6
Chlortalidone	T50.2X1	T50.2X2	T50.2X3	T50.2X4	T50.2X5	T50.2X6
Chlortetracycline	T36.4X1	T36.4X2	T36.4X3	T36.4X4	T36.4X5	T36.4X6
Chlorthalidone	T50.2X1	T50.2X2	T50.2X3	T50.2X4	T50.2X5	T50.2X6
Chlorthion	T60.0X1	T60.0X2	T60.0X3	T60.0X4	—	—
Chlorthiophos	T60.0X1	T60.0X2	T60.0X3	T60.0X4	—	—
Chlortrianisene	T38.5X1	T38.5X2	T38.5X3	T38.5X4	T38.5X5	T38.5X6
Chlor-Trimeton	T45.0X1	T45.0X2	T45.0X3	T45.0X4	T45.0X5	T45.0X6
Chlorzoxazone	T42.8X1	T42.8X2	T42.8X3	T42.8X4	T42.8X5	T42.8X6
Choke damp	T59.7X1	T59.7X2	T59.7X3	T59.7X4	—	—
Cholagogues	T47.5X1	T47.5X2	T47.5X3	T47.5X4	T47.5X5	T47.5X6
Cholebrine	T50.8X1	T50.8X2	T50.8X3	T50.8X4	T50.8X5	T50.8X6
Cholecalciferol	T45.2X1	T45.2X2	T45.2X3	T45.2X4	T45.2X5	T45.2X6
Cholecystokinin	T50.8X1	T50.8X2	T50.8X3	T50.8X4	T50.8X5	T50.8X6
Cholera vaccine	T50.A91	T50.A92	T50.A93	T50.A94	T50.A95	T50.A96
Choleretic	T47.5X1	T47.5X2	T47.5X3	T47.5X4	T47.5X5	T47.5X6
Cholesterol-lowering agents	T46.6X1	T46.6X2	T46.6X3	T46.6X4	T46.6X5	T46.6X6
Cholestyramine (resin)	T46.6X1	T46.6X2	T46.6X3	T46.6X4	T46.6X5	T46.6X6
Cholic acid	T47.5X1	T47.5X2	T47.5X3	T47.5X4	T47.5X5	T47.5X6
Choline	T48.6X1	T48.6X2	T48.6X3	T48.6X4	T48.6X5	T48.6X6
chloride	T50.991	T50.992	T50.993	T50.994	T50.995	T50.996
dihydrogen citrate	T50.991	T50.992	T50.993	T50.994	T50.995	T50.996
salicylate	T39.091	T39.092	T39.093	T39.094	T39.095	T39.096
theophyllinate	T48.6X1	T48.6X2	T48.6X3	T48.6X4	T48.6X5	T48.6X6
Cholinergic (drug) NEC	T44.1X1	T44.1X2	T44.1X3	T44.1X4	T44.1X5	T44.1X6
muscle tone enhancer	T44.1X1	T44.1X2	T44.1X3	T44.1X4	T44.1X5	T44.1X6
organophosphorus	T44.0X1	T44.0X2	T44.0X3	T44.0X4	T44.0X5	T44.0X6
insecticide	T60.0X1	T60.0X2	T60.0X3	T60.0X4	—	—
nerve gas	T59.891	T59.892	T59.893	T59.894	—	—
trimethyl ammonium propanediol	T44.1X1	T44.1X2	T44.1X3	T44.1X4	T44.1X5	T44.1X6
Cholinesterase reactivator	T50.6X1	T50.6X2	T50.6X3	T50.6X4	T50.6X5	T50.6X6
Cholografin	T50.8X1	T50.8X2	T50.8X3	T50.8X4	T50.8X5	T50.8X6
Chorionic gonadotropin	T38.891	T38.892	T38.893	T38.894	T38.895	T38.896
Chromate	T56.2X1	T56.2X2	T56.2X3	T56.2X4	—	—
dust or mist	T56.2X1	T56.2X2	T56.2X3	T56.2X4	—	—
lead — see also lead	T56.0X1	T56.0X2	T56.0X3	T56.0X4	—	—
paint	T56.0X1	T56.0X2	T56.0X3	T56.0X4	—	—
Chromic						
acid	T56.2X1	T56.2X2	T56.2X3	T56.2X4	—	—
dust or mist	T56.2X1	T56.2X2	T56.2X3	T56.2X4	—	—

Substance	Poisoning, Accidental (unintentional)	Poisoning, Intentional Self-harm	Poisoning, Assault	Poisoning, Undetermined	Adverse Effect	Under-dosing
Chromic — continued						
phosphate 32P	T45.1X1	T45.1X2	T45.1X3	T45.1X4	T45.1X5	T45.1X6
Chromium	T56.2X1	T56.2X2	T56.2X3	T56.2X4	—	—
compounds — see Chromate						
sesquioxide	T50.8X1	T50.8X2	T50.8X3	T50.8X4	T50.8X5	T50.8X6
Chromomycin A3	T45.1X1	T45.1X2	T45.1X3	T45.1X4	T45.1X5	T45.1X6
Chromonar	T46.3X1	T46.3X2	T46.3X3	T46.3X4	T46.3X5	T46.3X6
Chromyl chloride	T56.2X1	T56.2X2	T56.2X3	T56.2X4	—	—
Chrysarobin	T49.4X1	T49.4X2	T49.4X3	T49.4X4	T49.4X5	T49.4X6
Chrysazin	T47.2X1	T47.2X2	T47.2X3	T47.2X4	T47.2X5	T47.2X6
Chymar	T45.3X1	T45.3X2	T45.3X3	T45.3X4	T45.3X5	T45.3X6
ophthalmic preparation	T49.5X1	T49.5X2	T49.5X3	T49.5X4	T49.5X5	T49.5X6
Chymopapain	T45.3X1	T45.3X2	T45.3X3	T45.3X4	T45.3X5	T45.3X6
Chymotrypsin	T45.3X1	T45.3X2	T45.3X3	T45.3X4	T45.3X5	T45.3X6
ophthalmic preparation	T49.5X1	T49.5X2	T49.5X3	T49.5X4	T49.5X5	T49.5X6
Cianidanol	T50.991	T50.992	T50.993	T50.994	T50.995	T50.996
Cianopramine	T43.011	T43.012	T43.013	T43.014	T43.015	T43.016
Cibenzoline	T46.2X1	T46.2X2	T46.2X3	T46.2X4	T46.2X5	T46.2X6
Ciclacillin	T36.0X1	T36.0X2	T36.0X3	T36.0X4	T36.0X5	T36.0X6
Ciclobarbital — see Hexobarbital						
Ciclonicate	T46.7X1	T46.7X2	T46.7X3	T46.7X4	T46.7X5	T46.7X6
Ciclopirox (olamine)	T49.0X1	T49.0X2	T49.0X3	T49.0X4	T49.0X5	T49.0X6
Ciclosporin	T45.1X1	T45.1X2	T45.1X3	T45.1X4	T45.1X5	T45.1X6
Cicuta maculata or virosa	T62.2X1	T62.2X2	T62.2X3	T62.2X4	—	—
Cicutoxin	T62.2X1	T62.2X2	T62.2X3	T62.2X4	—	—
Cigarette lighter fluid	T52.0X1	T52.0X2	T52.0X3	T52.0X4	—	—
Cigarettes (tobacco)	T65.221	T65.222	T65.223	T65.224	—	—
Ciguatoxin	T61.01	T61.02	T61.03	T61.04	—	—
Cilazapril	T46.4X1	T46.4X2	T46.4X3	T46.4X4	T46.4X5	T46.4X6
Cimetidine	T47.0X1	T47.0X2	T47.0X3	T47.0X4	T47.0X5	T47.0X6
Cimetropium bromide	T44.3X1	T44.3X2	T44.3X3	T44.3X4	T44.3X5	T44.3X6
Cinchocaine	T41.3X1	T41.3X2	T41.3X3	T41.3X4	T41.3X5	T41.3X6
topical (surface)	T41.3X1	T41.3X2	T41.3X3	T41.3X4	T41.3X5	T41.3X6
Cinchona	T37.2X1	T37.2X2	T37.2X3	T37.2X4	T37.2X5	T37.2X6
Cinchonine alkaloids	T37.2X1	T37.2X2	T37.2X3	T37.2X4	T37.2X5	T37.2X6
Cinchophen	T50.4X1	T50.4X2	T50.4X3	T50.4X4	T50.4X5	T50.4X6
Cinepazide	T46.7X1	T46.7X2	T46.7X3	T46.7X4	T46.7X5	T46.7X6
Cinnamedrine	T48.5X1	T48.5X2	T48.5X3	T48.5X4	T48.5X5	T48.5X6
Cinnarizine	T45.0X1	T45.0X2	T45.0X3	T45.0X4	T45.0X5	T45.0X6
Cinoxacin	T37.8X1	T37.8X2	T37.8X3	T37.8X4	T37.8X5	T37.8X6
Ciprofibrate	T46.6X1	T46.6X2	T46.6X3	T46.6X4	T46.6X5	T46.6X6
Ciprofloxacin	T36.8X1	T36.8X2	T36.8X3	T36.8X4	T36.8X5	T36.8X6
Cisapride	T47.8X1	T47.8X2	T47.8X3	T47.8X4	T47.8X5	T47.8X6
Cisplatin	T45.1X1	T45.1X2	T45.1X3	T45.1X4	T45.1X5	T45.1X6
Citalopram	T43.221	T43.222	T43.223	T43.224	T43.225	T43.226
Citanest	T41.3X1	T41.3X2	T41.3X3	T41.3X4	T41.3X5	T41.3X6
infiltration (subcutaneous)	T41.3X1	T41.3X2	T41.3X3	T41.3X4	T41.3X5	T41.3X6
nerve block (peripheral) (plexus)	T41.3X1	T41.3X2	T41.3X3	T41.3X4	T41.3X5	T41.3X6
Citric acid	T47.5X1	T47.5X2	T47.5X3	T47.5X4	T47.5X5	T47.5X6
Citrovorum (factor)	T45.8X1	T45.8X2	T45.8X3	T45.8X4	T45.8X5	T45.8X6
Claviceps purpurea	T62.2X1	T62.2X2	T62.2X3	T62.2X4	—	—
Clavulanic acid	T36.1X1	T36.1X2	T36.1X3	T36.1X4	T36.1X5	T36.1X6
Cleaner, cleansing agent, type not specified	T65.891	T65.892	T65.893	T65.894		
of paint or varnish	T52.91	T52.92	T52.93	T52.94		
specified type NEC	T65.891	T65.892	T65.893	T65.894		
Clebopride	T47.8X1	T47.8X2	T47.8X3	T47.8X4	T47.8X5	T47.8X6
Clefamide	T37.3X1	T37.3X2	T37.3X3	T37.3X4	T37.3X5	T37.3X6
Clemastine	T45.0X1	T45.0X2	T45.0X3	T45.0X4	T45.0X5	T45.0X6
Clematis vitalba	T62.2X1	T62.2X2	T62.2X3	T62.2X4	—	—
Clemizole	T45.0X1	T45.0X2	T45.0X3	T45.0X4	T45.0X5	T45.0X6
penicillin	T36.0X1	T36.0X2	T36.0X3	T36.0X4	T36.0X5	T36.0X6
Clenbuterol	T48.6X1	T48.6X2	T48.6X3	T48.6X4	T48.6X5	T48.6X6
Clidinium bromide	T44.3X1	T44.3X2	T44.3X3	T44.3X4	T44.3X5	T44.3X6
Clindamycin	T36.8X1	T36.8X2	T36.8X3	T36.8X4	T36.8X5	T36.8X6
Clinofibrate	T46.6X1	T46.6X2	T46.6X3	T46.6X4	T46.6X5	T46.6X6
Clioquinol	T37.8X1	T37.8X2	T37.8X3	T37.8X4	T37.8X5	T37.8X6
Cliradon	T40.2X1	T40.2X2	T40.2X3	T40.2X4	—	—
Clobazam	T42.4X1	T42.4X2	T42.4X3	T42.4X4	T42.4X5	T42.4X6
Clobenzorex	T50.5X1	T50.5X2	T50.5X3	T50.5X4	T50.5X5	T50.5X6
Clobetasol	T49.0X1	T49.0X2	T49.0X3	T49.0X4	T49.0X5	T49.0X6
Clobetasone	T49.0X1	T49.0X2	T49.0X3	T49.0X4	T49.0X5	T49.0X6
Clobutinol	T48.3X1	T48.3X2	T48.3X3	T48.3X4	T48.3X5	T48.3X6
Clocortolone	T38.0X1	T38.0X2	T38.0X3	T38.0X4	T38.0X5	T38.0X6
Clodantoin	T49.0X1	T49.0X2	T49.0X3	T49.0X4	T49.0X5	T49.0X6
Clodronic acid	T50.991	T50.992	T50.993	T50.994	T50.995	T50.996
Clofazimine	T37.1X1	T37.1X2	T37.1X3	T37.1X4	T37.1X5	T37.1X6
Clofedanol	T48.3X1	T48.3X2	T48.3X3	T48.3X4	T48.3X5	T48.3X6
Clofenamide	T50.2X1	T50.2X2	T50.2X3	T50.2X4	T50.2X5	T50.2X6
Clofenotane	T49.0X1	T49.0X2	T49.0X3	T49.0X4	T49.0X5	T49.0X6
Clofezone	T39.2X1	T39.2X2	T39.2X3	T39.2X4	T39.2X5	T39.2X6
Clofibrate	T46.6X1	T46.6X2	T46.6X3	T46.6X4	T46.6X5	T46.6X6

Substance	Poisoning, Accidental (unintentional)	Poisoning, Intentional Self-harm	Poisoning, Assault	Poisoning, Undetermined	Adverse Effect	Under-dosing
Clofibride	T46.6X1	T46.6X2	T46.6X3	T46.6X4	T46.6X5	T46.6X6
Cloforex	T50.5X1	T50.5X2	T50.5X3	T50.5X4	T50.5X5	T50.5X6
Clomethiazole	T42.6X1	T42.6X2	T42.6X3	T42.6X4	T42.6X5	T42.6X6
Clometocillin	T36.0X1	T36.0X2	T36.0X3	T36.0X4	T36.0X5	T36.0X6
Clomifene	T38.5X1	T38.5X2	T38.5X3	T38.5X4	T38.5X5	T38.5X6
Clomiphene	T38.5X1	T38.5X2	T38.5X3	T38.5X4	T38.5X5	T38.5X6
Clomipramine	T43.011	T43.012	T43.013	T43.014	T43.015	T43.016
Clomocycline	T36.4X1	T36.4X2	T36.4X3	T36.4X4	T36.4X5	T36.4X6
Clonazepam	T42.4X1	T42.4X2	T42.4X3	T42.4X4	T42.4X5	T42.4X6
Clonidine	T46.5X1	T46.5X2	T46.5X3	T46.5X4	T46.5X5	T46.5X6
Clonixin	T39.8X1	T39.8X2	T39.8X3	T39.8X4	T39.8X5	T39.8X6
Clopamide	T50.2X1	T50.2X2	T50.2X3	T50.2X4	T50.2X5	T50.2X6
Clopenthixol	T43.4X1	T43.4X2	T43.4X3	T43.4X4	T43.4X5	T43.4X6
Cloperastine	T48.3X1	T48.3X2	T48.3X3	T48.3X4	T48.3X5	T48.3X6
Clophedianol	T48.3X1	T48.3X2	T48.3X3	T48.3X4	T48.3X5	T48.3X6
Cloponone	T36.2X1	T36.2X2	T36.2X3	T36.2X4	T36.2X5	T36.2X6
Cloprednol	T38.0X1	T38.0X2	T38.0X3	T38.0X4	T38.0X5	T38.0X6
Cloral betaine	T42.6X1	T42.6X2	T42.6X3	T42.6X4	T42.6X5	T42.6X6
Cloramfenicol	T36.2X1	T36.2X2	T36.2X3	T36.2X4	T36.2X5	T36.2X6
Clorazepate (dipotassium)	T42.4X1	T42.4X2	T42.4X3	T42.4X4	T42.4X5	T42.4X6
Clorexolone	T50.2X1	T50.2X2	T50.2X3	T50.2X4	T50.2X5	T50.2X6
Clorfenamine	T45.0X1	T45.0X2	T45.0X3	T45.0X4	T45.0X5	T45.0X6
Clorgiline	T43.1X1	T43.1X2	T43.1X3	T43.1X4	T43.1X5	T43.1X6
Clorotepine	T44.3X1	T44.3X2	T44.3X3	T44.3X4	T44.3X5	T44.3X6
Clorox (bleach)	T54.91	T54.92	T54.93	T54.94	—	—
Clorprenaline	T48.6X1	T48.6X2	T48.6X3	T48.6X4	T48.6X5	T48.6X6
Clortermine	T50.5X1	T50.5X2	T50.5X3	T50.5X4	T50.5X5	T50.5X6
Clotiapine	T43.591	T43.592	T43.593	T43.594	T43.595	T43.596
Clotiazepam	T42.4X1	T42.4X2	T42.4X3	T42.4X4	T42.4X5	T42.4X6
Clotibric acid	T46.6X1	T46.6X2	T46.6X3	T46.6X4	T46.6X5	T46.6X6
Clotrimazole	T49.0X1	T49.0X2	T49.0X3	T49.0X4	T49.0X5	T49.0X6
Cloxacillin	T36.0X1	T36.0X2	T36.0X3	T36.0X4	T36.0X5	T36.0X6
Cloxazolam	T42.4X1	T42.4X2	T42.4X3	T42.4X4	T42.4X5	T42.4X6
Cloxiquine	T49.0X1	T49.0X2	T49.0X3	T49.0X4	T49.0X5	T49.0X6
Clozapine	T42.4X1	T42.4X2	T42.4X3	T42.4X4	T42.4X5	T42.4X6
Coagulant NEC	T45.7X1	T45.7X2	T45.7X3	T45.7X4	T45.7X5	T45.7X6
Coal (carbon monoxide from) — see also Carbon, monoxide, coal	T58.2X1	T58.2X2	T58.2X3	T58.2X4	—	—
oil — see Kerosene						
tar	T49.1X1	T49.1X2	T49.1X3	T49.1X4	T49.1X5	T49.1X6
fumes	T59.891	T59.892	T59.893	T59.894	—	—
medicinal (ointment)	T49.4X1	T49.4X2	T49.4X3	T49.4X4	T49.4X5	T49.4X6
analgesics NEC	T39.2X1	T39.2X2	T39.2X3	T39.2X4	T39.2X5	T39.2X6
naphtha (solvent)	T52.0X1	T52.0X2	T52.0X3	T52.0X4	—	—
Cobalamine	T45.2X1	T45.2X2	T45.2X3	T45.2X4	T45.2X5	T45.2X6
Cobalt (nonmedicinal) (fumes) (industrial)	T56.891	T56.892	T56.893	T56.894	—	—
medicinal (trace) (chloride)	T45.8X1	T45.8X2	T45.8X3	T45.8X4	T45.8X5	T45.8X6
Cobra (venom)	T63.041	T63.042	T63.043	T63.044	—	—
Coca (leaf)	T40.5X1	T40.5X2	T40.5X3	T40.5X4	T40.5X5	T40.5X6
Cocaine	T40.5X1	T40.5X2	T40.5X3	T40.5X4	T40.5X5	T40.5X6
topical anesthetic	T41.3X1	T41.3X2	T41.3X3	T41.3X4	T41.3X5	T41.3X6
Cocarboxylase	T45.3X1	T45.3X2	T45.3X3	T45.3X4	T45.3X5	T45.3X6
Coccidioidin	T50.8X1	T50.8X2	T50.8X3	T50.8X4	T50.8X5	T50.8X6
Cocculus indicus	T62.1X1	T62.1X2	T62.1X3	T62.1X4	—	—
Cochineal	T65.6X1	T65.6X2	T65.6X3	T65.6X4	—	—
medicinal products	T50.991	T50.992	T50.993	T50.994	T50.995	T50.996
Codeine	T40.2X1	T40.2X2	T40.2X3	T40.2X4	T40.2X5	T40.2X6
Cod-liver oil	T45.2X1	T45.2X2	T45.2X3	T45.2X4	T45.2X5	T45.2X6
Coenzyme A	T50.991	T50.992	T50.993	T50.994	T50.995	T50.996
Coffee	T62.8X1	T62.8X2	T62.8X3	T62.8X4	—	—
Cogalactoisomerase	T50.991	T50.992	T50.993	T50.994	T50.995	T50.996
Cogentin	T44.3X1	T44.3X2	T44.3X3	T44.3X4	T44.3X5	T44.3X6
Coke fumes or gas (carbon monoxide)	T58.2X1	T58.2X2	T58.2X3	T58.2X4	—	—
industrial use	T58.8X1	T58.8X2	T58.8X3	T58.8X4	—	—
Colace	T47.4X1	T47.4X2	T47.4X3	T47.4X4	T47.4X5	T47.4X6
Colaspase	T45.1X1	T45.1X2	T45.1X3	T45.1X4	T45.1X5	T45.1X6
Colchicine	T50.4X1	T50.4X2	T50.4X3	T50.4X4	T50.4X5	T50.4X6
Colchicum	T62.2X1	T62.2X2	T62.2X3	T62.2X4	—	—
Cold cream	T49.3X1	T49.3X2	T49.3X3	T49.3X4	T49.3X5	T49.3X6
Colecalciferol	T45.2X1	T45.2X2	T45.2X3	T45.2X4	T45.2X5	T45.2X6
Colestipol	T46.6X1	T46.6X2	T46.6X3	T46.6X4	T46.6X5	T46.6X6
Colestyramine	T46.6X1	T46.6X2	T46.6X3	T46.6X4	T46.6X5	T46.6X6
Colimycin	T36.8X1	T36.8X2	T36.8X3	T36.8X4	T36.8X5	T36.8X6
Colistimethate	T36.8X1	T36.8X2	T36.8X3	T36.8X4	T36.8X5	T36.8X6
Colistin	T36.8X1	T36.8X2	T36.8X3	T36.8X4	T36.8X5	T36.8X6
sulfate (eye preparation)	T49.5X1	T49.5X2	T49.5X3	T49.5X4	T49.5X5	T49.5X6
Collagen	T50.991	T50.992	T50.993	T50.994	T50.995	T50.996
Collagenase	T49.4X1	T49.4X2	T49.4X3	T49.4X4	T49.4X5	T49.4X6
Collodion	T49.3X1	T49.3X2	T49.3X3	T49.3X4	T49.3X5	T49.3X6
Colocynth	T47.2X1	T47.2X2	T47.2X3	T47.2X4	T47.2X5	T47.2X6
Colophony adhesive	T49.3X1	T49.3X2	T49.3X3	T49.3X4	T49.3X5	T49.3X6
Colorant — see also Dye	T50.991	T50.992	T50.993	T50.994	T50.995	T50.996
Coloring matter — see Dye(s)						
Combustion gas (after combustion) — see Carbon, monoxide						
prior to combustion	T59.891	T59.892	T59.893	T59.894	—	—
Compazine	T43.3X1	T43.3X2	T43.3X3	T43.3X4	T43.3X5	T43.3X6
Compound						
1080 (sodium fluoroacetate)	T60.4X1	T60.4X2	T60.4X3	T60.4X4	—	—
269 (endrin)	T60.1X1	T60.1X2	T60.1X3	T60.1X4	—	—
3422 (parathion)	T60.0X1	T60.0X2	T60.0X3	T60.0X4	—	—
3911 (phorate)	T60.0X1	T60.0X2	T60.0X3	T60.0X4	—	—
3956 (toxaphene)	T60.1X1	T60.1X2	T60.1X3	T60.1X4	—	—
4049 (malathion)	T60.0X1	T60.0X2	T60.0X3	T60.0X4	—	—
4069 (malathion)	T60.0X1	T60.0X2	T60.0X3	T60.0X4	—	—
4124 (dicapthon)	T60.0X1	T60.0X2	T60.0X3	T60.0X4	—	—
42 (warfarin)	T60.4X1	T60.4X2	T60.4X3	T60.4X4	—	—
497 (dieldrin)	T60.1X1	T60.1X2	T60.1X3	T60.1X4	—	—
E (cortisone)	T38.0X1	T38.0X2	T38.0X3	T38.0X4	T38.0X5	T38.0X6
F (hydrocortisone)	T38.0X1	T38.0X2	T38.0X3	T38.0X4	T38.0X5	T38.0X6
Congener, anabolic	T38.7X1	T38.7X2	T38.7X3	T38.7X4	T38.7X5	T38.7X6
Congo red	T50.8X1	T50.8X2	T50.8X3	T50.8X4	T50.8X5	T50.8X6
Coniine, conine	T62.2X1	T62.2X2	T62.2X3	T62.2X4	—	—
Conium (maculatum)	T62.2X1	T62.2X2	T62.2X3	T62.2X4	—	—
Conjugated estrogenic substances	T38.5X1	T38.5X2	T38.5X3	T38.5X4	T38.5X5	T38.5X6
Contac	T48.5X1	T48.5X2	T48.5X3	T48.5X4	T48.5X5	T48.5X6
Contact lens solution	T49.5X1	T49.5X2	T49.5X3	T49.5X4	T49.5X5	T49.5X6
Contraceptive (oral)	T38.4X1	T38.4X2	T38.4X3	T38.4X4	T38.4X5	T38.4X6
vaginal	T49.8X1	T49.8X2	T49.8X3	T49.8X4	T49.8X5	T49.8X6
Contrast medium, radiography	T50.8X1	T50.8X2	T50.8X3	T50.8X4	T50.8X5	T50.8X6
Convallaria glycosides	T46.0X1	T46.0X2	T46.0X3	T46.0X4	T46.0X5	T46.0X6
Convallaria majalis	T62.2X1	T62.2X2	T62.2X3	T62.2X4	—	—
berry	T62.1X1	T62.1X2	T62.1X3	T62.1X4	—	—
Copperhead snake (bite) (venom)	T63.061	T63.062	T63.063	T63.064	—	—
Copper (dust) (fumes) (nonmedicinal) NEC	T56.4X1	T56.4X2	T56.4X3	T56.4X4	—	—
arsenate, arsenite	T57.0X1	T57.0X2	T57.0X3	T57.0X4	—	—
insecticide	T60.2X1	T60.2X2	T60.2X3	T60.2X4	—	—
emetic	T47.7X1	T47.7X2	T47.7X3	T47.7X4	T47.7X5	T47.7X6
fungicide	T60.3X1	T60.3X2	T60.3X3	T60.3X4	—	—
gluconate	T49.0X1	T49.0X2	T49.0X3	T49.0X4	T49.0X5	T49.0X6
insecticide	T60.2X1	T60.2X2	T60.2X3	T60.2X4	—	—
medicinal (trace)	T45.8X1	T45.8X2	T45.8X3	T45.8X4	T45.8X5	T45.8X6
oleate	T49.0X1	T49.0X2	T49.0X3	T49.0X4	T49.0X5	T49.0X6
sulfate	T56.4X1	T56.4X2	T56.4X3	T56.4X4	—	—
cupric	T56.4X1	T56.4X2	T56.4X3	T56.4X4	—	—
fungicide	T60.3X1	T60.3X2	T60.3X3	T60.3X4	—	—
medicinal						
ear	T49.6X1	T49.6X2	T49.6X3	T49.6X4	T49.6X5	T49.6X6
emetic	T47.7X1	T47.7X2	T47.7X3	T47.7X4	T47.7X5	T47.7X6
eye	T49.5X1	T49.5X2	T49.5X3	T49.5X4	T49.5X5	T49.5X6
cuprous	T56.4X1	T56.4X2	T56.4X3	T56.4X4	—	—
fungicide	T60.3X1	T60.3X2	T60.3X3	T60.3X4	—	—
medicinal						
ear	T49.6X1	T49.6X2	T49.6X3	T49.6X4	T49.6X5	T49.6X6
emetic	T47.7X1	T47.7X2	T47.7X3	T47.7X4	T47.7X5	T47.7X6
eye	T49.5X1	T49.5X2	T49.5X3	T49.5X4	T49.5X5	T49.5X6
Coral (sting)	T63.691	T63.692	T63.693	T63.694	—	—
snake (bite) (venom)	T63.021	T63.022	T63.023	T63.024	—	—
Corbadrine	T49.6X1	T49.6X2	T49.6X3	T49.6X4	T49.6X5	T49.6X6
Cordite	T65.891	T65.892	T65.893	T65.894	—	—
vapor	T59.891	T59.892	T59.893	T59.894	—	—
Cordran	T49.0X1	T49.0X2	T49.0X3	T49.0X4	T49.0X5	T49.0X6
Corn cures	T49.4X1	T49.4X2	T49.4X3	T49.4X4	T49.4X5	T49.4X6
Cornhusker's lotion	T49.3X1	T49.3X2	T49.3X3	T49.3X4	T49.3X5	T49.3X6
Corn starch	T49.3X1	T49.3X2	T49.3X3	T49.3X4	T49.3X5	T49.3X6
Coronary vasodilator NEC	T46.3X1	T46.3X2	T46.3X3	T46.3X4	T46.3X5	T46.3X6
Corrosive NEC	T54.91	T54.92	T54.93	T54.94	—	—
acid NEC	T54.2X1	T54.2X2	T54.2X3	T54.2X4	—	—
aromatics	T54.1X1	T54.1X2	T54.1X3	T54.1X4	—	—
disinfectant	T54.1X1	T54.1X2	T54.1X3	T54.1X4	—	—
fumes NEC	T54.91	T54.92	T54.93	T54.94	—	—
specified NEC	T54.91	T54.92	T54.93	T54.94	—	—
sublimate	T56.1X1	T56.1X2	T56.1X3	T56.1X4	—	—
Cortate	T38.0X1	T38.0X2	T38.0X3	T38.0X4	T38.0X5	T38.0X6
Cort-Dome	T38.0X1	T38.0X2	T38.0X3	T38.0X4	T38.0X5	T38.0X6
ENT agent	T49.6X1	T49.6X2	T49.6X3	T49.6X4	T49.6X5	T49.6X6
ophthalmic preparation	T49.5X1	T49.5X2	T49.5X3	T49.5X4	T49.5X5	T49.5X6

Substance	Poisoning, Accidental (unintentional)	Poisoning, Intentional Self-harm	Poisoning, Assault	Poisoning, Undetermined	Adverse Effect	Under-dosing
Cort-Dome — *continued*						
topical NEC	T49.0X1	T49.0X2	T49.0X3	T49.0X4	T49.0X5	T49.0X6
Cortef	T38.0X1	T38.0X2	T38.0X3	T38.0X4	T38.0X5	T38.0X6
ENT agent	T49.6X1	T49.6X2	T49.6X3	T49.6X4	T49.6X5	T49.6X6
ophthalmic preparation	T49.5X1	T49.5X2	T49.5X3	T49.5X4	T49.5X5	T49.5X6
topical NEC	T49.0X1	T49.0X2	T49.0X3	T49.0X4	T49.0X5	T49.0X6
Corticosteroid	T38.0X1	T38.0X2	T38.0X3	T38.0X4	T38.0X5	T38.0X6
ENT agent	T49.6X1	T49.6X2	T49.6X3	T49.6X4	T49.6X5	T49.6X6
mineral	T50.0X1	T50.0X2	T50.0X3	T50.0X4	T50.0X5	T50.0X6
ophthalmic	T49.5X1	T49.5X2	T49.5X3	T49.5X4	T49.5X5	T49.5X6
topical NEC	T49.0X1	T49.0X2	T49.0X3	T49.0X4	T49.0X5	T49.0X6
Corticotropin	T38.811	T38.812	T38.813	T38.814	T38.815	T38.816
Cortisol	T49.0X1	T49.0X2	T49.0X3	T49.0X4	T49.0X5	T49.0X6
ENT agent	T49.6X1	T49.6X2	T49.6X3	T49.6X4	T49.6X5	T49.6X6
ophthalmic preparation	T49.5X1	T49.5X2	T49.5X3	T49.5X4	T49.5X5	T49.5X6
topical NEC	T49.0X1	T49.0X2	T49.0X3	T49.0X4	T49.0X5	T49.0X6
Cortisone (acetate)	T38.0X1	T38.0X2	T38.0X3	T38.0X4	T38.0X5	T38.0X6
ENT agent	T49.6X1	T49.6X2	T49.6X3	T49.6X4	T49.6X5	T49.6X6
ophthalmic preparation	T49.5X1	T49.5X2	T49.5X3	T49.5X4	T49.5X5	T49.5X6
topical NEC	T49.0X1	T49.0X2	T49.0X3	T49.0X4	T49.0X5	T49.0X6
Cortivazol	T38.0X1	T38.0X2	T38.0X3	T38.0X4	T38.0X5	T38.0X6
Cortogen	T38.0X1	T38.0X2	T38.0X3	T38.0X4	T38.0X5	T38.0X6
ENT agent	T49.6X1	T49.6X2	T49.6X3	T49.6X4	T49.6X5	T49.6X6
ophthalmic preparation	T49.5X1	T49.5X2	T49.5X3	T49.5X4	T49.5X5	T49.5X6
Cortone	T38.0X1	T38.0X2	T38.0X3	T38.0X4	T38.0X5	T38.0X6
ENT agent	T49.6X1	T49.6X2	T49.6X3	T49.6X4	T49.6X5	T49.6X6
ophthalmic preparation	T49.5X1	T49.5X2	T49.5X3	T49.5X4	T49.5X5	T49.5X6
Cortril	T38.0X1	T38.0X2	T38.0X3	T38.0X4	T38.0X5	T38.0X6
ENT agent	T49.6X1	T49.6X2	T49.6X3	T49.6X4	T49.6X5	T49.6X6
ophthalmic preparation	T49.5X1	T49.5X2	T49.5X3	T49.5X4	T49.5X5	T49.5X6
topical NEC	T49.0X1	T49.0X2	T49.0X3	T49.0X4	T49.0X5	T49.0X6
Corynebacterium parvum	T45.1X1	T45.1X2	T45.1X3	T45.1X4	T45.1X5	T45.1X6
Cosmetic preparation	T49.8X1	T49.8X2	T49.8X3	T49.8X4	T49.8X5	T49.8X6
Cosmetics	T49.8X1	T49.8X2	T49.8X3	T49.8X4	T49.8X5	T49.8X6
Cosyntropin	T38.811	T38.812	T38.813	T38.814	T38.815	T38.816
Cotarnine	T45.7X1	T45.7X2	T45.7X3	T45.7X4	T45.7X5	T45.7X6
Co-trimoxazole	T36.8X1	T36.8X2	T36.8X3	T36.8X4	T36.8X5	T36.8X6
Cottonseed oil	T49.3X1	T49.3X2	T49.3X3	T49.3X4	T49.3X5	T49.3X6
Cough mixture (syrup)	T48.4X1	T48.4X2	T48.4X3	T48.4X4	T48.4X5	T48.4X6
containing opiates	T40.2X1	T40.2X2	T40.2X3	T40.2X4	T40.2X5	T40.2X6
expectorants	T48.4X1	T48.4X2	T48.4X3	T48.4X4	T48.4X5	T48.4X6
Coumadin	T45.511	T45.512	T45.513	T45.514	T45.515	T45.516
rodenticide	T60.4X1	T60.4X2	T60.4X3	T60.4X4	—	—
Coumaphos	T60.0X1	T60.0X2	T60.0X3	T60.0X4	—	—
Coumarin	T45.511	T45.512	T45.513	T45.514	T45.515	T45.516
Coumetarol	T45.511	T45.512	T45.513	T45.514	T45.515	T45.516
Cowbane	T62.2X1	T62.2X2	T62.2X3	T62.2X4	—	—
Cozyme	T45.2X1	T45.2X2	T45.2X3	T45.2X4	T45.2X5	T45.2X6
Crack	T40.5X1	T40.5X2	T40.5X3	T40.5X4	—	—
Crataegus extract	T46.0X1	T46.0X2	T46.0X3	T46.0X4	T46.0X5	T46.0X6
Creolin	T54.1X1	T54.1X2	T54.1X3	T54.1X4	—	—
disinfectant	T54.1X1	T54.1X2	T54.1X3	T54.1X4	—	—
Creosol (compound)	T49.0X1	T49.0X2	T49.0X3	T49.0X4	T49.0X5	T49.0X6
Creosote (coal tar)	T49.0X1	T49.0X2	T49.0X3	T49.0X4	T49.0X5	T49.0X6
(beechwood)						
medicinal (expectorant)	T48.4X1	T48.4X2	T48.4X3	T48.4X4	T48.4X5	T48.4X6
syrup	T48.4X1	T48.4X2	T48.4X3	T48.4X4	T48.4X5	T48.4X6
Cresol(s)	T49.0X1	T49.0X2	T49.0X3	T49.0X4	T49.0X5	T49.0X6
and soap solution	T49.0X1	T49.0X2	T49.0X3	T49.0X4	T49.0X5	T49.0X6
Cresyl acetate	T49.0X1	T49.0X2	T49.0X3	T49.0X4	T49.0X5	T49.0X6
Cresylic acid	T49.0X1	T49.0X2	T49.0X3	T49.0X4	T49.0X5	T49.0X6
Crimidine	T60.4X1	T60.4X2	T60.4X3	T60.4X4	—	—
Croconazole	T37.8X1	T37.8X2	T37.8X3	T37.8X4	T37.8X5	T37.8X6
Cromoglicic acid	T48.6X1	T48.6X2	T48.6X3	T48.6X4	T48.6X5	T48.6X6
Cromolyn	T48.6X1	T48.6X2	T48.6X3	T48.6X4	T48.6X5	T48.6X6
Cromonar	T46.3X1	T46.3X2	T46.3X3	T46.3X4	T46.3X5	T46.3X6
Cropropamide	T39.8X1	T39.8X2	T39.8X3	T39.8X4	T39.8X5	T39.8X6
with crotethamide	T50.7X1	T50.7X2	T50.7X3	T50.7X4	T50.7X5	T50.7X6
Crotamiton	T49.0X1	T49.0X2	T49.0X3	T49.0X4	T49.0X5	T49.0X6
Crotethamide	T39.8X1	T39.8X2	T39.8X3	T39.8X4	T39.8X5	T39.8X6
with cropropamide	T50.7X1	T50.7X2	T50.7X3	T50.7X4	T50.7X5	T50.7X6
Croton (oil)	T47.2X1	T47.2X2	T47.2X3	T47.2X4	T47.2X5	T47.2X6
chloral	T42.6X1	T42.6X2	T42.6X3	T42.6X4	T42.6X5	T42.6X6
Crude oil	T52.0X1	T52.0X2	T52.0X3	T52.0X4	—	—
Cryogenine	T39.8X1	T39.8X2	T39.8X3	T39.8X4	T39.8X5	T39.8X6
Cryolite (vapor)	T60.1X1	T60.1X2	T60.1X3	T60.1X4	—	—
insecticide	T60.1X1	T60.1X2	T60.1X3	T60.1X4	—	—
Cryptenamine (tannates)	T46.5X1	T46.5X2	T46.5X3	T46.5X4	T46.5X5	T46.5X6
Crystal violet	T49.0X1	T49.0X2	T49.0X3	T49.0X4	T49.0X5	T49.0X6
Cuckoopint	T62.2X1	T62.2X2	T62.2X3	T62.2X4	—	—
Cumetharol	T45.511	T45.512	T45.513	T45.514	T45.515	T45.516
Cupric						
acetate	T60.3X1	T60.3X2	T60.3X3	T60.3X4	—	—

Substance	Poisoning, Accidental (unintentional)	Poisoning, Intentional Self-harm	Poisoning, Assault	Poisoning, Undetermined	Adverse Effect	Under-dosing
Cupric — *continued*						
acetoarsenite	T57.0X1	T57.0X2	T57.0X3	T57.0X4	—	—
arsenate	T57.0X1	T57.0X2	T57.0X3	T57.0X4	—	—
gluconate	T49.0X1	T49.0X2	T49.0X3	T49.0X4	T49.0X5	T49.0X6
oleate	T49.0X1	T49.0X2	T49.0X3	T49.0X4	T49.0X5	T49.0X6
sulfate	T56.4X1	T56.4X2	T56.4X3	T56.4X4	—	—
Cuprous sulfate — *see also* Copper sulfate	T56.4X1	T56.4X2	T56.4X3	T56.4X4	—	—
Curare, curarine	T48.1X1	T48.1X2	T48.1X3	T48.1X4	T48.1X5	T48.1X6
Cyamemazine	T43.3X1	T43.3X2	T43.3X3	T43.3X4	T43.3X5	T43.3X6
Cyamopsis tetragonoloba	T46.6X1	T46.6X2	T46.6X3	T46.6X4	T46.6X5	T46.6X6
Cyanacetyl hydrazide	T37.1X1	T37.1X2	T37.1X3	T37.1X4	T37.1X5	T37.1X6
Cyanic acid (gas)	T59.891	T59.892	T59.893	T59.894	—	—
Cyanide(s) (compounds) (potassium) (sodium)	T65.0X1	T65.0X2	T65.0X3	T65.0X4	—	—
NEC						
dust or gas (inhalation) NEC	T57.3X1	T57.3X2	T57.3X3	T57.3X4	—	—
fumigant	T65.0X1	T65.0X2	T65.0X3	T65.0X4	—	—
hydrogen	T57.3X1	T57.3X2	T57.3X3	T57.3X4	—	—
mercuric — *see* Mercury						
pesticide (dust) (fumes)	T65.0X1	T65.0X2	T65.0X3	T65.0X4	—	—
Cyanoacrylate adhesive	T49.3X1	T49.3X2	T49.3X3	T49.3X4	T49.3X5	T49.3X6
Cyanocobalamin	T45.8X1	T45.8X2	T45.8X3	T45.8X4	T45.8X5	T45.8X6
Cyanogen (chloride) (gas)	T59.891	T59.892	T59.893	T59.894	—	—
NEC						
Cyclacillin	T36.0X1	T36.0X2	T36.0X3	T36.0X4	T36.0X5	T36.0X6
Cyclaine	T41.3X1	T41.3X2	T41.3X3	T41.3X4	T41.3X5	T41.3X6
Cyclamate	T50.991	T50.992	T50.993	T50.994	T50.995	T50.996
Cyclamen europaeum	T62.2X1	T62.2X2	T62.2X3	T62.2X4	—	—
Cyclandelate	T46.7X1	T46.7X2	T46.7X3	T46.7X4	T46.7X5	T46.7X6
Cyclazocine	T50.7X1	T50.7X2	T50.7X3	T50.7X4	T50.7X5	T50.7X6
Cyclizine	T45.0X1	T45.0X2	T45.0X3	T45.0X4	T45.0X5	T45.0X6
Cyclobarbital	T42.3X1	T42.3X2	T42.3X3	T42.3X4	T42.3X5	T42.3X6
Cyclobarbitone	T42.3X1	T42.3X2	T42.3X3	T42.3X4	T42.3X5	T42.3X6
Cyclobenzaprine	T48.1X1	T48.1X2	T48.1X3	T48.1X4	T48.1X5	T48.1X6
Cyclodrine	T44.3X1	T44.3X2	T44.3X3	T44.3X4	T44.3X5	T44.3X6
Cycloguanil embonate	T37.2X1	T37.2X2	T37.2X3	T37.2X4	T37.2X5	T37.2X6
Cyclohexane	T52.8X1	T52.8X2	T52.8X3	T52.8X4	—	—
Cyclohexanol	T51.8X1	T51.8X2	T51.8X3	T51.8X4	—	—
Cyclohexanone	T52.4X1	T52.4X2	T52.4X3	T52.4X4	—	—
Cycloheximide	T60.3X1	T60.3X2	T60.3X3	T60.3X4	—	—
Cyclohexyl acetate	T52.8X1	T52.8X2	T52.8X3	T52.8X4	—	—
Cycloleucin	T45.1X1	T45.1X2	T45.1X3	T45.1X4	T45.1X5	T45.1X6
Cyclomethycaine	T41.3X1	T41.3X2	T41.3X3	T41.3X4	T41.3X5	T41.3X6
Cyclopentamine	T44.4X1	T44.4X2	T44.4X3	T44.4X4	T44.4X5	T44.4X6
Cyclopenthiazide	T50.2X1	T50.2X2	T50.2X3	T50.2X4	T50.2X5	T50.2X6
Cyclopentolate	T44.3X1	T44.3X2	T44.3X3	T44.3X4	T44.3X5	T44.3X6
Cyclophosphamide	T45.1X1	T45.1X2	T45.1X3	T45.1X4	T45.1X5	T45.1X6
Cycloplegic drug	T49.5X1	T49.5X2	T49.5X3	T49.5X4	T49.5X5	T49.5X6
Cyclopropane	T41.291	T41.292	T41.293	T41.294	T41.295	T41.296
Cyclopyrabital	T39.8X1	T39.8X2	T39.8X3	T39.8X4	T39.8X5	T39.8X6
Cycloserine	T37.1X1	T37.1X2	T37.1X3	T37.1X4	T37.1X5	T37.1X6
Cyclosporin	T45.1X1	T45.1X2	T45.1X3	T45.1X4	T45.1X5	T45.1X6
Cyclothiazide	T50.2X1	T50.2X2	T50.2X3	T50.2X4	T50.2X5	T50.2X6
Cycrimine	T44.3X1	T44.3X2	T44.3X3	T44.3X4	T44.3X5	T44.3X6
Cyhalothrin	T60.1X1	T60.1X2	T60.1X3	T60.1X4	—	—
Cymarin	T46.0X1	T46.0X2	T46.0X3	T46.0X4	T46.0X5	T46.0X6
Cypermethrin	T60.1X1	T60.1X2	T60.1X3	T60.1X4	—	—
Cyphenothrin	T60.2X1	T60.2X2	T60.2X3	T60.2X4	—	—
Cyproheptadine	T45.0X1	T45.0X2	T45.0X3	T45.0X4	T45.0X5	T45.0X6
Cyproterone	T38.6X1	T38.6X2	T38.6X3	T38.6X4	T38.6X5	T38.6X6
Cysteamine	T50.6X1	T50.6X2	T50.6X3	T50.6X4	T50.6X5	T50.6X6
Cytarabine	T45.1X1	T45.1X2	T45.1X3	T45.1X4	T45.1X5	T45.1X6
Cytisus						
laburnum	T62.2X1	T62.2X2	T62.2X3	T62.2X4	—	—
scoparius	T62.2X1	T62.2X2	T62.2X3	T62.2X4	—	—
Cytochrome C	T47.5X1	T47.5X2	T47.5X3	T47.5X4	T47.5X5	T47.5X6
Cytomel	T38.1X1	T38.1X2	T38.1X3	T38.1X4	T38.1X5	T38.1X6
Cytosine arabinoside	T45.1X1	T45.1X2	T45.1X3	T45.1X4	T45.1X5	T45.1X6
Cytoxan	T45.1X1	T45.1X2	T45.1X3	T45.1X4	T45.1X5	T45.1X6
Cytozyme	T45.7X1	T45.7X2	T45.7X3	T45.7X4	T45.7X5	T45.7X6
S-Carboxymethylcysteine	T48.4X1	T48.4X2	T48.4X3	T48.4X4	T48.4X5	T48.4X6
Dacarbazine	T45.1X1	T45.1X2	T45.1X3	T45.1X4	T45.1X5	T45.1X6
Dactinomycin	T45.1X1	T45.1X2	T45.1X3	T45.1X4	T45.1X5	T45.1X6
DADPS	T37.1X1	T37.1X2	T37.1X3	T37.1X4	T37.1X5	T37.1X6
Dakin's solution	T49.0X1	T49.0X2	T49.0X3	T49.0X4	T49.0X5	T49.0X6
Dalapon (sodium)	T60.3X1	T60.3X2	T60.3X3	T60.3X4	—	—
Dalmane	T42.4X1	T42.4X2	T42.4X3	T42.4X4	T42.4X5	T42.4X6
Danazol	T38.6X1	T38.6X2	T38.6X3	T38.6X4	T38.6X5	T38.6X6
Danilone	T45.511	T45.512	T45.513	T45.514	T45.515	T45.516
Danthron	T47.2X1	T47.2X2	T47.2X3	T47.2X4	T47.2X5	T47.2X6
Dantrolene	T42.8X1	T42.8X2	T42.8X3	T42.8X4	T42.8X5	T42.8X6
Dantron	T47.2X1	T47.2X2	T47.2X3	T47.2X4	T47.2X5	T47.2X6

Additional Character May Be Required — Refer to the Tabular List for Character Selection ▽ **Subterms under main terms may continue to next column or page**

Substance	Poisoning, Accidental (unintentional)	Poisoning, Intentional Self-harm	Poisoning, Assault	Poisoning, Undetermined	Adverse Effect	Under-dosing
Daphne (gnidium) (mezereum)	T62.2X1	T62.2X2	T62.2X3	T62.2X4	—	—
berry	T62.1X1	T62.1X2	T62.1X3	T62.1X4	—	—
Dapsone	T37.1X1	T37.1X2	T37.1X3	T37.1X4	T37.1X5	T37.1X6
Daraprim	T37.2X1	T37.2X2	T37.2X3	T37.2X4	T37.2X5	T37.2X6
Darnel	T62.2X1	T62.2X2	T62.2X3	T62.2X4	—	—
Darvon	T39.8X1	T39.8X2	T39.8X3	T39.8X4	T39.8X5	T39.8X6
Daunomycin	T45.1X1	T45.1X2	T45.1X3	T45.1X4	T45.1X5	T45.1X6
Daunorubicin	T45.1X1	T45.1X2	T45.1X3	T45.1X4	T45.1X5	T45.1X6
DBI	T38.3X1	T38.3X2	T38.3X3	T38.3X4	T38.3X5	T38.3X6
D-Con	T60.91	T60.92	T60.93	T60.94	—	—
insecticide	T60.2X1	T60.2X2	T60.2X3	T60.2X4	—	—
rodenticide	T60.4X1	T60.4X2	T60.4X3	T60.4X4	—	—
DDAVP	T38.891	T38.892	T38.893	T38.894	T38.895	T38.896
DDE (bis(chlorophenyl)-dichloroethylene)	T60.2X1	T60.2X2	T60.2X3	T60.2X4	—	—
DDS	T37.1X1	T37.1X2	T37.1X3	T37.1X4	T37.1X5	T37.1X6
DDT (dust)	T60.1X1	T60.1X2	T60.1X3	T60.1X4	—	—
Deadly nightshade — see also Belladonna	T62.2X1	T62.2X2	T62.2X3	T62.2X4	—	—
berry	T62.1X1	T62.1X2	T62.1X3	T62.1X4	—	—
Deamino-D-arginine vasopressin	T38.891	T38.892	T38.893	T38.894	T38.895	T38.896
Deanol (aceglumate)	T50.991	T50.992	T50.993	T50.994	T50.995	T50.996
Debrisoquine	T46.5X1	T46.5X2	T46.5X3	T46.5X4	T46.5X5	T46.5X6
Decaborane	T57.8X1	T57.8X2	T57.8X3	T57.8X4	—	—
fumes	T59.891	T59.892	T59.893	T59.894	—	—
Decadron	T38.0X1	T38.0X2	T38.0X3	T38.0X4	T38.0X5	T38.0X6
ENT agent	T49.6X1	T49.6X2	T49.6X3	T49.6X4	T49.6X5	T49.6X6
ophthalmic preparation	T49.5X1	T49.5X2	T49.5X3	T49.5X4	T49.5X5	T49.5X6
topical NEC	T49.0X1	T49.0X2	T49.0X3	T49.0X4	T49.0X5	T49.0X6
Decahydronaphthalene	T52.8X1	T52.8X2	T52.8X3	T52.8X4	—	—
Decalin	T52.8X1	T52.8X2	T52.8X3	T52.8X4	—	—
Decamethonium (bromide)	T48.1X1	T48.1X2	T48.1X3	T48.1X4	T48.1X5	T48.1X6
Decholin	T47.5X1	T47.5X2	T47.5X3	T47.5X4	T47.5X5	T47.5X6
Declomycin	T36.4X1	T36.4X2	T36.4X3	T36.4X4	T36.4X5	T36.4X6
Decongestant, nasal (mucosa)	T48.5X1	T48.5X2	T48.5X3	T48.5X4	T48.5X5	T48.5X6
combination	T48.5X1	T48.5X2	T48.5X3	T48.5X4	T48.5X5	T48.5X6
Deet	T60.8X1	T60.8X2	T60.8X3	T60.8X4	—	—
Deferoxamine	T45.8X1	T45.8X2	T45.8X3	T45.8X4	T45.8X5	T45.8X6
Deflazacort	T38.0X1	T38.0X2	T38.0X3	T38.0X4	T38.0X5	T38.0X6
Deglycyrrhizinized extract of licorice	T48.4X1	T48.4X2	T48.4X3	T48.4X4	T48.4X5	T48.4X6
Dehydrocholic acid	T47.5X1	T47.5X2	T47.5X3	T47.5X4	T47.5X5	T47.5X6
Dehydroemetine	T37.3X1	T37.3X2	T37.3X3	T37.3X4	T37.3X5	T37.3X6
Dekalin	T52.8X1	T52.8X2	T52.8X3	T52.8X4	—	—
Delalutin	T38.5X1	T38.5X2	T38.5X3	T38.5X4	T38.5X5	T38.5X6
Delorazepam	T42.4X1	T42.4X2	T42.4X3	T42.4X4	T42.4X5	T42.4X6
Delphinium	T62.2X1	T62.2X2	T62.2X3	T62.2X4	—	—
Deltamethrin	T60.1X1	T60.1X2	T60.1X3	T60.1X4	—	—
Deltasone	T38.0X1	T38.0X2	T38.0X3	T38.0X4	T38.0X5	T38.0X6
Deltra	T38.0X1	T38.0X2	T38.0X3	T38.0X4	T38.0X5	T38.0X6
Delvinal	T42.3X1	T42.3X2	T42.3X3	T42.3X4	T42.3X5	T42.3X6
Demecarium (bromide)	T49.5X1	T49.5X2	T49.5X3	T49.5X4	T49.5X5	T49.5X6
Demeclocycline	T36.4X1	T36.4X2	T36.4X3	T36.4X4	T36.4X5	T36.4X6
Demecolcine	T45.1X1	T45.1X2	T45.1X3	T45.1X4	T45.1X5	T45.1X6
Demegestone	T38.5X1	T38.5X2	T38.5X3	T38.5X4	T38.5X5	T38.5X6
Demelanizing agents	T49.8X1	T49.8X2	T49.8X3	T49.8X4	T49.8X5	T49.8X6
Demephion -O and -S	T60.0X1	T60.0X2	T60.0X3	T60.0X4	—	—
Demerol	T40.2X1	T40.2X2	T40.2X3	T40.2X4	T40.2X5	T40.2X6
Demethylchlortetracycline	T36.4X1	T36.4X2	T36.4X3	T36.4X4	T36.4X5	T36.4X6
Demethyltetracycline	T36.4X1	T36.4X2	T36.4X3	T36.4X4	T36.4X5	T36.4X6
Demeton -O and -S	T60.0X1	T60.0X2	T60.0X3	T60.0X4	—	—
Demulcent (external)	T49.3X1	T49.3X2	T49.3X3	T49.3X4	T49.3X5	T49.3X6
specified NEC	T49.3X1	T49.3X2	T49.3X3	T49.3X4	T49.3X5	T49.3X6
Demulen	T38.4X1	T38.4X2	T38.4X3	T38.4X4	T38.4X5	T38.4X6
Denatured alcohol	T51.0X1	T51.0X2	T51.0X3	T51.0X4	—	—
Dendrid	T49.5X1	T49.5X2	T49.5X3	T49.5X4	T49.5X5	T49.5X6
Dental drug, topical application NEC	T49.7X1	T49.7X2	T49.7X3	T49.7X4	T49.7X5	T49.7X6
Dentifrice	T49.7X1	T49.7X2	T49.7X3	T49.7X4	T49.7X5	T49.7X6
Deodorant spray (feminine hygiene)	T49.8X1	T49.8X2	T49.8X3	T49.8X4	T49.8X5	T49.8X6
Deoxycortone	T50.0X1	T50.0X2	T50.0X3	T50.0X4	T50.0X5	T50.0X6
Deoxyribonuclease (pancreatic)	T45.3X1	T45.3X2	T45.3X3	T45.3X4	T45.3X5	T45.3X6
Depilatory	T49.4X1	T49.4X2	T49.4X3	T49.4X4	T49.4X5	T49.4X6
Deprenalin	T42.8X1	T42.8X2	T42.8X3	T42.8X4	T42.8X5	T42.8X6
Deprenyl	T42.8X1	T42.8X2	T42.8X3	T42.8X4	T42.8X5	T42.8X6
Depressant						
appetite (central)	T50.5X1	T50.5X2	T50.5X3	T50.5X4	T50.5X5	T50.5X6
cardiac	T46.2X1	T46.2X2	T46.2X3	T46.2X4	T46.2X5	T46.2X6

Substance	Poisoning, Accidental (unintentional)	Poisoning, Intentional Self-harm	Poisoning, Assault	Poisoning, Undetermined	Adverse Effect	Under-dosing
Depressant — continued						
central nervous system (anesthetic) — see also Central nervous system, depressants	T42.71	T42.72	T42.73	T42.74	T42.75	T42.76
general anesthetic	T41.201	T41.202	T41.203	T41.204	T41.205	T41.206
muscle tone	T42.8X1	T42.8X2	T42.8X3	T42.8X4	T42.8X5	T42.8X6
muscle tone, central	T42.8X1	T42.8X2	T42.8X3	T42.8X4	T42.8X5	T42.8X6
psychotherapeutic	T43.501	T43.502	T43.503	T43.504	T43.505	T43.506
Depressant, appetite	T50.5X1	T50.5X2	T50.5X3	T50.5X4	T50.5X5	T50.5X6
Deptropine	T45.0X1	T45.0X2	T45.0X3	T45.0X4	T45.0X5	T45.0X6
Dequalinium (chloride)	T49.0X1	T49.0X2	T49.0X3	T49.0X4	T49.0X5	T49.0X6
Derris root	T60.2X1	T60.2X2	T60.2X3	T60.2X4	—	—
Deserpidine	T46.5X1	T46.5X2	T46.5X3	T46.5X4	T46.5X5	T46.5X6
Desferrioxamine	T45.8X1	T45.8X2	T45.8X3	T45.8X4	T45.8X5	T45.8X6
Desipramine	T43.011	T43.012	T43.013	T43.014	T43.015	T43.016
Deslanoside	T46.0X1	T46.0X2	T46.0X3	T46.0X4	T46.0X5	T46.0X6
Desloughing agent	T49.4X1	T49.4X2	T49.4X3	T49.4X4	T49.4X5	T49.4X6
Desmethylimipramine	T43.011	T43.012	T43.013	T43.014	T43.015	T43.016
Desmopressin	T38.891	T38.892	T38.893	T38.894	T38.895	T38.896
Desocodeine	T40.2X1	T40.2X2	T40.2X3	T40.2X4	T40.2X5	T40.2X6
Desogestrel	T38.5X1	T38.5X2	T38.5X3	T38.5X4	T38.5X5	T38.5X6
Desomorphine	T40.2X1	T40.2X2	T40.2X3	T40.2X4	—	—
Desonide	T49.0X1	T49.0X2	T49.0X3	T49.0X4	T49.0X5	T49.0X6
Desoximetasone	T49.0X1	T49.0X2	T49.0X3	T49.0X4	T49.0X5	T49.0X6
Desoxycorticosteroid	T50.0X1	T50.0X2	T50.0X3	T50.0X4	T50.0X5	T50.0X6
Desoxycortone	T50.0X1	T50.0X2	T50.0X3	T50.0X4	T50.0X5	T50.0X6
Desoxyephedrine	T43.621	T43.622	T43.623	T43.624	T43.625	T43.626
Detaxtran	T46.6X1	T46.6X2	T46.6X3	T46.6X4	T46.6X5	T46.6X6
Detergent	T49.2X1	T49.2X2	T49.2X3	T49.2X4	T49.2X5	T49.2X6
external medication	T49.2X1	T49.2X2	T49.2X3	T49.2X4	T49.2X5	T49.2X6
local	T49.2X1	T49.2X2	T49.2X3	T49.2X4	T49.2X5	T49.2X6
medicinal	T49.2X1	T49.2X2	T49.2X3	T49.2X4	T49.2X5	T49.2X6
nonmedicinal	T55.1X1	T55.1X2	T55.1X3	T55.1X4	—	—
specified NEC	T55.1X1	T55.1X2	T55.1X3	T55.1X4	—	—
Deterrent, alcohol	T50.6X1	T50.6X2	T50.6X3	T50.6X4	T50.6X5	T50.6X6
Detoxifying agent	T50.6X1	T50.6X2	T50.6X3	T50.6X4	T50.6X5	T50.6X6
Detrothyronine	T38.1X1	T38.1X2	T38.1X3	T38.1X4	T38.1X5	T38.1X6
Dettol (external medication)	T49.0X1	T49.0X2	T49.0X3	T49.0X4	T49.0X5	T49.0X6
Dexamethasone	T38.0X1	T38.0X2	T38.0X3	T38.0X4	T38.0X5	T38.0X6
ENT agent	T49.6X1	T49.6X2	T49.6X3	T49.6X4	T49.6X5	T49.6X6
ophthalmic preparation	T49.5X1	T49.5X2	T49.5X3	T49.5X4	T49.5X5	T49.5X6
topical NEC	T49.0X1	T49.0X2	T49.0X3	T49.0X4	T49.0X5	T49.0X6
Dexamfetamine	T43.621	T43.622	T43.623	T43.624	T43.625	T43.626
Dexamphetamine	T43.621	T43.622	T43.623	T43.624	T43.625	T43.626
Dexbrompheniramine	T45.0X1	T45.0X2	T45.0X3	T45.0X4	T45.0X5	T45.0X6
Dexchlorpheniramine	T45.0X1	T45.0X2	T45.0X3	T45.0X4	T45.0X5	T45.0X6
Dexedrine	T43.621	T43.622	T43.623	T43.624	T43.625	T43.626
Dexetimide	T44.3X1	T44.3X2	T44.3X3	T44.3X4	T44.3X5	T44.3X6
Dexfenfluramine	T50.5X1	T50.5X2	T50.5X3	T50.5X4	T50.5X5	T50.5X6
Dexpanthenol	T45.2X1	T45.2X2	T45.2X3	T45.2X4	T45.2X5	T45.2X6
Dextran (40) (70) (150)	T45.8X1	T45.8X2	T45.8X3	T45.8X4	T45.8X5	T45.8X6
Dextriferron	T45.4X1	T45.4X2	T45.4X3	T45.4X4	T45.4X5	T45.4X6
Dextroamphetamine	T43.621	T43.622	T43.623	T43.624	T43.625	T43.626
Dextro calcium pantothenate	T45.2X1	T45.2X2	T45.2X3	T45.2X4	T45.2X5	T45.2X6
Dextromethorphan	T48.3X1	T48.3X2	T48.3X3	T48.3X4	T48.3X5	T48.3X6
Dextromoramide	T40.4X1	T40.4X2	T40.4X3	T40.4X4	—	—
topical	T49.8X1	T49.8X2	T49.8X3	T49.8X4	T49.8X5	T49.8X6
Dextro pantothenyl alcohol	T45.2X1	T45.2X2	T45.2X3	T45.2X4	T45.2X5	T45.2X6
Dextropropoxyphene	T40.4X1	T40.4X2	T40.4X3	T40.4X4	T40.4X5	T40.4X6
Dextrorphan	T40.2X1	T40.2X2	T40.2X3	T40.2X4	T40.2X5	T40.2X6
Dextrose	T50.3X1	T50.3X2	T50.3X3	T50.3X4	T50.3X5	T50.3X6
concentrated solution, intravenous	T46.8X1	T46.8X2	T46.8X3	T46.8X4	T46.8X5	T46.8X6
Dextrothyroxin	T38.1X1	T38.1X2	T38.1X3	T38.1X4	T38.1X5	T38.1X6
Dextrothyroxine sodium	T38.1X1	T38.1X2	T38.1X3	T38.1X4	T38.1X5	T38.1X6
DFP	T44.0X1	T44.0X2	T44.0X3	T44.0X4	T44.0X5	T44.0X6
DHE	T37.3X1	T37.3X2	T37.3X3	T37.3X4	T37.3X5	T37.3X6
45	T46.5X1	T46.5X2	T46.5X3	T46.5X4	T46.5X5	T46.5X6
Diabinese	T38.3X1	T38.3X2	T38.3X3	T38.3X4	T38.3X5	T38.3X6
Diacetone alcohol	T52.4X1	T52.4X2	T52.4X3	T52.4X4	—	—
Diacetyl monoxime	T50.991	T50.992	T50.993	T50.994	—	—
Diacetylmorphine	T40.1X1	T40.1X2	T40.1X3	T40.1X4	—	—
Diachylon plaster	T49.4X1	T49.4X2	T49.4X3	T49.4X4	T49.4X5	T49.4X6
Diaethylstilboestrolum	T38.5X1	T38.5X2	T38.5X3	T38.5X4	T38.5X5	T38.5X6
Diagnostic agent NEC	T50.8X1	T50.8X2	T50.8X3	T50.8X4	T50.8X5	T50.8X6
Dial (soap)	T49.2X1	T49.2X2	T49.2X3	T49.2X4	T49.2X5	T49.2X6
sedative	T42.3X1	T42.3X2	T42.3X3	T42.3X4	T42.3X5	T42.3X6
Dialkyl carbonate	T52.91	T52.92	T52.93	T52.94	—	—
Diallylbarbituric acid	T42.3X1	T42.3X2	T42.3X3	T42.3X4	T42.3X5	T42.3X6
Diallymal	T42.3X1	T42.3X2	T42.3X3	T42.3X4	T42.3X5	T42.3X6

Substance	Poisoning, Accidental (unintentional)	Poisoning, Intentional Self-harm	Poisoning, Assault	Poisoning, Undetermined	Adverse Effect	Under-dosing
Dialysis solution (intraperitoneal)	T50.3X1	T50.3X2	T50.3X3	T50.3X4	T50.3X5	T50.3X6
Diaminodiphenylsulfone	T37.1X1	T37.1X2	T37.1X3	T37.1X4	T37.1X5	T37.1X6
Diamorphine	T40.1X1	T40.1X2	T40.1X3	T40.1X4	—	—
Diamox	T50.2X1	T50.2X2	T50.2X3	T50.2X4	T50.2X5	T50.2X6
Diamthazole	T49.0X1	T49.0X2	T49.0X3	T49.0X4	T49.0X5	T49.0X6
Dianthone	T47.2X1	T47.2X2	T47.2X3	T47.2X4	T47.2X5	T47.2X6
Diaphenylsulfone	T37.0X1	T37.0X2	T37.0X3	T37.0X4	T37.0X5	T37.0X6
Diasone (sodium)	T37.1X1	T37.1X2	T37.1X3	T37.1X4	T37.1X5	T37.1X6
Diastase	T47.5X1	T47.5X2	T47.5X3	T47.5X4	T47.5X5	T47.5X6
Diatrizoate	T50.8X1	T50.8X2	T50.8X3	T50.8X4	T50.8X5	T50.8X6
Diazepam	T42.4X1	T42.4X2	T42.4X3	T42.4X4	T42.4X5	T42.4X6
Diazinon	T60.0X1	T60.0X2	T60.0X3	T60.0X4	—	—
Diazomethane (gas)	T59.891	T59.892	T59.893	T59.894	—	—
Diazoxide	T46.5X1	T46.5X2	T46.5X3	T46.5X4	T46.5X5	T46.5X6
Dibekacin	T36.5X1	T36.5X2	T36.5X3	T36.5X4	T36.5X5	T36.5X6
Dibenamine	T44.6X1	T44.6X2	T44.6X3	T44.6X4	T44.6X5	T44.6X6
Dibenzepin	T43.011	T43.012	T43.013	T43.014	T43.015	T43.016
Dibenzheptropine	T45.0X1	T45.0X2	T45.0X3	T45.0X4	T45.0X5	T45.0X6
Dibenzyline	T44.6X1	T44.6X2	T44.6X3	T44.6X4	T44.6X5	T44.6X6
Diborane (gas)	T59.891	T59.892	T59.893	T59.894	—	—
Dibromochloropropane	T60.8X1	T60.8X2	T60.8X3	T60.8X4	—	—
Dibromodulcitol	T45.1X1	T45.1X2	T45.1X3	T45.1X4	T45.1X5	T45.1X6
Dibromoethane	T53.6X1	T53.6X2	T53.6X3	T53.6X4	—	—
Dibromomannitol	T45.1X1	T45.1X2	T45.1X3	T45.1X4	T45.1X5	T45.1X6
Dibromopropamidine isethionate	T49.0X1	T49.0X2	T49.0X3	T49.0X4	T49.0X5	T49.0X6
Dibrompropamidine	T49.0X1	T49.0X2	T49.0X3	T49.0X4	T49.0X5	T49.0X6
Dibucaine	T41.3X1	T41.3X2	T41.3X3	T41.3X4	T41.3X5	T41.3X6
topical (surface)	T41.3X1	T41.3X2	T41.3X3	T41.3X4	T41.3X5	T41.3X6
Dibunate sodium	T48.3X1	T48.3X2	T48.3X3	T48.3X4	T48.3X5	T48.3X6
Dibutoline sulfate	T44.3X1	T44.3X2	T44.3X3	T44.3X4	T44.3X5	T44.3X6
Dicamba	T60.3X1	T60.3X2	T60.3X3	T60.3X4	—	—
Dicapthon	T60.0X1	T60.0X2	T60.0X3	T60.0X4	—	—
Dichlobenil	T60.3X1	T60.3X2	T60.3X3	T60.3X4	—	—
Dichlone	T60.3X1	T60.3X2	T60.3X3	T60.3X4	—	—
Dichloralphenozone	T42.6X1	T42.6X2	T42.6X3	T42.6X4	T42.6X5	T42.6X6
Dichlorbenzidine	T65.3X1	T65.3X2	T65.3X3	T65.3X4	—	—
Dichlorhydrin	T52.8X1	T52.8X2	T52.8X3	T52.8X4	—	—
Dichlorhydroxyquinoline	T37.8X1	T37.8X2	T37.8X3	T37.8X4	T37.8X5	T37.8X6
Dichlorobenzene	T53.7X1	T53.7X2	T53.7X3	T53.7X4	—	—
Dichlorobenzyl alcohol	T49.6X1	T49.6X2	T49.6X3	T49.6X4	T49.6X5	T49.6X6
Dichlorodifluoromethane	T53.5X1	T53.5X2	T53.5X3	T53.5X4	—	—
Dichloroethane	T52.8X1	T52.8X2	T52.8X3	T52.8X4	—	—
Dichloroethylene	T53.6X1	T53.6X2	T53.6X3	T53.6X4	—	—
Dichloroethyl sulfide, not in war	T59.891	T59.892	T59.893	T59.894	—	—
Dichloroformoxine, not in war	T59.891	T59.892	T59.893	T59.894	—	—
Dichlorohydrin, alpha-dichlorohydrin	T52.8X1	T52.8X2	T52.8X3	T52.8X4	—	—
Dichloromethane (solvent)	T53.4X1	T53.4X2	T53.4X3	T53.4X4	—	—
vapor	T53.4X1	T53.4X2	T53.4X3	T53.4X4	—	—
Dichloronaphthoquinone	T60.3X1	T60.3X2	T60.3X3	T60.3X4	—	—
Dichlorophen	T37.4X1	T37.4X2	T37.4X3	T37.4X4	T37.4X5	T37.4X6
Dichloropropene	T60.3X1	T60.3X2	T60.3X3	T60.3X4	—	—
Dichloropropionic acid	T60.3X1	T60.3X2	T60.3X3	T60.3X4	—	—
Dichlorphenamide	T50.2X1	T50.2X2	T50.2X3	T50.2X4	T50.2X5	T50.2X6
Dichlorvos	T60.0X1	T60.0X2	T60.0X3	T60.0X4	—	—
Diclofenac	T39.391	T39.392	T39.393	T39.394	T39.395	T39.396
Diclofenamide	T50.2X1	T50.2X2	T50.2X3	T50.2X4	T50.2X5	T50.2X6
Diclofensine	T43.291	T43.292	T43.293	T43.294	T43.295	T43.296
Diclonixine	T39.8X1	T39.8X2	T39.8X3	T39.8X4	T39.8X5	T39.8X6
Dicloxacillin	T36.0X1	T36.0X2	T36.0X3	T36.0X4	T36.0X5	T36.0X6
Dicophane	T49.0X1	T49.0X2	T49.0X3	T49.0X4	T49.0X5	T49.0X6
Dicoumarol, dicoumarin, dicumarol	T45.511	T45.512	T45.513	T45.514	T45.515	T45.516
Dicrotophos	T60.0X1	T60.0X2	T60.0X3	T60.0X4	—	—
Dicyanogen (gas)	T65.0X1	T65.0X2	T65.0X3	T65.0X4	—	—
Dicyclomine	T44.3X1	T44.3X2	T44.3X3	T44.3X4	T44.3X5	T44.3X6
Dicycloverine	T44.3X1	T44.3X2	T44.3X3	T44.3X4	T44.3X5	T44.3X6
Dideoxycytidine	T37.5X1	T37.5X2	T37.5X3	T37.5X4	T37.5X5	T37.5X6
Dideoxyinosine	T37.5X1	T37.5X2	T37.5X3	T37.5X4	T37.5X5	T37.5X6
Dieldrin (vapor)	T60.1X1	T60.1X2	T60.1X3	T60.1X4	—	—
Diemal	T42.3X1	T42.3X2	T42.3X3	T42.3X4	T42.3X5	T42.3X6
Dienestrol	T38.5X1	T38.5X2	T38.5X3	T38.5X4	T38.5X5	T38.5X6
Dienoestrol	T38.5X1	T38.5X2	T38.5X3	T38.5X4	T38.5X5	T38.5X6
Dietetic drug NEC	T50.901	T50.902	T50.903	T50.904	T50.905	T50.906
Diethazine	T42.8X1	T42.8X2	T42.8X3	T42.8X4	T42.8X5	T42.8X6
Diethyl						
barbituric acid	T42.3X1	T42.3X2	T42.3X3	T42.3X4	T42.3X5	T42.3X6
carbamazine	T37.4X1	T37.4X2	T37.4X3	T37.4X4	T37.4X5	T37.4X6
carbinol	T51.3X1	T51.3X2	T51.3X3	T51.3X4	—	—

Substance	Poisoning, Accidental (unintentional)	Poisoning, Intentional Self-harm	Poisoning, Assault	Poisoning, Undetermined	Adverse Effect	Under-dosing
Diethyl — *continued*						
carbonate	T52.8X1	T52.8X2	T52.8X3	T52.8X4	—	—
ether (vapor) — *see also* ether	T41.0X1	T41.0X2	T41.0X3	T41.0X4	T41.0X5	T41.0X6
oxide	T52.8X1	T52.8X2	T52.8X3	T52.8X4	—	—
propion	T50.5X1	T50.5X2	T50.5X3	T50.5X4	T50.5X5	T50.5X6
stilbestrol	T38.5X1	T38.5X2	T38.5X3	T38.5X4	T38.5X5	T38.5X6
toluamide (nonmedicinal)	T60.8X1	T60.8X2	T60.8X3	T60.8X4	—	—
medicinal	T49.3X1	T49.3X2	T49.3X3	T49.3X4	T49.3X5	T49.3X6
Diethylcarbamazine	T37.4X1	T37.4X2	T37.4X3	T37.4X4	T37.4X5	T37.4X6
Diethylene						
dioxide	T52.8X1	T52.8X2	T52.8X3	T52.8X4	—	—
glycol (monoacetate) (monobutyl ether) (monoethyl ether)	T52.3X1	T52.3X2	T52.3X3	T52.3X4	—	—
Diethylhexylphthalate	T65.891	T65.892	T65.893	T65.894	—	—
Diethylpropion	T50.5X1	T50.5X2	T50.5X3	T50.5X4	T50.5X5	T50.5X6
Diethylstilbestrol	T38.5X1	T38.5X2	T38.5X3	T38.5X4	T38.5X5	T38.5X6
Diethylstilboestrol	T38.5X1	T38.5X2	T38.5X3	T38.5X4	T38.5X5	T38.5X6
Diethylsulfone-diethylmethane	T42.6X1	T42.6X2	T42.6X3	T42.6X4	T42.6X5	T42.6X6
Diethyltoluamide	T49.0X1	T49.0X2	T49.0X3	T49.0X4	T49.0X5	T49.0X6
Diethyltryptamine (DET)	T40.991	T40.992	T40.993	T40.994	—	—
Difebarbamate	T42.3X1	T42.3X2	T42.3X3	T42.3X4	T42.3X5	T42.3X6
Difencloxazine	T40.2X1	T40.2X2	T40.2X3	T40.2X4	T40.2X5	T40.2X6
Difenidol	T45.0X1	T45.0X2	T45.0X3	T45.0X4	T45.0X5	T45.0X6
Difenoxin	T47.6X1	T47.6X2	T47.6X3	T47.6X4	T47.6X5	T47.6X6
Difetarsone	T37.3X1	T37.3X2	T37.3X3	T37.3X4	T37.3X5	T37.3X6
Diffusin	T45.3X1	T45.3X2	T45.3X3	T45.3X4	T45.3X5	T45.3X6
Diflorasone	T49.0X1	T49.0X2	T49.0X3	T49.0X4	T49.0X5	T49.0X6
Diflos	T44.0X1	T44.0X2	T44.0X3	T44.0X4	T44.0X5	T44.0X6
Diflubenzuron	T60.1X1	T60.1X2	T60.1X3	T60.1X4	—	—
Diflucortolone	T49.0X1	T49.0X2	T49.0X3	T49.0X4	T49.0X5	T49.0X6
Diflunisal	T39.091	T39.092	T39.093	T39.094	T39.095	T39.096
Difluoromethyldopa	T42.8X1	T42.8X2	T42.8X3	T42.8X4	T42.8X5	T42.8X6
Difluorophate	T44.0X1	T44.0X2	T44.0X3	T44.0X4	T44.0X5	T44.0X6
Digestant NEC	T47.5X1	T47.5X2	T47.5X3	T47.5X4	T47.5X5	T47.5X6
Digitalin (e)	T46.0X1	T46.0X2	T46.0X3	T46.0X4	T46.0X5	T46.0X6
Digitalis (leaf)(glycoside)	T46.0X1	T46.0X2	T46.0X3	T46.0X4	T46.0X5	T46.0X6
lanata	T46.0X1	T46.0X2	T46.0X3	T46.0X4	T46.0X5	T46.0X6
purpurea	T46.0X1	T46.0X2	T46.0X3	T46.0X4	T46.0X5	T46.0X6
Digitoxin	T46.0X1	T46.0X2	T46.0X3	T46.0X4	T46.0X5	T46.0X6
Digitoxose	T46.0X1	T46.0X2	T46.0X3	T46.0X4	T46.0X5	T46.0X6
Digoxin	T46.0X1	T46.0X2	T46.0X3	T46.0X4	T46.0X5	T46.0X6
Digoxine	T46.0X1	T46.0X2	T46.0X3	T46.0X4	T46.0X5	T46.0X6
Dihydralazine	T46.5X1	T46.5X2	T46.5X3	T46.5X4	T46.5X5	T46.5X6
Dihydrazine	T46.5X1	T46.5X2	T46.5X3	T46.5X4	T46.5X5	T46.5X6
Dihydrocodeine	T40.2X1	T40.2X2	T40.2X3	T40.2X4	T40.2X5	T40.2X6
Dihydrocodeinone	T40.2X1	T40.2X2	T40.2X3	T40.2X4	T40.2X5	T40.2X6
Dihydroergocornine	T46.7X1	T46.7X2	T46.7X3	T46.7X4	T46.7X5	T46.7X6
Dihydroergocristine (mesilate)	T46.7X1	T46.7X2	T46.7X3	T46.7X4	T46.7X5	T46.7X6
Dihydroergokryptine	T46.7X1	T46.7X2	T46.7X3	T46.7X4	T46.7X5	T46.7X6
Dihydroergotamine	T46.5X1	T46.5X2	T46.5X3	T46.5X4	T46.5X5	T46.5X6
Dihydroergotoxine	T46.7X1	T46.7X2	T46.7X3	T46.7X4	T46.7X5	T46.7X6
mesilate	T46.7X1	T46.7X2	T46.7X3	T46.7X4	T46.7X5	T46.7X6
Dihydrohydroxycodeinone	T40.2X1	T40.2X2	T40.2X3	T40.2X4	T40.2X5	T40.2X6
Dihydrohydroxymorphinone	T40.2X1	T40.2X2	T40.2X3	T40.2X4	T40.2X5	T40.2X6
Dihydroisocodeine	T40.2X1	T40.2X2	T40.2X3	T40.2X4	T40.2X5	T40.2X6
Dihydromorphine	T40.2X1	T40.2X2	T40.2X3	T40.2X4	—	—
Dihydromorphinone	T40.2X1	T40.2X2	T40.2X3	T40.2X4	T40.2X5	T40.2X6
Dihydrostreptomycin	T36.5X1	T36.5X2	T36.5X3	T36.5X4	T36.5X5	T36.5X6
Dihydrotachysterol	T45.2X1	T45.2X2	T45.2X3	T45.2X4	T45.2X5	T45.2X6
Dihydroxyaluminum aminoacetate	T47.1X1	T47.1X2	T47.1X3	T47.1X4	T47.1X5	T47.1X6
Dihydroxyaluminum sodium carbonate	T47.1X1	T47.1X2	T47.1X3	T47.1X4	T47.1X5	T47.1X6
Dihydroxyanthraquinone	T47.2X1	T47.2X2	T47.2X3	T47.2X4	T47.2X5	T47.2X6
Dihydroxycodeinone	T40.2X1	T40.2X2	T40.2X3	T40.2X4	T40.2X5	T40.2X6
Dihydroxypropyl theophylline	T50.2X1	T50.2X2	T50.2X3	T50.2X4	T50.2X5	T50.2X6
Diiodohydroxyquin	T37.8X1	T37.8X2	T37.8X3	T37.8X4	T37.8X5	T37.8X6
topical	T49.0X1	T49.0X2	T49.0X3	T49.0X4	T49.0X5	T49.0X6
Diiodohydroxyquinoline	T37.8X1	T37.8X2	T37.8X3	T37.8X4	T37.8X5	T37.8X6
Diiodotyrosine	T38.2X1	T38.2X2	T38.2X3	T38.2X4	T38.2X5	T38.2X6
Diisopromine	T44.3X1	T44.3X2	T44.3X3	T44.3X4	T44.3X5	T44.3X6
Diisopropylamine	T46.3X1	T46.3X2	T46.3X3	T46.3X4	T46.3X5	T46.3X6
Diisopropylfluorophosphonate	T44.0X1	T44.0X2	T44.0X3	T44.0X4	T44.0X5	T44.0X6
Dilantin	T42.0X1	T42.0X2	T42.0X3	T42.0X4	T42.0X5	T42.0X6
Dilaudid	T40.2X1	T40.2X2	T40.2X3	T40.2X4	T40.2X5	T40.2X6
Dilazep	T46.3X1	T46.3X2	T46.3X3	T46.3X4	T46.3X5	T46.3X6
Dill	T47.5X1	T47.5X2	T47.5X3	T47.5X4	T47.5X5	T47.5X6
Diloxanide	T37.3X1	T37.3X2	T37.3X3	T37.3X4	T37.3X5	T37.3X6
Diltiazem	T46.1X1	T46.1X2	T46.1X3	T46.1X4	T46.1X5	T46.1X6

354

Additional Character May Be Required — Refer to the Tabular List for Character Selection   ▽ Subterms under main terms may continue to next column or page

Substance	Poisoning, Accidental (unintentional)	Poisoning, Intentional Self-harm	Poisoning, Assault	Poisoning, Undetermined	Adverse Effect	Underdosing
Dimazole	T49.0X1	T49.0X2	T49.0X3	T49.0X4	T49.0X5	T49.0X6
Dimefline	T50.7X1	T50.7X2	T50.7X3	T50.7X4	T50.7X5	T50.7X6
Dimefox	T60.0X1	T60.0X2	T60.0X3	T60.0X4	—	—
Dimemorfan	T48.3X1	T48.3X2	T48.3X3	T48.3X4	T48.3X5	T48.3X6
Dimenhydrinate	T45.0X1	T45.0X2	T45.0X3	T45.0X4	T45.0X5	T45.0X6
Dimercaprol (British anti-lewisite)	T45.8X1	T45.8X2	T45.8X3	T45.8X4	T45.8X5	T45.8X6
Dimercaptopropanol	T45.8X1	T45.8X2	T45.8X3	T45.8X4	T45.8X5	T45.8X6
Dimestrol	T38.5X1	T38.5X2	T38.5X3	T38.5X4	T38.5X5	T38.5X6
Dimetane	T45.0X1	T45.0X2	T45.0X3	T45.0X4	T45.0X5	T45.0X6
Dimethicone	T47.1X1	T47.1X2	T47.1X3	T47.1X4	T47.1X5	T47.1X6
Dimethindene	T45.0X1	T45.0X2	T45.0X3	T45.0X4	T45.0X5	T45.0X6
Dimethisoquin	T49.1X1	T49.1X2	T49.1X3	T49.1X4	T49.1X5	T49.1X6
Dimethisterone	T38.5X1	T38.5X2	T38.5X3	T38.5X4	T38.5X5	T38.5X6
Dimethoate	T60.0X1	T60.0X2	T60.0X3	T60.0X4	—	—
Dimethocaine	T41.3X1	T41.3X2	T41.3X3	T41.3X4	T41.3X5	T41.3X6
Dimethoxanate	T48.3X1	T48.3X2	T48.3X3	T48.3X4	T48.3X5	T48.3X6
Dimethyl						
arsine, arsinic acid	T57.0X1	T57.0X2	T57.0X3	T57.0X4	—	—
carbinol	T51.2X1	T51.2X2	T51.2X3	T51.2X4	—	—
carbonate	T52.8X1	T52.8X2	T52.8X3	T52.8X4	—	—
diguanide	T38.3X1	T38.3X2	T38.3X3	T38.3X4	T38.3X5	T38.3X6
ketone	T52.4X1	T52.4X2	T52.4X3	T52.4X4	—	—
vapor	T52.4X1	T52.4X2	T52.4X3	T52.4X4	—	—
meperidine	T40.2X1	T40.2X2	T40.2X3	T40.2X4	T40.2X5	T40.2X6
parathion	T60.0X1	T60.0X2	T60.0X3	T60.0X4	—	—
phthlate	T49.3X1	T49.3X2	T49.3X3	T49.3X4	T49.3X5	T49.3X6
polysiloxane	T47.8X1	T47.8X2	T47.8X3	T47.8X4	T47.8X5	T47.8X6
sulfate (fumes)	T59.891	T59.892	T59.893	T59.894	—	—
liquid	T65.891	T65.892	T65.893	T65.894	—	—
sulfoxide (nonmedicinal)	T52.8X1	T52.8X2	T52.8X3	T52.8X4	—	—
medicinal	T49.4X1	T49.4X2	T49.4X3	T49.4X4	T49.4X5	T49.4X6
tryptamine	T40.991	T40.992	T40.993	T40.994	—	—
tubocurarine	T48.1X1	T48.1X2	T48.1X3	T48.1X4	T48.1X5	T48.1X6
Dimethylamine sulfate	T49.4X1	T49.4X2	T49.4X3	T49.4X4	T49.4X5	T49.4X6
Dimethylformamide	T52.8X1	T52.8X2	T52.8X3	T52.8X4	—	—
Dimethyltubocurarinium chloride	T48.1X1	T48.1X2	T48.1X3	T48.1X4	T48.1X5	T48.1X6
Dimeticone	T47.1X1	T47.1X2	T47.1X3	T47.1X4	T47.1X5	T47.1X6
Dimetilan	T60.0X1	T60.0X2	T60.0X3	T60.0X4	—	—
Dimetindene	T45.0X1	T45.0X2	T45.0X3	T45.0X4	T45.0X5	T45.0X6
Dimetotiazine	T43.3X1	T43.3X2	T43.3X3	T43.3X4	T43.3X5	T43.3X6
Dimorpholamine	T50.7X1	T50.7X2	T50.7X3	T50.7X4	T50.7X5	T50.7X6
Dimoxyline	T46.3X1	T46.3X2	T46.3X3	T46.3X4	T46.3X5	T46.3X6
Dinitrobenzene	T65.3X1	T65.3X2	T65.3X3	T65.3X4	—	—
vapor	T59.891	T59.892	T59.893	T59.894	—	—
Dinitrobenzol	T65.3X1	T65.3X2	T65.3X3	T65.3X4	—	—
vapor	T59.891	T59.892	T59.893	T59.894	—	—
Dinitrobutylphenol	T65.3X1	T65.3X2	T65.3X3	T65.3X4	—	—
Dinitro (-ortho-)cresol (pesticide) (spray)	T65.3X1	T65.3X2	T65.3X3	T65.3X4	—	—
Dinitrocyclohexylphenol	T65.3X1	T65.3X2	T65.3X3	T65.3X4	—	—
Dinitrophenol	T65.3X1	T65.3X2	T65.3X3	T65.3X4	—	—
Dinoprost	T48.0X1	T48.0X2	T48.0X3	T48.0X4	T48.0X5	T48.0X6
Dinoprostone	T48.0X1	T48.0X2	T48.0X3	T48.0X4	T48.0X5	T48.0X6
Dinoseb	T60.3X1	T60.3X2	T60.3X3	T60.3X4	—	—
Dioctyl sulfosuccinate (calcium) (sodium)	T47.4X1	T47.4X2	T47.4X3	T47.4X4	T47.4X5	T47.4X6
Diodone	T50.8X1	T50.8X2	T50.8X3	T50.8X4	T50.8X5	T50.8X6
Diodoquin	T37.8X1	T37.8X2	T37.8X3	T37.8X4	T37.8X5	T37.8X6
Dionin	T40.2X1	T40.2X2	T40.2X3	T40.2X4	T40.2X5	T40.2X6
Diosmin	T46.991	T46.992	T46.993	T46.994	T46.995	T46.996
Dioxane	T52.8X1	T52.8X2	T52.8X3	T52.8X4	—	—
Dioxathion	T60.0X1	T60.0X2	T60.0X3	T60.0X4	—	—
Dioxin	T53.7X1	T53.7X2	T53.7X3	T53.7X4	—	—
Dioxopromethazine	T43.3X1	T43.3X2	T43.3X3	T43.3X4	T43.3X5	T43.3X6
Dioxyline	T46.3X1	T46.3X2	T46.3X3	T46.3X4	T46.3X5	T46.3X6
Dipentene	T52.8X1	T52.8X2	T52.8X3	T52.8X4	—	—
Diperodon	T41.3X1	T41.3X2	T41.3X3	T41.3X4	T41.3X5	T41.3X6
Diphacinone	T60.4X1	T60.4X2	T60.4X3	T60.4X4	—	—
Diphemanil	T44.3X1	T44.3X2	T44.3X3	T44.3X4	T44.3X5	T44.3X6
metilsulfate	T44.3X1	T44.3X2	T44.3X3	T44.3X4	T44.3X5	T44.3X6
Diphenadione	T45.511	T45.512	T45.513	T45.514	T45.515	T45.516
rodenticide	T60.4X1	T60.4X2	T60.4X3	T60.4X4	—	—
Diphenhydramine	T45.0X1	T45.0X2	T45.0X3	T45.0X4	T45.0X5	T45.0X6
Diphenidol	T45.0X1	T45.0X2	T45.0X3	T45.0X4	T45.0X5	T45.0X6
Diphenoxylate	T47.6X1	T47.6X2	T47.6X3	T47.6X4	T47.6X5	T47.6X6
Diphenylamine	T65.3X1	T65.3X2	T65.3X3	T65.3X4	—	—
Diphenylbutazone	T39.2X1	T39.2X2	T39.2X3	T39.2X4	T39.2X5	T39.2X6
Diphenylchloroarsine, not in war	T57.0X1	T57.0X2	T57.0X3	T57.0X4	—	—
Diphenylhydantoin	T42.0X1	T42.0X2	T42.0X3	T42.0X4	T42.0X5	T42.0X6
Diphenylmethane dye	T52.1X1	T52.1X2	T52.1X3	T52.1X4	—	—

Substance	Poisoning, Accidental (unintentional)	Poisoning, Intentional Self-harm	Poisoning, Assault	Poisoning, Undetermined	Adverse Effect	Underdosing
Diphenylpyraline	T45.0X1	T45.0X2	T45.0X3	T45.0X4	T45.0X5	T45.0X6
Diphtheria						
antitoxin	T50.Z11	T50.Z12	T50.Z13	T50.Z14	T50.Z15	T50.Z16
toxoid	T50.A91	T50.A92	T50.A93	T50.A94	T50.A95	T50.A96
with tetanus toxoid	T50.A21	T50.A22	T50.A23	T50.A24	T50.A25	T50.A26
with pertussis component	T50.A11	T50.A12	T50.A13	T50.A14	T50.A15	T50.A16
vaccine	T50.A91	T50.A92	T50.A93	T50.A94	T50.A95	T50.A96
combination						
without pertussis	T50.A21	T50.A22	T50.A23	T50.A24	T50.A25	T50.A26
including pertussis	T50.A11	T50.A12	T50.A13	T50.A14	T50.A15	T50.A16
Diphylline	T50.2X1	T50.2X2	T50.2X3	T50.2X4	T50.2X5	T50.2X6
Dipipanone	T40.4X1	T40.4X2	T40.4X3	T40.4X4	—	—
Dipivefrine	T49.5X1	T49.5X2	T49.5X3	T49.5X4	T49.5X5	T49.5X6
Diplovax	T50.B91	T50.B92	T50.B93	T50.B94	T50.B95	T50.B96
Diprophylline	T50.2X1	T50.2X2	T50.2X3	T50.2X4	T50.2X5	T50.2X6
Dipropyline	T48.291	T48.292	T48.293	T48.294	T48.295	T48.296
Dipyridamole	T46.3X1	T46.3X2	T46.3X3	T46.3X4	T46.3X5	T46.3X6
Dipyrone	T39.2X1	T39.2X2	T39.2X3	T39.2X4	T39.2X5	T39.2X6
Diquat (dibromide)	T60.3X1	T60.3X2	T60.3X3	T60.3X4	—	—
Disinfectant	T65.891	T65.892	T65.893	T65.894	—	—
alkaline	T54.3X1	T54.3X2	T54.3X3	T54.3X4	—	—
aromatic	T54.1X1	T54.1X2	T54.1X3	T54.1X4	—	—
intestinal	T37.8X1	T37.8X2	T37.8X3	T37.8X4	T37.8X5	T37.8X6
Disipal	T42.8X1	T42.8X2	T42.8X3	T42.8X4	T42.8X5	T42.8X6
Disodium edetate	T50.6X1	T50.6X2	T50.6X3	T50.6X4	T50.6X5	T50.6X6
Disoprofol	T41.291	T41.292	T41.293	T41.294	T41.295	T41.296
Disopyramide	T46.2X1	T46.2X2	T46.2X3	T46.2X4	T46.2X5	T46.2X6
Distigmine (bromide)	T44.0X1	T44.0X2	T44.0X3	T44.0X4	T44.0X5	T44.0X6
Disulfamide	T50.2X1	T50.2X2	T50.2X3	T50.2X4	T50.2X5	T50.2X6
Disulfanilamide	T37.0X1	T37.0X2	T37.0X3	T37.0X4	T37.0X5	T37.0X6
Disulfiram	T50.6X1	T50.6X2	T50.6X3	T50.6X4	T50.6X5	T50.6X6
Disulfoton	T60.0X1	T60.0X2	T60.0X3	T60.0X4	—	—
Dithiazanine iodide	T37.4X1	T37.4X2	T37.4X3	T37.4X4	T37.4X5	T37.4X6
Dithiocarbamate	T60.0X1	T60.0X2	T60.0X3	T60.0X4	—	—
Dithranol	T49.4X1	T49.4X2	T49.4X3	T49.4X4	T49.4X5	T49.4X6
Diucardin	T50.2X1	T50.2X2	T50.2X3	T50.2X4	T50.2X5	T50.2X6
Diupres	T50.2X1	T50.2X2	T50.2X3	T50.2X4	T50.2X5	T50.2X6
Diuretic NEC	T50.2X1	T50.2X2	T50.2X3	T50.2X4	T50.2X5	T50.2X6
benzothiadiazine	T50.2X1	T50.2X2	T50.2X3	T50.2X4	T50.2X5	T50.2X6
carbonic acid anhydrase inhibitors	T50.2X1	T50.2X2	T50.2X3	T50.2X4	T50.2X5	T50.2X6
furfuryl NEC	T50.2X1	T50.2X2	T50.2X3	T50.2X4	T50.2X5	T50.2X6
loop (high-ceiling)	T50.1X1	T50.1X2	T50.1X3	T50.1X4	T50.1X5	T50.1X6
mercurial NEC	T50.2X1	T50.2X2	T50.2X3	T50.2X4	T50.2X5	T50.2X6
osmotic	T50.2X1	T50.2X2	T50.2X3	T50.2X4	T50.2X5	T50.2X6
purine NEC	T50.2X1	T50.2X2	T50.2X3	T50.2X4	T50.2X5	T50.2X6
saluretic NEC	T50.2X1	T50.2X2	T50.2X3	T50.2X4	T50.2X5	T50.2X6
sulfonamide	T50.2X1	T50.2X2	T50.2X3	T50.2X4	T50.2X5	T50.2X6
thiazide NEC	T50.2X1	T50.2X2	T50.2X3	T50.2X4	T50.2X5	T50.2X6
xanthine	T50.2X1	T50.2X2	T50.2X3	T50.2X4	T50.2X5	T50.2X6
Diurgin	T50.2X1	T50.2X2	T50.2X3	T50.2X4	T50.2X5	T50.2X6
Diuril	T50.2X1	T50.2X2	T50.2X3	T50.2X4	T50.2X5	T50.2X6
Diuron	T60.3X1	T60.3X2	T60.3X3	T60.3X4	—	—
Divalproex	T42.6X1	T42.6X2	T42.6X3	T42.6X4	T42.6X5	T42.6X6
Divinyl ether	T41.0X1	T41.0X2	T41.0X3	T41.0X4	T41.0X5	T41.0X6
Dixanthogen	T49.0X1	T49.0X2	T49.0X3	T49.0X4	T49.0X5	T49.0X6
Dixyrazine	T43.3X1	T43.3X2	T43.3X3	T43.3X4	T43.3X5	T43.3X6
D-lysergic acid diethylamide	T40.8X1	T40.8X2	T40.8X3	T40.8X4	—	—
DMCT	T36.4X1	T36.4X2	T36.4X3	T36.4X4	T36.4X5	T36.4X6
DMSO — see Dimethyl sulfoxide						
DNBP	T60.3X1	T60.3X2	T60.3X3	T60.3X4	—	—
DNOC	T65.3X1	T65.3X2	T65.3X3	T65.3X4	—	—
Dobutamine	T44.5X1	T44.5X2	T44.5X3	T44.5X4	T44.5X5	T44.5X6
DOCA	T38.0X1	T38.0X2	T38.0X3	T38.0X4	T38.0X5	T38.0X6
Docusate sodium	T47.4X1	T47.4X2	T47.4X3	T47.4X4	T47.4X5	T47.4X6
Dodicin	T49.0X1	T49.0X2	T49.0X3	T49.0X4	T49.0X5	T49.0X6
Dofamium chloride	T49.0X1	T49.0X2	T49.0X3	T49.0X4	T49.0X5	T49.0X6
Dolophine	T40.3X1	T40.3X2	T40.3X3	T40.3X4	T40.3X5	T40.3X6
Doloxene	T39.8X1	T39.8X2	T39.8X3	T39.8X4	T39.8X5	T39.8X6
Domestic gas (after combustion) — see Gas, utility						
prior to combustion	T59.891	T59.892	T59.893	T59.894	—	—
Domiodol	T48.4X1	T48.4X2	T48.4X3	T48.4X4	T48.4X5	T48.4X6
Domiphen (bromide)	T49.0X1	T49.0X2	T49.0X3	T49.0X4	T49.0X5	T49.0X6
Domperidone	T45.0X1	T45.0X2	T45.0X3	T45.0X4	T45.0X5	T45.0X6
Dopa	T42.8X1	T42.8X2	T42.8X3	T42.8X4	T42.8X5	T42.8X6
Dopamine	T44.991	T44.992	T44.993	T44.994	T44.995	T44.996
Doriden	T42.6X1	T42.6X2	T42.6X3	T42.6X4	T42.6X5	T42.6X6
Dormiral	T42.3X1	T42.3X2	T42.3X3	T42.3X4	T42.3X5	T42.3X6
Dormison	T42.6X1	T42.6X2	T42.6X3	T42.6X4	T42.6X5	T42.6X6
Dornase	T48.4X1	T48.4X2	T48.4X3	T48.4X4	T48.4X5	T48.4X6

Substance	Poisoning, Accidental (unintentional)	Poisoning, Intentional Self-harm	Poisoning, Assault	Poisoning, Undetermined	Adverse Effect	Under-dosing
Dorsacaine	T41.3X1	T41.3X2	T41.3X3	T41.3X4	T41.3X5	T41.3X6
Dosulepin	T43.011	T43.012	T43.013	T43.014	T43.015	T43.016
Dothiepin	T43.011	T43.012	T43.013	T43.014	T43.015	T43.016
Doxantrazole	T48.6X1	T48.6X2	T48.6X3	T48.6X4	T48.6X5	T48.6X6
Doxapram	T50.7X1	T50.7X2	T50.7X3	T50.7X4	T50.7X5	T50.7X6
Doxazosin	T44.6X1	T44.6X2	T44.6X3	T44.6X4	T44.6X5	T44.6X6
Doxepin	T43.011	T43.012	T43.013	T43.014	T43.015	T43.016
Doxifluridine	T45.1X1	T45.1X2	T45.1X3	T45.1X4	T45.1X5	T45.1X6
Doxorubicin	T45.1X1	T45.1X2	T45.1X3	T45.1X4	T45.1X5	T45.1X6
Doxycycline	T36.4X1	T36.4X2	T36.4X3	T36.4X4	T36.4X5	T36.4X6
Doxylamine	T45.0X1	T45.0X2	T45.0X3	T45.0X4	T45.0X5	T45.0X6
Dramamine	T45.0X1	T45.0X2	T45.0X3	T45.0X4	T45.0X5	T45.0X6
Drano (drain cleaner)	T54.3X1	T54.3X2	T54.3X3	T54.3X4	—	—
Dressing, live pulp	T49.7X1	T49.7X2	T49.7X3	T49.7X4	T49.7X5	T49.7X6
Drocode	T40.2X1	T40.2X2	T40.2X3	T40.2X4	T40.2X5	T40.2X6
Dromoran	T40.2X1	T40.2X2	T40.2X3	T40.2X4	T40.2X5	T40.2X6
Dromostanolone	T38.7X1	T38.7X2	T38.7X3	T38.7X4	T38.7X5	T38.7X6
Dronabinol	T40.7X1	T40.7X2	T40.7X3	T40.7X4	T40.7X5	T40.7X6
Droperidol	T43.591	T43.592	T43.593	T43.594	T43.595	T43.596
Dropropizine	T48.3X1	T48.3X2	T48.3X3	T48.3X4	T48.3X5	T48.3X6
Drostanolone	T38.7X1	T38.7X2	T38.7X3	T38.7X4	T38.7X5	T38.7X6
Drotaverine	T44.3X1	T44.3X2	T44.3X3	T44.3X4	T44.3X5	T44.3X6
Drotrecogin alfa	T45.511	T45.512	T45.513	T45.514	T45.515	T45.516
Drug NEC	T50.901	T50.902	T50.903	T50.904	T50.905	T50.906
specified NEC	T50.991	T50.992	T50.993	T50.994	T50.995	T50.996
DTIC	T45.1X1	T45.1X2	T45.1X3	T45.1X4	T45.1X5	T45.1X6
Duboisine	T44.3X1	T44.3X2	T44.3X3	T44.3X4	T44.3X5	T44.3X6
Dulcolax	T47.2X1	T47.2X2	T47.2X3	T47.2X4	T47.2X5	T47.2X6
Duponol (C) (EP)	T49.2X1	T49.2X2	T49.2X3	T49.2X4	T49.2X5	T49.2X6
Durabolin	T38.7X1	T38.7X2	T38.7X3	T38.7X4	T38.7X5	T38.7X6
Dyclone	T41.3X1	T41.3X2	T41.3X3	T41.3X4	T41.3X5	T41.3X6
Dyclonine	T41.3X1	T41.3X2	T41.3X3	T41.3X4	T41.3X5	T41.3X6
Dydrogesterone	T38.5X1	T38.5X2	T38.5X3	T38.5X4	T38.5X5	T38.5X6
Dye NEC	T65.6X1	T65.6X2	T65.6X3	T65.6X4	—	—
antiseptic	T49.0X1	T49.0X2	T49.0X3	T49.0X4	T49.0X5	T49.0X6
diagnostic agents	T50.8X1	T50.8X2	T50.8X3	T50.8X4	T50.8X5	T50.8X6
pharmaceutical NEC	T50.901	T50.902	T50.903	T50.904	T50.905	T50.906
Dyflos	T44.0X1	T44.0X2	T44.0X3	T44.0X4	T44.0X5	T44.0X6
Dymelor	T38.3X1	T38.3X2	T38.3X3	T38.3X4	T38.3X5	T38.3X6
Dynamite	T65.3X1	T65.3X2	T65.3X3	T65.3X4	—	—
fumes	T59.891	T59.892	T59.893	T59.894	—	—
Dyphylline	T44.3X1	T44.3X2	T44.3X3	T44.3X4	T44.3X5	T44.3X6
b-eucaine	T49.1X1	T49.1X2	T49.1X3	T49.1X4	T49.1X5	T49.1X6
Ear drug NEC	T49.6X1	T49.6X2	T49.6X3	T49.6X4	T49.6X5	T49.6X6
Ear preparations	T49.6X1	T49.6X2	T49.6X3	T49.6X4	T49.6X5	T49.6X6
Echothiophate, echothiophate, ecothiophate	T49.5X1	T49.5X2	T49.5X3	T49.5X4	T49.5X5	T49.5X6
Econazole	T49.0X1	T49.0X2	T49.0X3	T49.0X4	T49.0X5	T49.0X6
Ecothiopate iodide	T49.5X1	T49.5X2	T49.5X3	T49.5X4	T49.5X5	T49.5X6
Ecstasy	T43.621	T43.622	T43.623	T43.624	T43.625	T43.626
Ectylurea	T42.6X1	T42.6X2	T42.6X3	T42.6X4	T42.6X5	T42.6X6
Edathamil disodium	T45.8X1	T45.8X2	T45.8X3	T45.8X4	T45.8X5	T45.8X6
Edecrin	T50.1X1	T50.1X2	T50.1X3	T50.1X4	T50.1X5	T50.1X6
Edetate, disodium (calcium)	T45.8X1	T45.8X2	T45.8X3	T45.8X4	T45.8X5	T45.8X6
Edoxudine	T49.5X1	T49.5X2	T49.5X3	T49.5X4	T49.5X5	T49.5X6
Edrophonium	T44.0X1	T44.0X2	T44.0X3	T44.0X4	T44.0X5	T44.0X6
chloride	T44.0X1	T44.0X2	T44.0X3	T44.0X4	T44.0X5	T44.0X6
EDTA	T50.6X1	T50.6X2	T50.6X3	T50.6X4	T50.6X5	T50.6X6
Eflornithine	T37.2X1	T37.2X2	T37.2X3	T37.2X4	T37.2X5	T37.2X6
Efloxate	T46.3X1	T46.3X2	T46.3X3	T46.3X4	T46.3X5	T46.3X6
Elase	T49.8X1	T49.8X2	T49.8X3	T49.8X4	T49.8X5	T49.8X6
Elastase	T47.5X1	T47.5X2	T47.5X3	T47.5X4	T47.5X5	T47.5X6
Elaterium	T47.2X1	T47.2X2	T47.2X3	T47.2X4	T47.2X5	T47.2X6
Elcatonin	T50.991	T50.992	T50.993	T50.994	T50.995	T50.996
Elder	T62.2X1	T62.2X2	T62.2X3	T62.2X4	—	—
berry, (unripe)	T62.1X1	T62.1X2	T62.1X3	T62.1X4	—	—
Electrolyte balance drug	T50.3X1	T50.3X2	T50.3X3	T50.3X4	T50.3X5	T50.3X6
Electrolytes NEC	T50.3X1	T50.3X2	T50.3X3	T50.3X4	T50.3X5	T50.3X6
Electrolytic agent NEC	T50.3X1	T50.3X2	T50.3X3	T50.3X4	T50.3X5	T50.3X6
Elemental diet	T50.901	T50.902	T50.903	T50.904	T50.905	T50.906
Elliptinium acetate	T45.1X1	T45.1X2	T45.1X3	T45.1X4	T45.1X5	T45.1X6
Embramine	T45.0X1	T45.0X2	T45.0X3	T45.0X4	T45.0X5	T45.0X6
Emepronium (salts)	T44.3X1	T44.3X2	T44.3X3	T44.3X4	T44.3X5	T44.3X6
bromide	T44.3X1	T44.3X2	T44.3X3	T44.3X4	T44.3X5	T44.3X6
Emetic NEC	T47.7X1	T47.7X2	T47.7X3	T47.7X4	T47.7X5	T47.7X6
Emetine	T37.3X1	T37.3X2	T37.3X3	T37.3X4	T37.3X5	T37.3X6
Emollient NEC	T49.3X1	T49.3X2	T49.3X3	T49.3X4	T49.3X5	T49.3X6
Emorfazone	T39.8X1	T39.8X2	T39.8X3	T39.8X4	T39.8X5	T39.8X6
Emylcamate	T43.591	T43.592	T43.593	T43.594	T43.595	T43.596
Enalapril	T46.4X1	T46.4X2	T46.4X3	T46.4X4	T46.4X5	T46.4X6
Enalaprilat	T46.4X1	T46.4X2	T46.4X3	T46.4X4	T46.4X5	T46.4X6
Encainide	T46.2X1	T46.2X2	T46.2X3	T46.2X4	T46.2X5	T46.2X6
Endocaine	T41.3X1	T41.3X2	T41.3X3	T41.3X4	T41.3X5	T41.3X6
Endosulfan	T60.2X1	T60.2X2	T60.2X3	T60.2X4	—	—
Endothall	T60.3X1	T60.3X2	T60.3X3	T60.3X4	—	—
Endralazine	T46.5X1	T46.5X2	T46.5X3	T46.5X4	T46.5X5	T46.5X6
Endrin	T60.1X1	T60.1X2	T60.1X3	T60.1X4	—	—
Enflurane	T41.0X1	T41.0X2	T41.0X3	T41.0X4	T41.0X5	T41.0X6
Enhexymal	T42.3X1	T42.3X2	T42.3X3	T42.3X4	T42.3X5	T42.3X6
Enocitabine	T45.1X1	T45.1X2	T45.1X3	T45.1X4	T45.1X5	T45.1X6
Enovid	T38.4X1	T38.4X2	T38.4X3	T38.4X4	T38.4X5	T38.4X6
Enoxacin	T36.8X1	T36.8X2	T36.8X3	T36.8X4	T36.8X5	T36.8X6
Enoxaparin (sodium)	T45.511	T45.512	T45.513	T45.514	T45.515	T45.516
Enpiprazole	T43.591	T43.592	T43.593	T43.594	T43.595	T43.596
Enprofylline	T48.6X1	T48.6X2	T48.6X3	T48.6X4	T48.6X5	T48.6X6
Enprostil	T47.1X1	T47.1X2	T47.1X3	T47.1X4	T47.1X5	T47.1X6
Enterogastrone	T38.891	T38.892	T38.893	T38.894	T38.895	T38.896
ENT preparations (anti-infectives)	T49.6X1	T49.6X2	T49.6X3	T49.6X4	T49.6X5	T49.6X6
Enviomycin	T36.8X1	T36.8X2	T36.8X3	T36.8X4	T36.8X5	T36.8X6
Enzodase	T45.3X1	T45.3X2	T45.3X3	T45.3X4	T45.3X5	T45.3X6
Enzyme NEC	T45.3X1	T45.3X2	T45.3X3	T45.3X4	T45.3X5	T45.3X6
depolymerizing	T49.8X1	T49.8X2	T49.8X3	T49.8X4	T49.8X5	T49.8X6
fibrolytic	T45.3X1	T45.3X2	T45.3X3	T45.3X4	T45.3X5	T45.3X6
gastric	T47.5X1	T47.5X2	T47.5X3	T47.5X4	T47.5X5	T47.5X6
intestinal	T47.5X1	T47.5X2	T47.5X3	T47.5X4	T47.5X5	T47.5X6
local action	T49.4X1	T49.4X2	T49.4X3	T49.4X4	T49.4X5	T49.4X6
proteolytic	T49.4X1	T49.4X2	T49.4X3	T49.4X4	T49.4X5	T49.4X6
thrombolytic	T45.3X1	T45.3X2	T45.3X3	T45.3X4	T45.3X5	T45.3X6
EPAB	T41.3X1	T41.3X2	T41.3X3	T41.3X4	T41.3X5	T41.3X6
Epanutin	T42.0X1	T42.0X2	T42.0X3	T42.0X4	T42.0X5	T42.0X6
Ephedra	T44.991	T44.992	T44.993	T44.994	T44.995	T44.996
Ephedrine	T44.991	T44.992	T44.993	T44.994	T44.995	T44.996
Epichlorhydrin, epichlorohydrin	T52.8X1	T52.8X2	T52.8X3	T52.8X4	—	—
Epicillin	T36.0X1	T36.0X2	T36.0X3	T36.0X4	T36.0X5	T36.0X6
Epiestriol	T38.5X1	T38.5X2	T38.5X3	T38.5X4	T38.5X5	T38.5X6
Epilim — see Sodium valproate						
Epimestrol	T38.5X1	T38.5X2	T38.5X3	T38.5X4	T38.5X5	T38.5X6
Epinephrine	T44.5X1	T44.5X2	T44.5X3	T44.5X4	T44.5X5	T44.5X6
Epirubicin	T45.1X1	T45.1X2	T45.1X3	T45.1X4	T45.1X5	T45.1X6
Epitiostanol	T38.7X1	T38.7X2	T38.7X3	T38.7X4	T38.7X5	T38.7X6
Epitizide	T50.2X1	T50.2X2	T50.2X3	T50.2X4	T50.2X5	T50.2X6
EPN	T60.0X1	T60.0X2	T60.0X3	T60.0X4	—	—
EPO	T45.8X1	T45.8X2	T45.8X3	T45.8X4	T45.8X5	T45.8X6
Epoetin alpha	T45.8X1	T45.8X2	T45.8X3	T45.8X4	T45.8X5	T45.8X6
Epomediol	T50.991	T50.992	T50.993	T50.994	T50.995	T50.996
Epoprostenol	T45.521	T45.522	T45.523	T45.524	T45.525	T45.526
Epoxy resin	T65.891	T65.892	T65.893	T65.894	—	—
Eprazinone	T48.4X1	T48.4X2	T48.4X3	T48.4X4	T48.4X5	T48.4X6
Epsilon aminocaproic acid	T45.621	T45.622	T45.623	T45.624	T45.625	T45.626
Epsom salt	T47.3X1	T47.3X2	T47.3X3	T47.3X4	T47.3X5	T47.3X6
Eptazocine	T40.4X1	T40.4X2	T40.4X3	T40.4X4	T40.4X5	T40.4X6
Equanil	T43.591	T43.592	T43.593	T43.594	T43.595	T43.596
Equisetum	T62.2X1	T62.2X2	T62.2X3	T62.2X4	—	—
diuretic	T50.2X1	T50.2X2	T50.2X3	T50.2X4	T50.2X5	T50.2X6
Ergobasine	T48.0X1	T48.0X2	T48.0X3	T48.0X4	T48.0X5	T48.0X6
Ergocalciferol	T45.2X1	T45.2X2	T45.2X3	T45.2X4	T45.2X5	T45.2X6
Ergoloid mesylates	T46.7X1	T46.7X2	T46.7X3	T46.7X4	T46.7X5	T46.7X6
Ergometrine	T48.0X1	T48.0X2	T48.0X3	T48.0X4	T48.0X5	T48.0X6
Ergonovine	T48.0X1	T48.0X2	T48.0X3	T48.0X4	T48.0X5	T48.0X6
Ergot NEC	T64.81	T64.82	T64.83	T64.84	—	—
derivative	T48.0X1	T48.0X2	T48.0X3	T48.0X4	T48.0X5	T48.0X6
medicinal (alkaloids)	T48.0X1	T48.0X2	T48.0X3	T48.0X4	T48.0X5	T48.0X6
prepared	T48.0X1	T48.0X2	T48.0X3	T48.0X4	T48.0X5	T48.0X6
Ergotamine	T46.5X1	T46.5X2	T46.5X3	T46.5X4	T46.5X5	T46.5X6
Ergotocine	T48.0X1	T48.0X2	T48.0X3	T48.0X4	T48.0X5	T48.0X6
Ergotrate	T48.0X1	T48.0X2	T48.0X3	T48.0X4	T48.0X5	T48.0X6
Eritrityl tetranitrate	T46.3X1	T46.3X2	T46.3X3	T46.3X4	T46.3X5	T46.3X6
Erythrityl tetranitrate	T46.3X1	T46.3X2	T46.3X3	T46.3X4	T46.3X5	T46.3X6
Erythrol tetranitrate	T46.3X1	T46.3X2	T46.3X3	T46.3X4	T46.3X5	T46.3X6
Erythromycin (salts)	T36.3X1	T36.3X2	T36.3X3	T36.3X4	T36.3X5	T36.3X6
ophthalmic preparation	T49.5X1	T49.5X2	T49.5X3	T49.5X4	T49.5X5	T49.5X6
topical NEC	T49.0X1	T49.0X2	T49.0X3	T49.0X4	T49.0X5	T49.0X6
Erythropoietin	T45.8X1	T45.8X2	T45.8X3	T45.8X4	T45.8X5	T45.8X6
human	T45.8X1	T45.8X2	T45.8X3	T45.8X4	T45.8X5	T45.8X6
Escin	T46.991	T46.992	T46.993	T46.994	T46.995	T46.996
Esculin	T45.2X1	T45.2X2	T45.2X3	T45.2X4	T45.2X5	T45.2X6
Esculoside	T45.2X1	T45.2X2	T45.2X3	T45.2X4	T45.2X5	T45.2X6
ESDT (ether-soluble tar distillate)	T49.1X1	T49.1X2	T49.1X3	T49.1X4	T49.1X5	T49.1X6
Eserine	T49.5X1	T49.5X2	T49.5X3	T49.5X4	T49.5X5	T49.5X6
Esflurbiprofen	T39.311	T39.312	T39.313	T39.314	T39.315	T39.316
Eskabarb	T42.3X1	T42.3X2	T42.3X3	T42.3X4	T42.3X5	T42.3X6
Eskalith	T43.8X1	T43.8X2	T43.8X3	T43.8X4	T43.8X5	T43.8X6
Esmolol	T44.7X1	T44.7X2	T44.7X3	T44.7X4	T44.7X5	T44.7X6

Substance	Poisoning, Accidental (unintentional)	Poisoning, Intentional Self-harm	Poisoning, Assault	Poisoning, Undetermined	Adverse Effect	Under-dosing
Estanozolol	T38.7X1	T38.7X2	T38.7X3	T38.7X4	T38.7X5	T38.7X6
Estazolam	T42.4X1	T42.4X2	T42.4X3	T42.4X4	T42.4X5	T42.4X6
Estradiol	T38.5X1	T38.5X2	T38.5X3	T38.5X4	T38.5X5	T38.5X6
with testosterone	T38.7X1	T38.7X2	T38.7X3	T38.7X4	T38.7X5	T38.7X6
benzoate	T38.5X1	T38.5X2	T38.5X3	T38.5X4	T38.5X5	T38.5X6
Estramustine	T45.1X1	T45.1X2	T45.1X3	T45.1X4	T45.1X5	T45.1X6
Estriol	T38.5X1	T38.5X2	T38.5X3	T38.5X4	T38.5X5	T38.5X6
Estrogen	T38.5X1	T38.5X2	T38.5X3	T38.5X4	T38.5X5	T38.5X6
with progesterone	T38.5X1	T38.5X2	T38.5X3	T38.5X4	T38.5X5	T38.5X6
conjugated	T38.5X1	T38.5X2	T38.5X3	T38.5X4	T38.5X5	T38.5X6
Estrone	T38.5X1	T38.5X2	T38.5X3	T38.5X4	T38.5X5	T38.5X6
Estropipate	T38.5X1	T38.5X2	T38.5X3	T38.5X4	T38.5X5	T38.5X6
Etacrynate sodium	T50.1X1	T50.1X2	T50.1X3	T50.1X4	T50.1X5	T50.1X6
Etacrynic acid	T50.1X1	T50.1X2	T50.1X3	T50.1X4	T50.1X5	T50.1X6
Etafedrine	T48.6X1	T48.6X2	T48.6X3	T48.6X4	T48.6X5	T48.6X6
Etafenone	T46.3X1	T46.3X2	T46.3X3	T46.3X4	T46.3X5	T46.3X6
Etambutol	T37.1X1	T37.1X2	T37.1X3	T37.1X4	T37.1X5	T37.1X6
Etamiphyllin	T48.6X1	T48.6X2	T48.6X3	T48.6X4	T48.6X5	T48.6X6
Etamivan	T50.7X1	T50.7X2	T50.7X3	T50.7X4	T50.7X5	T50.7X6
Etamsylate	T45.7X1	T45.7X2	T45.7X3	T45.7X4	T45.7X5	T45.7X6
Etebenecid	T50.4X1	T50.4X2	T50.4X3	T50.4X4	T50.4X5	T50.4X6
Ethacridine	T49.0X1	T49.0X2	T49.0X3	T49.0X4	T49.0X5	T49.0X6
Ethacrynic acid	T50.1X1	T50.1X2	T50.1X3	T50.1X4	T50.1X5	T50.1X6
Ethadione	T42.2X1	T42.2X2	T42.2X3	T42.2X4	T42.2X5	T42.2X6
Ethambutol	T37.1X1	T37.1X2	T37.1X3	T37.1X4	T37.1X5	T37.1X6
Ethamide	T50.2X1	T50.2X2	T50.2X3	T50.2X4	T50.2X5	T50.2X6
Ethamivan	T50.7X1	T50.7X2	T50.7X3	T50.7X4	T50.7X5	T50.7X6
Ethamsylate	T45.7X1	T45.7X2	T45.7X3	T45.7X4	T45.7X5	T45.7X6
Ethanol	T51.0X1	T51.0X2	T51.0X3	T51.0X4	—	—
beverage	T51.0X1	T51.0X2	T51.0X3	T51.0X4	—	—
Ethanolamine oleate	T46.8X1	T46.8X2	T46.8X3	T46.8X4	T46.8X5	T46.8X6
Ethaverine	T44.3X1	T44.3X2	T44.3X3	T44.3X4	T44.3X5	T44.3X6
Ethchlorvynol	T42.6X1	T42.6X2	T42.6X3	T42.6X4	T42.6X5	T42.6X6
Ethebenecid	T50.4X1	T50.4X2	T50.4X3	T50.4X4	T50.4X5	T50.4X6
Ether (vapor)	T41.0X1	T41.0X2	T41.0X3	T41.0X4	T41.0X5	T41.0X6
anesthetic	T41.0X1	T41.0X2	T41.0X3	T41.0X4	T41.0X5	T41.0X6
divinyl	T41.0X1	T41.0X2	T41.0X3	T41.0X4	T41.0X5	T41.0X6
ethyl (medicinal)	T41.0X1	T41.0X2	T41.0X3	T41.0X4	T41.0X5	T41.0X6
nonmedicinal	T52.8X1	T52.8X2	T52.8X3	T52.8X4	—	—
petroleum — see Ligroin						
solvent	T52.8X1	T52.8X2	T52.8X3	T52.8X4	—	—
Ethiazide	T50.2X1	T50.2X2	T50.2X3	T50.2X4	T50.2X5	T50.2X6
Ethidium chloride (vapor)	T59.891	T59.892	T59.893	T59.894		
Ethinamate	T42.6X1	T42.6X2	T42.6X3	T42.6X4	T42.6X5	T42.6X6
Ethinylestradiol, ethinyloestradiol	T38.5X1	T38.5X2	T38.5X3	T38.5X4	T38.5X5	T38.5X6
with						
levonorgestrel	T38.4X1	T38.4X2	T38.4X3	T38.4X4	T38.4X5	T38.4X6
norethisterone	T38.4X1	T38.4X2	T38.4X3	T38.4X4	T38.4X5	T38.4X6
Ethiodized oil (131 I)	T50.8X1	T50.8X2	T50.8X3	T50.8X4	T50.8X5	T50.8X6
Ethion	T60.0X1	T60.0X2	T60.0X3	T60.0X4		
Ethionamide	T37.1X1	T37.1X2	T37.1X3	T37.1X4	T37.1X5	T37.1X6
Ethioniamide	T37.1X1	T37.1X2	T37.1X3	T37.1X4	T37.1X5	T37.1X6
Ethisterone	T38.5X1	T38.5X2	T38.5X3	T38.5X4	T38.5X5	T38.5X6
Ethobral	T42.3X1	T42.3X2	T42.3X3	T42.3X4	T42.3X5	T42.3X6
Ethocaine (infiltration) (topical)	T41.3X1	T41.3X2	T41.3X3	T41.3X4	T41.3X5	T41.3X6
nerve block (peripheral) (plexus)	T41.3X1	T41.3X2	T41.3X3	T41.3X4	T41.3X5	T41.3X6
spinal	T41.3X1	T41.3X2	T41.3X3	T41.3X4	T41.3X5	T41.3X6
Ethoheptazine	T40.4X1	T40.4X2	T40.4X3	T40.4X4	T40.4X5	T40.4X6
Ethopropazine	T44.3X1	T44.3X2	T44.3X3	T44.3X4	T44.3X5	T44.3X6
Ethosuximide	T42.2X1	T42.2X2	T42.2X3	T42.2X4	T42.2X5	T42.2X6
Ethotoin	T42.0X1	T42.0X2	T42.0X3	T42.0X4	T42.0X5	T42.0X6
Ethoxazene	T37.91	T37.92	T37.93	T37.94	T37.95	T37.96
Ethoxazorutoside	T46.991	T46.992	T46.993	T46.994	T46.995	T46.996
Ethoxzolamide	T50.2X1	T50.2X2	T50.2X3	T50.2X4	T50.2X5	T50.2X6
Ethyl						
acetate	T52.8X1	T52.8X2	T52.8X3	T52.8X4	—	—
alcohol	T51.0X1	T51.0X2	T51.0X3	T51.0X4	—	—
beverage	T51.0X1	T51.0X2	T51.0X3	T51.0X4	—	—
aldehyde (vapor)	T59.891	T59.892	T59.893	T59.894	—	—
liquid	T52.8X1	T52.8X2	T52.8X3	T52.8X4	—	—
aminobenzoate	T41.3X1	T41.3X2	T41.3X3	T41.3X4	T41.3X5	T41.3X6
aminophenothiazine	T43.3X1	T43.3X2	T43.3X3	T43.3X4	T43.3X5	T43.3X6
benzoate	T52.8X1	T52.8X2	T52.8X3	T52.8X4	—	—
biscoumacetate	T45.511	T45.512	T45.513	T45.514	T45.515	T45.516
bromide (anesthetic)	T41.0X1	T41.0X2	T41.0X3	T41.0X4	T41.0X5	T41.0X6
carbamate	T45.1X1	T45.1X2	T45.1X3	T45.1X4	T45.1X5	T45.1X6
carbinol	T51.3X1	T51.3X2	T51.3X3	T51.3X4	—	—
carbonate	T52.8X1	T52.8X2	T52.8X3	T52.8X4	—	—
chaulmoograte	T37.1X1	T37.1X2	T37.1X3	T37.1X4	T37.1X5	T37.1X6
chloride (anesthetic)	T41.0X1	T41.0X2	T41.0X3	T41.0X4	T41.0X5	T41.0X6

Substance	Poisoning, Accidental (unintentional)	Poisoning, Intentional Self-harm	Poisoning, Assault	Poisoning, Undetermined	Adverse Effect	Under-dosing
Ethyl — continued						
chloride — continued						
anesthetic (local)	T41.3X1	T41.3X2	T41.3X3	T41.3X4	T41.3X5	T41.3X6
inhaled	T41.0X1	T41.0X2	T41.0X3	T41.0X4	T41.0X5	T41.0X6
local	T49.4X1	T49.4X2	T49.4X3	T49.4X4	T49.4X5	T49.4X6
solvent	T53.6X1	T53.6X2	T53.6X3	T53.6X4		
dibunate	T48.3X1	T48.3X2	T48.3X3	T48.3X4	T48.3X5	T48.3X6
dichloroarsine (vapor)	T57.0X1	T57.0X2	T57.0X3	T57.0X4		
estranol	T38.7X1	T38.7X2	T38.7X3	T38.7X4	T38.7X5	T38.7X6
ether — see also ether	T52.8X1	T52.8X2	T52.8X3	T52.8X4		
formate NEC (solvent)	T52.0X1	T52.0X2	T52.0X3	T52.0X4		
fumarate	T49.4X1	T49.4X2	T49.4X3	T49.4X4	T49.4X5	T49.4X6
hydroxyisobutyrate NEC (solvent)	T52.8X1	T52.8X2	T52.8X3	T52.8X4		
iodoacetate	T59.3X1	T59.3X2	T59.3X3	T59.3X4		
lactate NEC (solvent)	T52.8X1	T52.8X2	T52.8X3	T52.8X4		
loflazepate	T42.4X1	T42.4X2	T42.4X3	T42.4X4	T42.4X5	T42.4X6
mercuric chloride	T56.1X1	T56.1X2	T56.1X3	T56.1X4		
methylcarbinol	T51.8X1	T51.8X2	T51.8X3	T51.8X4		
morphine	T40.2X1	T40.2X2	T40.2X3	T40.2X4	T40.2X5	T40.2X6
noradrenaline	T48.6X1	T48.6X2	T48.6X3	T48.6X4	T48.6X5	T48.6X6
oxybutyrate NEC (solvent)	T52.8X1	T52.8X2	T52.8X3	T52.8X4		
Ethylene (gas)	T59.891	T59.892	T59.893	T59.894		
anesthetic (general)	T41.0X1	T41.0X2	T41.0X3	T41.0X4	T41.0X5	T41.0X6
chlorohydrin	T52.8X1	T52.8X2	T52.8X3	T52.8X4		
vapor	T53.6X1	T53.6X2	T53.6X3	T53.6X4		
dichloride	T52.8X1	T52.8X2	T52.8X3	T52.8X4		
vapor	T53.6X1	T53.6X2	T53.6X3	T53.6X4		
dinitrate	T52.3X1	T52.3X2	T52.3X3	T52.3X4		
glycol(s)	T52.8X1	T52.8X2	T52.8X3	T52.8X4		
dinitrate	T52.3X1	T52.3X2	T52.3X3	T52.3X4		
monobutyl ether	T52.3X1	T52.3X2	T52.3X3	T52.3X4		
imine	T54.1X1	T54.1X2	T54.1X3	T54.1X4		
oxide (fumigant) (nonmedicinal)	T59.891	T59.892	T59.893	T59.894		
medicinal	T49.0X1	T49.0X2	T49.0X3	T49.0X4	T49.0X5	T49.0X6
Ethylenediaminetetra-acetic acid	T50.6X1	T50.6X2	T50.6X3	T50.6X4	T50.6X5	T50.6X6
Ethylenediamine theophylline	T48.6X1	T48.6X2	T48.6X3	T48.6X4	T48.6X5	T48.6X6
Ethylenedinitrilotetra-acetate	T50.6X1	T50.6X2	T50.6X3	T50.6X4	T50.6X5	T50.6X6
Ethylestrenol	T38.7X1	T38.7X2	T38.7X3	T38.7X4	T38.7X5	T38.7X6
Ethylhydroxycellulose	T47.4X1	T47.4X2	T47.4X3	T47.4X4	T47.4X5	T47.4X6
Ethylidene						
chloride NEC	T53.6X1	T53.6X2	T53.6X3	T53.6X4		
diacetate	T60.3X1	T60.3X2	T60.3X3	T60.3X4	—	—
dicoumarin	T45.511	T45.512	T45.513	T45.514	T45.515	T45.516
dicoumarol	T45.511	T45.512	T45.513	T45.514	T45.515	T45.516
diethyl ether	T52.0X1	T52.0X2	T52.0X3	T52.0X4	—	—
Ethylmorphine	T40.2X1	T40.2X2	T40.2X3	T40.2X4	T40.2X5	T40.2X6
Ethylnorepinephrine	T48.6X1	T48.6X2	T48.6X3	T48.6X4	T48.6X5	T48.6X6
Ethylparachlorophen-oxyisobutyrate	T46.6X1	T46.6X2	T46.6X3	T46.6X4	T46.6X5	T46.6X6
Ethynodiol	T38.4X1	T38.4X2	T38.4X3	T38.4X4	T38.4X5	T38.4X6
with mestranol diacetate	T38.4X1	T38.4X2	T38.4X3	T38.4X4	T38.4X5	T38.4X6
Etidocaine	T41.3X1	T41.3X2	T41.3X3	T41.3X4	T41.3X5	T41.3X6
infiltration (subcutaneous)	T41.3X1	T41.3X2	T41.3X3	T41.3X4	T41.3X5	T41.3X6
nerve (peripheral) (plexus)	T41.3X1	T41.3X2	T41.3X3	T41.3X4	T41.3X5	T41.3X6
Etidronate	T50.991	T50.992	T50.993	T50.994	T50.995	T50.996
Etidronic acid (disodium salt)	T50.991	T50.992	T50.993	T50.994	T50.995	T50.996
Etifoxine	T42.6X1	T42.6X2	T42.6X3	T42.6X4	T42.6X5	T42.6X6
Etilefrine	T44.4X1	T44.4X2	T44.4X3	T44.4X4	T44.4X5	T44.4X6
Etilfen	T42.3X1	T42.3X2	T42.3X3	T42.3X4	T42.3X5	T42.3X6
Etinodiol	T38.4X1	T38.4X2	T38.4X3	T38.4X4	T38.4X5	T38.4X6
Etiroxate	T46.6X1	T46.6X2	T46.6X3	T46.6X4	T46.6X5	T46.6X6
Etizolam	T42.4X1	T42.4X2	T42.4X3	T42.4X4	T42.4X5	T42.4X6
Etodolac	T39.391	T39.392	T39.393	T39.394	T39.395	T39.396
Etofamide	T37.3X1	T37.3X2	T37.3X3	T37.3X4	T37.3X5	T37.3X6
Etofibrate	T46.6X1	T46.6X2	T46.6X3	T46.6X4	T46.6X5	T46.6X6
Etofylline	T46.7X1	T46.7X2	T46.7X3	T46.7X4	T46.7X5	T46.7X6
clofibrate	T46.6X1	T46.6X2	T46.6X3	T46.6X4	T46.6X5	T46.6X6
Etoglucid	T45.1X1	T45.1X2	T45.1X3	T45.1X4	T45.1X5	T45.1X6
Etomidate	T41.1X1	T41.1X2	T41.1X3	T41.1X4	T41.1X5	T41.1X6
Etomide	T39.8X1	T39.8X2	T39.8X3	T39.8X4	T39.8X5	T39.8X6
Etomidoline	T44.3X1	T44.3X2	T44.3X3	T44.3X4	T44.3X5	T44.3X6
Etoposide	T45.1X1	T45.1X2	T45.1X3	T45.1X4	T45.1X5	T45.1X6
Etorphine	T40.2X1	T40.2X2	T40.2X3	T40.2X4	T40.2X5	T40.2X6
Etoval	T42.3X1	T42.3X2	T42.3X3	T42.3X4	T42.3X5	T42.3X6
Etozolin	T50.1X1	T50.1X2	T50.1X3	T50.1X4	T50.1X5	T50.1X6
Etretinate	T50.991	T50.992	T50.993	T50.994	T50.995	T50.996
Etryptamine	T43.691	T43.692	T43.693	T43.694	T43.695	T43.696
Etybenzatropine	T44.3X1	T44.3X2	T44.3X3	T44.3X4	T44.3X5	T44.3X6

Substance	Poisoning, Accidental (unintentional)	Poisoning, Intentional Self-harm	Poisoning, Assault	Poisoning, Undetermined	Adverse Effect	Under-dosing
Etynodiol	T38.4X1	T38.4X2	T38.4X3	T38.4X4	T38.4X5	T38.4X6
Eucaine	T41.3X1	T41.3X2	T41.3X3	T41.3X4	T41.3X5	T41.3X6
Eucalyptus oil	T49.7X1	T49.7X2	T49.7X3	T49.7X4	T49.7X5	T49.7X6
Eucatropine	T49.5X1	T49.5X2	T49.5X3	T49.5X4	T49.5X5	T49.5X6
Eucodal	T40.2X1	T40.2X2	T40.2X3	T40.2X4	T40.2X5	T40.2X6
Euneryl	T42.3X1	T42.3X2	T42.3X3	T42.3X4	T42.3X5	T42.3X6
Euphthalmine	T44.3X1	T44.3X2	T44.3X3	T44.3X4	T44.3X5	T44.3X6
Eurax	T49.0X1	T49.0X2	T49.0X3	T49.0X4	T49.0X5	T49.0X6
Euresol	T49.4X1	T49.4X2	T49.4X3	T49.4X4	T49.4X5	T49.4X6
Euthroid	T38.1X1	T38.1X2	T38.1X3	T38.1X4	T38.1X5	T38.1X6
Evans blue	T50.8X1	T50.8X2	T50.8X3	T50.8X4	T50.8X5	T50.8X6
Evipal	T42.3X1	T42.3X2	T42.3X3	T42.3X4	T42.3X5	T42.3X6
sodium	T41.1X1	T41.1X2	T41.1X3	T41.1X4	T41.1X5	T41.1X6
Evipan	T42.3X1	T42.3X2	T42.3X3	T42.3X4	T42.3X5	T42.3X6
sodium	T41.1X1	T41.1X2	T41.1X3	T41.1X4	T41.1X5	T41.1X6
Exalamide	T49.0X1	T49.0X2	T49.0X3	T49.0X4	T49.0X5	T49.0X6
Exalgin	T39.1X1	T39.1X2	T39.1X3	T39.1X4	T39.1X5	T39.1X6
Excipients, pharmaceutical	T50.901	T50.902	T50.903	T50.904	T50.905	T50.906
Exhaust gas (engine) (motor vehicle)	T58.01	T58.02	T58.03	T58.04	—	—
Ex-Lax (phenolphthalein)	T47.2X1	T47.2X2	T47.2X3	T47.2X4	T47.2X5	T47.2X6
Expectorant NEC	T48.4X1	T48.4X2	T48.4X3	T48.4X4	T48.4X5	T48.4X6
Extended insulin zinc suspension	T38.3X1	T38.3X2	T38.3X3	T38.3X4	T38.3X5	T38.3X6
External medications (skin) (mucous membrane)	T49.91	T49.92	T49.93	T49.94	T49.95	T49.96
dental agent	T49.7X1	T49.7X2	T49.7X3	T49.7X4	T49.7X5	T49.7X6
ENT agent	T49.6X1	T49.6X2	T49.6X3	T49.6X4	T49.6X5	T49.6X6
ophthalmic preparation	T49.5X1	T49.5X2	T49.5X3	T49.5X4	T49.5X5	T49.5X6
specified NEC	T49.8X1	T49.8X2	T49.8X3	T49.8X4	T49.8X5	T49.8X6
Extrapyramidal antagonist NEC	T44.3X1	T44.3X2	T44.3X3	T44.3X4	T44.3X5	T44.3X6
Eye agents (anti-infective)	T49.5X1	T49.5X2	T49.5X3	T49.5X4	T49.5X5	T49.5X6
Eye drug NEC	T49.5X1	T49.5X2	T49.5X3	T49.5X4	T49.5X5	T49.5X6
FAC (fluorouracil + doxorubicin + cyclophosphamide)	T45.1X1	T45.1X2	T45.1X3	T45.1X4	T45.1X5	T45.1X6
Factor						
I (fibrinogen)	T45.8X1	T45.8X2	T45.8X3	T45.8X4	T45.8X5	T45.8X6
III (thromboplastin)	T45.8X1	T45.8X2	T45.8X3	T45.8X4	T45.8X5	T45.8X6
VIII (antihemophilic Factor) (concentrate)	T45.8X1	T45.8X2	T45.8X3	T45.8X4	T45.8X5	T45.8X6
IX complex	T45.7X1	T45.7X2	T45.7X3	T45.7X4	T45.7X5	T45.7X6
human	T45.8X1	T45.8X2	T45.8X3	T45.8X4	T45.8X5	T45.8X6
Famotidine	T47.0X1	T47.0X2	T47.0X3	T47.0X4	T47.0X5	T47.0X6
Fat suspension, intravenous	T50.991	T50.992	T50.993	T50.994	T50.995	T50.996
Fazadinium bromide	T48.1X1	T48.1X2	T48.1X3	T48.1X4	T48.1X5	T48.1X6
Febarbamate	T42.3X1	T42.3X2	T42.3X3	T42.3X4	T42.3X5	T42.3X6
Fecal softener	T47.4X1	T47.4X2	T47.4X3	T47.4X4	T47.4X5	T47.4X6
Fedrilate	T48.3X1	T48.3X2	T48.3X3	T48.3X4	T48.3X5	T48.3X6
Felodipine	T46.1X1	T46.1X2	T46.1X3	T46.1X4	T46.1X5	T46.1X6
Felypressin	T38.891	T38.892	T38.893	T38.894	T38.895	T38.896
Femoxetine	T43.221	T43.222	T43.223	T43.224	T43.225	T43.226
Fenalcomine	T46.3X1	T46.3X2	T46.3X3	T46.3X4	T46.3X5	T46.3X6
Fenamisal	T37.1X1	T37.1X2	T37.1X3	T37.1X4	T37.1X5	T37.1X6
Fenazone	T39.2X1	T39.2X2	T39.2X3	T39.2X4	T39.2X5	T39.2X6
Fenbendazole	T37.4X1	T37.4X2	T37.4X3	T37.4X4	T37.4X5	T37.4X6
Fenbutrazate	T50.5X1	T50.5X2	T50.5X3	T50.5X4	T50.5X5	T50.5X6
Fencamfamine	T43.691	T43.692	T43.693	T43.694	T43.695	T43.696
Fendiline	T46.1X1	T46.1X2	T46.1X3	T46.1X4	T46.1X5	T46.1X6
Fenetylline	T43.691	T43.692	T43.693	T43.694	T43.695	T43.696
Fenflumizole	T39.391	T39.392	T39.393	T39.394	T39.395	T39.396
Fenfluramine	T50.5X1	T50.5X2	T50.5X3	T50.5X4	T50.5X5	T50.5X6
Fenobarbital	T42.3X1	T42.3X2	T42.3X3	T42.3X4	T42.3X5	T42.3X6
Fenofibrate	T46.6X1	T46.6X2	T46.6X3	T46.6X4	T46.6X5	T46.6X6
Fenoprofen	T39.311	T39.312	T39.313	T39.314	T39.315	T39.316
Fenoterol	T48.6X1	T48.6X2	T48.6X3	T48.6X4	T48.6X5	T48.6X6
Fenoverine	T44.3X1	T44.3X2	T44.3X3	T44.3X4	T44.3X5	T44.3X6
Fenoxazoline	T48.5X1	T48.5X2	T48.5X3	T48.5X4	T48.5X5	T48.5X6
Fenproporex	T50.5X1	T50.5X2	T50.5X3	T50.5X4	T50.5X5	T50.5X6
Fenquizone	T50.2X1	T50.2X2	T50.2X3	T50.2X4	T50.2X5	T50.2X6
Fentanyl	T40.4X1	T40.4X2	T40.4X3	T40.4X4	T40.4X5	T40.4X6
Fentazin	T43.3X1	T43.3X2	T43.3X3	T43.3X4	T43.3X5	T43.3X6
Fenthion	T60.0X1	T60.0X2	T60.0X3	T60.0X4	—	—
Fenticlor	T49.0X1	T49.0X2	T49.0X3	T49.0X4	T49.0X5	T49.0X6
Fenylbutazone	T39.2X1	T39.2X2	T39.2X3	T39.2X4	T39.2X5	T39.2X6
Feprazone	T39.2X1	T39.2X2	T39.2X3	T39.2X4	T39.2X5	T39.2X6
Fer de lance (bite) (venom)	T63.061	T63.062	T63.063	T63.064	—	—
Ferric — see also Iron						
chloride	T45.4X1	T45.4X2	T45.4X3	T45.4X4	T45.4X5	T45.4X6
citrate	T45.4X1	T45.4X2	T45.4X3	T45.4X4	T45.4X5	T45.4X6
hydroxide						
colloidal	T45.4X1	T45.4X2	T45.4X3	T45.4X4	T45.4X5	T45.4X6

Substance	Poisoning, Accidental (unintentional)	Poisoning, Intentional Self-harm	Poisoning, Assault	Poisoning, Undetermined	Adverse Effect	Under-dosing
Ferric — see also Iron — continued						
hydroxide — continued						
polymaltose	T45.4X1	T45.4X2	T45.4X3	T45.4X4	T45.4X5	T45.4X6
pyrophosphate	T45.4X1	T45.4X2	T45.4X3	T45.4X4	T45.4X5	T45.4X6
Ferritin	T45.4X1	T45.4X2	T45.4X3	T45.4X4	T45.4X5	T45.4X6
Ferrocholinate	T45.4X1	T45.4X2	T45.4X3	T45.4X4	T45.4X5	T45.4X6
Ferrodextrane	T45.4X1	T45.4X2	T45.4X3	T45.4X4	T45.4X5	T45.4X6
Ferropolimaler	T45.4X1	T45.4X2	T45.4X3	T45.4X4	T45.4X5	T45.4X6
Ferrous — see also Iron						
phosphate	T45.4X1	T45.4X2	T45.4X3	T45.4X4	T45.4X5	T45.4X6
salt	T45.4X1	T45.4X2	T45.4X3	T45.4X4	T45.4X5	T45.4X6
with folic acid	T45.4X1	T45.4X2	T45.4X3	T45.4X4	T45.4X5	T45.4X6
Ferrous fumerate, gluconate, lactate, salt NEC, sulfate (medicinal)	T45.4X1	T45.4X2	T45.4X3	T45.4X4	T45.4X5	T45.4X6
Ferrovanadium (fumes)	T59.891	T59.892	T59.893	T59.894	—	—
Ferrum — see Iron						
Fertilizers NEC	T65.891	T65.892	T65.893	T65.894	—	—
with herbicide mixture	T60.3X1	T60.3X2	T60.3X3	T60.3X4	—	—
Fetoxilate	T47.6X1	T47.6X2	T47.6X3	T47.6X4	T47.6X5	T47.6X6
Fiber, dietary	T47.4X1	T47.4X2	T47.4X3	T47.4X4	T47.4X5	T47.4X6
Fiberglass	T65.831	T65.832	T65.833	T65.834		
Fibrinogen (human)	T45.8X1	T45.8X2	T45.8X3	T45.8X4	T45.8X5	T45.8X6
Fibrinolysin (human)	T45.691	T45.692	T45.693	T45.694	T45.695	T45.696
Fibrinolysis						
affecting drug	T45.601	T45.602	T45.603	T45.604	T45.605	T45.606
inhibitor NEC	T45.621	T45.622	T45.623	T45.624	T45.625	T45.626
Fibrinolytic drug	T45.611	T45.612	T45.613	T45.614	T45.615	T45.616
Filix mas	T37.4X1	T37.4X2	T37.4X3	T37.4X4	T37.4X5	T37.4X6
Filtering cream	T49.3X1	T49.3X2	T49.3X3	T49.3X4	T49.3X5	T49.3X6
Fiorinal	T39.011	T39.012	T39.013	T39.014	T39.015	T39.016
Firedamp	T59.891	T59.892	T59.893	T59.894	—	—
Fish, noxious, nonbacterial	T61.91	T61.92	T61.93	T61.94	—	—
ciguatera	T61.01	T61.02	T61.03	T61.04	—	—
scombroid	T61.11	T61.12	T61.13	T61.14	—	—
shell	T61.781	T61.782	T61.783	T61.784	—	—
specified NEC	T61.771	T61.772	T61.773	T61.774	—	—
Flagyl	T37.3X1	T37.3X2	T37.3X3	T37.3X4	T37.3X5	T37.3X6
Flavine adenine dinucleotide	T45.2X1	T45.2X2	T45.2X3	T45.2X4	T45.2X5	T45.2X6
Flavodic acid	T46.991	T46.992	T46.993	T46.994	T46.995	T46.996
Flavoxate	T44.3X1	T44.3X2	T44.3X3	T44.3X4	T44.3X5	T44.3X6
Flaxedil	T48.1X1	T48.1X2	T48.1X3	T48.1X4	T48.1X5	T48.1X6
Flaxseed (medicinal)	T49.3X1	T49.3X2	T49.3X3	T49.3X4	T49.3X5	T49.3X6
Flecainide	T46.2X1	T46.2X2	T46.2X3	T46.2X4	T46.2X5	T46.2X6
Fleroxacin	T36.8X1	T36.8X2	T36.8X3	T36.8X4	T36.8X5	T36.8X6
Floctafenine	T39.8X1	T39.8X2	T39.8X3	T39.8X4	T39.8X5	T39.8X6
Flomax	T44.6X1	T44.6X2	T44.6X3	T44.6X4	T44.6X5	T44.6X6
Flomoxef	T36.1X1	T36.1X2	T36.1X3	T36.1X4	T36.1X5	T36.1X6
Flopropione	T44.3X1	T44.3X2	T44.3X3	T44.3X4	T44.3X5	T44.3X6
Florantyrone	T47.5X1	T47.5X2	T47.5X3	T47.5X4	T47.5X5	T47.5X6
Floraquin	T37.8X1	T37.8X2	T37.8X3	T37.8X4	T37.8X5	T37.8X6
Florinef	T38.0X1	T38.0X2	T38.0X3	T38.0X4	T38.0X5	T38.0X6
ENT agent	T49.6X1	T49.6X2	T49.6X3	T49.6X4	T49.6X5	T49.6X6
ophthalmic preparation	T49.5X1	T49.5X2	T49.5X3	T49.5X4	T49.5X5	T49.5X6
topical NEC	T49.0X1	T49.0X2	T49.0X3	T49.0X4	T49.0X5	T49.0X6
Flowers of sulfur	T49.4X1	T49.4X2	T49.4X3	T49.4X4	T49.4X5	T49.4X6
Floxuridine	T45.1X1	T45.1X2	T45.1X3	T45.1X4	T45.1X5	T45.1X6
Fluanisone	T43.4X1	T43.4X2	T43.4X3	T43.4X4	T43.4X5	T43.4X6
Flubendazole	T37.4X1	T37.4X2	T37.4X3	T37.4X4	T37.4X5	T37.4X6
Fluclorolone acetonide	T49.0X1	T49.0X2	T49.0X3	T49.0X4	T49.0X5	T49.0X6
Flucloxacillin	T36.0X1	T36.0X2	T36.0X3	T36.0X4	T36.0X5	T36.0X6
Fluconazole	T37.8X1	T37.8X2	T37.8X3	T37.8X4	T37.8X5	T37.8X6
Flucytosine	T37.8X1	T37.8X2	T37.8X3	T37.8X4	T37.8X5	T37.8X6
Fludeoxyglucose (18F)	T50.8X1	T50.8X2	T50.8X3	T50.8X4	T50.8X5	T50.8X6
Fludiazepam	T42.4X1	T42.4X2	T42.4X3	T42.4X4	T42.4X5	T42.4X6
Fludrocortisone	T50.0X1	T50.0X2	T50.0X3	T50.0X4	T50.0X5	T50.0X6
ENT agent	T49.6X1	T49.6X2	T49.6X3	T49.6X4	T49.6X5	T49.6X6
ophthalmic preparation	T49.5X1	T49.5X2	T49.5X3	T49.5X4	T49.5X5	T49.5X6
topical NEC	T49.0X1	T49.0X2	T49.0X3	T49.0X4	T49.0X5	T49.0X6
Fludroxycortide	T49.0X1	T49.0X2	T49.0X3	T49.0X4	T49.0X5	T49.0X6
Flufenamic acid	T39.391	T39.392	T39.393	T39.394	T39.395	T39.396
Fluindione	T45.511	T45.512	T45.513	T45.514	T45.515	T45.516
Flumequine	T37.8X1	T37.8X2	T37.8X3	T37.8X4	T37.8X5	T37.8X6
Flumethasone	T49.0X1	T49.0X2	T49.0X3	T49.0X4	T49.0X5	T49.0X6
Flumethiazide	T50.2X1	T50.2X2	T50.2X3	T50.2X4	T50.2X5	T50.2X6
Flumidin	T37.5X1	T37.5X2	T37.5X3	T37.5X4	T37.5X5	T37.5X6
Flunarizine	T46.7X1	T46.7X2	T46.7X3	T46.7X4	T46.7X5	T46.7X6
Flunidazole	T37.8X1	T37.8X2	T37.8X3	T37.8X4	T37.8X5	T37.8X6
Flunisolide	T48.6X1	T48.6X2	T48.6X3	T48.6X4	T48.6X5	T48.6X6
Flunitrazepam	T42.4X1	T42.4X2	T42.4X3	T42.4X4	T42.4X5	T42.4X6
Fluocinolone (acetonide)	T49.0X1	T49.0X2	T49.0X3	T49.0X4	T49.0X5	T49.0X6
Fluocinonide	T49.0X1	T49.0X2	T49.0X3	T49.0X4	T49.0X5	T49.0X6

Additional Character May Be Required — Refer to the Tabular List for Character Selection ▽ Subterms under main terms may continue to next column or page

Substance	Poisoning, Accidental (unintentional)	Poisoning, Intentional Self-harm	Poisoning, Assault	Poisoning, Undetermined	Adverse Effect	Under-dosing
Fluocortin (butyl)	T49.0X1	T49.0X2	T49.0X3	T49.0X4	T49.0X5	T49.0X6
Fluocortolone	T49.0X1	T49.0X2	T49.0X3	T49.0X4	T49.0X5	T49.0X6
Fluohydrocortisone	T38.0X1	T38.0X2	T38.0X3	T38.0X4	T38.0X5	T38.0X6
ENT agent	T49.6X1	T49.6X2	T49.6X3	T49.6X4	T49.6X5	T49.6X6
ophthalmic preparation	T49.5X1	T49.5X2	T49.5X3	T49.5X4	T49.5X5	T49.5X6
topical NEC	T49.0X1	T49.0X2	T49.0X3	T49.0X4	T49.0X5	T49.0X6
Fluonid	T49.0X1	T49.0X2	T49.0X3	T49.0X4	T49.0X5	T49.0X6
Fluopromazine	T43.3X1	T43.3X2	T43.3X3	T43.3X4	T43.3X5	T43.3X6
Fluoracetate	T60.8X1	T60.8X2	T60.8X3	T60.8X4	—	—
Fluorescein	T50.8X1	T50.8X2	T50.8X3	T50.8X4	T50.8X5	T50.8X6
Fluorhydrocortisone	T50.0X1	T50.0X2	T50.0X3	T50.0X4	T50.0X5	T50.0X6
Fluoride (nonmedicinal) (pesticide) (sodium) **NEC**	T60.8X1	T60.8X2	T60.8X3	T60.8X4	—	—
hydrogen — *see* Hydrofluoric acid						
medicinal NEC	T50.991	T50.992	T50.993	T50.994	T50.995	T50.996
dental use	T49.7X1	T49.7X2	T49.7X3	T49.7X4	T49.7X5	T49.7X6
not pesticide NEC	T54.91	T54.92	T54.93	T54.94	—	—
stannous	T49.7X1	T49.7X2	T49.7X3	T49.7X4	T49.7X5	T49.7X6
Fluorinated corticosteroids	T38.0X1	T38.0X2	T38.0X3	T38.0X4	T38.0X5	T38.0X6
Fluorine (gas)	T59.5X1	T59.5X2	T59.5X3	T59.5X4	—	—
salt — *see* Fluoride(s)						
Fluoristan	T49.7X1	T49.7X2	T49.7X3	T49.7X4	T49.7X5	T49.7X6
Fluormetholone	T49.0X1	T49.0X2	T49.0X3	T49.0X4	T49.0X5	T49.0X6
Fluoroacetate	T60.8X1	T60.8X2	T60.8X3	T60.8X4	—	—
Fluorocarbon monomer	T53.6X1	T53.6X2	T53.6X3	T53.6X4	—	—
Fluorocytosine	T37.8X1	T37.8X2	T37.8X3	T37.8X4	T37.8X5	T37.8X6
Fluorodeoxyuridine	T45.1X1	T45.1X2	T45.1X3	T45.1X4	T45.1X5	T45.1X6
Fluorometholone	T49.0X1	T49.0X2	T49.0X3	T49.0X4	T49.0X5	T49.0X6
ophthalmic preparation	T49.5X1	T49.5X2	T49.5X3	T49.5X4	T49.5X5	T49.5X6
Fluorophosphate insecticide	T60.0X1	T60.0X2	T60.0X3	T60.0X4	—	—
Fluorosol	T46.3X1	T46.3X2	T46.3X3	T46.3X4	T46.3X5	T46.3X6
Fluorouracil	T45.1X1	T45.1X2	T45.1X3	T45.1X4	T45.1X5	T45.1X6
Fluorphenylalanine	T49.5X1	T49.5X2	T49.5X3	T49.5X4	T49.5X5	T49.5X6
Fluothane	T41.0X1	T41.0X2	T41.0X3	T41.0X4	T41.0X5	T41.0X6
Fluoxetine	T43.221	T43.222	T43.223	T43.224	T43.225	T43.226
Fluoxymesterone	T38.7X1	T38.7X2	T38.7X3	T38.7X4	T38.7X5	T38.7X6
Flupenthixol	T43.4X1	T43.4X2	T43.4X3	T43.4X4	T43.4X5	T43.4X6
Flupentixol	T43.4X1	T43.4X2	T43.4X3	T43.4X4	T43.4X5	T43.4X6
Fluphenazine	T43.3X1	T43.3X2	T43.3X3	T43.3X4	T43.3X5	T43.3X6
Fluprednidene	T49.0X1	T49.0X2	T49.0X3	T49.0X4	T49.0X5	T49.0X6
Fluprednisolone	T38.0X1	T38.0X2	T38.0X3	T38.0X4	T38.0X5	T38.0X6
Fluradoline	T39.8X1	T39.8X2	T39.8X3	T39.8X4	T39.8X5	T39.8X6
Flurandrenolide	T49.0X1	T49.0X2	T49.0X3	T49.0X4	T49.0X5	T49.0X6
Flurandrenolone	T49.0X1	T49.0X2	T49.0X3	T49.0X4	T49.0X5	T49.0X6
Flurazepam	T42.4X1	T42.4X2	T42.4X3	T42.4X4	T42.4X5	T42.4X6
Flurbiprofen	T39.311	T39.312	T39.313	T39.314	T39.315	T39.316
Flurobate	T49.0X1	T49.0X2	T49.0X3	T49.0X4	T49.0X5	T49.0X6
Fluroxene	T41.0X1	T41.0X2	T41.0X3	T41.0X4	T41.0X5	T41.0X6
Fluspirilene	T43.591	T43.592	T43.593	T43.594	T43.595	T43.596
Flutamide	T38.6X1	T38.6X2	T38.6X3	T38.6X4	T38.6X5	T38.6X6
Flutazolam	T42.4X1	T42.4X2	T42.4X3	T42.4X4	T42.4X5	T42.4X6
Fluticasone propionate	T49.1X1	T49.1X2	T49.1X3	T49.1X4	T49.1X5	T49.1X6
Flutoprazepam	T42.4X1	T42.4X2	T42.4X3	T42.4X4	T42.4X5	T42.4X6
Flutropium bromide	T48.6X1	T48.6X2	T48.6X3	T48.6X4	T48.6X5	T48.6X6
Fluvoxamine	T43.221	T43.222	T43.223	T43.224	T43.225	T43.226
Folacin	T45.8X1	T45.8X2	T45.8X3	T45.8X4	T45.8X5	T45.8X6
Folic acid	T45.8X1	T45.8X2	T45.8X3	T45.8X4	T45.8X5	T45.8X6
with ferrous salt	T45.2X1	T45.2X2	T45.2X3	T45.2X4	T45.2X5	T45.2X6
antagonist	T45.1X1	T45.1X2	T45.1X3	T45.1X4	T45.1X5	T45.1X6
Folinic acid	T45.8X1	T45.8X2	T45.8X3	T45.8X4	T45.8X5	T45.8X6
Folium stramoniae	T48.6X1	T48.6X2	T48.6X3	T48.6X4	T48.6X5	T48.6X6
Follicle-stimulating hormone, human	T38.811	T38.812	T38.813	T38.814	T38.815	T38.816
Folpet	T60.3X1	T60.3X2	T60.3X3	T60.3X4	—	—
Fominoben	T48.3X1	T48.3X2	T48.3X3	T48.3X4	T48.3X5	T48.3X6
Food, foodstuffs, noxious, nonbacterial, NEC	T62.91	T62.92	T62.93	T62.94	—	—
berries	T62.1X1	T62.1X2	T62.1X3	T62.1X4	—	—
fish — *see also* Fish	T61.91	T61.92	T61.93	T61.94	—	—
mushrooms	T62.0X1	T62.0X2	T62.0X3	T62.0X4	—	—
plants	T62.2X1	T62.2X2	T62.2X3	T62.2X4	—	—
seafood	T61.91	T61.92	T61.93	T61.94	—	—
specified NEC	T61.8X1	T61.8X2	T61.8X3	T61.8X4	—	—
seeds	T62.2X1	T62.2X2	T62.2X3	T62.2X4	—	—
shellfish	T61.781	T61.782	T61.783	T61.784	—	—
specified NEC	T62.8X1	T62.8X2	T62.8X3	T62.8X4	—	—
Fool's parsley	T62.2X1	T62.2X2	T62.2X3	T62.2X4	—	—
Formaldehyde (solution), gas or vapor	T59.2X1	T59.2X2	T59.2X3	T59.2X4	—	—
fungicide	T60.3X1	T60.3X2	T60.3X3	T60.3X4	—	—
Formalin	T59.2X1	T59.2X2	T59.2X3	T59.2X4	—	—
Formalin — *continued*						
fungicide	T60.3X1	T60.3X2	T60.3X3	T60.3X4	—	—
vapor	T59.2X1	T59.2X2	T59.2X3	T59.2X4	—	—
Formic acid	T54.2X1	T54.2X2	T54.2X3	T54.2X4	—	—
vapor	T59.891	T59.892	T59.893	T59.894	—	—
Foscarnet sodium	T37.5X1	T37.5X2	T37.5X3	T37.5X4	T37.5X5	T37.5X6
Fosfestrol	T38.5X1	T38.5X2	T38.5X3	T38.5X4	T38.5X5	T38.5X6
Fosfomycin	T36.8X1	T36.8X2	T36.8X3	T36.8X4	T36.8X5	T36.8X6
Fosfonet sodium	T37.5X1	T37.5X2	T37.5X3	T37.5X4	T37.5X5	T37.5X6
Fosinopril	T46.4X1	T46.4X2	T46.4X3	T46.4X4	T46.4X5	T46.4X6
sodium	T46.4X1	T46.4X2	T46.4X3	T46.4X4	T46.4X5	T46.4X6
Fowler's solution	T57.0X1	T57.0X2	T57.0X3	T57.0X4	—	—
Foxglove	T62.2X1	T62.2X2	T62.2X3	T62.2X4	—	—
Framycetin	T36.5X1	T36.5X2	T36.5X3	T36.5X4	T36.5X5	T36.5X6
Frangula	T47.2X1	T47.2X2	T47.2X3	T47.2X4	T47.2X5	T47.2X6
extract	T47.2X1	T47.2X2	T47.2X3	T47.2X4	T47.2X5	T47.2X6
Frei antigen	T50.8X1	T50.8X2	T50.8X3	T50.8X4	T50.8X5	T50.8X6
Freon	T53.5X1	T53.5X2	T53.5X3	T53.5X4	—	—
Fructose	T50.3X1	T50.3X2	T50.3X3	T50.3X4	T50.3X5	T50.3X6
Frusemide	T50.1X1	T50.1X2	T50.1X3	T50.1X4	T50.1X5	T50.1X6
FSH	T38.811	T38.812	T38.813	T38.814	T38.815	T38.816
Ftorafur	T45.1X1	T45.1X2	T45.1X3	T45.1X4	T45.1X5	T45.1X6
Fuel						
automobile	T52.0X1	T52.0X2	T52.0X3	T52.0X4	—	—
exhaust gas, not in transit	T58.01	T58.02	T58.03	T58.04	—	—
vapor NEC	T52.0X1	T52.0X2	T52.0X3	T52.0X4	—	—
gas (domestic use) — *see also* Carbon, monoxide, fuel, utility	T59.891	T59.892	T59.893	T59.894	—	—
utility	T59.891	T59.892	T59.893	T59.894	—	—
incomplete combustion of — *see* Carbon, monoxide, fuel, utility						
in mobile container	T59.891	T59.892	T59.893	T59.894	—	—
piped (natural)	T59.891	T59.892	T59.893	T59.894	—	—
industrial, incomplete combustion	T58.8X1	T58.8X2	T58.8X3	T58.8X4	—	—
Fugillin	T36.8X1	T36.8X2	T36.8X3	T36.8X4	T36.8X5	T36.8X6
Fulminate of mercury	T56.1X1	T56.1X2	T56.1X3	T56.1X4	—	—
Fulvicin	T36.7X1	T36.7X2	T36.7X3	T36.7X4	T36.7X5	T36.7X6
Fumadil	T36.8X1	T36.8X2	T36.8X3	T36.8X4	T36.8X5	T36.8X6
Fumagillin	T36.8X1	T36.8X2	T36.8X3	T36.8X4	T36.8X5	T36.8X6
Fumaric acid	T49.4X1	T49.4X2	T49.4X3	T49.4X4	T49.4X5	T49.4X6
Fumes (from)	T59.91	T59.92	T59.93	T59.94	—	—
carbon monoxide — *see* Carbon, monoxide						
charcoal (domestic use) — *see* Charcoal, fumes						
chloroform — *see* Chloroform						
coke (in domestic stoves, fireplaces) — *see* Coke fumes						
corrosive NEC	T54.91	T54.92	T54.93	T54.94	—	—
ether — *see* ether						
freons	T53.5X1	T53.5X2	T53.5X3	T53.5X4	—	—
hydrocarbons	T59.891	T59.892	T59.893	T59.894	—	—
petroleum (liquefied)	T59.891	T59.892	T59.893	T59.894	—	—
distributed through pipes (pure or mixed with air)	T59.891	T59.892	T59.893	T59.894	—	—
lead — *see* lead						
metal — *see* Metals, or the specified metal						
nitrogen dioxide	T59.0X1	T59.0X2	T59.0X3	T59.0X4	—	—
pesticides — *see* Pesticides						
petroleum (liquefied)	T59.891	T59.892	T59.893	T59.894	—	—
distributed through pipes (pure or mixed with air)	T59.891	T59.892	T59.893	T59.894	—	—
polyester	T59.891	T59.892	T59.893	T59.894	—	—
specified source NEC — *see also* substance specified	T59.891	T59.892	T59.893	T59.894	—	—
sulfur dioxide	T59.1X1	T59.1X2	T59.1X3	T59.1X4	—	—
Fumigant NEC	T60.91	T60.92	T60.93	T60.94	—	—
Fungicide NEC (nonmedicinal)	T60.3X1	T60.3X2	T60.3X3	T60.3X4	—	—
Fungi, noxious, used as food	T62.0X1	T62.0X2	T62.0X3	T62.0X4	—	—
Fungizone	T36.7X1	T36.7X2	T36.7X3	T36.7X4	T36.7X5	T36.7X6
topical	T49.0X1	T49.0X2	T49.0X3	T49.0X4	T49.0X5	T49.0X6
Furacin	T49.0X1	T49.0X2	T49.0X3	T49.0X4	T49.0X5	T49.0X6
Furadantin	T37.91	T37.92	T37.93	T37.94	T37.95	T37.96
Furazolidone	T37.8X1	T37.8X2	T37.8X3	T37.8X4	T37.8X5	T37.8X6

Table of Drugs and Chemicals

Furazolium chloride — Ginger

Substance	Poisoning, Accidental (unintentional)	Poisoning, Intentional Self-harm	Poisoning, Assault	Poisoning, Undetermined	Adverse Effect	Under-dosing
Furazolium chloride	T49.0X1	T49.0X2	T49.0X3	T49.0X4	T49.0X5	T49.0X6
Furfural	T52.8X1	T52.8X2	T52.8X3	T52.8X4	—	—
Furnace (coal burning) (domestic), gas from	T58.2X1	T58.2X2	T58.2X3	T58.2X4	—	—
industrial	T58.8X1	T58.8X2	T58.8X3	T58.8X4	—	—
Furniture polish	T65.891	T65.892	T65.893	T65.894	—	—
Furosemide	T50.1X1	T50.1X2	T50.1X3	T50.1X4	T50.1X5	T50.1X6
Furoxone	T37.91	T37.92	T37.93	T37.94	T37.95	T37.96
Fursultiamine	T45.2X1	T45.2X2	T45.2X3	T45.2X4	T45.2X5	T45.2X6
Fusafungine	T36.8X1	T36.8X2	T36.8X3	T36.8X4	T36.8X5	T36.8X6
Fusel oil (any) (amyl) (butyl) (propyl), vapor	T51.3X1	T51.3X2	T51.3X3	T51.3X4	—	—
Fusidate (ethanolamine) (sodium)	T36.8X1	T36.8X2	T36.8X3	T36.8X4	T36.8X5	T36.8X6
Fusidic acid	T36.8X1	T36.8X2	T36.8X3	T36.8X4	T36.8X5	T36.8X6
Fytic acid, nonasodium	T50.6X1	T50.6X2	T50.6X3	T50.6X4	T50.6X5	T50.6X6
b-Galactosidase	T47.5X1	T47.5X2	T47.5X3	T47.5X4	T47.5X5	T47.5X6
GABA	T43.8X1	T43.8X2	T43.8X3	T43.8X4	T43.8X5	T43.8X6
Gadopentetic acid	T50.8X1	T50.8X2	T50.8X3	T50.8X4	T50.8X5	T50.8X6
Galactose	T50.3X1	T50.3X2	T50.3X3	T50.3X4	T50.3X5	T50.3X6
Galantamine	T44.0X1	T44.0X2	T44.0X3	T44.0X4	T44.0X5	T44.0X6
Gallamine (triethiodide)	T48.1X1	T48.1X2	T48.1X3	T48.1X4	T48.1X5	T48.1X6
Gallium citrate	T50.991	T50.992	T50.993	T50.994	T50.995	T50.996
Gallopamil	T46.1X1	T46.1X2	T46.1X3	T46.1X4	T46.1X5	T46.1X6
Gamboge	T47.2X1	T47.2X2	T47.2X3	T47.2X4	T47.2X5	T47.2X6
Gamimune	T50.Z11	T50.Z12	T50.Z13	T50.Z14	T50.Z15	T50.Z16
Gamma-aminobutyric acid	T43.8X1	T43.8X2	T43.8X3	T43.8X4	T43.8X5	T43.8X6
Gamma-benzene hexachloride (medicinal)	T49.0X1	T49.0X2	T49.0X3	T49.0X4	T49.0X5	T49.0X6
nonmedicinal, vapor	T53.6X1	T53.6X2	T53.6X3	T53.6X4	—	—
Gamma-BHC (medicinal) — see also Gamma-benzene hexachloride	T49.0X1	T49.0X2	T49.0X3	T49.0X4	T49.0X5	T49.0X6
Gamma globulin	T50.Z11	T50.Z12	T50.Z13	T50.Z14	T50.Z15	T50.Z16
Gamulin	T50.Z11	T50.Z12	T50.Z13	T50.Z14	T50.Z15	T50.Z16
Ganciclovir (sodium)	T37.5X1	T37.5X2	T37.5X3	T37.5X4	T37.5X5	T37.5X6
Ganglionic blocking drug NEC	T44.2X1	T44.2X2	T44.2X3	T44.2X4	T44.2X5	T44.2X6
specified NEC	T44.2X1	T44.2X2	T44.2X3	T44.2X4	T44.2X5	T44.2X6
Ganja	T40.7X1	T40.7X2	T40.7X3	T40.7X4	T40.7X5	T40.7X6
Garamycin	T36.5X1	T36.5X2	T36.5X3	T36.5X4	T36.5X5	T36.5X6
ophthalmic preparation	T49.5X1	T49.5X2	T49.5X3	T49.5X4	T49.5X5	T49.5X6
topical NEC	T49.0X1	T49.0X2	T49.0X3	T49.0X4	T49.0X5	T49.0X6
Gardenal	T42.3X1	T42.3X2	T42.3X3	T42.3X4	T42.3X5	T42.3X6
Gardepanyl	T42.3X1	T42.3X2	T42.3X3	T42.3X4	T42.3X5	T42.3X6
Gas	T59.91	T59.92	T59.93	T59.94	—	—
acetylene	T59.891	T59.892	T59.893	T59.894	—	—
incomplete combustion of	T58.11	T58.12	T58.13	T58.14	—	—
air contaminants, source or type not specified	T59.91	T59.92	T59.93	T59.94	—	—
anesthetic	T41.0X1	T41.0X2	T41.0X3	T41.0X4	T41.0X5	T41.0X6
blast furnace	T58.8X1	T58.8X2	T58.8X3	T58.8X4	—	—
butane — see butane						
carbon monoxide — see Carbon, monoxide						
chlorine	T59.4X1	T59.4X2	T59.4X3	T59.4X4	—	—
coal	T58.2X1	T58.2X2	T58.2X3	T58.2X4	—	—
cyanide	T57.3X1	T57.3X2	T57.3X3	T57.3X4	—	—
dicyanogen	T65.0X1	T65.0X2	T65.0X3	T65.0X4	—	—
domestic — see Domestic gas						
exhaust	T58.01	T58.02	T58.03	T58.04	—	—
from utility (for cooking, heating, or lighting) (after combustion) — see Carbon, monoxide, fuel, utility						
prior to combustion	T59.891	T59.892	T59.893	T59.894	—	—
from wood- or coal-burning stove or fireplace	T58.2X1	T58.2X2	T58.2X3	T58.2X4	—	—
fuel (domestic use) (after combustion) — see also Carbon, monoxide, fuel						
industrial use	T58.8X1	T58.8X2	T58.8X3	T58.8X4	—	—
prior to combustion	T59.891	T59.892	T59.893	T59.894	—	—
utility	T59.891	T59.892	T59.893	T59.894	—	—
incomplete combustion of — see Carbon, monoxide, fuel, utility						
in mobile container	T59.891	T59.892	T59.893	T59.894	—	—
piped (natural)	T59.891	T59.892	T59.893	T59.894	—	—
garage	T58.01	T58.02	T58.03	T58.04	—	—
hydrocarbon NEC	T59.891	T59.892	T59.893	T59.894	—	—

Substance	Poisoning, Accidental (unintentional)	Poisoning, Intentional Self-harm	Poisoning, Assault	Poisoning, Undetermined	Adverse Effect	Under-dosing
Gas — continued						
hydrocarbon — continued						
incomplete combustion of — see Carbon, monoxide, fuel, utility						
liquefied — see butane						
piped	T59.891	T59.892	T59.893	T59.894	—	—
hydrocyanic acid	T65.0X1	T65.0X2	T65.0X3	T65.0X4	—	—
illuminating (after combustion)	T58.11	T58.12	T58.13	T58.14	—	—
prior to combustion	T59.891	T59.892	T59.893	T59.894	—	—
incomplete combustion, any — see Carbon, monoxide						
kiln	T58.8X1	T58.8X2	T58.8X3	T58.8X4	—	—
lacrimogenic	T59.3X1	T59.3X2	T59.3X3	T59.3X4	—	—
liquefied petroleum — see butane						
marsh	T59.891	T59.892	T59.893	T59.894	—	—
motor exhaust, not in transit	T58.01	T58.02	T58.03	T58.04	—	—
mustard, not in war	T59.891	T59.892	T59.893	T59.894	—	—
natural	T59.891	T59.892	T59.893	T59.894	—	—
nerve, not in war	T59.91	T59.92	T59.93	T59.94	—	—
oil	T52.0X1	T52.0X2	T52.0X3	T52.0X4	—	—
petroleum (liquefied) (distributed in mobile containers)	T59.891	T59.892	T59.893	T59.894	—	—
piped (pure or mixed with air)	T59.891	T59.892	T59.893	T59.894	—	—
piped (manufactured) (natural) NEC	T59.891	T59.892	T59.893	T59.894	—	—
producer	T58.8X1	T58.8X2	T58.8X3	T58.8X4	—	—
propane — see propane						
refrigerant (chlorofluoro-carbon)	T53.5X1	T53.5X2	T53.5X3	T53.5X4	—	—
not chlorofluoro-carbon	T59.891	T59.892	T59.893	T59.894	—	—
sewer	T59.91	T59.92	T59.93	T59.94	—	—
specified source NEC	T59.91	T59.92	T59.93	T59.94	—	—
stove (after combustion)	T58.11	T58.12	T58.13	T58.14	—	—
prior to combustion	T59.891	T59.892	T59.893	T59.894	—	—
tear	T59.3X1	T59.3X2	T59.3X3	T59.3X4	—	—
therapeutic	T41.5X1	T41.5X2	T41.5X3	T41.5X4	T41.5X5	T41.5X6
utility (for cooking, heating, or lighting) (piped) NEC	T59.891	T59.892	T59.893	T59.894	—	—
incomplete combustion of — see Carbon, monoxide, fuel, utilty						
in mobile container	T59.891	T59.892	T59.893	T59.894	—	—
piped (natural)	T59.891	T59.892	T59.893	T59.894	—	—
water	T58.11	T58.12	T58.13	T58.14	—	—
incomplete combustion of — see Carbon, monoxide, fuel, utility						
Gaseous substance — see Gas						
Gasoline	T52.0X1	T52.0X2	T52.0X3	T52.0X4	—	—
vapor	T52.0X1	T52.0X2	T52.0X3	T52.0X4	—	—
Gastric enzymes	T47.5X1	T47.5X2	T47.5X3	T47.5X4	T47.5X5	T47.5X6
Gastrografin	T50.8X1	T50.8X2	T50.8X3	T50.8X4	T50.8X5	T50.8X6
Gastrointestinal drug	T47.91	T47.92	T47.93	T47.94	T47.95	T47.96
biological	T47.8X1	T47.8X2	T47.8X3	T47.8X4	T47.8X5	T47.8X6
specified NEC	T47.8X1	T47.8X2	T47.8X3	T47.8X4	T47.8X5	T47.8X6
Gaultheria procumbens	T62.2X1	T62.2X2	T62.2X3	T62.2X4	—	—
Gefarnate	T44.3X1	T44.3X2	T44.3X3	T44.3X4	T44.3X5	T44.3X6
Gelatin (intravenous)	T45.8X1	T45.8X2	T45.8X3	T45.8X4	T45.8X5	T45.8X6
absorbable (sponge)	T45.7X1	T45.7X2	T45.7X3	T45.7X4	T45.7X5	T45.7X6
Gelfilm	T49.8X1	T49.8X2	T49.8X3	T49.8X4	T49.8X5	T49.8X6
Gelfoam	T45.7X1	T45.7X2	T45.7X3	T45.7X4	T45.7X5	T45.7X6
Gelsemine	T50.991	T50.992	T50.993	T50.994	T50.995	T50.996
Gelsemium (sempervirens)	T62.2X1	T62.2X2	T62.2X3	T62.2X4	—	—
Gemeprost	T48.0X1	T48.0X2	T48.0X3	T48.0X4	T48.0X5	T48.0X6
Gemfibrozil	T46.6X1	T46.6X2	T46.6X3	T46.6X4	T46.6X5	T46.6X6
Gemonil	T42.3X1	T42.3X2	T42.3X3	T42.3X4	T42.3X5	T42.3X6
Gentamicin	T36.5X1	T36.5X2	T36.5X3	T36.5X4	T36.5X5	T36.5X6
ophthalmic preparation	T49.5X1	T49.5X2	T49.5X3	T49.5X4	T49.5X5	T49.5X6
topical NEC	T49.0X1	T49.0X2	T49.0X3	T49.0X4	T49.0X5	T49.0X6
Gentian	T47.5X1	T47.5X2	T47.5X3	T47.5X4	T47.5X5	T47.5X6
violet	T49.0X1	T49.0X2	T49.0X3	T49.0X4	T49.0X5	T49.0X6
Gepefrine	T44.4X1	T44.4X2	T44.4X3	T44.4X4	T44.4X5	T44.4X6
Gestonorone caproate	T38.5X1	T38.5X2	T38.5X3	T38.5X4	T38.5X5	T38.5X6
Gexane	T49.0X1	T49.0X2	T49.0X3	T49.0X4	T49.0X5	T49.0X6
Gila monster (venom)	T63.111	T63.112	T63.113	T63.114	—	—
Ginger	T47.5X1	T47.5X2	T47.5X3	T47.5X4	T47.5X5	T47.5X6
Jamaica — see Jamaica, ginger						

Substance	Poisoning, Accidental (unintentional)	Poisoning, Intentional Self-harm	Poisoning, Assault	Poisoning, Undetermined	Adverse Effect	Under-dosing
Gitalin	T46.0X1	T46.0X2	T46.0X3	T46.0X4	T46.0X5	T46.0X6
amorphous	T46.0X1	T46.0X2	T46.0X3	T46.0X4	T46.0X5	T46.0X6
Gitaloxin	T46.0X1	T46.0X2	T46.0X3	T46.0X4	T46.0X5	T46.0X6
Gitoxin	T46.0X1	T46.0X2	T46.0X3	T46.0X4	T46.0X5	T46.0X6
Glafenine	T39.8X1	T39.8X2	T39.8X3	T39.8X4	T39.8X5	T39.8X6
Glandular extract (medicinal) NEC	T50.Z91	T50.Z92	T50.Z93	T50.Z94	T50.Z95	T50.Z96
Glaucarubin	T37.3X1	T37.3X2	T37.3X3	T37.3X4	T37.3X5	T37.3X6
Glibenclamide	T38.3X1	T38.3X2	T38.3X3	T38.3X4	T38.3X5	T38.3X6
Glibornuride	T38.3X1	T38.3X2	T38.3X3	T38.3X4	T38.3X5	T38.3X6
Gliclazide	T38.3X1	T38.3X2	T38.3X3	T38.3X4	T38.3X5	T38.3X6
Glimidine	T38.3X1	T38.3X2	T38.3X3	T38.3X4	T38.3X5	T38.3X6
Glipizide	T38.3X1	T38.3X2	T38.3X3	T38.3X4	T38.3X5	T38.3X6
Gliquidone	T38.3X1	T38.3X2	T38.3X3	T38.3X4	T38.3X5	T38.3X6
Glisolamide	T38.3X1	T38.3X2	T38.3X3	T38.3X4	T38.3X5	T38.3X6
Glisoxepide	T38.3X1	T38.3X2	T38.3X3	T38.3X4	T38.3X5	T38.3X6
Globin zinc insulin	T38.3X1	T38.3X2	T38.3X3	T38.3X4	T38.3X5	T38.3X6
Globulin						
antilymphocytic	T50.Z11	T50.Z12	T50.Z13	T50.Z14	T50.Z15	T50.Z16
antirhesus	T50.Z11	T50.Z12	T50.Z13	T50.Z14	T50.Z15	T50.Z16
antivenin	T50.Z11	T50.Z12	T50.Z13	T50.Z14	T50.Z15	T50.Z16
antiviral	T50.Z11	T50.Z12	T50.Z13	T50.Z14	T50.Z15	T50.Z16
Glucagon	T38.3X1	T38.3X2	T38.3X3	T38.3X4	T38.3X5	T38.3X6
Glucocorticoids	T38.0X1	T38.0X2	T38.0X3	T38.0X4	T38.0X5	T38.0X6
Glucocorticosteroid	T38.0X1	T38.0X2	T38.0X3	T38.0X4	T38.0X5	T38.0X6
Gluconic acid	T50.991	T50.992	T50.993	T50.994	T50.995	T50.996
Glucosamine sulfate	T39.4X1	T39.4X2	T39.4X3	T39.4X4	T39.4X5	T39.4X6
Glucose	T50.3X1	T50.3X2	T50.3X3	T50.3X4	T50.3X5	T50.3X6
with sodium chloride	T50.3X1	T50.3X2	T50.3X3	T50.3X4	T50.3X5	T50.3X6
Glucosulfone sodium	T37.1X1	T37.1X2	T37.1X3	T37.1X4	T37.1X5	T37.1X6
Glucurolactone	T47.8X1	T47.8X2	T47.8X3	T47.8X4	T47.8X5	T47.8X6
Glue NEC	T52.8X1	T52.8X2	T52.8X3	T52.8X4	—	—
Glutamic acid	T47.5X1	T47.5X2	T47.5X3	T47.5X4	T47.5X5	T47.5X6
Glutaral (medicinal)	T49.0X1	T49.0X2	T49.0X3	T49.0X4	T49.0X5	T49.0X6
nonmedicinal	T65.891	T65.892	T65.893	T65.894	—	—
Glutaraldehyde (nonmedicinal)	T65.891	T65.892	T65.893	T65.894	—	—
medicinal	T49.0X1	T49.0X2	T49.0X3	T49.0X4	T49.0X5	T49.0X6
Glutathione	T50.6X1	T50.6X2	T50.6X3	T50.6X4	T50.6X5	T50.6X6
Glutethimide	T42.6X1	T42.6X2	T42.6X3	T42.6X4	T42.6X5	T42.6X6
Glyburide	T38.3X1	T38.3X2	T38.3X3	T38.3X4	T38.3X5	T38.3X6
Glycerin	T47.4X1	T47.4X2	T47.4X3	T47.4X4	T47.4X5	T47.4X6
Glycerol	T47.4X1	T47.4X2	T47.4X3	T47.4X4	T47.4X5	T47.4X6
borax	T49.6X1	T49.6X2	T49.6X3	T49.6X4	T49.6X5	T49.6X6
intravenous	T50.3X1	T50.3X2	T50.3X3	T50.3X4	T50.3X5	T50.3X6
iodinated	T48.4X1	T48.4X2	T48.4X3	T48.4X4	T48.4X5	T48.4X6
Glycerophosphate	T50.991	T50.992	T50.993	T50.994	T50.995	T50.996
Glyceryl						
gualacolate	T48.4X1	T48.4X2	T48.4X3	T48.4X4	T48.4X5	T48.4X6
nitrate	T46.3X1	T46.3X2	T46.3X3	T46.3X4	T46.3X5	T46.3X6
triacetate (topical)	T49.0X1	T49.0X2	T49.0X3	T49.0X4	T49.0X5	T49.0X6
trinitrate	T46.3X1	T46.3X2	T46.3X3	T46.3X4	T46.3X5	T46.3X6
Glycine	T50.3X1	T50.3X2	T50.3X3	T50.3X4	T50.3X5	T50.3X6
Glyclopyramide	T38.3X1	T38.3X2	T38.3X3	T38.3X4	T38.3X5	T38.3X6
Glycobiarsol	T37.3X1	T37.3X2	T37.3X3	T37.3X4	T37.3X5	T37.3X6
Glycols (ether)	T52.3X1	T52.3X2	T52.3X3	T52.3X4	—	—
Glyconiazide	T37.1X1	T37.1X2	T37.1X3	T37.1X4	T37.1X5	T37.1X6
Glycopyramide	T44.3X1	T44.3X2	T44.3X3	T44.3X4	T44.3X5	T44.3X6
Glycopyrronium	T44.3X1	T44.3X2	T44.3X3	T44.3X4	T44.3X5	T44.3X6
bromide	T44.3X1	T44.3X2	T44.3X3	T44.3X4	T44.3X5	T44.3X6
Glycoside, cardiac (stimulant)	T46.0X1	T46.0X2	T46.0X3	T46.0X4	T46.0X5	T46.0X6
Glycyclamide	T38.3X1	T38.3X2	T38.3X3	T38.3X4	T38.3X5	T38.3X6
Glycyrrhiza extract	T48.4X1	T48.4X2	T48.4X3	T48.4X4	T48.4X5	T48.4X6
Glycyrrhizic acid	T48.4X1	T48.4X2	T48.4X3	T48.4X4	T48.4X5	T48.4X6
Glycyrrhizinate potassium	T48.4X1	T48.4X2	T48.4X3	T48.4X4	T48.4X5	T48.4X6
Glymidine sodium	T38.3X1	T38.3X2	T38.3X3	T38.3X4	T38.3X5	T38.3X6
Glyphosate	T60.3X1	T60.3X2	T60.3X3	T60.3X4	—	—
Glyphylline	T48.6X1	T48.6X2	T48.6X3	T48.6X4	T48.6X5	T48.6X6
Gold						
colloidal (l98Au)	T45.1X1	T45.1X2	T45.1X3	T45.1X4	T45.1X5	T45.1X6
salts	T39.4X1	T39.4X2	T39.4X3	T39.4X4	T39.4X5	T39.4X6
Golden sulfide of antimony	T56.891	T56.892	T56.893	T56.894	—	—
Goldylocks	T62.2X1	T62.2X2	T62.2X3	T62.2X4	—	—
Gonadal tissue extract	T38.901	T38.902	T38.903	T38.904	T38.905	T38.906
female	T38.5X1	T38.5X2	T38.5X3	T38.5X4	T38.5X5	T38.5X6
male	T38.7X1	T38.7X2	T38.7X3	T38.7X4	T38.7X5	T38.7X6
Gonadorelin	T38.891	T38.892	T38.893	T38.894	T38.895	T38.896
Gonadotropin	T38.891	T38.892	T38.893	T38.894	T38.895	T38.896
chorionic	T38.891	T38.892	T38.893	T38.894	T38.895	T38.896
pituitary	T38.811	T38.812	T38.813	T38.814	T38.815	T38.816
Goserelin	T45.1X1	T45.1X2	T45.1X3	T45.1X4	T45.1X5	T45.1X6
Grain alcohol	T51.0X1	T51.0X2	T51.0X3	T51.0X4	—	—

Substance	Poisoning, Accidental (unintentional)	Poisoning, Intentional Self-harm	Poisoning, Assault	Poisoning, Undetermined	Adverse Effect	Under-dosing
Gramicidin	T49.0X1	T49.0X2	T49.0X3	T49.0X4	T49.0X5	T49.0X6
Granisetron	T45.0X1	T45.0X2	T45.0X3	T45.0X4	T45.0X5	T45.0X6
Gratiola officinalis	T62.2X1	T62.2X2	T62.2X3	T62.2X4	—	—
Grease	T65.891	T65.892	T65.893	T65.894	—	—
Green hellebore	T62.2X1	T62.2X2	T62.2X3	T62.2X4	—	—
Green soap	T49.2X1	T49.2X2	T49.2X3	T49.2X4	T49.2X5	T49.2X6
Grifulvin	T36.7X1	T36.7X2	T36.7X3	T36.7X4	T36.7X5	T36.7X6
Griseofulvin	T36.7X1	T36.7X2	T36.7X3	T36.7X4	T36.7X5	T36.7X6
Growth hormone	T38.811	T38.812	T38.813	T38.814	T38.815	T38.816
Guaiacol derivatives	T48.4X1	T48.4X2	T48.4X3	T48.4X4	T48.4X5	T48.4X6
Guaiac reagent	T50.991	T50.992	T50.993	T50.994	T50.995	T50.996
Guaifenesin	T48.4X1	T48.4X2	T48.4X3	T48.4X4	T48.4X5	T48.4X6
Guaimesal	T48.4X1	T48.4X2	T48.4X3	T48.4X4	T48.4X5	T48.4X6
Guaiphenesin	T48.4X1	T48.4X2	T48.4X3	T48.4X4	T48.4X5	T48.4X6
Guamecycline	T36.4X1	T36.4X2	T36.4X3	T36.4X4	T36.4X5	T36.4X6
Guanabenz	T46.5X1	T46.5X2	T46.5X3	T46.5X4	T46.5X5	T46.5X6
Guanacline	T46.5X1	T46.5X2	T46.5X3	T46.5X4	T46.5X5	T46.5X6
Guanadrel	T46.5X1	T46.5X2	T46.5X3	T46.5X4	T46.5X5	T46.5X6
Guanatol	T37.2X1	T37.2X2	T37.2X3	T37.2X4	T37.2X5	T37.2X6
Guanethidine	T46.5X1	T46.5X2	T46.5X3	T46.5X4	T46.5X5	T46.5X6
Guanfacine	T46.5X1	T46.5X2	T46.5X3	T46.5X4	T46.5X5	T46.5X6
Guano	T65.891	T65.892	T65.893	T65.894	—	—
Guanochlor	T46.5X1	T46.5X2	T46.5X3	T46.5X4	T46.5X5	T46.5X6
Guanoclor	T46.5X1	T46.5X2	T46.5X3	T46.5X4	T46.5X5	T46.5X6
Guanoctine	T46.5X1	T46.5X2	T46.5X3	T46.5X4	T46.5X5	T46.5X6
Guanoxabenz	T46.5X1	T46.5X2	T46.5X3	T46.5X4	T46.5X5	T46.5X6
Guanoxan	T46.5X1	T46.5X2	T46.5X3	T46.5X4	T46.5X5	T46.5X6
Guar gum (medicinal)	T46.6X1	T46.6X2	T46.6X3	T46.6X4	T46.6X5	T46.6X6
Hachimycin	T36.7X1	T36.7X2	T36.7X3	T36.7X4	T36.7X5	T36.7X6
Hair						
dye	T49.4X1	T49.4X2	T49.4X3	T49.4X4	T49.4X5	T49.4X6
preparation NEC	T49.4X1	T49.4X2	T49.4X3	T49.4X4	T49.4X5	T49.4X6
Halazepam	T42.4X1	T42.4X2	T42.4X3	T42.4X4	T42.4X5	T42.4X6
Halcinolone	T49.0X1	T49.0X2	T49.0X3	T49.0X4	T49.0X5	T49.0X6
Halcinonide	T49.0X1	T49.0X2	T49.0X3	T49.0X4	T49.0X5	T49.0X6
Halethazole	T49.0X1	T49.0X2	T49.0X3	T49.0X4	T49.0X5	T49.0X6
Hallucinogen NEC	T40.901	T40.902	T40.903	T40.904	T40.905	T40.906
Halofantrine	T37.2X1	T37.2X2	T37.2X3	T37.2X4	T37.2X5	T37.2X6
Halofenate	T46.6X1	T46.6X2	T46.6X3	T46.6X4	T46.6X5	T46.6X6
Halometasone	T49.0X1	T49.0X2	T49.0X3	T49.0X4	T49.0X5	T49.0X6
Haloperidol	T43.4X1	T43.4X2	T43.4X3	T43.4X4	T43.4X5	T43.4X6
Haloprogin	T49.0X1	T49.0X2	T49.0X3	T49.0X4	T49.0X5	T49.0X6
Halotex	T49.0X1	T49.0X2	T49.0X3	T49.0X4	T49.0X5	T49.0X6
Halothane	T41.0X1	T41.0X2	T41.0X3	T41.0X4	T41.0X5	T41.0X6
Haloxazolam	T42.4X1	T42.4X2	T42.4X3	T42.4X4	T42.4X5	T42.4X6
Halquinols	T49.0X1	T49.0X2	T49.0X3	T49.0X4	T49.0X5	T49.0X6
Hamamelis	T49.2X1	T49.2X2	T49.2X3	T49.2X4	T49.2X5	T49.2X6
Haptendextran	T45.8X1	T45.8X2	T45.8X3	T45.8X4	T45.8X5	T45.8X6
Harmonyl	T46.5X1	T46.5X2	T46.5X3	T46.5X4	T46.5X5	T46.5X6
Hartmann's solution	T50.3X1	T50.3X2	T50.3X3	T50.3X4	T50.3X5	T50.3X6
Hashish	T40.7X1	T40.7X2	T40.7X3	T40.7X4	T40.7X5	T40.7X6
Hawaiian Woodrose seeds	T40.991	T40.992	T40.993	T40.994	—	—
HCB	T60.3X1	T60.3X2	T60.3X3	T60.3X4	—	—
HCH	T53.6X1	T53.6X2	T53.6X3	T53.6X4	—	—
medicinal	T49.0X1	T49.0X2	T49.0X3	T49.0X4	T49.0X5	T49.0X6
HCN	T57.3X1	T57.3X2	T57.3X3	T57.3X4	—	—
Headache cures, drugs, powders NEC	T50.901	T50.902	T50.903	T50.904	T50.905	T50.906
Heavenly Blue (morning glory)	T40.991	T40.992	T40.993	T40.994	—	—
Heavy metal antidote	T45.8X1	T45.8X2	T45.8X3	T45.8X4	T45.8X5	T45.8X6
Hedaquinium	T49.0X1	T49.0X2	T49.0X3	T49.0X4	T49.0X5	T49.0X6
Hedge hyssop	T62.2X1	T62.2X2	T62.2X3	T62.2X4	—	—
Heet	T49.8X1	T49.8X2	T49.8X3	T49.8X4	T49.8X5	T49.8X6
Helenin	T37.4X1	T37.4X2	T37.4X3	T37.4X4	T37.4X5	T37.4X6
Helium (nonmedicinal) NEC	T59.891	T59.892	T59.893	T59.894	—	—
medicinal	T48.991	T48.992	T48.993	T48.994	T48.995	T48.996
Hellebore (black) (green) (white)	T62.2X1	T62.2X2	T62.2X3	T62.2X4	—	—
Hematin	T45.8X1	T45.8X2	T45.8X3	T45.8X4	T45.8X5	T45.8X6
Hematinic preparation	T45.8X1	T45.8X2	T45.8X3	T45.8X4	T45.8X5	T45.8X6
Hematological agent	T45.91	T45.92	T45.93	T45.94	T45.95	T45.96
specified NEC	T45.8X1	T45.8X2	T45.8X3	T45.8X4	T45.8X5	T45.8X6
Hemlock	T62.2X1	T62.2X2	T62.2X3	T62.2X4	—	—
Hemostatic	T45.621	T45.622	T45.623	T45.624	T45.625	T45.626
drug, systemic	T45.621	T45.622	T45.623	T45.624	T45.625	T45.626
Hemostyptic	T49.4X1	T49.4X2	T49.4X3	T49.4X4	T49.4X5	T49.4X6
Henbane	T62.2X1	T62.2X2	T62.2X3	T62.2X4	—	—
Heparin (sodium)	T45.511	T45.512	T45.513	T45.514	T45.515	T45.516
action reverser	T45.7X1	T45.7X2	T45.7X3	T45.7X4	T45.7X5	T45.7X6
Heparin-fraction	T45.511	T45.512	T45.513	T45.514	T45.515	T45.516
Heparinoid (systemic)	T45.511	T45.512	T45.513	T45.514	T45.515	T45.516

Substance	Poisoning, Accidental (unintentional)	Poisoning, Intentional Self-harm	Poisoning, Assault	Poisoning, Undetermined	Adverse Effect	Under-dosing
Hepatic secretion stimulant	T47.8X1	T47.8X2	T47.8X3	T47.8X4	T47.8X5	T47.8X6
Hepatitis B						
immune globulin	T50.Z11	T50.Z12	T50.Z13	T50.Z14	T50.Z15	T50.Z16
vaccine	T50.B91	T50.B92	T50.B93	T50.B94	T50.B95	T50.B96
Hepronicate	T46.7X1	T46.7X2	T46.7X3	T46.7X4	T46.7X5	T46.7X6
Heptabarb	T42.3X1	T42.3X2	T42.3X3	T42.3X4	T42.3X5	T42.3X6
Heptabarbital	T42.3X1	T42.3X2	T42.3X3	T42.3X4	T42.3X5	T42.3X6
Heptabarbitone	T42.3X1	T42.3X2	T42.3X3	T42.3X4	T42.3X5	T42.3X6
Heptachlor	T60.1X1	T60.1X2	T60.1X3	T60.1X4	—	—
Heptalgin	T40.2X1	T40.2X2	T40.2X3	T40.2X4	T40.2X5	T40.2X6
Heptaminol	T46.3X1	T46.3X2	T46.3X3	T46.3X4	T46.3X5	T46.3X6
Herbicide NEC	T60.3X1	T60.3X2	T60.3X3	T60.3X4	—	—
Heroin	T40.1X1	T40.1X2	T40.1X3	T40.1X4	—	—
Herplex	T49.5X1	T49.5X2	T49.5X3	T49.5X4	T49.5X5	T49.5X6
HES	T45.8X1	T45.8X2	T45.8X3	T45.8X4	T45.8X5	T45.8X6
Hesperidin	T46.991	T46.992	T46.993	T46.994	T46.995	T46.996
Hetacillin	T36.0X1	T36.0X2	T36.0X3	T36.0X4	T36.0X5	T36.0X6
Hetastarch	T45.8X1	T45.8X2	T45.8X3	T45.8X4	T45.8X5	T45.8X6
HETP	T60.0X1	T60.0X2	T60.0X3	T60.0X4	—	—
Hexachlorobenzene (vapor)	T60.3X1	T60.3X2	T60.3X3	T60.3X4	—	—
Hexachlorocyclohexane	T53.6X1	T53.6X2	T53.6X3	T53.6X4	—	—
Hexachlorophene	T49.0X1	T49.0X2	T49.0X3	T49.0X4	T49.0X5	T49.0X6
Hexadiline	T46.3X1	T46.3X2	T46.3X3	T46.3X4	T46.3X5	T46.3X6
Hexadimethrine (bromide)	T45.7X1	T45.7X2	T45.7X3	T45.7X4	T45.7X5	T45.7X6
Hexadylamine	T46.3X1	T46.3X2	T46.3X3	T46.3X4	T46.3X5	T46.3X6
Hexaethyl tetraphosphate	T60.0X1	T60.0X2	T60.0X3	T60.0X4	—	—
Hexafluorenium bromide	T48.1X1	T48.1X2	T48.1X3	T48.1X4	T48.1X5	T48.1X6
Hexafluronium (bromide)	T48.1X1	T48.1X2	T48.1X3	T48.1X4	T48.1X5	T48.1X6
Hexa-germ	T49.2X1	T49.2X2	T49.2X3	T49.2X4	T49.2X5	T49.2X6
Hexahydrobenzol	T52.8X1	T52.8X2	T52.8X3	T52.8X4	—	—
Hexahydrocresol(s)	T51.8X1	T51.8X2	T51.8X3	T51.8X4	—	—
arsenide	T57.0X1	T57.0X2	T57.0X3	T57.0X4	—	—
arseniurated	T57.0X1	T57.0X2	T57.0X3	T57.0X4	—	—
cyanide	T57.3X1	T57.3X2	T57.3X3	T57.3X4	—	—
gas	T59.891	T59.892	T59.893	T59.894	—	—
Fluoride (liquid)	T57.8X1	T57.8X2	T57.8X3	T57.8X4	—	—
vapor	T59.891	T59.892	T59.893	T59.894	—	—
phophorated	T60.0X1	T60.0X2	T60.0X3	T60.0X4	—	—
sulfate	T57.8X1	T57.8X2	T57.8X3	T57.8X4	—	—
sulfide (gas)	T59.6X1	T59.6X2	T59.6X3	T59.6X4	—	—
arseniurated	T57.0X1	T57.0X2	T57.0X3	T57.0X4	—	—
sulfurated	T57.8X1	T57.8X2	T57.8X3	T57.8X4	—	—
Hexahydrophenol	T51.8X1	T51.8X2	T51.8X3	T51.8X4	—	—
Hexalen	T51.8X1	T51.8X2	T51.8X3	T51.8X4	—	—
Hexamethonium bromide	T44.2X1	T44.2X2	T44.2X3	T44.2X4	T44.2X5	T44.2X6
Hexamethylene	T52.8X1	T52.8X2	T52.8X3	T52.8X4	—	—
Hexamethylmelamine	T45.1X1	T45.1X2	T45.1X3	T45.1X4	T45.1X5	T45.1X6
Hexamidine	T49.0X1	T49.0X2	T49.0X3	T49.0X4	T49.0X5	T49.0X6
Hexamine (mandelate)	T37.8X1	T37.8X2	T37.8X3	T37.8X4	T37.8X5	T37.8X6
Hexanone, 2-hexanone	T52.4X1	T52.4X2	T52.4X3	T52.4X4	—	—
Hexanuorenium	T48.1X1	T48.1X2	T48.1X3	T48.1X4	T48.1X5	T48.1X6
Hexapropymate	T42.6X1	T42.6X2	T42.6X3	T42.6X4	T42.6X5	T42.6X6
Hexasonium iodide	T44.3X1	T44.3X2	T44.3X3	T44.3X4	T44.3X5	T44.3X6
Hexcarbacholine bromide	T48.1X1	T48.1X2	T48.1X3	T48.1X4	T48.1X5	T48.1X6
Hexemal	T42.3X1	T42.3X2	T42.3X3	T42.3X4	T42.3X5	T42.3X6
Hexestrol	T38.5X1	T38.5X2	T38.5X3	T38.5X4	T38.5X5	T38.5X6
Hexethal (sodium)	T42.3X1	T42.3X2	T42.3X3	T42.3X4	T42.3X5	T42.3X6
Hexetidine	T37.8X1	T37.8X2	T37.8X3	T37.8X4	T37.8X5	T37.8X6
Hexobarbital	T42.3X1	T42.3X2	T42.3X3	T42.3X4	T42.3X5	T42.3X6
rectal	T41.291	T41.292	T41.293	T41.294	T41.295	T41.296
sodium	T41.1X1	T41.1X2	T41.1X3	T41.1X4	T41.1X5	T41.1X6
Hexobendine	T46.3X1	T46.3X2	T46.3X3	T46.3X4	T46.3X5	T46.3X6
Hexocyclium	T44.3X1	T44.3X2	T44.3X3	T44.3X4	T44.3X5	T44.3X6
metilsulfate	T44.3X1	T44.3X2	T44.3X3	T44.3X4	T44.3X5	T44.3X6
Hexoestrol	T38.5X1	T38.5X2	T38.5X3	T38.5X4	T38.5X5	T38.5X6
Hexone	T52.4X1	T52.4X2	T52.4X3	T52.4X4	—	—
Hexoprenaline	T48.6X1	T48.6X2	T48.6X3	T48.6X4	T48.6X5	T48.6X6
Hexylcaine	T41.3X1	T41.3X2	T41.3X3	T41.3X4	T41.3X5	T41.3X6
Hexylresorcinol	T52.2X1	T52.2X2	T52.2X3	T52.2X4	—	—
HGH (human growth hormone)	T38.811	T38.812	T38.813	T38.814	T38.815	T38.816
Hinkle's pills	T47.2X1	T47.2X2	T47.2X3	T47.2X4	T47.2X5	T47.2X6
Histalog	T50.8X1	T50.8X2	T50.8X3	T50.8X4	T50.8X5	T50.8X6
Histamine (phosphate)	T50.8X1	T50.8X2	T50.8X3	T50.8X4	T50.8X5	T50.8X6
Histoplasmin	T50.8X1	T50.8X2	T50.8X3	T50.8X4	T50.8X5	T50.8X6
Holly berries	T62.2X1	T62.2X2	T62.2X3	T62.2X4	—	—
Homatropine	T44.3X1	T44.3X2	T44.3X3	T44.3X4	T44.3X5	T44.3X6
methylbromide	T44.3X1	T44.3X2	T44.3X3	T44.3X4	T44.3X5	T44.3X6
Homochlorcyclizine	T45.0X1	T45.0X2	T45.0X3	T45.0X4	T45.0X5	T45.0X6
Homosalate	T49.3X1	T49.3X2	T49.3X3	T49.3X4	T49.3X5	T49.3X6
Homo-tet	T50.Z11	T50.Z12	T50.Z13	T50.Z14	T50.Z15	T50.Z16
Hormone	T38.801	T38.802	T38.803	T38.804	T38.805	T38.806

Substance	Poisoning, Accidental (unintentional)	Poisoning, Intentional Self-harm	Poisoning, Assault	Poisoning, Undetermined	Adverse Effect	Under-dosing
Hormone — continued						
adrenal cortical steroids	T38.0X1	T38.0X2	T38.0X3	T38.0X4	T38.0X5	T38.0X6
androgenic	T38.7X1	T38.7X2	T38.7X3	T38.7X4	T38.7X5	T38.7X6
anterior pituitary NEC	T38.811	T38.812	T38.813	T38.814	T38.815	T38.816
antidiabetic agents	T38.3X1	T38.3X2	T38.3X3	T38.3X4	T38.3X5	T38.3X6
antidiuretic	T38.891	T38.892	T38.893	T38.894	T38.895	T38.896
cancer therapy	T45.1X1	T45.1X2	T45.1X3	T45.1X4	T45.1X5	T45.1X6
follicle stimulating	T38.811	T38.812	T38.813	T38.814	T38.815	T38.816
gonadotropic	T38.891	T38.892	T38.893	T38.894	T38.895	T38.896
pituitary	T38.811	T38.812	T38.813	T38.814	T38.815	T38.816
growth	T38.811	T38.812	T38.813	T38.814	T38.815	T38.816
luteinizing	T38.811	T38.812	T38.813	T38.814	T38.815	T38.816
ovarian	T38.5X1	T38.5X2	T38.5X3	T38.5X4	T38.5X5	T38.5X6
oxytocic	T48.0X1	T48.0X2	T48.0X3	T48.0X4	T48.0X5	T48.0X6
parathyroid (derivatives)	T50.991	T50.992	T50.993	T50.994	T50.995	T50.996
pituitary (posterior) NEC	T38.891	T38.892	T38.893	T38.894	T38.895	T38.896
anterior	T38.811	T38.812	T38.813	T38.814	T38.815	T38.816
specified, NEC	T38.891	T38.892	T38.893	T38.894	T38.895	T38.896
thyroid	T38.1X1	T38.1X2	T38.1X3	T38.1X4	T38.1X5	T38.1X6
Hornet (sting)	T63.451	T63.452	T63.453	T63.454	—	—
Horse anti-human lymphocytic serum	T50.Z11	T50.Z12	T50.Z13	T50.Z14	T50.Z15	T50.Z16
Horticulture agent NEC	T65.91	T65.92	T65.93	T65.94	—	—
with pesticide	T60.91	T60.92	T60.93	T60.94	—	—
Human						
albumin	T45.8X1	T45.8X2	T45.8X3	T45.8X4	T45.8X5	T45.8X6
growth hormone (HGH)	T38.811	T38.812	T38.813	T38.814	T38.815	T38.816
immune serum	T50.Z11	T50.Z12	T50.Z13	T50.Z14	T50.Z15	T50.Z16
Hyaluronidase	T45.3X1	T45.3X2	T45.3X3	T45.3X4	T45.3X5	T45.3X6
Hyazyme	T45.3X1	T45.3X2	T45.3X3	T45.3X4	T45.3X5	T45.3X6
Hycodan	T40.2X1	T40.2X2	T40.2X3	T40.2X4	T40.2X5	T40.2X6
Hydantoin derivative NEC	T42.0X1	T42.0X2	T42.0X3	T42.0X4	T42.0X5	T42.0X6
Hydeltra	T38.0X1	T38.0X2	T38.0X3	T38.0X4	T38.0X5	T38.0X6
Hydergine	T44.6X1	T44.6X2	T44.6X3	T44.6X4	T44.6X5	T44.6X6
Hydrabamine penicillin	T36.0X1	T36.0X2	T36.0X3	T36.0X4	T36.0X5	T36.0X6
Hydralazine	T46.5X1	T46.5X2	T46.5X3	T46.5X4	T46.5X5	T46.5X6
Hydrargaphen	T49.0X1	T49.0X2	T49.0X3	T49.0X4	T49.0X5	T49.0X6
Hydrargyri aminochloridum	T49.0X1	T49.0X2	T49.0X3	T49.0X4	T49.0X5	T49.0X6
Hydrastine	T48.291	T48.292	T48.293	T48.294	T48.295	T48.296
Hydrazine	T54.1X1	T54.1X2	T54.1X3	T54.1X4	—	—
monoamine oxidase inhibitors	T43.1X1	T43.1X2	T43.1X3	T43.1X4	T43.1X5	T43.1X6
Hydrazoic acid, azides	T54.2X1	T54.2X2	T54.2X3	T54.2X4	—	—
Hydriodic acid	T48.4X1	T48.4X2	T48.4X3	T48.4X4	T48.4X5	T48.4X6
Hydrocarbon gas	T59.891	T59.892	T59.893	T59.894	—	—
incomplete combustion of — see Carbon, monoxide, fuel, utility						
liquefied (mobile container)	T59.891	T59.892	T59.893	T59.894	—	—
piped (natural)	T59.891	T59.892	T59.893	T59.894	—	—
Hydrochloric acid (liquid)	T54.2X1	T54.2X2	T54.2X3	T54.2X4	—	—
medicinal (digestant)	T47.5X1	T47.5X2	T47.5X3	T47.5X4	T47.5X5	T47.5X6
vapor	T59.891	T59.892	T59.893	T59.894	—	—
Hydrochlorothiazide	T50.2X1	T50.2X2	T50.2X3	T50.2X4	T50.2X5	T50.2X6
Hydrocodone	T40.2X1	T40.2X2	T40.2X3	T40.2X4	T40.2X5	T40.2X6
Hydrocortisone (derivatives)	T49.0X1	T49.0X2	T49.0X3	T49.0X4	T49.0X5	T49.0X6
aceponate	T49.0X1	T49.0X2	T49.0X3	T49.0X4	T49.0X5	T49.0X6
ENT agent	T49.6X1	T49.6X2	T49.6X3	T49.6X4	T49.6X5	T49.6X6
ophthalmic preparation	T49.5X1	T49.5X2	T49.5X3	T49.5X4	T49.5X5	T49.5X6
topical NEC	T49.0X1	T49.0X2	T49.0X3	T49.0X4	T49.0X5	T49.0X6
Hydrocortone	T38.0X1	T38.0X2	T38.0X3	T38.0X4	T38.0X5	T38.0X6
ENT agent	T49.6X1	T49.6X2	T49.6X3	T49.6X4	T49.6X5	T49.6X6
ophthalmic preparation	T49.5X1	T49.5X2	T49.5X3	T49.5X4	T49.5X5	T49.5X6
topical NEC	T49.0X1	T49.0X2	T49.0X3	T49.0X4	T49.0X5	T49.0X6
Hydrocyanic acid (liquid)	T57.3X1	T57.3X2	T57.3X3	T57.3X4	—	—
gas	T65.0X1	T65.0X2	T65.0X3	T65.0X4	—	—
Hydroflumethiazide	T50.2X1	T50.2X2	T50.2X3	T50.2X4	T50.2X5	T50.2X6
Hydrofluoric acid (liquid)	T54.2X1	T54.2X2	T54.2X3	T54.2X4	—	—
vapor	T59.891	T59.892	T59.893	T59.894	—	—
Hydrogen	T59.891	T59.892	T59.893	T59.894	—	—
arsenide	T57.0X1	T57.0X2	T57.0X3	T57.0X4	—	—
arseniureted	T57.0X1	T57.0X2	T57.0X3	T57.0X4	—	—
chloride	T57.8X1	T57.8X2	T57.8X3	T57.8X4	—	—
cyanide (salts)	T57.3X1	T57.3X2	T57.3X3	T57.3X4	—	—
gas	T57.3X1	T57.3X2	T57.3X3	T57.3X4	—	—
Fluoride	T59.5X1	T59.5X2	T59.5X3	T59.5X4	—	—
vapor	T59.5X1	T59.5X2	T59.5X3	T59.5X4	—	—
peroxide	T49.0X1	T49.0X2	T49.0X3	T49.0X4	T49.0X5	T49.0X6
phosphureted	T57.1X1	T57.1X2	T57.1X3	T57.1X4	—	—
sulfide	T59.6X1	T59.6X2	T59.6X3	T59.6X4	—	—
arseniureted	T57.0X1	T57.0X2	T57.0X3	T57.0X4	—	—
sulfureted	T59.6X1	T59.6X2	T59.6X3	T59.6X4	—	—

Substance	Poisoning, Accidental (unintentional)	Poisoning, Intentional Self-harm	Poisoning, Assault	Poisoning, Undetermined	Adverse Effect	Under-dosing
Hydromethylpyridine	T46.7X1	T46.7X2	T46.7X3	T46.7X4	T46.7X5	T46.7X6
Hydromorphinol	T40.2X1	T40.2X2	T40.2X3	T40.2X4	—	—
Hydromorphinone	T40.2X1	T40.2X2	T40.2X3	T40.2X4	T40.2X5	T40.2X6
Hydromorphone	T40.2X1	T40.2X2	T40.2X3	T40.2X4	T40.2X5	T40.2X6
Hydromox	T50.2X1	T50.2X2	T50.2X3	T50.2X4	T50.2X5	T50.2X6
Hydrophilic lotion	T49.3X1	T49.3X2	T49.3X3	T49.3X4	T49.3X5	T49.3X6
Hydroquinidine	T46.2X1	T46.2X2	T46.2X3	T46.2X4	T46.2X5	T46.2X6
Hydroquinone	T52.2X1	T52.2X2	T52.2X3	T52.2X4	—	—
vapor	T59.891	T59.892	T59.893	T59.894	—	—
Hydrosulfuric acid (gas)	T59.6X1	T59.6X2	T59.6X3	T59.6X4	—	—
Hydrotalcite	T47.1X1	T47.1X2	T47.1X3	T47.1X4	T47.1X5	T47.1X6
Hydrous wool fat	T49.3X1	T49.3X2	T49.3X3	T49.3X4	T49.3X5	T49.3X6
Hydroxide, caustic	T54.3X1	T54.3X2	T54.3X3	T54.3X4	—	—
Hydroxocobalamin	T45.8X1	T45.8X2	T45.8X3	T45.8X4	T45.8X5	T45.8X6
Hydroxyamphetamine	T49.5X1	T49.5X2	T49.5X3	T49.5X4	T49.5X5	T49.5X6
Hydroxycarbamide	T45.1X1	T45.1X2	T45.1X3	T45.1X4	T45.1X5	T45.1X6
Hydroxychloroquine	T37.8X1	T37.8X2	T37.8X3	T37.8X4	T37.8X5	T37.8X6
Hydroxydihydrocodeinone	T40.2X1	T40.2X2	T40.2X3	T40.2X4	T40.2X5	T40.2X6
Hydroxyestrone	T38.5X1	T38.5X2	T38.5X3	T38.5X4	T38.5X5	T38.5X6
Hydroxyethyl starch	T45.8X1	T45.8X2	T45.8X3	T45.8X4	T45.8X5	T45.8X6
Hydroxymethylpentanone	T52.4X1	T52.4X2	T52.4X3	T52.4X4	—	—
Hydroxyphenamate	T43.591	T43.592	T43.593	T43.594	T43.595	T43.596
Hydroxyphenylbutazone	T39.2X1	T39.2X2	T39.2X3	T39.2X4	T39.2X5	T39.2X6
Hydroxyprogesterone	T38.5X1	T38.5X2	T38.5X3	T38.5X4	T38.5X5	T38.5X6
caproate	T38.5X1	T38.5X2	T38.5X3	T38.5X4	T38.5X5	T38.5X6
Hydroxyquinoline (derivatives) NEC	T37.8X1	T37.8X2	T37.8X3	T37.8X4	T37.8X5	T37.8X6
Hydroxystilbamidine	T37.3X1	T37.3X2	T37.3X3	T37.3X4	T37.3X5	T37.3X6
Hydroxytoluene (nonmedicinal)	T54.0X1	T54.0X2	T54.0X3	T54.0X4	—	—
medicinal	T49.0X1	T49.0X2	T49.0X3	T49.0X4	T49.0X5	T49.0X6
Hydroxyurea	T45.1X1	T45.1X2	T45.1X3	T45.1X4	T45.1X5	T45.1X6
Hydroxyzine	T43.591	T43.592	T43.593	T43.594	T43.595	T43.596
Hyoscine	T44.3X1	T44.3X2	T44.3X3	T44.3X4	T44.3X5	T44.3X6
Hyoscyamine	T44.3X1	T44.3X2	T44.3X3	T44.3X4	T44.3X5	T44.3X6
Hyoscyamus	T44.3X1	T44.3X2	T44.3X3	T44.3X4	T44.3X5	T44.3X6
dry extract	T44.3X1	T44.3X2	T44.3X3	T44.3X4	T44.3X5	T44.3X6
Hypaque	T50.8X1	T50.8X2	T50.8X3	T50.8X4	T50.8X5	T50.8X6
Hypertussis	T50.Z11	T50.Z12	T50.Z13	T50.Z14	T50.Z15	T50.Z16
Hypnotic	T42.71	T42.72	T42.73	T42.74	T42.75	T42.76
anticonvulsant	T42.71	T42.72	T42.73	T42.74	T42.75	T42.76
specified NEC	T42.6X1	T42.6X2	T42.6X3	T42.6X4	T42.6X5	T42.6X6
Hypochlorite	T49.0X1	T49.0X2	T49.0X3	T49.0X4	T49.0X5	T49.0X6
Hypophysis, posterior	T38.891	T38.892	T38.893	T38.894	T38.895	T38.896
Hypotensive NEC	T46.5X1	T46.5X2	T46.5X3	T46.5X4	T46.5X5	T46.5X6
Hypromellose	T49.5X1	T49.5X2	T49.5X3	T49.5X4	T49.5X5	T49.5X6
Ibacitabine	T37.5X1	T37.5X2	T37.5X3	T37.5X4	T37.5X5	T37.5X6
Ibopamine	T44.991	T44.992	T44.993	T44.994	T44.995	T44.996
Ibufenac	T39.311	T39.312	T39.313	T39.314	T39.315	T39.316
Ibuprofen	T39.311	T39.312	T39.313	T39.314	T39.315	T39.316
Ibuproxam	T39.311	T39.312	T39.313	T39.314	T39.315	T39.316
Ibuterol	T48.6X1	T48.6X2	T48.6X3	T48.6X4	T48.6X5	T48.6X6
Ichthammol	T49.0X1	T49.0X2	T49.0X3	T49.0X4	T49.0X5	T49.0X6
Ichthyol	T49.4X1	T49.4X2	T49.4X3	T49.4X4	T49.4X5	T49.4X6
Idarubicin	T45.1X1	T45.1X2	T45.1X3	T45.1X4	T45.1X5	T45.1X6
Idrocilamide	T42.8X1	T42.8X2	T42.8X3	T42.8X4	T42.8X5	T42.8X6
Ifenprodil	T46.7X1	T46.7X2	T46.7X3	T46.7X4	T46.7X5	T46.7X6
Ifosfamide	T45.1X1	T45.1X2	T45.1X3	T45.1X4	T45.1X5	T45.1X6
Iletin	T38.3X1	T38.3X2	T38.3X3	T38.3X4	T38.3X5	T38.3X6
Ilex	T62.2X1	T62.2X2	T62.2X3	T62.2X4	—	—
Illuminating gas (after combustion)	T58.11	T58.12	T58.13	T58.14	—	—
prior to combustion	T59.891	T59.892	T59.893	T59.894	—	—
Ilopan	T45.2X1	T45.2X2	T45.2X3	T45.2X4	T45.2X5	T45.2X6
Iloprost	T46.7X1	T46.7X2	T46.7X3	T46.7X4	T46.7X5	T46.7X6
Ilotycin	T36.3X1	T36.3X2	T36.3X3	T36.3X4	T36.3X5	T36.3X6
ophthalmic preparation	T49.5X1	T49.5X2	T49.5X3	T49.5X4	T49.5X5	T49.5X6
topical NEC	T49.0X1	T49.0X2	T49.0X3	T49.0X4	T49.0X5	T49.0X6
Imidazole-4-carboxamide	T45.1X1	T45.1X2	T45.1X3	T45.1X4	T45.1X5	T45.1X6
Iminostilbene	T42.1X1	T42.1X2	T42.1X3	T42.1X4	T42.1X5	T42.1X6
Imipenem	T36.0X1	T36.0X2	T36.0X3	T36.0X4	T36.0X5	T36.0X6
Imipramine	T43.011	T43.012	T43.013	T43.014	T43.015	T43.016
Immuglobin	T50.Z11	T50.Z12	T50.Z13	T50.Z14	T50.Z15	T50.Z16
Immu-G	T50.Z11	T50.Z12	T50.Z13	T50.Z14	T50.Z15	T50.Z16
Immune						
globulin	T50.Z11	T50.Z12	T50.Z13	T50.Z14	T50.Z15	T50.Z16
serum globulin	T50.Z11	T50.Z12	T50.Z13	T50.Z14	T50.Z15	T50.Z16
Immunoglobin human	T50.Z11	T50.Z12	T50.Z13	T50.Z14	T50.Z15	T50.Z16
(intravenous) (normal)						
unmodified	T50.Z11	T50.Z12	T50.Z13	T50.Z14	T50.Z15	T50.Z16
Immunosuppressive drug	T45.1X1	T45.1X2	T45.1X3	T45.1X4	T45.1X5	T45.1X6
Immu-tetanus	T50.Z11	T50.Z12	T50.Z13	T50.Z14	T50.Z15	T50.Z16
Indalpine	T43.221	T43.222	T43.223	T43.224	T43.225	T43.226
Indanazoline	T48.5X1	T48.5X2	T48.5X3	T48.5X4	T48.5X5	T48.5X6

Substance	Poisoning, Accidental (unintentional)	Poisoning, Intentional Self-harm	Poisoning, Assault	Poisoning, Undetermined	Adverse Effect	Under-dosing
Indandione (derivatives)	T45.511	T45.512	T45.513	T45.514	T45.515	T45.516
Indapamide	T46.5X1	T46.5X2	T46.5X3	T46.5X4	T46.5X5	T46.5X6
Indendione (derivatives)	T45.511	T45.512	T45.513	T45.514	T45.515	T45.516
Indenolol	T44.7X1	T44.7X2	T44.7X3	T44.7X4	T44.7X5	T44.7X6
Inderal	T44.7X1	T44.7X2	T44.7X3	T44.7X4	T44.7X5	T44.7X6
Indian						
hemp	T40.7X1	T40.7X2	T40.7X3	T40.7X4	T40.7X5	T40.7X6
tobacco	T62.2X1	T62.2X2	T62.2X3	T62.2X4	—	—
Indigo carmine	T50.8X1	T50.8X2	T50.8X3	T50.8X4	T50.8X5	T50.8X6
Indobufen	T45.521	T45.522	T45.523	T45.524	T45.525	T45.526
Indocin	T39.2X1	T39.2X2	T39.2X3	T39.2X4	T39.2X5	T39.2X6
Indocyanine green	T50.8X1	T50.8X2	T50.8X3	T50.8X4	T50.8X5	T50.8X6
Indometacin	T39.391	T39.392	T39.393	T39.394	T39.395	T39.396
Indomethacin	T39.391	T39.392	T39.393	T39.394	T39.395	T39.396
farnesil	T39.4X1	T39.4X2	T39.4X3	T39.4X4	T39.4X5	T39.4X6
Indoramin	T44.6X1	T44.6X2	T44.6X3	T44.6X4	T44.6X5	T44.6X6
Industrial						
alcohol	T51.0X1	T51.0X2	T51.0X3	T51.0X4	—	—
fumes	T59.891	T59.892	T59.893	T59.894	—	—
solvents (fumes) (vapors)	T52.91	T52.92	T52.93	T52.94	—	—
Influenza vaccine	T50.B91	T50.B92	T50.B93	T50.B94	T50.B95	T50.B96
Ingested substance NEC	T65.91	T65.92	T65.93	T65.94	—	—
INH	T37.1X1	T37.1X2	T37.1X3	T37.1X4	T37.1X5	T37.1X6
Inhalation, gas (noxious) — see Gas						
Inhibitor						
angiotensin-converting enzyme	T46.4X1	T46.4X2	T46.4X3	T46.4X4	T46.4X5	T46.4X6
carbonic anhydrase	T50.2X1	T50.2X2	T50.2X3	T50.2X4	T50.2X5	T50.2X6
fibrinolysis	T45.621	T45.622	T45.623	T45.624	T45.625	T45.626
monoamine oxidase NEC	T43.1X1	T43.1X2	T43.1X3	T43.1X4	T43.1X5	T43.1X6
hydrazine	T43.1X1	T43.1X2	T43.1X3	T43.1X4	T43.1X5	T43.1X6
postsynaptic	T43.8X1	T43.8X2	T43.8X3	T43.8X4	T43.8X5	T43.8X6
prothrombin synthesis	T45.511	T45.512	T45.513	T45.514	T45.515	T45.516
Ink	T65.891	T65.892	T65.893	T65.894	—	—
Inorganic substance NEC	T57.91	T57.92	T57.93	T57.94	—	—
Inosine pranobex	T37.5X1	T37.5X2	T37.5X3	T37.5X4	T37.5X5	T37.5X6
Inositol	T50.991	T50.992	T50.993	T50.994	T50.995	T50.996
nicotinate	T46.7X1	T46.7X2	T46.7X3	T46.7X4	T46.7X5	T46.7X6
Inproquone	T45.1X1	T45.1X2	T45.1X3	T45.1X4	T45.1X5	T45.1X6
Insect (sting), venomous	T63.481	T63.482	T63.483	T63.484	—	—
ant	T63.421	T63.422	T63.423	T63.424	—	—
bee	T63.441	T63.442	T63.443	T63.444	—	—
caterpillar	T63.431	T63.432	T63.433	T63.434	—	—
hornet	T63.451	T63.452	T63.453	T63.454	—	—
wasp	T63.461	T63.462	T63.463	T63.464	—	—
Insecticide NEC	T60.91	T60.92	T60.93	T60.94	—	—
carbamate	T60.0X1	T60.0X2	T60.0X3	T60.0X4	—	—
chlorinated	T60.1X1	T60.1X2	T60.1X3	T60.1X4	—	—
mixed	T60.91	T60.92	T60.93	T60.94	—	—
organochlorine	T60.1X1	T60.1X2	T60.1X3	T60.1X4	—	—
organophosphorus	T60.0X1	T60.0X2	T60.0X3	T60.0X4	—	—
Insular tissue extract	T38.3X1	T38.3X2	T38.3X3	T38.3X4	T38.3X5	T38.3X6
Insulin (amorphous) (globin) (isophane) (Lente) (NPH) (Semilente) (Ultralente)	T38.3X1	T38.3X2	T38.3X3	T38.3X4	T38.3X5	T38.3X6
defalan	T38.3X1	T38.3X2	T38.3X3	T38.3X4	T38.3X5	T38.3X6
human	T38.3X1	T38.3X2	T38.3X3	T38.3X4	T38.3X5	T38.3X6
injection, soluble	T38.3X1	T38.3X2	T38.3X3	T38.3X4	T38.3X5	T38.3X6
biphasic	T38.3X1	T38.3X2	T38.3X3	T38.3X4	T38.3X5	T38.3X6
intermediate acting	T38.3X1	T38.3X2	T38.3X3	T38.3X4	T38.3X5	T38.3X6
protamine zinc	T38.3X1	T38.3X2	T38.3X3	T38.3X4	T38.3X5	T38.3X6
slow acting	T38.3X1	T38.3X2	T38.3X3	T38.3X4	T38.3X5	T38.3X6
zinc	T38.3X1	T38.3X2	T38.3X3	T38.3X4	T38.3X5	T38.3X6
protamine injection	T38.3X1	T38.3X2	T38.3X3	T38.3X4	T38.3X5	T38.3X6
suspension (amorphous) (crystalline)	T38.3X1	T38.3X2	T38.3X3	T38.3X4	T38.3X5	T38.3X6
Interferon (alpha) (beta) (gamma)	T37.5X1	T37.5X2	T37.5X3	T37.5X4	T37.5X5	T37.5X6
Intestinal motility control drug	T47.6X1	T47.6X2	T47.6X3	T47.6X4	T47.6X5	T47.6X6
biological	T47.8X1	T47.8X2	T47.8X3	T47.8X4	T47.8X5	T47.8X6
Intranarcon	T41.1X1	T41.1X2	T41.1X3	T41.1X4	T41.1X5	T41.1X6
Intravenous						
amino acids	T50.991	T50.992	T50.993	T50.994	T50.995	T50.996
fat suspension	T50.991	T50.992	T50.993	T50.994	T50.995	T50.996
Inulin	T50.8X1	T50.8X2	T50.8X3	T50.8X4	T50.8X5	T50.8X6
Invert sugar	T50.3X1	T50.3X2	T50.3X3	T50.3X4	T50.3X5	T50.3X6
Inza — see Naproxen						
Iobenzamic acid	T50.8X1	T50.8X2	T50.8X3	T50.8X4	T50.8X5	T50.8X6
Iocarmic acid	T50.8X1	T50.8X2	T50.8X3	T50.8X4	T50.8X5	T50.8X6
Iocetamic acid	T50.8X1	T50.8X2	T50.8X3	T50.8X4	T50.8X5	T50.8X6
Iodamide	T50.8X1	T50.8X2	T50.8X3	T50.8X4	T50.8X5	T50.8X6

Table of Drugs and Chemicals

Iodide NEC — Karaya

Substance	Poisoning, Accidental (unintentional)	Poisoning, Intentional Self-harm	Poisoning, Assault	Poisoning, Undetermined	Adverse Effect	Under-dosing
Iodide NEC — see also Iodine	T49.0X1	T49.0X2	T49.0X3	T49.0X4	T49.0X5	T49.0X6
mercury (ointment)	T49.0X1	T49.0X2	T49.0X3	T49.0X4	T49.0X5	T49.0X6
methylate	T49.0X1	T49.0X2	T49.0X3	T49.0X4	T49.0X5	T49.0X6
potassium (expectorant)	T48.4X1	T48.4X2	T48.4X3	T48.4X4	T48.4X5	T48.4X6
NEC						
Iodinated						
contrast medium	T50.8X1	T50.8X2	T50.8X3	T50.8X4	T50.8X5	T50.8X6
glycerol	T48.4X1	T48.4X2	T48.4X3	T48.4X4	T48.4X5	T48.4X6
human serum albumin (131I)	T50.8X1	T50.8X2	T50.8X3	T50.8X4	T50.8X5	T50.8X6
Iodine (antiseptic, external) (tincture) **NEC**	T49.0X1	T49.0X2	T49.0X3	T49.0X4	T49.0X5	T49.0X6
125 — see also Radiation sickness, and Exposure to radioactive isotopes	T50.8X1	T50.8X2	T50.8X3	T50.8X4	T50.8X5	T50.8X6
therapeutic	T50.991	T50.992	T50.993	T50.994	T50.995	T50.996
131 — see also Radiation sickness, and Exposure to radioactive isotopes	T50.8X1	T50.8X2	T50.8X3	T50.8X4	T50.8X5	T50.8X6
therapeutic	T38.2X1	T38.2X2	T38.2X3	T38.2X4	T38.2X5	T38.2X6
diagnostic	T50.8X1	T50.8X2	T50.8X3	T50.8X4	T50.8X5	T50.8X6
for thyroid conditions (antithyroid)	T38.2X1	T38.2X2	T38.2X3	T38.2X4	T38.2X5	T38.2X6
solution	T49.0X1	T49.0X2	T49.0X3	T49.0X4	T49.0X5	T49.0X6
vapor	T59.891	T59.892	T59.893	T59.894	—	—
Iodipamide	T50.8X1	T50.8X2	T50.8X3	T50.8X4	T50.8X5	T50.8X6
Iodized (poppy seed) oil	T50.8X1	T50.8X2	T50.8X3	T50.8X4	T50.8X5	T50.8X6
Iodobismitol	T37.8X1	T37.8X2	T37.8X3	T37.8X4	T37.8X5	T37.8X6
Iodochlorhydroxyquin	T37.8X1	T37.8X2	T37.8X3	T37.8X4	T37.8X5	T37.8X6
topical	T49.0X1	T49.0X2	T49.0X3	T49.0X4	T49.0X5	T49.0X6
Iodochlorhydroxyquinoline	T37.8X1	T37.8X2	T37.8X3	T37.8X4	T37.8X5	T37.8X6
Iodocholesterol (131I)	T50.8X1	T50.8X2	T50.8X3	T50.8X4	T50.8X5	T50.8X6
Iodoform	T49.0X1	T49.0X2	T49.0X3	T49.0X4	T49.0X5	T49.0X6
Iodohippuric acid	T50.8X1	T50.8X2	T50.8X3	T50.8X4	T50.8X5	T50.8X6
Iodopanoic acid	T50.8X1	T50.8X2	T50.8X3	T50.8X4	T50.8X5	T50.8X6
Iodophthalein (sodium)	T50.8X1	T50.8X2	T50.8X3	T50.8X4	T50.8X5	T50.8X6
Iodopyracet	T50.8X1	T50.8X2	T50.8X3	T50.8X4	T50.8X5	T50.8X6
Iodoquinol	T37.8X1	T37.8X2	T37.8X3	T37.8X4	T37.8X5	T37.8X6
Iodoxamic acid	T50.8X1	T50.8X2	T50.8X3	T50.8X4	T50.8X5	T50.8X6
Iofendylate	T50.8X1	T50.8X2	T50.8X3	T50.8X4	T50.8X5	T50.8X6
Ioglycamic acid	T50.8X1	T50.8X2	T50.8X3	T50.8X4	T50.8X5	T50.8X6
Iohexol	T50.8X1	T50.8X2	T50.8X3	T50.8X4	T50.8X5	T50.8X6
Ion exchange resin						
anion	T47.8X1	T47.8X2	T47.8X3	T47.8X4	T47.8X5	T47.8X6
cation	T50.3X1	T50.3X2	T50.3X3	T50.3X4	T50.3X5	T50.3X6
cholestyramine	T46.6X1	T46.6X2	T46.6X3	T46.6X4	T46.6X5	T46.6X6
intestinal	T47.8X1	T47.8X2	T47.8X3	T47.8X4	T47.8X5	T47.8X6
Iopamidol	T50.8X1	T50.8X2	T50.8X3	T50.8X4	T50.8X5	T50.8X6
Iopanoic acid	T50.8X1	T50.8X2	T50.8X3	T50.8X4	T50.8X5	T50.8X6
Iophenoic acid	T50.8X1	T50.8X2	T50.8X3	T50.8X4	T50.8X5	T50.8X6
Iopodate, sodium	T50.8X1	T50.8X2	T50.8X3	T50.8X4	T50.8X5	T50.8X6
Iopodic acid	T50.8X1	T50.8X2	T50.8X3	T50.8X4	T50.8X5	T50.8X6
Iopromide	T50.8X1	T50.8X2	T50.8X3	T50.8X4	T50.8X5	T50.8X6
Iopydol	T50.8X1	T50.8X2	T50.8X3	T50.8X4	T50.8X5	T50.8X6
Iotalamic acid	T50.8X1	T50.8X2	T50.8X3	T50.8X4	T50.8X5	T50.8X6
Iothalamate	T50.8X1	T50.8X2	T50.8X3	T50.8X4	T50.8X5	T50.8X6
Iothiouracil	T38.2X1	T38.2X2	T38.2X3	T38.2X4	T38.2X5	T38.2X6
Iotrol	T50.8X1	T50.8X2	T50.8X3	T50.8X4	T50.8X5	T50.8X6
Iotrolan	T50.8X1	T50.8X2	T50.8X3	T50.8X4	T50.8X5	T50.8X6
Iotroxate	T50.8X1	T50.8X2	T50.8X3	T50.8X4	T50.8X5	T50.8X6
Iotroxic acid	T50.8X1	T50.8X2	T50.8X3	T50.8X4	T50.8X5	T50.8X6
Ioversol	T50.8X1	T50.8X2	T50.8X3	T50.8X4	T50.8X5	T50.8X6
Ioxaglate	T50.8X1	T50.8X2	T50.8X3	T50.8X4	T50.8X5	T50.8X6
Ioxaglic acid	T50.8X1	T50.8X2	T50.8X3	T50.8X4	T50.8X5	T50.8X6
Ioxitalamic acid	T50.8X1	T50.8X2	T50.8X3	T50.8X4	T50.8X5	T50.8X6
Ipecac	T47.7X1	T47.7X2	T47.7X3	T47.7X4	T47.7X5	T47.7X6
Ipecacuanha	T48.4X1	T48.4X2	T48.4X3	T48.4X4	T48.4X5	T48.4X6
Ipodate, calcium	T50.8X1	T50.8X2	T50.8X3	T50.8X4	T50.8X5	T50.8X6
Ipral	T42.3X1	T42.3X2	T42.3X3	T42.3X4	T42.3X5	T42.3X6
Ipratropium (bromide)	T48.6X1	T48.6X2	T48.6X3	T48.6X4	T48.6X5	T48.6X6
Iproflavone	T46.3X1	T46.3X2	T46.3X3	T46.3X4	T46.3X5	T46.3X6
Iprindole	T43.011	T43.012	T43.013	T43.014	T43.015	T43.016
Iproclozide	T43.1X1	T43.1X2	T43.1X3	T43.1X4	T43.1X5	T43.1X6
Iprofenin	T50.8X1	T50.8X2	T50.8X3	T50.8X4	T50.8X5	T50.8X6
Iproheptine	T49.2X1	T49.2X2	T49.2X3	T49.2X4	T49.2X5	T49.2X6
Iproniazid	T43.1X1	T43.1X2	T43.1X3	T43.1X4	T43.1X5	T43.1X6
Iproplatin	T45.1X1	T45.1X2	T45.1X3	T45.1X4	T45.1X5	T45.1X6
Iproveratril	T46.1X1	T46.1X2	T46.1X3	T46.1X4	T46.1X5	T46.1X6
Iron (compounds) (medicinal)	T45.4X1	T45.4X2	T45.4X3	T45.4X4	T45.4X5	T45.4X6
NEC						
ammonium	T45.4X1	T45.4X2	T45.4X3	T45.4X4	T45.4X5	T45.4X6
dextran injection	T45.4X1	T45.4X2	T45.4X3	T45.4X4	T45.4X5	T45.4X6
nonmedicinal	T56.891	T56.892	T56.893	T56.894	—	—

Substance	Poisoning, Accidental (unintentional)	Poisoning, Intentional Self-harm	Poisoning, Assault	Poisoning, Undetermined	Adverse Effect	Under-dosing
Iron (compounds) (medicinal) **NEC** — continued						
salts	T45.4X1	T45.4X2	T45.4X3	T45.4X4	T45.4X5	T45.4X6
sorbitex	T45.4X1	T45.4X2	T45.4X3	T45.4X4	T45.4X5	T45.4X6
sorbitol citric acid complex	T45.4X1	T45.4X2	T45.4X3	T45.4X4	T45.4X5	T45.4X6
Irrigating fluid (vaginal)	T49.8X1	T49.8X2	T49.8X3	T49.8X4	T49.8X5	T49.8X6
eye	T49.5X1	T49.5X2	T49.5X3	T49.5X4	T49.5X5	T49.5X6
Isepamicin	T36.5X1	T36.5X2	T36.5X3	T36.5X4	T36.5X5	T36.5X6
Isoaminile (citrate)	T48.3X1	T48.3X2	T48.3X3	T48.3X4	T48.3X5	T48.3X6
Isoamyl nitrite	T46.3X1	T46.3X2	T46.3X3	T46.3X4	T46.3X5	T46.3X6
Isobenzan	T60.1X1	T60.1X2	T60.1X3	T60.1X4	—	—
Isobutyl acetate	T52.8X1	T52.8X2	T52.8X3	T52.8X4	—	—
Isocarboxazid	T43.1X1	T43.1X2	T43.1X3	T43.1X4	T43.1X5	T43.1X6
Isoconazole	T49.0X1	T49.0X2	T49.0X3	T49.0X4	T49.0X5	T49.0X6
Isocyanate	T65.0X1	T65.0X2	T65.0X3	T65.0X4	—	—
Isoephedrine	T44.991	T44.992	T44.993	T44.994	T44.995	T44.996
Isoetarine	T48.6X1	T48.6X2	T48.6X3	T48.6X4	T48.6X5	T48.6X6
Isoethadione	T42.2X1	T42.2X2	T42.2X3	T42.2X4	T42.2X5	T42.2X6
Isoetharine	T44.5X1	T44.5X2	T44.5X3	T44.5X4	T44.5X5	T44.5X6
Isoflurane	T41.0X1	T41.0X2	T41.0X3	T41.0X4	T41.0X5	T41.0X6
Isoflurophate	T44.0X1	T44.0X2	T44.0X3	T44.0X4	T44.0X5	T44.0X6
Isomaltose, ferric complex	T45.4X1	T45.4X2	T45.4X3	T45.4X4	T45.4X5	T45.4X6
Isometheptene	T44.3X1	T44.3X2	T44.3X3	T44.3X4	T44.3X5	T44.3X6
Isoniazid	T37.1X1	T37.1X2	T37.1X3	T37.1X4	T37.1X5	T37.1X6
with						
rifampicin	T36.6X1	T36.6X2	T36.6X3	T36.6X4	T36.6X5	T36.6X6
thioacetazone	T37.1X1	T37.1X2	T37.1X3	T37.1X4	T37.1X5	T37.1X6
Isonicotinic acid hydrazide	T37.1X1	T37.1X2	T37.1X3	T37.1X4	T37.1X5	T37.1X6
Isonipecaine	T40.4X1	T40.4X2	T40.4X3	T40.4X4	T40.4X5	T40.4X6
Isopentaquine	T37.2X1	T37.2X2	T37.2X3	T37.2X4	T37.2X5	T37.2X6
Isophane insulin	T38.3X1	T38.3X2	T38.3X3	T38.3X4	T38.3X5	T38.3X6
Isophorone	T65.891	T65.892	T65.893	T65.894	—	—
Isophosphamide	T45.1X1	T45.1X2	T45.1X3	T45.1X4	T45.1X5	T45.1X6
Isopregnenone	T38.5X1	T38.5X2	T38.5X3	T38.5X4	T38.5X5	T38.5X6
Isoprenaline	T48.6X1	T48.6X2	T48.6X3	T48.6X4	T48.6X5	T48.6X6
Isopromethazine	T43.3X1	T43.3X2	T43.3X3	T43.3X4	T43.3X5	T43.3X6
Isopropamide	T44.3X1	T44.3X2	T44.3X3	T44.3X4	T44.3X5	T44.3X6
iodide	T44.3X1	T44.3X2	T44.3X3	T44.3X4	T44.3X5	T44.3X6
Isopropanol	T51.2X1	T51.2X2	T51.2X3	T51.2X4	—	—
Isopropyl						
acetate	T52.8X1	T52.8X2	T52.8X3	T52.8X4	—	—
alcohol	T51.2X1	T51.2X2	T51.2X3	T51.2X4	—	—
medicinal	T49.4X1	T49.4X2	T49.4X3	T49.4X4	T49.4X5	T49.4X6
ether	T52.8X1	T52.8X2	T52.8X3	T52.8X4	—	—
Isopropylaminophenazone	T39.2X1	T39.2X2	T39.2X3	T39.2X4	T39.2X5	T39.2X6
Isoproterenol	T48.6X1	T48.6X2	T48.6X3	T48.6X4	T48.6X5	T48.6X6
Isosorbide dinitrate	T46.3X1	T46.3X2	T46.3X3	T46.3X4	T46.3X5	T46.3X6
Isothipendyl	T45.0X1	T45.0X2	T45.0X3	T45.0X4	T45.0X5	T45.0X6
Isotretinoin	T50.991	T50.992	T50.993	T50.994	T50.995	T50.996
Isoxazolyl penicillin	T36.0X1	T36.0X2	T36.0X3	T36.0X4	T36.0X5	T36.0X6
Isoxicam	T39.391	T39.392	T39.393	T39.394	T39.395	T39.396
Isoxsuprine	T46.7X1	T46.7X2	T46.7X3	T46.7X4	T46.7X5	T46.7X6
Ispagula	T47.4X1	T47.4X2	T47.4X3	T47.4X4	T47.4X5	T47.4X6
husk	T47.4X1	T47.4X2	T47.4X3	T47.4X4	T47.4X5	T47.4X6
Isradipine	T46.1X1	T46.1X2	T46.1X3	T46.1X4	T46.1X5	T46.1X6
I-thyroxine sodium	T38.1X1	T38.1X2	T38.1X3	T38.1X4	T38.1X5	T38.1X6
Itraconazole	T37.8X1	T37.8X2	T37.8X3	T37.8X4	T37.8X5	T37.8X6
Itramin tosilate	T46.3X1	T46.3X2	T46.3X3	T46.3X4	T46.3X5	T46.3X6
Ivermectin	T37.4X1	T37.4X2	T37.4X3	T37.4X4	T37.4X5	T37.4X6
Izoniazid	T37.1X1	T37.1X2	T37.1X3	T37.1X4	T37.1X5	T37.1X6
with thioacetazone	T37.1X1	T37.1X2	T37.1X3	T37.1X4	T37.1X5	T37.1X6
Jalap	T47.2X1	T47.2X2	T47.2X3	T47.2X4	T47.2X5	T47.2X6
Jamaica						
dogwood (bark)	T39.8X1	T39.8X2	T39.8X3	T39.8X4	T39.8X5	T39.8X6
ginger	T65.891	T65.892	T65.893	T65.894	—	—
root	T62.2X1	T62.2X2	T62.2X3	T62.2X4	—	—
Jatropha	T62.2X1	T62.2X2	T62.2X3	T62.2X4	—	—
curcas	T62.2X1	T62.2X2	T62.2X3	T62.2X4	—	—
Jectofer	T45.4X1	T45.4X2	T45.4X3	T45.4X4	T45.4X5	T45.4X6
Jellyfish (sting)	T63.621	T63.622	T63.623	T63.624	—	—
Jequirity (bean)	T62.2X1	T62.2X2	T62.2X3	T62.2X4	—	—
Jimson weed (stramonium)	T62.2X1	T62.2X2	T62.2X3	T62.2X4	—	—
seeds	T62.2X1	T62.2X2	T62.2X3	T62.2X4	—	—
Josamycin	T36.3X1	T36.3X2	T36.3X3	T36.3X4	T36.3X5	T36.3X6
Juniper tar	T49.1X1	T49.1X2	T49.1X3	T49.1X4	T49.1X5	T49.1X6
Kallidinogenase	T46.7X1	T46.7X2	T46.7X3	T46.7X4	T46.7X5	T46.7X6
Kallikrein	T46.7X1	T46.7X2	T46.7X3	T46.7X4	T46.7X5	T46.7X6
Kanamycin	T36.5X1	T36.5X2	T36.5X3	T36.5X4	T36.5X5	T36.5X6
Kantrex	T36.5X1	T36.5X2	T36.5X3	T36.5X4	T36.5X5	T36.5X6
Kaolin	T47.6X1	T47.6X2	T47.6X3	T47.6X4	T47.6X5	T47.6X6
light	T47.6X1	T47.6X2	T47.6X3	T47.6X4	T47.6X5	T47.6X6
Karaya (gum)	T47.4X1	T47.4X2	T47.4X3	T47.4X4	T47.4X5	T47.4X6

Additional Character May Be Required — Refer to the Tabular List for Character Selection   ▽ Subterms under main terms may continue to next column or page

Substance	Poisoning, Accidental (unintentional)	Poisoning, Intentional Self-harm	Poisoning, Assault	Poisoning, Undetermined	Adverse Effect	Under-dosing
Kebuzone	T39.2X1	T39.2X2	T39.2X3	T39.2X4	T39.2X5	T39.2X6
Kelevan	T60.1X1	T60.1X2	T60.1X3	T60.1X4	—	—
Kemithal	T41.1X1	T41.1X2	T41.1X3	T41.1X4	T41.1X5	T41.1X6
Kenacort	T38.0X1	T38.0X2	T38.0X3	T38.0X4	T38.0X5	T38.0X6
Keratolytic drug NEC	T49.4X1	T49.4X2	T49.4X3	T49.4X4	T49.4X5	T49.4X6
anthracene	T49.4X1	T49.4X2	T49.4X3	T49.4X4	T49.4X5	T49.4X6
Keratoplastic NEC	T49.4X1	T49.4X2	T49.4X3	T49.4X4	T49.4X5	T49.4X6
Kerosene, kerosine (fuel) (solvent) **NEC**	T52.0X1	T52.0X2	T52.0X3	T52.0X4	—	—
insecticide	T52.0X1	T52.0X2	T52.0X3	T52.0X4	—	—
vapor	T52.0X1	T52.0X2	T52.0X3	T52.0X4	—	—
Ketamine	T41.291	T41.292	T41.293	T41.294	T41.295	T41.296
Ketazolam	T42.4X1	T42.4X2	T42.4X3	T42.4X4	T42.4X5	T42.4X6
Ketazon	T39.2X1	T39.2X2	T39.2X3	T39.2X4	T39.2X5	T39.2X6
Ketobemidone	T40.4X1	T40.4X2	T40.4X3	T40.4X4	—	—
Ketoconazole	T49.0X1	T49.0X2	T49.0X3	T49.0X4	T49.0X5	T49.0X6
Ketols	T52.4X1	T52.4X2	T52.4X3	T52.4X4	—	—
Ketone oils	T52.4X1	T52.4X2	T52.4X3	T52.4X4	—	—
Ketoprofen	T39.311	T39.312	T39.313	T39.314	T39.315	T39.316
Ketorolac	T39.8X1	T39.8X2	T39.8X3	T39.8X4	T39.8X5	T39.8X6
Ketotifen	T45.0X1	T45.0X2	T45.0X3	T45.0X4	T45.0X5	T45.0X6
Khat	T43.691	T43.692	T43.693	T43.694	—	—
Khellin	T46.3X1	T46.3X2	T46.3X3	T46.3X4	T46.3X5	T46.3X6
Khelloside	T46.3X1	T46.3X2	T46.3X3	T46.3X4	T46.3X5	T46.3X6
Kiln gas or vapor (carbon monoxide)	T58.8X1	T58.8X2	T58.8X3	T58.8X4		
Kitasamycin	T36.3X1	T36.3X2	T36.3X3	T36.3X4	T36.3X5	T36.3X6
Konsyl	T47.4X1	T47.4X2	T47.4X3	T47.4X4	T47.4X5	T47.4X6
Kosam seed	T62.2X1	T62.2X2	T62.2X3	T62.2X4	—	—
Krait (venom)	T63.091	T63.092	T63.093	T63.094	—	—
Kwell (insecticide)	T60.1X1	T60.1X2	T60.1X3	T60.1X4	—	—
anti-infective (topical)	T49.0X1	T49.0X2	T49.0X3	T49.0X4	T49.0X5	T49.0X6
Labetalol	T44.8X1	T44.8X2	T44.8X3	T44.8X4	T44.8X5	T44.8X6
Laburnum (seeds)	T62.2X1	T62.2X2	T62.2X3	T62.2X4	—	—
leaves	T62.2X1	T62.2X2	T62.2X3	T62.2X4	—	—
Lachesine	T49.5X1	T49.5X2	T49.5X3	T49.5X4	T49.5X5	T49.5X6
Lacidipine	T46.5X1	T46.5X2	T46.5X3	T46.5X4	T46.5X5	T46.5X6
Lacquer	T65.6X1	T65.6X2	T65.6X3	T65.6X4	—	—
Lacrimogenic gas	T59.3X1	T59.3X2	T59.3X3	T59.3X4	—	—
Lactated potassic saline	T50.3X1	T50.3X2	T50.3X3	T50.3X4	T50.3X5	T50.3X6
Lactic acid	T49.8X1	T49.8X2	T49.8X3	T49.8X4	T49.8X5	T49.8X6
Lactobacillus						
acidophilus	T47.6X1	T47.6X2	T47.6X3	T47.6X4	T47.6X5	T47.6X6
compound	T47.6X1	T47.6X2	T47.6X3	T47.6X4	T47.6X5	T47.6X6
bifidus, lyophilized	T47.6X1	T47.6X2	T47.6X3	T47.6X4	T47.6X5	T47.6X6
bulgaricus	T47.6X1	T47.6X2	T47.6X3	T47.6X4	T47.6X5	T47.6X6
sporogenes	T47.6X1	T47.6X2	T47.6X3	T47.6X4	T47.6X5	T47.6X6
Lactoflavin	T45.2X1	T45.2X2	T45.2X3	T45.2X4	T45.2X5	T45.2X6
Lactose (as excipient)	T50.901	T50.902	T50.903	T50.904	T50.905	T50.906
Lactuca (virosa) (extract)	T42.6X1	T42.6X2	T42.6X3	T42.6X4	T42.6X5	T42.6X6
Lactucarium	T42.6X1	T42.6X2	T42.6X3	T42.6X4	T42.6X5	T42.6X6
Lactulose	T47.3X1	T47.3X2	T47.3X3	T47.3X4	T47.3X5	T47.3X6
Laevo — *see* Levo-						
Lanatosides	T46.0X1	T46.0X2	T46.0X3	T46.0X4	T46.0X5	T46.0X6
Lanolin	T49.3X1	T49.3X2	T49.3X3	T49.3X4	T49.3X5	T49.3X6
Largactil	T43.3X1	T43.3X2	T43.3X3	T43.3X4	T43.3X5	T43.3X6
Larkspur	T62.2X1	T62.2X2	T62.2X3	T62.2X4	—	—
Laroxyl	T43.011	T43.012	T43.013	T43.014	T43.015	T43.016
Lasix	T50.1X1	T50.1X2	T50.1X3	T50.1X4	T50.1X5	T50.1X6
Lassar's paste	T49.4X1	T49.4X2	T49.4X3	T49.4X4	T49.4X5	T49.4X6
Latamoxef	T36.1X1	T36.1X2	T36.1X3	T36.1X4	T36.1X5	T36.1X6
Latex	T65.811	T65.812	T65.813	T65.814	—	—
Lathyrus (seed)	T62.2X1	T62.2X2	T62.2X3	T62.2X4	—	—
Laudanum	T40.0X1	T40.0X2	T40.0X3	T40.0X4	T40.0X5	T40.0X6
Laudexium	T48.1X1	T48.1X2	T48.1X3	T48.1X4	T48.1X5	T48.1X6
Laughing gas	T41.0X1	T41.0X2	T41.0X3	T41.0X4	T41.0X5	T41.0X6
Laurel, black or cherry	T62.2X1	T62.2X2	T62.2X3	T62.2X4	—	—
Laurolinium	T49.0X1	T49.0X2	T49.0X3	T49.0X4	T49.0X5	T49.0X6
Lauryl sulfoacetate	T49.2X1	T49.2X2	T49.2X3	T49.2X4	T49.2X5	T49.2X6
Laxative NEC	T47.4X1	T47.4X2	T47.4X3	T47.4X4	T47.4X5	T47.4X6
osmotic	T47.3X1	T47.3X2	T47.3X3	T47.3X4	T47.3X5	T47.3X6
saline	T47.3X1	T47.3X2	T47.3X3	T47.3X4	T47.3X5	T47.3X6
stimulant	T47.2X1	T47.2X2	T47.2X3	T47.2X4	T47.2X5	T47.2X6
L-dopa	T42.8X1	T42.8X2	T42.8X3	T42.8X4	T42.8X5	T42.8X6
Lead (dust) (fumes) (vapor) **NEC**	T56.0X1	T56.0X2	T56.0X3	T56.0X4		
acetate	T49.2X1	T49.2X2	T49.2X3	T49.2X4	T49.2X5	T49.2X6
alkyl (fuel additive)	T56.0X1	T56.0X2	T56.0X3	T56.0X4	—	—
anti-infectives	T37.8X1	T37.8X2	T37.8X3	T37.8X4	T37.8X5	T37.8X6
antiknock compound (tetraethyl)	T56.0X1	T56.0X2	T56.0X3	T56.0X4	—	—

Substance	Poisoning, Accidental (unintentional)	Poisoning, Intentional Self-harm	Poisoning, Assault	Poisoning, Undetermined	Adverse Effect	Under-dosing
Lead (dust) (fumes) (vapor) **NEC** — *continued*						
arsenate, arsenite (dust)(herbicide) (insecticide) (vapor)	T57.0X1	T57.0X2	T57.0X3	T57.0X4	—	—
carbonate	T56.0X1	T56.0X2	T56.0X3	T56.0X4	—	—
paint	T56.0X1	T56.0X2	T56.0X3	T56.0X4	—	—
chromate	T56.0X1	T56.0X2	T56.0X3	T56.0X4	—	—
paint	T56.0X1	T56.0X2	T56.0X3	T56.0X4	—	—
dioxide	T56.0X1	T56.0X2	T56.0X3	T56.0X4	—	—
inorganic	T56.0X1	T56.0X2	T56.0X3	T56.0X4	—	—
iodide	T56.0X1	T56.0X2	T56.0X3	T56.0X4	—	—
pigment (paint)	T56.0X1	T56.0X2	T56.0X3	T56.0X4	—	—
monoxide (dust)	T56.0X1	T56.0X2	T56.0X3	T56.0X4	—	—
paint	T56.0X1	T56.0X2	T56.0X3	T56.0X4	—	—
organic	T56.0X1	T56.0X2	T56.0X3	T56.0X4	—	—
oxide	T56.0X1	T56.0X2	T56.0X3	T56.0X4	—	—
paint	T56.0X1	T56.0X2	T56.0X3	T56.0X4	—	—
paint	T56.0X1	T56.0X2	T56.0X3	T56.0X4	—	—
salts	T56.0X1	T56.0X2	T56.0X3	T56.0X4	—	—
specified compound NEC	T56.0X1	T56.0X2	T56.0X3	T56.0X4	—	—
tetra-ethyl	T56.0X1	T56.0X2	T56.0X3	T56.0X4	—	—
Lebanese red	T40.7X1	T40.7X2	T40.7X3	T40.7X4	T40.7X5	T40.7X6
Lefetamine	T39.8X1	T39.8X2	T39.8X3	T39.8X4	T39.8X5	T39.8X6
Lenperone	T43.4X1	T43.4X2	T43.4X3	T43.4X4	T43.4X5	T43.4X6
Lente lietin (insulin)	T38.3X1	T38.3X2	T38.3X3	T38.3X4	T38.3X5	T38.3X6
Leptazol	T50.7X1	T50.7X2	T50.7X3	T50.7X4	T50.7X5	T50.7X6
Leptophos	T60.0X1	T60.0X2	T60.0X3	T60.0X4	—	—
Leritine	T40.2X1	T40.2X2	T40.2X3	T40.2X4	T40.2X5	T40.2X6
Letosteine	T48.4X1	T48.4X2	T48.4X3	T48.4X4	T48.4X5	T48.4X6
Letter	T38.1X1	T38.1X2	T38.1X3	T38.1X4	T38.1X5	T38.1X6
Lettuce opium	T42.6X1	T42.6X2	T42.6X3	T42.6X4	T42.6X5	T42.6X6
Leucinocaine	T41.3X1	T41.3X2	T41.3X3	T41.3X4	T41.3X5	T41.3X6
Leucocianidol	T46.991	T46.992	T46.993	T46.994	T46.995	T46.996
Leucovorin (factor)	T45.8X1	T45.8X2	T45.8X3	T45.8X4	T45.8X5	T45.8X6
Leukeran	T45.1X1	T45.1X2	T45.1X3	T45.1X4	T45.1X5	T45.1X6
Leuprolide	T38.891	T38.892	T38.893	T38.894	T38.895	T38.896
Levalbuterol	T48.6X1	T48.6X2	T48.6X3	T48.6X4	T48.6X5	T48.6X6
Levallorphan	T50.7X1	T50.7X2	T50.7X3	T50.7X4	T50.7X5	T50.7X6
Levamisole	T37.4X1	T37.4X2	T37.4X3	T37.4X4	T37.4X5	T37.4X6
Levanil	T42.6X1	T42.6X2	T42.6X3	T42.6X4	T42.6X5	T42.6X6
Levarterenol	T44.4X1	T44.4X2	T44.4X3	T44.4X4	T44.4X5	T44.4X6
Levdropropizine	T48.3X1	T48.3X2	T48.3X3	T48.3X4	T48.3X5	T48.3X6
Levobunolol	T49.5X1	T49.5X2	T49.5X3	T49.5X4	T49.5X5	T49.5X6
Levocabastine (hydrochloride)	T45.0X1	T45.0X2	T45.0X3	T45.0X4	T45.0X5	T45.0X6
Levocarnitine	T50.991	T50.992	T50.993	T50.994	T50.995	T50.996
Levodopa	T42.8X1	T42.8X2	T42.8X3	T42.8X4	T42.8X5	T42.8X6
with carbidopa	T42.8X1	T42.8X2	T42.8X3	T42.8X4	T42.8X5	T42.8X6
Levo-dromoran	T40.2X1	T40.2X2	T40.2X3	T40.2X4	T40.2X5	T40.2X6
Levoglutamide	T50.991	T50.992	T50.993	T50.994	T50.995	T50.996
Levoid	T38.1X1	T38.1X2	T38.1X3	T38.1X4	T38.1X5	T38.1X6
Levo-isomethadone	T40.3X1	T40.3X2	T40.3X3	T40.3X4	T40.3X5	T40.3X6
Levomepromazine	T43.3X1	T43.3X2	T43.3X3	T43.3X4	T43.3X5	T43.3X6
Levonordefrin	T49.6X1	T49.6X2	T49.6X3	T49.6X4	T49.6X5	T49.6X6
Levonorgestrel	T38.4X1	T38.4X2	T38.4X3	T38.4X4	T38.4X5	T38.4X6
with ethinylestradiol	T38.5X1	T38.5X2	T38.5X3	T38.5X4	T38.5X5	T38.5X6
Levopromazine	T43.3X1	T43.3X2	T43.3X3	T43.3X4	T43.3X5	T43.3X6
Levoprome	T42.6X1	T42.6X2	T42.6X3	T42.6X4	T42.6X5	T42.6X6
Levopropoxyphene	T40.4X1	T40.4X2	T40.4X3	T40.4X4	T40.4X5	T40.4X6
Levopropylhexedrine	T50.5X1	T50.5X2	T50.5X3	T50.5X4	T50.5X5	T50.5X6
Levoproxyphylline	T48.6X1	T48.6X2	T48.6X3	T48.6X4	T48.6X5	T48.6X6
Levorphanol	T40.4X1	T40.4X2	T40.4X3	T40.4X4	T40.4X5	T40.4X6
Levothyroxine	T38.1X1	T38.1X2	T38.1X3	T38.1X4	T38.1X5	T38.1X6
sodium	T38.1X1	T38.1X2	T38.1X3	T38.1X4	T38.1X5	T38.1X6
Levsin	T44.3X1	T44.3X2	T44.3X3	T44.3X4	T44.3X5	T44.3X6
Levulose	T50.3X1	T50.3X2	T50.3X3	T50.3X4	T50.3X5	T50.3X6
Lewisite (gas), not in war	T57.0X1	T57.0X2	T57.0X3	T57.0X4	—	—
Librium	T42.4X1	T42.4X2	T42.4X3	T42.4X4	T42.4X5	T42.4X6
Lidex	T49.0X1	T49.0X2	T49.0X3	T49.0X4	T49.0X5	T49.0X6
Lidocaine	T41.3X1	T41.3X2	T41.3X3	T41.3X4	T41.3X5	T41.3X6
regional	T41.3X1	T41.3X2	T41.3X3	T41.3X4	T41.3X5	T41.3X6
spinal	T41.3X1	T41.3X2	T41.3X3	T41.3X4	T41.3X5	T41.3X6
Lidofenin	T50.8X1	T50.8X2	T50.8X3	T50.8X4	T50.8X5	T50.8X6
Lidoflazine	T46.1X1	T46.1X2	T46.1X3	T46.1X4	T46.1X5	T46.1X6
Lighter fluid	T52.0X1	T52.0X2	T52.0X3	T52.0X4	—	—
Lignin hemicellulose	T47.6X1	T47.6X2	T47.6X3	T47.6X4	T47.6X5	T47.6X6
Lignocaine	T41.3X1	T41.3X2	T41.3X3	T41.3X4	T41.3X5	T41.3X6
regional	T41.3X1	T41.3X2	T41.3X3	T41.3X4	T41.3X5	T41.3X6
spinal	T41.3X1	T41.3X2	T41.3X3	T41.3X4	T41.3X5	T41.3X6
Ligroin (e) (solvent)	T52.0X1	T52.0X2	T52.0X3	T52.0X4	—	—
vapor	T59.891	T59.892	T59.893	T59.894	—	—
Ligustrum vulgare	T62.2X1	T62.2X2	T62.2X3	T62.2X4	—	—

Substance	Poisoning, Accidental (unintentional)	Poisoning, Intentional Self-harm	Poisoning, Assault	Poisoning, Undetermined	Adverse Effect	Under-dosing
Lily of the valley	T62.2X1	T62.2X2	T62.2X3	T62.2X4	—	—
Lime (chloride)	T54.3X1	T54.3X2	T54.3X3	T54.3X4	—	—
Limonene	T52.8X1	T52.8X2	T52.8X3	T52.8X4	—	—
Lincomycin	T36.8X1	T36.8X2	T36.8X3	T36.8X4	T36.8X5	T36.8X6
Lindane (insecticide) (nonmedicinal) (vapor)	T53.6X1	T53.6X2	T53.6X3	T53.6X4	—	—
medicinal	T49.0X1	T49.0X2	T49.0X3	T49.0X4	T49.0X5	T49.0X6
Liniments NEC	T49.91	T49.92	T49.93	T49.94	T49.95	T49.96
Linoleic acid	T46.6X1	T46.6X2	T46.6X3	T46.6X4	T46.6X5	T46.6X6
Linolenic acid	T46.6X1	T46.6X2	T46.6X3	T46.6X4	T46.6X5	T46.6X6
Linseed	T47.4X1	T47.4X2	T47.4X3	T47.4X4	T47.4X5	T47.4X6
Liothyronine	T38.1X1	T38.1X2	T38.1X3	T38.1X4	T38.1X5	T38.1X6
Liotrix	T38.1X1	T38.1X2	T38.1X3	T38.1X4	T38.1X5	T38.1X6
Lipancreatin	T47.5X1	T47.5X2	T47.5X3	T47.5X4	T47.5X5	T47.5X6
Lipo-alprostadil	T46.7X1	T46.7X2	T46.7X3	T46.7X4	T46.7X5	T46.7X6
Lipo-Lutin	T38.5X1	T38.5X2	T38.5X3	T38.5X4	T38.5X5	T38.5X6
Lipotropic drug NEC	T50.901	T50.902	T50.903	T50.904	T50.905	T50.906
Liquefied petroleum gases	T59.891	T59.892	T59.893	T59.894	—	—
piped (pure or mixed with air)	T59.891	T59.892	T59.893	T59.894	—	—
Liquid						
paraffin	T47.4X1	T47.4X2	T47.4X3	T47.4X4	T47.4X5	T47.4X6
petrolatum	T47.4X1	T47.4X2	T47.4X3	T47.4X4	T47.4X5	T47.4X6
topical	T49.3X1	T49.3X2	T49.3X3	T49.3X4	T49.3X5	T49.3X6
specified NEC	T65.891	T65.892	T65.893	T65.894	—	—
substance	T65.91	T65.92	T65.93	T65.94	—	—
Liquor creosolis compositus	T65.891	T65.892	T65.893	T65.894	—	—
Liquorice	T48.4X1	T48.4X2	T48.4X3	T48.4X4	T48.4X5	T48.4X6
extract	T47.8X1	T47.8X2	T47.8X3	T47.8X4	T47.8X5	T47.8X6
Lisinopril	T46.4X1	T46.4X2	T46.4X3	T46.4X4	T46.4X5	T46.4X6
Lisuride	T42.8X1	T42.8X2	T42.8X3	T42.8X4	T42.8X5	T42.8X6
Lithane	T43.8X1	T43.8X2	T43.8X3	T43.8X4	T43.8X5	T43.8X6
Lithium	T56.891	T56.892	T56.893	T56.894	—	—
gluconate	T43.591	T43.592	T43.593	T43.594	T43.595	T43.596
salts (carbonate)	T43.591	T43.592	T43.593	T43.594	T43.595	T43.596
Lithonate	T43.8X1	T43.8X2	T43.8X3	T43.8X4	T43.8X5	T43.8X6
Liver						
extract	T45.8X1	T45.8X2	T45.8X3	T45.8X4	T45.8X5	T45.8X6
for parenteral use	T45.8X1	T45.8X2	T45.8X3	T45.8X4	T45.8X5	T45.8X6
fraction 1	T45.8X1	T45.8X2	T45.8X3	T45.8X4	T45.8X5	T45.8X6
hydrolysate	T45.8X1	T45.8X2	T45.8X3	T45.8X4	T45.8X5	T45.8X6
Lizard (bite) (venom)	T63.121	T63.122	T63.123	T63.124	—	—
LMD	T45.8X1	T45.8X2	T45.8X3	T45.8X4	T45.8X5	T45.8X6
Lobelia	T62.2X1	T62.2X2	T62.2X3	T62.2X4	—	—
Lobeline	T50.7X1	T50.7X2	T50.7X3	T50.7X4	T50.7X5	T50.7X6
Local action drug NEC	T49.8X1	T49.8X2	T49.8X3	T49.8X4	T49.8X5	T49.8X6
Locorten	T49.0X1	T49.0X2	T49.0X3	T49.0X4	T49.0X5	T49.0X6
Lofepramine	T43.011	T43.012	T43.013	T43.014	T43.015	T43.016
Lolium temulentum	T62.2X1	T62.2X2	T62.2X3	T62.2X4	—	—
Lomotil	T47.6X1	T47.6X2	T47.6X3	T47.6X4	T47.6X5	T47.6X6
Lomustine	T45.1X1	T45.1X2	T45.1X3	T45.1X4	T45.1X5	T45.1X6
Lonidamine	T45.1X1	T45.1X2	T45.1X3	T45.1X4	T45.1X5	T45.1X6
Loperamide	T47.6X1	T47.6X2	T47.6X3	T47.6X4	T47.6X5	T47.6X6
Loprazolam	T42.4X1	T42.4X2	T42.4X3	T42.4X4	T42.4X5	T42.4X6
Lorajmine	T46.2X1	T46.2X2	T46.2X3	T46.2X4	T46.2X5	T46.2X6
Loratidine	T45.0X1	T45.0X2	T45.0X3	T45.0X4	T45.0X5	T45.0X6
Lorazepam	T42.4X1	T42.4X2	T42.4X3	T42.4X4	T42.4X5	T42.4X6
Lorcainide	T46.2X1	T46.2X2	T46.2X3	T46.2X4	T46.2X5	T46.2X6
Lormetazepam	T42.4X1	T42.4X2	T42.4X3	T42.4X4	T42.4X5	T42.4X6
Lotions NEC	T49.91	T49.92	T49.93	T49.94	T49.95	T49.96
Lotusate	T42.3X1	T42.3X2	T42.3X3	T42.3X4	T42.3X5	T42.3X6
Lovastatin	T46.6X1	T46.6X2	T46.6X3	T46.6X4	T46.6X5	T46.6X6
Lowila	T49.2X1	T49.2X2	T49.2X3	T49.2X4	T49.2X5	T49.2X6
Loxapine	T43.591	T43.592	T43.593	T43.594	T43.595	T43.596
Lozenges (throat)	T49.6X1	T49.6X2	T49.6X3	T49.6X4	T49.6X5	T49.6X6
LSD	T40.8X1	T40.8X2	T40.8X3	T40.8X4	—	—
L-Tryptophan — *see* amino acid						
Lubricant, eye	T49.5X1	T49.5X2	T49.5X3	T49.5X4	T49.5X5	T49.5X6
Lubricating oil NEC	T52.0X1	T52.0X2	T52.0X3	T52.0X4	—	—
Lucanthone	T37.4X1	T37.4X2	T37.4X3	T37.4X4	T37.4X5	T37.4X6
Luminal	T42.3X1	T42.3X2	T42.3X3	T42.3X4	T42.3X5	T42.3X6
Lung irritant (gas) **NEC**	T59.91	T59.92	T59.93	T59.94	—	—
Luteinizing hormone	T38.811	T38.812	T38.813	T38.814	T38.815	T38.816
Lutocylol	T38.5X1	T38.5X2	T38.5X3	T38.5X4	T38.5X5	T38.5X6
Lutromone	T38.5X1	T38.5X2	T38.5X3	T38.5X4	T38.5X5	T38.5X6
Lututrin	T48.291	T48.292	T48.293	T48.294	T48.295	T48.296
Lye (concentrated)	T54.3X1	T54.3X2	T54.3X3	T54.3X4	—	—
Lygranum (skin test)	T50.8X1	T50.8X2	T50.8X3	T50.8X4	T50.8X5	T50.8X6
Lymecycline	T36.4X1	T36.4X2	T36.4X3	T36.4X4	T36.4X5	T36.4X6
Lymphogranuloma venereum antigen	T50.8X1	T50.8X2	T50.8X3	T50.8X4	T50.8X5	T50.8X6
Lynestrenol	T38.4X1	T38.4X2	T38.4X3	T38.4X4	T38.4X5	T38.4X6
Lyovac Sodium Edecrin	T50.1X1	T50.1X2	T50.1X3	T50.1X4	T50.1X5	T50.1X6
Lypressin	T38.891	T38.892	T38.893	T38.894	T38.895	T38.896
Lysergic acid diethylamide	T40.8X1	T40.8X2	T40.8X3	T40.8X4	—	—
Lysergide	T40.8X1	T40.8X2	T40.8X3	T40.8X4	—	—
Lysine vasopressin	T38.891	T38.892	T38.893	T38.894	T38.895	T38.896
Lysol	T54.1X1	T54.1X2	T54.1X3	T54.1X4	—	—
Lysozyme	T49.0X1	T49.0X2	T49.0X3	T49.0X4	T49.0X5	T49.0X6
Lytta (vitatta)	T49.8X1	T49.8X2	T49.8X3	T49.8X4	T49.8X5	T49.8X6
Mace	T59.3X1	T59.3X2	T59.3X3	T59.3X4	—	—
Macrogol	T50.991	T50.992	T50.993	T50.994	T50.995	T50.996
Macrolide						
anabolic drug	T38.7X1	T38.7X2	T38.7X3	T38.7X4	T38.7X5	T38.7X6
antibiotic	T36.3X1	T36.3X2	T36.3X3	T36.3X4	T36.3X5	T36.3X6
Mafenide	T49.0X1	T49.0X2	T49.0X3	T49.0X4	T49.0X5	T49.0X6
Magaldrate	T47.1X1	T47.1X2	T47.1X3	T47.1X4	T47.1X5	T47.1X6
Magic mushroom	T40.991	T40.992	T40.993	T40.994	—	—
Magnamycin	T36.8X1	T36.8X2	T36.8X3	T36.8X4	T36.8X5	T36.8X6
Magnesia magma	T47.1X1	T47.1X2	T47.1X3	T47.1X4	T47.1X5	T47.1X6
Magnesium NEC	T56.891	T56.892	T56.893	T56.894	—	—
carbonate	T47.1X1	T47.1X2	T47.1X3	T47.1X4	T47.1X5	T47.1X6
citrate	T47.4X1	T47.4X2	T47.4X3	T47.4X4	T47.4X5	T47.4X6
hydroxide	T47.1X1	T47.1X2	T47.1X3	T47.1X4	T47.1X5	T47.1X6
oxide	T47.1X1	T47.1X2	T47.1X3	T47.1X4	T47.1X5	T47.1X6
peroxide	T49.0X1	T49.0X2	T49.0X3	T49.0X4	T49.0X5	T49.0X6
salicylate	T39.091	T39.092	T39.093	T39.094	T39.095	T39.096
silicofluoride	T50.3X1	T50.3X2	T50.3X3	T50.3X4	T50.3X5	T50.3X6
sulfate	T47.4X1	T47.4X2	T47.4X3	T47.4X4	T47.4X5	T47.4X6
thiosulfate	T45.0X1	T45.0X2	T45.0X3	T45.0X4	T45.0X5	T45.0X6
trisilicate	T47.1X1	T47.1X2	T47.1X3	T47.1X4	T47.1X5	T47.1X6
Malathion (medicinal)	T49.0X1	T49.0X2	T49.0X3	T49.0X4	T49.0X5	T49.0X6
insecticide	T60.0X1	T60.0X2	T60.0X3	T60.0X4	—	—
Male fern extract	T37.4X1	T37.4X2	T37.4X3	T37.4X4	T37.4X5	T37.4X6
M-AMSA	T45.1X1	T45.1X2	T45.1X3	T45.1X4	T45.1X5	T45.1X6
Mandelic acid	T37.8X1	T37.8X2	T37.8X3	T37.8X4	T37.8X5	T37.8X6
Manganese (dioxide) (salts)	T57.2X1	T57.2X2	T57.2X3	T57.2X4	—	—
medicinal	T50.991	T50.992	T50.993	T50.994	T50.995	T50.996
Mannitol	T47.3X1	T47.3X2	T47.3X3	T47.3X4	T47.3X5	T47.3X6
hexanitrate	T46.3X1	T46.3X2	T46.3X3	T46.3X4	T46.3X5	T46.3X6
Mannomustine	T45.1X1	T45.1X2	T45.1X3	T45.1X4	T45.1X5	T45.1X6
MAO inhibitors	T43.1X1	T43.1X2	T43.1X3	T43.1X4	T43.1X5	T43.1X6
Mapharsen	T37.8X1	T37.8X2	T37.8X3	T37.8X4	T37.8X5	T37.8X6
Maphenide	T49.0X1	T49.0X2	T49.0X3	T49.0X4	T49.0X5	T49.0X6
Maprotiline	T43.021	T43.022	T43.023	T43.024	T43.025	T43.026
Marcaine	T41.3X1	T41.3X2	T41.3X3	T41.3X4	T41.3X5	T41.3X6
infiltration (subcutaneous)	T41.3X1	T41.3X2	T41.3X3	T41.3X4	T41.3X5	T41.3X6
nerve block (peripheral) (plexus)	T41.3X1	T41.3X2	T41.3X3	T41.3X4	T41.3X5	T41.3X6
Marezine	T45.0X1	T45.0X2	T45.0X3	T45.0X4	T45.0X5	T45.0X6
Marihuana	T40.7X1	T40.7X2	T40.7X3	T40.7X4	T40.7X5	T40.7X6
Marijuana	T40.7X1	T40.7X2	T40.7X3	T40.7X4	T40.7X5	T40.7X6
Marine (sting)	T63.691	T63.692	T63.693	T63.694	—	—
animals (sting)	T63.691	T63.692	T63.693	T63.694	—	—
plants (sting)	T63.711	T63.712	T63.713	T63.714	—	—
Marplan	T43.1X1	T43.1X2	T43.1X3	T43.1X4	T43.1X5	T43.1X6
Marsh gas	T59.891	T59.892	T59.893	T59.894	—	—
Marsilid	T43.1X1	T43.1X2	T43.1X3	T43.1X4	T43.1X5	T43.1X6
Matulane	T45.1X1	T45.1X2	T45.1X3	T45.1X4	T45.1X5	T45.1X6
Mazindol	T50.5X1	T50.5X2	T50.5X3	T50.5X4	T50.5X5	T50.5X6
MCPA	T60.3X1	T60.3X2	T60.3X3	T60.3X4	—	—
MDMA	T43.621	T43.622	T43.623	T43.624	T43.625	T43.626
Meadow saffron	T62.2X1	T62.2X2	T62.2X3	T62.2X4	—	—
Measles virus vaccine (attenuated)	T50.B91	T50.B92	T50.B93	T50.B94	T50.B95	T50.B96
Meat, noxious	T62.8X1	T62.8X2	T62.8X3	T62.8X4	—	—
Meballymal	T42.3X1	T42.3X2	T42.3X3	T42.3X4	T42.3X5	T42.3X6
Mebanazine	T43.1X1	T43.1X2	T43.1X3	T43.1X4	T43.1X5	T43.1X6
Mebaral	T42.3X1	T42.3X2	T42.3X3	T42.3X4	T42.3X5	T42.3X6
Mebendazole	T37.4X1	T37.4X2	T37.4X3	T37.4X4	T37.4X5	T37.4X6
Mebeverine	T44.3X1	T44.3X2	T44.3X3	T44.3X4	T44.3X5	T44.3X6
Mebhydrolin	T45.0X1	T45.0X2	T45.0X3	T45.0X4	T45.0X5	T45.0X6
Mebumal	T42.3X1	T42.3X2	T42.3X3	T42.3X4	T42.3X5	T42.3X6
Mebutamate	T43.591	T43.592	T43.593	T43.594	T43.595	T43.596
Mecamylamine	T44.2X1	T44.2X2	T44.2X3	T44.2X4	T44.2X5	T44.2X6
Mechlorethamine	T45.1X1	T45.1X2	T45.1X3	T45.1X4	T45.1X5	T45.1X6
Mecillinam	T36.0X1	T36.0X2	T36.0X3	T36.0X4	T36.0X5	T36.0X6
Meclizine (hydrochloride)	T45.0X1	T45.0X2	T45.0X3	T45.0X4	T45.0X5	T45.0X6
Meclocycline	T36.4X1	T36.4X2	T36.4X3	T36.4X4	T36.4X5	T36.4X6
Meclofenamate	T39.391	T39.392	T39.393	T39.394	T39.395	T39.396
Meclofenamic acid	T39.391	T39.392	T39.393	T39.394	T39.395	T39.396
Meclofenoxate	T43.691	T43.692	T43.693	T43.694	T43.695	T43.696
Meclozine	T45.0X1	T45.0X2	T45.0X3	T45.0X4	T45.0X5	T45.0X6
Mecobalamin	T45.8X1	T45.8X2	T45.8X3	T45.8X4	T45.8X5	T45.8X6
Mecoprop	T60.3X1	T60.3X2	T60.3X3	T60.3X4	—	—

Additional Character May Be Required — Refer to the Tabular List for Character Selection   ▽ Subterms under main terms may continue to next column or page

Substance	Poisoning, Accidental (unintentional)	Poisoning, Intentional Self-harm	Poisoning, Assault	Poisoning, Undetermined	Adverse Effect	Under-dosing
Mecrilate	T49.3X1	T49.3X2	T49.3X3	T49.3X4	T49.3X5	T49.3X6
Mecysteine	T48.4X1	T48.4X2	T48.4X3	T48.4X4	T48.4X5	T48.4X6
Medazepam	T42.4X1	T42.4X2	T42.4X3	T42.4X4	T42.4X5	T42.4X6
Medicament NEC	T50.901	T50.902	T50.903	T50.904	T50.905	T50.906
Medinal	T42.3X1	T42.3X2	T42.3X3	T42.3X4	T42.3X5	T42.3X6
Medomin	T42.3X1	T42.3X2	T42.3X3	T42.3X4	T42.3X5	T42.3X6
Medrogestone	T38.5X1	T38.5X2	T38.5X3	T38.5X4	T38.5X5	T38.5X6
Medroxalol	T44.8X1	T44.8X2	T44.8X3	T44.8X4	T44.8X5	T44.8X6
Medroxyprogesterone acetate (depot)	T38.5X1	T38.5X2	T38.5X3	T38.5X4	T38.5X5	T38.5X6
Medrysone	T49.0X1	T49.0X2	T49.0X3	T49.0X4	T49.0X5	T49.0X6
Mefenamic acid	T39.391	T39.392	T39.393	T39.394	T39.395	T39.396
Mefenorex	T50.5X1	T50.5X2	T50.5X3	T50.5X4	T50.5X5	T50.5X6
Mefloquine	T37.2X1	T37.2X2	T37.2X3	T37.2X4	T37.2X5	T37.2X6
Mefruside	T50.2X1	T50.2X2	T50.2X3	T50.2X4	T50.2X5	T50.2X6
Megahallucinogen	T40.901	T40.902	T40.903	T40.904	T40.905	T40.906
Megestrol	T38.5X1	T38.5X2	T38.5X3	T38.5X4	T38.5X5	T38.5X6
Meglumine						
antimoniate	T37.8X1	T37.8X2	T37.8X3	T37.8X4	T37.8X5	T37.8X6
diatrizoate	T50.8X1	T50.8X2	T50.8X3	T50.8X4	T50.8X5	T50.8X6
iodipamide	T50.8X1	T50.8X2	T50.8X3	T50.8X4	T50.8X5	T50.8X6
iotroxate	T50.8X1	T50.8X2	T50.8X3	T50.8X4	T50.8X5	T50.8X6
MEK (methyl ethyl ketone)	T52.4X1	T52.4X2	T52.4X3	T52.4X4	—	—
Meladinin	T49.3X1	T49.3X2	T49.3X3	T49.3X4	T49.3X5	T49.3X6
Meladrazine	T44.3X1	T44.3X2	T44.3X3	T44.3X4	T44.3X5	T44.3X6
Melaleuca alternifolia oil	T49.0X1	T49.0X2	T49.0X3	T49.0X4	T49.0X5	T49.0X6
Melanizing agents	T49.3X1	T49.3X2	T49.3X3	T49.3X4	T49.3X5	T49.3X6
Melanocyte-stimulating hormone	T38.891	T38.892	T38.893	T38.894	T38.895	T38.896
Melarsonyl potassium	T37.3X1	T37.3X2	T37.3X3	T37.3X4	T37.3X5	T37.3X6
Melarsoprol	T37.3X1	T37.3X2	T37.3X3	T37.3X4	T37.3X5	T37.3X6
Melia azedarach	T62.2X1	T62.2X2	T62.2X3	T62.2X4	—	—
Melitracen	T43.011	T43.012	T43.013	T43.014	T43.015	T43.016
Mellaril	T43.3X1	T43.3X2	T43.3X3	T43.3X4	T43.3X5	T43.3X6
Meloxine	T49.3X1	T49.3X2	T49.3X3	T49.3X4	T49.3X5	T49.3X6
Melperone	T43.4X1	T43.4X2	T43.4X3	T43.4X4	T43.4X5	T43.4X6
Melphalan	T45.1X1	T45.1X2	T45.1X3	T45.1X4	T45.1X5	T45.1X6
Memantine	T43.8X1	T43.8X2	T43.8X3	T43.8X4	T43.8X5	T43.8X6
Menadiol	T45.7X1	T45.7X2	T45.7X3	T45.7X4	T45.7X5	T45.7X6
sodium sulfate	T45.7X1	T45.7X2	T45.7X3	T45.7X4	T45.7X5	T45.7X6
Menadione	T45.7X1	T45.7X2	T45.7X3	T45.7X4	T45.7X5	T45.7X6
sodium bisulfite	T45.7X1	T45.7X2	T45.7X3	T45.7X4	T45.7X5	T45.7X6
Menaphthone	T45.7X1	T45.7X2	T45.7X3	T45.7X4	T45.7X5	T45.7X6
Menaquinone	T45.7X1	T45.7X2	T45.7X3	T45.7X4	T45.7X5	T45.7X6
Menatetrenone	T45.7X1	T45.7X2	T45.7X3	T45.7X4	T45.7X5	T45.7X6
Meningococcal vaccine	T50.A91	T50.A92	T50.A93	T50.A94	T50.A95	T50.A96
Menningovax (-AC) (-C)	T50.A91	T50.A92	T50.A93	T50.A94	T50.A95	T50.A96
Menotropins	T38.811	T38.812	T38.813	T38.814	T38.815	T38.816
Menthol	T48.5X1	T48.5X2	T48.5X3	T48.5X4	T48.5X5	T48.5X6
Mepacrine	T37.2X1	T37.2X2	T37.2X3	T37.2X4	T37.2X5	T37.2X6
Meparfynol	T42.6X1	T42.6X2	T42.6X3	T42.6X4	T42.6X5	T42.6X6
Mepartricin	T36.7X1	T36.7X2	T36.7X3	T36.7X4	T36.7X5	T36.7X6
Mepazine	T43.3X1	T43.3X2	T43.3X3	T43.3X4	T43.3X5	T43.3X6
Mepenzolate	T44.3X1	T44.3X2	T44.3X3	T44.3X4	T44.3X5	T44.3X6
bromide	T44.3X1	T44.3X2	T44.3X3	T44.3X4	T44.3X5	T44.3X6
Meperidine	T40.4X1	T40.4X2	T40.4X3	T40.4X4	T40.4X5	T40.4X6
Mephebarbital	T42.3X1	T42.3X2	T42.3X3	T42.3X4	T42.3X5	T42.3X6
Mephenamin (e)	T42.8X1	T42.8X2	T42.8X3	T42.8X4	T42.8X5	T42.8X6
Mephenesin	T42.8X1	T42.8X2	T42.8X3	T42.8X4	T42.8X5	T42.8X6
Mephenhydramine	T45.0X1	T45.0X2	T45.0X3	T45.0X4	T45.0X5	T45.0X6
Mephenoxalone	T42.8X1	T42.8X2	T42.8X3	T42.8X4	T42.8X5	T42.8X6
Mephentermine	T44.991	T44.992	T44.993	T44.994	T44.995	T44.996
Mephenytoin	T42.0X1	T42.0X2	T42.0X3	T42.0X4	T42.0X5	T42.0X6
with phenobarbital	T42.3X1	T42.3X2	T42.3X3	T42.3X4	T42.3X5	T42.3X6
Mephobarbital	T42.3X1	T42.3X2	T42.3X3	T42.3X4	T42.3X5	T42.3X6
Mephosfolan	T60.0X1	T60.0X2	T60.0X3	T60.0X4	—	—
Mepindolol	T44.7X1	T44.7X2	T44.7X3	T44.7X4	T44.7X5	T44.7X6
Mepiperphenidol	T44.3X1	T44.3X2	T44.3X3	T44.3X4	T44.3X5	T44.3X6
Mepitiostane	T38.7X1	T38.7X2	T38.7X3	T38.7X4	T38.7X5	T38.7X6
Mepivacaine	T41.3X1	T41.3X2	T41.3X3	T41.3X4	T41.3X5	T41.3X6
epidural	T41.3X1	T41.3X2	T41.3X3	T41.3X4	T41.3X5	T41.3X6
Meprednisone	T38.0X1	T38.0X2	T38.0X3	T38.0X4	T38.0X5	T38.0X6
Meprobam	T43.591	T43.592	T43.593	T43.594	T43.595	T43.596
Meprobamate	T43.591	T43.592	T43.593	T43.594	T43.595	T43.596
Meproscillarin	T46.0X1	T46.0X2	T46.0X3	T46.0X4	T46.0X5	T46.0X6
Meprylcaine	T41.3X1	T41.3X2	T41.3X3	T41.3X4	T41.3X5	T41.3X6
Meptazinol	T39.8X1	T39.8X2	T39.8X3	T39.8X4	T39.8X5	T39.8X6
Mepyramine	T45.0X1	T45.0X2	T45.0X3	T45.0X4	T45.0X5	T45.0X6
Mequitazine	T43.3X1	T43.3X2	T43.3X3	T43.3X4	T43.3X5	T43.3X6
Meralluride	T50.2X1	T50.2X2	T50.2X3	T50.2X4	T50.2X5	T50.2X6
Merbaphen	T50.2X1	T50.2X2	T50.2X3	T50.2X4	T50.2X5	T50.2X6
Merbromin	T49.0X1	T49.0X2	T49.0X3	T49.0X4	T49.0X5	T49.0X6
Mercaptobenzothiazole salts	T49.0X1	T49.0X2	T49.0X3	T49.0X4	T49.0X5	T49.0X6
Mercaptomerin	T50.2X1	T50.2X2	T50.2X3	T50.2X4	T50.2X5	T50.2X6
Mercaptopurine	T45.1X1	T45.1X2	T45.1X3	T45.1X4	T45.1X5	T45.1X6
Mercumatilin	T50.2X1	T50.2X2	T50.2X3	T50.2X4	T50.2X5	T50.2X6
Mercuramide	T50.2X1	T50.2X2	T50.2X3	T50.2X4	T50.2X5	T50.2X6
Mercurochrome	T49.0X1	T49.0X2	T49.0X3	T49.0X4	T49.0X5	T49.0X6
Mercurophylline	T50.2X1	T50.2X2	T50.2X3	T50.2X4	T50.2X5	T50.2X6
Mercury, mercurial, mercuric, mercurous (compounds) (cyanide) (fumes) (nonmedicinal) (vapor) NEC	T56.1X1	T56.1X2	T56.1X3	T56.1X4	—	—
ammoniated	T49.0X1	T49.0X2	T49.0X3	T49.0X4	T49.0X5	T49.0X6
anti-infective						
local	T49.0X1	T49.0X2	T49.0X3	T49.0X4	T49.0X5	T49.0X6
systemic	T37.8X1	T37.8X2	T37.8X3	T37.8X4	T37.8X5	T37.8X6
topical	T49.0X1	T49.0X2	T49.0X3	T49.0X4	T49.0X5	T49.0X6
chloride (ammoniated)	T49.0X1	T49.0X2	T49.0X3	T49.0X4	T49.0X5	T49.0X6
fungicide	T56.1X1	T56.1X2	T56.1X3	T56.1X4		
diuretic NEC	T50.2X1	T50.2X2	T50.2X3	T50.2X4	T50.2X5	T50.2X6
fungicide	T56.1X1	T56.1X2	T56.1X3	T56.1X4		
organic (fungicide)	T56.1X1	T56.1X2	T56.1X3	T56.1X4		
oxide, yellow	T49.0X1	T49.0X2	T49.0X3	T49.0X4	T49.0X5	T49.0X6
Mersalyl	T50.2X1	T50.2X2	T50.2X3	T50.2X4	T50.2X5	T50.2X6
Merthiolate	T49.0X1	T49.0X2	T49.0X3	T49.0X4	T49.0X5	T49.0X6
ophthalmic preparation	T49.5X1	T49.5X2	T49.5X3	T49.5X4	T49.5X5	T49.5X6
Meruvax	T50.B91	T50.B92	T50.B93	T50.B94	T50.B95	T50.B96
Mesalazine	T47.8X1	T47.8X2	T47.8X3	T47.8X4	T47.8X5	T47.8X6
Mescal buttons	T40.991	T40.992	T40.993	T40.994	—	—
Mescaline	T40.991	T40.992	T40.993	T40.994	—	—
Mesna	T48.4X1	T48.4X2	T48.4X3	T48.4X4	T48.4X5	T48.4X6
Mesoglycan	T46.6X1	T46.6X2	T46.6X3	T46.6X4	T46.6X5	T46.6X6
Mesoridazine	T43.3X1	T43.3X2	T43.3X3	T43.3X4	T43.3X5	T43.3X6
Mestanolone	T38.7X1	T38.7X2	T38.7X3	T38.7X4	T38.7X5	T38.7X6
Mesterolone	T38.7X1	T38.7X2	T38.7X3	T38.7X4	T38.7X5	T38.7X6
Mestranol	T38.5X1	T38.5X2	T38.5X3	T38.5X4	T38.5X5	T38.5X6
Mesulergine	T42.8X1	T42.8X2	T42.8X3	T42.8X4	T42.8X5	T42.8X6
Mesulfen	T49.0X1	T49.0X2	T49.0X3	T49.0X4	T49.0X5	T49.0X6
Mesuximide	T42.2X1	T42.2X2	T42.2X3	T42.2X4	T42.2X5	T42.2X6
Metabutethamine	T41.3X1	T41.3X2	T41.3X3	T41.3X4	T41.3X5	T41.3X6
Metactesylacetate	T49.0X1	T49.0X2	T49.0X3	T49.0X4	T49.0X5	T49.0X6
Metacycline	T36.4X1	T36.4X2	T36.4X3	T36.4X4	T36.4X5	T36.4X6
Metaldehyde (snail killer) NEC	T60.8X1	T60.8X2	T60.8X3	T60.8X4	—	—
Metals (heavy) (nonmedicinal)	T56.91	T56.92	T56.93	T56.94	—	—
dust, fumes, or vapor NEC	T56.91	T56.92	T56.93	T56.94	—	—
light NEC	T56.91	T56.92	T56.93	T56.94	—	—
dust, fumes, or vapor NEC	T56.91	T56.92	T56.93	T56.94	—	—
specified NEC	T56.891	T56.892	T56.893	T56.894	—	—
thallium	T56.811	T56.812	T56.813	T56.814	—	—
Metamfetamine	T43.621	T43.622	T43.623	T43.624	T43.625	T43.626
Metamizole sodium	T39.2X1	T39.2X2	T39.2X3	T39.2X4	T39.2X5	T39.2X6
Metampicillin	T36.0X1	T36.0X2	T36.0X3	T36.0X4	T36.0X5	T36.0X6
Metamucil	T47.4X1	T47.4X2	T47.4X3	T47.4X4	T47.4X5	T47.4X6
Metandienone	T38.7X1	T38.7X2	T38.7X3	T38.7X4	T38.7X5	T38.7X6
Metandrostenolone	T38.7X1	T38.7X2	T38.7X3	T38.7X4	T38.7X5	T38.7X6
Metaphen	T49.0X1	T49.0X2	T49.0X3	T49.0X4	T49.0X5	T49.0X6
Metaphos	T60.0X1	T60.0X2	T60.0X3	T60.0X4	—	—
Metapramine	T43.011	T43.012	T43.013	T43.014	T43.015	T43.016
Metaproterenol	T48.291	T48.292	T48.293	T48.294	T48.295	T48.296
Metaraminol	T44.4X1	T44.4X2	T44.4X3	T44.4X4	T44.4X5	T44.4X6
Metaxalone	T42.8X1	T42.8X2	T42.8X3	T42.8X4	T42.8X5	T42.8X6
Metenolone	T38.7X1	T38.7X2	T38.7X3	T38.7X4	T38.7X5	T38.7X6
Metergoline	T42.8X1	T42.8X2	T42.8X3	T42.8X4	T42.8X5	T42.8X6
Metescufylline	T46.991	T46.992	T46.993	T46.994	T46.995	T46.996
Metetoin	T42.0X1	T42.0X2	T42.0X3	T42.0X4	T42.0X5	T42.0X6
Metformin	T38.3X1	T38.3X2	T38.3X3	T38.3X4	T38.3X5	T38.3X6
Methacholine	T44.1X1	T44.1X2	T44.1X3	T44.1X4	T44.1X5	T44.1X6
Methacycline	T36.4X1	T36.4X2	T36.4X3	T36.4X4	T36.4X5	T36.4X6
Methadone	T40.3X1	T40.3X2	T40.3X3	T40.3X4	T40.3X5	T40.3X6
Methallenestril	T38.5X1	T38.5X2	T38.5X3	T38.5X4	T38.5X5	T38.5X6
Methallenoestril	T38.5X1	T38.5X2	T38.5X3	T38.5X4	T38.5X5	T38.5X6
Methamphetamine	T43.621	T43.622	T43.623	T43.624	T43.625	T43.626
Methampyrone	T39.2X1	T39.2X2	T39.2X3	T39.2X4	T39.2X5	T39.2X6
Methandienone	T38.7X1	T38.7X2	T38.7X3	T38.7X4	T38.7X5	T38.7X6
Methandriol	T38.7X1	T38.7X2	T38.7X3	T38.7X4	T38.7X5	T38.7X6
Methandrostenolone	T38.7X1	T38.7X2	T38.7X3	T38.7X4	T38.7X5	T38.7X6
Methane	T59.891	T59.892	T59.893	T59.894		
Methanethiol	T59.891	T59.892	T59.893	T59.894		
Methaniazide	T37.1X1	T37.1X2	T37.1X3	T37.1X4	T37.1X5	T37.1X6
Methanol (vapor)	T51.1X1	T51.1X2	T51.1X3	T51.1X4	—	—

Table of Drugs and Chemicals

Methantheline — Metrifonate

Substance	Poisoning, Accidental (unintentional)	Poisoning, Intentional Self-harm	Poisoning, Assault	Poisoning, Undetermined	Adverse Effect	Under-dosing
Methantheline	T44.3X1	T44.3X2	T44.3X3	T44.3X4	T44.3X5	T44.3X6
Methanthelinium bromide	T44.3X1	T44.3X2	T44.3X3	T44.3X4	T44.3X5	T44.3X6
Methaphenilene	T45.0X1	T45.0X2	T45.0X3	T45.0X4	T45.0X5	T45.0X6
Methapyrilene	T45.0X1	T45.0X2	T45.0X3	T45.0X4	T45.0X5	T45.0X6
Methaqualone (compound)	T42.6X1	T42.6X2	T42.6X3	T42.6X4	T42.6X5	T42.6X6
Metharbital	T42.3X1	T42.3X2	T42.3X3	T42.3X4	T42.3X5	T42.3X6
Methazolamide	T50.2X1	T50.2X2	T50.2X3	T50.2X4	T50.2X5	T50.2X6
Methdilazine	T43.3X1	T43.3X2	T43.3X3	T43.3X4	T43.3X5	T43.3X6
Methedrine	T43.621	T43.622	T43.623	T43.624	T43.625	T43.626
Methenamine (mandelate)	T37.8X1	T37.8X2	T37.8X3	T37.8X4	T37.8X5	T37.8X6
Methenolone	T38.7X1	T38.7X2	T38.7X3	T38.7X4	T38.7X5	T38.7X6
Methergine	T48.0X1	T48.0X2	T48.0X3	T48.0X4	T48.0X5	T48.0X6
Methetoin	T42.0X1	T42.0X2	T42.0X3	T42.0X4	T42.0X5	T42.0X6
Methiacil	T38.2X1	T38.2X2	T38.2X3	T38.2X4	T38.2X5	T38.2X6
Methicillin	T36.0X1	T36.0X2	T36.0X3	T36.0X4	T36.0X5	T36.0X6
Methimazole	T38.2X1	T38.2X2	T38.2X3	T38.2X4	T38.2X5	T38.2X6
Methiodal sodium	T50.8X1	T50.8X2	T50.8X3	T50.8X4	T50.8X5	T50.8X6
Methionine	T50.991	T50.992	T50.993	T50.994	T50.995	T50.996
Methisazone	T37.5X1	T37.5X2	T37.5X3	T37.5X4	T37.5X5	T37.5X6
Methisoprinol	T37.5X1	T37.5X2	T37.5X3	T37.5X4	T37.5X5	T37.5X6
Methitural	T42.3X1	T42.3X2	T42.3X3	T42.3X4	T42.3X5	T42.3X6
Methixene	T44.3X1	T44.3X2	T44.3X3	T44.3X4	T44.3X5	T44.3X6
Methobarbital, methobarbitone	T42.3X1	T42.3X2	T42.3X3	T42.3X4	T42.3X5	T42.3X6
Methocarbamol	T42.8X1	T42.8X2	T42.8X3	T42.8X4	T42.8X5	T42.8X6
skeletal muscle relaxant	T48.1X1	T48.1X2	T48.1X3	T48.1X4	T48.1X5	T48.1X6
Methohexital	T41.1X1	T41.1X2	T41.1X3	T41.1X4	T41.1X5	T41.1X6
Methohexitone	T41.1X1	T41.1X2	T41.1X3	T41.1X4	T41.1X5	T41.1X6
Methoin	T42.0X1	T42.0X2	T42.0X3	T42.0X4	T42.0X5	T42.0X6
Methopholine	T39.8X1	T39.8X2	T39.8X3	T39.8X4	T39.8X5	T39.8X6
Methopromazine	T43.3X1	T43.3X2	T43.3X3	T43.3X4	T43.3X5	T43.3X6
Methorate	T48.3X1	T48.3X2	T48.3X3	T48.3X4	T48.3X5	T48.3X6
Methoserpidine	T46.5X1	T46.5X2	T46.5X3	T46.5X4	T46.5X5	T46.5X6
Methotrexate	T45.1X1	T45.1X2	T45.1X3	T45.1X4	T45.1X5	T45.1X6
Methotrimeprazine	T43.3X1	T43.3X2	T43.3X3	T43.3X4	T43.3X5	T43.3X6
Methoxa-Dome	T49.3X1	T49.3X2	T49.3X3	T49.3X4	T49.3X5	T49.3X6
Methoxamine	T44.4X1	T44.4X2	T44.4X3	T44.4X4	T44.4X5	T44.4X6
Methoxsalen	T50.991	T50.992	T50.993	T50.994	T50.995	T50.996
Methoxyaniline	T65.3X1	T65.3X2	T65.3X3	T65.3X4	—	—
Methoxybenzyl penicillin	T36.0X1	T36.0X2	T36.0X3	T36.0X4	T36.0X5	T36.0X6
Methoxychlor	T53.7X1	T53.7X2	T53.7X3	T53.7X4	—	—
Methoxy-DDT	T53.7X1	T53.7X2	T53.7X3	T53.7X4	—	—
Methoxyflurane	T41.0X1	T41.0X2	T41.0X3	T41.0X4	T41.0X5	T41.0X6
Methoxyphenamine	T48.6X1	T48.6X2	T48.6X3	T48.6X4	T48.6X5	T48.6X6
Methoxypromazine	T43.3X1	T43.3X2	T43.3X3	T43.3X4	T43.3X5	T43.3X6
Methscopolamine bromide	T44.3X1	T44.3X2	T44.3X3	T44.3X4	T44.3X5	T44.3X6
Methsuximide	T42.2X1	T42.2X2	T42.2X3	T42.2X4	T42.2X5	T42.2X6
Methyclothiazide	T50.2X1	T50.2X2	T50.2X3	T50.2X4	T50.2X5	T50.2X6
Methyl						
acetate	T52.4X1	T52.4X2	T52.4X3	T52.4X4	—	—
acetone	T52.4X1	T52.4X2	T52.4X3	T52.4X4	—	—
acrylate	T65.891	T65.892	T65.893	T65.894	—	—
alcohol	T51.1X1	T51.1X2	T51.1X3	T51.1X4	—	—
aminophenol	T65.3X1	T65.3X2	T65.3X3	T65.3X4	—	—
amphetamine	T43.621	T43.622	T43.623	T43.624	T43.625	T43.626
androstanolone	T38.7X1	T38.7X2	T38.7X3	T38.7X4	T38.7X5	T38.7X6
atropine	T44.3X1	T44.3X2	T44.3X3	T44.3X4	T44.3X5	T44.3X6
benzene	T52.2X1	T52.2X2	T52.2X3	T52.2X4	—	—
benzoate	T52.8X1	T52.8X2	T52.8X3	T52.8X4	—	—
benzol	T52.2X1	T52.2X2	T52.2X3	T52.2X4	—	—
bromide (gas)	T59.891	T59.892	T59.893	T59.894	—	—
fumigant	T60.8X1	T60.8X2	T60.8X3	T60.8X4	—	—
butanol	T51.3X1	T51.3X2	T51.3X3	T51.3X4	—	—
carbinol	T51.1X1	T51.1X2	T51.1X3	T51.1X4	—	—
carbonate	T52.8X1	T52.8X2	T52.8X3	T52.8X4	—	—
CCNU	T45.1X1	T45.1X2	T45.1X3	T45.1X4	T45.1X5	T45.1X6
cellosolve	T52.91	T52.92	T52.93	T52.94	—	—
cellulose	T47.4X1	T47.4X2	T47.4X3	T47.4X4	T47.4X5	T47.4X6
chloride (gas)	T59.891	T59.892	T59.893	T59.894	—	—
chloroformate	T59.3X1	T59.3X2	T59.3X3	T59.3X4	—	—
cyclohexane	T52.8X1	T52.8X2	T52.8X3	T52.8X4	—	—
cyclohexanol	T51.8X1	T51.8X2	T51.8X3	T51.8X4	—	—
cyclohexanone	T52.8X1	T52.8X2	T52.8X3	T52.8X4	—	—
cyclohexyl acetate	T52.8X1	T52.8X2	T52.8X3	T52.8X4	—	—
demeton	T60.0X1	T60.0X2	T60.0X3	T60.0X4	—	—
dihydromorphinone	T40.2X1	T40.2X2	T40.2X3	T40.2X4	T40.2X5	T40.2X6
ergometrine	T48.0X1	T48.0X2	T48.0X3	T48.0X4	T48.0X5	T48.0X6
ergonovine	T48.0X1	T48.0X2	T48.0X3	T48.0X4	T48.0X5	T48.0X6
ethyl ketone	T52.4X1	T52.4X2	T52.4X3	T52.4X4	—	—
glucamine antimonate	T37.8X1	T37.8X2	T37.8X3	T37.8X4	T37.8X5	T37.8X6
hydrazine	T65.891	T65.892	T65.893	T65.894	—	—
iodide	T65.891	T65.892	T65.893	T65.894	—	—
isobutyl ketone	T52.4X1	T52.4X2	T52.4X3	T52.4X4	—	—
Methyl — continued						
isothiocyanate	T60.3X1	T60.3X2	T60.3X3	T60.3X4	—	—
mercaptan	T59.891	T59.892	T59.893	T59.894	—	—
morphine NEC	T40.2X1	T40.2X2	T40.2X3	T40.2X4	T40.2X5	T40.2X6
nicotinate	T49.4X1	T49.4X2	T49.4X3	T49.4X4	T49.4X5	T49.4X6
paraben	T49.0X1	T49.0X2	T49.0X3	T49.0X4	T49.0X5	T49.0X6
parafynol	T42.6X1	T42.6X2	T42.6X3	T42.6X4	T42.6X5	T42.6X6
parathion	T60.0X1	T60.0X2	T60.0X3	T60.0X4	—	—
peridol	T43.4X1	T43.4X2	T43.4X3	T43.4X4	T43.4X5	T43.4X6
phenidate	T43.631	T43.632	T43.633	T43.634	T43.635	T43.636
prednisolone	T38.0X1	T38.0X2	T38.0X3	T38.0X4	T38.0X5	T38.0X6
ENT agent	T49.6X1	T49.6X2	T49.6X3	T49.6X4	T49.6X5	T49.6X6
ophthalmic preparation	T49.5X1	T49.5X2	T49.5X3	T49.5X4	T49.5X5	T49.5X6
topical NEC	T49.0X1	T49.0X2	T49.0X3	T49.0X4	T49.0X5	T49.0X6
propylcarbinol	T51.3X1	T51.3X2	T51.3X3	T51.3X4	—	—
rosaniline NEC	T49.0X1	T49.0X2	T49.0X3	T49.0X4	T49.0X5	T49.0X6
salicylate	T49.2X1	T49.2X2	T49.2X3	T49.2X4	T49.2X5	T49.2X6
sulfate (fumes)	T59.891	T59.892	T59.893	T59.894	—	—
liquid	T52.8X1	T52.8X2	T52.8X3	T52.8X4	—	—
sulfonal	T42.6X1	T42.6X2	T42.6X3	T42.6X4	T42.6X5	T42.6X6
testosterone	T38.7X1	T38.7X2	T38.7X3	T38.7X4	T38.7X5	T38.7X6
thiouracil	T38.2X1	T38.2X2	T38.2X3	T38.2X4	T38.2X5	T38.2X6
Methylamphetamine	T43.621	T43.622	T43.623	T43.624	T43.625	T43.626
Methylated spirit	T51.1X1	T51.1X2	T51.1X3	T51.1X4	—	—
Methylatropine nitrate	T44.3X1	T44.3X2	T44.3X3	T44.3X4	T44.3X5	T44.3X6
Methylbenactyzium bromide	T44.3X1	T44.3X2	T44.3X3	T44.3X4	T44.3X5	T44.3X6
Methylbenzethonium chloride	T49.0X1	T49.0X2	T49.0X3	T49.0X4	T49.0X5	T49.0X6
Methylcellulose	T47.4X1	T47.4X2	T47.4X3	T47.4X4	T47.4X5	T47.4X6
laxative	T47.4X1	T47.4X2	T47.4X3	T47.4X4	T47.4X5	T47.4X6
Methylchlorophenoxyacetic acid	T60.3X1	T60.3X2	T60.3X3	T60.3X4	—	—
Methyldopa	T46.5X1	T46.5X2	T46.5X3	T46.5X4	T46.5X5	T46.5X6
Methyldopate	T46.5X1	T46.5X2	T46.5X3	T46.5X4	T46.5X5	T46.5X6
Methylene						
blue	T50.6X1	T50.6X2	T50.6X3	T50.6X4	T50.6X5	T50.6X6
chloride or dichloride (solvent) NEC	T53.4X1	T53.4X2	T53.4X3	T53.4X4	—	—
Methylenedioxyamphetamine	T43.621	T43.622	T43.623	T43.624	T43.625	T43.626
Methylenedioxymethamphetamine	T43.621	T43.622	T43.623	T43.624	T43.625	T43.626
Methylergometrine	T48.0X1	T48.0X2	T48.0X3	T48.0X4	T48.0X5	T48.0X6
Methylergonovine	T48.0X1	T48.0X2	T48.0X3	T48.0X4	T48.0X5	T48.0X6
Methylestrenolone	T38.5X1	T38.5X2	T38.5X3	T38.5X4	T38.5X5	T38.5X6
Methylethyl cellulose	T50.991	T50.992	T50.993	T50.994	T50.995	T50.996
Methylhexabital	T42.3X1	T42.3X2	T42.3X3	T42.3X4	T42.3X5	T42.3X6
Methylmorphine	T40.2X1	T40.2X2	T40.2X3	T40.2X4	T40.2X5	T40.2X6
Methylparaben (ophthalmic)	T49.5X1	T49.5X2	T49.5X3	T49.5X4	T49.5X5	T49.5X6
Methylparafynol	T42.6X1	T42.6X2	T42.6X3	T42.6X4	T42.6X5	T42.6X6
Methylpentynol, methylpenthynol	T42.6X1	T42.6X2	T42.6X3	T42.6X4	T42.6X5	T42.6X6
Methylphenidate	T43.631	T43.632	T43.633	T43.634	T43.635	T43.636
Methylphenobarbital	T42.3X1	T42.3X2	T42.3X3	T42.3X4	T42.3X5	T42.3X6
Methylpolysiloxane	T47.1X1	T47.1X2	T47.1X3	T47.1X4	T47.1X5	T47.1X6
Methylprednisolone — see Methyl, prednisolone						
Methylrosaniline	T49.0X1	T49.0X2	T49.0X3	T49.0X4	T49.0X5	T49.0X6
Methylrosanilinium chloride	T49.0X1	T49.0X2	T49.0X3	T49.0X4	T49.0X5	T49.0X6
Methyltestosterone	T38.7X1	T38.7X2	T38.7X3	T38.7X4	T38.7X5	T38.7X6
Methylthionine chloride	T50.6X1	T50.6X2	T50.6X3	T50.6X4	T50.6X5	T50.6X6
Methylthioninium chloride	T50.6X1	T50.6X2	T50.6X3	T50.6X4	T50.6X5	T50.6X6
Methylthiouracil	T38.2X1	T38.2X2	T38.2X3	T38.2X4	T38.2X5	T38.2X6
Methyprylon	T42.6X1	T42.6X2	T42.6X3	T42.6X4	T42.6X5	T42.6X6
Methysergide	T46.5X1	T46.5X2	T46.5X3	T46.5X4	T46.5X5	T46.5X6
Metiamide	T47.1X1	T47.1X2	T47.1X3	T47.1X4	T47.1X5	T47.1X6
Meticillin	T36.0X1	T36.0X2	T36.0X3	T36.0X4	T36.0X5	T36.0X6
Meticrane	T50.2X1	T50.2X2	T50.2X3	T50.2X4	T50.2X5	T50.2X6
Metildigoxin	T46.0X1	T46.0X2	T46.0X3	T46.0X4	T46.0X5	T46.0X6
Metipranolol	T49.5X1	T49.5X2	T49.5X3	T49.5X4	T49.5X5	T49.5X6
Metirosine	T46.5X1	T46.5X2	T46.5X3	T46.5X4	T46.5X5	T46.5X6
Metisazone	T37.5X1	T37.5X2	T37.5X3	T37.5X4	T37.5X5	T37.5X6
Metixene	T44.3X1	T44.3X2	T44.3X3	T44.3X4	T44.3X5	T44.3X6
Metizoline	T48.5X1	T48.5X2	T48.5X3	T48.5X4	T48.5X5	T48.5X6
Metoclopramide	T45.0X1	T45.0X2	T45.0X3	T45.0X4	T45.0X5	T45.0X6
Metofenazate	T43.3X1	T43.3X2	T43.3X3	T43.3X4	T43.3X5	T43.3X6
Metofoline	T39.8X1	T39.8X2	T39.8X3	T39.8X4	T39.8X5	T39.8X6
Metolazone	T50.2X1	T50.2X2	T50.2X3	T50.2X4	T50.2X5	T50.2X6
Metopon	T40.2X1	T40.2X2	T40.2X3	T40.2X4	T40.2X5	T40.2X6
Metoprine	T45.1X1	T45.1X2	T45.1X3	T45.1X4	T45.1X5	T45.1X6
Metoprolol	T44.7X1	T44.7X2	T44.7X3	T44.7X4	T44.7X5	T44.7X6
Metrifonate	T60.0X1	T60.0X2	T60.0X3	T60.0X4	—	—

Substance	Poisoning, Accidental (unintentional)	Poisoning, Intentional Self-harm	Poisoning, Assault	Poisoning, Undetermined	Adverse Effect	Under-dosing
Metrizamide	T50.8X1	T50.8X2	T50.8X3	T50.8X4	T50.8X5	T50.8X6
Metrizoic acid	T50.8X1	T50.8X2	T50.8X3	T50.8X4	T50.8X5	T50.8X6
Metronidazole	T37.8X1	T37.8X2	T37.8X3	T37.8X4	T37.8X5	T37.8X6
Metycaine	T41.3X1	T41.3X2	T41.3X3	T41.3X4	T41.3X5	T41.3X6
infiltration (subcutaneous)	T41.3X1	T41.3X2	T41.3X3	T41.3X4	T41.3X5	T41.3X6
nerve block (peripheral) (plexus)	T41.3X1	T41.3X2	T41.3X3	T41.3X4	T41.3X5	T41.3X6
topical (surface)	T41.3X1	T41.3X2	T41.3X3	T41.3X4	T41.3X5	T41.3X6
Metyrapone	T50.8X1	T50.8X2	T50.8X3	T50.8X4	T50.8X5	T50.8X6
Mevinphos	T60.0X1	T60.0X2	T60.0X3	T60.0X4	—	—
Mexazolam	T42.4X1	T42.4X2	T42.4X3	T42.4X4	T42.4X5	T42.4X6
Mexenone	T49.3X1	T49.3X2	T49.3X3	T49.3X4	T49.3X5	T49.3X6
Mexiletine	T46.2X1	T46.2X2	T46.2X3	T46.2X4	T46.2X5	T46.2X6
Mezereon	T62.2X1	T62.2X2	T62.2X3	T62.2X4	—	—
berries	T62.1X1	T62.1X2	T62.1X3	T62.1X4	—	—
Mezlocillin	T36.0X1	T36.0X2	T36.0X3	T36.0X4	T36.0X5	T36.0X6
Mianserin	T43.021	T43.022	T43.023	T43.024	T43.025	T43.026
Micatin	T49.0X1	T49.0X2	T49.0X3	T49.0X4	T49.0X5	T49.0X6
Miconazole	T49.0X1	T49.0X2	T49.0X3	T49.0X4	T49.0X5	T49.0X6
Micronomicin	T36.5X1	T36.5X2	T36.5X3	T36.5X4	T36.5X5	T36.5X6
Midazolam	T42.4X1	T42.4X2	T42.4X3	T42.4X4	T42.4X5	T42.4X6
Midecamycin	T36.3X1	T36.3X2	T36.3X3	T36.3X4	T36.3X5	T36.3X6
Mifepristone	T38.6X1	T38.6X2	T38.6X3	T38.6X4	T38.6X5	T38.6X6
Milk of magnesia	T47.1X1	T47.1X2	T47.1X3	T47.1X4	T47.1X5	T47.1X6
Millipede (tropical) (venomous)	T63.411	T63.412	T63.413	T63.414		
Miltown	T43.591	T43.592	T43.593	T43.594	T43.595	T43.596
Milverine	T44.3X1	T44.3X2	T44.3X3	T44.3X4	T44.3X5	T44.3X6
Minaprine	T43.291	T43.292	T43.293	T43.294	T43.295	T43.296
Minaxolone	T41.291	T41.292	T41.293	T41.294	T41.295	T41.296
Mineral						
acids	T54.2X1	T54.2X2	T54.2X3	T54.2X4	—	—
oil (laxative)(medicinal)	T47.4X1	T47.4X2	T47.4X3	T47.4X4	T47.4X5	T47.4X6
emulsion	T47.2X1	T47.2X2	T47.2X3	T47.2X4	T47.2X5	T47.2X6
nonmedicinal	T52.0X1	T52.0X2	T52.0X3	T52.0X4	—	—
topical	T49.3X1	T49.3X2	T49.3X3	T49.3X4	T49.3X5	T49.3X6
salt NEC	T50.3X1	T50.3X2	T50.3X3	T50.3X4	T50.3X5	T50.3X6
spirits	T52.0X1	T52.0X2	T52.0X3	T52.0X4	—	—
Mineralocorticosteroid	T50.0X1	T50.0X2	T50.0X3	T50.0X4	T50.0X5	T50.0X6
Minocycline	T36.4X1	T36.4X2	T36.4X3	T36.4X4	T36.4X5	T36.4X6
Minoxidil	T46.7X1	T46.7X2	T46.7X3	T46.7X4	T46.7X5	T46.7X6
Miokamycin	T36.3X1	T36.3X2	T36.3X3	T36.3X4	T36.3X5	T36.3X6
Miotic drug	T49.5X1	T49.5X2	T49.5X3	T49.5X4	T49.5X5	T49.5X6
Mipafox	T60.0X1	T60.0X2	T60.0X3	T60.0X4	—	—
Mirex	T60.1X1	T60.1X2	T60.1X3	T60.1X4	—	—
Mirtazapine	T43.021	T43.022	T43.023	T43.024	T43.025	T43.026
Misonidazole	T37.3X1	T37.3X2	T37.3X3	T37.3X4	T37.3X5	T37.3X6
Misoprostol	T47.1X1	T47.1X2	T47.1X3	T47.1X4	T47.1X5	T47.1X6
Mithramycin	T45.1X1	T45.1X2	T45.1X3	T45.1X4	T45.1X5	T45.1X6
Mitobronitol	T45.1X1	T45.1X2	T45.1X3	T45.1X4	T45.1X5	T45.1X6
Mitoguazone	T45.1X1	T45.1X2	T45.1X3	T45.1X4	T45.1X5	T45.1X6
Mitolactol	T45.1X1	T45.1X2	T45.1X3	T45.1X4	T45.1X5	T45.1X6
Mitomycin	T45.1X1	T45.1X2	T45.1X3	T45.1X4	T45.1X5	T45.1X6
Mitopodozide	T45.1X1	T45.1X2	T45.1X3	T45.1X4	T45.1X5	T45.1X6
Mitotane	T45.1X1	T45.1X2	T45.1X3	T45.1X4	T45.1X5	T45.1X6
Mitoxantrone	T45.1X1	T45.1X2	T45.1X3	T45.1X4	T45.1X5	T45.1X6
Mivacurium chloride	T48.1X1	T48.1X2	T48.1X3	T48.1X4	T48.1X5	T48.1X6
Miyari bacteria	T47.6X1	T47.6X2	T47.6X3	T47.6X4	T47.6X5	T47.6X6
Moclobemide	T43.1X1	T43.1X2	T43.1X3	T43.1X4	T43.1X5	T43.1X6
Moderil	T46.5X1	T46.5X2	T46.5X3	T46.5X4	T46.5X5	T46.5X6
Mofebutazone	T39.2X1	T39.2X2	T39.2X3	T39.2X4	T39.2X5	T39.2X6
Mogadon — see Nitrazepam						
Molindone	T43.591	T43.592	T43.593	T43.594	T43.595	T43.596
Molsidomine	T46.3X1	T46.3X2	T46.3X3	T46.3X4	T46.3X5	T46.3X6
Mometasone	T49.0X1	T49.0X2	T49.0X3	T49.0X4	T49.0X5	T49.0X6
Monistat	T49.0X1	T49.0X2	T49.0X3	T49.0X4	T49.0X5	T49.0X6
Monkshood	T62.2X1	T62.2X2	T62.2X3	T62.2X4	—	—
Monoamine oxidase inhibitor NEC	T43.1X1	T43.1X2	T43.1X3	T43.1X4	T43.1X5	T43.1X6
hydrazine	T43.1X1	T43.1X2	T43.1X3	T43.1X4	T43.1X5	T43.1X6
Monobenzone	T49.4X1	T49.4X2	T49.4X3	T49.4X4	T49.4X5	T49.4X6
Monochloroacetic acid	T60.3X1	T60.3X2	T60.3X3	T60.3X4	—	—
Monochlorobenzene	T53.7X1	T53.7X2	T53.7X3	T53.7X4	—	—
Monoethanolamine	T46.8X1	T46.8X2	T46.8X3	T46.8X4	T46.8X5	T46.8X6
oleate	T46.8X1	T46.8X2	T46.8X3	T46.8X4	T46.8X5	T46.8X6
Monooctanoin	T50.991	T50.992	T50.993	T50.994	T50.995	T50.996
Monophenylbutazone	T39.2X1	T39.2X2	T39.2X3	T39.2X4	T39.2X5	T39.2X6
Monosodium glutamate	T65.891	T65.892	T65.893	T65.894	—	—
Monosulfiram	T49.0X1	T49.0X2	T49.0X3	T49.0X4	T49.0X5	T49.0X6
Monoxide, carbon — see Carbon, monoxide						
Monoxidine hydrochloride	T46.1X1	T46.1X2	T46.1X3	T46.1X4	T46.1X5	T46.1X6
Monuron	T60.3X1	T60.3X2	T60.3X3	T60.3X4	—	—
Moperone	T43.4X1	T43.4X2	T43.4X3	T43.4X4	T43.4X5	T43.4X6
Mopidamol	T45.1X1	T45.1X2	T45.1X3	T45.1X4	T45.1X5	T45.1X6
MOPP (mechloreth-amine + vincristine + prednisone + procarba-zine)	T45.1X1	T45.1X2	T45.1X3	T45.1X4	T45.1X5	T45.1X6
Morfin	T40.2X1	T40.2X2	T40.2X3	T40.2X4	T40.2X5	T40.2X6
Morinamide	T37.1X1	T37.1X2	T37.1X3	T37.1X4	T37.1X5	T37.1X6
Morning glory seeds	T40.991	T40.992	T40.993	T40.994		
Moroxydine	T37.5X1	T37.5X2	T37.5X3	T37.5X4	T37.5X5	T37.5X6
Morphazinamide	T37.1X1	T37.1X2	T37.1X3	T37.1X4	T37.1X5	T37.1X6
Morphine	T40.2X1	T40.2X2	T40.2X3	T40.2X4	T40.2X5	T40.2X6
antagonist	T50.7X1	T50.7X2	T50.7X3	T50.7X4	T50.7X5	T50.7X6
Morpholinylethylmorphine	T40.2X1	T40.2X2	T40.2X3	T40.2X4	—	—
Morsuximide	T42.2X1	T42.2X2	T42.2X3	T42.2X4	T42.2X5	T42.2X6
Mosapramine	T43.591	T43.592	T43.593	T43.594	T43.595	T43.596
Moth balls — see also Pesticides	T60.2X1	T60.2X2	T60.2X3	T60.2X4	—	—
naphthalene	T60.2X1	T60.2X2	T60.2X3	T60.2X4	—	—
paradichlorobenzene	T60.1X1	T60.1X2	T60.1X3	T60.1X4	—	—
Motor exhaust gas	T58.02	T58.02	T58.03	T58.04	—	—
Mouthwash (antiseptic) (zinc chloride)	T49.6X1	T49.6X2	T49.6X3	T49.6X4	T49.6X5	T49.6X6
Moxastine	T45.0X1	T45.0X2	T45.0X3	T45.0X4	T45.0X5	T45.0X6
Moxaverine	T44.3X1	T44.3X2	T44.3X3	T44.3X4	T44.3X5	T44.3X6
Moxisylyte	T46.7X1	T46.7X2	T46.7X3	T46.7X4	T46.7X5	T46.7X6
Mucilage, plant	T47.4X1	T47.4X2	T47.4X3	T47.4X4	T47.4X5	T47.4X6
Mucolytic drug	T48.4X1	T48.4X2	T48.4X3	T48.4X4	T48.4X5	T48.4X6
Mucomyst	T48.4X1	T48.4X2	T48.4X3	T48.4X4	T48.4X5	T48.4X6
Mucous membrane agents (external)	T49.91	T49.92	T49.93	T49.94	T49.95	T49.96
specified NEC	T49.8X1	T49.8X2	T49.8X3	T49.8X4	T49.8X5	T49.8X6
Mumps						
immune globulin (human)	T50.Z11	T50.Z12	T50.Z13	T50.Z14	T50.Z15	T50.Z16
skin test antigen	T50.8X1	T50.8X2	T50.8X3	T50.8X4	T50.8X5	T50.8X6
vaccine	T50.B91	T50.B92	T50.B93	T50.B94	T50.B95	T50.B96
Mumpsvax	T50.B91	T50.B92	T50.B93	T50.B94	T50.B95	T50.B96
Mupirocin	T49.0X1	T49.0X2	T49.0X3	T49.0X4	T49.0X5	T49.0X6
Muriatic acid — see Hydrochloric acid						
Muromonab-CD3	T45.1X1	T45.1X2	T45.1X3	T45.1X4	T45.1X5	T45.1X6
Muscle-action drug NEC	T48.201	T48.202	T48.203	T48.204	T48.205	T48.206
Muscle affecting agents NEC	T48.201	T48.202	T48.203	T48.204	T48.205	T48.206
oxytocic	T48.0X1	T48.0X2	T48.0X3	T48.0X4	T48.0X5	T48.0X6
relaxants	T48.201	T48.202	T48.203	T48.204	T48.205	T48.206
central nervous system	T42.8X1	T42.8X2	T42.8X3	T42.8X4	T42.8X5	T42.8X6
skeletal	T48.1X1	T48.1X2	T48.1X3	T48.1X4	T48.1X5	T48.1X6
smooth	T44.3X1	T44.3X2	T44.3X3	T44.3X4	T44.3X5	T44.3X6
Muscle relaxant — see Relaxant, muscle						
Muscle-tone depressant, central NEC	T42.8X1	T42.8X2	T42.8X3	T42.8X4	T42.8X5	T42.8X6
specified NEC	T42.8X1	T42.8X2	T42.8X3	T42.8X4	T42.8X5	T42.8X6
Mushroom, noxious	T62.0X1	T62.0X2	T62.0X3	T62.0X4	—	—
Mussel, noxious	T61.781	T61.782	T61.783	T61.784	—	—
Mustard (emetic)	T47.7X1	T47.7X2	T47.7X3	T47.7X4	T47.7X5	T47.7X6
black	T47.7X1	T47.7X2	T47.7X3	T47.7X4	T47.7X5	T47.7X6
gas, not in war	T59.91	T59.92	T59.93	T59.94	—	—
nitrogen	T45.1X1	T45.1X2	T45.1X3	T45.1X4	T45.1X5	T45.1X6
Mustine	T45.1X1	T45.1X2	T45.1X3	T45.1X4	T45.1X5	T45.1X6
M-vac	T45.1X1	T45.1X2	T45.1X3	T45.1X4	T45.1X5	T45.1X6
Mycifradin	T36.5X1	T36.5X2	T36.5X3	T36.5X4	T36.5X5	T36.5X6
topical	T49.0X1	T49.0X2	T49.0X3	T49.0X4	T49.0X5	T49.0X6
Mycitracin	T36.8X1	T36.8X2	T36.8X3	T36.8X4	T36.8X5	T36.8X6
ophthalmic preparation	T49.5X1	T49.5X2	T49.5X3	T49.5X4	T49.5X5	T49.5X6
Mycostatin	T36.7X1	T36.7X2	T36.7X3	T36.7X4	T36.7X5	T36.7X6
topical	T49.0X1	T49.0X2	T49.0X3	T49.0X4	T49.0X5	T49.0X6
Mycotoxins	T64.81	T64.82	T64.83	T64.84	—	—
aflatoxin	T64.01	T64.02	T64.03	T64.04	—	—
specified NEC	T64.81	T64.82	T64.83	T64.84	—	—
Mydriacyl	T44.3X1	T44.3X2	T44.3X3	T44.3X4	T44.3X5	T44.3X6
Mydriatic drug	T49.5X1	T49.5X2	T49.5X3	T49.5X4	T49.5X5	T49.5X6
Myelobromal	T45.1X1	T45.1X2	T45.1X3	T45.1X4	T45.1X5	T45.1X6
Myleran	T45.1X1	T45.1X2	T45.1X3	T45.1X4	T45.1X5	T45.1X6
Myochrysin (e)	T39.2X1	T39.2X2	T39.2X3	T39.2X4	T39.2X5	T39.2X6
Myoneural blocking agents	T48.1X1	T48.1X2	T48.1X3	T48.1X4	T48.1X5	T48.1X6
Myralact	T49.0X1	T49.0X2	T49.0X3	T49.0X4	T49.0X5	T49.0X6
Myristica fragrans	T62.2X1	T62.2X2	T62.2X3	T62.2X4	—	—
Myristicin	T65.891	T65.892	T65.893	T65.894	—	—
Mysoline	T42.3X1	T42.3X2	T42.3X3	T42.3X4	T42.3X5	T42.3X6
Nabilone	T40.7X1	T40.7X2	T40.7X3	T40.7X4	T40.7X5	T40.7X6
Nabumetone	T39.391	T39.392	T39.393	T39.394	T39.395	T39.396
Nadolol	T44.7X1	T44.7X2	T44.7X3	T44.7X4	T44.7X5	T44.7X6

Table of Drugs and Chemicals

Nafcillin — Nitromersol

Substance	Poisoning, Accidental (unintentional)	Poisoning, Intentional Self-harm	Poisoning, Assault	Poisoning, Undetermined	Adverse Effect	Under-dosing
Nafcillin	T36.0X1	T36.0X2	T36.0X3	T36.0X4	T36.0X5	T36.0X6
Nafoxidine	T38.6X1	T38.6X2	T38.6X3	T38.6X4	T38.6X5	T38.6X6
Naftazone	T46.991	T46.992	T46.993	T46.994	T46.995	T46.996
Naftidrofuryl (oxalate)	T46.7X1	T46.7X2	T46.7X3	T46.7X4	T46.7X5	T46.7X6
Naftifine	T49.0X1	T49.0X2	T49.0X3	T49.0X4	T49.0X5	T49.0X6
Nail polish remover	T52.91	T52.92	T52.93	T52.94	—	—
Nalbuphine	T40.4X1	T40.4X2	T40.4X3	T40.4X4	T40.4X5	T40.4X6
Naled	T60.0X1	T60.0X2	T60.0X3	T60.0X4	—	—
Nalidixic acid	T37.8X1	T37.8X2	T37.8X3	T37.8X4	T37.8X5	T37.8X6
Nalorphine	T50.7X1	T50.7X2	T50.7X3	T50.7X4	T50.7X5	T50.7X6
Naloxone	T50.7X1	T50.7X2	T50.7X3	T50.7X4	T50.7X5	T50.7X6
Naltrexone	T50.7X1	T50.7X2	T50.7X3	T50.7X4	T50.7X5	T50.7X6
Namenda	T43.8X1	T43.8X2	T43.8X3	T43.8X4	T43.8X5	T43.8X6
Nandrolone	T38.7X1	T38.7X2	T38.7X3	T38.7X4	T38.7X5	T38.7X6
Naphazoline	T48.5X1	T48.5X2	T48.5X3	T48.5X4	T48.5X5	T48.5X6
Naphtha (painters')	T52.0X1	T52.0X2	T52.0X3	T52.0X4	—	—
(petroleum)						
solvent	T52.0X1	T52.0X2	T52.0X3	T52.0X4	—	—
vapor	T52.0X1	T52.0X2	T52.0X3	T52.0X4	—	—
Naphthalene	T60.2X1	T60.2X2	T60.2X3	T60.2X4	—	—
(non-chlorinated)						
chlorinated	T60.1X1	T60.1X2	T60.1X3	T60.1X4	—	—
vapor	T60.1X1	T60.1X2	T60.1X3	T60.1X4	—	—
insecticide or moth repellent	T60.2X1	T60.2X2	T60.2X3	T60.2X4	—	—
chlorinated	T60.1X1	T60.1X2	T60.1X3	T60.1X4	—	—
vapor	T60.2X1	T60.2X2	T60.2X3	T60.2X4	—	—
chlorinated	T60.1X1	T60.1X2	T60.1X3	T60.1X4	—	—
Naphthol	T65.891	T65.892	T65.893	T65.894	—	—
Naphthylamine	T65.891	T65.892	T65.893	T65.894	—	—
Naphthylthiourea (ANTU)	T60.4X1	T60.4X2	T60.4X3	T60.4X4	—	—
Naprosyn — see Naproxen						
Naproxen	T39.311	T39.312	T39.313	T39.314	T39.315	T39.316
Narcotic (drug)	T40.601	T40.602	T40.603	T40.604	T40.605	T40.606
analgesic NEC	T40.601	T40.602	T40.603	T40.604	T40.605	T40.606
antagonist	T50.7X1	T50.7X2	T50.7X3	T50.7X4	T50.7X5	T50.7X6
specified NEC	T40.691	T40.692	T40.693	T40.694	T40.695	T40.696
synthetic	T40.4X1	T40.4X2	T40.4X3	T40.4X4	T40.4X5	T40.4X6
Narcotine	T48.3X1	T48.3X2	T48.3X3	T48.3X4	T48.3X5	T48.3X6
Nardil	T43.1X1	T43.1X2	T43.1X3	T43.1X4	T43.1X5	T43.1X6
Nasal drug NEC	T49.6X1	T49.6X2	T49.6X3	T49.6X4	T49.6X5	T49.6X6
Natamycin	T49.0X1	T49.0X2	T49.0X3	T49.0X4	T49.0X5	T49.0X6
Natrium cyanide — see Cyanide(s)						
Natural						
blood (product)	T45.8X1	T45.8X2	T45.8X3	T45.8X4	T45.8X5	T45.8X6
gas (piped)	T59.891	T59.892	T59.893	T59.894	—	—
incomplete combustion	T58.11	T58.12	T58.13	T58.14	—	—
Nealbarbital	T42.3X1	T42.3X2	T42.3X3	T42.3X4	T42.3X5	T42.3X6
Nectadon	T48.3X1	T48.3X2	T48.3X3	T48.3X4	T48.3X5	T48.3X6
Nedocromil	T48.6X1	T48.6X2	T48.6X3	T48.6X4	T48.6X5	T48.6X6
Nefopam	T39.8X1	T39.8X2	T39.8X3	T39.8X4	T39.8X5	T39.8X6
Nematocyst (sting)	T63.691	T63.692	T63.693	T63.694	—	—
Nembutal	T42.3X1	T42.3X2	T42.3X3	T42.3X4	T42.3X5	T42.3X6
Nemonapride	T43.591	T43.592	T43.593	T43.594	T43.595	T43.596
Neoarsphenamine	T37.8X1	T37.8X2	T37.8X3	T37.8X4	T37.8X5	T37.8X6
Neocinchophen	T50.4X1	T50.4X2	T50.4X3	T50.4X4	T50.4X5	T50.4X6
Neomycin (derivatives)	T36.5X1	T36.5X2	T36.5X3	T36.5X4	T36.5X5	T36.5X6
with						
bacitracin	T49.0X1	T49.0X2	T49.0X3	T49.0X4	T49.0X5	T49.0X6
neostigmine	T44.0X1	T44.0X2	T44.0X3	T44.0X4	T44.0X5	T44.0X6
ENT agent	T49.6X1	T49.6X2	T49.6X3	T49.6X4	T49.6X5	T49.6X6
ophthalmic preparation	T49.5X1	T49.5X2	T49.5X3	T49.5X4	T49.5X5	T49.5X6
topical NEC	T49.0X1	T49.0X2	T49.0X3	T49.0X4	T49.0X5	T49.0X6
Neonal	T42.3X1	T42.3X2	T42.3X3	T42.3X4	T42.3X5	T42.3X6
Neoprontosil	T37.0X1	T37.0X2	T37.0X3	T37.0X4	T37.0X5	T37.0X6
Neosalvarsan	T37.8X1	T37.8X2	T37.8X3	T37.8X4	T37.8X5	T37.8X6
Neosilversalvarsan	T37.8X1	T37.8X2	T37.8X3	T37.8X4	T37.8X5	T37.8X6
Neosporin	T36.8X1	T36.8X2	T36.8X3	T36.8X4	T36.8X5	T36.8X6
ENT agent	T49.6X1	T49.6X2	T49.6X3	T49.6X4	T49.6X5	T49.6X6
opthalmic preparation	T49.5X1	T49.5X2	T49.5X3	T49.5X4	T49.5X5	T49.5X6
topical NEC	T49.0X1	T49.0X2	T49.0X3	T49.0X4	T49.0X5	T49.0X6
Neostigmine bromide	T44.0X1	T44.0X2	T44.0X3	T44.0X4	T44.0X5	T44.0X6
Neraval	T42.3X1	T42.3X2	T42.3X3	T42.3X4	T42.3X5	T42.3X6
Neravan	T42.3X1	T42.3X2	T42.3X3	T42.3X4	T42.3X5	T42.3X6
Nerium oleander	T62.2X1	T62.2X2	T62.2X3	T62.2X4	—	—
Nerve gas, not in war	T59.91	T59.92	T59.93	T59.94	—	—
Nesacaine	T41.3X1	T41.3X2	T41.3X3	T41.3X4	T41.3X5	T41.3X6
infiltration (subcutaneous)	T41.3X1	T41.3X2	T41.3X3	T41.3X4	T41.3X5	T41.3X6
nerve block (peripheral) (plexus)	T41.3X1	T41.3X2	T41.3X3	T41.3X4	T41.3X5	T41.3X6
Netilmicin	T36.5X1	T36.5X2	T36.5X3	T36.5X4	T36.5X5	T36.5X6
Neurobarb	T42.3X1	T42.3X2	T42.3X3	T42.3X4	T42.3X5	T42.3X6
Neuroleptic drug NEC	T43.501	T43.502	T43.503	T43.504	T43.505	T43.506
Neuromuscular blocking drug	T48.1X1	T48.1X2	T48.1X3	T48.1X4	T48.1X5	T48.1X6
Neutral insulin injection	T38.3X1	T38.3X2	T38.3X3	T38.3X4	T38.3X5	T38.3X6
Neutral spirits	T51.0X1	T51.0X2	T51.0X3	T51.0X4	—	—
beverage	T51.0X1	T51.0X2	T51.0X3	T51.0X4	—	—
Niacin	T46.7X1	T46.7X2	T46.7X3	T46.7X4	T46.7X5	T46.7X6
Niacinamide	T45.2X1	T45.2X2	T45.2X3	T45.2X4	T45.2X5	T45.2X6
Nialamide	T43.1X1	T43.1X2	T43.1X3	T43.1X4	T43.1X5	T43.1X6
Niaprazine	T42.6X1	T42.6X2	T42.6X3	T42.6X4	T42.6X5	T42.6X6
Nicametate	T46.7X1	T46.7X2	T46.7X3	T46.7X4	T46.7X5	T46.7X6
Nicardipine	T46.1X1	T46.1X2	T46.1X3	T46.1X4	T46.1X5	T46.1X6
Nicergoline	T46.7X1	T46.7X2	T46.7X3	T46.7X4	T46.7X5	T46.7X6
Nickel (carbonyl) (tetra-carbonyl)(fumes) (vapor)	T56.891	T56.892	T56.893	T56.894		
Nickelocene	T56.891	T56.892	T56.893	T56.894	—	—
Niclosamide	T37.4X1	T37.4X2	T37.4X3	T37.4X4	T37.4X5	T37.4X6
Nicofuranose	T46.7X1	T46.7X2	T46.7X3	T46.7X4	T46.7X5	T46.7X6
Nicomorphine	T40.2X1	T40.2X2	T40.2X3	T40.2X4	—	—
Nicorandil	T46.3X1	T46.3X2	T46.3X3	T46.3X4	T46.3X5	T46.3X6
Nicotiana (plant)	T62.2X1	T62.2X2	T62.2X3	T62.2X4	—	—
Nicotinamide	T45.2X1	T45.2X2	T45.2X3	T45.2X4	T45.2X5	T45.2X6
Nicotine (insecticide) (spray) (sulfate) NEC	T60.2X1	T60.2X2	T60.2X3	T60.2X4	—	—
from tobacco	T65.291	T65.292	T65.293	T65.294		
cigarettes	T65.221	T65.222	T65.223	T65.224		
not insecticide	T65.291	T65.292	T65.293	T65.294		
Nicotinic acid	T46.7X1	T46.7X2	T46.7X3	T46.7X4	T46.7X5	T46.7X6
Nicotinyl alcohol	T46.7X1	T46.7X2	T46.7X3	T46.7X4	T46.7X5	T46.7X6
Nicoumalone	T45.511	T45.512	T45.513	T45.514	T45.515	T45.516
Nifedipine	T46.1X1	T46.1X2	T46.1X3	T46.1X4	T46.1X5	T46.1X6
Nifenazone	T39.2X1	T39.2X2	T39.2X3	T39.2X4	T39.2X5	T39.2X6
Nifuraldezone	T37.91	T37.92	T37.93	T37.94	T37.95	T37.96
Nifuratel	T37.8X1	T37.8X2	T37.8X3	T37.8X4	T37.8X5	T37.8X6
Nifurtimox	T37.3X1	T37.3X2	T37.3X3	T37.3X4	T37.3X5	T37.3X6
Nifurtoinol	T37.8X1	T37.8X2	T37.8X3	T37.8X4	T37.8X5	T37.8X6
Nightshade, deadly (solanum) — see also Belladonna	T62.2X1	T62.2X2	T62.2X3	T62.2X4		
berry	T62.1X1	T62.1X2	T62.1X3	T62.1X4		
Nikethamide	T50.7X1	T50.7X2	T50.7X3	T50.7X4	T50.7X5	T50.7X6
Nilstat	T36.7X1	T36.7X2	T36.7X3	T36.7X4	T36.7X5	T36.7X6
topical	T49.0X1	T49.0X2	T49.0X3	T49.0X4	T49.0X5	T49.0X6
Nilutamide	T38.6X1	T38.6X2	T38.6X3	T38.6X4	T38.6X5	T38.6X6
Nimesulide	T39.391	T39.392	T39.393	T39.394	T39.395	T39.396
Nimetazepam	T42.4X1	T42.4X2	T42.4X3	T42.4X4	T42.4X5	T42.4X6
Nimodipine	T46.1X1	T46.1X2	T46.1X3	T46.1X4	T46.1X5	T46.1X6
Nimorazole	T37.3X1	T37.3X2	T37.3X3	T37.3X4	T37.3X5	T37.3X6
Nimustine	T45.1X1	T45.1X2	T45.1X3	T45.1X4	T45.1X5	T45.1X6
Niridazole	T37.4X1	T37.4X2	T37.4X3	T37.4X4	T37.4X5	T37.4X6
Nisentil	T40.2X1	T40.2X2	T40.2X3	T40.2X4	T40.2X5	T40.2X6
Nisoldipine	T46.1X1	T46.1X2	T46.1X3	T46.1X4	T46.1X5	T46.1X6
Nitramine	T65.3X1	T65.3X2	T65.3X3	T65.3X4	—	—
Nitrate, organic	T46.3X1	T46.3X2	T46.3X3	T46.3X4	T46.3X5	T46.3X6
Nitrazepam	T42.4X1	T42.4X2	T42.4X3	T42.4X4	T42.4X5	T42.4X6
Nitrefazole	T50.6X1	T50.6X2	T50.6X3	T50.6X4	T50.6X5	T50.6X6
Nitrendipine	T46.1X1	T46.1X2	T46.1X3	T46.1X4	T46.1X5	T46.1X6
Nitric						
acid (liquid)	T54.2X1	T54.2X2	T54.2X3	T54.2X4		
vapor	T59.891	T59.892	T59.893	T59.894	—	—
oxide (gas)	T59.0X1	T59.0X2	T59.0X3	T59.0X4	—	—
Nitrimidazine	T37.3X1	T37.3X2	T37.3X3	T37.3X4	T37.3X5	T37.3X6
Nitrite, amyl (medicinal) (vapor)	T46.3X1	T46.3X2	T46.3X3	T46.3X4	T46.3X5	T46.3X6
Nitroaniline	T65.3X1	T65.3X2	T65.3X3	T65.3X4	—	—
vapor	T59.891	T59.892	T59.893	T59.894	—	—
Nitrobenzene, nitrobenzol	T65.3X1	T65.3X2	T65.3X3	T65.3X4	—	—
vapor	T65.3X1	T65.3X2	T65.3X3	T65.3X4	—	—
Nitrocellulose	T65.891	T65.892	T65.893	T65.894	—	—
lacquer	T65.891	T65.892	T65.893	T65.894	—	—
Nitrodiphenyl	T65.3X1	T65.3X2	T65.3X3	T65.3X4	—	—
Nitrofural	T49.0X1	T49.0X2	T49.0X3	T49.0X4	T49.0X5	T49.0X6
Nitrofurantoin	T37.8X1	T37.8X2	T37.8X3	T37.8X4	T37.8X5	T37.8X6
Nitrofurazone	T49.0X1	T49.0X2	T49.0X3	T49.0X4	T49.0X5	T49.0X6
Nitrogen	T59.0X1	T59.0X2	T59.0X3	T59.0X4	—	—
mustard	T45.1X1	T45.1X2	T45.1X3	T45.1X4	T45.1X5	T45.1X6
Nitroglycerin, nitroglycerol (medicinal)	T46.3X1	T46.3X2	T46.3X3	T46.3X4	T46.3X5	T46.3X6
nonmedical	T65.5X1	T65.5X2	T65.5X3	T65.5X4		
fumes	T65.5X1	T65.5X2	T65.5X3	T65.5X4		
Nitroglycol	T52.3X1	T52.3X2	T52.3X3	T52.3X4		
Nitrohydrochloric acid	T54.2X1	T54.2X2	T54.2X3	T54.2X4	—	—
Nitromersol	T49.0X1	T49.0X2	T49.0X3	T49.0X4	T49.0X5	T49.0X6

Substance	Poisoning, Accidental (unintentional)	Poisoning, Intentional Self-harm	Poisoning, Assault	Poisoning, Undetermined	Adverse Effect	Under-dosing
Nitronaphthalene	T65.891	T65.892	T65.893	T65.894	—	—
Nitrophenol	T54.0X1	T54.0X2	T54.0X3	T54.0X4	—	—
Nitropropane	T52.8X1	T52.8X2	T52.8X3	T52.8X4	—	—
Nitroprusside	T46.5X1	T46.5X2	T46.5X3	T46.5X4	T46.5X5	T46.5X6
Nitrosodimethylamine	T65.3X1	T65.3X2	T65.3X3	T65.3X4	—	—
Nitrothiazol	T37.4X1	T37.4X2	T37.4X3	T37.4X4	T37.4X5	T37.4X6
Nitrotoluene, nitrotoluol	T65.3X1	T65.3X2	T65.3X3	T65.3X4	—	—
vapor	T65.3X1	T65.3X2	T65.3X3	T65.3X4	—	—
Nitrous						
acid (liquid)	T54.2X1	T54.2X2	T54.2X3	T54.2X4	—	—
fumes	T59.891	T59.892	T59.893	T59.894	—	—
ether spirit	T46.3X1	T46.3X2	T46.3X3	T46.3X4	T46.3X5	T46.3X6
oxide	T41.0X1	T41.0X2	T41.0X3	T41.0X4	T41.0X5	T41.0X6
Nitroxoline	T37.8X1	T37.8X2	T37.8X3	T37.8X4	T37.8X5	T37.8X6
Nitrozone	T49.0X1	T49.0X2	T49.0X3	T49.0X4	T49.0X5	T49.0X6
Nizatidine	T47.0X1	T47.0X2	T47.0X3	T47.0X4	T47.0X5	T47.0X6
Nizofenone	T43.8X1	T43.8X2	T43.8X3	T43.8X4	T43.8X5	T43.8X6
Noctec	T42.6X1	T42.6X2	T42.6X3	T42.6X4	T42.6X5	T42.6X6
Noludar	T42.6X1	T42.6X2	T42.6X3	T42.6X4	T42.6X5	T42.6X6
Nomegestrol	T38.5X1	T38.5X2	T38.5X3	T38.5X4	T38.5X5	T38.5X6
Nomifensine	T43.291	T43.292	T43.293	T43.294	T43.295	T43.296
Nonoxinol	T49.8X1	T49.8X2	T49.8X3	T49.8X4	T49.8X5	T49.8X6
Nonylphenoxy (polyethoxyethanol)	T49.8X1	T49.8X2	T49.8X3	T49.8X4	T49.8X5	T49.8X6
Noptil	T42.3X1	T42.3X2	T42.3X3	T42.3X4	T42.3X5	T42.3X6
Noradrenaline	T44.4X1	T44.4X2	T44.4X3	T44.4X4	T44.4X5	T44.4X6
Noramidopyrine	T39.2X1	T39.2X2	T39.2X3	T39.2X4	T39.2X5	T39.2X6
methanesulfonate sodium	T39.2X1	T39.2X2	T39.2X3	T39.2X4	T39.2X5	T39.2X6
Norbormide	T60.4X1	T60.4X2	T60.4X3	T60.4X4	—	—
Nordazepam	T42.4X1	T42.4X2	T42.4X3	T42.4X4	T42.4X5	T42.4X6
Norepinephrine	T44.4X1	T44.4X2	T44.4X3	T44.4X4	T44.4X5	T44.4X6
Norethandrolone	T38.7X1	T38.7X2	T38.7X3	T38.7X4	T38.7X5	T38.7X6
Norethindrone	T38.4X1	T38.4X2	T38.4X3	T38.4X4	T38.4X5	T38.4X6
Norethisterone (acetate) (enantate)	T38.4X1	T38.4X2	T38.4X3	T38.4X4	T38.4X5	T38.4X6
with ethinylestradiol	T38.5X1	T38.5X2	T38.5X3	T38.5X4	T38.5X5	T38.5X6
Noretynodrel	T38.5X1	T38.5X2	T38.5X3	T38.5X4	T38.5X5	T38.5X6
Norfenefrine	T44.4X1	T44.4X2	T44.4X3	T44.4X4	T44.4X5	T44.4X6
Norfloxacin	T36.8X1	T36.8X2	T36.8X3	T36.8X4	T36.8X5	T36.8X6
Norgestrel	T38.4X1	T38.4X2	T38.4X3	T38.4X4	T38.4X5	T38.4X6
Norgestrienone	T38.4X1	T38.4X2	T38.4X3	T38.4X4	T38.4X5	T38.4X6
Norlestrin	T38.4X1	T38.4X2	T38.4X3	T38.4X4	T38.4X5	T38.4X6
Norlutin	T38.4X1	T38.4X2	T38.4X3	T38.4X4	T38.4X5	T38.4X6
Normal serum albumin (human), salt-poor	T45.8X1	T45.8X2	T45.8X3	T45.8X4	T45.8X5	T45.8X6
Normethandrone	T38.5X1	T38.5X2	T38.5X3	T38.5X4	T38.5X5	T38.5X6
Normison — see Benzodiazepines						
Normorphine	T40.2X1	T40.2X2	T40.2X3	T40.2X4		
Norpseudoephedrine	T50.5X1	T50.5X2	T50.5X3	T50.5X4	T50.5X5	T50.5X6
Nortestosterone (furanpropionate)	T38.7X1	T38.7X2	T38.7X3	T38.7X4	T38.7X5	T38.7X6
Nortriptyline	T43.011	T43.012	T43.013	T43.014	T43.015	T43.016
Noscapine	T48.3X1	T48.3X2	T48.3X3	T48.3X4	T48.3X5	T48.3X6
Nose preparations	T49.6X1	T49.6X2	T49.6X3	T49.6X4	T49.6X5	T49.6X6
Novobiocin	T36.5X1	T36.5X2	T36.5X3	T36.5X4	T36.5X5	T36.5X6
Novocain (infiltration) (topical)	T41.3X1	T41.3X2	T41.3X3	T41.3X4	T41.3X5	T41.3X6
nerve block (peripheral) (plexus)	T41.3X1	T41.3X2	T41.3X3	T41.3X4	T41.3X5	T41.3X6
spinal	T41.3X1	T41.3X2	T41.3X3	T41.3X4	T41.3X5	T41.3X6
Noxious foodstuff	T62.91	T62.92	T62.93	T62.94		
specified NEC	T62.8X1	T62.8X2	T62.8X3	T62.8X4	—	—
Noxiptiline	T43.011	T43.012	T43.013	T43.014	T43.015	T43.016
Noxytiolin	T49.0X1	T49.0X2	T49.0X3	T49.0X4	T49.0X5	T49.0X6
NPH Iletin (insulin)	T38.3X1	T38.3X2	T38.3X3	T38.3X4	T38.3X5	T38.3X6
Numorphan	T40.2X1	T40.2X2	T40.2X3	T40.2X4	T40.2X5	T40.2X6
Nunol	T42.3X1	T42.3X2	T42.3X3	T42.3X4	T42.3X5	T42.3X6
Nupercaine (spinal anesthetic)	T41.3X1	T41.3X2	T41.3X3	T41.3X4	T41.3X5	T41.3X6
topical (surface)	T41.3X1	T41.3X2	T41.3X3	T41.3X4	T41.3X5	T41.3X6
Nutmeg oil (liniment)	T49.3X1	T49.3X2	T49.3X3	T49.3X4	T49.3X5	T49.3X6
Nutritional supplement	T50.901	T50.902	T50.903	T50.904	T50.905	T50.906
Nux vomica	T65.1X1	T65.1X2	T65.1X3	T65.1X4	—	—
Nydrazid	T37.1X1	T37.1X2	T37.1X3	T37.1X4	T37.1X5	T37.1X6
Nylidrin	T46.7X1	T46.7X2	T46.7X3	T46.7X4	T46.7X5	T46.7X6
Nystatin	T36.7X1	T36.7X2	T36.7X3	T36.7X4	T36.7X5	T36.7X6
topical	T49.0X1	T49.0X2	T49.0X3	T49.0X4	T49.0X5	T49.0X6
Nytol	T45.0X1	T45.0X2	T45.0X3	T45.0X4	T45.0X5	T45.0X6
Obidoxime chloride	T50.6X1	T50.6X2	T50.6X3	T50.6X4	T50.6X5	T50.6X6
Octafonium (chloride)	T49.3X1	T49.3X2	T49.3X3	T49.3X4	T49.3X5	T49.3X6
Octamethyl pyrophosphoramide	T60.0X1	T60.0X2	T60.0X3	T60.0X4	—	—
Octanoin	T50.991	T50.992	T50.993	T50.994	T50.995	T50.996
Octatropine methylbromide	T44.3X1	T44.3X2	T44.3X3	T44.3X4	T44.3X5	T44.3X6
Octotiamine	T45.2X1	T45.2X2	T45.2X3	T45.2X4	T45.2X5	T45.2X6
Octoxinol (9)	T49.8X1	T49.8X2	T49.8X3	T49.8X4	T49.8X5	T49.8X6
Octreotide	T38.991	T38.992	T38.993	T38.994	T38.995	T38.996
Octyl nitrite	T46.3X1	T46.3X2	T46.3X3	T46.3X4	T46.3X5	T46.3X6
Oestradiol	T38.5X1	T38.5X2	T38.5X3	T38.5X4	T38.5X5	T38.5X6
Oestriol	T38.5X1	T38.5X2	T38.5X3	T38.5X4	T38.5X5	T38.5X6
Oestrogen	T38.5X1	T38.5X2	T38.5X3	T38.5X4	T38.5X5	T38.5X6
Oestrone	T38.5X1	T38.5X2	T38.5X3	T38.5X4	T38.5X5	T38.5X6
Ofloxacin	T36.8X1	T36.8X2	T36.8X3	T36.8X4	T36.8X5	T36.8X6
Oil (of)	T65.891	T65.892	T65.893	T65.894		
bitter almond	T62.8X1	T62.8X2	T62.8X3	T62.8X4	—	—
cloves	T49.7X1	T49.7X2	T49.7X3	T49.7X4	T49.7X5	T49.7X6
colors	T65.6X1	T65.6X2	T65.6X3	T65.6X4	—	—
fumes	T59.891	T59.892	T59.893	T59.894	—	—
lubricating	T52.0X1	T52.0X2	T52.0X3	T52.0X4	—	—
Niobe	T52.8X1	T52.8X2	T52.8X3	T52.8X4	—	—
vitriol (liquid)	T54.2X1	T54.2X2	T54.2X3	T54.2X4	—	—
fumes	T54.2X1	T54.2X2	T54.2X3	T54.2X4	—	—
wintergreen (bitter) NEC	T49.3X1	T49.3X2	T49.3X3	T49.3X4	T49.3X5	T49.3X6
Oily preparation (for skin)	T49.3X1	T49.3X2	T49.3X3	T49.3X4	T49.3X5	T49.3X6
Ointment NEC	T49.3X1	T49.3X2	T49.3X3	T49.3X4	T49.3X5	T49.3X6
Olanzapine	T43.591	T43.592	T43.593	T43.594	T43.595	T43.596
Oleander	T62.2X1	T62.2X2	T62.2X3	T62.2X4	—	—
Oleandomycin	T36.3X1	T36.3X2	T36.3X3	T36.3X4	T36.3X5	T36.3X6
Oleandrin	T46.0X1	T46.0X2	T46.0X3	T46.0X4	T46.0X5	T46.0X6
Oleic acid	T46.6X1	T46.6X2	T46.6X3	T46.6X4	T46.6X5	T46.6X6
Oleovitamin A	T45.2X1	T45.2X2	T45.2X3	T45.2X4	T45.2X5	T45.2X6
Oleum ricini	T47.2X1	T47.2X2	T47.2X3	T47.2X4	T47.2X5	T47.2X6
Olive oil (medicinal) NEC	T47.4X1	T47.4X2	T47.4X3	T47.4X4	T47.4X5	T47.4X6
Olivomycin	T45.1X1	T45.1X2	T45.1X3	T45.1X4	T45.1X5	T45.1X6
Olsalazine	T47.8X1	T47.8X2	T47.8X3	T47.8X4	T47.8X5	T47.8X6
Omeprazole	T47.1X1	T47.1X2	T47.1X3	T47.1X4	T47.1X5	T47.1X6
OMPA	T60.0X1	T60.0X2	T60.0X3	T60.0X4	—	—
Oncovin	T45.1X1	T45.1X2	T45.1X3	T45.1X4	T45.1X5	T45.1X6
Ondansetron	T45.0X1	T45.0X2	T45.0X3	T45.0X4	T45.0X5	T45.0X6
Ophthaine	T41.3X1	T41.3X2	T41.3X3	T41.3X4	T41.3X5	T41.3X6
Ophthetic	T41.3X1	T41.3X2	T41.3X3	T41.3X4	T41.3X5	T41.3X6
Opiate NEC	T40.601	T40.602	T40.603	T40.604	T40.605	T40.606
antagonists	T50.7X1	T50.7X2	T50.7X3	T50.7X4	T50.7X5	T50.7X6
Opioid NEC	T40.2X1	T40.2X2	T40.2X3	T40.2X4	T40.2X5	T40.2X6
Opipramol	T43.011	T43.012	T43.013	T43.014	T43.015	T43.016
Opium alkaloids (total)	T40.0X1	T40.0X2	T40.0X3	T40.0X4	T40.0X5	T40.0X6
standardized powdered	T40.0X1	T40.0X2	T40.0X3	T40.0X4	T40.0X5	T40.0X6
tincture (camphorated)	T40.0X1	T40.0X2	T40.0X3	T40.0X4	T40.0X5	T40.0X6
Oracon	T38.4X1	T38.4X2	T38.4X3	T38.4X4	T38.4X5	T38.4X6
Oragrafin	T50.8X1	T50.8X2	T50.8X3	T50.8X4	T50.8X5	T50.8X6
Oral contraceptives	T38.4X1	T38.4X2	T38.4X3	T38.4X4	T38.4X5	T38.4X6
Oral rehydration salts	T50.3X1	T50.3X2	T50.3X3	T50.3X4	T50.3X5	T50.3X6
Orazamide	T50.991	T50.992	T50.993	T50.994	T50.995	T50.996
Orciprenaline	T48.291	T48.292	T48.293	T48.294	T48.295	T48.296
Organidin	T48.4X1	T48.4X2	T48.4X3	T48.4X4	T48.4X5	T48.4X6
Organonitrate NEC	T46.3X1	T46.3X2	T46.3X3	T46.3X4	T46.3X5	T46.3X6
Organophosphates	T60.0X1	T60.0X2	T60.0X3	T60.0X4	—	—
Orimune	T50.B91	T50.B92	T50.B93	T50.B94	T50.B95	T50.B96
Orinase	T38.3X1	T38.3X2	T38.3X3	T38.3X4	T38.3X5	T38.3X6
Ormeloxifene	T38.6X1	T38.6X2	T38.6X3	T38.6X4	T38.6X5	T38.6X6
Ornidazole	T37.3X1	T37.3X2	T37.3X3	T37.3X4	T37.3X5	T37.3X6
Ornithine aspartate	T50.991	T50.992	T50.993	T50.994	T50.995	T50.996
Ornoprostil	T47.1X1	T47.1X2	T47.1X3	T47.1X4	T47.1X5	T47.1X6
Orphenadrine (hydrochloride)	T42.8X1	T42.8X2	T42.8X3	T42.8X4	T42.8X5	T42.8X6
Ortal (sodium)	T42.3X1	T42.3X2	T42.3X3	T42.3X4	T42.3X5	T42.3X6
Orthoboric acid	T49.0X1	T49.0X2	T49.0X3	T49.0X4	T49.0X5	T49.0X6
ENT agent	T49.6X1	T49.6X2	T49.6X3	T49.6X4	T49.6X5	T49.6X6
ophthalmic preparation	T49.5X1	T49.5X2	T49.5X3	T49.5X4	T49.5X5	T49.5X6
Orthocaine	T41.3X1	T41.3X2	T41.3X3	T41.3X4	T41.3X5	T41.3X6
Orthodichlorobenzene	T53.7X1	T53.7X2	T53.7X3	T53.7X4	—	—
Ortho-Novum	T38.4X1	T38.4X2	T38.4X3	T38.4X4	T38.4X5	T38.4X6
Orthotolidine (reagent)	T54.2X1	T54.2X2	T54.2X3	T54.2X4	—	—
Osmic acid (liquid)	T54.2X1	T54.2X2	T54.2X3	T54.2X4	—	—
fumes	T54.2X1	T54.2X2	T54.2X3	T54.2X4	—	—
Osmotic diuretics	T50.2X1	T50.2X2	T50.2X3	T50.2X4	T50.2X5	T50.2X6
Otilonium bromide	T44.3X1	T44.3X2	T44.3X3	T44.3X4	T44.3X5	T44.3X6
Otorhinolaryngological drug NEC	T49.6X1	T49.6X2	T49.6X3	T49.6X4	T49.6X5	T49.6X6
Ouabain (e)	T46.0X1	T46.0X2	T46.0X3	T46.0X4	T46.0X5	T46.0X6
Ovarian						
hormone	T38.5X1	T38.5X2	T38.5X3	T38.5X4	T38.5X5	T38.5X6
stimulant	T38.5X1	T38.5X2	T38.5X3	T38.5X4	T38.5X5	T38.5X6
Ovral	T38.4X1	T38.4X2	T38.4X3	T38.4X4	T38.4X5	T38.4X6

Table of Drugs and Chemicals

Ovulen — Penicillinase

Substance	Poisoning, Accidental (unintentional)	Poisoning, Intentional Self-harm	Poisoning, Assault	Poisoning, Undetermined	Adverse Effect	Under-dosing
Ovulen	T38.4X1	T38.4X2	T38.4X3	T38.4X4	T38.4X5	T38.4X6
Oxacillin	T36.0X1	T36.0X2	T36.0X3	T36.0X4	T36.0X5	T36.0X6
Oxalic acid	T54.2X1	T54.2X2	T54.2X3	T54.2X4	—	—
ammonium salt	T50.991	T50.992	T50.993	T50.994	T50.995	T50.996
Oxamniquine	T37.4X1	T37.4X2	T37.4X3	T37.4X4	T37.4X5	T37.4X6
Oxanamide	T43.591	T43.592	T43.593	T43.594	T43.595	T43.596
Oxandrolone	T38.7X1	T38.7X2	T38.7X3	T38.7X4	T38.7X5	T38.7X6
Oxantel	T37.4X1	T37.4X2	T37.4X3	T37.4X4	T37.4X5	T37.4X6
Oxapium iodide	T44.3X1	T44.3X2	T44.3X3	T44.3X4	T44.3X5	T44.3X6
Oxaprotiline	T43.021	T43.022	T43.023	T43.024	T43.025	T43.026
Oxaprozin	T39.311	T39.312	T39.313	T39.314	T39.315	T39.316
Oxatomide	T45.0X1	T45.0X2	T45.0X3	T45.0X4	T45.0X5	T45.0X6
Oxazepam	T42.4X1	T42.4X2	T42.4X3	T42.4X4	T42.4X5	T42.4X6
Oxazimedrine	T50.5X1	T50.5X2	T50.5X3	T50.5X4	T50.5X5	T50.5X6
Oxazolam	T42.4X1	T42.4X2	T42.4X3	T42.4X4	T42.4X5	T42.4X6
Oxazolidine derivatives	T42.2X1	T42.2X2	T42.2X3	T42.2X4	T42.2X5	T42.2X6
Oxazolidinedione (derivative)	T42.2X1	T42.2X2	T42.2X3	T42.2X4	T42.2X5	T42.2X6
Ox bile extract	T47.5X1	T47.5X2	T47.5X3	T47.5X4	T47.5X5	T47.5X6
Oxcarbazepine	T42.1X1	T42.1X2	T42.1X3	T42.1X4	T42.1X5	T42.1X6
Oxedrine	T44.4X1	T44.4X2	T44.4X3	T44.4X4	T44.4X5	T44.4X6
Oxeladin (citrate)	T48.3X1	T48.3X2	T48.3X3	T48.3X4	T48.3X5	T48.3X6
Oxendolone	T38.5X1	T38.5X2	T38.5X3	T38.5X4	T38.5X5	T38.5X6
Oxetacaine	T41.3X1	T41.3X2	T41.3X3	T41.3X4	T41.3X5	T41.3X6
Oxethazine	T41.3X1	T41.3X2	T41.3X3	T41.3X4	T41.3X5	T41.3X6
Oxetorone	T39.8X1	T39.8X2	T39.8X3	T39.8X4	T39.8X5	T39.8X6
Oxiconazole	T49.0X1	T49.0X2	T49.0X3	T49.0X4	T49.0X5	T49.0X6
Oxidizing agent NEC	T54.91	T54.92	T54.93	T54.94	—	—
Oxipurinol	T50.4X1	T50.4X2	T50.4X3	T50.4X4	T50.4X5	T50.4X6
Oxitriptan	T43.291	T43.292	T43.293	T43.294	T43.295	T43.296
Oxitropium bromide	T48.6X1	T48.6X2	T48.6X3	T48.6X4	T48.6X5	T48.6X6
Oxodipine	T46.1X1	T46.1X2	T46.1X3	T46.1X4	T46.1X5	T46.1X6
Oxolamine	T48.3X1	T48.3X2	T48.3X3	T48.3X4	T48.3X5	T48.3X6
Oxolinic acid	T37.8X1	T37.8X2	T37.8X3	T37.8X4	T37.8X5	T37.8X6
Oxomemazine	T43.3X1	T43.3X2	T43.3X3	T43.3X4	T43.3X5	T43.3X6
Oxophenarsine	T37.3X1	T37.3X2	T37.3X3	T37.3X4	T37.3X5	T37.3X6
Oxprenolol	T44.7X1	T44.7X2	T44.7X3	T44.7X4	T44.7X5	T44.7X6
Oxsoralen	T49.3X1	T49.3X2	T49.3X3	T49.3X4	T49.3X5	T49.3X6
Oxtriphylline	T48.6X1	T48.6X2	T48.6X3	T48.6X4	T48.6X5	T48.6X6
Oxybate sodium	T41.291	T41.292	T41.293	T41.294	T41.295	T41.296
Oxybuprocaine	T41.3X1	T41.3X2	T41.3X3	T41.3X4	T41.3X5	T41.3X6
Oxybutynin	T44.3X1	T44.3X2	T44.3X3	T44.3X4	T44.3X5	T44.3X6
Oxychlorosene	T49.0X1	T49.0X2	T49.0X3	T49.0X4	T49.0X5	T49.0X6
Oxycodone	T40.2X1	T40.2X2	T40.2X3	T40.2X4	T40.2X5	T40.2X6
Oxyfedrine	T46.3X1	T46.3X2	T46.3X3	T46.3X4	T46.3X5	T46.3X6
Oxygen	T41.5X1	T41.5X2	T41.5X3	T41.5X4	T41.5X5	T41.5X6
Oxylone	T49.0X1	T49.0X2	T49.0X3	T49.0X4	T49.0X5	T49.0X6
ophthalmic preparation	T49.5X1	T49.5X2	T49.5X3	T49.5X4	T49.5X5	T49.5X6
Oxymesterone	T38.7X1	T38.7X2	T38.7X3	T38.7X4	T38.7X5	T38.7X6
Oxymetazoline	T48.5X1	T48.5X2	T48.5X3	T48.5X4	T48.5X5	T48.5X6
Oxymetholone	T38.7X1	T38.7X2	T38.7X3	T38.7X4	T38.7X5	T38.7X6
Oxymorphone	T40.2X1	T40.2X2	T40.2X3	T40.2X4	T40.2X5	T40.2X6
Oxypertine	T43.591	T43.592	T43.593	T43.594	T43.595	T43.596
Oxyphenbutazone	T39.2X1	T39.2X2	T39.2X3	T39.2X4	T39.2X5	T39.2X6
Oxyphencyclimine	T44.3X1	T44.3X2	T44.3X3	T44.3X4	T44.3X5	T44.3X6
Oxyphenisatine	T47.2X1	T47.2X2	T47.2X3	T47.2X4	T47.2X5	T47.2X6
Oxyphenonium bromide	T44.3X1	T44.3X2	T44.3X3	T44.3X4	T44.3X5	T44.3X6
Oxypolygelatin	T45.8X1	T45.8X2	T45.8X3	T45.8X4	T45.8X5	T45.8X6
Oxyquinoline (derivatives)	T37.8X1	T37.8X2	T37.8X3	T37.8X4	T37.8X5	T37.8X6
Oxytetracycline	T36.4X1	T36.4X2	T36.4X3	T36.4X4	T36.4X5	T36.4X6
Oxytocic drug NEC	T48.0X1	T48.0X2	T48.0X3	T48.0X4	T48.0X5	T48.0X6
Oxytocin (synthetic)	T48.0X1	T48.0X2	T48.0X3	T48.0X4	T48.0X5	T48.0X6
Ozone	T59.891	T59.892	T59.893	T59.894	—	—
PABA	T49.3X1	T49.3X2	T49.3X3	T49.3X4	T49.3X5	T49.3X6
Packed red cells	T45.8X1	T45.8X2	T45.8X3	T45.8X4	T45.8X5	T45.8X6
Padimate	T49.3X1	T49.3X2	T49.3X3	T49.3X4	T49.3X5	T49.3X6
Paint NEC	T65.6X1	T65.6X2	T65.6X3	T65.6X4	—	—
cleaner	T52.91	T52.92	T52.93	T52.94	—	—
fumes NEC	T59.891	T59.892	T59.893	T59.894	—	—
lead (fumes)	T56.0X1	T56.0X2	T56.0X3	T56.0X4	—	—
solvent NEC	T52.8X1	T52.8X2	T52.8X3	T52.8X4	—	—
stripper	T52.8X1	T52.8X2	T52.8X3	T52.8X4	—	—
Palfium	T40.2X1	T40.2X2	T40.2X3	T40.2X4	—	—
Palm kernel oil	T50.991	T50.992	T50.993	T50.994	T50.995	T50.996
Paludrine	T37.2X1	T37.2X2	T37.2X3	T37.2X4	T37.2X5	T37.2X6
PAM (pralidoxime)	T50.6X1	T50.6X2	T50.6X3	T50.6X4	T50.6X5	T50.6X6
Pamaquine (naphthoute)	T37.2X1	T37.2X2	T37.2X3	T37.2X4	T37.2X5	T37.2X6
Panadol	T39.1X1	T39.1X2	T39.1X3	T39.1X4	T39.1X5	T39.1X6
Pancreatic						
digestive secretion stimulant	T47.8X1	T47.8X2	T47.8X3	T47.8X4	T47.8X5	T47.8X6
dornase	T45.3X1	T45.3X2	T45.3X3	T45.3X4	T45.3X5	T45.3X6
Pancreatin	T47.5X1	T47.5X2	T47.5X3	T47.5X4	T47.5X5	T47.5X6
Pancrelipase	T47.5X1	T47.5X2	T47.5X3	T47.5X4	T47.5X5	T47.5X6
Pancuronium (bromide)	T48.1X1	T48.1X2	T48.1X3	T48.1X4	T48.1X5	T48.1X6
Pangamic acid	T45.2X1	T45.2X2	T45.2X3	T45.2X4	T45.2X5	T45.2X6
Panthenol	T45.2X1	T45.2X2	T45.2X3	T45.2X4	T45.2X5	T45.2X6
topical	T49.8X1	T49.8X2	T49.8X3	T49.8X4	T49.8X5	T49.8X6
Pantopon	T40.0X1	T40.0X2	T40.0X3	T40.0X4	T40.0X5	T40.0X6
Pantothenic acid	T45.2X1	T45.2X2	T45.2X3	T45.2X4	T45.2X5	T45.2X6
Panwarfin	T45.511	T45.512	T45.513	T45.514	T45.515	T45.516
Papain	T47.5X1	T47.5X2	T47.5X3	T47.5X4	T47.5X5	T47.5X6
digestant	T47.5X1	T47.5X2	T47.5X3	T47.5X4	T47.5X5	T47.5X6
Papaveretum	T40.0X1	T40.0X2	T40.0X3	T40.0X4	T40.0X5	T40.0X6
Papaverine	T44.3X1	T44.3X2	T44.3X3	T44.3X4	T44.3X5	T44.3X6
Para-acetamidophenol	T39.1X1	T39.1X2	T39.1X3	T39.1X4	T39.1X5	T39.1X6
Para-aminobenzoic acid	T49.3X1	T49.3X2	T49.3X3	T49.3X4	T49.3X5	T49.3X6
Para-aminophenol derivatives	T39.1X1	T39.1X2	T39.1X3	T39.1X4	T39.1X5	T39.1X6
Para-aminosalicylic acid	T37.1X1	T37.1X2	T37.1X3	T37.1X4	T37.1X5	T37.1X6
Paracetaldehyde	T42.6X1	T42.6X2	T42.6X3	T42.6X4	T42.6X5	T42.6X6
Paracetamol	T39.1X1	T39.1X2	T39.1X3	T39.1X4	T39.1X5	T39.1X6
Parachlorophenol (camphorated)	T49.0X1	T49.0X2	T49.0X3	T49.0X4	T49.0X5	T49.0X6
Paracodin	T40.2X1	T40.2X2	T40.2X3	T40.2X4	T40.2X5	T40.2X6
Paradione	T42.2X1	T42.2X2	T42.2X3	T42.2X4	T42.2X5	T42.2X6
Paraffin(s) (wax)	T52.0X1	T52.0X2	T52.0X3	T52.0X4	—	—
liquid (medicinal)	T47.4X1	T47.4X2	T47.4X3	T47.4X4	T47.4X5	T47.4X6
nonmedicinal	T52.0X1	T52.0X2	T52.0X3	T52.0X4	—	—
Paraformaldehyde	T60.3X1	T60.3X2	T60.3X3	T60.3X4	—	—
Paraldehyde	T42.6X1	T42.6X2	T42.6X3	T42.6X4	T42.6X5	T42.6X6
Paramethadione	T42.2X1	T42.2X2	T42.2X3	T42.2X4	T42.2X5	T42.2X6
Paramethasone	T38.0X1	T38.0X2	T38.0X3	T38.0X4	T38.0X5	T38.0X6
acetate	T49.0X1	T49.0X2	T49.0X3	T49.0X4	T49.0X5	T49.0X6
Paraoxon	T60.0X1	T60.0X2	T60.0X3	T60.0X4	—	—
Paraquat	T60.3X1	T60.3X2	T60.3X3	T60.3X4	—	—
Parasympatholytic NEC	T44.3X1	T44.3X2	T44.3X3	T44.3X4	T44.3X5	T44.3X6
Parasympathomimetic drug NEC	T44.1X1	T44.1X2	T44.1X3	T44.1X4	T44.1X5	T44.1X6
Parathion	T60.0X1	T60.0X2	T60.0X3	T60.0X4	—	—
Parathormone	T50.991	T50.992	T50.993	T50.994	T50.995	T50.996
Parathyroid extract	T50.991	T50.992	T50.993	T50.994	T50.995	T50.996
Paratyphoid vaccine	T50.A91	T50.A92	T50.A93	T50.A94	T50.A95	T50.A96
Paredrine	T44.4X1	T44.4X2	T44.4X3	T44.4X4	T44.4X5	T44.4X6
Paregoric	T40.0X1	T40.0X2	T40.0X3	T40.0X4	T40.0X5	T40.0X6
Pargyline	T46.5X1	T46.5X2	T46.5X3	T46.5X4	T46.5X5	T46.5X6
Paris green	T57.0X1	T57.0X2	T57.0X3	T57.0X4	—	—
insecticide	T57.0X1	T57.0X2	T57.0X3	T57.0X4	—	—
Parnate	T43.1X1	T43.1X2	T43.1X3	T43.1X4	T43.1X5	T43.1X6
Paromomycin	T36.5X1	T36.5X2	T36.5X3	T36.5X4	T36.5X5	T36.5X6
Paroxypropione	T45.1X1	T45.1X2	T45.1X3	T45.1X4	T45.1X5	T45.1X6
Parzone	T40.2X1	T40.2X2	T40.2X3	T40.2X4	T40.2X5	T40.2X6
PAS	T37.1X1	T37.1X2	T37.1X3	T37.1X4	T37.1X5	T37.1X6
Pasiniazid	T37.1X1	T37.1X2	T37.1X3	T37.1X4	T37.1X5	T37.1X6
PBB (polybrominated biphenyls)	T65.891	T65.892	T65.893	T65.894	—	—
PCB	T65.891	T65.892		T65.893	T65.894	—	—
PCP						
meaning pentachlorophenol	T60.1X1	T60.1X2	T60.1X3	T60.1X4	—	—
fungicide	T60.3X1	T60.3X2	T60.3X3	T60.3X4	—	—
herbicide	T60.3X1	T60.3X2	T60.3X3	T60.3X4	—	—
insecticide	T60.1X1	T60.1X2	T60.1X3	T60.1X4	—	—
meaning phencyclidine	T40.991	T40.992	T40.993	T40.994	—	—
Peach kernel oil (emulsion)	T47.4X1	T47.4X2	T47.4X3	T47.4X4	T47.4X5	T47.4X6
Peanut oil (emulsion) NEC	T47.4X1	T47.4X2	T47.4X3	T47.4X4	T47.4X5	T47.4X6
topical	T49.3X1	T49.3X2	T49.3X3	T49.3X4	T49.3X5	T49.3X6
Pearly Gates (morning glory seeds)	T40.991	T40.992	T40.993	T40.994	—	—
Pecazine	T43.3X1	T43.3X2	T43.3X3	T43.3X4	T43.3X5	T43.3X6
Pectin	T47.6X1	T47.6X2	T47.6X3	T47.6X4	T47.6X5	T47.6X6
Pefloxacin	T37.8X1	T37.8X2	T37.8X3	T37.8X4	T37.8X5	T37.8X6
Pegademase, bovine	T50.Z91	T50.Z92	T50.Z93	T50.Z94	T50.Z95	T50.Z96
Pelletierine tannate	T37.4X1	T37.4X2	T37.4X3	T37.4X4	T37.4X5	T37.4X6
Pemirolast (potassium)	T48.6X1	T48.6X2	T48.6X3	T48.6X4	T48.6X5	T48.6X6
Pemoline	T50.7X1	T50.7X2	T50.7X3	T50.7X4	T50.7X5	T50.7X6
Pempidine	T44.2X1	T44.2X2	T44.2X3	T44.2X4	T44.2X5	T44.2X6
Penamecillin	T36.0X1	T36.0X2	T36.0X3	T36.0X4	T36.0X5	T36.0X6
Penbutolol	T44.7X1	T44.7X2	T44.7X3	T44.7X4	T44.7X5	T44.7X6
Penethamate	T36.0X1	T36.0X2	T36.0X3	T36.0X4	T36.0X5	T36.0X6
Penfluridol	T43.591	T43.592	T43.593	T43.594	T43.595	T43.596
Penflutizide	T50.2X1	T50.2X2	T50.2X3	T50.2X4	T50.2X5	T50.2X6
Pengitoxin	T46.0X1	T46.0X2	T46.0X3	T46.0X4	T46.0X5	T46.0X6
Penicillamine	T50.6X1	T50.6X2	T50.6X3	T50.6X4	T50.6X5	T50.6X6
Penicillin (any)	T36.0X1	T36.0X2	T36.0X3	T36.0X4	T36.0X5	T36.0X6
Penicillinase	T45.3X1	T45.3X2	T45.3X3	T45.3X4	T45.3X5	T45.3X6

   Additional Character May Be Required — Refer to the Tabular List for Character Selection   ▽ **Subterms under main terms may continue to next column or page**

Substance	Poisoning, Accidental (unintentional)	Poisoning, Intentional Self-harm	Poisoning, Assault	Poisoning, Undetermined	Adverse Effect	Under-dosing
Penicilloyl polylysine	T50.8X1	T50.8X2	T50.8X3	T50.8X4	T50.8X5	T50.8X6
Penimepicycline	T36.4X1	T36.4X2	T36.4X3	T36.4X4	T36.4X5	T36.4X6
Pentachloroethane	T53.6X1	T53.6X2	T53.6X3	T53.6X4	—	—
Pentachloronaphthalene	T53.7X1	T53.7X2	T53.7X3	T53.7X4	—	—
Pentachlorophenol	T60.1X1	T60.1X2	T60.1X3	T60.1X4	—	—
(pesticide)						
fungicide	T60.3X1	T60.3X2	T60.3X3	T60.3X4	—	—
herbicide	T60.3X1	T60.3X2	T60.3X3	T60.3X4	—	—
insecticide	T60.1X1	T60.1X2	T60.1X3	T60.1X4	—	—
Pentaerythritol	T46.3X1	T46.3X2	T46.3X3	T46.3X4	T46.3X5	T46.3X6
chloral	T42.6X1	T42.6X2	T42.6X3	T42.6X4	T42.6X5	T42.6X6
tetranitrate NEC	T46.3X1	T46.3X2	T46.3X3	T46.3X4	T46.3X5	T46.3X6
Pentaerythrityl tetranitrate	T46.3X1	T46.3X2	T46.3X3	T46.3X4	T46.3X5	T46.3X6
Pentagastrin	T50.8X1	T50.8X2	T50.8X3	T50.8X4	T50.8X5	T50.8X6
Pentalin	T53.6X1	T53.6X2	T53.6X3	T53.6X4	—	—
Pentamethonium bromide	T44.2X1	T44.2X2	T44.2X3	T44.2X4	T44.2X5	T44.2X6
Pentamidine	T37.3X1	T37.3X2	T37.3X3	T37.3X4	T37.3X5	T37.3X6
Pentanol	T51.3X1	T51.3X2	T51.3X3	T51.3X4	—	—
Pentapyrrolinium (bitartrate)	T44.2X1	T44.2X2	T44.2X3	T44.2X4	T44.2X5	T44.2X6
Pentaquine	T37.2X1	T37.2X2	T37.2X3	T37.2X4	T37.2X5	T37.2X6
Pentazocine	T40.4X1	T40.4X2	T40.4X3	T40.4X4	T40.4X5	T40.4X6
Pentetrazole	T50.7X1	T50.7X2	T50.7X3	T50.7X4	T50.7X5	T50.7X6
Penthienate bromide	T44.3X1	T44.3X2	T44.3X3	T44.3X4	T44.3X5	T44.3X6
Pentifylline	T46.7X1	T46.7X2	T46.7X3	T46.7X4	T46.7X5	T46.7X6
Pentobarbital	T42.3X1	T42.3X2	T42.3X3	T42.3X4	T42.3X5	T42.3X6
sodium	T42.3X1	T42.3X2	T42.3X3	T42.3X4	T42.3X5	T42.3X6
Pentobarbitone	T42.3X1	T42.3X2	T42.3X3	T42.3X4	T42.3X5	T42.3X6
Pentolonium tartrate	T44.2X1	T44.2X2	T44.2X3	T44.2X4	T44.2X5	T44.2X6
Pentosan polysulfate (sodium)	T39.8X1	T39.8X2	T39.8X3	T39.8X4	T39.8X5	T39.8X6
Pentostatin	T45.1X1	T45.1X2	T45.1X3	T45.1X4	T45.1X5	T45.1X6
Pentothal	T41.1X1	T41.1X2	T41.1X3	T41.1X4	T41.1X5	T41.1X6
Pentoxifylline	T46.7X1	T46.7X2	T46.7X3	T46.7X4	T46.7X5	T46.7X6
Pentoxyverine	T48.3X1	T48.3X2	T48.3X3	T48.3X4	T48.3X5	T48.3X6
Pentrinat	T46.3X1	T46.3X2	T46.3X3	T46.3X4	T46.3X5	T46.3X6
Pentylenetetrazole	T50.7X1	T50.7X2	T50.7X3	T50.7X4	T50.7X5	T50.7X6
Pentylsalicylamide	T37.1X1	T37.1X2	T37.1X3	T37.1X4	T37.1X5	T37.1X6
Pentymal	T42.3X1	T42.3X2	T42.3X3	T42.3X4	T42.3X5	T42.3X6
Peplomycin	T45.1X1	T45.1X2	T45.1X3	T45.1X4	T45.1X5	T45.1X6
Peppermint (oil)	T47.5X1	T47.5X2	T47.5X3	T47.5X4	T47.5X5	T47.5X6
Pepsin	T47.5X1	T47.5X2	T47.5X3	T47.5X4	T47.5X5	T47.5X6
digestant	T47.5X1	T47.5X2	T47.5X3	T47.5X4	T47.5X5	T47.5X6
Pepstatin	T47.1X1	T47.1X2	T47.1X3	T47.1X4	T47.1X5	T47.1X6
Peptavlon	T50.8X1	T50.8X2	T50.8X3	T50.8X4	T50.8X5	T50.8X6
Perazine	T43.3X1	T43.3X2	T43.3X3	T43.3X4	T43.3X5	T43.3X6
Percaine (spinal)	T41.3X1	T41.3X2	T41.3X3	T41.3X4	T41.3X5	T41.3X6
topical (surface)	T41.3X1	T41.3X2	T41.3X3	T41.3X4	T41.3X5	T41.3X6
Perchloroethylene	T53.3X1	T53.3X2	T53.3X3	T53.3X4	—	—
medicinal	T37.4X1	T37.4X2	T37.4X3	T37.4X4	T37.4X5	T37.4X6
vapor	T53.3X1	T53.3X2	T53.3X3	T53.3X4	—	—
Percodan	T40.2X1	T40.2X2	T40.2X3	T40.2X4	T40.2X5	T40.2X6
Percogesic — see also acetaminophen	T45.0X1	T45.0X2	T45.0X3	T45.0X4	T45.0X5	T45.0X6
Percorten	T38.0X1	T38.0X2	T38.0X3	T38.0X4	T38.0X5	T38.0X6
Pergolide	T42.8X1	T42.8X2	T42.8X3	T42.8X4	T42.8X5	T42.8X6
Pergonal	T38.811	T38.812	T38.813	T38.814	T38.815	T38.816
Perhexilene	T46.3X1	T46.3X2	T46.3X3	T46.3X4	T46.3X5	T46.3X6
Perhexiline (maleate)	T46.3X1	T46.3X2	T46.3X3	T46.3X4	T46.3X5	T46.3X6
Periactin	T45.0X1	T45.0X2	T45.0X3	T45.0X4	T45.0X5	T45.0X6
Periciazine	T43.3X1	T43.3X2	T43.3X3	T43.3X4	T43.3X5	T43.3X6
Periclor	T42.6X1	T42.6X2	T42.6X3	T42.6X4	T42.6X5	T42.6X6
Perindopril	T46.4X1	T46.4X2	T46.4X3	T46.4X4	T46.4X5	T46.4X6
Perisoxal	T39.8X1	T39.8X2	T39.8X3	T39.8X4	T39.8X5	T39.8X6
Peritoneal dialysis solution	T50.3X1	T50.3X2	T50.3X3	T50.3X4	T50.3X5	T50.3X6
Peritrate	T46.3X1	T46.3X2	T46.3X3	T46.3X4	T46.3X5	T46.3X6
Perlapine	T42.4X1	T42.4X2	T42.4X3	T42.4X4	T42.4X5	T42.4X6
Permanganate	T65.891	T65.892	T65.893	T65.894	—	—
Permethrin	T60.1X1	T60.1X2	T60.1X3	T60.1X4	—	—
Pernocton	T42.3X1	T42.3X2	T42.3X3	T42.3X4	T42.3X5	T42.3X6
Pernoston	T42.3X1	T42.3X2	T42.3X3	T42.3X4	T42.3X5	T42.3X6
Peronine	T40.2X1	T40.2X2	T40.2X3	T40.2X4	—	—
Perphenazine	T43.3X1	T43.3X2	T43.3X3	T43.3X4	T43.3X5	T43.3X6
Pertofrane	T43.011	T43.012	T43.013	T43.014	T43.015	T43.016
Pertussis						
immune serum (human)	T50.Z11	T50.Z12	T50.Z13	T50.Z14	T50.Z15	T50.Z16
vaccine (with diphtheria toxoid)	T50.A11	T50.A12	T50.A13	T50.A14	T50.A15	T50.A16
(with tetanus toxoid)						
Peruvian balsam	T49.0X1	T49.0X2	T49.0X3	T49.0X4	T49.0X5	T49.0X6
Peruvoside	T46.0X1	T46.0X2	T46.0X3	T46.0X4	T46.0X5	T46.0X6
Pesticide (dust) (fumes) (vapor) NEC	T60.91	T60.92	T60.93	T60.94	—	—
Pesticide (dust) (fumes) (vapor) NEC — continued						
arsenic	T57.0X1	T57.0X2	T57.0X3	T57.0X4	—	—
chlorinated	T60.1X1	T60.1X2	T60.1X3	T60.1X4	—	—
cyanide	T65.0X1	T65.0X2	T65.0X3	T65.0X4	—	—
kerosene	T52.0X1	T52.0X2	T52.0X3	T52.0X4	—	—
mixture (of compounds)	T60.91	T60.92	T60.93	T60.94	—	—
naphthalene	T60.2X1	T60.2X2	T60.2X3	T60.2X4	—	—
organochlorine (compounds)	T60.1X1	T60.1X2	T60.1X3	T60.1X4	—	—
petroleum (distillate) (products) NEC	T60.8X1	T60.8X2	T60.8X3	T60.8X4	—	—
specified ingredient NEC	T60.8X1	T60.8X2	T60.8X3	T60.8X4	—	—
strychnine	T65.1X1	T65.1X2	T65.1X3	T65.1X4	—	—
thallium	T60.4X1	T60.4X2	T60.4X3	T60.4X4	—	—
Pethidine	T40.4X1	T40.4X2	T40.4X3	T40.4X4	T40.4X5	T40.4X6
Petrichloral	T42.6X1	T42.6X2	T42.6X3	T42.6X4	T42.6X5	T42.6X6
Petrol	T52.0X1	T52.0X2	T52.0X3	T52.0X4	—	—
vapor	T52.0X1	T52.0X2	T52.0X3	T52.0X4	—	—
Petrolatum	T49.3X1	T49.3X2	T49.3X3	T49.3X4	T49.3X5	T49.3X6
hydrophilic	T49.3X1	T49.3X2	T49.3X3	T49.3X4	T49.3X5	T49.3X6
liquid	T47.4X1	T47.4X2	T47.4X3	T47.4X4	T47.4X5	T47.4X6
topical	T49.3X1	T49.3X2	T49.3X3	T49.3X4	T49.3X5	T49.3X6
nonmedicinal	T52.0X1	T52.0X2	T52.0X3	T52.0X4	—	—
red veterinary	T49.3X1	T49.3X2	T49.3X3	T49.3X4	T49.3X5	T49.3X6
white	T49.3X1	T49.3X2	T49.3X3	T49.3X4	T49.3X5	T49.3X6
Petroleum (products) NEC	T52.0X1	T52.0X2	T52.0X3	T52.0X4	—	—
benzine(s) — see Ligroin						
ether — see Ligroin						
jelly — see Petrolatum						
naphtha — see Ligroin						
pesticide	T60.8X1	T60.8X2	T60.8X3	T60.8X4	—	—
solids	T52.0X1	T52.0X2	T52.0X3	T52.0X4	—	—
solvents	T52.0X1	T52.0X2	T52.0X3	T52.0X4	—	—
vapor	T52.0X1	T52.0X2	T52.0X3	T52.0X4	—	—
Peyote	T40.991	T40.992	T40.993	T40.994	—	—
Phanodorm, phanodorn	T42.3X1	T42.3X2	T42.3X3	T42.3X4	T42.3X5	T42.3X6
Phanquinone	T37.3X1	T37.3X2	T37.3X3	T37.3X4	T37.3X5	T37.3X6
Phanquone	T37.3X1	T37.3X2	T37.3X3	T37.3X4	T37.3X5	T37.3X6
Pharmaceutical						
adjunct NEC	T50.901	T50.902	T50.903	T50.904	T50.905	T50.906
excipient NEC	T50.901	T50.902	T50.903	T50.904	T50.905	T50.906
sweetener	T50.901	T50.902	T50.903	T50.904	T50.905	T50.906
viscous agent	T50.901	T50.902	T50.903	T50.904	T50.905	T50.906
Phemitone	T42.3X1	T42.3X2	T42.3X3	T42.3X4	T42.3X5	T42.3X6
Phenacaine	T41.3X1	T41.3X2	T41.3X3	T41.3X4	T41.3X5	T41.3X6
Phenacemide	T42.6X1	T42.6X2	T42.6X3	T42.6X4	T42.6X5	T42.6X6
Phenacetin	T39.1X1	T39.1X2	T39.1X3	T39.1X4	T39.1X5	T39.1X6
Phenadoxone	T40.2X1	T40.2X2	T40.2X3	T40.2X4	—	—
Phenaglycodol	T43.591	T43.592	T43.593	T43.594	T43.595	T43.596
Phenantoin	T42.0X1	T42.0X2	T42.0X3	T42.0X4	T42.0X5	T42.0X6
Phenaphthazine reagent	T50.991	T50.992	T50.993	T50.994	T50.995	T50.996
Phenazocine	T40.4X1	T40.4X2	T40.4X3	T40.4X4	T40.4X5	T40.4X6
Phenazone	T39.2X1	T39.2X2	T39.2X3	T39.2X4	T39.2X5	T39.2X6
Phenazopyridine	T39.8X1	T39.8X2	T39.8X3	T39.8X4	T39.8X5	T39.8X6
Phenbenicillin	T36.0X1	T36.0X2	T36.0X3	T36.0X4	T36.0X5	T36.0X6
Phenbutrazate	T50.5X1	T50.5X2	T50.5X3	T50.5X4	T50.5X5	T50.5X6
Phencyclidine	T40.991	T40.992	T40.993	T40.994	T40.995	T40.996
Phendimetrazine	T50.5X1	T50.5X2	T50.5X3	T50.5X4	T50.5X5	T50.5X6
Phenelzine	T43.1X1	T43.1X2	T43.1X3	T43.1X4	T43.1X5	T43.1X6
Phenemal	T42.3X1	T42.3X2	T42.3X3	T42.3X4	T42.3X5	T42.3X6
Phenergan	T42.6X1	T42.6X2	T42.6X3	T42.6X4	T42.6X5	T42.6X6
Pheneticillin	T36.0X1	T36.0X2	T36.0X3	T36.0X4	T36.0X5	T36.0X6
Pheneturide	T42.6X1	T42.6X2	T42.6X3	T42.6X4	T42.6X5	T42.6X6
Phenformin	T38.3X1	T38.3X2	T38.3X3	T38.3X4	T38.3X5	T38.3X6
Phenglutarimide	T44.3X1	T44.3X2	T44.3X3	T44.3X4	T44.3X5	T44.3X6
Phenicarbazide	T39.8X1	T39.8X2	T39.8X3	T39.8X4	T39.8X5	T39.8X6
Phenindamine	T45.0X1	T45.0X2	T45.0X3	T45.0X4	T45.0X5	T45.0X6
Phenindione	T45.511	T45.512	T45.513	T45.514	T45.515	T45.516
Pheniprazine	T43.1X1	T43.1X2	T43.1X3	T43.1X4	T43.1X5	T43.1X6
Pheniramine	T45.0X1	T45.0X2	T45.0X3	T45.0X4	T45.0X5	T45.0X6
Phenisatin	T47.2X1	T47.2X2	T47.2X3	T47.2X4	T47.2X5	T47.2X6
Phenmetrazine	T50.5X1	T50.5X2	T50.5X3	T50.5X4	T50.5X5	T50.5X6
Phenobal	T42.3X1	T42.3X2	T42.3X3	T42.3X4	T42.3X5	T42.3X6
Phenobarbital	T42.3X1	T42.3X2	T42.3X3	T42.3X4	T42.3X5	T42.3X6
with						
mephenytoin	T42.3X1	T42.3X2	T42.3X3	T42.3X4	T42.3X5	T42.3X6
phenytoin	T42.3X1	T42.3X2	T42.3X3	T42.3X4	T42.3X5	T42.3X6
sodium	T42.3X1	T42.3X2	T42.3X3	T42.3X4	T42.3X5	T42.3X6
Phenobarbitone	T42.3X1	T42.3X2	T42.3X3	T42.3X4	T42.3X5	T42.3X6
Phenobutiodil	T50.8X1	T50.8X2	T50.8X3	T50.8X4	T50.8X5	T50.8X6
Phenoctide	T49.0X1	T49.0X2	T49.0X3	T49.0X4	T49.0X5	T49.0X6
Phenol	T49.0X1	T49.0X2	T49.0X3	T49.0X4	T49.0X5	T49.0X6

Table of Drugs and Chemicals

Phenol — Plant

Substance	Poisoning, Accidental (unintentional)	Poisoning, Intentional Self-harm	Poisoning, Assault	Poisoning, Undetermined	Adverse Effect	Underdosing
Phenol — *continued*						
disinfectant	T54.0X1	T54.0X2	T54.0X3	T54.0X4	—	—
in oil injection	T46.8X1	T46.8X2	T46.8X3	T46.8X4	T46.8X5	T46.8X6
medicinal	T49.1X1	T49.1X2	T49.1X3	T49.1X4	T49.1X5	T49.1X6
nonmedicinal NEC	T54.0X1	T54.0X2	T54.0X3	T54.0X4	—	—
pesticide	T60.8X1	T60.8X2	T60.8X3	T60.8X4	—	—
red	T50.8X1	T50.8X2	T50.8X3	T50.8X4	T50.8X5	T50.8X6
Phenolic preparation	T49.1X1	T49.1X2	T49.1X3	T49.1X4	T49.1X5	T49.1X6
Phenolphthalein	T47.2X1	T47.2X2	T47.2X3	T47.2X4	T47.2X5	T47.2X6
Phenolsulfonphthalein	T50.8X1	T50.8X2	T50.8X3	T50.8X4	T50.8X5	T50.8X6
Phenomorphan	T40.2X1	T40.2X2	T40.2X3	T40.2X4	—	—
Phenonyl	T42.3X1	T42.3X2	T42.3X3	T42.3X4	T42.3X5	T42.3X6
Phenoperidine	T40.4X1	T40.4X2	T40.4X3	T40.4X4	—	—
Phenopyrazone	T46.991	T46.992	T46.993	T46.994	T46.995	T46.996
Phenoquin	T50.4X1	T50.4X2	T50.4X3	T50.4X4	T50.4X5	T50.4X6
Phenothiazine (psychotropic) **NEC**	T43.3X1	T43.3X2	T43.3X3	T43.3X4	T43.3X5	T43.3X6
insecticide	T60.2X1	T60.2X2	T60.2X3	T60.2X4	—	—
Phenothrin	T49.0X1	T49.0X2	T49.0X3	T49.0X4	T49.0X5	T49.0X6
Phenoxybenzamine	T46.7X1	T46.7X2	T46.7X3	T46.7X4	T46.7X5	T46.7X6
Phenoxyethanol	T49.0X1	T49.0X2	T49.0X3	T49.0X4	T49.0X5	T49.0X6
Phenoxymethyl penicillin	T36.0X1	T36.0X2	T36.0X3	T36.0X4	T36.0X5	T36.0X6
Phenprobamate	T42.8X1	T42.8X2	T42.8X3	T42.8X4	T42.8X5	T42.8X6
Phenprocoumon	T45.511	T45.512	T45.513	T45.514	T45.515	T45.516
Phensuximide	T42.2X1	T42.2X2	T42.2X3	T42.2X4	T42.2X5	T42.2X6
Phentermine	T50.5X1	T50.5X2	T50.5X3	T50.5X4	T50.5X5	T50.5X6
Phenthicillin	T36.0X1	T36.0X2	T36.0X3	T36.0X4	T36.0X5	T36.0X6
Phentolamine	T46.7X1	T46.7X2	T46.7X3	T46.7X4	T46.7X5	T46.7X6
Phenyl						
butazone	T39.2X1	T39.2X2	T39.2X3	T39.2X4	T39.2X5	T39.2X6
enediamine	T65.3X1	T65.3X2	T65.3X3	T65.3X4	—	—
hydrazine	T65.3X1	T65.3X2	T65.3X3	T65.3X4	—	—
antineoplastic	T45.1X1	T45.1X2	T45.1X3	T45.1X4	T45.1X5	T45.1X6
mercuric compounds — *see* Mercury						
salicylate	T49.3X1	T49.3X2	T49.3X3	T49.3X4	T49.3X5	T49.3X6
Phenylalanine mustard	T45.1X1	T45.1X2	T45.1X3	T45.1X4	T45.1X5	T45.1X6
Phenylbutazone	T39.2X1	T39.2X2	T39.2X3	T39.2X4	T39.2X5	T39.2X6
Phenylenediamine	T65.3X1	T65.3X2	T65.3X3	T65.3X4	—	—
Phenylephrine	T44.4X1	T44.4X2	T44.4X3	T44.4X4	T44.4X5	T44.4X6
Phenylethylbiguanide	T38.3X1	T38.3X2	T38.3X3	T38.3X4	T38.3X5	T38.3X6
Phenylmercuric						
acetate	T49.0X1	T49.0X2	T49.0X3	T49.0X4	T49.0X5	T49.0X6
borate	T49.0X1	T49.0X2	T49.0X3	T49.0X4	T49.0X5	T49.0X6
nitrate	T49.0X1	T49.0X2	T49.0X3	T49.0X4	T49.0X5	T49.0X6
Phenylmethylbarbitone	T42.3X1	T42.3X2	T42.3X3	T42.3X4	T42.3X5	T42.3X6
Phenylpropanol	T47.5X1	T47.5X2	T47.5X3	T47.5X4	T47.5X5	T47.5X6
Phenylpropanolamine	T44.991	T44.992	T44.993	T44.994	T44.995	T44.996
Phenylsulfthion	T60.0X1	T60.0X2	T60.0X3	T60.0X4	—	—
Phenyltoloxamine	T45.0X1	T45.0X2	T45.0X3	T45.0X4	T45.0X5	T45.0X6
Phenyramidol, phenyramidon	T39.8X1	T39.8X2	T39.8X3	T39.8X4	T39.8X5	T39.8X6
Phenytoin	T42.0X1	T42.0X2	T42.0X3	T42.0X4	T42.0X5	T42.0X6
with Phenobarbital	T42.3X1	T42.3X2	T42.3X3	T42.3X4	T42.3X5	T42.3X6
pHisoHex	T49.2X1	T49.2X2	T49.2X3	T49.2X4	T49.2X5	T49.2X6
Pholcodine	T48.3X1	T48.3X2	T48.3X3	T48.3X4	T48.3X5	T48.3X6
Pholedrine	T46.991	T46.992	T46.993	T46.994	T46.995	T46.996
Phorate	T60.0X1	T60.0X2	T60.0X3	T60.0X4	—	—
Phosdrin	T60.0X1	T60.0X2	T60.0X3	T60.0X4	—	—
Phosfolan	T60.0X1	T60.0X2	T60.0X3	T60.0X4	—	—
Phosgene (gas)	T59.891	T59.892	T59.893	T59.894	—	—
Phosphamidon	T60.0X1	T60.0X2	T60.0X3	T60.0X4	—	—
Phosphate	T65.891	T65.892	T65.893	T65.894	—	—
laxative	T47.4X1	T47.4X2	T47.4X3	T47.4X4	T47.4X5	T47.4X6
organic	T60.0X1	T60.0X2	T60.0X3	T60.0X4	—	—
solvent	T52.91	T52.92	T52.93	T52.94	—	—
tricresyl	T65.891	T65.892	T65.893	T65.894	—	—
Phosphine	T57.1X1	T57.1X2	T57.1X3	T57.1X4	—	—
fumigant	T57.1X1	T57.1X2	T57.1X3	T57.1X4	—	—
Phospholine	T49.5X1	T49.5X2	T49.5X3	T49.5X4	T49.5X5	T49.5X6
Phosphoric acid	T54.2X1	T54.2X2	T54.2X3	T54.2X4	—	—
Phosphorus (compound) **NEC**	T57.1X1	T57.1X2	T57.1X3	T57.1X4	—	—
pesticide	T60.0X1	T60.0X2	T60.0X3	T60.0X4	—	—
Phthalates	T65.891	T65.892	T65.893	T65.894	—	—
Phthalic anhydride	T65.891	T65.892	T65.893	T65.894	—	—
Phthalimidoglutarimide	T42.6X1	T42.6X2	T42.6X3	T42.6X4	T42.6X5	T42.6X6
Phthalylsulfathiazole	T37.0X1	T37.0X2	T37.0X3	T37.0X4	T37.0X5	T37.0X6
Phylloquinone	T45.7X1	T45.7X2	T45.7X3	T45.7X4	T45.7X5	T45.7X6
Physeptone	T40.3X1	T40.3X2	T40.3X3	T40.3X4	T40.3X5	T40.3X6
Physostigma venenosum	T62.2X1	T62.2X2	T62.2X3	T62.2X4	—	—
Physostigmine	T49.5X1	T49.5X2	T49.5X3	T49.5X4	T49.5X5	T49.5X6
Phytolacca decandra	T62.2X1	T62.2X2	T62.2X3	T62.2X4	—	—

Substance	Poisoning, Accidental (unintentional)	Poisoning, Intentional Self-harm	Poisoning, Assault	Poisoning, Undetermined	Adverse Effect	Underdosing
Phytolacca decandra — *continued*						
berries	T62.1X1	T62.1X2	T62.1X3	T62.1X4	—	—
Phytomenadione	T45.7X1	T45.7X2	T45.7X3	T45.7X4	T45.7X5	T45.7X6
Phytonadione	T45.7X1	T45.7X2	T45.7X3	T45.7X4	T45.7X5	T45.7X6
Picoperine	T48.3X1	T48.3X2	T48.3X3	T48.3X4	T48.3X5	T48.3X6
Picosulfate (sodium)	T47.2X1	T47.2X2	T47.2X3	T47.2X4	T47.2X5	T47.2X6
Picric (acid)	T54.2X1	T54.2X2	T54.2X3	T54.2X4	—	—
Picrotoxin	T50.7X1	T50.7X2	T50.7X3	T50.7X4	T50.7X5	T50.7X6
Piketoprofen	T49.0X1	T49.0X2	T49.0X3	T49.0X4	T49.0X5	T49.0X6
Pilocarpine	T44.1X1	T44.1X2	T44.1X3	T44.1X4	T44.1X5	T44.1X6
Pilocarpus (jaborandi) extract	T44.1X1	T44.1X2	T44.1X3	T44.1X4	T44.1X5	T44.1X6
Pilsicainide (hydrochloride)	T46.2X1	T46.2X2	T46.2X3	T46.2X4	T46.2X5	T46.2X6
Pimaricin	T36.7X1	T36.7X2	T36.7X3	T36.7X4	T36.7X5	T36.7X6
Pimeclone	T50.7X1	T50.7X2	T50.7X3	T50.7X4	T50.7X5	T50.7X6
Pimelic ketone	T52.8X1	T52.8X2	T52.8X3	T52.8X4	—	—
Pimethixene	T45.0X1	T45.0X2	T45.0X3	T45.0X4	T45.0X5	T45.0X6
Piminodine	T40.2X1	T40.2X2	T40.2X3	T40.2X4	T40.2X5	T40.2X6
Pimozide	T43.591	T43.592	T43.593	T43.594	T43.595	T43.596
Pinacidil	T46.5X1	T46.5X2	T46.5X3	T46.5X4	T46.5X5	T46.5X6
Pinaverium bromide	T44.3X1	T44.3X2	T44.3X3	T44.3X4	T44.3X5	T44.3X6
Pinazepam	T42.4X1	T42.4X2	T42.4X3	T42.4X4	T42.4X5	T42.4X6
Pindolol	T44.7X1	T44.7X2	T44.7X3	T44.7X4	T44.7X5	T44.7X6
Pindone	T60.4X1	T60.4X2	T60.4X3	T60.4X4	—	—
Pine oil (disinfectant)	T65.891	T65.892	T65.893	T65.894	—	—
Pinkroot	T37.4X1	T37.4X2	T37.4X3	T37.4X4	T37.4X5	T37.4X6
Pipadone	T40.2X1	T40.2X2	T40.2X3	T40.2X4	—	—
Pipamazine	T45.0X1	T45.0X2	T45.0X3	T45.0X4	T45.0X5	T45.0X6
Pipamperone	T43.4X1	T43.4X2	T43.4X3	T43.4X4	T43.4X5	T43.4X6
Pipazetate	T48.3X1	T48.3X2	T48.3X3	T48.3X4	T48.3X5	T48.3X6
Pipemidic acid	T37.8X1	T37.8X2	T37.8X3	T37.8X4	T37.8X5	T37.8X6
Pipenzolate bromide	T44.3X1	T44.3X2	T44.3X3	T44.3X4	T44.3X5	T44.3X6
Piperacetazine	T43.3X1	T43.3X2	T43.3X3	T43.3X4	T43.3X5	T43.3X6
Piperacillin	T36.0X1	T36.0X2	T36.0X3	T36.0X4	T36.0X5	T36.0X6
Piperazine	T37.4X1	T37.4X2	T37.4X3	T37.4X4	T37.4X5	T37.4X6
estrone sulfate	T38.5X1	T38.5X2	T38.5X3	T38.5X4	T38.5X5	T38.5X6
Piper cubeba	T62.2X1	T62.2X2	T62.2X3	T62.2X4	—	—
Piperidione	T48.3X1	T48.3X2	T48.3X3	T48.3X4	T48.3X5	T48.3X6
Piperidolate	T44.3X1	T44.3X2	T44.3X3	T44.3X4	T44.3X5	T44.3X6
Piperocaine	T41.3X1	T41.3X2	T41.3X3	T41.3X4	T41.3X5	T41.3X6
infiltration (subcutaneous)	T41.3X1	T41.3X2	T41.3X3	T41.3X4	T41.3X5	T41.3X6
nerve block (peripheral) (plexus)	T41.3X1	T41.3X2	T41.3X3	T41.3X4	T41.3X5	T41.3X6
topical (surface)	T41.3X1	T41.3X2	T41.3X3	T41.3X4	T41.3X5	T41.3X6
Piperonyl butoxide	T60.8X1	T60.8X2	T60.8X3	T60.8X4	—	—
Pipethanate	T44.3X1	T44.3X2	T44.3X3	T44.3X4	T44.3X5	T44.3X6
Pipobroman	T45.1X1	T45.1X2	T45.1X3	T45.1X4	T45.1X5	T45.1X6
Pipotiazine	T43.3X1	T43.3X2	T43.3X3	T43.3X4	T43.3X5	T43.3X6
Pipoxizine	T45.0X1	T45.0X2	T45.0X3	T45.0X4	T45.0X5	T45.0X6
Pipradrol	T43.691	T43.692	T43.693	T43.694	T43.695	T43.696
Piprinhydrinate	T45.0X1	T45.0X2	T45.0X3	T45.0X4	T45.0X5	T45.0X6
Pirarubicin	T45.1X1	T45.1X2	T45.1X3	T45.1X4	T45.1X5	T45.1X6
Pirazinamide	T37.1X1	T37.1X2	T37.1X3	T37.1X4	T37.1X5	T37.1X6
Pirbuterol	T48.6X1	T48.6X2	T48.6X3	T48.6X4	T48.6X5	T48.6X6
Pirenzepine	T47.1X1	T47.1X2	T47.1X3	T47.1X4	T47.1X5	T47.1X6
Piretanide	T50.1X1	T50.1X2	T50.1X3	T50.1X4	T50.1X5	T50.1X6
Piribedil	T42.8X1	T42.8X2	T42.8X3	T42.8X4	T42.8X5	T42.8X6
Piridoxilate	T46.3X1	T46.3X2	T46.3X3	T46.3X4	T46.3X5	T46.3X6
Piritramide	T40.4X1	T40.4X2	T40.4X3	T40.4X4	—	—
Piromidic acid	T37.8X1	T37.8X2	T37.8X3	T37.8X4	T37.8X5	T37.8X6
Piroxicam	T39.391	T39.392	T39.393	T39.394	T39.395	T39.396
beta-cyclodextrin complex	T39.8X1	T39.8X2	T39.8X3	T39.8X4	T39.8X5	T39.8X6
Pirozadil	T46.6X1	T46.6X2	T46.6X3	T46.6X4	T46.6X5	T46.6X6
Piscidia (bark) (erythrina)	T39.8X1	T39.8X2	T39.8X3	T39.8X4	T39.8X5	T39.8X6
Pitch	T65.891	T65.892	T65.893	T65.894	—	—
Pitkin's solution	T41.3X1	T41.3X2	T41.3X3	T41.3X4	T41.3X5	T41.3X6
Pitocin	T48.0X1	T48.0X2	T48.0X3	T48.0X4	T48.0X5	T48.0X6
Pitressin (tannate)	T38.891	T38.892	T38.893	T38.894	T38.895	T38.896
Pituitary extracts (posterior)	T38.891	T38.892	T38.893	T38.894	T38.895	T38.896
anterior	T38.811	T38.812	T38.813	T38.814	T38.815	T38.816
Pituitrin	T38.891	T38.892	T38.893	T38.894	T38.895	T38.896
Pivampicillin	T36.0X1	T36.0X2	T36.0X3	T36.0X4	T36.0X5	T36.0X6
Pivmecillinam	T36.0X1	T36.0X2	T36.0X3	T36.0X4	T36.0X5	T36.0X6
Placental hormone	T38.891	T38.892	T38.893	T38.894	T38.895	T38.896
Placidyl	T42.6X1	T42.6X2	T42.6X3	T42.6X4	T42.6X5	T42.6X6
Plague vaccine	T50.A91	T50.A92	T50.A93	T50.A94	T50.A95	T50.A96
Plant						
food or fertilizer NEC	T65.891	T65.892	T65.893	T65.894	—	—
containing herbicide	T60.3X1	T60.3X2	T60.3X3	T60.3X4	—	—
noxious, used as food	T62.2X1	T62.2X2	T62.2X3	T62.2X4	—	—
berries	T62.1X1	T62.1X2	T62.1X3	T62.1X4	—	—
seeds	T62.2X1	T62.2X2	T62.2X3	T62.2X4	—	—

Substance	Poisoning, Accidental (unintentional)	Poisoning, Intentional Self-harm	Poisoning, Assault	Poisoning, Undetermined	Adverse Effect	Under-dosing
Plant — *continued*						
noxious, used as food — *continued*						
specified type NEC	T62.2X1	T62.2X2	T62.2X3	T62.2X4	—	—
Plasma	T45.8X1	T45.8X2	T45.8X3	T45.8X4	T45.8X5	T45.8X6
expander NEC	T45.8X1	T45.8X2	T45.8X3	T45.8X4	T45.8X5	T45.8X6
protein fraction (human)	T45.8X1	T45.8X2	T45.8X3	T45.8X4	T45.8X5	T45.8X6
Plasmanate	T45.8X1	T45.8X2	T45.8X3	T45.8X4	T45.8X5	T45.8X6
Plasminogen (tissue)	T45.611	T45.612	T45.613	T45.614	T45.615	T45.616
activator						
Plaster dressing	T49.3X1	T49.3X2	T49.3X3	T49.3X4	T49.3X5	T49.3X6
Plastic dressing	T49.3X1	T49.3X2	T49.3X3	T49.3X4	T49.3X5	T49.3X6
Plegicil	T43.3X1	T43.3X2	T43.3X3	T43.3X4	T43.3X5	T43.3X6
Plicamycin	T45.1X1	T45.1X2	T45.1X3	T45.1X4	T45.1X5	T45.1X6
Podophyllotoxin	T49.8X1	T49.8X2	T49.8X3	T49.8X4	T49.8X5	T49.8X6
Podophyllum (resin)	T49.4X1	T49.4X2	T49.4X3	T49.4X4	T49.4X5	T49.4X6
Poisonous berries	T62.1X1	T62.1X2	T62.1X3	T62.1X4	—	—
Poison NEC	T65.91	T65.92	T65.93	T65.94	—	—
Pokeweed (any part)	T62.2X1	T62.2X2	T62.2X3	T62.2X4	—	—
Poldine metilsulfate	T44.3X1	T44.3X2	T44.3X3	T44.3X4	T44.3X5	T44.3X6
Polidexide (sulfate)	T46.6X1	T46.6X2	T46.6X3	T46.6X4	T46.6X5	T46.6X6
Polidocanol	T46.8X1	T46.8X2	T46.8X3	T46.8X4	T46.8X5	T46.8X6
Poliomyelitis vaccine	T50.B91	T50.B92	T50.B93	T50.B94	T50.B95	T50.B96
Polish (car) (floor) (furni-ture) (metal) (porcelain) (silver)	T65.891	T65.892	T65.893	T65.894	—	—
abrasive	T65.891	T65.892	T65.893	T65.894	—	—
porcelain	T65.891	T65.892	T65.893	T65.894	—	—
Poloxalkol	T47.4X1	T47.4X2	T47.4X3	T47.4X4	T47.4X5	T47.4X6
Poloxamer	T47.4X1	T47.4X2	T47.4X3	T47.4X4	T47.4X5	T47.4X6
Polyaminostyrene resins	T50.3X1	T50.3X2	T50.3X3	T50.3X4	T50.3X5	T50.3X6
Polycarbophil	T47.4X1	T47.4X2	T47.4X3	T47.4X4	T47.4X5	T47.4X6
Polychlorinated biphenyl	T65.891	T65.892	T65.893	T65.894	—	—
Polycycline	T36.4X1	T36.4X2	T36.4X3	T36.4X4	T36.4X5	T36.4X6
Polyester fumes	T59.891	T59.892	T59.893	T59.894	—	—
Polyester resin hardener	T52.91	T52.92	T52.93	T52.94	—	—
fumes	T59.891	T59.892	T59.893	T59.894	—	—
Polyestradiol phosphate	T38.5X1	T38.5X2	T38.5X3	T38.5X4	T38.5X5	T38.5X6
Polyethanolamine alkyl sulfate	T49.2X1	T49.2X2	T49.2X3	T49.2X4	T49.2X5	T49.2X6
Polyethylene adhesive	T49.3X1	T49.3X2	T49.3X3	T49.3X4	T49.3X5	T49.3X6
Polyferose	T45.4X1	T45.4X2	T45.4X3	T45.4X4	T45.4X5	T45.4X6
Polygeline	T45.8X1	T45.8X2	T45.8X3	T45.8X4	T45.8X5	T45.8X6
Polymyxin	T36.8X1	T36.8X2	T36.8X3	T36.8X4	T36.8X5	T36.8X6
B	T36.8X1	T36.8X2	T36.8X3	T36.8X4	T36.8X5	T36.8X6
ENT agent	T49.6X1	T49.6X2	T49.6X3	T49.6X4	T49.6X5	T49.6X6
ophthalmic preparation	T49.5X1	T49.5X2	T49.5X3	T49.5X4	T49.5X5	T49.5X6
topical NEC	T49.0X1	T49.0X2	T49.0X3	T49.0X4	T49.0X5	T49.0X6
E sulfate (eye preparation)	T49.5X1	T49.5X2	T49.5X3	T49.5X4	T49.5X5	T49.5X6
Polynoxylin	T49.0X1	T49.0X2	T49.0X3	T49.0X4	T49.0X5	T49.0X6
Polyoestradiol phosphate	T38.5X1	T38.5X2	T38.5X3	T38.5X4	T38.5X5	T38.5X6
Polyoxymethyleneurea	T49.0X1	T49.0X2	T49.0X3	T49.0X4	T49.0X5	T49.0X6
Polysilane	T47.8X1	T47.8X2	T47.8X3	T47.8X4	T47.8X5	T47.8X6
Polytetrafluoroethylene (inhaled)	T59.891	T59.892	T59.893	T59.894	—	—
Polythiazide	T50.2X1	T50.2X2	T50.2X3	T50.2X4	T50.2X5	T50.2X6
Polyvidone	T45.8X1	T45.8X2	T45.8X3	T45.8X4	T45.8X5	T45.8X6
Polyvinylpyrrolidone	T45.8X1	T45.8X2	T45.8X3	T45.8X4	T45.8X5	T45.8X6
Pontocaine (hydrochloride) (infiltration) (topical)	T41.3X1	T41.3X2	T41.3X3	T41.3X4	T41.3X5	T41.3X6
nerve block (peripheral) (plexus)	T41.3X1	T41.3X2	T41.3X3	T41.3X4	T41.3X5	T41.3X6
spinal	T41.3X1	T41.3X2	T41.3X3	T41.3X4	T41.3X5	T41.3X6
Porfiromycin	T45.1X1	T45.1X2	T45.1X3	T45.1X4	T45.1X5	T45.1X6
Posterior pituitary hormone NEC	T38.891	T38.892	T38.893	T38.894	T38.895	T38.896
Pot	T40.7X1	T40.7X2	T40.7X3	T40.7X4	T40.7X5	T40.7X6
Potash (caustic)	T54.3X1	T54.3X2	T54.3X3	T54.3X4	—	—
Potassic saline injection (lactated)	T50.3X1	T50.3X2	T50.3X3	T50.3X4	T50.3X5	T50.3X6
Potassium-removing resin	T50.3X1	T50.3X2	T50.3X3	T50.3X4	T50.3X5	T50.3X6
Potassium-retaining drug	T50.3X1	T50.3X2	T50.3X3	T50.3X4	T50.3X5	T50.3X6
Potassium (salts) NEC	T50.3X1	T50.3X2	T50.3X3	T50.3X4	T50.3X5	T50.3X6
aminobenzoate	T45.8X1	T45.8X2	T45.8X3	T45.8X4	T45.8X5	T45.8X6
aminosalicylate	T37.1X1	T37.1X2	T37.1X3	T37.1X4	T37.1X5	T37.1X6
antimony ' tartrate'	T37.8X1	T37.8X2	T37.8X3	T37.8X4	T37.8X5	T37.8X6
arsenite (solution)	T57.0X1	T57.0X2	T57.0X3	T57.0X4	—	—
bichromate	T56.2X1	T56.2X2	T56.2X3	T56.2X4	—	—
bisulfate	T47.3X1	T47.3X2	T47.3X3	T47.3X4	T47.3X5	T47.3X6
bromide	T42.6X1	T42.6X2	T42.6X3	T42.6X4	T42.6X5	T42.6X6
canreonate	T50.0X1	T50.0X2	T50.0X3	T50.0X4	T50.0X5	T50.0X6
carbonate	T54.3X1	T54.3X2	T54.3X3	T54.3X4	—	—
chlorate NEC	T65.891	T65.892	T65.893	T65.894	—	—
chloride	T50.3X1	T50.3X2	T50.3X3	T50.3X4	T50.3X5	T50.3X6

Substance	Poisoning, Accidental (unintentional)	Poisoning, Intentional Self-harm	Poisoning, Assault	Poisoning, Undetermined	Adverse Effect	Under-dosing
Potassium (salts) NEC — *continued*						
citrate	T50.991	T50.992	T50.993	T50.994	T50.995	T50.996
cyanide	T65.0X1	T65.0X2	T65.0X3	T65.0X4	—	—
ferric hexacyanoferrate (medicinal)	T50.6X1	T50.6X2	T50.6X3	T50.6X4	T50.6X5	T50.6X6
nonmedicinal	T65.891	T65.892	T65.893	T65.894	—	—
Fluoride	T57.8X1	T57.8X2	T57.8X3	T57.8X4	—	—
glucaldrate	T47.1X1	T47.1X2	T47.1X3	T47.1X4	T47.1X5	T47.1X6
hydroxide	T54.3X1	T54.3X2	T54.3X3	T54.3X4	—	—
iodate	T49.0X1	T49.0X2	T49.0X3	T49.0X4	T49.0X5	T49.0X6
iodide	T48.4X1	T48.4X2	T48.4X3	T48.4X4	T48.4X5	T48.4X6
nitrate	T57.8X1	T57.8X2	T57.8X3	T57.8X4	—	—
oxalate	T65.891	T65.892	T65.893	T65.894	—	—
perchlorate (nonmedicinal) NEC	T65.891	T65.892	T65.893	T65.894	—	—
antithyroid	T38.2X1	T38.2X2	T38.2X3	T38.2X4	T38.2X5	T38.2X6
medicinal	T38.2X1	T38.2X2	T38.2X3	T38.2X4	T38.2X5	T38.2X6
Permanganate (nonmedicinal)	T65.891	T65.892	T65.893	T65.894	—	—
medicinal	T49.0X1	T49.0X2	T49.0X3	T49.0X4	T49.0X5	T49.0X6
sulfate	T47.2X1	T47.2X2	T47.2X3	T47.2X4	T47.2X5	T47.2X6
Povidone	T45.8X1	T45.8X2	T45.8X3	T45.8X4	T45.8X5	T45.8X6
iodine	T49.0X1	T49.0X2	T49.0X3	T49.0X4	T49.0X5	T49.0X6
Practolol	T44.7X1	T44.7X2	T44.7X3	T44.7X4	T44.7X5	T44.7X6
Prajmalium bitartrate	T46.2X1	T46.2X2	T46.2X3	T46.2X4	T46.2X5	T46.2X6
Pralidoxime (iodide)	T50.6X1	T50.6X2	T50.6X3	T50.6X4	T50.6X5	T50.6X6
chloride	T50.6X1	T50.6X2	T50.6X3	T50.6X4	T50.6X5	T50.6X6
Pramiverine	T44.3X1	T44.3X2	T44.3X3	T44.3X4	T44.3X5	T44.3X6
Pramocaine	T49.1X1	T49.1X2	T49.1X3	T49.1X4	T49.1X5	T49.1X6
Pramoxine	T49.1X1	T49.1X2	T49.1X3	T49.1X4	T49.1X5	T49.1X6
Prasterone	T38.7X1	T38.7X2	T38.7X3	T38.7X4	T38.7X5	T38.7X6
Pravastatin	T46.6X1	T46.6X2	T46.6X3	T46.6X4	T46.6X5	T46.6X6
Prazepam	T42.4X1	T42.4X2	T42.4X3	T42.4X4	T42.4X5	T42.4X6
Praziquantel	T37.4X1	T37.4X2	T37.4X3	T37.4X4	T37.4X5	T37.4X6
Prazitone	T43.291	T43.292	T43.293	T43.294	T43.295	T43.296
Prazosin	T44.6X1	T44.6X2	T44.6X3	T44.6X4	T44.6X5	T44.6X6
Prednicarbate	T49.0X1	T49.0X2	T49.0X3	T49.0X4	T49.0X5	T49.0X6
Prednimustine	T45.1X1	T45.1X2	T45.1X3	T45.1X4	T45.1X5	T45.1X6
Prednisolone	T38.0X1	T38.0X2	T38.0X3	T38.0X4	T38.0X5	T38.0X6
ENT agent	T49.6X1	T49.6X2	T49.6X3	T49.6X4	T49.6X5	T49.6X6
ophthalmic preparation	T49.5X1	T49.5X2	T49.5X3	T49.5X4	T49.5X5	T49.5X6
steaglate	T49.0X1	T49.0X2	T49.0X3	T49.0X4	T49.0X5	T49.0X6
topical NEC	T49.0X1	T49.0X2	T49.0X3	T49.0X4	T49.0X5	T49.0X6
Prednisone	T38.0X1	T38.0X2	T38.0X3	T38.0X4	T38.0X5	T38.0X6
Prednylidene	T38.0X1	T38.0X2	T38.0X3	T38.0X4	T38.0X5	T38.0X6
Pregnandiol	T38.5X1	T38.5X2	T38.5X3	T38.5X4	T38.5X5	T38.5X6
Pregneninolone	T38.5X1	T38.5X2	T38.5X3	T38.5X4	T38.5X5	T38.5X6
Preludin	T43.691	T43.692	T43.693	T43.694	T43.695	T43.696
Premarin	T38.5X1	T38.5X2	T38.5X3	T38.5X4	T38.5X5	T38.5X6
Premedication anesthetic	T41.201	T41.202	T41.203	T41.204	T41.205	T41.206
Prenalterol	T44.5X1	T44.5X2	T44.5X3	T44.5X4	T44.5X5	T44.5X6
Prenoxdiazine	T48.3X1	T48.3X2	T48.3X3	T48.3X4	T48.3X5	T48.3X6
Prenylamine	T46.3X1	T46.3X2	T46.3X3	T46.3X4	T46.3X5	T46.3X6
Preparation H	T49.8X1	T49.8X2	T49.8X3	T49.8X4	T49.8X5	T49.8X6
Preparation, local	T49.4X1	T49.4X2	T49.4X3	T49.4X4	T49.4X5	T49.4X6
Preservative (nonmedicinal)	T65.891	T65.892	T65.893	T65.894	—	—
medicinal	T50.901	T50.902	T50.903	T50.904	T50.905	T50.906
wood	T60.91	T60.92	T60.93	T60.94	—	—
Prethcamide	T50.7X1	T50.7X2	T50.7X3	T50.7X4	T50.7X5	T50.7X6
Pride of China	T62.2X1	T62.2X2	T62.2X3	T62.2X4	—	—
Pridinol	T44.3X1	T44.3X2	T44.3X3	T44.3X4	T44.3X5	T44.3X6
Prifinium bromide	T44.3X1	T44.3X2	T44.3X3	T44.3X4	T44.3X5	T44.3X6
Prilocaine	T41.3X1	T41.3X2	T41.3X3	T41.3X4	T41.3X5	T41.3X6
infiltration (subcutaneous)	T41.3X1	T41.3X2	T41.3X3	T41.3X4	T41.3X5	T41.3X6
nerve block (peripheral) (plexus)	T41.3X1	T41.3X2	T41.3X3	T41.3X4	T41.3X5	T41.3X6
regional	T41.3X1	T41.3X2	T41.3X3	T41.3X4	T41.3X5	T41.3X6
Primaquine	T37.2X1	T37.2X2	T37.2X3	T37.2X4	T37.2X5	T37.2X6
Primidone	T42.6X1	T42.6X2	T42.6X3	T42.6X4	T42.6X5	T42.6X6
Primula (veris)	T62.2X1	T62.2X2	T62.2X3	T62.2X4	—	—
Prinadol	T40.2X1	T40.2X2	T40.2X3	T40.2X4	T40.2X5	T40.2X6
Priscol, Priscoline	T44.6X1	T44.6X2	T44.6X3	T44.6X4	T44.6X5	T44.6X6
Pristinamycin	T36.3X1	T36.3X2	T36.3X3	T36.3X4	T36.3X5	T36.3X6
Privet	T62.2X1	T62.2X2	T62.2X3	T62.2X4	—	—
berries	T62.1X1	T62.1X2	T62.1X3	T62.1X4	—	—
Privine	T44.4X1	T44.4X2	T44.4X3	T44.4X4	T44.4X5	T44.4X6
Pro-Banthine	T44.3X1	T44.3X2	T44.3X3	T44.3X4	T44.3X5	T44.3X6
Probarbital	T42.3X1	T42.3X2	T42.3X3	T42.3X4	T42.3X5	T42.3X6
Probenecid	T50.4X1	T50.4X2	T50.4X3	T50.4X4	T50.4X5	T50.4X6
Probucol	T46.6X1	T46.6X2	T46.6X3	T46.6X4	T46.6X5	T46.6X6
Procainamide	T46.2X1	T46.2X2	T46.2X3	T46.2X4	T46.2X5	T46.2X6
Procaine	T41.3X1	T41.3X2	T41.3X3	T41.3X4	T41.3X5	T41.3X6

Table of Drugs and Chemicals

Plant — Procaine

Substance	Poisoning, Accidental (unintentional)	Poisoning, Intentional Self-harm	Poisoning, Assault	Poisoning, Undetermined	Adverse Effect	Under-dosing
Procaine — continued						
benzylpenicillin	T36.0X1	T36.0X2	T36.0X3	T36.0X4	T36.0X5	T36.0X6
nerve block (periphreal) (plexus)	T41.3X1	T41.3X2	T41.3X3	T41.3X4	T41.3X5	T41.3X6
penicillin G	T36.0X1	T36.0X2	T36.0X3	T36.0X4	T36.0X5	T36.0X6
regional	T41.3X1	T41.3X2	T41.3X3	T41.3X4	T41.3X5	T41.3X6
spinal	T41.3X1	T41.3X2	T41.3X3	T41.3X4	T41.3X5	T41.3X6
Procalmidol	T43.591	T43.592	T43.593	T43.594	T43.595	T43.596
Procarbazine	T45.1X1	T45.1X2	T45.1X3	T45.1X4	T45.1X5	T45.1X6
Procaterol	T44.5X1	T44.5X2	T44.5X3	T44.5X4	T44.5X5	T44.5X6
Prochlorperazine	T43.3X1	T43.3X2	T43.3X3	T43.3X4	T43.3X5	T43.3X6
Procyclidine	T44.3X1	T44.3X2	T44.3X3	T44.3X4	T44.3X5	T44.3X6
Producer gas	T58.8X1	T58.8X2	T58.8X3	T58.8X4	—	—
Profadol	T40.4X1	T40.4X2	T40.4X3	T40.4X4	T40.4X5	T40.4X6
Profenamine	T44.3X1	T44.3X2	T44.3X3	T44.3X4	T44.3X5	T44.3X6
Profenil	T44.3X1	T44.3X2	T44.3X3	T44.3X4	T44.3X5	T44.3X6
Proflavine	T49.0X1	T49.0X2	T49.0X3	T49.0X4	T49.0X5	T49.0X6
Progabide	T42.6X1	T42.6X2	T42.6X3	T42.6X4	T42.6X5	T42.6X6
Progesterone	T38.5X1	T38.5X2	T38.5X3	T38.5X4	T38.5X5	T38.5X6
Progestin	T38.5X1	T38.5X2	T38.5X3	T38.5X4	T38.5X5	T38.5X6
oral contraceptive	T38.4X1	T38.4X2	T38.4X3	T38.4X4	T38.4X5	T38.4X6
Progestogen NEC	T38.5X1	T38.5X2	T38.5X3	T38.5X4	T38.5X5	T38.5X6
Progestone	T38.5X1	T38.5X2	T38.5X3	T38.5X4	T38.5X5	T38.5X6
Proglumide	T47.1X1	T47.1X2	T47.1X3	T47.1X4	T47.1X5	T47.1X6
Proguanil	T37.2X1	T37.2X2	T37.2X3	T37.2X4	T37.2X5	T37.2X6
Prolactin	T38.811	T38.812	T38.813	T38.814	T38.815	T38.816
Prolintane	T43.691	T43.692	T43.693	T43.694	T43.695	T43.696
Proloid	T38.1X1	T38.1X2	T38.1X3	T38.1X4	T38.1X5	T38.1X6
Proluton	T38.5X1	T38.5X2	T38.5X3	T38.5X4	T38.5X5	T38.5X6
Promacetin	T37.1X1	T37.1X2	T37.1X3	T37.1X4	T37.1X5	T37.1X6
Promazine	T43.3X1	T43.3X2	T43.3X3	T43.3X4	T43.3X5	T43.3X6
Promedol	T40.2X1	T40.2X2	T40.2X3	T40.2X4	—	—
Promegestone	T38.5X1	T38.5X2	T38.5X3	T38.5X4	T38.5X5	T38.5X6
Promethazine (teoclate)	T43.3X1	T43.3X2	T43.3X3	T43.3X4	T43.3X5	T43.3X6
Promin	T37.1X1	T37.1X2	T37.1X3	T37.1X4	T37.1X5	T37.1X6
Pronase	T45.3X1	T45.3X2	T45.3X3	T45.3X4	T45.3X5	T45.3X6
Pronestyl (hydrochloride)	T46.2X1	T46.2X2	T46.2X3	T46.2X4	T46.2X5	T46.2X6
Pronetalol	T44.7X1	T44.7X2	T44.7X3	T44.7X4	T44.7X5	T44.7X6
Prontosil	T37.0X1	T37.0X2	T37.0X4	T37.0X4	T37.0X5	T37.0X6
Propachlor	T60.3X1	T60.3X2	T60.3X3	T60.3X4	—	—
Propafenone	T46.2X1	T46.2X2	T46.2X3	T46.2X4	T46.2X5	T46.2X6
Propallylonal	T42.3X1	T42.3X2	T42.3X3	T42.3X4	T42.3X5	T42.3X6
Propamidine	T49.0X1	T49.0X2	T49.0X3	T49.0X4	T49.0X5	T49.0X6
Propane (distributed in mobile container)	T59.891	T59.892	T59.893	T59.894	—	—
distributed through pipes	T59.891	T59.892	T59.893	T59.894	—	—
incomplete combustion	T58.11	T58.12	T58.13	T58.14	—	—
Propanidid	T41.291	T41.292	T41.293	T41.294	T41.295	T41.296
Propanil	T60.3X1	T60.3X2	T60.3X3	T60.3X4	—	—
Propantheline	T44.3X1	T44.3X2	T44.3X3	T44.3X4	T44.3X5	T44.3X6
bromide	T44.3X1	T44.3X2	T44.3X3	T44.3X4	T44.3X5	T44.3X6
Proparacaine	T41.3X1	T41.3X2	T41.3X3	T41.3X4	T41.3X5	T41.3X6
Propatylnitrate	T46.3X1	T46.3X2	T46.3X3	T46.3X4	T46.3X5	T46.3X6
Propicillin	T36.0X1	T36.0X2	T36.0X3	T36.0X4	T36.0X5	T36.0X6
Propiolactone	T49.0X1	T49.0X2	T49.0X3	T49.0X4	T49.0X5	T49.0X6
Propiomazine	T45.0X1	T45.0X2	T45.0X3	T45.0X4	T45.0X5	T45.0X6
Propionaldehyde (medicinal)	T42.6X1	T42.6X2	T42.6X3	T42.6X4	T42.6X5	T42.6X6
Propionate (calcium) (sodium)	T49.0X1	T49.0X2	T49.0X3	T49.0X4	T49.0X5	T49.0X6
Propion gel	T49.0X1	T49.0X2	T49.0X3	T49.0X4	T49.0X5	T49.0X6
Propitocaine	T41.3X1	T41.3X2	T41.3X3	T41.3X4	T41.3X5	T41.3X6
infiltration (subcutaneous)	T41.3X1	T41.3X2	T41.3X3	T41.3X4	T41.3X5	T41.3X6
nerve block (peripheral) (plexus)	T41.3X1	T41.3X2	T41.3X3	T41.3X4	T41.3X5	T41.3X6
Propofol	T41.291	T41.292	T41.293	T41.294	T41.295	T41.296
Propoxur	T60.0X1	T60.0X2	T60.0X3	T60.0X4	—	—
Propoxycaine	T41.3X1	T41.3X2	T41.3X3	T41.3X4	T41.3X5	T41.3X6
infiltration (subcutaneous)	T41.3X1	T41.3X2	T41.3X3	T41.3X4	T41.3X5	T41.3X6
nerve block (peripheral) (plexus)	T41.3X1	T41.3X2	T41.3X3	T41.3X4	T41.3X5	T41.3X6
topical (surface)	T41.3X1	T41.3X2	T41.3X3	T41.3X4	T41.3X5	T41.3X6
Propoxyphene	T40.4X1	T40.4X2	T40.4X3	T40.4X4	T40.4X5	T40.4X6
Propranolol	T44.7X1	T44.7X2	T44.7X3	T44.7X4	T44.7X5	T44.7X6
Propyl						
alcohol	T51.3X1	T51.3X2	T51.3X3	T51.3X4	—	—
carbinol	T51.3X1	T51.3X2	T51.3X3	T51.3X4	—	—
hexadrine	T44.4X1	T44.4X2	T44.4X3	T44.4X4	—	—
iodone	T50.8X1	T50.8X2	T50.8X3	T50.8X4	T50.8X5	T50.8X6
thiouracil	T38.2X1	T38.2X2	T38.2X3	T38.2X4	T38.2X5	T38.2X6
Propylaminophenothiazine	T43.3X1	T43.3X2	T43.3X3	T43.3X4	T43.3X5	T43.3X6
Propylene	T59.891	T59.892	T59.893	T59.894	—	—
Propylhexedrine	T48.5X1	T48.5X2	T48.5X3	T48.5X4	T48.5X5	T48.5X6

Substance	Poisoning, Accidental (unintentional)	Poisoning, Intentional Self-harm	Poisoning, Assault	Poisoning, Undetermined	Adverse Effect	Under-dosing
Propyliodone	T50.8X1	T50.8X2	T50.8X3	T50.8X4	T50.8X5	T50.8X6
Propylparaben (ophthalmic)	T49.5X1	T49.5X2	T49.5X3	T49.5X4	T49.5X5	T49.5X6
Propylthiouracil	T38.2X1	T38.2X2	T38.2X3	T38.2X4	T38.2X5	T38.2X6
Propyphenazone	T39.2X1	T39.2X2	T39.2X3	T39.2X4	T39.2X5	T39.2X6
Proquazone	T39.391	T39.392	T39.393	T39.394	T39.395	T39.396
Proscillaridin	T46.0X1	T46.0X2	T46.0X3	T46.0X4	T46.0X5	T46.0X6
Prostacyclin	T45.521	T45.522	T45.523	T45.524	T45.525	T45.526
Prostaglandin (I2)	T45.521	T45.522	T45.523	T45.524	T45.525	T45.526
E1	T46.7X1	T46.7X2	T46.7X3	T46.7X4	T46.7X5	T46.7X6
E2	T48.0X1	T48.0X2	T48.0X3	T48.0X4	T48.0X5	T48.0X6
F2 alpha	T48.0X1	T48.0X2	T48.0X3	T48.0X4	T48.0X5	T48.0X6
Prostigmin	T44.0X1	T44.0X2	T44.0X3	T44.0X4	T44.0X5	T44.0X6
Prosultiamine	T45.2X1	T45.2X2	T45.2X3	T45.2X4	T45.2X5	T45.2X6
Protamine sulfate	T45.7X1	T45.7X2	T45.7X3	T45.7X4	T45.7X5	T45.7X6
zinc insulin	T38.3X1	T38.3X2	T38.3X3	T38.3X4	T38.3X5	T38.3X6
Protease	T47.5X1	T47.5X2	T47.5X3	T47.5X4	T47.5X5	T47.5X6
Protectant, skin NEC	T49.3X1	T49.3X2	T49.3X3	T49.3X4	T49.3X5	T49.3X6
Protein hydrolysate	T50.991	T50.992	T50.993	T50.994	T50.995	T50.996
Prothiaden — see Dothiepin hydrochloride						
Prothionamide	T37.1X1	T37.1X2	T37.1X3	T37.1X4	T37.1X5	T37.1X6
Prothipendyl	T43.591	T43.592	T43.593	T43.594	T43.595	T43.596
Prothoate	T60.0X1	T60.0X2	T60.0X3	T60.0X4	—	—
Prothrombin						
activator	T45.7X1	T45.7X2	T45.7X3	T45.7X4	T45.7X5	T45.7X6
synthesis inhibitor	T45.511	T45.512	T45.513	T45.514	T45.515	T45.516
Protionamide	T37.1X1	T37.1X2	T37.1X3	T37.1X4	T37.1X5	T37.1X6
Protirelin	T38.891	T38.892	T38.893	T38.894	T38.895	T38.896
Protokylol	T48.6X1	T48.6X2	T48.6X3	T48.6X4	T48.6X5	T48.6X6
Protopam	T50.6X1	T50.6X2	T50.6X3	T50.6X4	T50.6X5	T50.6X6
Protoveratrine(s) (A) (B)	T46.5X1	T46.5X2	T46.5X3	T46.5X4	T46.5X5	T46.5X6
Protriptyline	T43.011	T43.012	T43.013	T43.014	T43.015	T43.016
Provera	T38.5X1	T38.5X2	T38.5X3	T38.5X4	T38.5X5	T38.5X6
Provitamin A	T45.2X1	T45.2X2	T45.2X3	T45.2X4	T45.2X5	T45.2X6
Proxibarbal	T42.3X1	T42.3X2	T42.3X3	T42.3X4	T42.3X5	T42.3X6
Proxymetacaine	T41.3X1	T41.3X2	T41.3X3	T41.3X4	T41.3X5	T41.3X6
Proxyphylline	T48.6X1	T48.6X2	T48.6X3	T48.6X4	T48.6X5	T48.6X6
Prozac — see Fluoxetine hydrochloride						
Prunus						
laurocerasus	T62.2X1	T62.2X2	T62.2X3	T62.2X4		
virginiana	T62.2X1	T62.2X2	T62.2X3	T62.2X4		
Prussian blue						
commercial	T65.891	T65.892	T65.893	T65.894	—	—
therapeutic	T50.6X1	T50.6X2	T50.6X3	T50.6X4	T50.6X5	T50.6X6
Prussic acid	T65.0X1	T65.0X2	T65.0X3	T65.0X4	—	—
vapor	T57.3X1	T57.3X2	T57.3X3	T57.3X4	—	—
Pseudoephedrine	T44.991	T44.992	T44.993	T44.994	T44.995	T44.996
Psilocin	T40.991	T40.992	T40.993	T40.994		
Psilocybin	T40.991	T40.992	T40.993	T40.994		
Psilocybine	T40.991	T40.992	T40.993	T40.994		
Psoralene (nonmedicinal)	T65.891	T65.892	T65.893	T65.894	—	—
Psoralens (medicinal)	T50.991	T50.992	T50.993	T50.994	T50.995	T50.996
PSP (phenolsulfonphthalein)	T50.8X1	T50.8X2	T50.8X3	T50.8X4	T50.8X5	T50.8X6
Psychodysleptic drug NEC	T40.901	T40.902	T40.903	T40.904	T40.905	T40.906
Psychostimulant	T43.601	T43.602	T43.603	T43.604	T43.605	T43.606
amphetamine	T43.621	T43.622	T43.623	T43.624	T43.625	T43.626
caffeine	T43.611	T43.612	T43.613	T43.614	T43.615	T43.616
methylphenidate	T43.631	T43.632	T43.633	T43.634	T43.635	T43.636
specified NEC	T43.691	T43.692	T43.693	T43.694	T43.695	T43.696
Psychotherapeutic drug NEC	T43.91	T43.92	T43.93	T43.94	T43.95	T43.96
antidepressants — see also Antidepressant	T43.201	T43.202	T43.203	T43.204	T43.205	T43.206
specified NEC	T43.8X1	T43.8X2	T43.8X3	T43.8X4	T43.8X5	T43.8X6
tranquilizers NEC	T43.501	T43.502	T43.503	T43.504	T43.505	T43.506
Psychotomimetic agents	T40.901	T40.902	T40.903	T40.904	T40.905	T40.906
Psychotropic drug NEC	T43.91	T43.92	T43.93	T43.94	T43.95	T43.96
specified NEC	T43.8X1	T43.8X2	T43.8X3	T43.8X4	T43.8X5	T43.8X6
Psyllium hydrophilic mucilloid	T47.4X1	T47.4X2	T47.4X3	T47.4X4	T47.4X5	T47.4X6
Pteroylglutamic acid	T45.8X1	T45.8X2	T45.8X3	T45.8X4	T45.8X5	T45.8X6
Pteroyltriglutamate	T45.1X1	T45.1X2	T45.1X3	T45.1X4	T45.1X5	T45.1X6
PTFE — see Polytetrafluoroethylene						
Pulp						
devitalizing paste	T49.7X1	T49.7X2	T49.7X3	T49.7X4	T49.7X5	T49.7X6
dressing	T49.7X1	T49.7X2	T49.7X3	T49.7X4	T49.7X5	T49.7X6
Pulsatilla	T62.2X1	T62.2X2	T62.2X3	T62.2X4		
Pumpkin seed extract	T37.4X1	T37.4X2	T37.4X3	T37.4X4	T37.4X5	T37.4X6
Purex (bleach)	T54.91	T54.92	T54.93	T54.94		
Purgative NEC — see also Cathartic	T47.4X1	T47.4X2	T47.4X3	T47.4X4	T47.4X5	T47.4X6

Additional Character May Be Required — Refer to the Tabular List for Character Selection   ▽ **Subterms under main terms may continue to next column or page**

Substance	Poisoning, Accidental (unintentional)	Poisoning, Intentional Self-harm	Poisoning, Assault	Poisoning, Undetermined	Adverse Effect	Under-dosing
Purine analogue (antineoplastic)	T45.1X1	T45.1X2	T45.1X3	T45.1X4	T45.1X5	T45.1X6
Purine diuretics	T50.2X1	T50.2X2	T50.2X3	T50.2X4	T50.2X5	T50.2X6
Purinethol	T45.1X1	T45.1X2	T45.1X3	T45.1X4	T45.1X5	T45.1X6
PVP	T45.8X1	T45.8X2	T45.8X3	T45.8X4	T45.8X5	T45.8X6
Pyrabital	T39.8X1	T39.8X2	T39.8X3	T39.8X4	T39.8X5	T39.8X6
Pyramidon	T39.2X1	T39.2X2	T39.2X3	T39.2X4	T39.2X5	T39.2X6
Pyrantel	T37.4X1	T37.4X2	T37.4X3	T37.4X4	T37.4X5	T37.4X6
Pyrathiazine	T45.0X1	T45.0X2	T45.0X3	T45.0X4	T45.0X5	T45.0X6
Pyrazinamide	T37.1X1	T37.1X2	T37.1X3	T37.1X4	T37.1X5	T37.1X6
Pyrazinoic acid (amide)	T37.1X1	T37.1X2	T37.1X3	T37.1X4	T37.1X5	T37.1X6
Pyrazole (derivatives)	T39.2X1	T39.2X2	T39.2X3	T39.2X4	T39.2X5	T39.2X6
Pyrazolone analgesic NEC	T39.2X1	T39.2X2	T39.2X3	T39.2X4	T39.2X5	T39.2X6
Pyrethrin, pyrethrum (nonmedicinal)	T60.2X1	T60.2X2	T60.2X3	T60.2X4	—	—
Pyrethrum extract	T49.0X1	T49.0X2	T49.0X3	T49.0X4	T49.0X5	T49.0X6
Pyribenzamine	T45.0X1	T45.0X2	T45.0X3	T45.0X4	T45.0X5	T45.0X6
Pyridine	T52.8X1	T52.8X2	T52.8X3	T52.8X4	—	—
aldoxime methiodide	T50.6X1	T50.6X2	T50.6X3	T50.6X4	T50.6X5	T50.6X6
aldoxime methyl chloride	T50.6X1	T50.6X2	T50.6X3	T50.6X4	T50.6X5	T50.6X6
vapor	T59.891	T59.892	T59.893	T59.894	—	—
Pyridium	T39.8X1	T39.8X2	T39.8X3	T39.8X4	T39.8X5	T39.8X6
Pyridostigmine bromide	T44.0X1	T44.0X2	T44.0X3	T44.0X4	T44.0X5	T44.0X6
Pyridoxal phosphate	T45.2X1	T45.2X2	T45.2X3	T45.2X4	T45.2X5	T45.2X6
Pyridoxine	T45.2X1	T45.2X2	T45.2X3	T45.2X4	T45.2X5	T45.2X6
Pyrilamine	T45.0X1	T45.0X2	T45.0X3	T45.0X4	T45.0X5	T45.0X6
Pyrimethamine	T37.2X1	T37.2X2	T37.2X3	T37.2X4	T37.2X5	T37.2X6
with sulfadoxine	T37.2X1	T37.2X2	T37.2X3	T37.2X4	T37.2X5	T37.2X6
Pyrimidine antagonist	T45.1X1	T45.1X2	T45.1X3	T45.1X4	T45.1X5	T45.1X6
Pyriminil	T60.4X1	T60.4X2	T60.4X3	T60.4X4	—	—
Pyrithione zinc	T49.4X1	T49.4X2	T49.4X3	T49.4X4	T49.4X5	T49.4X6
Pyrithyldione	T42.6X1	T42.6X2	T42.6X3	T42.6X4	T42.6X5	T42.6X6
Pyrogallic acid	T49.0X1	T49.0X2	T49.0X3	T49.0X4	T49.0X5	T49.0X6
Pyrogallol	T49.0X1	T49.0X2	T49.0X3	T49.0X4	T49.0X5	T49.0X6
Pyroxylin	T49.3X1	T49.3X2	T49.3X3	T49.3X4	T49.3X5	T49.3X6
Pyrrobutamine	T45.0X1	T45.0X2	T45.0X3	T45.0X4	T45.0X5	T45.0X6
Pyrrolizidine alkaloids	T62.8X1	T62.8X2	T62.8X3	T62.8X4	—	—
Pyrvinium chloride	T37.4X1	T37.4X2	T37.4X3	T37.4X4	T37.4X5	T37.4X6
PZI	T38.3X1	T38.3X2	T38.3X3	T38.3X4	T38.3X5	T38.3X6
Quaalude	T42.6X1	T42.6X2	T42.6X3	T42.6X4	T42.6X5	T42.6X6
Quarternary ammonium						
anti-infective	T49.0X1	T49.0X2	T49.0X3	T49.0X4	T49.0X5	T49.0X6
ganglion blocking	T44.2X1	T44.2X2	T44.2X3	T44.2X4	T44.2X5	T44.2X6
parasympatholytic	T44.3X1	T44.3X2	T44.3X3	T44.3X4	T44.3X5	T44.3X6
Quazepam	T42.4X1	T42.4X2	T42.4X3	T42.4X4	T42.4X5	T42.4X6
Quicklime	T54.3X1	T54.3X2	T54.3X3	T54.3X4	—	—
Quillaja extract	T48.4X1	T48.4X2	T48.4X3	T48.4X4	T48.4X5	T48.4X6
Quinacrine	T37.2X1	T37.2X2	T37.2X3	T37.2X4	T37.2X5	T37.2X6
Quinaglute	T46.2X1	T46.2X2	T46.2X3	T46.2X4	T46.2X5	T46.2X6
Quinalbarbital	T42.3X1	T42.3X2	T42.3X3	T42.3X4	T42.3X5	T42.3X6
Quinalbarbitone sodium	T42.3X1	T42.3X2	T42.3X3	T42.3X4	T42.3X5	T42.3X6
Quinalphos	T60.0X1	T60.0X2	T60.0X3	T60.0X4	—	—
Quinapril	T46.4X1	T46.4X2	T46.4X3	T46.4X4	T46.4X5	T46.4X6
Quinestradiol	T38.5X1	T38.5X2	T38.5X3	T38.5X4	T38.5X5	T38.5X6
Quinestradol	T38.5X1	T38.5X2	T38.5X3	T38.5X4	T38.5X5	T38.5X6
Quinestrol	T38.5X1	T38.5X2	T38.5X3	T38.5X4	T38.5X5	T38.5X6
Quinethazone	T50.2X1	T50.2X2	T50.2X3	T50.2X4	T50.2X5	T50.2X6
Quingestanol	T38.4X1	T38.4X2	T38.4X3	T38.4X4	T38.4X5	T38.4X6
Quinidine	T46.2X1	T46.2X2	T46.2X3	T46.2X4	T46.2X5	T46.2X6
Quinine	T37.2X1	T37.2X2	T37.2X3	T37.2X4	T37.2X5	T37.2X6
Quiniobine	T37.8X1	T37.8X2	T37.8X3	T37.8X4	T37.8X5	T37.8X6
Quinisocaine	T49.1X1	T49.1X2	T49.1X3	T49.1X4	T49.1X5	T49.1X6
Quinocide	T37.2X1	T37.2X2	T37.2X3	T37.2X4	T37.2X5	T37.2X6
Quinoline (derivatives) NEC	T37.8X1	T37.8X2	T37.8X3	T37.8X4	T37.8X5	T37.8X6
Quinupramine	T43.011	T43.012	T43.013	T43.014	T43.015	T43.016
Quotane	T41.3X1	T41.3X2	T41.3X3	T41.3X4	T41.3X5	T41.3X6
Rabies						
immune globulin (human)	T50.Z11	T50.Z12	T50.Z13	T50.Z14	T50.Z15	T50.Z16
vaccine	T50.B91	T50.B92	T50.B93	T50.B94	T50.B95	T50.B96
Racemoramide	T40.2X1	T40.2X2	T40.2X3	T40.2X4	—	—
Racemorphan	T40.2X1	T40.2X2	T40.2X3	T40.2X4	T40.2X5	T40.2X6
Racepinefrin	T44.5X1	T44.5X2	T44.5X3	T44.5X4	T44.5X5	T44.5X6
Raclopride	T43.591	T43.592	T43.593	T43.594	T43.595	T43.596
Radiator alcohol	T51.1X1	T51.1X2	T51.1X3	T51.1X4	—	—
Radioactive drug NEC	T50.8X1	T50.8X2	T50.8X3	T50.8X4	T50.8X5	T50.8X6
Radio-opaque (drugs) (materials)	T50.8X1	T50.8X2	T50.8X3	T50.8X4	T50.8X5	T50.8X6
Ramifenazone	T39.2X1	T39.2X2	T39.2X3	T39.2X4	T39.2X5	T39.2X6
Ramipril	T46.4X1	T46.4X2	T46.4X3	T46.4X4	T46.4X5	T46.4X6
Ranitidine	T47.0X1	T47.0X2	T47.0X3	T47.0X4	T47.0X5	T47.0X6
Ranunculus	T62.2X1	T62.2X2	T62.2X3	T62.2X4	—	—
Rat poison NEC	T60.4X1	T60.4X2	T60.4X3	T60.4X4	—	—
Rattlesnake (venom)	T63.011	T63.012	T63.013	T63.014	—	—

Substance	Poisoning, Accidental (unintentional)	Poisoning, Intentional Self-harm	Poisoning, Assault	Poisoning, Undetermined	Adverse Effect	Under-dosing
Raubasine	T46.7X1	T46.7X2	T46.7X3	T46.7X4	T46.7X5	T46.7X6
Raudixin	T46.5X1	T46.5X2	T46.5X3	T46.5X4	T46.5X5	T46.5X6
Rautensin	T46.5X1	T46.5X2	T46.5X3	T46.5X4	T46.5X5	T46.5X6
Rautina	T46.5X1	T46.5X2	T46.5X3	T46.5X4	T46.5X5	T46.5X6
Rautotal	T46.5X1	T46.5X2	T46.5X3	T46.5X4	T46.5X5	T46.5X6
Rauwiloid	T46.5X1	T46.5X2	T46.5X3	T46.5X4	T46.5X5	T46.5X6
Rauwoldin	T46.5X1	T46.5X2	T46.5X3	T46.5X4	T46.5X5	T46.5X6
Rauwolfia (alkaloids)	T46.5X1	T46.5X2	T46.5X3	T46.5X4	T46.5X5	T46.5X6
Razoxane	T45.1X1	T45.1X2	T45.1X3	T45.1X4	T45.1X5	T45.1X6
Realgar	T57.0X1	T57.0X2	T57.0X3	T57.0X4	—	—
Recombinant (R) — see specific protein						
Red blood cells, packed	T45.8X1	T45.8X2	T45.8X3	T45.8X4	T45.8X5	T45.8X6
Red squill (scilliroside)	T60.4X1	T60.4X2	T60.4X3	T60.4X4	—	—
Reducing agent, industrial NEC	T65.891	T65.892	T65.893	T65.894	—	—
Refrigerant gas (chlorofluorocarbon)	T53.5X1	T53.5X2	T53.5X3	T53.5X4	—	—
not chlorofluorocarbon	T59.891	T59.892	T59.893	T59.894	—	—
Regroton	T50.2X1	T50.2X2	T50.2X3	T50.2X4	T50.2X5	T50.2X6
Rehydration salts (oral)	T50.3X1	T50.3X2	T50.3X3	T50.3X4	T50.3X5	T50.3X6
Rela	T42.8X1	T42.8X2	T42.8X3	T42.8X4	T42.8X5	T42.8X6
Relaxant, muscle						
anesthetic	T48.1X1	T48.1X2	T48.1X3	T48.1X4	T48.1X5	T48.1X6
central nervous system	T42.8X1	T42.8X2	T42.8X3	T42.8X4	T42.8X5	T42.8X6
skeletal NEC	T48.1X1	T48.1X2	T48.1X3	T48.1X4	T48.1X5	T48.1X6
smooth NEC	T44.3X1	T44.3X2	T44.3X3	T44.3X4	T44.3X5	T44.3X6
Remoxipride	T43.591	T43.592	T43.593	T43.594	T43.595	T43.596
Renese	T50.2X1	T50.2X2	T50.2X3	T50.2X4	T50.2X5	T50.2X6
Renografin	T50.8X1	T50.8X2	T50.8X3	T50.8X4	T50.8X5	T50.8X6
Replacement solution	T50.3X1	T50.3X2	T50.3X3	T50.3X4	T50.3X5	T50.3X6
Reproterol	T48.6X1	T48.6X2	T48.6X3	T48.6X4	T48.6X5	T48.6X6
Rescinnamine	T46.5X1	T46.5X2	T46.5X3	T46.5X4	T46.5X5	T46.5X6
Reserpin (e)	T46.5X1	T46.5X2	T46.5X3	T46.5X4	T46.5X5	T46.5X6
Resorcin, resorcinol (nonmedicinal)	T65.891	T65.892	T65.893	T65.894	—	—
medicinal	T49.4X1	T49.4X2	T49.4X3	T49.4X4	T49.4X5	T49.4X6
Respaire	T48.4X1	T48.4X2	T48.4X3	T48.4X4	T48.4X5	T48.4X6
Respiratory drug NEC	T48.901	T48.902	T48.903	T48.904	T48.905	T48.906
antiasthmatic NEC	T48.6X1	T48.6X2	T48.6X3	T48.6X4	T48.6X5	T48.6X6
anti-common-cold NEC	T48.5X1	T48.5X2	T48.5X3	T48.5X4	T48.5X5	T48.5X6
expectorant NEC	T48.4X1	T48.4X2	T48.4X3	T48.4X4	T48.4X5	T48.4X6
stimulant	T48.901	T48.902	T48.903	T48.904	T48.905	T48.906
Retinoic acid	T49.0X1	T49.0X2	T49.0X3	T49.0X4	T49.0X5	T49.0X6
Retinol	T45.2X1	T45.2X2	T45.2X3	T45.2X4	T45.2X5	T45.2X6
Rh (D) immune globulin (human)	T50.Z11	T50.Z12	T50.Z13	T50.Z14	T50.Z15	T50.Z16
Rhodine	T39.011	T39.012	T39.013	T39.014	T39.015	T39.016
RhoGAM	T50.Z11	T50.Z12	T50.Z13	T50.Z14	T50.Z15	T50.Z16
Rhubarb						
dry extract	T47.2X1	T47.2X2	T47.2X3	T47.2X4	T47.2X5	T47.2X6
tincture, compound	T47.2X1	T47.2X2	T47.2X3	T47.2X4	T47.2X5	T47.2X6
Ribavirin	T37.5X1	T37.5X2	T37.5X3	T37.5X4	T37.5X5	T37.5X6
Riboflavin	T45.2X1	T45.2X2	T45.2X3	T45.2X4	T45.2X5	T45.2X6
Ribostamycin	T36.5X1	T36.5X2	T36.5X3	T36.5X4	T36.5X5	T36.5X6
Ricin	T62.2X1	T62.2X2	T62.2X3	T62.2X4	—	—
Ricinus communis	T62.2X1	T62.2X2	T62.2X3	T62.2X4	—	—
Rickettsial vaccine NEC	T50.A91	T50.A92	T50.A93	T50.A94	T50.A95	T50.A96
Rifabutin	T36.6X1	T36.6X2	T36.6X3	T36.6X4	T36.6X5	T36.6X6
Rifamide	T36.6X1	T36.6X2	T36.6X3	T36.6X4	T36.6X5	T36.6X6
Rifampicin	T36.6X1	T36.6X2	T36.6X3	T36.6X4	T36.6X5	T36.6X6
with isoniazid	T37.1X1	T37.1X2	T37.1X3	T37.1X4	T37.1X5	T37.1X6
Rifampin	T36.6X1	T36.6X2	T36.6X3	T36.6X4	T36.6X5	T36.6X6
Rifamycin	T36.6X1	T36.6X2	T36.6X3	T36.6X4	T36.6X5	T36.6X6
Rifaximin	T36.6X1	T36.6X2	T36.6X3	T36.6X4	T36.6X5	T36.6X6
Rimantadine	T37.5X1	T37.5X2	T37.5X3	T37.5X4	T37.5X5	T37.5X6
Rimazolium metilsulfate	T39.8X1	T39.8X2	T39.8X3	T39.8X4	T39.8X5	T39.8X6
Rimifon	T37.1X1	T37.1X2	T37.1X3	T37.1X4	T37.1X5	T37.1X6
Rimiterol	T48.6X1	T48.6X2	T48.6X3	T48.6X4	T48.6X5	T48.6X6
Ringer (lactate) solution	T50.3X1	T50.3X2	T50.3X3	T50.3X4	T50.3X5	T50.3X6
Ristocetin	T36.8X1	T36.8X2	T36.8X3	T36.8X4	T36.8X5	T36.8X6
Ritalin	T43.631	T43.632	T43.633	T43.634	T43.635	T43.636
Ritodrine	T44.5X1	T44.5X2	T44.5X3	T44.5X4	T44.5X5	T44.5X6
Roach killer — see Insecticide						
Rociverine	T44.3X1	T44.3X2	T44.3X3	T44.3X4	T44.3X5	T44.3X6
Rocky Mountain spotted fever vaccine	T50.A91	T50.A92	T50.A93	T50.A94	T50.A95	T50.A96
Rodenticide NEC	T60.4X1	T60.4X2	T60.4X3	T60.4X4	—	—
Rohypnol	T42.4X1	T42.4X2	T42.4X3	T42.4X4	T42.4X5	T42.4X6
Rokitamycin	T36.3X1	T36.3X2	T36.3X3	T36.3X4	T36.3X5	T36.3X6
Rolaids	T47.1X1	T47.1X2	T47.1X3	T47.1X4	T47.1X5	T47.1X6
Rolitetracycline	T36.4X1	T36.4X2	T36.4X3	T36.4X4	T36.4X5	T36.4X6
Romilar	T48.3X1	T48.3X2	T48.3X3	T48.3X4	T48.3X5	T48.3X6

Substance	Poisoning, Accidental (unintentional)	Poisoning, Intentional Self-harm	Poisoning, Assault	Poisoning, Undetermined	Adverse Effect	Under-dosing
Ronifibrate	T46.6X1	T46.6X2	T46.6X3	T46.6X4	T46.6X5	T46.6X6
Rosaprostol	T47.1X1	T47.1X2	T47.1X3	T47.1X4	T47.1X5	T47.1X6
Rose bengal sodium (131I)	T50.8X1	T50.8X2	T50.8X3	T50.8X4	T50.8X5	T50.8X6
Rose water ointment	T49.3X1	T49.3X2	T49.3X3	T49.3X4	T49.3X5	T49.3X6
Rosoxacin	T37.8X1	T37.8X2	T37.8X3	T37.8X4	T37.8X5	T37.8X6
Rotenone	T60.2X1	T60.2X2	T60.2X3	T60.2X4	—	—
Rotoxamine	T45.0X1	T45.0X2	T45.0X3	T45.0X4	T45.0X5	T45.0X6
Rough-on-rats	T60.4X1	T60.4X2	T60.4X3	T60.4X4	—	—
Roxatidine	T47.0X1	T47.0X2	T47.0X3	T47.0X4	T47.0X5	T47.0X6
Roxithromycin	T36.3X1	T36.3X2	T36.3X3	T36.3X4	T36.3X5	T36.3X6
Rt-PA	T45.611	T45.612	T45.613	T45.614	T45.615	T45.616
Rubbing alcohol	T51.2X1	T51.2X2	T51.2X3	T51.2X4		
Rubefacient	T49.4X1	T49.4X2	T49.4X3	T49.4X4	T49.4X5	T49.4X6
Rubella vaccine	T50.B91	T50.B92	T50.B93	T50.B94	T50.B95	T50.B96
Rubeola vaccine	T50.B91	T50.B92	T50.B93	T50.B94	T50.B95	T50.B96
Rubidium chloride Rb82	T50.8X1	T50.8X2	T50.8X3	T50.8X4	T50.8X5	T50.8X6
Rubidomycin	T45.1X1	T45.1X2	T45.1X3	T45.1X4	T45.1X5	T45.1X6
Rue	T62.2X1	T62.2X2	T62.2X3	T62.2X4	—	—
Rufocromomycin	T45.1X1	T45.1X2	T45.1X3	T45.1X4	T45.1X5	T45.1X6
Russel's viper venin	T45.7X1	T45.7X2	T45.7X3	T45.7X4	T45.7X5	T45.7X6
Ruta (graveolens)	T62.2X1	T62.2X2	T62.2X3	T62.2X4		
Rutinum	T46.991	T46.992	T46.993	T46.994	T46.995	T46.996
Rutoside	T46.991	T46.992	T46.993	T46.994	T46.995	T46.996
b-sitosterol(s)	T46.6X1	T46.6X2	T46.6X3	T46.6X4	T46.6X5	T46.6X6
Sabadilla (plant)	T62.2X1	T62.2X2	T62.2X3	T62.2X4	—	—
pesticide	T60.2X1	T60.2X2	T60.2X3	T60.2X4	—	—
Saccharated iron oxide	T45.8X1	T45.8X2	T45.8X3	T45.8X4	T45.8X5	T45.8X6
Saccharin	T50.901	T50.902	T50.903	T50.904	T50.905	T50.906
Saccharomyces boulardii	T47.6X1	T47.6X2	T47.6X3	T47.6X4	T47.6X5	T47.6X6
Safflower oil	T46.6X1	T46.6X2	T46.6X3	T46.6X4	T46.6X5	T46.6X6
Safrazine	T43.1X1	T43.1X2	T43.1X3	T43.1X4	T43.1X5	T43.1X6
Salazosulfapyridine	T37.0X1	T37.0X2	T37.0X3	T37.0X4	T37.0X5	T37.0X6
Salbutamol	T48.6X1	T48.6X2	T48.6X3	T48.6X4	T48.6X5	T48.6X6
Salicylamide	T39.091	T39.092	T39.093	T39.094	T39.095	T39.096
Salicylate NEC	T39.091	T39.092	T39.093	T39.094	T39.095	T39.096
methyl	T49.3X1	T49.3X2	T49.3X3	T49.3X4	T49.3X5	T49.3X6
theobromine calcium	T50.2X1	T50.2X2	T50.2X3	T50.2X4	T50.2X5	T50.2X6
Salicylazosulfapyridine	T37.0X1	T37.0X2	T37.0X3	T37.0X4	T37.0X5	T37.0X6
Salicylhydroxamic acid	T49.0X1	T49.0X2	T49.0X3	T49.0X4	T49.0X5	T49.0X6
Salicylic acid	T49.4X1	T49.4X2	T49.4X3	T49.4X4	T49.4X5	T49.4X6
with benzoic acid	T49.4X1	T49.4X2	T49.4X3	T49.4X4	T49.4X5	T49.4X6
congeners	T39.091	T39.092	T39.093	T39.094	T39.095	T39.096
derivative	T39.091	T39.092	T39.093	T39.094	T39.095	T39.096
salts	T39.091	T39.092	T39.093	T39.094	T39.095	T39.096
Salinazid	T37.1X1	T37.1X2	T37.1X3	T37.1X4	T37.1X5	T37.1X6
Salmeterol	T48.6X1	T48.6X2	T48.6X3	T48.6X4	T48.6X5	T48.6X6
Salol	T49.3X1	T49.3X2	T49.3X3	T49.3X4	T49.3X5	T49.3X6
Salsalate	T39.091	T39.092	T39.093	T39.094	T39.095	T39.096
Salt-replacing drug	T50.901	T50.902	T50.903	T50.904	T50.905	T50.906
Salt-retaining mineralocorticoid	T50.0X1	T50.0X2	T50.0X3	T50.0X4	T50.0X5	T50.0X6
Salt substitute	T50.901	T50.902	T50.903	T50.904	T50.905	T50.906
Saluretic NEC	T50.2X1	T50.2X2	T50.2X3	T50.2X4	T50.2X5	T50.2X6
Saluron	T50.2X1	T50.2X2	T50.2X3	T50.2X4	T50.2X5	T50.2X6
Salvarsan 606 (neosilver) (silver)	T37.8X1	T37.8X2	T37.8X3	T37.8X4	T37.8X5	T37.8X6
Sambucus canadensis	T62.2X1	T62.2X2	T62.2X3	T62.2X4	—	—
berry	T62.1X1	T62.1X2	T62.1X3	T62.1X4	—	—
Sandril	T46.5X1	T46.5X2	T46.5X3	T46.5X4	T46.5X5	T46.5X6
Sanguinaria canadensis	T62.2X1	T62.2X2	T62.2X3	T62.2X4	—	—
Saniflush (cleaner)	T54.2X1	T54.2X2	T54.2X3	T54.2X4	—	—
Santonin	T37.4X1	T37.4X2	T37.4X3	T37.4X4	T37.4X5	T37.4X6
Santyl	T49.8X1	T49.8X2	T49.8X3	T49.8X4	T49.8X5	T49.8X6
Saralasin	T46.5X1	T46.5X2	T46.5X3	T46.5X4	T46.5X5	T46.5X6
Sarcolysin	T45.1X1	T45.1X2	T45.1X3	T45.1X4	T45.1X5	T45.1X6
Sarkomycin	T45.1X1	T45.1X2	T45.1X3	T45.1X4	T45.1X5	T45.1X6
Saroten	T43.011	T43.012	T43.013	T43.014	T43.015	T43.016
Saturnine — see Lead						
Savin (oil)	T49.4X1	T49.4X2	T49.4X3	T49.4X4	T49.4X5	T49.4X6
Scammony	T47.2X1	T47.2X2	T47.2X3	T47.2X4	T47.2X5	T47.2X6
Scarlet red	T49.8X1	T49.8X2	T49.8X3	T49.8X4	T49.8X5	T49.8X6
Scheele's green	T57.0X1	T57.0X2	T57.0X3	T57.0X4	—	—
insecticide	T57.0X1	T57.0X2	T57.0X3	T57.0X4	—	—
Schizontozide (blood) (tissue)	T37.2X1	T37.2X2	T37.2X3	T37.2X4	T37.2X5	T37.2X6
Schradan	T60.0X1	T60.0X2	T60.0X3	T60.0X4	—	—
Schweinfurth green	T57.0X1	T57.0X2	T57.0X3	T57.0X4	—	—
insecticide	T57.0X1	T57.0X2	T57.0X3	T57.0X4	—	—
Scilla, rat poison	T60.4X1	T60.4X2	T60.4X3	T60.4X4	—	—
Scillaren	T60.4X1	T60.4X2	T60.4X3	T60.4X4	—	—
Sclerosing agent	T46.8X1	T46.8X2	T46.8X3	T46.8X4	T46.8X5	T46.8X6
Scombrotoxin	T61.11	T61.12	T61.13	T61.14	—	—
Scopolamine	T44.3X1	T44.3X2	T44.3X3	T44.3X4	T44.3X5	T44.3X6

Substance	Poisoning, Accidental (unintentional)	Poisoning, Intentional Self-harm	Poisoning, Assault	Poisoning, Undetermined	Adverse Effect	Under-dosing
Scopolia extract	T44.3X1	T44.3X2	T44.3X3	T44.3X4	T44.3X5	T44.3X6
Scouring powder	T65.891	T65.892	T65.893	T65.894	—	—
Sea						
anemone (sting)	T63.631	T63.632	T63.633	T63.634	—	—
cucumber (sting)	T63.691	T63.692	T63.693	T63.694	—	—
snake (bite) (venom)	T63.091	T63.092	T63.093	T63.094	—	—
urchin spine (puncture)	T63.691	T63.692	T63.693	T63.694	—	—
Seafood	T61.91	T61.92	T61.93	T61.94	—	—
specified NEC	T61.8X1	T61.8X2	T61.8X3	T61.8X4	—	—
Secbutabarbital	T42.3X1	T42.3X2	T42.3X3	T42.3X4	T42.3X5	T42.3X6
Secbutabarbitone	T42.3X1	T42.3X2	T42.3X3	T42.3X4	T42.3X5	T42.3X6
Secnidazole	T37.3X1	T37.3X2	T37.3X3	T37.3X4	T37.3X5	T37.3X6
Secobarbital	T42.3X1	T42.3X2	T42.3X3	T42.3X4	T42.3X5	T42.3X6
Seconal	T42.3X1	T42.3X2	T42.3X3	T42.3X4	T42.3X5	T42.3X6
Secretin	T50.8X1	T50.8X2	T50.8X3	T50.8X4	T50.8X5	T50.8X6
Sedative NEC	T42.71	T42.72	T42.73	T42.74	T42.75	T42.76
mixed NEC	T42.6X1	T42.6X2	T42.6X3	T42.6X4	T42.6X5	T42.6X6
Sedormid	T42.6X1	T42.6X2	T42.6X3	T42.6X4	T42.6X5	T42.6X6
Seed disinfectant or dressing	T60.8X1	T60.8X2	T60.8X3	T60.8X4	—	—
Seeds (poisonous)	T62.2X1	T62.2X2	T62.2X3	T62.2X4		
Selegiline	T42.8X1	T42.8X2	T42.8X3	T42.8X4	T42.8X5	T42.8X6
Selenium NEC	T56.891	T56.892	T56.893	T56.894	—	—
disulfide or sulfide	T49.4X1	T49.4X2	T49.4X3	T49.4X4	T49.4X5	T49.4X6
fumes	T59.891	T59.892	T59.893	T59.894	—	—
sulfide	T49.4X1	T49.4X2	T49.4X3	T49.4X4	T49.4X5	T49.4X6
Selenomethionine (75Se)	T50.8X1	T50.8X2	T50.8X3	T50.8X4	T50.8X5	T50.8X6
Selsun	T49.4X1	T49.4X2	T49.4X3	T49.4X4	T49.4X5	T49.4X6
Semustine	T45.1X1	T45.1X2	T45.1X3	T45.1X4	T45.1X5	T45.1X6
Senega syrup	T48.4X1	T48.4X2	T48.4X3	T48.4X4	T48.4X5	T48.4X6
Senna	T47.2X1	T47.2X2	T47.2X3	T47.2X4	T47.2X5	T47.2X6
Sennoside A+B	T47.2X1	T47.2X2	T47.2X3	T47.2X4	T47.2X5	T47.2X6
Septisol	T49.2X1	T49.2X2	T49.2X3	T49.2X4	T49.2X5	T49.2X6
Seractide	T38.811	T38.812	T38.813	T38.814	T38.815	T38.816
Serax	T42.4X1	T42.4X2	T42.4X3	T42.4X4	T42.4X5	T42.4X6
Serenesil	T42.6X1	T42.6X2	T42.6X3	T42.6X4	T42.6X5	T42.6X6
Serenium (hydrochloride)	T37.91	T37.92	T37.93	T37.94	T37.95	T37.96
Serepax — see Oxazepam						
Sermorelin	T38.891	T38.892	T38.893	T38.894	T38.895	T38.896
Sernyl	T41.1X1	T41.1X2	T41.1X3	T41.1X4	T41.1X5	T41.1X6
Serotonin	T50.991	T50.992	T50.993	T50.994	T50.995	T50.996
Serpasil	T46.5X1	T46.5X2	T46.5X3	T46.5X4	T46.5X5	T46.5X6
Serrapeptase	T45.3X1	T45.3X2	T45.3X3	T45.3X4	T45.3X5	T45.3X6
Serum						
antibotulinus	T50.Z11	T50.Z12	T50.Z13	T50.Z14	T50.Z15	T50.Z16
anticytotoxic	T50.Z11	T50.Z12	T50.Z13	T50.Z14	T50.Z15	T50.Z16
antidiphtheria	T50.Z11	T50.Z12	T50.Z13	T50.Z14	T50.Z15	T50.Z16
antimeningococcus	T50.Z11	T50.Z12	T50.Z13	T50.Z14	T50.Z15	T50.Z16
anti-Rh	T50.Z11	T50.Z12	T50.Z13	T50.Z14	T50.Z15	T50.Z16
anti-snake-bite	T50.Z11	T50.Z12	T50.Z13	T50.Z14	T50.Z15	T50.Z16
antitetanic	T50.Z11	T50.Z12	T50.Z13	T50.Z14	T50.Z15	T50.Z16
antitoxic	T50.Z11	T50.Z12	T50.Z13	T50.Z14	T50.Z15	T50.Z16
complement (inhibitor)	T45.8X1	T45.8X2	T45.8X3	T45.8X4	T45.8X5	T45.8X6
convalescent	T50.Z11	T50.Z12	T50.Z13	T50.Z14	T50.Z15	T50.Z16
hemolytic complement	T45.8X1	T45.8X2	T45.8X3	T45.8X4	T45.8X5	T45.8X6
immune (human)	T50.Z11	T50.Z12	T50.Z13	T50.Z14	T50.Z15	T50.Z16
protective NEC	T50.Z11	T50.Z12	T50.Z13	T50.Z14	T50.Z15	T50.Z16
Setastine	T45.0X1	T45.0X2	T45.0X3	T45.0X4	T45.0X5	T45.0X6
Setoperone	T43.591	T43.592	T43.593	T43.594	T43.595	T43.596
Sewer gas	T59.91	T59.92	T59.93	T59.94	—	—
Shampoo	T55.0X1	T55.0X2	T55.0X3	T55.0X4	—	—
Shellfish, noxious, nonbacterial	T61.781	T61.782	T61.783	T61.784	—	—
Sildenafil	T46.7X1	T46.7X2	T46.7X3	T46.7X4	T46.7X5	T46.7X6
Silibinin	T50.991	T50.992	T50.993	T50.994	T50.995	T50.996
Silicone NEC	T65.891	T65.892	T65.893	T65.894	—	—
medicinal	T49.3X1	T49.3X2	T49.3X3	T49.3X4	T49.3X5	T49.3X6
Silvadene	T49.0X1	T49.0X2	T49.0X3	T49.0X4	T49.0X5	T49.0X6
Silver	T49.0X1	T49.0X2	T49.0X3	T49.0X4	T49.0X5	T49.0X6
anti-infectives	T49.0X1	T49.0X2	T49.0X3	T49.0X4	T49.0X5	T49.0X6
arsphenamine	T37.8X1	T37.8X2	T37.8X3	T37.8X4	T37.8X5	T37.8X6
colloidal	T49.0X1	T49.0X2	T49.0X3	T49.0X4	T49.0X5	T49.0X6
nitrate	T49.0X1	T49.0X2	T49.0X3	T49.0X4	T49.0X5	T49.0X6
ophthalmic preparation	T49.5X1	T49.5X2	T49.5X3	T49.5X4	T49.5X5	T49.5X6
toughened (keratolytic)	T49.4X1	T49.4X2	T49.4X3	T49.4X4	T49.4X5	T49.4X6
nonmedicinal (dust)	T56.891	T56.892	T56.893	T56.894	—	—
protein	T49.5X1	T49.5X2	T49.5X3	T49.5X4	T49.5X5	T49.5X6
salvarsan	T37.8X1	T37.8X2	T37.8X3	T37.8X4	T37.8X5	T37.8X6
sulfadiazine	T49.4X1	T49.4X2	T49.4X3	T49.4X4	T49.4X5	T49.4X6
Silymarin	T50.991	T50.992	T50.993	T50.994	T50.995	T50.996
Simaldrate	T47.1X1	T47.1X2	T47.1X3	T47.1X4	T47.1X5	T47.1X6
Simazine	T60.3X1	T60.3X2	T60.3X3	T60.3X4	—	—
Simethicone	T47.1X1	T47.1X2	T47.1X3	T47.1X4	T47.1X5	T47.1X6

Additional Character May Be Required — Refer to the Tabular List for Character Selection   ▽ Subterms under main terms may continue to next column or page

Substance	Poisoning, Accidental (unintentional)	Poisoning, Intentional Self-harm	Poisoning, Assault	Poisoning, Undetermined	Adverse Effect	Under-dosing
Simfibrate	T46.6X1	T46.6X2	T46.6X3	T46.6X4	T46.6X5	T46.6X6
Simvastatin	T46.6X1	T46.6X2	T46.6X3	T46.6X4	T46.6X5	T46.6X6
Sincalide	T50.8X1	T50.8X2	T50.8X3	T50.8X4	T50.8X5	T50.8X6
Sinequan	T43.011	T43.012	T43.013	T43.014	T43.015	T43.016
Singoserp	T46.5X1	T46.5X2	T46.5X3	T46.5X4	T46.5X5	T46.5X6
Sintrom	T45.511	T45.512	T45.513	T45.514	T45.515	T45.516
Sisomicin	T36.5X1	T36.5X2	T36.5X3	T36.5X4	T36.5X5	T36.5X6
Sitosterols	T46.6X1	T46.6X2	T46.6X3	T46.6X4	T46.6X5	T46.6X6
Skeletal muscle relaxants	T48.1X1	T48.1X2	T48.1X3	T48.1X4	T48.1X5	T48.1X6
Skin						
agents (external)	T49.91	T49.92	T49.93	T49.94	T49.95	T49.96
specified NEC	T49.8X1	T49.8X2	T49.8X3	T49.8X4	T49.8X5	T49.8X6
test antigen	T50.8X1	T50.8X2	T50.8X3	T50.8X4	T50.8X5	T50.8X6
Sleep-eze	T45.0X1	T45.0X2	T45.0X3	T45.0X4	T45.0X5	T45.0X6
Sleeping draught, pill	T42.71	T42.72	T42.73	T42.74	T42.75	T42.76
Smallpox vaccine	T50.B11	T50.B12	T50.B13	T50.B14	T50.B15	T50.B16
Smelter fumes NEC	T56.91	T56.92	T56.93	T56.94	—	—
Smog	T59.1X1	T59.1X2	T59.1X3	T59.1X4	—	—
Smoke NEC	T59.811	T59.812	T59.813	T59.814	—	—
Smooth muscle relaxant	T44.3X1	T44.3X2	T44.3X3	T44.3X4	T44.3X5	T44.3X6
Snail killer NEC	T60.8X1	T60.8X2	T60.8X3	T60.8X4	—	—
Snake venom or bite	T63.001	T63.002	T63.003	T63.004	—	—
hemocoagulase	T45.7X1	T45.7X2	T45.7X3	T45.7X4	T45.7X5	T45.7X6
Snuff	T65.211	T65.212	T65.213	T65.214	—	—
Soap (powder) (product)	T55.0X1	T55.0X2	T55.0X3	T55.0X4	—	—
enema	T47.4X1	T47.4X2	T47.4X3	T47.4X4	T47.4X5	T47.4X6
medicinal, soft	T49.2X1	T49.2X2	T49.2X3	T49.2X4	T49.2X5	T49.2X6
superfatted	T49.2X1	T49.2X2	T49.2X3	T49.2X4	T49.2X5	T49.2X6
Sobrerol	T48.4X1	T48.4X2	T48.4X3	T48.4X4	T48.4X5	T48.4X6
Soda (caustic)	T54.3X1	T54.3X2	T54.3X3	T54.3X4	—	—
bicarb	T47.1X1	T47.1X2	T47.1X3	T47.1X4	T47.1X5	T47.1X6
chlorinated — see Sodium, hypochlorite						
Sodium						
acetosulfone	T37.1X1	T37.1X2	T37.1X3	T37.1X4	T37.1X5	T37.1X6
acetrizoate	T50.8X1	T50.8X2	T50.8X3	T50.8X4	T50.8X5	T50.8X6
acid phosphate	T50.3X1	T50.3X2	T50.3X3	T50.3X4	T50.3X5	T50.3X6
alginate	T47.8X1	T47.8X2	T47.8X3	T47.8X4	T47.8X5	T47.8X6
amidotrizoate	T50.8X1	T50.8X2	T50.8X3	T50.8X4	T50.8X5	T50.8X6
aminopterin	T45.1X1	T45.1X2	T45.1X3	T45.1X4	T45.1X5	T45.1X6
amylosulfate	T47.8X1	T47.8X2	T47.8X3	T47.8X4	T47.8X5	T47.8X6
amytal	T42.3X1	T42.3X2	T42.3X3	T42.3X4	T42.3X5	T42.3X6
antimony gluconate	T37.3X1	T37.3X2	T37.3X3	T37.3X4	T37.3X5	T37.3X6
arsenate	T57.0X1	T57.0X2	T57.0X3	T57.0X4	—	—
aurothiomalate	T39.4X1	T39.4X2	T39.4X3	T39.4X4	T39.4X5	T39.4X6
aurothiosulfate	T39.4X1	T39.4X2	T39.4X3	T39.4X4	T39.4X5	T39.4X6
barbiturate	T42.3X1	T42.3X2	T42.3X3	T42.3X4	T42.3X5	T42.3X6
basic phosphate	T47.4X1	T47.4X2	T47.4X3	T47.4X4	T47.4X5	T47.4X6
bicarbonate	T47.1X1	T47.1X2	T47.1X3	T47.1X4	T47.1X5	T47.1X6
bichromate	T57.8X1	T57.8X2	T57.8X3	T57.8X4	—	—
biphosphate	T50.3X1	T50.3X2	T50.3X3	T50.3X4	T50.3X5	T50.3X6
bisulfate	T65.891	T65.892	T65.893	T65.894	—	—
borate						
cleanser	T57.8X1	T57.8X2	T57.8X3	T57.8X4	—	—
eye	T49.5X1	T49.5X2	T49.5X3	T49.5X4	T49.5X5	T49.5X6
therapeutic	T49.8X1	T49.8X2	T49.8X3	T49.8X4	T49.8X5	T49.8X6
bromide	T42.6X1	T42.6X2	T42.6X3	T42.6X4	T42.6X5	T42.6X6
cacodylate (nonmedicinal) NEC	T50.8X1	T50.8X2	T50.8X3	T50.8X4	T50.8X5	T50.8X6
anti-infective	T37.8X1	T37.8X2	T37.8X3	T37.8X4	T37.8X5	T37.8X6
herbicide	T60.3X1	T60.3X2	T60.3X3	T60.3X4	—	—
calcium edetate	T45.8X1	T45.8X2	T45.8X3	T45.8X4	T45.8X5	T45.8X6
carbonate NEC	T54.3X1	T54.3X2	T54.3X3	T54.3X4	—	—
chlorate NEC	T65.891	T65.892	T65.893	T65.894	—	—
herbicide	T54.91	T54.92	T54.93	T54.94	—	—
chloride	T50.3X1	T50.3X2	T50.3X3	T50.3X4	T50.3X5	T50.3X6
with glucose	T50.3X1	T50.3X2	T50.3X3	T50.3X4	T50.3X5	T50.3X6
chromate	T65.891	T65.892	T65.893	T65.894	—	—
citrate	T50.991	T50.992	T50.993	T50.994	T50.995	T50.996
cromoglicate	T48.6X1	T48.6X2	T48.6X3	T48.6X4	T48.6X5	T48.6X6
cyanide	T65.0X1	T65.0X2	T65.0X3	T65.0X4	—	—
cyclamate	T50.3X1	T50.3X2	T50.3X3	T50.3X4	T50.3X5	T50.3X6
dehydrocholate	T45.8X1	T45.8X2	T45.8X3	T45.8X4	T45.8X5	T45.8X6
diatrizoate	T50.8X1	T50.8X2	T50.8X3	T50.8X4	T50.8X5	T50.8X6
dibunate	T48.4X1	T48.4X2	T48.4X3	T48.4X4	T48.4X5	T48.4X6
dioctyl sulfosuccinate	T47.4X1	T47.4X2	T47.4X3	T47.4X4	T47.4X5	T47.4X6
dipantoyl ferrate	T45.8X1	T45.8X2	T45.8X3	T45.8X4	T45.8X5	T45.8X6
edetate	T45.8X1	T45.8X2	T45.8X3	T45.8X4	T45.8X5	T45.8X6
ethacrynate	T50.1X1	T50.1X2	T50.1X3	T50.1X4	T50.1X5	T50.1X6
feredetate	T45.8X1	T45.8X2	T45.8X3	T45.8X4	T45.8X5	T45.8X6
Fluoride — see Fluoride						
fluoroacetate (dust) (pesticide)	T60.4X1	T60.4X2	T60.4X3	T60.4X4	—	—
Sodium — *continued*						
free salt	T50.3X1	T50.3X2	T50.3X3	T50.3X4	T50.3X5	T50.3X6
fusidate	T36.8X1	T36.8X2	T36.8X3	T36.8X4	T36.8X5	T36.8X6
glucaldrate	T47.1X1	T47.1X2	T47.1X3	T47.1X4	T47.1X5	T47.1X6
glucosulfone	T37.1X1	T37.1X2	T37.1X3	T37.1X4	T37.1X5	T37.1X6
glutamate	T45.8X1	T45.8X2	T45.8X3	T45.8X4	T45.8X5	T45.8X6
hydrogen carbonate	T50.3X1	T50.3X2	T50.3X3	T50.3X4	T50.3X5	T50.3X6
hydroxide	T54.3X1	T54.3X2	T54.3X3	T54.3X4	—	—
hypochlorite (bleach) NEC	T54.3X1	T54.3X2	T54.3X3	T54.3X4	—	—
disinfectant	T54.3X1	T54.3X2	T54.3X3	T54.3X4	—	—
medicinal (anti-infective) (external)	T49.0X1	T49.0X2	T49.0X3	T49.0X4	T49.0X5	T49.0X6
vapor	T54.3X1	T54.3X2	T54.3X3	T54.3X4	—	—
hyposulfite	T49.0X1	T49.0X2	T49.0X3	T49.0X4	T49.0X5	T49.0X6
indigotin disulfonate	T50.8X1	T50.8X2	T50.8X3	T50.8X4	T50.8X5	T50.8X6
iodide	T50.991	T50.992	T50.993	T50.994	T50.995	T50.996
I-131	T50.8X1	T50.8X2	T50.8X3	T50.8X4	T50.8X5	T50.8X6
therapeutic	T38.2X1	T38.2X2	T38.2X3	T38.2X4	T38.2X5	T38.2X6
iodohippurate (131I)	T50.8X1	T50.8X2	T50.8X3	T50.8X4	T50.8X5	T50.8X6
iopodate	T50.8X1	T50.8X2	T50.8X3	T50.8X4	T50.8X5	T50.8X6
iothalamate	T50.8X1	T50.8X2	T50.8X3	T50.8X4	T50.8X5	T50.8X6
iron edetate	T45.4X1	T45.4X2	T45.4X3	T45.4X4	T45.4X5	T45.4X6
lactate (compound solution)	T45.8X1	T45.8X2	T45.8X3	T45.8X4	T45.8X5	T45.8X6
lauryl (sulfate)	T49.2X1	T49.2X2	T49.2X3	T49.2X4	T49.2X5	T49.2X6
L-triiodothyronine	T38.1X1	T38.1X2	T38.1X3	T38.1X4	T38.1X5	T38.1X6
magnesium citrate	T50.991	T50.992	T50.993	T50.994	T50.995	T50.996
mersalate	T50.2X1	T50.2X2	T50.2X3	T50.2X4	T50.2X5	T50.2X6
metasilicate	T65.891	T65.892	T65.893	T65.894	—	—
metrizoate	T50.8X1	T50.8X2	T50.8X3	T50.8X4	T50.8X5	T50.8X6
monofluoroacetate (pesticide)	T60.1X1	T60.1X2	T60.1X3	T60.1X4	—	—
morrhuate	T46.8X1	T46.8X2	T46.8X3	T46.8X4	T46.8X5	T46.8X6
nafcillin	T36.0X1	T36.0X2	T36.0X3	T36.0X4	T36.0X5	T36.0X6
nitrate (oxidizing agent)	T65.891	T65.892	T65.893	T65.894	—	—
nitrite	T50.6X1	T50.6X2	T50.6X3	T50.6X4	T50.6X5	T50.6X6
nitroferricyanide	T46.5X1	T46.5X2	T46.5X3	T46.5X4	T46.5X5	T46.5X6
nitroprusside	T46.5X1	T46.5X2	T46.5X3	T46.5X4	T46.5X5	T46.5X6
oxalate	T65.891	T65.892	T65.893	T65.894	—	—
oxide/peroxide	T65.891	T65.892	T65.893	T65.894	—	—
oxybate	T41.291	T41.292	T41.293	T41.294	T41.295	T41.296
para-aminohippurate	T50.8X1	T50.8X2	T50.8X3	T50.8X4	T50.8X5	T50.8X6
perborate (nonmedicinal) NEC	T65.891	T65.892	T65.893	T65.894	—	—
medicinal	T49.0X1	T49.0X2	T49.0X3	T49.0X4	T49.0X5	T49.0X6
soap	T55.0X1	T55.0X2	T55.0X3	T55.0X4	—	—
percarbonate — see Sodium, perborate						
pertechnetate Tc99m	T50.8X1	T50.8X2	T50.8X3	T50.8X4	T50.8X5	T50.8X6
phosphate						
cellulose	T45.8X1	T45.8X2	T45.8X3	T45.8X4	T45.8X5	T45.8X6
dibasic	T47.2X1	T47.2X2	T47.2X3	T47.2X4	T47.2X5	T47.2X6
monobasic	T47.2X1	T47.2X2	T47.2X3	T47.2X4	T47.2X5	T47.2X6
phytate	T50.6X1	T50.6X2	T50.6X3	T50.6X4	T50.6X5	T50.6X6
picosulfate	T47.2X1	T47.2X2	T47.2X3	T47.2X4	T47.2X5	T47.2X6
polyhydroxyaluminium monocarbonate	T47.1X1	T47.1X2	T47.1X3	T47.1X4	T47.1X5	T47.1X6
polystyrene sulfonate	T50.3X1	T50.3X2	T50.3X3	T50.3X4	T50.3X5	T50.3X6
propionate	T49.0X1	T49.0X2	T49.0X3	T49.0X4	T49.0X5	T49.0X6
propyl hydroxybenzoate	T50.991	T50.992	T50.993	T50.994	T50.995	T50.996
psylliate	T46.8X1	T46.8X2	T46.8X3	T46.8X4	T46.8X5	T46.8X6
removing resins	T50.3X1	T50.3X2	T50.3X3	T50.3X4	T50.3X5	T50.3X6
salicylate	T39.091	T39.092	T39.093	T39.094	T39.095	T39.096
salt NEC	T50.3X1	T50.3X2	T50.3X3	T50.3X4	T50.3X5	T50.3X6
selenate	T60.2X1	T60.2X2	T60.2X3	T60.2X4	—	—
stibogluconate	T37.3X1	T37.3X2	T37.3X3	T37.3X4	T37.3X5	T37.3X6
sulfate	T47.4X1	T47.4X2	T47.4X3	T47.4X4	T47.4X5	T47.4X6
sulfoxone	T37.1X1	T37.1X2	T37.1X3	T37.1X4	T37.1X5	T37.1X6
tetradecyl sulfate	T46.8X1	T46.8X2	T46.8X3	T46.8X4	T46.8X5	T46.8X6
thiopental	T41.1X1	T41.1X2	T41.1X3	T41.1X4	T41.1X5	T41.1X6
thiosalicylate	T39.091	T39.092	T39.093	T39.094	T39.095	T39.096
thiosulfate	T50.6X1	T50.6X2	T50.6X3	T50.6X4	T50.6X5	T50.6X6
tolbutamide	T38.3X1	T38.3X2	T38.3X3	T38.3X4	T38.3X5	T38.3X6
(L)-triiodothyronine	T38.1X1	T38.1X2	T38.1X3	T38.1X4	T38.1X5	T38.1X6
tyropanoate	T50.8X1	T50.8X2	T50.8X3	T50.8X4	T50.8X5	T50.8X6
valproate	T42.6X1	T42.6X2	T42.6X3	T42.6X4	T42.6X5	T42.6X6
versenate	T50.6X1	T50.6X2	T50.6X3	T50.6X4	T50.6X5	T50.6X6
Sodium-free salt	T50.901	T50.902	T50.903	T50.904	T50.905	T50.906
Sodium-removing resin	T50.3X1	T50.3X2	T50.3X3	T50.3X4	T50.3X5	T50.3X6
Soft soap	T55.0X1	T55.0X2	T55.0X3	T55.0X4	—	—
Solanine	T62.2X1	T62.2X2	T62.2X3	T62.2X4	—	—
berries	T62.1X1	T62.1X2	T62.1X3	T62.1X4	—	—
Solanum dulcamara	T62.2X1	T62.2X2	T62.2X3	T62.2X4	—	—

Table of Drugs and Chemicals

Solanum dulcamara — Sulfadiasulfone sodium

Substance	Poisoning, Accidental (unintentional)	Poisoning, Intentional Self-harm	Poisoning, Assault	Poisoning, Undetermined	Adverse Effect	Under-dosing
Solanum dulcamara — *continued*						
berries	T62.1X1	T62.1X2	T62.1X3	T62.1X4	—	—
Solapsone	T37.1X1	T37.1X2	T37.1X3	T37.1X4	T37.1X5	T37.1X6
Solar lotion	T49.3X1	T49.3X2	T49.3X3	T49.3X4	T49.3X5	T49.3X6
Solasulfone	T37.1X1	T37.1X2	T37.1X3	T37.1X4	T37.1X5	T37.1X6
Soldering fluid	T65.891	T65.892	T65.893	T65.894	—	—
Solid substance	T65.91	T65.92	T65.93	T65.94	—	—
specified NEC	T65.891	T65.892	T65.893	T65.894	—	—
Solvent, industrial NEC	T52.91	T52.92	T52.93	T52.94	—	—
naphtha	T52.0X1	T52.0X2	T52.0X3	T52.0X4	—	—
petroleum	T52.0X1	T52.0X2	T52.0X3	T52.0X4	—	—
specified NEC	T52.8X1	T52.8X2	T52.8X3	T52.8X4	—	—
Soma	T42.8X1	T42.8X2	T42.8X3	T42.8X4	T42.8X5	T42.8X6
Somatorelin	T38.891	T38.892	T38.893	T38.894	T38.895	T38.896
Somatostatin	T38.991	T38.992	T38.993	T38.994	T38.995	T38.996
Somatotropin	T38.811	T38.812	T38.813	T38.814	T38.815	T38.816
Somatrem	T38.811	T38.812	T38.813	T38.814	T38.815	T38.816
Somatropin	T38.811	T38.812	T38.813	T38.814	T38.815	T38.816
Sominex	T45.0X1	T45.0X2	T45.0X3	T45.0X4	T45.0X5	T45.0X6
Somnos	T42.6X1	T42.6X2	T42.6X3	T42.6X4	T42.6X5	T42.6X6
Somonal	T42.3X1	T42.3X2	T42.3X3	T42.3X4	T42.3X5	T42.3X6
Soneryl	T42.3X1	T42.3X2	T42.3X3	T42.3X4	T42.3X5	T42.3X6
Soothing syrup	T50.901	T50.902	T50.903	T50.904	T50.905	T50.906
Sopor	T42.6X1	T42.6X2	T42.6X3	T42.6X4	T42.6X5	T42.6X6
Soporific	T42.71	T42.72	T42.73	T42.74	T42.75	T42.76
Soporific drug	T42.71	T42.72	T42.73	T42.74	T42.75	T42.76
specified type NEC	T42.6X1	T42.6X2	T42.6X3	T42.6X4	T42.6X5	T42.6X6
Sorbide nitrate	T46.3X1	T46.3X2	T46.3X3	T46.3X4	T46.3X5	T46.3X6
Sorbitol	T47.4X1	T47.4X2	T47.4X3	T47.4X4	T47.4X5	T47.4X6
Sotalol	T44.7X1	T44.7X2	T44.7X3	T44.7X4	T44.7X5	T44.7X6
Sotradecol	T46.8X1	T46.8X2	T46.8X3	T46.8X4	T46.8X5	T46.8X6
Soysterol	T46.6X1	T46.6X2	T46.6X3	T46.6X4	T46.6X5	T46.6X6
Spacoline	T44.3X1	T44.3X2	T44.3X3	T44.3X4	T44.3X5	T44.3X6
Spanish fly	T49.8X1	T49.8X2	T49.8X3	T49.8X4	T49.8X5	T49.8X6
Sparine	T43.3X1	T43.3X2	T43.3X3	T43.3X4	T43.3X5	T43.3X6
Sparteine	T48.0X1	T48.0X2	T48.0X3	T48.0X4	T48.0X5	T48.0X6
Spasmolytic						
anticholinergics	T44.3X1	T44.3X2	T44.3X3	T44.3X4	T44.3X5	T44.3X6
autonomic	T44.3X1	T44.3X2	T44.3X3	T44.3X4	T44.3X5	T44.3X6
bronchial NEC	T48.6X1	T48.6X2	T48.6X3	T48.6X4	T48.6X5	T48.6X6
quaternary ammonium	T44.3X1	T44.3X2	T44.3X3	T44.3X4	T44.3X5	T44.3X6
skeletal muscle NEC	T48.1X1	T48.1X2	T48.1X3	T48.1X4	T48.1X5	T48.1X6
Spectinomycin	T36.5X1	T36.5X2	T36.5X3	T36.5X4	T36.5X5	T36.5X6
Speed	T43.621	T43.622	T43.623	T43.624	T43.625	T43.626
Spermicide	T49.8X1	T49.8X2	T49.8X3	T49.8X4	T49.8X5	T49.8X6
Spider (bite) (venom)	T63.391	T63.392	T63.393	T63.394	—	—
antivenin	T50.Z11	T50.Z12	T50.Z13	T50.Z14	T50.Z15	T50.Z16
Spigelia (root)	T37.4X1	T37.4X2	T37.4X3	T37.4X4	T37.4X5	T37.4X6
Spindle inactivator	T50.4X1	T50.4X2	T50.4X3	T50.4X4	T50.4X5	T50.4X6
Spiperone	T43.4X1	T43.4X2	T43.4X3	T43.4X4	T43.4X5	T43.4X6
Spiramycin	T36.3X1	T36.3X2	T36.3X3	T36.3X4	T36.3X5	T36.3X6
Spirapril	T46.4X1	T46.4X2	T46.4X3	T46.4X4	T46.4X5	T46.4X6
Spirilene	T43.591	T43.592	T43.593	T43.594	T43.595	T43.596
Spirit(s) (neutral) **NEC**	T51.0X1	T51.0X2	T51.0X3	T51.0X4	—	—
beverage	T51.0X1	T51.0X2	T51.0X3	T51.0X4	—	—
industrial	T51.0X1	T51.0X2	T51.0X3	T51.0X4	—	—
mineral	T52.0X1	T52.0X2	T52.0X3	T52.0X4	—	—
of salt — *see* Hydrochloric acid						
surgical	T51.0X1	T51.0X2	T51.0X3	T51.0X4	—	—
Spironolactone	T50.0X1	T50.0X2	T50.0X3	T50.0X4	T50.0X5	T50.0X6
Spiroperidol	T43.4X1	T43.4X2	T43.4X3	T43.4X4	T43.4X5	T43.4X6
Sponge, absorbable (gelatin)	T45.7X1	T45.7X2	T45.7X3	T45.7X4	T45.7X5	T45.7X6
Sporostacin	T49.0X1	T49.0X2	T49.0X3	T49.0X4	T49.0X5	T49.0X6
Spray (aerosol)	T65.91	T65.92	T65.93	T65.94	—	—
cosmetic	T65.891	T65.892	T65.893	T65.894	—	—
medicinal NEC	T50.901	T50.902	T50.903	T50.904	T50.905	T50.906
pesticides — *see* Pesticides						
specified content — *see* specific substance						
Spurge flax	T62.2X1	T62.2X2	T62.2X3	T62.2X4	—	—
Spurges	T62.2X1	T62.2X2	T62.2X3	T62.2X4	—	—
Sputum viscosity-lowering drug	T48.4X1	T48.4X2	T48.4X3	T48.4X4	T48.4X5	T48.4X6
Squill	T46.0X1	T46.0X2	T46.0X3	T46.0X4	T46.0X5	T46.0X6
rat poison	T60.4X1	T60.4X2	T60.4X3	T60.4X4	—	—
Squirting cucumber (cathartic)	T47.2X1	T47.2X2	T47.2X3	T47.2X4	T47.2X5	T47.2X6
Stains	T65.6X1	T65.6X2	T65.6X3	T65.6X4	—	—
Stannous fluoride	T49.7X1	T49.7X2	T49.7X3	T49.7X4	T49.7X5	T49.7X6
Stanolone	T38.7X1	T38.7X2	T38.7X3	T38.7X4	T38.7X5	T38.7X6
Stanozolol	T38.7X1	T38.7X2	T38.7X3	T38.7X4	T38.7X5	T38.7X6

Substance	Poisoning, Accidental (unintentional)	Poisoning, Intentional Self-harm	Poisoning, Assault	Poisoning, Undetermined	Adverse Effect	Under-dosing
Staphisagria or stavesacre (pediculicide)	T49.0X1	T49.0X2	T49.0X3	T49.0X4	T49.0X5	T49.0X6
Starch	T50.901	T50.902	T50.903	T50.904	T50.905	T50.906
Stelazine	T43.3X1	T43.3X2	T43.3X3	T43.3X4	T43.3X5	T43.3X6
Stemetil	T43.3X1	T43.3X2	T43.3X3	T43.3X4	T43.3X5	T43.3X6
Stepronin	T48.4X1	T48.4X2	T48.4X3	T48.4X4	T48.4X5	T48.4X6
Sterculia	T47.4X1	T47.4X2	T47.4X3	T47.4X4	T47.4X5	T47.4X6
Sternutator gas	T59.891	T59.892	T59.893	T59.894	—	—
Steroid	T38.0X1	T38.0X2	T38.0X3	T38.0X4	T38.0X5	T38.0X6
anabolic	T38.7X1	T38.7X2	T38.7X3	T38.7X4	T38.7X5	T38.7X6
androgenic	T38.7X1	T38.7X2	T38.7X3	T38.7X4	T38.7X5	T38.7X6
antineoplastic, hormone	T38.7X1	T38.7X2	T38.7X3	T38.7X4	T38.7X5	T38.7X6
estrogen	T38.5X1	T38.5X2	T38.5X3	T38.5X4	T38.5X5	T38.5X6
ENT agent	T49.6X1	T49.6X2	T49.6X3	T49.6X4	T49.6X5	T49.6X6
ophthalmic preparation	T49.5X1	T49.5X2	T49.5X3	T49.5X4	T49.5X5	T49.5X6
topical NEC	T49.0X1	T49.0X2	T49.0X3	T49.0X4	T49.0X5	T49.0X6
Stibine	T56.891	T56.892	T56.893	T56.894	—	—
Stibogluconate	T37.3X1	T37.3X2	T37.3X3	T37.3X4	T37.3X5	T37.3X6
Stibophen	T37.4X1	T37.4X2	T37.4X3	T37.4X4	T37.4X5	T37.4X6
Stilbamidine (isetionate)	T37.3X1	T37.3X2	T37.3X3	T37.3X4	T37.3X5	T37.3X6
Stilbestrol	T38.5X1	T38.5X2	T38.5X3	T38.5X4	T38.5X5	T38.5X6
Stilboestrol	T38.5X1	T38.5X2	T38.5X3	T38.5X4	T38.5X5	T38.5X6
Stimulant						
central nervous system — *see also* Psychostimulant						
analeptics	T50.7X1	T50.7X2	T50.7X3	T50.7X4	T50.7X5	T50.7X6
opiate antagonist	T50.7X1	T50.7X2	T50.7X3	T50.7X4	T50.7X5	T50.7X6
psychotherapeutic NEC — *see also* Psychotherapeutic drug	T43.601	T43.602	T43.603	T43.604	T43.605	T43.606
specified NEC	T43.691	T43.692	T43.693	T43.694	T43.695	T43.696
respiratory	T48.901	T48.902	T48.903	T48.904	T48.905	T48.906
Stone-dissolving drug	T50.901	T50.902	T50.903	T50.904	T50.905	T50.906
Storage battery (cells) (acid)	T54.2X1	T54.2X2	T54.2X3	T54.2X4	—	—
Stovaine	T41.3X1	T41.3X2	T41.3X3	T41.3X4	T41.3X5	T41.3X6
infiltration (subcutaneous)	T41.3X1	T41.3X2	T41.3X3	T41.3X4	T41.3X5	T41.3X6
nerve block (peripheral) (plexus)	T41.3X1	T41.3X2	T41.3X3	T41.3X4	T41.3X5	T41.3X6
spinal	T41.3X1	T41.3X2	T41.3X3	T41.3X4	T41.3X5	T41.3X6
topical (surface)	T41.3X1	T41.3X2	T41.3X3	T41.3X4	T41.3X5	T41.3X6
Stovarsal	T37.8X1	T37.8X2	T37.8X3	T37.8X4	T37.8X5	T37.8X6
Stove gas — *see* Gas, stove						
Stoxil	T49.5X1	T49.5X2	T49.5X3	T49.5X4	T49.5X5	T49.5X6
Stramonium	T48.6X1	T48.6X2	T48.6X3	T48.6X4	T48.6X5	T48.6X6
natural state	T62.2X1	T62.2X2	T62.2X3	T62.2X4	—	—
Streptodornase	T45.3X1	T45.3X2	T45.3X3	T45.3X4	T45.3X5	T45.3X6
Streptoduocin	T36.5X1	T36.5X2	T36.5X3	T36.5X4	T36.5X5	T36.5X6
Streptokinase	T45.611	T45.612	T45.613	T45.614	T45.615	T45.616
Streptomycin (derivative)	T36.5X1	T36.5X2	T36.5X3	T36.5X4	T36.5X5	T36.5X6
Streptonivicin	T36.5X1	T36.5X2	T36.5X3	T36.5X4	T36.5X5	T36.5X6
Streptovarycin	T36.5X1	T36.5X2	T36.5X3	T36.5X4	T36.5X5	T36.5X6
Streptozocin	T45.1X1	T45.1X2	T45.1X3	T45.1X4	T45.1X5	T45.1X6
Streptozotocin	T45.1X1	T45.1X2	T45.1X3	T45.1X4	T45.1X5	T45.1X6
Stripper (paint) (solvent)	T52.8X1	T52.8X2	T52.8X3	T52.8X4	—	—
Strobane	T60.1X1	T60.1X2	T60.1X3	T60.1X4	—	—
Strofantina	T46.0X1	T46.0X2	T46.0X3	T46.0X4	T46.0X5	T46.0X6
Strophanthin (g) (k)	T46.0X1	T46.0X2	T46.0X3	T46.0X4	T46.0X5	T46.0X6
Strophanthus	T46.0X1	T46.0X2	T46.0X3	T46.0X4	T46.0X5	T46.0X6
Strophantin	T46.0X1	T46.0X2	T46.0X3	T46.0X4	T46.0X5	T46.0X6
Strophantin-g	T46.0X1	T46.0X2	T46.0X3	T46.0X4	T46.0X5	T46.0X6
Strychnine (nonmedicinal) (pesticide) (salts)	T65.1X1	T65.1X2	T65.1X3	T65.1X4	—	—
medicinal	T48.291	T48.292	T48.293	T48.294	T48.295	T48.296
Strychnos (ignatii) — *see* Strychnine						
Styramate	T42.8X1	T42.8X2	T42.8X3	T42.8X4	T42.8X5	T42.8X6
Styrene	T65.891	T65.892	T65.893	T65.894	—	—
Succinimide, antiepileptic or anticonvulsant	T42.2X1	T42.2X2	T42.2X3	T42.2X4	T42.2X5	T42.2X6
mercuric — *see* Mercury						
Succinylcholine	T48.1X1	T48.1X2	T48.1X3	T48.1X4	T48.1X5	T48.1X6
Succinylsulfathiazole	T37.0X1	T37.0X2	T37.0X3	T37.0X4	T37.0X5	T37.0X6
Sucralfate	T47.1X1	T47.1X2	T47.1X3	T47.1X4	T47.1X5	T47.1X6
Sucrose	T50.3X1	T50.3X2	T50.3X3	T50.3X4	T50.3X5	T50.3X6
Sufentanil	T40.4X1	T40.4X2	T40.4X3	T40.4X4	T40.4X5	T40.4X6
Sulbactam	T36.0X1	T36.0X2	T36.0X3	T36.0X4	T36.0X5	T36.0X6
Sulbenicillin	T36.0X1	T36.0X2	T36.0X3	T36.0X4	T36.0X5	T36.0X6
Sulbentine	T49.0X1	T49.0X2	T49.0X3	T49.0X4	T49.0X5	T49.0X6
Sulfacetamide	T49.0X1	T49.0X2	T49.0X3	T49.0X4	T49.0X5	T49.0X6
ophthalmic preparation	T49.5X1	T49.5X2	T49.5X3	T49.5X4	T49.5X5	T49.5X6
Sulfachlorpyridazine	T37.0X1	T37.0X2	T37.0X3	T37.0X4	T37.0X5	T37.0X6
Sulfacitine	T37.0X1	T37.0X2	T37.0X3	T37.0X4	T37.0X5	T37.0X6
Sulfadiasulfone sodium	T37.0X1	T37.0X2	T37.0X3	T37.0X4	T37.0X5	T37.0X6

Substance	Poisoning, Accidental (unintentional)	Poisoning, Intentional Self-harm	Poisoning, Assault	Poisoning, Undetermined	Adverse Effect	Under-dosing
Sulfadiazine	T37.0X1	T37.0X2	T37.0X3	T37.0X4	T37.0X5	T37.0X6
silver (topical)	T49.0X1	T49.0X2	T49.0X3	T49.0X4	T49.0X5	T49.0X6
Sulfadimethoxine	T37.0X1	T37.0X2	T37.0X3	T37.0X4	T37.0X5	T37.0X6
Sulfadimidine	T37.0X1	T37.0X2	T37.0X3	T37.0X4	T37.0X5	T37.0X6
Sulfadoxine	T37.0X1	T37.0X2	T37.0X3	T37.0X4	T37.0X5	T37.0X6
with pyrimethamine	T37.2X1	T37.2X2	T37.2X3	T37.2X4	T37.2X5	T37.2X6
Sulfaethidole	T37.0X1	T37.0X2	T37.0X3	T37.0X4	T37.0X5	T37.0X6
Sulfafurazole	T37.0X1	T37.0X2	T37.0X3	T37.0X4	T37.0X5	T37.0X6
Sulfaguanidine	T37.0X1	T37.0X2	T37.0X3	T37.0X4	T37.0X5	T37.0X6
Sulfalene	T37.0X1	T37.0X2	T37.0X3	T37.0X4	T37.0X5	T37.0X6
Sulfaloxate	T37.0X1	T37.0X2	T37.0X3	T37.0X4	T37.0X5	T37.0X6
Sulfaloxic acid	T37.0X1	T37.0X2	T37.0X3	T37.0X4	T37.0X5	T37.0X6
Sulfamazone	T39.2X1	T39.2X2	T39.2X3	T39.2X4	T39.2X5	T39.2X6
Sulfamerazine	T37.0X1	T37.0X2	T37.0X3	T37.0X4	T37.0X5	T37.0X6
Sulfameter	T37.0X1	T37.0X2	T37.0X3	T37.0X4	T37.0X5	T37.0X6
Sulfamethazine	T37.0X1	T37.0X2	T37.0X3	T37.0X4	T37.0X5	T37.0X6
Sulfamethizole	T37.0X1	T37.0X2	T37.0X3	T37.0X4	T37.0X5	T37.0X6
Sulfamethoxazole	T37.0X1	T37.0X2	T37.0X3	T37.0X4	T37.0X5	T37.0X6
with trimethoprim	T36.8X1	T36.8X2	T36.8X3	T36.8X4	T36.8X5	T36.8X6
Sulfamethoxydiazine	T37.0X1	T37.0X2	T37.0X3	T37.0X4	T37.0X5	T37.0X6
Sulfamethoxypyridazine	T37.0X1	T37.0X2	T37.0X3	T37.0X4	T37.0X5	T37.0X6
Sulfamethylthiazole	T37.0X1	T37.0X2	T37.0X3	T37.0X4	T37.0X5	T37.0X6
Sulfametoxydiazine	T37.0X1	T37.0X2	T37.0X3	T37.0X4	T37.0X5	T37.0X6
Sulfamidopyrine	T39.2X1	T39.2X2	T39.2X3	T39.2X4	T39.2X5	T39.2X6
Sulfamonomethoxine	T37.0X1	T37.0X2	T37.0X3	T37.0X4	T37.0X5	T37.0X6
Sulfamoxole	T37.0X1	T37.0X2	T37.0X3	T37.0X4	T37.0X5	T37.0X6
Sulfamylon	T49.0X1	T49.0X2	T49.0X3	T49.0X4	T49.0X5	T49.0X6
Sulfan blue (diagnostic dye)	T50.8X1	T50.8X2	T50.8X3	T50.8X4	T50.8X5	T50.8X6
Sulfanilamide	T37.0X1	T37.0X2	T37.0X3	T37.0X4	T37.0X5	T37.0X6
Sulfanilylguanidine	T37.0X1	T37.0X2	T37.0X3	T37.0X4	T37.0X5	T37.0X6
Sulfaperin	T37.0X1	T37.0X2	T37.0X3	T37.0X4	T37.0X5	T37.0X6
Sulfaphenazole	T37.0X1	T37.0X2	T37.0X3	T37.0X4	T37.0X5	T37.0X6
Sulfaphenylthiazole	T37.0X1	T37.0X2	T37.0X3	T37.0X4	T37.0X5	T37.0X6
Sulfaproxyline	T37.0X1	T37.0X2	T37.0X3	T37.0X4	T37.0X5	T37.0X6
Sulfapyridine	T37.0X1	T37.0X2	T37.0X3	T37.0X4	T37.0X5	T37.0X6
Sulfapyrimidine	T37.0X1	T37.0X2	T37.0X3	T37.0X4	T37.0X5	T37.0X6
Sulfarsphenamine	T37.8X1	T37.8X2	T37.8X3	T37.8X4	T37.8X5	T37.8X6
Sulfasalazine	T37.0X1	T37.0X2	T37.0X3	T37.0X4	T37.0X5	T37.0X6
Sulfasuxidine	T37.0X1	T37.0X2	T37.0X3	T37.0X4	T37.0X5	T37.0X6
Sulfasymazine	T37.0X1	T37.0X2	T37.0X3	T37.0X4	T37.0X5	T37.0X6
Sulfated amylopectin	T47.8X1	T47.8X2	T47.8X3	T47.8X4	T47.8X5	T47.8X6
Sulfathiazole	T37.0X1	T37.0X2	T37.0X3	T37.0X4	T37.0X5	T37.0X6
Sulfatostearate	T49.2X1	T49.2X2	T49.2X3	T49.2X4	T49.2X5	T49.2X6
Sulfinpyrazone	T50.4X1	T50.4X2	T50.4X3	T50.4X4	T50.4X5	T50.4X6
Sulfiram	T49.0X1	T49.0X2	T49.0X3	T49.0X4	T49.0X5	T49.0X6
Sulfisomidine	T37.0X1	T37.0X2	T37.0X3	T37.0X4	T37.0X5	T37.0X6
Sulfisoxazole	T37.0X1	T37.0X2	T37.0X3	T37.0X4	T37.0X5	T37.0X6
ophthalmic preparation	T49.5X1	T49.5X2	T49.5X3	T49.5X4	T49.5X5	T49.5X6
Sulfobromophthalein (sodium)	T50.8X1	T50.8X2	T50.8X3	T50.8X4	T50.8X5	T50.8X6
Sulfobromphthalein	T50.8X1	T50.8X2	T50.8X3	T50.8X4	T50.8X5	T50.8X6
Sulfogaiacol	T48.4X1	T48.4X2	T48.4X3	T48.4X4	T48.4X5	T48.4X6
Sulfomyxin	T36.8X1	T36.8X2	T36.8X3	T36.8X4	T36.8X5	T36.8X6
Sulfonal	T42.6X1	T42.6X2	T42.6X3	T42.6X4	T42.6X5	T42.6X6
Sulfonamide NEC	T37.0X1	T37.0X2	T37.0X3	T37.0X4	T37.0X5	T37.0X6
eye	T49.5X1	T49.5X2	T49.5X3	T49.5X4	T49.5X5	T49.5X6
Sulfonazide	T37.1X1	T37.1X2	T37.1X3	T37.1X4	T37.1X5	T37.1X6
Sulfones	T37.1X1	T37.1X2	T37.1X3	T37.1X4	T37.1X5	T37.1X6
Sulfonethylmethane	T42.6X1	T42.6X2	T42.6X3	T42.6X4	T42.6X5	T42.6X6
Sulfonmethane	T42.6X1	T42.6X2	T42.6X3	T42.6X4	T42.6X5	T42.6X6
Sulfonphthal, sulfonphthol	T50.8X1	T50.8X2	T50.8X3	T50.8X4	T50.8X5	T50.8X6
Sulfonylurea derivatives, oral	T38.3X1	T38.3X2	T38.3X3	T38.3X4	T38.3X5	T38.3X6
Sulforidazine	T43.3X1	T43.3X2	T43.3X3	T43.3X4	T43.3X5	T43.3X6
Sulfoxone	T37.1X1	T37.1X2	T37.1X3	T37.1X4	T37.1X5	T37.1X6
Sulfuric acid	T54.2X1	T54.2X2	T54.2X3	T54.2X4	—	—
Sulfur, sulfurated, sulfuric, sulfurous, sulfuryl (compounds NEC) (medicinal)	T49.4X1	T49.4X2	T49.4X3	T49.4X4	T49.4X5	T49.4X6
acid	T54.2X1	T54.2X2	T54.2X3	T54.2X4	—	—
dioxide (gas)	T59.1X1	T59.1X2	T59.1X3	T59.1X4	—	—
ether — see Ether(s)						
hydrogen	T59.6X1	T59.6X2	T59.6X3	T59.6X4	—	—
medicinal (keratolytic) (ointment) NEC	T49.4X1	T49.4X2	T49.4X3	T49.4X4	T49.4X5	T49.4X6
ointment	T49.0X1	T49.0X2	T49.0X3	T49.0X4	T49.0X5	T49.0X6
pesticide (vapor)	T60.91	T60.92	T60.93	T60.94	—	—
vapor NEC	T59.891	T59.892	T59.893	T59.894	—	—
Sulglicotide	T47.1X1	T47.1X2	T47.1X3	T47.1X4	T47.1X5	T47.1X6
Sulindac	T39.391	T39.392	T39.393	T39.394	T39.395	T39.396
Sulisatin	T47.2X1	T47.2X2	T47.2X3	T47.2X4	T47.2X5	T47.2X6
Sulisobenzone	T49.3X1	T49.3X2	T49.3X3	T49.3X4	T49.3X5	T49.3X6
Sulkowitch's reagent	T50.8X1	T50.8X2	T50.8X3	T50.8X4	T50.8X5	T50.8X6
Sulmetozine	T44.3X1	T44.3X2	T44.3X3	T44.3X4	T44.3X5	T44.3X6
Suloctidil	T46.7X1	T46.7X2	T46.7X3	T46.7X4	T46.7X5	T46.7X6
Sulph- — see also Sulf-						
Sulphadiazine	T37.0X1	T37.0X2	T37.0X3	T37.0X4	T37.0X5	T37.0X6
Sulphadimethoxine	T37.0X1	T37.0X2	T37.0X3	T37.0X4	T37.0X5	T37.0X6
Sulphadimidine	T37.0X1	T37.0X2	T37.0X3	T37.0X4	T37.0X5	T37.0X6
Sulphadione	T37.1X1	T37.1X2	T37.1X3	T37.1X4	T37.1X5	T37.1X6
Sulphafurazole	T37.0X1	T37.0X2	T37.0X3	T37.0X4	T37.0X5	T37.0X6
Sulphamethizole	T37.0X1	T37.0X2	T37.0X3	T37.0X4	T37.0X5	T37.0X6
Sulphamethoxazole	T37.0X1	T37.0X2	T37.0X3	T37.0X4	T37.0X5	T37.0X6
Sulphan blue	T50.8X1	T50.8X2	T50.8X3	T50.8X4	T50.8X5	T50.8X6
Sulphaphenazole	T37.0X1	T37.0X2	T37.0X3	T37.0X4	T37.0X5	T37.0X6
Sulphapyridine	T37.0X1	T37.0X2	T37.0X3	T37.0X4	T37.0X5	T37.0X6
Sulphasalazine	T37.0X1	T37.0X2	T37.0X3	T37.0X4	T37.0X5	T37.0X6
Sulphinpyrazone	T50.4X1	T50.4X2	T50.4X3	T50.4X4	T50.4X5	T50.4X6
Sulpiride	T43.591	T43.592	T43.593	T43.594	T43.595	T43.596
Sulprostone	T48.0X1	T48.0X2	T48.0X3	T48.0X4	T48.0X5	T48.0X6
Sulpyrine	T39.2X1	T39.2X2	T39.2X3	T39.2X4	T39.2X5	T39.2X6
Sultamicillin	T36.0X1	T36.0X2	T36.0X3	T36.0X4	T36.0X5	T36.0X6
Sulthiame	T42.6X1	T42.6X2	T42.6X3	T42.6X4	T42.6X5	T42.6X6
Sultiame	T42.6X1	T42.6X2	T42.6X3	T42.6X4	T42.6X5	T42.6X6
Sultopride	T43.591	T43.592	T43.593	T43.594	T43.595	T43.596
Sumatriptan	T39.8X1	T39.8X2	T39.8X3	T39.8X4	T39.8X5	T39.8X6
Sunflower seed oil	T46.6X1	T46.6X2	T46.6X3	T46.6X4	T46.6X5	T46.6X6
Superinone	T48.4X1	T48.4X2	T48.4X3	T48.4X4	T48.4X5	T48.4X6
Suprofen	T39.311	T39.312	T39.313	T39.314	T39.315	T39.316
Suramin (sodium)	T37.4X1	T37.4X2	T37.4X3	T37.4X4	T37.4X5	T37.4X6
Surfacaine	T41.3X1	T41.3X2	T41.3X3	T41.3X4	T41.3X5	T41.3X6
Surital	T41.1X1	T41.1X2	T41.1X3	T41.1X4	T41.1X5	T41.1X6
Sutilains	T45.3X1	T45.3X2	T45.3X3	T45.3X4	T45.3X5	T45.3X6
Suxamethonium (chloride)	T48.1X1	T48.1X2	T48.1X3	T48.1X4	T48.1X5	T48.1X6
Suxethonium (chloride)	T48.1X1	T48.1X2	T48.1X3	T48.1X4	T48.1X5	T48.1X6
Suxibuzone	T39.2X1	T39.2X2	T39.2X3	T39.2X4	T39.2X5	T39.2X6
Sweetener	T50.901	T50.902	T50.903	T50.904	T50.905	T50.906
Sweet niter spirit	T46.3X1	T46.3X2	T46.3X3	T46.3X4	T46.3X5	T46.3X6
Sweet oil (birch)	T49.3X1	T49.3X2	T49.3X3	T49.3X4	T49.3X5	T49.3X6
Sym-dichloroethyl ether	T53.6X1	T53.6X2	T53.6X3	T53.6X4	—	—
Sympatholytic NEC	T44.8X1	T44.8X2	T44.8X3	T44.8X4	T44.8X5	T44.8X6
haloalkylamine	T44.8X1	T44.8X2	T44.8X3	T44.8X4	T44.8X5	T44.8X6
Sympathomimetic NEC	T44.901	T44.902	T44.903	T44.904	T44.905	T44.906
anti-common-cold	T48.5X1	T48.5X2	T48.5X3	T48.5X4	T48.5X5	T48.5X6
bronchodilator	T48.6X1	T48.6X2	T48.6X3	T48.6X4	T48.6X5	T48.6X6
specified NEC	T44.991	T44.992	T44.993	T44.994	T44.995	T44.996
Synagis	T50.B91	T50.B92	T50.B93	T50.B94	T50.B95	T50.B96
Synalar	T49.0X1	T49.0X2	T49.0X3	T49.0X4	T49.0X5	T49.0X6
Synthroid	T38.1X1	T38.1X2	T38.1X3	T38.1X4	T38.1X5	T38.1X6
Syntocinon	T48.0X1	T48.0X2	T48.0X3	T48.0X4	T48.0X5	T48.0X6
Syrosingopine	T46.5X1	T46.5X2	T46.5X3	T46.5X4	T46.5X5	T46.5X6
Systemic drug	T45.91	T45.92	T45.93	T45.94	T45.95	T45.96
specified NEC	T45.8X1	T45.8X2	T45.8X3	T45.8X4	T45.8X5	T45.8X6
Tablets — see also specified substance	T50.901	T50.902	T50.903	T50.904	T50.905	T50.906
Tace	T38.5X1	T38.5X2	T38.5X3	T38.5X4	T38.5X5	T38.5X6
Tacrine	T44.0X1	T44.0X2	T44.0X3	T44.0X4	T44.0X5	T44.0X6
Tadalafil	T46.7X1	T46.7X2	T46.7X3	T46.7X4	T46.7X5	T46.7X6
Talampicillin	T36.0X1	T36.0X2	T36.0X3	T36.0X4	T36.0X5	T36.0X6
Talbutal	T42.3X1	T42.3X2	T42.3X3	T42.3X4	T42.3X5	T42.3X6
Talc powder	T49.3X1	T49.3X2	T49.3X3	T49.3X4	T49.3X5	T49.3X6
Talcum	T49.3X1	T49.3X2	T49.3X3	T49.3X4	T49.3X5	T49.3X6
Taleranol	T38.6X1	T38.6X2	T38.6X3	T38.6X4	T38.6X5	T38.6X6
Tamoxifen	T38.6X1	T38.6X2	T38.6X3	T38.6X4	T38.6X5	T38.6X6
Tamsulosin	T44.6X1	T44.6X2	T44.6X3	T44.6X4	T44.6X5	T44.6X6
Tandearil, tanderil	T39.2X1	T39.2X2	T39.2X3	T39.2X4	T39.2X5	T39.2X6
Tannic acid	T49.2X1	T49.2X2	T49.2X3	T49.2X4	T49.2X5	T49.2X6
medicinal (astringent)	T49.2X1	T49.2X2	T49.2X3	T49.2X4	T49.2X5	T49.2X6
Tannin — see Tannic acid						
Tansy	T62.2X1	T62.2X2	T62.2X3	T62.2X4	—	—
TAO	T36.3X1	T36.3X2	T36.3X3	T36.3X4	T36.3X5	T36.3X6
Tapazole	T38.2X1	T38.2X2	T38.2X3	T38.2X4	T38.2X5	T38.2X6
Taractan	T43.591	T43.592	T43.593	T43.594	T43.595	T43.596
Tarantula (venomous)	T63.321	T63.322	T63.323	T63.324	—	—
Tartar emetic	T37.8X1	T37.8X2	T37.8X3	T37.8X4	T37.8X5	T37.8X6
Tartaric acid	T65.891	T65.892	T65.893	T65.894	—	—
Tartrated antimony (anti-infective)	T37.8X1	T37.8X2	T37.8X3	T37.8X4	T37.8X5	T37.8X6
Tartrate, laxative	T47.4X1	T47.4X2	T47.4X3	T47.4X4	T47.4X5	T47.4X6
Tar NEC	T52.0X1	T52.0X2	T52.0X3	T52.0X4	—	—
camphor	T60.1X1	T60.1X2	T60.1X3	T60.1X4	—	—
distillate	T49.1X1	T49.1X2	T49.1X3	T49.1X4	T49.1X5	T49.1X6
fumes	T59.891	T59.892	T59.893	T59.894	—	—
medicinal	T49.1X1	T49.1X2	T49.1X3	T49.1X4	T49.1X5	T49.1X6
ointment	T49.1X1	T49.1X2	T49.1X3	T49.1X4	T49.1X5	T49.1X6

Table of Drugs and Chemicals

Tauromustine — Thonzylamine

Substance	Poisoning, Accidental (unintentional)	Poisoning, Intentional Self-harm	Poisoning, Assault	Poisoning, Undetermined	Adverse Effect	Underdosing
Tauromustine	T45.1X1	T45.1X2	T45.1X3	T45.1X4	T45.1X5	T45.1X6
TCA — *see* Trichloroacetic acid						
TCDD	T53.7X1	T53.7X2	T53.7X3	T53.7X4	—	—
TDI (vapor)	T65.0X1	T65.0X2	T65.0X3	T65.0X4	—	—
Tear						
gas	T59.3X1	T59.3X2	T59.3X3	T59.3X4	—	—
solution	T49.5X1	T49.5X2	T49.5X3	T49.5X4	T49.5X5	T49.5X6
Teclothiazide	T50.2X1	T50.2X2	T50.2X3	T50.2X4	T50.2X5	T50.2X6
Teclozan	T37.3X1	T37.3X2	T37.3X3	T37.3X4	T37.3X5	T37.3X6
Tegafur	T45.1X1	T45.1X2	T45.1X3	T45.1X4	T45.1X5	T45.1X6
Tegretol	T42.1X1	T42.1X2	T42.1X3	T42.1X4	T42.1X5	T42.1X6
Teicoplanin	T36.8X1	T36.8X2	T36.8X3	T36.8X4	T36.8X5	T36.8X6
Telepaque	T50.8X1	T50.8X2	T50.8X3	T50.8X4	T50.8X5	T50.8X6
Tellurium	T56.891	T56.892	T56.893	T56.894	—	—
fumes	T56.891	T56.892	T56.893	T56.894	—	—
TEM	T45.1X1	T45.1X2	T45.1X3	T45.1X4	T45.1X5	T45.1X6
Temazepam	T42.4X1	T42.4X2	T42.4X3	T42.4X4	T42.4X5	T42.4X6
Temocillin	T36.0X1	T36.0X2	T36.0X3	T36.0X4	T36.0X5	T36.0X6
Tenamfetamine	T43.621	T43.622	T43.623	T43.624	T43.625	T43.626
Teniposide	T45.1X1	T45.1X2	T45.1X3	T45.1X4	T45.1X5	T45.1X6
Tenitramine	T46.3X1	T46.3X2	T46.3X3	T46.3X4	T46.3X5	T46.3X6
Tenoglicin	T48.4X1	T48.4X2	T48.4X3	T48.4X4	T48.4X5	T48.4X6
Tenonitrozole	T37.3X1	T37.3X2	T37.3X3	T37.3X4	T37.3X5	T37.3X6
Tenoxicam	T39.391	T39.392	T39.393	T39.394	T39.395	T39.396
TEPA	T45.1X1	T45.1X2	T45.1X3	T45.1X4	T45.1X5	T45.1X6
TEPP	T60.0X1	T60.0X2	T60.0X3	T60.0X4	—	—
Teprotide	T46.5X1	T46.5X2	T46.5X3	T46.5X4	T46.5X5	T46.5X6
Terazosin	T44.6X1	T44.6X2	T44.6X3	T44.6X4	T44.6X5	T44.6X6
Terbufos	T60.0X1	T60.0X2	T60.0X3	T60.0X4	—	—
Terbutaline	T48.6X1	T48.6X2	T48.6X3	T48.6X4	T48.6X5	T48.6X6
Terconazole	T49.0X1	T49.0X2	T49.0X3	T49.0X4	T49.0X5	T49.0X6
Terfenadine	T45.0X1	T45.0X2	T45.0X3	T45.0X4	T45.0X5	T45.0X6
Teriparatide (acetate)	T50.991	T50.992	T50.993	T50.994	T50.995	T50.996
Terizidone	T37.1X1	T37.1X2	T37.1X3	T37.1X4	T37.1X5	T37.1X6
Terlipressin	T38.891	T38.892	T38.893	T38.894	T38.895	T38.896
Terodiline	T46.3X1	T46.3X2	T46.3X3	T46.3X4	T46.3X5	T46.3X6
Teroxalene	T37.4X1	T37.4X2	T37.4X3	T37.4X4	T37.4X5	T37.4X6
Terpin (cis) **hydrate**	T48.4X1	T48.4X2	T48.4X3	T48.4X4	T48.4X5	T48.4X6
Terramycin	T36.4X1	T36.4X2	T36.4X3	T36.4X4	T36.4X5	T36.4X6
Tertatolol	T44.7X1	T44.7X2	T44.7X3	T44.7X4	T44.7X5	T44.7X6
Tessalon	T48.3X1	T48.3X2	T48.3X3	T48.3X4	T48.3X5	T48.3X6
Testolactone	T38.7X1	T38.7X2	T38.7X3	T38.7X4	T38.7X5	T38.7X6
Testosterone	T38.7X1	T38.7X2	T38.7X3	T38.7X4	T38.7X5	T38.7X6
Tetanus toxoid or vaccine	T50.A91	T50.A92	T50.A93	T50.A94	T50.A95	T50.A96
antitoxin	T50.Z11	T50.Z12	T50.Z13	T50.Z14	T50.Z15	T50.Z16
immune globulin (human)	T50.Z11	T50.Z12	T50.Z13	T50.Z14	T50.Z15	T50.Z16
toxoid	T50.A91	T50.A92	T50.A93	T50.A94	T50.A95	T50.A96
with diphtheria toxoid	T50.A21	T50.A22	T50.A23	T50.A24	T50.A25	T50.A26
with pertussis	T50.A11	T50.A12	T50.A13	T50.A14	T50.A15	T50.A16
Tetrabenazine	T43.591	T43.592	T43.593	T43.594	T43.595	T43.596
Tetracaine	T41.3X1	T41.3X2	T41.3X3	T41.3X4	T41.3X5	T41.3X6
nerve block (peripheral) (plexus)	T41.3X1	T41.3X2	T41.3X3	T41.3X4	T41.3X5	T41.3X6
regional	T41.3X1	T41.3X2	T41.3X3	T41.3X4	T41.3X5	T41.3X6
spinal	T41.3X1	T41.3X2	T41.3X3	T41.3X4	T41.3X5	T41.3X6
Tetrachlorethylene — *see* Tetrachloroethylene						
Tetrachlormethiazide	T50.2X1	T50.2X2	T50.2X3	T50.2X4	T50.2X5	T50.2X6
Tetrachloroethane	T53.6X1	T53.6X2	T53.6X3	T53.6X4	—	—
vapor	T53.6X1	T53.6X2	T53.6X3	T53.6X4	—	—
paint or varnish	T53.6X1	T53.6X2	T53.6X3	T53.6X4	—	—
Tetrachloroethylene (liquid)	T53.3X1	T53.3X2	T53.3X3	T53.3X4	—	—
medicinal	T37.4X1	T37.4X2	T37.4X3	T37.4X4	T37.4X5	T37.4X6
vapor	T53.3X1	T53.3X2	T53.3X3	T53.3X4	—	—
Tetrachloromethane — *see* Carbon tetrachloride						
Tetracosactide	T38.811	T38.812	T38.813	T38.814	T38.815	T38.816
Tetracosactrin	T38.811	T38.812	T38.813	T38.814	T38.815	T38.816
Tetracycline	T36.4X1	T36.4X2	T36.4X3	T36.4X4	T36.4X5	T36.4X6
ophthalmic preparation	T49.5X1	T49.5X2	T49.5X3	T49.5X4	T49.5X5	T49.5X6
topical NEC	T49.0X1	T49.0X2	T49.0X3	T49.0X4	T49.0X5	T49.0X6
Tetradifon	T60.8X1	T60.8X2	T60.8X3	T60.8X4	—	—
Tetradotoxin	T61.771	T61.772	T61.773	T61.774	—	—
Tetraethyl						
lead	T56.0X1	T56.0X2	T56.0X3	T56.0X4	—	—
pyrophosphate	T60.0X1	T60.0X2	T60.0X3	T60.0X4	—	—
Tetraethylammonium chloride	T44.2X1	T44.2X2	T44.2X3	T44.2X4	T44.2X5	T44.2X6
Tetraethylthiuram disulfide	T50.6X1	T50.6X2	T50.6X3	T50.6X4	T50.6X5	T50.6X6
Tetrahydroaminoacridine	T44.0X1	T44.0X2	T44.0X3	T44.0X4	T44.0X5	T44.0X6
Tetrahydrocannabinol	T40.7X1	T40.7X2	T40.7X3	T40.7X4	T40.7X5	T40.7X6
Tetrahydrofuran	T52.8X1	T52.8X2	T52.8X3	T52.8X4	—	—
Tetrahydronaphthalene	T52.8X1	T52.8X2	T52.8X3	T52.8X4	—	—
Tetrahydrozoline	T49.5X1	T49.5X2	T49.5X3	T49.5X4	T49.5X5	T49.5X6
Tetralin	T52.8X1	T52.8X2	T52.8X3	T52.8X4	—	—
Tetramethrin	T60.2X1	T60.2X2	T60.2X3	T60.2X4	—	—
Tetramethylthiuram (disulfide) NEC	T60.3X1	T60.3X2	T60.3X3	T60.3X4	—	—
medicinal	T49.0X1	T49.0X2	T49.0X3	T49.0X4	T49.0X5	T49.0X6
Tetramisole	T37.4X1	T37.4X2	T37.4X3	T37.4X4	T37.4X5	T37.4X6
Tetranicotinoyl fructose	T46.7X1	T46.7X2	T46.7X3	T46.7X4	T46.7X5	T46.7X6
Tetrazepam	T42.4X1	T42.4X2	T42.4X3	T42.4X4	T42.4X5	T42.4X6
Tetronal	T42.6X1	T42.6X2	T42.6X3	T42.6X4	T42.6X5	T42.6X6
Tetryl	T65.3X1	T65.3X2	T65.3X3	T65.3X4	—	—
Tetrylammonium chloride	T44.2X1	T44.2X2	T44.2X3	T44.2X4	T44.2X5	T44.2X6
Tetryzoline	T49.5X1	T49.5X2	T49.5X3	T49.5X4	T49.5X5	T49.5X6
Thalidomide	T45.1X1	T45.1X2	T45.1X3	T45.1X4	T45.1X5	T45.1X6
Thallium (compounds) (dust) NEC	T56.811	T56.812	T56.813	T56.814	—	—
pesticide	T60.4X1	T60.4X2	T60.4X3	T60.4X4	—	—
THC	T40.7X1	T40.7X2	T40.7X3	T40.7X4	T40.7X5	T40.7X6
Thebacon	T48.3X1	T48.3X2	T48.3X3	T48.3X4	T48.3X5	T48.3X6
Thebaine	T40.2X1	T40.2X2	T40.2X3	T40.2X4	T40.2X5	T40.2X6
Thenoic acid	T49.6X1	T49.6X2	T49.6X3	T49.6X4	T49.6X5	T49.6X6
Thenyldiamine	T45.0X1	T45.0X2	T45.0X3	T45.0X4	T45.0X5	T45.0X6
Theobromine (calcium salicylate)	T48.6X1	T48.6X2	T48.6X3	T48.6X4	T48.6X5	T48.6X6
sodium salicylate	T48.6X1	T48.6X2	T48.6X3	T48.6X4	T48.6X5	T48.6X6
Theophyllamine	T48.6X1	T48.6X2	T48.6X3	T48.6X4	T48.6X5	T48.6X6
Theophylline	T48.6X1	T48.6X2	T48.6X3	T48.6X4	T48.6X5	T48.6X6
aminobenzoic acid	T48.6X1	T48.6X2	T48.6X3	T48.6X4	T48.6X5	T48.6X6
ethylenediamine	T48.6X1	T48.6X2	T48.6X3	T48.6X4	T48.6X5	T48.6X6
piperazine	T48.6X1	T48.6X2	T48.6X3	T48.6X4	T48.6X5	T48.6X6
p-amino-benzoate						
Thiabendazole	T37.4X1	T37.4X2	T37.4X3	T37.4X4	T37.4X5	T37.4X6
Thialbarbital	T41.1X1	T41.1X2	T41.1X3	T41.1X4	T41.1X5	T41.1X6
Thiamazole	T38.2X1	T38.2X2	T38.2X3	T38.2X4	T38.2X5	T38.2X6
Thiambutosine	T37.1X1	T37.1X2	T37.1X3	T37.1X4	T37.1X5	T37.1X6
Thiamine	T45.2X1	T45.2X2	T45.2X3	T45.2X4	T45.2X5	T45.2X6
Thiamphenicol	T36.2X1	T36.2X2	T36.2X3	T36.2X4	T36.2X5	T36.2X6
Thiamylal	T41.1X1	T41.1X2	T41.1X3	T41.1X4	T41.1X5	T41.1X6
sodium	T41.1X1	T41.1X2	T41.1X3	T41.1X4	T41.1X5	T41.1X6
Thiazesim	T43.291	T43.292	T43.293	T43.294	T43.295	T43.296
Thiazides (diuretics)	T50.2X1	T50.2X2	T50.2X3	T50.2X4	T50.2X5	T50.2X6
Thiazinamium metilsulfate	T43.3X1	T43.3X2	T43.3X3	T43.3X4	T43.3X5	T43.3X6
Thiethylperazine	T43.3X1	T43.3X2	T43.3X3	T43.3X4	T43.3X5	T43.3X6
Thimerosal	T49.0X1	T49.0X2	T49.0X3	T49.0X4	T49.0X5	T49.0X6
ophthalmic preparation	T49.5X1	T49.5X2	T49.5X3	T49.5X4	T49.5X5	T49.5X6
Thioacetazone	T37.1X1	T37.1X2	T37.1X3	T37.1X4	T37.1X5	T37.1X6
with isoniazid	T37.1X1	T37.1X2	T37.1X3	T37.1X4	T37.1X5	T37.1X6
Thiobarbital sodium	T41.1X1	T41.1X2	T41.1X3	T41.1X4	T41.1X5	T41.1X6
Thiobarbiturate anesthetic	T41.1X1	T41.1X2	T41.1X3	T41.1X4	T41.1X5	T41.1X6
Thiobismol	T37.8X1	T37.8X2	T37.8X3	T37.8X4	T37.8X5	T37.8X6
Thiobutabarbital sodium	T41.1X1	T41.1X2	T41.1X3	T41.1X4	T41.1X5	T41.1X6
Thiocarbamate (insecticide)	T60.0X1	T60.0X2	T60.0X3	T60.0X4	—	—
Thiocarbamide	T38.2X1	T38.2X2	T38.2X3	T38.2X4	T38.2X5	T38.2X6
Thiocarbarsone	T37.8X1	T37.8X2	T37.8X3	T37.8X4	T37.8X5	T37.8X6
Thiocarlide	T37.1X1	T37.1X2	T37.1X3	T37.1X4	T37.1X5	T37.1X6
Thioctamide	T50.991	T50.992	T50.993	T50.994	T50.995	T50.996
Thioctic acid	T50.991	T50.992	T50.993	T50.994	T50.995	T50.996
Thiofos	T60.0X1	T60.0X2	T60.0X3	T60.0X4	—	—
Thioglycolate	T49.4X1	T49.4X2	T49.4X3	T49.4X4	T49.4X5	T49.4X6
Thioglycolic acid	T65.891	T65.892	T65.893	T65.894	—	—
Thioguanine	T45.1X1	T45.1X2	T45.1X3	T45.1X4	T45.1X5	T45.1X6
Thiomercaptomerin	T50.2X1	T50.2X2	T50.2X3	T50.2X4	T50.2X5	T50.2X6
Thiomerin	T50.2X1	T50.2X2	T50.2X3	T50.2X4	T50.2X5	T50.2X6
Thiomersal	T49.0X1	T49.0X2	T49.0X3	T49.0X4	T49.0X5	T49.0X6
Thionazin	T60.0X1	T60.0X2	T60.0X3	T60.0X4	—	—
Thiopental (sodium)	T41.1X1	T41.1X2	T41.1X3	T41.1X4	T41.1X5	T41.1X6
Thiopentone (sodium)	T41.1X1	T41.1X2	T41.1X3	T41.1X4	T41.1X5	T41.1X6
Thiopropazate	T43.3X1	T43.3X2	T43.3X3	T43.3X4	T43.3X5	T43.3X6
Thioproperazine	T43.3X1	T43.3X2	T43.3X3	T43.3X4	T43.3X5	T43.3X6
Thioridazine	T43.3X1	T43.3X2	T43.3X3	T43.3X4	T43.3X5	T43.3X6
Thiosinamine	T49.3X1	T49.3X2	T49.3X3	T49.3X4	T49.3X5	T49.3X6
Thiotepa	T45.1X1	T45.1X2	T45.1X3	T45.1X4	T45.1X5	T45.1X6
Thiothixene	T43.4X1	T43.4X2	T43.4X3	T43.4X4	T43.4X5	T43.4X6
Thiouracil (benzyl) (methyl) (propyl)	T38.2X1	T38.2X2	T38.2X3	T38.2X4	T38.2X5	T38.2X6
Thiourea	T38.2X1	T38.2X2	T38.2X3	T38.2X4	T38.2X5	T38.2X6
Thiphenamil	T44.3X1	T44.3X2	T44.3X3	T44.3X4	T44.3X5	T44.3X6
Thiram	T60.3X1	T60.3X2	T60.3X3	T60.3X4	—	—
medicinal	T49.2X1	T49.2X2	T49.2X3	T49.2X4	—	T49.2X6
Thonzylamine (systemic)	T45.0X1	T45.0X2	T45.0X3	T45.0X4	T45.0X5	T45.0X6
mucosal decongestant	T48.5X1	T48.5X2	T48.5X3	T48.5X4	T48.5X5	T48.5X6

Substance	Poisoning, Accidental (unintentional)	Poisoning, Intentional Self-harm	Poisoning, Assault	Poisoning, Undetermined	Adverse Effect	Under-dosing
Thorazine	T43.3X1	T43.3X2	T43.3X3	T43.3X4	T43.3X5	T43.3X6
Thorium dioxide suspension	T50.8X1	T50.8X2	T50.8X3	T50.8X4	T50.8X5	T50.8X6
Thornapple	T62.2X1	T62.2X2	T62.2X3	T62.2X4	—	—
Throat drug NEC	T49.6X1	T49.6X2	T49.6X3	T49.6X4	T49.6X5	T49.6X6
Thrombin	T45.7X1	T45.7X2	T45.7X3	T45.7X4	T45.7X5	T45.7X6
Thrombolysin	T45.611	T45.612	T45.613	T45.614	T45.615	T45.616
Thromboplastin	T45.7X1	T45.7X2	T45.7X3	T45.7X4	T45.7X5	T45.7X6
Thurfyl nicotinate	T46.7X1	T46.7X2	T46.7X3	T46.7X4	T46.7X5	T46.7X6
Thymol	T49.0X1	T49.0X2	T49.0X3	T49.0X4	T49.0X5	T49.0X6
Thymopentin	T37.5X1	T37.5X2	T37.5X3	T37.5X4	T37.5X5	T37.5X6
Thymoxamine	T46.7X1	T46.7X2	T46.7X3	T46.7X4	T46.7X5	T46.7X6
Thymus extract	T38.891	T38.892	T38.893	T38.894	T38.895	T38.896
Thyreotrophic hormone	T38.811	T38.812	T38.813	T38.814	T38.815	T38.816
Thyroglobulin	T38.1X1	T38.1X2	T38.1X3	T38.1X4	T38.1X5	T38.1X6
Thyroid (hormone)	T38.1X1	T38.1X2	T38.1X3	T38.1X4	T38.1X5	T38.1X6
Thyrolar	T38.1X1	T38.1X2	T38.1X3	T38.1X4	T38.1X5	T38.1X6
Thyrotrophin	T38.811	T38.812	T38.813	T38.814	T38.815	T38.816
Thyrotropic hormone	T38.811	T38.812	T38.813	T38.814	T38.815	T38.816
Thyroxine	T38.1X1	T38.1X2	T38.1X3	T38.1X4	T38.1X5	T38.1X6
Tiabendazole	T37.4X1	T37.4X2	T37.4X3	T37.4X4	T37.4X5	T37.4X6
Tiamizide	T50.2X1	T50.2X2	T50.2X3	T50.2X4	T50.2X5	T50.2X6
Tianeptine	T43.291	T43.292	T43.293	T43.294	T43.295	T43.296
Tiapamil	T46.1X1	T46.1X2	T46.1X3	T46.1X4	T46.1X5	T46.1X6
Tiapride	T43.591	T43.592	T43.593	T43.594	T43.595	T43.596
Tiaprofenic acid	T39.311	T39.312	T39.313	T39.314	T39.315	T39.316
Tiaramide	T39.8X1	T39.8X2	T39.8X3	T39.8X4	T39.8X5	T39.8X6
Ticarcillin	T36.0X1	T36.0X2	T36.0X3	T36.0X4	T36.0X5	T36.0X6
Ticlatone	T49.0X1	T49.0X2	T49.0X3	T49.0X4	T49.0X5	T49.0X6
Ticlopidine	T45.521	T45.522	T45.523	T45.524	T45.525	T45.526
Ticrynafen	T50.1X1	T50.1X2	T50.1X3	T50.1X4	T50.1X5	T50.1X6
Tidiacic	T50.991	T50.992	T50.993	T50.994	T50.995	T50.996
Tiemonium	T44.3X1	T44.3X2	T44.3X3	T44.3X4	T44.3X5	T44.3X6
iodide	T44.3X1	T44.3X2	T44.3X3	T44.3X4	T44.3X5	T44.3X6
Tienilic acid	T50.1X1	T50.1X2	T50.1X3	T50.1X4	T50.1X5	T50.1X6
Tifenamil	T44.3X1	T44.3X2	T44.3X3	T44.3X4	T44.3X5	T44.3X6
Tigan	T45.0X1	T45.0X2	T45.0X3	T45.0X4	T45.0X5	T45.0X6
Tigloidine	T44.3X1	T44.3X2	T44.3X3	T44.3X4	T44.3X5	T44.3X6
Tilactase	T47.5X1	T47.5X2	T47.5X3	T47.5X4	T47.5X5	T47.5X6
Tiletamine	T41.291	T41.292	T41.293	T41.294	T41.295	T41.296
Tilidine	T40.4X1	T40.4X2	T40.4X3	T40.4X4	—	—
Timepidium bromide	T44.3X1	T44.3X2	T44.3X3	T44.3X4	T44.3X5	T44.3X6
Timiperone	T43.4X1	T43.4X2	T43.4X3	T43.4X4	T43.4X5	T43.4X6
Timolol	T44.7X1	T44.7X2	T44.7X3	T44.7X4	T44.7X5	T44.7X6
Tincture, iodine — see Iodine						
Tindal	T43.3X1	T43.3X2	T43.3X3	T43.3X4	T43.3X5	T43.3X6
Tinidazole	T37.3X1	T37.3X2	T37.3X3	T37.3X4	T37.3X5	T37.3X6
Tinoridine	T39.8X1	T39.8X2	T39.8X3	T39.8X4	T39.8X5	T39.8X6
Tin (chloride) (dust) (oxide)	T56.6X1	T56.6X2	T56.6X3	T56.6X4	—	—
NEC anti-infectives	T37.8X1	T37.8X2	T37.8X3	T37.8X4	T37.8X5	T37.8X6
Tiocarlide	T37.1X1	T37.1X2	T37.1X3	T37.1X4	T37.1X5	T37.1X6
Tioclomarol	T45.511	T45.512	T45.513	T45.514	T45.515	T45.516
Tioconazole	T49.0X1	T49.0X2	T49.0X3	T49.0X4	T49.0X5	T49.0X6
Tioguanine	T45.1X1	T45.1X2	T45.1X3	T45.1X4	T45.1X5	T45.1X6
Tiopronin	T50.991	T50.992	T50.993	T50.994	T50.995	T50.996
Tiotixene	T43.4X1	T43.4X2	T43.4X3	T43.4X4	T43.4X5	T43.4X6
Tioxolone	T49.4X1	T49.4X2	T49.4X3	T49.4X4	T49.4X5	T49.4X6
Tipepidine	T48.3X1	T48.3X2	T48.3X3	T48.3X4	T48.3X5	T48.3X6
Tiquizium bromide	T44.3X1	T44.3X2	T44.3X3	T44.3X4	T44.3X5	T44.3X6
Tiratricol	T38.1X1	T38.1X2	T38.1X3	T38.1X4	T38.1X5	T38.1X6
Tisopurine	T50.4X1	T50.4X2	T50.4X3	T50.4X4	T50.4X5	T50.4X6
Titanium (compounds) (vapor)	T56.891	T56.892	T56.893	T56.894	—	—
dioxide	T49.3X1	T49.3X2	T49.3X3	T49.3X4	T49.3X5	T49.3X6
ointment	T49.3X1	T49.3X2	T49.3X3	T49.3X4	T49.3X5	T49.3X6
oxide	T49.3X1	T49.3X2	T49.3X3	T49.3X4	T49.3X5	T49.3X6
tetrachloride	T56.891	T56.892	T56.893	T56.894	—	—
Titanocene	T56.891	T56.892	T56.893	T56.894	—	—
Titroid	T38.1X1	T38.1X2	T38.1X3	T38.1X4	T38.1X5	T38.1X6
Tizanidine	T42.8X1	T42.8X2	T42.8X3	T42.8X4	T42.8X5	T42.8X6
TMTD	T60.3X1	T60.3X2	T60.3X3	T60.3X4	—	—
TNT (fumes)	T65.3X1	T65.3X2	T65.3X3	T65.3X4	—	—
Toadstool	T62.0X1	T62.0X2	T62.0X3	T62.0X4	—	—
Tobacco NEC	T65.291	T65.292	T65.293	T65.294	—	—
cigarettes	T65.221	T65.222	T65.223	T65.224	—	—
Indian	T62.2X1	T62.2X2	T62.2X3	T62.2X4	—	—
smoke, second-hand	T65.221	T65.222	T65.223	T65.224	—	—
Tobramycin	T36.5X1	T36.5X2	T36.5X3	T36.5X4	T36.5X5	T36.5X6
Tocainide	T46.2X1	T46.2X2	T46.2X3	T46.2X4	T46.2X5	T46.2X6
Tocoferol	T45.2X1	T45.2X2	T45.2X3	T45.2X4	T45.2X5	T45.2X6
Tocopherol	T45.2X1	T45.2X2	T45.2X3	T45.2X4	T45.2X5	T45.2X6
acetate	T45.2X1	T45.2X2	T45.2X3	T45.2X4	T45.2X5	T45.2X6
Tocosamine	T48.0X1	T48.0X2	T48.0X3	T48.0X4	T48.0X5	T48.0X6
Todralazine	T46.5X1	T46.5X2	T46.5X3	T46.5X4	T46.5X5	T46.5X6
Tofisopam	T42.4X1	T42.4X2	T42.4X3	T42.4X4	T42.4X5	T42.4X6
Tofranil	T43.011	T43.012	T43.013	T43.014	T43.015	T43.016
Toilet deodorizer	T65.891	T65.892	T65.893	T65.894	—	—
Tolamolol	T44.7X1	T44.7X2	T44.7X3	T44.7X4	T44.7X5	T44.7X6
Tolazamide	T38.3X1	T38.3X2	T38.3X3	T38.3X4	T38.3X5	T38.3X6
Tolazoline	T46.7X1	T46.7X2	T46.7X3	T46.7X4	T46.7X5	T46.7X6
Tolbutamide (sodium)	T38.3X1	T38.3X2	T38.3X3	T38.3X4	T38.3X5	T38.3X6
Tolciclate	T49.0X1	T49.0X2	T49.0X3	T49.0X4	T49.0X5	T49.0X6
Tolmetin	T39.391	T39.392	T39.393	T39.394	T39.395	T39.396
Tolnaftate	T49.0X1	T49.0X2	T49.0X3	T49.0X4	T49.0X5	T49.0X6
Tolonidine	T46.5X1	T46.5X2	T46.5X3	T46.5X4	T46.5X5	T46.5X6
Toloxatone	T42.6X1	T42.6X2	T42.6X3	T42.6X4	T42.6X5	T42.6X6
Tolperisone	T44.3X1	T44.3X2	T44.3X3	T44.3X4	T44.3X5	T44.3X6
Tolserol	T42.8X1	T42.8X2	T42.8X3	T42.8X4	T42.8X5	T42.8X6
Toluene (liquid)	T52.2X1	T52.2X2	T52.2X3	T52.2X4	—	—
diisocyanate	T65.0X1	T65.0X2	T65.0X3	T65.0X4	—	—
Toluidine	T65.891	T65.892	T65.893	T65.894	—	—
vapor	T59.891	T59.892	T59.893	T59.894	—	—
Toluol (liquid)	T52.2X1	T52.2X2	T52.2X3	T52.2X4	—	—
vapor	T52.2X1	T52.2X2	T52.2X3	T52.2X4	—	—
Toluylenediamine	T65.3X1	T65.3X2	T65.3X3	T65.3X4	—	—
Tolylene-2,4-diisocyanate	T65.0X1	T65.0X2	T65.0X3	T65.0X4	—	—
Tonic NEC	T50.901	T50.902	T50.903	T50.904	T50.905	T50.906
Topical action drug NEC	T49.91	T49.92	T49.93	T49.94	T49.95	T49.96
ear, nose or throat	T49.6X1	T49.6X2	T49.6X3	T49.6X4	T49.6X5	T49.6X6
eye	T49.5X1	T49.5X2	T49.5X3	T49.5X4	T49.5X5	T49.5X6
skin	T49.91	T49.92	T49.93	T49.94	T49.95	T49.96
specified NEC	T49.8X1	T49.8X2	T49.8X3	T49.8X4	T49.8X5	T49.8X6
Toquizine	T44.3X1	T44.3X2	T44.3X3	T44.3X4	T44.3X5	T44.3X6
Toremifene	T38.6X1	T38.6X2	T38.6X3	T38.6X4	T38.6X5	T38.6X6
Tosylchloramide sodium	T49.8X1	T49.8X2	T49.8X3	T49.8X4	T49.8X5	T49.8X6
Toxaphene (dust) (spray)	T60.1X1	T60.1X2	T60.1X3	T60.1X4	—	—
Toxin, diphtheria (Schick Test)	T50.8X1	T50.8X2	T50.8X3	T50.8X4	T50.8X5	T50.8X6
Toxoid						
combined	T50.A21	T50.A22	T50.A23	T50.A24	T50.A25	T50.A26
diphtheria	T50.A91	T50.A92	T50.A93	T50.A94	T50.A95	T50.A96
tetanus	T50.A91	T50.A92	T50.A93	T50.A94	T50.A95	T50.A96
Trace element NEC	T45.8X1	T45.8X2	T45.8X3	T45.8X4	T45.8X5	T45.8X6
Tractor fuel NEC	T52.0X1	T52.0X2	T52.0X3	T52.0X4	—	—
Tragacanth	T50.991	T50.992	T50.993	T50.994	T50.995	T50.996
Tramadol	T40.4X1	T40.4X2	T40.4X3	T40.4X4	T40.4X5	T40.4X6
Tramazoline	T48.5X1	T48.5X2	T48.5X3	T48.5X4	T48.5X5	T48.5X6
Tranexamic acid	T45.621	T45.622	T45.623	T45.624	T45.625	T45.626
Tranilast	T45.0X1	T45.0X2	T45.0X3	T45.0X4	T45.0X5	T45.0X6
Tranquilizer NEC	T43.501	T43.502	T43.503	T43.504	T43.505	T43.506
with hypnotic or sedative	T42.6X1	T42.6X2	T42.6X3	T42.6X4	T42.6X5	T42.6X6
benzodiazepine NEC	T42.4X1	T42.4X2	T42.4X3	T42.4X4	T42.4X5	T42.4X6
butyrophenone NEC	T43.4X1	T43.4X2	T43.4X3	T43.4X4	T43.4X5	T43.4X6
carbamate	T43.591	T43.592	T43.593	T43.594	T43.595	T43.596
dimethylamine	T43.3X1	T43.3X2	T43.3X3	T43.3X4	T43.3X5	T43.3X6
ethylamine	T43.3X1	T43.3X2	T43.3X3	T43.3X4	T43.3X5	T43.3X6
hydroxyzine	T43.591	T43.592	T43.593	T43.594	T43.595	T43.596
major NEC	T43.501	T43.502	T43.503	T43.504	T43.505	T43.506
penothiazine NEC	T43.3X1	T43.3X2	T43.3X3	T43.3X4	T43.3X5	T43.3X6
phenothiazine-based	T43.3X1	T43.3X2	T43.3X3	T43.3X4	T43.3X5	T43.3X6
piperazine NEC	T43.3X1	T43.3X2	T43.3X3	T43.3X4	T43.3X5	T43.3X6
piperidine	T43.3X1	T43.3X2	T43.3X3	T43.3X4	T43.3X5	T43.3X6
propylamine	T43.3X1	T43.3X2	T43.3X3	T43.3X4	T43.3X5	T43.3X6
specified NEC	T43.591	T43.592	T43.593	T43.594	T43.595	T43.596
thioxanthene NEC	T43.591	T43.592	T43.593	T43.594	T43.595	T43.596
Tranxene	T42.4X1	T42.4X2	T42.4X3	T42.4X4	T42.4X5	T42.4X6
Tranylcypromine	T43.1X1	T43.1X2	T43.1X3	T43.1X4	T43.1X5	T43.1X6
Trapidil	T46.3X1	T46.3X2	T46.3X3	T46.3X4	T46.3X5	T46.3X6
Trasentine	T44.3X1	T44.3X2	T44.3X3	T44.3X4	T44.3X5	T44.3X6
Travert	T50.3X1	T50.3X2	T50.3X3	T50.3X4	T50.3X5	T50.3X6
Trazodone	T43.211	T43.212	T43.213	T43.214	T43.215	T43.216
Trecator	T37.1X1	T37.1X2	T37.1X3	T37.1X4	T37.1X5	T37.1X6
Treosulfan	T45.1X1	T45.1X2	T45.1X3	T45.1X4	T45.1X5	T45.1X6
Tretamine	T45.1X1	T45.1X2	T45.1X3	T45.1X4	T45.1X5	T45.1X6
Tretinoin	T49.0X1	T49.0X2	T49.0X3	T49.0X4	T49.0X5	T49.0X6
Tretoquinol	T48.6X1	T48.6X2	T48.6X3	T48.6X4	T48.6X5	T48.6X6
Triacetin	T49.0X1	T49.0X2	T49.0X3	T49.0X4	T49.0X5	T49.0X6
Triacetoxyanthracene	T49.4X1	T49.4X2	T49.4X3	T49.4X4	T49.4X5	T49.4X6
Triacetyloleandomycin	T36.3X1	T36.3X2	T36.3X3	T36.3X4	T36.3X5	T36.3X6
Triamcinolone	T49.0X1	T49.0X2	T49.0X3	T49.0X4	T49.0X5	T49.0X6
ENT agent	T49.6X1	T49.6X2	T49.6X3	T49.6X4	T49.6X5	T49.6X6
hexacetonide	T49.0X1	T49.0X2	T49.0X3	T49.0X4	T49.0X5	T49.0X6
ophthalmic preparation	T49.5X1	T49.5X2	T49.5X3	T49.5X4	T49.5X5	T49.5X6
topical NEC	T49.0X1	T49.0X2	T49.0X3	T49.0X4	T49.0X5	T49.0X6
Triampyzine	T44.3X1	T44.3X2	T44.3X3	T44.3X4	T44.3X5	T44.3X6

▽ Subterms under main terms may continue to next column or page　　　Additional Character May Be Required — Refer to the Tabular List for Character Selection

Substance	Poisoning, Accidental (unintentional)	Poisoning, Intentional Self-harm	Poisoning, Assault	Poisoning, Undetermined	Adverse Effect	Under-dosing
Triamterene	T50.2X1	T50.2X2	T50.2X3	T50.2X4	T50.2X5	T50.2X6
Triazine (herbicide)	T60.3X1	T60.3X2	T60.3X3	T60.3X4	—	—
Triaziquone	T45.1X1	T45.1X2	T45.1X3	T45.1X4	T45.1X5	T45.1X6
Triazolam	T42.4X1	T42.4X2	T42.4X3	T42.4X4	T42.4X5	T42.4X6
Triazole (herbicide)	T60.3X1	T60.3X2	T60.3X3	T60.3X4	—	—
Tribenoside	T46.991	T46.992	T46.993	T46.994	T46.995	T46.996
Tribromacetaldehyde	T42.6X1	T42.6X2	T42.6X3	T42.6X4	T42.6X5	T42.6X6
Tribromoethanol, rectal	T41.291	T41.292	T41.293	T41.294	T41.295	T41.296
Tribromomethane	T42.6X1	T42.6X2	T42.6X3	T42.6X4	T42.6X5	T42.6X6
Trichlorethane	T53.2X1	T53.2X2	T53.2X3	T53.2X4	—	—
Trichlorethylene	T53.2X1	T53.2X2	T53.2X3	T53.2X4	—	—
Trichlorfon	T60.0X1	T60.0X2	T60.0X3	T60.0X4	—	—
Trichlormethiazide	T50.2X1	T50.2X2	T50.2X3	T50.2X4	T50.2X5	T50.2X6
Trichlormethine	T45.1X1	T45.1X2	T45.1X3	T45.1X4	T45.1X5	T45.1X6
Trichloroacetic acid, Trichloracetic acid	T54.2X1	T54.2X2	T54.2X3	T54.2X4	—	—
medicinal	T49.4X1	T49.4X2	T49.4X3	T49.4X4	T49.4X5	T49.4X6
Trichloroethane	T53.2X1	T53.2X2	T53.2X3	T53.2X4	—	—
Trichloroethanol	T42.6X1	T42.6X2	T42.6X3	T42.6X4	T42.6X5	T42.6X6
Trichloroethylene (liquid)	T53.2X1	T53.2X2	T53.2X3	T53.2X4	—	—
(vapor)						
anesthetic (gas)	T41.0X1	T41.0X2	T41.0X3	T41.0X4	T41.0X5	T41.0X6
vapor NEC	T53.2X1	T53.2X2	T53.2X3	T53.2X4	—	—
Trichloroethyl phosphate	T42.6X1	T42.6X2	T42.6X3	T42.6X4	T42.6X5	T42.6X6
Trichlorofluoromethane NEC	T53.5X1	T53.5X2	T53.5X3	T53.5X4	—	—
Trichloronate	T60.0X1	T60.0X2	T60.0X3	T60.0X4	—	—
Trichloropropane	T53.6X1	T53.6X2	T53.6X3	T53.6X4	—	—
Trichlorotriethylamine	T45.1X1	T45.1X2	T45.1X3	T45.1X4	T45.1X5	T45.1X6
Trichomonacides NEC	T37.3X1	T37.3X2	T37.3X3	T37.3X4	T37.3X5	T37.3X6
Trichomycin	T36.7X1	T36.7X2	T36.7X3	T36.7X4	T36.7X5	T36.7X6
Triclobisonium chloride	T49.0X1	T49.0X2	T49.0X3	T49.0X4	T49.0X5	T49.0X6
Triclocarban	T49.0X1	T49.0X2	T49.0X3	T49.0X4	T49.0X5	T49.0X6
Triclofos	T42.6X1	T42.6X2	T42.6X3	T42.6X4	T42.6X5	T42.6X6
Triclosan	T49.0X1	T49.0X2	T49.0X3	T49.0X4	T49.0X5	T49.0X6
Tricresyl phosphate	T65.891	T65.892	T65.893	T65.894	—	—
solvent	T52.91	T52.92	T52.93	T52.94	—	—
Tricyclamol chloride	T44.3X1	T44.3X2	T44.3X3	T44.3X4	T44.3X5	T44.3X6
Tridesilon	T49.0X1	T49.0X2	T49.0X3	T49.0X4	T49.0X5	T49.0X6
Tridihexethyl iodide	T44.3X1	T44.3X2	T44.3X3	T44.3X4	T44.3X5	T44.3X6
Tridione	T42.2X1	T42.2X2	T42.2X3	T42.2X4	T42.2X5	T42.2X6
Trientine	T45.8X1	T45.8X2	T45.8X3	T45.8X4	T45.8X5	T45.8X6
Triethanolamine NEC	T54.3X1	T54.3X2	T54.3X3	T54.3X4	—	—
detergent	T54.3X1	T54.3X2	T54.3X3	T54.3X4	—	—
trinitrate (biphosphate)	T46.3X1	T46.3X2	T46.3X3	T46.3X4	T46.3X5	T46.3X6
Triethanomelamine	T45.1X1	T45.1X2	T45.1X3	T45.1X4	T45.1X5	T45.1X6
Triethylenemelamine	T45.1X1	T45.1X2	T45.1X3	T45.1X4	T45.1X5	T45.1X6
Triethylenephosphoramide	T45.1X1	T45.1X2	T45.1X3	T45.1X4	T45.1X5	T45.1X6
Triethylenethiophosphoramide	T45.1X1	T45.1X2	T45.1X3	T45.1X4	T45.1X5	T45.1X6
Trifluoperazine	T43.3X1	T43.3X2	T43.3X3	T43.3X4	T43.3X5	T43.3X6
Trifluoroethyl vinyl ether	T41.0X1	T41.0X2	T41.0X3	T41.0X4	T41.0X5	T41.0X6
Trifluperidol	T43.4X1	T43.4X2	T43.4X3	T43.4X4	T43.4X5	T43.4X6
Triflupromazine	T43.3X1	T43.3X2	T43.3X3	T43.3X4	T43.3X5	T43.3X6
Trifluridine	T37.5X1	T37.5X2	T37.5X3	T37.5X4	T37.5X5	T37.5X6
Triflusal	T45.521	T45.522	T45.523	T45.524	T45.525	T45.526
Trihexyphenidyl	T44.3X1	T44.3X2	T44.3X3	T44.3X4	T44.3X5	T44.3X6
Triiodothyronine	T38.1X1	T38.1X2	T38.1X3	T38.1X4	T38.1X5	T38.1X6
Trilene	T41.0X1	T41.0X2	T41.0X3	T41.0X4	T41.0X5	T41.0X6
Trilostane	T38.991	T38.992	T38.993	T38.994	T38.995	T38.996
Trimebutine	T44.3X1	T44.3X2	T44.3X3	T44.3X4	T44.3X5	T44.3X6
Trimecaine	T41.3X1	T41.3X2	T41.3X3	T41.3X4	T41.3X5	T41.3X6
Trimeprazine (tartrate)	T44.3X1	T44.3X2	T44.3X3	T44.3X4	T44.3X5	T44.3X6
Trimetaphan camsilate	T44.2X1	T44.2X2	T44.2X3	T44.2X4	T44.2X5	T44.2X6
Trimetazidine	T46.7X1	T46.7X2	T46.7X3	T46.7X4	T46.7X5	T46.7X6
Trimethadione	T42.2X1	T42.2X2	T42.2X3	T42.2X4	T42.2X5	T42.2X6
Trimethaphan	T44.2X1	T44.2X2	T44.2X3	T44.2X4	T44.2X5	T44.2X6
Trimethidinium	T44.2X1	T44.2X2	T44.2X3	T44.2X4	T44.2X5	T44.2X6
Trimethobenzamide	T45.0X1	T45.0X2	T45.0X3	T45.0X4	T45.0X5	T45.0X6
Trimethoprim	T37.8X1	T37.8X2	T37.8X3	T37.8X4	T37.8X5	T37.8X6
with sulfamethoxazole	T36.8X1	T36.8X2	T36.8X3	T36.8X4	T36.8X5	T36.8X6
Trimethylcarbinol	T51.3X1	T51.3X2	T51.3X3	T51.3X4	—	—
Trimethylpsoralen	T49.3X1	T49.3X2	T49.3X3	T49.3X4	T49.3X5	T49.3X6
Trimeton	T45.0X1	T45.0X2	T45.0X3	T45.0X4	T45.0X5	T45.0X6
Trimetrexate	T45.1X1	T45.1X2	T45.1X3	T45.1X4	T45.1X5	T45.1X6
Trimipramine	T43.011	T43.012	T43.013	T43.014	T43.015	T43.016
Trimustine	T45.1X1	T45.1X2	T45.1X3	T45.1X4	T45.1X5	T45.1X6
Trinitrine	T46.3X1	T46.3X2	T46.3X3	T46.3X4	T46.3X5	T46.3X6
Trinitrobenzol	T65.3X1	T65.3X2	T65.3X3	T65.3X4	—	—
Trinitrophenol	T65.3X1	T65.3X2	T65.3X3	T65.3X4	—	—
Trinitrotoluene (fumes)	T65.3X1	T65.3X2	T65.3X3	T65.3X4	—	—
Trional	T42.6X1	T42.6X2	T42.6X3	T42.6X4	T42.6X5	T42.6X6
Triorthocresyl phosphate	T65.891	T65.892	T65.893	T65.894	—	—
Trioxide of arsenic	T57.0X1	T57.0X2	T57.0X3	T57.0X4	—	—

Substance	Poisoning, Accidental (unintentional)	Poisoning, Intentional Self-harm	Poisoning, Assault	Poisoning, Undetermined	Adverse Effect	Under-dosing
Trioxysalen	T49.4X1	T49.4X2	T49.4X3	T49.4X4	T49.4X5	T49.4X6
Tripamide	T50.2X1	T50.2X2	T50.2X3	T50.2X4	T50.2X5	T50.2X6
Triparanol	T46.6X1	T46.6X2	T46.6X3	T46.6X4	T46.6X5	T46.6X6
Tripelennamine	T45.0X1	T45.0X2	T45.0X3	T45.0X4	T45.0X5	T45.0X6
Triperiden	T44.3X1	T44.3X2	T44.3X3	T44.3X4	T44.3X5	T44.3X6
Triperidol	T43.4X1	T43.4X2	T43.4X3	T43.4X4	T43.4X5	T43.4X6
Triphenylphosphate	T65.891	T65.892	T65.893	T65.894	—	—
Triple						
bromides	T42.6X1	T42.6X2	T42.6X3	T42.6X4	T42.6X5	T42.6X6
carbonate	T47.1X1	T47.1X2	T47.1X3	T47.1X4	T47.1X5	T47.1X6
vaccine						
DPT	T50.A11	T50.A12	T50.A13	T50.A14	T50.A15	T50.A16
including pertussis	T50.A11	T50.A12	T50.A13	T50.A14	T50.A15	T50.A16
MMR	T50.B91	T50.B92	T50.B93	T50.B94	T50.B95	T50.B96
Triprolidine	T45.0X1	T45.0X2	T45.0X3	T45.0X4	T45.0X5	T45.0X6
Trisodium hydrogen edetate	T50.6X1	T50.6X2	T50.6X3	T50.6X4	T50.6X5	T50.6X6
Trisoralen	T49.3X1	T49.3X2	T49.3X3	T49.3X4	T49.3X5	T49.3X6
Trisulfapyrimidines	T37.0X1	T37.0X2	T37.0X3	T37.0X4	T37.0X5	T37.0X6
Trithiozine	T44.3X1	T44.3X2	T44.3X3	T44.3X4	T44.3X5	T44.3X6
Tritiozine	T44.3X1	T44.3X2	T44.3X3	T44.3X4	T44.3X5	T44.3X6
Tritoqualine	T45.0X1	T45.0X2	T45.0X3	T45.0X4	T45.0X5	T45.0X6
Trofosfamide	T45.1X1	T45.1X2	T45.1X3	T45.1X4	T45.1X5	T45.1X6
Troleandomycin	T36.3X1	T36.3X2	T36.3X3	T36.3X4	T36.3X5	T36.3X6
Trolnitrate (phosphate)	T46.3X1	T46.3X2	T46.3X3	T46.3X4	T46.3X5	T46.3X6
Tromantadine	T37.5X1	T37.5X2	T37.5X3	T37.5X4	T37.5X5	T37.5X6
Trometamol	T50.2X1	T50.2X2	T50.2X3	T50.2X4	T50.2X5	T50.2X6
Tromethamine	T50.2X1	T50.2X2	T50.2X3	T50.2X4	T50.2X5	T50.2X6
Tronothane	T41.3X1	T41.3X2	T41.3X3	T41.3X4	T41.3X5	T41.3X6
Tropacine	T44.3X1	T44.3X2	T44.3X3	T44.3X4	T44.3X5	T44.3X6
Tropatepine	T44.3X1	T44.3X2	T44.3X3	T44.3X4	T44.3X5	T44.3X6
Tropicamide	T44.3X1	T44.3X2	T44.3X3	T44.3X4	T44.3X5	T44.3X6
Trospium chloride	T44.3X1	T44.3X2	T44.3X3	T44.3X4	T44.3X5	T44.3X6
Troxerutin	T46.991	T46.992	T46.993	T46.994	T46.995	T46.996
Troxidone	T42.2X1	T42.2X2	T42.2X3	T42.2X4	T42.2X5	T42.2X6
Tryparsamide	T37.3X1	T37.3X2	T37.3X3	T37.3X4	T37.3X5	T37.3X6
Trypsin	T45.3X1	T45.3X2	T45.3X3	T45.3X4	T45.3X5	T45.3X6
Tryptizol	T43.011	T43.012	T43.013	T43.014	T43.015	T43.016
TSH	T38.811	T38.812	T38.813	T38.814	T38.815	T38.816
Tuaminoheptane	T48.5X1	T48.5X2	T48.5X3	T48.5X4	T48.5X5	T48.5X6
Tuberculin, purified protein derivative (PPD)	T50.8X1	T50.8X2	T50.8X3	T50.8X4	T50.8X5	T50.8X6
Tubocurare	T48.1X1	T48.1X2	T48.1X3	T48.1X4	T48.1X5	T48.1X6
Tubocurarine (chloride)	T48.1X1	T48.1X2	T48.1X3	T48.1X4	T48.1X5	T48.1X6
Tulobuterol	T48.6X1	T48.6X2	T48.6X3	T48.6X4	T48.6X5	T48.6X6
Turpentine (spirits of)	T52.8X1	T52.8X2	T52.8X3	T52.8X4	—	—
vapor	T52.8X1	T52.8X2	T52.8X3	T52.8X4	—	—
Tybamate	T43.591	T43.592	T43.593	T43.594	T43.595	T43.596
Tyloxapol	T48.4X1	T48.4X2	T48.4X3	T48.4X4	T48.4X5	T48.4X6
Tymazoline	T48.5X1	T48.5X2	T48.5X3	T48.5X4	T48.5X5	T48.5X6
Typhoid-paratyphoid vaccine	T50.A91	T50.A92	T50.A93	T50.A94	T50.A95	T50.A96
Typhus vaccine	T50.A91	T50.A92	T50.A93	T50.A94	T50.A95	T50.A96
Tyropanoate	T50.8X1	T50.8X2	T50.8X3	T50.8X4	T50.8X5	T50.8X6
Tyrothricin	T49.6X1	T49.6X2	T49.6X3	T49.6X4	T49.6X5	T49.6X6
ENT agent	T49.6X1	T49.6X2	T49.6X3	T49.6X4	T49.6X5	T49.6X6
ophthalmic preparation	T49.5X1	T49.5X2	T49.5X3	T49.5X4	T49.5X5	T49.5X6
Ufenamate	T39.391	T39.392	T39.393	T39.394	T39.395	T39.396
Ultraviolet light protectant	T49.3X1	T49.3X2	T49.3X3	T49.3X4	T49.3X5	T49.3X6
Undecenoic acid	T46.6X1	T46.6X2	T46.6X3	T46.6X4	T46.6X5	T46.6X6
Undecoylium	T49.0X1	T49.0X2	T49.0X3	T49.0X4	T49.0X5	T49.0X6
Undecylenic acid (derivatives)	T49.0X1	T49.0X2	T49.0X3	T49.0X4	T49.0X5	T49.0X6
Unna's boot	T49.3X1	T49.3X2	T49.3X3	T49.3X4	T49.3X5	T49.3X6
Unsaturated fatty acid	T46.6X1	T46.6X2	T46.6X3	T46.6X4	T46.6X5	T46.6X6
Uracil mustard	T45.1X1	T45.1X2	T45.1X3	T45.1X4	T45.1X5	T45.1X6
Uramustine	T45.1X1	T45.1X2	T45.1X3	T45.1X4	T45.1X5	T45.1X6
Urapidil	T46.5X1	T46.5X2	T46.5X3	T46.5X4	T46.5X5	T46.5X6
Urari	T48.1X1	T48.1X2	T48.1X3	T48.1X4	T48.1X5	T48.1X6
Urate oxidase	T50.4X1	T50.4X2	T50.4X3	T50.4X4	T50.4X5	T50.4X6
Urea	T47.3X1	T47.3X2	T47.3X3	T47.3X4	T47.3X5	T47.3X6
peroxide	T49.0X1	T49.0X2	T49.0X3	T49.0X4	T49.0X5	T49.0X6
stibamine	T37.4X1	T37.4X2	T37.4X3	T37.4X4	T37.4X5	T37.4X6
topical	T49.8X1	T49.8X2	T49.8X3	T49.8X4	T49.8X5	T49.8X6
Urethane	T45.1X1	T45.1X2	T45.1X3	T45.1X4	T45.1X5	T45.1X6
Urginea (maritima) (scilla) — see Squill						
Uric acid metabolism drug NEC	T50.4X1	T50.4X2	T50.4X3	T50.4X4	T50.4X5	T50.4X6
Uricosuric agent	T50.4X1	T50.4X2	T50.4X3	T50.4X4	T50.4X5	T50.4X6
Urinary anti-infective	T37.8X1	T37.8X2	T37.8X3	T37.8X4	T37.8X5	T37.8X6
Urofollitropin	T38.811	T38.812	T38.813	T38.814	T38.815	T38.816
Urokinase	T45.611	T45.612	T45.613	T45.614	T45.615	T45.616

Additional Character May Be Required — Refer to the Tabular List for Character Selection

Subterms under main terms may continue to next column or page

Substance	Poisoning, Accidental (unintentional)	Poisoning, Intentional Self-harm	Poisoning, Assault	Poisoning, Undetermined	Adverse Effect	Under-dosing
Urokon	T50.8X1	T50.8X2	T50.8X3	T50.8X4	T50.8X5	T50.8X6
Ursodeoxycholic acid	T50.991	T50.992	T50.993	T50.994	T50.995	T50.996
Ursodiol	T50.991	T50.992	T50.993	T50.994	T50.995	T50.996
Urtica	T62.2X1	T62.2X2	T62.2X3	T62.2X4	—	—
Utility gas — *see* Gas, utility						
Vaccine NEC	T50.Z91	T50.Z92	T50.Z93	T50.Z94	T50.Z95	T50.Z96
antineoplastic	T50.Z91	T50.Z92	T50.Z93	T50.Z94	T50.Z95	T50.Z96
bacterial NEC	T50.A91	T50.A92	T50.A93	T50.A94	T50.A95	T50.A96
with						
other bacterial	T50.A21	T50.A22	T50.A23	T50.A24	T50.A25	T50.A26
component						
pertussis component	T50.A11	T50.A12	T50.A13	T50.A14	T50.A15	T50.A16
viral-rickettsial	T50.A21	T50.A22	T50.A23	T50.A24	T50.A25	T50.A26
component						
mixed NEC	T50.A21	T50.A22	T50.A23	T50.A24	T50.A25	T50.A26
BCG	T50.A91	T50.A92	T50.A93	T50.A94	T50.A95	T50.A96
cholera	T50.A91	T50.A92	T50.A93	T50.A94	T50.A95	T50.A96
diphtheria	T50.A91	T50.A92	T50.A93	T50.A94	T50.A95	T50.A96
with tetanus	T50.A21	T50.A22	T50.A23	T50.A24	T50.A25	T50.A26
and pertussis	T50.A11	T50.A12	T50.A13	T50.A14	T50.A15	T50.A16
influenza	T50.B91	T50.B92	T50.B93	T50.B94	T50.B95	T50.B96
measles	T50.B91	T50.B92	T50.B93	T50.B94	T50.B95	T50.B96
with mumps and rubella	T50.B91	T50.B92	T50.B93	T50.B94	T50.B95	T50.B96
meningococcal	T50.A91	T50.A92	T50.A93	T50.A94	T50.A95	T50.A96
mumps	T50.B91	T50.B92	T50.B93	T50.B94	T50.B95	T50.B96
paratyphoid	T50.A91	T50.A92	T50.A93	T50.A94	T50.A95	T50.A96
pertussis	T50.A11	T50.A12	T50.A13	T50.A14	T50.A15	T50.A16
with diphtheria	T50.A11	T50.A12	T50.A13	T50.A14	T50.A15	T50.A16
and tetanus	T50.A11	T50.A12	T50.A13	T50.A14	T50.A15	T50.A16
with other component	T50.A11	T50.A12	T50.A13	T50.A14	T50.A15	T50.A16
plague	T50.A91	T50.A92	T50.A93	T50.A94	T50.A95	T50.A96
poliomyelitis	T50.B91	T50.B92	T50.B93	T50.B94	T50.B95	T50.B96
poliovirus	T50.B91	T50.B92	T50.B93	T50.B94	T50.B95	T50.B96
rabies	T50.B91	T50.B92	T50.B93	T50.B94	T50.B95	T50.B96
respiratory syncytial virus	T50.B91	T50.B92	T50.B93	T50.B94	T50.B95	T50.B96
rickettsial NEC	T50.A91	T50.A92	T50.A93	T50.A94	T50.A95	T50.A96
with						
bacterial component	T50.A21	T50.A22	T50.A23	T50.A24	T50.A25	T50.A26
Rocky Mountain spotted	T50.A91	T50.A92	T50.A93	T50.A94	T50.A95	T50.A96
fever						
rubella	T50.B91	T50.B92	T50.B93	T50.B94	T50.B95	T50.B96
sabin oral	T50.B91	T50.B92	T50.B93	T50.B94	T50.B95	T50.B96
smallpox	T50.B11	T50.B12	T50.B13	T50.B14	T50.B15	T50.B16
TAB	T50.A91	T50.A92	T50.A93	T50.A94	T50.A95	T50.A96
tetanus	T50.A91	T50.A92	T50.A93	T50.A94	T50.A95	T50.A96
typhoid	T50.A91	T50.A92	T50.A93	T50.A94	T50.A95	T50.A96
typhus	T50.A91	T50.A92	T50.A93	T50.A94	T50.A95	T50.A96
viral NEC	T50.B91	T50.B92	T50.B93	T50.B94	T50.B95	T50.B96
yellow fever	T50.B91	T50.B92	T50.B93	T50.B94	T50.B95	T50.B96
Vaccinia immune globulin	T50.Z11	T50.Z12	T50.Z13	T50.Z14	T50.Z15	T50.Z16
Vaginal contraceptives	T49.8X1	T49.8X2	T49.8X3	T49.8X4	T49.8X5	T49.8X6
Valerian						
root	T42.6X1	T42.6X2	T42.6X3	T42.6X4	T42.6X5	T42.6X6
tincture	T42.6X1	T42.6X2	T42.6X3	T42.6X4	T42.6X5	T42.6X6
Valethamate bromide	T44.3X1	T44.3X2	T44.3X3	T44.3X4	T44.3X5	T44.3X6
Valisone	T49.0X1	T49.0X2	T49.0X3	T49.0X4	T49.0X5	T49.0X6
Valium	T42.4X1	T42.4X2	T42.4X3	T42.4X4	T42.4X5	T42.4X6
Valmid	T42.6X1	T42.6X2	T42.6X3	T42.6X4	T42.6X5	T42.6X6
Valnoctamide	T42.6X1	T42.6X2	T42.6X3	T42.6X4	T42.6X5	T42.6X6
Valproate (sodium)	T42.6X1	T42.6X2	T42.6X3	T42.6X4	T42.6X5	T42.6X6
Valproic acid	T42.6X1	T42.6X2	T42.6X3	T42.6X4	T42.6X5	T42.6X6
Valpromide	T42.6X1	T42.6X2	T42.6X3	T42.6X4	T42.6X5	T42.6X6
Vanadium	T56.891	T56.892	T56.893	T56.894	—	—
Vancomycin	T36.8X1	T36.8X2	T36.8X3	T36.8X4	T36.8X5	T36.8X6
Vapor — *see also* Gas	T59.91	T59.92	T59.93	T59.94	—	—
kiln (carbon monoxide)	T58.8X1	T58.8X2	T58.8X3	T58.8X4	—	—
lead — *see* lead						
specified source NEC	T59.891	T59.892	T59.893	T59.894	—	—
Vardenafil	T46.7X1	T46.7X2	T46.7X3	T46.7X4	T46.7X5	T46.7X6
Varicose reduction drug	T46.8X1	T46.8X2	T46.8X3	T46.8X4	T46.8X5	T46.8X6
Varnish	T65.4X1	T65.4X2	T65.4X3	T65.4X4	—	—
cleaner	T52.91	T52.92	T52.93	T52.94	—	—
Vaseline	T49.3X1	T49.3X2	T49.3X3	T49.3X4	T49.3X5	T49.3X6
Vasodilan	T46.7X1	T46.7X2	T46.7X3	T46.7X4	T46.7X5	T46.7X6
Vasodilator						
coronary NEC	T46.3X1	T46.3X2	T46.3X3	T46.3X4	T46.3X5	T46.3X6
peripheral NEC	T46.7X1	T46.7X2	T46.7X3	T46.7X4	T46.7X5	T46.7X6
Vasopressin	T38.891	T38.892	T38.893	T38.894	T38.895	T38.896
Vasopressor drugs	T38.891	T38.892	T38.893	T38.894	T38.895	T38.896
Vecuronium bromide	T48.1X1	T48.1X2	T48.1X3	T48.1X4	T48.1X5	T48.1X6
Vegetable extract, astringent	T49.2X1	T49.2X2	T49.2X3	T49.2X4	T49.2X5	T49.2X6
Venlafaxine	T43.211	T43.212	T43.213	T43.214	T43.215	T43.216

Substance	Poisoning, Accidental (unintentional)	Poisoning, Intentional Self-harm	Poisoning, Assault	Poisoning, Undetermined	Adverse Effect	Under-dosing
Venom, venomous (bite) (sting)	T63.91	T63.92	T63.93	T63.94	—	—
amphibian NEC	T63.831	T63.832	T63.833	T63.834	—	—
animal NEC	T63.891	T63.892	T63.893	T63.894	—	—
ant	T63.421	T63.422	T63.423	T63.424	—	—
arthropod NEC	T63.481	T63.482	T63.483	T63.484	—	—
bee	T63.441	T63.442	T63.443	T63.444	—	—
centipede	T63.411	T63.412	T63.413	T63.414	—	—
fish	T63.591	T63.592	T63.593	T63.594	—	—
frog	T63.811	T63.812	T63.813	T63.814	—	—
hornet	T63.451	T63.452	T63.453	T63.454	—	—
insect NEC	T63.481	T63.482	T63.483	T63.484	—	—
lizard	T63.121	T63.122	T63.123	T63.124	—	—
marine						
animals	T63.691	T63.692	T63.693	T63.694	—	—
bluebottle	T63.611	T63.612	T63.613	T63.614	—	—
jellyfish NEC	T63.621	T63.622	T63.623	T63.624	—	—
Portugese Man-o-war	T63.611	T63.612	T63.613	T63.614	—	—
sea anemone	T63.631	T63.632	T63.633	T63.634	—	—
specified NEC	T63.691	T63.692	T63.693	T63.694	—	—
fish	T63.591	T63.592	T63.593	T63.594	—	—
plants	T63.711	T63.712	T63.713	T63.714	—	—
sting ray	T63.511	T63.512	T63.513	T63.514	—	—
millipede (tropical)	T63.411	T63.412	T63.413	T63.414	—	—
plant NEC	T63.791	T63.792	T63.793	T63.794	—	—
marine	T63.711	T63.712	T63.713	T63.714	—	—
reptile	T63.191	T63.192	T63.193	T63.194	—	—
gila monster	T63.111	T63.112	T63.113	T63.114	—	—
lizard NEC	T63.121	T63.122	T63.123	T63.124	—	—
scorpion	T63.2X1	T63.2X2	T63.2X3	T63.2X4	—	—
snake	T63.001	T63.002	T63.003	T63.004	—	—
African NEC	T63.081	T63.082	T63.083	T63.084	—	—
American (North) (South) NEC	T63.061	T63.062	T63.063	T63.064	—	—
Asian	T63.081	T63.082	T63.083	T63.084	—	—
Australian	T63.071	T63.072	T63.073	T63.074	—	—
cobra	T63.041	T63.042	T63.043	T63.044	—	—
coral snake	T63.021	T63.022	T63.023	T63.024	—	—
rattlesnake	T63.011	T63.012	T63.013	T63.014	—	—
specified NEC	T63.091	T63.092	T63.093	T63.094	—	—
taipan	T63.031	T63.032	T63.033	T63.034	—	—
specified NEC	T63.891	T63.892	T63.893	T63.894	—	—
spider	T63.301	T63.302	T63.303	T63.304	—	—
black widow	T63.311	T63.312	T63.313	T63.314	—	—
brown recluse	T63.331	T63.332	T63.333	T63.334	—	—
specified NEC	T63.391	T63.392	T63.393	T63.394	—	—
tarantula	T63.321	T63.322	T63.323	T63.324	—	—
sting ray	T63.511	T63.512	T63.513	T63.514	—	—
toad	T63.821	T63.822	T63.823	T63.824	—	—
wasp	T63.461	T63.462	T63.463	T63.464	—	—
Venous sclerosing drug NEC	T46.8X1	T46.8X2	T46.8X3	T46.8X4	T46.8X5	T46.8X6
Ventolin — *see* Albuterol						
Veramon	T42.3X1	T42.3X2	T42.3X3	T42.3X4	T42.3X5	T42.3X6
Verapamil	T46.1X1	T46.1X2	T46.1X3	T46.1X4	T46.1X5	T46.1X6
Veratrine	T46.5X1	T46.5X2	T46.5X3	T46.5X4	T46.5X5	T46.5X6
Veratrum						
album	T62.2X1	T62.2X2	T62.2X3	T62.2X4	—	—
alkaloids	T46.5X1	T46.5X2	T46.5X3	T46.5X4	T46.5X5	T46.5X6
viride	T62.2X1	T62.2X2	T62.2X3	T62.2X4	—	—
Verdigris	T60.3X1	T60.3X2	T60.3X3	T60.3X4	—	—
Veronal	T42.3X1	T42.3X2	T42.3X3	T42.3X4	T42.3X5	T42.3X6
Veroxil	T37.4X1	T37.4X2	T37.4X3	T37.4X4	T37.4X5	T37.4X6
Versenate	T50.6X1	T50.6X2	T50.6X3	T50.6X4	T50.6X5	T50.6X6
Versidyne	T39.8X1	T39.8X2	T39.8X3	T39.8X4	T39.8X5	T39.8X6
Vetrabutine	T48.0X1	T48.0X2	T48.0X3	T48.0X4	T48.0X5	T48.0X6
Vidarabine	T37.5X1	T37.5X2	T37.5X3	T37.5X4	T37.5X5	T37.5X6
Vienna						
green	T57.0X1	T57.0X2	T57.0X3	T57.0X4	—	—
insecticide	T60.2X1	T60.2X2	T60.2X3	T60.2X4	—	—
red	T57.0X1	T57.0X2	T57.0X3	T57.0X4	—	—
pharmaceutical dye	T50.991	T50.992	T50.993	T50.994	T50.995	T50.996
Vigabatrin	T42.6X1	T42.6X2	T42.6X3	T42.6X4	T42.6X5	T42.6X6
Viloxazine	T43.291	T43.292	T43.293	T43.294	T43.295	T43.296
Viminol	T39.8X1	T39.8X2	T39.8X3	T39.8X4	T39.8X5	T39.8X6
Vinbarbital, vinbarbitone	T42.3X1	T42.3X2	T42.3X3	T42.3X4	T42.3X5	T42.3X6
Vinblastine	T45.1X1	T45.1X2	T45.1X3	T45.1X4	T45.1X5	T45.1X6
Vinburnine	T46.7X1	T46.7X2	T46.7X3	T46.7X4	T46.7X5	T46.7X6
Vincamine	T45.1X1	T45.1X2	T45.1X3	T45.1X4	T45.1X5	T45.1X6
Vincristine	T45.1X1	T45.1X2	T45.1X3	T45.1X4	T45.1X5	T45.1X6
Vindesine	T45.1X1	T45.1X2	T45.1X3	T45.1X4	T45.1X5	T45.1X6
Vinesthene, vinethene	T41.0X1	T41.0X2	T41.0X3	T41.0X4	T41.0X5	T41.0X6
Vinorelbine tartrate	T45.1X1	T45.1X2	T45.1X3	T45.1X4	T45.1X5	T45.1X6

Substance	Poisoning, Accidental (unintentional)	Poisoning, Intentional Self-harm	Poisoning, Assault	Poisoning, Undetermined	Adverse Effect	Under-dosing
Vinpocetine	T46.7X1	T46.7X2	T46.7X3	T46.7X4	T46.7X5	T46.7X6
Vinyl						
acetate	T65.891	T65.892	T65.893	T65.894	—	—
bital	T42.3X1	T42.3X2	T42.3X3	T42.3X4	T42.3X5	T42.3X6
bromide	T65.891	T65.892	T65.893	T65.894	—	—
chloride	T59.891	T59.892	T59.893	T59.894	—	—
ether	T41.0X1	T41.0X2	T41.0X3	T41.0X4	T41.0X5	T41.0X6
Vinylbital	T42.3X1	T42.3X2	T42.3X3	T42.3X4	T42.3X5	T42.3X6
Vinylidene chloride	T65.891	T65.892	T65.893	T65.894	—	—
Vioform	T37.8X1	T37.8X2	T37.8X3	T37.8X4	T37.8X5	T37.8X6
topical	T49.0X1	T49.0X2	T49.0X3	T49.0X4	T49.0X5	T49.0X6
Viomycin	T36.8X1	T36.8X2	T36.8X3	T36.8X4	T36.8X5	T36.8X6
Viosterol	T45.2X1	T45.2X2	T45.2X3	T45.2X4	T45.2X5	T45.2X6
Viper (venom)	T63.091	T63.092	T63.093	T63.094		
Viprynium	T37.4X1	T37.4X2	T37.4X3	T37.4X4	T37.4X5	T37.4X6
Viquidil	T46.7X1	T46.7X2	T46.7X3	T46.7X4	T46.7X5	T46.7X6
Viral vaccine NEC	T50.B91	T50.B92	T50.B93	T50.B94	T50.B95	T50.B96
Virginiamycin	T36.8X1	T36.8X2	T36.8X3	T36.8X4	T36.8X5	T36.8X6
Virugon	T37.5X1	T37.5X2	T37.5X3	T37.5X4	T37.5X5	T37.5X6
Viscous agent	T50.901	T50.902	T50.903	T50.904	T50.905	T50.906
Visine	T49.5X1	T49.5X2	T49.5X3	T49.5X4	T49.5X5	T49.5X6
Visnadine	T46.3X1	T46.3X2	T46.3X3	T46.3X4	T46.3X5	T46.3X6
Vitamin NEC	T45.2X1	T45.2X2	T45.2X3	T45.2X4	T45.2X5	T45.2X6
A	T45.2X1	T45.2X2	T45.2X3	T45.2X4	T45.2X5	T45.2X6
B1	T45.2X1	T45.2X2	T45.2X3	T45.2X4	T45.2X5	T45.2X6
B2	T45.2X1	T45.2X2	T45.2X3	T45.2X4	T45.2X5	T45.2X6
B6	T45.2X1	T45.2X2	T45.2X3	T45.2X4	T45.2X5	T45.2X6
B12	T45.2X1	T45.2X2	T45.2X3	T45.2X4	T45.2X5	T45.2X6
B15	T45.2X1	T45.2X2	T45.2X3	T45.2X4	T45.2X5	T45.2X6
B NEC	T45.2X1	T45.2X2	T45.2X3	T45.2X4	T45.2X5	T45.2X6
nicotinic acid	T46.7X1	T46.7X2	T46.7X3	T46.7X4	T46.7X5	T46.7X6
C	T45.2X1	T45.2X2	T45.2X3	T45.2X4	T45.2X5	T45.2X6
D	T45.2X1	T45.2X2	T45.2X3	T45.2X4	T45.2X5	T45.2X6
D2	T45.2X1	T45.2X2	T45.2X3	T45.2X4	T45.2X5	T45.2X6
D3	T45.2X1	T45.2X2	T45.2X3	T45.2X4	T45.2X5	T45.2X6
E	T45.2X1	T45.2X2	T45.2X3	T45.2X4	T45.2X5	T45.2X6
E acetate	T45.2X1	T45.2X2	T45.2X3	T45.2X4	T45.2X5	T45.2X6
hematopoietic	T45.8X1	T45.8X2	T45.8X3	T45.8X4	T45.8X5	T45.8X6
K1	T45.7X1	T45.7X2	T45.7X3	T45.7X4	T45.7X5	T45.7X6
K2	T45.7X1	T45.7X2	T45.7X3	T45.7X4	T45.7X5	T45.7X6
K NEC	T45.7X1	T45.7X2	T45.7X3	T45.7X4	T45.7X5	T45.7X6
PP	T45.2X1	T45.2X2	T45.2X3	T45.2X4	T45.2X5	T45.2X6
ulceroprotectant	T47.1X1	T47.1X2	T47.1X3	T47.1X4	T47.1X5	T47.1X6
Vleminckx's solution	T49.4X1	T49.4X2	T49.4X3	T49.4X4	T49.4X5	T49.4X6
Voltaren — *see* Diclofenac sodium						
Warfarin	T45.511	T45.512	T45.513	T45.514	T45.515	T45.516
rodenticide	T60.4X1	T60.4X2	T60.4X3	T60.4X4	—	—
sodium	T60.4X1	T60.4X2	T60.4X3	T60.4X4	—	—
Wasp (sting)	T63.461	T63.462	T63.463	T63.464		
Water						
balance drug	T50.3X1	T50.3X2	T50.3X3	T50.3X4	T50.3X5	T50.3X6
distilled	T50.3X1	T50.3X2	T50.3X3	T50.3X4	T50.3X5	T50.3X6
gas — *see* Gas, water						
incomplete combustion of — *see* Carbon, monoxide, fuel, utility						
hemlock	T62.2X1	T62.2X2	T62.2X3	T62.2X4	—	—
moccasin (venom)	T63.061	T63.062	T63.063	T63.064	—	—
purified	T50.3X1	T50.3X2	T50.3X3	T50.3X4	T50.3X5	T50.3X6
Wax (paraffin) (petroleum)	T52.0X1	T52.0X2	T52.0X3	T52.0X4	—	—
automobile	T65.891	T65.892	T65.893	T65.894	—	—
floor	T52.0X1	T52.0X2	T52.0X3	T52.0X4	—	—
Weed killers NEC	T60.3X1	T60.3X2	T60.3X3	T60.3X4	—	—
Welldorm	T42.6X1	T42.6X2	T42.6X3	T42.6X4	T42.6X5	T42.6X6
White						
arsenic	T57.0X1	T57.0X2	T57.0X3	T57.0X4	—	—
hellebore	T62.2X1	T62.2X2	T62.2X3	T62.2X4	—	—
lotion (keratolytic)	T49.4X1	T49.4X2	T49.4X3	T49.4X4	T49.4X5	T49.4X6
spirit	T52.0X1	T52.0X2	T52.0X3	T52.0X4	—	—
Whitewash	T65.891	T65.892	T65.893	T65.894	—	—
Whole blood (human)	T45.8X1	T45.8X2	T45.8X3	T45.8X4	T45.8X5	T45.8X6
Wild						
black cherry	T62.2X1	T62.2X2	T62.2X3	T62.2X4	—	—
poisonous plants NEC	T62.2X1	T62.2X2	T62.2X3	T62.2X4	—	—
Window cleaning fluid	T65.891	T65.892	T65.893	T65.894	—	—
Wintergreen (oil)	T49.3X1	T49.3X2	T49.3X3	T49.3X4	T49.3X5	T49.3X6
Wisterine	T62.2X1	T62.2X2	T62.2X3	T62.2X4	—	—
Witch hazel	T49.2X1	T49.2X2	T49.2X3	T49.2X4	T49.2X5	T49.2X6
Wood alcohol or spirit	T51.1X1	T51.1X2	T51.1X3	T51.1X4		
Wool fat (hydrous)	T49.3X1	T49.3X2	T49.3X3	T49.3X4	T49.3X5	T49.3X6
Woorali	T48.1X1	T48.1X2	T48.1X3	T48.1X4	T48.1X5	T48.1X6
Wormseed, American	T37.4X1	T37.4X2	T37.4X3	T37.4X4	T37.4X5	T37.4X6

Substance	Poisoning, Accidental (unintentional)	Poisoning, Intentional Self-harm	Poisoning, Assault	Poisoning, Undetermined	Adverse Effect	Under-dosing
Xamoterol	T44.5X1	T44.5X2	T44.5X3	T44.5X4	T44.5X5	T44.5X6
Xanthine diuretics	T50.2X1	T50.2X2	T50.2X3	T50.2X4	T50.2X5	T50.2X6
Xanthinol nicotinate	T46.7X1	T46.7X2	T46.7X3	T46.7X4	T46.7X5	T46.7X6
Xanthotoxin	T49.3X1	T49.3X2	T49.3X3	T49.3X4	T49.3X5	T49.3X6
Xantinol nicotinate	T46.7X1	T46.7X2	T46.7X3	T46.7X4	T46.7X5	T46.7X6
Xantocillin	T36.0X1	T36.0X2	T36.0X3	T36.0X4	T36.0X5	T36.0X6
Xenon (127Xe) (133Xe)	T50.8X1	T50.8X2	T50.8X3	T50.8X4	T50.8X5	T50.8X6
Xenysalate	T49.4X1	T49.4X2	T49.4X3	T49.4X4	T49.4X5	T49.4X6
Xibornol	T37.8X1	T37.8X2	T37.8X3	T37.8X4	T37.8X5	T37.8X6
Xigris	T45.511	T45.512	T45.513	T45.514	T45.515	T45.516
Xipamide	T50.2X1	T50.2X2	T50.2X3	T50.2X4	T50.2X5	T50.2X6
Xylene (vapor)	T52.2X1	T52.2X2	T52.2X3	T52.2X4	—	—
Xylocaine (infiltration) (topical)	T41.3X1	T41.3X2	T41.3X3	T41.3X4	T41.3X5	T41.3X6
nerve block (peripheral) (plexus)	T41.3X1	T41.3X2	T41.3X3	T41.3X4	T41.3X5	T41.3X6
spinal	T41.3X1	T41.3X2	T41.3X3	T41.3X4	T41.3X5	T41.3X6
Xylol (vapor)	T52.2X1	T52.2X2	T52.2X3	T52.2X4	—	—
Xylometazoline	T48.5X1	T48.5X2	T48.5X3	T48.5X4	T48.5X5	T48.5X6
Yeast	T45.2X1	T45.2X2	T45.2X3	T45.2X4	T45.2X5	T45.2X6
dried	T45.2X1	T45.2X2	T45.2X3	T45.2X4	T45.2X5	T45.2X6
Yellow						
fever vaccine	T50.B91	T50.B92	T50.B93	T50.B94	T50.B95	T50.B96
jasmine	T62.2X1	T62.2X2	T62.2X3	T62.2X4		
phenolphthalein	T47.2X1	T47.2X2	T47.2X3	T47.2X4	T47.2X5	T47.2X6
Yew	T62.2X1	T62.2X2	T62.2X3	T62.2X4		
Yohimbic acid	T40.991	T40.992	T40.993	T40.994	T40.995	T40.996
Zactane	T39.8X1	T39.8X2	T39.8X3	T39.8X4	T39.8X5	T39.8X6
Zalcitabine	T37.5X1	T37.5X2	T37.5X3	T37.5X4	T37.5X5	T37.5X6
Zaroxolyn	T50.2X1	T50.2X2	T50.2X3	T50.2X4	T50.2X5	T50.2X6
Zephiran (topical)	T49.0X1	T49.0X2	T49.0X3	T49.0X4	T49.0X5	T49.0X6
ophthalmic preparation	T49.5X1	T49.5X2	T49.5X3	T49.5X4	T49.5X5	T49.5X6
Zeranol	T38.7X1	T38.7X2	T38.7X3	T38.7X4	T38.7X5	T38.7X6
Zerone	T51.1X1	T51.1X2	T51.1X3	T51.1X4		
Zidovudine	T37.5X1	T37.5X2	T37.5X3	T37.5X4	T37.5X5	T37.5X6
Zimeldine	T43.221	T43.222	T43.223	T43.224	T43.225	T43.226
Zinc (compounds) (fumes) (vapor)	T56.5X1	T56.5X2	T56.5X3	T56.5X4	—	—
NEC						
anti-infectives	T49.0X1	T49.0X2	T49.0X3	T49.0X4	T49.0X5	T49.0X6
antivaricose	T46.8X1	T46.8X2	T46.8X3	T46.8X4	T46.8X5	T46.8X6
bacitracin	T49.0X1	T49.0X2	T49.0X3	T49.0X4	T49.0X5	T49.0X6
chloride (mouthwash)	T49.6X1	T49.6X2	T49.6X3	T49.6X4	T49.6X5	T49.6X6
chromate	T56.5X1	T56.5X2	T56.5X3	T56.5X4	—	—
gelatin	T49.3X1	T49.3X2	T49.3X3	T49.3X4	T49.3X5	T49.3X6
oxide	T49.3X1	T49.3X2	T49.3X3	T49.3X4	T49.3X5	T49.3X6
plaster	T49.3X1	T49.3X2	T49.3X3	T49.3X4	T49.3X5	T49.3X6
peroxide	T49.0X1	T49.0X2	T49.0X3	T49.0X4	T49.0X5	T49.0X6
pesticides	T56.5X1	T56.5X2	T56.5X3	T56.5X4	—	—
phosphide	T60.4X1	T60.4X2	T60.4X3	T60.4X4	—	—
pyrithionate	T49.4X1	T49.4X2	T49.4X3	T49.4X4	T49.4X5	T49.4X6
stearate	T49.3X1	T49.3X2	T49.3X3	T49.3X4	T49.3X5	T49.3X6
sulfate	T49.5X1	T49.5X2	T49.5X3	T49.5X4	T49.5X5	T49.5X6
ENT agent	T49.6X1	T49.6X2	T49.6X3	T49.6X4	T49.6X5	T49.6X6
ophthalmic solution	T49.5X1	T49.5X2	T49.5X3	T49.5X4	T49.5X5	T49.5X6
topical NEC	T49.0X1	T49.0X2	T49.0X3	T49.0X4	T49.0X5	T49.0X6
undecylenate	T49.0X1	T49.0X2	T49.0X3	T49.0X4	T49.0X5	T49.0X6
Zineb	T60.0X1	T60.0X2	T60.0X3	T60.0X4	—	—
Zinostatin	T45.1X1	T45.1X2	T45.1X3	T45.1X4	T45.1X5	T45.1X6
Zipeprol	T48.3X1	T48.3X2	T48.3X3	T48.3X4	T48.3X5	T48.3X6
Zofenopril	T46.4X1	T46.4X2	T46.4X3	T46.4X4	T46.4X5	T46.4X6
Zolpidem	T42.6X1	T42.6X2	T42.6X3	T42.6X4	T42.6X5	T42.6X6
Zomepirac	T39.391	T39.392	T39.393	T39.394	T39.395	T39.396
Zopiclone	T42.6X1	T42.6X2	T42.6X3	T42.6X4	T42.6X5	T42.6X6
Zorubicin	T45.1X1	T45.1X2	T45.1X3	T45.1X4	T45.1X5	T45.1X6
Zotepine	T43.591	T43.592	T43.593	T43.594	T43.595	T43.596
Zovant	T45.511	T45.512	T45.513	T45.514	T45.515	T45.516
Zoxazolamine	T42.8X1	T42.8X2	T42.8X3	T42.8X4	T42.8X5	T42.8X6
Zuclopenthixol	T43.4X1	T43.4X2	T43.4X3	T43.4X4	T43.4X5	T43.4X6
Zygadenus (venenosus)	T62.2X1	T62.2X2	T62.2X3	T62.2X4		
Zyprexa	T43.591	T43.592	T43.593	T43.594	T43.595	T43.596

Additional Character May Be Required — Refer to the Tabular List for Character Selection ▼ Subterms under main terms may continue to next column or page

ICD-1Ø-CM Index to External Causes

A

Abandonment (causing exposure to weather conditions) (with intent to injure or kill) NEC X58 ☑
Abuse (adult) (child) (mental) (physical) (sexual) X58 ☑
Accident (to) X58 ☑
  aircraft (in transit) (powered) (*see also* Accident, transport, aircraft)
    due to, caused by cataclysm — *see* Forces of nature, by type
  animal-drawn vehicle — *see* Accident, transport, animal-drawn vehicle occupant
  animal-rider — *see* Accident, transport, animal-rider
  automobile — *see* Accident, transport, car occupant
  bare foot water skiier V94.4 ☑
  boat, boating (*see also* Accident, watercraft)
    striking swimmer
      powered V94.11 ☑
      unpowered V94.12 ☑
  bus — *see* Accident, transport, bus occupant
  cable car, not on rails V98.Ø ☑
    on rails — *see* Accident, transport, streetcar occupant
  car — *see* Accident, transport, car occupant
  caused by, due to
    animal NEC W64 ☑
    chain hoist W24.Ø ☑
    cold (excessive) — *see* Exposure, cold
    corrosive liquid, substance — *see* Table of Drugs and Chemicals
    cutting or piercing instrument — *see* Contact, with, by type of instrument
    drive belt W24.Ø ☑
    electric
      current — *see* Exposure, electric current
      motor (*see also* Contact, with, by type of machine) W31.3 ☑
        current (of) W86.8 ☑
    environmental factor NEC X58 ☑
    explosive material — *see* Explosion
    fire, flames — *see* Exposure, fire
    firearm missile — *see* Discharge, firearm by type
    heat (excessive) — *see* Heat
    hot — *see* Contact, with, hot
    ignition — *see* Ignition
    lifting device W24.Ø ☑
    lightning — *see* subcategory T75.Ø ☑
      causing fire — *see* Exposure, fire
    machine, machinery — *see* Contact, with, by type of machine
    natural factor NEC X58 ☑
    pulley (block) W24.Ø ☑
    radiation — *see* Radiation
    steam X13.1 ☑
      inhalation X13.Ø ☑
      pipe X16 ☑
    thunderbolt — *see* subcategory T75.Ø ☑
      causing fire — *see* Exposure, fire
    transmission device W24.1 ☑
  coach — *see* Accident, transport, bus occupant
  coal car — *see* Accident, transport, industrial vehicle occupant
  diving (*see also* Fall, into, water)
    with
      drowning or submersion — *see* Drowning
  forklift — *see* Accident, transport, industrial vehicle occupant
  heavy transport vehicle NOS — *see* Accident, transport, truck occupant
  ice yacht V98.2 ☑
  in
    medical, surgical procedure
      as, or due to misadventure — *see* Misadventure
      causing an abnormal reaction or later complication without mention of misadventure (*see also* Complication of or following, by type of procedure) Y84.9
  land yacht V98.1 ☑
  late effect of — *see* WØØ-X58 with 7th character S

Accident — *continued*
  logging car — *see* Accident, transport, industrial vehicle occupant
  machine, machinery (*see also* Contact, with, by type of machine)
    on board watercraft V93.69 ☑
      explosion — *see* Explosion, in, watercraft
      fire — *see* Burn, on board watercraft
      powered craft V93.63 ☑
        ferry boat V93.61 ☑
        fishing boat V93.62 ☑
        jetskis V93.63 ☑
        liner V93.61 ☑
        merchant ship V93.6Ø ☑
        passenger ship V93.61 ☑
        sailboat V93.64 ☑
  mine tram — *see* Accident, transport, industrial vehicle occupant
  mobility scooter (motorized) — *see* Accident, transport, pedestrian, conveyance, specified type NEC
  motor scooter — *see* Accident, transport, motorcyclist
  motor vehicle NOS (traffic) (*see also* Accident, transport) V89.2 ☑
    nontraffic V89.Ø ☑
    three-wheeled NOS — *see* Accident, transport, three-wheeled motor vehicle occupant
  motorcycle NOS — *see* Accident, transport, motorcyclist
  nonmotor vehicle NOS (nontraffic) (*see also* Accident, transport) V89.1 ☑
    traffic NOS V89.3 ☑
  nontraffic (victim's mode of transport NOS) V88.9 ☑
    collision (between) V88.7 ☑
      bus and truck V88.5 ☑
      car and:
        bus V88.3 ☑
        pickup V88.2 ☑
        three-wheeled motor vehicle V88.Ø ☑
        train V88.6 ☑
        truck V88.4 ☑
        two-wheeled motor vehicle V88.Ø ☑
        van V88.2 ☑
      specified vehicle NEC and:
        three-wheeled motor vehicle V88.1 ☑
        two-wheeled motor vehicle V88.1 ☑
    known mode of transport — *see* Accident, transport, by type of vehicle
    noncollision V88.8 ☑
  on board watercraft V93.89 ☑
    powered craft V93.83 ☑
      ferry boat V93.81 ☑
      fishing boat V93.82 ☑
      jetskis V93.83 ☑
      liner V93.81 ☑
      merchant ship V93.8Ø ☑
      passenger ship V93.81 ☑
    unpowered craft V93.88 ☑
      canoe V93.85 ☑
      inflatable V93.86 ☑
        in tow
          recreational V94.31 ☑
          specified NEC V94.32 ☑
      kayak V93.85 ☑
      sailboat V93.84 ☑
      surf-board V93.88 ☑
      water skis V93.87 ☑
      windsurfer V93.88 ☑
  parachutist V97.29 ☑
    entangled in object V97.21 ☑
    injured on landing V97.22 ☑
  pedal cycle — *see* Accident, transport, pedal cyclist
  pedestrian (on foot)
    with
      another pedestrian W51 ☑
        with fall WØ3 ☑
          due to ice or snow WØØ.Ø ☑
        on pedestrian conveyance NEC VØØ.Ø9 ☑
      roller skater (in-line) VØØ.Ø1 ☑
      skate boarder VØØ.Ø2 ☑
      transport vehicle — *see* Accident, transport

Accident — *continued*
  pedestrian — *continued*
    on pedestrian conveyance — *see* Accident, transport, pedestrian, conveyance
  pick-up truck or van — *see* Accident, transport, pickup truck occupant
  quarry truck — *see* Accident, transport, industrial vehicle occupant
  railway vehicle (any) (in motion) — *see* Accident, transport, railway vehicle occupant
    due to cataclysm — *see* Forces of nature, by type
  scooter (non-motorized) — *see* Accident, transport, pedestrian, conveyance, scooter
  sequelae of — *see* categories WØØ-X58 with 7th character S
  skateboard — *see* Accident, transport, pedestrian, conveyance, skateboard
  ski(ing) — *see* Accident, transport, pedestrian, conveyance
    lift V98.3 ☑
  specified cause NEC X58 ☑
  streetcar — *see* Accident, transport, streetcar occupant
  traffic (victim's mode of transport NOS) V87.9 ☑
    collision (between) V87.7 ☑
      bus and truck V87.5 ☑
      car and:
        bus V87.3 ☑
        pickup V87.2 ☑
        three-wheeled motor vehicle V87.Ø ☑
        train V87.6 ☑
        truck V87.4 ☑
        two-wheeled motor vehicle V87.Ø ☑
        van V87.2 ☑
      specified vehicle NEC and:
        three-wheeled motor vehicle V87.1 ☑
        two-wheeled motor vehicle V87.1 ☑
    known mode of transport — *see* Accident, transport, by type of vehicle
    noncollision V87.8 ☑
  transport (involving injury to) V99 ☑
    18 wheeler — *see* Accident, transport, truck occupant
    agricultural vehicle occupant (nontraffic) V84.9 ☑
      driver V84.5 ☑
      hanger-on V84.7 ☑
      passenger V84.6 ☑
      traffic V84.3 ☑
        driver V84.Ø ☑
        hanger-on V84.2 ☑
        passenger V84.1 ☑
      while boarding or alighting V84.4 ☑
    aircraft NEC V97.89 ☑
      military NEC V97.818 ☑
        with civlian aircraft V97.81Ø ☑
        civilian injured by V97.811 ☑
      occupant injured (in)
        nonpowered craft accident V96.9 ☑
          balloon V96.ØØ ☑
            collision V96.Ø3 ☑
            crash V96.Ø1 ☑
            explosion V96.Ø5 ☑
            fire V96.Ø4 ☑
            forced landing V96.Ø2 ☑
            specified type NEC V96.Ø9 ☑
          glider V96.2Ø ☑
            collision V96.23 ☑
            crash V96.21 ☑
            explosion V96.25 ☑
            fire V96.24 ☑
            forced landing V96.22 ☑
            specified type NEC V96.29 ☑
          hang glider V96.1Ø ☑
            collision V96.13 ☑
            crash V96.11 ☑
            explosion V96.15 ☑
            fire V96.14 ☑
            forced landing V96.12 ☑
            specified type NEC V96.19 ☑
          specified craft NEC V96.8 ☑
        powered craft accident V95.9 ☑

External Causes Index

Accident — Accident

Accident — *continued*
  transport — *continued*
    aircraft — *continued*
      occupant injured — *continued*
        powered craft accident — *continued*
          fixed wing NEC
            commercial V95.30 ☑
              collision V95.33 ☑
              crash V95.31 ☑
              explosion V95.35 ☑
              fire V95.34 ☑
              forced landing V95.32 ☑
              specified type NEC V95.39 ☑
            private V95.20 ☑
              collision V95.23 ☑
              crash V95.21 ☑
              explosion V95.25 ☑
              fire V95.24 ☑
              forced landing V95.22 ☑
              specified type NEC V95.29 ☑
          glider V95.10 ☑
            collision V95.13 ☑
            crash V95.11 ☑
            explosion V95.15 ☑
            fire V95.14 ☑
            forced landing V95.12 ☑
            specified type NEC V95.19 ☑
          helicopter V95.00 ☑
            collision V95.03 ☑
            crash V95.01 ☑
            explosion V95.05 ☑
            fire V95.04 ☑
            forced landing V95.02 ☑
            specified type NEC V95.09 ☑
          spacecraft V95.40 ☑
            collision V95.43 ☑
            crash V95.41 ☑
            explosion V95.45 ☑
            fire V95.44 ☑
            forced landing V95.42 ☑
            specified type NEC V95.49 ☑
          specified craft NEC V95.8 ☑
          ultralight V95.10 ☑
            collision V95.13 ☑
            crash V95.11 ☑
            explosion V95.15 ☑
            fire V95.14 ☑
            forced landing V95.12 ☑
            specified type NEC V95.19 ☑
        specified accident NEC V97.0 ☑
        while boarding or alighting V97.1 ☑
      person (injured by)
        falling from, in or on aircraft V97.0 ☑
        machinery on aircraft V97.89 ☑
        on ground with aircraft involvement V97.39 ☑
        rotating propeller V97.32 ☑
        struck by object falling from aircraft V97.31 ☑
        sucked into aircraft jet V97.33 ☑
        while boarding or alighting aircraft V97.1 ☑
      airport (battery-powered) passenger vehicle — *see* Accident, transport, industrial vehicle occupant
    all-terrain vehicle occupant (nontraffic) V86.99 ☑
      driver V86.59 ☑
      dune buggy — *see* Accident, transport, dune buggy occupant
      hanger-on V86.79 ☑
      passenger V86.69 ☑
      snowmobile — *see* Accident, transport, snowmobile occupant
      traffic V86.39 ☑
        driver V86.09 ☑
        hanger-on V86.29 ☑
        passenger V86.19 ☑
      while boarding or alighting V86.49 ☑
    ambulance occupant (traffic) V86.31 ☑
      driver V86.01 ☑
      hanger-on V86.21 ☑
      nontraffic V86.91 ☑
        driver V86.51 ☑
        hanger-on V86.71 ☑
        passenger V86.61 ☑
      passenger V86.11 ☑
      while boarding or alighting V86.41 ☑

Accident — *continued*
  transport — *continued*
    animal-drawn vehicle occupant (in) V80.929 ☑
      collision (with)
        animal V80.12 ☑
          being ridden V80.711 ☑
        animal-drawn vehicle V80.721 ☑
        bus V80.42 ☑
        car V80.42 ☑
        fixed or stationary object V80.82 ☑
        military vehicle V80.920 ☑
        nonmotor vehicle V80.791 ☑
        pedal cycle V80.22 ☑
        pedestrian V80.12 ☑
        pickup V80.42 ☑
        railway train or vehicle V80.62 ☑
        specified motor vehicle NEC V80.52 ☑
        streetcar V80.731 ☑
        truck V80.42 ☑
        two- or three-wheeled motor vehicle V80.32 ☑
        van V80.42 ☑
      noncollision V80.02 ☑
      specified circumstance NEC V80.928 ☑
    animal-rider V80.919 ☑
      collision (with)
        animal V80.11 ☑
          being ridden V80.710 ☑
        animal-drawn vehicle V80.720 ☑
        bus V80.41 ☑
        car V80.41 ☑
        fixed or stationary object V80.81 ☑
        military vehicle V80.910 ☑
        nonmotor vehicle V80.790 ☑
        pedal cycle V80.21 ☑
        pedestrian V80.11 ☑
        pickup V80.41 ☑
        railway train or vehicle V80.61 ☑
        specified motor vehicle NEC V80.51 ☑
        streetcar V80.730 ☑
        truck V80.41 ☑
        two- or three-wheeled motor vehicle V80.31 ☑
        van V80.41 ☑
      noncollision V80.018 ☑
        specified as horse rider V80.010 ☑
      specified circumstance NEC V80.918 ☑
    armored car — *see* Accident, transport, truck occupant
    battery-powered truck (baggage) (mail) — *see* Accident, transport, industrial vehicle occupant
    bus occupant V79.9 ☑
      collision (with)
        animal (traffic) V70.9 ☑
          being ridden (traffic) V76.9 ☑
            nontraffic V76.3 ☑
            while boarding or alighting V76.4 ☑
          nontraffic V70.3 ☑
          while boarding or alighting V70.4 ☑
        animal-drawn vehicle (traffic) V76.9 ☑
          nontraffic V76.3 ☑
          while boarding or alighting V76.4 ☑
        bus (traffic) V74.9 ☑
          nontraffic V74.3 ☑
          while boarding or alighting V74.4 ☑
        car (traffic) V73.9 ☑
          nontraffic V73.3 ☑
          while boarding or alighting V73.4 ☑
        motor vehicle NOS (traffic) V79.60 ☑
          nontraffic V79.20 ☑
          specified type NEC (traffic) V79.69 ☑
            nontraffic V79.29 ☑
        pedal cycle (traffic) V71.9 ☑
          nontraffic V71.3 ☑
          while boarding or alighting V71.4 ☑
        pickup truck (traffic) V73.9 ☑
          nontraffic V73.3 ☑
          while boarding or alighting V73.4 ☑
        railway vehicle (traffic) V75.9 ☑
          nontraffic V75.3 ☑
          while boarding or alighting V75.4 ☑
        specified vehicle NEC (traffic) V76.9 ☑
          nontraffic V76.3 ☑
          while boarding or alighting V76.4 ☑
        stationary object (traffic) V77.9 ☑

Accident — *continued*
  transport — *continued*
    bus occupant — *continued*
      collision — *continued*
        stationary object — *continued*
          nontraffic V77.3 ☑
          while boarding or alighting V77.4 ☑
        streetcar (traffic) V76.9 ☑
          nontraffic V76.3 ☑
          while boarding or alighting V76.4 ☑
        three wheeled motor vehicle (traffic) V72.9 ☑
          nontraffic V72.3 ☑
          while boarding or alighting V72.4 ☑
        truck (traffic) V74.9 ☑
          nontraffic V74.3 ☑
          while boarding or alighting V74.4 ☑
        two wheeled motor vehicle (traffic) V72.9 ☑
          nontraffic V72.3 ☑
          while boarding or alighting V72.4 ☑
        van (traffic) V73.9 ☑
          nontraffic V73.3 ☑
          while boarding or alighting V73.4 ☑
    driver
      collision (with)
        animal (traffic) V70.5 ☑
          being ridden (traffic) V76.5 ☑
          nontraffic V70.0 ☑
            nontraffic V76.0 ☑
        animal-drawn vehicle (traffic) V76.5 ☑
          nontraffic V76.0 ☑
        bus (traffic) V74.5 ☑
          nontraffic V74.0 ☑
        car (traffic) V73.5 ☑
          nontraffic V73.0 ☑
        motor vehicle NOS (traffic) V79.40 ☑
          nontraffic V79.00 ☑
            nontraffic V79.09 ☑
          specified type NEC (traffic) V79.49 ☑
        pedal cycle (traffic) V71.5 ☑
          nontraffic V71.0 ☑
        pickup truck (traffic) V73.5 ☑
          nontraffic V73.0 ☑
        railway vehicle (traffic) V75.5 ☑
          nontraffic V75.0 ☑
        specified vehicle NEC (traffic) V76.5 ☑
          nontraffic V76.0 ☑
        stationary object (traffic) V77.5 ☑
          nontraffic V77.0 ☑
        streetcar (traffic) V76.5 ☑
          nontraffic V76.0 ☑
        three wheeled motor vehicle (traffic) V72.5 ☑
          nontraffic V72.0 ☑
        truck (traffic) V74.5 ☑
          nontraffic V74.0 ☑
        two wheeled motor vehicle (traffic) V72.5 ☑
          nontraffic V72.0 ☑
        van (traffic) V73.5 ☑
          nontraffic V73.0 ☑
      noncollision accident (traffic) V78.5 ☑
        nontraffic V78.0 ☑
    hanger-on
      collision (with)
        animal (traffic) V70.7 ☑
          being ridden (traffic) V76.7 ☑
          nontraffic V70.2 ☑
            nontraffic V76.2 ☑
        animal-drawn vehicle (traffic) V76.7 ☑
          nontraffic V76.2 ☑
        bus (traffic) V74.7 ☑
          nontraffic V74.2 ☑
        car (traffic) V73.7 ☑
          nontraffic V73.2 ☑
        pedal cycle (traffic) V71.7 ☑
          nontraffic V71.2 ☑
        pickup truck (traffic) V73.7 ☑
          nontraffic V73.2 ☑
        railway vehicle (traffic) V75.7 ☑
          nontraffic V75.2 ☑
        specified vehicle NEC (traffic) V76.7 ☑
          nontraffic V76.2 ☑
        stationary object (traffic) V77.7 ☑
          nontraffic V77.2 ☑
        streetcar (traffic) V76.7 ☑

☑ **Additional Character Required** — Refer to the Tabular List for Character Selection   ▽ **Subterms under main terms may continue to next column or page**

Accident — *continued*
 transport — *continued*
  bus occupant — *continued*
   hanger-on — *continued*
    collision — *continued*
     streetcar — *continued*
      nontraffic V76.2 ☑
     three wheeled motor vehicle (traffic)
      V72.7 ☑
      nontraffic V72.2 ☑
     truck (traffic) V74.7 ☑
      nontraffic V74.2 ☑
     two wheeled motor vehicle (traffic)
      V72.7 ☑
      nontraffic V72.2 ☑
     van (traffic) V73.7 ☑
      nontraffic V73.2 ☑
    noncollision accident (traffic) V78.7 ☑
     nontraffic V78.2 ☑
   noncollision accident (traffic) V78.9 ☑
    nontraffic V78.3 ☑
    while boarding or alighting V78.4 ☑
   nontraffic V79.3 ☑
   passenger
    collision (with)
     animal (traffic) V70.6 ☑
      being ridden (traffic) V76.6 ☑
       nontraffic V70.1 ☑
        nontraffic V76.1 ☑
     animal-drawn vehicle (traffic) V76.6 ☑
      nontraffic V76.1 ☑
     bus (traffic) V74.6 ☑
      nontraffic V74.1 ☑
     car (traffic) V73.6 ☑
      nontraffic V73.1 ☑
     motor vehicle NOS (traffic) V79.50 ☑
      nontraffic V79.10 ☑
      specified type NEC (traffic) V79.59 ☑
       nontraffic V79.19 ☑
     pedal cycle (traffic) V71.6 ☑
      nontraffic V71.1 ☑
     pickup truck (traffic) V73.6 ☑
      nontraffic V73.1 ☑
     railway vehicle (traffic) V75.6 ☑
      nontraffic V75.1 ☑
     specified vehicle NEC (traffic) V76.6 ☑
      nontraffic V76.1 ☑
     stationary object (traffic) V77.6 ☑
      nontraffic V77.1 ☑
     streetcar (traffic) V76.6 ☑
      nontraffic V76.1 ☑
     three wheeled motor vehicle (traffic)
      V72.6 ☑
      nontraffic V72.1 ☑
     truck (traffic) V74.6 ☑
      nontraffic V74.1 ☑
     two wheeled motor vehicle (traffic)
      V72.6 ☑
      nontraffic V72.1 ☑
     van (traffic) V73.6 ☑
      nontraffic V73.1 ☑
    noncollision accident (traffic) V78.6 ☑
     nontraffic V78.1 ☑
   specified type NEC V79.88 ☑
    military vehicle V79.81 ☑
  cable car, not on rails V98.0 ☑
   on rails — *see* Accident, transport, streetcar
    occupant
  car occupant V49.9 ☑
   ambulance occupant — *see* Accident, transport,
    ambulance occupant
   collision (with)
    animal (traffic) V40.9 ☑
     being ridden (traffic) V46.9 ☑
      nontraffic V46.3 ☑
       while boarding or alighting V46.4 ☑
     nontraffic V40.3 ☑
     while boarding or alighting V40.4 ☑
    animal-drawn vehicle (traffic) V46.9 ☑
     nontraffic V46.3 ☑
     while boarding or alighting V46.4 ☑
    bus (traffic) V44.9 ☑
     nontraffic V44.3 ☑
     while boarding or alighting V44.4 ☑
    car (traffic) V43.92 ☑
     nontraffic V43.32 ☑

Accident — *continued*
 transport — *continued*
  car occupant — *continued*
   collision — *continued*
    car — *continued*
     while boarding or alighting V43.42 ☑
    motor vehicle NOS (traffic) V49.60 ☑
     nontraffic V49.20 ☑
     specified type NEC (traffic) V49.69 ☑
      nontraffic V49.29 ☑
    pedal cycle (traffic) V41.9 ☑
     nontraffic V41.3 ☑
     while boarding or alighting V41.4 ☑
    pickup truck (traffic) V43.93 ☑
     nontraffic V43.33 ☑
     while boarding or alighting V43.43 ☑
    railway vehicle (traffic) V45.9 ☑
     nontraffic V45.3 ☑
     while boarding or alighting V45.4 ☑
    specified vehicle NEC (traffic) V46.9 ☑
     nontraffic V46.3 ☑
     while boarding or alighting V46.4 ☑
    sport utility vehicle (traffic) V43.91 ☑
     nontraffic V43.31 ☑
     while boarding or alighting V43.41 ☑
    stationary object (traffic) V47.92 ☑
     nontraffic V47.32 ☑
     while boarding or alighting V47.4 ☑
    streetcar (traffic) V46.9 ☑
     nontraffic V46.3 ☑
     while boarding or alighting V46.4 ☑
    three wheeled motor vehicle (traffic)
     V42.9 ☑
     nontraffic V42.3 ☑
     while boarding or alighting V42.4 ☑
    truck (traffic) V44.9 ☑
     nontraffic V44.3 ☑
     while boarding or alighting V44.4 ☑
    two wheeled motor vehicle (traffic) V42.9 ☑
     nontraffic V42.3 ☑
     while boarding or alighting V42.4 ☑
    van (traffic) V43.94 ☑
     nontraffic V43.34 ☑
     while boarding or alighting V43.44 ☑
   driver
    collision (with)
     animal (traffic) V40.5 ☑
      being ridden (traffic) V46.5 ☑
       nontraffic V46.0 ☑
       nontraffic V40.0 ☑
     animal-drawn vehicle (traffic) V46.5 ☑
      nontraffic V46.0 ☑
     bus (traffic) V44.5 ☑
      nontraffic V44.0 ☑
     car (traffic) V43.52 ☑
      nontraffic V43.02 ☑
     motor vehicle NOS (traffic) V49.40 ☑
      nontraffic V49.00 ☑
      specified type NEC (traffic) V49.49 ☑
       nontraffic V49.09 ☑
     pedal cycle (traffic) V41.5 ☑
      nontraffic V41.0 ☑
     pickup truck (traffic) V43.53 ☑
      nontraffic V43.03 ☑
     railway vehicle (traffic) V45.5 ☑
      nontraffic V45.0 ☑
     specified vehicle NEC (traffic) V46.5 ☑
      nontraffic V46.0 ☑
     sport utility vehicle (traffic) V43.51 ☑
      nontraffic V43.01 ☑
     stationary object (traffic) V47.52 ☑
      nontraffic V47.02 ☑
     streetcar (traffic) V46.5 ☑
      nontraffic V46.0 ☑
     three wheeled motor vehicle (traffic)
      V42.5 ☑
      nontraffic V42.0 ☑
     truck (traffic) V44.5 ☑
      nontraffic V44.0 ☑
     two wheeled motor vehicle (traffic)
      V42.5 ☑
      nontraffic V42.0 ☑
     van (traffic) V43.54 ☑
      nontraffic V43.04 ☑
    noncollision accident (traffic) V48.5 ☑
     nontraffic V48.0 ☑

Accident — *continued*
 transport — *continued*
  car occupant — *continued*
   hanger-on
    collision (with)
     animal (traffic) V40.7 ☑
      being ridden (traffic) V46.7 ☑
       nontraffic V40.2 ☑
       nontraffic V46.2 ☑
     animal-drawn vehicle (traffic) V46.7 ☑
      nontraffic V46.2 ☑
     bus (traffic) V44.7 ☑
      nontraffic V44.2 ☑
     car (traffic) V43.72 ☑
      nontraffic V43.22 ☑
     pedal cycle (traffic) V41.7 ☑
      nontraffic V41.2 ☑
     pickup truck (traffic) V43.73 ☑
      nontraffic V43.23 ☑
     railway vehicle (traffic) V45.7 ☑
      nontraffic V45.2 ☑
     specified vehicle NEC (traffic) V46.7 ☑
      nontraffic V46.2 ☑
     sport utility vehicle (traffic) V43.71 ☑
      nontraffic V43.21 ☑
     stationary object (traffic) V47.7 ☑
      nontraffic V47.2 ☑
     streetcar (traffic) V46.7 ☑
      nontraffic V46.2 ☑
     three wheeled motor vehicle (traffic)
      V42.7 ☑
      nontraffic V42.2 ☑
     truck (traffic) V44.7 ☑
      nontraffic V44.2 ☑
     two wheeled motor vehicle (traffic)
      V42.7 ☑
      nontraffic V42.2 ☑
     van (traffic) V43.74 ☑
      nontraffic V43.24 ☑
    noncollision accident (traffic) V48.7 ☑
     nontraffic V48.2 ☑
   noncollision accident (traffic) V48.9 ☑
    nontraffic V48.3 ☑
    while boarding or alighting V48.4 ☑
   nontraffic V49.3 ☑
   passenger
    collision (with)
     animal (traffic) V40.6 ☑
      being ridden (traffic) V46.6 ☑
       nontraffic V46.1 ☑
       nontraffic V40.1 ☑
     animal-drawn vehicle (traffic) V46.6 ☑
      nontraffic V46.1 ☑
     bus (traffic) V44.6 ☑
      nontraffic V44.1 ☑
     car (traffic) V43.62 ☑
      nontraffic V43.12 ☑
     motor vehicle NOS (traffic) V49.50 ☑
      nontraffic V49.10 ☑
      specified type NEC (traffic) V49.59 ☑
       nontraffic V49.19 ☑
     pedal cycle (traffic) V41.6 ☑
      nontraffic V41.1 ☑
     pickup truck (traffic) V43.63 ☑
      nontraffic V43.13 ☑
     railway vehicle (traffic) V45.6 ☑
      nontraffic V45.1 ☑
     specified vehicle NEC (traffic) V46.6 ☑
      nontraffic V46.1 ☑
     sport utility vehicle (traffic) V43.61 ☑
      nontraffic V43.11 ☑
     stationary object (traffic) V47.62 ☑
      nontraffic V47.12 ☑
     streetcar (traffic) V46.6 ☑
      nontraffic V46.1 ☑
     three wheeled motor vehicle (traffic)
      V42.6 ☑
      nontraffic V42.1 ☑
     truck (traffic) V44.6 ☑
      nontraffic V44.1 ☑
     two wheeled motor vehicle (traffic)
      V42.6 ☑
      nontraffic V42.1 ☑
     van (traffic) V43.64 ☑
      nontraffic V43.14 ☑
    noncollision accident (traffic) V48.6 ☑

Accident — *continued*
  transport — *continued*
    car occupant — *continued*
      passenger — *continued*
        noncollision accident — *continued*
          nontraffic V48.1 ☑
      specified type NEC V49.88 ☑
        military vehicle V49.81 ☑
    coal car — *see* Accident, transport, industrial vehicle occupant
    construction vehicle occupant (nontraffic) V85.9 ☑
      driver V85.5 ☑
      hanger-on V85.7 ☑
      passenger V85.6 ☑
      traffic V85.3 ☑
        driver V85.0 ☑
        hanger-on V85.2 ☑
        passenger V85.1 ☑
      while boarding or alighting V85.4 ☑
    dirt bike rider — *see* Accident, transport, all-terrain vehicle occupant
    due to cataclysm — *see* Forces of nature, by type
    dune buggy occupant (nontraffic) V86.93 ☑
      driver V86.53 ☑
      hanger-on V86.73 ☑
      passenger V86.63 ☑
      traffic V86.33 ☑
        driver V86.03 ☑
        hanger-on V86.23 ☑
        passenger V86.13 ☑
      while boarding or alighting V86.43 ☑
    forklift — *see* Accident, transport, industrial vehicle occupant
    go cart — *see* Accident, transport, all-terrain vehicle occupant
    golf cart — *see* Accident, transport, all-terrain vehicle occupant
    heavy transport vehicle occupant — *see* Accident, transport, truck occupant
    ice yacht V98.2 ☑
    industrial vehicle occupant (nontraffic) V83.9 ☑
      driver V83.5 ☑
      hanger-on V83.7 ☑
      passenger V83.6 ☑
      traffic V83.3 ☑
        driver V83.0 ☑
        hanger-on V83.2 ☑
        passenger V83.1 ☑
      while boarding or alighting V83.4 ☑
    interurban electric car — *see* Accident, transport, streetcar
    land yacht V98.1 ☑
    logging car — *see* Accident, transport, industrial vehicle occupant
    military vehicle occupant (traffic) V86.34 ☑
      driver V86.04 ☑
      hanger-on V86.24 ☑
      nontraffic V86.94 ☑
        driver V86.54 ☑
        hanger-on V86.74 ☑
        passenger V86.64 ☑
      passenger V86.14 ☑
      while boarding or alighting V86.44 ☑
    mine tram — *see* Accident, transport, industrial vehicle occupant
    motor vehicle NEC occupant (traffic) V86.39 ☑
      driver V86.09 ☑
      hanger-on V86.29 ☑
      nontraffic V86.99 ☑
        driver V86.59 ☑
        hanger-on V86.79 ☑
        passenger V86.69 ☑
      passenger V86.19 ☑
      while boarding or alighting V86.49 ☑
    motorcoach — *see* Accident, transport, bus occupant
    motorcyclist V29.9 ☑
      collision (with)
        animal (traffic) V20.9 ☑
          being ridden (traffic) V26.9 ☑
            nontraffic V26.2 ☑
            while boarding or alighting V26.3 ☑
          nontraffic V20.2 ☑
          while boarding or alighting V20.3 ☑
        animal-drawn vehicle (traffic) V26.9 ☑
          nontraffic V26.2 ☑

Accident — *continued*
  transport — *continued*
    motorcyclist — *continued*
      collision — *continued*
        animal-drawn vehicle — *continued*
          while boarding or alighting V26.3 ☑
        bus (traffic) V24.9 ☑
          nontraffic V24.2 ☑
          while boarding or alighting V24.3 ☑
        car (traffic) V23.9 ☑
          nontraffic V23.2 ☑
          while boarding or alighting V23.3 ☑
        motor vehicle NOS (traffic) V29.60 ☑
          nontraffic V29.20 ☑
          specified type NEC (traffic) V29.69 ☑
            nontraffic V29.29 ☑
        pedal cycle (traffic) V21.9 ☑
          nontraffic V21.2 ☑
          while boarding or alighting V21.3 ☑
        pickup truck (traffic) V23.9 ☑
          nontraffic V23.2 ☑
          while boarding or alighting V23.3 ☑
        railway vehicle (traffic) V25.9 ☑
          nontraffic V25.2 ☑
          while boarding or alighting V25.3 ☑
        specified vehicle NEC (traffic) V26.9 ☑
          nontraffic V26.2 ☑
          while boarding or alighting V26.3 ☑
        stationary object (traffic) V27.9 ☑
          nontraffic V27.2 ☑
          while boarding or alighting V27.3 ☑
        streetcar (traffic) V26.9 ☑
          nontraffic V26.2 ☑
          while boarding or alighting V26.3 ☑
        three wheeled motor vehicle (traffic) V22.9 ☑
          nontraffic V22.2 ☑
          while boarding or alighting V22.3 ☑
        truck (traffic) V24.9 ☑
          nontraffic V24.2 ☑
          while boarding or alighting V24.3 ☑
        two wheeled motor vehicle (traffic) V22.9 ☑
          nontraffic V22.2 ☑
          while boarding or alighting V22.3 ☑
        van (traffic) V23.9 ☑
          nontraffic V23.2 ☑
          while boarding or alighting V23.3 ☑
      driver
        collision (with)
          animal (traffic) V20.4 ☑
            being ridden (traffic) V26.4 ☑
              nontraffic V26.0 ☑
            nontraffic V20.0 ☑
          animal-drawn vehicle (traffic) V26.4 ☑
            nontraffic V26.0 ☑
          bus (traffic) V24.4 ☑
            nontraffic V24.0 ☑
          car (traffic) V23.4 ☑
            nontraffic V23.0 ☑
          motor vehicle NOS (traffic) V29.40 ☑
            nontraffic V29.00 ☑
            specified type NEC (traffic) V29.49 ☑
              nontraffic V29.09 ☑
          pedal cycle (traffic) V21.4 ☑
            nontraffic V21.0 ☑
          pickup truck (traffic) V23.4 ☑
            nontraffic V23.0 ☑
          railway vehicle (traffic) V25.4 ☑
            nontraffic V25.0 ☑
          specified vehicle NEC (traffic) V26.4 ☑
            nontraffic V26.0 ☑
          stationary object (traffic) V27.4 ☑
            nontraffic V27.0 ☑
          streetcar (traffic) V26.4 ☑
            nontraffic V26.0 ☑
          three wheeled motor vehicle (traffic) V22.4 ☑
            nontraffic V22.0 ☑
          truck (traffic) V24.4 ☑
            nontraffic V24.0 ☑
          two wheeled motor vehicle (traffic) V22.4 ☑
            nontraffic V22.0 ☑
          van (traffic) V23.4 ☑
            nontraffic V23.0 ☑
        noncollision accident (traffic) V28.4 ☑

Accident — *continued*
  transport — *continued*
    motorcyclist — *continued*
      driver — *continued*
        noncollision accident — *continued*
          nontraffic V28.0 ☑
        noncollision accident (traffic) V28.9 ☑
          nontraffic V28.2 ☑
          while boarding or alighting V28.3 ☑
      nontraffic V29.3 ☑
      passenger
        collision (with)
          animal (traffic) V20.5 ☑
            being ridden (traffic) V26.5 ☑
              nontraffic V20.1 ☑
              nontraffic V26.1 ☑
          animal-drawn vehicle (traffic) V26.5 ☑
            nontraffic V26.1 ☑
          bus (traffic) V24.5 ☑
            nontraffic V24.1 ☑
          car (traffic) V23.5 ☑
            nontraffic V23.1 ☑
          motor vehicle NOS (traffic) V29.50 ☑
            nontraffic V29.10 ☑
            specified type NEC (traffic) V29.59 ☑
              nontraffic V29.19 ☑
          pedal cycle (traffic) V21.5 ☑
            nontraffic V21.1 ☑
          pickup truck (traffic) V23.5 ☑
            nontraffic V23.1 ☑
          railway vehicle (traffic) V25.5 ☑
            nontraffic V25.1 ☑
          specified vehicle NEC (traffic) V26.5 ☑
            nontraffic V26.1 ☑
          stationary object (traffic) V27.5 ☑
            nontraffic V27.1 ☑
          streetcar (traffic) V26.5 ☑
            nontraffic V26.1 ☑
          three wheeled motor vehicle (traffic) V22.5 ☑
            nontraffic V22.1 ☑
          truck (traffic) V24.5 ☑
            nontraffic V24.1 ☑
          two wheeled motor vehicle (traffic) V22.5 ☑
            nontraffic V22.1 ☑
          van (traffic) V23.5 ☑
            nontraffic V23.1 ☑
      noncollision accident (traffic) V28.5 ☑
        nontraffic V28.1 ☑
      specified type NEC V29.88 ☑
        military vehicle V29.81 ☑
    occupant (of)
      aircraft (powered) V95.9 ☑
        fixed wing
          commercial — *see* Accident, transport, aircraft, occupant, powered, fixed wing, commercial
          private — *see* Accident, transport, aircraft, occupant, powered, fixed wing, private
        nonpowered V96.9 ☑
        specified NEC V95.8 ☑
      airport battery-powered vehicle — *see* Accident, transport, industrial vehicle occupant
      all-terrain vehicle (ATV) — *see* Accident, transport, all-terrain vehicle occupant
      animal-drawn vehicle — *see* Accident, transport, animal-drawn vehicle occupant
      automobile — *see* Accident, transport, car occupant
      balloon V96.00 ☑
      battery-powered vehicle — *see* Accident, transport, industrial vehicle occupant
      bicycle — *see* Accident, transport, pedal cyclist
        motorized — *see* Accident, transport, motorcycle rider
      boat NEC — *see* Accident, watercraft
      bulldozer — *see* Accident, transport, construction vehicle occupant
      bus — *see* Accident, transport, bus occupant
      cable car (on rails) (*see also* Accident, transport, streetcar occupant)
        not on rails V98.0 ☑
      car (*see also* Accident, transport, car occupant)

☑ **Additional Character Required** — Refer to the Tabular List for Character Selection   🝾 **Subterms under main terms may continue to next column or page**

Accident — *continued*
  transport — *continued*
    occupant — *continued*
      car (*see also* Accident, transport, car occupant) — *continued*
        cable (on rails) (*see also* Accident, transport, streetcar occupant)
          not on rails V98.0 ☑
      coach — *see* Accident, transport, bus occupant
      coal-car — *see* Accident, transport, industrial vehicle occupant
      digger — *see* Accident, transport, construction vehicle occupant
      dump truck — *see* Accident, transport, construction vehicle occupant
      earth-leveler — *see* Accident, transport, construction vehicle occupant
      farm machinery (self-propelled) — *see* Accident, transport, agricultural vehicle occupant
      forklift — *see* Accident, transport, industrial vehicle occupant
      glider (unpowered) V96.20 ☑
        hang V96.10 ☑
        powered (microlight) (ultralight) — *see* Accident, transport, aircraft, occupant, powered, glider
      glider (unpowered) NEC V96.20 ☑
      hang-glider V96.10 ☑
      harvester — *see* Accident, transport, agricultural vehicle occupant
      heavy (transport) vehicle — *see* Accident, transport, truck occupant
      helicopter — *see* Accident, transport, aircraft, occupant, helicopter
      ice-yacht V98.2 ☑
      kite (carrying person) V96.8 ☑
      land-yacht V98.1 ☑
      logging car — *see* Accident, transport, industrial vehicle occupant
      mechanical shovel — *see* Accident, transport, construction vehicle occupant
      microlight — *see* Accident, transport, aircraft, occupant, powered, glider
      minibus — *see* Accident, transport, car occupant
      minivan — *see* Accident, transport, car occupant
      moped — *see* Accident, transport, motorcycle
      motor scooter — *see* Accident, transport, motorcycle
      motorcycle (with sidecar) — *see* Accident, transport, motorcycle
      pedal cycle (*see also* Accident, transport, pedal cyclist)
      pick-up (truck) — *see* Accident, transport, pickup truck occupant
      railway (train) (vehicle) (subterranean) (elevated) — *see* Accident, transport, railway vehicle occupant
      rickshaw — *see* Accident, transport, pedal cycle
        motorized — *see* Accident, transport, three-wheeled motor vehicle
        pedal driven — *see* Accident, transport, pedal cyclist
      road-roller — *see* Accident, transport, construction vehicle occupant
      ship NOS V94.9 ☑
      ski-lift (chair) (gondola) V98.3 ☑
      snowmobile — *see* Accident, transport, snowmobile occupant
      spacecraft, spaceship — *see* Accident, transport, aircraft, occupant, spacecraft
      sport utility vehicle — *see* Accident, transport, car occupant
      streetcar (interurban) (operating on public street or highway) — *see* Accident, transport, streetcar occupant
      SUV — *see* Accident, transport, car occupant
      téléférique V98.0 ☑
      three-wheeled vehicle (motorized) (*see also* Accident, transport, three-wheeled motor vehicle occupant)
        nonmotorized — *see* Accident, transport, pedal cycle
      tractor (farm) (and trailer) — *see* Accident, transport, agricultural vehicle occupant

Accident — *continued*
  transport — *continued*
    occupant — *continued*
      train — *see* Accident, transport, railway vehicle occupant
      tram — *see* Accident, transport, streetcar occupant
        in mine or quarry — *see* Accident, transport, industrial vehicle occupant
      tricycle — *see* Accident, transport, pedal cycle
        motorized — *see* Accident, transport, three-wheeled motor vehicle
      trolley — *see* Accident, transport, streetcar occupant
        in mine or quarry — *see* Accident, transport, industrial vehicle occupant
      tub, in mine or quarry — *see* Accident, transport, industrial vehicle occupant
      ultralight — *see* Accident, transport, aircraft, occupant, powered, glider
      van — *see* Accident, transport, van occupant
      vehicle NEC V89.9 ☑
        heavy transport — *see* Accident, transport, truck occupant
        motor (traffic) NEC V89.2 ☑
        nontraffic NEC V89.0 ☑
      watercraft NOS V94.9 ☑
        causing drowning B — *see* Drowning, resulting from accident to boat
    parachutist V97.29 ☑
      after accident to aircraft — *see* Accident, transport, aircraft
      entangled in object V97.21 ☑
      injured on landing V97.22 ☑
    pedal cyclist V19.9 ☑
      collision (with)
        animal (traffic) V10.9 ☑
          being ridden (traffic) V16.9 ☑
            nontraffic V16.2 ☑
            while boarding or alighting V16.3 ☑
          nontraffic V10.2 ☑
          while boarding or alighting V10.3 ☑
        animal-drawn vehicle (traffic) V16.9 ☑
          nontraffic V16.2 ☑
          while boarding or alighting V16.3 ☑
        bus (traffic) V14.9 ☑
          nontraffic V14.2 ☑
          while boarding or alighting V14.3 ☑
        car (traffic) V13.9 ☑
          nontraffic V13.2 ☑
          while boarding or alighting V13.3 ☑
        motor vehicle NOS (traffic) V19.60 ☑
          nontraffic V19.20 ☑
          specified type NEC (traffic) V19.69 ☑
            nontraffic V19.29 ☑
        pedal cycle (traffic) V11.9 ☑
          nontraffic V11.2 ☑
          while boarding or alighting V11.3 ☑
        pickup truck (traffic) V13.9 ☑
          nontraffic V13.2 ☑
          while boarding or alighting V13.3 ☑
        railway vehicle (traffic) V15.9 ☑
          nontraffic V15.2 ☑
          while boarding or alighting V15.3 ☑
        specified vehicle NEC (traffic) V16.9 ☑
          nontraffic V16.2 ☑
          while boarding or alighting V16.3 ☑
        stationary object (traffic) V17.9 ☑
          nontraffic V17.2 ☑
          while boarding or alighting V17.3 ☑
        streetcar (traffic) V16.9 ☑
          nontraffic V16.2 ☑
          while boarding or alighting V16.3 ☑
        three wheeled motor vehicle (traffic) V12.9 ☑
          nontraffic V12.2 ☑
          while boarding or alighting V12.3 ☑
        truck (traffic) V14.9 ☑
          nontraffic V14.2 ☑
          while boarding or alighting V14.3 ☑
        two wheeled motor vehicle (traffic) V12.9 ☑
          nontraffic V12.2 ☑
          while boarding or alighting V12.3 ☑
        van (traffic) V13.9 ☑
          nontraffic V13.2 ☑
          while boarding or alighting V13.3 ☑

Accident — *continued*
  transport — *continued*
    pedal cyclist — *continued*
      driver
        collision (with)
          animal (traffic) V10.4 ☑
            being ridden (traffic) V16.4 ☑
              nontraffic V16.0 ☑
            nontraffic V10.0 ☑
          animal-drawn vehicle (traffic) V16.4 ☑
            nontraffic V16.0 ☑
          bus (traffic) V14.4 ☑
            nontraffic V14.0 ☑
          car (traffic) V13.4 ☑
            nontraffic V13.0 ☑
          motor vehicle NOS (traffic) V19.40 ☑
            nontraffic V19.00 ☑
          specified type NEC (traffic) V19.49 ☑
            nontraffic V19.09 ☑
          pedal cycle (traffic) V11.4 ☑
            nontraffic V11.0 ☑
          pickup truck (traffic) V13.4 ☑
            nontraffic V13.0 ☑
          railway vehicle (traffic) V15.4 ☑
            nontraffic V15.0 ☑
          specified vehicle NEC (traffic) V16.4 ☑
            nontraffic V16.0 ☑
          stationary object (traffic) V17.4 ☑
            nontraffic V17.0 ☑
          streetcar (traffic) V16.4 ☑
            nontraffic V16.0 ☑
          three wheeled motor vehicle (traffic) V12.4 ☑
            nontraffic V12.0 ☑
          truck (traffic) V14.4 ☑
            nontraffic V14.0 ☑
          two wheeled motor vehicle (traffic) V12.4 ☑
            nontraffic V12.0 ☑
          van (traffic) V13.4 ☑
            nontraffic V13.0 ☑
        noncollision accident (traffic) V18.4 ☑
          nontraffic V18.0 ☑
      noncollision accident (traffic) V18.9 ☑
        nontraffic V18.2 ☑
        while boarding or alighting V18.3 ☑
      nontraffic V19.3 ☑
      passenger
        collision (with)
          animal (traffic) V10.5 ☑
            being ridden (traffic) V16.5 ☑
              nontraffic V10.1 ☑
                nontraffic V16.1 ☑
          animal-drawn vehicle (traffic) V16.5 ☑
            nontraffic V16.1 ☑
          bus (traffic) V14.5 ☑
            nontraffic V14.1 ☑
          car (traffic) V13.5 ☑
            nontraffic V13.1 ☑
          motor vehicle NOS (traffic) V19.50 ☑
            nontraffic V19.10 ☑
          specified type NEC (traffic) V19.59 ☑
            nontraffic V19.19 ☑
          pedal cycle (traffic) V11.5 ☑
            nontraffic V11.1 ☑
          pickup truck (traffic) V13.5 ☑
            nontraffic V13.1 ☑
          railway vehicle (traffic) V15.5 ☑
            nontraffic V15.1 ☑
          specified vehicle NEC (traffic) V16.5 ☑
            nontraffic V16.1 ☑
          stationary object (traffic) V17.5 ☑
            nontraffic V17.1 ☑
          streetcar (traffic) V16.5 ☑
            nontraffic V16.1 ☑
          three wheeled motor vehicle (traffic) V12.5 ☑
            nontraffic V12.1 ☑
          truck (traffic) V14.5 ☑
            nontraffic V14.1 ☑
          two wheeled motor vehicle (traffic) V12.5 ☑
            nontraffic V12.1 ☑
          van (traffic) V13.5 ☑
            nontraffic V13.1 ☑
        noncollision accident (traffic) V18.5 ☑

Accident — *continued*
  transport — *continued*
    pedal cyclist — *continued*
      passenger — *continued*
        noncollision accident — *continued*
          nontraffic V18.1 ☑
      specified type NEC V19.88 ☑
        military vehicle V19.81 ☑
    pedestrian
      conveyance (occupant) V09.9 ☑
        babystroller V00.828 ☑
          collision (with) V09.9 ☑
            animal being ridden or animal drawn
              vehicle V06.99 ☑
                nontraffic V06.09 ☑
                traffic V06.19 ☑
            bus or heavy transport V04.99 ☑
              nontraffic V04.09 ☑
              traffic V04.19 ☑
            car V03.99 ☑
              nontraffic V03.09 ☑
              traffic V03.19 ☑
            pedal cycle V01.99 ☑
              nontraffic V01.09 ☑
              traffic V01.19 ☑
            pick-up truck or van V03.99 ☑
              nontraffic V03.09 ☑
              traffic V03.19 ☑
            railway (train) (vehicle) V05.99 ☑
              nontraffic V05.09 ☑
              traffic V05.19 ☑
            stationary object V00.822 ☑
            streetcar V06.99 ☑
              nontraffic V06.09 ☑
              traffic V06.19 ☑
            two- or three-wheeled motor vehicle
              V02.99 ☑
              nontraffic V02.09 ☑
              traffic V02.19 ☑
            vehicle V09.9 ☑
              animal-drawn V06.99 ☑
                nontraffic V06.09 ☑
                traffic V06.19 ☑
              motor
                nontraffic V09.00 ☑
                traffic V09.20 ☑
          fall V00.821 ☑
          nontraffic V09.1 ☑
            involving motor vehicle NEC
              V09.00 ☑
          traffic V09.3 ☑
            involving motor vehicle NEC
              V09.20 ☑
        flat-bottomed NEC V00.388 ☑
          collision (with) V09.9 ☑
            animal being ridden or animal drawn
              vehicle V06.99 ☑
                nontraffic V06.09 ☑
                traffic V06.19 ☑
            bus or heavy transport V04.99 ☑
              nontraffic V04.09 ☑
              traffic V04.19 ☑
            car V03.99 ☑
              nontraffic V03.09 ☑
              traffic V03.19 ☑
            pedal cycle V01.99 ☑
              nontraffic V01.09 ☑
              traffic V01.19 ☑
            pick-up truck or van V03.99 ☑
              nontraffic V03.09 ☑
              traffic V03.19 ☑
            railway (train) (vehicle) V05.99 ☑
              nontraffic V05.09 ☑
              traffic V05.19 ☑
            stationary object V00.382 ☑
            streetcar V06.99 ☑
              nontraffic V06.09 ☑
              traffic V06.19 ☑
            two- or three-wheeled motor vehicle
              V02.99 ☑
              nontraffic V02.09 ☑
              traffic V02.19 ☑
            vehicle V09.9 ☑
              animal-drawn V06.99 ☑
                nontraffic V06.09 ☑
                traffic V06.19 ☑

Accident — *continued*
  transport — *continued*
    pedestrian — *continued*
      conveyance — *continued*
        flat-bottomed — *continued*
          collision — *continued*
            vehicle — *continued*
              motor
                nontraffic V09.00 ☑
                traffic V09.20 ☑
          fall V00.381 ☑
          nontraffic V09.1 ☑
            involving motor vehicle NEC
              V09.00 ☑
          snow
            board — *see* Accident, transport,
              pedestrian, conveyance, snow
              board
            ski — *see* Accident, transport,
              pedestrian, conveyance, skis
              (snow)
          traffic V09.3 ☑
            involving motor vehicle NEC
              V09.20 ☑
        gliding type NEC V00.288 ☑
          collision (with) V09.9 ☑
            animal being ridden or animal drawn
              vehicle V06.99 ☑
                nontraffic V06.09 ☑
                traffic V06.19 ☑
            bus or heavy transport V04.99 ☑
              nontraffic V04.09 ☑
              traffic V04.19 ☑
            car V03.99 ☑
              nontraffic V03.09 ☑
              traffic V03.19 ☑
            pedal cycle V01.99 ☑
              nontraffic V01.09 ☑
              traffic V01.19 ☑
            pick-up truck or van V03.99 ☑
              nontraffic V03.09 ☑
              traffic V03.19 ☑
            railway (train) (vehicle) V05.99 ☑
              nontraffic V05.09 ☑
              traffic V05.19 ☑
            stationary object V00.282 ☑
            streetcar V06.99 ☑
              nontraffic V06.09 ☑
              traffic V06.19 ☑
            two- or three-wheeled motor vehicle
              V02.99 ☑
              nontraffic V02.09 ☑
              traffic V02.19 ☑
            vehicle V09.9 ☑
              animal-drawn V06.99 ☑
                nontraffic V06.09 ☑
                traffic V06.19 ☑
              motor
                nontraffic V09.00 ☑
                traffic V09.20 ☑
          fall V00.281 ☑
          heelies — *see* Accident, transport,
            pedestrian, conveyance, heelies
          ice skate — *see* Accident, transport,
            pedestrian, conveyance, ice skate
          nontraffic V09.1 ☑
            involving motor vehicle NEC
              V09.00 ☑
          sled — *see* Accident, transport, pedestri-
            an, conveyance, sled
          traffic V09.3 ☑
            involving motor vehicle NEC
              V09.20 ☑
          wheelies — *see* Accident, transport,
            pedestrian, conveyance, heel-
            ies
        heelies V00.158 ☑
          colliding with stationary object
            V00.152 ☑
          fall V00.151 ☑
        ice skates V00.218 ☑
          collision (with) V09.9 ☑
            animal being ridden or animal drawn
              vehicle V06.99 ☑
                nontraffic V06.09 ☑
                traffic V06.19 ☑

Accident — *continued*
  transport — *continued*
    pedestrian — *continued*
      conveyance — *continued*
        ice skates — *continued*
          collision — *continued*
            bus or heavy transport V04.99 ☑
              nontraffic V04.09 ☑
              traffic V04.19 ☑
            car V03.99 ☑
              nontraffic V03.09 ☑
              traffic V03.19 ☑
            pedal cycle V01.99 ☑
              nontraffic V01.09 ☑
              traffic V01.19 ☑
            pick-up truck or van V03.99 ☑
              nontraffic V03.09 ☑
              traffic V03.19 ☑
            railway (train) (vehicle) V05.99 ☑
              nontraffic V05.09 ☑
              traffic V05.19 ☑
            stationary object V00.212 ☑
            streetcar V06.99 ☑
              nontraffic V06.09 ☑
              traffic V06.19 ☑
            two- or three-wheeled motor vehicle
              V02.99 ☑
              nontraffic V02.09 ☑
              traffic V02.19 ☑
            vehicle V09.9 ☑
              animal-drawn V06.99 ☑
                nontraffic V06.09 ☑
                traffic V06.19 ☑
              motor
                nontraffic V09.00 ☑
                traffic V09.20 ☑
          fall V00.211 ☑
          nontraffic V09.1 ☑
            involving motor vehicle NEC
              V09.00 ☑
          traffic V09.3 ☑
            involving motor vehicle NEC
              V09.20 ☑
        motorized mobility scooter V00.838 ☑
          collision with stationary object
            V00.832 ☑
          fall from V00.831 ☑
        nontraffic V09.1 ☑
          involving motor vehicle V09.00 ☑
            military V09.01 ☑
            specified type NEC V09.09 ☑
        roller skates (non in-line) V00.128 ☑
          collision (with) V09.9 ☑
            animal being ridden or animal drawn
              vehicle V06.91 ☑
                nontraffic V06.01 ☑
                traffic V06.11 ☑
            bus or heavy transport V04.91 ☑
              nontraffic V04.01 ☑
              traffic V04.11 ☑
            car V03.91 ☑
              nontraffic V03.01 ☑
              traffic V03.11 ☑
            pedal cycle V01.91 ☑
              nontraffic V01.01 ☑
              traffic V01.11 ☑
            pick-up truck or van V03.91 ☑
              nontraffic V03.01 ☑
              traffic V03.11 ☑
            railway (train) (vehicle) V05.91 ☑
              nontraffic V05.01 ☑
              traffic V05.11 ☑
            stationary object V00.122 ☑
            streetcar V06.91 ☑
              nontraffic V06.01 ☑
              traffic V06.11 ☑
            two- or three-wheeled motor vehicle
              V02.91 ☑
              nontraffic V02.01 ☑
              traffic V02.11 ☑
            vehicle V09.9 ☑
              animal-drawn V06.91 ☑
                nontraffic V06.01 ☑
                traffic V06.11 ☑
              motor
                nontraffic V09.00 ☑

   ☑ **Additional Character Required** — Refer to the Tabular List for Character Selection   ▽ Subterms under main terms may continue to next column or page

Accident — *continued*
  transport — *continued*
    pedestrian — *continued*
      conveyance — *continued*
        roller skates — *continued*
          collision — *continued*
            vehicle — *continued*
              motor — *continued*
                traffic V09.20 ☑
          fall V00.121 ☑
          in-line V00.118 ☑
            collision — *see also* Accident, transport, pedestrian, conveyance occupant, roller skates, collision
              with stationary object V00.112 ☑
            fall V00.111 ☑
            nontraffic V09.1 ☑
              involving motor vehicle NEC V09.00 ☑
            traffic V09.3 ☑
              involving motor vehicle NEC V09.20 ☑
          rolling shoes V00.158 ☑
            colliding with stationary object V00.152 ☑
            fall V00.151 ☑
          rolling type NEC V00.188 ☑
            collision (with) V09.9 ☑
              animal being ridden or animal drawn vehicle V06.99 ☑
                nontraffic V06.09 ☑
                traffic V06.19 ☑
              bus or heavy transport V04.99 ☑
                nontraffic V04.09 ☑
                traffic V04.19 ☑
              car V03.99 ☑
                nontraffic V03.09 ☑
                traffic V03.19 ☑
              pedal cycle V01.99 ☑
                nontraffic V01.09 ☑
                traffic V01.19 ☑
              pick-up truck or van V03.99 ☑
                nontraffic V03.09 ☑
                traffic V03.19 ☑
              railway (train) (vehicle) V05.99 ☑
                nontraffic V05.09 ☑
                traffic V05.19 ☑
              stationary object V00.182 ☑
              streetcar V06.99 ☑
                nontraffic V06.09 ☑
                traffic V06.19 ☑
              two- or three-wheeled motor vehicle V02.99 ☑
                nontraffic V02.09 ☑
                traffic V02.19 ☑
              vehicle V09.9 ☑
                animal-drawn V06.99 ☑
                  nontraffic V06.09 ☑
                  traffic V06.19 ☑
                motor
                  nontraffic V09.00 ☑
                  traffic V09.20 ☑
            fall V00.181 ☑
          in-line roller skate — *see* Accident, transport, pedestrian, conveyance, roller skate, in-line
          nontraffic V09.1 ☑
            involving motor vehicle NEC V09.00 ☑
          roller skate — *see* Accident, transport, pedestrian, conveyance, roller skate
          scooter (non-motorized) — *see* Accident, transport, pedestrian, conveyance, scooter
          skateboard — *see* Accident, transport, pedestrian, conveyance, skateboard
          traffic V09.3 ☑
            involving motor vehicle NEC V09.20 ☑
        scooter (non-motorized) V00.148 ☑
          collision (with) V09.9 ☑
            animal being ridden or animal drawn vehicle V06.99 ☑

Accident — *continued*
  transport — *continued*
    pedestrian — *continued*
      conveyance — *continued*
        scooter — *continued*
          collision — *continued*
            animal being ridden or animal drawn vehicle — *continued*
              nontraffic V06.09 ☑
              traffic V06.19 ☑
            bus or heavy transport V04.99 ☑
              nontraffic V04.09 ☑
              traffic V04.19 ☑
            car V03.99 ☑
              nontraffic V03.09 ☑
              traffic V03.19 ☑
            pedal cycle V01.99 ☑
              nontraffic V01.09 ☑
              traffic V01.19 ☑
            pick-up truck or van V03.99 ☑
              nontraffic V03.09 ☑
              traffic V03.19 ☑
            railway (train) (vehicle) V05.99 ☑
              nontraffic V05.09 ☑
              traffic V05.19 ☑
            stationary object V00.142 ☑
            streetcar V06.99 ☑
              nontraffic V06.09 ☑
              traffic V06.19 ☑
            two- or three-wheeled motor vehicle V02.99 ☑
              nontraffic V02.09 ☑
              traffic V02.19 ☑
            vehicle V09.9 ☑
              animal-drawn V06.99 ☑
                nontraffic V06.09 ☑
                traffic V06.19 ☑
              motor
                nontraffic V09.00 ☑
                traffic V09.20 ☑
          fall V00.141 ☑
          nontraffic V09.1 ☑
            involving motor vehicle NEC V09.00 ☑
          traffic V09.3 ☑
            involving motor vehicle NEC V09.20 ☑
        skate board V00.138 ☑
          collision (with) V09.9 ☑
            animal being ridden or animal drawn vehicle V06.92 ☑
              nontraffic V06.02 ☑
              traffic V06.12 ☑
            bus or heavy transport V04.92 ☑
              nontraffic V04.02 ☑
              traffic V04.12 ☑
            car V03.92 ☑
              nontraffic V03.02 ☑
              traffic V03.12 ☑
            pedal cycle V01.92 ☑
              nontraffic V01.02 ☑
              traffic V01.12 ☑
            pick-up truck or van V03.92 ☑
              nontraffic V03.02 ☑
              traffic V03.12 ☑
            railway (train) (vehicle) V05.92 ☑
              nontraffic V05.02 ☑
              traffic V05.12 ☑
            stationary object V00.132 ☑
            streetcar V06.92 ☑
              nontraffic V06.02 ☑
              traffic V06.12 ☑
            two- or three-wheeled motor vehicle V02.92 ☑
              nontraffic V02.02 ☑
              traffic V02.12 ☑
            vehicle V09.9 ☑
              animal-drawn V06.92 ☑
                nontraffic V06.02 ☑
                traffic V06.12 ☑
              motor
                nontraffic V09.00 ☑
                traffic V09.20 ☑
          fall V00.131 ☑
          nontraffic V09.1 ☑

Accident — *continued*
  transport — *continued*
    pedestrian — *continued*
      conveyance — *continued*
        skate board — *continued*
          nontraffic — *continued*
            involving motor vehicle NEC V09.00 ☑
          traffic V09.3 ☑
            involving motor vehicle NEC V09.20 ☑
        skis (snow) V00.328 ☑
          collision (with) V09.9 ☑
            animal being ridden or animal drawn vehicle V06.99 ☑
              nontraffic V06.09 ☑
              traffic V06.19 ☑
            bus or heavy transport V04.99 ☑
              nontraffic V04.09 ☑
              traffic V04.19 ☑
            car V03.99 ☑
              nontraffic V03.09 ☑
              traffic V03.19 ☑
            pedal cycle V01.99 ☑
              nontraffic V01.09 ☑
              traffic V01.19 ☑
            pick-up truck or van V03.99 ☑
              nontraffic V03.09 ☑
              traffic V03.19 ☑
            railway (train) (vehicle) V05.99 ☑
              nontraffic V05.09 ☑
              traffic V05.19 ☑
            stationary object V00.322 ☑
            streetcar V06.99 ☑
              nontraffic V06.09 ☑
              traffic V06.19 ☑
            two- or three-wheeled motor vehicle V02.99 ☑
              nontraffic V02.09 ☑
              traffic V02.19 ☑
            vehicle V09.9 ☑
              animal-drawn V06.99 ☑
                nontraffic V06.09 ☑
                traffic V06.19 ☑
              motor
                nontraffic V09.00 ☑
                traffic V09.20 ☑
          fall V00.321 ☑
          nontraffic V09.1 ☑
            involving motor vehicle NEC V09.00 ☑
          traffic V09.3 ☑
            involving motor vehicle NEC V09.20 ☑
        sled V00.228 ☑
          collision (with) V09.9 ☑
            animal being ridden or animal drawn vehicle V06.99 ☑
              nontraffic V06.09 ☑
              traffic V06.19 ☑
            bus or heavy transport V04.99 ☑
              nontraffic V04.09 ☑
              traffic V04.19 ☑
            car V03.99 ☑
              nontraffic V03.09 ☑
              traffic V03.19 ☑
            pedal cycle V01.99 ☑
              nontraffic V01.09 ☑
              traffic V01.19 ☑
            pick-up truck or van V03.99 ☑
              nontraffic V03.09 ☑
              traffic V03.19 ☑
            railway (train) (vehicle) V05.99 ☑
              nontraffic V05.09 ☑
              traffic V05.19 ☑
            stationary object V00.222 ☑
            streetcar V06.99 ☑
              nontraffic V06.09 ☑
              traffic V06.19 ☑
            two- or three-wheeled motor vehicle V02.99 ☑
              nontraffic V02.09 ☑
              traffic V02.19 ☑
            vehicle V09.9 ☑
              animal-drawn V06.99 ☑
                nontraffic V06.09 ☑

Accident — *continued*
- transport — *continued*
  - pedestrian — *continued*
    - conveyance — *continued*
      - sled — *continued*
        - collision — *continued*
          - vehicle — *continued*
            - animal-drawn — *continued*
              - traffic V06.19 ✔
            - motor
              - nontraffic V09.00 ✔
              - traffic V09.20 ✔
        - fall V00.221 ✔
        - nontraffic V09.1 ✔
          - involving motor vehicle NEC V09.00 ✔
        - traffic V09.3 ✔
          - involving motor vehicle NEC V09.20 ✔
      - snow board V00.318 ✔
        - collision (with) V09.9 ✔
          - animal being ridden or animal drawn vehicle V06.99 ✔
            - nontraffic V06.09 ✔
            - traffic V06.19 ✔
          - bus or heavy transport V04.99 ✔
            - nontraffic V04.09 ✔
            - traffic V04.19 ✔
          - car V03.99 ✔
            - nontraffic V03.09 ✔
            - traffic V03.19 ✔
          - pedal cycle V01.99 ✔
            - nontraffic V01.09 ✔
            - traffic V01.19 ✔
          - pick-up truck or van V03.99 ✔
            - nontraffic V03.09 ✔
            - traffic V03.19 ✔
          - railway (train) (vehicle) V05.99 ✔
            - nontraffic V05.09 ✔
            - traffic V05.19 ✔
          - stationary object V00.312 ✔
          - streetcar V06.99 ✔
            - nontraffic V06.09 ✔
            - traffic V06.19 ✔
          - two- or three-wheeled motor vehicle V02.99 ✔
            - nontraffic V02.09 ✔
            - traffic V02.19 ✔
          - vehicle V09.9 ✔
            - animal-drawn V06.99 ✔
              - nontraffic V06.09 ✔
              - traffic V06.19 ✔
            - motor
              - nontraffic V09.00 ✔
              - traffic V09.20 ✔
        - fall V00.311 ✔
        - nontraffic V09.1 ✔
          - involving motor vehicle NEC V09.00 ✔
        - traffic V09.3 ✔
          - involving motor vehicle NEC V09.20 ✔
      - specified type NEC V00.898 ✔
        - collision (with) V09.9 ✔
          - animal being ridden or animal drawn vehicle V06.99 ✔
            - nontraffic V06.09 ✔
            - traffic V06.19 ✔
          - bus or heavy transport V04.99 ✔
            - nontraffic V04.09 ✔
            - traffic V04.19 ✔
          - car V03.99 ✔
            - nontraffic V03.09 ✔
            - traffic V03.19 ✔
          - pedal cycle V01.99 ✔
            - nontraffic V01.09 ✔
            - traffic V01.19 ✔
          - pick-up truck or van V03.99 ✔
            - nontraffic V03.09 ✔
            - traffic V03.19 ✔
          - railway (train) (vehicle) V05.99 ✔
            - nontraffic V05.09 ✔
            - traffic V05.19 ✔
          - stationary object V00.892 ✔
          - streetcar V06.99 ✔
            - nontraffic V06.09 ✔

Accident — *continued*
- transport — *continued*
  - pedestrian — *continued*
    - conveyance — *continued*
      - specified type — *continued*
        - collision — *continued*
          - streetcar — *continued*
            - traffic V06.19 ✔
          - two- or three-wheeled motor vehicle V02.99 ✔
            - nontraffic V02.09 ✔
            - traffic V02.19 ✔
          - vehicle V09.9 ✔
            - animal-drawn V06.99 ✔
              - nontraffic V06.09 ✔
              - traffic V06.19 ✔
            - motor
              - nontraffic V09.00 ✔
              - traffic V09.20 ✔
        - fall V00.891 ✔
        - nontraffic V09.1 ✔
          - involving motor vehicle NEC V09.00 ✔
        - traffic V09.3 ✔
          - involving motor vehicle NEC V09.20 ✔
      - traffic V09.3 ✔
        - involving motor vehicle V09.20 ✔
          - military V09.21 ✔
          - specified type NEC V09.29 ✔
    - wheelchair (powered) V00.818 ✔
      - collision (with) V09.9 ✔
        - animal being ridden or animal drawn vehicle V06.99 ✔
          - nontraffic V06.09 ✔
          - traffic V06.19 ✔
        - bus or heavy transport V04.99 ✔
          - nontraffic V04.09 ✔
          - traffic V04.19 ✔
        - car V03.99 ✔
          - nontraffic V03.09 ✔
          - traffic V03.19 ✔
        - pedal cycle V01.99 ✔
          - nontraffic V01.09 ✔
          - traffic V01.19 ✔
        - pick-up truck or van V03.99 ✔
          - nontraffic V03.09 ✔
          - traffic V03.19 ✔
        - railway (train) (vehicle) V05.99 ✔
          - nontraffic V05.09 ✔
          - traffic V05.19 ✔
        - stationary object V00.812 ✔
        - streetcar V06.99 ✔
          - nontraffic V06.09 ✔
          - traffic V06.19 ✔
        - two- or three-wheeled motor vehicle V02.99 ✔
          - nontraffic V02.09 ✔
          - traffic V02.19 ✔
        - vehicle V09.9 ✔
          - animal-drawn V06.99 ✔
            - nontraffic V06.09 ✔
            - traffic V06.19 ✔
          - motor
            - nontraffic V09.00 ✔
            - traffic V09.20 ✔
      - fall V00.811 ✔
      - nontraffic V09.1 ✔
        - involving motor vehicle NEC V09.00 ✔
      - traffic V09.3 ✔
        - involving motor vehicle NEC V09.20 ✔
    - wheeled shoe V00.158 ✔
      - colliding with stationary object V00.152 ✔
      - fall V00.151 ✔
    - on foot (*see also* Accident, pedestrian)
      - collision (with)
        - animal being ridden or animal drawn vehicle V06.90 ✔
          - nontraffic V06.00 ✔
          - traffic V06.10 ✔
        - bus or heavy transport V04.90 ✔
          - nontraffic V04.00 ✔
          - traffic V04.10 ✔

Accident — *continued*
- transport — *continued*
  - pedestrian — *continued*
    - on foot (*see also* Accident, pedestrian) — *continued*
      - collision — *continued*
        - car V03.90 ✔
          - nontraffic V03.00 ✔
          - traffic V03.10 ✔
        - pedal cycle V01.90 ✔
          - nontraffic V01.00 ✔
          - traffic V01.10 ✔
        - pick-up truck or van V03.90 ✔
          - nontraffic V03.00 ✔
          - traffic V03.10 ✔
        - railway (train) (vehicle) V05.90 ✔
          - nontraffic V05.00 ✔
          - traffic V05.10 ✔
        - streetcar V06.90 ✔
          - nontraffic V06.00 ✔
          - traffic V06.10 ✔
        - two- or three-wheeled motor vehicle V02.90 ✔
          - nontraffic V02.00 ✔
          - traffic V02.10 ✔
        - vehicle V09.9 ✔
          - animal-drawn V06.90 ✔
            - nontraffic V06.00 ✔
            - traffic V06.10 ✔
          - motor
            - nontraffic V09.00 ✔
            - traffic V09.20 ✔
      - nontraffic V09.1 ✔
        - involving motor vehicle V09.00 ✔
          - military V09.01 ✔
          - specified type NEC V09.09 ✔
      - traffic V09.3 ✔
        - involving motor vehicle V09.20 ✔
          - military V09.21 ✔
          - specified type NEC V09.29 ✔
    - person NEC (unknown way or transportation) V99 ✔
    - collision (between)
      - bus (with)
        - heavy transport vehicle (traffic) V87.5 ✔
          - nontraffic V88.5 ✔
      - car (with)
        - bus (traffic) V87.3 ✔
          - nontraffic V88.3 ✔
        - heavy transport vehicle (traffic) V87.4 ✔
          - nontraffic V88.4 ✔
          - nontraffic V88.5 ✔
        - pick-up truck or van (traffic) V87.2 ✔
          - nontraffic V88.2 ✔
        - train or railway vehicle (traffic) V87.6 ✔
          - nontraffic V88.6 ✔
        - two-or three-wheeled motor vehicle (traffic) V87.0 ✔
          - nontraffic V88.0 ✔
      - motor vehicle (traffic) NEC V87.7 ✔
        - nontraffic V88.7 ✔
      - two-or three-wheeled vehicle (with) (traffic) motor vehicle NEC V87.1 ✔
        - nontraffic V88.1 ✔
      - nonmotor vehicle (collision) (noncollision) (traffic) V87.9 ✔
        - nontraffic V88.9 ✔
    - pickup truck occupant V59.9 ✔
      - collision (with)
        - animal (traffic) V50.9 ✔
          - being ridden (traffic) V56.9 ✔
            - nontraffic V56.3 ✔
            - while boarding or alighting V56.4 ✔
          - nontraffic V50.3 ✔
          - while boarding or alighting V50.4 ✔
        - animal-drawn vehicle (traffic) V56.9 ✔
          - nontraffic V56.3 ✔
          - while boarding or alighting V56.4 ✔
        - bus (traffic) V54.9 ✔
          - nontraffic V54.3 ✔
          - while boarding or alighting V54.4 ✔
        - car (traffic) V53.9 ✔
          - nontraffic V53.3 ✔
          - while boarding or alighting V53.4 ✔
        - motor vehicle NOS (traffic) V59.60 ✔
          - nontraffic V59.20 ✔

Accident — *continued*
- transport — *continued*
  - pickup truck occupant — *continued*
    - collision — *continued*
      - motor vehicle — *continued*
        - specified type NEC (traffic) V59.69 ☑
        - nontraffic V59.29 ☑
      - pedal cycle (traffic) V51.9 ☑
        - nontraffic V51.3 ☑
        - while boarding or alighting V51.4 ☑
      - pickup truck (traffic) V53.9 ☑
        - nontraffic V53.3 ☑
        - while boarding or alighting V53.4 ☑
      - railway vehicle (traffic) V55.9 ☑
        - nontraffic V55.3 ☑
        - while boarding or alighting V55.4 ☑
      - specified vehicle NEC (traffic) V56.9 ☑
        - nontraffic V56.3 ☑
        - while boarding or alighting V56.4 ☑
      - stationary object (traffic) V57.9 ☑
        - nontraffic V57.3 ☑
        - while boarding or alighting V57.4 ☑
      - streetcar (traffic) V56.9 ☑
        - nontraffic V56.3 ☑
        - while boarding or alighting V56.4 ☑
      - three wheeled motor vehicle (traffic) V52.9 ☑
        - nontraffic V52.3 ☑
        - while boarding or alighting V52.4 ☑
      - truck (traffic) V54.9 ☑
        - nontraffic V54.3 ☑
        - while boarding or alighting V54.4 ☑
      - two wheeled motor vehicle (traffic) V52.9 ☑
        - nontraffic V52.3 ☑
        - while boarding or alighting V52.4 ☑
      - van (traffic) V53.9 ☑
        - nontraffic V53.3 ☑
        - while boarding or alighting V53.4 ☑
    - driver
      - collision (with)
        - animal (traffic) V50.5 ☑
          - being ridden (traffic) V56.5 ☑
            - nontraffic V56.0 ☑
          - nontraffic V50.0 ☑
        - animal-drawn vehicle (traffic) V56.5 ☑
          - nontraffic V56.0 ☑
        - bus (traffic) V54.5 ☑
          - nontraffic V54.0 ☑
        - car (traffic) V53.5 ☑
          - nontraffic V53.0 ☑
        - motor vehicle NOS (traffic) V59.40 ☑
          - nontraffic V59.00 ☑
          - specified type NEC (traffic) V59.49 ☑
            - nontraffic V59.09 ☑
        - pedal cycle (traffic) V51.5 ☑
          - nontraffic V51.0 ☑
        - pickup truck (traffic) V53.5 ☑
          - nontraffic V53.0 ☑
        - railway vehicle (traffic) V55.5 ☑
          - nontraffic V55.0 ☑
        - specified vehicle NEC (traffic) V56.5 ☑
          - nontraffic V56.0 ☑
        - stationary object (traffic) V57.5 ☑
          - nontraffic V57.0 ☑
        - streetcar (traffic) V56.5 ☑
          - nontraffic V56.0 ☑
        - three wheeled motor vehicle (traffic) V52.5 ☑
          - nontraffic V52.0 ☑
        - truck (traffic) V54.5 ☑
          - nontraffic V54.0 ☑
        - two wheeled motor vehicle (traffic) V52.5 ☑
          - nontraffic V52.0 ☑
        - van (traffic) V53.5 ☑
          - nontraffic V53.0 ☑
      - noncollision accident (traffic) V58.5 ☑
        - nontraffic V58.0 ☑
    - hanger-on
      - collision (with)
        - animal (traffic) V50.7 ☑
          - being ridden (traffic) V56.7 ☑
            - nontraffic V50.2 ☑
              - nontraffic V56.2 ☑
          - animal-drawn vehicle (traffic) V56.7 ☑
            - nontraffic V56.2 ☑

Accident — *continued*
- transport — *continued*
  - pickup truck occupant — *continued*
    - hanger-on — *continued*
      - collision — *continued*
        - bus (traffic) V54.7 ☑
          - nontraffic V54.2 ☑
        - car (traffic) V53.7 ☑
          - nontraffic V53.2 ☑
        - pedal cycle (traffic) V51.7 ☑
          - nontraffic V51.2 ☑
        - pickup truck (traffic) V53.7 ☑
          - nontraffic V53.2 ☑
        - railway vehicle (traffic) V55.7 ☑
          - nontraffic V55.2 ☑
        - specified vehicle NEC (traffic) V56.7 ☑
          - nontraffic V56.2 ☑
        - stationary object (traffic) V57.7 ☑
          - nontraffic V57.2 ☑
        - streetcar (traffic) V56.7 ☑
          - nontraffic V56.2 ☑
        - three wheeled motor vehicle (traffic) V52.7 ☑
          - nontraffic V52.2 ☑
        - truck (traffic) V54.7 ☑
          - nontraffic V54.2 ☑
        - two wheeled motor vehicle (traffic) V52.7 ☑
          - nontraffic V52.2 ☑
        - van (traffic) V53.7 ☑
          - nontraffic V53.2 ☑
      - noncollision accident (traffic) V58.7 ☑
        - nontraffic V58.2 ☑
    - noncollision accident (traffic) V58.9 ☑
      - nontraffic V58.3 ☑
      - while boarding or alighting V58.4 ☑
    - nontraffic V59.3 ☑
    - passenger
      - collision (with)
        - animal (traffic) V50.6 ☑
          - being ridden (traffic) V56.6 ☑
            - nontraffic V50.1 ☑
              - nontraffic V56.1 ☑
          - animal-drawn vehicle (traffic) V56.6 ☑
            - nontraffic V56.1 ☑
        - bus (traffic) V54.6 ☑
          - nontraffic V54.1 ☑
        - car (traffic) V53.6 ☑
          - nontraffic V53.1 ☑
        - motor vehicle NOS (traffic) V59.50 ☑
          - nontraffic V59.10 ☑
            - nontraffic V59.19 ☑
          - specified type NEC (traffic) V59.59 ☑
        - pedal cycle (traffic) V51.6 ☑
          - nontraffic V51.1 ☑
        - pickup truck (traffic) V53.6 ☑
          - nontraffic V53.1 ☑
        - railway vehicle (traffic) V55.6 ☑
          - nontraffic V55.1 ☑
        - specified vehicle NEC (traffic) V56.6 ☑
          - nontraffic V56.1 ☑
        - stationary object (traffic) V57.6 ☑
          - nontraffic V57.1 ☑
        - streetcar (traffic) V56.6 ☑
          - nontraffic V56.1 ☑
        - three wheeled motor vehicle (traffic) V52.6 ☑
          - nontraffic V52.1 ☑
        - truck (traffic) V54.6 ☑
          - nontraffic V54.1 ☑
        - two wheeled motor vehicle (traffic) V52.6 ☑
          - nontraffic V52.1 ☑
        - van (traffic) V53.6 ☑
          - nontraffic V53.1 ☑
      - noncollision accident (traffic) V58.6 ☑
        - nontraffic V58.1 ☑
    - specified type NEC V59.88 ☑
    - military vehicle V59.81 ☑
  - quarry truck — *see* Accident, transport, industrial vehicle occupant
  - race car — *see* Accident, transport, motor vehicle NEC occupant
  - railway vehicle occupant V81.9 ☑
    - collision (with) V81.3 ☑

Accident — *continued*
- transport — *continued*
  - railway vehicle occupant — *continued*
    - collision — *continued*
      - motor vehicle (non-military) (traffic) V81.1 ☑
        - military V81.83 ☑
        - nontraffic V81.0 ☑
      - rolling stock V81.2 ☑
      - specified object NEC V81.3 ☑
    - during derailment V81.7 ☑
      - with antecedent collision B — *see* Accident, transport, railway vehicle occupant, collision
    - explosion V81.81 ☑
    - fall (in railway vehicle) V81.5 ☑
      - during derailment V81.7 ☑
        - with antecedent collision B — *see* Accident, transport, railway vehicle occupant, collision
      - from railway vehicle V81.6 ☑
        - during derailment V81.7 ☑
          - with antecedent collision B — *see* Accident, transport, railway vehicle occupant, collision
      - while boarding or alighting V81.4 ☑
    - fire V81.81 ☑
    - object falling onto train V81.82 ☑
    - specified type NEC V81.89 ☑
    - while boarding or alighting V81.4 ☑
  - ski lift V98.3 ☑
  - snowmobile occupant (nontraffic) V86.92 ☑
    - driver V86.52 ☑
    - hanger-on V86.72 ☑
    - passenger V86.62 ☑
    - traffic V86.32 ☑
      - driver V86.02 ☑
      - hanger-on V86.22 ☑
      - passenger V86.12 ☑
    - while boarding or alighting V86.42 ☑
  - specified NEC V98.8 ☑
  - sport utility vehicle occupant (*see also* Accident, transport, car occupant)
    - collision (with)
      - stationary object (traffic) V47.91 ☑
        - nontraffic V47.31 ☑
    - driver
      - collision (with)
        - stationary object (traffic) V47.51 ☑
          - nontraffic V47.01 ☑
    - passenger
      - collision (with)
        - stationary object (traffic) V47.61 ☑
          - nontraffic V47.11 ☑
  - streetcar occupant V82.9 ☑
    - collision (with) V82.3 ☑
      - motor vehicle (traffic) V82.1 ☑
        - nontraffic V82.0 ☑
      - rolling stock V82.2 ☑
    - during derailment V82.7 ☑
      - with antecedent collision B — *see* Accident, transport, streetcar occupant, collision
    - fall (in streetcar) V82.5 ☑
      - during derailment V82.7 ☑
        - with antecedent collision B — *see* Accident, transport, streetcar occupant, collision
      - from streetcar V82.6 ☑
        - during derailment V82.7 ☑
          - with antecedent collision B — *see* Accident, transport, streetcar occupant, collision
      - while boarding or alighting V82.4 ☑
    - while boarding or alighting V82.4 ☑
    - specified type NEC V82.8 ☑
    - while boarding or alighting V82.4 ☑
  - three-wheeled motor vehicle occupant V39.9 ☑
    - collision (with)
      - animal (traffic) V30.9 ☑
        - being ridden (traffic) V36.9 ☑
          - nontraffic V36.3 ☑
            - while boarding or alighting V36.4 ☑
        - nontraffic V30.3 ☑
          - while boarding or alighting V30.4 ☑
      - animal-drawn vehicle (traffic) V36.9 ☑
        - nontraffic V36.3 ☑

Accident — *continued*
transport — *continued*
  three-wheeled motor vehicle occupant — *continued*
    collision — *continued*
      animal-drawn vehicle — *continued*
        while boarding or alighting V36.4 ☑
      bus (traffic) V34.9 ☑
        nontraffic V34.3 ☑
        while boarding or alighting V34.4 ☑
      car (traffic) V33.9 ☑
        nontraffic V33.3 ☑
        while boarding or alighting V33.4 ☑
      motor vehicle NOS (traffic) V39.60 ☑
        nontraffic V39.20 ☑
        specified type NEC (traffic) V39.69 ☑
          nontraffic V39.29 ☑
      pedal cycle (traffic) V31.9 ☑
        nontraffic V31.3 ☑
        while boarding or alighting V31.4 ☑
      pickup truck (traffic) V33.9 ☑
        nontraffic V33.3 ☑
        while boarding or alighting V33.4 ☑
      railway vehicle (traffic) V35.9 ☑
        nontraffic V35.3 ☑
        while boarding or alighting V35.4 ☑
      specified vehicle NEC (traffic) V36.9 ☑
        nontraffic V36.3 ☑
        while boarding or alighting V36.4 ☑
      stationary object (traffic) V37.9 ☑
        nontraffic V37.3 ☑
        while boarding or alighting V37.4 ☑
      streetcar (traffic) V36.9 ☑
        nontraffic V36.3 ☑
        while boarding or alighting V36.4 ☑
      three wheeled motor vehicle (traffic) V32.9 ☑
        nontraffic V32.3 ☑
        while boarding or alighting V32.4 ☑
      truck (traffic) V34.9 ☑
        nontraffic V34.3 ☑
        while boarding or alighting V34.4 ☑
      two wheeled motor vehicle (traffic) V32.9 ☑
        nontraffic V32.3 ☑
        while boarding or alighting V32.4 ☑
      van (traffic) V33.9 ☑
        nontraffic V33.3 ☑
        while boarding or alighting V33.4 ☑
    driver
      collision (with)
        animal (traffic) V30.5 ☑
          being ridden (traffic) V36.5 ☑
            nontraffic V36.0 ☑
          nontraffic V30.0 ☑
        animal-drawn vehicle (traffic) V36.5 ☑
          nontraffic V36.0 ☑
        bus (traffic) V34.5 ☑
          nontraffic V34.0 ☑
        car (traffic) V33.5 ☑
          nontraffic V33.0 ☑
        motor vehicle NOS (traffic) V39.40 ☑
          nontraffic V39.00 ☑
        specified type NEC (traffic) V39.49 ☑
          nontraffic V39.09 ☑
        pedal cycle (traffic) V31.5 ☑
          nontraffic V31.0 ☑
        pickup truck (traffic) V33.5 ☑
          nontraffic V33.0 ☑
        railway vehicle (traffic) V35.5 ☑
          nontraffic V35.0 ☑
        specified vehicle NEC (traffic) V36.5 ☑
          nontraffic V36.0 ☑
        stationary object (traffic) V37.5 ☑
          nontraffic V37.0 ☑
        streetcar (traffic) V36.5 ☑
          nontraffic V36.0 ☑
        three wheeled motor vehicle (traffic) V32.5 ☑
          nontraffic V32.0 ☑
        truck (traffic) V34.5 ☑
          nontraffic V34.0 ☑
        two wheeled motor vehicle (traffic) V32.5 ☑
          nontraffic V32.0 ☑
        van (traffic) V33.5 ☑
          nontraffic V33.0 ☑

Accident — *continued*
transport — *continued*
  three-wheeled motor vehicle occupant — *continued*
    driver — *continued*
      noncollision accident (traffic) V38.5 ☑
        nontraffic V38.0 ☑
    hanger-on
      collision (with)
        animal (traffic) V30.7 ☑
          being ridden (traffic) V36.7 ☑
            nontraffic V36.2 ☑
          nontraffic V30.2 ☑
        animal-drawn vehicle (traffic) V36.7 ☑
          nontraffic V36.2 ☑
        bus (traffic) V34.7 ☑
          nontraffic V34.2 ☑
        car (traffic) V33.7 ☑
          nontraffic V33.2 ☑
        pedal cycle (traffic) V31.7 ☑
          nontraffic V31.2 ☑
        pickup truck (traffic) V33.7 ☑
          nontraffic V33.2 ☑
        railway vehicle (traffic) V35.7 ☑
          nontraffic V35.2 ☑
        specified vehicle NEC (traffic) V36.7 ☑
          nontraffic V36.2 ☑
        stationary object (traffic) V37.7 ☑
          nontraffic V37.2 ☑
        streetcar (traffic) V36.7 ☑
          nontraffic V36.2 ☑
        three wheeled motor vehicle (traffic) V32.7 ☑
          nontraffic V32.2 ☑
        truck (traffic) V34.7 ☑
          nontraffic V34.2 ☑
        two wheeled motor vehicle (traffic) V32.7 ☑
          nontraffic V32.2 ☑
        van (traffic) V33.7 ☑
          nontraffic V33.2 ☑
      noncollision accident (traffic) V38.7 ☑
        nontraffic V38.2 ☑
    noncollision accident (traffic) V38.9 ☑
      nontraffic V38.3 ☑
      while boarding or alighting V38.4 ☑
    nontraffic V39.3 ☑
    passenger
      collision (with)
        animal (traffic) V30.6 ☑
          being ridden (traffic) V36.6 ☑
            nontraffic V36.1 ☑
          nontraffic V30.1 ☑
        animal-drawn vehicle (traffic) V36.6 ☑
          nontraffic V36.1 ☑
        bus (traffic) V34.6 ☑
          nontraffic V34.1 ☑
        car (traffic) V33.6 ☑
          nontraffic V33.1 ☑
        motor vehicle NOS (traffic) V39.50 ☑
          nontraffic V39.10 ☑
        specified type NEC (traffic) V39.59 ☑
          nontraffic V39.19 ☑
        pedal cycle (traffic) V31.6 ☑
          nontraffic V31.1 ☑
        pickup truck (traffic) V33.6 ☑
          nontraffic V33.1 ☑
        railway vehicle (traffic) V35.6 ☑
          nontraffic V35.1 ☑
        specified vehicle NEC (traffic) V36.6 ☑
          nontraffic V36.1 ☑
        stationary object (traffic) V37.6 ☑
          nontraffic V37.1 ☑
        streetcar (traffic) V36.6 ☑
          nontraffic V36.1 ☑
        three wheeled motor vehicle (traffic) V32.6 ☑
          nontraffic V32.1 ☑
        truck (traffic) V34.6 ☑
          nontraffic V34.1 ☑
        two wheeled motor vehicle (traffic) V32.6 ☑
          nontraffic V32.1 ☑
        van (traffic) V33.6 ☑
          nontraffic V33.1 ☑
      noncollision accident (traffic) V38.6 ☑

Accident — *continued*
transport — *continued*
  three-wheeled motor vehicle occupant — *continued*
    passenger — *continued*
      noncollision accident — *continued*
        nontraffic V38.1 ☑
    specified type NEC V39.89 ☑
    military vehicle V39.81 ☑
  tractor (farm) (and trailer) — *see* Accident, transport, agricultural vehicle occupant
  tram — *see* Accident, transport, streetcar
    in mine or quarry — *see* Accident, transport, industrial vehicle occupant
  trolley — *see* Accident, transport, streetcar
    in mine or quarry — *see* Accident, transport, industrial vehicle occupant
  truck (heavy) occupant V69.9 ☑
    collision (with)
      animal (traffic) V60.9 ☑
        being ridden (traffic) V66.9 ☑
          nontraffic V66.3 ☑
          while boarding or alighting V66.4 ☑
        nontraffic V60.3 ☑
        while boarding or alighting V60.4 ☑
      animal-drawn vehicle (traffic) V66.9 ☑
        nontraffic V66.3 ☑
        while boarding or alighting V66.4 ☑
      bus (traffic) V64.9 ☑
        nontraffic V64.3 ☑
        while boarding or alighting V64.4 ☑
      car (traffic) V63.9 ☑
        nontraffic V63.3 ☑
        while boarding or alighting V63.4 ☑
      motor vehicle NOS (traffic) V69.60 ☑
        nontraffic V69.20 ☑
        specified type NEC (traffic) V69.69 ☑
          nontraffic V69.29 ☑
      pedal cycle (traffic) V61.9 ☑
        nontraffic V61.3 ☑
        while boarding or alighting V61.4 ☑
      pickup truck (traffic) V63.9 ☑
        nontraffic V63.3 ☑
        while boarding or alighting V63.4 ☑
      railway vehicle (traffic) V65.9 ☑
        nontraffic V65.3 ☑
        while boarding or alighting V65.4 ☑
      specified vehicle NEC (traffic) V66.9 ☑
        nontraffic V66.3 ☑
        while boarding or alighting V66.4 ☑
      stationary object (traffic) V67.9 ☑
        nontraffic V67.3 ☑
        while boarding or alighting V67.4 ☑
      streetcar (traffic) V66.9 ☑
        nontraffic V66.3 ☑
        while boarding or alighting V66.4 ☑
      three wheeled motor vehicle (traffic) V62.9 ☑
        nontraffic V62.3 ☑
        while boarding or alighting V62.4 ☑
      truck (traffic) V64.9 ☑
        nontraffic V64.3 ☑
        while boarding or alighting V64.4 ☑
      two wheeled motor vehicle (traffic) V62.9 ☑
        nontraffic V62.3 ☑
        while boarding or alighting V62.4 ☑
      van (traffic) V63.9 ☑
        nontraffic V63.3 ☑
        while boarding or alighting V63.4 ☑
    driver
      collision (with)
        animal (traffic) V60.5 ☑
          being ridden (traffic) V66.5 ☑
            nontraffic V60.0 ☑
              nontraffic V66.0 ☑
        animal-drawn vehicle (traffic) V66.5 ☑
          nontraffic V66.0 ☑
        bus (traffic) V64.5 ☑
          nontraffic V64.0 ☑
        car (traffic) V63.5 ☑
          nontraffic V63.0 ☑
        motor vehicle NOS (traffic) V69.40 ☑
          nontraffic V69.00 ☑
        specified type NEC (traffic) V69.49 ☑
          nontraffic V69.09 ☑
        pedal cycle (traffic) V61.5 ☑

Accident — *continued*
 transport — *continued*
  truck occupant — *continued*
   driver — *continued*
    collision — *continued*
     pedal cycle — *continued*
      nontraffic V61.0 ☑
     pickup truck (traffic) V63.5 ☑
      nontraffic V63.0 ☑
     railway vehicle (traffic) V65.5 ☑
      nontraffic V65.0 ☑
     specified vehicle NEC (traffic) V66.5 ☑
      nontraffic V66.0 ☑
     stationary object (traffic) V67.5 ☑
      nontraffic V67.0 ☑
     streetcar (traffic) V66.5 ☑
      nontraffic V66.0 ☑
     three wheeled motor vehicle (traffic)
       V62.5 ☑
      nontraffic V62.0 ☑
     truck (traffic) V64.5 ☑
      nontraffic V64.0 ☑
     two wheeled motor vehicle (traffic)
       V62.5 ☑
      nontraffic V62.0 ☑
     van (traffic) V63.5 ☑
      nontraffic V63.0 ☑
    noncollision accident (traffic) V68.5 ☑
     nontraffic V68.0 ☑
   dump — *see* Accident, transport, construction
     vehicle occupant
   hanger-on
    collision (with)
     animal (traffic) V60.7 ☑
      being ridden (traffic) V66.7 ☑
       nontraffic V66.2 ☑
      nontraffic V60.2 ☑
     animal-drawn vehicle (traffic) V66.7 ☑
      nontraffic V66.2 ☑
     bus (traffic) V64.7 ☑
      nontraffic V64.2 ☑
     car (traffic) V63.7 ☑
      nontraffic V63.2 ☑
     pedal cycle (traffic) V61.7 ☑
      nontraffic V61.2 ☑
     pickup truck (traffic) V63.7 ☑
      nontraffic V63.2 ☑
     railway vehicle (traffic) V65.7 ☑
      nontraffic V65.2 ☑
     specified vehicle NEC (traffic) V66.7 ☑
      nontraffic V66.2 ☑
     stationary object (traffic) V67.7 ☑
      nontraffic V67.2 ☑
     streetcar (traffic) V66.7 ☑
      nontraffic V66.2 ☑
     three wheeled motor vehicle (traffic)
       V62.7 ☑
      nontraffic V62.2 ☑
     truck (traffic) V64.7 ☑
      nontraffic V64.2 ☑
     two wheeled motor vehicle (traffic)
       V62.7 ☑
      nontraffic V62.2 ☑
     van (traffic) V63.7 ☑
      nontraffic V63.2 ☑
    noncollision accident (traffic) V68.7 ☑
     nontraffic V68.2 ☑
   noncollision accident (traffic) V68.9 ☑
    nontraffic V68.3 ☑
    while boarding or alighting V68.4 ☑
   nontraffic V69.3 ☑
   passenger
    collision (with)
     animal (traffic) V60.6 ☑
      being ridden (traffic) V66.6 ☑
       nontraffic V60.1 ☑
      nontraffic V66.1 ☑
     animal-drawn vehicle (traffic) V66.6 ☑
      nontraffic V66.1 ☑
     bus (traffic) V64.6 ☑
      nontraffic V64.1 ☑
     car (traffic) V63.6 ☑
      nontraffic V63.1 ☑
     motor vehicle NOS (traffic) V69.50 ☑
      nontraffic V69.10 ☑
       specified type NEC (traffic) V69.59 ☑

Accident — *continued*
 transport — *continued*
  truck occupant — *continued*
   passenger — *continued*
    collision — *continued*
     motor vehicle — *continued*
      specified type — *continued*
       nontraffic V69.19 ☑
     pedal cycle (traffic) V61.6 ☑
      nontraffic V61.1 ☑
     pickup truck (traffic) V63.6 ☑
      nontraffic V63.1 ☑
     railway vehicle (traffic) V65.6 ☑
      nontraffic V65.1 ☑
     specified vehicle NEC (traffic) V66.6 ☑
      nontraffic V66.1 ☑
     stationary object (traffic) V67.6 ☑
      nontraffic V67.1 ☑
     streetcar (traffic) V66.6 ☑
      nontraffic V66.1 ☑
     three wheeled motor vehicle (traffic)
       V62.6 ☑
      nontraffic V62.1 ☑
     truck (traffic) V64.6 ☑
      nontraffic V64.1 ☑
     two wheeled motor vehicle (traffic)
       V62.6 ☑
      nontraffic V62.1 ☑
     van (traffic) V63.6 ☑
      nontraffic V63.1 ☑
    noncollision accident (traffic) V68.6 ☑
     nontraffic V68.1 ☑
   pickup — *see* Accident, transport, pickup truck
     occupant
   specified type NEC V69.88 ☑
    military vehicle V69.81 ☑
 van occupant V59.9 ☑
  collision (with)
   animal (traffic) V50.9 ☑
    being ridden (traffic) V56.9 ☑
     nontraffic V56.3 ☑
     while boarding or alighting V56.4 ☑
    nontraffic V50.3 ☑
    while boarding or alighting V50.4 ☑
   animal-drawn vehicle (traffic) V56.9 ☑
    nontraffic V56.3 ☑
    while boarding or alighting V56.4 ☑
   bus (traffic) V54.9 ☑
    nontraffic V54.3 ☑
    while boarding or alighting V54.4 ☑
   car (traffic) V53.9 ☑
    nontraffic V53.3 ☑
    while boarding or alighting V53.4 ☑
   motor vehicle NOS (traffic) V59.60 ☑
    nontraffic V59.20 ☑
    specified type NEC (traffic) V59.69 ☑
     nontraffic V59.29 ☑
   pedal cycle (traffic) V51.9 ☑
    nontraffic V51.3 ☑
    while boarding or alighting V51.4 ☑
   pickup truck (traffic) V53.9 ☑
    nontraffic V53.3 ☑
    while boarding or alighting V53.4 ☑
   railway vehicle (traffic) V55.9 ☑
    nontraffic V55.3 ☑
    while boarding or alighting V55.4 ☑
   specified vehicle NEC (traffic) V56.9 ☑
    nontraffic V56.3 ☑
    while boarding or alighting V56.4 ☑
   stationary object (traffic) V57.9 ☑
    nontraffic V57.3 ☑
    while boarding or alighting V57.4 ☑
   streetcar (traffic) V56.9 ☑
    nontraffic V56.3 ☑
    while boarding or alighting V56.4 ☑
   three wheeled motor vehicle (traffic)
     V52.9 ☑
    nontraffic V52.3 ☑
    while boarding or alighting V52.4 ☑
   truck (traffic) V54.9 ☑
    nontraffic V54.3 ☑
    while boarding or alighting V54.4 ☑
   two wheeled motor vehicle (traffic) V52.9 ☑
    nontraffic V52.3 ☑
    while boarding or alighting V52.4 ☑
   van (traffic) V53.9 ☑

Accident — *continued*
 transport — *continued*
  van occupant — *continued*
   collision — *continued*
    van — *continued*
     nontraffic V53.3 ☑
     while boarding or alighting V53.4 ☑
   driver
    collision (with)
     animal (traffic) V50.5 ☑
      being ridden (traffic) V56.5 ☑
       nontraffic V56.0 ☑
      nontraffic V50.0 ☑
     animal-drawn vehicle (traffic) V56.5 ☑
      nontraffic V56.0 ☑
     bus (traffic) V54.5 ☑
      nontraffic V54.0 ☑
     car (traffic) V53.5 ☑
      nontraffic V53.0 ☑
     motor vehicle NOS (traffic) V59.40 ☑
      nontraffic V59.00 ☑
      specified type NEC (traffic) V59.49 ☑
       nontraffic V59.09 ☑
     pedal cycle (traffic) V51.5 ☑
      nontraffic V51.0 ☑
     pickup truck (traffic) V53.5 ☑
      nontraffic V53.0 ☑
     railway vehicle (traffic) V55.5 ☑
      nontraffic V55.0 ☑
     specified vehicle NEC (traffic) V56.5 ☑
      nontraffic V56.0 ☑
     stationary object (traffic) V57.5 ☑
      nontraffic V57.0 ☑
     streetcar (traffic) V56.5 ☑
      nontraffic V56.0 ☑
     three wheeled motor vehicle (traffic)
       V52.5 ☑
      nontraffic V52.0 ☑
     truck (traffic) V54.5 ☑
      nontraffic V54.0 ☑
     two wheeled motor vehicle (traffic)
       V52.5 ☑
      nontraffic V52.0 ☑
     van (traffic) V53.5 ☑
      nontraffic V53.0 ☑
    noncollision accident (traffic) V58.5 ☑
     nontraffic V58.0 ☑
   hanger-on
    collision (with)
     animal (traffic) V50.7 ☑
      being ridden (traffic) V56.7 ☑
       nontraffic V50.2 ☑
       nontraffic V56.2 ☑
     animal-drawn vehicle (traffic) V56.7 ☑
      nontraffic V56.2 ☑
     bus (traffic) V54.7 ☑
      nontraffic V54.2 ☑
     car (traffic) V53.7 ☑
      nontraffic V53.2 ☑
     pedal cycle (traffic) V51.7 ☑
      nontraffic V51.2 ☑
     pickup truck (traffic) V53.7 ☑
      nontraffic V53.2 ☑
     railway vehicle (traffic) V55.7 ☑
      nontraffic V55.2 ☑
     specified vehicle NEC (traffic) V56.7 ☑
      nontraffic V56.2 ☑
     stationary object (traffic) V57.7 ☑
      nontraffic V57.2 ☑
     streetcar (traffic) V56.7 ☑
      nontraffic V56.2 ☑
     three wheeled motor vehicle (traffic)
       V52.7 ☑
      nontraffic V52.2 ☑
     truck (traffic) V54.7 ☑
      nontraffic V54.2 ☑
     two wheeled motor vehicle (traffic)
       V52.7 ☑
      nontraffic V52.2 ☑
     van (traffic) V53.7 ☑
      nontraffic V53.2 ☑
    noncollision accident (traffic) V58.7 ☑
     nontraffic V58.2 ☑
   noncollision accident (traffic) V58.9 ☑
    nontraffic V58.3 ☑
    while boarding or alighting V58.4 ☑

Accident — *continued*
  transport — *continued*
    van occupant — *continued*
      nontraffic V59.3 ☑
      passenger
        collision (with)
          animal (traffic) V50.6 ☑
            being ridden (traffic) V56.6 ☑
            nontraffic V50.1 ☑
              nontraffic V56.1 ☑
          animal-drawn vehicle (traffic) V56.6 ☑
            nontraffic V56.1 ☑
          bus (traffic) V54.6 ☑
            nontraffic V54.1 ☑
          car (traffic) V53.6 ☑
            nontraffic V53.1 ☑
          motor vehicle NOS (traffic) V59.50 ☑
            nontraffic V59.10 ☑
            specified type NEC (traffic) V59.59 ☑
              nontraffic V59.19 ☑
          pedal cycle (traffic) V51.6 ☑
            nontraffic V51.1 ☑
          pickup truck (traffic) V53.6 ☑
            nontraffic V53.1 ☑
          railway vehicle (traffic) V55.6 ☑
            nontraffic V55.1 ☑
          specified vehicle NEC (traffic) V56.6 ☑
            nontraffic V56.1 ☑
          stationary object (traffic) V57.6 ☑
            nontraffic V57.1 ☑
          streetcar (traffic) V56.6 ☑
            nontraffic V56.1 ☑
          three wheeled motor vehicle (traffic)
            V52.6 ☑
            nontraffic V52.1 ☑
          truck (traffic) V54.6 ☑
            nontraffic V54.1 ☑
          two wheeled motor vehicle (traffic)
            V52.6 ☑
            nontraffic V52.1 ☑
          van (traffic) V53.6 ☑
            nontraffic V53.1 ☑
        noncollision accident (traffic) V58.6 ☑
          nontraffic V58.1 ☑
      specified type NEC V59.88 ☑
      military vehicle V59.81 ☑
    watercraft occupant — *see* Accident, watercraft
  vehicle NEC V89.9 ☑
    animal-drawn NEC — *see* Accident, transport, animal-drawn vehicle occupant
    special
      agricultural — *see* Accident, transport, agricultural vehicle occupant
      construction — *see* Accident, transport, construction vehicle occupant
      industrial — *see* Accident, transport, industrial vehicle occupant
      three-wheeled NEC (motorized) — *see* Accident, transport, three-wheeled motor vehicle occupant
  watercraft V94.9 ☑
    causing
      drowning B — *see* Drowning, due to, accident to, watercraft
      injury NEC V91.89 ☑
        crushed between craft and object V91.19 ☑
          powered craft V91.13 ☑
            ferry boat V91.11 ☑
            fishing boat V91.12 ☑
            jetskis V91.13 ☑
            liner V91.11 ☑
            merchant ship V91.10 ☑
            passenger ship V91.11 ☑
          unpowered craft V91.18 ☑
            canoe V91.15 ☑
            inflatable V91.16 ☑
            kayak V91.15 ☑
            sailboat V91.14 ☑
            surf-board V91.18 ☑
            windsurfer V91.18 ☑
        fall on board V91.29 ☑
          powered craft V91.23 ☑
            ferry boat V91.21 ☑
            fishing boat V91.22 ☑
            jetskis V91.23 ☑
            liner V91.21 ☑

Accident — *continued*
  watercraft — *continued*
    causing — *continued*
      injury — *continued*
        fall on board — *continued*
          powered craft — *continued*
            merchant ship V91.20 ☑
            passenger ship V91.21 ☑
          unpowered craft
            canoe V91.25 ☑
            inflatable V91.26 ☑
            kayak V91.25 ☑
            sailboat V91.24 ☑
        fire on board causing burn V91.09 ☑
          powered craft V91.03 ☑
            ferry boat V91.01 ☑
            fishing boat V91.02 ☑
            jetskis V91.03 ☑
            liner V91.01 ☑
            merchant ship V91.00 ☑
            passenger ship V91.01 ☑
          unpowered craft V91.08 ☑
            canoe V91.05 ☑
            inflatable V91.06 ☑
            kayak V91.05 ☑
            sailboat V91.04 ☑
            surf-board V91.08 ☑
            water skis V91.07 ☑
            windsurfer V91.08 ☑
        hit by falling object V91.39 ☑
          powered craft V91.33 ☑
            ferry boat V91.31 ☑
            fishing boat V91.32 ☑
            jetskis V91.33 ☑
            liner V91.31 ☑
            merchant ship V91.30 ☑
            passenger ship V91.31 ☑
          unpowered craft V91.38 ☑
            canoe V91.35 ☑
            inflatable V91.36 ☑
            kayak V91.35 ☑
            sailboat V91.34 ☑
            surf-board V91.38 ☑
            water skis V91.37 ☑
            windsurfer V91.38 ☑
        specified type NEC V91.89 ☑
          powered craft V91.83 ☑
            ferry boat V91.81 ☑
            fishing boat V91.82 ☑
            jetskis V91.83 ☑
            liner V91.81 ☑
            merchant ship V91.80 ☑
            passenger ship V91.81 ☑
          unpowered craft V91.88 ☑
            canoe V91.85 ☑
            inflatable V91.86 ☑
            kayak V91.85 ☑
            sailboat V91.84 ☑
            surf-board V91.88 ☑
            water skis V91.87 ☑
            windsurfer V91.88 ☑
      due to, caused by cataclysm — *see* Forces of nature, by type
      military NEC V94.818 ☑
        with civilian watercraft V94.810 ☑
        civilian in water injured by V94.811 ☑
      nonpowered, struck by
        nonpowered vessel V94.22 ☑
        powered vessel V94.21 ☑
      specified type NEC V94.89 ☑
      striking swimmer
        powered V94.11 ☑
        unpowered V94.12 ☑
Acid throwing (assault) Y08.89 ☑
Activity (involving) (of victim at time of event) Y93.9
  aerobic and step exercise (class) Y93.A3 (*following* Y93.7)
  alpine skiing Y93.23
  animal care NEC Y93.K9 (*following* Y93.7)
  arts and handcrafts NEC Y93.D9 (*following* Y93.7)
  athletics played as a team or group NEC Y93.69
  athletics played individually NEC Y93.59
  athletics NEC Y93.79
  baking Y93.G3 (*following* Y93.7)
  ballet Y93.41
  barbells Y93.B3 (*following* Y93.7)

Activity — *continued*
  BASE (Building, Antenna, Span, Earth) jumping Y93.33
  baseball Y93.64
  basketball Y93.67
  bathing (personal) Y93.E1 (*following* Y93.7)
  beach volleyball Y93.68
  bike riding Y93.55
  boogie boarding Y93.18
  bowling Y93.54
  boxing Y93.71
  brass instrument playing Y93.J4 (*following* Y93.7)
  building construction Y93.H3 (*following* Y93.7)
  bungee jumping Y93.34
  calisthenics Y93.A2 (*following* Y93.7)
  canoeing (in calm and turbulent water) Y93.16
  capture the flag Y93.6A
  cardiorespiratory exercise NEC Y93.A9 (*following* Y93.7)
  caregiving (providing) NEC Y93.F9 (*following* Y93.7)
    bathing Y93.F1 (*following* Y93.7)
    lifting Y93.F2 (*following* Y93.7)
  cellular
    communication device Y93.C2 (*following* Y93.7)
    telephone Y93.C2 (*following* Y93.7)
  challenge course Y93.A5 (*following* Y93.7)
  cheerleading Y93.45
  circuit training Y93.A4 (*following* Y93.7)
  cleaning
    floor Y93.E5 (*following* Y93.7)
  climbing NEC Y93.39
    mountain Y93.31
    rock Y93.31
    wall Y93.31
  clothing care and maintenance NEC Y93.E9 (*following* Y93.7)
  combatives Y93.75
  computer
    keyboarding Y93.C1 (*following* Y93.7)
    technology NEC Y93.C9 (*following* Y93.7)
  confidence course Y93.A5 (*following* Y93.7)
  construction (building) Y93.H3 (*following* Y93.7)
  cooking and baking Y93.G3 (*following* Y93.7)
  cool down exercises Y93.A2 (*following* Y93.7)
  cricket Y93.69
  crocheting Y93.D1 (*following* Y93.7)
  cross country skiing Y93.24
  dancing (all types) Y93.41
  digging
    dirt Y93.H1 (*following* Y93.7)
  dirt digging Y93.H1 (*following* Y93.7)
  dishwashing Y93.G1 (*following* Y93.7)
  diving (platform) (springboard) Y93.12
    underwater Y93.15
  dodge ball Y93.6A
  downhill skiing Y93.23
  drum playing Y93.J2 (*following* Y93.7)
  dumbbells Y93.B3 (*following* Y93.7)
  electronic
    devices NEC Y93.C9 (*following* Y93.7)
      hand held interactive Y93.C2 (*following* Y93.7)
    game playing (using) (with)
      interactive device Y93.C2 (*following* Y93.7)
      keyboard or other stationary device Y93.C1 (*following* Y93.7)
  elliptical machine Y93.A1 (*following* Y93.7)
  exercise(s)
    machines ((primarily) for)
      cardiorespiratory conditioning Y93.A1 (*following* Y93.7)
      muscle strengthening Y93.B1 (*following* Y93.7)
    muscle strengthening (non-machine) NEC Y93.B9 (*following* Y93.7)
  external motion NEC Y93.I9 (*following* Y93.7)
    rollercoaster Y93.I1 (*following* Y93.7)
  field hockey Y93.65
  figure skating (pairs) (singles) Y93.21
  flag football Y93.62
  floor mopping and cleaning Y93.E5 (*following* Y93.7)
  food preparation and clean up Y93.G1 (*following* Y93.7)
  football (American) NOS Y93.61
    flag Y93.62
    tackle Y93.61
    touch Y93.62
  four square Y93.6A
  free weights Y93.B3 (*following* Y93.7)
  frisbee (ultimate) Y93.74
  furniture
    building Y93.D3 (*following* Y93.7)
    finishing Y93.D3 (*following* Y93.7)

Activity — *continued*
  furniture — *continued*
    repair Y93.D3 (*following* Y93.7)
  game playing (electronic)
    using interactive device Y93.C2 (*following* Y93.7)
    using keyboard or other stationary device Y93.C1 (*following* Y93.7)
  gardening Y93.H2 (*following* Y93.7)
  golf Y93.53
  grass drills Y93.A6 (*following* Y93.7)
  grilling and smoking food Y93.G2 (*following* Y93.7)
  grooming and shearing an animal Y93.K3 (*following* Y93.7)
  guerilla drills Y93.A6 (*following* Y93.7)
  gymnastics (rhythmic) Y93.43
  hand held interactive electronic device Y93.C2 (*following* Y93.7)
  handball Y93.73
  handcrafts NEC Y93.D9 (*following* Y93.7)
  hang gliding Y93.35
  hiking (on level or elevated terrain) Y93.Ø1
  hockey (ice) Y93.22
    field Y93.65
  horseback riding Y93.52
  household (interior) maintenance NEC Y93.E9 (*following* Y93.7)
  ice NEC Y93.29
    dancing Y93.21
    hockey Y93.22
    skating Y93.21
  inline roller skating Y93.51
  ironing Y93.E4 (*following* Y93.7)
  judo Y93.75
  jumping jacks Y93.A2 (*following* Y93.7)
  jumping rope Y93.56
  jumping (off) NEC Y93.39
    BASE (Building, Antenna, Span, Earth) Y93.33
    bungee Y93.34
    jacks Y93.A2 (*following* Y93.7)
    rope Y93.56
  karate Y93.75
  kayaking (in calm and turbulent water) Y93.16
  keyboarding (computer) Y93.C1 (*following* Y93.7)
  kickball Y93.6A
  knitting Y93.D1 (*following* Y93.7)
  lacrosse Y93.65
  land maintenance NEC Y93.H9 (*following* Y93.7)
  landscaping Y93.H2 (*following* Y93.7)
  laundry Y93.E2 (*following* Y93.7)
  machines (exercise)
    primarily for cardiorespiratory conditioning Y93.A1 (*following* Y93.7)
    primarily for muscle strengthening Y93.B1 (*following* Y93.7)
  maintenance
    exterior building NEC Y93.H9 (*following* Y93.7)
    household (interior) NEC Y93.E9 (*following* Y93.7)
    land Y93.H9 (*following* Y93.7)
    property Y93.H9 (*following* Y93.7)
  marching (on level or elevated terrain) Y93.Ø1
  martial arts Y93.75
  microwave oven Y93.G3 (*following* Y93.7)
  milking an animal Y93.K2 (*following* Y93.7)
  mopping (floor) Y93.E5 (*following* Y93.7)
  mountain climbing Y93.31
  muscle strengthening
    exercises (non-machine) NEC Y93.B9 (*following* Y93.7)
    machines Y93.B1 (*following* Y93.7)
  musical keyboard (electronic) playing Y93.J1 (*following* Y93.7)
  nordic skiing Y93.24
  obstacle course Y93.A5 (*following* Y93.7)
  oven (microwave) Y93.G3 (*following* Y93.7)
  packing up and unpacking in moving to a new residence Y93.E6 (*following* Y93.7)
  parasailing Y93.19
  percussion instrument playing NEC Y93.J2 (*following* Y93.7)
  personal
    bathing and showering Y93.E1 (*following* Y93.7)
    hygiene NEC Y93.E8 (*following* Y93.7)
    showering Y93.E1 (*following* Y93.7)
  physical games generally associated with school recess, summer camp and children Y93.6A
  physical training NEC Y93.A9 (*following* Y93.7)
  piano playing Y93.J1 (*following* Y93.7)
  pilates Y93.B4 (*following* Y93.7)

Activity — *continued*
  platform diving Y93.12
  playing musical instrument
    brass instrument Y93.J4 (*following* Y93.7)
    drum Y93.J2 (*following* Y93.7)
    musical keyboard (electronic) Y93.J1 (*following* Y93.7)
    percussion instrument NEC Y93.J2 (*following* Y93.7)
    piano Y93.J1 (*following* Y93.7)
    string instrument Y93.J3 (*following* Y93.7)
    winds instrument Y93.J4 (*following* Y93.7)
  property maintenance
    exterior NEC Y93.H9 (*following* Y93.7)
    interior NEC Y93.E9 (*following* Y93.7)
  pruning (garden and lawn) Y93.H2 (*following* Y93.7)
  pull-ups Y93.B2 (*following* Y93.7)
  push-ups Y93.B2 (*following* Y93.7)
  racquetball Y93.73
  rafting (in calm and turbulent water) Y93.16
  raking (leaves) Y93.H1 (*following* Y93.7)
  rappelling Y93.32
  refereeing a sports activity Y93.81
  residential relocation Y93.E6 (*following* Y93.7)
  rhythmic gymnastics Y93.43
  rhythmic movement NEC Y93.49
  riding
    horseback Y93.52
    rollercoaster Y93.I1 (*following* Y93.7)
  rock climbing Y93.31
  roller skating (inline) Y93.51
  rollercoaster riding Y93.I1 (*following* Y93.7)
  rough housing and horseplay Y93.83
  rowing (in calm and turbulent water) Y93.16
  rugby Y93.63
  running Y93.Ø2
  SCUBA diving Y93.15
  sewing Y93.D2 (*following* Y93.7)
  shoveling Y93.H1 (*following* Y93.7)
    dirt Y93.H1 (*following* Y93.7)
    snow Y93.H1 (*following* Y93.7)
  showering (personal) Y93.E1 (*following* Y93.7)
  sit-ups Y93.B2 (*following* Y93.7)
  skateboarding Y93.51
  skating (ice) Y93.21
    roller Y93.51
  skiing (alpine) (downhill) Y93.23
    cross country Y93.24
    nordic Y93.24
    water Y93.17
  sledding (snow) Y93.23
  sleeping (sleep) Y93.84
  smoking and grilling food Y93.G2 (*following* Y93.7)
  snorkeling Y93.15
  snow NEC Y93.29
    boarding Y93.23
    shoveling Y93.H1 (*following* Y93.7)
    sledding Y93.23
    tubing Y93.23
  soccer Y93.66
  softball Y93.64
  specified NEC Y93.89
  spectator at an event Y93.82
  sports NEC Y93.79
    sports played as a team or group NEC Y93.69
    sports played individually NEC Y93.59
  springboard diving Y93.12
  squash Y93.73
  stationary bike Y93.A1 (*following* Y93.7)
  step (stepping) exercise (class) Y93.A3 (*following* Y93.7)
  stepper machine Y93.A1 (*following* Y93.7)
  stove Y93.G3 (*following* Y93.7)
  string instrument playing Y93.J3 (*following* Y93.7)
  surfing Y93.18
    wind Y93.18
  swimming Y93.11
  tackle football Y93.61
  tap dancing Y93.41
  tennis Y93.73
  tobogganing Y93.23
  touch football Y93.62
  track and field events (non-running) Y93.57
    running Y93.Ø2
  trampoline Y93.44
  treadmill Y93.A1 (*following* Y93.7)
  trimming shrubs Y93.H2 (*following* Y93.7)
  tubing (in calm and turbulent water) Y93.16
    snow Y93.23
  ultimate frisbee Y93.74

Activity — *continued*
  underwater diving Y93.15
  unpacking in moving to a new residence Y93.E6 (*following* Y93.7)
  use of stove, oven and microwave oven Y93.G3 (*following* Y93.7)
  vacuuming Y93.E3 (*following* Y93.7)
  volleyball (beach) (court) Y93.68
  wake boarding Y93.17
  walking (on level or elevated terrain) Y93.Ø1
    an animal Y93.K1 (*following* Y93.7)
  walking an animal Y93.K1 (*following* Y93.7)
  wall climbing Y93.31
  warm up and cool down exercises Y93.A2 (*following* Y93.7)
  water NEC Y93.19
    aerobics Y93.14
    craft NEC Y93.19
    exercise Y93.14
    polo Y93.13
    skiing Y93.17
    sliding Y93.18
    survival training and testing Y93.19
  weeding (garden and lawn) Y93.H2 (*following* Y93.7)
  wind instrument playing Y93.J4 (*following* Y93.7)
  windsurfing Y93.18
  wrestling Y93.72
  yoga Y93.42
Adverse effect of drugs — *see* Table of Drugs and Chemicals
Aerosinusitis — *see* Air, pressure
After-effect, late — *see* Sequelae
Air
  blast in war operations — *see* War operations, air blast
  pressure
    change, rapid
      during
        ascent W94.29 ☑
          while (in) (surfacing from)
            aircraft W94.23 ☑
            deep water diving W94.21 ☑
            underground W94.22 ☑
        descent W94.39 ☑
          in
            aircraft W94.31 ☑
            water W94.32 ☑
    high, prolonged W94.Ø ☑
    low, prolonged W94.12 ☑
      due to residence or long visit at high altitude W94.11 ☑
Alpine sickness W94.11 ☑
Altitude sickness W94.11 ☑
Anaphylactic shock, anaphylaxis — *see* Table of Drugs and Chemicals
Andes disease W94.11 ☑
Arachnidism, arachnoidism X58 ☑
Arson (with intent to injure or kill) X97 ☑
Asphyxia, asphyxiation
  by
    food (bone) (seed) — *see* categories T17 and T18 ☑
    gas (*see also* Table of Drugs and Chemicals)
      legal
        execution — *see* Legal, intervention, gas
        intervention — *see* Legal, intervention, gas
  from
    fire (*see also* Exposure, fire)
      in war operations — *see* War operations, fire
    ignition — *see* Ignition
    vomitus T17.81 ☑
  in war operations — *see* War operations, restriction of airway
Aspiration
  food (any type) (into respiratory tract) (with asphyxia, obstruction respiratory tract, suffocation) — *see* categories T17 and T18 ☑
  foreign body — *see* Foreign body, aspiration
  vomitus (with asphyxia, obstruction respiratory tract, suffocation) T17.81 ☑
Assassination (attempt) — *see* Assault
Assault (homicidal) (by) (in) YØ9
  arson X97 ☑
  bite (of human being) YØ4.1 ☑
  bodily force YØ4.8 ☑
    bite YØ4.1 ☑
    bumping into YØ4.2 ☑
    sexual — *see* subcategories T74.Ø, T76.Ø ☑

Assault — *continued*
- bodily force — *continued*
  - unarmed fight Y04.0 ☑
- bomb X96.9 ☑
  - antipersonnel X96.0 ☑
  - fertilizer X96.3 ☑
  - gasoline X96.1 ☑
  - letter X96.2 ☑
  - petrol X96.1 ☑
  - pipe X96.3 ☑
  - specified NEC X96.8 ☑
- brawl (hand) (fists) (foot) (unarmed) Y04.0 ☑
- burning, burns (by fire) NEC X97 ☑
  - acid Y08.89 ☑
  - caustic, corrosive substance Y08.89 ☑
  - chemical from swallowing caustic, corrosive substance — *see* Table of Drugs and Chemicals
  - cigarette(s) X97 ☑
  - hot object X98.9 ☑
    - fluid NEC X98.2 ☑
    - household appliance X98.3 ☑
    - specified NEC X98.8 ☑
    - steam X98.0 ☑
    - tap water X98.1 ☑
    - vapors X98.0 ☑
  - scalding — *see* Assault, burning
  - steam X98.0 ☑
  - vitriol Y08.89 ☑
- caustic, corrosive substance (gas) Y08.89 ☑
- crashing of
  - aircraft Y08.81 ☑
  - motor vehicle Y03.8 ☑
    - pushed in front of Y02.0 ☑
    - run over Y03.0 ☑
    - specified NEC Y03.8 ☑
- cutting or piercing instrument X99.9 ☑
  - dagger X99.2 ☑
  - glass X99.0 ☑
  - knife X99.1 ☑
  - specified NEC X99.8 ☑
  - sword X99.2 ☑
- dagger X99.2 ☑
- drowning (in) X92.9 ☑
  - bathtub X92.0 ☑
  - natural water X92.3 ☑
  - specified NEC X92.8 ☑
  - swimming pool X92.1 ☑
    - following fall X92.2 ☑
- dynamite X96.8 ☑
- explosive(s) (material) X96.9 ☑
- fight (hand) (fists) (foot) (unarmed) Y04.0 ☑
  - with weapon — *see* Assault, by type of weapon
- fire X97 ☑
- firearm X95.9 ☑
  - airgun X95.01 ☑
  - handgun X93 ☑
  - hunting rifle X94.1 ☑
  - larger X94.9 ☑
    - specified NEC X94.8 ☑
  - machine gun X94.2 ☑
  - shotgun X94.0 ☑
  - specified NEC X95.8 ☑
- from high place Y01 ☑
- gunshot (wound) NEC — *see* Assault, firearm, by type
- incendiary device X97 ☑
- injury Y09
  - to child due to criminal abortion attempt NEC Y08.89 ☑
- knife X99.1 ☑
- late effect of — *see* categories X92-Y08 with 7th character S
- placing before moving object NEC Y02.8 ☑
  - motor vehicle Y02.0 ☑
- poisoning — *see* categories T36-T65 with 7th character S
- puncture, any part of body — *see* Assault, cutting or piercing instrument
- pushing
  - before moving object NEC Y02.8 ☑
    - motor vehicle Y02.0 ☑
    - subway train Y02.1 ☑
    - train Y02.1 ☑
  - from high place Y01 ☑
- rape T74.2- ☑
- scalding — *see* Assault, burning

Assault — *continued*
- sequelae of — *see* categories X92-Y08 with 7th character S
- sexual (by bodily force) T74.2- ☑
- shooting — *see* Assault, firearm
- specified means NEC Y08.89 ☑
- stab, any part of body — *see* Assault, cutting or piercing instrument
- steam X98.0 ☑
- striking against
  - other person Y04.2 ☑
  - sports equipment Y08.09 ☑
    - baseball bat Y08.02 ☑
    - hockey stick Y08.01 ☑
- struck by
  - sports equipment Y08.09 ☑
    - baseball bat Y08.02 ☑
    - hockey stick Y08.01 ☑
- submersion — *see* Assault, drowning
- violence Y09
- weapon Y09
  - blunt Y00 ☑
  - cutting or piercing — *see* Assault, cutting or piercing instrument
  - firearm — *see* Assault, firearm
- wound Y09
  - cutting — *see* Assault, cutting or piercing instrument
  - gunshot — *see* Assault, firearm
  - knife X99.1 ☑
  - piercing — *see* Assault, cutting or piercing instrument
  - puncture — *see* Assault, cutting or piercing instrument
  - stab — *see* Assault, cutting or piercing instrument

Attack by mammals NEC W55.89 ☑
Avalanche — *see* Landslide
Aviator's disease — *see* Air, pressure

B

Barotitis, barodontalgia, barosinusitis, barotrauma (otitic) (sinus) — *see* Air, pressure
Battered (baby) (child) (person) (syndrome) X58 ☑
Bayonet wound W26.1 ☑
- in
  - legal intervention — *see* Legal, intervention, sharp object, bayonet
  - war operations — *see* War operations, combat
- stated as undetermined whether accidental or intentional Y28.8 ☑
- suicide (attempt) X78.2 ☑
Bean in nose — *see* categories T17 and T18 ☑
Bed set on fire NEC — *see* Exposure, fire, uncontrolled, building, bed
Beheading (by guillotine)
- homicide X99.9 ☑
- legal execution — *see* Legal, intervention
Bending, injury in — *see* Overexertion
Bends — *see* Air, pressure, change
Bite, bitten by
- alligator W58.01 ☑
- arthropod (nonvenomous) NEC W57 ☑
- bull W55.21 ☑
- cat W55.01 ☑
- cow W55.21 ☑
- crocodile W58.11 ☑
- dog W54.0 ☑
- goat W55.31 ☑
- hoof stock NEC W55.31 ☑
- horse W55.11 ☑
- human being (accidentally) W50.3 ☑
  - with intent to injure or kill Y04.1 ☑
  - as, or caused by, a crowd or human stampede (with fall) W52 ☑
  - assault Y04.1 ☑
  - homicide (attempt) Y04.1 ☑
  - in
    - fight Y04.1 ☑
- insect (nonvenomous) W57 ☑
- lizard (nonvenomous) W59.01 ☑
- mammal NEC W55.81 ☑
- mammal NEC W55.81 ☑
  - marine W56.31 ☑
- marine animal (nonvenomous) W56.81 ☑
- millipede W57 ☑

Bite, bitten by — *continued*
- moray eel W56.51 ☑
- mouse W53.01 ☑
- person(s) (accidentally) W50.3 ☑
  - with intent to injure or kill Y04.1 ☑
  - as, or caused by, a crowd or human stampede (with fall) W52 ☑
  - assault Y04.1 ☑
  - homicide (attempt) Y04.1 ☑
  - in
    - fight Y04.1 ☑
- pig W55.41 ☑
- raccoon W55.51 ☑
- rat W53.11 ☑
- reptile W59.81 ☑
  - lizard W59.01 ☑
  - snake W59.11 ☑
  - turtle W59.21 ☑
    - terrestrial W59.81 ☑
- rodent W53.81 ☑
  - mouse W53.01 ☑
  - rat W53.11 ☑
  - specified NEC W53.81 ☑
  - squirrel W53.21 ☑
- shark W56.41 ☑
- sheep W55.31 ☑
- snake (nonvenomous) W59.11 ☑
- spider (nonvenomous) W57 ☑
- squirrel W53.21 ☑
Blast (air) in war operations — *see* War operations, blast
Blizzard X37.2 ☑
Blood alcohol level Y90.9
- less than 20mg/100ml Y90.0
- 20-39mg/100ml Y90.1
- 40-59mg/100ml Y90.2
- 60-79mg/100ml Y90.3
- 80-99mg/100ml Y90.4
- 100-119mg/100ml Y90.5
- 120-199mg/100ml Y90.6
- 200-239mg/100ml Y90.7
- presence in blood, level not specified Y90.9
Blow X58 ☑
- by law-enforcing agent, police (on duty) — *see* Legal, intervention, manhandling
- blunt object — *see* Legal, intervention, blunt object
Blowing up — *see* Explosion
Brawl (hand) (fists) (foot) Y04.0 ☑
Breakage (accidental) (part of)
- ladder (causing fall) W11 ☑
- scaffolding (causing fall) W12 ☑
Broken
- glass, contact with — *see* Contact, with, glass
- power line (causing electric shock) W85 ☑
Bumping against, into (accidentally)
- object NEC W22.8 ☑
  - with fall — *see* Fall, due to, bumping against, object
  - caused by crowd or human stampede (with fall) W52 ☑
  - sports equipment W21.9 ☑
- person(s) W51 ☑
  - with fall W03 ☑
    - due to ice or snow W00.0 ☑
  - assault Y04.2 ☑
  - caused by, a crowd or human stampede (with fall) W52 ☑
  - homicide (attempt) Y04.2 ☑
  - sports equipment W21.9 ☑
Burn, burned, burning (accidental) (by) (from) (on)
- acid NEC — *see* Table of Drugs and Chemicals
- bed linen — *see* Exposure, fire, uncontrolled, in building, bed
- blowtorch X08.8 ☑
  - with ignition of clothing NEC X06.2 ☑
    - nightwear X05 ☑
- bonfire, campfire (controlled) (*see also* Exposure, fire, controlled, not in building)
  - uncontrolled — *see* Exposure, fire, uncontrolled, not in building
- candle X08.8 ☑
  - with ignition of clothing NEC X06.2 ☑
    - nightwear X05 ☑
- caustic liquid, substance (external) (internal) NEC — *see* Table of Drugs and Chemicals
- chemical (external) (internal) (*see also* Table of Drugs and Chemicals)

Burn, burned, burning — *continued*
  chemical (*see also* Table of Drugs and Chemicals) — *continued*
    in war operations — *see* War operations. fire
  cigar(s) or cigarette(s) X08.8 ☑
    with ignition of clothing NEC X06.2 ☑
      nightwear X05 ☑
  clothes, clothing NEC (from controlled fire) X06.2 ☑
    with conflagration — *see* Exposure, fire, uncontrolled, building
    not in building or structure — *see* Exposure, fire, uncontrolled, not in building
  cooker (hot) X15.8 ☑
    stated as undetermined whether accidental or intentional Y27.3 ☑
    suicide (attempt) X77.3 ☑
  electric blanket X16 ☑
  engine (hot) X17 ☑
  fire, flames — *see* Exposure, fire
  flare, Very pistol — *see* Discharge, firearm NEC
  heat
    from appliance (electrical) (household) X15.8 ☑
      cooker X15.8 ☑
      hotplate X15.2 ☑
      kettle X15.8 ☑
      light bulb X15.8 ☑
      saucepan X15.3 ☑
      skillet X15.3 ☑
      stated as undetermined whether accidental or intentional Y27.3 ☑
      stove X15.0 ☑
      suicide (attempt) X77.3 ☑
      toaster X15.1 ☑
    in local application or packing during medical or surgical procedure Y63.5
  heating
    appliance, radiator or pipe X16 ☑
  homicide (attempt) — *see* Assault, burning
  hot
    air X14.1 ☑
    cooker X15.8 ☑
    drink X10.0 ☑
    engine X17 ☑
    fat X10.2 ☑
    fluid NEC X12 ☑
    food X10.1 ☑
    gases X14.1 ☑
    heating appliance X16 ☑
    household appliance NEC X15.8 ☑
    kettle X15.8 ☑
    liquid NEC X12 ☑
    machinery X17 ☑
    metal (molten) (liquid) NEC X18 ☑
    object (not producing fire or flames) NEC X19 ☑
    oil (cooking) X10.2 ☑
    pipe(s) X16 ☑
    radiator X16 ☑
    saucepan (glass) (metal) X15.3 ☑
    stove (kitchen) X15.0 ☑
    substance NEC X19 ☑
      caustic or corrosive NEC — *see* Table of Drugs and Chemicals
    toaster X15.1 ☑
    tool X17 ☑
    vapor X13.1 ☑
    water (tap) — *see* Contact, with, hot, tap water
  hotplate X15.2 ☑
    suicide (attempt) X77.3 ☑
  ignition — *see* Ignition
  in war operations — *see* War operations, fire
  inflicted by other person X97 ☑
    by hot objects, hot vapor, and steam — *see* Assault, burning, hot object
  internal, from swallowed caustic, corrosive liquid, substance — *see* Table of Drugs and Chemicals
  iron (hot) X15.8 ☑
    stated as undetermined whether accidental or intentional Y27.3 ☑
    suicide (attempt) X77.3 ☑
  kettle (hot) X15.8 ☑
    stated as undetermined whether accidental or intentional Y27.3 ☑
    suicide (attempt) X77.3 ☑
  lamp (flame) X08.8 ☑
    with ignition of clothing NEC X06.2 ☑
      nightwear X05 ☑

Burn, burned, burning — *continued*
  lighter (cigar) (cigarette) X08.8 ☑
    with ignition of clothing NEC X06.2 ☑
      nightwear X05 ☑
  lightning — *see* subcategory T75.0 ☑
    causing fire — *see* Exposure, fire
  liquid (boiling) (hot) NEC X12 ☑
    stated as undetermined whether accidental or intentional Y27.2 ☑
    suicide (attempt) X77.2 ☑
  local application of externally applied substance in medical or surgical care Y63.5
  machinery (hot) X17 ☑
  matches X08.8 ☑
    with ignition of clothing NEC X06.2 ☑
      nightwear X05 ☑
  mattress — *see* Exposure, fire, uncontrolled, building, bed
  medicament, externally applied Y63.5
  metal (hot) (liquid) (molten) NEC X18 ☑
  nightwear (nightclothes, nightdress, gown, pajamas, robe) X05 ☑
  object (hot) NEC X19 ☑
  on board watercraft
    due to
      accident to watercraft V91.09 ☑
        powered craft V91.03 ☑
          ferry boat V91.01 ☑
          fishing boat V91.02 ☑
          jetskis V91.03 ☑
          liner V91.01 ☑
          merchant ship V91.00 ☑
          passenger ship V91.01 ☑
        unpowered craft V91.08 ☑
          canoe V91.05 ☑
          inflatable V91.06 ☑
          kayak V91.05 ☑
          sailboat V91.04 ☑
          surf-board V91.08 ☑
          water skis V91.07 ☑
          windsurfer V91.08 ☑
      fire on board V93.09 ☑
        ferry boat V93.01 ☑
        fishing boat V93.02 ☑
        jetskis V93.03 ☑
        liner V93.01 ☑
        merchant ship V93.00 ☑
        passenger ship V93.01 ☑
        powered craft NEC V93.03 ☑
        sailboat V93.04 ☑
      specified heat source NEC on board V93.19 ☑
        ferry boat V93.11 ☑
        fishing boat V93.12 ☑
        jetskis V93.13 ☑
        liner V93.11 ☑
        merchant ship V93.10 ☑
        passenger ship V93.11 ☑
        powered craft NEC V93.13 ☑
        sailboat V93.14 ☑
  pipe (hot) X16 ☑
    smoking X08.8 ☑
      with ignition of clothing NEC X06.2 ☑
        nightwear X05 ☑
  powder — *see* Powder burn
  radiator (hot) X16 ☑
  saucepan (hot) (glass) (metal) X15.3 ☑
    stated as undetermined whether accidental or intentional Y27.3 ☑
    suicide (attempt) X77.3 ☑
  self-inflicted X76 ☑
    stated as undetermined whether accidental or intentional Y26 ☑
  stated as undetermined whether accidental or intentional Y27.0 ☑
  steam X13.1 ☑
    pipe X16 ☑
      stated as undetermined whether accidental or intentional Y27.8 ☑
    stated as undetermined whether accidental or intentional Y27.0 ☑
    suicide (attempt) X77.0 ☑
  stove (hot) (kitchen) X15.0 ☑
    stated as undetermined whether accidental or intentional Y27.3 ☑
    suicide (attempt) X77.3 ☑
  substance (hot) NEC X19 ☑

Burn, burned, burning — *continued*
  substance — *continued*
    boiling X12 ☑
    stated as undetermined whether accidental or intentional Y27.2 ☑
    suicide (attempt) X77.2 ☑
    molten (metal) X18 ☑
  suicide (attempt) NEC X76 ☑
    hot
      household appliance X77.3 ☑
      object X77.9 ☑
  therapeutic misadventure
    heat in local application or packing during medical or surgical procedure Y63.5
    overdose of radiation Y63.2
  toaster (hot) X15.1 ☑
    stated as undetermined whether accidental or intentional Y27.3 ☑
    suicide (attempt) X77.3 ☑
  tool (hot) X17 ☑
  torch, welding X08.8 ☑
    with ignition of clothing NEC X06.2 ☑
      nightwear X05 ☑
  trash fire (controlled) — *see* Exposure, fire, controlled, not in building
    uncontrolled — *see* Exposure, fire, uncontrolled, not in building
  vapor (hot) X13.1 ☑
    stated as undetermined whether accidental or intentional Y27.0 ☑
    suicide (attempt) X77.0 ☑
  Very pistol — *see* Discharge, firearm NEC
Butted by animal W55.82 ☑
  bull W55.22 ☑
  cow W55.22 ☑
  goat W55.32 ☑
  horse W55.12 ☑
  pig W55.42 ☑
  sheep W55.32 ☑

C

Caisson disease — *see* Air, pressure, change
Campfire (exposure to) (controlled) (*see also* Exposure, fire, controlled, not in building)
  uncontrolled — *see* Exposure, fire, uncontrolled, not in building
Capital punishment (any means) — *see* Legal, intervention
Car sickness T75.3 ☑
Casualty (not due to war) NEC X58 ☑
  war — *see* War operations
Cat
  bite W55.01 ☑
  scratch W55.03 ☑
Cataclysm, cataclysmic (any injury) NEC — *see* Forces of nature
Catching fire — *see* Exposure, fire
Caught
  between
    folding object W23.0 ☑
    objects (moving) (stationary and moving) W23.0 ☑
      and machinery — *see* Contact, with, by type of machine
    stationary W23.1 ☑
    sliding door and door frame W23.0 ☑
  by, in
    machinery (moving parts of) — *see* Contact, with, by type of machine
    washing-machine wringer W23.0 ☑
  under packing crate (due to losing grip) W23.1 ☑
Cave-in caused by cataclysmic earth surface movement or eruption — *see* Landslide
Change(s) in air pressure — *see* Air, pressure, change
Choked, choking (on) (any object except food or vomitus)
  food (bone) (seed) — *see* categories T17 and T18 ☑
  vomitus T17.81- ☑
Civil insurrection — *see* War operations
Cloudburst (any injury) X37.8 ☑
Cold, exposure to (accidental) (excessive) (extreme) (natural) (place) NEC — *see* Exposure, cold
Collapse
  building W20.1 ☑
    burning (uncontrolled fire) X00.2 ☑

Collapse — *continued*
  dam or man-made structure (causing earth movement)
      X36.0 ✓
  machinery — *see* Contact, with, by type of machine
  structure W20.1 ✓
      burning (uncontrolled fire) X00.2 ✓
Collision (accidental) NEC (*see also* Accident, transport)
      V89.9 ✓
  pedestrian W51 ✓
      with fall W03 ✓
          due to ice or snow W00.0 ✓
          involving pedestrian conveyance — *see* Accident, transport, pedestrian, conveyance
      and
          crowd or human stampede (with fall) W52 ✓
          object W22.8 ✓
              with fall — *see* Fall, due to, bumping against, object
  person(s) — *see* Collision, pedestrian
  transport vehicle NEC V89.9 ✓
      and
          avalanche, fallen or not moving — *see* Accident, transport
          falling or moving — *see* Landslide
          landslide, fallen or not moving — *see* Accident, transport
          falling or moving — *see* Landslide
  due to cataclysm — *see* Forces of nature, by type
  intentional, purposeful suicide (attempt) — *see* Suicide, collision
Combustion, spontaneous — *see* Ignition
Complication (delayed) **of or following** (medical or surgical procedure) Y84.9
  with misadventure — *see* Misadventure
  amputation of limb(s) Y83.5
  anastomosis (arteriovenous) (blood vessel) (gastrojejunal) (tendon) (natural or artificial material) Y83.2
  aspiration (of fluid) Y84.4
      tissue Y84.8
  biopsy Y84.8
  blood
      sampling Y84.7
      transfusion
          procedure Y84.8
  bypass Y83.2
  catheterization (urinary) Y84.6
      cardiac Y84.0
  colostomy Y83.3
  cystostomy Y83.3
  dialysis (kidney) Y84.1
  drug — *see* Table of Drugs and Chemicals
  due to misadventure — *see* Misadventure
  duodenostomy Y83.3
  electroshock therapy Y84.3
  external stoma, creation of Y83.3
  formation of external stoma Y83.3
  gastrostomy Y83.3
  graft Y83.2
  hypothermia (medically-induced) Y84.8
  implant, implantation (of)
      artificial
          internal device (cardiac pacemaker) (electrodes in brain) (heart valve prosthesis) (orthopedic) Y83.1
          material or tissue (for anastomosis or bypass) Y83.2
              with creation of external stoma Y83.3
          natural tissues (for anastomosis or bypass) Y83.2
              with creation of external stoma Y83.3
  infusion
      procedure Y84.8
  injection — *see* Table of Drugs and Chemicals
      procedure Y84.8
  insertion of gastric or duodenal sound Y84.5
  insulin-shock therapy Y84.3
  paracentesis (abdominal) (thoracic) (aspirative) Y84.4
  procedures other than surgical operation — *see* Complication of or following, by type of procedure
  radiological procedure or therapy Y84.2
  removal of organ (partial) (total) NEC Y83.6
  sampling
      blood Y84.7
      fluid NEC Y84.4
      tissue Y84.8
  shock therapy Y84.3

Complication (delayed) **of or following** — *continued*
  surgical operation NEC (*see also* Complication of or following, by type of operation) Y83.9
      reconstructive NEC Y83.4
          with
              anastomosis, bypass or graft Y83.2
              formation of external stoma Y83.3
      specified NEC Y83.8
  transfusion (*see also* Table of Drugs and Chemicals)
      procedure Y84.8
  transplant, transplantation (heart) (kidney) (liver) (whole organ, any) Y83.0
      partial organ Y83.4
  ureterostomy Y83.3
  vaccination (*see also* Table of Drugs and Chemicals)
      procedure Y84.8
Compression
  divers' squeeze — *see* Air, pressure, change
  trachea by
      food (lodged in esophagus) — *see* categories T17 and T18 ✓
      vomitus (lodged in esophagus) T17.81- ✓
Conflagration — *see* Exposure, fire, uncontrolled
Constriction (external)
  hair W49.01 ✓
  jewelry W49.04 ✓
  ring W49.04 ✓
  rubber band W49.03 ✓
  specified item NEC W49.09 ✓
  string W49.02 ✓
  thread W49.02 ✓
Contact (accidental)
  with
      abrasive wheel (metalworking) W31.1 ✓
      alligator W58.09 ✓
          bite W58.01 ✓
          crushing W58.03 ✓
          strike W58.02 ✓
      amphibian W62.9 ✓
          frog W62.0 ✓
          toad W62.1 ✓
      animal (nonvenomous) NEC W64 ✓
          marine W56.89 ✓
              bite W56.81 ✓
              dolphin — *see* Contact, with, dolphin
              fish NEC — *see* Contact, with, fish
              mammal — *see* Contact, with, mammal, marine
              orca — *see* Contact, with, orca
              sea lion — *see* Contact, with, sea lion
              shark — *see* Contact, with, shark
              strike W56.82 ✓
      animate mechanical force NEC W64 ✓
      arrow W21.89 ✓
          not thrown, projected or falling W45.8 ✓
      arthropods (nonvenomous) W57 ✓
      axe W27.0 ✓
      band-saw (industrial) W31.2 ✓
      bayonet — *see* Bayonet wound
      bee(s) X58 ✓
      bench-saw (industrial) W31.2 ✓
      bird W61.99 ✓
          bite W61.91 ✓
          chicken — *see* Contact, with, chicken
          duck — *see* Contact, with, duck
          goose — *see* Contact, with, goose
          macaw — *see* Contact, with, macaw
          parrot — *see* Contact, with, parrot
          psittacine — *see* Contact, with, psittacine
          strike W61.92 ✓
          turkey — *see* Contact, with, turkey
      blender W29.0 ✓
      boiling water X12 ✓
          stated as undetermined whether accidental or intentional Y27.2 ✓
          suicide (attempt) X77.2 ✓
      bore, earth-drilling or mining (land) (seabed) W31.0 ✓
      buffalo — *see* Contact, with, hoof stock NEC
      bull W55.29 ✓
          bite W55.21 ✓
          gored W55.22 ✓
          strike W55.22 ✓
      bumper cars W31.81 ✓
      camel — *see* Contact, with, hoof stock NEC

Contact — *continued*
  with — *continued*
      can
          lid W45.2 ✓
          opener W27.4 ✓
              powered W29.0 ✓
      cat W55.09 ✓
          bite W55.01 ✓
          scratch W55.03 ✓
      caterpillar (venomous) X58 ✓
      centipede (venomous) X58 ✓
      chain
          hoist W24.0 ✓
              agricultural operations W30.89 ✓
          saw W29.3 ✓
      chicken W61.39 ✓
          peck W61.33 ✓
          strike W61.32 ✓
      chisel W27.0 ✓
      circular saw W31.2 ✓
      cobra X58 ✓
      combine (harvester) W30.0 ✓
      conveyer belt W24.1 ✓
      cooker (hot) X15.8 ✓
          stated as undetermined whether accidental or intentional Y27.3 ✓
          suicide (attempt) X77.3 ✓
      coral X58 ✓
      cotton gin W31.82 ✓
      cow W55.29 ✓
          bite W55.21 ✓
          strike W55.22 ✓
      crane W24.0 ✓
          agricultural operations W30.89 ✓
      crocodile W58.19 ✓
          bite W58.11 ✓
          crushing W58.13 ✓
          strike W58.12 ✓
      dagger W26.1 ✓
          stated as undetermined whether accidental or intentional Y28.2 ✓
          suicide (attempt) X78.2 ✓
      dairy equipment W31.82 ✓
      dart W21.89 ✓
          not thrown, projected or falling W45.8 ✓
      deer — *see* Contact, with, hoof stock NEC
      derrick W24.0 ✓
          agricultural operations W30.89 ✓
              hay W30.2 ✓
      dog W54.8 ✓
          bite W54.0 ✓
          strike W54.1 ✓
      dolphin W56.09 ✓
          bite W56.01 ✓
          strike W56.02 ✓
      donkey — *see* Contact, with, hoof stock NEC
      drill (powered) W29.8 ✓
          earth (land) (seabed) W31.0 ✓
          nonpowered W27.8 ✓
      drive belt W24.0 ✓
          agricultural operations W30.89 ✓
      dry ice — *see* Exposure, cold, man-made
      dryer (clothes) (powered) (spin) W29.2 ✓
      duck W61.69 ✓
          bite W61.61 ✓
          strike W61.62 ✓
      earth (-)
          drilling machine (industrial) W31.0 ✓
          scraping machine in stationary use W31.83 ✓
      edge of stiff paper W45.1 ✓
      electric
          beater W29.0 ✓
          blanket X16 ✓
          fan W29.2 ✓
              commercial W31.82 ✓
          knife W29.1 ✓
          mixer W29.0 ✓
      elevator (building) W24.0 ✓
          agricultural operations W30.89 ✓
              grain W30.3 ✓
      engine(s), hot NEC X17 ✓
      excavating machine W31.0 ✓
      farm machine W30.9 ✓
      feces — *see* Contact, with, by type of animal
      fer de lance X58 ✓

Contact — *continued*
　with — *continued*
　　fish W56.59 ☑
　　　bite W56.51 ☑
　　　shark — *see* Contact, with, shark
　　　strike W56.52 ☑
　　flying horses W31.81 ☑
　　forging (metalworking) machine W31.1 ☑
　　fork W27.4 ☑
　　forklift (truck) W24.0 ☑
　　　agricultural operations W30.89 ☑
　　frog W62.0 ☑
　　garden
　　　cultivator (powered) W29.3 ☑
　　　　riding W30.89 ☑
　　　fork W27.1 ☑
　　gas turbine W31.3 ☑
　　Gila monster X58 ☑
　　giraffe — *see* Contact, with, hoof stock NEC
　　glass (sharp) (broken) W25 ☑
　　　with subsequent fall W18.02 ☑
　　　assault X99.0 ☑
　　　due to fall — *see* Fall, by type
　　　stated as undetermined whether accidental or intentional Y28.0 ☑
　　　suicide (attempt) X78.0 ☑
　　goat W55.39 ☑
　　　bite W55.31 ☑
　　　strike W55.32 ☑
　　goose W61.59 ☑
　　　bite W61.51 ☑
　　　strike W61.52 ☑
　　hand
　　　saw W27.0 ☑
　　　tool (not powered) NEC W27.8 ☑
　　　　powered W29.8 ☑
　　harvester W30.0 ☑
　　hay-derrick W30.2 ☑
　　heating
　　　appliance (hot) X16 ☑
　　　pad (electric) X16 ☑
　　heat NEC X19 ☑
　　　from appliance (electrical) (household) — *see* Contact, with, hot, household appliance
　　　heating appliance X16 ☑
　　hedge-trimmer (powered) W29.3 ☑
　　hoe W27.1 ☑
　　hoist (chain) (shaft) NEC W24.0 ☑
　　　agricultural W30.89 ☑
　　hoof stock NEC W55.39 ☑
　　　bite W55.31 ☑
　　　strike W55.32 ☑
　　hornet(s) X58 ☑
　　horse W55.19 ☑
　　　bite W55.11 ☑
　　　strike W55.12 ☑
　　hot
　　　air X14.1 ☑
　　　　inhalation X14.0 ☑
　　　cooker X15.8 ☑
　　　drinks X10.0 ☑
　　　engine X17 ☑
　　　fats X10.2 ☑
　　　fluids NEC X12 ☑
　　　　assault X98.2 ☑
　　　　suicide (attempt) X77.2 ☑
　　　　undetermined whether accidental or intentional Y27.2 ☑
　　　food X10.1 ☑
　　　gases X14.1 ☑
　　　　inhalation X14.0 ☑
　　　heating appliance X16 ☑
　　　household appliance X15.8 ☑
　　　　assault X98.3 ☑
　　　　cooker X15.8 ☑
　　　　hotplate X15.2 ☑
　　　　kettle X15.8 ☑
　　　　light bulb X15.8 ☑
　　　　object NEC X19 ☑
　　　　　assault X98.8 ☑
　　　　　stated as undetermined whether accidental or intentional Y27.9 ☑
　　　　　suicide (attempt) X77.8 ☑
　　　　saucepan X15.3 ☑
　　　　skillet X15.3 ☑

Contact — *continued*
　with — *continued*
　　hot — *continued*
　　　household appliance — *continued*
　　　　stated as undetermined whether accidental or intentional Y27.3 ☑
　　　　stove X15.0 ☑
　　　　suicide (attempt) X77.3 ☑
　　　　toaster X15.1 ☑
　　　kettle X15.8 ☑
　　　light bulb X15.8 ☑
　　　liquid NEC (*see also* Burn) X12 ☑
　　　　drinks X10.0 ☑
　　　　stated as undetermined whether accidental or intentional Y27.2 ☑
　　　　suicide (attempt) X77.2 ☑
　　　　tap water X11.8 ☑
　　　　　stated as undetermined whether accidental or intentional Y27.1 ☑
　　　　　suicide (attempt) X77.1 ☑
　　　machinery X17 ☑
　　　metal (molten) (liquid) NEC X18 ☑
　　　object (not producing fire or flames) NEC X19 ☑
　　　oil (cooking) X10.2 ☑
　　　pipe X16 ☑
　　　plate X15.2 ☑
　　　radiator X16 ☑
　　　saucepan (glass) (metal) X15.3 ☑
　　　skillet X15.3 ☑
　　　stove (kitchen) X15.0 ☑
　　　substance NEC X19 ☑
　　　tap-water X11.8 ☑
　　　　assault X98.1 ☑
　　　　heated on stove X12 ☑
　　　　　stated as undetermined whether accidental or intentional Y27.2 ☑
　　　　　suicide (attempt) X77.2 ☑
　　　　in bathtub X11.0 ☑
　　　　running X11.1 ☑
　　　　stated as undetermined whether accidental or intentional Y27.1 ☑
　　　　suicide (attempt) X77.1 ☑
　　　toaster X15.1 ☑
　　　tool X17 ☑
　　　vapors X13.1 ☑
　　　　inhalation X13.0 ☑
　　　water (tap) X11.8 ☑
　　　　boiling X12 ☑
　　　　　stated as undetermined whether accidental or intentional Y27.2 ☑
　　　　　suicide (attempt) X77.2 ☑
　　　　heated on stove X12 ☑
　　　　　stated as undetermined whether accidental or intentional Y27.2 ☑
　　　　　suicide (attempt) X77.2 ☑
　　　　in bathtub X11.0 ☑
　　　　running X11.1 ☑
　　　　stated as undetermined whether accidental or intentional Y27.1 ☑
　　　　suicide (attempt) X77.1 ☑
　　hotplate X15.2 ☑
　　ice-pick W27.4 ☑
　　insect (nonvenomous) NEC W57 ☑
　　kettle (hot) X15.8 ☑
　　knife W26.0 ☑
　　　assault X99.1 ☑
　　　electric W29.1 ☑
　　　stated as undetermined whether accidental or intentional Y28.1 ☑
　　　suicide (attempt) X78.1 ☑
　　lathe (metalworking) W31.1 ☑
　　　turnings W45.8 ☑
　　　woodworking W31.2 ☑
　　lawnmower (powered) (ridden) W28 ☑
　　　causing electrocution W86.8 ☑
　　　　suicide (attempt) X83.1 ☑
　　　unpowered W27.1 ☑
　　lift, lifting (devices) W24.0 ☑
　　　agricultural operations W30.89 ☑
　　　shaft W24.0 ☑
　　liquefied gas — *see* Exposure, cold, man-made
　　liquid air, hydrogen, nitrogen — *see* Exposure, cold, man-made
　　lizard (nonvenomous) W59.09 ☑
　　　bite W59.01 ☑
　　　strike W59.02 ☑

Contact — *continued*
　with — *continued*
　　llama — *see* Contact, with, hoof stock NEC
　　macaw W61.19 ☑
　　　bite W61.11 ☑
　　　strike W61.12 ☑
　　machine, machinery W31.9 ☑
　　　abrasive wheel W31.1 ☑
　　　agricultural including animal-powered W30.9 ☑
　　　　combine harvester W30.0 ☑
　　　　grain storage elevator W30.3 ☑
　　　　hay derrick W30.2 ☑
　　　　power take-off device W30.1 ☑
　　　　reaper W30.0 ☑
　　　　specified NEC W30.89 ☑
　　　　thresher W30.0 ☑
　　　　transport vehicle, stationary W30.81 ☑
　　　band saw W31.2 ☑
　　　bench saw W31.2 ☑
　　　circular saw W31.2 ☑
　　　commercial NEC W31.82 ☑
　　　drilling, metal (industrial) W31.1 ☑
　　　earth-drilling W31.0 ☑
　　　earthmoving or scraping W31.89 ☑
　　　excavating W31.89 ☑
　　　forging machine W31.1 ☑
　　　gas turbine W31.3 ☑
　　　hot X17 ☑
　　　internal combustion engine W31.3 ☑
　　　land drill W31.0 ☑
　　　lathe W31.1 ☑
　　　lifting (devices) W24.0 ☑
　　　metal drill W31.1 ☑
　　　metalworking (industrial) W31.1 ☑
　　　milling, metal W31.1 ☑
　　　mining W31.0 ☑
　　　molding W31.2 ☑
　　　overhead plane W31.2 ☑
　　　power press, metal W31.1 ☑
　　　prime mover W31.3 ☑
　　　printing W31.89 ☑
　　　radial saw W31.2 ☑
　　　recreational W31.81 ☑
　　　roller-coaster W31.81 ☑
　　　rolling mill, metal W31.1 ☑
　　　sander W31.2 ☑
　　　seabed drill W31.0 ☑
　　　shaft
　　　　hoist W31.0 ☑
　　　　lift W31.0 ☑
　　　specified NEC W31.89 ☑
　　　spinning W31.89 ☑
　　　steam engine W31.3 ☑
　　　transmission W24.1 ☑
　　　undercutter W31.0 ☑
　　　water driven turbine W31.3 ☑
　　　weaving W31.89 ☑
　　　woodworking or forming (industrial) W31.2 ☑
　　mammal (feces) (urine) W55.89 ☑
　　　bull — *see* Contact, with, bull
　　　cat — *see* Contact, with, cat
　　　cow — *see* Contact, with, cow
　　　goat — *see* Contact, with, goat
　　　hoof stock — *see* Contact, with, hoof stock
　　　horse — *see* Contact, with, horse
　　　marine W56.39 ☑
　　　　dolphin — *see* Contact, with, dolphin
　　　　orca — *see* Contact, with, orca
　　　　sea lion — *see* Contact, with, sea lion
　　　　specified NEC W56.39 ☑
　　　　　bite W56.31 ☑
　　　　　strike W56.32 ☑
　　　pig — *see* Contact, with, pig
　　　raccoon — *see* Contact, with, raccoon
　　　rodent — *see* Contact, with, rodent
　　　sheep — *see* Contact, with, sheep
　　　specified NEC W55.89 ☑
　　　　bite W55.81 ☑
　　　　strike W55.82 ☑
　　marine
　　　animal W56.89 ☑
　　　　bite W56.81 ☑
　　　　dolphin — *see* Contact, with, dolphin
　　　　fish NEC — *see* Contact, with, fish

Contact — continued
  with — continued
    marine — continued
      animal — continued
        mammal — see Contact, with, mammal, marine
        orca — see Contact, with, orca
        sea lion — see Contact, with, sea lion
        shark — see Contact, with, shark
        strike W56.82 ✓
    meat
      grinder (domestic) W29.0 ✓
        industrial W31.82 ✓
        nonpowered W27.4 ✓
      slicer (domestic) W29.0 ✓
        industrial W31.82 ✓
    merry go round W31.81 ✓
    metal, hot (liquid) (molten) NEC X18 ✓
    millipede W57 ✓
    nail W45.0 ✓
      gun W29.4 ✓
    needle (sewing) W27.3 ✓
      hypodermic W46.0 ✓
        contaminated W46.1 ✓
    object (blunt) NEC
      hot NEC X19 ✓
      legal intervention — see Legal, intervention, blunt object
      sharp NEC W45.8 ✓
        inflicted by other person NEC W45.8 ✓
          stated as
            intentional homicide (attempt) — see Assault, cutting or piercing instrument
        legal intervention — see Legal, intervention, sharp object
        self-inflicted X78.9 ✓
    orca W56.29 ✓
      bite W56.21 ✓
      strike W56.22 ✓
    overhead plane W31.2 ✓
    paper (as sharp object) W45.1 ✓
    paper-cutter W27.5 ✓
    parrot W61.09 ✓
      bite W61.01 ✓
      strike W61.02 ✓
    pig W55.49 ✓
      bite W55.41 ✓
      strike W55.42 ✓
    pipe, hot X16 ✓
    pitchfork W27.1 ✓
    plane (metal) (wood) W27.0 ✓
      overhead W31.2 ✓
    plant thorns, spines, sharp leaves or other mechanisms W60 ✓
    powered
      garden cultivator W29.3 ✓
      household appliance, implement, or machine W29.8 ✓
      saw (industrial) W31.2 ✓
        hand W29.8 ✓
    printing machine W31.89 ✓
    psittacine bird W61.29 ✓
      bite W61.21 ✓
      macaw — see Contact, with, macaw
      parrot — see Contact, with, parrot
      strike W61.22 ✓
    pulley (block) (transmission) W24.0 ✓
      agricultural operations W30.89 ✓
    raccoon W55.59 ✓
      bite W55.51 ✓
      strike W55.52 ✓
    radial-saw (industrial) W31.2 ✓
    radiator (hot) X16 ✓
    rake W27.1 ✓
    rattlesnake X58 ✓
    reaper W30.0 ✓
    reptile W59.89 ✓
      lizard — see Contact, with, lizard
      snake — see Contact, with, snake
      specified NEC W59.89 ✓
        bite W59.81 ✓
        crushing W59.83 ✓
        strike W59.82 ✓
      turtle — see Contact, with, turtle
    rivet gun (powered) W29.4 ✓

Contact — continued
  with — continued
    road scraper — see Accident, transport, construction vehicle
    rodent (feces) (urine) W53.89 ✓
      bite W53.81 ✓
      mouse W53.09 ✓
        bite W53.01 ✓
      rat W53.19 ✓
        bite W53.11 ✓
      specified NEC W53.89 ✓
        bite W53.81 ✓
      squirrel W53.29 ✓
        bite W53.21 ✓
    roller coaster W31.81 ✓
    rope NEC W24.0 ✓
      agricultural operations W30.89 ✓
    saliva — see Contact, with, by type of animal
    sander W29.8 ✓
      industrial W31.2 ✓
    saucepan (hot) (glass) (metal) X15.3 ✓
    saw W27.0 ✓
      band (industrial) W31.2 ✓
      bench (industrial) W31.2 ✓
      chain W29.3 ✓
      hand W27.0 ✓
    sawing machine, metal W31.1 ✓
    scissors W27.2 ✓
    scorpion X58 ✓
    screwdriver W27.0 ✓
      powered W29.8 ✓
    sea
      anemone, cucumber or urchin (spine) X58 ✓
      lion W56.19 ✓
        bite W56.11 ✓
        strike W56.12 ✓
      serpent — see Contact, with, snake, by type
    sewing-machine (electric) (powered) W29.2 ✓
      not powered W27.8 ✓
    shaft (hoist) (lift) (transmission) NEC W24.0 ✓
      agricultural W30.89 ✓
    shark W56.49 ✓
      bite W56.41 ✓
      strike W56.42 ✓
    shears (hand) W27.2 ✓
      powered (industrial) W31.1 ✓
        domestic W29.2 ✓
    sheep W55.39 ✓
      bite W55.31 ✓
      strike W55.32 ✓
    shovel W27.8 ✓
      steam — see Accident, transport, construction vehicle
    snake (nonvenomous) W59.19 ✓
      bite W59.11 ✓
      crushing W59.13 ✓
      strike W59.12 ✓
    spade W27.1 ✓
    spider (venomous) X58 ✓
    spin-drier W29.2 ✓
    spinning machine W31.89 ✓
    splinter W45.8 ✓
    sports equipment W21.9 ✓
    staple gun (powered) W29.8 ✓
    steam X13.1 ✓
      engine W31.3 ✓
      inhalation X13.0 ✓
      pipe X16 ✓
      shovel W31.89 ✓
    stove (hot) (kitchen) X15.0 ✓
    substance, hot NEC X19 ✓
      molten (metal) X18 ✓
    sword W26.1 ✓
      assault X99.2 ✓
      stated as undetermined whether accidental or intentional Y28.2 ✓
      suicide (attempt) X78.2 ✓
    tarantula X58 ✓
    thresher W30.0 ✓
    tin can lid W45.2 ✓
    toad W62.1 ✓
    toaster (hot) X15.1 ✓
    tool W27.8 ✓
      hand (not powered) W27.8 ✓
        auger W27.0 ✓

Contact — continued
  with — continued
    tool — continued
      hand — continued
        axe W27.0 ✓
        can opener W27.4 ✓
        chisel W27.0 ✓
        fork W27.4 ✓
        garden W27.1 ✓
        handsaw W27.0 ✓
        hoe W27.1 ✓
        ice-pick W27.4 ✓
        kitchen utensil W27.4 ✓
        manual
          lawn mower W27.1 ✓
          sewing machine W27.8 ✓
        meat grinder W27.4 ✓
        needle (sewing) W27.3 ✓
          hypodermic W46.0 ✓
            contaminated W46.1 ✓
        paper cutter W27.5 ✓
        pitchfork W27.1 ✓
        rake W27.1 ✓
        scissors W27.2 ✓
        screwdriver W27.0 ✓
        specified NEC W27.8 ✓
        workbench W27.0 ✓
      hot X17 ✓
      powered W29.8 ✓
        blender W29.0 ✓
          commercial W31.82 ✓
        can opener W29.0 ✓
          commercial W31.82 ✓
        chainsaw W29.3 ✓
        clothes dryer W29.2 ✓
          commercial W31.82 ✓
        dishwasher W29.2 ✓
          commercial W31.82 ✓
        edger W29.3 ✓
        electric fan W29.2 ✓
          commercial W31.82 ✓
        electric knife W29.1 ✓
        food processor W29.0 ✓
          commercial W31.82 ✓
        garbage disposal W29.0 ✓
          commercial W31.82 ✓
        garden tool W29.3 ✓
        hedge trimmer W29.3 ✓
        ice maker W29.0 ✓
          commercial W31.82 ✓
        kitchen appliance W29.0 ✓
          commercial W31.82 ✓
        lawn mower W28 ✓
        meat grinder W29.0 ✓
          commercial W31.82 ✓
        mixer W29.0 ✓
          commercial W31.82 ✓
        rototiller W29.3 ✓
        sewing machine W29.2 ✓
          commercial W31.82 ✓
        washing machine W29.2 ✓
          commercial W31.82 ✓
    transmission device (belt, cable, chain, gear, pinion, shaft) W24.1 ✓
      agricultural operations W30.89 ✓
    turbine (gas) (water-driven) W31.3 ✓
    turkey W61.49 ✓
      peck W61.43 ✓
      strike W61.42 ✓
    turtle (nonvenomous) W59.29 ✓
      bite W59.21 ✓
      strike W59.22 ✓
      terrestrial W59.89 ✓
        bite W59.81 ✓
        crushing W59.83 ✓
        strike W59.82 ✓
    under-cutter W31.0 ✓
    urine — see Contact, with, by type of animal
    vehicle
      agricultural use (transport) — see Accident, transport, agricultural vehicle
        not on public highway W30.81 ✓
      industrial use (transport) — see Accident, transport, industrial vehicle
        not on public highway W31.83 ✓

✓ Additional Character Required — Refer to the Tabular List for Character Selection   ▽ Subterms under main terms may continue to next column or page

Contact — *continued*
  with — *continued*
    vehicle — *continued*
      off-road use (transport) — *see* Accident, transport, all-terrain or off-road vehicle
        not on public highway W31.83 ☑
      special construction use (transport) — *see* Accident, transport, construction vehicle
        not on public highway W31.83 ☑
    venomous
      animal X58 ☑
      arthropods X58 ☑
      lizard X58 ☑
      marine animal NEC X58 ☑
      marine plant NEC X58 ☑
      millipedes (tropical) X58 ☑
      plant(s) X58 ☑
      snake X58 ☑
      spider X58 ☑
      viper X58 ☑
    washing-machine (powered) W29.2 ☑
    wasp X58 ☑
    weaving-machine W31.89 ☑
    winch W24.0 ☑
      agricultural operations W30.89 ☑
    wire NEC W24.0 ☑
      agricultural operations W30.89 ☑
    wood slivers W45.8 ☑
    yellow jacket X58 ☑
    zebra — *see* Contact, with, hoof stock NEC
Coup de soleil X32 ☑
Crash
  aircraft (in transit) (powered) V95.9 ☑
    balloon V96.01 ☑
    fixed wing NEC (private) V95.21 ☑
      commercial V95.31 ☑
    glider V96.21 ☑
      hang V96.11 ☑
      powered V95.11 ☑
    helicopter V95.01 ☑
    in war operations — *see* War operations, destruction of aircraft
    microlight V95.11 ☑
    nonpowered V96.9 ☑
      specified NEC V96.8 ☑
    powered NEC V95.8 ☑
    stated as
      homicide (attempt) Y08.81 ☑
      suicide (attempt) X83.0 ☑
    ultralight V95.11 ☑
  spacecraft V95.41 ☑
  transport vehicle NEC (*see also* Accident, transport) V89.9 ☑
    homicide (attempt) Y03.8 ☑
    motor NEC (traffic) V89.2 ☑
      homicide (attempt) Y03.8 ☑
      suicide (attempt) — *see* Suicide, collision
Cruelty (mental) (physical) (sexual) X58 ☑
Crushed (accidentally) X58 ☑
  between objects (moving) (stationary and moving) W23.0 ☑
    stationary W23.1 ☑
  by
    alligator W58.03 ☑
    avalanche NEC — *see* Landslide
    cave-in W20.0 ☑
      caused by cataclysmic earth surface movement — *see* Landslide
    crocodile W58.13 ☑
    crowd or human stampede W52 ☑
    falling
      aircraft V97.39 ☑
        in war operations — *see* War operations, destruction of aircraft
      earth, material W20.0 ☑
        caused by cataclysmic earth surface movement — *see* Landslide
      object NEC W20.8 ☑
    landslide NEC — *see* Landslide
    lizard (nonvenomous) W59.09 ☑
    machinery — *see* Contact, with, by type of machine
    reptile NEC W59.89 ☑
    snake (nonvenomous) W59.13 ☑
  in
    machinery — *see* Contact, with, by type of machine

Cut, cutting (any part of body) (accidental) (*see also* Contact, with, by object or machine)
  during medical or surgical treatment as misadventure — *see* Index to Diseases and Injuries, Complications
  homicide (attempt) — *see* Assault, cutting or piercing instrument
  inflicted by other person — *see* Assault, cutting or piercing instrument
  legal
    execution — *see* Legal, intervention
    intervention — *see* Legal, intervention, sharp object
  machine NEC (*see also* Contact, with, by type of machine) W31.9 ☑
  self-inflicted — *see* Suicide, cutting or piercing instrument
  suicide (attempt) — *see* Suicide, cutting or piercing instrument
Cyclone (any injury) X37.1 ☑

D

Decapitation (accidental circumstances) NEC X58 ☑
  homicide X99.9 ☑
  legal execution — *see* Legal, intervention
Dehydration from lack of water X58 ☑
Deprivation X58 ☑
Derailment (accidental)
  railway (rolling stock) (train) (vehicle) (without antecedent collision) V81.7 ☑
    with antecedent collision — *see* Accident, transport, railway vehicle occupant
  streetcar (without antecedent collision) V82.7 ☑
    with antecedent collision — *see* Accident, transport, streetcar occupant
Descent
  parachute (voluntary) (without accident to aircraft) V97.29 ☑
    due to accident to aircraft — *see* Accident, transport, aircraft
Desertion X58 ☑
Destitution X58 ☑
Disability, late effect or sequela of injury — *see* Sequelae
Discharge (accidental)
  airgun W34.010 ☑
    assault X95.01 ☑
    homicide (attempt) X95.01 ☑
    stated as undetermined whether accidental or intentional Y24.0 ☑
    suicide (attempt) X74.01 ☑
  BB gun — *see* Discharge, airgun
  firearm (accidental) W34.00 ☑
    assault X95.9 ☑
    handgun (pistol) (revolver) W32.0 ☑
      assault X93 ☑
      homicide (attempt) X93 ☑
      legal intervention — *see* Legal, intervention, firearm, handgun
      stated as undetermined whether accidental or intentional Y22 ☑
      suicide (attempt) X72 ☑
    homicide (attempt) X95.9 ☑
    hunting rifle W33.02 ☑
      assault X94.1 ☑
      homicide (attempt) X94.1 ☑
      legal intervention
        injuring
          bystander Y35.032 ☑
          law enforcement personnel Y35.031 ☑
          suspect Y35.033 ☑
      stated as undetermined whether accidental or intentional Y23.1 ☑
      suicide (attempt) X73.1 ☑
    larger W33.00 ☑
      assault X94.9 ☑
      homicide (attempt) X94.9 ☑
      hunting rifle — *see* Discharge, firearm, hunting rifle
      legal intervention — *see* Legal, intervention, firearm by type of firearm
      machine gun — *see* Discharge, firearm, machine gun
      shotgun — *see* Discharge, firearm, shotgun
      specified NEC W33.09 ☑

Discharge — *continued*
  firearm — *continued*
    larger — *continued*
      specified — *continued*
        assault X94.8 ☑
        homicide (attempt) X94.8 ☑
        legal intervention
          injuring
            bystander Y35.092 ☑
            law enforcement personnel Y35.091 ☑
            suspect Y35.093 ☑
        stated as undetermined whether accidental or intentional Y23.8 ☑
        suicide (attempt) X73.8 ☑
      stated as undetermined whether accidental or intentional Y23.9 ☑
      suicide (attempt) X73.9 ☑
      legal intervention
        injuring
          bystander Y35.002 ☑
          law enforcement personnel Y35.001 ☑
          suspect Y35.03 ☑
        using rubber bullet
          injuring
            bystander Y35.042 ☑
            law enforcement personnel Y35.041 ☑
            suspect Y35.043 ☑
    machine gun W33.03 ☑
      assault X94.2 ☑
      homicide (attempt) X94.2 ☑
      legal intervention — *see* Legal, intervention, firearm, machine gun
      stated as undetermined whether accidental or intentional Y23.3 ☑
      suicide (attempt) X73.2 ☑
    pellet gun — *see* Discharge, airgun
    shotgun W33.01 ☑
      assault X94.0 ☑
      homicide (attempt) X94.0 ☑
      legal intervention — *see* Legal, intervention, firearm, specified NEC
      stated as undetermined whether accidental or intentional Y23.0 ☑
      suicide (attempt) X73.0 ☑
    specified NEC W34.09 ☑
      assault X95.8 ☑
      homicide (attempt) X95.8 ☑
      legal intervention — *see* Legal, intervention, firearm, specified NEC
      stated as undetermined whether accidental or intentional Y24.8 ☑
      suicide (attempt) X74.8 ☑
    stated as undetermined whether accidental or intentional Y24.9 ☑
    suicide (attempt) X74.9 ☑
    Very pistol W34.09 ☑
      assault X95.8 ☑
      homicide (attempt) X95.8 ☑
      stated as undetermined whether accidental or intentional Y24.8 ☑
      suicide (attempt) X74.8 ☑
  firework(s) W39 ☑
    stated as undetermined whether accidental or intentional Y25 ☑
  gas-operated gun NEC W34.018 ☑
    airgun — *see* Discharge, airgun
    assault X95.09 ☑
    homicide (attempt) X95.09 ☑
    paintball gun — *see* Discharge, paintball gun
    stated as undetermined whether accidental or intentional Y24.8 ☑
    suicide (attempt) X74.09 ☑
  gun NEC (*see also* Discharge, firearm NEC)
    air — *see* Discharge, airgun
    BB — *see* Discharge, airgun
    for single hand use — *see* Discharge, firearm, handgun
    hand — *see* Discharge, firearm, handgun
    machine — *see* Discharge, firearm, machine gun
    other specified — *see* Discharge, firearm NEC
    paintball — *see* Discharge, paintball gun
    pellet — *see* Discharge, airgun
  handgun — *see* Discharge, firearm, handgun
  machine gun — *see* Discharge, firearm, machine gun
  paintball gun W34.011 ☑

Discharge — continued
    paintball gun — continued
        assault X95.02 ☑
        homicide (attempt) X95.02 ☑
        stated as undetermined whether accidental or in-
            tentional Y24.8 ☑
        suicide (attempt) X74.02 ☑
    pistol — see Discharge, firearm, handgun
        flare — see Discharge, firearm, Very pistol
    pellet — see Discharge, airgun
    Very — see Discharge, firearm, Very pistol
    revolver — see Discharge, firearm, handgun
    rifle (hunting) — see Discharge, firearm, hunting rifle
    shotgun — see Discharge, firearm, shotgun
    spring-operated gun NEC W34.018 ☑
        assault X95.09 ☑
        homicide (attempt) X95.09 ☑
        stated as undetermined whether accidental or in-
            tentional Y24.8 ☑
        suicide (attempt) X74.09 ☑
Disease
    Andes W94.11 ☑
    aviator's — see Air, pressure
    range W94.11 ☑
Diver's disease, palsy, paralysis, squeeze — see Air,
        pressure
Diving (into water) — see Accident, diving
Dog bite W54.0 ☑
Dragged by transport vehicle NEC (see also Accident,
        transport) V09.9 ☑
Drinking poison (accidental) — see Table of Drugs and
        Chemicals
Dropped (accidentally) **while being carried or support-
        ed by other person** W04 ☑
Drowning (accidental) W74 ☑
    assault X92.9 ☑
    due to
        accident (to)
            machinery — see Contact, with, by type of
                machine
            watercraft V90.89 ☑
                burning V90.29 ☑
                    powered V90.23 ☑
                        fishing boat V90.22 ☑
                        jetskis V90.23 ☑
                        merchant ship V90.20 ☑
                        passenger ship V90.21 ☑
                    unpowered V90.28 ☑
                        canoe V90.25 ☑
                        inflatable V90.26 ☑
                        kayak V90.25 ☑
                        sailboat V90.24 ☑
                        water skis V90.27 ☑
                crushed V90.39 ☑
                    powered V90.33 ☑
                        fishing boat V90.32 ☑
                        jetskis V90.33 ☑
                        merchant ship V90.30 ☑
                        passenger ship V90.31 ☑
                    unpowered V90.38 ☑
                        canoe V90.35 ☑
                        inflatable V90.36 ☑
                        kayak V90.35 ☑
                        sailboat V90.34 ☑
                        water skis V90.37 ☑
                overturning V90.09 ☑
                    powered V90.03 ☑
                        fishing boat V90.02 ☑
                        jetskis V90.03 ☑
                        merchant ship V90.00 ☑
                        passenger ship V90.01 ☑
                    unpowered V90.08 ☑
                        canoe V90.05 ☑
                        inflatable V90.06 ☑
                        kayak V90.05 ☑
                        sailboat V90.04 ☑
                sinking V90.19 ☑
                    powered V90.13 ☑
                        fishing boat V90.12 ☑
                        jetskis V90.13 ☑
                        merchant ship V90.10 ☑
                        passenger ship V90.11 ☑
                    unpowered V90.18 ☑
                        canoe V90.15 ☑
                        inflatable V90.16 ☑
                        kayak V90.15 ☑

Drowning — continued
    due to — continued
        accident — continued
            watercraft — continued
                sinking — continued
                    unpowered — continued
                        sailboat V90.14 ☑
                    specified type NEC V90.89 ☑
                    powered V90.83 ☑
                        fishing boat V90.82 ☑
                        jetskis V90.83 ☑
                        merchant ship V90.80 ☑
                        passenger ship V90.81 ☑
                    unpowered V90.88 ☑
                        canoe V90.85 ☑
                        inflatable V90.86 ☑
                        kayak V90.85 ☑
                        sailboat V90.84 ☑
                        water skis V90.87 ☑
    avalanche — see Landslide
    cataclysmic
        earth surface movement NEC — see Forces of
            nature, earth movement
        storm — see Forces of nature, cataclysmic
            storm
    cloudburst X37.8 ☑
    cyclone X37.1 ☑
    fall overboard (from) V92.09 ☑
        powered craft V92.03 ☑
            ferry boat V92.01 ☑
            fishing boat V92.02 ☑
            jetskis V92.03 ☑
            liner V92.01 ☑
            merchant ship V92.00 ☑
            passenger ship V92.01 ☑
        resulting from
            accident to watercraft — see Drowning, due
                to, accident to, watercraft
            being washed overboard (from) V92.29 ☑
                powered craft V92.23 ☑
                    ferry boat V92.21 ☑
                    fishing boat V92.22 ☑
                    jetskis V92.23 ☑
                    liner V92.21 ☑
                    merchant ship V92.20 ☑
                    passenger ship V92.21 ☑
                unpowered craft V92.28 ☑
                    canoe V92.25 ☑
                    inflatable V92.26 ☑
                    kayak V92.25 ☑
                    sailboat V92.24 ☑
                    surf-board V92.28 ☑
                    water skis V92.27 ☑
                    windsurfer V92.28 ☑
            motion of watercraft V92.19 ☑
                powered craft V92.13 ☑
                    ferry boat V92.11 ☑
                    fishing boat V92.12 ☑
                    jetskis V92.13 ☑
                    liner V92.11 ☑
                    merchant ship V92.10 ☑
                    passenger ship V92.11 ☑
                unpowered craft
                    canoe V92.15 ☑
                    inflatable V92.16 ☑
                    kayak V92.15 ☑
                    sailboat V92.14 ☑
        unpowered craft V92.08 ☑
            canoe V92.05 ☑
            inflatable V92.06 ☑
            kayak V92.05 ☑
            sailboat V92.04 ☑
            surf-board V92.08 ☑
            water skis V92.07 ☑
            windsurfer V92.08 ☑
    hurricane X37.0 ☑
    jumping into water from watercraft (involved in
        accident) (see also Drowning, due to, acci-
        dent to, watercraft)
        without accident to or on watercraft
            W16.711 ☑
    tidal wave NEC — see Forces of nature, tidal wave
    torrential rain X37.8 ☑

Drowning — continued
    following
        fall
            into
                bathtub W16.211 ☑
                bucket W16.221 ☑
                fountain — see Drowning, following, fall,
                    into, water, specified NEC
                quarry — see Drowning, following, fall, into,
                    water, specified NEC
                reservoir — see Drowning, following, fall,
                    into, water, specified NEC
                swimming-pool W16.011 ☑
                    stated as undetermined whether acciden-
                        tal or intentional Y21.3 ☑
                    striking
                        bottom W16.021 ☑
                        wall W16.031 ☑
                    suicide (attempt) X71.2 ☑
                water NOS W16.41 ☑
                    natural (lake) (open sea) (river) (stream)
                        (pond) W16.111 ☑
                        striking
                            bottom W16.121 ☑
                            side W16.131 ☑
                    specified NEC W16.311 ☑
                        striking
                            bottom W16.321 ☑
                            wall W16.331 ☑
        overboard NEC — see Drowning, due to, fall
            overboard
        jump or dive
            from boat W16.711 ☑
                striking bottom W16.721 ☑
            into
                fountain — see Drowning, following, jump
                    or dive, into, water, specified NEC
                quarry — see Drowning, following, jump or
                    dive, into, water, specified NEC
                reservoir — see Drowning, following, jump
                    or dive, into, water, specified NEC
                swimming-pool W16.511 ☑
                    striking
                        bottom W16.521 ☑
                        wall W16.531 ☑
                    suicide (attempt) X71.2 ☑
                water NOS W16.91 ☑
                    natural (lake) (open sea) (river) (stream)
                        (pond) W16.611 ☑
                    specified NEC W16.811 ☑
                        bottom W16.821 ☑
                        striking
                            bottom W16.821 ☑
                            wall W16.831 ☑
                        striking
                            bottom W16.821 ☑
                            wall W16.831 ☑
                        striking bottom W16.621 ☑
    homicide (attempt) X92.9 ☑
    in
        bathtub (accidental) W65 ☑
            assault X92.0 ☑
            following fall W16.211 ☑
                stated as undetermined whether accidental
                    or intentional Y21.1 ☑
            stated as undetermined whether accidental or
                intentional Y21.0 ☑
            suicide (attempt) X71.0 ☑
        lake — see Drowning, in, natural water
        natural water (lake) (open sea) (river) (stream)
            (pond) W69 ☑
            assault X92.3 ☑
            following
                dive or jump W16.611 ☑
                    striking bottom W16.621 ☑
                fall W16.111 ☑
                    striking
                        bottom W16.121 ☑
                        side W16.131 ☑
            stated as undetermined whether accidental or
                intentional Y21.4 ☑
            suicide (attempt) X71.3 ☑
        quarry — see Drowning, in, specified place NEC
        quenching tank — see Drowning, in, specified
            place NEC
        reservoir — see Drowning, in, specified place NEC

Drowning — *continued*
  in — *continued*
    river — *see* Drowning, in, natural water
    sea — *see* Drowning, in, natural water
    specified place NEC W73 ☑
      assault X92.8 ☑
      following
        dive or jump W16.811 ☑
          striking
            bottom W16.821 ☑
            wall W16.831 ☑
        fall W16.311 ☑
          striking
            bottom W16.321 ☑
            wall W16.331 ☑
      stated as undetermined whether accidental or
        intentional Y21.8 ☑
      suicide (attempt) X71.8 ☑
    stream — *see* Drowning, in, natural water
    swimming-pool W67 ☑
      assault X92.1 ☑
        following fall X92.2 ☑
      following
        dive or jump W16.511 ☑
          striking
            bottom W16.521 ☑
            wall W16.531 ☑
        fall W16.011 ☑
          striking
            bottom W16.021 ☑
            wall W16.031 ☑
      stated as undetermined whether accidental or
        intentional Y21.2 ☑
      following fall Y21.3 ☑
      suicide (attempt) X71.1 ☑
        following fall X71.2 ☑
    war operations — *see* War operations, restriction
      of airway
  resulting from accident to watercraft — *see* Drowning,
    due to, accident, watercraft
  self-inflicted X71.9 ☑
  stated as undetermined whether accidental or inten-
    tional Y21.9 ☑
  suicide (attempt) X71.9 ☑

E

Earth falling (on) W20.0 ☑
  caused by cataclysmic earth surface movement or
    eruption — *see* Landslide
Earth (surface) movement NEC — *see* Forces of nature,
  earth movement
Earthquake (any injury) X34 ☑
Effect(s) (adverse) **of**
  air pressure (any) — *see* Air, pressure
  cold, excessive (exposure to) — *see* Exposure, cold
  heat (excessive) — *see* Heat
  hot place (weather) B — *see* Heat
  insolation X30 ☑
  late — *see* Sequelae
  motion — *see* Motion
  nuclear explosion or weapon in war operations — *see*
    War operations, nuclear weapon
  radiation — *see* Radiation
  travel — *see* Travel
Electric shock (accidental) (by) (in) — *see* Exposure,
  electric current
Electrocution (accidental) — *see* Exposure, electric current
Endotracheal tube wrongly placed during anesthetic
  procedure
Entanglement
  in
    bed linen, causing suffocation T71 ☑
    wheel of pedal cycle V19.88 ☑
Entry of foreign body or material — *see* Foreign body
Environmental pollution related condition — *see*
  category Z57
Execution, legal (any method) — *see* Legal, intervention
Exhaustion
  cold — *see* Exposure, cold
  due to excessive exertion — *see* Overexertion
  heat — *see* Heat
Explosion (accidental) (of) (with secondary fire) W40.9 ☑
  acetylene W40.1 ☑
  aerosol can W36.1 ☑

Explosion — *continued*
  air tank (compressed) (in machinery) W36.2 ☑
  aircraft (in transit) (powered) NEC V95.9 ☑
    balloon V96.05 ☑
    fixed wing NEC (private) V95.25 ☑
      commercial V95.35 ☑
    glider V96.25 ☑
      hang V96.15 ☑
      powered V95.15 ☑
    helicopter V95.05 ☑
    in war operations — *see* War operations, destruc-
      tion of aircraft
    microlight V95.15 ☑
    nonpowered V96.9 ☑
      specified NEC V96.8 ☑
    powered NEC V95.8 ☑
    stated as
      homicide (attempt) Y03.8 ☑
      suicide (attempt) X83.0 ☑
    ultralight V95.15 ☑
  anesthetic gas in operating room W40.1 ☑
  antipersonnel bomb W40.8 ☑
    assault X96.0 ☑
    homicide (attempt) X96.0 ☑
    suicide (attempt) X75 ☑
  assault X96.9 ☑
  bicycle tire W37.0 ☑
  blasting (cap) (materials) W40.0 ☑
  boiler (machinery), not on transport vehicle W35 ☑
    on watercraft — *see* Explosion, in, watercraft
  butane W40.1 ☑
  caused by other person X96.9 ☑
  coal gas W40.1 ☑
  detonator W40.0 ☑
  dump (munitions) W40.8 ☑
  dynamite W40.0 ☑
    in
      assault X96.8 ☑
      homicide (attempt) X96.8 ☑
      legal intervention
        injuring
          bystander Y35.112 ☑
          law enforcement personnel Y35.111 ☑
          suspect Y35.113 ☑
      suicide (attempt) X75 ☑
  explosive (material) W40.9 ☑
    gas W40.1 ☑
    in blasting operation W40.0 ☑
    specified NEC W40.8 ☑
      in
        assault X96.8 ☑
        homicide (attempt) X96.8 ☑
        legal intervention
          injuring
            bystander Y35.192 ☑
            law enforcement personnel
              Y35.191 ☑
            suspect Y35.193 ☑
        suicide (attempt) X75 ☑
  factory (munitions) W40.8 ☑
  fertilizer bomb W40.8 ☑
    assault X96.3 ☑
    homicide (attempt) X96.3 ☑
    suicide (attempt) X75 ☑
  fire-damp W40.1 ☑
  firearm (parts) NEC W34.19 ☑
    airgun W34.110 ☑
    BB gun W34.110 ☑
    gas, air or spring-operated gun NEC W34.118 ☑
    hangun W32.1 ☑
    hunting rifle W33.12 ☑
    larger firearm W33.10 ☑
      specified NEC W33.19 ☑
    machine gun W33.13 ☑
    paintball gun W34.111 ☑
    pellet gun W34.110 ☑
    shotgun W33.11 ☑
    Very pistol [flare] W34.19 ☑
  fireworks W39 ☑
  gas (coal) (explosive) W40.1 ☑
    cylinder W36.9 ☑
      aerosol can W36.1 ☑
      air tank W36.2 ☑
      pressurized W36.3 ☑
      specified NEC W36.8 ☑

Explosion — *continued*
  gasoline (fumes) (tank) not in moving motor vehicle
    W40.1 ☑
    bomb W40.8 ☑
      assault X96.1 ☑
      homicide (attempt) X96.1 ☑
      suicide (attempt) X75 ☑
    in motor vehicle — *see* Accident, transport, by type
      of vehicle
  grain store W40.8 ☑
  grenade W40.8 ☑
    in
      assault X96.8 ☑
      homicide (attempt) X96.8 ☑
      legal intervention
        injuring
          bystander Y35.192 ☑
          law enforcement personnel Y35.191 ☑
          suspect Y35.193 ☑
      suicide (attempt) X75 ☑
  handgun (parts) — *see* Explosion, firearm, hangun
    (parts)
  homicide (attempt) X96.9 ☑
    antipersonnel bomb — *see* Explosion, antiperson-
      nel bomb
    fertilizer bomb — *see* Explosion, fertilizer bomb
    gasoline bomb — *see* Explosion, gasoline bomb
    letter bomb — *see* Explosion, letter bomb
    pipe bomb — *see* Explosion, pipe bomb
    specified NEC X96.8 ☑
  hose, pressurized W37.8 ☑
  hot water heater, tank (in machinery) W35 ☑
    on watercraft — *see* Explosion, in, watercraft
  in, on
    dump W40.8 ☑
    factory W40.8 ☑
    mine (of explosive gases) NEC W40.1 ☑
    watercraft W93.59 ☑
      powered craft V93.53 ☑
        ferry boat V93.51 ☑
        fishing boat V93.52 ☑
        jetskis V93.53 ☑
        liner V93.51 ☑
        merchant ship V93.50 ☑
        passenger ship V93.51 ☑
        sailboat V93.54 ☑
  letter bomb W40.8 ☑
    assault X96.2 ☑
    homicide (attempt) X96.2 ☑
    suicide (attempt) X75 ☑
  machinery (*see also* Contact, with, by type of machine)
    on board watercraft — *see* Explosion, in, watercraft
    pressure vessel — *see* Explosion, by type of vessel
  methane W40.1 ☑
  mine W40.1 ☑
  missile NEC W40.8 ☑
  mortar bomb W40.8 ☑
    in
      assault X96.8 ☑
      homicide (attempt) X96.8 ☑
      legal intervention
        injuring
          bystander Y35.192 ☑
          law enforcement personnel Y35.191 ☑
          suspect Y35.193 ☑
      suicide (attempt) X75 ☑
  munitions (dump) (factory) W40.8 ☑
  pipe, pressurized W37.8 ☑
    bomb W40.8 ☑
      assault X96.4 ☑
      homicide (attempt) X96.4 ☑
      suicide (attempt) X75 ☑
  pressure, pressurized
    cooker W38 ☑
    gas tank (in machinery) W36.3 ☑
    hose W37.8 ☑
    pipe W37.8 ☑
    specified device NEC W38 ☑
    tire W37.8 ☑
      bicycle W37.0 ☑
    vessel (in machinery) W38 ☑
  propane W40.1 ☑
  self-inflicted X75 ☑
  shell (artillery) NEC W40.8 ☑
    during war operations — *see* War operations, ex-
      plosion

Explosion — *continued*
  shell — *continued*
    in
      legal intervention
        injuring
          bystander Y35.122 ☑
          law enforcement personnel Y35.121 ☑
          suspect Y35.123 ☑
      war — *see* War operations, explosion
  spacecraft V95.45 ☑
  stated as undetermined whether accidental or intentional Y25 ☑
  steam or water lines (in machinery) W37.8 ☑
  stove W40.9 ☑
  suicide (attempt) X75 ☑
  tire, pressurized W37.8 ☑
    bicycle W37.0 ☑
  undetermined whether accidental or intentional Y25 ☑
  vehicle tire NEC W37.8 ☑
    bicycle W37.0 ☑
  war operations — *see* War operations, explosion
Exposure (to) X58 ☑
  air pressure change — *see* Air, pressure
  cold (accidental) (excessive) (extreme) (natural) (place) X31 ☑
    assault Y08.89 ☑
    due to
      man-made conditions W93.8 ☑
        dry ice (contact) W93.01 ☑
          inhalation W93.02 ☑
        liquid air (contact) (hydrogen) (nitrogen) W93.11 ☑
          inhalation W93.12 ☑
        refrigeration unit (deep freeze) W93.2 ☑
      suicide (attempt) X83.2 ☑
      weather (conditions) X31 ☑
    homicide (attempt) Y08.89 ☑
    self-inflicted X83.2 ☑
  due to abandonment or neglect X58 ☑
  electric current W86.8 ☑
    appliance (faulty) W86.8 ☑
      domestic W86.0 ☑
    caused by other person Y08.89 ☑
    conductor (faulty) W86.1 ☑
    control apparatus (faulty) W86.1 ☑
    electric power generating plant, distribution station W86.1 ☑
    electroshock gun — *see* Exposure, electric current, taser
    high-voltage cable W85 ☑
    homicide (attempt) Y08.89 ☑
    legal execution — *see* Legal, intervention, specified means NEC
    lightning — *see* subcategory T75.0 ☑
    live rail W86.8 ☑
    misadventure in medical or surgical procedure in electroshock therapy Y63.4
    motor (electric) (faulty) W86.8 ☑
      domestic W86.0 ☑
    self-inflicted X83.1 ☑
    specified NEC W86.8 ☑
      domestic W86.0 ☑
    stun gun — *see* Exposure, electric current, taser
    suicide (attempt) X83.1 ☑
    taser W86.8 ☑
      assault Y08.89 ☑
      legal intervention — *see* category Y35 ☑
      self-harm (intentional) X83.8 ☑
      undetermined intent Y33 ☑
    third rail W86.8 ☑
    transformer (faulty) W86.1 ☑
    transmission lines W85 ☑
  environmental tobacco smoke X58 ☑
  excessive
    cold — *see* Exposure, cold
    heat (natural) NEC X30 ☑
      man-made W92 ☑
  factor(s) NOS X58 ☑
    environmental NEC X58 ☑
      man-made NEC W99 ☑
      natural NEC — *see* Forces of nature
    specified NEC X58 ☑
  fire, flames (accidental) X08.8 ☑
    assault X97 ☑

Exposure — *continued*
  fire, flames — *continued*
    campfire — *see* Exposure, fire, controlled, not in building
    controlled (in)
      with ignition (of) clothing (*see also* Ignition, clothes) X06.2 ☑
        nightwear X05 ☑
      bonfire — *see* Exposure, fire, controlled, not in building
      brazier (in building or structure) (*see also* Exposure, fire, controlled, building)
        not in building or structure — *see* Exposure, fire, controlled, not in building
      building or structure X02.0 ☑
        with
          fall from building X02.3 ☑
          from building X02.5 ☑
          injury due to building collapse X02.2 ☑
          smoke inhalation X02.1 ☑
        hit by object from building X02.4 ☑
        specified mode of injury NEC X02.8 ☑
      fireplace, furnace or stove — *see* Exposure, fire, controlled, building
      not in building or structure X03.0 ☑
        with
          fall X03.3 ☑
          smoke inhalation X03.1 ☑
        hit by object X03.4 ☑
        specified mode of injury NEC X03.8 ☑
      trash — *see* Exposure, fire, controlled, not in building
    fireplace — *see* Exposure, fire, controlled, building
    fittings or furniture (in building or structure) (uncontrolled) — *see* Exposure, fire, uncontrolled, building
    forest (uncontrolled) — *see* Exposure, fire, uncontrolled, not in building
    grass (uncontrolled) — *see* Exposure, fire, uncontrolled, not in building
    hay (uncontrolled) — *see* Exposure, fire, uncontrolled, not in building
    homicide (attempt) X97 ☑
    ignition of highly flammable material X04 ☑
    in, of, on, starting in
      machinery — *see* Contact, with, by type of machine
      motor vehicle (in motion) (*see also* Accident, transport, occupant by type of vehicle) V87.8 ☑
        with collision — *see* Collision
      railway rolling stock, train, vehicle V81.81 ☑
        with collision — *see* Accident, transport, railway vehicle occupant
      street car (in motion) V82.8 ☑
        with collision — *see* Accident, transport, streetcar occupant
      transport vehicle NEC (*see also* Accident, transport)
        with collision — *see* Collision
      war operations (*see also* War operations, fire)
        from nuclear explosion — *see* War operations, nuclear weapons
      watercraft (in transit) (not in transit) V91.09 ☑
        localized — *see* Burn, on board watercraft, due to, fire on board
        powered craft V91.03 ☑
          ferry boat V91.01 ☑
          fishing boat V91.02 ☑
          jet skis V91.03 ☑
          liner V91.01 ☑
          merchant ship V91.00 ☑
          passenger ship V91.01 ☑
        unpowered craft V91.08 ☑
          canoe V91.05 ☑
          inflatable V91.06 ☑
          kayak V91.05 ☑
          sailboat V91.04 ☑
          surf-board V91.08 ☑
          waterskis V91.07 ☑
          windsurfer V91.08 ☑
    lumber (uncontrolled) — *see* Exposure, fire, uncontrolled, not in building
    mine (uncontrolled) — *see* Exposure, fire, uncontrolled, not in building

Exposure — *continued*
  fire, flames — *continued*
    prairie (uncontrolled) — *see* Exposure, fire, uncontrolled, not in building
    resulting from
      explosion — *see* Explosion
      lightning X08.8 ☑
    self-inflicted X76 ☑
    specified NEC X08.8 ☑
    started by other person X97 ☑
    stated as undetermined whether accidental or intentional Y26 ☑
    stove — *see* Exposure, fire, controlled, building
    suicide (attempt) X76 ☑
    tunnel (uncontrolled) — *see* Exposure, fire, uncontrolled, not in building
    uncontrolled
      in building or structure X00.0 ☑
        with
          fall from building X00.3 ☑
          injury due to building collapse X00.2 ☑
          jump from building X00.5 ☑
          smoke inhalation X00.1 ☑
        bed X08.00 ☑
          due to
            cigarette X08.01 ☑
            specified material NEC X08.09 ☑
        furniture NEC X08.20 ☑
          due to
            cigarette X08.21 ☑
            specified material NEC X08.29 ☑
        hit by object from building X00.4 ☑
        sofa X08.10 ☑
          due to
            cigarette X08.11 ☑
            specified material NEC X08.19 ☑
        specified mode of injury NEC X00.8 ☑
      not in building or structure (any) X01.0 ☑
        with
          fall X01.3 ☑
          smoke inhalation X01.1 ☑
        hit by object X01.4 ☑
        specified mode of injury NEC X01.8 ☑
    undetermined whether accidental or intentional Y26 ☑
  forces of nature NEC — *see* Forces of nature
  G-forces (abnormal) W49.9 ☑
  gravitational forces (abnormal) W49.9 ☑
  heat (natural) NEC — *see* Heat
  high-pressure jet (hydraulic) (pneumatic) W49.9 ☑
  hydraulic jet W49.9 ☑
  inanimate mechanical force W49.9 ☑
  jet, high-pressure (hydraulic) (pneumatic) W49.9 ☑
  lightning — *see* subcategory T75.0 ☑
    causing fire — *see* Exposure, fire
  mechanical forces NEC W49.9 ☑
    animate NEC W64 ☑
    inanimate NEC W49.9 ☑
  noise W42.9 ☑
    supersonic W42.0 ☑
  noxious substance — *see* Table of Drugs and Chemicals
  pneumatic jet W49.9 ☑
  prolonged in deep-freeze unit or refrigerator W93.2 ☑
  radiation — *see* Radiation
  smoke (*see also* Exposure, fire)
    tobacco, second hand Z77.22
  specified factors NEC X58 ☑
  sunlight X32 ☑
    man-made (sun lamp) W89.8 ☑
      tanning bed W89.1 ☑
  supersonic waves W42.0 ☑
  transmission line(s), electric W85 ☑
  vibration W49.9 ☑
  waves
    infrasound W49.9 ☑
    sound W42.9 ☑
    supersonic W42.0 ☑
  weather NEC — *see* Forces of nature
External cause status Y99.9
  child assisting in compensated work for family Y99.8
  civilian activity done for financial or other compensation Y99.0
  civilian activity done for income or pay Y99.0
  family member assisting in compensated work for other family member Y99.8

External cause status — *continued*
  hobby not done for income Y99.8
  leisure activity Y99.8
  military activity Y99.1
  off-duty activity of military personnel Y99.8
  recreation or sport not for income or while a student
    Y99.8
  specified NEC Y99.8
  student activity Y99.8
  volunteer activity Y99.2

F

Factors, supplemental
  alcohol
    blood level
      less than 20mg/100ml Y90.0
      20-39mg/100ml Y90.1
      40-59mg/100ml Y90.2
      60-79mg/100ml Y90.3
      80-99mg/100ml Y90.4
      100-119mg/100ml Y90.5
      120-199mg/100ml Y90.6
      200-239mg/100ml Y90.7
      240mg/100ml or more Y90.8
      presence in blood, level not specified Y90.9
    presence in blood, but level not specified Y90.9
  environmental-pollution-related condition- see Z57 ☑
  nosocomial condition Y95
  work-related condition Y99.0
Failure
  in suture or ligature during surgical procedure Y65.2
  mechanical, of instrument or apparatus (any) (during
    any medical or surgical procedure) Y65.8
  sterile precautions (during medical and surgical care)
    — *see* Misadventure, failure, sterile precautions,
    by type of procedure
  to
    introduce tube or instrument Y65.4
      endotracheal tube during anesthesia Y65.3
    make curve (transport vehicle) NEC — *see* Accident,
      transport
    remove tube or instrument Y65.4
Fall, falling (accidental) W19 ☑
  building W20.1 ☑
  burning (uncontrolled fire) X00.3 ☑
  down
    embankment W17.81 ☑
    escalator W10.0 ☑
    hill W17.81 ☑
    ladder W11 ☑
    ramp W10.2 ☑
    stairs, steps W10.9 ☑
  due to
    bumping against
      object W18.00 ☑
        sharp glass W18.02 ☑
        specified NEC W18.09 ☑
        sports equipment W18.01 ☑
      person W03 ☑
        due to ice or snow W00.0 ☑
        on pedestrian conveyance — *see* Accident,
          transport, pedestrian, conveyance
    collision with another person W03 ☑
      due to ice or snow W00.0 ☑
      involving pedestrian conveyance — *see* Acci-
        dent, transport, pedestrian, conveyance
    grocery cart tipping over W17.82 ☑
    ice or snow W00.9 ☑
      from one level to another W00.2 ☑
      on stairs or steps W00.1 ☑
      involving pedestrian conveyance — *see* Acci-
        dent, transport, pedestrian, conveyance
      on same level W00.0 ☑
    slipping (on moving sidewalk) W01.0 ☑
      with subsequent striking against object
        W01.10 ☑
        furniture W01.190 ☑
        sharp object W01.119 ☑
          glass W01.110 ☑
          power tool or machine W01.111 ☑
          specified NEC W01.118 ☑
        specified NEC W01.198 ☑
    striking against
      object W18.00 ☑
        sharp glass W18.02 ☑
        specified NEC W18.09 ☑

Fall, falling — *continued*
  due to — *continued*
    striking against — *continued*
      object — *continued*
        sports equipment W18.01 ☑
        person W03 ☑
          due to ice or snow W00.0 ☑
          on pedestrian conveyance — *see* Accident,
            transport, pedestrian, conveyance
  earth (with asphyxia or suffocation (by pressure)) —
    see Earth, falling
  from, off, out of
    aircraft NEC (with accident to aircraft NEC) V97.0 ☑
      while boarding or alighting V97.1 ☑
    balcony W13.0 ☑
    bed W06 ☑
    boat, ship, watercraft NEC (with drowning or sub-
      mersion) — *see* Drowning, due to, fall over-
      board
      with hitting bottom or object V94.0 ☑
    bridge W13.1 ☑
    building W13.9 ☑
      burning (uncontrolled fire) X00.3 ☑
    cavity W17.2 ☑
    chair W07 ☑
    cherry picker W17.89 ☑
    cliff W15 ☑
    dock W17.4 ☑
    embankment W17.81 ☑
    escalator W10.0 ☑
    flagpole W13.8 ☑
    furniture NEC W08 ☑
    grocery cart W17.82 ☑
    haystack W17.89 ☑
    high place NEC W17.89 ☑
      stated as undetermined whether accidental or
        intentional Y30 ☑
    hole W17.2 ☑
    incline W10.2 ☑
    ladder W11 ☑
    lifting device W17.89 ☑
    machine, machinery (*see also* Contact, with, by
      type of machine)
      not in operation W17.89 ☑
    manhole W17.1 ☑
    mobile elevated work platform [MEWP] W17.89 ☑
    motorized mobility scooter W05.2 ☑
    one level to another NEC W17.89 ☑
      intentional, purposeful, suicide (attempt)
        X80 ☑
      stated as undetermined whether accidental or
        intentional Y30 ☑
    pit W17.2 ☑
    playground equipment W09.8 ☑
      jungle gym W09.2 ☑
      slide W09.0 ☑
      swing W09.1 ☑
    quarry W17.89 ☑
    railing W13.9 ☑
    ramp W10.2 ☑
    roof W13.2 ☑
    scaffolding W12 ☑
    scooter (nonmotorized) W05.1 ☑
      motorized mobility W05.2 ☑
    sky lift W17.89 ☑
    stairs, steps W10.9 ☑
      curb W10.1 ☑
      due to ice or snow W00.1 ☑
      escalator W10.0 ☑
      incline W10.2 ☑
      ramp W10.2 ☑
      sidewalk curb W10.1 ☑
      specified NEC W10.8 ☑
    stepladder W11 ☑
    storm drain W17.1 ☑
    streetcar NEC V82.6 ☑
      with antecedent collision — *see* Accident,
        transport, streetcar occupant
      while boarding or alighting V82.4 ☑
    structure NEC W13.8 ☑
      burning (uncontrolled fire) X00.3 ☑
    table W08 ☑
    toilet W18.11 ☑
      with subsequent striking against object
        W18.12 ☑
    train NEC V81.6 ☑

Fall, falling — *continued*
  from, off, out of — *continued*
    train — *continued*
      during derailment (without antecedent colli-
        sion) V81.7 ☑
      with antecedent collision — *see* Accident,
        transport, railway vehicle occupant
      while boarding or alighting V81.4 ☑
    transport vehicle after collision — *see* Accident,
      transport, by type of vehicle, collision
    tree W14 ☑
    vehicle (in motion) NEC (*see also* Accident, trans-
      port) V89.9 ☑
      motor NEC (*see also* Accident, transport, occu-
        pant, by type of vehicle) V87.8 ☑
      stationary W17.89 ☑
        while boarding or alighting B — *see* Acci-
          dent, transport, by type of vehicle,
          while boarding or alighting
    viaduct W13.8 ☑
    wall W13.8 ☑
    watercraft (*see also* Drowning, due to, fall over-
      board)
      with hitting bottom or object V94.0 ☑
    well W17.0 ☑
    wheelchair, non-moving W05.0 ☑
      powered — *see* Accident, transport, pedestrian,
        conveyance occupant, specified type NEC
    window W13.4 ☑
  in, on
    aircraft NEC V97.0 ☑
      with accident to aircraft V97.0 ☑
      while boarding or alighting V97.1 ☑
    bathtub (empty) W18.2 ☑
      filled W16.212 ☑
        causing drowning W16.211 ☑
    escalator W10.0 ☑
    incline W10.2 ☑
    ladder W11 ☑
    machine, machinery — *see* Contact, with, by type
      of machine
    object, edged, pointed or sharp (with cut) — *see*
      Fall, by type
    playground equipment W09.8 ☑
      jungle gym W09.2 ☑
      slide W09.0 ☑
      swing W09.1 ☑
    ramp W10.2 ☑
    scaffolding W12 ☑
    shower W18.2 ☑
      causing drowning W16.211 ☑
    staircase, stairs, steps W10.9 ☑
      curb W10.1 ☑
      due to ice or snow W00.1 ☑
      escalator W10.0 ☑
      incline W10.2 ☑
      specified NEC W10.8 ☑
    streetcar (without antecedent collision) V82.5 ☑
      with antecedent collision — *see* Accident,
        transport, streetcar occupant
      while boarding or alighting V82.4 ☑
    train (without antecedent collision) V81.5 ☑
      with antecedent collision — *see* Accident,
        transport, railway vehicle occupant
      during derailment (without antecedent colli-
        sion) V81.7 ☑
      with antecedent collision — *see* Accident,
        transport, railway vehicle occupant
      while boarding or alighting V81.4 ☑
    transport vehicle after collision — *see* Accident,
      transport, by type of vehicle, collision
    watercraft V93.39 ☑
      due to
        accident to craft V91.29 ☑
          powered craft V91.23 ☑
            ferry boat V91.21 ☑
            fishing boat V91.22 ☑
            jetskis V91.23 ☑
            liner V91.21 ☑
            merchant ship V91.20 ☑
            passenger ship V91.21 ☑
          unpowered craft
            canoe V91.25 ☑
            inflatable V91.26 ☑
            kayak V91.25 ☑
            sailboat V91.24 ☑

Fall, falling — continued
  in, on — continued
    watercraft — continued
      powered craft V93.33 ☑
        ferry boat V93.31 ☑
        fishing boat V93.32 ☑
        jetskis V93.33 ☑
        liner V93.31 ☑
        merchant ship V93.30 ☑
        passenger ship V93.31 ☑
      unpowered craft V93.38 ☑
        canoe V93.35 ☑
        inflatable V93.36 ☑
        kayak V93.35 ☑
        sailboat V93.34 ☑
        surf-board V93.38 ☑
        windsurfer V93.38 ☑
  into
    cavity W17.2 ☑
    dock W17.4 ☑
    fire — see Exposure, fire, by type
    haystack W17.89 ☑
    hole W17.2 ☑
    lake — see Fall, into, water
    lake — see Fall, into, water
    manhole W17.1 ☑
    moving part of machinery — see Contact, with, by
        type of machine
    ocean — see Fall, into, water
    opening in surface NEC W17.89 ☑
    pit W17.2 ☑
    pond — see Fall, into, water
    quarry W17.89 ☑
    river — see Fall, into, water
    shaft W17.89 ☑
    storm drain W17.1 ☑
    stream — see Fall, into, water
    swimming pool (see also Fall, into, water, in,
        swimming pool)
      empty W17.3 ☑
    tank W17.89 ☑
    water W16.42 ☑
      causing drowning W16.41 ☑
      from watercraft — see Drowning, due to, fall
          overboard
      hitting diving board W21.4 ☑
      in
        bathtub W16.212 ☑
          causing drowning W16.211 ☑
        bucket W16.222 ☑
          causing drowning W16.221 ☑
        natural body of water W16.112 ☑
          causing drowning W16.111 ☑
          striking
            bottom W16.122 ☑
              causing drowning W16.121 ☑
              causing drowning W16.131 ☑
            side W16.132 ☑
        specified water NEC W16.312 ☑
          causing drowning W16.311 ☑
          striking
            bottom W16.322 ☑
              causing drowning W16.321 ☑
            wall W16.332 ☑
              causing drowning W16.331 ☑
        swimming pool W16.012 ☑
          causing drowning W16.011 ☑
          striking
            bottom W16.022 ☑
              causing drowning W16.031 ☑
            wall W16.032 ☑
              causing drowning W16.021 ☑
        utility bucket W16.222 ☑
          causing drowning W16.221 ☑
    well W17.0 ☑
  involving
    bed W06 ☑
    chair W07 ☑
    furniture NEC W08 ☑
    glass — see Fall, by type
    playground equipment W09.8 ☑
      jungle gym W09.2 ☑
      slide W09.0 ☑
      swing W09.1 ☑
    roller blades — see Accident, transport, pedestrian,
        conveyance

Fall, falling — continued
  involving — continued
    skateboard(s) — see Accident, transport, pedestri-
        an, conveyance
    skates (ice) (in line) (roller) — see Accident, trans-
        port, pedestrian, conveyance
    skis — see Accident, transport, pedestrian, con-
        veyance
    table W08 ☑
    wheelchair, non-moving W05.0 ☑
      powered — see Accident, transport, pedestrian,
          conveyance, specified type NEC
  object — see Struck by, object, falling
  off
    toilet W18.11 ☑
      with subsequent striking against object
          W18.12 ☑
  on same level W18.30 ☑
    due to
      specified NEC W18.39 ☑
      stepping on an object W18.31 ☑
  out of
    bed W06 ☑
    building NEC W13.8 ☑
    chair W07 ☑
    furniture NEC W08 ☑
    wheelchair, non-moving W05.0 ☑
      powered — see Accident, transport, pedestrian,
          conveyance, specified type NEC
    window W13.4 ☑
  over
    animal W01.0 ☑
    cliff W15 ☑
    embankment W17.81 ☑
    small object W01.0 ☑
  rock W20.8 ☑
  same level W18.30 ☑
    from
      being crushed, pushed, or stepped on by a
          crowd or human stampede W52 ☑
      collision, pushing, shoving, by or with other
          person W03 ☑
      slipping, stumbling, tripping W01.0 ☑
    involving ice or snow W00.0 ☑
      involving skates (ice) (roller), skateboard, skis
          — see Accident, transport, pedestrian,
          conveyance
  snowslide (avalanche) — see Landslide
  stone W20.8 ☑
  structure W20.1 ☑
    burning (uncontrolled fire) X00.3 ☑
  through
    bridge W13.1 ☑
    floor W13.3 ☑
    roof W13.2 ☑
    wall W13.8 ☑
    window W13.4 ☑
  timber W20.8 ☑
  tree (caused by lightning) W20.8 ☑
  while being carried or supported by other person(s)
      W04 ☑
Fallen on by
  animal (not being ridden) NEC W55.89 ☑
Felo-de-se — see Suicide
Fight (hand) (fists) (foot) — see Assault, fight
Fire (accidental) — see Exposure, fire
Firearm discharge — see Discharge, firearm
**Fireball effects from nuclear explosion in war oper-
    ations** — see War operations, nuclear weapons
Fireworks (explosion) W39 ☑
Flash burns from explosion — see Explosion
Flood (any injury) (caused by) X38 ☑
  collapse of man-made structure causing earth move-
      ment X36.0 ☑
  tidal wave — see Forces of nature, tidal wave
Food (any type) **in**
  air passages (with asphyxia, obstruction, or suffoca-
      tion) — see categories T17 and T18
  alimentary tract causing asphyxia (due to compression
      of trachea) — see categories T17 and T18
Forces of nature X39.8 ☑
  avalanche X36.1 ☑
    causing transport accident — see Accident, trans-
        port, by type of vehicle
  blizzard X37.2 ☑
  cataclysmic storm X37.9 ☑

Forces of nature — continued
  cataclysmic storm — continued
    with flood X38 ☑
    blizzard X37.2 ☑
    cloudburst X37.8 ☑
    cyclone X37.1 ☑
    dust storm X37.3 ☑
    hurricane X37.0 ☑
    specified storm NEC X37.8 ☑
    storm surge X37.0 ☑
    tornado X37.1 ☑
    twister X37.1 ☑
    typhoon X37.0 ☑
  cloudburst X37.8 ☑
  cold (natural) X31 ☑
  cyclone X37.1 ☑
  dam collapse causing earth movement X36.0 ☑
  dust storm X37.3 ☑
  earth movement X36.1 ☑
    caused by dam or structure collapse X36.0 ☑
    earthquake X34 ☑
  earthquake X34 ☑
  flood (caused by) X38 ☑
    dam collapse X36.0 ☑
    tidal wave B — see Forces of nature, tidal wave
  heat (natural) X30 ☑
  hurricane X37.0 ☑
  landslide X36.1 ☑
    causing transport accident — see Accident, trans-
        port, by type of vehicle
  lightning — see subcategory T75.0 ☑
    causing fire — see Exposure, fire
  mudslide X36.1 ☑
    causing transport accident — see Accident, trans-
        port, by type of vehicle
  radiation (natural) X39.08 ☑
    radon X39.01 ☑
  radon X39.01 ☑
  specified force NEC X39.8 ☑
  storm surge X37.0 ☑
  structure collapse causing earth movement X36.0 ☑
  sunlight X32 ☑
  tidal wave X37.41 ☑
    due to
      earthquake X37.41 ☑
      landslide X37.43 ☑
      storm X37.42 ☑
      volcanic eruption X37.41 ☑
  tornado X37.1 ☑
  tsunami X37.41 ☑
  twister X37.1 ☑
  typhoon X37.0 ☑
  volcanic eruption X35 ☑
Foreign body
  aspiration — see Index to Diseases and Injuries, For-
      eign body, respiratory tract
  entering through skin W45.8 ☑
    can lid W45.2 ☑
    nail W45.0 ☑
    paper W45.1 ☑
    specified NEC W45.8 ☑
    splinter W45.8 ☑
Forest fire (exposure to) — see Exposure, fire, uncon-
    trolled, not in building
Found injured X58 ☑
  from exposure (to) — see Exposure
  on
    highway, road(way), street V89.9 ☑
    railway right of way V81.9 ☑
Fracture (circumstances unknown or unspecified) X58 ☑
  due to specified cause NEC X58 ☑
Freezing — see Exposure, cold
Frostbite X31 ☑
  due to man-made conditions — see Exposure, cold,
      man-made
Frozen — see Exposure, cold

G

Gored by bull W55.22 ☑
Gunshot wound W34.00 ☑

H

Hailstones, injured by X39.8 ☑

☑ **Additional Character Required** — Refer to the Tabular List for Character Selection   ▽ Subterms under main terms may continue to next column or page

Hanged herself or himself — *see* Hanging, self-inflicted
Hanging (accidental) (*see also* category) T71 ☑
  legal execution — *see* Legal, intervention, specified
    means NEC
Heat (effects of) (excessive) X30 ☑
  due to
    man-made conditions W92 ☑
      on board watercraft V93.29 ☑
        fishing boat V93.22 ☑
        merchant ship V93.20 ☑
        passenger ship V93.21 ☑
        sailboat V93.24 ☑
        specified powered craft NEC V93.23 ☑
    weather (conditions) X30 ☑
  from
    electric heating apparatus causing burning X16 ☑
    nuclear explosion in war operations — *see* War
      operations, nuclear weapons
  inappropriate in local application or packing in medical
    or surgical procedure Y63.5
Hemorrhage
  delayed following medical or surgical treatment
    without mention of misadventure — *see* Index
    to Diseases and Injuries, Complication(s)
  during medical or surgical treatment as misadventure
    — *see* Index to Diseases and Injuries, Complica-
    tion(s)
High
  altitude (effects) — *see* Air, pressure, low
  level of radioactivity, effects — *see* Radiation
  pressure (effects) — *see* Air, pressure, high
  temperature, effects — *see* Heat
Hit, hitting (accidental) by — *see* Struck by
Hitting against — *see* Striking against
Homicide (attempt) (justifiable) — *see* Assault
Hot
  place, effects (*see also* Heat)
  weather, effects X30 ☑
House fire (uncontrolled) — *see* Exposure, fire, uncon-
  trolled, building
Humidity, causing problem X39.8 ☑
Hunger X58 ☑
Hurricane (any injury) X37.0 ☑
Hypobarism, hypobaropathy — *see* Air, pressure, low

Ictus
  caloris (*see also* Heat)
  solaris X30 ☑
Ignition (accidental) (*see also* Exposure, fire) X08.8 ☑
  anesthetic gas in operating room W40.1 ☑
  apparel X06.2 ☑
    from highly flammable material X04 ☑
    nightwear X05 ☑
  bed linen (sheets) (spreads) (pillows) (mattress) — *see*
    Exposure, fire, uncontrolled, building, bed
  benzine X04 ☑
  clothes, clothing NEC (from controlled fire) X06.2 ☑
    from
      highly flammable material X04 ☑
  ether X04 ☑
    in operating room W40.1 ☑
  explosive material — *see* Explosion
  gasoline X04 ☑
  jewelry (plastic) (any) X06.0 ☑
  kerosene X04 ☑
  material
    explosive — *see* Explosion
    highly flammable with secondary explosion X04 ☑
  nightwear X05 ☑
  paraffin X04 ☑
  petrol X04 ☑
Immersion (accidental) (*see also* Drowning)
  hand or foot due to cold (excessive) X31 ☑
Implantation of quills of porcupine W55.89 ☑
Inanition (from) (hunger) X58 ☑
  thirst X58 ☑
Inappropriate operation performed
  correct operation on wrong side or body part (wrong
    side) (wrong site) Y65.53
  operation intended for another patient done on wrong
    patient Y65.52
  wrong operation performed on correct patient Y65.51
Inattention after, at birth (homicidal intent) (infantici-
  dal intent) X58 ☑

Incident, adverse
  device
    anesthesiology Y70.8
      accessory Y70.2
      diagnostic Y70.0
      miscellaneous Y70.8
      monitoring Y70.0
      prosthetic Y70.2
      rehabilitative Y70.1
      surgical Y70.3
      therapeutic Y70.1
    cardiovascular Y71.8
      accessory Y71.2
      diagnostic Y71.0
      miscellaneous Y71.8
      monitoring Y71.0
      prosthetic Y71.2
      rehabilitative Y71.1
      surgical Y71.3
      therapeutic Y71.1
    gastroenterology Y73.8
      accessory Y73.2
      diagnostic Y73.0
      miscellaneous Y73.8
      monitoring Y73.0
      prosthetic Y73.2
      rehabilitative Y73.1
      surgical Y73.3
      therapeutic Y73.1
    general
      hospital Y74.8
        accessory Y74.2
        diagnostic Y74.0
        miscellaneous Y74.8
        monitoring Y74.0
        prosthetic Y74.2
        rehabilitative Y74.1
        surgical Y74.3
        therapeutic Y74.1
      surgical Y81.8
        accessory Y81.2
        diagnostic Y81.0
        miscellaneous Y81.8
        monitoring Y81.0
        prosthetic Y81.2
        rehabilitative Y81.1
        surgical Y81.3
        therapeutic Y81.1
    gynecological Y76.8
      accessory Y76.2
      diagnostic Y76.0
      miscellaneous Y76.8
      monitoring Y76.0
      prosthetic Y76.2
      rehabilitative Y76.1
      surgical Y76.3
      therapeutic Y76.1
    medical Y82.9
      specified type NEC Y82.8
    neurological Y75.8
      accessory Y75.2
      diagnostic Y75.0
      miscellaneous Y75.8
      monitoring Y75.0
      prosthetic Y75.2
      rehabilitative Y75.1
      surgical Y75.3
      therapeutic Y75.1
    obstetrical Y76.8
      accessory Y76.2
      diagnostic Y76.0
      miscellaneous Y76.8
      monitoring Y76.0
      prosthetic Y76.2
      rehabilitative Y76.1
      surgical Y76.3
      therapeutic Y76.1
    ophthalmic Y77.8
      accessory Y77.2
      diagnostic Y77.0
      miscellaneous Y77.8
      monitoring Y77.0
      prosthetic Y77.2
      rehabilitative Y77.1
      surgical Y77.3
      therapeutic Y77.1
    orthopedic Y79.8
      accessory Y79.2

Incident, adverse — *continued*
  device — *continued*
    orthopedic — *continued*
      diagnostic Y79.0
      miscellaneous Y79.8
      monitoring Y79.0
      prosthetic Y79.2
      rehabilitative Y79.1
      surgical Y79.3
      therapeutic Y79.1
    otorhinolaryngological Y72.8
      accessory Y72.2
      diagnostic Y72.0
      miscellaneous Y72.8
      monitoring Y72.0
      prosthetic Y72.2
      rehabilitative Y72.1
      surgical Y72.3
      therapeutic Y72.1
    personal use Y74.8
      accessory Y74.2
      diagnostic Y74.0
      miscellaneous Y74.8
      monitoring Y74.0
      prosthetic Y74.2
      rehabilitative Y74.1
      surgical Y74.3
      therapeutic Y74.1
    physical medicine Y80.8
      accessory Y80.2
      diagnostic Y80.0
      miscellaneous Y80.8
      monitoring Y80.0
      prosthetic Y80.2
      rehabilitative Y80.1
      surgical Y80.3
      therapeutic Y80.1
    plastic surgical Y81.8
      accessory Y81.2
      diagnostic Y81.0
      miscellaneous Y81.8
      monitoring Y81.0
      prosthetic Y81.2
      rehabilitative Y81.1
      surgical Y81.3
      therapeutic Y81.1
    radiological Y78.8
      accessory Y78.2
      diagnostic Y78.0
      miscellaneous Y78.8
      monitoring Y78.0
      prosthetic Y78.2
      rehabilitative Y78.1
      surgical Y78.3
      therapeutic Y78.1
    urology Y73.8
      accessory Y73.2
      diagnostic Y73.0
      miscellaneous Y73.8
      monitoring Y73.0
      prosthetic Y73.2
      rehabilitative Y73.1
      surgical Y73.3
      therapeutic Y73.1
Incineration (accidental) — *see* Exposure, fire
Infanticide — *see* Assault
Infrasound waves (causing injury) W49.9 ☑
Ingestion
  foreign body (causing injury) (with obstruction) — *see*
    Foreign body, alimentary canal
  poisonous
    plant(s) X58 ☑
    substance NEC — *see* Table of Drugs and Chemicals
Inhalation
  excessively cold substance, man-made — *see* Expo-
    sure, cold, man-made
  food (any type) (into respiratory tract) (with asphyxia,
    obstruction respiratory tract, suffocation) — *see*
    categories T17 and T18 ☑
  foreign body — *see* Foreign body, aspiration
  gastric contents (with asphyxia, obstruction respiratory
    passage, suffocation) T17.81- ☑
  hot air or gases X14.0 ☑
  liquid air, hydrogen, nitrogen W93.12 ☑
    suicide (attempt) X83.2 ☑
  steam X13.0 ☑
    assault X98.0 —

Inhalation — continued
  steam — continued
    stated as undetermined whether accidental or intentional Y27.0 ☑
    suicide (attempt) X77.0 ☑
  toxic gas — see Table of Drugs and Chemicals
  vomitus (with asphyxia, obstruction respiratory passage, suffocation) T17.81- ☑
Injury, injured (accidental(ly)) NOS X58 ☑
  by, caused by, from
    assault — see Assault
    law-enforcing agent, police, in course of legal intervention — see Legal intervention
    suicide (attempt) X83.8 ☑
  due to, in
    civil insurrection — see War operations
    fight (see also Assault, fight) Y04.0 ☑
    war operations — see War operations
  homicide (see also Assault) Y09
  inflicted (by)
    in course of arrest (attempted), suppression of disturbance, maintenance of order, by law-enforcing agents — see Legal intervention
    other person
      stated as
        accidental X58 ☑
        intentional, homicide (attempt) — see Assault
        undetermined whether accidental or intentional Y33 ☑
  purposely (inflicted) by other person(s) — see Assault
  self-inflicted X83.8 ☑
    stated as accidental X58 ☑
  specified cause NEC X58 ☑
  undetermined whether accidental or intentional Y33 ☑
Insolation, effects X30 ☑
Insufficient nourishment X58 ☑
Interruption of respiration (by)
  food (lodged in esophagus) — see categories T17 and T18 ☑
  vomitus (lodged in esophagus) T17.81- ☑
Intervention, legal — see Legal intervention
Intoxication
  drug — see Table of Drugs and Chemicals
  poison — see Table of Drugs and Chemicals

J

Jammed (accidentally)
  between objects (moving) (stationary and moving) W23.0 ☑
    stationary W23.1 ☑
Jumped, jumping
  before moving object NEC X81.8 ☑
    motor vehicle X81.0 ☑
    subway train X81.1 ☑
    train X81.1 ☑
    undetermined whether accidental or intentional Y31 ☑
  from
    boat (into water) voluntarily, without accident (to or on boat) W16.712 ☑
      with
        accident to or on boat — see Accident, watercraft
        drowning or submersion W16.711 ☑
          suicide (attempt) X71.3 ☑
        striking bottom W16.722 ☑
          causing drowning W16.721 ☑
    building (see also Jumped, from, high place) W13.9 ☑
      burning (uncontrolled fire) X00.5 ☑
    high place NEC W17.89 ☑
      suicide (attempt) X80 ☑
      undetermined whether accidental or intentional Y30 ☑
    structure (see also Jumped, from, high place) W13.9 ☑
      burning (uncontrolled fire) X00.5 ☑
  into water W16.92 ☑
    causing drowning W16.91 ☑
    from, off watercraft — see Jumped, from, boat
    in
      natural body W16.612 ☑
        causing drowning W16.611 ☑

Jumped, jumping — continued
  into water — continued
    in — continued
      natural body — continued
        striking bottom W16.622 ☑
          causing drowning W16.621 ☑
      specified place NEC W16.812 ☑
        causing drowning W16.811 ☑
        striking
          bottom W16.822 ☑
            causing drowning W16.821 ☑
          wall W16.832 ☑
            causing drowning W16.831 ☑
      swimming pool W16.512 ☑
        causing drowning W16.511 ☑
        striking
          bottom W16.522 ☑
            causing drowning W16.521 ☑
          wall W16.532 ☑
            causing drowning W16.531 ☑
    suicide (attempt) X71.3 ☑

K

Kicked by
  animal NEC W55.82 ☑
  person(s) (accidentally) W50.1 ☑
    with intent to injure or kill Y04.0 ☑
    as, or caused by, a crowd or human stampede (with fall) W52 ☑
    assault Y04.0 ☑
    homicide (attempt) Y04.0 ☑
    in
      fight Y04.0 ☑
      legal intervention
        injuring
          bystander Y35.812 ☑
          law enforcement personnel Y35.811 ☑
          suspect Y35.813 ☑
Kicking against
  object W22.8 ☑
    sports equipment W21.9 ☑
    stationary wW22.09
      sports equipment W21.89 ☑
  person — see Striking against, person
  sports equipment W21.9 ☑
Killed, killing (accidentally) NOS (see also Injury) X58 ☑
  in
    action — see War operations
    brawl, fight (hand) (fists) (foot) Y04.0 ☑
      by weapon (see also Assault)
        cutting, piercing — see Assault, cutting or piercing instrument
        firearm — see Discharge, firearm, by type, homicide
  self
    stated as
      accident NOS X58 ☑
      suicide — see Suicide
      undetermined whether accidental or intentional Y33 ☑
Knocked down (accidentally) (by) NOS X58 ☑
  animal (not being ridden) NEC (see also Struck by, by type of animal)
  crowd or human stampede W52 ☑
  person W51 ☑
    in brawl, fight Y04.0 ☑
  transport vehicle NEC (see also Accident, transport) V09.9 ☑

L

Laceration NEC — see Injury
Lack of
  care (helpless person) (infant) (newborn) X58 ☑
  food except as result of abandonment or neglect X58 ☑
    due to abandonment or neglect X58 ☑
  water except as result of transport accident X58 ☑
    due to transport accident B — see Accident, transport, by type
    helpless person, infant, newborn X58 ☑
Landslide (falling on transport vehicle) X36.1 ☑
  caused by collapse of man-made structure X36.0 ☑
Late effect — see Sequelae

Legal
  execution (any method) — see Legal, intervention
  intervention (by)
    baton — see Legal, intervention, blunt object, baton
    bayonet — see Legal, intervention, sharp object, bayonet
    blow — see Legal, intervention, manhandling
    blunt object
      baton
        injuring
          bystander Y35.312 ☑
          law enforcement personnel Y35.311 ☑
          suspect Y35.313 ☑
      injuring
        bystander Y35.302 ☑
        law enforcement personnel Y35.301 ☑
        suspect Y35.303 ☑
      specified NEC
        injuring
          bystander Y35.392 ☑
          law enforcement personnel Y35.391 ☑
          suspect Y35.393 ☑
      stave
        injuring
          bystander Y35.392 ☑
          law enforcement personnel Y35.391 ☑
          suspect Y35.393 ☑
    bomb — see Legal, intervention, explosive
    cutting or piercing instrument — see Legal, intervention, sharp object
    dynamite — see Legal, intervention, explosive, dynamite
    explosive(s)
      dynamite
        injuring
          bystander Y35.112 ☑
          law enforcement personnel Y35.111 ☑
          suspect Y35.113 ☑
      grenade
        injuring
          bystander Y35.192 ☑
          law enforcement personnel Y35.191 ☑
          suspect Y35.193 ☑
      injuring
        bystander Y35.102 ☑
        law enforcement personnel Y35.101 ☑
        suspect Y35.103 ☑
      mortar bomb
        injuring
          bystander Y35.192 ☑
          law enforcement personnel Y35.191 ☑
          suspect Y35.193 ☑
      shell
        injuring
          bystander Y35.122 ☑
          law enforcement personnel Y35.121 ☑
          suspect Y35.123 ☑
      specified NEC
        injuring
          bystander Y35.192 ☑
          law enforcement personnel Y35.191 ☑
          suspect Y35.193 ☑
    firearm(s) (discharge)
      handgun
        injuring
          bystander Y35.022 ☑
          law enforcement personnel Y35.021 ☑
          suspect Y35.023 ☑
      injuring
        bystander Y35.002 ☑
        law enforcement personnel Y35.001 ☑
        suspect Y35.003 ☑
      machine gun
        injuring
          bystander Y35.012 ☑
          law enforcement personnel Y35.011 ☑
          suspect Y35.013 ☑
      rifle pellet
        injuring
          bystander Y35.032 ☑
          law enforcement personnel Y35.031 ☑
          suspect Y35.033 ☑
      rubber bullet
        injuring
          bystander Y35.042 ☑
          law enforcement personnel Y35.041 ☑

☑ Additional Character Required — Refer to the Tabular List for Character Selection ☒ Subterms under main terms may continue to next column or page

Legal — *continued*
  intervention — *continued*
    firearm(s) — *continued*
      rubber bullet — *continued*
        injuring — *continued*
          suspect Y35.043 ☑
      shotgun — *see* Legal, intervention, firearm, specified NEC
      specified NEC
        injuring
          bystander Y35.092 ☑
          law enforcement personnel Y35.091 ☑
          suspect Y35.093 ☑
    gas (asphyxiation) (poisoning)
      injuring
        bystander Y35.202 ☑
        law enforcement personnel Y35.201 ☑
        suspect Y35.203 ☑
      specified NEC
        injuring
          bystander Y35.292 ☑
          law enforcement personnel Y35.291 ☑
          suspect Y35.293 ☑
      tear gas
        injuring
          bystander Y35.212 ☑
          law enforcement personnel Y35.211 ☑
          suspect Y35.213 ☑
    grenade — *see* Legal, intervention, explosive, grenade
    injuring
      bystander Y35.92 ☑
      law enforcement personnel Y35.91 ☑
      suspect Y35.93 ☑
    late effect (of) — *see with 7th character S Y35* ☑
    manhandling
      injuring
        bystander Y35.812 ☑
        law enforcement personnel Y35.811 ☑
        suspect Y35.813 ☑
    sequelae (of) — *see with 7th character S Y35* ☑
    sharp objects
      bayonet
        injuring
          bystander Y35.412 ☑
          law enforcement personnel Y35.411 ☑
          suspect Y35.413 ☑
      injuring
        bystander Y35.402 ☑
        law enforcement personnel Y35.401 ☑
        suspect Y35.403 ☑
      specified NEC
        injuring
          bystander Y35.492 ☑
          law enforcement personnel Y35.491 ☑
          suspect Y35.493 ☑
    specified means NEC
      injuring
        bystander Y35.892 ☑
        law enforcement personnel Y35.891 ☑
        suspect Y35.893 ☑
    stabbing — *see* Legal, intervention, sharp object
    stave — *see* Legal, intervention, blunt object, stave
    tear gas — *see* Legal, intervention, gas, tear gas
    truncheon — *see* Legal, intervention, blunt object, stave

Lightning (shock) (stroke) (struck by) — *see* subcategory T75.0 ☑
  causing fire — *see* Exposure, fire
Loss of control (transport vehicle) NEC — *see* Accident, transport
Lost at sea NOS — *see* Drowning, due to, fall overboard
Low
  pressure (effects) — *see* Air, pressure, low
  temperature (effects) — *see* Exposure, cold
Lying before train, vehicle or other moving object X81.8 ☑
  subway train X81.1 ☑
  train X81.1 ☑
  undetermined whether accidental or intentional Y31 ☑
Lynching — *see* Assault

M

Malfunction (mechanism or component) (of)
  firearm W34.10 ☑
    airgun W34.110 ☑
    BB gun W34.110 ☑
    gas, air or spring-operated gun NEC W34.118 ☑
    handgun W32.1 ☑
    hunting rifle W33.12 ☑
    larger firearm W33.10 ☑
      specified NEC W33.19 ☑
    machine gun W33.13 ☑
    paintball gun W34.111 ☑
    pellet gun W34.110 ☑
    shotgun W33.11 ☑
    specified NEC W34.19 ☑
    Very pistol [flare] W34.19 ☑
  handgun — *see* Malfunction, firearm, handgun
Maltreatment — *see* Perpetrator
Mangled (accidentally) NOS X58 ☑
Manhandling (in brawl, fight) Y04.0 ☑
  legal intervention — *see* Legal, intervention, manhandling
Manslaughter (nonaccidental) — *see* Assault
Mauled by animal NEC W55.89 ☑
Medical procedure, complication of (delayed or as an abnormal reaction without mention of misadventure) — *see* Complication of or following, by specified type of procedure
  due to or as a result of misadventure — *see* Misadventure
Melting (due to fire) (*see also* Exposure, fire)
  apparel NEC X06.3 ☑
  clothes, clothing NEC X06.3 ☑
    nightwear X05 ☑
  fittings or furniture (burning building) (uncontrolled fire) X00.8 ☑
  nightwear X05 ☑
  plastic jewelry X06.1 ☑
Mental cruelty X58 ☑
Military operations (injuries to military and civilians occuring during peacetime on military property and during routine military exercises and operations) (by) (from) (involving) Y37.90- ☑
  air blast Y37.20- ☑
  aircraft
    destruction — *see* Military operations, destruction of aircraft
  airway restriction — *see* Military operations, restriction of airways
  asphyxiation — *see* Military operations, restriction of airways
  biological weapons Y37.6X- ☑
  blast Y37.20- ☑
  blast fragments Y37.20- ☑
  blast wave Y37.20- ☑
  blast wind Y37.20- ☑
  bomb Y37.20- ☑
    dirty Y37.50- ☑
    gasoline Y37.31- ☑
    incendiary Y37.31- ☑
    petrol Y37.31- ☑
  bullet Y37.43- ☑
    incendiary Y37.32- ☑
    rubber Y37.41- ☑
  chemical weapons Y37.7X- ☑
  combat
    hand to hand (unarmed) combat Y37.44- ☑
    using blunt or piercing object Y37.45- ☑
  conflagration — *see* Military operations, fire
  conventional warfare NEC Y37.49- ☑
  depth-charge Y37.01- ☑
  destruction of aircraft Y37.10- ☑
    due to
      air to air missile Y37.11- ☑
      collision with other aircraft Y37.12- ☑
      detonation (accidental) of onboard munitions and explosives Y37.14- ☑
      enemy fire or explosives Y37.11- ☑
      explosive placed on aircraft Y37.11- ☑
      onboard fire Y37.13- ☑
      rocket propelled grenade [RPG] Y37.11- ☑
      small arms fire Y37.11- ☑
      surface to air missile Y37.11- ☑
    specified NEC Y37.19- ☑

Military operations — *continued*
  detonation (accidental) of
    onboard marine weapons Y37.05- ☑
    own munitions or munitions launch device Y37.24- ☑
  dirty bomb Y37.50- ☑
  explosion (of) Y37.20- ☑
    aerial bomb Y37.21- ☑
    bomb NOS (*see also* Military operations, bomb(s)) Y37.20- ☑
    fragments Y37.20- ☑
    grenade Y37.29- ☑
    guided missile Y37.22- ☑
    improvised explosive device [IED] (person-borne) (roadside) (vehicle-borne) Y37.23- ☑
    land mine Y37.29- ☑
    marine mine (at sea) (in harbor) Y37.02- ☑
    marine weapon Y37.00- ☑
      specified NEC Y37.09- ☑
    own munitions or munitions launch device (accidental) Y37.24- ☑
    sea-based artillery shell Y37.03- ☑
    specified NEC Y37.29- ☑
    torpedo Y37.04- ☑
  fire Y37.30- ☑
    specified NEC Y37.39- ☑
  firearms
    discharge Y37.43- ☑
    pellets Y37.42- ☑
  flamethrower Y37.33- ☑
  fragments (from) (of)
    improvised explosive device [IED] (person-borne) (roadside) (vehicle-borne) Y37.26- ☑
    munitions Y37.25- ☑
    specified NEC Y37.29- ☑
    weapons Y37.27- ☑
  friendly fire Y37.92- ☑
  hand to hand (unarmed) combat Y37.44- ☑
  hot substances — *see* Military operations, fire
  incendiary bullet Y37.32- ☑
  nuclear weapon (effects of) Y37.50- ☑
    acute radiation exposure Y37.54- ☑
    blast pressure Y37.51- ☑
    direct blast Y37.51- ☑
    direct heat Y37.53- ☑
    fallout exposure Y37.54- ☑
    fireball Y37.53- ☑
    indirect blast (struck or crushed by blast debris) (being thrown by blast) Y37.52- ☑
    ionizing radiation (immediate exposure) Y37.54- ☑
    nuclear radiation Y37.54- ☑
    radiation
      ionizing (immediate exposure) Y37.54- ☑
      nuclear Y37.54- ☑
      thermal Y37.53- ☑
    secondary effects Y37.54- ☑
    specified NEC Y37.59- ☑
    thermal radiation Y37.53- ☑
  restriction of air (airway)
    intentional Y37.46- ☑
    unintentional Y37.47- ☑
  rubber bullets Y37.41- ☑
  shrapnel NOS Y37.29- ☑
  suffocation — *see* Military operations, restriction of airways
  unconventional warfare NEC Y37.7X- ☑
  underwater blast NOS Y37.00- ☑
  warfare
    conventional NEC Y37.49- ☑
    unconventional NEC Y37.7X- ☑
  weapon of mass destruction [WMD] Y37.91- ☑
  weapons
    biological weapons Y37.6X- ☑
    chemical Y37.7X- ☑
    nuclear (effects of) Y37.50- ☑
      acute radiation exposure Y37.54- ☑
      blast pressure Y37.51- ☑
      direct blast Y37.51- ☑
      direct heat Y37.53- ☑
      fallout exposure Y37.54- ☑
      fireball Y37.53- ☑
      indirect blast (struck or crushed by blast debris) (being thrown by blast) Y37.52- ☑
      radiation
        ionizing (immediate exposure) Y37.54- ☑
        nuclear Y37.54- ☑

Military operations — continued
  weapons — continued
    nuclear — continued
      radiation — continued
        thermal Y37.53- ☑
      secondary effects Y37.54- ☑
      specified NEC Y37.59- ☑
    of mass destruction [WMD] Y37.91- ☑
Misadventure(s) **to patient**(s) **during surgical or medical care** Y69
  contaminated medical or biological substance (blood, drug, fluid) Y64.9
    administered (by) NEC Y64.9
      immunization Y64.1
      infusion Y64.0
      injection Y64.1
      specified means NEC Y64.8
      transfusion Y64.0
      vaccination Y64.1
  excessive amount of blood or other fluid during transfusion or infusion Y63.0
  failure
    in dosage Y63.9
      electroshock therapy Y63.4
      inappropriate temperature (too hot or too cold) in local application and packing Y63.5
      infusion
        excessive amount of fluid Y63.0
        incorrect dilution of fluid Y63.1
      insulin-shock therapy Y63.4
      nonadministration of necessary drug or biological substance Y63.6
      overdose — see Table of Drugs and Chemicals
      radiation, in therapy Y63.2
      radiation
        overdose Y63.2
      specified procedure NEC Y63.8
      transfusion
        excessive amount of blood Y63.0
    mechanical, of instrument or apparatus (any) (during any procedure) Y65.8
    sterile precautions (during procedure) Y62.9
      aspiration of fluid or tissue (by puncture or catheterization, except heart) Y62.6
      biopsy (except needle aspiration) Y62.8
        needle (aspirating) Y62.6
      blood sampling Y62.6
      catheterization Y62.6
        heart Y62.5
      dialysis (kidney) Y62.2
      endoscopic examination Y62.4
      enema Y62.8
      immunization Y62.3
      infusion Y62.1
      injection Y62.3
      needle biopsy Y62.6
      paracentesis (abdominal) (thoracic) Y62.6
      perfusion Y62.2
      puncture (lumbar) Y62.6
      removal of catheter or packing Y62.8
      specified procedure NEC Y62.8
      surgical operation Y62.0
      transfusion Y62.1
      vaccination Y62.3
    suture or ligature during surgical procedure Y65.2
    to introduce or to remove tube or instrument B — see Failure, to
  hemorrhage — see Index to Diseases and Injuries, Complication(s)
  inadvertent exposure of patient to radiation Y63.3
  inappropriate
    operation performed — see Inappropriate operation performed
    temperature (too hot or too cold) in local application or packing Y63.5
  infusion (see also Misadventure, by type, infusion) Y69
    excessive amount of fluid Y63.0
    incorrect dilution of fluid Y63.1
    wrong fluid Y65.1
  mismatched blood in transfusion Y65.0
  nonadministration of necessary drug or biological substance Y63.6
  overdose — see Table of Drugs and Chemicals
    radiation (in therapy) Y63.2
  perforation — see Index to Diseases and Injuries, Complication(s)
  performance of inappropriate operation — see Inappropriate operation performed

Misadventure(s) **to patient**(s) **during surgical or medical care** — continued
  puncture — see Index to Diseases and Injuries, Complication(s)
  specified type NEC Y65.8
    failure
      suture or ligature during surgical operation Y65.2
      to introduce or to remove tube or instrument B — see Failure, to
    infusion of wrong fluid Y65.1
    performance of inappropriate operation — see Inappropriate operation performed
    transfusion of mismatched blood Y65.0
    wrong
      fluid in infusion Y65.1
      placement of endotracheal tube during anesthetic procedure Y65.3
  transfusion — see Misadventure, by type, transfusion
    excessive amount of blood Y63.0
    mismatched blood Y65.0
  wrong
    drug given in error — see Table of Drugs and Chemicals
    fluid in infusion Y65.1
    placement of endotracheal tube during anesthetic procedure Y65.3
Mismatched blood in transfusion Y65.0
Motion sickness T75.3 ☑
Mountain sickness W94.11 ☑
Mudslide (of cataclysmic nature) — see Landslide
Murder (attempt) — see Assault

N

Nail, contact with W45.0 ☑
  gun W29.4 ☑
Neglect (criminal) (homicidal intent) X58 ☑
Noise (causing injury) (pollution) W42.9 ☑
  supersonic W42.0 ☑
Nonadministration (of)
  drug or biological substance (necessary) Y63.6
  surgical and medical care Y66
Nosocomial condition Y95

O

Object
  falling
    from, in, on, hitting
      machinery — see Contact, with, by type of machine
    set in motion by
      accidental explosion or rupture of pressure vessel W38 ☑
      firearm — see Discharge, firearm, by type
      machine(ry) — see Contact, with, by type of machine
Overdose (drug) — see Table of Drugs and Chemicals
  radiation Y63.2
Overexertion — see category Y93 ☑
Overexposure (accidental) (to)
  cold (see also Exposure, cold) X31 ☑
    due to man-made conditions — see Exposure, cold, man-made
  heat (see also Heat) X30 ☑
  radiation — see Radiation
  radioactivity W88.0 ☑
  sun (sunburn) X32 ☑
  weather NEC — see Forces of nature
  wind NEC — see Forces of nature
Overheated — see Heat
Overturning (accidental)
  machinery — see Contact, with, by type of machine
  transport vehicle NEC (see also Accident, transport) V89.9 ☑
  watercraft (causing drowning, submersion) (see also Drowning, due to, accident to, watercraft, overturning)
    causing injury except drowning or submersion B — see Accident, watercraft, causing, injury NEC

P

Parachute descent (voluntary) (without accident to aircraft) V97.29 ☑
  due to accident to aircraft — see Accident, transport, aircraft
Pecked by bird W61.99 ☑
Perforation during medical or surgical treatment as misadventure — see Index to Diseases and Injuries, Complication(s)
Perpetrator, perpetration, of assault, maltreatment and neglect (by) Y07.9
  boyfriend Y07.03
  brother Y07.410
    stepbrother Y07.435
  coach Y07.53
  cousin
    female Y07.491
    male Y07.490
  daycare provider Y07.519
    at-home
      adult care Y07.512
      childcare Y07.510
    care center
      adult care Y07.513
      childcare Y07.511
  family member NEC Y07.499
  father Y07.11
    adoptive Y07.13
    foster Y07.420
    stepfather Y07.430
  foster father Y07.420
  foster mother Y07.421
  girl friend Y07.04
  healthcare provider Y07.529
    mental health Y07.521
    specified NEC Y07.528
  husband Y07.01
  instructor Y07.53
  mother Y07.12
    adoptive Y07.14
    foster Y07.421
    stepmother Y07.433
  nonfamily member Y07.50
    specified NEC Y07.59
  nurse Y07.528
  occupational therapist Y07.528
  partner of parent
    female Y07.434
    male Y07.432
  physical therapist Y07.528
  sister Y07.411
  speech therapist Y07.528
  stepbrother Y07.435
  stepfather Y07.430
  stepmother Y07.433
  stepsister Y07.436
  teacher Y07.53
  wife Y07.02
Piercing — see Contact, with, by type of object or machine
Pinched
  between objects (moving) (stationary and moving) W23.0 ☑
    stationary W23.1 ☑
Pinned under machine(ry) — see Contact, with, by type of machine
Place of occurrence Y92.9
  abandoned house Y92.89
  airplane Y92.813
  airport Y92.520
  ambulatory health services establishment NEC Y92.538
  ambulatory surgery center Y92.530
  amusement park Y92.831
  apartment (co-op) — see Place of occurrence, residence, apartment
  assembly hall Y92.29
  bank Y92.510
  barn Y92.71
  baseball field Y92.320
  basketball court Y92.310
  beach Y92.832
  boarding house — see Place of occurrence, residence, boarding house
  boat Y92.814
  bowling alley Y92.39
  bridge Y92.89

Place of occurrence — *continued*
building under construction Y92.61
bus Y92.811
    station Y92.521
cafe Y92.511
campsite Y92.833
campus — *see* Place of occurrence, school
canal Y92.89
car Y92.810
casino Y92.59
children's home — *see* Place of occurrence, residence,
    institutional, orphanage
church Y92.22
cinema Y92.26
clubhouse Y92.29
coal pit Y92.64
college (community) Y92.214
condominium — *see* Place of occurrence, residence,
    apartment
construction area — *see* Place of occurrence, industrial
    and construction area
convalescent home — *see* Place of occurrence, resi-
    dence, institutional, nursing home
court-house Y92.240
cricket ground Y92.328
cultural building Y92.258
    art gallery Y92.250
    museum Y92.251
    music hall Y92.252
    opera house Y92.253
    specified NEC Y92.258
    theater Y92.254
dancehall Y92.252
day nursery Y92.210
dentist office Y92.531
derelict house Y92.89
desert Y92.820
dockyard Y92.62
dock NOS Y92.89
doctor's office Y92.531
dormitory — *see* Place of occurrence, residence, insti-
    tutional, school dormitory
dry dock Y92.62
factory (building) (premises) Y92.63
farm (land under cultivation) (outbuildings) Y92.79
    barn Y92.71
    chicken coop Y92.72
    field Y92.73
    hen house Y92.72
    house — *see* Place of occurrence, residence, house
    orchard Y92.74
    specified NEC Y92.79
football field Y92.321
forest Y92.821
freeway Y92.411
gallery Y92.250
garage (commercial) Y92.59
    boarding house Y92.044
    military base Y92.135
    mobile home Y92.025
    nursing home Y92.124
    orphanage Y92.114
    private house Y92.015
    reform school Y92.155
gas station Y92.524
gasworks Y92.69
golf course Y92.39
gravel pit Y92.64
grocery Y92.512
gymnasium Y92.39
handball court Y92.318
harbor Y92.89
harness racing course Y92.39
healthcare provider office Y92.531
highway (interstate) Y92.411
hill Y92.828
hockey rink Y92.330
home — *see* Place of occurrence, residence
hospice — *see* Place of occurrence, residence, institu-
    tional, nursing home
hospital Y92.239
    cafeteria Y92.233
    corridor Y92.232
    operating room Y92.234
    patient
        bathroom Y92.231
        room Y92.230
    specified NEC Y92.238

Place of occurrence — *continued*
hotel Y92.59
house (*see also* Place of occurrence, residence)
    abandoned Y92.89
    under construction Y92.61
industrial and construction area (yard) Y92.69
    building under construction Y92.61
    dock Y92.62
    dry dock Y92.62
    factory Y92.63
    gasworks Y92.69
    mine Y92.64
    oil rig Y92.65
    pit Y92.64
    power station Y92.69
    shipyard Y92.62
    specified NEC Y92.69
    tunnel under construction Y92.69
    workshop Y92.69
kindergarten Y92.211
lacrosse field Y92.328
lake Y92.828
library Y92.241
mall Y92.59
market Y92.512
marsh Y92.828
military
    base — *see* Place of occurrence, residence, institu-
        tional, military base
    training ground Y92.84
mine Y92.64
mosque Y92.22
motel Y92.59
motorway (interstate) Y92.411
mountain Y92.828
movie-house Y92.26
museum Y92.251
music-hall Y92.252
not applicable Y92.9
nuclear power station Y92.69
nursing home — *see* Place of occurrence, residence,
    institutional, nursing home
office building Y92.59
offshore installation Y92.65
oil rig Y92.65
old people's home — *see* Place of occurrence, resi-
    dence, institutional, specified NEC
opera-house Y92.253
orphanage — *see* Place of occurrence, residence, insti-
    tutional, orphanage
outpatient surgery center Y92.530
park (public) Y92.830
    amusement Y92.831
parking garage Y92.89
    lot Y92.481
pavement Y92.480
physician office Y92.531
polo field Y92.328
pond Y92.828
post office Y92.242
power station Y92.69
prairie Y92.828
prison — *see* Place of occurrence, residence, institu-
    tional, prison
public
    administration building Y92.248
        city hall Y92.243
        courthouse Y92.240
        library Y92.241
        post office Y92.242
        specified NEC Y92.248
    building NEC Y92.29
    hall Y92.29
    place NOS Y92.89
race course Y92.39
radio station Y92.59
railway line (bridge) Y92.85
ranch (outbuildings) — *see* Place of occurrence, farm
recreation area Y92.838
    amusement park Y92.831
    beach Y92.832
    campsite Y92.833
    park (public) Y92.830
    seashore Y92.832
    specified NEC Y92.838
reform school - — *see* Place of occurrence, residence,
    institutional, reform school
religious institution Y92.22

Place of occurrence — *continued*
residence (non-institutional) (private) Y92.009
    apartment Y92.039
        bathroom Y92.031
        bedroom Y92.032
        kitchen Y92.030
        specified NEC Y92.038
    bathroom Y92.002
    bedroom Y92.003
    boarding house Y92.049
        bathroom Y92.041
        bedroom Y92.042
        driveway Y92.043
        garage Y92.044
        garden Y92.046
        kitchen Y92.040
        specified NEC Y92.048
        swimming pool Y92.045
        yard Y92.046
    dining room Y92.001
    garden Y92.007
    home Y92.009
    house, single family Y92.019
        bathroom Y92.012
        bedroom Y92.013
        dining room Y92.011
        driveway Y92.014
        garage Y92.015
        garden Y92.017
        kitchen Y92.010
        specified NEC Y92.018
        swimming pool Y92.016
        yard Y92.017
    institutional Y92.10
        children's home — *see* Place of occurrence,
            residence, institutional, orphanage
        hospice — *see* Place of occurrence, residence,
            institutional, nursing home
        military base Y92.139
            barracks Y92.133
            garage Y92.135
            garden Y92.137
            kitchen Y92.130
            mess hall Y92.131
            specified NEC Y92.138
            swimming pool Y92.136
            yard Y92.137
        nursing home Y92.129
            bathroom Y92.121
            bedroom Y92.122
            driveway Y92.123
            garage Y92.124
            garden Y92.126
            kitchen Y92.120
            specified NEC Y92.128
            swimming pool Y92.125
            yard Y92.126
        orphanage Y92.119
            bathroom Y92.111
            bedroom Y92.112
            driveway Y92.113
            garage Y92.114
            garden Y92.116
            kitchen Y92.110
            specified NEC Y92.118
            swimming pool Y92.115
            yard Y92.116
        prison Y92.149
            bathroom Y92.142
            cell Y92.143
            courtyard Y92.147
            dining room Y92.141
            kitchen Y92.140
            specified NEC Y92.148
            swimming pool Y92.146
        reform school Y92.159
            bathroom Y92.152
            bedroom Y92.153
            dining room Y92.151
            driveway Y92.154
            garage Y92.155
            garden Y92.157
            kitchen Y92.150
            specified NEC Y92.158
            swimming pool Y92.156
            yard Y92.157
        school dormitory Y92.169
            bathroom Y92.162

Place of occurrence — *continued*
  residence — *continued*
    institutional — *continued*
      school dormitory — *continued*
        bedroom Y92.163
        dining room Y92.161
        kitchen Y92.160
        specified NEC Y92.168
      specified NEC Y92.199
        bathroom Y92.192
        bedroom Y92.193
        dining room Y92.191
        driveway Y92.194
        garage Y92.195
        garden Y92.197
        kitchen Y92.190
        specified NEC Y92.198
        swimming pool Y92.196
        yard Y92.197
    kitchen Y92.000
    mobile home Y92.029
      bathroom Y92.022
      bedroom Y92.023
      dining room Y92.021
      driveway Y92.024
      garage Y92.025
      garden Y92.027
      kitchen Y92.020
      specified NEC Y92.028
      swimming pool Y92.026
      yard Y92.027
    specified place in residence NEC Y92.009
    specified residence type NEC Y92.099
      bathroom Y92.091
      bedroom Y92.092
      driveway Y92.093
      garage Y92.094
      garden Y92.096
      kitchen Y92.090
      specified NEC Y92.098
      swimming pool Y92.095
      yard Y92.096
  restaurant Y92.511
  riding school Y92.39
  river Y92.828
  road Y92.488
  rodeo ring Y92.39
  rugby field Y92.328
  same day surgery center Y92.530
  sand pit Y92.64
  school (private) (public) (state) Y92.219
    college Y92.214
    daycare center Y92.210
    elementary school Y92.211
    high school Y92.213
    kindergarten Y92.211
    middle school Y92.212
    specified NEC Y92.218
    trace school Y92.215
    university Y92.214
    vocational school Y92.215
  sea (shore) Y92.832
  senior citizen center Y92.29
  service area
    airport Y92.520
    bus station Y92.521
    gas station Y92.524
    highway rest stop Y92.523
    railway station Y92.522
  shipyard Y92.62
  shop (commercial) Y92.513
  sidewalk Y92.480
  silo Y92.79
  skating rink (roller) Y92.331
    ice Y92.330
  slaughter house Y92.86
  soccer field Y92.322
  specified place NEC Y92.89
  sports area Y92.39
    athletic
      court Y92.318
        basketball Y92.310
        specified NEC Y92.318
        squash Y92.311
        tennis Y92.312
      field Y92.328
        baseball Y92.320
        cricket ground Y92.328

Place of occurrence — *continued*
  sports area — *continued*
    athletic — *continued*
      field — *continued*
        football Y92.321
        hockey Y92.328
        soccer Y92.322
        specified NEC Y92.328
    golf course Y92.39
    gymnasium Y92.39
    riding school Y92.39
    skating rink (roller) Y92.331
      ice Y92.330
    stadium Y92.39
    swimming pool Y92.34
  squash court Y92.311
  stadium Y92.39
  steeplechasing course Y92.39
  store Y92.512
  stream Y92.828
  street and highway Y92.410
    bike path Y92.482
    freeway Y92.411
    highway ramp Y92.415
    interstate highway Y92.411
    local residential or business street Y92.414
    motorway Y92.411
    parking lot Y92.481
    parkway Y92.412
    sidewalk Y92.480
    specified NEC Y92.488
    state road Y92.413
  subway car Y92.816
  supermarket Y92.512
  swamp Y92.828
  swimming pool (public) Y92.34
    private (at) Y92.095
      boarding house Y92.045
      military base Y92.136
      mobile home Y92.026
      nursing home Y92.125
      orphanage Y92.115
      prison Y92.146
      reform school Y92.156
      single family residence Y92.016
  synagogue Y92.22
  television station Y92.59
  tennis court Y92.312
  theater Y92.254
  trade area Y92.59
    bank Y92.510
    cafe Y92.511
    casino Y92.59
    garage Y92.59
    hotel Y92.59
    market Y92.512
    office building Y92.59
    radio station Y92.59
    restaurant Y92.511
    shop Y92.513
    shopping mall Y92.59
    store Y92.512
    supermarket Y92.512
    television station Y92.59
    warehouse Y92.59
  trailer park, residential — *see* Place of occurrence, residence, mobile home
  trailer site NOS Y92.89
  train Y92.815
    station Y92.522
  truck Y92.812
  tunnel under construction Y92.69
  university Y92.214
  urgent (health) care center Y92.532
  vehicle (transport) Y92.818
    airplane Y92.813
    boat Y92.814
    bus Y92.811
    car Y92.810
    specified NEC Y92.818
    subway car Y92.816
    train Y92.815
    truck Y92.812
  warehouse Y92.59
  water reservoir Y92.89
  wilderness area Y92.828
    desert Y92.820
    forest Y92.821

Place of occurrence — *continued*
  wilderness area — *continued*
    marsh Y92.828
    mountain Y92.828
    prairie Y92.828
    specified NEC Y92.828
    swamp Y92.828
  workshop Y92.69
  yard, private Y92.096
    boarding house Y92.046
    mobile home Y92.027
    single family house Y92.017
  youth center Y92.29
  zoo (zoological garden) Y92.834
Plumbism — *see* Table of Drugs and Chemicals, lead
Poisoning (accidental) (by) (*see also* Table of Drugs and Chemicals)
  by plant, thorns, spines, sharp leaves or other mechanisms NEC X58 ☑
  carbon monoxide
    generated by
      motor vehicle — *see* Accident, transport
      watercraft (in transit) (not in transit) V93.89 ☑
        ferry boat V93.81 ☑
        fishing boat V93.82 ☑
        jet skis V93.83 ☑
        liner V93.81 ☑
        merchant ship V93.80 ☑
        passenger ship V93.81 ☑
        powered craft NEC V93.83 ☑
  caused by injection of poisons into skin by plant thorns, spines, sharp leaves X58 ☑
    marine or sea plants (venomous) X58 ☑
  execution — *see* Legal, intervention, gas
  intervention
    by gas — *see* Legal, intervention, gas
    other specified means — *see* Legal, intervention, specified means NEC
  exhaust gas
    generated by
      motor vehicle — *see* Accident, transport
      watercraft (in transit) (not in transit) V93.89 ☑
        ferry boat V93.81 ☑
        fishing boat V93.82 ☑
        jet skis V93.83 ☑
        liner V93.81 ☑
        merchant ship V93.80 ☑
        passenger ship V93.81 ☑
        powered craft NEC V93.83 ☑
  fumes or smoke due to
    explosion (*see also* Explosion) W40.9 ☑
    fire — *see* Exposure, fire
    ignition — *see* Ignition
  gas
    in legal intervention — *see* Legal, intervention, gas
    legal execution — *see* Legal, intervention, gas
  in war operations — *see* War operations
  legal
Powder burn (by) (from)
  airgun W34.110 ☑
  BB gun W34.110 ☑
  firearm NEC W34.19 ☑
  gas, air or spring-operated gun NEC W34.118 ☑
  handgun W32.1 ☑
  hunting rifle W33.12 ☑
  larger firearm W33.10 ☑
    specified NEC W33.19 ☑
  machine gun W33.13 ☑
  paintball gun W34.111 ☑
  pellet gun W34.110 ☑
  shotgun W33.11 ☑
  Very pistol [flare] W34.19 ☑
Premature cessation (of) **surgical and medical care** Y66
Privation (food) (water) X58 ☑
Procedure (operation)
  correct, on wrong side or body part (wrong side) (wrong site) Y65.53
  intended for another patient done on wrong patient Y65.52
  performed on patient not scheduled for surgery Y65.52
  performed on wrong patient Y65.52
  wrong, performed on correct patient Y65.51
Prolonged
  sitting in transport vehicle — *see* Travel, by type of vehicle

☑ **Additional Character Required** — Refer to the Tabular List for Character Selection   ▽ Subterms under main terms may continue to next column or page

Prolonged — *continued*
  stay in
    high altitude as cause of anoxia, barodontalgia,
      barotitis or hypoxia W94.11 ☑
    weightless environment X52 ☑
Pulling, excessive — *see* Overexertion
Puncture, puncturing (*see also* Contact, with, by type
  of object or machine)
  by
    plant thorns, spines, sharp leaves or other mecha-
      nisms NEC W60 ☑
    during medical or surgical treatment as misadventure
      — *see* Index to Diseases and Injuries, Complica-
      tion(s)
Pushed, pushing (accidental) (injury in) (overexertion)
  (*see also* Overexertion)
  by other person(s) (accidental) W51 ☑
    with fall W03 ☑
      due to ice or snow W00.0 ☑
    as, or caused by, a crowd or human stampede (with
      fall) W52 ☑
    before moving object NEC Y02.8 ☑
      motor vehicle Y02.0 ☑
      subway train Y02.1 ☑
      train Y02.1 ☑
    from
      high place NEC
        in accidental circumstances W17.89 ☑
        stated as
          intentional, homicide (attempt) Y01 ☑
          undetermined whether accidental or
            intentional Y30 ☑
      transport vehicle NEC (*see also* Accident, trans-
        port) V89.9 ☑
        stated as
          intentional, homicide (attempt)
            Y08.89 ☑

R

Radiation (exposure to)
  arc lamps W89.0 ☑
  atomic power plant (malfunction) NEC W88.1 ☑
  complication of or abnormal reaction to medical radio-
    therapy Y84.2
  electromagnetic, ionizing W88.0 ☑
  gamma rays W88.1 ☑
  in
    war operations (from or following nuclear explo-
      sion) — *see* War operations
  inadvertent exposure of patient (receiving test or
    therapy) Y63.3
  infrared (heaters and lamps) W90.1 ☑
    excessive heat from W92 ☑
  ionized, ionizing (particles, artificially accelerated)
    radioisotopes W88.1 ☑
    specified NEC W88.8 ☑
    x-rays W88.0 ☑
  isotopes, radioactive — *see* Radiation, radioactive
    isotopes
  laser(s) W90.2 ☑
    in war operations — *see* War operations
    misadventure in medical care Y63.2
  light sources (man-made visible and ultraviolet)
    W89.9 ☑
    natural X32 ☑
    specified NEC W89.8 ☑
    tanning bed W89.1 ☑
    welding light W89.0 ☑
  man-made visible light W89.9 ☑
    specified NEC W89.8 ☑
    tanning bed W89.1 ☑
    welding light W89.0 ☑
  microwave W90.8 ☑
  misadventure in medical or surgical procedure Y63.2
  natural NEC X39.08 ☑
    radon X39.01 ☑
  overdose (in medical or surgical procedure) Y63.2
  radar W90.0 ☑
  radioactive isotopes (any) W88.1 ☑
    atomic power plant malfunction W88.1 ☑
    misadventure in medical or surgical treatment
      Y63.2
  radiofrequency W90.0 ☑
  radium NEC W88.1 ☑
  sun X32 ☑

Radiation — *continued*
  ultraviolet (light) (man-made) W89.9 ☑
    natural X32 ☑
    specified NEC W89.8 ☑
    tanning bed W89.1 ☑
    welding light W89.0 ☑
  welding arc, torch, or light W89.0 ☑
    excessive heat from W92 ☑
  x-rays (hard) (soft) W88.0 ☑
Range disease W94.11 ☑
Rape (attempted) T74.2-
Rat bite W53.11 ☑
Reaction, abnormal to medical procedure (*see also*
  Complication of or following, by type of procedure)
  Y84.9
  with misadventure — *see* Misadventure
  biologicals — *see* Table of Drugs and Chemicals
  drugs — *see* Table of Drugs and Chemicals
  vaccine — *see* Table of Drugs and Chemicals
Recoil
  airgun W34.110 ☑
  BB gun W34.110 ☑
  firearm NEC W34.19 ☑
  gas, air or spring-operated gun NEC W34.118 ☑
  handgun W32.1 ☑
  hunting rifle W33.12 ☑
  larger firearm W33.10 ☑
    specified NEC W33.19 ☑
  machine gun W33.13 ☑
  paintball gun W34.111 ☑
  pellet W34.110 ☑
  shotgun W33.11 ☑
  Very pistol [flare] W34.19 ☑
Reduction in
  atmospheric pressure — *see* Air, pressure, change
Rock falling on or hitting (accidentally) (person)
  W20.8 ☑
  in cave-in W20.0 ☑
Run over (accidentally) (by)
  animal (not being ridden) NEC W55.89 ☑
  machinery — *see* Contact, with, by specified type of
    machine
  transport vehicle NEC (*see also* Accident, transport)
    V09.9 ☑
    intentional homicide (attempt) Y03.0 ☑
    motor NEC V09.20 ☑
      intentional homicide (attempt) Y03.0 ☑
Running
  before moving object X81.8 ☑
  motor vehicle X81.0 ☑
Running off, away
  animal (being ridden) (*see also* Accident, transport)
    V80.918 ☑
    not being ridden W55.89 ☑
  animal-drawn vehicle NEC (*see also* Accident, trans-
    port) V80.928 ☑
  highway, road(way), street
    transport vehicle NEC (*see also* Accident, transport)
      V89.9 ☑
Rupture pressurized devices — *see* Explosion, by type
  of device

S

Saturnism — *see* Table of Drugs and Chemicals, lead
Scald, scalding (accidental) (by) (from) (in) X19 ☑
  air (hot) X14.1 ☑
  gases (hot) X14.1 ☑
  homicide (attempt) — *see* Assault, burning, hot object
  inflicted by other person
    stated as intentional, homicide (attempt) — *see*
      Assault, burning, hot object
  liquid (boiling) (hot) NEC X12 ☑
    stated as undetermined whether accidental or in-
      tentional Y27.2 ☑
    suicide (attempt) X77.2 ☑
  local application of externally applied substance in
    medical or surgical care Y63.5
  metal (molten) (liquid) (hot) NEC X18 ☑
  self-inflicted X77.9 ☑
  stated as undetermined whether accidental or inten-
    tional Y27.8 ☑
  steam X13.1 ☑
    assault X98.0 ☑
    stated as undetermined whether accidental or in-
      tentional Y27.0 ☑

Scald, scalding — *continued*
  steam — *continued*
    suicide (attempt) X77.0 ☑
  suicide (attempt) X77.9 ☑
  vapor (hot) X13.1 ☑
    assault X98.0 ☑
    stated as undetermined whether accidental or in-
      tentional Y27.0 ☑
    suicide (attempt) X77.0 ☑
Scratched by
  cat W55.03 ☑
  person(s) (accidentally) W50.4 ☑
    with intent to injure or kill Y04.0 ☑
    as, or caused by, a crowd or human stampede (with
      fall) W52 ☑
    assault Y04.0 ☑
    homicide (attempt) Y04.0 ☑
    in
      fight Y04.0 ☑
      legal intervention
        injuring
          bystander Y35.892 ☑
          law enforcement personnel Y35.891 ☑
          suspect Y35.893 ☑
Seasickness T75.3
Self-harm NEC (*see also* External cause by type, undetermined whether accidental or intentional)
  intentional — *see* Suicide
  poisoning NEC — *see* Table of Drugs and Chemicals,
    poisoning, accidental
Self-inflicted (injury) **NEC** (*see also* External cause by
  type, undetermined whether accidental or intentional)
  intentional — *see* Suicide
  poisoning NEC — *see* Table of Drugs and Chemicals,
    poisoning, accidental
Sequelae (of)
  accident NEC — *see* W00-X58 with 7th character S
  assault (homicidal) (any means) — *see* X92-Y08 with
    7th character S
  homicide, attempt (any means) — *see* X92-Y08 with
    7th character S
  injury undetermined whether accidentally or purposely
    inflicted — *see* Y21-Y33 with 7th character S
  intentional self-harm (classifiable to X71-X83) — *see*
    X71-X83 with 7th character S
  legal intervention — *see* with 7th character S Y35 ☑
  motor vehicle accident — *see* V00-V99 with 7th char-
    acter S
  suicide, attempt (any means) — *see* X71-X83 with 7th
    character S
  transport accident — *see* V00-V99 with 7th character
    S
  war operations — *see* War operations
Shock
  electric — *see* Exposure, electric current
  from electric appliance (any) (faulty) W86.8 ☑
    domestic W86.0 ☑
    suicide (attempt) X83.1 ☑
Shooting, shot (accidental(ly)) (*see also* Discharge,
  firearm, by type)
  herself or himself — *see* Discharge, firearm by type,
    self-inflicted
  homicide (attempt) — *see* Discharge, firearm by type,
    homicide
  in war operations — *see* War operations
  inflicted by other person — *see* Discharge, firearm by
    type, homicide
    accidental — *see* Discharge, firearm, by type of
      firearm
  legal
    execution — *see* Legal, intervention, firearm
    intervention — *see* Legal, intervention, firearm
  self-inflicted — *see* Discharge, firearm by type, suicide
    accidental — *see* Discharge, firearm, by type of
      firearm
  suicide (attempt) — *see* Discharge, firearm by type,
    suicide
Shoving (accidentally) **by other person** — *see* Pushed,
  by other person
Sickness
  alpine W94.11 ☑
  motion — *see* Motion
  mountain W94.11 ☑

Sinking (accidental)
  watercraft (causing drowning, submersion) (see also
    Drowning, due to, accident to, watercraft, sink-
    ing)
    causing injury except drowning or submersion B
      — see Accident, watercraft, causing, injury
      NEC
Siriasis X32 ☑
Slashed wrists — see Cut, self-inflicted
Slipping (accidental) (on same level) (with fall) W01.0 ☑
  without fall W18.40 ☑
    due to
      specified NEC W18.49 ☑
      stepping from one level to another W18.43 ☑
      stepping into hole or opening W18.42 ☑
      stepping on object W18.41 ☑
  on
    ice W00.0 ☑
      with skates — see Accident, transport, pedestri-
      an, conveyance
    mud W01.0 ☑
    oil W01.0 ☑
    snow W00.0 ☑
      with skis — see Accident, transport, pedestrian,
      conveyance
    surface (slippery) (wet) NEC W01.0 ☑
Sliver, wood, contact with W45.8 ☑
Smoldering (due to fire) — see Exposure, fire
Sodomy (attempted) **by force** T74.2 ☑
Sound waves (causing injury) W42.9 ☑
  supersonic W42.0 ☑
Splinter, contact with W45.8 ☑
Stab, stabbing B — see Cut
Starvation X58 ☑
Status of external cause Y99.9
  child assisting in compensated work for family Y99.8
  civilian activity done for financial or other compensa-
    tion Y99.0
  civilian activity done for income or pay Y99.0
  family member assisting in compensated work for
    other family member Y99.8
  hobby not done for income Y99.8
  leisure activity Y99.8
  military activity Y99.1
  off-duty activity of military personnel Y99.8
  recreation or sport not for income or while a student
    Y99.8
  specified NEC Y99.8
  student activity Y99.8
  volunteer activity Y99.2
Stepped on
  by
    animal (not being ridden) NEC W55.89 ☑
    crowd or human stampede W52 ☑
    person W50.0 ☑
Stepping on
  object W22.8 ☑
    with fall W18.31 ☑
    sports equipment W21.9 ☑
    stationary W22.09 ☑
      sports equipment W21.89 ☑
  person W51 ☑
    by crowd or human stampede W52 ☑
  sports equipment W21.9 ☑
Sting
  arthropod, nonvenomous W57 ☑
  insect, nonvenomous W57 ☑
Storm (cataclysmic) B — see Forces of nature, cataclysmic
  storm
Straining, excessive — see Overexertion
Strangling — see Strangulation
Strangulation (accidental) T71 ☑
Strenuous movements — see Repetitive movements
Striking against
  airbag (automobile) W22.10 ☑
    driver side W22.11 ☑
    front passenger side W22.12 ☑
    specified NEC W22.19 ☑
  bottom when
    diving or jumping into water (in) W16.822 ☑
      causing drowning W16.821 ☑
      from boat W16.722 ☑
        causing drowning W16.721 ☑
      natural body W16.622 ☑
        causing drowning W16.821 ☑
      swimming pool W16.522 ☑

Striking against — continued
  bottom when — continued
    diving or jumping into water — continued
      swimming pool — continued
        causing drowning W16.521 ☑
      falling into water (in) W16.322 ☑
        causing drowning W16.321 ☑
      fountain — see Striking against, bottom when,
        falling into water, specified NEC
      natural body W16.122 ☑
        causing drowning W16.121 ☑
      reservoir — see Striking against, bottom when,
        falling into water, specified NEC
      specified NEC W16.322 ☑
        causing drowning W16.321 ☑
      swimming pool W16.022 ☑
        causing drowning W16.021 ☑
  diving board (swimming-pool) W21.4 ☑
  object W22.8 ☑
    with
      drowning or submersion — see Drowning
    fall — see Fall, due to, bumping against, object
    caused by crowd or human stampede (with fall)
      W52 ☑
    furniture W22.03 ☑
    lamppost W22.02 ☑
    sports equipment W21.9 ☑
    stationary W22.09 ☑
      sports equipment W21.89 ☑
    wall W22.01 ☑
  person(s) W51 ☑
    with fall W03 ☑
      due to ice or snow W00.0 ☑
    as, or caused by, a crowd or human stampede (with
      fall) W52 ☑
    assault Y04.2 ☑
    homicide (attempt) Y04.2 ☑
  sports equipment W21.9 ☑
  wall (when) W22.01 ☑
    diving or jumping into water (in) W16.832 ☑
      causing drowning W16.831 ☑
      swimming pool W16.532 ☑
        causing drowning W16.531 ☑
      falling into water (in) W16.332 ☑
        causing drowning W16.331 ☑
      fountain — see Striking against, wall when,
        falling into water, specified NEC
      natural body W16.132 ☑
        causing drowning W16.131 ☑
      reservoir — see Striking against, wall when,
        falling into water, specified NEC
      specified NEC W16.332 ☑
        causing drowning W16.331 ☑
      swimming pool W16.032 ☑
        causing drowning W16.031 ☑
    swimming pool (when) W22.042 ☑
      causing drowning W22.041 ☑
      diving or jumping into water W16.532 ☑
        causing drowning W16.531 ☑
      falling into water W16.032 ☑
        causing drowning W16.031 ☑
Struck (accidentally) **by**
  airbag (automobile) W22.10 ☑
    driver side W22.11 ☑
    front passenger side W22.12 ☑
    specified NEC W22.19 ☑
  alligator W58.02 ☑
  animal (not being ridden) NEC W55.89 ☑
  avalanche — see Landslide
  ball (hit) (thrown) W21.00 ☑
    assault Y08.09 ☑
    baseball W21.03 ☑
    basketball W21.05 ☑
    football W21.01 ☑
    golf ball W21.04 ☑
    soccer W21.02 ☑
    softball W21.07 ☑
    specified NEC W21.09 ☑
    volleyball W21.06 ☑
  bat or racquet
    baseball bat W21.11 ☑
      assault Y08.02 ☑
    golf club W21.13 ☑
      assault Y08.09 ☑
    specified NEC W21.19 ☑
      assault Y08.09 ☑

Struck (accidentally) **by** — continued
  bat or racquet — continued
    tennis racquet W21.12 ☑
      assault Y08.09 ☑
  bullet (see also Discharge, firearm by type)
    in war operations — see War operations
  crocodile W58.12 ☑
  dog W54.1 ☑
  flare, Very pistol — see Discharge, firearm NEC
  hailstones X39.8 ☑
  hockey (ice)
    field
      puck W21.221 ☑
      stick W21.211 ☑
    puck W21.220 ☑
    stick W21.210 ☑
      assault Y08.01 ☑
  landslide — see Landslide
  law-enforcement agent (on duty) — see Legal, inter-
    vention, manhandling
    with blunt object — see Legal, intervention, blunt
      object
  lightning T75.0 ☑
    causing fire — see Exposure, fire
  machine — see Contact, with, by type of machine
  mammal NEC W55.89 ☑
    marine W56.32 ☑
  marine animal W56.82 ☑
  missile
    firearm — see Discharge, firearm by type
    in war operations — see War operations, missile
  object W22.8 ☑
    blunt W22.8 ☑
      assault Y00 ☑
      suicide (attempt) X79 ☑
      undetermined whether accidental or intention-
        al Y29 ☑
    falling W20.8 ☑
      from, in, on
        building W20.1 ☑
          burning (uncontrolled fire) X00.4 ☑
      cataclysmic
        earth surface movement NEC — see
          Landslide
        storm — see Forces of nature, cata-
          clysmic storm
      cave-in W20.0 ☑
      earthquake X34 ☑
      machine (in operation) — see Contact, with,
        by type of machine
      structure W20.1 ☑
        burning X00.4 ☑
      transport vehicle (in motion) — see Acci-
        dent, transport, by type of vehicle
      watercraft V93.49 ☑
        due to
          accident to craft V91.39 ☑
            powered craft V91.33 ☑
            ferry boat V91.31 ☑
            fishing boat V91.32 ☑
            jetskis V91.33 ☑
            liner V91.31 ☑
            merchant ship V91.30 ☑
            passenger ship V91.31 ☑
            unpowered craft V91.38 ☑
              canoe V91.35 ☑
              inflatable V91.36 ☑
              kayak V91.35 ☑
              sailboat V91.34 ☑
              surf-board V91.38 ☑
              windsurfer V91.38 ☑
          powered craft V93.43 ☑
            ferry boat V93.41 ☑
            fishing boat V93.42 ☑
            jetskis V93.43 ☑
            liner V93.41 ☑
            merchant ship V93.40 ☑
            passenger ship V93.41 ☑
            unpowered craft V93.48 ☑
              sailboat V93.44 ☑
              surf-board V93.48 ☑
              windsurfer V93.48 ☑
    moving NEC W20.8 ☑
    projected W20.8 ☑
      assault Y00 ☑
      in sports W21.9 ☑

Struck (accidentally) **by** — continued
　object — continued
　　projected — continued
　　　in sports — continued
　　　　assault Y08.09 ☑
　　　　ball W21.00 ☑
　　　　　baseball W21.03 ☑
　　　　　basketball W21.05 ☑
　　　　　football W21.01 ☑
　　　　　golf ball W21.04 ☑
　　　　　soccer W21.02 ☑
　　　　　softball W21.07 ☑
　　　　　specified NEC W21.09 ☑
　　　　　volleyball W21.06 ☑
　　　　bat or racquet
　　　　　baseball bat W21.11 ☑
　　　　　　assault Y08.02 ☑
　　　　　golf club W21.13 ☑
　　　　　　assault Y08.09 ☑
　　　　　specified NEC W21.19 ☑
　　　　　　assault Y08.09 ☑
　　　　　tennis racquet W21.12 ☑
　　　　　　assault Y08.09 ☑
　　　　hockey (ice)
　　　　　field
　　　　　　puck W21.221 ☑
　　　　　　stick W21.211 ☑
　　　　　puck W21.220 ☑
　　　　　stick W21.210 ☑
　　　　　　assault Y08.01 ☑
　　　　specified NEC W21.89 ☑
　　set in motion by explosion — see Explosion
　　thrown W20.8 ☑
　　　assault Y00 ☑
　　　in sports W21.9 ☑
　　　　assault Y08.09 ☑
　　　　ball W21.00 ☑
　　　　　baseball W21.03 ☑
　　　　　basketball W21.05 ☑
　　　　　football W21.01 ☑
　　　　　golf ball W21.04 ☑
　　　　　soccer W21.02 ☑
　　　　　soft ball W21.07 ☑
　　　　　specified NEC W21.09 ☑
　　　　　volleyball W21.06 ☑
　　　　bat or racquet
　　　　　baseball bat W21.11 ☑
　　　　　　assault Y08.02 ☑
　　　　　golf club W21.13 ☑
　　　　　　assault Y08.09 ☑
　　　　　specified NEC W21.19 ☑
　　　　　　assault Y08.09 ☑
　　　　　tennis racquet W21.12 ☑
　　　　　　assault Y08.09 ☑
　　　　hockey (ice)
　　　　　field
　　　　　　puck W21.221 ☑
　　　　　　stick W21.211 ☑
　　　　　puck W21.220 ☑
　　　　　stick W21.210 ☑
　　　　　　assault Y08.01 ☑
　　　　specified NEC W21.89 ☑
　other person(s) W50.0 ☑
　　with
　　　blunt object W22.8 ☑
　　　　intentional, homicide (attempt) Y00 ☑
　　　　sports equipment W21.9 ☑
　　　　undetermined whether accidental or intentional Y29 ☑
　　　fall W03 ☑
　　　　due to ice or snow W00.0 ☑
　　as, or caused by, a crowd or human stampede (with fall) W52 ☑
　　assault Y04.2 ☑
　　homicide (attempt) Y04.2 ☑
　　in legal intervention
　　　injuring
　　　　bystander Y35.812 ☑
　　　　law enforcement personnel Y35.811 ☑
　　　　suspect Y35.813 ☑
　　　sports equipment W21.9 ☑
　　police (on duty) — see Legal, intervention, manhandling
　　　with blunt object — see Legal, intervention, blunt object
　　sports equipment W21.9 ☑

Struck (accidentally) **by** — continued
　sports equipment — continued
　　assault Y08.09 ☑
　　ball W21.00 ☑
　　　baseball W21.03 ☑
　　　basketball W21.05 ☑
　　　football W21.01 ☑
　　　golf ball W21.04 ☑
　　　soccer W21.02 ☑
　　　soft ball W21.07 ☑
　　　specified NEC W21.09 ☑
　　　volleyball W21.06 ☑
　　bat or racquet
　　　baseball bat W21.11 ☑
　　　　assault Y08.02 ☑
　　　golf club W21.13 ☑
　　　　assault Y08.09 ☑
　　　specified NEC W21.19 ☑
　　　tennis racquet W21.12 ☑
　　　　assault Y08.09 ☑
　　cleats (shoe) W21.31 ☑
　　foot wear NEC W21.39 ☑
　　football helmet W21.81 ☑
　　hockey (ice)
　　　field
　　　　puck W21.221 ☑
　　　　stick W21.211 ☑
　　　puck W21.220 ☑
　　　stick W21.210 ☑
　　　　assault Y08.01 ☑
　　skate blades W21.32 ☑
　　specified NEC W21.89 ☑
　　　assault Y08.09 ☑
　thunderbolt — see subcategory T75.0 ☑
　　causing fire — see Exposure, fire
　transport vehicle NEC (see also Accident, transport) V09.9 ☑
　　intentional, homicide (attempt) Y03.0 ☑
　　motor NEC (see also Accident, transport) V09.20 ☑
　　　homicide Y03.0 ☑
　vehicle (transport) NEC — see Accident, transport, by type of vehicle
　　stationary (falling from jack, hydraulic lift, ramp) W20.8 ☑

Stumbling
　without fall W18.40 ☑
　　due to
　　　specified NEC W18.49 ☑
　　　stepping from one level to another W18.43 ☑
　　　stepping into hole or opening W18.42 ☑
　　　stepping on object W18.41 ☑
　　over
　　　animal NEC W01.0 ☑
　　　　with fall W18.09 ☑
　　　carpet, rug or (small) object W22.8 ☑
　　　　with fall W18.09 ☑
　　　person W51 ☑
　　　　with fall W03 ☑
　　　　　due to ice or snow W00.0 ☑
Submersion (accidental) — see Drowning
Suffocation (accidental) (by external means) (by pressure) (mechanical) (see also category) T71 ☑
　due to, by
　　avalanche — see Landslide
　　explosion — see Explosion
　　fire — see Exposure, fire
　　food, any type (aspiration) (ingestion) (inhalation) — see categories T17 and T18 ☑
　　ignition — see Ignition
　　landslide — see Landslide
　　machine(ry) — see Contact, with, by type of machine
　　vomitus (aspiration) (inhalation) T17.81- ☑
　in
　　burning building X00.8 ☑
Suicide, suicidal (attempted) (by) X83.8 ☑
　blunt object X79 ☑
　burning, burns X76 ☑
　　hot object X77.9 ☑
　　　fluid NEC X77.2 ☑
　　　household appliance X77.3 ☑
　　　specified NEC X77.8 ☑
　　　steam X77.0 ☑
　　　tap water X77.1 ☑
　　　vapors X77.0 ☑
　caustic substance — see Table of Drugs and Chemicals

Suicide, suicidal — continued
　cold, extreme X83.2 ☑
　collision of motor vehicle with
　　motor vehicle X82.0 ☑
　　specified NEC X82.8 ☑
　　train X82.1 ☑
　　tree X82.2 ☑
　crashing of aircraft X83.0 ☑
　cut (any part of body) X78.9 ☑
　cutting or piercing instrument X78.9 ☑
　　dagger X78.2 ☑
　　glass X78.0 ☑
　　knife X78.1 ☑
　　specified NEC X78.8 ☑
　　sword X78.2 ☑
　drowning (in) X71.9 ☑
　　bathtub X71.0 ☑
　　natural water X71.3 ☑
　　specified NEC X71.8 ☑
　　swimming pool X71.1 ☑
　　　following fall X71.2 ☑
　electrocution X83.1 ☑
　explosive(s) (material) X75 ☑
　fire, flames X76 ☑
　firearm X74.9 ☑
　　airgun X74.01 ☑
　　handgun X72 ☑
　　hunting rifle X73.1 ☑
　　larger X73.9 ☑
　　　specified NEC X73.8 ☑
　　machine gun X73.2 ☑
　　shotgun X73.0 ☑
　　specified NEC X74.8 ☑
　hanging X83.8 ☑
　hot object — see Suicide, burning, hot object
　jumping
　　before moving object X81.8 ☑
　　　motor vehicle X81.0 ☑
　　　subway train X81.1 ☑
　　　train X81.1 ☑
　　from high place X80 ☑
　late effect of attempt — see X71-X83 with 7th character S
　lying before moving object, train, vehicle X81.8 ☑
　poisoning — see Table of Drugs and Chemicals
　puncture (any part of body) — see Suicide, cutting or piercing instrument
　scald — see Suicide, burning, hot object
　sequelae of attempt — see X71-X83 with 7th character S
　sharp object (any) — see Suicide, cutting or piercing instrument
　shooting — see Suicide, firearm
　specified means NEC X83.8 ☑
　stab (any part of body) — see Suicide, cutting or piercing instrument
　steam, hot vapors X77.0 ☑
　strangulation X83.8 ☑
　submersion — see Suicide, drowning
　suffocation X83.8 ☑
　wound NEC X83.8 ☑
Sunstroke X32 ☑
Supersonic waves (causing injury) W42.0 ☑
Surgical procedure, complication of (delayed or as an abnormal reaction without mention of misadventure) (see also Complication of or following, by type of procedure)
　due to or as a result of misadventure — see Misadventure
Swallowed, swallowing
　foreign body — see Foreign body, alimentary canal
　poison — see Table of Drugs and Chemicals
　substance
　　caustic or corrosive — see Table of Drugs and Chemicals
　　poisonous — see Table of Drugs and Chemicals

T

Tackle in sport W03 ☑
Terrorism (involving) Y38.80 ☑
　biological weapons Y38.6X- ☑
　chemical weapons Y38.7X- ☑
　conflagration Y38.3X- ☑
　explosion Y38.2X- ☑
　　destruction of aircraft Y38.1X- ☑

Terrorism — *continued*
　explosion — *continued*
　　marine weapons Y38.0X- ☑
　　fire Y38.3X- ☑
　　firearms Y38.4X- ☑
　　hot substances Y38.5X- ☑
　　nuclear weapons Y38.5X- ☑
　　specified method NEC Y38.89- ☑
Thirst X58 ☑
Threat to breathing
　aspiration — *see* Aspiration
　due to cave-in, falling earth or substance NEC T71 ☑
Thrown (accidentally)
　against part (any) of or object in transport vehicle (in motion) NEC (*see also* Accident, transport)
　from
　　high place, homicide (attempt) Y01 ☑
　　machinery — *see* Contact, with, by type of machine
　　transport vehicle NEC (*see also* Accident, transport) V89.9 ☑
　off — *see* Thrown, from
Thunderbolt — *see* subcategory T75.0 ☑
　causing fire — *see* Exposure, fire
Tidal wave (any injury) NEC — *see* Forces of nature, tidal wave
Took
　overdose (drug) — *see* Table of Drugs and Chemicals
　poison — *see* Table of Drugs and Chemicals
Tornado (any injury) X37.1 ☑
Torrential rain (any injury) X37.8 ☑
Torture X58 ☑
Trampled by animal NEC W55.89 ☑
Trapped (accidentally)
　between objects (moving) (stationary and moving) — *see* Caught
　by part (any) of
　　motorcycle V29.88 ☑
　　pedal cycle V19.88 ☑
　　transport vehicle NEC (*see also* Accident, transport) V89.9 ☑
Travel (effects) (sickness) T75.3 ☑
Tree falling on or hitting (accidentally) (person) W20.8 ☑
Tripping
　without fall W18.40 ☑
　　due to
　　　specified NEC W18.49 ☑
　　　stepping from one level to another W18.43 ☑
　　　stepping into hole or opening W18.42 ☑
　　　stepping on object W18.41 ☑
　　over
　　　animal W01.0 ☑
　　　　with fall W01.0 ☑
　　　carpet, rug or (small) object W22.8 ☑
　　　　with fall W18.09 ☑
　　　person W51 ☑
　　　　with fall W03 ☑
　　　　　due to ice or snow W00.0 ☑
Twisted by person(s) (accidentally) W50.2 ☑
　with intent to injure or kill Y04.0 ☑
　as, or caused by, a crowd or human stampede (with fall) W52 ☑
　assault Y04.0 ☑
　homicide (attempt) Y04.0 ☑
　in
　　fight Y04.0 ☑
　　legal intervention — *see* Legal, intervention, manhandling
Twisting, excessive — *see* Overexertion

U

Underdosing of necessary drugs, medicaments or biological substances Y63.6
Undetermined intent (contact) (exposure)
　automobile collision Y32 ☑
　blunt object Y29 ☑
　drowning (submersion) (in) Y21.9 ☑
　　bathtub Y21.0 ☑
　　　after fall Y21.1 ☑
　　natural water (lake) (ocean) (pond) (river) (stream) Y21.4 ☑
　　specified place NEC Y21.8 ☑
　　swimming pool Y21.2 ☑
　　　after fall Y21.3 ☑
　explosive material Y25 ☑

Undetermined intent — *continued*
　fall, jump or push from high place Y30 ☑
　falling, lying or running before moving object Y31 ☑
　fire Y26 ☑
　firearm discharge Y24.9 ☑
　　airgun (BB) (pellet) Y24.0 ☑
　　handgun (pistol) (revolver) Y22 ☑
　　hunting rifle Y23.1 ☑
　　larger Y23.9 ☑
　　　hunting rifle Y23.1 ☑
　　　machine gun Y23.3 ☑
　　　military Y23.2 ☑
　　　shotgun Y23.0 ☑
　　　specified type NEC Y23.8 ☑
　　machine gun Y23.3 ☑
　　military Y23.2 ☑
　　shotgun Y23.0 ☑
　　specified type NEC Y24.8 ☑
　　Very pistol Y24.8 ☑
　hot object Y27.9 ☑
　　fluid NEC Y27.2 ☑
　　household appliance Y27.3 ☑
　　specified object NEC Y27.8 ☑
　　steam Y27.0 ☑
　　tap water Y27.1 ☑
　　vapor Y27.0 ☑
　jump, fall or push from high place Y30 ☑
　lying, falling or running before moving object Y31 ☑
　motor vehicle crash Y32 ☑
　push, fall or jump from high place Y30 ☑
　running, falling or lying before moving object Y31 ☑
　sharp object Y28.9 ☑
　　dagger Y28.2 ☑
　　glass Y28.0 ☑
　　knife Y28.1 ☑
　　specified object NEC Y28.8 ☑
　　sword Y28.2 ☑
　smoke Y26 ☑
　specified event NEC Y33 ☑

V

Vibration (causing injury) W49.9 ☑
Victim (of)
　avalanche — *see* Landslide
　earth movements NEC — *see* Forces of nature, earth movement
　earthquake X34 ☑
　flood — *see* Flood
　landslide — *see* Landslide
　lightning — *see* subcategory T75.0 ☑
　　causing fire — *see* Exposure, fire
　storm (cataclysmic) NEC — *see* Forces of nature, cataclysmic storm
　volcanic eruption X35 ☑
Volcanic eruption (any injury) X35 ☑
Vomitus, gastric contents in air passages (with asphyxia, obstruction or suffocation) T17.81- ☑

W

Walked into stationary object (any) W22.09 ☑
　furniture W22.03 ☑
　lamppost W22.02 ☑
　wall W22.01 ☑
War operations (injuries to military personnel and civilians during war, civil insurrection and peacekeeping missions) (by) (from) (involving) Y36.90 ☑
　after cessation of hostilities Y36.89- ☑
　　explosion (of)
　　　bomb placed during war operations Y36.82- ☑
　　　mine placed during war operations Y36.81- ☑
　　　specified NEC Y36.88- ☑
　air blast Y36.20- ☑
　aircraft
　　destruction — *see* War operations, destruction of aircraft
　　airway restriction — *see* War operations, restriction of airways
　　asphyxiation — *see* War operations, restriction of airways
　biological weapons Y36.6X- ☑
　blast Y36.20- ☑
　blast fragments Y36.20- ☑
　blast wave Y36.20- ☑

War operations — *continued*
　blast wind Y36.20- ☑
　bomb Y36.20- ☑
　　dirty Y36.50- ☑
　　gasoline Y36.31- ☑
　　incendiary Y36.31- ☑
　　petrol Y36.31- ☑
　bullet Y36.43- ☑
　　incendiary Y36.32- ☑
　　rubber Y36.41- ☑
　chemical weapons Y36.7X- ☑
　combat
　　hand to hand (unarmed) combat Y36.44- ☑
　　using blunt or piercing object Y36.45- ☑
　conflagration — *see* War operations, fire
　conventional warfare NEC Y36.49- ☑
　depth-charge Y36.01- ☑
　destruction of aircraft Y36.10- ☑
　　due to
　　　air to air missile Y36.11- ☑
　　　collision with other aircraft Y36.12- ☑
　　　detonation (accidental) of onboard munitions and explosives Y36.14- ☑
　　　enemy fire or explosives Y36.11- ☑
　　　explosive placed on aircraft Y36.11- ☑
　　　onboard fire Y36.13- ☑
　　　rocket propelled grenade [RPG] Y36.11- ☑
　　　small arms fire Y36.11- ☑
　　　surface to air missile Y36.11- ☑
　　specified NEC Y36.19- ☑
　detonation (accidental) of
　　onboard marine weapons Y36.05- ☑
　　own munitions or munitions launch device Y36.24- ☑
　dirty bomb Y36.50- ☑
　explosion (of) Y36.20- ☑
　　aerial bomb Y36.21- ☑
　　after cessation of hostilities
　　　bomb placed during war operations Y36.82- ☑
　　　mine placed during war operations Y36.81- ☑
　　bomb NOS (*see also* War operations, bomb(s)) Y36.20- ☑
　　fragments Y36.20- ☑
　　grenade Y36.29- ☑
　　guided missile Y36.22- ☑
　　improvised explosive device [IED] (person-borne) (roadside) (vehicle-borne) Y36.23- ☑
　　land mine Y36.29- ☑
　　marine mine (at sea) (in harbor) Y36.02- ☑
　　marine weapon Y36.00- ☑
　　　specified NEC Y36.09- ☑
　　own munitions or munitions launch device (accidental) Y36.24- ☑
　　sea-based artillery shell Y36.03- ☑
　　specified NEC Y36.29- ☑
　　torpedo Y36.04- ☑
　fire Y36.30- ☑
　　specified NEC Y36.39- ☑
　firearms
　　discharge Y36.43- ☑
　　pellets Y36.42- ☑
　flamethrower Y36.33- ☑
　fragments (from) (of)
　　improvised explosive device [IED] (person-borne) (roadside) (vehicle-borne) Y36.26- ☑
　　munitions Y36.25- ☑
　　specified NEC Y36.29- ☑
　　weapons Y36.27- ☑
　friendly fire Y36.92 ☑
　hand to hand (unarmed) combat Y36.44- ☑
　hot substances — *see* War operations, fire
　incendiary bullet Y36.32- ☑
　nuclear weapon (effects of) Y36.50- ☑
　　acute radiation exposure Y36.54- ☑
　　blast pressure Y36.51- ☑
　　direct blast Y36.51- ☑
　　direct heat Y36.53- ☑
　　fallout exposure Y36.54- ☑
　　fireball Y36.53- ☑
　　indirect blast (struck or crushed by blast debris) (being thrown by blast) Y36.52- ☑
　　ionizing radiation (immediate exposure) Y36.54- ☑
　　nuclear radiation Y36.54- ☑
　　radiation
　　　ionizing (immediate exposure) Y36.54- ☑
　　　nuclear Y36.54- ☑

War operations — *continued*
  nuclear weapon — *continued*
    radiation — *continued*
      thermal Y36.53- ☑
    secondary effects Y36.54- ☑
    specified NEC Y36.59- ☑
    thermal radiation Y36.53- ☑
  restriction of air (airway)
    intentional Y36.46- ☑
    unintentional Y36.47- ☑
  rubber bullets Y36.41- ☑
  shrapnel NOS Y36.29- ☑
  suffocation — *see* War operations, restriction of airways
  unconventional warfare NEC Y36.7X- ☑
  underwater blast NOS Y36.00- ☑
  warfare
    conventional NEC Y36.49- ☑
    unconventional NEC Y36.7X- ☑
  weapon of mass destruction [WMD] Y36.91 ☑

War operations — *continued*
  weapons
    biological weapons Y36.6X- ☑
    chemical Y36.7X- ☑
    nuclear (effects of) Y36.50- ☑
      acute radiation exposure Y36.54- ☑
      blast pressure Y36.51- ☑
      direct blast Y36.51- ☑
      direct heat Y36.53- ☑
      fallout exposure Y36.54- ☑
      fireball Y36.53- ☑
      indirect blast (struck or crushed by blast debris) (being thrown by blast) Y36.52- ☑
      radiation
        ionizing (immediate exposure) Y36.54- ☑
        nuclear Y36.54- ☑
        thermal Y36.53- ☑
      secondary effects Y36.54- ☑
      specified NEC Y36.59- ☑
    of mass destruction [WMD] Y36.91 ☑

Washed
  away by flood — *see* Flood
  off road by storm (transport vehicle) — *see* Forces of nature, cataclysmic storm
Weather exposure NEC — *see* Forces of nature
Weightlessness (causing injury) (effects of) (in spacecraft, real or simulated) X52 ☑
Work related condition Y99.0
Wound (accidental) NEC (*see also* Injury) X58 ☑
  battle (*see also* War operations) Y36.90 ☑
  gunshot — *see* Discharge, firearm by type
Wreck transport vehicle NEC (*see also* Accident, transport) V89.9 ☑
Wrong
  device implanted into correct surgical site Y65.51
  fluid in infusion Y65.1
  patient, procedure performed on Y65.52
  procedure (operation) on correct patient Y65.51

Chapter 1. Certain Infectious and Parasitic Diseases (A00-B99)

INCLUDES diseases generally recognized as communicable or transmissible

Use additional code to identify resistance to antimicrobial drugs (Z16.-)

EXCLUDES 1 certain localized infections—see body system-related chapters

EXCLUDES 2 carrier or suspected carrier of infectious disease (Z22.-)

infectious and parasitic diseases specific to the perinatal period (P35-P39)

infectious and parasitic diseases complicating pregnancy, childbirth and the puerperium (O98.-)

influenza and other acute respiratory infections (J00-J22)

This chapter contains the following blocks:

A00-A09	Intestinal infectious diseases
A15-A19	Tuberculosis
A20-A28	Certain zoonotic bacterial diseases
A30-A49	Other bacterial diseases
A50-A64	Infections with a predominantly sexual mode of transmission
A65-A69	Other spirochetal diseases
A70-A74	Other diseases caused by chlamydiae
A75-A79	Rickettsioses
A80-A89	Viral infections of the central nervous system
A90-A99	Arthropod-borne viral fevers and viral hemorrhagic fevers
B00-B09	Viral infections characterized by skin and mucous membrane lesions
B10	Other human herpesviruses
B15-B19	Viral hepatitis
B20	Human immunodeficiency virus [HIV] disease
B25-B34	Other viral diseases
B35-B49	Mycoses
B50-B64	Protozoal diseases
B65-B83	Helminthiases
B85-B89	Pediculosis, acariasis and other infestations
B90-B94	Sequelae of infectious and parasitic diseases
B95-B97	Bacterial and viral infectious agents
B99	Other infectious diseases

Intestinal Infectious Diseases (A00-A09)

A00 Cholera

A00.0 Cholera due to Vibrio cholerae 01, biovar cholerae
Classical cholera

A00.1 Cholera due to Vibrio cholerae 01, biovar eltor
Cholera eltor

A00.9 Cholera, unspecified

A01 Typhoid and paratyphoid fevers

A01.0 Typhoid fever
Infection due to Salmonella typhi

A01.00 Typhoid fever, unspecified

A01.01 Typhoid meningitis

A01.02 Typhoid fever with heart involvement
Typhoid endocarditis
Typhoid myocarditis

A01.03 Typhoid pneumonia

A01.04 Typhoid arthritis

A01.05 Typhoid osteomyelitis

A01.09 Typhoid fever with other complications

A01.1 Paratyphoid fever A

A01.2 Paratyphoid fever B

A01.3 Paratyphoid fever C

A01.4 Paratyphoid fever, unspecified
Infection due to Salmonella paratyphi NOS

A02 Other salmonella infections
INCLUDES infection or foodborne intoxication due to any Salmonella species other than S. typhi and S. paratyphi

A02.0 Salmonella enteritis
Salmonellosis

A02.1 Salmonella sepsis

A02.2 Localized salmonella infections

A02.20 Localized salmonella infection, unspecified

A02.21 Salmonella meningitis

A02.22 Salmonella pneumonia

A02.23 Salmonella arthritis

A02.24 Salmonella osteomyelitis

A02.25 Salmonella pyelonephritis
Salmonella tubulo-interstitial nephropathy

A02.29 Salmonella with other localized infection

A02.8 Other specified salmonella infections

A02.9 Salmonella infection, unspecified

A03 Shigellosis

A03.0 Shigellosis due to Shigella dysenteriae
Group A shigellosis [Shiga-Kruse dysentery]

A03.1 Shigellosis due to Shigella flexneri
Group B shigellosis

A03.2 Shigellosis due to Shigella boydii
Group C shigellosis

A03.3 Shigellosis due to Shigella sonnei
Group D shigellosis

A03.8 Other shigellosis

A03.9 Shigellosis, unspecified
Bacillary dysentery NOS

A04 Other bacterial intestinal infections
EXCLUDES 1 bacterial foodborne intoxications, NEC (A05.-)
tuberculous enteritis (A18.32)

A04.0 Enteropathogenic Escherichia coli infection

A04.1 Enterotoxigenic Escherichia coli infection

A04.2 Enteroinvasive Escherichia coli infection

A04.3 Enterohemorrhagic Escherichia coli infection

A04.4 Other intestinal Escherichia coli infections
Escherichia coli enteritis NOS

A04.5 Campylobacter enteritis

A04.6 Enteritis due to Yersinia enterocolitica
EXCLUDES 1 extraintestinal yersiniosis (A28.2)

A04.7 Enterocolitis due to Clostridium difficile
Foodborne intoxication by Clostridium difficile
Pseudomembraneous colitis

A04.8 Other specified bacterial intestinal infections

A04.9 Bacterial intestinal infection, unspecified
Bacterial enteritis NOS

A05 Other bacterial foodborne intoxications, not elsewhere classified
EXCLUDES 1 Clostridium difficile foodborne intoxication and infection (A04.7)
Escherichia coli infection (A04.0-A04.4)
listeriosis (A32.-)
salmonella foodborne intoxication and infection (A02.-)
toxic effect of noxious foodstuffs (T61-T62)

A05.0 Foodborne staphylococcal intoxication

A05.1 Botulism food poisoning
Botulism NOS
Classical foodborne intoxication due to Clostridium botulinum
EXCLUDES 1 infant botulism (A48.51)
wound botulism (A48.52)

A05.2 Foodborne Clostridium perfringens [Clostridium welchii] intoxication
Enteritis necroticans
Pig-bel

A05.3 Foodborne Vibrio parahaemolyticus intoxication

A05.4 Foodborne Bacillus cereus intoxication

A05.5 Foodborne Vibrio vulnificus intoxication

A05.8 Other specified bacterial foodborne intoxications

A05.9 Bacterial foodborne intoxication, unspecified

A06 Amebiasis
INCLUDES infection due to Entamoeba histolytica
EXCLUDES 1 other protozoal intestinal diseases (A07.-)
EXCLUDES 2 acanthamebiasis (B60.1-)
Naegleriasis (B60.2)

A06.0 Acute amebic dysentery
Acute amebiasis
Intestinal amebiasis NOS

A06.1 Chronic intestinal amebiasis

A06.2 Amebic nondysenteric colitis

A06.3 Ameboma of intestine
Ameboma NOS

A06.4 Amebic liver abscess
Hepatic amebiasis

A06.5 Amebic lung abscess
Amebic abscess of lung (and liver)

A06.6 Amebic brain abscess
Amebic abscess of brain (and liver) (and lung)

☑ Additional Character Required   Xtension Alert   Unspecified Code   Other Specified Code   Manifestation Code   ►◄ Revised Text   ● New Code   ▲ Revised Code Title

ICD-10-CM 2014 (Draft)

423

A06.7   Cutaneous **amebiasis**

✓5ᵗʰ **A06.8**   **Amebic infection of other sites**

    A06.81   **Amebic** cystitis

    A06.82   Other **amebic** genitourinary **infections**
      Amebic balanitis
      Amebic vesiculitis
      Amebic vulvovaginitis

    A06.89   **Other amebic infections**
      Amebic appendicitis
      Amebic splenic abscess

A06.9   **Amebiasis, unspecified**

✓4ᵗʰ **A07**   **Other protozoal intestinal diseases**

A07.0   **Balantidiasis**
    Balantidial dysentery

A07.1   **Giardiasis [lambliasis]**

A07.2   **Cryptosporidiosis**

A07.3   **Isosporiasis**
    Infection due to Isospora belli and Isospora hominis
    Intestinal coccidiosis
    Isosporosis

A07.4   **Cyclosporiasis**

A07.8   **Other specified protozoal intestinal diseases**
    Intestinal microsporidiosis
    Intestinal trichomoniasis
    Sarcocystosis
    Sarcosporidiosis

A07.9   **Protozoal intestinal disease, unspecified**
    Flagellate diarrhea   Protozoal diarrhea
    Protozoal colitis   Protozoal dysentery

✓4ᵗʰ **A08**   **Viral and other specified intestinal infections**
    EXCLUDES 1   *influenza with involvement of gastrointestinal tract (J09.X3, J10.2, J11.2)*

A08.0   **Rotaviral enteritis**

✓5ᵗʰ **A08.1**   **Acute gastroenteropathy due to Norwalk agent and other small round viruses**

    A08.11   **Acute gastroenteropathy due to** Norwalk agent
      Acute gastroenteropathy due to Norovirus
      Acute gastroenteropathy due to Norwalk-like agent

    A08.19   **Acute gastroenteropathy due to** other small round **viruses**
      Acute gastroenteropathy due to small round virus [SRV] NOS

A08.2   **Adenoviral enteritis**

✓5ᵗʰ **A08.3**   **Other viral enteritis**

    A08.31   Calicivirus **enteritis**

    A08.32   Astrovirus **enteritis**

    A08.39   **Other viral enteritis**
      Coxsackie virus enteritis
      Echovirus enteritis
      Enterovirus enteritis NEC
      Torovirus enteritis

A08.4   **Viral intestinal infection, unspecified**
    Viral enteritis NOS
    Viral gastroenteritis NOS
    Viral gastroenteropathy NOS

A08.8   **Other specified intestinal infections**

A09   **Infectious gastroenteritis and colitis, unspecified**
    Infectious colitis NOS
    Infectious enteritis NOS
    Infectious gastroenteritis NOS
    EXCLUDES 1   *colitis NOS (K52.9)*
      diarrhea NOS (R19.7)
      enteritis NOS (K52.9)
      gastroenteritis NOS (K52.9)
      noninfective gastroenteritis and colitis, unspecified (K52.9)

Tuberculosis (A15-A19)

INCLUDES   infections due to Mycobacterium tuberculosis and Mycobacterium bovis
EXCLUDES 1   *congenital tuberculosis (P37.0)*
    nonspecific reaction to test for tuberculosis without active tuberculosis (R76.1-)
    pneumoconiosis associated with tuberculosis, any type in A15 (J65)
    positive PPD (R76.11)
    positive tuberculin skin test without active tuberculosis (R76.11)
    sequelae of tuberculosis (B90.-)
    silicotuberculosis (J65)

✓4ᵗʰ **A15**   **Respiratory tuberculosis**

A15.0   **Tuberculosis of** lung
    Tuberculous bronchiectasis
    Tuberculous fibrosis of lung
    Tuberculous pneumonia
    Tuberculous pneumothorax

A15.4   **Tuberculosis of** intrathoracic lymph nodes
    Tuberculosis of hilar lymph nodes
    Tuberculosis of mediastinal lymph nodes
    Tuberculosis of tracheobronchial lymph nodes
    EXCLUDES 1   *tuberculosis specified as primary (A15.7)*

A15.5   **Tuberculosis of larynx, trachea and bronchus**
    Tuberculosis of bronchus
    Tuberculosis of glottis
    Tuberculosis of larynx
    Tuberculosis of trachea

A15.6   **Tuberculous** pleurisy
    Tuberculosis of pleura Tuberculous empyema
    EXCLUDES 1   *primary respiratory tuberculosis (A15.7)*

A15.7   **Primary respiratory tuberculosis**

A15.8   **Other respiratory tuberculosis**
    Mediastinal tuberculosis
    Nasopharyngeal tuberculosis
    Tuberculosis of nose
    Tuberculosis of sinus [any nasal]

A15.9   **Respiratory tuberculosis unspecified**

✓4ᵗʰ **A17**   **Tuberculosis of** nervous system

A17.0   **Tuberculous** meningitis
    Tuberculosis of meninges (cerebral)(spinal)
    Tuberculous leptomeningitis
    EXCLUDES 1   *tuberculous meningoencephalitis (A17.82)*

A17.1   Meningeal **tuberculoma**
    Tuberculoma of meninges (cerebral) (spinal)
    EXCLUDES 2   *tuberculoma of brain and spinal cord (A17.81)*

✓5ᵗʰ **A17.8**   Other **tuberculosis of nervous system**

    A17.81   **Tuberculoma of** brain and spinal cord
      Tuberculous abscess of brain and spinal cord

    A17.82   **Tuberculous** meningoencephalitis
      Tuberculous myelitis

    A17.83   **Tuberculous** neuritis
      Tuberculous mononeuropathy

    A17.89   **Other tuberculosis of nervous system**
      Tuberculous polyneuropathy

A17.9   **Tuberculosis of nervous system, unspecified**

✓4ᵗʰ **A18**   **Tuberculosis of** other organs

✓5ᵗʰ **A18.0**   **Tuberculosis of** bones and joints

    A18.01   **Tuberculosis of** spine
      Pott's disease or curvature of spine
      Tuberculous arthritis
      Tuberculous osteomyelitis of spine
      Tuberculous spondylitis

    A18.02   **Tuberculous arthritis of other joints**
      Tuberculosis of hip (joint)
      Tuberculosis of knee (joint)

    A18.03   **Tuberculosis of** other bones
      Tuberculous mastoiditis
      Tuberculous osteomyelitis

    A18.09   **Other musculoskeletal tuberculosis**
      Tuberculous myositis
      Tuberculous synovitis
      Tuberculous tenosynovitis

✓5ᵗʰ **A18.1**   **Tuberculosis of** genitourinary system

    A18.10   **Tuberculosis of genitourinary system, unspecified**

    A18.11   **Tuberculosis of** kidney and ureter

    A18.12   **Tuberculosis of** bladder

EXCLUDES 1 Not coded here   EXCLUDES 2 Not included here   N Newborn Age: 0   P Pediatric Age: 0-17   M Maternity Age: 12-55   A Adult Age: 15-124

424   ICD-10-CM 2014 (Draft)

A18.13 Tuberculosis of other urinary organs
Tuberculous urethritis

A18.14 Tuberculosis of prostate   🄰♂

A18.15 Tuberculosis of other male genital organs ♂

A18.16 Tuberculosis of cervix ♀

A18.17 Tuberculous female pelvic inflammatory disease ♀
Tuberculous endometritis
Tuberculous oophoritis and salpingitis

A18.18 Tuberculosis of other female genital organs ♀
Tuberculous ulceration of vulva

A18.2 Tuberculous peripheral lymphadenopathy
Tuberculous adenitis
EXCLUDES 2 tuberculosis of bronchial and mediastinal lymph nodes (A15.4)
tuberculosis of mesenteric and retroperitoneal lymph nodes (A18.39)
tuberculous tracheobronchial adenopathy (A15.4)

✓5th **A18.3 Tuberculosis of** intestines, peritoneum and mesenteric glands

A18.31 Tuberculous peritonitis
Tuberculous ascites

A18.32 Tuberculous enteritis
Tuberculosis of anus and rectum
Tuberculosis of intestine (large) (small)

A18.39 Retroperitoneal tuberculosis
Tuberculosis of mesenteric glands
Tuberculosis of retroperitoneal (lymph glands)

A18.4 Tuberculosis of skin and subcutaneous tissue
Erythema induratum, tuberculous
Lupus excedens
Lupus vulgaris NOS
Lupus vulgaris of eyelid
Scrofuloderma
Tuberculosis of external ear
EXCLUDES 2 lupus erythematosus (L93.-)
lupus NOS (M32.9)
systemic (M32.-)

✓5th **A18.5 Tuberculosis of** eye
EXCLUDES 2 lupus vulgaris of eyelid (A18.4)

A18.50 Tuberculosis of eye, unspecified

A18.51 Tuberculous episcleritis

A18.52 Tuberculous keratitis
Tuberculous interstitial keratitis
Tuberculous keratoconjunctivitis (interstitial) (phlyctenular)

A18.53 Tuberculous chorioretinitis

A18.54 Tuberculous iridocyclitis

A18.59 Other tuberculosis of eye
Tuberculous conjunctivitis

A18.6 Tuberculosis of (inner) (middle) ear
Tuberculous otitis media
EXCLUDES 2 tuberculosis of external ear (A18.4)
tuberculous mastoiditis (A18.03)

A18.7 Tuberculosis of adrenal glands
Tuberculous Addison's disease

✓5th **A18.8 Tuberculosis of** other specified organs

A18.81 Tuberculosis of thyroid gland

A18.82 Tuberculosis of other endocrine glands
Tuberculosis of pituitary gland
Tuberculosis of thymus gland

A18.83 Tuberculosis of digestive tract organs, not elsewhere classified
EXCLUDES 1 tuberculosis of intestine (A18.32)

A18.84 Tuberculosis of heart
Tuberculous cardiomyopathy
Tuberculous endocarditis
Tuberculous myocarditis
Tuberculous pericarditis

A18.85 Tuberculosis of spleen

A18.89 Tuberculosis of other sites
Tuberculosis of muscle
Tuberculous cerebral arteritis

✓4th **A19 Miliary tuberculosis**
INCLUDES disseminated tuberculosis
generalized tuberculosis
tuberculous polyserositis

A19.0 Acute miliary tuberculosis of a single specified site

A19.1 Acute miliary tuberculosis of multiple sites

A19.2 Acute miliary tuberculosis, unspecified

A19.8 Other miliary tuberculosis

A19.9 Miliary tuberculosis, unspecified

Certain zoonotic bacterial diseases (A20-A28)

✓4th **A20 Plague**
INCLUDES infection due to Yersinia pestis

A20.0 Bubonic plague

A20.1 Cellulocutaneous plague

A20.2 Pneumonic plague

A20.3 Plague meningitis

A20.7 Septicemic plague

A20.8 Other forms of plague
Abortive plague
Asymptomatic plague
Pestis minor

A20.9 Plague, unspecified

✓4th **A21 Tularemia**
INCLUDES deer-fly fever
infection due to Francisella tularensis
rabbit fever

A21.0 Ulceroglandular tularemia

A21.1 Oculoglandular tularemia
Ophthalmic tularemia

A21.2 Pulmonary tularemia

A21.3 Gastrointestinal tularemia
Abdominal tularemia

A21.7 Generalized tularemia

A21.8 Other forms of tularemia

A21.9 Tularemia, unspecified

✓4th **A22 Anthrax**
INCLUDES infection due to Bacillus anthracis

A22.0 Cutaneous anthrax
Malignant carbuncle
Malignant pustule

A22.1 Pulmonary anthrax
Inhalation anthrax
Ragpicker's disease
Woolsorter's disease

A22.2 Gastrointestinal anthrax

A22.7 Anthrax sepsis

A22.8 Other forms of anthrax
Anthrax meningitis

A22.9 Anthrax, unspecified

✓4th **A23 Brucellosis**
Malta fever
Mediterranean fever
Undulant fever

A23.0 Brucellosis due to Brucella melitensis

A23.1 Brucellosis due to Brucella abortus

A23.2 Brucellosis due to Brucella suis

A23.3 Brucellosis due to Brucella canis

A23.8 Other brucellosis

A23.9 Brucellosis, unspecified

✓4th **A24 Glanders and melioidosis**

A24.0 Glanders
Infection due to Pseudomonas mallei
Malleus

A24.1 Acute and fulminating melioidosis
Melioidosis pneumonia
Melioidosis sepsis

A24.2 Subacute and chronic melioidosis

A24.3 Other melioidosis

A24.9 Melioidosis, unspecified
Infection due to Pseudomonas pseudomallei NOS
Whitmore's disease

✓4th **A25 Rat-bite fevers**

A25.0 Spirillosis
Sodoku

A25.1 Streptobacillosis
Epidemic arthritic erythema
Haverhill fever
Streptobacillary rat-bite fever

A25.9 Rat-bite fever, unspecified

Certain Infectious and Parasitic Diseases

A26–A39.53

√4ᵗʰ **A26** **Erysipeloid**

  A26.Ø **Cutaneous erysipeloid**
    Erythema migrans

  A26.7 **Erysipelothrix sepsis**

  A26.8 **Other forms of erysipeloid**

  A26.9 **Erysipeloid, unspecified**

√4ᵗʰ **A27** **Leptospirosis**

  A27.Ø **Leptospirosis icterohemorrhagica**
    Leptospiral or spirochetal jaundice (hemorrhagic)
    Weil's disease

  √5ᵗʰ **A27.8** **Other forms of leptospirosis**

    A27.81 **Aseptic meningitis in leptospirosis**

    A27.89 **Other forms of leptospirosis**

  A27.9 **Leptospirosis, unspecified**

√4ᵗʰ **A28** **Other zoonotic bacterial diseases, not elsewhere classified**

  A28.Ø **Pasteurellosis**

  A28.1 **Cat-scratch disease**
    Cat-scratch fever

  A28.2 **Extraintestinal yersiniosis**
    EXCLUDES 1   enteritis due to Yersinia enterocolitica (AØ4.6)
                    plague (A2Ø.-)

  A28.8 **Other specified zoonotic bacterial diseases, not elsewhere classified**

  A28.9 **Zoonotic bacterial disease, unspecified**

Other bacterial diseases (A3Ø-A49)

√4ᵗʰ **A3Ø** **Leprosy [Hansen's disease]**
  INCLUDES infection due to Mycobacterium leprae
  EXCLUDES 1 sequelae of leprosy (B92)

  A3Ø.Ø **Indeterminate leprosy**
    I leprosy

  A3Ø.1 **Tuberculoid leprosy**
    TT leprosy

  A3Ø.2 **Borderline tuberculoid leprosy**
    BT leprosy

  A3Ø.3 **Borderline leprosy**
    BB leprosy

  A3Ø.4 **Borderline lepromatous leprosy**
    BL leprosy

  A3Ø.5 **Lepromatous leprosy**
    LL leprosy

  A3Ø.8 **Other forms of leprosy**

  A3Ø.9 **Leprosy, unspecified**

√4ᵗʰ **A31** **Infection due to other mycobacteria**
  EXCLUDES 2 leprosy (A3Ø.-)
          tuberculosis (A15-A19)

  A31.Ø **Pulmonary mycobacterial infection**
    Infection due to Mycobacterium avium
    Infection due to Mycobacterium intracellulare [Battey bacillus]
    Infection due to Mycobacterium kansasii

  A31.1 **Cutaneous mycobacterial infection**
    Buruli ulcer
    Infection due to Mycobacterium marinum
    Infection due to Mycobacterium ulcerans

  A31.2 **Disseminated mycobacterium avium-intracellulare complex (DMAC)**
    MAC sepsis

  A31.8 **Other mycobacterial infections**

  A31.9 **Mycobacterial infection, unspecified**
    Atypical mycobacterial infection NOS
    Mycobacteriosis NOS

√4ᵗʰ **A32** **Listeriosis**
  INCLUDES listerial foodborne infection
  EXCLUDES 1 neonatal (disseminated) listeriosis (P37.2)

  A32.Ø **Cutaneous listeriosis**

  √5ᵗʰ **A32.1** **Listerial meningitis and meningoencephalitis**

    A32.11 **Listerial meningitis**

    A32.12 **Listerial meningoencephalitis**

  A32.7 **Listerial sepsis**

  √5ᵗʰ **A32.8** **Other forms of listeriosis**

    A32.81 **Oculoglandular listeriosis**

    A32.82 **Listerial endocarditis**

    A32.89 **Other forms of listeriosis**
      Listerial cerebral arteritis

  A32.9 **Listeriosis, unspecified**

A33 **Tetanus neonatorum**   N

A34 **Obstetrical tetanus**   M♀

A35 **Other tetanus**
  Tetanus NOS
  EXCLUDES 1 obstetrical tetanus (A34)
          tetanus neonatorum (A33)

√4ᵗʰ **A36** **Diphtheria**

  A36.Ø **Pharyngeal diphtheria**
    Diphtheritic membranous angina
    Tonsillar diphtheria

  A36.1 **Nasopharyngeal diphtheria**

  A36.2 **Laryngeal diphtheria**
    Diphtheritic laryngotracheitis

  A36.3 **Cutaneous diphtheria**
    EXCLUDES 2 erythrasma (LØ8.1)

  √5ᵗʰ **A36.8** **Other diphtheria**

    A36.81 **Diphtheritic cardiomyopathy**
      Diphtheritic myocarditis

    A36.82 **Diphtheritic radiculomyelitis**

    A36.83 **Diphtheritic polyneuritis**

    A36.84 **Diphtheritic tubulo-interstitial nephropathy**

    A36.85 **Diphtheritic cystitis**

    A36.86 **Diphtheritic conjunctivitis**

    A36.89 **Other diphtheritic complications**
      Diphtheritic peritonitis

  A36.9 **Diphtheria, unspecified**

√4ᵗʰ **A37** **Whooping cough**

  √5ᵗʰ **A37.Ø** **Whooping cough due to Bordetella pertussis**

    A37.ØØ **Whooping cough due to Bordetella pertussis without pneumonia**

    A37.Ø1 **Whooping cough due to Bordetella pertussis with pneumonia**

  √5ᵗʰ **A37.1** **Whooping cough due to Bordetella parapertussis**

    A37.1Ø **Whooping cough due to Bordetella parapertussis without pneumonia**

    A37.11 **Whooping cough due to Bordetella parapertussis with pneumonia**

  √5ᵗʰ **A37.8** **Whooping cough due to other Bordetella species**

    A37.8Ø **Whooping cough due to other Bordetella species without pneumonia**

    A37.81 **Whooping cough due to other Bordetella species with pneumonia**

  √5ᵗʰ **A37.9** **Whooping cough, unspecified species**

    A37.9Ø **Whooping cough, unspecified species without pneumonia**

    A37.91 **Whooping cough, unspecified species with pneumonia**

√4ᵗʰ **A38** **Scarlet fever**
  INCLUDES scarlatina
  EXCLUDES 2 streptococcal sore throat (JØ2.Ø)

  A38.Ø **Scarlet fever with otitis media**

  A38.1 **Scarlet fever with myocarditis**

  A38.8 **Scarlet fever with other complications**

  A38.9 **Scarlet fever, uncomplicated**
    Scarlet fever, NOS

√4ᵗʰ **A39** **Meningococcal infection**

  A39.Ø **Meningococcal meningitis**

  A39.1 **Waterhouse-Friderichsen syndrome**
    Meningococcal hemorrhagic adrenalitis
    Meningococcic adrenal syndrome

  A39.2 **Acute meningococcemia**

  A39.3 **Chronic meningococcemia**

  A39.4 **Meningococcemia, unspecified**

  √5ᵗʰ **A39.5** **Meningococcal heart disease**

    A39.5Ø **Meningococcal carditis, unspecified**

    A39.51 **Meningococcal endocarditis**

    A39.52 **Meningococcal myocarditis**

    A39.53 **Meningococcal pericarditis**

EXCLUDES 1 Not coded here   EXCLUDES 2 Not included here   N Newborn Age: Ø   P Pediatric Age: Ø-17   M Maternity Age: 12-55   A Adult Age: 15-124

Certain Infectious and Parasitic Diseases

A39.8–A49.9

☑5ᵗʰ **A39.8 Other meningococcal infections**
    A39.81 Meningococcal encephalitis
    A39.82 Meningococcal retrobulbar neuritis
    A39.83 Meningococcal arthritis
    A39.84 Postmeningococcal arthritis
    A39.89 Other meningococcal infections
      Meningococcal conjunctivitis
A39.9 Meningococcal infection, unspecified
    Meningococcal disease NOS

☑4ᵗʰ **A40 Streptococcal sepsis**
  Code first: postprocedural streptococcal sepsis (T81.4)
    streptococcal sepsis during labor (O75.3)
    streptococcal sepsis following abortion or ectopic or molar pregnancy (O03-O07, O08.0)
    streptococcal sepsis following immunization (T88.0)
    streptococcal sepsis following infusion, transfusion or therapeutic injection (T80.2-)
  EXCLUDES 1 neonatal (P36.0-P36.1)
    puerperal sepsis (O85)
    sepsis due to Streptococcus, group D (A41.81)
A40.0 Sepsis due to streptococcus, group A
A40.1 Sepsis due to streptococcus, group B
A40.3 Sepsis due to Streptococcus pneumoniae
    Pneumococcal sepsis
A40.8 Other streptococcal sepsis
A40.9 Streptococcal sepsis, unspecified

☑4ᵗʰ **A41 Other sepsis**
  Code first: postprocedural sepsis (T81.4)
    sepsis during labor (O75.3)
    sepsis following abortion, ectopic or molar pregnancy (O03-O07, O08.0)
    sepsis following immunization (T88.0)
    sepsis following infusion, transfusion or therapeutic injection (T80.2-)
  EXCLUDES 1 bacteremia NOS (R78.81)
    neonatal (P36.-)
    puerperal sepsis (O85)
    sepsis NOS (A41.9)
    streptococcal sepsis (A40.-)
  EXCLUDES 2 sepsis (due to) (in) actinomycotic (A42.7)
    sepsis (due to) (in) anthrax (A22.7)
    sepsis (due to) (in) candidal (B37.7)
    sepsis (due to) (in) Erysipelothrix (A26.7)
    sepsis (due to) (in) extraintestinal yersiniosis (A28.2)
    sepsis (due to) (in) gonococcal (A54.86)
    sepsis (due to) (in) herpesviral (B00.7)
    sepsis (due to) (in) listerial (A32.7)
    sepsis (due to) (in) melioidosis (A24.1)
    sepsis (due to) (in) meningococcal (A39.2-A39.4)
    sepsis (due to) (in) plague (A20.7)
    sepsis (due to) (in) tularemia (A21.7)
    toxic shock syndrome (A48.3)
☑5ᵗʰ **A41.0 Sepsis due to Staphylococcus aureus**
    A41.01 Sepsis due to methicillin susceptible Staphylococcus aureus
      MSSA sepsis
      Staphylococcus aureus sepsis NOS
    A41.02 Sepsis due to methicillin resistant Staphylococcus aureus
A41.1 Sepsis due to other specified staphylococcus
    Coagulase negative staphylococcus sepsis
A41.2 Sepsis due to unspecified staphylococcus
A41.3 Sepsis due to Hemophilus influenzae
A41.4 Sepsis due to anaerobes
  EXCLUDES 1 gas gangrene (A48.0)
☑5ᵗʰ **A41.5 Sepsis due to other Gram-negative organisms**
    A41.50 Gram-negative sepsis, unspecified
      Gram-negative sepsis NOS
    A41.51 Sepsis due to Escherichia coli [E. coli]
    A41.52 Sepsis due to Pseudomonas
      Pseudomonas aeroginosa
    A41.53 Sepsis due to Serratia
    A41.59 Other Gram-negative sepsis
☑5ᵗʰ **A41.8 Other specified sepsis**
    A41.81 Sepsis due to Enterococcus
    A41.89 Other specified sepsis

A41.9 Sepsis, unspecified organism
    Septicemia NOS

☑4ᵗʰ **A42 Actinomycosis**
  EXCLUDES 1 actinomycetoma (B47.1)
A42.0 Pulmonary actinomycosis
A42.1 Abdominal actinomycosis
A42.2 Cervicofacial actinomycosis
A42.7 Actinomycotic sepsis
☑5ᵗʰ **A42.8 Other forms of actinomycosis**
    A42.81 Actinomycotic meningitis
    A42.82 Actinomycotic encephalitis
    A42.89 Other forms of actinomycosis
A42.9 Actinomycosis, unspecified

☑4ᵗʰ **A43 Nocardiosis**
A43.0 Pulmonary nocardiosis
A43.1 Cutaneous nocardiosis
A43.8 Other forms of nocardiosis
A43.9 Nocardiosis, unspecified

☑4ᵗʰ **A44 Bartonellosis**
A44.0 Systemic bartonellosis
    Oroya fever
A44.1 Cutaneous and mucocutaneous bartonellosis
    Verruga peruana
A44.8 Other forms of bartonellosis
A44.9 Bartonellosis, unspecified

A46 Erysipelas
  EXCLUDES 1 postpartum or puerperal erysipelas (O86.89)

☑4ᵗʰ **A48 Other bacterial diseases, not elsewhere classified**
  EXCLUDES 1 actinomycetoma (B47.1)
A48.0 Gas gangrene
    Clostridial cellulitis
    Clostridial myonecrosis
A48.1 Legionnaires' disease
A48.2 Nonpneumonic Legionnaires' disease [Pontiac fever]
A48.3 Toxic shock syndrome
    Use additional code to identify the organism (B95, B96)
  EXCLUDES 1 endotoxic shock NOS (R57.8)
    sepsis NOS (A41.9)
A48.4 Brazilian purpuric fever
    Systemic Hemophilus aegyptius infection
☑5ᵗʰ **A48.5 Other specified botulism**
    Non-foodborne intoxication due to toxins of Clostridium botulinum [C. botulinum]
  EXCLUDES 1 food poisoning due to toxins of Clostridium botulinum (A05.1)
    A48.51 Infant botulism P
    A48.52 Wound botulism
      Non-foodborne botulism NOS
      Use additional code for associated wound
A48.8 Other specified bacterial diseases

☑4ᵗʰ **A49 Bacterial infection of unspecified site**
  EXCLUDES 1 bacterial agents as the cause of diseases classified elsewhere (B95-B96)
    chlamydial infection NOS (A74.9)
    meningococcal infection NOS (A39.9)
    rickettsial infection NOS (A79.9)
    spirochetal infection NOS (A69.9)
☑5ᵗʰ **A49.0 Staphylococcal infection, unspecified site**
    A49.01 Methicillin susceptible Staphylococcus aureus infection, unspecified site
      Methicillin susceptible Staphylococcus aureus (MSSA) infection
      Staphylococcus aureus infection NOS
    A49.02 Methicillin resistant Staphylococcus aureus infection, unspecified site
      Methicillin resistant Staphylococcus aureus (MRSA) infection
A49.1 Streptococcal infection, unspecified site
A49.2 Hemophilus influenzae infection, unspecified site
A49.3 Mycoplasma infection, unspecified site
A49.8 Other bacterial infections of unspecified site
A49.9 Bacterial infection, unspecified
  EXCLUDES 1 bacteremia NOS (R78.81)

Infections with a predominantly sexual mode of transmission (A50-A64)

EXCLUDES 1   *human immunodeficiency virus [HIV] disease (B20)*
nonspecific and nongonococcal urethritis (N34.1)
Reiter's disease (M02.3-)

√4th **A50**   **Congenital syphilis**

√5th   **A50.0**   **Early congenital syphilis, symptomatic**
Any congenital syphilitic condition specified as early or manifest less than two years after birth.

     A50.01   **Early congenital syphilitic oculopathy**

     A50.02   **Early congenital syphilitic osteochondropathy**

     A50.03   **Early congenital syphilitic pharyngitis**
Early congenital syphilitic laryngitis

     A50.04   **Early congenital syphilitic pneumonia**

     A50.05   **Early congenital syphilitic rhinitis**

     A50.06   **Early cutaneous congenital syphilis**

     A50.07   **Early mucocutaneous congenital syphilis**

     A50.08   **Early visceral congenital syphilis**

     A50.09   **Other early congenital syphilis, symptomatic**

  A50.1   **Early congenital syphilis, latent**
Congenital syphilis without clinical manifestations, with positive serological reaction and negative spinal fluid test, less than two years after birth.

  A50.2   **Early congenital syphilis, unspecified**
Congenital syphilis NOS less than two years after birth.

√5th   **A50.3**   **Late congenital syphilitic oculopathy**
EXCLUDES 1   *Hutchinson's triad (A50.53)*

     A50.30   **Late congenital syphilitic oculopathy, unspecified**

     A50.31   **Late congenital syphilitic interstitial keratitis**

     A50.32   **Late congenital syphilitic chorioretinitis**

     A50.39   **Other late congenital syphilitic oculopathy**

√5th   **A50.4**   **Late congenital neurosyphilis [juvenile neurosyphilis]**
Use additional code to identify any associated mental disorder
EXCLUDES 1   *Hutchinson's triad (A50.53)*

     A50.40   **Late congenital neurosyphilis, unspecified**
Juvenile neurosyphilis NOS

     A50.41   **Late congenital syphilitic meningitis**

     A50.42   **Late congenital syphilitic encephalitis**

     A50.43   **Late congenital syphilitic polyneuropathy**

     A50.44   **Late congenital syphilitic optic nerve atrophy**

     A50.45   **Juvenile general paresis**
Dementia paralytica juvenilis
Juvenile tabetoparetic neurosyphilis

     A50.49   **Other late congenital neurosyphilis**
Juvenile tabes dorsalis

√5th   **A50.5**   **Other late congenital syphilis, symptomatic**
Any congenital syphilitic condition specified as late or manifest two years or more after birth.

     A50.51   **Clutton's joints**

     A50.52   **Hutchinson's teeth**

     A50.53   **Hutchinson's triad**

     A50.54   **Late congenital cardiovascular syphilis**

     A50.55   **Late congenital syphilitic arthropathy**

     A50.56   **Late congenital syphilitic osteochondropathy**

     A50.57   **Syphilitic saddle nose**

     A50.59   **Other late congenital syphilis, symptomatic**

  A50.6   **Late congenital syphilis, latent**
Congenital syphilis without clinical manifestations, with positive serological reaction and negative spinal fluid test, two years or more after birth.

  A50.7   **Late congenital syphilis, unspecified**
Congenital syphilis NOS two years or more after birth.

  A50.9   **Congenital syphilis, unspecified**

√4th **A51**   **Early syphilis**

  A51.0   **Primary genital syphilis**
Syphilitic chancre NOS

  A51.1   **Primary anal syphilis**

  A51.2   **Primary syphilis of other sites**

√5th   **A51.3**   **Secondary syphilis of skin and mucous membranes**

     A51.31   **Condyloma latum**

     A51.32   **Syphilitic alopecia**

     A51.39   **Other secondary syphilis of skin**
Syphilitic leukoderma
Syphilitic mucous patch
EXCLUDES 1   *late syphilitic leukoderma (A52.79)*

√5th   **A51.4**   **Other secondary syphilis**

     A51.41   **Secondary syphilitic meningitis**

     A51.42   **Secondary syphilitic female pelvic disease**   ♀

     A51.43   **Secondary syphilitic oculopathy**
Secondary syphilitic chorioretinitis
Secondary syphilitic iridocyclitis, iritis
Secondary syphilitic uveitis

     A51.44   **Secondary syphilitic nephritis**

     A51.45   **Secondary syphilitic hepatitis**

     A51.46   **Secondary syphilitic osteopathy**

     A51.49   **Other secondary syphilitic conditions**
Secondary syphilitic lymphadenopathy
Secondary syphilitic myositis

  A51.5   **Early syphilis, latent**
Syphilis (acquired) without clinical manifestations, with positive serological reaction and negative spinal fluid test, less than two years after infection.

  A51.9   **Early syphilis, unspecified**

√4th **A52**   **Late syphilis**

√5th   **A52.0**   **Cardiovascular and cerebrovascular syphilis**

     A52.00   **Cardiovascular syphilis, unspecified**

     A52.01   **Syphilitic aneurysm of aorta**

     A52.02   **Syphilitic aortitis**

     A52.03   **Syphilitic endocarditis**
Syphilitic aortic valve incompetence or stenosis
Syphilitic mitral valve stenosis
Syphilitic pulmonary valve regurgitation

     A52.04   **Syphilitic cerebral arteritis**

     A52.05   **Other cerebrovascular syphilis**
Syphilitic cerebral aneurysm (ruptured) (non-ruptured)
Syphilitic cerebral thrombosis

     A52.06   **Other syphilitic heart involvement**
Syphilitic coronary artery disease
Syphilitic myocarditis
Syphilitic pericarditis

     A52.09   **Other cardiovascular syphilis**

√5th   **A52.1**   **Symptomatic neurosyphilis**

     A52.10   **Symptomatic neurosyphilis, unspecified**

     A52.11   **Tabes dorsalis**
Locomotor ataxia (progressive)
Tabetic neurosyphilis

     A52.12   **Other cerebrospinal syphilis**

     A52.13   **Late syphilitic meningitis**

     A52.14   **Late syphilitic encephalitis**

     A52.15   **Late syphilitic neuropathy**
Late syphilitic acoustic neuritis
Late syphilitic optic (nerve) atrophy
Late syphilitic polyneuropathy
Late syphilitic retrobulbar neuritis

     A52.16   **Charcôt's arthropathy (tabetic)**

     A52.17   **General paresis**
Dementia paralytica

     A52.19   **Other symptomatic neurosyphilis**
Syphilitic parkinsonism

  A52.2   **Asymptomatic neurosyphilis**

  A52.3   **Neurosyphilis, unspecified**
Gumma (syphilitic)
Syphilis (late)
Syphiloma

√5th   **A52.7**   **Other symptomatic late syphilis**

     A52.71   **Late syphilitic oculopathy**
Late syphilitic chorioretinitis
Late syphilitic episcleritis

     A52.72   **Syphilis of lung and bronchus**

     A52.73   **Symptomatic late syphilis of other respiratory organs**

     A52.74   **Syphilis of liver and other viscera**
Late syphilitic peritonitis

     A52.75   **Syphilis of kidney and ureter**
Syphilitic glomerular disease

EXCLUDES 1 Not coded here   EXCLUDES 2 Not included here   N Newborn Age: 0   P Pediatric Age: 0-17   M Maternity Age: 12-55   A Adult Age: 15-124

428   ICD-10-CM 2014 (Draft)

A52.76 Other genitourinary **symptomatic late syphilis**
Late syphilitic female pelvic inflammatory disease

A52.77 **Syphilis of** bone and joint

A52.78 **Syphilis of other** musculoskeletal tissue
Late syphilitic bursitis
Syphilis [stage unspecified] of bursa
Syphilis [stage unspecified] of muscle
Syphilis [stage unspecified] of synovium
Syphilis [stage unspecified] of tendon

A52.79 Other symptomatic late syphilis
Late syphilitic leukoderma
Syphilis of adrenal gland
Syphilis of pituitary gland
Syphilis of thyroid gland
Syphilitic splenomegaly
EXCLUDES 1 *syphilitic leukoderma (secondary) (A51.39)*

A52.8 **Late syphilis,** latent
Syphilis (acquired) without clinical manifestations, with positive serological reaction and negative spinal fluid test, two years or more after infection

A52.9 Late syphilis, unspecified

✓4th **A53** Other and unspecified **syphilis**

A53.0 Latent **syphilis, unspecified as early or late**
Latent syphilis NOS
Positive serological reaction for syphilis

A53.9 Syphilis, unspecified
Infection due to Treponema pallidum NOS
Syphilis (acquired) NOS
EXCLUDES 1 *syphilis NOS under two years of age (A50.2)*

✓4th **A54** Gonococcal infection

✓5th A54.0 **Gonococcal infection of** lower genitourinary tract without periurethral or accessory gland abscess
EXCLUDES 1 *gonococcal infection with genitourinary gland abscess (A54.1)*
gonococcal infection with periurethral abscess (A54.1)

A54.00 **Gonococcal infection of lower genitourinary tract, unspecified**

A54.01 **Gonococcal** cystitis and urethritis, unspecified

A54.02 **Gonococcal** vulvovaginitis, unspecified   ♀

A54.03 **Gonococcal** cervicitis, unspecified   ♀

A54.09 Other gonococcal infection of lower genitourinary tract

A54.1 Gonococcal infection of lower genitourinary tract with periurethral and accessory gland abscess
Gonococcal Bartholin's gland abscess

✓5th A54.2 **Gonococcal** pelviperitonitis **and other** gonococcal genitourinary infection

A54.21 **Gonococcal infection of** kidney and ureter

A54.22 **Gonococcal** prostatitis   ♂

A54.23 **Gonococcal infection of** other male genital organs ♂
Gonococcal epididymitis
Gonococcal orchitis

A54.24 **Gonococcal** female pelvic inflammatory disease ♀
Gonococcal pelviperitonitis
EXCLUDES 1 *gonococcal peritonitis (A54.85)*

A54.29 Other gonococcal genitourinary infections

✓5th A54.3 **Gonococcal infection of** eye

A54.30 **Gonococcal infection of eye, unspecified**

A54.31 **Gonococcal** conjunctivitis
Ophthalmia neonatorum due to gonococcus

A54.32 **Gonococcal** iridocyclitis

A54.33 **Gonococcal** keratitis

A54.39 Other gonococcal eye infection
Gonococcal endophthalmia

✓5th A54.4 **Gonococcal infection of** musculoskeletal system

A54.40 **Gonococcal infection of musculoskeletal system, unspecified**

A54.41 **Gonococcal** spondylopathy

A54.42 **Gonococcal** arthritis
EXCLUDES 2 *gonococcal infection of spine (A54.41)*

A54.43 **Gonococcal** osteomyelitis
EXCLUDES 2 *gonococcal infection of spine (A54.41)*

A54.49 **Gonococcal infection of** other **musculoskeletal tissue**
Gonococcal bursitis
Gonococcal myositis
Gonococcal synovitis
Gonococcal tenosynovitis

A54.5 **Gonococcal** pharyngitis

A54.6 **Gonococcal infection of** anus and rectum

✓5th A54.8 Other **gonococcal infections**

A54.81 **Gonococcal** meningitis

A54.82 **Gonococcal** brain abscess

A54.83 **Gonococcal** heart infection
Gonococcal endocarditis
Gonococcal myocarditis
Gonococcal pericarditis

A54.84 **Gonococcal** pneumonia

A54.85 **Gonococcal** peritonitis
EXCLUDES 1 *gonococcal pelviperitonitis (A54.24)*

A54.86 **Gonococcal** sepsis

A54.89 Other gonococcal infections
Gonococcal keratoderma
Gonococcal lymphadenitis

A54.9 **Gonococcal infection,** unspecified

A55 Chlamydial lymphogranuloma (venereum)
Climatic or tropical bubo
Durand-Nicolas-Favre disease
Esthiomene
Lymphogranuloma inguinale

✓4th **A56** Other sexually transmitted chlamydial diseases
INCLUDES sexually transmitted diseases due to Chlamydia trachomatis
EXCLUDES 1 *neonatal chlamydial conjunctivitis (P39.1)*
neonatal chlamydial pneumonia (P23.1)
EXCLUDES 2 *chlamydial lymphogranuloma (A55)*
conditions classified to A74-

✓5th A56.0 **Chlamydial infection of** lower genitourinary tract

A56.00 **Chlamydial infection of lower genitourinary tract, unspecified**

A56.01 **Chlamydial** cystitis and urethritis

A56.02 **Chlamydial** vulvovaginitis   ♀

A56.09 **Other chlamydial infection of lower genitourinary tract**
Chlamydial cervicitis

✓5th A56.1 **Chlamydial infection of** pelviperitoneum and other genitourinary organs

A56.11 **Chlamydial** female pelvic inflammatory **disease** ♀

A56.19 Other chlamydial genitourinary infection
Chlamydial epididymitis
Chlamydial orchitis

A56.2 Chlamydial infection of genitourinary tract, unspecified

A56.3 **Chlamydial infection of** anus and rectum

A56.4 **Chlamydial infection of** pharynx

A56.8 Sexually transmitted chlamydial infection of other sites

A57 Chancroid
Ulcus molle

A58 Granuloma inguinale
Donovanosis

✓4th **A59** Trichomoniasis
EXCLUDES 2 *intestinal trichomoniasis (A07.8)*

✓5th A59.0 Urogenital **trichomoniasis**

A59.00 **Urogenital trichomoniasis, unspecified**
Fluor (vaginalis) due to Trichomonas
Leukorrhea (vaginalis) due to Trichomonas

A59.01 **Trichomonal** vulvovaginitis   ♀

A59.02 **Trichomonal** prostatitis   ♂

A59.03 **Trichomonal** cystitis and urethritis

A59.09 **Other urogenital trichomoniasis**
Trichomonas cervicitis

A59.8 Trichomoniasis of other sites

A59.9 Trichomoniasis, unspecified

✓4th **A60** Anogenital herpesviral [herpes simplex] infections

✓5th A60.0 **Herpesviral infection of** genitalia and urogenital tract

A60.00 **Herpesviral infection of urogenital system, unspecified**

A60.01 **Herpesviral infection of** penis   ♂

A60.02 **Herpesviral infection of** other male genital organs   ♂

A60.03 **Herpesviral** cervicitis   ♀

✓ Additional Character Required   ✓x7th Xtension Alert   Unspecified Code   Other Specified Code   Manifestation Code   ▶◀ Revised Text   ● New Code   ▲ Revised Code Title

ICD-10-CM 2014 (Draft)   **429**

Certain Infectious and Parasitic Diseases

A60.04–A75.1

A60.04　Herpesviral vulvovaginitis ♀
　　　Herpesviral [herpes simplex] ulceration
　　　Herpesviral [herpes simplex] vaginitis
　　　Herpesviral [herpes simplex] vulvitis

A60.09　Herpesviral infection of other urogenital tract

A60.1　Herpesviral infection of perianal skin and rectum

A60.9　Anogenital herpesviral infection, unspecified

✓4ᵗʰ **A63　Other predominantly sexually transmitted diseases, not elsewhere classified**
　　EXCLUDES 2　*molluscum contagiosum (B08.1)*
　　　　　　papilloma of cervix (D26.0)

A63.0　Anogenital (venereal) warts
　　　Anogenital warts due to (human) papillomavirus [HPV]
　　　Condyloma acuminatum

A63.8　Other specified predominantly sexually transmitted diseases

A64　Unspecified sexually transmitted disease

Other spirochetal diseases (A65-A69)
　　EXCLUDES 2　*leptospirosis (A27.-)*
　　　　　　syphilis (A50-A53)

A65　Nonvenereal syphilis
　　Bejel　　　　　　Njovera
　　Endemic syphilis

✓4ᵗʰ **A66　Yaws**
　　INCLUDES　bouba
　　　　　frambesia (tropica)
　　　　　pian

A66.0　Initial lesions of yaws
　　　Chancre of yaws
　　　Frambesia, initial or primary
　　　Initial frambesial ulcer
　　　Mother yaw

A66.1　Multiple papillomata and wet crab yaws
　　　Frambesioma
　　　Pianoma
　　　Plantar or palmar papilloma of yaws

A66.2　Other early skin lesions of yaws
　　　Cutaneous yaws, less than five years after infection
　　　Early yaws (cutaneous) (macular) (maculopapular) (micropapular) (papular)
　　　Frambeside of early yaws

A66.3　Hyperkeratosis of yaws
　　　Ghoul hand
　　　Hyperkeratosis, palmar or plantar (early) (late) due to yaws
　　　Worm-eaten soles

A66.4　Gummata and ulcers of yaws
　　　Gummatous frambeside
　　　Nodular late yaws (ulcerated)

A66.5　Gangosa
　　　Rhinopharyngitis mutilans

A66.6　Bone and joint lesions of yaws
　　　Yaws ganglion　　　　Yaws hydrarthrosis
　　　Yaws goundou　　　　Yaws osteitis
　　　Yaws gumma, bone　　Yaws periostitis (hypertrophic)
　　　Yaws gummatous osteitis or periostitis

A66.7　Other manifestations of yaws
　　　Juxta-articular nodules of yaws
　　　Mucosal yaws

A66.8　Latent yaws
　　　Yaws without clinical manifestations, with positive serology

A66.9　Yaws, unspecified

✓4ᵗʰ **A67　Pinta [carate]**

A67.0　Primary lesions of pinta
　　　Chancre (primary) of pinta
　　　Papule (primary) of pinta

A67.1　Intermediate lesions of pinta
　　　Erythematous plaques of pinta
　　　Hyperchromic lesions of pinta
　　　Hyperkeratosis of pinta
　　　Pintids

A67.2　Late lesions of pinta
　　　Achromic skin lesions of pinta
　　　Cicatricial skin lesions of pinta
　　　Dyschromic skin lesions of pinta

A67.3　Mixed lesions of pinta
　　　Achromic with hyperchromic skin lesions of pinta [carate]

A67.9　Pinta, unspecified

✓4ᵗʰ **A68　Relapsing fevers**
　　INCLUDES　recurrent fever
　　EXCLUDES 2　*Lyme disease (A69.2-)*

A68.0　Louse-borne relapsing fever
　　　Relapsing fever due to Borrelia recurrentis

A68.1　Tick-borne relapsing fever
　　　Relapsing fever due to any Borrelia species other than Borrelia recurrentis

A68.9　Relapsing fever, unspecified

✓4ᵗʰ **A69　Other spirochetal infections**

A69.0　Necrotizing ulcerative stomatitis
　　　Cancrum oris
　　　Fusospirochetal gangrene
　　　Noma
　　　Stomatitis gangrenosa

A69.1　Other Vincent's infections
　　　Fusospirochetal pharyngitis
　　　Necrotizing ulcerative (acute) gingivitis
　　　Necrotizing ulcerative (acute) gingivostomatitis
　　　Spirochetal stomatitis
　　　Trench mouth
　　　Vincent's angina
　　　Vincent's gingivitis

✓5ᵗʰ **A69.2　Lyme disease**
　　　Erythema chronicum migrans due to Borrelia burgdorferi

A69.20　Lyme disease, unspecified

A69.21　Meningitis due to Lyme disease

A69.22　Other neurologic disorders in Lyme disease
　　　Cranial neuritis
　　　Meningoencephalitis
　　　Polyneuropathy

A69.23　Arthritis due to Lyme disease

A69.29　Other conditions associated with Lyme disease
　　　Myopericarditis due to Lyme disease

A69.8　Other specified spirochetal infections

A69.9　Spirochetal infection, unspecified

Other diseases caused by chlamydiae (A70-A74)
　　EXCLUDES 1　*sexually transmitted chlamydial diseases (A55-A56)*

A70　Chlamydia psittaci infections
　　　Ornithosis
　　　Parrot fever
　　　Psittacosis

✓4ᵗʰ **A71　Trachoma**
　　EXCLUDES 1　*sequelae of trachoma (B94.0)*

A71.0　Initial stage of trachoma
　　　Trachoma dubium

A71.1　Active stage of trachoma
　　　Granular conjunctivitis (trachomatous)
　　　Trachomatous follicular conjunctivitis
　　　Trachomatous pannus

A71.9　Trachoma, unspecified

✓4ᵗʰ **A74　Other diseases caused by chlamydiae**
　　EXCLUDES 1　*neonatal chlamydial conjunctivitis (P39.1)*
　　　　　　neonatal chlamydial pneumonia (P23.1)
　　　　　　Reiter's disease (M02.3-)
　　　　　　sexually transmitted chlamydial diseases (A55-A56)
　　EXCLUDES 2　*chlamydial pneumonia (J16.0)*

A74.0　Chlamydial conjunctivitis
　　　Paratrachoma

✓5ᵗʰ **A74.8　Other chlamydial diseases**

A74.81　Chlamydial peritonitis

A74.89　Other chlamydial diseases

A74.9　Chlamydial infection, unspecified
　　　Chlamydiosis NOS

Rickettsioses (A75-A79)

✓4ᵗʰ **A75　Typhus fever**
　　EXCLUDES 1　*rickettsiosis due to Ehrlichia sennetsu (A79.81)*

A75.0　Epidemic louse-borne typhus fever due to Rickettsia prowazekii
　　　Classical typhus (fever)
　　　Epidemic (louse-borne) typhus

A75.1　Recrudescent typhus [Brill's disease]
　　　Brill-Zinsser disease

EXCLUDES 1 Not coded here　　　EXCLUDES 2 Not included here　　　N Newborn Age: 0　　　P Pediatric Age: 0-17　　　M Maternity Age: 12-55　　　A Adult Age: 15-124

430　　　ICD-10-CM 2014 (Draft)

A75.2 Typhus fever due to Rickettsia typhi
   Murine (flea-borne) typhus

A75.3 Typhus fever due to Rickettsia tsutsugamushi
   Scrub (mite-borne) typhus
   Tsutsugamushi fever

A75.9 Typhus fever, unspecified
   Typhus (fever) NOS

√4ᵗʰ **A77 Spotted fever [tick-borne rickettsioses]**

A77.0 Spotted fever due to Rickettsia rickettsii
   Rocky Mountain spotted fever
   Sao Paulo fever

A77.1 Spotted fever due to Rickettsia conorii
   African tick typhus
   Boutonneuse fever
   India tick typhus
   Kenya tick typhus
   Marseilles fever
   Mediterranean tick fever

A77.2 Spotted fever due to Rickettsia siberica
   North Asian tick fever
   Siberian tick typhus

A77.3 Spotted fever due to Rickettsia australis
   Queensland tick typhus

√5ᵗʰ **A77.4 Ehrlichiosis**
   EXCLUDES 1 *Rickettsiosis due to Ehrlichia sennetsu (A79.81)*

A77.40 Ehrlichiosis, unspecified

A77.41 Ehrlichiosis chafeensis [E. chafeensis]

A77.49 Other ehrlichiosis

A77.8 Other spotted fevers

A77.9 Spotted fever, unspecified
   Tick-borne typhus NOS

A78 Q fever
   Infection due to Coxiella burnetii
   Nine Mile fever
   Quadrilateral fever

√4ᵗʰ **A79 Other rickettsioses**

A79.0 Trench fever
   Quintan fever
   Wolhynian fever

A79.1 Rickettsialpox due to Rickettsia akari
   Kew Garden fever
   Vesicular rickettsiosis

√5ᵗʰ **A79.8 Other specified rickettsioses**

A79.81 Rickettsiosis due to Ehrlichia sennetsu

A79.89 Other specified rickettsioses

A79.9 Rickettsiosis, unspecified
   Rickettsial infection NOS

Viral and prion infections of the central nervous system (A80-A89)

EXCLUDES 1 *postpolio syndrome (G14)*
   sequelae of poliomyelitis (B91)
   sequelae of viral encephalitis (B94.1)

√4ᵗʰ **A80 Acute poliomyelitis**

A80.0 Acute paralytic poliomyelitis, vaccine-associated

A80.1 Acute paralytic poliomyelitis, wild virus, imported

A80.2 Acute paralytic poliomyelitis, wild virus, indigenous

√5ᵗʰ **A80.3 Acute paralytic poliomyelitis, other and unspecified**

A80.30 Acute paralytic poliomyelitis, unspecified

A80.39 Other acute paralytic poliomyelitis

A80.4 Acute nonparalytic poliomyelitis

A80.9 Acute poliomyelitis, unspecified

√4ᵗʰ **A81 Atypical virus infections of central nervous system**
   INCLUDES diseases of the central nervous system caused by prions
   Use additional code to identify:
      dementia with behavioral disturbance (F02.81)
      dementia without behavioral disturbance (F02.80)

√5ᵗʰ **A81.0 Creutzfeldt-Jakob disease**

A81.00 Creutzfeldt-Jakob disease, unspecified
   Jakob-Creutzfeldt disease, unspecified

A81.01 Variant Creutzfeldt-Jakob disease
   vCJD

A81.09 Other Creutzfeldt-Jakob disease
   CJD
   Familial Creutzfeldt-Jakob disease
   Iatrogenic Creutzfeldt-Jakob disease
   Sporadic Creutzfeldt-Jakob disease
   Subacute spongiform encephalopathy (with dementia)

A81.1 Subacute sclerosing panencephalitis
   Dawson's inclusion body encephalitis
   Van Bogaert's sclerosing leukoencephalopathy

A81.2 Progressive multifocal leukoencephalopathy
   Multifocal leukoencephalopathy NOS

√5ᵗʰ **A81.8 Other atypical virus infections of central nervous system**

A81.81 Kuru

A81.82 Gerstmann-Sträussler-Scheinker syndrome
   GSS syndrome

A81.83 Fatal familial insomnia
   FFI

A81.89 Other atypical virus infections of central nervous system

A81.9 Atypical virus infection of central nervous system, unspecified
   Prion diseases of the central nervous system NOS

√4ᵗʰ **A82 Rabies**

A82.0 Sylvatic rabies

A82.1 Urban rabies

A82.9 Rabies, unspecified

√4ᵗʰ **A83 Mosquito-borne viral encephalitis**
   INCLUDES mosquito-borne viral meningoencephalitis
   EXCLUDES 2 *Venezuelan equine encephalitis (A92.2)*
      West Nile fever (A92.3-)
      West Nile virus (A92.3-)

A83.0 Japanese encephalitis

A83.1 Western equine encephalitis

A83.2 Eastern equine encephalitis

A83.3 St Louis encephalitis

A83.4 Australian encephalitis
   Kunjin virus disease

A83.5 California encephalitis
   California meningoencephalitis
   La Crosse encephalitis

A83.6 Rocio virus disease

A83.8 Other mosquito-borne viral encephalitis

A83.9 Mosquito-borne viral encephalitis, unspecified

√4ᵗʰ **A84 Tick-borne viral encephalitis**
   INCLUDES tick-borne viral meningoencephalitis

A84.0 Far Eastern tick-borne encephalitis [Russian spring-summer encephalitis]

A84.1 Central European tick-borne encephalitis

A84.8 Other tick-borne viral encephalitis
   Louping ill
   Powassan virus disease

A84.9 Tick-borne viral encephalitis, unspecified

√4ᵗʰ **A85 Other viral encephalitis, not elsewhere classified**
   INCLUDES specified viral encephalomyelitis NEC
      specified viral meningoencephalitis NEC
   EXCLUDES 1 *benign myalgic encephalomyelitis (G93.3)*
      encephalitis due to cytomegalovirus (B25.8)
      encephalitis due to herpesvirus NEC (B10.0-)
      encephalitis due to herpesvirus [herpes simplex] (B00.4)
      encephalitis due to measles virus (B05.0)
      encephalitis due to mumps virus (B26.2)
      encephalitis due to poliomyelitis virus (A80.-)
      encephalitis due to zoster (B02.0
      lymphocytic choriomeningitis (A87.2)

A85.0 Enteroviral encephalitis
   Enteroviral encephalomyelitis

A85.1 Adenoviral encephalitis
   Adenoviral meningoencephalitis

A85.2 Arthropod-borne viral encephalitis, unspecified
   EXCLUDES 1 *West nile virus with encephalitis (A92.31)*

A85.8 Other specified viral encephalitis
   Encephalitis lethargica
   Von Economo-Cruchet disease

☑ Additional Character Required   ᴠ⁷ᵗʰ Xtension Alert   Unspecified Code   Other Specified Code   Manifestation Code   ▶◀ Revised Text   ● New Code   ▲ Revised Code Title

ICD-10-CM 2014 (Draft)   **431**

A86 Unspecified viral encephalitis
Viral encephalomyelitis NOS
Viral meningoencephalitis NOS

✓4ᵗʰ **A87 Viral meningitis**
EXCLUDES 1 *meningitis due to herpesvirus [herpes simplex] (B00.3)*
meningitis due to measles virus (B05.1)
meningitis due to mumps virus (B26.1)
meningitis due to poliomyelitis virus (A80.-)
meningitis due to zoster (B02.1)

A87.0 Enteroviral meningitis
Coxsackievirus meningitis
Echovirus meningitis

A87.1 Adenoviral meningitis

A87.2 Lymphocytic choriomeningitis
Lymphocytic meningoencephalitis

A87.8 Other viral meningitis

A87.9 Viral meningitis, unspecified

✓4ᵗʰ **A88 Other viral infections of central nervous system, not elsewhere classified**
EXCLUDES 1 *viral encephalitis NOS (A86)*
viral meningitis NOS (A87.9)

A88.0 Enteroviral exanthematous fever [Boston exanthem]

A88.1 Epidemic vertigo

A88.8 Other specified viral infections of central nervous system

A89 Unspecified viral infection of central nervous system

Arthropod-borne viral fevers and viral hemorrhagic fevers (A90-A99)

A90 Dengue fever [classical dengue]
EXCLUDES 1 *dengue hemorrhagic fever (A91)*

A91 Dengue hemorrhagic fever

✓4ᵗʰ **A92 Other mosquito-borne viral fevers**
EXCLUDES 1 *Ross River disease (B33.1)*

A92.0 Chikungunya virus disease
Chikungunya (hemorrhagic) fever

A92.1 O'nyong-nyong fever

A92.2 Venezuelan equine fever
Venezuelan equine encephalitis
Venezuelan equine encephalomyelitis virus disease

✓5ᵗʰ **A92.3 West Nile virus infection**
West Nile fever

A92.30 West Nile virus infection, unspecified
West Nile fever NOS
West Nile fever without complications
West Nile virus NOS

A92.31 West Nile virus infection with encephalitis
West Nile encephalitis
West Nile encephalomyelitis

A92.32 West Nile virus infection with other neurologic manifestation
Use additional code to specify the neurologic manifestation

A92.39 West Nile virus infection with other complications
Use additional code to specify the other conditions

A92.4 Rift Valley fever

A92.8 Other specified mosquito-borne viral fevers

A92.9 Mosquito-borne viral fever, unspecified

✓4ᵗʰ **A93 Other arthropod-borne viral fevers, not elsewhere classified**

A93.0 Oropouche virus disease
Oropouche fever

A93.1 Sandfly fever
Pappataci fever
Phlebotomus fever

A93.2 Colorado tick fever

A93.8 Other specified arthropod-borne viral fevers
Piry virus disease
Vesicular stomatitis virus disease [Indiana fever]

A94 Unspecified arthropod-borne viral fever
Arboviral fever NOS
Arbovirus infection NOS

✓4ᵗʰ **A95 Yellow fever**

A95.0 Sylvatic yellow fever
Jungle yellow fever

A95.1 Urban yellow fever

A95.9 Yellow fever, unspecified

✓4ᵗʰ **A96 Arenaviral hemorrhagic fever**

A96.0 Junin hemorrhagic fever
Argentinian hemorrhagic fever

A96.1 Machupo hemorrhagic fever
Bolivian hemorrhagic fever

A96.2 Lassa fever

A96.8 Other arenaviral hemorrhagic fevers

A96.9 Arenaviral hemorrhagic fever, unspecified

✓4ᵗʰ **A98 Other viral hemorrhagic fevers, not elsewhere classified**
EXCLUDES 1 *chikungunya hemorrhagic fever (A92.0)*
dengue hemorrhagic fever (A91)

A98.0 Crimean-Congo hemorrhagic fever
Central Asian hemorrhagic fever

A98.1 Omsk hemorrhagic fever

A98.2 Kyasanur Forest disease

A98.3 Marburg virus disease

A98.4 Ebola virus disease

A98.5 Hemorrhagic fever with renal syndrome
Epidemic hemorrhagic fever
Korean hemorrhagic fever
Russian hemorrhagic fever
Hantaan virus disease
Hantavirus disease with renal manifestations
Nephropathia epidemica
Songo fever
EXCLUDES 1 *hantavirus (cardio)-pulmonary syndrome (B33.4)*

A98.8 Other specified viral hemorrhagic fevers

A99 Unspecified viral hemorrhagic fever

Viral infections characterized by skin and mucous membrane lesions (B00-B09)

✓4ᵗʰ **B00 Herpesviral [herpes simplex] infections**
EXCLUDES 1 *congenital herpesviral infections (P35.2)*
EXCLUDES 2 *anogenital herpesviral infection (A60.-)*
gammaherpesviral mononucleosis (B27.0-)
herpangina (B08.5)

B00.0 Eczema herpeticum
Kaposi's varicelliform eruption

B00.1 Herpesviral vesicular dermatitis
Herpes simplex facialis
Herpes simplex labialis
Herpes simplex otitis externa
Vesicular dermatitis of ear
Vesicular dermatitis of lip

B00.2 Herpesviral gingivostomatitis and pharyngotonsillitis
Herpesviral pharyngitis

B00.3 Herpesviral meningitis

B00.4 Herpesviral encephalitis
Herpesviral meningoencephalitis
Simian B disease
EXCLUDES 1 *herpesviral encephalitis due to herpesvirus 6 and 7 (B10.01, B10.09)*
non-simplex herpesviral encephalitis (B10.0-)

✓5ᵗʰ **B00.5 Herpesviral ocular disease**

B00.50 Herpesviral ocular disease, unspecified

B00.51 Herpesviral iridocyclitis
Herpesviral iritis
Herpesviral uveitis, anterior

B00.52 Herpesviral keratitis
Herpesviral keratoconjunctivitis

B00.53 Herpesviral conjunctivitis

B00.59 Other herpesviral disease of eye
Herpesviral dermatitis of eyelid

B00.7 Disseminated herpesviral disease
Herpesviral sepsis

✓5ᵗʰ **B00.8 Other forms of herpesviral infections**

B00.81 Herpesviral hepatitis

B00.82 Herpes simplex myelitis

B00.89 Other herpesviral infection
Herpesviral whitlow

B00.9 Herpesviral infection, unspecified
Herpes simplex infection NOS

EXCLUDES 1 Not coded here   *EXCLUDES 2* Not included here   Ⓝ Newborn Age: 0   Ⓟ Pediatric Age: 0-17   Ⓜ Maternity Age: 12-55   Ⓐ Adult Age: 15-124

432   ICD-10-CM 2014 (Draft)

Certain Infectious and Parasitic Diseases

B01–B09

☑4ᵗʰ **B01 Varicella [chickenpox]**

B01.0 Varicella meningitis

☑5ᵗʰ **B01.1 Varicella** encephalitis, myelitis and encephalomyelitis
Postchickenpox encephalitis, myelitis and encephalomyelitis

B01.11 Varicella encephalitis and encephalomyelitis
Postchickenpox encephalitis and encephalomyelitis

B01.12 Varicella myelitis
Postchickenpox myelitis

B01.2 Varicella pneumonia

☑5ᵗʰ **B01.8 Varicella with** other complications

B01.81 Varicella keratitis

B01.89 Other varicella complications

B01.9 Varicella without complication
Varicella NOS

☑4ᵗʰ **B02 Zoster [herpes zoster]**

INCLUDES shingles
zona

B02.0 Zoster encephalitis
Zoster meningoencephalitis

B02.1 Zoster meningitis

☑5ᵗʰ **B02.2 Zoster with** other nervous system **involvement**

B02.21 Postherpetic geniculate ganglionitis

B02.22 Postherpetic trigeminal neuralgia

B02.23 Postherpetic polyneuropathy

B02.24 Postherpetic myelitis
Herpes zoster myelitis

B02.29 Other postherpetic nervous system involvement
Postherpetic radiculopathy

☑5ᵗʰ **B02.3 Zoster** ocular **disease**

B02.30 Zoster ocular disease, unspecified

B02.31 Zoster conjunctivitis

B02.32 Zoster iridocyclitis

B02.33 Zoster keratitis
Herpes zoster keratoconjunctivitis

B02.34 Zoster scleritis

B02.39 Other herpes zoster eye disease
Zoster blepharitis

B02.7 Disseminated zoster

B02.8 Zoster with other complications
Herpes zoster otitis externa

B02.9 Zoster without complications
Zoster NOS

B03 Smallpox

NOTE In 1980 the 33rd World Health Assembly declared that smallpox had been eradicated.
The classification is maintained for surveillance purposes.

B04 Monkeypox

☑4ᵗʰ **B05 Measles**

INCLUDES morbilli
EXCLUDES 1 subacute sclerosing panencephalitis (A81.1)

B05.0 Measles complicated by encephalitis
Postmeasles encephalitis

B05.1 Measles complicated by meningitis
Postmeasles meningitis

B05.2 Measles complicated by pneumonia
Postmeasles pneumonia

B05.3 Measles complicated by otitis media
Postmeasles otitis media

B05.4 Measles with intestinal **complications**

☑5ᵗʰ **B05.8 Measles with** other complications

B05.81 Measles keratitis and keratoconjunctivitis

B05.89 Other measles complications

B05.9 Measles without complication
Measles NOS

☑4ᵗʰ **B06 Rubella [German measles]**

EXCLUDES 1 congenital rubella (P35.0)

☑5ᵗʰ **B06.0 Rubella with** neurological complications

B06.00 Rubella with neurological complication, unspecified

B06.01 Rubella encephalitis
Rubella meningoencephalitis

B06.02 Rubella meningitis

B06.09 Other neurological complications of rubella

☑5ᵗʰ **B06.8 Rubella with** other complications

B06.81 Rubella pneumonia

B06.82 Rubella arthritis

B06.89 Other rubella complications

B06.9 Rubella without complication
Rubella NOS

☑4ᵗʰ **B07 Viral warts**

INCLUDES verruca simplex
verruca vulgaris
viral warts due to human papillomavirus
EXCLUDES 2 anogenital (venereal) warts (A63.0)
papilloma of bladder (D41.4)
papilloma of cervix (D26.0)
papilloma larynx (D14.1)

B07.0 Plantar wart
Verruca plantaris

B07.8 Other viral warts
Common wart
Flat wart
Verruca plana

B07.9 Viral wart, unspecified

☑4ᵗʰ **B08 Other viral infections characterized by skin and mucous membrane lesions, not elsewhere classified**

EXCLUDES 1 vesicular stomatitis virus disease (A93.8)

☑5ᵗʰ **B08.0 Other orthopoxvirus infections**

EXCLUDES 2 monkeypox (B04)

☑6ᵗʰ **B08.01 Cowpox and vaccinia not from vaccine**

B08.010 Cowpox

B08.011 Vaccinia not from vaccine
EXCLUDES 1 vaccinia (from vaccination) (generalized) (T88.1)

B08.02 Orf virus disease
Contagious pustular dermatitis
Ecthyma contagiosum

B08.03 Pseudocowpox [milker's node]

B08.04 Paravaccinia, unspecified

B08.09 Other orthopoxvirus infections
Orthopoxvirus infection NOS

B08.1 Molluscum contagiosum

☑5ᵗʰ **B08.2 Exanthema subitum [sixth disease]**
Roseola infantum

B08.20 Exanthema subitum [sixth disease], unspecified P
Roseola infantum, unspecified

B08.21 Exanthema subitum [sixth disease] due to human P **herpesvirus 6**
Roseola infantum due to human herpesvirus 6

B08.22 Exanthema subitum [sixth disease] due to human P **herpesvirus 7**
Roseola infantum due to human herpesvirus 7

B08.3 Erythema infectiosum [fifth disease]

B08.4 Enteroviral vesicular stomatitis with exanthem
Hand, foot and mouth disease

B08.5 Enteroviral vesicular pharyngitis
Herpangina

☑5ᵗʰ **B08.6 Parapoxvirus infections**

B08.60 Parapoxvirus infection, unspecified

B08.61 Bovine stomatitis

B08.62 Sealpox

B08.69 Other parapoxvirus infections

☑5ᵗʰ **B08.7 Yatapoxvirus infections**

B08.70 Yatapoxvirus infection, unspecified

B08.71 Tanapox virus disease

B08.72 Yaba pox virus disease
Yaba monkey tumor disease

B08.79 Other yatapoxvirus infections

B08.8 Other specified viral infections characterized by skin and mucous membrane lesions
Enteroviral lymphonodular pharyngitis
Foot-and-mouth disease
Poxvirus NEC

B09 Unspecified viral infection characterized by skin and mucous membrane lesions
Viral enanthema NOS
Viral exanthema NOS

☑ Additional Character Required   ⁵ˣ⁷ᵗʰ Xtension Alert   Unspecified Code   Other Specified Code   Manifestation Code   ▶◀ Revised Text   ● New Code   ▲ Revised Code Title

ICD-10-CM 2014 (Draft)   **433**

B10–B27.82

Other human herpesviruses (B10)

B10 Other human herpesviruses

EXCLUDES 2 cytomegalovirus (B25.9)
Epstein-Barr virus (B27.0-)
herpes NOS (B00.9)
herpes simplex (B00.-)
herpes zoster (B02.-)
human herpesvirus NOS (B00.-)
human herpesvirus 1 and 2 (B00.-)
human herpesvirus 3 (B01.-, B02.-)
human herpesvirus 4 (B27.0-)
human herpesvirus 5 (B25.-)
varicella (B01.-)
zoster (B02.-)

B10.0 Other human herpesvirus encephalitis

EXCLUDES 2 herpes encephalitis NOS (B00.4)
herpes simplex encephalitis (B00.4)
human herpesvirus encephalitis (B00.4)
simian B herpes virus encephalitis (B00.4)

B10.01 Human herpesvirus 6 encephalitis

B10.09 Other human herpesvirus encephalitis
Human herpesvirus 7 encephalitis

B10.8 Other human herpesvirus infection

B10.81 Human herpesvirus 6 infection

B10.82 Human herpesvirus 7 infection

B10.89 Other human herpesvirus infection
Human herpesvirus 8 infection
Kaposi's sarcoma-associated herpesvirus infection

Viral hepatitis (B15-B19)

EXCLUDES 1 sequelae of viral hepatitis (B94.2)
EXCLUDES 2 cytomegaloviral hepatitis (B25.1)
herpesviral [herpes simplex] hepatitis (B00.81)

B15 Acute hepatitis A

B15.0 Hepatitis A with hepatic coma

B15.9 Hepatitis A without hepatic coma
Hepatitis A (acute)(viral) NOS

B16 Acute hepatitis B

B16.0 Acute hepatitis B with delta-agent with hepatic coma

B16.1 Acute hepatitis B with delta-agent without hepatic coma

B16.2 Acute hepatitis B without delta-agent with hepatic coma

B16.9 Acute hepatitis B without delta-agent and without hepatic coma
Hepatitis B (acute) (viral) NOS

B17 Other acute viral hepatitis

B17.0 Acute delta-(super) infection of hepatitis B carrier

B17.1 Acute hepatitis C

B17.10 Acute hepatitis C without hepatic coma
Acute hepatitis C NOS

B17.11 Acute hepatitis C with hepatic coma

B17.2 Acute hepatitis E

B17.8 Other specified acute viral hepatitis
Hepatitis non-A non-B (acute) (viral) NEC

B17.9 Acute viral hepatitis, unspecified
Acute hepatitis NOS

B18 Chronic viral hepatitis

B18.0 Chronic viral hepatitis B with delta-agent

B18.1 Chronic viral hepatitis B without delta-agent
Chronic (viral) hepatitis B

B18.2 Chronic viral hepatitis C

B18.8 Other chronic viral hepatitis

B18.9 Chronic viral hepatitis, unspecified

B19 Unspecified viral hepatitis

B19.0 Unspecified viral hepatitis with hepatic coma

B19.1 Unspecified viral hepatitis B

B19.10 Unspecified viral hepatitis B without hepatic coma
Unspecified viral hepatitis B NOS

B19.11 Unspecified viral hepatitis B with hepatic coma

B19.2 Unspecified viral hepatitis C

B19.20 Unspecified viral hepatitis C without hepatic coma
Viral hepatitis C NOS

B19.21 Unspecified viral hepatitis C with hepatic coma

B19.9 Unspecified viral hepatitis without hepatic coma
Viral hepatitis NOS

Human immunodeficiency virus [HIV] disease (B20)

B20 Human immunodeficiency virus [HIV] disease

INCLUDES acquired immune deficiency syndrome [AIDS]
AIDS-related complex [ARC]
HIV infection, symptomatic

Code first human immunodeficiency virus [HIV] disease complicating pregnancy, childbirth and the puerperium, if applicable (O98.7-)
Use additional code(s) to identify all manifestations of HIV infection

EXCLUDES 1 asymptomatic human immunodeficiency virus [HIV] infection status (Z21)
exposure to HIV virus (Z20.6)
inconclusive serologic evidence of HIV (R75)

Other viral diseases (B25-B34)

B25 Cytomegaloviral disease

EXCLUDES 1 congenital cytomegalovirus infection (P35.1)
cytomegaloviral mononucleosis (B27.1-)

B25.0 Cytomegaloviral pneumonitis

B25.1 Cytomegaloviral hepatitis

B25.2 Cytomegaloviral pancreatitis

B25.8 Other cytomegaloviral diseases
Cytomegaloviral encephalitis

B25.9 Cytomegaloviral disease, unspecified

B26 Mumps

INCLUDES epidemic parotitis
infectious parotitis

B26.0 Mumps orchitis

B26.1 Mumps meningitis

B26.2 Mumps encephalitis

B26.3 Mumps pancreatitis

B26.8 Mumps with other complications

B26.81 Mumps hepatitis

B26.82 Mumps myocarditis

B26.83 Mumps nephritis

B26.84 Mumps polyneuropathy

B26.85 Mumps arthritis

B26.89 Other mumps complications

B26.9 Mumps without complication
Mumps NOS
Mumps parotitis NOS

B27 Infectious mononucleosis

INCLUDES glandular fever
monocytic angina
Pfeiffer's disease

B27.0 Gammaherpesviral mononucleosis
Mononucleosis due to Epstein-Barr virus

B27.00 Gammaherpesviral mononucleosis without complication

B27.01 Gammaherpesviral mononucleosis with polyneuropathy

B27.02 Gammaherpesviral mononucleosis with meningitis

B27.09 Gammaherpesviral mononucleosis with other complications
Hepatomegaly in gammaherpesviral mononucleosis

B27.1 Cytomegaloviral mononucleosis

B27.10 Cytomegaloviral mononucleosis without complications

B27.11 Cytomegaloviral mononucleosis with polyneuropathy

B27.12 Cytomegaloviral mononucleosis with meningitis

B27.19 Cytomegaloviral mononucleosis with other complication
Hepatomegaly in cytomegaloviral mononucleosis

B27.8 Other infectious mononucleosis

B27.80 Other infectious mononucleosis without complication

B27.81 Other infectious mononucleosis with polyneuropathy

B27.82 Other infectious mononucleosis with meningitis

B27.89 Other infectious mononucleosis with other complication
Hepatomegaly in other infectious mononucleosis

√5ᵗʰ **B27.9 Infectious mononucleosis, unspecified**

B27.90 Infectious mononucleosis, unspecified without complication

B27.91 Infectious mononucleosis, unspecified with polyneuropathy

B27.92 Infectious mononucleosis, unspecified with meningitis

B27.99 Infectious mononucleosis, unspecified with other complication
Hepatomegaly in unspecified infectious mononucleosis

√4ᵗʰ **B30 Viral conjunctivitis**
EXCLUDES 1 herpesviral [herpes simplex] ocular disease (B00.5)
ocular zoster (B02.3)

B30.0 Keratoconjunctivitis due to adenovirus
Epidemic keratoconjunctivitis
Shipyard eye

B30.1 Conjunctivitis due to adenovirus
Acute adenoviral follicular conjunctivitis
Swimming-pool conjunctivitis

B30.2 Viral pharyngoconjunctivitis

B30.3 Acute epidemic hemorrhagic conjunctivitis (enteroviral)
Conjunctivitis due to coxsackievirus 24
Conjunctivitis due to enterovirus 70
Hemorrhagic conjunctivitis (acute)(epidemic)

B30.8 Other viral conjunctivitis
Newcastle conjunctivitis

B30.9 Viral conjunctivitis, unspecified

√4ᵗʰ **B33 Other viral diseases, not elsewhere classified**

B33.0 Epidemic myalgia
Bornholm disease

B33.1 Ross River disease
Epidemic polyarthritis and exanthema
Ross River fever

√5ᵗʰ **B33.2 Viral carditis**
Coxsackie (virus) carditis

B33.20 Viral carditis, unspecified

B33.21 Viral endocarditis

B33.22 Viral myocarditis

B33.23 Viral pericarditis

B33.24 Viral cardiomyopathy

B33.3 Retrovirus infections, not elsewhere classified
Retrovirus infection NOS

B33.4 Hantavirus (cardio)-pulmonary syndrome [HPS] [HCPS]
Hantavirus disease with pulmonary manifestations
Sin nombre virus disease
Use additional code to identify any associated acute kidney failure (N17.9)
EXCLUDES 1 hantavirus disease with renal manifestations (A98.5)
hemorrhagic fever with renal manifestations (A98.5)

B33.8 Other specified viral diseases
EXCLUDES 1 anogenital human papillomavirus infection (A63.0)
viral warts due to human papillomavirus infection (B07)

√4ᵗʰ **B34 Viral infection of unspecified site**
EXCLUDES 1 anogenital human papillomavirus infection (A63.0)
cytomegaloviral disease NOS (B25.9)
herpesvirus [herpes simplex] infection NOS (B00.9)
retrovirus infection NOS (B33.3)
viral agents as the cause of diseases classified elsewhere (B97.-)
viral warts due to human papillomavirus infection (B07)

B34.0 Adenovirus infection, unspecified

B34.1 Enterovirus infection, unspecified
Coxsackievirus infection NOS
Echovirus infection NOS

B34.2 Coronavirus infection, unspecified
EXCLUDES 1 pneumonia due to SARS-associated coronavirus (J12.81)

B34.3 Parvovirus infection, unspecified

B34.4 Papovavirus infection, unspecified

B34.8 Other viral infections of unspecified site

B34.9 Viral infection, unspecified
Viremia NOS

Mycoses (B35-B49)
EXCLUDES 2 hypersensitivity pneumonitis due to organic dust (J67.-)
mycosis fungoides (C84.0-)

√4ᵗʰ **B35 Dermatophytosis**
INCLUDES favus
infections due to species of Epidermophyton, Micro-sporum and Trichophyton
tinea, any type except those in B36-

B35.0 Tinea barbae and tinea capitis
Beard ringworm
Kerion
Scalp ringworm
Sycosis, mycotic

B35.1 Tinea unguium
Dermatophytic onychia
Dermatophytosis of nail
Onychomycosis
Ringworm of nails

B35.2 Tinea manuum
Dermatophytosis of hand
Hand ringworm

B35.3 Tinea pedis
Athlete's foot
Dermatophytosis of foot
Foot ringworm

B35.4 Tinea corporis
Ringworm of the body

B35.5 Tinea imbricata
Tokelau

B35.6 Tinea cruris
Dhobi itch
Groin ringworm
Jock itch

B35.8 Other dermatophytoses
Disseminated dermatophytosis
Granulomatous dermatophytosis

B35.9 Dermatophytosis, unspecified
Ringworm NOS

√4ᵗʰ **B36 Other superficial mycoses**

B36.0 Pityriasis versicolor
Tinea flava
Tinea versicolor

B36.1 Tinea nigra
Keratomycosis nigricans palmaris
Microsporosis nigra
Pityriasis nigra

B36.2 White piedra
Tinea blanca

B36.3 Black piedra

B36.8 Other specified superficial mycoses

B36.9 Superficial mycosis, unspecified

√4ᵗʰ **B37 Candidiasis**
INCLUDES candidosis
moniliasis
EXCLUDES 1 neonatal candidiasis (P37.5)

B37.0 Candidal stomatitis
Oral thrush

B37.1 Pulmonary candidiasis
Candidal bronchitis
Candidal pneumonia

B37.2 Candidiasis of skin and nail
Candidal onychia
Candidal paronychia
EXCLUDES 2 diaper dermatitis (L22)

B37.3 Candidiasis of vulva and vagina ♀
Candidal vulvovaginitis
Monilial vulvovaginitis
Vaginal thrush

√5ᵗʰ **B37.4 Candidiasis of other urogenital sites**

B37.41 Candidal cystitis and urethritis

B37.42 Candidal balanitis

B37.49 Other urogenital candidiasis
Candidal pyelonephritis

B37.5 Candidal meningitis

B37.6 Candidal endocarditis

B37.7 Candidal sepsis
Disseminated candidiasis
Systemic candidiasis

☑ Additional Character Required   ✗7ᵗʰ Xtension Alert   Unspecified Code   Other Specified Code   Manifestation Code   ▶◀ Revised Text   ● New Code   ▲ Revised Code Title

Certain Infectious and Parasitic Diseases

B37.8–B49

✓5ᵗʰ **B37.8 Candidiasis of** other sites

    B37.81 Candidal esophagitis

    B37.82 Candidal enteritis
        Candidal proctitis

    B37.83 Candidal cheilitis

    B37.84 Candidal otitis externa

    B37.89 Other sites of candidiasis
        Candidal osteomyelitis

  B37.9 Candidiasis, unspecified
    Thrush NOS

✓4ᵗʰ **B38 Coccidioidomycosis**

  B38.0 Acute pulmonary coccidioidomycosis

  B38.1 Chronic pulmonary coccidioidomycosis

  B38.2 Pulmonary coccidioidomycosis, unspecified

  B38.3 Cutaneous coccidioidomycosis

  B38.4 Coccidioidomycosis meningitis

  B38.7 Disseminated coccidioidomycosis
    Generalized coccidioidomycosis

✓5ᵗʰ **B38.8 Other forms of coccidioidomycosis**

    B38.81 Prostatic coccidioidomycosis ♂

    B38.89 Other forms of coccidioidomycosis

  B38.9 Coccidioidomycosis, unspecified

✓4ᵗʰ **B39 Histoplasmosis**

  Code first associated AIDS (B20)
  Use additional code for any associated manifestations, such as:
    endocarditis (I39)
    meningitis (G02)
    pericarditis (I32)
    retinitits (H32)

  B39.0 Acute pulmonary histoplasmosis capsulati

  B39.1 Chronic pulmonary histoplasmosis capsulati

  B39.2 Pulmonary histoplasmosis capsulati, unspecified

  B39.3 Disseminated histoplasmosis capsulati
    Generalized histoplasmosis capsulati

  B39.4 Histoplasmosis capsulati, unspecified
    American histoplasmosis

  B39.5 Histoplasmosis duboisii
    African histoplasmosis

  B39.9 Histoplasmosis, unspecified

✓4ᵗʰ **B40 Blastomycosis**

  EXCLUDES 1 Brazilian blastomycosis (B41.-)
        keloidal blastomycosis (B48.0)

  B40.0 Acute pulmonary blastomycosis

  B40.1 Chronic pulmonary blastomycosis

  B40.2 Pulmonary blastomycosis, unspecified

  B40.3 Cutaneous blastomycosis

  B40.7 Disseminated blastomycosis
    Generalized blastomycosis

✓5ᵗʰ **B40.8 Other forms of blastomycosis**

    B40.81 Blastomycotic meningoencephalitis
        Meningomyelitis due to blastomycosis

    B40.89 Other forms of blastomycosis

  B40.9 Blastomycosis, unspecified

✓4ᵗʰ **B41 Paracoccidioidomycosis**

  INCLUDES Brazilian blastomycosis
        Lutz' disease

  B41.0 Pulmonary paracoccidioidomycosis

  B41.7 Disseminated paracoccidioidomycosis
    Generalized paracoccidioidomycosis

  B41.8 Other forms of paracoccidioidomycosis

  B41.9 Paracoccidioidomycosis, unspecified

✓4ᵗʰ **B42 Sporotrichosis**

  B42.0 Pulmonary sporotrichosis

  B42.1 Lymphocutaneous sporotrichosis

  B42.7 Disseminated sporotrichosis
    Generalized sporotrichosis

✓5ᵗʰ **B42.8 Other forms of sporotrichosis**

    B42.81 Cerebral sporotrichosis
        Meningitis due to sporotrichosis

    B42.82 Sporotrichosis arthritis

    B42.89 Other forms of sporotrichosis

  B42.9 Sporotrichosis, unspecified

✓4ᵗʰ **B43 Chromomycosis and pheomycotic abscess**

  B43.0 Cutaneous chromomycosis
    Dermatitis verrucosa

  B43.1 Pheomycotic brain abscess
    Cerebral chromomycosis

  B43.2 Subcutaneous pheomycotic abscess and cyst

  B43.8 Other forms of chromomycosis

  B43.9 Chromomycosis, unspecified

✓4ᵗʰ **B44 Aspergillosis**

  INCLUDES aspergilloma

  B44.0 Invasive pulmonary aspergillosis

  B44.1 Other pulmonary aspergillosis

  B44.2 Tonsillar aspergillosis

  B44.7 Disseminated aspergillosis
    Generalized aspergillosis

✓5ᵗʰ **B44.8 Other forms of aspergillosis**

    B44.81 Allergic bronchopulmonary aspergillosis

    B44.89 Other forms of aspergillosis

  B44.9 Aspergillosis, unspecified

✓4ᵗʰ **B45 Cryptococcosis**

  B45.0 Pulmonary cryptococcosis

  B45.1 Cerebral cryptococcosis
    Cryptococcal meningitis
    Cryptococcosis meningocerebralis

  B45.2 Cutaneous cryptococcosis

  B45.3 Osseous cryptococcosis

  B45.7 Disseminated cryptococcosis
    Generalized cryptococcosis

  B45.8 Other forms of cryptococcosis

  B45.9 Cryptococcosis, unspecified

✓4ᵗʰ **B46 Zygomycosis**

  B46.0 Pulmonary mucormycosis

  B46.1 Rhinocerebral mucormycosis

  B46.2 Gastrointestinal mucormycosis

  B46.3 Cutaneous mucormycosis
    Subcutaneous mucormycosis

  B46.4 Disseminated mucormycosis
    Generalized mucormycosis

  B46.5 Mucormycosis, unspecified

  B46.8 Other zygomycoses
    Entomophthoromycosis

  B46.9 Zygomycosis, unspecified
    Phycomycosis NOS

✓4ᵗʰ **B47 Mycetoma**

  B47.0 Eumycetoma
    Madura foot, mycotic
    Maduromycosis

  B47.1 Actinomycetoma

  B47.9 Mycetoma, unspecified
    Madura foot NOS

✓4ᵗʰ **B48 Other mycoses, not elsewhere classified**

  B48.0 Lobomycosis
    Keloidal blastomycosis
    Lobo's disease

  B48.1 Rhinosporidiosis

  B48.2 Allescheriasis
    Infection due to Pseudallescheria boydii
    EXCLUDES 1 eumycetoma (B47.0)

  B48.3 Geotrichosis
    Geotrichum stomatitis

  B48.4 Penicillosis

  B48.8 Other specified mycoses
    Adiaspiromycosis
    Infection of tissue and organs by Alternaria
    Infection of tissue and organs by Drechslera
    Infection of tissue and organs by Fusarium
    Infection of tissue and organs by saprophytic fungi NEC

B49 Unspecified mycosis
  Fungemia NOS

EXCLUDES 1 Not coded here   **EXCLUDES 2** Not included here   **N** Newborn Age: 0   **P** Pediatric Age: 0-17   **M** Maternity Age: 12-55   **A** Adult Age: 15-124

Protozoal diseases (B50-B64)

EXCLUDES1   amebiasis (A06.-)
other protozoal intestinal diseases (A07.-)

✓4th **B50**   **Plasmodium falciparum malaria**
   INCLUDES   mixed infections of Plasmodium falciparum with any other Plasmodium species

   B50.0   **Plasmodium falciparum malaria with cerebral complications**
     Cerebral malaria NOS

   B50.8   **Other severe and complicated Plasmodium falciparum malaria**
     Severe or complicated Plasmodium falciparum malaria NOS

   B50.9   **Plasmodium falciparum malaria, unspecified**

✓4th **B51**   **Plasmodium vivax malaria**
   INCLUDES   mixed infections of Plasmodium vivax with other Plasmodium species, except Plasmodium falciparum
     EXCLUDES1   plasmodium vivax with Plasmodium falciparum (B50.-)

   B51.0   **Plasmodium vivax malaria with rupture of spleen**

   B51.8   **Plasmodium vivax malaria with other complications**

   B51.9   **Plasmodium vivax malaria without complication**
     Plasmodium vivax malaria NOS

✓4th **B52**   **Plasmodium malariae malaria**
   INCLUDES   mixed infections of Plasmodium malariae with other Plasmodium species, except Plasmodium falciparum and Plasmodium vivax
     EXCLUDES1   Plasmodium falciparum (B50.-)
     Plasmodium vivax (B51.-)

   B52.0   **Plasmodium malariae malaria with nephropathy**

   B52.8   **Plasmodium malariae malaria with other complications**

   B52.9   **Plasmodium malariae malaria without complication**
     Plasmodium malariae malaria NOS

✓4th **B53**   **Other specified malaria**

   B53.0   **Plasmodium ovale malaria**
     EXCLUDES1   Plasmodium ovale with Plasmodium falciparum (B50.-)
     Plasmodium ovale with Plasmodium malariae (B52.-)
     Plasmodium ovale with Plasmodium vivax (B51.-)

   B53.1   **Malaria due to simian plasmodia**
     EXCLUDES1   Malaria due to simian plasmodia with Plasmodium falciparum (B50.-)
     Malaria du e to simian plasmodia with Plasmodium malariae (B52.-)
     Malaria due to simian plasmodia with Plasmodium ovale (B53.0)
     Malaria due to simian plasmodia with Plasmodium vivax (B51.-)

   B53.8   **Other malaria, not elsewhere classified**

   B54   **Unspecified malaria**

✓4th **B55**   **Leishmaniasis**

   B55.0   **Visceral leishmaniasis**
     Kala-azar
     Post-kala-azar dermal leishmaniasis

   B55.1   **Cutaneous leishmaniasis**

   B55.2   **Mucocutaneous leishmaniasis**

   B55.9   **Leishmaniasis, unspecified**

✓4th **B56**   **African trypanosomiasis**

   B56.0   **Gambiense trypanosomiasis**
     Infection due to Trypanosoma brucei gambiense
     West African sleeping sickness

   B56.1   **Rhodesiense trypanosomiasis**
     East African sleeping sickness
     Infection due to Trypanosoma brucei rhodesiense

   B56.9   **African trypanosomiasis, unspecified**
     Sleeping sickness NOS

✓4th **B57**   **Chagas' disease**
   INCLUDES   American trypanosomiasis
     infection due to Trypanosoma cruzi

   B57.0   **Acute Chagas' disease with heart involvement**
     Acute Chagas' disease with myocarditis

   B57.1   **Acute Chagas' disease without heart involvement**
     Acute Chagas' disease NOS

   B57.2   **Chagas' disease (chronic) with heart involvement**
     American trypanosomiasis NOS
     Chagas' disease (chronic) NOS
     Chagas' disease (chronic) with myocarditis
     Trypanosomiasis NOS

✓5th **B57.3**   **Chagas' disease (chronic) with digestive system involvement**

   B57.30   **Chagas' disease with digestive system involvement, unspecified**

   B57.31   **Megaesophagus in Chagas' disease**

   B57.32   **Megacolon in Chagas' disease**

   B57.39   **Other digestive system involvement in Chagas' disease**

✓5th **B57.4**   **Chagas' disease (chronic) with nervous system involvement**

   B57.40   **Chagas' disease with nervous system involvement, unspecified**

   B57.41   **Meningitis in Chagas' disease**

   B57.42   **Meningoencephalitis in Chagas' disease**

   B57.49   **Other nervous system involvement in Chagas' disease**

   B57.5   **Chagas' disease (chronic) with other organ involvement**

✓4th **B58**   **Toxoplasmosis**
   INCLUDES   infection due to Toxoplasma gondii
     EXCLUDES1   congenital toxoplasmosis (P37.1)

✓5th **B58.0**   **Toxoplasma oculopathy**

   B58.00   **Toxoplasma oculopathy, unspecified**

   B58.01   **Toxoplasma chorioretinitis**

   B58.09   **Other toxoplasma oculopathy**
     Toxoplasma uveitis

   B58.1   **Toxoplasma hepatitis**

   B58.2   **Toxoplasma meningoencephalitis**

   B58.3   **Pulmonary toxoplasmosis**

✓5th **B58.8**   **Toxoplasmosis with other organ involvement**

   B58.81   **Toxoplasma myocarditis**

   B58.82   **Toxoplasma myositis**

   B58.83   **Toxoplasma tubulo-interstitial nephropathy**
     Toxoplasma pyelonephritis

   B58.89   **Toxoplasmosis with other organ involvement**

   B58.9   **Toxoplasmosis, unspecified**

   B59   **Pneumocystosis**
     Pneumonia due to Pneumocystis carinii
     Pneumonia due to Pneumocystis jiroveci

✓4th **B60**   **Other protozoal diseases, not elsewhere classified**
     EXCLUDES1   cryptosporidiosis (A07.2)
     intestinal microsporidiosis (A07.8)
     isosporiasis (A07.3)

   B60.0   **Babesiosis**
     Piroplasmosis

✓5th **B60.1**   **Acanthamebiasis**

   B60.10   **Acanthamebiasis, unspecified**

   B60.11   **Meningoencephalitis due to Acanthamoeba (culbertsoni)**

   B60.12   **Conjunctivitis due to Acanthamoeba**

   B60.13   **Keratoconjunctivitis due to Acanthamoeba**

   B60.19   **Other acanthamebic disease**

   B60.2   **Naegleriasis**
     Primary amebic meningoencephalitis

   B60.8   **Other specified protozoal diseases**
     Microsporidiosis

   B64   **Unspecified protozoal disease**

Helminthiases (B65-B83)

✓4th **B65**   **Schistosomiasis [bilharziasis]**
   INCLUDES   snail fever

   B65.0   **Schistosomiasis due to Schistosoma haematobium [urinary schistosomiasis]**

   B65.1   **Schistosomiasis due to Schistosoma mansoni [intestinal schistosomiasis]**

   B65.2   **Schistosomiasis due to Schistosoma japonicum**
     Asiatic schistosomiasis

   B65.3   **Cercarial dermatitis**
     Swimmer's itch

   B65.8   **Other schistosomiasis**
     Infection due to Schistosoma intercalatum
     Infection due to Schistosoma mattheei
     Infection due to Schistosoma mekongi

   B65.9   **Schistosomiasis, unspecified**

✔ Additional Character Required   ✓7th Xtension Alert   Unspecified Code   Other Specified Code   Manifestation Code   ►◄ Revised Text   ● New Code   ▲ Revised Code Title

Certain Infectious and Parasitic Diseases

B66–B78.9

✓4th **B66 Other fluke infections**

B66.0 Opisthorchiasis
Infection due to cat liver fluke
Infection due to Opisthorchis (felineus)(viverrini)

B66.1 Clonorchiasis
Chinese liver fluke disease
Infection due to Clonorchis sinensis
Oriental liver fluke disease

B66.2 Dicroceliasis
Infection due to Dicrocoelium dendriticum
Lancet fluke infection

B66.3 Fascioliasis
Infection due to Fasciola gigantica
Infection due to Fasciola hepatica
Infection due to Fasciola indica
Sheep liver fluke disease

B66.4 Paragonimiasis
Infection due to Paragonimus species
Lung fluke disease
Pulmonary distomiasis

B66.5 Fasciolopsiasis
Infection due to Fasciolopsis buski
Intestinal distomiasis

B66.8 Other specified fluke infections
Echinostomiasis
Heterophyiasis
Metagonimiasis
Nanophyetiasis
Watsoniasis

B66.9 Fluke infection, unspecified

✓4th **B67 Echinococcosis**
INCLUDES hydatidosis

B67.0 Echinococcus granulosus infection of liver

B67.1 Echinococcus granulosus infection of lung

B67.2 Echinococcus granulosus infection of bone

✓5th **B67.3 Echinococcus granulosus infection, other and multiple sites**

B67.31 Echinococcus granulosus infection, thyroid gland

B67.32 Echinococcus granulosus infection, multiple sites

B67.39 Echinococcus granulosus infection, other sites

B67.4 Echinococcus granulosus infection, unspecified
Dog tapeworm (infection)

B67.5 Echinococcus multilocularis infection of liver

✓5th **B67.6 Echinococcus multilocularis infection, other and multiple sites**

B67.61 Echinococcus multilocularis infection, multiple sites

B67.69 Echinococcus multilocularis infection, other sites

B67.7 Echinococcus multilocularis infection, unspecified

B67.8 Echinococcosis, unspecified, of liver

✓5th **B67.9 Echinococcosis, other and unspecified**

B67.90 Echinococcosis, unspecified
Echinococcosis NOS

B67.99 Other echinococcosis

✓4th **B68 Taeniasis**
EXCLUDES 1 cysticercosis (B69.-)

B68.0 Taenia solium taeniasis
Pork tapeworm (infection)

B68.1 Taenia saginata taeniasis
Beef tapeworm (infection)
Infection due to adult tapeworm Taenia saginata

B68.9 Taeniasis, unspecified

✓4th **B69 Cysticercosis**
INCLUDES cysticerciasis infection due to larval form of Taenia solium

B69.0 Cysticercosis of central nervous system

B69.1 Cysticercosis of eye

✓5th **B69.8 Cysticercosis of other sites**

B69.81 Myositis in cysticercosis

B69.89 Cysticercosis of other sites

B69.9 Cysticercosis, unspecified

✓4th **B70 Diphyllobothriasis and sparganosis**

B70.0 Diphyllobothriasis
Diphyllobothrium (adult) (latum) (pacificum) infection
Fish tapeworm (infection)
EXCLUDES 2 larval diphyllobothriasis (B70.1)

B70.1 Sparganosis
Infection due to Sparganum (mansoni) (proliferum)
Infection due to Spirometra larva
Larval diphyllobothriasis
Spirometrosis

✓4th **B71 Other cestode infections**

B71.0 Hymenolepiasis
Dwarf tapeworm infection
Rat tapeworm (infection)

B71.1 Dipylidiasis

B71.8 Other specified cestode infections
Coenurosis

B71.9 Cestode infection, unspecified
Tapeworm (infection) NOS

B72 Dracunculiasis
INCLUDES guinea worm infection
infection due to Dracunculus medinensis

✓4th **B73 Onchocerciasis**
INCLUDES onchocerca volvulus infection
onchocercosis
river blindness

✓5th **B73.0 Onchocerciasis with eye disease**

B73.00 Onchocerciasis with eye involvement, unspecified

B73.01 Onchocerciasis with endophthalmitis

B73.02 Onchocerciasis with glaucoma

B73.09 Onchocerciasis with other eye involvement
Infestation of eyelid due to onchocerciasis

B73.1 Onchocerciasis without eye disease

✓4th **B74 Filariasis**
EXCLUDES 2 onchocerciasis (B73)
tropical (pulmonary) eosinophilia NOS (J82)

B74.0 Filariasis due to Wuchereria bancrofti
Bancroftian elephantiasis
Bancroftian filariasis

B74.1 Filariasis due to Brugia malayi

B74.2 Filariasis due to Brugia timori

B74.3 Loiasis
Calabar swelling
Eyeworm disease of Africa
Loa loa infection

B74.4 Mansonelliasis
Infection due to Mansonella ozzardi
Infection due to Mansonella perstans
Infection due to Mansonella streptocerca

B74.8 Other filariases
Dirofilariasis

B74.9 Filariasis, unspecified

B75 Trichinellosis
INCLUDES infection due to Trichinella species
trichiniasis

✓4th **B76 Hookworm diseases**
INCLUDES uncinariasis

B76.0 Ancylostomiasis
Infection due to Ancylostoma species

B76.1 Necatoriasis
Infection due to Necator americanus

B76.8 Other hookworm diseases

B76.9 Hookworm disease, unspecified
Cutaneous larva migrans NOS

✓4th **B77 Ascariasis**
INCLUDES ascaridiasis
roundworm infection

B77.0 Ascariasis with intestinal complications

✓5th **B77.8 Ascariasis with other complications**

B77.81 Ascariasis pneumonia

B77.89 Ascariasis with other complications

B77.9 Ascariasis, unspecified

✓4th **B78 Strongyloidiasis**
EXCLUDES 1 trichostrongyliasis (B81.2)

B78.0 Intestinal strongyloidiasis

B78.1 Cutaneous strongyloidiasis

B78.7 Disseminated strongyloidiasis

B78.9 Strongyloidiasis, unspecified

B79 Trichuriasis
> INCLUDES trichocephaliasis
> whipworm (disease)(infection)

B80 Enterobiasis
> INCLUDES oxyuriasis
> pinworm infection
> threadworm infection

✓4th **B81 Other intestinal helminthiases, not elsewhere classified**
> EXCLUDES 1 angiostrongyliasis due to Parastrongylus cantonensis (B83.2)

B81.0 Anisakiasis
> Infection due to Anisakis larva

B81.1 Intestinal capillariasis
> Capillariasis NOS
> Infection due to Capillaria philippinensis
> EXCLUDES 2 hepatic capillariasis (B83.8)

B81.2 Trichostrongyliasis

B81.3 Intestinal angiostrongyliasis
> Angiostrongyliasis due to Parastrongylus costaricensis

B81.4 Mixed intestinal helminthiases
> Infection due to intestinal helminths classified to more than one of the categories B65.0-B81.3 and B81.8
> Mixed helminthiasis NOS

B81.8 Other specified intestinal helminthiases
> Infection due to Oesophagostomum species [esophagostomiasis]
> Infection due to Ternidens diminutus [ternidensiasis]

✓4th **B82 Unspecified intestinal parasitism**

B82.0 Intestinal helminthiasis, unspecified

B82.9 Intestinal parasitism, unspecified

✓4th **B83 Other helminthiases**
> EXCLUDES 1 capillariasis NOS (B81.1)
> EXCLUDES 2 intestinal capillariasis (B81.1)

B83.0 Visceral larva migrans
> Toxocariasis

B83.1 Gnathostomiasis
> Wandering swelling

B83.2 Angiostrongyliasis due to Parastrongylus cantonensis
> Eosinophilic meningoencephalitis due to Parastrongylus cantonensis
> EXCLUDES 2 intestinal angiostrongyliasis (B81.3)

B83.3 Syngamiasis
> Syngamosis

B83.4 Internal hirudiniasis
> EXCLUDES 2 external hirudiniasis (B88.3)

B83.8 Other specified helminthiases
> Acanthocephaliasis
> Gongylonemiasis
> Hepatic capillariasis
> Metastrongyliasis
> Thelaziasis

B83.9 Helminthiasis, unspecified
> Worms NOS
> EXCLUDES 1 intestinal helminthiasis NOS (B82.0)

Pediculosis, acariasis and other infestations (B85-B89)

✓4th **B85 Pediculosis and phthiriasis**

B85.0 Pediculosis due to Pediculus humanus capitis
> Head-louse infestation

B85.1 Pediculosis due to Pediculus humanus corporis
> Body-louse infestation

B85.2 Pediculosis, unspecified

B85.3 Phthiriasis
> Infestation by crab-louse
> Infestation by Phthirus pubis

B85.4 Mixed pediculosis and phthiriasis
> Infestation classifiable to more than one of the categories B85.0-B85.3

B86 Scabies
> Sarcoptic itch

✓4th **B87 Myiasis**
> INCLUDES infestation by larva of flies

B87.0 Cutaneous myiasis
> Creeping myiasis

B87.1 Wound myiasis
> Traumatic myiasis

B87.2 Ocular myiasis

B87.3 Nasopharyngeal myiasis
> Laryngeal myiasis

B87.4 Aural myiasis

✓5th **B87.8 Myiasis of other sites**

B87.81 Genitourinary myiasis

B87.82 Intestinal myiasis

B87.89 Myiasis of other sites

B87.9 Myiasis, unspecified

✓4th **B88 Other infestations**

B88.0 Other acariasis
> Acarine dermatitis
> Dermatitis due to Demodex species
> Dermatitis due to Dermanyssus gallinae
> Dermatitis due to Liponyssoides sanguineus
> Trombiculosis
> EXCLUDES 2 scabies (B86)

B88.1 Tungiasis [sandflea infestation]

B88.2 Other arthropod infestations
> Scarabiasis

B88.3 External hirudiniasis
> Leech infestation NOS
> EXCLUDES 2 internal hirudiniasis (B83.4)

B88.8 Other specified infestations
> Ichthyoparasitism due to Vandellia cirrhosa
> Linguatulosis
> Porocephaliasis

B88.9 Infestation, unspecified
> Infestation (skin) NOS
> Infestation by mites NOS
> Skin parasites NOS

B89 Unspecified parasitic disease

Sequelae of infectious and parasitic diseases (B90-B94)

Categories B90-B94 are to be used to indicate conditions in categories A00-B89 as the cause of sequelae, which are themselves classified elsewhere. The "sequelae" include conditions specified as such; they also include residuals of diseases classifiable to the above categories if there is evidence that the disease itself is no longer present. Codes from these categories are not to be used for chronic infections. Code chronic current infections to active infectious disease as appropriate.

Code first condition resulting from (sequela) the infectious or parasitic disease

✓4th **B90 Sequelae of tuberculosis**

B90.0 Sequelae of central nervous system tuberculosis

B90.1 Sequelae of genitourinary tuberculosis

B90.2 Sequelae of tuberculosis of bones and joints

B90.8 Sequelae of tuberculosis of other organs
> EXCLUDES 2 sequelae of respiratory tuberculosis (B90.9)

B90.9 Sequelae of respiratory and unspecified tuberculosis
> Sequelae of tuberculosis NOS

B91 Sequelae of poliomyelitis
> EXCLUDES 1 postpolio syndrome (G14)

B92 Sequelae of leprosy

✓4th **B94 Sequelae of other and unspecified infectious and parasitic diseases**

B94.0 Sequelae of trachoma

B94.1 Sequelae of viral encephalitis

B94.2 Sequelae of viral hepatitis

B94.8 Sequelae of other specified infectious and parasitic diseases

B94.9 Sequelae of unspecified infectious and parasitic disease

Bacterial and viral infectious agents (B95-B97)

> NOTE These categories are provided for use as supplementary or additional codes to identify the infectious agent(s) in diseases classified elsewhere.

✓4th **B95 Streptococcus, Staphylococcus, and Enterococcus as the cause of diseases classified elsewhere**

B95.0 Streptococcus, group A, as the cause of diseases classified elsewhere

B95.1 Streptococcus, group B, as the cause of diseases classified elsewhere

B95.2 Enterococcus as the cause of diseases classified elsewhere

✓ Additional Character Required   ✓x7th Xtension Alert   Unspecified Code   Other Specified Code   Manifestation Code   ►◄ Revised Text   ● New Code   ▲ Revised Code Title

ICD-10-CM 2014 (Draft)   439

Certain Infectious and Parasitic Diseases

B95.3–B99.9

B95.3   Streptococcus pneumoniae as the cause of diseases classified elsewhere

B95.4   Other streptococcus as the cause of diseases classified elsewhere

B95.5   Unspecified streptococcus as the cause of diseases classified elsewhere

✓5ᵗʰ B95.6   Staphylococcus aureus as the cause of diseases classified elsewhere

    B95.61   Methicillin susceptible Staphylococcus aureus infection as the cause of diseases classified elsewhere

      Methicillin susceptible Staphylococcus aureus (MSSA) infection as the cause of diseases classified elsewhere

      Staphylococcus aureus infection NOS as the cause of diseases classified elsewhere

    B95.62   Methicillin resistant Staphylococcus aureus infection as the cause of diseases classified elsewhere

      Methicillin resistant Staphylococcus aureus (MRSA) infection as the cause of diseases classified elsewhere

B95.7   Other staphylococcus as the cause of diseases classified elsewhere

B95.8   Unspecified staphylococcus as the cause of diseases classified elsewhere

✓4ᵗʰ **B96**   Other bacterial agents as the cause of diseases classified elsewhere

B96.0   Mycoplasma pneumoniae [M. pneumoniae] as the cause of diseases classified elsewhere

    Pleuro-pneumonia-like-organism [PPLO]

B96.1   Klebsiella pneumoniae [K. pneumoniae] as the cause of diseases classified elsewhere

✓5ᵗʰ B96.2   Escherichia coli [E. coli] as the cause of diseases classified elsewhere

    B96.20   Unspecified Escherichia coli [E. coli] as the cause of diseases classified elsewhere

      Escherichia coli [E. coli] NOS

    B96.21   Shiga toxin-producing Escherichia coli [E. coli] (STEC) O157 as the cause of diseases classified elsewhere

      E. coli O157:H- (nonmotile) with confirmation of Shiga toxin

      E. coli O157 with confirmation of Shiga toxin when H antigen is unknown, or is not H7

      O157:H7 Escherichia coli [E.coli] with or without confirmation of Shiga toxin-production

      Shiga toxin-producing Escherichia coli [E.coli] O157:H7 with or without confirmation of Shiga toxin-production

      STEC O157:H7 with or without confirmation of Shiga toxin-production

    B96.22   Other specified Shiga toxin-producing Escherichia coli [E. coli] (STEC) as the cause of diseases classified elsewhere

      Non-O157 Shiga toxin-producing Escherichia coli [E.coli]

      Non-O157 Shiga toxin-producing Escherichia coli [E.coli] with known O group

    B96.23   Unspecified Shiga toxin-producing Escherichia coli [E. coli] (STEC) as the cause of diseases classified elsewhere

      Shiga toxin-producing Escherichia coli [E. coli] with unspecified O group

      STEC NOS

    B96.29   Other Escherichia coli [E. coli] as the cause of diseases classified elsewhere

      Non-Shiga toxin-producing E. coli

B96.3   Hemophilus influenzae [H. influenzae] as the cause of diseases classified elsewhere

B96.4   Proteus (mirabilis) (morganii) as the cause of diseases classified elsewhere

B96.5   Pseudomonas (aeruginosa) (mallei) (pseudomallei) as the cause of diseases classified elsewhere

B96.6   Bacteroides fragilis [B. fragilis] as the cause of diseases classified elsewhere

B96.7   Clostridium perfringens [C. perfringens] as the cause of diseases classified elsewhere

✓5ᵗʰ B96.8   Other specified bacterial agents as the cause of diseases classified elsewhere

    B96.81   Helicobacter pylori [H. pylori] as the cause of diseases classified elsewhere

    B96.82   Vibrio vulnificus as the cause of diseases classified elsewhere

    B96.89   Other specified bacterial agents as the cause of diseases classified elsewhere

✓4ᵗʰ **B97**   Viral agents as the cause of diseases classified elsewhere

B97.0   Adenovirus as the cause of diseases classified elsewhere

✓5ᵗʰ B97.1   Enterovirus as the cause of diseases classified elsewhere

    B97.10   Unspecified enterovirus as the cause of diseases classified elsewhere

    B97.11   Coxsackievirus as the cause of diseases classified elsewhere

    B97.12   Echovirus as the cause of diseases classified elsewhere

    B97.19   Other enterovirus as the cause of diseases classified elsewhere

✓5ᵗʰ B97.2   Coronavirus as the cause of diseases classified elsewhere

    B97.21   SARS-associated coronavirus as the cause of diseases classified elsewhere

      EXCLUDES 1   pneumonia due to SARS-associated coronavirus (J12.81)

    B97.29   Other coronavirus as the cause of diseases classified elsewhere

✓5ᵗʰ B97.3   Retrovirus as the cause of diseases classified elsewhere

    EXCLUDES 1   human immunodeficiency virus [HIV} disease (B20)

    B97.30   Unspecified retrovirus as the cause of diseases classified elsewhere

    B97.31   Lentivirus as the cause of diseases classified elsewhere

    B97.32   Oncovirus as the cause of diseases classified elsewhere

    B97.33   Human T-cell lymphotrophic virus, type I [HTLV-I] as the cause of diseases classified elsewhere

    B97.34   Human T-cell lymphotrophic virus, type II [HTLV-II] as the cause of diseases classified elsewhere

    B97.35   Human immunodeficiency virus, type 2 [HIV 2] as the cause of diseases classified elsewhere

    B97.39   Other retrovirus as the cause of diseases classified elsewhere

B97.4   Respiratory syncytial virus as the cause of diseases classified elsewhere

B97.5   Reovirus as the cause of diseases classified elsewhere

B97.6   Parvovirus as the cause of diseases classified elsewhere

B97.7   Papillomavirus as the cause of diseases classified elsewhere

✓5ᵗʰ B97.8   Other viral agents as the cause of diseases classified elsewhere

    B97.81   Human metapneumovirus as the cause of diseases classified elsewhere

    B97.89   Other viral agents as the cause of diseases classified elsewhere

Other infectious diseases (B99)

✓4ᵗʰ **B99**   Other and unspecified infectious diseases

B99.8   Other infectious disease

B99.9   Unspecified infectious disease

EXCLUDES 1 Not coded here   EXCLUDES 2 Not included here   N Newborn Age: 0   P Pediatric Age: 0-17   M Maternity Age: 12-55   A Adult Age: 15-124

440   ICD-10-CM 2014 (Draft)

Chapter 2. Neoplasms (C00-D49)

This chapter contains the following broad groups of neoplasms:

C00-C14	Malignant neoplasms of lip, oral cavity and pharynx
C15-C26	Malignant neoplasms of digestive organs
C30-C39	Malignant neoplasms of respiratory and intrathoracic organs
C40-C41	Malignant neoplasms of bone and articular cartilage
C43-C44	Melanoma and other malignant neoplasms of skin
C45-C49	Malignant neoplasms of mesothelial and soft tissue
C50	Malignant neoplasms of breast
C51-C58	Malignant neoplasms of female genital organs
C60-C63	Malignant neoplasms of male genital organs
C64-C68	Malignant neoplasms of urinary tract
C69-C72	Malignant neoplasms of eye, brain and other parts of central nervous system
C73-C75	Malignant neoplasms of thyroid and other endocrine glands
C7A	Malignant neuroendocrine tumors
C7B	Secondary neuroendocrine tumors
C76-C80	Malignant neoplasms of ill-defined, other secondary and unspecified sites
C81-C96	Malignant neoplasms of lymphoid, hematopoietic and related tissue
D00-D09	In situ neoplasms
D10-D36	Benign neoplasms, except benign neuroendocrine tumors
D3A	Benign neuroendocrine tumors
D37-D48	Neoplasms of uncertain behavior, polycythemia vera and myelodysplastic syndromes
D49	Neoplasms of unspecified behavior

NOTE

Functional activity

All neoplasms are classified in this chapter, whether they are functionally active or not. An additional code from Chapter 4 may be used, to identify functional activity associated with any neoplasm.

Morphology [Histology]

Chapter 2 classifies neoplasms primarily by site (topography), with broad groupings for behavior, malignant, in situ, benign, etc. The Table of Neoplasms should be used to identify the correct topography code. In a few cases, such as for malignant melanoma and certain neuroendocrine tumors, the morphology (histologic type) is included in the category and codes.

Primary malignant neoplasms overlapping site boundaries

A primary malignant neoplasm that overlaps two or more contiguous (next to each other) sites should be classified to the subcategory/code .8 ("overlapping lesion"), unless the combination is specifically indexed elsewhere. For multiple neoplasms of the same site that are not contiguous, such as tumors in different quadrants of the same breast, codes for each site should be assigned.

Malignant neoplasm of ectopic tissue

Malignant neoplasms of ectopic tissue are to be coded to the site mentioned, e.g., ectopic pancreatic malignant neoplasms are coded to pancreas, unspecified (C25.9).

MALIGNANT NEOPLASMS (C00-C96)

NOTE Malignant neoplasms, stated or presumed to be primary (of specified sites), and certain specified histologies, except neuroendocrine, and of lymphoid, hematopoietic and related tissue (C00-C75).

Malignant neoplasms of lip, oral cavity and pharynx (C00-C14)

✓4th C00 Malignant neoplasm of lip
  EXCLUDES 1 malignant melanoma of lip (C43.0)
    Merkel cell carcinoma of lip (C4A.0)
    other and unspecified malignant neoplasm of skin of lip (C44.0-)
  Use additional code to identify:
    alcohol abuse and dependence (F10.-)
    history of tobacco use (Z87.891)
    tobacco dependence (F17.-)
    tobacco use (Z72.0)

  C00.0 Malignant neoplasm of external upper lip
    Malignant neoplasm of lipstick area of upper lip
    Malignant neoplasm of upper lip NOS
    Malignant neoplasm of vermilion border of upper lip

  C00.1 Malignant neoplasm of external lower lip
    Malignant neoplasm of lower lip NOS
    Malignant neoplasm of lipstick area of lower lip
    Malignant neoplasm of vermilion border of lower lip

  C00.2 Malignant neoplasm of external lip, unspecified
    Malignant neoplasm of vermilion border of lip NOS

  C00.3 Malignant neoplasm of upper lip, inner aspect
    Malignant neoplasm of buccal aspect of upper lip
    Malignant neoplasm of frenulum of upper lip
    Malignant neoplasm of mucosa of upper lip
    Malignant neoplasm of oral aspect of upper lip

  C00.4 Malignant neoplasm of lower lip, inner aspect
    Malignant neoplasm of buccal aspect of lower lip
    Malignant neoplasm of frenulum of lower lip
    Malignant neoplasm of mucosa of lower lip
    Malignant neoplasm of oral aspect of lower lip

  C00.5 Malignant neoplasm of lip, unspecified, inner aspect
    Malignant neoplasm of buccal aspect of lip, unspecified
    Malignant neoplasm of frenulum of lip, unspecified
    Malignant neoplasm of mucosa of lip, unspecified
    Malignant neoplasm of oral aspect of lip, unspecified

  C00.6 Malignant neoplasm of commissure of lip, unspecified

  C00.8 Malignant neoplasm of overlapping sites of lip

  C00.9 Malignant neoplasm of lip, unspecified

C01 Malignant neoplasm of base of tongue
  Malignant neoplasm of dorsal surface of base of tongue
  Malignant neoplasm of fixed part of tongue NOS
  Malignant neoplasm of posterior third of tongue
  Use additional code to identify:
    alcohol abuse and dependence (F10.-)
    history of tobacco use (Z87.891)
    tobacco dependence (F17.-)
    tobacco use (Z72.0)

✓4th C02 Malignant neoplasm of other and unspecified parts of tongue
  Use additional code to identify:
    alcohol abuse and dependence (F10.-)
    history of tobacco use (Z87.891)
    tobacco dependence (F17.-)
    tobacco use (Z72.0)

  C02.0 Malignant neoplasm of dorsal surface of tongue
    Malignant neoplasm of anterior two-thirds of tongue, dorsal surface
    EXCLUDES 2 malignant neoplasm of dorsal surface of base of tongue (C01)

  C02.1 Malignant neoplasm of border of tongue
    Malignant neoplasm of tip of tongue

  C02.2 Malignant neoplasm of ventral surface of tongue
    Malignant neoplasm of anterior two-thirds of tongue, ventral surface
    Malignant neoplasm of frenulum linguae

  C02.3 Malignant neoplasm of anterior two-thirds of tongue, part unspecified
    Malignant neoplasm of middle third of tongue NOS
    Malignant neoplasm of mobile part of tongue NOS

  C02.4 Malignant neoplasm of lingual tonsil
    EXCLUDES 2 malignant neoplasm of tonsil NOS (C09.9)

  C02.8 Malignant neoplasm of overlapping sites of tongue
    Malignant neoplasm of two or more contiguous sites of tongue

  C02.9 Malignant neoplasm of tongue, unspecified

✓4th C03 Malignant neoplasm of gum
  INCLUDES malignant neoplasm of alveolar (ridge) mucosa
    malignant neoplasm of gingiva
  EXCLUDES 2 malignant odontogenic neoplasms (C41.0-C41.1)
  Use additional code to identify:
    alcohol abuse and dependence (F10.-)
    history of tobacco use (Z87.891)
    tobacco dependence (F17.-)
    tobacco use (Z72.0)

  C03.0 Malignant neoplasm of upper gum

  C03.1 Malignant neoplasm of lower gum

  C03.9 Malignant neoplasm of gum, unspecified

✓4th C04 Malignant neoplasm of floor of mouth
  Use additional code to identify:
    alcohol abuse and dependence (F10.-)
    history of tobacco use (Z87.891)
    tobacco dependence (F17.-)
    tobacco use (Z72.0)

  C04.0 Malignant neoplasm of anterior floor of mouth
    Malignant neoplasm of anterior to the premolar-canine junction

  C04.1 Malignant neoplasm of lateral floor of mouth

  C04.8 Malignant neoplasm of overlapping sites of floor of mouth

  C04.9 Malignant neoplasm of floor of mouth, unspecified

Neoplasms

C05–C12

✓4th **C05 Malignant neoplasm of palate**

EXCLUDES 1   *Kaposi's sarcoma of palate (C46.2)*

Use additional code to identify:
  alcohol abuse and dependence (F10.-)
  history of tobacco use (Z87.891)
  tobacco dependence (F17.-)
  tobacco use (Z72.0)

C05.0 Malignant neoplasm of hard palate

C05.1 Malignant neoplasm of soft palate

EXCLUDES 2   *malignant neoplasm of nasopharyngeal surface of soft palate (C11.3)*

C05.2 Malignant neoplasm of uvula

C05.8 Malignant neoplasm of overlapping sites of palate

C05.9 Malignant neoplasm of palate, unspecified
  Malignant neoplasm of roof of mouth

✓4th **C06 Malignant neoplasm of other and unspecified parts of mouth**

Use additional code to identify:
  alcohol abuse and dependence (F10.-)
  history of tobacco use (Z87.891)
  tobacco dependence (F17.-)
  tobacco use (Z72.0)

C06.0 Malignant neoplasm of cheek mucosa
  Malignant neoplasm of buccal mucosa NOS
  Malignant neoplasm of internal cheek

C06.1 Malignant neoplasm of vestibule of mouth
  Malignant neoplasm of buccal sulcus (upper) (lower)
  Malignant neoplasm of labial sulcus (upper) (lower)

C06.2 Malignant neoplasm of retromolar area

✓5th **C06.8 Malignant neoplasm of overlapping sites of other and unspecified parts of mouth**

  C06.80 Malignant neoplasm of overlapping sites of unspecified parts of mouth

  C06.89 Malignant neoplasm of overlapping sites of other parts of mouth
    "book leaf" neoplasm [ventral surface of tongue and floor of mouth]

C06.9 Malignant neoplasm of mouth, unspecified
  Malignant neoplasm of minor salivary gland, unspecified site
  Malignant neoplasm of oral cavity NOS

C07 Malignant neoplasm of parotid gland

Use additional code to identify:
  alcohol abuse and dependence (F10.-)
  exposure to environmental tobacco smoke (Z77.22)
  exposure to tobacco smoke in the perinatal period (P96.81)
  history of tobacco use (Z87.891)
  occupational exposure to environmental tobacco smoke (Z57.31)
  tobacco dependence (F17.-)
  tobacco use (Z72.0)

✓4th **C08 Malignant neoplasm of other and unspecified major salivary glands**

INCLUDES   malignant neoplasm of salivary ducts

EXCLUDES 1   *malignant neoplasms of specified minor salivary glands which are classified according to their anatomical location*

EXCLUDES 2   *malignant neoplasms of minor salivary glands NOS (C06.9)*
    malignant neoplasm of parotid gland (C07)

Use additional code to identify:
  alcohol abuse and dependence (F10.-)
  exposure to environmental tobacco smoke (Z77.22)
  exposure to tobacco smoke in the perinatal period (P96.81)
  history of tobacco use (Z87.891)
  occupational exposure to environmental tobacco smoke (Z57.31)
  tobacco dependence (F17.-)
  tobacco use (Z72.0)

C08.0 Malignant neoplasm of submandibular gland
  Malignant neoplasm of submaxillary gland

C08.1 Malignant neoplasm of sublingual gland

C08.9 Malignant neoplasm of major salivary gland, unspecified
  Malignant neoplasm of salivary gland (major) NOS

✓4th **C09 Malignant neoplasm of tonsil**

EXCLUDES 2   *malignant neoplasm of lingual tonsil (C02.4)*
    malignant neoplasm of pharyngeal tonsil (C11.1)

Use additional code to identify:
  alcohol abuse and dependence (F10.-)
  exposure to environmental tobacco smoke (Z77.22)
  exposure to tobacco smoke in the perinatal period (P96.81)
  history of tobacco use (Z87.891)
  occupational exposure to environmental tobacco smoke (Z57.31)
  tobacco dependence (F17.-)
  tobacco use (Z72.0)

C09.0 Malignant neoplasm of tonsillar fossa

C09.1 Malignant neoplasm of tonsillar pillar (anterior) (posterior)

C09.8 Malignant neoplasm of overlapping sites of tonsil

C09.9 Malignant neoplasm of tonsil, unspecified
  Malignant neoplasm of tonsil NOS
  Malignant neoplasm of faucial tonsils
  Malignant neoplasm of palatine tonsils

✓4th **C10 Malignant neoplasm of oropharynx**

EXCLUDES 2   *malignant neoplasm of tonsil (C09.-)*

Use additional code to identify:
  alcohol abuse and dependence (F10.-)
  exposure to environmental tobacco smoke (Z77.22)
  exposure to tobacco smoke in the perinatal period (P96.81)
  history of tobacco use (Z87.891)
  occupational exposure to environmental tobacco smoke (Z57.31)
  tobacco dependence (F17.-)
  tobacco use (Z72.0)

C10.0 Malignant neoplasm of vallecula

C10.1 Malignant neoplasm of anterior surface of epiglottis
  Malignant neoplasm of epiglottis, free border [margin]
  Malignant neoplasm of glossoepiglottic fold(s)

EXCLUDES 2   *malignant neoplasm of epiglottis (suprahyoid portion) NOS (C32.1)*

C10.2 Malignant neoplasm of lateral wall of oropharynx

C10.3 Malignant neoplasm of posterior wall of oropharynx

C10.4 Malignant neoplasm of branchial cleft
  Malignant neoplasm of branchial cyst [site of neoplasm]

C10.8 Malignant neoplasm of overlapping sites of oropharynx
  Malignant neoplasm of junctional region of oropharynx

C10.9 Malignant neoplasm of oropharynx, unspecified

✓4th **C11 Malignant neoplasm of nasopharynx**

Use additional code to identify:
  exposure to environmental tobacco smoke (Z77.22)
  exposure to tobacco smoke in the perinatal period (P96.81)
  history of tobacco use (Z87.891)
  occupational exposure to environmental tobacco smoke (Z57.31)
  tobacco dependence (F17.-)
  tobacco use (Z72.0)

C11.0 Malignant neoplasm of superior wall of nasopharynx
  Malignant neoplasm of roof of nasopharynx

C11.1 Malignant neoplasm of posterior wall of nasopharynx
  Malignant neoplasm of adenoid
  Malignant neoplasm of pharyngeal tonsil

C11.2 Malignant neoplasm of lateral wall of nasopharynx
  Malignant neoplasm of fossa of Rosenmüller
  Malignant neoplasm of opening of auditory tube
  Malignant neoplasm of pharyngeal recess

C11.3 Malignant neoplasm of anterior wall of nasopharynx
  Malignant neoplasm of floor of nasopharynx
  Malignant neoplasm of nasopharyngeal (anterior) (posterior) surface of soft palate
  Malignant neoplasm of posterior margin of nasal choana
  Malignant neoplasm of posterior margin of nasal septum

C11.8 Malignant neoplasm of overlapping sites of nasopharynx

C11.9 Malignant neoplasm of nasopharynx, unspecified
  Malignant neoplasm of nasopharyngeal wall NOS

C12 Malignant neoplasm of pyriform sinus
  Malignant neoplasm of pyriform fossa

Use additional code to identify:
  exposure to environmental tobacco smoke (Z77.22)
  exposure to tobacco smoke in the perinatal period (P96.81)
  history of tobacco use (Z87.891)
  occupational exposure to environmental tobacco smoke (Z57.31)
  tobacco dependence (F17.-)
  tobacco use (Z72.0)

EXCLUDES 1 Not coded here   EXCLUDES 2 Not included here   N Newborn Age: 0   P Pediatric Age: 0-17   M Maternity Age: 12-55   A Adult Age: 15-124

442   ICD-10-CM 2014 (Draft)

✓4ᵗʰ **C13** **Malignant neoplasm of** hypopharynx
     EXCLUDES 2   *malignant neoplasm of pyriform sinus (C12)*
     Use additional code to identify:
       exposure to environmental tobacco smoke (Z77.22)
       exposure to tobacco smoke in the perinatal period (P96.81)
       history of tobacco use (Z87.891)
       occupational exposure to environmental tobacco smoke (Z57.31)
       tobacco dependence (F17.-)
       tobacco use (Z72.0)

   C13.0 **Malignant neoplasm of** postcricoid region

   C13.1 **Malignant neoplasm of** aryepiglottic fold, hypopharyngeal **aspect**
       Malignant neoplasm of aryepiglottic fold, marginal zone
       Malignant neoplasm of aryepiglottic fold NOS
       Malignant neoplasm of interarytenoid fold, marginal zone
       Malignant neoplasm of interarytenoid fold NOS
       EXCLUDES 2   *malignant neoplasm of aryepiglottic fold or interarytenoid fold, laryngeal aspect (C32.1)*

   C13.2 **Malignant neoplasm of** posterior wall **of hypopharynx**

   C13.8 **Malignant neoplasm of** overlapping sites **of hypopharynx**

   C13.9 **Malignant neoplasm of hypopharynx, unspecified**
       Malignant neoplasm of hypopharyngeal wall NOS

✓4ᵗʰ **C14** **Malignant neoplasm of** other and ill-defined sites in the lip, oral **cavity and pharynx**
     EXCLUDES 1   *malignant neoplasm of oral cavity NOS (C06.9)*
     Use additional code to identify:
       alcohol abuse and dependence (F10.-)
       exposure to environmental tobacco smoke (Z77.22)
       exposure to tobacco smoke in the perinatal period (P96.81)
       history of tobacco use (Z87.891)
       occupational exposure to environmental tobacco smoke (Z57.31)
       tobacco dependence (F17.-)
       tobacco use (Z72.0)

   C14.0 **Malignant neoplasm of pharynx, unspecified**

   C14.2 **Malignant neoplasm of** Waldeyer's ring

   C14.8 **Malignant neoplasm of** overlapping sites **of lip, oral cavity and pharynx**
       Primary malignant neoplasm of two or more contiguous sites of lip, oral cavity and pharynx
       EXCLUDES 1   *"book leaf" neoplasm [ventral surface of tongue and floor of mouth] (C06.89)*

Malignant neoplasms of digestive organs (C15-C26)
     EXCLUDES 1   *Kaposi's sarcoma of gastrointestinal sites (C46.4)*

✓4ᵗʰ **C15** **Malignant neoplasm of** esophagus
     Use additional code to identify:
       alcohol abuse and dependence (F10.-)

   C15.3 **Malignant neoplasm of** upper third **of esophagus**

   C15.4 **Malignant neoplasm of** middle third **of esophagus**

   C15.5 **Malignant neoplasm of** lower third **of esophagus**
       EXCLUDES 1   *malignant neoplasm of cardio-esophageal junction (C16.0)*

   C15.8 **Malignant neoplasm of** overlapping sites **of esophagus**

   C15.9 **Malignant neoplasm of esophagus, unspecified**

✓4ᵗʰ **C16** **Malignant neoplasm of** stomach
     Use additional code to identify:
       alcohol abuse and dependence (F10.-)
     EXCLUDES 2   *malignant carcinoid tumor of the stomach (C7A.092)*

   C16.0 **Malignant neoplasm of** cardia
       Malignant neoplasm of cardiac orifice
       Malignant neoplasm of cardio-esophageal junction
       Malignant neoplasm of esophagus and stomach
       Malignant neoplasm of gastro-esophageal junction

   C16.1 **Malignant neoplasm of** fundus **of stomach**

   C16.2 **Malignant neoplasm of** body **of stomach**

   C16.3 **Malignant neoplasm of** pyloric **antrum**
       Malignant neoplasm of gastric antrum

   C16.4 **Malignant neoplasm of** pylorus
       Malignant neoplasm of prepylorus
       Malignant neoplasm of pyloric canal

   C16.5 **Malignant neoplasm of** lesser curvature **of stomach, unspecified**
       Malignant neoplasm of lesser curvature of stomach, not classifiable to C16.1-C16.4

   C16.6 **Malignant neoplasm of** greater curvature **of stomach, unspecified**
       Malignant neoplasm of greater curvature of stomach, not classifiable to C16.0-C16.4

   C16.8 **Malignant neoplasm of** overlapping sites **of stomach**

   C16.9 **Malignant neoplasm of stomach, unspecified**
       Gastric cancer NOS

✓4ᵗʰ **C17** **Malignant neoplasm of** small intestine
     EXCLUDES 1   *malignant carcinoid tumors of the small intestine (C7A.01)*

   C17.0 **Malignant neoplasm of** duodenum

   C17.1 **Malignant neoplasm of** jejunum

   C17.2 **Malignant neoplasm of** ileum
       EXCLUDES 1   *malignant neoplasm of ileocecal valve (C18.0)*

   C17.3 **Meckel's diverticulum, malignant**
       EXCLUDES 1   *Meckel's diverticulum, congenital (Q43.0)*

   C17.8 **Malignant neoplasm of** overlapping sites **of small intestine**

   C17.9 **Malignant neoplasm of small intestine, unspecified**

✓4ᵗʰ **C18** **Malignant neoplasm of** colon
     EXCLUDES 1   *malignant carcinoid tumors of the colon (C7A.02-)*

   C18.0 **Malignant neoplasm of** cecum
       Malignant neoplasm of ileocecal valve

   C18.1 **Malignant neoplasm of** appendix

   C18.2 **Malignant neoplasm of** ascending colon

   C18.3 **Malignant neoplasm of** hepatic flexure

   C18.4 **Malignant neoplasm of** transverse colon

   C18.5 **Malignant neoplasm of** splenic flexure

   C18.6 **Malignant neoplasm of** descending colon

   C18.7 **Malignant neoplasm of** sigmoid colon
       Malignant neoplasm of sigmoid (flexure)
       EXCLUDES 1   *malignant neoplasm of rectosigmoid junction (C19)*

   C18.8 **Malignant neoplasm of** overlapping sites **of colon**

   C18.9 **Malignant neoplasm of colon, unspecified**
       Malignant neoplasm of large intestine NOS

C19 **Malignant neoplasm of** rectosigmoid junction
     Malignant neoplasm of colon with rectum
     Malignant neoplasm of rectosigmoid (colon)
     EXCLUDES 1   *malignant carcinoid tumors of the colon (C7A.02-)*

C20 **Malignant neoplasm of** rectum
     Malignant neoplasm of rectal ampulla
     EXCLUDES 1   *malignant carcinoid tumor of the rectum (C7A.026)*

✓4ᵗʰ **C21** **Malignant neoplasm of** anus and anal canal
     EXCLUDES 2   *malignant carcinoid tumors of the colon (C7A.02-)*
       other and unspecified malignant neoplasm of anal margin (C44.500, C44.510, C44.520, C44.590)
       other and unspecified malignant neoplasm of anal skin (C44.500, C44.510, C44.520, C44.590)
       other and unspecified malignant neoplasm of perianal skin (C44.500, C44.510, C44.520, C44.590)

   C21.0 **Malignant neoplasm of anus, unspecified**

   C21.1 **Malignant neoplasm of** anal canal
       Malignant neoplasm of anal sphincter

   C21.2 **Malignant neoplasm of** cloacogenic zone

   C21.8 **Malignant neoplasm of** overlapping sites **of rectum, anus and anal canal**
       Malignant neoplasm of anorectal junction
       Malignant neoplasm of anorectum
       Primary malignant neoplasm of two or more contiguous sites of rectum, anus and anal canal

✓4ᵗʰ **C22** **Malignant neoplasm of** liver and intrahepatic bile ducts
     EXCLUDES 1   *malignant neoplasm of biliary tract NOS (C24.9)*
       secondary malignant neoplasm of liver and intrahepatic bile duct (C78.7)
     Use additional code to identify:
       alcohol abuse and dependence (F10.-)
       hepatitis B (B16.-, B18.0-B18.1)
       hepatitis C (B17.1-, B18.2)

   C22.0 **Liver cell carcinoma**
       Hepatocellular carcinoma
       Hepatoma

   C22.1 **Intrahepatic bile duct carcinoma**
       Cholangiocarcinoma
       EXCLUDES 1   *malignant neoplasm of hepatic duct (C24.0)*

   C22.2 **Hepatoblastoma**

   C22.3 **Angiosarcoma of liver**
       Kupffer cell sarcoma

   C22.4 **Other sarcomas of liver**

   C22.7 **Other specified carcinomas of liver**

   C22.8 **Malignant neoplasm of liver, primary, unspecified as to type**

☑ Additional Character Required   ✗7ᵗʰ Xtension Alert   Unspecified Code   Other Specified Code   Manifestation Code   ▶◀ Revised Text   ● New Code   ▲ Revised Code Title

Neoplasms

C22.9 Malignant neoplasm of liver, not specified as primary or secondary

C23 Malignant neoplasm of gallbladder

☑4ᵗʰ **C24 Malignant neoplasm of other and unspecified parts of biliary tract**
> EXCLUDES 1 malignant neoplasm of intrahepatic bile duct (C22.1)

C24.0 Malignant neoplasm of extrahepatic bile duct
Malignant neoplasm of biliary duct or passage NOS
Malignant neoplasm of common bile duct
Malignant neoplasm of cystic duct
Malignant neoplasm of hepatic duct

C24.1 Malignant neoplasm of ampulla of Vater

C24.8 Malignant neoplasm of overlapping sites of biliary tract
Malignant neoplasm involving both intrahepatic and extrahepatic bile ducts
Primary malignant neoplasm of two or more contiguous sites of biliary tract

C24.9 Malignant neoplasm of biliary tract, unspecified

☑4ᵗʰ **C25 Malignant neoplasm of pancreas**
Use additional code to identify:
alcohol abuse and dependence (F10.-)

C25.0 Malignant neoplasm of head of pancreas

C25.1 Malignant neoplasm of body of pancreas

C25.2 Malignant neoplasm of tail of pancreas

C25.3 Malignant neoplasm of pancreatic duct

C25.4 Malignant neoplasm of endocrine pancreas
Malignant neoplasm of islets of Langerhans
Use additional code to identify any functional activity

C25.7 Malignant neoplasm of other parts of pancreas
Malignant neoplasm of neck of pancreas

C25.8 Malignant neoplasm of overlapping sites of pancreas

C25.9 Malignant neoplasm of pancreas, unspecified

☑4ᵗʰ **C26 Malignant neoplasm of other and ill-defined digestive organs**
> EXCLUDES 1 malignant neoplasm of peritoneum and retroperitoneum (C48.-)

C26.0 Malignant neoplasm of intestinal tract, part unspecified
Malignant neoplasm of intestine NOS

C26.1 Malignant neoplasm of spleen
> EXCLUDES 1 Hodgkin lymphoma (C81.-)
> non-Hodgkin lymphoma (C82-C85)

C26.9 Malignant neoplasm of ill-defined sites within the digestive system
Malignant neoplasm of alimentary canal or tract NOS
Malignant neoplasm of gastrointestinal tract NOS
> EXCLUDES 1 malignant neoplasm of abdominal NOS (C76.2)
> malignant neoplasm of intra-abdominal NOS (C76.2)

Malignant neoplasms of respiratory and intrathoracic organs (C30-C39)

> INCLUDES malignant neoplasm of middle ear
> EXCLUDES 1 mesothelioma (C45.-)

☑4ᵗʰ **C30 Malignant neoplasm of nasal cavity and middle ear**

C30.0 Malignant neoplasm of nasal cavity
Malignant neoplasm of cartilage of nose
Malignant neoplasm of nasal concha
Malignant neoplasm of internal nose
Malignant neoplasm of septum of nose
Malignant neoplasm of vestibule of nose
> EXCLUDES 1 malignant melanoma of skin of nose (C43.31)
> malignant neoplasm of nasal bone (C41.0)
> malignant neoplasm of nose NOS (C76.0)
> malignant neoplasm of olfactory bulb (C72.2-)
> malignant neoplasm of posterior margin of nasal septum and choana (C11.3)
> malignant neoplasm of turbinates (C41.0)
> other and unspecified malignant neoplasm of skin of nose (C44.301, C44.311, C44.321, C44.391)

C30.1 Malignant neoplasm of middle ear
Malignant neoplasm of antrum tympanicum
Malignant neoplasm of auditory tube
Malignant neoplasm of eustachian tube
Malignant neoplasm of inner ear
Malignant neoplasm of mastoid air cells
Malignant neoplasm of tympanic cavity
> EXCLUDES 1 malignant melanoma of skin of (external) ear (C43.2-)
> malignant neoplasm of auricular canal (external) (C43.2-,C44.2-)
> malignant neoplasm of bone of ear (meatus) (C41.0)
> malignant neoplasm of cartilage of ear (C49.0)
> other and unspecified malignant neoplasm of skin of (external) ear (C44.2-)

☑4ᵗʰ **C31 Malignant neoplasm of accessory sinuses**

C31.0 Malignant neoplasm of maxillary sinus
Malignant neoplasm of antrum (Highmore) (maxillary)

C31.1 Malignant neoplasm of ethmoidal sinus

C31.2 Malignant neoplasm of frontal sinus

C31.3 Malignant neoplasm of sphenoid sinus

C31.8 Malignant neoplasm of overlapping sites of accessory sinuses

C31.9 Malignant neoplasm of accessory sinus, unspecified

☑4ᵗʰ **C32 Malignant neoplasm of larynx**
Use additional code to identify:
alcohol abuse and dependence (F10.-)
exposure to environmental tobacco smoke (Z77.22)
exposure to tobacco smoke in the perinatal period (P96.81)
history of tobacco use (Z87.891)
occupational exposure to environmental tobacco smoke (Z57.31)
tobacco dependence (F17.-)
tobacco use (Z72.0)

C32.0 Malignant neoplasm of glottis
Malignant neoplasm of intrinsic larynx
Malignant neoplasm of laryngeal commissure (anterior)(posterior)
Malignant neoplasm of vocal cord (true) NOS

C32.1 Malignant neoplasm of supraglottis
Malignant neoplasm of aryepiglottic fold or interarytenoid fold, laryngeal aspect
Malignant neoplasm of epiglottis (suprahyoid portion) NOS
Malignant neoplasm of extrinsic larynx
Malignant neoplasm of false vocal cord
Malignant neoplasm of posterior (laryngeal) surface of epiglottis
Malignant neoplasm of ventricular bands
> EXCLUDES 2 malignant neoplasm of anterior surface of epiglottis (C10.1)
> malignant neoplasm of aryepiglottic fold or interarytenoid fold, hypopharyngeal aspect (C13.1)
> malignant neoplasm of aryepiglottic fold or interarytenoid fold, marginal zone (C13.1)
> malignant neoplasm of aryepiglottic fold or interarytenoid fold NOS (C13.1)

C32.2 Malignant neoplasm of subglottis

C32.3 Malignant neoplasm of laryngeal cartilage

C32.8 Malignant neoplasm of overlapping sites of larynx

C32.9 Malignant neoplasm of larynx, unspecified

C33 Malignant neoplasm of trachea
Use additional code to identify:
exposure to environmental tobacco smoke (Z77.22)
exposure to tobacco smoke in the perinatal period (P96.81)
history of tobacco use (Z87.891)
occupational exposure to environmental tobacco smoke (Z57.31)
tobacco dependence (F17.-)
tobacco use (Z72.0)

☑4ᵗʰ **C34 Malignant neoplasm of bronchus and lung**
> EXCLUDES 1 Kaposi's sarcoma of lung (C46.5-)
> malignant carcinoid tumor of the bronchus and lung (C7A.090)
Use additional code to identify:
exposure to environmental tobacco smoke (Z77.22)
exposure to tobacco smoke in the perinatal period (P96.81)
history of tobacco use (Z87.891)
occupational exposure to environmental tobacco smoke (Z57.31)
tobacco dependence (F17.-)
tobacco use (Z72.0)

☑5ᵗʰ **C34.0 Malignant neoplasm of main bronchus**
Malignant neoplasm of carina
Malignant neoplasm of hilus (of lung)

C34.00 Malignant neoplasm of unspecified main bronchus

C34.01 Malignant neoplasm of right main bronchus

EXCLUDES 1 Not coded here   EXCLUDES 2 Not included here   N Newborn Age: 0   P Pediatric Age: 0-17   M Maternity Age: 12-55   A Adult Age: 15-124

444   ICD-10-CM 2014 (Draft)

C34.02 Malignant neoplasm of left main bronchus

☑5ᵗʰ **C34.1 Malignant neoplasm of upper lobe, bronchus or lung**

    C34.10 **Malignant neoplasm of upper lobe, unspecified bronchus or lung**

    C34.11 **Malignant neoplasm of upper lobe, right bronchus or lung**

    C34.12 **Malignant neoplasm of upper lobe, left bronchus or lung**

  C34.2 Malignant neoplasm of middle lobe, bronchus or lung

☑5ᵗʰ **C34.3 Malignant neoplasm of lower lobe, bronchus or lung**

    C34.30 **Malignant neoplasm of lower lobe, unspecified bronchus or lung**

    C34.31 **Malignant neoplasm of lower lobe, right bronchus or lung**

    C34.32 **Malignant neoplasm of lower lobe, left bronchus or lung**

☑5ᵗʰ **C34.8 Malignant neoplasm of overlapping sites of bronchus and lung**

    C34.80 **Malignant neoplasm of overlapping sites of unspecified bronchus and lung**

    C34.81 **Malignant neoplasm of overlapping sites of right bronchus and lung**

    C34.82 **Malignant neoplasm of overlapping sites of left bronchus and lung**

☑5ᵗʰ **C34.9 Malignant neoplasm of unspecified part of bronchus or lung**

    C34.90 **Malignant neoplasm of unspecified part of unspecified bronchus or lung**
      Lung cancer NOS

    C34.91 **Malignant neoplasm of unspecified part of right bronchus or lung**

    C34.92 **Malignant neoplasm of unspecified part of left bronchus or lung**

C37 Malignant neoplasm of thymus
    EXCLUDES 1 *malignant carcinoid tumor of the thymus (C7A.091)*

☑4ᵗʰ **C38 Malignant neoplasm of heart, mediastinum and pleura**
    EXCLUDES 1 *mesothelioma (C45.-)*

  C38.0 Malignant neoplasm of heart
    Malignant neoplasm of pericardium
    EXCLUDES 1 *malignant neoplasm of great vessels (C49.3)*

  C38.1 Malignant neoplasm of anterior mediastinum

  C38.2 Malignant neoplasm of posterior mediastinum

  C38.3 Malignant neoplasm of mediastinum, part unspecified

  C38.4 Malignant neoplasm of pleura

  C38.8 Malignant neoplasm of overlapping sites of heart, mediastinum and pleura

☑4ᵗʰ **C39 Malignant neoplasm of other and ill-defined sites in the respiratory system and intrathoracic organs**
    EXCLUDES 1 *intrathoracic malignant neoplasm NOS (C76.1)*
         thoracic malignant neoplasm NOS (C76.1)
    Use additional code to identify:
    exposure to environmental tobacco smoke (Z77.22)
    exposure to tobacco smoke in the perinatal period (P96.81)
    history of tobacco use (Z87.891)
    occupational exposure to environmental tobacco smoke (Z57.31)
    tobacco dependence (F17.-)
    tobacco use (Z72.0)

  C39.0 Malignant neoplasm of upper respiratory tract, part unspecified

  C39.9 Malignant neoplasm of lower respiratory tract, part unspecified
    Malignant neoplasm of respiratory tract NOS

Malignant neoplasms of bone and articular cartilage (C40-C41)

  INCLUDES malignant neoplasm of cartilage (articular) (joint)
         malignant neoplasm of periosteum
  EXCLUDES 1 *malignant neoplasm of bone marrow NOS (C96.9)*
         malignant neoplasm of synovia (C49.-)

☑4ᵗʰ **C40 Malignant neoplasm of bone and articular cartilage of limbs**
    Use additional code to identify major osseous defect, if applicable (M89.7-)

☑5ᵗʰ **C40.0 Malignant neoplasm of scapula and long bones of upper limb**

    C40.00 **Malignant neoplasm of scapula and long bones of unspecified upper limb**

    C40.01 **Malignant neoplasm of scapula and long bones of right upper limb**

C40.02 **Malignant neoplasm of scapula and long bones of left upper limb**

☑5ᵗʰ **C40.1 Malignant neoplasm of short bones of upper limb**

    C40.10 **Malignant neoplasm of short bones of unspecified upper limb**

    C40.11 **Malignant neoplasm of short bones of right upper limb**

    C40.12 **Malignant neoplasm of short bones of left upper limb**

☑5ᵗʰ **C40.2 Malignant neoplasm of long bones of lower limb**

    C40.20 **Malignant neoplasm of long bones of unspecified lower limb**

    C40.21 **Malignant neoplasm of long bones of right lower limb**

    C40.22 **Malignant neoplasm of long bones of left lower limb**

☑5ᵗʰ **C40.3 Malignant neoplasm of short bones of lower limb**

    C40.30 **Malignant neoplasm of short bones of unspecified lower limb**

    C40.31 **Malignant neoplasm of short bones of right lower limb**

    C40.32 **Malignant neoplasm of short bones of left lower limb**

☑5ᵗʰ **C40.8 Malignant neoplasm of overlapping sites of bone and articular cartilage of limb**

    C40.80 **Malignant neoplasm of overlapping sites of bone and articular cartilage of unspecified limb**

    C40.81 **Malignant neoplasm of overlapping sites of bone and articular cartilage of right limb**

    C40.82 **Malignant neoplasm of overlapping sites of bone and articular cartilage of left limb**

☑5ᵗʰ **C40.9 Malignant neoplasm of unspecified bones and articular cartilage of limb**

    C40.90 **Malignant neoplasm of unspecified bones and articular cartilage of unspecified limb**

    C40.91 **Malignant neoplasm of unspecified bones and articular cartilage of right limb**

    C40.92 **Malignant neoplasm of unspecified bones and articular cartilage of left limb**

☑4ᵗʰ **C41 Malignant neoplasm of bone and articular cartilage of other and unspecified sites**
    EXCLUDES 1 *malignant neoplasm of bones of limbs (C40.-)*
         malignant neoplasm of cartilage of ear (C49.0)
         malignant neoplasm of cartilage of eyelid (C49.0)
         malignant neoplasm of cartilage of larynx (C32.3)
         malignant neoplasm of cartilage of limbs (C40.-)
         malignant neoplasm of cartilage of nose (C30.0)

  C41.0 Malignant neoplasm of bones of skull and face
    Malignant neoplasm of maxilla (superior)
    Malignant neoplasm of orbital bone
    EXCLUDES 2 *carcinoma, any type except intraosseous or*
         odontogenic of:
           maxillary sinus (C31.0)
           upper jaw (C03.0)
         malignant neoplasm of jaw bone (lower) (C41.1)

  C41.1 Malignant neoplasm of mandible
    Malignant neoplasm of inferior maxilla
    Malignant neoplasm of lower jaw bone
    EXCLUDES 2 *carcinoma, any type except intraosseous or*
         odontogenic of:
           jaw NOS (C03.9)
           lower (C03.1)
         malignant neoplasm of upper jaw bone (C41.0)

  C41.2 Malignant neoplasm of vertebral column
    EXCLUDES 1 *malignant neoplasm of sacrum and coccyx (C41.4)*

  C41.3 Malignant neoplasm of ribs, sternum and clavicle

  C41.4 Malignant neoplasm of pelvic bones, sacrum and coccyx

  C41.9 Malignant neoplasm of bone and articular cartilage, unspecified

☑ Additional Character Required   ☑7ᵗʰ Xtension Alert   Unspecified Code   Other Specified Code   Manifestation Code   ▶◀ Revised Text   ● New Code   ▲ Revised Code Title

ICD-10-CM 2014 (Draft)   445

Neoplasms

C43–C44.192

Melanoma and other malignant neoplasms of skin (C43-C44)

✓4ᵗʰ C43 Malignant melanoma of skin
> *EXCLUDES 1*   melanoma in situ (D03.-)
> *EXCLUDES 2*   malignant melanoma of skin of genital organs (C51-C52, C60.-, C63.-)
>   Merkel cell carcinoma (C4A.-)
>   sites other than skin—code to malignant neoplasm of the site

C43.0 Malignant melanoma of lip
> *EXCLUDES 1*   malignant neoplasm of vermilion border of lip (C00.0-C00.2)

✓5ᵗʰ C43.1 Malignant melanoma of eyelid, including canthus
- **C43.10 Malignant melanoma of unspecified eyelid, including canthus**
- **C43.11 Malignant melanoma of right eyelid, including canthus**
- **C43.12 Malignant melanoma of left eyelid, including canthus**

✓5ᵗʰ C43.2 Malignant melanoma of ear and external auricular canal
- **C43.20 Malignant melanoma of unspecified ear and external auricular canal**
- **C43.21 Malignant melanoma of right ear and external auricular canal**
- **C43.22 Malignant melanoma of left ear and external auricular canal**

✓5ᵗʰ C43.3 Malignant melanoma of other and unspecified parts of face
- **C43.30 Malignant melanoma of unspecified part of face**
- **C43.31 Malignant melanoma of nose**
- **C43.39 Malignant melanoma of other parts of face**

C43.4 Malignant melanoma of scalp and neck

✓5ᵗʰ C43.5 Malignant melanoma of trunk
> *EXCLUDES 2*   malignant neoplasm of anus NOS (C21.0)
>   malignant neoplasm of scrotum (C63.2)
- **C43.51 Malignant melanoma of anal skin**
  Malignant melanoma of anal margin
  Malignant melanoma of perianal skin
- **C43.52 Malignant melanoma of skin of breast**
- **C43.59 Malignant melanoma of other part of trunk**

✓5ᵗʰ C43.6 Malignant melanoma of upper limb, including shoulder
- **C43.60 Malignant melanoma of unspecified upper limb, including shoulder**
- **C43.61 Malignant melanoma of right upper limb, including shoulder**
- **C43.62 Malignant melanoma of left upper limb, including shoulder**

✓5ᵗʰ C43.7 Malignant melanoma of lower limb, including hip
- **C43.70 Malignant melanoma of unspecified lower limb, including hip**
- **C43.71 Malignant melanoma of right lower limb, including hip**
- **C43.72 Malignant melanoma of left lower limb, including hip**

C43.8 Malignant melanoma of overlapping sites of skin

C43.9 Malignant melanoma of skin, unspecified
  Malignant melanoma of unspecified site of skin

✓4ᵗʰ C4A Merkel cell carcinoma

C4A.0 Merkel cell carcinoma of lip
> *EXCLUDES 1*   malignant neoplasm of vermilion border of lip (C00.0-C00.2)

✓5ᵗʰ C4A.1 Merkel cell carcinoma of eyelid, including canthus
- **C4A.10 Merkel cell carcinoma of unspecified eyelid, including canthus**
- **C4A.11 Merkel cell carcinoma of right eyelid, including canthus**
- **C4A.12 Merkel cell carcinoma of left eyelid, including canthus**

✓5ᵗʰ C4A.2 Merkel cell carcinoma of ear and external auricular canal
- **C4A.20 Merkel cell carcinoma of unspecified ear and external auricular canal**
- **C4A.21 Merkel cell carcinoma of right ear and external auricular canal**
- **C4A.22 Merkel cell carcinoma of left ear and external auricular canal**

✓5ᵗʰ C4A.3 Merkel cell carcinoma of other and unspecified parts of face
- **C4A.30 Merkel cell carcinoma of unspecified part of face**
- **C4A.31 Merkel cell carcinoma of nose**
- **C4A.39 Merkel cell carcinoma of other parts of face**

C4A.4 Merkel cell carcinoma of scalp and neck

✓5ᵗʰ C4A.5 Merkel cell carcinoma of trunk
> *EXCLUDES 2*   malignant neoplasm of anus NOS (C21.0)
>   malignant neoplasm of scrotum (C63.2)
- **C4A.51 Merkel cell carcinoma of anal skin**
  Merkel cell carcinoma of anal margin
  Merkel cell carcinoma of perianal skin
- **C4A.52 Merkel cell carcinoma of skin of breast**
- **C4A.59 Merkel cell carcinoma of other part of trunk**

✓5ᵗʰ C4A.6 Merkel cell carcinoma of upper limb, including shoulder
- **C4A.60 Merkel cell carcinoma of unspecified upper limb, including shoulder**
- **C4A.61 Merkel cell carcinoma of right upper limb, including shoulder**
- **C4A.62 Merkel cell carcinoma of left upper limb, including shoulder**

✓5ᵗʰ C4A.7 Merkel cell carcinoma of lower limb, including hip
- **C4A.70 Merkel cell carcinoma of unspecified lower limb, including hip**
- **C4A.71 Merkel cell carcinoma of right lower limb, including hip**
- **C4A.72 Merkel cell carcinoma of left lower limb, including hip**

C4A.8 Merkel cell carcinoma of overlapping sites

C4A.9 Merkel cell carcinoma, unspecified
  Merkel cell carcinoma of unspecified site

✓4ᵗʰ C44 Other and unspecified malignant neoplasm of skin
> *INCLUDES*   malignant neoplasm of sebaceous glands
>   malignant neoplasm of sweat glands
> *EXCLUDES 1*   Kaposi's sarcoma of skin (C46.0)
>   malignant melanoma of skin (C43.-)
>   malignant neoplasm of skin of genital organs (C51-C52, C60-, C63.2)
>   Merkel cell carcinoma (C4A.-)

✓5ᵗʰ C44.0 Other and unspecified malignant neoplasm of skin of lip
> *EXCLUDES 1*   malignant neoplasm of lip (C00.-)
- **C44.00 Unspecified malignant neoplasm of skin of lip**
- **C44.01 Basal cell carcinoma of skin of lip**
- **C44.02 Squamous cell carcinoma of skin of lip**
- **C44.09 Other specified malignant neoplasm of skin of lip**

✓5ᵗʰ C44.1 Other and unspecified malignant neoplasm of skin of eyelid, including canthus
> *EXCLUDES 1*   connective tissue of eyelid (C49.0)
- **✓6ᵗʰ C44.10 Unspecified malignant neoplasm of skin of eyelid, including canthus**
  - **C44.101 Unspecified malignant neoplasm of skin of unspecified eyelid, including canthus**
  - **C44.102 Unspecified malignant neoplasm of skin of right eyelid, including canthus**
  - **C44.109 Unspecified malignant neoplasm of skin of left eyelid, including canthus**
- **✓6ᵗʰ C44.11 Basal cell carcinoma of skin of eyelid, including canthus**
  - **C44.111 Basal cell carcinoma of skin of unspecified eyelid, including canthus**
  - **C44.112 Basal cell carcinoma of skin of right eyelid, including canthus**
  - **C44.119 Basal cell carcinoma of skin of left eyelid, including canthus**
- **✓6ᵗʰ C44.12 Squamous cell carcinoma of skin of eyelid, including canthus**
  - **C44.121 Squamous cell carcinoma of skin of unspecified eyelid, including canthus**
  - **C44.122 Squamous cell carcinoma of skin of right eyelid, including canthus**
  - **C44.129 Squamous cell carcinoma of skin of left eyelid, including canthus**
- **✓6ᵗʰ C44.19 Other specified malignant neoplasm of skin of eyelid, including canthus**
  - **C44.191 Other specified malignant neoplasm of skin of unspecified eyelid, including canthus**
  - **C44.192 Other specified malignant neoplasm of skin of right eyelid, including canthus**

EXCLUDES 1 Not coded here   *EXCLUDES 2* Not included here   N Newborn Age: 0   P Pediatric Age: 0-17   M Maternity Age: 12-55   A Adult Age: 15-124

446   ICD-10-CM 2014 (Draft)

C44.199 Other specified malignant neoplasm of skin of left eyelid, including canthus

✓5ᵗʰ **C44.2** Other and unspecified malignant neoplasm of skin of ear and external auricular canal

> EXCLUDES 1　connective tissue of ear (C49.0)

✓6ᵗʰ **C44.20** Unspecified malignant neoplasm of skin of ear and external auricular canal

C44.201 Unspecified malignant neoplasm of skin of unspecified ear and external auricular canal

C44.202 Unspecified malignant neoplasm of skin of right ear and external auricular canal

C44.209 Unspecified malignant neoplasm of skin of left ear and external auricular canal

✓6ᵗʰ **C44.21** Basal cell carcinoma of skin of ear and external auricular canal

C44.211 Basal cell carcinoma of skin of unspecified ear and external auricular canal

C44.212 Basal cell carcinoma of skin of right ear and external auricular canal

C44.219 Basal cell carcinoma of skin of left ear and external auricular canal

✓6ᵗʰ **C44.22** Squamous cell carcinoma of skin of ear and external auricular canal

C44.221 Squamous cell carcinoma of skin of unspecified ear and external auricular canal

C44.222 Squamous cell carcinoma of skin of right ear and external auricular canal

C44.229 Squamous cell carcinoma of skin of left ear and external auricular canal

✓6ᵗʰ **C44.29** Other specified malignant neoplasm of skin of ear and external auricular canal

C44.291 Other specified malignant neoplasm of skin of unspecified ear and external auricular canal

C44.292 Other specified malignant neoplasm of skin of right ear and external auricular canal

C44.299 Other specified malignant neoplasm of skin of left ear and external auricular canal

✓5ᵗʰ **C44.3** Other and unspecified malignant neoplasm of skin of other and unspecified parts of face

✓6ᵗʰ **C44.30** Unspecified malignant neoplasm of skin of other and unspecified parts of face

C44.300 Unspecified malignant neoplasm of skin of unspecified part of face

C44.301 Unspecified malignant neoplasm of skin of nose

C44.309 Unspecified malignant neoplasm of skin of other parts of face

✓6ᵗʰ **C44.31** Basal cell carcinoma of skin of other and unspecified parts of face

C44.310 Basal cell carcinoma of skin of unspecified parts of face

C44.311 Basal cell carcinoma of skin of nose

C44.319 Basal cell carcinoma of skin of other parts of face

✓6ᵗʰ **C44.32** Squamous cell carcinoma of skin of other and unspecified parts of face

C44.320 Squamous cell carcinoma of skin of unspecified parts of face

C44.321 Squamous cell carcinoma of skin of nose

C44.329 Squamous cell carcinoma of skin of other parts of face

✓6ᵗʰ **C44.39** Other specified malignant neoplasm of skin of other and unspecified parts of face

C44.390 Other specified malignant neoplasm of skin of unspecified parts of face

C44.391 Other specified malignant neoplasm of skin of nose

C44.399 Other specified malignant neoplasm of skin of other parts of face

✓5ᵗʰ **C44.4** Other and unspecified malignant neoplasm of skin of scalp and neck

C44.40 Unspecified malignant neoplasm of skin of scalp and neck

C44.41 Basal cell carcinoma of skin of scalp and neck

C44.42 Squamous cell carcinoma of skin of scalp and neck

C44.49 Other specified malignant neoplasm of skin of scalp and neck

✓5ᵗʰ **C44.5** Other and unspecified malignant neoplasm of skin of trunk

> EXCLUDES 1　anus NOS (C21.0)
> 　　　　　　scrotum (C63.2)

✓6ᵗʰ **C44.50** Unspecified malignant neoplasm of skin of trunk

C44.500 Unspecified malignant neoplasm of anal skin

Unspecified malignant neoplasm of anal margin

Unspecified malignant neoplasm of perianal skin

C44.501 Unspecified malignant neoplasm of skin of breast

C44.509 Unspecified malignant neoplasm of skin of other part of trunk

✓6ᵗʰ **C44.51** Basal cell carcinoma of skin of trunk

C44.510 Basal cell carcinoma of anal skin

Basal cell carcinoma of anal margin

Basal cell carcinoma of perianal skin

C44.511 Basal cell carcinoma of skin of breast

C44.519 Basal cell carcinoma of skin of other part of trunk

✓6ᵗʰ **C44.52** Squamous cell carcinoma of skin of trunk

C44.520 Squamous cell carcinoma of anal skin

Squamous cell carcinoma of anal margin

Squamous cell carcinoma of perianal skin

C44.521 Squamous cell carcinoma of skin of breast

C44.529 Squamous cell carcinoma of skin of other part of trunk

✓6ᵗʰ **C44.59** Other specified malignant neoplasm of skin of trunk

C44.590 Other specified malignant neoplasm of anal skin

Other specified malignant neoplasm of anal margin

Other specified malignant neoplasm of perianal skin

C44.591 Other specified malignant neoplasm of skin of breast

C44.599 Other specified malignant neoplasm of skin of other part of trunk

✓5ᵗʰ **C44.6** Other and unspecified malignant neoplasm of skin of upper limb, including shoulder

✓6ᵗʰ **C44.60** Unspecified malignant neoplasm of skin of upper limb, including shoulder

C44.601 Unspecified malignant neoplasm of skin of unspecified upper limb, including shoulder

C44.602 Unspecified malignant neoplasm of skin of right upper limb, including shoulder

C44.609 Unspecified malignant neoplasm of skin of left upper limb, including shoulder

✓6ᵗʰ **C44.61** Basal cell carcinoma of skin of upper limb, including shoulder

C44.611 Basal cell carcinoma of skin of unspecified upper limb, including shoulder

C44.612 Basal cell carcinoma of skin of right upper limb, including shoulder

C44.619 Basal cell carcinoma of skin of left upper limb, including shoulder

✓6ᵗʰ **C44.62** Squamous cell carcinoma of skin of upper limb, including shoulder

C44.621 Squamous cell carcinoma of skin of unspecified upper limb, including shoulder

C44.622 Squamous cell carcinoma of skin of right upper limb, including shoulder

C44.629 Squamous cell carcinoma of skin of left upper limb, including shoulder

✓6ᵗʰ **C44.69** Other specified malignant neoplasm of skin of upper limb, including shoulder

C44.691 Other specified malignant neoplasm of skin of unspecified upper limb, including shoulder

C44.692 Other specified malignant neoplasm of skin of right upper limb, including shoulder

---

✓ Additional Character Required　　✓x7ᵗʰ Xtension Alert　　Unspecified Code　　Other Specified Code　　Manifestation Code　　►◄ Revised Text　　● New Code　　▲ Revised Code Title

Neoplasms

C44.699–C48.8

C44.699 Other specified malignant neoplasm of skin of left upper limb, including shoulder

✓5ᵗʰ **C44.7** Other and unspecified malignant neoplasm of skin of lower limb, including hip

  ✓6ᵗʰ **C44.70** Unspecified malignant neoplasm of skin of lower limb, including hip

    C44.701 Unspecified malignant neoplasm of skin of unspecified lower limb, including hip

    C44.702 Unspecified malignant neoplasm of skin of right lower limb, including hip

    C44.709 Unspecified malignant neoplasm of skin of left lower limb, including hip

  ✓6ᵗʰ **C44.71** Basal cell carcinoma of skin of lower limb, including hip

    C44.711 Basal cell carcinoma of skin of unspecified lower limb, including hip

    C44.712 Basal cell carcinoma of skin of right lower limb, including hip

    C44.719 Basal cell carcinoma of skin of left lower limb, including hip

  ✓6ᵗʰ **C44.72** Squamous cell carcinoma of skin of lower limb, including hip

    C44.721 Squamous cell carcinoma of skin of unspecified lower limb, including hip

    C44.722 Squamous cell carcinoma of skin of right lower limb, including hip

    C44.729 Squamous cell carcinoma of skin of left lower limb, including hip

  ✓6ᵗʰ **C44.79** Other specified malignant neoplasm of skin of lower limb, including hip

    C44.791 Other specified malignant neoplasm of skin of unspecified lower limb, including hip

    C44.792 Other specified malignant neoplasm of skin of right lower limb, including hip

    C44.799 Other specified malignant neoplasm of skin of left lower limb, including hip

✓5ᵗʰ **C44.8** Other and unspecified malignant neoplasm of overlapping sites of skin

  C44.80 Unspecified malignant neoplasm of overlapping sites of skin

  C44.81 Basal cell carcinoma of overlapping sites of skin

  C44.82 Squamous cell carcinoma of overlapping sites of skin

  C44.89 Other specified malignant neoplasm of overlapping sites of skin

✓5ᵗʰ **C44.9** Other and unspecified malignant neoplasm of skin, unspecified

  C44.90 Unspecified malignant neoplasm of skin, unspecified

    Malignant neoplasm of unspecified site of skin

  C44.91 Basal cell carcinoma of skin, unspecified

  C44.92 Squamous cell carcinoma of skin, unspecified

  C44.99 Other specified malignant neoplasm of skin, unspecified

Malignant neoplasms of mesothelial and soft tissue (C45-C49)

✓4ᵗʰ **C45** **Mesothelioma**

C45.0 Mesothelioma of pleura

  EXCLUDES 1   other malignant neoplasm of pleura (C38.4)

C45.1 Mesothelioma of peritoneum

  Mesothelioma of cul-de-sac
  Mesothelioma of mesentery
  Mesothelioma of mesocolon
  Mesothelioma of omentum
  Mesothelioma of peritoneum (parietal) (pelvic)
  EXCLUDES 1   other malignant neoplasm of soft tissue of peritoneum (C48.-)

C45.2 Mesothelioma of pericardium

  EXCLUDES 1   other malignant neoplasm of pericardium (C38.0)

C45.7 Mesothelioma of other sites

C45.9 Mesothelioma, unspecified

✓4ᵗʰ **C46** **Kaposi's sarcoma**

Code first any human immunodeficiency virus [HIV] disease (B20)

C46.0 Kaposi's sarcoma of skin

C46.1 Kaposi's sarcoma of soft tissue

  Kaposi's sarcoma of blood vessel
  Kaposi's sarcoma of connective tissue
  Kaposi's sarcoma of fascia
  Kaposi's sarcoma of ligament
  Kaposi's sarcoma of lymphatic(s) NEC
  Kaposi's sarcoma of muscle
  EXCLUDES 2   Kaposi's sarcoma of lymph glands and nodes (C46.3)

C46.2 Kaposi's sarcoma of palate

C46.3 Kaposi's sarcoma of lymph nodes

C46.4 Kaposi's sarcoma of gastrointestinal sites

✓5ᵗʰ **C46.5** Kaposi's sarcoma of lung

  C46.50 Kaposi's sarcoma of unspecified lung

  C46.51 Kaposi's sarcoma of right lung

  C46.52 Kaposi's sarcoma of left lung

C46.7 Kaposi's sarcoma of other sites

C46.9 Kaposi's sarcoma, unspecified

  Kaposi's sarcoma of unspecified site

✓4ᵗʰ **C47** **Malignant neoplasm of peripheral nerves and autonomic nervous system**

  INCLUDES   malignant neoplasm of sympathetic and parasympathetic nerves and ganglia

  EXCLUDES 1   Kaposi's sarcoma of soft tissue (C46.1)

C47.0 Malignant neoplasm of peripheral nerves of head, face and neck

  EXCLUDES 1   malignant neoplasm of peripheral nerves of orbit (C69.6-)

✓5ᵗʰ **C47.1** Malignant neoplasm of peripheral nerves of upper limb, including shoulder

  C47.10 Malignant neoplasm of peripheral nerves of unspecified upper limb, including shoulder

  C47.11 Malignant neoplasm of peripheral nerves of right upper limb, including shoulder

  C47.12 Malignant neoplasm of peripheral nerves of left upper limb, including shoulder

✓5ᵗʰ **C47.2** Malignant neoplasm of peripheral nerves of lower limb, including hip

  C47.20 Malignant neoplasm of peripheral nerves of unspecified lower limb, including hip

  C47.21 Malignant neoplasm of peripheral nerves of right lower limb, including hip

  C47.22 Malignant neoplasm of peripheral nerves of left lower limb, including hip

C47.3 Malignant neoplasm of peripheral nerves of thorax

C47.4 Malignant neoplasm of peripheral nerves of abdomen

C47.5 Malignant neoplasm of peripheral nerves of pelvis

C47.6 Malignant neoplasm of peripheral nerves of trunk, unspecified

  Malignant neoplasm of peripheral nerves of unspecified part of trunk

C47.8 Malignant neoplasm of overlapping sites of peripheral nerves and autonomic nervous system

C47.9 Malignant neoplasm of peripheral nerves and autonomic nervous system, unspecified

  Malignant neoplasm of unspecified site of peripheral nerves and autonomic nervous system

✓4ᵗʰ **C48** **Malignant neoplasm of retroperitoneum and peritoneum**

  EXCLUDES 1   Kaposi's sarcoma of connective tissue (C46.1)
                 mesothelioma (C45.-)

C48.0 Malignant neoplasm of retroperitoneum

C48.1 Malignant neoplasm of specified parts of peritoneum

  Malignant neoplasm of cul-de-sac
  Malignant neoplasm of mesentery
  Malignant neoplasm of mesocolon
  Malignant neoplasm of omentum
  Malignant neoplasm of parietal peritoneum
  Malignant neoplasm of pelvic peritoneum

C48.2 Malignant neoplasm of peritoneum, unspecified

C48.8 Malignant neoplasm of overlapping sites of retroperitoneum and peritoneum

---

EXCLUDES 1 Not coded here   EXCLUDES 2 Not included here   N Newborn Age: 0   P Pediatric Age: 0-17   M Maternity Age: 12-55   A Adult Age: 15-124

Neoplasms

✓4ᵗʰ **C49 Malignant neoplasm of** other connective and soft tissue

INCLUDES malignant neoplasm of blood vessel
malignant neoplasm of bursa
malignant neoplasm of cartilage
malignant neoplasm of fascia
malignant neoplasm of fat
malignant neoplasm of ligament, except uterine
malignant neoplasm of lymphatic vessel
malignant neoplasm of muscle
malignant neoplasm of synovia
malignant neoplasm of tendon (sheath)

EXCLUDES 1 malignant neoplasm of cartilage (of):
articular (C40-C41)
larynx (C32.3)
nose (C30.0)
malignant neoplasm of connective tissue of breast (C50.-)

EXCLUDES 2 Kaposi's sarcoma of soft tissue (C46.1)
malignant neoplasm of heart (C38.0)
malignant neoplasm of peripheral nerves and autonomic
nervous system (C47.-)
malignant neoplasm of peritoneum (C48.2)
malignant neoplasm of retroperitoneum (C48.0)
malignant neoplasm of uterine ligament (C57.3)
mesothelioma (C45.-)

C49.0 Malignant neoplasm of connective and soft tissue of head, face and neck
Malignant neoplasm of connective tissue of ear
Malignant neoplasm of connective tissue of eyelid
EXCLUDES 1 connective tissue of orbit (C69.6-)

✓5ᵗʰ **C49.1 Malignant neoplasm of connective and soft tissue of** upper limb, including shoulder

C49.10 Malignant neoplasm of connective and soft tissue of unspecified upper limb, including shoulder

C49.11 Malignant neoplasm of connective and soft tissue of right upper limb, including shoulder

C49.12 Malignant neoplasm of connective and soft tissue of left upper limb, including shoulder

✓5ᵗʰ **C49.2 Malignant neoplasm of connective and soft tissue of** lower limb, including hip

C49.20 Malignant neoplasm of connective and soft tissue of unspecified lower limb, including hip

C49.21 Malignant neoplasm of connective and soft tissue of right lower limb, including hip

C49.22 Malignant neoplasm of connective and soft tissue of left lower limb, including hip

C49.3 Malignant neoplasm of connective and soft tissue of thorax
Malignant neoplasm of axilla
Malignant neoplasm of diaphragm
Malignant neoplasm of great vessels
EXCLUDES 1 malignant neoplasm of breast (C50.-)
malignant neoplasm of heart (C38.0)
malignant neoplasm of mediastinum (C38.1-C38.3)
malignant neoplasm of thymus (C37)

C49.4 Malignant neoplasm of connective and soft tissue of abdomen
Malignant neoplasm of abdominal wall
Malignant neoplasm of hypochondrium

C49.5 Malignant neoplasm of connective and soft tissue of pelvis
Malignant neoplasm of buttock
Malignant neoplasm of groin
Malignant neoplasm of perineum

C49.6 Malignant neoplasm of connective and soft tissue of trunk, unspecified
Malignant neoplasm of back NOS

C49.8 Malignant neoplasm of overlapping sites **of connective and soft tissue**
Primary malignant neoplasm of two or more contiguous sites of connective and soft tissue

C49.9 Malignant neoplasm of connective and soft tissue, unspecified

Malignant neoplasms of breast (C50)

✓4ᵗʰ **C50 Malignant neoplasm of** breast
INCLUDES connective tissue of breast
Paget's disease of breast
Paget's disease of nipple
Use additional code to identify estrogen receptor status (Z17.0, Z17.1)
EXCLUDES 1 skin of breast (C44.501, C44.511, C44.521, C44.591)

✓5ᵗʰ **C50.0 Malignant neoplasm of** nipple and areola

✓6ᵗʰ **C50.01 Malignant neoplasm of nipple and areola,** female

C50.011 Malignant neoplasm of nipple and areola, right female breast ♀

C50.012 Malignant neoplasm of nipple and areola, left female breast ♀

C50.019 Malignant neoplasm of nipple and areola, unspecified female breast ♀

✓6ᵗʰ **C50.02 Malignant neoplasm of nipple and areola,** male

C50.021 Malignant neoplasm of nipple and areola, right male breast ♂

C50.022 Malignant neoplasm of nipple and areola, left male breast ♂

C50.029 Malignant neoplasm of nipple and areola, unspecified male breast ♂

✓5ᵗʰ **C50.1 Malignant neoplasm of** central portion of breast

✓6ᵗʰ **C50.11 Malignant neoplasm of central portion of breast,** female

C50.111 Malignant neoplasm of central portion of right female breast ♀

C50.112 Malignant neoplasm of central portion of left female breast ♀

C50.119 Malignant neoplasm of central portion of unspecified female breast ♀

✓6ᵗʰ **C50.12 Malignant neoplasm of central portion of breast,** male

C50.121 Malignant neoplasm of central portion of right male breast ♂

C50.122 Malignant neoplasm of central portion of left male breast ♂

C50.129 Malignant neoplasm of central portion of unspecified male breast ♂

✓5ᵗʰ **C50.2 Malignant neoplasm of** upper-inner quadrant of breast

✓6ᵗʰ **C50.21 Malignant neoplasm of upper-inner quadrant of breast,** female

C50.211 Malignant neoplasm of upper-inner quadrant of right female breast ♀

C50.212 Malignant neoplasm of upper-inner quadrant of left female breast ♀

C50.219 Malignant neoplasm of upper-inner quadrant of unspecified female breast ♀

✓6ᵗʰ **C50.22 Malignant neoplasm of upper-inner quadrant of breast,** male

C50.221 Malignant neoplasm of upper-inner quadrant of right male breast ♂

C50.222 Malignant neoplasm of upper-inner quadrant of left male breast ♂

C50.229 Malignant neoplasm of upper-inner quadrant of unspecified male breast ♂

✓5ᵗʰ **C50.3 Malignant neoplasm of** lower-inner quadrant of breast

✓6ᵗʰ **C50.31 Malignant neoplasm of lower-inner quadrant of breast,** female

C50.311 Malignant neoplasm of lower-inner quadrant of right female breast ♀

C50.312 Malignant neoplasm of lower-inner quadrant of left female breast ♀

C50.319 Malignant neoplasm of lower-inner quadrant of unspecified female breast ♀

✓6ᵗʰ **C50.32 Malignant neoplasm of lower-inner quadrant of breast,** male

C50.321 Malignant neoplasm of lower-inner quadrant of right male breast ♂

C50.322 Malignant neoplasm of lower-inner quadrant of left male breast ♂

C50.329 Malignant neoplasm of lower-inner quadrant of unspecified male breast ♂

Neoplasms

C50.4–C57.7

√5th **C50.4 Malignant neoplasm of** upper-outer quadrant **of breast**

  √6th **C50.41 Malignant neoplasm of upper-outer quadrant of breast,** female

    C50.411 Malignant neoplasm of upper-outer quadrant of right female breast ♀

    C50.412 Malignant neoplasm of upper-outer quadrant of left female breast ♀

    C50.419 Malignant neoplasm of upper-outer quadrant of unspecified female breast ♀

  √6th **C50.42 Malignant neoplasm of upper-outer quadrant of breast,** male

    C50.421 Malignant neoplasm of upper-outer quadrant of right male breast ♂

    C50.422 Malignant neoplasm of upper-outer quadrant of left male breast ♂

    C50.429 Malignant neoplasm of upper-outer quadrant of unspecified male breast ♂

√5th **C50.5 Malignant neoplasm of** lower-outer quadrant **of breast**

  √6th **C50.51 Malignant neoplasm of lower-outer quadrant of breast,** female

    C50.511 Malignant neoplasm of lower-outer quadrant of right female breast ♀

    C50.512 Malignant neoplasm of lower-outer quadrant of left female breast ♀

    C50.519 Malignant neoplasm of lower-outer quadrant of unspecified female breast ♀

  √6th **C50.52 Malignant neoplasm of lower-outer quadrant of breast,** male

    C50.521 Malignant neoplasm of lower-outer quadrant of right male breast ♂

    C50.522 Malignant neoplasm of lower-outer quadrant of left male breast ♂

    C50.529 Malignant neoplasm of lower-outer quadrant of unspecified male breast ♂

√5th **C50.6 Malignant neoplasm of** axillary tail **of breast**

  √6th **C50.61 Malignant neoplasm of axillary tail of breast,** female

    C50.611 Malignant neoplasm of axillary tail of right female breast ♀

    C50.612 Malignant neoplasm of axillary tail of left female breast ♀

    C50.619 Malignant neoplasm of axillary tail of unspecified female breast ♀

  √6th **C50.62 Malignant neoplasm of axillary tail of breast,** male

    C50.621 Malignant neoplasm of axillary tail of right male breast ♂

    C50.622 Malignant neoplasm of axillary tail of left male breast ♂

    C50.629 Malignant neoplasm of axillary tail of unspecified male breast ♂

√5th **C50.8 Malignant neoplasm of** overlapping sites **of breast**

  √6th **C50.81 Malignant neoplasm of overlapping sites of breast,** female

    C50.811 Malignant neoplasm of overlapping sites of right female breast ♀

    C50.812 Malignant neoplasm of overlapping sites of left female breast ♀

    C50.819 Malignant neoplasm of overlapping sites of unspecified female breast ♀

  √6th **C50.82 Malignant neoplasm of overlapping sites of breast,** male

    C50.821 Malignant neoplasm of overlapping sites of right male breast ♂

    C50.822 Malignant neoplasm of overlapping sites of left male breast ♂

    C50.829 Malignant neoplasm of overlapping sites of unspecified male breast ♂

√5th **C50.9 Malignant neoplasm of breast of** unspecified site

  √6th **C50.91 Malignant neoplasm of breast of unspecified site,** female

    C50.911 Malignant neoplasm of unspecified site of right female breast ♀

    C50.912 Malignant neoplasm of unspecified site of left female breast ♀

    C50.919 Malignant neoplasm of unspecified site of unspecified female breast ♀

  √6th **C50.92 Malignant neoplasm of breast of unspecified site,** male

    C50.921 Malignant neoplasm of unspecified site of right male breast ♂

    C50.922 Malignant neoplasm of unspecified site of left male breast ♂

    C50.929 Malignant neoplasm of unspecified site of unspecified male breast ♂

Malignant neoplasms of female genital organs (C51-C58)

INCLUDES   malignant neoplasm of skin of female genital organs

√4th **C51 Malignant neoplasm of** vulva

  EXCLUDES 1   carcinoma in situ of vulva (D07.1)

  C51.0 Malignant neoplasm of labium majus ♀
    Malignant neoplasm of Bartholin's [greater vestibular] gland

  C51.1 Malignant neoplasm of labium minus ♀

  C51.2 Malignant neoplasm of clitoris ♀

  C51.8 Malignant neoplasm of overlapping sites **of vulva** ♀

  C51.9 Malignant neoplasm of vulva, unspecified ♀
    Malignant neoplasm of external female genitalia NOS
    Malignant neoplasm of pudendum

C52 Malignant neoplasm of vagina ♀
  EXCLUDES 1   carcinoma in situ of vagina (D07.2)

√4th **C53 Malignant neoplasm of** cervix uteri
  EXCLUDES 1   carcinoma in situ of cervix uteri (D06.-)

  C53.0 Malignant neoplasm of endocervix ♀

  C53.1 Malignant neoplasm of exocervix ♀

  C53.8 Malignant neoplasm of overlapping sites **of cervix uteri** ♀

  C53.9 Malignant neoplasm of cervix uteri, unspecified ♀

√4th **C54 Malignant neoplasm of** corpus uteri

  C54.0 Malignant neoplasm of isthmus uteri ♀
    Malignant neoplasm of lower uterine segment

  C54.1 Malignant neoplasm of endometrium ♀

  C54.2 Malignant neoplasm of myometrium ♀

  C54.3 Malignant neoplasm of fundus uteri ♀

  C54.8 Malignant neoplasm of overlapping sites **of corpus uteri** ♀

  C54.9 Malignant neoplasm of corpus uteri, unspecified ♀

C55 Malignant neoplasm of uterus, part unspecified ♀

√4th **C56 Malignant neoplasm of** ovary
  Use additional code to identify any functional activity

  C56.1 Malignant neoplasm of right **ovary** ♀

  C56.2 Malignant neoplasm of left **ovary** ♀

  C56.9 Malignant neoplasm of unspecified ovary ♀

√4th **C57 Malignant neoplasm of** other and unspecified female genital **organs**

  √5th **C57.0 Malignant neoplasm of** fallopian tube
    Malignant neoplasm of oviduct
    Malignant neoplasm of uterine tube

    C57.00 Malignant neoplasm of unspecified fallopian tube ♀

    C57.01 Malignant neoplasm of right fallopian tube ♀

    C57.02 Malignant neoplasm of left fallopian tube ♀

  √5th **C57.1 Malignant neoplasm of** broad ligament

    C57.10 Malignant neoplasm of unspecified broad ligament ♀

    C57.11 Malignant neoplasm of right broad ligament ♀

    C57.12 Malignant neoplasm of left broad ligament ♀

  √5th **C57.2 Malignant neoplasm of** round ligament

    C57.20 Malignant neoplasm of unspecified round ligament ♀

    C57.21 Malignant neoplasm of right round ligament ♀

    C57.22 Malignant neoplasm of left round ligament ♀

  C57.3 Malignant neoplasm of parametrium ♀
    Malignant neoplasm of uterine ligament NOS

  C57.4 Malignant neoplasm of uterine adnexa, unspecified ♀

  C57.7 Malignant neoplasm of other specified female genital organs ♀
    Malignant neoplasm of wolffian body or duct

EXCLUDES 1 Not coded here   EXCLUDES 2 Not included here   N Newborn Age: 0   P Pediatric Age: 0-17   M Maternity Age: 12-55   A Adult Age: 15-124

450   ICD-10-CM 2014 (Draft)

C57.8 Malignant neoplasm of overlapping sites **of female genital organs** ♀
  Primary malignant neoplasm of two or more contiguous sites of the female genital organs whose point of origin cannot be determined
  Primary tubo-ovarian malignant neoplasm whose point of origin cannot be determined
  Primary utero-ovarian malignant neoplasm whose point of origin cannot be determined

C57.9 Malignant neoplasm of female genital organ, unspecified ♀
  Malignant neoplasm of female genitourinary tract NOS

C58 Malignant neoplasm of placenta ♀
  INCLUDES choriocarcinoma NOS
    chorionepithelioma NOS
  EXCLUDES 1 *chorioadenoma (destruens) (D39.2)*
    hydatidiform mole NOS (O01.9)
    invasive hydatidiform mole (D39.2)
    male choriocarcinoma NOS (C62.9-)
    malignant hydatidiform mole (D39.2)

Malignant neoplasms of male genital organs (C60-C63)
INCLUDES malignant neoplasm of skin of male genital organs

✓4ᵗʰ **C60 Malignant neoplasm of** penis

C60.0 Malignant neoplasm of prepuce ♂
  Malignant neoplasm of foreskin

C60.1 Malignant neoplasm of glans penis ♂

C60.2 Malignant neoplasm of body **of penis** ♂
  Malignant neoplasm of corpus cavernosum

C60.8 Malignant neoplasm of overlapping sites **of penis** ♂

C60.9 Malignant neoplasm of penis, unspecified ♂
  Malignant neoplasm of skin of penis NOS

C61 Malignant neoplasm of prostate ♂
  EXCLUDES 1 *malignant neoplasm of seminal vesicle (C63.7)*

✓4ᵗʰ **C62 Malignant neoplasm of** testis
  Use additional code to identify any functional activity

✓5ᵗʰ **C62.0 Malignant neoplasm of** undescended **testis**
  Malignant neoplasm of ectopic testis
  Malignant neoplasm of retained testis

C62.00 Malignant neoplasm of unspecified undescended ♂ **testis**

C62.01 Malignant neoplasm of undescended right **testis** ♂

C62.02 Malignant neoplasm of undescended left **testis** ♂

✓5ᵗʰ **C62.1 Malignant neoplasm of** descended **testis**
  Malignant neoplasm of scrotal testis

C62.10 Malignant neoplasm of unspecified descended ♂ **testis**

C62.11 Malignant neoplasm of descended right **testis** ♂

C62.12 Malignant neoplasm of descended left **testis** ♂

✓5ᵗʰ **C62.9 Malignant neoplasm of testis,** unspecified whether descended or undescended

C62.90 Malignant neoplasm of unspecified testis, unspecified whether descended or undescended ♂
  Malignant neoplasm of testis NOS

C62.91 Malignant neoplasm of right **testis, unspecified whether descended or undescended** ♂

C62.92 Malignant neoplasm of left **testis, unspecified whether descended or undescended** ♂

✓4ᵗʰ **C63 Malignant neoplasm of** other and unspecified male genital organs

✓5ᵗʰ **C63.0 Malignant neoplasm of** epididymis

C63.00 Malignant neoplasm of unspecified epididymis ♂

C63.01 Malignant neoplasm of right **epididymis** ♂

C63.02 Malignant neoplasm of left **epididymis** ♂

✓5ᵗʰ **C63.1 Malignant neoplasm of** spermatic cord

C63.10 Malignant neoplasm of unspecified spermatic cord ♂

C63.11 Malignant neoplasm of right **spermatic cord** ♂

C63.12 Malignant neoplasm of left **spermatic cord** ♂

C63.2 Malignant neoplasm of scrotum ♂
  Malignant neoplasm of skin of scrotum

C63.7 Malignant neoplasm of other specified **male genital organs** ♂
  Malignant neoplasm of seminal vesicle
  Malignant neoplasm of tunica vaginalis

C63.8 Malignant neoplasm of overlapping sites **of male genital organs** ♂
  Primary malignant neoplasm of two or more contiguous sites of male genital organs whose point of origin cannot be determined

C63.9 Malignant neoplasm of male genital organ, unspecified ♂
  Malignant neoplasm of male genitourinary tract NOS

Malignant neoplasms of urinary tract (C64-C68)

✓4ᵗʰ **C64 Malignant neoplasm of** kidney, except renal pelvis
  EXCLUDES 1 *malignant carcinoid tumor of the kidney (C7A.093)*
    malignant neoplasm of renal calyces (C65.-)
    malignant neoplasm of renal pelvis (C65.-)

C64.1 Malignant neoplasm of right **kidney, except renal pelvis**

C64.2 Malignant neoplasm of left **kidney, except renal pelvis**

C64.9 Malignant neoplasm of unspecified kidney, except renal pelvis

✓4ᵗʰ **C65 Malignant neoplasm of** renal pelvis
  INCLUDES malignant neoplasm of pelviureteric junction
    malignant neoplasm of renal calyces

C65.1 Malignant neoplasm of right **renal pelvis**

C65.2 Malignant neoplasm of left **renal pelvis**

C65.9 Malignant neoplasm of unspecified renal pelvis

✓4ᵗʰ **C66 Malignant neoplasm of** ureter
  EXCLUDES 1 *malignant neoplasm of ureteric orifice of bladder (C67.6)*

C66.1 Malignant neoplasm of right **ureter**

C66.2 Malignant neoplasm of left **ureter**

C66.9 Malignant neoplasm of unspecified ureter

✓4ᵗʰ **C67 Malignant neoplasm of** bladder

C67.0 Malignant neoplasm of trigone **of bladder**

C67.1 Malignant neoplasm of dome **of bladder**

C67.2 Malignant neoplasm of lateral wall **of bladder**

C67.3 Malignant neoplasm of anterior wall **of bladder**

C67.4 Malignant neoplasm of posterior wall **of bladder**

C67.5 Malignant neoplasm of bladder neck
  Malignant neoplasm of internal urethral orifice

C67.6 Malignant neoplasm of ureteric orifice

C67.7 Malignant neoplasm of urachus

C67.8 Malignant neoplasm of overlapping sites **of bladder**

C67.9 Malignant neoplasm of bladder, unspecified

✓4ᵗʰ **C68 Malignant neoplasm of** other and unspecified urinary organs
  EXCLUDES 1 *malignant neoplasm of female genitourinary tract NOS (C57.9)*
    malignant neoplasm of male genitourinary tract NOS (C63.9)

C68.0 Malignant neoplasm of urethra
  EXCLUDES 1 *malignant neoplasm of urethral orifice of bladder (C67.5)*

C68.1 Malignant neoplasm of paraurethral glands

C68.8 Malignant neoplasm of overlapping sites **of urinary organs**
  Primary malignant neoplasm of two or more contiguous sites of urinary organs whose point of origin cannot be determined

C68.9 Malignant neoplasm of urinary organ, unspecified
  Malignant neoplasm of urinary system NOS

Malignant neoplasms of eye, brain and other parts of central nervous system (C69-C72)

✓4ᵗʰ **C69 Malignant neoplasm of** eye and adnexa
  EXCLUDES 1 *malignant neoplasm of connective tissue of eyelid (C49.0)*
    malignant neoplasm of eyelid (skin) (C43.1-, C44.1-)
    malignant neoplasm of optic nerve (C72.3-)

✓5ᵗʰ **C69.0 Malignant neoplasm of** conjunctiva

C69.00 Malignant neoplasm of unspecified conjunctiva

C69.01 Malignant neoplasm of right **conjunctiva**

C69.02 Malignant neoplasm of left **conjunctiva**

✓5ᵗʰ **C69.1 Malignant neoplasm of** cornea

C69.10 Malignant neoplasm of unspecified cornea

C69.11 Malignant neoplasm of right **cornea**

C69.12 Malignant neoplasm of left **cornea**

✓ Additional Character Required   ✓7ᵗʰ Xtension Alert   Unspecified Code   Other Specified Code   Manifestation Code   ▶◀ Revised Text   ● New Code   ▲ Revised Code Title

ICD-10-CM 2014 (Draft)   **451**

Neoplasms

C69.2–C75.9

✓5ᵗʰ **C69.2 Malignant neoplasm of** retina
- EXCLUDES 1   dark area on retina (D49.81)
  - neoplasm of unspecified behavior of retina and choroid (D49.81)
  - retinal freckle (D49.81)
- **C69.20 Malignant neoplasm of unspecified retina**
- **C69.21 Malignant neoplasm of** right **retina**
- **C69.22 Malignant neoplasm of** left **retina**

✓5ᵗʰ **C69.3 Malignant neoplasm of** choroid
- **C69.30 Malignant neoplasm of unspecified choroid**
- **C69.31 Malignant neoplasm of** right **choroid**
- **C69.32 Malignant neoplasm of** left **choroid**

✓5ᵗʰ **C69.4 Malignant neoplasm of** ciliary body
- **C69.40 Malignant neoplasm of unspecified ciliary body**
- **C69.41 Malignant neoplasm of** right **ciliary body**
- **C69.42 Malignant neoplasm of** left **ciliary body**

✓5ᵗʰ **C69.5 Malignant neoplasm of** lacrimal gland and duct
- Malignant neoplasm of lacrimal sac
- Malignant neoplasm of nasolacrimal duct
- **C69.50 Malignant neoplasm of unspecified lacrimal gland and duct**
- **C69.51 Malignant neoplasm of** right **lacrimal gland and duct**
- **C69.52 Malignant neoplasm of** left **lacrimal gland and duct**

✓5ᵗʰ **C69.6 Malignant neoplasm of** orbit
- Malignant neoplasm of connective tissue of orbit
- Malignant neoplasm of extraocular muscle
- Malignant neoplasm of peripheral nerves of orbit
- Malignant neoplasm of retrobulbar tissue
- Malignant neoplasm of retro-ocular tissue
- EXCLUDES 1   malignant neoplasm of orbital bone (C41.0)
- **C69.60 Malignant neoplasm of unspecified orbit**
- **C69.61 Malignant neoplasm of** right **orbit**
- **C69.62 Malignant neoplasm of** left **orbit**

✓5ᵗʰ **C69.8 Malignant neoplasm of** overlapping sites of eye and adnexa
- **C69.80 Malignant neoplasm of overlapping sites of unspecified eye and adnexa**
- **C69.81 Malignant neoplasm of overlapping sites of** right **eye and adnexa**
- **C69.82 Malignant neoplasm of overlapping sites of** left **eye and adnexa**

✓5ᵗʰ **C69.9 Malignant neoplasm of** unspecified **site of eye**
- Malignant neoplasm of eyeball
- **C69.90 Malignant neoplasm of unspecified site of unspecified eye**
- **C69.91 Malignant neoplasm of unspecified site of** right **eye**
- **C69.92 Malignant neoplasm of unspecified site of** left **eye**

✓4ᵗʰ **C70 Malignant neoplasm of** meninges
- **C70.0 Malignant neoplasm of** cerebral **meninges**
- **C70.1 Malignant neoplasm of** spinal **meninges**
- **C70.9 Malignant neoplasm of meninges, unspecified**

✓4ᵗʰ **C71 Malignant neoplasm of** brain
- EXCLUDES 1   malignant neoplasm of cranial nerves (C72.2-C72.5)
  - retrobulbar malignant neoplasm (C69.6-)
- **C71.0 Malignant neoplasm of** cerebrum, except lobes and ventricles
  - Malignant neoplasm of supratentorial NOS
- **C71.1 Malignant neoplasm of** frontal **lobe**
- **C71.2 Malignant neoplasm of** temporal **lobe**
- **C71.3 Malignant neoplasm of** parietal **lobe**
- **C71.4 Malignant neoplasm of** occipital **lobe**
- **C71.5 Malignant neoplasm of** cerebral **ventricle**
  - EXCLUDES 1   malignant neoplasm of fourth cerebral ventricle (C71.7)
- **C71.6 Malignant neoplasm of** cerebellum
- **C71.7 Malignant neoplasm of** brain stem
  - Malignant neoplasm of fourth cerebral ventricle
  - Infratentorial malignant neoplasm NOS
- **C71.8 Malignant neoplasm of** overlapping sites **of brain**
- **C71.9 Malignant neoplasm of brain, unspecified**

✓4ᵗʰ **C72 Malignant neoplasm of** spinal cord, cranial nerves and other parts of central nervous system
- EXCLUDES 1   malignant neoplasm of meninges (C70.-)
  - malignant neoplasm of peripheral nerves and autonomic nervous system (C47.-)
- **C72.0 Malignant neoplasm of** spinal cord

- **C72.1 Malignant neoplasm of** cauda equina

✓5ᵗʰ **C72.2 Malignant neoplasm of** olfactory nerve
- Malignant neoplasm of olfactory bulb
- **C72.20 Malignant neoplasm of unspecified olfactory nerve**
- **C72.21 Malignant neoplasm of** right **olfactory nerve**
- **C72.22 Malignant neoplasm of** left **olfactory nerve**

✓5ᵗʰ **C72.3 Malignant neoplasm of** optic nerve
- **C72.30 Malignant neoplasm of unspecified optic nerve**
- **C72.31 Malignant neoplasm of** right **optic nerve**
- **C72.32 Malignant neoplasm of** left **optic nerve**

✓5ᵗʰ **C72.4 Malignant neoplasm of** acoustic nerve
- **C72.40 Malignant neoplasm of unspecified acoustic nerve**
- **C72.41 Malignant neoplasm of** right **acoustic nerve**
- **C72.42 Malignant neoplasm of** left **acoustic nerve**

✓5ᵗʰ **C72.5 Malignant neoplasm of** other and unspecified cranial nerves
- **C72.50 Malignant neoplasm of unspecified cranial nerve**
  - Malignant neoplasm of cranial nerve NOS
- **C72.59 Malignant neoplasm of other cranial nerves**
- **C72.9 Malignant neoplasm of central nervous system, unspecified**
  - Malignant neoplasm of unspecified site of central nervous system
  - Malignant neoplasm of nervous system NOS

Malignant neoplasms of thyroid and other endocrine glands (C73-C75)

C73 Malignant neoplasm of thyroid gland
- Use additional code to identify any functional activity

✓4ᵗʰ **C74 Malignant neoplasm of** adrenal gland

✓5ᵗʰ **C74.0 Malignant neoplasm of** cortex **of adrenal gland**
- **C74.00 Malignant neoplasm of cortex of unspecified adrenal gland**
- **C74.01 Malignant neoplasm of cortex of** right **adrenal gland**
- **C74.02 Malignant neoplasm of cortex of** left **adrenal gland**

✓5ᵗʰ **C74.1 Malignant neoplasm of** medulla **of adrenal gland**
- **C74.10 Malignant neoplasm of medulla of unspecified adrenal gland**
- **C74.11 Malignant neoplasm of medulla of** right **adrenal gland**
- **C74.12 Malignant neoplasm of medulla of** left **adrenal gland**

✓5ᵗʰ **C74.9 Malignant neoplasm of** unspecified part **of adrenal gland**
- **C74.90 Malignant neoplasm of unspecified part of unspecified adrenal gland**
- **C74.91 Malignant neoplasm of unspecified part of** right **adrenal gland**
- **C74.92 Malignant neoplasm of unspecified part of** left **adrenal gland**

✓4ᵗʰ **C75 Malignant neoplasm of** other endocrine glands and related structures
- EXCLUDES 1   malignant carcinoid tumors (C7A.0-)
  - malignant neoplasm of adrenal gland (C74.-)
  - malignant neoplasm of endocrine pancreas (C25.4)
  - malignant neoplasm of islets of Langerhans (C25.4)
  - malignant neoplasm of ovary (C56.-)
  - malignant neoplasm of testis (C62.-)
  - malignant neoplasm of thymus (C37)
  - malignant neoplasm of thyroid gland (C73)
  - malignant neuroendocrine tumors (C7A.-)
- **C75.0 Malignant neoplasm of** parathyroid **gland**
- **C75.1 Malignant neoplasm of** pituitary **gland**
- **C75.2 Malignant neoplasm of** craniopharyngeal **duct**
- **C75.3 Malignant neoplasm of** pineal **gland**
- **C75.4 Malignant neoplasm of** carotid body
- **C75.5 Malignant neoplasm of** aortic body and other paraganglia
- **C75.8 Malignant neoplasm with** pluriglandular involvement, unspecified
- **C75.9 Malignant neoplasm of endocrine gland, unspecified**

EXCLUDES 1 Not coded here   EXCLUDES 2 Not included here   N Newborn Age: 0   P Pediatric Age: 0-17   M Maternity Age: 12-55   A Adult Age: 15-124

Malignant neuroendocrine tumors (C7A)

☑4ᵗʰ **C7A Malignant** neuroendocrine tumors

Code also any associated multiple endocrine neoplasia [MEN] syndromes (E31.2-)

Use additional code to identify any associated endocrine syndrome, such as:

carcinoid syndrome (E34.0)

EXCLUDES 2   malignant pancreatic islet cell tumors (C25.4)

Merkel cell carcinoma (C4A.-)

☑5ᵗʰ **C7A.0 Malignant** carcinoid tumors

     C7A.00 Malignant carcinoid tumor of unspecified site

☑6ᵗʰ   **C7A.01 Malignant carcinoid tumors of the** small intestine

       C7A.010 Malignant carcinoid tumor of the duodenum

       C7A.011 Malignant carcinoid tumor of the jejunum

       C7A.012 Malignant carcinoid tumor of the ileum

       C7A.019 Malignant carcinoid tumor of the small intestine, unspecified portion

☑6ᵗʰ   **C7A.02 Malignant carcinoid tumors of the** appendix, large intestine, and rectum

       C7A.020 Malignant carcinoid tumor of the appendix

       C7A.021 Malignant carcinoid tumor of the cecum

       C7A.022 Malignant carcinoid tumor of the ascending colon

       C7A.023 Malignant carcinoid tumor of the transverse colon

       C7A.024 Malignant carcinoid tumor of the descending colon

       C7A.025 Malignant carcinoid tumor of the sigmoid colon

       C7A.026 Malignant carcinoid tumor of the rectum

       C7A.029 Malignant carcinoid tumor of the large intestine, unspecified portion

         Malignant carcinoid tumor of the colon NOS

☑6ᵗʰ   **C7A.09 Malignant carcinoid tumors of** other sites

       C7A.090 Malignant carcinoid tumor of the bronchus and lung

       C7A.091 Malignant carcinoid tumor of the thymus

       C7A.092 Malignant carcinoid tumor of the stomach

       C7A.093 Malignant carcinoid tumor of the kidney

       C7A.094 Malignant carcinoid tumor of the foregut NOS

       C7A.095 Malignant carcinoid tumor of the midgut NOS

       C7A.096 Malignant carcinoid tumor of the hindgut NOS

       C7A.098 Malignant carcinoid tumors of other sites

C7A.1 Malignant poorly differentiated **neuroendocrine tumors**

     High grade neuroendocrine carcinoma, any site

     Malignant poorly differentiated neuroendocrine tumor NOS

     Malignant poorly differentiated neuroendocrine carcinoma, any site

C7A.8 Other malignant neuroendocrine tumors

Secondary neuroendocrine tumors (C7B)

☑4ᵗʰ **C7B Secondary** neuroendocrine tumors

Use additional code to identify any functional activity

☑5ᵗʰ **C7B.0 Secondary** carcinoid tumors

     C7B.00 Secondary carcinoid tumors, unspecified site

     C7B.01 Secondary carcinoid tumors of distant lymph nodes

     C7B.02 Secondary carcinoid tumors of liver

     C7B.03 Secondary carcinoid tumors of bone

     C7B.04 Secondary carcinoid tumors of peritoneum

       Mesentery metastasis of carcinoid tumor

     C7B.09 Secondary carcinoid tumors of other sites

C7B.1 Secondary Merkel cell carcinoma

     Merkel cell carcinoma nodal presentation

     Merkel cell carcinoma visceral metastatic presentation

C7B.8 Other secondary neuroendocrine tumors

Malignant neoplasms of ill-defined, other secondary and unspecified sites (C76-C80)

☑4ᵗʰ **C76 Malignant neoplasm of** other and ill-defined sites

EXCLUDES 1   malignant neoplasm of female genitourinary tract NOS (C57.9)

malignant neoplasm of male genitourinary tract NOS (C63.9)

malignant neoplasm of lymphoid, hematopoietic and related tissue (C81-C96)

malignant neoplasm of skin (C44.-)

malignant neoplasm of unspecified site NOS (C80.1)

C76.0 Malignant neoplasm of head, face and neck

     Malignant neoplasm of cheek NOS

     Malignant neoplasm of nose NOS

C76.1 Malignant neoplasm of thorax

     Intrathoracic malignant neoplasm NOS

     Malignant neoplasm of axilla NOS

     Thoracic malignant neoplasm NOS

C76.2 Malignant neoplasm of abdomen

C76.3 Malignant neoplasm of pelvis

     Malignant neoplasm of groin NOS

     Malignant neoplasm of sites overlapping systems within the pelvis

     Rectovaginal (septum) malignant neoplasm

     Rectovesical (septum) malignant neoplasm

☑5ᵗʰ **C76.4 Malignant neoplasm of** upper limb

     C76.40 Malignant neoplasm of unspecified upper limb

     C76.41 Malignant neoplasm of right upper limb

     C76.42 Malignant neoplasm of left upper limb

☑5ᵗʰ **C76.5 Malignant neoplasm of** lower limb

     C76.50 Malignant neoplasm of unspecified lower limb

     C76.51 Malignant neoplasm of right lower limb

     C76.52 Malignant neoplasm of left lower limb

C76.8 Malignant neoplasm of other specified ill-defined sites

     Malignant neoplasm of overlapping ill-defined sites

☑4ᵗʰ **C77 Secondary and unspecified** malignant neoplasm of lymph nodes

EXCLUDES 1   malignant neoplasm of lymph nodes, specified as primary (C81-C86, C88, C96.-)

mesentery metastasis of carcinoid tumor (C7B.04)

secondary carcinoid tumors of distant lymph nodes (C7B.01)

C77.0 Secondary and unspecified malignant neoplasm of lymph nodes of head, face and neck

     Secondary and unspecified malignant neoplasm of supraclavicular lymph nodes

C77.1 Secondary and unspecified malignant neoplasm of intrathoracic lymph nodes

C77.2 Secondary and unspecified malignant neoplasm of intra-abdominal lymph nodes

C77.3 Secondary and unspecified malignant neoplasm of axilla and upper limb lymph nodes

     Secondary and unspecified malignant neoplasm of pectoral lymph nodes

C77.4 Secondary and unspecified malignant neoplasm of inguinal and lower limb lymph nodes

C77.5 Secondary and unspecified malignant neoplasm of intrapelvic lymph nodes

C77.8 Secondary and unspecified malignant neoplasm of lymph nodes of multiple regions

C77.9 Secondary and unspecified malignant neoplasm of lymph node, unspecified

☑4ᵗʰ **C78 Secondary malignant neoplasm of respiratory and digestive organs**

EXCLUDES 1   lymph node metastases (C77.0)

secondary carcinoid tumors of liver (C7B.02)

secondary carcinoid tumors of peritoneum (C7B.04)

☑5ᵗʰ **C78.0 Secondary malignant neoplasm of lung**

     C78.00 Secondary malignant neoplasm of unspecified lung

     C78.01 Secondary malignant neoplasm of right lung

     C78.02 Secondary malignant neoplasm of left lung

C78.1 Secondary malignant neoplasm of mediastinum

C78.2 Secondary malignant neoplasm of pleura

☑5ᵗʰ **C78.3 Secondary malignant neoplasm of** other and unspecified respiratory organs

     C78.30 Secondary malignant neoplasm of unspecified respiratory organ

     C78.39 Secondary malignant neoplasm of other respiratory organs

C78.4 Secondary malignant neoplasm of small intestine

Neoplasms

C7A–C78.4

Neoplasms

C78.5–C81.22

C78.5 Secondary malignant neoplasm of large intestine and rectum

C78.6 Secondary malignant neoplasm of retroperitoneum and peritoneum

C78.7 Secondary malignant neoplasm of liver and intrahepatic bile duct

☑5ᵗʰ **C78.8** Secondary malignant neoplasm of other and unspecified digestive organs

   C78.80 Secondary malignant neoplasm of unspecified digestive organ

   C78.89 Secondary malignant neoplasm of other digestive organs

☑4ᵗʰ **C79** Secondary malignant neoplasm of other and unspecified sites

   EXCLUDES 1 *lymph node metastases (C77.0)*
   secondary carcinoid tumors (C7B.-)
   secondary neuroendocrine tumors (C7B.-)

☑5ᵗʰ **C79.0** Secondary malignant neoplasm of kidney and renal pelvis

   C79.00 Secondary malignant neoplasm of unspecified kidney and renal pelvis

   C79.01 Secondary malignant neoplasm of right kidney and renal pelvis

   C79.02 Secondary malignant neoplasm of left kidney and renal pelvis

☑5ᵗʰ **C79.1** Secondary malignant neoplasm of bladder and other and unspecified urinary organs

   C79.10 Secondary malignant neoplasm of unspecified urinary organs

   C79.11 Secondary malignant neoplasm of bladder

   C79.19 Secondary malignant neoplasm of other urinary organs

C79.2 Secondary malignant neoplasm of skin

   EXCLUDES 1 *secondary Merkel cell carcinoma (C7B.1)*

☑5ᵗʰ **C79.3** Secondary malignant neoplasm of brain and cerebral meninges

   C79.31 Secondary malignant neoplasm of brain

   C79.32 Secondary malignant neoplasm of cerebral meninges

☑5ᵗʰ **C79.4** Secondary malignant neoplasm of other and unspecified parts of nervous system

   C79.40 Secondary malignant neoplasm of unspecified part of nervous system

   C79.49 Secondary malignant neoplasm of other parts of nervous system

☑5ᵗʰ **C79.5** Secondary malignant neoplasm of bone and bone marrow

   EXCLUDES 1 *secondary carcinoid tumors of bone (C7B.03)*

   C79.51 Secondary malignant neoplasm of bone

   C79.52 Secondary malignant neoplasm of bone marrow

☑5ᵗʰ **C79.6** Secondary malignant neoplasm of ovary

   C79.60 Secondary malignant neoplasm of unspecified ovary ♀

   C79.61 Secondary malignant neoplasm of right ovary ♀

   C79.62 Secondary malignant neoplasm of left ovary ♀

☑5ᵗʰ **C79.7** Secondary malignant neoplasm of adrenal gland

   C79.70 Secondary malignant neoplasm of unspecified adrenal gland

   C79.71 Secondary malignant neoplasm of right adrenal gland

   C79.72 Secondary malignant neoplasm of left adrenal gland

☑5ᵗʰ **C79.8** Secondary malignant neoplasm of other specified sites

   C79.81 Secondary malignant neoplasm of breast

   C79.82 Secondary malignant neoplasm of genital organs

   C79.89 Secondary malignant neoplasm of other specified sites

C79.9 Secondary malignant neoplasm of unspecified site
   Metastatic cancer NOS
   Metastatic disease NOS

   EXCLUDES 1 *carcinomatosis NOS (C80.0)*
   generalized cancer NOS (C80.0)
   malignant (primary) neoplasm of unspecified site (C80.1)

☑4ᵗʰ **C80** Malignant neoplasm without specification of site

   EXCLUDES 1 *malignant carcinoid tumor of unspecified site (C7A.00)*
   malignant neoplasm of specified multiple sites—code to each site

C80.0 Disseminated malignant neoplasm, unspecified
   Carcinomatosis NOS
   Generalized cancer, unspecified site (primary) (secondary)
   Generalized malignancy, unspecified site (primary) (secondary)

C80.1 Malignant (primary) neoplasm, unspecified
   Cancer NOS
   Cancer unspecified site (primary)
   Carcinoma unspecified site (primary)
   Malignancy unspecified site (primary)

   EXCLUDES 1 *secondary malignant neoplasm of unspecified site (C79.9)*

C80.2 Malignant neoplasm associated with transplanted organ
   Code first complication of transplanted organ (T86.-)
   Use additional code to identify the specific malignancy

Malignant neoplasms of lymphoid, hematopoietic and related tissue (C81-C96)

   EXCLUDES 2 *Kaposi's sarcoma of lymph nodes (C46.3)*
   secondary and unspecified neoplasm of lymph nodes (C77.-)
   secondary neoplasm of bone marrow (C79.52)
   secondary neoplasm of spleen (C78.89)

☑4ᵗʰ **C81** Hodgkin lymphoma

   EXCLUDES 1 *personal history of Hodgkin lymphoma (Z85.71)*

☑5ᵗʰ **C81.0** Nodular lymphocyte predominant Hodgkin lymphoma

   C81.00 Nodular lymphocyte predominant Hodgkin lymphoma, unspecified site

   C81.01 Nodular lymphocyte predominant Hodgkin lymphoma, lymph nodes of head, face, and neck

   C81.02 Nodular lymphocyte predominant Hodgkin lymphoma, intrathoracic lymph nodes

   C81.03 Nodular lymphocyte predominant Hodgkin lymphoma, intra-abdominal lymph nodes

   C81.04 Nodular lymphocyte predominant Hodgkin lymphoma, lymph nodes of axilla and upper limb

   C81.05 Nodular lymphocyte predominant Hodgkin lymphoma, lymph nodes of inguinal region and lower limb

   C81.06 Nodular lymphocyte predominant Hodgkin lymphoma, intrapelvic lymph nodes

   C81.07 Nodular lymphocyte predominant Hodgkin lymphoma, spleen

   C81.08 Nodular lymphocyte predominant Hodgkin lymphoma, lymph nodes of multiple sites

   C81.09 Nodular lymphocyte predominant Hodgkin lymphoma, extranodal and solid organ sites

☑5ᵗʰ **C81.1** Nodular sclerosis classical Hodgkin lymphoma

   C81.10 Nodular sclerosis classical Hodgkin lymphoma, unspecified site

   C81.11 Nodular sclerosis classical Hodgkin lymphoma, lymph nodes of head, face, and neck

   C81.12 Nodular sclerosis classical Hodgkin lymphoma, intrathoracic lymph nodes

   C81.13 Nodular sclerosis classical Hodgkin lymphoma, intra-abdominal lymph nodes

   C81.14 Nodular sclerosis classical Hodgkin lymphoma, lymph nodes of axilla and upper limb

   C81.15 Nodular sclerosis classical Hodgkin lymphoma, lymph nodes of inguinal region and lower limb

   C81.16 Nodular sclerosis classical Hodgkin lymphoma, intrapelvic lymph nodes

   C81.17 Nodular sclerosis classical Hodgkin lymphoma, spleen

   C81.18 Nodular sclerosis classical Hodgkin lymphoma, lymph nodes of multiple sites

   C81.19 Nodular sclerosis classical Hodgkin lymphoma, extranodal and solid organ sites

☑5ᵗʰ **C81.2** Mixed cellularity classical Hodgkin lymphoma

   C81.20 Mixed cellularity classical Hodgkin lymphoma, unspecified site

   C81.21 Mixed cellularity classical Hodgkin lymphoma, lymph nodes of head, face, and neck

   C81.22 Mixed cellularity classical Hodgkin lymphoma, intrathoracic lymph nodes

EXCLUDES 1 Not coded here   EXCLUDES 2 Not included here   N Newborn Age: 0   P Pediatric Age: 0-17   M Maternity Age: 12-55   A Adult Age: 15-124

454   ICD-10-CM 2014 (Draft)

C81.23　**Mixed cellularity classical Hodgkin lymphoma, intra-abdominal lymph nodes**

C81.24　**Mixed cellularity classical Hodgkin lymphoma, lymph nodes of** axilla and upper limb

C81.25　**Mixed cellularity classical Hodgkin lymphoma, lymph nodes of** inguinal region and lower limb

C81.26　**Mixed cellularity classical Hodgkin lymphoma, intrapelvic lymph nodes**

C81.27　**Mixed cellularity classical Hodgkin lymphoma, spleen**

C81.28　**Mixed cellularity classical Hodgkin lymphoma, lymph nodes of** multiple sites

C81.29　**Mixed cellularity classical Hodgkin lymphoma, extranodal and solid organ sites**

✓5ᵗʰ **C81.3　Lymphocyte-depleted classical Hodgkin lymphoma**

C81.30　**Lymphocyte-depleted classical Hodgkin lymphoma, unspecified site**

C81.31　**Lymphocyte-depleted classical Hodgkin lymphoma, lymph nodes of** head, face, and neck

C81.32　**Lymphocyte-depleted classical Hodgkin lymphoma, intrathoracic lymph nodes**

C81.33　**Lymphocyte-depleted classical Hodgkin lymphoma, intra-abdominal lymph nodes**

C81.34　**Lymphocyte-depleted classical Hodgkin lymphoma, lymph nodes of** axilla and upper limb

C81.35　**Lymphocyte-depleted classical Hodgkin lymphoma, lymph nodes of** inguinal region and lower limb

C81.36　**Lymphocyte-depleted classical Hodgkin lymphoma, intrapelvic lymph nodes**

C81.37　**Lymphocyte-depleted classical Hodgkin lymphoma, spleen**

C81.38　**Lymphocyte-depleted classical Hodgkin lymphoma, lymph nodes of** multiple sites

C81.39　**Lymphocyte-depleted classical Hodgkin lymphoma, extranodal and solid organ sites**

✓5ᵗʰ **C81.4　Lymphocyte-rich classical Hodgkin lymphoma**

EXCLUDES 1　*nodular lymphocyte predominant Hodgkin lymphoma (C81.0-)*

C81.40　**Lymphocyte-rich classical Hodgkin lymphoma, unspecified site**

C81.41　**Lymphocyte-rich classical Hodgkin lymphoma, lymph nodes of** head, face, and neck

C81.42　**Lymphocyte-rich classical Hodgkin lymphoma, intrathoracic lymph nodes**

C81.43　**Lymphocyte-rich classical Hodgkin lymphoma, intra-abdominal lymph nodes**

C81.44　**Lymphocyte-rich classical Hodgkin lymphoma, lymph nodes of** axilla and upper limb

C81.45　**Lymphocyte-rich classical Hodgkin lymphoma, lymph nodes of** inguinal region and lower limb

C81.46　**Lymphocyte-rich classical Hodgkin lymphoma, intrapelvic lymph nodes**

C81.47　**Lymphocyte-rich classical Hodgkin lymphoma, spleen**

C81.48　**Lymphocyte-rich classical Hodgkin lymphoma, lymph nodes of** multiple sites

C81.49　**Lymphocyte-rich classical Hodgkin lymphoma, extranodal and solid organ sites**

✓5ᵗʰ **C81.7　Other classical Hodgkin lymphoma**
Classical Hodgkin lymphoma NOS

C81.70　**Other classical Hodgkin lymphoma, unspecified site**

C81.71　**Other classical Hodgkin lymphoma, lymph nodes of** head, face, and neck

C81.72　**Other classical Hodgkin lymphoma, intrathoracic lymph nodes**

C81.73　**Other classical Hodgkin lymphoma, intra-abdominal lymph nodes**

C81.74　**Other classical Hodgkin lymphoma, lymph nodes of** axilla and upper limb

C81.75　**Other classical Hodgkin lymphoma, lymph nodes of** inguinal region and lower limb

C81.76　**Other classical Hodgkin lymphoma, intrapelvic lymph nodes**

C81.77　**Other classical Hodgkin lymphoma,** spleen

C81.78　**Other classical Hodgkin lymphoma, lymph nodes of** multiple sites

C81.79　**Other classical Hodgkin lymphoma,** extranodal and solid organ sites

✓5ᵗʰ **C81.9　Hodgkin lymphoma,** unspecified

C81.90　**Hodgkin lymphoma, unspecified, unspecified site**

C81.91　**Hodgkin lymphoma, unspecified, lymph nodes of** head, face, and neck

C81.92　**Hodgkin lymphoma, unspecified, intrathoracic lymph nodes**

C81.93　**Hodgkin lymphoma, unspecified, intra-abdominal lymph nodes**

C81.94　**Hodgkin lymphoma, unspecified, lymph nodes of** axilla and upper limb

C81.95　**Hodgkin lymphoma, unspecified, lymph nodes of** inguinal region and lower limb

C81.96　**Hodgkin lymphoma, unspecified, intrapelvic lymph nodes**

C81.97　**Hodgkin lymphoma, unspecified,** spleen

C81.98　**Hodgkin lymphoma, unspecified, lymph nodes of** multiple sites

C81.99　**Hodgkin lymphoma, unspecified,** extranodal and solid organ sites

✓4ᵗʰ **C82　Follicular lymphoma**
INCLUDES　follicular lymphoma with or without diffuse areas
EXCLUDES 1　*mature T/NK-cell lymphomas (C84.-)*
personal history of non-Hodgkin lymphoma (Z85.72)

✓5ᵗʰ **C82.0　Follicular lymphoma** grade I

C82.00　**Follicular lymphoma grade I, unspecified site**

C82.01　**Follicular lymphoma grade I, lymph nodes of** head, face, and neck

C82.02　**Follicular lymphoma grade I, intrathoracic lymph nodes**

C82.03　**Follicular lymphoma grade I, intra-abdominal lymph nodes**

C82.04　**Follicular lymphoma grade I, lymph nodes of** axilla and upper limb

C82.05　**Follicular lymphoma grade I, lymph nodes of** inguinal region and lower limb

C82.06　**Follicular lymphoma grade I, intrapelvic lymph nodes**

C82.07　**Follicular lymphoma grade I,** spleen

C82.08　**Follicular lymphoma grade I, lymph nodes of** multiple sites

C82.09　**Follicular lymphoma grade I,** extranodal and solid organ sites

✓5ᵗʰ **C82.1　Follicular lymphoma** grade II

C82.10　**Follicular lymphoma grade II, unspecified site**

C82.11　**Follicular lymphoma grade II, lymph nodes of** head, face, and neck

C82.12　**Follicular lymphoma grade II, intrathoracic lymph nodes**

C82.13　**Follicular lymphoma grade II, intra-abdominal lymph nodes**

C82.14　**Follicular lymphoma grade II, lymph nodes of** axilla and upper limb

C82.15　**Follicular lymphoma grade II, lymph nodes of** inguinal region and lower limb

C82.16　**Follicular lymphoma grade II, intrapelvic lymph nodes**

C82.17　**Follicular lymphoma grade II,** spleen

C82.18　**Follicular lymphoma grade II, lymph nodes of** multiple sites

C82.19　**Follicular lymphoma grade II,** extranodal and solid organ sites

✓5ᵗʰ **C82.2　Follicular lymphoma** grade III, unspecified

C82.20　**Follicular lymphoma grade III, unspecified, unspecified site**

C82.21　**Follicular lymphoma grade III, unspecified, lymph nodes of** head, face, and neck

C82.22　**Follicular lymphoma grade III, unspecified, intrathoracic lymph nodes**

Follicular lymphoma grade III, unspecified, intra-abdominal lymph nodes

C82.24　**Follicular lymphoma grade III, unspecified, lymph nodes of** axilla and upper limb

C82.25　**Follicular lymphoma grade III, unspecified, lymph nodes of** inguinal region and lower limb

---

☑ Additional Character Required　🔲7ᵗʰ Xtension Alert　Unspecified Code　Other Specified Code　Manifestation Code　▶◀ Revised Text　● New Code　▲ Revised Code Title

ICD-10-CM 2014 (Draft)　　　　　　　　　　　　　　　　　455

Neoplasms

C81.23–C82.25

Neoplasms

C82.26–C83.09

C82.26   Follicular lymphoma grade III, unspecified, intrapelvic **lymph nodes**

C82.27   Follicular lymphoma grade III, unspecified, spleen

C82.28   Follicular lymphoma grade III, unspecified, lymph nodes of **multiple sites**

C82.29   Follicular lymphoma grade III, unspecified, extranodal and solid organ sites

✓5ᵗʰ **C82.3**   Follicular lymphoma grade IIIa

C82.30   Follicular lymphoma grade IIIa, unspecified site

C82.31   Follicular lymphoma grade IIIa, lymph nodes of head, face, and neck

C82.32   Follicular lymphoma grade IIIa, intrathoracic **lymph nodes**

C82.33   Follicular lymphoma grade IIIa, intra-abdominal **lymph nodes**

C82.34   Follicular lymphoma grade IIIa, lymph nodes of axilla and upper limb

C82.35   Follicular lymphoma grade IIIa, lymph nodes of inguinal region and lower limb

C82.36   Follicular lymphoma grade IIIa, intrapelvic **lymph nodes**

C82.37   Follicular lymphoma grade IIIa, spleen

C82.38   Follicular lymphoma grade IIIa, lymph nodes of **multiple sites**

C82.39   Follicular lymphoma grade IIIa, extranodal and solid organ sites

✓5ᵗʰ **C82.4**   Follicular lymphoma grade IIIb

C82.40   Follicular lymphoma grade IIIb, unspecified site

C82.41   Follicular lymphoma grade IIIb, lymph nodes of head, face, and neck

C82.42   Follicular lymphoma grade IIIb, intrathoracic **lymph nodes**

C82.43   Follicular lymphoma grade IIIb, intra-abdominal **lymph nodes**

C82.44   Follicular lymphoma grade IIIb, lymph nodes of axilla and upper limb

C82.45   Follicular lymphoma grade IIIb, lymph nodes of inguinal region and lower limb

C82.46   Follicular lymphoma grade IIIb, intrapelvic **lymph nodes**

C82.47   Follicular lymphoma grade IIIb, spleen

C82.48   Follicular lymphoma grade IIIb, lymph nodes of **multiple sites**

C82.49   Follicular lymphoma grade IIIb, extranodal and solid organ sites

✓5ᵗʰ **C82.5**   Diffuse follicle center **lymphoma**

C82.50   Diffuse follicle center lymphoma, unspecified site

C82.51   Diffuse follicle center lymphoma, lymph nodes of head, face, and neck

C82.52   Diffuse follicle center lymphoma, intrathoracic **lymph nodes**

C82.53   Diffuse follicle center lymphoma, intra-abdominal **lymph nodes**

C82.54   Diffuse follicle center lymphoma, lymph nodes of axilla and upper limb

C82.55   Diffuse follicle center lymphoma, lymph nodes of inguinal region and lower limb

C82.56   Diffuse follicle center lymphoma, intrapelvic **lymph nodes**

C82.57   Diffuse follicle center lymphoma, spleen

C82.58   Diffuse follicle center lymphoma, lymph nodes of **multiple sites**

C82.59   Diffuse follicle center lymphoma, extranodal and solid organ sites

✓5ᵗʰ **C82.6**   Cutaneous follicle center **lymphoma**

C82.60   Cutaneous follicle center lymphoma, unspecified site

C82.61   Cutaneous follicle center lymphoma, lymph nodes of head, face, and neck

C82.62   Cutaneous follicle center lymphoma, intrathoracic **lymph nodes**

C82.63   Cutaneous follicle center lymphoma, intra-abdominal **lymph nodes**

C82.64   Cutaneous follicle center lymphoma, lymph nodes of axilla and upper limb

C82.65   Cutaneous follicle center lymphoma, lymph nodes of inguinal region and lower limb

C82.66   Cutaneous follicle center lymphoma, intrapelvic lymph nodes

C82.67   Cutaneous follicle center lymphoma, spleen

C82.68   Cutaneous follicle center lymphoma, lymph nodes of **multiple sites**

C82.69   Cutaneous follicle center lymphoma, extranodal and solid organ sites

✓5ᵗʰ **C82.8**   Other types of follicular lymphoma

C82.80   Other types of follicular lymphoma, unspecified site

C82.81   Other types of follicular lymphoma, lymph nodes of head, face, and neck

C82.82   Other types of follicular lymphoma, intrathoracic lymph nodes

C82.83   Other types of follicular lymphoma, intra-abdominal lymph nodes

C82.84   Other types of follicular lymphoma, lymph nodes of axilla and upper limb

C82.85   Other types of follicular lymphoma, lymph nodes of inguinal region and lower limb

C82.86   Other types of follicular lymphoma, intrapelvic lymph nodes

C82.87   Other types of follicular lymphoma, spleen

C82.88   Other types of follicular lymphoma, lymph nodes of multiple sites

C82.89   Other types of follicular lymphoma, extranodal and solid organ sites

✓5ᵗʰ **C82.9**   Follicular lymphoma, unspecified

C82.90   Follicular lymphoma, unspecified, unspecified site

C82.91   Follicular lymphoma, unspecified, lymph nodes of head, face, and neck

C82.92   Follicular lymphoma, unspecified, intrathoracic lymph nodes

C82.93   Follicular lymphoma, unspecified, intra-abdominal lymph nodes

C82.94   Follicular lymphoma, unspecified, lymph nodes of axilla and upper limb

C82.95   Follicular lymphoma, unspecified, lymph nodes of inguinal region and lower limb

C82.96   Follicular lymphoma, unspecified, intrapelvic lymph nodes

C82.97   Follicular lymphoma, unspecified, spleen

C82.98   Follicular lymphoma, unspecified, lymph nodes of multiple sites

C82.99   Follicular lymphoma, unspecified, extranodal and solid organ sites

✓4ᵗʰ **C83**   Non-follicular **lymphoma**

    EXCLUDES 1   personal history of non-Hodgkin lymphoma (Z85.72)

✓5ᵗʰ **C83.0**   Small cell B-cell **lymphoma**

    Lymphoplasmacytic lymphoma
    Nodal marginal zone lymphoma
    Non-leukemic variant of B-CLL
    Splenic marginal zone lymphoma

    EXCLUDES 1   chronic lymphocytic leukemia (C91.1)
              mature T/NK-cell lymphomas (C84.-)
              Waldenström macroglobulinemia (C88.Ø)

C83.00   Small cell B-cell lymphoma, unspecified site

C83.01   Small cell B-cell lymphoma, lymph nodes of head, face, and neck

C83.02   Small cell B-cell lymphoma, intrathoracic **lymph nodes**

C83.03   Small cell B-cell lymphoma, intra-abdominal **lymph nodes**

C83.04   Small cell B-cell lymphoma, lymph nodes of axilla and upper limb

C83.05   Small cell B-cell lymphoma, lymph nodes of inguinal region and lower limb

C83.06   Small cell B-cell lymphoma, intrapelvic lymph nodes

C83.07   Small cell B-cell lymphoma, spleen

C83.08   Small cell B-cell lymphoma, lymph nodes of multiple sites

C83.09   Small cell B-cell lymphoma, extranodal and solid organ sites

---

EXCLUDES 1 Not coded here   *EXCLUDES 2* Not included here   **N** Newborn Age: Ø   **P** Pediatric Age: Ø-17   **M** Maternity Age: 12-55   **A** Adult Age: 15-124

✓5th **C83.1** Mantle cell **lymphoma**
Centrocytic lymphoma
Malignant lymphomatous polyposis

C83.10 Mantle cell lymphoma, unspecified site

C83.11 Mantle cell lymphoma, lymph nodes of head, face, and neck

C83.12 Mantle cell lymphoma, intrathoracic lymph nodes

C83.13 Mantle cell lymphoma, intra-abdominal lymph nodes

C83.14 Mantle cell lymphoma, lymph nodes of axilla and upper limb

C83.15 Mantle cell lymphoma, lymph nodes of inguinal region and lower limb

C83.16 Mantle cell lymphoma, intrapelvic lymph nodes

C83.17 Mantle cell lymphoma, spleen

C83.18 Mantle cell lymphoma, lymph nodes of multiple sites

C83.19 Mantle cell lymphoma, extranodal and solid organ sites

✓5th **C83.3** Diffuse large B-cell **lymphoma**
Anaplastic diffuse large B-cell lymphoma
CD30-positive diffuse large B-cell lymphoma
Centroblastic diffuse large B-cell lymphoma
Diffuse large B-cell lymphoma, subtype not specified
Immunoblastic diffuse large B-cell lymphoma
Plasmablastic diffuse large B-cell lymphoma
T-cell rich diffuse large B-cell lymphoma
EXCLUDES 1　mediastinal (thymic) large B-cell lymphoma (C85.2-)
mature T/NK-cell lymphomas (C84.-)

C83.30 Diffuse large B-cell lymphoma, unspecified site

C83.31 Diffuse large B-cell lymphoma, lymph nodes of head, face, and neck

C83.32 Diffuse large B-cell lymphoma, intrathoracic lymph nodes

C83.33 Diffuse large B-cell lymphoma, intra-abdominal lymph nodes

C83.34 Diffuse large B-cell lymphoma, lymph nodes of axilla and upper limb

C83.35 Diffuse large B-cell lymphoma, lymph nodes of inguinal region and lower limb

C83.36 Diffuse large B-cell lymphoma, intrapelvic lymph nodes

C83.37 Diffuse large B-cell lymphoma, spleen

C83.38 Diffuse large B-cell lymphoma, lymph nodes of multiple sites

C83.39 Diffuse large B-cell lymphoma, extranodal and solid organ sites

✓5th **C83.5** Lymphoblastic (diffuse) **lymphoma**
B-precursor lymphoma
Lymphoblastic B-cell lymphoma
Lymphoblastic lymphoma NOS
Lymphoblastic T-cell lymphoma
T-precursor lymphoma

C83.50 Lymphoblastic (diffuse) lymphoma, unspecified site

C83.51 Lymphoblastic (diffuse) lymphoma, lymph nodes of head, face, and neck

C83.52 Lymphoblastic (diffuse) lymphoma, intrathoracic lymph nodes

C83.53 Lymphoblastic (diffuse) lymphoma, intra-abdominal lymph nodes

C83.54 Lymphoblastic (diffuse) lymphoma, lymph nodes of axilla and upper limb

C83.55 Lymphoblastic (diffuse) lymphoma, lymph nodes of inguinal region and lower limb

C83.56 Lymphoblastic (diffuse) lymphoma, intrapelvic lymph nodes

C83.57 Lymphoblastic (diffuse) lymphoma, spleen

C83.58 Lymphoblastic (diffuse) lymphoma, lymph nodes of multiple sites

C83.59 Lymphoblastic (diffuse) lymphoma, extranodal and solid organ sites

✓5th **C83.7** Burkitt **lymphoma**
Atypical Burkitt lymphoma
Burkitt-like lymphoma
EXCLUDES 1　mature B-cell leukemia Burkitt type (C91.A-)

C83.70 Burkitt lymphoma, unspecified site

C83.71 Burkitt lymphoma, lymph nodes of head, face, and neck

C83.72 Burkitt lymphoma, intrathoracic lymph nodes

C83.73 Burkitt lymphoma, intra-abdominal lymph nodes

C83.74 Burkitt lymphoma, lymph nodes of axilla and upper limb

C83.75 Burkitt lymphoma, lymph nodes of inguinal region and lower limb

C83.76 Burkitt lymphoma, intrapelvic lymph nodes

C83.77 Burkitt lymphoma, spleen

C83.78 Burkitt lymphoma, lymph nodes of multiple sites

C83.79 Burkitt lymphoma, extranodal and solid organ sites

✓5th **C83.8** Other non-follicular **lymphoma**
Intravascular large B-cell lymphoma
Lymphoid granulomatosis
Primary effusion B-cell lymphoma
EXCLUDES 1　mediastinal (thymic) large B-cell lymphoma (C85.2-)
T-cell rich B-cell lymphoma (C83.3-)

C83.80 Other non-follicular lymphoma, unspecified site

C83.81 Other non-follicular lymphoma, lymph nodes of head, face, and neck

C83.82 Other non-follicular lymphoma, intrathoracic lymph nodes

C83.83 Other non-follicular lymphoma, intra-abdominal lymph nodes

C83.84 Other non-follicular lymphoma, lymph nodes of axilla and upper limb

C83.85 Other non-follicular lymphoma, lymph nodes of inguinal region and lower limb

C83.86 Other non-follicular lymphoma, intrapelvic lymph nodes

C83.87 Other non-follicular lymphoma, spleen

C83.88 Other non-follicular lymphoma, lymph nodes of multiple sites

C83.89 Other non-follicular lymphoma, extranodal and solid organ sites

✓5th **C83.9** Non-follicular (diffuse) lymphoma, unspecified

C83.90 Non-follicular (diffuse) lymphoma, unspecified, unspecified site

C83.91 Non-follicular (diffuse) lymphoma, unspecified, lymph nodes of head, face, and neck

C83.92 Non-follicular (diffuse) lymphoma, unspecified, intrathoracic lymph nodes

C83.93 Non-follicular (diffuse) lymphoma, unspecified, intra-abdominal lymph nodes

C83.94 Non-follicular (diffuse) lymphoma, unspecified, lymph nodes of axilla and upper limb

C83.95 Non-follicular (diffuse) lymphoma, unspecified, lymph nodes of inguinal region and lower limb

C83.96 Non-follicular (diffuse) lymphoma, unspecified, intrapelvic lymph nodes

C83.97 Non-follicular (diffuse) lymphoma, unspecified, spleen

C83.98 Non-follicular (diffuse) lymphoma, unspecified, lymph nodes of multiple sites

C83.99 Non-follicular (diffuse) lymphoma, unspecified, extranodal and solid organ sites

✓4th **C84** **Mature T/NK-cell lymphomas**
EXCLUDES 1　personal history of non-Hodgkin lymphoma (Z85.72)

✓5th **C84.0** **Mycosis fungoides**
EXCLUDES 1　peripheral T-cell lymphoma, not classified (C84.4-)

C84.00 Mycosis fungoides, unspecified site

C84.01 Mycosis fungoides, lymph nodes of head, face, and neck

C84.02 Mycosis fungoides, intrathoracic lymph nodes

C84.03 Mycosis fungoides, intra-abdominal lymph nodes

C84.04 Mycosis fungoides, lymph nodes of axilla and upper limb

C84.05 Mycosis fungoides, lymph nodes of inguinal region and lower limb

C84.06 Mycosis fungoides, intrapelvic lymph nodes

C84.07 Mycosis fungoides, spleen

C84.08 Mycosis fungoides, lymph nodes of multiple sites

C84.09 Mycosis fungoides, extranodal and solid organ sites

✓5th **C84.1** Sézary disease

C84.10 Sézary disease, unspecified site

C84.11 Sézary disease, lymph nodes of head, face, and neck

✓ Additional Character Required　　✓x7th Xtension Alert　　Unspecified Code　　Other Specified Code　　Manifestation Code　　▶◀ Revised Text　　● New Code　　▲ Revised Code Title

ICD-10-CM 2014 (Draft)　　　　　　　　　　　　　　　　　　　　　　　　　　　　　　457

Neoplasms

C84.12 Sézary disease, intrathoracic lymph nodes

C84.13 Sézary disease, intra-abdominal lymph nodes

C84.14 Sézary disease, lymph nodes of axilla and upper limb

C84.15 Sézary disease, lymph nodes of inguinal region and lower limb

C84.16 Sézary disease, intrapelvic lymph nodes

C84.17 Sézary disease, spleen

C84.18 Sézary disease, lymph nodes of multiple sites

C84.19 Sézary disease, extranodal and solid organ sites

✓5ᵗʰ **C84.4** Peripheral T-cell lymphoma, not classified
Lennert's lymphoma
Lymphoepithelioid lymphoma
Mature T-cell lymphoma, not elsewhere classified

     C84.40 Peripheral T-cell lymphoma, not classified, unspecified site

     C84.41 Peripheral T-cell lymphoma, not classified, lymph nodes of head, face, and neck

     C84.42 Peripheral T-cell lymphoma, not classified, intrathoracic lymph nodes

     C84.43 Peripheral T-cell lymphoma, not classified, intra-abdominal lymph nodes

     C84.44 Peripheral T-cell lymphoma, not classified, lymph nodes of axilla and upper limb

     C84.45 Peripheral T-cell lymphoma, not classified, lymph nodes of inguinal region and lower limb

     C84.46 Peripheral T-cell lymphoma, not classified, intrapelvic lymph nodes

     C84.47 Peripheral T-cell lymphoma, not classified, spleen

     C84.48 Peripheral T-cell lymphoma, not classified, lymph nodes of multiple sites

     C84.49 Peripheral T-cell lymphoma, not classified, extranodal and solid organ sites

✓5ᵗʰ **C84.6** Anaplastic large cell lymphoma, ALK-positive
Anaplastic large cell lymphoma, CD30-positive

     C84.60 Anaplastic large cell lymphoma, ALK-positive, unspecified site

     C84.61 Anaplastic large cell lymphoma, ALK-positive, lymph nodes of head, face, and neck

     C84.62 Anaplastic large cell lymphoma, ALK-positive, intrathoracic lymph nodes

     C84.63 Anaplastic large cell lymphoma, ALK-positive, intra-abdominal lymph nodes

     C84.64 Anaplastic large cell lymphoma, ALK-positive, lymph nodes of axilla and upper limb

     C84.65 Anaplastic large cell lymphoma, ALK-positive, lymph nodes of inguinal region and lower limb

     C84.66 Anaplastic large cell lymphoma, ALK-positive, intrapelvic lymph nodes

     C84.67 Anaplastic large cell lymphoma, ALK-positive, spleen

     C84.68 Anaplastic large cell lymphoma, ALK-positive, lymph nodes of multiple sites

     C84.69 Anaplastic large cell lymphoma, ALK-positive, extranodal and solid organ sites

✓5ᵗʰ **C84.7** Anaplastic large cell lymphoma, ALK-negative
EXCLUDES 1   primary cutaneous CD30-positive T-cell proliferations (C86.6-)

     C84.70 Anaplastic large cell lymphoma, ALK-negative, unspecified site

     C84.71 Anaplastic large cell lymphoma, ALK-negative, lymph nodes of head, face, and neck

     C84.72 Anaplastic large cell lymphoma, ALK-negative, intrathoracic lymph nodes

     C84.73 Anaplastic large cell lymphoma, ALK-negative, intra-abdominal lymph nodes

     C84.74 Anaplastic large cell lymphoma, ALK-negative, lymph nodes of axilla and upper limb

     C84.75 Anaplastic large cell lymphoma, ALK-negative, lymph nodes of inguinal region and lower limb

     C84.76 Anaplastic large cell lymphoma, ALK-negative, intrapelvic lymph nodes

     C84.77 Anaplastic large cell lymphoma, ALK-negative, spleen

     C84.78 Anaplastic large cell lymphoma, ALK-negative, lymph nodes of multiple sites

     C84.79 Anaplastic large cell lymphoma, ALK-negative, extranodal and solid organ sites

✓5ᵗʰ **C84.A** Cutaneous T-cell lymphoma, unspecified

     C84.A0 Cutaneous T-cell lymphoma, unspecified, unspecified site

     C84.A1 Cutaneous T-cell lymphoma, unspecified lymph nodes of head, face, and neck

     C84.A2 Cutaneous T-cell lymphoma, unspecified, intrathoracic lymph nodes

     C84.A3 Cutaneous T-cell lymphoma, unspecified, intra-abdominal lymph nodes

     C84.A4 Cutaneous T-cell lymphoma, unspecified, lymph nodes of axilla and upper limb

     C84.A5 Cutaneous T-cell lymphoma, unspecified, lymph nodes of inguinal region and lower limb

     C84.A6 Cutaneous T-cell lymphoma, unspecified, intrapelvic lymph nodes

     C84.A7 Cutaneous T-cell lymphoma, unspecified, spleen

     C84.A8 Cutaneous T-cell lymphoma, unspecified, lymph nodes of multiple sites

     C84.A9 Cutaneous T-cell lymphoma, unspecified, extranodal and solid organ sites

✓5ᵗʰ **C84.Z** Other mature T/NK-cell lymphomas

     NOTE   If T-cell lineage or involvement is mentioned in conjunction with a specific lymphoma, code to the more specific description.

     EXCLUDES 1   angioimmunoblastic T-cell lymphoma (C86.5)
blastic NK-cell lymphoma (C86.4)
enteropathy-type T-cell lymphoma (C86.2)
extranodal NK-cell lymphoma, nasal type (C86.0)
hepatosplenic T-cell lymphoma (C86.1)
primary cutaneous CD30-positive T-cell proliferations (C86.6)
subcutaneous panniculitis-like T-cell lymphoma (C86.3)
T-cell leukemia (C91.1-)

     C84.Z0 Other mature T/NK-cell lymphomas, unspecified site

     C84.Z1 Other mature T/NK-cell lymphomas, lymph nodes of head, face, and neck

     C84.Z2 Other mature T/NK-cell lymphomas, intrathoracic lymph nodes

     C84.Z3 Other mature T/NK-cell lymphomas, intra-abdominal lymph nodes

     C84.Z4 Other mature T/NK-cell lymphomas, lymph nodes of axilla and upper limb

     C84.Z5 Other mature T/NK-cell lymphomas, lymph nodes of inguinal region and lower limb

     C84.Z6 Other mature T/NK-cell lymphomas, intrapelvic lymph nodes

     C84.Z7 Other mature T/NK-cell lymphomas, spleen

     C84.Z8 Other mature T/NK-cell lymphomas, lymph nodes of multiple sites

     C84.Z9 Other mature T/NK-cell lymphomas, extranodal and solid organ sites

✓5ᵗʰ **C84.9** Mature T/NK-cell lymphomas, unspecified
NK/T cell lymphoma NOS
EXCLUDES 1   mature T-cell lymphoma, not elsewhere classified (C84.4-)

     C84.90 Mature T/NK-cell lymphomas, unspecified, unspecified site

     C84.91 Mature T/NK-cell lymphomas, unspecified, lymph nodes of head, face, and neck

     C84.92 Mature T/NK-cell lymphomas, unspecified, intrathoracic lymph nodes

     C84.93 Mature T/NK-cell lymphomas, unspecified, intra-abdominal lymph nodes

     C84.94 Mature T/NK-cell lymphomas, unspecified, lymph nodes of axilla and upper limb

     C84.95 Mature T/NK-cell lymphomas, unspecified, lymph nodes of inguinal region and lower limb

     C84.96 Mature T/NK-cell lymphomas, unspecified, intrapelvic lymph nodes

     C84.97 Mature T/NK-cell lymphomas, unspecified, spleen

     C84.98 Mature T/NK-cell lymphomas, unspecified, lymph nodes of multiple sites

     C84.99 Mature T/NK-cell lymphomas, unspecified, extranodal and solid organ sites

---

EXCLUDES 1 Not coded here   EXCLUDES 2 Not included here   N Newborn Age: 0   P Pediatric Age: 0-17   M Maternity Age: 12-55   A Adult Age: 15-124

458   ICD-10-CM 2014 (Draft)

C85 Other specified and unspecified types of non-Hodgkin lymphoma

EXCLUDES 1 *other specified types of T/NK-cell lymphoma (C86.-)*
personal history of non-Hodgkin lymphoma (Z85.72)

C85.1 Unspecified B-cell lymphoma

NOTE If B-cell lineage or involvement is mentioned in conjunction with a specific lymphoma, code to the more specific description.

C85.10 Unspecified B-cell lymphoma, unspecified site

C85.11 Unspecified B-cell lymphoma, lymph nodes of head, face, and neck

C85.12 Unspecified B-cell lymphoma, intrathoracic lymph nodes

C85.13 Unspecified B-cell lymphoma, intra-abdominal lymph nodes

C85.14 Unspecified B-cell lymphoma, lymph nodes of axilla and upper limb

C85.15 Unspecified B-cell lymphoma, lymph nodes of inguinal region and lower limb

C85.16 Unspecified B-cell lymphoma, intrapelvic lymph nodes

C85.17 Unspecified B-cell lymphoma, spleen

C85.18 Unspecified B-cell lymphoma, lymph nodes of multiple sites

C85.19 Unspecified B-cell lymphoma, extranodal and solid organ sites

C85.2 Mediastinal (thymic) large B-cell lymphoma

C85.20 Mediastinal (thymic) large B-cell lymphoma, unspecified site

C85.21 Mediastinal (thymic) large B-cell lymphoma, lymph nodes of head, face, and neck

C85.22 Mediastinal (thymic) large B-cell lymphoma, intrathoracic lymph nodes

C85.23 Mediastinal (thymic) large B-cell lymphoma, intra-abdominal lymph nodes

C85.24 Mediastinal (thymic) large B-cell lymphoma, lymph nodes of axilla and upper limb

C85.25 Mediastinal (thymic) large B-cell lymphoma, lymph nodes of inguinal region and lower limb

C85.26 Mediastinal (thymic) large B-cell lymphoma, intrapelvic lymph nodes

C85.27 Mediastinal (thymic) large B-cell lymphoma, spleen

C85.28 Mediastinal (thymic) large B-cell lymphoma, lymph nodes of multiple sites

C85.29 Mediastinal (thymic) large B-cell lymphoma, extranodal and solid organ sites

C85.8 Other specified types of non-Hodgkin lymphoma

C85.80 Other specified types of non-Hodgkin lymphoma, unspecified site

C85.81 Other specified types of non-Hodgkin lymphoma, lymph nodes of head, face, and neck

C85.82 Other specified types of non-Hodgkin lymphoma, intrathoracic lymph nodes

C85.83 Other specified types of non-Hodgkin lymphoma, intra-abdominal lymph nodes

C85.84 Other specified types of non-Hodgkin lymphoma, lymph nodes of axilla and upper limb

C85.85 Other specified types of non-Hodgkin lymphoma, lymph nodes of inguinal region and lower limb

C85.86 Other specified types of non-Hodgkin lymphoma, intrapelvic lymph nodes

C85.87 Other specified types of non-Hodgkin lymphoma, spleen

C85.88 Other specified types of non-Hodgkin lymphoma, lymph nodes of multiple sites

C85.89 Other specified types of non-Hodgkin lymphoma, extranodal and solid organ sites

C85.9 Non-Hodgkin lymphoma, unspecified

Lymphoma NOS
Malignant lymphoma NOS
Non-Hodgkin lymphoma NOS

C85.90 Non-Hodgkin lymphoma, unspecified, unspecified site

C85.91 Non-Hodgkin lymphoma, unspecified, lymph nodes of head, face, and neck

C85.92 Non-Hodgkin lymphoma, unspecified, intrathoracic lymph nodes

C85.93 Non-Hodgkin lymphoma, unspecified, intra-abdominal lymph nodes

C85.94 Non-Hodgkin lymphoma, unspecified, lymph nodes of axilla and upper limb

C85.95 Non-Hodgkin lymphoma, unspecified, lymph nodes of inguinal region and lower limb

C85.96 Non-Hodgkin lymphoma, unspecified, intrapelvic lymph nodes

C85.97 Non-Hodgkin lymphoma, unspecified, spleen

C85.98 Non-Hodgkin lymphoma, unspecified, lymph nodes of multiple sites

C85.99 Non-Hodgkin lymphoma, unspecified, extranodal and solid organ sites

C86 Other specified types of T/NK-cell lymphoma

EXCLUDES 1 *anaplastic large cell lymphoma, ALK negative (C84.7-)*
anaplastic large cell lymphoma, ALK positive (C84.6-)
mature T/NK-cell lymphomas (C84.-)
other specified types of non-Hodgkin lymphoma (C85.8-)

C86.0 Extranodal NK/T-cell lymphoma, nasal type

C86.1 Hepatosplenic T-cell lymphoma
Alpha-beta and gamma delta types

C86.2 Enteropathy-type (intestinal) T-cell lymphoma
Enteropathy associated T-cell lymphoma

C86.3 Subcutaneous panniculitis-like T-cell lymphoma

C86.4 Blastic NK-cell lymphoma

C86.5 Angioimmunoblastic T-cell lymphoma
Angioimmunoblastic lymphadenopathy with dysproteinemia [AILD]

C86.6 Primary cutaneous CD30-positive T-cell proliferations
Lymphomatoid papulosis
Primary cutaneous anaplastic large cell lymphoma
Primary cutaneous CD30-positive large T-cell lymphoma

C88 Malignant immunoproliferative diseases and certain other B-cell lymphomas

EXCLUDES 1 *B-cell lymphoma, unspecified (C85.1-)*
personal history of other malignant neoplasms of lymphoid, hematopoietic and related tissues (Z85.79)

C88.0 Waldenström macroglobulinemia
Lymphoplasmacytic lymphoma with IgM-production
Macroglobulinemia (idiopathic) (primary)
EXCLUDES 1 *small cell B-cell lymphoma (C83.0)*

C88.2 Heavy chain disease
Franklin disease
Gamma heavy chain disease
Mu heavy chain disease

C88.3 Immunoproliferative small intestinal disease
Alpha heavy chain disease
Mediterranean lymphoma

C88.4 Extranodal marginal zone B-cell lymphoma of mucosa-associated lymphoid tissue [MALT-lymphoma]
Lymphoma of skin-associated lymphoid tissue [SALT-lymphoma]
Lymphoma of bronchial-associated lymphoid tissue [BALT-lymphoma]
EXCLUDES 1 *high malignant (diffuse large B-cell) lymphoma (C83.3-)*

C88.8 Other malignant immunoproliferative diseases

C88.9 Malignant immunoproliferative disease, unspecified
Immunoproliferative disease NOS

C90 Multiple myeloma and malignant plasma cell neoplasms

EXCLUDES 1 *personal history of other malignant neoplasms of lymphoid, hematopoietic and related tissues (Z85.79)*

C90.0 Multiple myeloma
Kahler's disease   Myelomatosis
Medullary plasmacytoma   Plasma cell myeloma
EXCLUDES 1 *solitary myeloma (C90.3-)*
solitary plasmactyoma (C90.3-)

C90.00 Multiple myeloma not having achieved remission
Multiple myeloma with failed remission
Multiple myeloma NOS

C90.01 Multiple myeloma in remission

C90.02 Multiple myeloma in relapse

C90.1 Plasma cell leukemia
Plasmacytic leukemia

C90.10 Plasma cell leukemia not having achieved remission
Plasma cell leukemia with failed remission
Plasma cell leukemia NOS

✓ Additional Character Required   ✓x7ᵗʰ Xtension Alert   Unspecified Code   Other Specified Code   Manifestation Code   ►◄ Revised Text   ● New Code   ▲ Revised Code Title

C90.11   **Plasma cell leukemia** in remission

C90.12   **Plasma cell leukemia** in relapse

✓5th **C90.2** **Extramedullary plasmacytoma**

  C90.20   **Extramedullary plasmacytoma** not having achieved remission

    Extramedullary plasmacytoma with failed remission

    Extramedullary plasmacytoma NOS

  C90.21   **Extramedullary plasmacytoma** in remission

  C90.22   **Extramedullary plasmacytoma** in relapse

✓5th **C90.3** **Solitary plasmacytoma**

  Localized malignant plasma cell tumor NOS

  Plasmacytoma NOS

  Solitary myeloma

  C90.30   **Solitary plasmacytoma** not having achieved remission

    Solitary plasmacytoma with failed remission

    Solitary plasmacytoma NOS

  C90.31   **Solitary plasmacytoma** in remission

  C90.32   **Solitary plasmacytoma** in relapse

✓4th **C91** **Lymphoid leukemia**

  EXCLUDES 1   personal history of leukemia (Z85.6)

✓5th **C91.0** **Acute lymphoblastic leukemia [ALL]**

  NOTE   Code C91.0 should only be used for T-cell and B-cell precursor leukemia.

  C91.00   **Acute lymphoblastic leukemia** not having achieved remission

    Acute lymphoblastic leukemia with failed remission

    Acute lymphoblastic leukemia NOS

  C91.01   **Acute lymphoblastic leukemia,** in remission

  C91.02   **Acute lymphoblastic leukemia,** in relapse

✓5th **C91.1** **Chronic lymphocytic leukemia of B-cell type**

  Lymphoplasmacytic leukemia

  Richter syndrome

  EXCLUDES 1   lymphoplasmacytic lymphoma (C83.0-)

  C91.10   **Chronic lymphocytic leukemia of B-cell type** not having achieved remission

    Chronic lymphocytic leukemia of B-cell type with failed remission

    Chronic lymphocytic leukemia of B-cell type NOS

  C91.11   **Chronic lymphocytic leukemia of B-cell type** in remission

  C91.12   **Chronic lymphocytic leukemia of B-cell type** in relapse

✓5th **C91.3** **Prolymphocytic leukemia of B-cell type**

  C91.30   **Prolymphocytic leukemia of B-cell type** not having achieved remission

    Prolymphocytic leukemia of B-cell type with failed remission

    Prolymphocytic leukemia of B-cell type NOS

  C91.31   **Prolymphocytic leukemia of B-cell type,** in remission

  C91.32   **Prolymphocytic leukemia of B-cell type,** in relapse

✓5th **C91.4** **Hairy cell leukemia**

  Leukemic reticuloendotheliosis

  C91.40   **Hairy cell leukemia** not having achieved remission

    Hairy cell leukemia with failed remission

    Hairy cell leukemia NOS

  C91.41   **Hairy cell leukemia,** in remission

  C91.42   **Hairy cell leukemia,** in relapse

✓5th **C91.5** **Adult T-cell lymphoma/leukemia (HTLV-1-associated)**

  Acute variant of adult T-cell lymphoma/leukemia (HTLV-1-associated)

  Chronic variant of adult T-cell lymphoma/leukemia (HTLV-1-associated)

  Lymphomatoid variant of adult T-cell lymphoma/leukemia (HTLV-1-associated)

  Smouldering variant of adult T-cell lymphoma/leukemia (HTLV-1-associated)

  C91.50   **Adult T-cell lymphoma/leukemia (HTLV-1-associated)** not having achieved remission   🅰

    Adult T-cell lymphoma/leukemia (HTLV-1-associated) with failed remission

    Adult T-cell lymphoma/leukemia (HTLV-1-associated) NOS

  C91.51   **Adult T-cell lymphoma/leukemia (HTLV-1-associated), in remission**   🅰

  C91.52   **Adult T-cell lymphoma/leukemia (HTLV-1-associated), in relapse**   🅰

✓5th **C91.6** **Prolymphocytic leukemia of T-cell type**

  C91.60   **Prolymphocytic leukemia of T-cell type** not having achieved remission

    Prolymphocytic leukemia of T-cell type with failed remission

    Prolymphocytic leukemia of T-cell type NOS

  C91.61   **Prolymphocytic leukemia of T-cell type, in remission**

  C91.62   **Prolymphocytic leukemia of T-cell type, in relapse**

✓5th **C91.A** **Mature B-cell leukemia Burkitt-type**

  EXCLUDES 1   Burkitt lymphoma (C83.7-)

  C91.A0   **Mature B-cell leukemia Burkitt-type** not having achieved remission

    Mature B-cell leukemia Burkitt-type with failed remission

    Mature B-cell leukemia Burkitt-type NOS

  C91.A1   **Mature B-cell leukemia Burkitt-type, in remission**

  C91.A2   **Mature B-cell leukemia Burkitt-type, in relapse**

✓5th **C91.Z** **Other lymphoid leukemia**

  T-cell large granular lymphocytic leukemia (associated with rheumatoid arthritis)

  C91.Z0   **Other lymphoid leukemia** not having achieved remission

    Other lymphoid leukemia with failed remission

    Other lymphoid leukemia NOS

  C91.Z1   **Other lymphoid leukemia, in remission**

  C91.Z2   **Other lymphoid leukemia, in relapse**

✓5th **C91.9** **Lymphoid leukemia, unspecified**

  C91.90   **Lymphoid leukemia, unspecified** not having achieved remission

    Lymphoid leukemia with failed remission

    Lymphoid leukemia NOS

  C91.91   **Lymphoid leukemia, unspecified, in remission**

  C91.92   **Lymphoid leukemia, unspecified, in relapse**

✓4th **C92** **Myeloid leukemia**

  INCLUDES   granulocytic leukemia

    myelogenous leukemia

  EXCLUDES 1   personal history of leukemia (Z85.6)

✓5th **C92.0** **Acute myeloblastic leukemia**

  Acute myeloblastic leukemia, minimal differentiation

  Acute myeloblastic leukemia (with maturation)

  Acute myeloblastic leukemia 1/ETO

  Acute myeloblastic leukemia M0

  Acute myeloblastic leukemia M1

  Acute myeloblastic leukemia M2

  Acute myeloblastic leukemia with t(8;21)

  Acute myeloblastic leukemia (without a FAB classification) NOS

  Refractory anemia with excess blasts in transformation [RAEB T]

  EXCLUDES 1   acute exacerbation of chronic myeloid leukemia (C92.10)

    refractory anemia with excess of blasts not in transformation (D46.2-)

  C92.00   **Acute myeloblastic leukemia,** not having achieved remission

    Acute myeloblastic leukemia with failed remission

    Acute myeloblastic leukemia NOS

  C92.01   **Acute myeloblastic leukemia, in remission**

  C92.02   **Acute myeloblastic leukemia, in relapse**

✓5th **C92.1** **Chronic myeloid leukemia, BCR/ABL-positive**

  Chronic myelogenous leukemia, Philadelphia chromosome (Ph1) positive

  Chronic myelogenous leukemia, t(9;22) (q34;q11)

  Chronic myelogenous leukemia with crisis of blast cells

  EXCLUDES 1   atypical chronic myeloid leukemia BCR/ABL-negative (C92.2-)

    chronic myelomonocytic leukemia (C93.1-)

    chronic myeloproliferative disease (D47.1)

  C92.10   **Chronic myeloid leukemia, BCR/ABL-positive,** not having achieved remission

    Chronic myeloid leukemia, BCR/ABL-positive with failed remission

    Chronic myeloid leukemia, BCR/ABL-positive NOS

  C92.11   **Chronic myeloid leukemia, BCR/ABL-positive,** in remission

  C92.12   **Chronic myeloid leukemia, BCR/ABL-positive,** in relapse

---

EXCLUDES 1 Not coded here   *EXCLUDES 2* Not included here   🅝 Newborn Age: 0   🅟 Pediatric Age: 0-17   🅜 Maternity Age: 12-55   🅐 Adult Age: 15-124

460   ICD-10-CM 2014 (Draft)

√5ᵗʰ **C92.2** Atypical chronic **myeloid leukemia, BCR/ABL-negative**

C92.20 **Atypical chronic myeloid leukemia, BCR/ABL-negative, not having achieved remission**
Atypical chronic myeloid leukemia, BCR/ABL-negative with failed remission
Atypical chronic myeloid leukemia, BCR/ABL-negative NOS

C92.21 **Atypical chronic myeloid leukemia, BCR/ABL-negative, in remission**

C92.22 **Atypical chronic myeloid leukemia, BCR/ABL-negative, in relapse**

√5ᵗʰ **C92.3** Myeloid sarcoma
A malignant tumor of immature myeloid cells
Chloroma
Granulocytic sarcoma

C92.30 **Myeloid sarcoma, not having achieved remission**
Myeloid sarcoma with failed remission
Myeloid sarcoma NOS

C92.31 **Myeloid sarcoma, in remission**

C92.32 **Myeloid sarcoma, in relapse**

√5ᵗʰ **C92.4** Acute promyelocytic **leukemia**
AML M3
AML Me with t(15;17) and variants

C92.40 **Acute promyelocytic leukemia, not having achieved remission**
Acute promyelocytic leukemia with failed remission
Acute promyelocytic leukemia NOS

C92.41 **Acute promyelocytic leukemia, in remission**

C92.42 **Acute promyelocytic leukemia, in relapse**

√5ᵗʰ **C92.5** Acute myelomonocytic **leukemia**
AML M4
AML M4 Eo with inv(16) or t(16;16)

C92.50 **Acute myelomonocytic leukemia, not having achieved remission**
Acute myelomonocytic leukemia with failed remission
Acute myelomonocytic leukemia NOS

C92.51 **Acute myelomonocytic leukemia, in remission**

C92.52 **Acute myelomonocytic leukemia, in relapse**

√5ᵗʰ **C92.6** Acute myeloid **leukemia with** 11q23-abnormality
Acute myeloid leukemia with variation of MLL-gene

C92.60 **Acute myeloid leukemia with 11q23-abnormality not having achieved remission**
Acute myeloid leukemia with 11q23-abnormality with failed remission
Acute myeloid leukemia with 11q23-abnormality NOS

C92.61 **Acute myeloid leukemia with 11q23-abnormality in remission**

C92.62 **Acute myeloid leukemia with 11q23-abnormality in relapse**

√5ᵗʰ **C92.A** Acute myeloid **leukemia with** multilineage dysplasia
Acute myeloid leukemia with dysplasia of remaining hematopoesis and/or myelodysplastic disease in its history

C92.A0 **Acute myeloid leukemia with multilineage dysplasia, not having achieved remission**
Acute myeloid leukemia with multilineage dysplasia with failed remission
Acute myeloid leukemia with multilineage dysplasia NOS

C92.A1 **Acute myeloid leukemia with multilineage dysplasia, in remission**

C92.A2 **Acute myeloid leukemia with multilineage dysplasia, in relapse**

√5ᵗʰ **C92.Z** Other myeloid leukemia

C92.Z0 **Other myeloid leukemia not having achieved remission**
Myeloid leukemia NEC with failed remission
Myeloid leukemia NEC

C92.Z1 **Other myeloid leukemia, in remission**

C92.Z2 **Other myeloid leukemia, in relapse**

√5ᵗʰ **C92.9** Myeloid leukemia, unspecified

C92.90 **Myeloid leukemia, unspecified, not having achieved remission**
Myeloid leukemia, unspecified with failed remission
Myeloid leukemia, unspecified NOS

C92.91 **Myeloid leukemia, unspecified in remission**

C92.92 **Myeloid leukemia, unspecified in relapse**

√4ᵗʰ **C93** Monocytic leukemia
INCLUDES monocytoid leukemia
EXCLUDES1 personal history of leukemia (Z85.6)

√5ᵗʰ **C93.0** Acute **monoblastic/monocytic leukemia**
AML M5　　AML M5b
AML M5a

C93.00 **Acute monoblastic/monocytic leukemia, not having achieved remission**
Acute monoblastic/monocytic leukemia with failed remission
Acute monoblastic/monocytic leukemia NOS

C93.01 **Acute monoblastic/monocytic leukemia, in remission**

C93.02 **Acute monoblastic/monocytic leukemia, in relapse**

√5ᵗʰ **C93.1** Chronic **myelomonocytic leukemia**
Chronic monocytic leukemia
CMML-1
CMML-2
CMML with eosinophilia

C93.10 **Chronic myelomonocytic leukemia not having achieved remission**
Chronic myelomonocytic leukemia with failed remission
Chronic myelomonocytic leukemia NOS

C93.11 **Chronic myelomonocytic leukemia, in remission**

C93.12 **Chronic myelomonocytic leukemia, in relapse**

√5ᵗʰ **C93.3** Juvenile **myelomonocytic leukemia**

C93.30 **Juvenile myelomonocytic leukemia, not having achieved remission** P
Juvenile myelomonocytic leukemia with failed remission
Juvenile myelomonocytic leukemia NOS

C93.31 **Juvenile myelomonocytic leukemia, in remission** P

C93.32 **Juvenile myelomonocytic leukemia, in relapse** P

√5ᵗʰ **C93.Z** Other **monocytic leukemia**

C93.Z0 **Other monocytic leukemia, not having achieved remission**
Other monocytic leukemia NOS

C93.Z1 **Other monocytic leukemia, in remission**

C93.Z2 **Other monocytic leukemia, in relapse**

√5ᵗʰ **C93.9** Monocytic leukemia, unspecified

C93.90 **Monocytic leukemia, unspecified, not having achieved remission**
Monocytic leukemia, unspecified with failed remission
Monocytic leukemia, unspecified NOS

C93.91 **Monocytic leukemia, unspecified in remission**

C93.92 **Monocytic leukemia, unspecified in relapse**

√4ᵗʰ **C94** Other **leukemias of** specified cell type
EXCLUDES1 leukemic reticuloendotheliosis (C91.4-)
myelodysplastic syndromes (D46.-)
personal history of leukemia (Z85.6)
plasma cell leukemia (C90.1-)

√5ᵗʰ **C94.0** Acute **erythroid leukemia**
Acute myeloid leukemia M6(a)(b)
Erythroleukemia

C94.00 **Acute erythroid leukemia, not having achieved remission**
Acute erythroid leukemia with failed remission
Acute erythroid leukemia NOS

C94.01 **Acute erythroid leukemia, in remission**

C94.02 **Acute erythroid leukemia, in relapse**

√5ᵗʰ **C94.2** Acute **megakaryoblastic leukemia**
Acute myeloid leukemia M7
Acute megakaryocytic leukemia

C94.20 **Acute megakaryoblastic leukemia not having achieved remission**
Acute megakaryoblastic leukemia with failed remission
Acute megakaryoblastic leukemia NOS

C94.21 **Acute megakaryoblastic leukemia, in remission**

C94.22 **Acute megakaryoblastic leukemia, in relapse**

√5ᵗʰ **C94.3** Mast cell leukemia

C94.30 **Mast cell leukemia not having achieved remission**
Mast cell leukemia with failed remission
Mast cell leukemia NOS

C94.31 **Mast cell leukemia, in remission**

C94.32 **Mast cell leukemia, in relapse**

Neoplasms

C94.4–D01.5

✓5ᵗʰ **C94.4 Acute panmyelosis with myelofibrosis**
Acute myelofibrosis
EXCLUDES 1   myelofibrosis NOS (D75.81)
secondary myelofibrosis NOS (D75.81)

     C94.40 Acute panmyelosis with myelofibrosis not having achieved remission
Acute myelofibrosis NOS
Acute panmyelosis with myelofibrosis with failed remission
Acute panmyelosis NOS

     C94.41 Acute panmyelosis with myelofibrosis, in remission

     C94.42 Acute panmyelosis with myelofibrosis, in relapse

    C94.6 Myelodysplastic disease, not classified
Myeloproliferative disease, not classified

✓5ᵗʰ **C94.8 Other specified leukemias**
Aggressive NK-cell leukemia
Acute basophilic leukemia

     C94.80 Other specified leukemias not having achieved remission
Other specified leukemia with failed remission
Other specified leukemias NOS

     C94.81 Other specified leukemias, in remission

     C94.82 Other specified leukemias, in relapse

✓4ᵗʰ **C95 Leukemia of** unspecified cell type
EXCLUDES 1   personal history of leukemia (Z85.6)

✓5ᵗʰ **C95.0 Acute leukemia of unspecified cell type**
Acute bilineal leukemia
Acute mixed lineage leukemia
Biphenotypic acute leukemia
Stem cell leukemia of unclear lineage
EXCLUDES 1   acute exacerbation of unspecified chronic leukemia (C95.10)

     C95.00 Acute leukemia of unspecified cell type not having achieved remission
Acute leukemia of unspecified cell type with failed remission
Acute leukemia NOS

     C95.01 Acute leukemia of unspecified cell type, in remission

     C95.02 Acute leukemia of unspecified cell type, in relapse

✓5ᵗʰ **C95.1 Chronic leukemia of unspecified cell type**

     C95.10 Chronic leukemia of unspecified cell type not having achieved remission
Chronic leukemia of unspecified cell type with failed remission
Chronic leukemia NOS

     C95.11 Chronic leukemia of unspecified cell type, in remission

     C95.12 Chronic leukemia of unspecified cell type, in relapse

✓5ᵗʰ **C95.9 Leukemia,** unspecified

     C95.90 Leukemia, unspecified not having achieved remission
Leukemia, unspecified with failed remission
Leukemia NOS

     C95.91 Leukemia, unspecified, in remission

     C95.92 Leukemia, unspecified, in relapse

✓4ᵗʰ **C96 Other and unspecified malignant neoplasms of lymphoid, hematopoietic and related tissue**
EXCLUDES 1   personal history of other malignant neoplasms of lymphoid, hematopoietic and related tissues (Z85.79)

    C96.0 Multifocal and multisystemic (disseminated) Langerhans-cell histiocytosis
Histiocytosis X, multisystemic
Letterer-Siwe disease
EXCLUDES 1   adult pulmonary Langerhans cell histiocytosis (J84.82)
multifocal and unisystemic Langerhans-cell histiocytosis (C96.5)
unifocal Langerhans-cell histiocytosis (C96.6)

    C96.2 Malignant mast cell tumor
Aggressive systemic mastocytosis
Mast cell sarcoma
EXCLUDES 1   indolent mastocytosis (D47.0)
mast cell leukemia (C94.30)
mastocytosis (congenital) (cutaneous) (Q82.2)

    C96.4 Sarcoma of dendritic cells (accessory cells)
Follicular dendritic cell sarcoma
Interdigitating dendritic cell sarcoma
Langerhans cell sarcoma

    C96.5 Multifocal and unisystemic Langerhans-cell histiocytosis
Hand-Schüller-Christian disease
Histiocytosis X, multifocal
EXCLUDES 1   multifocal and multisystemic (disseminated) Langerhans-cell histiocytosis (C96.0)
unifocal Langerhans-cell histiocytosis (C96.6)

    C96.6 Unifocal Langerhans-cell histiocytosis
Eosinophilic granuloma
Histiocytosis X, unifocal
Histiocytosis X NOS
Langerhans-cell histiocytosis NOS
EXCLUDES 1   multifocal and multisysemic (disseminated) Langerhans-cell histiocytosis (C96.0)
multifocal and unisystemic Langerhans-cell histiocytosis (C96.5)

    C96.A Histiocytic sarcoma
Malignant histiocytosis

    C96.Z Other specified malignant neoplasms of lymphoid, hematopoietic and related tissue

    C96.9 Malignant neoplasm of lymphoid, hematopoietic and related tissue, unspecified

In situ neoplasms (D00-D09)

INCLUDES   Bowen's disease
erythroplasia
grade III intraepithelial neoplasia
Queyrat's erythroplasia

✓4ᵗʰ **D00 Carcinoma in situ of** oral cavity, esophagus and stomach
EXCLUDES 1   melanoma in situ (D03.-)

✓5ᵗʰ **D00.0 Carcinoma in situ of** lip, oral cavity and pharynx
EXCLUDES 1   carcinoma in situ of aryepiglottic fold or interarytenoid fold, laryngeal aspect (D02.0)
carcinoma in situ of epiglottis NOS (D02.0)
carcinoma in situ of epiglottis suprahyoid portion (D02.0)
carcinoma in situ of skin of lip (D03.0, D04.0)
Use additional code to identify:
exposure to environmental tobacco smoke (Z77.22)
exposure to tobacco smoke in the perinatal period (P96.81)
history of tobacco use (Z87.891)
occupational exposure to environmental tobacco smoke (Z57.31)
tobacco dependence (F17.-)
tobacco use (Z72.0)

     D00.00 Carcinoma in situ of oral cavity, unspecified site

     D00.01 Carcinoma in situ of labial mucosa and vermilion border

     D00.02 Carcinoma in situ of buccal mucosa

     D00.03 Carcinoma in situ of gingiva and edentulous alveolar ridge

     D00.04 Carcinoma in situ of soft palate

     D00.05 Carcinoma in situ of hard palate

     D00.06 Carcinoma in situ of floor of mouth

     D00.07 Carcinoma in situ of tongue

     D00.08 Carcinoma in situ of pharynx
Carcinoma in situ of aryepiglottic fold NOS
Carcinoma in situ of hypopharyngeal aspect of aryepiglottic fold
Carcinoma in situ of marginal zone of aryepiglottic fold

    D00.1 Carcinoma in situ of esophagus

    D00.2 Carcinoma in situ of stomach

✓4ᵗʰ **D01 Carcinoma in situ of** other and unspecified digestive organs
EXCLUDES 1   melanoma in situ (D03.-)

    D01.0 Carcinoma in situ of colon
EXCLUDES 1   carcinoma in situ of rectosigmoid junction (D01.1)

    D01.1 Carcinoma in situ of rectosigmoid junction

    D01.2 Carcinoma in situ of rectum

    D01.3 Carcinoma in situ of anus and anal canal
EXCLUDES 1   carcinoma in situ of anal margin (D04.5)
carcinoma in situ of anal skin (D04.5)
carcinoma in situ of perianal skin (D04.5)

✓5ᵗʰ **D01.4 Carcinoma in situ of other and unspecified parts of** intestine
EXCLUDES 1   carcinoma in situ of ampulla of Vater (D01.5)

     D01.40 Carcinoma in situ of unspecified part of intestine

     D01.49 Carcinoma in situ of other parts of intestine

    D01.5 Carcinoma in situ of liver, gallbladder and bile ducts
Carcinoma in situ of ampulla of Vater

EXCLUDES 1 Not coded here   *EXCLUDES 2* Not included here   **N** Newborn Age: 0   **P** Pediatric Age: 0-17   **M** Maternity Age: 12-55   **A** Adult Age: 15-124

462   ICD-10-CM 2014 (Draft)

D01.7 Carcinoma in situ of other specified digestive organs
Carcinoma in situ of pancreas

D01.9 Carcinoma in situ of digestive organ, unspecified

✓4ᵗʰ **D02 Carcinoma in situ of middle ear and respiratory system**
EXCLUDES 1　melanoma in situ (D03.-)
Use additional code to identify:
exposure to environmental tobacco smoke (Z77.22)
exposure to tobacco smoke in the perinatal period (P96.81)
history of tobacco use (Z87.891)
occupational exposure to environmental tobacco smoke (Z57.31)
tobacco dependence (F17.-)
tobacco use (Z72.0)

D02.0 Carcinoma in situ of larynx
Carcinoma in situ of aryepiglottic fold or interarytenoid fold, laryngeal aspect
Carcinoma in situ of epiglottis (suprahyoid portion)
EXCLUDES 1　carcinoma in situ of aryepiglottic fold or interarytenoid fold NOS (D00.08)
carcinoma in situ of hypopharyngeal aspect (D00.08)
carcinoma in situ of marginal zone (D00.08)

D02.1 Carcinoma in situ of trachea

✓5ᵗʰ **D02.2 Carcinoma in situ of bronchus and lung**
D02.20 Carcinoma in situ of unspecified bronchus and lung
D02.21 Carcinoma in situ of right bronchus and lung
D02.22 Carcinoma in situ of left bronchus and lung

D02.3 Carcinoma in situ of other parts of respiratory system
Carcinoma in situ of accessory sinuses
Carcinoma in situ of middle ear
Carcinoma in situ of nasal cavities
EXCLUDES 1　carcinoma in situ of ear (external) (skin) (D04.2-)
carcinoma in situ of nose NOS (D09.8)
carcinoma in situ of skin of nose (D04.3)

D02.4 Carcinoma in situ of respiratory system, unspecified

✓4ᵗʰ **D03 Melanoma in situ**

D03.0 Melanoma in situ of lip

✓5ᵗʰ **D03.1 Melanoma in situ of eyelid, including canthus**
D03.10 Melanoma in situ of unspecified eyelid, including canthus
D03.11 Melanoma in situ of right eyelid, including canthus
D03.12 Melanoma in situ of left eyelid, including canthus

✓5ᵗʰ **D03.2 Melanoma in situ of ear and external auricular canal**
D03.20 Melanoma in situ of unspecified ear and external auricular canal
D03.21 Melanoma in situ of right ear and external auricular canal
D03.22 Melanoma in situ of left ear and external auricular canal

✓5ᵗʰ **D03.3 Melanoma in situ of other and unspecified parts of face**
D03.30 Melanoma in situ of unspecified part of face
D03.39 Melanoma in situ of other parts of face

D03.4 Melanoma in situ of scalp and neck

✓5ᵗʰ **D03.5 Melanoma in situ of trunk**
D03.51 Melanoma in situ of anal skin
Melanoma in situ of anal margin
Melanoma in situ of perianal skin
D03.52 Melanoma in situ of breast (skin) (soft tissue)
D03.59 Melanoma in situ of other part of trunk

✓5ᵗʰ **D03.6 Melanoma in situ of upper limb, including shoulder**
D03.60 Melanoma in situ of unspecified upper limb, including shoulder
D03.61 Melanoma in situ of right upper limb, including shoulder
D03.62 Melanoma in situ of left upper limb, including shoulder

✓5ᵗʰ **D03.7 Melanoma in situ of lower limb, including hip**
D03.70 Melanoma in situ of unspecified lower limb, including hip
D03.71 Melanoma in situ of right lower limb, including hip
D03.72 Melanoma in situ of left lower limb, including hip

D03.8 Melanoma in situ of other sites
Melanoma in situ of scrotum
EXCLUDES 1　carcinoma in situ of scrotum (D07.61)

D03.9 Melanoma in situ, unspecified

✓4ᵗʰ **D04 Carcinoma in situ of skin**
EXCLUDES 1　erythroplasia of Queyrat (penis) NOS (D07.4)
melanoma in situ (D03.-)

D04.0 Carcinoma in situ of skin of lip
EXCLUDES 1　carcinoma in situ of vermilion border of lip (D00.01)

✓5ᵗʰ **D04.1 Carcinoma in situ of skin of eyelid, including canthus**
D04.10 Carcinoma in situ of skin of unspecified eyelid, including canthus
D04.11 Carcinoma in situ of skin of right eyelid, including canthus
D04.12 Carcinoma in situ of skin of left eyelid, including canthus

✓5ᵗʰ **D04.2 Carcinoma in situ of skin of ear and external auricular canal**
D04.20 Carcinoma in situ of skin of unspecified ear and external auricular canal
D04.21 Carcinoma in situ of skin of right ear and external auricular canal
D04.22 Carcinoma in situ of skin of left ear and external auricular canal

✓5ᵗʰ **D04.3 Carcinoma in situ of skin of other and unspecified parts of face**
D04.30 Carcinoma in situ of skin of unspecified part of face
D04.39 Carcinoma in situ of skin of other parts of face

D04.4 Carcinoma in situ of skin of scalp and neck

D04.5 Carcinoma in situ of skin of trunk
Carcinoma in situ of anal margin
Carcinoma in situ of anal skin
Carcinoma in situ of perianal skin
Carcinoma in situ of skin of breast
EXCLUDES 1　carcinoma in situ of anus NOS (D01.3)
carcinoma in situ of scrotum (D07.61)
carcinoma in situ of skin of genital organs (D07.-)

✓5ᵗʰ **D04.6 Carcinoma in situ of skin of upper limb, including shoulder**
D04.60 Carcinoma in situ of skin of unspecified upper limb, including shoulder
D04.61 Carcinoma in situ of skin of right upper limb, including shoulder
D04.62 Carcinoma in situ of skin of left upper limb, including shoulder

✓5ᵗʰ **D04.7 Carcinoma in situ of skin of lower limb, including hip**
D04.70 Carcinoma in situ of skin of unspecified lower limb, including hip
D04.71 Carcinoma in situ of skin of right lower limb, including hip
D04.72 Carcinoma in situ of skin of left lower limb, including hip

D04.8 Carcinoma in situ of skin of other sites

D04.9 Carcinoma in situ of skin, unspecified

✓4ᵗʰ **D05 Carcinoma in situ of breast**
EXCLUDES 1　carcinoma in situ of skin of breast (D04.5)
melanoma in situ of breast (skin) (D03.5)
Paget's disease of breast or nipple (C50.-)

✓5ᵗʰ **D05.0 Lobular carcinoma in situ of breast**
D05.00 Lobular carcinoma in situ of unspecified breast
D05.01 Lobular carcinoma in situ of right breast
D05.02 Lobular carcinoma in situ of left breast

✓5ᵗʰ **D05.1 Intraductal carcinoma in situ of breast**
D05.10 Intraductal carcinoma in situ of unspecified breast
D05.11 Intraductal carcinoma in situ of right breast
D05.12 Intraductal carcinoma in situ of left breast

✓5ᵗʰ **D05.8 Other specified type of carcinoma in situ of breast**
D05.80 Other specified type of carcinoma in situ of unspecified breast
D05.81 Other specified type of carcinoma in situ of right breast
D05.82 Other specified type of carcinoma in situ of left breast

✓5ᵗʰ **D05.9 Unspecified type of carcinoma in situ of breast**
D05.90 Unspecified type of carcinoma in situ of unspecified breast
D05.91 Unspecified type of carcinoma in situ of right breast
D05.92 Unspecified type of carcinoma in situ of left breast

D01.7–D05.92

✓ Additional Character Required　　ᵛˣ⁷ᵗʰ Xtension Alert　　Unspecified Code　　Other Specified Code　　Manifestation Code　　►◄ Revised Text　　● New Code　　▲ Revised Code Title

Neoplasms

D06–D13.2

✓4ᵗʰ **D06 Carcinoma in situ of cervix uteri**
> INCLUDES   cervical adenocarcinoma in situ
> cervical intraepithelial glandular neoplasia
> cervical intraepithelial neoplasia III [CIN III]
> severe dysplasia of cervix uteri
>
> EXCLUDES 1   cervical intraepithelial neoplasia II [CIN II] (N87.1)
> cytologic evidence of malignancy of cervix without histologic confirmation (R87.614)
> high grade squamous intraepithelial lesion (HGSIL) of cervix (R87.613)
> melanoma in situ of cervix (D03.5)
> moderate cervical dysplasia (N87.1)

D06.0 Carcinoma in situ of endocervix   ♀

D06.1 Carcinoma in situ of exocervix   ♀

D06.7 Carcinoma in situ of other parts of cervix   ♀

D06.9 Carcinoma in situ of cervix, unspecified   ♀

✓4ᵗʰ **D07 Carcinoma in situ of other and unspecified genital organs**
> EXCLUDES 1   melanoma in situ of trunk (D03.5)

D07.0 Carcinoma in situ of endometrium   ♀

D07.1 Carcinoma in situ of vulva   ♀
> Severe dysplasia of vulva
> Vulvar intraepithelial neoplasia III [VIN III]
> EXCLUDES 1   moderate dysplasia of vulva (N90.1)
> vulvar intraepithelial neoplasia II [VIN II] (N90.1)

D07.2 Carcinoma in situ of vagina   ♀
> Severe dysplasia of vagina
> Vaginal intraepithelial neoplasia III [VAIN III]
> EXCLUDES 1   moderate dysplasia of vagina (N89.1)
> vaginal intraepithelial neoplasia II [VIN II] (N89.1)

✓5ᵗʰ **D07.3 Carcinoma in situ of other and unspecified female genital organs**

     D07.30 Carcinoma in situ of unspecified female genital organs   ♀

     D07.39 Carcinoma in situ of other female genital organs   ♀

D07.4 Carcinoma in situ of penis   ♂
> Erythroplasia of Queyrat NOS

D07.5 Carcinoma in situ of prostate   ♂
> Prostatic intraepithelial neoplasia III (PIN III)
> Severe dysplasia of prostate
> EXCLUDES 1   dysplasia (mild) (moderate) of prostate (N42.3)

✓5ᵗʰ **D07.6 Carcinoma in situ of other and unspecified male genital organs**

     D07.60 Carcinoma in situ of unspecified male genital organs   ♂

     D07.61 Carcinoma in situ of scrotum   ♂

     D07.69 Carcinoma in situ of other male genital organs   ♂

✓4ᵗʰ **D09 Carcinoma in situ of other and unspecified sites**
> EXCLUDES 1   melanoma in situ (D03.-)

D09.0 Carcinoma in situ of bladder

✓5ᵗʰ **D09.1 Carcinoma in situ of other and unspecified urinary organs**

     D09.10 Carcinoma in situ of unspecified urinary organ

     D09.19 Carcinoma in situ of other urinary organs

✓5ᵗʰ **D09.2 Carcinoma in situ of eye**
> EXCLUDES 1   carcinoma in situ of skin of eyelid (D04.1-)

     D09.20 Carcinoma in situ of unspecified eye

     D09.21 Carcinoma in situ of right eye

     D09.22 Carcinoma in situ of left eye

D09.3 Carcinoma in situ of thyroid and other endocrine glands
> EXCLUDES 1   carcinoma in situ of endocrine pancreas (D01.7)
> carcinoma in situ of ovary (D07.39)
> carcinoma in situ of testis (D07.69)

D09.8 Carcinoma in situ of other specified sites

D09.9 Carcinoma in situ, unspecified

Benign neoplasms, except benign neuroendocrine tumors (D10-D36)

✓4ᵗʰ **D10 Benign neoplasm of mouth and pharynx**

D10.0 Benign neoplasm of lip
> Benign neoplasm of lip (frenulum) (inner aspect) (mucosa) (vermilion border)
> EXCLUDES 1   benign neoplasm of skin of lip (D22.0, D23.0)

D10.1 Benign neoplasm of tongue
> Benign neoplasm of lingual tonsil

D10.2 Benign neoplasm of floor of mouth

✓5ᵗʰ **D10.3 Other and unspecified parts of mouth**

     D10.30 Benign neoplasm of unspecified part of mouth

     D10.39 Benign neoplasm of other parts of mouth
> Benign neoplasm of minor salivary gland NOS
> EXCLUDES 1   benign odontogenic neoplasms (D16.4-D16.5)
> benign neoplasm of mucosa of lip (D10.0)
> benign neoplasm of nasopharyngeal surface of soft palate (D10.6)

D10.4 Benign neoplasm of tonsil
> Benign neoplasm of tonsil (faucial) (palatine)
> EXCLUDES 1   benign neoplasm of lingual tonsil (D10.1)
> benign neoplasm of pharyngeal tonsil (D10.6)
> benign neoplasm of tonsillar fossa (D10.5)
> benign neoplasm of tonsillar pillars (D10.5)

D10.5 Benign neoplasm of other parts of oropharynx
> Benign neoplasm of epiglottis, anterior aspect
> Benign neoplasm of tonsillar fossa
> Benign neoplasm of tonsillar pillars
> Benign neoplasm of vallecula
> EXCLUDES 1   benign neoplasm of epiglottis NOS (D14.1)
> benign neoplasm of epiglottis, suprahyoid portion (D14.1)

D10.6 Benign neoplasm of nasopharynx
> Benign neoplasm of pharyngeal tonsil
> Benign neoplasm of posterior margin of septum and choanae

D10.7 Benign neoplasm of hypopharynx

D10.9 Benign neoplasm of pharynx, unspecified

✓4ᵗʰ **D11 Benign neoplasm of major salivary glands**
> EXCLUDES 1   benign neoplasms of specified minor salivary glands which are classified according to their anatomical location
> benign neoplasms of minor salivary glands NOS (D10.39)

D11.0 Benign neoplasm of parotid gland

D11.7 Benign neoplasm of other major salivary glands
> Benign neoplasm of sublingual salivary gland
> Benign neoplasm of submandibular salivary gland

D11.9 Benign neoplasm of major salivary gland, unspecified

✓4ᵗʰ **D12 Benign neoplasm of colon, rectum, anus and anal canal**
> EXCLUDES 1   benign carcinoid tumors of the large intestine, and rectum (D3A.02-)

D12.0 Benign neoplasm of cecum
> Benign neoplasm of ileocecal valve

D12.1 Benign neoplasm of appendix
> EXCLUDES 1   benign carcinoid tumor of the appendix (D3A.020)

D12.2 Benign neoplasm of ascending colon

D12.3 Benign neoplasm of transverse colon
> Benign neoplasm of hepatic flexure
> Benign neoplasm of splenic flexure

D12.4 Benign neoplasm of descending colon

D12.5 Benign neoplasm of sigmoid colon

D12.6 Benign neoplasm of colon, unspecified
> Adenomatosis of colon
> Benign neoplasm of large intestine NOS
> Polyposis (hereditary) of colon
> EXCLUDES 1   inflammatory polyp of colon (K51.4-)
> polyp of colon NOS (K63.5)

D12.7 Benign neoplasm of rectosigmoid junction

D12.8 Benign neoplasm of rectum
> EXCLUDES 1   benign carcinoid tumor of the rectum (D3A.026)

D12.9 Benign neoplasm of anus and anal canal
> Benign neoplasm of anus NOS
> EXCLUDES 1   benign neoplasm of anal margin (D22.5, D23.5)
> benign neoplasm of anal skin (D22.5, D23.5)
> benign neoplasm of perianal skin (D22.5, D23.5)

✓4ᵗʰ **D13 Benign neoplasm of other and ill-defined parts of digestive system**
> EXCLUDES 1   benign stromal tumors of digestive system (D21.4)

D13.0 Benign neoplasm of esophagus

D13.1 Benign neoplasm of stomach
> EXCLUDES 1   benign carcinoid tumor of the stomach (D3A.092)

D13.2 Benign neoplasm of duodenum
> EXCLUDES 1   benign carcinoid tumor of the duodenum (D3A.010)

EXCLUDES 1 Not coded here   EXCLUDES 2 Not included here   N Newborn Age: 0   P Pediatric Age: 0-17   M Maternity Age: 12-55   A Adult Age: 15-124

464   ICD-10-CM 2014 (Draft)

✓5th **D13.3 Benign neoplasm of other and unspecified parts of** small
intestine

> EXCLUDES 1 *benign carcinoid tumors of the small intestine
> (D3A.01-)*
> *benign neoplasm of ileocecal valve (D12.0)*

**D13.30 Benign neoplasm of unspecified part of small
intestine**

D13.39 Benign neoplasm of other parts of small intestine

D13.4 Benign neoplasm of liver
Benign neoplasm of intrahepatic bile ducts

D13.5 Benign neoplasm of extrahepatic bile ducts

D13.6 Benign neoplasm of pancreas

> EXCLUDES 1 *benign neoplasm of endocrine pancreas (D13.7)*

D13.7 Benign neoplasm of endocrine pancreas
Islet cell tumor
Benign neoplasm of islets of Langerhans
Use additional code to identify any functional activity

D13.9 Benign neoplasm of ill-defined sites **within the digestive
system**
Benign neoplasm of digestive system NOS
Benign neoplasm of intestine NOS
Benign neoplasm of spleen

✓4th **D14 Benign neoplasm of** middle ear and respiratory system

D14.0 Benign neoplasm of middle ear, nasal cavity and accessory
sinuses
Benign neoplasm of cartilage of nose

> EXCLUDES 1 *benign neoplasm of auricular canal (external) (D22.2-,
> D23.2-)*
> *benign neoplasm of bone of ear (D16.4)*
> *benign neoplasm of bone of nose (D16.4)*
> *benign neoplasm of cartilage of ear (D21.0)*
> *benign neoplasm of ear (external)(skin) (D22.2-,
> D23.2-)*
> *benign neoplasm of nose NOS (D36.7)*
> *benign neoplasm of skin of nose (D22.39, D23.39)*
> *benign neoplasm of olfactory bulb (D33.3)*
> *benign neoplasm of posterior margin of septum and
> choanae (D10.6)*
> *polyp of accessory sinus (J33.8)*
> *polyp of ear (middle) (H74.4)*
> *polyp of nasal (cavity) (J33.-)*

D14.1 Benign neoplasm of larynx
Adenomatous polyp of larynx
Benign neoplasm of epiglottis (suprahyoid portion)

> EXCLUDES 1 *benign neoplasm of epiglottis, anterior aspect (D10.5)*
> *polyp (nonadenomatous) of vocal cord or larynx (J38.1)*

D14.2 Benign neoplasm of trachea

✓5th **D14.3 Benign neoplasm of** bronchus and lung

> EXCLUDES 1 *benign carcinoid tumor of the bronchus and lung
> (D3A.090)*

D14.30 Benign neoplasm of unspecified bronchus and lung

D14.31 Benign neoplasm of right **bronchus and lung**

D14.32 Benign neoplasm of left **bronchus and lung**

D14.4 Benign neoplasm of respiratory system, unspecified

✓4th **D15 Benign neoplasm of** other and unspecified intrathoracic organs

> EXCLUDES 1 *benign neoplasm of mesothelial tissue (D19.-)*

D15.0 Benign neoplasm of thymus

> EXCLUDES 1 *benign carcinoid tumor of the thymus (D3A.091)*

D15.1 Benign neoplasm of heart

> EXCLUDES 1 *benign neoplasm of great vessels (D21.3)*

D15.2 Benign neoplasm of mediastinum

D15.7 Benign neoplasm of other specified intrathoracic organs

D15.9 Benign neoplasm of intrathoracic organ, unspecified

✓4th **D16 Benign neoplasm of** bone and articular cartilage

> EXCLUDES 1 *benign neoplasm of connective tissue of ear (D21.0)*
> *benign neoplasm of connective tissue of eyelid (D21.0)*
> *benign neoplasm of connective tissue of larynx (D14.1)*
> *benign neoplasm of connective tissue of nose (D14.0)*
> *benign neoplasm of synovia (D21.-)*

✓5th **D16.0 Benign neoplasm of** scapula and long bones of upper limb

**D16.00 Benign neoplasm of scapula and long bones of
unspecified upper limb**

D16.01 Benign neoplasm of scapula and long bones of right
upper limb

D16.02 Benign neoplasm of scapula and long bones of left
upper limb

✓5th **D16.1 Benign neoplasm of** short bones of upper limb

**D16.10 Benign neoplasm of short bones of unspecified
upper limb**

D16.11 Benign neoplasm of short bones of right **upper limb**

D16.12 Benign neoplasm of short bones of left **upper limb**

✓5th **D16.2 Benign neoplasm of** long bones of lower limb

**D16.20 Benign neoplasm of long bones of unspecified lower
limb**

D16.21 Benign neoplasm of long bones of right **lower limb**

D16.22 Benign neoplasm of long bones of left **lower limb**

✓5th **D16.3 Benign neoplasm of** short bones of lower limb

**D16.30 Benign neoplasm of short bones of unspecified
lower limb**

D16.31 Benign neoplasm of short bones of right **lower limb**

D16.32 Benign neoplasm of short bones of left **lower limb**

D16.4 Benign neoplasm of bones of skull and face
Benign neoplasm of maxilla (superior)
Benign neoplasm of orbital bone
Keratocyst of maxilla
Keratocystic odontogenic tumor of maxilla

> EXCLUDES 1 *benign neoplasm of lower jaw bone (D16.5)*

D16.5 Benign neoplasm of lower jaw bone
Keratocyst of mandible
Keratocystic odontogenic tumor of mandible

D16.6 Benign neoplasm of vertebral column

> EXCLUDES 1 *benign neoplasm of sacrum and coccyx (D16.8)*

D16.7 Benign neoplasm of ribs, sternum and clavicle

D16.8 Benign neoplasm of pelvic bones, sacrum and coccyx

D16.9 Benign neoplasm of bone and articular cartilage, unspecified

✓4th **D17 Benign** lipomatous neoplasm

D17.0 Benign lipomatous neoplasm of skin and subcutaneous tissue
of head, face and neck

D17.1 Benign lipomatous neoplasm of skin and subcutaneous tissue
of trunk

✓5th **D17.2 Benign lipomatous neoplasm of** skin and subcutaneous tissue
of limb

**D17.20 Benign lipomatous neoplasm of skin and
subcutaneous tissue of unspecified limb**

**D17.21 Benign lipomatous neoplasm of skin and
subcutaneous tissue of** right **arm**

**D17.22 Benign lipomatous neoplasm of skin and
subcutaneous tissue of** left **arm**

**D17.23 Benign lipomatous neoplasm of skin and
subcutaneous tissue of** right **leg**

**D17.24 Benign lipomatous neoplasm of skin and
subcutaneous tissue of** left **leg**

✓5th **D17.3 Benign lipomatous neoplasm of** skin and subcutaneous tissue
of other and unspecified sites

**D17.30 Benign lipomatous neoplasm of skin and
subcutaneous tissue of unspecified sites**

**D17.39 Benign lipomatous neoplasm of skin and
subcutaneous tissue of other sites**

D17.4 Benign lipomatous neoplasm of intrathoracic organs

D17.5 Benign lipomatous neoplasm of intra-abdominal organs

> EXCLUDES 1 *benign lipomatous neoplasm of peritoneum and
> retroperitoneum (D17.79)*

D17.6 Benign lipomatous neoplasm of spermatic cord   ♂

✓5th **D17.7 Benign lipomatous neoplasm of** other sites

D17.71 Benign lipomatous neoplasm of kidney

D17.72 Benign lipomatous neoplasm of other genitourinary
organ

D17.79 Benign lipomatous neoplasm of other sites
Benign lipomatous neoplasm of peritoneum
Benign lipomatous neoplasm of retroperitoneum

D17.9 Benign lipomatous neoplasm, unspecified
Lipoma NOS

✓4th **D18 Hemangioma and lymphangioma, any site**

> EXCLUDES 1 *benign neoplasm of glomus jugulare (D35.6)*
> *blue or pigmented nevus (D22.-)*
> *nevus NOS (D22.-)*
> *vascular nevus (Q82.5)*

✓5th **D18.0 Hemangioma**
Angioma NOS
Cavernous nevus

D18.00 Hemangioma unspecified site

✓ Additional Character Required   ✓x7th Xtension Alert   Unspecified Code   Other Specified Code   Manifestation Code   ▶◀ Revised Text   ● New Code   ▲ Revised Code Title

ICD-10-CM 2014 (Draft)   **465**

Neoplasms

D18.01–D23.39

D18.01 **Hemangioma of** skin and subcutaneous tissue

D18.02 **Hemangioma of** intracranial structures

D18.03 **Hemangioma of** intra-abdominal structures

D18.09 **Hemangioma of other sites**

D18.1 **Lymphangioma, any site**

✓4ᵗʰ **D19 Benign neoplasm of** mesothelial tissue

D19.0 **Benign neoplasm of mesothelial tissue of** pleura

D19.1 **Benign neoplasm of mesothelial tissue of** peritoneum

D19.7 **Benign neoplasm of mesothelial tissue of other sites**

D19.9 **Benign neoplasm of mesothelial tissue, unspecified**
Benign mesothelioma NOS

✓4ᵗʰ **D20 Benign neoplasm of soft tissue of** retroperitoneum and peritoneum

EXCLUDES 1 *benign lipomatous neoplasm of peritoneum and retroperitoneum (D17.79)*
benign neoplasm of mesothelial tissue (D19.-)

D20.0 **Benign neoplasm of soft tissue of** retroperitoneum

D20.1 **Benign neoplasm of soft tissue of** peritoneum

✓4ᵗʰ **D21 Other benign neoplasms of** connective and other soft tissue

INCLUDES benign neoplasm of blood vessel
benign neoplasm of bursa
benign neoplasm of cartilage
benign neoplasm of fascia
benign neoplasm of fat
benign neoplasm of ligament, except uterine
benign neoplasm of lymphatic channel
benign neoplasm of muscle
benign neoplasm of synovia
benign neoplasm of tendon (sheath)
benign stromal tumors

EXCLUDES 1 *benign neoplasm of articular cartilage (D16.-)*
benign neoplasm of cartilage of larynx (D14.1)
benign neoplasm of cartilage of nose (D14.0)
benign neoplasm of connective tissue of breast (D24.-)
benign neoplasm of peripheral nerves and autonomic nervous system (D36.1-)
benign neoplasm of peritoneum (D20.1)
benign neoplasm of retroperitoneum (D20.0)
benign neoplasm of uterine ligament, any (D28.2)
benign neoplasm of vascular tissue (D18.-)
hemangioma (D18.0-)
lipomatous neoplasm (D17.-)
lymphangioma (D18.1)
uterine leiomyoma (D25.-)

D21.0 **Benign neoplasm of connective and other soft tissue of** head, face and neck
Benign neoplasm of connective tissue of ear
Benign neoplasm of connective tissue of eyelid

EXCLUDES 1 *benign neoplasm of connective tissue of orbit (D31.6-)*

✓5ᵗʰ D21.1 **Benign neoplasm of connective and other soft tissue of** upper limb, including shoulder

D21.10 **Benign neoplasm of connective and other soft tissue of unspecified upper limb, including shoulder**

D21.11 **Benign neoplasm of connective and other soft tissue of** right **upper limb, including shoulder**

D21.12 **Benign neoplasm of connective and other soft tissue of** left **upper limb, including shoulder**

✓5ᵗʰ D21.2 **Benign neoplasm of connective and other soft tissue of** lower limb, including hip

D21.20 **Benign neoplasm of connective and other soft tissue of unspecified lower limb, including hip**

D21.21 **Benign neoplasm of connective and other soft tissue of** right **lower limb, including hip**

D21.22 **Benign neoplasm of connective and other soft tissue of** left **lower limb, including hip**

D21.3 **Benign neoplasm of connective and other soft tissue of** thorax
Benign neoplasm of axilla
Benign neoplasm of diaphragm
Benign neoplasm of great vessels

EXCLUDES 1 *benign neoplasm of heart (D15.1)*
benign neoplasm of mediastinum (D15.2)
benign neoplasm of thymus (D15.0)

D21.4 **Benign neoplasm of connective and other soft tissue of** abdomen
Benign stromal tumors of abdomen

D21.5 **Benign neoplasm of connective and other soft tissue of** pelvis

EXCLUDES 1 *benign neoplasm of any uterine ligament (D28.2)*
uterine leiomyoma (D25.-)

D21.6 **Benign neoplasm of connective and other soft tissue of trunk, unspecified**
Benign neoplasm of back NOS

D21.9 **Benign neoplasm of connective and other soft tissue, unspecified**

✓4ᵗʰ **D22 Melanocytic nevi**

INCLUDES atypical nevus
blue hairy pigmented nevus
nevus NOS

D22.0 **Melanocytic nevi of** lip

✓5ᵗʰ D22.1 **Melanocytic nevi of** eyelid, including canthus

D22.10 **Melanocytic nevi of unspecified eyelid, including canthus**

D22.11 **Melanocytic nevi of** right **eyelid, including canthus**

D22.12 **Melanocytic nevi of** left **eyelid, including canthus**

✓5ᵗʰ D22.2 **Melanocytic nevi of** ear and external auricular canal

D22.20 **Melanocytic nevi of unspecified ear and external auricular canal**

D22.21 **Melanocytic nevi of** right **ear and external auricular canal**

D22.22 **Melanocytic nevi of** left **ear and external auricular canal**

✓5ᵗʰ D22.3 **Melanocytic nevi of** other and unspecified parts of face

D22.30 **Melanocytic nevi of unspecified part of face**

D22.39 **Melanocytic nevi of other parts of face**

D22.4 **Melanocytic nevi of** scalp and neck

D22.5 **Melanocytic nevi of** trunk
Melanocytic nevi of anal margin
Melanocytic nevi of anal skin
Melanocytic nevi of perianal skin
Melanocytic nevi of skin of breast

✓5ᵗʰ D22.6 **Melanocytic nevi of** upper limb, including shoulder

D22.60 **Melanocytic nevi of unspecified upper limb, including shoulder**

D22.61 **Melanocytic nevi of** right **upper limb, including shoulder**

D22.62 **Melanocytic nevi of** left **upper limb, including shoulder**

✓5ᵗʰ D22.7 **Melanocytic nevi of** lower limb, including hip

D22.70 **Melanocytic nevi of unspecified lower limb, including hip**

D22.71 **Melanocytic nevi of** right **lower limb, including hip**

D22.72 **Melanocytic nevi of** left **lower limb, including hip**

D22.9 **Melanocytic nevi, unspecified**

✓4ᵗʰ **D23 Other benign neoplasms of** skin

INCLUDES benign neoplasm of hair follicles
benign neoplasm of sebaceous glands
benign neoplasm of sweat glands

EXCLUDES 1 *benign lipomatous neoplasms of skin (D17.0-D17.3)*
melanocytic nevi (D22.-)

D23.0 **Other benign neoplasm of skin of lip**

EXCLUDES 1 *benign neoplasm of vermilion border of lip (D10.0)*

✓5ᵗʰ D23.1 **Other benign neoplasm of skin of** eyelid, including canthus

D23.10 **Other benign neoplasm of skin of unspecified eyelid, including canthus**

D23.11 **Other benign neoplasm of skin of** right **eyelid, including canthus**

D23.12 **Other benign neoplasm of skin of** left **eyelid, including canthus**

✓5ᵗʰ D23.2 **Other benign neoplasm of skin of** ear and external auricular canal

D23.20 **Other benign neoplasm of skin of unspecified ear and external auricular canal**

D23.21 **Other benign neoplasm of skin of** right **ear and external auricular canal**

D23.22 **Other benign neoplasm of skin of** left **ear and external auricular canal**

✓5ᵗʰ D23.3 **Other benign neoplasm of skin of** other and unspecified parts of face

D23.30 **Other benign neoplasm of skin of unspecified part of face**

D23.39 **Other benign neoplasm of skin of other parts of face**

EXCLUDES 1 Not coded here   EXCLUDES 2 Not included here   N Newborn Age: 0   P Pediatric Age: 0-17   M Maternity Age: 12-55   A Adult Age: 15-124

D23.4 Other benign neoplasm of skin of scalp and neck

D23.5 Other benign neoplasm of skin of trunk
Other benign neoplasm of anal margin
Other benign neoplasm of anal skin
Other benign neoplasm of perianal skin
Other benign neoplasm of skin of breast
　EXCLUDES 1 　*benign neoplasm of anus NOS (D12.9)*

✓5th **D23.6** Other benign neoplasm of skin of upper limb, including shoulder
　　D23.60 Other benign neoplasm of skin of unspecified upper limb, including shoulder
　　D23.61 Other benign neoplasm of skin of right upper limb, including shoulder
　　D23.62 Other benign neoplasm of skin of left upper limb, including shoulder

✓5th **D23.7** Other benign neoplasm of skin of lower limb, including hip
　　D23.70 Other benign neoplasm of skin of unspecified lower limb, including hip
　　D23.71 Other benign neoplasm of skin of right lower limb, including hip
　　D23.72 Other benign neoplasm of skin of left lower limb, including hip

D23.9 Other benign neoplasm of skin, unspecified

✓4th **D24** Benign neoplasm of breast
　INCLUDES 　benign neoplasm of connective tissue of breast
　　　　　benign neoplasm of soft parts of breast
　　　　　fibroadenoma of breast
　EXCLUDES 2 　*adenofibrosis of breast (N60.2)*
　　　　　benign cyst of breast (N60.-)
　　　　　benign mammary dysplasia (N60.-)
　　　　　benign neoplasm of skin of breast (D22.5, D23.5)
　　　　　fibrocystic disease of breast (N60.-)
D24.1 Benign neoplasm of right breast
D24.2 Benign neoplasm of left breast
D24.9 Benign neoplasm of unspecified breast

✓4th **D25** Leiomyoma of uterus
　INCLUDES 　uterine fibroid
　　　　　uterine fibromyoma
　　　　　uterine myoma
D25.0 Submucous leiomyoma of uterus ♀
D25.1 Intramural leiomyoma of uterus ♀
　　Interstitial leiomyoma of uterus
D25.2 Subserosal leiomyoma of uterus ♀
　　Subperitoneal leiomyoma of uterus
D25.9 Leiomyoma of uterus, unspecified ♀

✓4th **D26** Other benign neoplasms of uterus
D26.0 Other benign neoplasm of cervix uteri ♀
D26.1 Other benign neoplasm of corpus uteri ♀
D26.7 Other benign neoplasm of other parts of uterus ♀
D26.9 Other benign neoplasm of uterus, unspecified ♀

✓4th **D27** Benign neoplasm of ovary
　Use additional code to identify any functional activity
　EXCLUDES 2 　*corpus albicans cyst (N83.2)*
　　　　　corpus luteum cyst (N83.1)
　　　　　endometrial cyst (N80.1)
　　　　　follicular (atretic) cyst (N83.0)
　　　　　graafian follicle cyst (N83.0)
　　　　　ovarian cyst NEC (N83.2)
　　　　　ovarian retention cyst (N83.2)
D27.0 Benign neoplasm of right ovary ♀
D27.1 Benign neoplasm of left ovary ♀
D27.9 Benign neoplasm of unspecified ovary ♀

✓4th **D28** Benign neoplasm of other and unspecified female genital organs
　INCLUDES 　adenomatous polyp
　　　　　benign neoplasm of skin of female genital organs
　　　　　benign teratoma
　EXCLUDES 1 　*epoophoron cyst (Q50.5)*
　　　　　fimbrial cyst (Q50.4)
　　　　　Gartner's duct cyst (Q52.4)
　　　　　parovarian cyst (Q50.5)
D28.0 Benign neoplasm of vulva ♀
D28.1 Benign neoplasm of vagina ♀
D28.2 Benign neoplasm of uterine tubes and ligaments ♀
　　Benign neoplasm of fallopian tube
　　Benign neoplasm of uterine ligament (broad) (round)

D28.7 Benign neoplasm of other specified female genital organs ♀
D28.9 Benign neoplasm of female genital organ, unspecified ♀

✓4th **D29** Benign neoplasm of male genital organs
　INCLUDES 　benign neoplasm of skin of male genital organs
D29.0 Benign neoplasm of penis ♂
D29.1 Benign neoplasm of prostate ♂
　EXCLUDES 1 　*enlarged prostate (N40.-)*
✓5th **D29.2** Benign neoplasm of testis
　Use additional code to identify any functional activity
　　D29.20 Benign neoplasm of unspecified testis ♂
　　D29.21 Benign neoplasm of right testis ♂
　　D29.22 Benign neoplasm of left testis ♂
✓5th **D29.3** Benign neoplasm of epididymis
　　D29.30 Benign neoplasm of unspecified epididymis ♂
　　D29.31 Benign neoplasm of right epididymis ♂
　　D29.32 Benign neoplasm of left epididymis ♂
D29.4 Benign neoplasm of scrotum
　　Benign neoplasm of skin of scrotum
D29.8 Benign neoplasm of other specified male genital organs ♂
　　Benign neoplasm of seminal vesicle
　　Benign neoplasm of spermatic cord
　　Benign neoplasm of tunica vaginalis
D29.9 Benign neoplasm of male genital organ, unspecified ♂

✓4th **D30** Benign neoplasm of urinary organs
✓5th **D30.0** Benign neoplasm of kidney
　EXCLUDES 1 　*benign carcinoid tumor of the kidney (D3A.093)*
　　　　　benign neoplasm of renal calyces (D30.1-)
　　　　　benign neoplasm of renal pelvis (D30.1-)
　　D30.00 Benign neoplasm of unspecified kidney
　　D30.01 Benign neoplasm of right kidney
　　D30.02 Benign neoplasm of left kidney
✓5th **D30.1** Benign neoplasm of renal pelvis
　　D30.10 Benign neoplasm of unspecified renal pelvis
　　D30.11 Benign neoplasm of right renal pelvis
　　D30.12 Benign neoplasm of left renal pelvis
✓5th **D30.2** Benign neoplasm of ureter
　EXCLUDES 1 　*benign neoplasm of ureteric orifice of bladder (D30.3)*
　　D30.20 Benign neoplasm of unspecified ureter
　　D30.21 Benign neoplasm of right ureter
　　D30.22 Benign neoplasm of left ureter
D30.3 Benign neoplasm of bladder
　　Benign neoplasm of ureteric orifice of bladder
　　Benign neoplasm of urethral orifice of bladder
D30.4 Benign neoplasm of urethra
　EXCLUDES 1 　*benign neoplasm of urethral orifice of bladder (D30.3)*
D30.8 Benign neoplasm of other specified urinary organs
　　Benign neoplasm of paraurethral glands
D30.9 Benign neoplasm of urinary organ, unspecified
　　Benign neoplasm of urinary system NOS

✓4th **D31** Benign neoplasm of eye and adnexa
　EXCLUDES 1 　*benign neoplasm of connective tissue of eyelid (D21.0)*
　　　　　benign neoplasm of optic nerve (D33.3)
　　　　　benign neoplasm of skin of eyelid (D22.1-, D23.1-)
✓5th **D31.0** Benign neoplasm of conjunctiva
　　D31.00 Benign neoplasm of unspecified conjunctiva
　　D31.01 Benign neoplasm of right conjunctiva
　　D31.02 Benign neoplasm of left conjunctiva
✓5th **D31.1** Benign neoplasm of cornea
　　D31.10 Benign neoplasm of unspecified cornea
　　D31.11 Benign neoplasm of right cornea
　　D31.12 Benign neoplasm of left cornea
✓5th **D31.2** Benign neoplasm of retina
　EXCLUDES 1 　*dark area on retina (D49.81)*
　　　　　hemangioma of retina (D49.81)
　　　　　neoplasm of unspecified behavior of retina and choroid (D49.81)
　　　　　retinal freckle (D49.81)
　　D31.20 Benign neoplasm of unspecified retina
　　D31.21 Benign neoplasm of right retina
　　D31.22 Benign neoplasm of left retina
✓5th **D31.3** Benign neoplasm of choroid
　　D31.30 Benign neoplasm of unspecified choroid

☑ Additional Character Required　　✓7th Xtension Alert　　Unspecified Code　　Other Specified Code　　Manifestation Code　　►◄ Revised Text　　● New Code　　▲ Revised Code Title

Neoplasms

D31.31–D3A.029

D31.31   Benign neoplasm of right choroid
D31.32   Benign neoplasm of left choroid

✓5ᵗʰ D31.4 **Benign neoplasm of ciliary body**

D31.40   Benign neoplasm of unspecified ciliary body
D31.41   Benign neoplasm of right ciliary body
D31.42   Benign neoplasm of left ciliary body

✓5ᵗʰ D31.5 **Benign neoplasm of lacrimal gland and duct**
Benign neoplasm of lacrimal sac
Benign neoplasm of nasolacrimal duct

D31.50   Benign neoplasm of unspecified lacrimal gland and duct
D31.51   Benign neoplasm of right lacrimal gland and duct
D31.52   Benign neoplasm of left lacrimal gland and duct

✓5ᵗʰ D31.6 **Benign neoplasm of unspecified site of orbit**
Benign neoplasm of connective tissue of orbit
Benign neoplasm of extraocular muscle
Benign neoplasm of peripheral nerves of orbit
Benign neoplasm of retrobulbar tissue
Benign neoplasm of retro-ocular tissue
EXCLUDES 1   benign neoplasm of orbital bone (D16.4)

D31.60   Benign neoplasm of unspecified site of unspecified orbit
D31.61   Benign neoplasm of unspecified site of right orbit
D31.62   Benign neoplasm of unspecified site of left orbit

✓5ᵗʰ D31.9 **Benign neoplasm of unspecified part of eye**
Benign neoplasm of eyeball

D31.90   Benign neoplasm of unspecified part of unspecified eye
D31.91   Benign neoplasm of unspecified part of right eye
D31.92   Benign neoplasm of unspecified part of left eye

✓4ᵗʰ **D32 Benign neoplasm of meninges**

D32.0   **Benign neoplasm of cerebral meninges**
D32.1   **Benign neoplasm of spinal meninges**
D32.9   **Benign neoplasm of meninges, unspecified**
Meningioma NOS

✓4ᵗʰ **D33 Benign neoplasm of brain and other parts of central nervous system**
EXCLUDES 1   angioma (D18.0-)
benign neoplasm of meninges (D32.-)
benign neoplasm of peripheral nerves and autonomic nervous system (D36.1-)
hemangioma (D18.0-)
neurofibromatosis (Q85.0-)
retro-ocular benign neoplasm (D31.6-)

D33.0   **Benign neoplasm of brain, supratentorial**
Benign neoplasm of cerebral ventricle
Benign neoplasm of cerebrum
Benign neoplasm of frontal lobe
Benign neoplasm of occipital lobe
Benign neoplasm of parietal lobe
Benign neoplasm of temporal lobe
EXCLUDES 1   benign neoplasm of fourth ventricle (D33.1)

D33.1   **Benign neoplasm of brain, infratentorial**
Benign neoplasm of brain stem
Benign neoplasm of cerebellum
Benign neoplasm of fourth ventricle

D33.2   **Benign neoplasm of brain, unspecified**
D33.3   **Benign neoplasm of cranial nerves**
Benign neoplasm of olfactory bulb
D33.4   **Benign neoplasm of spinal cord**
D33.7   **Benign neoplasm of other specified parts of central nervous system**
D33.9   **Benign neoplasm of central nervous system, unspecified**
Benign neoplasm of nervous system (central) NOS

D34 Benign neoplasm of thyroid gland
Use additional code to identify any functional activity

✓4ᵗʰ **D35 Benign neoplasm of other and unspecified endocrine glands**
Use additional code to identify any functional activity
EXCLUDES 1   benign neoplasm of endocrine pancreas (D13.7)
benign neoplasm of ovary (D27.-)
benign neoplasm of testis (D29.2-)
benign neoplasm of thymus (D15.0)

✓5ᵗʰ D35.0 **Benign neoplasm of adrenal gland**
D35.00   Benign neoplasm of unspecified adrenal gland
D35.01   Benign neoplasm of right adrenal gland

D35.02   Benign neoplasm of left adrenal gland
D35.1   **Benign neoplasm of parathyroid gland**
D35.2   **Benign neoplasm of pituitary gland**
D35.3   **Benign neoplasm of craniopharyngeal duct**
D35.4   **Benign neoplasm of pineal gland**
D35.5   **Benign neoplasm of carotid body**
D35.6   **Benign neoplasm of aortic body and other paraganglia**
Benign tumor of glomus jugulare
D35.7   **Benign neoplasm of other specified endocrine glands**
D35.9   **Benign neoplasm of endocrine gland, unspecified**
Benign neoplasm of unspecified endocrine gland

✓4ᵗʰ **D36 Benign neoplasm of other and unspecified sites**

D36.0   **Benign neoplasm of lymph nodes**
EXCLUDES 1   lymphangioma (D18.1)

✓5ᵗʰ D36.1 **Benign neoplasm of peripheral nerves and autonomic nervous system**
EXCLUDES 1   benign neoplasm of peripheral nerves of orbit (D31.6-)
neurofibromatosis (Q85.0-)

D36.10   Benign neoplasm of peripheral nerves and autonomic nervous system, unspecified
D36.11   Benign neoplasm of peripheral nerves and autonomic nervous system of face, head, and neck
D36.12   Benign neoplasm of peripheral nerves and autonomic nervous system, upper limb, including shoulder
D36.13   Benign neoplasm of peripheral nerves and autonomic nervous system of lower limb, including hip
D36.14   Benign neoplasm of peripheral nerves and autonomic nervous system of thorax
D36.15   Benign neoplasm of peripheral nerves and autonomic nervous system of abdomen
D36.16   Benign neoplasm of peripheral nerves and autonomic nervous system of pelvis
D36.17   Benign neoplasm of peripheral nerves and autonomic nervous system of trunk, unspecified

D36.7   **Benign neoplasm of other specified sites**
Benign neoplasm of nose NOS
D36.9   **Benign neoplasm, unspecified site**

Benign neuroendocrine tumors (D3A)

✓4ᵗʰ **D3A Benign neuroendocrine tumors**
Code also any associated multiple endocrine neoplasia [MEN] syndromes (E31.2-)
Use additional code to identify any associated endocrine syndrome, such as:
carcinoid syndrome (E34.0)
EXCLUDES 2   benign pancreatic islet cell tumors (D13.7)

✓5ᵗʰ D3A.0 **Benign carcinoid tumors**

D3A.00   **Benign carcinoid tumor of unspecified site**
Carcinoid tumor NOS

✓6ᵗʰ D3A.01 **Benign carcinoid tumors of the small intestine**
D3A.010   Benign carcinoid tumor of the duodenum
D3A.011   Benign carcinoid tumor of the jejunum
D3A.012   Benign carcinoid tumor of the ileum
D3A.019   Benign carcinoid tumor of the small intestine, unspecified portion

✓6ᵗʰ D3A.02 **Benign carcinoid tumors of the appendix, large intestine, and rectum**
D3A.020   Benign carcinoid tumor of the appendix
D3A.021   Benign carcinoid tumor of the cecum
D3A.022   Benign carcinoid tumor of the ascending colon
D3A.023   Benign carcinoid tumor of the transverse colon
D3A.024   Benign carcinoid tumor of the descending colon
D3A.025   Benign carcinoid tumor of the sigmoid colon
D3A.026   Benign carcinoid tumor of the rectum
D3A.029   Benign carcinoid tumor of the large intestine, unspecified portion
Benign carcinoid tumor of the colon NOS

EXCLUDES 1 Not coded here   EXCLUDES 2 Not included here   N Newborn Age: 0   P Pediatric Age: 0-17   M Maternity Age: 12-55   A Adult Age: 15-124

468   ICD-10-CM 2014 (Draft)

✓6ᵗʰ **D3A.09** **Benign carcinoid tumors of** other sites

D3A.090 **Benign carcinoid tumor of the** bronchus and lung

D3A.091 **Benign carcinoid tumor of the** thymus

D3A.092 **Benign carcinoid tumor of the** stomach

D3A.093 **Benign carcinoid tumor of the** kidney

D3A.094 **Benign carcinoid tumor of the** foregut NOS

D3A.095 **Benign carcinoid tumor of the** midgut NOS

D3A.096 **Benign carcinoid tumor of the** hindgut NOS

D3A.098 **Benign carcinoid tumors of other sites**

D3A.8 **Other benign neuroendocrine tumors**
Neuroendocrine tumor NOS

Neoplasms of uncertain behavior, polycythemia vera and myelodysplastic syndromes (D37-D48)

NOTE Categories D37-D44, and D48 classify by site neoplasms of uncertain behavior, i.e., histologic confirmation whether the neoplasm is malignant or benign cannot be made.

EXCLUDES 1 neoplasms of unspecified behavior (D49.-)

✓4ᵗʰ **D37** **Neoplasm of uncertain behavior of** oral cavity and digestive organs
EXCLUDES 1 stromal tumors of uncertain behavior of digestive system (D48.1)

✓5ᵗʰ **D37.0** **Neoplasm of uncertain behavior of** lip, oral cavity and pharynx
EXCLUDES 1 neoplasm of uncertain behavior of aryepiglottic fold or interarytenoid fold, laryngeal aspect (D38.0)
neoplasm of uncertain behavior of epiglottis NOS (D38.0)
neoplasm of uncertain behavior of skin of lip (D48.5)
neoplasm of uncertain behavior of suprahyoid portion of epiglottis (D38.0)

D37.01 **Neoplasm of uncertain behavior of** lip
Neoplasm of uncertain behavior of vermilion border of lip

D37.02 **Neoplasm of uncertain behavior of** tongue

✓6ᵗʰ **D37.03** **Neoplasm of uncertain behavior of the** major salivary glands

D37.030 **Neoplasm of uncertain behavior of the** parotid salivary glands

D37.031 **Neoplasm of uncertain behavior of the** sublingual salivary glands

D37.032 **Neoplasm of uncertain behavior of the** submandibular salivary glands

D37.039 **Neoplasm of uncertain behavior of the** major salivary glands, unspecified

D37.04 **Neoplasm of uncertain behavior of the** minor salivary glands
Neoplasm of uncertain behavior of submucosal salivary glands of lip
Neoplasm of uncertain behavior of submucosal salivary glands of cheek
Neoplasm of uncertain behavior of submucosal salivary glands of hard palate
Neoplasm of uncertain behavior of submucosal salivary glands of soft palate

D37.05 **Neoplasm of uncertain behavior of** pharynx
Neoplasm of uncertain behavior of aryepiglottic fold of pharynx NOS
Neoplasm of uncertain behavior of hypopharyngeal aspect of aryepiglottic fold of pharynx
Neoplasm of uncertain behavior of marginal zone of aryepiglottic fold of pharynx

D37.09 **Neoplasm of uncertain behavior of other specified sites of the oral cavity**

D37.1 **Neoplasm of uncertain behavior of** stomach

D37.2 **Neoplasm of uncertain behavior of** small intestine

D37.3 **Neoplasm of uncertain behavior of** appendix

D37.4 **Neoplasm of uncertain behavior of** colon

D37.5 **Neoplasm of uncertain behavior of** rectum
Neoplasm of uncertain behavior of rectosigmoid junction

D37.6 **Neoplasm of uncertain behavior of** liver, gallbladder and bile ducts
Neoplasm of uncertain behavior of ampulla of Vater

D37.8 **Neoplasm of uncertain behavior of other specified digestive organs**
Neoplasm of uncertain behavior of anal canal
Neoplasm of uncertain behavior of anal sphincter
Neoplasm of uncertain behavior of anus NOS
Neoplasm of uncertain behavior of esophagus
Neoplasm of uncertain behavior of intestine NOS
Neoplasm of uncertain behavior of pancreas
EXCLUDES 1 neoplasm of uncertain behavior of anal margin (D48.5)
neoplasm of uncertain behavior of anal skin (D48.5)
neoplasm of uncertain behavior of perianal skin (D48.5)

D37.9 **Neoplasm of uncertain behavior of digestive organ, unspecified**

✓4ᵗʰ **D38** **Neoplasm of uncertain behavior of** middle ear and respiratory and intrathoracic organs
EXCLUDES 1 neoplasm of uncertain behavior of heart (D48.7)

D38.0 **Neoplasm of uncertain behavior of** larynx
Neoplasm of uncertain behavior of aryepiglottic fold or interarytenoid fold, laryngeal aspect
Neoplasm of uncertain behavior of epiglottis (suprahyoid portion)
EXCLUDES 1 neoplasm of uncertain behavior of aryepiglottic fold or interarytenoid fold NOS (D37.05)
neoplasm of uncertain behavior of hypopharyngeal aspect of aryepiglottic fold (D37.05)
neoplasm of uncertain behavior of marginal zone of aryepiglottic fold (D37.05)

D38.1 **Neoplasm of uncertain behavior of** trachea, bronchus and lung

D38.2 **Neoplasm of uncertain behavior of** pleura

D38.3 **Neoplasm of uncertain behavior of** mediastinum

D38.4 **Neoplasm of uncertain behavior of** thymus

D38.5 **Neoplasm of uncertain behavior of other respiratory organs**
Neoplasm of uncertain behavior of accessory sinuses
Neoplasm of uncertain behavior of cartilage of nose
Neoplasm of uncertain behavior of middle ear
Neoplasm of uncertain behavior of nasal cavities
EXCLUDES 1 neoplasm of uncertain behavior of ear (external) (skin) (D48.5)
neoplasm of uncertain behavior of nose NOS (D48.7)
neoplasm of uncertain behavior of skin of nose (D48.5)

D38.6 **Neoplasm of uncertain behavior of respiratory organ, unspecified**

✓4ᵗʰ **D39** **Neoplasm of uncertain behavior of** female genital organs

D39.0 **Neoplasm of uncertain behavior of** uterus ♀

✓5ᵗʰ **D39.1** **Neoplasm of uncertain behavior of** ovary
Use additional code to identify any functional activity

D39.10 **Neoplasm of uncertain behavior of unspecified ovary** ♀

D39.11 **Neoplasm of uncertain behavior of** right ovary ♀

D39.12 **Neoplasm of uncertain behavior of** left ovary ♀

D39.2 **Neoplasm of uncertain behavior of** placenta ♀
Chorioadenoma destruens
Invasive hydatidiform mole
Malignant hydatidiform mole
EXCLUDES 1 hydatidiform mole NOS (O01.9)

D39.8 **Neoplasm of uncertain behavior of other specified female genital organs** ♀
Neoplasm of uncertain behavior of skin of female genital organs

D39.9 **Neoplasm of uncertain behavior of female genital organ, unspecified** ♀

✓4ᵗʰ **D40** **Neoplasm of uncertain behavior of** male genital organs

D40.0 **Neoplasm of uncertain behavior of** prostate ♂

✓5ᵗʰ **D40.1** **Neoplasm of uncertain behavior of** testis

D40.10 **Neoplasm of uncertain behavior of unspecified testis** ♂

D40.11 **Neoplasm of uncertain behavior of** right testis ♂

D40.12 **Neoplasm of uncertain behavior of** left testis ♂

D40.8 **Neoplasm of uncertain behavior of other specified male genital organs** ♂
Neoplasm of uncertain behavior of skin of male genital organs

D40.9 **Neoplasm of uncertain behavior of male genital organ, unspecified** ♂

✓4th **D41 Neoplasm of uncertain behavior of urinary organs**

  ✓5th **D41.0 Neoplasm of uncertain behavior of kidney**
     EXCLUDES 1   *neoplasm of uncertain behavior of renal pelvis (D41.1-)*

     D41.00 Neoplasm of uncertain behavior of unspecified kidney
     D41.01 Neoplasm of uncertain behavior of right kidney
     D41.02 Neoplasm of uncertain behavior of left kidney

  ✓5th **D41.1 Neoplasm of uncertain behavior of renal pelvis**

     D41.10 Neoplasm of uncertain behavior of unspecified renal pelvis
     D41.11 Neoplasm of uncertain behavior of right renal pelvis
     D41.12 Neoplasm of uncertain behavior of left renal pelvis

  ✓5th **D41.2 Neoplasm of uncertain behavior of ureter**

     D41.20 Neoplasm of uncertain behavior of unspecified ureter
     D41.21 Neoplasm of uncertain behavior of right ureter
     D41.22 Neoplasm of uncertain behavior of left ureter

  D41.3 Neoplasm of uncertain behavior of urethra
  D41.4 Neoplasm of uncertain behavior of bladder
  D41.8 Neoplasm of uncertain behavior of other specified urinary organs
  D41.9 Neoplasm of uncertain behavior of unspecified urinary organ

✓4th **D42 Neoplasm of uncertain behavior of meninges**
  D42.0 Neoplasm of uncertain behavior of cerebral meninges
  D42.1 Neoplasm of uncertain behavior of spinal meninges
  D42.9 Neoplasm of uncertain behavior of meninges, unspecified

✓4th **D43 Neoplasm of uncertain behavior of brain and central nervous system**
   EXCLUDES 1   *neoplasm of uncertain behavior of peripheral nerves and autonomic nervous system (D48.2)*

  D43.0 Neoplasm of uncertain behavior of brain, supratentorial
     Neoplasm of uncertain behavior of cerebral ventricle
     Neoplasm of uncertain behavior of cerebrum
     Neoplasm of uncertain behavior of frontal lobe
     Neoplasm of uncertain behavior of occipital lobe
     Neoplasm of uncertain behavior of parietal lobe
     Neoplasm of uncertain behavior of temporal lobe
     EXCLUDES 1   *neoplasm of uncertain behavior of fourth ventricle (D43.1)*

  D43.1 Neoplasm of uncertain behavior of brain, infratentorial
     Neoplasm of uncertain behavior of brain stem
     Neoplasm of uncertain behavior of cerebellum
     Neoplasm of uncertain behavior of fourth ventricle

  D43.2 Neoplasm of uncertain behavior of brain, unspecified
  D43.3 Neoplasm of uncertain behavior of cranial nerves
  D43.4 Neoplasm of uncertain behavior of spinal cord
  D43.8 Neoplasm of uncertain behavior of other specified parts of central nervous system
  D43.9 Neoplasm of uncertain behavior of central nervous system, unspecified
     Neoplasm of uncertain behavior of nervous system (central) NOS

✓4th **D44 Neoplasm of uncertain behavior of endocrine glands**
   EXCLUDES 1   *multiple endocrine adenomatosis (E31.2-)*
     multiple endocrine neoplasia (E31.2-)
     neoplasm of uncertain behavior of endocrine pancreas (D37.8)
     neoplasm of uncertain behavior of ovary (D39.1-)
     neoplasm of uncertain behavior of testis (D40.1-)
     neoplasm of uncertain behavior of thymus (D38.4)

  D44.0 Neoplasm of uncertain behavior of thyroid gland
  ✓5th **D44.1 Neoplasm of uncertain behavior of adrenal gland**
     Use additional code to identify any functional activity

     D44.10 Neoplasm of uncertain behavior of unspecified adrenal gland
     D44.11 Neoplasm of uncertain behavior of right adrenal gland
     D44.12 Neoplasm of uncertain behavior of left adrenal gland

  D44.2 Neoplasm of uncertain behavior of parathyroid gland
  D44.3 Neoplasm of uncertain behavior of pituitary gland
     Use additional code to identify any functional activity
  D44.4 Neoplasm of uncertain behavior of craniopharyngeal duct
  D44.5 Neoplasm of uncertain behavior of pineal gland
  D44.6 Neoplasm of uncertain behavior of carotid body

  D44.7 Neoplasm of uncertain behavior of aortic body and other paraganglia
  D44.9 Neoplasm of uncertain behavior of unspecified endocrine gland

D45 Polycythemia vera
   EXCLUDES 1   *familial polycythemia (D75.0)*
     secondary polycythemia (D75.1)

✓4th **D46 Myelodysplastic syndromes**
   Use additional code for adverse effect, if applicable, to identify drug (T36-T50 with fifth or sixth character 5)
   EXCLUDES 2   *drug-induced aplastic anemia (D61.1)*

  D46.0 Refractory anemia without ring sideroblasts, so stated
     Refractory anemia without sideroblasts, without excess of blasts
  D46.1 Refractory anemia with ring sideroblasts
     RARS
  ✓5th **D46.2 Refractory anemia with excess of blasts**

     D46.20 Refractory anemia with excess of blasts, unspecified
     RAEB NOS
     D46.21 Refractory anemia with excess of blasts 1
     RAEB 1
     D46.22 Refractory anemia with excess of blasts 2
     RAEB 2

  D46.A Refractory cytopenia with multilineage dysplasia
  D46.B Refractory cytopenia with multilineage dysplasia and ring sideroblasts
     RCMD RS
  D46.C Myelodysplastic syndrome with isolated del(5q) chromosomal abnormality
     Myelodysplastic syndrome with 5q deletion
     5q minus syndrome NOS
  D46.4 Refractory anemia, unspecified
  D46.Z Other myelodysplastic syndromes
     EXCLUDES 1   *chronic myelomonocytic leukemia (C93.1-)*
  D46.9 Myelodysplastic syndrome, unspecified
     Myelodysplasia NOS

✓4th **D47 Other neoplasms of uncertain behavior of lymphoid, hematopoietic and related tissue**

  D47.0 Histiocytic and mast cell tumors of uncertain behavior
     Indolent systemic mastocytosis
     Mast cell tumor NOS
     Mastocytoma NOS
     EXCLUDES 1   *malignant mast cell tumor (C96.2)*
     mastocytosis (congenital) (cutaneous) (Q82.2)

  D47.1 Chronic myeloproliferative disease
     Chronic neutrophilic leukemia
     Myeloproliferative disease, unspecified
     EXCLUDES 1   *atypical chronic myeloid leukemia BCR/ABL-negative (C92.2-)*
     chronic myeloid leukemia BCR/ABL-positive (C92.1-)
     myelofibrosis NOS (D75.81)
     myelophthisic anemia (D61.82)
     myelophthisis (D61.82)
     secondary myelofibrosis NOS (D75.81)

  D47.2 Monoclonal gammopathy
     Monoclonal gammopathy of undetermined significance [MGUS]
  D47.3 Essential (hemorrhagic) thrombocythemia
     Essential thrombocytosis
     Idiopathic hemorrhagic thrombocythemia
  D47.4 Osteomyelofibrosis
     Chronic idiopathic myelofibrosis
     Myelofibrosis (idiopathic) (with myeloid metaplasia)
     Myelosclerosis (megakaryocytic) with myeloid metaplasia
     Secondary myelofibrosis in myeloproliferative disease
     EXCLUDES 1   *acute myelofibrosis (C94.4-)*

  ✓5th **D47.Z Other specified neoplasms of uncertain behavior of lymphoid, hematopoietic and related tissue**

     D47.Z1 Post-transplant lymphoproliferative disorder (PTLD)
     Code first complications of transplanted organs and tissue (T86.-)
     D47.Z9 Other specified neoplasms of uncertain behavior of lymphoid, hematopoietic and related tissue
     Histiocytic tumors of uncertain behavior

  D47.9 Neoplasm of uncertain behavior of lymphoid, hematopoietic and related tissue, unspecified
     Lymphoproliferative disease NOS

EXCLUDES 1 Not coded here   EXCLUDES 2 Not included here   N Newborn Age: 0   P Pediatric Age: 0-17   M Maternity Age: 12-55   A Adult Age: 15-124

470   ICD-10-CM 2014 (Draft)

☑4ᵗʰ D48 Neoplasm of uncertain behavior of other and unspecified sites
> EXCLUDES 1 *neurofibromatosis (nonmalignant) (Q85.0-)*

D48.0 Neoplasm of uncertain behavior of bone and articular cartilage
> EXCLUDES 1 *neoplasm of uncertain behavior of cartilage of ear (D48.1)*
> *neoplasm of uncertain behavior of cartilage of larynx (D38.0)*
> *neoplasm of uncertain behavior of cartilage of nose (D38.5)*
> *neoplasm of uncertain behavior of connective tissue of eyelid (D48.1)*
> *neoplasm of uncertain behavior of synovia (D48.1)*

D48.1 Neoplasm of uncertain behavior of connective and other soft tissue
Neoplasm of uncertain behavior of connective tissue of ear
Neoplasm of uncertain behavior of connective tissue of eyelid
Stromal tumors of uncertain behavior of digestive system
> EXCLUDES 1 *neoplasm of uncertain behavior of articular cartilage (D48.0)*
> *neoplasm of uncertain behavior of cartilage of larynx (D38.0)*
> *neoplasm of uncertain behavior of cartilage of nose (D38.5)*
> *neoplasm of uncertain behavior of connective tissue of breast (D48.6-)*

D48.2 Neoplasm of uncertain behavior of peripheral nerves and autonomic nervous system
> EXCLUDES 1 *neoplasm of uncertain behavior of peripheral nerves of orbit (D48.7)*

D48.3 Neoplasm of uncertain behavior of retroperitoneum

D48.4 Neoplasm of uncertain behavior of peritoneum

D48.5 Neoplasm of uncertain behavior of skin
Neoplasm of uncertain behavior of anal margin
Neoplasm of uncertain behavior of anal skin
Neoplasm of uncertain behavior of perianal skin
Neoplasm of uncertain behavior of skin of breast
> EXCLUDES 1 *neoplasm of uncertain behavior of anus NOS (D37.8)*
> *neoplasm of uncertain behavior of skin of genital organs (D39.8, D40.8)*
> *neoplasm of uncertain behavior of vermilion border of lip (D37.0)*

☑5ᵗʰ D48.6 Neoplasm of uncertain behavior of breast
Neoplasm of uncertain behavior of connective tissue of breast
Cystosarcoma phyllodes
> EXCLUDES 1 *neoplasm of uncertain behavior of skin of breast (D48.5)*

D48.60 Neoplasm of uncertain behavior of unspecified breast

D48.61 Neoplasm of uncertain behavior of right breast

D48.62 Neoplasm of uncertain behavior of left breast

D48.7 Neoplasm of uncertain behavior of other specified sites
Neoplasm of uncertain behavior of eye
Neoplasm of uncertain behavior of heart
Neoplasm of uncertain behavior of peripheral nerves of orbit
> EXCLUDES 1 *neoplasm of uncertain behavior of connective tissue (D48.1)*
> *neoplasm of uncertain behavior of skin of eyelid (D48.5)*

D48.9 Neoplasm of uncertain behavior, unspecified

Neoplasms of uncertain behavior (D49)

☑4ᵗʰ D49 Neoplasms of unspecified behavior
> NOTE Category D49 classifies by site neoplasms of unspecified morphology and behavior. The term "mass", unless otherwise stated, is not to be regarded as a neoplastic growth.
> INCLUDES "growth" NOS
> neoplasm NOS
> new growth NOS
> tumor NOS
> EXCLUDES 1 *neoplasms of uncertain behavior (D37-D44, D48)*

D49.0 Neoplasm of unspecified behavior of digestive system
> EXCLUDES 1 *neoplasm of unspecified behavior of margin of anus (D49.2)*
> *neoplasm of unspecified behavior of perianal skin (D49.2)*
> *neoplasm of unspecified behavior of skin of anus (D49.2)*

D49.1 Neoplasm of unspecified behavior of respiratory system

D49.2 Neoplasm of unspecified behavior of bone, soft tissue, and skin
> EXCLUDES 1 *neoplasm of unspecified behavior of anal canal (D49.0)*
> *neoplasm of unspecified behavior of anus NOS (D49.0)*
> *neoplasm of unspecified behavior of bone marrow (D49.89)*
> *neoplasm of unspecified behavior of cartilage of larynx (D49.1)*
> *neoplasm of unspecified behavior of cartilage of nose (D49.1)*
> *neoplasm of unspecified behavior of connective tissue of breast (D49.3)*
> *neoplasm of unspecified behavior of skin of genital organs (D49.5)*
> *neoplasm of unspecified behavior of vermilion border of lip (D49.0)*

D49.3 Neoplasm of unspecified behavior of breast
> EXCLUDES 1 *neoplasm of unspecified behavior of skin of breast (D49.2)*

D49.4 Neoplasm of unspecified behavior of bladder

D49.5 Neoplasm of unspecified behavior of other genitourinary organs

D49.6 Neoplasm of unspecified behavior of brain
> EXCLUDES 1 *neoplasm of unspecified behavior of cerebral meninges (D49.7)*
> *neoplasm of unspecified behavior of cranial nerves (D49.7)*

D49.7 Neoplasm of unspecified behavior of endocrine glands and other parts of nervous system
> EXCLUDES 1 *neoplasm of unspecified behavior of peripheral, sympathetic, and parasympathetic nerves and ganglia (D49.2)*

☑5ᵗʰ D49.8 Neoplasm of unspecified behavior of other specified sites
> EXCLUDES 1 *neoplasm of unspecified behavior of eyelid (skin) (D49.2)*
> *neoplasm of unspecified behavior of eyelid cartilage (D49.2)*
> *neoplasm of unspecified behavior of great vessels (D49.2)*
> *neoplasm of unspecified behavior of optic nerve (D49.7)*

D49.81 Neoplasm of unspecified behavior of retina and choroid
Dark area on retina
Retinal freckle

D49.89 Neoplasm of unspecified behavior of other specified sites

D49.9 Neoplasm of unspecified behavior of unspecified site

Chapter 3. Diseases of the Blood and Blood-forming Organs and Certain Disorders Involving the Immune Mechanism (D50-D89)

EXCLUDES 2　autoimmune disease (systemic) NOS (M35.9)
certain conditions originating in the perinatal period (P00-P96)
complications of pregnancy, childbirth and the puerperium (O00-O9A)
congenital malformations, deformations and chromosomal abnormalities (Q00-Q99)
endocrine, nutritional and metabolic diseases (E00-E88)
human immunodeficiency virus [HIV] disease (B20)
injury, poisoning and certain other consequences of external causes (S00-T88)
neoplasms (C00-D49)
symptoms, signs and abnormal clinical and laboratory findings, not elsewhere classified (R00-R94)

This chapter contains the following blocks:
D50-D53　Nutritional anemias
D55-D59　Hemolytic anemias
D60-D64　Aplastic and other anemias and other bone marrow failure syndromes
D65-D69　Coagulation defects, purpura and other hemorrhagic conditions
D70-D77　Other disorders of blood and blood-forming organs
D78　　　Intraoperative and postprocedural complications of the spleen
D80-D89　Certain disorders involving the immune mechanism

Nutritional anemias (D50-D53)

✓4th **D50　Iron deficiency anemia**
　　INCLUDES　asiderotic anemia
　　　　　　　hypochromic anemia

　D50.0　Iron deficiency anemia secondary to blood loss (chronic)
　　　Posthemorrhagic anemia (chronic)
　　　EXCLUDES 1　acute posthemorrhagic anemia (D62)
　　　　　　　　congenital anemia from fetal blood loss (P61.3)

　D50.1　Sideropenic dysphagia
　　　Kelly-Paterson syndrome
　　　Plummer-Vinson syndrome

　D50.8　Other iron deficiency anemias
　　　Iron deficiency anemia due to inadequate dietary iron intake

　D50.9　Iron deficiency anemia, unspecified

✓4th **D51　Vitamin B12 deficiency anemia**
　　EXCLUDES 1　vitamin B12 deficiency (E53.8)

　D51.0　Vitamin B12 deficiency anemia due to intrinsic factor deficiency
　　　Addison anemia
　　　Biermer anemia
　　　Pernicious (congenital) anemia
　　　Congenital intrinsic factor deficiency

　D51.1　Vitamin B12 deficiency anemia due to selective vitamin B12 malabsorption with proteinuria
　　　Imerslund (Gräsbeck) syndrome
　　　Megaloblastic hereditary anemia

　D51.2　Transcobalamin II deficiency

　D51.3　Other dietary vitamin B12 deficiency anemia
　　　Vegan anemia

　D51.8　Other vitamin B12 deficiency anemias

　D51.9　Vitamin B12 deficiency anemia, unspecified

✓4th **D52　Folate deficiency anemia**
　　EXCLUDES 1　folate deficiency without anemia (E53.8)

　D52.0　Dietary folate deficiency anemia
　　　Nutritional megaloblastic anemia

　D52.1　Drug-induced folate deficiency anemia
　　　Use additional code for adverse effect, if applicable, to identify drug (T36-T50 with fifth or sixth character 5)

　D52.8　Other folate deficiency anemias

　D52.9　Folate deficiency anemia, unspecified
　　　Folic acid deficiency anemia NOS

✓4th **D53　Other nutritional anemias**
　　INCLUDES　megaloblastic anemia unresponsive to vitamin B12 or folate therapy

　D53.0　Protein deficiency anemia
　　　Amino-acid deficiency anemia
　　　Orotaciduric anemia
　　　EXCLUDES 1　Lesch-Nyhan syndrome (E79.1)

　D53.1　Other megaloblastic anemias, not elsewhere classified
　　　Megaloblastic anemia NOS
　　　EXCLUDES 1　Di Guglielmo's disease (C94.0)

　D53.2　Scorbutic anemia
　　　EXCLUDES 1　scurvy (E54)

　D53.8　Other specified nutritional anemias
　　　Anemia associated with deficiency of copper
　　　Anemia associated with deficiency of molybdenum
　　　Anemia associated with deficiency of zinc
　　　EXCLUDES 1　nutritional deficiencies without anemia, such as:
　　　　　　　　copper deficiency NOS (E61.0)
　　　　　　　　molybdenum deficiency NOS (E61.5)
　　　　　　　　zinc deficiency NOS (E60)

　D53.9　Nutritional anemia, unspecified
　　　Simple chronic anemia
　　　EXCLUDES 1　anemia NOS (D64.9)

Hemolytic anemias (D55-D59)

✓4th **D55　Anemia due to enzyme disorders**
　　EXCLUDES 1　drug-induced enzyme deficiency anemia (D59.2)

　D55.0　Anemia due to glucose-6-phosphate dehydrogenase [G6PD] deficiency
　　　Favism
　　　G6PD deficiency anemia

　D55.1　Anemia due to other disorders of glutathione metabolism
　　　Anemia (due to) enzyme deficiencies, except G6PD, related to the hexose monophosphate [HMP] shunt pathway
　　　Anemia (due to) hemolytic nonspherocytic (hereditary), type I

　D55.2　Anemia due to disorders of glycolytic enzymes
　　　Hemolytic nonspherocytic (hereditary) anemia, type II
　　　Hexokinase deficiency anemia
　　　Pyruvate kinase [PK] deficiency anemia
　　　Triose-phosphate isomerase deficiency anemia
　　　EXCLUDES 1　disorders of glycolysis not associated with anemia (E74.8)

　D55.3　Anemia due to disorders of nucleotide metabolism

　D55.8　Other anemias due to enzyme disorders

　D55.9　Anemia due to enzyme disorder, unspecified

✓4th **D56　Thalassemia**
　　EXCLUDES 1　sickle-cell thalassemia (D57.4-)

　D56.0　Alpha thalassemia
　　　Alpha thalassemia major
　　　Hemoglobin H Constant Spring
　　　Hemoglobin H disease
　　　Hydrops fetalis due to alpha thalassemia
　　　Severe alpha thalassemia
　　　Triple gene defect alpha thalassemia
　　　Use additional code, if applicable, for hydrops fetalis due to alpha thalassemia (P56.99)
　　　EXCLUDES 1　alpha thalassemia trait or minor (D56.3)
　　　　　　　　asymptomatic alpha thalassemia (D56.3)
　　　　　　　　hydrops fetalis due to isoimmunization (P56.0)
　　　　　　　　hydrops fetalis not due to immune hemolysis (P83.2)

　D56.1　Beta thalassemia
　　　Beta thalassemia major
　　　Cooley's anemia
　　　Homozygous beta thalassemia
　　　Severe beta thalassemia
　　　Thalassemia intermedia
　　　Thalassemia major
　　　EXCLUDES 1　beta thalassemia minor (D56.3)
　　　　　　　　beta thalassemia trait (D56.3)
　　　　　　　　delta-beta thalassemia (D56.2)
　　　　　　　　hemoglobin E-beta thalassemia (D56.5)
　　　　　　　　sickle-cell beta thalassemia (D57.4-)

　D56.2　Delta-beta thalassemia
　　　Homozygous delta-beta thalassemia
　　　EXCLUDES 1　delta-beta thalassemia minor (D56.3)
　　　　　　　　delta-beta thalassemia trait (D56.3)

　D56.3　Thalassemia minor
　　　Alpha thalassemia minor
　　　Alpha thalassemia silent carrier
　　　Alpha thalassemia trait
　　　Beta thalassemia minor
　　　Beta thalassemia trait
　　　Delta-beta thalassemia minor
　　　Delta-beta thalassemia trait
　　　Thalassemia trait NOS
　　　EXCLUDES 1　alpha thalassemia (D56.0)
　　　　　　　　beta thalassemia (D56.1)
　　　　　　　　delta-beta thalassemia (D56.2)
　　　　　　　　hemoglobin E-beta thalassemia (D56.5)
　　　　　　　　sickle-cell trait (D57.3)

D56.4   Hereditary persistence of fetal hemoglobin [HPFH]

D56.5   Hemoglobin E-beta thalassemia
> EXCLUDES 1   *beta thalassemia (D56.1)*
> *beta thalassemia minor (D56.3)*
> *beta thalassemia trait (D56.3)*
> *delta-beta thalassemia (D56.2)*
> *delta-beta thalassemia trait (D56.3)*
> *hemoglobin E disease (D58.2)*
> *other hemoglobinopathies (D58.2)*
> *sickle-cell beta thalassemia (D57.4-)*

D56.8   Other thalassemias
Dominant thalassemia
Hemoglobin C thalassemia
Mixed thalassemia
Thalassemia with other hemoglobinopathy
> EXCLUDES 1   *hemoglobin C disease (D58.2)*
> *hemoglobin E disease (D58.2)*
> *other hemoglobinopathies (D58.2)*
> *sickle-cell anemia (D57.-)*
> *sickle-cell thalassemia (D57.4)*

D56.9   Thalassemia, unspecified
Mediterranean anemia (with other hemoglobinopathy)

✓4th **D57**   **Sickle-cell disorders**
Use additional code for any associated fever (R50.81)
> EXCLUDES 1   *other hemoglobinopathies (D58.-)*

✓5th **D57.0**   **Hb-SS disease with crisis**
Sickle-cell disease NOS with crisis
Hb-SS disease with vasoocclusive pain

     D57.00   Hb-SS disease with crisis, unspecified

     D57.01   Hb-SS disease with acute chest syndrome

     D57.02   Hb-SS disease with splenic sequestration

D57.1   **Sickle-cell disease without crisis**
Hb-SS disease without crisis
Sickle-cell anemia NOS
Sickle-cell disease NOS
Sickle-cell disorder NOS

✓5th **D57.2**   **Sickle-cell/Hb-C disease**
Hb-SC disease
Hb-S/Hb-C disease

     D57.20   Sickle-cell/Hb-C disease without crisis

     ✓6th **D57.21**   Sickle-cell/Hb-C disease with crisis

         D57.211   Sickle-cell/Hb-C disease with acute chest syndrome

         D57.212   Sickle-cell/Hb-C disease with splenic sequestration

         D57.219   Sickle-cell/Hb-C disease with crisis, unspecified
Sickle-cell/Hb-C disease with crisis NOS

D57.3   **Sickle-cell trait**
Hb-S trait
Heterozygous hemoglobin S

✓5th **D57.4**   **Sickle-cell thalassemia**
Sickle-cell beta thalassemia
Thalassemia Hb-S disease

     D57.40   Sickle-cell thalassemia without crisis
Microdrepanocytosis
Sickle-cell thalassemia NOS

     ✓6th **D57.41**   Sickle-cell thalassemia with crisis
Sickle-cell thalassemia with vasoocclusive pain

         D57.411   Sickle-cell thalassemia with acute chest syndrome

         D57.412   Sickle-cell thalassemia with splenic sequestration

         D57.419   Sickle-cell thalassemia with crisis, unspecified
Sickle-cell thalassemia with crisis NOS

✓5th **D57.8**   **Other sickle-cell disorders**
Hb-SD disease
Hb-SE disease

     D57.80   Other sickle-cell disorders without crisis

     ✓6th **D57.81**   Other sickle-cell disorders with crisis

         D57.811   Other sickle-cell disorders with acute chest syndrome

         D57.812   Other sickle-cell disorders with splenic sequestration

         D57.819   Other sickle-cell disorders with crisis, unspecified
Other sickle-cell disorders with crisis NOS

✓4th **D58**   **Other hereditary hemolytic anemias**
> EXCLUDES 1   *hemolytic anemia of the newborn (P55.-)*

D58.0   Hereditary spherocytosis
Acholuric (familial) jaundice
Congenital (spherocytic) hemolytic icterus
Minkowski-Chauffard syndrome

D58.1   Hereditary elliptocytosis
Elliptocytosis (congenital)
Ovalocytosis (congenital) (hereditary)

D58.2   Other hemoglobinopathies
Abnormal hemoglobin NOS
Congenital Heinz body anemia
Hb-C disease
Hb-D disease
Hb-E disease
Hemoglobinopathy NOS
Unstable hemoglobin hemolytic disease
> EXCLUDES 1   *familial polycythemia (D75.0)*
> *Hb-M disease (D74.0)*
> *hemoglobin E-beta thalassemia (D56.5)*
> *hereditary persistence of fetal hemoglobin [HPFH] (D56.4)*
> *high-altitude polycythemia (D75.1)*
> *methemoglobinemia (D74.-)*
> *other hemoglobinopathies with thalassemia (D56.8)*

D58.8   Other specified hereditary hemolytic anemias
Stomatocytosis

D58.9   Hereditary hemolytic anemia, unspecified

✓4th **D59**   **Acquired hemolytic anemia**

D59.0   Drug-induced autoimmune hemolytic anemia
Use additional code for adverse effect, if applicable, to identify drug (T36-T50 with fifth or sixth character 5)

D59.1   Other autoimmune hemolytic anemias
Autoimmune hemolytic disease (cold type) (warm type)
Chronic cold hemagglutinin disease
Cold agglutinin disease
Cold agglutinin hemoglobinuria
Cold type (secondary) (symptomatic) hemolytic anemia
Warm type (secondary) (symptomatic) hemolytic anemia
> EXCLUDES 1   *Evans syndrome (D69.41)*
> *hemolytic disease of newborn (P55.-)*
> *paroxysmal cold hemoglobinuria (D59.6)*

D59.2   Drug-induced nonautoimmune hemolytic anemia
Drug-induced enzyme deficiency anemia
Use additional code for adverse effect, if applicable, to identify drug (T36-T50 with fifth or sixth character 5)

D59.3   Hemolytic-uremic syndrome
Use additional code to identify associated:
E. coli infection (B96.2-)
Pneumococcal pneumonia (J13)
Shigella dysenteriae (A03.9)

D59.4   Other nonautoimmune hemolytic anemias
Mechanical hemolytic anemia
Microangiopathic hemolytic anemia
Toxic hemolytic anemia

D59.5   Paroxysmal nocturnal hemoglobinuria [Marchiafava-Micheli]
> EXCLUDES 1   *hemoglobinuria NOS (R82.3)*

D59.6   Hemoglobinuria due to hemolysis from other external causes
Hemoglobinuria from exertion
March hemoglobinuria
Paroxysmal cold hemoglobinuria
Use additional code (Chapter 20) to identify external cause
> EXCLUDES 1   *hemoglobinuria NOS (R82.3)*

D59.8   Other acquired hemolytic anemias

D59.9   Acquired hemolytic anemia, unspecified
Idiopathic hemolytic anemia, chronic

Aplastic and other anemias and other bone marrow failure syndromes (D60-D64)

✓4th **D60**   **Acquired pure red cell aplasia [erythroblastopenia]**
> INCLUDES   red cell aplasia (acquired) (adult) (with thymoma)
> EXCLUDES 1   *congenital red cell aplasia (D61.01)*

D60.0   Chronic acquired pure red cell aplasia

D60.1   Transient acquired pure red cell aplasia

D60.8   Other acquired pure red cell aplasias

D60.9   Acquired pure red cell aplasia, unspecified

Diseases of the Blood and Blood-forming Organs   **D61–D68.0**

✓4th **D61 Other aplastic anemias and other bone marrow failure syndromes**
> EXCLUDES 1   neutropenia (D70.-)

✓5th **D61.0 Constitutional aplastic anemia**

D61.01 Constitutional (pure) red blood cell aplasia
Blackfan-Diamond syndrome
Congenital (pure) red cell aplasia
Familial hypoplastic anemia
Primary (pure) red cell aplasia
Red cell (pure) aplasia of infants
> EXCLUDES 1   acquired red cell aplasia (D60.9)

D61.09 Other constitutional aplastic anemia
Fanconi's anemia
Pancytopenia with malformations

D61.1 Drug-induced aplastic anemia
Use additional code for adverse effect, if applicable, to identify drug (T36-T50 with fifth or sixth character 5)

D61.2 Aplastic anemia due to other external agents
Code first, if applicable, toxic effects of substances chiefly nonmedicinal as to source (T51-T65)

D61.3 Idiopathic aplastic anemia

✓5th **D61.8 Other specified aplastic anemias and other bone marrow failure syndromes**

✓6th **D61.81 Pancytopenia**
> EXCLUDES 1   pancytopenia (due to) (with) aplastic anemia (D61.9)
> pancytopenia (due to) (with) bone marrow infiltration (D61.82)
> pancytopenia (due to) (with) congenital (pure) red cell aplasia (D61.01)
> pancytopenia (due to) (with) hairy cell leukemia (C91.4-)
> pancytopenia (due to) (with) human immunodeficiency virus disease (B20)
> pancytopenia (due to) (with) leukoerythroblastic anemia (D61.82)
> pancytopenia (due to) (with) myelodysplastic syndromes (D46.-)
> pancytopenia (due to) (with) myeloproliferative disease (D47.1)

D61.810 Antineoplastic chemotherapy induced pancytopenia
> EXCLUDES 2   aplastic anemia due to antineoplastic chemotherapy (D61.1)

D61.811 Other drug-induced pancytopenia
> EXCLUDES 2   aplastic anemia due to drugs (D61.1)

D61.818 Other pancytopenia

D61.82 Myelophthisis
Leukoerythroblastic anemia
Myelophthisic anemia
Panmyelophthisis
Code also the underlying disorder, such as:
malignant neoplasm of breast (C50.-)
tuberculosis (A15.-)
> EXCLUDES 1   idiopathic myelofibrosis (D47.1)
> myelofibrosis NOS (D75.81)
> myelofibrosis with myeloid metaplasia (D47.4)
> primary myelofibrosis (D47.1)
> secondary myelofibrosis (D75.81)

D61.89 Other specified aplastic anemias and other bone marrow failure syndromes

D61.9 Aplastic anemia, unspecified
Hypoplastic anemia NOS
Medullary hypoplasia

D62 Acute posthemorrhagic anemia
> EXCLUDES 1   anemia due to chronic blood loss (D50.0)
> blood loss anemia NOS (D50.0)
> congenital anemia from fetal blood loss (P61.3)

✓4th **D63 Anemia in chronic diseases classified elsewhere**

D63.0 Anemia in neoplastic disease
Code first neoplasm (C00-D49)
> EXCLUDES 1   anemia due to antineoplastic chemotherapy (D64.81)
> aplastic anemia due to antineoplastic chemotherapy (D61.1)

D63.1 Anemia in chronic kidney disease
Erythropoietin resistant anemia (EPO resistant anemia)
Code first underlying chronic kidney disease (CKD) (N18.-)

D63.8 Anemia in other chronic diseases classified elsewhere
Code first underlying disease, such as:
diphyllobothriasis (B70.0)
hookworm disease (B76.0-B76.9)
hypothyroidism (E00.0-E03.9)
malaria (B50.0-B54)
symptomatic late syphilis (A52.79)
tuberculosis (A18.89)

✓4th **D64 Other anemias**
> EXCLUDES 1   refractory anemia (D46.-)
> refractory anemia with excess blasts in transformation [RAEB T] (C92.0-)

D64.0 Hereditary sideroblastic anemia
Sex-linked hypochromic sideroblastic anemia

D64.1 Secondary sideroblastic anemia due to disease
Code first underlying disease

D64.2 Secondary sideroblastic anemia due to drugs and toxins
Code first poisoning due to drug or toxin, if applicable (T36-T65 with fifth or sixth character 1-4 or 6)
Use additional code for adverse effect, if applicable, to identify drug (T36-T50 with fifth or sixth character 5)

D64.3 Other sideroblastic anemias
Sideroblastic anemia NOS
Pyridoxine-responsive sideroblastic anemia NEC

D64.4 Congenital dyserythropoietic anemia
Dyshematopoietic anemia (congenital)
> EXCLUDES 1   Blackfan-Diamond syndrome (D61.01)
> Di Guglielmo's disease (C94.0)

✓5th **D64.8 Other specified anemias**

D64.81 Anemia due to antineoplastic chemotherapy
Antineoplastic chemotherapy induced anemia
> EXCLUDES 1   anemia in neoplastic disease (D63.0)
> aplastic anemia due to antineoplastic chemotherapy (D61.1)

D64.89 Other specified anemias
Infantile pseudoleukemia

D64.9 Anemia, unspecified

Coagulation defects, purpura and other hemorrhagic conditions (D65-D69)

D65 Disseminated intravascular coagulation [defibrination syndrome]
Afibrinogenemia, acquired
Consumption coagulopathy
Diffuse or disseminated intravascular coagulation [DIC]
Fibrinolytic hemorrhage, acquired
Fibrinolytic purpura
Purpura fulminans
> EXCLUDES 1   disseminated intravascular coagulation (complicating):
> abortion or ectopic or molar pregnancy (O00-O07, O08.1)
> in newborn (P60)
> pregnancy, childbirth and the puerperium (O45.0, O46.0, O67.0, O72.3)

D66 Hereditary factor VIII deficiency
Classical hemophilia
Deficiency factor VIII (with functional defect)
Hemophilia NOS
Hemophilia A
> EXCLUDES 1   factor VIII deficiency with vascular defect (D68.0)

D67 Hereditary factor IX deficiency
Christmas disease
Factor IX deficiency (with functional defect)
Hemophilia B
Plasma thromboplastin component [PTC] deficiency

✓4th **D68 Other coagulation defects**
> EXCLUDES 1   abnormal coagulation profile (R79.1)
> coagulation defects complicating abortion or ectopic or molar pregnancy (O00-O07, O08.1)
> coagulation defects complicating pregnancy, childbirth and the puerperium (O45.0, O46.0, O67.0, O72.3)

D68.0 Von Willebrand's disease
Angiohemophilia
Factor VIII deficiency with vascular defect
Vascular hemophilia
> EXCLUDES 1   capillary fragility (hereditary) (D69.8)
> factor VIII deficiency NOS (D66)
> factor VIII deficiency with functional defect (D66)

EXCLUDES 1 Not coded here   EXCLUDES 2 Not included here   N Newborn Age: 0   P Pediatric Age: 0-17   M Maternity Age: 12-55   A Adult Age: 15-124

474   ICD-10-CM 2014 (Draft)

D68.1 **Hereditary factor XI** deficiency
　　Hemophilia C
　　Plasma thromboplastin antecedent [PTA] deficiency
　　Rosenthal's disease

D68.2 **Hereditary deficiency of other clotting factors**
　　AC globulin deficiency
　　Congenital afibrinogenemia
　　Deficiency of factor I [fibrinogen]
　　Deficiency of factor II [prothrombin]
　　Deficiency of factor V [labile]
　　Deficiency of factor VII [stable]
　　Deficiency of factor X [Stuart-Prower]
　　Deficiency of factor XII [Hageman]
　　Deficiency of factor XIII [fibrin stabilizing]
　　Dysfibrinogenemia (congenital)
　　Hypoproconvertinemia
　　Owren's disease
　　Proaccelerin deficiency

✓5ᵗʰ **D68.3** **Hemorrhagic disorder due to circulating anticoagulants**

　✓6ᵗʰ **D68.31** **Hemorrhagic disorder due to intrinsic circulating anticoagulants, antibodies, or inhibitors**

　　D68.311 **Acquired hemophilia**
　　　　Autoimmune hemophilia
　　　　Autoimmune inhibitors to clotting factors
　　　　Secondary hemophilia

　　D68.312 **Antiphospholipid antibody with hemorrhagic disorder**
　　　　Lupus anticoagulant (LAC) with hemorrhagic disorder
　　　　Systemic lupus erythematosus [SLE] inhibitor with hemorrhagic disorder
　　　　EXCLUDES 1　*antiphospholipid antibody, finding without diagnosis (R76.0)*
　　　　　　antiphospholipid antibody syndrome (D68.61)
　　　　　　antiphospholipid antibody with hypercoagulable state (D68.61)
　　　　　　lupus anticoagulant (LAC) finding without diagnosis (R76.0)
　　　　　　lupus anticoagulant (LAC) with hypercoagulable state (D68.62)
　　　　　　systemic lupus erythematosus [SLE] inhibitor finding without diagnosis (R76.0)
　　　　　　systemic lupus erythematosus [SLE] inhibitor with hypercoagulable state (D68.62)

　　D68.318 **Other hemorrhagic disorder due to intrinsic circulating anticoagulants, antibodies, or inhibitors**
　　　　Antithromboplastinemia
　　　　Antithromboplastinogenemia
　　　　Hemorrhagic disorder due to intrinsic increase in antithrombin
　　　　Hemorrhagic disorder due to intrinsic increase in anti-VIIIa
　　　　Hemorrhagic disorder due to intrinsic increase in anti-IXa
　　　　Hemorrhagic disorder due to intrinsic increase in anti-XIa

　D68.32 **Hemorrhagic disorder due to extrinsic circulating anticoagulants**
　　　Drug-induced hemorrhagic disorder
　　　Hemorrhagic disorder due to increase in anti-IIa
　　　Hemorrhagic disorder due to increase in anti-Xa
　　　Hyperheparinemia
　　　Use additional code for adverse effect, if applicable, to identify drug (T45.515, T45.525)

D68.4 **Acquired coagulation factor deficiency**
　　Deficiency of coagulation factor due to liver disease
　　Deficiency of coagulation factor due to vitamin K deficiency
　　EXCLUDES 1　*vitamin K deficiency of newborn (P53)*

✓5ᵗʰ **D68.5** **Primary thrombophilia**
　　Primary hypercoagulable states
　　EXCLUDES 1　*antiphospholipid syndrome (D68.61)*
　　　　lupus anticoagulant (D68.62)
　　　　secondary activated protein C resistance (D68.69)
　　　　secondary antiphospholipid antibody syndrome (D68.69)
　　　　secondary lupus anticoagulant with hypercoagulable state (D68.69)
　　　　secondary systemic lupus erythematosus [SLE] inhibitor with hypercoagulable state (D68.69)
　　　　systemic lupus erythematosus [SLE] inhibitor finding without diagnosis (R76.0)
　　　　systemic lupus erythematosus [SLE] inhibitor with hemorrhagic disorder (D68.312)
　　　　thrombotic thrombocytopenic purpura (M31.1)

　D68.51 **Activated protein C resistance**
　　　Factor V Leiden mutation

　D68.52 **Prothrombin gene mutation**

　D68.59 **Other primary thrombophilia**
　　　Antithrombin III deficiency　　Protein C deficiency
　　　Hypercoagulable state NOS　　Protein S deficiency
　　　Primary hypercoagulable　　　Thrombophilia NOS
　　　　state NEC
　　　Primary thrombophilia NEC

✓5ᵗʰ **D68.6** **Other thrombophilia**
　　Other hypercoagulable states
　　EXCLUDES 1　*diffuse or disseminated intravascular coagulation [DIC] (D65)*
　　　　heparin induced thrombocytopenia (HIT) (D75.82)
　　　　hyperhomocysteinemia (E72.11)

　D68.61 **Antiphospholipid syndrome**
　　　Anticardiolipin syndrome
　　　Antiphospholipid antibody syndrome
　　　EXCLUDES 1　*antiphospholipid antibody, finding without diagnosis (R76.0)*
　　　　antiphospholipid antibody with hemorrhagic disorder (D68.312)
　　　　lupus anticoagulant syndrome (D68.62)

　D68.62 **Lupus anticoagulant syndrome**
　　　Lupus anticoagulant
　　　Presence of systemic lupus erythematosus [SLE] inhibitor
　　　EXCLUDES 1　*anticardiolipin syndrome (D68.61)*
　　　　antiphospholipid syndrome (D68.61)
　　　　lupus anticoagulant (LAC) finding without diagnosis (R79.0)
　　　　lupus anticoagulant (LAC) with hemorrhagic disorder (D68.312)

　D68.69 **Other thrombophilia**
　　　Hypercoagulable states NEC
　　　Secondary hypercoagulable state NOS

　D68.8 **Other specified coagulation defects**
　　　EXCLUDES 1　*hemorrhagic disease of newborn (P53)*

　D68.9 **Coagulation defect, unspecified**

✓4ᵗʰ **D69** **Purpura and other hemorrhagic conditions**
　　EXCLUDES 1　*benign hypergammaglobulinemic purpura (D89.0)*
　　　　cryoglobulinemic purpura (D89.1)
　　　　essential (hemorrhagic) thrombocythemia (D47.3)
　　　　hemorrhagic thrombocythemia (D47.3)
　　　　purpura fulminans (D65)
　　　　thrombotic thrombocytopenic purpura (M31.1)
　　　　Waldenström hypergammaglobulinemic purpura (D89.0)

　D69.0 **Allergic purpura**
　　　Allergic vasculitis
　　　Nonthrombocytopenic hemorrhagic purpura
　　　Nonthrombocytopenic idiopathic purpura
　　　Purpura anaphylactoid
　　　Purpura Henoch(-Schönlein)
　　　Purpura rheumatica
　　　Vascular purpura
　　　EXCLUDES 1　*thrombocytopenic hemorrhagic purpura (D69.3)*

　D69.1 **Qualitative platelet defects**
　　　Bernard-Soulier [giant platelet] syndrome
　　　Glanzmann's disease
　　　Grey platelet syndrome
　　　Thromboasthenia (hemorrhagic) (hereditary)
　　　Thrombocytopathy
　　　EXCLUDES 1　*von Willebrand's disease (D68.0)*

　D69.2 **Other nonthrombocytopenic purpura**
　　　Purpura NOS　　　Senile purpura
　　　Purpura simplex

✓ Additional Character Required　　✓x7ᵗʰ Xtension Alert　　Unspecified Code　　Other Specified Code　　Manifestation Code　　▶◀ Revised Text　　● New Code　　▲ Revised Code Title

Diseases of the Blood and Blood-forming Organs

D69.3–D73.81

D69.3 Immune thrombocytopenic purpura
Hemorrhagic (thrombocytopenic) purpura
Idiopathic thrombocytopenic purpura
Tidal platelet dysgenesis

√5ᵗʰ **D69.4 Other primary thrombocytopenia**
EXCLUDES 1   *transient neonatal thrombocytopenia (P61.0)*
Wiskott-Aldrich syndrome (D82.0)

D69.41 Evans syndrome

D69.42 Congenital and hereditary thrombocytopenia purpura
Congenital thrombocytopenia
Hereditary thrombocytopenia
Code first congenital or hereditary disorder, such as:
thrombocytopenia with absent radius (TAR syndrome) (Q87.2)

D69.49 Other primary thrombocytopenia
Megakaryocytic hypoplasia
Primary thrombocytopenia NOS

√5ᵗʰ **D69.5 Secondary thrombocytopenia**
EXCLUDES 1   *heparin induced thrombocytopenia (HIT) (D75.82)*
transient thrombocytopenia of newborn (P61.0)

D69.51 Posttransfusion purpura
Posttransfusion purpura from whole blood (fresh) or blood products
PTP

D69.59 Other secondary thrombocytopenia

D69.6 Thrombocytopenia, unspecified

D69.8 Other specified hemorrhagic conditions
Capillary fragility (hereditary)   Vascular pseudohemophilia

D69.9 Hemorrhagic condition, unspecified

Other disorders of blood and blood-forming organs (D70-D77)

√4ᵗʰ **D70 Neutropenia**
INCLUDES   agranulocytosis
decreased absolute neurophile count (ANC)
Use additional code for any associated:
fever (R50.81)
mucositis (J34.81, K12.3-, K92.81, N76.81)
EXCLUDES 1   *neutropenic splenomegaly (D73.81)*
transient neonatal neutropenia (P61.5)

D70.0 Congenital agranulocytosis
Congenital neutropenia
Infantile genetic agranulocytosis
Kostmann's disease

D70.1 Agranulocytosis secondary to cancer chemotherapy
Use additional code for adverse effect, if applicable, to identify drug (T45.1X5)
Code also underlying neoplasm

D70.2 Other drug-induced agranulocytosis
Use additional code for adverse effect, if applicable, to identify drug (T36-T50 with fifth or sixth character 5)

D70.3 Neutropenia due to infection

D70.4 Cyclic neutropenia
Cyclic hematopoiesis
Periodic neutropenia

D70.8 Other neutropenia

D70.9 Neutropenia, unspecified

D71 Functional disorders of polymorphonuclear neutrophils
Cell membrane receptor complex [CR3] defect
Chronic (childhood) granulomatous disease
Congenital dysphagocytosis
Progressive septic granulomatosis

√4ᵗʰ **D72 Other disorders of white blood cells**
EXCLUDES 1   *basophilia (D72.824)*
immunity disorders (D80-D89)
neutropenia (D70)
preleukemia (syndrome) (D46.9)

D72.0 Genetic anomalies of leukocytes
Alder (granulation) (granulocyte) anomaly
Alder syndrome
Hereditary leukocytic hypersegmentation
Hereditary leukocytic hyposegmentation
Hereditary leukomelanopathy
May-Hegglin (granulation) (granulocyte) anomaly
May-Hegglin syndrome
Pelger-Huët (granulation) (granulocyte) anomaly
Pelger-Huët syndrome
EXCLUDES 1   *Chédiak (-Steinbrinck)-Higashi syndrome (E70.330)*

D72.1 Eosinophilia
Allergic eosinophilia
Hereditary eosinophilia
EXCLUDES 1   *Löffler's syndrome (J82)*
pulmonary eosinophilia (J82)

√5ᵗʰ **D72.8 Other specified disorders of white blood cells**
EXCLUDES 1   *leukemia (C91-C95)*

√6ᵗʰ **D72.81 Decreased white blood cell count**
EXCLUDES 1   *neutropenia (D70.-)*

D72.810 Lymphocytopenia
Decreased lymphocytes

D72.818 Other decreased white blood cell count
Basophilic leukopenia
Eosinophilic leukopenia
Monocytopenia
Other decreased leukocytes
Plasmacytopenia

D72.819 Decreased white blood cell count, unspecified
Decreased leukocytes, unspecified
Leukocytopenia, unspecified
Leukopenia
EXCLUDES 1   *malignant leukopenia (D70.9)*

√6ᵗʰ **D72.82 Elevated white blood cell count**
EXCLUDES 1   *eosinophilia (D72.1)*

D72.820 Lymphocytosis (symptomatic)
Elevated lymphocytes

D72.821 Monocytosis (symptomatic)
EXCLUDES 1   *infectious mononucleosis (B27.-)*

D72.822 Plasmacytosis

D72.823 Leukemoid reaction
Basophilic leukemoid reaction
Leukemoid reaction NOS
Lymphocytic leukemoid reaction
Monocytic leukemoid reaction
Myelocytic leukemoid reaction
Neutrophilic leukemoid reaction

D72.824 Basophilia

D72.825 Bandemia
Bandemia without diagnosis of specific infection
EXCLUDES 1   *confirmed infection—code to infection*
leukemia (C91.-, C92.-, C93.-, C94.-, C95.-)

D72.828 Other elevated white blood cell count

D72.829 Elevated white blood cell count, unspecified
Elevated leukocytes, unspecified
Leukocytosis, unspecified

D72.89 Other specified disorders of white blood cells
Abnormality of white blood cells NEC

D72.9 Disorder of white blood cells, unspecified
Abnormal leukocyte differential NOS

√4ᵗʰ **D73 Diseases of spleen**

D73.0 Hyposplenism
Atrophy of spleen
EXCLUDES 1   *asplenia (congenital) (Q89.01)*
postsurgical absence of spleen (Z90.81)

D73.1 Hypersplenism
EXCLUDES 1   *neutropenic splenomegaly (D73.81)*
primary splenic neutropenia (D73.81)
splenitis, splenomegaly in late syphilis (A52.79)
splenitis, splenomegaly in tuberculosis (A18.85)
splenomegaly NOS (R16.1)
splenomegaly congenital (Q89.0)

D73.2 Chronic congestive splenomegaly

D73.3 Abscess of spleen

D73.4 Cyst of spleen

D73.5 Infarction of spleen
Splenic rupture, nontraumatic
Torsion of spleen
EXCLUDES 1   *rupture of spleen due to Plasmodium vivax malaria (B51.0)*
traumatic rupture of spleen (S36.03-)

√5ᵗʰ **D73.8 Other diseases of spleen**

D73.81 Neutropenic splenomegaly
Werner-Schultz disease

EXCLUDES 1 Not coded here   EXCLUDES 2 Not included here   N Newborn Age: 0   P Pediatric Age: 0-17   M Maternity Age: 12-55   A Adult Age: 15-124

476   ICD-10-CM 2014 (Draft)

D73.89 Other diseases of spleen
Fibrosis of spleen NOS
Perisplenitis
Splenitis NOS

D73.9 Disease of spleen, unspecified

✓4ᵗʰ **D74 Methemoglobinemia**

D74.0 Congenital methemoglobinemia
Congenital NADH-methemoglobin reductase deficiency
Hemoglobin-M [Hb-M] disease
Methemoglobinemia, hereditary

D74.8 Other methemoglobinemias
Acquired methemoglobinemia (with sulfhemoglobinemia)
Toxic methemoglobinemia

D74.9 Methemoglobinemia, unspecified

✓4ᵗʰ **D75 Other and unspecified diseases of blood and blood-forming organs**
EXCLUDES 2   acute lymphadenitis (L04.-)
chronic lymphadenitis (I88.1)
enlarged lymph nodes (R59.-)
hypergammaglobulinemia NOS (D89.2)
lymphadenitis NOS (I88.9)
mesenteric lymphadenitis (acute) (chronic) (I88.0)

D75.0 Familial erythrocytosis
Benign polycythemia
Familial polycythemia
EXCLUDES 1   hereditary ovalocytosis (D58.1)

D75.1 Secondary polycythemia
Acquired polycythemia
Emotional polycythemia
Erythrocytosis NOS
Hypoxemic polycythemia
Nephrogenous polycythemia
Polycythemia due to erythropoietin
Polycythemia due to fall in plasma volume
Polycythemia due to high altitude
Polycythemia due to stress
Polycythemia NOS
Relative polycythemia
EXCLUDES 1   polycythemia neonatorum (P61.1)
polycythemia vera (D45)

✓5ᵗʰ **D75.8 Other specified diseases of blood and blood-forming organs**

D75.81 Myelofibrosis
Myelofibrosis NOS
Secondary myelofibrosis NOS
Code first the underlying disorder, such as:
malignant neoplasm of breast (C50.-)
Use additional code, if applicable, for associated
therapy-related myelodysplastic syndrome
(D46.-)
Use additional code for adverse effect, if applicable, to
identify drug (T45.1X5)
EXCLUDES 1   acute myelofibrosis (C94.4-)
idiopathic myelofibrosis (D47.1)
leukoerythroblastic anemia (D61.82)
myelofibrosis with myeloid metaplasia
(D47.4)
myelophthisic anemia (D61.82)
myelophthisis (D61.82)
primary myelofibrosis (D47.1)

D75.82 Heparin induced thrombocytopenia (HIT)

D75.89 Other specified diseases of blood and blood-forming organs

D75.9 Disease of blood and blood-forming organs, unspecified

✓4ᵗʰ **D76 Other specified diseases with participation of lymphoreticular and reticulohistiocytic tissue**
EXCLUDES 1   (Abt-) Letterer-Siwe disease (C96.0)
eosinophilic granuloma (C96.6)
Hand-Schüller-Christian disease (C96.5)
histiocytic sarcoma (C96.A)
histiocytosis X, multifocal (C96.5)
histiocytosis X, unifocal (C96.6)
malignant histiocytosis (C96.A)
Langerhans-cell histiocytosis, multifocal (C96.5)
Langerhans-cell histiocytosis NOS (C96.6)
Langerhans-cell histiocytosis, unifocal (C96.6)
leukemic reticuloendotheliosis or reticulosis (C91.4-)
lipomelanotic reticuloendotheliosis or reticulosis (I89.8)

D76.1 Hemophagocytic lymphohistiocytosis
Familial hemophagocytic reticulosis
Histiocytoses of mononuclear phagocytes

D76.2 Hemophagocytic syndrome, infection-associated
Use additional code to identify infectious agent or disease

D76.3 Other histiocytosis syndromes
Reticulohistiocytoma (giant-cell)
Sinus histiocytosis with massive lymphadenopathy
Xanthogranuloma

D77 Other disorders of blood and blood-forming organs in diseases classified elsewhere
Code first underlying disease, such as:
amyloidosis (E85.-)
congenital early syphilis (A50.-)
echinococcosis (B67.0-B67.9)
malaria (B50.0-B54)
schistosomiasis [bilharziasis] (B65.0-B65.9)
vitamin C deficiency (E54)
EXCLUDES 1   rupture of spleen due to Plasmodium vivax malaria (B51.0)
splenitis, splenomegaly in late syphilis (A52.79)
splenitis, splenomegaly in tuberculosis (A18.85)

Intraoperative and postprocedural complications of the spleen (D78)

✓4ᵗʰ **D78 Intraoperative and postprocedural complications of the spleen**

✓5ᵗʰ **D78.0 Intraoperative hemorrhage and hematoma of the spleen complicating a procedure**
EXCLUDES 1   intraoperative hemorrhage and hematoma of the
spleen due to accidental puncture or laceration
during a procedure (D78.1-)

D78.01 Intraoperative hemorrhage and hematoma of the spleen complicating a procedure on the spleen

D78.02 Intraoperative hemorrhage and hematoma of the spleen complicating other procedure

✓5ᵗʰ **D78.1 Accidental puncture and laceration of the spleen during a procedure**

D78.11 Accidental puncture and laceration of the spleen during a procedure on the spleen

D78.12 Accidental puncture and laceration of the spleen during other procedure

✓5ᵗʰ **D78.2 Postprocedural hemorrhage and hematoma of the spleen following a procedure**

D78.21 Postprocedural hemorrhage and hematoma of the spleen following a procedure on the spleen

D78.22 Postprocedural hemorrhage and hematoma of the spleen following other procedure

✓5ᵗʰ **D78.8 Other intraoperative and postprocedural complications of the spleen**
Use additional code, if applicable, to further specify disorder

D78.81 Other intraoperative complications of the spleen

D78.89 Other postprocedural complications of the spleen

Certain disorders involving the immune mechanism (D80-D89)
INCLUDES   defects in the complement system
immunodeficiency disorders, except human immunodeficiency virus
[HIV] disease
sarcoidosis
EXCLUDES 1   autoimmune disease (systemic) NOS (M35.9)
functional disorders of polymorphonuclear neutrophils (D71)
human immunodeficiency virus [HIV] disease (B20)

✓4ᵗʰ **D80 Immunodeficiency with predominantly antibody defects**

D80.0 Hereditary hypogammaglobulinemia
Autosomal recessive agammaglobulinemia (Swiss type)
X-linked agammaglobulinemia [Bruton] (with growth hormone
deficiency)

D80.1 Nonfamilial hypogammaglobulinemia
Agammaglobulinemia with immunoglobulin-bearing
B-lymphocytes
Common variable agammaglobulinemia [CVAgamma]
Hypogammaglobulinemia NOS

D80.2 Selective deficiency of immunoglobulin A [IgA]

D80.3 Selective deficiency of immunoglobulin G [IgG] subclasses

D80.4 Selective deficiency of immunoglobulin M [IgM]

D80.5 Immunodeficiency with increased immunoglobulin M [IgM]

D80.6 Antibody deficiency with near-normal immunoglobulins or with hyperimmunoglobulinemia

D80.7 Transient hypogammaglobulinemia of infancy   N

D80.8 Other immunodeficiencies with predominantly antibody defects
Kappa light chain deficiency

✓ Additional Character Required   ✓x7ᵗʰ Xtension Alert   Unspecified Code   Other Specified Code   Manifestation Code   ►◄ Revised Text   ● New Code   ▲ Revised Code Title

ICD-10-CM 2014 (Draft)   **477**

D80.9 Immunodeficiency with predominantly antibody defects, unspecified

✓4ᵗʰ **D81** **Combined immunodeficiencies**
> EXCLUDES 1 *autosomal recessive agammaglobulinemia (Swiss type) (D80.0)*

D81.0 Severe combined immunodeficiency [SCID] with reticular dysgenesis

D81.1 Severe combined immunodeficiency [SCID] with low T- and B-cell numbers

D81.2 Severe combined immunodeficiency [SCID] with low or normal B-cell numbers

D81.3 Adenosine deaminase [ADA] deficiency

D81.4 Nezelof's syndrome

D81.5 Purine nucleoside phosphorylase [PNP] deficiency

D81.6 Major histocompatibility complex class I deficiency
> Bare lymphocyte syndrome

D81.7 Major histocompatibility complex class II deficiency

✓5ᵗʰ **D81.8** Other combined immunodeficiencies

   ✓6ᵗʰ **D81.81** Biotin-dependent carboxylase deficiency
> Multiple carboxylase deficiency
> EXCLUDES 1 *biotin-dependent carboxylase deficiency due to dietary deficiency of biotin (E53.8)*

     D81.810 Biotinidase deficiency

     D81.818 Other biotin-dependent carboxylase deficiency
> Holocarboxylase synthetase deficiency
> Other multiple carboxylase deficiency

     D81.819 Biotin-dependent carboxylase deficiency, unspecified
> Multiple carboxylase deficiency, unspecified

   D81.89 Other combined immunodeficiencies

D81.9 Combined immunodeficiency, unspecified
> Severe combined immunodeficiency disorder [SCID] NOS

✓4ᵗʰ **D82** **Immunodeficiency associated with other major defects**
> EXCLUDES 1 *ataxia telangiectasia [Louis-Bar] (G11.3)*

D82.0 Wiskott-Aldrich syndrome
> Immunodeficiency with thrombocytopenia and eczema

D82.1 Di George's syndrome
> Pharyngeal pouch syndrome   Thymic aplasia or hypoplasia
> Thymic alymphoplasia   with immunodeficiency

D82.2 Immunodeficiency with short-limbed stature

D82.3 Immunodeficiency following hereditary defective response to Epstein-Barr virus
> X-linked lymphoproliferative disease

D82.4 Hyperimmunoglobulin E [IgE] syndrome

D82.8 Immunodeficiency associated with other specified major defects

D82.9 Immunodeficiency associated with major defect, unspecified

✓4ᵗʰ **D83** **Common variable immunodeficiency**

D83.0 Common variable immunodeficiency with predominant abnormalities of B-cell numbers and function

D83.1 Common variable immunodeficiency with predominant immunoregulatory T-cell disorders

D83.2 Common variable immunodeficiency with autoantibodies to B- or T-cells

D83.8 Other common variable immunodeficiencies

D83.9 Common variable immunodeficiency, unspecified

✓4ᵗʰ **D84** **Other immunodeficiencies**

D84.0 Lymphocyte function antigen-1 [LFA-1] defect

D84.1 Defects in the complement system
> C1 esterase inhibitor [C1-INH] deficiency

D84.8 Other specified immunodeficiencies

D84.9 Immunodeficiency, unspecified

✓4ᵗʰ **D86** **Sarcoidosis**

D86.0 Sarcoidosis of lung

D86.1 Sarcoidosis of lymph nodes

D86.2 Sarcoidosis of lung with sarcoidosis of lymph nodes

D86.3 Sarcoidosis of skin

✓5ᵗʰ **D86.8** Sarcoidosis of other sites

   D86.81 Sarcoid meningitis

   D86.82 Multiple cranial nerve palsies in sarcoidosis

   D86.83 Sarcoid iridocyclitis

   D86.84 Sarcoid pyelonephritis
> Tubulo-interstitial nephropathy in sarcoidosis

   D86.85 Sarcoid myocarditis

   D86.86 Sarcoid arthropathy
> Polyarthritis in sarcoidosis

   D86.87 Sarcoid myositis

   D86.89 Sarcoidosis of other sites
> Hepatic granuloma   Uveoparotid fever [Heerfordt]

D86.9 Sarcoidosis, unspecified

✓4ᵗʰ **D89** **Other disorders involving the immune mechanism, not elsewhere classified**
> EXCLUDES 1 *hyperglobulinemia NOS (R77.1)*
> *monoclonal gammopathy (of undetermined significance) (D47.2)*
> EXCLUDES 2 *transplant failure and rejection (T86.-)*

D89.0 Polyclonal hypergammaglobulinemia
> Benign hypergammaglobulinemic purpura
> Polyclonal gammopathy NOS

D89.1 Cryoglobulinemia
> Cryoglobulinemic purpura   Mixed cryoglobulinemia
> Cryoglobulinemic vasculitis   Primary cryoglobulinemia
> Essential cryoglobulinemia   Secondary cryoglobulinemia
> Idiopathic cryoglobulinemia

D89.2 Hypergammaglobulinemia, unspecified

D89.3 Immune reconstitution syndrome
> Immune reconstitution inflammatory syndrome [IRIS]
> Use additional code for adverse effect, if applicable, to identify drug (T36-T50 with fifth or sixth character 5)

✓5ᵗʰ **D89.8** Other specified disorders involving the immune mechanism, not elsewhere classified

   ✓6ᵗʰ **D89.81** Graft-versus-host disease
> Code first underlying cause, such as:
> complications of transplanted organs and tissue (T86.-)
> complications of blood transfusion (T80.89)
> Use additional code to identify associated manifestations, such as:
> desquamative dermatitis (L30.8)
> diarrhea (R19.7)
> elevated bilirubin (R17)
> hair loss (L65.9)

     D89.810 Acute graft-versus-host disease

     D89.811 Chronic graft-versus-host disease

     D89.812 Acute on chronic graft-versus-host disease

     D89.813 Graft-versus-host disease, unspecified

   D89.82 Autoimmune lymphoproliferative syndrome [ALPS]

   D89.89 Other specified disorders involving the immune mechanism, not elsewhere classified
> EXCLUDES 1 *human immunodeficiency virus disease (B20)*

D89.9 Disorder involving the immune mechanism, unspecified
> Immune disease NOS

EXCLUDES 1 Not coded here   EXCLUDES 2 Not included here   N Newborn Age: 0   P Pediatric Age: 0-17   M Maternity Age: 12-55   A Adult Age: 15-124

478   ICD-10-CM 2014 (Draft)

Chapter 4. Endocrine, Nutritional and Metabolic Diseases (E00-E89)

NOTE All neoplasms, whether functionally active or not, are classified in Chapter 2. Appropriate codes in this chapter (i.e. E05.8, E07.0, E16-E31, E34-) may be used as additional codes to indicate either functional activity by neoplasms and ectopic endocrine tissue or hyperfunction and hypofunction of endocrine glands associated with neoplasms and other conditions classified elsewhere.

EXCLUDES 1 *transitory endocrine and metabolic disorders specific to newborn (P70-P74)*

This chapter contains the following blocks:

E00-E07 Disorders of thyroid gland
E08-E13 Diabetes mellitus
E15-E16 Other disorders of glucose regulation and pancreatic internal secretion
E20-E35 Disorders of other endocrine glands
E36 Intraoperative complications of endocrine system
E40-E46 Malnutrition
E50-E64 Other nutritional deficiencies
E65-E68 Overweight, obesity and other hyperalimentation
E70-E88 Metabolic disorders
E89 Postprocedural endocrine and metabolic complications and disorders, not elsewhere classified

Disorders of thyroid gland (E00-E07)

☑4ᵗʰ E00 Congenital iodine-deficiency syndrome
Use additional code (F70-F79) to identify associated intellectual disabilities
EXCLUDES 1 *subclinical iodine-deficiency hypothyroidism (E02)*

E00.0 Congenital iodine-deficiency syndrome, neurological type
Endemic cretinism, neurological type

E00.1 Congenital iodine-deficiency syndrome, myxedematous type
Endemic hypothyroid cretinism
Endemic cretinism, myxedematous type

E00.2 Congenital iodine-deficiency syndrome, mixed type
Endemic cretinism, mixed type

E00.9 Congenital iodine-deficiency syndrome, unspecified
Congenital iodine-deficiency hypothyroidism NOS
Endemic cretinism NOS

☑4ᵗʰ E01 Iodine-deficiency related thyroid disorders and allied conditions
EXCLUDES 1 *congenital iodine-deficiency syndrome (E00.-)*
subclinical iodine-deficiency hypothyroidism (E02)

E01.0 Iodine-deficiency related diffuse (endemic) goiter

E01.1 Iodine-deficiency related multinodular (endemic) goiter
Iodine-deficiency related nodular goiter

E01.2 Iodine-deficiency related (endemic) goiter, unspecified
Endemic goiter NOS

E01.8 Other iodine-deficiency related thyroid disorders and allied conditions
Acquired iodine-deficiency hypothyroidism NOS

E02 Subclinical iodine-deficiency hypothyroidism

☑4ᵗʰ E03 Other hypothyroidism
EXCLUDES 1 *iodine-deficiency related hypothyroidism (E00-E02)*
postprocedural hypothyroidism (E89.0)

E03.0 Congenital hypothyroidism with diffuse goiter
Congenital parenchymatous goiter (nontoxic)
Congenital goiter (nontoxic) NOS
EXCLUDES 1 *transitory congenital goiter with normal function (P72.0)*

E03.1 Congenital hypothyroidism without goiter
Aplasia of thyroid (with myxedema)
Congenital atrophy of thyroid
Congenital hypothyroidism NOS

E03.2 Hypothyroidism due to medicaments and other exogenous substances
Code first poisoning due to drug or toxin, if applicable (T36-T65 with fifth or sixth character 1-4 or 6)
Use additional code for adverse effect, if applicable, to identify drug (T36-T50 with fifth or sixth character 5)

E03.3 Postinfectious hypothyroidism

E03.4 Atrophy of thyroid (acquired)
EXCLUDES 1 *congenital atrophy of thyroid (E03.1)*

E03.5 Myxedema coma

E03.8 Other specified hypothyroidism

E03.9 Hypothyroidism, unspecified
Myxedema NOS

☑4ᵗʰ E04 Other nontoxic goiter
EXCLUDES 1 *congenital goiter (NOS) (diffuse) (parenchymatous) (E03.0)*
iodine-deficiency related goiter (E00-E02)

E04.0 Nontoxic diffuse goiter
Diffuse (colloid) nontoxic goiter
Simple nontoxic goiter

E04.1 Nontoxic single thyroid nodule
Colloid nodule (cystic) (thyroid)
Nontoxic uninodular goiter
Thyroid (cystic) nodule NOS

E04.2 Non toxic multinodular goiter
Cystic goiter NOS
Multinodular (cystic) goiter NOS

E04.8 Other specified nontoxic goiter

E04.9 Nontoxic goiter, unspecified
Goiter NOS
Nodular goiter (nontoxic) NOS

☑4ᵗʰ E05 Thyrotoxicosis [hyperthyroidism]
EXCLUDES 1 *chronic thyroiditis with transient thyrotoxicosis (E06.2)*
neonatal thyrotoxicosis (P72.1)

☑5ᵗʰ E05.0 Thyrotoxicosis with diffuse goiter
Exophthalmic or toxic   Graves' disease
goiter NOS   Toxic diffuse goiter

E05.00 Thyrotoxicosis with diffuse goiter without thyrotoxic crisis or storm

E05.01 Thyrotoxicosis with diffuse goiter with thyrotoxic crisis or storm

☑5ᵗʰ E05.1 Thyrotoxicosis with toxic single thyroid nodule
Thyrotoxicosis with toxic uninodular goiter

E05.10 Thyrotoxicosis with toxic single thyroid nodule without thyrotoxic crisis or storm

E05.11 Thyrotoxicosis with toxic single thyroid nodule with thyrotoxic crisis or storm

☑5ᵗʰ E05.2 Thyrotoxicosis with toxic multinodular goiter
Toxic nodular goiter NOS

E05.20 Thyrotoxicosis with toxic multinodular goiter without thyrotoxic crisis or storm

E05.21 Thyrotoxicosis with toxic multinodular goiter with thyrotoxic crisis or storm

☑5ᵗʰ E05.3 Thyrotoxicosis from ectopic thyroid tissue

E05.30 Thyrotoxicosis from ectopic thyroid tissue without thyrotoxic crisis or storm

E05.31 Thyrotoxicosis from ectopic thyroid tissue with thyrotoxic crisis or storm

☑5ᵗʰ E05.4 Thyrotoxicosis factitia

E05.40 Thyrotoxicosis factitia without thyrotoxic crisis or storm

E05.41 Thyrotoxicosis factitia with thyrotoxic crisis or storm

☑5ᵗʰ E05.8 Other thyrotoxicosis
Overproduction of thyroid-stimulating hormone

E05.80 Other thyrotoxicosis without thyrotoxic crisis or storm

E05.81 Other thyrotoxicosis with thyrotoxic crisis or storm

☑5ᵗʰ E05.9 Thyrotoxicosis, unspecified
Hyperthyroidism NOS

E05.90 Thyrotoxicosis, unspecified without thyrotoxic crisis or storm

E05.91 Thyrotoxicosis, unspecified with thyrotoxic crisis or storm

☑4ᵗʰ E06 Thyroiditis
EXCLUDES 1 *postpartum thyroiditis (O90.5)*

E06.0 Acute thyroiditis
Abscess of thyroid   Suppurative thyroiditis
Pyogenic thyroiditis
Use additional code (B95-B97) to identify infectious agent

E06.1 Subacute thyroiditis
de Quervain thyroiditis   Nonsuppurative thyroiditis
Giant-cell thyroiditis   Viral thyroiditis
Granulomatous thyroiditis
EXCLUDES 1 *autoimmune thyroiditis (E06.3)*

E06.2 Chronic thyroiditis with transient thyrotoxicosis
EXCLUDES 1 *autoimmune thyroiditis (E06.3)*

E06.3 Autoimmune thyroiditis
Hashimoto's thyroiditis   Lymphocytic thyroiditis
Hashitoxicosis (transient)   Struma lymphomatosa
Lymphadenoid goiter

☑ Additional Character Required   ☑7ᵗʰ Xtension Alert   Unspecified Code   Other Specified Code   Manifestation Code   ►◄ Revised Text   ● New Code   ▲ Revised Code Title

E06.4   **Drug-induced thyroiditis**
Use additional code for adverse effect, if applicable, to identify drug (T36-T50 with fifth or sixth character 5)

E06.5   **Other chronic thyroiditis**
Chronic fibrous thyroiditis
Chronic thyroiditis NOS
Ligneous thyroiditis
Riedel thyroiditis

E06.9   **Thyroiditis, unspecified**

✓4th **E07**   **Other disorders of thyroid**

E07.0   **Hypersecretion of calcitonin**
C-cell hyperplasia of thyroid
Hypersecretion of thyrocalcitonin

E07.1   **Dyshormogenetic goiter**
Familial dyshormogenetic goiter
Pendred's syndrome
EXCLUDES 1   *transitory congenital goiter with normal function (P72.0)*

✓5th **E07.8**   **Other specified disorders of thyroid**

E07.81   **Sick-euthyroid syndrome**
Euthyroid sick-syndrome

E07.89   **Other specified disorders of thyroid**
Abnormality of thyroid-binding globulin
Hemorrhage of thyroid
Infarction of thyroid

E07.9   **Disorder of thyroid, unspecified**

Diabetes mellitus (E08-E13)

✓4th **E08**   **Diabetes mellitus due to underlying condition**
Code first the underlying condition, such as:
congenital rubella (P35.0)
cushing's syndrome (E24.-)
cystic fibrosis (E84.-)
malignant neoplasm (C00-C96)
malnutrition (E40-E46)
pancreatitis and other diseases of the pancreas (K85.-, K86.-)
Use additional code to identify any insulin use (Z79.4)
EXCLUDES 1   *drug or chemical induced diabetes mellitus (E09.-)*
gestational diabetes (O24.4-)
neonatal diabetes mellitus (P70.2)
postpancreatectomy diabetes mellitus (E13.-)
postprocedural diabetes mellitus (E13.-)
secondary diabetes mellitus NEC (E13.-)
type 1 diabetes mellitus (E10.-)
type 2 diabetes mellitus (E11.-)

✓5th **E08.0**   **Diabetes mellitus due to underlying condition with hyperosmolarity**

E08.00   **Diabetes mellitus due to underlying condition with hyperosmolarity without nonketotic hyperglycemic-hyperosmolar coma (NKHHC)**

E08.01   **Diabetes mellitus due to underlying condition with hyperosmolarity with coma**

✓5th **E08.1**   **Diabetes mellitus due to underlying condition with ketoacidosis**

E08.10   **Diabetes mellitus due to underlying condition with ketoacidosis without coma**

E08.11   **Diabetes mellitus due to underlying condition with ketoacidosis with coma**

✓5th **E08.2**   **Diabetes mellitus due to underlying condition with kidney complications**

E08.21   **Diabetes mellitus due to underlying condition with diabetic nephropathy**
Diabetes mellitus due to underlying condition with intercapillary glomerulosclerosis
Diabetes mellitus due to underlying condition with intracapillary glomerulonephrosis
Diabetes mellitus due to underlying condition with Kimmelstiel-Wilson disease

E08.22   **Diabetes mellitus due to underlying condition with diabetic chronic kidney disease**
Use additional code to identify stage of chronic kidney disease (N18.1-N18.6)

E08.29   **Diabetes mellitus due to underlying condition with other diabetic kidney complication**
Renal tubular degeneration in diabetes mellitus due to underlying condition

✓5th **E08.3**   **Diabetes mellitus due to underlying condition with ophthalmic complications**

✓6th **E08.31**   **Diabetes mellitus due to underlying condition with unspecified diabetic retinopathy**

E08.311   **Diabetes mellitus due to underlying condition with unspecified diabetic retinopathy with macular edema**

E08.319   **Diabetes mellitus due to underlying condition with unspecified diabetic retinopathy without macular edema**

✓6th **E08.32**   **Diabetes mellitus due to underlying condition with mild nonproliferative diabetic retinopathy**
Diabetes mellitus due to underlying condition with nonproliferative diabetic retinopathy NOS

E08.321   **Diabetes mellitus due to underlying condition with mild nonproliferative diabetic retinopathy with macular edema**

E08.329   **Diabetes mellitus due to underlying condition with mild nonproliferative diabetic retinopathy without macular edema**

✓6th **E08.33**   **Diabetes mellitus due to underlying condition with moderate nonproliferative diabetic retinopathy**

E08.331   **Diabetes mellitus due to underlying condition with moderate nonproliferative diabetic retinopathy with macular edema**

E08.339   **Diabetes mellitus due to underlying condition with moderate nonproliferative diabetic retinopathy without macular edema**

✓6th **E08.34**   **Diabetes mellitus due to underlying condition with severe nonproliferative diabetic retinopathy**

E08.341   **Diabetes mellitus due to underlying condition with severe nonproliferative diabetic retinopathy with macular edema**

E08.349   **Diabetes mellitus due to underlying condition with severe nonproliferative diabetic retinopathy without macular edema**

✓6th **E08.35**   **Diabetes mellitus due to underlying condition with proliferative diabetic retinopathy**

E08.351   **Diabetes mellitus due to underlying condition with proliferative diabetic retinopathy with macular edema**

E08.359   **Diabetes mellitus due to underlying condition with proliferative diabetic retinopathy without macular edema**

E08.36   **Diabetes mellitus due to underlying condition with diabetic cataract**

E08.39   **Diabetes mellitus due to underlying condition with other diabetic ophthalmic complication**
Use additional code to identify manifestation, such as: diabetic glaucoma (H40-H42)

✓5th **E08.4**   **Diabetes mellitus due to underlying condition with neurological complications**

E08.40   **Diabetes mellitus due to underlying condition with diabetic neuropathy, unspecified**

E08.41   **Diabetes mellitus due to underlying condition with diabetic mononeuropathy**

E08.42   **Diabetes mellitus due to underlying condition with diabetic polyneuropathy**
Diabetes mellitus due to underlying condition with diabetic neuralgia

E08.43   **Diabetes mellitus due to underlying condition with diabetic autonomic (poly)neuropathy**
Diabetes mellitus due to underlying condition with diabetic gastroparesis

E08.44   **Diabetes mellitus due to underlying condition with diabetic amyotrophy**

E08.49   **Diabetes mellitus due to underlying condition with other diabetic neurological complication**

✓5th **E08.5**   **Diabetes mellitus due to underlying condition with circulatory complications**

E08.51   **Diabetes mellitus due to underlying condition with diabetic peripheral angiopathy without gangrene**

E08.52   **Diabetes mellitus due to underlying condition with diabetic peripheral angiopathy with gangrene**
Diabetes mellitus due to underlying condition with diabetic gangrene

E08.59   **Diabetes mellitus due to underlying condition with other circulatory complications**

EXCLUDES 1 Not coded here   EXCLUDES 2 Not included here   N Newborn Age: 0   P Pediatric Age: 0-17   M Maternity Age: 12-55   A Adult Age: 15-124

480   ICD-10-CM 2014 (Draft)

✓5ᵗʰ **E08.6 Diabetes mellitus due to underlying condition with** other specified complications

  ✓6ᵗʰ **E08.61 Diabetes mellitus due to underlying condition with** diabetic arthropathy

    E08.610 Diabetes mellitus due to underlying condition with diabetic neuropathic arthropathy
      Diabetes mellitus due to underlying condition with Charcôt's joints

    E08.618 Diabetes mellitus due to underlying condition with other diabetic arthropathy

  ✓6ᵗʰ **E08.62 Diabetes mellitus due to underlying condition with** skin complications

    E08.620 Diabetes mellitus due to underlying condition with diabetic dermatitis
      Diabetes mellitus due to underlying condition with diabetic necrobiosis lipoidica

    E08.621 Diabetes mellitus due to underlying condition with foot ulcer
      Use additional code to identify site of ulcer (L97.4-, L97.5-)

    E08.622 Diabetes mellitus due to underlying condition with other skin ulcer
      Use additional code to identify site of ulcer (L97.1-L97.9, L98.41-L98.49)

    E08.628 Diabetes mellitus due to underlying condition with other skin complications

  ✓6ᵗʰ **E08.63 Diabetes mellitus due to underlying condition with** oral complications

    E08.630 Diabetes mellitus due to underlying condition with periodontal disease

    E08.638 Diabetes mellitus due to underlying condition with other oral complications

  ✓6ᵗʰ **E08.64 Diabetes mellitus due to underlying condition with** hypoglycemia

    E08.641 Diabetes mellitus due to underlying condition with hypoglycemia with coma

    E08.649 Diabetes mellitus due to underlying condition with hypoglycemia without coma

  E08.65 Diabetes mellitus due to underlying condition with hyperglycemia

  E08.69 Diabetes mellitus due to underlying condition with other specified complication
    Use additional code to identify complication

E08.8 Diabetes mellitus due to underlying condition with unspecified complications

E08.9 Diabetes mellitus due to underlying condition without complications

✓4ᵗʰ **E09 Drug or chemical induced diabetes mellitus**
  Code first poisoning due to drug or toxin, if applicable (T36-T65 with fifth or sixth character 1-4 or 6)
  Use additional code for adverse effect, if applicable, to identify drug (T36-T50 with fifth or sixth character 5)
  Use additional code to identify any insulin use (Z79.4)
  EXCLUDES 1 *diabetes mellitus due to underlying condition (E08.-)*
    gestational diabetes (O24.4-)
    neonatal diabetes mellitus (P70.2)
    postpancreatectomy diabetes mellitus (E13.-)
    postprocedural diabetes mellitus (E13.-)
    secondary diabetes mellitus NEC (E13.-)
    type 1 diabetes mellitus (E10.-)
    type 2 diabetes mellitus (E11.-)

  ✓5ᵗʰ **E09.0 Drug or chemical induced diabetes mellitus with** hyperosmolarity

    E09.00 Drug or chemical induced diabetes mellitus with hyperosmolarity without nonketotic hyperglycemic-hyperosmolar coma **(NKHHC)**

    E09.01 Drug or chemical induced diabetes mellitus with hyperosmolarity with coma

  ✓5ᵗʰ **E09.1 Drug or chemical induced diabetes mellitus with** ketoacidosis

    E09.10 Drug or chemical induced diabetes mellitus with ketoacidosis without coma

    E09.11 Drug or chemical induced diabetes mellitus with ketoacidosis with coma

✓5ᵗʰ **E09.2 Drug or chemical induced diabetes mellitus with** kidney complications

  E09.21 Drug or chemical induced diabetes mellitus with diabetic nephropathy
    Drug or chemical induced diabetes mellitus with intercapillary glomerulosclerosis
    Drug or chemical induced diabetes mellitus with intracapillary glomerulonephrosis
    Drug or chemical induced diabetes mellitus with Kimmelstiel-Wilson disease

  E09.22 Drug or chemical induced diabetes mellitus with diabetic chronic kidney disease
    Use additional code to identify stage of chronic kidney disease (N18.1-N18.6)

  E09.29 Drug or chemical induced diabetes mellitus with other diabetic kidney complication
    Drug or chemical induced diabetes mellitus with renal tubular degeneration

✓5ᵗʰ **E09.3 Drug or chemical induced diabetes mellitus with** ophthalmic complications

  ✓6ᵗʰ **E09.31 Drug or chemical induced diabetes mellitus with** unspecified diabetic retinopathy

    E09.311 Drug or chemical induced diabetes mellitus with unspecified diabetic retinopathy with macular edema

    E09.319 Drug or chemical induced diabetes mellitus with unspecified diabetic retinopathy without macular edema

  ✓6ᵗʰ **E09.32 Drug or chemical induced diabetes mellitus with** mild nonproliferative **diabetic retinopathy**
    Drug or chemical induced diabetes mellitus with nonproliferative diabetic retinopathy NOS

    E09.321 Drug or chemical induced diabetes mellitus with mild nonproliferative diabetic retinopathy with macular edema

    E09.329 Drug or chemical induced diabetes mellitus with mild nonproliferative diabetic retinopathy without macular edema

  ✓6ᵗʰ **E09.33 Drug or chemical induced diabetes mellitus with** moderate nonproliferative **diabetic retinopathy**

    E09.331 Drug or chemical induced diabetes mellitus with moderate nonproliferative diabetic retinopathy with macular edema

    E09.339 Drug or chemical induced diabetes mellitus with moderate nonproliferative diabetic retinopathy without macular edema

  ✓6ᵗʰ **E09.34 Drug or chemical induced diabetes mellitus with** severe nonproliferative **diabetic retinopathy**

    E09.341 Drug or chemical induced diabetes mellitus with severe nonproliferative diabetic retinopathy with macular edema

    E09.349 Drug or chemical induced diabetes mellitus with severe nonproliferative diabetic retinopathy without macular edema

  ✓6ᵗʰ **E09.35 Drug or chemical induced diabetes mellitus with** proliferative **diabetic retinopathy**

    E09.351 Drug or chemical induced diabetes mellitus with proliferative diabetic retinopathy with macular edema

    E09.359 Drug or chemical induced diabetes mellitus with proliferative diabetic retinopathy without macular edema

  E09.36 Drug or chemical induced diabetes mellitus with diabetic cataract

  E09.39 Drug or chemical induced diabetes mellitus with other diabetic ophthalmic complication
    Use additional code to identify manifestation, such as: diabetic glaucoma (H40-H42)

✓5ᵗʰ **E09.4 Drug or chemical induced diabetes mellitus with** neurological complications

  E09.40 Drug or chemical induced diabetes mellitus with neurological complications with diabetic neuropathy, unspecified

  E09.41 Drug or chemical induced diabetes mellitus with neurological complications with diabetic mononeuropathy

E09.42 Drug or chemical induced diabetes mellitus with neurological complications with diabetic polyneuropathy
Drug or chemical induced diabetes mellitus with diabetic neuralgia

E09.43 Drug or chemical induced diabetes mellitus with neurological complications with diabetic autonomic (poly)neuropathy
Drug or chemical induced diabetes mellitus with diabetic gastroparesis

E09.44 Drug or chemical induced diabetes mellitus with neurological complications with diabetic amyotrophy

E09.49 Drug or chemical induced diabetes mellitus with neurological complications with other diabetic neurological complication

√5ᵗʰ **E09.5 Drug or chemical induced diabetes mellitus with circulatory complications**

E09.51 Drug or chemical induced diabetes mellitus with diabetic peripheral angiopathy without gangrene

E09.52 Drug or chemical induced diabetes mellitus with diabetic peripheral angiopathy with gangrene
Drug or chemical induced diabetes mellitus with diabetic gangrene

E09.59 Drug or chemical induced diabetes mellitus with other circulatory complications

√5ᵗʰ **E09.6 Drug or chemical induced diabetes mellitus with other specified complications**

√6ᵗʰ **E09.61 Drug or chemical induced diabetes mellitus with diabetic arthropathy**

E09.610 Drug or chemical induced diabetes mellitus with diabetic neuropathic arthropathy
Drug or chemical induced diabetes mellitus with Charcôt's joints

E09.618 Drug or chemical induced diabetes mellitus with other diabetic arthropathy

√6ᵗʰ **E09.62 Drug or chemical induced diabetes mellitus with skin complications**

E09.620 Drug or chemical induced diabetes mellitus with diabetic dermatitis
Drug or chemical induced diabetes mellitus with diabetic necrobiosis lipoidica

E09.621 Drug or chemical induced diabetes mellitus with foot ulcer
Use additional code to identify site of ulcer (L97.4-, L97.5-)

E09.622 Drug or chemical induced diabetes mellitus with other skin ulcer
Use additional code to identify site of ulcer (L97.1-L97.9, L98.41-L98.49)

E09.628 Drug or chemical induced diabetes mellitus with other skin complications

√6ᵗʰ **E09.63 Drug or chemical induced diabetes mellitus with oral complications**

E09.630 Drug or chemical induced diabetes mellitus with periodontal disease

E09.638 Drug or chemical induced diabetes mellitus with other oral complications

√6ᵗʰ **E09.64 Drug or chemical induced diabetes mellitus with hypoglycemia**

E09.641 Drug or chemical induced diabetes mellitus with hypoglycemia with coma

E09.649 Drug or chemical induced diabetes mellitus with hypoglycemia without coma

E09.65 Drug or chemical induced diabetes mellitus with hyperglycemia

E09.69 Drug or chemical induced diabetes mellitus with other specified complication
Use additional code to identify complication

E09.8 Drug or chemical induced diabetes mellitus with unspecified complications

E09.9 Drug or chemical induced diabetes mellitus without complications

√4ᵗʰ **E10 Type 1 diabetes mellitus**
INCLUDES   brittle diabetes (mellitus)
diabetes (mellitus) due to autoimmune process
diabetes (mellitus) due to immune mediated pancreatic islet beta-cell destruction
idiopathic diabetes (mellitus)
juvenile onset diabetes (mellitus)
ketosis-prone diabetes (mellitus)

EXCLUDES 1   *diabetes mellitus due to underlying condition (E08.-)*
drug or chemical induced diabetes mellitus (E09.-)
gestational diabetes (O24.4-)
hyperglycemia NOS (R73.9)
neonatal diabetes mellitus (P70.2)
postpancreatectomy diabetes mellitus (E13.-)
postprocedural diabetes mellitus (E13.-)
secondary diabetes mellitus NEC (E13.-)
type 2 diabetes mellitus (E11.-)

√5ᵗʰ **E10.1 Type 1 diabetes mellitus with ketoacidosis**

E10.10 Type 1 diabetes mellitus with ketoacidosis without coma

E10.11 Type 1 diabetes mellitus with ketoacidosis with coma

√5ᵗʰ **E10.2 Type 1 diabetes mellitus with kidney complications**

E10.21 Type 1 diabetes mellitus with diabetic nephropathy
Type 1 diabetes mellitus with intercapillary glomerulosclerosis
Type 1 diabetes mellitus with intracapillary glomerulonephrosis
Type 1 diabetes mellitus with Kimmelstiel-Wilson disease

E10.22 Type 1 diabetes mellitus with diabetic chronic kidney disease
Use additional code to identify stage of chronic kidney disease (N18.1-N18.6)

E10.29 Type 1 diabetes mellitus with other diabetic kidney complication
Type 1 diabetes mellitus with renal tubular degeneration

√5ᵗʰ **E10.3 Type 1 diabetes mellitus with ophthalmic complications**

√6ᵗʰ **E10.31 Type 1 diabetes mellitus with unspecified diabetic retinopathy**

E10.311 Type 1 diabetes mellitus with unspecified diabetic retinopathy with macular edema

E10.319 Type 1 diabetes mellitus with unspecified diabetic retinopathy without macular edema

√6ᵗʰ **E10.32 Type 1 diabetes mellitus with mild nonproliferative diabetic retinopathy**
Type 1 diabetes mellitus with nonproliferative diabetic retinopathy NOS

E10.321 Type 1 diabetes mellitus with mild nonproliferative diabetic retinopathy with macular edema

E10.329 Type 1 diabetes mellitus with mild nonproliferative diabetic retinopathy without macular edema

√6ᵗʰ **E10.33 Type 1 diabetes mellitus with moderate nonproliferative diabetic retinopathy**

E10.331 Type 1 diabetes mellitus with moderate nonproliferative diabetic retinopathy with macular edema

E10.339 Type 1 diabetes mellitus with moderate nonproliferative diabetic retinopathy without macular edema

√6ᵗʰ **E10.34 Type 1 diabetes mellitus with severe nonproliferative diabetic retinopathy**

E10.341 Type 1 diabetes mellitus with severe nonproliferative diabetic retinopathy with macular edema

E10.349 Type 1 diabetes mellitus with severe nonproliferative diabetic retinopathy without macular edema

√6ᵗʰ **E10.35 Type 1 diabetes mellitus with proliferative diabetic retinopathy**

E10.351 Type 1 diabetes mellitus with proliferative diabetic retinopathy with macular edema

EXCLUDES 1 Not coded here   EXCLUDES 2 Not included here   N Newborn Age: 0   P Pediatric Age: 0-17   M Maternity Age: 12-55   A Adult Age: 15-124

482   ICD-10-CM 2014 (Draft)

E10.359 Type 1 diabetes mellitus with proliferative diabetic retinopathy without macular edema

E10.36 Type 1 diabetes mellitus with diabetic cataract

E10.39 Type 1 diabetes mellitus with other diabetic ophthalmic complication
Use additional code to identify manifestation, such as: diabetic glaucoma (H40-H42)

✓5th **E10.4** Type 1 diabetes mellitus with neurological complications

E10.40 Type 1 diabetes mellitus with diabetic neuropathy, unspecified

E10.41 Type 1 diabetes mellitus with diabetic mononeuropathy

E10.42 Type 1 diabetes mellitus with diabetic polyneuropathy
Type 1 diabetes mellitus with diabetic neuralgia

E10.43 Type 1 diabetes mellitus with diabetic autonomic (poly)neuropathy
Type 1 diabetes mellitus with diabetic gastroparesis

E10.44 Type 1 diabetes mellitus with diabetic amyotrophy

E10.49 Type 1 diabetes mellitus with other diabetic neurological complication

✓5th **E10.5** Type 1 diabetes mellitus with circulatory complications

E10.51 Type 1 diabetes mellitus with diabetic peripheral angiopathy without gangrene

E10.52 Type 1 diabetes mellitus with diabetic peripheral angiopathy with gangrene
Type 1 diabetes mellitus with diabetic gangrene

E10.59 Type 1 diabetes mellitus with other circulatory complications

✓5th **E10.6** Type 1 diabetes mellitus with other specified complications

✓6th **E10.61** Type 1 diabetes mellitus with diabetic arthropathy

E10.610 Type 1 diabetes mellitus with diabetic neuropathic arthropathy
Type 1 diabetes mellitus with Charcôt's joints

E10.618 Type 1 diabetes mellitus with other diabetic arthropathy

✓6th **E10.62** Type 1 diabetes mellitus with skin complications

E10.620 Type 1 diabetes mellitus with diabetic dermatitis
Type 1 diabetes mellitus with diabetic necrobiosis lipoidica

E10.621 Type 1 diabetes mellitus with foot ulcer
Use additional code to identify site of ulcer (L97.4-, L97.5-)

E10.622 Type 1 diabetes mellitus with other skin ulcer
Use additional code to identify site of ulcer (L97.1-L97.9, L98.41-L98.49)

E10.628 Type 1 diabetes mellitus with other skin complications

✓6th **E10.63** Type 1 diabetes mellitus with oral complications

E10.630 Type 1 diabetes mellitus with periodontal disease

E10.638 Type 1 diabetes mellitus with other oral complications

✓6th **E10.64** Type 1 diabetes mellitus with hypoglycemia

E10.641 Type 1 diabetes mellitus with hypoglycemia with coma

E10.649 Type 1 diabetes mellitus with hypoglycemia without coma

E10.65 Type 1 diabetes mellitus with hyperglycemia

E10.69 Type 1 diabetes mellitus with other specified complication
Use additional code to identify complication

E10.8 Type 1 diabetes mellitus with unspecified complications

E10.9 Type 1 diabetes mellitus without complications

✓4th **E11** Type 2 diabetes mellitus
INCLUDES diabetes (mellitus) due to insulin secretory defect
diabetes NOS
insulin resistant diabetes (mellitus)
Use additional code to identify any insulin use (Z79.4)
EXCLUDES 1 diabetes mellitus due to underlying condition (E08.-)
drug or chemical induced diabetes mellitus (E09.-)
gestational diabetes (O24.4-)
neonatal diabetes mellitus (P70.2)
postpancreatectomy diabetes mellitus (E13.-)
postprocedural diabetes mellitus (E13.-)
secondary diabetes mellitus NEC (E13.-)
type 1 diabetes mellitus (E10.-)

✓5th **E11.0** Type 2 diabetes mellitus with hyperosmolarity

E11.00 Type 2 diabetes mellitus with hyperosmolarity without nonketotic hyperglycemic-hyperosmolar coma (NKHHC)

E11.01 Type 2 diabetes mellitus with hyperosmolarity with coma

✓5th **E11.2** Type 2 diabetes mellitus with kidney complications

E11.21 Type 2 diabetes mellitus with diabetic nephropathy
Type 2 diabetes mellitus with intercapillary glomerulosclerosis
Type 2 diabetes mellitus with intracapillary glomerulonephrosis
Type 2 diabetes mellitus with Kimmelstiel-Wilson disease

E11.22 Type 2 diabetes mellitus with diabetic chronic kidney disease
Use additional code to identify stage of chronic kidney disease (N18.1-N18.6)

E11.29 Type 2 diabetes mellitus with other diabetic kidney complication
Type 2 diabetes mellitus with renal tubular degeneration

✓5th **E11.3** Type 2 diabetes mellitus with ophthalmic complications

✓6th **E11.31** Type 2 diabetes mellitus with unspecified diabetic retinopathy

E11.311 Type 2 diabetes mellitus with unspecified diabetic retinopathy with macular edema

E11.319 Type 2 diabetes mellitus with unspecified diabetic retinopathy without macular edema

✓6th **E11.32** Type 2 diabetes mellitus with mild nonproliferative diabetic retinopathy
Type 2 diabetes mellitus with nonproliferative diabetic retinopathy NOS

E11.321 Type 2 diabetes mellitus with mild nonproliferative diabetic retinopathy with macular edema

E11.329 Type 2 diabetes mellitus with mild nonproliferative diabetic retinopathy without macular edema

✓6th **E11.33** Type 2 diabetes mellitus with moderate nonproliferative diabetic retinopathy

E11.331 Type 2 diabetes mellitus with moderate nonproliferative diabetic retinopathy with macular edema

E11.339 Type 2 diabetes mellitus with moderate nonproliferative diabetic retinopathy without macular edema

✓6th **E11.34** Type 2 diabetes mellitus with severe nonproliferative diabetic retinopathy

E11.341 Type 2 diabetes mellitus with severe nonproliferative diabetic retinopathy with macular edema

E11.349 Type 2 diabetes mellitus with severe nonproliferative diabetic retinopathy without macular edema

✓6th **E11.35** Type 2 diabetes mellitus with proliferative diabetic retinopathy

E11.351 Type 2 diabetes mellitus with proliferative diabetic retinopathy with macular edema

E11.359 Type 2 diabetes mellitus with proliferative diabetic retinopathy without macular edema

E11.36 Type 2 diabetes mellitus with diabetic cataract

Endocrine, Nutritional and Metabolic Diseases

E11.39–E13.349

E11.39 **Type 2 diabetes mellitus with other diabetic ophthalmic complication**
> Use additional code to identify manifestation, such as: diabetic glaucoma (H40-H42)

✓5th **E11.4** **Type 2 diabetes mellitus with neurological complications**

    E11.40 **Type 2 diabetes mellitus with diabetic neuropathy, unspecified**

    E11.41 **Type 2 diabetes mellitus with diabetic mononeuropathy**

    E11.42 **Type 2 diabetes mellitus with diabetic polyneuropathy**
> Type 2 diabetes mellitus with diabetic neuralgia

    E11.43 **Type 2 diabetes mellitus with diabetic autonomic (poly)neuropathy**
> Type 2 diabetes mellitus with diabetic gastroparesis

    E11.44 **Type 2 diabetes mellitus with diabetic amyotrophy**

    E11.49 **Type 2 diabetes mellitus with other diabetic neurological complication**

✓5th **E11.5** **Type 2 diabetes mellitus with circulatory complications**

    E11.51 **Type 2 diabetes mellitus with diabetic peripheral angiopathy without gangrene**

    E11.52 **Type 2 diabetes mellitus with diabetic peripheral angiopathy with gangrene**
> Type 2 diabetes mellitus with diabetic gangrene

    E11.59 **Type 2 diabetes mellitus with other circulatory complications**

✓5th **E11.6** **Type 2 diabetes mellitus with other specified complications**

  ✓6th **E11.61** **Type 2 diabetes mellitus with diabetic arthropathy**

    E11.610 **Type 2 diabetes mellitus with diabetic neuropathic arthropathy**
> Type 2 diabetes mellitus with Charcôt's joints

    E11.618 **Type 2 diabetes mellitus with other diabetic arthropathy**

  ✓6th **E11.62** **Type 2 diabetes mellitus with skin complications**

    E11.620 **Type 2 diabetes mellitus with diabetic dermatitis**
> Type 2 diabetes mellitus with diabetic necrobiosis lipoidica

    E11.621 **Type 2 diabetes mellitus with foot ulcer**
> Use additional code to identify site of ulcer (L97.4-, L97.5-)

    E11.622 **Type 2 diabetes mellitus with other skin ulcer**
> Use additional code to identify site of ulcer (L97.1-L97.9, L98.41-L98.49)

    E11.628 **Type 2 diabetes mellitus with other skin complications**

  ✓6th **E11.63** **Type 2 diabetes mellitus with oral complications**

    E11.630 **Type 2 diabetes mellitus with periodontal disease**

    E11.638 **Type 2 diabetes mellitus with other oral complications**

  ✓6th **E11.64** **Type 2 diabetes mellitus with hypoglycemia**

    E11.641 **Type 2 diabetes mellitus with hypoglycemia with coma**

    E11.649 **Type 2 diabetes mellitus with hypoglycemia without coma**

    E11.65 **Type 2 diabetes mellitus with hyperglycemia**

    E11.69 **Type 2 diabetes mellitus with other specified complication**
> Use additional code to identify complication

E11.8 **Type 2 diabetes mellitus with unspecified complications**

E11.9 **Type 2 diabetes mellitus without complications**

✓4th **E13** **Other specified diabetes mellitus**
> Diabetes mellitus due to genetic defects of beta-cell function
> Diabetes mellitus due to genetic defects in insulin action
> Postpancreatectomy diabetes mellitus
> Postprocedural diabetes mellitus
> Secondary diabetes mellitus NEC
> Use additional code to identify any insulin use (Z79.4)

> *EXCLUDES 1*   *diabetes (mellitus) due to autoimmune process (E10.-)*
> *diabetes (mellitus) due to immune mediated pancreatic islet beta-cell destruction (E10.-)*
> *diabetes mellitus due to underlying condition (E08.-)*
> *drug or chemical induced diabetes mellitus (E09.-)*
> *gestational diabetes (O24.4-)*
> *neonatal diabetes mellitus (P70.2)*
> *type 2 diabetes mellitus (E11.-)*

✓5th **E13.0** **Other specified diabetes mellitus with hyperosmolarity**

    E13.00 **Other specified diabetes mellitus with hyperosmolarity without nonketotic hyperglycemic-hyperosmolar coma (NKHHC)**

    E13.01 **Other specified diabetes mellitus with hyperosmolarity with coma**

✓5th **E13.1** **Other specified diabetes mellitus with ketoacidosis**

    E13.10 **Other specified diabetes mellitus with ketoacidosis without coma**

    E13.11 **Other specified diabetes mellitus with ketoacidosis with coma**

✓5th **E13.2** **Other specified diabetes mellitus with kidney complications**

    E13.21 **Other specified diabetes mellitus with diabetic nephropathy**
> Other specified diabetes mellitus with intercapillary glomerulosclerosis
> Other specified diabetes mellitus with intracapillary glomerulonephrosis
> Other specified diabetes mellitus with Kimmelstiel-Wilson disease

    E13.22 **Other specified diabetes mellitus with diabetic chronic kidney disease**
> Use additional code to identify stage of chronic kidney disease (N18.1-N18.6)

    E13.29 **Other specified diabetes mellitus with other diabetic kidney complication**
> Other specified diabetes mellitus with renal tubular degeneration

✓5th **E13.3** **Other specified diabetes mellitus with ophthalmic complications**

  ✓6th **E13.31** **Other specified diabetes mellitus with unspecified diabetic retinopathy**

    E13.311 **Other specified diabetes mellitus with unspecified diabetic retinopathy with macular edema**

    E13.319 **Other specified diabetes mellitus with unspecified diabetic retinopathy without macular edema**

  ✓6th **E13.32** **Other specified diabetes mellitus with mild nonproliferative diabetic retinopathy**
> Other specified diabetes mellitus with nonproliferative diabetic retinopathy NOS

    E13.321 **Other specified diabetes mellitus with mild nonproliferative diabetic retinopathy with macular edema**

    E13.329 **Other specified diabetes mellitus with mild nonproliferative diabetic retinopathy without macular edema**

  ✓6th **E13.33** **Other specified diabetes mellitus with moderate nonproliferative diabetic retinopathy**

    E13.331 **Other specified diabetes mellitus with moderate nonproliferative diabetic retinopathy with macular edema**

    E13.339 **Other specified diabetes mellitus with moderate nonproliferative diabetic retinopathy without macular edema**

  ✓6th **E13.34** **Other specified diabetes mellitus with severe nonproliferative diabetic retinopathy**

    E13.341 **Other specified diabetes mellitus with severe nonproliferative diabetic retinopathy with macular edema**

    E13.349 **Other specified diabetes mellitus with severe nonproliferative diabetic retinopathy without macular edema**

EXCLUDES 1 Not coded here   *EXCLUDES 2* Not included here   N Newborn Age: 0   P Pediatric Age: 0-17   M Maternity Age: 12-55   A Adult Age: 15-124

484   ICD-10-CM 2014 (Draft)

✓6th **E13.35** **Other specified diabetes mellitus with proliferative diabetic retinopathy**

E13.351 **Other specified diabetes mellitus with proliferative diabetic retinopathy with macular edema**

E13.359 **Other specified diabetes mellitus with proliferative diabetic retinopathy without macular edema**

E13.36 **Other specified diabetes mellitus with diabetic cataract**

E13.39 **Other specified diabetes mellitus with other diabetic ophthalmic complication**

Use additional code to identify manifestation, such as: diabetic glaucoma (H40-H42)

✓5th **E13.4** **Other specified diabetes mellitus with neurological complications**

E13.40 **Other specified diabetes mellitus with diabetic neuropathy, unspecified**

E13.41 **Other specified diabetes mellitus with diabetic mononeuropathy**

E13.42 **Other specified diabetes mellitus with diabetic polyneuropathy**

Other specified diabetes mellitus with diabetic neuralgia

E13.43 **Other specified diabetes mellitus with diabetic autonomic (poly)neuropathy**

Other specified diabetes mellitus with diabetic gastroparesis

E13.44 **Other specified diabetes mellitus with diabetic amyotrophy**

E13.49 **Other specified diabetes mellitus with other diabetic neurological complication**

✓5th **E13.5** **Other specified diabetes mellitus with circulatory complications**

E13.51 **Other specified diabetes mellitus with diabetic peripheral angiopathy without gangrene**

E13.52 **Other specified diabetes mellitus with diabetic peripheral angiopathy with gangrene**

Other specified diabetes mellitus with diabetic gangrene

E13.59 **Other specified diabetes mellitus with other circulatory complications**

✓5th **E13.6** **Other specified diabetes mellitus with other specified complications**

✓6th **E13.61** **Other specified diabetes mellitus with diabetic arthropathy**

E13.610 **Other specified diabetes mellitus with diabetic neuropathic arthropathy**

Other specified diabetes mellitus with Charcôt's joints

E13.618 **Other specified diabetes mellitus with other diabetic arthropathy**

✓6th **E13.62** **Other specified diabetes mellitus with skin complications**

E13.620 **Other specified diabetes mellitus with diabetic dermatitis**

Other specified diabetes mellitus with diabetic necrobiosis lipoidica

E13.621 **Other specified diabetes mellitus with foot ulcer**

Use additional code to identify site of ulcer (L97.4-, L97.5-)

E13.622 **Other specified diabetes mellitus with other skin ulcer**

Use additional code to identify site of ulcer (L97.1-L97.9, L98.41-L98.49)

E13.628 **Other specified diabetes mellitus with other skin complications**

✓6th **E13.63** **Other specified diabetes mellitus with oral complications**

E13.630 **Other specified diabetes mellitus with periodontal disease**

E13.638 **Other specified diabetes mellitus with other oral complications**

✓6th **E13.64** **Other specified diabetes mellitus with hypoglycemia**

E13.641 **Other specified diabetes mellitus with hypoglycemia with coma**

E13.649 **Other specified diabetes mellitus with hypoglycemia without coma**

E13.65 **Other specified diabetes mellitus with hyperglycemia**

E13.69 **Other specified diabetes mellitus with other specified complication**

Use additional code to identify complication

E13.8 **Other specified diabetes mellitus with unspecified complications**

E13.9 **Other specified diabetes mellitus without complications**

Other disorders of glucose regulation and pancreatic internal secretion (E15-E16)

E15 **Nondiabetic hypoglycemic coma**

INCLUDES drug-induced insulin coma in nondiabetic
hyperinsulinism with hypoglycemic coma
hypoglycemic coma NOS

✓4th **E16** **Other disorders of pancreatic internal secretion**

E16.0 **Drug-induced hypoglycemia without coma**

Use additional code for adverse effect, if applicable, to identify drug (T36-T50 with fifth or sixth character 5)

E16.1 **Other hypoglycemia**

Functional hyperinsulinism
Functional nonhyperinsulinemic hypoglycemia
Hyperinsulinism NOS
Hyperplasia of pancreatic islet beta cells NOS

EXCLUDES 1 *hypoglycemia in infant of diabetic mother (P70.1)*
neonatal hypoglycemia (P70.4)

E16.2 **Hypoglycemia, unspecified**

E16.3 **Increased secretion of glucagon**

Hyperplasia of pancreatic endocrine cells with glucagon excess

E16.4 **Increased secretion of gastrin**

Hypergastrinemia
Hyperplasia of pancreatic endocrine cells with gastrin excess
Zollinger-Ellison syndrome

E16.8 **Other specified disorders of pancreatic internal secretion**

Increased secretion from endocrine pancreas of growth hormone-releasing hormone
Increased secretion from endocrine pancreas of pancreatic polypeptide
Increased secretion from endocrine pancreas of somatostatin
Increased secretion from endocrine pancreas of vasoactive-intestinal polypeptide

E16.9 **Disorder of pancreatic internal secretion, unspecified**

Islet-cell hyperplasia NOS
Pancreatic endocrine cell hyperplasia NOS

Disorders of other endocrine glands (E20-E35)

EXCLUDES 1 *galactorrhea (N64.3)*
gynecomastia (N62)

✓4th **E20** **Hypoparathyroidism**

EXCLUDES 1 *Di George's syndrome (D82.1)*
postprocedural hypoparathyroidism (E89.2)
tetany NOS (R29.0)
transitory neonatal hypoparathyroidism (P71.4)

E20.0 **Idiopathic hypoparathyroidism**

E20.1 **Pseudohypoparathyroidism**

E20.8 **Other hypoparathyroidism**

E20.9 **Hypoparathyroidism, unspecified**

Parathyroid tetany

✓4th **E21** **Hyperparathyroidism and other disorders of parathyroid gland**

EXCLUDES 1 *adult osteomalacia (M83.-)*
ectopic hyperparathyroidism (E34.2)
familial hypocalciuric hypercalcemia (E83.52)
hungry bone syndrome (E83.81)
infantile and juvenile osteomalacia (E55.0)

E21.0 **Primary hyperparathyroidism**

Hyperplasia of parathyroid
Osteitis fibrosa cystica generalisata [von Recklinghausen's disease of bone]

E21.1 **Secondary hyperparathyroidism, not elsewhere classified**

EXCLUDES 1 *secondary hyperparathyroidism of renal origin (N25.81)*

E21.2 **Other hyperparathyroidism**

Tertiary hyperparathyroidism

EXCLUDES 1 *familial hypocalciuric hypercalcemia (E83.52)*

E21.3 **Hyperparathyroidism, unspecified**

E21.4 **Other specified disorders of parathyroid gland**

E21.5 **Disorder of parathyroid gland, unspecified**

✓ Additional Character Required   ✓x7th Xtension Alert   Unspecified Code   Other Specified Code   Manifestation Code   ►◄ Revised Text   ● New Code   ▲ Revised Code Title

Endocrine, Nutritional and Metabolic Diseases

E22–E28.2

✓4ᵗʰ **E22 Hyperfunction of pituitary gland**

EXCLUDES 1 *Cushing's syndrome (E24.-)*
Nelson's syndrome (E24.1)
overproduction of ACTH not associated with Cushing's disease (E27.0)
overproduction of pituitary ACTH (E24.0)
overproduction of thyroid-stimulating hormone (E05.8-)

E22.0 Acromegaly and pituitary gigantism
Overproduction of growth hormone
EXCLUDES 1 *constitutional gigantism (E34.4)*
constitutional tall stature (E34.4)
increased secretion from endocrine pancreas of growth hormone-releasing hormone (E16.8)

E22.1 Hyperprolactinemia
Use additional code for adverse effect, if applicable, to identify drug (T36-T50 with fifth or sixth character 5)

E22.2 Syndrome of inappropriate secretion of antidiuretic hormone

E22.8 Other hyperfunction of pituitary gland
Central precocious puberty

E22.9 Hyperfunction of pituitary gland, unspecified

✓4ᵗʰ **E23 Hypofunction and other disorders of the pituitary gland**

INCLUDES the listed conditions whether the disorder is in the pituitary or the hypothalamus
EXCLUDES 1 *postprocedural hypopituitarism (E89.3)*

E23.0 Hypopituitarism
Fertile eunuch syndrome
Hypogonadotropic hypogonadism
Idiopathic growth hormone deficiency
Isolated deficiency of gonadotropin
Isolated deficiency of growth hormone
Isolated deficiency of pituitary hormone
Kallmann's syndrome
Lorain-Levi short stature
Necrosis of pituitary gland (postpartum)
Panhypopituitarism
Pituitary cachexia
Pituitary insufficiency NOS
Pituitary short stature
Sheehan's syndrome
Simmonds' disease

E23.1 Drug-induced hypopituitarism
Use additional code for adverse effect, if applicable, to identify drug (T36-T50 with fifth or sixth character 5)

E23.2 Diabetes insipidus
EXCLUDES 1 *nephrogenic diabetes insipidus (N25.1)*

E23.3 Hypothalamic dysfunction, not elsewhere classified
EXCLUDES 1 *Prader-Willi syndrome (Q87.1)*
Russell-Silver syndrome (Q87.1)

E23.6 Other disorders of pituitary gland
Abscess of pituitary
Adiposogenital dystrophy

E23.7 Disorder of pituitary gland, unspecified

✓4ᵗʰ **E24 Cushing's syndrome**
EXCLUDES 1 *congenital adrenal hyperplasia (E25.0)*

E24.0 Pituitary-dependent Cushing's disease
Overproduction of pituitary ACTH
Pituitary-dependent hypercorticolism

E24.1 Nelson's syndrome

E24.2 Drug-induced Cushing's syndrome
Use additional code for adverse effect, if applicable, to identify drug (T36-T50 with fifth or sixth character 5)

E24.3 Ectopic ACTH syndrome

E24.4 Alcohol-induced pseudo-Cushing's syndrome

E24.8 Other Cushing's syndrome

E24.9 Cushing's syndrome, unspecified

✓4ᵗʰ **E25 Adrenogenital disorders**
Adrenogenital syndromes, virilizing or feminizing, whether acquired or due to adrenal hyperplasia
Consequent on inborn enzyme defects in hormone synthesis
Female adrenal pseudohermaphroditism
Female heterosexual precocious pseudopuberty
Male isosexual precocious pseudopuberty
Male macrogenitosomia praecox
Male sexual precocity with adrenal hyperplasia
Male virilization (female)
EXCLUDES 1 *indeterminate sex and pseudohermaphroditism (Q56)*
chromosomal abnormalities (Q90-Q99)

E25.0 Congenital adrenogenital disorders associated with enzyme deficiency
Congenital adrenal hyperplasia
21-Hydroxylase deficiency
Salt-losing congenital adrenal hyperplasia

E25.8 Other adrenogenital disorders
Idiopathic adrenogenital disorder
Use additional code for adverse effect, if applicable, to identify drug (T36-T50 with fifth or sixth character 5)

E25.9 Adrenogenital disorder, unspecified
Adrenogenital syndrome NOS

✓4ᵗʰ **E26 Hyperaldosteronism**

✓5ᵗʰ **E26.0 Primary hyperaldosteronism**

E26.01 Conn's syndrome
Code also adrenal adenoma (D35.0-)

E26.02 Glucocorticoid-remediable aldosteronism
Familial aldosteronism type I

E26.09 Other primary hyperaldosteronism
Primary aldosteronism due to adrenal hyperplasia (bilateral)

E26.1 Secondary hyperaldosteronism

✓5ᵗʰ **E26.8 Other hyperaldosteronism**

E26.81 Bartter's syndrome

E26.89 Other hyperaldosteronism

E26.9 Hyperaldosteronism, unspecified
Aldosteronism NOS
Hyperaldosteronism NOS

✓4ᵗʰ **E27 Other disorders of adrenal gland**

E27.0 Other adrenocortical overactivity
Overproduction of ACTH, not associated with Cushing's disease
Premature adrenarche
EXCLUDES 1 *Cushing's syndrome (E24.-)*

E27.1 Primary adrenocortical insufficiency
Addison's disease
Autoimmune adrenalitis
EXCLUDES 1 *Addison only phenotype adrenoleukodystrophy (E71.528)*
amyloidosis (E85.-)
tuberculous Addison's disease (A18.7)
Waterhouse-Friderichsen syndrome (A39.1)

E27.2 Addisonian crisis
Adrenal crisis
Adrenocortical crisis

E27.3 Drug-induced adrenocortical insufficiency
Use additional code for adverse effect, if applicable, to identify drug (T36-T50 with fifth or sixth character 5)

✓5ᵗʰ **E27.4 Other and unspecified adrenocortical insufficiency**
EXCLUDES 1 *adrenoleukodystrophy [Addison-Schilder] (E71.528)*
Waterhouse-Friderichsen syndrome (A39.1)

E27.40 Unspecified adrenocortical insufficiency
Adrenocortical insufficiency NOS
Hypoaldosteronism

E27.49 Other adrenocortical insufficiency
Adrenal hemorrhage
Adrenal infarction

E27.5 Adrenomedullary hyperfunction
Adrenomedullary hyperplasia
Catecholamine hypersecretion

E27.8 Other specified disorders of adrenal gland
Abnormality of cortisol-binding globulin

E27.9 Disorder of adrenal gland, unspecified

✓4ᵗʰ **E28 Ovarian dysfunction**
EXCLUDES 1 *isolated gonadotropin deficiency (E23.0)*
postprocedural ovarian failure (E89.4-)

E28.0 Estrogen excess ♀
Use additional code for adverse effect, if applicable, to identify drug (T36-T50 with fifth or sixth character 5)

E28.1 Androgen excess
Hypersecretion of ovarian androgens
Use additional code for adverse effect, if applicable, to identify drug (T36-T50 with fifth or sixth character 5)

E28.2 Polycystic ovarian syndrome ♀
Sclerocystic ovary syndrome
Stein-Leventhal syndrome

EXCLUDES 1 Not coded here   **EXCLUDES 2** Not included here   **N** Newborn Age: 0   **P** Pediatric Age: 0-17   **M** Maternity Age: 12-55   **A** Adult Age: 15-124

486   ICD-10-CM 2014 (Draft)

✓5ᵗʰ **E28.3 Primary ovarian failure** ♀
> *EXCLUDES 1* *pure gonadal dysgenesis (Q99.1)*
> *Turner's syndrome (Q96.-)*

✓6ᵗʰ **E28.31 Premature menopause**
  E28.310 Symptomatic premature menopause Ⓐ♀
  > Symptoms such as flushing, sleeplessness, headache, lack of concentration, associated with premature menopause

  E28.319 Asymptomatic premature menopause Ⓐ♀
  > Premature menopause NOS

E28.39 Other primary ovarian failure ♀
> Decreased estrogen
> Resistant ovary syndrome

E28.8 Other ovarian dysfunction ♀
> Ovarian hyperfunction NOS
> *EXCLUDES 1* *postprocedural ovarian failure (E89.4-)*

E28.9 Ovarian dysfunction, unspecified ♀

✓4ᵗʰ **E29 Testicular dysfunction**
> *EXCLUDES 1* *androgen insensitivity syndrome (E34.5-)*
> *azoospermia or oligospermia NOS (N46.0-N46.1)*
> *isolated gonadotropin deficiency (E23.0)*
> *Klinefelter's syndrome (Q98.0-Q98.2, Q98.4)*

E29.0 Testicular hyperfunction ♂
> Hypersecretion of testicular hormones

E29.1 Testicular hypofunction ♂
> Defective biosynthesis of testicular androgen NOS
> 5-delta-Reductase deficiency (with male pseudohermaphroditism)
> Testicular hypogonadism NOS
> Use additional code for adverse effect, if applicable, to identify drug (T36-T50 with fifth or sixth character 5)
> *EXCLUDES 1* *postprocedural testicular hypofunction (E89.5)*

E29.8 Other testicular dysfunction ♂

E29.9 Testicular dysfunction, unspecified ♂

✓4ᵗʰ **E30 Disorders of puberty, not elsewhere classified**

E30.0 Delayed puberty
> Constitutional delay of puberty
> Delayed sexual development

E30.1 Precocious puberty ℙ
> Precocious menstruation
> *EXCLUDES 1* *Albright (-McCune) (-Sternberg) syndrome (Q78.1)*
> *central precocious puberty (E22.8)*
> *congenital adrenal hyperplasia (E25.0)*
> *female heterosexual precocious pseudopuberty (E25.-)*
> *male isosexual precocious pseudopuberty (E25.-)*

E30.8 Other disorders of puberty ℙ
> Premature thelarche

E30.9 Disorder of puberty, unspecified

✓4ᵗʰ **E31 Polyglandular dysfunction**
> *EXCLUDES 1* *ataxia telangiectasia [Louis-Bar] (G11.3)*
> *dystrophia myotonica [Steinert] (G71.11)*
> *pseudohypoparathyroidism (E20.1)*

E31.0 Autoimmune polyglandular failure
> Schmidt's syndrome

E31.1 Polyglandular hyperfunction
> *EXCLUDES 1* *multiple endocrine adenomatosis (E31.2-)*
> *multiple endocrine neoplasia (E31.2-)*

✓5ᵗʰ **E31.2 Multiple endocrine neoplasia [MEN] syndromes**
> Multiple endocrine adenomatosis
> Code also any associated malignancies and other conditions associated with the syndromes

  E31.20 Multiple endocrine neoplasia [MEN] syndrome, unspecified
  > Multiple endocrine adenomatosis NOS
  > Multiple endocrine neoplasia [MEN] syndrome NOS

  E31.21 Multiple endocrine neoplasia [MEN] type I
  > Wermer's syndrome

  E31.22 Multiple endocrine neoplasia [MEN] type IIA
  > Sipple's syndrome

  E31.23 Multiple endocrine neoplasia [MEN] type IIB

E31.8 Other polyglandular dysfunction

E31.9 Polyglandular dysfunction, unspecified

✓4ᵗʰ **E32 Diseases of thymus**
> *EXCLUDES 1* *aplasia or hypoplasia of thymus with immunodeficiency (D82.1)*
> *myasthenia gravis (G70.0)*

E32.0 Persistent hyperplasia of thymus
> Hypertrophy of thymus

E32.1 Abscess of thymus

E32.8 Other diseases of thymus
> *EXCLUDES 1* *aplasia or hypoplasia with immunodeficiency (D82.1)*
> *thymoma (D15.0)*

E32.9 Disease of thymus, unspecified

✓4ᵗʰ **E34 Other endocrine disorders**
> *EXCLUDES 1* *pseudohypoparathyroidism (E20.1)*

E34.0 Carcinoid syndrome
> **NOTE** May be used as an additional code to identify functional activity associated with a carcinoid tumor.

E34.1 Other hypersecretion of intestinal hormones

E34.2 Ectopic hormone secretion, not elsewhere classified
> *EXCLUDES 1* *ectopic ACTH syndrome (E24.3)*

E34.3 Short stature due to endocrine disorder
> Constitutional short stature
> Laron-type short stature
> *EXCLUDES 1* *achondroplastic short stature (Q77.4)*
> *hypochondroplastic short stature (Q77.4)*
> *nutritional short stature (E45)*
> *pituitary short stature (E23.0)*
> *progeria (E34.8)*
> *renal short stature (N25.0)*
> *Russell-Silver syndrome (Q87.1)*
> *short-limbed stature with immunodeficiency (D82.2)*
> *short stature in specific dysmorphic syndromes— code to syndrome—see Alphabetical Index*
> *short stature NOS (R62.52)*

E34.4 Constitutional tall stature
> Constitutional gigantism

✓5ᵗʰ **E34.5 Androgen insensitivity syndrome**
  E34.50 Androgen insensitivity syndrome, unspecified
  > Androgen insensitivity NOS

  E34.51 Complete androgen insensitivity syndrome
  > Complete androgen insensitivity
  > de Quervain syndrome
  > Goldberg-Maxwell syndrome

  E34.52 Partial androgen insensitivity syndrome
  > Partial androgen insensitivity
  > Reifenstein syndrome

E34.8 Other specified endocrine disorders
> Pineal gland dysfunction
> Progeria
> *EXCLUDES 2* *pseudohypoparathyroidism (E20.1)*

E34.9 Endocrine disorder, unspecified
> Endocrine disturbance NOS
> Hormone disturbance NOS

E35 Disorders of endocrine glands in diseases classified elsewhere
> *Code first underlying disease, such as:*
> *late congenital syphilis of thymus gland [Dubois disease] (A50.5)*
> Use additional code, if applicable, to identify:
> sequelae of tuberculosis of other organs (B90.8)
> *EXCLUDES 1* *Echinococcus granulosus infection of thyroid gland (B67.3)*
> *meningococcal hemorrhagic adrenalitis (A39.1)*
> *syphilis of endocrine gland (A52.79)*
> *tuberculosis of adrenal gland, except calcification (A18.7)*
> *tuberculosis of endocrine gland NEC (A18.82)*
> *tuberculosis of thyroid gland (A18.81)*
> *Waterhouse-Friderichsen syndrome (A39.1)*

✓4ᵗʰ **E36 Intraoperative complications of endocrine system**
> *EXCLUDES 2* *postprocedural endocrine and metabolic complications and disorders, not elsewhere classified (E89.-)*

✓5ᵗʰ **E36.0 Intraoperative hemorrhage and hematoma of an endocrine system organ or structure complicating a procedure**
> *EXCLUDES 1* *intraoperative hemorrhage and hematoma of an endocrine system organ or structure due to accidental puncture or laceration during a procedure (E36.1-)*

  E36.01 Intraoperative hemorrhage and hematoma of an endocrine system organ or structure complicating an endocrine system procedure

  E36.02 Intraoperative hemorrhage and hematoma of an endocrine system organ or structure complicating other procedure

---

✓ Additional Character Required   ✓x7ᵗʰ Xtension Alert   Unspecified Code   Other Specified Code   Manifestation Code   ►◄ Revised Text   ● New Code   ▲ Revised Code Title

ICD-10-CM 2014 (Draft)   487

Endocrine, Nutritional and Metabolic Diseases

E28.3–E36.02

Endocrine, Nutritional and Metabolic Diseases

E36.1–E61.9

√5ᵗʰ **E36.1**   **Accidental puncture and laceration** of an endocrine system organ or structure during a procedure

     E36.11   Accidental puncture and laceration of an endocrine system organ or structure during an **endocrine system procedure**

     E36.12   Accidental puncture and laceration of an endocrine system organ or structure during **other procedure**

E36.8   **Other intraoperative complications of endocrine system**
     Use additional code, if applicable, to further specify disorder

Malnutrition (E40-E46)

EXCLUDES 1   intestinal malabsorption (K90.-)
     sequelae of protein-calorie malnutrition (E64.0)
EXCLUDES 2   nutritional anemias (D50-D53)
     starvation (T73.0)

E40   **Kwashiorkor**
     Severe malnutrition with nutritional edema with dyspigmentation of skin and hair
     EXCLUDES 1   marasmic kwashiorkor (E42)

E41   **Nutritional marasmus**
     Severe malnutrition with marasmus
     EXCLUDES 1   marasmic kwashiorkor (E42)

E42   **Marasmic kwashiorkor**
     Intermediate form severe protein-calorie malnutrition
     Severe protein-calorie malnutrition with signs of both kwashiorkor and marasmus

E43   **Unspecified severe protein-calorie malnutrition**
     Starvation edema

√4ᵗʰ **E44**   **Protein-calorie malnutrition of moderate and mild degree**
     E44.0   **Moderate** protein-calorie malnutrition
     E44.1   **Mild** protein-calorie malnutrition

E45   **Retarded development following protein-calorie malnutrition**
     Nutritional short stature
     Nutritional stunting
     Physical retardation due to malnutrition

E46   **Unspecified protein-calorie malnutrition**
     Malnutrition NOS
     Protein-calorie imbalance NOS
     EXCLUDES 1   nutritional deficiency NOS (E63.9)

Other nutritional deficiencies (E50-E64)

EXCLUDES 2   nutritional anemias (D50-D53)

√4ᵗʰ **E50**   **Vitamin A deficiency**
     EXCLUDES 1   sequelae of vitamin A deficiency (E64.1)

     E50.0   **Vitamin A deficiency with conjunctival xerosis**
     E50.1   **Vitamin A deficiency with Bitot's spot and conjunctival xerosis**
         Bitot's spot in the young child
     E50.2   **Vitamin A deficiency with corneal xerosis**
     E50.3   **Vitamin A deficiency with corneal ulceration and xerosis**
     E50.4   **Vitamin A deficiency with keratomalacia**
     E50.5   **Vitamin A deficiency with night blindness**
     E50.6   **Vitamin A deficiency with xerophthalmic scars of cornea**
     E50.7   **Other ocular manifestations of vitamin A deficiency**
         Xerophthalmia NOS
     E50.8   **Other manifestations of vitamin A deficiency**
         Follicular keratosis
         Xeroderma
     E50.9   **Vitamin A deficiency, unspecified**
         Hypovitaminosis A NOS

√4ᵗʰ **E51**   **Thiamine deficiency**
     EXCLUDES 1   sequelae of thiamine deficiency (E64.8)

     √5ᵗʰ **E51.1**   **Beriberi**
         E51.11   **Dry beriberi**
             Beriberi NOS
             Beriberi with polyneuropathy
         E51.12   **Wet beriberi**
             Beriberi with cardiovascular manifestations
             Cardiovascular beriberi
             Shoshin disease

     E51.2   **Wernicke's encephalopathy**
     E51.8   **Other manifestations of thiamine deficiency**
     E51.9   **Thiamine deficiency, unspecified**

E52   **Niacin deficiency [pellagra]**
     Niacin (-tryptophan) deficiency
     Nicotinamide deficiency
     Pellagra (alcoholic)
     EXCLUDES 1   sequelae of niacin deficiency (E64.8)

√4ᵗʰ **E53**   **Deficiency of other B group vitamins**
     EXCLUDES 1   sequelae of vitamin B deficiency (E64.8)

     E53.0   **Riboflavin deficiency**
         Ariboflavinosis
         Vitamin B2 deficiency
     E53.1   **Pyridoxine deficiency**
         Vitamin B6 deficiency
         EXCLUDES 1   pyridoxine-responsive sideroblastic anemia (D64.3)
     E53.8   **Deficiency of other specified B group vitamins**
         Biotin deficiency   Folic acid deficiency
         Cyanocobalamin deficiency   Pantothenic acid deficiency
         Folate deficiency   Vitamin B12 deficiency
         EXCLUDES 1   folate deficiency anemia (D52.-)
             vitamin B12 deficiency anemia (D51.-)
     E53.9   **Vitamin B deficiency, unspecified**

E54   **Ascorbic acid deficiency**
     Deficiency of vitamin C
     Scurvy
     EXCLUDES 1   scorbutic anemia (D53.2)
         sequelae of vitamin C deficiency (E64.2)

√4ᵗʰ **E55**   **Vitamin D deficiency**
     EXCLUDES 1   adult osteomalacia (M83.-)
         osteoporosis (M80.-)
         sequelae of rickets (E64.3)

     E55.0   **Rickets, active**
         Infantile osteomalacia
         Juvenile osteomalacia
         EXCLUDES 1   celiac rickets (K90.0)
             Crohn's rickets (K50.-)
             hereditary vitamin D-dependent rickets (E83.32)
             inactive rickets (E64.3)
             renal rickets (N25.0)
             sequelae of rickets (E64.3)
             vitamin D-resistant rickets (E83.31)
     E55.9   **Vitamin D deficiency, unspecified**
         Avitaminosis D

√4ᵗʰ **E56**   **Other vitamin deficiencies**
     EXCLUDES 1   sequelae of other vitamin deficiencies (E64.8)

     E56.0   **Deficiency of vitamin E**
     E56.1   **Deficiency of vitamin K**
         EXCLUDES 1   deficiency of coagulation factor due to vitamin K deficiency (D68.4)
             vitamin K deficiency of newborn (P53)
     E56.8   **Deficiency of other vitamins**
     E56.9   **Vitamin deficiency, unspecified**

E58   **Dietary calcium deficiency**
     EXCLUDES 1   disorders of calcium metabolism (E83.5-)
         sequelae of calcium deficiency (E64.8)

E59   **Dietary selenium deficiency**
     Keshan disease
     EXCLUDES 1   sequelae of selenium deficiency (E64.8)

E60   **Dietary zinc deficiency**

√4ᵗʰ **E61**   **Deficiency of other nutrient elements**
     Use additional code for adverse effect, if applicable, to identify drug (T36-T50 with fifth or sixth character 5)
     EXCLUDES 1   disorders of mineral metabolism (E83.-)
         iodine deficiency related thyroid disorders (E00-E02)
         sequelae of malnutrition and other nutritional deficiencies (E64.-)

     E61.0   **Copper deficiency**
     E61.1   **Iron deficiency**
         EXCLUDES 1   iron deficiency anemia (D50.-)
     E61.2   **Magnesium deficiency**
     E61.3   **Manganese deficiency**
     E61.4   **Chromium deficiency**
     E61.5   **Molybdenum deficiency**
     E61.6   **Vanadium deficiency**
     E61.7   **Deficiency of multiple nutrient elements**
     E61.8   **Deficiency of other specified nutrient elements**
     E61.9   **Deficiency of nutrient element, unspecified**

EXCLUDES 1 Not coded here   *EXCLUDES 2* Not included here   N Newborn Age: 0   P Pediatric Age: 0-17   M Maternity Age: 12-55   A Adult Age: 15-124

488   ICD-10-CM 2014 (Draft)

☑4ᵗʰ **E63 Other nutritional deficiencies**
> EXCLUDES1   dehydration (E86.0)
> failure to thrive, adult (R62.7)
> failure to thrive, child (R62.51)
> feeding problems in newborn (P92.-)
> sequelae of malnutrition and other nutritional deficiencies (E64.-)

E63.0 Essential fatty acid [EFA] deficiency

E63.1 Imbalance of constituents of food intake

E63.8 Other specified nutritional deficiencies

E63.9 Nutritional deficiency, unspecified

☑4ᵗʰ **E64 Sequelae of malnutrition and other nutritional deficiencies**
> NOTE   This category is to be used to indicate conditions in categories E43, E44, E46, E50-E63 as the cause of sequelae, which are themselves classified elsewhere. The 'sequelae' include conditions specified as such; they also include the late effects of diseases classifiable to the above categories if the disease itself is no longer present.
>
> Code first condition resulting from (sequela) of malnutrition and other nutritional deficiencies

E64.0 Sequelae of protein-calorie malnutrition
> EXCLUDES2   retarded development following protein-calorie malnutrition (E45)

E64.1 Sequelae of vitamin A deficiency

E64.2 Sequelae of vitamin C deficiency

E64.3 Sequelae of rickets

E64.8 Sequelae of other nutritional deficiencies

E64.9 Sequelae of unspecified nutritional deficiency

Overweight, obesity and other hyperalimentation (E65-E68)

E65 Localized adiposity
> Fat pad

☑4ᵗʰ **E66 Overweight and obesity**
> Code first obesity complicating pregnancy, childbirth and the puerperium, if applicable (O99.21-)
> Use additional code to identify body mass index (BMI), if known (Z68.-)
> EXCLUDES1   adiposogenital dystrophy (E23.6)
> lipomatosis NOS (E88.2)
> lipomatosis dolorosa [Dercum] (E88.2)
> Prader-Willi syndrome (Q87.1)

☑5ᵗʰ **E66.0 Obesity due to excess calories**

E66.01 Morbid (severe) obesity due to excess calories
> EXCLUDES1   morbid (severe) obesity with alveolar hypoventilation (E66.2)

E66.09 Other obesity due to excess calories

E66.1 Drug-induced obesity
> Use additional code for adverse effect, if applicable, to identify drug (T36-T50 with fifth or sixth character 5)

E66.2 Morbid (severe) obesity with alveolar hypoventilation
> Pickwickian syndrome

E66.3 Overweight

E66.8 Other obesity

E66.9 Obesity, unspecified
> Obesity NOS

☑4ᵗʰ **E67 Other hyperalimentation**
> EXCLUDES1   hyperalimentation NOS (R63.2)
> sequelae of hyperalimentation (E68)

E67.0 Hypervitaminosis A

E67.1 Hypercarotinemia

E67.2 Megavitamin-B6 syndrome

E67.3 Hypervitaminosis D

E67.8 Other specified hyperalimentation

E68 Sequelae of hyperalimentation
> Code first condition resulting from (sequela) of hyperalimentation

Metabolic disorders (E70-E88)

> EXCLUDES1   androgen insensitivity syndrome (E34.5-)
> congenital adrenal hyperplasia (E25.0)
> Ehlers-Danlos syndrome (Q79.6)
> hemolytic anemias attributable to enzyme disorders (D55.-)
> Marfan's syndrome (Q87.4)
> 5-alpha-reductase deficiency (E29.1)

☑4ᵗʰ **E70 Disorders of aromatic amino-acid metabolism**

E70.0 Classical phenylketonuria

E70.1 Other hyperphenylalaninemias

☑5ᵗʰ **E70.2 Disorders of tyrosine metabolism**
> EXCLUDES1   transitory tyrosinemia of newborn (P74.5)

E70.20 Disorder of tyrosine metabolism, unspecified

E70.21 Tyrosinemia
> Hypertyrosinemia

E70.29 Other disorders of tyrosine metabolism
> Alkaptonuria   Ochronosis

☑5ᵗʰ **E70.3 Albinism**

E70.30 Albinism, unspecified

☑6ᵗʰ **E70.31 Ocular albinism**

E70.310 X-linked ocular albinism

E70.311 Autosomal recessive ocular albinism

E70.318 Other ocular albinism

E70.319 Ocular albinism, unspecified

☑6ᵗʰ **E70.32 Oculocutaneous albinism**
> EXCLUDES1   Chediak-Higashi syndrome (E70.330)
> Hermansky-Pudlak syndrome (E70.331)

E70.320 Tyrosinase negative oculocutaneous albinism
> Albinism I
> Oculocutaneous albinism ty-neg

E70.321 Tyrosinase positive oculocutaneous albinism
> Albinism II
> Oculocutaneous albinism ty-pos

E70.328 Other oculocutaneous albinism
> Cross syndrome

E70.329 Oculocutaneous albinism, unspecified

☑6ᵗʰ **E70.33 Albinism with hematologic abnormality**

E70.330 Chediak-Higashi syndrome

E70.331 Hermansky-Pudlak syndrome

E70.338 Other albinism with hematologic abnormality

E70.339 Albinism with hematologic abnormality, unspecified

E70.39 Other specified albinism
> Piebaldism

☑5ᵗʰ **E70.4 Disorders of histidine metabolism**

E70.40 Disorders of histidine metabolism, unspecified

E70.41 Histidinemia

E70.49 Other disorders of histidine metabolism

E70.5 Disorders of tryptophan metabolism

E70.8 Other disorders of aromatic amino-acid metabolism

E70.9 Disorder of aromatic amino-acid metabolism, unspecified

☑4ᵗʰ **E71 Disorders of branched-chain amino-acid metabolism and fatty-acid metabolism**

E71.0 Maple-syrup-urine disease

☑5ᵗʰ **E71.1 Other disorders of branched-chain amino-acid metabolism**

☑6ᵗʰ **E71.11 Branched-chain organic acidurias**

E71.110 Isovaleric acidemia

E71.111 3-methylglutaconic aciduria

E71.118 Other branched-chain organic acidurias

☑6ᵗʰ **E71.12 Disorders of propionate metabolism**

E71.120 Methylmalonic acidemia

E71.121 Propionic acidemia

E71.128 Other disorders of propionate metabolism

E71.19 Other disorders of branched-chain amino-acid metabolism
> Hyperleucine-isoleucinemia
> Hypervalinemia

E71.2 Disorder of branched-chain amino-acid metabolism, unspecified

☑ Additional Character Required   ˣ⁷ᵗʰ Xtension Alert   Unspecified Code   Other Specified Code   Manifestation Code   ▶◀ Revised Text   ● New Code   ▲ Revised Code Title

ICD-10-CM 2014 (Draft)   **489**

√5th **E71.3** **Disorders of fatty-acid metabolism**
 EXCLUDES 1 *peroxisomal disorders (E71.5)*
 Refsum's disease (G60.1)
 Schilder's disease (G37.0)
 EXCLUDES 2 *carnitine deficiency due to inborn error of metabolism (E71.42)*

E71.30 **Disorder of fatty-acid metabolism, unspecified**

√6th **E71.31** **Disorders of fatty-acid oxidation**

E71.310 **Long chain/very long chain acyl CoA dehydrogenase deficiency**
 LCAD VLCAD

E71.311 **Medium chain acyl CoA dehydrogenase deficiency**
 MCAD

E71.312 **Short chain acyl CoA dehydrogenase deficiency**
 SCAD

E71.313 **Glutaric aciduria type II**
 Glutaric aciduria type II A
 Glutaric aciduria type II B
 Glutaric aciduria type II C
 EXCLUDES 1 *glutaric aciduria (type 1) NOS (E72.3)*

E71.314 **Muscle carnitine palmitoyltransferase deficiency**

E71.318 **Other disorders of fatty-acid oxidation**

E71.32 **Disorders of ketone metabolism**

E71.39 **Other disorders of fatty-acid metabolism**

√5th **E71.4** **Disorders of carnitine metabolism**
 EXCLUDES 1 *muscle carnitine palmitoyltransferase deficiency (E71.314)*

E71.40 **Disorder of carnitine metabolism, unspecified**

E71.41 **Primary carnitine deficiency**

E71.42 **Carnitine deficiency due to inborn errors of metabolism**
 Code also associated inborn error or metabolism

E71.43 **Iatrogenic carnitine deficiency**
 Carnitine deficiency due to hemodialysis
 Carnitine deficiency due to Valproic acid therapy

√6th **E71.44** **Other secondary carnitine deficiency**

E71.440 **Ruvalcaba-Myhre-Smith syndrome**

E71.448 **Other secondary carnitine deficiency**

√5th **E71.5** **Peroxisomal disorders**
 EXCLUDES 1 *Schilder's disease (G37.0)*

E71.50 **Peroxisomal disorder, unspecified**

√6th **E71.51** **Disorders of peroxisome biogenesis**
 Group 1 peroxisomal disorders
 EXCLUDES 1 *Refsum's disease (G60.1)*

E71.510 **Zellweger syndrome**

E71.511 **Neonatal adrenoleukodystrophy** N
 EXCLUDES 1 *X-linked adrenoleuko- dystrophy (E71.52-)*

E71.518 **Other disorders of peroxisome biogenesis**

√6th **E71.52** **X-linked adrenoleukodystrophy**

E71.520 **Childhood cerebral X-linked adrenoleukodystrophy**

E71.521 **Adolescent X-linked adrenoleukodystrophy**

E71.522 **Adrenomyeloneuropathy**

E71.528 **Other X-linked adrenoleukodystrophy**
 Addison only phenotype adrenoleukodystrophy
 Addison-Schilder adrenoleukodystrophy

E71.529 **X-linked adrenoleukodystrophy, unspecified type**

E71.53 **Other group 2 peroxisomal disorders**

√6th **E71.54** **Other peroxisomal disorders**

E71.540 **Rhizomelic chondrodysplasia punctata**
 EXCLUDES 1 *chondrodysplasia punctata NOS (Q77.3)*

E71.541 **Zellweger-like syndrome**

E71.542 **Other group 3 peroxisomal disorders**

E71.548 **Other peroxisomal disorders**

√4th **E72** **Other disorders of amino-acid metabolism**
 EXCLUDES 1 *disorders of:*
 aromatic amino-acid metabolism (E70.-)
 branched-chain amino-acid metabolism (E71.0-E71.2)
 fatty-acid metabolism (E71.3)
 purine and pyrimidine metabolism (E79.-)
 gout (M1A.-, M10.-)

√5th **E72.0** **Disorders of amino-acid transport**
 EXCLUDES 1 *disorders of tryptophan metabolism (E70.5)*

E72.00 **Disorders of amino-acid transport, unspecified**

E72.01 **Cystinuria**

E72.02 **Hartnup's disease**

E72.03 **Lowe's syndrome**
 Use additional code for associated glaucoma (H42)

E72.04 **Cystinosis**
 Fanconi (-de Toni) (-Debré) syndrome with cystinosis
 EXCLUDES 1 *Fanconi (-de Toni) (-Debré) syndrome without cystinosis (E72.09)*

E72.09 **Other disorders of amino-acid transport**
 Fanconi (-de Toni) (-Debré) syndrome, unspecified

√5th **E72.1** **Disorders of sulfur-bearing amino-acid metabolism**
 EXCLUDES 1 *cystinosis (E72.04)*
 cystinuria (E72.01)
 transcobalamin II deficiency (D51.2)

E72.10 **Disorders of sulfur-bearing amino-acid metabolism, unspecified**

E72.11 **Homocystinuria**
 Cystathionine synthase deficiency

E72.12 **Methylenetetrahydrofolate reductase deficiency**

E72.19 **Other disorders of sulfur-bearing amino-acid metabolism**
 Cystathioninuria
 Methioninemia
 Sulfite oxidase deficiency

√5th **E72.2** **Disorders of urea cycle metabolism**
 EXCLUDES 1 *disorders of ornithine metabolism (E72.4)*

E72.20 **Disorder of urea cycle metabolism, unspecified**
 Hyperammonemia
 EXCLUDES 1 *hyperammonemia- hyperornithinemia- homocitrullinemia syndrome (E72.4)*
 transient hyperammonemia of newborn (P74.6)

E72.21 **Argininemia**

E72.22 **Arginosuccinic aciduria**

E72.23 **Citrullinemia**

E72.29 **Other disorders of urea cycle metabolism**

E72.3 **Disorders of lysine and hydroxylysine metabolism**
 Glutaric aciduria NOS   Hydroxylysinemia
 Glutaric aciduria (type I)   Hyperlysinemia
 EXCLUDES 1 *glutaric aciduria type II (E71.313)*
 Refsum's disease (G60.1)
 Zellweger syndrome (E71.510)

E72.4 **Disorders of ornithine metabolism**
 Hyperammonemia-hyperornithinemia-homocitrullinemia syndrome
 Ornithinemia (types I, II)
 Ornithine transcarbamylase deficiency
 EXCLUDES 1 *hereditary choroidal dystrophy (H31.2-)*

√5th **E72.5** **Disorders of glycine metabolism**

E72.50 **Disorder of glycine metabolism, unspecified**

E72.51 **Non-ketotic hyperglycinemia**

E72.52 **Trimethylaminuria**

E72.53 **Hyperoxaluria**
 Oxalosis
 Oxaluria

E72.59 **Other disorders of glycine metabolism**
 D-glycericacidemia
 Hyperhydroxyprolinemia
 Hyperprolinemia (types I, II)
 Sarcosinemia

E72.8 **Other specified disorders of amino-acid metabolism**
 Disorders of beta-amino-acid metabolism
 Disorders of gamma-glutamyl cycle

E72.9 **Disorder of amino-acid metabolism, unspecified**

√4th **E73** **Lactose intolerance**

E73.0 **Congenital lactase deficiency**

E73.1 **Secondary lactase deficiency**

EXCLUDES 1 Not coded here   EXCLUDES 2 Not included here   N Newborn Age: 0   P Pediatric Age: 0-17   M Maternity Age: 12-55   A Adult Age: 15-124

490   ICD-10-CM 2014 (Draft)

E73.8 **Other lactose intolerance**

E73.9 **Lactose intolerance, unspecified**

✓4th **E74 Other disorders of carbohydrate metabolism**
> EXCLUDES 1 *diabetes mellitus (E08-E13)*
> *hypoglycemia NOS (E16.2)*
> *increased secretion of glucagon (E16.3)*
> *mucopolysaccharidosis (E76.0-E76.3)*

✓5th E74.0 **Glycogen storage disease**

E74.00 **Glycogen storage disease, unspecified**

E74.01 **von Gierke disease**
Type I glycogen storage disease

E74.02 **Pompe disease**
Cardiac glycogenosis
Type II glycogen storage disease

E74.03 **Cori disease**
Forbes disease
Type III glycogen storage disease

E74.04 **McArdle disease**
Type V glycogen storage disease

E74.09 **Other glycogen storage disease**
Andersen disease
Hers disease
Tauri disease
Glycogen storage disease, types 0, IV, VI-XI
Liver phosphorylase deficiency
Muscle phosphofructokinase deficiency

✓5th E74.1 **Disorders of fructose metabolism**
> EXCLUDES 1 *muscle phosphofructokinase deficiency (E74.09)*

E74.10 **Disorder of fructose metabolism, unspecified**

E74.11 **Essential fructosuria**
Fructokinase deficiency

E74.12 **Hereditary fructose intolerance**
Fructosemia

E74.19 **Other disorders of fructose metabolism**
Fructose-1, 6-diphosphatase deficiency

✓5th E74.2 **Disorders of galactose metabolism**

E74.20 **Disorders of galactose metabolism, unspecified**

E74.21 **Galactosemia**

E74.29 **Other disorders of galactose metabolism**
Galactokinase deficiency

✓5th E74.3 **Other disorders of intestinal carbohydrate absorption**
> EXCLUDES 2 *lactose intolerance (E73.-)*

E74.31 **Sucrase-isomaltase deficiency**

E74.39 **Other disorders of intestinal carbohydrate absorption**
Disorder of intestinal carbohydrate absorption NOS
Glucose-galactose malabsorption
Sucrase deficiency

E74.4 **Disorders of pyruvate metabolism and gluconeogenesis**
Deficiency of phosphoenolpyruvate carboxykinase
Deficiency of pyruvate carboxylase
Deficiency of pyruvate dehydrogenase
> EXCLUDES 1 *disorders of pyruvate metabolism and gluconeogenesis*
> *with anemia (D55.-)*
> *Leigh's syndrome (G31.82)*

E74.8 **Other specified disorders of carbohydrate metabolism**
Essential pentosuria
Renal glycosuria

E74.9 **Disorder of carbohydrate metabolism, unspecified**

✓4th **E75 Disorders of sphingolipid metabolism and other lipid storage disorders**
> EXCLUDES 1 *mucolipidosis, types I-III (E77.0-E77.1)*
> *Refsum's disease (G60.1)*

✓5th E75.0 **GM2 gangliosidosis**

E75.00 **GM2 gangliosidosis, unspecified**

E75.01 **Sandhoff disease**

E75.02 **Tay-Sachs disease**

E75.09 **Other GM2 gangliosidosis**
Adult GM2 gangliosidosis
Juvenile GM2 gangliosidosis

✓5th E75.1 **Other and unspecified gangliosidosis**

E75.10 **Unspecified gangliosidosis**
Gangliosidosis NOS

E75.11 **Mucolipidosis IV**

E75.19 **Other gangliosidosis**
GM1 gangliosidosis
GM3 gangliosidosis

✓5th E75.2 **Other sphingolipidosis**
> EXCLUDES 1 *adrenoleukodystrophy [Addison-Schilder] (E71.528)*

E75.21 **Fabry (-Anderson) disease**

E75.22 **Gaucher disease**

E75.23 **Krabbe disease**

✓6th E75.24 **Niemann-Pick disease**

E75.240 **Niemann-Pick disease** type A

E75.241 **Niemann-Pick disease** type B

E75.242 **Niemann-Pick disease** type C

E75.243 **Niemann-Pick disease** type D

E75.248 **Other Niemann-Pick disease**

E75.249 **Niemann-Pick disease, unspecified**

E75.25 **Metachromatic leukodystrophy**

E75.29 **Other sphingolipidosis**
Farber's syndrome
Sulfatase deficiency
Sulfatide lipidosis

E75.3 **Sphingolipidosis, unspecified**

E75.4 **Neuronal ceroid lipofuscinosis**
Batten disease   Kufs disease
Bielschowsky-Jansky disease   Spielmeyer-Vogt disease

E75.5 **Other lipid storage disorders**
Cerebrotendinous cholesterosis [van Bogaert-Scherer-Epstein]
Wolman's disease

E75.6 **Lipid storage disorder, unspecified**

✓4th **E76 Disorders of glycosaminoglycan metabolism**

✓5th E76.0 **Mucopolysaccharidosis, type I**

E76.01 **Hurler's syndrome**

E76.02 **Hurler-Scheie syndrome**

E76.03 **Scheie's syndrome**

E76.1 **Mucopolysaccharidosis, type II**
Hunter's syndrome

✓5th E76.2 **Other mucopolysaccharidoses**

✓6th E76.21 **Morquio mucopolysaccharidoses**

E76.210 **Morquio A mucopolysaccharidoses**
Classic Morquio syndrome
Morquio syndrome A
Mucopolysaccharidosis, type IVA

E76.211 **Morquio B mucopolysaccharidoses**
Morquio-like mucopolysaccharidoses
Morquio-like syndrome
Morquio syndrome B
Mucopolysaccharidosis, type IVB

E76.219 **Morquio mucopolysaccharidoses, unspecified**
Morquio syndrome
Mucopolysaccharidosis, type IV

E76.22 **Sanfilippo mucopolysaccharidoses**
Mucopolysaccharidosis, type III (A) (B) (C) (D)
Sanfilippo A syndrome
Sanfilippo B syndrome
Sanfilippo C syndrome
Sanfilippo D syndrome

E76.29 **Other mucopolysaccharidoses**
beta-Glucuronidase deficiency
Maroteaux-Lamy (mild) (severe) syndrome
Mucopolysaccharidosis, types VI, VII

E76.3 **Mucopolysaccharidosis, unspecified**

E76.8 **Other disorders of glycosaminoglycan metabolism**

E76.9 **Glucosaminoglycan metabolism disorder, unspecified**

✓4th **E77 Disorders of glycoprotein metabolism**

E77.0 **Defects in post-translational modification of lysosomal enzymes**
Mucolipidosis II [I-cell disease]
Mucolipidosis III [pseudo-Hurler polydystrophy]

E77.1 **Defects in glycoprotein degradation**
Aspartylglucosaminuria
Fucosidosis
Mannosidosis
Sialidosis [mucolipidosis I]

E77.8 **Other disorders of glycoprotein metabolism**

E77.9 **Disorder of glycoprotein metabolism, unspecified**

✓ Additional Character Required   ✓x7th Xtension Alert   Unspecified Code   Other Specified Code   Manifestation Code   ►◄ Revised Text   ● New Code   ▲ Revised Code Title

✓4ᵗʰ **E78** **Disorders of** lipoprotein metabolism and other lipidemias
  EXCLUDES 1 *sphingolipidosis (E75.0-E75.3)*

E78.0 **Pure hypercholesterolemia**
  Familial hypercholesterolemia
  Fredrickson's hyperlipoproteinemia, type IIa
  Hyperbetalipoproteinemia
  Hyperlipidemia, Group A
  Low-density-lipoprotein-type [LDL] hyperlipoproteinemia

E78.1 **Pure hyperglyceridemia**
  Elevated fasting triglycerides
  Endogenous hyperglyceridemia
  Fredrickson's hyperlipoproteinemia, type IV
  Hyperlipidemia, group B
  Hyperprebetalipoproteinemia
  Very-low-density-lipoprotein-type [VLDL] hyperlipoproteinemia

E78.2 **Mixed hyperlipidemia**
  Broad- or floating-betalipoproteinemia
  Combined hyperlipidemia NOS
  Elevated cholesterol with elevated triglycerides NEC
  Fredrickson's hyperlipoproteinemia, type IIb or III
  Hyperbetalipoproteinemia with prebetalipoproteinemia
  Hypercholesteremia with endogenous hyperglyceridemia
  Hyperlipidemia, group C
  Tubo-eruptive xanthoma
  Xanthoma tuberosum
    EXCLUDES 1 *cerebrotendinous cholesterosis [van Bogaert-Scherer-Epstein] (E75.5)*
                familial combined hyperlipidemia (E78.4)

E78.3 **Hyperchylomicronemia**
  Chylomicron retention disease
  Fredrickson's hyperlipoproteinemia, type I or V
  Hyperlipidemia, group D
  Mixed hyperglyceridemia

E78.4 **Other hyperlipidemia**
  Familial combined hyperlipidemia

E78.5 **Hyperlipidemia, unspecified**

E78.6 **Lipoprotein deficiency**
  Abetalipoproteinemia
  Depressed HDL cholesterol
  High-density lipoprotein deficiency
  Hypoalphalipoproteinemia
  Hypobetalipoproteinemia (familial)
  Lecithin cholesterol acyltransferase deficiency
  Tangier disease

✓5ᵗʰ **E78.7** **Disorders of** bile acid and cholesterol **metabolism**
  EXCLUDES 1 *Niemann-Pick disease type C (E75.242)*

E78.70 **Disorder of bile acid and cholesterol metabolism, unspecified**

E78.71 **Barth syndrome**

E78.72 **Smith-Lemli-Opitz syndrome**

E78.79 **Other disorders of bile acid and cholesterol metabolism**

✓5ᵗʰ **E78.8** **Other disorders of lipoprotein metabolism**

E78.81 **Lipoid dermatoarthritis**

E78.89 **Other lipoprotein metabolism disorders**

E78.9 **Disorder of lipoprotein metabolism, unspecified**

✓4ᵗʰ **E79** **Disorders of** purine and pyrimidine **metabolism**
  EXCLUDES 1 *Ataxia-telangiectasia (G11.3)*
             Bloom's syndrome (Q82.8)
             Cockayne's syndrome (Q87.1)
             calculus of kidney (N20.0)
             combined immunodeficiency disorders (D81.-)
             Fanconi's anemia (D61.09)
             gout (M1A.-, M10.-)
             orotaciduric anemia (D53.0)
             progeria (E34.8)
             Werner's syndrome (E34.8)
             xeroderma pigmentosum (Q82.1)

E79.0 **Hyperuricemia without signs of inflammatory arthritis and tophaceous disease**
  Asymptomatic hyperuricemia

E79.1 **Lesch-Nyhan syndrome**
  HGPRT deficiency

E79.2 **Myoadenylate deaminase deficiency**

E79.8 **Other disorders of purine and pyrimidine metabolism**
  Hereditary xanthinuria

E79.9 **Disorder of purine and pyrimidine metabolism, unspecified**

✓4ᵗʰ **E80** **Disorders of** porphyrin and bilirubin **metabolism**
  INCLUDES defects of catalase and peroxidase

E80.0 **Hereditary erythropoietic porphyria**
  Congenital erythropoietic porphyria
  Erythropoietic protoporphyria

E80.1 **Porphyria cutanea tarda**

✓5ᵗʰ **E80.2** **Other and unspecified porphyria**

E80.20 **Unspecified porphyria**
  Porphyria NOS

E80.21 **Acute intermittent (hepatic) porphyria**

E80.29 **Other porphyria**
  Hereditary coproporphyria

E80.3 **Defects of catalase and peroxidase**
  Acatalasia [Takahara]

E80.4 **Gilbert syndrome**

E80.5 **Crigler-Najjar syndrome**

E80.6 **Other disorders of bilirubin metabolism**
  Dubin-Johnson syndrome
  Rotor's syndrome

E80.7 **Disorder of bilirubin metabolism, unspecified**

✓4ᵗʰ **E83** **Disorders of** mineral **metabolism**
  EXCLUDES 1 *dietary mineral deficiency (E58-E61)*
             parathyroid disorders (E20-E21)
             vitamin D deficiency (E55.-)

✓5ᵗʰ **E83.0** **Disorders of** copper **metabolism**

E83.00 **Disorder of copper metabolism, unspecified**

E83.01 **Wilson's disease**
  Code also associated Kayser Fleischer ring (H18.04-)

E83.09 **Other disorders of copper metabolism**
  Menkes' (kinky hair) (steely hair) disease

✓5ᵗʰ **E83.1** **Disorders of** iron **metabolism**
  EXCLUDES 1 *iron deficiency anemia (D50.-)*
             sideroblastic anemia (D64.0-D64.3)

E83.10 **Disorder of iron metabolism, unspecified**

✓6ᵗʰ **E83.11** **Hemochromatosis**

E83.110 **Hereditary hemochromatosis**
  Bronzed diabetes
  Pigmentary cirrhosis (of liver)
  Primary (hereditary) hemochromatosis

E83.111 **Hemochromatosis due to repeated red blood cell transfusions**
  Iron overload due to repeated red blood cell transfusions
  Transfusion (red blood cell) associated hemochromatosis

E83.118 **Other hemochromatosis**

E83.119 **Hemochromatosis, unspecified**

E83.19 **Other disorders of iron metabolism**
  Use additional code, if applicable, for idiopathic pulmonary hemosiderosis (J84.03)

E83.2 **Disorders of zinc metabolism**
  Acrodermatitis enteropathica

✓5ᵗʰ **E83.3** **Disorders of** phosphorus **metabolism and** phosphatases
  EXCLUDES 1 *adult osteomalacia (M83.-)*
             osteoporosis (M80.-)

E83.30 **Disorder of phosphorus metabolism, unspecified**

E83.31 **Familial hypophosphatemia**
  Vitamin D-resistant osteomalacia
  Vitamin D-resistant rickets
    EXCLUDES 1 *vitamin D-deficiency rickets (E55.0)*

E83.32 **Hereditary vitamin D-dependent rickets (type 1) (type 2)**
  25-hydroxyvitamin D 1-alpha-hydroxylase deficiency
  Pseudovitamin D deficiency
  Vitamin D receptor defect

E83.39 **Other disorders of phosphorus metabolism**
  Acid phosphatase deficiency
  Hypophosphatasia

✓5ᵗʰ **E83.4** **Disorders of** magnesium **metabolism**

E83.40 **Disorders of magnesium metabolism, unspecified**

E83.41 **Hypermagnesemia**

E83.42 **Hypomagnesemia**

E83.49 **Other disorders of magnesium metabolism**

√5th **E83.5** **Disorders of calcium metabolism**

> EXCLUDES 1 *chondrocalcinosis (M11.1-M11.2)*
> *hungry bone syndrome (E83.81)*
> *hyperparathyroidism (E21.0-E21.3)*

E83.50 **Unspecified disorder of calcium metabolism**

E83.51 **Hypocalcemia**

E83.52 **Hypercalcemia**
Familial hypocalciuric hypercalcemia

E83.59 **Other disorders of calcium metabolism**
Idiopathic hypercalciuria

√5th **E83.8** **Other disorders of mineral metabolism**

E83.81 **Hungry bone syndrome**

E83.89 **Other disorders of mineral metabolism**

E83.9 **Disorder of mineral metabolism, unspecified**

√4th **E84** **Cystic fibrosis**

> INCLUDES mucoviscidosis

E84.0 **Cystic fibrosis with pulmonary manifestations**
Use additional code to identify any infectious organism present, such as:
Pseudomonas (B96.5)

√5th **E84.1** **Cystic fibrosis with intestinal manifestations**

E84.11 **Meconium ileus in cystic fibrosis**   N

> EXCLUDES 1 *meconium ileus not due to cystic fibrosis (P76.0)*

E84.19 **Cystic fibrosis with other intestinal manifestations**
Distal intestinal obstruction syndrome

E84.8 **Cystic fibrosis with other manifestations**

E84.9 **Cystic fibrosis, unspecified**

√4th **E85** **Amyloidosis**

> EXCLUDES 1 *Alzheimer's disease (G30.0-)*

E85.0 **Non-neuropathic heredofamilial amyloidosis**
Familial Mediterranean fever
Hereditary amyloid nephropathy

E85.1 **Neuropathic heredofamilial amyloidosis**
Amyloid polyneuropathy (Portuguese)
AHA: 2012, Q4, 99

E85.2 **Heredofamilial amyloidosis, unspecified**

E85.3 **Secondary systemic amyloidosis**
Hemodialysis-associated amyloidosis

E85.4 **Organ-limited amyloidosis**
Localized amyloidosis

E85.8 **Other amyloidosis**

E85.9 **Amyloidosis, unspecified**

√4th **E86** **Volume depletion**

> EXCLUDES 1 *dehydration of newborn (P74.1)*
> *hypovolemic shock NOS (R57.1)*
> *postprocedural hypovolemic shock (T81.19)*
> *traumatic hypovolemic shock (T79.4)*

E86.0 **Dehydration**

E86.1 **Hypovolemia**
Depletion of volume of plasma

E86.9 **Volume depletion, unspecified**

√4th **E87** **Other disorders of fluid, electrolyte and acid-base balance**

> EXCLUDES 1 *diabetes insipidus (E23.2)*
> *electrolyte imbalance associated with hyperemesis gravidarum (O21.1)*
> *electrolyte imbalance following ectopic or molar pregnancy (O08.5)*
> *familial periodic paralysis (G72.3)*

E87.0 **Hyperosmolality and hypernatremia**
Sodium [Na] excess
Sodium [Na] overload

E87.1 **Hypo-osmolality and hyponatremia**
Sodium [Na] deficiency

> EXCLUDES 1 *syndrome of inappropriate secretion of antidiuretic hormone (E22.2)*

E87.2 **Acidosis**
Acidosis NOS   Metabolic acidosis
Lactic acidosis   Respiratory acidosis

> EXCLUDES 1 *diabetic acidosis—see categories E08-E10, E13 with ketoacidosis*

E87.3 **Alkalosis**
Alkalosis NOS   Respiratory alkalosis
Metabolic alkalosis

E87.4 **Mixed disorder of acid-base balance**

E87.5 **Hyperkalemia**
Potassium [K] excess   Potassium [K] overload

E87.6 **Hypokalemia**
Potassium [K] deficiency

√5th **E87.7** **Fluid overload**

> EXCLUDES 1 *edema NOS (R60.9)*
> *fluid retention (R60.9)*

E87.70 **Fluid overload, unspecified**

E87.71 **Transfusion associated circulatory overload**
Fluid overload due to transfusion (blood) (blood components)
TACO

E87.79 **Other fluid overload**

E87.8 **Other disorders of electrolyte and fluid balance, not elsewhere classified**
Electrolyte imbalance NOS
Hyperchloremia
Hypochloremia

√4th **E88** **Other and unspecified metabolic disorders**
Use additional codes for associated conditions

> EXCLUDES 1 *histiocytosis X (chronic) (C96.6)*

√5th **E88.0** **Disorders of plasma-protein metabolism, not elsewhere classified**

> EXCLUDES 1 *disorder of lipoprotein metabolism (E78.-)*
> *monoclonal gammopathy (of undetermined significance) (D47.2)*
> *polyclonal hypergammaglobulinemia (D89.0)*
> *Waldenström's macroglobulinemia (C88.0)*

E88.01 **Alpha-1-antitrypsin deficiency**
AAT deficiency

E88.09 **Other disorders of plasma-protein metabolism, not elsewhere classified**
Bisalbuminemia

E88.1 **Lipodystrophy, not elsewhere classified**
Lipodystrophy NOS

> EXCLUDES 1 *Whipple's disease (K90.81)*

E88.2 **Lipomatosis, not elsewhere classified**
Lipomatosis NOS
Lipomatosis (Check) dolorosa [Dercum]

E88.3 **Tumor lysis syndrome**
Tumor lysis syndrome (spontaneous)
Tumor lysis syndrome following antineoplastic drug chemotherapy
Use additional code for adverse effect, if applicable, to identify drug (T45.1X5)

√5th **E88.4** **Mitochondrial metabolism disorders**

> EXCLUDES 1 *disorders of pyruvate metabolism (E74.4)*
> *Kearns-Sayre syndrome (H49.81)*
> *Leber's disease (H47.22)*
> *Leigh's encephalopathy (G31.82)*
> *Mitochondrial myopathy, NEC (G71.3)*
> *Reye's syndrome (G93.7)*

E88.40 **Mitochondrial metabolism disorder, unspecified**

E88.41 **MELAS syndrome**
Mitochondrial myopathy, encephalopathy, lactic acidosis and stroke-like episodes

E88.42 **MERRF syndrome**
Myoclonic epilepsy associated with ragged-red fibers
Code also myoclonic epilepsy (G40.3-)

E88.49 **Other mitochondrial metabolism disorders**

√5th **E88.8** **Other specified metabolic disorders**

E88.81 **Metabolic syndrome**
Dysmetabolic syndrome X
Use additional codes for associated manifestations, such as:
obesity (E66.-)

E88.89 **Other specified metabolic disorders**
Launois-Bensaude adenolipomatosis

> EXCLUDES 1 *adult pulmonary Langerhans cell histiocytosis (J84.82)*

E88.9 **Metabolic disorder, unspecified**

☑ Additional Character Required   √x7th Xtension Alert   Unspecified Code   Other Specified Code   Manifestation Code   ▶◀ Revised Text   ● New Code   ▲ Revised Code Title

Endocrine, Nutritional and Metabolic Diseases

E89–E89.89

√4ᵗʰ **E89 Postprocedural endocrine and metabolic complications and disorders, not elsewhere classified**
   EXCLUDES 2 intraoperative complications of endocrine system organ or structure (E36.0-, E36.1-, E36.8)

E89.0 Postprocedural hypothyroidism
Postirradiation hypothyroidism
Postsurgical hypothyroidism

E89.1 Postprocedural hypoinsulinemia
Postpancreatectomy hyperglycemia
Postsurgical hypoinsulinemia
Use additional code, if applicable, to identify:
  acquired absence of pancreas (Z90.41-)
  diabetes mellitus (postpancreatectomy) (postprocedural) (E13.-)
  insulin use (Z79.4)
  EXCLUDES 1 transient postprocedural hyperglycemia (R73.9)
     transient postprocedural hypoglycemia (E16.2)

E89.2 Postprocedural hypoparathyroidism
Parathyroprival tetany

E89.3 Postprocedural hypopituitarism
Postirradiation hypopituitarism

√5ᵗʰ **E89.4 Postprocedural ovarian failure**
  E89.40 Asymptomatic postprocedural ovarian failure ♀
    Postprocedural ovarian failure NOS
  E89.41 Symptomatic postprocedural ovarian failure ♀
    Symptoms such as flushing, sleeplessness, headache, lack of concentration, associated with postprocedural menopause

E89.5 Postprocedural testicular hypofunction ♂
E89.6 Postprocedural adrenocortical (-medullary) hypofunction
√5ᵗʰ **E89.8 Other postprocedural endocrine and metabolic complications and disorders**
  √6ᵗʰ **E89.81 Postprocedural hemorrhage and hematoma of an endocrine system organ or structure following a procedure**
    E89.810 Postprocedural hemorrhage and hematoma of an endocrine system organ or structure following an endocrine system procedure
    E89.811 Postprocedural hemorrhage and hematoma of an endocrine system organ or structure following other procedure
  E89.89 Other postprocedural endocrine and metabolic complications and disorders
    Use additional code, if applicable, to further specify disorder

Chapter 5. Mental, Behavioral, and Neurodevelopmental Disorders (F01-F99)

INCLUDES disorders of psychological development
EXCLUDES 2 symptoms, signs and abnormal clinical laboratory findings, not elsewhere classified (R00-R99)

This chapter contains the following blocks:

F01-F09 Mental disorders due to known physiological conditions
F10-F19 Mental and behavioral disorders due to psychoactive substance use
F20-F29 Schizophrenia, schizotypal, delusional, and other non-mood psychotic disorders
F30-F39 Mood [affective] disorders
F40-F48 Anxiety, dissociative, stress-related, somatoform and other nonpsychotic mental disorders
F50-F59 Behavioral syndromes associated with physiological disturbances and physical factors
F60-F69 Disorders of adult personality and behavior
F70-F79 Intellectual disabilities
F80-F89 Pervasive and specific developmental disorders
F90-F98 Behavioral and emotional disorders with onset usually occurring in childhood and adolescence
F99 Unspecified mental disorder

Mental disorders due to known physiological conditions (F01-F09)

NOTE This block comprises a range of mental disorders grouped together on the basis of their having in common a demonstrable etiology in cerebral disease, brain injury, or other insult leading to cerebral dysfunction. The dysfunction may be primary, as in diseases, injuries, and insults that affect the brain directly and selectively; or secondary, as in systemic diseases and disorders that attack the brain only as one of the multiple organs or systems of the body that are involved.

√4th **F01 Vascular dementia**
Vascular dementia as a result of infarction of the brain due to vascular disease, including hypertensive cerebrovascular disease.
INCLUDES arteriosclerotic dementia
Code first the underlying physiological condition or sequelae of cerebrovascular disease.

√5th **F01.5 Vascular dementia**

F01.50 Vascular dementia without behavioral disturbance A

F01.51 Vascular dementia with behavioral disturbance A
Vascular dementia with aggressive behavior
Vascular dementia with combative behavior
Vascular dementia with violent behavior
Use additional code, if applicable, to identify wandering in vascular dementia (Z91.83)

√4th **F02 Dementia in other diseases classified elsewhere**
Code first the underlying physiological condition, such as:
Alzheimer's (G30.-)
cerebral lipidosis (E75.4)
Creutzfeldt-Jakob disease (A81.0-)
dementia with Lewy bodies (G31.83)
epilepsy and recurrent seizures (G40.-)
frontotemporal dementia (G31.09)
hepatolenticular degeneration (E83.0)
human immunodeficiency virus [HIV] disease (B20)
hypercalcemia (E83.52)
hypothyroidism, acquired (E00-E03.-)
intoxications (T36-T65)
Jakob-Creutzfeldt disease (A81.0-)
multiple sclerosis (G35)
neurosyphilis (A52.17)
niacin deficiency [pellagra] (E52)
Parkinson's disease (G20)
Pick's disease (G31.01)
polyarteritis nodosa (M30.0)
systemic lupus erythematosus (M32.-)
trypanosomiasis (B56.-, B57.-)
vitamin B deficiency (E53.8)
EXCLUDES 1 dementia with Parkinsonism (G31.83)
EXCLUDES 2 dementia in alcohol and psychoactive substance disorders (F10-F19, with .17, .27, .97)
vascular dementia (F01.5-)

√5th **F02.8 Dementia in other diseases classified elsewhere**

F02.80 Dementia in other diseases classified elsewhere without behavioral disturbance
Dementia in other diseases classified elsewhere NOS

F02.81 Dementia in other diseases classified elsewhere with behavioral disturbance
Dementia in other diseases classified elsewhere with aggressive behavior
Dementia in other diseases classified elsewhere with combative behavior
Dementia in other diseases classified elsewhere with violent behavior
Use additional code, if applicable, to identify wandering in dementia in conditions classified elsewhere (Z91.83)

√4th **F03 Unspecified dementia**
Presenile dementia NOS
Presenile psychosis NOS
Primary degenerative dementia NOS
Senile dementia NOS
Senile dementia depressed or paranoid type
Senile psychosis NOS
EXCLUDES 1 senility NOS (R41.81)
EXCLUDES 2 mild memory disturbance due to known physiological condition (F06.8)
senile dementia with delirium or acute confusional state (F05)

√5th **F03.9 Unspecified dementia**

F03.90 Unspecified dementia without behavioral disturbance A
Dementia NOS
AHA: 2012, Q4, 92

F03.91 Unspecified dementia with behavioral disturbance A
Unspecified dementia with aggressive behavior
Unspecified dementia with combative behavior
Unspecified dementia with violent behavior
Use additional code, if applicable, to identify wandering in unspecified dementia (Z91.83)

F04 Amnestic disorder due to known physiological condition
Korsakov's psychosis or syndrome, nonalcoholic
Code first the underlying physiological condition
EXCLUDES 1 amnesia NOS (R41.3)
anterograde amnesia (R41.1)
dissociative amnesia (F44.0)
retrograde amnesia (R41.2)
EXCLUDES 2 alcohol-induced or unspecified Korsakov's syndrome (F10.26, F10.96)
Korsakov's syndrome induced by other psychoactive substances (F13.26, F13.96, F19.16, F19.26, F19.96)

F05 Delirium due to known physiological condition
Acute or subacute brain syndrome
Acute or subacute confusional state (nonalcoholic)
Acute or subacute infective psychosis
Acute or subacute organic reaction
Acute or subacute psycho-organic syndrome
Delirium of mixed etiology
Delirium superimposed on dementia
Sundowning
Code first the underlying physiological condition
EXCLUDES 1 delirium NOS (R41.0)
EXCLUDES 2 delirium tremens alcohol-induced or unspecified (F10.231, F10.921)

√4th **F06 Other mental disorders due to known physiological condition**
INCLUDES mental disorders due to endocrine disorder
mental disorders due to exogenous hormone
mental disorders due to exogenous toxic substance
mental disorders due to primary cerebral disease
mental disorders due to somatic illness
mental disorders due to systemic disease affecting the brain
Code first the underlying physiological condition
EXCLUDES 1 unspecified dementia (F03)
EXCLUDES 2 delirium due to known physiological condition (F05)
dementia as classified in F01-F02
other mental disorders associated with alcohol and other psychoactive substances (F10-F19)

F06.0 Psychotic disorder with hallucinations **due to known physiological condition**
Organic hallucinatory state (nonalcoholic)
EXCLUDES 2 hallucinations and perceptual disturbance induced by alcohol and other psychoactive substances (F10-F19 with .151, .251, .951)
schizophrenia (F20.-)

F06.1 **Catatonic** disorder due to known physiological condition
> **EXCLUDES 1** *catatonic stupor (R40.1)*
> *stupor NOS (R40.1)*
> **EXCLUDES 2** *catatonic schizophrenia (F20.2)*
> *dissociative stupor (F44.2)*

F06.2 **Psychotic** disorder **with delusions** due to known physiological condition
> Paranoid and paranoid-hallucinatory organic states
> Schizophrenia-like psychosis in epilepsy
> **EXCLUDES 2** *alcohol and drug-induced psychotic disorder (F10-F19 with .150, .250, .950)*
> *brief psychotic disorder (F23)*
> *delusional disorder (F22)*
> *schizophrenia (F20.-)*

✓5th **F06.3** **Mood** disorder due to known physiological condition
> **EXCLUDES 2** *mood disorders due to alcohol and other psychoactive substances (F10-F19 with .14, .24, .94)*
> *mood disorders, not due to known physiological condition or unspecified (F30-F39)*

    F06.30 **Mood disorder due to known physiological condition, unspecified**

    F06.31 **Mood disorder due to known physiological condition with depressive features**

    F06.32 **Mood disorder due to known physiological condition with major depressive-like episode**

    F06.33 **Mood disorder due to known physiological condition with manic features**

    F06.34 **Mood disorder due to known physiological condition with mixed features**

F06.4 **Anxiety** disorder due to known physiological condition
> **EXCLUDES 2** *anxiety disorders due to alcohol and other psychoactive substances (F10-F19 with .180, .280, .980)*
> *anxiety disorders, not due to known physiological condition or unspecified (F40.-, F41.-)*

F06.8 **Other specified mental disorders due to known physiological condition**
> Epileptic psychosis NOS
> Organic dissociative disorder
> Organic emotionally labile [asthenic] disorder

✓4th **F07** **Personality** and behavioral disorders due to known physiological condition
> Code first the underlying physiological condition

    F07.0 **Personality** change due to known physiological condition
> Frontal lobe syndrome
> Limbic epilepsy personality syndrome
> Lobotomy syndrome
> Organic personality disorder
> Organic pseudopsychopathic personality
> Organic pseudoretarded personality
> Postleucotomy syndrome
> Code first underlying physiological condition
> **EXCLUDES 1** *mild cognitive impairment (G31.84)*
> *postconcussional syndrome (F07.81)*
> *postencephalitic syndrome (F07.89)*
> *signs and symptoms involving emotional state (R45.-)*
> **EXCLUDES 2** *specific personality disorder (F60.-)*

✓5th **F07.8** **Other personality and behavioral disorders due to known physiological condition**

    F07.81 **Postconcussional** syndrome
> Postcontusional syndrome (encephalopathy)
> Post-traumatic brain syndrome, nonpsychotic
> Use additional code to identify associated post-traumatic headache, if applicable (G44.3-)
> **EXCLUDES 1** *current concussion (brain) (S06.0-)*
> *postencephalitic syndrome (F07.89)*

    F07.89 **Other personality and behavioral disorders due to known physiological condition**
> Postencephalitic syndrome
> Right hemispheric organic affective disorder

F07.9 **Unspecified personality and behavioral disorder due to known physiological condition**
> Organic psychosyndrome

F09 **Unspecified mental disorder due to known physiological condition**
> Mental disorder NOS due to known physiological condition
> Organic brain syndrome NOS
> Organic mental disorder NOS
> Organic psychosis NOS
> Symptomatic psychosis NOS
> Code first the underlying physiological condition
> **EXCLUDES 1** *psychosis NOS (F29)*

Mental and behavioral disorders due to psychoactive substance use (F10-F19)

✓4th **F10** **Alcohol** related disorders
> Use additional code for blood alcohol level, if applicable (Y90.-)

✓5th   **F10.1** **Alcohol** abuse
> **EXCLUDES 1** *alcohol dependence (F10.2-)*
> *alcohol use, unspecified (F10.9-)*

    F10.10 **Alcohol abuse, uncomplicated**

✓6th   **F10.12** **Alcohol abuse with intoxication**

        F10.120 **Alcohol abuse with intoxication, uncomplicated**

        F10.121 **Alcohol abuse with intoxication delirium**

        F10.129 **Alcohol abuse with intoxication, unspecified**

    F10.14 **Alcohol abuse with alcohol-induced mood disorder**

✓6th   **F10.15** **Alcohol abuse with alcohol-induced psychotic disorder**

        F10.150 **Alcohol abuse with alcohol-induced psychotic disorder with delusions**

        F10.151 **Alcohol abuse with alcohol-induced psychotic disorder with hallucinations**

        F10.159 **Alcohol abuse with alcohol-induced psychotic disorder, unspecified**

✓6th   **F10.18** **Alcohol abuse with other alcohol-induced disorders**

        F10.180 **Alcohol abuse with alcohol-induced anxiety disorder**

        F10.181 **Alcohol abuse with alcohol-induced sexual dysfunction**

        F10.182 **Alcohol abuse with alcohol-induced sleep disorder**

        F10.188 **Alcohol abuse with other alcohol-induced disorder**

    F10.19 **Alcohol abuse with unspecified alcohol-induced disorder**

✓5th   **F10.2** **Alcohol** dependence
> **EXCLUDES 1** *alcohol abuse (F10.1-)*
> *alcohol use, unspecified (F10.9-)*
> **EXCLUDES 2** *toxic effect of alcohol (T51.0-)*

    F10.20 **Alcohol dependence, uncomplicated**

    F10.21 **Alcohol dependence, in remission**

✓6th   **F10.22** **Alcohol dependence with intoxication**
> Acute drunkenness (in alcoholism)
> **EXCLUDES 1** *alcohol dependence with withdrawal (F10.23-)*

        F10.220 **Alcohol dependence with intoxication, uncomplicated**

        F10.221 **Alcohol dependence with intoxication delirium**

        F10.229 **Alcohol dependence with intoxication, unspecified**

✓6th   **F10.23** **Alcohol dependence with withdrawal**
> **EXCLUDES 1** *Alcohol dependence with intoxication (F10.22-)*

        F10.230 **Alcohol dependence with withdrawal, uncomplicated**

        F10.231 **Alcohol dependence with withdrawal delirium**

        F10.232 **Alcohol dependence with withdrawal with perceptual disturbance**

        F10.239 **Alcohol dependence with withdrawal, unspecified**

    F10.24 **Alcohol dependence with alcohol-induced mood disorder**

✓6th   **F10.25** **Alcohol dependence with alcohol-induced psychotic disorder**

        F10.250 **Alcohol dependence with alcohol-induced psychotic disorder with delusions**

        F10.251 **Alcohol dependence with alcohol-induced psychotic disorder with hallucinations**

        F10.259 **Alcohol dependence with alcohol-induced psychotic disorder, unspecified**

    F10.26 **Alcohol dependence with alcohol-induced persisting amnestic disorder**

    F10.27 **Alcohol dependence with alcohol-induced persisting dementia**

EXCLUDES 1 Not coded here   **EXCLUDES 2** Not included here   **N** Newborn Age: 0   **P** Pediatric Age: 0-17   **M** Maternity Age: 12-55   **A** Adult Age: 15-124

496   ICD-10-CM 2014 (Draft)

✓6th **F10.28 Alcohol dependence with** other **alcohol-induced disorders**

F10.280 Alcohol dependence with alcohol-induced anxiety **disorder**

F10.281 Alcohol dependence with alcohol-induced sexual dysfunction

F10.282 Alcohol dependence with alcohol-induced sleep **disorder**

F10.288 Alcohol dependence with other alcohol-induced disorder

F10.29 Alcohol dependence with unspecified alcohol-induced disorder

✓5th **F10.9 Alcohol** use, unspecified

EXCLUDES 1 *alcohol abuse (F10.1-)*
alcohol dependence (F10.2-)

✓6th **F10.92 Alcohol use, unspecified with** intoxication

F10.920 Alcohol use, unspecified with intoxication, uncomplicated

F10.921 Alcohol use, unspecified with intoxication delirium

F10.929 Alcohol use, unspecified with intoxication, unspecified

F10.94 Alcohol use, unspecified with alcohol-induced mood disorder

✓6th **F10.95 Alcohol use, unspecified with alcohol-induced** psychotic disorder

F10.950 Alcohol use, unspecified with alcohol-induced psychotic disorder with delusions

F10.951 Alcohol use, unspecified with alcohol-induced psychotic disorder with hallucinations

F10.959 Alcohol use, unspecified with alcohol-induced psychotic disorder, unspecified

F10.96 Alcohol use, unspecified with alcohol-induced persisting amnestic disorder

F10.97 Alcohol use, unspecified with alcohol-induced persisting dementia

✓6th **F10.98 Alcohol use,** unspecified **with other alcohol-induced** disorders

F10.980 Alcohol use, unspecified with alcohol-induced anxiety disorder

F10.981 Alcohol use, unspecified with alcohol-induced sexual dysfunction

F10.982 Alcohol use, unspecified with alcohol-induced sleep disorder

F10.988 Alcohol use, unspecified with other alcohol-induced disorder

F10.99 Alcohol use, unspecified with unspecified alcohol-induced disorder

✓4th **F11 Opioid** related disorders

✓5th **F11.1 Opioid** abuse

EXCLUDES 1 *opioid dependence (F11.2-)*
opioid use, unspecified (F11.9-)

F11.10 Opioid abuse, uncomplicated

✓6th **F11.12 Opioid abuse with** intoxication

F11.120 Opioid abuse with intoxication, uncomplicated

F11.121 Opioid abuse with intoxication delirium

F11.122 Opioid abuse with intoxication with perceptual disturbance

F11.129 Opioid abuse with intoxication, unspecified

F11.14 Opioid abuse with opioid-induced mood disorder

✓6th **F11.15 Opioid abuse with opioid-induced** psychotic disorder

F11.150 Opioid abuse with opioid-induced psychotic disorder with delusions

F11.151 Opioid abuse with opioid-induced psychotic disorder with hallucinations

F11.159 Opioid abuse with opioid-induced psychotic disorder, unspecified

✓6th **F11.18 Opioid abuse with** other **opioid-induced disorder**

F11.181 Opioid abuse with opioid-induced sexual dysfunction

F11.182 Opioid abuse with opioid-induced sleep disorder

F11.188 Opioid abuse with other opioid-induced disorder

F11.19 Opioid abuse with unspecified opioid-induced disorder

✓5th **F11.2 Opioid** dependence

EXCLUDES 1 *opioid abuse (F11.1-)*
opioid use, unspecified (F11.9-)
EXCLUDES 2 *opioid poisoning (T40.0-T40.2-)*

F11.20 Opioid dependence, uncomplicated

F11.21 Opioid dependence, in remission

✓6th **F11.22 Opioid dependence with** intoxication

EXCLUDES 1 *opioid dependence with withdrawal (F11.23)*

F11.220 Opioid dependence with intoxication, uncomplicated

F11.221 Opioid dependence with intoxication delirium

F11.222 Opioid dependence with intoxication with perceptual disturbance

F11.229 Opioid dependence with intoxication, unspecified

F11.23 Opioid dependence with withdrawal

EXCLUDES 1 *opioid dependence with intoxication (F11.22-)*

F11.24 Opioid dependence with opioid-induced mood disorder

✓6th **F11.25 Opioid dependence with opioid-induced** psychotic disorder

F11.250 Opioid dependence with opioid-induced psychotic disorder with delusions

F11.251 Opioid dependence with opioid-induced psychotic disorder with hallucinations

F11.259 Opioid dependence with opioid-induced psychotic disorder, unspecified

✓6th **F11.28 Opioid dependence with** other **opioid-induced disorder**

F11.281 Opioid dependence with opioid-induced sexual dysfunction

F11.282 Opioid dependence with opioid-induced sleep disorder

F11.288 Opioid dependence with other opioid-induced disorder

F11.29 Opioid dependence with unspecified opioid-induced disorder

✓5th **F11.9 Opioid use,** unspecified

EXCLUDES 1 *opioid abuse (F11.1-)*
opioid dependence (F11.2-)

F11.90 Opioid use, unspecified, uncomplicated

✓6th **F11.92 Opioid use, unspecified with** intoxication

EXCLUDES 1 *opioid use, unspecified with withdrawal (F11.93)*

F11.920 Opioid use, unspecified with intoxication, uncomplicated

F11.921 Opioid use, unspecified with intoxication delirium

F11.922 Opioid use, unspecified with intoxication with perceptual disturbance

F11.929 Opioid use, unspecified with intoxication, unspecified

F11.93 Opioid use, unspecified with withdrawal

EXCLUDES 1 *opioid use, unspecified with intoxication (F11.92-)*

F11.94 Opioid use, unspecified with opioid-induced mood disorder

✓6th **F11.95 Opioid use, unspecified with opioid-induced** psychotic disorder

F11.950 Opioid use, unspecified with opioid-induced psychotic disorder with delusions

F11.951 Opioid use, unspecified with opioid-induced psychotic disorder with hallucinations

F11.959 Opioid use, unspecified with opioid-induced psychotic disorder, unspecified

---

☑ Additional Character Required   ✓x7th Xtension Alert   Unspecified Code   Other Specified Code   Manifestation Code   ▶◀ Revised Text   ● New Code   ▲ Revised Code Title

✓6ᵗʰ **F11.98** **Opioid use, unspecified with** other specified opioid-induced disorder

F11.981 Opioid use, unspecified with opioid-induced sexual dysfunction

F11.982 Opioid use, unspecified with opioid-induced sleep disorder

F11.988 Opioid use, unspecified with other opioid-induced disorder

F11.99 Opioid use, unspecified with unspecified opioid-induced disorder

✓4ᵗʰ **F12** **Cannabis** related disorders

INCLUDES   marijuana

✓5ᵗʰ **F12.1** **Cannabis** abuse

EXCLUDES 1   cannabis dependence (F12.2-)
cannabis use, unspecified (F12.9-)

F12.10 **Cannabis abuse,** uncomplicated

✓6ᵗʰ **F12.12** **Cannabis abuse with** intoxication

F12.120 Cannabis abuse with intoxication, uncomplicated

F12.121 Cannabis abuse with intoxication delirium

F12.122 Cannabis abuse with intoxication with perceptual disturbance

F12.129 Cannabis abuse with intoxication, unspecified

✓6ᵗʰ **F12.15** **Cannabis abuse with** psychotic disorder

F12.150 Cannabis abuse with psychotic disorder with delusions

F12.151 Cannabis abuse with psychotic disorder with hallucinations

F12.159 Cannabis abuse with psychotic disorder, unspecified

✓6ᵗʰ **F12.18** **Cannabis abuse with** other cannabis-induced disorder

F12.180 Cannabis abuse with cannabis-induced anxiety disorder

F12.188 Cannabis abuse with other cannabis-induced disorder

F12.19 Cannabis abuse with unspecified cannabis-induced disorder

✓5ᵗʰ **F12.2** **Cannabis** dependence

EXCLUDES 1   cannabis abuse (F12.1-)
cannabis use, unspecified (F12.9-)

EXCLUDES 2   cannabis poisoning (T40.7-)

F12.20 **Cannabis dependence,** uncomplicated

F12.21 **Cannabis dependence,** in remission

✓6ᵗʰ **F12.22** **Cannabis dependence with** intoxication

F12.220 Cannabis dependence with intoxication, uncomplicated

F12.221 Cannabis dependence with intoxication delirium

F12.222 Cannabis dependence with intoxication with perceptual disturbance

F12.229 Cannabis dependence with intoxication, unspecified

✓6ᵗʰ **F12.25** **Cannabis dependence with** psychotic disorder

F12.250 Cannabis dependence with psychotic disorder with delusions

F12.251 Cannabis dependence with psychotic disorder with hallucinations

F12.259 Cannabis dependence with psychotic disorder, unspecified

✓6ᵗʰ **F12.28** **Cannabis dependence with** other cannabis-induced disorder

F12.280 Cannabis dependence with cannabis-induced anxiety disorder

F12.288 Cannabis dependence with other cannabis-induced disorder

F12.29 Cannabis dependence with unspecified cannabis-induced disorder

✓5ᵗʰ **F12.9** **Cannabis use,** unspecified

EXCLUDES 1   cannabis abuse (F12.1-)
cannabis dependence (F12.2-)

F12.90 **Cannabis use, unspecified,** uncomplicated

✓6ᵗʰ **F12.92** **Cannabis use, unspecified with** intoxication

F12.920 Cannabis use, unspecified with intoxication, uncomplicated

F12.921 Cannabis use, unspecified with intoxication delirium

F12.922 Cannabis use, unspecified with intoxication with perceptual disturbance

F12.929 Cannabis use, unspecified with intoxication, unspecified

✓6ᵗʰ **F12.95** **Cannabis use, unspecified with** psychotic disorder

F12.950 Cannabis use, unspecified with psychotic disorder with delusions

F12.951 Cannabis use, unspecified with psychotic disorder with hallucinations

F12.959 Cannabis use, unspecified with psychotic disorder, unspecified

✓6ᵗʰ **F12.98** **Cannabis use, unspecified with** other cannabis-induced disorder

F12.980 Cannabis use, unspecified with anxiety disorder

F12.988 Cannabis use, unspecified with other cannabis-induced disorder

F12.99 Cannabis use, unspecified with unspecified cannabis-induced disorder

✓4ᵗʰ **F13** **Sedative, hypnotic, or anxiolytic** related disorders

✓5ᵗʰ **F13.1** **Sedative, hypnotic or anxiolytic-related** abuse

EXCLUDES 1   sedative, hypnotic or anxiolytic-related dependence (F13.2-)
sedative, hypnotic, or anxiolytic use, unspecified (F13.9-)

F13.10 Sedative, hypnotic or anxiolytic abuse, uncomplicated

✓6ᵗʰ **F13.12** Sedative, hypnotic or anxiolytic abuse with intoxication

F13.120 Sedative, hypnotic or anxiolytic abuse with intoxication, uncomplicated

F13.121 Sedative, hypnotic or anxiolytic abuse with intoxication delirium

F13.129 Sedative, hypnotic or anxiolytic abuse with intoxication, unspecified

F13.14 Sedative, hypnotic or anxiolytic abuse with sedative, hypnotic or anxiolytic-induced mood disorder

✓6ᵗʰ **F13.15** Sedative, hypnotic or anxiolytic abuse with sedative, hypnotic or anxiolytic-induced psychotic disorder

F13.150 Sedative, hypnotic or anxiolytic abuse with sedative, hypnotic or anxiolytic-induced psychotic disorder with delusions

F13.151 Sedative, hypnotic or anxiolytic abuse with sedative, hypnotic or anxiolytic-induced psychotic disorder with hallucinations

F13.159 Sedative, hypnotic or anxiolytic abuse with sedative, hypnotic or anxiolytic-induced psychotic disorder, unspecified

✓6ᵗʰ **F13.18** Sedative, hypnotic or anxiolytic abuse with other sedative, hypnotic or anxiolytic-induced disorders

F13.180 Sedative, hypnotic or anxiolytic abuse with sedative, hypnotic or anxiolytic-induced anxiety disorder

F13.181 Sedative, hypnotic or anxiolytic abuse with sedative, hypnotic or anxiolytic-induced sexual dysfunction

F13.182 Sedative, hypnotic or anxiolytic abuse with sedative, hypnotic or anxiolytic-induced sleep disorder

F13.188 Sedative, hypnotic or anxiolytic abuse with other sedative, hypnotic or anxiolytic-induced disorder

F13.19 Sedative, hypnotic or anxiolytic abuse with unspecified sedative, hypnotic or anxiolytic-induced disorder

✓5ᵗʰ **F13.2** **Sedative, hypnotic or anxiolytic-related** dependence

EXCLUDES 1   sedative, hypnotic or anxiolytic-related abuse (F13.1-)
sedative, hypnotic, or anxiolytic use, unspecified (F13.9-)

EXCLUDES 2   sedative, hypnotic, or anxiolytic poisoning (T42.-)

F13.20 Sedative, hypnotic or anxiolytic dependence, uncomplicated

F13.21 Sedative, hypnotic or anxiolytic dependence, in remission

---

EXCLUDES 1 Not coded here   EXCLUDES 2 Not included here   N Newborn Age: 0   P Pediatric Age: 0–17   M Maternity Age: 12–55   A Adult Age: 15–124

498   ICD-10-CM 2014 (Draft)

√6ᵗʰ **F13.22 Sedative, hypnotic or anxiolytic dependence with intoxication**
> EXCLUDES 1 *sedative, hypnotic or anxiolytic dependence with withdrawal (F13.23-)*

F13.220 Sedative, hypnotic or anxiolytic dependence with intoxication, uncomplicated

F13.221 Sedative, hypnotic or anxiolytic dependence with intoxication delirium

F13.229 Sedative, hypnotic or anxiolytic dependence with intoxication, unspecified

√6ᵗʰ **F13.23 Sedative, hypnotic or anxiolytic dependence with withdrawal**
> EXCLUDES 1 *sedative, hypnotic or anxiolytic dependence with intoxication (F13.22-)*

F13.230 Sedative, hypnotic or anxiolytic dependence with withdrawal, uncomplicated

F13.231 Sedative, hypnotic or anxiolytic dependence with withdrawal delirium

F13.232 Sedative, hypnotic or anxiolytic dependence with withdrawal with perceptual disturbance

F13.239 Sedative, hypnotic or anxiolytic dependence with withdrawal, unspecified

F13.24 Sedative, hypnotic or anxiolytic dependence with sedative, hypnotic or anxiolytic-induced mood disorder

√6ᵗʰ **F13.25 Sedative, hypnotic or anxiolytic dependence with sedative, hypnotic or anxiolytic-induced psychotic disorder**

F13.250 Sedative, hypnotic or anxiolytic dependence with sedative, hypnotic or anxiolytic-induced psychotic disorder with delusions

F13.251 Sedative, hypnotic or anxiolytic dependence with sedative, hypnotic or anxiolytic-induced psychotic disorder with hallucinations

F13.259 Sedative, hypnotic or anxiolytic dependence with sedative, hypnotic or anxiolytic-induced psychotic disorder, unspecified

F13.26 Sedative, hypnotic or anxiolytic dependence with sedative, hypnotic or anxiolytic-induced persisting amnestic disorder

F13.27 Sedative, hypnotic or anxiolytic dependence with sedative, hypnotic or anxiolytic-induced persisting dementia

√6ᵗʰ **F13.28 Sedative, hypnotic or anxiolytic dependence with other sedative, hypnotic or anxiolytic-induced disorders**

F13.280 Sedative, hypnotic or anxiolytic dependence with sedative, hypnotic or anxiolytic-induced anxiety disorder

F13.281 Sedative, hypnotic or anxiolytic dependence with sedative, hypnotic or anxiolytic-induced sexual dysfunction

F13.282 Sedative, hypnotic or anxiolytic dependence with sedative, hypnotic or anxiolytic-induced sleep disorder

F13.288 Sedative, hypnotic or anxiolytic dependence with other sedative, hypnotic or anxiolytic-induced disorder

F13.29 Sedative, hypnotic or anxiolytic dependence with unspecified sedative, hypnotic or anxiolytic-induced disorder

√5ᵗʰ **F13.9 Sedative, hypnotic or anxiolytic-related use, unspecified**
> EXCLUDES 1 *sedative, hypnotic or anxiolytic-related abuse (F13.1-)*
> *sedative, hypnotic or anxiolytic-related dependence (F13.2-)*

F13.90 Sedative, hypnotic, or anxiolytic use, unspecified, uncomplicated

√6ᵗʰ **F13.92 Sedative, hypnotic or anxiolytic use, unspecified with intoxication**
> EXCLUDES 1 *sedative, hypnotic or anxiolytic use, unspecified with withdrawal (F13.93-)*

F13.920 Sedative, hypnotic or anxiolytic use, unspecified with intoxication, uncomplicated

F13.921 Sedative, hypnotic or anxiolytic use, unspecified with intoxication delirium

F13.929 Sedative, hypnotic or anxiolytic use, unspecified with intoxication, unspecified

√6ᵗʰ **F13.93 Sedative, hypnotic or anxiolytic use, unspecified with withdrawal**
> EXCLUDES 1 *sedative, hypnotic or anxiolytic use, unspecified with intoxication (F13.92-)*

F13.930 Sedative, hypnotic or anxiolytic use, unspecified with withdrawal, uncomplicated

F13.931 Sedative, hypnotic or anxiolytic use, unspecified with withdrawal delirium

F13.932 Sedative, hypnotic or anxiolytic use, unspecified with withdrawal with perceptual disturbances

F13.939 Sedative, hypnotic or anxiolytic use, unspecified with withdrawal, unspecified

F13.94 Sedative, hypnotic or anxiolytic use, unspecified with sedative, hypnotic or anxiolytic-induced mood disorder

√6ᵗʰ **F13.95 Sedative, hypnotic or anxiolytic use, unspecified with sedative, hypnotic or anxiolytic-induced psychotic disorder**

F13.950 Sedative, hypnotic or anxiolytic use, unspecified with sedative, hypnotic or anxiolytic-induced psychotic disorder with delusions

F13.951 Sedative, hypnotic or anxiolytic use, unspecified with sedative, hypnotic or anxiolytic-induced psychotic disorder with hallucinations

F13.959 Sedative, hypnotic or anxiolytic use, unspecified with sedative, hypnotic or anxiolytic-induced psychotic disorder, unspecified

F13.96 Sedative, hypnotic or anxiolytic use, unspecified with sedative, hypnotic or anxiolytic-induced persisting amnestic disorder

F13.97 Sedative, hypnotic or anxiolytic use, unspecified with sedative, hypnotic or anxiolytic-induced persisting dementia

√6ᵗʰ **F13.98 Sedative, hypnotic or anxiolytic use, unspecified with other sedative, hypnotic or anxiolytic-induced disorders**

F13.980 Sedative, hypnotic or anxiolytic use, unspecified with sedative, hypnotic or anxiolytic-induced anxiety disorder

F13.981 Sedative, hypnotic or anxiolytic use, unspecified with sedative, hypnotic or anxiolytic-induced sexual dysfunction

F13.982 Sedative, hypnotic or anxiolytic use, unspecified with sedative, hypnotic or anxiolytic-induced sleep disorder

F13.988 Sedative, hypnotic or anxiolytic use, unspecified with other sedative, hypnotic or anxiolytic-induced disorder

F13.99 Sedative, hypnotic or anxiolytic use, unspecified with unspecified sedative, hypnotic or anxiolytic-induced disorder

√4ᵗʰ **F14 Cocaine related disorders**
> EXCLUDES 2 *other stimulant-related disorders (F15.-)*

√5ᵗʰ **F14.1 Cocaine abuse**
> EXCLUDES 1 *cocaine dependence (F14.2-)*
> *cocaine use, unspecified (F14.9-)*

F14.10 Cocaine abuse, uncomplicated

√6ᵗʰ **F14.12 Cocaine abuse with intoxication**

F14.120 Cocaine abuse with intoxication, uncomplicated

F14.121 Cocaine abuse with intoxication with delirium

F14.122 Cocaine abuse with intoxication with perceptual disturbance

F14.129 Cocaine abuse with intoxication, unspecified

F14.14 Cocaine abuse with cocaine-induced mood disorder

☑6ᵗʰ **F14.15** Cocaine abuse with cocaine-induced psychotic disorder

F14.150 Cocaine abuse with cocaine-induced psychotic disorder with delusions

F14.151 Cocaine abuse with cocaine-induced psychotic disorder with hallucinations

F14.159 Cocaine abuse with cocaine-induced psychotic disorder, unspecified

☑6ᵗʰ **F14.18** Cocaine abuse with other cocaine-induced disorder

F14.180 Cocaine abuse with cocaine-induced anxiety disorder

F14.181 Cocaine abuse with cocaine-induced sexual dysfunction

F14.182 Cocaine abuse with cocaine-induced sleep disorder

F14.188 Cocaine abuse with other cocaine-induced disorder

F14.19 Cocaine abuse with unspecified cocaine-induced disorder

☑5ᵗʰ **F14.2** Cocaine dependence
> EXCLUDES 1   cocaine abuse (F14.1-)
>   cocaine use, unspecified (F14.9-)
> EXCLUDES 2   cocaine poisoning (T40.5-)

F14.20 Cocaine dependence, uncomplicated

F14.21 Cocaine dependence, in remission

☑6ᵗʰ **F14.22** Cocaine dependence with intoxication
> EXCLUDES 1   cocaine dependence with withdrawal (F14.23)

F14.220 Cocaine dependence with intoxication, uncomplicated

F14.221 Cocaine dependence with intoxication delirium

F14.222 Cocaine dependence with intoxication with perceptual disturbance

F14.229 Cocaine dependence with intoxication, unspecified

F14.23 Cocaine dependence with withdrawal
> EXCLUDES 1   cocaine dependence with intoxication (F14.22-)

F14.24 Cocaine dependence with cocaine-induced mood disorder

☑6ᵗʰ **F14.25** Cocaine dependence with cocaine-induced psychotic disorder

F14.250 Cocaine dependence with cocaine-induced psychotic disorder with delusions

F14.251 Cocaine dependence with cocaine-induced psychotic disorder with hallucinations

F14.259 Cocaine dependence with cocaine-induced psychotic disorder, unspecified

☑6ᵗʰ **F14.28** Cocaine dependence with other cocaine-induced disorder

F14.280 Cocaine dependence with cocaine-induced anxiety disorder

F14.281 Cocaine dependence with cocaine-induced sexual dysfunction

F14.282 Cocaine dependence with cocaine-induced sleep disorder

F14.288 Cocaine dependence with other cocaine-induced disorder

F14.29 Cocaine dependence with unspecified cocaine-induced disorder

☑5ᵗʰ **F14.9** Cocaine use, unspecified
> EXCLUDES 1   cocaine abuse (F14.1-)
>   cocaine dependence (F14.2-)

F14.90 Cocaine use, unspecified, uncomplicated

☑6ᵗʰ **F14.92** Cocaine use, unspecified with intoxication

F14.920 Cocaine use, unspecified with intoxication, uncomplicated

F14.921 Cocaine use, unspecified with intoxication delirium

F14.922 Cocaine use, unspecified with intoxication with perceptual disturbance

F14.929 Cocaine use, unspecified with intoxication, unspecified

F14.94 Cocaine use, unspecified with cocaine-induced mood disorder

☑6ᵗʰ **F14.95** Cocaine use, unspecified with cocaine-induced psychotic disorder

F14.950 Cocaine use, unspecified with cocaine-induced psychotic disorder with delusions

F14.951 Cocaine use, unspecified with cocaine-induced psychotic disorder with hallucinations

F14.959 Cocaine use, unspecified with cocaine-induced psychotic disorder, unspecified

☑6ᵗʰ **F14.98** Cocaine use, unspecified with other specified cocaine-induced disorder

F14.980 Cocaine use, unspecified with cocaine-induced anxiety disorder

F14.981 Cocaine use, unspecified with cocaine-induced sexual dysfunction

F14.982 Cocaine use, unspecified with cocaine-induced sleep disorder

F14.988 Cocaine use, unspecified with other cocaine-induced disorder

F14.99 Cocaine use, unspecified with unspecified cocaine-induced disorder

☑4ᵗʰ **F15** Other stimulant related disorders
> INCLUDES   amphetamine-related disorders
>   caffeine
> EXCLUDES 2   cocaine-related disorders (F14.-)

☑5ᵗʰ **F15.1** Other stimulant abuse
> EXCLUDES 1   other stimulant dependence (F15.2-)
>   other stimulant use, unspecified (F15.9-)

F15.10 Other stimulant abuse, uncomplicated

☑6ᵗʰ **F15.12** Other stimulant abuse with intoxication

F15.120 Other stimulant abuse with intoxication, uncomplicated

F15.121 Other stimulant abuse with intoxication delirium

F15.122 Other stimulant abuse with intoxication with perceptual disturbance

F15.129 Other stimulant abuse with intoxication, unspecified

F15.14 Other stimulant abuse with stimulant-induced mood disorder

☑6ᵗʰ **F15.15** Other stimulant abuse with stimulant-induced psychotic disorder

F15.150 Other stimulant abuse with stimulant-induced psychotic disorder with delusions

F15.151 Other stimulant abuse with stimulant-induced psychotic disorder with hallucinations

F15.159 Other stimulant abuse with stimulant-induced psychotic disorder, unspecified

☑6ᵗʰ **F15.18** Other stimulant abuse with other stimulant-induced disorder

F15.180 Other stimulant abuse with stimulant-induced anxiety disorder

F15.181 Other stimulant abuse with stimulant-induced sexual dysfunction

F15.182 Other stimulant abuse with stimulant-induced sleep disorder

F15.188 Other stimulant abuse with other stimulant-induced disorder

F15.19 Other stimulant abuse with unspecified stimulant-induced disorder

☑5ᵗʰ **F15.2** Other stimulant dependence
> EXCLUDES 1   other stimulant abuse (F15.1-)
>   other stimulant use, unspecified (F15.9-)

F15.20 Other stimulant dependence, uncomplicated

F15.21 Other stimulant dependence, in remission

EXCLUDES 1 Not coded here   EXCLUDES 2 Not included here   N Newborn Age: 0   P Pediatric Age: 0-17   M Maternity Age: 12-55   A Adult Age: 15-124

500   ICD-10-CM 2014 (Draft)

✓6th **F15.22 Other stimulant dependence with** intoxication
EXCLUDES1 *other stimulant dependence with withdrawal (F15.23)*

F15.220 Other stimulant dependence with intoxication, uncomplicated

F15.221 Other stimulant dependence with intoxication delirium

F15.222 Other stimulant dependence with intoxication with perceptual disturbance

F15.229 Other stimulant dependence with intoxication, unspecified

F15.23 Other stimulant dependence with withdrawal
EXCLUDES1 *other stimulant dependence with intoxication (F15.22-)*

F15.24 Other stimulant dependence with stimulant-induced mood disorder

✓6th **F15.25 Other stimulant dependence with stimulant-induced** psychotic disorder

F15.250 Other stimulant dependence with stimulant-induced psychotic disorder with delusions

F15.251 Other stimulant dependence with stimulant-induced psychotic disorder with hallucinations

F15.259 Other stimulant dependence with stimulant-induced psychotic disorder, unspecified

✓6th **F15.28 Other stimulant dependence with** other stimulant-induced disorder

F15.280 Other stimulant dependence with stimulant-induced anxiety disorder

F15.281 Other stimulant dependence with stimulant-induced sexual dysfunction

F15.282 Other stimulant dependence with stimulant-induced sleep disorder

F15.288 Other stimulant dependence with other stimulant-induced disorder

F15.29 Other stimulant dependence with unspecified stimulant-induced disorder

✓5th **F15.9 Other stimulant use,** unspecified
EXCLUDES1 *other stimulant abuse (F15.1-)*
other stimulant dependence (F15.2-)

F15.90 Other stimulant use, unspecified, uncomplicated

✓6th **F15.92 Other stimulant use, unspecified** with intoxication
EXCLUDES1 *other stimulant use, unspecified with withdrawal (F15.93)*

F15.920 Other stimulant use, unspecified with intoxication, uncomplicated

F15.921 Other stimulant use, unspecified with intoxication delirium

F15.922 Other stimulant use, unspecified with intoxication with perceptual disturbance

F15.929 Other stimulant use, unspecified with intoxication, unspecified

F15.93 Other stimulant use, unspecified with withdrawal
EXCLUDES1 *other stimulant use, unspecified with intoxication (F15.92-)*

F15.94 Other stimulant use, unspecified with stimulant-induced mood disorder

✓6th **F15.95 Other stimulant use, unspecified with stimulant-induced** psychotic disorder

F15.950 Other stimulant use, unspecified with stimulant-induced psychotic disorder with delusions

F15.951 Other stimulant use, unspecified with stimulant-induced psychotic disorder with hallucinations

F15.959 Other stimulant use, unspecified with stimulant-induced psychotic disorder, unspecified

✓6th **F15.98 Other stimulant use, unspecified with** other stimulant-induced disorder

F15.980 Other stimulant use, unspecified with stimulant-induced anxiety disorder

F15.981 Other stimulant use, unspecified with stimulant-induced sexual dysfunction

F15.982 Other stimulant use, unspecified with stimulant-induced sleep disorder

F15.988 Other stimulant use, unspecified with other stimulant-induced disorder

F15.99 Other stimulant use, unspecified with unspecified stimulant-induced disorder

✓4th **F16 Hallucinogen related disorders**
INCLUDES ecstasy
PCP
phencyclidine

✓5th **F16.1 Hallucinogen** abuse
EXCLUDES1 *hallucinogen dependence (F16.2-)*
hallucinogen use, unspecified (F16.9-)

F16.10 Hallucinogen abuse, uncomplicated

✓6th **F16.12 Hallucinogen abuse with** intoxication

F16.120 Hallucinogen abuse with intoxication, uncomplicated

F16.121 Hallucinogen abuse with intoxication with delirium

F16.122 Hallucinogen abuse with intoxication with perceptual disturbance

F16.129 Hallucinogen abuse with intoxication, unspecified

F16.14 Hallucinogen abuse with hallucinogen-induced mood disorder

✓6th **F16.15 Hallucinogen abuse with hallucinogen-induced** psychotic disorder

F16.150 Hallucinogen abuse with hallucinogen-induced psychotic disorder with delusions

F16.151 Hallucinogen abuse with hallucinogen-induced psychotic disorder with hallucinations

F16.159 Hallucinogen abuse with hallucinogen-induced psychotic disorder, unspecified

✓6th **F16.18 Hallucinogen abuse with** other hallucinogen-induced disorder

F16.180 Hallucinogen abuse with hallucinogen-induced anxiety disorder

F16.183 Hallucinogen abuse with hallucinogen persisting perception disorder (flashbacks)

F16.188 Hallucinogen abuse with other hallucinogen-induced disorder

F16.19 Hallucinogen abuse with unspecified hallucinogen-induced disorder

✓5th **F16.2 Hallucinogen** dependence
EXCLUDES1 *hallucinogen abuse (F16.1-)*
hallucinogen use, unspecified (F16.9-)

F16.20 Hallucinogen dependence, uncomplicated

F16.21 Hallucinogen dependence, in remission

✓6th **F16.22 Hallucinogen dependence with** intoxication

F16.220 Hallucinogen dependence with intoxication, uncomplicated

F16.221 Hallucinogen dependence with intoxication with delirium

F16.229 Hallucinogen dependence with intoxication, unspecified

F16.24 Hallucinogen dependence with hallucinogen-induced mood disorder

✓6th **F16.25 Hallucinogen dependence with hallucinogen-induced** psychotic disorder

F16.250 Hallucinogen dependence with hallucinogen-induced psychotic disorder with delusions

F16.251 Hallucinogen dependence with hallucinogen-induced psychotic disorder with hallucinations

F16.259 Hallucinogen dependence with hallucinogen-induced psychotic disorder, unspecified

✓6th **F16.28 Hallucinogen dependence with** other hallucinogen-induced disorder

F16.280 Hallucinogen dependence with hallucinogen-induced anxiety disorder

F16.283 Hallucinogen dependence with hallucinogen persisting perception disorder (flashbacks)

Mental, Behavioral, and Neurodevelopmental Disorders

F16.288–F18.27

F16.288 Hallucinogen dependence with other hallucinogen-induced disorder

F16.29 Hallucinogen dependence with unspecified hallucinogen-induced disorder

✓5th **F16.9** Hallucinogen use, unspecified
> EXCLUDES 1   hallucinogen abuse (F16.1-)
> hallucinogen dependence (F16.2-)

F16.90 Hallucinogen use, unspecified, uncomplicated

✓6th **F16.92** Hallucinogen use, unspecified with intoxication

F16.920 Hallucinogen use, unspecified with intoxication, uncomplicated

F16.921 Hallucinogen use, unspecified with intoxication with delirium

F16.929 Hallucinogen use, unspecified with intoxication, unspecified

F16.94 Hallucinogen use, unspecified with hallucinogen-induced mood disorder

✓6th **F16.95** Hallucinogen use, unspecified with hallucinogen-induced psychotic disorder

F16.950 Hallucinogen use, unspecified with hallucinogen-induced psychotic disorder with delusions

F16.951 Hallucinogen use, unspecified with hallucinogen-induced psychotic disorder with hallucinations

F16.959 Hallucinogen use, unspecified with hallucinogen-induced psychotic disorder, unspecified

✓6th **F16.98** Hallucinogen use, unspecified with other specified hallucinogen-induced disorder

F16.980 Hallucinogen use, unspecified with hallucinogen-induced anxiety disorder

F16.983 Hallucinogen use, unspecified with hallucinogen persisting perception disorder (flashbacks)

F16.988 Hallucinogen use, unspecified with other hallucinogen-induced disorder

F16.99 Hallucinogen use, unspecified with unspecified hallucinogen-induced disorder

✓4th **F17** Nicotine dependence
> EXCLUDES 1   history of tobacco dependence (Z87.891)
> tobacco use NOS (Z72.0)
> EXCLUDES 2   tobacco use (smoking) during pregnancy, childbirth and the puerperium (O99.33-)
> toxic effect of nicotine (T65.2-)

✓5th **F17.2** Nicotine dependence

✓6th **F17.20** Nicotine dependence, unspecified

F17.200 Nicotine dependence, unspecified, uncomplicated

F17.201 Nicotine dependence, unspecified, in remission

F17.203 Nicotine dependence unspecified, with withdrawal

F17.208 Nicotine dependence, unspecified, with other nicotine-induced disorders

F17.209 Nicotine dependence, unspecified, with unspecified nicotine-induced disorders

✓6th **F17.21** Nicotine dependence, cigarettes

F17.210 Nicotine dependence, cigarettes, uncomplicated

F17.211 Nicotine dependence, cigarettes, in remission

F17.213 Nicotine dependence, cigarettes, with withdrawal

F17.218 Nicotine dependence, cigarettes, with other nicotine-induced disorders

F17.219 Nicotine dependence, cigarettes, with unspecified nicotine-induced disorders

✓6th **F17.22** Nicotine dependence, chewing tobacco

F17.220 Nicotine dependence, chewing tobacco, uncomplicated

F17.221 Nicotine dependence, chewing tobacco, in remission

F17.223 Nicotine dependence, chewing tobacco, with withdrawal

F17.228 Nicotine dependence, chewing tobacco, with other nicotine-induced disorders

F17.229 Nicotine dependence, chewing tobacco, with unspecified nicotine-induced disorders

✓6th **F17.29** Nicotine dependence, other tobacco product

F17.290 Nicotine dependence, other tobacco product, uncomplicated

F17.291 Nicotine dependence, other tobacco product, in remission

F17.293 Nicotine dependence, other tobacco product, with withdrawal

F17.298 Nicotine dependence, other tobacco product, with other nicotine-induced disorders

F17.299 Nicotine dependence, other tobacco product, with unspecified nicotine-induced disorders

✓4th **F18** Inhalant related disorders
> INCLUDES   volatile solvents

✓5th **F18.1** Inhalant abuse
> EXCLUDES 1   inhalant dependence (F18.2-)
> inhalant use, unspecified (F18.9-)

F18.10 Inhalant abuse, uncomplicated

✓6th **F18.12** Inhalant abuse with intoxication

F18.120 Inhalant abuse with intoxication, uncomplicated

F18.121 Inhalant abuse with intoxication delirium

F18.129 Inhalant abuse with intoxication, unspecified

F18.14 Inhalant abuse with inhalant-induced mood disorder

✓6th **F18.15** Inhalant abuse with inhalant-induced psychotic disorder

F18.150 Inhalant abuse with inhalant-induced psychotic disorder with delusions

F18.151 Inhalant abuse with inhalant-induced psychotic disorder with hallucinations

F18.159 Inhalant abuse with inhalant-induced psychotic disorder, unspecified

F18.17 Inhalant abuse with inhalant-induced dementia

✓6th **F18.18** Inhalant abuse with other inhalant-induced disorders

F18.180 Inhalant abuse with inhalant-induced anxiety disorder

F18.188 Inhalant abuse with other inhalant-induced disorder

F18.19 Inhalant abuse with unspecified inhalant-induced disorder

✓5th **F18.2** Inhalant dependence
> EXCLUDES 1   inhalant abuse (F18.1-)
> inhalant use, unspecified (F18.9-)

F18.20 Inhalant dependence, uncomplicated

F18.21 Inhalant dependence, in remission

✓6th **F18.22** Inhalant dependence with intoxication

F18.220 Inhalant dependence with intoxication, uncomplicated

F18.221 Inhalant dependence with intoxication delirium

F18.229 Inhalant dependence with intoxication, unspecified

F18.24 Inhalant dependence with inhalant-induced mood disorder

✓6th **F18.25** Inhalant dependence with inhalant-induced psychotic disorder

F18.250 Inhalant dependence with inhalant-induced psychotic disorder with delusions

F18.251 Inhalant dependence with inhalant-induced psychotic disorder with hallucinations

F18.259 Inhalant dependence with inhalant-induced psychotic disorder, unspecified

F18.27 Inhalant dependence with inhalant-induced dementia

EXCLUDES 1 Not coded here   EXCLUDES 2 Not included here   N Newborn Age: 0   P Pediatric Age: 0-17   M Maternity Age: 12-55   A Adult Age: 15-124

502   ICD-10-CM 2014 (Draft)

✓6th **F18.28 Inhalant dependence with** other **inhalant-induced disorders**

F18.280 **Inhalant dependence with inhalant-induced** anxiety disorder

F18.288 **Inhalant dependence with other inhalant-induced disorder**

F18.29 **Inhalant dependence with unspecified inhalant-induced disorder**

✓5th **F18.9 Inhalant use,** unspecified

EXCLUDES1 *inhalant abuse (F18.1-)*
inhalant dependence (F18.2-)

F18.90 **Inhalant use, unspecified,** uncomplicated

✓6th **F18.92 Inhalant use, unspecified with** intoxication

F18.920 **Inhalant use, unspecified with intoxication,** uncomplicated

F18.921 **Inhalant use, unspecified with intoxication with** delirium

F18.929 **Inhalant use, unspecified with intoxication,** unspecified

F18.94 **Inhalant use, unspecified with inhalant-induced** mood disorder

✓6th **F18.95 Inhalant use, unspecified with inhalant-induced** psychotic disorder

F18.950 **Inhalant use, unspecified with inhalant-induced psychotic disorder** with delusions

F18.951 **Inhalant use, unspecified with inhalant-induced psychotic disorder with** hallucinations

F18.959 **Inhalant use, unspecified with inhalant-induced psychotic disorder, unspecified**

F18.97 **Inhalant use, unspecified with inhalant-induced** persisting dementia

✓6th **F18.98 Inhalant use, unspecified with** other **inhalant-induced disorders**

F18.980 **Inhalant use, unspecified with inhalant-induced** anxiety disorder

F18.988 **Inhalant use, unspecified with other inhalant-induced disorder**

F18.99 **Inhalant use, unspecified with unspecified inhalant-induced disorder**

✓4th **F19 Other psychoactive substance related disorders**

INCLUDES polysubstance drug use (indiscriminate drug use)

✓5th **F19.1 Other psychoactive substance** abuse

EXCLUDES1 *other psychoactive substance dependence (F19.2-)*
other psychoactive substance use, unspecified (F19.9-)

F19.10 **Other psychoactive substance abuse,** uncomplicated

✓6th **F19.12 Other psychoactive substance abuse with** intoxication

F19.120 **Other psychoactive substance abuse with intoxication,** uncomplicated

F19.121 **Other psychoactive substance abuse with intoxication** delirium

F19.122 **Other psychoactive substance abuse with intoxication with** perceptual disturbances

F19.129 **Other psychoactive substance abuse with intoxication, unspecified**

F19.14 **Other psychoactive substance abuse with psychoactive substance-induced** mood disorder

✓6th **F19.15 Other psychoactive substance abuse with psychoactive substance-induced** psychotic disorder

F19.150 **Other psychoactive substance abuse with psychoactive substance-induced psychotic disorder with** delusions

F19.151 **Other psychoactive substance abuse with psychoactive substance-induced psychotic disorder with** hallucinations

F19.159 **Other psychoactive substance abuse with psychoactive substance-induced psychotic disorder, unspecified**

F19.16 **Other psychoactive substance abuse with psychoactive substance-induced** persisting amnestic disorder

F19.17 **Other psychoactive substance abuse with psychoactive substance-induced** persisting dementia

✓6th **F19.18 Other psychoactive substance abuse with** other **psychoactive substance-induced disorders**

F19.180 **Other psychoactive substance abuse with psychoactive substance-induced** anxiety disorder

F19.181 **Other psychoactive substance abuse with psychoactive substance-induced** sexual dysfunction

F19.182 **Other psychoactive substance abuse with psychoactive substance-induced** sleep disorder

F19.188 **Other psychoactive substance abuse with other psychoactive substance-induced disorder**

F19.19 **Other psychoactive substance abuse with unspecified psychoactive substance-induced disorder**

✓5th **F19.2 Other psychoactive substance** dependence

EXCLUDES1 *other psychoactive substance abuse (F19.1-)*
other psychoactive substance use, unspecified (F19.9-)

F19.20 **Other psychoactive substance dependence,** uncomplicated

F19.21 **Other psychoactive substance dependence,** in remission

✓6th **F19.22 Other psychoactive substance dependence with** intoxication

EXCLUDES1 *other psychoactive substance dependence with withdrawal (F19.23-)*

F19.220 **Other psychoactive substance dependence with intoxication,** uncomplicated

F19.221 **Other psychoactive substance dependence with intoxication** delirium

F19.222 **Other psychoactive substance dependence with intoxication with** perceptual disturbance

F19.229 **Other psychoactive substance dependence with intoxication, unspecified**

✓6th **F19.23 Other psychoactive substance dependence with** withdrawal

EXCLUDES1 *other psychoactive substance dependence with intoxication (F19.22-)*

F19.230 **Other psychoactive substance dependence with withdrawal,** uncomplicated

F19.231 **Other psychoactive substance dependence with withdrawal** delirium

F19.232 **Other psychoactive substance dependence with withdrawal with** perceptual disturbance

F19.239 **Other psychoactive substance dependence with withdrawal, unspecified**

F19.24 **Other psychoactive substance dependence with psychoactive substance-induced** mood disorder

✓6th **F19.25 Other psychoactive substance dependence with psychoactive substance-induced** psychotic disorder

F19.250 **Other psychoactive substance dependence with psychoactive substance-induced psychotic disorder with** delusions

F19.251 **Other psychoactive substance dependence with psychoactive substance-induced psychotic disorder with** hallucinations

F19.259 **Other psychoactive substance dependence with psychoactive substance-induced psychotic disorder, unspecified**

F19.26 **Other psychoactive substance dependence with psychoactive substance-induced** persisting amnestic disorder

F19.27 **Other psychoactive substance dependence with psychoactive substance-induced** persisting dementia

✓6th **F19.28 Other psychoactive substance dependence with** other **psychoactive substance-induced disorders**

F19.280 **Other psychoactive substance dependence with psychoactive substance-induced** anxiety disorder

Mental, Behavioral, and Neurodevelopmental Disorders

F18.28–F19.280

F19.281 Other psychoactive substance dependence with psychoactive substance-induced sexual dysfunction

F19.282 Other psychoactive substance dependence with psychoactive substance-induced sleep disorder

F19.288 Other psychoactive substance dependence with other psychoactive substance-induced disorder

F19.29 Other psychoactive substance dependence with unspecified psychoactive substance-induced disorder

√5th **F19.9** Other psychoactive substance use, unspecified
> EXCLUDES 1   other psychoactive substance abuse (F19.1-)
> other psychoactive substance dependence (F19.2-)

F19.90 Other psychoactive substance use, unspecified, uncomplicated

√6th **F19.92** Other psychoactive substance use, unspecified with intoxication
> EXCLUDES 1   other psychoactive substance use, unspecified with withdrawal (F19.93)

F19.920 Other psychoactive substance use, unspecified with intoxication, uncomplicated

F19.921 Other psychoactive substance use, unspecified with intoxication with delirium

F19.922 Other psychoactive substance use, unspecified with intoxication with perceptual disturbance

F19.929 Other psychoactive substance use, unspecified with intoxication, unspecified

√6th **F19.93** Other psychoactive substance use, unspecified with withdrawal
> EXCLUDES 1   other psychoactive substance use, unspecified with intoxication (F19.92-)

F19.930 Other psychoactive substance use, unspecified with withdrawal, uncomplicated

F19.931 Other psychoactive substance use, unspecified with withdrawal delirium

F19.932 Other psychoactive substance use, unspecified with withdrawal with perceptual disturbance

F19.939 Other psychoactive substance use, unspecified with withdrawal, unspecified

F19.94 Other psychoactive substance use, unspecified with psychoactive substance-induced mood disorder

√6th **F19.95** Other psychoactive substance use, unspecified with psychoactive substance-induced psychotic disorder

F19.950 Other psychoactive substance use, unspecified with psychoactive substance-induced psychotic disorder with delusions

F19.951 Other psychoactive substance use, unspecified with psychoactive substance-induced psychotic disorder with hallucinations

F19.959 Other psychoactive substance use, unspecified with psychoactive substance-induced psychotic disorder, unspecified

F19.96 Other psychoactive substance use, unspecified with psychoactive substance-induced persisting amnestic disorder

F19.97 Other psychoactive substance use, unspecified with psychoactive substance-induced persisting dementia

√6th **F19.98** Other psychoactive substance use, unspecified with other psychoactive substance-induced disorders

F19.980 Other psychoactive substance use, unspecified with psychoactive substance-induced anxiety disorder

F19.981 Other psychoactive substance use, unspecified with psychoactive substance-induced sexual dysfunction

F19.982 Other psychoactive substance use, unspecified with psychoactive substance-induced sleep disorder

F19.988 Other psychoactive substance use, unspecified with other psychoactive substance-induced disorder

F19.99 Other psychoactive substance use, unspecified with unspecified psychoactive substance-induced disorder

Schizophrenia, schizotypal, delusional, and other non-mood psychotic disorders (F20-F29)

√4th **F20** Schizophrenia
> EXCLUDES 1   brief psychotic disorder (F23)
> cyclic schizophrenia (F25.0)
> mood [affective] disorders with psychotic symptoms (F30.2, F31.2, F31.5, F31.64, F32.3, F33.3)
> schizoaffective disorder (F25.-)
> schizophrenic reaction NOS (F23)
> EXCLUDES 2   schizophrenic reaction in:
> alcoholism (F10.15-, F10.25-, F10.95-)
> brain disease (F06.2)
> epilepsy (F06.2)
> psychoactive drug use (F11-F19 with .15, .25, .95)
> schizotypal disorder (F21)

F20.0 Paranoid schizophrenia
Paraphrenic schizophrenia
> EXCLUDES 1   involutional paranoid state (F22)
> paranoia (F22)

F20.1 Disorganized schizophrenia
Hebephrenic schizophrenia
Hebephrenia

F20.2 Catatonic schizophrenia
Schizophrenic catalepsy
Schizophrenic catatonia
Schizophrenic flexibilitas cerea
> EXCLUDES 1   catatonic stupor (R40.1)

F20.3 Undifferentiated schizophrenia
Atypical schizophrenia
> EXCLUDES 1   acute schizophrenia-like psychotic disorder (F23)
> EXCLUDES 2   post-schizophrenic depression (F32.8)

F20.5 Residual schizophrenia
Restzustand (schizophrenic)
Schizophrenic residual state

√5th **F20.8** Other schizophrenia

F20.81 Schizophreniform disorder
Schizophreniform psychosis NOS

F20.89 Other schizophrenia
Cenesthopathic schizophrenia
Simple schizophrenia

F20.9 Schizophrenia, unspecified

F21 Schizotypal disorder
Borderline schizophrenia
Latent schizophrenia
Latent schizophrenic reaction
Prepsychotic schizophrenia
Prodromal schizophrenia
Pseudoneurotic schizophrenia
Pseudopsychopathic schizophrenia
Schizotypal personality disorder
> EXCLUDES 2   Asperger's syndrome (F84.5)
> schizoid personality disorder (F60.1)

F22 Delusional disorders
Delusional dysmorphophobia
Involutional paranoid state
Paranoia
Paranoia querulans
Paranoid psychosis
Paranoid state
Paraphrenia (late)
Sensitiver Beziehungswahn
> EXCLUDES 1   mood [affective] disorders with psychotic symptoms (F30.2, F31.2, F31.5, F31.64, F32.3, F33.3)
> paranoid schizophrenia (F20.0)
> EXCLUDES 2   paranoid personality disorder (F60.0)
> paranoid psychosis, psychogenic (F23)
> paranoid reaction (F23)

F23 Brief psychotic disorder
Paranoid reaction
Psychogenic paranoid psychosis
> EXCLUDES 2   mood [affective] disorders with psychotic symptoms (F30.2, F31.2, F31.5, F31.64, F32.3, F33.3)

F24 Shared psychotic disorder
Folie à deux
Induced paranoid disorder
Induced psychotic disorder

EXCLUDES 1 Not coded here   EXCLUDES 2 Not included here   N Newborn Age: 0   P Pediatric Age: 0-17   M Maternity Age: 12-55   A Adult Age: 15-124

504   ICD-10-CM 2014 (Draft)

☑️4th F25 Schizoaffective disorders

> **EXCLUDES 1** *mood [affective] disorders with psychotic symptoms (F30.2, F31.2, F31.5, F31.64, F32.3, F33.3)*
> *schizophrenia (F20.-)*

F25.0 Schizoaffective disorder, bipolar type
Cyclic schizophrenia
Schizoaffective disorder, manic type
Schizoaffective disorder, mixed type
Schizoaffective psychosis, bipolar type
Schizophreniform psychosis, manic type

F25.1 Schizoaffective disorder, depressive type
Schizoaffective psychosis, depressive type
Schizophreniform psychosis, depressive type

F25.8 Other schizoaffective disorders

F25.9 Schizoaffective disorder, unspecified
Schizoaffective psychosis NOS

F28 Other psychotic disorder not due to a substance or known physiological condition
Chronic hallucinatory psychosis

F29 Unspecified psychosis not due to a substance or known physiological condition
Psychosis NOS

> **EXCLUDES 1** *mental disorder NOS (F99)*
> *unspecified mental disorder due to known physiological condition (F09)*

Mood [affective] disorders (F30-F39)

☑️4th F30 Manic episode

> **INCLUDES** bipolar disorder, single manic episode
> mixed affective episode

> **EXCLUDES 1** *bipolar disorder (F31.-)*
> *major depressive disorder, single episode (F32.-)*
> *major depressive disorder, recurrent (F33.-)*

☑️5th F30.1 Manic episode without psychotic symptoms

     F30.10 Manic episode without psychotic symptoms, unspecified

     F30.11 Manic episode without psychotic symptoms, mild

     F30.12 Manic episode without psychotic symptoms, moderate

     F30.13 Manic episode, severe, without psychotic symptoms

F30.2 Manic episode, severe with psychotic symptoms
Manic stupor
Mania with mood-congruent psychotic symptoms
Mania with mood-incongruent psychotic symptoms

F30.3 Manic episode in partial remission

F30.4 Manic episode in full remission

F30.8 Other manic episodes
Hypomania

F30.9 Manic episode, unspecified
Mania NOS

☑️4th F31 Bipolar disorder

> **INCLUDES** manic-depressive illness
> manic-depressive psychosis
> manic-depressive reaction

> **EXCLUDES 1** *bipolar disorder, single manic episode (F30.-)*
> *major depressive disorder, single episode (F32.-)*
> *major depressive disorder, recurrent (F33.-)*

> **EXCLUDES 2** *cyclothymia (F34.0)*

F31.0 Bipolar disorder, current episode hypomanic

☑️5th F31.1 Bipolar disorder, current episode manic without psychotic features

     F31.10 Bipolar disorder, current episode manic without psychotic features, unspecified

     F31.11 Bipolar disorder, current episode manic without psychotic features, mild

     F31.12 Bipolar disorder, current episode manic without psychotic features, moderate

     F31.13 Bipolar disorder, current episode manic without psychotic features, severe

F31.2 Bipolar disorder, current episode manic severe with psychotic features
Bipolar disorder, current episode manic with mood-congruent psychotic symptoms
Bipolar disorder, current episode manic with mood-incongruent psychotic symptoms

☑️5th F31.3 Bipolar disorder, current episode depressed, mild or moderate severity

     F31.30 Bipolar disorder, current episode depressed, mild or moderate severity, unspecified

     F31.31 Bipolar disorder, current episode depressed, mild

     F31.32 Bipolar disorder, current episode depressed, moderate

F31.4 Bipolar disorder, current episode depressed, severe, without psychotic features

F31.5 Bipolar disorder, current episode depressed, severe, with psychotic features
Bipolar disorder, current episode depressed with mood-incongruent psychotic symptoms
Bipolar disorder, current episode depressed with mood-congruent psychotic symptoms

☑️5th F31.6 Bipolar disorder, current episode mixed

     F31.60 Bipolar disorder, current episode mixed, unspecified

     F31.61 Bipolar disorder, current episode mixed, mild

     F31.62 Bipolar disorder, current episode mixed, moderate

     F31.63 Bipolar disorder, current episode mixed, severe, without psychotic features

     F31.64 Bipolar disorder, current episode mixed, severe, with psychotic features
Bipolar disorder, current episode mixed with mood-congruent psychotic symptoms
Bipolar disorder, current episode mixed with mood-incongruent psychotic symptoms

☑️5th F31.7 Bipolar disorder, currently in remission

     F31.70 Bipolar disorder, currently in remission, most recent episode unspecified

     F31.71 Bipolar disorder, in partial remission, most recent episode hypomanic

     F31.72 Bipolar disorder, in full remission, most recent episode hypomanic

     F31.73 Bipolar disorder, in partial remission, most recent episode manic

     F31.74 Bipolar disorder, in full remission, most recent episode manic

     F31.75 Bipolar disorder, in partial remission, most recent episode depressed

     F31.76 Bipolar disorder, in full remission, most recent episode depressed

     F31.77 Bipolar disorder, in partial remission, most recent episode mixed

     F31.78 Bipolar disorder, in full remission, most recent episode mixed

☑️5th F31.8 Other bipolar disorders

     F31.81 Bipolar II disorder

     F31.89 Other bipolar disorder
Recurrent manic episodes NOS

F31.9 Bipolar disorder, unspecified

☑️4th F32 Major depressive disorder, single episode

> **INCLUDES** single episode of agitated depression
> single episode of depressive reaction
> single episode of major depression
> single episode of psychogenic depression
> single episode of reactive depression
> single episode of vital depression

> **EXCLUDES 1** *bipolar disorder (F31.-)*
> *manic episode (F30.-)*
> *recurrent depressive disorder (F33.-)*

> **EXCLUDES 2** *adjustment disorder (F43.2)*

F32.0 Major depressive disorder, single episode, mild

F32.1 Major depressive disorder, single episode, moderate

F32.2 Major depressive disorder, single episode, severe without psychotic features

F32.3 Major depressive disorder, single episode, severe with psychotic features
Single episode of major depression with mood-congruent psychotic symptoms
Single episode of major depression with mood-incongruent psychotic symptoms
Single episode of major depression with psychotic symptoms
Single episode of psychogenic depressive psychosis
Single episode of psychotic depression
Single episode of reactive depressive psychosis

F32.4 Major depressive disorder, single episode, in partial remission

☑️ Additional Character Required   ✓x7th Xtension Alert   Unspecified Code   Other Specified Code   Manifestation Code   ▶◀ Revised Text   ● New Code   ▲ Revised Code Title

ICD-10-CM 2014 (Draft)   **505**

Mental, Behavioral, and Neurodevelopmental Disorders

F32.5–F43.0

F32.5 Major depressive disorder, single episode, in full remission

F32.8 Other depressive episodes
Atypical depression
Post-schizophrenic depression
Single episode of 'masked' depression NOS

F32.9 Major depressive disorder, single episode, unspecified
Depression NOS
Depressive disorder NOS
Major depression NOS

✓4th **F33** Major depressive disorder, recurrent
Recurrent episodes of depressive reaction
Recurrent episodes of endogenous depression
Recurrent episodes of major depression
Recurrent episodes of psychogenic depression
Recurrent episodes of reactive depression
Recurrent episodes of seasonal depressive disorder
Recurrent episodes of vital depression
EXCLUDES 1 bipolar disorder (F31.-)
manic episode (F30.-)

F33.0 Major depressive disorder, recurrent, mild

F33.1 Major depressive disorder, recurrent, moderate

F33.2 Major depressive disorder, recurrent, severe without psychotic features

F33.3 Major depressive disorder, recurrent, severe with psychotic symptoms
Endogenous depression with psychotic symptoms
Recurrent severe episodes of major depression with mood-congruent psychotic symptoms
Recurrent severe episodes of major depression with mood-incongruent psychotic symptoms
Recurrent severe episodes of major depression with psychotic symptoms
Recurrent severe episodes of psychogenic depressive psychosis
Recurrent severe episodes of psychotic depression
Recurrent severe episodes of reactive depressive psychosis

✓5th **F33.4** Major depressive disorder, recurrent, in remission

F33.40 Major depressive disorder, recurrent, in remission, unspecified

F33.41 Major depressive disorder, recurrent, in partial remission

F33.42 Major depressive disorder, recurrent, in full remission

F33.8 Other recurrent depressive disorders
Recurrent brief depressive episodes

F33.9 Major depressive disorder, recurrent, unspecified
Monopolar depression NOS

✓4th **F34** Persistent mood [affective] disorders

F34.0 Cyclothymic disorder
Affective personality disorder
Cycloid personality
Cyclothymia
Cyclothymic personality

F34.1 Dysthymic disorder
Depressive neurosis
Depressive personality disorder
Dysthymia
Neurotic depression
Persistent anxiety depression
EXCLUDES 2 anxiety depression (mild or not persistent) (F41.8)

F34.8 Other persistent mood [affective] disorders

F34.9 Persistent mood [affective] disorder, unspecified

F39 Unspecified mood [affective] disorder
Affective psychosis NOS

Anxiety, dissociative, stress-related, somatoform and other nonpsychotic mental disorders (F40-F48)

✓4th **F40** Phobic anxiety disorders

✓5th **F40.0** Agoraphobia

F40.00 Agoraphobia, unspecified

F40.01 Agoraphobia with panic disorder
Panic disorder with agoraphobia
EXCLUDES 1 panic disorder without agoraphobia (F41.0)

F40.02 Agoraphobia without panic disorder

✓5th **F40.1** Social phobias
Anthropophobia
Social anxiety disorder of childhood
Social neurosis

F40.10 Social phobia, unspecified

F40.11 Social phobia, generalized

✓5th **F40.2** Specific (isolated) phobias
EXCLUDES 2 dysmorphophobia (nondelusional) (F45.22)
nosophobia (F45.22)

✓6th **F40.21** Animal type phobia

F40.210 Arachnophobia
Fear of spiders

F40.218 Other animal type phobia

✓6th **F40.22** Natural environment type phobia

F40.220 Fear of thunderstorms

F40.228 Other natural environment type phobia

✓6th **F40.23** Blood, injection, injury type phobia

F40.230 Fear of blood

F40.231 Fear of injections and transfusions

F40.232 Fear of other medical care

F40.233 Fear of injury

✓6th **F40.24** Situational type phobia

F40.240 Claustrophobia

F40.241 Acrophobia

F40.242 Fear of bridges

F40.243 Fear of flying

F40.248 Other situational type phobia

✓6th **F40.29** Other specified phobia

F40.290 Androphobia
Fear of men

F40.291 Gynephobia
Fear of women

F40.298 Other specified phobia

F40.8 Other phobic anxiety disorders
Phobic anxiety disorder of childhood

F40.9 Phobic anxiety disorder, unspecified
Phobia NOS
Phobic state NOS

✓4th **F41** Other anxiety disorders
EXCLUDES 2 anxiety in:
acute stress reaction (F43.0)
transient adjustment reaction (F43.2)
neurasthenia (F48.8)
psychophysiologic disorders (F45.-)
separation anxiety (F93.0)

F41.0 Panic disorder [episodic paroxysmal anxiety] without agoraphobia
Panic attack   Panic state
EXCLUDES 1 panic disorder with agoraphobia (F40.01)

F41.1 Generalized anxiety disorder
Anxiety neurosis   Anxiety state
Anxiety reaction   Overanxious disorder
EXCLUDES 2 neurasthenia (F48.8)

F41.3 Other mixed anxiety disorders

F41.8 Other specified anxiety disorders
Anxiety depression (mild or not persistent)
Anxiety hysteria
Mixed anxiety and depressive disorder

F41.9 Anxiety disorder, unspecified
Anxiety NOS

F42 Obsessive-compulsive disorder
Anancastic neurosis
Obsessive-compulsive neurosis
EXCLUDES 2 obsessive-compulsive personality (disorder) (F60.5)
obsessive-compulsive symptoms occurring in depression (F32-F33)
obsessive-compulsive symptoms occurring in schizophrenia (F20.-)

✓4th **F43** Reaction to severe stress, and adjustment disorders

F43.0 Acute stress reaction
Acute crisis reaction
Acute reaction to stress
Combat and operational stress reaction
Combat fatigue
Crisis state
Psychic shock

EXCLUDES 1 Not coded here   EXCLUDES 2 Not included here   N Newborn Age: 0   P Pediatric Age: 0-17   M Maternity Age: 12-55   A Adult Age: 15-124

506   ICD-10-CM 2014 (Draft)

✓5th F43.1 Post-traumatic stress disorder (PTSD)
Traumatic neurosis
- **F43.10 Post-traumatic stress disorder, unspecified**
- **F43.11 Post-traumatic stress disorder, acute**
- **F43.12 Post-traumatic stress disorder, chronic**

✓5th F43.2 Adjustment disorders
Culture shock
Grief reaction
Hospitalism in children
EXCLUDES 2 *separation anxiety disorder of childhood (F93.0)*
- **F43.20 Adjustment disorder, unspecified**
- **F43.21 Adjustment disorder with depressed mood**
- **F43.22 Adjustment disorder with anxiety**
- **F43.23 Adjustment disorder with mixed anxiety and depressed mood**
- **F43.24 Adjustment disorder with disturbance of conduct**
- **F43.25 Adjustment disorder with mixed disturbance of emotions and conduct**
- **F43.29 Adjustment disorder with other symptoms**

F43.8 Other reactions to severe stress

F43.9 Reaction to severe stress, unspecified

✓4th F44 Dissociative and conversion disorders
INCLUDES conversion hysteria
conversion reaction
hysteria
hysterical psychosis
EXCLUDES 2 *malingering [conscious simulation] (Z76.5)*

F44.0 Dissociative amnesia
EXCLUDES 1 *amnesia NOS (R41.3)*
anterograde amnesia (R41.1)
retrograde amnesia (R41.2)
EXCLUDES 2 *alcohol-or other psychoactive substance-induced amnestic disorder (F10, F13, F19 with .26, .96)*
amnestic disorder due to known physiological condition (F04)
postictal amnesia in epilepsy (G40.-)

F44.1 Dissociative fugue
EXCLUDES 2 *postictal fugue in epilepsy (G40.-)*

F44.2 Dissociative stupor
EXCLUDES 1 *catatonic stupor (R40.1)*
stupor NOS (R40.1)
EXCLUDES 2 *catatonic disorder due to known physiological condition (F06.1)*
depressive stupor (F32, F33)
manic stupor (F30, F31)

F44.4 Conversion disorder with motor symptom or deficit
Dissociative motor disorders
Psychogenic aphonia
Psychogenic dysphonia

F44.5 Conversion disorder with seizures or convulsions
Dissociative convulsions

F44.6 Conversion disorder with sensory symptom or deficit
Dissociative anesthesia and sensory loss
Psychogenic deafness

F44.7 Conversion disorder with mixed symptom presentation

✓5th F44.8 Other dissociative and conversion disorders
- **F44.81 Dissociative identity disorder**
Multiple personality disorder
- **F44.89 Other dissociative and conversion disorders**
Ganser's syndrome
Psychogenic confusion
Psychogenic twilight state
Trance and possession disorders

F44.9 Dissociative and conversion disorder, unspecified
Dissociative disorder NOS

✓4th F45 Somatoform disorders
EXCLUDES 2 *dissociative and conversion disorders (F44.-)*
factitious disorders (F68.1-)
hair-plucking (F63.3)
lalling (F80.0)
lisping (F80.0)
malingering [conscious simulation] (Z76.5)
nail-biting (F98.8)
psychological or behavioral factors associated with disorders or diseases classified elsewhere (F54)
sexual dysfunction, not due to a substance or known physiological condition (F52.-)
thumb-sucking (F98.8)
tic disorders (in childhood and adolescence) (F95.-)
Tourette's syndrome (F95.2)
trichotillomania (F63.3)

F45.0 Somatization disorder
Briquet's disorder
Multiple psychosomatic disorder

F45.1 Undifferentiated somatoform disorder
Undifferentiated psychosomatic disorder

✓5th F45.2 Hypochondriacal disorders
EXCLUDES 2 *delusional dysmorphophobia (F22)*
fixed delusions about bodily functions or shape (F22)
- **F45.20 Hypochondriacal disorder, unspecified**
- **F45.21 Hypochondriasis**
Hypochondriacal neurosis
- **F45.22 Body dysmorphic disorder**
Dysmorphophobia (nondelusional)
Nosophobia
- **F45.29 Other hypochondriacal disorders**

✓5th F45.4 Pain disorders related to psychological factors
EXCLUDES 1 *pain NOS (R52)*
- **F45.41 Pain disorder exclusively related to psychological factors**
Somatoform pain disorder (persistent)
- **F45.42 Pain disorder with related psychological factors**
Code also associated acute or chronic pain (G89.-)

F45.8 Other somatoform disorders
Psychogenic dysmenorrhea
Psychogenic dysphagia, including "globus hystericus"
Psychogenic pruritus
Psychogenic torticollis
Somatoform autonomic dysfunction
Teeth grinding
EXCLUDES 1 *sleep related teeth grinding (G47.63)*

F45.9 Somatoform disorder, unspecified
Psychosomatic disorder NOS

✓4th F48 Other nonpsychotic mental disorders

F48.1 Depersonalization-derealization syndrome

F48.2 Pseudobulbar affect
Involuntary emotional expression disorder
Code first underlying cause, if known, such as:
amyotrophic lateral sclerosis (G12.21)
multiple sclerosis (G35)
sequelae of cerebrovascular disease (I69.-)
sequelae of traumatic intracranial injury (S06.-)

F48.8 Other specified nonpsychotic mental disorders
Dhat syndrome
Neurasthenia
Occupational neurosis, including writer's cramp
Psychasthenia
Psychasthenic neurosis
Psychogenic syncope

F48.9 Nonpsychotic mental disorder, unspecified
Neurosis NOS

Behavioral syndromes associated with physiological disturbances and physical factors (F50-F59)

✓4th F50 Eating disorders
EXCLUDES 1 *anorexia NOS (R63.0)*
feeding difficulties (R63.3)
polyphagia (R63.2)
EXCLUDES 2 *feeding disorder in infancy or childhood (F98.2-)*

✓5th F50.0 Anorexia nervosa
EXCLUDES 1 *loss of appetite (R63.0)*
psychogenic loss of appetite (F50.8)
- **F50.00 Anorexia nervosa, unspecified**
- **F50.01 Anorexia nervosa, restricting type**

Mental, Behavioral, and Neurodevelopmental Disorders

F50.02–F60.0

F50.02 Anorexia nervosa, binge eating/purging type
    EXCLUDES 1 *bulimia nervosa (F50.2)*

F50.2 Bulimia nervosa
    Bulimia NOS
    Hyperorexia nervosa
    EXCLUDES 1 *anorexia nervosa, binge eating/purging type (F50.02)*

F50.8 Other eating disorders
    Pica in adults
    Psychogenic loss of appetite
    EXCLUDES 2 *pica of infancy and childhood (F98.3)*

F50.9 Eating disorder, unspecified
    Atypical anorexia nervosa
    Atypical bulimia nervosa

✓4th **F51 Sleep disorders not due to a substance or known physiological condition**
    EXCLUDES 2 *organic sleep disorders (G47.-)*

  ✓5th **F51.0 Insomnia not due to a substance or known physiological condition**
      EXCLUDES 2 *alcohol related insomnia (F10.182, F10.282, F10.982)*
          drug-related insomnia (F11.182, F11.282, F11.982, F13.182, F13.282, F13.982, F14.182, F14.282, F14.982, F15.182, F15.282, F15.982, F19.182, F19.282, F19.982)
          insomnia NOS (G47.0-)
          insomnia due to known physiological condition (G47.0-)
          organic insomnia (G47.0-)
          sleep deprivation (Z72.820)

    F51.01 Primary insomnia
      Idiopathic insomnia

    F51.02 Adjustment insomnia

    F51.03 Paradoxical insomnia

    F51.04 Psychophysiologic insomnia

    F51.05 Insomnia due to other mental disorder
      Code also associated mental disorder

    F51.09 Other insomnia not due to a substance or known physiological condition

  ✓5th **F51.1 Hypersomnia not due to a substance or known physiological condition**
      EXCLUDES 2 *alcohol related hypersomnia (F10.182, F10.282, F10.982)*
          drug-related hypersomnia (F11.182, F11.282, F11.982, F13.182, F13.282, F13.982, F14.182, F14.282, F14.982, F15.182, F15.282, F15.982, F19.182, F19.282, F19.982)
          hypersomnia NOS (G47.10)
          hypersomnia due to known physiological condition (G47.10)
          idiopathic hypersomnia (G47.11, G47.12)
          narcolepsy (G47.4-)

    F51.11 Primary hypersomnia
    F51.12 Insufficient sleep syndrome
      EXCLUDES 1 *sleep deprivation (Z72.820)*

    F51.13 Hypersomnia due to other mental disorder
      Code also associated mental disorder

    F51.19 Other hypersomnia not due to a substance or known physiological condition

  F51.3 Sleepwalking [somnambulism]
  F51.4 Sleep terrors [night terrors]
  F51.5 Nightmare disorder
    Dream anxiety disorder

  F51.8 Other sleep disorders not due to a substance or known physiological condition

  F51.9 Sleep disorder not due to a substance or known physiological condition, unspecified
    Emotional sleep disorder NOS

✓4th **F52 Sexual dysfunction not due to a substance or known physiological condition**
    EXCLUDES 2 *Dhat syndrome (F48.8)*

  F52.0 Hypoactive sexual desire disorder
    Anhedonia (sexual)
    Lack or loss of sexual desire
    EXCLUDES 1 *decreased libido (R68.82)*

  F52.1 Sexual aversion disorder
    Sexual aversion and lack of sexual enjoyment

  F52.2 Sexual arousal disorders
    Failure of genital response

    F52.21 Male erectile disorder   ♂
      Psychogenic impotence
      EXCLUDES 1 *impotence of organic origin (N52.-)*
          impotence NOS (N52.-)

    F52.22 Female sexual arousal disorder   ♀
      Frigidity

  ✓5th **F52.3 Orgasmic disorder**
    Inhibited orgasm
    Psychogenic anorgasmy

    F52.31 Female orgasmic disorder   ♀
    F52.32 Male orgasmic disorder   ♂

  F52.4 Premature ejaculation   ♂

  F52.5 Vaginismus not due to a substance or known physiological condition   ♀
    Psychogenic vaginismus
    EXCLUDES 2 *vaginismus (due to a known physiological condition) (N94.2)*

  F52.6 Dyspareunia not due to a substance or known physiological condition   ♀
    Psychogenic dyspareunia
    EXCLUDES 2 *dyspareunia (due to a known physiological condition) (N94.1)*

  F52.8 Other sexual dysfunction not due to a substance or known physiological condition
    Excessive sexual drive
    Nymphomania
    Satyriasis

  F52.9 Unspecified sexual dysfunction not due to a substance or known physiological condition
    Sexual dysfunction NOS

F53 Puerperal psychosis   ♀
  Postpartum depression
  EXCLUDES 1 *mood disorders with psychotic features (F30.2, F31.2, F31.5, F31.64, F32.3, F33.3)*
      postpartum dysphoria (O90.6)
      psychosis in schizophrenia, schizotypal, delusional, and other psychotic disorders (F20-F29)

F54 Psychological and behavioral factors associated with disorders or diseases classified elsewhere
  Psychological factors affecting physical conditions
  Code first the associated physical disorder, such as:
    asthma (J45.-)
    dermatitis (L23-L25)
    gastric ulcer (K25.-)
    mucous colitis (K58.-)
    ulcerative colitis (K51.-)
    urticaria (L50.-)
  EXCLUDES 2 *tension-type headache (G44.2)*

✓4th **F55 Abuse of non-psychoactive substances**
  EXCLUDES 2 *abuse of psychoactive substances (F10-F19)*

  F55.0 Abuse of antacids
  F55.1 Abuse of herbal or folk remedies
  F55.2 Abuse of laxatives
  F55.3 Abuse of steroids or hormones
  F55.4 Abuse of vitamins
  F55.8 Abuse of other non-psychoactive substances

F59 Unspecified behavioral syndromes associated with physiological disturbances and physical factors
  Psychogenic physiological dysfunction NOS

Disorders of adult personality and behavior (F60-F69)

✓4th **F60 Specific personality disorders**

  F60.0 Paranoid personality disorder
    Expansive paranoid personality (disorder)
    Fanatic personality (disorder)
    Querulant personality (disorder)
    Paranoid personality (disorder)
    Sensitive paranoid personality (disorder)
    EXCLUDES 2 *paranoia (F22)*
      paranoia querulans (F22)
      paranoid psychosis (F22)
      paranoid schizophrenia (F20.0)
      paranoid state (F22)

EXCLUDES 1 Not coded here   EXCLUDES 2 Not included here   N Newborn Age: 0   P Pediatric Age: 0-17   M Maternity Age: 12-55   A Adult Age: 15-124

F60.1 Schizoid personality disorder
EXCLUDES 2 *Asperger's syndrome (F84.5)*
delusional disorder (F22)
schizoid disorder of childhood (F84.5)
schizophrenia (F20.-)
schizotypal disorder (F21)

F60.2 Antisocial personality disorder
Amoral personality (disorder)
Asocial personality (disorder)
Dissocial personality disorder
Psychopathic personality (disorder)
Sociopathic personality (disorder)
EXCLUDES 1 *conduct disorders (F91.-)*
EXCLUDES 2 *borderline personality disorder (F60.3)*

F60.3 Borderline personality disorder
Aggressive personality (disorder)
Emotionally unstable personality disorder
Explosive personality (disorder)
EXCLUDES 2 *antisocial personality disorder (F60.2)*

F60.4 Histrionic personality disorder
Hysterical personality (disorder)
Psychoinfantile personality (disorder)

F60.5 Obsessive-compulsive personality disorder
Anankastic personality (disorder)
Compulsive personality (disorder)
Obsessional personality (disorder)
EXCLUDES 2 *obsessive-compulsive disorder (F42)*

F60.6 Avoidant personality disorder
Anxious personality disorder

F60.7 Dependent personality disorder
Asthenic personality (disorder)
Inadequate personality (disorder)
Passive personality (disorder)

F60.8 Other specific personality disorders
F60.81 Narcissistic personality disorder
F60.89 Other specific personality disorders
Eccentric personality disorder
"Haltlose" type personality disorder
Immature personality disorder
Passive-aggressive personality disorder
Psychoneurotic personality disorder
Self-defeating personality disorder

F60.9 Personality disorder, unspecified
Character disorder NOS
Character neurosis NOS
Pathological personality NOS

F63 Impulse disorders
EXCLUDES 2 *habitual excessive use of alcohol or psychoactive substances (F10-F19)*
impulse disorders involving sexual behavior (F65.-)

F63.0 Pathological gambling
Compulsive gambling
EXCLUDES 1 *gambling and betting NOS (Z72.6)*
EXCLUDES 2 *excessive gambling by manic patients (F30, F31)*
gambling in antisocial personality disorder (F60.2)

F63.1 Pyromania
Pathological fire-setting
EXCLUDES 2 *fire-setting (by) (in):*
adult with antisocial personality disorder (F60.2)
alcohol or psychoactive substance intoxication (F10-F19)
conduct disorders (F91.-)
mental disorders due to known physiological condition (F01-F09)
schizophrenia (F20.-)

F63.2 Kleptomania
Pathological stealing
EXCLUDES 1 *shoplifting as the reason for observation for suspected mental disorder (Z03.8)*
EXCLUDES 2 *depressive disorder with stealing (F31-F33)*
stealing due to underlying mental condition—code to mental condition
stealing in mental disorders due to known physiological condition (F01-F09)

F63.3 Trichotillomania
Hair plucking
EXCLUDES 2 *other stereotyped movement disorder (F98.4)*

F63.8 Other impulse disorders
F63.81 Intermittent explosive disorder
F63.89 Other impulse disorders

F63.9 Impulse disorder, unspecified
Impulse control disorder NOS

F64 Gender identity disorders
F64.1 Gender identity disorder in adolescence and adulthood
Dual role transvestism
Transsexualism
Use additional code to identify sex reassignment status (Z87.890)
EXCLUDES 1 *gender identity disorder in childhood (F64.2)*
EXCLUDES 2 *fetishistic transvestism (F65.1)*

F64.2 Gender identity disorder of childhood P
EXCLUDES 1 *gender identity disorder in adolescence and adulthood (F64.1)*
EXCLUDES 2 *sexual maturation disorder (F66)*

F64.8 Other gender identity disorders
F64.9 Gender identity disorder, unspecified
Gender-role disorder NOS

F65 Paraphilias
F65.0 Fetishism
F65.1 Transvestic fetishism
Fetishistic transvestism
F65.2 Exhibitionism
F65.3 Voyeurism
F65.4 Pedophilia
F65.5 Sadomasochism
F65.50 Sadomasochism, unspecified
F65.51 Sexual masochism
F65.52 Sexual sadism
F65.8 Other paraphilias
F65.81 Frotteurism
F65.89 Other paraphilias
Necrophilia
F65.9 Paraphilia, unspecified
Sexual deviation NOS

F66 Other sexual disorders
Sexual maturation disorder
Sexual relationship disorder

F68 Other disorders of adult personality and behavior
F68.1 Factitious disorder
Compensation neurosis
Elaboration of physical symptoms for psychological reasons
Hospital hopper syndrome
Münchhausen's syndrome
Peregrinating patient
EXCLUDES 2 *factitial dermatitis (L98.1)*
person feigning illness (with obvious motivation) (Z76.5)

F68.10 Factitious disorder, unspecified
F68.11 Factitious disorder with predominantly psychological signs and symptoms
F68.12 Factitious disorder with predominantly physical signs and symptoms
F68.13 Factitious disorder with combined psychological and physical signs and symptoms

F68.8 Other specified disorders of adult personality and behavior

F69 Unspecified disorder of adult personality and behavior A

Intellectual Disabilities (F70-F79)
Code first any associated physical or developmental disorders
EXCLUDES 1 *borderline intellectual functioning, IQ above 70 to 84 (R41.83)*

F70 Mild intellectual disabilities
IQ level 50-55 to approximately 70
Mild mental subnormality

F71 Moderate intellectual disabilities
IQ level 35-40 to 50-55
Moderate mental subnormality

F72 Severe intellectual disabilities
IQ 20-25 to 35-40
Severe mental subnormality

F73 Profound intellectual disabilities
IQ level below 20-25
Profound mental subnormality

F78 Other intellectual disabilities

F79 Unspecified intellectual disabilities
Mental deficiency NOS
Mental subnormality NOS

Pervasive and specific developmental disorders (F80-F89)

☑4ᵗʰ F80 Specific developmental disorders of speech and language

F80.0 Phonological disorder
Dyslalia
Functional speech articulation disorder
Lalling
Lisping
Phonological developmental disorder
Speech articulation developmental disorder
EXCLUDES 1 speech articulation impairment due to aphasia NOS (R47.01)
speech articulation impairment due to apraxia (R48.2)
EXCLUDES 2 speech articulation impairment due to hearing loss (F80.4)
speech articulation impairment due to intellectual disabilities (F70-F79)
speech articulation impairment with expressive language developmental disorder (F80.1)
speech articulation impairment with mixed receptive expressive language developmental disorder (F80.2)

F80.1 Expressive language disorder
Developmental dysphasia or aphasia, expressive type
EXCLUDES 1 dysphasia and aphasia NOS (R47.-)
mixed receptive-expressive language disorder (F80.2)
EXCLUDES 2 acquired aphasia with epilepsy [Landau-Kleffner] (G40.80-)
intellectual disabilities (F70-F79)
pervasive developmental disorders (F84.-)
selective mutism (F94.0)

F80.2 Mixed receptive-expressive language disorder
Developmental dysphasia or aphasia, receptive type
Developmental Wernicke's aphasia
EXCLUDES 1 central auditory processing disorder (H93.25)
dysphasia or aphasia NOS (R47.-)
expressive language disorder (F80.1)
expressive type dysphasia or aphasia (F80.1)
word deafness (H93.25)
EXCLUDES 2 acquired aphasia with epilepsy [Landau-Kleffner] (G40.80-)
intellectual disabilities (F70-F79)
pervasive developmental disorders (F84.-)
selective mutism (F94.0)

F80.4 Speech and language development delay due to hearing loss
Code also type of hearing loss (H90.-, H91.-)

☑5ᵗʰ F80.8 Other developmental disorders of speech and language

F80.81 Childhood onset fluency disorder
Cluttering NOS
Stuttering NOS
EXCLUDES 1 adult onset fluency disorder (F98.5)
fluency disorder in conditions classified elsewhere (R47.82)
fluency disorder (stuttering) following cerebrovascular disease (I69. with final characters-23)

F80.89 Other developmental disorders of speech and language

F80.9 Developmental disorder of speech and language, unspecified
Communication disorder NOS
Language disorder NOS

☑4ᵗʰ F81 Specific developmental disorders of scholastic skills

F81.0 Specific reading disorder
"Backward reading"
Developmental dyslexia
Specific reading retardation
EXCLUDES 1 alexia NOS (R48.0)
dyslexia NOS (R48.0)

F81.2 Mathematics disorder
Developmental acalculia
Developmental arithmetical disorder
Developmental Gerstmann's syndrome
EXCLUDES 1 acalculia NOS (R48.8)
EXCLUDES 2 arithmetical difficulties associated with a reading disorder (F81.0)
arithmetical difficulties associated with a spelling disorder (F81.81)
arithmetical difficulties due to inadequate teaching (Z55.8)

☑5ᵗʰ F81.8 Other developmental disorders of scholastic skills

F81.81 Disorder of written expression
Specific spelling disorder

F81.89 Other developmental disorders of scholastic skills

F81.9 Developmental disorder of scholastic skills, unspecified
Knowledge acquisition disability NOS
Learning disability NOS
Learning disorder NOS

F82 Specific developmental disorder of motor function
Clumsy child syndrome
Developmental coordination disorder
Developmental dyspraxia
EXCLUDES 1 abnormalities of gait and mobility (R26.-)
lack of coordination (R27.-)
EXCLUDES 2 lack of coordination secondary to intellectual disabilities (F70-F79)

☑4ᵗʰ F84 Pervasive developmental disorders
Use additional code to identify any associated medical condition and intellectual disabilities

F84.0 Autistic disorder
Infantile autism
Infantile psychosis
Kanner's syndrome
EXCLUDES 1 Asperger's syndrome (F84.5)

F84.2 Rett's syndrome
EXCLUDES 1 Asperger's syndrome (F84.5)
Autistic disorder (F84.0)
Other childhood disintegrative disorder (F84.3)

F84.3 Other childhood disintegrative disorder   **P**
Dementia infantilis
Disintegrative psychosis
Heller's syndrome
Symbiotic psychosis
Use additional code to identify any associated neurological condition
EXCLUDES 1 Asperger's syndrome (F84.5)
Autistic disorder (F84.0)
Rett's syndrome (F84.2)

F84.5 Asperger's syndrome
Asperger's disorder
Autistic psychopathy
Schizoid disorder of childhood

F84.8 Other pervasive developmental disorders
Overactive disorder associated with intellectual disabilities and stereotyped movements

F84.9 Pervasive developmental disorder, unspecified
Atypical autism

F88 Other disorders of psychological development
Developmental agnosia

F89 Unspecified disorder of psychological development
Developmental disorder NOS

Behavioral and emotional disorders with onset usually occurring in childhood and adolescence (F90-F98)

NOTE Codes within categories F90-F98 may be used regardless of the age of a patient. These disorders generally have onset within the childhood or adolescent years, but may continue throughout life or not be diagnosed until adulthood.

☑4ᵗʰ F90 Attention-deficit hyperactivity disorders
INCLUDES attention deficit disorder with hyperactivity
attention deficit syndrome with hyperactivity
EXCLUDES 2 anxiety disorders (F40.-, F41.-)
mood [affective] disorders (F30-F39)
pervasive developmental disorders (F84.-)
schizophrenia (F20.-)

F90.0 Attention-deficit hyperactivity disorder, predominantly inattentive type

EXCLUDES 1 Not coded here   *EXCLUDES 2* Not included here   **N** Newborn Age: 0   **P** Pediatric Age: 0-17   **M** Maternity Age: 12-55   **A** Adult Age: 15-124

510   ICD-10-CM 2014 (Draft)

F90.1 **Attention-deficit hyperactivity disorder, predominantly hyperactive type**

F90.2 **Attention-deficit hyperactivity disorder, combined type**

F90.8 **Attention-deficit hyperactivity disorder, other type**

F90.9 **Attention-deficit hyperactivity disorder, unspecified type**
  Attention-deficit hyperactivity disorder of childhood or adolescence NOS
  Attention-deficit hyperactivity disorder NOS

✓4ᵗʰ **F91 Conduct disorders**
  EXCLUDES 1 antisocial behavior (Z72.81-)
    antisocial personality disorder (F60.2)
  EXCLUDES 2 conduct problems associated with attention-deficit hyperactivity disorder (F90.-)
    mood [affective] disorders (F30-F39)
    pervasive developmental disorders (F84.-)
    schizophrenia (F20.-)

  F91.0 **Conduct disorder confined to family context**

  F91.1 **Conduct disorder, childhood-onset type**
    Unsocialized conduct disorder
    Conduct disorder, solitary aggressive type
    Unsocialized aggressive disorder

  F91.2 **Conduct disorder, adolescent-onset type**
    Socialized conduct disorder
    Conduct disorder, group type

  F91.3 **Oppositional defiant disorder**

  F91.8 **Other conduct disorders**

  F91.9 **Conduct disorder, unspecified**
    Behavioral disorder NOS
    Conduct disorder NOS
    Disruptive behavior disorder NOS

✓4ᵗʰ **F93 Emotional disorders with onset specific to childhood**

  F93.0 **Separation anxiety disorder of childhood** Ⓟ
    EXCLUDES 2 mood [affective] disorders (F30-F39)
      nonpsychotic mental disorders (F40-F48)
      phobic anxiety disorder of childhood (F40.8)
      social phobia (F40.1)

  F93.8 **Other childhood emotional disorders** Ⓟ
    Identity disorder
    EXCLUDES 2 gender identity disorder of childhood (F64.2)

  F93.9 **Childhood emotional disorder, unspecified** Ⓟ

✓4ᵗʰ **F94 Disorders of social functioning with onset specific to childhood and adolescence**

  F94.0 **Selective mutism**
    Elective mutism
    EXCLUDES 2 pervasive developmental disorders (F84.-)
      schizophrenia (F20.-)
      specific developmental disorders of speech and language (F80.-)
      transient mutism as part of separation anxiety in young children (F93.0)

  F94.1 **Reactive attachment disorder of childhood** Ⓟ
    Use additional code to identify any associated failure to thrive or growth retardation
    EXCLUDES 1 disinhibited attachment disorder of childhood (F94.1)
      normal variation in pattern of selective attachment
    EXCLUDES 2 Asperger's syndrome (F84.5)
      maltreatment syndromes (T74.-)
      sexual or physical abuse in childhood, resulting in psychosocial problems (Z62.81-)

  F94.2 **Disinhibited attachment disorder of childhood** Ⓟ
    Affectionless psychopathy
    Institutional syndrome
    EXCLUDES 1 reactive attachment disorder of childhood (F94.1)
    EXCLUDES 2 Asperger's syndrome (F84.5)
      attention-deficit hyperactivity disorders (F90.-)
      hospitalism in children (F43.2-)

  F94.8 **Other childhood disorders of social functioning** Ⓟ

  F94.9 **Childhood disorder of social functioning, unspecified** Ⓟ

✓4ᵗʰ **F95 Tic disorder**

  F95.0 **Transient tic disorder**

  F95.1 **Chronic motor or vocal tic disorder**

  F95.2 **Tourette's disorder**
    Combined vocal and multiple motor tic disorder [de la Tourette]
    Tourette's syndrome

  F95.8 **Other tic disorders**

  F95.9 **Tic disorder, unspecified**
    Tic NOS

✓4ᵗʰ **F98 Other behavioral and emotional disorders with onset usually occurring in childhood and adolescence**
  EXCLUDES 2 breath-holding spells (R06.89)
    gender identity disorder of childhood (F64.2)
    Kleine-Levin syndrome (G47.13)
    obsessive-compulsive disorder (F42)
    sleep disorders not due to a substance or known physiological condition (F51.-)

  F98.0 **Enuresis not due to a substance or known physiological condition**
    Enuresis (primary) (secondary) of nonorganic origin
    Functional enuresis
    Psychogenic enuresis
    Urinary incontinence of nonorganic origin
    EXCLUDES 1 enuresis NOS (R32)

  F98.1 **Encopresis not due to a substance or known physiological condition**
    Functional encopresis
    Incontinence of feces of nonorganic origin
    Psychogenic encopresis
    Use additional code to identify the cause of any coexisting constipation
    EXCLUDES 1 encopresis NOS (R15.-)

✓5ᵗʰ F98.2 **Other feeding disorders of infancy and childhood**
    EXCLUDES 1 feeding difficulties (R63.3)
    EXCLUDES 2 anorexia nervosa and other eating disorders (F50.-)
      feeding problems of newborn (P92.-)
      pica of infancy or childhood (F98.3)

    F98.21 **Rumination disorder of infancy** Ⓟ

    F98.29 **Other feeding disorders of infancy and early childhood** Ⓟ

  F98.3 **Pica of infancy and childhood** Ⓟ

  F98.4 **Stereotyped movement disorders**
    Stereotype/habit disorder
    EXCLUDES 1 abnormal involuntary movements (R25.-)
    EXCLUDES 2 compulsions in obsessive-compulsive disorder (F42)
      hair plucking (F63.3)
      movement disorders of organic origin (G20-G25)
      nail-biting (F98.8)
      nose-picking (F98.8)
      stereotypies that are part of a broader psychiatric condition (F01-F95)
      thumb-sucking (F98.8)
      tic disorders (F95.-)
      trichotillomania (F63.3)

  F98.5 **Adult onset fluency disorder**
    EXCLUDES 1 childhood onset fluency disorder (F80.81)
      dysphasia (R47.02)
      fluency disorder in conditions classified elsewhere (R47.82)
      fluency disorder (stuttering) following cerebrovascular disease (I69. with final characters -23)
      tic disorders (F95.-)

  F98.8 **Other specified behavioral and emotional disorders with** Ⓟ **onset usually occurring in childhood and adolescence**
    Excessive masturbation
    Nail-biting
    Nose-picking
    Thumb-sucking

  F98.9 **Unspecified behavioral and emotional disorders with** Ⓟ **onset usually occurring in childhood and adolescence**

Unspecified mental disorder (F99)

F99 Mental disorder, not otherwise specified
  Mental illness NOS
  EXCLUDES 1 unspecified mental disorder due to known physiological condition (F09)

✓ Additional Character Required ✓x7ᵗʰ Xtension Alert Unspecified Code Other Specified Code Manifestation Code ►◄ Revised Text ● New Code ▲ Revised Code Title

Diseases of the Nervous System

G00–G04.39

Chapter 6. Diseases of the Nervous System (G00-G99)

EXCLUDES 2   certain conditions originating in the perinatal period (P04-P96)
certain infectious and parasitic diseases (A00-B99)
complications of pregnancy, childbirth and the puerperium (O00-O9A)
congenital malformations, deformations, and chromosomal abnormalities (Q00-Q99)
endocrine, nutritional and metabolic diseases (E00-E88)
injury, poisoning and certain other consequences of external causes (S00-T88)
neoplasms (C00-D49)
symptoms, signs and abnormal clinical and laboratory findings, not elsewhere classified (R00-R94)

This chapter contains the following blocks:

G00-G09   Inflammatory diseases of the central nervous system
G10-G14   Systemic atrophies primarily affecting the central nervous system
G20-G26   Extrapyramidal and movement disorders
G30-G32   Other degenerative diseases of the nervous system
G35-G37   Demyelinating diseases of the central nervous system
G40-G47   Episodic and paroxysmal disorders
G50-G59   Nerve, nerve root and plexus disorders
G60-G65   Polyneuropathies and other disorders of the peripheral nervous system
G70-G73   Diseases of myoneural junction and muscle
G80-G83   Cerebral palsy and other paralytic syndromes
G89-G99   Other disorders of the nervous system

Inflammatory diseases of the central nervous system (G00-G09)

G00   Bacterial meningitis, not elsewhere classified
    INCLUDES   bacterial arachnoiditis
           bacterial leptomeningitis
           bacterial meningitis
           bacterial pachymeningitis
    EXCLUDES 1   bacterial:
           meningoencephalitis (G04.2)
           meningomyelitis (G04.2)

G00.0   Hemophilus meningitis
    Meningitis due to Hemophilus influenzae

G00.1   Pneumococcal meningitis

G00.2   Streptococcal meningitis
    Use additional code to further identify organism (B95.0-B95.5)

G00.3   Staphylococcal meningitis
    Use additional code to further identify organism (B95.61-B95.8)

G00.8   Other bacterial meningitis
    Meningitis due to Escherichia coli
    Meningitis due to Friedländer's bacillus
    Meningitis due to Klebsiella
    Use additional code to further identify organism (B96.-)

G00.9   Bacterial meningitis, unspecified
    Meningitis due to gram-negative bacteria, unspecified
    Purulent meningitis NOS
    Pyogenic meningitis NOS
    Suppurative meningitis NOS

G01   Meningitis in bacterial diseases classified elsewhere
    Code first underlying disease
    EXCLUDES 1   meningitis (in):
           gonococcal (A54.81)
           leptospirosis (A27.81)
           listeriosis (A32.11)
           Lyme disease (A69.21)
           meningococcal (A39.0)
           neurosyphilis (A52.13)
           tuberculosis (A17.0)
           meningoencephalitis and meningomyelitis in bacterial diseases classified elsewhere (G05)

G02   Meningitis in other infectious and parasitic diseases classified elsewhere
    Code first underlying disease, such as:
    African trypanosomiasis (B56.-)
    poliovirus infection (A80.-)
    EXCLUDES 1   candidal meningitis (B37.5)
           coccidioidomycosis meningitis (B38.4)
           cryptococcal meningitis (B45.1)
           herpesviral [herpes simplex] meningitis (B00.3)
           infectious mononucleosis complicated by meningitis (B27.- with fourth character 2)
           measles complicated by meningitis (B05.1)
           meningoencephalitis and meningomyelitis in other infectious and parasitic diseases classified elsewhere (G05)
           mumps meningitis (B26.1)
           rubella meningitis (B06.02)
           varicella [chickenpox] meningitis (B01.0)
           zoster meningitis (B02.1)

G03   Meningitis due to other and unspecified causes
    INCLUDES   arachnoiditis NOS
           leptomeningitis NOS
           meningitis NOS
           pachymeningitis NOS
    EXCLUDES 1   meningoencephalitis (G04.-)
           meningomyelitis (G04.-)

G03.0   Nonpyogenic meningitis
    Aseptic meningitis
    Nonbacterial meningitis

G03.1   Chronic meningitis

G03.2   Benign recurrent meningitis [Mollaret]

G03.8   Meningitis due to other specified causes

G03.9   Meningitis, unspecified
    Arachnoiditis (spinal) NOS

G04   Encephalitis, myelitis and encephalomyelitis
    INCLUDES   acute ascending myelitis
           meningoencephalitis
           meningomyelitis
    EXCLUDES 1   encephalopathy NOS (G93.40)
    EXCLUDES 2   acute transverse myelitis (G37.3-)
           alcoholic encephalopathy (G31.2)
           benign myalgic encephalomyelitis (G93.3)
           multiple sclerosis (G35)
           subacute necrotizing myelitis (G37.4)
           toxic encephalitis (G92)
           toxic encephalopathy (G92)

G04.0   Acute disseminated encephalitis and encephalomyelitis (ADEM)
    EXCLUDES 1   acute necrotizing hemorrhagic encephalopathy (G04.3-)
           other noninfectious acute disseminated encephalomyelitis (noninfectious ADEM) (G04.81)

G04.00   Acute disseminated encephalitis and encephalomyelitis, unspecified

G04.01   Postinfectious acute disseminated encephalitis and encephalomyelitis (postinfectious ADEM)
    EXCLUDES 1   post chickenpox encephalitis (B01.1)
           post measles encephalitis (B05.0)
           post measles myelitis (B05.1)

G04.02   Postimmunization acute disseminated encephalitis, myelitis and encephalomyelitis
    Encephalitis, postimmunization
    Encephalomyelitis, postimmunization

G04.1   Tropical spastic paraplegia

G04.2   Bacterial meningoencephalitis and meningomyelitis, not elsewhere classified

G04.3   Acute necrotizing hemorrhagic encephalopathy
    EXCLUDES 1   acute disseminated encephalitis and encephalomyelitis (G04.0-)

G04.30   Acute necrotizing hemorrhagic encephalopathy, unspecified

G04.31   Postinfectious acute necrotizing hemorrhagic encephalopathy

G04.32   Postimmunization acute necrotizing hemorrhagic encephalopathy

G04.39   Other acute necrotizing hemorrhagic encephalopathy
    Code also underlying etiology, if applicable

EXCLUDES 1 Not coded here   *EXCLUDES 2* Not included here   N Newborn Age: 0   P Pediatric Age: 0-17   M Maternity Age: 12-55   A Adult Age: 15-124

512   ICD-10-CM 2014 (Draft)

✓5th **G04.8   Other encephalitis, myelitis and encephalomyelitis**
Code also any associated seizure (G40.-, R56.9)

G04.81   Other encephalitis and encephalomyelitis
Noninfectious acute disseminated encephalomyelitis (noninfectious ADEM)

G04.89   Other myelitis

✓5th **G04.9   Encephalitis, myelitis and encephalomyelitis, unspecified**

G04.90   Encephalitis and encephalomyelitis, unspecified
Ventriculitis (cerebral) NOS

G04.91   Myelitis, unspecified

✓4th **G05   Encephalitis, myelitis and encephalomyelitis in diseases classified elsewhere**
Code first underlying disease, such as:
human immunodeficiency virus [HIV] disease (B20)
poliovirus (A80.-)
suppurative otitis media (H66.01-H66.4)
trichinellosis (B75)

EXCLUDES 1   *adenoviral encephalitis, myelitis and encephalomyelitis (A85.1)*
congenital toxoplasmosis encephalitis, myelitis and encephalomyelitis (P37.1)
cytomegaloviral encephalitis, myelitis and encephalomyelitis (B25.8)
encephalitis, myelitis and encephalomyelitis (in) measles (B05.0)
encephalitis, myelitis and encephalomyelitis (in) systemic lupus erythematosus (M32.19)
enteroviral encephalitis, myelitis and encephalomyelitis (A85.0)
eosinophilic meningoencephalitis (B83.2)
herpesviral [herpes simplex] encephalitis, myelitis and encephalomyelitis (B00.4)
listerial encephalitis, myelitis and encephalomyelitis (A32.12)
meningococcal encephalitis, myelitis and encephalomyelitis (A39.81)
mumps encephalitis, myelitis and encephalomyelitis (B26.2)
postchickenpox encephalitis, myelitis and encephalomyelitis (B01.1-)
rubella encephalitis, myelitis and encephalomyelitis (B06.01)
toxoplasmosis encephalitis, myelitis and encephalomyelitis (B58.2)
zoster encephalitis, myelitis and encephalomyelitis (B02.0)

G05.3   Encephalitis and encephalomyelitis in diseases classified elsewhere
Meningoencephalitis in diseases classified elsewhere

G05.4   Myelitis in diseases classified elsewhere
Meningomyelitis in diseases classified elsewhere

✓4th **G06   Intracranial and intraspinal abscess and granuloma**
Use additional code (B95-B97) to identify infectious agent

G06.0   Intracranial abscess and granuloma
Brain [any part] abscess (embolic)
Cerebellar abscess (embolic)
Cerebral abscess (embolic)
Intracranial epidural abscess or granuloma
Intracranial extradural abscess or granuloma
Intracranial subdural abscess or granuloma
Otogenic abscess (embolic)

EXCLUDES 1   *tuberculous intracranial abscess and granuloma (A17.81)*

G06.1   Intraspinal abscess and granuloma
Abscess (embolic) of spinal cord [any part]
Intraspinal epidural abscess or granuloma
Intraspinal extradural abscess or granuloma
Intraspinal subdural abscess or granuloma

EXCLUDES 1   *tuberculous intraspinal abscess and granuloma (A17.81)*

G06.2   Extradural and subdural abscess, unspecified

G07   Intracranial and intraspinal abscess and granuloma in diseases classified elsewhere
Code first underlying disease, such as:
schistosomiasis granuloma of brain (B65.-)

EXCLUDES 1   *abscess of brain:*
amebic (A06.6)
chromomycotic (B43.1)
gonococcal (A54.82)
tuberculous (A17.81)
tuberculoma of meninges (A17.1)

G08   Intracranial and intraspinal phlebitis and thrombophlebitis
Septic embolism of intracranial or intraspinal venous sinuses and veins
Septic endophlebitis of intracranial or intraspinal venous sinuses and veins
Septic phlebitis of intracranial or intraspinal venous sinuses and veins
Septic thrombophlebitis of intracranial or intraspinal venous sinuses and veins
Septic thrombosis of intracranial or intraspinal venous sinuses and veins

EXCLUDES 1   *intracranial phlebitis and thrombophlebitis complicating:*
abortion, ectopic or molar pregnancy (O00-O07, O08.7)
pregnancy, childbirth and the puerperium (O22.5, O87.3)

EXCLUDES 2   *intracranial phlebitis and thrombophlebitis complicating nonpyogenic intraspinal phlebitis and thrombophlebitis (G95.1)*

G09   Sequelae of inflammatory diseases of central nervous system
NOTE   Category G09 is to be used to indicate conditions whose primary classification is to G00-G08 as the cause of sequelae, themselves classifiable elsewhere. The "sequelae" include conditions specified as residuals.
Code first condition resulting from (sequela) of inflammatory diseases of central nervous system

Systemic atrophies primarily affecting the central nervous system (G10-G14)

G10   Huntington's disease
Huntington's chorea
Huntington's dementia

✓4th **G11   Hereditary ataxia**
EXCLUDES 2   *cerebral palsy (G80.-)*
hereditary and idiopathic neuropathy (G60.-)
metabolic disorders (E70-E88)

G11.0   Congenital nonprogressive ataxia

G11.1   Early-onset cerebellar ataxia
Early-onset cerebellar ataxia with essential tremor
Early-onset cerebellar ataxia with myoclonus [Hunt's ataxia]
Early-onset cerebellar ataxia with retained tendon reflexes
Friedreich's ataxia (autosomal recessive)
X-linked recessive spinocerebellar ataxia

G11.2   Late-onset cerebellar ataxia   A

G11.3   Cerebellar ataxia with defective DNA repair
Ataxia telangiectasia [Louis-Bar]
EXCLUDES 2   *Cockayne's syndrome (Q87.1)*
other disorders of purine and pyrimidine metabolism (E79.-)
xeroderma pigmentosum (Q82.1)

G11.4   Hereditary spastic paraplegia

G11.8   Other hereditary ataxias

G11.9   Hereditary ataxia, unspecified
Hereditary cerebellar ataxia NOS
Hereditary cerebellar degeneration
Hereditary cerebellar disease
Hereditary cerebellar syndrome

✓4th **G12   Spinal muscular atrophy and related syndromes**

G12.0   Infantile spinal muscular atrophy, type I [Werdnig-Hoffman]

G12.1   Other inherited spinal muscular atrophy
Adult form spinal muscular atrophy
Childhood form, type II spinal muscular atrophy
Distal spinal muscular atrophy
Juvenile form, type III spinal muscular atrophy [Kugelberg-Welander]
Progressive bulbar palsy of childhood [Fazio-Londe]
Scapuloperoneal form spinal muscular atrophy

✓5th **G12.2   Motor neuron disease**

G12.20   Motor neuron disease, unspecified

G12.21   Amyotrophic lateral sclerosis   A
Progressive spinal muscle atrophy

G12.22   Progressive bulbar palsy

G12.29   Other motor neuron disease
Familial motor neuron disease
Primary lateral sclerosis

G12.8   Other spinal muscular atrophies and related syndromes

G12.9   Spinal muscular atrophy, unspecified

Diseases of the Nervous System

G13–G25.81

☑4ᵗʰ **G13 Systemic atrophies primarily affecting central nervous system in diseases classified elsewhere**

G13.0 Paraneoplastic neuromyopathy and neuropathy
Carcinomatous neuromyopathy
Sensorial paraneoplastic neuropathy [Denny Brown]
Code first underlying neoplasm (C00-D49)

G13.1 Other systemic atrophy primarily affecting central nervous system in neoplastic disease
Paraneoplastic limbic encephalopathy
Code first underlying neoplasm (C00-D49)

G13.2 Systemic atrophy primarily affecting the central nervous system in myxedema
Code first underlying disease, such as:
hypothyroidism (E03.-)
myxedematous congenital iodine deficiency (E00.1)

G13.8 Systemic atrophy primarily affecting central nervous system in other diseases classified elsewhere
Code first underlying disease

G14 Postpolio syndrome
Postpolio myelitic syndrome
EXCLUDES 1 *sequelae of poliomyelitis (B91)*

Extrapyramidal and movement disorders (G20-G26)

G20 Parkinson's disease
Hemiparkinsonism
Idiopathic Parkinsonism or Parkinson's disease
Paralysis agitans
Parkinsonism or Parkinson's disease NOS
Primary Parkinsonism or Parkinson's disease
EXCLUDES 1 *dementia with Parkinsonism (G31.83)*

☑4ᵗʰ **G21 Secondary parkinsonism**
EXCLUDES 1 *dementia with Parkinsonism (G31.83)*
Huntington's disease (G10)
Shy-Drager syndrome (G90.3)
syphilitic Parkinsonism (A52.19)

G21.0 Malignant neuroleptic syndrome
Use additional code for adverse effect, if applicable, to identify drug (T43.3X5, T43.4X5, T43.505, T43.595)
EXCLUDES 1 *neuroleptic induced parkinsonism (G21.11)*

☑5ᵗʰ **G21.1 Other drug-induced secondary parkinsonism**

G21.11 Neuroleptic induced parkinsonism
Use additional code for adverse effect, if applicable, to identify drug (T43.3X5, T43.4X5, T43.505, T43.595)
EXCLUDES 1 *malignant neuroleptic syndrome (G21.0)*

G21.19 Other drug induced secondary parkinsonism
Use additional code for adverse effect, if applicable, to identify drug (T36-T50 with fifth or sixth character 5)

G21.2 Secondary parkinsonism due to other external agents
Code first (T51-T65) to identify external agent

G21.3 Postencephalitic parkinsonism

G21.4 Vascular parkinsonism

G21.8 Other secondary parkinsonism

G21.9 Secondary parkinsonism, unspecified

☑4ᵗʰ **G23 Other degenerative diseases of basal ganglia**
EXCLUDES 2 *multi-system degeneration of the autonomic nervous system (G90.3)*

G23.0 Hallervorden-Spatz disease
Pigmentary pallidal degeneration

G23.1 Progressive supranuclear ophthalmoplegia [Steele-Richardson-Olszewski]
Progressive supranuclear palsy

G23.2 Striatonigral degeneration

G23.8 Other specified degenerative diseases of basal ganglia
Calcification of basal ganglia

G23.9 Degenerative disease of basal ganglia, unspecified

☑4ᵗʰ **G24 Dystonia**
INCLUDES dyskinesia
EXCLUDES 2 *athetoid cerebral palsy (G80.3)*

☑5ᵗʰ **G24.0 Drug induced dystonia**
Use additional code code for adverse effect, if applicable, to identify drug (T36-T50 with fifth or sixth character5)

G24.01 Drug induced subacute dyskinesia
Drug induced blepharospasm
Drug induced orofacial dyskinesia
Neuroleptic induced tardive dyskinesia
Tardive dyskinesia

G24.02 Drug induced acute dystonia
Acute dystonic reaction to drugs
Neuroleptic induced acute dystonia

G24.09 Other drug induced dystonia

G24.1 Genetic torsion dystonia
Dystonia deformans progressiva
Dystonia musculorum deformans
Familial torsion dystonia
Idiopathic familial dystonia
Idiopathic (torsion) dystonia NOS
(Schwalbe-) Ziehen-Oppenheim disease

G24.2 Idiopathic nonfamilial dystonia

G24.3 Spasmodic torticollis
EXCLUDES 1 *congenital torticollis (Q68.0)*
hysterical torticollis (F44.4)
ocular torticollis (R29.891)
psychogenic torticollis (F45.8)
torticollis NOS (M43.6)
traumatic recurrent torticollis (S13.4)

G24.4 Idiopathic orofacial dystonia
Orofacial dyskinesia
EXCLUDES 1 *drug induced orofacial dyskinesia (G24.01)*

G24.5 Blepharospasm
EXCLUDES 1 *drug induced blepharospasm (G24.01)*

G24.8 Other dystonia
Acquired torsion dystonia NOS

G24.9 Dystonia, unspecified
Dyskinesia NOS

☑4ᵗʰ **G25 Other extrapyramidal and movement disorders**
EXCLUDES 2 *sleep related movement disorders (G47.6-)*

G25.0 Essential tremor
Familial tremor
EXCLUDES 1 *tremor NOS (R25.1)*

G25.1 Drug-induced tremor
Use additional code for adverse effect, if applicable, to identify drug (T36-T50 with fifth or sixth character 5)

G25.2 Other specified forms of tremor
Intention tremor

G25.3 Myoclonus
Drug-induced myoclonus
Palatal myoclonus
Use additional code for adverse effect, if applicable, to identify drug (T36-T50 with fifth or sixth character 5)
EXCLUDES 1 *facial myokymia (G51.4)*
myoclonic epilepsy (G40.-)

G25.4 Drug-induced chorea
Use additional code for adverse effect, if applicable, to identify drug (T36-T50 with fifth or sixth character 5)

G25.5 Other chorea
Chorea NOS
EXCLUDES 1 *chorea NOS with heart involvement (I02.0)*
Huntington's chorea (G10)
rheumatic chorea (I02.-)
Sydenham's chorea (I02.-)

☑5ᵗʰ **G25.6 Drug induced tics and other tics of organic origin**

G25.61 Drug induced tics
Use additional code for adverse effect, if applicable, to identify drug (T36-T50 with fifth or sixth character 5)

G25.69 Other tics of organic origin
EXCLUDES 1 *habit spasm (F95.9)*
tic NOS (F95.9)
Tourette's syndrome (F95.2)

☑5ᵗʰ **G25.7 Other and unspecified drug induced movement disorders**
Use additional code for adverse effect, if applicable, to identify drug (T36-T50 with fifth or sixth character 5)

G25.70 Drug induced movement disorder, unspecified

G25.71 Drug induced akathisia
Drug induced acathisia
Neuroleptic induced acute akathisia

G25.79 Other drug induced movement disorders

☑5ᵗʰ **G25.8 Other specified extrapyramidal and movement disorders**

G25.81 Restless legs syndrome

EXCLUDES 1 Not coded here   EXCLUDES 2 Not included here   N Newborn Age: 0   P Pediatric Age: 0-17   M Maternity Age: 12-55   A Adult Age: 15-124

514   ICD-10-CM 2014 (Draft)

Diseases of the Nervous System

G25.82–G37.9

    G25.82 Stiff-man syndrome

    G25.83 Benign shuddering attacks

    G25.89 Other specified extrapyramidal and movement disorders

  G25.9 Extrapyramidal and movement disorder, unspecified

G26 *Extrapyramidal and movement disorders in diseases classified elsewhere*

    Code first underlying disease

Other degenerative diseases of the nervous system (G30-G32)

✓4ᵗʰ **G30 Alzheimer's disease**

    INCLUDES Alzheimer's dementia senile and presenile forms

    Use additional code to identify:
      delirium, if applicable (F05)
      dementia with behavioral disturbance (F02.81)
      dementia without behavioral disturbance (F02.80)

    EXCLUDES 1 senile degeneration of brain NEC (G31.1)
      senile dementia NOS (F03)
      senility NOS (R41.81)

  G30.0 Alzheimer's disease with early onset

  G30.1 Alzheimer's disease with late onset   Ⓐ

  G30.8 Other Alzheimer's disease

  G30.9 Alzheimer's disease, unspecified

    AHA: 2012, Q4, 95

✓4ᵗʰ **G31 Other degenerative diseases of nervous system, not elsewhere classified**

    Use additional code to identify:
      dementia with behavioral disturbance (F02.81)
      dementia without behavioral disturbance (F02.80)

    EXCLUDES 2 Reye's syndrome (G93.7)

✓5ᵗʰ **G31.0 Frontotemporal dementia**

  G31.01 Pick's disease
    Primary progressive aphasia
    Progressive isolated aphasia

  G31.09 Other frontotemporal dementia
    Frontal dementia

  G31.1 Senile degeneration of brain, not elsewhere classified
    EXCLUDES 1 Alzheimer's disease (G30.-)
      senility NOS (R41.81)

  G31.2 Degeneration of nervous system due to alcohol
    Alcoholic cerebellar ataxia
    Alcoholic cerebellar degeneration
    Alcoholic cerebral degeneration
    Alcoholic encephalopathy
    Dysfunction of the autonomic nervous system due to alcohol
    Code also associated alcoholism (F10.-)

✓5ᵗʰ **G31.8 Other specified degenerative diseases of nervous system**

  G31.81 Alpers disease
    Grey-matter degeneration

  G31.82 Leigh's disease
    Subacute necrotizing encephalopathy

  G31.83 Dementia with Lewy bodies
    Dementia with Parkinsonism
    Lewy body dementia
    Lewy body disease

  G31.84 Mild cognitive impairment, so stated
    EXCLUDES 1 age related cognitive decline (R41.81)
      altered mental status (R41.82)
      cerebral degeneration (G31.9)
      change in mental status (R41.82)
      cognitive deficits following (sequelae of)
        cerebral hemorrhage or infarction
        (I69.01, I69.11, I69.21, I69.31, I69.81, I69.91)
      cognitive impairment due to intracranial or
        head injury (S06.-)
      dementia (F01.-, F02.-, F03)
      mild memory disturbance (F06.8)
      neurologic neglect syndrome (R41.4)
      personality change, nonpsychotic (F68.8)

  G31.85 Corticobasal degeneration

  G31.89 Other specified degenerative diseases of nervous system

  G31.9 Degenerative disease of nervous system, unspecified

✓4ᵗʰ **G32 Other degenerative disorders of nervous system in diseases classified elsewhere**

  G32.0 *Subacute combined degeneration of spinal cord in diseases classified elsewhere*
    Dana-Putnam syndrome
    Sclerosis of spinal cord (combined) (dorsolateral) (posterolateral)

    Code first underlying disease, such as:
      vitamin B12 deficiency (E53.8)
      vitamin B12 deficiency:
        anemia (D51.9)
        dietary (D51.3)
        pernicious (D51.0)

    EXCLUDES 1 syphilitic combined degeneration of spinal cord (A52.11)

✓5ᵗʰ **G32.8 Other specified degenerative disorders of nervous system in diseases classified elsewhere**

    Code first underlying disease, such as:
      amyloidosis cerebral degeneration (E85.-)
      cerebral degeneration (due to) hypothyroidism (E00.0-E03.9)
      cerebral degeneration (due to) neoplasm (C00-D49)
      cerebral degeneration (due to) vitamin B deficiency, except thiamine (E52-E53.-)

    EXCLUDES 1 superior hemorrhagic polioencephalitis [Wernicke's encephalopathy] (E51.2)

  G32.81 *Cerebellar ataxia in diseases classified elsewhere*
    Code first underlying disease, such as:
      celiac disease (with gluten ataxia) (K90.0)
      cerebellar ataxia (in) neoplastic disease
        (paraneoplastic cerebellar degeneration) (C00-D49)
      non-celiac gluten ataxia (M35.9)

    EXCLUDES 1 systemic atrophy primarily affecting the central nervous system in alcoholic cerebellar ataxia (G31.2)
      systemic atrophy primarily affecting the central nervous system in myxedema (G13.2)

  G32.89 *Other specified degenerative disorders of nervous system in diseases classified elsewhere*
    Degenerative encephalopathy in diseases classified elsewhere

Demyelinating diseases of the central nervous system (G35-G37)

  G35 Multiple sclerosis
    Disseminated multiple sclerosis
    Generalized multiple sclerosis
    Multiple sclerosis NOS
    Multiple sclerosis of brain stem
    Multiple sclerosis of cord

✓4ᵗʰ **G36 Other acute disseminated demyelination**
    EXCLUDES 1 postinfectious encephalitis and encephalomyelitis NOS (G04.01)

  G36.0 Neuromyelitis optica [Devic]
    Demyelination in optic neuritis
    EXCLUDES 1 optic neuritis NOS (H46)

  G36.1 Acute and subacute hemorrhagic leukoencephalitis [Hurst]

  G36.8 Other specified acute disseminated demyelination

  G36.9 Acute disseminated demyelination, unspecified

✓4ᵗʰ **G37 Other demyelinating diseases of central nervous system**

  G37.0 Diffuse sclerosis of central nervous system
    Periaxial encephalitis
    Schilder's disease
    EXCLUDES 1 X linked adrenoleukodystrophy (E71.52-)

  G37.1 Central demyelination of corpus callosum

  G37.2 Central pontine myelinolysis

  G37.3 Acute transverse myelitis in demyelinating disease of central nervous system
    Acute transverse myelitis NOS
    Acute transverse myelopathy
    EXCLUDES 1 multiple sclerosis (G35)
      neuromyelitis optica [Devic] (G36.0)

  G37.4 Subacute necrotizing myelitis of central nervous system

  G37.5 Concentric sclerosis [Balo] of central nervous system

  G37.8 Other specified demyelinating diseases of central nervous system

  G37.9 Demyelinating disease of central nervous system, unspecified

✓ Additional Character Required   ✓x7ᵗʰ Xtension Alert   Unspecified Code   Other Specified Code   Manifestation Code   ▶◀ Revised Text   ● New Code   ▲ Revised Code Title

ICD-10-CM 2014 (Draft)   515

Diseases of the Nervous System

G40–G40.A11

Episodic and paroxysmal disorders (G40-G47)

☑4ᵗʰ **G40 Epilepsy and recurrent seizures**

> **NOTE** The following terms are to be considered equivalent to intractable: pharmacoresistant (pharmacologically resistant), treatment resistant, refractory (medically) and poorly controlled.

> **EXCLUDES 1** *conversion disorder with seizures (F44.5)*
> *convulsions NOS (R56.9)*
> *hippocampal sclerosis (G93.81)*
> *mesial temporal sclerosis (G93.81)*
> *post traumatic seizures (R56.1)*
> *seizure (convulsive) NOS (R56.9)*
> *seizure of newborn (P90)*
> *temporal sclerosis (G93.81)*
> *Todd's paralysis (G83.8)*

☑5ᵗʰ **G40.0 Localization-related (focal) (partial) idiopathic epilepsy and epileptic syndromes with seizures of localized onset**
Benign childhood epilepsy with centrotemporal EEG spikes
Childhood epilepsy with occipital EEG paroxysms

> **EXCLUDES 1** *adult onset localization-related epilepsy (G40.1-, G40.2-)*

☑6ᵗʰ **G40.00 Localization-related (focal) (partial) idiopathic epilepsy and epileptic syndromes with seizures of localized onset, not intractable**
Localization-related (focal) (partial) idiopathic epilepsy and epileptic syndromes with seizures of localized onset without intractability

G40.001 Localization-related (focal) (partial) idiopathic epilepsy and epileptic syndromes with seizures of localized onset, not intractable, with status epilepticus

G40.009 Localization-related (focal) (partial) idiopathic epilepsy and epileptic syndromes with seizures of localized onset, not intractable, without status epilepticus
Localization-related (focal) (partial) idiopathic epilepsy and epileptic syndromes with seizures of localized onset NOS

☑6ᵗʰ **G40.01 Localization-related (focal) (partial) idiopathic epilepsy and epileptic syndromes with seizures of localized onset, intractable**

G40.011 Localization-related (focal) (partial) idiopathic epilepsy and epileptic syndromes with seizures of localized onset, intractable, with status epilepticus

G40.019 Localization-related (focal) (partial) idiopathic epilepsy and epileptic syndromes with seizures of localized onset, intractable, without status epilepticus

☑5ᵗʰ **G40.1 Localization-related (focal) (partial) symptomatic epilepsy and epileptic syndromes with simple partial seizures**
Attacks without alteration of consciousness
Epilepsia partialis continua [Kozhevnikof]
Simple partial seizures developing into secondarily generalized seizures

☑6ᵗʰ **G40.10 Localization-related (focal) (partial) symptomatic epilepsy and epileptic syndromes with simple partial seizures, not intractable**
Localization-related (focal) (partial) symptomatic epilepsy and epileptic syndromes with simple partial seizures without intractability

G40.101 Localization-related (focal) (partial) symptomatic epilepsy and epileptic syndromes with simple partial seizures, not intractable, with status epilepticus

G40.109 Localization-related (focal) (partial) symptomatic epilepsy and epileptic syndromes with simple partial seizures, not intractable, without status epilepticus
Localization-related (focal) (partial) symptomatic epilepsy and epileptic syndromes with simple partial seizures NOS

☑6ᵗʰ **G40.11 Localization-related (focal) (partial) symptomatic epilepsy and epileptic syndromes with simple partial seizures, intractable**

G40.111 Localization-related (focal) (partial) symptomatic epilepsy and epileptic syndromes with simple partial seizures, intractable, with status epilepticus

G40.119 Localization-related (focal) (partial) symptomatic epilepsy and epileptic syndromes with simple partial seizures, intractable, without status epilepticus

☑5ᵗʰ **G40.2 Localization-related (focal) (partial) symptomatic epilepsy and epileptic syndromes with complex partial seizures**
Attacks with alteration of consciousness, often with automatisms
Complex partial seizures developing into secondarily generalized seizures

☑6ᵗʰ **G40.20 Localization-related (focal) (partial) symptomatic epilepsy and epileptic syndromes with complex partial seizures, not intractable**
Localization-related (focal) (partial) symptomatic epilepsy and epileptic syndromes with complex partial seizures without intractability

G40.201 Localization-related (focal) (partial) symptomatic epilepsy and epileptic syndromes with complex partial seizures, not intractable, with status epilepticus

G40.209 Localization-related (focal) (partial) symptomatic epilepsy and epileptic syndromes with complex partial seizures, not intractable, without status epilepticus
Localization-related (focal) (partial) symptomatic epilepsy and epileptic syndromes with complex partial seizures NOS

☑6ᵗʰ **G40.21 Localization-related (focal) (partial) symptomatic epilepsy and epileptic syndromes with complex partial seizures, intractable**

G40.211 Localization-related (focal) (partial) symptomatic epilepsy and epileptic syndromes with complex partial seizures, intractable, with status epilepticus

G40.219 Localization-related (focal) (partial) symptomatic epilepsy and epileptic syndromes with complex partial seizures, intractable, without status epilepticus

☑5ᵗʰ **G40.3 Generalized idiopathic epilepsy and epileptic syndromes**
Code also MERRF syndrome, if applicable (E88.42)

☑6ᵗʰ **G40.30 Generalized idiopathic epilepsy and epileptic syndromes, not intractable**
Generalized idiopathic epilepsy and epileptic syndromes without intractability

G40.301 Generalized idiopathic epilepsy and epileptic syndromes, not intractable, with status epilepticus

G40.309 Generalized idiopathic epilepsy and epileptic syndromes, not intractable, without status epilepticus
Generalized idiopathic epilepsy and epileptic syndromes NOS

☑6ᵗʰ **G40.31 Generalized idiopathic epilepsy and epileptic syndromes, intractable**

G40.311 Generalized idiopathic epilepsy and epileptic syndromes, intractable, with status epilepticus

G40.319 Generalized idiopathic epilepsy and epileptic syndromes, intractable, without status epilepticus

☑5ᵗʰ **G40.A Absence epileptic syndrome**
Childhood absence epilepsy [pyknolepsy]
Juvenile absence epilepsy
Absence epileptic syndrome, NOS

☑6ᵗʰ **G40.A0 Absence epileptic syndrome, not intractable**

G40.A01 Absence epileptic syndrome, not intractable, with status epilepticus

G40.A09 Absence epileptic syndrome, not intractable, without status epilepticus

☑6ᵗʰ **G40.A1 Absence epileptic syndrome, intractable**

G40.A11 Absence epileptic syndrome, intractable, with status epilepticus

EXCLUDES 1 Not coded here   **EXCLUDES 2** Not included here   N Newborn Age: 0   P Pediatric Age: 0-17   M Maternity Age: 12-55   A Adult Age: 15-124

516   ICD-10-CM 2014 (Draft)

G40.A19   **Absence epileptic syndrome, intractable, without status epilepticus**

☑5ᵗʰ   **G40.B**   Juvenile myoclonic epilepsy [impulsive petit mal]

   ☑6ᵗʰ   **G40.B0**   **Juvenile myoclonic epilepsy, not intractable**

     G40.B01   **Juvenile myoclonic epilepsy, not intractable, with status epilepticus**

     G40.B09   **Juvenile myoclonic epilepsy, not intractable, without status epilepticus**

   ☑6ᵗʰ   **G40.B1**   **Juvenile myoclonic epilepsy, intractable**

     G40.B11   **Juvenile myoclonic epilepsy, intractable, with status epilepticus**

     G40.B19   **Juvenile myoclonic epilepsy, intractable, without status epilepticus**

☑5ᵗʰ   **G40.4**   **Other generalized epilepsy and epileptic syndromes**

     Epilepsy with grand mal seizures on awakening
     Epilepsy with myoclonic absences
     Epilepsy with myoclonic-astatic seizures
     Grand mal seizure NOS
     Nonspecific atonic epileptic seizures
     Nonspecific clonic epileptic seizures
     Nonspecific myoclonic epileptic seizures
     Nonspecific tonic epileptic seizures
     Nonspecific tonic-clonic epileptic seizures
     Symptomatic early myoclonic encephalopathy

   ☑6ᵗʰ   **G40.40**   **Other generalized epilepsy and epileptic syndromes, not intractable**

     Other generalized epilepsy and epileptic syndromes without intractability
     Other generalized epilepsy and epileptic syndromes NOS

     G40.401   **Other generalized epilepsy and epileptic syndromes, not intractable, with status epilepticus**

     G40.409   **Other generalized epilepsy and epileptic syndromes, not intractable, without status epilepticus**

   ☑6ᵗʰ   **G40.41**   **Other generalized epilepsy and epileptic syndromes, intractable**

     G40.411   **Other generalized epilepsy and epileptic syndromes, intractable, with status epilepticus**

     G40.419   **Other generalized epilepsy and epileptic syndromes, intractable, without status epilepticus**

☑5ᵗʰ   **G40.5**   **Epileptic seizures related to external causes**

     Epileptic seizures related to alcohol
     Epileptic seizures related to drugs
     Epileptic seizures related to hormonal changes
     Epileptic seizures related to sleep deprivation
     Epileptic seizures related to stress
     Use additional code for adverse effect, if applicable, to identify drug (T36-T50 with fifth or sixth character 5)
     Code also, if applicable, associated epilepsy and recurrent seizures (G40.-)

   ☑6ᵗʰ   **G40.50**   **Epileptic seizures related to external causes, not intractable**

     G40.501   **Epileptic seizures related to external causes, not intractable, with status epilepticus**

     G40.509   **Epileptic seizures related to external causes, not intractable, without status epilepticus**

       Epileptic seizures related to external causes, NOS

☑5ᵗʰ   **G40.8**   **Other epilepsy and recurrent seizures**

     Epilepsies and epileptic syndromes undetermined as to whether they are focal or generalized
     Landau-Kleffner syndrome

   ☑6ᵗʰ   **G40.80**   **Other epilepsy**

     G40.801   **Other epilepsy, not intractable, with status epilepticus**

       Other epilepsy without intractability with status epilepticus

     G40.802   **Other epilepsy, not intractable, without status epilepticus**

       Other epilepsy without intractability without status epilepticus

     G40.803   **Other epilepsy, intractable, with status epilepticus**

     G40.804   **Other epilepsy, intractable, without status epilepticus**

   ☑6ᵗʰ   **G40.81**   **Lennox-Gastaut syndrome**

     G40.811   **Lennox-Gastaut syndrome, not intractable, with status epilepticus**

     G40.812   **Lennox-Gastaut syndrome, not intractable, without status epilepticus**

     G40.813   **Lennox-Gastaut syndrome, intractable, with status epilepticus**

     G40.814   **Lennox-Gastaut syndrome, intractable, without status epilepticus**

   ☑6ᵗʰ   **G40.82**   **Epileptic spasms**

     Infantile spasms
     Salaam attacks
     West's syndrome

     G40.821   **Epileptic spasms, not intractable, with status epilepticus**

     G40.822   **Epileptic spasms, not intractable, without status epilepticus**

     G40.823   **Epileptic spasms, intractable, with status epilepticus**

     G40.824   **Epileptic spasms, intractable, without status epilepticus**

   G40.89   **Other seizures**

     EXCLUDES 1   *post traumatic seizures (R56.1)*
             recurrent seizures NOS (G40.909)
             seizure NOS (R56.9)

☑5ᵗʰ   **G40.9**   **Epilepsy, unspecified**

   ☑6ᵗʰ   **G40.90**   **Epilepsy, unspecified, not intractable**

     Epilepsy, unspecified, without intractability

     G40.901   **Epilepsy, unspecified, not intractable, with status epilepticus**

     G40.909   **Epilepsy, unspecified, not intractable, without status epilepticus**

       Epilepsy NOS
       Epileptic convulsions NOS
       Epileptic fits NOS
       Epileptic seizures NOS
       Recurrent seizures NOS
       Seizure disorder NOS

   ☑6ᵗʰ   **G40.91**   **Epilepsy, unspecified, intractable**

     Intractable seizure disorder NOS

     G40.911   **Epilepsy, unspecified, intractable, with status epilepticus**

     G40.919   **Epilepsy, unspecified, intractable, without status epilepticus**

☑4ᵗʰ   **G43**   **Migraine**

   NOTE   The following terms are to be considered equivalent to intractable: pharmacoresistant (pharmacologically resistant), treatment resistant, refractory (medically) and poorly controlled.

     Use additional code f.or adverse effect, if applicable, to identify drug (T36-T50 with fifth or sixth character 5)

   EXCLUDES 1   *headache NOS (R51)*
             lower half migraine (G44.00)
   EXCLUDES 2   *headache syndromes (G44.-)*

☑5ᵗʰ   **G43.0**   **Migraine without aura**

     Common migraine
     EXCLUDES 1   *chronic migraine without aura (G43.7-)*

   ☑6ᵗʰ   **G43.00**   **Migraine without aura, not intractable**

     Migraine without aura without mention of refractory migraine

     G43.001   **Migraine without aura, not intractable, with status migrainosus**

     G43.009   **Migraine without aura, not intractable, without status migrainosus**

       Migraine without aura NOS

   ☑6ᵗʰ   **G43.01**   **Migraine without aura, intractable**

     Migraine without aura with refractory migraine

     G43.011   **Migraine without aura, intractable, with status migrainosus**

     G43.019   **Migraine without aura, intractable, without status migrainosus**

☑ Additional Character Required   ✓x7ᵗʰ *X*tension Alert   Unspecified Code   Other Specified Code   Manifestation Code   ◄► Revised Text   ● New Code   ▲ Revised Code Title

ICD-10-CM 2014 (Draft)   **517**

✓5th **G43.1** **Migraine** with aura
Basilar migraine
Classical migraine
Migraine equivalents
Migraine preceded or accompanied by transient focal
    neurological phenomena
Migraine triggered seizures
Migraine with acute-onset aura
Migraine with aura without headache (migraine equivalents)
Migraine with prolonged aura
Migraine with typical aura
Retinal migraine
Code also any associated seizure (G40.-, R56.9)
EXCLUDES 1   persistent migraine aura (G43.5-, G43.6-)

    ✓6th **G43.10** **Migraine with aura,** not intractable
Migraine with aura without mention of refractory
migraine

        G43.101 **Migraine with aura, not intractable,** with
status migrainosus

        G43.109 **Migraine with aura, not intractable,**
without status migrainosus
Migraine with aura NOS

    ✓6th **G43.11** **Migraine with aura,** intractable
Migraine with aura with refractory migraine

        G43.111 **Migraine with aura, intractable,** with
status migrainosus

        G43.119 **Migraine with aura, intractable,** without
status migrainosus

✓5th **G43.4** **Hemiplegic migraine**
Familial migraine
Sporadic migraine

    ✓6th **G43.40** **Hemiplegic migraine,** not intractable
Hemiplegic migraine without refractory migraine

        G43.401 **Hemiplegic migraine, not intractable,** with
status migrainosus

        G43.409 **Hemiplegic migraine, not intractable,**
without status migrainosus
Hemiplegic migraine NOS

    ✓6th **G43.41** **Hemiplegic migraine,** intractable
Hemiplegic migraine with refractory migraine

        G43.411 **Hemiplegic migraine, intractable,** with
status migrainosus

        G43.419 **Hemiplegic migraine, intractable,** without
status migrainosus

✓5th **G43.5** **Persistent migraine** aura without cerebral infarction

    ✓6th **G43.50** **Persistent migraine aura without cerebral infarction,**
not intractable
Persistent migraine aura without cerebral infarction,
without refractory migraine

        G43.501 **Persistent migraine aura without cerebral
infarction, not intractable,** with status
migrainosus

        G43.509 **Persistent migraine aura without cerebral
infarction, not intractable,** without status
migrainosus
Persistent migraine aura NOS

    ✓6th **G43.51** **Persistent migraine aura without cerebral infarction,**
intractable
Persistent migraine aura without cerebral infarction,
with refractory migraine

        G43.511 **Persistent migraine aura without cerebral
infarction, intractable,** with status
migrainosus

        G43.519 **Persistent migraine aura without cerebral
infarction, intractable,** without status
migrainosus

✓5th **G43.6** **Persistent migraine** aura with cerebral infarction
Code also the type of cerebral infarction (I63.-)

    ✓6th **G43.60** **Persistent migraine aura with cerebral infarction,**
not intractable
Persistent migraine aura with cerebral infarction,
without refractory migraine

        G43.601 **Persistent migraine aura with cerebral
infarction, not intractable,** with status
migrainosus

        G43.609 **Persistent migraine aura with cerebral
infarction, not intractable,** without status
migrainosus

    ✓6th **G43.61** **Persistent migraine aura with cerebral infarction,**
intractable
Persistent migraine aura with cerebral infarction, with
refractory migraine

        G43.611 **Persistent migraine aura with cerebral
infarction, intractable,** with status
migrainosus

        G43.619 **Persistent migraine aura with cerebral
infarction, intractable,** without status
migrainosus

✓5th **G43.7** **Chronic migraine** without aura
Transformed migraine
EXCLUDES 1   migraine without aura (G43.0-)

    ✓6th **G43.70** **Chronic migraine without aura,** not intractable
Chronic migraine without aura, without refractory
migraine

        G43.701 **Chronic migraine without aura, not
intractable,** with status migrainosus

        G43.709 **Chronic migraine without aura, not
intractable,** without status migrainosus
Chronic migraine without aura NOS

    ✓6th **G43.71** **Chronic migraine without aura,** intractable
Chronic migraine without aura, with refractory
migraine

        G43.711 **Chronic migraine without aura,
intractable,** with status migrainosus

        G43.719 **Chronic migraine without aura,
intractable,** without status migrainosus

✓5th **G43.A** **Cyclical vomiting**

    G43.A0 **Cyclical vomiting,** not intractable
Cyclical vomiting, without refractory migraine

    G43.A1 **Cyclical vomiting,** intractable
Cyclical vomiting, with refractory migraine

✓5th **G43.B** **Ophthalmoplegic migraine**

    G43.B0 **Ophthalmoplegic migraine,** not intractable
Ophthalmoplegic migraine, without refractory
migraine

    G43.B1 **Ophthalmoplegic migraine,** intractable
Ophthalmoplegic migraine, with refractory migraine

✓5th **G43.C** **Periodic headache syndromes in child or adult**

    G43.C0 **Periodic headache syndromes in child or adult,** not
intractable
Periodic headache syndromes in child or adult,
without refractory migraine

    G43.C1 **Periodic headache syndromes in child or adult,**
intractable
Periodic headache syndromes in child or adult, with
refractory migraine

✓5th **G43.D** **Abdominal migraine**

    G43.D0 **Abdominal migraine,** not intractable
Abdominal migraine, without refractory migraine

    G43.D1 **Abdominal migraine,** intractable
Abdominal migraine, with refractory migraine

✓5th **G43.8** **Other migraine**

    ✓6th **G43.80** **Other migraine,** not intractable
Other migraine, without refractory migraine

        G43.801 **Other migraine, not intractable,** with
status migrainosus

        G43.809 **Other migraine, not intractable,** without
status migrainosus

    ✓6th **G43.81** **Other migraine,** intractable
Other migraine, with refractory migraine

        G43.811 **Other migraine, intractable,** with status
migrainosus

        G43.819 **Other migraine, intractable,** without
status migrainosus

    ✓6th **G43.82** **Menstrual migraine,** not intractable
Menstrual headache, not intractable
Menstrual migraine, without refractory migraine
Menstrually related migraine, not intractable
Pre-menstrual headache, not intractable
Pre-menstrual migraine, not intractable
Pure menstrual migraine, not intractable
Code also associated premenstrual tension syndrome
(N94.3)

        G43.821 **Menstrual migraine, not intractable,** ♀
with status migrainosus

EXCLUDES 1 Not coded here   EXCLUDES 2 Not included here   N Newborn Age: 0   P Pediatric Age: 0-17   M Maternity Age: 12-55   A Adult Age: 15-124

518   ICD-10-CM 2014 (Draft)

G43.829　Menstrual migraine, not intractable, ♀
without status migrainosus
Menstrual migraine NOS

✓6th G43.83　Menstrual **migraine,** intractable
Menstrual headache, intractable
Menstrual migraine, with refractory migraine
Menstrually related migraine, intractable
Pre-menstrual headache, intractable
Pre-menstrual migraine, intractable
Pure menstrual migraine, intractable
Code also associated premenstrual tension syndrome
(N94.3)

G43.831　Menstrual migraine, intractable, with ♀
status migrainosus

G43.839　Menstrual migraine, intractable, ♀
without status migrainosus

✓5th G43.9　Migraine, unspecified

✓6th G43.90　Migraine, unspecified, not intractable
Migraine, unspecified, without refractory migraine

G43.901　Migraine, unspecified, not intractable, with status migrainosus
Status migrainosus NOS

G43.909　Migraine, unspecified, not intractable, without status migrainosus
Migraine NOS

✓6th G43.91　Migraine, unspecified, intractable
Migraine, unspecified, with refractory migraine

G43.911　Migraine, unspecified, intractable, with status migrainosus

G43.919　Migraine, unspecified, intractable, without status migrainosus

✓4th **G44**　Other headache **syndromes**
EXCLUDES 1　headache NOS (R51)
EXCLUDES 2　atypical facial pain (G50.1)
headache due to lumbar puncture (G97.1)
migraines (G43.-)
trigeminal neuralgia (G50.0)

✓5th **G44.0**　Cluster headaches and other trigeminal autonomic cephalgias (TAC)

✓6th G44.00　Cluster headache syndrome, unspecified
Ciliary neuralgia
Cluster headache NOS
Histamine cephalgia
Lower half migraine
Migrainous neuralgia

G44.001　Cluster headache syndrome, unspecified, intractable

G44.009　Cluster headache syndrome, unspecified, not intractable
Cluster headache syndrome NOS

✓6th G44.01　Episodic **cluster headache**
G44.011　Episodic cluster headache, intractable
G44.019　Episodic cluster headache, not intractable
Episodic cluster headache NOS

✓6th G44.02　Chronic **cluster headache**
G44.021　Chronic cluster headache, intractable
G44.029　Chronic cluster headache, not intractable
Chronic cluster headache NOS

✓6th G44.03　Episodic **paroxysmal hemicrania**
Paroxysmal hemicrania NOS

G44.031　Episodic paroxysmal hemicrania, intractable

G44.039　Episodic paroxysmal hemicrania, not intractable
Episodic paroxysmal hemicrania NOS

✓6th G44.04　Chronic **paroxysmal hemicrania**
G44.041　Chronic paroxysmal hemicrania, intractable

G44.049　Chronic paroxysmal hemicrania, not intractable
Chronic paroxysmal hemicrania NOS

✓6th G44.05　Short lasting unilateral **neuralgiform headache with conjunctival injection and tearing (SUNCT)**
G44.051　Short lasting unilateral neuralgiform headache with conjunctival injection and tearing (SUNCT), intractable

G44.059　Short lasting unilateral neuralgiform headache with conjunctival injection and tearing (SUNCT), not intractable
Short lasting unilateral neuralgiform headache with conjunctival injection and tearing (SUNCT) NOS

✓6th G44.09　Other trigeminal autonomic cephalgias (TAC)
G44.091　Other trigeminal autonomic cephalgias (TAC), intractable

G44.099　Other trigeminal autonomic cephalgias syndrome (TAC), not intractable

G44.1　Vascular **headache, not elsewhere classified**
EXCLUDES 2　cluster headache (G44.0)
complicated headache syndromes (G44.5-)
drug-induced headache (G44.4-)
migraine (G43.-)
other specified headache syndromes (G44.8-)
post-traumatic headache (G44.3-)
tension-type headache (G44.2-)

✓5th G44.2　Tension-type **headache**
✓6th G44.20　Tension-type headache, unspecified
G44.201　Tension-type headache, unspecified, intractable

G44.209　Tension-type headache, unspecified, not intractable
Tension headache NOS

✓6th G44.21　Episodic **tension-type headache**
G44.211　Episodic tension-type headache, intractable

G44.219　Episodic tension-type headache, not intractable
Episodic tension-type headache NOS

✓6th G44.22　Chronic **tension-type headache**
G44.221　Chronic tension-type headache, intractable

G44.229　Chronic tension-type headache, not intractable
Chronic tension-type headache NOS

✓5th G44.3　Post-traumatic **headache**
✓6th G44.30　Post-traumatic headache, unspecified
G44.301　Post-traumatic headache, unspecified, intractable

G44.309　Post-traumatic headache, unspecified, not intractable
Post-traumatic headache NOS

✓6th G44.31　Acute **post-traumatic headache**
G44.311　Acute post-traumatic headache, intractable

G44.319　Acute post-traumatic headache, not intractable
Acute post-traumatic headache NOS

✓6th G44.32　Chronic **post-traumatic headache**
G44.321　Chronic post-traumatic headache, intractable

G44.329　Chronic post-traumatic headache, not intractable
Chronic post-traumatic headache NOS

✓5th G44.4　Drug-induced **headache, not elsewhere classified**
Medication overuse headache
Use additional code for adverse effect, if applicable, to identify drug (T36-T50 with fifth or sixth character 5)

G44.40　Drug-induced headache, not elsewhere classified, not intractable

G44.41　Drug-induced headache, not elsewhere classified, intractable

✓5th G44.5　Complicated **headache syndromes**
G44.51　Hemicrania continua
G44.52　New daily persistent headache (NDPH)
G44.53　Primary **thunderclap headache**
G44.59　Other complicated headache syndrome

✓5th G44.8　Other specified **headache syndromes**
G44.81　Hypnic **headache**
G44.82　Headache associated with **sexual activity**
Orgasmic headache
Preorgasmic headache

G44.83　Primary **cough headache**
G44.84　Primary **exertional headache**

✓ Additional Character Required　　✓x7th Xtension Alert　　Unspecified Code　　Other Specified Code　　Manifestation Code　　▶◀ Revised Text　　● New Code　　▲ Revised Code Title

G44.85   Primary stabbing headache

G44.89   Other headache syndrome

☑4th **G45**   **Transient cerebral ischemic attacks and related syndromes**

> EXCLUDES 1   neonatal cerebral ischemia (P91.0)
> transient retinal artery occlusion (H34.0-)

G45.0   Vertebro-basilar artery syndrome

G45.1   Carotid artery syndrome (hemispheric)

G45.2   Multiple and bilateral precerebral artery syndromes

G45.3   Amaurosis fugax

G45.4   Transient global amnesia

> EXCLUDES 1   amnesia NOS (R41.3)

G45.8   Other transient cerebral ischemic attacks and related syndromes

G45.9   Transient cerebral ischemic attack, unspecified
Spasm of cerebral artery
TIA
Transient cerebral ischemia NOS

☑4th **G46**   **Vascular syndromes of brain in cerebrovascular diseases**
Code first underlying cerebrovascular disease (I60-I69)

G46.0   Middle cerebral artery syndrome

G46.1   Anterior cerebral artery syndrome

G46.2   Posterior cerebral artery syndrome

G46.3   Brain stem stroke syndrome
Benedikt syndrome
Claude syndrome
Foville syndrome
Millard-Gubler syndrome
Wallenberg syndrome
Weber syndrome

G46.4   Cerebellar stroke syndrome

G46.5   Pure motor lacunar syndrome

G46.6   Pure sensory lacunar syndrome

G46.7   Other lacunar syndromes

G46.8   Other vascular syndromes of brain in cerebrovascular diseases

☑4th **G47**   **Sleep disorders**

> EXCLUDES 2   nightmares (F51.5)
> nonorganic sleep disorders (F51.-)
> sleep terrors (F51.4)
> sleepwalking (F51.3)

☑5th **G47.0**   Insomnia

> EXCLUDES 2   alcohol related insomnia (F10.182, F10.282, F10.982)
> drug-related insomnia (F11.182, F11.282, F11.982,
>   F13.182, F13.282, F13.982, F14.182,
>   F14.282, F14.982, F15.182, F15.282, F15.982,
>   F19.182, F19.282, F19.982)
> idiopathic insomnia (F51.01)
> insomnia due to a mental disorder (F51.05)
> insomnia not due to a substance or known
>   physiological condition (F51.0-)
> nonorganic insomnia (F51.0-)
> primary insomnia (F51.01)
> sleep apnea (G47.3-)

G47.00   Insomnia, unspecified
Insomnia NOS

G47.01   Insomnia due to medical condition
Code also associated medical condition

G47.09   Other insomnia

☑5th **G47.1**   Hypersomnia

> EXCLUDES 2   alcohol-related hypersomnia (F10.182, F10.282,
>   F10.982)
> drug-related hypersomnia (F11.182, F11.282, F11.982,
>   F13.182, F13.282, F13.982, F14.182, F14.282,
>   F14.982, F15.182, F15.282, F15.982, F19.182,
>   F19.282, F19.982)
> hypersomnia due to a mental disorder (F51.13)
> hypersomnia not due to a substance or known
>   physiological condition (F51.1-)
> primary hypersomnia (F51.11)
> sleep apnea (G47.3-)

G47.10   Hypersomnia, unspecified
Hypersomnia NOS

G47.11   Idiopathic hypersomnia with long sleep time
Idiopathic hypersomnia NOS

G47.12   Idiopathic hypersomnia without long sleep time

G47.13   Recurrent hypersomnia
Kleine-Levin syndrome
Menstrual related hypersomnia

G47.14   Hypersomnia due to medical condition
Code also associated medical condition

G47.19   Other hypersomnia

☑5th **G47.2**   Circadian rhythm sleep disorders
Disorders of the sleep wake schedule
Inversion of nyctohemeral rhythm
Inversion of sleep rhythm

G47.20   Circadian rhythm sleep disorder, unspecified type
Sleep wake schedule disorder NOS

G47.21   Circadian rhythm sleep disorder, delayed sleep phase type
Delayed sleep phase syndrome

G47.22   Circadian rhythm sleep disorder, advanced sleep phase type

G47.23   Circadian rhythm sleep disorder, irregular sleep wake type
Irregular sleep-wake pattern

G47.24   Circadian rhythm sleep disorder, free running type

G47.25   Circadian rhythm sleep disorder, jet lag type

G47.26   Circadian rhythm sleep disorder, shift work type

G47.27   *Circadian rhythm sleep disorder in conditions classified elsewhere*
Code first underlying condition

G47.29   Other circadian rhythm sleep disorder

☑5th **G47.3**   Sleep apnea
Code also any associated underlying condition

> EXCLUDES 1   apnea NOS (R06.81)
> Cheyne-Stokes breathing (R06.3)
> pickwickian syndrome (E66.2)
> sleep apnea of newborn (P28.3)

G47.30   Sleep apnea, unspecified
Sleep apnea NOS

G47.31   Primary central sleep apnea

G47.32   High altitude periodic breathing

G47.33   Obstructive sleep apnea (adult) (pediatric)

> EXCLUDES 1   obstructive sleep apnea of newborn (P28.3)

G47.34   Idiopathic sleep related nonobstructive alveolar hypoventilation
Sleep related hypoxia

G47.35   Congenital central alveolar hypoventilation syndrome

G47.36   *Sleep related hypoventilation in conditions classified elsewhere*
Sleep related hypoxemia in conditions classified elsewhere
Code first underlying condition

G47.37   *Central sleep apnea in conditions classified elsewhere*
Code first underlying condition

G47.39   Other sleep apnea

☑5th **G47.4**   Narcolepsy and cataplexy

☑6th **G47.41**   Narcolepsy

G47.411   Narcolepsy with cataplexy

G47.419   Narcolepsy without cataplexy
Narcolepsy NOS

☑6th **G47.42**   Narcolepsy in conditions classified elsewhere
Code first underlying condition

G47.421   *Narcolepsy in conditions classified elsewhere with cataplexy*

G47.429   *Narcolepsy in conditions classified elsewhere without cataplexy*

☑5th **G47.5**   Parasomnia

> EXCLUDES 1   alcohol induced parasomnia (F10.182, F10.282,
>   F10.982)
> drug induced parasomnia (F11.182, F11.282, F11.982,
>   F13.182, F13.282, F13.982, F14.182, F14.282,
>   F14.982, F15.182, F15.282, F15.982, F19.182,
>   F19.282, F19.982)
> parasomnia not due to a substance or known
>   physiological condition (F51.8)

G47.50   Parasomnia, unspecified
Parasomnia NOS

G47.51   Confusional arousals

G47.52   REM sleep behavior disorder

G47.53   Recurrent isolated sleep paralysis

EXCLUDES 1 Not coded here   EXCLUDES 2 Not included here   N Newborn Age: 0   P Pediatric Age: 0-17   M Maternity Age: 12-55   A Adult Age: 15-124

520   ICD-10-CM 2014 (Draft)

G47.54 **Parasomnia in conditions classified elsewhere**
Code first underlying condition

G47.59 **Other parasomnia**

√5ᵗʰ **G47.6 Sleep related movement disorders**
EXCLUDES 2 *restless legs syndrome (G25.81)*

G47.61 **Periodic limb movement disorder**

G47.62 **Sleep related leg cramps**

G47.63 **Sleep related bruxism**
EXCLUDES 1 *psychogenic bruxism (F45.8)*

G47.69 **Other sleep related movement disorders**

G47.8 **Other sleep disorders**

G47.9 **Sleep disorder, unspecified**
Sleep disorder NOS

Nerve, nerve root and plexus disorders (G50-G59)

EXCLUDES 1 *current traumatic nerve, nerve root and plexus disorders—see Injury, nerve by body region*
neuralgia NOS (M79.2)
neuritis NOS (M79.2)
peripheral neuritis in pregnancy (O26.82-)
radiculitis NOS (M54.1-)

√4ᵗʰ **G50 Disorders of trigeminal nerve**
INCLUDES disorders of 5th cranial nerve

G50.0 **Trigeminal neuralgia**
Syndrome of paroxysmal facial pain
Tic douloureux

G50.1 **Atypical facial pain**

G50.8 **Other disorders of trigeminal nerve**

G50.9 **Disorder of trigeminal nerve, unspecified**

√4ᵗʰ **G51 Facial nerve disorders**
INCLUDES disorders of 7th cranial nerve

G51.0 **Bell's palsy**
Facial palsy

G51.1 **Geniculate ganglionitis**
EXCLUDES 1 *postherpetic geniculate ganglionitis (B02.21)*

G51.2 **Melkersson's syndrome**
Melkersson-Rosenthal syndrome

G51.3 **Clonic hemifacial spasm**

G51.4 **Facial myokymia**

G51.8 **Other disorders of facial nerve**

G51.9 **Disorder of facial nerve, unspecified**

√4ᵗʰ **G52 Disorders of other cranial nerves**
EXCLUDES 2 *disorders of acoustic [8th] nerve (H93.3)*
disorders of optic [2nd] nerve (H46, H47.0)
paralytic strabismus due to nerve palsy (H49.0-H49.2)

G52.0 **Disorders of olfactory nerve**
Disorders of 1st cranial nerve

G52.1 **Disorders of glossopharyngeal nerve**
Disorder of 9th cranial nerve
Glossopharyngeal neuralgia

G52.2 **Disorders of vagus nerve**
Disorders of pneumogastric [10th] nerve

G52.3 **Disorders of hypoglossal nerve**
Disorders of 12th cranial nerve

G52.7 **Disorders of multiple cranial nerves**
Polyneuritis cranialis

G52.8 **Disorders of other specified cranial nerves**

G52.9 **Cranial nerve disorder, unspecified**

G53 Cranial nerve disorders in diseases classified elsewhere
Code first underlying disease, such as:
neoplasm (C00-D49)
EXCLUDES 1 *multiple cranial nerve palsy in sarcoidosis (D86.82)*
multiple cranial nerve palsy in syphilis (A52.15)
postherpetic geniculate ganglionitis (B02.21)
postherpetic trigeminal neuralgia (B02.22)

√4ᵗʰ **G54 Nerve root and plexus disorders**
EXCLUDES 1 *current traumatic nerve root and plexus disorders—see nerve injury by body region*
intervertebral disc disorders (M50-M51)
neuralgia or neuritis NOS (M79.2)
neuritis or radiculitis brachial NOS (M54.13)
neuritis or radiculitis lumbar NOS (M54.16)
neuritis or radiculitis lumbosacral NOS (M54.17)
neuritis or radiculitis thoracic NOS (M54.14)
radiculitis NOS (M54.10)
radiculopathy NOS (M54.10)
spondylosis (M47.-)

G54.0 **Brachial plexus disorders**
Thoracic outlet syndrome

G54.1 **Lumbosacral plexus disorders**

G54.2 **Cervical root disorders, not elsewhere classified**

G54.3 **Thoracic root disorders, not elsewhere classified**

G54.4 **Lumbosacral root disorders, not elsewhere classified**

G54.5 **Neuralgic amyotrophy**
Parsonage-Aldren-Turner syndrome
Shoulder-girdle neuritis
EXCLUDES 1 *neuralgic amyotrophy in diabetes mellitus (E08-E13 with .44)*

G54.6 **Phantom limb syndrome with pain**

G54.7 **Phantom limb syndrome without pain**
Phantom limb syndrome NOS

G54.8 **Other nerve root and plexus disorders**

G54.9 **Nerve root and plexus disorder, unspecified**

G55 Nerve root and plexus compressions in diseases classified elsewhere
Code first underlying disease, such as:
neoplasm (C00-D49)
EXCLUDES 1 *nerve root compression (due to) (in) ankylosing spondylitis (M45.-)*
nerve root compression (due to) (in) dorsopathies (M53.-, M54.-)
nerve root compression (due to) (in) intervertebral disc disorders (M50.1-, M51.1-)
nerve root compression (due to) (in) spondylopathies (M46.-, M48.-)
nerve root compression (due to) (in) spondylosis (M47.0-M47.2-)

√4ᵗʰ **G56 Mononeuropathies of upper limb**
EXCLUDES 1 *current traumatic nerve disorder—see nerve injury by body region*

√5ᵗʰ **G56.0 Carpal tunnel syndrome**

G56.00 **Carpal tunnel syndrome, unspecified upper limb**

G56.01 **Carpal tunnel syndrome, right upper limb**

G56.02 **Carpal tunnel syndrome, left upper limb**

√5ᵗʰ **G56.1 Other lesions of median nerve**

G56.10 **Other lesions of median nerve, unspecified upper limb**

G56.11 **Other lesions of median nerve, right upper limb**

G56.12 **Other lesions of median nerve, left upper limb**

√5ᵗʰ **G56.2 Lesion of ulnar nerve**
Tardy ulnar nerve palsy

G56.20 **Lesion of ulnar nerve, unspecified upper limb**

G56.21 **Lesion of ulnar nerve, right upper limb**

G56.22 **Lesion of ulnar nerve, left upper limb**

√5ᵗʰ **G56.3 Lesion of radial nerve**

G56.30 **Lesion of radial nerve, unspecified upper limb**

G56.31 **Lesion of radial nerve, right upper limb**

G56.32 **Lesion of radial nerve, left upper limb**

√5ᵗʰ **G56.4 Causalgia of upper limb**
Complex regional pain syndrome II of upper limb
EXCLUDES 1 *complex regional pain syndrome I of lower limb (G90.52-)*
complex regional pain syndrome I of upper limb (G90.51-)
complex regional pain syndrome II of lower limb (G57.7-)
reflex sympathetic dystrophy of lower limb (G90.52-)
reflex sympathetic dystrophy of upper limb (G90.51-)

G56.40 **Causalgia of unspecified upper limb**

G56.41 **Causalgia of right upper limb**

G56.42 **Causalgia of left upper limb**

G47.54–G56.42

☑ Additional Character Required   √ᴸ7ᵗʰ Xtension Alert   Unspecified Code   Other Specified Code   Manifestation Code   ►◄ Revised Text   ● New Code   ▲ Revised Code Title

ICD-10-CM 2014 (Draft)   **521**

Diseases of the Nervous System

G56.8–G62.9

√5ᵗʰ **G56.8** Other specified mononeuropathies of upper limb
Interdigital neuroma of upper limb

    G56.80 Other specified mononeuropathies of unspecified upper limb

    G56.81 Other specified mononeuropathies of right upper limb

    G56.82 Other specified mononeuropathies of left upper limb

√5ᵗʰ **G56.9** Unspecified mononeuropathy of upper limb

    G56.90 Unspecified mononeuropathy of unspecified upper limb

    G56.91 Unspecified mononeuropathy of right upper limb

    G56.92 Unspecified mononeuropathy of left upper limb

√4ᵗʰ **G57** Mononeuropathies of lower limb

    EXCLUDES 1 current traumatic nerve disorder—see nerve injury by body region

√5ᵗʰ **G57.0** Lesion of sciatic nerve

    EXCLUDES 1 sciatica NOS (M54.3-)
    EXCLUDES 2 sciatica attributed to intervertebral disc disorder (M51.1-)

    G57.00 Lesion of sciatic nerve, unspecified lower limb

    G57.01 Lesion of sciatic nerve, right lower limb

    G57.02 Lesion of sciatic nerve, left lower limb

√5ᵗʰ **G57.1** Meralgia paresthetica
Lateral cutaneous nerve of thigh syndrome

    G57.10 Meralgia paresthetica, unspecified lower limb

    G57.11 Meralgia paresthetica, right lower limb

    G57.12 Meralgia paresthetica, left lower limb

√5ᵗʰ **G57.2** Lesion of femoral nerve

    G57.20 Lesion of femoral nerve, unspecified lower limb

    G57.21 Lesion of femoral nerve, right lower limb

    G57.22 Lesion of femoral nerve, left lower limb

√5ᵗʰ **G57.3** Lesion of lateral popliteal nerve
Peroneal nerve palsy

    G57.30 Lesion of lateral popliteal nerve, unspecified lower limb

    G57.31 Lesion of lateral popliteal nerve, right lower limb

    G57.32 Lesion of lateral popliteal nerve, left lower limb

√5ᵗʰ **G57.4** Lesion of medial popliteal nerve

    G57.40 Lesion of medial popliteal nerve, unspecified lower limb

    G57.41 Lesion of medial popliteal nerve, right lower limb

    G57.42 Lesion of medial popliteal nerve, left lower limb

√5ᵗʰ **G57.5** Tarsal tunnel syndrome

    G57.50 Tarsal tunnel syndrome, unspecified lower limb

    G57.51 Tarsal tunnel syndrome, right lower limb

    G57.52 Tarsal tunnel syndrome, left lower limb

√5ᵗʰ **G57.6** Lesion of plantar nerve
Morton's metatarsalgia

    G57.60 Lesion of plantar nerve, unspecified lower limb

    G57.61 Lesion of plantar nerve, right lower limb

    G57.62 Lesion of plantar nerve, left lower limb

√5ᵗʰ **G57.7** Causalgia of lower limb
Complex regional pain syndrome II of lower limb

    EXCLUDES 1 complex regional pain syndrome I of lower limb (G90.52-)
    complex regional pain syndrome I of upper limb (G90.51-)
    complex regional pain syndrome II of upper limb (G56.4-)
    reflex sympathetic dystrophy of lower limb (G90.52-)
    reflex sympathetic dystrophy of upper limb (G90.51-)

    G57.70 Causalgia of unspecified lower limb

    G57.71 Causalgia of right lower limb

    G57.72 Causalgia of left lower limb

√5ᵗʰ **G57.8** Other specified mononeuropathies of lower limb
Interdigital neuroma of lower limb

    G57.80 Other specified mononeuropathies of unspecified lower limb

    G57.81 Other specified mononeuropathies of right lower limb

    G57.82 Other specified mononeuropathies of left lower limb

√5ᵗʰ **G57.9** Unspecified mononeuropathy of lower limb

    G57.90 Unspecified mononeuropathy of unspecified lower limb

    G57.91 Unspecified mononeuropathy of right lower limb

    G57.92 Unspecified mononeuropathy of left lower limb

√4ᵗʰ **G58** Other mononeuropathies

    G58.0 Intercostal neuropathy

    G58.7 Mononeuritis multiplex

    G58.8 Other specified mononeuropathies

    G58.9 Mononeuropathy, unspecified

G59 **Mononeuropathy in diseases classified elsewhere**
Code first underlying disease

    EXCLUDES 1 diabetic mononeuropathy (E08-E13 with .41)
    syphilitic nerve paralysis (A52.19)
    syphilitic neuritis (A52.15)
    tuberculous mononeuropathy (A17.83)

Polyneuropathies and other disorders of the peripheral nervous system (G60-G65)

EXCLUDES 1 neuralgia NOS (M79.2)
neuritis NOS (M79.2)
peripheral neuritis in pregnancy (O26.82-)
radiculitis NOS (M54.10)

√4ᵗʰ **G60** Hereditary and idiopathic neuropathy

    G60.0 Hereditary motor and sensory neuropathy
Charcôt-Marie-Tooth disease
Déjérine-Sottas disease
Hereditary motor and sensory neuropathy, types I-IV
Hypertrophic neuropathy of infancy
Peroneal muscular atrophy (axonal type) (hypertrophic type)
Roussy-Levy syndrome

    G60.1 Refsum's disease
Infantile Refsum disease

    G60.2 Neuropathy in association with hereditary ataxia

    G60.3 Idiopathic progressive neuropathy

    G60.8 Other hereditary and idiopathic neuropathies
Dominantly inherited sensory neuropathy
Morvan's disease
Nelaton's syndrome
Recessively inherited sensory neuropathy

    G60.9 Hereditary and idiopathic neuropathy, unspecified

√4ᵗʰ **G61** Inflammatory polyneuropathy

    G61.0 Guillain-Barre syndrome
Acute (post-)infective polyneuritis
Miller Fisher syndrome

    G61.1 Serum neuropathy
Use additional code for adverse effect, if applicable, to identify serum (T50.-)

√5ᵗʰ   **G61.8** Other inflammatory polyneuropathies

        G61.81 Chronic inflammatory demyelinating polyneuritis

        G61.89 Other inflammatory polyneuropathies

    G61.9 Inflammatory polyneuropathy, unspecified

√4ᵗʰ **G62** Other and unspecified polyneuropathies

    G62.0 Drug-induced polyneuropathy
Use additional code for adverse effect, if applicable, to identify drug (T36-T50 with fifth or sixth character 5)

    G62.1 Alcoholic polyneuropathy

    G62.2 Polyneuropathy due to other toxic agents
Code first (T51-T65) to identify toxic agent

√5ᵗʰ   **G62.8** Other specified polyneuropathies

        G62.81 Critical illness polyneuropathy
Acute motor neuropathy

        G62.82 Radiation-induced polyneuropathy
Use additional external cause code (W88-W90, X39.0-) to identify cause

        G62.89 Other specified polyneuropathies

    G62.9 Polyneuropathy, unspecified
Neuropathy NOS

EXCLUDES 1 Not coded here   *EXCLUDES 2* Not included here   N Newborn Age: 0   P Pediatric Age: 0-17   M Maternity Age: 12-55   A Adult Age: 15-124

522   ICD-10-CM 2014 (Draft)

G63 Polyneuropathy in diseases classified elsewhere

Code first underlying disease, such as:
amyloidosis (E85.-)
endocrine disease, except diabetes (E00-E07, E15-E16, E20-E34)
metabolic diseases (E70-E88)
neoplasm (C00-D49)
nutritional deficiency (E40-E64)

EXCLUDES 1   polyneuropathy (in):
diabetes mellitus (E08-E13 with .42)
diphtheria (A36.83)
infectious mononucleosis (B27.0-B27.9 with 1)
Lyme disease (A69.22)
mumps (B26.84)
postherpetic (B02.23)
rheumatoid arthritis (M05.33)
scleroderma (M34.83)
systemic lupus erythematosus (M32.19)

AHA: 2012, Q4, 99

G64 Other disorders of peripheral nervous system
Disorder of peripheral nervous system NOS

☑4th **G65 Sequelae of inflammatory and toxic polyneuropathies**

Code first condition resulting from (sequela) of inflammatory and toxic polyneuropathies

G65.0 Sequelae of Guillain-Barré syndrome

G65.1 Sequelae of other inflammatory polyneuropathy

G65.2 Sequelae of toxic polyneuropathy

Diseases of myoneural junction and muscle (G70-G73)

☑4th **G70 Myasthenia gravis and other myoneural disorders**

EXCLUDES 1   botulism (A05.1, A48.51-A48.52)
transient neonatal myasthenia gravis (P94.0)

☑5th **G70.0 Myasthenia gravis**

G70.00 Myasthenia gravis without (acute) exacerbation
Myasthenia gravis NOS

G70.01 Myasthenia gravis with (acute) exacerbation
Myasthenia gravis in crisis

G70.1 Toxic myoneural disorders
Code first (T51-T65) to identify toxic agent

G70.2 Congenital and developmental myasthenia

☑5th **G70.8 Other specified myoneural disorders**

G70.80 Lambert-Eaton syndrome, unspecified
Lambert-Eaton syndrome NOS

G70.81 Lambert-Eaton syndrome in disease classified elsewhere
Code first underlying disease
EXCLUDES 1   Lambert-Eaton syndrome in neoplastic disease (G73.1)

G70.89 Other specified myoneural disorders

G70.9 Myoneural disorder, unspecified

☑4th **G71 Primary disorders of muscles**

EXCLUDES 2   arthrogryposis multiplex congenita (Q74.3)
metabolic disorders (E70-E88)
myositis (M60.-)

G71.0 Muscular dystrophy
Autosomal recessive, childhood type, muscular dystrophy resembling Duchenne or Becker muscular dystrophy
Benign [Becker] muscular dystrophy
Benign scapuloperoneal muscular dystrophy with early contractures [Emery-Dreifuss]
Congenital muscular dystrophy NOS
Congenital muscular dystrophy with specific morphological abnormalities of the muscle fiber
Distal muscular dystrophy
Facioscapulohumeral muscular dystrophy
Limb-girdle muscular dystrophy
Ocular muscular dystrophy
Oculopharyngeal muscular dystrophy
Scapuloperoneal muscular dystrophy
Severe [Duchenne] muscular dystrophy

☑5th **G71.1 Myotonic disorders**

G71.11 Myotonic muscular dystrophy
Dystrophia myotonica [Steinert]
Myotonia atrophica
Myotonic dystrophy
Proximal myotonic myopathy (PROMM)
Steinert disease

G71.12 Myotonia congenita
Acetazolamide responsive myotonia congenita
Dominant myotonia congenita [Thomsen disease]
Myotonia levior
Recessive myotonia congenita [Becker disease]

G71.13 Myotonic chondrodystrophy
Chondrodystrophic myotonia
Congenital myotonic chondrodystrophy
Schwartz-Jampel disease

G71.14 Drug induced myotonia
Use additional code for adverse effect, if applicable, to identify drug (T36-T50 with fifth or sixth character 5)

G71.19 Other specified myotonic disorders
Myotonia fluctuans
Myotonia permanens
Neuromyotonia [Isaacs]
Paramyotonia congenita (of von Eulenburg)
Pseudomyotonia
Symptomatic myotonia

G71.2 Congenital myopathies
Central core disease
Fiber-type disproportion
Minicore disease
Multicore disease
Myotubular (centronuclear) myopathy
Nemaline myopathy
EXCLUDES 1   arthrogryposis multiplex congenita (Q74.3)

G71.3 Mitochondrial myopathy, not elsewhere classified
EXCLUDES 1   Kearns-Sayre syndrome (H49.81)
Leber's disease (H47.21)
Leigh's encephalopathy (G31.82)
mitochondrial metabolism disorders (E88.4-)
Reye's syndrome (G93.7)

G71.8 Other primary disorders of muscles

G71.9 Primary disorder of muscle, unspecified
Hereditary myopathy NOS

☑4th **G72 Other and unspecified myopathies**
EXCLUDES 1   arthrogryposis multiplex congenita (Q74.3)
dermatopolymyositis (M33.-)
ischemic infarction of muscle (M62.2-)
myositis (M60.-)
polymyositis (M33.2-)

G72.0 Drug-induced myopathy
Use additional code for adverse effect, if applicable, to identify drug (T36-T50 with fifth or sixth character 5)

G72.1 Alcoholic myopathy
Use additional code to identify alcoholism (F10.-)

G72.2 Myopathy due to other toxic agents
Code first (T51-T65) to identify toxic agent

G72.3 Periodic paralysis
Familial periodic paralysis
Hyperkalemic periodic paralysis (familial)
Hypokalemic periodic paralysis (familial)
Myotonic periodic paralysis (familial)
Normokalemic paralysis (familial)
Potassium sensitive periodic paralysis
EXCLUDES 1   paramyotonia congenita (of von Eulenburg) (G71.19)

☑5th **G72.4 Inflammatory and immune myopathies, not elsewhere classified**

G72.41 Inclusion body myositis [IBM]

G72.49 Other inflammatory and immune myopathies, not elsewhere classified
Inflammatory myopathy NOS

☑5th **G72.8 Other specified myopathies**

G72.81 Critical illness myopathy
Acute necrotizing myopathy
Acute quadriplegic myopathy
Intensive care (ICU) myopathy
Myopathy of critical illness

G72.89 Other specified myopathies

G72.9 Myopathy, unspecified

☑4th **G73 Disorders of myoneural junction and muscle in diseases classified elsewhere**

G73.1 Lambert-Eaton syndrome in neoplastic disease
Code first underlying neoplasm (C00-D49)
EXCLUDES 1   Lambert-Eaton syndrome not associated with neoplasm (G70.80-G70.81)

☑ Additional Character Required   ✗7th Xtension Alert   Unspecified Code   Other Specified Code   Manifestation Code   ▶◀ Revised Text   ● New Code   ▲ Revised Code Title

Diseases of the Nervous System

G73.3–G83.5

G73.3 Myasthenic syndromes in other diseases classified elsewhere
Code first underlying disease, such as:
neoplasm (C00-D49)
thyrotoxicosis (E05.-)

G73.7 Myopathy in diseases classified elsewhere
Code first underlying disease, such as:
hyperparathyroidism (E21.0, E21.3)
hypoparathyroidism (E20.-)
glycogen storage disease (E74.0)
lipid storage disorders (E75.-)
EXCLUDES 1 myopathy in:
rheumatoid arthritis (M05.4-)
sarcoidosis (D86.87)
scleroderma (M34.82)
sicca syndrome [Sjögren] (M35.03)
systemic lupus erythematosus (M32.19)

Cerebral palsy and other paralytic syndromes (G80-G83)

G80 Cerebral palsy
EXCLUDES 1 hereditary spastic paraplegia (G11.4)

G80.0 Spastic quadriplegic cerebral palsy
Congenital spastic paralysis (cerebral)

G80.1 Spastic diplegic cerebral palsy
Spastic cerebral palsy NOS

G80.2 Spastic hemiplegic cerebral palsy

G80.3 Athetoid cerebral palsy
Double athetosis (syndrome)
Dyskinetic cerebral palsy
Dystonic cerebral palsy
Vogt disease

G80.4 Ataxic cerebral palsy

G80.8 Other cerebral palsy
Mixed cerebral palsy syndromes

G80.9 Cerebral palsy, unspecified
Cerebral palsy NOS

G81 Hemiplegia and hemiparesis
NOTE This category is to be used only when hemiplegia (complete)(incomplete) is reported without further specification, or is stated to be old or longstanding but of unspecified cause. The category is also for use in multiple coding to identify these types of hemiplegia resulting from any cause.
EXCLUDES 1 congenital cerebral palsy (G80.-)
hemiplegia and hemiparesis due to sequela of cerebrovascular disease (I69.05-, I69.15-, I69.25-, I69.35-, I69.85-, I69.95-)

G81.0 Flaccid hemiplegia
G81.00 Flaccid hemiplegia affecting unspecified side
G81.01 Flaccid hemiplegia affecting right dominant side
G81.02 Flaccid hemiplegia affecting left dominant side
G81.03 Flaccid hemiplegia affecting right nondominant side
G81.04 Flaccid hemiplegia affecting left nondominant side

G81.1 Spastic hemiplegia
G81.10 Spastic hemiplegia affecting unspecified side
G81.11 Spastic hemiplegia affecting right dominant side
G81.12 Spastic hemiplegia affecting left dominant side
G81.13 Spastic hemiplegia affecting right nondominant side
G81.14 Spastic hemiplegia affecting left nondominant side

G81.9 Hemiplegia, unspecified
G81.90 Hemiplegia, unspecified affecting unspecified side
G81.91 Hemiplegia, unspecified affecting right dominant side
G81.92 Hemiplegia, unspecified affecting left dominant side
G81.93 Hemiplegia, unspecified affecting right nondominant side
G81.94 Hemiplegia, unspecified affecting left nondominant side

G82 Paraplegia (paraparesis) and quadriplegia (quadriparesis)
NOTE This category is to be used only when the listed conditions are reported without further specification, or are stated to be old or longstanding but of unspecified cause. The category is also for use in multiple coding to identify these conditions resulting from any cause
EXCLUDES 1 congenital cerebral palsy (G80.-)
functional quadriplegia (R53.2)
hysterical paralysis (F44.4)

G82.2 Paraplegia
Paralysis of both lower limbs NOS
Paraparesis (lower) NOS
Paraplegia (lower) NOS
G82.20 Paraplegia, unspecified
G82.21 Paraplegia, complete
G82.22 Paraplegia, incomplete

G82.5 Quadriplegia
G82.50 Quadriplegia, unspecified
G82.51 Quadriplegia, C1-C4 complete
G82.52 Quadriplegia, C1-C4 incomplete
G82.53 Quadriplegia, C5-C7 complete
G82.54 Quadriplegia, C5-C7 incomplete

G83 Other paralytic syndromes
NOTE This category is to be used only when the listed conditions are reported without further specification, or are stated to be old or longstanding but of unspecified cause. The category is also for use in multiple coding to identify these conditions resulting from any cause.
INCLUDES paralysis (complete) (incomplete), except as in G80-G82

G83.0 Diplegia of upper limbs
Diplegia (upper)
Paralysis of both upper limbs

G83.1 Monoplegia of lower limb
Paralysis of lower limb
EXCLUDES 1 monoplegia of lower limbs due to sequela of cerebrovascular disease (I69.04-, I69.14-, I69.24-, I69.34-, I69.84-, I69.94-)
G83.10 Monoplegia of lower limb affecting unspecified side
G83.11 Monoplegia of lower limb affecting right dominant side
G83.12 Monoplegia of lower limb affecting left dominant side
G83.13 Monoplegia of lower limb affecting right nondominant side
G83.14 Monoplegia of lower limb affecting left nondominant side

G83.2 Monoplegia of upper limb
Paralysis of upper limb
EXCLUDES 1 monoplegia of upper limbs due to sequela of cerebrovascular disease (I69.03-, I69.13-, I69.23-, I69.33-, I69.83-, I69.93-)
G83.20 Monoplegia of upper limb affecting unspecified side
G83.21 Monoplegia of upper limb affecting right dominant side
G83.22 Monoplegia of upper limb affecting left dominant side
G83.23 Monoplegia of upper limb affecting right nondominant side
G83.24 Monoplegia of upper limb affecting left nondominant side

G83.3 Monoplegia, unspecified
G83.30 Monoplegia, unspecified affecting unspecified side
G83.31 Monoplegia, unspecified affecting right dominant side
G83.32 Monoplegia, unspecified affecting left dominant side
G83.33 Monoplegia, unspecified affecting right nondominant side
G83.34 Monoplegia, unspecified affecting left nondominant side

G83.4 Cauda equina syndrome
Neurogenic bladder due to cauda equina syndrome
EXCLUDES 1 cord bladder NOS (G95.89)
neurogenic bladder NOS (N31.9)

G83.5 Locked-in state

✓5th **G83.8 Other specified paralytic syndromes**

> *EXCLUDES 1* *paralytic syndromes due to current spinal cord injury—code to spinal cord injury (S14, S24, S34)*

G83.81 Brown-Séquard syndrome

G83.82 Anterior cord syndrome

G83.83 Posterior cord syndrome

G83.84 Todd's paralysis (postepileptic)

G83.89 Other specified paralytic syndromes

G83.9 Paralytic syndrome, unspecified

Other disorders of the nervous system (G89-G99)

✓4th **G89 Pain, not elsewhere classified**

> Code also related psychological factors associated with pain (F45.42)
>
> *EXCLUDES 1* *generalized pain NOS (R52)*
> *pain disorders exclusively related to psychological factors (F45.41)*
> *pain NOS (R52)*
>
> *EXCLUDES 2* *atypical face pain (G50.1)*
> *headache syndromes (G44.-)*
> *localized pain, unspecified type—code to pain by site, such as:*
> *abdomen pain (R10.-)*
> *back pain (M54.9)*
> *breast pain (N64.4)*
> *chest pain (R07.1-R07.9)*
> *ear pain (H92.0-)*
> *eye pain (H57.1)*
> *headache (R51)*
> *joint pain (M25.5-)*
> *limb pain (M79.6-)*
> *lumbar region pain (M54.5)*
> *painful urination (R30.9)*
> *pelvic and perineal pain (R10.2)*
> *renal colic (N23)*
> *shoulder pain (M25.51-)*
> *spine pain (M54.-)*
> *throat pain (R07.0)*
> *tongue pain (K14.6)*
> *tooth pain (K08.8)*
> *migraines (G43.-)*
> *myalgia (M79.1)*
> *pain from prosthetic devices, implants, and grafts (T82.84, T83.84, T84.84, T85.84)*
> *phantom limb syndrome with pain (G54.6)*
> *vulvar vestibulitis (N94.810)*
> *vulvodynia (N94.81-)*

G89.0 Central pain syndrome

> Déjérine-Roussy syndrome
> Myelopathic pain syndrome
> Thalamic pain syndrome (hyperesthetic)

✓5th **G89.1 Acute pain, not elsewhere classified**

G89.11 Acute pain due to trauma

G89.12 Acute post-thoracotomy pain
> Post-thoracotomy pain NOS

G89.18 Other acute postprocedural pain
> Postoperative pain NOS
> Postprocedural pain NOS

✓5th **G89.2 Chronic pain, not elsewhere classified**

> *EXCLUDES 1* *causalgia, lower limb (G57.7-)*
> *causalgia, upper limb (G56.4-)*
> *central pain syndrome (G89.0)*
> *chronic pain syndrome (G89.4)*
> *complex regional pain syndrome II, lower limb (G57.7-)*
> *complex regional pain syndrome II, upper limb (G56.4-)*
> *neoplasm related chronic pain (G89.3)*
> *reflex sympathetic dystrophy (G90.5-)*

G89.21 Chronic pain due to trauma

G89.22 Chronic post-thoracotomy pain

G89.28 Other chronic postprocedural pain
> Other chronic postoperative pain

G89.29 Other chronic pain

G89.3 Neoplasm related pain (acute) (chronic)
> Cancer associated pain
> Pain due to malignancy (primary) (secondary)
> Tumor associated pain

G89.4 Chronic pain syndrome
> Chronic pain associated with significant psychosocial dysfunction

✓4th **G90 Disorders of autonomic nervous system**

> *EXCLUDES 1* *dysfunction of the autonomic nervous system due to alcohol (G31.2)*

✓5th **G90.0 Idiopathic peripheral autonomic neuropathy**

G90.01 Carotid sinus syncope
> Carotid sinus syndrome

G90.09 Other idiopathic peripheral autonomic neuropathy
> Idiopathic peripheral autonomic neuropathy NOS

G90.1 Familial dysautonomia [Riley-Day]

G90.2 Horner's syndrome
> Bernard(-Horner) syndrome
> Cervical sympathetic dystrophy or paralysis

G90.3 Multi-system degeneration of the autonomic nervous system
> Neurogenic orthostatic hypotension [Shy-Drager]
>
> *EXCLUDES 1* *orthostatic hypotension NOS (I95.1)*

G90.4 Autonomic dysreflexia
> Use additional code to identify the cause, such as:
> fecal impaction (K56.41)
> pressure ulcer (pressure area) (L89.-)
> urinary tract infection (N39.0)

✓5th **G90.5 Complex regional pain syndrome I (CRPS I)**
> Reflex sympathetic dystrophy
>
> *EXCLUDES 1* *causalgia of lower limb (G57.7-)*
> *causalgia of upper limb (G56.4-)*
> *complex regional pain syndrome II of lower limb (G57.7-)*
> *complex regional pain syndrome II of upper limb (G56.4-)*

G90.50 Complex regional pain syndrome I, unspecified

✓6th **G90.51 Complex regional pain syndrome I of upper limb**

G90.511 Complex regional pain syndrome I of right upper limb

G90.512 Complex regional pain syndrome I of left upper limb

G90.513 Complex regional pain syndrome I of upper limb, bilateral

G90.519 Complex regional pain syndrome I of unspecified upper limb

✓6th **G90.52 Complex regional pain syndrome I of lower limb**

G90.521 Complex regional pain syndrome I of right lower limb

G90.522 Complex regional pain syndrome I of left lower limb

G90.523 Complex regional pain syndrome I of lower limb, bilateral

G90.529 Complex regional pain syndrome I of unspecified lower limb

G90.59 Complex regional pain syndrome I of other specified site

G90.8 Other disorders of autonomic nervous system

G90.9 Disorder of the autonomic nervous system, unspecified

✓4th **G91 Hydrocephalus**

> *INCLUDES* acquired hydrocephalus
>
> *EXCLUDES 1* *Arnold-Chiari syndrome with hydrocephalus (Q07.-)*
> *congenital hydrocephalus (Q03.-)*
> *spina bifida with hydrocephalus (Q05.-)*

G91.0 Communicating hydrocephalus
> Secondary normal pressure hydrocephalus

G91.1 Obstructive hydrocephalus

G91.2 (Idiopathic) normal pressure hydrocephalus
> Normal pressure hydrocephalus NOS

G91.3 Post-traumatic hydrocephalus, unspecified

G91.4 Hydrocephalus in diseases classified elsewhere
> Code first underlying condition, such as:
> congenital syphilis (A50.4-)
> neoplasm (C00-D49)
>
> *EXCLUDES 1* *hydrocephalus due to congenital toxoplasmosis (P37.1)*

G91.8 Other hydrocephalus

G91.9 Hydrocephalus, unspecified

G92 Toxic encephalopathy
> Toxic encephalitis
> Toxic metabolic encephalopathy
> Code first (T51-T65) to identify toxic agent

✓ Additional Character Required   ✓7th *X*tension Alert   Unspecified Code   Other Specified Code   Manifestation Code   ►◄ Revised Text   ● New Code   ▲ Revised Code Title

ICD-10-CM 2014 (Draft)   **525**

Diseases of the Nervous System

G83.8–G92

√4th **G93 Other disorders of brain**

G93.0 Cerebral cysts
Arachnoid cyst
Porencephalic cyst, acquired
EXCLUDES 1 *acquired periventricular cysts of newborn (P91.1)*
congenital cerebral cysts (Q04.6)

G93.1 Anoxic brain damage, not elsewhere classified
EXCLUDES 1 *cerebral anoxia due to anesthesia during labor and delivery (O74.3)*
cerebral anoxia due to anesthesia during the puerperium (O89.2)
neonatal anoxia (P84)

G93.2 Benign intracranial hypertension
EXCLUDES 1 *hypertensive encephalopathy (I67.4)*

G93.3 Postviral fatigue syndrome
Benign myalgic encephalomyelitis
EXCLUDES 1 *chronic fatigue syndrome NOS (R53.82)*

√5th **G93.4 Other and unspecified encephalopathy**
EXCLUDES 1 *alcoholic encephalopathy (G31.2)*
encephalopathy in diseases classified elsewhere (G94)
hypertensive encephalopathy (I67.4)
toxic (metabolic) encephalopathy (G92)

G93.40 Encephalopathy, unspecified

G93.41 Metabolic encephalopathy
Septic encephalopathy

G93.49 Other encephalopathy
Encephalopathy NEC

G93.5 Compression of brain
Arnold-Chiari type 1 compression of brain
Compression of brain (stem)
Herniation of brain (stem)
EXCLUDES 1 *diffuse traumatic compression of brain (S06.2-)*
focal traumatic compression of brain (S06.3-)

G93.6 Cerebral edema
EXCLUDES 1 *cerebral edema due to birth injury (P11.0)*
traumatic cerebral edema (S06.1-)

G93.7 Reye's syndrome   P
Code first (T39.0-), if salicylates-induced

√5th **G93.8 Other specified disorders of brain**

G93.81 Temporal sclerosis
Hippocampal sclerosis
Mesial temporal sclerosis

G93.82 Brain death

G93.89 Other specified disorders of brain
Postradiation encephalopathy

G93.9 Disorder of brain, unspecified

G94 Other disorders of brain in diseases classified elsewhere
Code first underlying disease
EXCLUDES 1 *encephalopathy in congenital syphilis (A50.49)*
encephalopathy in influenza (J09.X9, J10.81, J11.81)
encephalopathy in syphilis (A52.19)
hydrocephalus in diseases classified elsewhere (G91.4)

√4th **G95 Other and unspecified diseases of spinal cord**
EXCLUDES 2 *myelitis (G04.-)*

G95.0 Syringomyelia and syringobulbia

√5th **G95.1 Vascular myelopathies**
EXCLUDES 2 *intraspinal phlebitis and thrombophlebitis, except non-pyogenic (G08)*

G95.11 Acute infarction of spinal cord (embolic) (nonembolic)
Anoxia of spinal cord
Arterial thrombosis of spinal cord

G95.19 Other vascular myelopathies
Edema of spinal cord
Hematomyelia
Nonpyogenic intraspinal phlebitis and thrombophlebitis
Subacute necrotic myelopathy

√5th **G95.2 Other and unspecified cord compression**

G95.20 Unspecified cord compression

G95.29 Other cord compression

√5th **G95.8 Other specified diseases of spinal cord**
EXCLUDES 1 *neurogenic bladder NOS (N31.9)*
neurogenic bladder due to cauda equina syndrome (G83.4)
neuromuscular dysfunction of bladder without spinal cord lesion (N31.-)

G95.81 Conus medullaris syndrome

G95.89 Other specified diseases of spinal cord
Cord bladder NOS
Drug-induced myelopathy
Radiation-induced myelopathy
EXCLUDES 1 *myelopathy NOS (G95.9)*

G95.9 Disease of spinal cord, unspecified
Myelopathy NOS

√4th **G96 Other disorders of central nervous system**

G96.0 Cerebrospinal fluid leak
EXCLUDES 1 *cerebrospinal fluid leak from spinal puncture (G97.0)*

√5th **G96.1 Disorders of meninges, not elsewhere classified**

G96.11 Dural tear
EXCLUDES 1 *accidental puncture or laceration of dura during a procedure (G97.41)*

G96.12 Meningeal adhesions (cerebral) (spinal)

G96.19 Other disorders of meninges, not elsewhere classified

G96.8 Other specified disorders of central nervous system

G96.9 Disorder of central nervous system, unspecified

√4th **G97 Intraoperative and postprocedural complications and disorders of nervous system, not elsewhere classified**
EXCLUDES 2 *intraoperative and postprocedural cerebrovascular infarction (I97.81-, I97.82-)*

G97.0 Cerebrospinal fluid leak from spinal puncture

G97.1 Other reaction to spinal and lumbar puncture
Headache due to lumbar puncture

G97.2 Intracranial hypotension following ventricular shunting

√5th **G97.3 Intraoperative hemorrhage and hematoma of a nervous system organ or structure complicating a procedure**
EXCLUDES 1 *intraoperative hemorrhage and hematoma of a nervous system organ or structure due to accidental puncture and laceration during a procedure (G97.4-)*

G97.31 Intraoperative hemorrhage and hematoma of a nervous system organ or structure complicating a nervous system procedure

G97.32 Intraoperative hemorrhage and hematoma of a nervous system organ or structure complicating other procedure

√5th **G97.4 Accidental puncture and laceration of a nervous system organ or structure during a procedure**

G97.41 Accidental puncture or laceration of dura during a procedure
Incidental (inadvertent) durotomy

G97.48 Accidental puncture and laceration of other nervous system organ or structure during a nervous system procedure

G97.49 Accidental puncture and laceration of other nervous system organ or structure during other procedure

√5th **G97.5 Postprocedural hemorrhage and hematoma of a nervous system organ or structure following a procedure**

G97.51 Postprocedural hemorrhage and hematoma of a nervous system organ or structure following a nervous system procedure

G97.52 Postprocedural hemorrhage and hematoma of a nervous system organ or structure following other procedure

√5th **G97.8 Other intraoperative and postprocedural complications and disorders of nervous system**
Use additional code to further specify disorder

G97.81 Other intraoperative complications of nervous system

G97.82 Other postprocedural complications and disorders of nervous system

√4th **G98 Other disorders of nervous system not elsewhere classified**
INCLUDES nervous system disorder NOS

G98.0 Neurogenic arthritis, not elsewhere classified
Nonsyphilitic neurogenic arthropathy NEC
Nonsyphilitic neurogenic spondylopathy NEC
EXCLUDES 1 *spondylopathy (in):*
syringomyelia and syringobulbia (G95.0)
tabes dorsalis (A52.11)

G98.8 Other disorders of nervous system
Nervous system disorder NOS

EXCLUDES 1 Not coded here   *EXCLUDES 2* Not included here   N Newborn Age: 0   P Pediatric Age: 0-17   M Maternity Age: 12-55   A Adult Age: 15-124

526   ICD-10-CM 2014 (Draft)

☑4ᵗʰ **G99　Other disorders of nervous system in diseases classified elsewhere**

　　G99.0　Autonomic neuropathy in diseases classified elsewhere

　　　　Code first underlying disease, such as:
　　　　　amyloidosis (E85.-)
　　　　　gout (M1A.-, M10.-)
　　　　　hyperthyroidism (E05.-)

　　　　EXCLUDES 1　diabetic autonomic neuropathy (E08-E13 with .43)

　　G99.2　Myelopathy in diseases classified elsewhere

　　　　Code first underlying disease, such as:
　　　　　neoplasm (C00-D49)

　　　　EXCLUDES 1　myelopathy in:
　　　　　intervertebral disease (M50.0-, M51.0-)
　　　　　spondylosis (M47.0-, M47.1-)

　　G99.8　Other specified disorders of nervous system in diseases classified elsewhere

　　　　Code first underlying disorder, such as:
　　　　　amyloidosis (E85.-)
　　　　　avitaminosis (E56.9)

　　　　EXCLUDES 1　nervous system involvement in:
　　　　　cysticercosis (B69.0)
　　　　　rubella (B06.0-)
　　　　　syphilis (A52.1-)

☑ Additional Character Required　　　x7ᵗʰ Xtension Alert　　Unspecified Code　　Other Specified Code　　Manifestation Code　　▶◀ Revised Text　　● New Code　　▲ Revised Code Title

ICD-10-CM 2014 (Draft)　　　　　　　　　　　　　　　　　　　　　　　　　　　　　　　　527

Chapter 7. Diseases of the Eye and Adnexa (H00-H59)

NOTE   Use an external cause code following the code for the eye condition, if applicable, to identify the cause of the eye condition.

EXCLUDES 2   *certain conditions originating in the perinatal period (P04-P96)*
certain infectious and parasitic diseases (A00-B99)
complications of pregnancy, childbirth and the puerperium (O00-O9A)
congenital malformations, deformations, and chromosomal abnormalities (Q00-Q99)
diabetes mellitus related eye conditions (E09.3-, E10.3-, E11.3-, E13.3-)
endocrine, nutritional and metabolic diseases (E00-E88)
injury (trauma) of eye and orbit (S05.-)
injury, poisoning and certain other consequences of external causes (S00-T88)
neoplasms (C00-D49)
symptoms, signs and abnormal clinical and laboratory findings, not elsewhere classified (R00-R94)
syphilis related eye disorders (A50.01, A50.3-, A51.43, A52.71)

This chapter contains the following blocks:

H00-H05	Disorders of eyelid, lacrimal system and orbit
H10-H11	Disorders of conjunctiva
H15-H22	Disorders of sclera, cornea, iris and ciliary body
H25-H28	Disorders of lens
H30-H36	Disorders of choroid and retina
H40-H42	Glaucoma
H43-H44	Disorders of vitreous body and globe
H46-H47	Disorders of optic nerve and visual pathways
H49-H52	Disorders of ocular muscles, binocular movement, accommodation and refraction
H53-H54	Visual disturbances and blindness
H55-H57	Other disorders of eye and adnexa
H59	Intraoperative and postprocedural complications and disorders of eye and adnexa, not elsewhere classified

Disorders of eyelid, lacrimal system and orbit (H00-H5)

EXCLUDES 2   *open wound of eyelid (S01.1-)*
superficial injury of eyelid (S00.1-, S00.2-)

✓4th H00   Hordeolum and chalazion

     ✓5th H00.0   Hordeolum (externum) (internum) of eyelid

         ✓6th H00.01   Hordeolum externum
             Hordeolum NOS
             Stye

             H00.011   Hordeolum externum right upper eyelid
             H00.012   Hordeolum externum right lower eyelid
             H00.013   Hordeolum externum right eye, unspecified eyelid
             H00.014   Hordeolum externum left upper eyelid
             H00.015   Hordeolum externum left lower eyelid
             H00.016   Hordeolum externum left eye, unspecified eyelid
             H00.019   Hordeolum externum unspecified eye, unspecified eyelid

         ✓6th H00.02   Hordeolum internum
             Infection of meibomian gland

             H00.021   Hordeolum internum right upper eyelid
             H00.022   Hordeolum internum right lower eyelid
             H00.023   Hordeolum internum right eye, unspecified eyelid
             H00.024   Hordeolum internum left upper eyelid
             H00.025   Hordeolum internum left lower eyelid
             H00.026   Hordeolum internum left eye, unspecified eyelid
             H00.029   Hordeolum internum unspecified eye, unspecified eyelid

         ✓6th H00.03   Abscess of eyelid
             Furuncle of eyelid

             H00.031   Abscess of right upper eyelid
             H00.032   Abscess of right lower eyelid
             H00.033   Abscess of eyelid right eye, unspecified eyelid
             H00.034   Abscess of left upper eyelid
             H00.035   Abscess of left lower eyelid
             H00.036   Abscess of eyelid left eye, unspecified eyelid
             H00.039   Abscess of eyelid unspecified eye, unspecified eyelid

     ✓5th H00.1   Chalazion
         Meibomian (gland) cyst
         EXCLUDES 2   *infected meibomian gland (H00.02-)*

         H00.11   Chalazion right upper eyelid
         H00.12   Chalazion right lower eyelid
         H00.13   Chalazion right eye, unspecified eyelid
         H00.14   Chalazion left upper eyelid
         H00.15   Chalazion left lower eyelid
         H00.16   Chalazion left eye, unspecified eyelid
         H00.19   Chalazion unspecified eye, unspecified eyelid

✓4th H01   Other inflammation of eyelid

     ✓5th H01.0   Blepharitis
         EXCLUDES 1   *blepharoconjunctivitis (H10.5-)*

         ✓6th H01.00   Unspecified blepharitis
             H01.001   Unspecified blepharitis right upper eyelid
             H01.002   Unspecified blepharitis right lower eyelid
             H01.003   Unspecified blepharitis right eye, unspecified eyelid
             H01.004   Unspecified blepharitis left upper eyelid
             H01.005   Unspecified blepharitis left lower eyelid
             H01.006   Unspecified blepharitis left eye, unspecified eyelid
             H01.009   Unspecified blepharitis unspecified eye, unspecified eyelid

         ✓6th H01.01   Ulcerative blepharitis
             H01.011   Ulcerative blepharitis right upper eyelid
             H01.012   Ulcerative blepharitis right lower eyelid
             H01.013   Ulcerative blepharitis right eye, unspecified eyelid
             H01.014   Ulcerative blepharitis left upper eyelid
             H01.015   Ulcerative blepharitis left lower eyelid
             H01.016   Ulcerative blepharitis left eye, unspecified eyelid
             H01.019   Ulcerative blepharitis unspecified eye, unspecified eyelid

         ✓6th H01.02   Squamous blepharitis
             H01.021   Squamous blepharitis right upper eyelid
             H01.022   Squamous blepharitis right lower eyelid
             H01.023   Squamous blepharitis right eye, unspecified eyelid
             H01.024   Squamous blepharitis left upper eyelid
             H01.025   Squamous blepharitis left lower eyelid
             H01.026   Squamous blepharitis left eye, unspecified eyelid
             H01.029   Squamous blepharitis unspecified eye, unspecified eyelid

     ✓5th H01.1   Noninfectious dermatoses of eyelid

         ✓6th H01.11   Allergic dermatitis of eyelid
             Contact dermatitis of eyelid

             H01.111   Allergic dermatitis of right upper eyelid
             H01.112   Allergic dermatitis of right lower eyelid
             H01.113   Allergic dermatitis of right eye, unspecified eyelid
             H01.114   Allergic dermatitis of left upper eyelid
             H01.115   Allergic dermatitis of left lower eyelid
             H01.116   Allergic dermatitis of left eye, unspecified eyelid
             H01.119   Allergic dermatitis of unspecified eye, unspecified eyelid

         ✓6th H01.12   Discoid lupus erythematosus of eyelid
             H01.121   Discoid lupus erythematosus of right upper eyelid
             H01.122   Discoid lupus erythematosus of right lower eyelid
             H01.123   Discoid lupus erythematosus of right eye, unspecified eyelid
             H01.124   Discoid lupus erythematosus of left upper eyelid
             H01.125   Discoid lupus erythematosus of left lower eyelid
             H01.126   Discoid lupus erythematosus of left eye, unspecified eyelid
             H01.129   Discoid lupus erythematosus of unspecified eye, unspecified eyelid

EXCLUDES 1 Not coded here   **EXCLUDES 2** Not included here   **N** Newborn Age: 0   **P** Pediatric Age: 0-17   **M** Maternity Age: 12-55   **A** Adult Age: 15-124

528   ICD-10-CM 2014 (Draft)

☑6ᵗʰ **H01.13 Eczematous dermatitis of eyelid**

H01.131 Eczematous dermatitis of right upper eyelid

H01.132 Eczematous dermatitis of right lower eyelid

H01.133 Eczematous dermatitis of right eye, unspecified eyelid

H01.134 Eczematous dermatitis of left upper eyelid

H01.135 Eczematous dermatitis of left lower eyelid

H01.136 Eczematous dermatitis of left eye, unspecified eyelid

H01.139 Eczematous dermatitis of unspecified eye, unspecified eyelid

☑6ᵗʰ **H01.14 Xeroderma of eyelid**

H01.141 Xeroderma of right upper eyelid

H01.142 Xeroderma of right lower eyelid

H01.143 Xeroderma of right eye, unspecified eyelid

H01.144 Xeroderma of left upper eyelid

H01.145 Xeroderma of left lower eyelid

H01.146 Xeroderma of left eye, unspecified eyelid

H01.149 Xeroderma of unspecified eye, unspecified eyelid

H01.8 Other specified inflammations of eyelid

H01.9 Unspecified inflammation of eyelid
Inflammation of eyelid NOS

☑4ᵗʰ **H02 Other disorders of eyelid**
EXCLUDES 1 *congenital malformations of eyelid (Q10.0-Q10.3)*

☑5ᵗʰ **H02.0 Entropion and trichiasis of eyelid**

☑6ᵗʰ **H02.00 Unspecified entropion of eyelid**

H02.001 Unspecified entropion of right upper eyelid

H02.002 Unspecified entropion of right lower eyelid

H02.003 Unspecified entropion of right eye, unspecified eyelid

H02.004 Unspecified entropion of left upper eyelid

H02.005 Unspecified entropion of left lower eyelid

H02.006 Unspecified entropion of left eye, unspecified eyelid

H02.009 Unspecified entropion of unspecified eye, unspecified eyelid

☑6ᵗʰ **H02.01 Cicatricial entropion of eyelid**

H02.011 Cicatricial entropion of right upper eyelid

H02.012 Cicatricial entropion of right lower eyelid

H02.013 Cicatricial entropion of right eye, unspecified eyelid

H02.014 Cicatricial entropion of left upper eyelid

H02.015 Cicatricial entropion of left lower eyelid

H02.016 Cicatricial entropion of left eye, unspecified eyelid

H02.019 Cicatricial entropion of unspecified eye, unspecified eyelid

☑6ᵗʰ **H02.02 Mechanical entropion of eyelid**

H02.021 Mechanical entropion of right upper eyelid

H02.022 Mechanical entropion of right lower eyelid

H02.023 Mechanical entropion of right eye, unspecified eyelid

H02.024 Mechanical entropion of left upper eyelid

H02.025 Mechanical entropion of left lower eyelid

H02.026 Mechanical entropion of left eye, unspecified eyelid

H02.029 Mechanical entropion of unspecified eye, unspecified eyelid

☑6ᵗʰ **H02.03 Senile entropion of eyelid**

H02.031 Senile entropion of right upper **eyelid** Ⓐ

H02.032 Senile entropion of right lower **eyelid** Ⓐ

H02.033 Senile entropion of right eye, unspecified eyelid Ⓐ

H02.034 Senile entropion of left upper **eyelid** Ⓐ

H02.035 Senile entropion of left lower **eyelid** Ⓐ

H02.036 Senile entropion of left eye, unspecified eyelid Ⓐ

H02.039 Senile entropion of unspecified eye, unspecified eyelid Ⓐ

☑6ᵗʰ **H02.04 Spastic entropion of eyelid**

H02.041 Spastic entropion of right upper eyelid

H02.042 Spastic entropion of right lower eyelid

H02.043 Spastic entropion of right eye, unspecified eyelid

H02.044 Spastic entropion of left upper eyelid

H02.045 Spastic entropion of left lower eyelid

H02.046 Spastic entropion of left eye, unspecified eyelid

H02.049 Spastic entropion of unspecified eye, unspecified eyelid

☑6ᵗʰ **H02.05 Trichiasis without entropian**

H02.051 Trichiasis without entropian right upper eyelid

H02.052 Trichiasis without entropian right lower eyelid

H02.053 Trichiasis without entropian right eye, unspecified eyelid

H02.054 Trichiasis without entropian left upper eyelid

H02.055 Trichiasis without entropian left lower eyelid

H02.056 Trichiasis without entropian left eye, unspecified eyelid

H02.059 Trichiasis without entropian unspecified eye, unspecified eyelid

☑5ᵗʰ **H02.1 Ectropion of eyelid**

☑6ᵗʰ **H02.10 Unspecified ectropion of eyelid**

H02.101 Unspecified ectropion of right upper eyelid

H02.102 Unspecified ectropion of right lower eyelid

H02.103 Unspecified ectropion of right eye, unspecified eyelid

H02.104 Unspecified ectropion of left upper eyelid

H02.105 Unspecified ectropion of left lower eyelid

H02.106 Unspecified ectropion of left eye, unspecified eyelid

H02.109 Unspecified ectropion of unspecified eye, unspecified eyelid

☑6ᵗʰ **H02.11 Cicatricial ectropion of eyelid**

H02.111 Cicatricial ectropion of right upper eyelid

H02.112 Cicatricial ectropion of right lower eyelid

H02.113 Cicatricial ectropion of right eye, unspecified eyelid

H02.114 Cicatricial ectropion of left upper eyelid

H02.115 Cicatricial ectropion of left lower eyelid

H02.116 Cicatricial ectropion of left eye, unspecified eyelid

H02.119 Cicatricial ectropion of unspecified eye, unspecified eyelid

☑6ᵗʰ **H02.12 Mechanical ectropion of eyelid**

H02.121 Mechanical ectropion of right upper eyelid

H02.122 Mechanical ectropion of right lower eyelid

H02.123 Mechanical ectropion of right eye, unspecified eyelid

H02.124 Mechanical ectropion of left upper eyelid

H02.125 Mechanical ectropion of left lower eyelid

H02.126 Mechanical ectropion of left eye, unspecified eyelid

H02.129 Mechanical ectropion of unspecified eye, unspecified eyelid

☑6ᵗʰ **H02.13 Senile ectropion of eyelid**

H02.131 Senile ectropion of right upper eyelid Ⓐ

H02.132 Senile ectropion of right lower eyelid Ⓐ

H02.133 Senile ectropion of right eye, unspecified eyelid Ⓐ

H02.134 Senile ectropion of left upper eyelid Ⓐ

H02.135 Senile ectropion of left lower eyelid Ⓐ

H02.136 Senile ectropion of left eye, unspecified eyelid Ⓐ

H02.139 Senile ectropion of unspecified eye, unspecified eyelid Ⓐ

☑6ᵗʰ **H02.14 Spastic ectropion of eyelid**

H02.141 Spastic ectropion of right upper eyelid

H02.142 Spastic ectropion of right lower eyelid

☑ Additional Character Required   ☑x7ᵗʰ Xtension Alert   Unspecified Code   Other Specified Code   Manifestation Code   ▶◀ Revised Text   ● New Code   ▲ Revised Code Title

Diseases of the Eye and Adnexa

H02.143–H02.65

H02.143   **Spastic ectropion of** right eye, unspecified **eyelid**

H02.144   **Spastic ectropion of** left upper **eyelid**

H02.145   **Spastic ectropion of** left lower **eyelid**

H02.146   **Spastic ectropion of** left eye, unspecified **eyelid**

H02.149   **Spastic ectropion of unspecified eye, unspecified eyelid**

√5ᵗʰ   **H02.2   Lagophthalmos**

   √6ᵗʰ   **H02.20   Unspecified lagophthalmos**

H02.201   **Unspecified lagophthalmos** right upper eyelid

H02.202   **Unspecified lagophthalmos** right lower eyelid

H02.203   **Unspecified lagophthalmos** right eye, unspecified eyelid

H02.204   **Unspecified lagophthalmos** left upper eyelid

H02.205   **Unspecified lagophthalmos** left lower eyelid

H02.206   **Unspecified lagophthalmos** left eye, unspecified eyelid

H02.209   **Unspecified lagophthalmos unspecified eye, unspecified eyelid**

   √6ᵗʰ   **H02.21   Cicatricial lagophthalmos**

H02.211   **Cicatricial lagophthalmos** right upper eyelid

H02.212   **Cicatricial lagophthalmos** right lower eyelid

H02.213   **Cicatricial lagophthalmos** right eye, unspecified eyelid

H02.214   **Cicatricial lagophthalmos** left upper **eyelid**

H02.215   **Cicatricial lagophthalmos** left lower **eyelid**

H02.216   **Cicatricial lagophthalmos** left eye, unspecified eyelid

H02.219   **Cicatricial lagophthalmos unspecified eye, unspecified eyelid**

   √6ᵗʰ   **H02.22   Mechanical lagophthalmos**

H02.221   **Mechanical lagophthalmos** right upper eyelid

H02.222   **Mechanical lagophthalmos** right lower eyelid

H02.223   **Mechanical lagophthalmos** right eye, unspecified eyelid

H02.224   **Mechanical lagophthalmos** left upper eyelid

H02.225   **Mechanical lagophthalmos** left lower eyelid

H02.226   **Mechanical lagophthalmos** left eye, unspecified eyelid

H02.229   **Mechanical lagophthalmos unspecified eye, unspecified eyelid**

   √6ᵗʰ   **H02.23   Paralytic lagophthalmos**

H02.231   **Paralytic lagophthalmos** right upper eyelid

H02.232   **Paralytic lagophthalmos** right lower eyelid

H02.233   **Paralytic lagophthalmos** right eye, unspecified eyelid

H02.234   **Paralytic lagophthalmos** left upper **eyelid**

H02.235   **Paralytic lagophthalmos** left lower **eyelid**

H02.236   **Paralytic lagophthalmos** left eye, unspecified eyelid

H02.239   **Paralytic lagophthalmos unspecified eye, unspecified eyelid**

√5ᵗʰ   **H02.3   Blepharochalasis**

Pseudoptosis

H02.30   **Blepharochalasis unspecified eye, unspecified eyelid**

H02.31   **Blepharochalasis** right upper **eyelid**

H02.32   **Blepharochalasis** right lower **eyelid**

H02.33   **Blepharochalasis** right eye, unspecified eyelid

H02.34   **Blepharochalasis** left upper **eyelid**

H02.35   **Blepharochalasis** left lower **eyelid**

H02.36   **Blepharochalasis** left eye, unspecified eyelid

√5ᵗʰ   **H02.4   Ptosis of eyelid**

   √6ᵗʰ   **H02.40   Unspecified ptosis of eyelid**

H02.401   **Unspecified ptosis of** right **eyelid**

H02.402   **Unspecified ptosis of** left **eyelid**

H02.403   **Unspecified ptosis of** bilateral **eyelids**

H02.409   **Unspecified ptosis of unspecified eyelid**

   √6ᵗʰ   **H02.41   Mechanical ptosis of eyelid**

H02.411   **Mechanical ptosis of** right **eyelid**

H02.412   **Mechanical ptosis of** left **eyelid**

H02.413   **Mechanical ptosis of** bilateral **eyelids**

H02.419   **Mechanical ptosis of unspecified eyelid**

   √6ᵗʰ   **H02.42   Myogenic ptosis of eyelid**

H02.421   **Myogenic ptosis of** right **eyelid**

H02.422   **Myogenic ptosis of** left **eyelid**

H02.423   **Myogenic ptosis of** bilateral **eyelids**

H02.429   **Myogenic ptosis of unspecified eyelid**

   √6ᵗʰ   **H02.43   Paralytic ptosis of eyelid**

Neurogenic ptosis of eyelid

H02.431   **Paralytic ptosis of** right **eyelid**

H02.432   **Paralytic ptosis of** left **eyelid**

H02.433   **Paralytic ptosis of** bilateral **eyelids**

H02.439   **Paralytic ptosis unspecified eyelid**

√5ᵗʰ   **H02.5   Other disorders affecting eyelid function**

EXCLUDES 2   *blepharospasm (G24.5)*

organic tic (G25.69)

psychogenic tic (F95.-)

   √6ᵗʰ   **H02.51   Abnormal innervation syndrome**

H02.511   **Abnormal innervation syndrome** right upper **eyelid**

H02.512   **Abnormal innervation syndrome** right lower **eyelid**

H02.513   **Abnormal innervation syndrome** right eye, unspecified eyelid

H02.514   **Abnormal innervation syndrome** left upper **eyelid**

H02.515   **Abnormal innervation syndrome** left lower **eyelid**

H02.516   **Abnormal innervation syndrome** left eye, unspecified eyelid

H02.519   **Abnormal innervation syndrome unspecified eye, unspecified eyelid**

   √6ᵗʰ   **H02.52   Blepharophimosis**

Ankyloblepharon

H02.521   **Blepharophimosis** right upper **eyelid**

H02.522   **Blepharophimosis** right lower **eyelid**

H02.523   **Blepharophimosis** right eye, unspecified eyelid

H02.524   **Blepharophimosis** left upper **eyelid**

H02.525   **Blepharophimosis** left lower **eyelid**

H02.526   **Blepharophimosis** left eye, unspecified eyelid

H02.529   **Blepharophimosis unspecified eye, unspecified lid**

   √6ᵗʰ   **H02.53   Eyelid retraction**

Eyelid lag

H02.531   **Eyelid retraction** right upper **eyelid**

H02.532   **Eyelid retraction** right lower **eyelid**

H02.533   **Eyelid retraction** right eye, unspecified eyelid

H02.534   **Eyelid retraction** left upper **eyelid**

H02.535   **Eyelid retraction** left lower **eyelid**

H02.536   **Eyelid retraction** left eye, unspecified eyelid

H02.539   **Eyelid retraction unspecified eye, unspecified lid**

H02.59   **Other disorders affecting eyelid function**

Deficient blink reflex

Sensory disorders

√5ᵗʰ   **H02.6   Xanthelasma of eyelid**

H02.60   **Xanthelasma of unspecified eye, unspecified eyelid**

H02.61   **Xanthelasma of** right upper **eyelid**

H02.62   **Xanthelasma of** right lower **eyelid**

H02.63   **Xanthelasma of** right eye, unspecified eyelid

H02.64   **Xanthelasma of** left upper **eyelid**

H02.65   **Xanthelasma of** left lower **eyelid**

EXCLUDES 1 Not coded here   EXCLUDES 2 Not included here   N Newborn Age: 0   P Pediatric Age: 0-17   M Maternity Age: 12-55   A Adult Age: 15-124

530   ICD-10-CM 2014 (Draft)

Diseases of the Eye and Adnexa

H02.66–H04.001

H02.66   Xanthelasma of left eye, unspecified eyelid

✓5ᵗʰ H02.7   Other and unspecified degenerative disorders of eyelid and periocular area

   H02.70   Unspecified degenerative disorders of eyelid and periocular area

   ✓6ᵗʰ H02.71   Chloasma of eyelid and periocular area
      Dyspigmentation of eyelid
      Hyperpigmentation of eyelid

      H02.711   Chloasma of right upper eyelid and periocular area
      H02.712   Chloasma of right lower eyelid and periocular area
      H02.713   Chloasma of right eye, unspecified eyelid and periocular area
      H02.714   Chloasma of left upper eyelid and periocular area
      H02.715   Chloasma of left lower eyelid and periocular area
      H02.716   Chloasma of left eye, unspecified eyelid and periocular area
      H02.719   Chloasma of unspecified eye, unspecified eyelid and periocular area

   ✓6ᵗʰ H02.72   Madarosis of eyelid and periocular area
      Hypotrichosis of eyelid

      H02.721   Madarosis of right upper eyelid and periocular area
      H02.722   Madarosis of right lower eyelid and periocular area
      H02.723   Madarosis of right eye, unspecified eyelid and periocular area
      H02.724   Madarosis of left upper eyelid and periocular area
      H02.725   Madarosis of left lower eyelid and periocular area
      H02.726   Madarosis of left eye, unspecified eyelid and periocular area
      H02.729   Madarosis of unspecified eye, unspecified eyelid and periocular area

   ✓6ᵗʰ H02.73   Vitiligo of eyelid and periocular area
      Hypopigmentation of eyelid

      H02.731   Vitiligo of right upper eyelid and periocular area
      H02.732   Vitiligo of right lower eyelid and periocular area
      H02.733   Vitiligo of right eye, unspecified eyelid and periocular area
      H02.734   Vitiligo of left upper eyelid and periocular area
      H02.735   Vitiligo of left lower eyelid and periocular area
      H02.736   Vitiligo of left eye, unspecified eyelid and periocular area
      H02.739   Vitiligo of unspecified eye, unspecified eyelid and periocular area

   H02.79   Other degenerative disorders of eyelid and periocular area

✓5ᵗʰ H02.8   Other specified disorders of eyelid

   ✓6ᵗʰ H02.81   Retained foreign body in eyelid
      Use additional code to identify the type of retained foreign body (Z18.-)
      EXCLUDES 1   laceration of eyelid with foreign body (S01.12-)
        retained intraocular foreign body (H44.6-, H44.7-)
        superficial foreign body of eyelid and periocular area (S00.25-)

      H02.811   Retained foreign body in right upper eyelid
      H02.812   Retained foreign body in right lower eyelid
      H02.813   Retained foreign body in right eye, unspecified eyelid
      H02.814   Retained foreign body in left upper eyelid
      H02.815   Retained foreign body in left lower eyelid
      H02.816   Retained foreign body in left eye, unspecified eyelid
      H02.819   Retained foreign body in unspecified eye, unspecified eyelid

   ✓6ᵗʰ H02.82   Cysts of eyelid
      Sebaceous cyst of eyelid

      H02.821   Cysts of right upper eyelid
      H02.822   Cysts of right lower eyelid
      H02.823   Cysts of right eye, unspecified eyelid
      H02.824   Cysts of left upper eyelid
      H02.825   Cysts of left lower eyelid
      H02.826   Cysts of left eye, unspecified eyelid
      H02.829   Cysts of unspecified eye, unspecified eyelid

   ✓6ᵗʰ H02.83   Dermatochalasis of eyelid
      H02.831   Dermatochalasis of right upper eyelid
      H02.832   Dermatochalasis of right lower eyelid
      H02.833   Dermatochalasis of right eye, unspecified eyelid
      H02.834   Dermatochalasis of left upper eyelid
      H02.835   Dermatochalasis of left lower eyelid
      H02.836   Dermatochalasis of left eye, unspecified eyelid
      H02.839   Dermatochalasis of unspecified eye, unspecified eyelid

   ✓6ᵗʰ H02.84   Edema of eyelid
      Hyperemia of eyelid

      H02.841   Edema of right upper eyelid
      H02.842   Edema of right lower eyelid
      H02.843   Edema of right eye, unspecified eyelid
      H02.844   Edema of left upper eyelid
      H02.845   Edema of left lower eyelid
      H02.846   Edema of left eye, unspecified eyelid
      H02.849   Edema of unspecified eye, unspecified eyelid

   ✓6ᵗʰ H02.85   Elephantiasis of eyelid
      H02.851   Elephantiasis of right upper eyelid
      H02.852   Elephantiasis of right lower eyelid
      H02.853   Elephantiasis of right eye, unspecified eyelid
      H02.854   Elephantiasis of left upper eyelid
      H02.855   Elephantiasis of left lower eyelid
      H02.856   Elephantiasis of left eye, unspecified eyelid
      H02.859   Elephantiasis of unspecified eye, unspecified eyelid

   ✓6ᵗʰ H02.86   Hypertrichosis of eyelid
      H02.861   Hypertrichosis of right upper eyelid
      H02.862   Hypertrichosis of right lower eyelid
      H02.863   Hypertrichosis of right eye, unspecified eyelid
      H02.864   Hypertrichosis of left upper eyelid
      H02.865   Hypertrichosis of left lower eyelid
      H02.866   Hypertrichosis of left eye, unspecified eyelid
      H02.869   Hypertrichosis of unspecified eye, unspecified eyelid

   ✓6ᵗʰ H02.87   Vascular anomalies of eyelid
      H02.871   Vascular anomalies of right upper eyelid
      H02.872   Vascular anomalies of right lower eyelid
      H02.873   Vascular anomalies of right eye, unspecified eyelid
      H02.874   Vascular anomalies of left upper eyelid
      H02.875   Vascular anomalies of left lower eyelid
      H02.876   Vascular anomalies of left eye, unspecified eyelid
      H02.879   Vascular anomalies of unspecified eye, unspecified eyelid

   H02.89   Other specified disorders of eyelid
      Hemorrhage of eyelid

H02.9   Unspecified disorder of eyelid
   Disorder of eyelid NOS

✓4ᵗʰ H04   Disorders of lacrimal system
   EXCLUDES 1   congenital malformations of lacrimal system (Q10.4-Q10.6)

   ✓5ᵗʰ H04.0   Dacryoadenitis

      ✓6ᵗʰ H04.00   Unspecified dacryoadenitis
         H04.001   Unspecified dacryoadenitis, right lacrimal gland

✓ Additional Character Required   ✓ˣ7ᵗʰ Xtension Alert   Unspecified Code   Other Specified Code   Manifestation Code   ►◄ Revised Text   ● New Code   ▲ Revised Code Title

ICD-10-CM 2014 (Draft)   581

Diseases of the Eye and Adnexa

H04.002–H04.419

H04.002   Unspecified dacryoadenitis, left lacrimal gland

H04.003   Unspecified dacryoadenitis, bilateral lacrimal glands

H04.009   Unspecified dacryoadenitis, unspecified lacrimal gland

✓6th H04.01   Acute dacryoadenitis

H04.011   Acute dacryoadenitis, right lacrimal gland

H04.012   Acute dacryoadenitis, left lacrimal gland

H04.013   Acute dacryoadenitis, bilateral lacrimal glands

H04.019   Acute dacryoadenitis, unspecified lacrimal gland

✓6th H04.02   Chronic dacryoadenitis

H04.021   Chronic dacryoadenitis, right lacrimal gland

H04.022   Chronic dacryoadenitis, left lacrimal gland

H04.023   Chronic dacryoadenitis, bilateral lacrimal glands

H04.029   Chronic dacryoadenitis, unspecified lacrimal gland

✓6th H04.03   Chronic enlargement of lacrimal gland

H04.031   Chronic enlargement of right lacrimal gland

H04.032   Chronic enlargement of left lacrimal gland

H04.033   Chronic enlargement of bilateral lacrimal glands

H04.039   Chronic enlargement of unspecified lacrimal gland

✓5th H04.1   Other disorders of lacrimal gland

✓6th H04.11   Dacryops

H04.111   Dacryops of right lacrimal gland

H04.112   Dacryops of left lacrimal gland

H04.113   Dacryops of bilateral lacrimal glands

H04.119   Dacryops of unspecified lacrimal gland

✓6th H04.12   Dry eye syndrome
Tear film insufficiency, NOS

H04.121   Dry eye syndrome of right lacrimal gland

H04.122   Dry eye syndrome of left lacrimal gland

H04.123   Dry eye syndrome of bilateral lacrimal glands

H04.129   Dry eye syndrome of unspecified lacrimal gland

✓6th H04.13   Lacrimal cyst
Lacrimal cystic degeneration

H04.131   Lacrimal cyst, right lacrimal gland

H04.132   Lacrimal cyst, left lacrimal gland

H04.133   Lacrimal cyst, bilateral lacrimal glands

H04.139   Lacrimal cyst, unspecified lacrimal gland

✓6th H04.14   Primary lacrimal gland atrophy

H04.141   Primary lacrimal gland atrophy, right lacrimal gland

H04.142   Primary lacrimal gland atrophy, left lacrimal gland

H04.143   Primary lacrimal gland atrophy, bilateral lacrimal glands

H04.149   Primary lacrimal gland atrophy, unspecified lacrimal gland

✓6th H04.15   Secondary lacrimal gland atrophy

H04.151   Secondary lacrimal gland atrophy, right lacrimal gland

H04.152   Secondary lacrimal gland atrophy, left lacrimal gland

H04.153   Secondary lacrimal gland atrophy, bilateral lacrimal glands

H04.159   Secondary lacrimal gland atrophy, unspecified lacrimal gland

✓6th H04.16   Lacrimal gland dislocation

H04.161   Lacrimal gland dislocation, right lacrimal gland

H04.162   Lacrimal gland dislocation, left lacrimal gland

H04.163   Lacrimal gland dislocation, bilateral lacrimal glands

H04.169   Lacrimal gland dislocation, unspecified lacrimal gland

H04.19   Other specified disorders of lacrimal gland

✓5th H04.2   Epiphora

✓6th H04.20   Unspecified epiphora

H04.201   Unspecified epiphora, right lacrimal gland

H04.202   Unspecified epiphora, left lacrimal gland

H04.203   Unspecified epiphora, bilateral lacrimal glands

H04.209   Unspecified epiphora, unspecified lacrimal gland

✓6th H04.21   Epiphora due to excess lacrimation

H04.211   Epiphora due to excess lacrimation, right lacrimal gland

H04.212   Epiphora due to excess lacrimation, left lacrimal gland

H04.213   Epiphora due to excess lacrimation, bilateral lacrimal glands

H04.219   Epiphora due to excess lacrimation, unspecified lacrimal gland

✓6th H04.22   Epiphora due to insufficient drainage

H04.221   Epiphora due to insufficient drainage, right lacrimal gland

H04.222   Epiphora due to insufficient drainage, left lacrimal gland

H04.223   Epiphora due to insufficient drainage, bilateral lacrimal glands

H04.229   Epiphora due to insufficient drainage, unspecified lacrimal gland

✓5th H04.3   Acute and unspecified inflammation of lacrimal passages

    EXCLUDES 1   neonatal dacryocystitis (P39.1)

✓6th H04.30   Unspecified dacryocystitis

H04.301   Unspecified dacryocystitis of right lacrimal passage

H04.302   Unspecified dacryocystitis of left lacrimal passage

H04.303   Unspecified dacryocystitis of bilateral lacrimal passages

H04.309   Unspecified dacryocystitis of unspecified lacrimal passage

✓6th H04.31   Phlegmonous dacryocystitis

H04.311   Phlegmonous dacryocystitis of right lacrimal passage

H04.312   Phlegmonous dacryocystitis of left lacrimal passage

H04.313   Phlegmonous dacryocystitis of bilateral lacrimal passages

H04.319   Phlegmonous dacryocystitis of unspecified lacrimal passage

✓6th H04.32   Acute dacryocystitis
Acute dacryopericystitis

H04.321   Acute dacryocystitis of right lacrimal passage

H04.322   Acute dacryocystitis of left lacrimal passage

H04.323   Acute dacryocystitis of bilateral lacrimal passages

H04.329   Acute dacryocystitis of unspecified lacrimal passage

✓6th H04.33   Acute lacrimal canaliculitis

H04.331   Acute lacrimal canaliculitis of right lacrimal passage

H04.332   Acute lacrimal canaliculitis of left lacrimal passage

H04.333   Acute lacrimal canaliculitis of bilateral lacrimal passages

H04.339   Acute lacrimal canaliculitis of unspecified lacrimal passage

✓5th H04.4   Chronic inflammation of lacrimal passages

✓6th H04.41   Chronic dacryocystitis

H04.411   Chronic dacryocystitis of right lacrimal passage

H04.412   Chronic dacryocystitis of left lacrimal passage

H04.413   Chronic dacryocystitis of bilateral lacrimal passages

H04.419   Chronic dacryocystitis of unspecified lacrimal passage

EXCLUDES 1 Not coded here   *EXCLUDES 2* Not included here   N Newborn Age: 0   P Pediatric Age: 0-17   M Maternity Age: 12-55   A Adult Age: 15-124

532   ICD-10-CM 2014 (Draft)

☑6ᵗʰ **H04.42** Chronic lacrimal canaliculitis
- **H04.421** Chronic lacrimal canaliculitis of right lacrimal passage
- **H04.422** Chronic lacrimal canaliculitis of left lacrimal passage
- **H04.423** Chronic lacrimal canaliculitis of bilateral lacrimal passages
- **H04.429** Chronic lacrimal canaliculitis of unspecified lacrimal passage

☑6ᵗʰ **H04.43** Chronic lacrimal mucocele
- **H04.431** Chronic lacrimal mucocele of right lacrimal passage
- **H04.432** Chronic lacrimal mucocele of left lacrimal passage
- **H04.433** Chronic lacrimal mucocele of bilateral lacrimal passages
- **H04.439** Chronic lacrimal mucocele of unspecified lacrimal passage

☑5ᵗʰ **H04.5** Stenosis and insufficiency of lacrimal passages

☑6ᵗʰ **H04.51** Dacryolith
- **H04.511** Dacryolith of right lacrimal passage
- **H04.512** Dacryolith of left lacrimal passage
- **H04.513** Dacryolith of bilateral lacrimal passages
- **H04.519** Dacryolith of unspecified lacrimal passage

☑6ᵗʰ **H04.52** Eversion of lacrimal punctum
- **H04.521** Eversion of right lacrimal punctum
- **H04.522** Eversion of left lacrimal punctum
- **H04.523** Eversion of bilateral lacrimal punctum
- **H04.529** Eversion of unspecified lacrimal punctum

☑6ᵗʰ **H04.53** Neonatal obstruction of nasolacrimal duct

     EXCLUDES 1   *congenital stenosis and stricture of lacrimal duct (Q10.5)*
- **H04.531** Neonatal obstruction of right nasolacrimal duct   Ⓝ
- **H04.532** Neonatal obstruction of left nasolacrimal duct   Ⓝ
- **H04.533** Neonatal obstruction of bilateral nasolacrimal duct   Ⓝ
- **H04.539** Neonatal obstruction of unspecified nasolacrimal duct   Ⓝ

☑6ᵗʰ **H04.54** Stenosis of lacrimal canaliculi
- **H04.541** Stenosis of right lacrimal canaliculi
- **H04.542** Stenosis of left lacrimal canaliculi
- **H04.543** Stenosis of bilateral lacrimal canaliculi
- **H04.549** Stenosis of unspecified lacrimal canaliculi

☑6ᵗʰ **H04.55** Acquired stenosis of nasolacrimal duct
- **H04.551** Acquired stenosis of right nasolacrimal duct
- **H04.552** Acquired stenosis of left nasolacrimal duct
- **H04.553** Acquired stenosis of bilateral nasolacrimal duct
- **H04.559** Acquired stenosis of unspecified nasolacrimal duct

☑6ᵗʰ **H04.56** Stenosis of lacrimal punctum
- **H04.561** Stenosis of right lacrimal punctum
- **H04.562** Stenosis of left lacrimal punctum
- **H04.563** Stenosis of bilateral lacrimal punctum
- **H04.569** Stenosis of unspecified lacrimal punctum

☑6ᵗʰ **H04.57** Stenosis of lacrimal sac
- **H04.571** Stenosis of right lacrimal sac
- **H04.572** Stenosis of left lacrimal sac
- **H04.573** Stenosis of bilateral lacrimal sac
- **H04.579** Stenosis of unspecified lacrimal sac

☑5ᵗʰ **H04.6** Other changes of lacrimal passages

☑6ᵗʰ **H04.61** Lacrimal fistula
- **H04.611** Lacrimal fistula right lacrimal passage
- **H04.612** Lacrimal fistula left lacrimal passage
- **H04.613** Lacrimal fistula bilateral lacrimal passages
- **H04.619** Lacrimal fistula unspecified lacrimal passage

     H04.69 Other changes of lacrimal passages

☑5ᵗʰ **H04.8** Other disorders of lacrimal system

☑6ᵗʰ **H04.81** Granuloma of lacrimal passages
- **H04.811** Granuloma of right lacrimal passage

- **H04.812** Granuloma of left lacrimal passage
- **H04.813** Granuloma of bilateral lacrimal passages
- **H04.819** Granuloma of unspecified lacrimal passage

     H04.89 Other disorders of lacrimal system

     H04.9 Disorder of lacrimal system, unspecified

☑4ᵗʰ **H05** **Disorders of orbit**

     EXCLUDES 1   *congenital malformation of orbit (Q10.7)*

☑5ᵗʰ **H05.0** Acute inflammation of orbit

     H05.00 Unspecified acute inflammation of orbit

☑6ᵗʰ **H05.01** Cellulitis of orbit
     Abscess of orbit
- **H05.011** Cellulitis of right orbit
- **H05.012** Cellulitis of left orbit
- **H05.013** Cellulitis of bilateral orbits
- **H05.019** Cellulitis of unspecified orbit

☑6ᵗʰ **H05.02** Osteomyelitis of orbit
- **H05.021** Osteomyelitis of right orbit
- **H05.022** Osteomyelitis of left orbit
- **H05.023** Osteomyelitis of bilateral orbits
- **H05.029** Osteomyelitis of unspecified orbit

☑6ᵗʰ **H05.03** Periostitis of orbit
- **H05.031** Periostitis of right orbit
- **H05.032** Periostitis of left orbit
- **H05.033** Periostitis of bilateral orbits
- **H05.039** Periostitis of unspecified orbit

☑6ᵗʰ **H05.04** Tenonitis of orbit
- **H05.041** Tenonitis of right orbit
- **H05.042** Tenonitis of left orbit
- **H05.043** Tenonitis of bilateral orbits
- **H05.049** Tenonitis of unspecified orbit

☑5ᵗʰ **H05.1** Chronic inflammatory disorders of orbit

     H05.10 Unspecified chronic inflammatory disorders of orbit

☑6ᵗʰ **H05.11** Granuloma of orbit
     Pseudotumor (inflammatory) of orbit
- **H05.111** Granuloma of right orbit
- **H05.112** Granuloma of left orbit
- **H05.113** Granuloma of bilateral orbits
- **H05.119** Granuloma of unspecified orbit

☑6ᵗʰ **H05.12** Orbital myositis
- **H05.121** Orbital myositis, right orbit
- **H05.122** Orbital myositis, left orbit
- **H05.123** Orbital myositis, bilateral
- **H05.129** Orbital myositis, unspecified orbit

☑5ᵗʰ **H05.2** Exophthalmic conditions

     H05.20 Unspecified exophthalmos

☑6ᵗʰ **H05.21** Displacement (lateral) of globe
- **H05.211** Displacement (lateral) of globe, right eye
- **H05.212** Displacement (lateral) of globe, left eye
- **H05.213** Displacement (lateral) of globe, bilateral
- **H05.219** Displacement (lateral) of globe, unspecified eye

☑6ᵗʰ **H05.22** Edema of orbit
     Orbital congestion
- **H05.221** Edema of right orbit
- **H05.222** Edema of left orbit
- **H05.223** Edema of bilateral orbit
- **H05.229** Edema of unspecified orbit

☑6ᵗʰ **H05.23** Hemorrhage of orbit
- **H05.231** Hemorrhage of right orbit
- **H05.232** Hemorrhage of left orbit
- **H05.233** Hemorrhage of bilateral orbit
- **H05.239** Hemorrhage of unspecified orbit

☑6ᵗʰ **H05.24** Constant exophthalmos
- **H05.241** Constant exophthalmos, right eye
- **H05.242** Constant exophthalmos, left eye
- **H05.243** Constant exophthalmos, bilateral
- **H05.249** Constant exophthalmos, unspecified eye

☑6ᵗʰ **H05.25** Intermittent exophthalmos
- **H05.251** Intermittent exophthalmos, right eye
- **H05.252** Intermittent exophthalmos, left eye

☑ Additional Character Required   ✓x7ᵗʰ Xtension Alert   Unspecified Code   Other Specified Code   Manifestation Code   ►◄ Revised Text   ● New Code   ▲ Revised Code Title

Diseases of the Eye and Adnexa

H05.253–H10.222

H05.253   Intermittent exophthalmos, bilateral

H05.259   Intermittent exophthalmos, unspecified eye

✓6ᵗʰ   **H05.26   Pulsating exophthalmos**

H05.261   Pulsating exophthalmos, right eye

H05.262   Pulsating exophthalmos, left eye

H05.263   Pulsating exophthalmos, bilateral

H05.269   Pulsating exophthalmos, unspecified eye

✓5ᵗʰ   **H05.3   Deformity of orbit**

EXCLUDES 1   congenital deformity of orbit (Q10.7)

hypertelorism (Q75.2)

H05.30   **Unspecified deformity of orbit**

✓6ᵗʰ   **H05.31   Atrophy of orbit**

H05.311   Atrophy of right orbit

H05.312   Atrophy of left orbit

H05.313   Atrophy of bilateral orbit

H05.319   Atrophy of unspecified orbit

✓6ᵗʰ   **H05.32   Deformity of orbit due to bone disease**

Code also associated bone disease

H05.321   Deformity of right orbit due to bone disease

H05.322   Deformity of left orbit due to bone disease

H05.323   Deformity of bilateral orbits due to bone disease

H05.329   Deformity of unspecified orbit due to bone disease

✓6ᵗʰ   **H05.33   Deformity of orbit due to trauma or surgery**

H05.331   Deformity of right orbit due to trauma or surgery

H05.332   Deformity of left orbit due to trauma or surgery

H05.333   Deformity of bilateral orbits due to trauma or surgery

H05.339   Deformity of unspecified orbit due to trauma or surgery

✓6ᵗʰ   **H05.34   Enlargement of orbit**

H05.341   Enlargement of right orbit

H05.342   Enlargement of left orbit

H05.343   Enlargement of bilateral orbits

H05.349   Enlargement of unspecified orbit

✓6ᵗʰ   **H05.35   Exostosis of orbit**

H05.351   Exostosis of right orbit

H05.352   Exostosis of left orbit

H05.353   Exostosis of bilateral orbits

H05.359   Exostosis of unspecified orbit

✓5ᵗʰ   **H05.4   Enophthalmos**

✓6ᵗʰ   **H05.40   Unspecified enophthalmos**

H05.401   Unspecified enophthalmos, right eye

H05.402   Unspecified enophthalmos, left eye

H05.403   Unspecified enophthalmos, bilateral

H05.409   Unspecified enophthalmos, unspecified eye

✓6ᵗʰ   **H05.41   Enophthalmos due to atrophy of orbital tissue**

H05.411   Enophthalmos due to atrophy of orbital tissue, right eye

H05.412   Enophthalmos due to atrophy of orbital tissue, left eye

H05.413   Enophthalmos due to atrophy of orbital tissue, bilateral

H05.419   Enophthalmos due to atrophy of orbital tissue, unspecified eye

✓6ᵗʰ   **H05.42   Enophthalmos due to trauma or surgery**

H05.421   Enophthalmos due to trauma or surgery, right eye

H05.422   Enophthalmos due to trauma or surgery, left eye

H05.423   Enophthalmos due to trauma or surgery, bilateral

H05.429   Enophthalmos due to trauma or surgery, unspecified eye

✓5ᵗʰ   **H05.5   Retained (old) foreign body following penetrating wound of orbit**

Use additional code to identify the type of retained foreign body (Z18.-)

Retrobulbar foreign body

EXCLUDES 1   current penetrating wound of orbit (S05.4-)

EXCLUDES 2   retained foreign body of eyelid (H02.81-)

retained intraocular foreign body (H44.6-, H44.7-)

H05.50   **Retained (old) foreign body following penetrating wound of unspecified orbit**

H05.51   **Retained (old) foreign body following penetrating wound of right orbit**

H05.52   **Retained (old) foreign body following penetrating wound of left orbit**

H05.53   **Retained (old) foreign body following penetrating wound of bilateral orbits**

✓5ᵗʰ   **H05.8   Other disorders of orbit**

✓6ᵗʰ   **H05.81   Cyst of orbit**

Encephalocele of orbit

H05.811   Cyst of right orbit

H05.812   Cyst of left orbit

H05.813   Cyst of bilateral orbits

H05.819   Cyst of unspecified orbit

✓6ᵗʰ   **H05.82   Myopathy of extraocular muscles**

H05.821   Myopathy of extraocular muscles, right orbit

H05.822   Myopathy of extraocular muscles, left orbit

H05.823   Myopathy of extraocular muscles, bilateral

H05.829   Myopathy of extraocular muscles, unspecified orbit

H05.89   **Other disorders of orbit**

H05.9   **Unspecified disorder of orbit**

Disorders of conjunctiva (H10-H11)

✓4ᵗʰ   **H10   Conjunctivitis**

EXCLUDES 1   keratoconjunctivitis (H16.2-)

✓5ᵗʰ   **H10.0   Mucopurulent conjunctivitis**

✓6ᵗʰ   **H10.01   Acute follicular conjunctivitis**

H10.011   Acute follicular conjunctivitis, right eye

H10.012   Acute follicular conjunctivitis, left eye

H10.013   Acute follicular conjunctivitis, bilateral

H10.019   Acute follicular conjunctivitis, unspecified eye

✓6ᵗʰ   **H10.02   Other mucopurulent conjunctivitis**

H10.021   Other mucopurulent conjunctivitis, right eye

H10.022   Other mucopurulent conjunctivitis, left eye

H10.023   Other mucopurulent conjunctivitis, bilateral

H10.029   Other mucopurulent conjunctivitis, unspecified eye

✓5ᵗʰ   **H10.1   Acute atopic conjunctivitis**

Acute papillary conjunctivitis

H10.10   **Acute atopic conjunctivitis, unspecified eye**

H10.11   **Acute atopic conjunctivitis, right eye**

H10.12   **Acute atopic conjunctivitis, left eye**

H10.13   **Acute atopic conjunctivitis, bilateral**

✓5ᵗʰ   **H10.2   Other acute conjunctivitis**

✓6ᵗʰ   **H10.21   Acute toxic conjunctivitis**

Acute chemical conjunctivitis

Code first (T51-T65) to identify chemical and intent

EXCLUDES 1   burn and corrosion of eye and adnexa (T26.-)

H10.211   Acute toxic conjunctivitis, right eye

H10.212   Acute toxic conjunctivitis, left eye

H10.213   Acute toxic conjunctivitis, bilateral

H10.219   Acute toxic conjunctivitis, unspecified eye

✓6ᵗʰ   **H10.22   Pseudomembranous conjunctivitis**

H10.221   Pseudomembranous conjunctivitis, right eye

H10.222   Pseudomembranous conjunctivitis, left eye

EXCLUDES 1 Not coded here   *EXCLUDES 2* Not included here   N Newborn Age: 0   P Pediatric Age: 0-17   M Maternity Age: 12-55   A Adult Age: 15-124

534   ICD-10-CM 2014 (Draft)

H10.223　Pseudomembranous conjunctivitis, bilateral
H10.229　Pseudomembranous conjunctivitis, unspecified eye

√6th H10.23　Serous conjunctivitis, except viral
　　EXCLUDES 1　viral conjunctivitis (B30.-)
H10.231　Serous conjunctivitis, except viral, right eye
H10.232　Serous conjunctivitis, except viral, left eye
H10.233　Serous conjunctivitis, except viral, bilateral
H10.239　Serous conjunctivitis, except viral, unspecified eye

√5th H10.3　Unspecified acute conjunctivitis
　　EXCLUDES 1　ophthalmia neonatorum NOS (P39.1)
H10.30　Unspecified acute conjunctivitis, unspecified eye
H10.31　Unspecified acute conjunctivitis, right eye
H10.32　Unspecified acute conjunctivitis, left eye
H10.33　Unspecified acute conjunctivitis, bilateral

√5th H10.4　Chronic conjunctivitis
√6th H10.40　Unspecified chronic conjunctivitis
H10.401　Unspecified chronic conjunctivitis, right eye
H10.402　Unspecified chronic conjunctivitis, left eye
H10.403　Unspecified chronic conjunctivitis, bilateral
H10.409　Unspecified chronic conjunctivitis, unspecified eye

√6th H10.41　Chronic giant papillary conjunctivitis
H10.411　Chronic giant papillary conjunctivitis, right eye
H10.412　Chronic giant papillary conjunctivitis, left eye
H10.413　Chronic giant papillary conjunctivitis, bilateral
H10.419　Chronic giant papillary conjunctivitis, unspecified eye

√6th H10.42　Simple chronic conjunctivitis
H10.421　Simple chronic conjunctivitis, right eye
H10.422　Simple chronic conjunctivitis, left eye
H10.423　Simple chronic conjunctivitis, bilateral
H10.429　Simple chronic conjunctivitis, unspecified eye

√6th H10.43　Chronic follicular conjunctivitis
H10.431　Chronic follicular conjunctivitis, right eye
H10.432　Chronic follicular conjunctivitis, left eye
H10.433　Chronic follicular conjunctivitis, bilateral
H10.439　Chronic follicular conjunctivitis, unspecified eye

H10.44　Vernal conjunctivitis
　　EXCLUDES 1　vernal keratoconjunctivitis with limbar and corneal involvement (H16.26-)

H10.45　Other chronic allergic conjunctivitis

√5th H10.5　Blepharoconjunctivitis
√6th H10.50　Unspecified blepharoconjunctivitis
H10.501　Unspecified blepharoconjunctivitis, right eye
H10.502　Unspecified blepharoconjunctivitis, left eye
H10.503　Unspecified blepharoconjunctivitis, bilateral
H10.509　Unspecified blepharoconjunctivitis, unspecified eye

√6th H10.51　Ligneous conjunctivitis
H10.511　Ligneous conjunctivitis, right eye
H10.512　Ligneous conjunctivitis, left eye
H10.513　Ligneous conjunctivitis, bilateral
H10.519　Ligneous conjunctivitis, unspecified eye

√6th H10.52　Angular blepharoconjunctivitis
H10.521　Angular blepharoconjunctivitis, right eye
H10.522　Angular blepharoconjunctivitis, left eye
H10.523　Angular blepharoconjunctivitis, bilateral
H10.529　Angular blepharoconjunctivitis, unspecified eye

√6th H10.53　Contact blepharoconjunctivitis
H10.531　Contact blepharoconjunctivitis, right eye
H10.532　Contact blepharoconjunctivitis, left eye
H10.533　Contact blepharoconjunctivitis, bilateral
H10.539　Contact blepharoconjunctivitis, unspecified eye

√5th H10.8　Other conjunctivitis
√6th H10.81　Pingueculitis
　　EXCLUDES 1　pinguecula (H11.15-)
H10.811　Pingueculitis, right eye
H10.812　Pingueculitis, left eye
H10.813　Pingueculitis, bilateral
H10.819　Pingueculitis, unspecified eye

H10.89　Other conjunctivitis

H10.9　Unspecified conjunctivitis

√4th H11　Other disorders of conjunctiva
　　EXCLUDES 1　keratoconjunctivitis (H16.2-)

√5th H11.0　Pterygium of eye
　　EXCLUDES 1　pseudopterygium (H11.81-)
√6th H11.00　Unspecified pterygium of eye
H11.001　Unspecified pterygium of right eye
H11.002　Unspecified pterygium of left eye
H11.003　Unspecified pterygium of eye, bilateral
H11.009　Unspecified pterygium of unspecified eye

√6th H11.01　Amyloid pterygium
H11.011　Amyloid pterygium of right eye
H11.012　Amyloid pterygium of left eye
H11.013　Amyloid pterygium of eye, bilateral
H11.019　Amyloid pterygium of unspecified eye

√6th H11.02　Central pterygium of eye
H11.021　Central pterygium of right eye
H11.022　Central pterygium of left eye
H11.023　Central pterygium of eye, bilateral
H11.029　Central pterygium of unspecified eye

√6th H11.03　Double pterygium of eye
H11.031　Double pterygium of right eye
H11.032　Double pterygium of left eye
H11.033　Double pterygium of eye, bilateral
H11.039　Double pterygium of unspecified eye

√6th H11.04　Peripheral pterygium of eye, stationary
H11.041　Peripheral pterygium, stationary, right eye
H11.042　Peripheral pterygium, stationary, left eye
H11.043　Peripheral pterygium, stationary, bilateral
H11.049　Peripheral pterygium, stationary, unspecified eye

√6th H11.05　Peripheral pterygium of eye, progressive
H11.051　Peripheral pterygium, progressive, right eye
H11.052　Peripheral pterygium, progressive, left eye
H11.053　Peripheral pterygium, progressive, bilateral
H11.059　Peripheral pterygium, progressive, unspecified eye

√6th H11.06　Recurrent pterygium of eye
H11.061　Recurrent pterygium of right eye
H11.062　Recurrent pterygium of left eye
H11.063　Recurrent pterygium of eye, bilateral
H11.069　Recurrent pterygium of unspecified eye

√5th H11.1　Conjunctival degenerations and deposits
　　EXCLUDES 2　pseudopterygium (H11.81)
H11.10　Unspecified conjunctival degenerations
√6th H11.11　Conjunctival deposits
H11.111　Conjunctival deposits, right eye
H11.112　Conjunctival deposits, left eye
H11.113　Conjunctival deposits, bilateral
H11.119　Conjunctival deposits, unspecified eye

√6th H11.12　Conjunctival concretions
H11.121　Conjunctival concretions, right eye
H11.122　Conjunctival concretions, left eye
H11.123　Conjunctival concretions, bilateral

Diseases of the Eye and Adnexa

H11.129-H15.109

H11.129   Conjunctival concretions, unspecified eye

✓6th H11.13   Conjunctival pigmentations
Conjunctival argyrosis [argyria]
H11.131   Conjunctival pigmentations, right eye
H11.132   Conjunctival pigmentations, left eye
H11.133   Conjunctival pigmentations, bilateral
H11.139   Conjunctival pigmentations, unspecified eye

✓6th H11.14   Conjunctival xerosis, unspecified
EXCLUDES1   xerosis of conjunctiva due to vitamin A deficiency (E50.0, E50.1)
H11.141   Conjunctival xerosis, unspecified, right eye
H11.142   Conjunctival xerosis , unspecified, left eye
H11.143   Conjunctival xerosis, unspecified, bilateral
H11.149   Conjunctival xerosis, unspecified, unspecified eye

✓6th H11.15   Pinguecula
EXCLUDES1   pingueculitis (H10.81-)
H11.151   Pinguecula, right eye
H11.152   Pinguecula, left eye
H11.153   Pinguecula, bilateral
H11.159   Pinguecula, unspecified eye

✓5th H11.2   Conjunctival scars
✓6th H11.21   Conjunctival adhesions and strands (localized)
H11.211   Conjunctival adhesions and strands (localized), right eye
H11.212   Conjunctival adhesions and strands (localized), left eye
H11.213   Conjunctival adhesions and strands (localized), bilateral
H11.219   Conjunctival adhesions and strands (localized), unspecified eye

✓6th H11.22   Conjunctival granuloma
H11.221   Conjunctival granuloma, right eye
H11.222   Conjunctival granuloma, left eye
H11.223   Conjunctival granuloma, bilateral
H11.229   Conjunctival granuloma, unspecified

✓6th H11.23   Symblepharon
H11.231   Symblepharon, right eye
H11.232   Symblepharon, left eye
H11.233   Symblepharon, bilateral
H11.239   Symblepharon, unspecified eye

✓6th H11.24   Scarring of conjunctiva
H11.241   Scarring of conjunctiva, right eye
H11.242   Scarring of conjunctiva, left eye
H11.243   Scarring of conjunctiva, bilateral
H11.249   Scarring of conjunctiva, unspecified eye

✓5th H11.3   Conjunctival hemorrhage
Subconjunctival hemorrhage
H11.30   Conjunctival hemorrhage, unspecified eye
H11.31   Conjunctival hemorrhage, right eye
H11.32   Conjunctival hemorrhage, left eye
H11.33   Conjunctival hemorrhage, bilateral

✓5th H11.4   Other conjunctival vascular disorders and cysts
✓6th H11.41   Vascular abnormalities of conjunctiva
Conjunctival aneurysm
H11.411   Vascular abnormalities of conjunctiva, right eye
H11.412   Vascular abnormalities of conjunctiva, left eye
H11.413   Vascular abnormalities of conjunctiva, bilateral
H11.419   Vascular abnormalities of conjunctiva, unspecified eye

✓6th H11.42   Conjunctival edema
H11.421   Conjunctival edema, right eye
H11.422   Conjunctival edema, left eye
H11.423   Conjunctival edema, bilateral
H11.429   Conjunctival edema, unspecified eye

✓6th H11.43   Conjunctival hyperemia
H11.431   Conjunctival hyperemia, right eye
H11.432   Conjunctival hyperemia, left eye
H11.433   Conjunctival hyperemia, bilateral

H11.439   Conjunctival hyperemia, unspecified eye

✓6th H11.44   Conjunctival cysts
H11.441   Conjunctival cysts, right eye
H11.442   Conjunctival cysts, left eye
H11.443   Conjunctival cysts, bilateral
H11.449   Conjunctival cysts, unspecified eye

✓5th H11.8   Other specified disorders of conjunctiva
✓6th H11.81   Pseudopterygium of conjunctiva
H11.811   Pseudopterygium of conjunctiva, right eye
H11.812   Pseudopterygium of conjunctiva, left eye
H11.813   Pseudopterygium of conjunctiva, bilateral
H11.819   Pseudopterygium of conjunctiva, unspecified eye

✓6th H11.82   Conjunctivochalasis
H11.821   Conjunctivochalasis, right eye
H11.822   Conjunctivochalasis, left eye
H11.823   Conjunctivochalasis, bilateral
H11.829   Conjunctivochalasis, unspecified eye
H11.89   Other specified disorders of conjunctiva
H11.9   Unspecified disorder of conjunctiva

Disorders of sclera, cornea, iris and ciliary body (H15-H22)

✓4th H15   Disorders of sclera
✓5th H15.0   Scleritis
✓6th H15.00   Unspecified scleritis
H15.001   Unspecified scleritis, right eye
H15.002   Unspecified scleritis, left eye
H15.003   Unspecified scleritis, bilateral
H15.009   Unspecified scleritis, unspecified eye

✓6th H15.01   Anterior scleritis
H15.011   Anterior scleritis, right eye
H15.012   Anterior scleritis, left eye
H15.013   Anterior scleritis, bilateral
H15.019   Anterior scleritis, unspecified eye

✓6th H15.02   Brawny scleritis
H15.021   Brawny scleritis, right eye
H15.022   Brawny scleritis, left eye
H15.023   Brawny scleritis, bilateral
H15.029   Brawny scleritis, unspecified eye

✓6th H15.03   Posterior scleritis
Sclerotenonitis
H15.031   Posterior scleritis, right eye
H15.032   Posterior scleritis, left eye
H15.033   Posterior scleritis, bilateral
H15.039   Posterior scleritis, unspecified eye

✓6th H15.04   Scleritis with corneal involvement
H15.041   Scleritis with corneal involvement, right eye
H15.042   Scleritis with corneal involvement, left eye
H15.043   Scleritis with corneal involvement, bilateral
H15.049   Scleritis with corneal involvement, unspecified eye

✓6th H15.05   Scleromalacia perforans
H15.051   Scleromalacia perforans, right eye
H15.052   Scleromalacia perforans, left eye
H15.053   Scleromalacia perforans, bilateral
H15.059   Scleromalacia perforans, unspecified eye

✓6th H15.09   Other scleritis
Scleral abscess
H15.091   Other scleritis, right eye
H15.092   Other scleritis, left eye
H15.093   Other scleritis, bilateral
H15.099   Other scleritis, unspecified eye

✓5th H15.1   Episcleritis
✓6th H15.10   Unspecified episcleritis
H15.101   Unspecified episcleritis, right eye
H15.102   Unspecified episcleritis, left eye
H15.103   Unspecified episcleritis, bilateral
H15.109   Unspecified episcleritis, unspecified eye

☑6th **H15.11 Episcleritis** periodica fugax
- **H15.111 Episcleritis periodica fugax, right** eye
- **H15.112 Episcleritis periodica fugax, left** eye
- **H15.113 Episcleritis periodica fugax, bilateral**
- **H15.119 Episcleritis periodica fugax, unspecified eye**

☑6th **H15.12 Nodular** episcleritis
- **H15.121 Nodular episcleritis, right** eye
- **H15.122 Nodular episcleritis, left** eye
- **H15.123 Nodular episcleritis, bilateral**
- **H15.129 Nodular episcleritis, unspecified eye**

☑5th **H15.8 Other disorders of sclera**

EXCLUDES 2 *blue sclera (Q13.5)*
degenerative myopia (H44.2-)

☑6th **H15.81 Equatorial** staphyloma
- **H15.811 Equatorial staphyloma, right** eye
- **H15.812 Equatorial staphyloma, left** eye
- **H15.813 Equatorial staphyloma, bilateral**
- **H15.819 Equatorial staphyloma, unspecified eye**

☑6th **H15.82 Localized anterior** staphyloma
- **H15.821 Localized anterior staphyloma, right** eye
- **H15.822 Localized anterior staphyloma, left** eye
- **H15.823 Localized anterior staphyloma, bilateral**
- **H15.829 Localized anterior staphyloma, unspecified eye**

☑6th **H15.83 Staphyloma posticum**
- **H15.831 Staphyloma posticum, right** eye
- **H15.832 Staphyloma posticum, left** eye
- **H15.833 Staphyloma posticum, bilateral**
- **H15.839 Staphyloma posticum, unspecified eye**

☑6th **H15.84 Scleral** ectasia
- **H15.841 Scleral ectasia, right** eye
- **H15.842 Scleral ectasia, left** eye
- **H15.843 Scleral ectasia, bilateral**
- **H15.849 Scleral ectasia, unspecified eye**

☑6th **H15.85 Ring** staphyloma
- **H15.851 Ring staphyloma, right** eye
- **H15.852 Ring staphyloma, left** eye
- **H15.853 Ring staphyloma, bilateral**
- **H15.859 Ring staphyloma, unspecified eye**

H15.89 Other disorders of sclera

H15.9 Unspecified disorder of sclera

☑4th **H16 Keratitis**

☑5th **H16.0 Corneal ulcer**

☑6th **H16.00 Unspecified corneal ulcer**
- **H16.001 Unspecified corneal ulcer, right** eye
- **H16.002 Unspecified corneal ulcer, left** eye
- **H16.003 Unspecified corneal ulcer, bilateral**
- **H16.009 Unspecified corneal ulcer, unspecified eye**

☑6th **H16.01 Central** corneal ulcer
- **H16.011 Central corneal ulcer, right** eye
- **H16.012 Central corneal ulcer, left** eye
- **H16.013 Central corneal ulcer, bilateral**
- **H16.019 Central corneal ulcer, unspecified eye**

☑6th **H16.02 Ring** corneal ulcer
- **H16.021 Ring corneal ulcer, right** eye
- **H16.022 Ring corneal ulcer, left** eye
- **H16.023 Ring corneal ulcer, bilateral**
- **H16.029 Ring corneal ulcer, unspecified eye**

☑6th **H16.03 Corneal ulcer** with hypopyon
- **H16.031 Corneal ulcer with hypopyon, right** eye
- **H16.032 Corneal ulcer with hypopyon, left** eye
- **H16.033 Corneal ulcer with hypopyon, bilateral**
- **H16.039 Corneal ulcer with hypopyon, unspecified eye**

☑6th **H16.04 Marginal** corneal ulcer
- **H16.041 Marginal corneal ulcer, right** eye
- **H16.042 Marginal corneal ulcer, left** eye
- **H16.043 Marginal corneal ulcer, bilateral**
- **H16.049 Marginal corneal ulcer, unspecified eye**

☑6th **H16.05 Mooren's** corneal ulcer
- **H16.051 Mooren's corneal ulcer, right** eye
- **H16.052 Mooren's corneal ulcer, left** eye
- **H16.053 Mooren's corneal ulcer, bilateral**
- **H16.059 Mooren's corneal ulcer, unspecified eye**

☑6th **H16.06 Mycotic** corneal ulcer
- **H16.061 Mycotic corneal ulcer, right** eye
- **H16.062 Mycotic corneal ulcer, left** eye
- **H16.063 Mycotic corneal ulcer, bilateral**
- **H16.069 Mycotic corneal ulcer, unspecified eye**

☑6th **H16.07 Perforated** corneal ulcer
- **H16.071 Perforated corneal ulcer, right** eye
- **H16.072 Perforated corneal ulcer, left** eye
- **H16.073 Perforated corneal ulcer, bilateral**
- **H16.079 Perforated corneal ulcer, unspecified eye**

☑5th **H16.1 Other and unspecified superficial keratitis without conjunctivitis**

☑6th **H16.10 Unspecified superficial keratitis**
- **H16.101 Unspecified superficial keratitis, right** eye
- **H16.102 Unspecified superficial keratitis, left** eye
- **H16.103 Unspecified superficial keratitis, bilateral**
- **H16.109 Unspecified superficial keratitis, unspecified eye**

☑6th **H16.11 Macular** keratitis
Areolar keratitis
Nummular keratitis
Stellate keratitis
Striate keratitis
- **H16.111 Macular keratitis, right** eye
- **H16.112 Macular keratitis, left** eye
- **H16.113 Macular keratitis, bilateral**
- **H16.119 Macular keratitis, unspecified eye**

☑6th **H16.12 Filamentary** keratitis
- **H16.121 Filamentary keratitis, right** eye
- **H16.122 Filamentary keratitis, left** eye
- **H16.123 Filamentary keratitis, bilateral**
- **H16.129 Filamentary keratitis, unspecified eye**

☑6th **H16.13 Photokeratitis**
Snow blindness
Welders keratitis
- **H16.131 Photokeratitis, right** eye
- **H16.132 Photokeratitis, left** eye
- **H16.133 Photokeratitis, bilateral**
- **H16.139 Photokeratitis, unspecified eye**

☑6th **H16.14 Punctate** keratitis
- **H16.141 Punctate keratitis, right** eye
- **H16.142 Punctate keratitis, left** eye
- **H16.143 Punctate keratitis, bilateral**
- **H16.149 Punctate keratitis, unspecified eye**

☑5th **H16.2 Keratoconjunctivitis**

☑6th **H16.20 Unspecified keratoconjunctivitis**
Superficial keratitis with conjunctivitis NOS
- **H16.201 Unspecified keratoconjunctivitis, right** eye
- **H16.202 Unspecified keratoconjunctivitis, left** eye
- **H16.203 Unspecified keratoconjunctivitis, bilateral**
- **H16.209 Unspecified keratoconjunctivitis, unspecified eye**

☑6th **H16.21 Exposure** keratoconjunctivitis
- **H16.211 Exposure keratoconjunctivitis, right** eye
- **H16.212 Exposure keratoconjunctivitis, left** eye
- **H16.213 Exposure keratoconjunctivitis, bilateral**
- **H16.219 Exposure keratoconjunctivitis, unspecified eye**

☑6th **H16.22 Keratoconjunctivitis sicca, not specified as Sjögren's**

EXCLUDES 1 *Sjögren's syndrome (M35.01)*
- **H16.221 Keratoconjunctivitis sicca, not specified as Sjögren's, right** eye
- **H16.222 Keratoconjunctivitis sicca, not specified as Sjögren's, left** eye
- **H16.223 Keratoconjunctivitis sicca, not specified as Sjögren's, bilateral**
- **H16.229 Keratoconjunctivitis sicca, not specified as Sjögren's, unspecified eye**

☑ Additional Character Required   v x7th *Xtension Alert*   Unspecified Code   Other Specified Code   Manifestation Code   ►◄ Revised Text   ● New Code   ▲ Revised Code Title

√6th **H16.23 Neurotrophic keratoconjunctivitis**
- H16.231 Neurotrophic keratoconjunctivitis, right eye
- H16.232 Neurotrophic keratoconjunctivitis, left eye
- H16.233 Neurotrophic keratoconjunctivitis, bilateral
- H16.239 Neurotrophic keratoconjunctivitis, unspecified eye

√6th **H16.24 Ophthalmia nodosa**
- H16.241 Ophthalmia nodosa, right eye
- H16.242 Ophthalmia nodosa, left eye
- H16.243 Ophthalmia nodosa, bilateral
- H16.249 Ophthalmia nodosa, unspecified eye

√6th **H16.25 Phlyctenular keratoconjunctivitis**
- H16.251 Phlyctenular keratoconjunctivitis, right eye
- H16.252 Phlyctenular keratoconjunctivitis, left eye
- H16.253 Phlyctenular keratoconjunctivitis, bilateral
- H16.259 Phlyctenular keratoconjunctivitis, unspecified eye

√6th **H16.26 Vernal keratoconjunctivitis, with limbar and corneal involvement**
> EXCLUDES1 vernal conjunctivitis without limbar and corneal involvement (H10.44)
- H16.261 Vernal keratoconjunctivitis, with limbar and corneal involvement, right eye
- H16.262 Vernal keratoconjunctivitis, with limbar and corneal involvement, left eye
- H16.263 Vernal keratoconjunctivitis, with limbar and corneal involvement, bilateral
- H16.269 Vernal keratoconjunctivitis, with limbar and corneal involvement, unspecified eye

√6th **H16.29 Other keratoconjunctivitis**
- H16.291 Other keratoconjunctivitis, right eye
- H16.292 Other keratoconjunctivitis, left eye
- H16.293 Other keratoconjunctivitis, bilateral
- H16.299 Other keratoconjunctivitis, unspecified eye

√5th **H16.3 Interstitial and deep keratitis**

√6th **H16.30 Unspecified interstitial keratitis**
- H16.301 Unspecified interstitial keratitis, right eye
- H16.302 Unspecified interstitial keratitis, left eye
- H16.303 Unspecified interstitial keratitis, bilateral
- H16.309 Unspecified interstitial keratitis, unspecified eye

√6th **H16.31 Corneal abscess**
- H16.311 Corneal abscess, right eye
- H16.312 Corneal abscess, left eye
- H16.313 Corneal abscess, bilateral
- H16.319 Corneal abscess, unspecified eye

√6th **H16.32 Diffuse interstitial keratitis**
Cogan's syndrome
- H16.321 Diffuse interstitial keratitis, right eye
- H16.322 Diffuse interstitial keratitis, left eye
- H16.323 Diffuse interstitial keratitis, bilateral
- H16.329 Diffuse interstitial keratitis, unspecified eye

√6th **H16.33 Sclerosing keratitis**
- H16.331 Sclerosing keratitis, right eye
- H16.332 Sclerosing keratitis, left eye
- H16.333 Sclerosing keratitis, bilateral
- H16.339 Sclerosing keratitis, unspecified eye

√6th **H16.39 Other interstitial and deep keratitis**
- H16.391 Other interstitial and deep keratitis, right eye
- H16.392 Other interstitial and deep keratitis, left eye
- H16.393 Other interstitial and deep keratitis, bilateral
- H16.399 Other interstitial and deep keratitis, unspecified eye

√5th **H16.4 Corneal neovascularization**

√6th **H16.40 Unspecified corneal neovascularization**
- H16.401 Unspecified corneal neovascularization, right eye
- H16.402 Unspecified corneal neovascularization, left eye
- H16.403 Unspecified corneal neovascularization, bilateral
- H16.409 Unspecified corneal neovascularization, unspecified eye

√6th **H16.41 Ghost vessels (corneal)**
- H16.411 Ghost vessels (corneal), right eye
- H16.412 Ghost vessels (corneal), left eye
- H16.413 Ghost vessels (corneal), bilateral
- H16.419 Ghost vessels (corneal), unspecified eye

√6th **H16.42 Pannus (corneal)**
- H16.421 Pannus (corneal), right eye
- H16.422 Pannus (corneal), left eye
- H16.423 Pannus (corneal), bilateral
- H16.429 Pannus (corneal), unspecified eye

√6th **H16.43 Localized vascularization of cornea**
- H16.431 Localized vascularization of cornea, right eye
- H16.432 Localized vascularization of cornea, left eye
- H16.433 Localized vascularization of cornea, bilateral
- H16.439 Localized vascularization of cornea, unspecified eye

√6th **H16.44 Deep vascularization of cornea**
- H16.441 Deep vascularization of cornea, right eye
- H16.442 Deep vascularization of cornea, left eye
- H16.443 Deep vascularization of cornea, bilateral
- H16.449 Deep vascularization of cornea, unspecified eye

H16.8 Other keratitis

H16.9 Unspecified keratitis

√4th **H17 Corneal scars and opacities**

√5th **H17.0 Adherent leukoma**
- H17.00 Adherent leukoma, unspecified eye
- H17.01 Adherent leukoma, right eye
- H17.02 Adherent leukoma, left eye
- H17.03 Adherent leukoma, bilateral

√5th **H17.1 Central corneal opacity**
- H17.10 Central corneal opacity, unspecified eye
- H17.11 Central corneal opacity, right eye
- H17.12 Central corneal opacity, left eye
- H17.13 Central corneal opacity, bilateral

√5th **H17.8 Other corneal scars and opacities**

√6th **H17.81 Minor opacity of cornea**
Corneal nebula
- H17.811 Minor opacity of cornea, right eye
- H17.812 Minor opacity of cornea, left eye
- H17.813 Minor opacity of cornea, bilateral
- H17.819 Minor opacity of cornea, unspecified eye

√6th **H17.82 Peripheral opacity of cornea**
- H17.821 Peripheral opacity of cornea, right eye
- H17.822 Peripheral opacity of cornea, left eye
- H17.823 Peripheral opacity of cornea, bilateral
- H17.829 Peripheral opacity of cornea, unspecified eye

- H17.89 Other corneal scars and opacities

H17.9 Unspecified corneal scar and opacity

√4th **H18 Other disorders of cornea**

√5th **H18.0 Corneal pigmentations and deposits**

√6th **H18.00 Unspecified corneal deposit**
- H18.001 Unspecified corneal deposit, right eye
- H18.002 Unspecified corneal deposit, left eye
- H18.003 Unspecified corneal deposit, bilateral
- H18.009 Unspecified corneal deposit, unspecified eye

EXCLUDES1 Not coded here   EXCLUDES2 Not included here   N Newborn Age: 0   P Pediatric Age: 0-17   M Maternity Age: 12-55   A Adult Age: 15-124

538   ICD-10-CM 2014 (Draft)

✓6th **H18.01　Anterior corneal pigmentations**
　　　　　Staehli's line
　　　H18.011　Anterior corneal pigmentations, right eye
　　　H18.012　Anterior corneal pigmentations, left eye
　　　H18.013　Anterior corneal pigmentations, bilateral
　　　H18.019　Anterior corneal pigmentations, unspecified eye

✓6th **H18.02　Argentous corneal deposits**
　　　H18.021　Argentous corneal deposits, right eye
　　　H18.022　Argentous corneal deposits, left eye
　　　H18.023　Argentous corneal deposits, bilateral
　　　H18.029　Argentous corneal deposits, unspecified eye

✓6th **H18.03　Corneal deposits in metabolic disorders**
　　　　　Code also associated metabolic disorder
　　　H18.031　Corneal deposits in metabolic disorders, right eye
　　　H18.032　Corneal deposits in metabolic disorders, left eye
　　　H18.033　Corneal deposits in metabolic disorders, bilateral
　　　H18.039　Corneal deposits in metabolic disorders, unspecified eye

✓6th **H18.04　Kayser-Fleischer ring**
　　　　　Code also associated Wilson's disease (E83.01)
　　　H18.041　Kayser-Fleischer ring, right eye
　　　H18.042　Kayser-Fleischer ring, left eye
　　　H18.043　Kayser-Fleischer ring, bilateral
　　　H18.049　Kayser-Fleischer ring, unspecified eye

✓6th **H18.05　Posterior corneal pigmentations**
　　　　　Krukenberg's spindle
　　　H18.051　Posterior corneal pigmentations, right eye
　　　H18.052　Posterior corneal pigmentations, left eye
　　　H18.053　Posterior corneal pigmentations, bilateral
　　　H18.059　Posterior corneal pigmentations, unspecified eye

✓6th **H18.06　Stromal corneal pigmentations**
　　　　　Hematocornea
　　　H18.061　Stromal corneal pigmentations, right eye
　　　H18.062　Stromal corneal pigmentations, left eye
　　　H18.063　Stromal corneal pigmentations, bilateral
　　　H18.069　Stromal corneal pigmentations, unspecified eye

✓5th **H18.1　Bullous keratopathy**
　　　H18.10　Bullous keratopathy, unspecified eye
　　　H18.11　Bullous keratopathy, right eye
　　　H18.12　Bullous keratopathy, left eye
　　　H18.13　Bullous keratopathy, bilateral

✓5th **H18.2　Other and unspecified corneal edema**
　　　H18.20　Unspecified corneal edema

✓6th **H18.21　Corneal edema secondary to contact lens**
　　　　　EXCLUDES 2　*other corneal disorders due to contact lens (H18.82-)*
　　　H18.211　Corneal edema secondary to contact lens, right eye
　　　H18.212　Corneal edema secondary to contact lens, left eye
　　　H18.213　Corneal edema secondary to contact lens, bilateral
　　　H18.219　Corneal edema secondary to contact lens, unspecified eye

✓6th **H18.22　Idiopathic corneal edema**
　　　H18.221　Idiopathic corneal edema, right eye
　　　H18.222　Idiopathic corneal edema, left eye
　　　H18.223　Idiopathic corneal edema, bilateral
　　　H18.229　Idiopathic corneal edema, unspecified eye

✓6th **H18.23　Secondary corneal edema**
　　　H18.231　Secondary corneal edema, right eye
　　　H18.232　Secondary corneal edema, left eye
　　　H18.233　Secondary corneal edema, bilateral
　　　H18.239　Secondary corneal edema, unspecified eye

✓5th **H18.3　Changes of corneal membranes**
　　　H18.30　Unspecified corneal membrane change

✓6th **H18.31　Folds and rupture in Bowman's membrane**
　　　H18.311　Folds and rupture in Bowman's membrane, right eye
　　　H18.312　Folds and rupture in Bowman's membrane, left eye
　　　H18.313　Folds and rupture in Bowman's membrane, bilateral
　　　H18.319　Folds and rupture in Bowman's membrane, unspecified eye

✓6th **H18.32　Folds in Descemet's membrane**
　　　H18.321　Folds in Descemet's membrane, right eye
　　　H18.322　Folds in Descemet's membrane, left eye
　　　H18.323　Folds in Descemet's membrane, bilateral
　　　H18.329　Folds in Descemet's membrane, unspecified eye

✓6th **H18.33　Rupture in Descemet's membrane**
　　　H18.331　Rupture in Descemet's membrane, right eye
　　　H18.332　Rupture in Descemet's membrane, left eye
　　　H18.333　Rupture in Descemet's membrane, bilateral
　　　H18.339　Rupture in Descemet's membrane, unspecified eye

✓5th **H18.4　Corneal degeneration**
　　　　　EXCLUDES 1　*Mooren's ulcer (H16.0-)*
　　　　　　　　　　　recurrent erosion of cornea (H18.83-)
　　　H18.40　Unspecified corneal degeneration

✓6th **H18.41　Arcus senilis**
　　　　　Senile corneal changes
　　　H18.411　Arcus senilis, right eye
　　　H18.412　Arcus senilis, left eye
　　　H18.413　Arcus senilis, bilateral
　　　H18.419　Arcus senilis, unspecified eye

✓6th **H18.42　Band keratopathy**
　　　H18.421　Band keratopathy, right eye
　　　H18.422　Band keratopathy, left eye
　　　H18.423　Band keratopathy, bilateral
　　　H18.429　Band keratopathy, unspecified eye

　　　H18.43　Other calcerous corneal degeneration

✓6th **H18.44　Keratomalacia**
　　　　　EXCLUDES 1　*keratomalacia due to vitamin A deficiency (E50.4)*
　　　H18.441　Keratomalacia, right eye
　　　H18.442　Keratomalacia, left eye
　　　H18.443　Keratomalacia, bilateral
　　　H18.449　Keratomalacia, unspecified eye

✓6th **H18.45　Nodular corneal degeneration**
　　　H18.451　Nodular corneal degeneration, right eye
　　　H18.452　Nodular corneal degeneration, left eye
　　　H18.453　Nodular corneal degeneration, bilateral
　　　H18.459　Nodular corneal degeneration, unspecified eye

✓6th **H18.46　Peripheral corneal degeneration**
　　　H18.461　Peripheral corneal degeneration, right eye
　　　H18.462　Peripheral corneal degeneration, left eye
　　　H18.463　Peripheral corneal degeneration, bilateral
　　　H18.469　Peripheral corneal degeneration, unspecified eye

　　　H18.49　Other corneal degeneration

✓5th **H18.5　Hereditary corneal dystrophies**
　　　H18.50　Unspecified hereditary corneal dystrophies
　　　H18.51　Endothelial corneal dystrophy
　　　　　Fuchs' dystrophy
　　　H18.52　Epithelial (juvenile) corneal dystrophy
　　　H18.53　Granular corneal dystrophy
　　　H18.54　Lattice corneal dystrophy
　　　H18.55　Macular corneal dystrophy
　　　H18.59　Other hereditary corneal dystrophies

✓5th **H18.6　Keratoconus**
✓6th **H18.60　Keratoconus, unspecified**
　　　H18.601　Keratoconus, unspecified, right eye
　　　H18.602　Keratoconus, unspecified, left eye

H18.603   Keratoconus, unspecified, bilateral
H18.609   Keratoconus, unspecified, unspecified eye

✓6ᵗʰ H18.61   Keratoconus, stable
H18.611   Keratoconus, stable, right eye
H18.612   Keratoconus, stable, left eye
H18.613   Keratoconus, stable, bilateral
H18.619   Keratoconus, stable, unspecified eye

✓6ᵗʰ H18.62   Keratoconus, unstable
    Acute hydrops
H18.621   Keratoconus, unstable, right eye
H18.622   Keratoconus, unstable, left eye
H18.623   Keratoconus, unstable, bilateral
H18.629   Keratoconus, unstable, unspecified eye

✓5ᵗʰ H18.7   Other and unspecified corneal deformities
    EXCLUDES 1   congenital malformations of cornea (Q13.3-Q13.4)
H18.70   Unspecified corneal deformity

✓6ᵗʰ H18.71   Corneal ectasia
H18.711   Corneal ectasia, right eye
H18.712   Corneal ectasia, left eye
H18.713   Corneal ectasia, bilateral
H18.719   Corneal ectasia, unspecified eye

✓6ᵗʰ H18.72   Corneal staphyloma
H18.721   Corneal staphyloma, right eye
H18.722   Corneal staphyloma, left eye
H18.723   Corneal staphyloma, bilateral
H18.729   Corneal staphyloma, unspecified eye

✓6ᵗʰ H18.73   Descemetocele
H18.731   Descemetocele, right eye
H18.732   Descemetocele, left eye
H18.733   Descemetocele, bilateral
H18.739   Descemetocele, unspecified eye

✓6ᵗʰ H18.79   Other corneal deformities
H18.791   Other corneal deformities, right eye
H18.792   Other corneal deformities, left eye
H18.793   Other corneal deformities, bilateral
H18.799   Other corneal deformities, unspecified eye

✓5ᵗʰ H18.8   Other specified disorders of cornea
✓6ᵗʰ H18.81   Anesthesia and hypoesthesia of cornea
H18.811   Anesthesia and hypoesthesia of cornea, right eye
H18.812   Anesthesia and hypoesthesia of cornea, left eye
H18.813   Anesthesia and hypoesthesia of cornea, bilateral
H18.819   Anesthesia and hypoesthesia of cornea, unspecified eye

✓6ᵗʰ H18.82   Corneal disorder due to contact lens
    EXCLUDES 2   corneal edema due to contact lens (H18.21-)
H18.821   Corneal disorder due to contact lens, right eye
H18.822   Corneal disorder due to contact lens, left eye
H18.823   Corneal disorder due to contact lens, bilateral
H18.829   Corneal disorder due to contact lens, unspecified eye

✓6ᵗʰ H18.83   Recurrent erosion of cornea
H18.831   Recurrent erosion of cornea, right eye
H18.832   Recurrent erosion of cornea, left eye
H18.833   Recurrent erosion of cornea, bilateral
H18.839   Recurrent erosion of cornea, unspecified eye

✓6ᵗʰ H18.89   Other specified disorders of cornea
H18.891   Other specified disorders of cornea, right eye
H18.892   Other specified disorders of cornea, left eye
H18.893   Other specified disorders of cornea, bilateral
H18.899   Other specified disorders of cornea, unspecified eye

H18.9   Unspecified disorder of cornea

✓4ᵗʰ H20   Iridocyclitis
✓5ᵗʰ H20.0   Acute and subacute iridocyclitis
    Acute anterior uveitis
    Acute cyclitis
    Acute iritis
    Subacute anterior uveitis
    Subacute cyclitis
    Subacute iritis
    EXCLUDES 1   iridocyclitis, iritis, uveitis (due to) (in) diabetes mellitus (E08-E13 with .39)
        iridocyclitis, iritis, uveitis (due to) (in) diphtheria (A36.89)
        iridocyclitis, iritis, uveitis (due to) (in) gonococcal (A54.32)
        iridocyclitis, iritis, uveitis (due to) (in) herpes (simplex) (B00.51)
        iridocyclitis, iritis, uveitis (due to) (in) herpes zoster (B02.32)
        iridocyclitis, iritis, uveitis (due to) (in) late congenital syphilis (A50.39)
        iridocyclitis, iritis, uveitis (due to) (in) late syphilis (A52.71)
        iridocyclitis, iritis, uveitis (due to) (in) sarcoidosis (D86.83)
        iridocyclitis, iritis, uveitis (due to) (in) syphilis (A51.43)
        iridocyclitis, iritis, uveitis (due to) (in) toxoplasmosis (B58.09)
        iridocyclitis, iritis, uveitis (due to) (in) tuberculosis (A18.54)

H20.00   Unspecified acute and subacute iridocyclitis

✓6ᵗʰ H20.01   Primary iridocyclitis
H20.011   Primary iridocyclitis, right eye
H20.012   Primary iridocyclitis, left eye
H20.013   Primary iridocyclitis, bilateral
H20.019   Primary iridocyclitis, unspecified eye

✓6ᵗʰ H20.02   Recurrent acute iridocyclitis
H20.021   Recurrent acute iridocyclitis, right eye
H20.022   Recurrent acute iridocyclitis, left eye
H20.023   Recurrent acute iridocyclitis, bilateral
H20.029   Recurrent acute iridocyclitis, unspecified eye

✓6ᵗʰ H20.03   Secondary infectious iridocyclitis
H20.031   Secondary infectious iridocyclitis, right eye
H20.032   Secondary infectious iridocyclitis, left eye
H20.033   Secondary infectious iridocyclitis, bilateral
H20.039   Secondary infectious iridocyclitis, unspecified eye

✓6ᵗʰ H20.04   Secondary noninfectious iridocyclitis
H20.041   Secondary noninfectious iridocyclitis, right eye
H20.042   Secondary noninfectious iridocyclitis, left eye
H20.043   Secondary noninfectious iridocyclitis, bilateral
H20.049   Secondary noninfectious iridocyclitis, unspecified eye

✓6ᵗʰ H20.05   Hypopyon
H20.051   Hypopyon, right eye
H20.052   Hypopyon, left eye
H20.053   Hypopyon, bilateral
H20.059   Hypopyon, unspecified eye

✓5ᵗʰ H20.1   Chronic iridocyclitis
    Use additional code for any associated cataract (H26.21-)
    EXCLUDES 2   posterior cyclitis (H30.2-)
H20.10   Chronic iridocyclitis, unspecified eye
H20.11   Chronic iridocyclitis, right eye
H20.12   Chronic iridocyclitis, left eye
H20.13   Chronic iridocyclitis, bilateral

✓5ᵗʰ H20.2   Lens-induced iridocyclitis
H20.20   Lens-induced iridocyclitis, unspecified eye
H20.21   Lens-induced iridocyclitis, right eye
H20.22   Lens-induced iridocyclitis, left eye
H20.23   Lens-induced iridocyclitis, bilateral

EXCLUDES 1 Not coded here   EXCLUDES 2 Not included here   N Newborn Age: 0   P Pediatric Age: 0-17   M Maternity Age: 12-55   A Adult Age: 15-124

540   ICD-10-CM 2014 (Draft)

✓5ᵗʰ **H20.8**   **Other iridocyclitis**
    EXCLUDES 2   *glaucomatocyclitis crises (H40.4-)*
              posterior cyclitis (H30.2-)
              sympathetic uveitis (H44.13-)

    ✓6ᵗʰ **H20.81**   **Fuchs' heterochromic cyclitis**
        H20.811   **Fuchs' heterochromic cyclitis, right eye**
        H20.812   **Fuchs' heterochromic cyclitis, left eye**
        H20.813   **Fuchs' heterochromic cyclitis, bilateral**
        H20.819   **Fuchs' heterochromic cyclitis, unspecified eye**

    ✓6ᵗʰ **H20.82**   **Vogt-Koyanagi syndrome**
        H20.821   **Vogt-Koyanagi syndrome, right eye**
        H20.822   **Vogt-Koyanagi syndrome, left eye**
        H20.823   **Vogt-Koyanagi syndrome, bilateral**
        H20.829   **Vogt-Koyanagi syndrome, unspecified eye**

H20.9   **Unspecified iridocyclitis**
    Uveitis NOS

✓4ᵗʰ **H21**   **Other disorders of iris and ciliary body**
    EXCLUDES 2   *sympathetic uveitis (H44.1-)*

✓5ᵗʰ **H21.0**   **Hyphema**
    EXCLUDES 1   *traumatic hyphema (S05.1-)*

     H21.00   **Hyphema, unspecified eye**
     H21.01   **Hyphema, right eye**
     H21.02   **Hyphema, left eye**
     H21.03   **Hyphema, bilateral**

✓5ᵗʰ **H21.1**   **Other vascular disorders of iris and ciliary body**
    Neovascularization of iris or ciliary body
    Rubeosis iridis
    Rubeosis of iris

    ✓6ᵗʰ **H21.1X**   **Other vascular disorders of iris and ciliary body**
        H21.1X1   **Other vascular disorders of iris and ciliary body, right eye**
        H21.1X2   **Other vascular disorders of iris and ciliary body, left eye**
        H21.1X3   **Other vascular disorders of iris and ciliary body, bilateral**
        H21.1X9   **Other vascular disorders of iris and ciliary body, unspecified eye**

✓5ᵗʰ **H21.2**   **Degeneration of iris and ciliary body**

    ✓6ᵗʰ **H21.21**   **Degeneration of chamber angle**
        H21.211   **Degeneration of chamber angle, right eye**
        H21.212   **Degeneration of chamber angle, left eye**
        H21.213   **Degeneration of chamber angle, bilateral**
        H21.219   **Degeneration of chamber angle, unspecified eye**

    ✓6ᵗʰ **H21.22**   **Degeneration of ciliary body**
        H21.221   **Degeneration of ciliary body, right eye**
        H21.222   **Degeneration of ciliary body, left eye**
        H21.223   **Degeneration of ciliary body, bilateral**
        H21.229   **Degeneration of ciliary body, unspecified eye**

    ✓6ᵗʰ **H21.23**   **Degeneration of iris (pigmentary)**
        Translucency of iris
        H21.231   **Degeneration of iris (pigmentary), right eye**
        H21.232   **Degeneration of iris (pigmentary), left eye**
        H21.233   **Degeneration of iris (pigmentary), bilateral**
        H21.239   **Degeneration of iris (pigmentary), unspecified eye**

    ✓6ᵗʰ **H21.24**   **Degeneration of pupillary margin**
        H21.241   **Degeneration of pupillary margin, right eye**
        H21.242   **Degeneration of pupillary margin, left eye**
        H21.243   **Degeneration of pupillary margin, bilateral**
        H21.249   **Degeneration of pupillary margin, unspecified eye**

    ✓6ᵗʰ **H21.25**   **Iridoschisis**
        H21.251   **Iridoschisis, right eye**
        H21.252   **Iridoschisis, left eye**
        H21.253   **Iridoschisis, bilateral**
        H21.259   **Iridoschisis, unspecified eye**

    ✓6ᵗʰ **H21.26**   **Iris atrophy (essential) (progressive)**
        H21.261   **Iris atrophy (essential) (progressive), right eye**
        H21.262   **Iris atrophy (essential) (progressive), left eye**
        H21.263   **Iris atrophy (essential) (progressive), bilateral**
        H21.269   **Iris atrophy (essential) (progressive), unspecified eye**

    ✓6ᵗʰ **H21.27**   **Miotic pupillary cyst**
        H21.271   **Miotic pupillary cyst, right eye**
        H21.272   **Miotic pupillary cyst, left eye**
        H21.273   **Miotic pupillary cyst, bilateral**
        H21.279   **Miotic pupillary cyst, unspecified eye**

    H21.29   **Other iris atrophy**

✓5ᵗʰ **H21.3**   **Cyst of iris, ciliary body and anterior chamber**
    EXCLUDES 2   *miotic pupillary cyst (H21.27-)*

    ✓6ᵗʰ **H21.30**   **Idiopathic cysts of iris, ciliary body or anterior chamber**
        Cyst of iris, ciliary body or anterior chamber NOS
        H21.301   **Idiopathic cysts of iris, ciliary body or anterior chamber, right eye**
        H21.302   **Idiopathic cysts of iris, ciliary body or anterior chamber, left eye**
        H21.303   **Idiopathic cysts of iris, ciliary body or anterior chamber, bilateral**
        H21.309   **Idiopathic cysts of iris, ciliary body or anterior chamber, unspecified eye**

    ✓6ᵗʰ **H21.31**   **Exudative cysts of iris or anterior chamber**
        H21.311   **Exudative cysts of iris or anterior chamber, right eye**
        H21.312   **Exudative cysts of iris or anterior chamber, left eye**
        H21.313   **Exudative cysts of iris or anterior chamber, bilateral**
        H21.319   **Exudative cysts of iris or anterior chamber, unspecified eye**

    ✓6ᵗʰ **H21.32**   **Implantation cysts of iris, ciliary body or anterior chamber**
        H21.321   **Implantation cysts of iris, ciliary body or anterior chamber, right eye**
        H21.322   **Implantation cysts of iris, ciliary body or anterior chamber, left eye**
        H21.323   **Implantation cysts of iris, ciliary body or anterior chamber, bilateral**
        H21.329   **Implantation cysts of iris, ciliary body or anterior chamber, unspecified eye**

    ✓6ᵗʰ **H21.33**   **Parasitic cyst of iris, ciliary body or anterior chamber**
        H21.331   **Parasitic cyst of iris, ciliary body or anterior chamber, right eye**
        H21.332   **Parasitic cyst of iris, ciliary body or anterior chamber, left eye**
        H21.333   **Parasitic cyst of iris, ciliary body or anterior chamber, bilateral**
        H21.339   **Parasitic cyst of iris, ciliary body or anterior chamber, unspecified eye**

    ✓6ᵗʰ **H21.34**   **Primary cyst of pars plana**
        H21.341   **Primary cyst of pars plana, right eye**
        H21.342   **Primary cyst of pars plana, left eye**
        H21.343   **Primary cyst of pars plana, bilateral**
        H21.349   **Primary cyst of pars plana, unspecified eye**

    ✓6ᵗʰ **H21.35**   **Exudative cyst of pars plana**
        H21.351   **Exudative cyst of pars plana, right eye**
        H21.352   **Exudative cyst of pars plana, left eye**
        H21.353   **Exudative cyst of pars plana, bilateral**
        H21.359   **Exudative cyst of pars plana, unspecified eye**

✓5ᵗʰ **H21.4**   **Pupillary membranes**
    Iris bombé   Pupillary seclusion
    Pupillary occlusion
    EXCLUDES 1   *congenital pupillary membranes (Q13.8)*

     H21.40   **Pupillary membranes, unspecified eye**
     H21.41   **Pupillary membranes, right eye**
     H21.42   **Pupillary membranes, left eye**
     H21.43   **Pupillary membranes, bilateral**

✓ Additional Character Required   ✓x7ᵗʰ Xtension Alert   Unspecified Code   Other Specified Code   Manifestation Code   ▶◀ Revised Text   ● New Code   ▲ Revised Code Title

ICD-10-CM 2014 (Draft)   **541**

Diseases of the Eye and Adnexa

H21.5–H26.013

✓5th **H21.5 Other and unspecified adhesions and disruptions of iris and ciliary body**
EXCLUDES1 *corectopia (Q13.2)*

✓6th **H21.50 Unspecified adhesions of iris**
Synechia (iris) NOS
- H21.501 Unspecified adhesions of iris, right eye
- H21.502 Unspecified adhesions of iris, left eye
- H21.503 Unspecified adhesions of iris, bilateral
- H21.509 Unspecified adhesions of iris and ciliary body, unspecified eye

✓6th **H21.51 Anterior synechiae (iris)**
- H21.511 Anterior synechiae (iris), right eye
- H21.512 Anterior synechiae (iris), left eye
- H21.513 Anterior synechiae (iris), bilateral
- H21.519 Anterior synechiae (iris), unspecified eye

✓6th **H21.52 Goniosynechiae**
- H21.521 Goniosynechiae, right eye
- H21.522 Goniosynechiae, left eye
- H21.523 Goniosynechiae, bilateral
- H21.529 Goniosynechiae, unspecified eye

✓6th **H21.53 Iridodialysis**
- H21.531 Iridodialysis, right eye
- H21.532 Iridodialysis, left eye
- H21.533 Iridodialysis, bilateral
- H21.539 Iridodialysis, unspecified eye

✓6th **H21.54 Posterior synechiae (iris)**
- H21.541 Posterior synechiae (iris), right eye
- H21.542 Posterior synechiae (iris), left eye
- H21.543 Posterior synechiae (iris), bilateral
- H21.549 Posterior synechiae (iris), unspecified eye

✓6th **H21.55 Recession of chamber angle**
- H21.551 Recession of chamber angle, right eye
- H21.552 Recession of chamber angle, left eye
- H21.553 Recession of chamber angle, bilateral
- H21.559 Recession of chamber angle, unspecified eye

✓6th **H21.56 Pupillary abnormalities**
Deformed pupil
Ectopic pupil
Rupture of sphincter, pupil
EXCLUDES1 *congenital deformity of pupil (Q13.2-)*
- H21.561 Pupillary abnormality, right eye
- H21.562 Pupillary abnormality, left eye
- H21.563 Pupillary abnormality, bilateral
- H21.569 Pupillary abnormality, unspecified eye

✓5th **H21.8 Other specified disorders of iris and ciliary body**
H21.81 Floppy iris syndrome
Intraoperative floppy iris syndrome (IFIS)
Use additional code for adverse effect, if applicable, to identify drug (T36-T50 with fifth or sixth character 5)
H21.82 Plateau iris syndrome (post-iridectomy) (postprocedural)
H21.89 Other specified disorders of iris and ciliary body
H21.9 Unspecified disorder of iris and ciliary body

H22 Disorders of iris and ciliary body in diseases classified elsewhere
Code first underlying disease, such as:
gout (M1A.-, M10.-)
leprosy (A30.-)
parasitic disease (B89)

Disorders of lens (H25-H28)

✓4th **H25 Age-related cataract**
Senile cataract
EXCLUDES2 *capsular glaucoma with pseudoexfoliation of lens (H40.1-)*

✓5th **H25.0 Age-related incipient cataract**

✓6th **H25.01 Cortical age-related cataract**
- H25.011 Cortical age-related cataract, right eye A
- H25.012 Cortical age-related cataract, left eye A
- H25.013 Cortical age-related cataract, bilateral A
- H25.019 Cortical age-related cataract, unspecified eye A

✓6th **H25.03 Anterior subcapsular polar age-related cataract**
- H25.031 Anterior subcapsular polar age-related cataract, right eye A
- H25.032 Anterior subcapsular polar age-related cataract, left eye A
- H25.033 Anterior subcapsular polar age-related cataract, bilateral A
- H25.039 Anterior subcapsular polar age-related cataract, unspecified eye A

✓6th **H25.04 Posterior subcapsular polar age-related cataract**
- H25.041 Posterior subcapsular polar age-related cataract, right eye A
- H25.042 Posterior subcapsular polar age-related cataract, left eye A
- H25.043 Posterior subcapsular polar age-related cataract, bilateral A
- H25.049 Posterior subcapsular polar age-related cataract, unspecified eye A

✓6th **H25.09 Other age-related incipient cataract**
Coronary age-related cataract
Punctate age-related cataract
Water clefts
- H25.091 Other age-related incipient cataract, right eye A
- H25.092 Other age-related incipient cataract, left eye A
- H25.093 Other age-related incipient cataract, bilateral A
- H25.099 Other age-related incipient cataract, unspecified eye A

✓5th **H25.1 Age-related nuclear cataract**
Cataracta brunescens
Nuclear sclerosis cataract
- H25.10 Age-related nuclear cataract, unspecified eye A
- H25.11 Age-related nuclear cataract, right eye A
- H25.12 Age-related nuclear cataract, left eye A
- H25.13 Age-related nuclear cataract, bilateral A

✓5th **H25.2 Age-related cataract, morgagnian type**
Age-related hypermature cataract
- H25.20 Age-related cataract, morgagnian type, unspecified eye A
- H25.21 Age-related cataract, morgagnian type, right eye A
- H25.22 Age-related cataract, morgagnian type, left eye A
- H25.23 Age-related cataract, morgagnian type, bilateral A

✓5th **H25.8 Other age-related cataract**
✓6th **H25.81 Combined forms of age-related cataract**
- H25.811 Combined forms of age-related cataract, right eye A
- H25.812 Combined forms of age-related cataract, left eye A
- H25.813 Combined forms of age-related cataract, bilateral A
- H25.819 Combined forms of age-related cataract, unspecified eye A
H25.89 Other age-related cataract A
H25.9 Unspecified age-related cataract A

✓4th **H26 Other cataract**
EXCLUDES1 *congenital cataract (Q12.0)*

✓5th **H26.0 Infantile and juvenile cataract**
✓6th **H26.00 Unspecified infantile and juvenile cataract**
- H26.001 Unspecified infantile and juvenile cataract, right eye P
- H26.002 Unspecified infantile and juvenile cataract, left eye P
- H26.003 Unspecified infantile and juvenile cataract, bilateral P
- H26.009 Unspecified infantile and juvenile cataract, unspecified eye P

✓6th **H26.01 Infantile and juvenile cortical, lamellar, or zonular cataract**
- H26.011 Infantile and juvenile cortical, lamellar, or zonular cataract, right eye P
- H26.012 Infantile and juvenile cortical, lamellar, or zonular cataract, left eye P
- H26.013 Infantile and juvenile cortical, lamellar, or zonular cataract, bilateral P

EXCLUDES1 Not coded here   EXCLUDES2 Not included here   N Newborn Age: 0   P Pediatric Age: 0-17   M Maternity Age: 12-55   A Adult Age: 15-124

542   ICD-10-CM 2014 (Draft)

H26.019 Infantile and juvenile cortical, lamellar, ℙ
or zonular cataract, unspecified eye

✓6ᵗʰ H26.03 Infantile and juvenile nuclear cataract
H26.031 Infantile and juvenile nuclear cataract, ℙ
right eye
H26.032 Infantile and juvenile nuclear cataract, ℙ
left eye
H26.033 Infantile and juvenile nuclear cataract, ℙ
bilateral
H26.039 Infantile and juvenile nuclear cataract, ℙ
unspecified eye

✓6ᵗʰ H26.04 Anterior subcapsular polar infantile and juvenile
cataract
H26.041 Anterior subcapsular polar infantile ℙ
and juvenile cataract, right eye
H26.042 Anterior subcapsular polar infantile ℙ
and juvenile cataract, left eye
H26.043 Anterior subcapsular polar infantile ℙ
and juvenile cataract, bilateral
H26.049 Anterior subcapsular polar infantile
and juvenile cataract, unspecified eye

✓6ᵗʰ H26.05 Posterior subcapsular polar infantile and juvenile
cataract
H26.051 Posterior subcapsular polar infantile ℙ
and juvenile cataract, right eye
H26.052 Posterior subcapsular polar infantile ℙ
and juvenile cataract, left eye
H26.053 Posterior subcapsular polar infantile ℙ
and juvenile cataract, bilateral
H26.059 Posterior subcapsular polar infantile ℙ
and juvenile cataract, unspecified eye

✓6ᵗʰ H26.06 Combined forms of infantile and juvenile cataract
H26.061 Combined forms of infantile and ℙ
juvenile cataract, right eye
H26.062 Combined forms of infantile and ℙ
juvenile cataract, left eye
H26.063 Combined forms of infantile and ℙ
juvenile cataract, bilateral
H26.069 Combined forms of infantile and ℙ
juvenile cataract, unspecified eye

H26.09 Other infantile and juvenile cataract ℙ

✓5ᵗʰ H26.1 Traumatic cataract
Use additional code (Chapter 20) to identify external cause

✓6ᵗʰ H26.10 Unspecified traumatic cataract
H26.101 Unspecified traumatic cataract, right eye
H26.102 Unspecified traumatic cataract, left eye
H26.103 Unspecified traumatic cataract, bilateral
H26.109 Unspecified traumatic cataract,
unspecified eye

✓6ᵗʰ H26.11 Localized traumatic opacities
H26.111 Localized traumatic opacities, right eye
H26.112 Localized traumatic opacities, left eye
H26.113 Localized traumatic opacities, bilateral
H26.119 Localized traumatic opacities, unspecified
eye

✓6ᵗʰ H26.12 Partially resolved traumatic cataract
H26.121 Partially resolved traumatic cataract, right
eye
H26.122 Partially resolved traumatic cataract, left
eye
H26.123 Partially resolved traumatic cataract,
bilateral
H26.129 Partially resolved traumatic cataract,
unspecified eye

✓6ᵗʰ H26.13 Total traumatic cataract
H26.131 Total traumatic cataract, right eye
H26.132 Total traumatic cataract, left eye
H26.133 Total traumatic cataract, bilateral
H26.139 Total traumatic cataract, unspecified eye

✓5ᵗʰ H26.2 Complicated cataract
H26.20 Unspecified complicated cataract
Cataracta complicata NOS

✓6ᵗʰ H26.21 Cataract with neovascularization
Code also associated condition, such as:
chronic iridocyclitis (H20.1-)

H26.211 Cataract with neovascularization, right
eye
H26.212 Cataract with neovascularization, left eye
H26.213 Cataract with neovascularization, bilateral
H26.219 Cataract with neovascularization,
unspecified eye

✓6ᵗʰ H26.22 Cataract secondary to ocular disorders
(degenerative) (inflammatory)
Code also associated ocular disorder
H26.221 Cataract secondary to ocular disorders
(degenerative) (inflammatory), right eye
H26.222 Cataract secondary to ocular disorders
(degenerative) (inflammatory), left eye
H26.223 Cataract secondary to ocular disorders
(degenerative) (inflammatory), bilateral
H26.229 Cataract secondary to ocular disorders
(degenerative) (inflammatory),
unspecified eye

✓6ᵗʰ H26.23 Glaucomatous flecks (subcapsular)
Code first underlying glaucoma (H40-H42)
H26.231 Glaucomatous flecks (subcapsular), right
eye
H26.232 Glaucomatous flecks (subcapsular), left
eye
H26.233 Glaucomatous flecks (subcapsular),
bilateral
H26.239 Glaucomatous flecks (subcapsular),
unspecified eye

✓5ᵗʰ H26.3 Drug-induced cataract
Toxic cataract
Use additional code for adverse effect, if applicable, to identify
drug (T36-T50 with fifth or sixth character 5)
H26.30 Drug-induced cataract, unspecified eye
H26.31 Drug-induced cataract, right eye
H26.32 Drug-induced cataract, left eye
H26.33 Drug-induced cataract, bilateral

✓5ᵗʰ H26.4 Secondary cataract
H26.40 Unspecified secondary cataract
✓6ᵗʰ H26.41 Soemmering's ring
H26.411 Soemmering's ring, right eye
H26.412 Soemmering's ring, left eye
H26.413 Soemmering's ring, bilateral
H26.419 Soemmering's ring, unspecified eye
✓6ᵗʰ H26.49 Other secondary cataract
H26.491 Other secondary cataract, right eye
H26.492 Other secondary cataract, left eye
H26.493 Other secondary cataract, bilateral
H26.499 Other secondary cataract, unspecified eye

H26.8 Other specified cataract
H26.9 Unspecified cataract

✓4ᵗʰ H27 Other disorders of lens
EXCLUDES 1 congenital lens malformations (Q12.-)
mechanical complications of intraocular lens implant (T85.2)
pseudophakia (Z96.1)

✓5ᵗʰ H27.0 Aphakia
Acquired absence of lens
Acquired aphakia
Aphakia due to trauma
EXCLUDES 1 cataract extraction status (Z98.4-)
congenital absence of lens (Q12.3)
congenital aphakia (Q12.3)
H27.00 Aphakia, unspecified eye
H27.01 Aphakia, right eye
H27.02 Aphakia, left eye
H27.03 Aphakia, bilateral

✓5ᵗʰ H27.1 Dislocation of lens
H27.10 Unspecified dislocation of lens
✓6ᵗʰ H27.11 Subluxation of lens
H27.111 Subluxation of lens, right eye
H27.112 Subluxation of lens, left eye
H27.113 Subluxation of lens, bilateral
H27.119 Subluxation of lens, unspecified eye
✓6ᵗʰ H27.12 Anterior dislocation of lens
H27.121 Anterior dislocation of lens, right eye
H27.122 Anterior dislocation of lens, left eye

Diseases of the Eye and Adnexa

H27.123–H30.892

H27.123   Anterior dislocation of lens, bilateral
H27.129   Anterior dislocation of lens, unspecified eye

✓6ᵗʰ H27.13   Posterior dislocation of lens
H27.131   Posterior dislocation of lens, right eye
H27.132   Posterior dislocation of lens, left eye
H27.133   Posterior dislocation of lens, bilateral
H27.139   Posterior dislocation of lens, unspecified eye

H27.8   Other specified disorders of lens
H27.9   Unspecified disorder of lens

H28   *Cataract in diseases classified elsewhere*
Code first underlying disease, such as:
hypoparathyroidism (E20.-)
myotonia (G71.1-)
myxedema (E03.-)
protein-calorie malnutrition (E40-E46)
EXCLUDES 1   cataract in diabetes mellitus (E08.36, E09.36, E10.36, E11.36, E13.36)

Disorders of choroid and retina (H30-H36)

✓4ᵗʰ H30   Chorioretinal inflammation

✓5ᵗʰ H30.0   Focal chorioretinal inflammation
Focal chorioretinitis
Focal choroiditis
Focal retinitis
Focal retinochoroiditis

✓6ᵗʰ H30.00   Unspecified focal chorioretinal inflammation
Focal chorioretinitis NOS
Focal choroiditis NOS
Focal retinitis NOS
Focal retinochoroiditis NOS
H30.001   Unspecified focal chorioretinal inflammation, right eye
H30.002   Unspecified focal chorioretinal inflammation, left eye
H30.003   Unspecified focal chorioretinal inflammation, bilateral
H30.009   Unspecified focal chorioretinal inflammation, unspecified eye

✓6ᵗʰ H30.01   Focal chorioretinal inflammation, juxtapapillary
H30.011   Focal chorioretinal inflammation, juxtapapillary, right eye
H30.012   Focal chorioretinal inflammation, juxtapapillary, left eye
H30.013   Focal chorioretinal inflammation, juxtapapillary, bilateral
H30.019   Focal chorioretinal inflammation, juxtapapillary, unspecified eye

✓6ᵗʰ H30.02   Focal chorioretinal inflammation of posterior pole
H30.021   Focal chorioretinal inflammation of posterior pole, right eye
H30.022   Focal chorioretinal inflammation of posterior pole, left eye
H30.023   Focal chorioretinal inflammation of posterior pole, bilateral
H30.029   Focal chorioretinal inflammation of posterior pole, unspecified eye

✓6ᵗʰ H30.03   Focal chorioretinal inflammation, peripheral
H30.031   Focal chorioretinal inflammation, peripheral, right eye
H30.032   Focal chorioretinal inflammation, peripheral, left eye
H30.033   Focal chorioretinal inflammation, peripheral, bilateral
H30.039   Focal chorioretinal inflammation, peripheral, unspecified eye

✓6ᵗʰ H30.04   Focal chorioretinal inflammation, macular or paramacular
H30.041   Focal chorioretinal inflammation, macular or paramacular, right eye
H30.042   Focal chorioretinal inflammation, macular or paramacular, left eye
H30.043   Focal chorioretinal inflammation, macular or paramacular, bilateral
H30.049   Focal chorioretinal inflammation, macular or paramacular, unspecified eye

✓5ᵗʰ H30.1   Disseminated chorioretinal inflammation
Disseminated chorioretinitis
Disseminated choroiditis
Disseminated retinitis
Disseminated retinochoroiditis
EXCLUDES 2   exudative retinopathy (H35.02-)

✓6ᵗʰ H30.10   Unspecified disseminated chorioretinal inflammation
Disseminated chorioretinitis NOS
Disseminated choroiditis NOS
Disseminated retinitis NOS
Disseminated retinochoroiditis NOS
H30.101   Unspecified disseminated chorioretinal inflammation, right eye
H30.102   Unspecified disseminated chorioretinal inflammation, left eye
H30.103   Unspecified disseminated chorioretinal inflammation, bilateral
H30.109   Unspecified disseminated chorioretinal inflammation, unspecified eye

✓6ᵗʰ H30.11   Disseminated chorioretinal inflammation of posterior pole
H30.111   Disseminated chorioretinal inflammation of posterior pole, right eye
H30.112   Disseminated chorioretinal inflammation of posterior pole, left eye
H30.113   Disseminated chorioretinal inflammation of posterior pole, bilateral
H30.119   Disseminated chorioretinal inflammation of posterior pole, unspecified eye

✓6ᵗʰ H30.12   Disseminated chorioretinal inflammation, peripheral
H30.121   Disseminated chorioretinal inflammation, peripheral right eye
H30.122   Disseminated chorioretinal inflammation, peripheral, left eye
H30.123   Disseminated chorioretinal inflammation, peripheral, bilateral
H30.129   Disseminated chorioretinal inflammation, peripheral, unspecified eye

✓6ᵗʰ H30.13   Disseminated chorioretinal inflammation, generalized
H30.131   Disseminated chorioretinal inflammation, generalized, right eye
H30.132   Disseminated chorioretinal inflammation, generalized, left eye
H30.133   Disseminated chorioretinal inflammation, generalized, bilateral
H30.139   Disseminated chorioretinal inflammation, generalized, unspecified eye

✓6ᵗʰ H30.14   Acute posterior multifocal placoid pigment epitheliopathy
H30.141   Acute posterior multifocal placoid pigment epitheliopathy, right eye
H30.142   Acute posterior multifocal placoid pigment epitheliopathy, left eye
H30.143   Acute posterior multifocal placoid pigment epitheliopathy, bilateral
H30.149   Acute posterior multifocal placoid pigment epitheliopathy, unspecified eye

✓5ᵗʰ H30.2   Posterior cyclitis
Pars planitis
H30.20   Posterior cyclitis, unspecified eye
H30.21   Posterior cyclitis, right eye
H30.22   Posterior cyclitis, left eye
H30.23   Posterior cyclitis, bilateral

✓5ᵗʰ H30.8   Other chorioretinal inflammations
✓6ᵗʰ H30.81   Harada's disease
H30.811   Harada's disease, right eye
H30.812   Harada's disease, left eye
H30.813   Harada's disease, bilateral
H30.819   Harada's disease, unspecified eye
✓6ᵗʰ H30.89   Other chorioretinal inflammations
H30.891   Other chorioretinal inflammations, right eye
H30.892   Other chorioretinal inflammations, left eye

H30.893 Other chorioretinal inflammations, bilateral

H30.899 Other chorioretinal inflammations, unspecified eye

√5ᵗʰ **H30.9 Unspecified chorioretinal inflammation**
Chorioretinitis NOS Retinitis NOS
Choroiditis NOS Retinochoroiditis NOS
Neuroretinitis NOS

H30.90 Unspecified chorioretinal inflammation, unspecified eye

H30.91 Unspecified chorioretinal inflammation, right eye

H30.92 Unspecified chorioretinal inflammation, left eye

H30.93 Unspecified chorioretinal inflammation, bilateral

√4ᵗʰ **H31 Other disorders of choroid**

√5ᵗʰ **H31.0 Chorioretinal scars**
EXCLUDES 2 postsurgical chorioretinal scars (H59.81-)

√6ᵗʰ **H31.00 Unspecified chorioretinal scars**

H31.001 Unspecified chorioretinal scars, right eye

H31.002 Unspecified chorioretinal scars, left eye

H31.003 Unspecified chorioretinal scars, bilateral

H31.009 Unspecified chorioretinal scars, unspecified eye

√6ᵗʰ **H31.01 Macula scars of posterior pole (postinflammatory) (post-traumatic)**
EXCLUDES 1 postprocedural chorioretinal scar (H59.81-)

H31.011 Macula scars of posterior pole (postinflammatory) (post-traumatic), right eye

H31.012 Macula scars of posterior pole (postinflammatory) (post-traumatic), left eye

H31.013 Macula scars of posterior pole (postinflammatory) (post-traumatic), bilateral

H31.019 Macula scars of posterior pole (postinflammatory) (post-traumatic), unspecified eye

√6ᵗʰ **H31.02 Solar retinopathy**

H31.021 Solar retinopathy, right eye

H31.022 Solar retinopathy, left eye

H31.023 Solar retinopathy, bilateral

H31.029 Solar retinopathy, unspecified eye

√6ᵗʰ **H31.09 Other chorioretinal scars**

H31.091 Other chorioretinal scars, right eye

H31.092 Other chorioretinal scars, left eye

H31.093 Other chorioretinal scars, bilateral

H31.099 Other chorioretinal scars, unspecified eye

√5ᵗʰ **H31.1 Choroidal degeneration**
EXCLUDES 2 angioid streaks of macula (H35.33)

√6ᵗʰ **H31.10 Unspecified choroidal degeneration**
Choroidal sclerosis NOS

H31.101 Choroidal degeneration, unspecified, right eye

H31.102 Choroidal degeneration, unspecified, left eye

H31.103 Choroidal degeneration, unspecified, bilateral

H31.109 Choroidal degeneration, unspecified, unspecified eye

√6ᵗʰ **H31.11 Age-related choroidal atrophy**

H31.111 Age-related choroidal atrophy, right eye A

H31.112 Age-related choroidal atrophy, left eye A

H31.113 Age-related choroidal atrophy, bilateral A

H31.119 Age-related choroidal atrophy, unspecified eye A

√6ᵗʰ **H31.12 Diffuse secondary atrophy of choroid**

H31.121 Diffuse secondary atrophy of choroid, right eye

H31.122 Diffuse secondary atrophy of choroid, left eye

H31.123 Diffuse secondary atrophy of choroid, bilateral

H31.129 Diffuse secondary atrophy of choroid, unspecified eye

√5ᵗʰ **H31.2 Hereditary choroidal dystrophy**
EXCLUDES 2 hyperornithinemia (E72.4)
ornithinemia (E72.4)

H31.20 Hereditary choroidal dystrophy, unspecified

H31.21 Choroideremia

H31.22 Choroidal dystrophy (central areolar) (generalized) (peripapillary)

H31.23 Gyrate atrophy, choroid

H31.29 Other hereditary choroidal dystrophy

√5ᵗʰ **H31.3 Choroidal hemorrhage and rupture**

√6ᵗʰ **H31.30 Unspecified choroidal hemorrhage**

H31.301 Unspecified choroidal hemorrhage, right eye

H31.302 Unspecified choroidal hemorrhage, left eye

H31.303 Unspecified choroidal hemorrhage, bilateral

H31.309 Unspecified choroidal hemorrhage, unspecified eye

√6ᵗʰ **H31.31 Expulsive choroidal hemorrhage**

H31.311 Expulsive choroidal hemorrhage, right eye

H31.312 Expulsive choroidal hemorrhage, left eye

H31.313 Expulsive choroidal hemorrhage, bilateral

H31.319 Expulsive choroidal hemorrhage, unspecified eye

√6ᵗʰ **H31.32 Choroidal rupture**

H31.321 Choroidal rupture, right eye

H31.322 Choroidal rupture, left eye

H31.323 Choroidal rupture, bilateral

H31.329 Choroidal rupture, unspecified eye

√5ᵗʰ **H31.4 Choroidal detachment**

√6ᵗʰ **H31.40 Unspecified choroidal detachment**

H31.401 Unspecified choroidal detachment, right eye

H31.402 Unspecified choroidal detachment, left eye

H31.403 Unspecified choroidal detachment, bilateral

H31.409 Unspecified choroidal detachment, unspecified eye

√6ᵗʰ **H31.41 Hemorrhagic choroidal detachment**

H31.411 Hemorrhagic choroidal detachment, right eye

H31.412 Hemorrhagic choroidal detachment, left eye

H31.413 Hemorrhagic choroidal detachment, bilateral

H31.419 Hemorrhagic choroidal detachment, unspecified eye

√6ᵗʰ **H31.42 Serous choroidal detachment**

H31.421 Serous choroidal detachment, right eye

H31.422 Serous choroidal detachment, left eye

H31.423 Serous choroidal detachment, bilateral

H31.429 Serous choroidal detachment, unspecified eye

H31.8 Other specified disorders of choroid

H31.9 Unspecified disorder of choroid

H32 Chorioretinal disorders in diseases classified elsewhere
Code first underlying disease, such as:
congenital toxoplasmosis (P37.1)
histoplasmosis (B39.-)
leprosy (A30.-)
EXCLUDES 1 chorioretinitis (in):
toxoplasmosis (acquired) (B58.01)
tuberculosis (A18.53)

√4ᵗʰ **H33 Retinal detachments and breaks**
EXCLUDES 1 detachment of retinal pigment epithelium (H35.72-, H35.73-)

√5ᵗʰ **H33.0 Retinal detachment with retinal break**
Rhegmatogenous retinal detachment
EXCLUDES 1 serous retinal detachment (without retinal break) (H33.2-)

√6ᵗʰ **H33.00 Unspecified retinal detachment with retinal break**

H33.001 Unspecified retinal detachment with retinal break, right eye

Diseases of the Eye and Adnexa

H33.002–H34.233

H33.002   **Unspecified retinal detachment with retinal break, left eye**

H33.003   **Unspecified retinal detachment with retinal break, bilateral**

H33.009   **Unspecified retinal detachment with retinal break, unspecified eye**

✓6ᵗʰ   **H33.01   Retinal detachment with single break**

H33.011   **Retinal detachment with single break, right eye**

H33.012   **Retinal detachment with single break, left eye**

H33.013   **Retinal detachment with single break, bilateral**

H33.019   **Retinal detachment with single break, unspecified eye**

✓6ᵗʰ   **H33.02   Retinal detachment with multiple breaks**

H33.021   **Retinal detachment with multiple breaks, right eye**

H33.022   **Retinal detachment with multiple breaks, left eye**

H33.023   **Retinal detachment with multiple breaks, bilateral**

H33.029   **Retinal detachment with multiple breaks, unspecified eye**

✓6ᵗʰ   **H33.03   Retinal detachment with giant retinal tear**

H33.031   **Retinal detachment with giant retinal tear, right eye**

H33.032   **Retinal detachment with giant retinal tear, left eye**

H33.033   **Retinal detachment with giant retinal tear, bilateral**

H33.039   **Retinal detachment with giant retinal tear, unspecified eye**

✓6ᵗʰ   **H33.04   Retinal detachment with retinal dialysis**

H33.041   **Retinal detachment with retinal dialysis, right eye**

H33.042   **Retinal detachment with retinal dialysis, left eye**

H33.043   **Retinal detachment with retinal dialysis, bilateral**

H33.049   **Retinal detachment with retinal dialysis, unspecified eye**

✓6ᵗʰ   **H33.05   Total retinal detachment**

H33.051   **Total retinal detachment, right eye**

H33.052   **Total retinal detachment, left eye**

H33.053   **Total retinal detachment, bilateral**

H33.059   **Total retinal detachment, unspecified eye**

✓5ᵗʰ   **H33.1   Retinoschisis and retinal cysts**

EXCLUDES 1   congenital retinoschisis (Q14.1)
microcystoid degeneration of retina (H35.42-)

✓6ᵗʰ   **H33.10   Unspecified retinoschisis**

H33.101   **Unspecified retinoschisis, right eye**

H33.102   **Unspecified retinoschisis, left eye**

H33.103   **Unspecified retinoschisis, bilateral**

H33.109   **Unspecified retinoschisis, unspecified eye**

✓6ᵗʰ   **H33.11   Cyst of ora serrata**

H33.111   **Cyst of ora serrata, right eye**

H33.112   **Cyst of ora serrata, left eye**

H33.113   **Cyst of ora serrata, bilateral**

H33.119   **Cyst of ora serrata, unspecified eye**

✓6ᵗʰ   **H33.12   Parasitic cyst of retina**

H33.121   **Parasitic cyst of retina, right eye**

H33.122   **Parasitic cyst of retina, left eye**

H33.123   **Parasitic cyst of retina, bilateral**

H33.129   **Parasitic cyst of retina, unspecified eye**

✓6ᵗʰ   **H33.19   Other retinoschisis and retinal cysts**

Pseudocyst of retina

H33.191   **Other retinoschisis and retinal cysts, right eye**

H33.192   **Other retinoschisis and retinal cysts, left eye**

H33.193   **Other retinoschisis and retinal cysts, bilateral**

H33.199   **Other retinoschisis and retinal cysts, unspecified eye**

✓5ᵗʰ   **H33.2   Serous retinal detachment**

Retinal detachment NOS
Retinal detachment without retinal break

EXCLUDES 1   central serous chorioretinopathy (H35.71-)

H33.20   **Serous retinal detachment, unspecified eye**

H33.21   **Serous retinal detachment, right eye**

H33.22   **Serous retinal detachment, left eye**

H33.23   **Serous retinal detachment, bilateral**

✓5ᵗʰ   **H33.3   Retinal breaks without detachment**

EXCLUDES 1   chorioretinal scars after surgery for detachment (H59.81-)
peripheral retinal degeneration without break (H35.4-)

✓6ᵗʰ   **H33.30   Unspecified retinal break**

H33.301   **Unspecified retinal break, right eye**

H33.302   **Unspecified retinal break, left eye**

H33.303   **Unspecified retinal break, bilateral**

H33.309   **Unspecified retinal break, unspecified eye**

✓6ᵗʰ   **H33.31   Horseshoe tear of retina without detachment**

Operculum of retina without detachment

H33.311   **Horseshoe tear of retina without detachment, right eye**

H33.312   **Horseshoe tear of retina without detachment, left eye**

H33.313   **Horseshoe tear of retina without detachment, bilateral**

H33.319   **Horseshoe tear of retina without detachment, unspecified eye**

✓6ᵗʰ   **H33.32   Round hole of retina without detachment**

H33.321   **Round hole, right eye**

H33.322   **Round hole, left eye**

H33.323   **Round hole, bilateral**

H33.329   **Round hole, unspecified eye**

✓6ᵗʰ   **H33.33   Multiple defects of retina without detachment**

H33.331   **Multiple defects of retina without detachment, right eye**

H33.332   **Multiple defects of retina without detachment, left eye**

H33.333   **Multiple defects of retina without detachment, bilateral**

H33.339   **Multiple defects of retina without detachment, unspecified eye**

✓5ᵗʰ   **H33.4   Traction detachment of retina**

Proliferative vitreo-retinopathy with retinal detachment

H33.40   **Traction detachment of retina, unspecified eye**

H33.41   **Traction detachment of retina, right eye**

H33.42   **Traction detachment of retina, left eye**

H33.43   **Traction detachment of retina, bilateral**

H33.8   **Other retinal detachments**

✓4ᵗʰ   **H34   Retinal vascular occlusions**

EXCLUDES 1   amaurosis fugax (G45.3)

✓5ᵗʰ   **H34.0   Transient retinal artery occlusion**

H34.00   **Transient retinal artery occlusion, unspecified eye**

H34.01   **Transient retinal artery occlusion, right eye**

H34.02   **Transient retinal artery occlusion, left eye**

H34.03   **Transient retinal artery occlusion, bilateral**

✓5ᵗʰ   **H34.1   Central retinal artery occlusion**

H34.10   **Central retinal artery occlusion, unspecified eye**

H34.11   **Central retinal artery occlusion, right eye**

H34.12   **Central retinal artery occlusion, left eye**

H34.13   **Central retinal artery occlusion, bilateral**

✓5ᵗʰ   **H34.2   Other retinal artery occlusions**

✓6ᵗʰ   **H34.21   Partial retinal artery occlusion**

Hollenhorst's plaque
Retinal microembolism

H34.211   **Partial retinal artery occlusion, right eye**

H34.212   **Partial retinal artery occlusion, left eye**

H34.213   **Partial retinal artery occlusion, bilateral**

H34.219   **Partial retinal artery occlusion, unspecified eye**

✓6ᵗʰ   **H34.23   Retinal artery branch occlusion**

H34.231   **Retinal artery branch occlusion, right eye**

H34.232   **Retinal artery branch occlusion, left eye**

H34.233   **Retinal artery branch occlusion, bilateral**

EXCLUDES 1 Not coded here   *EXCLUDES 2* Not included here   **N** Newborn Age: 0   **P** Pediatric Age: 0-17   **M** Maternity Age: 12-55   **A** Adult Age: 15-124

H34.239　Retinal artery branch occlusion, unspecified eye

✓5ᵗʰ **H34.8　Other retinal vascular occlusions**

　✓6ᵗʰ **H34.81　Central retinal vein occlusion**
　　H34.811　Central retinal vein occlusion, right eye
　　H34.812　Central retinal vein occlusion, left eye
　　H34.813　Central retinal vein occlusion, bilateral
　　H34.819　Central retinal vein occlusion, unspecified eye

　✓6ᵗʰ **H34.82　Venous engorgement**
　　　Incipient retinal vein occlusion
　　　Partial retinal vein occlusion
　　H34.821　Venous engorgement, right eye
　　H34.822　Venous engorgement, left eye
　　H34.823　Venous engorgement, bilateral
　　H34.829　Venous engorgement, unspecified eye

　✓6ᵗʰ **H34.83　Tributary (branch) retinal vein occlusion**
　　H34.831　Tributary (branch) retinal vein occlusion, right eye
　　H34.832　Tributary (branch) retinal vein occlusion, left eye
　　H34.833　Tributary (branch) retinal vein occlusion, bilateral
　　H34.839　Tributary (branch) retinal vein occlusion, unspecified eye

　H34.9　Unspecified retinal vascular occlusion

✓4ᵗʰ **H35　Other retinal disorders**

　EXCLUDES 2　*diabetic retinal disorders (E08.311- E08.359, E09.311- E09.359, E10.311- E10.359, E11.311- E11.359, E13.311- E13.359)*

　✓5ᵗʰ **H35.0　Background retinopathy and retinal vascular changes**
　　　Code also any associated hypertension (I10.-)

　　H35.00　Unspecified background retinopathy

　✓6ᵗʰ **H35.01　Changes in retinal vascular appearance**
　　　Retinal vascular sheathing
　　H35.011　Changes in retinal vascular appearance, right eye
　　H35.012　Changes in retinal vascular appearance, left eye
　　H35.013　Changes in retinal vascular appearance, bilateral
　　H35.019　Changes in retinal vascular appearance, unspecified eye

　✓6ᵗʰ **H35.02　Exudative retinopathy**
　　　Coats retinopathy
　　H35.021　Exudative retinopathy, right eye
　　H35.022　Exudative retinopathy, left eye
　　H35.023　Exudative retinopathy, bilateral
　　H35.029　Exudative retinopathy, unspecified eye

　✓6ᵗʰ **H35.03　Hypertensive retinopathy**
　　H35.031　Hypertensive retinopathy, right eye
　　H35.032　Hypertensive retinopathy, left eye
　　H35.033　Hypertensive retinopathy, bilateral
　　H35.039　Hypertensive retinopathy, unspecified eye

　✓6ᵗʰ **H35.04　Retinal micro-aneurysms, unspecified**
　　H35.041　Retinal micro-aneurysms, unspecified, right eye
　　H35.042　Retinal micro-aneurysms, unspecified, left eye
　　H35.043　Retinal micro-aneurysms, unspecified, bilateral
　　H35.049　Retinal micro-aneurysms, unspecified, unspecified eye

　✓6ᵗʰ **H35.05　Retinal neovascularization, unspecified**
　　H35.051　Retinal neovascularization, unspecified, right eye
　　H35.052　Retinal neovascularization, unspecified, left eye
　　H35.053　Retinal neovascularization, unspecified, bilateral
　　H35.059　Retinal neovascularization, unspecified, unspecified eye

　✓6ᵗʰ **H35.06　Retinal vasculitis**
　　　Eales disease　　Retinal perivasculitis
　　H35.061　Retinal vasculitis, right eye
　　H35.062　Retinal vasculitis, left eye
　　H35.063　Retinal vasculitis, bilateral
　　H35.069　Retinal vasculitis, unspecified eye

　✓6ᵗʰ **H35.07　Retinal telangiectasis**
　　H35.071　Retinal telangiectasis, right eye
　　H35.072　Retinal telangiectasis, left eye
　　H35.073　Retinal telangiectasis, bilateral
　　H35.079　Retinal telangiectasis, unspecified eye

　H35.09　Other intraretinal microvascular abnormalities
　　　Retinal varices

　✓5ᵗʰ **H35.1　Retinopathy of prematurity**

　✓6ᵗʰ **H35.10　Retinopathy of prematurity, unspecified**
　　　Retinopathy of prematurity NOS
　　H35.101　Retinopathy of prematurity, unspecified, right eye
　　H35.102　Retinopathy of prematurity, unspecified, left eye
　　H35.103　Retinopathy of prematurity, unspecified, bilateral
　　H35.109　Retinopathy of prematurity, unspecified, unspecified eye

　✓6ᵗʰ **H35.11　Retinopathy of prematurity, stage 0**
　　H35.111　Retinopathy of prematurity, stage 0, right eye
　　H35.112　Retinopathy of prematurity, stage 0, left eye
　　H35.113　Retinopathy of prematurity, stage 0, bilateral
　　H35.119　Retinopathy of prematurity, stage 0, unspecified eye

　✓6ᵗʰ **H35.12　Retinopathy of prematurity, stage 1**
　　H35.121　Retinopathy of prematurity, stage 1, right eye
　　H35.122　Retinopathy of prematurity, stage 1, left eye
　　H35.123　Retinopathy of prematurity, stage 1, bilateral
　　H35.129　Retinopathy of prematurity, stage 1, unspecified eye

　✓6ᵗʰ **H35.13　Retinopathy of prematurity, stage 2**
　　H35.131　Retinopathy of prematurity, stage 2, right eye
　　H35.132　Retinopathy of prematurity, stage 2, left eye
　　H35.133　Retinopathy of prematurity, stage 2, bilateral
　　H35.139　Retinopathy of prematurity, stage 2, unspecified eye

　✓6ᵗʰ **H35.14　Retinopathy of prematurity, stage 3**
　　H35.141　Retinopathy of prematurity, stage 3, right eye
　　H35.142　Retinopathy of prematurity, stage 3, left eye
　　H35.143　Retinopathy of prematurity, stage 3, bilateral
　　H35.149　Retinopathy of prematurity, stage 3, unspecified eye

　✓6ᵗʰ **H35.15　Retinopathy of prematurity, stage 4**
　　H35.151　Retinopathy of prematurity, stage 4, right eye
　　H35.152　Retinopathy of prematurity, stage 4, left eye
　　H35.153　Retinopathy of prematurity, stage 4, bilateral
　　H35.159　Retinopathy of prematurity, stage 4, unspecified eye

　✓6ᵗʰ **H35.16　Retinopathy of prematurity, stage 5**
　　H35.161　Retinopathy of prematurity, stage 5, right eye
　　H35.162　Retinopathy of prematurity, stage 5, left eye
　　H35.163　Retinopathy of prematurity, stage 5, bilateral
　　H35.169　Retinopathy of prematurity, stage 5, unspecified eye

H35.17 Retrolental fibroplasia
- H35.171 Retrolental fibroplasia, right eye
- H35.172 Retrolental fibroplasia, left eye
- H35.173 Retrolental fibroplasia, bilateral
- H35.179 Retrolental fibroplasia, unspecified eye

H35.2 Other non-diabetic proliferative retinopathy
Proliferative vitreo-retinopathy
EXCLUDES 1 proliferative vitreo-retinopathy with retinal detachment (H33.4-)
- H35.20 Other non-diabetic proliferative retinopathy, unspecified eye
- H35.21 Other non-diabetic proliferative retinopathy, right eye
- H35.22 Other non-diabetic proliferative retinopathy, left eye
- H35.23 Other non-diabetic proliferative retinopathy, bilateral

H35.3 Degeneration of macula and posterior pole
- H35.30 Unspecified macular degeneration A
  Age-related macular degeneration
- H35.31 Nonexudative age-related macular degeneration A
  Atrophic age-related macular degeneration
- H35.32 Exudative age-related macular degeneration A
- H35.33 Angioid streaks of macula
- H35.34 Macular cyst, hole, or pseudohole
  - H35.341 Macular cyst, hole, or pseudohole, right eye
  - H35.342 Macular cyst, hole, or pseudohole, left eye
  - H35.343 Macular cyst, hole, or pseudohole, bilateral
  - H35.349 Macular cyst, hole, or pseudohole, unspecified eye
- H35.35 Cystoid macular degeneration
  EXCLUDES 1 cystoid macular edema following cataract surgery (H59.03-)
  - H35.351 Cystoid macular degeneration, right eye
  - H35.352 Cystoid macular degeneration, left eye
  - H35.353 Cystoid macular degeneration, bilateral
  - H35.359 Cystoid macular degeneration, unspecified eye
- H35.36 Drusen (degenerative) of macula
  - H35.361 Drusen (degenerative) of macula, right eye
  - H35.362 Drusen (degenerative) of macula, left eye
  - H35.363 Drusen (degenerative) of macula, bilateral
  - H35.369 Drusen (degenerative) of macula, unspecified eye
- H35.37 Puckering of macula
  - H35.371 Puckering of macula, right eye
  - H35.372 Puckering of macula, left eye
  - H35.373 Puckering of macula, bilateral
  - H35.379 Puckering of macula, unspecified eye
- H35.38 Toxic maculopathy
  Code first poisoning due to drug or toxin, if applicable (T36-T65 with fifth or sixth character 1-4 or 6)
  Use additional code for adverse effect, if applicable, to identify drug (T36-T50 with fifth or sixth character 5)
  - H35.381 Toxic maculopathy, right eye
  - H35.382 Toxic maculopathy, left eye
  - H35.383 Toxic maculopathy, bilateral
  - H35.389 Toxic maculopathy, unspecified eye

H35.4 Peripheral retinal degeneration
EXCLUDES 1 hereditary retinal degeneration (dystrophy) (H35.5-)
peripheral retinal degeneration with retinal break (H33.3-)
- H35.40 Unspecified peripheral retinal degeneration
- H35.41 Lattice degeneration of retina
  Palisade degeneration of retina
  - H35.411 Lattice degeneration of retina, right eye
  - H35.412 Lattice degeneration of retina, left eye
  - H35.413 Lattice degeneration of retina, bilateral
  - H35.419 Lattice degeneration of retina, unspecified eye

H35.42 Microcystoid degeneration of retina
- H35.421 Microcystoid degeneration of retina, right eye
- H35.422 Microcystoid degeneration of retina, left eye
- H35.423 Microcystoid degeneration of retina, bilateral
- H35.429 Microcystoid degeneration of retina, unspecified eye

H35.43 Paving stone degeneration of retina
- H35.431 Paving stone degeneration of retina, right eye
- H35.432 Paving stone degeneration of retina, left eye
- H35.433 Paving stone degeneration of retina, bilateral
- H35.439 Paving stone degeneration of retina, unspecified eye

H35.44 Age-related reticular degeneration of retina
- H35.441 Age-related reticular degeneration of retina, right eye A
- H35.442 Age-related reticular degeneration of retina, left eye A
- H35.443 Age-related reticular degeneration of retina, bilateral A
- H35.449 Age-related reticular degeneration of retina, unspecified eye A

H35.45 Secondary pigmentary degeneration
- H35.451 Secondary pigmentary degeneration, right eye
- H35.452 Secondary pigmentary degeneration, left eye
- H35.453 Secondary pigmentary degeneration, bilateral
- H35.459 Secondary pigmentary degeneration, unspecified eye

H35.46 Secondary vitreoretinal degeneration
- H35.461 Secondary vitreoretinal degeneration, right eye
- H35.462 Secondary vitreoretinal degeneration, left eye
- H35.463 Secondary vitreoretinal degeneration, bilateral
- H35.469 Secondary vitreoretinal degeneration, unspecified eye

H35.5 Hereditary retinal dystrophy
EXCLUDES 1 dystrophies primarily involving Bruch's membrane (H31.1-)
- H35.50 Unspecified hereditary retinal dystrophy
- H35.51 Vitreoretinal dystrophy
- H35.52 Pigmentary retinal dystrophy
  Albipunctate retinal dystrophy
  Retinitis pigmentosa
  Tapetoretinal dystrophy
- H35.53 Other dystrophies primarily involving the sensory retina
  Stargardt's disease
- H35.54 Dystrophies primarily involving the retinal pigment epithelium
  Vitelliform retinal dystrophy

H35.6 Retinal hemorrhage
- H35.60 Retinal hemorrhage, unspecified eye
- H35.61 Retinal hemorrhage, right eye
- H35.62 Retinal hemorrhage, left eye
- H35.63 Retinal hemorrhage, bilateral

H35.7 Separation of retinal layers
EXCLUDES 1 retinal detachment (serous) (H33.2-)
rhegmatogenous retinal detachment (H33.0-)
- H35.70 Unspecified separation of retinal layers
- H35.71 Central serous chorioretinopathy
  - H35.711 Central serous chorioretinopathy, right eye
  - H35.712 Central serous chorioretinopathy, left eye
  - H35.713 Central serous chorioretinopathy, bilateral
  - H35.719 Central serous chorioretinopathy, unspecified eye

√6th **H35.72** Serous **detachment of retinal pigment epithelium**

    H35.721 **Serous detachment of retinal pigment epithelium,** right **eye**

    H35.722 **Serous detachment of retinal pigment epithelium,** left **eye**

    H35.723 **Serous detachment of retinal pigment epithelium,** bilateral

    H35.729 **Serous detachment of retinal pigment epithelium, unspecified eye**

√6th **H35.73** Hemorrhagic **detachment of retinal pigment epithelium**

    H35.731 **Hemorrhagic detachment of retinal pigment epithelium,** right **eye**

    H35.732 **Hemorrhagic detachment of retinal pigment epithelium,** left **eye**

    H35.733 **Hemorrhagic detachment of retinal pigment epithelium,** bilateral

    H35.739 **Hemorrhagic detachment of retinal pigment epithelium, unspecified eye**

√5th **H35.8 Other specified retinal disorders**

    EXCLUDES 2   *retinal hemorrhage (H35.6-)*

  H35.81 **Retinal edema**

    Retinal cotton wool spots

  H35.82 **Retinal ischemia**

  H35.89 Other specified retinal disorders

  H35.9 **Unspecified retinal disorder**

H36 *Retinal disorders in diseases classified elsewhere*

    Code first underlying disease, such as:
    lipid storage disorders (E75.-)
    sickle-cell disorders (D57.-)

    EXCLUDES 1   *arteriosclerotic retinopathy (H35.0-)*
                 diabetic retinopathy (E08.3-, E09.3-, E10.3-, E11.3-, E13.3-)

Glaucoma (H40-H42)

√4th **H40** **Glaucoma**

    EXCLUDES 1   *absolute glaucoma (H44.51-)*
                  congenital glaucoma (Q15.0)
                  traumatic glaucoma due to birth injury (P15.3)

√5th **H40.0** **Glaucoma** suspect

 √6th **H40.00** **Preglaucoma,** unspecified

    H40.001 **Preglaucoma, unspecified,** right **eye**

    H40.002 **Preglaucoma, unspecified,** left **eye**

    H40.003 **Preglaucoma, unspecified,** bilateral

    H40.009 **Preglaucoma, unspecified, unspecified eye**

 √6th **H40.01** Open angle **with borderline findings,** low risk

    Open angle, low risk

    H40.011 **Open angle with borderline findings, low risk,** right **eye**

    H40.012 **Open angle with borderline findings, low risk,** left **eye**

    H40.013 **Open angle with borderline findings, low risk,** bilateral

    H40.019 **Open angle with borderline findings, low risk, unspecified eye**

 √6th **H40.02** Open angle **with borderline findings,** high risk

    Open angle, high risk

    H40.021 **Open angle with borderline findings, high risk,** right **eye**

    H40.022 **Open angle with borderline findings, high risk,** left **eye**

    H40.023 **Open angle with borderline findings, high risk,** bilateral

    H40.029 **Open angle with borderline findings, high risk, unspecified eye**

 √6th **H40.03** **Anatomical narrow angle**

    Primary angle closure suspect

    H40.031 **Anatomical narrow angle,** right **eye**

    H40.032 **Anatomical narrow angle,** left **eye**

    H40.033 **Anatomical narrow angle,** bilateral

    H40.039 Anatomical narrow angle, unspecified eye

 √6th **H40.04** **Steroid responder**

    H40.041 **Steroid responder,** right **eye**

    H40.042 **Steroid responder,** left **eye**

    H40.043 **Steroid responder,** bilateral

    H40.049 **Steroid responder, unspecified eye**

 √6th **H40.05** Ocular hypertension

    H40.051 **Ocular hypertension,** right **eye**

    H40.052 **Ocular hypertension,** left **eye**

    H40.053 **Ocular hypertension,** bilateral

    H40.059 Ocular hypertension, unspecified eye

 √6th **H40.06** **Primary angle** closure **without glaucoma damage**

    H40.061 **Primary angle closure without glaucoma damage,** right **eye**

    H40.062 **Primary angle closure without glaucoma damage,** left **eye**

    H40.063 **Primary angle closure without glaucoma damage,** bilateral

    H40.069 **Primary angle closure without glaucoma damage, unspecified eye**

√5th **H40.1** **Open-angle glaucoma**

    One of the following 7th characters is to be assigned to each code in subcategories H40.10, H40.11, H40.12-, H40.13-, and H40.14- to designate the stage of glaucoma.
    0   stage unspecified
    1   mild stage
    2   moderate stage
    3   severe stage
    4   indeterminate stage

 √x7th **H40.10** **Unspecified open-angle glaucoma**

 √x7th **H40.11** **Primary open-angle glaucoma**

    Chronic simple glaucoma

 √6th **H40.12** **Low-tension glaucoma**

  √7th **H40.121** **Low-tension glaucoma,** right **eye**

  √7th **H40.122** **Low-tension glaucoma,** left **eye**

  √7th **H40.123** **Low-tension glaucoma,** bilateral

  √7th **H40.129** **Low-tension glaucoma, unspecified eye**

 √6th **H40.13** **Pigmentary glaucoma**

  √7th **H40.131** **Pigmentary glaucoma,** right **eye**

  √7th **H40.132** **Pigmentary glaucoma,** left **eye**

  √7th **H40.133** **Pigmentary glaucoma,** bilateral

  √7th **H40.139** Pigmentary glaucoma, unspecified eye

 √6th **H40.14** **Capsular glaucoma with pseudoexfoliation** of lens

  √7th **H40.141** **Capsular glaucoma with pseudoexfoliation of lens,** right **eye**

  √7th **H40.142** **Capsular glaucoma with pseudoexfoliation of lens,** left **eye**

  √7th **H40.143** **Capsular glaucoma with pseudoexfoliation of lens,** bilateral

  √7th **H40.149** Capsular glaucoma with pseudoexfoliation of lens, unspecified eye

 √6th **H40.15** **Residual stage** of open-angle glaucoma

    H40.151 **Residual stage of open-angle glaucoma,** right **eye**

    H40.152 **Residual stage of open-angle glaucoma,** left **eye**

    H40.153 **Residual stage of open-angle glaucoma,** bilateral

    H40.159 Residual stage of open-angle glaucoma, unspecified eye

√5th **H40.2** **Primary angle-closure glaucoma**

    One of the following 7th characters is to be assigned to each code in subcategories H40.20 and H40.22- to designate the stage of glaucoma.
    0   stage unspecified
    1   mild stage
    2   moderate stage
    3   severe stage
    4   indeterminate stage

    EXCLUDES 1   *aqueous misdirection (H40.83-)*
                  malignant glaucoma (H40.83-)

 √x7th **H40.20** **Unspecified primary angle-closure glaucoma**

 √6th **H40.21** **Acute** angle-closure **glaucoma**

    Acute angle-closure glaucoma attack
    Acute angle-closure glaucoma crisis

    H40.211 **Acute angle-closure glaucoma,** right **eye**

    H40.212 **Acute angle-closure glaucoma,** left **eye**

    H40.213 **Acute angle-closure glaucoma,** bilateral

√ Additional Character Required   √x7th *X*tension Alert   Unspecified Code   Other Specified Code   Manifestation Code   ►◄ Revised Text   ● New Code   ▲ Revised Code Title

ICD-10-CM 2014 (Draft)   **549**

H40.219 **Acute angle-closure glaucoma, unspecified eye**

√6ᵗʰ H40.22 Chronic **angle-closure glaucoma**
Chronic primary angle-closure glaucoma

√7ᵗʰ H40.221 Chronic angle-closure glaucoma, right **eye**

√7ᵗʰ H40.222 Chronic angle-closure glaucoma, left **eye**

√7ᵗʰ H40.223 Chronic angle-closure glaucoma, bilateral

√7ᵗʰ H40.229 **Chronic angle-closure glaucoma, unspecified eye**

√6ᵗʰ H40.23 Intermittent **angle-closure glaucoma**

H40.231 Intermittent angle-closure glaucoma, right **eye**

H40.232 Intermittent angle-closure glaucoma, left **eye**

H40.233 Intermittent angle-closure glaucoma, bilateral

H40.239 **Intermittent angle-closure glaucoma, unspecified eye**

√6ᵗʰ H40.24 Residual stage **of angle-closure glaucoma**

H40.241 Residual stage of angle-closure glaucoma, right **eye**

H40.242 Residual stage of angle-closure glaucoma, left **eye**

H40.243 Residual stage of angle-closure glaucoma, bilateral

H40.249 **Residual stage of angle-closure glaucoma, unspecified eye**

√5ᵗʰ H40.3 Glaucoma secondary **to eye** trauma
Code also underlying condition

One of the following 7th characters is to be assigned to each code in subcategory H40.3- to designate the stage of glaucoma.
Ø   stage unspecified
1   mild stage
2   moderate stage
3   severe stage
4   indeterminate stage

√x7ᵗʰ H40.30 **Glaucoma secondary to eye trauma, unspecified eye**

√x7ᵗʰ H40.31 **Glaucoma secondary to eye trauma,** right **eye**

√x7ᵗʰ H40.32 **Glaucoma secondary to eye trauma,** left **eye**

√x7ᵗʰ H40.33 **Glaucoma secondary to eye trauma,** bilateral

√5ᵗʰ H40.4 Glaucoma secondary **to eye** inflammation
Code also underlying condition

One of the following 7th characters is to be assigned to each code in subcategory H40.4- to designate the stage of glaucoma.
Ø   stage unspecified
1   mild stage
2   moderate stage
3   severe stage
4   indeterminate stage

√x7ᵗʰ H40.40 **Glaucoma secondary to eye inflammation, unspecified eye**

√x7ᵗʰ H40.41 **Glaucoma secondary to eye inflammation,** right **eye**

√x7ᵗʰ H40.42 **Glaucoma secondary to eye inflammation,** left **eye**

√x7ᵗʰ H40.43 **Glaucoma secondary to eye inflammation,** bilateral

√5ᵗʰ H40.5 Glaucoma secondary **to other** eye disorders
Code also underlying eye disorder

One of the following 7th characters is to be assigned to each code in subcategory H40.5- to designate the stage of glaucoma.
Ø   stage unspecified
1   mild stage
2   moderate stage
3   severe stage
4   indeterminate stage

√x7ᵗʰ H40.50 **Glaucoma secondary to other eye disorders, unspecified eye**

√x7ᵗʰ H40.51 **Glaucoma secondary to other eye disorders,** right **eye**

√x7ᵗʰ H40.52 **Glaucoma secondary to other eye disorders,** left **eye**

√x7ᵗʰ H40.53 **Glaucoma secondary to other eye disorders, bilateral**

√5ᵗʰ H40.6 Glaucoma secondary **to drugs**
Use additional code for adverse effect, if applicable, to identify drug (T36-T50 with fifth or sixth character 5)

One of the following 7th characters is to be assigned to each code in subcategory H40.6- to designate the stage of glaucoma.
Ø   stage unspecified
1   mild stage
2   moderate stage
3   severe stage
4   indeterminate stage

√x7ᵗʰ H40.60 **Glaucoma secondary to drugs, unspecified eye**

√x7ᵗʰ H40.61 **Glaucoma secondary to drugs,** right **eye**

√x7ᵗʰ H40.62 **Glaucoma secondary to drugs,** left **eye**

√x7ᵗʰ H40.63 **Glaucoma secondary to drugs,** bilateral

√5ᵗʰ H40.8 Other **glaucoma**

√6ᵗʰ H40.81 **Glaucoma with** increased episcleral venous pressure

H40.811 **Glaucoma with increased episcleral venous pressure,** right **eye**

H40.812 **Glaucoma with increased episcleral venous pressure,** left **eye**

H40.813 **Glaucoma with increased episcleral venous pressure,** bilateral

H40.819 **Glaucoma with increased episcleral venous pressure, unspecified eye**

√6ᵗʰ H40.82 **Hypersecretion glaucoma**

H40.821 **Hypersecretion glaucoma,** right **eye**

H40.822 **Hypersecretion glaucoma,** left **eye**

H40.823 **Hypersecretion glaucoma,** bilateral

H40.829 **Hypersecretion glaucoma, unspecified eye**

√6ᵗʰ H40.83 **Aqueous misdirection**
Malignant glaucoma

H40.831 **Aqueous misdirection,** right **eye**

H40.832 **Aqueous misdirection,** left **eye**

H40.833 **Aqueous misdirection,** bilateral

H40.839 **Aqueous misdirection, unspecified eye**

H40.89 **Other specified glaucoma**

H40.9 **Unspecified glaucoma**

H42   *Glaucoma in diseases classified elsewhere*
Code first underlying condition, such as:
amyloidosis (E85.-)
aniridia (Q13.1)
Lowe's syndrome (E72.03)
Reiger's anomaly (Q13.81)
specified metabolic disorder (E70-E88)
EXCLUDES 1   *glaucoma (in):*
diabetes mellitus (E08.39, E09.39, E10.39, E11.39, E13.39)
onchocerciasis (B73.02)
syphilis (A52.71)
tuberculous (A18.59)

Disorders of vitreous body and globe (H43-H44)

√4ᵗʰ **H43**   **Disorders of vitreous body**

√5ᵗʰ H43.0 **Vitreous** prolapse
EXCLUDES 1   *vitreous syndrome following cataract surgery (H59.0-)*
traumatic vitreous prolapse (S05.2-)

H43.00 **Vitreous prolapse, unspecified eye**

H43.01 **Vitreous prolapse,** right **eye**

H43.02 **Vitreous prolapse,** left **eye**

H43.03 **Vitreous prolapse,** bilateral

√5ᵗʰ H43.1 **Vitreous** hemorrhage

H43.10 **Vitreous hemorrhage, unspecified eye**

H43.11 **Vitreous hemorrhage,** right **eye**

H43.12 **Vitreous hemorrhage,** left **eye**

H43.13 **Vitreous hemorrhage,** bilateral

√5ᵗʰ H43.2 **Crystalline deposits** in vitreous body

H43.20 **Crystalline deposits in vitreous body, unspecified eye**

H43.21 **Crystalline deposits in vitreous body,** right **eye**

H43.22 **Crystalline deposits in vitreous body,** left **eye**

H43.23 **Crystalline deposits in vitreous body,** bilateral

EXCLUDES 1 Not coded here   EXCLUDES 2 Not included here   N Newborn Age: 0   P Pediatric Age: 0-17   M Maternity Age: 12-55   A Adult Age: 15-124

550   ICD-10-CM 2014 (Draft)

Diseases of the Eye and Adnexa

☑5ᵗʰ H43.3 Other vitreous opacities
☑6ᵗʰ H43.31 Vitreous membranes and strands
  H43.311 Vitreous membranes and strands, right eye
  H43.312 Vitreous membranes and strands, left eye
  H43.313 Vitreous membranes and strands, bilateral
  H43.319 Vitreous membranes and strands, unspecified eye
☑6ᵗʰ H43.39 Other vitreous opacities
  Vitreous floaters
  H43.391 Other vitreous opacities, right eye
  H43.392 Other vitreous opacities, left eye
  H43.393 Other vitreous opacities, bilateral
  H43.399 Other vitreous opacities, unspecified eye
☑5ᵗʰ H43.8 Other disorders of vitreous body
  EXCLUDES 1 proliferative vitreo-retinopathy with retinal detachment (H33.4-)
  EXCLUDES 2 vitreous abscess (H44.02-)
☑6ᵗʰ H43.81 Vitreous degeneration
  Vitreous detachment
  H43.811 Vitreous degeneration, right eye
  H43.812 Vitreous degeneration, left eye
  H43.813 Vitreous degeneration, bilateral
  H43.819 Vitreous degeneration, unspecified eye
☑6ᵗʰ H43.82 Vitreomacular adhesion
  Vitreomacular traction
  H43.821 Vitreomacular adhesion, right eye ▲
  H43.822 Vitreomacular adhesion, left eye ▲
  H43.823 Vitreomacular adhesion, bilateral ▲
  H43.829 Vitreomacular adhesion, unspecified eye ▲
  H43.89 Other disorders of vitreous body
  H43.9 Unspecified disorder of vitreous body
☑4ᵗʰ H44 Disorders of globe
  INCLUDES disorders affecting multiple structures of eye
☑5ᵗʰ H44.0 Purulent endophthalmitis
  Use additional code to identify organism
  EXCLUDES 1 bleb associated endophthalmitis (H59.4-)
☑6ᵗʰ H44.00 Unspecified purulent endophthalmitis
  H44.001 Unspecified purulent endophthalmitis, right eye
  H44.002 Unspecified purulent endophthalmitis, left eye
  H44.003 Unspecified purulent endophthalmitis, bilateral
  H44.009 Unspecified purulent endophthalmitis, unspecified eye
☑6ᵗʰ H44.01 Panophthalmitis (acute)
  H44.011 Panophthalmitis (acute), right eye
  H44.012 Panophthalmitis (acute), left eye
  H44.013 Panophthalmitis (acute), bilateral
  H44.019 Panophthalmitis (acute), unspecified eye
☑6ᵗʰ H44.02 Vitreous abscess (chronic)
  H44.021 Vitreous abscess (chronic), right eye
  H44.022 Vitreous abscess (chronic), left eye
  H44.023 Vitreous abscess (chronic), bilateral
  H44.029 Vitreous abscess (chronic), unspecified eye
☑5ᵗʰ H44.1 Other endophthalmitis
  EXCLUDES 1 bleb associated endophthalmitis (H59.4-)
  EXCLUDES 2 ophthalmia nodosa (H16.2-)
☑6ᵗʰ H44.11 Panuveitis
  H44.111 Panuveitis, right eye
  H44.112 Panuveitis, left eye
  H44.113 Panuveitis, bilateral
  H44.119 Panuveitis, unspecified eye
☑6ᵗʰ H44.12 Parasitic endophthalmitis, unspecified
  H44.121 Parasitic endophthalmitis, unspecified, right eye
  H44.122 Parasitic endophthalmitis, unspecified, left eye
  H44.123 Parasitic endophthalmitis, unspecified, bilateral

  H44.129 Parasitic endophthalmitis, unspecified, unspecified eye
☑6ᵗʰ H44.13 Sympathetic uveitis
  H44.131 Sympathetic uveitis, right eye
  H44.132 Sympathetic uveitis, left eye
  H44.133 Sympathetic uveitis, bilateral
  H44.139 Sympathetic uveitis, unspecified eye
  H44.19 Other endophthalmitis
☑5ᵗʰ H44.2 Degenerative myopia
  Malignant myopia
  H44.20 Degenerative myopia, unspecified eye
  H44.21 Degenerative myopia, right eye
  H44.22 Degenerative myopia, left eye
  H44.23 Degenerative myopia, bilateral
☑5ᵗʰ H44.3 Other and unspecified degenerative disorders of globe
  H44.30 Unspecified degenerative disorder of globe
☑6ᵗʰ H44.31 Chalcosis
  H44.311 Chalcosis, right eye
  H44.312 Chalcosis, left eye
  H44.313 Chalcosis, bilateral
  H44.319 Chalcosis, unspecified eye
☑6ᵗʰ H44.32 Siderosis of eye
  H44.321 Siderosis of eye, right eye
  H44.322 Siderosis of eye, left eye
  H44.323 Siderosis of eye, bilateral
  H44.329 Siderosis of eye, unspecified eye
☑6ᵗʰ H44.39 Other degenerative disorders of globe
  H44.391 Other degenerative disorders of globe, right eye
  H44.392 Other degenerative disorders of globe, left eye
  H44.393 Other degenerative disorders of globe, bilateral
  H44.399 Other degenerative disorders of globe, unspecified eye
☑5ᵗʰ H44.4 Hypotony of eye
  H44.40 Unspecified hypotony of eye
☑6ᵗʰ H44.41 Flat anterior chamber hypotony of eye
  H44.411 Flat anterior chamber hypotony of right eye
  H44.412 Flat anterior chamber hypotony of left eye
  H44.413 Flat anterior chamber hypotony of eye, bilateral
  H44.419 Flat anterior chamber hypotony of unspecified eye
☑6ᵗʰ H44.42 Hypotony of eye due to ocular fistula
  H44.421 Hypotony of right eye due to ocular fistula
  H44.422 Hypotony of left eye due to ocular fistula
  H44.423 Hypotony of eye due to ocular fistula, bilateral
  H44.429 Hypotony of unspecified eye due to ocular fistula
☑6ᵗʰ H44.43 Hypotony of eye due to other ocular disorders
  H44.431 Hypotony of eye due to other ocular disorders, right eye
  H44.432 Hypotony of eye due to other ocular disorders, left eye
  H44.433 Hypotony of eye due to other ocular disorders, bilateral
  H44.439 Hypotony of eye due to other ocular disorders, unspecified eye
☑6ᵗʰ H44.44 Primary hypotony of eye
  H44.441 Primary hypotony of right eye
  H44.442 Primary hypotony of left eye
  H44.443 Primary hypotony of eye, bilateral
  H44.449 Primary hypotony of unspecified eye
☑5ᵗʰ H44.5 Degenerated conditions of globe
  H44.50 Unspecified degenerated conditions of globe
☑6ᵗʰ H44.51 Absolute glaucoma
  H44.511 Absolute glaucoma, right eye
  H44.512 Absolute glaucoma, left eye
  H44.513 Absolute glaucoma, bilateral
  H44.519 Absolute glaucoma, unspecified eye

✓6th **H44.52 Atrophy of globe**
Phthisis bulbi

     H44.521 **Atrophy of globe, right eye**
     H44.522 **Atrophy of globe, left eye**
     H44.523 **Atrophy of globe, bilateral**
     H44.529 **Atrophy of globe, unspecified eye**

✓6th **H44.53 Leucocoria**

     H44.531 **Leucocoria, right eye**
     H44.532 **Leucocoria, left eye**
     H44.533 **Leucocoria, bilateral**
     H44.539 **Leucocoria, unspecified eye**

✓5th **H44.6 Retained (old) intraocular foreign body, magnetic**
Use additional code to identify magnetic foreign body (Z18.11)

EXCLUDES 1   *current intraocular foreign body (S05.-)*
EXCLUDES 2   *retained foreign body in eyelid (H02.81-)*
          retained (old) foreign body following penetrating wound of orbit (H05.5-)
          retained (old) intraocular foreign body, nonmagnetic (H44.7-)

✓6th **H44.60 Unspecified retained (old) intraocular foreign body, magnetic**

     H44.601 **Unspecified retained (old) intraocular foreign body, magnetic, right eye**
     H44.602 **Unspecified retained (old) intraocular foreign body, magnetic, left eye**
     H44.603 **Unspecified retained (old) intraocular foreign body, magnetic, bilateral**
     H44.609 **Unspecified retained (old) intraocular foreign body, magnetic, unspecified eye**

✓6th **H44.61 Retained (old) magnetic foreign body in anterior chamber**

     H44.611 **Retained (old) magnetic foreign body in anterior chamber, right eye**
     H44.612 **Retained (old) magnetic foreign body in anterior chamber, left eye**
     H44.613 **Retained (old) magnetic foreign body in anterior chamber, bilateral**
     H44.619 **Retained (old) magnetic foreign body in anterior chamber, unspecified eye**

✓6th **H44.62 Retained (old) magnetic foreign body in iris or ciliary body**

     H44.621 **Retained (old) magnetic foreign body in iris or ciliary body, right eye**
     H44.622 **Retained (old) magnetic foreign body in iris or ciliary body, left eye**
     H44.623 **Retained (old) magnetic foreign body in iris or ciliary body, bilateral**
     H44.629 **Retained (old) magnetic foreign body in iris or ciliary body, unspecified eye**

✓6th **H44.63 Retained (old) magnetic foreign body in lens**

     H44.631 **Retained (old) magnetic foreign body in lens, right eye**
     H44.632 **Retained (old) magnetic foreign body in lens, left eye**
     H44.633 **Retained (old) magnetic foreign body in lens, bilateral**
     H44.639 **Retained (old) magnetic foreign body in lens, unspecified eye**

✓6th **H44.64 Retained (old) magnetic foreign body in posterior wall of globe**

     H44.641 **Retained (old) magnetic foreign body in posterior wall of globe, right eye**
     H44.642 **Retained (old) magnetic foreign body in posterior wall of globe, left eye**
     H44.643 **Retained (old) magnetic foreign body in posterior wall of globe, bilateral**
     H44.649 **Retained (old) magnetic foreign body in posterior wall of globe, unspecified eye**

✓6th **H44.65 Retained (old) magnetic foreign body in vitreous body**

     H44.651 **Retained (old) magnetic foreign body in vitreous body, right eye**
     H44.652 **Retained (old) magnetic foreign body in vitreous body, left eye**
     H44.653 **Retained (old) magnetic foreign body in vitreous body, bilateral**

     H44.659 **Retained (old) magnetic foreign body in vitreous body, unspecified eye**

✓6th **H44.69 Retained (old) intraocular foreign body, magnetic, in other or multiple sites**

     H44.691 **Retained (old) intraocular foreign body, magnetic, in other or multiple sites, right eye**
     H44.692 **Retained (old) intraocular foreign body, magnetic, in other or multiple sites, left eye**
     H44.693 **Retained (old) intraocular foreign body, magnetic, in other or multiple sites, bilateral**
     H44.699 **Retained (old) intraocular foreign body, magnetic, in other or multiple sites, unspecified eye**

✓5th **H44.7 Retained (old) intraocular foreign body, nonmagnetic**
Use additional code to identify nonmagnetic foreign body (Z18.01-Z18.10, Z18.12, Z18.2-Z18.9)

EXCLUDES 1   *current intraocular foreign body (S05.-)*
EXCLUDES 2   *retained foreign body in eyelid (H02.81-)*
          retained (old) foreign body following penetrating wound of orbit (H05.5-)
          retained (old) intraocular foreign body, magnetic (H44.6-)

✓6th **H44.70 Unspecified retained (old) intraocular foreign body, nonmagnetic**

     H44.701 **Unspecified retained (old) intraocular foreign body, nonmagnetic, right eye**
     H44.702 **Unspecified retained (old) intraocular foreign body, nonmagnetic, left eye**
     H44.703 **Unspecified retained (old) intraocular foreign body, nonmagnetic, bilateral**
     H44.709 **Unspecified retained (old) intraocular foreign body, nonmagnetic, unspecified eye**
          Retained (old) intraocular foreign body NOS

✓6th **H44.71 Retained (nonmagnetic) (old) foreign body in anterior chamber**

     H44.711 **Retained (nonmagnetic) (old) foreign body in anterior chamber, right eye**
     H44.712 **Retained (nonmagnetic) (old) foreign body in anterior chamber, left eye**
     H44.713 **Retained (nonmagnetic) (old) foreign body in anterior chamber, bilateral**
     H44.719 **Retained (nonmagnetic) (old) foreign body in anterior chamber, unspecified eye**

✓6th **H44.72 Retained (nonmagnetic) (old) foreign body in iris or ciliary body**

     H44.721 **Retained (nonmagnetic) (old) foreign body in iris or ciliary body, right eye**
     H44.722 **Retained (nonmagnetic) (old) foreign body in iris or ciliary body, left eye**
     H44.723 **Retained (nonmagnetic) (old) foreign body in iris or ciliary body, bilateral**
     H44.729 **Retained (nonmagnetic) (old) foreign body in iris or ciliary body, unspecified eye**

✓6th **H44.73 Retained (nonmagnetic) (old) foreign body in lens**

     H44.731 **Retained (nonmagnetic) (old) foreign body in lens, right eye**
     H44.732 **Retained (nonmagnetic) (old) foreign body in lens, left eye**
     H44.733 **Retained (nonmagnetic) (old) foreign body in lens, bilateral**
     H44.739 **Retained (nonmagnetic) (old) foreign body in lens, unspecified eye**

✓6th **H44.74 Retained (nonmagnetic) (old) foreign body in posterior wall of globe**

     H44.741 **Retained (nonmagnetic) (old) foreign body in posterior wall of globe, right eye**
     H44.742 **Retained (nonmagnetic) (old) foreign body in posterior wall of globe, left eye**
     H44.743 **Retained (nonmagnetic) (old) foreign body in posterior wall of globe, bilateral**
     H44.749 **Retained (nonmagnetic) (old) foreign body in posterior wall of globe, unspecified eye**

EXCLUDES 1 Not coded here   EXCLUDES 2 Not included here   N Newborn Age: 0   P Pediatric Age: 0-17   M Maternity Age: 12-55   A Adult Age: 15-124

552   ICD-10-CM 2014 (Draft)

✓6ᵗʰ **H44.75** Retained (nonmagnetic) (old) foreign body in vitreous body

     H44.751 Retained (nonmagnetic) (old) foreign body in vitreous body, **right eye**

     H44.752 Retained (nonmagnetic) (old) foreign body in vitreous body, **left eye**

     H44.753 Retained (nonmagnetic) (old) foreign body in vitreous body, **bilateral**

     H44.759 Retained (nonmagnetic) (old) foreign body in vitreous body, unspecified eye

✓6ᵗʰ **H44.79** Retained (old) intraocular foreign body, nonmagnetic, in other or multiple sites

     H44.791 Retained (old) intraocular foreign body, nonmagnetic, in other or multiple sites, **right eye**

     H44.792 Retained (old) intraocular foreign body, nonmagnetic, in other or multiple sites, **left eye**

     H44.793 Retained (old) intraocular foreign body, nonmagnetic, in other or multiple sites, **bilateral**

     H44.799 Retained (old) intraocular foreign body, nonmagnetic, in other or multiple sites, unspecified eye

✓5ᵗʰ **H44.8** Other disorders of globe

   ✓6ᵗʰ **H44.81** Hemophthalmos

     H44.811 Hemophthalmos, **right eye**

     H44.812 Hemophthalmos, **left eye**

     H44.813 Hemophthalmos, **bilateral**

     H44.819 Hemophthalmos, unspecified eye

   ✓6ᵗʰ **H44.82** Luxation of globe

     H44.821 Luxation of globe, **right eye**

     H44.822 Luxation of globe, **left eye**

     H44.823 Luxation of globe, **bilateral**

     H44.829 Luxation of globe, unspecified eye

   H44.89 Other disorders of globe

  H44.9 Unspecified disorder of globe

Disorders of optic nerve and visual pathways (H46-H47)

✓4ᵗʰ **H46** Optic neuritis

   EXCLUDES 2   *ischemic optic neuropathy (H47.01-)*
            neuromyelitis optica [Devic] (G36.0)

  ✓5ᵗʰ **H46.0** Optic papillitis

    H46.00 Optic papillitis, unspecified eye

    H46.01 Optic papillitis, **right eye**

    H46.02 Optic papillitis, **left eye**

    H46.03 Optic papillitis, **bilateral**

  ✓5ᵗʰ **H46.1** Retrobulbar neuritis

    Retrobulbar neuritis NOS

    EXCLUDES 1   *syphilitic retrobulbar neuritis (A52.15)*

    H46.10 Retrobulbar neuritis, unspecified eye

    H46.11 Retrobulbar neuritis, **right eye**

    H46.12 Retrobulbar neuritis, **left eye**

    H46.13 Retrobulbar neuritis, **bilateral**

  H46.2 Nutritional optic neuropathy

  H46.3 Toxic optic neuropathy

    Code first (T51-T65) to identify cause

  H46.8 Other optic neuritis

  H46.9 Unspecified optic neuritis

✓4ᵗʰ **H47** Other disorders of optic [2nd] nerve and visual pathways

  ✓5ᵗʰ **H47.0** Disorders of optic nerve, not elsewhere classified

   ✓6ᵗʰ **H47.01** Ischemic optic neuropathy

     H47.011 Ischemic optic neuropathy, **right eye**

     H47.012 Ischemic optic neuropathy, **left eye**

     H47.013 Ischemic optic neuropathy, **bilateral**

     H47.019 Ischemic optic neuropathy, unspecified eye

   ✓6ᵗʰ **H47.02** Hemorrhage in optic nerve sheath

     H47.021 Hemorrhage in optic nerve sheath, **right eye**

     H47.022 Hemorrhage in optic nerve sheath, **left eye**

     H47.023 Hemorrhage in optic nerve sheath, **bilateral**

     H47.029 Hemorrhage in optic nerve sheath, unspecified eye

   ✓6ᵗʰ **H47.03** Optic nerve hypoplasia

     H47.031 Optic nerve hypoplasia, **right eye**

     H47.032 Optic nerve hypoplasia, **left eye**

     H47.033 Optic nerve hypoplasia, **bilateral**

     H47.039 Optic nerve hypoplasia, unspecified eye

   ✓6ᵗʰ **H47.09** Other disorders of optic nerve, not elsewhere classified

     Compression of optic nerve

     H47.091 Other disorders of optic nerve, not elsewhere classified, **right eye**

     H47.092 Other disorders of optic nerve, not elsewhere classified, **left eye**

     H47.093 Other disorders of optic nerve, not elsewhere classified, **bilateral**

     H47.099 Other disorders of optic nerve, not elsewhere classified, unspecified eye

  ✓5ᵗʰ **H47.1** Papilledema

    H47.10 Unspecified papilledema

    H47.11 Papilledema associated with increased intracranial pressure

    H47.12 Papilledema associated with decreased ocular pressure

    H47.13 Papilledema associated with retinal disorder

   ✓6ᵗʰ **H47.14** Foster-Kennedy syndrome

     H47.141 Foster-Kennedy syndrome, **right eye**

     H47.142 Foster-Kennedy syndrome, **left eye**

     H47.143 Foster-Kennedy syndrome, **bilateral**

     H47.149 Foster-Kennedy syndrome, unspecified eye

  ✓5ᵗʰ **H47.2** Optic atrophy

    H47.20 Unspecified optic atrophy

   ✓6ᵗʰ **H47.21** Primary optic atrophy

     H47.211 Primary optic atrophy, **right eye**

     H47.212 Primary optic atrophy, **left eye**

     H47.213 Primary optic atrophy, **bilateral**

     H47.219 Primary optic atrophy, unspecified eye

   H47.22 Hereditary optic atrophy

     Leber's optic atrophy

   ✓6ᵗʰ **H47.23** Glaucomatous optic atrophy

     H47.231 Glaucomatous optic atrophy, **right eye**

     H47.232 Glaucomatous optic atrophy, **left eye**

     H47.233 Glaucomatous optic atrophy, **bilateral**

     H47.239 Glaucomatous optic atrophy, unspecified eye

   ✓6ᵗʰ **H47.29** Other optic atrophy

     Temporal pallor of optic disc

     H47.291 Other optic atrophy, **right eye**

     H47.292 Other optic atrophy, **left eye**

     H47.293 Other optic atrophy, **bilateral**

     H47.299 Other optic atrophy, unspecified eye

  ✓5ᵗʰ **H47.3** Other disorders of optic disc

   ✓6ᵗʰ **H47.31** Coloboma of optic disc

     H47.311 Coloboma of optic disc, **right eye**

     H47.312 Coloboma of optic disc, **left eye**

     H47.313 Coloboma of optic disc, **bilateral**

     H47.319 Coloboma of optic disc, unspecified eye

   ✓6ᵗʰ **H47.32** Drusen of optic disc

     H47.321 Drusen of optic disc, **right eye**

     H47.322 Drusen of optic disc, **left eye**

     H47.323 Drusen of optic disc, **bilateral**

     H47.329 Drusen of optic disc, unspecified eye

   ✓6ᵗʰ **H47.33** Pseudopapilledema of optic disc

     H47.331 Pseudopapilledema of optic disc, **right eye**

     H47.332 Pseudopapilledema of optic disc, **left eye**

     H47.333 Pseudopapilledema of optic disc, **bilateral**

     H47.339 Pseudopapilledema of optic disc, unspecified eye

   ✓6ᵗʰ **H47.39** Other disorders of optic disc

     H47.391 Other disorders of optic disc, **right eye**

     H47.392 Other disorders of optic disc, **left eye**

     H47.393 Other disorders of optic disc, **bilateral**

✓ Additional Character Required   ✓x7ᵗʰ Xtension Alert   Unspecified Code   Other Specified Code   Manifestation Code   ▶◀ Revised Text   ● New Code   ▲ Revised Code Title

ICD-10-CM 2014 (Draft)   **553**

Diseases of the Eye and Adnexa

H47.399–H50.032

H47.399   **Other disorders of optic disc, unspecified eye**

✓5ᵗʰ **H47.4**   **Disorders of optic chiasm**
Code also underlying condition

H47.41   **Disorders of optic chiasm in (due to)** inflammatory disorders

H47.42   **Disorders of optic chiasm in (due to)** neoplasm

H47.43   **Disorders of optic chiasm in (due to)** vascular disorders

H47.49   **Disorders of optic chiasm in (due to) other disorders**

✓5ᵗʰ **H47.5**   **Disorders of other visual pathways**
Disorders of optic tracts, geniculate nuclei and optic radiations
Code also underlying condition

✓6ᵗʰ **H47.51**   **Disorders of visual pathways in (due to) inflammatory disorders**

H47.511   **Disorders of visual pathways in (due to) inflammatory disorders, right side**

H47.512   **Disorders of visual pathways in (due to) inflammatory disorders, left side**

H47.519   **Disorders of visual pathways in (due to) inflammatory disorders, unspecified side**

✓6ᵗʰ **H47.52**   **Disorders of visual pathways in (due to) neoplasm**

H47.521   **Disorders of visual pathways in (due to) neoplasm, right side**

H47.522   **Disorders of visual pathways in (due to) neoplasm, left side**

H47.529   **Disorders of visual pathways in (due to) neoplasm, unspecified side**

✓6ᵗʰ **H47.53**   **Disorders of visual pathways in (due to) vascular disorders**

H47.531   **Disorders of visual pathways in (due to) vascular disorders, right side**

H47.532   **Disorders of visual pathways in (due to) vascular disorders, left side**

H47.539   **Disorders of visual pathways in (due to) vascular disorders, unspecified side**

✓5ᵗʰ **H47.6**   **Disorders of visual cortex**
Code also underlying condition
EXCLUDES 1   injury to visual cortex S04.04

✓6ᵗʰ **H47.61**   **Cortical blindness**

H47.611   **Cortical blindness, right side of brain**

H47.612   **Cortical blindness, left side of brain**

H47.619   **Cortical blindness, unspecified side of brain**

✓6ᵗʰ **H47.62**   **Disorders of visual cortex in (due to) inflammatory disorders**

H47.621   **Disorders of visual cortex in (due to) inflammatory disorders, right side of brain**

H47.622   **Disorders of visual cortex in (due to) inflammatory disorders, left side of brain**

H47.629   **Disorders of visual cortex in (due to) inflammatory disorders, unspecified side of brain**

✓6ᵗʰ **H47.63**   **Disorders of visual cortex in (due to) neoplasm**

H47.631   **Disorders of visual cortex in (due to) neoplasm, right side of brain**

H47.632   **Disorders of visual cortex in (due to) neoplasm, left side of brain**

H47.639   **Disorders of visual cortex in (due to) neoplasm, unspecified side of brain**

✓6ᵗʰ **H47.64**   **Disorders of visual cortex in (due to) vascular disorders**

H47.641   **Disorders of visual cortex in (due to) vascular disorders, right side of brain**

H47.642   **Disorders of visual cortex in (due to) vascular disorders, left side of brain**

H47.649   **Disorders of visual cortex in (due to) vascular disorders, unspecified side of brain**

H47.9   **Unspecified disorder of visual pathways**

Disorders of ocular muscles, binocular movement, accommodation and refraction (H49-H52)

EXCLUDES 2   nystagmus and other irregular eye movements (H55)

✓4ᵗʰ **H49**   **Paralytic strabismus**
EXCLUDES 2   internal ophthalmoplegia (H52.51-)
internuclear ophthalmoplegia (H51.2-)
progressive supranuclear ophthalmoplegia (G23.1)

✓5ᵗʰ **H49.0**   **Third [oculomotor] nerve palsy**

H49.00   **Third [oculomotor] nerve palsy, unspecified eye**

H49.01   **Third [oculomotor] nerve palsy, right eye**

H49.02   **Third [oculomotor] nerve palsy, left eye**

H49.03   **Third [oculomotor] nerve palsy, bilateral**

✓5ᵗʰ **H49.1**   **Fourth [trochlear] nerve palsy**

H49.10   **Fourth [trochlear] nerve palsy, unspecified eye**

H49.11   **Fourth [trochlear] nerve palsy, right eye**

H49.12   **Fourth [trochlear] nerve palsy, left eye**

H49.13   **Fourth [trochlear] nerve palsy, bilateral**

✓5ᵗʰ **H49.2**   **Sixth [abducent] nerve palsy**

H49.20   **Sixth [abducent] nerve palsy, unspecified eye**

H49.21   **Sixth [abducent] nerve palsy, right eye**

H49.22   **Sixth [abducent] nerve palsy, left eye**

H49.23   **Sixth [abducent] nerve palsy, bilateral**

✓5ᵗʰ **H49.3**   **Total (external) ophthalmoplegia**

H49.30   **Total (external) ophthalmoplegia, unspecified eye**

H49.31   **Total (external) ophthalmoplegia, right eye**

H49.32   **Total (external) ophthalmoplegia, left eye**

H49.33   **Total (external) ophthalmoplegia, bilateral**

✓5ᵗʰ **H49.4**   **Progressive external ophthalmoplegia**
EXCLUDES 1   Kearns-Sayre syndrome (H49.81-)

H49.40   **Progressive external ophthalmoplegia, unspecified eye**

H49.41   **Progressive external ophthalmoplegia, right eye**

H49.42   **Progressive external ophthalmoplegia, left eye**

H49.43   **Progressive external ophthalmoplegia, bilateral**

✓5ᵗʰ **H49.8**   **Other paralytic strabismus**

✓6ᵗʰ **H49.81**   **Kearns-Sayre syndrome**
Progressive external ophthalmoplegia with pigmentary retinopathy
Use additional code for other manifestation, such as: heart block (I45.9)

H49.811   **Kearns-Sayre syndrome, right eye**

H49.812   **Kearns-Sayre syndrome, left eye**

H49.813   **Kearns-Sayre syndrome, bilateral**

H49.819   **Kearns-Sayre syndrome, unspecified eye**

✓6ᵗʰ **H49.88**   **Other paralytic strabismus**
External ophthalmoplegia NOS

H49.881   **Other paralytic strabismus, right eye**

H49.882   **Other paralytic strabismus, left eye**

H49.883   **Other paralytic strabismus, bilateral**

H49.889   **Other paralytic strabismus, unspecified eye**

H49.9   **Unspecified paralytic strabismus**

✓4ᵗʰ **H50**   **Other strabismus**

✓5ᵗʰ **H50.0**   **Esotropia**
Convergent concomitant strabismus
EXCLUDES 1   intermittent esotropia (H50.31-, H50.32)

H50.00   **Unspecified esotropia**

✓6ᵗʰ **H50.01**   **Monocular esotropia**

H50.011   **Monocular esotropia, right eye**

H50.012   **Monocular esotropia, left eye**

✓6ᵗʰ **H50.02**   **Monocular esotropia with A pattern**

H50.021   **Monocular esotropia with A pattern, right eye**

H50.022   **Monocular esotropia with A pattern, left eye**

✓6ᵗʰ **H50.03**   **Monocular esotropia with V pattern**

H50.031   **Monocular esotropia with V pattern, right eye**

H50.032   **Monocular esotropia with V pattern, left eye**

EXCLUDES 1   Not coded here   EXCLUDES 2   Not included here   N Newborn Age: 0   P Pediatric Age: 0-17   M Maternity Age: 12-55   A Adult Age: 15-124

554   ICD-10-CM 2014 (Draft)

✓6ᵗʰ **H50.04 Monocular esotropia with** other noncomitancies
  H50.041 Monocular esotropia with other noncomitancies, right eye
  H50.042 Monocular esotropia with other noncomitancies, left eye
 H50.05 Alternating **esotropia**
 H50.06 Alternating **esotropia with** A pattern
 H50.07 Alternating **esotropia with** V pattern
 H50.08 Alternating **esotropia with other** noncomitancies

✓5ᵗʰ **H50.1 Exotropia**
 Divergent concomitant strabismus
 EXCLUDES1 intermittent exotropia (H50.33-, H50.34)
 H50.10 Unspecified exotropia
✓6ᵗʰ **H50.11** Monocular **exotropia**
  H50.111 Monocular exotropia, right eye
  H50.112 Monocular exotropia, left eye
✓6ᵗʰ **H50.12 Monocular exotropia with** A pattern
  H50.121 Monocular exotropia with A pattern, right eye
  H50.122 Monocular exotropia with A pattern, left eye
✓6ᵗʰ **H50.13 Monocular exotropia with** V pattern
  H50.131 Monocular exotropia with V pattern, right eye
  H50.132 Monocular exotropia with V pattern, left eye
✓6ᵗʰ **H50.14 Monocular exotropia with** other noncomitancies
  H50.141 Monocular exotropia with other noncomitancies, right eye
  H50.142 Monocular exotropia with other noncomitancies, left eye
 H50.15 Alternating **exotropia**
 H50.16 Alternating **exotropia with** A pattern
 H50.17 Alternating **exotropia with** V pattern
 H50.18 Alternating **exotropia with other** noncomitancies

✓5ᵗʰ **H50.2 Vertical strabismus**
 Hypertropia
 H50.21 Vertical strabismus, right eye
 H50.22 Vertical strabismus, left eye

✓5ᵗʰ **H50.3 Intermittent heterotropia**
 H50.30 Unspecified intermittent heterotropia
✓6ᵗʰ **H50.31 Intermittent** monocular esotropia
  H50.311 Intermittent monocular esotropia, right eye
  H50.312 Intermittent monocular esotropia, left eye
 H50.32 Intermittent alternating **esotropia**
✓6ᵗʰ **H50.33 Intermittent** monocular exotropia
  H50.331 Intermittent monocular exotropia, right eye
  H50.332 Intermittent monocular exotropia, left eye
 H50.34 Intermittent alternating **exotropia**

✓5ᵗʰ **H50.4 Other and unspecified heterotropia**
 H50.40 Unspecified heterotropia
✓6ᵗʰ **H50.41** Cyclotropia
  H50.411 Cyclotropia, right eye
  H50.412 Cyclotropia, left eye
 H50.42 Monofixation **syndrome**
 H50.43 Accommodative component in esotropia

✓5ᵗʰ **H50.5 Heterophoria**
 H50.50 Unspecified heterophoria
 H50.51 Esophoria
 H50.52 Exophoria
 H50.53 Vertical **heterophoria**
 H50.54 Cyclophoria
 H50.55 Alternating **heterophoria**

✓5ᵗʰ **H50.6 Mechanical strabismus**
 H50.60 Mechanical strabismus, unspecified
✓6ᵗʰ **H50.61** Brown's sheath **syndrome**
  H50.611 Brown's sheath syndrome, right eye
  H50.612 Brown's sheath syndrome, left eye

 H50.69 Other mechanical strabismus
  Strabismus due to adhesions
  Traumatic limitation of duction of eye muscle
✓5ᵗʰ **H50.8 Other specified strabismus**
✓6ᵗʰ **H50.81 Duane's syndrome**
  H50.811 Duane's syndrome, right eye
  H50.812 Duane's syndrome, left eye
 H50.89 Other specified strabismus
 H50.9 Unspecified strabismus

✓4ᵗʰ **H51 Other disorders of binocular movement**
 H51.0 Palsy (spasm) of conjugate gaze
✓5ᵗʰ **H51.1 Convergence insufficiency and excess**
 H51.11 Convergence insufficiency
 H51.12 Convergence excess
✓5ᵗʰ **H51.2 Internuclear ophthalmoplegia**
 H51.20 Internuclear ophthalmoplegia, unspecified eye
 H51.21 Internuclear ophthalmoplegia, right eye
 H51.22 Internuclear ophthalmoplegia, left eye
 H51.23 Internuclear ophthalmoplegia, bilateral
 H51.8 Other specified disorders of binocular movement
 H51.9 Unspecified disorder of binocular movement

✓4ᵗʰ **H52 Disorders of refraction and accommodation**
✓5ᵗʰ **H52.0 Hypermetropia**
 H52.00 Hypermetropia, unspecified eye
 H52.01 Hypermetropia, right **eye**
 H52.02 Hypermetropia, left **eye**
 H52.03 Hypermetropia, bilateral
✓5ᵗʰ **H52.1 Myopia**
 EXCLUDES1 degenerative myopia (H44.2-)
 H52.10 Myopia, unspecified eye
 H52.11 Myopia, right eye
 H52.12 Myopia, left eye
 H52.13 Myopia, bilateral
✓5ᵗʰ **H52.2 Astigmatism**
✓6ᵗʰ **H52.20** Unspecified **astigmatism**
  H52.201 Unspecified astigmatism, right eye
  H52.202 Unspecified astigmatism, left eye
  H52.203 Unspecified astigmatism, bilateral
  H52.209 Unspecified astigmatism, unspecified eye
✓6ᵗʰ **H52.21** Irregular **astigmatism**
  H52.211 Irregular astigmatism, right eye
  H52.212 Irregular astigmatism, left eye
  H52.213 Irregular astigmatism, bilateral
  H52.219 Irregular astigmatism, unspecified eye
✓6ᵗʰ **H52.22** Regular **astigmatism**
  H52.221 Regular astigmatism, right eye
  H52.222 Regular astigmatism, left eye
  H52.223 Regular astigmatism, bilateral
  H52.229 Regular astigmatism, unspecified eye
✓5ᵗʰ **H52.3 Anisometropia and aniseikonia**
 H52.31 Anisometropia
 H52.32 Aniseikonia
 H52.4 Presbyopia
✓5ᵗʰ **H52.5 Disorders of accommodation**
✓6ᵗʰ **H52.51** Internal ophthalmoplegia (complete) (total)
  H52.511 Internal ophthalmoplegia (complete) (total), right eye
  H52.512 Internal ophthalmoplegia (complete) (total), left eye
  H52.513 Internal ophthalmoplegia (complete) (total), bilateral
  H52.519 Internal ophthalmoplegia (complete) (total), unspecified eye
✓6ᵗʰ **H52.52** Paresis **of accommodation**
  H52.521 Paresis of accommodation, right eye
  H52.522 Paresis of accommodation, left eye
  H52.523 Paresis of accommodation, bilateral
  H52.529 Paresis of accommodation, unspecified eye

✓ Additional Character Required ✓x7ᵗʰ Xtension Alert Unspecified Code Other Specified Code Manifestation Code ▶◀ Revised Text ● New Code ▲ Revised Code Title

ICD-10-CM 2014 (Draft) 555

Diseases of the Eye and Adnexa

H52.53–H53.61

√6ᵗʰ **H52.53 Spasm** of accommodation
  H52.531 Spasm of accommodation, right **eye**
  H52.532 Spasm of accommodation, left **eye**
  H52.533 Spasm of accommodation, bilateral
  H52.539 Spasm of accommodation, unspecified eye

H52.6 Other disorders of refraction

H52.7 Unspecified disorder of refraction

Visual disturbances and blindness (H53-H54)

√4ᵗʰ **H53 Visual disturbances**

√5ᵗʰ **H53.0 Amblyopia ex anopsia**
  EXCLUDES1 amblyopia due to vitamin A deficiency (E50.5)

√6ᵗʰ **H53.00 Unspecified amblyopia**
  H53.001 Unspecified amblyopia, right eye
  H53.002 Unspecified amblyopia, left eye
  H53.003 Unspecified amblyopia, bilateral
  H53.009 Unspecified amblyopia, unspecified eye

√6ᵗʰ **H53.01 Deprivation amblyopia**
  H53.011 Deprivation amblyopia, right eye
  H53.012 Deprivation amblyopia, left eye
  H53.013 Deprivation amblyopia, bilateral
  H53.019 Deprivation amblyopia, unspecified eye

√6ᵗʰ **H53.02 Refractive amblyopia**
  H53.021 Refractive amblyopia, right eye
  H53.022 Refractive amblyopia, left eye
  H53.023 Refractive amblyopia, bilateral
  H53.029 Refractive amblyopia, unspecified eye

√6ᵗʰ **H53.03 Strabismic amblyopia**
  EXCLUDES1 strabismus (H50.-)
  H53.031 Strabismic amblyopia, right eye
  H53.032 Strabismic amblyopia, left eye
  H53.033 Strabismic amblyopia, bilateral
  H53.039 Strabismic amblyopia, unspecified eye

√5ᵗʰ **H53.1 Subjective visual disturbances**
  EXCLUDES1 subjective visual disturbances due to vitamin A deficiency (E50.5)
    visual hallucinations (R44.1)

  H53.10 Unspecified subjective visual disturbances

  H53.11 Day blindness
    Hemeralopia

√6ᵗʰ **H53.12 Transient visual loss**
  Scintillating scotoma
  EXCLUDES1 amaurosis fugax (G45.3-)
    transient retinal artery occlusion (H34.0-)
  H53.121 Transient visual loss, right eye
  H53.122 Transient visual loss, left eye
  H53.123 Transient visual loss, bilateral
  H53.129 Transient visual loss, unspecified eye

√6ᵗʰ **H53.13 Sudden visual loss**
  H53.131 Sudden visual loss, right eye
  H53.132 Sudden visual loss, left eye
  H53.133 Sudden visual loss, bilateral
  H53.139 Sudden visual loss, unspecified eye

√6ᵗʰ **H53.14 Visual discomfort**
  Asthenopia
  Photophobia
  H53.141 Visual discomfort, right eye
  H53.142 Visual discomfort, left eye
  H53.143 Visual discomfort, bilateral
  H53.149 Visual discomfort, unspecified

  H53.15 Visual distortions of shape and size
    Metamorphopsia

  H53.16 Psychophysical visual disturbances

  H53.19 Other subjective visual disturbances
    Visual halos

H53.2 Diplopia
  Double vision

√5ᵗʰ **H53.3 Other and unspecified disorders of binocular vision**
  H53.30 Unspecified disorder of binocular vision
  H53.31 Abnormal retinal correspondence
  H53.32 Fusion with defective stereopsis
  H53.33 Simultaneous visual perception without fusion

  H53.34 Suppression of binocular vision

√5ᵗʰ **H53.4 Visual field defects**
  H53.40 Unspecified visual field defects

√6ᵗʰ **H53.41 Scotoma involving central area**
  Central scotoma
  H53.411 Scotoma involving central area, right eye
  H53.412 Scotoma involving central area, left eye
  H53.413 Scotoma involving central area, bilateral
  H53.419 Scotoma involving central area, unspecified eye

√6ᵗʰ **H53.42 Scotoma of blind spot area**
  Enlarged blind spot
  H53.421 Scotoma of blind spot area, right eye
  H53.422 Scotoma of blind spot area, left eye
  H53.423 Scotoma of blind spot area, bilateral
  H53.429 Scotoma of blind spot area, unspecified eye

√6ᵗʰ **H53.43 Sector or arcuate defects**
  Arcuate scotoma
  Bjerrum scotoma
  H53.431 Sector or arcuate defects, right eye
  H53.432 Sector or arcuate defects, left eye
  H53.433 Sector or arcuate defects, bilateral
  H53.439 Sector or arcuate defects, unspecified eye

√6ᵗʰ **H53.45 Other localized visual field defect**
  Peripheral visual field defect
  Ring scotoma NOS
  Scotoma NOS
  H53.451 Other localized visual field defect, right eye
  H53.452 Other localized visual field defect, left eye
  H53.453 Other localized visual field defect, bilateral
  H53.459 Other localized visual field defect, unspecified eye

√6ᵗʰ **H53.46 Homonymous bilateral field defects**
  Homonymous hemianopia
  Homonymous hemianopsia
  Quadrant anopia
  Quadrant anopsia
  H53.461 Homonymous bilateral field defects, right side
  H53.462 Homonymous bilateral field defects, left side
  H53.469 Homonymous bilateral field defects, unspecified side
    Homonymous bilateral field defects NOS

  H53.47 Heteronymous bilateral field defects
    Heteronymous hemianop(s)ia

√6ᵗʰ **H53.48 Generalized contraction of visual field**
  H53.481 Generalized contraction of visual field, right eye
  H53.482 Generalized contraction of visual field, left eye
  H53.483 Generalized contraction of visual field, bilateral
  H53.489 Generalized contraction of visual field, unspecified eye

√5ᵗʰ **H53.5 Color vision deficiencies**
  Color blindness
  EXCLUDES2 day blindness (H53.11)
  H53.50 Unspecified color vision deficiencies
    Color blindness NOS
  H53.51 Achromatopsia
  H53.52 Acquired color vision deficiency
  H53.53 Deuteranomaly
    Deuteranopia
  H53.54 Protanomaly
    Protanopia
  H53.55 Tritanomaly
    Tritanopia
  H53.59 Other color vision deficiencies

√5ᵗʰ **H53.6 Night blindness**
  EXCLUDES1 night blindness due to vitamin A deficiency (E50.5)
  H53.60 Unspecified night blindness
  H53.61 Abnormal dark adaptation curve

H53.62 Acquired **night blindness**
H53.63 Congenital **night blindness**
H53.69 Other **night blindness**
✓5ᵗʰ **H53.7** Vision **sensitivity** deficiencies
H53.71 Glare **sensitivity**
H53.72 Impaired contrast **sensitivity**
H53.8 Other visual disturbances
H53.9 Unspecified visual disturbance

✓4ᵗʰ **H54** **Blindness and low vision**
> NOTE For definition of visual impairment categories see table below
> Code first any associated underlying cause of the blindness
> EXCLUDES 1 *amaurosis fugax (G45.3)*

H54.0 **Blindness,** both eyes
> Visual impairment categories 3, 4, 5 in both eyes.

✓5ᵗʰ **H54.1** **Blindness,** one eye, low vision other eye
> Visual impairment categories 3, 4, 5 in one eye, with categories 1 or 2 in the other eye.
H54.10 **Blindness, one eye, low vision other eye, unspecified eyes**
H54.11 **Blindness,** right eye, low vision left eye
H54.12 **Blindness,** left eye, low vision right eye

H54.2 Low vision, both eyes
> Visual impairment categories 1 or 2 in both eyes.

H54.3 Unqualified visual loss, both eyes
> Visual impairment category 9 in both eyes.

✓5ᵗʰ **H54.4** **Blindness,** one eye
> Visual impairment categories 3, 4, 5 in one eye [normal vision in other eye]
H54.40 **Blindness, one eye, unspecified eye**
H54.41 **Blindness,** right eye, normal vision left eye
H54.42 **Blindness,** left eye, normal vision right eye

✓5ᵗʰ **H54.5** Low vision, one eye
> Visual impairment categories 1 or 2 in one eye [normal vision in other eye].
H54.50 **Low vision, one eye, unspecified eye**
H54.51 Low vision, right eye, normal vision left eye
H54.52 Low vision, left eye, normal vision right eye

✓5ᵗʰ **H54.6** Unqualified visual loss, one eye
> Visual impairment category 9 in one eye [normal vision in other eye].
H54.60 **Unqualified visual loss, one eye, unspecified**
H54.61 Unqualified visual loss, right eye, normal vision left eye
H54.62 Unqualified visual loss, left eye, normal vision right eye

H54.7 Unspecified visual loss
> Visual impairment category 9 NOS

H54.8 Legal blindness, as defined in USA
> Blindness NOS according to USA definition
> EXCLUDES 1 *legal blindness with specification of impairment level (H54.0-H54.7)*

> NOTE The following table gives a classification of severity of visual impairment recommended by a WHO Study Group on the Prevention of Blindness, Geneva, 6-10 November 1972.
>
> The term "low vision" in category H54 comprises categories 1 and 2 of the table, the term "blindness" categories 3, 4 and 5, and the term "unqualified visual loss" category 9.
>
> If the extent of the visual field is taken into account, patients with a field no greater than 10 but greater than 5 around central fixation should be placed in category 3 and patients with a field no greater than 5 around central fixation should be placed in 4, even if the central acuity is not impaired.

Category of visual impairment	Visual acuity with best possible correction	
	Maximum less than:	**Minimum equal to or better than:**
1	6/18 3/10 (0.3) 20/70	6/60 1/10 (0.1) 20/200
2	6/60 1/10 (0.1) 20/200	3/60 1/20 (0.5) 20/400
3	3/60 1/20 (0.05) 20/400	1/60 (finger counting at one meter) 1/50 (0.02) 5/300 (20/1200)
4	1/60 (finger counting at one meter) 1/50 (0.02) 5/300	Light perception
5	No light perception	
9	Undetermined or unspecified	

Other disorders of eye and adnexa (H55-H59)

✓4ᵗʰ **H55** **Nystagmus and other irregular eye movements**
✓5ᵗʰ **H55.0** Nystagmus
H55.00 **Unspecified nystagmus**
H55.01 Congenital **nystagmus**
H55.02 Latent **nystagmus**
H55.03 Visual deprivation **nystagmus**
H55.04 Dissociated **nystagmus**
H55.09 **Other forms of nystagmus**
✓5ᵗʰ **H55.8** Other irregular eye movements
H55.81 Saccadic eye movements
H55.89 **Other irregular eye movements**

✓4ᵗʰ **H57** **Other disorders of eye and adnexa**
✓5ᵗʰ **H57.0** Anomalies of pupillary function
H57.00 **Unspecified anomaly of pupillary function**
H57.01 Argyll Robertson pupil, atypical
> EXCLUDES 1 *syphilitic Argyll Robertson pupil (A52.19)*
H57.02 Anisocoria
H57.03 Miosis
H57.04 Mydriasis
✓6ᵗʰ **H57.05** Tonic pupil
H57.051 Tonic pupil, right eye
H57.052 Tonic pupil, left eye
H57.053 Tonic pupil, bilateral
H57.059 **Tonic pupil, unspecified eye**
H57.09 **Other anomalies of pupillary function**
✓5ᵗʰ **H57.1** Ocular pain
H57.10 **Ocular pain, unspecified eye**
H57.11 Ocular pain, right eye
H57.12 Ocular pain, left eye
H57.13 Ocular pain, bilateral
H57.8 **Other specified disorders of eye and adnexa**
H57.9 **Unspecified disorder of eye and adnexa**

✓4ᵗʰ **H59** **Intraoperative and postprocedural complications and disorders of eye and adnexa, not elsewhere classified**
> EXCLUDES 1 *mechanical complication of intraocular lens (T85.2)*
> *mechanical complication of other ocular prosthetic devices, implants and grafts (T85.3)*
> *pseudophakia (Z96.1)*
> *secondary cataracts (H26.4-)*
✓5ᵗʰ **H59.0** Disorders of the eye following cataract surgery
✓6ᵗʰ **H59.01** Keratopathy (bullous aphakic) following cataract surgery
> Vitreal corneal syndrome
> Vitreous (touch) syndrome
H59.011 Keratopathy (bullous aphakic) following cataract surgery, right eye
H59.012 Keratopathy (bullous aphakic) following cataract surgery, left eye

---

✓ Additional Character Required   ✓x7ᵗʰ Xtension Alert   Unspecified Code   Other Specified Code   Manifestation Code   ▶◀ Revised Text   ● New Code   ▲ Revised Code Title

Diseases of the Eye and Adnexa

H59.013 Keratopathy (bullous aphakic) following cataract surgery, bilateral

H59.019 Keratopathy (bullous aphakic) following cataract surgery, unspecified eye

√6th **H59.02** Cataract (lens) fragments in eye following cataract surgery

H59.021 Cataract (lens) fragments in eye following cataract surgery, right eye

H59.022 Cataract (lens) fragments in eye following cataract surgery, left eye

H59.023 Cataract (lens) fragments in eye following cataract surgery, bilateral

H59.029 Cataract (lens) fragments in eye following cataract surgery, unspecified eye

√6th **H59.03** Cystoid macular edema following cataract surgery

H59.031 Cystoid macular edema following cataract surgery, right eye

H59.032 Cystoid macular edema following cataract surgery, left eye

H59.033 Cystoid macular edema following cataract surgery, bilateral

H59.039 Cystoid macular edema following cataract surgery, unspecified eye

√6th **H59.09** Other disorders of the eye following cataract surgery

H59.091 Other disorders of the right eye following cataract surgery

H59.092 Other disorders of the left eye following cataract surgery

H59.093 Other disorders of the eye following cataract surgery, bilateral

H59.099 Other disorders of unspecified eye following cataract surgery

√5th **H59.1** Intraoperative hemorrhage and hematoma of eye and adnexa complicating a procedure

> EXCLUDES 1   intraoperative hemorrhage and hematoma of eye and adnexa due to accidental puncture or laceration during a procedure (H59.2-)

√6th **H59.11** Intraoperative hemorrhage and hematoma of eye and adnexa complicating an ophthalmic procedure

H59.111 Intraoperative hemorrhage and hematoma of right eye and adnexa complicating an ophthalmic procedure

H59.112 Intraoperative hemorrhage and hematoma of left eye and adnexa complicating an ophthalmic procedure

H59.113 Intraoperative hemorrhage and hematoma of eye and adnexa complicating an ophthalmic procedure, bilateral

H59.119 Intraoperative hemorrhage and hematoma of unspecified eye and adnexa complicating an ophthalmic procedure

√6th **H59.12** Intraoperative hemorrhage and hematoma of eye and adnexa complicating other procedure

H59.121 Intraoperative hemorrhage and hematoma of right eye and adnexa complicating other procedure

H59.122 Intraoperative hemorrhage and hematoma of left eye and adnexa complicating other procedure

H59.123 Intraoperative hemorrhage and hematoma of eye and adnexa complicating other procedure, bilateral

H59.129 Intraoperative hemorrhage and hematoma of unspecified eye and adnexa complicating other procedure

√5th **H59.2** Accidental puncture and laceration of eye and adnexa during a procedure

√6th **H59.21** Accidental puncture and laceration of eye and adnexa during an ophthalmic procedure

H59.211 Accidental puncture and laceration of right eye and adnexa during an ophthalmic procedure

H59.212 Accidental puncture and laceration of left eye and adnexa during an ophthalmic procedure

H59.213 Accidental puncture and laceration of eye and adnexa during an ophthalmic procedure, bilateral

H59.219 Accidental puncture and laceration of unspecified eye and adnexa during an ophthalmic procedure

√6th **H59.22** Accidental puncture and laceration of eye and adnexa during other procedure

H59.221 Accidental puncture and laceration of right eye and adnexa during other procedure

H59.222 Accidental puncture and laceration of left eye and adnexa during other procedure

H59.223 Accidental puncture and laceration of eye and adnexa during other procedure, bilateral

H59.229 Accidental puncture and laceration of unspecified eye and adnexa during other procedure

√5th **H59.3** Postprocedural hemorrhage and hematoma of eye and adnexa following a procedure

√6th **H59.31** Postprocedural hemorrhage and hematoma of eye and adnexa following an ophthalmic procedure

H59.311 Postprocedural hemorrhage and hematoma of right eye and adnexa following an ophthalmic procedure

H59.312 Postprocedural hemorrhage and hematoma of left eye and adnexa following an ophthalmic procedure

H59.313 Postprocedural hemorrhage and hematoma of eye and adnexa following an ophthalmic procedure, bilateral

H59.319 Postprocedural hemorrhage and hematoma of unspecified eye and adnexa following an ophthalmic procedure

√6th **H59.32** Postprocedural hemorrhage and hematoma of eye and adnexa following other procedure

H59.321 Postprocedural hemorrhage and hematoma of right eye and adnexa following other procedure

H59.322 Postprocedural hemorrhage and hematoma of left eye and adnexa following other procedure

H59.323 Postprocedural hemorrhage and hematoma of eye and adnexa following other procedure, bilateral

H59.329 Postprocedural hemorrhage and hematoma of unspecified eye and adnexa following other procedure

√5th **H59.4** Inflammation (infection) of postprocedural bleb

Postprocedural blebitis

> EXCLUDES 1   filtering (vitreous) bleb after glaucoma surgery status (Z98.83)

H59.40 Inflammation (infection) of postprocedural bleb, unspecified

H59.41 Inflammation (infection) of postprocedural bleb, stage 1

H59.42 Inflammation (infection) of postprocedural bleb, stage 2

H59.43 Inflammation (infection) of postprocedural bleb, stage 3

Bleb endophthalmitis

√5th **H59.8** Other intraoperative and postprocedural complications and disorders of eye and adnexa, not elsewhere classified

√6th **H59.81** Chorioretinal scars after surgery for detachment

H59.811 Chorioretinal scars after surgery for detachment, right eye

H59.812 Chorioretinal scars after surgery for detachment, left eye

H59.813 Chorioretinal scars after surgery for detachment, bilateral

H59.819 Chorioretinal scars after surgery for detachment, unspecified eye

H59.88 Other intraoperative complications of eye and adnexa, not elsewhere classified

H59.89 Other postprocedural complications and disorders of eye and adnexa, not elsewhere classified

EXCLUDES 1 Not coded here   EXCLUDES 2 Not included here   N Newborn Age: 0   P Pediatric Age: 0-17   M Maternity Age: 12-55   A Adult Age: 15-124

558   ICD-10-CM 2014 (Draft)

Chapter 8. Diseases of the Ear and Mastoid Process (H60-H95)

> **NOTE** Use an external cause code following the code for the ear condition, if applicable, to identify the cause of the ear condition.
>
> **EXCLUDES 2** *certain conditions originating in the perinatal period (P04-P96)*
> *certain infectious and parasitic diseases (A00-B99)*
> *complications of pregnancy, childbirth and the puerperium (O00-O9A)*
> *congenital malformations, deformations and chromosomal abnormalities (Q00-Q99)*
> *endocrine, nutritional and metabolic diseases (E00-E88)*
> *injury, poisoning and certain other consequences of external causes (S00-T88)*
> *neoplasms (C00-D49)*
> *symptoms, signs and abnormal clinical and laboratory findings, not elsewhere classified (R00-R94)*

This chapter contains the following blocks:
H60-H62 Diseases of external ear
H65-H75 Diseases of middle ear and mastoid
H80-H83 Diseases of inner ear
H90-H94 Other disorders of ear
H95 Intraoperative and postprocedural complications and disorders of ear and mastoid process, not elsewhere classified

Diseases of external ear (H60-H62)

√4th **H60 Otitis externa**

√5th **H60.0 Abscess of external ear**
Boil of external ear
Carbuncle of auricle or external auditory canal
Furuncle of external ear

H60.00 Abscess of external ear, unspecified ear
H60.01 Abscess of right external ear
H60.02 Abscess of left external ear
H60.03 Abscess of external ear, bilateral

√5th **H60.1 Cellulitis of external ear**
Cellulitis of auricle
Cellulitis of external auditory canal

H60.10 Cellulitis of external ear, unspecified ear
H60.11 Cellulitis of right external ear
H60.12 Cellulitis of left external ear
H60.13 Cellulitis of external ear, bilateral

√5th **H60.2 Malignant otitis externa**
H60.20 Malignant otitis externa, unspecified ear
H60.21 Malignant otitis externa, right ear
H60.22 Malignant otitis externa, left ear
H60.23 Malignant otitis externa, bilateral

√5th **H60.3 Other infective otitis externa**

√6th **H60.31 Diffuse otitis externa**
H60.311 Diffuse otitis externa, right ear
H60.312 Diffuse otitis externa, left ear
H60.313 Diffuse otitis externa, bilateral
H60.319 Diffuse otitis externa, unspecified ear

√6th **H60.32 Hemorrhagic otitis externa**
H60.321 Hemorrhagic otitis externa, right ear
H60.322 Hemorrhagic otitis externa, left ear
H60.323 Hemorrhagic otitis externa, bilateral
H60.329 Hemorrhagic otitis externa, unspecified ear

√6th **H60.33 Swimmer's ear**
H60.331 Swimmer's ear, right ear
H60.332 Swimmer's ear, left ear
H60.333 Swimmer's ear, bilateral
H60.339 Swimmer's ear, unspecified ear

√6th **H60.39 Other infective otitis externa**
H60.391 Other infective otitis externa, right ear
H60.392 Other infective otitis externa, left ear
H60.393 Other infective otitis externa, bilateral
H60.399 Other infective otitis externa, unspecified ear

√5th **H60.4 Cholesteatoma of external ear**
Keratosis obturans of external ear (canal)
> **EXCLUDES 2** *cholesteatoma of middle ear (H71.-)*
> *recurrent cholesteatoma of postmastoidectomy cavity (H95.0-)*

H60.40 Cholesteatoma of external ear, unspecified ear

H60.41 Cholesteatoma of right external ear
H60.42 Cholesteatoma of left external ear
H60.43 Cholesteatoma of external ear, bilateral

√5th **H60.5 Acute noninfective otitis externa**

√6th **H60.50 Unspecified acute noninfective otitis externa**
Acute otitis externa NOS
H60.501 Unspecified acute noninfective otitis externa, right ear
H60.502 Unspecified acute noninfective otitis externa, left ear
H60.503 Unspecified acute noninfective otitis externa, bilateral
H60.509 Unspecified acute noninfective otitis externa, unspecified ear

√6th **H60.51 Acute actinic otitis externa**
H60.511 Acute actinic otitis externa, right ear
H60.512 Acute actinic otitis externa, left ear
H60.513 Acute actinic otitis externa, bilateral
H60.519 Acute actinic otitis externa, unspecified ear

√6th **H60.52 Acute chemical otitis externa**
H60.521 Acute chemical otitis externa, right ear
H60.522 Acute chemical otitis externa, left ear
H60.523 Acute chemical otitis externa, bilateral
H60.529 Acute chemical otitis externa, unspecified ear

√6th **H60.53 Acute contact otitis externa**
H60.531 Acute contact otitis externa, right ear
H60.532 Acute contact otitis externa, left ear
H60.533 Acute contact otitis externa, bilateral
H60.539 Acute contact otitis externa, unspecified ear

√6th **H60.54 Acute eczematoid otitis externa**
H60.541 Acute eczematoid otitis externa, right ear
H60.542 Acute eczematoid otitis externa, left ear
H60.543 Acute eczematoid otitis externa, bilateral
H60.549 Acute eczematoid otitis externa, unspecified ear

√6th **H60.55 Acute reactive otitis externa**
H60.551 Acute reactive otitis externa, right ear
H60.552 Acute reactive otitis externa, left ear
H60.553 Acute reactive otitis externa, bilateral
H60.559 Acute reactive otitis externa, unspecified ear

√6th **H60.59 Other noninfective acute otitis externa**
H60.591 Other noninfective acute otitis externa, right ear
H60.592 Other noninfective acute otitis externa, left ear
H60.593 Other noninfective acute otitis externa, bilateral
H60.599 Other noninfective acute otitis externa, unspecified ear

√5th **H60.6 Unspecified chronic otitis externa**
H60.60 Unspecified chronic otitis externa, unspecified ear
H60.61 Unspecified chronic otitis externa, right ear
H60.62 Unspecified chronic otitis externa, left ear
H60.63 Unspecified chronic otitis externa, bilateral

√5th **H60.8 Other otitis externa**
√6th **H60.8X Other otitis externa**
H60.8X1 Other otitis externa, right ear
H60.8X2 Other otitis externa, left ear
H60.8X3 Other otitis externa, bilateral
H60.8X9 Other otitis externa, unspecified ear

√5th **H60.9 Unspecified otitis externa**
H60.90 Unspecified otitis externa, unspecified ear
H60.91 Unspecified otitis externa, right ear
H60.92 Unspecified otitis externa, left ear
H60.93 Unspecified otitis externa, bilateral

☑ Additional Character Required   √7th Xtension Alert   Unspecified Code   Other Specified Code   Manifestation Code   ►◄ Revised Text   ● New Code   ▲ Revised Code Title

H61 Other disorders of external ear

H61.0 Chondritis and perichondritis of external ear
Chondrodermatitis nodularis chronica helicis
Perichondritis of auricle
Perichondritis of pinna

H61.00 Unspecified perichondritis of external ear
H61.001 Unspecified perichondritis of right external ear
H61.002 Unspecified perichondritis of left external ear
H61.003 Unspecified perichondritis of external ear, bilateral
H61.009 Unspecified perichondritis of external ear, unspecified ear

H61.01 Acute perichondritis of external ear
H61.011 Acute perichondritis of right external ear
H61.012 Acute perichondritis of left external ear
H61.013 Acute perichondritis of external ear, bilateral
H61.019 Acute perichondritis of external ear, unspecified ear

H61.02 Chronic perichondritis of external ear
H61.021 Chronic perichondritis of right external ear
H61.022 Chronic perichondritis of left external ear
H61.023 Chronic perichondritis of external ear, bilateral
H61.029 Chronic perichondritis of external ear, unspecified ear

H61.03 Chondritis of external ear
Chondritis of auricle
Chondritis of pinna
H61.031 Chondritis of right external ear
H61.032 Chondritis of left external ear
H61.033 Chondritis of external ear, bilateral
H61.039 Chondritis of external ear, unspecified ear

H61.1 Noninfective disorders of pinna
EXCLUDES 2   cauliflower ear (M95.1-)
gouty tophi of ear (M1A.-)

H61.10 Unspecified noninfective disorders of pinna
Disorder of pinna NOS
H61.101 Unspecified noninfective disorders of pinna, right ear
H61.102 Unspecified noninfective disorders of pinna, left ear
H61.103 Unspecified noninfective disorders of pinna, bilateral
H61.109 Unspecified noninfective disorders of pinna, unspecified ear

H61.11 Acquired deformity of pinna
Acquired deformity of auricle
EXCLUDES 2   cauliflower ear (M95.1-)
H61.111 Acquired deformity of pinna, right ear
H61.112 Acquired deformity of pinna, left ear
H61.113 Acquired deformity of pinna, bilateral
H61.119 Acquired deformity of pinna, unspecified ear

H61.12 Hematoma of pinna
Hematoma of auricle
H61.121 Hematoma of pinna, right ear
H61.122 Hematoma of pinna, left ear
H61.123 Hematoma of pinna, bilateral
H61.129 Hematoma of pinna, unspecified ear

H61.19 Other noninfective disorders of pinna
H61.191 Noninfective disorders of pinna, right ear
H61.192 Noninfective disorders of pinna, left ear
H61.193 Noninfective disorders of pinna, bilateral
H61.199 Noninfective disorders of pinna, unspecified ear

H61.2 Impacted cerumen
Wax in ear
H61.20 Impacted cerumen, unspecified ear
H61.21 Impacted cerumen, right ear
H61.22 Impacted cerumen, left ear
H61.23 Impacted cerumen, bilateral

H61.3 Acquired stenosis of external ear canal
Collapse of external ear canal
EXCLUDES 1   postprocedural stenosis of external ear canal (H95.81-)

H61.30 Acquired stenosis of external ear canal, unspecified
H61.301 Acquired stenosis of right external ear canal, unspecified
H61.302 Acquired stenosis of left external ear canal, unspecified
H61.303 Acquired stenosis of external ear canal, unspecified, bilateral
H61.309 Acquired stenosis of external ear canal, unspecified, unspecified ear

H61.31 Acquired stenosis of external ear canal secondary to trauma
H61.311 Acquired stenosis of right external ear canal secondary to trauma
H61.312 Acquired stenosis of left external ear canal secondary to trauma
H61.313 Acquired stenosis of external ear canal secondary to trauma, bilateral
H61.319 Acquired stenosis of external ear canal secondary to trauma, unspecified ear

H61.32 Acquired stenosis of external ear canal secondary to inflammation and infection
H61.321 Acquired stenosis of right external ear canal secondary to inflammation and infection
H61.322 Acquired stenosis of left external ear canal secondary to inflammation and infection
H61.323 Acquired stenosis of external ear canal secondary to inflammation and infection, bilateral
H61.329 Acquired stenosis of external ear canal secondary to inflammation and infection, unspecified ear

H61.39 Other acquired stenosis of external ear canal
H61.391 Other acquired stenosis of right external ear canal
H61.392 Other acquired stenosis of left external ear canal
H61.393 Other acquired stenosis of external ear canal, bilateral
H61.399 Other acquired stenosis of external ear canal, unspecified ear

H61.8 Other specified disorders of external ear

H61.81 Exostosis of external canal
H61.811 Exostosis of right external canal
H61.812 Exostosis of left external canal
H61.813 Exostosis of external canal, bilateral
H61.819 Exostosis of external canal, unspecified ear

H61.89 Other specified disorders of external ear
H61.891 Other specified disorders of right external ear
H61.892 Other specified disorders of left external ear
H61.893 Other specified disorders of external ear, bilateral
H61.899 Other specified disorders of external ear, unspecified ear

H61.9 Disorder of external ear, unspecified
H61.90 Disorder of external ear, unspecified, unspecified ear
H61.91 Disorder of right external ear, unspecified
H61.92 Disorder of left external ear, unspecified
H61.93 Disorder of external ear, unspecified, bilateral

H62 Disorders of external ear in diseases classified elsewhere

H62.4 Otitis externa in other diseases classified elsewhere
Code first underlying disease, such as:
erysipelas (A46)
impetigo (L01.0)
EXCLUDES 1   otitis externa (in):
candidiasis (B37.84)
herpes viral [herpes simplex] (B00.1)
herpes zoster (B02.8)

H62.40 Otitis externa in other diseases classified elsewhere, unspecified ear

EXCLUDES 1 Not coded here   EXCLUDES 2 Not included here   N Newborn Age: 0   P Pediatric Age: 0-17   M Maternity Age: 12-55   A Adult Age: 15-124

560   ICD-10-CM 2014 (Draft)

H62.41   *Otitis externa in other diseases classified elsewhere, right ear*

H62.42   *Otitis externa in other diseases classified elsewhere, left ear*

H62.43   *Otitis externa in other diseases classified elsewhere, bilateral*

√5th **H62.8** **Other disorders of external ear in diseases classified elsewhere**

Code first underlying disease, such as:
gout (M1A-, M10.-)

√6th **H62.8X** **Other disorders of external ear in diseases classified elsewhere**

H62.8X1   *Other disorders of right external ear in diseases classified elsewhere*

H62.8X2   *Other disorders of left external ear in diseases classified elsewhere*

H62.8X3   *Other disorders of external ear in diseases classified elsewhere, bilateral*

H62.8X9   *Other disorders of external ear in diseases classified elsewhere, unspecified ear*

Diseases of middle ear and mastoid (H65-H75)

√4th **H65** **Nonsuppurative otitis media**

INCLUDES   nonsuppurative otitis media with myringitis

Use additional code for any associated perforated tympanic membrane (H72.-)

Use additional code to identify:
exposure to environmental tobacco smoke (Z77.22)
exposure to tobacco smoke in the perinatal period (P96.81)
history of tobacco use (Z87.891)
occupational exposure to environmental tobacco smoke (Z57.31)
tobacco dependence (F17.-)
tobacco use (Z72.0)

√5th **H65.0** **Acute serous otitis media**

Acute and subacute secretory otitis

H65.00   **Acute serous otitis media, unspecified ear**

H65.01   **Acute serous otitis media, right ear**

H65.02   **Acute serous otitis media, left ear**

H65.03   **Acute serous otitis media, bilateral**

H65.04   **Acute serous otitis media, recurrent, right ear**

H65.05   **Acute serous otitis media, recurrent, left ear**

H65.06   **Acute serous otitis media, recurrent, bilateral**

H65.07   **Acute serous otitis media, recurrent, unspecified ear**

√5th **H65.1** **Other acute nonsuppurative otitis media**

EXCLUDES 1   *otitic barotrauma (T70.0)*
otitis media (acute) NOS (H66.9)

√6th **H65.11** **Acute and subacute allergic otitis media (mucoid) (sanguinous) (serous)**

H65.111   **Acute and subacute allergic otitis media (mucoid) (sanguinous) (serous), right ear**

H65.112   **Acute and subacute allergic otitis media (mucoid) (sanguinous) (serous), left ear**

H65.113   **Acute and subacute allergic otitis media (mucoid) (sanguinous) (serous), bilateral**

H65.114   **Acute and subacute allergic otitis media (mucoid) (sanguinous) (serous), recurrent, right ear**

H65.115   **Acute and subacute allergic otitis media (mucoid) (sanguinous) (serous), recurrent, left ear**

H65.116   **Acute and subacute allergic otitis media (mucoid) (sanguinous) (serous), recurrent, bilateral**

H65.117   **Acute and subacute allergic otitis media (mucoid) (sanguinous) (serous), recurrent, unspecified ear**

H65.119   **Acute and subacute allergic otitis media (mucoid) (sanguinous) (serous), unspecified ear**

√6th **H65.19** **Other acute nonsuppurative otitis media**

Acute and subacute mucoid otitis media
Acute and subacute nonsuppurative otitis media NOS
Acute and subacute sanguinous otitis media
Acute and subacute seromucinous otitis media

H65.191   **Other acute nonsuppurative otitis media, right ear**

H65.192   **Other acute nonsuppurative otitis media, left ear**

H65.193   **Other acute nonsuppurative otitis media, bilateral**

H65.194   **Other acute nonsuppurative otitis media, recurrent, right ear**

H65.195   **Other acute nonsuppurative otitis media, recurrent, left ear**

H65.196   **Other acute nonsuppurative otitis media, recurrent, bilateral**

H65.197   **Other acute nonsuppurative otitis media recurrent, unspecified ear**

H65.199   **Other acute nonsuppurative otitis media, unspecified ear**

√5th **H65.2** **Chronic serous otitis media**

Chronic tubotympanic catarrh

H65.20   **Chronic serous otitis media, unspecified ear**

H65.21   **Chronic serous otitis media, right ear**

H65.22   **Chronic serous otitis media, left ear**

H65.23   **Chronic serous otitis media, bilateral**

√5th **H65.3** **Chronic mucoid otitis media**

Chronic mucinous otitis media
Chronic secretory otitis media
Glue ear
Chronic transudative otitis media

EXCLUDES 1   *adhesive middle ear disease (H74.1)*

H65.30   **Chronic mucoid otitis media, unspecified ear**

H65.31   **Chronic mucoid otitis media, right ear**

H65.32   **Chronic mucoid otitis media, left ear**

H65.33   **Chronic mucoid otitis media, bilateral**

√5th **H65.4** **Other chronic nonsuppurative otitis media**

√6th **H65.41** **Chronic allergic otitis media**

H65.411   **Chronic allergic otitis media, right ear**

H65.412   **Chronic allergic otitis media, left ear**

H65.413   **Chronic allergic otitis media, bilateral**

H65.419   **Chronic allergic otitis media, unspecified ear**

√6th **H65.49** **Other chronic nonsuppurative otitis media**

Chronic exudative otitis media
Chronic nonsuppurative otitis media NOS
Chronic otitis media with effusion (nonpurulent)
Chronic seromucinous otitis media

H65.491   **Other chronic nonsuppurative otitis media, right ear**

H65.492   **Other chronic nonsuppurative otitis media, left ear**

H65.493   **Other chronic nonsuppurative otitis media, bilateral**

H65.499   **Other chronic nonsuppurative otitis media, unspecified ear**

√5th **H65.9** **Unspecified nonsuppurative otitis media**

Allergic otitis media NOS
Catarrhal otitis media NOS
Exudative otitis media NOS
Mucoid otitis media NOS
Otitis media with effusion (nonpurulent) NOS

Secretory otitis media NOS
Seromucinous otitis media NOS
Serous otitis media NOS
Transudative otitis media NOS

H65.90   **Unspecified nonsuppurative otitis media, unspecified ear**

H65.91   **Unspecified nonsuppurative otitis media, right ear**

H65.92   **Unspecified nonsuppurative otitis media, left ear**

H65.93   **Unspecified nonsuppurative otitis media, bilateral**

√4th **H66** **Suppurative and unspecified otitis media**

INCLUDES   suppurative and unspecified otitis media with myringitis

Use additional code to identify:
exposure to environmental tobacco smoke (Z77.22)
exposure to tobacco smoke in the perinatal period (P96.81)
history of tobacco use (Z87.891)
occupational exposure to environmental tobacco smoke (Z57.31)
tobacco dependence (F17.-)
tobacco use (Z72.0)

√5th **H66.0** **Acute suppurative otitis media**

√6th **H66.00** **Acute suppurative otitis media without spontaneous rupture of ear drum**

H66.001   **Acute suppurative otitis media without spontaneous rupture of ear drum, right ear**

☑ Additional Character Required   √x7th Xtension Alert   Unspecified Code   Other Specified Code   Manifestation Code   ►◄ Revised Text   ● New Code   ▲ Revised Code Title

ICD-10-CM 2014 (Draft)   **561**

Diseases of the Ear and Mastoid Process

H66.002–H68.112

H66.002 Acute suppurative otitis media without spontaneous rupture of ear drum, left ear

H66.003 Acute suppurative otitis media without spontaneous rupture of ear drum, bilateral

H66.004 Acute suppurative otitis media without spontaneous rupture of ear drum, recurrent, right ear

H66.005 Acute suppurative otitis media without spontaneous rupture of ear drum, recurrent, left ear

H66.006 Acute suppurative otitis media without spontaneous rupture of ear drum, recurrent, bilateral

H66.007 Acute suppurative otitis media without spontaneous rupture of ear drum, recurrent, unspecified ear

H66.009 Acute suppurative otitis media without spontaneous rupture of ear drum, unspecified ear

√6ᵗʰ **H66.01** Acute suppurative otitis media with spontaneous rupture of ear drum

H66.011 Acute suppurative otitis media with spontaneous rupture of ear drum, right ear

H66.012 Acute suppurative otitis media with spontaneous rupture of ear drum, left ear

H66.013 Acute suppurative otitis media with spontaneous rupture of ear drum, bilateral

H66.014 Acute suppurative otitis media with spontaneous rupture of ear drum, recurrent, right ear

H66.015 Acute suppurative otitis media with spontaneous rupture of ear drum, recurrent, left ear

H66.016 Acute suppurative otitis media with spontaneous rupture of ear drum, recurrent, bilateral

H66.017 Acute suppurative otitis media with spontaneous rupture of ear drum, recurrent, unspecified ear

H66.019 Acute suppurative otitis media with spontaneous rupture of ear drum, unspecified ear

√5ᵗʰ **H66.1** Chronic tubotympanic suppurative otitis media
Benign chronic suppurative otitis media
Chronic tubotympanic disease
Use additional code for any associated perforated tympanic membrane (H72.-)

H66.10 Chronic tubotympanic suppurative otitis media, unspecified

H66.11 Chronic tubotympanic suppurative otitis media, right ear

H66.12 Chronic tubotympanic suppurative otitis media, left ear

H66.13 Chronic tubotympanic suppurative otitis media, bilateral

√5ᵗʰ **H66.2** Chronic atticoantral suppurative otitis media
Chronic atticoantral disease
Use additional code for any associated perforated tympanic membrane (H72.-)

H66.20 Chronic atticoantral suppurative otitis media, unspecified ear

H66.21 Chronic atticoantral suppurative otitis media, right ear

H66.22 Chronic atticoantral suppurative otitis media, left ear

H66.23 Chronic atticoantral suppurative otitis media, bilateral

√5ᵗʰ **H66.3** Other chronic suppurative otitis media
Chronic suppurative otitis media NOS
Use additional code for any associated perforated tympanic membrane (H72.-)
EXCLUDES 1   tuberculous otitis media (A18.6)

√6ᵗʰ **H66.3X** Other chronic suppurative otitis media

H66.3X1 Other chronic suppurative otitis media, right ear

H66.3X2 Other chronic suppurative otitis media, left ear

H66.3X3 Other chronic suppurative otitis media, bilateral

H66.3X9 Other chronic suppurative otitis media, unspecified ear

√5ᵗʰ **H66.4** Suppurative otitis media, unspecified
Purulent otitis media NOS
Use additional code for any associated perforated tympanic membrane (H72.-)

H66.40 Suppurative otitis media, unspecified, unspecified ear

H66.41 Suppurative otitis media, unspecified, right ear

H66.42 Suppurative otitis media, unspecified, left ear

H66.43 Suppurative otitis media, unspecified, bilateral

√5ᵗʰ **H66.9** Otitis media, unspecified
Otitis media NOS
Acute otitis media NOS
Chronic otitis media NOS
Use additional code for any associated perforated tympanic membrane (H72.-)

H66.90 Otitis media, unspecified, unspecified ear

H66.91 Otitis media, unspecified, right ear

H66.92 Otitis media, unspecified, left ear

H66.93 Otitis media, unspecified, bilateral

√4ᵗʰ **H67** Otitis media in diseases classified elsewhere
Code first underlying disease, such as:
viral disease NEC (B00-B34)
Use additional code for any associated perforated tympanic membrane (H72.-)
EXCLUDES 1   otitis media in:
influenza (J09.X9, J10.83, J11.83)
measles (B05.3)
scarlet fever (A38.0)
tuberculosis (A18.6)

H67.1 Otitis media in diseases classified elsewhere, right ear

H67.2 Otitis media in diseases classified elsewhere, left ear

H67.3 Otitis media in diseases classified elsewhere, bilateral

H67.9 Otitis media in diseases classified elsewhere, unspecified ear

√4ᵗʰ **H68** Eustachian salpingitis and obstruction

√5ᵗʰ **H68.0** Eustachian salpingitis

√6ᵗʰ **H68.00** Unspecified Eustachian salpingitis

H68.001 Unspecified Eustachian salpingitis, right ear

H68.002 Unspecified Eustachian salpingitis, left ear

H68.003 Unspecified Eustachian salpingitis, bilateral

H68.009 Unspecified Eustachian salpingitis, unspecified ear

√6ᵗʰ **H68.01** Acute Eustachian salpingitis

H68.011 Acute Eustachian salpingitis, right ear

H68.012 Acute Eustachian salpingitis, left ear

H68.013 Acute Eustachian salpingitis, bilateral

H68.019 Acute Eustachian salpingitis, unspecified ear

√6ᵗʰ **H68.02** Chronic Eustachian salpingitis

H68.021 Chronic Eustachian salpingitis, right ear

H68.022 Chronic Eustachian salpingitis, left ear

H68.023 Chronic Eustachian salpingitis, bilateral

H68.029 Chronic Eustachian salpingitis, unspecified ear

√5ᵗʰ **H68.1** Obstruction of Eustachian tube
Stenosis of Eustachian tube   Stricture of Eustachian tube

√6ᵗʰ **H68.10** Unspecified obstruction of Eustachian tube

H68.101 Unspecified obstruction of Eustachian tube, right ear

H68.102 Unspecified obstruction of Eustachian tube, left ear

H68.103 Unspecified obstruction of Eustachian tube, bilateral

H68.109 Unspecified obstruction of Eustachian tube, unspecified ear

√6ᵗʰ **H68.11** Osseous obstruction of Eustachian tube

H68.111 Osseous obstruction of Eustachian tube, right ear

H68.112 Osseous obstruction of Eustachian tube, left ear

EXCLUDES 1 Not coded here   EXCLUDES 2 Not included here   N Newborn Age: 0   P Pediatric Age: 0-17   M Maternity Age: 12-55   A Adult Age: 15-124

562   ICD-10-CM 2014 (Draft)

H68.113 Osseous obstruction of Eustachian tube, bilateral

H68.119 **Osseous obstruction of Eustachian tube, unspecified ear**

√6th H68.12 **Intrinsic cartilagenous obstruction of Eustachian tube**

H68.121 **Intrinsic cartilagenous obstruction of Eustachian tube, right ear**

H68.122 **Intrinsic cartilagenous obstruction of Eustachian tube, left ear**

H68.123 **Intrinsic cartilagenous obstruction of Eustachian tube, bilateral**

H68.129 **Intrinsic cartilagenous obstruction of Eustachian tube, unspecified ear**

√6th H68.13 **Extrinsic cartilagenous obstruction of Eustachian tube**
Compression of Eustachian tube

H68.131 **Extrinsic cartilagenous obstruction of Eustachian tube, right ear**

H68.132 **Extrinsic cartilagenous obstruction of Eustachian tube, left ear**

H68.133 **Extrinsic cartilagenous obstruction of Eustachian tube, bilateral**

H68.139 **Extrinsic cartilagenous obstruction of Eustachian tube, unspecified ear**

√4th H69 **Other and unspecified disorders of Eustachian tube**

√5th H69.0 Patulous Eustachian tube

H69.00 Patulous Eustachian tube, unspecified ear

H69.01 Patulous Eustachian tube, right ear

H69.02 Patulous Eustachian tube, left ear

H69.03 Patulous Eustachian tube, bilateral

√5th H69.8 Other specified disorders of Eustachian tube

H69.80 **Other specified disorders of Eustachian tube, unspecified ear**

H69.81 **Other specified disorders of Eustachian tube, right ear**

H69.82 **Other specified disorders of Eustachian tube, left ear**

H69.83 **Other specified disorders of Eustachian tube, bilateral**

√5th H69.9 Unspecified Eustachian tube disorder

H69.90 **Unspecified Eustachian tube disorder, unspecified ear**

H69.91 Unspecified Eustachian tube disorder, right ear

H69.92 Unspecified Eustachian tube disorder, left ear

H69.93 **Unspecified Eustachian tube disorder, bilateral**

√4th H70 **Mastoiditis and related conditions**

√5th H70.0 Acute mastoiditis
Abscess of mastoid
Empyema of mastoid

√6th H70.00 **Acute mastoiditis without complications**

H70.001 **Acute mastoiditis without complications, right ear**

H70.002 **Acute mastoiditis without complications, left ear**

H70.003 **Acute mastoiditis without complications, bilateral**

H70.009 **Acute mastoiditis without complications, unspecified ear**

√6th H70.01 Subperiosteal abscess of mastoid

H70.011 Subperiosteal abscess of mastoid, right ear

H70.012 Subperiosteal abscess of mastoid, left ear

H70.013 **Subperiosteal abscess of mastoid, bilateral**

H70.019 **Subperiosteal abscess of mastoid, unspecified ear**

√6th H70.09 Acute mastoiditis with other complications

H70.091 Acute mastoiditis with other complications, right ear

H70.092 Acute mastoiditis with other complications, left ear

H70.093 Acute mastoiditis with other complications, bilateral

H70.099 **Acute mastoiditis with other complications, unspecified ear**

√5th H70.1 Chronic mastoiditis
Caries of mastoid
Fistula of mastoid
EXCLUDES 1 *tuberculous mastoiditis (A18.03)*

H70.10 **Chronic mastoiditis, unspecified ear**

H70.11 Chronic mastoiditis, right ear

H70.12 Chronic mastoiditis, left ear

H70.13 Chronic mastoiditis, bilateral

√5th H70.2 Petrositis
Inflammation of petrous bone

√6th H70.20 Unspecified petrositis

H70.201 Unspecified petrositis, right ear

H70.202 Unspecified petrositis, left ear

H70.203 Unspecified petrositis, bilateral

H70.209 **Unspecified petrositis, unspecified ear**

√6th H70.21 Acute petrositis

H70.211 Acute petrositis, right ear

H70.212 Acute petrositis, left ear

H70.213 Acute petrositis, bilateral

H70.219 **Acute petrositis, unspecified ear**

√6th H70.22 Chronic petrositis

H70.221 Chronic petrositis, right ear

H70.222 Chronic petrositis, left ear

H70.223 Chronic petrositis, bilateral

H70.229 **Chronic petrositis, unspecified ear**

√5th H70.8 Other mastoiditis and related conditions
EXCLUDES 1 *preauricular sinus and cyst (Q18.1)*
sinus, fistula, and cyst of branchial cleft (Q18.0)

√6th H70.81 Postauricular fistula

H70.811 Postauricular fistula, right ear

H70.812 Postauricular fistula, left ear

H70.813 Postauricular fistula, bilateral

H70.819 **Postauricular fistula, unspecified ear**

√6th H70.89 Other mastoiditis and related conditions

H70.891 **Other mastoiditis and related conditions, right ear**

H70.892 **Other mastoiditis and related conditions, left ear**

H70.893 **Other mastoiditis and related conditions, bilateral**

H70.899 **Other mastoiditis and related conditions, unspecified ear**

√5th H70.9 Unspecified mastoiditis

H70.90 **Unspecified mastoiditis, unspecified ear**

H70.91 **Unspecified mastoiditis, right ear**

H70.92 **Unspecified mastoiditis, left ear**

H70.93 **Unspecified mastoiditis, bilateral**

√4th H71 Cholesteatoma of middle ear
EXCLUDES 2 *cholesteatoma of external ear (H60.4-)*
recurrent cholesteatoma of postmastoidectomy cavity (H95.0-)

√5th H71.0 Cholesteatoma of attic

H71.00 **Cholesteatoma of attic, unspecified ear**

H71.01 **Cholesteatoma of attic, right ear**

H71.02 **Cholesteatoma of attic, left ear**

H71.03 **Cholesteatoma of attic, bilateral**

√5th H71.1 Cholesteatoma of tympanum

H71.10 **Cholesteatoma of tympanum, unspecified ear**

H71.11 Cholesteatoma of tympanum, right ear

H71.12 Cholesteatoma of tympanum, left ear

H71.13 Cholesteatoma of tympanum, bilateral

√5th H71.2 Cholesteatoma of mastoid

H71.20 **Cholesteatoma of mastoid, unspecified ear**

H71.21 Cholesteatoma of mastoid, right ear

H71.22 Cholesteatoma of mastoid, left ear

H71.23 Cholesteatoma of mastoid, bilateral

√5th H71.3 Diffuse cholesteatosis

H71.30 **Diffuse cholesteatosis, unspecified ear**

H71.31 Diffuse cholesteatosis, right ear

H71.32 Diffuse cholesteatosis, left ear

H71.33 Diffuse cholesteatosis, bilateral

☑ Additional Character Required   √x7th Xtension Alert   Unspecified Code   Other Specified Code   Manifestation Code   ►◄ Revised Text   ● New Code   ▲ Revised Code Title

✓5ᵗʰ **H71.9** Unspecified **cholesteatoma**
  H71.90 Unspecified cholesteatoma, unspecified ear
  H71.91 Unspecified cholesteatoma, right ear
  H71.92 Unspecified cholesteatoma, left ear
  H71.93 Unspecified cholesteatoma, bilateral

✓4ᵗʰ **H72** **Perforation of tympanic membrane**
  INCLUDES   persistent post-traumatic perforation of ear drum
         postinflammatory perforation of ear drum
  Code first any associated otitis media (H65.-, H66.1-, H66.2-, H66.3-,
    H66.4-, H66.9-, H67-)
  EXCLUDES 1   acute suppurative otitis media with rupture of the tympanic
         membrane (H66.01-)
         traumatic rupture of ear drum (S09.2-)

✓5ᵗʰ **H72.0** Central **perforation of tympanic membrane**
  H72.00 **Central perforation of tympanic membrane, unspecified ear**
  H72.01 Central perforation of tympanic membrane, right ear
  H72.02 Central perforation of tympanic membrane, left ear
  H72.03 Central perforation of tympanic membrane, bilateral

✓5ᵗʰ **H72.1** Attic **perforation of tympanic membrane**
  Perforation of pars flaccida
  H72.10 **Attic perforation of tympanic membrane, unspecified ear**
  H72.11 Attic perforation of tympanic membrane, right ear
  H72.12 Attic perforation of tympanic membrane, left ear
  H72.13 Attic perforation of tympanic membrane, bilateral

✓5ᵗʰ **H72.2** Other marginal perforations of tympanic membrane
  ✓6ᵗʰ **H72.2X** Other marginal **perforations of tympanic membrane**
    H72.2X1 **Other marginal perforations of tympanic membrane, right ear**
    H72.2X2 **Other marginal perforations of tympanic membrane, left ear**
    H72.2X3 **Other marginal perforations of tympanic membrane, bilateral**
    H72.2X9 **Other marginal perforations of tympanic membrane, unspecified ear**

✓5ᵗʰ **H72.8** Other perforations of tympanic membrane
  ✓6ᵗʰ **H72.81** Multiple **perforations of tympanic membrane**
    H72.811 **Multiple perforations of tympanic membrane, right ear**
    H72.812 **Multiple perforations of tympanic membrane, left ear**
    H72.813 **Multiple perforations of tympanic membrane, bilateral**
    H72.819 **Multiple perforations of tympanic membrane, unspecified ear**
  ✓6ᵗʰ **H72.82** Total **perforations of tympanic membrane**
    H72.821 **Total perforations of tympanic membrane, right ear**
    H72.822 **Total perforations of tympanic membrane, left ear**
    H72.823 **Total perforations of tympanic membrane, bilateral**
    H72.829 **Total perforations of tympanic membrane, unspecified ear**

✓5ᵗʰ **H72.9** Unspecified **perforation of tympanic membrane**
  H72.90 **Unspecified perforation of tympanic membrane, unspecified ear**
  H72.91 **Unspecified perforation of tympanic membrane, right ear**
  H72.92 **Unspecified perforation of tympanic membrane, left ear**
  H72.93 **Unspecified perforation of tympanic membrane, bilateral**

✓4ᵗʰ **H73** **Other disorders of tympanic membrane**
  ✓5ᵗʰ **H73.0** Acute **myringitis**
    EXCLUDES 1   acute myringitis with otitis media (H65, H66)
    ✓6ᵗʰ **H73.00** Unspecified **acute myringitis**
      Acute tympanitis NOS
      H73.001 Acute myringitis, right ear
      H73.002 Acute myringitis, left ear
      H73.003 Acute myringitis, bilateral
      H73.009 **Acute myringitis, unspecified ear**

  ✓6ᵗʰ **H73.01** Bullous **myringitis**
    H73.011 Bullous myringitis, right ear
    H73.012 Bullous myringitis, left ear
    H73.013 Bullous myringitis, bilateral
    H73.019 **Bullous myringitis, unspecified ear**
  ✓6ᵗʰ **H73.09** Other **acute myringitis**
    H73.091 **Other acute myringitis, right ear**
    H73.092 **Other acute myringitis, left ear**
    H73.093 **Other acute myringitis, bilateral**
    H73.099 **Other acute myringitis, unspecified ear**

✓5ᵗʰ **H73.1** Chronic **myringitis**
  Chronic tympanitis
  EXCLUDES 1   chronic myringitis with otitis media (H65, H66)
  H73.10 **Chronic myringitis, unspecified ear**
  H73.11 **Chronic myringitis, right ear**
  H73.12 **Chronic myringitis, left ear**
  H73.13 **Chronic myringitis, bilateral**

✓5ᵗʰ **H73.2** Unspecified **myringitis**
  H73.20 **Unspecified myringitis, unspecified ear**
  H73.21 **Unspecified myringitis, right ear**
  H73.22 **Unspecified myringitis, left ear**
  H73.23 **Unspecified myringitis, bilateral**

✓5ᵗʰ **H73.8** Other specified disorders of tympanic membrane
  ✓6ᵗʰ **H73.81** Atrophic flaccid **tympanic membrane**
    H73.811 **Atrophic flaccid tympanic membrane, right ear**
    H73.812 **Atrophic flaccid tympanic membrane, left ear**
    H73.813 **Atrophic flaccid tympanic membrane, bilateral**
    H73.819 **Atrophic flaccid tympanic membrane, unspecified ear**
  ✓6ᵗʰ **H73.82** Atrophic nonflaccid **tympanic membrane**
    H73.821 **Atrophic nonflaccid tympanic membrane, right ear**
    H73.822 **Atrophic nonflaccid tympanic membrane, left ear**
    H73.823 **Atrophic nonflaccid tympanic membrane, bilateral**
    H73.829 **Atrophic nonflaccid tympanic membrane, unspecified ear**
  ✓6ᵗʰ **H73.89** Other specified disorders of tympanic membrane
    H73.891 **Other specified disorders of tympanic membrane, right ear**
    H73.892 **Other specified disorders of tympanic membrane, left ear**
    H73.893 **Other specified disorders of tympanic membrane, bilateral**
    H73.899 **Other specified disorders of tympanic membrane, unspecified ear**

✓5ᵗʰ **H73.9** Unspecified disorder of tympanic membrane
  H73.90 **Unspecified disorder of tympanic membrane, unspecified ear**
  H73.91 **Unspecified disorder of tympanic membrane, right ear**
  H73.92 **Unspecified disorder of tympanic membrane, left ear**
  H73.93 **Unspecified disorder of tympanic membrane, bilateral**

✓4ᵗʰ **H74** **Other disorders of middle ear mastoid**
  EXCLUDES 2   mastoiditis (H70.-)
  ✓5ᵗʰ **H74.0** Tympanosclerosis
    H74.01 Tympanosclerosis, right ear
    H74.02 Tympanosclerosis, left ear
    H74.03 Tympanosclerosis, bilateral
    H74.09 **Tympanosclerosis, unspecified ear**
  ✓5ᵗʰ **H74.1** Adhesive middle ear disease
    Adhesive otitis
    EXCLUDES 1   glue ear (H65.3-)
    H74.11 Adhesive right middle ear disease
    H74.12 Adhesive left middle ear disease
    H74.13 Adhesive middle ear disease, bilateral
    H74.19 **Adhesive middle ear disease, unspecified ear**

✓5ᵗʰ **H74.2 Discontinuity and dislocation of ear ossicles**
- H74.20 **Discontinuity and dislocation of ear ossicles, unspecified ear**
- H74.21 **Discontinuity and dislocation of right ear ossicles**
- H74.22 **Discontinuity and dislocation of left ear ossicles**
- H74.23 **Discontinuity and dislocation of ear ossicles, bilateral**

✓5ᵗʰ **H74.3 Other acquired abnormalities of ear ossicles**
- ✓6ᵗʰ H74.31 **Ankylosis of ear ossicles**
  - H74.311 **Ankylosis of ear ossicles, right ear**
  - H74.312 **Ankylosis of ear ossicles, left ear**
  - H74.313 **Ankylosis of ear ossicles, bilateral**
  - H74.319 **Ankylosis of ear ossicles, unspecified ear**
- ✓6ᵗʰ H74.32 **Partial loss of ear ossicles**
  - H74.321 **Partial loss of ear ossicles, right ear**
  - H74.322 **Partial loss of ear ossicles, left ear**
  - H74.323 **Partial loss of ear ossicles, bilateral**
  - H74.329 **Partial loss of ear ossicles, unspecified ear**
- ✓6ᵗʰ H74.39 **Other acquired abnormalities of ear ossicles**
  - H74.391 **Other acquired abnormalities of right ear ossicles**
  - H74.392 **Other acquired abnormalities of left ear ossicles**
  - H74.393 **Other acquired abnormalities of ear ossicles, bilateral**
  - H74.399 **Other acquired abnormalities of ear ossicles, unspecified ear**

✓5ᵗʰ **H74.4 Polyp of middle ear**
- H74.40 **Polyp of middle ear, unspecified ear**
- H74.41 **Polyp of right middle ear**
- H74.42 **Polyp of left middle ear**
- H74.43 **Polyp of middle ear, bilateral**

✓5ᵗʰ **H74.8 Other specified disorders of middle ear and mastoid**
- ✓6ᵗʰ H74.8X **Other specified disorders of middle ear and mastoid**
  - H74.8X1 **Other specified disorders of right middle ear and mastoid**
  - H74.8X2 **Other specified disorders of left middle ear and mastoid**
  - H74.8X3 **Other specified disorders of middle ear and mastoid, bilateral**
  - H74.8X9 **Other specified disorders of middle ear and mastoid, unspecified ear**

✓5ᵗʰ **H74.9 Unspecified disorder of middle ear and mastoid**
- H74.90 **Unspecified disorder of middle ear and mastoid, unspecified ear**
- H74.91 **Unspecified disorder of right middle ear and mastoid**
- H74.92 **Unspecified disorder of left middle ear and mastoid**
- H74.93 **Unspecified disorder of middle ear and mastoid, bilateral**

✓4ᵗʰ **H75 Other disorders of middle ear and mastoid in diseases classified elsewhere**
Code first underlying disease

✓5ᵗʰ **H75.0 Mastoiditis in infectious and parasitic diseases classified elsewhere**
EXCLUDES 1   mastoiditis (in):
 syphilis (A52.77)
 tuberculosis (A18.03)
- H75.00 *Mastoiditis in infectious and parasitic diseases classified elsewhere, unspecified ear*
- H75.01 *Mastoiditis in infectious and parasitic diseases classified elsewhere, right ear*
- H75.02 *Mastoiditis in infectious and parasitic diseases classified elsewhere, left ear*
- H75.03 *Mastoiditis in infectious and parasitic diseases classified elsewhere, bilateral*

✓5ᵗʰ **H75.8 Other specified disorders of middle ear and mastoid in diseases classified elsewhere**
- H75.80 *Other specified disorders of middle ear and mastoid in diseases classified elsewhere, unspecified ear*
- H75.81 *Other specified disorders of right middle ear and mastoid in diseases classified elsewhere*
- H75.82 *Other specified disorders of left middle ear and mastoid in diseases classified elsewhere*
- H75.83 *Other specified disorders of middle ear and mastoid in diseases classified elsewhere, bilateral*

Diseases of inner ear (H80-H83)

✓4ᵗʰ **H80 Otosclerosis**
INCLUDES   Otospongiosis

✓5ᵗʰ **H80.0 Otosclerosis involving oval window, nonobliterative**
- H80.00 **Otosclerosis involving oval window, nonobliterative, unspecified ear**
- H80.01 **Otosclerosis involving oval window, nonobliterative, right ear**
- H80.02 **Otosclerosis involving oval window, nonobliterative, left ear**
- H80.03 **Otosclerosis involving oval window, nonobliterative, bilateral**

✓5ᵗʰ **H80.1 Otosclerosis involving oval window, obliterative**
- H80.10 **Otosclerosis involving oval window, obliterative, unspecified ear**
- H80.11 **Otosclerosis involving oval window, obliterative, right ear**
- H80.12 **Otosclerosis involving oval window, obliterative, left ear**
- H80.13 **Otosclerosis involving oval window, obliterative, bilateral**

✓5ᵗʰ **H80.2 Cochlear otosclerosis**
Otosclerosis involving otic capsule
Otosclerosis involving round window
- H80.20 **Cochlear otosclerosis, unspecified ear**
- H80.21 **Cochlear otosclerosis, right ear**
- H80.22 **Cochlear otosclerosis, left ear**
- H80.23 **Cochlear otosclerosis, bilateral**

✓5ᵗʰ **H80.8 Other otosclerosis**
- H80.80 **Other otosclerosis, unspecified ear**
- H80.81 **Other otosclerosis, right ear**
- H80.82 **Other otosclerosis, left ear**
- H80.83 **Other otosclerosis, bilateral**

✓5ᵗʰ **H80.9 Unspecified otosclerosis**
- H80.90 **Unspecified otosclerosis, unspecified ear**
- H80.91 **Unspecified otosclerosis, right ear**
- H80.92 **Unspecified otosclerosis, left ear**
- H80.93 **Unspecified otosclerosis, bilateral**

✓4ᵗʰ **H81 Disorders of vestibular function**
EXCLUDES 1   epidemic vertigo (A88.1)
 vertigo NOS (R42)

✓5ᵗʰ **H81.0 Ménière's disease**
Labyrinthine hydrops
Ménière's syndrome or vertigo
- H81.01 **Ménière's disease, right ear**
- H81.02 **Ménière's disease, left ear**
- H81.03 **Ménière's disease, bilateral**
- H81.09 **Ménière's disease, unspecified ear**

✓5ᵗʰ **H81.1 Benign paroxysmal vertigo**
- H81.10 **Benign paroxysmal vertigo, unspecified ear**
- H81.11 **Benign paroxysmal vertigo, right ear**
- H81.12 **Benign paroxysmal vertigo, left ear**
- H81.13 **Benign paroxysmal vertigo, bilateral**

✓5ᵗʰ **H81.2 Vestibular neuronitis**
- H81.20 **Vestibular neuronitis, unspecified ear**
- H81.21 **Vestibular neuronitis, right ear**
- H81.22 **Vestibular neuronitis, left ear**
- H81.23 **Vestibular neuronitis, bilateral**

✓5ᵗʰ **H81.3 Other peripheral vertigo**
- ✓6ᵗʰ H81.31 **Aural vertigo**
  - H81.311 **Aural vertigo, right ear**
  - H81.312 **Aural vertigo, left ear**
  - H81.313 **Aural vertigo, bilateral**
  - H81.319 **Aural vertigo, unspecified ear**
- ✓6ᵗʰ H81.39 **Other peripheral vertigo**
  Lermoyez' syndrome
  Otogenic vertigo
  Peripheral vertigo NOS
  - H81.391 **Other peripheral vertigo, right ear**

Diseases of the Ear and Mastoid Process

H81.392–H91.21

         H81.392   **Other peripheral vertigo, left ear**
         H81.393   **Other peripheral vertigo, bilateral**
         H81.399   **Other peripheral vertigo, unspecified ear**

✓5th **H81.4 Vertigo of central origin**
     Central positional nystagmus
         H81.41   **Vertigo of central origin, right ear**
         H81.42   **Vertigo of central origin, left ear**
         H81.43   **Vertigo of central origin, bilateral**
         H81.49   **Vertigo of central origin, unspecified ear**

✓5th **H81.8 Other disorders of vestibular function**
     ✓6th **H81.8X Other disorders of vestibular function**
         H81.8X1   **Other disorders of vestibular function, right ear**
         H81.8X2   **Other disorders of vestibular function, left ear**
         H81.8X3   **Other disorders of vestibular function, bilateral**
         H81.8X9   **Other disorders of vestibular function, unspecified ear**

✓5th **H81.9 Unspecified disorder of vestibular function**
     Vertiginous syndrome NOS
         H81.90   **Unspecified disorder of vestibular function, unspecified ear**
         H81.91   **Unspecified disorder of vestibular function, right ear**
         H81.92   **Unspecified disorder of vestibular function, left ear**
         H81.93   **Unspecified disorder of vestibular function, bilateral**

✓4th **H82 Vertiginous syndromes in diseases classified elsewhere**
     Code first underlying disease
     EXCLUDES 1 *epidemic vertigo (A88.1)*
     H82.1 Vertiginous syndromes in diseases classified elsewhere, right ear
     H82.2 Vertiginous syndromes in diseases classified elsewhere, left ear
     H82.3 Vertiginous syndromes in diseases classified elsewhere, bilateral
     H82.9 Vertiginous syndromes in diseases classified elsewhere, unspecified ear

✓4th **H83 Other diseases of inner ear**
     ✓5th **H83.0 Labyrinthitis**
         H83.01   **Labyrinthitis, right ear**
         H83.02   **Labyrinthitis, left ear**
         H83.03   **Labyrinthitis, bilateral**
         H83.09   **Labyrinthitis, unspecified ear**

     ✓5th **H83.1 Labyrinthine fistula**
         H83.11   **Labyrinthine fistula, right ear**
         H83.12   **Labyrinthine fistula, left ear**
         H83.13   **Labyrinthine fistula, bilateral**
         H83.19   **Labyrinthine fistula, unspecified ear**

     ✓5th **H83.2 Labyrinthine dysfunction**
     Labyrinthine hypersensitivity
     Labyrinthine hypofunction
     Labyrinthine loss of function
     ✓6th **H83.2X Labyrinthine dysfunction**
         H83.2X1   **Labyrinthine dysfunction, right ear**
         H83.2X2   **Labyrinthine dysfunction, left ear**
         H83.2X3   **Labyrinthine dysfunction, bilateral**
         H83.2X9   **Labyrinthine dysfunction, unspecified ear**

     ✓5th **H83.3 Noise effects on inner ear**
     Acoustic trauma of inner ear
     Noise-induced hearing loss of inner ear
     ✓6th **H83.3X Noise effects on inner ear**
         H83.3X1   **Noise effects on right inner ear**
         H83.3X2   **Noise effects on left inner ear**
         H83.3X3   **Noise effects on inner ear, bilateral**
         H83.3X9   **Noise effects on inner ear, unspecified ear**

     ✓5th **H83.8 Other specified diseases of inner ear**
     ✓6th **H83.8X Other specified diseases of inner ear**
         H83.8X1   **Other specified diseases of right inner ear**
         H83.8X2   **Other specified diseases of left inner ear**
         H83.8X3   **Other specified diseases of inner ear, bilateral**
         H83.8X9   **Other specified diseases of inner ear, unspecified ear**

✓5th **H83.9 Unspecified disease of inner ear**
         H83.90   **Unspecified disease of inner ear, unspecified ear**
         H83.91   **Unspecified disease of right inner ear**
         H83.92   **Unspecified disease of left inner ear**
         H83.93   **Unspecified disease of inner ear, bilateral**

Other disorders of ear (H90-H94)

✓4th **H90 Conductive and sensorineural hearing loss**
     EXCLUDES 1 *deaf nonspeaking NEC (H91.3)*
         deafness NOS (H91.9-)
         hearing loss NOS (H91.9-)
         noise-induced hearing loss (H83.3-)
         ototoxic hearing loss (H91.0-)
         sudden (idiopathic) hearing loss (H91.2-)
     H90.0 Conductive hearing loss, bilateral

     ✓5th **H90.1 Conductive hearing loss, unilateral with unrestricted hearing on the contralateral side**
         H90.11   **Conductive hearing loss, unilateral, right ear, with unrestricted hearing on the contralateral side**
         H90.12   **Conductive hearing loss, unilateral, left ear, with unrestricted hearing on the contralateral side**

     H90.2 Conductive hearing loss, unspecified
     Conductive deafness NOS

     H90.3 Sensorineural hearing loss, bilateral

     ✓5th **H90.4 Sensorineural hearing loss, unilateral with unrestricted hearing on the contralateral side**
         H90.41   **Sensorineural hearing loss, unilateral, right ear, with unrestricted hearing on the contralateral side**
         H90.42   **Sensorineural hearing loss, unilateral, left ear, with unrestricted hearing on the contralateral side**

     H90.5 Unspecified sensorineural hearing loss
     Central hearing loss NOS
     Congenital deafness NOS
     Neural hearing loss NOS
     Perceptive hearing loss NOS
     Sensorineural deafness NOS
     Sensory hearing loss NOS
     EXCLUDES 1 *abnormal auditory perception (H93.2-)*
         psychogenic deafness (F44.6)

     H90.6 Mixed conductive and sensorineural hearing loss, bilateral

     ✓5th **H90.7 Mixed conductive and sensorineural hearing loss, unilateral with unrestricted hearing on the contralateral side**
         H90.71   **Mixed conductive and sensorineural hearing loss, unilateral, right ear, with unrestricted hearing on the contralateral side**
         H90.72   **Mixed conductive and sensorineural hearing loss, unilateral, left ear, with unrestricted hearing on the contralateral side**

     H90.8 Mixed conductive and sensorineural hearing loss, unspecified

✓4th **H91 Other and unspecified hearing loss**
     EXCLUDES 1 *abnormal auditory perception (H93.2-)*
         hearing loss as classified in H90-
         impacted cerumen (H61.2-)
         noise-induced hearing loss (H83.3-)
         psychogenic deafness (F44.6)
         transient ischemic deafness (H93.01-)

     ✓5th **H91.0 Ototoxic hearing loss**
     Code first poisoning due to drug or toxin, if applicable (T36-T65 with fifth or sixth character 1-4 or 6)
     Use additional code for adverse effect, if applicable, to identify drug (T36-T50 with fifth or sixth character 5)
         H91.01   **Ototoxic hearing loss, right ear**
         H91.02   **Ototoxic hearing loss, left ear**
         H91.03   **Ototoxic hearing loss, bilateral**
         H91.09   **Ototoxic hearing loss, unspecified ear**

     ✓5th **H91.1 Presbycusis**
     Presbyacusia
         H91.10   **Presbycusis, unspecified ear**
         H91.11   **Presbycusis, right ear**
         H91.12   **Presbycusis, left ear**
         H91.13   **Presbycusis, bilateral**

     ✓5th **H91.2 Sudden idiopathic hearing loss**
     Sudden hearing loss NOS
         H91.20   **Sudden idiopathic hearing loss, unspecified ear**
         H91.21   **Sudden idiopathic hearing loss, right ear**

EXCLUDES 1 Not coded here   **EXCLUDES 2** Not included here   N Newborn Age: 0   P Pediatric Age: 0-17   M Maternity Age: 12-55   A Adult Age: 15-124

566   ICD-10-CM 2014 (Draft)

H91.22 **Sudden idiopathic hearing loss,** left ear
H91.23 **Sudden idiopathic hearing loss,** bilateral
H91.3 **Deaf nonspeaking, not elsewhere classified**
☑5ᵗʰ H91.8 **Other specified hearing loss**
 ☑6ᵗʰ H91.8X **Other specified hearing loss**
 H91.8X1 **Other specified hearing loss,** right ear
 H91.8X2 **Other specified hearing loss,** left ear
 H91.8X3 **Other specified hearing loss,** bilateral
 H91.8X9 **Other specified hearing loss, unspecified ear**
☑5ᵗʰ H91.9 **Unspecified hearing loss**
 Deafness NOS
 High frequency deafness
 Low frequency deafness
 H91.90 **Unspecified hearing loss, unspecified ear**
 H91.91 **Unspecified hearing loss,** right ear
 H91.92 **Unspecified hearing loss,** left ear
 H91.93 **Unspecified hearing loss,** bilateral
☑4ᵗʰ H92 **Otalgia and effusion of ear**
 ☑5ᵗʰ H92.0 **Otalgia**
 H92.01 **Otalgia,** right ear
 H92.02 **Otalgia,** left ear
 H92.03 **Otalgia,** bilateral
 H92.09 **Otalgia, unspecified ear**
 ☑5ᵗʰ H92.1 **Otorrhea**
 EXCLUDES 1 *leakage of cerebrospinal fluid through ear (G96.0)*
 H92.10 **Otorrhea, unspecified ear**
 H92.11 **Otorrhea,** right ear
 H92.12 **Otorrhea,** left ear
 H92.13 **Otorrhea,** bilateral
 ☑5ᵗʰ H92.2 **Otorrhagia**
 EXCLUDES 1 *traumatic otorrhagia—code to injury*
 H92.20 **Otorrhagia, unspecified ear**
 H92.21 **Otorrhagia,** right ear
 H92.22 **Otorrhagia,** left ear
 H92.23 **Otorrhagia,** bilateral
☑4ᵗʰ H93 **Other disorders of ear, not elsewhere classified**
 ☑5ᵗʰ H93.0 **Degenerative and vascular disorders of ear**
 EXCLUDES 1 *presbycusis (H91.1)*
 ☑6ᵗʰ H93.01 **Transient ischemic deafness**
 H93.011 **Transient ischemic deafness,** right ear
 H93.012 **Transient ischemic deafness,** left ear
 H93.013 **Transient ischemic deafness,** bilateral
 H93.019 **Transient ischemic deafness, unspecified ear**
 ☑6ᵗʰ H93.09 **Unspecified degenerative and vascular disorders of ear**
 H93.091 **Unspecified degenerative and vascular disorders of** right **ear**
 H93.092 **Unspecified degenerative and vascular disorders of** left **ear**
 H93.093 **Unspecified degenerative and vascular disorders of ear,** bilateral
 H93.099 **Unspecified degenerative and vascular disorders of unspecified ear**
 ☑5ᵗʰ H93.1 **Tinnitus**
 H93.11 **Tinnitus,** right ear
 H93.12 **Tinnitus,** left ear
 H93.13 **Tinnitus,** bilateral
 H93.19 **Tinnitus, unspecified ear**
 ☑5ᵗʰ H93.2 **Other abnormal auditory perceptions**
 EXCLUDES 2 *auditory hallucinations (R44.0)*
 ☑6ᵗʰ H93.21 **Auditory recruitment**
 H93.211 **Auditory recruitment,** right ear
 H93.212 **Auditory recruitment,** left ear
 H93.213 **Auditory recruitment,** bilateral
 H93.219 **Auditory recruitment, unspecified ear**
 ☑6ᵗʰ H93.22 **Diplacusis**
 H93.221 **Diplacusis,** right ear
 H93.222 **Diplacusis,** left ear
 H93.223 **Diplacusis,** bilateral

H93.229 **Diplacusis, unspecified ear**
☑6ᵗʰ H93.23 **Hyperacusis**
 H93.231 **Hyperacusis,** right ear
 H93.232 **Hyperacusis,** left ear
 H93.233 **Hyperacusis,** bilateral
 H93.239 **Hyperacusis, unspecified ear**
☑6ᵗʰ H93.24 **Temporary auditory threshold shift**
 H93.241 **Temporary auditory threshold shift,** right ear
 H93.242 **Temporary auditory threshold shift,** left ear
 H93.243 **Temporary auditory threshold shift,** bilateral
 H93.249 **Temporary auditory threshold shift, unspecified ear**
 H93.25 **Central auditory processing disorder**
 Congenital auditory imperception
 Word deafness
 EXCLUDES 1 *mixed receptive-expressive language disorder (F80.2)*
☑6ᵗʰ H93.29 **Other abnormal auditory perceptions**
 H93.291 **Other abnormal auditory perceptions,** right **ear**
 H93.292 **Other abnormal auditory perceptions,** left **ear**
 H93.293 **Other abnormal auditory perceptions,** bilateral
 H93.299 **Other abnormal auditory perceptions, unspecified ear**
☑5ᵗʰ H93.3 **Disorders of acoustic nerve**
 Disorder of 8th cranial nerve
 EXCLUDES 1 *acoustic neuroma (D33.3)*
 syphilitic acoustic neuritis (A52.15)
 ☑6ᵗʰ H93.3X **Disorders of acoustic nerve**
 H93.3X1 **Disorders of** right **acoustic nerve**
 H93.3X2 **Disorders of** left **acoustic nerve**
 H93.3X3 **Disorders of** bilateral **acoustic nerves**
 H93.3X9 **Disorders of unspecified acoustic nerve**
☑5ᵗʰ H93.8 **Other specified disorders of ear**
 ☑6ᵗʰ H93.8X **Other specified disorders of ear**
 H93.8X1 **Other specified disorders of** right **ear**
 H93.8X2 **Other specified disorders of** left **ear**
 H93.8X3 **Other specified disorders of ear,** bilateral
 H93.8X9 **Other specified disorders of ear, unspecified ear**
☑5ᵗʰ H93.9 **Unspecified disorder of ear**
 H93.90 **Unspecified disorder of ear, unspecified ear**
 H93.91 **Unspecified disorder of** right **ear**
 H93.92 **Unspecified disorder of** left **ear**
 H93.93 **Unspecified disorder of ear,** bilateral
☑4ᵗʰ H94 **Other disorders of ear in diseases classified elsewhere**
 ☑5ᵗʰ H94.0 **Acoustic neuritis in infectious and parasitic diseases classified elsewhere**
 Code first underlying disease, such as:
 parasitic disease (B65-B89)
 EXCLUDES 1 *acoustic neuritis (in):*
 herpes zoster (B02.29)
 syphilis (A52.15)
 H94.00 *Acoustic neuritis in infectious and parasitic diseases classified elsewhere, unspecified ear*
 H94.01 *Acoustic neuritis in infectious and parasitic diseases classified elsewhere, right ear*
 H94.02 *Acoustic neuritis in infectious and parasitic diseases classified elsewhere, left ear*
 H94.03 *Acoustic neuritis in infectious and parasitic diseases classified elsewhere, bilateral*
 ☑5ᵗʰ H94.8 **Other specified disorders of ear in diseases classified elsewhere**
 Code first underlying disease, such as:
 congenital syphilis (A50.0)
 EXCLUDES 1 *aural myiasis (B87.4)*
 syphilitic labyrinthitis (A52.79)
 H94.80 *Other specified disorders of ear in diseases classified elsewhere, unspecified ear*

H94.81   *Other specified disorders of right ear in diseases classified elsewhere*

H94.82   *Other specified disorders of left ear in diseases classified elsewhere*

H94.83   *Other specified disorders of ear in diseases classified elsewhere, bilateral*

Intraoperative and postprocedural complications and disorders of ear and mastoid process, not elsewhere classified (H95)

✓4th **H95   Intraoperative and postprocedural complications and disorders of ear and mastoid process, not elsewhere classified**

✓5th **H95.0   Recurrent cholesteatoma of postmastoidectomy cavity**

    H95.00   **Recurrent cholesteatoma of postmastoidectomy cavity, unspecified ear**

    H95.01   **Recurrent cholesteatoma of postmastoidectomy cavity, right ear**

    H95.02   **Recurrent cholesteatoma of postmastoidectomy cavity, left ear**

    H95.03   **Recurrent cholesteatoma of postmastoidectomy cavity, bilateral ears**

✓5th **H95.1   Other disorders of ear and mastoid process following mastoidectomy**

  ✓6th **H95.11   Chronic inflammation of postmastoidectomy cavity**

    H95.111   **Chronic inflammation of postmastoidectomy cavity, right ear**

    H95.112   **Chronic inflammation of postmastoidectomy cavity, left ear**

    H95.113   **Chronic inflammation of postmastoidectomy cavity, bilateral ears**

    H95.119   **Chronic inflammation of postmastoidectomy cavity, unspecified ear**

  ✓6th **H95.12   Granulation of postmastoidectomy cavity**

    H95.121   **Granulation of postmastoidectomy cavity, right ear**

    H95.122   **Granulation of postmastoidectomy cavity, left ear**

    H95.123   **Granulation of postmastoidectomy cavity, bilateral ears**

    H95.129   **Granulation of postmastoidectomy cavity, unspecified ear**

  ✓6th **H95.13   Mucosal cyst of postmastoidectomy cavity**

    H95.131   **Mucosal cyst of postmastoidectomy cavity, right ear**

    H95.132   **Mucosal cyst of postmastoidectomy cavity, left ear**

    H95.133   **Mucosal cyst of postmastoidectomy cavity, bilateral ears**

    H95.139   **Mucosal cyst of postmastoidectomy cavity, unspecified ear**

  ✓6th **H95.19   Other disorders following mastoidectomy**

    H95.191   **Other disorders following mastoidectomy, right ear**

    H95.192   **Other disorders following mastoidectomy, left ear**

    H95.193   **Other disorders following mastoidectomy, bilateral ears**

    H95.199   **Other disorders following mastoidectomy, unspecified ear**

✓5th **H95.2   Intraoperative hemorrhage and hematoma of ear and mastoid process complicating a procedure**

    EXCLUDES 1   *intraoperative hemorrhage and hematoma of ear and mastoid process due to accidental puncture or laceration during a procedure (H95.3-)*

    H95.21   **Intraoperative hemorrhage and hematoma of ear and mastoid process complicating a procedure on the ear and mastoid process**

    H95.22   **Intraoperative hemorrhage and hematoma of ear and mastoid process complicating other procedure**

✓5th **H95.3   Accidental puncture and laceration of ear and mastoid process during a procedure**

    H95.31   **Accidental puncture and laceration of the ear and mastoid process during a procedure on the ear and mastoid process**

    H95.32   **Accidental puncture and laceration of the ear and mastoid process during other procedure**

✓5th **H95.4   Postprocedural hemorrhage and hematoma of ear and mastoid process following a procedure**

    H95.41   **Postprocedural hemorrhage and hematoma of ear and mastoid process following a procedure on the ear and mastoid process**

    H95.42   **Postprocedural hemorrhage and hematoma of ear and mastoid process following other procedure**

✓5th **H95.8   Other intraoperative and postprocedural complications and disorders of the ear and mastoid process, not elsewhere classified**

    EXCLUDES 2   *postprocedural complications and disorders following mastoidectomy (H95.0-, H95.1-)*

  ✓6th **H95.81   Postprocedural stenosis of external ear canal**

    H95.811   **Postprocedural stenosis of right external ear canal**

    H95.812   **Postprocedural stenosis of left external ear canal**

    H95.813   **Postprocedural stenosis of external ear canal, bilateral**

    H95.819   **Postprocedural stenosis of unspecified external ear canal**

    H95.88   **Other intraoperative complications and disorders of the ear and mastoid process, not elsewhere classified**

      Use additional code, if applicable, to further specify disorder

    H95.89   **Other postprocedural complications and disorders of the ear and mastoid process, not elsewhere classified**

      Use additional code, if applicable, to further specify disorder

EXCLUDES 1 Not coded here   EXCLUDES 2 Not included here   N Newborn Age: 0   P Pediatric Age: 0-17   M Maternity Age: 12-55   A Adult Age: 15-124

568   ICD-10-CM 2014 (Draft)

Chapter 9. Diseases of the Circulatory System (I00-I99)

EXCLUDES 2   certain conditions originating in the perinatal period (P04-P96)
certain infectious and parasitic diseases (A00-B99)
complications of pregnancy, childbirth and the puerperium (O00-O9A)
congenital malformations, deformations, and chromosomal abnormalities (Q00-Q99)
endocrine, nutritional and metabolic diseases (E00-E88)
injury, poisoning and certain other consequences of external causes (S00-T88)
neoplasms (C00-D49)
symptoms, signs and abnormal clinical and laboratory findings, not elsewhere classified (R00-R94)
systemic connective tissue disorders (M30-M36)
transient cerebral ischemic attacks and related syndromes (G45.-)

This chapter contains the following blocks:
I00-I02   Acute rheumatic fever
I05-I09   Chronic rheumatic heart diseases
I10-I15   Hypertensive diseases
I20-I25   Ischemic heart diseases
I26-I28   Pulmonary heart disease and diseases of pulmonary circulation
I30-I52   Other forms of heart disease
I60-I69   Cerebrovascular diseases
I70-I79   Diseases of arteries, arterioles and capillaries
I80-I89   Diseases of veins, lymphatic vessels and lymph nodes, not elsewhere classified
I95-I99   Other and unspecified disorders of the circulatory system

Acute rheumatic fever (I00-I02)

I00   **Rheumatic fever without heart involvement**
    INCLUDES   arthritis, rheumatic, acute or subacute
    EXCLUDES 1   rheumatic fever with heart involvement (I01.0-I01.9)

✓4ᵗʰ **I01**   **Rheumatic fever with heart involvement**
    EXCLUDES 1   chronic diseases of rheumatic origin (I05-I09) unless rheumatic fever is also present or there is evidence of reactivation or activity of the rheumatic process.

   I01.0   **Acute rheumatic pericarditis**
     Any condition in I00 with pericarditis
     Rheumatic pericarditis (acute)
     EXCLUDES 1   acute pericarditis not specified as rheumatic (I30.-)

   I01.1   **Acute rheumatic endocarditis**
     Any condition in I00 with endocarditis or valvulitis
     Acute rheumatic valvulitis

   I01.2   **Acute rheumatic myocarditis**
     Any condition in I00 with myocarditis

   I01.8   **Other acute rheumatic heart disease**
     Any condition in I00 with other or multiple types of heart involvement
     Acute rheumatic pancarditis

   I01.9   **Acute rheumatic heart disease, unspecified**
     Any condition in I00 with unspecified type of heart involvement
     Rheumatic carditis, acute
     Rheumatic heart disease, active or acute

✓4ᵗʰ **I02**   **Rheumatic chorea**
    INCLUDES   Sydenham's chorea
    EXCLUDES 1   chorea NOS (G25.5)
              Huntington's chorea (G10)

   I02.0   **Rheumatic chorea with heart involvement**
     Chorea NOS with heart involvement
     Rheumatic chorea with heart involvement of any type classifiable under I01-

   I02.9   **Rheumatic chorea without heart involvement**
     Rheumatic chorea NOS

Chronic rheumatic heart diseases (I05-I09)

✓4ᵗʰ **I05**   **Rheumatic mitral valve diseases**
    INCLUDES   conditions classifiable to both I05.0 and I05.2-I05.9, whether specified as rheumatic or not
    EXCLUDES 1   mitral valve disease specified as nonrheumatic (I34.-)
            mitral valve disease with aortic and/or tricuspid valve involvement (I08.-)

   I05.0   **Rheumatic mitral stenosis**
     Mitral (valve) obstruction (rheumatic)

   I05.1   **Rheumatic mitral insufficiency**
     Rheumatic mitral incompetence
     Rheumatic mitral regurgitation
     EXCLUDES 1   mitral insufficiency not specified as rheumatic (I34.0)

   I05.2   **Rheumatic mitral stenosis with insufficiency**
     Rheumatic mitral stenosis with incompetence or regurgitation

   I05.8   **Other rheumatic mitral valve diseases**
     Rheumatic mitral (valve) failure

   I05.9   **Rheumatic mitral valve disease, unspecified**
     Rheumatic mitral (valve) disorder (chronic) NOS

✓4ᵗʰ **I06**   **Rheumatic aortic valve diseases**
    EXCLUDES 1   aortic valve disease not specified as rheumatic (I35.-)
            aortic valve disease with mitral and/or tricuspid valve involvement (I08.-)

   I06.0   **Rheumatic aortic stenosis**
     Rheumatic aortic (valve) obstruction

   I06.1   **Rheumatic aortic insufficiency**
     Rheumatic aortic incompetence
     Rheumatic aortic regurgitation

   I06.2   **Rheumatic aortic stenosis with insufficiency**
     Rheumatic aortic stenosis with incompetence or regurgitation

   I06.8   **Other rheumatic aortic valve diseases**

   I06.9   **Rheumatic aortic valve disease, unspecified**
     Rheumatic aortic (valve) disease NOS

✓4ᵗʰ **I07**   **Rheumatic tricuspid valve diseases**
    INCLUDES   rheumatic tricuspid valve diseases specified as rheumatic or unspecified
    EXCLUDES 1   tricuspid valve disease specified as nonrheumatic (I36.-)
            tricuspid valve disease with aortic and/or mitral valve involvement (I08.-)

   I07.0   **Rheumatic tricuspid stenosis**
     Tricuspid (valve) stenosis (rheumatic)

   I07.1   **Rheumatic tricuspid insufficiency**
     Tricuspid (valve) insufficiency (rheumatic)

   I07.2   **Rheumatic tricuspid stenosis and insufficiency**

   I07.8   **Other rheumatic tricuspid valve diseases**

   I07.9   **Rheumatic tricuspid valve disease, unspecified**
     Rheumatic tricuspid valve disorder NOS

✓4ᵗʰ **I08**   **Multiple valve diseases**
    INCLUDES   multiple valve diseases specified as rheumatic or unspecified
    EXCLUDES 1   endocarditis, valve unspecified (I38)
            multiple valve disease specified a nonrheumatic (I34.-, I35.-, I36.-, I37.-, I38.-, Q22.-, Q23.-, Q24.8-)
            rheumatic valve disease NOS (I09.1)

   I08.0   **Rheumatic disorders of both mitral and aortic valves**
     Involvement of both mitral and aortic valves specified as rheumatic or unspecified

   I08.1   **Rheumatic disorders of both mitral and tricuspid valves**

   I08.2   **Rheumatic disorders of both aortic and tricuspid valves**

   I08.3   **Combined rheumatic disorders of mitral, aortic and tricuspid valves**

   I08.8   **Other rheumatic multiple valve diseases**

   I08.9   **Rheumatic multiple valve disease, unspecified**

✓4ᵗʰ **I09**   **Other rheumatic heart diseases**
   I09.0   **Rheumatic myocarditis**
     EXCLUDES 1   myocarditis not specified as rheumatic (I51.4)

   I09.1   **Rheumatic diseases of endocardium, valve unspecified**
     Rheumatic endocarditis (chronic)
     Rheumatic valvulitis (chronic)
     EXCLUDES 1   endocarditis, valve unspecified (I38)

   I09.2   **Chronic rheumatic pericarditis**
     Adherent pericardium, rheumatic
     Chronic rheumatic mediastinopericarditis
     Chronic rheumatic myopericarditis
     EXCLUDES 1   chronic pericarditis not specified as rheumatic (I31.-)

✓5ᵗʰ   **I09.8**   **Other specified rheumatic heart diseases**
     I09.81   **Rheumatic heart failure**
       Use additional code to identify type of heart failure (I50.-)

     I09.89   **Other specified rheumatic heart diseases**
       Rheumatic disease of pulmonary valve

   I09.9   **Rheumatic heart disease, unspecified**
     Rheumatic carditis
     EXCLUDES 1   rheumatoid carditis (M05.31)

✓ Additional Character Required   ✓x7ᵗʰ Xtension Alert   Unspecified Code   Other Specified Code   Manifestation Code   ▶◀ Revised Text   ● New Code   ▲ Revised Code Title

Hypertensive diseases (I10-I15)

Use additional code to identify:
exposure to environmental tobacco smoke (Z77.22)
history of tobacco use (Z87.891)
occupational exposure to environmental tobacco smoke (Z57.31)
tobacco dependence (F17.-)
tobacco use (Z72.0)
EXCLUDES1 *hypertensive disease complicating pregnancy, childbirth and the puerperium (O10-O11, O13-O16)*
neonatal hypertension (P29.2)
primary pulmonary hypertension (I27.0)

I10 Essential (primary) hypertension
INCLUDES high blood pressure
hypertension (arterial) (benign) (essential) (malignant) (primary) (systemic)
EXCLUDES1 *hypertensive disease complicating pregnancy, childbirth and the puerperium (O10-O11, O13-O16)*
EXCLUDES2 *essential (primary) hypertension involving vessels of brain (I60-I69)*
essential (primary) hypertension involving vessels of eye (H35.0-)

✓4th **I11 Hypertensive heart disease**
INCLUDES any condition in I51.4-I51.9 due to hypertension

I11.0 Hypertensive heart disease with heart failure
Hypertensive heart failure
Use additional code to identify type of heart failure (I50.-)

I11.9 Hypertensive heart disease without heart failure
Hypertensive heart disease NOS

✓4th **I12 Hypertensive chronic kidney disease**
INCLUDES any condition in N18- and N26- due to hypertension
arteriosclerosis of kidney
arteriosclerotic nephritis (chronic) (interstitial)
hypertensive nephropathy
nephrosclerosis
EXCLUDES1 *hypertension due to kidney disease (I15.0, I15.1)*
renovascular hypertension (I15.0)
secondary hypertension (I15.-)
EXCLUDES2 *acute kidney failure (N17.-)*

I12.0 Hypertensive chronic kidney disease with stage 5 chronic kidney disease or end stage renal disease
Use additional code to identify the stage of chronic kidney disease (N18.5, N18.6)

I12.9 Hypertensive chronic kidney disease with stage 1 through stage 4 chronic kidney disease, or unspecified chronic kidney disease
Hypertensive chronic kidney disease NOS
Hypertensive renal disease NOS
Use additional code to identify the stage of chronic kidney disease (N18.1-N18.4, N18.9)

✓4th **I13 Hypertensive heart and chronic kidney disease**
INCLUDES any condition in I11- with any condition in I12-
cardiorenal disease
cardiovascular renal disease

I13.0 Hypertensive heart and chronic kidney disease with heart failure and stage 1 through stage 4 chronic kidney disease, or unspecified chronic kidney disease
Use additional code to identify type of heart failure (I50.-)
Use additional code to identify stage of chronic kidney disease (N18.1-N18.4, N18.9)

✓5th **I13.1 Hypertensive heart and chronic kidney disease without heart failure**

I13.10 Hypertensive heart and chronic kidney disease without heart failure, with stage 1 through stage 4 chronic kidney disease, or unspecified chronic kidney disease
Hypertensive heart disease and hypertensive chronic kidney disease NOS
Use additional code to identify the stage of chronic kidney disease (N18.1-N18.4, N18.9)

I13.11 Hypertensive heart and chronic kidney disease without heart failure, with stage 5 chronic kidney disease, or end stage renal disease
Use additional code to identify the stage of chronic kidney disease (N18.5, N18.6)

I13.2 Hypertensive heart and chronic kidney disease with heart failure and with stage 5 chronic kidney disease, or end stage renal disease
Use additional code to identify type of heart failure (I50.-)
Use additional code to identify the stage of chronic kidney disease (N18.5, N18.6)

✓4th **I15 Secondary hypertension**
Code also underlying condition
EXCLUDES1 *postprocedural hypertension (I97.3)*
EXCLUDES2 *secondary hypertension involving vessels of brain (I60-I69)*
secondary hypertension involving vessels of eye (H35.0-)

I15.0 Renovascular hypertension
I15.1 Hypertension secondary to other renal disorders
I15.2 Hypertension secondary to endocrine disorders
I15.8 Other secondary hypertension
I15.9 Secondary hypertension, unspecified

Ischemic heart diseases (I20-I25)

Use additional code to identify presence of hypertension (I10-I15)

✓4th **I20 Angina pectoris**
Use additional code to identify:
exposure to environmental tobacco smoke (Z77.22)
history of tobacco use (Z87.891)
occupational exposure to environmental tobacco smoke (Z57.31)
tobacco dependence (F17.-)
tobacco use (Z72.0)
EXCLUDES1 *angina pectoris with atherosclerotic heart disease of native coronary arteries (I25.1-)*
atherosclerosis of coronary artery bypass graft(s) and coronary artery of transplanted heart with angina pectoris (I25.7-)
postinfarction angina (I23.7)

I20.0 Unstable angina
Accelerated angina
Crescendo angina
De novo effort angina
Intermediate coronary syndrome
Preinfarction syndrome
Worsening effort angina

I20.1 Angina pectoris with documented spasm
Angiospastic angina
Prinzmetal angina
Spasm-induced angina
Variant angina

I20.8 Other forms of angina pectoris
Angina equivalent
Angina of effort
Coronary slow flow syndrome
Stenocardia
Use additional code(s) for symptoms associated with angina equivalent

I20.9 Angina pectoris, unspecified
Angina NOS
Anginal syndrome
Cardiac angina
Ischemic chest pain

✓4th **I21 ST elevation (STEMI) and non-ST elevation (NSTEMI) myocardial infarction**
INCLUDES cardiac infarction
coronary (artery) embolism
coronary (artery) occlusion
coronary (artery) rupture
coronary (artery) thrombosis
infarction of heart, myocardium, or ventricle
myocardial infarction specified as acute or with a stated duration of 4 weeks (28 days) or less from onset
Use additional code, if applicable, to identify:
exposure to environmental tobacco smoke (Z77.22)
history of tobacco use (Z87.891)
occupational exposure to environmental tobacco smoke (Z57.31)
status post administration of tPA (rtPA) in a different facility within the last 24 hours prior to admission to current facility (Z92.82)
tobacco dependence (F17.-)
tobacco use (Z72.0)
EXCLUDES2 *old myocardial infarction (I25.2)*
postmyocardial infarction syndrome (I24.1)
subsequent myocardial infarction (I22.-)
AHA: 2012, Q4, 96, 102-103

✓5th **I21.0 ST elevation (STEMI) myocardial infarction of anterior wall**

I21.01 ST elevation (STEMI) myocardial infarction involving left main coronary artery

I21.02 ST elevation (STEMI) myocardial infarction involving left anterior descending coronary artery
ST elevation (STEMI) myocardial infarction involving diagonal coronary artery

I21.09   **ST elevation (STEMI) myocardial infarction involving other coronary artery of anterior wall**
Acute transmural myocardial infarction of anterior wall
Anteroapical transmural (Q wave) infarction (acute)
Anterolateral transmural (Q wave) infarction (acute)
Anteroseptal transmural (Q wave) infarction (acute)
Transmural (Q wave) infarction (acute) (of) anterior (wall) NOS
AHA: 2012, Q4, 102-103

☑5ᵗʰ **I21.1**   **ST elevation (STEMI) myocardial infarction of inferior wall**

I21.11   **ST elevation (STEMI) myocardial infarction involving right coronary artery**
Inferoposterior transmural (Q wave) infarction (acute)

I21.19   **ST elevation (STEMI) myocardial infarction involving other coronary artery of inferior wall**
Acute transmural myocardial infarction of inferior wall
Inferolateral transmural (Q wave) infarction (acute)
Transmural (Q wave) infarction (acute) (of) diaphragmatic wall
Transmural (Q wave) infarction (acute) (of) inferior (wall) NOS
EXCLUDES 2   *ST elevation (STEMI) myocardial infarction involving left circumflex coronary artery (I21.21)*
AHA: 2012, Q4, 102

☑5ᵗʰ **I21.2**   **ST elevation (STEMI) myocardial infarction of other sites**

I21.21   **ST elevation (STEMI) myocardial infarction involving left circumflex coronary artery**
ST elevation (STEMI) myocardial infarction involving oblique marginal coronary artery

I21.29   **ST elevation (STEMI) myocardial infarction involving other sites**
Acute transmural myocardial infarction of other sites
Apical-lateral transmural (Q wave) infarction (acute)
Basal-lateral transmural (Q wave) infarction (acute)
High lateral transmural (Q wave) infarction (acute)
Lateral (wall) NOS transmural (Q wave) infarction (acute)
Posterior (true) transmural (Q wave) infarction (acute)
Posterobasal transmural (Q wave) infarction (acute)
Posterolateral transmural (Q wave) infarction (acute)
Posteroseptal transmural (Q wave) infarction (acute)
Septal transmural (Q wave) infarction (acute) NOS

I21.3   **ST elevation (STEMI) myocardial infarction of unspecified site**
Acute transmural myocardial infarction of unspecified site
Myocardial infarction (acute) NOS
Transmural (Q wave) myocardial infarction NOS

I21.4   **Non-ST elevation (NSTEMI) myocardial infarction**
Acute subendocardial myocardial infarction
Non-Q wave myocardial infarction NOS
Nontransmural myocardial infarction NOS

☑4ᵗʰ **I22**   **Subsequent ST elevation (STEMI) and non-ST elevation (NSTEMI) myocardial infarction**
INCLUDES   acute myocardial infarction occurring within four weeks (28 days) of a previous acute myocardial infarction, regardless of site
cardiac infarction
coronary (artery) embolism
coronary (artery) occlusion
coronary (artery) rupture
coronary (artery) thrombosis
infarction of heart, myocardium, or ventricle
recurrent myocardial infarction
reinfarction of myocardium
rupture of heart, myocardium, or ventricle
Use additional code, if applicable, to identify:
exposure to environmental tobacco smoke (Z77.22)
history of tobacco use (Z87.891)
occupational exposure to environmental tobacco smoke (Z57.31)
status post administration of tPA (rtPA) in a different facility within the last 24 hours prior to admission to current facility (Z92.82)
tobacco dependence (F17.-)
tobacco use (Z72.0)
AHA: 2012, Q4, 97, 102-103

I22.0   **Subsequent ST elevation (STEMI) myocardial infarction of anterior wall**
Subsequent acute transmural myocardial infarction of anterior wall
Subsequent transmural (Q wave) infarction (acute) (of) anterior (wall) NOS
Subsequent anteroapical transmural (Q wave) infarction (acute)
Subsequent anterolateral transmural (Q wave) infarction (acute)
Subsequent anteroseptal transmural (Q wave) infarction (acute)

I22.1   **Subsequent ST elevation (STEMI) myocardial infarction of inferior wall**
Subsequent acute transmural myocardial infarction of inferior wall
Subsequent transmural (Q wave) infarction (acute) (of) diaphragmatic wall
Subsequent transmural (Q wave) infarction (acute) (of) inferior (wall) NOS
Subsequent inferolateral transmural (Q wave) infarction (acute)
Subsequent inferoposterior transmural (Q wave) infarction (acute)
AHA: 2012, Q4, 102

I22.2   **Subsequent non-ST elevation (NSTEMI) myocardial infarction**
Subsequent acute subendocardial myocardial infarction
Subsequent non-Q wave myocardial infarction NOS
Subsequent nontransmural myocardial infarction NOS

I22.8   **Subsequent ST elevation (STEMI) myocardial infarction of other sites**
Subsequent acute transmural myocardial infarction of other sites
Subsequent apical-lateral transmural (Q wave) myocardial infarction (acute)
Subsequent basal-lateral transmural (Q wave) myocardial infarction (acute)
Subsequent high lateral transmural (Q wave) myocardial infarction (acute)
Subsequent transmural (Q wave) myocardial infarction (acute) (of) lateral (wall) NOS
Subsequent posterior (true) transmural (Q wave) myocardial infarction (acute)
Subsequent posterobasal transmural (Q wave) myocardial infarction (acute)
Subsequent posterolateral transmural (Q wave) myocardial infarction (acute)
Subsequent posteroseptal transmural (Q wave) myocardial infarction (acute)
Subsequent septal NOS transmural (Q wave) myocardial infarction (acute)

I22.9   **Subsequent ST elevation (STEMI) myocardial infarction of unspecified site**
Subsequent acute myocardial infarction of unspecified site
Subsequent myocardial infarction (acute) NOS

☑4ᵗʰ **I23**   **Certain current complications following ST elevation (STEMI) and non-ST elevation (NSTEMI) myocardial infarction (within the 28 day period)**

I23.0   **Hemopericardium as current complication following acute myocardial infarction**   🅰
EXCLUDES 1   *hemopericardium not specified as current complication following acute myocardial infarction (I31.2)*

I23.1   **Atrial septal defect as current complication following acute myocardial infarction**   🅰
EXCLUDES 1   *acquired atrial septal defect not specified as current complication following acute myocardial infarction (I51.0)*

I23.2   **Ventricular septal defect as current complication following acute myocardial infarction**   🅰
EXCLUDES 1   *acquired ventricular septal defect not specified as current complication following acute myocardial infarction (I51.0)*

I23.3   **Rupture of cardiac wall without hemopericardium as current complication following acute myocardial infarction**   🅰

I23.4   **Rupture of chordae tendineae as current complication following acute myocardial infarction**   🅰
EXCLUDES 1   *rupture of chordae tendineae not specified as current complication following acute myocardial infarction (I51.1)*

I23.5   **Rupture of papillary muscle as current complication following acute myocardial infarction**   🅰
EXCLUDES 1   *rupture of papillary muscle not specified as current complication following acute myocardial infarction (I51.2)*

I23.6   **Thrombosis of atrium, auricular appendage, and ventricle as current complications following acute myocardial infarction**   🅰
EXCLUDES 1   *thrombosis of atrium, auricular appendage, and ventricle not specified as current complication following acute myocardial infarction (I51.3)*

I23.7   **Postinfarction angina**   🅰

I23.8   **Other current complications following acute myocardial infarction**   🅰

Diseases of the Circulatory System

I24–I25.718

√4th **I24** **Other acute ischemic heart diseases**
  EXCLUDES 1   *angina pectoris (I20.-)*
           transient myocardial ischemia in newborn (P29.4)

I24.0 **Acute coronary thrombosis not resulting in myocardial infarction**
  Acute coronary (artery) (vein) embolism not resulting in myocardial infarction
  Acute coronary (artery) (vein) occlusion not resulting in myocardial infarction
  Acute coronary (artery) (vein) thromboembolism not resulting in myocardial infarction
  EXCLUDES 1   *atherosclerotic heart disease (I25.1-)*

I24.1 **Dressler's syndrome**
  Postmyocardial infarction syndrome
  EXCLUDES 1   *postinfarction angina (I23.7)*

I24.8 **Other forms of acute ischemic heart disease**

I24.9 **Acute ischemic heart disease, unspecified**
  EXCLUDES 1   *ischemic heart disease (chronic) NOS (I25.9)*

√4th **I25** **Chronic ischemic heart disease**
  Use additional code to identify:
  chronic total occlusion of coronary artery (I25.82)
  exposure to environmental tobacco smoke (Z77.22)
  history of tobacco use (Z87.891)
  occupational exposure to environmental tobacco smoke (Z57.31)
  tobacco dependence (F17.-)
  tobacco use (Z72.0)

I25.1 **Atherosclerotic heart disease of native coronary artery**
  Atherosclerotic cardiovascular disease
  Coronary (artery) atheroma
  Coronary (artery) atherosclerosis
  Coronary (artery) disease
  Coronary (artery) sclerosis
  Use additional code, if applicable, to identify:
  coronary atherosclerosis due to calcified coronary lesion (I25.84)
  coronary atherosclerosis due to lipid rich plaque (I25.83)
  EXCLUDES 2   *atheroembolism (I75.-)*
           atherosclerosis of coronary artery bypass graft(s) and transplanted heart (I25.7-)

  I25.10 **Atherosclerotic heart disease of native coronary artery without angina pectoris** A
      Atherosclerotic heart disease NOS
      AHA: 2012, Q4, 92

√6th **I25.11** **Atherosclerotic heart disease of native coronary artery with angina pectoris**
      I25.110 **Atherosclerotic heart disease of native coronary artery with unstable angina pectoris** A
        EXCLUDES 1   *unstable angina without atherosclerotic heart disease (I20.0)*
      I25.111 **Atherosclerotic heart disease of native coronary artery with angina pectoris with documented spasm** A
        EXCLUDES 1   *angina pectoris with documented spasm without atherosclerotic heart disease (I20.1)*
      I25.118 **Atherosclerotic heart disease of native coronary artery with other forms of angina pectoris** A
        EXCLUDES 1   *other forms of angina pectoris without atherosclerotic heart disease (I20.8)*
      I25.119 **Atherosclerotic heart disease of native coronary artery with unspecified angina pectoris** A
        Atherosclerotic heart disease with angina NOS
        Atherosclerotic heart disease with ischemic chest pain
        EXCLUDES 1   *unspecified angina pectoris without atherosclerotic heart disease (I20.9)*

I25.2 **Old myocardial infarction**
  Healed myocardial infarction
  Past myocardial infarction diagnosed by ECG or other investigation, but currently presenting no symptoms

I25.3 **Aneurysm of heart**
  Mural aneurysm
  Ventricular aneurysm

√5th **I25.4** **Coronary artery aneurysm and dissection**

  I25.41 **Coronary artery aneurysm**
      Coronary arteriovenous fistula, acquired
      EXCLUDES 1   *congenital coronary (artery) aneurysm (Q24.5)*

  I25.42 **Coronary artery dissection**

I25.5 **Ischemic cardiomyopathy**
  EXCLUDES 2   *coronary atherosclerosis (I25.1-, I25.7-)*

I25.6 **Silent myocardial ischemia**

√5th **I25.7** **Atherosclerosis of coronary artery bypass graft(s) and coronary artery of transplanted heart with angina pectoris**
  Use additional code, if applicable, to identify:
  coronary atherosclerosis due to calcified coronary lesion (I25.84)
  coronary atherosclerosis due to lipid rich plaque (I25.83)
  EXCLUDES 1   *atherosclerosis of bypass graft(s) of transplanted heart without angina pectoris (I25.812)*
       atherosclerosis of coronary artery bypass graft(s) without angina pectoris (I25.810)
       atherosclerosis of native coronary artery of transplanted heart without angina pectoris (I25.811)
       embolism or thrombus of coronary artery bypass graft(s) (T82.8-)

√6th **I25.70** **Atherosclerosis of coronary artery bypass graft(s), unspecified, with angina pectoris**
      I25.700 **Atherosclerosis of coronary artery bypass graft(s), unspecified, with unstable angina pectoris** A
        EXCLUDES 1   *unstable angina pectoris without atherosclerosis of coronary artery bypass graft (I20.0)*
      I25.701 **Atherosclerosis of coronary artery bypass graft(s), unspecified, with angina pectoris with documented spasm** A
        EXCLUDES 1   *angina pectoris with documented spasm without atherosclerosis of coronary artery bypass graft (I20.1)*
      I25.708 **Atherosclerosis of coronary artery bypass graft(s), unspecified, with other forms of angina pectoris** A
        EXCLUDES 1   *other forms of angina pectoris without atherosclerosis of coronary artery bypass graft (I20.8)*
      I25.709 **Atherosclerosis of coronary artery bypass graft(s), unspecified, with unspecified angina pectoris** A
        EXCLUDES 1   *unspecified angina pectoris without atherosclerosis of coronary artery bypass graft (I20.9)*

√6th **I25.71** **Atherosclerosis of autologous vein coronary artery bypass graft(s) with angina pectoris**
      I25.710 **Atherosclerosis of autologous vein coronary artery bypass graft(s) with unstable angina pectoris** A
        EXCLUDES 1   *unstable angina without atherosclerosis of autologous vein coronary artery bypass graft(s) (I20.0)*
      I25.711 **Atherosclerosis of autologous vein coronary artery bypass graft(s) with angina pectoris with documented spasm** A
        EXCLUDES 1   *angina pectoris with documented spasm without atherosclerosis of autologous vein coronary artery bypass graft(s) (I20.1)*
      I25.718 **Atherosclerosis of autologous vein coronary artery bypass graft(s) with other forms of angina pectoris** A
        EXCLUDES 1   *other forms of angina pectoris without atherosclerosis of autologous vein coronary artery bypass graft(s) (I20.8)*

EXCLUDES 1 Not coded here   EXCLUDES 2 Not included here   N Newborn Age: 0   P Pediatric Age: 0-17   M Maternity Age: 12-55   A Adult Age: 15-124

572   ICD-10-CM 2014 (Draft)

I25.719 **Atherosclerosis of autologous vein coronary artery bypass graft(s) with unspecified angina pectoris** △
> EXCLUDES 1 *unspecified angina pectoris without atherosclerosis of autologous vein coronary artery bypass graft(s) (I20.9)*

✓6ᵗʰ **I25.72** **Atherosclerosis of autologous artery coronary artery bypass graft(s) with angina pectoris**
> Atherosclerosis of internal mammary artery graft with angina pectoris

I25.720 **Atherosclerosis of autologous artery coronary artery bypass graft(s) with unstable angina pectoris** △
> EXCLUDES 1 *unstable angina without atherosclerosis of autologous artery coronary artery bypass graft(s) (I20.0)*

I25.721 **Atherosclerosis of autologous artery coronary artery bypass graft(s) with angina pectoris with documented spasm** △
> EXCLUDES 1 *angina pectoris with documented spasm without atherosclerosis of autologous artery coronary artery bypass graft(s) (I20.1)*

I25.728 **Atherosclerosis of autologous artery coronary artery bypass graft(s) with other forms of angina pectoris** △
> EXCLUDES 1 *other forms of angina pectoris without atherosclerosis of autologous artery coronary artery bypass graft(s) (I20.8)*

I25.729 **Atherosclerosis of autologous artery coronary artery bypass graft(s) with unspecified angina pectoris** △
> EXCLUDES 1 *unspecified angina pectoris without atherosclerosis of autologous artery coronary artery bypass graft(s) (I20.9)*

✓6ᵗʰ **I25.73** **Atherosclerosis of nonautologous biological coronary artery bypass graft(s) with angina pectoris**

I25.730 **Atherosclerosis of nonautologous biological coronary artery bypass graft(s) with unstable angina pectoris** △
> EXCLUDES 1 *unstable angina without atherosclerosis of nonautologous biological coronary artery bypass graft(s) (I20.0)*

I25.731 **Atherosclerosis of nonautologous biological coronary artery bypass graft(s) with angina pectoris with documented spasm** △
> EXCLUDES 1 *angina pectoris with documented spasm without atherosclerosis of nonautologous biological coronary artery bypass graft(s) (I20.1)*

I25.738 **Atherosclerosis of nonautologous biological coronary artery bypass graft(s) with other forms of angina pectoris** △
> EXCLUDES 1 *other forms of angina pectoris without atherosclerosis of nonautologous biological coronary artery bypass graft(s) (I20.8)*

I25.739 **Atherosclerosis of nonautologous biological coronary artery bypass graft(s) with unspecified angina pectoris** △
> EXCLUDES 1 *unspecified angina pectoris without atherosclerosis of nonautologous biological coronary artery bypass graft(s) (I20.9)*

✓6ᵗʰ **I25.75** **Atherosclerosis of native coronary artery of transplanted heart with angina pectoris**
> EXCLUDES 1 *atherosclerosis of native coronary artery of transplanted heart without angina pectoris (I25.811)*

I25.750 **Atherosclerosis of native coronary artery of transplanted heart with unstable angina**

I25.751 **Atherosclerosis of native coronary artery of transplanted heart with angina pectoris with documented spasm**

I25.758 **Atherosclerosis of native coronary artery of transplanted heart with other forms of angina pectoris**

I25.759 **Atherosclerosis of native coronary artery of transplanted heart with unspecified angina pectoris**

✓6ᵗʰ **I25.76** **Atherosclerosis of bypass graft of coronary artery of transplanted heart with angina pectoris**
> EXCLUDES 1 *atherosclerosis of bypass graft of coronary artery of transplanted heart without angina pectoris (I25.812)*

I25.760 **Atherosclerosis of bypass graft of coronary artery of transplanted heart with unstable angina** △

I25.761 **Atherosclerosis of bypass graft of coronary artery of transplanted heart with angina pectoris with documented spasm** △

I25.768 **Atherosclerosis of bypass graft of coronary artery of transplanted heart with other forms of angina pectoris** △

I25.769 **Atherosclerosis of bypass graft of coronary artery of transplanted heart with unspecified angina pectoris** △

✓6ᵗʰ **I25.79** **Atherosclerosis of other coronary artery bypass graft(s) with angina pectoris**

I25.790 **Atherosclerosis of other coronary artery bypass graft(s) with unstable angina pectoris** △
> EXCLUDES 1 *unstable angina without atherosclerosis of other coronary artery bypass graft(s) (I20.0)*

I25.791 **Atherosclerosis of other coronary artery bypass graft(s) with angina pectoris with documented spasm** △
> EXCLUDES 1 *angina pectoris with documented spasm without atherosclerosis of other coronary artery bypass graft(s) (I20.1)*

I25.798 **Atherosclerosis of other coronary artery bypass graft(s) with other forms of angina pectoris** △
> EXCLUDES 1 *other forms of angina pectoris without atherosclerosis of other coronary artery bypass graft(s)(I20.8)*

I25.799 **Atherosclerosis of other coronary artery bypass graft(s) with unspecified angina pectoris** △
> EXCLUDES 1 *unspecified angina pectoris without atherosclerosis of other coronary artery bypass graft(s) (I20.9)*

✓5ᵗʰ **I25.8** **Other forms of chronic ischemic heart disease**

✓6ᵗʰ **I25.81** **Atherosclerosis of other coronary vessels without angina pectoris**
> Use additional code, if applicable, to identify:
> coronary atherosclerosis due to calcified coronary lesion (I25.84)
> coronary atherosclerosis due to lipid rich plaque (I25.83)
> EXCLUDES 1 *atherosclerotic heart disease of native coronary artery without angina pectoris (I25.10)*

I25.810 **Atherosclerosis of coronary artery bypass graft(s) without angina pectoris** △
> Atherosclerosis of coronary artery bypass graft NOS
> EXCLUDES 1 *atherosclerosis of coronary bypass graft(s) with angina pectoris (I25.70--I25.73-, I25.79-)*

☑ Additional Character Required   ✓x7ᵗʰ Xtension Alert   Unspecified Code   Other Specified Code   Manifestation Code   ▶◀ Revised Text   ● New Code   ▲ Revised Code Title

ICD-10-CM 2014 (Draft)   573

I25.811   Atherosclerosis of native coronary artery of transplanted heart without angina pectoris
Atherosclerosis of native coronary artery of transplanted heart NOS
EXCLUDES 1   *atherosclerosis of native coronary artery of transplanted heart with angina pectoris (I25.75-)*

I25.812   Atherosclerosis of bypass graft of coronary artery of transplanted heart without angina pectoris   A
Atherosclerosis of bypass graft of transplanted heart NOS
EXCLUDES 1   *atherosclerosis of bypass graft of transplanted heart with angina pectoris (I25.76)*

I25.82   Chronic total occlusion of coronary artery
Complete occlusion of coronary artery
Total occlusion of coronary artery
Code first coronary atherosclerosis (I25.1-, I25.7-, I25.81-)
EXCLUDES 1   *acute coronary occulsion with myocardial infarction (I21.-, I22.-)*
acute coronary occulsion without myocardial infarction (I24.0)

I25.83   Coronary atherosclerosis due to lipid rich plaque   A
Code first coronary atherosclerosis (I25.1-, I25.7-, I25.81-)

I25.84   Coronary atherosclerosis due to calcified coronary lesion
Coronary atherosclerosis due to severely calcified coronary lesion
Code first coronary atherosclerosis (I25.1-, I25.7-, I25.81-)

I25.89   Other forms of chronic ischemic heart disease

I25.9   Chronic ischemic heart disease, unspecified
Ischemic heart disease (chronic) NOS

Pulmonary heart disease and diseases of pulmonary circulation (I26-I28)

✓4ᵗʰ **I26   Pulmonary embolism**
Pulmonary (acute) (artery)(vein) infarction
Pulmonary (acute) (artery)(vein) thromboembolism
Pulmonary (acute) (artery)(vein) thrombosis
EXCLUDES 2   *chronic pulmonary embolism (I27.82)*
personal history of pulmonary embolism (Z86.711)
pulmonary embolism due to trauma (T79.0, T79.1)
pulmonary embolism due to complications of surgical and medical care (T80.0, T81.7-, T82.8-)
pulmonary embolism complicating abortion, ectopic or molar pregnancy (O00-O07, O08.2)
pulmonary embolism complicating pregnancy, childbirth and the puerperium (O88.-)
septic (non-pulmonary) arterial embolism (I76)

✓5ᵗʰ **I26.0   Pulmonary embolism with acute cor pulmonale**

I26.01   Septic pulmonary embolism with acute cor pulmonale
Code first underlying infection

I26.02   Saddle embolus of pulmonary artery with acute cor pulmonale

I26.09   Other pulmonary embolism with acute cor pulmonale
Acute cor pulmonale NOS

✓5ᵗʰ **I26.9   Pulmonary embolism without acute cor pulmonale**

I26.90   Septic pulmonary embolism without acute cor pulmonale
Code first underlying infection

I26.92   Saddle embolus of pulmonary artery without acute cor pulmonale

I26.99   Other pulmonary embolism without acute cor pulmonale
Acute pulmonary embolism NOS
Pulmonary embolism NOS

✓4ᵗʰ **I27   Other pulmonary heart diseases**

I27.0   Primary pulmonary hypertension
EXCLUDES 1   *pulmonary hypertension NOS (I27.2)*
secondary pulmonary hypertension (I27.2)

I27.1   Kyphoscoliotic heart disease

I27.2   Other secondary pulmonary hypertension
Pulmonary hypertension NOS
Code also associated underlying condition

✓5ᵗʰ **I27.8   Other specified pulmonary heart diseases**

I27.81   Cor pulmonale (chronic)
Cor pulmonale NOS
EXCLUDES 1   *acute cor pulmonale (I26.0-)*

I27.82   Chronic pulmonary embolism
Use additional code, if applicable, for associated long-term (current) use of anticoagulants (Z79.01)
EXCLUDES 1   *personal history of pulmonary embolism (Z86.711)*

I27.89   Other specified pulmonary heart diseases
Eisenmenger's complex
Eisenmenger's syndrome
EXCLUDES 1   *Eisenmenger's defect (Q21.8)*

I27.9   Pulmonary heart disease, unspecified
Chronic cardiopulmonary disease

✓4ᵗʰ **I28   Other diseases of pulmonary vessels**

I28.0   Arteriovenous fistula of pulmonary vessels
EXCLUDES 1   *congenital arteriovenous fistula (Q25.72)*

I28.1   Aneurysm of pulmonary artery
EXCLUDES 1   *congenital aneurysm (Q25.79)*
congenital arteriovenous aneurysm (Q25.72)

I28.8   Other diseases of pulmonary vessels
Pulmonary arteritis
Pulmonary endarteritis
Rupture of pulmonary vessels
Stenosis of pulmonary vessels
Stricture of pulmonary vessels

I28.9   Disease of pulmonary vessels, unspecified

Other forms of heart disease (I30-I52)

✓4ᵗʰ **I30   Acute pericarditis**
INCLUDES   acute mediastinopericarditis
acute myopericarditis
acute pericardial effusion
acute pleuropericarditis
acute pneumopericarditis
EXCLUDES 1   *Dressler's syndrome (I24.1)*
rheumatic pericarditis (acute) (I01.0)

I30.0   Acute nonspecific idiopathic pericarditis

I30.1   Infective pericarditis
Pneumococcal pericarditis
Pneumopyopericardium
Purulent pericarditis
Pyopericarditis
Pyopericardium
Pyopneumopericardium
Staphylococcal pericarditis
Streptococcal pericarditis
Suppurative pericarditis
Viral pericarditis
Use additional code (B95-B97) to identify infectious agent

I30.8   Other forms of acute pericarditis

I30.9   Acute pericarditis, unspecified

✓4ᵗʰ **I31   Other diseases of pericardium**
EXCLUDES 1   *diseases of pericardium specified as rheumatic (I09.2)*
postcardiotomy syndrome (I97.0)
traumatic injury to pericardium (S26.-)

I31.0   Chronic adhesive pericarditis
Accretio cordis
Adherent pericardium
Adhesive mediastinopericarditis

I31.1   Chronic constrictive pericarditis
Concretio cordis
Pericardial calcification

I31.2   Hemopericardium, not elsewhere classified
EXCLUDES 1   *hemopericardium as current complication following acute myocardial infarction (I23.0)*

I31.3   Pericardial effusion (noninflammatory)
Chylopericardium
EXCLUDES 1   *acute pericardial effusion (I30.9)*

I31.4   Cardiac tamponade
Code first underlying cause

EXCLUDES 1 Not coded here   EXCLUDES 2 Not included here   N Newborn Age: 0   P Pediatric Age: 0-17   M Maternity Age: 12-55   A Adult Age: 15-124

574   ICD-10-CM 2014 (Draft)

I31.8 Other specified diseases of pericardium
Epicardial plaques
Focal pericardial adhesions

I31.9 Disease of pericardium, unspecified
Pericarditis (chronic) NOS

I32 Pericarditis in diseases classified elsewhere
Code first underlying disease
EXCLUDES 1 *pericarditis (in):*
coxsackie (virus) (B33.23)
gonococcal (A54.83)
meningococcal (A39.53)
rheumatoid (arthritis) (M05.31)
syphilitic (A52.06)
systemic lupus erythematosus (M32.12)
tuberculosis (A18.84)

✓4ᵗʰ **I33 Acute and subacute endocarditis**
EXCLUDES 1 *acute rheumatic endocarditis (I01.1)*
endocarditis NOS (I38)

I33.0 Acute and subacute infective endocarditis
Bacterial endocarditis (acute) (subacute)
Infective endocarditis (acute) (subacute) NOS
Endocarditis lenta (acute) (subacute)
Malignant endocarditis (acute) (subacute)
Purulent endocarditis (acute) (subacute)
Septic endocarditis (acute) (subacute)
Ulcerative endocarditis (acute) (subacute)
Vegetative endocarditis (acute) (subacute)
Use additional code (B95-B97) to identify infectious agent

I33.9 Acute and subacute endocarditis, unspecified
Acute endocarditis NOS
Acute myoendocarditis NOS
Acute periendocarditis NOS
Subacute endocarditis NOS
Subacute myoendocarditis NOS
Subacute periendocarditis NOS

✓4ᵗʰ **I34 Nonrheumatic mitral valve disorders**
EXCLUDES 1 *mitral valve disease (I05.9)*
mitral valve failure (I05.8)
mitral valve stenosis (I05.0)
mitral valve disorder of unspecified cause with diseases of aortic and/or tricuspid valve(s) (I08.-)
mitral valve disorder of unspecified cause with mitral stenosis or obstruction (I05.0)
mitral valve disorder specified as congenital (Q23.2, Q23.3)
mitral valve disorder specified as rheumatic (I05.-)

I34.0 Nonrheumatic mitral (valve) insufficiency
Nonrheumatic mitral (valve) incompetence NOS
Nonrheumatic mitral (valve) regurgitation NOS

I34.1 Nonrheumatic mitral (valve) prolapse
Floppy nonrheumatic mitral valve syndrome
EXCLUDES 1 *Marfan's syndrome (Q87.4-)*

I34.2 Nonrheumatic mitral (valve) stenosis

I34.8 Other nonrheumatic mitral valve disorders

I34.9 Nonrheumatic mitral valve disorder, unspecified

✓4ᵗʰ **I35 Nonrheumatic aortic valve disorders**
EXCLUDES 1 *aortic valve disorder of unspecified cause but with diseases of mitral and/or tricuspid valve(s) (I08.-)*
aortic valve disorder specified as congenital (Q23.0, Q23.1)
aortic valve disorder specified as rheumatic (I06.-)
hypertrophic subaortic stenosis (I42.1)

I35.0 Nonrheumatic aortic (valve) stenosis

I35.1 Nonrheumatic aortic (valve) insufficiency
Nonrheumatic aortic (valve) incompetence NOS
Nonrheumatic aortic (valve) regurgitation NOS

I35.2 Nonrheumatic aortic (valve) stenosis with insufficiency

I35.8 Other nonrheumatic aortic valve disorders

I35.9 Nonrheumatic aortic valve disorder, unspecified

✓4ᵗʰ **I36 Nonrheumatic tricuspid valve disorders**
EXCLUDES 1 *tricuspid valve disorders of unspecified cause (I07.-)*
tricuspid valve disorders specified as congenital (Q22.4, Q22.8, Q22.9)
tricuspid valve disorders specified as rheumatic (I07.-)
tricuspid valve disorders with aortic and/or mitral valve involvement (I08.-)

I36.0 Nonrheumatic tricuspid (valve) stenosis

I36.1 Nonrheumatic tricuspid (valve) insufficiency
Nonrheumatic tricuspid (valve) incompetence
Nonrheumatic tricuspid (valve) regurgitation

I36.2 Nonrheumatic tricuspid (valve) stenosis with insufficiency

I36.8 Other nonrheumatic tricuspid valve disorders

I36.9 Nonrheumatic tricuspid valve disorder, unspecified

✓4ᵗʰ **I37 Nonrheumatic pulmonary valve disorders**
EXCLUDES 1 *pulmonary valve disorder specified as congenital (Q22.1, Q22.2, Q22.3)*
pulmonary valve disorder specified as rheumatic (I09.89)

I37.0 Nonrheumatic pulmonary valve stenosis

I37.1 Nonrheumatic pulmonary valve insufficiency
Nonrheumatic pulmonary valve incompetence
Nonrheumatic pulmonary valve regurgitation

I37.2 Nonrheumatic pulmonary valve stenosis with insufficiency

I37.8 Other nonrheumatic pulmonary valve disorders

I37.9 Nonrheumatic pulmonary valve disorder, unspecified

I38 Endocarditis, valve unspecified
INCLUDES endocarditis (chronic) NOS
valvular incompetence NOS
valvular insufficiency NOS
valvular regurgitation NOS
valvular stenosis NOS
valvulitis (chronic) NOS
EXCLUDES 1 *congenital insufficiency of cardiac valve NOS (Q24.8)*
congenital stenosis of cardiac valve NOS (Q24.8)
endocardial fibroelastosis (I42.4)
endocarditis specified as rheumatic (I09.1)

I39 Endocarditis and heart valve disorders in diseases classified elsewhere
Code first underlying disease, such as:
Q fever (A78)
EXCLUDES 1 *endocardial involvement in:*
candidiasis (B37.6)
gonococcal infection (A54.83)
Libman-Sacks disease (M32.11)
listerosis (A32.82)
meningococcal infection (A39.51)
rheumatoid arthritis (M05.31)
syphilis (A52.03)
tuberculosis (A18.84)
typhoid fever (A01.02)

✓4ᵗʰ **I40 Acute myocarditis**
INCLUDES subacute myocarditis
EXCLUDES 1 *acute rheumatic myocarditis (I01.2)*

I40.0 Infective myocarditis
Septic myocarditis
Use additional code (B95-B97) to identify infectious agent

I40.1 Isolated myocarditis
Fiedler's myocarditis
Giant cell myocarditis
Idiopathic myocarditis

I40.8 Other acute myocarditis

I40.9 Acute myocarditis, unspecified

I41 Myocarditis in diseases classified elsewhere
Code first underlying disease, such as:
typhus (A75.0-A75.9)
EXCLUDES 1 *myocarditis (in):*
Chagas' disease (chronic) (B57.2)
acute (B57.0)
coxsackie (virus) infection (B33.22)
diphtheritic (A36.81)
gonococcal (A54.83)
influenzal (J09.X9, J10.82, J11.82)
meningococcal (A39.52)
mumps (B26.82)
rheumatoid arthritis (M05.31)
sarcoid (D86.85)
syphilis (A52.06)
toxoplasmosis (B58.81)
tuberculous (A18.84)

✓4ᵗʰ **I42 Cardiomyopathy**
INCLUDES myocardiopathy
Code first pre-existing cardiomyopathy complicating pregnancy and puerperium (O99.4)
EXCLUDES 1 *ischemic cardiomyopathy (I25.5)*
peripartum cardiomyopathy (O90.3)
EXCLUDES 2 *ventricular hypertrophy (I51.7)*

I42.0 Dilated cardiomyopathy
Congestive cardiomyopathy

I42.1 Obstructive hypertrophic cardiomyopathy
Hypertrophic subaortic stenosis (idiopathic)

✓ Additional Character Required   ✓x7ᵗʰ Xtension Alert   Unspecified Code   Other Specified Code   Manifestation Code   ▶◀ Revised Text   ● New Code   ▲ Revised Code Title

I42.2 **Other hypertrophic cardiomyopathy**
Nonobstructive hypertrophic cardiomyopathy

I42.3 **Endomyocardial (eosinophilic) disease**
Endomyocardial (tropical) fibrosis
Löffler's endocarditis

I42.4 **Endocardial fibroelastosis**
Congenital cardiomyopathy
Elastomyofibrosis

I42.5 **Other restrictive cardiomyopathy**
Constrictive cardiomyopathy NOS

I42.6 **Alcoholic cardiomyopathy**
Code also presence of alcoholism (F10.-)

I42.7 **Cardiomyopathy due to drug and external agent**
Code first poisoning due to drug or toxin, if applicable (T36-T65 with fifth or sixth character 1-4 or 6)
Use additional code for adverse effect, if applicable, to identify drug (T36-T50 with fifth or sixth character 5)

I42.8 **Other cardiomyopathies**

I42.9 **Cardiomyopathy, unspecified**
Cardiomyopathy (primary) (secondary) NOS

I43 *Cardiomyopathy in diseases classified elsewhere*
Code first underlying disease, such as:
amyloidosis (E85.-)
glycogen storage disease (E74.0)
gout (M10.0-)
thyrotoxicosis (E05.0-E05.9-)
EXCLUDES 1 *cardiomyopathy (in):*
coxsackie (virus) (B33.24)
diphtheria (A36.81)
sarcoidosis (D86.85)
tuberculosis (A18.84)

✓4th **I44** **Atrioventricular and left bundle-branch block**

I44.0 **Atrioventricular block, first degree**

I44.1 **Atrioventricular block, second degree**
Atrioventricular block, type I and II
Möbitz block, type I and II
Second degree block, type I and II
Wenckebach's block

I44.2 **Atrioventricular block, complete**
Complete heart block NOS
Third degree block

✓5th **I44.3** **Other and unspecified atrioventricular block**
Atrioventricular block NOS

I44.30 **Unspecified atrioventricular block**

I44.39 **Other atrioventricular block**

I44.4 **Left anterior fascicular block**

I44.5 **Left posterior fascicular block**

✓5th **I44.6** **Other and unspecified fascicular block**

I44.60 **Unspecified fascicular block**
Left bundle-branch hemiblock NOS

I44.69 **Other fascicular block**

I44.7 **Left bundle-branch block, unspecified**

✓4th **I45** **Other conduction disorders**

I45.0 **Right fascicular block**

✓5th **I45.1** **Other and unspecified right bundle-branch block**

I45.10 **Unspecified right bundle-branch block**
Right bundle-branch block NOS

I45.19 **Other right bundle-branch block**

I45.2 **Bifascicular block**

I45.3 **Trifascicular block**

I45.4 **Nonspecific intraventricular block**
Bundle-branch block NOS

I45.5 **Other specified heart block**
Sinoatrial block
Sinoauricular block
EXCLUDES 1 *heart block NOS (I45.9)*

I45.6 **Pre-excitation syndrome**
Accelerated atrioventricular conduction
Accessory atrioventricular conduction
Anomalous atrioventricular excitation
Lown-Ganong-Levine syndrome
Pre-excitation atrioventricular conduction
Wolff-Parkinson-White syndrome

✓5th **I45.8** **Other specified conduction disorders**

I45.81 **Long QT syndrome**

I45.89 **Other specified conduction disorders**
Atrioventricular [AV] dissociation
Interference dissociation
Isorhythmic dissociation
Nonparoxysmal AV nodal tachycardia

I45.9 **Conduction disorder, unspecified**
Heart block NOS
Stokes-Adams syndrome

✓4th **I46** **Cardiac arrest**
EXCLUDES 1 *cardiogenic shock (R57.0)*

I46.2 **Cardiac arrest due to underlying cardiac condition**
Code first underlying cardiac condition

I46.8 **Cardiac arrest due to other underlying condition**
Code first underlying condition

I46.9 **Cardiac arrest, cause unspecified**

✓4th **I47** **Paroxysmal tachycardia**
Code first tachycardia complicating:
abortion or ectopic or molar pregnancy (O00-O07, O08.8)
obstetric surgery and procedures (O75.4)
EXCLUDES 1 *tachycardia NOS (R00.0)*
sinoauricular tachycardia NOS (R00.0)
sinus [sinusal] tachycardia NOS (R00.0)

I47.0 **Re-entry ventricular arrhythmia**

I47.1 **Supraventricular tachycardia**
Atrial (paroxysmal) tachycardia
Atrioventricular [AV] (paroxysmal) tachycardia
Atrioventricular re-entrant (nodal) tachycardia [AVNRT] [AVRT]
Junctional (paroxysmal) tachycardia
Nodal (paroxysmal) tachycardia

I47.2 **Ventricular tachycardia**

I47.9 **Paroxysmal tachycardia, unspecified**
Bouveret (-Hoffman) syndrome

✓4th **I48** **Atrial fibrillation and flutter**

I48.0 **Paroxysmal atrial fibrillation**

I48.1 **Persistent atrial fibrillation**

I48.2 **Chronic atrial fibrillation**
Permanent atrial fibrillation

I48.3 **Typical atrial flutter**
Type I atrial flutter

I48.4 **Atypical atrial flutter**
Type II atrial flutter

✓5th **I48.9** **Unspecified atrial fibrillation and atrial flutter**

I48.91 **Unspecified atrial fibrillation**

I48.92 **Unspecified atrial flutter**

✓4th **I49** **Other cardiac arrhythmias**
Code first cardiac arrhythmia complicating:
abortion or ectopic or molar pregnancy (O00-O07, O08.8)
obstetric surgery and procedures (O75.4)
EXCLUDES 1 *bradycardia NOS (R00.1)*
neonatal dysrhythmia (P29.1-)
sinoatrial bradycardia (R00.1)
sinus bradycardia (R00.1)
vagal bradycardia (R00.1)

✓5th **I49.0** **Ventricular fibrillation and flutter**

I49.01 **Ventricular fibrillation**

I49.02 **Ventricular flutter**

I49.1 **Atrial premature depolarization**
Atrial premature beats

I49.2 **Junctional premature depolarization**

I49.3 **Ventricular premature depolarization**

✓5th **I49.4** **Other and unspecified premature depolarization**

I49.40 **Unspecified premature depolarization**
Premature beats NOS

I49.49 **Other premature depolarization**
Ectopic beats   Extrasystolic arrhythmias
Extrasystoles   Premature contractions

I49.5 **Sick sinus syndrome**
Tachycardia-bradycardia syndrome

I49.8 **Other specified cardiac arrhythmias**
Coronary sinus rhythm disorder
Ectopic rhythm disorder
Nodal rhythm disorder

I49.9 **Cardiac arrhythmia, unspecified**
Arrhythmia (cardiac) NOS

EXCLUDES 1 Not coded here   **EXCLUDES 2** Not included here   **N** Newborn Age: 0   **P** Pediatric Age: 0-17   **M** Maternity Age: 12-55   **A** Adult Age: 15-124

☑4th **I50   Heart failure**
Code first:
heart failure complicating abortion or ectopic or molar pregnancy (O00-O07, O08.8)
heart failure following surgery (I97.13-)
heart failure due to hypertension (I11.0)
heart failure due to hypertension with chronic kidney disease (I13.-)
obstetric surgery and procedures (O75.4)
rheumatic heart failure (I09.81)
EXCLUDES 1   cardiac arrest (I46.-)
neonatal cardiac failure (P29.0)

I50.1   Left ventricular failure
Cardiac asthma
Edema of lung with heart disease NOS
Edema of lung with heart failure
Left heart failure
Pulmonary edema with heart disease NOS
Pulmonary edema with heart failure
EXCLUDES 1   edema of lung without heart disease or heart failure (J81.-)
pulmonary edema without heart disease or failure (J81.-)

☑5th **I50.2   Systolic (congestive) heart failure**
EXCLUDES 1   combined systolic (congestive) and diastolic (congestive) heart failure (I50.4-)

I50.20   Unspecified systolic (congestive) heart failure
I50.21   Acute systolic (congestive) heart failure
I50.22   Chronic systolic (congestive) heart failure
I50.23   Acute on chronic systolic (congestive) heart failure

☑5th **I50.3   Diastolic (congestive) heart failure**
EXCLUDES 1   combined systolic (congestive) and diastolic (congestive) heart failure (I50.4-)

I50.30   Unspecified diastolic (congestive) heart failure
I50.31   Acute diastolic (congestive) heart failure
I50.32   Chronic diastolic (congestive) heart failure
I50.33   Acute on chronic diastolic (congestive) heart failure

☑5th **I50.4   Combined systolic (congestive) and diastolic (congestive) heart failure**
I50.40   Unspecified combined systolic (congestive) and diastolic (congestive) heart failure
I50.41   Acute combined systolic (congestive) and diastolic (congestive) heart failure
I50.42   Chronic combined systolic (congestive) and diastolic (congestive) heart failure
I50.43   Acute on chronic combined systolic (congestive) and diastolic (congestive) heart failure

I50.9   Heart failure, unspecified
Biventricular (heart) failure NOS
Cardiac, heart or myocardial failure NOS
Congestive heart disease
Congestive heart failure NOS
Right ventricular failure (secondary to left heart failure)
EXCLUDES 1   fluid overload (E87.70)
AHA: 2012, Q4, 92

☑4th **I51   Complications and ill-defined descriptions of heart disease**
EXCLUDES 1   any condition in I51.4-I51.9 due to hypertension (I11.-)
any condition in I51.4-I51.9 due to hypertension and chronic kidney disease (I13.-)
heart disease specified as rheumatic (I00-I09)

I51.0   Cardiac septal defect, acquired   Ⓐ
Acquired septal atrial defect (old)
Acquired septal auricular defect (old)
Acquired septal ventricular defect (old)
EXCLUDES 1   cardiac septal defect as current complication following acute myocardial infarction (I23.1, I23.2)

I51.1   Rupture of chordae tendineae, not elsewhere classified
EXCLUDES 1   rupture of chordae tendineae as current complication following acute myocardial infarction (I23.4)

I51.2   Rupture of papillary muscle, not elsewhere classified
EXCLUDES 1   rupture of papillary muscle as current complication following acute myocardial infarction (I23.5)

I51.3   Intracardiac thrombosis, not elsewhere classified   Ⓐ
Apical thrombosis (old)
Atrial thrombosis (old)
Auricular thrombosis (old)
Mural thrombosis (old)
Ventricular thrombosis (old)
EXCLUDES 1   intracardiac thrombosis as current complication following acute myocardial infarction (I23.6)

I51.4   Myocarditis, unspecified
Chronic (interstitial) myocarditis
Myocardial fibrosis
Myocarditis NOS
EXCLUDES 1   acute or subacute myocarditis (I40.-)

I51.5   Myocardial degeneration
Fatty degeneration of heart or myocardium
Myocardial disease
Senile degeneration of heart or myocardium

I51.7   Cardiomegaly
Cardiac dilatation
Cardiac hypertrophy
Ventricular dilatation

☑5th **I51.8   Other ill-defined heart diseases**
I51.81   Takotsubo syndrome
Reversible left ventricular dysfunction following sudden emotional stress
Stress induced cardiomyopathy
Takotsubo cardiomyopathy
Transient left ventricular apical ballooning syndrome

I51.89   Other ill-defined heart diseases
Carditis (acute)(chronic)
Pancarditis (acute)(chronic)

I51.9   Heart disease, unspecified

I52   Other heart disorders in diseases classified elsewhere
Code first underlying disease, such as:
congenital syphilis (A50.5)
mucopolysaccharidosis (E76.3)
schistosomiasis (B65.0-B65.9)
EXCLUDES 1   heart disease (in):
gonococcal infection (A54.83)
meningococcal infection (A39.50)
rheumatoid arthritis (M05.31)
syphilis (A52.06)

Cerebrovascular diseases (I60-I69)

Use additional code to identify presence of:
alcohol abuse and dependence (F10.-)
exposure to environmental tobacco smoke (Z77.22)
history of tobacco use (Z87.891)
hypertension (I10-I15)
occupational exposure to environmental tobacco smoke (Z57.31)
tobacco dependence (F17.-)
tobacco use (Z72.0)
EXCLUDES 1   transient cerebral ischemic attacks and related syndromes (G45.-)
traumatic intracranial hemorrhage (S06.-)
AHA: 2012, Q4, 91-92

☑4th **I60   Nontraumatic subarachnoid hemorrhage**
INCLUDES   ruptured cerebral aneurysm
EXCLUDES 1   sequelae of subarachnoid hemorrhage (I69.0-)
syphilitic ruptured cerebral aneurysm (A52.05)

☑5th **I60.0   Nontraumatic subarachnoid hemorrhage from carotid siphon and bifurcation**
I60.00   Nontraumatic subarachnoid hemorrhage from unspecified carotid siphon and bifurcation
I60.01   Nontraumatic subarachnoid hemorrhage from right carotid siphon and bifurcation
I60.02   Nontraumatic subarachnoid hemorrhage from left carotid siphon and bifurcation

☑5th **I60.1   Nontraumatic subarachnoid hemorrhage from middle cerebral artery**
I60.10   Nontraumatic subarachnoid hemorrhage from unspecified middle cerebral artery
I60.11   Nontraumatic subarachnoid hemorrhage from right middle cerebral artery
I60.12   Nontraumatic subarachnoid hemorrhage from left middle cerebral artery

☑5th **I60.2   Nontraumatic subarachnoid hemorrhage from anterior communicating artery**
I60.20   Nontraumatic subarachnoid hemorrhage from unspecified anterior communicating artery
I60.21   Nontraumatic subarachnoid hemorrhage from right anterior communicating artery
I60.22   Nontraumatic subarachnoid hemorrhage from left anterior communicating artery

☑5th **I60.3   Nontraumatic subarachnoid hemorrhage from posterior communicating artery**
I60.30   Nontraumatic subarachnoid hemorrhage from unspecified posterior communicating artery

---

☑ Additional Character Required   ✓x7th Xtension Alert   Unspecified Code   Other Specified Code   Manifestation Code   ►◄ Revised Text   ● New Code   ▲ Revised Code Title

I60.31 Nontraumatic subarachnoid hemorrhage from right posterior communicating artery

I60.32 Nontraumatic subarachnoid hemorrhage from left posterior communicating artery

I60.4 Nontraumatic subarachnoid hemorrhage from basilar artery

✓5ᵗʰ **I60.5** Nontraumatic subarachnoid hemorrhage from vertebral artery

I60.50 Nontraumatic subarachnoid hemorrhage from unspecified vertebral artery

I60.51 Nontraumatic subarachnoid hemorrhage from right vertebral artery

I60.52 Nontraumatic subarachnoid hemorrhage from left vertebral artery

I60.6 Nontraumatic subarachnoid hemorrhage from other intracranial arteries

I60.7 Nontraumatic subarachnoid hemorrhage from unspecified intracranial artery

Ruptured (congenital) berry aneurysm
Ruptured (congenital) cerebral aneurysm
Subarachnoid hemorrhage (nontraumatic) from cerebral artery NOS
Subarachnoid hemorrhage (nontraumatic) from communicating artery NOS

EXCLUDES 1 berry aneurysm, nonruptured (I67.1)

I60.8 Other nontraumatic subarachnoid hemorrhage
Meningeal hemorrhage
Rupture of cerebral arteriovenous malformation

I60.9 Nontraumatic subarachnoid hemorrhage, unspecified

✓4ᵗʰ **I61** Nontraumatic intracerebral hemorrhage
EXCLUDES 1 sequelae of intracerebral hemorrhage (I69.1-)

I61.0 Nontraumatic intracerebral hemorrhage in hemisphere, subcortical
Deep intracerebral hemorrhage (nontraumatic)

I61.1 Nontraumatic intracerebral hemorrhage in hemisphere, cortical
Cerebral lobe hemorrhage (nontraumatic)
Superficial intracerebral hemorrhage (nontraumatic)

I61.2 Nontraumatic intracerebral hemorrhage in hemisphere, unspecified

I61.3 Nontraumatic intracerebral hemorrhage in brain stem

I61.4 Nontraumatic intracerebral hemorrhage in cerebellum

I61.5 Nontraumatic intracerebral hemorrhage, intraventricular

I61.6 Nontraumatic intracerebral hemorrhage, multiple localized

I61.8 Other nontraumatic intracerebral hemorrhage

I61.9 Nontraumatic intracerebral hemorrhage, unspecified

✓4ᵗʰ **I62** Other and unspecified nontraumatic intracranial hemorrhage
EXCLUDES 1 sequelae of intracranial hemorrhage (I69.2)

✓5ᵗʰ **I62.0** Nontraumatic subdural hemorrhage

I62.00 Nontraumatic subdural hemorrhage, unspecified

I62.01 Nontraumatic acute subdural hemorrhage

I62.02 Nontraumatic subacute subdural hemorrhage

I62.03 Nontraumatic chronic subdural hemorrhage

I62.1 Nontraumatic extradural hemorrhage
Nontraumatic epidural hemorrhage

I62.9 Nontraumatic intracranial hemorrhage, unspecified

✓4ᵗʰ **I63** Cerebral infarction
INCLUDES occlusion and stenosis of cerebral and precerebral arteries, resulting in cerebral infarction
Use additional code, if applicable, to identify status post administration of tPA (rtPA) in a different facility within the last 24 hours prior to admission to current facility (Z92.82)
EXCLUDES 1 sequelae of cerebral infarction (I69.3-)

✓5ᵗʰ **I63.0** Cerebral infarction due to thrombosis of precerebral arteries

I63.00 Cerebral infarction due to thrombosis of unspecified precerebral artery

✓6ᵗʰ **I63.01** Cerebral infarction due to thrombosis of vertebral artery

I63.011 Cerebral infarction due to thrombosis of right vertebral artery

I63.012 Cerebral infarction due to thrombosis of left vertebral artery

I63.019 Cerebral infarction due to thrombosis of unspecified vertebral artery

I63.02 Cerebral infarction due to thrombosis of basilar artery

✓6ᵗʰ **I63.03** Cerebral infarction due to thrombosis of carotid artery

I63.031 Cerebral infarction due to thrombosis of right carotid artery

I63.032 Cerebral infarction due to thrombosis of left carotid artery

I63.039 Cerebral infarction due to thrombosis of unspecified carotid artery

I63.09 Cerebral infarction due to thrombosis of other precerebral artery

✓5ᵗʰ **I63.1** Cerebral infarction due to embolism of precerebral arteries

I63.10 Cerebral infarction due to embolism of unspecified precerebral artery

✓6ᵗʰ **I63.11** Cerebral infarction due to embolism of vertebral artery

I63.111 Cerebral infarction due to embolism of right vertebral artery

I63.112 Cerebral infarction due to embolism of left vertebral artery

I63.119 Cerebral infarction due to embolism of unspecified vertebral artery

I63.12 Cerebral infarction due to embolism of basilar artery

✓6ᵗʰ **I63.13** Cerebral infarction due to embolism of carotid artery

I63.131 Cerebral infarction due to embolism of right carotid artery

I63.132 Cerebral infarction due to embolism of left carotid artery

I63.139 Cerebral infarction due to embolism of unspecified carotid artery

I63.19 Cerebral infarction due to embolism of other precerebral artery

✓5ᵗʰ **I63.2** Cerebral infarction due to unspecified occlusion or stenosis of precerebral arteries

I63.20 Cerebral infarction due to unspecified occlusion or stenosis of unspecified precerebral arteries

✓6ᵗʰ **I63.21** Cerebral infarction due to unspecified occlusion or stenosis of vertebral arteries

I63.211 Cerebral infarction due to unspecified occlusion or stenosis of right vertebral arteries

I63.212 Cerebral infarction due to unspecified occlusion or stenosis of left vertebral arteries

I63.219 Cerebral infarction due to unspecified occlusion or stenosis of unspecified vertebral arteries

I63.22 Cerebral infarction due to unspecified occlusion or stenosis of basilar arteries

✓6ᵗʰ **I63.23** Cerebral infarction due to unspecified occlusion or stenosis of carotid arteries

I63.231 Cerebral infarction due to unspecified occlusion or stenosis of right carotid arteries

I63.232 Cerebral infarction due to unspecified occlusion or stenosis of left carotid arteries

I63.239 Cerebral infarction due to unspecified occlusion or stenosis of unspecified carotid arteries

I63.29 Cerebral infarction due to unspecified occlusion or stenosis of other precerebral arteries

✓5ᵗʰ **I63.3** Cerebral infarction due to thrombosis of cerebral arteries

I63.30 Cerebral infarction due to thrombosis of unspecified cerebral artery

✓6ᵗʰ **I63.31** Cerebral infarction due to thrombosis of middle cerebral artery

I63.311 Cerebral infarction due to thrombosis of right middle cerebral artery

I63.312 Cerebral infarction due to thrombosis of left middle cerebral artery

I63.319 Cerebral infarction due to thrombosis of unspecified middle cerebral artery

✓6ᵗʰ **I63.32** Cerebral infarction due to thrombosis of anterior cerebral artery

I63.321 Cerebral infarction due to thrombosis of right anterior cerebral artery

I63.322 Cerebral infarction due to thrombosis of left anterior cerebral artery

---

EXCLUDES 1 Not coded here **EXCLUDES 2** Not included here **N** Newborn Age: 0 **P** Pediatric Age: 0-17 **M** Maternity Age: 12-55 **A** Adult Age: 15-124

I63.329   **Cerebral infarction due to thrombosis of unspecified anterior cerebral artery**

✓6ᵗʰ **I63.33**   Cerebral infarction due to thrombosis of posterior cerebral artery

    I63.331   Cerebral infarction due to thrombosis of right posterior cerebral artery

    I63.332   Cerebral infarction due to thrombosis of left posterior cerebral artery

    I63.339   **Cerebral infarction due to thrombosis of unspecified posterior cerebral artery**

✓6ᵗʰ **I63.34**   Cerebral infarction due to thrombosis of cerebellar artery

    I63.341   Cerebral infarction due to thrombosis of right cerebellar artery

    I63.342   Cerebral infarction due to thrombosis of left cerebellar artery

    I63.349   **Cerebral infarction due to thrombosis of unspecified cerebellar artery**

    I63.39   **Cerebral infarction due to thrombosis of other cerebral artery**

✓5ᵗʰ **I63.4**   Cerebral infarction due to embolism of cerebral arteries

    I63.4Ø   **Cerebral infarction due to embolism of unspecified cerebral artery**

✓6ᵗʰ **I63.41**   Cerebral infarction due to embolism of middle cerebral artery

    I63.411   Cerebral infarction due to embolism of right middle cerebral artery

    I63.412   Cerebral infarction due to embolism of left middle cerebral artery

    I63.419   **Cerebral infarction due to embolism of unspecified middle cerebral artery**

✓6ᵗʰ **I63.42**   Cerebral infarction due to embolism of anterior cerebral artery

    I63.421   Cerebral infarction due to embolism of right anterior cerebral artery

    I63.422   Cerebral infarction due to embolism of left anterior cerebral artery

    I63.429   **Cerebral infarction due to embolism of unspecified anterior cerebral artery**

✓6ᵗʰ **I63.43**   Cerebral infarction due to embolism of posterior cerebral artery

    I63.431   Cerebral infarction due to embolism of right posterior cerebral artery

    I63.432   Cerebral infarction due to embolism of left posterior cerebral artery

    I63.439   **Cerebral infarction due to embolism of unspecified posterior cerebral artery**

✓6ᵗʰ **I63.44**   Cerebral infarction due to embolism of cerebellar artery

    I63.441   Cerebral infarction due to embolism of right cerebellar artery

    I63.442   Cerebral infarction due to embolism of left cerebellar artery

    I63.449   **Cerebral infarction due to embolism of unspecified cerebellar artery**

    I63.49   **Cerebral infarction due to embolism of other cerebral artery**

✓5ᵗʰ **I63.5**   Cerebral infarction due to unspecified occlusion or stenosis of cerebral arteries

    I63.5Ø   **Cerebral infarction due to unspecified occlusion or stenosis of unspecified cerebral artery**

✓6ᵗʰ **I63.51**   Cerebral infarction due to unspecified occlusion or stenosis of middle cerebral artery

    I63.511   Cerebral infarction due to unspecified occlusion or stenosis of right middle cerebral artery

    I63.512   Cerebral infarction due to unspecified occlusion or stenosis of left middle cerebral artery

    I63.519   **Cerebral infarction due to unspecified occlusion or stenosis of unspecified middle cerebral artery**

✓6ᵗʰ **I63.52**   Cerebral infarction due to unspecified occlusion or stenosis of anterior cerebral artery

    I63.521   Cerebral infarction due to unspecified occlusion or stenosis of right anterior cerebral artery

I63.522   Cerebral infarction due to unspecified occlusion or stenosis of left anterior cerebral artery

I63.529   **Cerebral infarction due to unspecified occlusion or stenosis of unspecified anterior cerebral artery**

✓6ᵗʰ **I63.53**   Cerebral infarction due to unspecified occlusion or stenosis of posterior cerebral artery

    I63.531   Cerebral infarction due to unspecified occlusion or stenosis of right posterior cerebral artery

    I63.532   Cerebral infarction due to unspecified occlusion or stenosis of left posterior cerebral artery

    I63.539   **Cerebral infarction due to unspecified occlusion or stenosis of unspecified posterior cerebral artery**

✓6ᵗʰ **I63.54**   Cerebral infarction due to unspecified occlusion or stenosis of cerebellar artery

    I63.541   Cerebral infarction due to unspecified occlusion or stenosis of right cerebellar artery

    I63.542   Cerebral infarction due to unspecified occlusion or stenosis of left cerebellar artery

    I63.549   **Cerebral infarction due to unspecified occlusion or stenosis of unspecified cerebellar artery**

    I63.59   **Cerebral infarction due to unspecified occlusion or stenosis of other cerebral artery**

I63.6   Cerebral infarction due to cerebral venous thrombosis, nonpyogenic

I63.8   **Other cerebral infarction**

I63.9   **Cerebral infarction, unspecified**
    Stroke NOS

✓4ᵗʰ **I65**   **Occlusion and stenosis of precerebral arteries, not resulting in cerebral infarction**
    INCLUDES   embolism of precerebral artery
             narrowing of precerebral artery
             obstruction (complete) (partial) of precerebral artery
             thrombosis of precerebral artery
    EXCLUDES 1   *insufficiency, NOS, of precerebral artery (G45.-)*
             insufficiency of precerebral arteries causing cerebral infarction (I63.Ø-I63.2)

✓5ᵗʰ **I65.Ø**   **Occlusion and stenosis of vertebral artery**

    I65.Ø1   Occlusion and stenosis of right vertebral artery

    I65.Ø2   Occlusion and stenosis of left vertebral artery

    I65.Ø3   Occlusion and stenosis of bilateral vertebral arteries

    I65.Ø9   **Occlusion and stenosis of unspecified vertebral artery**

I65.1   **Occlusion and stenosis of basilar artery**

✓5ᵗʰ **I65.2**   **Occlusion and stenosis of carotid artery**

    I65.21   Occlusion and stenosis of right carotid artery

    I65.22   Occlusion and stenosis of left carotid artery

    I65.23   Occlusion and stenosis of bilateral carotid arteries

    I65.29   **Occlusion and stenosis of unspecified carotid artery**

I65.8   **Occlusion and stenosis of other precerebral arteries**

I65.9   **Occlusion and stenosis of unspecified precerebral artery**
    Occlusion and stenosis of precerebral artery NOS

✓4ᵗʰ **I66**   **Occlusion and stenosis of cerebral arteries, not resulting in cerebral infarction**
    INCLUDES   embolism of cerebral artery
             narrowing of cerebral artery
             obstruction (complete) (partial) of cerebral artery
             thrombosis of cerebral artery
    EXCLUDES 1   *occlusion and stenosis of cerebral artery causing cerebral infarction (I63.3-I63.5)*

✓5ᵗʰ **I66.Ø**   **Occlusion and stenosis of middle cerebral artery**

    I66.Ø1   Occlusion and stenosis of right middle cerebral artery

    I66.Ø2   Occlusion and stenosis of left middle cerebral artery

    I66.Ø3   Occlusion and stenosis of bilateral middle cerebral arteries

    I66.Ø9   **Occlusion and stenosis of unspecified middle cerebral artery**

☑ Additional Character Required   x7ᵗʰ Xtension Alert   Unspecified Code   Other Specified Code   Manifestation Code   ►◄ Revised Text   ● New Code   ▲ Revised Code Title

ICD-1Ø-CM 2Ø14 (Draft)   **579**

Diseases of the Circulatory System

I66.1–I69.052

✓5ᵗʰ **I66.1** **Occlusion and stenosis of** anterior **cerebral artery**

I66.11 **Occlusion and stenosis of** right **anterior cerebral artery**

I66.12 **Occlusion and stenosis of** left **anterior cerebral artery**

I66.13 **Occlusion and stenosis of** bilateral **anterior cerebral arteries**

I66.19 **Occlusion and stenosis of unspecified anterior cerebral artery**

✓5ᵗʰ **I66.2** **Occlusion and stenosis of** posterior **cerebral artery**

I66.21 **Occlusion and stenosis of** right **posterior cerebral artery**

I66.22 **Occlusion and stenosis of** left **posterior cerebral artery**

I66.23 **Occlusion and stenosis of** bilateral **posterior cerebral arteries**

I66.29 **Occlusion and stenosis of unspecified posterior cerebral artery**

I66.3 **Occlusion and stenosis of** cerebellar **arteries**

I66.8 **Occlusion and stenosis of other cerebral arteries**
Occlusion and stenosis of perforating arteries

I66.9 **Occlusion and stenosis of unspecified cerebral artery**

✓4ᵗʰ **I67** **Other cerebrovascular diseases**
EXCLUDES 1   *sequelae of the listed conditions (I69.8)*

I67.0 **Dissection of cerebral arteries, nonruptured**
EXCLUDES 1   *ruptured cerebral arteries (I60.7)*

I67.1 **Cerebral aneurysm, nonruptured**
Cerebral aneurysm NOS
Cerebral arteriovenous fistula, acquired
Internal carotid artery aneurysm, intracranial portion
Internal carotid artery aneurysm, NOS
EXCLUDES 1   *congenital cerebral aneurysm, nonruptured (Q28.-)*
ruptured cerebral aneurysm (I60.7)

I67.2 **Cerebral atherosclerosis**   Ⓐ
Atheroma of cerebral and precerebral arteries

I67.3 **Progressive vascular leukoencephalopathy**
Binswanger's disease

I67.4 **Hypertensive encephalopathy**

I67.5 **Moyamoya disease**

I67.6 **Nonpyogenic thrombosis of intracranial venous system**
Nonpyogenic thrombosis of cerebral vein
Nonpyogenic thrombosis of intracranial venous sinus
EXCLUDES 1   *nonpyogenic thrombosis of intracranial venous system causing infarction (I63.6)*

I67.7 **Cerebral arteritis, not elsewhere classified**
Granulomatous angiitis of the nervous system
EXCLUDES 1   *allergic granulomatous angiitis (M30.1)*

✓5ᵗʰ **I67.8** **Other specified cerebrovascular diseases**

I67.81 **Acute cerebrovascular insufficiency**
Acute cerebrovascular insufficiency unspecified as to location or reversibility

I67.82 **Cerebral ischemia**
Chronic cerebral ischemia

I67.83 **Posterior reversible encephalopathy syndrome**
PRES

✓6ᵗʰ **I67.84** **Cerebral vasospasm and vasoconstriction**

I67.841 **Reversible cerebrovascular vasoconstriction syndrome**
Call-Fleming syndrome
Code first underlying condition, if applicable, such as eclampsia (O15.00-O15.9)

I67.848 **Other cerebrovascular vasospasm and vasoconstriction**

I67.89 **Other cerebrovascular disease**

I67.9 **Cerebrovascular disease, unspecified**

✓4ᵗʰ **I68** **Cerebrovascular disorders in diseases classified elsewhere**

I68.0 *Cerebral amyloid angiopathy*
Code first underlying amyloidosis (E85.-)

I68.2 *Cerebral arteritis in other diseases classified elsewhere*
Code first underlying disease
EXCLUDES 1   *cerebral arteritis (in):*
listerosis (A32.89)
systemic lupus erythematosus (M32.19)
syphilis (A52.04)
tuberculosis (A18.89)

I68.8 *Other cerebrovascular disorders in diseases classified elsewhere*
Code first underlying disease
EXCLUDES 1   *syphilitic cerebral aneurysm (A52.05)*

✓4ᵗʰ **I69** **Sequelae of cerebrovascular disease**
NOTE   Category I69 is to be used to indicate conditions in I60-I67 as the cause of sequelae. The "sequelae" include conditions specified as such or as residuals which may occur at any time after the onset of the causal condition
EXCLUDES 1   *personal history of cerebral infarction without residual deficit (Z86.73)*
personal history of prolonged reversible ischemic neurologic deficit (PRIND) (Z86.73)
personal history of reversible ischemic neurologcial deficit (RIND) (Z86.73)
sequelae of traumatic intracranial injury (S06.-)
transient ischemic attack (TIA) (G45.9)
AHA: 2012, Q4, 106

✓5ᵗʰ **I69.0** **Sequelae of nontraumatic** subarachnoid **hemorrhage**

I69.00 **Unspecified sequelae of nontraumatic subarachnoid hemorrhage**

I69.01 **Cognitive deficits** following nontraumatic subarachnoid hemorrhage

✓6ᵗʰ **I69.02** **Speech** and language deficits **following nontraumatic subarachnoid hemorrhage**

I69.020 **Aphasia** following nontraumatic subarachnoid hemorrhage

I69.021 **Dysphasia** following nontraumatic subarachnoid hemorrhage

I69.022 **Dysarthria** following nontraumatic subarachnoid hemorrhage

I69.023 **Fluency disorder** following nontraumatic subarachnoid hemorrhage
Stuttering following nontraumatic subarachnoid hemorrhage

I69.028 **Other speech and language deficits following nontraumatic subarachnoid hemorrhage**

✓6ᵗʰ **I69.03** **Monoplegia** of upper limb **following nontraumatic subarachnoid hemorrhage**

I69.031 **Monoplegia of upper limb following nontraumatic subarachnoid hemorrhage affecting** right dominant **side**

I69.032 **Monoplegia of upper limb following nontraumatic subarachnoid hemorrhage affecting** left dominant **side**

I69.033 **Monoplegia of upper limb following nontraumatic subarachnoid hemorrhage affecting** right non-dominant **side**

I69.034 **Monoplegia of upper limb following nontraumatic subarachnoid hemorrhage affecting** left non-dominant **side**

I69.039 **Monoplegia of upper limb following nontraumatic subarachnoid hemorrhage affecting unspecified side**

✓6ᵗʰ **I69.04** **Monoplegia** of lower limb **following nontraumatic subarachnoid hemorrhage**

I69.041 **Monoplegia of lower limb following nontraumatic subarachnoid hemorrhage affecting** right dominant **side**

I69.042 **Monoplegia of lower limb following nontraumatic subarachnoid hemorrhage affecting** left dominant **side**

I69.043 **Monoplegia of lower limb following nontraumatic subarachnoid hemorrhage affecting** right non-dominant **side**

I69.044 **Monoplegia of lower limb following nontraumatic subarachnoid hemorrhage affecting** left non-dominant **side**

I69.049 **Monoplegia of lower limb following nontraumatic subarachnoid hemorrhage affecting unspecified side**

✓6ᵗʰ **I69.05** **Hemiplegia and hemiparesis** following **nontraumatic subarachnoid hemorrhage**

I69.051 **Hemiplegia and hemiparesis following nontraumatic subarachnoid hemorrhage affecting** right dominant **side**

I69.052 **Hemiplegia and hemiparesis following nontraumatic subarachnoid hemorrhage affecting** left dominant **side**

EXCLUDES 1 Not coded here   EXCLUDES 2 Not included here   Ⓝ Newborn Age: 0   Ⓟ Pediatric Age: 0-17   Ⓜ Maternity Age: 12-55   Ⓐ Adult Age: 15-124

I69.053   **Hemiplegia and hemiparesis following nontraumatic subarachnoid hemorrhage affecting right non-dominant side**

I69.054   **Hemiplegia and hemiparesis following nontraumatic subarachnoid hemorrhage affecting left non-dominant side**

I69.059   **Hemiplegia and hemiparesis following nontraumatic subarachnoid hemorrhage affecting unspecified side**

☑6ᵗʰ **I69.06**   **Other paralytic syndrome following nontraumatic subarachnoid hemorrhage**
     Use additional code to identify type of paralytic syndrome, such as:
     locked-in state (G83.5)
     quadriplegia (G82.5-)

     EXCLUDES 1   *hemiplegia/hemiparesis following nontraumatic subarachnoid hemorrhage (I69.05-)*
           monoplegia of lower limb following nontraumatic subarachnoid hemorrhage (I69.04-)
           monoplegia of upper limb following nontraumatic subarachnoid hemorrhage (I69.03-)

I69.061   **Other paralytic syndrome following nontraumatic subarachnoid hemorrhage affecting right dominant side**

I69.062   **Other paralytic syndrome following nontraumatic subarachnoid hemorrhage affecting left dominant side**

I69.063   **Other paralytic syndrome following nontraumatic subarachnoid hemorrhage affecting right non-dominant side**

I69.064   **Other paralytic syndrome following nontraumatic subarachnoid hemorrhage affecting left non-dominant side**

I69.065   **Other paralytic syndrome following nontraumatic subarachnoid hemorrhage, bilateral**

I69.069   **Other paralytic syndrome following nontraumatic subarachnoid hemorrhage affecting unspecified side**

☑6ᵗʰ **I69.09**   **Other sequelae of nontraumatic subarachnoid hemorrhage**

I69.090   **Apraxia following nontraumatic subarachnoid hemorrhage**

I69.091   **Dysphagia following nontraumatic subarachnoid hemorrhage**
     Use additional code to identify the type of dysphagia, if known (R13.1-)

I69.092   **Facial weakness following nontraumatic subarachnoid hemorrhage**
     Facial droop following nontraumatic subarachnoid hemorrhage

I69.093   **Ataxia following nontraumatic subarachnoid hemorrhage**

I69.098   **Other sequelae following nontraumatic subarachnoid hemorrhage**
     Alterations of sensation following nontraumatic subarachnoid hemorrhage
     Disturbance of vision following nontraumatic subarachnoid hemorrhage
     Use additional code to identify the sequelae

☑5ᵗʰ **I69.1**   **Sequelae of nontraumatic intracerebral hemorrhage**

I69.10   **Unspecified sequelae of nontraumatic intracerebral hemorrhage**

I69.11   **Cognitive deficits following nontraumatic intracerebral hemorrhage**

☑6ᵗʰ **I69.12**   **Speech and language deficits following nontraumatic intracerebral hemorrhage**

I69.120   **Aphasia following nontraumatic intracerebral hemorrhage**

I69.121   **Dysphasia following nontraumatic intracerebral hemorrhage**

I69.122   **Dysarthria following nontraumatic intracerebral hemorrhage**

I69.123   **Fluency disorder following nontraumatic intracerebral hemorrhage**
     Stuttering following nontraumatic subarachnoid hemorrhage

I69.128   **Other speech and language deficits following nontraumatic intracerebral hemorrhage**

☑6ᵗʰ **I69.13**   **Monoplegia of upper limb following nontraumatic intracerebral hemorrhage**

I69.131   **Monoplegia of upper limb following nontraumatic intracerebral hemorrhage affecting right dominant side**

I69.132   **Monoplegia of upper limb following nontraumatic intracerebral hemorrhage affecting left dominant side**

I69.133   **Monoplegia of upper limb following nontraumatic intracerebral hemorrhage affecting right non-dominant side**

I69.134   **Monoplegia of upper limb following nontraumatic intracerebral hemorrhage affecting left non-dominant side**

I69.139   **Monoplegia of upper limb following nontraumatic intracerebral hemorrhage affecting unspecified side**

☑6ᵗʰ **I69.14**   **Monoplegia of lower limb following nontraumatic intracerebral hemorrhage**

I69.141   **Monoplegia of lower limb following nontraumatic intracerebral hemorrhage affecting right dominant side**

I69.142   **Monoplegia of lower limb following nontraumatic intracerebral hemorrhage affecting left dominant side**

I69.143   **Monoplegia of lower limb following nontraumatic intracerebral hemorrhage affecting right non-dominant side**

I69.144   **Monoplegia of lower limb following nontraumatic intracerebral hemorrhage affecting left non-dominant side**

I69.149   **Monoplegia of lower limb following nontraumatic intracerebral hemorrhage affecting unspecified side**

☑6ᵗʰ **I69.15**   **Hemiplegia and hemiparesis following nontraumatic intracerebral hemorrhage**

I69.151   **Hemiplegia and hemiparesis following nontraumatic intracerebral hemorrhage affecting right dominant side**

I69.152   **Hemiplegia and hemiparesis following nontraumatic intracerebral hemorrhage affecting left dominant side**

I69.153   **Hemiplegia and hemiparesis following nontraumatic intracerebral hemorrhage affecting right non-dominant side**

I69.154   **Hemiplegia and hemiparesis following nontraumatic intracerebral hemorrhage affecting left non-dominant side**

I69.159   **Hemiplegia and hemiparesis following nontraumatic intracerebral hemorrhage affecting unspecified side**

☑6ᵗʰ **I69.16**   **Other paralytic syndrome following nontraumatic intracerebral hemorrhage**
     Use additional code to identify type of paralytic syndrome, such as:
     locked-in state (G83.5)
     quadriplegia (G82.5-)

     EXCLUDES 1   *hemiplegia/hemiparesis following nontraumatic intracerebral hemorrhage (I69.15-)*
           monoplegia of lower limb following nontraumatic intracerebral hemorrhage (I69.14-)
           monoplegia of upper limb following nontraumatic intracerebral hemorrhage (I69.13-)

I69.161   **Other paralytic syndrome following nontraumatic intracerebral hemorrhage affecting right dominant side**

I69.162   **Other paralytic syndrome following nontraumatic intracerebral hemorrhage affecting left dominant side**

I69.163   **Other paralytic syndrome following nontraumatic intracerebral hemorrhage affecting right non-dominant side**

I69.164   **Other paralytic syndrome following nontraumatic intracerebral hemorrhage affecting left non-dominant side**

☑ Additional Character Required   ✓x7ᵗʰ Xtension Alert   Unspecified Code   Other Specified Code   Manifestation Code   ►◄ Revised Text   ● New Code   ▲ Revised Code Title

ICD-10-CM 2014 (Draft)   581

Diseases of the Circulatory System

I69.165–I69.31

I69.165   **Other paralytic syndrome following nontraumatic intracerebral hemorrhage, bilateral**

I69.169   **Other paralytic syndrome following nontraumatic intracerebral hemorrhage affecting unspecified side**

✓6th **I69.19**   Other sequelae of nontraumatic intracerebral hemorrhage

I69.190   **Apraxia following nontraumatic intracerebral hemorrhage**

I69.191   **Dysphagia following nontraumatic intracerebral hemorrhage**
    Use additional code to identify the type of dysphagia, if known (R13.1-)

I69.192   **Facial weakness following nontraumatic intracerebral hemorrhage**
    Facial droop following nontraumatic intracerebral hemorrhage

I69.193   **Ataxia following nontraumatic intracerebral hemorrhage**

I69.198   **Other sequelae of nontraumatic intracerebral hemorrhage**
    Alteration of sensations following nontraumatic intracerebral hemorrhage
    Disturbance of vision following nontraumatic intracerebral hemorrhage
    Use additional code to identify the sequelae

✓5th **I69.2**   **Sequelae of other nontraumatic intracranial hemorrhage**

I69.20   **Unspecified sequelae of other nontraumatic intracranial hemorrhage**

I69.21   **Cognitive deficits following other nontraumatic intracranial hemorrhage**

✓6th **I69.22**   **Speech and language deficits following other nontraumatic intracranial hemorrhage**

I69.220   **Aphasia following other nontraumatic intracranial hemorrhage**

I69.221   **Dysphasia following other nontraumatic intracranial hemorrhage**

I69.222   **Dysarthria following other nontraumatic intracranial hemorrhage**

I69.223   **Fluency disorder following other nontraumatic intracranial hemorrhage**
    Stuttering following nontraumatic subarachnoid hemorrhage

I69.228   **Other speech and language deficits following other nontraumatic intracranial hemorrhage**

✓6th **I69.23**   Monoplegia of upper limb following other nontraumatic intracranial hemorrhage

I69.231   **Monoplegia of upper limb following other nontraumatic intracranial hemorrhage affecting right dominant side**

I69.232   **Monoplegia of upper limb following other nontraumatic intracranial hemorrhage affecting left dominant side**

I69.233   **Monoplegia of upper limb following other nontraumatic intracranial hemorrhage affecting right non-dominant side**

I69.234   **Monoplegia of upper limb following other nontraumatic intracranial hemorrhage affecting left non-dominant side**

I69.239   **Monoplegia of upper limb following other nontraumatic intracranial hemorrhage affecting unspecified side**

✓6th **I69.24**   Monoplegia of lower limb following other nontraumatic intracranial hemorrhage

I69.241   **Monoplegia of lower limb following other nontraumatic intracranial hemorrhage affecting right dominant side**

I69.242   **Monoplegia of lower limb following other nontraumatic intracranial hemorrhage affecting left dominant side**

I69.243   **Monoplegia of lower limb following other nontraumatic intracranial hemorrhage affecting right non-dominant side**

I69.244   **Monoplegia of lower limb following other nontraumatic intracranial hemorrhage affecting left non-dominant side**

I69.249   **Monoplegia of lower limb following other nontraumatic intracranial hemorrhage affecting unspecified side**

✓6th **I69.25**   Hemiplegia and hemiparesis following other nontraumatic intracranial hemorrhage

I69.251   **Hemiplegia and hemiparesis following other nontraumatic intracranial hemorrhage affecting right dominant side**

I69.252   **Hemiplegia and hemiparesis following other nontraumatic intracranial hemorrhage affecting left dominant side**

I69.253   **Hemiplegia and hemiparesis following other nontraumatic intracranial hemorrhage affecting right non-dominant side**

I69.254   **Hemiplegia and hemiparesis following other nontraumatic intracranial hemorrhage affecting left non-dominant side**

I69.259   **Hemiplegia and hemiparesis following other nontraumatic intracranial hemorrhage affecting unspecified side**

✓6th **I69.26**   Other paralytic syndrome following other nontraumatic intracranial hemorrhage
    Use additional code to identify type of paralytic syndrome, such as:
    locked-in state (G83.5)
    quadriplegia (G82.5-)

EXCLUDES 1   hemiplegia/hemiparesis following other nontraumatic intracranial hemorrhage (I69.25-)
    monoplegia of lower limb following other nontraumatic intracranial hemorrhage (I69.24-)
    monoplegia of upper limb following other nontraumatic intracranial hemorrhage (I69.23-)

I69.261   **Other paralytic syndrome following other nontraumatic intracranial hemorrhage affecting right dominant side**

I69.262   **Other paralytic syndrome following other nontraumatic intracranial hemorrhage affecting left dominant side**

I69.263   **Other paralytic syndrome following other nontraumatic intracranial hemorrhage affecting right non-dominant side**

I69.264   **Other paralytic syndrome following other nontraumatic intracranial hemorrhage affecting left non-dominant side**

I69.265   **Other paralytic syndrome following other nontraumatic intracranial hemorrhage, bilateral**

I69.269   **Other paralytic syndrome following other nontraumatic intracranial hemorrhage affecting unspecified side**

✓6th **I69.29**   Other sequelae of other nontraumatic intracranial hemorrhage

I69.290   **Apraxia following other nontraumatic intracranial hemorrhage**

I69.291   **Dysphagia following other nontraumatic intracranial hemorrhage**
    Use additional code to identify the type of dysphagia, if known (R13.1-)

I69.292   **Facial weakness following other nontraumatic intracranial hemorrhage**
    Facial droop following other nontraumatic intracranial hemorrhage

I69.293   **Ataxia following other nontraumatic intracranial hemorrhage**

I69.298   **Other sequelae of other nontraumatic intracranial hemorrhage**
    Alteration of sensation following other nontraumatic intracranial hemorrhage
    Disturbance of vision following other nontraumatic intracranial hemorrhage
    Use additional code to identify the sequelae

✓5th **I69.3**   **Sequelae of cerebral infarction**
    Sequelae of stroke NOS
    AHA: 2012, Q4, 92, 94

I69.30   **Unspecified sequelae of cerebral infarction**

I69.31   **Cognitive deficits following cerebral infarction**

EXCLUDES 1 Not coded here   EXCLUDES 2 Not included here   N Newborn Age: 0   P Pediatric Age: 0-17   M Maternity Age: 12-55   A Adult Age: 15-124

582   ICD-10-CM 2014 (Draft)

☑6ᵗʰ I69.32 Speech and language deficits following cerebral infarction

I69.320 Aphasia following cerebral infarction

I69.321 Dysphasia following cerebral infarction
AHA: 2012, Q4, 91

I69.322 Dysarthria following cerebral infarction

I69.323 Fluency disorder following cerebral infarction
Stuttering following nontraumatic subarachnoid hemorrhage

I69.328 Other speech and language deficits following cerebral infarction

☑6ᵗʰ I69.33 Monoplegia of upper limb following cerebral infarction

I69.331 Monoplegia of upper limb following cerebral infarction affecting right dominant side

I69.332 Monoplegia of upper limb following cerebral infarction affecting left dominant side

I69.333 Monoplegia of upper limb following cerebral infarction affecting right non-dominant side

I69.334 Monoplegia of upper limb following cerebral infarction affecting left non-dominant side

I69.339 Monoplegia of upper limb following cerebral infarction affecting unspecified side

☑6ᵗʰ I69.34 Monoplegia of lower limb following cerebral infarction

I69.341 Monoplegia of lower limb following cerebral infarction affecting right dominant side

I69.342 Monoplegia of lower limb following cerebral infarction affecting left dominant side

I69.343 Monoplegia of lower limb following cerebral infarction affecting right non-dominant side

I69.344 Monoplegia of lower limb following cerebral infarction affecting left non-dominant side

I69.349 Monoplegia of lower limb following cerebral infarction affecting unspecified side

☑6ᵗʰ I69.35 Hemiplegia and hemiparesis following cerebral infarction

I69.351 Hemiplegia and hemiparesis following cerebral infarction affecting right dominant side

I69.352 Hemiplegia and hemiparesis following cerebral infarction affecting left dominant side

I69.353 Hemiplegia and hemiparesis following cerebral infarction affecting right non-dominant side

I69.354 Hemiplegia and hemiparesis following cerebral infarction affecting left non-dominant side
AHA: 2012, Q4, 91

I69.359 Hemiplegia and hemiparesis following cerebral infarction affecting unspecified side

☑6ᵗʰ I69.36 Other paralytic syndrome following cerebral infarction
Use additional code to identify type of paralytic syndrome, such as:
locked-in state (G83.5)
quadriplegia (G82.5-)
EXCLUDES 1 *hemiplegia/hemiparesis following cerebral infarction (I69.35-)*
monoplegia of lower limb following cerebral infarction (I69.34-)
monoplegia of upper limb following cerebral infarction (I69.33-)

I69.361 Other paralytic syndrome following cerebral infarction affecting right dominant side

I69.362 Other paralytic syndrome following cerebral infarction affecting left dominant side

I69.363 Other paralytic syndrome following cerebral infarction affecting right non-dominant side

I69.364 Other paralytic syndrome following cerebral infarction affecting left non-dominant side

I69.365 Other paralytic syndrome following cerebral infarction, bilateral

I69.369 Other paralytic syndrome following cerebral infarction affecting unspecified side

☑6ᵗʰ I69.39 Other sequelae of cerebral infarction

I69.390 Apraxia following cerebral infarction

I69.391 Dysphagia following cerebral infarction
Use additional code to identify the type of dysphagia, if known (R13.1-)

I69.392 Facial weakness following cerebral infarction
Facial droop following cerebral infarction

I69.393 Ataxia following cerebral infarction

I69.398 Other sequelae of cerebral infarction
Alteration of sensation following cerebral infarction
Disturbance of vision following cerebral infarction
Use additional code to identify the sequelae

☑5ᵗʰ I69.8 Sequelae of other cerebrovascular diseases
EXCLUDES 1 *sequelae of traumatic intracranial injury (S06.-)*

I69.80 Unspecified sequelae of other cerebrovascular disease

I69.81 Cognitive deficits following other cerebrovascular disease

☑6ᵗʰ I69.82 Speech and language deficits following other cerebrovascular disease

I69.820 Aphasia following other cerebrovascular disease

I69.821 Dysphasia following other cerebrovascular disease

I69.822 Dysarthria following other cerebrovascular disease

I69.823 Fluency disorder following other cerebrovascular disease
Stuttering following nontraumatic subarachnoid hemorrhage

I69.828 Other speech and language deficits following other cerebrovascular disease

☑6ᵗʰ I69.83 Monoplegia of upper limb following other cerebrovascular disease

I69.831 Monoplegia of upper limb following other cerebrovascular disease affecting right dominant side

I69.832 Monoplegia of upper limb following other cerebrovascular disease affecting left dominant side

I69.833 Monoplegia of upper limb following other cerebrovascular disease affecting right non-dominant side

I69.834 Monoplegia of upper limb following other cerebrovascular disease affecting left non-dominant side

I69.839 Monoplegia of upper limb following other cerebrovascular disease affecting unspecified side

☑6ᵗʰ I69.84 Monoplegia of lower limb following other cerebrovascular disease

I69.841 Monoplegia of lower limb following other cerebrovascular disease affecting right dominant side

I69.842 Monoplegia of lower limb following other cerebrovascular disease affecting left dominant side

I69.843 Monoplegia of lower limb following other cerebrovascular disease affecting right non-dominant side

---

☑ Additional Character Required   √×7ᵗʰ *X*tension Alert   Unspecified Code   Other Specified Code   Manifestation Code   ►◄ Revised Text   ● New Code   ▲ Revised Code Title

Diseases of the Circulatory System

I69.844–I69.96

I69.844   **Monoplegia of lower limb following other cerebrovascular disease affecting left non-dominant side**

I69.849   **Monoplegia of lower limb following other cerebrovascular disease affecting unspecified side**

✓6ᵗʰ I69.85   Hemiplegia and hemiparesis following other cerebrovascular disease

I69.851   **Hemiplegia and hemiparesis following other cerebrovascular disease affecting right dominant side**

I69.852   **Hemiplegia and hemiparesis following other cerebrovascular disease affecting left dominant side**

I69.853   **Hemiplegia and hemiparesis following other cerebrovascular disease affecting right non-dominant side**

I69.854   **Hemiplegia and hemiparesis following other cerebrovascular disease affecting left non-dominant side**

I69.859   **Hemiplegia and hemiparesis following other cerebrovascular disease affecting unspecified side**

✓6ᵗʰ I69.86   Other paralytic syndrome following other cerebrovascular disease

Use additional code to identify type of paralytic syndrome, such as:
locked-in state (G83.5)
quadriplegia (G82.5-)

EXCLUDES 1   hemiplegia/hemiparesis following other cerebrovascular disease (I69.85-)
monoplegia of lower limb following other cerebrovascular disease (I69.84-)
monoplegia of upper limb following other cerebrovascular disease (I69.83-)

I69.861   **Other paralytic syndrome following other cerebrovascular disease affecting right dominant side**

I69.862   **Other paralytic syndrome following other cerebrovascular disease affecting left dominant side**

I69.863   **Other paralytic syndrome following other cerebrovascular disease affecting right non-dominant side**

I69.864   **Other paralytic syndrome following other cerebrovascular disease affecting left non-dominant side**

I69.865   **Other paralytic syndrome following other cerebrovascular disease, bilateral**

I69.869   **Other paralytic syndrome following other cerebrovascular disease affecting unspecified side**

✓6ᵗʰ I69.89   Other sequelae of other cerebrovascular disease

I69.890   Apraxia following other cerebrovascular disease

I69.891   Dysphagia following other cerebrovascular disease
Use additional code to identify the type of dysphagia, if known (R13.1-)

I69.892   Facial weakness following other cerebrovascular disease
Facial droop following other cerebrovascular disease

I69.893   Ataxia following other cerebrovascular disease

I69.898   **Other sequelae of other cerebrovascular disease**
Alteration of sensation following other cerebrovascular disease
Disturbance of vision following other cerebrovascular disease
Use additional code to identify the sequelae

✓5ᵗʰ I69.9   Sequelae of unspecified cerebrovascular diseases
EXCLUDES 1   sequelae of stroke (I69.3)
sequelae of traumatic intracranial injury (S06.-)

I69.90   **Unspecified sequelae of unspecified cerebrovascular disease**

I69.91   Cognitive deficits following unspecified cerebrovascular disease

✓5ᵗʰ I69.92   Speech and language deficits following unspecified cerebrovascular disease

I69.920   Aphasia following unspecified cerebrovascular disease

I69.921   Dysphasia following unspecified cerebrovascular disease

I69.922   Dysarthria following unspecified cerebrovascular disease

I69.923   Fluency disorder following unspecified cerebrovascular disease
Stuttering following nontraumatic subarachnoid hemorrhage

I69.928   **Other speech and language deficits following unspecified cerebrovascular disease**

✓6ᵗʰ I69.93   Monoplegia of upper limb following unspecified cerebrovascular disease

I69.931   **Monoplegia of upper limb following unspecified cerebrovascular disease affecting right dominant side**

I69.932   **Monoplegia of upper limb following unspecified cerebrovascular disease affecting left dominant side**

I69.933   **Monoplegia of upper limb following unspecified cerebrovascular disease affecting right non-dominant side**

I69.934   **Monoplegia of upper limb following unspecified cerebrovascular disease affecting left non-dominant side**

I69.939   **Monoplegia of upper limb following unspecified cerebrovascular disease affecting unspecified side**

✓6ᵗʰ I69.94   Monoplegia of lower limb following unspecified cerebrovascular disease

I69.941   **Monoplegia of lower limb following unspecified cerebrovascular disease affecting right dominant side**

I69.942   **Monoplegia of lower limb following unspecified cerebrovascular disease affecting left dominant side**

I69.943   **Monoplegia of lower limb following unspecified cerebrovascular disease affecting right non-dominant side**

I69.944   **Monoplegia of lower limb following unspecified cerebrovascular disease affecting left non-dominant side**

I69.949   **Monoplegia of lower limb following unspecified cerebrovascular disease affecting unspecified side**

✓6ᵗʰ I69.95   Hemiplegia and hemiparesis following unspecified cerebrovascular disease

I69.951   **Hemiplegia and hemiparesis following unspecified cerebrovascular disease affecting right dominant side**

I69.952   **Hemiplegia and hemiparesis following unspecified cerebrovascular disease affecting left dominant side**

I69.953   **Hemiplegia and hemiparesis following unspecified cerebrovascular disease affecting right non-dominant side**

I69.954   **Hemiplegia and hemiparesis following unspecified cerebrovascular disease affecting left non-dominant side**

I69.959   **Hemiplegia and hemiparesis following unspecified cerebrovascular disease affecting unspecified side**

✓6ᵗʰ I69.96   Other paralytic syndrome following unspecified cerebrovascular disease
Use additional code to identify type of paralytic syndrome, such as:
locked-in state (G83.5)
quadriplegia (G82.5-)

EXCLUDES 1   hemiplegia/hemiparesis following unspecified cerebrovascular disease (I69.95-)
monoplegia of lower limb following unspecified cerebrovascular disease (I69.94-)
monoplegia of upper limb following unspecified cerebrovascular disease (I69.93-)

EXCLUDES 1 Not coded here   *EXCLUDES 2* Not included here   N Newborn Age: 0   P Pediatric Age: 0-17   M Maternity Age: 12-55   A Adult Age: 15-124

584   ICD-10-CM 2014 (Draft)

I69.961 Other paralytic syndrome following unspecified cerebrovascular disease affecting right dominant side

I69.962 Other paralytic syndrome following unspecified cerebrovascular disease affecting left dominant side

I69.963 Other paralytic syndrome following unspecified cerebrovascular disease affecting right non-dominant side

I69.964 Other paralytic syndrome following unspecified cerebrovascular disease affecting left non-dominant side

I69.965 Other paralytic syndrome following unspecified cerebrovascular disease, bilateral

I69.969 Other paralytic syndrome following unspecified cerebrovascular disease affecting unspecified side

√6ᵗʰ **I69.99** Other sequelae of unspecified cerebrovascular disease

I69.990 Apraxia following unspecified cerebrovascular disease

I69.991 Dysphagia following unspecified cerebrovascular disease
Use additional code to identify the type of dysphagia, if known (R13.1-)

I69.992 Facial weakness following unspecified cerebrovascular disease
Facial droop following unspecified cerebrovascular disease

I69.993 Ataxia following unspecified cerebrovascular disease

I69.998 Other sequelae following unspecified cerebrovascular disease
Alteration in sensation following unspecified cerebrovascular disease
Disturbance of vision following unspecified cerebrovascular disease
Use additional code to identify the sequelae

Diseases of arteries, arterioles and capillaries (I70-I79)

√4ᵗʰ **I70 Atherosclerosis**
INCLUDES arteriolosclerosis
arterial degeneration
arteriosclerosis
arteriosclerotic vascular disease
arteriovascular degeneration
atheroma
endarteritis deformans or obliterans
senile arteritis
senile endarteritis
vascular degeneration
Use additional code to identify:
exposure to environmental tobacco smoke (Z77.22)
history of tobacco use (Z87.891)
occupational exposure to environmental tobacco smoke (Z57.31)
tobacco dependence (F17.-)
tobacco use (Z72.0)
EXCLUDES 2 arteriosclerotic cardiovascular disease (I25.1-)
arteriosclerotic heart disease (I25.1-)
atheroembolism (I75.-)
cerebral atherosclerosis (I67.2)
coronary atherosclerosis (I25.1-)
mesenteric atherosclerosis (K55.1)
precerebral atherosclerosis (I67.2)
primary pulmonary atherosclerosis (I27.0)

I70.0 Atherosclerosis of aorta A

I70.1 Atherosclerosis of renal artery A
Goldblatt's kidney
EXCLUDES 2 atherosclerosis of renal arterioles (I12.-)

√5ᵗʰ **I70.2 Atherosclerosis of native arteries of the extremities**
Mönckeberg's (medial) sclerosis
Use additional code, if applicable, to identify chronic total occlusion of artery of extremity (I70.92)
EXCLUDES 2 atherosclerosis of bypass graft of extremities (I70.30-I70.79)

√6ᵗʰ **I70.20** Unspecified atherosclerosis of native arteries of extremities

I70.201 Unspecified atherosclerosis of native arteries of extremities, right leg A

I70.202 Unspecified atherosclerosis of native arteries of extremities, left leg A

I70.203 Unspecified atherosclerosis of native arteries of extremities, bilateral legs A

I70.208 Unspecified atherosclerosis of native arteries of extremities, other extremity A

I70.209 Unspecified atherosclerosis of native arteries of extremities, unspecified extremity A

√6ᵗʰ **I70.21** Atherosclerosis of native arteries of extremities with intermittent claudication

I70.211 Atherosclerosis of native arteries of extremities with intermittent claudication, right leg A

I70.212 Atherosclerosis of native arteries of extremities with intermittent claudication, left leg A

I70.213 Atherosclerosis of native arteries of extremities with intermittent claudication, bilateral legs A

I70.218 Atherosclerosis of native arteries of extremities with intermittent claudication, other extremity A

I70.219 Atherosclerosis of native arteries of extremities with intermittent claudication, unspecified extremity A

√6ᵗʰ **I70.22** Atherosclerosis of native arteries of extremities with rest pain
Includes any condition classifiable to I70.21-

I70.221 Atherosclerosis of native arteries of extremities with rest pain, right leg A

I70.222 Atherosclerosis of native arteries of extremities with rest pain, left leg A

I70.223 Atherosclerosis of native arteries of extremities with rest pain, bilateral legs A

I70.228 Atherosclerosis of native arteries of extremities with rest pain, other extremity A

I70.229 Atherosclerosis of native arteries of extremities with rest pain, unspecified extremity A

√6ᵗʰ **I70.23** Atherosclerosis of native arteries of right leg with ulceration
Includes any condition classifiable to I70.211 and I70.221
Use additional code to identify severity of ulcer (L97.-)

I70.231 Atherosclerosis of native arteries of right leg with ulceration of thigh A

I70.232 Atherosclerosis of native arteries of right leg with ulceration of calf A

I70.233 Atherosclerosis of native arteries of right leg with ulceration of ankle A

I70.234 Atherosclerosis of native arteries of right leg with ulceration of heel and midfoot A
Atherosclerosis of native arteries of right leg with ulceration of plantar surface of midfoot

I70.235 Atherosclerosis of native arteries of right leg with ulceration of other part of foot A
Atherosclerosis of native arteries of right leg extremities with ulceration of toe

I70.238 Atherosclerosis of native arteries of right leg with ulceration of other part of lower right leg A

I70.239 Atherosclerosis of native arteries of right leg with ulceration of unspecified site A

√6ᵗʰ **I70.24** Atherosclerosis of native arteries of left leg with ulceration
Includes any condition classifiable to I70.212 and I70.222
Use additional code to identify severity of ulcer (L97.-)

I70.241 Atherosclerosis of native arteries of left leg with ulceration of thigh A

I70.242 Atherosclerosis of native arteries of left leg with ulceration of calf A

I70.243 Atherosclerosis of native arteries of left leg with ulceration of ankle A

√ Additional Character Required   √x7ᵗʰ Xtension Alert   Unspecified Code   Other Specified Code   Manifestation Code   ►◄ Revised Text   ● New Code   ▲ Revised Code Title

I70.244   Atherosclerosis of native arteries of left 🄰 leg with ulceration of heel and midfoot
> Atherosclerosis of native arteries of left leg with ulceration of plantar surface of midfoot

I70.245   Atherosclerosis of native arteries of left 🄰 leg with ulceration of other part of foot
> Atherosclerosis of native arteries of left leg extremities with ulceration of toe

I70.248   Atherosclerosis of native arteries of left 🄰 leg with ulceration of other part of lower left leg

I70.249   Atherosclerosis of native arteries of left 🄰 leg with ulceration of unspecified site

I70.25   Atherosclerosis of native arteries of other 🄰 extremities with ulceration
> Includes any condition classifiable to I70.218 and I70.228
> Use additional code to identify the severity of the ulcer (L98.49-)

√6ᵗʰ I70.26   Atherosclerosis of native arteries of extremities with gangrene
> Includes any condition classifiable to I70.21-, I70.22-, I70.23-, I70.24-, and I70.25-
> Use additional code to identify the severity of any ulcer (L97.-, L98.49-), if applicable

I70.261   Atherosclerosis of native arteries of 🄰 extremities with gangrene, right leg

I70.262   Atherosclerosis of native arteries of 🄰 extremities with gangrene, left leg

I70.263   Atherosclerosis of native arteries of 🄰 extremities with gangrene, bilateral legs

I70.268   Atherosclerosis of native arteries of 🄰 extremities with gangrene, other extremity

I70.269   Atherosclerosis of native arteries of 🄰 extremities with gangrene, unspecified extremity

√6ᵗʰ I70.29   Other atherosclerosis of native arteries of extremities

I70.291   Other atherosclerosis of native arteries 🄰 of extremities, right leg

I70.292   Other atherosclerosis of native arteries 🄰 of extremities, left leg

I70.293   Other atherosclerosis of native arteries 🄰 of extremities, bilateral legs

I70.298   Other atherosclerosis of native arteries 🄰 of extremities, other extremity

I70.299   Other atherosclerosis of native arteries 🄰 of extremities, unspecified extremity

√5ᵗʰ I70.3   Atherosclerosis of unspecified type of bypass graft(s) of the extremities
> Use additional code, if applicable, to identify chronic total occlusion of artery of extremity (I70.92)
> EXCLUDES 1   embolism or thrombus of bypass graft(s) of extremities (T82.8-)

√6ᵗʰ I70.30   Unspecified atherosclerosis of unspecified type of bypass graft(s) of the extremities

I70.301   Unspecified atherosclerosis of 🄰 unspecified type of bypass graft(s) of the extremities, right leg

I70.302   Unspecified atherosclerosis of 🄰 unspecified type of bypass graft(s) of the extremities, left leg

I70.303   Unspecified atherosclerosis of 🄰 unspecified type of bypass graft(s) of the extremities, bilateral legs

I70.308   Unspecified atherosclerosis of 🄰 unspecified type of bypass graft(s) of the extremities, other extremity

I70.309   Unspecified atherosclerosis of 🄰 unspecified type of bypass graft(s) of the extremities, unspecified extremity

√6ᵗʰ I70.31   Atherosclerosis of unspecified type of bypass graft(s) of the extremities with intermittent claudication

I70.311   Atherosclerosis of unspecified type of 🄰 bypass graft(s) of the extremities with intermittent claudication, right leg

I70.312   Atherosclerosis of unspecified type of 🄰 bypass graft(s) of the extremities with intermittent claudication, left leg

I70.313   Atherosclerosis of unspecified type of 🄰 bypass graft(s) of the extremities with intermittent claudication, bilateral legs

I70.318   Atherosclerosis of unspecified type of 🄰 bypass graft(s) of the extremities with intermittent claudication, other extremity

I70.319   Atherosclerosis of unspecified type of 🄰 bypass graft(s) of the extremities with intermittent claudication, unspecified extremity

√6ᵗʰ I70.32   Atherosclerosis of unspecified type of bypass graft(s) of the extremities with rest pain
> Includes any condition classifiable to I70.31-

I70.321   Atherosclerosis of unspecified type of 🄰 bypass graft(s) of the extremities with rest pain, right leg

I70.322   Atherosclerosis of unspecified type of 🄰 bypass graft(s) of the extremities with rest pain, left leg

I70.323   Atherosclerosis of unspecified type of 🄰 bypass graft(s) of the extremities with rest pain, bilateral legs

I70.328   Atherosclerosis of unspecified type of 🄰 bypass graft(s) of the extremities with rest pain, other extremity

I70.329   Atherosclerosis of unspecified type of 🄰 bypass graft(s) of the extremities with rest pain, unspecified extremity

√6ᵗʰ I70.33   Atherosclerosis of unspecified type of bypass graft(s) of the right leg with ulceration
> Includes any condition classifiable to I70.311 and I70.321
> Use additional code to identify severity of ulcer (L97.-)

I70.331   Atherosclerosis of unspecified type of 🄰 bypass graft(s) of the right leg with ulceration of thigh

I70.332   Atherosclerosis of unspecified type of 🄰 bypass graft(s) of the right leg with ulceration of calf

I70.333   Atherosclerosis of unspecified type of 🄰 bypass graft(s) of the right leg with ulceration of ankle

I70.334   Atherosclerosis of unspecified type of 🄰 bypass graft(s) of the right leg with ulceration of heel and midfoot
> Atherosclerosis of unspecified type of bypass graft(s) of right leg with ulceration of plantar surface of midfoot

I70.335   Atherosclerosis of unspecified type of 🄰 bypass graft(s) of the right leg with ulceration of other part of foot
> Atherosclerosis of unspecified type of bypass graft(s) of the right leg with ulceration of toe

I70.338   Atherosclerosis of unspecified type of 🄰 bypass graft(s) of the right leg with ulceration of other part of lower leg

I70.339   Atherosclerosis of unspecified type of 🄰 bypass graft(s) of the right leg with ulceration of unspecified site

√6ᵗʰ I70.34   Atherosclerosis of unspecified type of bypass graft(s) of the left leg with ulceration
> Includes any condition classifiable to I70.312 and I70.322
> Use additional code to identify severity of ulcer (L97.-)

I70.341   Atherosclerosis of unspecified type of 🄰 bypass graft(s) of the left leg with ulceration of thigh

I70.342   Atherosclerosis of unspecified type of 🄰 bypass graft(s) of the left leg with ulceration of calf

I70.343   Atherosclerosis of unspecified type of 🄰 bypass graft(s) of the left leg with ulceration of ankle

EXCLUDES 1 Not coded here   EXCLUDES 2 Not included here   🅽 Newborn Age: 0   🅿 Pediatric Age: 0-17   🅼 Maternity Age: 12-55   🄰 Adult Age: 15-124

586   ICD-10-CM 2014 (Draft)

I70.344 Atherosclerosis of unspecified type of bypass graft(s) of the left leg with ulceration of heel and midfoot ▲

Atherosclerosis of unspecified type of bypass graft(s) of left leg with ulceration of plantar surface of midfoot

I70.345 Atherosclerosis of unspecified type of bypass graft(s) of the left leg with ulceration of other part of foot ▲

Atherosclerosis of unspecified type of bypass graft(s) of the left leg with ulceration of toe

I70.348 Atherosclerosis of unspecified type of bypass graft(s) of the left leg with ulceration of other part of lower leg ▲

I70.349 Atherosclerosis of unspecified type of bypass graft(s) of the left leg with ulceration of unspecified site ▲

I70.35 Atherosclerosis of unspecified type of bypass graft(s) of other extremity with ulceration ▲

Includes any condition classifiable to I70.318 and I70.328
Use additional code to identify severity of ulcer (L98.49-)

√6ᵗʰ I70.36 Atherosclerosis of unspecified type of bypass graft(s) of the extremities with gangrene

Includes any condition classifiable to I70.31-, I70.32-, I70.33-, I70.34-, I70.35
Use additional code to identify the severity of any ulcer (L97.-, L98.49-), if applicable

I70.361 Atherosclerosis of unspecified type of bypass graft(s) of the extremities with gangrene, right leg ▲

I70.362 Atherosclerosis of unspecified type of bypass graft(s) of the extremities with gangrene, left leg ▲

I70.363 Atherosclerosis of unspecified type of bypass graft(s) of the extremities with gangrene, bilateral legs ▲

I70.368 Atherosclerosis of unspecified type of bypass graft(s) of the extremities with gangrene, other extremity ▲

I70.369 Atherosclerosis of unspecified type of bypass graft(s) of the extremities with gangrene, unspecified extremity ▲

√6ᵗʰ I70.39 Other atherosclerosis of unspecified type of bypass graft(s) of the extremities

I70.391 Other atherosclerosis of unspecified type of bypass graft(s) of the extremities, right leg ▲

I70.392 Other atherosclerosis of unspecified type of bypass graft(s) of the extremities, left leg ▲

I70.393 Other atherosclerosis of unspecified type of bypass graft(s) of the extremities, bilateral legs ▲

I70.398 Other atherosclerosis of unspecified type of bypass graft(s) of the extremities, other extremity ▲

I70.399 Other atherosclerosis of unspecified type of bypass graft(s) of the extremities, unspecified extremity ▲

√5ᵗʰ I70.4 Atherosclerosis of autologous vein bypass graft(s) of the extremities

Use additional code, if applicable, to identify chronic total occlusion of artery of extremity (I70.92)

√6ᵗʰ I70.40 Unspecified atherosclerosis of autologous vein bypass graft(s) of the extremities

I70.401 Unspecified atherosclerosis of autologous vein bypass graft(s) of the extremities, right leg ▲

I70.402 Unspecified atherosclerosis of autologous vein bypass graft(s) of the extremities, left leg ▲

I70.403 Unspecified atherosclerosis of autologous vein bypass graft(s) of the extremities, bilateral legs ▲

I70.408 Unspecified atherosclerosis of autologous vein bypass graft(s) of the extremities, other extremity ▲

I70.409 Unspecified atherosclerosis of autologous vein bypass graft(s) of the extremities, unspecified extremity ▲

√6ᵗʰ I70.41 Atherosclerosis of autologous vein bypass graft(s) of the extremities with intermittent claudication

I70.411 Atherosclerosis of autologous vein bypass graft(s) of the extremities with intermittent claudication, right leg ▲

I70.412 Atherosclerosis of autologous vein bypass graft(s) of the extremities with intermittent claudication, left leg ▲

I70.413 Atherosclerosis of autologous vein bypass graft(s) of the extremities with intermittent claudication, bilateral legs ▲

I70.418 Atherosclerosis of autologous vein bypass graft(s) of the extremities with intermittent claudication, other extremity ▲

I70.419 Atherosclerosis of autologous vein bypass graft(s) of the extremities with intermittent claudication, unspecified extremity ▲

√6ᵗʰ I70.42 Atherosclerosis of autologous vein bypass graft(s) of the extremities with rest pain

Includes any condition classifiable to I70.41-

I70.421 Atherosclerosis of autologous vein bypass graft(s) of the extremities with rest pain, right leg ▲

I70.422 Atherosclerosis of autologous vein bypass graft(s) of the extremities with rest pain, left leg ▲

I70.423 Atherosclerosis of autologous vein bypass graft(s) of the extremities with rest pain, bilateral legs ▲

I70.428 Atherosclerosis of autologous vein bypass graft(s) of the extremities with rest pain, other extremity ▲

I70.429 Atherosclerosis of autologous vein bypass graft(s) of the extremities with rest pain, unspecified extremity ▲

√6ᵗʰ I70.43 Atherosclerosis of autologous vein bypass graft(s) of the right leg with ulceration

Includes any condition classifiable to I70.411 and I70.421
Use additional code to identify severity of ulcer (L97.-)

I70.431 Atherosclerosis of autologous vein bypass graft(s) of the right leg with ulceration of thigh ▲

I70.432 Atherosclerosis of autologous vein bypass graft(s) of the right leg with ulceration of calf ▲

I70.433 Atherosclerosis of autologous vein bypass graft(s) of the right leg with ulceration of ankle ▲

I70.434 Atherosclerosis of autologous vein bypass graft(s) of the right leg with ulceration of heel and midfoot ▲

Atherosclerosis of autologous vein bypass graft(s) of right leg with ulceration of plantar surface of midfoot

I70.435 Atherosclerosis of autologous vein bypass graft(s) of the right leg with ulceration of other part of foot ▲

Atherosclerosis of autologous vein bypass graft(s) of right leg with ulceration of toe

I70.438 Atherosclerosis of autologous vein bypass graft(s) of the right leg with ulceration of other part of lower leg ▲

I70.439 Atherosclerosis of autologous vein bypass graft(s) of the right leg with ulceration of unspecified site ▲

√6ᵗʰ I70.44 Atherosclerosis of autologous vein bypass graft(s) of the left leg with ulceration

Includes any condition classifiable to I70.412 and I70.422
Use additional code to identify severity of ulcer (L97.-)

I70.441 Atherosclerosis of autologous vein bypass graft(s) of the left leg with ulceration of thigh ▲

I70.442 Atherosclerosis of autologous vein bypass graft(s) of the left leg with ulceration of calf ▲

Diseases of the Circulatory System

I70.443–I70.538

I70.443   **Atherosclerosis of autologous vein bypass graft(s) of the left leg with ulceration of** ankle   Ⓐ

I70.444   **Atherosclerosis of autologous vein bypass graft(s) of the left leg with ulceration of** heel and midfoot   Ⓐ
Atherosclerosis of autologous vein bypass graft(s) of left leg with ulceration of plantar surface of midfoot

I70.445   **Atherosclerosis of autologous vein bypass graft(s) of the left leg with ulceration of other** part of foot   Ⓐ
Atherosclerosis of autologous vein bypass graft(s) of left leg with ulceration of toe

I70.448   **Atherosclerosis of autologous vein bypass graft(s) of the left leg with ulceration of other** part of lower leg   Ⓐ

I70.449   **Atherosclerosis of autologous vein bypass graft(s) of the left leg with ulceration of unspecified site**   Ⓐ

I70.45   **Atherosclerosis of autologous vein bypass graft(s) of other extremity with** ulceration   Ⓐ
Includes any condition classifiable to I70.418, I70.428, and I70.438
Use additional code to identify severity of ulcer (L98.49)

✓6ᵗʰ **I70.46**   **Atherosclerosis of autologous vein bypass graft(s) of the extremities with** gangrene
Includes any condition classifiable to I70.41-, I70.42-, and I70.43-, I70.44-, I70.45
Use additional code to identify the severity of any ulcer (L97.-, L98.49-), if applicable

I70.461   **Atherosclerosis of autologous vein bypass graft(s) of the extremities with gangrene,** right leg   Ⓐ

I70.462   **Atherosclerosis of autologous vein bypass graft(s) of the extremities with gangrene,** left leg   Ⓐ

I70.463   **Atherosclerosis of autologous vein bypass graft(s) of the extremities with gangrene,** bilateral legs   Ⓐ

I70.468   **Atherosclerosis of autologous vein bypass graft(s) of the extremities with gangrene, other extremity**   Ⓐ

I70.469   **Atherosclerosis of autologous vein bypass graft(s) of the extremities with gangrene, unspecified extremity**   Ⓐ

✓6ᵗʰ **I70.49**   Other **atherosclerosis of autologous vein bypass graft(s) of the extremities**

I70.491   **Other atherosclerosis of autologous vein bypass graft(s) of the extremities,** right leg   Ⓐ

I70.492   **Other atherosclerosis of autologous vein bypass graft(s) of the extremities,** left leg   Ⓐ

I70.493   **Other atherosclerosis of autologous vein bypass graft(s) of the extremities,** bilateral legs   Ⓐ

I70.498   **Other atherosclerosis of autologous vein bypass graft(s) of the extremities, other extremity**   Ⓐ

I70.499   **Other atherosclerosis of autologous vein bypass graft(s) of the extremities, unspecified extremity**   Ⓐ

✓5ᵗʰ **I70.5**   **Atherosclerosis of** nonautologous biological bypass graft(s) **of the** extremities
Use additional code, if applicable, to identify chronic total occlusion of artery of extremity (I70.92)

✓6ᵗʰ **I70.50**   Unspecified **atherosclerosis of nonautologous biological bypass graft(s) of the extremities**

I70.501   **Unspecified atherosclerosis of nonautologous biological bypass graft(s) of the extremities,** right leg   Ⓐ

I70.502   **Unspecified atherosclerosis of nonautologous biological bypass graft(s) of the extremities,** left leg   Ⓐ

I70.503   **Unspecified atherosclerosis of nonautologous biological bypass graft(s) of the extremities,** bilateral legs   Ⓐ

I70.508   **Unspecified atherosclerosis of nonautologous biological bypass graft(s) of the extremities, other extremity**   Ⓐ

I70.509   **Unspecified atherosclerosis of nonautologous biological bypass graft(s) of the extremities, unspecified extremity**   Ⓐ

✓6ᵗʰ **I70.51**   **Atherosclerosis of nonautologous biological bypass graft(s) of the extremities with** intermittent claudication

I70.511   **Atherosclerosis of nonautologous biological bypass graft(s) of the extremities with intermittent claudication,** right leg   Ⓐ

I70.512   **Atherosclerosis of nonautologous biological bypass graft(s) of the extremities with intermittent claudication,** left leg   Ⓐ

I70.513   **Atherosclerosis of nonautologous biological bypass graft(s) of the extremities with intermittent claudication,** bilateral legs   Ⓐ

I70.518   **Atherosclerosis of nonautologous biological bypass graft(s) of the extremities with intermittent claudication, other extremity**   Ⓐ

I70.519   **Atherosclerosis of nonautologous biological bypass graft(s) of the extremities with intermittent claudication, unspecified extremity**   Ⓐ

✓6ᵗʰ **I70.52**   **Atherosclerosis of nonautologous biological bypass graft(s) of the extremities with** rest pain
Includes any condition classifiable to I70.51-

I70.521   **Atherosclerosis of nonautologous biological bypass graft(s) of the extremities with rest pain,** right leg   Ⓐ

I70.522   **Atherosclerosis of nonautologous biological bypass graft(s) of the extremities with rest pain,** left leg   Ⓐ

I70.523   **Atherosclerosis of nonautologous biological bypass graft(s) of the extremities with rest pain,** bilateral legs   Ⓐ

I70.528   **Atherosclerosis of nonautologous biological bypass graft(s) of the extremities with rest pain, other extremity**   Ⓐ

I70.529   **Atherosclerosis of nonautologous biological bypass graft(s) of the extremities with rest pain, unspecified extremity**   Ⓐ

✓6ᵗʰ **I70.53**   **Atherosclerosis of nonautologous biological bypass graft(s) of the** right leg **with** ulceration
Includes any condition classifiable to I70.511 and I70.521
Use additional code to identify severity of ulcer (L97.-)

I70.531   **Atherosclerosis of nonautologous biological bypass graft(s) of the right leg with ulceration of** thigh   Ⓐ

I70.532   **Atherosclerosis of nonautologous biological bypass graft(s) of the right leg with ulceration of** calf   Ⓐ

I70.533   **Atherosclerosis of nonautologous biological bypass graft(s) of the right leg with ulceration of** ankle   Ⓐ

I70.534   **Atherosclerosis of nonautologous biological bypass graft(s) of the right leg with ulceration of** heel and midfoot   Ⓐ
Atherosclerosis of nonautologous biological bypass graft(s) of right leg with ulceration of plantar surface of midfoot

I70.535   **Atherosclerosis of nonautologous biological bypass graft(s) of the right leg with ulceration of other** part of foot   Ⓐ
Atherosclerosis of nonautologous biological bypass graft(s) of the right leg with ulceration of toe

I70.538   **Atherosclerosis of nonautologous biological bypass graft(s) of the right leg with ulceration of other** part of lower leg   Ⓐ

EXCLUDES 1 Not coded here   **EXCLUDES 2** Not included here   Ⓝ Newborn Age: 0   Ⓟ Pediatric Age: 0-17   Ⓜ Maternity Age: 12-55   Ⓐ Adult Age: 15-124

588   ICD-10-CM 2014 (Draft)

I70.539 Atherosclerosis of nonautologous ⒶΑ
biological bypass graft(s) of the right leg
with ulceration of unspecified site

✓6ᵗʰ **I70.54** Atherosclerosis of nonautologous biological bypass
graft(s) of the left leg with ulceration
Includes any condition classifiable to I70.512 and
I70.522
Use additional code to identify severity of ulcer (L97.-)

I70.541 Atherosclerosis of nonautologous Ⓐ
biological bypass graft(s) of the left leg
with ulceration of thigh

I70.542 Atherosclerosis of nonautologous Ⓐ
biological bypass graft(s) of the left leg
with ulceration of calf

I70.543 Atherosclerosis of nonautologous Ⓐ
biological bypass graft(s) of the left leg
with ulceration of ankle

I70.544 Atherosclerosis of nonautologous Ⓐ
biological bypass graft(s) of the left leg
with ulceration of heel and midfoot
Atherosclerosis of nonautologous
biological bypass graft(s) of left leg
with ulceration of plantar surface of
midfoot

I70.545 Atherosclerosis of nonautologous Ⓐ
biological bypass graft(s) of the left leg
with ulceration of other part of foot
Atherosclerosis of nonautologous
biological bypass graft(s) of the left leg
with ulceration of toe

I70.548 Atherosclerosis of nonautologous Ⓐ
biological bypass graft(s) of the left leg
with ulceration of other part of lower leg

I70.549 Atherosclerosis of nonautologous Ⓐ
biological bypass graft(s) of the left leg
with ulceration of unspecified site

I70.55 Atherosclerosis of nonautologous biological Ⓐ
bypass graft(s) of other extremity with ulceration
Includes any condition classifiable to I70.518, I70.528,
and I70.538
Use additional code to identify severity of ulcer
(L98.49)

✓6ᵗʰ **I70.56** Atherosclerosis of nonautologous biological bypass
graft(s) of the extremities with gangrene
Includes any condition classifiable to I70.51-, I70.52-,
and I70.53-, I70.54-, I70.55
Use additional code to identify the severity of any
ulcer (L97.-, L98.49-), if applicable

I70.561 Atherosclerosis of nonautologous Ⓐ
biological bypass graft(s) of the
extremities with gangrene, right leg

I70.562 Atherosclerosis of nonautologous Ⓐ
biological bypass graft(s) of the
extremities with gangrene, left leg

I70.563 Atherosclerosis of nonautologous Ⓐ
biological bypass graft(s) of the
extremities with gangrene, bilateral legs

I70.568 Atherosclerosis of nonautologous Ⓐ
biological bypass graft(s) of the
extremities with gangrene, other
extremity

I70.569 Atherosclerosis of nonautologous Ⓐ
biological bypass graft(s) of the
extremities with gangrene, unspecified
extremity

✓6ᵗʰ **I70.59** Other atherosclerosis of nonautologous biological
bypass graft(s) of the extremities

I70.591 Other atherosclerosis of nonautologous Ⓐ
biological bypass graft(s) of the
extremities, right leg

I70.592 Other atherosclerosis of nonautologous Ⓐ
biological bypass graft(s) of the
extremities, left leg

I70.593 Other atherosclerosis of nonautologous Ⓐ
biological bypass graft(s) of the
extremities, bilateral legs

I70.598 Other atherosclerosis of nonautologous Ⓐ
biological bypass graft(s) of the
extremities, other extremity

I70.599 Other atherosclerosis of nonautologous Ⓐ
biological bypass graft(s) of the
extremities, unspecified extremity

✓5ᵗʰ **I70.6** Atherosclerosis of nonbiological bypass graft(s) of the
extremities
Use additional code, if applicable, to identify chronic total
occlusion of artery of extremity (I70.92)

✓6ᵗʰ **I70.60** Unspecified atherosclerosis of nonbiological bypass
graft(s) of the extremities

I70.601 Unspecified atherosclerosis of Ⓐ
nonbiological bypass graft(s) of the
extremities, right leg

I70.602 Unspecified atherosclerosis of Ⓐ
nonbiological bypass graft(s) of the
extremities, left leg

I70.603 Unspecified atherosclerosis of Ⓐ
nonbiological bypass graft(s) of the
extremities, bilateral legs

I70.608 Unspecified atherosclerosis of Ⓐ
nonbiological bypass graft(s) of the
extremities, other extremity

I70.609 Unspecified atherosclerosis of Ⓐ
nonbiological bypass graft(s) of the
extremities, unspecified extremity

✓6ᵗʰ **I70.61** Atherosclerosis of nonbiological bypass graft(s) of
the extremities with intermittent claudication

I70.611 Atherosclerosis of nonbiological bypass Ⓐ
graft(s) of the extremities with
intermittent claudication, right leg

I70.612 Atherosclerosis of nonbiological bypass Ⓐ
graft(s) of the extremities with
intermittent claudication, left leg

I70.613 Atherosclerosis of nonbiological bypass Ⓐ
graft(s) of the extremities with
intermittent claudication, bilateral legs

I70.618 Atherosclerosis of nonbiological bypass Ⓐ
graft(s) of the extremities with
intermittent claudication, other extremity

I70.619 Atherosclerosis of nonbiological bypass Ⓐ
graft(s) of the extremities with
intermittent claudication, unspecified
extremity

✓6ᵗʰ **I70.62** Atherosclerosis of nonbiological bypass graft(s) of
the extremities with rest pain
Includes any condition classifiable to I70.61-

I70.621 Atherosclerosis of nonbiological bypass Ⓐ
graft(s) of the extremities with rest pain,
right leg

I70.622 Atherosclerosis of nonbiological bypass Ⓐ
graft(s) of the extremities with rest pain,
left leg

I70.623 Atherosclerosis of nonbiological bypass Ⓐ
graft(s) of the extremities with rest pain,
bilateral legs

I70.628 Atherosclerosis of nonbiological bypass Ⓐ
graft(s) of the extremities with rest pain,
other extremity

I70.629 Atherosclerosis of nonbiological bypass Ⓐ
graft(s) of the extremities with rest pain,
unspecified extremity

✓6ᵗʰ **I70.63** Atherosclerosis of nonbiological bypass graft(s) of
the right leg with ulceration
Includes any condition classifiable to I70.611 and
I70.621
Use additional code to identify severity of ulcer (L97.-)

I70.631 Atherosclerosis of nonbiological bypass Ⓐ
graft(s) of the right leg with ulceration of
thigh

I70.632 Atherosclerosis of nonbiological bypass Ⓐ
graft(s) of the right leg with ulceration of
calf

I70.633 Atherosclerosis of nonbiological bypass Ⓐ
graft(s) of the right leg with ulceration of
ankle

I70.634 Atherosclerosis of nonbiological bypass Ⓐ
graft(s) of the right leg with ulceration of
heel and midfoot
Atherosclerosis of nonbiological bypass
graft(s) of right leg with ulceration of
plantar surface of midfoot

I70.635   **Atherosclerosis of nonbiological bypass** Ⓐ **graft(s) of the right leg with ulceration of other part of foot**
    Atherosclerosis of nonbiological bypass graft(s) of the right leg with ulceration of toe

I70.638   **Atherosclerosis of nonbiological bypass** Ⓐ **graft(s) of the right leg with ulceration of other part of lower leg**

I70.639   **Atherosclerosis of nonbiological bypass** Ⓐ **graft(s) of the right leg with ulceration of unspecified site**

√6ᵗʰ **I70.64**   **Atherosclerosis of nonbiological bypass graft(s) of the left leg with ulceration**
    Includes any condition classifiable to I70.612 and I70.622
    Use additional code to identify severity of ulcer (L97.-)

I70.641   **Atherosclerosis of nonbiological bypass** Ⓐ **graft(s) of the left leg with ulceration of thigh**

I70.642   **Atherosclerosis of nonbiological bypass** Ⓐ **graft(s) of the left leg with ulceration of calf**

I70.643   **Atherosclerosis of nonbiological bypass** Ⓐ **graft(s) of the left leg with ulceration of ankle**

I70.644   **Atherosclerosis of nonbiological bypass** Ⓐ **graft(s) of the left leg with ulceration of heel and midfoot**
    Atherosclerosis of nonbiological bypass graft(s) of left leg with ulceration of plantar surface of midfoot

I70.645   **Atherosclerosis of nonbiological** Ⓐ **bypassgraft(s) of the left leg with ulceration of other part of foot**
    Atherosclerosis of nonbiological bypass graft(s) of the left leg with ulceration of toe

I70.648   **Atherosclerosis of nonbiological** Ⓐ **bypass graft(s) of the left leg with ulceration of other part of lower leg**

I70.649   **Atherosclerosis of nonbiological** Ⓐ **bypass graft(s) of the left leg with ulceration of unspecified site**

I70.65   **Atherosclerosis of nonbiological bypass graft(s)** Ⓐ **of other extremity with ulceration**
    Includes any condition classifiable to I70.618 and I70.628
    Use additional code to identify severity of ulcer (L98.49)

√6ᵗʰ **I70.66**   **Atherosclerosis of nonbiological bypass graft(s) of the extremities with gangrene**
    Includes any condition classifiable to I70.61-, I70.62-, I70.63-, I70.64-, I70.65
    Use additional code to identify the severity of any ulcer (L97.-, L98.49-), if applicable

I70.661   **Atherosclerosis of nonbiological bypass** Ⓐ **graft(s) of the extremities with gangrene, right leg**

I70.662   **Atherosclerosis of nonbiological bypass** Ⓐ **graft(s) of the extremities with gangrene, left leg**

I70.663   **Atherosclerosis of nonbiological bypass** Ⓐ **graft(s) of the extremities with gangrene, bilateral legs**

I70.668   **Atherosclerosis of nonbiological bypass** Ⓐ **graft(s) of the extremities with gangrene, other extremity**

I70.669   **Atherosclerosis of nonbiological bypass** Ⓐ **graft(s) of the extremities with gangrene, unspecified extremity**

√6ᵗʰ **I70.69**   **Other atherosclerosis of nonbiological bypass graft(s) of the extremities**

I70.691   **Other atherosclerosis of nonbiological** Ⓐ **bypass graft(s) of the extremities, right leg**

I70.692   **Other atherosclerosis of nonbiological** Ⓐ **bypass graft(s) of the extremities, left leg**

I70.693   **Other atherosclerosis of nonbiological** Ⓐ **bypass graft(s) of the extremities, bilateral legs**

I70.698   **Other atherosclerosis of nonbiological** Ⓐ **bypass graft(s) of the extremities, other extremity**

I70.699   **Other atherosclerosis of nonbiological** Ⓐ **bypass graft(s) of the extremities, unspecified extremity**

√5ᵗʰ **I70.7**   **Atherosclerosis of other type of bypass graft(s) of the extremities**
    Use additional code, if applicable, to identify chronic total occlusion of artery of extremity (I70.92)

√6ᵗʰ **I70.70**   **Unspecified atherosclerosis of other type of bypass graft(s) of the extremities**

I70.701   **Unspecified atherosclerosis of other** Ⓐ **type of bypass graft(s) of the extremities, right leg**

I70.702   **Unspecified atherosclerosis of other** Ⓐ **type of bypass graft(s) of the extremities, left leg**

I70.703   **Unspecified atherosclerosis of other** Ⓐ **type of bypass graft(s) of the extremities, bilateral legs**

I70.708   **Unspecified atherosclerosis of other** Ⓐ **type of bypass graft(s) of the extremities, other extremity**

I70.709   **Unspecified atherosclerosis of other** Ⓐ **type of bypass graft(s) of the extremities, unspecified extremity**

√6ᵗʰ **I70.71**   **Atherosclerosis of other type of bypass graft(s) of the extremities with intermittent claudication**

I70.711   **Atherosclerosis of other type of bypass** Ⓐ **graft(s) of the extremities with intermittent claudication, right leg**

I70.712   **Atherosclerosis of other type of bypass** Ⓐ **graft(s) of the extremities with intermittent claudication, left leg**

I70.713   **Atherosclerosis of other type of bypass** Ⓐ **graft(s) of the extremities with intermittent claudication, bilateral legs**

I70.718   **Atherosclerosis of other type of bypass** Ⓐ **graft(s) of the extremities with intermittent claudication, other extremity**

I70.719   **Atherosclerosis of other type of bypass** Ⓐ **graft(s) of the extremities with intermittent claudication, unspecified extremity**

√6ᵗʰ **I70.72**   **Atherosclerosis of other type of bypass graft(s) of the extremities with rest pain**
    Includes any condition classifiable to I70.71-

I70.721   **Atherosclerosis of other type of bypass** Ⓐ **graft(s) of the extremities with rest pain, right leg**

I70.722   **Atherosclerosis of other type of bypass** Ⓐ **graft(s) of the extremities with rest pain, left leg**

I70.723   **Atherosclerosis of other type of bypass** Ⓐ **graft(s) of the extremities with rest pain, bilateral legs**

I70.728   **Atherosclerosis of other type of bypass** Ⓐ **graft(s) of the extremities with rest pain, other extremity**

I70.729   **Atherosclerosis of other type of bypass** Ⓐ **graft(s) of the extremities with rest pain, unspecified extremity**

√6ᵗʰ **I70.73**   **Atherosclerosis of other type of bypass graft(s) of the right leg with ulceration**
    Includes any condition classifiable to I70.711 and I70.721
    Use additional code to identify severity of ulcer (L97.-)

I70.731   **Atherosclerosis of other type of bypass** Ⓐ **graft(s) of the right leg with ulceration of thigh**

I70.732   **Atherosclerosis of other type of bypass** Ⓐ **graft(s) of the right leg with ulceration of calf**

I70.733   **Atherosclerosis of other type of bypass** Ⓐ **graft(s) of the right leg with ulceration of ankle**

EXCLUDES 1 Not coded here   *EXCLUDES 2* Not included here   Ⓝ Newborn Age: 0   Ⓟ Pediatric Age: 0-17   Ⓜ Maternity Age: 12-55   Ⓐ Adult Age: 15-124

590   ICD-10-CM 2014 (Draft)

I70.734   **Atherosclerosis of other type of bypass** △
graft(s) of the right leg with ulceration
of heel and midfoot
    Atherosclerosis of other type of bypass
graft(s) of right leg with ulceration of
plantar surface of midfoot

I70.735   **Atherosclerosis of other type of bypass** △
graft(s) of the right leg with ulceration
of other part of foot
    Atherosclerosis of other type of bypass
graft(s) of right leg with ulceration of
toe

I70.738   **Atherosclerosis of other type of bypass** △
graft(s) of the right leg with ulceration
of other part of lower leg

I70.739   **Atherosclerosis of other type of bypass** △
graft(s) of the right leg with ulceration
of unspecified site

✓6ᵗʰ **I70.74**   **Atherosclerosis of other type of bypass graft(s) of**
the left leg with ulceration
    Includes any condition classifiable to I70.712 and
I70.722
    Use additional code to identify severity of ulcer (L97.-)

I70.741   **Atherosclerosis of other type of bypass** △
graft(s) of the left leg with ulceration
of thigh

I70.742   **Atherosclerosis of other type of bypass** △
graft(s) of the left leg with ulceration
of calf

I70.743   **Atherosclerosis of other type of bypass** △
graft(s) of the left leg with ulceration
of ankle

I70.744   **Atherosclerosis of other type of bypass** △
graft(s) of the left leg with ulceration
of heel and midfoot
    Atherosclerosis of other type of bypass
graft(s) of left leg with ulceration of
plantar surface of midfoot

I70.745   **Atherosclerosis of other type of bypass** △
graft(s) of the left leg with ulceration
of other part of foot
    Atherosclerosis of other type of bypass
graft(s) of left leg with ulceration of
toe

I70.748   **Atherosclerosis of other type of bypass** △
graft(s) of the left leg with ulceration
of other part of lower leg

I70.749   **Atherosclerosis of other type of bypass** △
graft(s) of the left leg with ulceration
of unspecified site

I70.75   **Atherosclerosis of other type of bypass graft(s)** △
of other extremity with ulceration
    Includes any condition classifiable to I70.718 and
I70.728
    Use additional code to identify severity of ulcer
(L98.49)

✓6ᵗʰ **I70.76**   **Atherosclerosis of other type of bypass graft(s) of**
the extremities with gangrene
    Includes any condition classifiable to I70.71-, I70.72-,
I70.73-, I70.74-, I70.75
    Use additional code to identify the severity of any
ulcer (L97.-, L98.49-), if applicable

I70.761   **Atherosclerosis of other type of bypass** △
graft(s) of the extremities with gangrene,
right leg

I70.762   **Atherosclerosis of other type of bypass** △
graft(s) of the extremities with gangrene,
left leg

I70.763   **Atherosclerosis of other type of bypass** △
graft(s) of the extremities with gangrene,
bilateral legs

I70.768   **Atherosclerosis of other type of bypass** △
graft(s) of the extremities with gangrene,
other extremity

I70.769   **Atherosclerosis of other type of bypass** △
graft(s) of the extremities with gangrene,
unspecified extremity

✓6ᵗʰ **I70.79**   Other atherosclerosis of other type of bypass graft(s)
of the extremities

I70.791   **Other atherosclerosis of other type of** △
bypass graft(s) of the extremities,
right leg

I70.792   **Other atherosclerosis of other type of** △
bypass graft(s) of the extremities, left leg

I70.793   **Other atherosclerosis of other type of** △
bypass graft(s) of the extremities,
bilateral legs

I70.798   **Other atherosclerosis of other type of** △
bypass graft(s) of the extremities, other
extremity

I70.799   **Other atherosclerosis of other type of** △
bypass graft(s) of the extremities,
unspecified extremity

I70.8   **Atherosclerosis of other arteries** △

✓5ᵗʰ **I70.9**   **Other and unspecified atherosclerosis**

I70.90   **Unspecified atherosclerosis** △

I70.91   **Generalized atherosclerosis** △

I70.92   **Chronic total occlusion of artery of the extremities** △
    Complete occlusion of artery of the extremities
    Total occlusion of artery of the extremities
    Code first atherosclerosis of arteries of the extremities
(I70.2-, I70.3-, I70.4-, I70.5-, I70.6-, I70.7-)

✓4ᵗʰ **I71**   **Aortic aneurysm and dissection**
    EXCLUDES 1   *aortic ectasia (I77.81-)*
             syphilitic aortic aneurysm (A52.01)
             traumatic aortic aneurysm (S25.09, S35.09)

✓5ᵗʰ **I71.0**   **Dissection of aorta**

I71.00   **Dissection of unspecified site of aorta**

I71.01   **Dissection of thoracic aorta**

I71.02   **Dissection of abdominal aorta**

I71.03   **Dissection of thoracoabdominal aorta**

I71.1   **Thoracic aortic aneurysm, ruptured**

I71.2   **Thoracic aortic aneurysm, without rupture**

I71.3   **Abdominal aortic aneurysm, ruptured**

I71.4   **Abdominal aortic aneurysm, without rupture**

I71.5   **Thoracoabdominal aortic aneurysm, ruptured**

I71.6   **Thoracoabdominal aortic aneurysm, without rupture**

I71.8   **Aortic aneurysm of unspecified site, ruptured**
    Rupture of aorta NOS

I71.9   **Aortic aneurysm of unspecified site, without rupture**
    Aneurysm of aorta
    Dilatation of aorta
    Hyaline necrosis of aorta

✓4ᵗʰ **I72**   **Other aneurysm**
    INCLUDES   aneurysm (cirsoid) (false) (ruptured)
    EXCLUDES 2   *acquired aneurysm (I77.0)*
             aneurysm (of) aorta (I71.-)
             aneurysm (of) arteriovenous NOS (Q27.3-)
             carotid artery dissection (I77.71)
             cerebral (nonruptured) aneurysm (I67.1)
             coronary aneurysm (I25.4)
             coronary artery dissection (I25.42)
             dissection of artery NEC (I77.79)
             heart aneurysm (I25.3)
             iliac artery dissection (I77.72)
             pulmonary artery aneurysm (I28.1)
             renal artery dissection (I77.73)
             retinal aneurysm (H35.0)
             ruptured cerebral aneurysm (I60.7)
             varicose aneurysm (I77.0)
             vertebral artery dissection (I77.74)

I72.0   **Aneurysm of carotid artery**
    Aneurysm of common carotid artery
    Aneurysm of external carotid artery
    Aneurysm of internal carotid artery, extracranial portion
    EXCLUDES 1   *aneurysm of internal carotid artery, intracranial portion (I67.1)*
             aneurysm of internal carotid artery NOS (I67.1)

I72.1   **Aneurysm of artery of upper extremity**

I72.2   **Aneurysm of renal artery**

I72.3   **Aneurysm of iliac artery**

I72.4   **Aneurysm of artery of lower extremity**

I72.8   **Aneurysm of other specified arteries**

I72.9   **Aneurysm of unspecified site**

✔ Additional Character Required   √x7ᵗʰ Xtension Alert   Unspecified Code   Other Specified Code   Manifestation Code   ▶◀ Revised Text   ● New Code   ▲ Revised Code Title

Diseases of the Circulatory System

I73–I77.9

✓4ᵗʰ **I73 Other peripheral vascular diseases**
 EXCLUDES 2   chilblains (T69.1)
 frostbite (T33- T34)
 immersion hand or foot (T69.0-)
 spasm of cerebral artery (G45.9)

✓5ᵗʰ **I73.0 Raynaud's syndrome**
 Raynaud's disease
 Raynaud's phenomenon (secondary)

     I73.00 Raynaud's syndrome without gangrene

     I73.01 Raynaud's syndrome with gangrene

   I73.1 Thromboangiitis obliterans [Buerger's disease]

✓5ᵗʰ **I73.8 Other specified peripheral vascular diseases**
 EXCLUDES 1   diabetic (peripheral) angiopathy (E08-E13 with .51-.52)

     I73.81 Erythromelalgia

     I73.89 Other specified peripheral vascular diseases
 Acrocyanosis
 Erythrocyanosis
 Simple acroparesthesia [Schultze's type]
 Vasomotor acroparesthesia [Nothnagel's type]

   I73.9 Peripheral vascular disease, unspecified
 Intermittent claudication
 Peripheral angiopathy NOS
 Spasm of artery
 EXCLUDES 1   atherosclerosis of the extremities (I70.2--I70.7-)

✓4ᵗʰ **I74 Arterial embolism and thrombosis**
 Embolic infarction
 Embolic occlusion
 Thrombotic infarction
 Thrombotic occlusion
 Code first:
 embolism and thrombosis complicating abortion or ectopic or molar
 pregnancy (O00-O07, O08.2)
 embolism and thrombosis complicating pregnancy, childbirth and
 the puerperium (O88.-)
 EXCLUDES 2   atheroembolism (I75.-)
 basilar embolism and thrombosis (I63.0-I63.2, I65.1)
 carotid embolism and thrombosis (I63.0-I63.2, I65.2)
 cerebral embolism and thrombosis (I63.3-I63.5, I66-)
 coronary embolism and thrombosis (I21-I25)
 mesenteric embolism and thrombosis (K55.0)
 ophthalmic embolism and thrombosis (H34.-)
 precerebral embolism and thrombosis NOS (I63.0-I63.2, I65.9)
 pulmonary embolism and thrombosis (I26.-)
 renal embolism and thrombosis (N28.0)
 retinal embolism and thrombosis (H34.-)
 septic embolism and thrombosis (I76)
 vertebral embolism and thrombosis (I63.0-I63.2, I65.0)

✓5ᵗʰ **I74.0 Embolism and thrombosis of** abdominal aorta

     I74.01 Saddle embolus of abdominal aorta

     I74.09 Other arterial **embolism and thrombosis of abdominal aorta**
 Aortic bifurcation syndrome
 Aortoiliac obstruction
 Leriche's syndrome

✓5ᵗʰ **I74.1 Embolism and thrombosis of** other and unspecified parts **of aorta**

     I74.10 Embolism and thrombosis of unspecified parts of aorta

     I74.11 Embolism and thrombosis of thoracic **aorta**

     I74.19 Embolism and thrombosis of other parts of aorta

   I74.2 Embolism and thrombosis of arteries of the upper extremities

   I74.3 Embolism and thrombosis of arteries of the lower extremities

   I74.4 Embolism and thrombosis of arteries of extremities, unspecified
 Peripheral arterial embolism NOS

   I74.5 Embolism and thrombosis of iliac **artery**

   I74.8 Embolism and thrombosis of other arteries

   I74.9 Embolism and thrombosis of unspecified artery

✓4ᵗʰ **I75 Atheroembolism**
 Atherothrombotic microembolism
 Cholesterol embolism

✓5ᵗʰ **I75.0 Atheroembolism of** extremities

✓6ᵗʰ **I75.01 Atheroembolism of** upper **extremity**

     I75.011 Atheroembolism of right upper extremity

     I75.012 Atheroembolism of left upper extremity

     I75.013 Atheroembolism of bilateral upper extremity

     I75.019 Atheroembolism of unspecified upper extremity

✓6ᵗʰ **I75.02 Atheroembolism of lower extremity**

     I75.021 Atheroembolism of right lower extremity

     I75.022 Atheroembolism of left lower extremity

     I75.023 Atheroembolism of bilateral lower extremities

     I75.029 Atheroembolism of unspecified lower extremity

✓5ᵗʰ **I75.8 Atheroembolism of** other sites

     I75.81 Atheroembolism of kidney
 Use additional code for any associated acute kidney
 failure and chronic kidney disease (N17.-, N18.-)

     I75.89 Atheroembolism of other site

I76 Septic arterial embolism
 Code first underlying infection, such as:
 infective endocarditis (I33.0)
 lung abscess (J85.-)
 Use additional code to identify the site of the embolism (I74.-)
 EXCLUDES 2   septic pulmonary embolism (I26.01, I26.90)

✓4ᵗʰ **I77 Other disorders of arteries and arterioles**
 EXCLUDES 2   collagen (vascular) diseases (M30-M36)
 hypersensitivity angiitis (M31.0)
 pulmonary artery (I28.-)

   I77.0 Arteriovenous fistula, acquired
 Aneurysmal varix
 Arteriovenous aneurysm, acquired
 EXCLUDES 1   arteriovenous aneurysm NOS (Q27.3-)
 presence of arteriovenous shunt (fistula) for dialysis
 (Z99.2)
 traumatic—see injury of blood vessel by body region
 EXCLUDES 2   cerebral (I67.1)
 coronary (I25.4)

   I77.1 Stricture of artery
 Narrowing of artery

   I77.2 Rupture of artery
 Erosion of artery
 Fistula of artery
 Ulcer of artery
 EXCLUDES 1   traumatic rupture of artery—see injury of blood vessel
 by body region

   I77.3 Arterial fibromuscular dysplasia
 Fibromuscular hyperplasia (of) carotid artery
 Fibromuscular hyperplasia (of) renal artery

   I77.4 Celiac artery compression syndrome

   I77.5 Necrosis of artery

   I77.6 Arteritis, unspecified
 Aortitis NOS
 Endarteritis NOS
 EXCLUDES 1   arteritis or endarteritis:
 aortic arch (M31.4)
 cerebral NEC (I67.7)
 coronary (I25.89)
 deformans (I70.-)
 giant cell (M31.5., M31.6)
 obliterans (I70.-)
 senile (I70.-)

✓5ᵗʰ **I77.7 Other arterial dissection**
 EXCLUDES 2   dissection of aorta (I71.0-)
 dissection of coronary artery (I25.42)

     I77.71 Dissection of carotid **artery**

     I77.72 Dissection of iliac **artery**

     I77.73 Dissection of renal **artery**

     I77.74 Dissection of vertebral **artery**

     I77.79 Dissection of other artery

✓5ᵗʰ **I77.8 Other specified disorders of arteries and arterioles**

✓6ᵗʰ **I77.81 Aortic ectasia**
 Ectasis aorta
 EXCLUDES 1   aortic aneurysm and dissection (I71.0-)

     I77.810 Thoracic aortic ectasia

     I77.811 Abdominal aortic ectasia

     I77.812 Thoracoabdominal aortic ectasia

     I77.819 Aortic ectasia, unspecified site

     I77.89 Other specified disorders of arteries and arterioles

   I77.9 Disorder of arteries and arterioles, unspecified

EXCLUDES 1 Not coded here   EXCLUDES 2 Not included here   N Newborn Age: 0   P Pediatric Age: 0-17   M Maternity Age: 12-55   A Adult Age: 15-124

✓4th **I78　Diseases of capillaries**

I78.0　Hereditary hemorrhagic telangiectasia
　　　　Rendu-Osler-Weber disease

I78.1　Nevus, non-neoplastic
　　　　Araneus nevus
　　　　Senile nevus
　　　　Spider nevus
　　　　Stellar nevus
　　　　EXCLUDES 1　*nevus NOS (D22.-)*
　　　　　　　　　　vascular NOS (Q82.5)
　　　　EXCLUDES 2　*blue nevus (D22.-)*
　　　　　　　　　　flammeus nevus (Q82.5)
　　　　　　　　　　hairy nevus (D22.-)
　　　　　　　　　　melanocytic nevus (D22.-)
　　　　　　　　　　pigmented nevus (D22.-)
　　　　　　　　　　portwine nevus (Q82.5)
　　　　　　　　　　sanguineous nevus (Q82.5)
　　　　　　　　　　strawberry nevus (Q82.5)
　　　　　　　　　　verrucous nevus (Q82.5)

I78.8　Other diseases of capillaries

I78.9　Disease of capillaries, unspecified

✓4th **I79　Disorders of arteries, arterioles and capillaries in diseases classified elsewhere**

I79.0　Aneurysm of aorta in diseases classified elsewhere
　　　　Code first underlying disease
　　　　EXCLUDES 1　*syphilitic aneurysm (A52.01)*

I79.1　Aortitis in diseases classified elsewhere
　　　　Code first underlying disease
　　　　EXCLUDES 1　*syphilitic aortitis (A52.02)*

I79.8　Other disorders of arteries, arterioles and capillaries in diseases classified elsewhere
　　　　Code first underlying disease, such as:
　　　　　　amyloidosis (E85.-)
　　　　EXCLUDES 1　*diabetic (peripheral) angiopathy (E08-E13 with .51-.52)*
　　　　　　　　　　syphilitic endarteritis (A52.09)
　　　　　　　　　　tuberculous endarteritis (A18.89)

Diseases of veins, lymphatic vessels and lymph nodes, not elsewhere classified. (I80-I89)

✓4th **I80　Phlebitis and thrombophlebitis**
　　　　INCLUDES　endophlebitis
　　　　　　　　　inflammation, vein
　　　　　　　　　periphlebitis
　　　　　　　　　suppurative phlebitis
　　　　Code first:
　　　　　　phlebitis and thrombophlebitis complicating abortion, ectopic or molar pregnancy (O00-O07, O08.7)
　　　　　　phlebitis and thrombophlebitis complicating pregnancy, childbirth and the puerperium (O22.-, O87.-)
　　　　EXCLUDES 1　*venous embolism and thrombosis of lower extremities ((I82.4-, I82.5-, I82.81-)*

✓5th **I80.0　Phlebitis and thrombophlebitis of superficial vessels of lower extremities**
　　　　Phlebitis and thrombophlebitis of femoropopliteal vein

I80.00　Phlebitis and thrombophlebitis of superficial vessels of unspecified lower extremity

I80.01　Phlebitis and thrombophlebitis of superficial vessels of right lower extremity

I80.02　Phlebitis and thrombophlebitis of superficial vessels of left lower extremity

I80.03　Phlebitis and thrombophlebitis of superficial vessels of lower extremities, bilateral

✓5th **I80.1　Phlebitis and thrombophlebitis of femoral vein**

I80.10　Phlebitis and thrombophlebitis of unspecified femoral vein

I80.11　Phlebitis and thrombophlebitis of right femoral vein

I80.12　Phlebitis and thrombophlebitis of left femoral vein

I80.13　Phlebitis and thrombophlebitis of femoral vein, bilateral

✓5th **I80.2　Phlebitis and thrombophlebitis of other and unspecified deep vessels of lower extremities**

✓6th **I80.20　Phlebitis and thrombophlebitis of unspecified deep vessels of lower extremities**

I80.201　Phlebitis and thrombophlebitis of unspecified deep vessels of right lower extremity

I80.202　Phlebitis and thrombophlebitis of unspecified deep vessels of left lower extremity

I80.203　Phlebitis and thrombophlebitis of unspecified deep vessels of lower extremities, bilateral

I80.209　Phlebitis and thrombophlebitis of unspecified deep vessels of unspecified lower extremity

✓6th **I80.21　Phlebitis and thrombophlebitis of iliac vein**

I80.211　Phlebitis and thrombophlebitis of right iliac vein

I80.212　Phlebitis and thrombophlebitis of left iliac vein

I80.213　Phlebitis and thrombophlebitis of iliac vein, bilateral

I80.219　Phlebitis and thrombophlebitis of unspecified iliac vein

✓6th **I80.22　Phlebitis and thrombophlebitis of popliteal vein**

I80.221　Phlebitis and thrombophlebitis of right popliteal vein

I80.222　Phlebitis and thrombophlebitis of left popliteal vein

I80.223　Phlebitis and thrombophlebitis of popliteal vein, bilateral

I80.229　Phlebitis and thrombophlebitis of unspecified popliteal vein

✓6th **I80.23　Phlebitis and thrombophlebitis of tibial vein**

I80.231　Phlebitis and thrombophlebitis of right tibial vein

I80.232　Phlebitis and thrombophlebitis of left tibial vein

I80.233　Phlebitis and thrombophlebitis of tibial vein, bilateral

I80.239　Phlebitis and thrombophlebitis of unspecified tibial vein

✓6th **I80.29　Phlebitis and thrombophlebitis of other deep vessels of lower extremities**

I80.291　Phlebitis and thrombophlebitis of other deep vessels of right lower extremity

I80.292　Phlebitis and thrombophlebitis of other deep vessels of left lower extremity

I80.293　Phlebitis and thrombophlebitis of other deep vessels of lower extremities, bilateral

I80.299　Phlebitis and thrombophlebitis of other deep vessels of unspecified lower extremity

I80.3　Phlebitis and thrombophlebitis of lower extremities, unspecified

I80.8　Phlebitis and thrombophlebitis of other sites

I80.9　Phlebitis and thrombophlebitis of unspecified site

I81　Portal vein thrombosis
　　　　Portal (vein) obstruction
　　　　EXCLUDES 2　*hepatic vein thrombosis (I82.0)*
　　　　　　　　　　phlebitis of portal vein (K75.1)

✓4th **I82　Other venous embolism and thrombosis**
　　　　Code first venous embolism and thrombosis complicating:
　　　　　　abortion, ectopic or molar pregnancy (O00-O07, O08.7)
　　　　　　pregnancy, childbirth and the puerperium (O22.-, O87.-)
　　　　EXCLUDES 2　*venous embolism and thrombosis (of):*
　　　　　　　　　　cerebral (I63.6, I67.6)
　　　　　　　　　　coronary (I21-I25)
　　　　　　　　　　intracranial and intraspinal, septic or NOS (G08)
　　　　　　　　　　intracranial, nonpyogenic (I67.6)
　　　　　　　　　　intraspinal, nonpyogenic (G95.1)
　　　　　　　　　　mesenteric (K55.0)
　　　　　　　　　　portal (I81)
　　　　　　　　　　pulmonary (I26.-)

I82.0　Budd-Chiari syndrome
　　　　Hepatic vein thrombosis

I82.1　Thrombophlebitis migrans

✓5th **I82.2　Embolism and thrombosis of vena cava and other thoracic veins**

✓6th **I82.21　Embolism and thrombosis of superior vena cava**

I82.210　Acute embolism and thrombosis of superior vena cava
　　　　Embolism and thrombosis of superior vena cava NOS

✓ Additional Character Required　　✓x7th Xtension Alert　　Unspecified Code　　Other Specified Code　　Manifestation Code　　▶◀ Revised Text　　● New Code　　▲ Revised Code Title

    I82.211 Chronic embolism and thrombosis of superior vena cava

✓6ᵗʰ **I82.22** Embolism and thrombosis of inferior vena cava

    I82.220 Acute embolism and thrombosis of inferior vena cava
         Embolism and thrombosis of inferior vena cava NOS

    I82.221 Chronic embolism and thrombosis of inferior vena cava

✓6ᵗʰ **I82.29** Embolism and thrombosis of other thoracic veins
     Embolism and thrombosis of brachiocephalic (innominate) vein

    I82.290 Acute embolism and thrombosis of other thoracic veins

    I82.291 Chronic embolism and thrombosis of other thoracic veins

I82.3 Embolism and thrombosis of renal vein

✓5ᵗʰ **I82.4** Acute embolism and thrombosis of deep veins of lower extremity

✓6ᵗʰ **I82.40** Acute embolism and thrombosis of unspecified deep veins of lower extremity
     Deep vein thrombosis NOS
     DVT NOS

    EXCLUDES 1   acute embolism and thrombosis of unspecified deep veins of distal lower extremity (I82.4Z-)
         acute embolism and thrombosis of unspecified deep veins of proximal lower extremity (I82.4Y-)

    I82.401 Acute embolism and thrombosis of unspecified deep veins of right lower extremity

    I82.402 Acute embolism and thrombosis of unspecified deep veins of left lower extremity

    I82.403 Acute embolism and thrombosis of unspecified deep veins of lower extremity, bilateral

    I82.409 Acute embolism and thrombosis of unspecified deep veins of unspecified lower extremity

✓6ᵗʰ **I82.41** Acute embolism and thrombosis of femoral vein

    I82.411 Acute embolism and thrombosis of right femoral vein

    I82.412 Acute embolism and thrombosis of left femoral vein

    I82.413 Acute embolism and thrombosis of femoral vein, bilateral

    I82.419 Acute embolism and thrombosis of unspecified femoral vein

✓6ᵗʰ **I82.42** Acute embolism and thrombosis of iliac vein

    I82.421 Acute embolism and thrombosis of right iliac vein

    I82.422 Acute embolism and thrombosis of left iliac vein

    I82.423 Acute embolism and thrombosis of iliac vein, bilateral

    I82.429 Acute embolism and thrombosis of unspecified iliac vein

✓6ᵗʰ **I82.43** Acute embolism and thrombosis of popliteal vein

    I82.431 Acute embolism and thrombosis of right popliteal vein

    I82.432 Acute embolism and thrombosis of left popliteal vein

    I82.433 Acute embolism and thrombosis of popliteal vein, bilateral

    I82.439 Acute embolism and thrombosis of unspecified popliteal vein

✓6ᵗʰ **I82.44** Acute embolism and thrombosis of tibial vein

    I82.441 Acute embolism and thrombosis of right tibial vein

    I82.442 Acute embolism and thrombosis of left tibial vein

    I82.443 Acute embolism and thrombosis of tibial vein, bilateral

    I82.449 Acute embolism and thrombosis of unspecified tibial vein

✓6ᵗʰ **I82.49** Acute embolism and thrombosis of other specified deep vein of lower extremity

    I82.491 Acute embolism and thrombosis of other specified deep vein of right lower extremity

    I82.492 Acute embolism and thrombosis of other specified deep vein of left lower extremity

    I82.493 Acute embolism and thrombosis of other specified deep vein of lower extremity, bilateral

    I82.499 Acute embolism and thrombosis of other specified deep vein of unspecified lower extremity

✓6ᵗʰ **I82.4Y** Acute embolism and thrombosis of unspecified deep veins of proximal lower extremity
     Acute embolism and thrombosis of deep vein of thigh NOS
     Acute embolism and thrombosis of deep vein of upper leg NOS

    I82.4Y1 Acute embolism and thrombosis of unspecified deep veins of right proximal lower extremity

    I82.4Y2 Acute embolism and thrombosis of unspecified deep veins of left proximal lower extremity

    I82.4Y3 Acute embolism and thrombosis of unspecified deep veins of proximal lower extremity, bilateral

    I82.4Y9 Acute embolism and thrombosis of unspecified deep veins of unspecified proximal lower extremity

✓6ᵗʰ **I82.4Z** Acute embolism and thrombosis of unspecified deep veins of distal lower extremity
     Acute embolism and thrombosis of deep vein of calf NOS
     Acute embolism and thrombosis of deep vein of lower leg NOS

    I82.4Z1 Acute embolism and thrombosis of unspecified deep veins of right distal lower extremity

    I82.4Z2 Acute embolism and thrombosis of unspecified deep veins of left distal lower extremity

    I82.4Z3 Acute embolism and thrombosis of unspecified deep veins of distal lower extremity, bilateral

    I82.4Z9 Acute embolism and thrombosis of unspecified deep veins of unspecified distal lower extremity

✓5ᵗʰ **I82.5** Chronic embolism and thrombosis of deep veins of lower extremity
     Use additional code, if applicable, for associated long-term (current) use of anticoagulants (Z79.01)

    EXCLUDES 1   personal history of venous embolism and thrombosis (Z86.718)

✓6ᵗʰ **I82.50** Chronic embolism and thrombosis of unspecified deep veins of lower extremity

    EXCLUDES 1   chronic embolism and thrombosis of unspecified deep veins of distal lower extremity (I82.5Z-)
         chronic embolism and thrombosis of unspecified deep veins of proximal lower extremity (I82.5Y-)

    I82.501 Chronic embolism and thrombosis of unspecified deep veins of right lower extremity

    I82.502 Chronic embolism and thrombosis of unspecified deep veins of left lower extremity

    I82.503 Chronic embolism and thrombosis of unspecified deep veins of lower extremity, bilateral

    I82.509 Chronic embolism and thrombosis of unspecified deep veins of unspecified lower extremity

✓6ᵗʰ **I82.51** Chronic embolism and thrombosis of femoral vein

    I82.511 Chronic embolism and thrombosis of right femoral vein

    I82.512 Chronic embolism and thrombosis of left femoral vein

---

EXCLUDES 1 Not coded here   *EXCLUDES 2* Not included here   **N** Newborn Age: 0   **P** Pediatric Age: 0-17   **M** Maternity Age: 12-55   **A** Adult Age: 15-124

594   ICD-10-CM 2014 (Draft)

I82.513 **Chronic embolism and thrombosis of femoral vein,** bilateral

I82.519 **Chronic embolism and thrombosis of unspecified femoral vein**

✓6ᵗʰ I82.52 Chronic embolism and thrombosis of iliac vein

I82.521 **Chronic embolism and thrombosis of** right **iliac vein**

I82.522 **Chronic embolism and thrombosis of** left **iliac vein**

I82.523 **Chronic embolism and thrombosis of iliac vein,** bilateral

I82.529 **Chronic embolism and thrombosis of unspecified iliac vein**

✓6ᵗʰ I82.53 Chronic embolism and thrombosis of popliteal vein

I82.531 **Chronic embolism and thrombosis of** right **popliteal vein**

I82.532 **Chronic embolism and thrombosis of** left **popliteal vein**

I82.533 **Chronic embolism and thrombosis of popliteal vein,** bilateral

I82.539 **Chronic embolism and thrombosis of unspecified popliteal vein**

✓6ᵗʰ I82.54 Chronic embolism and thrombosis of tibial vein

I82.541 **Chronic embolism and thrombosis of** right **tibial vein**

I82.542 **Chronic embolism and thrombosis of** left **tibial vein**

I82.543 **Chronic embolism and thrombosis of tibial vein,** bilateral

I82.549 **Chronic embolism and thrombosis of unspecified tibial vein**

✓6ᵗʰ I82.59 Chronic embolism and thrombosis of other specified deep vein of lower extremity

I82.591 **Chronic embolism and thrombosis of other specified deep vein of** right **lower extremity**

I82.592 **Chronic embolism and thrombosis of other specified deep vein of** left **lower extremity**

I82.593 **Chronic embolism and thrombosis of other specified deep vein of lower extremity,** bilateral

I82.599 **Chronic embolism and thrombosis of other specified deep vein of unspecified lower extremity**

✓6ᵗʰ I82.5Y Chronic embolism and thrombosis of unspecified deep veins of proximal lower extremity
Chronic embolism and thrombosis of deep veins of thigh NOS
Chronic embolism and thrombosis of deep veins of upper leg NOS

I82.5Y1 **Chronic embolism and thrombosis of unspecified deep veins of** right **proximal lower extremity**

I82.5Y2 **Chronic embolism and thrombosis of unspecified deep veins of** left **proximal lower extremity**

I82.5Y3 **Chronic embolism and thrombosis of unspecified deep veins of proximal lower extremity,** bilateral

I82.5Y9 **Chronic embolism and thrombosis of unspecified deep veins of unspecified proximal lower extremity**

✓6ᵗʰ I82.5Z Chronic embolism and thrombosis of unspecified deep veins of distal lower extremity
Chronic embolism and thrombosis of deep veins of calf NOS
Chronic embolism and thrombosis of deep veins of lower leg NOS

I82.5Z1 **Chronic embolism and thrombosis of unspecified deep veins of** right **distal lower extremity**

I82.5Z2 **Chronic embolism and thrombosis of unspecified deep veins of** left **distal lower extremity**

I82.5Z3 **Chronic embolism and thrombosis of unspecified deep veins of distal lower extremity,** bilateral

I82.5Z9 **Chronic embolism and thrombosis of unspecified deep veins of unspecified distal lower extremity**

✓5ᵗʰ I82.6 Acute embolism and thrombosis of veins of upper extremity

✓6ᵗʰ I82.6Ø Acute embolism and thrombosis of unspecified veins of upper extremity

I82.6Ø1 **Acute embolism and thrombosis of unspecified veins of** right **upper extremity**

I82.6Ø2 **Acute embolism and thrombosis of unspecified veins of** left **upper extremity**

I82.6Ø3 **Acute embolism and thrombosis of unspecified veins of upper extremity,** bilateral

I82.6Ø9 **Acute embolism and thrombosis of unspecified veins of unspecified upper extremity**

✓6ᵗʰ I82.61 Acute embolism and thrombosis of superficial veins of upper extremity
Acute embolism and thrombosis of antecubital vein
Acute embolism and thrombosis of basilic vein
Acute embolism and thrombosis of cephalic vein

I82.611 **Acute embolism and thrombosis of superficial veins of** right **upper extremity**

I82.612 **Acute embolism and thrombosis of superficial veins of** left **upper extremity**

I82.613 **Acute embolism and thrombosis of superficial veins of upper extremity,** bilateral

I82.619 **Acute embolism and thrombosis of superficial veins of unspecified upper extremity**

✓6ᵗʰ I82.62 Acute embolism and thrombosis of deep veins of upper extremity
Acute embolism and thrombosis of brachial vein
Acute embolism and thrombosis of radial vein
Acute embolism and thrombosis of ulnar vein

I82.621 **Acute embolism and thrombosis of deep veins of** right **upper extremity**

I82.622 **Acute embolism and thrombosis of deep veins of** left **upper extremity**

I82.623 **Acute embolism and thrombosis of deep veins of upper extremity,** bilateral

I82.629 **Acute embolism and thrombosis of deep veins of unspecified upper extremity**

✓5ᵗʰ I82.7 Chronic embolism and thrombosis of veins of upper extremity
Use additional code, if applicable, for associated long-term (current) use of anticoagulants (Z79.Ø1)
EXCLUDES 1   personal history of venous embolism and thrombosis (Z86.718)

✓6ᵗʰ I82.7Ø Chronic embolism and thrombosis of unspecified veins of upper extremity

I82.7Ø1 **Chronic embolism and thrombosis of unspecified veins of** right **upper extremity**

I82.7Ø2 **Chronic embolism and thrombosis of unspecified veins of** left **upper extremity**

I82.7Ø3 **Chronic embolism and thrombosis of unspecified veins of upper extremity,** bilateral

I82.7Ø9 **Chronic embolism and thrombosis of unspecified veins of unspecified upper extremity**

✓6ᵗʰ I82.71 Chronic embolism and thrombosis of superficial veins of upper extremity
Chronic embolism and thrombosis of antecubital vein
Chronic embolism and thrombosis of basilic vein
Chronic embolism and thrombosis of cephalic vein

I82.711 **Chronic embolism and thrombosis of superficial veins of** right **upper extremity**

I82.712 **Chronic embolism and thrombosis of superficial veins of** left **upper extremity**

I82.713 **Chronic embolism and thrombosis of superficial veins of upper extremity,** bilateral

I82.719 **Chronic embolism and thrombosis of superficial veins of unspecified upper extremity**

Diseases of the Circulatory System

I82.72-I83.022

✓6ᵗʰ I82.72 Chronic embolism and thrombosis of deep veins of upper extremity
Chronic embolism and thrombosis of brachial vein
Chronic embolism and thrombosis of radial vein
Chronic embolism and thrombosis of ulnar vein

- **I82.721** Chronic embolism and thrombosis of deep veins of right upper extremity
- **I82.722** Chronic embolism and thrombosis of deep veins of left upper extremity
- **I82.723** Chronic embolism and thrombosis of deep veins of upper extremity, bilateral
- **I82.729** Chronic embolism and thrombosis of deep veins of unspecified upper extremity

✓5ᵗʰ I82.A Embolism and thrombosis of axillary vein

✓6ᵗʰ I82.A1 Acute embolism and thrombosis of axillary vein
- **I82.A11** Acute embolism and thrombosis of right axillary vein
- **I82.A12** Acute embolism and thrombosis of left axillary vein
- **I82.A13** Acute embolism and thrombosis of axillary vein, bilateral
- **I82.A19** Acute embolism and thrombosis of unspecified axillary vein

✓6ᵗʰ I82.A2 Chronic embolism and thrombosis of axillary vein
- **I82.A21** Chronic embolism and thrombosis of right axillary vein
- **I82.A22** Chronic embolism and thrombosis of left axillary vein
- **I82.A23** Chronic embolism and thrombosis of axillary vein, bilateral
- **I82.A29** Chronic embolism and thrombosis of unspecified axillary vein

✓5ᵗʰ I82.B Embolism and thrombosis of subclavian vein

✓6ᵗʰ I82.B1 Acute embolism and thrombosis of subclavian vein
- **I82.B11** Acute embolism and thrombosis of right subclavian vein
- **I82.B12** Acute embolism and thrombosis of left subclavian vein
- **I82.B13** Acute embolism and thrombosis of subclavian vein, bilateral
- **I82.B19** Acute embolism and thrombosis of unspecified subclavian vein

✓6ᵗʰ I82.B2 Chronic embolism and thrombosis of subclavian vein
- **I82.B21** Chronic embolism and thrombosis of right subclavian vein
- **I82.B22** Chronic embolism and thrombosis of left subclavian vein
- **I82.B23** Chronic embolism and thrombosis of subclavian vein, bilateral
- **I82.B29** Chronic embolism and thrombosis of unspecified subclavian vein

✓5ᵗʰ I82.C Embolism and thrombosis of internal jugular vein

✓6ᵗʰ I82.C1 Acute embolism and thrombosis of internal jugular vein
- **I82.C11** Acute embolism and thrombosis of right internal jugular vein
- **I82.C12** Acute embolism and thrombosis of left internal jugular vein
- **I82.C13** Acute embolism and thrombosis of internal jugular vein, bilateral
- **I82.C19** Acute embolism and thrombosis of unspecified internal jugular vein

✓6ᵗʰ I82.C2 Chronic embolism and thrombosis of internal jugular vein
- **I82.C21** Chronic embolism and thrombosis of right internal jugular vein
- **I82.C22** Chronic embolism and thrombosis of left internal jugular vein
- **I82.C23** Chronic embolism and thrombosis of internal jugular vein, bilateral
- **I82.C29** Chronic embolism and thrombosis of unspecified internal jugular vein

✓5ᵗʰ I82.8 Embolism and thrombosis of other specified veins
Use additional code, if applicable, for associated long-term (current) use of anticoagulants (Z79.01)

✓6ᵗʰ I82.81 Embolism and thrombosis of superficial veins of lower extremities
Embolism and thrombosis of saphenous vein (greater) (lesser)
- **I82.811** Embolism and thrombosis of superficial veins of right lower extremities
- **I82.812** Embolism and thrombosis of superficial veins of left lower extremities
- **I82.813** Embolism and thrombosis of superficial veins of lower extremities, bilateral
- **I82.819** Embolism and thrombosis of superficial veins of unspecified lower extremities

✓6ᵗʰ I82.89 Embolism and thrombosis of other specified veins
- **I82.890** Acute embolism and thrombosis of other specified veins
- **I82.891** Chronic embolism and thrombosis of other specified veins

✓5ᵗʰ I82.9 Embolism and thrombosis of unspecified vein
- **I82.90** Acute embolism and thrombosis of unspecified vein
Embolism of vein NOS
Thrombosis (vein) NOS
- **I82.91** Chronic embolism and thrombosis of unspecified vein

✓4ᵗʰ I83 Varicose veins of lower extremities
EXCLUDES 1 varicose veins complicating pregnancy (O22.0-)
varicose veins complicating the puerperium (O87.4)

✓5ᵗʰ I83.0 Varicose veins of lower extremities with ulcer
Use additional code to identify severity of ulcer (L97.-)

✓6ᵗʰ I83.00 Varicose veins of unspecified lower extremity with ulcer
- **I83.001** Varicose veins of unspecified lower extremity with ulcer of thigh 🅰
- **I83.002** Varicose veins of unspecified lower extremity with ulcer of calf 🅰
- **I83.003** Varicose veins of unspecified lower extremity with ulcer of ankle 🅰
- **I83.004** Varicose veins of unspecified lower extremity with ulcer of heel and midfoot 🅰
Varicose veins of unspecified lower extremity with ulcer of plantar surface of midfoot
- **I83.005** Varicose veins of unspecified lower extremity with ulcer other part of foot 🅰
Varicose veins of unspecified lower extremity with ulcer of toe
- **I83.008** Varicose veins of unspecified lower extremity with ulcer other part of lower leg 🅰
- **I83.009** Varicose veins of unspecified lower extremity with ulcer of unspecified site 🅰

✓6ᵗʰ I83.01 Varicose veins of right lower extremity with ulcer
- **I83.011** Varicose veins of right lower extremity with ulcer of thigh 🅰
- **I83.012** Varicose veins of right lower extremity with ulcer of calf 🅰
- **I83.013** Varicose veins of right lower extremity with ulcer of ankle 🅰
- **I83.014** Varicose veins of right lower extremity with ulcer of heel and midfoot 🅰
Varicose veins of right lower extremity with ulcer of plantar surface of midfoot
- **I83.015** Varicose veins of right lower extremity with ulcer other part of foot 🅰
Varicose veins of right lower extremity with ulcer of toe
- **I83.018** Varicose veins of right lower extremity with ulcer other part of lower leg 🅰
- **I83.019** Varicose veins of right lower extremity with ulcer of unspecified site 🅰

✓6ᵗʰ I83.02 Varicose veins of left lower extremity with ulcer
- **I83.021** Varicose veins of left lower extremity with ulcer of thigh 🅰
- **I83.022** Varicose veins of left lower extremity with ulcer of calf 🅰

I83.Ø23 **Varicose veins of left lower extremity with ulcer of** ankle [A]

I83.Ø24 **Varicose veins of left lower extremity with ulcer of** heel and midfoot [A]
Varicose veins of left lower extremity with ulcer of plantar surface of midfoot

I83.Ø25 **Varicose veins of left lower extremity with ulcer other** part of foot [A]
Varicose veins of left lower extremity with ulcer of toe

I83.Ø28 **Varicose veins of left lower extremity with ulcer other** part of lower leg [A]

I83.Ø29 **Varicose veins of left lower extremity with ulcer of unspecified site** [A]

✓5th **I83.1 Varicose veins of lower extremities with** inflammation
Stasis dermatitis

I83.1Ø **Varicose veins of unspecified lower extremity with inflammation** [A]

I83.11 **Varicose veins of** right **lower extremity with inflammation** [A]

I83.12 **Varicose veins of** left **lower extremity with inflammation** [A]

✓5th **I83.2 Varicose veins of lower extremities with both** ulcer and inflammation
Use additional code to identify severity of ulcer (L97.-)

✓6th I83.2Ø **Varicose veins of** unspecified **lower extremity with both ulcer and inflammation**

I83.2Ø1 **Varicose veins of unspecified lower extremity with both ulcer of** thigh **and inflammation** [A]

I83.2Ø2 **Varicose veins of unspecified lower extremity with both ulcer of** calf **and inflammation** [A]

I83.2Ø3 **Varicose veins of unspecified lower extremity with both ulcer of** ankle **and inflammation** [A]

I83.2Ø4 **Varicose veins of unspecified lower extremity with both ulcer of** heel and midfoot **and inflammation** [A]
Varicose veins of unspecified lower extremity with both ulcer of plantar surface of midfoot and inflammation

I83.2Ø5 **Varicose veins of unspecified lower extremity with both ulcer of other** part of foot **and inflammation** [A]
Varicose veins of unspecified lower extremity with both ulcer of toe and inflammation

I83.2Ø8 **Varicose veins of unspecified lower extremity with both ulcer of other** part of lower extremity **and inflammation** [A]

I83.2Ø9 **Varicose veins of unspecified lower extremity with both ulcer of unspecified site and inflammation** [A]

✓6th I83.21 **Varicose veins of** right **lower extremity with both ulcer and inflammation**

I83.211 **Varicose veins of right lower extremity with both ulcer of** thigh **and inflammation** [A]

I83.212 **Varicose veins of right lower extremity with both ulcer of** calf **and inflammation** [A]

I83.213 **Varicose veins of right lower extremity with both ulcer of** ankle **and inflammation** [A]

I83.214 **Varicose veins of right lower extremity with both ulcer of** heel and midfoot **and inflammation** [A]
Varicose veins of right lower extremity with both ulcer of plantar surface of midfoot and inflammation

I83.215 **Varicose veins of right lower extremity with both ulcer other** part of foot **and inflammation** [A]
Varicose veins of right lower extremity with both ulcer of toe and inflammation

I83.218 **Varicose veins of right lower extremity with both ulcer of other** part of lower extremity **and inflammation** [A]

I83.219 **Varicose veins of right lower extremity with both ulcer of unspecified site and inflammation** [A]

✓6th **I83.22 Varicose veins of** left **lower extremity with both ulcer and inflammation**

I83.221 **Varicose veins of left lower extremity with both ulcer of** thigh **and inflammation** [A]

I83.222 **Varicose veins of left lower extremity with both ulcer of** calf **and inflammation** [A]

I83.223 **Varicose veins of left lower extremity with both ulcer of** ankle **and inflammation** [A]

I83.224 **Varicose veins of left lower extremity with both ulcer of** heel and midfoot **and inflammation** [A]
Varicose veins of left lower extremity with both ulcer of plantar surface of midfoot and inflammation

I83.225 **Varicose veins of left lower extremity with both ulcer other** part of foot **and inflammation** [A]
Varicose veins of left lower extremity with both ulcer of toe and inflammation

I83.228 **Varicose veins of left lower extremity with both ulcer of other** part of lower extremity **and inflammation** [A]

I83.229 **Varicose veins of left lower extremity with both ulcer of unspecified site and inflammation** [A]

✓5th **I83.8 Varicose veins of lower extremities with** other complications

✓6th I83.81 **Varicose veins of lower extremities with** pain

I83.811 **Varicose veins of** right **lower extremities with pain** [A]

I83.812 **Varicose veins of** left **lower extremities with pain** [A]

I83.813 **Varicose veins of** bilateral **lower extremities with pain** [A]

I83.819 **Varicose veins of unspecified lower extremities with pain** [A]

✓6th I83.89 **Varicose veins of lower extremities with** other complications
Varicose veins of lower extremities with edema
Varicose veins of lower extremities with swelling

I83.891 **Varicose veins of** right **lower extremities with other complications** [A]

I83.892 **Varicose veins of** left **lower extremities with other complications** [A]

I83.893 **Varicose veins of** bilateral **lower extremities with other complications** [A]

I83.899 **Varicose veins of unspecified lower extremities with other complications** [A]

✓5th **I83.9 Asymptomatic varicose veins of lower extremities**
Phlebectasia of lower extremities
Varicose veins of lower extremities
Varix of lower extremities

I83.9Ø **Asymptomatic varicose veins of unspecified lower extremity** [A]
Varicose veins NOS

I83.91 **Asymptomatic varicose veins of** right **lower extremity** [A]

I83.92 **Asymptomatic varicose veins of** left **lower extremity** [A]

I83.93 **Asymptomatic varicose veins of** bilateral **lower extremities** [A]

✓4th **I85 Esophageal varices**
Use additional code to identify:
alcohol abuse and dependence (F1Ø.-)

✓5th **I85.Ø Esophageal varices**
Idiopathic esophageal varices
Primary esophageal varices

I85.ØØ **Esophageal varices** without bleeding
Esophageal varices NOS

I85.Ø1 **Esophageal varices** with bleeding

✓5th **I85.1 Secondary esophageal varices**
Esophageal varices secondary to alcoholic liver disease
Esophageal varices secondary to cirrhosis of liver
Esophageal varices secondary to schistosomiasis
Esophageal varices secondary to toxic liver disease
Code first underlying disease

I85.1Ø **Secondary esophageal varices** without bleeding

I85.11 **Secondary esophageal varices** with bleeding

Diseases of the Circulatory System

I86–I87.393

✓4th **I86　Varicose veins of other sites**
> EXCLUDES 1　*varicose veins of unspecified site (I83.9-)*
> EXCLUDES 2　*retinal varices (H35.0-)*

I86.0　Sublingual varices

I86.1　Scrotal varices　　　　　　　　　　　　　♂
> Varicocele

I86.2　Pelvic varices

I86.3　Vulval varices　　　　　　　　　　　　　♀
> EXCLUDES 1　*vulval varices complicating childbirth and the puerperium (O87.8)*
> *vulval varices complicating pregnancy (O22.1-)*

I86.4　Gastric varices

I86.8　Varicose veins of other specified sites　　Ⓐ
> Varicose ulcer of nasal septum

✓4th **I87　Other disorders of veins**

✓5th **I87.0　Postthrombotic syndrome**
> Chronic venous hypertension due to deep vein thrombosis
> Postphlebitic syndrome
> EXCLUDES 1　*chronic venous hypertension without deep vein thrombosis (I87.3-)*

✓6th **I87.00　Postthrombotic syndrome without complications**
> Asymptomatic postthrombotic syndrome

I87.001　Postthrombotic syndrome without complications of right lower extremity

I87.002　Postthrombotic syndrome without complications of left lower extremity

I87.003　Postthrombotic syndrome without complications of bilateral lower extremity

I87.009　Postthrombotic syndrome without complications of unspecified extremity
> Postthrombotic syndrome NOS

✓6th **I87.01　Postthrombotic syndrome with ulcer**
> Use additional code to specify site and severity of ulcer (L97.-)

I87.011　Postthrombotic syndrome with ulcer of right lower extremity

I87.012　Postthrombotic syndrome with ulcer of left lower extremity

I87.013　Postthrombotic syndrome with ulcer of bilateral lower extremity

I87.019　Postthrombotic syndrome with ulcer of unspecified lower extremity

✓6th **I87.02　Postthrombotic syndrome with inflammation**

I87.021　Postthrombotic syndrome with inflammation of right lower extremity

I87.022　Postthrombotic syndrome with inflammation of left lower extremity

I87.023　Postthrombotic syndrome with inflammation of bilateral lower extremity

I87.029　Postthrombotic syndrome with inflammation of unspecified lower extremity

✓6th **I87.03　Postthrombotic syndrome with ulcer and inflammation**
> Use additional code to specify site and severity of ulcer (L97.-)

I87.031　Postthrombotic syndrome with ulcer and inflammation of right lower extremity

I87.032　Postthrombotic syndrome with ulcer and inflammation of left lower extremity

I87.033　Postthrombotic syndrome with ulcer and inflammation of bilateral lower extremity

I87.039　Postthrombotic syndrome with ulcer and inflammation of unspecified lower extremity

✓6th **I87.09　Postthrombotic syndrome with other complications**

I87.091　Postthrombotic syndrome with other complications of right lower extremity

I87.092　Postthrombotic syndrome with other complications of left lower extremity

I87.093　Postthrombotic syndrome with other complications of bilateral lower extremity

I87.099　Postthrombotic syndrome with other complications of unspecified lower extremity

I87.1　Compression of vein
> Stricture of vein
> Vena cava syndrome (inferior) (superior)
> EXCLUDES 2　*compression of pulmonary vein (I28.8)*

I87.2　Venous insufficiency (chronic) (peripheral)

✓5th **I87.3　Chronic venous hypertension (idiopathic)**
> Stasis edema
> EXCLUDES 1　*chronic venous hypertension due to deep vein thrombosis (I87.0-)*
> *varicose veins of lower extremities (I83.-)*

✓6th **I87.30　Chronic venous hypertension (idiopathic) without complications**
> Asymptomatic chronic venous hypertension (idiopathic)

I87.301　Chronic venous hypertension (idiopathic) without complications of right lower extremity

I87.302　Chronic venous hypertension (idiopathic) without complications of left lower extremity

I87.303　Chronic venous hypertension (idiopathic) without complications of bilateral lower extremity

I87.309　Chronic venous hypertension (idiopathic) without complications of unspecified lower extremity
> Chronic venous hypertension NOS

✓6th **I87.31　Chronic venous hypertension (idiopathic) with ulcer**
> Use additional code to specify site and severity of ulcer (L97.-)

I87.311　Chronic venous hypertension (idiopathic) with ulcer of right lower extremity

I87.312　Chronic venous hypertension (idiopathic) with ulcer of left lower extremity

I87.313　Chronic venous hypertension (idiopathic) with ulcer of bilateral lower extremity

I87.319　Chronic venous hypertension (idiopathic) with ulcer of unspecified lower extremity

✓6th **I87.32　Chronic venous hypertension (idiopathic) with inflammation**

I87.321　Chronic venous hypertension (idiopathic) with inflammation of right lower extremity

I87.322　Chronic venous hypertension (idiopathic) with inflammation of left lower extremity

I87.323　Chronic venous hypertension (idiopathic) with inflammation of bilateral lower extremity

I87.329　Chronic venous hypertension (idiopathic) with inflammation of unspecified lower extremity

✓6th **I87.33　Chronic venous hypertension (idiopathic) with ulcer and inflammation**
> Use additional code to specify site and severity of ulcer (L97.-)

I87.331　Chronic venous hypertension (idiopathic) with ulcer and inflammation of right lower extremity

I87.332　Chronic venous hypertension (idiopathic) with ulcer and inflammation of left lower extremity

I87.333　Chronic venous hypertension (idiopathic) with ulcer and inflammation of bilateral lower extremity

I87.339　Chronic venous hypertension (idiopathic) with ulcer and inflammation of unspecified lower extremity

✓6th **I87.39　Chronic venous hypertension (idiopathic) with other complications**

I87.391　Chronic venous hypertension (idiopathic) with other complications of right lower extremity

I87.392　Chronic venous hypertension (idiopathic) with other complications of left lower extremity

I87.393　Chronic venous hypertension (idiopathic) with other complications of bilateral lower extremity

EXCLUDES 1 Not coded here　　EXCLUDES 2 Not included here　　N Newborn Age: 0　　P Pediatric Age: 0-17　　M Maternity Age: 12-55　　Ⓐ Adult Age: 15-124

598　　　　　　　　　　　　　　　　　　　　　　　　ICD-10-CM 2014 (Draft)

I87.399 **Chronic venous hypertension (idiopathic) with other complications of unspecified lower extremity**

I87.8 **Other specified disorders of veins**
Phlebosclerosis
Venofibrosis

I87.9 **Disorder of vein, unspecified**

√4th **I88** **Nonspecific lymphadenitis**
EXCLUDES 1 *acute lymphadenitis, except mesenteric (L04.-)*
enlarged lymph nodes NOS (R59.-)
human immunodeficiency virus [HIV] disease resulting in generalized lymphadenopathy (B20)

I88.0 **Nonspecific mesenteric lymphadenitis**
Mesenteric lymphadenitis (acute)(chronic)

I88.1 **Chronic lymphadenitis, except mesenteric**
Adenitis
Lymphadenitis

I88.8 **Other nonspecific lymphadenitis**

I88.9 **Nonspecific lymphadenitis, unspecified**
Lymphadenitis NOS

√4th **I89** **Other noninfective disorders of lymphatic vessels and lymph nodes**
EXCLUDES 1 *chylocele, tunica vaginalis (nonfilarial) NOS (N50.8)*
enlarged lymph nodes NOS (R59.-)
filarial chylocele (B74.-)
hereditary lymphedema (Q82.0)

I89.0 **Lymphedema, not elsewhere classified**
Elephantiasis (nonfilarial) NOS
Lymphangiectasis
Obliteration, lymphatic vessel
Praecox lymphedema
Secondary lymphedema
EXCLUDES 1 *postmastectomy lymphedema (I97.2)*

I89.1 **Lymphangitis**
Chronic lymphangitis
Lymphangitis NOS
Subacute lymphangitis
EXCLUDES 1 *acute lymphangitis (L03.-)*

I89.8 **Other specified noninfective disorders of lymphatic vessels and lymph nodes**
Chylocele (nonfilarial)
Chylous ascites
Chylous cyst
Lipomelanotic reticulosis
Lymph node or vessel fistula
Lymph node or vessel infarction
Lymph node or vessel rupture

I89.9 **Noninfective disorder of lymphatic vessels and lymph nodes, unspecified**
Disease of lymphatic vessels NOS

Other and unspecified disorders of the circulatory system (I95-I99)

√4th **I95** **Hypotension**
EXCLUDES 1 *cardiovascular collapse (R57.9)*
maternal hypotension syndrome (O26.5-)
nonspecific low blood pressure reading NOS (R03.1)

I95.0 **Idiopathic hypotension**

I95.1 **Orthostatic hypotension**
Hypotension, postural
EXCLUDES 1 *neurogenic orthostatic hypotension [Shy-Drager] (G90.3)*
orthostatic hypotension due to drugs (I95.2)

I95.2 **Hypotension due to drugs**
Orthostatic hypotension due to drugs
Use additional code for adverse effect, if applicable, to identify drug (T36-T50 with fifth or sixth character 5)

I95.3 **Hypotension of hemodialysis**
Intra-dialytic hypotension

√5th **I95.8** **Other hypotension**

I95.81 **Postprocedural hypotension**

I95.89 **Other hypotension**
Chronic hypotension

I95.9 **Hypotension, unspecified**

I96 **Gangrene, not elsewhere classified**
Gangrenous cellulitis
EXCLUDES 1 *gangrene in atherosclerosis of native arteries of the extremities (I70.26)*
gangrene in diabetes mellitus (E08-E13)
gangrene in hernia (K40.1, K40.4, K41.1, K41.4, K42.1, K43.1-, K44.1, K45.1, K46.1)
gangrene in other peripheral vascular diseases (I73.-)
gangrene of certain specified sites—see Alphabetical Index
gas gangrene (A48.0)
pyoderma gangrenosum (L88)

√4th **I97** **Intraoperative and postprocedural complications and disorders of circulatory system, not elsewhere classified**
EXCLUDES 2 *postprocedural shock (T81.1-)*

I97.0 **Postcardiotomy syndrome**

√5th **I97.1** **Other postprocedural cardiac functional disturbances**
EXCLUDES 2 *acute pulmonary insufficiency following thoracic surgery (J95.1)*
intraoperative cardiac functional disturbances (I97.7-)

√6th **I97.11** **Postprocedural cardiac insufficiency**

I97.110 **Postprocedural cardiac insufficiency following cardiac surgery**

I97.111 **Postprocedural cardiac insufficiency following other surgery**

√6th **I97.12** **Postprocedural cardiac arrest**

I97.120 **Postprocedural cardiac arrest following cardiac surgery**

I97.121 **Postprocedural cardiac arrest following other surgery**

√6th **I97.13** **Postprocedural heart failure**
Use additional code to identify the heart failure (I50.-)

I97.130 **Postprocedural heart failure following cardiac surgery**

I97.131 **Postprocedural heart failure following other surgery**

√6th **I97.19** **Other postprocedural cardiac functional disturbances**
Use additional code, if applicable, to further specify disorder

I97.190 **Other postprocedural cardiac functional disturbances following cardiac surgery**

I97.191 **Other postprocedural cardiac functional disturbances following other surgery**

I97.2 **Postmastectomy lymphedema syndrome** ▲
Elephantiasis due to mastectomy
Obliteration of lymphatic vessels

I97.3 **Postprocedural hypertension**

√5th **I97.4** **Intraoperative hemorrhage and hematoma of a circulatory system organ or structure complicating a procedure**
EXCLUDES 1 *intraoperative hemorrhage and hematoma of a circulatory system organ or structure due to accidental puncture and laceration during a procedure (I97.5-)*
EXCLUDES 2 *intraoperative cerebrovascular hemorrhage complicating a procedure (G97.3-)*

√6th **I97.41** **Intraoperative hemorrhage and hematoma of a circulatory system organ or structure complicating a circulatory system procedure**

I97.410 **Intraoperative hemorrhage and hematoma of a circulatory system organ or structure complicating a cardiac catheterization**

I97.411 **Intraoperative hemorrhage and hematoma of a circulatory system organ or structure complicating a cardiac bypass**

I97.418 **Intraoperative hemorrhage and hematoma of a circulatory system organ or structure complicating other circulatory system procedure**

I97.42 **Intraoperative hemorrhage and hematoma of a circulatory system organ or structure complicating other procedure**

√5th **I97.5** **Accidental puncture and laceration of a circulatory system organ or structure during a procedure**
EXCLUDES 2 *accidental puncture and laceration of brain during a procedure (G97.4-)*

I97.51 **Accidental puncture and laceration of a circulatory system organ or structure during a circulatory system procedure**

✓ Additional Character Required   √x7th Xtension Alert   Unspecified Code   Other Specified Code   Manifestation Code   ►◄ Revised Text   ● New Code   ▲ Revised Code Title

ICD-10-CM 2014 (Draft)   599

Diseases of the Circulatory System

I97.52–I99.9

I97.52   **Accidental puncture and laceration of a circulatory system organ or structure during** other procedure

☑5ᵗʰ **I97.6**   **Postprocedural hemorrhage and hematoma of a circulatory system organ or structure following a procedure**

> *EXCLUDES 2*   *postprocedural cerebrovascular hemorrhage complicating a procedure (G97.5-)*

    ☑6ᵗʰ **I97.61**   **Postprocedural hemorrhage and hematoma of a circulatory system organ or structure following a** circulatory system procedure

       I97.610   **Postprocedural hemorrhage and hematoma of a circulatory system organ or structure following a** cardiac catheterization

       I97.611   **Postprocedural hemorrhage and hematoma of a circulatory system organ or structure following** cardiac bypass

       I97.618   **Postprocedural hemorrhage and hematoma of a circulatory system organ or structure following** other circulatory system procedure

    I97.62   **Postprocedural hemorrhage and hematoma of a circulatory system organ or structure following other procedure**

☑5ᵗʰ **I97.7**   **Intraoperative** cardiac **functional disturbances**

> *EXCLUDES 2*   *acute pulmonary insufficiency following thoracic surgery (J95.1)*
> *postprocedural cardiac functional disturbances (I97.1-)*

    ☑6ᵗʰ **I97.71**   **Intraoperative** cardiac arrest

       I97.710   **Intraoperative cardiac arrest during** cardiac surgery

       I97.711   **Intraoperative cardiac arrest during** other surgery

    ☑6ᵗʰ **I97.79**   **Other** intraoperative cardiac functional disturbances
      Use additional code, if applicable, to further specify disorder

       I97.790   **Other intraoperative cardiac functional disturbances during** cardiac surgery

       I97.791   **Other intraoperative cardiac functional disturbances during other surgery**

☑5ᵗʰ **I97.8**   **Other intraoperative and postprocedural complications and disorders of the circulatory system, not elsewhere classified**
    Use additional code, if applicable, to further specify disorder

    ☑6ᵗʰ **I97.81**   **Intraoperative** cerebrovascular infarction

       I97.810   **Intraoperative cerebrovascular infarction during** cardiac surgery

       I97.811   **Intraoperative cerebrovascular infarction during** other surgery

    ☑6ᵗʰ **I97.82**   **Postprocedural** cerebrovascular infarction

       I97.820   **Postprocedural cerebrovascular infarction during** cardiac surgery

       I97.821   **Postprocedural cerebrovascular infarction during** other surgery

    I97.88   **Other** intraoperative **complications of the circulatory system, not elsewhere classified**

    I97.89   **Other** postprocedural **complications and disorders of the circulatory system, not elsewhere classified**

☑4ᵗʰ **I99**   **Other and unspecified disorders of circulatory system**

    I99.8   **Other disorder of circulatory system**

    I99.9   **Unspecified disorder of circulatory system**

EXCLUDES 1 Not coded here   *EXCLUDES 2* Not included here   N Newborn Age: 0   P Pediatric Age: 0-17   M Maternity Age: 12-55   A Adult Age: 15-124

600   ICD-10-CM 2014 (Draft)

Chapter 10. Diseases of the Respiratory System (J00-J99)

NOTE When a respiratory condition is described as occurring in more than one site and is not specifically indexed, it should be classified to the lower anatomic site (e.g. tracheobronchitis to bronchitis in J40).

Use additional code, where applicable, to identify:
exposure to environmental tobacco smoke (Z77.22)
exposure to tobacco smoke in the perinatal period (P96.81)
history of tobacco use (Z87.891)
occupational exposure to environmental tobacco smoke (Z57.31)
tobacco dependence (F17.-)
tobacco use (Z72.0)

EXCLUDES 2 *certain conditions originating in the perinatal period (P04-P96)*
certain infectious and parasitic diseases (A00-B99)
complications of pregnancy, childbirth and the puerperium (O00-O9A)
congenital malformations, deformations and chromosomal abnormalities (Q00-Q99)
endocrine, nutritional and metabolic diseases (E00-E88)
injury, poisoning and certain other consequences of external causes (S00-T88)
neoplasms (C00-D49)
smoke inhalation (T59.81-)
symptoms, signs and abnormal clinical and laboratory findings, not elsewhere classified (R00-R94)

This chapter contains the following blocks:
J00-J06　　Acute upper respiratory infections
J09-J18　　Influenza and pneumonia
J20-J22　　Other acute lower respiratory infections
J30-J39　　Other diseases of upper respiratory tract
J40-J47　　Chronic lower respiratory diseases
J60-J70　　Lung diseases due to external agents
J80-J84　　Other respiratory diseases principally affecting the interstitium
J85-J86　　Suppurative and necrotic conditions of the lower respiratory tract
J90-J94　　Other diseases of the pleura
J95　　　　Intraoperative and postprocedural complications and disorders of respiratory system, not elsewhere classified
J96-J99　　Other diseases of the respiratory system

Acute upper respiratory infections (J00-J06)

EXCLUDES 1 *influenza virus with other respiratory manifestations (J09.X2, J10.1, J11.1)*

EXCLUDES 2 *chronic obstructive pulmonary disease with acute lower respiratory infection (J44.0)*

J00　Acute nasopharyngitis (common cold)
Acute rhinitis
Coryza (acute)
Infective nasopharyngitis NOS
Infective rhinitis
Nasal catarrh, acute
Nasopharyngitis NOS

EXCLUDES 1 *acute pharyngitis (J02.-)*
acute sore throat NOS (J02.9)
pharyngitis NOS (J02.9)
rhinitis NOS (J31.0)
sore throat NOS (J02.9)

EXCLUDES 2 *allergic rhinitis (J30.1-J30.9)*
chronic pharyngitis (J31.2)
chronic rhinitis (J31.0)
chronic sore throat (J31.2)
nasopharyngitis, chronic (J31.1)
vasomotor rhinitis (J30.0)

☑4th J01　Acute sinusitis
INCLUDES acute abscess of sinus
acute empyema of sinus
acute infection of sinus
acute inflammation of sinus
acute suppuration of sinus

Use additional code (B95-B97) to identify infectious agent

EXCLUDES 1 *sinusitis NOS (J32.9)*
EXCLUDES 2 *chronic sinusitis (J32.0-J32.8)*

☑5th J01.0　Acute maxillary sinusitis
Acute antritis
J01.00　Acute maxillary sinusitis, unspecified
J01.01　Acute recurrent maxillary sinusitis

☑5th J01.1　Acute frontal sinusitis
J01.10　Acute frontal sinusitis, unspecified
J01.11　Acute recurrent frontal sinusitis

☑5th J01.2　Acute ethmoidal sinusitis
J01.20　Acute ethmoidal sinusitis, unspecified

J01.21　Acute recurrent ethmoidal sinusitis

☑5th J01.3　Acute sphenoidal sinusitis
J01.30　Acute sphenoidal sinusitis, unspecified
J01.31　Acute recurrent sphenoidal sinusitis

☑5th J01.4　Acute pansinusitis
J01.40　Acute pansinusitis, unspecified
J01.41　Acute recurrent pansinusitis

☑5th J01.8　Other acute sinusitis
J01.80　Other acute sinusitis
Acute sinusitis involving more than one sinus but not pansinusitis
J01.81　Other acute recurrent sinusitis
Acute recurrent sinusitis involving more than one sinus but not pansinusitis

☑5th J01.9　Acute sinusitis, unspecified
J01.90　Acute sinusitis, unspecified
J01.91　Acute recurrent sinusitis, unspecified

☑4th J02　Acute pharyngitis
INCLUDES acute sore throat
EXCLUDES 1 *acute laryngopharyngitis (J06.0)*
peritonsillar abscess (J36)
pharyngeal abscess (J39.1)
retropharyngeal abscess (J39.0)
EXCLUDES 2 *chronic pharyngitis (J31.2)*

J02.0　Streptococcal pharyngitis
Septic pharyngitis
Streptococcal sore throat
EXCLUDES 2 *scarlet fever (A38.-)*

J02.8　Acute pharyngitis due to other specified organisms
Use additional code (B95-B97) to identify infectious agent
EXCLUDES 1 *acute pharyngitis due to coxsackie virus (B08.5)*
acute pharyngitis due to gonococcus (A54.5)
acute pharyngitis due to herpes [simplex] virus (B00.2)
acute pharyngitis due to infectious mononucleosis (B27.-)
enteroviral vesicular pharyngitis (B08.5)

J02.9　Acute pharyngitis, unspecified
Gangrenous pharyngitis (acute)
Infective pharyngitis (acute) NOS
Pharyngitis (acute) NOS
Sore throat (acute) NOS
Suppurative pharyngitis (acute)
Ulcerative pharyngitis (acute)

☑4th J03　Acute tonsillitis
EXCLUDES 1 *acute sore throat (J02.-)*
hypertrophy of tonsils (J35.1)
peritonsillar abscess (J36)
sore throat NOS (J02.9)
streptococcal sore throat (J02.0)
EXCLUDES 2 *chronic tonsillitis (J35.0)*

☑5th J03.0　Streptococcal tonsillitis
J03.00　Acute streptococcal tonsillitis, unspecified
J03.01　Acute recurrent streptococcal tonsillitis

☑5th J03.8　Acute tonsillitis due to other specified organisms
Use additional code (B95-B97) to identify infectious agent
EXCLUDES 1 *diphtheritic tonsillitis (A36.0)*
herpesviral pharyngotonsillitis (B00.2)
streptococcal tonsillitis (J03.0)
tuberculous tonsillitis (A15.8)
Vincent's tonsillitis (A69.1)

J03.80　Acute tonsillitis due to other specified organisms
J03.81　Acute recurrent tonsillitis due to other specified organisms

☑5th J03.9　Acute tonsillitis, unspecified
Follicular tonsillitis (acute)
Gangrenous tonsillitis (acute)
Infective tonsillitis (acute)
Tonsillitis (acute) NOS
Ulcerative tonsillitis (acute)
J03.90　Acute tonsillitis, unspecified
J03.91　Acute recurrent tonsillitis, unspecified

Diseases of the Respiratory System

J04–J11.08

☑4ᵗʰ **J04 Acute laryngitis and tracheitis**
Use additional code (B95-B97) to identify infectious agent
EXCLUDES 1 acute obstructive laryngitis [croup] and epiglottitis (J05.-)
EXCLUDES 2 laryngismus (stridulus) (J38.5)

J04.0 Acute laryngitis
Edematous laryngitis (acute)
Laryngitis (acute) NOS
Subglottic laryngitis (acute)
Suppurative laryngitis (acute)
Ulcerative laryngitis (acute)
EXCLUDES 1 acute obstructive laryngitis (J05.0)
EXCLUDES 2 chronic laryngitis (J37.0)

☑5ᵗʰ **J04.1 Acute tracheitis**
Acute viral tracheitis
Catarrhal tracheitis (acute)
Tracheitis (acute) NOS
EXCLUDES 2 chronic tracheitis (J42)
J04.10 Acute tracheitis without obstruction
J04.11 Acute tracheitis with obstruction

J04.2 Acute laryngotracheitis
Laryngotracheitis NOS
Tracheitis (acute) with laryngitis (acute)
EXCLUDES 1 acute obstructive laryngotracheitis (J05.0)
EXCLUDES 2 chronic laryngotracheitis (J37.1)

☑5ᵗʰ **J04.3 Supraglottitis, unspecified**
J04.30 Supraglottitis, unspecified, without obstruction
J04.31 Supraglottitis, unspecified, with obstruction

☑4ᵗʰ **J05 Acute obstructive laryngitis [croup] and epiglottitis**
Use additional code (B95-B97) to identify infectious agent
J05.0 Acute obstructive laryngitis [croup]
Obstructive laryngitis (acute) NOS
Obstructive laryngotracheitis NOS

☑5ᵗʰ **J05.1 Acute epiglottitis**
EXCLUDES 2 epiglottitis, chronic (J37.0)
J05.10 Acute epiglottitis without obstruction
Epiglottitis NOS
J05.11 Acute epiglottitis with obstruction

☑4ᵗʰ **J06 Acute upper respiratory infections of multiple and unspecified sites**
EXCLUDES 1 acute respiratory infection NOS (J22)
streptococcal pharyngitis (J02.0)3
J06.0 Acute laryngopharyngitis
J06.9 Acute upper respiratory infection, unspecified
Upper respiratory disease, acute
Upper respiratory infection NOS

Influenza and pneumonia (J09-J18)
EXCLUDES 2 allergic or eosinophilic pneumonia (J82)
aspiration pneumonia NOS (J69.0)
congenital pneumonia (P23.9)
lipid pneumonia (J69.1)
meconium pneumonia (P24.01)
neonatal aspiration pneumonia (P24.-)
pneumonia due to solids and liquids (J69.-)
rheumatic pneumonia (I00)
ventilator associated pneumonia (J95.851)

☑4ᵗʰ **J09 Influenza due to certain identified influenza viruses**
EXCLUDES 1 seasonal influenza due to other identified influenza virus (J10.-)
seasonal influenza due to unidentified influenza virus (J11.-)

☑5ᵗʰ **J09.X Influenza due to identified novel influenza A virus**
Avian influenza
Bird influenza
Influenza A/H5N1
Influenza of other animal origin, not bird or swine
Swine influenza virus (viruses that normally cause infections in pigs)
J09.X1 Influenza due to identified novel influenza A virus with pneumonia
Code also, if applicable, associated:
lung abscess (J85.1)
other specified type of pneumonia

J09.X2 Influenza due to identified novel influenza A virus with other respiratory manifestations
Influenza due to identified novel influenza A virus NOS
Influenza due to identified novel influenza A virus with laryngitis
Influenza due to identified novel influenza A virus with pharyngitis
Influenza due to identified novel influenza A virus with upper respiratory symptoms
Use additional code, if applicable, for associated:
pleural effusion (J91.8)
sinusitis (J01.-)

J09.X3 Influenza due to identified novel influenza A virus with gastrointestinal manifestations
Influenza due to identified novel influenza A virus gastroenteritis
EXCLUDES 1 'intestinal flu' [viral gastroenteritis] (A08.-)

J09.X9 Influenza due to identified novel influenza A virus with other manifestations
Influenza due to identified novel influenza A virus with encephalopathy
Influenza due to identified novel influenza A virus with myocarditis
Influenza due to identified novel influenza A virus with otitis media
Use additional code to identify manifestation

☑4ᵗʰ **J10 Influenza due to other identified influenza virus**
EXCLUDES 1 influenza due to avian influenza virus (J09.X-)
influenza due to swine flu (J09.X-)
influenza due to unidentifed influenza virus (J11.-)

☑5ᵗʰ **J10.0 Influenza due to other identified influenza virus with pneumonia**
Code also associated lung abscess, if applicable (J85.1)
J10.00 Influenza due to other identified influenza virus with unspecified type of pneumonia
J10.01 Influenza due to other identified influenza virus with the same other identified influenza virus pneumonia
J10.08 Influenza due to other identified influenza virus with other specified pneumonia
Code also other specified type of pneumonia

J10.1 Influenza due to other identified influenza virus with other respiratory manifestations
Influenza due to other identified influenza virus NOS
Influenza due to other identified influenza virus with laryngitis
Influenza due to other identified influenza virus with pharyngitis
Influenza due to other identified influenza virus with upper respiratory symptoms
Use additional code for associated pleural effusion, if applicable (J91.8)
Use additional code for associated sinusitis, if applicable (J01.-)

J10.2 Influenza due to other identified influenza virus with gastrointestinal manifestations
Influenza due to other identified influenza virus gastroenteritis
EXCLUDES 1 'intestinal flu' [viral gastroenteritis] (A08.-)

☑5ᵗʰ **J10.8 Influenza due to other identified influenza virus with other manifestations**
J10.81 Influenza due to other identified influenza virus with encephalopathy
J10.82 Influenza due to other identified influenza virus with myocarditis
J10.83 Influenza due to other identified influenza virus with otitis media
Use additional code for any associated perforated tympanic membrane (H72.-)
J10.89 Influenza due to other identified influenza virus with other manifestations
Use additional codes to identify the manifestations

☑4ᵗʰ **J11 Influenza due to unidentified influenza virus**
☑5ᵗʰ **J11.0 Influenza due to unidentified influenza virus with pneumonia**
Code also associated lung abscess, if applicable (J85.1)
J11.00 Influenza due to unidentified influenza virus with unspecified type of pneumonia
Influenza with pneumonia NOS
J11.08 Influenza due to unidentified influenza virus with specified pneumonia
Code also other specified type of pneumonia

J11.1 Influenza due to unidentified influenza virus with other respiratory manifestations
Influenza NOS
Influenzal laryngitis NOS
Influenzal pharyngitis NOS
Influenza with upper respiratory symptoms NOS
Use additional code for associated pleural effusion, if applicable (J91.8)
Use additional code for associated sinusitis, if applicable (J01.-)

J11.2 Influenza due to unidentified influenza virus with gastrointestinal manifestations
Influenza gastroenteritis NOS
EXCLUDES 1 'intestinal flu' [viral gastroenteritis] (A08.-)

✓5ᵗʰ **J11.8 Influenza due to unidentified influenza virus with other manifestations**

    J11.81 Influenza due to unidentified influenza virus with encephalopathy
Influenzal encephalopathy NOS

    J11.82 Influenza due to unidentified influenza virus with myocarditis
Influenzal myocarditis NOS

    J11.83 Influenza due to unidentified influenza virus with otitis media
Influenzal otitis media NOS
Use additional code for any associated perforated tympanic membrane (H72.-)

    J11.89 Influenza due to unidentified influenza virus with other manifestations
Use additional codes to identify the manifestations

✓4ᵗʰ **J12 Viral pneumonia, not elsewhere classified**
INCLUDES bronchopneumonia due to viruses other than influenza viruses
Code first associated influenza, if applicable (J09.X1, J10.0-, J11.0-)
Code also associated abscess, if applicable (J85.1)
EXCLUDES 1 aspiration pneumonia due to anesthesia during labor and delivery (O74.0)
aspiration pneumonia due to anesthesia during pregnancy (O29)
aspiration pneumonia due to anesthesia during puerperium (O89.0)
aspiration pneumonia due to solids and liquids (J69.-)
aspiration pneumonia NOS (J69.0)
congenital pneumonia (P23.0)
congenital rubella pneumonitis (P35.0)
interstitial pneumonia NOS (J84.9)
lipid pneumonia (J69.1)
neonatal aspiration pneumonia (P24.-)

J12.0 Adenoviral pneumonia

J12.1 Respiratory syncytial virus pneumonia

J12.2 Parainfluenza virus pneumonia

J12.3 Human metapneumovirus pneumonia

✓5ᵗʰ **J12.8 Other viral pneumonia**

    J12.81 Pneumonia due to SARS-associated coronavirus
Severe acute respiratory syndrome NOS

    J12.89 Other viral pneumonia

J12.9 Viral pneumonia, unspecified

J13 Pneumonia due to Streptococcus pneumoniae
Bronchopneumonia due to S. pneumoniae
Code first associated influenza, if applicable (J09.X1, J10.0-, J11.0-)
Code also associated lung abscess, if applicable (J85.1)
EXCLUDES 1 congenital pneumonia due to S. pneumoniae (P23.6)
lobar pneumonia, unspecified organism (J18.1)
pneumonia due to other streptococci (J15.3-J15.4)

J14 Pneumonia due to Hemophilus influenzae
Bronchopneumonia due to H. influenzae
Code first associated influenza, if applicable (J09.X1, J10.0-, J11.0-)
Code also associated lung abscess, if applicable (J85.1)
EXCLUDES 1 congenital pneumonia due to H. influenzae (P23.6)

✓4ᵗʰ **J15 Bacterial pneumonia, not elsewhere classified**
Bronchopneumonia due to bacteria other than S. pneumoniae and H. influenzae
Code first associated influenza, if applicable (J09.X1, J10.0-, J11.0-)
Code also associated lung abscess, if applicable (J85.1)
EXCLUDES 1 chlamydial pneumonia (J16.0)
congenital pneumonia (P23.-)
Legionnaires' disease (A48.1)
spirochetal pneumonia (A69.8)

J15.0 Pneumonia due to Klebsiella pneumoniae

J15.1 Pneumonia due to Pseudomonas

✓5ᵗʰ **J15.2 Pneumonia due to staphylococcus**

    J15.20 Pneumonia due to staphylococcus, unspecified

✓6ᵗʰ   **J15.21 Pneumonia due to Staphylococcus aureus**

       J15.211 Pneumonia due to methicillin susceptible Staphylococcus aureus
MSSA pneumonia
Pneumonia due to Staphylococcus aureus NOS

       J15.212 Pneumonia due to methicillin resistant Staphylococcus aureus

    J15.29 Pneumonia due to other staphylococcus

J15.3 Pneumonia due to streptococcus, group B

J15.4 Pneumonia due to other streptococci
EXCLUDES 1 pneumonia due to streptococcus, group B (J15.3)
pneumonia due to Streptococcus pneumoniae (J13)

J15.5 Pneumonia due to Escherichia coli

J15.6 Pneumonia due to other aerobic Gram-negative bacteria
Pneumonia due to Serratia marcescens

J15.7 Pneumonia due to Mycoplasma pneumoniae

J15.8 Pneumonia due to other specified bacteria

J15.9 Unspecified bacterial pneumonia
Pneumonia due to gram-positive bacteria

✓4ᵗʰ **J16 Pneumonia due to other infectious organisms, not elsewhere classified**
Code first associated influenza, if applicable (J09.X1, J10.0-, J11.0-)
Code also associated lung abscess, if applicable (J85.1)
EXCLUDES 1 congenital pneumonia (P23.-)
ornithosis (A70)
pneumocystosis (B59)
pneumonia NOS (J18.9)

J16.0 Chlamydial pneumonia

J16.8 Pneumonia due to other specified infectious organisms

J17 Pneumonia in diseases classified elsewhere
Code first underlying disease, such as:
Q fever (A78)
rheumatic fever (I00)
schistosomiasis (B65.0-B65.9)
EXCLUDES 1 candidial pneumonia (B37.1)
chlamydial pneumonia (J16.0)
gonorrheal pneumonia (A54.84)
histoplasmosis pneumonia (B39.0-B39.2)
measles pneumonia (B05.2)
nocardiosis pneumonia (A43.0)
pneumocystosis (B59)
pneumonia due to Pneumocystis carinii (B59)
pneumonia due to Pneumocystis jiroveci (B59)
pneumonia in actinomycosis (A42.0)
pneumonia in anthrax (A22.1)
pneumonia in ascariasis (B77.81)
pneumonia in aspergillosis (B44.0-B44.1)
pneumonia in coccidioidomycosis (B38.0-B38.2)
pneumonia in cytomegalovirus disease (B25.0)
pneumonia in toxoplasmosis (B58.3)
rubella pneumonia (B06.81)
salmonella pneumonia (A02.22)
spirochetal infection NEC with pneumonia (A69.8)
tularemia pneumonia (A21.2)
typhoid fever with pneumonia (A01.03)
varicella pneumonia (B01.2)
whooping cough with pneumonia (A37 with fifth-character 1)

☑ Additional Character Required   ✔x7ᵗʰ Xtension Alert   Unspecified Code   Other Specified Code   Manifestation Code   ▶◀ Revised Text   ● New Code   ▲ Revised Code Title

✓4th **J18** **Pneumonia, unspecified organism**
Code first associated influenza, if applicable (J09.X1, J10.0-, J11.0-)
EXCLUDES 1   abscess of lung with pneumonia (J85.1)
aspiration pneumonia due to anesthesia during labor and delivery (O74.0)
aspiration pneumonia due to anesthesia during pregnancy (O29)
aspiration pneumonia due to anesthesia during puerperium (O89.0)
aspiration pneumonia due to solids and liquids (J69.-)
aspiration pneumonia NOS (J69.0)
congenital pneumonia (P23.0)
drug-induced interstitial lung disorder (J70.2-J70.4)
interstitial pneumonia NOS (J84.9)
lipid pneumonia (J69.1)
neonatal aspiration pneumonia (P24.-)
pneumonitis due to external agents (J67-J70)
pneumonitis due to fumes and vapors (J68.0)
usual interstitial pneumonia (J84.17)

J18.0 **Bronchopneumonia, unspecified organism**
EXCLUDES 1   hypostatic bronchopneumonia (J18.2)
lipid pneumonia (J69.1)
EXCLUDES 2   acute bronchiolitis (J21.-)
chronic bronchiolitis (J44.9)

J18.1 **Lobar pneumonia, unspecified organism**

J18.2 **Hypostatic pneumonia, unspecified organism**
Hypostatic bronchopneumonia
Passive pneumonia

J18.8 **Other pneumonia, unspecified organism**

J18.9 **Pneumonia, unspecified organism**
AHA: 2012, Q4, 94

Other acute lower respiratory infections (J20-J22)
EXCLUDES 2   chronic obstructive pulmonary disease with acute lower respiratory infection (J44.0)

✓4th **J20** **Acute bronchitis**
INCLUDES   acute and subacute bronchitis (with) bronchospasm
acute and subacute bronchitis (with) tracheitis
acute and subacute bronchitis (with) tracheobronchitis, acute
acute and subacute fibrinous bronchitis
acute and subacute membranous bronchitis
acute and subacute purulent bronchitis
acute and subacute septic bronchitis
EXCLUDES 1   bronchitis NOS (J40)
tracheobronchitis NOS (J40)
EXCLUDES 2   acute bronchitis with bronchiectasis (J47.0)
acute bronchitis with chronic obstructive asthma (J44.0)
acute bronchitis with chronic obstructive pulmonary disease (J44.0)
allergic bronchitis NOS (J45.909)
bronchitis due to chemicals, fumes and vapors (J68.0)
chronic bronchitis NOS (J42)
chronic mucopurulent bronchitis (J41.1)
chronic obstructive bronchitis (J44.-)
chronic obstructive tracheobronchitis (J44.-)
chronic simple bronchitis (J41.0)
chronic tracheobronchitis (J42)

J20.0 **Acute bronchitis due to Mycoplasma pneumoniae**
J20.1 **Acute bronchitis due to Hemophilus influenzae**
J20.2 **Acute bronchitis due to streptococcus**
J20.3 **Acute bronchitis due to coxsackievirus**
J20.4 **Acute bronchitis due to parainfluenza virus**
J20.5 **Acute bronchitis due to respiratory syncytial virus**
J20.6 **Acute bronchitis due to rhinovirus**
J20.7 **Acute bronchitis due to echovirus**
J20.8 **Acute bronchitis due to other specified organisms**
J20.9 **Acute bronchitis, unspecified**

✓4th **J21** **Acute bronchiolitis**
Acute bronchiolitis with bronchospasm
EXCLUDES 2   respiratory bronchiolitis interstitial lung disease (J84.115)

J21.0 **Acute bronchiolitis due to respiratory syncytial virus**
J21.1 **Acute bronchiolitis due to human metapneumovirus**
J21.8 **Acute bronchiolitis due to other specified organisms**
J21.9 **Acute bronchiolitis, unspecified**
Bronchiolitis (acute)
EXCLUDES 1   chronic bronchiolitis (J44.-)

J22 **Unspecified acute lower respiratory infection**
Acute (lower) respiratory (tract) infection NOS
EXCLUDES 1   upper respiratory infection (acute) (J06.9)

Other diseases of upper respiratory tract (J30-J39)

✓4th **J30** **Vasomotor and allergic rhinitis**
INCLUDES   spasmodic rhinorrhea
EXCLUDES 1   allergic rhinitis with asthma (bronchial) (J45.909)
rhinitis NOS (J31.0)

J30.0 **Vasomotor rhinitis**
J30.1 **Allergic rhinitis due to pollen**
Allergy NOS due to pollen
Hay fever
Pollinosis
J30.2 **Other seasonal allergic rhinitis**
J30.5 **Allergic rhinitis due to food**
✓5th **J30.8** **Other allergic rhinitis**
  J30.81 **Allergic rhinitis due to animal (cat) (dog) hair and dander**
  J30.89 **Other allergic rhinitis**
    Perennial allergic rhinitis
J30.9 **Allergic rhinitis, unspecified**

✓4th **J31** **Chronic rhinitis, nasopharyngitis and pharyngitis**
Use additional code to identify:
exposure to environmental tobacco smoke (Z77.22)
exposure to tobacco smoke in the perinatal period (P96.81)
history of tobacco use (Z87.891)
occupational exposure to environmental tobacco smoke (Z57.31)
tobacco dependence (F17.-)
tobacco use (Z72.0)

J31.0 **Chronic rhinitis**
Atrophic rhinitis (chronic)
Granulomatous rhinitis (chronic)
Hypertrophic rhinitis (chronic)
Obstructive rhinitis (chronic)
Ozena
Purulent rhinitis (chronic)
Rhinitis (chronic) NOS
Ulcerative rhinitis (chronic)
EXCLUDES 1   allergic rhinitis (J30.1-J30.9)
vasomotor rhinitis (J30.0)

J31.1 **Chronic nasopharyngitis**
EXCLUDES 2   acute nasopharyngitis (J00)

J31.2 **Chronic pharyngitis**
Atrophic pharyngitis (chronic)
Chronic sore throat
Granular pharyngitis (chronic)
Hypertrophic pharyngitis (chronic)
EXCLUDES 2   acute pharyngitis (J02.9)

✓4th **J32** **Chronic sinusitis**
INCLUDES   sinus abscess
sinus empyema
sinus infection
sinus suppuration
Use additional code to identify:
exposure to environmental tobacco smoke (Z77.22)
exposure to tobacco smoke in the perinatal period (P96.81)
history of tobacco use (Z87.891)
infectious agent (B95-B97)
occupational exposure to environmental tobacco smoke (Z57.31)
tobacco dependence (F17.-)
tobacco use (Z72.0)
EXCLUDES 2   acute sinusitis (J01.-)

J32.0 **Chronic maxillary sinusitis**
Antritis (chronic)
Maxillary sinusitis NOS
J32.1 **Chronic frontal sinusitis**
Frontal sinusitis NOS
J32.2 **Chronic ethmoidal sinusitis**
Ethmoidal sinusitis NOS
EXCLUDES 1   Woakes' ethmoiditis (J33.1)
J32.3 **Chronic sphenoidal sinusitis**
Sphenoidal sinusitis NOS
J32.4 **Chronic pansinusitis**
Pansinusitis NOS
J32.8 **Other chronic sinusitis**
Sinusitis (chronic) involving more than one sinus but not pansinusitis

J32.9   Chronic sinusitis, unspecified
Sinusitis (chronic) NOS

✓4ᵗʰ **J33   Nasal polyp**
Use additional code to identify:
exposure to environmental tobacco smoke (Z77.22)
exposure to tobacco smoke in the perinatal period (P96.81)
history of tobacco use (Z87.891)
occupational exposure to environmental tobacco smoke (Z57.31)
tobacco dependence (F17.-)
tobacco use (Z72.0)
EXCLUDES 1   adenomatous polyps (D14.0)

J33.0   Polyp of nasal cavity
Choanal polyp
Nasopharyngeal polyp

J33.1   Polypoid sinus degeneration
Woakes' syndrome or ethmoiditis

J33.8   Other polyp of sinus
Accessory polyp of sinus
Ethmoidal polyp of sinus
Maxillary polyp of sinus
Sphenoidal polyp of sinus

J33.9   Nasal polyp, unspecified

✓4ᵗʰ **J34   Other and unspecified disorders of nose and nasal sinuses**
EXCLUDES 2   varicose ulcer of nasal septum (I86.8)

J34.0   Abscess, furuncle and carbuncle of nose
Cellulitis of nose
Necrosis of nose
Ulceration of nose

J34.1   Cyst and mucocele of nose and nasal sinus

J34.2   Deviated nasal septum
Deflection or deviation of septum (nasal) (acquired)
EXCLUDES 1   congenital deviated nasal septum (Q67.4)

J34.3   Hypertrophy of nasal turbinates

✓5ᵗʰ **J34.8   Other specified disorders of nose and nasal sinuses**

J34.81   Nasal mucositis (ulcerative)
Code also type of associated therapy, such as:
antineoplastic and immunosuppressive drugs
(T45.1X-)
radiological procedure and radiotherapy (Y84.2)
EXCLUDES 2   gastrointestinal mucositis (ulcerative)
(K92.81)
mucositis (ulcerative) of vagina and vulva
(N76.81)
oral mucositis (ulcerative) (K12.3-)

J34.89   Other specified disorders of nose and nasal sinuses
Perforation of nasal septum NOS
Rhinolith

J34.9   Unspecified disorder of nose and nasal sinuses

✓4ᵗʰ **J35   Chronic diseases of tonsils and adenoids**
Use additional code to identify:
exposure to environmental tobacco smoke (Z77.22)
exposure to tobacco smoke in the perinatal period (P96.81)
history of tobacco use (Z87.891)
occupational exposure to environmental tobacco smoke (Z57.31)
tobacco dependence (F17.-)
tobacco use (Z72.0)

✓5ᵗʰ **J35.0   Chronic tonsillitis and adenoiditis**
EXCLUDES 2   acute tonsillitis (J03.-)

J35.01   Chronic tonsillitis

J35.02   Chronic adenoiditis

J35.03   Chronic tonsillitis and adenoiditis

J35.1   Hypertrophy of tonsils
Enlargement of tonsils
EXCLUDES 1   hypertrophy of tonsils with tonsillitis (J35.0-)

J35.2   Hypertrophy of adenoids
Enlargement of adenoids
EXCLUDES 1   hypertrophy of adenoids with adenoiditis (J35.0-)

J35.3   Hypertrophy of tonsils with hypertrophy of adenoids
EXCLUDES 1   hypertrophy of tonsils and adenoids with tonsillitis and
adenoiditis (J35.03)

J35.8   Other chronic diseases of tonsils and adenoids
Adenoid vegetations
Amygdalolith
Calculus, tonsil
Cicatrix of tonsil (and adenoid)
Tonsillar tag
Ulcer of tonsil

J35.9   Chronic disease of tonsils and adenoids, unspecified
Disease (chronic) of tonsils and adenoids NOS

J36   Peritonsillar abscess
INCLUDES   abscess of tonsil
peritonsillar cellulitis
quinsy
Use additional code (B95-B97) to identify infectious agent
EXCLUDES 1   acute tonsillitis (J03.-)
chronic tonsillitis (J35.0)
retropharyngeal abscess (J39.0)
tonsillitis NOS (J03.9-)

✓4ᵗʰ **J37   Chronic laryngitis and laryngotracheitis**
Use additional code to identify:
exposure to environmental tobacco smoke (Z77.22)
exposure to tobacco smoke in the perinatal period (P96.81)
history of tobacco use (Z87.891)
infectious agent (B95-B97)
occupational exposure to environmental tobacco smoke (Z57.31)
tobacco dependence (F17.-)
tobacco use (Z72.0)

J37.0   Chronic laryngitis
Catarrhal laryngitis
Hypertrophic laryngitis
Sicca laryngitis
EXCLUDES 2   acute laryngitis (J04.0)
obstructive (acute) laryngitis (J05.0)

J37.1   Chronic laryngotracheitis
Laryngitis, chronic, with tracheitis (chronic)
Tracheitis, chronic, with laryngitis
EXCLUDES 2   chronic tracheitis (J42)
EXCLUDES 2   acute laryngotracheitis (J04.2)
acute tracheitis (J04.1)

✓4ᵗʰ **J38   Diseases of vocal cords and larynx, not elsewhere classified**
Use additional code to identify:
exposure to environmental tobacco smoke (Z77.22)
exposure to tobacco smoke in the perinatal period (P96.81)
history of tobacco use (Z87.891)
occupational exposure to environmental tobacco smoke (Z57.31)
tobacco dependence (F17.-)
tobacco use (Z72.0)
EXCLUDES 1   congenital laryngeal stridor (P28.89)
obstructive laryngitis (acute) (J05.0)
postprocedural subglottic stenosis (J95.5)
stridor (R06.1)
ulcerative laryngitis (J04.0)

✓5ᵗʰ **J38.0   Paralysis of vocal cords and larynx**
Laryngoplegia
Paralysis of glottis

J38.00   Paralysis of vocal cords and larynx, unspecified

J38.01   Paralysis of vocal cords and larynx, unilateral

J38.02   Paralysis of vocal cords and larynx, bilateral

J38.1   Polyp of vocal cord and larynx
EXCLUDES 1   adenomatous polyps (D14.1)

J38.2   Nodules of vocal cords
Chorditis (fibrinous)(nodosa)(tuberosa)
Singer's nodes
Teacher's nodes

J38.3   Other diseases of vocal cords
Abscess of vocal cords
Cellulitis of vocal cords
Granuloma of vocal cords
Leukokeratosis of vocal cords
Leukoplakia of vocal cords

J38.4   Edema of larynx
Edema (of) glottis
Subglottic edema
Supraglottic edema
EXCLUDES 1   acute obstructive laryngitis [croup] (J05.0)
edematous laryngitis (J04.0)

J38.5   Laryngeal spasm
Laryngismus (stridulus)

J38.6   Stenosis of larynx

J38.7   Other diseases of larynx

Abscess of larynx	Pachyderma of larynx
Cellulitis of larynx	Perichondritis of larynx
Disease of larynx NOS	Ulcer of larynx
Necrosis of larynx	

✓ Additional Character Required   ✓x7ᵗʰ Xtension Alert   Unspecified Code   Other Specified Code   Manifestation Code   ▶◀ Revised Text   ● New Code   ▲ Revised Code Title

ICD-10-CM 2014 (Draft)   605

✓4ᵗʰ **J39   Other diseases of upper respiratory tract**
> EXCLUDES 1   *acute respiratory infection NOS (J22)*
> *acute upper respiratory infection (J06.9)*
> *upper respiratory inflammation due to chemicals, gases, fumes or vapors (J68.2)*

J39.0   Retropharyngeal and parapharyngeal abscess
Peripharyngeal abscess
> EXCLUDES 1   *peritonsillar abscess (J36)*

J39.1   Other abscess of pharynx
Cellulitis of pharynx
Nasopharyngeal abscess

J39.2   Other diseases of pharynx
Cyst of pharynx
Edema of pharynx
> EXCLUDES 2   *chronic pharyngitis (J31.2)*
> *ulcerative pharyngitis (J02.9)*

J39.3   Upper respiratory tract hypersensitivity reaction, site unspecified
> EXCLUDES 1   *hypersensitivity reaction of upper respiratory tract, such as:*
> *extrinsic allergic alveolitis (J67.9)*
> *pneumoconiosis (J60-J67.9)*

J39.8   Other specified diseases of upper respiratory tract

J39.9   Disease of upper respiratory tract, unspecified

Chronic lower respiratory diseases (J40-J47)

> EXCLUDES 1   *bronchitis due to chemicals, gases, fumes and vapors (J68.0)*
> EXCLUDES 2   *cystic fibrosis (E84.-)*

J40   Bronchitis, not specified as acute or chronic
Bronchitis NOS
Bronchitis with tracheitis NOS
Catarrhal bronchitis
Tracheobronchitis NOS
Use additional code to identify:
  exposure to environmental tobacco smoke (Z77.22)
  exposure to tobacco smoke in the perinatal period (P96.81)
  history of tobacco use (Z87.891)
  occupational exposure to environmental tobacco smoke (Z57.31)
  tobacco dependence (F17.-)
  tobacco use (Z72.0)
> EXCLUDES 1   *acute bronchitis (J20.-)*
> *allergic bronchitis NOS (J45.909)*
> *asthmatic bronchitis NOS (J45.9-)*
> *bronchitis due to chemicals, gases, fumes and vapors (J68.0)*

✓4ᵗʰ **J41   Simple and mucopurulent chronic bronchitis**
Use additional code to identify:
  exposure to environmental tobacco smoke (Z77.22)
  exposure to tobacco smoke in the perinatal period (P96.81)
  history of tobacco use (Z87.891)
  occupational exposure to environmental tobacco smoke (Z57.31)
  tobacco dependence (F17.-)
  tobacco use (Z72.0)
> EXCLUDES 1   *chronic bronchitis NOS (J42)*
> *chronic obstructive bronchitis (J44.-)*

J41.0   Simple chronic bronchitis

J41.1   Mucopurulent chronic bronchitis

J41.8   Mixed simple and mucopurulent chronic bronchitis

J42   Unspecified chronic bronchitis
Chronic bronchitis NOS
Chronic tracheitis
Chronic tracheobronchitis
Use additional code to identify:
  exposure to environmental tobacco smoke (Z77.22)
  exposure to tobacco smoke in the perinatal period (P96.81)
  history of tobacco use (Z87.891)
  occupational exposure to environmental tobacco smoke (Z57.31)
  tobacco dependence (F17.-)
  tobacco use (Z72.0)
> EXCLUDES 1   *chronic asthmatic bronchitis (J44.-)*
> *chronic bronchitis with airways obstruction (J44.-)*
> *chronic emphysematous bronchitis (J44.-)*
> *chronic obstructive pulmonary disease NOS (J44.9)*
> *simple and mucopurulent chronic bronchitis (J41.-)*

✓4ᵗʰ **J43   Emphysema**
Use additional code to identify:
  exposure to environmental tobacco smoke (Z77.22)
  history of tobacco use (Z87.891)
  occupational exposure to environmental tobacco smoke (Z57.31)
  tobacco dependence (F17.-)
  tobacco use (Z72.0)
> EXCLUDES 1   *compensatory emphysema (J98.3)*
> *emphysema due to inhalation of chemicals, gases, fumes or vapors (J68.4)*
> *emphysema with chronic (obstructive) bronchitis (J44.-)*
> *emphysematous (obstructive) bronchitis (J44.-)*
> *interstitial emphysema (J98.2)*
> *mediastinal emphysema (J98.2)*
> *neonatal interstitial emphysema (P25.0)*
> *surgical (subcutaneous) emphysema (T81.82)*
> *traumatic subcutaneous emphysema (T79.7)*

J43.0   Unilateral pulmonary emphysema [MacLeod's syndrome]
Swyer-James syndrome
Unilateral emphysema
Unilateral hyperlucent lung
Unilateral pulmonary artery functional hypoplasia
Unilateral transparency of lung

J43.1   Panlobular emphysema
Panacinar emphysema

J43.2   Centrilobular emphysema

J43.8   Other emphysema

J43.9   Emphysema, unspecified
Bullous emphysema (lung)(pulmonary)
Emphysema (lung)(pulmonary) NOS
Emphysematous bleb
Vesicular emphysema (lung)(pulmonary)

✓4ᵗʰ **J44   Other chronic obstructive pulmonary disease**
> INCLUDES   asthma with chronic obstructive pulmonary disease
> chronic asthmatic (obstructive) bronchitis
> chronic bronchitis with airways obstruction
> chronic bronchitis with emphysema
> chronic emphysematous bronchitis
> chronic obstructive asthma
> chronic obstructive bronchitis
> chronic obstructive tracheobronchitis

Code also type of asthma, if applicable (J45.-)
Use additional code to identify:
  exposure to environmental tobacco smoke (Z77.22)
  history of tobacco use (Z87.891)
  occupational exposure to environmental tobacco smoke (Z57.31)
  tobacco dependence (F17.-)
  tobacco use (Z72.0)
> EXCLUDES 1   *bronchiectasis (J47.-)*
> *chronic bronchitis NOS (J42)*
> *chronic simple and mucopurulent bronchitis (J41.-)*
> *chronic tracheitis (J42)*
> *chronic tracheobronchitis (J42)*
> *emphysema without chronic bronchitis (J43.-)*
> *lung diseases due to external agents (J60-J70)*

J44.0   Chronic obstructive pulmonary disease with acute lower respiratory infection
Use additional code to identify the infection

J44.1   Chronic obstructive pulmonary disease with (acute) exacerbation
Decompensated COPD
Decompensated COPD with (acute) exacerbation
> EXCLUDES 2   *chronic obstructive pulmonary disease [COPD] with acute bronchitis (J44.0)*

J44.9   Chronic obstructive pulmonary disease, unspecified
Chronic obstructive airway disease NOS
Chronic obstructive lung disease NOS

EXCLUDES 1 Not coded here   EXCLUDES 2 Not included here   N Newborn Age: 0   P Pediatric Age: 0-17   M Maternity Age: 12-55   A Adult Age: 15-124

606   ICD-10-CM 2014 (Draft)

✓4th J45 Asthma
Allergic (predominantly) asthma
Allergic bronchitis NOS
Allergic rhinitis with asthma
Atopic asthma
Extrinsic allergic asthma
Hay fever with asthma
Idiosyncratic asthma
Intrinsic nonallergic asthma
Nonallergic asthma

Use additional code to identify:
exposure to environmental tobacco smoke (Z77.22)
exposure to tobacco smoke in the perinatal period (P96.81)
history of tobacco use (Z87.891)
occupational exposure to environmental tobacco smoke (Z57.31)
tobacco dependence (F17.-)
tobacco use (Z72.0)

EXCLUDES 1　detergent asthma (J69.8)
eosinophilic asthma (J82)
lung diseases due to external agents (J60-J70)
miner's asthma (J60)
wheezing NOS (R06.2)
wood asthma (J67.8)

EXCLUDES 2　asthma with chronic obstructive pulmonary disease (J44.9)
chronic asthmatic (obstructive) bronchitis (J44.9)
chronic obstructive asthma (J44.9)

✓5th J45.2 Mild intermittent asthma
J45.20　Mild intermittent asthma, uncomplicated
Mild intermittent asthma NOS
J45.21　Mild intermittent asthma with (acute) exacerbation
J45.22　Mild intermittent asthma with status asthmaticus

✓5th J45.3 Mild persistent asthma
J45.30　Mild persistent asthma, uncomplicated
Mild persistent asthma NOS
J45.31　Mild persistent asthma with (acute) exacerbation
J45.32　Mild persistent asthma with status asthmaticus

✓5th J45.4 Moderate persistent asthma
J45.40　Moderate persistent asthma, uncomplicated
Moderate persistent asthma NOS
J45.41　Moderate persistent asthma with (acute) exacerbation
J45.42　Moderate persistent asthma with status asthmaticus

✓5th J45.5 Severe persistent asthma
J45.50　Severe persistent asthma, uncomplicated
Severe persistent asthma NOS
J45.51　Severe persistent asthma with (acute) exacerbation
J45.52　Severe persistent asthma with status asthmaticus

✓5th J45.9 Other and unspecified asthma
✓6th J45.90 Unspecified asthma
Asthmatic bronchitis NOS
Childhood asthma NOS
Late onset asthma
J45.901　Unspecified asthma with (acute) exacerbation
J45.902　Unspecified asthma with status asthmaticus
J45.909　Unspecified asthma, uncomplicated
Asthma NOS
✓6th J45.99 Other asthma
J45.990　Exercise induced bronchospasm
J45.991　Cough variant asthma
J45.998　Other asthma

✓4th J47 Bronchiectasis
INCLUDES　bronchiolectasis
Use additional code to identify:
exposure to environmental tobacco smoke (Z77.22)
exposure to tobacco smoke in the perinatal period (P96.81)
history of tobacco use (Z87.891)
occupational exposure to environmental tobacco smoke (Z57.31)
tobacco dependence (F17.-)
tobacco use (Z72.0)
EXCLUDES 1　congenital bronchiectasis (Q33.4)
tuberculous bronchiectasis (current disease) (A15.0)

J47.0 Bronchiectasis with acute lower respiratory infection
Bronchiectasis with acute bronchitis

J47.1 Bronchiectasis with (acute) exacerbation

J47.9 Bronchiectasis, uncomplicated
Bronchiectasis NOS

Lung diseases due to external agents (J60-J70)
EXCLUDES 2　asthma (J45.-)
malignant neoplasm of bronchus and lung (C34.-)

J60 Coalworker's pneumoconiosis　　　A
Anthracosilicosis　　　Black lung disease
Anthracosis　　　Coalworker's lung
EXCLUDES 1　coalworker pneumoconiosis with tuberculosis, any type in A15 (J65)

J61 Pneumoconiosis due to asbestos and other mineral fibers　A
Asbestosis
EXCLUDES 1　pleural plaque with asbestosis (J92.0)
pneumoconiosis with tuberculosis, any type in A15 (J65)

✓4th J62 Pneumoconiosis due to dust containing silica
INCLUDES　silicotic fibrosis (massive) of lung
EXCLUDES 1　pneumoconiosis with tuberculosis, any type in A15 (J65)

J62.0 Pneumoconiosis due to talc dust

J62.8 Pneumoconiosis due to other dust containing silica
Silicosis NOS

✓4th J63 Pneumoconiosis due to other inorganic dusts
EXCLUDES 1　pneumoconiosis with tuberculosis, any type in A15 (J65)

J63.0 Aluminosis (of lung)
J63.1 Bauxite fibrosis (of lung)
J63.2 Berylliosis
J63.3 Graphite fibrosis (of lung)
J63.4 Siderosis
J63.5 Stannosis
J63.6 Pneumoconiosis due to other specified inorganic dusts

J64 Unspecified pneumoconiosis
EXCLUDES 1　pneumonoconiosis with tuberculosis, any type in A15 (J65)

J65 Pneumoconiosis associated with tuberculosis
Any condition in J60-J64 with tuberculosis, any type in A15
silicotuberculosis

✓4th J66 Airway disease due to specific organic dust
EXCLUDES 2　allergic alveolitis (J67.-)
asbestosis (J61)
bagassosis (J67.1)
farmer's lung (J67.0)
hypersensitivity pneumonitis due to organic dust (J67.-)
reactive airways dysfunction syndrome (J68.3)

J66.0 Byssinosis
Airway disease due to cotton dust
J66.1 Flax-dressers' disease
J66.2 Cannabinosis
J66.8 Airway disease due to other specific organic dusts

✓4th J67 Hypersensitivity pneumonitis due to organic dust
INCLUDES　allergic alveolitis and pneumonitis due to inhaled organic dust and particles of fungal, actinomycetic or other origin
EXCLUDES 1　pneumonitis due to inhalation of chemicals, gases, fumes or vapors (J68.0)

J67.0 Farmer's lung
Harvester's lung　　　Moldy hay disease
Haymaker's lung

J67.1 Bagassosis
Bagasse disease　　　Bagasse pneumonitis

J67.2 Bird fancier's lung
Budgerigar fancier's disease or lung
Pigeon fancier's disease or lung

J67.3 Suberosis
Corkhandler's disease or lung
Corkworker's disease or lung

J67.4 Maltworker's lung
Alveolitis due to Aspergillus clavatus

J67.5 Mushroom-worker's lung

J67.6 Maple-bark-stripper's lung
Alveolitis due to Cryptostroma corticale
Cryptostromosis

J67.7 Air conditioner and humidifier lung
Allergic alveolitis due to fungal, thermophilic actinomycetes and other organisms growing in ventilation [air conditioning] systems

J67.8 Hypersensitivity pneumonitis due to other organic dusts
Cheese-washer's lung　　　Furrier's lung
Coffee-worker's lung　　　Sequoiosis
Fish-meal worker's lung

✓ Additional Character Required　　✓x7th Xtension Alert　　Unspecified Code　　Other Specified Code　　Manifestation Code　　►◄ Revised Text　　● New Code　　▲ Revised Code Title

Diseases of the Respiratory System

J67.9   **Hypersensitivity pneumonitis due to unspecified organic dust**
     Allergic alveolitis (extrinsic) NOS
     Hypersensitivity pneumonitis NOS

√4th **J68**   **Respiratory conditions due to inhalation of chemicals, gases, fumes and vapors**
     Code first (T51-T65) to identify cause
     Use additional code to identify associated respiratory conditions, such as:
     acute respiratory failure (J96.0-)

J68.0   **Bronchitis and pneumonitis due to chemicals, gases, fumes and vapors**
     Chemical bronchitis (acute)

J68.1   **Pulmonary edema due to chemicals, gases, fumes and vapors**
     Chemical pulmonary edema (acute) (chronic)
     EXCLUDES 1   *pulmonary edema (acute) (chronic) NOS (J81.-)*

J68.2   **Upper respiratory inflammation due to chemicals, gases, fumes and vapors, not elsewhere classified**

J68.3   **Other acute and subacute respiratory conditions due to chemicals, gases, fumes and vapors**
     Reactive airways dysfunction syndrome

J68.4   **Chronic respiratory conditions due to chemicals, gases, fumes and vapors**
     Emphysema (diffuse) (chronic) due to inhalation of chemicals, gases, fumes and vapors
     Obliterative bronchiolitis (chronic) (subacute) due to inhalation of chemicals, gases, fumes and vapors
     Pulmonary fibrosis (chronic) due to inhalation of chemicals, gases, fumes and vapors
     EXCLUDES 1   *chronic pulmonary edema due to chemicals, gases, fumes and vapors (J68.1)*

J68.8   **Other respiratory conditions due to chemicals, gases, fumes and vapors**

J68.9   **Unspecified respiratory condition due to chemicals, gases, fumes and vapors**

√4th **J69**   **Pneumonitis due to solids and liquids**
     EXCLUDES 1   *neonatal aspiration syndromes (P24.-)*
                postprocedural pneumonitis (J95.4)

J69.0   **Pneumonitis due to inhalation of food and vomit**
     Aspiration pneumonia NOS
     Aspiration pneumonia (due to) food (regurgitated)
     Aspiration pneumonia (due to) gastric secretions
     Aspiration pneumonia (due to) milk
     Aspiration pneumonia (due to) vomit
     Code also any associated foreign body in respiratory tract (T17.-)
     EXCLUDES 1   *chemical pneumonitis due to anesthesia (J95.4)*
                obstetric aspiration pneumonia (O74.0)

J69.1   **Pneumonitis due to inhalation of oils and essences**
     Exogenous lipoid pneumonia
     Lipid pneumonia NOS
     Code first (T51-T65) to identify substance
     EXCLUDES 1   *endogenous lipoid pneumonia (J84.89)*

J69.8   **Pneumonitis due to inhalation of other solids and liquids**
     Pneumonitis due to aspiration of blood
     Pneumonitis due to aspiration of detergent
     Code first (T51-T65) to identify substance

√4th **J70**   **Respiratory conditions due to other external agents**

J70.0   **Acute pulmonary manifestations due to radiation**
     Radiation pneumonitis
     Use additional code (W88-W90, X39.0-) to identify the external cause

J70.1   **Chronic and other pulmonary manifestations due to radiation**
     Fibrosis of lung following radiation
     Use additional code (W88-W90, X39.0-) to identify the external cause

J70.2   **Acute drug-induced interstitial lung disorders**
     Use additional code for adverse effect, if applicable, to identify drug (T36-T50 with fifth or sixth character 5)
     EXCLUDES 1   *interstitial pneumonia NOS (J84.9)*
                lymphoid interstitial pneumonia (J84.2)

J70.3   **Chronic drug-induced interstitial lung disorders**
     Use additional code for adverse effect, if applicable, to identify drug (T36-T50 with fifth or sixth character 5)
     EXCLUDES 1   *interstitial pneumonia NOS (J84.9)*
                lymphoid interstitial pneumonia (J84.2)

J70.4   **Drug-induced interstitial lung disorders, unspecified**
     Use additional code for adverse effect, if applicable, to identify drug (T36-T50 with fifth or sixth character 5)
     EXCLUDES 1   *interstitial pneumonia NOS (J84.9)*
                lymphoid interstitial pneumonia (J84.2)

J70.5   **Respiratory conditions due to smoke inhalation**
     Smoke inhalation NOS
     EXCLUDES 1   *smoke inhalation due to chemicals, gases, fumes and vapors (J68.9)*

J70.8   **Respiratory conditions due to other specified external agents**
     Code first (T51-T65) to identify the external agent

J70.9   **Respiratory conditions due to unspecified external agent**
     Code first (T51-T65) to identify the external agent

Other respiratory diseases principally affecting the interstitium (J80-J84)

J80   **Acute respiratory distress syndrome**
     Acute respiratory distress syndrome in adult or child
     Adult hyaline membrane disease
     EXCLUDES 1   *respiratory distress syndrome in newborn (perinatal) (P22.0)*

√4th **J81**   **Pulmonary edema**
     Use additional code to identify:
     exposure to environmental tobacco smoke (Z77.22)
     history of tobacco use (Z87.891)
     occupational exposure to environmental tobacco smoke (Z57.31)
     tobacco dependence (F17.-)
     tobacco use (Z72.0)
     EXCLUDES 1   *chemical (acute) pulmonary edema (J68.1)*
                hypostatic pneumonia (J18.2)
                passive pneumonia (J18.2)
                pulmonary edema due to external agents (J60-J70)
                pulmonary edema with heart disease NOS (I50.1)
                pulmonary edema with heart failure (I50.1)

J81.0   **Acute pulmonary edema**
     Acute edema of lung

J81.1   **Chronic pulmonary edema**
     Pulmonary congestion (chronic) (passive)
     Pulmonary edema NOS

J82   **Pulmonary eosinophilia, not elsewhere classified**
     Allergic pneumonia
     Eosinophilic asthma
     Eosinophilic pneumonia
     Löffler's pneumonia
     Tropical (pulmonary) eosinophilia NOS
     EXCLUDES 1   *pulmonary eosinophilia due to aspergillosis (B44.-)*
                pulmonary eosinophilia due to drugs (J70.2-J70.4)
                pulmonary eosinophilia due to specified parasitic infection (B50-B83)
                pulmonary eosinophilia due to systemic connective tissue disorders (M30-M36)
                pulmonary infiltrate NOS (R91.8)

√4th **J84**   **Other interstitial pulmonary diseases**
     EXCLUDES 1   *drug-induced interstitial lung disorders (J70.2-J70.4)*
                interstitial emphysema (J98.2)
                lung diseases due to external agents (J60-J70)

√5th **J84.0**   **Alveolar and parieto-alveolar conditions**

J84.01   **Alveolar proteinosis**

J84.02   **Pulmonary alveolar microlithiasis**

J84.03   ***Idiopathic pulmonary hemosiderosis***
     Essential brown induration of lung
     Code first underlying disease, such as:
       disorders of iron metabolism (E83.1-)
     EXCLUDES 1   *acute idiopathic pulmonary hemorrhage in infants [AIPHI] (R04.81)*

J84.09   **Other alveolar and parieto-alveolar conditions**

√5th **J84.1**   **Other interstitial pulmonary diseases with fibrosis**
     EXCLUDES 1   *pulmonary fibrosis (chronic) due to inhalation of chemicals, gases, fumes or vapors (J68.4)*
                pulmonary fibrosis (chronic) following radiation (J70.1)

J84.10   **Pulmonary fibrosis, unspecified**
     Capillary fibrosis of lung
     Cirrhosis of lung (chronic) NOS
     Fibrosis of lung (atrophic) (chronic) (confluent) (massive) (perialveolar) (peribronchial) NOS
     Induration of lung (chronic) NOS
     Postinflammatory pulmonary fibrosis

√6th **J84.11**   **Idiopathic interstitial pneumonia**
     EXCLUDES 1   *lymphoid interstitial pneumonia (J84.2)*
                pneumocystis pneumonia (B59)

J84.111   **Idiopathic interstitial pneumonia, not otherwise specified**

J84.112   **Idiopathic pulmonary fibrosis**
     Cryptogenic fibrosing alveolitis
     Idiopathic fibrosing alveolitis

EXCLUDES 1 Not coded here   *EXCLUDES 2* Not included here   N Newborn Age: 0   P Pediatric Age: 0-17   M Maternity Age: 12-55   A Adult Age: 15-124

608   ICD-10-CM 2014 (Draft)

J84.113　Idiopathic non-specific interstitial pneumonitis
　　EXCLUDES 1 non-specific interstitial pneumonia NOS, or due to known underlying cause (J84.89)

J84.114　Acute interstitial pneumonitis
　　Hamman-Rich syndrome
　　EXCLUDES 1 pneumocystis pneumonia (B59)

J84.115　Respiratory bronchiolitis interstitial lung disease

J84.116　Cryptogenic organizing pneumonia
　　EXCLUDES 1 organizing pneumonia NOS, or due to known underlying cause (J84.89)

J84.117　Desquamative interstitial pneumonia

J84.17　Other interstitial pulmonary diseases with fibrosis in diseases classified elsewhere
　　Interstitial pneumonia (nonspecific) (usual) due to collagen vascular disease
　　Interstitial pneumonia (nonspecific) (usual) in diseases classified elsewhere
　　Organizing pneumonia due to collagen vascular disease
　　Organizing pneumonia in diseases classified elsewhere
　　Code first underlying disease, such as:
　　　progressive systemic sclerosis (M34.0)
　　　rheumatoid arthritis (M05.00-M06.9)
　　　systemic lupus erythematosis (M32.0-M32.9)

J84.2　Lymphoid interstitial pneumonia
　　Lymphoid interstitial pneumonitis

☑5ᵗʰ **J84.8　Other specified interstitial pulmonary diseases**
　　EXCLUDES 1 exogenous lipoid pneumonia (J69.1)
　　　unspecified lipoid pneumonia (J69.1)

J84.81　Lymphangioleiomyomatosis　♀
　　Lymphangiomyomatosis

J84.82　Adult pulmonary Langerhans cell histiocytosis　Ⓐ
　　Adult PLCH

J84.83　Surfactant mutations of the lung

☑6ᵗʰ **J84.84　Other interstitial lung diseases of childhood**
　　J84.841　Neuroendocrine cell hyperplasia of infancy
　　J84.842　Pulmonary interstitial glycogenosis
　　J84.843　Alveolar capillary dysplasia with vein misalignment
　　J84.848　Other interstitial lung diseases of childhood

J84.89　Other specified interstitial pulmonary diseases
　　Endogenous lipoid pneumonia
　　Interstitial pneumonitis
　　Non-specific interstitial pneumonitis NOS
　　Organizing pneumonia due to known underlying cause
　　Organizing pneumonia NOS
　　Code first, if applicable:
　　　poisoning due to drug or toxin (T51-T65 with fifth or sixth character to indicate intent), for toxic pneumonopathy
　　underlying cause of pneumonopathy, if known
　　Use additional code, for adverse effect, to identify drug (T36-T50 with fifth or sixth character 5), if drug-induced
　　EXCLUDES 1 cryptogenic organizing pneumonia (J84.116)
　　　idiopathic non-specific interstitial pneumonitis (J84.113)
　　　lipoid pneumonia, exogenous or unspecified (J69.1)
　　　lymphoid interstitial pneumonia (J84.2)

J84.9　Interstitial pulmonary disease, unspecified
　　Interstitial pneumonia NOS

Suppurative and necrotic conditions of the lower respiratory tract (J85-J86)

☑4ᵗʰ **J85　Abscess of lung and mediastinum**
　　Use additional code (B95-B97) to identify infectious agent.

J85.0　Gangrene and necrosis of lung

J85.1　Abscess of lung with pneumonia
　　Code also the type of pneumonia

J85.2　Abscess of lung without pneumonia
　　Abscess of lung NOS

J85.3　Abscess of mediastinum

☑4ᵗʰ **J86　Pyothorax**
　　Use additional code (B95-B97) to identify infectious agent
　　EXCLUDES 1 abscess of lung (J85.-)
　　　pyothorax due to tuberculosis (A15.6)

J86.0　Pyothorax with fistula
　　Bronchocutaneous fistula
　　Bronchopleural fistula
　　Hepatopleural fistula
　　Mediastinal fistula
　　Pleural fistula
　　Thoracic fistula
　　Any condition classifiable to J86.9 with fistula

J86.9　Pyothorax without fistula
　　Abscess of pleura　　　　　　Pyopneumothorax
　　Abscess of thorax　　　　　　Septic pleurisy
　　Empyema (chest) (lung) (pleura)　Seropurulent pleurisy
　　Fibrinopurulent pleurisy　　　Suppurative pleurisy
　　Purulent pleurisy

Other diseases of the pleura (J90-J94)

J90　Pleural effusion, not elsewhere classified
　　Encysted pleurisy
　　Pleural effusion NOS
　　Pleurisy with effusion (exudative) (serous)
　　EXCLUDES 1 chylous (pleural) effusion (J94.0)
　　　malignant pleural effusion (J91.0))
　　　pleurisy NOS (R09.1)
　　　tuberculous pleural effusion (A15.6)

☑4ᵗʰ **J91　Pleural effusion in conditions classified elsewhere**
　　EXCLUDES 2 pleural effusion in heart failure (I50.-)
　　　pleural effusion in systemic lupus erythematosus (M32.13)

J91.0　Malignant pleural effusion
　　Code first underlying neoplasm

J91.8　Pleural effusion in other conditions classified elsewhere
　　Code first underlying disease, such as:
　　　filariasis (B74.0-B74.9)
　　　influenza (J09.X2, J10.1, J11.1)

☑4ᵗʰ **J92　Pleural plaque**
　　INCLUDES pleural thickening

J92.0　Pleural plaque with presence of asbestos

J92.9　Pleural plaque without asbestos
　　Pleural plaque NOS

☑4ᵗʰ **J93　Pneumothorax and air leak**
　　EXCLUDES 1 congenital or perinatal pneumothorax (P25.1)
　　　postprocedural air leak (J95.812)
　　　postprocedural pneumothorax (J95.811)
　　　traumatic pneumothorax (S27.0)
　　　tuberculous (current disease) pneumothorax (A15.-)
　　　pyopneumothorax (J86.-)

J93.0　Spontaneous tension pneumothorax

☑5ᵗʰ **J93.1　Other spontaneous pneumothorax**
　　J93.11　Primary spontaneous pneumothorax
　　J93.12　Secondary spontaneous pneumothorax
　　　Code first underlying condition, such as:
　　　　catamenial pneumothorax due to endometriosis (N80.8)
　　　　cystic fibrosis (E84.-)
　　　　eosinophilic pneumonia (J82)
　　　　lymphangioleiomyomatosis (J84.81)
　　　　malignant neoplasm of bronchus and lung (C34.-)
　　　　Marfan's syndrome (Q87.4)
　　　　pneumonia due to Pneumocystis carinii (B59)
　　　　secondary malignant neoplasm of lung (C78.0-)
　　　　spontaneous rupture of the esophagus (K22.3)

☑5ᵗʰ **J93.8　Other pneumothorax and air leak**
　　J93.81　Chronic pneumothorax
　　J93.82　Other air leak
　　　Persistent air leak
　　J93.83　Other pneumothorax
　　　Acute pneumothorax
　　　Spontaneous pneumothorax NOS

J93.9　Pneumothorax, unspecified
　　Pneumothorax NOS

☑ Additional Character Required　　✓x7ᵗʰ Xtension Alert　　Unspecified Code　　Other Specified Code　　Manifestation Code　　►◄ Revised Text　　● New Code　　▲ Revised Code Title

Diseases of the Respiratory System

J94–J96.22

☑4th **J94 Other pleural conditions**
   EXCLUDES 1 *pleurisy NOS (R09.1)*
     traumatic hemopneumothorax (S27.2)
     traumatic hemothorax (S27.1)
     tuberculous pleural conditions (current disease) (A15.-)

  J94.0 Chylous effusion
    Chyliform effusion

  J94.1 Fibrothorax

  J94.2 Hemothorax
    Hemopneumothorax

  J94.8 Other specified pleural conditions
    Hydropneumothorax
    Hydrothorax

  J94.9 Pleural condition, unspecified

Intraoperative and postprocedural complications and disorders of respiratory system, not elsewhere classified (J95)

☑4th **J95 Intraoperative and postprocedural complications and disorders of respiratory system, not elsewhere classified**
   EXCLUDES 2 *aspiration pneumonia (J69.-)*
    emphysema (subcutaneous) resulting from a procedure (T81.82)
    hypostatic pneumonia (J18.2)
    pulmonary manifestations due to radiation (J70.0- J70.1)

 ☑5th **J95.0 Tracheostomy complications**
   J95.00 Unspecified tracheostomy complication
   J95.01 Hemorrhage from tracheostomy stoma
   J95.02 Infection of tracheostomy stoma
     Use additional code to identify type of infection, such as:
      cellulitis of neck (L03.8)
      sepsis (A40, A41-)
   J95.03 Malfunction of tracheostomy stoma
     Mechanical complication of tracheostomy stoma
     Obstruction of tracheostomy airway
     Tracheal stenosis due to tracheostomy
   J95.04 Tracheo-esophageal fistula following tracheostomy
   J95.09 Other tracheostomy complication

  J95.1 Acute pulmonary insufficiency following thoracic surgery
   EXCLUDES 2 *functional disturbances following cardiac surgery (I97.0, I97.1-)*

  J95.2 Acute pulmonary insufficiency following nonthoracic surgery
   EXCLUDES 2 *functional disturbances following cardiac surgery (I97.0, I97.1-)*

  J95.3 Chronic pulmonary insufficiency following surgery
   EXCLUDES 2 *functional disturbances following cardiac surgery (I97.0, I97.1-)*

  J95.4 Chemical pneumonitis due to anesthesia
    Mendelson's syndrome
    Postprocedural aspiration pneumonia
    Use additional code for adverse effect, if applicable, to identify drug (T41.- with fifth or sixth character 5)
   EXCLUDES 1 *aspiration pneumonitis due to anesthesia complicating labor and delivery (O74.0)*
    aspiration pneumonitis due to anesthesia complicating pregnancy (O29)
    aspiration pneumonitis due to anesthesia complicating the puerperium (O89.01)

  J95.5 Postprocedural subglottic stenosis

 ☑5th **J95.6 Intraoperative hemorrhage and hematoma of a respiratory system organ or structure complicating a procedure**
   EXCLUDES 1 *intraoperative hemorrhage and hematoma of a respiratory system organ or structure due to accidental puncture and laceration during procedure (J95.7-)*
   J95.61 Intraoperative hemorrhage and hematoma of a respiratory system organ or structure complicating a respiratory system procedure
   J95.62 Intraoperative hemorrhage and hematoma of a respiratory system organ or structure complicating other procedure

 ☑5th **J95.7 Accidental puncture and laceration of a respiratory system organ or structure during a procedure**
   EXCLUDES 2 *postprocedural pneumothorax (J95.811)*
   J95.71 Accidental puncture and laceration of a respiratory system organ or structure during a respiratory system procedure

   J95.72 Accidental puncture and laceration of a respiratory system organ or structure during other procedure

 ☑5th **J95.8 Other intraoperative and postprocedural complications and disorders of respiratory system, not elsewhere classified**
  ☑6th **J95.81 Postprocedural pneumothorax and air leak**
    J95.811 Postprocedural pneumothorax
    J95.812 Postprocedural air leak
  ☑6th **J95.82 Postprocedural respiratory failure**
   EXCLUDES 1 *respiratory failure in other conditions (J96.-)*
    J95.821 Acute postprocedural respiratory failure
     Postprocedural respiratory failure NOS
    J95.822 Acute and chronic postprocedural respiratory failure
  ☑6th **J95.83 Postprocedural hemorrhage and hematoma of a respiratory system organ or structure following a procedure**
    J95.830 Postprocedural hemorrhage and hematoma of a respiratory system organ or structure following a respiratory system procedure
    J95.831 Postprocedural hemorrhage and hematoma of a respiratory system organ or structure following other procedure
   J95.84 Transfusion-related acute lung injury (TRALI)
  ☑6th **J95.85 Complication of respirator [ventilator]**
    J95.850 Mechanical complication of respirator
     EXCLUDES 1 *encounter for respirator [ventilator] dependence during power failure (Z99.12)*
    J95.851 Ventilator associated pneumonia
     Ventilator associated pneumonitis
     Use additional code to identify the organism, if known (B95.-, B96.-, B97.-)
     EXCLUDES 1 *ventilator lung in newborn (P27.8)*
    J95.859 Other complication of respirator [ventilator]
   J95.88 Other intraoperative complications of respiratory system, not elsewhere classified
   J95.89 Other postprocedural complications and disorders of respiratory system, not elsewhere classified
     Use additional code to identify disorder, such as:
      aspiration pneumonia (J69.-)
      bacterial or viral pneumonia (J12-J18)
     EXCLUDES 2 *acute pulmonary insufficiency following thoracic surgery (J95.1)*
     postprocedural subglottic stenosis (J95.5)

Other diseases of the respiratory system (J96-J99)

☑4th **J96 Respiratory failure, not elsewhere classified**
   EXCLUDES 1 *acute respiratory distress syndrome (J80)*
    cardiorespiratory failure (R09.2)
    newborn respiratory distress syndrome (P22.0)
    postprocedural respiratory failure (J95.82-)
    respiratory arrest (R09.2)
    respiratory arrest of newborn (P28.81)
    respiratory failure of newborn (P28.5)

 ☑5th **J96.0 Acute respiratory failure**
   J96.00 Acute respiratory failure, unspecified whether with hypoxia or hypercapnia
   J96.01 Acute respiratory failure with hypoxia
   J96.02 Acute respiratory failure with hypercapnia

 ☑5th **J96.1 Chronic respiratory failure**
   J96.10 Chronic respiratory failure, unspecified whether with hypoxia or hypercapnia
   J96.11 Chronic respiratory failure with hypoxia
   J96.12 Chronic respiratory failure with hypercapnia

 ☑5th **J96.2 Acute and chronic respiratory failure**
    Acute on chronic respiratory failure
   J96.20 Acute and chronic respiratory failure, unspecified whether with hypoxia or hypercapnia
   J96.21 Acute and chronic respiratory failure with hypoxia
   J96.22 Acute and chronic respiratory failure with hypercapnia

✓5th **J96.9 Respiratory failure, unspecified**

    J96.90 Respiratory failure, unspecified, unspecified whether with hypoxia or hypercapnia

    J96.91 Respiratory failure, unspecified with hypoxia

    J96.92 Respiratory failure, unspecified with hypercapnia

✓4th **J98 Other respiratory disorders**

Use additional code to identify:
exposure to environmental tobacco smoke (Z77.22)
exposure to tobacco smoke in the perinatal period (P96.81)
history of tobacco use (Z87.891)
occupational exposure to environmental tobacco smoke (Z57.31)
tobacco dependence (F17.-)
tobacco use (Z72.0)

EXCLUDES 1 newborn apnea (P28.4)
newborn sleep apnea (P28.3)
EXCLUDES 2 apnea NOS (R06.81)
sleep apnea (G47.3-)

✓5th **J98.0 Diseases of bronchus, not elsewhere classified**

    J98.01 Acute bronchospasm

    EXCLUDES 1 acute bronchiolitis with bronchospasm (J21.-)
acute bronchitis with bronchospasm (J20.-)
asthma (J45.-)
exercise induced bronchospasm (J45.990)

    J98.09 Other diseases of bronchus, not elsewhere classified

Broncholithiasis
Calcification of bronchus
Stenosis of bronchus
Tracheobronchial collapse
Tracheobronchial dyskinesia
Ulcer of bronchus

✓5th **J98.1 Pulmonary collapse**

EXCLUDES 1 therapeutic collapse of lung status (Z98.3)

    J98.11 Atelectasis

EXCLUDES 1 newborn atelectasis
tuberculous atelectasis (current disease) (A15)

    J98.19 Other pulmonary collapse

J98.2 Interstitial emphysema

Mediastinal emphysema
EXCLUDES 1 emphysema NOS (J43.9)
emphysema in newborn (P25.0)
surgical emphysema (subcutaneous) (T81.82)
traumatic subcutaneous emphysema (T79.7)

J98.3 Compensatory emphysema

J98.4 Other disorders of lung

Calcification of lung
Cystic lung disease (acquired)
Lung disease NOS
Pulmolithiasis
EXCLUDES 1 acute interstitial pneumonitis (J84.114)
pulmonary insufficiency following surgery (J95.1-J95.2)

J98.5 Diseases of mediastinum, not elsewhere classified

Fibrosis of mediastinum
Hernia of mediastinum
Retraction of mediastinum
Mediastinitis
EXCLUDES 2 abscess of mediastinum (J85.3)

J98.6 Disorders of diaphragm

Diaphragmatitis
Paralysis of diaphragm
Relaxation of diaphragm
EXCLUDES 1 congenital malformation of diaphragm NEC (Q79.1)
congenital diaphragmatic hernia (Q79.0)
EXCLUDES 2 diaphragmatic hernia (K44.-)

J98.8 Other specified respiratory disorders

J98.9 Respiratory disorder, unspecified

Respiratory disease (chronic) NOS

J99 Respiratory disorders in diseases classified elsewhere

Code first underlying disease, such as:
amyloidosis (E85.-)
ankylosing spondylitis (M45)
congenital syphilis (A50.5)
cryoglobulinemia (D89.1)
early congenital syphilis (A50.0)
schistosomiasis (B65.0-B65.9)
EXCLUDES 1 respiratory disorders in:
amebiasis (A06.5)
blastomycosis (B40.0-B40.2)
candidiasis (B37.1)
coccidioidomycosis (B38.0-B38.2)
cystic fibrosis with pulmonary manifestations (E84.0)
dermatomyositis (M33.01, M33.11)
histoplasmosis (B39.0-B39.2)
late syphilis (A52.72, A52.73)
polymyositis (M33.21)
sicca syndrome (M35.02)
systemic lupus erythematosus (M32.13)
systemic sclerosis (M34.81)
Wegener's granulomatosis (M31.30-M31.31)

Chapter 11. Diseases of the Digestive System (K00-K95)

EXCLUDES 2   certain conditions originating in the perinatal period (P04-P96)
certain infectious and parasitic diseases (A00-B99)
complications of pregnancy, childbirth and the puerperium (O00-O9A)
congenital malformations, deformations and chromosomal abnormalities (Q00-Q99)
endocrine, nutritional and metabolic diseases (E00-E88)
injury, poisoning and certain other consequences of external causes (S00-T88)
neoplasms (C00-D49)
symptoms, signs and abnormal clinical and laboratory findings, not elsewhere classified (R00-R94)

This chapter contains the following blocks:
K00-K14   Diseases of oral cavity and salivary glands
K20-K31   Diseases of esophagus, stomach and duodenum
K35-K38   Diseases of appendix
K40-K46   Hernia
K50-K52   Noninfective enteritis and colitis
K55-K64   Other diseases of intestines
K65-K68   Diseases of peritoneum and retroperitoneum
K70-K77   Diseases of liver
K80-K87   Disorders of gallbladder, biliary tract and pancreas
K90-K95   Other diseases of the digestive system

Diseases of oral cavity and salivary glands (K00-K14)

K00   Disorders of tooth development and eruption
EXCLUDES 2   embedded and impacted teeth (K01.-)

K00.0   Anodontia
Hypodontia
Oligodontia
EXCLUDES 1   acquired absence of teeth (K08.1-)

K00.1   Supernumerary teeth
Distomolar
Fourth molar
Mesiodens
Paramolar
Supplementary teeth
EXCLUDES 2   supernumerary roots (K00.2)

K00.2   Abnormalities of size and form of teeth
Concrescence of teeth
Dens evaginatus
Dens in dente
Dens invaginatus
Enamel pearls
Fusion of teeth
Gemination of teeth
Macrodontia
Microdontia
Peg-shaped [conical] teeth
Supernumerary roots
Taurodontism
Tuberculum paramolare
EXCLUDES 1   abnormalities of teeth due to congenital syphilis (A50.5)
tuberculum Carabelli, which is regarded as a normal variation and should not be coded

K00.3   Mottled teeth
Dental fluorosis
Mottling of enamel
Nonfluoride enamel opacities
EXCLUDES 2   deposits [accretions] on teeth (K03.6)

K00.4   Disturbances in tooth formation
Aplasia and hypoplasia of cementum
Dilaceration of tooth
Enamel hypoplasia (neonatal) (postnatal) (prenatal)
Regional odontodysplasia
Turner's tooth
EXCLUDES 1   Hutchinson's teeth and mulberry molars in congenital syphilis (A50.5)
EXCLUDES 2   mottled teeth (K00.3)

K00.5   Hereditary disturbances in tooth structure, not elsewhere classified
Amelogenesis imperfecta
Dentinogenesis imperfecta
Odontogenesis imperfecta
Dentinal dysplasia
Shell teeth

K00.6   Disturbances in tooth eruption
Dentia praecox
Natal tooth
Neonatal tooth
Premature eruption of tooth
Premature shedding of primary [deciduous] tooth
Prenatal teeth
Retained [persistent] primary tooth
EXCLUDES 2   embedded and impacted teeth (K01.-)

K00.7   Teething syndrome

K00.8   Other disorders of tooth development
Color changes during tooth formation
Intrinsic staining of teeth NOS
EXCLUDES 2   posteruptive color changes (K03.7)

K00.9   Disorder of tooth development, unspecified
Disorder of odontogenesis NOS

K01   Embedded and impacted teeth
EXCLUDES 1   abnormal position of fully erupted teeth (M26.3-)

K01.0   Embedded teeth

K01.1   Impacted teeth

K02   Dental caries
Dental cavities
Tooth decay

K02.3   Arrested dental caries
Arrested coronal and root caries

K02.5   Dental caries on pit and fissure surface
Dental caries on chewing surface of tooth

K02.51   Dental caries on pit and fissure surface limited to enamel
White spot lesions [initial caries] on pit and fissure surface of tooth

K02.52   Dental caries on pit and fissure surface penetrating into dentin

K02.53   Dental caries on pit and fissure surface penetrating into pulp

K02.6   Dental caries on smooth surface

K02.61   Dental caries on smooth surface limited to enamel
White spot lesions [initial caries] on smooth surface of tooth

K02.62   Dental caries on smooth surface penetrating into dentin

K02.63   Dental caries on smooth surface penetrating into pulp

K02.7   Dental root caries

K02.9   Dental caries, unspecified

K03   Other diseases of hard tissues of teeth
EXCLUDES 2   bruxism (F45.8)
dental caries (K02.-)
teeth-grinding NOS (F45.8)

K03.0   Excessive attrition of teeth
Approximal wear of teeth
Occlusal wear of teeth

K03.1   Abrasion of teeth
Dentifrice abrasion of teeth
Habitual abrasion of teeth
Occupational abrasion of teeth
Ritual abrasion of teeth
Traditional abrasion of teeth
Wedge defect NOS

K03.2   Erosion of teeth
Erosion of teeth due to diet
Erosion of teeth due to drugs and medicaments
Erosion of teeth due to persistent vomiting
Erosion of teeth NOS
Idiopathic erosion of teeth
Occupational erosion of teeth

K03.3   Pathological resorption of teeth
Internal granuloma of pulp
Resorption of teeth (external)

K03.4   Hypercementosis
Cementation hyperplasia

K03.5   Ankylosis of teeth

K03.6　Deposits [accretions] on teeth
　　Betel deposits [accretions] on teeth
　　Black deposits [accretions] on teeth
　　Extrinsic staining of teeth NOS
　　Green deposits [accretions] on teeth
　　Materia alba deposits [accretions] on teeth
　　Orange deposits [accretions] on teeth
　　Staining of teeth NOS
　　Subgingival dental calculus
　　Supragingival dental calculus
　　Tobacco deposits [accretions] on teeth

K03.7　Posteruptive color changes of dental hard tissues
　　EXCLUDES 2　deposits [accretions] on teeth (K03.6)

✓5ᵗʰ **K03.8　Other specified diseases of hard tissues of teeth**
　　K03.81　Cracked tooth
　　　　EXCLUDES 1　asymptomatic craze lines in enamel—omit code
　　　　　　broken or fractured tooth due to trauma (S02.5)
　　K03.89　Other specified diseases of hard tissues of teeth

K03.9　Disease of hard tissues of teeth, unspecified

✓4ᵗʰ **K04　Diseases of pulp and periapical tissues**
　　K04.0　Pulpitis
　　　　Acute pulpitis
　　　　Chronic (hyperplastic) (ulcerative) pulpitis
　　　　Irreversible pulpitis
　　　　Reversible pulpitis

　　K04.1　Necrosis of pulp
　　　　Pulpal gangrene

　　K04.2　Pulp degeneration
　　　　Denticles
　　　　Pulpal calcifications
　　　　Pulpal stones

　　K04.3　Abnormal hard tissue formation in pulp
　　　　Secondary or irregular dentine

　　K04.4　Acute apical periodontitis of pulpal origin
　　　　Acute apical periodontitis NOS
　　　　EXCLUDES 1　acute periodontitis (K05.2-)

　　K04.5　Chronic apical periodontitis
　　　　Apical or periapical granuloma
　　　　Apical periodontitis NOS
　　　　EXCLUDES 1　chronic periodontitis (K05.3-)

　　K04.6　Periapical abscess with sinus
　　　　Dental abscess with sinus
　　　　Dentoalveolar abscess with sinus

　　K04.7　Periapical abscess without sinus
　　　　Dental abscess without sinus
　　　　Dentoalveolar abscess without sinus
　　　　Periapical abscess without sinus

　　K04.8　Radicular cyst
　　　　Apical (periodontal) cyst
　　　　Periapical cyst
　　　　Residual radicular cyst
　　　　EXCLUDES 2　lateral periodontal cyst (K09.0)

✓5ᵗʰ **K04.9　Other and unspecified diseases of pulp and periapical tissues**
　　K04.90　Unspecified diseases of pulp and periapical tissues
　　K04.99　Other diseases of pulp and periapical tissues

✓4ᵗʰ **K05　Gingivitis and periodontal diseases**
　　Use additional code to identify:
　　　　alcohol abuse and dependence (F10.-)
　　　　exposure to environmental tobacco smoke (Z77.22)
　　　　exposure to tobacco smoke in the perinatal period (P96.81)
　　　　history of tobacco use (Z87.891)
　　　　occupational exposure to environmental tobacco smoke (Z57.31)
　　　　tobacco dependence (F17.-)
　　　　tobacco use (Z72.0)

✓5ᵗʰ **K05.0　Acute gingivitis**
　　　　EXCLUDES 1　acute necrotizing ulcerative gingivitis (A69.1)
　　　　　　herpesviral [herpes simplex] gingivostomatitis (B00.2)
　　K05.00　Acute gingivitis, plaque induced
　　　　Acute gingivitis NOS
　　K05.01　Acute gingivitis, non-plaque induced

✓5ᵗʰ **K05.1　Chronic gingivitis**
　　　　Desquamative gingivitis (chronic)
　　　　Gingivitis (chronic) NOS
　　　　Hyperplastic gingivitis (chronic)
　　　　Simple marginal gingivitis (chronic)
　　　　Ulcerative gingivitis (chronic)

　　K05.10　Chronic gingivitis, plaque induced
　　　　Chronic gingivitis NOS
　　　　Gingivitis NOS
　　K05.11　Chronic gingivitis, non-plaque induced

✓5ᵗʰ **K05.2　Aggressive periodontitis**
　　　　Acute pericoronitis
　　　　EXCLUDES 1　acute apical periodontitis (K04.4)
　　　　　　periapical abscess (K04.7)
　　　　　　periapical abscess with sinus (K04.6)
　　K05.20　Aggressive periodontitis, unspecified
　　K05.21　Aggressive periodontitis, localized
　　　　Periodontal abscess
　　K05.22　Aggressive periodontitis, generalized

✓5ᵗʰ **K05.3　Chronic periodontitis**
　　　　Chronic pericoronitis
　　　　Complex periodontitis
　　　　Periodontitis NOS
　　　　Simplex periodontitis
　　　　EXCLUDES 1　chronic apical periodontitis (K04.5)
　　K05.30　Chronic periodontitis, unspecified
　　K05.31　Chronic periodontitis, localized
　　K05.32　Chronic periodontitis, generalized

　　K05.4　Periodontosis
　　　　Juvenile periodontosis

　　K05.5　Other periodontal diseases
　　　　EXCLUDES 2　leukoplakia of gingiva (K13.21)

　　K05.6　Periodontal disease, unspecified

✓4ᵗʰ **K06　Other disorders of gingiva and edentulous alveolar ridge**
　　EXCLUDES 2　acute gingivitis (K05.0)
　　　　atrophy of edentulous alveolar ridge (K08.2)
　　　　chronic gingivitis (K05.1)
　　　　gingivitis NOS (K05.1)

　　K06.0　Gingival recession
　　　　Gingival recession (generalized) (localized) (postinfective) (postprocedural)

　　K06.1　Gingival enlargement
　　　　Gingival fibromatosis

　　K06.2　Gingival and edentulous alveolar ridge lesions associated with trauma
　　　　Irritative hyperplasia of edentulous ridge [denture hyperplasia]
　　　　Use additional code (Chapter 20) to identify external cause or denture status (Z97.2)

　　K06.8　Other specified disorders of gingiva and edentulous alveolar ridge
　　　　Fibrous epulis
　　　　Flabby alveolar ridge
　　　　Giant cell epulis
　　　　Peripheral giant cell granuloma of gingiva
　　　　Pyogenic granuloma of gingiva
　　　　EXCLUDES 2　gingival cyst (K09.0)

　　K06.9　Disorder of gingiva and edentulous alveolar ridge, unspecified

✓4ᵗʰ **K08　Other disorders of teeth and supporting structures**
　　EXCLUDES 2　dentofacial anomalies [including malocclusion] (M26.-)
　　　　disorders of jaw (M27.-)

　　K08.0　Exfoliation of teeth due to systemic causes
　　　　Code also underlying systemic condition

✓5ᵗʰ **K08.1　Complete loss of teeth**
　　　　Acquired loss of teeth, complete
　　　　EXCLUDES 1　congenital absence of teeth (K00.0)
　　　　　　exfoliation of teeth due to systemic causes (K08.0)
　　　　　　partial loss of teeth (K08.4-)

✓6ᵗʰ **K08.10　Complete loss of teeth, unspecified cause**
　　K08.101　Complete loss of teeth, unspecified cause, class I
　　K08.102　Complete loss of teeth, unspecified cause, class II
　　K08.103　Complete loss of teeth, unspecified cause, class III
　　K08.104　Complete loss of teeth, unspecified cause, class IV
　　K08.109　Complete loss of teeth, unspecified cause, unspecified class
　　　　Edentulism NOS

✓6ᵗʰ **K08.11　Complete loss of teeth due to trauma**
　　K08.111　Complete loss of teeth due to trauma, class I

☑ Additional Character Required　　ᵛˣ⁷ᵗʰ Xtension Alert　　**Unspecified Code**　　Other Specified Code　　Manifestation Code　　►◄ Revised Text　　● New Code　　▲ Revised Code Title

Diseases of the Digestive System

K08.112–K08.59

K08.112 Complete loss of teeth due to trauma, class II

K08.113 Complete loss of teeth due to trauma, class III

K08.114 Complete loss of teeth due to trauma, class IV

K08.119 Complete loss of teeth due to trauma, unspecified class

√6th **K08.12** Complete loss of teeth due to periodontal diseases

K08.121 Complete loss of teeth due to periodontal diseases, class I

K08.122 Complete loss of teeth due to periodontal diseases, class II

K08.123 Complete loss of teeth due to periodontal diseases, class III

K08.124 Complete loss of teeth due to periodontal diseases, class IV

K08.129 Complete loss of teeth due to periodontal diseases, unspecified class

√6th **K08.13** Complete loss of teeth due to caries

K08.131 Complete loss of teeth due to caries, class I

K08.132 Complete loss of teeth due to caries, class II

K08.133 Complete loss of teeth due to caries, class III

K08.134 Complete loss of teeth due to caries, class IV

K08.139 Complete loss of teeth due to caries, unspecified class

√6th **K08.19** Complete loss of teeth due to other specified cause

K08.191 Complete loss of teeth due to other specified cause, class I

K08.192 Complete loss of teeth due to other specified cause, class II

K08.193 Complete loss of teeth due to other specified cause, class III

K08.194 Complete loss of teeth due to other specified cause, class IV

K08.199 Complete loss of teeth due to other specified cause, unspecified class

√5th **K08.2** Atrophy of edentulous alveolar ridge

K08.20 Unspecified atrophy of edentulous alveolar ridge
Atrophy of the mandible NOS
Atrophy of the maxilla NOS

K08.21 Minimal atrophy of the mandible
Minimal atrophy of the edentulous mandible

K08.22 Moderate atrophy of the mandible
Moderate atrophy of the edentulous mandible

K08.23 Severe atrophy of the mandible
Severe atrophy of the edentulous mandible

K08.24 Minimal atrophy of maxilla
Minimal atrophy of the edentulous maxilla

K08.25 Moderate atrophy of the maxilla
Moderate atrophy of the edentulous maxilla

K08.26 Severe atrophy of the maxilla
Severe atrophy of the edentulous maxilla

K08.3 Retained dental root

√5th **K08.4** Partial loss of teeth
Acquired loss of teeth, partial
EXCLUDES 1 complete loss of teeth (K08.1-)
congenital absence of teeth (K00.0)
EXCLUDES 2 exfoliation of teeth due to systemic causes (K08.0)

√6th **K08.40** Partial loss of teeth, unspecified cause

K08.401 Partial loss of teeth, unspecified cause, class I

K08.402 Partial loss of teeth, unspecified cause, class II

K08.403 Partial loss of teeth, unspecified cause, class III

K08.404 Partial loss of teeth, unspecified cause, class IV

K08.409 Partial loss of teeth, unspecified cause, unspecified class
Tooth extraction status NOS

√6th **K08.41** Partial loss of teeth due to trauma

K08.411 Partial loss of teeth due to trauma, class I

K08.412 Partial loss of teeth due to trauma, class II

K08.413 Partial loss of teeth due to trauma, class III

K08.414 Partial loss of teeth due to trauma, class IV

K08.419 Partial loss of teeth due to trauma, unspecified class

√6th **K08.42** Partial loss of teeth due to periodontal diseases

K08.421 Partial loss of teeth due to periodontal diseases, class I

K08.422 Partial loss of teeth due to periodontal diseases, class II

K08.423 Partial loss of teeth due to periodontal diseases, class III

K08.424 Partial loss of teeth due to periodontal diseases, class IV

K08.429 Partial loss of teeth due to periodontal diseases, unspecified class

√6th **K08.43** Partial loss of teeth due to caries

K08.431 Partial loss of teeth due to caries, class I

K08.432 Partial loss of teeth due to caries, class II

K08.433 Partial loss of teeth due to caries, class III

K08.434 Partial loss of teeth due to caries, class IV

K08.439 Partial loss of teeth due to caries, unspecified class

√6th **K08.49** Partial loss of teeth due to other specified cause

K08.491 Partial loss of teeth due to other specified cause, class I

K08.492 Partial loss of teeth due to other specified cause, class II

K08.493 Partial loss of teeth due to other specified cause, class III

K08.494 Partial loss of teeth due to other specified cause, class IV

K08.499 Partial loss of teeth due to other specified cause, unspecified class

√5th **K08.5** Unsatisfactory restoration of tooth
Defective bridge, crown, filling
Defective dental restoration
EXCLUDES 1 dental restoration status (Z98.811)
EXCLUDES 2 endosseous dental implant failure (M27.6-)
unsatisfactory endodontic treatment (M27.5-)

K08.50 Unsatisfactory restoration of tooth, unspecified
Defective dental restoration NOS

K08.51 Open restoration margins of tooth
Dental restoration failure of marginal integrity
Open margin on tooth restoration
Poor gingival margin to tooth restoration

K08.52 Unrepairable overhanging of dental restorative materials
Overhanging of tooth restoration

√6th **K08.53** Fractured dental restorative material
EXCLUDES 1 cracked tooth (K03.81)
traumatic fracture of tooth (S02.5)

K08.530 Fractured dental restorative material without loss of material

K08.531 Fractured dental restorative material with loss of material

K08.539 Fractured dental restorative material, unspecified

K08.54 Contour of existing restoration of tooth biologically incompatible with oral health
Dental restoration failure of periodontal anatomical integrity
Unacceptable contours of existing restoration of tooth
Unacceptable morphology of existing restoration of tooth

K08.55 Allergy to existing dental restorative material
Use additional code to identify the specific type of allergy

K08.56 Poor aesthetic of existing restoration of tooth
Dental restoration aesthetically inadequate or displeasing

K08.59 Other unsatisfactory restoration of tooth
Other defective dental restoration

EXCLUDES 1 Not coded here   EXCLUDES 2 Not included here   N Newborn Age: 0   P Pediatric Age: 0-17   M Maternity Age: 12-55   A Adult Age: 15-124

614   ICD-10-CM 2014 (Draft)

K08.8 **Other specified disorders of teeth and supporting structures**
Enlargement of alveolar ridge NOS
Irregular alveolar process
Toothache NOS

K08.9 **Disorder of teeth and supporting structures, unspecified**

☑4th **K09** **Cysts of oral region, not elsewhere classified**
INCLUDES lesions showing histological features both of aneurysmal cyst and of another fibro-osseous lesion
EXCLUDES 2 cysts of jaw (M27.0-, M27.4-)
radicular cyst (K04.8)

K09.0 Developmental odontogenic **cysts**
Dentigerous cyst
Eruption cyst
Follicular cyst
Gingival cyst
Lateral periodontal cyst
Primordial cyst
EXCLUDES 2 keratocysts (D16.4, D16.5)
odontogenic keratocystic tumors (D16.4, D16.5)

K09.1 Developmental (nonodontogenic) **cysts of oral region**
Cyst (of) incisive canal
Cyst (of) palatine of papilla
Globulomaxillary cyst
Median palatal cyst
Nasoalveolar cyst
Nasolabial cyst
Nasopalatine duct cyst

K09.8 **Other cysts of oral region, not elsewhere classified**
Dermoid cyst
Epidermoid cyst
Lymphoepithelial cyst
Epstein's pearl

K09.9 **Cyst of oral region, unspecified**

☑4th **K11** **Diseases of salivary glands**
Use additional code to identify:
alcohol abuse and dependence (F10.-)
exposure to environmental tobacco smoke (Z77.22)
exposure to tobacco smoke in the perinatal period (P96.81)
history of tobacco use (Z87.891)
occupational exposure to environmental tobacco smoke (Z57.31)
tobacco dependence (F17.-)
tobacco use (Z72.0)

K11.0 Atrophy **of salivary gland**

K11.1 Hypertrophy **of salivary gland**

☑5th **K11.2** Sialoadenitis
Parotitis
EXCLUDES 1 epidemic parotitis (B26.-)
mumps (B26.-)
uveoparotid fever [Heerfordt] (D86.89)

K11.20 **Sialoadenitis, unspecified**

K11.21 Acute **sialoadenitis**
EXCLUDES 1 acute recurrent sialoadenitis (K11.22)

K11.22 Acute recurrent **sialoadenitis**

K11.23 Chronic **sialoadenitis**

K11.3 Abscess **of salivary gland**

K11.4 Fistula **of salivary gland**
EXCLUDES 1 congenital fistula of salivary gland (Q38.4)

K11.5 Sialolithiasis
Calculus of salivary gland or duct
Stone of salivary gland or duct

K11.6 Mucocele **of salivary gland**
Mucous extravasation cyst of salivary gland
Mucous retention cyst of salivary gland
Ranula

K11.7 Disturbances of salivary **secretion**
Hypoptyalism
Ptyalism
Xerostomia
EXCLUDES 2 dry mouth NOS (R68.2)

K11.8 **Other diseases of salivary glands**
Benign lymphoepithelial lesion of salivary gland
Mikulicz' disease
Necrotizing sialometaplasia
Sialectasia
Stenosis of salivary duct
Stricture of salivary duct
EXCLUDES 1 sicca syndrome [Sjögren] (M35.0-)

K11.9 **Disease of salivary gland, unspecified**
Sialoadenopathy NOS

☑4th **K12** **Stomatitis and related lesions**
Use additional code to identify:
alcohol abuse and dependence (F10.-)
exposure to environmental tobacco smoke (Z77.22)
exposure to tobacco smoke in the perinatal period (P96.81)
history of tobacco use (Z87.891)
occupational exposure to environmental tobacco smoke (Z57.31)
tobacco dependence (F17.-)
tobacco use (Z72.0)
EXCLUDES 1 cancrum oris (A69.0)
cheilitis (K13.0)
gangrenous stomatitis (A69.0)
herpesviral [herpes simplex] gingivostomatitis (B00.2)
noma (A69.0)

K12.0 **Recurrent oral aphthae**
Aphthous stomatitis (major) (minor)
Bednar's aphthae
Periadenitis mucosa necrotica recurrens
Recurrent aphthous ulcer
Stomatitis herpetiformis

K12.1 **Other forms of stomatitis**
Stomatitis NOS   Ulcerative stomatitis
Denture stomatitis   Vesicular stomatitis
EXCLUDES 1 acute necrotizing ulcerative stomatitis (A69.1)
Vincent's stomatitis (A69.1)

K12.2 **Cellulitis and abscess of mouth**
Cellulitis of mouth (floor)
Submandibular abscess
EXCLUDES 2 abscess of salivary gland (K11.3)
abscess of tongue (K14.0)
periapical abscess (K04.6-K04.7)
periodontal abscess (K05.21)
peritonsillar abscess (J36)

☑5th **K12.3** **Oral mucositis (ulcerative)**
Mucositis (oral) (oropharyneal)
EXCLUDES 2 gastrointestinal mucositis (ulcerative) (K92.81)
mucositis (ulcerative) of vagina and vulva (N76.81)
nasal mucositis (ulcerative) (J34.81)

K12.30 **Oral mucositis (ulcerative), unspecified**

K12.31 **Oral mucositis (ulcerative) due to** antineoplastic therapy
Use additional code for adverse effect, if applicable, to identify antineoplastic and immunosuppressive drugs (T45.1X5)
Use additional code for other antineoplastic therapy, such as:
radiological procedure and radiotherapy (Y84.2)

K12.32 **Oral mucositis (ulcerative) due to** other drugs
Use additional code for adverse effect, if applicable, to identify drug (T36-T50 with fifth or sixth character 5)

K12.33 **Oral mucositis (ulcerative) due to** radiation
Use additional external cause code (W88-W90, X39.0-) to identify cause

K12.39 **Other oral mucositis (ulcerative)**
Viral oral mucositis (ulcerative)

☑ Additional Character Required   •x 7th Xtension Alert   Unspecified Code   Other Specified Code   Manifestation Code   ►◄ Revised Text   ● New Code   ▲ Revised Code Title

ICD-10-CM 2014 (Draft)   615

Diseases of the Digestive System

K13–K22.2

✓4ᵗʰ K13 Other diseases of lip and oral mucosa
INCLUDES epithelial disturbances of tongue
Use additional code to identify:
   alcohol abuse and dependence (F10.-)
   exposure to environmental tobacco smoke (Z77.22)
   exposure to tobacco smoke in the perinatal period (P96.81)
   history of tobacco use (Z87.891)
   occupational exposure to environmental tobacco smoke (Z57.31)
   tobacco dependence (F17.-)
   tobacco use (Z72.0)
   EXCLUDES 2 certain disorders of gingiva and edentulous alveolar ridge
      (K05-K06)
      cysts of oral region (K09.-)
      diseases of tongue (K14.-)
      stomatitis and related lesions (K12.-)

K13.0 Diseases of lips
Abscess of lips	Exfoliative cheilitis
Angular cheilitis	Fistula of lips
Cellulitis of lips	Glandular cheilitis
Cheilitis NOS	Hypertrophy of lips
Cheilodynia	Perlèche NEC
Cheilosis	

   EXCLUDES 1 ariboflavinosis (E53.0)
      cheilitis due to radiation-related disorders (L55-L59)
      congenital fistula of lips (Q38.0)
      congenital hypertrophy of lips (Q18.6)
      Perlèche due to candidiasis (B37.83)
      Perlèche due to riboflavin deficiency (E53.0)

K13.1 Cheek and lip biting

✓5ᵗʰ K13.2 Leukoplakia and other disturbances of oral epithelium, including tongue
   EXCLUDES 1 carcinoma in situ of oral epithelium (D00.0-)
      hairy leukoplakia (K13.3)

K13.21 Leukoplakia of oral mucosa, including tongue
   Leukokeratosis of oral mucosa
   Leukoplakia of gingiva, lips, tongue
   EXCLUDES 1 hairy leukoplakia (K13.3)
      leukokeratosis nicotina palati (K13.24)

K13.22 Minimal keratinized residual ridge mucosa
   Minimal keratinization of alveolar ridge mucosa

K13.23 Excessive keratinized residual ridge mucosa
   Excessive keratinization of alveolar ridge mucosa

K13.24 Leukokeratosis nicotina palati
   Smoker's palate

K13.29 Other disturbances of oral epithelium, including tongue
   Erythroplakia of mouth or tongue
   Focal epithelial hyperplasia of mouth or tongue
   Leukoedema of mouth or tongue
   Other oral epithelium disturbances

K13.3 Hairy leukoplakia

K13.4 Granuloma and granuloma-like lesions of oral mucosa
Eosinophilic granuloma	Verrucous xanthoma
Granuloma pyogenicum	

K13.5 Oral submucous fibrosis
   Submucous fibrosis of tongue

K13.6 Irritative hyperplasia of oral mucosa
   EXCLUDES 2 irritative hyperplasia of edentulous ridge [denture
      hyperplasia] (K06.2)

✓5ᵗʰ K13.7 Other and unspecified lesions of oral mucosa
K13.70 Unspecified lesions of oral mucosa
K13.79 Other lesions of oral mucosa
   Focal oral mucinosis

✓4ᵗʰ K14 Diseases of tongue
Use additional code to identify:
   alcohol abuse and dependence (F10.-)
   exposure to environmental tobacco smoke (Z77.22)
   history of tobacco use (Z87.891)
   occupational exposure to environmental tobacco smoke (Z57.31)
   tobacco dependence (F17.-)
   tobacco use (Z72.0)
   EXCLUDES 2 erythroplakia (K13.29)
      focal epithelial hyperplasia (K13.29)
      leukedema of tongue (K13.29)
      leukoplakia of tongue (K13.21)
      hairy leukoplakia (K13.3)
      macroglossia (congenital) (Q38.2)
      submucous fibrosis of tongue (K13.5)

K14.0 Glossitis
   Abscess of tongue   Ulceration (traumatic) of tongue
   EXCLUDES 1 atrophic glossitis (K14.4)

K14.1 Geographic tongue
   Benign migratory glossitis
   Glossitis areata exfoliativa

K14.2 Median rhomboid glossitis

K14.3 Hypertrophy of tongue papillae
   Black hairy tongue
   Coated tongue
   Hypertrophy of foliate papillae
   Lingua villosa nigra

K14.4 Atrophy of tongue papillae
   Atrophic glossitis

K14.5 Plicated tongue
   Fissured tongue
   Furrowed tongue
   Scrotal tongue
   EXCLUDES 1 fissured tongue, congenital (Q38.3)

K14.6 Glossodynia
   Glossopyrosis
   Painful tongue

K14.8 Other diseases of tongue
   Atrophy of tongue
   Crenated tongue
   Enlargement of tongue
   Glossocele
   Glossoptosis
   Hypertrophy of tongue

K14.9 Disease of tongue, unspecified
   Glossopathy NOS

Diseases of esophagus, stomach and duodenum (K20-K31)
   EXCLUDES 2 hiatus hernia (K44.-)

✓4ᵗʰ K20 Esophagitis
Use additional code to identify:
   alcohol abuse and dependence (F10.-)
   EXCLUDES 1 erosion of esophagus (K22.1-)
      esophagitis with gastro-esophageal reflux disease (K21.0)
      reflux esophagitis (K21.0)
      ulcerative esophagitis (K22.1-)
   EXCLUDES 2 eosinophilic gastritis or gastroenteritis (K52.81)

K20.0 Eosinophilic esophagitis

K20.8 Other esophagitis
   Abscess of esophagus

K20.9 Esophagitis, unspecified
   Esophagitis NOS

✓4ᵗʰ K21 Gastro-esophageal reflux disease
   EXCLUDES 1 newborn esophageal reflux (P78.83)

K21.0 Gastro-esophageal reflux disease with esophagitis
   Reflux esophagitis

K21.9 Gastro-esophageal reflux disease without esophagitis
   Esophageal reflux NOS

✓4ᵗʰ K22 Other diseases of esophagus
   EXCLUDES 2 esophageal varices (I85.-)

K22.0 Achalasia of cardia
   Achalasia NOS
   Cardiospasm
   EXCLUDES 1 congenital cardiospasm (Q39.5)

✓5ᵗʰ K22.1 Ulcer of esophagus
   Barrett's ulcer
   Erosion of esophagus
   Fungal ulcer of esophagus
   Peptic ulcer of esophagus
   Ulcer of esophagus due to ingestion of chemicals
   Ulcer of esophagus due to ingestion of drugs and medicaments
   Ulcerative esophagitis
   Code first poisoning due to drug or toxin, if applicable (T36-T65
      with fifth or sixth character 1-4 or 6)
   Use additional code for adverse effect, if applicable, to identify
      drug (T36-T50 with fifth or sixth character 5)
   EXCLUDES 1 Barrett's esophagus (K22.7-)

K22.10 Ulcer of esophagus without bleeding
   Ulcer of esophagus NOS

K22.11 Ulcer of esophagus with bleeding
   EXCLUDES 2 bleeding esophageal varices (I85.01, I85.11)

K22.2 Esophageal obstruction
   Compression of esophagus
   Constriction of esophagus
   Stenosis of esophagus
   Stricture of esophagus
   EXCLUDES 1 congenital stenosis or stricture of esophagus (Q39.3)

EXCLUDES 1 Not coded here   EXCLUDES 2 Not included here   N Newborn Age: 0   P Pediatric Age: 0-17   M Maternity Age: 12-55   A Adult Age: 15-124

616   ICD-10-CM 2014 (Draft)

K22.3 Perforation of esophagus
Rupture of esophagus
EXCLUDES 1 *traumatic perforation of (thoracic) esophagus (S27.8-)*

K22.4 Dyskinesia of esophagus
Corkscrew esophagus
Diffuse esophageal spasm
Spasm of esophagus
EXCLUDES 1 *cardiospasm (K22.0)*

K22.5 Diverticulum of esophagus, acquired
Esophageal pouch, acquired
EXCLUDES 1 *diverticulum of esophagus (congenital) (Q39.6)*

K22.6 Gastro-esophageal laceration-hemorrhage syndrome
Mallory-Weiss syndrome

✓5th **K22.7 Barrett's esophagus**
Barrett's disease
Barrett's syndrome
EXCLUDES 1 *Barrett's ulcer (K22.1)*
malignant neoplasm of esophagus (C15.-)

K22.70 Barrett's esophagus without dysplasia
Barrett's esophagus NOS

✓6th **K22.71 Barrett's esophagus with dysplasia**
K22.710 Barrett's esophagus with low grade dysplasia
K22.711 Barrett's esophagus with high grade dysplasia
K22.719 Barrett's esophagus with dysplasia, unspecified

K22.8 Other specified diseases of esophagus
Hemorrhage of esophagus NOS
EXCLUDES 2 *esophageal varices (I85.-)*
Paterson-Kelly syndrome (D50.1)

K22.9 Disease of esophagus, unspecified

K23 Disorders of esophagus in diseases classified elsewhere
Code first underlying disease, such as:
congenital syphilis (A50.5)
EXCLUDES 1 *late syphilis (A52.79)*
megaesophagus due to Chagas' disease (B57.31)
tuberculosis (A18.83)

✓4th **K25 Gastric ulcer**
INCLUDES erosion (acute) of stomach
pylorus ulcer (peptic)
stomach ulcer (peptic)
Use additional code to identify:
alcohol abuse and dependence (F10.-)
EXCLUDES 1 *acute gastritis (K29.0-)*
peptic ulcer NOS (K27.-)

K25.0 Acute gastric ulcer with hemorrhage
K25.1 Acute gastric ulcer with perforation
K25.2 Acute gastric ulcer with both hemorrhage and perforation
K25.3 Acute gastric ulcer without hemorrhage or perforation
K25.4 Chronic or unspecified gastric ulcer with hemorrhage
K25.5 Chronic or unspecified gastric ulcer with perforation
K25.6 Chronic or unspecified gastric ulcer with both hemorrhage and perforation
K25.7 Chronic gastric ulcer without hemorrhage or perforation
K25.9 Gastric ulcer, unspecified as acute or chronic, without hemorrhage or perforation

✓4th **K26 Duodenal ulcer**
INCLUDES erosion (acute) of duodenum
duodenum ulcer (peptic)
postpyloric ulcer (peptic)
Use additional code to identify:
alcohol abuse and dependence (F10.-)
EXCLUDES 1 *peptic ulcer NOS (K27.-)*

K26.0 Acute duodenal ulcer with hemorrhage
K26.1 Acute duodenal ulcer with perforation
K26.2 Acute duodenal ulcer with both hemorrhage and perforation
K26.3 Acute duodenal ulcer without hemorrhage or perforation
K26.4 Chronic or unspecified duodenal ulcer with hemorrhage
K26.5 Chronic or unspecified duodenal ulcer with perforation
K26.6 Chronic or unspecified duodenal ulcer with both hemorrhage and perforation
K26.7 Chronic duodenal ulcer without hemorrhage or perforation
K26.9 Duodenal ulcer, unspecified as acute or chronic, without hemorrhage or perforation

✓4th **K27 Peptic ulcer, site unspecified**
INCLUDES gastroduodenal ulcer NOS
peptic ulcer NOS
Use additional code to identify:
alcohol abuse and dependence (F10.-)
EXCLUDES 1 *peptic ulcer of newborn (P78.82)*

K27.0 Acute peptic ulcer, site unspecified, with hemorrhage
K27.1 Acute peptic ulcer, site unspecified, with perforation
K27.2 Acute peptic ulcer, site unspecified, with both hemorrhage and perforation
K27.3 Acute peptic ulcer, site unspecified, without hemorrhage or perforation
K27.4 Chronic or unspecified peptic ulcer, site unspecified, with hemorrhage
K27.5 Chronic or unspecified peptic ulcer, site unspecified, with perforation
K27.6 Chronic or unspecified peptic ulcer, site unspecified, with both hemorrhage and perforation
K27.7 Chronic peptic ulcer, site unspecified, without hemorrhage or perforation
K27.9 Peptic ulcer, site unspecified, unspecified as acute or chronic, without hemorrhage or perforation

✓4th **K28 Gastrojejunal ulcer**
INCLUDES anastomotic ulcer (peptic) or erosion
gastrocolic ulcer (peptic) or erosion
gastrointestinal ulcer (peptic) or erosion
gastrojejunal ulcer (peptic) or erosion
jejunal ulcer (peptic) or erosion
marginal ulcer (peptic) or erosion
stomal ulcer (peptic) or erosion
Use additional code to identify:
alcohol abuse and dependence (F10.-)
EXCLUDES 1 *primary ulcer of small intestine (K63.3)*

K28.0 Acute gastrojejunal ulcer with hemorrhage
K28.1 Acute gastrojejunal ulcer with perforation
K28.2 Acute gastrojejunal ulcer with both hemorrhage and perforation
K28.3 Acute gastrojejunal ulcer without hemorrhage or perforation
K28.4 Chronic or unspecified gastrojejunal ulcer with hemorrhage
K28.5 Chronic or unspecified gastrojejunal ulcer with perforation
K28.6 Chronic or unspecified gastrojejunal ulcer with both hemorrhage and perforation
K28.7 Chronic gastrojejunal ulcer without hemorrhage or perforation
K28.9 Gastrojejunal ulcer, unspecified as acute or chronic, without hemorrhage or perforation

✓4th **K29 Gastritis and duodenitis**
EXCLUDES 1 *eosinophilic gastritis or gastroenteritis (K52.81)*
Zollinger-Ellison syndrome (E16.4)

✓5th **K29.0 Acute gastritis**
Use additional code to identify:
alcohol abuse and dependence (F10.-)
EXCLUDES 1 *erosion (acute) of stomach (K25.-)*
K29.00 Acute gastritis without bleeding
K29.01 Acute gastritis with bleeding

✓5th **K29.2 Alcoholic gastritis**
Use additional code to identify:
alcohol abuse and dependence (F10.-)
K29.20 Alcoholic gastritis without bleeding
K29.21 Alcoholic gastritis with bleeding

✓5th **K29.3 Chronic superficial gastritis**
K29.30 Chronic superficial gastritis without bleeding
K29.31 Chronic superficial gastritis with bleeding

✓5th **K29.4 Chronic atrophic gastritis**
Gastric atrophy
K29.40 Chronic atrophic gastritis without bleeding
K29.41 Chronic atrophic gastritis with bleeding

✓5th **K29.5 Unspecified chronic gastritis**
Chronic antral gastritis
Chronic fundal gastritis
K29.50 Unspecified chronic gastritis without bleeding
K29.51 Unspecified chronic gastritis with bleeding

(right margin) Diseases of the Digestive System
*(right margin)* K22.3–K29.51

✓ Additional Character Required   √x7th Xtension Alert   Unspecified Code   Other Specified Code   Manifestation Code   ►◄ Revised Text   ● New Code   ▲ Revised Code Title

Diseases of the Digestive System

K29.6–K40.21

✓5ᵗʰ **K29.6** Other **gastritis**
Giant hypertrophic gastritis
Granulomatous gastritis
Ménétrier's disease

    K29.60 **Other gastritis** without bleeding

    K29.61 **Other gastritis** with bleeding

✓5ᵗʰ **K29.7** Gastritis, unspecified

    K29.70 **Gastritis, unspecified,** without bleeding

    K29.71 **Gastritis, unspecified,** with bleeding

✓5ᵗʰ **K29.8** Duodenitis

    K29.80 **Duodenitis** without bleeding

    K29.81 **Duodenitis** with bleeding

✓5ᵗʰ **K29.9** Gastroduodenitis, unspecified

    K29.90 **Gastroduodenitis, unspecified,** without bleeding

    K29.91 **Gastroduodenitis, unspecified,** with bleeding

K30 **Functional dyspepsia**
Indigestion
   EXCLUDES1   *dyspepsia NOS (R10.13)*
      heartburn (R12)
      nervous dyspepsia (F45.8)
      neurotic dyspepsia (F45.8)
      psychogenic dyspepsia (F45.8)

✓4ᵗʰ **K31** **Other diseases of stomach and duodenum**
   INCLUDES   functional disorders of stomach
   EXCLUDES2   *diabetic gastroparesis (E08.43, E09.43, E10.43, E11.43, E13.43)*
      diverticulum of duodenum (K57.00-K57.13)

K31.0 **Acute dilatation of stomach**
Acute distention of stomach

K31.1 **Adult hypertrophic pyloric stenosis**   A
Pyloric stenosis NOS
   EXCLUDES1   *congenital or infantile pyloric stenosis (Q40.0)*

K31.2 **Hourglass stricture and stenosis of stomach**
   EXCLUDES1   *congenital hourglass stomach (Q40.2)*
      hourglass contraction of stomach (K31.89)

K31.3 **Pylorospasm, not elsewhere classified**
   EXCLUDES1   *congenital or infantile pylorospasm (Q40.0)*
      neurotic pylorospasm (F45.8)
      psychogenic pylorospasm (F45.8)

K31.4 **Gastric diverticulum**
   EXCLUDES1   *congenital diverticulum of stomach (Q40.2)*

K31.5 **Obstruction of duodenum**
Constriction of duodenum
Duodenal ileus (chronic)
Stenosis of duodenum
Stricture of duodenum
Volvulus of duodenum
   EXCLUDES1   *congenital stenosis of duodenum (Q41.0)*

K31.6 **Fistula of stomach and duodenum**
Gastrocolic fistula
Gastrojejunocolic fistula

K31.7 **Polyp of stomach and duodenum**
   EXCLUDES1   *adenomatous polyp of stomach (D13.1)*

✓5ᵗʰ **K31.8** Other specified diseases of stomach and duodenum

   ✓6ᵗʰ **K31.81** Angiodysplasia of stomach and duodenum

     K31.811 **Angiodysplasia of stomach and duodenum** with bleeding

     K31.819 **Angiodysplasia of stomach and duodenum** without bleeding
Angiodysplasia of stomach and duodenum NOS

   K31.82 **Dieulafoy lesion (hemorrhagic) of stomach and duodenum**
     EXCLUDES2   *Dieulafoy lesion of intestine (K63.81)*

   K31.83 **Achlorhydria**

   K31.84 **Gastroparesis**
Gastroparalysis
Code first underlying disease, if known, such as:
   anorexia nervosa (F50.0-)
   diabetes mellitus (E08.43, E09.43, E10.43, E11.43, E13.43)
   scleroderma (M34.-)

   K31.89 **Other diseases of stomach and duodenum**

K31.9 **Disease of stomach and duodenum, unspecified**

Diseases of appendix (K35-K38)

✓4ᵗʰ **K35** Acute **appendicitis**

K35.2 **Acute appendicitis with generalized peritonitis**
Appendicitis (acute) with generalized (diffuse) peritonitis following rupture or perforation of appendix
Perforated appendix NOS
Ruptured appendix NOS

K35.3 **Acute appendicitis with localized peritonitis**
Acute appendicitis with or without perforation or rupture NOS
Acute appendicitis with or without perforation or rupture with localized peritonitis
Acute appendicitis with peritoneal abscess

✓5ᵗʰ **K35.8** Other **and unspecified acute appendicitis**

   K35.80 **Unspecified acute appendicitis**
Acute appendicitis NOS
Acute appendicitis without (localized) (generalized) peritonitis

   K35.89 **Other acute appendicitis**

K36 **Other appendicitis**
Chronic appendicitis
Recurrent appendicitis

K37 **Unspecified appendicitis**
   EXCLUDES1   *unspecified appendicitis with peritonitis (K35.2-K35.3)*

✓4ᵗʰ **K38** **Other diseases of appendix**

K38.0 **Hyperplasia of appendix**

K38.1 **Appendicular concretions**
Fecalith of appendix
Stercolith of appendix

K38.2 **Diverticulum of appendix**

K38.3 **Fistula of appendix**

K38.8 **Other specified diseases of appendix**
Intussusception of appendix

K38.9 **Disease of appendix, unspecified**

Hernia (K40-K46)

   NOTE   Hernia with both gangrene and obstruction is classified to hernia with gangrene.
   INCLUDES   acquired hernia
      congenital [except diaphragmatic or hiatus] hernia
      recurrent hernia

✓4ᵗʰ **K40** **Inguinal hernia**
   INCLUDES   bubonocele
      direct inguinal hernia
      double inguinal hernia
      indirect inguinal hernia
      inguinal hernia NOS
      oblique inguinal hernia
      scrotal hernia

✓5ᵗʰ **K40.0** Bilateral **inguinal hernia, with obstruction, without gangrene**
Inguinal hernia (bilateral) causing obstruction without gangrene
Incarcerated inguinal hernia (bilateral) without gangrene
Irreducible inguinal hernia (bilateral) without gangrene
Strangulated inguinal hernia (bilateral) without gangrene

   K40.00 **Bilateral inguinal hernia, with obstruction, without gangrene,** not specified as recurrent
Bilateral inguinal hernia, with obstruction, without gangrene NOS

   K40.01 **Bilateral inguinal hernia, with obstruction, without gangrene,** recurrent

✓5ᵗʰ **K40.1** Bilateral **inguinal hernia, with gangrene**

   K40.10 **Bilateral inguinal hernia, with gangrene,** not specified as recurrent
Bilateral inguinal hernia, with gangrene NOS

   K40.11 **Bilateral inguinal hernia, with gangrene,** recurrent

✓5ᵗʰ **K40.2** Bilateral **inguinal hernia, without obstruction or gangrene**

   K40.20 **Bilateral inguinal hernia, without obstruction or gangrene,** not specified as recurrent
Bilateral inguinal hernia NOS

   K40.21 **Bilateral inguinal hernia, without obstruction or gangrene,** recurrent

EXCLUDES1 Not coded here   EXCLUDES2 Not included here   N Newborn Age: 0   P Pediatric Age: 0-17   M Maternity Age: 12-55   A Adult Age: 15-124

618   ICD-10-CM 2014 (Draft)

✓5ᵗʰ **K40.3** Unilateral **inguinal hernia,** with obstruction, without gangrene
  Inguinal hernia (unilateral) causing obstruction without gangrene
  Incarcerated inguinal hernia (unilateral) without gangrene
  Irreducible inguinal hernia (unilateral) without gangrene
  Strangulated inguinal hernia (unilateral) without gangrene

  K40.30 **Unilateral inguinal hernia, with obstruction, without gangrene,** not specified as recurrent
    Inguinal hernia, with obstruction NOS
    Unilateral inguinal hernia, with obstruction, without gangrene NOS

  K40.31 **Unilateral inguinal hernia, with obstruction, without gangrene,** recurrent

✓5ᵗʰ **K40.4** Unilateral **inguinal hernia,** with gangrene

  K40.40 **Unilateral inguinal hernia, with gangrene,** not specified as recurrent
    Inguinal hernia with gangrene NOS
    Unilateral inguinal hernia with gangrene NOS

  K40.41 **Unilateral inguinal hernia, with gangrene,** recurrent

✓5ᵗʰ **K40.9** Unilateral **inguinal hernia,** without obstruction or gangrene

  K40.90 **Unilateral inguinal hernia, without obstruction or gangrene,** not specified as recurrent
    Inguinal hernia NOS
    Unilateral inguinal hernia NOS

  K40.91 **Unilateral inguinal hernia, without obstruction or gangrene,** recurrent

✓4ᵗʰ **K41** Femoral **hernia**

✓5ᵗʰ **K41.0** Bilateral **femoral hernia,** with obstruction, without gangrene
  Femoral hernia (bilateral) causing obstruction, without gangrene
  Incarcerated femoral hernia (bilateral), without gangrene
  Irreducible femoral hernia (bilateral), without gangrene
  Strangulated femoral hernia (bilateral), without gangrene

  K41.00 **Bilateral femoral hernia, with obstruction, without gangrene,** not specified as recurrent
    Bilateral femoral hernia, with obstruction, without gangrene NOS

  K41.01 **Bilateral femoral hernia, with obstruction, without gangrene,** recurrent

✓5ᵗʰ **K41.1** Bilateral **femoral hernia,** with gangrene

  K41.10 **Bilateral femoral hernia, with gangrene,** not specified as recurrent
    Bilateral femoral hernia, with gangrene NOS

  K41.11 **Bilateral femoral hernia, with gangrene,** recurrent

✓5ᵗʰ **K41.2** Bilateral **femoral hernia,** without obstruction or gangrene

  K41.20 **Bilateral femoral hernia, without obstruction or gangrene,** not specified as recurrent
    Bilateral femoral hernia NOS

  K41.21 **Bilateral femoral hernia, without obstruction or gangrene,** recurrent

✓5ᵗʰ **K41.3** Unilateral **femoral hernia,** with obstruction, without gangrene
  Femoral hernia (unilateral) causing obstruction, without gangrene
  Incarcerated femoral hernia (unilateral), without gangrene
  Irreducible femoral hernia (unilateral), without gangrene
  Strangulated femoral hernia (unilateral), without gangrene

  K41.30 **Unilateral femoral hernia, with obstruction, without gangrene,** not specified as recurrent
    Femoral hernia, with obstruction NOS
    Unilateral femoral hernia, with obstruction NOS

  K41.31 **Unilateral femoral hernia, with obstruction, without gangrene,** recurrent

✓5ᵗʰ **K41.4** Unilateral **femoral hernia,** with gangrene

  K41.40 **Unilateral femoral hernia, with gangrene,** not specified as recurrent
    Femoral hernia with gangrene NOS
    Unilateral femoral hernia, with gangrene NOS

  K41.41 **Unilateral femoral hernia, with gangrene,** recurrent

✓5ᵗʰ **K41.9** Unilateral **femoral hernia,** without obstruction or gangrene

  K41.90 **Unilateral femoral hernia, without obstruction or gangrene,** not specified as recurrent
    Femoral hernia NOS
    Unilateral femoral hernia NOS

  K41.91 **Unilateral femoral hernia, without obstruction or gangrene,** recurrent

✓4ᵗʰ **K42** Umbilical **hernia**
  INCLUDES paraumbilical hernia
  EXCLUDES 1 *omphalocele (Q79.2)*

  K42.0 **Umbilical hernia** with obstruction, without gangrene
    Umbilical hernia causing obstruction, without gangrene
    Incarcerated umbilical hernia, without gangrene
    Irreducible umbilical hernia, without gangrene
    Strangulated umbilical hernia, without gangrene

  K42.1 **Umbilical hernia** with gangrene
    Gangrenous umbilical hernia

  K42.9 **Umbilical hernia** without obstruction or gangrene
    Umbilical hernia NOS

✓4ᵗʰ **K43** Ventral **hernia**

  K43.0 **Incisional hernia with obstruction,** without gangrene
    Incisional hernia causing obstruction, without gangrene
    Incarcerated incisional hernia, without gangrene
    Irreducible incisional hernia, without gangrene
    Strangulated incisional hernia, without gangrene

  K43.1 **Incisional hernia** with gangrene
    Gangrenous incisional hernia

  K43.2 **Incisional hernia** without obstruction or gangrene
    Incisional hernia NOS

  K43.3 **Parastomal hernia with obstruction,** without gangrene
    Incarcerated parastomal hernia, without gangrene
    Irreducible parastomal hernia, without gangrene
    Parastomal hernia causing obstruction, without gangrene
    Strangulated parastomal hernia, without gangrene

  K43.4 **Parastomal hernia** with gangrene
    Gangrenous parastomal hernia

  K43.5 **Parastomal hernia** without obstruction or gangrene
    Parastomal hernia NOS

  K43.6 **Other and unspecified ventral hernia with obstruction, without gangrene**
    Epigastric hernia causing obstruction, without gangrene
    Hypogastric hernia causing obstruction, without gangrene
    Incarcerated epigastric hernia without gangrene
    Incarcerated hypogastric hernia without gangrene
    Incarcerated midline hernia without gangrene
    Incarcerated spigelian hernia without gangrene
    Incarcerated subxiphoid hernia without gangrene
    Irreducible epigastric hernia without gangrene
    Irreducible hypogastric hernia without gangrene
    Irreducible midline hernia without gangrene
    Irreducible spigelian hernia without gangrene
    Irreducible subxiphoid hernia without gangrene
    Midline hernia causing obstruction, without gangrene
    Spigelian hernia causing obstruction, without gangrene
    Strangulated epigastric hernia without gangrene
    Strangulated hypogastric hernia without gangrene
    Strangulated midline hernia without gangrene
    Strangulated spigelian hernia without gangrene
    Strangulated subxiphoid hernia without gangrene
    Subxiphoid hernia causing obstruction, without gangrene

  K43.7 **Other and unspecified ventral hernia** with gangrene
    Any condition listed under K43.6 specified as gangrenous

  K43.9 **Ventral hernia** without obstruction or gangrene
    Epigastric hernia
    Ventral hernia NOS

✓4ᵗʰ **K44** Diaphragmatic **hernia**
  INCLUDES hiatus hernia (esophageal) (sliding)
      paraesophageal hernia
  EXCLUDES 1 *congenital diaphragmatic hernia (Q79.0)*
      congenital hiatus hernia (Q40.1)

  K44.0 **Diaphragmatic hernia** with obstruction, without gangrene
    Diaphragmatic hernia causing obstruction
    Incarcerated diaphragmatic hernia
    Irreducible diaphragmatic hernia
    Strangulated diaphragmatic hernia

  K44.1 **Diaphragmatic hernia** with gangrene
    Gangrenous diaphragmatic hernia

  K44.9 **Diaphragmatic hernia** without obstruction or gangrene
    Diaphragmatic hernia NOS

☑ Additional Character Required ✓x7ᵗʰ Xtension Alert Unspecified Code Other Specified Code Manifestation Code ▶◀ Revised Text ● New Code ▲ Revised Code Title

Diseases of the Digestive System

K45–K51.214

✓4ᵗʰ **K45** **Other abdominal hernia**
     INCLUDES   abdominal hernia, specified site NEC
          lumbar hernia
          obturator hernia
          pudendal hernia
          retroperitoneal hernia
          sciatic hernia

    K45.0 **Other specified abdominal hernia** with obstruction, without gangrene
         Other specified abdominal hernia causing obstruction
         Other specified incarcerated abdominal hernia
         Other specified irreducible abdominal hernia
         Other specified strangulated abdominal hernia

    K45.1 **Other specified abdominal hernia** with gangrene
         Any condition listed under K4 specified as gangrenous

    K45.8 **Other specified abdominal hernia** without obstruction or gangrene

✓4ᵗʰ **K46** **Unspecified abdominal hernia**
     INCLUDES   enterocele
          epiplocele
          hernia NOS
          interstitial hernia
          intestinal hernia
          intra-abdominal hernia
     EXCLUDES 1   *vaginal enterocele (N81.5)*

    K46.0 **Unspecified abdominal hernia** with obstruction, without gangrene
         Unspecified abdominal hernia causing obstruction
         Unspecified incarcerated abdominal hernia
         Unspecified irreducible abdominal hernia
         Unspecified strangulated abdominal hernia

    K46.1 **Unspecified abdominal hernia** with gangrene
         Any condition listed under K46 specified as gangrenous

    K46.9 **Unspecified abdominal hernia** without obstruction or gangrene
         Abdominal hernia NOS

Noninfective enteritis and colitis (K50-K52)

     INCLUDES   noninfective inflammatory bowel disease
     EXCLUDES 1   *irritable bowel syndrome (K58.-)*
              megacolon (K59.3)

✓4ᵗʰ **K50** **Crohn's disease [regional enteritis]**
     INCLUDES   granulomatous enteritis
     EXCLUDES 1   *ulcerative colitis (K51.-)*
     Use additional code to identify manifestations, such as:
         pyoderma gangrenosum (L88)
     AHA: 2012, Q4, 104

✓5ᵗʰ   **K50.0** **Crohn's disease of** small intestine
         Crohn's disease [regional enteritis] of duodenum
         Crohn's disease [regional enteritis] of ileum
         Crohn's disease [regional enteritis] of jejunum
         Regional ileitis
         Terminal ileitis
       EXCLUDES 1   *Crohn's disease of both small and large intestine (K50.8-)*

     K50.00 **Crohn's disease of small intestine** without complications

✓6ᵗʰ   **K50.01** **Crohn's disease of small intestine** with complications
        K50.011 **Crohn's disease of small intestine with** rectal bleeding
        K50.012 **Crohn's disease of small intestine with** intestinal obstruction
        K50.013 **Crohn's disease of small intestine with** fistula
        K50.014 **Crohn's disease of small intestine with** abscess
            AHA: 2012, Q4, 104
        K50.018 **Crohn's disease of small intestine with other complication**
        K50.019 **Crohn's disease of small intestine with unspecified complications**

✓5ᵗʰ   **K50.1** **Crohn's disease of** large intestine
         Crohn's disease [regional enteritis] of colon
         Crohn's disease [regional enteritis] of large bowel
         Crohn's disease [regional enteritis] of rectum
         Granulomatous colitis
         Regional colitis
       EXCLUDES 1   *Crohn's disease of both small and large intestine (K50.8)*

     K50.10 **Crohn's disease of large intestine** without complications

✓6ᵗʰ   **K50.11** **Crohn's disease of large intestine** with complications
        K50.111 **Crohn's disease of large intestine with** rectal bleeding
        K50.112 **Crohn's disease of large intestine with** intestinal obstruction
        K50.113 **Crohn's disease of large intestine with** fistula
        K50.114 **Crohn's disease of large intestine with** abscess
        K50.118 **Crohn's disease of large intestine with other complication**
        K50.119 **Crohn's disease of large intestine with unspecified complications**

✓5ᵗʰ   **K50.8** **Crohn's disease of** both small and large intestine
     K50.80 **Crohn's disease of both small and large intestine** without complications

✓6ᵗʰ   **K50.81** **Crohn's disease of both small and large intestine** with complications
        K50.811 **Crohn's disease of both small and large intestine with** rectal bleeding
        K50.812 **Crohn's disease of both small and large intestine with** intestinal obstruction
        K50.813 **Crohn's disease of both small and large intestine with** fistula
        K50.814 **Crohn's disease of both small and large intestine with** abscess
        K50.818 **Crohn's disease of both small and large intestine with other complication**
        K50.819 **Crohn's disease of both small and large intestine with unspecified complications**

✓5ᵗʰ   **K50.9** **Crohn's disease,** unspecified
     K50.90 **Crohn's disease, unspecified,** without complications
         Crohn's disease NOS
         Regional enteritis NOS

✓6ᵗʰ   **K50.91** **Crohn's disease, unspecified,** with complications
        K50.911 **Crohn's disease, unspecified,** with rectal bleeding
        K50.912 **Crohn's disease, unspecified,** with intestinal obstruction
        K50.913 **Crohn's disease, unspecified,** with fistula
        K50.914 **Crohn's disease, unspecified,** with abscess
        K50.918 **Crohn's disease, unspecified, with other complication**
        K50.919 **Crohn's disease, unspecified, with unspecified complications**

✓4ᵗʰ **K51** **Ulcerative colitis**
     Use additional code to identify manifestations, such as:
         pyoderma gangrenosum (L88)
     EXCLUDES 1   *Crohn's disease [regional enteritis] (K50.-)*

✓5ᵗʰ   **K51.0** **Ulcerative (chronic)** pancolitis
         Backwash ileitis
     K51.00 **Ulcerative (chronic) pancolitis** without complications
         Ulcerative (chronic) pancolitis NOS

✓6ᵗʰ   **K51.01** **Ulcerative (chronic) pancolitis** with complications
        K51.011 **Ulcerative (chronic) pancolitis with** rectal bleeding
        K51.012 **Ulcerative (chronic) pancolitis with** intestinal obstruction
        K51.013 **Ulcerative (chronic) pancolitis with** fistula
        K51.014 **Ulcerative (chronic) pancolitis with** abscess
        K51.018 **Ulcerative (chronic) pancolitis with other complication**
        K51.019 **Ulcerative (chronic) pancolitis with unspecified complications**

✓5ᵗʰ   **K51.2** **Ulcerative (chronic)** proctitis
     K51.20 **Ulcerative (chronic) proctitis** without complications
         Ulcerative (chronic) proctitis NOS

✓6ᵗʰ   **K51.21** **Ulcerative (chronic) proctitis** with complications
        K51.211 **Ulcerative (chronic) proctitis with** rectal bleeding
        K51.212 **Ulcerative (chronic) proctitis with** intestinal obstruction
        K51.213 **Ulcerative (chronic) proctitis with** fistula
        K51.214 **Ulcerative (chronic) proctitis with** abscess

---

EXCLUDES 1 Not coded here   EXCLUDES 2 Not included here   N Newborn Age: 0   P Pediatric Age: 0-17   M Maternity Age: 12-55   A Adult Age: 15-124

620   ICD-10-CM 2014 (Draft)

K51.218 **Ulcerative (chronic) proctitis with other complication**

K51.219 **Ulcerative (chronic) proctitis with unspecified complications**

✓5th **K51.3** Ulcerative (chronic) rectosigmoiditis

K51.30 **Ulcerative (chronic) rectosigmoiditis** without complications
Ulcerative (chronic) rectosigmoiditis NOS

✓6th **K51.31** Ulcerative (chronic) rectosigmoiditis with complications

K51.311 **Ulcerative (chronic) rectosigmoiditis with** rectal bleeding

K51.312 **Ulcerative (chronic) rectosigmoiditis with** intestinal obstruction

K51.313 **Ulcerative (chronic) rectosigmoiditis with** fistula

K51.314 **Ulcerative (chronic) rectosigmoiditis with** abscess

K51.318 **Ulcerative (chronic) rectosigmoiditis with other complication**

K51.319 **Ulcerative (chronic) rectosigmoiditis with unspecified complications**

✓5th **K51.4** Inflammatory polyps of colon
EXCLUDES 1 *adenomatous polyp of colon (D12.6)*
polyposis of colon (D12.6)
polyps of colon NOS (K63.5)

K51.40 **Inflammatory polyps of colon** without complications
Inflammatory polyps of colon NOS

✓6th **K51.41** Inflammatory polyps of colon with complications

K51.411 **Inflammatory polyps of colon with** rectal bleeding

K51.412 **Inflammatory polyps of colon with** intestinal obstruction

K51.413 **Inflammatory polyps of colon with** fistula
K51.414 **Inflammatory polyps of colon with** abscess
K51.418 **Inflammatory polyps of colon with other complication**

K51.419 **Inflammatory polyps of colon with unspecified complications**

✓5th **K51.5** Left sided colitis
Left hemicolitis

K51.50 **Left sided colitis** without complications
Left sided colitis NOS

✓6th **K51.51** Left sided colitis with complications
K51.511 **Left sided colitis with** rectal bleeding
K51.512 **Left sided colitis with** intestinal obstruction
K51.513 **Left sided colitis with** fistula
K51.514 **Left sided colitis with** abscess
K51.518 **Left sided colitis with other complication**
K51.519 **Left sided colitis with unspecified complications**

✓5th **K51.8** Other ulcerative colitis
K51.80 **Other ulcerative colitis** without complications
✓6th **K51.81** Other ulcerative colitis with complications
K51.811 **Other ulcerative colitis with** rectal bleeding
K51.812 **Other ulcerative colitis with** intestinal obstruction
K51.813 **Other ulcerative colitis with** fistula
K51.814 **Other ulcerative colitis with** abscess
K51.818 **Other ulcerative colitis with other complication**
K51.819 **Other ulcerative colitis with unspecified complications**

✓5th **K51.9** Ulcerative colitis, unspecified
K51.90 **Ulcerative colitis, unspecified,** without complications
✓6th **K51.91** Ulcerative colitis, unspecified, with complications
K51.911 **Ulcerative colitis, unspecified with** rectal bleeding
K51.912 **Ulcerative colitis, unspecified with** intestinal obstruction
K51.913 **Ulcerative colitis, unspecified with** fistula
K51.914 **Ulcerative colitis, unspecified with** abscess

K51.918 **Ulcerative colitis, unspecified with other complication**
K51.919 **Ulcerative colitis, unspecified with unspecified complications**

✓4th **K52** Other and unspecified noninfective gastroenteritis and colitis

K52.0 **Gastroenteritis and colitis due to** radiation

K52.1 **Toxic gastroenteritis and colitis**
Drug-induced gastroenteritis and colitis
Code first (T51-T65) to identify toxic agent
Use additional code for adverse effect, if applicable, to identify drug (T36-T50 with fifth or sixth character 5)

K52.2 **Allergic and dietetic gastroenteritis and colitis**
Food hypersensitivity gastroenteritis or colitis
Use additional code to identify type of food allergy (Z91.01-, Z91.02-)

✓5th **K52.8** Other specified noninfective gastroenteritis and colitis
K52.81 **Eosinophilic gastritis or gastroenteritis**
Eosinophilic enteritis
EXCLUDES 1 *eosinophilic esophagitis (K20.0)*

K52.82 **Eosinophilic colitis**
K52.89 **Other specified noninfective gastroenteritis and colitis**
Collagenous colitis
Lymphocytic colitis
Microscopic colitis (collagenous or lymphocytic)

K52.9 **Noninfective gastroenteritis and colitis, unspecified**
Colitis NOS   Ileitis NOS
Enteritis NOS   Jejunitis NOS
Gastroenteritis NOS   Sigmoiditis NOS
EXCLUDES 1 *diarrhea NOS (R19.7)*
functional diarrhea (K59.1)
infectious gastroenteritis and colitis NOS (A09)
neonatal diarrhea (noninfective) (P78.3)
psychogenic diarrhea (F45.8)

Other diseases of intestines (K55-K64)

✓4th **K55** Vascular disorders of intestine
EXCLUDES 1 *necrotizing enterocolitis of newborn (P77.-)*

K55.0 **Acute vascular disorders of intestine**
Acute fulminant ischemic colitis
Acute intestinal infarction
Acute small intestine ischemia
Infarction of appendices epiploicae
Mesenteric (artery) (vein) embolism
Mesenteric (artery) (vein) infarction
Mesenteric (artery) (vein) thrombosis
Necrosis of intestine
Subacute ischemic colitis

K55.1 **Chronic vascular disorders of intestine**
Chronic ischemic colitis   Mesenteric atherosclerosis
Chronic ischemic enteritis Mesenteric vascular
Chronic ischemic enterocolitis   insufficiency
Ischemic stricture of intestine

✓5th **K55.2** Angiodysplasia of colon
K55.20 **Angiodysplasia of colon** without hemorrhage
K55.21 **Angiodysplasia of colon** with hemorrhage

K55.8 **Other vascular disorders of intestine**
K55.9 **Vascular disorder of intestine, unspecified**
Ischemic colitis
Ischemic enteritis
Ischemic enterocolitis

✓4th **K56** Paralytic ileus and intestinal obstruction without hernia
EXCLUDES 1 *congenital stricture or stenosis of intestine (Q41-Q42)*
cystic fibrosis with meconium ileus (E84.11)
intestinal obstruction with hernia (K40-K46)
ischemic stricture of intestine (K55.1)
meconium ileus NOS (P76.0)
neonatal intestinal obstructions classifiable to P76-
obstruction of duodenum (K31.5)
postprocedural intestinal obstruction (K91.3)
stenosis of anus or rectum (K62.4)

K56.0 **Paralytic ileus**
Paralysis of bowel
Paralysis of colon
Paralysis of intestine
EXCLUDES 1 *gallstone ileus (K56.3)*
ileus NOS (K56.7)
obstructive ileus NOS (K56.69)

☑ Additional Character Required   ✓x7th Xtension Alert   Unspecified Code   Other Specified Code   Manifestation Code   ▶◀ Revised Text   ● New Code   ▲ Revised Code Title

Diseases of the Digestive System

K56.1–K59.4

K56.1 Intussusception
Intussusception or invagination of bowel
Intussusception or invagination of colon
Intussusception or invagination of intestine
Intussusception or invagination of rectum
EXCLUDES 2 *intussusception of appendix (K38.8)*

K56.2 Volvulus
Strangulation of colon or intestine
Torsion of colon or intestine
Twist of colon or intestine
EXCLUDES 2 *volvulus of duodenum (K31.5)*

K56.3 Gallstone ileus
Obstruction of intestine by gallstone

✓5th **K56.4 Other impaction of intestine**

     K56.41 Fecal impaction
         EXCLUDES 1 *constipation (K59.0-)*
                  incomplete defecation (R15.0)

     K56.49 Other impaction of intestine

K56.5 Intestinal adhesions [bands] with obstruction (postprocedural) (postinfection)
Abdominal hernia due to adhesions with obstruction
Peritoneal adhesions [bands] with intestinal obstruction (postprocedural) (postinfection)

✓5th **K56.6 Other and unspecified intestinal obstruction**

     K56.60 Unspecified intestinal obstruction
         Intestinal obstruction NOS
         EXCLUDES 1 *intestinal obstruction due to specified condition—code to condition*

     K56.69 Other intestinal obstruction
         Enterostenosis NOS
         Obstructive ileus NOS
         Occlusion of colon or intestine NOS
         Stenosis of colon or intestine NOS
         Stricture of colon or intestine NOS
         EXCLUDES 1 *intestinal obstruction due to specified condition—code to condition*

K56.7 Ileus, unspecified
EXCLUDES 1 *obstructive ileus (K56.69)*

✓4th **K57 Diverticular disease of intestine**
EXCLUDES 1 *congenital diverticulum of intestine (Q43.8)*
Meckel's diverticulum (Q43.0)
EXCLUDES 2 *diverticulum of appendix (K38.2)*

✓5th **K57.0 Diverticulitis of small intestine with perforation and abscess**
Diverticulitis of small intestine with peritonitis
EXCLUDES 1 *diverticulitis of both small and large intestine with perforation and abscess (K57.4-)*

     K57.00 Diverticulitis of small intestine with perforation and abscess without bleeding

     K57.01 Diverticulitis of small intestine with perforation and abscess with bleeding

✓5th **K57.1 Diverticular disease of small intestine without perforation or abscess**
EXCLUDES 1 *diverticular disease of both small and large intestine without perforation or abscess (K57.5-)*

     K57.10 Diverticulosis of small intestine without perforation or abscess without bleeding
         Diverticular disease of small intestine NOS

     K57.11 Diverticulosis of small intestine without perforation or abscess with bleeding

     K57.12 Diverticulitis of small intestine without perforation or abscess without bleeding

     K57.13 Diverticulitis of small intestine without perforation or abscess with bleeding

✓5th **K57.2 Diverticulitis of large intestine with perforation and abscess**
Diverticulitis of colon with peritonitis
EXCLUDES 1 *diverticulitis of both small and large intestine with perforation and abscess (K57.4-)*

     K57.20 Diverticulitis of large intestine with perforation and abscess without bleeding

     K57.21 Diverticulitis of large intestine with perforation and abscess with bleeding

✓5th **K57.3 Diverticular disease of large intestine without perforation or abscess**
EXCLUDES 1 *diverticular disease of both small and large intestine without perforation or abscess (K57.5-)*

     K57.30 Diverticulosis of large intestine without perforation or abscess without bleeding
         Diverticular disease of colon NOS

     K57.31 Diverticulosis of large intestine without perforation or abscess with bleeding

     K57.32 Diverticulitis of large intestine without perforation or abscess without bleeding

     K57.33 Diverticulitis of large intestine without perforation or abscess with bleeding

✓5th **K57.4 Diverticulitis of both small and large intestine with perforation and abscess**
Diverticulitis of both small and large intestine with peritonitis

     K57.40 Diverticulitis of both small and large intestine with perforation and abscess without bleeding

     K57.41 Diverticulitis of both small and large intestine with perforation and abscess with bleeding

✓5th **K57.5 Diverticular disease of both small and large intestine without perforation or abscess**

     K57.50 Diverticulosis of both small and large intestine without perforation or abscess without bleeding
         Diverticular disease of both small and large intestine NOS

     K57.51 Diverticulosis of both small and large intestine without perforation or abscess with bleeding

     K57.52 Diverticulitis of both small and large intestine without perforation or abscess without bleeding

     K57.53 Diverticulitis of both small and large intestine without perforation or abscess with bleeding

✓5th **K57.8 Diverticulitis of intestine, part unspecified, with perforation and abscess**
Diverticulitis of intestine NOS with peritonitis

     K57.80 Diverticulitis of intestine, part unspecified, with perforation and abscess without bleeding

     K57.81 Diverticulitis of intestine, part unspecified, with perforation and abscess with bleeding

✓5th **K57.9 Diverticular disease of intestine, part unspecified, without perforation or abscess**

     K57.90 Diverticulosis of intestine, part unspecified, without perforation or abscess without bleeding
         Diverticular disease of intestine NOS

     K57.91 Diverticulosis of intestine, part unspecified, without perforation or abscess with bleeding

     K57.92 Diverticulitis of intestine, part unspecified, without perforation or abscess without bleeding

     K57.93 Diverticulitis of intestine, part unspecified, without perforation or abscess with bleeding

✓4th **K58 Irritable bowel syndrome**
INCLUDES irritable colon
           spastic colon

K58.0 Irritable bowel syndrome with diarrhea

K58.9 Irritable bowel syndrome without diarrhea
Irritable bowel syndrome NOS

✓4th **K59 Other functional intestinal disorders**
EXCLUDES 1 *change in bowel habit NOS (R19.4)*
intestinal malabsorption (K90.-)
psychogenic intestinal disorders (F45.8)
EXCLUDES 2 *functional disorders of stomach (K31.-)*

✓5th **K59.0 Constipation**
EXCLUDES 1 *fecal impaction (K56.41)*
incomplete defecation (R15.0)

     K59.00 Constipation, unspecified
     K59.01 Slow transit constipation
     K59.02 Outlet dysfunction constipation
     K59.09 Other constipation

K59.1 Functional diarrhea
EXCLUDES 1 *diarrhea NOS (R19.7)*
irritable bowel syndrome with diarrhea (K58.0)

K59.2 Neurogenic bowel, not elsewhere classified

K59.3 Megacolon, not elsewhere classified
Dilatation of colon
Toxic megacolon
Code first (T51-T65) to identify toxic agent
EXCLUDES 1 *congenital megacolon (aganglionic) (Q43.1)*
megacolon (due to) (in) Chagas' disease (B57.32)
megacolon (due to) (in) Clostridium difficile (A04.7)
megacolon (due to) (in) Hirschsprung's disease (Q43.1)

K59.4 Anal spasm
Proctalgia fugax

EXCLUDES 1 Not coded here   *EXCLUDES 2* Not included here   N Newborn Age: 0   P Pediatric Age: 0-17   M Maternity Age: 12-55   A Adult Age: 15-124

622   ICD-10-CM 2014 (Draft)

K59.8 Other specified functional intestinal disorders
  Atony of colon
  Pseudo-obstruction (acute) (chronic) of intestine

K59.9 Functional intestinal disorder, unspecified

✓4ᵗʰ **K60 Fissure and fistula of anal and rectal regions**
  EXCLUDES 1 *fissure and fistula of anal and rectal regions with abscess or*
        cellulitis (K61.-)
  EXCLUDES 2 *anal sphincter tear (healed) (nontraumatic) (old) (K62.81)*

K60.0 Acute anal fissure

K60.1 Chronic anal fissure

K60.2 Anal fissure, unspecified

K60.3 Anal fistula

K60.4 Rectal fistula
  Fistula of rectum to skin
  EXCLUDES 1 *rectovaginal fistula (N82.3)*
        vesicorectal fistual (N32.1)

K60.5 Anorectal fistula

✓4ᵗʰ **K61 Abscess of anal and rectal regions**
  INCLUDES abscess of anal and rectal regions
        cellulitis of anal and rectal regions

K61.0 Anal abscess
  Perianal abscess
  EXCLUDES 1 *intrasphincteric abscess (K61.4)*

K61.1 Rectal abscess
  Perirectal abscess
  EXCLUDES 1 *ischiorectal abscess (K61.3)*
  AHA: 2012, Q4, 104

K61.2 Anorectal abscess

K61.3 Ischiorectal abscess
  Abscess of ischiorectal fossa

K61.4 Intrasphincteric abscess

✓4ᵗʰ **K62 Other diseases of anus and rectum**
  INCLUDES anal canal
  EXCLUDES 2 *colostomy and enterostomy malfunction (K94.0-, K94.1-)*
        fecal incontinence (R15.-)
        hemorrhoids (K64.-)

K62.0 Anal polyp

K62.1 Rectal polyp
  EXCLUDES 1 *adenomatous polyp (D12.8)*

K62.2 Anal prolapse
  Prolapse of anal canal

K62.3 Rectal prolapse
  Prolapse of rectal mucosa

K62.4 Stenosis of anus and rectum
  Stricture of anus (sphincter)

K62.5 Hemorrhage of anus and rectum
  EXCLUDES 1 *gastrointestinal bleeding NOS (K92.2)*
        melena (K92.1)
        neonatal rectal hemorrhage (P54.2)

K62.6 Ulcer of anus and rectum
  Solitary ulcer of anus and rectum
  Stercoral ulcer of anus and rectum
  EXCLUDES 1 *fissure and fistula of anus and rectum (K60.-)*
        ulcerative colitis (K51.-)

K62.7 Radiation proctitis
  Use additional code to identify the type of radiation (W90.-)

✓5ᵗʰ **K62.8 Other specified diseases of anus and rectum**
  EXCLUDES 2 *ulcerative proctitis (K51.2)*

  K62.81 Anal sphincter tear (healed) (nontraumatic) (old)
    Tear of anus, nontraumatic
    Use additional code for any associated fecal
        incontinence (R15.-)
    EXCLUDES 2 *anal fissure (K60.-)*
          anal sphincter tear (healed) (old)
            complicating delivery (O34.7-)
          traumatic tear of anal sphincter (S31.831)

K62.82 Dysplasia of anus
  Anal intraepithelial neoplasia I and II (AIN I and II)
      (histologically confirmed)
  Dysplasia of anus NOS
  Mild and moderate dysplasia of anus (histologically
      confirmed)
  EXCLUDES 1 *abnormal results from anal cytologic*
        examination without histologic
        confirmation (R85.61-)
        anal intraepithelial neoplasia III (D01.3)
        carcinoma in situ of anus (D01.3)
        HGSIL of anus (R85.613)
        severe dysplasia of anus (D01.3)

K62.89 Other specified diseases of anus and rectum
  Proctitis NOS
  Use additional code for any associated fecal
      incontinence (R15.-)

K62.9 Disease of anus and rectum, unspecified

✓4ᵗʰ **K63 Other diseases of intestine**

K63.0 Abscess of intestine
  EXCLUDES 1 *abscess of intestine with Crohn's disease (K50.014,*
        K50.114, K50.814, K50.914)
        abscess of intestine with diverticular disease (K57.0,
        K57.2, K57.4, K57.8)
        abscess of intestine with ulcerative colitis (K51.014,
        K51.214, K51.314, K51.414, K51.514, K51.814,
        K51.914)
  EXCLUDES 2 *abscess of anal and rectal regions (K61.-)*
        abscess of appendix (K35.3)

K63.1 Perforation of intestine (nontraumatic)
  Perforation (nontraumatic) of rectum
  EXCLUDES 1 *perforation (nontraumatic) of duodenum (K26.-)*
        perforation (nontraumatic) of intestine with
        diverticular disease (K57.0, K57.2, K57.4, K57.8)
  EXCLUDES 2 *perforation (nontraumatic) of appendix (K35.2, K35.3)*

K63.2 Fistula of intestine
  EXCLUDES 1 *fistula of duodenum (K31.6)*
        fistula of intestine with Crohn's disease (K50.013,
        K50.113, K50.813, K50.913)
        fistula of intestine with ulcerative colitis (K51.013,
        K51.213, K51.313, K51.413, K51.513, K51.813,
        K51.913)
  EXCLUDES 2 *fistula of anal and rectal regions (K60.-)*
        fistula of appendix (K38.3)
        intestinal-genital fistula, female (N82.2-N82.4)
        vesicointestinal fistula (N32.1)

K63.3 Ulcer of intestine
  Primary ulcer of small intestine
  EXCLUDES 1 *duodenal ulcer (K26.-)*
        gastrointestinal ulcer (K28.-)
        gastrojejunal ulcer (K28.-)
        jejunal ulcer (K28.-)
        peptic ulcer, site unspecified (K27.-)
        ulcer of intestine with perforation (K63.1)
        ulcer of anus or rectum (K62.6)
        ulcerative colitis (K51.-)

K63.4 Enteroptosis

K63.5 Polyp of colon
  EXCLUDES 1 *adenomatous polyp of colon (D12.6)*
        inflammatory polyp of colon (K51.4-)
        polyposis of colon (D12.6)

✓5ᵗʰ **K63.8 Other specified diseases of intestine**

  K63.81 Dieulafoy lesion of intestine
    EXCLUDES 2 *Dieulafoy lesion of stomach and duodenum*
          (K31.82)

  K63.89 Other specified diseases of intestine

K63.9 Disease of intestine, unspecified

✓4ᵗʰ **K64 Hemorrhoids and perianal venous thrombosis**
  INCLUDES piles
  EXCLUDES 1 *hemorrhoids complicating childbirth and the puerperium*
        (O87.2)
        hemorrhoids complicating pregnancy (O22.4)

K64.0 First degree hemorrhoids
  Grade/stage I hemorrhoids
  Hemorrhoids (bleeding) without prolapse outside of anal canal

K64.1 Second degree hemorrhoids
  Grade/stage II hemorrhoids
  Hemorrhoids (bleeding) that prolapse with straining, but retract
      spontaneously

☑ Additional Character Required   ᵛˣ⁷ᵗʰ Xtension Alert   Unspecified Code   Other Specified Code   Manifestation Code   ▶◀ Revised Text   ● New Code   ▲ Revised Code Title

ICD-10-CM 2014 (Draft)   **623**

Diseases of the Digestive System

K64.2–K71.3

K64.2 Third degree **hemorrhoids**
Grade/stage III hemorrhoids
Hemorrhoids (bleeding) that prolapse with straining and require manual replacement back inside anal canal

K64.3 Fourth degree **hemorrhoids**
Grade/stage IV hemorrhoids
Hemorrhoids (bleeding) with prolapsed tissue that cannot be manually replaced

K64.4 Residual **hemorrhoidal skin tags**
External hemorrhoids, NOS
Skin tags of anus

K64.5 Perianal venous thrombosis
External hemorrhoids with thrombosis
Perianal hematoma
Thrombosed hemorrhoids NOS

K64.8 Other hemorrhoids
Internal hemorrhoids, without mention of degree
Prolapsed hemorrhoids, degree not specified

K64.9 Unspecified hemorrhoids
Hemorrhoids (bleeding) NOS
Hemorrhoids (bleeding) without mention of degree

Diseases of peritoneum and retroperitoneum (K65–K68)

✓4ᵗʰ K65 Peritonitis
Use additional code (B95-B97), to identify infectious agent
EXCLUDES 1   *acute appendicitis with generalized peritonitis (K35.2)*
aseptic peritonitis (T81.6)
benign paroxysmal peritonitis (E85.0)
chemical peritonitis (T81.6)
diverticulitis of both small and large intestine with peritonitis (K57.4-)
diverticulitis of colon with peritonitis (K57.2-)
diverticulitis of intestine, NOS, with peritonitis (K57.8-)
diverticulitis of small intestine with peritonitis (K57.0-)
gonococcal peritonitis (A54.85)
neonatal peritonitis (P78.0-P78.1)
pelvic peritonitis, female (N73.3-N73.5)
periodic familial peritonitis (E85.0)
peritonitis due to talc or other foreign substance (T81.6)
peritonitis in chlamydia (A74.81)
peritonitis in diphtheria (A36.89)
peritonitis in syphilis (late) (A52.74)
peritonitis in tuberculosis (A18.31)
peritonitis with or following abortion or ectopic or molar pregnancy (O00-O07, O08.0)
peritonitis with or following appendicitis (K35.-)
peritonitis with or following diverticular disease of intestine (K57.-)
puerperal peritonitis (O85)
retroperitoneal infections (K68.-)

K65.0 Generalized (acute) peritonitis
Pelvic peritonitis (acute), male
Subphrenic peritonitis (acute)
Suppurative peritonitis (acute)

K65.1 Peritoneal **abscess**
Abdominopelvic abscess   Subdiaphragmatic abscess
Abscess (of) omentum   Subhepatic abscess
Abscess (of) peritoneum   Subphrenic abscess
Mesenteric abscess
Retrocecal abscess

K65.2 Spontaneous bacterial **peritonitis**
EXCLUDES 1   *bacterial peritonitis NOS (K65.9)*

K65.3 Choleperitonitis
Peritonitis due to bile

K65.4 Sclerosing mesenteritis
Fat necrosis of peritoneum
(Idiopathic) sclerosing mesenteric fibrosis
Mesenteric lipodystrophy
Mesenteric panniculitis
Retractile mesenteritis

K65.8 Other peritonitis
Chronic proliferative peritonitis
Peritonitis due to urine

K65.9 Peritonitis, unspecified
Bacterial peritonitis NOS

✓4ᵗʰ K66 Other disorders of peritoneum
EXCLUDES 2   *ascites (R18.-)*
peritoneal effusion (chronic) (R18.8)

K66.0 Peritoneal adhesions (postprocedural) (postinfection)
Adhesions (of) abdominal (wall)   Adhesions (of) omentum
Adhesions (of) diaphragm   Adhesions (of) stomach
Adhesions (of) intestine   Adhesive bands
Adhesions (of) male pelvis   Mesenteric adhesions
EXCLUDES 1   *female pelvic adhesions [bands] (N73.6)*
peritoneal adhesions with intestinal obstruction (K56.5)

K66.1 Hemoperitoneum
EXCLUDES 1   *traumatic hemoperitoneum (S36.8-)*

K66.8 Other specified disorders of peritoneum

K66.9 Disorder of peritoneum, unspecified

K67 *Disorders of peritoneum in infectious diseases classified elsewhere*
Code first underlying disease, such as :
congenital syphilis (A50.0)
helminthiasis (B65.0-B83.9)
EXCLUDES 1   *peritonitis in chlamydia (A74.81)*
peritonitis in diphtheria (A36.89)
peritonitis in gonococcal (A54.85)
peritonitis in syphilis (late) (A52.74)
peritonitis in tuberculosis (A18.31)

✓4ᵗʰ K68 Disorders of retroperitoneum

✓5ᵗʰ K68.1 Retroperitoneal abscess

K68.11 Postprocedural **retroperitoneal abscess**

K68.12 Psoas muscle **abscess**

K68.19 Other **retroperitoneal abscess**

K68.9 Other disorders of retroperitoneum

Diseases of liver (K70–K77)

EXCLUDES 1   *jaundice NOS (R17)*
EXCLUDES 2   *hemochromatosis (E83.11-)*
Reye's syndrome (G93.7)
vira lhepatitis (B15-B19)
Wilson's disease (E83.0)

✓4ᵗʰ K70 Alcoholic liver disease
Use additional code to identify:
alcohol abuse and dependence (F10.-)

K70.0 Alcoholic **fatty liver**   A

✓5ᵗʰ K70.1 Alcoholic **hepatitis**

K70.10 Alcoholic hepatitis **without ascites**   A

K70.11 Alcoholic hepatitis **with ascites**   A

K70.2 Alcoholic **fibrosis and sclerosis of liver**   A

✓5ᵗʰ K70.3 Alcoholic **cirrhosis of liver**
Alcoholic cirrhosis NOS

K70.30 Alcoholic cirrhosis of liver **without ascites**   A

K70.31 Alcoholic cirrhosis of liver **with ascites**   A

✓5ᵗʰ K70.4 Alcoholic **hepatic failure**
Acute alcoholic hepatic failure
Alcoholic hepatic failure NOS
Chronic alcoholic hepatic failure
Subacute alcoholic hepatic failure

K70.40 Alcoholic hepatic failure **without coma**   A

K70.41 Alcoholic hepatic failure **with coma**   A

K70.9 Alcoholic liver disease, unspecified   A

✓4ᵗʰ K71 Toxic liver disease
INCLUDES   drug-induced idiosyncratic (unpredictable) liver disease
drug-induced toxic (predictable) liver disease
Code first poisoning due to drug or toxin, if applicable (T36-T65 with fifth or sixth character 1-4 or 6)
Use additional code for adverse effect, if applicable, to identify drug (T36-T50 with fifth or sixth character 5)
EXCLUDES 2   *alcoholic liver disease (K70.-)*
Budd-Chiari syndrome (I82.0)

K71.0 Toxic liver disease with **cholestasis**
Cholestasis with hepatocyte injury
"Pure" cholestasis

✓5ᵗʰ K71.1 Toxic liver disease with **hepatic necrosis**
Hepatic failure (acute) (chronic) due to drugs

K71.10 Toxic liver disease with hepatic necrosis, **without coma**

K71.11 Toxic liver disease with hepatic necrosis, **with coma**

K71.2 Toxic liver disease with **acute hepatitis**

K71.3 Toxic liver disease with **chronic persistent hepatitis**

EXCLUDES 1 Not coded here   EXCLUDES 2 Not included here   N Newborn Age: 0   P Pediatric Age: 0-17   M Maternity Age: 12-55   A Adult Age: 15-124

624   ICD-10-CM 2014 (Draft)

K71.4   **Toxic liver disease with** chronic lobular hepatitis

✓5ᵗʰ **K71.5**   **Toxic liver disease with** chronic active hepatitis
           Toxic liver disease with lupoid hepatitis

      K71.50   **Toxic liver disease with chronic active hepatitis** without ascites

      K71.51   **Toxic liver disease with chronic active hepatitis** with ascites

K71.6   **Toxic liver disease with** hepatitis, not elsewhere classified

K71.7   **Toxic liver disease with** fibrosis and cirrhosis **of liver**

K71.8   Toxic liver disease with other disorders of liver
           Toxic liver disease with focal nodular hyperplasia
           Toxic liver disease with hepatic granulomas
           Toxic liver disease with peliosis hepatis
           Toxic liver disease with veno-occlusive disease of liver

K71.9   **Toxic liver disease, unspecified**

✓4ᵗʰ **K72**   **Hepatic failure, not elsewhere classified**
     INCLUDES   acute hepatitis NEC, with hepatic failure
           fulminant hepatitis NEC, with hepatic failure
           hepatic encephalopathy NOS
           liver (cell) necrosis with hepatic failure
           malignant hepatitis NEC, with hepatic failure
           yellow liver atrophy or dystrophy
     EXCLUDES 1   alcoholic hepatic failure (K70.4)
           hepatic failure with toxic liver disease (K71.1-)
           icterus of newborn (P55-P59)
           postprocedural hepatic failure (K91.82)
           viral hepatitis with hepatic coma (B15-B19)
     EXCLUDES 2   hepatic failure complicating abortion or ectopic or molar pregnancy (O00-O07, O08.8)
           hepatic failure complicating pregnancy, childbirth and the puerperium (O26.6-)

✓5ᵗʰ **K72.0**   **Acute and subacute** hepatic failure

      K72.00   **Acute and subacute hepatic failure** without coma

      K72.01   **Acute and subacute hepatic failure** with coma

✓5ᵗʰ **K72.1**   **Chronic** hepatic failure

      K72.10   **Chronic hepatic failure** without coma

      K72.11   **Chronic hepatic failure** with coma

✓5ᵗʰ **K72.9**   **Hepatic failure,** unspecified

      K72.90   **Hepatic failure, unspecified** without coma

      K72.91   **Hepatic failure, unspecified** with coma
           Hepatic coma NOS

✓4ᵗʰ **K73**   **Chronic hepatitis, not elsewhere classified**
     EXCLUDES 1   alcoholic hepatitis (chronic) (K70.1-)
           drug-induced hepatitis (chronic) (K71.-)
           granulomatous hepatitis (chronic) NEC (K75.3)
           reactive, nonspecific hepatitis (chronic) (K75.2)
           viral hepatitis (chronic) (B15-B19)

K73.0   **Chronic** persistent **hepatitis, not elsewhere classified**

K73.1   **Chronic** lobular **hepatitis, not elsewhere classified**

K73.2   **Chronic** active **hepatitis, not elsewhere classified**

K73.8   **Other chronic hepatitis, not elsewhere classified**

K73.9   **Chronic hepatitis, unspecified**

✓4ᵗʰ **K74**   **Fibrosis and cirrhosis of liver**
     Code also, if applicable, viral hepatitis (acute) (chronic) (B15-B19)
     EXCLUDES 1   alcoholic cirrhosis (of liver) (K70.3)
           alcoholic fibrosis of liver (K70.2)
           cardiac sclerosis of liver (K76.1)
           cirrhosis (of liver) with toxic liver disease (K71.7)
           congenital cirrhosis (of liver) (P78.81)
           pigmentary cirrhosis (of liver) (E83.110)

K74.0   **Hepatic** fibrosis

K74.1   **Hepatic** sclerosis

K74.2   **Hepatic** fibrosis with hepatic sclerosis

K74.3   Primary **biliary cirrhosis**
           Chronic nonsuppurative destructive cholangitis

K74.4   Secondary **biliary cirrhosis**

K74.5   **Biliary cirrhosis, unspecified**

✓5ᵗʰ **K74.6**   **Other and unspecified cirrhosis of liver**

      K74.60   **Unspecified cirrhosis of liver**
           Cirrhosis (of liver) NOS

      K74.69   Other cirrhosis of liver
           Cryptogenic cirrhosis (of liver)
           Macronodular cirrhosis (of liver)
           Micronodular cirrhosis (of liver)
           Mixed type cirrhosis (of liver)
           Portal cirrhosis (of liver)
           Postnecrotic cirrhosis (of liver)

✓4ᵗʰ **K75**   **Other inflammatory liver diseases**
     EXCLUDES 2   toxic liver disease (K71.-)

K75.0   **Abscess of liver**
           Cholangitic hepatic abscess
           Hematogenic hepatic abscess
           Hepatic abscess NOS
           Lymphogenic hepatic abscess
           Pylephlebitic hepatic abscess
     EXCLUDES 1   amebic liver abscess (A06.4)
           cholangitis without liver abscess (K83.0)
           pylephlebitis without liver abscess (K75.1)

K75.1   **Phlebitis of portal vein**
           Pylephlebitis
     EXCLUDES 1   pylephlebitic liver abscess (K75.0)

K75.2   **Nonspecific reactive hepatitis**
     EXCLUDES 1   acute or subacute hepatitis (K72.0-)
           chronic hepatitis NEC (K73.-)
           viral hepatitis (B15-B19)

K75.3   **Granulomatous hepatitis, not elsewhere classified**
     EXCLUDES 1   acute or subacute hepatitis (K72.0-)
           chronic hepatitis NEC (K73.-)
           viral hepatitis (B15-B19)

K75.4   **Autoimmune hepatitis**
           Lupoid hepatitis NEC

✓5ᵗʰ **K75.8**   **Other specified inflammatory liver diseases**

      K75.81   **Nonalcoholic steatohepatitis (NASH)**

      K75.89   **Other specified inflammatory liver diseases**

K75.9   **Inflammatory liver disease, unspecified**
           Hepatitis NOS
     EXCLUDES 1   acute or subacute hepatitis (K72.0-)
           chronic hepatitis NEC (K73.-)
           viral hepatitis (B15-B19)

✓4ᵗʰ **K76**   **Other diseases of liver**
     EXCLUDES 2   alcoholic liver disease (K70.-)
           amyloid degeneration of liver (E85.-)
           cystic disease of liver (congenital) (Q44.6)
           hepatic vein thrombosis (I82.0)
           hepatomegaly NOS (R16.0)
           pigmentary cirrhosis (of liver) (E83.110)
           portal vein thrombosis (I81)
           toxic liver disease (K71.-)

K76.0   **Fatty (change of) liver, not elsewhere classified**
           Nonalcoholic fatty liver disease (NAFLD)
     EXCLUDES 1   nonalcoholic steatohepatitis (NASH) (K75.81)

K76.1   **Chronic passive congestion of liver**
           Cardiac cirrhosis
           Cardiac sclerosis

K76.2   **Central hemorrhagic necrosis of liver**
     EXCLUDES 1   liver necrosis with hepatic failure (K72.-)

K76.3   **Infarction of liver**

K76.4   **Peliosis hepatis**
           Hepatic angiomatosis

K76.5   **Hepatic veno-occlusive disease**
     EXCLUDES 1   Budd-Chiari syndrome (I82.0)

K76.6   **Portal hypertension**
     Use additional code for any associated complications, such as:
           portal hypertensive gastropathy (K31.89)

K76.7   **Hepatorenal syndrome**
     EXCLUDES 1   hepatorenal syndrome following labor and delivery (O90.4)
           postprocedural hepatorenal syndrome (K91.82)

✓5ᵗʰ **K76.8**   **Other specified diseases of liver**

      K76.81   **Hepatopulmonary syndrome**
           Code first underlying liver disease, such as:
             alcoholic cirrhosis of liver (K70.3-)
             cirrhosis of liver without mention of alcohol (K74.6-)

      K76.89   **Other specified diseases of liver**
           Cyst (simple) of liver
           Focal nodular hyperplasia of liver
           Hepatoptosis

K76.9   **Liver disease, unspecified**

☑ Additional Character Required   ᴠˣ⁷ᵗʰ Xtension Alert   **Unspecified Code**   Other Specified Code   Manifestation Code   ►◄ Revised Text   ● New Code   ▲ Revised Code Title

Diseases of the Digestive System

K77–K82.3

K77 Liver disorders in diseases classified elsewhere

Code first underlying disease, such as:
amyloidosis (E85.-)
congenital syphilis (A50.0, A50.5)
congenital toxoplasmosis (P37.1)
schistosomiasis (B65.0-B65.9)

EXCLUDES 1   alcoholic hepatitis (K70.1-)
alcoholic liver disease (K70-.)
cytomegaloviral hepatitis (B25.1)
herpesviral [herpes simplex] hepatitis (B00.81)
infectious mononucleosis with liver disease
(B27.0-B27.9 with .9)
mumps hepatitis (B26.81)
sarcoidosis with liver disease (D86.89)
secondary syphilis with liver disease (A51.45)
syphilis (late) with liver disease (A52.74)
toxoplasmosis (acquired) hepatitis (B58.1)
tuberculosis with liver disease (A18.83)

Disorders of gallbladder, biliary tract and pancreas (K80-K87)

✓4th K80 Cholelithiasis

EXCLUDES 1   retained cholelithiasis following cholecystectomy (K91.86)

✓5th K80.0 Calculus of gallbladder with acute cholecystitis
Any condition listed in K80.2 with acute cholecystitis

K80.00 Calculus of gallbladder with acute cholecystitis without obstruction

K80.01 Calculus of gallbladder with acute cholecystitis with obstruction

✓5th K80.1 Calculus of gallbladder with other cholecystitis

K80.10 Calculus of gallbladder with chronic cholecystitis without obstruction
Cholelithiasis with cholecystitis NOS

K80.11 Calculus of gallbladder with chronic cholecystitis with obstruction

K80.12 Calculus of gallbladder with acute and chronic cholecystitis without obstruction

K80.13 Calculus of gallbladder with acute and chronic cholecystitis with obstruction

K80.18 Calculus of gallbladder with other cholecystitis without obstruction

K80.19 Calculus of gallbladder with other cholecystitis with obstruction

✓5th K80.2 Calculus of gallbladder without cholecystitis
Cholecystolithiasis without cholecystitis
Cholelithiasis (without cholecystitis)
Colic (recurrent) of gallbladder (without cholecystitis)
Gallstone (impacted) of cystic duct (without cholecystitis)
Gallstone (impacted) of gallbladder (without cholecystitis)

K80.20 Calculus of gallbladder without cholecystitis without obstruction

K80.21 Calculus of gallbladder without cholecystitis with obstruction

✓5th K80.3 Calculus of bile duct with cholangitis
Any condition listed in K80.5 with cholangitis

K80.30 Calculus of bile duct with cholangitis, unspecified, without obstruction

K80.31 Calculus of bile duct with cholangitis, unspecified, with obstruction

K80.32 Calculus of bile duct with acute cholangitis without obstruction

K80.33 Calculus of bile duct with acute cholangitis with obstruction

K80.34 Calculus of bile duct with chronic cholangitis without obstruction

K80.35 Calculus of bile duct with chronic cholangitis with obstruction

K80.36 Calculus of bile duct with acute and chronic cholangitis without obstruction

K80.37 Calculus of bile duct with acute and chronic cholangitis with obstruction

✓5th K80.4 Calculus of bile duct with cholecystitis
Any condition listed in K80.5 with cholecystitis (with cholangitis)

K80.40 Calculus of bile duct with cholecystitis, unspecified, without obstruction

K80.41 Calculus of bile duct with cholecystitis, unspecified, with obstruction

K80.42 Calculus of bile duct with acute cholecystitis without obstruction

K80.43 Calculus of bile duct with acute cholecystitis with obstruction

K80.44 Calculus of bile duct with chronic cholecystitis without obstruction

K80.45 Calculus of bile duct with chronic cholecystitis with obstruction

K80.46 Calculus of bile duct with acute and chronic cholecystitis without obstruction

K80.47 Calculus of bile duct with acute and chronic cholecystitis with obstruction

✓5th K80.5 Calculus of bile duct without cholangitis or cholecystitis
Choledocholithiasis (without cholangitis or cholecystitis)
Gallstone (impacted) of bile duct NOS (without cholangitis or cholecystitis)
Gallstone (impacted) of common duct (without cholangitis or cholecystitis)
Gallstone (impacted) of hepatic duct (without cholangitis or cholecystitis)
Hepatic cholelithiasis (without cholangitis or cholecystitis)
Hepatic colic (recurrent) (without cholangitis or cholecystitis)

K80.50 Calculus of bile duct without cholangitis or cholecystitis without obstruction

K80.51 Calculus of bile duct without cholangitis or cholecystitis with obstruction

✓5th K80.6 Calculus of gallbladder and bile duct with cholecystitis

K80.60 Calculus of gallbladder and bile duct with cholecystitis, unspecified, without obstruction

K80.61 Calculus of gallbladder and bile duct with cholecystitis, unspecified, with obstruction

K80.62 Calculus of gallbladder and bile duct with acute cholecystitis without obstruction

K80.63 Calculus of gallbladder and bile duct with acute cholecystitis with obstruction

K80.64 Calculus of gallbladder and bile duct with chronic cholecystitis without obstruction

K80.65 Calculus of gallbladder and bile duct with chronic cholecystitis with obstruction

K80.66 Calculus of gallbladder and bile duct with acute and chronic cholecystitis without obstruction

K80.67 Calculus of gallbladder and bile duct with acute and chronic cholecystitis with obstruction

✓5th K80.7 Calculus of gallbladder and bile duct without cholecystitis

K80.70 Calculus of gallbladder and bile duct without cholecystitis without obstruction

K80.71 Calculus of gallbladder and bile duct without cholecystitis with obstruction

✓5th K80.8 Other cholelithiasis

K80.80 Other cholelithiasis without obstruction

K80.81 Other cholelithiasis with obstruction

✓4th K81 Cholecystitis

EXCLUDES 1   cholecystitis with cholelithiasis (K80.-)

K81.0 Acute cholecystitis
Abscess of gallbladder
Angiocholecystitis
Emphysematous (acute) cholecystitis
Empyema of gallbladder
Gangrene of gallbladder
Gangrenous cholecystitis
Suppurative cholecystitis

K81.1 Chronic cholecystitis

K81.2 Acute cholecystitis with chronic cholecystitis

K81.9 Cholecystitis, unspecified

✓4th K82 Other diseases of gallbladder

EXCLUDES 1   nonvisualization of gallbladder (R93.2)
postcholecystectomy syndrome (K91.5)

K82.0 Obstruction of gallbladder
Occlusion of cystic duct or gallbladder without cholelithiasis
Stenosis of cystic duct or gallbladder without cholelithiasis
Stricture of cystic duct or gallbladder without cholelithiasis
EXCLUDES 1   obstruction of gallbladder with cholelithiasis (K80.-)

K82.1 Hydrops of gallbladder
Mucocele of gallbladder

K82.2 Perforation of gallbladder
Rupture of cystic duct or gallbladder

K82.3 Fistula of gallbladder
Cholecystocolic fistula
Cholecystoduodenal fistula

EXCLUDES 1 Not coded here   **EXCLUDES 2** Not included here   N Newborn Age: 0   P Pediatric Age: 0-17   M Maternity Age: 12-55   A Adult Age: 15-124

626   ICD-10-CM 2014 (Draft)

K82.4 Cholesterolosis of gallbladder
Strawberry gallbladder
EXCLUDES 1 *cholesterolosis of gallbladder with cholecystitis (K81.-)*
cholesterolosis of gallbladder with cholelithiasis (K80.-)

K82.8 Other specified diseases of gallbladder
Adhesions of cystic duct or gallbladder
Atrophy of cystic duct or gallbladder
Cyst of cystic duct or gallbladder
Dyskinesia of cystic duct or gallbladder
Hypertrophy of cystic duct or gallbladder
Nonfunctioning of cystic duct or gallbladder
Ulcer of cystic duct or gallbladder

K82.9 Disease of gallbladder, unspecified

✓4ᵗʰ **K83 Other diseases of biliary tract**
EXCLUDES 1 *postcholecystectomy syndrome (K91.5)*
EXCLUDES 2 *conditions involving the gallbladder (K81-K82)*
conditions involving the cystic duct (K81-K82)

K83.0 Cholangitis
Ascending cholangitis
Cholangitis NOS
Primary cholangitis
Recurrent cholangitis
Sclerosing cholangitis
Secondary cholangitis
Stenosing cholangitis
Suppurative cholangitis
EXCLUDES 1 *cholangitic liver abscess (K75.0)*
cholangitis with choledocholithiasis (K80.3-, K80.4-)
chronic nonsuppurative destructive cholangitis (K74.3)

K83.1 Obstruction of bile duct
Occlusion of bile duct without cholelithiasis
Stenosis of bile duct without cholelithiasis
Stricture of bile duct without cholelithiasis
EXCLUDES 1 *congenital obstruction of bile duct (Q44.3)*
obstruction of bile duct with cholelithiasis (K80.-)

K83.2 Perforation of bile duct
Rupture of bile duct

K83.3 Fistula of bile duct
Choledochoduodenal fistula

K83.4 Spasm of sphincter of Oddi

K83.5 Biliary cyst

K83.8 Other specified diseases of biliary tract
Adhesions of biliary tract
Atrophy of biliary tract
Hypertrophy of biliary tract
Ulcer of biliary tract

K83.9 Disease of biliary tract, unspecified

✓4ᵗʰ **K85 Acute pancreatitis**
Abscess of pancreas
Acute necrosis of pancreas
Acute (recurrent) pancreatitis
Gangrene of (gangrenous) pancreas
Hemorrhagic pancreatitis
Infective necrosis of pancreas
Subacute pancreatitis
Suppurative pancreatitis

K85.0 Idiopathic acute pancreatitis

K85.1 Biliary acute pancreatitis
Gallstone pancreatitis

K85.2 Alcohol induced acute pancreatitis
EXCLUDES 2 *alcohol induced chronic pancreatitis (K86.0)*

K85.3 Drug induced acute pancreatitis
Use additional code for adverse effect, if applicable, to identify drug (T36-T50 with fifth or sixth character 5)
Use additional code to identify drug abuse and dependence (F11.-F17.-)

K85.8 Other acute pancreatitis

K85.9 Acute pancreatitis, unspecified
Pancreatitis NOS

✓4ᵗʰ **K86 Other diseases of pancreas**
EXCLUDES 2 *fibrocystic disease of pancreas (E84.-)*
islet cell tumor (of pancreas) (D13.7)
pancreatic steatorrhea (K90.3)

K86.0 Alcohol-induced chronic pancreatitis
Use additional code to identify:
alcohol abuse and dependence (F10.-)
EXCLUDES 2 *alcohol induced acute pancreatitis (K85.2)*

K86.1 Other chronic pancreatitis
Chronic pancreatitis NOS
Infectious chronic pancreatitis
Recurrent chronic pancreatitis
Relapsing chronic pancreatitis

K86.2 Cyst of pancreas

K86.3 Pseudocyst of pancreas

K86.8 Other specified diseases of pancreas
Aseptic pancreatic necrosis
Atrophy of pancreas
Calculus of pancreas
Cirrhosis of pancreas
Fibrosis of pancreas
Pancreatic fat necrosis
Pancreatic infantilism
Pancreatic necrosis NOS

K86.9 Disease of pancreas, unspecified

K87 *Disorders of gallbladder, biliary tract and pancreas in diseases classified elsewhere*
Code first underlying disease
EXCLUDES 1 *cytomegaloviral pancreatitis (B25.2)*
mumps pancreatitis (B26.3)
syphilitic gallbladder (A52.74)
syphilitic pancreas (A52.74)
tuberculosis of gallbladder (A18.83)
tuberculosis of pancreas (A18.83)

Other diseases of the digestive system (K90-K95)

✓4ᵗʰ **K90 Intestinal malabsorption**
EXCLUDES 1 *intestinal malabsorption following gastrointestinal surgery (K91.2)*

K90.0 Celiac disease
Gluten-sensitive enteropathy
Idiopathic steatorrhea
Nontropical sprue
Use additional code for associated disorders including:
dermatitis herpetiformis (L13.0)
gluten ataxia (G32.81)

K90.1 Tropical sprue
Sprue NOS
Tropical steatorrhea

K90.2 Blind loop syndrome, not elsewhere classified
Blind loop syndrome NOS
EXCLUDES 1 *congenital blind loop syndrome (Q43.8)*
postsurgical blind loop syndrome (K91.2)

K90.3 Pancreatic steatorrhea

K90.4 Malabsorption due to intolerance, not elsewhere classified
Malabsorption due to intolerance to carbohydrate
Malabsorption due to intolerance to fat
Malabsorption due to intolerance to protein
Malabsorption due to intolerance to starch
EXCLUDES 2 *gluten-sensitive enteropathy (K90.0)*
lactose intolerance (E73.-)

✓5ᵗʰ **K90.8 Other intestinal malabsorption**

K90.81 Whipple's disease

K90.89 Other intestinal malabsorption

K90.9 Intestinal malabsorption, unspecified

✓4ᵗʰ **K91 Intraoperative and postprocedural complications and disorders of digestive system, not elsewhere classified**
EXCLUDES 2 *complications of artificial opening of digestive system (K94.-)*
complications of bariatric procedures (K95.-)
gastrojejunal ulcer (K28.-)
postprocedural (radiation) retroperitoneal abscess (K68.11)
radiation colitis (K52.0)
radiation gastroenteritis (K52.0)
radiation proctitis (K62.7)

K91.0 Vomiting following gastrointestinal surgery

K91.1 Postgastric surgery syndromes
Dumping syndrome
Postgastrectomy syndrome
Postvagotomy syndrome

K91.2 Postsurgical malabsorption, not elsewhere classified
Postsurgical blind loop syndrome
EXCLUDES 1 *malabsorption osteomalacia in adults (M83.2)*
malabsorption osteoporosis, postsurgical (M80.8-, M81.8)

K91.3 Postprocedural intestinal obstruction

K91.5 Postcholecystectomy syndrome

☑ Additional Character Required   ✓x7ᵗʰ Xtension Alert   Unspecified Code   Other Specified Code   Manifestation Code   ►◄ Revised Text   ● New Code   ▲ Revised Code Title

ICD-10-CM 2014 (Draft)   **627**

✓5ᵗʰ **K91.6** Intraoperative hemorrhage and hematoma of a digestive system organ or structure complicating a procedure
- EXCLUDES 1   *intraoperative hemorrhage and hematoma of a digestive system organ or structure due to accidental puncture and laceration during a procedure (K91.7-)*
- **K91.61** Intraoperative hemorrhage and hematoma of a digestive system organ or structure complicating a digestive sytem procedure
- **K91.62** Intraoperative hemorrhage and hematoma of a digestive system organ or structure complicating other procedure

✓5ᵗʰ **K91.7** Accidental puncture and laceration of a digestive system organ or structure during a procedure
- **K91.71** Accidental puncture and laceration of a digestive system organ or structure during a digestive system procedure
- **K91.72** Accidental puncture and laceration of a digestive system organ or structure during other procedure

✓5ᵗʰ **K91.8** Other intraoperative and postprocedural complications and disorders of digestive system
- **K91.81** Other intraoperative complications of digestive system
- **K91.82** Postprocedural hepatic failure
- **K91.83** Postprocedural hepatorenal syndrome
- ✓6ᵗʰ **K91.84** Postprocedural hemorrhage and hematoma of a digestive system organ or structure following a procedure
  - **K91.84Ø** Postprocedural hemorrhage and hematoma of a digestive system organ or structure following a digestive system procedure
  - **K91.841** Postprocedural hemorrhage and hematoma of a digestive system organ or structure following other procedure
- ✓6ᵗʰ **K91.85** Complications of intestinal pouch
  - **K91.85Ø** Pouchitis
    - Inflammation of internal ileoanal pouch
  - **K91.858** Other complications of intestinal pouch
- **K91.86** Retained cholelithiasis following cholecystectomy
- **K91.89** Other postprocedural complications and disorders of digestive system
  - Use additional code, if applicable, to further specify disorder
  - EXCLUDES 2   *postprocedural retroperitoneal abscess (K68.11)*

✓4ᵗʰ **K92** Other diseases of digestive system
- EXCLUDES 1   *neonatal gastrointestinal hemorrhage (P54.Ø-P54.3)*
- **K92.Ø** Hematemesis
- **K92.1** Melena
  - EXCLUDES 1   *occult blood in feces (R19.5)*
- **K92.2** Gastrointestinal hemorrhage, unspecified
  - Gastric hemorrhage NOS
  - Intestinal hemorrhage NOS
  - EXCLUDES 1   *acute hemorrhagic gastritis (K29.Ø1)*
    hemorrhage of anus and rectum (K62.5)
    angiodysplasia of stomach with hemorrhage (K31.811)
    diverticular disease with hemorrhage (K57.-)
    gastritis and duodenitis with hemorrhage (K29.-)
    peptic ulcer with hemorrhage (K25-K28)
- ✓5ᵗʰ **K92.8** Other specified diseases of the digestive system
  - **K92.81** Gastrointestinal mucositis (ulcerative)
    - Code also type of associated therapy, such as:
      antineoplastic and immunosuppressive drugs (T45.1X-)
      radiological procedure and radiotherapy (Y84.2)
    - EXCLUDES 2   *mucositis (ulcerative) of vagina and vulva (N76.81)*
      nasal mucositis (ulcerative) (J34.81)
      oral mucositis (ulcerative) (K12.3-)
  - **K92.89** Other specified diseases of the digestive system
- **K92.9** Disease of digestive system, unspecified

✓4ᵗʰ **K94** Complications of artificial openings of the digestive system
- ✓5ᵗʰ **K94.Ø** Colostomy complications
  - **K94.ØØ** Colostomy complication, unspecified
  - **K94.Ø1** Colostomy hemorrhage
  - **K94.Ø2** Colostomy infection
    - Use additional code to specify type of infection, such as:
      cellulitis of abdominal wall (LØ3.311)
      sepsis (A4Ø, A41)
  - **K94.Ø3** Colostomy malfunction
    - Mechanical complication of colostomy
  - **K94.Ø9** Other complications of colostomy
- ✓5ᵗʰ **K94.1** Enterostomy complications
  - **K94.1Ø** Enterostomy complication, unspecified
  - **K94.11** Enterostomy hemorrhage
  - **K94.12** Enterostomy infection
    - Use additional code to specify type of infection, such as:
      cellulitis of abdominal wall (LØ3.311)
      sepsis (A4Ø-, A41-)
  - **K94.13** Enterostomy malfunction
    - Mechanical complication of enterostomy
  - **K94.19** Other complications of enterostomy
- ✓5ᵗʰ **K94.2** Gastrostomy complications
  - **K94.2Ø** Gastrostomy complication, unspecified
  - **K94.21** Gastrostomy hemorrhage
  - **K94.22** Gastrostomy infection
    - Use additional code to specify type of infection, such as:
      cellulitis of abdominal wall (LØ3.311)
      sepsis (A4Ø-, A41-)
  - **K94.23** Gastrostomy malfunction
    - Mechanical complication of gastrostomy
  - **K94.29** Other complications of gastrostomy
- ✓5ᵗʰ **K94.3** Esophagostomy complications
  - **K94.3Ø** Esophagostomy complications, unspecified
  - **K94.31** Esophagostomy hemorrhage
  - **K94.32** Esophagostomy infection
    - Use additional code to identify the infection
  - **K94.33** Esophagostomy malfunction
    - Mechanical complication of esophagostomy
  - **K94.39** Other complications of esophagostom

✓4ᵗʰ **K95** Complications of bariatric procedures
- ✓5ᵗʰ **K95.Ø** Complications of gastric band procedure
  - **K95.Ø1** Infection due to gastric band procedure
    - Use additional code to specify type of infection or organism, such as:
      bacterial and viral infectious agents (B95.-, B96.-)
      cellulitis of abdominal wall (LØ3.311)
      sepsis (A4Ø.-, A41.-)
  - **K95.Ø9** Other complications of gastric band procedure
    - Use additional code, if applicable, to further specify complication
- ✓5ᵗʰ **K95.8** Complications of other bariatric procedure
  - EXCLUDES 1   *complications of gastric band surgery (K95.Ø-)*
  - **K95.81** Infection due to other bariatric procedure
    - Use additional code to specify type of infection or organism, such as:
      bacterial and viral infectious agents (B95.-, B96.-)
      cellulitis of abdominal wall (LØ3.311)
      sepsis (A4Ø.-, A41.-)
  - **K95.89** Other complications of other bariatric procedure
    - Use additional code, if applicable, to further specify complication

EXCLUDES 1 Not coded here   EXCLUDES 2 Not included here   N Newborn Age: Ø   P Pediatric Age: Ø-17   M Maternity Age: 12-55   A Adult Age: 15-124

628   ICD-1Ø-CM 2Ø14 (Draft)

Chapter 12. Diseases of the Skin and Subcutaneous Tissue (L00-L99)

EXCLUDES 2   certain conditions originating in the perinatal period (P04-P96)
certain infectious and parasitic diseases (A00-B99)
complications of pregnancy, childbirth and the puerperium (O00-O9A)
congenital malformations, deformations, and chromosomal abnormalities (Q00-Q99)
endocrine, nutritional and metabolic diseases (E00-E88)
lipomelanotic reticulosis (I89.8)
neoplasms (C00-D49)
symptoms, signs and abnormal clinical and laboratory findings, not elsewhere classified (R00-R94)
systemic connective tissue disorders (M30-M36)
viral warts (B07.-)

This chapter contains the following blocks:

L00-L08	Infections of the skin and subcutaneous tissue
L10-L14	Bullous disorders
L20-L30	Dermatitis and eczema
L40-L45	Papulosquamous disorders
L49-L54	Urticaria and erythema
L55-L59	Radiation-related disorders of the skin and subcutaneous tissue
L60-L75	Disorders of skin appendages
L76	Intraoperative and postprocedural complications of skin and subcutaneous tissue
L80-L99	Other disorders of the skin and subcutaneous tissue

Infections of the skin and subcutaneous tissue (L00-L08)

Use additional code (B95-B97) to identify infectious agent

EXCLUDES 2   hordeolum (H00.0)
infective dermatitis (L30.3)
local infections of skin classified in Chapter 1
lupus panniculitis (L93.2)
panniculitis NOS (M79.3)
panniculitis of neck and back (M54.0-)
Perlèche NOS (K13.0)
Perlèche due to candidiasis (B37.0)
Perlèche due to riboflavin deficiency (E53.0)
pyogenic granuloma (L98.0)
relapsing panniculitis [Weber-Christian] (M35.6)
viral warts (B07.-)
zoster (B02.-)

L00   Staphylococcal scalded skin syndrome
Ritter's disease
Use additional code to identify percentage of skin exfoliation (L49.-)
EXCLUDES 1   bullous impetigo (L01.03)
pemphigus neonatorum (L01.03)
toxic epidermal necrolysis [Lyell] (L51.2)

√4th **L01   Impetigo**
EXCLUDES 1   impetigo herpetiformis (L40.1)

√5th **L01.0   Impetigo**
Impetigo contagiosa   Impetigo vulgaris

L01.00   Impetigo, unspecified
Impetigo NOS

L01.01   Non-bullous impetigo

L01.02   Bockhart's impetigo
Impetigo follicularis   Superficial pustular
Perifolliculitis NOS   perifolliculitis

L01.03   Bullous impetigo
Impetigo neonatorum   Pemphigus neonatorum

L01.09   Other impetigo
Ulcerative impetigo

L01.1   Impetiginization of other dermatoses

√4th **L02   Cutaneous abscess, furuncle and carbuncle**
Use additional code to identify organism (B95-B96)
EXCLUDES 2   abscess of anus and rectal regions (K61.-)
abscess of female genital organs (external) (N76.4)
abscess of male genital organs (external) (N48.2, N49-)

√5th **L02.0   Cutaneous abscess, furuncle and carbuncle of face**
EXCLUDES 2   abscess of ear, external (H60.0)
abscess of eyelid (H00.0)
abscess of head [any part, except face] (L02.8)
abscess of lacrimal gland (H04.0)
abscess of lacrimal passages (H04.3)
abscess of mouth (K12.2)
abscess of nose (J34.0)
abscess of orbit (H05.0)
submandibular abscess (K12.2)

L02.01   Cutaneous abscess of face

L02.02   Furuncle of face
Boil of face
Folliculitis of face

L02.03   Carbuncle of face

√5th **L02.1   Cutaneous abscess, furuncle and carbuncle of neck**

L02.11   Cutaneous abscess of neck

L02.12   Furuncle of neck
Boil of neck
Folliculitis of neck

L02.13   Carbuncle of neck

√5th **L02.2   Cutaneous abscess, furuncle and carbuncle of trunk**
EXCLUDES 1   non-newborn omphalitis (L08.82)
omphalitis of newborn (P38.-)
EXCLUDES 2   abscess of breast (N61)
abscess of buttocks (L02.3)
abscess of female external genital organs (N76.4)
abscess of hip (L02.4)
abscess of male external genital organs (N48.2, N49-)

√6th **L02.21   Cutaneous abscess of trunk**

L02.211   Cutaneous abscess of abdominal wall

L02.212   Cutaneous abscess of back [any part, except buttock]

L02.213   Cutaneous abscess of chest wall

L02.214   Cutaneous abscess of groin

L02.215   Cutaneous abscess of perineum

L02.216   Cutaneous abscess of umbilicus

L02.219   Cutaneous abscess of trunk, unspecified

√6th **L02.22   Furuncle of trunk**
Boil of trunk
Folliculitis of trunk

L02.221   Furuncle of abdominal wall

L02.222   Furuncle of back [any part, except buttock]

L02.223   Furuncle of chest wall

L02.224   Furuncle of groin

L02.225   Furuncle of perineum

L02.226   Furuncle of umbilicus

L02.229   Furuncle of trunk, unspecified

√6th **L02.23   Carbuncle of trunk**

L02.231   Carbuncle of abdominal wall

L02.232   Carbuncle of back [any part, except buttock]

L02.233   Carbuncle of chest wall

L02.234   Carbuncle of groin

L02.235   Carbuncle of perineum

L02.236   Carbuncle of umbilicus

L02.239   Carbuncle of trunk, unspecified

√5th **L02.3   Cutaneous abscess, furuncle and carbuncle of buttock**
EXCLUDES 1   pilonidal cyst with abscess (L05.01)

L02.31   Cutaneous abscess of buttock
Cutaneous abscess of gluteal region

L02.32   Furuncle of buttock
Boil of buttock
Folliculitis of buttock
Furuncle of gluteal region

L02.33   Carbuncle of buttock
Carbuncle of gluteal region

√5th **L02.4   Cutaneous abscess, furuncle and carbuncle of limb**
EXCLUDES 2   cutaneous abscess, furuncle and carbuncle of groin (L02.214, L02.224, L02.234)
cutaneous abscess, furuncle and carbuncle of hand (L02.5-)
cutaneous abscess, furuncle and carbuncle of foot (L02.6-)

√6th **L02.41   Cutaneous abscess of limb**

L02.411   Cutaneous abscess of right axilla

L02.412   Cutaneous abscess of left axilla

L02.413   Cutaneous abscess of right upper limb

L02.414   Cutaneous abscess of left upper limb

L02.415   Cutaneous abscess of right lower limb

L02.416   Cutaneous abscess of left lower limb

L02.419   Cutaneous abscess of limb, unspecified

√6th **L02.42   Furuncle of limb**
Boil of limb
Folliculitis of limb

L02.421   Furuncle of right axilla

☑ Additional Character Required   XTension Alert   Unspecified Code   Other Specified Code   Manifestation Code   ▶◀ Revised Text   ● New Code   ▲ Revised Code Title

ICD-10-CM 2014 (Draft)   629

L02.422 Furuncle of left axilla
L02.423 Furuncle of right upper limb
L02.424 Furuncle of left upper limb
L02.425 Furuncle of right lower limb
L02.426 Furuncle of left lower limb
L02.429 Furuncle of limb, unspecified

✓6th L02.43 Carbuncle of limb
L02.431 Carbuncle of right axilla
L02.432 Carbuncle of left axilla
L02.433 Carbuncle of right upper limb
L02.434 Carbuncle of left upper limb
L02.435 Carbuncle of right lower limb
L02.436 Carbuncle of left lower limb
L02.439 Carbuncle of limb, unspecified

✓5th L02.5 Cutaneous abscess, furuncle and carbuncle of hand
✓6th L02.51 Cutaneous abscess of hand
L02.511 Cutaneous abscess of right hand
L02.512 Cutaneous abscess of left hand
L02.519 Cutaneous abscess of unspecified hand

✓6th L02.52 Furuncle hand
Boil of hand
Folliculitis of hand
L02.521 Furuncle right hand
L02.522 Furuncle left hand
L02.529 Furuncle unspecified hand

✓6th L02.53 Carbuncle of hand
L02.531 Carbuncle of right hand
L02.532 Carbuncle of left hand
L02.539 Carbuncle of unspecified hand

✓5th L02.6 Cutaneous abscess, furuncle and carbuncle of foot
✓6th L02.61 Cutaneous abscess of foot
L02.611 Cutaneous abscess of right foot
L02.612 Cutaneous abscess of left foot
L02.619 Cutaneous abscess of unspecified foot

✓6th L02.62 Furuncle of foot
Boil of foot
Folliculitis of foot
L02.621 Furuncle of right foot
L02.622 Furuncle of left foot
L02.629 Furuncle of unspecified foot

✓6th L02.63 Carbuncle of foot
L02.631 Carbuncle of right foot
L02.632 Carbuncle of left foot
L02.639 Carbuncle of unspecified foot

✓5th L02.8 Cutaneous abscess, furuncle and carbuncle of other sites
✓6th L02.81 Cutaneous abscess of other sites
L02.811 Cutaneous abscess of head [any part, except face]
L02.818 Cutaneous abscess of other sites

✓6th L02.82 Furuncle of other sites
Boil of other sites
Folliculitis of other sites
L02.821 Furuncle of head [any part, except face]
L02.828 Furuncle of other sites

✓6th L02.83 Carbuncle of other sites
L02.831 Carbuncle of head [any part, except face]
L02.838 Carbuncle of other sites

✓5th L02.9 Cutaneous abscess, furuncle and carbuncle, unspecified
L02.91 Cutaneous abscess, unspecified
L02.92 Furuncle, unspecified
Boil NOS
Furunculosis NOS
L02.93 Carbuncle, unspecified

✓4th L03 Cellulitis and acute lymphangitis
EXCLUDES 2 cellulitis of anal and rectal region (K61.-)
cellulitis of external auditory canal (H60.1)
cellulitis of eyelid (H00.03-)
cellulitis of female external genital organs (N76.4)
cellulitis of lacrimal apparatus (H04.3)
cellulitis of male external genital organs (N48.2, N49-)
cellulitis of mouth (K12.2)
cellulitis of nose (J34.0)
eosinophilic cellulitis [Wells] (L98.3)
febrile neutrophilic dermatosis [Sweet] (L98.2)
lymphangitis (chronic) (subacute) (I89.1)

✓5th L03.0 Cellulitis and acute lymphangitis of finger and toe
Infection of nail
Onychia
Paronychia
Perionychia

✓6th L03.01 Cellulitis of finger
Felon
Whitlow
EXCLUDES 1 herpetic whitlow (B00.89)
L03.011 Cellulitis of right finger
L03.012 Cellulitis of left finger
L03.019 Cellulitis of unspecified finger

✓6th L03.02 Acute lymphangitis of finger
Hangnail with lymphangitis of finger
L03.021 Acute lymphangitis of right finger
L03.022 Acute lymphangitis of left finger
L03.029 Acute lymphangitis of unspecified finger

✓6th L03.03 Cellulitis of toe
L03.031 Cellulitis of right toe
L03.032 Cellulitis of left toe
L03.039 Cellulitis of unspecified toe

✓6th L03.04 Acute lymphangitis of toe
Hangnail with lymphangitis of toe
L03.041 Acute lymphangitis of right toe
L03.042 Acute lymphangitis of left toe
L03.049 Acute lymphangitis of unspecified toe

✓5th L03.1 Cellulitis and acute lymphangitis of other parts of limb
✓6th L03.11 Cellulitis of other parts of limb
EXCLUDES 2 cellulitis of fingers (L03.01-)
cellulitis of toes (L03.03-)
groin (L03.314)
L03.111 Cellulitis of right axilla
L03.112 Cellulitis of left axilla
L03.113 Cellulitis of right upper limb
L03.114 Cellulitis of left upper limb
L03.115 Cellulitis of right lower limb
L03.116 Cellulitis of left lower limb
L03.119 Cellulitis of unspecified part of limb

✓6th L03.12 Acute lymphangitis of other parts of limb
EXCLUDES 2 acute lymphangitis of fingers (L03.02-)
acute lymphangitis of groin (L03.324)
acute lymphangitis of toes (L03.04-)
L03.121 Acute lymphangitis of right axilla
L03.122 Acute lymphangitis of left axilla
L03.123 Acute lymphangitis of right upper limb
L03.124 Acute lymphangitis of left upper limb
L03.125 Acute lymphangitis of right lower limb
L03.126 Acute lymphangitis of left lower limb
L03.129 Acute lymphangitis of unspecified part of limb

✓5th L03.2 Cellulitis and acute lymphangitis of face and neck
✓6th L03.21 Cellulitis and acute lymphangitis of face
L03.211 Cellulitis of face
EXCLUDES 2 cellulitis of ear (H60.1-)
cellulitis of eyelid (H00.03-)
cellulitis of head (L03.811)
cellulitis of lacrimal apparatus (H04.3)
cellulitis of lip (K13.0)
cellulitis of mouth (K12.2)
cellulitis of nose (internal) (J34.0)
cellulitis of orbit (H05.0)
cellulitis of scalp (L03.811)
L03.212 Acute lymphangitis of face

☑6ᵗʰ **L03.22** Cellulitis and acute lymphangitis of neck
- **L03.221** Cellulitis of neck
- **L03.222** Acute lymphangitis of neck

☑5ᵗʰ **L03.3** Cellulitis and acute lymphangitis of trunk

☑6ᵗʰ **L03.31** Cellulitis of trunk
EXCLUDES 2 cellulitis of anal and rectal regions (K61.-)
cellulitis of breast NOS (N61)
cellulitis of female external genital organs (N76.4)
cellulitis of male external genital organs (N48.2, N49-)
omphalitis of newborn (P38.-)
puerperal cellulitis of breast (O91.2)
- **L03.311** Cellulitis of abdominal wall
  EXCLUDES 2 cellulitis of umbilicus (L03.316)
  cellulitis of groin (L03.314)
- **L03.312** Cellulitis of back [any part except buttock]
- **L03.313** Cellulitis of chest wall
- **L03.314** Cellulitis of groin
- **L03.315** Cellulitis of perineum
- **L03.316** Cellulitis of umbilicus
- **L03.317** Cellulitis of buttock
- **L03.319** Cellulitis of trunk, unspecified

☑6ᵗʰ **L03.32** Acute lymphangitis of trunk
- **L03.321** Acute lymphangitis of abdominal wall
- **L03.322** Acute lymphangitis of back [any part except buttock]
- **L03.323** Acute lymphangitis of chest wall
- **L03.324** Acute lymphangitis of groin
- **L03.325** Acute lymphangitis of perineum
- **L03.326** Acute lymphangitis of umbilicus
- **L03.327** Acute lymphangitis of buttock
- **L03.329** Acute lymphangitis of trunk, unspecified

☑5ᵗʰ **L03.8** Cellulitis and acute lymphangitis of other sites

☑6ᵗʰ **L03.81** Cellulitis of other sites
- **L03.811** Cellulitis of head [any part, except face]
  Cellulitis of scalp
  EXCLUDES 2 cellulitis of face (L03.211)
- **L03.818** Cellulitis of other sites

☑6ᵗʰ **L03.89** Acute lymphangitis of other sites
- **L03.891** Acute lymphangitis of head [any part, except face]
- **L03.898** Acute lymphangitis of other sites

☑5ᵗʰ **L03.9** Cellulitis and acute lymphangitis, unspecified
- **L03.90** Cellulitis, unspecified
- **L03.91** Acute lymphangitis, unspecified
  EXCLUDES 1 lymphangitis NOS (I89.1)

☑4ᵗʰ **L04 Acute lymphadenitis**
INCLUDES abscess (acute) of lymph nodes, except mesenteric
acute lymphadenitis, except mesenteric
EXCLUDES 1 chronic or subacute lymphadenitis, except mesenteric (I88.1)
enlarged lymph nodes (R59.-)
human immunodeficiency virus [HIV] disease resulting in generalized lymphadenopathy (B20)
lymphadenitis NOS (I88.9)
nonspecific mesenteric lymphadenitis (I88.0)

- **L04.0** Acute lymphadenitis of face, head and neck
- **L04.1** Acute lymphadenitis of trunk
- **L04.2** Acute lymphadenitis of upper limb
  Acute lymphadenitis of axilla
  Acute lymphadenitis of shoulder
- **L04.3** Acute lymphadenitis of lower limb
  Acute lymphadenitis of hip
  EXCLUDES 2 acute lymphadenitis of groin (L04.1)
- **L04.8** Acute lymphadenitis of other sites
- **L04.9** Acute lymphadenitis, unspecified

☑4ᵗʰ **L05 Pilonidal cyst and sinus**

☑5ᵗʰ **L05.0** Pilonidal cyst and sinus with abscess
- **L05.01** Pilonidal cyst with abscess
  Parasacral dimple with abscess
  Pilonidal abscess
  Pilonidal dimple with abscess
  Postanal dimple with abscess

- **L05.02** Pilonidal sinus with abscess
  Coccygeal fistula with abscess
  Coccygeal sinus with abscess
  Pilonidal fistula with abscess

☑5ᵗʰ **L05.9** Pilonidal cyst and sinus without abscess
- **L05.91** Pilonidal cyst without abscess
  Parasacral dimple
  Pilonidal dimple
  Postanal dimple
  Pilonidal cyst NOS
- **L05.92** Pilonidal sinus without abscess
  Coccygeal fistula
  Coccygeal sinus without abscess
  Pilonidal fistula

☑4ᵗʰ **L08 Other local infections of skin and subcutaneous tissue**
- **L08.0** Pyoderma
  Dermatitis gangrenosa
  Purulent dermatitis
  Septic dermatitis
  Suppurative dermatitis
  EXCLUDES 1 pyoderma gangrenosum (L88)
  pyoderma vegetans (L08.81)
- **L08.1** Erythrasma

☑5ᵗʰ **L08.8** Other specified local infections of the skin and subcutaneous tissue
- **L08.81** Pyoderma vegetans
  EXCLUDES 1 pyoderma gangrenosum (L88)
  pyoderma NOS (L08.0)
- **L08.82** Omphalitis not of newborn
  EXCLUDES 1 omphalitis of newborn (P38.-)
- **L08.89** Other specified local infections of the skin and subcutaneous tissue
- **L08.9** Local infection of the skin and subcutaneous tissue, unspecified

Bullous disorders (L10-L14)
EXCLUDES 1 benign familial pemphigus [Hailey-Hailey] (Q82.8)
staphylococcal scalded skin syndrome (L00)
toxic epidermal necrolysis [Lyell] (L51.2)

☑4ᵗʰ **L10 Pemphigus**
EXCLUDES 1 pemphigus neonatorum (L01.03)
- **L10.0** Pemphigus vulgaris
- **L10.1** Pemphigus vegetans
- **L10.2** Pemphigus foliaceous
- **L10.3** Brazilian pemphigus [fogo selvagem]
- **L10.4** Pemphigus erythematosus
  Senear-Usher syndrome
- **L10.5** Drug-induced pemphigus
  Use additional code for adverse effect, if applicable, to identify drug (T36-T50 with fifth or sixth character 5)

☑5ᵗʰ **L10.8** Other pemphigus
- **L10.81** Paraneoplastic pemphigus
- **L10.89** Other pemphigus
- **L10.9** Pemphigus, unspecified

☑4ᵗʰ **L11 Other acantholytic disorders**
- **L11.0** Acquired keratosis follicularis
  EXCLUDES 1 keratosis follicularis (congenital) [Darier-White] (Q82.8)
- **L11.1** Transient acantholytic dermatosis [Grover]
- **L11.8** Other specified acantholytic disorders
- **L11.9** Acantholytic disorder, unspecified

☑4ᵗʰ **L12 Pemphigoid**
EXCLUDES 1 herpes gestationis (O26.4-)
impetigo herpetiformis (L40.1)
- **L12.0** Bullous pemphigoid
- **L12.1** Cicatricial pemphigoid
  Benign mucous membrane pemphigoid
- **L12.2** Chronic bullous disease of childhood P
  Juvenile dermatitis herpetiformis

☑5ᵗʰ **L12.3** Acquired epidermolysis bullosa
EXCLUDES 1 epidermolysis bullosa (congenital) (Q81.-)
- **L12.30** Acquired epidermolysis bullosa, unspecified
- **L12.31** Epidermolysis bullosa due to drug
  Use additional code for adverse effect, if applicable, to identify drug (T36-T50 with fifth or sixth character 5)

☑ Additional Character Required ✗7ᵗʰ Xtension Alert Unspecified Code Other Specified Code Manifestation Code ►◄ Revised Text ● New Code ▲ Revised Code Title

ICD-10-CM 2014 (Draft) 631

Diseases of the Skin and Subcutaneous Tissue

L12.35–L25.2

L12.35   Other acquired epidermolysis bullosa
L12.8   Other pemphigoid
L12.9   Pemphigoid, unspecified

✓4ᵗʰ **L13**   Other bullous disorders

L13.0   Dermatitis herpetiformis
      Duhring's disease
      Hydroa herpetiformis
      EXCLUDES 1   *juvenile dermatitis herpetiformis (L12.2)*
              senile dermatitis herpetiformis (L12.0)

L13.1   Subcorneal pustular dermatitis
      Sneddon-Wilkinson disease

L13.8   Other specified bullous disorders

L13.9   Bullous disorder, unspecified

L14   *Bullous disorders in diseases classified elsewhere*
      Code first underlying disease

Dermatitis and eczema (L20-L30)

NOTE   In this block the terms dermatitis and eczema are used synonymously and interchangeably.

EXCLUDES 2   *chronic (childhood) granulomatous disease (D71)*
      dermatitis gangrenosa (L08.0)
      dermatitis herpetiformis (L13.0)
      dry skin dermatitis (L85.3)
      factitial dermatitis (L98.1)
      perioral dermatitis (L71.0)
      radiation-related disorders of the skin and subcutaneous tissue (L55-L59)
      stasis dermatitis (I83.1-I83.2)

✓4ᵗʰ **L20**   Atopic dermatitis

L20.0   Besnier's prurigo

✓5ᵗʰ **L20.8**   Other atopic dermatitis
      EXCLUDES 2   *circumscribed neurodermatitis (L28.0)*

      L20.81   Atopic neurodermatitis
              Diffuse neurodermatitis

      L20.82   Flexural eczema

      L20.83   Infantile (acute) (chronic) eczema   P

      L20.84   Intrinsic (allergic) eczema

      L20.89   Other atopic dermatitis

L20.9   Atopic dermatitis, unspecified

✓4ᵗʰ **L21**   Seborrheic dermatitis
      EXCLUDES 2   *infective dermatitis (L30.3)*
              seborrheic keratosis (L82.-)

L21.0   Seborrhea capitis   P
      Cradle cap

L21.1   Seborrheic infantile dermatitis   P

L21.8   Other seborrheic dermatitis

L21.9   Seborrheic dermatitis, unspecified
      Seborrhea NOS

L22   Diaper dermatitis
      Diaper erythema
      Diaper rash
      Psoriasiform diaper rash

✓4ᵗʰ **L23**   Allergic contact dermatitis
      EXCLUDES 1   *allergy NOS (T78.40)*
              contact dermatitis NOS (L25.9)
              dermatitis NOS (L30.9)
      EXCLUDES 2   *dermatitis due to substances taken internally (L27.-)*
              dermatitis of eyelid (H01.1-)
              diaper dermatitis (L22)
              eczema of external ear (H60.5-)
              irritant contact dermatitis (L24.-)
              perioral dermatitis (L71.0)
              radiation-related disorders of the skin and subcutaneous tissue (L55-L59)

L23.0   Allergic contact dermatitis due to metals
      Allergic contact dermatitis due to chromium
      Allergic contact dermatitis due to nickel

L23.1   Allergic contact dermatitis due to adhesives

L23.2   Allergic contact dermatitis due to cosmetics

L23.3   Allergic contact dermatitis due to drugs in contact with skin
      Use additional code for adverse effect, if applicable, to identify drug (T36-T50 with fifth or sixth character 5)
      EXCLUDES 2   *dermatitis due to ingested drugs and medicaments (L27.0-L27.1)*

L23.4   Allergic contact dermatitis due to dyes

L23.5   Allergic contact dermatitis due to other chemical products
      Allergic contact dermatitis due to cement
      Allergic contact dermatitis due to insecticide
      Allergic contact dermatitis due to plastic
      Allergic contact dermatitis due to rubber

L23.6   Allergic contact dermatitis due to food in contact with the skin
      EXCLUDES 2   *dermatitis due to ingested food (L27.2)*

L23.7   Allergic contact dermatitis due to plants, except food
      EXCLUDES 2   *allergy NOS due to pollen (J30.1)*

✓5ᵗʰ **L23.8**   Allergic contact dermatitis due to other agents

      L23.81   Allergic contact dermatitis due to animal (cat) (dog) dander
              Allergic contact dermatitis due to animal (cat) (dog) hair

      L23.89   Allergic contact dermatitis due to other agents

L23.9   Allergic contact dermatitis, unspecified cause
      Allergic contact eczema NOS

✓4ᵗʰ **L24**   Irritant contact dermatitis
      EXCLUDES 1   *allergy NOS (T78.40)*
              contact dermatitis NOS (L25.9)
              dermatitis NOS (L30.9)
      EXCLUDES 2   *allergic contact dermatitis (L23.-)*
              dermatitis due to substances taken internally (L27.-)
              dermatitis of eyelid (H01.1-)
              diaper dermatitis (L22)
              eczema of external ear (H60.5-)
              perioral dermatitis (L71.0)
              radiation-related disorders of the skin and subcutaneous tissue (L55-L59)

L24.0   Irritant contact dermatitis due to detergents

L24.1   Irritant contact dermatitis due to oils and greases

L24.2   Irritant contact dermatitis due to solvents
      Irritant contact dermatitis due to chlorocompound
      Irritant contact dermatitis due to cyclohexane
      Irritant contact dermatitis due to ester
      Irritant contact dermatitis due to glycol
      Irritant contact dermatitis due to hydrocarbon
      Irritant contact dermatitis due to ketone

L24.3   Irritant contact dermatitis due to cosmetics

L24.4   Irritant contact dermatitis due to drugs in contact with skin
      Use additional code for adverse effect, if applicable, to identify drug (T36-T50 with fifth or sixth character 5)

L24.5   Irritant contact dermatitis due to other chemical products
      Irritant contact dermatitis due to cement
      Irritant contact dermatitis due to insecticide
      Irritant contact dermatitis due to plastic
      Irritant contact dermatitis due to rubber

L24.6   Irritant contact dermatitis due to food in contact with skin
      EXCLUDES 2   *dermatitis due to ingested food (L27.2)*

L24.7   Irritant contact dermatitis due to plants, except food
      EXCLUDES 2   *allergy NOS to pollen (J30.1)*

✓5ᵗʰ **L24.8**   Irritant contact dermatitis due to other agents

      L24.81   Irritant contact dermatitis due to metals
              Irritant contact dermatitis due to chromium
              Irritant contact dermatitis due to nickel

      L24.89   Irritant contact dermatitis due to other agents
              Irritant contact dermatitis due to dyes

L24.9   Irritant contact dermatitis, unspecified cause
      Irritant contact eczema NOS

✓4ᵗʰ **L25**   Unspecified contact dermatitis
      EXCLUDES 1   *allergic contact dermatitis (L23.-)*
              allergy NOS (T78.40)
              dermatitis NOS (L30.9)
              irritant contact dermatitis (L24.-)
      EXCLUDES 2   *dermatitis due to ingested substances (L27.-)*
              dermatitis of eyelid (H01.1-)
              eczema of external ear (H60.5-)
              perioral dermatitis (L71.0)
              radiation-related disorders of the skin and subcutaneous tissue (L55-L59)

L25.0   Unspecified contact dermatitis due to cosmetics

L25.1   Unspecified contact dermatitis due to drugs in contact with skin
      Use additional code for adverse effect, if applicable, to identify drug (T36-T50 with fifth or sixth character 5)
      EXCLUDES 2   *dermatitis due to ingested drugs and medicaments (L27.0-L27.1)*

L25.2   Unspecified contact dermatitis due to dyes

EXCLUDES 1 Not coded here   EXCLUDES 2 Not included here   N Newborn Age: 0   P Pediatric Age: 0-17   M Maternity Age: 12-55   A Adult Age: 15-124

632   ICD-10-CM 2014 (Draft)

L25.3 **Unspecified contact dermatitis due to** other chemical products
  Unspecified contact dermatitis due to cement
  Unspecified contact dermatitis due to insecticide

L25.4 **Unspecified contact dermatitis due to** food in contact with skin
  EXCLUDES 2   *dermatitis due to ingested food (L27.2)*

L25.5 **Unspecified contact dermatitis due to** plants, except food
  EXCLUDES 1   *nettle rash (L50.9)*
  EXCLUDES 2   *allergy NOS due to pollen (J30.1)*

L25.8 **Unspecified contact dermatitis due to other** agents

L25.9 **Unspecified contact dermatitis, unspecified cause**
  Contact dermatitis (occupational) NOS
  Contact eczema (occupational) NOS

L26 **Exfoliative** dermatitis
  Hebra's pityriasis
  EXCLUDES 1   *Ritter's disease (L00)*

✓4ᵗʰ **L27** **Dermatitis** due to substances taken internally
  EXCLUDES 1   *allergy NOS (T78.40)*
  EXCLUDES 2   *adverse food reaction, except dermatitis (T78.0-T78.1)*
      contact dermatitis (L23-L25)
      drug photoallergic response (L56.1)
      drug phototoxic response (L56.0)
      urticaria (L50.-)

L27.0 **Generalized** skin eruption due to drugs and medicaments taken internally
  Use additional code for adverse effect, if applicable, to identify drug (T36-T50 with fifth or sixth character 5)

L27.1 **Localized** skin eruption due to drugs and medicaments taken internally
  Use additional code for adverse effect, if applicable, to identify drug (T36-T50 with fifth or sixth character 5)

L27.2 **Dermatitis** due to ingested food
  EXCLUDES 2   *dermatitis due to food in contact with skin (L23.6, L24.6, L25.4)*

L27.8 **Dermatitis due to other substances taken internally**

L27.9 **Dermatitis due to unspecified substance taken internally**

✓4ᵗʰ **L28** **Lichen simplex chronicus and prurigo**

L28.0 **Lichen simplex chronicus**
  Circumscribed neurodermatitis
  Lichen NOS

L28.1 **Prurigo nodularis**

L28.2 **Other prurigo**
  Prurigo NOS
  Prurigo Hebra
  Prurigo mitis
  Urticaria papulosa

✓4ᵗʰ **L29** **Pruritus**
  EXCLUDES 1   *neurotic excoriation (L98.1)*
      psychogenic pruritus (F45.8)

L29.0 **Pruritus** ani

L29.1 **Pruritus** scroti   ♂

L29.2 **Pruritus** vulvae   ♀

L29.3 **Anogenital** pruritus, unspecified

L29.8 **Other pruritus**

L29.9 **Pruritus, unspecified**
  Itch NOS

✓4ᵗʰ **L30** **Other and unspecified dermatitis**
  EXCLUDES 2   *contact dermatitis (L23-L25)*
      dry skin dermatitis (L85.3)
      small plaque parapsoriasis (L41.3)
      stasis dermatitis (I83.1-.2)

L30.0 **Nummular dermatitis**

L30.1 **Dyshidrosis [pompholyx]**

L30.2 **Cutaneous autosensitization**
  Candidid [levurid]
  Dermatophytid
  Eczematid

L30.3 **Infective dermatitis**
  Infectious eczematoid dermatitis

L30.4 **Erythema intertrigo**

L30.5 **Pityriasis alba**

L30.8 **Other specified dermatitis**

L30.9 **Dermatitis, unspecified**
  Eczema NOS

Papulosquamous disorders (L40-L45)

✓4ᵗʰ **L40** **Psoriasis**

L40.0 **Psoriasis** vulgaris
  Nummular psoriasis
  Plaque psoriasis

L40.1 **Generalized pustular psoriasis**
  Impetigo herpetiformis
  Von Zumbusch's disease

L40.2 **Acrodermatitis continua**

L40.3 **Pustulosis palmaris et plantaris**

L40.4 **Guttate** psoriasis

✓5ᵗʰ **L40.5** **Arthropathic** psoriasis

L40.50 **Arthropathic psoriasis, unspecified**

L40.51 **Distal interphalangeal** psoriatic arthropathy

L40.52 **Psoriatic arthritis** mutilans

L40.53 **Psoriatic** spondylitis

L40.54 **Psoriatic** juvenile arthropathy

L40.59 **Other psoriatic arthropathy**

L40.8 **Other psoriasis**
  Flexural psoriasis

L40.9 **Psoriasis, unspecified**

✓4ᵗʰ **L41** **Parapsoriasis**
  EXCLUDES 1   *poikiloderma vasculare atrophicans (L94.5)*

L41.0 **Pityriasis lichenoides et varioliformis acuta**
  Mucha-Habermann disease

L41.1 **Pityriasis lichenoides chronica**

L41.3 **Small plaque parapsoriasis**

L41.4 **Large plaque parapsoriasis**

L41.5 **Retiform parapsoriasis**

L41.8 **Other parapsoriasis**

L41.9 **Parapsoriasis, unspecified**

L42 **Pityriasis rosea**

✓4ᵗʰ **L43** **Lichen planus**
  EXCLUDES 1   *lichen planopilaris (L66.1)*

L43.0 **Hypertrophic** lichen planus

L43.1 **Bullous** lichen planus

L43.2 **Lichenoid** drug reaction
  Use additional code for adverse effect, if applicable, to identify drug (T36-T50 with fifth or sixth character 5)

L43.3 **Subacute (active) lichen planus**
  Lichen planus tropicus

L43.8 **Other lichen planus**

L43.9 **Lichen planus, unspecified**

✓4ᵗʰ **L44** **Other papulosquamous disorders**

L44.0 **Pityriasis rubra pilaris**

L44.1 **Lichen nitidus**

L44.2 **Lichen striatus**

L44.3 **Lichen ruber moniliformis**

L44.4 **Infantile papular acrodermatitis [Gianotti-Crosti]**   ℗

L44.8 **Other specified papulosquamous disorders**

L44.9 **Papulosquamous disorder, unspecified**

L45 *Papulosquamous disorders in diseases classified elsewhere*
  Code first underlying disease

Urticaria and erythema (L49-L54)

  EXCLUDES 1   *Lyme disease (A69.2-)*
      rosacea (L71.-)

✓4ᵗʰ **L49** **Exfoliation due to erythematous conditions according to extent of body surface involved**
  Code first erythematous condition causing exfoliation, such as:
    Ritter's disease (L00)
    (Staphylococcal) scalded skin syndrom (L00)
    Stevens-Johnson syndrome (L51.1)
    Stevens-Johnson syndrome-toxic epidermal necrolysis overlap syndrome (L51.3)
    toxic epidermal necrolysis (L51.2)

L49.0 **Exfoliation due to erythematous condition involving less than 10 percent of body surface**
  Exfoliation due to erythematous condition NOS

L49.1 **Exfoliation due to erythematous condition involving 10-19 percent of body surface**

☑ Additional Character Required   ✓x7ᵗʰ Xtension Alert   Unspecified Code   Other Specified Code   Manifestation Code   ▶◀ Revised Text   ● New Code   ▲ Revised Code Title

Diseases of the Skin and Subcutaneous Tissue

L49.2   **Exfoliation due to erythematous condition involving** 20-29 **percent of body surface**

L49.3   **Exfoliation due to erythematous condition involving** 30-39 **percent of body surface**

L49.4   **Exfoliation due to erythematous condition involving** 40-49 **percent of body surface**

L49.5   **Exfoliation due to erythematous condition involving** 50-59 **percent of body surface**

L49.6   **Exfoliation due to erythematous condition involving** 60-69 **percent of body surface**

L49.7   **Exfoliation due to erythematous condition involving** 70-79 **percent of body surface**

L49.8   **Exfoliation due to erythematous condition involving** 80-89 **percent of body surface**

L49.9   **Exfoliation due to erythematous condition involving** 90 or **more percent of body surface**

✓4ᵗʰ **L50**   **Urticaria**
> EXCLUDES 1   *allergic contact dermatitis (L23.-)*
> *angioneurotic edema (T78.3)*
> *giant urticaria (T78.3)*
> *hereditary angio-edema (D84.1)*
> *Quincke's edema (T78.3)*
> *serum urticaria (T80.6-)*
> *solar urticaria (L56.3)*
> *urticaria neonatorum (P83.8)*
> *urticaria papulosa (L28.2)*
> *urticaria pigmentosa (Q82.2)*

L50.0   **Allergic urticaria**

L50.1   **Idiopathic urticaria**

L50.2   **Urticaria due to cold and heat**

L50.3   **Dermatographic urticaria**

L50.4   **Vibratory urticaria**

L50.5   **Cholinergic urticaria**

L50.6   **Contact urticaria**

L50.8   **Other urticaria**
> Chronic urticaria
> Recurrent periodic urticaria

L50.9   **Urticaria, unspecified**

✓4ᵗʰ **L51**   **Erythema multiforme**
> Use additional code for adverse effect, if applicable, to identify drug (T36-T50 with fifth or sixth character 5)
> Use additional code to identify associated manifestations, such as:
> arthropathy associated with dermatological disorders (M14.8-)
> conjunctival edema (H11.42)
> conjunctivitis (H10.22-)
> corneal scars and opacities (H17.-)
> corneal ulcer (H16.0-)
> edema of eyelid (H02.84)
> inflammation of eyelid (H01.8)
> keratoconjunctivitis sicca (H16.22-)
> mechanical lagophthalmos (H02.22-)
> stomatitis (K12.-)
> symblepharon (H11.23-)
> Use additional code to identify percentage of skin exfoliation (L49.-)
> EXCLUDES 1   *staphylococcal scalded skin syndrome (L00)*
> *Ritter's disease (L00)*

L51.0   **Nonbullous erythema multiforme**

L51.1   **Stevens-Johnson syndrome**

L51.2   **Toxic epidermal necrolysis [Lyell]**

L51.3   **Stevens-Johnson syndrome-toxic epidermal necrolysis overlap syndrome**
> SJS-TEN overlap syndrome

L51.8   **Other erythema multiforme**

L51.9   **Erythema multiforme, unspecified**
> Erythema iris
> Erythema multiforme major NOS
> Erythema multiforme minor NOS
> Herpes iris

L52   **Erythema nodosum**
> EXCLUDES 1   *tuberculous erythema nodosum (A18.4)*

✓4ᵗʰ **L53**   **Other erythematous conditions**
> EXCLUDES 1   *erythema ab igne (L59.0)*
> *erythema due to external agents in contact with skin (L23-L25)*
> *erythema intertrigo (L30.4)*

L53.0   **Toxic erythema**
> Code first poisoning due to drug or toxin, if applicable (T36-T65 with fifth or sixth character 1-4 or 6)
> Use additional code for adverse effect, if applicable, to identify drug (T36-T50 with fifth or sixth character 5)
> EXCLUDES 1   *neonatal erythema toxicum (P83.1)*

L53.1   **Erythema annulare centrifugum**

L53.2   **Erythema marginatum**

L53.3   **Other chronic figurate erythema**

L53.8   **Other specified erythematous conditions**

L53.9   **Erythematous condition, unspecified**
> Erythema NOS
> Erythroderma NOS

L54   *Erythema in diseases classified elsewhere*
> *Code first underlying disease*

Radiation-related disorders of the skin and subcutaneous tissue (L55-L59)

✓4ᵗʰ **L55**   **Sunburn**

L55.0   **Sunburn of first degree**

L55.1   **Sunburn of second degree**

L55.2   **Sunburn of third degree**

L55.9   **Sunburn, unspecified**

✓4ᵗʰ **L56**   **Other acute skin changes due to ultraviolet radiation**
> Use additional code to identify the source of the ultraviolet radiation (W89, X32)

L56.0   **Drug phototoxic response**
> Use additional code for adverse effect, if applicable, to identify drug (T36-T50 with fifth or sixth character 5)

L56.1   **Drug photoallergic response**
> Use additional code for adverse effect, if applicable, to identify drug (T36-T50 with fifth or sixth character 5)

L56.2   **Photocontact dermatitis [berloque dermatitis]**

L56.3   **Solar urticaria**

L56.4   **Polymorphous light eruption**

L56.5   **Disseminated superficial actinic porokeratosis (DSAP)**

L56.8   **Other specified acute skin changes due to ultraviolet radiation**

L56.9   **Acute skin change due to ultraviolet radiation, unspecified**

✓4ᵗʰ **L57**   **Skin changes due to chronic exposure to nonionizing radiation**
> Use additional code to identify the source of the ultraviolet radiation (W89, X32)

L57.0   **Actinic keratosis**
> Keratosis NOS
> Senile keratosis
> Solar keratosis

L57.1   **Actinic reticuloid**

L57.2   **Cutis rhomboidalis nuchae**

L57.3   **Poikiloderma of Civatte**

L57.4   **Cutis laxa senilis**
> Elastosis senilis

L57.5   **Actinic granuloma**

L57.8   **Other skin changes due to chronic exposure to nonionizing radiation**
> Farmer's skin
> Sailor's skin
> Solar dermatitis

L57.9   **Skin changes due to chronic exposure to nonionizing radiation, unspecified**

✓4ᵗʰ **L58**   **Radiodermatitis**
> Use additional code to identify the source of the radiation (W88, W90)

L58.0   **Acute radiodermatitis**

L58.1   **Chronic radiodermatitis**

L58.9   **Radiodermatitis, unspecified**

✓4ᵗʰ **L59**   **Other disorders of skin and subcutaneous tissue related to radiation**

L59.0   **Erythema ab igne [dermatitis ab igne]**

L59.8   **Other specified disorders of the skin and subcutaneous tissue related to radiation**

EXCLUDES 1 Not coded here   EXCLUDES 2 Not included here   N Newborn Age: 0   P Pediatric Age: 0-17   M Maternity Age: 12-55   A Adult Age: 15-124

634   ICD-10-CM 2014 (Draft)

L59.9   **Disorder of the skin and subcutaneous tissue related to radiation, unspecified**

Disorders of skin appendages (L60-L75)

EXCLUDES 1   congenital malformations of integument (Q84.-)

✓4th **L60**   **Nail disorders**

     EXCLUDES 2   clubbing of nails (R68.3)
               onychia and paronychia (L03.0-)

     L60.0   **Ingrowing nail**

     L60.1   **Onycholysis**

     L60.2   **Onychogryphosis**

     L60.3   **Nail dystrophy**

     L60.4   **Beau's lines**

     L60.5   **Yellow nail syndrome**

     L60.8   **Other nail disorders**

     L60.9   **Nail disorder, unspecified**

L62   *Nail disorders in diseases classified elsewhere*

     Code first underlying disease, such as:
        pachydermoperiostosis (M89.4-)

✓4th **L63**   **Alopecia areata**

     L63.0   **Alopecia (capitis) totalis**

     L63.1   **Alopecia universalis**

     L63.2   **Ophiasis**

     L63.8   **Other alopecia areata**

     L63.9   **Alopecia areata, unspecified**

✓4th **L64**   **Androgenic alopecia**

     INCLUDES   male-pattern baldness

     L64.0   **Drug-induced androgenic alopecia**

         Use additional code for adverse effect, if applicable, to identify drug (T36-T50 with fifth or sixth character 5)

     L64.8   **Other androgenic alopecia**

     L64.9   **Androgenic alopecia, unspecified**

✓4th **L65**   **Other nonscarring hair loss**

     Use additional code for adverse effect, if applicable, to identify drug (T36-T50 with fifth or sixth character 5)

     EXCLUDES 1   trichotillomania (F63.3)

     L65.0   **Telogen effluvium**

     L65.1   **Anagen effluvium**

     L65.2   **Alopecia mucinosa**

     L65.8   **Other specified nonscarring hair loss**

     L65.9   **Nonscarring hair loss, unspecified**
         Alopecia NOS

✓4th **L66**   **Cicatricial alopecia [scarring hair loss]**

     L66.0   **Pseudopelade**

     L66.1   **Lichen planopilaris**
         Follicular lichen planus

     L66.2   **Folliculitis decalvans**

     L66.3   **Perifolliculitis capitis abscedens**

     L66.4   **Folliculitis ulerythematosa reticulata**

     L66.8   **Other cicatricial alopecia**

     L66.9   **Cicatricial alopecia, unspecified**

✓4th **L67**   **Hair color and hair shaft abnormalities**

     EXCLUDES 1   monilethrix (Q84.1)
               pili annulati (Q84.1)
               telogen effluvium (L65.0)

     L67.0   **Trichorrhexis nodosa**

     L67.1   **Variations in hair color**
         Canities
         Greyness, hair (premature)
         Heterochromia of hair
         Poliosis circumscripta, acquired
         Poliosis NOS

     L67.8   **Other hair color and hair shaft abnormalities**
         Fragilitas crinium

     L67.9   **Hair color and hair shaft abnormality, unspecified**

✓4th **L68**   **Hypertrichosis**

     INCLUDES   excess hair

     EXCLUDES 1   congenital hypertrichosis (Q84.2)
               persistent lanugo (Q84.2)

     L68.0   **Hirsutism**

     L68.1   **Acquired hypertrichosis lanuginosa**

     L68.2   **Localized hypertrichosis**

     L68.3   **Polytrichia**

     L68.8   **Other hypertrichosis**

     L68.9   **Hypertrichosis, unspecified**

✓4th **L70**   **Acne**

     EXCLUDES 2   acne keloid (L73.0)

     L70.0   **Acne vulgaris**

     L70.1   **Acne conglobata**

     L70.2   **Acne varioliformis**
         Acne necrotica miliaris

     L70.3   **Acne tropica**

     L70.4   **Infantile acne**   P

     L70.5   **Acné excoriée des jeunes filles**
         Picker's acne

     L70.8   **Other acne**

     L70.9   **Acne, unspecified**

✓4th **L71**   **Rosacea**

     Use additional code for adverse effect, if applicable, to identify drug (T36-T50 with fifth or sixth character 5)

     L71.0   **Perioral dermatitis**

     L71.1   **Rhinophyma**

     L71.8   **Other rosacea**

     L71.9   **Rosacea, unspecified**

✓4th **L72**   **Follicular cysts of skin and subcutaneous tissue**

     L72.0   **Epidermal cyst**

     ✓5th **L72.1**   **Pilar and trichodermal cyst**

         L72.11   **Pilar cyst**

         L72.12   **Trichodermal cyst**
              Trichilemmal (proliferating) cyst

     L72.2   **Steatocystoma multiplex**

     L72.3   **Sebaceous cyst**

         EXCLUDES 2   pilar cyst (L72.11)
                     trichilemmal (proliferating) cyst (L72.12)

     L72.8   **Other follicular cysts of the skin and subcutaneous tissue**

     L72.9   **Follicular cyst of the skin and subcutaneous tissue, unspecified**

✓4th **L73**   **Other follicular disorders**

     L73.0   **Acne keloid**

     L73.1   **Pseudofolliculitis barbae**

     L73.2   **Hidradenitis suppurativa**

     L73.8   **Other specified follicular disorders**
         Sycosis barbae

     L73.9   **Follicular disorder, unspecified**

✓4th **L74**   **Eccrine sweat disorders**

     EXCLUDES 2   generalized hyperhidrosis (R61)

     L74.0   **Miliaria rubra**

     L74.1   **Miliaria crystallina**

     L74.2   **Miliaria profunda**
         Miliaria tropicalis

     L74.3   **Miliaria, unspecified**

     L74.4   **Anhidrosis**
         Hypohidrosis

     ✓5th **L74.5**   **Focal hyperhidrosis**

         ✓6th **L74.51**   **Primary focal hyperhidrosis**

              L74.510   **Primary focal hyperhidrosis, axilla**

              L74.511   **Primary focal hyperhidrosis, face**

              L74.512   **Primary focal hyperhidrosis, palms**

              L74.513   **Primary focal hyperhidrosis, soles**

              L74.519   **Primary focal hyperhidrosis, unspecified**

         L74.52   **Secondary focal hyperhidrosis**
              Frey's syndrome

     L74.8   **Other eccrine sweat disorders**

     L74.9   **Eccrine sweat disorder, unspecified**
         Sweat gland disorder NOS

✓4th **L75**   **Apocrine sweat disorders**

     EXCLUDES 1   dyshidrosis (L30.1)
               hidradenitis suppurativa (L73.2)

     L75.0   **Bromhidrosis**

     L75.1   **Chromhidrosis**

     L75.2   **Apocrine miliaria**
         Fox-Fordyce disease

     L75.8   **Other apocrine sweat disorders**

✓ Additional Character Required   ✓x7th Xtension Alert   Unspecified Code   Other Specified Code   Manifestation Code   ►◄ Revised Text   ● New Code   ▲ Revised Code Title

Diseases of the Skin and Subcutaneous Tissue

L75.9–L89.004

L75.9   **Apocrine sweat disorder, unspecified**

Intraoperative and postprocedural complications of skin and subcutaneous tissue (L76)

☑4ᵗʰ **L76**   **Intraoperative and postprocedural complications of skin and subcutaneous tissue**

    ☑5ᵗʰ **L76.0**   Intraoperative hemorrhage and hematoma of skin and subcutaneous tissue complicating a procedure

       EXCLUDES 1   *intraoperative hemorrhage and hematoma of skin and subcutaneous tissue due to accidental puncture and laceration during a procedure (L76.1-)*

       L76.01   **Intraoperative hemorrhage and hematoma of skin and subcutaneous tissue complicating a dermatologic procedure**

       L76.02   **Intraoperative hemorrhage and hematoma of skin and subcutaneous tissue complicating other procedure**

    ☑5ᵗʰ **L76.1**   Accidental puncture and laceration of skin and subcutaneous tissue during a procedure

       L76.11   **Accidental puncture and laceration of skin and subcutaneous tissue during a dermatologic procedure**

       L76.12   **Accidental puncture and laceration of skin and subcutaneous tissue during other procedure**

    ☑5ᵗʰ **L76.2**   Postprocedural hemorrhage and hematoma of skin and subcutaneous tissue following a procedure

       L76.21   **Postprocedural hemorrhage and hematoma of skin and subcutaneous tissue following a dermatologic procedure**

       L76.22   **Postprocedural hemorrhage and hematoma of skin and subcutaneous tissue following other procedure**

    ☑5ᵗʰ **L76.8**   Other intraoperative and postprocedural complications of skin and subcutaneous tissue

       Use additional code, if applicable, to further specify disorder

       L76.81   **Other intraoperative complications of skin and subcutaneous tissue**

       L76.82   **Other postprocedural complications of skin and subcutaneous tissue**

Other disorders of the skin and subcutaneous tissue (L80-L99)

L80   **Vitiligo**

    EXCLUDES 2   *vitiligo of eyelids (H02.73-)*
                vitiligo of vulva (N90.89)

☑4ᵗʰ **L81**   **Other disorders of pigmentation**

    EXCLUDES 1   *birthmark NOS (Q82.5)*
                Peutz-Jeghers syndrome (Q85.8)

    EXCLUDES 2   *nevus—see Alphabetical Index*

    L81.0   **Postinflammatory hyperpigmentation**

    L81.1   **Chloasma**

    L81.2   **Freckles**

    L81.3   **Café au lait spots**

    L81.4   **Other melanin hyperpigmentation**
           Lentigo

    L81.5   **Leukoderma, not elsewhere classified**

    L81.6   **Other disorders of diminished melanin formation**

    L81.7   **Pigmented purpuric dermatosis**
           Angioma serpiginosum

    L81.8   **Other specified disorders of pigmentation**
           Iron pigmentation
           Tattoo pigmentation

    L81.9   **Disorder of pigmentation, unspecified**

☑4ᵗʰ **L82**   **Seborrheic keratosis**

    INCLUDES   dermatosis papulosa nigra
               Leser-Trélat disease

    EXCLUDES 2   *seborrheic dermatitis (L21.-)*

    L82.0   **Inflamed seborrheic keratosis**

    L82.1   **Other seborrheic keratosis**
           Seborrheic keratosis NOS

L83   **Acanthosis nigricans**
       Confluent and reticulated papillomatosis

L84   **Corns and callosities**
       Callus
       Clavus

☑4ᵗʰ **L85**   **Other epidermal thickening**

    EXCLUDES 2   *hypertrophic disorders of the skin (L91.-)*

    L85.0   **Acquired ichthyosis**
       EXCLUDES 1   *congenital ichthyosis (Q80.-)*

    L85.1   **Acquired keratosis [keratoderma] palmaris et plantaris**
       EXCLUDES 1   *inherited keratosis palmaris et plantaris (Q82.8)*

    L85.2   **Keratosis punctata (palmaris et plantaris)**

    L85.3   **Xerosis cutis**
       Dry skin dermatitis

    L85.8   **Other specified epidermal thickening**
       Cutaneous horn

    L85.9   **Epidermal thickening, unspecified**

L86   ***Keratoderma in diseases classified elsewhere***

    Code first underlying disease, such as:
       Reiter's disease (M02.3-)

    EXCLUDES 1   *gonococcal keratoderma (A54.89)*
                gonococcal keratosis (A54.89)
                keratoderma due to vitamin A deficiency (E50.8)
                keratosis due to vitamin A deficiency (E50.8)
                xeroderma due to vitamin A deficiency (E50.8)

☑4ᵗʰ **L87**   **Transepidermal elimination disorders**

    EXCLUDES 1   *granuloma annulare (perforating) (L92.0)*

    L87.0   **Keratosis follicularis et parafollicularis in cutem penetrans**
       Kyrle disease
       Hyperkeratosis follicularis penetrans

    L87.1   **Reactive perforating collagenosis**

    L87.2   **Elastosis perforans serpiginosa**

    L87.8   **Other transepidermal elimination disorders**

    L87.9   **Transepidermal elimination disorder, unspecified**

L88   **Pyoderma gangrenosum**
       Phagedenic pyoderma
    EXCLUDES 1   *dermatitis gangrenosa (L08.0)*

☑4ᵗʰ **L89**   **Pressure ulcer**
       Bed sore
       Decubitus ulcer
       Plaster ulcer
       Pressure area
       Pressure sore
       Code first any associated gangrene (I96)

    EXCLUDES 2   *decubitus (trophic) ulcer of cervix (uteri) (N86)*
                diabetic ulcers (E08.621, E08.622, E09.621, E09.622, E10.621, E10.622, E11.621, E11.622, E13.621, E13.622)
                non-pressure chronic ulcer of skin (L97.-)
                skin infections (L00-L08)
                varicose ulcer (I83.0, I83.2)

    ☑5ᵗʰ **L89.0**   Pressure ulcer of elbow

       ☑6ᵗʰ **L89.00**   **Pressure ulcer of unspecified elbow**

          L89.000   **Pressure ulcer of unspecified elbow, unstageable**

          L89.001   **Pressure ulcer of unspecified elbow, stage 1**
             Healing pressure ulcer of unspecified elbow, stage 1
             Pressure pre-ulcer skin changes limited to persistent focal edema, unspecified elbow

          L89.002   **Pressure ulcer of unspecified elbow, stage 2**
             Healing pressure ulcer of unspecified elbow, stage 2
             Pressure ulcer with abrasion, blister, partial thickness skin loss involving epidermis and/or dermis, unspecified elbow

          L89.003   **Pressure ulcer of unspecified elbow, stage 3**
             Healing pressure ulcer of unspecified elbow, stage 3
             Pressure ulcer with full thickness skin loss involving damage or necrosis of subcutaneous tissue, unspecified elbow

          L89.004   **Pressure ulcer of unspecified elbow, stage 4**
             Healing pressure ulcer of unspecified elbow, stage 4
             Pressure ulcer with necrosis of soft tissues through to underlying muscle, tendon, or bone, unspecified elbow

---

EXCLUDES 1 Not coded here   EXCLUDES 2 Not included here   N Newborn Age: 0   P Pediatric Age: 0-17   M Maternity Age: 12-55   A Adult Age: 15-124

636   ICD-10-CM 2014 (Draft)

L89.009   **Pressure ulcer of unspecified elbow, unspecified stage**
    Healing pressure ulcer of elbow NOS
    Healing pressure ulcer of unspecified elbow, unspecified stage

✓6ᵗʰ **L89.01**   **Pressure ulcer of right elbow**

L89.010   **Pressure ulcer of right elbow, unstageable**

L89.011   **Pressure ulcer of right elbow, stage 1**
    Healing pressure ulcer of right elbow, stage 1
    Pressure pre-ulcer skin changes limited to persistent focal edema, right elbow

L89.012   **Pressure ulcer of right elbow, stage 2**
    Healing pressure ulcer of right elbow, stage 2
    Pressure ulcer with abrasion, blister, partial thickness skin loss involving epidermis and/or dermis, right elbow

L89.013   **Pressure ulcer of right elbow, stage 3**
    Healing pressure ulcer of right elbow, stage 3
    Pressure ulcer with full thickness skin loss involving damage or necrosis of subcutaneous tissue, right elbow

L89.014   **Pressure ulcer of right elbow, stage 4**
    Healing pressure ulcer of right elbow, stage 4
    Pressure ulcer with necrosis of soft tissues through to underlying muscle, tendon, or bone, right elbow

L89.019   **Pressure ulcer of right elbow, unspecified stage**
    Healing pressure right of elbow NOS
    Healing pressure ulcer of unspecified elbow, unspecified stage

✓6ᵗʰ **L89.02**   **Pressure ulcer of left elbow**

L89.020   **Pressure ulcer of left elbow, unstageable**

L89.021   **Pressure ulcer of left elbow, stage 1**
    Healing pressure ulcer of left elbow, stage 1
    Pressure pre-ulcer skin changes limited to persistent focal edema, left elbow

L89.022   **Pressure ulcer of left elbow, stage 2**
    Healing pressure ulcer of left elbow, stage 2
    Pressure ulcer with abrasion, blister, partial thickness skin loss involving epidermis and/or dermis, left elbow

L89.023   **Pressure ulcer of left elbow, stage 3**
    Healing pressure ulcer of left elbow, stage 3
    Pressure ulcer with full thickness skin loss involving damage or necrosis of subcutaneous tissue, left elbow

L89.024   **Pressure ulcer of left elbow, stage 4**
    Healing pressure ulcer of left elbow, stage 4
    Pressure ulcer with necrosis of soft tissues through to underlying muscle, tendon, or bone, left elbow

L89.029   **Pressure ulcer of left elbow, unspecified stage**
    Healing pressure ulcer of left of elbow NOS
    Healing pressure ulcer of unspecified elbow, unspecified stage

✓5ᵗʰ **L89.1**   **Pressure ulcer of back**

✓6ᵗʰ **L89.10**   **Pressure ulcer of unspecified part of back**

L89.100   **Pressure ulcer of unspecified part of back, unstageable**

L89.101   **Pressure ulcer of unspecified part of back, stage 1**
    Healing pressure ulcer of unspecified part of back, stage 1
    Pressure pre-ulcer skin changes limited to persistent focal edema, unspecified part of back

L89.102   **Pressure ulcer of unspecified part of back, stage 2**
    Healing pressure ulcer of unspecified part of back, stage 2
    Pressure ulcer with abrasion, blister, partial thickness skin loss involving epidermis and/or dermis, unspecified part of back

L89.103   **Pressure ulcer of unspecified part of back, stage 3**
    Healing pressure ulcer of unspecified part of back, stage 3
    Pressure ulcer with full thickness skin loss involving damage or necrosis of subcutaneous tissue, unspecified part of back

L89.104   **Pressure ulcer of unspecified part of back, stage 4**
    Healing pressure ulcer of unspecified part of back, stage 4
    Pressure ulcer with necrosis of soft tissues through to underlying muscle, tendon, or bone, unspecified part of back

L89.109   **Pressure ulcer of unspecified part of back, unspecified stage**
    Healing pressure ulcer of unspecified part of back NOS
    Healing pressure ulcer of unspecified part of back, unspecified stage

✓6ᵗʰ **L89.11**   **Pressure ulcer of right upper back**
    Pressure ulcer of right shoulder blade

L89.110   **Pressure ulcer of right upper back, unstageable**

L89.111   **Pressure ulcer of right upper back, stage 1**
    Healing pressure ulcer of right upper back, stage 1
    Pressure pre-ulcer skin changes limited to persistent focal edema, right upper back

L89.112   **Pressure ulcer of right upper back, stage 2**
    Healing pressure ulcer of right upper back, stage 2
    Pressure ulcer with abrasion, blister, partial thickness skin loss involving epidermis and/or dermis, right upper back

L89.113   **Pressure ulcer of right upper back, stage 3**
    Healing pressure ulcer of right upper back, stage 3
    Pressure ulcer with full thickness skin loss involving damage or necrosis of subcutaneous tissue, right upper back

L89.114   **Pressure ulcer of right upper back, stage 4**
    Healing pressure ulcer of right upper back, stage 4
    Pressure ulcer with necrosis of soft tissues through to underlying muscle, tendon, or bone, right upper back

L89.119   **Pressure ulcer of right upper back, unspecified stage**
    Healing pressure ulcer of right upper back NOS
    Healing pressure ulcer of right upper back, unspecified stage

✓6ᵗʰ **L89.12**   **Pressure ulcer of left upper back**
    Pressure ulcer of left shoulder blade

L89.120   **Pressure ulcer of left upper back, unstageable**

L89.121   **Pressure ulcer of left upper back, stage 1**
    Healing pressure ulcer of left upper back, stage 1
    Pressure pre-ulcer skin changes limited to persistent focal edema, left upper back

L89.122   **Pressure ulcer of left upper back, stage 2**
    Healing pressure ulcer of left upper back, stage 2
    Pressure ulcer with abrasion, blister, partial thickness skin loss involving epidermis and/or dermis, left upper back

L89.123   **Pressure ulcer of left upper back, stage 3**
    Healing pressure ulcer of left upper back, stage 3
    Pressure ulcer with full thickness skin loss involving damage or necrosis of subcutaneous tissue, left upper back

L89.124   **Pressure ulcer of left upper back, stage 4**
    Healing pressure ulcer of left upper back, stage 4
    Pressure ulcer with necrosis of soft tissues through to underlying muscle, tendon, or bone, left upper back

✓ Additional Character Required   ✗x7ᵗʰ Xtension Alert   Unspecified Code   Other Specified Code   Manifestation Code   ▶◀ Revised Text   ● New Code   ▲ Revised Code Title

ICD-10-CM 2014 (Draft)

637

Diseases of the Skin and Subcutaneous Tissue

L89.129–L89.214

L89.129 **Pressure ulcer of left upper back, unspecified stage**
　　Healing pressure ulcer of left upper back NOS
　　Healing pressure ulcer of left upper back, unspecified stage

√6ᵗʰ **L89.13** **Pressure ulcer of right lower back**

L89.130 **Pressure ulcer of right lower back, unstageable**

L89.131 **Pressure ulcer of right lower back, stage 1**
　　Healing pressure ulcer of right lower back, stage 1
　　Pressure pre-ulcer skin changes limited to persistent focal edema, right lower back

L89.132 **Pressure ulcer of right lower back, stage 2**
　　Healing pressure ulcer of right lower back, stage 2
　　Pressure ulcer with abrasion, blister, partial thickness skin loss involving epidermis and/or dermis, right lower back

L89.133 **Pressure ulcer of right lower back, stage 3**
　　Healing pressure ulcer of right lower back, stage 3
　　Pressure ulcer with full thickness skin loss involving damage or necrosis of subcutaneous tissue, right lower back

L89.134 **Pressure ulcer of right lower back, stage 4**
　　Healing pressure ulcer of right lower back, stage 4
　　Pressure ulcer with necrosis of soft tissues through to underlying muscle, tendon, or bone, right lower back

L89.139 **Pressure ulcer of right lower back, unspecified stage**
　　Healing pressure ulcer of right lower back NOS
　　Healing pressure ulcer of right lower back, unspecified stage

√6ᵗʰ **L89.14** **Pressure ulcer of left lower back**

L89.140 **Pressure ulcer of left lower back, unstageable**

L89.141 **Pressure ulcer of left lower back, stage 1**
　　Healing pressure ulcer of left lower back, stage 1
　　Pressure pre-ulcer skin changes limited to persistent focal edema, left lower back

L89.142 **Pressure ulcer of left lower back, stage 2**
　　Healing pressure ulcer of left lower back, stage 2
　　Pressure ulcer with abrasion, blister, partial thickness skin loss involving epidermis and/or dermis, left lower back

L89.143 **Pressure ulcer of left lower back, stage 3**
　　Healing pressure ulcer of left lower back, stage 3
　　Pressure ulcer with full thickness skin loss involving damage or necrosis of subcutaneous tissue, left lower back

L89.144 **Pressure ulcer of left lower back, stage 4**
　　Healing pressure ulcer of left lower back, stage 4
　　Pressure ulcer with necrosis of soft tissues through to underlying muscle, tendon, or bone, left lower back

L89.149 **Pressure ulcer of left lower back, unspecified stage**
　　Healing pressure ulcer of left lower back NOS
　　Healing pressure ulcer of left lower back, unspecified stage

√6ᵗʰ **L89.15** **Pressure ulcer of sacral region**
　　Pressure ulcer of coccyx
　　Pressure ulcer of tailbone

L89.150 **Pressure ulcer of sacral region, unstageable**

L89.151 **Pressure ulcer of sacral region, stage 1**
　　Healing pressure ulcer of sacral region, stage 1
　　Pressure pre-ulcer skin changes limited to persistent focal edema, sacral region

L89.152 **Pressure ulcer of sacral region, stage 2**
　　Healing pressure ulcer of sacral region, stage 2
　　Pressure ulcer with abrasion, blister, partial thickness skin loss involving epidermis and/or dermis, sacral region

L89.153 **Pressure ulcer of sacral region, stage 3**
　　Healing pressure ulcer of sacral region, stage 3
　　Pressure ulcer with full thickness skin loss involving damage or necrosis of subcutaneous tissue, sacral region

L89.154 **Pressure ulcer of sacral region, stage 4**
　　Healing pressure ulcer of sacral region, stage 4
　　Pressure ulcer with necrosis of soft tissues through to underlying muscle, tendon, or bone, sacral region

L89.159 **Pressure ulcer of sacral region, unspecified stage**
　　Healing pressure ulcer of sacral region NOS
　　Healing pressure ulcer of sacral region, unspecified stage

√5ᵗʰ **L89.2** **Pressure ulcer of hip**

√6ᵗʰ **L89.20** **Pressure ulcer of unspecified hip**

L89.200 **Pressure ulcer of unspecified hip, unstageable**

L89.201 **Pressure ulcer of unspecified hip, stage 1**
　　Healing pressure ulcer of unspecified hip, stage 1
　　Pressure pre-ulcer skin changes limited to persistent focal edema, unspecified hip

L89.202 **Pressure ulcer of unspecified hip, stage 2**
　　Healing pressure ulcer of unspecified hip, stage 2
　　Pressure ulcer with abrasion, blister, partial thickness skin loss involving epidermis and/or dermis, unspecified hip

L89.203 **Pressure ulcer of unspecified hip, stage 3**
　　Healing pressure ulcer of unspecified hip, stage 3
　　Pressure ulcer with full thickness skin loss involving damage or necrosis of subcutaneous tissue, unspecified hip

L89.204 **Pressure ulcer of unspecified hip, stage 4**
　　Healing pressure ulcer of unspecified hip, stage 4
　　Pressure ulcer with necrosis of soft tissues through to underlying muscle, tendon, or bone, unspecified hip

L89.209 **Pressure ulcer of unspecified hip, unspecified stage**
　　Healing pressure ulcer of unspecified hip NOS
　　Healing pressure ulcer of unspecified hip, unspecified stage

√6ᵗʰ **L89.21** **Pressure ulcer of right hip**

L89.210 **Pressure ulcer of right hip, unstageable**

L89.211 **Pressure ulcer of right hip, stage 1**
　　Healing pressure ulcer of right hip, stage 1
　　Pressure pre-ulcer skin changes limited to persistent focal edema, right hip

L89.212 **Pressure ulcer of right hip, stage 2**
　　Healing pressure ulcer of right hip, stage 2
　　Pressure ulcer with abrasion, blister, partial thickness skin loss involving epidermis and/or dermis, right hip

L89.213 **Pressure ulcer of right hip, stage 3**
　　Healing pressure ulcer of right hip, stage 3
　　Pressure ulcer with full thickness skin loss involving damage or necrosis of subcutaneous tissue, right hip

L89.214 **Pressure ulcer of right hip, stage 4**
　　Healing pressure ulcer of right hip, stage 4
　　Pressure ulcer with necrosis of soft tissues through to underlying muscle, tendon, or bone, right hip

---

EXCLUDES 1 Not coded here　　　**EXCLUDES 2** Not included here　　　**N** Newborn Age: 0　　　**P** Pediatric Age: 0-17　　　**M** Maternity Age: 12-55　　　**A** Adult Age: 15-124

638   ICD-10-CM 2014 (Draft)

L89.219 Pressure ulcer of right hip, unspecified stage
Healing pressure ulcer of right hip NOS
Healing pressure ulcer of right hip, unspecified stage

✓6ᵗʰ **L89.22 Pressure ulcer of left hip**

L89.220 Pressure ulcer of left hip, unstageable

L89.221 Pressure ulcer of left hip, stage 1
Healing pressure ulcer of left hip, stage 1
Pressure pre-ulcer skin changes limited to persistent focal edema, left hip

L89.222 Pressure ulcer of left hip, stage 2
Healing pressure ulcer of left hip, stage 2
Pressure ulcer with abrasion, blister, partial thickness skin loss involving epidermis and/or dermis, left hip

L89.223 Pressure ulcer of left hip, stage 3
Healing pressure ulcer of left hip, stage 3
Pressure ulcer with full thickness skin loss involving damage or necrosis of subcutaneous tissue, left hip

L89.224 Pressure ulcer of left hip, stage 4
Healing pressure ulcer of left hip, stage 4
Pressure ulcer with necrosis of soft tissues through to underlying muscle, tendon, or bone, left hip

L89.229 Pressure ulcer of left hip, unspecified stage
Healing pressure ulcer of left hip NOS
Healing pressure ulcer of left hip, unspecified stage

✓5ᵗʰ **L89.3 Pressure ulcer of buttock**

✓6ᵗʰ **L89.30 Pressure ulcer of unspecified buttock**

L89.300 Pressure ulcer of unspecified buttock, unstageable

L89.301 Pressure ulcer of unspecified buttock, stage 1
Healing pressure ulcer of unspecified buttock, stage 1
Pressure pre-ulcer skin changes limited to persistent focal edema, unspecified buttock

L89.302 Pressure ulcer of unspecified buttock, stage 2
Healing pressure ulcer of unspecified buttock, stage 2
Pressure ulcer with abrasion, blister, partial thickness skin loss involving epidermis and/or dermis, unspecified buttock

L89.303 Pressure ulcer of unspecified buttock, stage 3
Healing pressure ulcer of unspecified buttock, stage 3
Pressure ulcer with full thickness skin loss involving damage or necrosis of subcutaneous tissue, unspecified buttock

L89.304 Pressure ulcer of unspecified buttock, stage 4
Healing pressure ulcer of unspecified buttock, stage 4
Pressure ulcer with necrosis of soft tissues through to underlying muscle, tendon, or bone, unspecified buttock

L89.309 Pressure ulcer of unspecified buttock, unspecified stage
Healing pressure ulcer of unspecified buttock NOS
Healing pressure ulcer of unspecified buttock, unspecified stage

✓6ᵗʰ **L89.31 Pressure ulcer of right buttock**

L89.310 Pressure ulcer of right buttock, unstageable

L89.311 Pressure ulcer of right buttock, stage 1
Healing pressure ulcer of right buttock, stage 1
Pressure pre-ulcer skin changes limited to persistent focal edema, right buttock

L89.312 Pressure ulcer of right buttock, stage 2
Healing pressure ulcer of right buttock, stage 2
Pressure ulcer with abrasion, blister, partial thickness skin loss involving epidermis and/or dermis, right buttock

L89.313 Pressure ulcer of right buttock, stage 3
Healing pressure ulcer of right buttock, stage 3
Pressure ulcer with full thickness skin loss involving damage or necrosis of subcutaneous tissue, right buttock

L89.314 Pressure ulcer of right buttock, stage 4
Healing pressure ulcer of right buttock, stage 4
Pressure ulcer with necrosis of soft tissues through to underlying muscle, tendon, or bone, right buttock

L89.319 Pressure ulcer of right buttock, unspecified stage
Healing pressure ulcer of right buttock NOS
Healing pressure ulcer of right buttock, unspecified stage

✓6ᵗʰ **L89.32 Pressure ulcer of left buttock**

L89.320 Pressure ulcer of left buttock, unstageable

L89.321 Pressure ulcer of left buttock, stage 1
Healing pressure ulcer of left buttock, stage 1
Pressure pre-ulcer skin changes limited to persistent focal edema, left buttock

L89.322 Pressure ulcer of left buttock, stage 2
Healing pressure ulcer of left buttock, stage 2
Pressure ulcer with abrasion, blister, partial thickness skin loss involving epidermis and/or dermis, left buttock

L89.323 Pressure ulcer of left buttock, stage 3
Healing pressure ulcer of left buttock, stage 3
Pressure ulcer with full thickness skin loss involving damage or necrosis of subcutaneous tissue, left buttock

L89.324 Pressure ulcer of left buttock, stage 4
Healing pressure ulcer of left buttock, stage 4
Pressure ulcer with necrosis of soft tissues through to underlying muscle, tendon, or bone, left buttock

L89.329 Pressure ulcer of left buttock, unspecified stage
Healing pressure ulcer of left buttock NOS
Healing pressure ulcer of left buttock, unspecified stage

✓5ᵗʰ **L89.4 Pressure ulcer of contiguous site of back, buttock and hip**

L89.40 Pressure ulcer of contiguous site of back, buttock and hip, unspecified stage
Healing pressure ulcer of contiguous site of back, buttock and hip NOS
Healing pressure ulcer of contiguous site of back, buttock and hip, unspecified stage

L89.41 Pressure ulcer of contiguous site of back, buttock and hip, stage 1
Healing pressure ulcer of contiguous site of back, buttock and hip, stage 1
Pressure pre-ulcer skin changes limited to persistent focal edema, contiguous site of back, buttock and hip

L89.42 Pressure ulcer of contiguous site of back, buttock and hip, stage 2
Healing pressure ulcer of contiguous site of back, buttock and hip, stage 2
Pressure ulcer with abrasion, blister, partial thickness skin loss involving epidermis and/or dermis, contiguous site of back, buttock and hip

L89.43 Pressure ulcer of contiguous site of back, buttock and hip, stage 3
Healing pressure ulcer of contiguous site of back, buttock and hip, stage 3
Pressure ulcer with full thickness skin loss involving damage or necrosis of subcutaneous tissue, contiguous site of back, buttock and hip

✓ Additional Character Required   ✓x7ᵗʰ Xtension Alert   Unspecified Code   Other Specified Code   Manifestation Code   ►◄ Revised Text   ● New Code   ▲ Revised Code Title

ICD-10-CM 2014 (Draft)   639

Diseases of the Skin and Subcutaneous Tissue

L89.44–L89.613

L89.44 **Pressure ulcer of contiguous site of back, buttock and hip, stage 4**
Healing pressure ulcer of contiguous site of back, buttock and hip, stage 4
Pressure ulcer with necrosis of soft tissues through to underlying muscle, tendon, or bone, contiguous site of back, buttock and hip

L89.45 **Pressure ulcer of contiguous site of back, buttock and hip, unstageable**

✓5th **L89.5** **Pressure ulcer of ankle**

  ✓6th **L89.50** **Pressure ulcer of unspecified ankle**

    L89.500 **Pressure ulcer of unspecified ankle, unstageable**

    L89.501 **Pressure ulcer of unspecified ankle, stage 1**
Healing pressure ulcer of unspecified ankle, stage 1
Pressure pre-ulcer skin changes limited to persistent focal edema, unspecified ankle

    L89.502 **Pressure ulcer of unspecified ankle, stage 2**
Healing pressure ulcer of unspecified ankle, stage 2
Pressure ulcer with abrasion, blister, partial thickness skin loss involving epidermis and/or dermis, unspecified ankle

    L89.503 **Pressure ulcer of unspecified ankle, stage 3**
Healing pressure ulcer of unspecified ankle, stage 3
Pressure ulcer with full thickness skin loss involving damage or necrosis of subcutaneous tissue, unspecified ankle

    L89.504 **Pressure ulcer of unspecified ankle, stage 4**
Healing pressure ulcer of unspecified ankle, stage 4
Pressure ulcer with necrosis of soft tissues through to underlying muscle, tendon, or bone, unspecified ankle

    L89.509 **Pressure ulcer of unspecified ankle, unspecified stage**
Healing pressure ulcer of unspecified ankle NOS
Healing pressure ulcer of unspecified ankle, unspecified stage

  ✓6th **L89.51** **Pressure ulcer of right ankle**

    L89.510 **Pressure ulcer of right ankle, unstageable**

    L89.511 **Pressure ulcer of right ankle, stage 1**
Healing pressure ulcer of right ankle, stage 1
Pressure pre-ulcer skin changes limited to persistent focal edema, right ankle

    L89.512 **Pressure ulcer of right ankle, stage 2**
Healing pressure ulcer of right ankle, stage 2
Pressure ulcer with abrasion, blister, partial thickness skin loss involving epidermis and/or dermis, right ankle

    L89.513 **Pressure ulcer of right ankle, stage 3**
Healing pressure ulcer of right ankle, stage 3
Pressure ulcer with full thickness skin loss involving damage or necrosis of subcutaneous tissue, right ankle

    L89.514 **Pressure ulcer of right ankle, stage 4**
Healing pressure ulcer of right ankle, stage 4
Pressure ulcer with necrosis of soft tissues through to underlying muscle, tendon, or bone, right ankle

    L89.519 **Pressure ulcer of right ankle, unspecified stage**
Healing pressure ulcer of right ankle NOS
Healing pressure ulcer of right ankle, unspecified stage

  ✓6th **L89.52** **Pressure ulcer of left ankle**

    L89.520 **Pressure ulcer of left ankle, unstageable**

    L89.521 **Pressure ulcer of left ankle, stage 1**
Healing pressure ulcer of left ankle, stage 1
Pressure pre-ulcer skin changes limited to persistnt focal edema, left ankle

    L89.522 **Pressure ulcer of left ankle, stage 2**
Healing pressure ulcer of left ankle, stage 2
Pressure ulcer with abrasion, blister, partial thickness skin loss involving epidermis and/or dermis, left ankle

    L89.523 **Pressure ulcer of left ankle, stage 3**
Healing pressure ulcer of left ankle, stage 3
Pressure ulcer with full thickness skin loss involving damage or necrosis of subcutaneous tissue, left ankle

    L89.524 **Pressure ulcer of left ankle, stage 4**
Healing pressure ulcer of left ankle, stage 4
Pressure ulcer with necrosis of soft tissues through to underlying muscle, tendon, or bone, left ankle

    L89.529 **Pressure ulcer of left ankle, unspecified stage**
Healing pressure ulcer of left ankle NOS
Healing pressure ulcer of left ankle, unspecified stage

✓5th **L89.6** **Pressure ulcer of heel**

  ✓6th **L89.60** **Pressure ulcer of unspecified heel**

    L89.600 **Pressure ulcer of unspecified heel, unstageable**

    L89.601 **Pressure ulcer of unspecified heel, stage 1**
Healing pressure ulcer of unspecified heel, stage 1
Pressure pre-ulcer skin changes limited to persistent focal edema, unspecified heel

    L89.602 **Pressure ulcer of unspecified heel, stage 2**
Healing pressure ulcer of unspecified heel, stage 2
Pressure ulcer with abrasion, blister, partial thickness skin loss involving epidermis and/or dermis, unspecified heel

    L89.603 **Pressure ulcer of unspecified heel, stage 3**
Healing pressure ulcer of unspecified heel, stage 3
Pressure ulcer with full thickness skin loss involving damage or necrosis of subcutaneous tissue, unspecified heel

    L89.604 **Pressure ulcer of unspecified heel, stage 4**
Healing pressure ulcer of unspecified heel, stage 4
Pressure ulcer with necrosis of soft tissues through to underlying muscle, tendon, or bone, unspecified heel

    L89.609 **Pressure ulcer of unspecified heel, unspecified stage**
Healing pressure ulcer of unspecified heel NOS
Healing pressure ulcer of unspecified heel, unspecified stage

  ✓6th **L89.61** **Pressure ulcer of right heel**

    L89.610 **Pressure ulcer of right heel, unstageable**

    L89.611 **Pressure ulcer of right heel, stage 1**
Healing pressure ulcer of right heel, stage 1
Pressure pre-ulcer skin changes limited to persistent focal edema, right heel

    L89.612 **Pressure ulcer of right heel, stage 2**
Healing pressure ulcer of right heel, stage 2
Pressure ulcer with abrasion, blister, partial thickness skin loss involving epidermis and/or dermis, right heel

    L89.613 **Pressure ulcer of right heel, stage 3**
Healing pressure ulcer of right heel, stage 3
Pressure ulcer with full thickness skin loss involving damage or necrosis of subcutaneous tissue, right heel

---

EXCLUDES 1 Not coded here   *EXCLUDES 2* Not included here   N Newborn Age: 0   P Pediatric Age: 0-17   M Maternity Age: 12-55   A Adult Age: 15-124

L89.614 Pressure ulcer of right heel, stage 4
Healing pressure ulcer of right heel, stage 4
Pressure ulcer with necrosis of soft tissues through to underlying muscle, tendon, or bone, right heel

L89.619 Pressure ulcer of right heel, unspecified stage
Healing pressure ulcer of right heel NOS
Healing pressure ulcer of unspecified heel, right stage

√6th **L89.62 Pressure ulcer of left heel**

L89.620 Pressure ulcer of left heel, unstageable

L89.621 Pressure ulcer of left heel, stage 1
Healing pressure ulcer of left heel, stage 1
Pressure pre-ulcer skin changes limited to persistent focal edema, left heel

L89.622 Pressure ulcer of left heel, stage 2
Healing pressure ulcer of left heel, stage 2
Pressure ulcer with abrasion, blister, partial thickness skin loss involving epidermis and/or dermis, left heel

L89.623 Pressure ulcer of left heel, stage 3
Healing pressure ulcer of left heel, stage 3
Pressure ulcer with full thickness skin loss involving damage or necrosis of subcutaneous tissue, left heel

L89.624 Pressure ulcer of left heel, stage 4
Healing pressure ulcer of left heel, stage 4
Pressure ulcer with necrosis of soft tissues through to underlying muscle, tendon, or bone, left heel

L89.629 Pressure ulcer of left heel, unspecified stage
Healing pressure ulcer of left heel NOS
Healing pressure ulcer of left heel, unspecified stage

√5th **L89.8 Pressure ulcer of other site**

√6th **L89.81 Pressure ulcer of head**
Pressure ulcer of face

L89.810 Pressure ulcer of head, unstageable

L89.811 Pressure ulcer of head, stage 1
Healing pressure ulcer of head, stage 1
Pressure pre-ulcer skin changes limited to persistent focal edema, head

L89.812 Pressure ulcer of head, stage 2
Healing pressure ulcer of head, stage 2
Pressure ulcer with abrasion, blister, partial thickness skin loss involving epidermis and/or dermis, head

L89.813 Pressure ulcer of head, stage 3
Healing pressure ulcer of head, stage 3
Pressure ulcer with full thickness skin loss involving damage or necrosis of subcutaneous tissue, head

L89.814 Pressure ulcer of head, stage 4
Healing pressure ulcer of head, stage 4
Pressure ulcer with necrosis of soft tissues through to underlying muscle, tendon, or bone, head

L89.819 Pressure ulcer of head, unspecified stage
Healing pressure ulcer of head NOS
Healing pressure ulcer of head, unspecified stage

√6th **L89.89 Pressure ulcer of other site**

L89.890 Pressure ulcer of other site, unstageable

L89.891 Pressure ulcer of other site, stage 1
Healing pressure ulcer of other site, stage 1
Pressure pre-ulcer skin changes limited to persistent focal edema, other site

L89.892 Pressure ulcer of other site, stage 2
Healing pressure ulcer of other site, stage 2
Pressure ulcer with abrasion, blister, partial thickness skin loss involving epidermis and/or dermis, other site

L89.893 Pressure ulcer of other site, stage 3
Healing pressure ulcer of other site, stage 3
Pressure ulcer with full thickness skin loss involving damage or necrosis of subcutaneous tissue, other site

L89.894 Pressure ulcer of other site, stage 4
Healing pressure ulcer of other site, stage 4
Pressure ulcer with necrosis of soft tissues through to underlying muscle, tendon, or bone, other site

L89.899 Pressure ulcer of other site, unspecified stage
Healing pressure ulcer of other site NOS
Healing pressure ulcer of other site, unspecified stage

√5th **L89.9 Pressure ulcer of unspecified site**

L89.90 Pressure ulcer of unspecified site, unspecified stage
Healing pressure ulcer of unspecified site NOS
Healing pressure ulcer of unspecified site, unspecified stage

L89.91 Pressure ulcer of unspecified site, stage 1
Healing pressure ulcer of unspecified site, stage 1
Pressure pre-ulcer skin changes limited to persistent focal edema, unspecified site

L89.92 Pressure ulcer of unspecified site, stage 2
Healing pressure ulcer of unspecified site, stage 2
Pressure ulcer with abrasion, blister, partial thickness skin loss involving epidermis and/or dermis, unspecified site

L89.93 Pressure ulcer of unspecified site, stage 3
Healing pressure ulcer of unspecified site, stage 3
Pressure ulcer with full thickness skin loss involving damage or necrosis of subcutaneous tissue, unspecified site

L89.94 Pressure ulcer of unspecified site, stage 4
Healing pressure ulcer of unspecified site, stage 4
Pressure ulcer with necrosis of soft tissues through to underlying muscle, tendon, or bone, unspecified site

L89.95 Pressure ulcer of unspecified site, unstageable

√4th **L90 Atrophic disorders of skin**

L90.0 Lichen sclerosus et atrophicus
EXCLUDES 2 lichen sclerosus of external female genital organs (N90.4)
lichen sclerosus of external male genital organs (N48.0)

L90.1 Anetoderma of Schweninger-Buzzi

L90.2 Anetoderma of Jadassohn-Pellizzari

L90.3 Atrophoderma of Pasini and Pierini

L90.4 Acrodermatitis chronica atrophicans

L90.5 Scar conditions and fibrosis of skin
Adherent scar (skin)
Cicatrix
Disfigurement of skin due to scar
Fibrosis of skin NOS
Scar NOS
EXCLUDES 2 hypertrophic scar (L91.0)
keloid scar (L91.0)

L90.6 Striae atrophicae

L90.8 Other atrophic disorders of skin

L90.9 Atrophic disorder of skin, unspecified

√4th **L91 Hypertrophic disorders of skin**

L91.0 Hypertrophic scar
Keloid
Keloid scar
EXCLUDES 2 acne keloid (L73.0)
scar NOS (L90.5)

L91.8 Other hypertrophic disorders of the skin

L91.9 Hypertrophic disorder of the skin, unspecified

√4th **L92 Granulomatous disorders of skin and subcutaneous tissue**
EXCLUDES 2 actinic granuloma (L57.5)

L92.0 Granuloma annulare
Perforating granuloma annulare

L92.1 Necrobiosis lipoidica, not elsewhere classified
EXCLUDES 1 necrobiosis lipoidica associated with diabetes mellitus (E08-E13 with .620)

L92.2 Granuloma faciale [eosinophilic granuloma of skin]

L92.3　Foreign body granuloma of the skin and subcutaneous tissue
　　　Use additional code to identify the type of retained foreign body (Z18.-)

L92.8　Other granulomatous disorders of the skin and subcutaneous tissue

L92.9　Granulomatous disorder of the skin and subcutaneous tissue, unspecified

✓4th **L93　Lupus erythematosus**
　　　Use additional code for adverse effect, if applicable, to identify drug (T36-T5Ø with fifth or sixth character 5)
　　　EXCLUDES 1　lupus exedens (A18.4)
　　　　　　　　lupus vulgaris (A18.4)
　　　　　　　　scleroderma (M34.-)
　　　　　　　　systemic lupus erythematosus (M32.-)

L93.Ø　Discoid lupus erythematosus
　　　Lupus erythematosus NOS

L93.1　Subacute cutaneous lupus erythematosus

L93.2　Other local lupus erythematosus
　　　Lupus erythematosus profundus
　　　Lupus panniculitis

✓4th **L94　Other localized connective tissue disorders**
　　　EXCLUDES 1　systemic connective tissue disorders (M3Ø-M36)

L94.Ø　Localized scleroderma [morphea]
　　　Circumscribed scleroderma

L94.1　Linear scleroderma
　　　En coup de sabre lesion

L94.2　Calcinosis cutis

L94.3　Sclerodactyly

L94.4　Gottron's papules

L94.5　Poikiloderma vasculare atrophicans

L94.6　Ainhum

L94.8　Other specified localized connective tissue disorders

L94.9　Localized connective tissue disorder, unspecified

✓4th **L95　Vasculitis limited to skin, not elsewhere classified**
　　　EXCLUDES 1　angioma serpiginosum (L81.7)
　　　　　　　　Henoch(-Schönlein) purpura (D69.Ø)
　　　　　　　　hypersensitivity angiitis (M31.Ø)
　　　　　　　　lupus panniculitis (L93.2)
　　　　　　　　panniculitis NOS (M79.3)
　　　　　　　　panniculitis of neck and back (M54.Ø-)
　　　　　　　　polyarteritis nodosa (M3Ø.Ø)
　　　　　　　　relapsing panniculitis (M35.6)
　　　　　　　　rheumatoid vasculitis (MØ5.2)
　　　　　　　　serum sickness (T8Ø.6-)
　　　　　　　　urticaria (L5Ø.-)
　　　　　　　　Wegener's granulomatosis (M31.3-)

L95.Ø　Livedoid vasculitis
　　　Atrophie blanche (en plaque)

L95.1　Erythema elevatum diutinum

L95.8　Other vasculitis limited to the skin

L95.9　Vasculitis limited to the skin, unspecified

✓4th **L97　Non-pressure chronic ulcer of lower limb, not elsewhere classified**
　　　INCLUDES　chronic ulcer of skin of lower limb NOS
　　　　　　　non-healing ulcer of skin
　　　　　　　non-infected sinus of skin
　　　　　　　trophic ulcer NOS
　　　　　　　tropical ulcer NOS
　　　　　　　ulcer of skin of lower limb NOS
　　　Code first any associated underlying condition, such as:
　　　　　atherosclerosis of the lower extremities (I7Ø.23-, I7Ø.24-, I7Ø.33-, I7Ø.34-, I7Ø.43-, I7Ø.44-, I7Ø.53-, I7Ø.54-, I7Ø.63-, I7Ø.64-, I7Ø.73-, I7Ø.74-)
　　　　　chronic venous hypertension (I87.31-, I87.33-)
　　　　　diabetic ulcers (EØ8.621, EØ8.622, EØ9.621, EØ9.622, E1Ø.621, E1Ø.622, E11.621, E11.622, E13.621, E13.622)
　　　　　postphlebitic syndrome (I87.Ø1-, I87.Ø3-)
　　　　　postthrombotic syndrome (I87.Ø1-, I87.Ø3-)
　　　　　varicose ulcer (I83.Ø-, I83.2-)
　　　Code first any associated gangrene (I96)
　　　EXCLUDES 2　pressure ulcer (pressure area) (L89.-)
　　　　　　　　skin infections (LØØ-LØ8)
　　　　　　　　specific infections classified to AØØ-B99

✓5th **L97.1　Non-pressure chronic ulcer of thigh**

✓6th **L97.1Ø　Non-pressure chronic ulcer of unspecified thigh**

L97.1Ø1　Non-pressure chronic ulcer of unspecified thigh limited to breakdown of skin

L97.1Ø2　Non-pressure chronic ulcer of unspecified thigh with fat layer exposed

L97.1Ø3　Non-pressure chronic ulcer of unspecified thigh with necrosis of muscle

L97.1Ø4　Non-pressure chronic ulcer of unspecified thigh with necrosis of bone

L97.1Ø9　Non-pressure chronic ulcer of unspecified thigh with unspecified severity

✓6th **L97.11　Non-pressure chronic ulcer of right thigh**

L97.111　Non-pressure chronic ulcer of right thigh limited to breakdown of skin

L97.112　Non-pressure chronic ulcer of right thigh with fat layer exposed

L97.113　Non-pressure chronic ulcer of right thigh with necrosis of muscle

L97.114　Non-pressure chronic ulcer of right thigh with necrosis of bone

L97.119　Non-pressure chronic ulcer of right thigh with unspecified severity

✓6th **L97.12　Non-pressure chronic ulcer of left thigh**

L97.121　Non-pressure chronic ulcer of left thigh limited to breakdown of skin

L97.122　Non-pressure chronic ulcer of left thigh with fat layer exposed

L97.123　Non-pressure chronic ulcer of left thigh with necrosis of muscle

L97.124　Non-pressure chronic ulcer of left thigh with necrosis of bone

L97.129　Non-pressure chronic ulcer of left thigh with unspecified severity

✓5th **L97.2　Non-pressure chronic ulcer of calf**

✓6th **L97.2Ø　Non-pressure chronic ulcer of unspecified calf**

L97.2Ø1　Non-pressure chronic ulcer of unspecified calf limited to breakdown of skin

L97.2Ø2　Non-pressure chronic ulcer of unspecified calf with fat layer exposed

L97.2Ø3　Non-pressure chronic ulcer of unspecified calf with necrosis of muscle

L97.2Ø4　Non-pressure chronic ulcer of unspecified calf with necrosis of bone

L97.2Ø9　Non-pressure chronic ulcer of unspecified calf with unspecified severity

✓6th **L97.21　Non-pressure chronic ulcer of right calf**

L97.211　Non-pressure chronic ulcer of right calf limited to breakdown of skin

L97.212　Non-pressure chronic ulcer of right calf with fat layer exposed

L97.213　Non-pressure chronic ulcer of right calf with necrosis of muscle

L97.214　Non-pressure chronic ulcer of right calf with necrosis of bone

L97.219　Non-pressure chronic ulcer of right calf with unspecified severity

✓6th **L97.22　Non-pressure chronic ulcer of left calf**

L97.221　Non-pressure chronic ulcer of left calf limited to breakdown of skin

L97.222　Non-pressure chronic ulcer of left calf with fat layer exposed

L97.223　Non-pressure chronic ulcer of left calf with necrosis of muscle

L97.224　Non-pressure chronic ulcer of left calf with necrosis of bone

L97.229　Non-pressure chronic ulcer of left calf with unspecified severity

✓5th **L97.3　Non-pressure chronic ulcer of ankle**

✓6th **L97.3Ø　Non-pressure chronic ulcer of unspecified ankle**

L97.3Ø1　Non-pressure chronic ulcer of unspecified ankle limited to breakdown of skin

L97.3Ø2　Non-pressure chronic ulcer of unspecified ankle with fat layer exposed

L97.3Ø3　Non-pressure chronic ulcer of unspecified ankle with necrosis of muscle

L97.3Ø4　Non-pressure chronic ulcer of unspecified ankle with necrosis of bone

L97.3Ø9　Non-pressure chronic ulcer of unspecified ankle with unspecified severity

EXCLUDES 1 Not coded here　　　EXCLUDES 2 Not included here　　　N Newborn Age: Ø　　　P Pediatric Age: Ø-17　　　M Maternity Age: 12-55　　　A Adult Age: 15-124

642　　　ICD-1Ø-CM 2Ø14 (Draft)

√6ᵗʰ **L97.31** Non-pressure chronic ulcer of right ankle

L97.311 Non-pressure chronic ulcer of right ankle limited to breakdown of skin

L97.312 Non-pressure chronic ulcer of right ankle with fat layer exposed

L97.313 Non-pressure chronic ulcer of right ankle with necrosis of muscle

L97.314 Non-pressure chronic ulcer of right ankle with necrosis of bone

L97.319 Non-pressure chronic ulcer of right ankle with unspecified severity

√6ᵗʰ **L97.32** Non-pressure chronic ulcer of left ankle

L97.321 Non-pressure chronic ulcer of left ankle limited to breakdown of skin

L97.322 Non-pressure chronic ulcer of left ankle with fat layer exposed

L97.323 Non-pressure chronic ulcer of left ankle with necrosis of muscle

L97.324 Non-pressure chronic ulcer of left ankle with necrosis of bone

L97.329 Non-pressure chronic ulcer of left ankle with unspecified severity

√5ᵗʰ **L97.4** Non-pressure chronic ulcer of heel and midfoot
Non-pressure chronic ulcer of plantar surface of midfoot

√6ᵗʰ **L97.40** Non-pressure chronic ulcer of unspecified heel and midfoot

L97.401 Non-pressure chronic ulcer of unspecified heel and midfoot limited to breakdown of skin

L97.402 Non-pressure chronic ulcer of unspecified heel and midfoot with fat layer exposed

L97.403 Non-pressure chronic ulcer of unspecified heel and midfoot with necrosis of muscle

L97.404 Non-pressure chronic ulcer of unspecified heel and midfoot with necrosis of bone

L97.409 Non-pressure chronic ulcer of unspecified heel and midfoot with unspecified severity

√6ᵗʰ **L97.41** Non-pressure chronic ulcer of right heel and midfoot

L97.411 Non-pressure chronic ulcer of right heel and midfoot limited to breakdown of skin

L97.412 Non-pressure chronic ulcer of right heel and midfoot with fat layer exposed

L97.413 Non-pressure chronic ulcer of right heel and midfoot with necrosis of muscle

L97.414 Non-pressure chronic ulcer of right heel and midfoot with necrosis of bone

L97.419 Non-pressure chronic ulcer of right heel and midfoot with unspecified severity

√6ᵗʰ **L97.42** Non-pressure chronic ulcer of left heel and midfoot

L97.421 Non-pressure chronic ulcer of left heel and midfoot limited to breakdown of skin

L97.422 Non-pressure chronic ulcer of left heel and midfoot with fat layer exposed

L97.423 Non-pressure chronic ulcer of left heel and midfoot with necrosis of muscle

L97.424 Non-pressure chronic ulcer of left heel and midfoot with necrosis of bone

L97.429 Non-pressure chronic ulcer of left heel and midfoot with unspecified severity

√5ᵗʰ **L97.5** Non-pressure chronic ulcer of other part of foot
Non-pressure chronic ulcer of toe

√6ᵗʰ **L97.50** Non-pressure chronic ulcer of other part of unspecified foot

L97.501 Non-pressure chronic ulcer of other part of unspecified foot limited to breakdown of skin

L97.502 Non-pressure chronic ulcer of other part of unspecified foot with fat layer exposed

L97.503 Non-pressure chronic ulcer of other part of unspecified foot with necrosis of muscle

L97.504 Non-pressure chronic ulcer of other part of unspecified foot with necrosis of bone

L97.509 Non-pressure chronic ulcer of other part of unspecified foot with unspecified severity

√6ᵗʰ **L97.51** Non-pressure chronic ulcer of other part of right foot

L97.511 Non-pressure chronic ulcer of other part of right foot limited to breakdown of skin

L97.512 Non-pressure chronic ulcer of other part of right foot with fat layer exposed

L97.513 Non-pressure chronic ulcer of other part of right foot with necrosis of muscle

L97.514 Non-pressure chronic ulcer of other part of right foot with necrosis of bone

L97.519 Non-pressure chronic ulcer of other part of right foot with unspecified severity

√6ᵗʰ **L97.52** Non-pressure chronic ulcer of other part of left foot

L97.521 Non-pressure chronic ulcer of other part of left foot limited to breakdown of skin

L97.522 Non-pressure chronic ulcer of other part of left foot with fat layer exposed

L97.523 Non-pressure chronic ulcer of other part of left foot with necrosis of muscle

L97.524 Non-pressure chronic ulcer of other part of left foot with necrosis of bone

L97.529 Non-pressure chronic ulcer of other part of left foot with unspecified severity

√5ᵗʰ **L97.8** Non-pressure chronic ulcer of other part of lower leg

√6ᵗʰ **L97.80** Non-pressure chronic ulcer of other part of unspecified lower leg

L97.801 Non-pressure chronic ulcer of other part of unspecified lower leg limited to breakdown of skin

L97.802 Non-pressure chronic ulcer of other part of unspecified lower leg with fat layer exposed

L97.803 Non-pressure chronic ulcer of other part of unspecified lower leg with necrosis of muscle

L97.804 Non-pressure chronic ulcer of other part of unspecified lower leg with necrosis of bone

L97.809 Non-pressure chronic ulcer of other part of unspecified lower leg with unspecified severity

√6ᵗʰ **L97.81** Non-pressure chronic ulcer of other part of right lower leg

L97.811 Non-pressure chronic ulcer of other part of right lower leg limited to breakdown of skin

L97.812 Non-pressure chronic ulcer of other part of right lower leg with fat layer exposed

L97.813 Non-pressure chronic ulcer of other part of right lower leg with necrosis of muscle

L97.814 Non-pressure chronic ulcer of other part of right lower leg with necrosis of bone

L97.819 Non-pressure chronic ulcer of other part of right lower leg with unspecified severity

√6ᵗʰ **L97.82** Non-pressure chronic ulcer of other part of left lower leg

L97.821 Non-pressure chronic ulcer of other part of left lower leg limited to breakdown of skin

L97.822 Non-pressure chronic ulcer of other part of left lower leg with fat layer exposed

L97.823 Non-pressure chronic ulcer of other part of left lower leg with necrosis of muscle

L97.824 Non-pressure chronic ulcer of other part of left lower leg with necrosis of bone

L97.829 Non-pressure chronic ulcer of other part of left lower leg with unspecified severity

√5ᵗʰ **L97.9** Non-pressure chronic ulcer of unspecified part of lower leg

√6ᵗʰ **L97.90** Non-pressure chronic ulcer of unspecified part of unspecified lower leg

L97.901 Non-pressure chronic ulcer of unspecified part of unspecified lower leg limited to breakdown of skin

L97.902 Non-pressure chronic ulcer of unspecified part of unspecified lower leg with fat layer exposed

L97.903 Non-pressure chronic ulcer of unspecified part of unspecified lower leg with necrosis of muscle

L97.904 Non-pressure chronic ulcer of unspecified part of unspecified lower leg with necrosis of bone

L97.909 Non-pressure chronic ulcer of unspecified part of unspecified lower leg with unspecified severity

☑6ᵗʰ **L97.91** Non-pressure chronic ulcer of unspecified part of right lower leg

    L97.911 Non-pressure chronic ulcer of unspecified part of right lower leg limited to breakdown of skin

    L97.912 Non-pressure chronic ulcer of unspecified part of right lower leg with fat layer exposed

    L97.913 Non-pressure chronic ulcer of unspecified part of right lower leg with necrosis of muscle

    L97.914 Non-pressure chronic ulcer of unspecified part of right lower leg with necrosis of bone

    L97.919 Non-pressure chronic ulcer of unspecified part of right lower leg with unspecified severity

☑6ᵗʰ **L97.92** Non-pressure chronic ulcer of unspecified part of left lower leg

    L97.921 Non-pressure chronic ulcer of unspecified part of left lower leg limited to breakdown of skin

    L97.922 Non-pressure chronic ulcer of unspecified part of left lower leg with fat layer exposed

    L97.923 Non-pressure chronic ulcer of unspecified part of left lower leg with necrosis of muscle

    L97.924 Non-pressure chronic ulcer of unspecified part of left lower leg with necrosis of bone

    L97.929 Non-pressure chronic ulcer of unspecified part of left lower leg with unspecified severity

☑4ᵗʰ **L98** **Other disorders of skin and subcutaneous tissue, not elsewhere classified**

  L98.0 **Pyogenic granuloma**
    EXCLUDES 2 *pyogenic granuloma of gingiva (K06.8)*
    pyogenic granuloma of maxillary alveolar ridge (K04.5)
    pyogenic granuloma of oral mucosa (K13.4)

  L98.1 **Factitial dermatitis**
    Neurotic excoriation

  L98.2 **Febrile neutrophilic dermatosis [Sweet]**

  L98.3 **Eosinophilic cellulitis [Wells]**

☑5ᵗʰ **L98.4** **Non-pressure chronic ulcer of skin, not elsewhere classified**
    Chronic ulcer of skin NOS
    Tropical ulcer NOS
    Ulcer of skin NOS
    EXCLUDES 2 *pressure ulcer (pressure area) (L89.-)*
    gangrene (I96)
    skin infections (L00-L08)
    specific infections classified to A00-B99
    ulcer of lower limb NEC (L97.-)
    varicose ulcer (I83.0-I82.2)

☑6ᵗʰ **L98.41** **Non-pressure chronic ulcer of buttock**

    L98.411 Non-pressure chronic ulcer of buttock limited to breakdown of skin

    L98.412 Non-pressure chronic ulcer of buttock with fat layer exposed

    L98.413 Non-pressure chronic ulcer of buttock with necrosis of muscle

    L98.414 Non-pressure chronic ulcer of buttock with necrosis of bone

    L98.419 Non-pressure chronic ulcer of buttock with unspecified severity

☑6ᵗʰ **L98.42** Non-pressure chronic ulcer of back

    L98.421 Non-pressure chronic ulcer of back limited to breakdown of skin

    L98.422 Non-pressure chronic ulcer of back with fat layer exposed

    L98.423 Non-pressure chronic ulcer of back with necrosis of muscle

    L98.424 Non-pressure chronic ulcer of back with necrosis of bone

    L98.429 Non-pressure chronic ulcer of back with unspecified severity

☑6ᵗʰ **L98.49** Non-pressure chronic ulcer of skin of other sites
    Non-pressure chronic ulcer of skin NOS

    L98.491 Non-pressure chronic ulcer of skin of other sites limited to breakdown of skin

    L98.492 Non-pressure chronic ulcer of skin of other sites with fat layer exposed

    L98.493 Non-pressure chronic ulcer of skin of other sites with necrosis of muscle

    L98.494 Non-pressure chronic ulcer of skin of other sites with necrosis of bone

    L98.499 Non-pressure chronic ulcer of skin of other sites with unspecified severity

  L98.5 **Mucinosis of the skin**
    Focal mucinosis
    Lichen myxedematosus
    Reticular erythematous mucinosis
    EXCLUDES 1 *focal oral mucinosis (K13.79)*
    myxedema (E03.9)

  L98.6 **Other infiltrative disorders of the skin and subcutaneous tissue**
    EXCLUDES 1 *hyalinosis cutis et mucosae (E78.89)*

  L98.8 **Other specified disorders of the skin and subcutaneous tissue**

  L98.9 **Disorder of the skin and subcutaneous tissue, unspecified**

L99 ***Other disorders of skin and subcutaneous tissue in diseases classified elsewhere***
  Code first underlying disease, such as:
    amyloidosis (E85.-)
    EXCLUDES 1 *skin disorders in diabetes (E08-E13 with .62)*
    skin disorders in gonorrhea (A54.89)
    skin disorders in syphilis (A51.31, A52.79)

Chapter 13. Diseases of the Musculoskeletal System and Connective Tissue (M00-M99)

NOTE Use an external cause code following the code for the musculoskeletal condition, if applicable, to identify the cause of the musculoskeletal condition.

EXCLUDES 2 *arthropathic psoriasis (L40.5-)*
certain conditions originating in the perinatal period (P04-P96)
certain infectious and parasitic diseases (A00-B99)
compartment syndrome (traumatic) (T79.A-)
complications of pregnancy, childbirth and the puerperium (O00-O9A)
congenital malformations, deformations, and chromosomal abnormalities (Q00-Q99)
endocrine, nutritional and metabolic diseases (E00-E88)
injury, poisoning and certain other consequences of external causes (S00-T88)
neoplasms (C00-D49)
symptoms, signs and abnormal clinical and laboratory findings, not elsewhere classified (R00-R94)

This chapter contains the following blocks:

M00-M02   Infectious arthropathies
M05-M14   Inflammatory polyarthropathies
M15-M19   Osteoarthritis
M20-M25   Other joint disorders
M26-M27   Dentofacial anomalies [including malocclusion] and other disorders of jaw
M30-M36   Systemic connective tissue disorders
M40-M43   Deforming dorsopathies
M45-M49   Spondylopathies
M50-M54   Other dorsopathies
M60-M63   Disorders of muscles
M65-M67   Disorders of synovium and tendon
M70-M79   Other soft tissue disorders
M80-M85   Disorders of bone density and structure
M86-M90   Other osteopathies
M91-M94   Chondropathies
M95   Other disorders of the musculoskeletal system and connective tissue
M96   Intraoperative and postprocedural complications and disorders of musculoskeletal system, not elsewhere classified
M99   Biomechanical lesions, not elsewhere classified

ARTHROPATHIES (M00-M25)

INCLUDES disorders affecting predominantly peripheral (limb) joints

Infectious arthropathies (M00-M02)

This block comprises arthropathies due to microbiological agents. Distinction is made between the following types of etiological relationship:

a) direct infection of joint, where organisms invade synovial tissue and microbial antigen is present in the joint;

b) indirect infection, which may be of two types: a reactive arthropathy, where microbial infection of the body is established but neither organisms nor antigens can be identified in the joint, and a postinfective arthropathy, where microbial antigen is present but recovery of an organism is inconstant and evidence of local multiplication is lacking.

✓4th **M00 Pyogenic arthritis**

  ✓5th **M00.0 Staphylococcal arthritis and polyarthritis**
    Use additional code (B95.61-B95.8) to identify bacterial agent
    EXCLUDES 2 *infection and inflammatory reaction due to internal joint prosthesis (T84.5-)*

    M00.00 Staphylococcal arthritis, unspecified joint

    ✓6th **M00.01 Staphylococcal arthritis, shoulder**
      M00.011 Staphylococcal arthritis, right shoulder
      M00.012 Staphylococcal arthritis, left shoulder
      M00.019 Staphylococcal arthritis, unspecified shoulder

    ✓6th **M00.02 Staphylococcal arthritis, elbow**
      M00.021 Staphylococcal arthritis, right elbow
      M00.022 Staphylococcal arthritis, left elbow
      M00.029 Staphylococcal arthritis, unspecified elbow

    ✓6th **M00.03 Staphylococcal arthritis, wrist**
      Staphylococcal arthritis of carpal bones
      M00.031 Staphylococcal arthritis, right wrist
      M00.032 Staphylococcal arthritis, left wrist
      M00.039 Staphylococcal arthritis, unspecified wrist

✓6th **M00.04 Staphylococcal arthritis, hand**
    Staphylococcal arthritis of metacarpus and phalanges
    M00.041 Staphylococcal arthritis, right hand
    M00.042 Staphylococcal arthritis, left hand
    M00.049 Staphylococcal arthritis, unspecified hand

✓6th **M00.05 Staphylococcal arthritis, hip**
    M00.051 Staphylococcal arthritis, right hip
    M00.052 Staphylococcal arthritis, left hip
    M00.059 Staphylococcal arthritis, unspecified hip

✓6th **M00.06 Staphylococcal arthritis, knee**
    M00.061 Staphylococcal arthritis, right knee
    M00.062 Staphylococcal arthritis, left knee
    M00.069 Staphylococcal arthritis, unspecified knee

✓6th **M00.07 Staphylococcal arthritis, ankle and foot**
    Staphylococcal arthritis, tarsus, metatarsus and phalanges
    M00.071 Staphylococcal arthritis, right ankle and foot
    M00.072 Staphylococcal arthritis, left ankle and foot
    M00.079 Staphylococcal arthritis, unspecified ankle and foot

  M00.08 Staphylococcal arthritis, vertebrae

  M00.09 Staphylococcal polyarthritis

✓5th **M00.1 Pneumococcal arthritis and polyarthritis**

  M00.10 Pneumococcal arthritis, unspecified joint

✓6th **M00.11 Pneumococcal arthritis, shoulder**
    M00.111 Pneumococcal arthritis, right shoulder
    M00.112 Pneumococcal arthritis, left shoulder
    M00.119 Pneumococcal arthritis, unspecified shoulder

✓6th **M00.12 Pneumococcal arthritis, elbow**
    M00.121 Pneumococcal arthritis, right elbow
    M00.122 Pneumococcal arthritis, left elbow
    M00.129 Pneumococcal arthritis, unspecified elbow

✓6th **M00.13 Pneumococcal arthritis, wrist**
    Pneumococcal arthritis of carpal bones
    M00.131 Pneumococcal arthritis, right wrist
    M00.132 Pneumococcal arthritis, left wrist
    M00.139 Pneumococcal arthritis, unspecified wrist

✓6th **M00.14 Pneumococcal arthritis, hand**
    Pneumococcal arthritis of metacarpus and phalanges
    M00.141 Pneumococcal arthritis, right hand
    M00.142 Pneumococcal arthritis, left hand
    M00.149 Pneumococcal arthritis, unspecified hand

✓6th **M00.15 Pneumococcal arthritis, hip**
    M00.151 Pneumococcal arthritis, right hip
    M00.152 Pneumococcal arthritis, left hip
    M00.159 Pneumococcal arthritis, unspecified hip

✓6th **M00.16 Pneumococcal arthritis, knee**
    M00.161 Pneumococcal arthritis, right knee
    M00.162 Pneumococcal arthritis, left knee
    M00.169 Pneumococcal arthritis, unspecified knee

✓6th **M00.17 Pneumococcal arthritis, ankle and foot**
    Pneumococcal arthritis, tarsus, metatarsus and phalanges
    M00.171 Pneumococcal arthritis, right ankle and foot
    M00.172 Pneumococcal arthritis, left ankle and foot
    M00.179 Pneumococcal arthritis, unspecified ankle and foot

  M00.18 Pneumococcal arthritis, vertebrae

  M00.19 Pneumococcal polyarthritis

✓5th **M00.2 Other streptococcal arthritis and polyarthritis**
    Use additional code (B95.0-B95.2, B95.4-B95.5) to identify bacterial agent

  M00.20 Other streptococcal arthritis, unspecified joint

✓6th **M00.21 Other streptococcal arthritis, shoulder**
    M00.211 Other streptococcal arthritis, right shoulder
    M00.212 Other streptococcal arthritis, left shoulder
    M00.219 Other streptococcal arthritis, unspecified shoulder

Diseases of the Musculoskeletal System and Connective Tissue

M00.22–M01.X49

√6ᵗʰ **M00.22 Other streptococcal arthritis,** elbow
     M00.221 Other streptococcal arthritis, right elbow
     M00.222 Other streptococcal arthritis, left elbow
     M00.229 Other streptococcal arthritis, unspecified elbow

√6ᵗʰ **M00.23 Other streptococcal arthritis,** wrist
     Other streptococcal arthritis of carpal bones
     M00.231 Other streptococcal arthritis, right wrist
     M00.232 Other streptococcal arthritis, left wrist
     M00.239 Other streptococcal arthritis, unspecified wrist

√6ᵗʰ **M00.24 Other streptococcal arthritis,** hand
     Other streptococcal arthritis metacarpus and phalanges
     M00.241 Other streptococcal arthritis, right hand
     M00.242 Other streptococcal arthritis, left hand
     M00.249 Other streptococcal arthritis, unspecified hand

√6ᵗʰ **M00.25 Other streptococcal arthritis,** hip
     M00.251 Other streptococcal arthritis, right hip
     M00.252 Other streptococcal arthritis, left hip
     M00.259 Other streptococcal arthritis, unspecified hip

√6ᵗʰ **M00.26 Other streptococcal arthritis,** knee
     M00.261 Other streptococcal arthritis, right knee
     M00.262 Other streptococcal arthritis, left knee
     M00.269 Other streptococcal arthritis, unspecified knee

√6ᵗʰ **M00.27 Other streptococcal arthritis,** ankle and foot
     Other streptococcal arthritis, tarsus, metatarsus and phalanges
     M00.271 Other streptococcal arthritis, right ankle and foot
     M00.272 Other streptococcal arthritis, left ankle and foot
     M00.279 Other streptococcal arthritis, unspecified ankle and foot

     M00.28 Other streptococcal arthritis, vertebrae
     M00.29 Other streptococcal polyarthritis

√5ᵗʰ **M00.8 Arthritis and polyarthritis due to other bacteria**
     Use additional code (B96) to identify bacteria
     M00.80 Arthritis due to other bacteria, unspecified joint

√6ᵗʰ **M00.81 Arthritis due to other bacteria,** shoulder
     M00.811 Arthritis due to other bacteria, right shoulder
     M00.812 Arthritis due to other bacteria, left shoulder
     M00.819 Arthritis due to other bacteria, unspecified shoulder

√6ᵗʰ **M00.82 Arthritis due to other bacteria,** elbow
     M00.821 Arthritis due to other bacteria, right elbow
     M00.822 Arthritis due to other bacteria, left elbow
     M00.829 Arthritis due to other bacteria, unspecified elbow

√6ᵗʰ **M00.83 Arthritis due to other bacteria,** wrist
     Arthritis due to other bacteria, carpal bones
     M00.831 Arthritis due to other bacteria, right wrist
     M00.832 Arthritis due to other bacteria, left wrist
     M00.839 Arthritis due to other bacteria, unspecified wrist

√6ᵗʰ **M00.84 Arthritis due to other bacteria,** hand
     Arthritis due to other bacteria, metacarpus and phalanges
     M00.841 Arthritis due to other bacteria, right hand
     M00.842 Arthritis due to other bacteria, left hand
     M00.849 Arthritis due to other bacteria, unspecified hand

√6ᵗʰ **M00.85 Arthritis due to other bacteria,** hip
     M00.851 Arthritis due to other bacteria, right hip
     M00.852 Arthritis due to other bacteria, left hip
     M00.859 Arthritis due to other bacteria, unspecified hip

√6ᵗʰ **M00.86 Arthritis due to other bacteria,** knee
     M00.861 Arthritis due to other bacteria, right knee
     M00.862 Arthritis due to other bacteria, left knee

     M00.869 Arthritis due to other bacteria, unspecified knee

√6ᵗʰ **M00.87 Arthritis due to other bacteria,** ankle and foot
     Arthritis due to other bacteria, tarsus, metatarsus, and phalanges
     M00.871 Arthritis due to other bacteria, right ankle and foot
     M00.872 Arthritis due to other bacteria, left ankle and foot
     M00.879 Arthritis due to other bacteria, unspecified ankle and foot

     M00.88 Arthritis due to other bacteria, vertebrae
     M00.89 Polyarthritis due to other bacteria

M00.9 Pyogenic arthritis, unspecified
     Infective arthritis NOS

√4ᵗʰ **M01 Direct infections of joint in infectious and parasitic diseases classified elsewhere**
     Code first underlying disease, such as:
     leprosy [Hansen's disease] (A30.-)
     mycoses (B35-B49)
     O'nyong-nyong fever (A92.1)
     paratyphoid fever (A01.1-A01.4)

     EXCLUDES 1   *arthropathy in Lyme disease (A69.23)*
         gonococcal arthritis (A54.42)
         meningococcal arthritis (A39.83)
         mumps arthritis (B26.85)
         postinfective arthropathy (M02.-)
         postmeningococcal arthritis (A39.84)
         reactive arthritis (M02.3)
         rubella arthritis (B06.82)
         sarcoidosis arthritis (D86.86)
         typhoid fever arthritis (A01.04)
         tuberculosis arthritis (A18.01-A18.02)

√5ᵗʰ **M01.X Direct infection of joint in infectious and parasitic diseases classified elsewhere**

     M01.X0 Direct infection of unspecified joint in infectious and parasitic diseases classified elsewhere

√6ᵗʰ *M01.X1 Direct infection of shoulder joint in infectious and parasitic diseases classified elsewhere*
     M01.X11 Direct infection of right shoulder in infectious and parasitic diseases classified elsewhere
     M01.X12 Direct infection of left shoulder in infectious and parasitic diseases classified elsewhere
     M01.X19 Direct infection of unspecified shoulder in infectious and parasitic diseases classified elsewhere

√6ᵗʰ *M01.X2 Direct infection of elbow in infectious and parasitic diseases classified elsewhere*
     M01.X21 Direct infection of right elbow in infectious and parasitic diseases classified elsewhere
     M01.X22 Direct infection of left elbow in infectious and parasitic diseases classified elsewhere
     M01.X29 Direct infection of unspecified elbow in infectious and parasitic diseases classified elsewhere

√6ᵗʰ *M01.X3 Direct infection of wrist in infectious and parasitic diseases classified elsewhere*
     Direct infection of carpal bones in infectious and parasitic diseases classified elsewhere
     M01.X31 Direct infection of right wrist in infectious and parasitic diseases classified elsewhere
     M01.X32 Direct infection of left wrist in infectious and parasitic diseases classified elsewhere
     M01.X39 Direct infection of unspecified wrist in infectious and parasitic diseases classified elsewhere

√6ᵗʰ *M01.X4 Direct infection of hand in infectious and parasitic diseases classified elsewhere*
     Direct infection of metacarpus and phalanges in infectious and parasitic diseases classified elsewhere
     M01.X41 Direct infection of right hand in infectious and parasitic diseases classified elsewhere
     M01.X42 Direct infection of left hand in infectious and parasitic diseases classified elsewhere
     M01.X49 Direct infection of unspecified hand in infectious and parasitic diseases classified elsewhere

---

EXCLUDES 1 Not coded here   **EXCLUDES 2** Not included here   N Newborn Age: 0   P Pediatric Age: 0-17   M Maternity Age: 12-55   A Adult Age: 15-124

646   ICD-10-CM 2014 (Draft)

√6ᵗʰ **M01.X5 Direct infection of hip in infectious and parasitic diseases classified elsewhere**

M01.X51 Direct infection of right hip in infectious and parasitic diseases classified elsewhere

M01.X52 Direct infection of left hip in infectious and parasitic diseases classified elsewhere

M01.X59 Direct infection of unspecified hip in infectious and parasitic diseases classified elsewhere

√6ᵗʰ **M01.X6 Direct infection of knee in infectious and parasitic diseases classified elsewhere**

M01.X61 Direct infection of right knee in infectious and parasitic diseases classified elsewhere

M01.X62 Direct infection of left knee in infectious and parasitic diseases classified elsewhere

M01.X69 Direct infection of unspecified knee in infectious and parasitic diseases classified elsewhere

√6ᵗʰ **M01.X7 Direct infection of ankle and foot in infectious and parasitic diseases classified elsewhere**

Direct infection of tarsus, metatarsus and phalanges in infectious and parasitic diseases classified elsewhere

M01.X71 Direct infection of right ankle and foot in infectious and parasitic diseases classified elsewhere

M01.X72 Direct infection of left ankle and foot in infectious and parasitic diseases classified elsewhere

M01.X79 Direct infection of unspecified ankle and foot in infectious and parasitic diseases classified elsewhere

M01.X8 Direct infection of vertebrae in infectious and parasitic diseases classified elsewhere

M01.X9 Direct infection of multiple joints in infectious and parasitic diseases classified elsewhere

√4ᵗʰ **M02 Postinfective and reactive arthropathies**

Code first underlying disease, such as:
congenital syphilis [Clutton's joints] (A50.5)
enteritis due to Yersinia enterocolitica (A04.6)
infective endocarditis (I33.0)
viral hepatitis (B15-B19)

EXCLUDES 1 *Behçet's disease (M35.2)*
direct infections of joint in infectious and parasitic diseases classified elsewhere (M01.-)
postmeningococcal arthritis (A39.84)
mumps arthritis (B26.85)
rheumatic fever (I00)
rubella arthritis (B06.82)
syphilis arthritis (late) (A52.77)
tabetic arthropathy [Charcôt's] (A52.16)

√5ᵗʰ **M02.0 Arthropathy following intestinal bypass**

M02.00 Arthropathy following intestinal bypass, unspecified site

√6ᵗʰ **M02.01 Arthropathy following intestinal bypass, shoulder**

M02.011 Arthropathy following intestinal bypass, right shoulder

M02.012 Arthropathy following intestinal bypass, left shoulder

M02.019 Arthropathy following intestinal bypass, unspecified shoulder

√6ᵗʰ **M02.02 Arthropathy following intestinal bypass, elbow**

M02.021 Arthropathy following intestinal bypass, right elbow

M02.022 Arthropathy following intestinal bypass, left elbow

M02.029 Arthropathy following intestinal bypass, unspecified elbow

√6ᵗʰ **M02.03 Arthropathy following intestinal bypass, wrist**

Arthropathy following intestinal bypass, carpal bones

M02.031 Arthropathy following intestinal bypass, right wrist

M02.032 Arthropathy following intestinal bypass, left wrist

M02.039 Arthropathy following intestinal bypass, unspecified wrist

√6ᵗʰ **M02.04 Arthropathy following intestinal bypass, hand**

Arthropathy following intestinal bypass, metacarpals and phalanges

M02.041 Arthropathy following intestinal bypass, right hand

M02.042 Arthropathy following intestinal bypass, left hand

M02.049 Arthropathy following intestinal bypass, unspecified hand

√6ᵗʰ **M02.05 Arthropathy following intestinal bypass, hip**

M02.051 Arthropathy following intestinal bypass, right hip

M02.052 Arthropathy following intestinal bypass, left hip

M02.059 Arthropathy following intestinal bypass, unspecified hip

√6ᵗʰ **M02.06 Arthropathy following intestinal bypass, knee**

M02.061 Arthropathy following intestinal bypass, right knee

M02.062 Arthropathy following intestinal bypass, left knee

M02.069 Arthropathy following intestinal bypass, unspecified knee

√6ᵗʰ **M02.07 Arthropathy following intestinal bypass, ankle and foot**

Arthropathy following intestinal bypass, tarsus, metatarsus and phalanges

M02.071 Arthropathy following intestinal bypass, right ankle and foot

M02.072 Arthropathy following intestinal bypass, left ankle and foot

M02.079 Arthropathy following intestinal bypass, unspecified ankle and foot

M02.08 Arthropathy following intestinal bypass, vertebrae

M02.09 Arthropathy following intestinal bypass, multiple sites

√5ᵗʰ **M02.1 Postdysenteric arthropathy**

M02.10 Postdysenteric arthropathy, unspecified site

√6ᵗʰ **M02.11 Postdysenteric arthropathy, shoulder**

M02.111 Postdysenteric arthropathy, right shoulder

M02.112 Postdysenteric arthropathy, left shoulder

M02.119 Postdysenteric arthropathy, unspecified shoulder

√6ᵗʰ **M02.12 Postdysenteric arthropathy, elbow**

M02.121 Postdysenteric arthropathy, right elbow

M02.122 Postdysenteric arthropathy, left elbow

M02.129 Postdysenteric arthropathy, unspecified elbow

√6ᵗʰ **M02.13 Postdysenteric arthropathy, wrist**

Postdysenteric arthropathy, carpal bones

M02.131 Postdysenteric arthropathy, right wrist

M02.132 Postdysenteric arthropathy, left wrist

M02.139 Postdysenteric arthropathy, unspecified wrist

√6ᵗʰ **M02.14 Postdysenteric arthropathy, hand**

Postdysenteric arthropathy, metacarpus and phalanges

M02.141 Postdysenteric arthropathy, right hand

M02.142 Postdysenteric arthropathy, left hand

M02.149 Postdysenteric arthropathy, unspecified hand

√6ᵗʰ **M02.15 Postdysenteric arthropathy, hip**

M02.151 Postdysenteric arthropathy, right hip

M02.152 Postdysenteric arthropathy, left hip

M02.159 Postdysenteric arthropathy, unspecified hip

√6ᵗʰ **M02.16 Postdysenteric arthropathy, knee**

M02.161 Postdysenteric arthropathy, right knee

M02.162 Postdysenteric arthropathy, left knee

M02.169 Postdysenteric arthropathy, unspecified knee

☑ Additional Character Required   √x7ᵗʰ Xtension Alert   Unspecified Code   Other Specified Code   Manifestation Code   ▶◀ Revised Text   ● New Code   ▲ Revised Code Title

ICD-10-CM 2014 (Draft)   647

✓6ᵗʰ **M02.17 Postdysenteric arthropathy,** ankle and foot
Postdysenteric arthropathy, tarsus, metatarsus and phalanges
    M02.171 Postdysenteric arthropathy, right ankle and foot
    M02.172 Postdysenteric arthropathy, left ankle and foot
    M02.179 Postdysenteric arthropathy, unspecified ankle and foot
    M02.18 Postdysenteric arthropathy, vertebrae
    M02.19 Postdysenteric arthropathy, multiple sites

✓5ᵗʰ **M02.2 Postimmunization arthropathy**
    M02.20 Postimmunization arthropathy, unspecified site
✓6ᵗʰ **M02.21 Postimmunization arthropathy,** shoulder
    M02.211 Postimmunization arthropathy, right shoulder
    M02.212 Postimmunization arthropathy, left shoulder
    M02.219 Postimmunization arthropathy, unspecified shoulder
✓6ᵗʰ **M02.22 Postimmunization arthropathy,** elbow
    M02.221 Postimmunization arthropathy, right elbow
    M02.222 Postimmunization arthropathy, left elbow
    M02.229 Postimmunization arthropathy, unspecified elbow
✓6ᵗʰ **M02.23 Postimmunization arthropathy,** wrist
Postimmunization arthropathy, carpal bones
    M02.231 Postimmunization arthropathy, right wrist
    M02.232 Postimmunization arthropathy, left wrist
    M02.239 Postimmunization arthropathy, unspecified wrist
✓6ᵗʰ **M02.24 Postimmunization arthropathy,** hand
Postimmunization arthropathy, metacarpus and phalanges
    M02.241 Postimmunization arthropathy, right hand
    M02.242 Postimmunization arthropathy, left hand
    M02.249 Postimmunization arthropathy, unspecified hand
✓6ᵗʰ **M02.25 Postimmunization arthropathy,** hip
    M02.251 Postimmunization arthropathy, right hip
    M02.252 Postimmunization arthropathy, left hip
    M02.259 Postimmunization arthropathy, unspecified hip
✓6ᵗʰ **M02.26 Postimmunization arthropathy,** knee
    M02.261 Postimmunization arthropathy, right knee
    M02.262 Postimmunization arthropathy, left knee
    M02.269 Postimmunization arthropathy, unspecified knee
✓6ᵗʰ **M02.27 Postimmunization arthropathy,** ankle and foot
Postimmunization arthropathy, tarsus, metatarsus and phalanges
    M02.271 Postimmunization arthropathy, right ankle and foot
    M02.272 Postimmunization arthropathy, left ankle and foot
    M02.279 Postimmunization arthropathy, unspecified ankle and foot
    M02.28 Postimmunization arthropathy, vertebrae
    M02.29 Postimmunization arthropathy, multiple sites

✓5ᵗʰ **M02.3 Reiter's disease**
Reactive arthritis
    M02.30 Reiter's disease, unspecified site
✓6ᵗʰ **M02.31 Reiter's disease,** shoulder
    M02.311 Reiter's disease, right shoulder
    M02.312 Reiter's disease, left shoulder
    M02.319 Reiter's disease, unspecified shoulder
✓6ᵗʰ **M02.32 Reiter's disease,** elbow
    M02.321 Reiter's disease, right elbow
    M02.322 Reiter's disease, left elbow
    M02.329 Reiter's disease, unspecified elbow

✓6ᵗʰ **M02.33 Reiter's disease,** wrist
Reiter's disease, carpal bones
    M02.331 Reiter's disease, right wrist
    M02.332 Reiter's disease, left wrist
    M02.339 Reiter's disease, unspecified wrist
✓6ᵗʰ **M02.34 Reiter's disease,** hand
Reiter's disease, metacarpus and phalanges
    M02.341 Reiter's disease, right hand
    M02.342 Reiter's disease, left hand
    M02.349 Reiter's disease, unspecified hand
✓6ᵗʰ **M02.35 Reiter's disease,** hip
    M02.351 Reiter's disease, right hip
    M02.352 Reiter's disease, left hip
    M02.359 Reiter's disease, unspecified hip
✓6ᵗʰ **M02.36 Reiter's disease,** knee
    M02.361 Reiter's disease, right knee
    M02.362 Reiter's disease, left knee
    M02.369 Reiter's disease, unspecified knee
✓6ᵗʰ **M02.37 Reiter's disease,** ankle and foot
Reiter's disease, tarsus, metatarsus and phalanges
    M02.371 Reiter's disease, right ankle and foot
    M02.372 Reiter's disease, left ankle and foot
    M02.379 Reiter's disease, unspecified ankle and foot
    M02.38 Reiter's disease, vertebrae
    M02.39 Reiter's disease, multiple sites

✓5ᵗʰ **M02.8 Other reactive arthropathies**
    M02.80 Other reactive arthropathies, unspecified site
✓6ᵗʰ **M02.81 Other reactive arthropathies,** shoulder
    M02.811 Other reactive arthropathies, right shoulder
    M02.812 Other reactive arthropathies, left shoulder
    M02.819 Other reactive arthropathies, unspecified shoulder
✓6ᵗʰ **M02.82 Other reactive arthropathies,** elbow
    M02.821 Other reactive arthropathies, right elbow
    M02.822 Other reactive arthropathies, left elbow
    M02.829 Other reactive arthropathies, unspecified elbow
✓6ᵗʰ **M02.83 Other reactive arthropathies,** wrist
Other reactive arthropathies, carpal bones
    M02.831 Other reactive arthropathies, right wrist
    M02.832 Other reactive arthropathies, left wrist
    M02.839 Other reactive arthropathies, unspecified wrist
✓6ᵗʰ **M02.84 Other reactive arthropathies,** hand
Other reactive arthropathies, metacarpus and phalanges
    M02.841 Other reactive arthropathies, right hand
    M02.842 Other reactive arthropathies, left hand
    M02.849 Other reactive arthropathies, unspecified hand
✓6ᵗʰ **M02.85 Other reactive arthropathies,** hip
    M02.851 Other reactive arthropathies, right hip
    M02.852 Other reactive arthropathies, left hip
    M02.859 Other reactive arthropathies, unspecified hip
✓6ᵗʰ **M02.86 Other reactive arthropathies,** knee
    M02.861 Other reactive arthropathies, right knee
    M02.862 Other reactive arthropathies, left knee
    M02.869 Other reactive arthropathies, unspecified knee
✓6ᵗʰ **M02.87 Other reactive arthropathies,** ankle and foot
Other reactive arthropathies, tarsus, metatarsus and phalanges
    M02.871 Other reactive arthropathies, right ankle and foot
    M02.872 Other reactive arthropathies, left ankle and foot
    M02.879 Other reactive arthropathies, unspecified ankle and foot
    M02.88 Other reactive arthropathies, vertebrae
    M02.89 Other reactive arthropathies, multiple sites
M02.9 Reactive arthropathy, unspecified

EXCLUDES 1 Not coded here   **EXCLUDES 2** Not included here   **N** Newborn Age: 0   **P** Pediatric Age: 0-17   **M** Maternity Age: 12-55   **A** Adult Age: 15-124

648   ICD-10-CM 2014 (Draft)

Inflammatory polyarthropathies (M05-M14)

☑4ᵗʰ **M05 Rheumatoid arthritis with rheumatoid factor**
　　EXCLUDES 1　*rheumatic fever (I00)*
　　　　　　　　juvenile rheumatoid arthritis (M08.-)
　　　　　　　　rheumatoid arthritis of spine (M45.-)

　☑5ᵗʰ **M05.0　Felty's syndrome**
　　　　　　Rheumatoid arthritis with splenoadenomegaly and leukopenia
　　　　M05.00　Felty's syndrome, unspecified site
　　　☑6ᵗʰ **M05.01　Felty's syndrome, shoulder**
　　　　　　M05.011　Felty's syndrome, right shoulder
　　　　　　M05.012　Felty's syndrome, left shoulder
　　　　　　M05.019　Felty's syndrome, unspecified shoulder
　　　☑6ᵗʰ **M05.02　Felty's syndrome, elbow**
　　　　　　M05.021　Felty's syndrome, right elbow
　　　　　　M05.022　Felty's syndrome, left elbow
　　　　　　M05.029　Felty's syndrome, unspecified elbow
　　　☑6ᵗʰ **M05.03　Felty's syndrome, wrist**
　　　　　　　Felty's syndrome, carpal bones
　　　　　　M05.031　Felty's syndrome, right wrist
　　　　　　M05.032　Felty's syndrome, left wrist
　　　　　　M05.039　Felty's syndrome, unspecified wrist
　　　☑6ᵗʰ **M05.04　Felty's syndrome, hand**
　　　　　　　Felty's syndrome, metacarpus and phalanges
　　　　　　M05.041　Felty's syndrome, right hand
　　　　　　M05.042　Felty's syndrome, left hand
　　　　　　M05.049　Felty's syndrome, unspecified hand
　　　☑6ᵗʰ **M05.05　Felty's syndrome, hip**
　　　　　　M05.051　Felty's syndrome, right hip
　　　　　　M05.052　Felty's syndrome, left hip
　　　　　　M05.059　Felty's syndrome, unspecified hip
　　　☑6ᵗʰ **M05.06　Felty's syndrome, knee**
　　　　　　M05.061　Felty's syndrome, right knee
　　　　　　M05.062　Felty's syndrome, left knee
　　　　　　M05.069　Felty's syndrome, unspecified knee
　　　☑6ᵗʰ **M05.07　Felty's syndrome, ankle and foot**
　　　　　　　Felty's syndrome, tarsus, metatarsus and phalanges
　　　　　　M05.071　Felty's syndrome, right ankle and foot
　　　　　　M05.072　Felty's syndrome, left ankle and foot
　　　　　　M05.079　Felty's syndrome, unspecified ankle and foot
　　　　M05.09　Felty's syndrome, multiple sites
　☑5ᵗʰ **M05.1　Rheumatoid lung disease with rheumatoid arthritis**
　　　　M05.10　Rheumatoid lung disease with rheumatoid arthritis of unspecified site
　　　☑6ᵗʰ **M05.11　Rheumatoid lung disease with rheumatoid arthritis of shoulder**
　　　　　　M05.111　Rheumatoid lung disease with rheumatoid arthritis of right shoulder
　　　　　　M05.112　Rheumatoid lung disease with rheumatoid arthritis of left shoulder
　　　　　　M05.119　Rheumatoid lung disease with rheumatoid arthritis of unspecified shoulder
　　　☑6ᵗʰ **M05.12　Rheumatoid lung disease with rheumatoid arthritis of elbow**
　　　　　　M05.121　Rheumatoid lung disease with rheumatoid arthritis of right elbow
　　　　　　M05.122　Rheumatoid lung disease with rheumatoid arthritis of left elbow
　　　　　　M05.129　Rheumatoid lung disease with rheumatoid arthritis of unspecified elbow
　　　☑6ᵗʰ **M05.13　Rheumatoid lung disease with rheumatoid arthritis of wrist**
　　　　　　　Rheumatoid lung disease with rheumatoid arthritis, carpal bones
　　　　　　M05.131　Rheumatoid lung disease with rheumatoid arthritis of right wrist
　　　　　　M05.132　Rheumatoid lung disease with rheumatoid arthritis of left wrist
　　　　　　M05.139　Rheumatoid lung disease with rheumatoid arthritis of unspecified wrist

　　　☑6ᵗʰ **M05.14　Rheumatoid lung disease with rheumatoid arthritis of hand**
　　　　　　　Rheumatoid lung disease with rheumatoid arthritis, metacarpus and phalanges
　　　　　　M05.141　Rheumatoid lung disease with rheumatoid arthritis of right hand
　　　　　　M05.142　Rheumatoid lung disease with rheumatoid arthritis of left hand
　　　　　　M05.149　Rheumatoid lung disease with rheumatoid arthritis of unspecified hand
　　　☑6ᵗʰ **M05.15　Rheumatoid lung disease with rheumatoid arthritis of hip**
　　　　　　M05.151　Rheumatoid lung disease with rheumatoid arthritis of right hip
　　　　　　M05.152　Rheumatoid lung disease with rheumatoid arthritis of left hip
　　　　　　M05.159　Rheumatoid lung disease with rheumatoid arthritis of unspecified hip
　　　☑6ᵗʰ **M05.16　Rheumatoid lung disease with rheumatoid arthritis of knee**
　　　　　　M05.161　Rheumatoid lung disease with rheumatoid arthritis of right knee
　　　　　　M05.162　Rheumatoid lung disease with rheumatoid arthritis of left knee
　　　　　　M05.169　Rheumatoid lung disease with rheumatoid arthritis of unspecified knee
　　　☑6ᵗʰ **M05.17　Rheumatoid lung disease with rheumatoid arthritis of ankle and foot**
　　　　　　　Rheumatoid lung disease with rheumatoid arthritis, tarsus, metatarsus and phalanges
　　　　　　M05.171　Rheumatoid lung disease with rheumatoid arthritis of right ankle and foot
　　　　　　M05.172　Rheumatoid lung disease with rheumatoid arthritis of left ankle and foot
　　　　　　M05.179　Rheumatoid lung disease with rheumatoid arthritis of unspecified ankle and foot
　　　　M05.19　Rheumatoid lung disease with rheumatoid arthritis of multiple sites
　☑5ᵗʰ **M05.2　Rheumatoid vasculitis with rheumatoid arthritis**
　　　　M05.20　Rheumatoid vasculitis with rheumatoid arthritis of unspecified site
　　　☑6ᵗʰ **M05.21　Rheumatoid vasculitis with rheumatoid arthritis of shoulder**
　　　　　　M05.211　Rheumatoid vasculitis with rheumatoid arthritis of right shoulder
　　　　　　M05.212　Rheumatoid vasculitis with rheumatoid arthritis of left shoulder
　　　　　　M05.219　Rheumatoid vasculitis with rheumatoid arthritis of unspecified shoulder
　　　☑6ᵗʰ **M05.22　Rheumatoid vasculitis with rheumatoid arthritis of elbow**
　　　　　　M05.221　Rheumatoid vasculitis with rheumatoid arthritis of right elbow
　　　　　　M05.222　Rheumatoid vasculitis with rheumatoid arthritis of left elbow
　　　　　　M05.229　Rheumatoid vasculitis with rheumatoid arthritis of unspecified elbow
　　　☑6ᵗʰ **M05.23　Rheumatoid vasculitis with rheumatoid arthritis of wrist**
　　　　　　　Rheumatoid vasculitis with rheumatoid arthritis, carpal bones
　　　　　　M05.231　Rheumatoid vasculitis with rheumatoid arthritis of right wrist
　　　　　　M05.232　Rheumatoid vasculitis with rheumatoid arthritis of left wrist
　　　　　　M05.239　Rheumatoid vasculitis with rheumatoid arthritis of unspecified wrist
　　　☑6ᵗʰ **M05.24　Rheumatoid vasculitis with rheumatoid arthritis of hand**
　　　　　　　Rheumatoid vasculitis with rheumatoid arthritis, metacarpus and phalanges
　　　　　　M05.241　Rheumatoid vasculitis with rheumatoid arthritis of right hand
　　　　　　M05.242　Rheumatoid vasculitis with rheumatoid arthritis of left hand
　　　　　　M05.249　Rheumatoid vasculitis with rheumatoid arthritis of unspecified hand

☑ Additional Character Required　　✗7ᵗʰ Xtension Alert　　Unspecified Code　　Other Specified Code　　Manifestation Code　　►◄ Revised Text　　● New Code　　▲ Revised Code Title

ICD-10-CM 2014 (Draft)　　　　　　　　　　　　　　　　　　　　　　　　　　　　　　　　**649**

Diseases of the Musculoskeletal System and Connective Tissue

M05.25–M05.469

✓6ᵗʰ **M05.25** Rheumatoid vasculitis with rheumatoid arthritis of hip

   M05.251 Rheumatoid vasculitis with rheumatoid arthritis of right hip

   M05.252 Rheumatoid vasculitis with rheumatoid arthritis of left hip

   M05.259 Rheumatoid vasculitis with rheumatoid arthritis of unspecified hip

✓6ᵗʰ **M05.26** Rheumatoid vasculitis with rheumatoid arthritis of knee

   M05.261 Rheumatoid vasculitis with rheumatoid arthritis of right knee

   M05.262 Rheumatoid vasculitis with rheumatoid arthritis of left knee

   M05.269 Rheumatoid vasculitis with rheumatoid arthritis of unspecified knee

✓6ᵗʰ **M05.27** Rheumatoid vasculitis with rheumatoid arthritis of ankle and foot

   Rheumatoid vasculitis with rheumatoid arthritis, tarsus, metatarsus and phalanges

   M05.271 Rheumatoid vasculitis with rheumatoid arthritis of right ankle and foot

   M05.272 Rheumatoid vasculitis with rheumatoid arthritis of left ankle and foot

   M05.279 Rheumatoid vasculitis with rheumatoid arthritis of unspecified ankle and foot

  M05.29 Rheumatoid vasculitis with rheumatoid arthritis of multiple sites

✓5ᵗʰ **M05.3** Rheumatoid heart disease with rheumatoid arthritis

   Rheumatoid carditis   Rheumatoid myocarditis

   Rheumatoid endocarditis   Rheumatoid pericarditis

  M05.30 Rheumatoid heart disease with rheumatoid arthritis of unspecified site

✓6ᵗʰ **M05.31** Rheumatoid heart disease with rheumatoid arthritis of shoulder

   M05.311 Rheumatoid heart disease with rheumatoid arthritis of right shoulder

   M05.312 Rheumatoid heart disease with rheumatoid arthritis of left shoulder

   M05.319 Rheumatoid heart disease with rheumatoid arthritis of unspecified shoulder

✓6ᵗʰ **M05.32** Rheumatoid heart disease with rheumatoid arthritis of elbow

   M05.321 Rheumatoid heart disease with rheumatoid arthritis of right elbow

   M05.322 Rheumatoid heart disease with rheumatoid arthritis of left elbow

   M05.329 Rheumatoid heart disease with rheumatoid arthritis of unspecified elbow

✓6ᵗʰ **M05.33** Rheumatoid heart disease with rheumatoid arthritis of wrist

   Rheumatoid heart disease with rheumatoid arthritis, carpal bones

   M05.331 Rheumatoid heart disease with rheumatoid arthritis of right wrist

   M05.332 Rheumatoid heart disease with rheumatoid arthritis of left wrist

   M05.339 Rheumatoid heart disease with rheumatoid arthritis of unspecified wrist

✓6ᵗʰ **M05.34** Rheumatoid heart disease with rheumatoid arthritis of hand

   Rheumatoid heart disease with rheumatoid arthritis, metacarpus and phalanges

   M05.341 Rheumatoid heart disease with rheumatoid arthritis of right hand

   M05.342 Rheumatoid heart disease with rheumatoid arthritis of left hand

   M05.349 Rheumatoid heart disease with rheumatoid arthritis of unspecified hand

✓6ᵗʰ **M05.35** Rheumatoid heart disease with rheumatoid arthritis of hip

   M05.351 Rheumatoid heart disease with rheumatoid arthritis of right hip

   M05.352 Rheumatoid heart disease with rheumatoid arthritis of left hip

   M05.359 Rheumatoid heart disease with rheumatoid arthritis of unspecified hip

✓6ᵗʰ **M05.36** Rheumatoid heart disease with rheumatoid arthritis of knee

   M05.361 Rheumatoid heart disease with rheumatoid arthritis of right knee

   M05.362 Rheumatoid heart disease with rheumatoid arthritis of left knee

   M05.369 Rheumatoid heart disease with rheumatoid arthritis of unspecified knee

✓6ᵗʰ **M05.37** Rheumatoid heart disease with rheumatoid arthritis of ankle and foot

   Rheumatoid heart disease with rheumatoid arthritis, tarsus, metatarsus and phalanges

   M05.371 Rheumatoid heart disease with rheumatoid arthritis of right ankle and foot

   M05.372 Rheumatoid heart disease with rheumatoid arthritis of left ankle and foot

   M05.379 Rheumatoid heart disease with rheumatoid arthritis of unspecified ankle and foot

  M05.39 Rheumatoid heart disease with rheumatoid arthritis of multiple sites

✓5ᵗʰ **M05.4** Rheumatoid myopathy with rheumatoid arthritis

  M05.40 Rheumatoid myopathy with rheumatoid arthritis of unspecified site

✓6ᵗʰ **M05.41** Rheumatoid myopathy with rheumatoid arthritis of shoulder

   M05.411 Rheumatoid myopathy with rheumatoid arthritis of right shoulder

   M05.412 Rheumatoid myopathy with rheumatoid arthritis of left shoulder

   M05.419 Rheumatoid myopathy with rheumatoid arthritis of unspecified shoulder

✓6ᵗʰ **M05.42** Rheumatoid myopathy with rheumatoid arthritis of elbow

   M05.421 Rheumatoid myopathy with rheumatoid arthritis of right elbow

   M05.422 Rheumatoid myopathy with rheumatoid arthritis of left elbow

   M05.429 Rheumatoid myopathy with rheumatoid arthritis of unspecified elbow

✓6ᵗʰ **M05.43** Rheumatoid myopathy with rheumatoid arthritis of wrist

   Rheumatoid myopathy with rheumatoid arthritis, carpal bones

   M05.431 Rheumatoid myopathy with rheumatoid arthritis of right wrist

   M05.432 Rheumatoid myopathy with rheumatoid arthritis of left wrist

   M05.439 Rheumatoid myopathy with rheumatoid arthritis of unspecified wrist

✓6ᵗʰ **M05.44** Rheumatoid myopathy with rheumatoid arthritis of hand

   Rheumatoid myopathy with rheumatoid arthritis, metacarpus and phalanges

   M05.441 Rheumatoid myopathy with rheumatoid arthritis of right hand

   M05.442 Rheumatoid myopathy with rheumatoid arthritis of left hand

   M05.449 Rheumatoid myopathy with rheumatoid arthritis of unspecified hand

✓6ᵗʰ **M05.45** Rheumatoid myopathy with rheumatoid arthritis of hip

   M05.451 Rheumatoid myopathy with rheumatoid arthritis of right hip

   M05.452 Rheumatoid myopathy with rheumatoid arthritis of left hip

   M05.459 Rheumatoid myopathy with rheumatoid arthritis of unspecified hip

✓6ᵗʰ **M05.46** Rheumatoid myopathy with rheumatoid arthritis of knee

   M05.461 Rheumatoid myopathy with rheumatoid arthritis of right knee

   M05.462 Rheumatoid myopathy with rheumatoid arthritis of left knee

   M05.469 Rheumatoid myopathy with rheumatoid arthritis of unspecified knee

EXCLUDES 1 Not coded here   EXCLUDES 2 Not included here   N Newborn Age: 0   P Pediatric Age: 0-17   M Maternity Age: 12-55   A Adult Age: 15-124

650   ICD-10-CM 2014 (Draft)

✓6th **M05.47 Rheumatoid myopathy with rheumatoid arthritis of ankle and foot**
Rheumatoid myopathy with rheumatoid arthritis, tarsus, metatarsus and phalanges
- M05.471 Rheumatoid myopathy with rheumatoid arthritis of right ankle and foot
- M05.472 Rheumatoid myopathy with rheumatoid arthritis of left ankle and foot
- M05.479 Rheumatoid myopathy with rheumatoid arthritis of unspecified ankle and foot

M05.49 Rheumatoid myopathy with rheumatoid arthritis of multiple sites

✓5th **M05.5 Rheumatoid polyneuropathy with rheumatoid arthritis**
- M05.50 Rheumatoid polyneuropathy with rheumatoid arthritis of unspecified site

✓6th **M05.51 Rheumatoid polyneuropathy with rheumatoid arthritis of shoulder**
- M05.511 Rheumatoid polyneuropathy with rheumatoid arthritis of right shoulder
- M05.512 Rheumatoid polyneuropathy with rheumatoid arthritis of left shoulder
- M05.519 Rheumatoid polyneuropathy with rheumatoid arthritis of unspecified shoulder

✓6th **M05.52 Rheumatoid polyneuropathy with rheumatoid arthritis of elbow**
- M05.521 Rheumatoid polyneuropathy with rheumatoid arthritis of right elbow
- M05.522 Rheumatoid polyneuropathy with rheumatoid arthritis of left elbow
- M05.529 Rheumatoid polyneuropathy with rheumatoid arthritis of unspecified elbow

✓6th **M05.53 Rheumatoid polyneuropathy with rheumatoid arthritis of wrist**
Rheumatoid polyneuropathy with rheumatoid arthritis, carpal bones
- M05.531 Rheumatoid polyneuropathy with rheumatoid arthritis of right wrist
- M05.532 Rheumatoid polyneuropathy with rheumatoid arthritis of left wrist
- M05.539 Rheumatoid polyneuropathy with rheumatoid arthritis of unspecified wrist

✓6th **M05.54 Rheumatoid polyneuropathy with rheumatoid arthritis of hand**
Rheumatoid polyneuropathy with rheumatoid arthritis, metacarpus and phalanges
- M05.541 Rheumatoid polyneuropathy with rheumatoid arthritis of right hand
- M05.542 Rheumatoid polyneuropathy with rheumatoid arthritis of left hand
- M05.549 Rheumatoid polyneuropathy with rheumatoid arthritis of unspecified hand

✓6th **M05.55 Rheumatoid polyneuropathy with rheumatoid arthritis of hip**
- M05.551 Rheumatoid polyneuropathy with rheumatoid arthritis of right hip
- M05.552 Rheumatoid polyneuropathy with rheumatoid arthritis of left hip
- M05.559 Rheumatoid polyneuropathy with rheumatoid arthritis of unspecified hip

✓6th **M05.56 Rheumatoid polyneuropathy with rheumatoid arthritis of knee**
- M05.561 Rheumatoid polyneuropathy with rheumatoid arthritis of right knee
- M05.562 Rheumatoid polyneuropathy with rheumatoid arthritis of left knee
- M05.569 Rheumatoid polyneuropathy with rheumatoid arthritis of unspecified knee

✓6th **M05.57 Rheumatoid polyneuropathy with rheumatoid arthritis of ankle and foot**
Rheumatoid polyneuropathy with rheumatoid arthritis, tarsus, metatarsus and phalanges
- M05.571 Rheumatoid polyneuropathy with rheumatoid arthritis of right ankle and foot
- M05.572 Rheumatoid polyneuropathy with rheumatoid arthritis of left ankle and foot

- M05.579 Rheumatoid polyneuropathy with rheumatoid arthritis of unspecified ankle and foot

M05.59 Rheumatoid polyneuropathy with rheumatoid arthritis of multiple sites

✓5th **M05.6 Rheumatoid arthritis with involvement of other organs and systems**
- M05.60 Rheumatoid arthritis of unspecified site with involvement of other organs and systems

✓6th **M05.61 Rheumatoid arthritis of shoulder with involvement of other organs and systems**
- M05.611 Rheumatoid arthritis of right shoulder with involvement of other organs and systems
- M05.612 Rheumatoid arthritis of left shoulder with involvement of other organs and systems
- M05.619 Rheumatoid arthritis of unspecified shoulder with involvement of other organs and systems

✓6th **M05.62 Rheumatoid arthritis of elbow with involvement of other organs and systems**
- M05.621 Rheumatoid arthritis of right elbow with involvement of other organs and systems
- M05.622 Rheumatoid arthritis of left elbow with involvement of other organs and systems
- M05.629 Rheumatoid arthritis of unspecified elbow with involvement of other organs and systems

✓6th **M05.63 Rheumatoid arthritis of wrist with involvement of other organs and systems**
Rheumatoid arthritis of carpal bones with involvement of other organs and systems
- M05.631 Rheumatoid arthritis of right wrist with involvement of other organs and systems
- M05.632 Rheumatoid arthritis of left wrist with involvement of other organs and systems
- M05.639 Rheumatoid arthritis of unspecified wrist with involvement of other organs and systems

✓6th **M05.64 Rheumatoid arthritis of hand with involvement of other organs and systems**
Rheumatoid arthritis of metacarpus and phalanges with involvement of other organs and systems
- M05.641 Rheumatoid arthritis of right hand with involvement of other organs and systems
- M05.642 Rheumatoid arthritis of left hand with involvement of other organs and systems
- M05.649 Rheumatoid arthritis of unspecified hand with involvement of other organs and systems

✓6th **M05.65 Rheumatoid arthritis of hip with involvement of other organs and systems**
- M05.651 Rheumatoid arthritis of right hip with involvement of other organs and systems
- M05.652 Rheumatoid arthritis of left hip with involvement of other organs and systems
- M05.659 Rheumatoid arthritis of unspecified hip with involvement of other organs and systems

✓6th **M05.66 Rheumatoid arthritis of knee with involvement of other organs and systems**
- M05.661 Rheumatoid arthritis of right knee with involvement of other organs and systems
- M05.662 Rheumatoid arthritis of left knee with involvement of other organs and systems
- M05.669 Rheumatoid arthritis of unspecified knee with involvement of other organs and systems

✓6th **M05.67 Rheumatoid arthritis of ankle and foot with involvement of other organs and systems**
Rheumatoid arthritis of tarsus, metatarsus and phalanges with involvement of other organs and systems
- M05.671 Rheumatoid arthritis of right ankle and foot with involvement of other organs and systems
- M05.672 Rheumatoid arthritis of left ankle and foot with involvement of other organs and systems

M05.679 Rheumatoid arthritis of unspecified ankle and foot with involvement of other organs and systems

M05.69 Rheumatoid arthritis of multiple sites with involvement of other organs and systems

✓5ᵗʰ **M05.7** Rheumatoid arthritis with rheumatoid factor without organ or systems involvement

M05.70 Rheumatoid arthritis with rheumatoid factor of unspecified site without organ or systems involvement

✓6ᵗʰ **M05.71** Rheumatoid arthritis with rheumatoid factor of shoulder without organ or systems involvement

M05.711 Rheumatoid arthritis with rheumatoid factor of right shoulder without organ or systems involvement

M05.712 Rheumatoid arthritis with rheumatoid factor of left shoulder without organ or systems involvement

M05.719 Rheumatoid arthritis with rheumatoid factor of unspecified shoulder without organ or systems involvement

✓6ᵗʰ **M05.72** Rheumatoid arthritis with rheumatoid factor of elbow without organ or systems involvement

M05.721 Rheumatoid arthritis with rheumatoid factor of right elbow without organ or systems involvement

M05.722 Rheumatoid arthritis with rheumatoid factor of left elbow without organ or systems involvement

M05.729 Rheumatoid arthritis with rheumatoid factor of unspecified elbow without organ or systems involvement

✓6ᵗʰ **M05.73** Rheumatoid arthritis with rheumatoid factor of wrist without organ or systems involvement

M05.731 Rheumatoid arthritis with rheumatoid factor of right wrist without organ or systems involvement

M05.732 Rheumatoid arthritis with rheumatoid factor of left wrist without organ or systems involvement

M05.739 Rheumatoid arthritis with rheumatoid factor of unspecified wrist without organ or systems involvement

✓6ᵗʰ **M05.74** Rheumatoid arthritis with rheumatoid factor of hand without organ or systems involvement

M05.741 Rheumatoid arthritis with rheumatoid factor of right hand without organ or systems involvement

M05.742 Rheumatoid arthritis with rheumatoid factor of left hand without organ or systems involvement

M05.749 Rheumatoid arthritis with rheumatoid factor of unspecified hand without organ or systems involvement

✓6ᵗʰ **M05.75** Rheumatoid arthritis with rheumatoid factor of hip without organ or systems involvement

M05.751 Rheumatoid arthritis with rheumatoid factor of right hip without organ or systems involvement

M05.752 Rheumatoid arthritis with rheumatoid factor of left hip without organ or systems involvement

M05.759 Rheumatoid arthritis with rheumatoid factor of unspecified hip without organ or systems involvement

✓6ᵗʰ **M05.76** Rheumatoid arthritis with rheumatoid factor of knee without organ or systems involvement

M05.761 Rheumatoid arthritis with rheumatoid factor of right knee without organ or systems involvement

M05.762 Rheumatoid arthritis with rheumatoid factor of left knee without organ or systems involvement

M05.769 Rheumatoid arthritis with rheumatoid factor of unspecified knee without organ or systems involvement

✓6ᵗʰ **M05.77** Rheumatoid arthritis with rheumatoid factor of ankle and foot without organ or systems involvement

M05.771 Rheumatoid arthritis with rheumatoid factor of right ankle and foot without organ or systems involvement

M05.772 Rheumatoid arthritis with rheumatoid factor of left ankle and foot without organ or systems involvement

M05.779 Rheumatoid arthritis with rheumatoid factor of unspecified ankle and foot without organ or systems involvement

M05.79 Rheumatoid arthritis with rheumatoid factor of multiple sites without organ or systems involvement

✓5ᵗʰ **M05.8** Other rheumatoid arthritis with rheumatoid factor

M05.80 Other rheumatoid arthritis with rheumatoid factor of unspecified site

✓6ᵗʰ **M05.81** Other rheumatoid arthritis with rheumatoid factor of shoulder

M05.811 Other rheumatoid arthritis with rheumatoid factor of right shoulder

M05.812 Other rheumatoid arthritis with rheumatoid factor of left shoulder

M05.819 Other rheumatoid arthritis with rheumatoid factor of unspecified shoulder

✓6ᵗʰ **M05.82** Other rheumatoid arthritis with rheumatoid factor of elbow

M05.821 Other rheumatoid arthritis with rheumatoid factor of right elbow

M05.822 Other rheumatoid arthritis with rheumatoid factor of left elbow

M05.829 Other rheumatoid arthritis with rheumatoid factor of unspecified elbow

✓6ᵗʰ **M05.83** Other rheumatoid arthritis with rheumatoid factor of wrist

M05.831 Other rheumatoid arthritis with rheumatoid factor of right wrist

M05.832 Other rheumatoid arthritis with rheumatoid factor of left wrist

M05.839 Other rheumatoid arthritis with rheumatoid factor of unspecified wrist

✓6ᵗʰ **M05.84** Other rheumatoid arthritis with rheumatoid factor of hand

M05.841 Other rheumatoid arthritis with rheumatoid factor of right hand

M05.842 Other rheumatoid arthritis with rheumatoid factor of left hand

M05.849 Other rheumatoid arthritis with rheumatoid factor of unspecified hand

✓6ᵗʰ **M05.85** Other rheumatoid arthritis with rheumatoid factor of hip

M05.851 Other rheumatoid arthritis with rheumatoid factor of right hip

M05.852 Other rheumatoid arthritis with rheumatoid factor of left hip

M05.859 Other rheumatoid arthritis with rheumatoid factor of unspecified hip

✓6ᵗʰ **M05.86** Other rheumatoid arthritis with rheumatoid factor of knee

M05.861 Other rheumatoid arthritis with rheumatoid factor of right knee

M05.862 Other rheumatoid arthritis with rheumatoid factor of left knee

M05.869 Other rheumatoid arthritis with rheumatoid factor of unspecified knee

✓6ᵗʰ **M05.87** Other rheumatoid arthritis with rheumatoid factor of ankle and foot

M05.871 Other rheumatoid arthritis with rheumatoid factor of right ankle and foot

M05.872 Other rheumatoid arthritis with rheumatoid factor of left ankle and foot

M05.879 Other rheumatoid arthritis with rheumatoid factor of unspecified ankle and foot

M05.89 Other rheumatoid arthritis with rheumatoid factor of multiple sites

M05.9 Rheumatoid arthritis with rheumatoid factor, unspecified

EXCLUDES 1 Not coded here   EXCLUDES 2 Not included here   N Newborn Age: 0   P Pediatric Age: 0-17   M Maternity Age: 12-55   A Adult Age: 15-124

652   ICD-10-CM 2014 (Draft)

☑4ᵗʰ M06 Other rheumatoid arthritis

  ☑5ᵗʰ **M06.0 Rheumatoid arthritis** without rheumatoid factor

    M06.00 Rheumatoid arthritis without rheumatoid factor, unspecified site

    ☑6ᵗʰ **M06.01 Rheumatoid arthritis without rheumatoid factor, shoulder**

      M06.011 Rheumatoid arthritis without rheumatoid factor, right shoulder

      M06.012 Rheumatoid arthritis without rheumatoid factor, left shoulder

      M06.019 Rheumatoid arthritis without rheumatoid factor, unspecified shoulder

    ☑6ᵗʰ **M06.02 Rheumatoid arthritis without rheumatoid factor, elbow**

      M06.021 Rheumatoid arthritis without rheumatoid factor, right elbow

      M06.022 Rheumatoid arthritis without rheumatoid factor, left elbow

      M06.029 Rheumatoid arthritis without rheumatoid factor, unspecified elbow

    ☑6ᵗʰ **M06.03 Rheumatoid arthritis without rheumatoid factor, wrist**

      M06.031 Rheumatoid arthritis without rheumatoid factor, right wrist

      M06.032 Rheumatoid arthritis without rheumatoid factor, left wrist

      M06.039 Rheumatoid arthritis without rheumatoid factor, unspecified wrist

    ☑6ᵗʰ **M06.04 Rheumatoid arthritis without rheumatoid factor, hand**

      M06.041 Rheumatoid arthritis without rheumatoid factor, right hand

      M06.042 Rheumatoid arthritis without rheumatoid factor, left hand

      M06.049 Rheumatoid arthritis without rheumatoid factor, unspecified hand

    ☑6ᵗʰ **M06.05 Rheumatoid arthritis without rheumatoid factor, hip**

      M06.051 Rheumatoid arthritis without rheumatoid factor, right hip

      M06.052 Rheumatoid arthritis without rheumatoid factor, left hip

      M06.059 Rheumatoid arthritis without rheumatoid factor, unspecified hip

    ☑6ᵗʰ **M06.06 Rheumatoid arthritis without rheumatoid factor, knee**

      M06.061 Rheumatoid arthritis without rheumatoid factor, right knee

      M06.062 Rheumatoid arthritis without rheumatoid factor, left knee

      M06.069 Rheumatoid arthritis without rheumatoid factor, unspecified knee

    ☑6ᵗʰ **M06.07 Rheumatoid arthritis without rheumatoid factor, ankle and foot**

      M06.071 Rheumatoid arthritis without rheumatoid factor, right ankle and foot

      M06.072 Rheumatoid arthritis without rheumatoid factor, left ankle and foot

      M06.079 Rheumatoid arthritis without rheumatoid factor, unspecified ankle and foot

    M06.08 Rheumatoid arthritis without rheumatoid factor, vertebrae

    M06.09 Rheumatoid arthritis without rheumatoid factor, multiple sites

  M06.1 Adult-onset Still's disease Ⓐ

    EXCLUDES 1 Still's disease NOS (M08.2-)

  ☑5ᵗʰ **M06.2 Rheumatoid bursitis**

    M06.20 Rheumatoid bursitis, unspecified site

    ☑6ᵗʰ **M06.21 Rheumatoid bursitis, shoulder**

      M06.211 Rheumatoid bursitis, right shoulder

      M06.212 Rheumatoid bursitis, left shoulder

      M06.219 Rheumatoid bursitis, unspecified shoulder

    ☑6ᵗʰ **M06.22 Rheumatoid bursitis, elbow**

      M06.221 Rheumatoid bursitis, right elbow

      M06.222 Rheumatoid bursitis, left elbow

      M06.229 Rheumatoid bursitis, unspecified elbow

    ☑6ᵗʰ **M06.23 Rheumatoid bursitis, wrist**

      M06.231 Rheumatoid bursitis, right wrist

      M06.232 Rheumatoid bursitis, left wrist

      M06.239 Rheumatoid bursitis, unspecified wrist

    ☑6ᵗʰ **M06.24 Rheumatoid bursitis, hand**

      M06.241 Rheumatoid bursitis, right hand

      M06.242 Rheumatoid bursitis, left hand

      M06.249 Rheumatoid bursitis, unspecified hand

    ☑6ᵗʰ **M06.25 Rheumatoid bursitis, hip**

      M06.251 Rheumatoid bursitis, right hip

      M06.252 Rheumatoid bursitis, left hip

      M06.259 Rheumatoid bursitis, unspecified hip

    ☑6ᵗʰ **M06.26 Rheumatoid bursitis, knee**

      M06.261 Rheumatoid bursitis, right knee

      M06.262 Rheumatoid bursitis, left knee

      M06.269 Rheumatoid bursitis, unspecified knee

    ☑6ᵗʰ **M06.27 Rheumatoid bursitis, ankle and foot**

      M06.271 Rheumatoid bursitis, right ankle and foot

      M06.272 Rheumatoid bursitis, left ankle and foot

      M06.279 Rheumatoid bursitis, unspecified ankle and foot

    M06.28 Rheumatoid bursitis, vertebrae

    M06.29 Rheumatoid bursitis, multiple sites

  ☑5ᵗʰ **M06.3 Rheumatoid nodule**

    M06.30 Rheumatoid nodule, unspecified site

    ☑6ᵗʰ **M06.31 Rheumatoid nodule, shoulder**

      M06.311 Rheumatoid nodule, right shoulder

      M06.312 Rheumatoid nodule, left shoulder

      M06.319 Rheumatoid nodule, unspecified shoulder

    ☑6ᵗʰ **M06.32 Rheumatoid nodule, elbow**

      M06.321 Rheumatoid nodule, right elbow

      M06.322 Rheumatoid nodule, left elbow

      M06.329 Rheumatoid nodule, unspecified elbow

    ☑6ᵗʰ **M06.33 Rheumatoid nodule, wrist**

      M06.331 Rheumatoid nodule, right wrist

      M06.332 Rheumatoid nodule, left wrist

      M06.339 Rheumatoid nodule, unspecified wrist

    ☑6ᵗʰ **M06.34 Rheumatoid nodule, hand**

      M06.341 Rheumatoid nodule, right hand

      M06.342 Rheumatoid nodule, left hand

      M06.349 Rheumatoid nodule, unspecified hand

    ☑6ᵗʰ **M06.35 Rheumatoid nodule, hip**

      M06.351 Rheumatoid nodule, right hip

      M06.352 Rheumatoid nodule, left hip

      M06.359 Rheumatoid nodule, unspecified hip

    ☑6ᵗʰ **M06.36 Rheumatoid nodule, knee**

      M06.361 Rheumatoid nodule, right knee

      M06.362 Rheumatoid nodule, left knee

      M06.369 Rheumatoid nodule, unspecified knee

    ☑6ᵗʰ **M06.37 Rheumatoid nodule, ankle and foot**

      M06.371 Rheumatoid nodule, right ankle and foot

      M06.372 Rheumatoid nodule, left ankle and foot

      M06.379 Rheumatoid nodule, unspecified ankle and foot

    M06.38 Rheumatoid nodule, vertebrae

    M06.39 Rheumatoid nodule, multiple sites

  M06.4 Inflammatory polyarthropathy

    EXCLUDES 1 polyarthritis NOS (M13.0)

  ☑5ᵗʰ **M06.8 Other specified rheumatoid arthritis**

    M06.80 Other specified rheumatoid arthritis, unspecified site

    ☑6ᵗʰ **M06.81 Other specified rheumatoid arthritis, shoulder**

      M06.811 Other specified rheumatoid arthritis, right shoulder

      M06.812 Other specified rheumatoid arthritis, left shoulder

      M06.819 Other specified rheumatoid arthritis, unspecified shoulder

    ☑6ᵗʰ **M06.82 Other specified rheumatoid arthritis, elbow**

      M06.821 Other specified rheumatoid arthritis, right elbow

---

☑ Additional Character Required √x7ᵗʰ Xtension Alert Unspecified Code Other Specified Code Manifestation Code ►◄ Revised Text ● New Code ▲ Revised Code Title

M06.822 **Other specified rheumatoid arthritis, left elbow**

M06.829 **Other specified rheumatoid arthritis, unspecified elbow**

✓6ᵗʰ M06.83 Other specified rheumatoid arthritis, wrist

M06.831 **Other specified rheumatoid arthritis, right wrist**

M06.832 **Other specified rheumatoid arthritis, left wrist**

M06.839 **Other specified rheumatoid arthritis, unspecified wrist**

✓6ᵗʰ M06.84 Other specified rheumatoid arthritis, hand

M06.841 **Other specified rheumatoid arthritis, right hand**

M06.842 **Other specified rheumatoid arthritis, left hand**

M06.849 **Other specified rheumatoid arthritis, unspecified hand**

✓6ᵗʰ M06.85 Other specified rheumatoid arthritis, hip

M06.851 **Other specified rheumatoid arthritis, right hip**

M06.852 **Other specified rheumatoid arthritis, left hip**

M06.859 **Other specified rheumatoid arthritis, unspecified hip**

✓6ᵗʰ M06.86 Other specified rheumatoid arthritis, knee

M06.861 **Other specified rheumatoid arthritis, right knee**

M06.862 **Other specified rheumatoid arthritis, left knee**

M06.869 **Other specified rheumatoid arthritis, unspecified knee**

✓6ᵗʰ M06.87 Other specified rheumatoid arthritis, ankle and foot

M06.871 **Other specified rheumatoid arthritis, right ankle and foot**

M06.872 **Other specified rheumatoid arthritis, left ankle and foot**

M06.879 **Other specified rheumatoid arthritis, unspecified ankle and foot**

M06.88 **Other specified rheumatoid arthritis, vertebrae**

M06.89 **Other specified rheumatoid arthritis, multiple sites**

M06.9 **Rheumatoid arthritis, unspecified**

✓4ᵗʰ **M07 Enteropathic arthropathies**

Code also associated enteropathy, such as:
regional enteritis [Crohn's disease] (K50.-)
ulcerative colitis (K51.-)

EXCLUDES 1 psoriatic arthropathies (L40.5-)

✓5ᵗʰ M07.6 Enteropathic arthropathies

M07.60 **Enteropathic arthropathies, unspecified site**

✓6ᵗʰ M07.61 Enteropathic arthropathies, shoulder

M07.611 **Enteropathic arthropathies, right shoulder**

M07.612 **Enteropathic arthropathies, left shoulder**

M07.619 **Enteropathic arthropathies, unspecified shoulder**

✓6ᵗʰ M07.62 Enteropathic arthropathies, elbow

M07.621 **Enteropathic arthropathies, right elbow**

M07.622 **Enteropathic arthropathies, left elbow**

M07.629 **Enteropathic arthropathies, unspecified elbow**

✓6ᵗʰ M07.63 Enteropathic arthropathies, wrist

M07.631 **Enteropathic arthropathies, right wrist**

M07.632 **Enteropathic arthropathies, left wrist**

M07.639 **Enteropathic arthropathies, unspecified wrist**

✓6ᵗʰ M07.64 Enteropathic arthropathies, hand

M07.641 **Enteropathic arthropathies, right hand**

M07.642 **Enteropathic arthropathies, left hand**

M07.649 **Enteropathic arthropathies, unspecified hand**

✓6ᵗʰ M07.65 Enteropathic arthropathies, hip

M07.651 **Enteropathic arthropathies, right hip**

M07.652 **Enteropathic arthropathies, left hip**

M07.659 **Enteropathic arthropathies, unspecified hip**

✓6ᵗʰ M07.66 Enteropathic arthropathies, knee

M07.661 **Enteropathic arthropathies, right knee**

M07.662 **Enteropathic arthropathies, left knee**

M07.669 **Enteropathic arthropathies, unspecified knee**

✓6ᵗʰ M07.67 Enteropathic arthropathies, ankle and foot

M07.671 **Enteropathic arthropathies, right ankle and foot**

M07.672 **Enteropathic arthropathies, left ankle and foot**

M07.679 **Enteropathic arthropathies, unspecified ankle and foot**

M07.68 **Enteropathic arthropathies, vertebrae**

M07.69 **Enteropathic arthropathies, multiple sites**

✓4ᵗʰ **M08 Juvenile arthritis**

Code also any associated underlying condition, such as:
regional enteritis [Crohn's disease] (K50.-)
ulcerative colitis (K51.-)

EXCLUDES 1 arthropathy in Whipple's disease (M14.8)
Felty's syndrome (M05.0)
juvenile dermatomyositis (M33.0-)
psoriatic juvenile arthropathy (L40.54)

✓5ᵗʰ M08.0 Unspecified juvenile rheumatoid arthritis

Juvenile rheumatoid arthritis with or without rheumatoid factor

M08.00 **Unspecified juvenile rheumatoid arthritis of unspecified site**

✓6ᵗʰ M08.01 Unspecified juvenile rheumatoid arthritis, shoulder

M08.011 **Unspecified juvenile rheumatoid arthritis, right shoulder**

M08.012 **Unspecified juvenile rheumatoid arthritis, left shoulder**

M08.019 **Unspecified juvenile rheumatoid arthritis, unspecified shoulder**

✓6ᵗʰ M08.02 Unspecified juvenile rheumatoid arthritis of elbow

M08.021 **Unspecified juvenile rheumatoid arthritis, right elbow**

M08.022 **Unspecified juvenile rheumatoid arthritis, left elbow**

M08.029 **Unspecified juvenile rheumatoid arthritis, unspecified elbow**

✓6ᵗʰ M08.03 Unspecified juvenile rheumatoid arthritis, wrist

M08.031 **Unspecified juvenile rheumatoid arthritis, right wrist**

M08.032 **Unspecified juvenile rheumatoid arthritis, left wrist**

M08.039 **Unspecified juvenile rheumatoid arthritis, unspecified wrist**

✓6ᵗʰ M08.04 Unspecified juvenile rheumatoid arthritis, hand

M08.041 **Unspecified juvenile rheumatoid arthritis, right hand**

M08.042 **Unspecified juvenile rheumatoid arthritis, left hand**

M08.049 **Unspecified juvenile rheumatoid arthritis, unspecified hand**

✓6ᵗʰ M08.05 Unspecified juvenile rheumatoid arthritis, hip

M08.051 **Unspecified juvenile rheumatoid arthritis, right hip**

M08.052 **Unspecified juvenile rheumatoid arthritis, left hip**

M08.059 **Unspecified juvenile rheumatoid arthritis, unspecified hip**

✓6ᵗʰ M08.06 Unspecified juvenile rheumatoid arthritis, knee

M08.061 **Unspecified juvenile rheumatoid arthritis, right knee**

M08.062 **Unspecified juvenile rheumatoid arthritis, left knee**

M08.069 **Unspecified juvenile rheumatoid arthritis, unspecified knee**

✓6ᵗʰ M08.07 Unspecified juvenile rheumatoid arthritis, ankle and foot

M08.071 **Unspecified juvenile rheumatoid arthritis, right ankle and foot**

M08.072 **Unspecified juvenile rheumatoid arthritis, left ankle and foot**

M08.079 **Unspecified juvenile rheumatoid arthritis, unspecified ankle and foot**

M08.08 **Unspecified juvenile rheumatoid arthritis, vertebrae**

EXCLUDES 1 Not coded here   EXCLUDES 2 Not included here   N Newborn Age: 0   P Pediatric Age: 0-17   M Maternity Age: 12-55   A Adult Age: 15-124

654   ICD-10-CM 2014 (Draft)

      M08.09 **Unspecified juvenile rheumatoid arthritis, multiple sites**

  M08.1 **Juvenile ankylosing spondylitis**

      EXCLUDES1 *ankylosing spondylitis in adults (M45.0-)*

✓5ᵗʰ M08.2 **Juvenile rheumatoid arthritis with systemic onset**
      Still's disease NOS
      EXCLUDES1 *adult-onset Still's disease (M06.1-)*

      M08.20 **Juvenile rheumatoid arthritis with systemic onset, unspecified site**

✓6ᵗʰ M08.21 **Juvenile rheumatoid arthritis with systemic onset, shoulder**

          M08.211 **Juvenile rheumatoid arthritis with systemic onset, right shoulder**

          M08.212 **Juvenile rheumatoid arthritis with systemic onset, left shoulder**

          M08.219 **Juvenile rheumatoid arthritis with systemic onset, unspecified shoulder**

✓6ᵗʰ M08.22 **Juvenile rheumatoid arthritis with systemic onset, elbow**

          M08.221 **Juvenile rheumatoid arthritis with systemic onset, right elbow**

          M08.222 **Juvenile rheumatoid arthritis with systemic onset, left elbow**

          M08.229 **Juvenile rheumatoid arthritis with systemic onset, unspecified elbow**

✓6ᵗʰ M08.23 **Juvenile rheumatoid arthritis with systemic onset, wrist**

          M08.231 **Juvenile rheumatoid arthritis with systemic onset, right wrist**

          M08.232 **Juvenile rheumatoid arthritis with systemic onset, left wrist**

          M08.239 **Juvenile rheumatoid arthritis with systemic onset, unspecified wrist**

✓6ᵗʰ M08.24 **Juvenile rheumatoid arthritis with systemic onset, hand**

          M08.241 **Juvenile rheumatoid arthritis with systemic onset, right hand**

          M08.242 **Juvenile rheumatoid arthritis with systemic onset, left hand**

          M08.249 **Juvenile rheumatoid arthritis with systemic onset, unspecified hand**

✓6ᵗʰ M08.25 **Juvenile rheumatoid arthritis with systemic onset, hip**

          M08.251 **Juvenile rheumatoid arthritis with systemic onset, right hip**

          M08.252 **Juvenile rheumatoid arthritis with systemic onset, left hip**

          M08.259 **Juvenile rheumatoid arthritis with systemic onset, unspecified hip**

✓6ᵗʰ M08.26 **Juvenile rheumatoid arthritis with systemic onset, knee**

          M08.261 **Juvenile rheumatoid arthritis with systemic onset, right knee**

          M08.262 **Juvenile rheumatoid arthritis with systemic onset, left knee**

          M08.269 **Juvenile rheumatoid arthritis with systemic onset, unspecified knee**

✓6ᵗʰ M08.27 **Juvenile rheumatoid arthritis with systemic onset, ankle and foot**

          M08.271 **Juvenile rheumatoid arthritis with systemic onset, right ankle and foot**

          M08.272 **Juvenile rheumatoid arthritis with systemic onset, left ankle and foot**

          M08.279 **Juvenile rheumatoid arthritis with systemic onset, unspecified ankle and foot**

      M08.28 **Juvenile rheumatoid arthritis with systemic onset, vertebrae**

      M08.29 **Juvenile rheumatoid arthritis with systemic onset, multiple sites**

  M08.3 **Juvenile rheumatoid polyarthritis (seronegative)**

✓5ᵗʰ M08.4 **Pauciarticular juvenile rheumatoid arthritis**

      M08.40 **Pauciarticular juvenile rheumatoid arthritis, unspecified site**

✓6ᵗʰ M08.41 **Pauciarticular juvenile rheumatoid arthritis, shoulder**

          M08.411 **Pauciarticular juvenile rheumatoid arthritis, right shoulder**

          M08.412 **Pauciarticular juvenile rheumatoid arthritis, left shoulder**

          M08.419 **Pauciarticular juvenile rheumatoid arthritis, unspecified shoulder**

✓6ᵗʰ M08.42 **Pauciarticular juvenile rheumatoid arthritis, elbow**

          M08.421 **Pauciarticular juvenile rheumatoid arthritis, right elbow**

          M08.422 **Pauciarticular juvenile rheumatoid arthritis, left elbow**

          M08.429 **Pauciarticular juvenile rheumatoid arthritis, unspecified elbow**

✓6ᵗʰ M08.43 **Pauciarticular juvenile rheumatoid arthritis, wrist**

          M08.431 **Pauciarticular juvenile rheumatoid arthritis, right wrist**

          M08.432 **Pauciarticular juvenile rheumatoid arthritis, left wrist**

          M08.439 **Pauciarticular juvenile rheumatoid arthritis, unspecified wrist**

✓6ᵗʰ M08.44 **Pauciarticular juvenile rheumatoid arthritis, hand**

          M08.441 **Pauciarticular juvenile rheumatoid arthritis, right hand**

          M08.442 **Pauciarticular juvenile rheumatoid arthritis, left hand**

          M08.449 **Pauciarticular juvenile rheumatoid arthritis, unspecified hand**

✓6ᵗʰ M08.45 **Pauciarticular juvenile rheumatoid arthritis, hip**

          M08.451 **Pauciarticular juvenile rheumatoid arthritis, right hip**

          M08.452 **Pauciarticular juvenile rheumatoid arthritis, left hip**

          M08.459 **Pauciarticular juvenile rheumatoid arthritis, unspecified hip**

✓6ᵗʰ M08.46 **Pauciarticular juvenile rheumatoid arthritis, knee**

          M08.461 **Pauciarticular juvenile rheumatoid arthritis, right knee**

          M08.462 **Pauciarticular juvenile rheumatoid arthritis, left knee**

          M08.469 **Pauciarticular juvenile rheumatoid arthritis, unspecified knee**

✓6ᵗʰ M08.47 **Pauciarticular juvenile rheumatoid arthritis, ankle and foot**

          M08.471 **Pauciarticular juvenile rheumatoid arthritis, right ankle and foot**

          M08.472 **Pauciarticular juvenile rheumatoid arthritis, left ankle and foot**

          M08.479 **Pauciarticular juvenile rheumatoid arthritis, unspecified ankle and foot**

      M08.48 **Pauciarticular juvenile rheumatoid arthritis, vertebrae**

✓5ᵗʰ M08.8 **Other juvenile arthritis**

      M08.80 **Other juvenile arthritis, unspecified site**

✓6ᵗʰ M08.81 **Other juvenile arthritis, shoulder**

          M08.811 **Other juvenile arthritis, right shoulder**

          M08.812 **Other juvenile arthritis, left shoulder**

          M08.819 **Other juvenile arthritis, unspecified shoulder**

✓6ᵗʰ M08.82 **Other juvenile arthritis, elbow**

          M08.821 **Other juvenile arthritis, right elbow**

          M08.822 **Other juvenile arthritis, left elbow**

          M08.829 **Other juvenile arthritis, unspecified elbow**

✓6ᵗʰ M08.83 **Other juvenile arthritis, wrist**

          M08.831 **Other juvenile arthritis, right wrist**

          M08.832 **Other juvenile arthritis, left wrist**

          M08.839 **Other juvenile arthritis, unspecified wrist**

✓6ᵗʰ M08.84 **Other juvenile arthritis, hand**

          M08.841 **Other juvenile arthritis, right hand**

          M08.842 **Other juvenile arthritis, left hand**

          M08.849 **Other juvenile arthritis, unspecified hand**

✓6ᵗʰ M08.85 **Other juvenile arthritis, hip**

          M08.851 **Other juvenile arthritis, right hip**

          M08.852 **Other juvenile arthritis, left hip**

          M08.859 **Other juvenile arthritis, unspecified hip**

✓6ᵗʰ M08.86 **Other juvenile arthritis, knee**

          M08.861 **Other juvenile arthritis, right knee**

          M08.862 **Other juvenile arthritis, left knee**

✅ Additional Character Required   ✔7ᵗʰ Xtension Alert   Unspecified Code   Other Specified Code   Manifestation Code   ▶◀ Revised Text   ● New Code   ▲ Revised Code Title

ICD-10-CM 2014 (Draft)   **655**

Diseases of the Musculoskeletal System and Connective Tissue

M08.869–M1A.171

M08.869 **Other juvenile arthritis, unspecified knee**

✓6ᵗʰ M08.87 Other juvenile arthritis, **ankle and foot**

M08.871 **Other juvenile arthritis, right ankle and foot**

M08.872 **Other juvenile arthritis, left ankle and foot**

M08.879 **Other juvenile arthritis, unspecified ankle and foot**

M08.88 **Other juvenile arthritis, other specified site**
Other juvenile arthritis, vertebrae

M08.89 **Other juvenile arthritis, multiple sites**

✓5ᵗʰ M08.9 **Juvenile arthritis, unspecified**

EXCLUDES 1   *juvenile rheumatoid arthritis, unspecified (M08.0-)*

M08.90 **Juvenile arthritis, unspecified, unspecified site**

✓6ᵗʰ M08.91 Juvenile arthritis, unspecified, **shoulder**

M08.911 Juvenile arthritis, unspecified, **right shoulder**

M08.912 Juvenile arthritis, unspecified, **left shoulder**

M08.919 **Juvenile arthritis, unspecified, unspecified shoulder**

✓6ᵗʰ M08.92 Juvenile arthritis, unspecified, **elbow**

M08.921 Juvenile arthritis, unspecified, **right elbow**

M08.922 Juvenile arthritis, unspecified, **left elbow**

M08.929 **Juvenile arthritis, unspecified, unspecified elbow**

✓6ᵗʰ M08.93 Juvenile arthritis, unspecified, **wrist**

M08.931 Juvenile arthritis, unspecified, **right wrist**

M08.932 Juvenile arthritis, unspecified, **left wrist**

M08.939 **Juvenile arthritis, unspecified, unspecified wrist**

✓6ᵗʰ M08.94 Juvenile arthritis, unspecified, **hand**

M08.941 Juvenile arthritis, unspecified, **right hand**

M08.942 Juvenile arthritis, unspecified, **left hand**

M08.949 **Juvenile arthritis, unspecified, unspecified hand**

✓6ᵗʰ M08.95 Juvenile arthritis, unspecified, **hip**

M08.951 Juvenile arthritis, unspecified, **right hip**

M08.952 Juvenile arthritis, unspecified, **left hip**

M08.959 **Juvenile arthritis, unspecified, unspecified hip**

✓6ᵗʰ M08.96 Juvenile arthritis, unspecified, **knee**

M08.961 Juvenile arthritis, unspecified, **right knee**

M08.962 Juvenile arthritis, unspecified, **left knee**

M08.969 **Juvenile arthritis, unspecified, unspecified knee**

✓6ᵗʰ M08.97 Juvenile arthritis, unspecified, **ankle and foot**

M08.971 **Juvenile arthritis, unspecified, right ankle and foot**

M08.972 **Juvenile arthritis, unspecified, left ankle and foot**

M08.979 **Juvenile arthritis, unspecified, unspecified ankle and foot**

M08.98 Juvenile arthritis, unspecified, **vertebrae**

M08.99 Juvenile arthritis, unspecified, **multiple sites**

✓4ᵗʰ **M1A Chronic gout**

Use additional code to identify:
autonomic neuropathy in diseases classified elsewhere (G99.0)
calculus of urinary tract in diseases classified elsewhere (N22)
cardiomyopathy in diseases classified elsewhere (I43)
disorders of external ear in diseases classified elsewhere (H61.1-, H62.8-)
disorders of iris and ciliary body in diseases classified elsewhere (H22)
glomerular disorders in diseases classified elsewhere (N08)

The appropriate 7th character is to be added to each code from category M1A.
0   without tophus (tophi)
1   with tophus (tophi)

EXCLUDES 1   *acute gout (M10.-)*
gout NOS (M10.-)

✓5ᵗʰ **M1A.0 Idiopathic chronic gout**
Chronic gouty bursitis   Primary chronic gout

✓x7ᵗʰ **M1A.00 Idiopathic chronic gout, unspecified site**

✓6ᵗʰ **M1A.01 Idiopathic chronic gout, shoulder**

✓7ᵗʰ **M1A.011 Idiopathic chronic gout, right shoulder**

✓7ᵗʰ M1A.012 **Idiopathic chronic gout, left shoulder**

✓7ᵗʰ M1A.019 **Idiopathic chronic gout, unspecified shoulder**

✓6ᵗʰ M1A.02 **Idiopathic chronic gout, elbow**

✓7ᵗʰ M1A.021 **Idiopathic chronic gout, right elbow**

✓7ᵗʰ M1A.022 **Idiopathic chronic gout, left elbow**

✓7ᵗʰ M1A.029 **Idiopathic chronic gout, unspecified elbow**

✓6ᵗʰ M1A.03 **Idiopathic chronic gout, wrist**

✓7ᵗʰ M1A.031 **Idiopathic chronic gout, right wrist**

✓7ᵗʰ M1A.032 **Idiopathic chronic gout, left wrist**

✓7ᵗʰ M1A.039 **Idiopathic chronic gout, unspecified wrist**

✓6ᵗʰ M1A.04 **Idiopathic chronic gout, hand**

✓7ᵗʰ M1A.041 **Idiopathic chronic gout, right hand**

✓7ᵗʰ M1A.042 **Idiopathic chronic gout, left hand**

✓7ᵗʰ M1A.049 **Idiopathic chronic gout, unspecified hand**

✓6ᵗʰ M1A.05 **Idiopathic chronic gout, hip**

✓7ᵗʰ M1A.051 **Idiopathic chronic gout, right hip**

✓7ᵗʰ M1A.052 **Idiopathic chronic gout, left hip**

✓7ᵗʰ M1A.059 **Idiopathic chronic gout, unspecified hip**

✓6ᵗʰ M1A.06 **Idiopathic chronic gout, knee**

✓7ᵗʰ M1A.061 **Idiopathic chronic gout, right knee**

✓7ᵗʰ M1A.062 **Idiopathic chronic gout, left knee**

✓7ᵗʰ M1A.069 **Idiopathic chronic gout, unspecified knee**

✓6ᵗʰ M1A.07 **Idiopathic chronic gout, ankle and foot**

✓7ᵗʰ M1A.071 **Idiopathic chronic gout, right ankle and foot**

✓7ᵗʰ M1A.072 **Idiopathic chronic gout, left ankle and foot**

✓7ᵗʰ M1A.079 **Idiopathic chronic gout, unspecified ankle and foot**

✓x7ᵗʰ M1A.08 **Idiopathic chronic gout, vertebrae**

✓x7ᵗʰ M1A.09 **Idiopathic chronic gout, multiple sites**

✓5ᵗʰ M1A.1 **Lead-induced chronic gout**
Code first: toxic effects of lead and its compounds (T56.0-)

✓x7ᵗʰ **M1A.10 Lead-induced chronic gout, unspecified site**

✓6ᵗʰ **M1A.11 Lead-induced chronic gout, shoulder**

✓7ᵗʰ M1A.111 Lead-induced chronic gout, **right shoulder**

✓7ᵗʰ M1A.112 Lead-induced chronic gout, **left shoulder**

✓7ᵗʰ M1A.119 **Lead-induced chronic gout, unspecified shoulder**

✓6ᵗʰ **M1A.12 Lead-induced chronic gout, elbow**

✓7ᵗʰ M1A.121 Lead-induced chronic gout, **right elbow**

✓7ᵗʰ M1A.122 Lead-induced chronic gout, **left elbow**

✓7ᵗʰ M1A.129 **Lead-induced chronic gout, unspecified elbow**

✓6ᵗʰ **M1A.13 Lead-induced chronic gout, wrist**

✓7ᵗʰ M1A.131 Lead-induced chronic gout, **right wrist**

✓7ᵗʰ M1A.132 Lead-induced chronic gout, **left wrist**

✓7ᵗʰ M1A.139 **Lead-induced chronic gout, unspecified wrist**

✓6ᵗʰ **M1A.14 Lead-induced chronic gout, hand**

✓7ᵗʰ M1A.141 Lead-induced chronic gout, **right hand**

✓7ᵗʰ M1A.142 Lead-induced chronic gout, **left hand**

✓7ᵗʰ M1A.149 **Lead-induced chronic gout, unspecified hand**

✓6ᵗʰ **M1A.15 Lead-induced chronic gout, hip**

✓7ᵗʰ M1A.151 Lead-induced chronic gout, **right hip**

✓7ᵗʰ M1A.152 Lead-induced chronic gout, **left hip**

✓7ᵗʰ M1A.159 **Lead-induced chronic gout, unspecified hip**

✓6ᵗʰ **M1A.16 Lead-induced chronic gout, knee**

✓7ᵗʰ M1A.161 Lead-induced chronic gout, **right knee**

✓7ᵗʰ M1A.162 Lead-induced chronic gout, **left knee**

✓7ᵗʰ M1A.169 **Lead-induced chronic gout, unspecified knee**

✓6ᵗʰ **M1A.17 Lead-induced chronic gout, ankle and foot**

✓7ᵗʰ M1A.171 Lead-induced chronic gout, **right ankle and foot**

EXCLUDES 1 Not coded here   EXCLUDES 2 Not included here   N Newborn Age: 0   P Pediatric Age: 0-17   M Maternity Age: 12-55   A Adult Age: 15-124

656   ICD-10-CM 2014 (Draft)

√7th **M1A.172** Lead-induced chronic gout, left ankle and foot

√7th **M1A.179** Lead-induced chronic gout, unspecified ankle and foot

√x7th **M1A.18** Lead-induced chronic gout, vertebrae

√x7th **M1A.19** Lead-induced chronic gout, multiple sites

√5th **M1A.2** Drug-induced chronic gout
Use additional code for adverse effect, if applicable, to identify drug (T36-T50 with fifth or sixth character 5)

√x7th **M1A.20** Drug-induced chronic gout, unspecified site

√6th **M1A.21** Drug-induced chronic gout, shoulder

√7th **M1A.211** Drug-induced chronic gout, right shoulder

√7th **M1A.212** Drug-induced chronic gout, left shoulder

√7th **M1A.219** Drug-induced chronic gout, unspecified shoulder

√6th **M1A.22** Drug-induced chronic gout, elbow

√7th **M1A.221** Drug-induced chronic gout, right elbow

√7th **M1A.222** Drug-induced chronic gout, left elbow

√7th **M1A.229** Drug-induced chronic gout, unspecified elbow

√6th **M1A.23** Drug-induced chronic gout, wrist

√7th **M1A.231** Drug-induced chronic gout, right wrist

√7th **M1A.232** Drug-induced chronic gout, left wrist

√7th **M1A.239** Drug-induced chronic gout, unspecified wrist

√6th **M1A.24** Drug-induced chronic gout, hand

√7th **M1A.241** Drug-induced chronic gout, right hand

√7th **M1A.242** Drug-induced chronic gout, left hand

√7th **M1A.249** Drug-induced chronic gout, unspecified hand

√6th **M1A.25** Drug-induced chronic gout, hip

√7th **M1A.251** Drug-induced chronic gout, right hip

√7th **M1A.252** Drug-induced chronic gout, left hip

√7th **M1A.259** Drug-induced chronic gout, unspecified hip

√6th **M1A.26** Drug-induced chronic gout, knee

√7th **M1A.261** Drug-induced chronic gout, right knee

√7th **M1A.262** Drug-induced chronic gout, left knee

√7th **M1A.269** Drug-induced chronic gout, unspecified knee

√6th **M1A.27** Drug-induced chronic gout, ankle and foot

√7th **M1A.271** Drug-induced chronic gout, right ankle and foot

√7th **M1A.272** Drug-induced chronic gout, left ankle and foot

√7th **M1A.279** Drug-induced chronic gout, unspecified ankle and foot

√x7th **M1A.28** Drug-induced chronic gout, vertebrae

√x7th **M1A.29** Drug-induced chronic gout, multiple sites

√5th **M1A.3** Chronic gout due to renal impairment
Code first associated renal disease

√x7th **M1A.30** Chronic gout due to renal impairment, unspecified site

√6th **M1A.31** Chronic gout due to renal impairment, shoulder

√7th **M1A.311** Chronic gout due to renal impairment, right shoulder

√7th **M1A.312** Chronic gout due to renal impairment, left shoulder

√7th **M1A.319** Chronic gout due to renal impairment, unspecified shoulder

√6th **M1A.32** Chronic gout due to renal impairment, elbow

√7th **M1A.321** Chronic gout due to renal impairment, right elbow

√7th **M1A.322** Chronic gout due to renal impairment, left elbow

√7th **M1A.329** Chronic gout due to renal impairment, unspecified elbow

√6th **M1A.33** Chronic gout due to renal impairment, wrist

√7th **M1A.331** Chronic gout due to renal impairment, right wrist

√7th **M1A.332** Chronic gout due to renal impairment, left wrist

√7th **M1A.339** Chronic gout due to renal impairment, unspecified wrist

√6th **M1A.34** Chronic gout due to renal impairment, hand

√7th **M1A.341** Chronic gout due to renal impairment, right hand

√7th **M1A.342** Chronic gout due to renal impairment, left hand

√7th **M1A.349** Chronic gout due to renal impairment, unspecified hand

√6th **M1A.35** Chronic gout due to renal impairment, hip

√7th **M1A.351** Chronic gout due to renal impairment, right hip

√7th **M1A.352** Chronic gout due to renal impairment, left hip

√7th **M1A.359** Chronic gout due to renal impairment, unspecified hip

√6th **M1A.36** Chronic gout due to renal impairment, knee

√7th **M1A.361** Chronic gout due to renal impairment, right knee

√7th **M1A.362** Chronic gout due to renal impairment, left knee

√7th **M1A.369** Chronic gout due to renal impairment, unspecified knee

√6th **M1A.37** Chronic gout due to renal impairment, ankle and foot

√7th **M1A.371** Chronic gout due to renal impairment, right ankle and foot

√7th **M1A.372** Chronic gout due to renal impairment, left ankle and foot

√7th **M1A.379** Chronic gout due to renal impairment, unspecified ankle and foot

√x7th **M1A.38** Chronic gout due to renal impairment, vertebrae

√x7th **M1A.39** Chronic gout due to renal impairment, multiple sites

√5th **M1A.4** Other secondary chronic gout
Code first associated condition

√x7th **M1A.40** Other secondary chronic gout, unspecified site

√6th **M1A.41** Other secondary chronic gout, shoulder

√7th **M1A.411** Other secondary chronic gout, right shoulder

√7th **M1A.412** Other secondary chronic gout, left shoulder

√7th **M1A.419** Other secondary chronic gout, unspecified shoulder

√6th **M1A.42** Other secondary chronic gout, elbow

√7th **M1A.421** Other secondary chronic gout, right elbow

√7th **M1A.422** Other secondary chronic gout, left elbow

√7th **M1A.429** Other secondary chronic gout, unspecified elbow

√6th **M1A.43** Other secondary chronic gout, wrist

√7th **M1A.431** Other secondary chronic gout, right wrist

√7th **M1A.432** Other secondary chronic gout, left wrist

√7th **M1A.439** Other secondary chronic gout, unspecified wrist

√6th **M1A.44** Other secondary chronic gout, hand

√7th **M1A.441** Other secondary chronic gout, right hand

√7th **M1A.442** Other secondary chronic gout, left hand

√7th **M1A.449** Other secondary chronic gout, unspecified hand

√6th **M1A.45** Other secondary chronic gout, hip

√7th **M1A.451** Other secondary chronic gout, right hip

√7th **M1A.452** Other secondary chronic gout, left hip

√7th **M1A.459** Other secondary chronic gout, unspecified hip

√6th **M1A.46** Other secondary chronic gout, knee

√7th **M1A.461** Other secondary chronic gout, right knee

√7th **M1A.462** Other secondary chronic gout, left knee

√7th **M1A.469** Other secondary chronic gout, unspecified knee

Diseases of the Musculoskeletal System and Connective Tissue

M1A.47–M10.332

✓6ᵗʰ **M1A.47 Other secondary chronic gout, ankle and foot**
- ✓7ᵗʰ **M1A.471 Other secondary chronic gout, right ankle and foot**
- ✓7ᵗʰ **M1A.472 Other secondary chronic gout, left ankle and foot**
- ✓7ᵗʰ **M1A.479 Other secondary chronic gout, unspecified ankle and foot**

✓x7ᵗʰ **M1A.48 Other secondary chronic gout, vertebrae**

✓x7ᵗʰ **M1A.49 Other secondary chronic gout, multiple sites**

✓x7ᵗʰ **M1A.9 Chronic gout, unspecified**

✓4ᵗʰ **M10 Gout**

Acute gout   Gout NOS
Gout attack   Podagra
Gout flare

Use additional code to identify:
autonomic neuropathy in diseases classified elsewhere (G99.0)
calculus of urinary tract in diseases classified elsewhere (N22)
cardiomyopathy in diseases classified elsewhere (I43)
disorders of external ear in diseases classified elsewhere (H61.1-, H62.8-)
disorders of iris and ciliary body in diseases classified elsewhere (H22)
glomerular disorders in diseases classified elsewhere (N08)

EXCLUDES 1   chronic gout (M1A.-)

✓5ᵗʰ **M10.0 Idiopathic gout**
Gouty bursitis
Primary gout

- **M10.00 Idiopathic gout, unspecified site**
- ✓6ᵗʰ **M10.01 Idiopathic gout, shoulder**
  - **M10.011 Idiopathic gout, right shoulder**
  - **M10.012 Idiopathic gout, left shoulder**
  - **M10.019 Idiopathic gout, unspecified shoulder**
- ✓6ᵗʰ **M10.02 Idiopathic gout, elbow**
  - **M10.021 Idiopathic gout, right elbow**
  - **M10.022 Idiopathic gout, left elbow**
  - **M10.029 Idiopathic gout, unspecified elbow**
- ✓6ᵗʰ **M10.03 Idiopathic gout, wrist**
  - **M10.031 Idiopathic gout, right wrist**
  - **M10.032 Idiopathic gout, left wrist**
  - **M10.039 Idiopathic gout, unspecified wrist**
- ✓6ᵗʰ **M10.04 Idiopathic gout, hand**
  - **M10.041 Idiopathic gout, right hand**
  - **M10.042 Idiopathic gout, left hand**
  - **M10.049 Idiopathic gout, unspecified hand**
- ✓6ᵗʰ **M10.05 Idiopathic gout, hip**
  - **M10.051 Idiopathic gout, right hip**
  - **M10.052 Idiopathic gout, left hip**
  - **M10.059 Idiopathic gout, unspecified hip**
- ✓6ᵗʰ **M10.06 Idiopathic gout, knee**
  - **M10.061 Idiopathic gout, right knee**
  - **M10.062 Idiopathic gout, left knee**
  - **M10.069 Idiopathic gout, unspecified knee**
- ✓6ᵗʰ **M10.07 Idiopathic gout, ankle and foot**
  - **M10.071 Idiopathic gout, right ankle and foot**
  - **M10.072 Idiopathic gout, left ankle and foot**
  - **M10.079 Idiopathic gout, unspecified ankle and foot**
- **M10.08 Idiopathic gout, vertebrae**
- **M10.09 Idiopathic gout, multiple sites**

✓5ᵗʰ **M10.1 Lead-induced gout**
Code first: toxic effects of lead and its compounds (T56.0-)

- **M10.10 Lead-induced gout, unspecified site**
- ✓6ᵗʰ **M10.11 Lead-induced gout, shoulder**
  - **M10.111 Lead-induced gout, right shoulder**
  - **M10.112 Lead-induced gout, left shoulder**
  - **M10.119 Lead-induced gout, unspecified shoulder**
- ✓6ᵗʰ **M10.12 Lead-induced gout, elbow**
  - **M10.121 Lead-induced gout, right elbow**
  - **M10.122 Lead-induced gout, left elbow**
  - **M10.129 Lead-induced gout, unspecified elbow**
- ✓6ᵗʰ **M10.13 Lead-induced gout, wrist**
  - **M10.131 Lead-induced gout, right wrist**
  - **M10.132 Lead-induced gout, left wrist**
  - **M10.139 Lead-induced gout, unspecified wrist**

✓6ᵗʰ **M10.14 Lead-induced gout, hand**
- **M10.141 Lead-induced gout, right hand**
- **M10.142 Lead-induced gout, left hand**
- **M10.149 Lead-induced gout, unspecified hand**

✓6ᵗʰ **M10.15 Lead-induced gout, hip**
- **M10.151 Lead-induced gout, right hip**
- **M10.152 Lead-induced gout, left hip**
- **M10.159 Lead-induced gout, unspecified hip**

✓6ᵗʰ **M10.16 Lead-induced gout, knee**
- **M10.161 Lead-induced gout, right knee**
- **M10.162 Lead-induced gout, left knee**
- **M10.169 Lead-induced gout, unspecified knee**

✓6ᵗʰ **M10.17 Lead-induced gout, ankle and foot**
- **M10.171 Lead-induced gout, right ankle and foot**
- **M10.172 Lead-induced gout, left ankle and foot**
- **M10.179 Lead-induced gout, unspecified ankle and foot**

- **M10.18 Lead-induced gout, vertebrae**
- **M10.19 Lead-induced gout, multiple sites**

✓5ᵗʰ **M10.2 Drug-induced gout**
Use additional code for adverse effect, if applicable, to identify drug (T36-T50 with fifth or sixth character 5)

- **M10.20 Drug-induced gout, unspecified site**
- ✓6ᵗʰ **M10.21 Drug-induced gout, shoulder**
  - **M10.211 Drug-induced gout, right shoulder**
  - **M10.212 Drug-induced gout, left shoulder**
  - **M10.219 Drug-induced gout, unspecified shoulder**
- ✓6ᵗʰ **M10.22 Drug-induced gout, elbow**
  - **M10.221 Drug-induced gout, right elbow**
  - **M10.222 Drug-induced gout, left elbow**
  - **M10.229 Drug-induced gout, unspecified elbow**
- ✓6ᵗʰ **M10.23 Drug-induced gout, wrist**
  - **M10.231 Drug-induced gout, right wrist**
  - **M10.232 Drug-induced gout, left wrist**
  - **M10.239 Drug-induced gout, unspecified wrist**
- ✓6ᵗʰ **M10.24 Drug-induced gout, hand**
  - **M10.241 Drug-induced gout, right hand**
  - **M10.242 Drug-induced gout, left hand**
  - **M10.249 Drug-induced gout, unspecified hand**
- ✓6ᵗʰ **M10.25 Drug-induced gout, hip**
  - **M10.251 Drug-induced gout, right hip**
  - **M10.252 Drug-induced gout, left hip**
  - **M10.259 Drug-induced gout, unspecified hip**
- ✓6ᵗʰ **M10.26 Drug-induced gout, knee**
  - **M10.261 Drug-induced gout, right knee**
  - **M10.262 Drug-induced gout, left knee**
  - **M10.269 Drug-induced gout, unspecified knee**
- ✓6ᵗʰ **M10.27 Drug-induced gout, ankle and foot**
  - **M10.271 Drug-induced gout, right ankle and foot**
  - **M10.272 Drug-induced gout, left ankle and foot**
  - **M10.279 Drug-induced gout, unspecified ankle and foot**
- **M10.28 Drug-induced gout, vertebrae**
- **M10.29 Drug-induced gout, multiple sites**

✓5ᵗʰ **M10.3 Gout due to renal impairment**
Code first associated renal disease

- **M10.30 Gout due to renal impairment, unspecified site**
- ✓6ᵗʰ **M10.31 Gout due to renal impairment, shoulder**
  - **M10.311 Gout due to renal impairment, right shoulder**
  - **M10.312 Gout due to renal impairment, left shoulder**
  - **M10.319 Gout due to renal impairment, unspecified shoulder**
- ✓6ᵗʰ **M10.32 Gout due to renal impairment, elbow**
  - **M10.321 Gout due to renal impairment, right elbow**
  - **M10.322 Gout due to renal impairment, left elbow**
  - **M10.329 Gout due to renal impairment, unspecified elbow**
- ✓6ᵗʰ **M10.33 Gout due to renal impairment, wrist**
  - **M10.331 Gout due to renal impairment, right wrist**
  - **M10.332 Gout due to renal impairment, left wrist**

EXCLUDES 1 Not coded here   *EXCLUDES 2* Not included here   **N** Newborn Age: 0   **P** Pediatric Age: 0-17   **M** Maternity Age: 12-55   **A** Adult Age: 15-124

658   ICD-10-CM 2014 (Draft)

    M10.339 Gout due to renal impairment, unspecified wrist

✓6ᵗʰ M10.34 Gout due to renal impairment, hand
    M10.341 Gout due to renal impairment, right hand
    M10.342 Gout due to renal impairment, left hand
    M10.349 Gout due to renal impairment, unspecified hand

✓6ᵗʰ M10.35 Gout due to renal impairment, hip
    M10.351 Gout due to renal impairment, right hip
    M10.352 Gout due to renal impairment, left hip
    M10.359 Gout due to renal impairment, unspecified hip

✓6ᵗʰ M10.36 Gout due to renal impairment, knee
    M10.361 Gout due to renal impairment, right knee
    M10.362 Gout due to renal impairment, left knee
    M10.369 Gout due to renal impairment, unspecified knee

✓6ᵗʰ M10.37 Gout due to renal impairment, ankle and foot
    M10.371 Gout due to renal impairment, right ankle and foot
    M10.372 Gout due to renal impairment, left ankle and foot
    M10.379 Gout due to renal impairment, unspecified ankle and foot

    M10.38 Gout due to renal impairment, vertebrae
    M10.39 Gout due to renal impairment, multiple sites

✓5ᵗʰ M10.4 Other secondary gout
    Code first associated condition
    M10.40 Other secondary gout, unspecified site

✓6ᵗʰ M10.41 Other secondary gout, shoulder
    M10.411 Other secondary gout, right shoulder
    M10.412 Other secondary gout, left shoulder
    M10.419 Other secondary gout, unspecified shoulder

✓6ᵗʰ M10.42 Other secondary gout, elbow
    M10.421 Other secondary gout, right elbow
    M10.422 Other secondary gout, left elbow
    M10.429 Other secondary gout, unspecified elbow

✓6ᵗʰ M10.43 Other secondary gout, wrist
    M10.431 Other secondary gout, right wrist
    M10.432 Other secondary gout, left wrist
    M10.439 Other secondary gout, unspecified wrist

✓6ᵗʰ M10.44 Other secondary gout, hand
    M10.441 Other secondary gout, right hand
    M10.442 Other secondary gout, left hand
    M10.449 Other secondary gout, unspecified hand

✓6ᵗʰ M10.45 Other secondary gout, hip
    M10.451 Other secondary gout, right hip
    M10.452 Other secondary gout, left hip
    M10.459 Other secondary gout, unspecified hip

✓6ᵗʰ M10.46 Other secondary gout, knee
    M10.461 Other secondary gout, right knee
    M10.462 Other secondary gout, left knee
    M10.469 Other secondary gout, unspecified knee

✓6ᵗʰ M10.47 Other secondary gout, ankle and foot
    M10.471 Other secondary gout, right ankle and foot
    M10.472 Other secondary gout, left ankle and foot
    M10.479 Other secondary gout, unspecified ankle and foot

    M10.48 Other secondary gout, vertebrae
    M10.49 Other secondary gout, multiple sites

M10.9 Gout, unspecified
    Gout NOS

✓4ᵗʰ **M11** **Other crystal arthropathies**

✓5ᵗʰ M11.0 Hydroxyapatite deposition disease
    M11.00 Hydroxyapatite deposition disease, unspecified site

✓6ᵗʰ M11.01 Hydroxyapatite deposition disease, shoulder
    M11.011 Hydroxyapatite deposition disease, right shoulder
    M11.012 Hydroxyapatite deposition disease, left shoulder

    M11.019 Hydroxyapatite deposition disease, unspecified shoulder

✓6ᵗʰ M11.02 Hydroxyapatite deposition disease, elbow
    M11.021 Hydroxyapatite deposition disease, right elbow
    M11.022 Hydroxyapatite deposition disease, left elbow
    M11.029 Hydroxyapatite deposition disease, unspecified elbow

✓6ᵗʰ M11.03 Hydroxyapatite deposition disease, wrist
    M11.031 Hydroxyapatite deposition disease, right wrist
    M11.032 Hydroxyapatite deposition disease, left wrist
    M11.039 Hydroxyapatite deposition disease, unspecified wrist

✓6ᵗʰ M11.04 Hydroxyapatite deposition disease, hand
    M11.041 Hydroxyapatite deposition disease, right hand
    M11.042 Hydroxyapatite deposition disease, left hand
    M11.049 Hydroxyapatite deposition disease, unspecified hand

✓6ᵗʰ M11.05 Hydroxyapatite deposition disease, hip
    M11.051 Hydroxyapatite deposition disease, right hip
    M11.052 Hydroxyapatite deposition disease, left hip
    M11.059 Hydroxyapatite deposition disease, unspecified hip

✓6ᵗʰ M11.06 Hydroxyapatite deposition disease, knee
    M11.061 Hydroxyapatite deposition disease, right knee
    M11.062 Hydroxyapatite deposition disease, left knee
    M11.069 Hydroxyapatite deposition disease, unspecified knee

✓6ᵗʰ M11.07 Hydroxyapatite deposition disease, ankle and foot
    M11.071 Hydroxyapatite deposition disease, right ankle and foot
    M11.072 Hydroxyapatite deposition disease, left ankle and foot
    M11.079 Hydroxyapatite deposition disease, unspecified ankle and foot

    M11.08 Hydroxyapatite deposition disease, vertebrae
    M11.09 Hydroxyapatite deposition disease, multiple sites

✓5ᵗʰ M11.1 Familial chondrocalcinosis
    M11.10 Familial chondrocalcinosis, unspecified site

✓6ᵗʰ M11.11 Familial chondrocalcinosis, shoulder
    M11.111 Familial chondrocalcinosis, right shoulder
    M11.112 Familial chondrocalcinosis, left shoulder
    M11.119 Familial chondrocalcinosis, unspecified shoulder

✓6ᵗʰ M11.12 Familial chondrocalcinosis, elbow
    M11.121 Familial chondrocalcinosis, right elbow
    M11.122 Familial chondrocalcinosis, left elbow
    M11.129 Familial chondrocalcinosis, unspecified elbow

✓6ᵗʰ M11.13 Familial chondrocalcinosis, wrist
    M11.131 Familial chondrocalcinosis, right wrist
    M11.132 Familial chondrocalcinosis, left wrist
    M11.139 Familial chondrocalcinosis, unspecified wrist

✓6ᵗʰ M11.14 Familial chondrocalcinosis, hand
    M11.141 Familial chondrocalcinosis, right hand
    M11.142 Familial chondrocalcinosis, left hand
    M11.149 Familial chondrocalcinosis, unspecified hand

✓6ᵗʰ M11.15 Familial chondrocalcinosis, hip
    M11.151 Familial chondrocalcinosis, right hip
    M11.152 Familial chondrocalcinosis, left hip
    M11.159 Familial chondrocalcinosis, unspecified hip

✓6ᵗʰ M11.16 Familial chondrocalcinosis, knee
    M11.161 Familial chondrocalcinosis, right knee

M11.162   Familial chondrocalcinosis, left knee
M11.169   Familial chondrocalcinosis, unspecified knee

✓6th M11.17   Familial chondrocalcinosis, ankle and foot
M11.171   Familial chondrocalcinosis, right ankle and foot
M11.172   Familial chondrocalcinosis, left ankle and foot
M11.179   Familial chondrocalcinosis, unspecified ankle and foot

M11.18   Familial chondrocalcinosis, vertebrae
M11.19   Familial chondrocalcinosis, multiple sites

✓5th M11.2   Other chondrocalcinosis
Chondrocalcinosis NOS
M11.20   Other chondrocalcinosis, unspecified site

✓6th M11.21   Other chondrocalcinosis, shoulder
M11.211   Other chondrocalcinosis, right shoulder
M11.212   Other chondrocalcinosis, left shoulder
M11.219   Other chondrocalcinosis, unspecified shoulder

✓6th M11.22   Other chondrocalcinosis, elbow
M11.221   Other chondrocalcinosis, right elbow
M11.222   Other chondrocalcinosis, left elbow
M11.229   Other chondrocalcinosis, unspecified elbow

✓6th M11.23   Other chondrocalcinosis, wrist
M11.231   Other chondrocalcinosis, right wrist
M11.232   Other chondrocalcinosis, left wrist
M11.239   Other chondrocalcinosis, unspecified wrist

✓6th M11.24   Other chondrocalcinosis, hand
M11.241   Other chondrocalcinosis, right hand
M11.242   Other chondrocalcinosis, left hand
M11.249   Other chondrocalcinosis, unspecified hand

✓6th M11.25   Other chondrocalcinosis, hip
M11.251   Other chondrocalcinosis, right hip
M11.252   Other chondrocalcinosis, left hip
M11.259   Other chondrocalcinosis, unspecified hip

✓6th M11.26   Other chondrocalcinosis, knee
M11.261   Other chondrocalcinosis, right knee
M11.262   Other chondrocalcinosis, left knee
M11.269   Other chondrocalcinosis, unspecified knee

✓6th M11.27   Other chondrocalcinosis, ankle and foot
M11.271   Other chondrocalcinosis, right ankle and foot
M11.272   Other chondrocalcinosis, left ankle and foot
M11.279   Other chondrocalcinosis, unspecified ankle and foot

M11.28   Other chondrocalcinosis, vertebrae
M11.29   Other chondrocalcinosis, multiple sites

✓5th M11.8   Other specified crystal arthropathies
M11.80   Other specified crystal arthropathies, unspecified site

✓6th M11.81   Other specified crystal arthropathies, shoulder
M11.811   Other specified crystal arthropathies, right shoulder
M11.812   Other specified crystal arthropathies, left shoulder
M11.819   Other specified crystal arthropathies, unspecified shoulder

✓6th M11.82   Other specified crystal arthropathies, elbow
M11.821   Other specified crystal arthropathies, right elbow
M11.822   Other specified crystal arthropathies, left elbow
M11.829   Other specified crystal arthropathies, unspecified elbow

✓6th M11.83   Other specified crystal arthropathies, wrist
M11.831   Other specified crystal arthropathies, right wrist
M11.832   Other specified crystal arthropathies, left wrist

M11.839   Other specified crystal arthropathies, unspecified wrist

✓6th M11.84   Other specified crystal arthropathies, hand
M11.841   Other specified crystal arthropathies, right hand
M11.842   Other specified crystal arthropathies, left hand
M11.849   Other specified crystal arthropathies, unspecified hand

✓6th M11.85   Other specified crystal arthropathies, hip
M11.851   Other specified crystal arthropathies, right hip
M11.852   Other specified crystal arthropathies, left hip
M11.859   Other specified crystal arthropathies, unspecified hip

✓6th M11.86   Other specified crystal arthropathies, knee
M11.861   Other specified crystal arthropathies, right knee
M11.862   Other specified crystal arthropathies, left knee
M11.869   Other specified crystal arthropathies, unspecified knee

✓6th M11.87   Other specified crystal arthropathies, ankle and foot
M11.871   Other specified crystal arthropathies, right ankle and foot
M11.872   Other specified crystal arthropathies, left ankle and foot
M11.879   Other specified crystal arthropathies, unspecified ankle and foot

M11.88   Other specified crystal arthropathies, vertebrae
M11.89   Other specified crystal arthropathies, multiple sites

M11.9   Crystal arthropathy, unspecified

✓4th M12   Other and unspecified arthropathy
EXCLUDES 1   arthrosis (M15-M19)
cricoarytenoid arthropathy (J38.7)

✓5th M12.0   Chronic postrheumatic arthropathy [Jaccoud]
M12.00   Chronic postrheumatic arthropathy [Jaccoud], unspecified site

✓6th M12.01   Chronic postrheumatic arthropathy [Jaccoud], shoulder
M12.011   Chronic postrheumatic arthropathy [Jaccoud], right shoulder
M12.012   Chronic postrheumatic arthropathy [Jaccoud], left shoulder
M12.019   Chronic postrheumatic arthropathy [Jaccoud], unspecified shoulder

✓6th M12.02   Chronic postrheumatic arthropathy [Jaccoud], elbow
M12.021   Chronic postrheumatic arthropathy [Jaccoud], right elbow
M12.022   Chronic postrheumatic arthropathy [Jaccoud], left elbow
M12.029   Chronic postrheumatic arthropathy [Jaccoud], unspecified elbow

✓6th M12.03   Chronic postrheumatic arthropathy [Jaccoud], wrist
M12.031   Chronic postrheumatic arthropathy [Jaccoud], right wrist
M12.032   Chronic postrheumatic arthropathy [Jaccoud], left wrist
M12.039   Chronic postrheumatic arthropathy [Jaccoud], unspecified wrist

✓6th M12.04   Chronic postrheumatic arthropathy [Jaccoud], hand
M12.041   Chronic postrheumatic arthropathy [Jaccoud], right hand
M12.042   Chronic postrheumatic arthropathy [Jaccoud], left hand
M12.049   Chronic postrheumatic arthropathy [Jaccoud], unspecified hand

✓6th M12.05   Chronic postrheumatic arthropathy [Jaccoud], hip
M12.051   Chronic postrheumatic arthropathy [Jaccoud], right hip
M12.052   Chronic postrheumatic arthropathy [Jaccoud], left hip
M12.059   Chronic postrheumatic arthropathy [Jaccoud], unspecified hip

✓6th **M12.06 Chronic postrheumatic arthropathy [Jaccoud], knee**
    M12.061 **Chronic postrheumatic arthropathy [Jaccoud], right knee**
    M12.062 **Chronic postrheumatic arthropathy [Jaccoud], left knee**
    M12.069 **Chronic postrheumatic arthropathy [Jaccoud], unspecified knee**

✓6th **M12.07 Chronic postrheumatic arthropathy [Jaccoud], ankle and foot**
    M12.071 **Chronic postrheumatic arthropathy [Jaccoud], right ankle and foot**
    M12.072 **Chronic postrheumatic arthropathy [Jaccoud], left ankle and foot**
    M12.079 **Chronic postrheumatic arthropathy [Jaccoud], unspecified ankle and foot**

M12.08 Chronic postrheumatic arthropathy [Jaccoud], other specified site
    Chronic postrheumatic arthropathy [Jaccoud], vertebrae

M12.09 Chronic postrheumatic arthropathy [Jaccoud], multiple sites

✓5th **M12.1 Kaschin-Beck disease**
    Osteochondroarthrosis deformans endemica

M12.10 Kaschin-Beck disease, unspecified site

✓6th **M12.11 Kaschin-Beck disease, shoulder**
    M12.111 **Kaschin-Beck disease, right shoulder**
    M12.112 **Kaschin-Beck disease, left shoulder**
    M12.119 **Kaschin-Beck disease, unspecified shoulder**

✓6th **M12.12 Kaschin-Beck disease, elbow**
    M12.121 **Kaschin-Beck disease, right elbow**
    M12.122 **Kaschin-Beck disease, left elbow**
    M12.129 **Kaschin-Beck disease, unspecified elbow**

✓6th **M12.13 Kaschin-Beck disease, wrist**
    M12.131 **Kaschin-Beck disease, right wrist**
    M12.132 **Kaschin-Beck disease, left wrist**
    M12.139 **Kaschin-Beck disease, unspecified wrist**

✓6th **M12.14 Kaschin-Beck disease, hand**
    M12.141 **Kaschin-Beck disease, right hand**
    M12.142 **Kaschin-Beck disease, left hand**
    M12.149 **Kaschin-Beck disease, unspecified hand**

✓6th **M12.15 Kaschin-Beck disease, hip**
    M12.151 **Kaschin-Beck disease, right hip**
    M12.152 **Kaschin-Beck disease, left hip**
    M12.159 **Kaschin-Beck disease, unspecified hip**

✓6th **M12.16 Kaschin-Beck disease, knee**
    M12.161 **Kaschin-Beck disease, right knee**
    M12.162 **Kaschin-Beck disease, left knee**
    M12.169 **Kaschin-Beck disease, unspecified knee**

✓6th **M12.17 Kaschin-Beck disease, ankle and foot**
    M12.171 **Kaschin-Beck disease, right ankle and foot**
    M12.172 **Kaschin-Beck disease, left ankle and foot**
    M12.179 **Kaschin-Beck disease, unspecified ankle and foot**

M12.18 Kaschin-Beck disease, vertebrae

M12.19 Kaschin-Beck disease, multiple sites

✓5th **M12.2 Villonodular synovitis (pigmented)**

M12.20 Villonodular synovitis (pigmented), unspecified site

✓6th **M12.21 Villonodular synovitis (pigmented), shoulder**
    M12.211 **Villonodular synovitis (pigmented), right shoulder**
    M12.212 **Villonodular synovitis (pigmented), left shoulder**
    M12.219 **Villonodular synovitis (pigmented), unspecified shoulder**

✓6th **M12.22 Villonodular synovitis (pigmented), elbow**
    M12.221 **Villonodular synovitis (pigmented), right elbow**
    M12.222 **Villonodular synovitis (pigmented), left elbow**
    M12.229 **Villonodular synovitis (pigmented), unspecified elbow**

✓6th **M12.23 Villonodular synovitis (pigmented), wrist**
    M12.231 **Villonodular synovitis (pigmented), right wrist**
    M12.232 **Villonodular synovitis (pigmented), left wrist**
    M12.239 **Villonodular synovitis (pigmented), unspecified wrist**

✓6th **M12.24 Villonodular synovitis (pigmented), hand**
    M12.241 **Villonodular synovitis (pigmented), right hand**
    M12.242 **Villonodular synovitis (pigmented), left hand**
    M12.249 **Villonodular synovitis (pigmented), unspecified hand**

✓6th **M12.25 Villonodular synovitis (pigmented), hip**
    M12.251 **Villonodular synovitis (pigmented), right hip**
    M12.252 **Villonodular synovitis (pigmented), left hip**
    M12.259 **Villonodular synovitis (pigmented), unspecified hip**

✓6th **M12.26 Villonodular synovitis (pigmented), knee**
    M12.261 **Villonodular synovitis (pigmented), right knee**
    M12.262 **Villonodular synovitis (pigmented), left knee**
    M12.269 **Villonodular synovitis (pigmented), unspecified knee**

✓6th **M12.27 Villonodular synovitis (pigmented), ankle and foot**
    M12.271 **Villonodular synovitis (pigmented), right ankle and foot**
    M12.272 **Villonodular synovitis (pigmented), left ankle and foot**
    M12.279 **Villonodular synovitis (pigmented), unspecified ankle and foot**

M12.28 Villonodular synovitis (pigmented), other specified site
    Villonodular synovitis (pigmented), vertebrae

M12.29 Villonodular synovitis (pigmented), multiple sites

✓5th **M12.3 Palindromic rheumatism**

M12.30 Palindromic rheumatism, unspecified site

✓6th **M12.31 Palindromic rheumatism, shoulder**
    M12.311 **Palindromic rheumatism, right shoulder**
    M12.312 **Palindromic rheumatism, left shoulder**
    M12.319 **Palindromic rheumatism, unspecified shoulder**

✓6th **M12.32 Palindromic rheumatism, elbow**
    M12.321 **Palindromic rheumatism, right elbow**
    M12.322 **Palindromic rheumatism, left elbow**
    M12.329 **Palindromic rheumatism, unspecified elbow**

✓6th **M12.33 Palindromic rheumatism, wrist**
    M12.331 **Palindromic rheumatism, right wrist**
    M12.332 **Palindromic rheumatism, left wrist**
    M12.339 **Palindromic rheumatism, unspecified wrist**

✓6th **M12.34 Palindromic rheumatism, hand**
    M12.341 **Palindromic rheumatism, right hand**
    M12.342 **Palindromic rheumatism, left hand**
    M12.349 **Palindromic rheumatism, unspecified hand**

✓6th **M12.35 Palindromic rheumatism, hip**
    M12.351 **Palindromic rheumatism, right hip**
    M12.352 **Palindromic rheumatism, left hip**
    M12.359 **Palindromic rheumatism, unspecified hip**

✓6th **M12.36 Palindromic rheumatism, knee**
    M12.361 **Palindromic rheumatism, right knee**
    M12.362 **Palindromic rheumatism, left knee**
    M12.369 **Palindromic rheumatism, unspecified knee**

✓6th **M12.37 Palindromic rheumatism, ankle and foot**
    M12.371 **Palindromic rheumatism, right ankle and foot**
    M12.372 **Palindromic rheumatism, left ankle and foot**

✔ Additional Character Required   ✓x7th Xtension Alert   Unspecified Code   Other Specified Code   Manifestation Code   ►◄ Revised Text   ● New Code   ▲ Revised Code Title

M12.379   **Palindromic rheumatism, unspecified ankle and foot**

M12.38   **Palindromic rheumatism,** other specified site
     Palindromic rheumatism, vertebrae

M12.39   **Palindromic rheumatism,** multiple sites

✓5ᵗʰ M12.4   **Intermittent hydrarthrosis**

     M12.40   **Intermittent hydrarthrosis, unspecified site**

✓6ᵗʰ M12.41   **Intermittent hydrarthrosis,** shoulder
     M12.411   **Intermittent hydrarthrosis,** right **shoulder**
     M12.412   **Intermittent hydrarthrosis,** left **shoulder**
     M12.419   **Intermittent hydrarthrosis, unspecified shoulder**

✓6ᵗʰ M12.42   **Intermittent hydrarthrosis,** elbow
     M12.421   **Intermittent hydrarthrosis,** right **elbow**
     M12.422   **Intermittent hydrarthrosis,** left **elbow**
     M12.429   **Intermittent hydrarthrosis, unspecified elbow**

✓6ᵗʰ M12.43   **Intermittent hydrarthrosis,** wrist
     M12.431   **Intermittent hydrarthrosis,** right **wrist**
     M12.432   **Intermittent hydrarthrosis,** left **wrist**
     M12.439   **Intermittent hydrarthrosis, unspecified wrist**

✓6ᵗʰ M12.44   **Intermittent hydrarthrosis,** hand
     M12.441   **Intermittent hydrarthrosis,** right **hand**
     M12.442   **Intermittent hydrarthrosis,** left **hand**
     M12.449   **Intermittent hydrarthrosis, unspecified hand**

✓6ᵗʰ M12.45   **Intermittent hydrarthrosis,** hip
     M12.451   **Intermittent hydrarthrosis,** right **hip**
     M12.452   **Intermittent hydrarthrosis,** left **hip**
     M12.459   **Intermittent hydrarthrosis, unspecified hip**

✓6ᵗʰ M12.46   **Intermittent hydrarthrosis,** knee
     M12.461   **Intermittent hydrarthrosis,** right **knee**
     M12.462   **Intermittent hydrarthrosis,** left **knee**
     M12.469   **Intermittent hydrarthrosis, unspecified knee**

✓6ᵗʰ M12.47   **Intermittent hydrarthrosis,** ankle and foot
     M12.471   **Intermittent hydrarthrosis,** right **ankle and foot**
     M12.472   **Intermittent hydrarthrosis,** left **ankle and foot**
     M12.479   **Intermittent hydrarthrosis, unspecified ankle and foot**

M12.48   **Intermittent hydrarthrosis,** other site

M12.49   **Intermittent hydrarthrosis,** multiple sites

✓5ᵗʰ M12.5   **Traumatic arthropathy**

     EXCLUDES 1   current injury–see Alphabetic Index
         post-traumatic osteoarthritis of first carpometacarpal joint (M18.2-M18.3)
         post-traumatic osteoarthritis of hip (M16.4-M16.5)
         post-traumatic osteoarthritis of knee (M17.2-M17.3)
         post-traumatic osteoarthritis NOS (M19.1-)
         post-traumatic osteoarthritis of other single joints (M19.1-)

     M12.50   **Traumatic arthropathy, unspecified**

✓6ᵗʰ M12.51   **Traumatic arthropathy,** shoulder
     M12.511   **Traumatic arthropathy,** right **shoulder**
     M12.512   **Traumatic arthropathy,** left **shoulder**
     M12.519   **Traumatic arthropathy, unspecified shoulder**

✓6ᵗʰ M12.52   **Traumatic arthropathy,** elbow
     M12.521   **Traumatic arthropathy,** right **elbow**
     M12.522   **Traumatic arthropathy,** left **elbow**
     M12.529   **Traumatic arthropathy, unspecified elbow**

✓6ᵗʰ M12.53   **Traumatic arthropathy,** wrist
     M12.531   **Traumatic arthropathy,** right **wrist**
     M12.532   **Traumatic arthropathy,** left **wrist**
     M12.539   **Traumatic arthropathy, unspecified wrist**

✓6ᵗʰ M12.54   **Traumatic arthropathy,** hand
     M12.541   **Traumatic arthropathy,** right **hand**
     M12.542   **Traumatic arthropathy,** left **hand**
     M12.549   **Traumatic arthropathy, unspecified hand**

✓6ᵗʰ M12.55   **Traumatic arthropathy,** hip

M12.551   **Traumatic arthropathy,** right **hip**
M12.552   **Traumatic arthropathy,** left **hip**
M12.559   **Traumatic arthropathy, unspecified hip**

✓6ᵗʰ M12.56   **Traumatic arthropathy,** knee
     M12.561   **Traumatic arthropathy,** right **knee**
     M12.562   **Traumatic arthropathy,** left **knee**
     M12.569   **Traumatic arthropathy, unspecified knee**

✓6ᵗʰ M12.57   **Traumatic arthropathy,** ankle and foot
     M12.571   **Traumatic arthropathy,** right **ankle and foot**
     M12.572   **Traumatic arthropathy,** left **ankle and foot**
     M12.579   **Traumatic arthropathy, unspecified ankle and foot**

M12.58   **Traumatic arthropathy,** other specified site
     Traumatic arthropathy, vertebrae

M12.59   **Traumatic arthropathy,** multiple sites

✓5ᵗʰ M12.8   **Other specific arthropathies, not elsewhere classified**
     Transient arthropathy

     M12.80   **Other specific arthropathies, not elsewhere classified, unspecified**

✓6ᵗʰ M12.81   **Other specific arthropathies, not elsewhere classified,** shoulder
     M12.811   **Other specific arthropathies, not elsewhere classified,** right **shoulder**
     M12.812   **Other specific arthropathies, not elsewhere classified,** left **shoulder**
     M12.819   **Other specific arthropathies, not elsewhere classified, unspecified shoulder**

✓6ᵗʰ M12.82   **Other specific arthropathies, not elsewhere classified,** elbow
     M12.821   **Other specific arthropathies, not elsewhere classified,** right **elbow**
     M12.822   **Other specific arthropathies, not elsewhere classified,** left **elbow**
     M12.829   **Other specific arthropathies, not elsewhere classified, unspecified elbow**

✓6ᵗʰ M12.83   **Other specific arthropathies, not elsewhere classified,** wrist
     M12.831   **Other specific arthropathies, not elsewhere classified,** right **wrist**
     M12.832   **Other specific arthropathies, not elsewhere classified,** left **wrist**
     M12.839   **Other specific arthropathies, not elsewhere classified, unspecified wrist**

✓6ᵗʰ M12.84   **Other specific arthropathies, not elsewhere classified,** hand
     M12.841   **Other specific arthropathies, not elsewhere classified,** right **hand**
     M12.842   **Other specific arthropathies, not elsewhere classified,** left **hand**
     M12.849   **Other specific arthropathies, not elsewhere classified, unspecified hand**

✓6ᵗʰ M12.85   **Other specific arthropathies, not elsewhere classified,** hip
     M12.851   **Other specific arthropathies, not elsewhere classified,** right **hip**
     M12.852   **Other specific arthropathies, not elsewhere classified,** left **hip**
     M12.859   **Other specific arthropathies, not elsewhere classified, unspecified hip**

✓6ᵗʰ M12.86   **Other specific arthropathies, not elsewhere classified,** knee
     M12.861   **Other specific arthropathies, not elsewhere classified,** right **knee**
     M12.862   **Other specific arthropathies, not elsewhere classified,** left **knee**
     M12.869   **Other specific arthropathies, not elsewhere classified, unspecified knee**

✓6ᵗʰ M12.87   **Other specific arthropathies, not elsewhere classified,** ankle and foot
     M12.871   **Other specific arthropathies, not elsewhere classified,** right **ankle and foot**
     M12.872   **Other specific arthropathies, not elsewhere classified,** left **ankle and foot**
     M12.879   **Other specific arthropathies, not elsewhere classified, unspecified ankle and foot**

EXCLUDES 1 Not coded here   **EXCLUDES 2** Not included here   N Newborn Age: 0   P Pediatric Age: 0-17   M Maternity Age: 12-55   A Adult Age: 15-124

662   ICD-10-CM 2014 (Draft)

M12.88 **Other specific arthropathies, not elsewhere classified,** other specified site
  Other specific arthropathies, not elsewhere classified, vertebrae

M12.89 **Other specific arthropathies, not elsewhere classified,** multiple sites

M12.9 **Arthropathy, unspecified**

✓4th **M13 Other arthritis**
  EXCLUDES 1   arthrosis (M15-M19)
         osteoarthritis (M15-M19)

M13.0 **Polyarthritis, unspecified**

✓5th M13.1 **Monoarthritis, not elsewhere classified**
  M13.10 **Monoarthritis, not elsewhere classified, unspecified**

  ✓6th M13.11 **Monoarthritis, not elsewhere classified,** shoulder
    M13.111 **Monoarthritis, not elsewhere classified, right shoulder**
    M13.112 **Monoarthritis, not elsewhere classified, left shoulder**
    M13.119 **Monoarthritis, not elsewhere classified, unspecified shoulder**

  ✓6th M13.12 **Monoarthritis, not elsewhere classified,** elbow
    M13.121 **Monoarthritis, not elsewhere classified, right elbow**
    M13.122 **Monoarthritis, not elsewhere classified, left elbow**
    M13.129 **Monoarthritis, not elsewhere classified, unspecified elbow**

  ✓6th M13.13 **Monoarthritis, not elsewhere classified,** wrist
    M13.131 **Monoarthritis, not elsewhere classified, right wrist**
    M13.132 **Monoarthritis, not elsewhere classified, left wrist**
    M13.139 **Monoarthritis, not elsewhere classified, unspecified wrist**

  ✓6th M13.14 **Monoarthritis, not elsewhere classified,** hand
    M13.141 **Monoarthritis, not elsewhere classified, right hand**
    M13.142 **Monoarthritis, not elsewhere classified, left hand**
    M13.149 **Monoarthritis, not elsewhere classified, unspecified hand**

  ✓6th M13.15 **Monoarthritis, not elsewhere classified,** hip
    M13.151 **Monoarthritis, not elsewhere classified, right hip**
    M13.152 **Monoarthritis, not elsewhere classified, left hip**
    M13.159 **Monoarthritis, not elsewhere classified, unspecified hip**

  ✓6th M13.16 **Monoarthritis, not elsewhere classified,** knee
    M13.161 **Monoarthritis, not elsewhere classified, right knee**
    M13.162 **Monoarthritis, not elsewhere classified, left knee**
    M13.169 **Monoarthritis, not elsewhere classified, unspecified knee**

  ✓6th M13.17 **Monoarthritis, not elsewhere classified,** ankle and foot
    M13.171 **Monoarthritis, not elsewhere classified, right ankle and foot**
    M13.172 **Monoarthritis, not elsewhere classified, left ankle and foot**
    M13.179 **Monoarthritis, not elsewhere classified, unspecified ankle and foot**

✓5th M13.8 **Other specified arthritis**
  Allergic arthritis
  EXCLUDES 1   osteoarthritis (M15-M19)

  M13.80 **Other specified arthritis, unspecified site**

  ✓6th M13.81 **Other specified arthritis,** shoulder
    M13.811 **Other specified arthritis, right shoulder**
    M13.812 **Other specified arthritis, left shoulder**
    M13.819 **Other specified arthritis, unspecified shoulder**

  ✓6th M13.82 **Other specified arthritis,** elbow
    M13.821 **Other specified arthritis, right elbow**
    M13.822 **Other specified arthritis, left elbow**

M13.829 **Other specified arthritis, unspecified elbow**

✓6th M13.83 **Other specified arthritis,** wrist
  M13.831 **Other specified arthritis, right wrist**
  M13.832 **Other specified arthritis, left wrist**
  M13.839 **Other specified arthritis, unspecified wrist**

✓6th M13.84 **Other specified arthritis,** hand
  M13.841 **Other specified arthritis, right hand**
  M13.842 **Other specified arthritis, left hand**
  M13.849 **Other specified arthritis, unspecified hand**

✓6th M13.85 **Other specified arthritis,** hip
  M13.851 **Other specified arthritis, right hip**
  M13.852 **Other specified arthritis, left hip**
  M13.859 **Other specified arthritis, unspecified hip**

✓6th M13.86 **Other specified arthritis,** knee
  M13.861 **Other specified arthritis, right knee**
  M13.862 **Other specified arthritis, left knee**
  M13.869 **Other specified arthritis, unspecified knee**

✓6th M13.87 **Other specified arthritis,** ankle and foot
  M13.871 **Other specified arthritis, right ankle and foot**
  M13.872 **Other specified arthritis, left ankle and foot**
  M13.879 **Other specified arthritis, unspecified ankle and foot**

M13.88 **Other specified arthritis,** other site
M13.89 **Other specified arthritis,** multiple sites

✓4th **M14 Arthropathies in other diseases classified elsewhere**
  EXCLUDES 1   arthropathy in:
    diabetes mellitus (E08-E13 with .61-)
    hematological disorders (M36.2-M36.3)
    hypersensitivity reactions (M36.4)
    neoplastic disease (M36.1)
    neurosyphillis (A52.16)
    sarcoidosis (D86.86)
    enteropathic arthropathies (M07.-)
    juvenile psoriatic arthropathy (L40.54)
    lipoid dermatoarthritis (E78.81)

✓5th M14.6 **Charcôt's joint**
  Neuropathic arthropathy
  EXCLUDES 1   Charcôt's joint in diabetes mellitus (E08-E13 with .610)
         Charcôt's joint in tabes dorsalis (A52.16)

  M14.60 **Charcôt's joint, unspecified site**

  ✓6th M14.61 **Charcôt's joint,** shoulder
    M14.611 **Charcôt's joint, right shoulder**
    M14.612 **Charcôt's joint, left shoulder**
    M14.619 **Charcôt's joint, unspecified shoulder**

  ✓6th M14.62 **Charcôt's joint,** elbow
    M14.621 **Charcôt's joint, right elbow**
    M14.622 **Charcôt's joint, left elbow**
    M14.629 **Charcôt's joint, unspecified elbow**

  ✓6th M14.63 **Charcôt's joint,** wrist
    M14.631 **Charcôt's joint, right wrist**
    M14.632 **Charcôt's joint, left wrist**
    M14.639 **Charcôt's joint, unspecified wrist**

  ✓6th M14.64 **Charcôt's joint,** hand
    M14.641 **Charcôt's joint, right hand**
    M14.642 **Charcôt's joint, left hand**
    M14.649 **Charcôt's joint, unspecified hand**

  ✓6th M14.65 **Charcôt's joint,** hip
    M14.651 **Charcôt's joint, right hip**
    M14.652 **Charcôt's joint, left hip**
    M14.659 **Charcôt's joint, unspecified hip**

  ✓6th M14.66 **Charcôt's joint,** knee
    M14.661 **Charcôt's joint, right knee**
    M14.662 **Charcôt's joint, left knee**
    M14.669 **Charcôt's joint, unspecified knee**

  ✓6th M14.67 **Charcôt's joint,** ankle and foot
    M14.671 **Charcôt's joint, right ankle and foot**
    M14.672 **Charcôt's joint, left ankle and foot**
    M14.679 **Charcôt's joint, unspecified ankle and foot**

  M14.68 **Charcôt's joint,** vertebrae
  M14.69 **Charcôt's joint,** multiple sites

☑ Additional Character Required   ✓x7th Xtension Alert   Unspecified Code   Other Specified Code   Manifestation Code   ►◄ Revised Text   ● New Code   ▲ Revised Code Title

Diseases of the Musculoskeletal System and Connective Tissue

M14.8–M18.12

✓5ᵗʰ **M14.8 Arthropathies in other specified diseases classified elsewhere**

Code first underlying disease, such as:
amyloidosis (E85.-)
erythema multiforme (L51.-)
erythema nodosum (L52)
hemochromatosis (E83.11-)
hyperparathyroidism (E21.-)
hypothyroidism (E00-E03)
sickle-cell disorders (D57.-)
thyrotoxicosis [hyperthyroidism] (E05.-)
Whipple's disease (K90.81)

M14.80 Arthropathies in other specified diseases classified elsewhere, unspecified site

✓6ᵗʰ **M14.81 Arthropathies in other specified diseases classified elsewhere, shoulder**

M14.811 Arthropathies in other specified diseases classified elsewhere, right shoulder

M14.812 Arthropathies in other specified diseases classified elsewhere, left shoulder

M14.819 Arthropathies in other specified diseases classified elsewhere, unspecified shoulder

✓6ᵗʰ **M14.82 Arthropathies in other specified diseases classified elsewhere, elbow**

M14.821 Arthropathies in other specified diseases classified elsewhere, right elbow

M14.822 Arthropathies in other specified diseases classified elsewhere, left elbow

M14.829 Arthropathies in other specified diseases classified elsewhere, unspecified elbow

✓6ᵗʰ **M14.83 Arthropathies in other specified diseases classified elsewhere, wrist**

M14.831 Arthropathies in other specified diseases classified elsewhere, right wrist

M14.832 Arthropathies in other specified diseases classified elsewhere, left wrist

M14.839 Arthropathies in other specified diseases classified elsewhere, unspecified wrist

✓6ᵗʰ **M14.84 Arthropathies in other specified diseases classified elsewhere, hand**

M14.841 Arthropathies in other specified diseases classified elsewhere, right hand

M14.842 Arthropathies in other specified diseases classified elsewhere, left hand

M14.849 Arthropathies in other specified diseases classified elsewhere, unspecified hand

✓6ᵗʰ **M14.85 Arthropathies in other specified diseases classified elsewhere, hip**

M14.851 Arthropathies in other specified diseases classified elsewhere, right hip

M14.852 Arthropathies in other specified diseases classified elsewhere, right hip

M14.859 Arthropathies in other specified diseases classified elsewhere, unspecified hip

✓6ᵗʰ **M14.86 Arthropathies in other specified diseases classified elsewhere, knee**

M14.861 Arthropathies in other specified diseases classified elsewhere, right knee

M14.862 Arthropathies in other specified diseases classified elsewhere, left knee

M14.869 Arthropathies in other specified diseases classified elsewhere, unspecified knee

✓6ᵗʰ **M14.87 Arthropathies in other specified diseases classified elsewhere, ankle and foot**

M14.871 Arthropathies in other specified diseases classified elsewhere, right ankle and foot

M14.872 Arthropathies in other specified diseases classified elsewhere, left ankle and foot

M14.879 Arthropathies in other specified diseases classified elsewhere, unspecified ankle and foot

M14.88 Arthropathies in other specified diseases classified elsewhere, vertebrae

M14.89 Arthropathies in other specified diseases classified elsewhere, multiple sites

Osteoarthritis (M15-M19)

EXCLUDES 2 osteoarthritis of spine (M47.-)

✓4ᵗʰ **M15 Polyosteoarthritis**

INCLUDES arthritis of multiple sites
EXCLUDES 1 bilateral involvement of single joint (M16-M19)

M15.0 Primary generalized (osteo)arthritis

M15.1 Heberden's nodes (with arthropathy)
Interphalangeal distal osteoarthritis

M15.2 Bouchard's nodes (with arthropathy)
Juxtaphalangeal distal osteoarthritis

M15.3 Secondary multiple arthritis
Post-traumatic polyosteoarthritis

M15.4 Erosive (osteo)arthritis

M15.8 Other polyosteoarthritis

M15.9 Polyosteoarthritis, unspecified
Generalized osteoarthritis NOS

✓4ᵗʰ **M16 Osteoarthritis of hip**

M16.0 Bilateral primary osteoarthritis of hip

✓5ᵗʰ **M16.1 Unilateral primary osteoarthritis of hip**
Primary osteoarthritis of hip NOS

M16.10 Unilateral primary osteoarthritis, unspecified hip

M16.11 Unilateral primary osteoarthritis, right hip

M16.12 Unilateral primary osteoarthritis, left hip

M16.2 Bilateral osteoarthritis resulting from hip dysplasia

✓5ᵗʰ **M16.3 Unilateral osteoarthritis resulting from hip dysplasia**
Dysplastic osteoarthritis of hip NOS

M16.30 Unilateral osteoarthritis resulting from hip dysplasia, unspecified hip

M16.31 Unilateral osteoarthritis resulting from hip dysplasia, right hip

M16.32 Unilateral osteoarthritis resulting from hip dysplasia, left hip

M16.4 Bilateral post-traumatic osteoarthritis of hip

✓5ᵗʰ **M16.5 Unilateral post-traumatic osteoarthritis of hip**
Post-traumatic osteoarthritis of hip NOS

M16.50 Unilateral post-traumatic osteoarthritis, unspecified hip

M16.51 Unilateral post-traumatic osteoarthritis, right hip

M16.52 Unilateral post-traumatic osteoarthritis, left hip

M16.6 Other bilateral secondary osteoarthritis of hip

M16.7 Other unilateral secondary osteoarthritis of hip
Secondary osteoarthritis of hip NOS

M16.9 Osteoarthritis of hip, unspecified

✓4ᵗʰ **M17 Osteoarthritis of knee**

M17.0 Bilateral primary osteoarthritis of knee

✓5ᵗʰ **M17.1 Unilateral primary osteoarthritis of knee**
Primary osteoarthritis of knee NOS

M17.10 Unilateral primary osteoarthritis, unspecified knee

M17.11 Unilateral primary osteoarthritis, right knee

M17.12 Unilateral primary osteoarthritis, left knee

M17.2 Bilateral post-traumatic osteoarthritis of knee

✓5ᵗʰ **M17.3 Unilateral post-traumatic osteoarthritis of knee**
Post-traumatic osteoarthritis of knee NOS

M17.30 Unilateral post-traumatic osteoarthritis, unspecified knee

M17.31 Unilateral post-traumatic osteoarthritis, right knee

M17.32 Unilateral post-traumatic osteoarthritis, left knee

M17.4 Other bilateral secondary osteoarthritis of knee

M17.5 Other unilateral secondary osteoarthritis of knee
Secondary osteoarthritis of knee NOS

M17.9 Osteoarthritis of knee, unspecified

✓4ᵗʰ **M18 Osteoarthritis of first carpometacarpal joint**

M18.0 Bilateral primary osteoarthritis of first carpometacarpal joints

✓5ᵗʰ **M18.1 Unilateral primary osteoarthritis of first carpometacarpal joint**
Primary osteoarthritis of first carpometacarpal joint NOS

M18.10 Unilateral primary osteoarthritis of first carpometacarpal joint, unspecified hand

M18.11 Unilateral primary osteoarthritis of first carpometacarpal joint, right hand

M18.12 Unilateral primary osteoarthritis of first carpometacarpal joint, left hand

EXCLUDES 1 Not coded here   EXCLUDES 2 Not included here   N Newborn Age: 0   P Pediatric Age: 0-17   M Maternity Age: 12-55   A Adult Age: 15-124

664   ICD-10-CM 2014 (Draft)

M18.2 Bilateral post-traumatic osteoarthritis of first carpometacarpal joints

✓5th M18.3 Unilateral post-traumatic osteoarthritis of first carpometacarpal joint
    Post-traumatic osteoarthritis of first carpometacarpal joint NOS

    M18.30 Unilateral post-traumatic osteoarthritis of first carpometacarpal joint, unspecified hand

    M18.31 Unilateral post-traumatic osteoarthritis of first carpometacarpal joint, right hand

    M18.32 Unilateral post-traumatic osteoarthritis of first carpometacarpal joint, left hand

M18.4 Other bilateral secondary osteoarthritis of first carpometacarpal joints

✓5th M18.5 Other unilateral secondary osteoarthritis of first carpometacarpal joint
    Secondary osteoarthritis of first carpometacarpal joint NOS

    M18.50 Other unilateral secondary osteoarthritis of first carpometacarpal joint, unspecified hand

    M18.51 Other unilateral secondary osteoarthritis of first carpometacarpal joint, right hand

    M18.52 Other unilateral secondary osteoarthritis of first carpometacarpal joint, left hand

M18.9 Osteoarthritis of first carpometacarpal joint, unspecified

✓4th M19 Other and unspecified osteoarthritis
    EXCLUDES 1   polyarthritis (M15.-)
    EXCLUDES 2   arthrosis of spine (M47.-)
                 hallux rigidus (M20.2)
                 osteoarthritis of spine (M47.-)

✓5th M19.0 Primary osteoarthritis of other joints

    ✓6th M19.01 Primary osteoarthritis, shoulder
        M19.011 Primary osteoarthritis, right shoulder
        M19.012 Primary osteoarthritis, left shoulder
        M19.019 Primary osteoarthritis, unspecified shoulder

    ✓6th M19.02 Primary osteoarthritis, elbow
        M19.021 Primary osteoarthritis, right elbow
        M19.022 Primary osteoarthritis, left elbow
        M19.029 Primary osteoarthritis, unspecified elbow

    ✓6th M19.03 Primary osteoarthritis, wrist
        M19.031 Primary osteoarthritis, right wrist
        M19.032 Primary osteoarthritis, left wrist
        M19.039 Primary osteoarthritis, unspecified wrist

    ✓6th M19.04 Primary osteoarthritis, hand
        EXCLUDES 2   primary osteoarthritis of first carpometacarpal joint (M18.0-, M18.1-)
        M19.041 Primary osteoarthritis, right hand
        M19.042 Primary osteoarthritis, left hand
        M19.049 Primary osteoarthritis, unspecified hand

    ✓6th M19.07 Primary osteoarthritis ankle and foot
        M19.071 Primary osteoarthritis, right ankle and foot
        M19.072 Primary osteoarthritis, left ankle and foot
        M19.079 Primary osteoarthritis, unspecified ankle and foot

✓5th M19.1 Post-traumatic osteoarthritis of other joints

    ✓6th M19.11 Post-traumatic osteoarthritis, shoulder
        M19.111 Post-traumatic osteoarthritis, right shoulder
        M19.112 Post-traumatic osteoarthritis, left shoulder
        M19.119 Post-traumatic osteoarthritis, unspecified shoulder

    ✓6th M19.12 Post-traumatic osteoarthritis, elbow
        M19.121 Post-traumatic osteoarthritis, right elbow
        M19.122 Post-traumatic osteoarthritis, left elbow
        M19.129 Post-traumatic osteoarthritis, unspecified elbow

    ✓6th M19.13 Post-traumatic osteoarthritis, wrist
        M19.131 Post-traumatic osteoarthritis, right wrist
        M19.132 Post-traumatic osteoarthritis, left wrist
        M19.139 Post-traumatic osteoarthritis, unspecified wrist

✓6th M19.14 Post-traumatic osteoarthritis, hand
    EXCLUDES 2   post-traumatic osteoarthritis of first carpometacarpal joint (M18.2-, M18.3-)
    M19.141 Post-traumatic osteoarthritis, right hand
    M19.142 Post-traumatic osteoarthritis, left hand
    M19.149 Post-traumatic osteoarthritis, unspecified hand

✓6th M19.17 Post-traumatic osteoarthritis, ankle and foot
    M19.171 Post-traumatic osteoarthritis, right ankle and foot
    M19.172 Post-traumatic osteoarthritis, left ankle and foot
    M19.179 Post-traumatic osteoarthritis, unspecified ankle and foot

✓5th M19.2 Secondary osteoarthritis of other joints

    ✓6th M19.21 Secondary osteoarthritis, shoulder
        M19.211 Secondary osteoarthritis, right shoulder
        M19.212 Secondary osteoarthritis, left shoulder
        M19.219 Secondary osteoarthritis, unspecified shoulder

    ✓6th M19.22 Secondary osteoarthritis, elbow
        M19.221 Secondary osteoarthritis, right elbow
        M19.222 Secondary osteoarthritis, left elbow
        M19.229 Secondary osteoarthritis, unspecified elbow

    ✓6th M19.23 Secondary osteoarthritis, wrist
        M19.231 Secondary osteoarthritis, right wrist
        M19.232 Secondary osteoarthritis, left wrist
        M19.239 Secondary osteoarthritis, unspecified wrist

    ✓6th M19.24 Secondary osteoarthritis, hand
        M19.241 Secondary osteoarthritis, right hand
        M19.242 Secondary osteoarthritis, left hand
        M19.249 Secondary osteoarthritis, unspecified hand

    ✓6th M19.27 Secondary osteoarthritis, ankle and foot
        M19.271 Secondary osteoarthritis, right ankle and foot
        M19.272 Secondary osteoarthritis, left ankle and foot
        M19.279 Secondary osteoarthritis, unspecified ankle and foot

✓5th M19.9 Osteoarthritis, unspecified site
    M19.90 Unspecified osteoarthritis, unspecified site
        Arthrosis NOS   Osteoarthritis NOS
        Arthritis NOS

    M19.91 Primary osteoarthritis, unspecified site
        Primary osteoarthritis NOS

    M19.92 Post-traumatic osteoarthritis, unspecified site
        Post-traumatic osteoarthritis NOS

    M19.93 Secondary osteoarthritis, unspecified site
        Secondary osteoarthritis NOS

Other joint disorders (M20-M25)

EXCLUDES 2   joints of the spine (M40-M54)

✓4th M20 Acquired deformities of fingers and toes
    EXCLUDES 1   acquired absence of fingers and toes (Z89.-)
                 congenital absence of fingers and toes (Q71.3-, Q72.3-)
                 congenital deformities and malformations of fingers and toes (Q66-, Q68-Q70, Q74.-)

✓5th M20.0 Deformity of finger(s)
    EXCLUDES 1   clubbing of fingers (R68.3)
                 palmar fascial fibromatosis [Dupuytren] (M72.0)
                 trigger finger (M65.3)

    ✓6th M20.00 Unspecified deformity of finger(s)
        M20.001 Unspecified deformity of right finger(s)
        M20.002 Unspecified deformity of left finger(s)
        M20.009 Unspecified deformity of unspecified finger(s)

    ✓6th M20.01 Mallet finger
        M20.011 Mallet finger of right finger(s)
        M20.012 Mallet finger of left finger(s)
        M20.019 Mallet finger of unspecified finger(s)

    ✓6th M20.02 Boutonnière deformity
        M20.021 Boutonnière deformity of right finger(s)

✓ Additional Character Required   ✓x7th Xtension Alert   Unspecified Code   Other Specified Code   Manifestation Code   ▶◀ Revised Text   ● New Code   ▲ Revised Code Title

ICD-10-CM 2014 (Draft)   665

Diseases of the Musculoskeletal System and Connective Tissue

M20.022–M21.259

M20.022   Boutonnière deformity of left finger(s)
M20.029   Boutonnière deformity of unspecified finger(s)

✓6ᵗʰ **M20.03 Swan-neck deformity**
M20.031   Swan-neck deformity of right finger(s)
M20.032   Swan-neck deformity of left finger(s)
M20.039   Swan-neck deformity of unspecified finger(s)

✓6ᵗʰ **M20.09 Other deformity of finger(s)**
M20.091   Other deformity of right finger(s)
M20.092   Other deformity of left finger(s)
M20.099   Other deformity of finger(s), unspecified finger(s)

✓5ᵗʰ **M20.1 Hallux valgus (acquired)**
Bunion
M20.10   Hallux valgus (acquired), unspecified foot
M20.11   Hallux valgus (acquired), right foot
M20.12   Hallux valgus (acquired), left foot

✓5ᵗʰ **M20.2 Hallux rigidus**
M20.20   Hallux rigidus, unspecified foot
M20.21   Hallux rigidus, right foot
M20.22   Hallux rigidus, left foot

✓5ᵗʰ **M20.3 Hallux varus (acquired)**
M20.30   Hallux varus (acquired), unspecified foot
M20.31   Hallux varus (acquired), right foot
M20.32   Hallux varus (acquired), left foot

✓5ᵗʰ **M20.4 Other hammer toe(s) (acquired)**
M20.40   Other hammer toe(s) (acquired), unspecified foot
M20.41   Other hammer toe(s) (acquired), right foot
M20.42   Other hammer toe(s) (acquired), left foot

✓5ᵗʰ **M20.5 Other deformities of toe(s) (acquired)**
✓6ᵗʰ **M20.5X Other deformities of toe(s) (acquired)**
M20.5X1   Other deformities of toe(s) (acquired), right foot
M20.5X2   Other deformities of toe(s) (acquired), left foot
M20.5X9   Other deformities of toe(s) (acquired), unspecified foot

✓5ᵗʰ **M20.6 Acquired deformities of toe(s), unspecified**
M20.60   Acquired deformities of toe(s), unspecified, unspecified foot
M20.61   Acquired deformities of toe(s), unspecified, right foot
M20.62   Acquired deformities of toe(s), unspecified, left foot

✓4ᵗʰ **M21 Other acquired deformities of limbs**
EXCLUDES 1   *acquired absence of limb (Z89.-)*
congenital absence of limbs (Q71-Q73)
congenital deformities and malformations of limbs (Q65-Q66, Q68-Q74)
EXCLUDES 2   *acquired deformities of fingers or toes (M20.-)*
coxa plana (M91.2)

✓5ᵗʰ **M21.0 Valgus deformity, not elsewhere classified**
EXCLUDES 1   *metatarsus valgus (Q66.6)*
talipes calcaneovalgus (Q66.4)
M21.00   Valgus deformity, not elsewhere classified, unspecified site

✓6ᵗʰ **M21.02 Valgus deformity, not elsewhere classified, elbow**
Cubitus valgus
M21.021   Valgus deformity, not elsewhere classified, right elbow
M21.022   Valgus deformity, not elsewhere classified, left elbow
M21.029   Valgus deformity, not elsewhere classified, unspecified elbow

✓6ᵗʰ **M21.05 Valgus deformity, not elsewhere classified, hip**
M21.051   Valgus deformity, not elsewhere classified, right hip
M21.052   Valgus deformity, not elsewhere classified, left hip
M21.059   Valgus deformity, not elsewhere classified, unspecified hip

✓6ᵗʰ **M21.06 Valgus deformity, not elsewhere classified, knee**
Genu valgum   Knock knee
M21.061   Valgus deformity, not elsewhere classified, right knee
M21.062   Valgus deformity, not elsewhere classified, left knee
M21.069   Valgus deformity, not elsewhere classified, unspecified knee

✓6ᵗʰ **M21.07 Valgus deformity, not elsewhere classified, ankle**
M21.071   Valgus deformity, not elsewhere classified, right ankle
M21.072   Valgus deformity, not elsewhere classified, left ankle
M21.079   Valgus deformity, not elsewhere classified, unspecified ankle

✓5ᵗʰ **M21.1 Varus deformity, not elsewhere classified**
EXCLUDES 1   *metatarsus varus (Q66.2)*
tibia vara (M92.5)
M21.10   Varus deformity, not elsewhere classified, unspecified site

✓6ᵗʰ **M21.12 Varus deformity, not elsewhere classified, elbow**
Cubitus varus, elbow
M21.121   Varus deformity, not elsewhere classified, right elbow
M21.122   Varus deformity, not elsewhere classified, left elbow
M21.129   Varus deformity, not elsewhere classified, unspecified elbow

✓6ᵗʰ **M21.15 Varus deformity, not elsewhere classified, hip**
M21.151   Varus deformity, not elsewhere classified, right hip
M21.152   Varus deformity, not elsewhere classified, left hip
M21.159   Varus deformity, not elsewhere classified, unspecified

✓6ᵗʰ **M21.16 Varus deformity, not elsewhere classified, knee**
Bow leg
Genu varum
M21.161   Varus deformity, not elsewhere classified, right knee
M21.162   Varus deformity, not elsewhere classified, left knee
M21.169   Varus deformity, not elsewhere classified, unspecified knee

✓6ᵗʰ **M21.17 Varus deformity, not elsewhere classified, ankle**
M21.171   Varus deformity, not elsewhere classified, right ankle
M21.172   Varus deformity, not elsewhere classified, left ankle
M21.179   Varus deformity, not elsewhere classified, unspecified ankle

✓5ᵗʰ **M21.2 Flexion deformity**
M21.20   Flexion deformity, unspecified site
✓6ᵗʰ **M21.21 Flexion deformity, shoulder**
M21.211   Flexion deformity, right shoulder
M21.212   Flexion deformity, left shoulder
M21.219   Flexion deformity, unspecified shoulder

✓6ᵗʰ **M21.22 Flexion deformity, elbow**
M21.221   Flexion deformity, right elbow
M21.222   Flexion deformity, left elbow
M21.229   Flexion deformity, unspecified elbow

✓6ᵗʰ **M21.23 Flexion deformity, wrist**
M21.231   Flexion deformity, right wrist
M21.232   Flexion deformity, left wrist
M21.239   Flexion deformity, unspecified wrist

✓6ᵗʰ **M21.24 Flexion deformity, finger joints**
M21.241   Flexion deformity, right finger joints
M21.242   Flexion deformity, left finger joints
M21.249   Flexion deformity, unspecified finger joints

✓6ᵗʰ **M21.25 Flexion deformity, hip**
M21.251   Flexion deformity, right hip
M21.252   Flexion deformity, left hip
M21.259   Flexion deformity, unspecified hip

EXCLUDES 1 Not coded here   EXCLUDES 2 Not included here   N Newborn Age: 0   P Pediatric Age: 0-17   M Maternity Age: 12-55   A Adult Age: 15-124

666   ICD-10-CM 2014 (Draft)

√6th **M21.26 Flexion deformity, knee**
- M21.261 Flexion deformity, right knee
- M21.262 Flexion deformity, left knee
- M21.269 Flexion deformity, unspecified knee

√6th **M21.27 Flexion deformity, ankle and toes**
- M21.271 Flexion deformity, right ankle and toes
- M21.272 Flexion deformity, left ankle and toes
- M21.279 Flexion deformity, unspecified ankle and toes

√5th **M21.3 Wrist or foot drop (acquired)**

√6th **M21.33 Wrist drop (acquired)**
- M21.331 Wrist drop, right wrist
- M21.332 Wrist drop, left wrist
- M21.339 Wrist drop, unspecified wrist

√6th **M21.37 Foot drop (acquired)**
- M21.371 Foot drop, right foot
- M21.372 Foot drop, left foot
- M21.379 Foot drop, unspecified foot

√5th **M21.4 Flat foot [pes planus] (acquired)**
> EXCLUDES 1 congenital pes planus (Q66.5-)
- M21.40 Flat foot [pes planus] (acquired), unspecified foot
- M21.41 Flat foot [pes planus] (acquired), right foot
- M21.42 Flat foot [pes planus] (acquired), left foot

√5th **M21.5 Acquired clawhand, clubhand, clawfoot and clubfoot**
> EXCLUDES 1 clubfoot, not specified as acquired (Q66.89)

√6th **M21.51 Acquired clawhand**
- M21.511 Acquired clawhand, right hand
- M21.512 Acquired clawhand, left hand
- M21.519 Acquired clawhand, unspecified hand

√6th **M21.52 Acquired clubhand**
- M21.521 Acquired clubhand, right hand
- M21.522 Acquired clubhand, left hand
- M21.529 Acquired clubhand, unspecified hand

√6th **M21.53 Acquired clawfoot**
- M21.531 Acquired clawfoot, right foot
- M21.532 Acquired clawfoot, left foot
- M21.539 Acquired clawfoot, unspecified foot

√6th **M21.54 Acquired clubfoot**
- M21.541 Acquired clubfoot, right foot
- M21.542 Acquired clubfoot, left foot
- M21.549 Acquired clubfoot, unspecified foot

√5th **M21.6 Other acquired deformities of foot**
> EXCLUDES 2 deformities of toe (acquired) (M20.1-M20.6)

√6th **M21.6X Other acquired deformities of foot**
- M21.6X1 Other acquired deformities of right foot
- M21.6X2 Other acquired deformities of left foot
- M21.6X9 Other acquired deformities of unspecified foot

√5th **M21.7 Unequal limb length (acquired)**
> NOTE The site used should correspond to the shorter limb.
- M21.70 Unequal limb length (acquired), unspecified site

√6th **M21.72 Unequal limb length (acquired), humerus**
- M21.721 Unequal limb length (acquired), right humerus
- M21.722 Unequal limb length (acquired), left humerus
- M21.729 Unequal limb length (acquired), unspecified humerus

√6th **M21.73 Unequal limb length (acquired), ulna and radius**
- M21.731 Unequal limb length (acquired), right ulna
- M21.732 Unequal limb length (acquired), left ulna
- M21.733 Unequal limb length (acquired), right radius
- M21.734 Unequal limb length (acquired), left radius
- M21.739 Unequal limb length (acquired), unspecified ulna and radius

√6th **M21.75 Unequal limb length (acquired), femur**
- M21.751 Unequal limb length (acquired), right femur
- M21.752 Unequal limb length (acquired), left femur
- M21.759 Unequal limb length (acquired), unspecified femur

√6th **M21.76 Unequal limb length (acquired), tibia and fibula**
- M21.761 Unequal limb length (acquired), right tibia
- M21.762 Unequal limb length (acquired), left tibia
- M21.763 Unequal limb length (acquired), right fibula
- M21.764 Unequal limb length (acquired), left fibula
- M21.769 Unequal limb length (acquired), unspecified tibia and fibula

√5th **M21.8 Other specified acquired deformities of limbs**
> EXCLUDES 2 coxa plana (M91.2)
- M21.80 Other specified acquired deformities of unspecified limb

√6th **M21.82 Other specified acquired deformities of upper arm**
- M21.821 Other specified acquired deformities of right upper arm
- M21.822 Other specified acquired deformities of left upper arm
- M21.829 Other specified acquired deformities of unspecified upper arm

√6th **M21.83 Other specified acquired deformities of forearm**
- M21.831 Other specified acquired deformities of right forearm
- M21.832 Other specified acquired deformities of left forearm
- M21.839 Other specified acquired deformities of unspecified forearm

√6th **M21.85 Other specified acquired deformities of thigh**
- M21.851 Other specified acquired deformities of right thigh
- M21.852 Other specified acquired deformities of left thigh
- M21.859 Other specified acquired deformities of unspecified thigh

√6th **M21.86 Other specified acquired deformities of lower leg**
- M21.861 Other specified acquired deformities of right lower leg
- M21.862 Other specified acquired deformities of left lower leg
- M21.869 Other specified acquired deformities of unspecified lower leg

√5th **M21.9 Unspecified acquired deformity of limb and hand**
- M21.90 Unspecified acquired deformity of unspecified limb

√6th **M21.92 Unspecified acquired deformity of upper arm**
- M21.921 Unspecified acquired deformity of right upper arm
- M21.922 Unspecified acquired deformity of left upper arm
- M21.929 Unspecified acquired deformity of unspecified upper arm

√6th **M21.93 Unspecified acquired deformity of forearm**
- M21.931 Unspecified acquired deformity of right forearm
- M21.932 Unspecified acquired deformity of left forearm
- M21.939 Unspecified acquired deformity of unspecified forearm

√6th **M21.94 Unspecified acquired deformity of hand**
- M21.941 Unspecified acquired deformity of hand, right hand
- M21.942 Unspecified acquired deformity of hand, left hand
- M21.949 Unspecified acquired deformity of hand, unspecified hand

√6th **M21.95 Unspecified acquired deformity of thigh**
- M21.951 Unspecified acquired deformity of right thigh
- M21.952 Unspecified acquired deformity of left thigh
- M21.959 Unspecified acquired deformity of unspecified thigh

√6th **M21.96 Unspecified acquired deformity of lower leg**
- M21.961 Unspecified acquired deformity of right lower leg
- M21.962 Unspecified acquired deformity of left lower leg

☑ Additional Character Required   √x7th Xtension Alert   Unspecified Code   Other Specified Code   Manifestation Code   ▶◀ Revised Text   ● New Code   ▲ Revised Code Title

ICD-10-CM 2014 (Draft)   667

Diseases of the Musculoskeletal System and Connective Tissue

M21.969–M23.212

M21.969   Unspecified acquired deformity of unspecified lower leg

☑4ᵗʰ **M22**   **Disorder of patella**
> EXCLUDES 1   *traumatic dislocation of patella (S83.0-)*

☑5ᵗʰ **M22.0**   **Recurrent dislocation** of patella
- **M22.00**   **Recurrent dislocation of patella, unspecified knee**
- **M22.01**   **Recurrent dislocation of patella, right knee**
- **M22.02**   **Recurrent dislocation of patella, left knee**

☑5ᵗʰ **M22.1**   **Recurrent subluxation** of patella
> Incomplete dislocation of patella
- **M22.10**   **Recurrent subluxation of patella, unspecified knee**
- **M22.11**   **Recurrent subluxation of patella, right knee**
- **M22.12**   **Recurrent subluxation of patella, left knee**

☑5ᵗʰ **M22.2**   **Patellofemoral disorders**
> ☑6ᵗʰ **M22.2X**   **Patellofemoral disorders**
> - **M22.2X1**   **Patellofemoral disorders, right knee**
> - **M22.2X2**   **Patellofemoral disorders, left knee**
> - **M22.2X9**   **Patellofemoral disorders, unspecified knee**

☑5ᵗʰ **M22.3**   **Other derangements** of patella
> ☑6ᵗʰ **M22.3X**   **Other derangements of patella**
> - **M22.3X1**   **Other derangements of patella, right knee**
> - **M22.3X2**   **Other derangements of patella, left knee**
> - **M22.3X9**   **Other derangements of patella, unspecified knee**

☑5ᵗʰ **M22.4**   **Chondromalacia patellae**
- **M22.40**   **Chondromalacia patellae, unspecified knee**
- **M22.41**   **Chondromalacia patellae, right knee**
- **M22.42**   **Chondromalacia patellae, left knee**

☑5ᵗʰ **M22.8**   **Other disorders** of patella
> ☑6ᵗʰ **M22.8X**   **Other disorders of patella**
> - **M22.8X1**   **Other disorders of patella, right knee**
> - **M22.8X2**   **Other disorders of patella, left knee**
> - **M22.8X9**   **Other disorders of patella, unspecified knee**

☑5ᵗʰ **M22.9**   **Unspecified disorder of patella**
- **M22.90**   **Unspecified disorder of patella, unspecified knee**
- **M22.91**   **Unspecified disorder of patella, right knee**
- **M22.92**   **Unspecified disorder of patella, left knee**

☑4ᵗʰ **M23**   **Internal derangement of knee**
> EXCLUDES 1   *ankylosis (M24.66)*
> *current injury—see injury of knee and lower leg (S80-S89)*
> *deformity of knee (M21.-)*
> *osteochondritis dissecans (M93.2)*
> *recurrent dislocation or subluxation of joints (M24.4)*
> *recurrent dislocation or subluxation of patella (M22.0-M22.1)*

☑5ᵗʰ **M23.0**   **Cystic meniscus**
> ☑6ᵗʰ **M23.00**   **Cystic meniscus, unspecified meniscus**
> > Cystic meniscus, unspecified lateral meniscus
> > Cystic meniscus, unspecified medial meniscus
> - **M23.000**   **Cystic meniscus, unspecified lateral meniscus, right knee**
> - **M23.001**   **Cystic meniscus, unspecified lateral meniscus, left knee**
> - **M23.002**   **Cystic meniscus, unspecified lateral meniscus, unspecified knee**
> - **M23.003**   **Cystic meniscus, unspecified medial meniscus, right knee**
> - **M23.004**   **Cystic meniscus, unspecified medial meniscus, left knee**
> - **M23.005**   **Cystic meniscus, unspecified medial meniscus, unspecified knee**
> - **M23.006**   **Cystic meniscus, unspecified meniscus, right knee**
> - **M23.007**   **Cystic meniscus, unspecified meniscus, left knee**
> - **M23.009**   **Cystic meniscus, unspecified meniscus, unspecified knee**
>
> ☑6ᵗʰ **M23.01**   **Cystic meniscus, anterior horn of medial meniscus**
> - **M23.011**   **Cystic meniscus, anterior horn of medial meniscus, right knee**
> - **M23.012**   **Cystic meniscus, anterior horn of medial meniscus, left knee**

M23.019   **Cystic meniscus, anterior horn of medial meniscus, unspecified knee**

☑6ᵗʰ **M23.02**   **Cystic meniscus, posterior horn of medial meniscus**
- **M23.021**   **Cystic meniscus, posterior horn of medial meniscus, right knee**
- **M23.022**   **Cystic meniscus, posterior horn of medial meniscus, left knee**
- **M23.029**   **Cystic meniscus, posterior horn of medial meniscus, unspecified knee**

☑6ᵗʰ **M23.03**   **Cystic meniscus, other medial meniscus**
- **M23.031**   **Cystic meniscus, other medial meniscus, right knee**
- **M23.032**   **Cystic meniscus, other medial meniscus, left knee**
- **M23.039**   **Cystic meniscus, other medial meniscus, unspecified knee**

☑6ᵗʰ **M23.04**   **Cystic meniscus, anterior horn of lateral meniscus**
- **M23.041**   **Cystic meniscus, anterior horn of lateral meniscus, right knee**
- **M23.042**   **Cystic meniscus, anterior horn of lateral meniscus, left knee**
- **M23.049**   **Cystic meniscus, anterior horn of lateral meniscus, unspecified knee**

☑6ᵗʰ **M23.05**   **Cystic meniscus, posterior horn of lateral meniscus**
- **M23.051**   **Cystic meniscus, posterior horn of lateral meniscus, right knee**
- **M23.052**   **Cystic meniscus, posterior horn of lateral meniscus, left knee**
- **M23.059**   **Cystic meniscus, posterior horn of lateral meniscus, unspecified knee**

☑6ᵗʰ **M23.06**   **Cystic meniscus, other lateral meniscus**
- **M23.061**   **Cystic meniscus, other lateral meniscus, right knee**
- **M23.062**   **Cystic meniscus, other lateral meniscus, left knee**
- **M23.069**   **Cystic meniscus, other lateral meniscus, unspecified knee**

☑5ᵗʰ **M23.2**   **Derangement of meniscus due to old tear or injury**
> Old bucket-handle tear
> ☑6ᵗʰ **M23.20**   **Derangement of unspecified meniscus due to old tear or injury**
> > Derangement of unspecified lateral meniscus due to old tear or injury
> > Derangement of unspecified medial meniscus due to old tear or injury
> - **M23.200**   **Derangement of unspecified lateral meniscus due to old tear or injury, right knee**
> - **M23.201**   **Derangement of unspecified lateral meniscus due to old tear or injury, left knee**
> - **M23.202**   **Derangement of unspecified lateral meniscus due to old tear or injury, unspecified knee**
> - **M23.203**   **Derangement of unspecified medial meniscus due to old tear or injury, right knee**
> - **M23.204**   **Derangement of unspecified medial meniscus due to old tear or injury, left knee**
> - **M23.205**   **Derangement of unspecified medial meniscus due to old tear or injury, unspecified knee**
> - **M23.206**   **Derangement of unspecified meniscus due to old tear or injury, right knee**
> - **M23.207**   **Derangement of unspecified meniscus due to old tear or injury, left knee**
> - **M23.209**   **Derangement of unspecified meniscus due to old tear or injury, unspecified knee**
>
> ☑6ᵗʰ **M23.21**   **Derangement of anterior horn of medial meniscus due to old tear or injury**
> - **M23.211**   **Derangement of anterior horn of medial meniscus due to old tear or injury, right knee**
> - **M23.212**   **Derangement of anterior horn of medial meniscus due to old tear or injury, left knee**

EXCLUDES 1 Not coded here   EXCLUDES 2 Not included here   N Newborn Age: 0   P Pediatric Age: 0-17   M Maternity Age: 12-55   A Adult Age: 15-124

668   ICD-10-CM 2014 (Draft)

M23.219   Derangement of anterior horn of medial meniscus due to old tear or injury, unspecified knee

✓6ᵗʰ M23.22   Derangement of posterior horn of medial meniscus due to old tear or injury

M23.221   Derangement of posterior horn of medial meniscus due to old tear or injury, right knee

M23.222   Derangement of posterior horn of medial meniscus due to old tear or injury, left knee

M23.229   Derangement of posterior horn of medial meniscus due to old tear or injury, unspecified knee

✓6ᵗʰ M23.23   Derangement of other medial meniscus due to old tear or injury

M23.231   Derangement of other medial meniscus due to old tear or injury, right knee

M23.232   Derangement of other medial meniscus due to old tear or injury, left knee

M23.239   Derangement of other medial meniscus due to old tear or injury, unspecified knee

✓6ᵗʰ M23.24   Derangement of anterior horn of lateral meniscus due to old tear or injury

M23.241   Derangement of anterior horn of lateral meniscus due to old tear or injury, right knee

M23.242   Derangement of anterior horn of lateral meniscus due to old tear or injury, left knee

M23.249   Derangement of anterior horn of lateral meniscus due to old tear or injury, unspecified knee

✓6ᵗʰ M23.25   Derangement of posterior horn of lateral meniscus due to old tear or injury

M23.251   Derangement of posterior horn of lateral meniscus due to old tear or injury, right knee

M23.252   Derangement of posterior horn of lateral meniscus due to old tear or injury, left knee

M23.259   Derangement of posterior horn of lateral meniscus due to old tear or injury, unspecified knee

✓6ᵗʰ M23.26   Derangement of other lateral meniscus due to old tear or injury

M23.261   Derangement of other lateral meniscus due to old tear or injury, right knee

M23.262   Derangement of other lateral meniscus due to old tear or injury, left knee

M23.269   Derangement of other lateral meniscus due to old tear or injury, unspecified knee

✓5ᵗʰ M23.3   Other meniscus derangements
Degenerate meniscus
Detached meniscus
Retained meniscus

✓6ᵗʰ M23.30   Other meniscus derangements, unspecified meniscus
Other meniscus derangements, unspecified lateral meniscus
Other meniscus derangements, unspecified medial meniscus

M23.300   Other meniscus derangements, unspecified lateral meniscus, right knee

M23.301   Other meniscus derangements, unspecified lateral meniscus, left knee

M23.302   Other meniscus derangements, unspecified lateral meniscus, unspecified knee

M23.303   Other meniscus derangements, unspecified medial meniscus, right knee

M23.304   Other meniscus derangements, unspecified medial meniscus, left knee

M23.305   Other meniscus derangements, unspecified medial meniscus, unspecified knee

M23.306   Other meniscus derangements, unspecified meniscus, right knee

M23.307   Other meniscus derangements, unspecified meniscus, left knee

M23.309   Other meniscus derangements, unspecified meniscus, unspecified knee

✓6ᵗʰ M23.31   Other meniscus derangements, anterior horn of medial meniscus

M23.311   Other meniscus derangements, anterior horn of medial meniscus, right knee

M23.312   Other meniscus derangements, anterior horn of medial meniscus, left knee

M23.319   Other meniscus derangements, anterior horn of medial meniscus, unspecified knee

✓6ᵗʰ M23.32   Other meniscus derangements, posterior horn of medial meniscus

M23.321   Other meniscus derangements, posterior horn of medial meniscus, right knee

M23.322   Other meniscus derangements, posterior horn of medial meniscus, left knee

M23.329   Other meniscus derangements, posterior horn of medial meniscus, unspecified knee

✓6ᵗʰ M23.33   Other meniscus derangements, other medial meniscus

M23.331   Other meniscus derangements, other medial meniscus, right knee

M23.332   Other meniscus derangements, other medial meniscus, left knee

M23.339   Other meniscus derangements, other medial meniscus, unspecified knee

✓6ᵗʰ M23.34   Other meniscus derangements, anterior horn of lateral meniscus

M23.341   Other meniscus derangements, anterior horn of lateral meniscus, right knee

M23.342   Other meniscus derangements, anterior horn of lateral meniscus, left knee

M23.349   Other meniscus derangements, anterior horn of lateral meniscus, unspecified knee

✓6ᵗʰ M23.35   Other meniscus derangements, posterior horn of lateral meniscus

M23.351   Other meniscus derangements, posterior horn of lateral meniscus, right knee

M23.352   Other meniscus derangements, posterior horn of lateral meniscus, left knee

M23.359   Other meniscus derangements, posterior horn of lateral meniscus, unspecified knee

✓6ᵗʰ M23.36   Other meniscus derangements, other lateral meniscus

M23.361   Other meniscus derangements, other lateral meniscus, right knee

M23.362   Other meniscus derangements, other lateral meniscus, left knee

M23.369   Other meniscus derangements, other lateral meniscus, unspecified knee

✓5ᵗʰ M23.4   Loose body in knee

M23.40   Loose body in knee, unspecified knee

M23.41   Loose body in knee, right knee

M23.42   Loose body in knee, left knee

✓5ᵗʰ M23.5   Chronic instability of knee

M23.50   Chronic instability of knee, unspecified knee

M23.51   Chronic instability of knee, right knee

M23.52   Chronic instability of knee, left knee

✓5ᵗʰ M23.6   Other spontaneous disruption of ligament(s) of knee

✓6ᵗʰ M23.60   Other spontaneous disruption of unspecified ligament of knee

M23.601   Other spontaneous disruption of unspecified ligament of right knee

M23.602   Other spontaneous disruption of unspecified ligament of left knee

M23.609   Other spontaneous disruption of unspecified ligament of unspecified knee

✓6ᵗʰ M23.61   Other spontaneous disruption of anterior cruciate ligament of knee

M23.611   Other spontaneous disruption of anterior cruciate ligament of right knee

M23.612   Other spontaneous disruption of anterior cruciate ligament of left knee

M23.619   Other spontaneous disruption of anterior cruciate ligament of unspecified knee

☑ Additional Character Required   ✓ₓ7ᵗʰ Xtension Alert   Unspecified Code   Other Specified Code   Manifestation Code   ▶◀ Revised Text   ● New Code   ▲ Revised Code Title

ICD-10-CM 2014 (Draft)   669

✓6ᵗʰ **M23.62 Other spontaneous disruption of posterior cruciate ligament of knee**
     M23.621 Other spontaneous disruption of posterior cruciate ligament of right knee
     M23.622 Other spontaneous disruption of posterior cruciate ligament of left knee
     M23.629 Other spontaneous disruption of posterior cruciate ligament of unspecified knee

✓6ᵗʰ **M23.63 Other spontaneous disruption of medial collateral ligament of knee**
     M23.631 Other spontaneous disruption of medial collateral ligament of right knee
     M23.632 Other spontaneous disruption of medial collateral ligament of left knee
     M23.639 Other spontaneous disruption of medial collateral ligament of unspecified knee

✓6ᵗʰ **M23.64 Other spontaneous disruption of lateral collateral ligament of knee**
     M23.641 Other spontaneous disruption of lateral collateral ligament of right knee
     M23.642 Other spontaneous disruption of lateral collateral ligament of left knee
     M23.649 Other spontaneous disruption of lateral collateral ligament of unspecified knee

✓6ᵗʰ **M23.67 Other spontaneous disruption of capsular ligament of knee**
     M23.671 Other spontaneous disruption of capsular ligament of right knee
     M23.672 Other spontaneous disruption of capsular ligament of left knee
     M23.679 Other spontaneous disruption of capsular ligament of unspecified knee

✓5ᵗʰ **M23.8 Other internal derangements of knee**
     Laxity of ligament of knee
     Snapping knee

✓6ᵗʰ **M23.8X Other internal derangements of knee**
     M23.8X1 Other internal derangements of right knee
     M23.8X2 Other internal derangements of left knee
     M23.8X9 Other internal derangements of unspecified knee

✓5ᵗʰ **M23.9 Unspecified internal derangement of knee**
     M23.90 Unspecified internal derangement of unspecified knee
     M23.91 Unspecified internal derangement of right knee
     M23.92 Unspecified internal derangement of left knee

✓4ᵗʰ **M24 Other specific joint derangements**
     EXCLUDES 1   current injury—see injury of joint by body region
     EXCLUDES 2   ganglion (M67.4)
                 snapping knee (M23.8-)
                 temporomandibular joint disorders (M26.6-)

✓5ᵗʰ **M24.0 Loose body in joint**
     EXCLUDES 2   loose body in knee (M23.4)
     M24.00 Loose body in unspecified joint

✓6ᵗʰ **M24.01 Loose body in shoulder**
     M24.011 Loose body in right shoulder
     M24.012 Loose body in left shoulder
     M24.019 Loose body in unspecified shoulder

✓6ᵗʰ **M24.02 Loose body in elbow**
     M24.021 Loose body in right elbow
     M24.022 Loose body in left elbow
     M24.029 Loose body in unspecified elbow

✓6ᵗʰ **M24.03 Loose body in wrist**
     M24.031 Loose body in right wrist
     M24.032 Loose body in left wrist
     M24.039 Loose body in unspecified wrist

✓6ᵗʰ **M24.04 Loose body in finger joints**
     M24.041 Loose body in right finger joint(s)
     M24.042 Loose body in left finger joint(s)
     M24.049 Loose body in unspecified finger joint(s)

✓6ᵗʰ **M24.05 Loose body in hip**
     M24.051 Loose body in right hip
     M24.052 Loose body in left hip
     M24.059 Loose body in unspecified hip

✓6ᵗʰ **M24.07 Loose body in ankle and toe joints**
     M24.071 Loose body in right ankle
     M24.072 Loose body in left ankle
     M24.073 Loose body in unspecified ankle
     M24.074 Loose body in right toe joint(s)
     M24.075 Loose body in left toe joint(s)
     M24.076 Loose body in unspecified toe joints
     M24.08 Loose body, other site

✓5ᵗʰ **M24.1 Other articular cartilage disorders**
     EXCLUDES 2   chondrocalcinosis (M11.1, M11.2-)
                 internal derangement of knee (M23.-)
                 metastatic calcification (E83.5)
                 ochronosis (E70.2)
     M24.10 Other articular cartilage disorders, unspecified site

✓6ᵗʰ **M24.11 Other articular cartilage disorders, shoulder**
     M24.111 Other articular cartilage disorders, right shoulder
     M24.112 Other articular cartilage disorders, left shoulder
     M24.119 Other articular cartilage disorders, unspecified shoulder

✓6ᵗʰ **M24.12 Other articular cartilage disorders, elbow**
     M24.121 Other articular cartilage disorders, right elbow
     M24.122 Other articular cartilage disorders, left elbow
     M24.129 Other articular cartilage disorders, unspecified elbow

✓6ᵗʰ **M24.13 Other articular cartilage disorders, wrist**
     M24.131 Other articular cartilage disorders, right wrist
     M24.132 Other articular cartilage disorders, left wrist
     M24.139 Other articular cartilage disorders, unspecified wrist

✓6ᵗʰ **M24.14 Other articular cartilage disorders, hand**
     M24.141 Other articular cartilage disorders, right hand
     M24.142 Other articular cartilage disorders, left hand
     M24.149 Other articular cartilage disorders, unspecified hand

✓6ᵗʰ **M24.15 Other articular cartilage disorders, hip**
     M24.151 Other articular cartilage disorders, right hip
     M24.152 Other articular cartilage disorders, left hip
     M24.159 Other articular cartilage disorders, unspecified hip

✓6ᵗʰ **M24.17 Other articular cartilage disorders, ankle and foot**
     M24.171 Other articular cartilage disorders, right ankle
     M24.172 Other articular cartilage disorders, left ankle
     M24.173 Other articular cartilage disorders, unspecified ankle
     M24.174 Other articular cartilage disorders, right foot
     M24.175 Other articular cartilage disorders, left foot
     M24.176 Other articular cartilage disorders, unspecified foot

✓5ᵗʰ **M24.2 Disorder of ligament**
     Instability secondary to old ligament injury
     Ligamentous laxity NOS
     EXCLUDES 1   familial ligamentous laxity (M35.7)
     EXCLUDES 2   internal derangement of knee (M23.5-M23.89)
     M24.20 Disorder of ligament, unspecified site

✓6ᵗʰ **M24.21 Disorder of ligament, shoulder**
     M24.211 Disorder of ligament, right shoulder
     M24.212 Disorder of ligament, left shoulder
     M24.219 Disorder of ligament, unspecified shoulder

✓6ᵗʰ **M24.22 Disorder of ligament, elbow**
     M24.221 Disorder of ligament, right elbow
     M24.222 Disorder of ligament, left elbow
     M24.229 Disorder of ligament, unspecified elbow

EXCLUDES 1 Not coded here   *EXCLUDES 2* Not included here   N Newborn Age: 0   P Pediatric Age: 0-17   M Maternity Age: 12-55   A Adult Age: 15-124

670   ICD-10-CM 2014 (Draft)

√6ᵗʰ **M24.23** Disorder of ligament, wrist
    M24.231 Disorder of ligament, right wrist
    M24.232 Disorder of ligament, left wrist
    M24.239 Disorder of ligament, unspecified wrist

√6ᵗʰ **M24.24** Disorder of ligament, hand
    M24.241 Disorder of ligament, right hand
    M24.242 Disorder of ligament, left hand
    M24.249 Disorder of ligament, unspecified hand

√6ᵗʰ **M24.25** Disorder of ligament, hip
    M24.251 Disorder of ligament, right hip
    M24.252 Disorder of ligament, left hip
    M24.259 Disorder of ligament, unspecified hip

√6ᵗʰ **M24.27** Disorder of ligament, ankle and foot
    M24.271 Disorder of ligament, right ankle
    M24.272 Disorder of ligament, left ankle
    M24.273 Disorder of ligament, unspecified ankle
    M24.274 Disorder of ligament, right foot
    M24.275 Disorder of ligament, left foot
    M24.276 Disorder of ligament, unspecified foot

M24.28 Disorder of ligament, vertebrae

√5ᵗʰ **M24.3** Pathological dislocation of joint, not elsewhere classified
    EXCLUDES 1 *congenital dislocation or displacement of joint—see congenital malformations and deformations of the musculoskeletal system (Q65-Q79)*
        current injury—see injury of joints and ligaments by body region
        recurrent dislocation of joint (M24.4-)

    M24.30 Pathological dislocation of unspecified joint, not elsewhere classified

√6ᵗʰ **M24.31** Pathological dislocation of shoulder, not elsewhere classified
    M24.311 Pathological dislocation of right shoulder, not elsewhere classified
    M24.312 Pathological dislocation of left shoulder, not elsewhere classified
    M24.319 Pathological dislocation of unspecified shoulder, not elsewhere classified

√6ᵗʰ **M24.32** Pathological dislocation of elbow, not elsewhere classified
    M24.321 Pathological dislocation of right elbow, not elsewhere classified
    M24.322 Pathological dislocation of left elbow, not elsewhere classified
    M24.329 Pathological dislocation of unspecified elbow, not elsewhere classified

√6ᵗʰ **M24.33** Pathological dislocation of wrist, not elsewhere classified
    M24.331 Pathological dislocation of right wrist, not elsewhere classified
    M24.332 Pathological dislocation of left wrist, not elsewhere classified
    M24.339 Pathological dislocation of unspecified wrist, not elsewhere classified

√6ᵗʰ **M24.34** Pathological dislocation of hand, not elsewhere classified
    M24.341 Pathological dislocation of right hand, not elsewhere classified
    M24.342 Pathological dislocation of left hand, not elsewhere classified
    M24.349 Pathological dislocation of unspecified hand, not elsewhere classified

√6ᵗʰ **M24.35** Pathological dislocation of hip, not elsewhere classified
    M24.351 Pathological dislocation of right hip, not elsewhere classified
    M24.352 Pathological dislocation of left hip, not elsewhere classified
    M24.359 Pathological dislocation of unspecified hip, not elsewhere classified

√6ᵗʰ **M24.36** Pathological dislocation of knee, not elsewhere classified
    M24.361 Pathological dislocation of right knee, not elsewhere classified
    M24.362 Pathological dislocation of left knee, not elsewhere classified

    M24.369 Pathological dislocation of unspecified knee, not elsewhere classified

√6ᵗʰ **M24.37** Pathological dislocation of ankle and foot, not elsewhere classified
    M24.371 Pathological dislocation of right ankle, not elsewhere classified
    M24.372 Pathological dislocation of left ankle, not elsewhere classified
    M24.373 Pathological dislocation of unspecified ankle, not elsewhere classified
    M24.374 Pathological dislocation of right foot, not elsewhere classified
    M24.375 Pathological dislocation of left foot, not elsewhere classified
    M24.376 Pathological dislocation of unspecified foot, not elsewhere classified

√5ᵗʰ **M24.4** Recurrent dislocation of joint
    Recurrent subluxation of joint
    EXCLUDES 2 *recurrent dislocation of patella (M22.0-M22.1)*
        recurrent vertebral dislocation (M43.3-, M43.4, M43.5-)

    M24.40 Recurrent dislocation, unspecified joint

√6ᵗʰ **M24.41** Recurrent dislocation, shoulder
    M24.411 Recurrent dislocation, right shoulder
    M24.412 Recurrent dislocation, left shoulder
    M24.419 Recurrent dislocation, unspecified shoulder

√6ᵗʰ **M24.42** Recurrent dislocation, elbow
    M24.421 Recurrent dislocation, right elbow
    M24.422 Recurrent dislocation, left elbow
    M24.429 Recurrent dislocation, unspecified elbow

√6ᵗʰ **M24.43** Recurrent dislocation, wrist
    M24.431 Recurrent dislocation, right wrist
    M24.432 Recurrent dislocation, left wrist
    M24.439 Recurrent dislocation, unspecified wrist

√6ᵗʰ **M24.44** Recurrent dislocation, hand and finger(s)
    M24.441 Recurrent dislocation, right hand
    M24.442 Recurrent dislocation, left hand
    M24.443 Recurrent dislocation, unspecified hand
    M24.444 Recurrent dislocation, right finger
    M24.445 Recurrent dislocation, left finger
    M24.446 Recurrent dislocation, unspecified finger

√6ᵗʰ **M24.45** Recurrent dislocation, hip
    M24.451 Recurrent dislocation, right hip
    M24.452 Recurrent dislocation, left hip
    M24.459 Recurrent dislocation, unspecified hip

√6ᵗʰ **M24.46** Recurrent dislocation, knee
    M24.461 Recurrent dislocation, right knee
    M24.462 Recurrent dislocation, left knee
    M24.469 Recurrent dislocation, unspecified knee

√6ᵗʰ **M24.47** Recurrent dislocation, ankle, foot and toes
    M24.471 Recurrent dislocation, right ankle
    M24.472 Recurrent dislocation, left ankle
    M24.473 Recurrent dislocation, unspecified ankle
    M24.474 Recurrent dislocation, right foot
    M24.475 Recurrent dislocation, left foot
    M24.476 Recurrent dislocation, unspecified foot
    M24.477 Recurrent dislocation, right toe(s)
    M24.478 Recurrent dislocation, left toe(s)
    M24.479 Recurrent dislocation, unspecified toe(s)

√5ᵗʰ **M24.5** Contracture of joint
    EXCLUDES 1 *contracture of muscle without contracture of joint (M62.4-)*
        contracture of tendon (sheath) without contracture of joint (M62.4-)
        Dupuytren's contracture (M72.0)
    EXCLUDES 2 *acquired deformities of limbs (M20-M21)*

    M24.50 Contracture, unspecified joint

√6ᵗʰ **M24.51** Contracture, shoulder
    M24.511 Contracture, right shoulder
    M24.512 Contracture, left shoulder
    M24.519 Contracture, unspecified shoulder

√6ᵗʰ **M24.52** Contracture, elbow
    M24.521 Contracture, right elbow
    M24.522 Contracture, left elbow

☑ Additional Character Required   √x7ᵗʰ Xtension Alert   Unspecified Code   Other Specified Code   Manifestation Code   ►◄ Revised Text   ● New Code   ▲ Revised Code Title

Diseases of the Musculoskeletal System and Connective Tissue

M24.529–M25.039

M24.529   **Contracture, unspecified elbow**

✓6ᵗʰ **M24.53**   Contracture, wrist
- M24.531   Contracture, right wrist
- M24.532   Contracture, left wrist
- M24.539   **Contracture, unspecified wrist**

✓6ᵗʰ **M24.54**   Contracture, hand
- M24.541   Contracture, right hand
- M24.542   Contracture, left hand
- M24.549   **Contracture, unspecified hand**

✓6ᵗʰ **M24.55**   Contracture, hip
- M24.551   Contracture, right hip
- M24.552   Contracture, left hip
- M24.559   **Contracture, unspecified hip**

✓6ᵗʰ **M24.56**   Contracture, knee
- M24.561   Contracture, right knee
- M24.562   Contracture, left knee
- M24.569   **Contracture, unspecified knee**

✓6ᵗʰ **M24.57**   Contracture, ankle and foot
- M24.571   **Contracture, right ankle**
- M24.572   **Contracture, left ankle**
- M24.573   **Contracture, unspecified ankle**
- M24.574   **Contracture, right foot**
- M24.575   **Contracture, left foot**
- M24.576   **Contracture, unspecified foot**

✓5ᵗʰ **M24.6**   **Ankylosis of joint**
> *EXCLUDES 1*   stiffness of joint without ankylosis (M25.6-)
> *EXCLUDES 2*   spine (M43.2-)

M24.60   **Ankylosis, unspecified joint**

✓6ᵗʰ **M24.61**   Ankylosis, shoulder
- M24.611   Ankylosis, right shoulder
- M24.612   Ankylosis, left shoulder
- M24.619   **Ankylosis, unspecified shoulder**

✓6ᵗʰ **M24.62**   Ankylosis, elbow
- M24.621   Ankylosis, right elbow
- M24.622   Ankylosis, left elbow
- M24.629   **Ankylosis, unspecified elbow**

✓6ᵗʰ **M24.63**   Ankylosis, wrist
- M24.631   Ankylosis, right wrist
- M24.632   Ankylosis, left wrist
- M24.639   **Ankylosis, unspecified wrist**

✓6ᵗʰ **M24.64**   Ankylosis, hand
- M24.641   Ankylosis, right hand
- M24.642   Ankylosis, left hand
- M24.649   **Ankylosis, unspecified hand**

✓6ᵗʰ **M24.65**   Ankylosis, hip
- M24.651   Ankylosis, right hip
- M24.652   Ankylosis, left hip
- M24.659   **Ankylosis, unspecified hip**

✓6ᵗʰ **M24.66**   Ankylosis, knee
- M24.661   Ankylosis, right knee
- M24.662   Ankylosis, left knee
- M24.669   **Ankylosis, unspecified knee**

✓6ᵗʰ **M24.67**   Ankylosis, ankle and foot
- M24.671   Ankylosis, right ankle
- M24.672   Ankylosis, left ankle
- M24.673   **Ankylosis, unspecified ankle**
- M24.674   Ankylosis, right foot
- M24.675   Ankylosis, left foot
- M24.676   **Ankylosis, unspecified foot**

M24.7   **Protrusio acetabuli**

✓5ᵗʰ **M24.8**   **Other specific joint derangements, not elsewhere classified**
> *EXCLUDES 2*   iliotibial band syndrome (M76.3)

M24.80   **Other specific joint derangements of unspecified joint, not elsewhere classified**

✓6ᵗʰ **M24.81**   Other specific joint derangements of shoulder, not elsewhere classified
- M24.811   **Other specific joint derangements of right shoulder, not elsewhere classified**
- M24.812   **Other specific joint derangements of left shoulder, not elsewhere classified**

- M24.819   **Other specific joint derangements of unspecified shoulder, not elsewhere classified**

✓6ᵗʰ **M24.82**   Other specific joint derangements of elbow, not elsewhere classified
- M24.821   **Other specific joint derangements of right elbow, not elsewhere classified**
- M24.822   **Other specific joint derangements of left elbow, not elsewhere classified**
- M24.829   **Other specific joint derangements of unspecified elbow, not elsewhere classified**

✓6ᵗʰ **M24.83**   Other specific joint derangements of wrist, not elsewhere classified
- M24.831   **Other specific joint derangements of right wrist, not elsewhere classified**
- M24.832   **Other specific joint derangements of left wrist, not elsewhere classified**
- M24.839   **Other specific joint derangements of unspecified wrist, not elsewhere classified**

✓6ᵗʰ **M24.84**   Other specific joint derangements of hand, not elsewhere classified
- M24.841   **Other specific joint derangements of right hand, not elsewhere classified**
- M24.842   **Other specific joint derangements of left hand, not elsewhere classified**
- M24.849   **Other specific joint derangements of unspecified hand, not elsewhere classified**

✓6ᵗʰ **M24.85**   Other specific joint derangements of hip, not elsewhere classified
> Irritable hip
- M24.851   **Other specific joint derangements of right hip, not elsewhere classified**
- M24.852   **Other specific joint derangements of left hip, not elsewhere classified**
- M24.859   **Other specific joint derangements of unspecified hip, not elsewhere classified**

✓6ᵗʰ **M24.87**   Other specific joint derangements of ankle and foot, not elsewhere classified
- M24.871   **Other specific joint derangements of right ankle, not elsewhere classified**
- M24.872   **Other specific joint derangements of left ankle, not elsewhere classified**
- M24.873   **Other specific joint derangements of unspecified ankle, not elsewhere classified**
- M24.874   **Other specific joint derangements of right foot, not elsewhere classified**
- M24.875   **Other specific joint derangements left foot, not elsewhere classified**
- M24.876   **Other specific joint derangements of unspecified foot, not elsewhere classified**

M24.9   **Joint derangement, unspecified**

M25   **Other joint disorder, not elsewhere classified**
> *EXCLUDES 2*   abnormality of gait and mobility (R26.-)
> acquired deformities of limb (M20-M21)
> calcification of bursa (M71.4-)
> calcification of shoulder (joint) (M75.3)
> calcification of tendon (M65.2-)
> difficulty in walking (R26.2)
> temporomandibular joint disorder (M26.6-)

✓5ᵗʰ **M25.0**   **Hemarthrosis**
> *EXCLUDES 1*   current injury—see injury of joint by body region
> hemophilic arthropathy (M36.2)

M25.00   **Hemarthrosis, unspecified joint**

✓6ᵗʰ **M25.01**   Hemarthrosis, shoulder
- M25.011   Hemarthrosis, right shoulder
- M25.012   Hemarthrosis, left shoulder
- M25.019   **Hemarthrosis, unspecified shoulder**

✓6ᵗʰ **M25.02**   Hemarthrosis, elbow
- M25.021   Hemarthrosis, right elbow
- M25.022   Hemarthrosis, left elbow
- M25.029   **Hemarthrosis, unspecified elbow**

✓6ᵗʰ **M25.03**   Hemarthrosis, wrist
- M25.031   Hemarthrosis, right wrist
- M25.032   Hemarthrosis, left wrist
- M25.039   **Hemarthrosis, unspecified wrist**

EXCLUDES 1 Not coded here   *EXCLUDES 2* Not included here   N Newborn Age: 0   P Pediatric Age: 0-17   M Maternity Age: 12-55   A Adult Age: 15-124

672   ICD-10-CM 2014 (Draft)

✓6th **M25.04** Hemarthrosis, hand
- M25.041 Hemarthrosis, right hand
- M25.042 Hemarthrosis, left hand
- M25.049 Hemarthrosis, unspecified hand

✓6th **M25.05** Hemarthrosis, hip
- M25.051 Hemarthrosis, right hip
- M25.052 Hemarthrosis, left hip
- M25.059 Hemarthrosis, unspecified hip

✓6th **M25.06** Hemarthrosis, knee
- M25.061 Hemarthrosis, right knee
- M25.062 Hemarthrosis, left knee
- M25.069 Hemarthrosis, unspecified knee

✓6th **M25.07** Hemarthrosis, ankle and foot
- M25.071 Hemarthrosis, right ankle
- M25.072 Hemarthrosis, left ankle
- M25.073 Hemarthrosis, unspecified ankle
- M25.074 Hemarthrosis, right foot
- M25.075 Hemarthrosis, left foot
- M25.076 Hemarthrosis, unspecified foot

M25.08 Hemarthrosis, other specified site
     Hemarthrosis, vertebrae

✓5th **M25.1 Fistula of joint**

M25.10 Fistula, unspecified joint

✓6th **M25.11** Fistula, shoulder
- M25.111 Fistula, right shoulder
- M25.112 Fistula, left shoulder
- M25.119 Fistula, unspecified shoulder

✓6th **M25.12** Fistula, elbow
- M25.121 Fistula, right elbow
- M25.122 Fistula, left elbow
- M25.129 Fistula, unspecified elbow

✓6th **M25.13** Fistula, wrist
- M25.131 Fistula, right wrist
- M25.132 Fistula, left wrist
- M25.139 Fistula, unspecified wrist

✓6th **M25.14** Fistula, hand
- M25.141 Fistula, right hand
- M25.142 Fistula, left hand
- M25.149 Fistula, unspecified hand

✓6th **M25.15** Fistula, hip
- M25.151 Fistula, right hip
- M25.152 Fistula, left hip
- M25.159 Fistula, unspecified hip

✓6th **M25.16** Fistula, knee
- M25.161 Fistula, right knee
- M25.162 Fistula, left knee
- M25.169 Fistula, unspecified knee

✓6th **M25.17** Fistula, ankle and foot
- M25.171 Fistula, right ankle
- M25.172 Fistula, left ankle
- M25.173 Fistula, unspecified ankle
- M25.174 Fistula, right foot
- M25.175 Fistula, left foot
- M25.176 Fistula, unspecified foot

M25.18 Fistula, other specified site
     Fistula, vertebrae

✓5th **M25.2 Flail joint**

M25.20 Flail joint, unspecified joint

✓6th **M25.21** Flail joint, shoulder
- M25.211 Flail joint, right shoulder
- M25.212 Flail joint, left shoulder
- M25.219 Flail joint, unspecified shoulder

✓6th **M25.22** Flail joint, elbow
- M25.221 Flail joint, right elbow
- M25.222 Flail joint, left elbow
- M25.229 Flail joint, unspecified elbow

✓6th **M25.23** Flail joint, wrist
- M25.231 Flail joint, right wrist
- M25.232 Flail joint, left wrist
- M25.239 Flail joint, unspecified wrist

✓6th **M25.24** Flail joint, hand
- M25.241 Flail joint, right hand
- M25.242 Flail joint, left hand
- M25.249 Flail joint, unspecified hand

✓6th **M25.25** Flail joint, hip
- M25.251 Flail joint, right hip
- M25.252 Flail joint, left hip
- M25.259 Flail joint, unspecified hip

✓6th **M25.26** Flail joint, knee
- M25.261 Flail joint, right knee
- M25.262 Flail joint, left knee
- M25.269 Flail joint, unspecified knee

✓6th **M25.27** Flail joint, ankle and foot
- M25.271 Flail joint, right ankle and foot
- M25.272 Flail joint, left ankle and foot
- M25.279 Flail joint, unspecified ankle and foot

M25.28 Flail joint, other site

✓5th **M25.3 Other instability of joint**

> **EXCLUDES 1**   instability of joint secondary to old ligament injury (M24.2-)
> instability of joint secondary to removal of joint prosthesis (M96.8-)
>
> **EXCLUDES 2**   spinal instabilities (M53.2-)

M25.30 Other instability, unspecified joint

✓6th **M25.31** Other instability, shoulder
- M25.311 Other instability, right shoulder
- M25.312 Other instability, left shoulder
- M25.319 Other instability, unspecified shoulder

✓6th **M25.32** Other instability, elbow
- M25.321 Other instability, right elbow
- M25.322 Other instability, left elbow
- M25.329 Other instability, unspecified elbow

✓6th **M25.33** Other instability, wrist
- M25.331 Other instability, right wrist
- M25.332 Other instability, left wrist
- M25.339 Other instability, unspecified wrist

✓6th **M25.34** Other instability, hand
- M25.341 Other instability, right hand
- M25.342 Other instability, left hand
- M25.349 Other instability, unspecified hand

✓6th **M25.35** Other instability, hip
- M25.351 Other instability, right hip
- M25.352 Other instability, left hip
- M25.359 Other instability, unspecified hip

✓6th **M25.36** Other instability, knee
- M25.361 Other instability, right knee
- M25.362 Other instability, left knee
- M25.369 Other instability, unspecified knee

✓6th **M25.37** Other instability, ankle and foot
- M25.371 Other instability, right ankle
- M25.372 Other instability, left ankle
- M25.373 Other instability, unspecified ankle
- M25.374 Other instability, right foot
- M25.375 Other instability, left foot
- M25.376 Other instability, unspecified foot

✓5th **M25.4 Effusion of joint**

> **EXCLUDES 1**   hydrarthrosis in yaws (A66.6)
> intermittent hydrarthrosis (M12.4-)
> other infective (teno)synovitis (M65.1-)

M25.40 Effusion, unspecified joint

✓6th **M25.41** Effusion, shoulder
- M25.411 Effusion, right shoulder
- M25.412 Effusion, left shoulder
- M25.419 Effusion, unspecified shoulder

✓6th **M25.42** Effusion, elbow
- M25.421 Effusion, right elbow
- M25.422 Effusion, left elbow
- M25.429 Effusion, unspecified elbow

✓6th **M25.43** Effusion, wrist
- M25.431 Effusion, right wrist
- M25.432 Effusion, left wrist
- M25.439 Effusion, unspecified wrist

☑ Additional Character Required   ✓x7th Xtension Alert   Unspecified Code   Other Specified Code   Manifestation Code   ►◄ Revised Text   ● New Code   ▲ Revised Code Title

✓6ᵗʰ **M25.44 Effusion,** hand
  M25.441 Effusion, right hand
  M25.442 Effusion, left hand
  M25.449 Effusion, unspecified hand

✓6ᵗʰ **M25.45 Effusion,** hip
  M25.451 Effusion, right hip
  M25.452 Effusion, left hip
  M25.459 Effusion, unspecified hip

✓6ᵗʰ **M25.46 Effusion,** knee
  M25.461 Effusion, right knee
  M25.462 Effusion, left knee
  M25.469 Effusion, unspecified knee

✓6ᵗʰ **M25.47 Effusion,** ankle and foot
  M25.471 Effusion, right ankle
  M25.472 Effusion, left ankle
  M25.473 Effusion, unspecified ankle
  M25.474 Effusion, right foot
  M25.475 Effusion, left foot
  M25.476 Effusion, unspecified foot

M25.48 Effusion, other site

✓5ᵗʰ **M25.5 Pain in joint**
  EXCLUDES 2 pain in hand (M79.64-)
  pain in fingers (M79.64-)
  pain in foot (M79.67-)
  pain in limb (M79.6-)
  pain in toes (M79.67-)

M25.50 Pain in unspecified joint

✓6ᵗʰ **M25.51 Pain in** shoulder
  M25.511 Pain in right shoulder
  M25.512 Pain in left shoulder
  M25.519 Pain in unspecified shoulder

✓6ᵗʰ **M25.52 Pain in** elbow
  M25.521 Pain in right elbow
  M25.522 Pain in left elbow
  M25.529 Pain in unspecified elbow

✓6ᵗʰ **M25.53 Pain in** wrist
  M25.531 Pain in right wrist
  M25.532 Pain in left wrist
  M25.539 Pain in unspecified wrist

✓6ᵗʰ **M25.55 Pain in** hip
  M25.551 Pain in right hip
  M25.552 Pain in left hip
  M25.559 Pain in unspecified hip

✓6ᵗʰ **M25.56 Pain in** knee
  M25.561 Pain in right knee
  M25.562 Pain in left knee
  M25.569 Pain in unspecified knee

✓6ᵗʰ **M25.57 Pain in** ankle and joints of foot
  M25.571 Pain in right ankle and joints of right foot
  M25.572 Pain in left ankle and joints of left foot
  M25.579 Pain in unspecified ankle and joints of unspecified foot

✓5ᵗʰ **M25.6 Stiffness of joint, not elsewhere classified**
  EXCLUDES 1 ankylosis of joint (M24.6-)
  contracture of joint (M24.5-)

M25.60 Stiffness of unspecified joint, not elsewhere classified

✓6ᵗʰ **M25.61 Stiffness of** shoulder, not elsewhere classified
  M25.611 Stiffness of right shoulder, not elsewhere classified
  M25.612 Stiffness of left shoulder, not elsewhere classified
  M25.619 Stiffness of unspecified shoulder, not elsewhere classified

✓6ᵗʰ **M25.62 Stiffness of** elbow, not elsewhere classified
  M25.621 Stiffness of right elbow, not elsewhere classified
  M25.622 Stiffness of left elbow, not elsewhere classified
  M25.629 Stiffness of unspecified elbow, not elsewhere classified

✓6ᵗʰ **M25.63 Stiffness of** wrist, not elsewhere classified
  M25.631 Stiffness of right wrist, not elsewhere classified
  M25.632 Stiffness of left wrist, not elsewhere classified
  M25.639 Stiffness of unspecified wrist, not elsewhere classified

✓6ᵗʰ **M25.64 Stiffness of** hand, not elsewhere classified
  M25.641 Stiffness of right hand, not elsewhere classified
  M25.642 Stiffness of left hand, not elsewhere classified
  M25.649 Stiffness of unspecified hand, not elsewhere classified

✓6ᵗʰ **M25.65 Stiffness of** hip, not elsewhere classified
  M25.651 Stiffness of right hip, not elsewhere classified
  M25.652 Stiffness of left hip, not elsewhere classified
  M25.659 Stiffness of unspecified hip, not elsewhere classified

✓6ᵗʰ **M25.66 Stiffness of** knee, not elsewhere classified
  M25.661 Stiffness of right knee, not elsewhere classified
  M25.662 Stiffness of left knee, not elsewhere classified
  M25.669 Stiffness of unspecified knee, not elsewhere classified

✓6ᵗʰ **M25.67 Stiffness of** ankle and foot, not elsewhere classified
  M25.671 Stiffness of right ankle, not elsewhere classified
  M25.672 Stiffness of left ankle, not elsewhere classified
  M25.673 Stiffness of unspecified ankle, not elsewhere classified
  M25.674 Stiffness of right foot, not elsewhere classified
  M25.675 Stiffness of left foot, not elsewhere classified
  M25.676 Stiffness of unspecified foot, not elsewhere classified

✓5ᵗʰ **M25.7 Osteophyte**
  M25.70 Osteophyte, unspecified joint

✓6ᵗʰ **M25.71 Osteophyte,** shoulder
  M25.711 Osteophyte, right shoulder
  M25.712 Osteophyte, left shoulder
  M25.719 Osteophyte, unspecified shoulder

✓6ᵗʰ **M25.72 Osteophyte,** elbow
  M25.721 Osteophyte, right elbow
  M25.722 Osteophyte, left elbow
  M25.729 Osteophyte, unspecified elbow

✓6ᵗʰ **M25.73 Osteophyte,** wrist
  M25.731 Osteophyte, right wrist
  M25.732 Osteophyte, left wrist
  M25.739 Osteophyte, unspecified wrist

✓6ᵗʰ **M25.74 Osteophyte,** hand
  M25.741 Osteophyte, right hand
  M25.742 Osteophyte, left hand
  M25.749 Osteophyte, unspecified hand

✓6ᵗʰ **M25.75 Osteophyte,** hip
  M25.751 Osteophyte, right hip
  M25.752 Osteophyte, left hip
  M25.759 Osteophyte, unspecified hip

✓6ᵗʰ **M25.76 Osteophyte,** knee
  M25.761 Osteophyte, right knee
  M25.762 Osteophyte, left knee
  M25.769 Osteophyte, unspecified knee

✓6ᵗʰ **M25.77 Osteophyte,** ankle and foot
  M25.771 Osteophyte, right ankle
  M25.772 Osteophyte, left ankle
  M25.773 Osteophyte, unspecified ankle
  M25.774 Osteophyte, right foot
  M25.775 Osteophyte, left foot
  M25.776 Osteophyte, unspecified foot

EXCLUDES 1 Not coded here   **EXCLUDES 2** Not included here   N Newborn Age: 0   P Pediatric Age: 0-17   M Maternity Age: 12-55   A Adult Age: 15-124

674   ICD-10-CM 2014 (Draft)

M25.78 **Osteophyte**, vertebrae

√5th M25.8 **Other specified joint disorders**

　　M25.80 **Other specified joint disorders, unspecified joint**

　√6th M25.81 **Other specified joint disorders**, shoulder

　　　M25.811 **Other specified joint disorders**, right shoulder

　　　M25.812 **Other specified joint disorders**, left shoulder

　　　M25.819 **Other specified joint disorders, unspecified shoulder**

　√6th M25.82 **Other specified joint disorders**, elbow

　　　M25.821 **Other specified joint disorders**, right elbow

　　　M25.822 **Other specified joint disorders**, left elbow

　　　M25.829 **Other specified joint disorders, unspecified elbow**

　√6th M25.83 **Other specified joint disorders**, wrist

　　　M25.831 **Other specified joint disorders**, right wrist

　　　M25.832 **Other specified joint disorders**, left wrist

　　　M25.839 **Other specified joint disorders, unspecifiedwrist**

　√6th M25.84 **Other specified joint disorders**, hand

　　　M25.841 **Other specified joint disorders**, right hand

　　　M25.842 **Other specified joint disorders**, left hand

　　　M25.849 **Other specified joint disorders, unspecified hand**

　√6th M25.85 **Other specified joint disorders**, hip

　　　M25.851 **Other specified joint disorders**, right hip

　　　M25.852 **Other specified joint disorders**, left hip

　　　M25.859 **Other specified joint disorders, unspecified hip**

　√6th M25.86 **Other specified joint disorders**, knee

　　　M25.861 **Other specified joint disorders**, right knee

　　　M25.862 **Other specified joint disorders**, left knee

　　　M25.869 **Other specified joint disorders, unspecified knee**

　√6th M25.87 **Other specified joint disorders**, ankle and foot

　　　M25.871 **Other specified joint disorders**, right ankle and foot

　　　M25.872 **Other specified joint disorders**, left ankle and foot

　　　M25.879 **Other specified joint disorders, unspecified ankle and foot**

M25.9 **Joint disorder, unspecified**

Dentofacial anomalies [including malocclusion] and other disorders of jaw (M26-M27)

EXCLUDES 1 *hemifacial atrophy or hypertrophy (Q67.4)*
unilateral condylar hyperplasia or hypoplasia (M27.8)

√4th **M26 Dentofacial anomalies [including malocclusion]**

　√5th M26.0 **Major anomalies of jaw size**

　　EXCLUDES 1 *acromegaly (E22.0)*
　　　Robin's syndrome (Q87.0)

　　M26.00 **Unspecified anomaly of jaw size**

　　M26.01 **Maxillary hyperplasia**

　　M26.02 **Maxillary hypoplasia**

　　M26.03 **Mandibular hyperplasia**

　　M26.04 **Mandibular hypoplasia**

　　M26.05 **Macrogenia**

　　M26.06 **Microgenia**

　　M26.07 **Excessive tuberosity of jaw**
　　　Entire maxillary tuberosity

　　M26.09 **Other specified anomalies of jaw size**

　√5th M26.1 **Anomalies of jaw-cranial base relationship**

　　M26.10 **Unspecified anomaly of jaw-cranial base relationship**

　　M26.11 **Maxillary asymmetry**

　　M26.12 **Other jaw asymmetry**

　　M26.19 **Other specified anomalies of jaw-cranial base relationship**

　√5th M26.2 **Anomalies of dental arch relationship**

　　M26.20 **Unspecified anomaly of dental arch relationship**

　√6th M26.21 **Malocclusion, Angle's class**

　　M26.211 **Malocclusion, Angle's class I**
　　　Neutro-occlusion

　　M26.212 **Malocclusion, Angle's class II**
　　　Disto-occlusion Division I
　　　Disto-occlusion Division II

　　M26.213 **Malocclusion, Angle's class III**
　　　Mesio-occlusion

　　M26.219 **Malocclusion, Angle's class, unspecified**

　√6th M26.22 **Open occlusal relationship**

　　M26.220 **Open** anterior **occlusal relationship**
　　　Anterior openbite

　　M26.221 **Open** posterior **occlusal relationship**
　　　Posterior openbite

　M26.23 **Excessive horizontal overlap**
　　Excessive horizontal overjet

　M26.24 **Reverse articulation**
　　Crossbite (anterior) (posterior)

　M26.25 **Anomalies of interarch distance**

　M26.29 **Other anomalies of dental arch relationship**
　　Midline deviation of dental arch
　　Overbite (excessive) deep
　　Overbite (excessive) horizontal
　　Overbite (excessive) vertical
　　Posterior lingual occlusion of mandibular teeth

√5th M26.3 **Anomalies of tooth position of fully erupted tooth or teeth**
　EXCLUDES 2 *embedded and impacted teeth (K01.-)*

　M26.30 **Unspecified anomaly of tooth position of fully erupted tooth or teeth**
　　Abnormal spacing of fully erupted tooth or teeth NOS
　　Displacement of fully erupted tooth or teeth NOS
　　Transposition of fully erupted tooth or teeth NOS

　M26.31 **Crowding of fully erupted teeth**

　M26.32 **Excessive spacing of fully erupted teeth**
　　Diastema of fully erupted tooth or teeth NOS

　M26.33 **Horizontal displacement of fully erupted tooth or teeth**
　　Tipped tooth or teeth
　　Tipping of fully erupted tooth

　M26.34 **Vertical displacement of fully erupted tooth or teeth**
　　Extruded tooth
　　Infraeruption of tooth or teeth
　　Supraeruption of tooth or teeth

　M26.35 **Rotation of fully erupted tooth or teeth**

　M26.36 **Insufficient interocclusal distance of fully erupted teeth (ridge)**
　　Lack of adequate intermaxillary vertical dimension of fully erupted teeth

　M26.37 **Excessive interocclusal distance of fully erupted teeth**
　　Excessive intermaxillary vertical dimension of fully erupted teeth
　　Loss of occlusal vertical dimension of fully erupted teeth

　M26.39 **Other anomalies of tooth position of fully erupted tooth or teeth**

M26.4 **Malocclusion, unspecified**

√5th M26.5 **Dentofacial functional abnormalities**
　EXCLUDES 1 *bruxism (F45.8)*
　　teeth-grinding NOS (F45.8)

　M26.50 **Dentofacial functional abnormalities, unspecified**

　M26.51 **Abnormal jaw closure**

　M26.52 **Limited mandibular range of motion**

　M26.53 **Deviation in opening and closing of the mandible**

　M26.54 **Insufficient anterior guidance**
　　Insufficient anterior occlusal guidance

　M26.55 **Centric occlusion maximum intercuspation discrepancy**
　　EXCLUDES 1 *centric occlusion NOS (M26.59)*

　M26.56 **Non-working side interference**
　　Balancing side interference

　M26.57 **Lack of posterior occlusal support**

　M26.59 **Other dentofacial functional abnormalities**
　　Centric occlusion (of teeth) NOS
　　Malocclusion due to abnormal swallowing
　　Malocclusion due to mouth breathing
　　Malocclusion due to tongue, lip or finger habits

Diseases of the Musculoskeletal System and Connective Tissue

M26.6–M32.0

✓5ᵗʰ **M26.6 Temporomandibular joint disorders**
> EXCLUDES 2   *current temporomandibular joint dislocation (S03.0)*
> *current temporomandibular joint sprain (S03.4)*

M26.60 Temporomandibular joint disorder, unspecified

M26.61 Adhesions and ankylosis of temporomandibular joint

M26.62 Arthralgia of temporomandibular joint

M26.63 Articular disc disorder of temporomandibular joint

M26.69 Other specified disorders of temporomandibular joint

✓5ᵗʰ **M26.7 Dental alveolar anomalies**

M26.70 Unspecified alveolar anomaly

M26.71 Alveolar maxillary hyperplasia

M26.72 Alveolar mandibular hyperplasia

M26.73 Alveolar maxillary hypoplasia

M26.74 Alveolar mandibular hypoplasia

M26.79 Other specified alveolar anomalies

✓5ᵗʰ **M26.8 Other dentofacial anomalies**

M26.81 Anterior soft tissue impingement
Anterior soft tissue impingement on teeth

M26.82 Posterior soft tissue impingement
Posterior soft tissue impingement on teeth

M26.89 Other dentofacial anomalies

M26.9 Dentofacial anomaly, unspecified

✓4ᵗʰ **M27 Other diseases of jaws**

M27.0 Developmental disorders of jaws
Latent bone cyst of jaw   Torus mandibularis
Stafne's cyst   Torus palatinus

M27.1 Giant cell granuloma, central
Giant cell granuloma NOS
> EXCLUDES 1   *peripheral giant cell granuloma (K06.8)*

M27.2 Inflammatory conditions of jaws
Osteitis of jaw(s)   Periostitis jaw(s)
Osteomyelitis (neonatal) jaw(s)   Sequestrum of jaw bone
Osteoradionecrosis jaw(s)
Use additional code (W88-W90, X39.0) to identify radiation, if radiation-induced
> EXCLUDES 2   *osteonecrosis of jaw due to drug (M87.180)*

M27.3 Alveolitis of jaws
Alveolar osteitis
Dry socket

✓5ᵗʰ **M27.4 Other and unspecified cysts of jaw**
> EXCLUDES 1   *cysts of oral region (K09.-)*
> *latent bone cyst of jaw (M27.0)*
> *Stafne's cyst (M27.0)*

M27.40 Unspecified cyst of jaw
Cyst of jaw NOS

M27.49 Other cysts of jaw
Aneurysmal cyst of jaw
Hemorrhagic cyst of jaw
Traumatic cyst of jaw

✓5ᵗʰ **M27.5 Periradicular pathology associated with previous endodontic treatment**

M27.51 Perforation of root canal space due to endodontic treatment

M27.52 Endodontic overfill

M27.53 Endodontic underfill

M27.59 Other periradicular pathology associated with previous endodontic treatment

✓5ᵗʰ **M27.6 Endosseous dental implant failure**

M27.61 Osseointegration failure of dental implant
Hemorrhagic complications of dental implant placement
Iatrogenic osseointegration failure of dental implant
Osseointegration failure of dental implant due to complications of systemic disease
Osseointegration failure of dental implant due to poor bone quality
Pre-integration failure of dental implant NOS
Pre-osseointegration failure of dental implant

M27.62 Post-osseointegration biological failure of dental implant
Failure of dental implant due to lack of attached gingiva
Failure of dental implant due to occlusal trauma (caused by poor prosthetic design)
Failure of dental implant due to parafunctional habits
Failure of dental implant due to periodontal infection (peri-implantitis)
Failure of dental implant due to poor oral hygiene
Iatrogenic post-osseointegration failure of dental implant
Post-osseointegration failure of dental implant due to complications of systemic disease

M27.63 Post-osseointegration mechanical failure of dental implant
Failure of dental prosthesis causing loss of dental implant
Fracture of dental implant
> EXCLUDES 2   *cracked tooth (K03.81)*
> *fractured dental restorative material with loss of material (K08.531)*
> *fractured dental restorative material without loss of material (K08.530)*
> *fractured tooth (S02.5)*

M27.69 Other endosseous dental implant failure
Dental implant failure NOS

M27.8 Other specified diseases of jaws
Cherubism   Unilateral condylar hyperplasia
Exostosis   Unilateral condylar hypoplasia
Fibrous dysplasia
> EXCLUDES 1   *jaw pain (R68.84)*

M27.9 Disease of jaws, unspecified

Systemic connective tissue disorders (M30-M36)

> INCLUDES   autoimmune disease NOS
> collagen (vascular) disease NOS
> systemic autoimmune disease
> systemic collagen (vascular) disease
> EXCLUDES 1   *autoimmune disease, single organ or single cell-type—code to relevant condition category*

✓4ᵗʰ **M30 Polyarteritis nodosa and related conditions**
> EXCLUDES 1   *microscopic polyarteritis (M31.7)*

M30.0 Polyarteritis nodosa

M30.1 Polyarteritis with lung involvement [Churg-Strauss]
Allergic granulomatous angiitis

M30.2 Juvenile polyarteritis

M30.3 Mucocutaneous lymph node syndrome [Kawasaki]

M30.8 Other conditions related to polyarteritis nodosa
Polyangiitis overlap syndrome

✓4ᵗʰ **M31 Other necrotizing vasculopathies**

M31.0 Hypersensitivity angiitis
Goodpasture's syndrome

M31.1 Thrombotic microangiopathy
Thrombotic thrombocytopenic purpura

M31.2 Lethal midline granuloma

✓5ᵗʰ **M31.3 Wegener's granulomatosis**
Necrotizing respiratory granulomatosis

M31.30 Wegener's granulomatosis without renal involvement
Wegener's granulomatosis NOS

M31.31 Wegener's granulomatosis with renal involvement

M31.4 Aortic arch syndrome [Takayasu]

M31.5 Giant cell arteritis with polymyalgia rheumatica

M31.6 Other giant cell arteritis

M31.7 Microscopic polyangiitis
Microscopic polyarteritis
> EXCLUDES 1   *polyarteritis nodosa (M30.0)*

M31.8 Other specified necrotizing vasculopathies
Hypocomplementemic vasculitis
Septic vasculitis

M31.9 Necrotizing vasculopathy, unspecified

✓4ᵗʰ **M32 Systemic lupus erythematosus (SLE)**
> EXCLUDES 1   *lupus erythematosus (discoid) (NOS) (L93.0)*

M32.0 Drug-induced systemic lupus erythematosus
Use additional code for adverse effect, if applicable, to identify drug (T36-T50 with fifth or sixth character 5)

EXCLUDES 1 Not coded here   EXCLUDES 2 Not included here   N Newborn Age: 0   P Pediatric Age: 0-17   M Maternity Age: 12-55   A Adult Age: 15-124

676   ICD-10-CM 2014 (Draft)

✓5th **M32.1 Systemic lupus erythematosus** with organ or system involvement

    M32.10 Systemic lupus erythematosus, organ or system involvement unspecified

    M32.11 Endocarditis in systemic lupus erythematosus
        Libman-Sacks disease

    M32.12 Pericarditis in systemic lupus erythematosus
        Lupus pericarditis

    M32.13 Lung involvement in systemic lupus erythematosus
        Pleural effusion due to systemic lupus erythematosus

    M32.14 Glomerular disease in systemic lupus erythematosus
        Lupus renal disease NOS

    M32.15 Tubulo-interstitial nephropathy in systemic lupus erythematosus

    M32.19 Other organ or system involvement in systemic lupus erythematosus

  M32.8 Other forms of systemic lupus erythematosus

  M32.9 Systemic lupus erythematosus, unspecified
    SLE NOS
    Systemic lupus erythematosus NOS
    Systemic lupus erythematosus without organ involvement

✓4th **M33 Dermatopolymyositis**

  ✓5th **M33.0 Juvenile dermatopolymyositis**

    M33.00 Juvenile dermatopolymyositis, organ involvement unspecified

    M33.01 Juvenile dermatopolymyositis with respiratory involvement

    M33.02 Juvenile dermatopolymyositis with myopathy

    M33.09 Juvenile dermatopolymyositis with other organ involvement

  ✓5th **M33.1 Other dermatopolymyositis**

    M33.10 Other dermatopolymyositis, organ involvement unspecified

    M33.11 Other dermatopolymyositis with respiratory involvement

    M33.12 Other dermatopolymyositis with myopathy

    M33.19 Other dermatopolymyositis with other organ involvement

  ✓5th **M33.2 Polymyositis**

    M33.20 Polymyositis, organ involvement unspecified

    M33.21 Polymyositis with respiratory involvement

    M33.22 Polymyositis with myopathy

    M33.29 Polymyositis with other organ involvement

  ✓5th **M33.9 Dermatopolymyositis, unspecified**

    M33.90 Dermatopolymyositis, unspecified, organ involvement unspecified

    M33.91 Dermatopolymyositis, unspecified with respiratory involvement

    M33.92 Dermatopolymyositis, unspecified with myopathy

    M33.99 Dermatopolymyositis, unspecified with other organ involvement

✓4th **M34 Systemic sclerosis [scleroderma]**
  EXCLUDES 1 circumscribed scleroderma (L94.0)
          neonatal scleroderma (P83.8)

  M34.0 Progressive systemic sclerosis

  M34.1 CR(E)ST syndrome
    Combination of calcinosis, Raynaud's phenomenon, esophageal dysfunction, sclerodactyly, telangiectasia

  M34.2 Systemic sclerosis induced by drug and chemical
    Code first poisoning due to drug or toxin, if applicable (T36-T65 with fifth or sixth character 1-4 or 6)
    Use additional code for adverse effect, if applicable, to identify drug (T36-T50 with fifth or sixth character 5)

  ✓5th **M34.8 Other forms of systemic sclerosis**

    M34.81 Systemic sclerosis with lung involvement

    M34.82 Systemic sclerosis with myopathy

    M34.83 Systemic sclerosis with polyneuropathy

    M34.89 Other systemic sclerosis

  M34.9 Systemic sclerosis, unspecified

✓4th **M35 Other systemic involvement of connective tissue**
  EXCLUDES 1 reactive perforating collagenosis (L87.1)

  ✓5th **M35.0 Sicca syndrome [Sjögren]**

    M35.00 Sicca syndrome, unspecified

    M35.01 Sicca syndrome with keratoconjunctivitis

    M35.02 Sicca syndrome with lung involvement

    M35.03 Sicca syndrome with myopathy

    M35.04 Sicca syndrome with tubulo-interstitial nephropathy
        Renal tubular acidosis in sicca syndrome

    M35.09 Sicca syndrome with other organ involvement

  M35.1 Other overlap syndromes
    Mixed connective tissue disease
    EXCLUDES 1 polyangiitis overlap syndrome (M30.8)

  M35.2 Behçet's disease

  M35.3 Polymyalgia rheumatica
    EXCLUDES 1 polymyalgia rheumatica with giant cell arteritis (M31.5)

  M35.4 Diffuse (eosinophilic) fasciitis

  M35.5 Multifocal fibrosclerosis

  M35.6 Relapsing panniculitis [Weber-Christian]
    EXCLUDES 1 lupus panniculitis (L93.2)
          panniculitis NOS (M79.3-)

  M35.7 Hypermobility syndrome
    Familial ligamentous laxity
    EXCLUDES 1 Ehlers-Danlos syndrome (Q79.6)
          ligamentous laxity, NOS (M24.2-)

  M35.8 Other specified systemic involvement of connective tissue

  M35.9 Systemic involvement of connective tissue, unspecified
    Autoimmune disease (systemic) NOS
    Collagen (vascular) disease NOS

✓4th **M36 Systemic disorders of connective tissue in diseases classified elsewhere**
  EXCLUDES 2 arthropathies in diseases classified elsewhere (M14.-)

  M36.0 Dermato(poly)myositis in neoplastic disease
    Code first underlying neoplasm (C00-D49)

  M36.1 Arthropathy in neoplastic disease
    Code first underlying neoplasm, such as:
      leukemia (C91-C95)
      malignant histiocytosis (C96.A)
      multiple myeloma (C90.0)

  M36.2 Hemophilic arthropathy
    Hemarthrosis in hemophilic arthropathy
    Code first underlying disease, such as:
      factor VIII deficiency (D66)
      with vascular defect (D68.0)
      factor IX deficiency (D67)
      hemophilia (classical) (D66)
      hemophilia B (D67)
      hemophilia C (D68.1)

  M36.3 Arthropathy in other blood disorders

  M36.4 Arthropathy in hypersensitivity reactions classified elsewhere
    Code first underlying disease, such as:
      Henoch (-Schönlein) purpura (D69.0)
      serum sickness (T80.6-)

  M36.8 Systemic disorders of connective tissue in other diseases classified elsewhere
    Code first underlying disease, such as:
      alkaptonuria (E70.2)
      hypogammaglobulinemia (D80.-)
      ochronosis (E70.2)

DORSOPATHIES (M40-M54)

Deforming dorsopathies (M40-M43)

✓4th **M40 Kyphosis and lordosis**
  EXCLUDES 1 congenital kyphosis and lordosis (Q76.4)
          kyphoscoliosis (M41.-)
          postprocedural kyphosis and lordosis (M96.-)

  ✓5th **M40.0 Postural kyphosis**
    EXCLUDES 1 osteochondrosis of spine (M42.-)

    M40.00 Postural kyphosis, site unspecified

    M40.03 Postural kyphosis, cervicothoracic region

    M40.04 Postural kyphosis, thoracic region

    M40.05 Postural kyphosis, thoracolumbar region

  ✓5th **M40.1 Other secondary kyphosis**

    M40.10 Other secondary kyphosis, site unspecified

    M40.12 Other secondary kyphosis, cervical region

    M40.13 Other secondary kyphosis, cervicothoracic region

    M40.14 Other secondary kyphosis, thoracic region

    M40.15 Other secondary kyphosis, thoracolumbar region

✓ Additional Character Required   ✓x7th Xtension Alert   Unspecified Code   Other Specified Code   Manifestation Code   ►◄ Revised Text   ● New Code   ▲ Revised Code Title

✓5th **M40.2 Other and unspecified kyphosis**

   ✓6th **M40.20** Unspecified kyphosis
- M40.202 **Unspecified kyphosis, cervical region**
- M40.203 **Unspecified kyphosis, cervicothoracic region**
- M40.204 **Unspecified kyphosis, thoracic region**
- M40.205 **Unspecified kyphosis, thoracolumbar region**
- M40.209 **Unspecified kyphosis, site unspecified**

   ✓6th **M40.29** Other kyphosis
- M40.292 **Other kyphosis, cervical region**
- M40.293 **Other kyphosis, cervicothoracic region**
- M40.294 **Other kyphosis, thoracic region**
- M40.295 **Other kyphosis, thoracolumbar region**
- M40.299 **Other kyphosis, site unspecified**

✓5th **M40.3 Flatback syndrome**
- M40.30 **Flatback syndrome, site unspecified**
- M40.35 **Flatback syndrome, thoracolumbar region**
- M40.36 **Flatback syndrome, lumbar region**
- M40.37 **Flatback syndrome, lumbosacral region**

✓5th **M40.4 Postural lordosis**
   Acquired lordosis
- M40.40 **Postural lordosis, site unspecified**
- M40.45 **Postural lordosis, thoracolumbar region**
- M40.46 **Postural lordosis, lumbar region**
- M40.47 **Postural lordosis, lumbosacral region**

✓5th **M40.5 Lordosis, unspecified**
- M40.50 **Lordosis, unspecified, site unspecified**
- M40.55 **Lordosis, unspecified, thoracolumbar region**
- M40.56 **Lordosis, unspecified, lumbar region**
- M40.57 **Lordosis, unspecified, lumbosacral region**

✓4th **M41 Scoliosis**
   INCLUDES kyphoscoliosis
   EXCLUDES 1 congenital scoliosis NOS (Q67.5)
      congenital scoliosis due to bony malformation (Q76.3)
      kyphoscoliotic heart disease (I27.1)
      postprocedural scoliosis (M96.-)
      postural congenital scoliosis (Q67.5)

✓5th **M41.0 Infantile idiopathic scoliosis**
- M41.00 **Infantile idiopathic scoliosis, site unspecified**
- M41.02 **Infantile idiopathic scoliosis, cervical region**
- M41.03 **Infantile idiopathic scoliosis, cervicothoracic region**
- M41.04 **Infantile idiopathic scoliosis, thoracic region**
- M41.05 **Infantile idiopathic scoliosis, thoracolumbar region**
- M41.06 **Infantile idiopathic scoliosis, lumbar region**
- M41.07 **Infantile idiopathic scoliosis, lumbosacral region**
- M41.08 **Infantile idiopathic scoliosis, sacral and sacrococcygeal region**

✓5th **M41.1 Juvenile and adolescent idiopathic scoliosis**

   ✓6th **M41.11** Juvenile idiopathic scoliosis
- M41.112 **Juvenile idiopathic scoliosis, cervical region**
- M41.113 **Juvenile idiopathic scoliosis, cervicothoracic region**
- M41.114 **Juvenile idiopathic scoliosis, thoracic region**
- M41.115 **Juvenile idiopathic scoliosis, thoracolumbar region**
- M41.116 **Juvenile idiopathic scoliosis, lumbar region**
- M41.117 **Juvenile idiopathic scoliosis, lumbosacral region**
- M41.119 **Juvenile idiopathic scoliosis, site unspecified**

   ✓6th **M41.12** Adolescent scoliosis
- M41.122 **Adolescent idiopathic scoliosis, cervical region**
- M41.123 **Adolescent idiopathic scoliosis, cervicothoracic region**
- M41.124 **Adolescent idiopathic scoliosis, thoracic region**
- M41.125 **Adolescent idiopathic scoliosis, thoracolumbar region**
- M41.126 **Adolescent idiopathic scoliosis, lumbar region**
- M41.127 **Adolescent idiopathic scoliosis, lumbosacral region**
- M41.129 **Adolescent idiopathic scoliosis, site unspecified**

✓5th **M41.2 Other idiopathic scoliosis**
- M41.20 **Other idiopathic scoliosis, site unspecified**
- M41.22 **Other idiopathic scoliosis, cervical region**
- M41.23 **Other idiopathic scoliosis, cervicothoracic region**
- M41.24 **Other idiopathic scoliosis, thoracic region**
- M41.25 **Other idiopathic scoliosis, thoracolumbar region**
- M41.26 **Other idiopathic scoliosis, lumbar region**
- M41.27 **Other idiopathic scoliosis, lumbosacral region**

✓5th **M41.3 Thoracogenic scoliosis**
- M41.30 **Thoracogenic scoliosis, site unspecified**
- M41.34 **Thoracogenic scoliosis, thoracic region**
- M41.35 **Thoracogenic scoliosis, thoracolumbar region**

✓5th **M41.4 Neuromuscular scoliosis**
   Scoliosis secondary to cerebral palsy, Friedreich's ataxia, poliomyelitis and other neuromuscular disorders
   Code also underlying condition
- M41.40 **Neuromuscular scoliosis, site unspecified**
- M41.41 **Neuromuscular scoliosis, occipito-atlanto-axial region**
- M41.42 **Neuromuscular scoliosis, cervical region**
- M41.43 **Neuromuscular scoliosis, cervicothoracic region**
- M41.44 **Neuromuscular scoliosis, thoracic region**
- M41.45 **Neuromuscular scoliosis, thoracolumbar region**
- M41.46 **Neuromuscular scoliosis, lumbar region**
- M41.47 **Neuromuscular scoliosis, lumbosacral region**

✓5th **M41.5 Other secondary scoliosis**
- M41.50 **Other secondary scoliosis, site unspecified**
- M41.52 **Other secondary scoliosis, cervical region**
- M41.53 **Other secondary scoliosis, cervicothoracic region**
- M41.54 **Other secondary scoliosis, thoracic region**
- M41.55 **Other secondary scoliosis, thoracolumbar region**
- M41.56 **Other secondary scoliosis, lumbar region**
- M41.57 **Other secondary scoliosis, lumbosacral region**

✓5th **M41.8 Other forms of scoliosis**
- M41.80 **Other forms of scoliosis, site unspecified**
- M41.82 **Other forms of scoliosis, cervical region**
- M41.83 **Other forms of scoliosis, cervicothoracic region**
- M41.84 **Other forms of scoliosis, thoracic region**
- M41.85 **Other forms of scoliosis, thoracolumbar region**
- M41.86 **Other forms of scoliosis, lumbar region**
- M41.87 **Other forms of scoliosis, lumbosacral region**

- M41.9 **Scoliosis, unspecified**

✓4th **M42 Spinal osteochondrosis**

✓5th **M42.0 Juvenile osteochondrosis of spine**
   Calvé's disease
   Scheuermann's disease
   EXCLUDES 1 postural kyphosis (M40.0)
- M42.00 **Juvenile osteochondrosis of spine, site unspecified**
- M42.01 **Juvenile osteochondrosis of spine, occipito-atlanto-axial region**
- M42.02 **Juvenile osteochondrosis of spine, cervical region**
- M42.03 **Juvenile osteochondrosis of spine, cervicothoracic region**
- M42.04 **Juvenile osteochondrosis of spine, thoracic region**
- M42.05 **Juvenile osteochondrosis of spine, thoracolumbar region**
- M42.06 **Juvenile osteochondrosis of spine, lumbar region**
- M42.07 **Juvenile osteochondrosis of spine, lumbosacral region**
- M42.08 **Juvenile osteochondrosis of spine, sacral and sacrococcygeal region**
- M42.09 **Juvenile osteochondrosis of spine, multiple sites in spine**

✓5th **M42.1 Adult osteochondrosis of spine**
- M42.10 **Adult osteochondrosis of spine, site unspecified** A

EXCLUDES 1 Not coded here   EXCLUDES 2 Not included here   N Newborn Age: 0   P Pediatric Age: 0-17   M Maternity Age: 12-55   A Adult Age: 15-124

M42.11 **Adult osteochondrosis of spine, occipito-atlanto-axial region** △

M42.12 **Adult osteochondrosis of spine, cervical region** △

M42.13 **Adult osteochondrosis of spine, cervicothoracic region** △

M42.14 **Adult osteochondrosis of spine, thoracic region** △

M42.15 **Adult osteochondrosis of spine, thoracolumbar region** △

M42.16 **Adult osteochondrosis of spine, lumbar region** △

M42.17 **Adult osteochondrosis of spine, lumbosacral region** △

M42.18 **Adult osteochondrosis of spine, sacral and sacrococcygeal region** △

M42.19 **Adult osteochondrosis of spine, multiple sites in spine** △

M42.9 **Spinal osteochondrosis, unspecified**

☑4ᵗʰ **M43 Other deforming dorsopathies**

    EXCLUDES 1   *congenital spondylolysis and spondylolisthesis (Q76.2)*
      hemivertebra (Q76.3-Q76.4)
      Klippel-Feil syndrome (Q76.1)
      lumbarization and sacralization (Q76.4)
      platyspondylisis (Q76.4)
      spina bifida occulta (Q76.0)
      spinal curvature in osteoporosis (M80.-)
      spinal curvature in Paget's disease of bone [osteitis deformans] (M88.-)

☑5ᵗʰ **M43.0 Spondylolysis**

    EXCLUDES 1   *congenital spondylolysis (Q76.2)*
      spondylolisthesis (M43.1)

    M43.00 **Spondylolysis, site unspecified**

    M43.01 **Spondylolysis, occipito-atlanto-axial region**

    M43.02 **Spondylolysis, cervical region**

    M43.03 **Spondylolysis, cervicothoracic region**

    M43.04 **Spondylolysis, thoracic region**

    M43.05 **Spondylolysis, thoracolumbar region**

    M43.06 **Spondylolysis, lumbar region**

    M43.07 **Spondylolysis, lumbosacral region**

    M43.08 **Spondylolysis, sacral and sacrococcygeal region**

    M43.09 **Spondylolysis, multiple sites in spine**

☑5ᵗʰ **M43.1 Spondylolisthesis**

    EXCLUDES 1   *acute traumatic of lumbosacral region (S33.1)*
      acute traumatic of sites other than lumbosacral— code to Fracture, vertebra, by region
      congenital spondylolisthesis (Q76.2)

    M43.10 **Spondylolisthesis, site unspecified**

    M43.11 **Spondylolisthesis, occipito-atlanto-axial region**

    M43.12 **Spondylolisthesis, cervical region**

    M43.13 **Spondylolisthesis, cervicothoracic region**

    M43.14 **Spondylolisthesis, thoracic region**

    M43.15 **Spondylolisthesis, thoracolumbar region**

    M43.16 **Spondylolisthesis, lumbar region**

    M43.17 **Spondylolisthesis, lumbosacral region**

    M43.18 **Spondylolisthesis, sacral and sacrococcygeal region**

    M43.19 **Spondylolisthesis, multiple sites in spine**

☑5ᵗʰ **M43.2 Fusion of spine**

    Ankylosis of spinal joint

    EXCLUDES 1   *ankylosing spondylitis (M45.0-)*
      congenital fusion of spine (Q76.4)

    EXCLUDES 2   *arthrodesis status (Z98.1)*
      pseudoarthrosis after fusion or arthrodesis (M96.0)

    M43.20 **Fusion of spine, site unspecified**

    M43.21 **Fusion of spine, occipito-atlanto-axial region**

    M43.22 **Fusion of spine, cervical region**

    M43.23 **Fusion of spine, cervicothoracic region**

    M43.24 **Fusion of spine, thoracic region**

    M43.25 **Fusion of spine, thoracolumbar region**

    M43.26 **Fusion of spine, lumbar region**

    M43.27 **Fusion of spine, lumbosacral region**

    M43.28 **Fusion of spine, sacral and sacrococcygeal region**

M43.3 **Recurrent atlantoaxial dislocation with myelopathy**

M43.4 **Other recurrent atlantoaxial dislocation**

☑5ᵗʰ **M43.5 Other recurrent vertebral dislocation**

    EXCLUDES 1   *biomechanical lesions NEC (M99.-)*

☑6ᵗʰ **M43.5X Other recurrent vertebral dislocation**

    M43.5X2 **Other recurrent vertebral dislocation, cervical region**

    M43.5X3 **Other recurrent vertebral dislocation, cervicothoracic region**

    M43.5X4 **Other recurrent vertebral dislocation, thoracic region**

    M43.5X5 **Other recurrent vertebral dislocation, thoracolumbar region**

    M43.5X6 **Other recurrent vertebral dislocation, lumbar region**

    M43.5X7 **Other recurrent vertebral dislocation, lumbosacral region**

    M43.5X8 **Other recurrent vertebral dislocation, sacral and sacrococcygeal region**

    M43.5X9 **Other recurrent vertebral dislocation, site unspecified**

M43.6 **Torticollis**

    EXCLUDES 1   *congenital (sternomastoid) torticollis (Q68.0)*
      current injury—see Injury, of spine, by body region
      ocular torticollis (R29.891)
      psychogenic torticollis (F45.8)
      spasmodic torticollis (G24.3)
      torticollis due to birth injury (P15.2)

☑5ᵗʰ **M43.8 Other specified deforming dorsopathies**

    EXCLUDES 2   *kyphosis and lordosis (M40.-)*
      scoliosis (M41.-)

☑6ᵗʰ **M43.8X Other specified deforming dorsopathies**

    M43.8X1 **Other specified deforming dorsopathies, occipito-atlanto-axial region**

    M43.8X2 **Other specified deforming dorsopathies, cervical region**

    M43.8X3 **Other specified deforming dorsopathies, cervicothoracic region**

    M43.8X4 **Other specified deforming dorsopathies, thoracic region**

    M43.8X5 **Other specified deforming dorsopathies, thoracolumbar region**

    M43.8X6 **Other specified deforming dorsopathies, lumbar region**

    M43.8X7 **Other specified deforming dorsopathies, lumbosacral region**

    M43.8X8 **Other specified deforming dorsopathies, sacral and sacrococcygeal region**

    M43.8X9 **Other specified deforming dorsopathies, site unspecified**

M43.9 **Deforming dorsopathy, unspecified**
    Curvature of spine NOS

Spondylopathies (M45-M49)

☑4ᵗʰ **M45 Ankylosing spondylitis**
    Rheumatoid arthritis of spine

    EXCLUDES 1   *arthropathy in Reiter's disease (M02.3-)*
      juvenile (ankylosing) spondylitis (M08.1)

    EXCLUDES 2   *Behçet's disease (M35.2)*

M45.0 **Ankylosing spondylitis of multiple sites in spine**

M45.1 **Ankylosing spondylitis of occipito-atlanto-axial region**

M45.2 **Ankylosing spondylitis of cervical region**

M45.3 **Ankylosing spondylitis of cervicothoracic region**

M45.4 **Ankylosing spondylitis of thoracic region**

M45.5 **Ankylosing spondylitis of thoracolumbar region**

M45.6 **Ankylosing spondylitis lumbar region**

M45.7 **Ankylosing spondylitis of lumbosacral region**

M45.8 **Ankylosing spondylitis sacral and sacrococcygeal region**

M45.9 **Ankylosing spondylitis of unspecified sites in spine**

☑4ᵗʰ **M46 Other inflammatory spondylopathies**

☑5ᵗʰ **M46.0 Spinal enthesopathy**
    Disorder of ligamentous or muscular attachments of spine

    M46.00 **Spinal enthesopathy, site unspecified**

    M46.01 **Spinal enthesopathy, occipito-atlanto-axial region**

    M46.02 **Spinal enthesopathy, cervical region**

    M46.03 **Spinal enthesopathy, cervicothoracic region**

    M46.04 **Spinal enthesopathy, thoracic region**

M46.05	Spinal enthesopathy, **thoracolumbar** region
M46.06	Spinal enthesopathy, **lumbar** region
M46.07	Spinal enthesopathy, **lumbosacral** region
M46.08	Spinal enthesopathy, **sacral and sacrococcygeal region**
M46.09	Spinal enthesopathy, **multiple sites** in spine
M46.1	Sacroiliitis, not elsewhere classified
✓5ᵗʰ M46.2	Osteomyelitis of vertebra
M46.20	**Osteomyelitis of vertebra, site unspecified**
M46.21	Osteomyelitis of vertebra, **occipito-atlanto-axial** region
M46.22	Osteomyelitis of vertebra, **cervical** region
M46.23	Osteomyelitis of vertebra, **cervicothoracic** region
M46.24	Osteomyelitis of vertebra, **thoracic** region
M46.25	Osteomyelitis of vertebra, **thoracolumbar** region
M46.26	Osteomyelitis of vertebra, **lumbar** region
M46.27	Osteomyelitis of vertebra, **lumbosacral** region
M46.28	Osteomyelitis of vertebra, **sacral and sacrococcygeal region**
✓5ᵗʰ M46.3	Infection of intervertebral disc (pyogenic)
Use additional code (B95-B97) to identify infectious agent
M46.30	**Infection of intervertebral disc (pyogenic), site unspecified**
M46.31	Infection of intervertebral disc (pyogenic), **occipito-atlanto-axial** region
M46.32	Infection of intervertebral disc (pyogenic), **cervical** region
M46.33	Infection of intervertebral disc (pyogenic), **cervicothoracic** region
M46.34	Infection of intervertebral disc (pyogenic), **thoracic** region
M46.35	Infection of intervertebral disc (pyogenic), **thoracolumbar** region
M46.36	Infection of intervertebral disc (pyogenic), **lumbar** region
M46.37	Infection of intervertebral disc (pyogenic), **lumbosacral** region
M46.38	Infection of intervertebral disc (pyogenic), **sacral and sacrococcygeal** region
M46.39	Infection of intervertebral disc (pyogenic), **multiple sites** in spine
✓5ᵗʰ M46.4	Discitis, unspecified
M46.40	**Discitis, unspecified, site unspecified**
M46.41	Discitis, unspecified, **occipito-atlanto-axial region**
M46.42	Discitis, unspecified, **cervical region**
M46.43	Discitis, unspecified, **cervicothoracic region**
M46.44	Discitis, unspecified, **thoracic region**
M46.45	Discitis, unspecified, **thoracolumbar region**
M46.46	Discitis, unspecified, **lumbar region**
M46.47	Discitis, unspecified, **lumbosacral region**
M46.48	Discitis, unspecified, **sacral and sacrococcygeal region**
M46.49	Discitis, unspecified, **multiple sites** in spine
✓5ᵗʰ M46.5	Other infective spondylopathies
M46.50	**Other infective spondylopathies, site unspecified**
M46.51	Other infective spondylopathies, **occipito-atlanto-axial region**
M46.52	Other infective spondylopathies, **cervical region**
M46.53	Other infective spondylopathies, **cervicothoracic region**
M46.54	Other infective spondylopathies, **thoracic region**
M46.55	Other infective spondylopathies, **thoracolumbar region**
M46.56	Other infective spondylopathies, **lumbar region**
M46.57	Other infective spondylopathies, **lumbosacral region**
M46.58	Other infective spondylopathies, **sacral and sacrococcygeal region**
M46.59	Other infective spondylopathies, **multiple sites** in spine
✓5ᵗʰ M46.8	Other specified inflammatory spondylopathies
M46.80	**Other specified inflammatory spondylopathies, site unspecified**

M46.81	**Other specified inflammatory spondylopathies, occipito-atlanto-axial region**
M46.82	**Other specified inflammatory spondylopathies, cervical region**
M46.83	**Other specified inflammatory spondylopathies, cervicothoracic region**
M46.84	**Other specified inflammatory spondylopathies, thoracic region**
M46.85	**Other specified inflammatory spondylopathies, thoracolumbar region**
M46.86	**Other specified inflammatory spondylopathies, lumbar region**
M46.87	**Other specified inflammatory spondylopathies, lumbosacral region**
M46.88	**Other specified inflammatory spondylopathies, sacral and sacrococcygeal region**
M46.89	**Other specified inflammatory spondylopathies, multiple sites** in spine
✓5ᵗʰ M46.9	Unspecified inflammatory spondylopathy
M46.90	**Unspecified inflammatory spondylopathy, site unspecified**
M46.91	**Unspecified inflammatory spondylopathy, occipito-atlanto-axial region**
M46.92	**Unspecified inflammatory spondylopathy, cervical region**
M46.93	**Unspecified inflammatory spondylopathy, cervicothoracic region**
M46.94	**Unspecified inflammatory spondylopathy, thoracic region**
M46.95	**Unspecified inflammatory spondylopathy, thoracolumbar region**
M46.96	**Unspecified inflammatory spondylopathy, lumbar region**
M46.97	**Unspecified inflammatory spondylopathy, lumbosacral region**
M46.98	**Unspecified inflammatory spondylopathy, sacral and sacrococcygeal region**
M46.99	**Unspecified inflammatory spondylopathy, multiple sites** in spine
✓4ᵗʰ **M47	Spondylosis**
INCLUDES	arthrosis or osteoarthritis of spine
degeneration of facet joints
✓5ᵗʰ M47.0	Anterior spinal and vertebral artery compression syndromes
✓6ᵗʰ M47.01	Anterior spinal artery compression syndromes
M47.011	Anterior spinal artery compression syndromes, occipito-atlanto-axial region
M47.012	Anterior spinal artery compression syndromes, cervical region
M47.013	Anterior spinal artery compression syndromes, cervicothoracic region
M47.014	Anterior spinal artery compression syndromes, thoracic region
M47.015	Anterior spinal artery compression syndromes, thoracolumbar region
M47.016	Anterior spinal artery compression syndromes, lumbar region
M47.019	**Anterior spinal artery compression syndromes, site unspecified**
✓6ᵗʰ M47.02	Vertebral artery compression syndromes
M47.021	Vertebral artery compression syndromes, occipito-atlanto-axial region
M47.022	Vertebral artery compression syndromes, cervical region
M47.029	**Vertebral artery compression syndromes, site unspecified**
✓5ᵗʰ M47.1	Other spondylosis with myelopathy
Spondylogenic compression of spinal cord
EXCLUDES 1	vertebral subluxation (M43.3-M43.5X9)
M47.10	Other spondylosis with myelopathy, site unspecified
M47.11	Other spondylosis with myelopathy, **occipito-atlanto-axial region**
M47.12	Other spondylosis with myelopathy, **cervical region**
M47.13	Other spondylosis with myelopathy, **cervicothoracic region**
M47.14	Other spondylosis with myelopathy, **thoracic region**

M47.15 **Other spondylosis with myelopathy,** thoracolumbar region

M47.16 **Other spondylosis with myelopathy,** lumbar **region**

√5ᵗʰ M47.2 Other spondylosis with radiculopathy

M47.20 **Other spondylosis with radiculopathy, site unspecified**

M47.21 **Other spondylosis with radiculopathy,** occipito-atlanto-axial **region**

M47.22 **Other spondylosis with radiculopathy,** cervical region

M47.23 **Other spondylosis with radiculopathy,** cervicothoracic **region**

M47.24 **Other spondylosis with radiculopathy,** thoracic region

M47.25 **Other spondylosis with radiculopathy,** thoracolumbar **region**

M47.26 **Other spondylosis with radiculopathy,** lumbar region

M47.27 **Other spondylosis with radiculopathy,** lumbosacral region

M47.28 **Other spondylosis with radiculopathy,** sacral and sacrococcygeal **region**

√5ᵗʰ M47.8 Other spondylosis

√6ᵗʰ M47.81 **Spondylosis** without myelopathy or radiculopathy

M47.811 **Spondylosis without myelopathy or radiculopathy,** occipito-atlanto-axial **region**

M47.812 **Spondylosis without myelopathy or radiculopathy,** cervical **region**

M47.813 **Spondylosis without myelopathy or radiculopathy,** cervicothoracic **region**

M47.814 **Spondylosis without myelopathy or radiculopathy,** thoracic **region**

M47.815 **Spondylosis without myelopathy or radiculopathy,** thoracolumbar **region**

M47.816 **Spondylosis without myelopathy or radiculopathy,** lumbar **region**

M47.817 **Spondylosis without myelopathy or radiculopathy,** lumbosacral **region**

M47.818 **Spondylosis without myelopathy or radiculopathy,** sacral and sacrococcygeal **region**

M47.819 **Spondylosis without myelopathy or radiculopathy, site unspecified**

√6ᵗʰ M47.89 **Other** spondylosis

M47.891 **Other spondylosis,** occipito-atlanto-axial **region**

M47.892 **Other spondylosis,** cervical region

M47.893 **Other spondylosis,** cervicothoracic **region**

M47.894 **Other spondylosis,** thoracic **region**

M47.895 **Other spondylosis,** thoracolumbar **region**

M47.896 **Other spondylosis,** lumbar **region**

M47.897 **Other spondylosis,** lumbosacral **region**

M47.898 **Other spondylosis,** sacral and sacrococcygeal **region**

M47.899 **Other spondylosis, site unspecified**

M47.9 **Spondylosis, unspecified**

√4ᵗʰ **M48 Other spondylopathies**

√5ᵗʰ M48.0 Spinal stenosis
Caudal stenosis

M48.00 **Spinal stenosis, site unspecified**

M48.01 **Spinal stenosis,** occipito-atlanto-axial region

M48.02 **Spinal stenosis,** cervical **region**

M48.03 **Spinal stenosis,** cervicothoracic region

M48.04 **Spinal stenosis,** thoracic region

M48.05 **Spinal stenosis,** thoracolumbar region

M48.06 **Spinal stenosis,** lumbar region

M48.07 **Spinal stenosis,** lumbosacral region

M48.08 **Spinal stenosis,** sacral and sacrococcygeal **region**

√5ᵗʰ M48.1 Ankylosing hyperostosis [Forestier]
Diffuse idiopathic skeletal hyperostosis [DISH]

M48.10 **Ankylosing hyperostosis [Forestier], site unspecified**

M48.11 **Ankylosing hyperostosis [Forestier],** occipito-atlanto-axial **region**

M48.12 **Ankylosing hyperostosis [Forestier],** cervical region

M48.13 **Ankylosing hyperostosis [Forestier],** cervicothoracic **region**

M48.14 **Ankylosing hyperostosis [Forestier],** thoracic region

M48.15 **Ankylosing hyperostosis [Forestier],** thoracolumbar region

M48.16 **Ankylosing hyperostosis [Forestier],** lumbar region

M48.17 **Ankylosing hyperostosis [Forestier],** lumbosacral region

M48.18 **Ankylosing hyperostosis [Forestier],** sacral and sacrococcygeal **region**

M48.19 **Ankylosing hyperostosis [Forestier],** multiple sites in spine

√5ᵗʰ M48.2 Kissing spine

M48.20 **Kissing spine, site unspecified**

M48.21 **Kissing spine,** occipito-atlanto-axial **region**

M48.22 **Kissing spine,** cervical **region**

M48.23 **Kissing spine,** cervicothoracic region

M48.24 **Kissing spine,** thoracic region

M48.25 **Kissing spine,** thoracolumbar **region**

M48.26 **Kissing spine,** lumbar **region**

M48.27 **Kissing spine,** lumbosacral **region**

√5ᵗʰ M48.3 Traumatic spondylopathy

M48.30 **Traumatic spondylopathy, site unspecified**

M48.31 **Traumatic spondylopathy,** occipito-atlanto-axial **region**

M48.32 **Traumatic spondylopathy,** cervical **region**

M48.33 **Traumatic spondylopathy,** cervicothoracic **region**

M48.34 **Traumatic spondylopathy,** thoracic **region**

M48.35 **Traumatic spondylopathy,** thoracolumbar **region**

M48.36 **Traumatic spondylopathy,** lumbar **region**

M48.37 **Traumatic spondylopathy,** lumbosacral **region**

M48.38 **Traumatic spondylopathy,** sacral and sacrococcygeal **region**

√5ᵗʰ M48.4 Fatigue fracture of vertebra
Stress fracture of vertebra

EXCLUDES 1 *pathological fracture NOS (M84.4-)*
pathological fracture of vertebra due to neoplasm (M84.58)
pathological fracture of vertebra due to other diagnosis (M84.68)
pathological fracture of vertebra due to osteoporosis (M80.-)
traumatic fracture of vertebrae (S12.0-S12.3-, S22.0-, S32.0-)

The appropriate 7th character is to be added to each code from subcategory M48.4.
A   initial encounter for fracture
D   subsequent encounter for fracture with routine healing
G   subsequent encounter for fracture with delayed healing
S   sequela of fracture

√x7ᵗʰ M48.40 **Fatigue fracture of vertebra, site unspecified**

√x7ᵗʰ M48.41 **Fatigue fracture of vertebra,** occipito-atlanto-axial region

√x7ᵗʰ M48.42 **Fatigue fracture of vertebra,** cervical region

√x7ᵗʰ M48.43 **Fatigue fracture of vertebra,** cervicothoracic region

√x7ᵗʰ M48.44 **Fatigue fracture of vertebra,** thoracic region

√x7ᵗʰ M48.45 **Fatigue fracture of vertebra,** thoracolumbar region

√x7ᵗʰ M48.46 **Fatigue fracture of vertebra,** lumbar region

√x7ᵗʰ M48.47 **Fatigue fracture of vertebra,** lumbosacral region

√x7ᵗʰ M48.48 **Fatigue fracture of vertebra,** sacral and sacrococcygeal region

✓ Additional Character Required   √x7ᵗʰ Xtension Alert   Unspecified Code   Other Specified Code   Manifestation Code   ▶◀ Revised Text   ● New Code   ▲ Revised Code Title

ICD-10-CM 2014 (Draft)   681

✓5ᵗʰ **M48.5 Collapsed vertebra, not elsewhere classified**
Collapsed vertebra NOS
Wedging of vertebra NOS

EXCLUDES 1 *current injury—see Injury of spine, by body region*
fatigue fracture of vertebra (M48.4)
pathological fracture of vertebra due to neoplasm
(M84.58)
pathological fracture of vertebra due to other diagnosis
(M84.68)
pathological fracture of vertebra due to osteoporosis
(M80.-)
pathological fracture NOS (M84.4-)
stress fracture of vertebra (M48.4-)
traumatic fracture of vertebra (S12-, S22-, S32-)

The appropriate 7th character is to be added to each code
from subcategory M48.5.
A   initial encounter for fracture
D   subsequent encounter for fracture with routine healing
G   subsequent encounter for fracture with delayed healing
S   sequela of fracture

✓x 7ᵗʰ **M48.50 Collapsed vertebra, not elsewhere classified, site unspecified**

✓x 7ᵗʰ **M48.51 Collapsed vertebra, not elsewhere classified, occipito-atlanto-axial region**

✓x 7ᵗʰ **M48.52 Collapsed vertebra, not elsewhere classified, cervical region**

✓x 7ᵗʰ **M48.53 Collapsed vertebra, not elsewhere classified, cervicothoracic region**

✓x 7ᵗʰ **M48.54 Collapsed vertebra, not elsewhere classified, thoracic region**

✓x 7ᵗʰ **M48.55 Collapsed vertebra, not elsewhere classified, thoracolumbar region**

✓x 7ᵗʰ **M48.56 Collapsed vertebra, not elsewhere classified, lumbar region**

✓x 7ᵗʰ **M48.57 Collapsed vertebra, not elsewhere classified, lumbosacral region**

✓x 7ᵗʰ **M48.58 Collapsed vertebra, not elsewhere classified, sacral and sacrococcygeal region**

✓5ᵗʰ **M48.8 Other specified spondylopathies**
Ossification of posterior longitudinal ligament

✓6ᵗʰ **M48.8X Other specified spondylopathies**

M48.8X1 Other specified spondylopathies, occipito-atlanto-axial region

M48.8X2 Other specified spondylopathies, cervical region

M48.8X3 Other specified spondylopathies, cervicothoracic region

M48.8X4 Other specified spondylopathies, thoracic region

M48.8X5 Other specified spondylopathies, thoracolumbar region

M48.8X6 Other specified spondylopathies, lumbar region

M48.8X7 Other specified spondylopathies, lumbosacral region

M48.8X8 Other specified spondylopathies, sacral and sacrococcygeal region

M48.8X9 Other specified spondylopathies, site unspecified

M48.9 Spondylopathy, unspecified

✓4ᵗʰ **M49 Spondylopathies in diseases classified elsewhere**
Curvature of spine in diseases classified elsewhere
Deformity of spine in diseases classified elsewhere
Kyphosis in diseases classified elsewhere
Scoliosis in diseases classified elsewhere
Spondylopathy in diseases classified elsewhere

EXCLUDES 1 *curvature of spine in tuberculosis [Pott's] (A18.01)*
enteropathic arthropathies (M07.-)
gonococcal spondylitis (A54.41)
neuropathic [tabes dorsalis] spondylitis (A52.11)
neuropathic spondylopathy in syringomyelia (G95.0)
neuropathic spondylopathy in tabes dorsalis (A52.11)
nonsyphilitic neuropathic spondylopathy NEC (G98.0)
spondylitis in syphilis (acquired) (A52.77)
tuberculous spondylitis (A18.01)
typhoid fever spondylitis (A01.05)

Code first underlying disease, such as:
brucellosis (A23.-)
Charcôt-Marie-Tooth disease (G60.0)
enterobacterial infections (A01-A04)
osteitis fibrosa cystica (E21.0)

✓5ᵗʰ **M49.8 Spondylopathy in diseases classified elsewhere**

M49.80 Spondylopathy in diseases classified elsewhere, site unspecified

M49.81 Spondylopathy in diseases classified elsewhere, occipito-atlanto-axial region

M49.82 Spondylopathy in diseases classified elsewhere, cervical region

M49.83 Spondylopathy in diseases classified elsewhere, cervicothoracic region

M49.84 Spondylopathy in diseases classified elsewhere, thoracic region

M49.85 Spondylopathy in diseases classified elsewhere, thoracolumbar region

M49.86 Spondylopathy in diseases classified elsewhere, lumbar region

M49.87 Spondylopathy in diseases classified elsewhere, lumbosacral region

M49.88 Spondylopathy in diseases classified elsewhere, sacral and sacrococcygeal region

M49.89 Spondylopathy in diseases classified elsewhere, multiple sites in spine

Other dorsopathies (M50-M54)

EXCLUDES 1 *current injury—see injury of spine by body region*
discitis NOS (M46.4-)

✓4ᵗʰ **M50 Cervical disc disorders**
INCLUDES cervicothoracic disc disorders with cervicalgia
cervicothoracic disc disorders
NOTE Code to the most superior level of disorder.

✓5ᵗʰ **M50.0 Cervical disc disorder with myelopathy**

M50.00 Cervical disc disorder with myelopathy, unspecified cervical region

M50.01 Cervical disc disorder with myelopathy, high cervical region
C2-C3 disc disorder with myelopathy
C3-C4 disc disorder with myelopathy

M50.02 Cervical disc disorder with myelopathy, mid-cervical region
C4-C5 disc disorder with myelopathy
C5-C6 disc disorder with myelopathy
C6-C7 disc disorder with myelopathy

M50.03 Cervical disc disorder with myelopathy, cervicothoracic region
C7-T1 disc disorder with myelopathy

✓5ᵗʰ **M50.1 Cervical disc disorder with radiculopathy**
EXCLUDES 2 *brachial radiculitis NOS (M54.13)*

M50.10 Cervical disc disorder with radiculopathy, unspecified cervical region

M50.11 Cervical disc disorder with radiculopathy, high cervical region
C2-C3 disc disorder with radiculopathy
C3 radiculopathy due to disc disorder
C3-C4 disc disorder with radiculopathy
C4 radiculopathy due to disc disorder

EXCLUDES 1 Not coded here   **EXCLUDES 2** Not included here   **N** Newborn Age: 0   **P** Pediatric Age: 0-17   **M** Maternity Age: 12-55   **A** Adult Age: 15-124

682   ICD-10-CM 2014 (Draft)

M50.12 **Cervical disc disorder with radiculopathy, mid-cervical region**
C4-C5 disc disorder with radiculopathy
C5 radiculopathy due to disc disorder
C5-C6 disc disorder with radiculopathy
C6 radiculopathy due to disc disorder
C6-C7 disc disorder with radiculopathy
C7 radiculopathy due to disc disorder

M50.13 **Cervical disc disorder with radiculopathy, cervicothoracic region**
C7-T1 disc disorder with radiculopathy
C8 radiculopathy due to disc disorder

√5th **M50.2** Other cervical disc displacement

M50.20 **Other cervical disc displacement, unspecified cervical region**

M50.21 **Other cervical disc displacement, high cervical region**
Other C2-C3 cervical disc displacement
Other C3-C4 cervical disc displacement

M50.22 **Other cervical disc displacement, mid-cervical region**
Other C4-C5 cervical disc displacement
Other C5-C6 cervical disc displacement
Other C6-C7 cervical disc displacement

M50.23 **Other cervical disc displacement, cervicothoracic region**
Other C7-T1 cervical disc displacement

√5th **M50.3** Other cervical disc degeneration

M50.30 **Other cervical disc degeneration, unspecified cervical region**

M50.31 **Other cervical disc degeneration, high cervical region**
Other C2-C3 cervical disc degeneration
Other C3-C4 cervical disc degeneration

M50.32 **Other cervical disc degeneration, mid-cervical region**
Other C4-C5 cervical disc degeneration
Other C5-C6 cervical disc degeneration
Other C6-C7 cervical disc degeneration

M50.33 **Other cervical disc degeneration, cervicothoracic region**
Other C7-T1 cervical disc degeneration

√5th **M50.8** Other cervical disc disorders

M50.80 **Other cervical disc disorders, unspecified cervical region**

M50.81 **Other cervical disc disorders, high cervical region**
Other C2-C3 cervical disc disorders
Other C3-C4 cervical disc disorders

M50.82 **Other cervical disc disorders, mid-cervical region**
Other C4-C5 cervical disc disorders
Other C5-C6 cervical disc disorders
Other C6-C7 cervical disc disorders

M50.83 **Other cervical disc disorders, cervicothoracic region**
Other C7-T1 cervical disc disorders

√5th **M50.9** Cervical disc disorder, unspecified

M50.90 **Cervical disc disorder, unspecified, unspecified cervical region**

M50.91 **Cervical disc disorder, unspecified, high cervical region**
C2-C3 cervical disc disorder, unspecified
C3-C4 cervical disc disorder, unspecified

M50.92 **Cervical disc disorder, unspecified, mid-cervical region**
C4-C5 cervical disc disorder, unspecified
C5-C6 cervical disc disorder, unspecified
C6-C7 cervical disc disorder, unspecified

M50.93 **Cervical disc disorder, unspecified, cervicothoracic region**
C7-T1 cervical disc disorder, unspecified

√4th **M51 Thoracic, thoracolumbar, and lumbosacral intervertebral disc disorders**
EXCLUDES 2 *cervical and cervicothoracic disc disorders (M50.-)*
sacral and sacrococcygeal disorders (M53.3)

√5th **M51.0** Thoracic, thoracolumbar and lumbosacral intervertebral disc disorders with myelopathy

M51.04 **Intervertebral disc disorders with myelopathy, thoracic region**

M51.05 **Intervertebral disc disorders with myelopathy, thoracolumbar region**

M51.06 **Intervertebral disc disorders with myelopathy, lumbar region**

√5th **M51.1** Thoracic, thoracolumbar and lumbosacral intervertebral disc disorders with radiculopathy
Sciatica due to intervertebral disc disorder
EXCLUDES 1 *lumbar radiculitis NOS (M54.16)*
sciatica NOS (M54.3)

M51.14 **Intervertebral disc disorders with radiculopathy, thoracic region**

M51.15 **Intervertebral disc disorders with radiculopathy, thoracolumbar region**

M51.16 **Intervertebral disc disorders with radiculopathy, lumbar region**

M51.17 **Intervertebral disc disorders with radiculopathy, lumbosacral region**

√5th **M51.2** Other thoracic, thoracolumbar and lumbosacral intervertebral disc displacement
Lumbago due to displacement of intervertebral disc

M51.24 **Other intervertebral disc displacement, thoracic region**

M51.25 **Other intervertebral disc displacement, thoracolumbar region**

M51.26 **Other intervertebral disc displacement, lumbar region**

M51.27 **Other intervertebral disc displacement, lumbosacral region**

√5th **M51.3** Other thoracic, thoracolumbar and lumbosacral intervertebral disc degeneration

M51.34 **Other intervertebral disc degeneration, thoracic region**

M51.35 **Other intervertebral disc degeneration, thoracolumbar region**

M51.36 **Other intervertebral disc degeneration, lumbar region**

M51.37 **Other intervertebral disc degeneration, lumbosacral region**

√5th **M51.4** Schmorl's nodes

M51.44 **Schmorl's nodes, thoracic region**

M51.45 **Schmorl's nodes, thoracolumbar region**

M51.46 **Schmorl's nodes, lumbar region**

M51.47 **Schmorl's nodes, lumbosacral region**

√5th **M51.8** Other thoracic, thoracolumbar and lumbosacral intervertebral disc disorders

M51.84 **Other intervertebral disc disorders, thoracic region**

M51.85 **Other intervertebral disc disorders, thoracolumbar region**

M51.86 **Other intervertebral disc disorders, lumbar region**

M51.87 **Other intervertebral disc disorders, lumbosacral region**

M51.9 **Unspecified thoracic, thoracolumbar and lumbosacral intervertebral disc disorder**

√4th **M53 Other and unspecified dorsopathies, not elsewhere classified**

M53.0 **Cervicocranial syndrome**
Posterior cervical sympathetic syndrome

M53.1 **Cervicobrachial syndrome**
EXCLUDES 2 *cervical disc disorder (M50.-)*
thoracic outlet syndrome (G54.0)

√5th **M53.2** Spinal instabilities

√6th **M53.2X** Spinal instabilities

M53.2X1 **Spinal instabilities, occipito-atlanto-axial region**

M53.2X2 **Spinal instabilities, cervical region**

M53.2X3 **Spinal instabilities, cervicothoracic region**

M53.2X4 **Spinal instabilities, thoracic region**

M53.2X5 **Spinal instabilities, thoracolumbar region**

M53.2X6 **Spinal instabilities, lumbar region**

M53.2X7 **Spinal instabilities, lumbosacral region**

M53.2X8 **Spinal instabilities, sacral and sacrococcygeal region**

M53.2X9 **Spinal instabilities, site unspecified**

M53.3 **Sacrococcygeal disorders, not elsewhere classified**
Coccygodynia

√5th **M53.8** Other specified dorsopathies

M53.80 **Other specified dorsopathies, site unspecified**

M53.81 Other specified dorsopathies, occipito-atlanto-axial region

M53.82 Other specified dorsopathies, cervical region

M53.83 Other specified dorsopathies, cervicothoracic region

M53.84 Other specified dorsopathies, thoracic region

M53.85 Other specified dorsopathies, thoracolumbar region

M53.86 Other specified dorsopathies, lumbar region

M53.87 Other specified dorsopathies, lumbosacral region

M53.88 Other specified dorsopathies, sacral and sacrococcygeal region

M53.9 Dorsopathy, unspecified

√4th **M54 Dorsalgia**

     EXCLUDES 1   psychogenic dorsalgia (F45.41)

√5th **M54.0 Panniculitis affecting regions of neck and back**

     EXCLUDES 1   lupus panniculitis (L93.2)
           panniculitis NOS (M79.3)
           relapsing [Weber-Christian] panniculitis (M35.6)

M54.00 Panniculitis affecting regions of neck and back, site unspecified

M54.01 Panniculitis affecting regions of neck and back, occipito-atlanto-axial region

M54.02 Panniculitis affecting regions of neck and back, cervical region

M54.03 Panniculitis affecting regions of neck and back, cervicothoracic region

M54.04 Panniculitis affecting regions of neck and back, thoracic region

M54.05 Panniculitis affecting regions of neck and back, thoracolumbar region

M54.06 Panniculitis affecting regions of neck and back, lumbar region

M54.07 Panniculitis affecting regions of neck and back, lumbosacral region

M54.08 Panniculitis affecting regions of neck and back, sacral and sacrococcygeal region

M54.09 Panniculitis affecting regions, neck and back, multiple sites in spine

√5th **M54.1 Radiculopathy**

     Brachial neuritis or radiculitis NOS
     Lumbar neuritis or radiculitis NOS
     Lumbosacral neuritis or radiculitis NOS
     Thoracic neuritis or radiculitis NOS
     Radiculitis NOS

     EXCLUDES 1   neuralgia and neuritis NOS (M79.2)
           radiculopathy with cervical disc disorder (M50.1)
           radiculopathy with lumbar and other intervertebral disc disorder (M51.1-)
           radiculopathy with spondylosis (M47.2-)

M54.10 Radiculopathy, site unspecified

M54.11 Radiculopathy, occipito-atlanto-axial region

M54.12 Radiculopathy, cervical region

M54.13 Radiculopathy, cervicothoracic region

M54.14 Radiculopathy, thoracic region

M54.15 Radiculopathy, thoracolumbar region

M54.16 Radiculopathy, lumbar region

M54.17 Radiculopathy, lumbosacral region

M54.18 Radiculopathy, sacral and sacrococcygeal region

M54.2 Cervicalgia

     EXCLUDES 1   cervicalgia due to intervertebral cervical disc disorder (M50.-)

√5th **M54.3 Sciatica**

     EXCLUDES 1   lesion of sciatic nerve (G57.0)
           sciatica due to intervertebral disc disorder (M51.1-)
           sciatica with lumbago (M54.4-)

M54.30 Sciatica, unspecified side

M54.31 Sciatica, right side

M54.32 Sciatica, left side

√5th **M54.4 Lumbago with sciatica**

     EXCLUDES 1   lumbago with sciatica due to intervertebral disc disorder (M51.1-)

M54.40 Lumbago with sciatica, unspecified side

M54.41 Lumbago with sciatica, right side

M54.42 Lumbago with sciatica, left side

M54.5 Low back pain

     Loin pain
     Lumbago NOS

     EXCLUDES 1   low back strain (S39.012)
           lumbago due to intervertebral disc displacement (M51.2-)
           lumbago with sciatica (M54.4-)

M54.6 Pain in thoracic spine

     EXCLUDES 1   pain in thoracic spine due to intervertebral disc disorder (M51.-)

√5th **M54.8 Other dorsalgia**

     EXCLUDES 1   dorsalgia in thoracic region (M54.6)
           low back pain (M54.5)

M54.81 Occipital neuralgia

M54.89 Other dorsalgia

M54.9 Dorsalgia, unspecified

     Backache NOS   Back pain NOS

SOFT TISSUE DISORDERS (M60-M79)

Disorders of muscles (M60-M63)

     EXCLUDES 1   dermatopolymyositis (M33.-)
           muscular dystrophies and myopathies (G71-G72)
           myopathy in amyloidosis (E85.-)
           myopathy in polyarteritis nodosa (M30.0)
           myopathy in rheumatoid arthritis (M05.32)
           myopathy in scleroderma (M34.-)
           myopathy in Sjögren's syndrome (M35.03)
           myopathy in systemic lupus erythematosus (M32.-)

√4th **M60 Myositis**

     EXCLUDES 2   inclusion body myositis [IBM] (G72.41)

√5th **M60.0 Infective myositis**

     Tropical pyomyositis
     Use additional code (B95-B97) to identify infectious agent

√6th **M60.00 Infective myositis, unspecified site**

     M60.000 Infective myositis, unspecified right arm
           Infective myositis, right upper limb NOS

     M60.001 Infective myositis, unspecified left arm
           Infective myositis, left upper limb NOS

     M60.002 Infective myositis, unspecified arm
           Infective myositis, upper limb NOS

     M60.003 Infective myositis, unspecified right leg
           Infective myositis, right lower limb NOS

     M60.004 Infective myositis, unspecified left leg
           Infective myositis, left lower limb NOS

     M60.005 Infective myositis, unspecified leg
           Infective myositis, lower limb NOS

     M60.009 Infective myositis, unspecified site

√6th **M60.01 Infective myositis, shoulder**

     M60.011 Infective myositis, right shoulder
     M60.012 Infective myositis, left shoulder
     M60.019 Infective myositis, unspecified shoulder

√6th **M60.02 Infective myositis, upper arm**

     M60.021 Infective myositis, right upper arm
     M60.022 Infective myositis, left upper arm
     M60.029 Infective myositis, unspecified upper arm

√6th **M60.03 Infective myositis, forearm**

     M60.031 Infective myositis, right forearm
     M60.032 Infective myositis, left forearm
     M60.039 Infective myositis, unspecified forearm

√6th **M60.04 Infective myositis, hand and fingers**

     M60.041 Infective myositis, right hand
     M60.042 Infective myositis, left hand
     M60.043 Infective myositis, unspecified hand
     M60.044 Infective myositis, right finger(s)
     M60.045 Infective myositis, left finger(s)
     M60.046 Infective myositis, unspecified finger(s)

√6th **M60.05 Infective myositis, thigh**

     M60.051 Infective myositis, right thigh
     M60.052 Infective myositis, left thigh
     M60.059 Infective myositis, unspecified thigh

√6th **M60.06 Infective myositis, lower leg**

     M60.061 Infective myositis, right lower leg
     M60.062 Infective myositis, left lower leg
     M60.069 Infective myositis, unspecified lower leg

EXCLUDES 1 Not coded here   EXCLUDES 2 Not included here   N Newborn Age: 0   P Pediatric Age: 0-17   M Maternity Age: 12-55   A Adult Age: 15-124

684   ICD-10-CM 2014 (Draft)

☑️6th **M60.07** Infective myositis, ankle, foot and toes
     M60.070 Infective myositis, right ankle
     M60.071 Infective myositis, left ankle
     M60.072 Infective myositis, unspecified ankle
     M60.073 Infective myositis, right foot
     M60.074 Infective myositis, left foot
     M60.075 Infective myositis, unspecified foot
     M60.076 Infective myositis, right toe(s)
     M60.077 Infective myositis, left toe(s)
     M60.078 Infective myositis, unspecified toe(s)
   M60.08 Infective myositis, other site
   M60.09 Infective myositis, multiple sites
☑️5th **M60.1** Interstitial myositis
   M60.10 Interstitial myositis of unspecified site
☑️6th **M60.11** Interstitial myositis, shoulder
     M60.111 Interstitial myositis, right shoulder
     M60.112 Interstitial myositis, left shoulder
     M60.119 Interstitial myositis, unspecified shoulder
☑️6th **M60.12** Interstitial myositis, upper arm
     M60.121 Interstitial myositis, right upper arm
     M60.122 Interstitial myositis, left upper arm
     M60.129 Interstitial myositis, unspecified upper arm
☑️6th **M60.13** Interstitial myositis, forearm
     M60.131 Interstitial myositis, right forearm
     M60.132 Interstitial myositis, left forearm
     M60.139 Interstitial myositis, unspecified forearm
☑️6th **M60.14** Interstitial myositis, hand
     M60.141 Interstitial myositis, right hand
     M60.142 Interstitial myositis, left hand
     M60.149 Interstitial myositis, unspecified hand
☑️6th **M60.15** Interstitial myositis, thigh
     M60.151 Interstitial myositis, right thigh
     M60.152 Interstitial myositis, left thigh
     M60.159 Interstitial myositis, unspecified thigh
☑️6th **M60.16** Interstitial myositis, lower leg
     M60.161 Interstitial myositis, right lower leg
     M60.162 Interstitial myositis, left lower leg
     M60.169 Interstitial myositis, unspecified lower leg
☑️6th **M60.17** Interstitial myositis, ankle and foot
     M60.171 Interstitial myositis, right ankle and foot
     M60.172 Interstitial myositis, left ankle and foot
     M60.179 Interstitial myositis, unspecified ankle and foot
   M60.18 Interstitial myositis, other site
   M60.19 Interstitial myositis, multiple sites
☑️5th **M60.2** Foreign body granuloma of soft tissue, not elsewhere classified
     Use additional code to identify the type of retained foreign body (Z18.-)
     EXCLUDES 1   foreign body granuloma of skin and subcutaneous tissue (L92.3)
   M60.20 Foreign body granuloma of soft tissue, not elsewhere classified, unspecified site
☑️6th **M60.21** Foreign body granuloma of soft tissue, not elsewhere classified, shoulder
     M60.211 Foreign body granuloma of soft tissue, not elsewhere classified, right shoulder
     M60.212 Foreign body granuloma of soft tissue, not elsewhere classified, left shoulder
     M60.219 Foreign body granuloma of soft tissue, not elsewhere classified, unspecified shoulder
☑️6th **M60.22** Foreign body granuloma of soft tissue, not elsewhere classified, upper arm
     M60.221 Foreign body granuloma of soft tissue, not elsewhere classified, right upper arm
     M60.222 Foreign body granuloma of soft tissue, not elsewhere classified, left upper arm
     M60.229 Foreign body granuloma of soft tissue, not elsewhere classified, unspecified upper arm

☑️6th **M60.23** Foreign body granuloma of soft tissue, not elsewhere classified, forearm
     M60.231 Foreign body granuloma of soft tissue, not elsewhere classified, right forearm
     M60.232 Foreign body granuloma of soft tissue, not elsewhere classified, left forearm
     M60.239 Foreign body granuloma of soft tissue, not elsewhere classified, unspecified forearm
☑️6th **M60.24** Foreign body granuloma of soft tissue, not elsewhere classified, hand
     M60.241 Foreign body granuloma of soft tissue, not elsewhere classified, right hand
     M60.242 Foreign body granuloma of soft tissue, not elsewhere classified, left hand
     M60.249 Foreign body granuloma of soft tissue, not elsewhere classified, unspecified hand
☑️6th **M60.25** Foreign body granuloma of soft tissue, not elsewhere classified, thigh
     M60.251 Foreign body granuloma of soft tissue, not elsewhere classified, right thigh
     M60.252 Foreign body granuloma of soft tissue, not elsewhere classified, left thigh
     M60.259 Foreign body granuloma of soft tissue, not elsewhere classified, unspecified thigh
☑️6th **M60.26** Foreign body granuloma of soft tissue, not elsewhere classified, lower leg
     M60.261 Foreign body granuloma of soft tissue, not elsewhere classified, right lower leg
     M60.262 Foreign body granuloma of soft tissue, not elsewhere classified, left lower leg
     M60.269 Foreign body granuloma of soft tissue, not elsewhere classified, unspecified lower leg
☑️6th **M60.27** Foreign body granuloma of soft tissue, not elsewhere classified, ankle and foot
     M60.271 Foreign body granuloma of soft tissue, not elsewhere classified, right ankle and foot
     M60.272 Foreign body granuloma of soft tissue, not elsewhere classified, left ankle and foot
     M60.279 Foreign body granuloma of soft tissue, not elsewhere classified, unspecified ankle and foot
   M60.28 Foreign body granuloma of soft tissue, not elsewhere classified, other site
☑️5th **M60.8** Other myositis
   M60.80 Other myositis, unspecified site
☑️6th **M60.81** Other myositis shoulder
     M60.811 Other myositis, right shoulder
     M60.812 Other myositis, left shoulder
     M60.819 Other myositis, unspecified shoulder
☑️6th **M60.82** Other myositis, upper arm
     M60.821 Other myositis, right upper arm
     M60.822 Other myositis, left upper arm
     M60.829 Other myositis, unspecified upper arm
☑️6th **M60.83** Other myositis, forearm
     M60.831 Other myositis, right forearm
     M60.832 Other myositis, left forearm
     M60.839 Other myositis, unspecified forearm
☑️6th **M60.84** Other myositis, hand
     M60.841 Other myositis, right hand
     M60.842 Other myositis, left hand
     M60.849 Other myositis, unspecified hand
☑️6th **M60.85** Other myositis, thigh
     M60.851 Other myositis, right thigh
     M60.852 Other myositis, left thigh
     M60.859 Other myositis, unspecified thigh
☑️6th **M60.86** Other myositis, lower leg
     M60.861 Other myositis, right lower leg
     M60.862 Other myositis, left lower leg
     M60.869 Other myositis, unspecified lower leg
☑️6th **M60.87** Other myositis, ankle and foot
     M60.871 Other myositis, right ankle and foot
     M60.872 Other myositis, left ankle and foot
     M60.879 Other myositis, unspecified ankle and foot
   M60.88 Other myositis, other site
   M60.89 Other myositis, multiple sites

☑️ Additional Character Required   ✓x7th Xtension Alert   Unspecified Code   Other Specified Code   Manifestation Code   ▶◀ Revised Text   ● New Code   ▲ Revised Code Title

M60.9 Myositis, unspecified

✓4ᵗʰ **M61** Calcification and ossification of muscle

✓5ᵗʰ **M61.0** Myositis ossificans traumatica

M61.00 Myositis ossificans traumatica, unspecified site

✓6ᵗʰ **M61.01** Myositis ossificans traumatica, shoulder

M61.011 Myositis ossificans traumatica, right shoulder

M61.012 Myositis ossificans traumatica, left shoulder

M61.019 Myositis ossificans traumatica, unspecified shoulder

✓6ᵗʰ **M61.02** Myositis ossificans traumatica, upper arm

M61.021 Myositis ossificans traumatica, right upper arm

M61.022 Myositis ossificans traumatica, left upper arm

M61.029 Myositis ossificans traumatica, unspecified upper arm

✓6ᵗʰ **M61.03** Myositis ossificans traumatica, forearm

M61.031 Myositis ossificans traumatica, right forearm

M61.032 Myositis ossificans traumatica, left forearm

M61.039 Myositis ossificans traumatica, unspecified forearm

✓6ᵗʰ **M61.04** Myositis ossificans traumatica, hand

M61.041 Myositis ossificans traumatica, right hand

M61.042 Myositis ossificans traumatica, left hand

M61.049 Myositis ossificans traumatica, unspecified hand

✓6ᵗʰ **M61.05** Myositis ossificans traumatica, thigh

M61.051 Myositis ossificans traumatica, right thigh

M61.052 Myositis ossificans traumatica, left thigh

M61.059 Myositis ossificans traumatica, unspecified thigh

✓6ᵗʰ **M61.06** Myositis ossificans traumatica, lower leg

M61.061 Myositis ossificans traumatica, right lower leg

M61.062 Myositis ossificans traumatica, left lower leg

M61.069 Myositis ossificans traumatica, unspecified lower leg

✓6ᵗʰ **M61.07** Myositis ossificans traumatica, ankle and foot

M61.071 Myositis ossificans traumatica, right ankle and foot

M61.072 Myositis ossificans traumatica, left ankle and foot

M61.079 Myositis ossificans traumatica, unspecified ankle and foot

M61.08 Myositis ossificans traumatica, other site

M61.09 Myositis ossificans traumatica, multiple sites

✓5ᵗʰ **M61.1** Myositis ossificans progressiva

Fibrodysplasia ossificans progressiva

M61.10 Myositis ossificans progressiva, unspecified site

✓6ᵗʰ **M61.11** Myositis ossificans progressiva, shoulder

M61.111 Myositis ossificans progressiva, right shoulder

M61.112 Myositis ossificans progressiva, left shoulder

M61.119 Myositis ossificans progressiva, unspecified shoulder

✓6ᵗʰ **M61.12** Myositis ossificans progressiva, upper arm

M61.121 Myositis ossificans progressiva, right upper arm

M61.122 Myositis ossificans progressiva, left upper arm

M61.129 Myositis ossificans progressiva, unspecified arm

✓6ᵗʰ **M61.13** Myositis ossificans progressiva, forearm

M61.131 Myositis ossificans progressiva, right forearm

M61.132 Myositis ossificans progressiva, left forearm

M61.139 Myositis ossificans progressiva, unspecified forearm

✓6ᵗʰ **M61.14** Myositis ossificans progressiva, hand and finger(s)

M61.141 Myositis ossificans progressiva, right hand

M61.142 Myositis ossificans progressiva, left hand

M61.143 Myositis ossificans progressiva, unspecified hand

M61.144 Myositis ossificans progressiva, right finger(s)

M61.145 Myositis ossificans progressiva, left finger(s)

M61.146 Myositis ossificans progressiva, unspecified finger(s)

✓6ᵗʰ **M61.15** Myositis ossificans progressiva, thigh

M61.151 Myositis ossificans progressiva, right thigh

M61.152 Myositis ossificans progressiva, left thigh

M61.159 Myositis ossificans progressiva, unspecified thigh

✓6ᵗʰ **M61.16** Myositis ossificans progressiva, lower leg

M61.161 Myositis ossificans progressiva, right lower leg

M61.162 Myositis ossificans progressiva, left lower leg

M61.169 Myositis ossificans progressiva, unspecified lower leg

✓6ᵗʰ **M61.17** Myositis ossificans progressiva, ankle, foot and toe(s)

M61.171 Myositis ossificans progressiva, right ankle

M61.172 Myositis ossificans progressiva, left ankle

M61.173 Myositis ossificans progressiva, unspecified ankle

M61.174 Myositis ossificans progressiva, right foot

M61.175 Myositis ossificans progressiva, left foot

M61.176 Myositis ossificans progressiva, unspecified foot

M61.177 Myositis ossificans progressiva, right toe(s)

M61.178 Myositis ossificans progressiva, left toe(s)

M61.179 Myositis ossificans progressiva, unspecified toe(s)

M61.18 Myositis ossificans progressiva, other site

M61.19 Myositis ossificans progressiva, multiple sites

✓5ᵗʰ **M61.2** Paralytic calcification and ossification of muscle

Myositis ossificans associated with quadriplegia or paraplegia

M61.20 Paralytic calcification and ossification of muscle, unspecified site

✓6ᵗʰ **M61.21** Paralytic calcification and ossification of muscle, shoulder

M61.211 Paralytic calcification and ossification of muscle, right shoulder

M61.212 Paralytic calcification and ossification of muscle, left shoulder

M61.219 Paralytic calcification and ossification of muscle, unspecified shoulder

✓6ᵗʰ **M61.22** Paralytic calcification and ossification of muscle, upper arm

M61.221 Paralytic calcification and ossification of muscle, right upper arm

M61.222 Paralytic calcification and ossification of muscle, left upper arm

M61.229 Paralytic calcification and ossification of muscle, unspecified upper arm

✓6ᵗʰ **M61.23** Paralytic calcification and ossification of muscle, forearm

M61.231 Paralytic calcification and ossification of muscle, right forearm

M61.232 Paralytic calcification and ossification of muscle, left forearm

M61.239 Paralytic calcification and ossification of muscle, unspecified forearm

✓6ᵗʰ **M61.24** Paralytic calcification and ossification of muscle, hand

M61.241 Paralytic calcification and ossification of muscle, right hand

---

EXCLUDES 1 Not coded here   EXCLUDES 2 Not included here   N Newborn Age: 0   P Pediatric Age: 0-17   M Maternity Age: 12-55   A Adult Age: 15-124

686   ICD-10-CM 2014 (Draft)

M61.242   Paralytic calcification and ossification of muscle, left hand

M61.249   Paralytic calcification and ossification of muscle, unspecified hand

√6ᵗʰ M61.25   Paralytic calcification and ossification of muscle, thigh

M61.251   Paralytic calcification and ossification of muscle, right thigh

M61.252   Paralytic calcification and ossification of muscle, left thigh

M61.259   Paralytic calcification and ossification of muscle, unspecified thigh

√6ᵗʰ M61.26   Paralytic calcification and ossification of muscle, lower leg

M61.261   Paralytic calcification and ossification of muscle, right lower leg

M61.262   Paralytic calcification and ossification of muscle, left lower leg

M61.269   Paralytic calcification and ossification of muscle, unspecified lower leg

√6ᵗʰ M61.27   Paralytic calcification and ossification of muscle, ankle and foot

M61.271   Paralytic calcification and ossification of muscle, right ankle and foot

M61.272   Paralytic calcification and ossification of muscle, left ankle and foot

M61.279   Paralytic calcification and ossification of muscle, unspecified ankle and foot

M61.28   Paralytic calcification and ossification of muscle, other site

M61.29   Paralytic calcification and ossification of muscle, multiple sites

√5ᵗʰ M61.3   Calcification and ossification of muscles associated with burns

Myositis ossificans associated with burns

M61.30   Calcification and ossification of muscles associated with burns, unspecified site

√6ᵗʰ M61.31   Calcification and ossification of muscles associated with burns, shoulder

M61.311   Calcification and ossification of muscles associated with burns, right shoulder

M61.312   Calcification and ossification of muscles associated with burns, left shoulder

M61.319   Calcification and ossification of muscles associated with burns, unspecified shoulder

√6ᵗʰ M61.32   Calcification and ossification of muscles associated with burns, upper arm

M61.321   Calcification and ossification of muscles associated with burns, right upper arm

M61.322   Calcification and ossification of muscles associated with burns, left upper arm

M61.329   Calcification and ossification of muscles associated with burns, unspecified upper arm

√6ᵗʰ M61.33   Calcification and ossification of muscles associated with burns, forearm

M61.331   Calcification and ossification of muscles associated with burns, right forearm

M61.332   Calcification and ossification of muscles associated with burns, left forearm

M61.339   Calcification and ossification of muscles associated with burns, unspecified forearm

√6ᵗʰ M61.34   Calcification and ossification of muscles associated with burns, hand

M61.341   Calcification and ossification of muscles associated with burns, right hand

M61.342   Calcification and ossification of muscles associated with burns, left hand

M61.349   Calcification and ossification of muscles associated with burns, unspecified hand

√6ᵗʰ M61.35   Calcification and ossification of muscles associated with burns, thigh

M61.351   Calcification and ossification of muscles associated with burns, right thigh

M61.352   Calcification and ossification of muscles associated with burns, left thigh

M61.359   Calcification and ossification of muscles associated with burns, unspecified thigh

√6ᵗʰ M61.36   Calcification and ossification of muscles associated with burns, lower leg

M61.361   Calcification and ossification of muscles associated with burns, right lower leg

M61.362   Calcification and ossification of muscles associated with burns, left lower leg

M61.369   Calcification and ossification of muscles associated with burns, unspecified lower leg

√6ᵗʰ M61.37   Calcification and ossification of muscles associated with burns, ankle and foot

M61.371   Calcification and ossification of muscles associated with burns, right ankle and foot

M61.372   Calcification and ossification of muscles associated with burns, left ankle and foot

M61.379   Calcification and ossification of muscles associated with burns, unspecified ankle and foot

M61.38   Calcification and ossification of muscles associated with burns, other site

M61.39   Calcification and ossification of muscles associated with burns, multiple sites

√5ᵗʰ M61.4   Other calcification of muscle

EXCLUDES 1   calcific tendinitis NOS (M65.2-)
calcific tendinitis of shoulder (M75.3)

M61.40   Other calcification of muscle, unspecified site

√6ᵗʰ M61.41   Other calcification of muscle, shoulder

M61.411   Other calcification of muscle, right shoulder

M61.412   Other calcification of muscle, left shoulder

M61.419   Other calcification of muscle, unspecified shoulder

√6ᵗʰ M61.42   Other calcification of muscle, upper arm

M61.421   Other calcification of muscle, right upper arm

M61.422   Other calcification of muscle, left upper arm

M61.429   Other calcification of muscle, unspecified upper arm

√6ᵗʰ M61.43   Other calcification of muscle, forearm

M61.431   Other calcification of muscle, right forearm

M61.432   Other calcification of muscle, left forearm

M61.439   Other calcification of muscle, unspecified forearm

√6ᵗʰ M61.44   Other calcification of muscle, hand

M61.441   Other calcification of muscle, right hand

M61.442   Other calcification of muscle, left hand

M61.449   Other calcification of muscle, unspecified hand

√6ᵗʰ M61.45   Other calcification of muscle, thigh

M61.451   Other calcification of muscle, right thigh

M61.452   Other calcification of muscle, left thigh

M61.459   Other calcification of muscle, unspecified thigh

√6ᵗʰ M61.46   Other calcification of muscle, lower leg

M61.461   Other calcification of muscle, right lower leg

M61.462   Other calcification of muscle, left lower leg

M61.469   Other calcification of muscle, unspecified lower leg

√6ᵗʰ M61.47   Other calcification of muscle, ankle and foot

M61.471   Other calcification of muscle, right ankle and foot

M61.472   Other calcification of muscle, left ankle and foot

M61.479   Other calcification of muscle, unspecified ankle and foot

M61.48   Other calcification of muscle, other site

M61.49   Other calcification of muscle, multiple sites

√5ᵗʰ M61.5   Other ossification of muscle

M61.50   Other ossification of muscle, unspecified site

✓ Additional Character Required   √x7ᵗʰ Xtension Alert   Unspecified Code   Other Specified Code   Manifestation Code   ►◄ Revised Text   ● New Code   ▲ Revised Code Title

ICD-10-CM 2014 (Draft)   687

Diseases of the Musculoskeletal System and Connective Tissue

M61.51–M62.161

√6ᵗʰ **M61.51 Other ossification of muscle, shoulder**
- **M61.511 Other ossification of muscle, right shoulder**
- **M61.512 Other ossification of muscle, left shoulder**
- **M61.519 Other ossification of muscle, unspecified shoulder**

√6ᵗʰ **M61.52 Other ossification of muscle, upper arm**
- **M61.521 Other ossification of muscle, right upper arm**
- **M61.522 Other ossification of muscle, left upper arm**
- **M61.529 Other ossification of muscle, unspecified upper arm**

√6ᵗʰ **M61.53 Other ossification of muscle, forearm**
- **M61.531 Other ossification of muscle, right forearm**
- **M61.532 Other ossification of muscle, left forearm**
- **M61.539 Other ossification of muscle, unspecified forearm**

√6ᵗʰ **M61.54 Other ossification of muscle, hand**
- **M61.541 Other ossification of muscle, right hand**
- **M61.542 Other ossification of muscle, left hand**
- **M61.549 Other ossification of muscle, unspecified hand**

√6ᵗʰ **M61.55 Other ossification of muscle, thigh**
- **M61.551 Other ossification of muscle, right thigh**
- **M61.552 Other ossification of muscle, left thigh**
- **M61.559 Other ossification of muscle, unspecified thigh**

√6ᵗʰ **M61.56 Other ossification of muscle, lower leg**
- **M61.561 Other ossification of muscle, right lower leg**
- **M61.562 Other ossification of muscle, left lower leg**
- **M61.569 Other ossification of muscle, unspecified lower leg**

√6ᵗʰ **M61.57 Other ossification of muscle, ankle and foot**
- **M61.571 Other ossification of muscle, right ankle and foot**
- **M61.572 Other ossification of muscle, left ankle and foot**
- **M61.579 Other ossification of muscle, unspecified ankle and foot**

M61.58 Other ossification of muscle, other site

M61.59 Other ossification of muscle, multiple sites

M61.9 Calcification and ossification of muscle, unspecified

√4ᵗʰ **M62 Other disorders of muscle**
- *EXCLUDES 1*   alcoholic myopathy (G72.1)
- cramp and spasm (R25.2)
- drug-induced myopathy (G72.0)
- myalgia (M79.1)
- stiff-man syndrome (G25.82)
- *EXCLUDES 2*   nontraumatic hematoma of muscle (M79.81)

√5ᵗʰ **M62.0 Separation of muscle (nontraumatic)**
- Diastasis of muscle
- *EXCLUDES 1*   diastasis recti complicating pregnancy, labor and delivery (O71.8)
- traumatic separation of muscle—see strain of muscle by body region

M62.00 Separation of muscle (nontraumatic), unspecified site

√6ᵗʰ **M62.01 Separation of muscle (nontraumatic), shoulder**
- **M62.011 Separation of muscle (nontraumatic), right shoulder**
- **M62.012 Separation of muscle (nontraumatic), left shoulder**
- **M62.019 Separation of muscle (nontraumatic), unspecified shoulder**

√6ᵗʰ **M62.02 Separation of muscle (nontraumatic), upper arm**
- **M62.021 Separation of muscle (nontraumatic), right upper arm**
- **M62.022 Separation of muscle (nontraumatic), left upper arm**
- **M62.029 Separation of muscle (nontraumatic), unspecified upper arm**

√6ᵗʰ **M62.03 Separation of muscle (nontraumatic), forearm**
- **M62.031 Separation of muscle (nontraumatic), right forearm**
- **M62.032 Separation of muscle (nontraumatic), left forearm**
- **M62.039 Separation of muscle (nontraumatic), unspecified forearm**

√6ᵗʰ **M62.04 Separation of muscle (nontraumatic), hand**
- **M62.041 Separation of muscle (nontraumatic), right hand**
- **M62.042 Separation of muscle (nontraumatic), left hand**
- **M62.049 Separation of muscle (nontraumatic), unspecified hand**

√6ᵗʰ **M62.05 Separation of muscle (nontraumatic), thigh**
- **M62.051 Separation of muscle (nontraumatic), right thigh**
- **M62.052 Separation of muscle (nontraumatic), left thigh**
- **M62.059 Separation of muscle (nontraumatic), unspecified thigh**

√6ᵗʰ **M62.06 Separation of muscle (nontraumatic), lower leg**
- **M62.061 Separation of muscle (nontraumatic), right lower leg**
- **M62.062 Separation of muscle (nontraumatic), left lower leg**
- **M62.069 Separation of muscle (nontraumatic), unspecified lower leg**

√6ᵗʰ **M62.07 Separation of muscle (nontraumatic), ankle and foot**
- **M62.071 Separation of muscle (nontraumatic), right ankle and foot**
- **M62.072 Separation of muscle (nontraumatic), left ankle and foot**
- **M62.079 Separation of muscle (nontraumatic), unspecified ankle and foot**

M62.08 Separation of muscle (nontraumatic), other site

√5ᵗʰ **M62.1 Other rupture of muscle (nontraumatic)**
- *EXCLUDES 1*   traumatic rupture of muscle—see strain of muscle by body region
- *EXCLUDES 2*   rupture of tendon (M66.-)

M62.10 Other rupture of muscle (nontraumatic), unspecified site

√6ᵗʰ **M62.11 Other rupture of muscle (nontraumatic), shoulder**
- **M62.111 Other rupture of muscle (nontraumatic), right shoulder**
- **M62.112 Other rupture of muscle (nontraumatic), left shoulder**
- **M62.119 Other rupture of muscle (nontraumatic), unspecified shoulder**

√6ᵗʰ **M62.12 Other rupture of muscle (nontraumatic), upper arm**
- **M62.121 Other rupture of muscle (nontraumatic), right upper arm**
- **M62.122 Other rupture of muscle (nontraumatic), left upper arm**
- **M62.129 Other rupture of muscle (nontraumatic), unspecified upper arm**

√6ᵗʰ **M62.13 Other rupture of muscle (nontraumatic), forearm**
- **M62.131 Other rupture of muscle (nontraumatic), right forearm**
- **M62.132 Other rupture of muscle (nontraumatic), left forearm**
- **M62.139 Other rupture of muscle (nontraumatic), unspecified forearm**

√6ᵗʰ **M62.14 Other rupture of muscle (nontraumatic), hand**
- **M62.141 Other rupture of muscle (nontraumatic), right hand**
- **M62.142 Other rupture of muscle (nontraumatic), left hand**
- **M62.149 Other rupture of muscle (nontraumatic), unspecified hand**

√6ᵗʰ **M62.15 Other rupture of muscle (nontraumatic), thigh**
- **M62.151 Other rupture of muscle (nontraumatic), right thigh**
- **M62.152 Other rupture of muscle (nontraumatic), left thigh**
- **M62.159 Other rupture of muscle (nontraumatic), unspecified thigh**

√6ᵗʰ **M62.16 Other rupture of muscle (nontraumatic), lower leg**
- **M62.161 Other rupture of muscle (nontraumatic), right lower leg**

EXCLUDES 1 Not coded here   *EXCLUDES 2* Not included here   N Newborn Age: 0   P Pediatric Age: 0-17   M Maternity Age: 12-55   A Adult Age: 15-124

688   ICD-10-CM 2014 (Draft)

M62.162 **Other rupture of muscle (nontraumatic), left lower leg**

M62.169 **Other rupture of muscle (nontraumatic), unspecified lower leg**

☑6ᵗʰ M62.17 Other rupture of muscle (nontraumatic), ankle and foot

M62.171 **Other rupture of muscle (nontraumatic), right ankle and foot**

M62.172 **Other rupture of muscle (nontraumatic), left ankle and foot**

M62.179 **Other rupture of muscle (nontraumatic), unspecified ankle and foot**

M62.18 **Other rupture of muscle (nontraumatic), other site**

☑5ᵗʰ M62.2 Nontraumatic ischemic infarction of muscle

EXCLUDES 1   *compartment syndrome (traumatic) (T79.A-)*
nontraumatic compartment syndrome (M79.A-)
rhabdomyolysis (M62.82)
traumatic ischemia of muscle (T79.6)
Volkmann's ischemic contracture (T79.6)

M62.20 **Nontraumatic ischemic infarction of muscle, unspecified site**

☑6ᵗʰ M62.21 Nontraumatic ischemic infarction of muscle, shoulder

M62.211 Nontraumatic ischemic infarction of muscle, right shoulder

M62.212 Nontraumatic ischemic infarction of muscle, left shoulder

M62.219 **Nontraumatic ischemic infarction of muscle, unspecified shoulder**

☑6ᵗʰ M62.22 Nontraumatic ischemic infarction of muscle, upper arm

M62.221 Nontraumatic ischemic infarction of muscle, right upper arm

M62.222 Nontraumatic ischemic infarction of muscle, left upper arm

M62.229 **Nontraumatic ischemic infarction of muscle, unspecified upper arm**

☑6ᵗʰ M62.23 Nontraumatic ischemic infarction of muscle, forearm

M62.231 Nontraumatic ischemic infarction of muscle, right forearm

M62.232 Nontraumatic ischemic infarction of muscle, left forearm

M62.239 **Nontraumatic ischemic infarction of muscle, unspecified forearm**

☑6ᵗʰ M62.24 Nontraumatic ischemic infarction of muscle, hand

M62.241 Nontraumatic ischemic infarction of muscle, right hand

M62.242 Nontraumatic ischemic infarction of muscle, left hand

M62.249 **Nontraumatic ischemic infarction of muscle, unspecified hand**

☑6ᵗʰ M62.25 Nontraumatic ischemic infarction of muscle, thigh

M62.251 Nontraumatic ischemic infarction of muscle, right thigh

M62.252 Nontraumatic ischemic infarction of muscle, left thigh

M62.259 **Nontraumatic ischemic infarction of muscle, unspecified thigh**

☑6ᵗʰ M62.26 Nontraumatic ischemic infarction of muscle, lower leg

M62.261 Nontraumatic ischemic infarction of muscle, right lower leg

M62.262 Nontraumatic ischemic infarction of muscle, left lower leg

M62.269 **Nontraumatic ischemic infarction of muscle, unspecified lower leg**

☑6ᵗʰ M62.27 Nontraumatic ischemic infarction of muscle, ankle and foot

M62.271 Nontraumatic ischemic infarction of muscle, right ankle and foot

M62.272 Nontraumatic ischemic infarction of muscle, left ankle and foot

M62.279 **Nontraumatic ischemic infarction of muscle, unspecified ankle and foot**

M62.28 **Nontraumatic ischemic infarction of muscle, other site**

M62.3 Immobility syndrome (paraplegic)

☑5ᵗʰ M62.4 Contracture of muscle
Contracture of tendon (sheath)
EXCLUDES 1   *contracture of joint (M24.5-)*

M62.40 **Contracture of muscle, unspecified site**

☑6ᵗʰ M62.41 Contracture of muscle, shoulder

M62.411 Contracture of muscle, right shoulder

M62.412 Contracture of muscle, left shoulder

M62.419 **Contracture of muscle, unspecified shoulder**

☑6ᵗʰ M62.42 Contracture of muscle, upper arm

M62.421 Contracture of muscle, right upper arm

M62.422 Contracture of muscle, left upper arm

M62.429 **Contracture of muscle, unspecified upper arm**

☑6ᵗʰ M62.43 Contracture of muscle, forearm

M62.431 Contracture of muscle, right forearm

M62.432 Contracture of muscle, left forearm

M62.439 **Contracture of muscle, unspecified forearm**

☑6ᵗʰ M62.44 Contracture of muscle, hand

M62.441 Contracture of muscle, right hand

M62.442 Contracture of muscle, left hand

M62.449 **Contracture of muscle, unspecified hand**

☑6ᵗʰ M62.45 Contracture of muscle, thigh

M62.451 Contracture of muscle, right thigh

M62.452 Contracture of muscle, left thigh

M62.459 **Contracture of muscle, unspecified thigh**

☑6ᵗʰ M62.46 Contracture of muscle, lower leg

M62.461 Contracture of muscle, right lower leg

M62.462 Contracture of muscle, left lower leg

M62.469 **Contracture of muscle, unspecified lower leg**

☑6ᵗʰ M62.47 Contracture of muscle, ankle and foot

M62.471 Contracture of muscle, right ankle and foot

M62.472 Contracture of muscle, left ankle and foot

M62.479 **Contracture of muscle, unspecified ankle and foot**

M62.48 **Contracture of muscle, other site**

M62.49 **Contracture of muscle, multiple sites**

☑5ᵗʰ M62.5 Muscle wasting and atrophy, not elsewhere classified
Disuse atrophy NEC
EXCLUDES 1   *neuralgic amyotrophy (G54.5)*
progressive muscular atrophy (G12.29)
EXCLUDES 2   *pelvic muscle wasting (N81.84)*

M62.50 **Muscle wasting and atrophy, not elsewhere classified, unspecified site**

☑6ᵗʰ M62.51 Muscle wasting and atrophy, not elsewhere classified, shoulder

M62.511 Muscle wasting and atrophy, not elsewhere classified, right shoulder

M62.512 Muscle wasting and atrophy, not elsewhere classified, left shoulder

M62.519 **Muscle wasting and atrophy, not elsewhere classified, unspecified shoulder**

☑6ᵗʰ M62.52 Muscle wasting and atrophy, not elsewhere classified, upper arm

M62.521 Muscle wasting and atrophy, not elsewhere classified, right upper arm

M62.522 Muscle wasting and atrophy, not elsewhere classified, left upper arm

M62.529 **Muscle wasting and atrophy, not elsewhere classified, unspecified upper arm**

☑6ᵗʰ M62.53 Muscle wasting and atrophy, not elsewhere classified, forearm

M62.531 Muscle wasting and atrophy, not elsewhere classified, right forearm

M62.532 Muscle wasting and atrophy, not elsewhere classified, left forearm

M62.539 **Muscle wasting and atrophy, not elsewhere classified, unspecified forearm**

☑ Additional Character Required   ☑7ᵗʰ Xtension Alert   Unspecified Code   Other Specified Code   Manifestation Code   ▶◀ Revised Text   ● New Code   ▲ Revised Code Title

ICD-10-CM 2014 (Draft)   689

√6ᵗʰ **M62.54 Muscle wasting and atrophy, not elsewhere classified, hand**

     M62.541 Muscle wasting and atrophy, not elsewhere classified, right hand

     M62.542 Muscle wasting and atrophy, not elsewhere classified, left hand

     M62.549 Muscle wasting and atrophy, not elsewhere classified, unspecified hand

√6ᵗʰ **M62.55 Muscle wasting and atrophy, not elsewhere classified, thigh**

     M62.551 Muscle wasting and atrophy, not elsewhere classified, right thigh

     M62.552 Muscle wasting and atrophy, not elsewhere classified, left thigh

     M62.559 Muscle wasting and atrophy, not elsewhere classified, unspecified thigh

√6ᵗʰ **M62.56 Muscle wasting and atrophy, not elsewhere classified, lower leg**

     M62.561 Muscle wasting and atrophy, not elsewhere classified, right lower leg

     M62.562 Muscle wasting and atrophy, not elsewhere classified, left lower leg

     M62.569 Muscle wasting and atrophy, not elsewhere classified, unspecified lower leg

√6ᵗʰ **M62.57 Muscle wasting and atrophy, not elsewhere classified, ankle and foot**

     M62.571 Muscle wasting and atrophy, not elsewhere classified, right ankle and foot

     M62.572 Muscle wasting and atrophy, not elsewhere classified, left ankle and foot

     M62.579 Muscle wasting and atrophy, not elsewhere classified, unspecified ankle and foot

   M62.58 Muscle wasting and atrophy, not elsewhere classified, other site

   M62.59 Muscle wasting and atrophy, not elsewhere classified, multiple sites

√5ᵗʰ **M62.8 Other specified disorders of muscle**

     EXCLUDES 2   *nontraumatic hematoma of muscle (M79.81)*

   M62.81 Muscle weakness (generalized)

   M62.82 Rhabdomyolysis

     EXCLUDES 1   *traumatic rhabdomyolysis (T79.6)*

√6ᵗʰ   **M62.83 Muscle spasm**

     M62.83Ø Muscle spasm of back

     M62.831 Muscle spasm of calf
          Charley-horse

     M62.838 Other muscle spasm

   M62.89 Other specified disorders of muscle
         Muscle (sheath) hernia

   M62.9 Disorder of muscle, unspecified

√4ᵗʰ **M63 Disorders of muscle in diseases classified elsewhere**

     EXCLUDES 1   *myopathy in cysticercosis (B69.81)*
          myopathy in endocrine diseases (G73.7)
          myopathy in metabolic diseases (G73.7)
          myopathy in sarcoidosis (D86.87)
          myopathy in secondary syphilis (A51.49)
          myopathy in syphilis (late) (A52.78)
          myopathy in toxoplasmosis (B58.82)
          myopathy in tuberculosis (A18.Ø9)

     Code first underlying disease, such as:
         leprosy (A3Ø.-)
         neoplasm (C49-, C79.89, D21-, D48.1)
         schistosomiasis (B65.-)
         trichinellosis (B75)

√5ᵗʰ **M63.8 Disorders of muscle in diseases classified elsewhere**

     M63.8Ø *Disorders of muscle in diseases classified elsewhere, unspecified site*

√6ᵗʰ   **M63.81 Disorders of muscle in diseases classified elsewhere, shoulder**

     M63.811 *Disorders of muscle in diseases classified elsewhere, right shoulder*

     M63.812 *Disorders of muscle in diseases classified elsewhere, left shoulder*

     M63.819 *Disorders of muscle in diseases classified elsewhere, unspecified shoulder*

√6ᵗʰ **M63.82 Disorders of muscle in diseases classified elsewhere, upper arm**

     M63.821 *Disorders of muscle in diseases classified elsewhere, right upper arm*

     M63.822 *Disorders of muscle in diseases classified elsewhere, left upper arm*

     M63.829 *Disorders of muscle in diseases classified elsewhere, unspecified upper arm*

√6ᵗʰ **M63.83 Disorders of muscle in diseases classified elsewhere, forearm**

     M63.831 *Disorders of muscle in diseases classified elsewhere, right forearm*

     M63.832 *Disorders of muscle in diseases classified elsewhere, left forearm*

     M63.839 *Disorders of muscle in diseases classified elsewhere, unspecified forearm*

√6ᵗʰ **M63.84 Disorders of muscle in diseases classified elsewhere, hand**

     M63.841 *Disorders of muscle in diseases classified elsewhere, right hand*

     M63.842 *Disorders of muscle in diseases classified elsewhere, left hand*

     M63.849 *Disorders of muscle in diseases classified elsewhere, unspecified hand*

√6ᵗʰ **M63.85 Disorders of muscle in diseases classified elsewhere, thigh**

     M63.851 *Disorders of muscle in diseases classified elsewhere, right thigh*

     M63.852 *Disorders of muscle in diseases classified elsewhere, left thigh*

     M63.859 *Disorders of muscle in diseases classified elsewhere, unspecified thigh*

√6ᵗʰ **M63.86 Disorders of muscle in diseases classified elsewhere, lower leg**

     M63.861 *Disorders of muscle in diseases classified elsewhere, right lower leg*

     M63.862 *Disorders of muscle in diseases classified elsewhere, left lower leg*

     M63.869 *Disorders of muscle in diseases classified elsewhere, unspecified lower leg*

√6ᵗʰ **M63.87 Disorders of muscle in diseases classified elsewhere, ankle and foot**

     M63.871 *Disorders of muscle in diseases classified elsewhere, right ankle and foot*

     M63.872 *Disorders of muscle in diseases classified elsewhere, left ankle and foot*

     M63.879 *Disorders of muscle in diseases classified elsewhere, unspecified ankle and foot*

   M63.88 *Disorders of muscle in diseases classified elsewhere, other site*

   M63.89 *Disorders of muscle in diseases classified elsewhere, multiple sites*

Disorders of synovium and tendon (M65-M67)

√4ᵗʰ **M65 Synovitis and tenosynovitis**

     EXCLUDES 1   *chronic crepitant synovitis of hand and wrist (M7Ø.Ø-)*
          current injury—see injury of ligament or tendon by body region
          soft tissue disorders related to use, overuse and pressure (M7Ø.-)

√5ᵗʰ **M65.Ø Abscess of tendon sheath**

     Use additional code (B95-B96) to identify bacterial agent.

   M65.ØØ Abscess of tendon sheath, unspecified site

√6ᵗʰ   **M65.Ø1 Abscess of tendon sheath, shoulder**

     M65.Ø11 Abscess of tendon sheath, right shoulder

     M65.Ø12 Abscess of tendon sheath, left shoulder

     M65.Ø19 Abscess of tendon sheath, unspecified shoulder

√6ᵗʰ   **M65.Ø2 Abscess of tendon sheath, upper arm**

     M65.Ø21 Abscess of tendon sheath, right upper arm

     M65.Ø22 Abscess of tendon sheath, left upper arm

     M65.Ø29 Abscess of tendon sheath, unspecified upper arm

√6ᵗʰ   **M65.Ø3 Abscess of tendon sheath, forearm**

     M65.Ø31 Abscess of tendon sheath, right forearm

     M65.Ø32 Abscess of tendon sheath, left forearm

     M65.Ø39 Abscess of tendon sheath, unspecified forearm

EXCLUDES 1 Not coded here   EXCLUDES 2 Not included here   N Newborn Age: Ø   P Pediatric Age: Ø-17   M Maternity Age: 12-55   A Adult Age: 15-124

690   ICD-1Ø-CM 2Ø14 (Draft)

☑ 6th **M65.04** Abscess of tendon sheath, hand
  M65.041 Abscess of tendon sheath, right hand
  M65.042 Abscess of tendon sheath, left hand
  M65.049 Abscess of tendon sheath, unspecified hand

☑ 6th **M65.05** Abscess of tendon sheath, thigh
  M65.051 Abscess of tendon sheath, right thigh
  M65.052 Abscess of tendon sheath, left thigh
  M65.059 Abscess of tendon sheath, unspecified thigh

☑ 6th **M65.06** Abscess of tendon sheath, lower leg
  M65.061 Abscess of tendon sheath, right lower leg
  M65.062 Abscess of tendon sheath, left lower leg
  M65.069 Abscess of tendon sheath, unspecified lower leg

☑ 6th **M65.07** Abscess of tendon sheath, ankle and foot
  M65.071 Abscess of tendon sheath, right ankle and foot
  M65.072 Abscess of tendon sheath, left ankle and foot
  M65.079 Abscess of tendon sheath, unspecified ankle and foot

 M65.08 Abscess of tendon sheath, other site

☑ 5th **M65.1** Other infective (teno)synovitis
 M65.10 Other infective (teno)synovitis, unspecified site

☑ 6th **M65.11** Other infective (teno)synovitis, shoulder
  M65.111 Other infective (teno)synovitis, right shoulder
  M65.112 Other infective (teno)synovitis, left shoulder
  M65.119 Other infective (teno)synovitis, unspecified shoulder

☑ 6th **M65.12** Other infective (teno)synovitis, elbow
  M65.121 Other infective (teno)synovitis, right elbow
  M65.122 Other infective (teno)synovitis, left elbow
  M65.129 Other infective (teno)synovitis, unspecified elbow

☑ 6th **M65.13** Other infective (teno)synovitis, wrist
  M65.131 Other infective (teno)synovitis, right wrist
  M65.132 Other infective (teno)synovitis, left wrist
  M65.139 Other infective (teno)synovitis, unspecified wrist

☑ 6th **M65.14** Other infective (teno)synovitis, hand
  M65.141 Other infective (teno)synovitis, right hand
  M65.142 Other infective (teno)synovitis, left hand
  M65.149 Other infective (teno)synovitis, unspecified hand

☑ 6th **M65.15** Other infective (teno)synovitis, hip
  M65.151 Other infective (teno)synovitis, right hip
  M65.152 Other infective (teno)synovitis, left hip
  M65.159 Other infective (teno)synovitis, unspecified hip

☑ 6th **M65.16** Other infective (teno)synovitis, knee
  M65.161 Other infective (teno)synovitis, right knee
  M65.162 Other infective (teno)synovitis, left knee
  M65.169 Other infective (teno)synovitis, unspecified knee

☑ 6th **M65.17** Other infective (teno)synovitis, ankle and foot
  M65.171 Other infective (teno)synovitis, right ankle and foot
  M65.172 Other infective (teno)synovitis, left ankle and foot
  M65.179 Other infective (teno)synovitis, unspecified ankle and foot

 M65.18 Other infective (teno)synovitis, other site
 M65.19 Other infective (teno)synovitis, multiple sites

☑ 5th **M65.2** Calcific tendinitis
  EXCLUDES 1 tendinitis as classified in M75-M77
      calcified tendinitis of shoulder (M75.3)
 M65.20 Calcific tendinitis, unspecified site

☑ 6th **M65.22** Calcific tendinitis, upper arm
  M65.221 Calcific tendinitis, right upper arm
  M65.222 Calcific tendinitis, left upper arm

  M65.229 Calcific tendinitis, unspecified upper arm

☑ 6th **M65.23** Calcific tendinitis, forearm
  M65.231 Calcific tendinitis, right forearm
  M65.232 Calcific tendinitis, left forearm
  M65.239 Calcific tendinitis, unspecified forearm

☑ 6th **M65.24** Calcific tendinitis, hand
  M65.241 Calcific tendinitis, right hand
  M65.242 Calcific tendinitis, left hand
  M65.249 Calcific tendinitis, unspecified hand

☑ 6th **M65.25** Calcific tendinitis, thigh
  M65.251 Calcific tendinitis, right thigh
  M65.252 Calcific tendinitis, left thigh
  M65.259 Calcific tendinitis, unspecified thigh

☑ 6th **M65.26** Calcific tendinitis, lower leg
  M65.261 Calcific tendinitis, right lower leg
  M65.262 Calcific tendinitis, left lower leg
  M65.269 Calcific tendinitis, unspecified lower leg

☑ 6th **M65.27** Calcific tendinitis, ankle and foot
  M65.271 Calcific tendinitis, right ankle and foot
  M65.272 Calcific tendinitis, left ankle and foot
  M65.279 Calcific tendinitis, unspecified ankle and foot

 M65.28 Calcific tendinitis, other site
 M65.29 Calcific tendinitis, multiple sites

M65.3 Trigger finger
  Nodular tendinous disease
 M65.30 Trigger finger, unspecified finger

☑ 6th **M65.31** Trigger thumb
  M65.311 Trigger thumb, right thumb
  M65.312 Trigger thumb, left thumb
  M65.319 Trigger thumb, unspecified thumb

☑ 6th **M65.32** Trigger finger, index finger
  M65.321 Trigger finger, right index finger
  M65.322 Trigger finger, left index finger
  M65.329 Trigger finger, unspecified index finger

☑ 6th **M65.33** Trigger finger, middle finger
  M65.331 Trigger finger, right middle finger
  M65.332 Trigger finger, left middle finger
  M65.339 Trigger finger, unspecified middle finger

☑ 6th **M65.34** Trigger finger, ring finger
  M65.341 Trigger finger, right ring finger
  M65.342 Trigger finger, left ring finger
  M65.349 Trigger finger, unspecified ring finger

☑ 6th **M65.35** Trigger finger, little finger
  M65.351 Trigger finger, right little finger
  M65.352 Trigger finger, left little finger
  M65.359 Trigger finger, unspecified little finger

M65.4 Radial styloid tenosynovitis [de Quervain]

☑ 5th **M65.8** Other synovitis and tenosynovitis
 M65.80 Other synovitis and tenosynovitis, unspecified site

☑ 6th **M65.81** Other synovitis and tenosynovitis, shoulder
  M65.811 Other synovitis and tenosynovitis, right shoulder
  M65.812 Other synovitis and tenosynovitis, left shoulder
  M65.819 Other synovitis and tenosynovitis, unspecified shoulder

☑ 6th **M65.82** Other synovitis and tenosynovitis, upper arm
  M65.821 Other synovitis and tenosynovitis, right upper arm
  M65.822 Other synovitis and tenosynovitis, left upper arm
  M65.829 Other synovitis and tenosynovitis, unspecified upper arm

☑ 6th **M65.83** Other synovitis and tenosynovitis, forearm
  M65.831 Other synovitis and tenosynovitis, right forearm
  M65.832 Other synovitis and tenosynovitis, left forearm
  M65.839 Other synovitis and tenosynovitis, unspecified forearm

✓6ᵗʰ **M65.84 Other synovitis and tenosynovitis,** hand
    M65.841 Other synovitis and tenosynovitis, right hand
    M65.842 Other synovitis and tenosynovitis, left hand
    M65.849 Other synovitis and tenosynovitis, unspecified hand

✓6ᵗʰ **M65.85 Other synovitis and tenosynovitis,** thigh
    M65.851 Other synovitis and tenosynovitis, right thigh
    M65.852 Other synovitis and tenosynovitis, left thigh
    M65.859 Other synovitis and tenosynovitis, unspecified thigh

✓6ᵗʰ **M65.86 Other synovitis and tenosynovitis,** lower leg
    M65.861 Other synovitis and tenosynovitis, right **lower leg**
    M65.862 Other synovitis and tenosynovitis, left **lower leg**
    M65.869 Other synovitis and tenosynovitis, unspecified lower leg

✓6ᵗʰ **M65.87 Other synovitis and tenosynovitis,** ankle and foot
    M65.871 Other synovitis and tenosynovitis, right **ankle and foot**
    M65.872 Other synovitis and tenosynovitis, left **ankle and foot**
    M65.879 Other synovitis and tenosynovitis, unspecified ankle and foot

M65.88 Other synovitis and tenosynovitis, other site
M65.89 Other synovitis and tenosynovitis, multiple sites

M65.9 Synovitis and tenosynovitis, unspecified

✓4ᵗʰ **M66 Spontaneous rupture of synovium and tendon**
    INCLUDES rupture that occurs when a normal force is applied to tissues that are inferred to have less than normal strength
    EXCLUDES 2 rotator cuff syndrome (M75.1-)
    rupture where an abnormal force is applied to normal tissue—see injury of tendon by body region

M66.0 Rupture of popliteal cyst

✓5ᵗʰ **M66.1 Rupture of** synovium
    Rupture of synovial cyst
    EXCLUDES 2 rupture of popliteal cyst (M66.0)

    M66.10 Rupture of synovium, unspecified joint

✓6ᵗʰ **M66.11 Rupture of synovium,** shoulder
    M66.111 Rupture of synovium, right **shoulder**
    M66.112 Rupture of synovium, left **shoulder**
    M66.119 Rupture of synovium, unspecified shoulder

✓6ᵗʰ **M66.12 Rupture of synovium,** elbow
    M66.121 Rupture of synovium, right **elbow**
    M66.122 Rupture of synovium, left **elbow**
    M66.129 Rupture of synovium, unspecified elbow

✓6ᵗʰ **M66.13 Rupture of synovium,** wrist
    M66.131 Rupture of synovium, right **wrist**
    M66.132 Rupture of synovium, left **wrist**
    M66.139 Rupture of synovium, unspecified wrist

✓6ᵗʰ **M66.14 Rupture of synovium,** hand and fingers
    M66.141 Rupture of synovium, right hand
    M66.142 Rupture of synovium, left hand
    M66.143 Rupture of synovium, unspecified hand
    M66.144 Rupture of synovium, right finger(s)
    M66.145 Rupture of synovium, left finger(s)
    M66.146 Rupture of synovium, unspecified finger(s)

✓6ᵗʰ **M66.15 Rupture of synovium,** hip
    M66.151 Rupture of synovium, right **hip**
    M66.152 Rupture of synovium, left **hip**
    M66.159 Rupture of synovium, unspecified hip

✓6ᵗʰ **M66.17 Rupture of synovium,** ankle, foot and toes
    M66.171 Rupture of synovium, right ankle
    M66.172 Rupture of synovium, left ankle
    M66.173 Rupture of synovium, unspecified ankle
    M66.174 Rupture of synovium, right foot
    M66.175 Rupture of synovium, left foot
    M66.176 Rupture of synovium, unspecified foot

    M66.177 Rupture of synovium, right toe(s)
    M66.178 Rupture of synovium, left toe(s)
    M66.179 Rupture of synovium, unspecified toe(s)

    M66.18 Rupture of synovium, other site

✓5ᵗʰ **M66.2 Spontaneous rupture of** extensor tendons
    M66.20 Spontaneous rupture of extensor tendons, unspecified site

✓6ᵗʰ **M66.21 Spontaneous rupture of extensor tendons,** shoulder
    M66.211 Spontaneous rupture of extensor tendons, right **shoulder**
    M66.212 Spontaneous rupture of extensor tendons, left **shoulder**
    M66.219 Spontaneous rupture of extensor tendons, unspecified shoulder

✓6ᵗʰ **M66.22 Spontaneous rupture of extensor tendons,** upper arm
    M66.221 Spontaneous rupture of extensor tendons, right **upper arm**
    M66.222 Spontaneous rupture of extensor tendons, left **upper arm**
    M66.229 Spontaneous rupture of extensor tendons, unspecified upper arm

✓6ᵗʰ **M66.23 Spontaneous rupture of extensor tendons,** forearm
    M66.231 Spontaneous rupture of extensor tendons, right **forearm**
    M66.232 Spontaneous rupture of extensor tendons, left **forearm**
    M66.239 Spontaneous rupture of extensor tendons, unspecified forearm

✓6ᵗʰ **M66.24 Spontaneous rupture of extensor tendons,** hand
    M66.241 Spontaneous rupture of extensor tendons, right **hand**
    M66.242 Spontaneous rupture of extensor tendons, left **hand**
    M66.249 Spontaneous rupture of extensor tendons, unspecified hand

✓6ᵗʰ **M66.25 Spontaneous rupture of extensor tendons,** thigh
    M66.251 Spontaneous rupture of extensor tendons, right **thigh**
    M66.252 Spontaneous rupture of extensor tendons, left **thigh**
    M66.259 Spontaneous rupture of extensor tendons, unspecified thigh

✓6ᵗʰ **M66.26 Spontaneous rupture of extensor tendons,** lower leg
    M66.261 Spontaneous rupture of extensor tendons, right **lower leg**
    M66.262 Spontaneous rupture of extensor tendons, left **lower leg**
    M66.269 Spontaneous rupture of extensor tendons, unspecified lower leg

✓6ᵗʰ **M66.27 Spontaneous rupture of extensor tendons,** ankle and foot
    M66.271 Spontaneous rupture of extensor tendons, right **ankle and foot**
    M66.272 Spontaneous rupture of extensor tendons, left **ankle and foot**
    M66.279 Spontaneous rupture of extensor tendons, unspecified ankle and foot

    M66.28 Spontaneous rupture of extensor tendons, other site
    M66.29 Spontaneous rupture of extensor tendons, multiple sites

✓5ᵗʰ **M66.3 Spontaneous rupture of** flexor tendons
    M66.30 Spontaneous rupture of flexor tendons, unspecified site

✓6ᵗʰ **M66.31 Spontaneous rupture of flexor tendons,** shoulder
    M66.311 Spontaneous rupture of flexor tendons, right **shoulder**
    M66.312 Spontaneous rupture of flexor tendons, left **shoulder**
    M66.319 Spontaneous rupture of flexor tendons, unspecified shoulder

✓6ᵗʰ **M66.32 Spontaneous rupture of flexor tendons,** upper arm
    M66.321 Spontaneous rupture of flexor tendons, right **upper arm**
    M66.322 Spontaneous rupture of flexor tendons, left **upper arm**

EXCLUDES 1 Not coded here   **EXCLUDES 2** Not included here   N Newborn Age: 0   P Pediatric Age: 0-17   M Maternity Age: 12-55   A Adult Age: 15-124

692   ICD-10-CM 2014 (Draft)

M66.329 Spontaneous rupture of flexor tendons, unspecified upper arm

✓6ᵗʰ **M66.33** Spontaneous rupture of flexor tendons, forearm

     M66.331 Spontaneous rupture of flexor tendons, right forearm

     M66.332 Spontaneous rupture of flexor tendons, left forearm

     M66.339 Spontaneous rupture of flexor tendons, unspecified forearm

✓6ᵗʰ **M66.34** Spontaneous rupture of flexor tendons, hand

     M66.341 Spontaneous rupture of flexor tendons, right hand

     M66.342 Spontaneous rupture of flexor tendons, left hand

     M66.349 Spontaneous rupture of flexor tendons, unspecified hand

✓6ᵗʰ **M66.35** Spontaneous rupture of flexor tendons, thigh

     M66.351 Spontaneous rupture of flexor tendons, right thigh

     M66.352 Spontaneous rupture of flexor tendons, left thigh

     M66.359 Spontaneous rupture of flexor tendons, unspecified thigh

✓6ᵗʰ **M66.36** Spontaneous rupture of flexor tendons, lower leg

     M66.361 Spontaneous rupture of flexor tendons, right lower leg

     M66.362 Spontaneous rupture of flexor tendons, left lower leg

     M66.369 Spontaneous rupture of flexor tendons, unspecified lower leg

✓6ᵗʰ **M66.37** Spontaneous rupture of flexor tendons, ankle and foot

     M66.371 Spontaneous rupture of flexor tendons, right ankle and foot

     M66.372 Spontaneous rupture of flexor tendons, left ankle and foot

     M66.379 Spontaneous rupture of flexor tendons, unspecified ankle and foot

     M66.38 Spontaneous rupture of flexor tendons, other site

     M66.39 Spontaneous rupture of flexor tendons, multiple sites

✓5ᵗʰ **M66.8** Spontaneous rupture of other tendons

     M66.80 Spontaneous rupture of other tendons, unspecified site

✓6ᵗʰ **M66.81** Spontaneous rupture of other tendons, shoulder

     M66.811 Spontaneous rupture of other tendons, right shoulder

     M66.812 Spontaneous rupture of other tendons, left shoulder

     M66.819 Spontaneous rupture of other tendons, unspecified shoulder

✓6ᵗʰ **M66.82** Spontaneous rupture of other tendons, upper arm

     M66.821 Spontaneous rupture of other tendons, right upper arm

     M66.822 Spontaneous rupture of other tendons, left upper arm

     M66.829 Spontaneous rupture of other tendons, unspecified upper arm

✓6ᵗʰ **M66.83** Spontaneous rupture of other tendons, forearm

     M66.831 Spontaneous rupture of other tendons, right forearm

     M66.832 Spontaneous rupture of other tendons, left forearm

     M66.839 Spontaneous rupture of other tendons, unspecified forearm

✓6ᵗʰ **M66.84** Spontaneous rupture of other tendons, hand

     M66.841 Spontaneous rupture of other tendons, right hand

     M66.842 Spontaneous rupture of other tendons, left hand

     M66.849 Spontaneous rupture of other tendons, unspecified hand

✓6ᵗʰ **M66.85** Spontaneous rupture of other tendons, thigh

     M66.851 Spontaneous rupture of other tendons, right thigh

     M66.852 Spontaneous rupture of other tendons, left thigh

     M66.859 Spontaneous rupture of other tendons, unspecified thigh

✓6ᵗʰ **M66.86** Spontaneous rupture of other tendons, lower leg

     M66.861 Spontaneous rupture of other tendons, right lower leg

     M66.862 Spontaneous rupture of other tendons, left lower leg

     M66.869 Spontaneous rupture of other tendons, unspecified lower leg

✓6ᵗʰ **M66.87** Spontaneous rupture of other tendons, ankle and foot

     M66.871 Spontaneous rupture of other tendons, right ankle and foot

     M66.872 Spontaneous rupture of other tendons, left ankle and foot

     M66.879 Spontaneous rupture of other tendons, unspecified ankle and foot

     M66.88 Spontaneous rupture of other tendons, other

     M66.89 Spontaneous rupture of other tendons, multiple sites

M66.9 Spontaneous rupture of unspecified tendon
     Rupture at musculotendinous junction, nontraumatic

✓4ᵗʰ **M67** **Other disorders of synovium and tendon**
     EXCLUDES 1   *palmar fascial fibromatosis [Dupuytren] (M72.0)*
               tendinitis NOS (M77.9-)
               xanthomatosis localized to tendons (E78.2)

✓5ᵗʰ **M67.0** Short Achilles tendon (acquired)

     M67.00 Short Achilles tendon (acquired), unspecified ankle

     M67.01 Short Achilles tendon (acquired), right ankle

     M67.02 Short Achilles tendon (acquired), left ankle

✓5ᵗʰ **M67.2** Synovial hypertrophy, not elsewhere classified
     EXCLUDES 1   *villonodular synovitis (pigmented) (M12.2-)*

     M67.20 Synovial hypertrophy, not elsewhere classified, unspecified site

✓6ᵗʰ **M67.21** Synovial hypertrophy, not elsewhere classified, shoulder

     M67.211 Synovial hypertrophy, not elsewhere classified, right shoulder

     M67.212 Synovial hypertrophy, not elsewhere classified, left shoulder

     M67.219 Synovial hypertrophy, not elsewhere classified, unspecified shoulder

✓6ᵗʰ **M67.22** Synovial hypertrophy, not elsewhere classified, upper arm

     M67.221 Synovial hypertrophy, not elsewhere classified, right upper arm

     M67.222 Synovial hypertrophy, not elsewhere classified, left upper arm

     M67.229 Synovial hypertrophy, not elsewhere classified, unspecified upper arm

✓6ᵗʰ **M67.23** Synovial hypertrophy, not elsewhere classified, forearm

     M67.231 Synovial hypertrophy, not elsewhere classified, right forearm

     M67.232 Synovial hypertrophy, not elsewhere classified, left forearm

     M67.239 Synovial hypertrophy, not elsewhere classified, unspecified forearm

✓6ᵗʰ **M67.24** Synovial hypertrophy, not elsewhere classified, hand

     M67.241 Synovial hypertrophy, not elsewhere classified, right hand

     M67.242 Synovial hypertrophy, not elsewhere classified, left hand

     M67.249 Synovial hypertrophy, not elsewhere classified, unspecified hand

✓6ᵗʰ **M67.25** Synovial hypertrophy, not elsewhere classified, thigh

     M67.251 Synovial hypertrophy, not elsewhere classified, right thigh

     M67.252 Synovial hypertrophy, not elsewhere classified, left thigh

     M67.259 Synovial hypertrophy, not elsewhere classified, unspecified thigh

☑ Additional Character Required   ✓x7ᵗʰ Xtension Alert   Unspecified Code   Other Specified Code   Manifestation Code   ►◄ Revised Text   ● New Code   ▲ Revised Code Title

ICD-10-CM 2014 (Draft)   **693**

√6ᵗʰ **M67.26 Synovial hypertrophy, not elsewhere classified, lower leg**
    M67.261 Synovial hypertrophy, not elsewhere classified, right lower leg
    M67.262 Synovial hypertrophy, not elsewhere classified, left lower leg
    M67.269 Synovial hypertrophy, not elsewhere classified, unspecified lower leg

√6ᵗʰ **M67.27 Synovial hypertrophy, not elsewhere classified, ankle and foot**
    M67.271 Synovial hypertrophy, not elsewhere classified, right ankle and foot
    M67.272 Synovial hypertrophy, not elsewhere classified, left ankle and foot
    M67.279 Synovial hypertrophy, not elsewhere classified, unspecified ankle and foot

    M67.28 Synovial hypertrophy, not elsewhere classified, other site
    M67.29 Synovial hypertrophy, not elsewhere classified, multiple sites

√5ᵗʰ **M67.3 Transient synovitis**
    Toxic synovitis
    EXCLUDES 1   palindromic rheumatism (M12.3-)

    M67.30 Transient synovitis, unspecified site

√6ᵗʰ **M67.31 Transient synovitis, shoulder**
    M67.311 Transient synovitis, right shoulder
    M67.312 Transient synovitis, left shoulder
    M67.319 Transient synovitis, unspecified shoulder

√6ᵗʰ **M67.32 Transient synovitis, elbow**
    M67.321 Transient synovitis, right elbow
    M67.322 Transient synovitis, left elbow
    M67.329 Transient synovitis, unspecified elbow

√6ᵗʰ **M67.33 Transient synovitis, wrist**
    M67.331 Transient synovitis, right wrist
    M67.332 Transient synovitis, left wrist
    M67.339 Transient synovitis, unspecified wrist

√6ᵗʰ **M67.34 Transient synovitis, hand**
    M67.341 Transient synovitis, right hand
    M67.342 Transient synovitis, left hand
    M67.349 Transient synovitis, unspecified hand

√6ᵗʰ **M67.35 Transient synovitis, hip**
    M67.351 Transient synovitis, right hip
    M67.352 Transient synovitis, left hip
    M67.359 Transient synovitis, unspecified hip

√6ᵗʰ **M67.36 Transient synovitis, knee**
    M67.361 Transient synovitis, right knee
    M67.362 Transient synovitis, left knee
    M67.369 Transient synovitis, unspecified knee

√6ᵗʰ **M67.37 Transient synovitis, ankle and foot**
    M67.371 Transient synovitis, right ankle and foot
    M67.372 Transient synovitis, left ankle and foot
    M67.379 Transient synovitis, unspecified ankle and foot

    M67.38 Transient synovitis, other site
    M67.39 Transient synovitis, multiple sites

√5ᵗʰ **M67.4 Ganglion**
    Ganglion of joint or tendon (sheath)
    EXCLUDES 1   ganglion in yaws (A66.6)
    EXCLUDES 2   cyst of bursa (M71.2-M71.3)
             cyst of synovium (M71.2-M71.3)

    M67.40 Ganglion, unspecified site

√6ᵗʰ **M67.41 Ganglion, shoulder**
    M67.411 Ganglion, right shoulder
    M67.412 Ganglion, left shoulder
    M67.419 Ganglion, unspecified shoulder

√6ᵗʰ **M67.42 Ganglion, elbow**
    M67.421 Ganglion, right elbow
    M67.422 Ganglion, left elbow
    M67.429 Ganglion, unspecified elbow

√6ᵗʰ **M67.43 Ganglion, wrist**
    M67.431 Ganglion, right wrist
    M67.432 Ganglion, left wrist
    M67.439 Ganglion, unspecified wrist

√6ᵗʰ **M67.44 Ganglion, hand**
    M67.441 Ganglion, right hand
    M67.442 Ganglion, left hand
    M67.449 Ganglion, unspecified hand

√6ᵗʰ **M67.45 Ganglion, hip**
    M67.451 Ganglion, right hip
    M67.452 Ganglion, left hip
    M67.459 Ganglion, unspecified hip

√6ᵗʰ **M67.46 Ganglion, knee**
    M67.461 Ganglion, right knee
    M67.462 Ganglion, left knee
    M67.469 Ganglion, unspecified knee

√6ᵗʰ **M67.47 Ganglion, ankle and foot**
    M67.471 Ganglion, right ankle and foot
    M67.472 Ganglion, left ankle and foot
    M67.479 Ganglion, unspecified ankle and foot

    M67.48 Ganglion, other site
    M67.49 Ganglion, multiple sites

√5ᵗʰ **M67.5 Plica syndrome**
    Plica knee
    M67.50 Plica syndrome, unspecified knee
    M67.51 Plica syndrome, right knee
    M67.52 Plica syndrome, left knee

√5ᵗʰ **M67.8 Other specified disorders of synovium and tendon**
    M67.80 Other specified disorders of synovium and tendon, unspecified site

√6ᵗʰ **M67.81 Other specified disorders of synovium and tendon, shoulder**
    M67.811 Other specified disorders of synovium, right shoulder
    M67.812 Other specified disorders of synovium, left shoulder
    M67.813 Other specified disorders of tendon, right shoulder
    M67.814 Other specified disorders of tendon, left shoulder
    M67.819 Other specified disorders of synovium and tendon, unspecified shoulder

√6ᵗʰ **M67.82 Other specified disorders of synovium and tendon, elbow**
    M67.821 Other specified disorders of synovium, right elbow
    M67.822 Other specified disorders of synovium, left elbow
    M67.823 Other specified disorders of tendon, right elbow
    M67.824 Other specified disorders of tendon, left elbow
    M67.829 Other specified disorders of synovium and tendon, unspecified elbow

√6ᵗʰ **M67.83 Other specified disorders of synovium and tendon, wrist**
    M67.831 Other specified disorders of synovium, right wrist
    M67.832 Other specified disorders of synovium, left wrist
    M67.833 Other specified disorders of tendon, right wrist
    M67.834 Other specified disorders of tendon, left wrist
    M67.839 Other specified disorders of synovium and tendon, unspecified forearm

√6ᵗʰ **M67.84 Other specified disorders of synovium and tendon, hand**
    M67.841 Other specified disorders of synovium, right hand
    M67.842 Other specified disorders of synovium, left hand
    M67.843 Other specified disorders of tendon, right hand
    M67.844 Other specified disorders of tendon, left hand
    M67.849 Other specified disorders of synovium and tendon, unspecified hand

EXCLUDES 1 Not coded here   EXCLUDES 2 Not included here   N Newborn Age: 0   P Pediatric Age: 0-17   M Maternity Age: 12-55   A Adult Age: 15-124

694   ICD-10-CM 2014 (Draft)

✓6ᵗʰ **M67.85** Other specified disorders of synovium and tendon, hip

    M67.851 Other specified disorders of synovium, right hip

    M67.852 Other specified disorders of synovium, left hip

    M67.853 Other specified disorders of tendon, right hip

    M67.854 Other specified disorders of tendon, left hip

    M67.859 Other specified disorders of synovium and tendon, unspecified hip

✓6ᵗʰ **M67.86** Other specified disorders of synovium and tendon, knee

    M67.861 Other specified disorders of synovium, right knee

    M67.862 Other specified disorders of synovium, left knee

    M67.863 Other specified disorders of tendon, right knee

    M67.864 Other specified disorders of tendon, left knee

    M67.869 Other specified disorders of synovium and tendon, unspecified knee

✓6ᵗʰ **M67.87** Other specified disorders of synovium and tendon, ankle and foot

    M67.871 Other specified disorders of synovium, right ankle and foot

    M67.872 Other specified disorders of synovium, left ankle and foot

    M67.873 Other specified disorders of tendon, right ankle and foot

    M67.874 Other specified disorders of tendon, left ankle and foot

    M67.879 Other specified disorders of synovium and tendon, unspecified ankle and foot

    M67.88 Other specified disorders of synovium and tendon, other site

    M67.89 Other specified disorders of synovium and tendon, multiple sites

✓5ᵗʰ **M67.9** Unspecified disorder of synovium and tendon

    M67.90 Unspecified disorder of synovium and tendon, unspecified site

✓6ᵗʰ **M67.91** Unspecified disorder of synovium and tendon, shoulder

    M67.911 Unspecified disorder of synovium and tendon, right shoulder

    M67.912 Unspecified disorder of synovium and tendon, left shoulder

    M67.919 Unspecified disorder of synovium and tendon, unspecified shoulder

✓6ᵗʰ **M67.92** Unspecified disorder of synovium and tendon, upper arm

    M67.921 Unspecified disorder of synovium and tendon, right upper arm

    M67.922 Unspecified disorder of synovium and tendon, left upper arm

    M67.929 Unspecified disorder of synovium and tendon, unspecified upper arm

✓6ᵗʰ **M67.93** Unspecified disorder of synovium and tendon, forearm

    M67.931 Unspecified disorder of synovium and tendon, right forearm

    M67.932 Unspecified disorder of synovium and tendon, left forearm

    M67.939 Unspecified disorder of synovium and tendon, unspecified forearm

✓6ᵗʰ **M67.94** Unspecified disorder of synovium and tendon, hand

    M67.941 Unspecified disorder of synovium and tendon, right hand

    M67.942 Unspecified disorder of synovium and tendon, left hand

    M67.949 Unspecified disorder of synovium and tendon, unspecified hand

✓6ᵗʰ **M67.95** Unspecified disorder of synovium and tendon, thigh

    M67.951 Unspecified disorder of synovium and tendon, right thigh

    M67.952 Unspecified disorder of synovium and tendon, left thigh

    M67.959 Unspecified disorder of synovium and tendon, unspecified thigh

✓6ᵗʰ **M67.96** Unspecified disorder of synovium and tendon, lower leg

    M67.961 Unspecified disorder of synovium and tendon, right lower leg

    M67.962 Unspecified disorder of synovium and tendon, left lower leg

    M67.969 Unspecified disorder of synovium and tendon, unspecified lower leg

✓6ᵗʰ **M67.97** Unspecified disorder of synovium and tendon, ankle and foot

    M67.971 Unspecified disorder of synovium and tendon, right ankle and foot

    M67.972 Unspecified disorder of synovium and tendon, left ankle and foot

    M67.979 Unspecified disorder of synovium and tendon, unspecified ankle and foot

    M67.98 Unspecified disorder of synovium and tendon, other site

    M67.99 Unspecified disorder of synovium and tendon, multiple sites

Other soft tissue disorders (M70-M79)

✓4ᵗʰ **M70 Soft tissue disorders related to use, overuse and pressure**

    INCLUDES soft tissue disorders of occupational origin

    EXCLUDES 1 bursitis NOS (M71.9-)

    EXCLUDES 2 bursitis of shoulder (M75.5)
         enthesopathies (M76-M77)
         pressure ulcer (pressure area) (L89.-)

    Use additional external cause code to identify activity causing disorder (Y93.-)

✓5ᵗʰ **M70.0** Crepitant synovitis (acute) (chronic) of hand and wrist

✓6ᵗʰ   **M70.03** Crepitant synovitis (acute) (chronic), wrist

    M70.031 Crepitant synovitis (acute) (chronic), right wrist

    M70.032 Crepitant synovitis (acute) (chronic), left wrist

    M70.039 Crepitant synovitis (acute) (chronic), unspecified wrist

✓6ᵗʰ   **M70.04** Crepitant synovitis (acute) (chronic), hand

    M70.041 Crepitant synovitis (acute) (chronic), right hand

    M70.042 Crepitant synovitis (acute) (chronic), left hand

    M70.049 Crepitant synovitis (acute) (chronic), unspecified hand

✓5ᵗʰ **M70.1** Bursitis of hand

    M70.10 Bursitis, unspecified hand

    M70.11 Bursitis, right hand

    M70.12 Bursitis, left hand

✓5ᵗʰ **M70.2** Olecranon bursitis

    M70.20 Olecranon bursitis, unspecified elbow

    M70.21 Olecranon bursitis, right elbow

    M70.22 Olecranon bursitis, left elbow

✓5ᵗʰ **M70.3** Other bursitis of elbow

    M70.30 Other bursitis of elbow, unspecified elbow

    M70.31 Other bursitis of elbow, right elbow

    M70.32 Other bursitis of elbow, left elbow

✓5ᵗʰ **M70.4** Prepatellar bursitis

    M70.40 Prepatellar bursitis, unspecified knee

    M70.41 Prepatellar bursitis, right knee

    M70.42 Prepatellar bursitis, left knee

✓5ᵗʰ **M70.5** Other bursitis of knee

    M70.50 Other bursitis of knee, unspecified knee

    M70.51 Other bursitis of knee, right knee

    M70.52 Other bursitis of knee, left knee

✓5ᵗʰ **M70.6** Trochanteric bursitis

    Trochanteric tendinitis

    M70.60 Trochanteric bursitis, unspecified hip

    M70.61 Trochanteric bursitis, right hip

    M70.62 Trochanteric bursitis, left hip

☑ Additional Character Required   ✓x7ᵗʰ Xtension Alert   Unspecified Code   Other Specified Code   Manifestation Code   ▶◀ Revised Text   ● New Code   ▲ Revised Code Title

ICD-10-CM 2014 (Draft)   **695**

✓5ᵗʰ **M70.7 Other bursitis of hip**
Ischial bursitis

    M70.70 Other bursitis of hip, unspecified hip

    M70.71 Other bursitis of hip, right hip

    M70.72 Other bursitis of hip, left hip

✓5ᵗʰ **M70.8 Other soft tissue disorders related to use, overuse and pressure**

    M70.80 Other soft tissue disorders related to use, overuse and pressure of unspecified site

  ✓6ᵗʰ **M70.81 Other soft tissue disorders related to use, overuse and pressure of shoulder**

    M70.811 Other soft tissue disorders related to use, overuse and pressure, right shoulder

    M70.812 Other soft tissue disorders related to use, overuse and pressure, left shoulder

    M70.819 Other soft tissue disorders related to use, overuse and pressure, unspecified shoulder

  ✓6ᵗʰ **M70.82 Other soft tissue disorders related to use, overuse and pressure of upper arm**

    M70.821 Other soft tissue disorders related to use, overuse and pressure, right upper arm

    M70.822 Other soft tissue disorders related to use, overuse and pressure, left upper arm

    M70.829 Other soft tissue disorders related to use, overuse and pressure, unspecified upper arms

  ✓6ᵗʰ **M70.83 Other soft tissue disorders related to use, overuse and pressure of forearm**

    M70.831 Other soft tissue disorders related to use, overuse and pressure, right forearm

    M70.832 Other soft tissue disorders related to use, overuse and pressure, left forearm

    M70.839 Other soft tissue disorders related to use, overuse and pressure, unspecified forearm

  ✓6ᵗʰ **M70.84 Other soft tissue disorders related to use, overuse and pressure of hand**

    M70.841 Other soft tissue disorders related to use, overuse and pressure, right hand

    M70.842 Other soft tissue disorders related to use, overuse and pressure, left hand

    M70.849 Other soft tissue disorders related to use, overuse and pressure, unspecified hand

  ✓6ᵗʰ **M70.85 Other soft tissue disorders related to use, overuse and pressure of thigh**

    M70.851 Other soft tissue disorders related to use, overuse and pressure, right thigh

    M70.852 Other soft tissue disorders related to use, overuse and pressure, left thigh

    M70.859 Other soft tissue disorders related to use, overuse and pressure, unspecified thigh

  ✓6ᵗʰ **M70.86 Other soft tissue disorders related to use, overuse and pressure lower leg**

    M70.861 Other soft tissue disorders related to use, overuse and pressure, right lower leg

    M70.862 Other soft tissue disorders related to use, overuse and pressure, left lower leg

    M70.869 Other soft tissue disorders related to use, overuse and pressure, unspecified leg

  ✓6ᵗʰ **M70.87 Other soft tissue disorders related to use, overuse and pressure of ankle and foot**

    M70.871 Other soft tissue disorders related to use, overuse and pressure, right ankle and foot

    M70.872 Other soft tissue disorders related to use, overuse and pressure, left ankle and foot

    M70.879 Other soft tissue disorders related to use, overuse and pressure, unspecified ankle and foot

    M70.88 Other soft tissue disorders related to use, overuse and pressure other site

    M70.89 Other soft tissue disorders related to use, overuse and pressure multiple sites

✓5ᵗʰ **M70.9 Unspecified soft tissue disorder related to use, overuse and pressure**

    M70.90 Unspecified soft tissue disorder related to use, overuse and pressure of unspecified site

  ✓6ᵗʰ **M70.91 Unspecified soft tissue disorder related to use, overuse and pressure of shoulder**

    M70.911 Unspecified soft tissue disorder related to use, overuse and pressure, right shoulder

    M70.912 Unspecified soft tissue disorder related to use, overuse and pressure, left shoulder

    M70.919 Unspecified soft tissue disorder related to use, overuse and pressure, unspecified shoulder

  ✓6ᵗʰ **M70.92 Unspecified soft tissue disorder related to use, overuse and pressure of upper arm**

    M70.921 Unspecified soft tissue disorder related to use, overuse and pressure, right upper arm

    M70.922 Unspecified soft tissue disorder related to use, overuse and pressure, left upper arm

    M70.929 Unspecified soft tissue disorder related to use, overuse and pressure, unspecified upper arm

  ✓6ᵗʰ **M70.93 Unspecified soft tissue disorder related to use, overuse and pressure of forearm**

    M70.931 Unspecified soft tissue disorder related to use, overuse and pressure, right forearm

    M70.932 Unspecified soft tissue disorder related to use, overuse and pressure, left forearm

    M70.939 Unspecified soft tissue disorder related to use, overuse and pressure, unspecified forearm

  ✓6ᵗʰ **M70.94 Unspecified soft tissue disorder related to use, overuse and pressure of hand**

    M70.941 Unspecified soft tissue disorder related to use, overuse and pressure, right hand

    M70.942 Unspecified soft tissue disorder related to use, overuse and pressure, left hand

    M70.949 Unspecified soft tissue disorder related to use, overuse and pressure, unspecified hand

  ✓6ᵗʰ **M70.95 Unspecified soft tissue disorder related to use, overuse and pressure of thigh**

    M70.951 Unspecified soft tissue disorder related to use, overuse and pressure, right thigh

    M70.952 Unspecified soft tissue disorder related to use, overuse and pressure, left thigh

    M70.959 Unspecified soft tissue disorder related to use, overuse and pressure, unspecified thigh

  ✓6ᵗʰ **M70.96 Unspecified soft tissue disorder related to use, overuse and pressure lower leg**

    M70.961 Unspecified soft tissue disorder related to use, overuse and pressure, right lower leg

    M70.962 Unspecified soft tissue disorder related to use, overuse and pressure, left lower leg

    M70.969 Unspecified soft tissue disorder related to use, overuse and pressure, unspecified lower leg

  ✓6ᵗʰ **M70.97 Unspecified soft tissue disorder related to use, overuse and pressure of ankle and foot**

    M70.971 Unspecified soft tissue disorder related to use, overuse and pressure, right ankle and foot

    M70.972 Unspecified soft tissue disorder related to use, overuse and pressure, left ankle and foot

    M70.979 Unspecified soft tissue disorder related to use, overuse and pressure, unspecified ankle and foot

    M70.98 Unspecified soft tissue disorder related to use, overuse and pressure other

    M70.99 Unspecified soft tissue disorder related to use, overuse and pressure multiple sites

✓4ᵗʰ **M71 Other bursopathies**

    EXCLUDES 1 bunion (M20.1)
bursitis related to use, overuse or pressure (M70.-)
enthesopathies (M76-M77)

✓5ᵗʰ **M71.0 Abscess of bursa**
Use additional code (B95.-, B96.-) to identify causative organism

    M71.00 Abscess of bursa, unspecified site

EXCLUDES 1 Not coded here   **EXCLUDES 2** Not included here   **N** Newborn Age: 0   **P** Pediatric Age: 0-17   **M** Maternity Age: 12-55   **A** Adult Age: 15-124

696   ICD-10-CM 2014 (Draft)

√6th **M71.01** Abscess of bursa, shoulder
    M71.011 Abscess of bursa, right shoulder
    M71.012 Abscess of bursa, left shoulder
    M71.019 Abscess of bursa, unspecified shoulder

√6th **M71.02** Abscess of bursa, elbow
    M71.021 Abscess of bursa, right elbow
    M71.022 Abscess of bursa, left elbow
    M71.029 Abscess of bursa, unspecified elbow

√6th **M71.03** Abscess of bursa, wrist
    M71.031 Abscess of bursa, right wrist
    M71.032 Abscess of bursa, left wrist
    M71.039 Abscess of bursa, unspecified wrist

√6th **M71.04** Abscess of bursa, hand
    M71.041 Abscess of bursa, right hand
    M71.042 Abscess of bursa, left hand
    M71.049 Abscess of bursa, unspecified hand

√6th **M71.05** Abscess of bursa, hip
    M71.051 Abscess of bursa, right hip
    M71.052 Abscess of bursa, left hip
    M71.059 Abscess of bursa, unspecified hip

√6th **M71.06** Abscess of bursa, knee
    M71.061 Abscess of bursa, right knee
    M71.062 Abscess of bursa, left knee
    M71.069 Abscess of bursa, unspecified knee

√6th **M71.07** Abscess of bursa, ankle and foot
    M71.071 Abscess of bursa, right ankle and foot
    M71.072 Abscess of bursa, left ankle and foot
    M71.079 Abscess of bursa, unspecified ankle and foot

    M71.08 Abscess of bursa, other site

    M71.09 Abscess of bursa, multiple sites

√5th **M71.1** Other infective bursitis
    Use additional code (B95.-, B96.-) to identify causative organism
    M71.10 Other infective bursitis, unspecified site

√6th **M71.11** Other infective bursitis, shoulder
    M71.111 Other infective bursitis, right shoulder
    M71.112 Other infective bursitis, left shoulder
    M71.119 Other infective bursitis, unspecified shoulder

√6th **M71.12** Other infective bursitis, elbow
    M71.121 Other infective bursitis, right elbow
    M71.122 Other infective bursitis, left elbow
    M71.129 Other infective bursitis, unspecified elbow

√6th **M71.13** Other infective bursitis, wrist
    M71.131 Other infective bursitis, right wrist
    M71.132 Other infective bursitis, left wrist
    M71.139 Other infective bursitis, unspecified wrist

√6th **M71.14** Other infective bursitis, hand
    M71.141 Other infective bursitis, right hand
    M71.142 Other infective bursitis, left hand
    M71.149 Other infective bursitis, unspecified hand

√6th **M71.15** Other infective bursitis, hip
    M71.151 Other infective bursitis, right hip
    M71.152 Other infective bursitis, left hip
    M71.159 Other infective bursitis, unspecified hip

√6th **M71.16** Other infective bursitis, knee
    M71.161 Other infective bursitis, right knee
    M71.162 Other infective bursitis, left knee
    M71.169 Other infective bursitis, unspecified knee

√6th **M71.17** Other infective bursitis, ankle and foot
    M71.171 Other infective bursitis, right ankle and foot
    M71.172 Other infective bursitis, left ankle and foot
    M71.179 Other infective bursitis, unspecified ankle and foot

    M71.18 Other infective bursitis, other site

    M71.19 Other infective bursitis, multiple sites

√5th **M71.2** Synovial cyst of popliteal space [Baker]
    EXCLUDES 1   synovial cyst of popliteal space with rupture (M66.0)

    M71.20 Synovial cyst of popliteal space [Baker], unspecified knee

    M71.21 Synovial cyst of popliteal space [Baker], right knee

    M71.22 Synovial cyst of popliteal space [Baker], left knee

√5th **M71.3** Other bursal cyst
    Synovial cyst NOS
    EXCLUDES 1   synovial cyst with rupture (M66.1-)

    M71.30 Other bursal cyst, unspecified site

√6th **M71.31** Other bursal cyst, shoulder
    M71.311 Other bursal cyst, right shoulder
    M71.312 Other bursal cyst, left shoulder
    M71.319 Other bursal cyst, unspecified shoulder

√6th **M71.32** Other bursal cyst, elbow
    M71.321 Other bursal cyst, right elbow
    M71.322 Other bursal cyst, left elbow
    M71.329 Other bursal cyst, unspecified elbow

√6th **M71.33** Other bursal cyst, wrist
    M71.331 Other bursal cyst, right wrist
    M71.332 Other bursal cyst, left wrist
    M71.339 Other bursal cyst, unspecified wrist

√6th **M71.34** Other bursal cyst, hand
    M71.341 Other bursal cyst, right hand
    M71.342 Other bursal cyst, left hand
    M71.349 Other bursal cyst, unspecified hand

√6th **M71.35** Other bursal cyst, hip
    M71.351 Other bursal cyst, right hip
    M71.352 Other bursal cyst, left hip
    M71.359 Other bursal cyst, unspecified hip

√6th **M71.37** Other bursal cyst, ankle and foot
    M71.371 Other bursal cyst, right ankle and foot
    M71.372 Other bursal cyst, left ankle and foot
    M71.379 Other bursal cyst, unspecified ankle and foot

    M71.38 Other bursal cyst, other site

    M71.39 Other bursal cyst, multiple sites

√5th **M71.4** Calcium deposit in bursa
    EXCLUDES 2   calcium deposit in bursa of shoulder (M75.3)

    M71.40 Calcium deposit in bursa, unspecified site

√6th **M71.42** Calcium deposit in bursa, elbow
    M71.421 Calcium deposit in bursa, right elbow
    M71.422 Calcium deposit in bursa, left elbow
    M71.429 Calcium deposit in bursa, unspecified elbow

√6th **M71.43** Calcium deposit in bursa, wrist
    M71.431 Calcium deposit in bursa, right wrist
    M71.432 Calcium deposit in bursa, left wrist
    M71.439 Calcium deposit in bursa, unspecified wrist

√6th **M71.44** Calcium deposit in bursa, hand
    M71.441 Calcium deposit in bursa, right hand
    M71.442 Calcium deposit in bursa, left hand
    M71.449 Calcium deposit in bursa, unspecified hand

√6th **M71.45** Calcium deposit in bursa, hip
    M71.451 Calcium deposit in bursa, right hip
    M71.452 Calcium deposit in bursa, left hip
    M71.459 Calcium deposit in bursa, unspecified hip

√6th **M71.46** Calcium deposit in bursa, knee
    M71.461 Calcium deposit in bursa, right knee
    M71.462 Calcium deposit in bursa, left knee
    M71.469 Calcium deposit in bursa, unspecified knee

√6th **M71.47** Calcium deposit in bursa, ankle and foot
    M71.471 Calcium deposit in bursa, right ankle and foot
    M71.472 Calcium deposit in bursa, left ankle and foot
    M71.479 Calcium deposit in bursa, unspecified ankle and foot

    M71.48 Calcium deposit in bursa, other site

    M71.49 Calcium deposit in bursa, multiple sites

☑ Additional Character Required   √x7th Xtension Alert   Unspecified Code   Other Specified Code   Manifestation Code   ►◄ Revised Text   ● New Code   ▲ Revised Code Title

✓5ᵗʰ **M71.5 Other bursitis, not elsewhere classified**
 EXCLUDES 1 bursitis NOS (M71.9-)
 EXCLUDES 2 bursitis of shoulder (M75.5)
  bursitis of tibial collateral [Pellegrini-Stieda] (M76.4)

 M71.50 Other bursitis, not elsewhere classified, unspecified site

 ✓6ᵗʰ **M71.52 Other bursitis, not elsewhere classified, elbow**
  M71.521 Other bursitis, not elsewhere classified, right elbow
  M71.522 Other bursitis, not elsewhere classified, left elbow
  M71.529 Other bursitis, not elsewhere classified, unspecified elbow

 ✓6ᵗʰ **M71.53 Other bursitis, not elsewhere classified, wrist**
  M71.531 Other bursitis, not elsewhere classified, right wrist
  M71.532 Other bursitis, not elsewhere classified, left wrist
  M71.539 Other bursitis, not elsewhere classified, unspecified wrist

 ✓6ᵗʰ **M71.54 Other bursitis, not elsewhere classified, hand**
  M71.541 Other bursitis, not elsewhere classified, right hand
  M71.542 Other bursitis, not elsewhere classified, left hand
  M71.549 Other bursitis, not elsewhere classified, unspecified hand

 ✓6ᵗʰ **M71.55 Other bursitis, not elsewhere classified, hip**
  M71.551 Other bursitis, not elsewhere classified, right hip
  M71.552 Other bursitis, not elsewhere classified, left hip
  M71.559 Other bursitis, not elsewhere classified, unspecified hip

 ✓6ᵗʰ **M71.56 Other bursitis, not elsewhere classified, knee**
  M71.561 Other bursitis, not elsewhere classified, right knee
  M71.562 Other bursitis, not elsewhere classified, left knee
  M71.569 Other bursitis, not elsewhere classified, unspecified knee

 ✓6ᵗʰ **M71.57 Other bursitis, not elsewhere classified, ankle and foot**
  M71.571 Other bursitis, not elsewhere classified, right ankle and foot
  M71.572 Other bursitis, not elsewhere classified, left ankle and foot
  M71.579 Other bursitis, not elsewhere classified, unspecified ankle and foot

 M71.58 Other bursitis, not elsewhere classified, other site

✓5ᵗʰ **M71.8 Other specified bursopathies**
 M71.80 Other specified bursopathies, unspecified site

 ✓6ᵗʰ **M71.81 Other specified bursopathies, shoulder**
  M71.811 Other specified bursopathies, right shoulder
  M71.812 Other specified bursopathies, left shoulder
  M71.819 Other specified bursopathies, unspecified shoulder

 ✓6ᵗʰ **M71.82 Other specified bursopathies, elbow**
  M71.821 Other specified bursopathies, right elbow
  M71.822 Other specified bursopathies, left elbow
  M71.829 Other specified bursopathies, unspecified elbow

 ✓6ᵗʰ **M71.83 Other specified bursopathies, wrist**
  M71.831 Other specified bursopathies, right wrist
  M71.832 Other specified bursopathies, left wrist
  M71.839 Other specified bursopathies, unspecified wrist

 ✓6ᵗʰ **M71.84 Other specified bursopathies, hand**
  M71.841 Other specified bursopathies, right hand
  M71.842 Other specified bursopathies, left hand
  M71.849 Other specified bursopathies, unspecified hand

 ✓6ᵗʰ **M71.85 Other specified bursopathies, hip**
  M71.851 Other specified bursopathies, right hip
  M71.852 Other specified bursopathies, left hip
  M71.859 Other specified bursopathies, unspecified hip

 ✓6ᵗʰ **M71.86 Other specified bursopathies, knee**
  M71.861 Other specified bursopathies, right knee
  M71.862 Other specified bursopathies, left knee
  M71.869 Other specified bursopathies, unspecified knee

 ✓6ᵗʰ **M71.87 Other specified bursopathies, ankle and foot**
  M71.871 Other specified bursopathies, right ankle and footq
  M71.872 Other specified bursopathies, left ankle and foot
  M71.879 Other specified bursopathies, unspecified ankle and foot

 M71.88 Other specified bursopathies, other site
 M71.89 Other specified bursopathies, multiple sites

M71.9 Bursopathy, unspecified
 Bursitis NOS

✓4ᵗʰ **M72 Fibroblastic disorders**
 EXCLUDES 2 retroperitoneal fibromatosis (D48.3)

 M72.0 Palmar fascial fibromatosis [Dupuytren] 🄐

 M72.1 Knuckle pads

 M72.2 Plantar fascial fibromatosis
  Plantar fasciitis

 M72.4 Pseudosarcomatous fibromatosis
  Nodular fasciitis

 M72.6 Necrotizing fasciitis
  Use additional code (B95.-, B96.-) to identify causative organism

 M72.8 Other fibroblastic disorders
  Abscess of fascia
  Fasciitis NEC
  Other infective fasciitis
  Use additional code to (B95.-, B96.-) identify causative organism
  EXCLUDES 1 diffuse (eosinophilic) fasciitis (M35.4)
   necrotizing fasciitis (M72.6)
   nodular fasciitis (M72.4)
   perirenal fasciitis NOS (N13.5)
   perirenal fasciitis with infection (N13.6)
   plantar fasciitis (M72.2)

 M72.9 Fibroblastic disorder, unspecified
  Fasciitis NOS
  Fibromatosis NOS

✓4ᵗʰ **M75 Shoulder lesions**
 EXCLUDES 2 shoulder-hand syndrome (M89.0-)

 ✓5ᵗʰ **M75.0 Adhesive capsulitis of shoulder**
  Frozen shoulder
  Periarthritis of shoulder
  M75.00 Adhesive capsulitis of unspecified shoulder
  M75.01 Adhesive capsulitis of right shoulder
  M75.02 Adhesive capsulitis of left shoulder

 ✓5ᵗʰ **M75.1 Rotator cuff tear or rupture, not specified as traumatic**
  Rotator cuff syndrome
  Supraspinatus syndrome
  Supraspinatus tear or rupture, not specified as traumatic
  EXCLUDES 1 tear of rotator cuff, traumatic (S46.01-)

  ✓6ᵗʰ **M75.10 Unspecified rotator cuff tear or rupture, not specified as traumatic**
   M75.100 Unspecified rotator cuff tear or rupture of unspecified shoulder, not specified as traumatic
   M75.101 Unspecified rotator cuff tear or rupture of right shoulder, not specified as traumatic
   M75.102 Unspecified rotator cuff tear or rupture of left shoulder, not specified as traumatic

  ✓6ᵗʰ **M75.11 Incomplete rotator cuff tear or rupture not specified as traumatic**
   M75.110 Incomplete rotator cuff tear or rupture of unspecified shoulder, not specified as traumatic
   M75.111 Incomplete rotator cuff tear or rupture of right shoulder, not specified as traumatic
   M75.112 Incomplete rotator cuff tear or rupture of left shoulder, not specified as traumatic

EXCLUDES 1 Not coded here   *EXCLUDES 2* Not included here   N Newborn Age: 0   P Pediatric Age: 0-17   M Maternity Age: 12-55   A Adult Age: 15-124

698   ICD-10-CM 2014 (Draft)

√6ᵗʰ **M75.12** Complete **rotator cuff tear or rupture not specified as traumatic**

M75.120 Complete rotator cuff tear or rupture of unspecified shoulder, not specified as traumatic

M75.121 Complete rotator cuff tear or rupture of right shoulder, not specified as traumatic

M75.122 Complete rotator cuff tear or rupture of left shoulder, not specified as traumatic

√5ᵗʰ **M75.2** Bicipital **tendinitis**

M75.20 Bicipital **tendinitis, unspecified shoulder**

M75.21 Bicipital tendinitis, right shoulder

M75.22 Bicipital tendinitis, left shoulder

√5ᵗʰ **M75.3** Calcific **tendinitis of shoulder**
Calcified bursa of shoulder

M75.30 Calcific **tendinitis of unspecified shoulder**

M75.31 Calcific tendinitis of right shoulder

M75.32 Calcific tendinitis of left shoulder

√5ᵗʰ **M75.4** Impingement syndrome **of shoulder**

M75.40 Impingement syndrome **of unspecified shoulder**

M75.41 Impingement syndrome of right shoulder

M75.42 Impingement syndrome of left shoulder

√5ᵗʰ **M75.5** Bursitis **of shoulder**

M75.50 Bursitis **of unspecified shoulder**

M75.51 Bursitis of right shoulder

M75.52 Bursitis of left shoulder

√5ᵗʰ **M75.8** Other shoulder lesions

M75.80 Other shoulder lesions, unspecified shoulder

M75.81 Other shoulder lesions, right shoulder

M75.82 Other shoulder lesions, left shoulder

√5ᵗʰ **M75.9** Shoulder lesion, unspecified

M75.90 Shoulder lesion, unspecified, unspecified shoulder

M75.91 Shoulder lesion, unspecified, right shoulder

M75.92 Shoulder lesion, unspecified, left shoulder

√4ᵗʰ **M76** Enthesopathies, lower limb, excluding foot
EXCLUDES 2 *bursitis due to use, overuse and pressure (M70.-)*
enthesopathies of ankle and foot (M77.5-)

√5ᵗʰ **M76.0** Gluteal **tendinitis**

M76.00 Gluteal tendinitis, unspecified hip

M76.01 Gluteal tendinitis, right hip

M76.02 Gluteal tendinitis, left hip

√5ᵗʰ **M76.1** Psoas **tendinitis**

M76.10 Psoas tendinitis, unspecified hip

M76.11 Psoas tendinitis, right hip

M76.12 Psoas tendinitis, left hip

√5ᵗʰ **M76.2** Iliac crest **spur**

M76.20 Iliac crest spur, unspecified hip

M76.21 Iliac crest spur, right hip

M76.22 Iliac crest spur, left hip

√5ᵗʰ **M76.3** Iliotibial band **syndrome**

M76.30 Iliotibial band syndrome, unspecified leg

M76.31 Iliotibial band syndrome, right leg

M76.32 Iliotibial band syndrome, left leg

√5ᵗʰ **M76.4** Tibial collateral **bursitis [Pellegrini-Stieda]**

M76.40 Tibial collateral bursitis [Pellegrini-Stieda], unspecified leg

M76.41 Tibial collateral bursitis [Pellegrini-Stieda], right leg

M76.42 Tibial collateral bursitis [Pellegrini-Stieda], left leg

√5ᵗʰ **M76.5** Patellar **tendinitis**

M76.50 Patellar tendinitis, unspecified knee

M76.51 Patellar tendinitis, right knee

M76.52 Patellar tendinitis, left knee

√5ᵗʰ **M76.6** Achilles **tendinitis**
Achilles bursitis

M76.60 Achilles tendinitis, unspecified leg

M76.61 Achilles tendinitis, right leg

M76.62 Achilles tendinitis, left leg

√5ᵗʰ **M76.7** Peroneal **tendinitis**

M76.70 Peroneal tendinitis, unspecified leg

M76.71 Peroneal tendinitis, right leg

M76.72 Peroneal tendinitis, left leg

√5ᵗʰ **M76.8** Other specified enthesopathies of lower limb, excluding foot

√6ᵗʰ **M76.81** Anterior tibial syndrome

M76.811 Anterior tibial syndrome, right leg

M76.812 Anterior tibial syndrome, left leg

M76.819 Anterior tibial syndrome, unspecified leg

√6ᵗʰ **M76.82** Posterior tibial tendinitis

M76.821 Posterior tibial tendinitis, right leg

M76.822 Posterior tibial tendinitis, left leg

M76.829 Posterior tibial tendinitis, unspecified leg

√6ᵗʰ **M76.89** Other specified enthesopathies of lower limb, excluding foot

M76.891 Other specified enthesopathies of right lower limb, excluding foot

M76.892 Other specified enthesopathies of left lower limb, excluding foot

M76.899 Other specified enthesopathies of unspecified lower limb, excluding foot

M76.9 Unspecified enthesopathy, lower limb, excluding foot

√4ᵗʰ **M77** Other enthesopathies
EXCLUDES 1 *bursitis NOS (M71.9-)*
EXCLUDES 2 *bursitis due to use, overuse and pressure (M70.-)*
osteophyte (M25.7)
spinal enthesopathy (M46.0-)

√5ᵗʰ **M77.0** Medial **epicondylitis**

M77.00 Medial **epicondylitis, unspecified elbow**

M77.01 Medial epicondylitis, right elbow

M77.02 Medial epicondylitis, left elbow

√5ᵗʰ **M77.1** Lateral **epicondylitis**
Tennis elbow

M77.10 Lateral **epicondylitis, unspecified elbow**

M77.11 Lateral epicondylitis, right elbow

M77.12 Lateral epicondylitis, left elbow

√5ᵗʰ **M77.2** Periarthritis **of wrist**

M77.20 Periarthritis, unspecified wrist

M77.21 Periarthritis, right wrist

M77.22 Periarthritis, left wrist

√5ᵗʰ **M77.3** Calcaneal **spur**

M77.30 Calcaneal spur, unspecified foot

M77.31 Calcaneal spur, right foot

M77.32 Calcaneal spur, left foot

√5ᵗʰ **M77.4** Metatarsalgia
EXCLUDES 1 *Morton's metatarsalgia (G57.6)*

M77.40 Metatarsalgia, unspecified foot

M77.41 Metatarsalgia, right foot

M77.42 Metatarsalgia, left foot

√5ᵗʰ **M77.5** Other enthesopathy of foot

M77.50 Other enthesopathy of unspecified foot

M77.51 Other enthesopathy of right foot

M77.52 Other enthesopathy of left foot

M77.8 Other enthesopathies, not elsewhere classified

M77.9 Enthesopathy, unspecified
Bone spur NOS   Periarthritis NOS
Capsulitis NOS   Tendinitis NOS

√4ᵗʰ **M79** Other and unspecified soft tissue disorders, not elsewhere classified
EXCLUDES 1 *psychogenic rheumatism (F45.8)*
soft tissue pain, psychogenic (F45.41)

M79.0 Rheumatism, unspecified
EXCLUDES 1 *fibromyalgia (M79.7)*
palindromic rheumatism (M12.3-)

M79.1 Myalgia
Myofascial pain syndrome
EXCLUDES 1 *fibromyalgia (M79.7)*
myositis (M60.-)

M79.2 Neuralgia and neuritis, unspecified
EXCLUDES 1 *brachial radiculitis NOS (M54.1)*
lumbosacral radiculitis NOS (M54.1)
mononeuropathies (G56-G58)
radiculitis NOS (M54.1)
sciatica (M54.3-M54.4)

M79.3 Panniculitis, unspecified

> *EXCLUDES 1* lupus panniculitis (L93.2)
> neck and back panniculitis (M54.0-)
> relapsing [Weber-Christian] panniculitis (M35.6)

M79.4 Hypertrophy of (infrapatellar) fat pad

M79.5 Residual foreign body in soft tissue

> *EXCLUDES 1* foreign body granuloma of skin and subcutaneous
> tissue (L92.3)
> foreign body granuloma of soft tissue (M60.2-)

✓5th M79.6 Pain in limb, hand, foot, fingers and toes

> *EXCLUDES 2* pain in joint (M25.5-)

✓6th M79.60 Pain in limb, unspecified

M79.601 Pain in right arm
Pain in right upper limb NOS

M79.602 Pain in left arm
Pain in left upper limb NOS

M79.603 Pain in arm, unspecified
Pain in upper limb NOS

M79.604 Pain in right leg
Pain in right lower limb NOS

M79.605 Pain in left leg
Pain in left lower limb NOS

M79.606 Pain in leg, unspecified
Pain in lower limb NOS

M79.609 Pain in unspecified limb
Pain in limb NOS

✓6th M79.62 Pain in upper arm
Pain in axillary region

M79.621 Pain in right upper arm
M79.622 Pain in left upper arm
M79.629 Pain in unspecified upper arm

✓6th M79.63 Pain in forearm

M79.631 Pain in right forearm
M79.632 Pain in left forearm
M79.639 Pain in unspecified forearm

✓6th M79.64 Pain in hand and fingers

M79.641 Pain in right hand
M79.642 Pain in left hand
M79.643 Pain in unspecified hand
M79.644 Pain in right finger(s)
M79.645 Pain in left finger(s)
M79.646 Pain in unspecified finger(s)

✓6th M79.65 Pain in thigh

M79.651 Pain in right thigh
M79.652 Pain in left thigh
M79.659 Pain in unspecified thigh

✓6th M79.66 Pain in lower leg

M79.661 Pain in right lower leg
M79.662 Pain in left lower leg
M79.669 Pain in unspecified lower leg

✓6th M79.67 Pain in foot and toes

M79.671 Pain in right foot
M79.672 Pain in left foot
M79.673 Pain in unspecified foot
M79.674 Pain in right toe(s)
M79.675 Pain in left toe(s)
M79.676 Pain in unspecified toe(s)

M79.7 Fibromyalgia
Fibromyositis   Myofibrositis
Fibrositis

✓5th M79.A Nontraumatic compartment syndrome

> Code first, if applicable, associated postprocedural complication
> *EXCLUDES 1* compartment syndrome NOS (T79.A-)
> fibromyalgia (M79.7)
> nontraumatic ischemic infarction of muscle (M62.2-)
> traumatic compartment syndrome (T79.A-)

✓6th M79.A1 Nontraumatic compartment syndrome of upper extremity
Nontraumatic compartment syndrome of shoulder, arm, forearm, wrist, hand, and fingers

M79.A11 Nontraumatic compartment syndrome of right upper extremity
M79.A12 Nontraumatic compartment syndrome of left upper extremity

M79.A19 Nontraumatic compartment syndrome of unspecified upper extremity

✓6th M79.A2 Nontraumatic compartment syndrome of lower extremity
Nontraumatic compartment syndrome of hip, buttock, thigh, leg, foot, and toes

M79.A21 Nontraumatic compartment syndrome of right lower extremity
M79.A22 Nontraumatic compartment syndrome of left lower extremity
M79.A29 Nontraumatic compartment syndrome of unspecified lower extremity

M79.A3 Nontraumatic compartment syndrome of abdomen
M79.A9 Nontraumatic compartment syndrome of other sites

✓5th M79.8 Other specified soft tissue disorders

M79.81 Nontraumatic hematoma of soft tissue
Nontraumatic hematoma of muscle
Nontraumatic seroma of muscle and soft tissue

M79.89 Other specified soft tissue disorders
Polyalgia

M79.9 Soft tissue disorder, unspecified

OSTEOPATHIES AND CHONDROPATHIES (M80-M94)

Disorders of bone density and structure (M80-M85)

✓4th M80 Osteoporosis with current pathological fracture

> *INCLUDES* osteoporosis with current fragility fracture
> Use additional code to identify major osseous defect, if applicable (M89.7-)
> *EXCLUDES 1* collapsed vertebra NOS (M48.5)
> pathological fracture NOS (M84.4)
> wedging of vertebra NOS (M48.5)
> *EXCLUDES 2* personal history of (healed) osteoporosis fracture (Z87.310)

The appropriate 7th character is to be added to each code from category M80.
A   initial encounter for fracture
D   subsequent encounter for fracture with routine healing
G   subsequent encounter for fracture with delayed healing
K   subsequent encounter for fracture with nonunion
P   subsequent encounter for fracture with malunion
S   sequela

✓5th M80.0 Age-related osteoporosis with current pathological fracture
Involutional osteoporosis with current pathological fracture
Osteoporosis NOS with current pathological fracture
Postmenopausal osteoporosis with current pathological fracture
Senile osteoporosis with current pathological fracture

✓x7th M80.00 Age-related osteoporosis with current pathological fracture, unspecified site Ⓐ

✓6th M80.01 Age-related osteoporosis with current pathological fracture, shoulder

✓7th M80.011 Age-related osteoporosis with current pathological fracture, right shoulder Ⓐ
✓7th M80.012 Age-related osteoporosis with current pathological fracture, left shoulder Ⓐ
✓7th M80.019 Age-related osteoporosis with current pathological fracture, unspecified shoulder Ⓐ

✓6th M80.02 Age-related osteoporosis with current pathological fracture, humerus

✓7th M80.021 Age-related osteoporosis with current pathological fracture, right humerus Ⓐ
✓7th M80.022 Age-related osteoporosis with current pathological fracture, left humerus Ⓐ
✓7th M80.029 Age-related osteoporosis with current pathological fracture, unspecified humerus Ⓐ

✓6th M80.03 Age-related osteoporosis with current pathological fracture, forearm
Age-related osteoporosis with current pathological fracture of wrist

✓7th M80.031 Age-related osteoporosis with current pathological fracture, right forearm Ⓐ
✓7th M80.032 Age-related osteoporosis with current pathological fracture, left forearm Ⓐ
✓7th M80.039 Age-related osteoporosis with current pathological fracture, unspecified forearm Ⓐ

√6th **M80.04** **Age-related osteoporosis with current pathological fracture, hand**

√7th **M80.041** Age-related osteoporosis with current pathological fracture, right hand Ⓐ

√7th **M80.042** Age-related osteoporosis with current pathological fracture, left hand Ⓐ

√7th **M80.049** Age-related osteoporosis with current pathological fracture, unspecified hand Ⓐ

√6th **M80.05** **Age-related osteoporosis with current pathological fracture, femur**
Age-related osteoporosis with current pathological fracture of hip

√7th **M80.051** Age-related osteoporosis with current pathological fracture, right femur Ⓐ

√7th **M80.052** Age-related osteoporosis with current pathological fracture, left femur Ⓐ

√7th **M80.059** Age-related osteoporosis with current pathological fracture, unspecified femur Ⓐ

√6th **M80.06** **Age-related osteoporosis with current pathological fracture, lower leg**

√7th **M80.061** Age-related osteoporosis with current pathological fracture, right lower leg Ⓐ

√7th **M80.062** Age-related osteoporosis with current pathological fracture, left lower leg Ⓐ

√7th **M80.069** Age-related osteoporosis with current pathological fracture, unspecified lower leg Ⓐ

√6th **M80.07** **Age-related osteoporosis with current pathological fracture, ankle and foot**

√7th **M80.071** Age-related osteoporosis with current pathological fracture, right ankle and foot Ⓐ

√7th **M80.072** Age-related osteoporosis with current pathological fracture, left ankle and foot Ⓐ

√7th **M80.079** Age-related osteoporosis with current pathological fracture, unspecified ankle and foot Ⓐ

√x7th **M80.08** **Age-related osteoporosis with current pathological fracture, vertebra(e)** Ⓐ

√5th **M80.8** **Other osteoporosis with current pathological fracture**
Drug-induced osteoporosis with current pathological fracture
Idiopathic osteoporosis with current pathological fracture
Osteoporosis of disuse with current pathological fracture
Postoophorectomy osteoporosis with current pathological fracture
Postsurgical malabsorption osteoporosis with current pathological fracture
Post-traumatic osteoporosis with current pathological fracture
Use additional code for adverse effect, if applicable, to identify drug (T36-T50 with fifth or sixth character 5)

√x7th **M80.80** **Other osteoporosis with current pathological fracture, unspecified site**

√6th **M80.81** **Other osteoporosis with pathological fracture, shoulder**

√7th **M80.811** Other osteoporosis with current pathological fracture, right shoulder

√7th **M80.812** Other osteoporosis with current pathological fracture, left shoulder

√7th **M80.819** Other osteoporosis with current pathological fracture, unspecified shoulder

√6th **M80.82** **Other osteoporosis with current pathological fracture, humerus**

√7th **M80.821** Other osteoporosis with current pathological fracture, right humerus

√7th **M80.822** Other osteoporosis with current pathological fracture, left humerus

√7th **M80.829** Other osteoporosis with current pathological fracture, unspecified humerus

√6th **M80.83** **Other osteoporosis with current pathological fracture, forearm**
Other osteoporosis with current pathological fracture of wrist

√7th **M80.831** Other osteoporosis with current pathological fracture, right forearm

√7th **M80.832** Other osteoporosis with current pathological fracture, left forearm

√7th **M80.839** Other osteoporosis with current pathological fracture, unspecified forearm

√6th **M80.84** **Other osteoporosis with current pathological fracture, hand**

√7th **M80.841** Other osteoporosis with current pathological fracture, right hand

√7th **M80.842** Other osteoporosis with current pathological fracture, left hand

√7th **M80.849** Other osteoporosis with current pathological fracture, unspecified hand

√6th **M80.85** **Other osteoporosis with current pathological fracture, femur**
Other osteoporosis with current pathological fracture of hip

√7th **M80.851** Other osteoporosis with current pathological fracture, right femur

√7th **M80.852** Other osteoporosis with current pathological fracture, left femur

√7th **M80.859** Other osteoporosis with current pathological fracture, unspecified femur

√6th **M80.86** **Other osteoporosis with current pathological fracture, lower leg**

√7th **M80.861** Other osteoporosis with current pathological fracture, right lower leg

√7th **M80.862** Other osteoporosis with current pathological fracture, left lower leg

√7th **M80.869** Other osteoporosis with current pathological fracture, unspecified lower leg

√6th **M80.87** **Other osteoporosis with current pathological fracture, ankle and foot**

√7th **M80.871** Other osteoporosis with current pathological fracture, right ankle and foot

√7th **M80.872** Other osteoporosis with current pathological fracture, left ankle and foot

√7th **M80.879** Other osteoporosis with current pathological fracture, unspecified ankle and foot

√x7th **M80.88** **Other osteoporosis with current pathological fracture, vertebra(e)**

√4th **M81** **Osteoporosis without current pathological fracture**
Use additional code to identify:
major osseous defect, if applicable (M89.7-)
personal history of (healed) osteoporosis fracture, if applicable (Z87.310)

EXCLUDES 1 osteoporosis with current pathological fracture (M80.-)
Sudeck's atrophy (M89.0)

M81.0 **Age-related osteoporosis without current pathological fracture** Ⓐ
Involutional osteoporosis without current pathological fracture
Osteoporosis NOS
Postmenopausal osteoporosis without current pathological fracture
Senile osteoporosis without current pathological fracture

M81.6 **Localized osteoporosis [Lequesne]**
EXCLUDES 1 Sudeck's atrophy (M89.0)

M81.8 **Other osteoporosis without current pathological fracture**
Drug-induced osteoporosis without current pathological fracture
Idiopathic osteoporosis without current pathological fracture
Osteoporosis of disuse without current pathological fracture
Postoophorectomy osteoporosis without current pathological fracture
Postsurgical malabsorption osteoporosis without current pathological fracture
Post-traumatic osteoporosis without current pathological fracture
Use additional code for adverse effect, if applicable, to identify drug (T36-T50 with fifth or sixth character 5)

√4th **M83** **Adult osteomalacia**
EXCLUDES 1 infantile and juvenile osteomalacia (E55.0)
renal osteodystrophy (N25.0)
rickets (active) (E55.0)
rickets (active) sequelae (E64.3)
vitamin D-resistant osteomalacia (E83.3)
vitamin D-resistant rickets (active) (E83.3)

M83.0 **Puerperal osteomalacia** Ⓜ♀

M83.1 **Senile osteomalacia** Ⓐ

Diseases of the Musculoskeletal System and Connective Tissue

M83.2–M84.472

M83.2 Adult osteomalacia due to malabsorption 🅐
    Postsurgical malabsorption osteomalacia in adults

M83.3 Adult osteomalacia due to malnutrition 🅐

M83.4 Aluminum bone disease

M83.5 Other drug-induced **osteomalacia in adults** 🅐
    Use additional code for adverse effect, if applicable, to identify
      drug (T36-T50 with fifth or sixth character 5)

M83.8 Other adult osteomalacia 🅐

M83.9 Adult osteomalacia, unspecified 🅐

✓4ᵗʰ **M84 Disorder of continuity of bone**
    EXCLUDES 2   *traumatic fracture of bone-see fracture, by site*

✓5ᵗʰ **M84.3 Stress fracture**
    Fatigue fracture   Stress fracture NOS
    March fracture   Stress reaction
    Use additional external cause code(s) to identify the cause of the
      stress fracture
    EXCLUDES 1   *pathological fracture NOS (M84.4-)*
           pathological fracture due to osteoporosis (M80.-)
           traumatic fracture (S12-, S22-, S32-, S42-, S52-, S62-,
             S72-, S82-, S92-)
    EXCLUDES 2   *personal history of (healed) stress (fatigue) fracture*
           (Z87.312)
           stress fracture of vertebra (M48.4-)

    The appropriate 7th character is to be added to each code
    from subcategory M84.3.
    A   initial encounter for fracture
    D   subsequent encounter for fracture with routine healing
    G   subsequent encounter for fracture with delayed healing
    K   subsequent encounter for fracture with nonunion
    P   subsequent encounter for fracture with malunion
    S   sequela

✓x7ᵗʰ **M84.30 Stress fracture, unspecified site**

✓6ᵗʰ **M84.31 Stress fracture, shoulder**
    ✓7ᵗʰ **M84.311 Stress fracture, right shoulder**
    ✓7ᵗʰ **M84.312 Stress fracture, left shoulder**
    ✓7ᵗʰ **M84.319 Stress fracture, unspecified shoulder**

✓6ᵗʰ **M84.32 Stress fracture, humerus**
    ✓7ᵗʰ **M84.321 Stress fracture, right humerus**
    ✓7ᵗʰ **M84.322 Stress fracture, left humerus**
    ✓7ᵗʰ **M84.329 Stress fracture, unspecified humerus**

✓6ᵗʰ **M84.33 Stress fracture, ulna and radius**
    ✓7ᵗʰ **M84.331 Stress fracture, right ulna**
    ✓7ᵗʰ **M84.332 Stress fracture, left ulna**
    ✓7ᵗʰ **M84.333 Stress fracture, right radius**
    ✓7ᵗʰ **M84.334 Stress fracture, left radius**
    ✓7ᵗʰ **M84.339 Stress fracture, unspecified ulna and
                 radius**

✓6ᵗʰ **M84.34 Stress fracture, hand and fingers**
    ✓7ᵗʰ **M84.341 Stress fracture, right hand**
    ✓7ᵗʰ **M84.342 Stress fracture, left hand**
    ✓7ᵗʰ **M84.343 Stress fracture, unspecified hand**
    ✓7ᵗʰ **M84.344 Stress fracture, right finger(s)**
    ✓7ᵗʰ **M84.345 Stress fracture, left finger(s)**
    ✓7ᵗʰ **M84.346 Stress fracture, unspecified finger(s)**

✓6ᵗʰ **M84.35 Stress fracture, pelvis and femur**
    Stress fracture, hip
    ✓7ᵗʰ **M84.350 Stress fracture, pelvis**
    ✓7ᵗʰ **M84.351 Stress fracture, right femur**
    ✓7ᵗʰ **M84.352 Stress fracture, left femur**
    ✓7ᵗʰ **M84.353 Stress fracture, unspecified femur**
    ✓7ᵗʰ **M84.359 Stress fracture, hip, unspecified**

✓6ᵗʰ **M84.36 Stress fracture, tibia and fibula**
    ✓7ᵗʰ **M84.361 Stress fracture, right tibia**
    ✓7ᵗʰ **M84.362 Stress fracture, left tibia**
    ✓7ᵗʰ **M84.363 Stress fracture, right fibula**
    ✓7ᵗʰ **M84.364 Stress fracture, left fibula**
    ✓7ᵗʰ **M84.369 Stress fracture, unspecified tibia and
                 fibula**

✓6ᵗʰ **M84.37 Stress fracture, ankle, foot and toes**
    ✓7ᵗʰ **M84.371 Stress fracture, right ankle**
    ✓7ᵗʰ **M84.372 Stress fracture, left ankle**

✓7ᵗʰ **M84.373 Stress fracture, unspecified ankle**
✓7ᵗʰ **M84.374 Stress fracture, right foot**
✓7ᵗʰ **M84.375 Stress fracture, left foot**
✓7ᵗʰ **M84.376 Stress fracture, unspecified foot**
✓7ᵗʰ **M84.377 Stress fracture, right toe(s)**
✓7ᵗʰ **M84.378 Stress fracture, left toe(s)**
✓7ᵗʰ **M84.379 Stress fracture, unspecified toe(s)**

✓x7ᵗʰ **M84.38 Stress fracture, other site**
    EXCLUDES 2   *stress fracture of vertebra (M48.4-)*

✓5ᵗʰ **M84.4 Pathological fracture,** not elsewhere classified
    Chronic fracture
    Pathological fracture NOS
    EXCLUDES 1   *collapsed vertebra NEC (M48.5)*
           pathological fracture in neoplastic disease (M84.5-)
           pathological fracture in osteoporosis (M80.-)
           pathological fracture in other disease (M84.6-)
           stress fracture (M84.3-)
           traumatic fracture (S12.-, S22.-, S32.-, S42.-, S52.-, S62.-,
             S72.-, S82.-, S92.-)
    EXCLUDES 2   *personal history of (healed) pathological fracture*
           (Z87.311)

    The appropriate 7th character is to be added to each code
    from subcategory M84.4.
    A   initial encounter for fracture
    D   subsequent encounter for fracture with routine healing
    G   subsequent encounter for fracture with delayed healing
    K   subsequent encounter for fracture with nonunion
    P   subsequent encounter for fracture with malunion
    S   sequela

✓x7ᵗʰ **M84.40 Pathological fracture, unspecified site**

✓6ᵗʰ **M84.41 Pathological fracture,** shoulder
    ✓7ᵗʰ **M84.411 Pathological fracture, right shoulder**
    ✓7ᵗʰ **M84.412 Pathological fracture, left shoulder**
    ✓7ᵗʰ **M84.419 Pathological fracture, unspecified
                 shoulder**

✓6ᵗʰ **M84.42 Pathological fracture,** humerus
    ✓7ᵗʰ **M84.421 Pathological fracture, right humerus**
    ✓7ᵗʰ **M84.422 Pathological fracture, left humerus**
    ✓7ᵗʰ **M84.429 Pathological fracture, unspecified
                 humerus**

✓6ᵗʰ **M84.43 Pathological fracture,** ulna and radius
    ✓7ᵗʰ **M84.431 Pathological fracture, right ulna**
    ✓7ᵗʰ **M84.432 Pathological fracture, left ulna**
    ✓7ᵗʰ **M84.433 Pathological fracture, right radius**
    ✓7ᵗʰ **M84.434 Pathological fracture, left radius**
    ✓7ᵗʰ **M84.439 Pathological fracture, unspecified ulna
                 and radius**

✓6ᵗʰ **M84.44 Pathological fracture,** hand and fingers
    ✓7ᵗʰ **M84.441 Pathological fracture, right hand**
    ✓7ᵗʰ **M84.442 Pathological fracture, left hand**
    ✓7ᵗʰ **M84.443 Pathological fracture, unspecified hand**
    ✓7ᵗʰ **M84.444 Pathological fracture, right finger(s)**
    ✓7ᵗʰ **M84.445 Pathological fracture, left finger(s)**
    ✓7ᵗʰ **M84.446 Pathological fracture, unspecified
                 finger(s)**

✓6ᵗʰ **M84.45 Pathological fracture,** femur and pelvis
    ✓7ᵗʰ **M84.451 Pathological fracture, right femur**
    ✓7ᵗʰ **M84.452 Pathological fracture, left femur**
    ✓7ᵗʰ **M84.453 Pathological fracture, unspecified femur**
    ✓7ᵗʰ **M84.454 Pathological fracture, pelvis**
    ✓7ᵗʰ **M84.459 Pathological fracture, hip, unspecified**

✓6ᵗʰ **M84.46 Pathological fracture,** tibia and fibula
    ✓7ᵗʰ **M84.461 Pathological fracture, right tibia**
    ✓7ᵗʰ **M84.462 Pathological fracture, left tibia**
    ✓7ᵗʰ **M84.463 Pathological fracture, right fibula**
    ✓7ᵗʰ **M84.464 Pathological fracture, left fibula**
    ✓7ᵗʰ **M84.469 Pathological fracture, unspecified tibia
                 and fibula**

✓6ᵗʰ **M84.47 Pathological fracture,** ankle, foot and toes
    ✓7ᵗʰ **M84.471 Pathological fracture, right ankle**
    ✓7ᵗʰ **M84.472 Pathological fracture, left ankle**

EXCLUDES 1   Not coded here   EXCLUDES 2   Not included here   🅝 Newborn Age: 0   🅟 Pediatric Age: 0-17   🅜 Maternity Age: 12-55   🅐 Adult Age: 15-124

702   ICD-10-CM 2014 (Draft)

✓7ᵗʰ **M84.473** **Pathological fracture, unspecified** ankle

✓7ᵗʰ **M84.474** **Pathological fracture,** right foot

✓7ᵗʰ **M84.475** **Pathological fracture,** left foot

✓7ᵗʰ **M84.476** **Pathological fracture, unspecified** foot

✓7ᵗʰ **M84.477** **Pathological fracture,** right toe(s)

✓7ᵗʰ **M84.478** **Pathological fracture,** left toe(s)

✓7ᵗʰ **M84.479** **Pathological fracture, unspecified** toe(s)

✓x7ᵗʰ **M84.48** **Pathological fracture, other site**

✓5ᵗʰ **M84.5** **Pathological fracture in** neoplastic disease
Code also underlying neoplasm

The appropriate 7th character is to be added to each code from subcategory M84.5.
A   initial encounter for fracture
D   subsequent encounter for fracture with routine healing
G   subsequent encounter for fracture with delayed healing
K   subsequent encounter for fracture with nonunion
P   subsequent encounter for fracture with malunion
S   sequela

✓7ᵗʰ **M84.50** **Pathological fracture in neoplastic disease, unspecified site**

✓6ᵗʰ **M84.51** **Pathological fracture in neoplastic disease,** shoulder

✓7ᵗʰ **M84.511** **Pathological fracture in neoplastic disease,** right **shoulder**

✓7ᵗʰ **M84.512** **Pathological fracture in neoplastic disease,** left **shoulder**

✓7ᵗʰ **M84.519** **Pathological fracture in neoplastic disease, unspecified shoulder**

✓6ᵗʰ **M84.52** **Pathological fracture in neoplastic disease,** humerus

✓7ᵗʰ **M84.521** **Pathological fracture in neoplastic disease,** right **humerus**

✓7ᵗʰ **M84.522** **Pathological fracture in neoplastic disease,** left **humerus**

✓7ᵗʰ **M84.529** **Pathological fracture in neoplastic disease, unspecified humerus**

✓6ᵗʰ **M84.53** **Pathological fracture in neoplastic disease, ulna and radius**

✓7ᵗʰ **M84.531** **Pathological fracture in neoplastic disease,** right **ulna**

✓7ᵗʰ **M84.532** **Pathological fracture in neoplastic disease,** left **ulna**

✓7ᵗʰ **M84.533** **Pathological fracture in neoplastic disease,** right **radius**

✓7ᵗʰ **M84.534** **Pathological fracture in neoplastic disease,** left **radius**

✓7ᵗʰ **M84.539** **Pathological fracture in neoplastic disease, unspecified ulna and radius**

✓6ᵗʰ **M84.54** **Pathological fracture in neoplastic disease,** hand

✓7ᵗʰ **M84.541** **Pathological fracture in neoplastic disease,** right **hand**

✓7ᵗʰ **M84.542** **Pathological fracture in neoplastic disease,** left **hand**

✓7ᵗʰ **M84.549** **Pathological fracture in neoplastic disease, unspecified hand**

✓6ᵗʰ **M84.55** **Pathological fracture in neoplastic disease, pelvis and femur**

✓7ᵗʰ **M84.550** **Pathological fracture in neoplastic disease,** pelvis

✓7ᵗʰ **M84.551** **Pathological fracture in neoplastic disease,** right **femur**

✓7ᵗʰ **M84.552** **Pathological fracture in neoplastic disease,** left **femur**

✓7ᵗʰ **M84.553** **Pathological fracture in neoplastic disease, unspecified** femur

✓7ᵗʰ **M84.559** **Pathological fracture in neoplastic disease, hip, unspecified**

✓6ᵗʰ **M84.56** **Pathological fracture in neoplastic disease, tibia and fibula**

✓7ᵗʰ **M84.561** **Pathological fracture in neoplastic disease,** right **tibia**

✓7ᵗʰ **M84.562** **Pathological fracture in neoplastic disease,** left **tibia**

✓7ᵗʰ **M84.563** **Pathological fracture in neoplastic disease,** right **fibula**

✓7ᵗʰ **M84.564** **Pathological fracture in neoplastic disease,** left **fibula**

✓7ᵗʰ **M84.569** **Pathological fracture in neoplastic disease, unspecified tibia and fibula**

✓6ᵗʰ **M84.57** **Pathological fracture in neoplastic disease,** ankle and foot

✓7ᵗʰ **M84.571** **Pathological fracture in neoplastic disease,** right **ankle**

✓7ᵗʰ **M84.572** **Pathological fracture in neoplastic disease,** left **ankle**

✓7ᵗʰ **M84.573** **Pathological fracture in neoplastic disease, unspecified** ankle

✓7ᵗʰ **M84.574** **Pathological fracture in neoplastic disease,** right **foot**

✓7ᵗʰ **M84.575** **Pathological fracture in neoplastic disease,** left **foot**

✓7ᵗʰ **M84.576** **Pathological fracture in neoplastic disease, unspecified** foot

✓x7ᵗʰ **M84.58** **Pathological fracture in neoplastic disease, other specified site**
Pathological fracture in neoplastic disease, vertebrae

✓5ᵗʰ **M84.6** **Pathological fracture** in other disease
Code also underlying condition
EXCLUDES 1 pathological fracture in osteoporosis (M80.-)

The appropriate 7th character is to be added to each code from subcategory M84.6.
A   initial encounter for fracture
D   subsequent encounter for fracture with routine healing
G   subsequent encounter for fracture with delayed healing
K   subsequent encounter for fracture with nonunion
P   subsequent encounter for fracture with malunion
S   sequela

✓x7ᵗʰ **M84.60** **Pathological fracture in other disease, unspecified site**

✓6ᵗʰ **M84.61** **Pathological fracture in other disease,** shoulder

✓7ᵗʰ **M84.611** **Pathological fracture in other disease,** right **shoulder**

✓7ᵗʰ **M84.612** **Pathological fracture in other disease,** left **shoulder**

✓7ᵗʰ **M84.619** **Pathological fracture in other disease, unspecified shoulder**

✓6ᵗʰ **M84.62** **Pathological fracture in other disease,** humerus

✓7ᵗʰ **M84.621** **Pathological fracture in other disease,** right **humerus**

✓7ᵗʰ **M84.622** **Pathological fracture in other disease,** left **humerus**

✓7ᵗʰ **M84.629** **Pathological fracture in other disease, unspecified humerus**

✓6ᵗʰ **M84.63** **Pathological fracture in other disease,** ulna and radius

✓7ᵗʰ **M84.631** **Pathological fracture in other disease,** right **ulna**

✓7ᵗʰ **M84.632** **Pathological fracture in other disease,** left **ulna**

✓7ᵗʰ **M84.633** **Pathological fracture in other disease,** right **radius**

✓7ᵗʰ **M84.634** **Pathological fracture in other disease,** left **radius**

✓7ᵗʰ **M84.639** **Pathological fracture in other disease, unspecified ulna and radius**

✓6ᵗʰ **M84.64** **Pathological fracture in other disease,** hand

✓7ᵗʰ **M84.641** **Pathological fracture in other disease,** right **hand**

✓7ᵗʰ **M84.642** **Pathological fracture in other disease,** left **hand**

✓7ᵗʰ **M84.649** **Pathological fracture in other disease, unspecified hand**

✓6ᵗʰ **M84.65** **Pathological fracture in other disease,** pelvis and femur

✓7ᵗʰ **M84.650** **Pathological fracture in other disease,** pelvis

✓7ᵗʰ **M84.651** **Pathological fracture in other disease,** right femur

✓7ᵗʰ **M84.652** **Pathological fracture in other disease,** left femur

Diseases of the Musculoskeletal System and Connective Tissue

M84.653–M85.08

√7ᵗʰ **M84.653 Pathological fracture in other disease, unspecified** femur

√7ᵗʰ **M84.659 Pathological fracture in other disease, hip, unspecified**

√6ᵗʰ **M84.66 Pathological fracture in other disease,** tibia and fibula

   √7ᵗʰ **M84.661 Pathological fracture in other disease, right tibia**

   √7ᵗʰ **M84.662 Pathological fracture in other disease, left tibia**

   √7ᵗʰ **M84.663 Pathological fracture in other disease, right fibula**

   √7ᵗʰ **M84.664 Pathological fracture in other disease, left fibula**

   √7ᵗʰ **M84.669 Pathological fracture in other disease, unspecified tibia and fibula**

√6ᵗʰ **M84.67 Pathological fracture in other disease, ankle and foot**

   √7ᵗʰ **M84.671 Pathological fracture in other disease, right ankle**

   √7ᵗʰ **M84.672 Pathological fracture in other disease, left ankle**

   √7ᵗʰ **M84.673 Pathological fracture in other disease, unspecified** ankle

   √7ᵗʰ **M84.674 Pathological fracture in other disease, right foot**

   √7ᵗʰ **M84.675 Pathological fracture in other disease, left foot**

   √7ᵗʰ **M84.676 Pathological fracture in other disease, unspecified** foot

√x7ᵗʰ **M84.68 Pathological fracture in other disease, other site**

√5ᵗʰ **M84.8 Other disorders of continuity of bone**

   M84.80 Other disorders of continuity of bone, unspecified site

  √6ᵗʰ **M84.81 Other disorders of continuity of bone,** shoulder

    M84.811 Other disorders of continuity of bone, right shoulder

    M84.812 Other disorders of continuity of bone, left shoulder

    M84.819 Other disorders of continuity of bone, unspecified shoulder

  √6ᵗʰ **M84.82 Other disorders of continuity of bone,** humerus

    M84.821 Other disorders of continuity of bone, right humerus

    M84.822 Other disorders of continuity of bone, left humerus

    M84.829 Other disorders of continuity of bone, unspecified humerus

  √6ᵗʰ **M84.83 Other disorders of continuity of bone, ulna and radius**

    M84.831 Other disorders of continuity of bone, right ulna

    M84.832 Other disorders of continuity of bone, left ulna

    M84.833 Other disorders of continuity of bone, right radius

    M84.834 Other disorders of continuity of bone, left radius

    M84.839 Other disorders of continuity of bone, unspecified ulna and radius

  √6ᵗʰ **M84.84 Other disorders of continuity of bone,** hand

    M84.841 Other disorders of continuity of bone, right hand

    M84.842 Other disorders of continuity of bone, left hand

    M84.849 Other disorders of continuity of bone, unspecified hand

  √6ᵗʰ **M84.85 Other disorders of continuity of bone,** pelvic region and thigh

    M84.851 Other disorders of continuity of bone, right pelvic region and thigh

    M84.852 Other disorders of continuity of bone, left pelvic region and thigh

    M84.859 Other disorders of continuity of bone, unspecified pelvic region and thigh

√6ᵗʰ **M84.86 Other disorders of continuity of bone,** tibia and fibula

   M84.861 Other disorders of continuity of bone, right tibia

   M84.862 Other disorders of continuity of bone, left tibia

   M84.863 Other disorders of continuity of bone, right fibula

   M84.864 Other disorders of continuity of bone, left fibula

   M84.869 Other disorders of continuity of bone, unspecified tibia and fibula

√6ᵗʰ **M84.87 Other disorders of continuity of bone,** ankle and foot

   M84.871 Other disorders of continuity of bone, right ankle and foot

   M84.872 Other disorders of continuity of bone, left ankle and foot

   M84.879 Other disorders of continuity of bone, unspecified ankle and foot

  M84.88 Other disorders of continuity of bone, other site

M84.9 Disorder of continuity of bone, unspecified

√4ᵗʰ **M85 Other disorders of bone density and structure**

  EXCLUDES 1   *osteogenesis imperfecta (Q78.0)*
           osteopetrosis (Q78.2)
           osteopoikilosis (Q78.8)
           polyostotic fibrous dysplasia (Q78.1)

√5ᵗʰ **M85.0 Fibrous dysplasia (monostotic)**

  EXCLUDES 2   *fibrous dysplasia of jaw (M27.8)*

  M85.00 Fibrous dysplasia (monostotic), unspecified site

  √6ᵗʰ **M85.01 Fibrous dysplasia (monostotic),** shoulder

    M85.011 Fibrous dysplasia (monostotic), right shoulder

    M85.012 Fibrous dysplasia (monostotic), left shoulder

    M85.019 Fibrous dysplasia (monostotic), unspecified shoulder

  √6ᵗʰ **M85.02 Fibrous dysplasia (monostotic),** upper arm

    M85.021 Fibrous dysplasia (monostotic), right upper arm

    M85.022 Fibrous dysplasia (monostotic), left upper arm

    M85.029 Fibrous dysplasia (monostotic), unspecified upper arm

  √6ᵗʰ **M85.03 Fibrous dysplasia (monostotic),** forearm

    M85.031 Fibrous dysplasia (monostotic), right forearm

    M85.032 Fibrous dysplasia (monostotic), left forearm

    M85.039 Fibrous dysplasia (monostotic), unspecified forearm

  √6ᵗʰ **M85.04 Fibrous dysplasia (monostotic),** hand

    M85.041 Fibrous dysplasia (monostotic), right hand

    M85.042 Fibrous dysplasia (monostotic), left hand

    M85.049 Fibrous dysplasia (monostotic), unspecified hand

  √6ᵗʰ **M85.05 Fibrous dysplasia (monostotic),** thigh

    M85.051 Fibrous dysplasia (monostotic), right thigh

    M85.052 Fibrous dysplasia (monostotic), left thigh

    M85.059 Fibrous dysplasia (monostotic), unspecified thigh

  √6ᵗʰ **M85.06 Fibrous dysplasia (monostotic),** lower leg

    M85.061 Fibrous dysplasia (monostotic), right lower leg

    M85.062 Fibrous dysplasia (monostotic), left lower leg

    M85.069 Fibrous dysplasia (monostotic), unspecified lower leg

  √6ᵗʰ **M85.07 Fibrous dysplasia (monostotic),** ankle and foot

    M85.071 Fibrous dysplasia (monostotic), right ankle and foot

    M85.072 Fibrous dysplasia (monostotic), left ankle and foot

    M85.079 Fibrous dysplasia (monostotic), unspecified ankle and foot

  M85.08 Fibrous dysplasia (monostotic), other site

EXCLUDES 1 Not coded here   EXCLUDES 2 Not included here   N Newborn Age: 0   P Pediatric Age: 0-17   M Maternity Age: 12-55   A Adult Age: 15-124

704   ICD-10-CM 2014 (Draft)

M85.09 Fibrous dysplasia (monostotic), multiple sites

√5ᵗʰ M85.1 Skeletal fluorosis

M85.10 Skeletal fluorosis, unspecified site

√6ᵗʰ M85.11 Skeletal fluorosis, shoulder
- M85.111 Skeletal fluorosis, right shoulder
- M85.112 Skeletal fluorosis, left shoulder
- M85.119 Skeletal fluorosis, unspecified shoulder

√6ᵗʰ M85.12 Skeletal fluorosis, upper arm
- M85.121 Skeletal fluorosis, right upper arm
- M85.122 Skeletal fluorosis, left upper arm
- M85.129 Skeletal fluorosis, unspecified upper arm

√6ᵗʰ M85.13 Skeletal fluorosis, forearm
- M85.131 Skeletal fluorosis, right forearm
- M85.132 Skeletal fluorosis, left forearm
- M85.139 Skeletal fluorosis, unspecified forearm

√6ᵗʰ M85.14 Skeletal fluorosis, hand
- M85.141 Skeletal fluorosis, right hand
- M85.142 Skeletal fluorosis, left hand
- M85.149 Skeletal fluorosis, unspecified hand

√6ᵗʰ M85.15 Skeletal fluorosis, thigh
- M85.151 Skeletal fluorosis, right thigh
- M85.152 Skeletal fluorosis, left thigh
- M85.159 Skeletal fluorosis, unspecified thigh

√6ᵗʰ M85.16 Skeletal fluorosis, lower leg
- M85.161 Skeletal fluorosis, right lower leg
- M85.162 Skeletal fluorosis, left lower leg
- M85.169 Skeletal fluorosis, unspecified lower leg

√6ᵗʰ M85.17 Skeletal fluorosis, ankle and foot
- M85.171 Skeletal fluorosis, right ankle and foot
- M85.172 Skeletal fluorosis, left ankle and foot
- M85.179 Skeletal fluorosis, unspecified ankle and foot

M85.18 Skeletal fluorosis, other site

M85.19 Skeletal fluorosis, multiple sites

M85.2 Hyperostosis of skull

√5ᵗʰ M85.3 Osteitis condensans

M85.30 Osteitis condensans, unspecified site

√6ᵗʰ M85.31 Osteitis condensans, shoulder
- M85.311 Osteitis condensans, right shoulder
- M85.312 Osteitis condensans, left shoulder
- M85.319 Osteitis condensans, unspecified shoulder

√6ᵗʰ M85.32 Osteitis condensans, upper arm
- M85.321 Osteitis condensans, right upper arm
- M85.322 Osteitis condensans, left upper arm
- M85.329 Osteitis condensans, unspecified upper arm

√6ᵗʰ M85.33 Osteitis condensans, forearm
- M85.331 Osteitis condensans, right forearm
- M85.332 Osteitis condensans, left forearm
- M85.339 Osteitis condensans, unspecified forearm

√6ᵗʰ M85.34 Osteitis condensans, hand
- M85.341 Osteitis condensans, right hand
- M85.342 Osteitis condensans, left hand
- M85.349 Osteitis condensans, unspecified hand

√6ᵗʰ M85.35 Osteitis condensans, thigh
- M85.351 Osteitis condensans, right thigh
- M85.352 Osteitis condensans, left thigh
- M85.359 Osteitis condensans, unspecified thigh

√6ᵗʰ M85.36 Osteitis condensans, lower leg
- M85.361 Osteitis condensans, right lower leg
- M85.362 Osteitis condensans, left lower leg
- M85.369 Osteitis condensans, unspecified lower leg

√6ᵗʰ M85.37 Osteitis condensans, ankle and foot
- M85.371 Osteitis condensans, right ankle and foot
- M85.372 Osteitis condensans, left ankle and foot
- M85.379 Osteitis condensans, unspecified ankle and foot

M85.38 Osteitis condensans, other site

M85.39 Osteitis condensans, multiple sites

√5ᵗʰ M85.4 Solitary bone cyst
EXCLUDES 2 solitary cyst of jaw (M27.4)

M85.40 Solitary bone cyst, unspecified site

√6ᵗʰ M85.41 Solitary bone cyst, shoulder
- M85.411 Solitary bone cyst, right shoulder
- M85.412 Solitary bone cyst, left shoulder
- M85.419 Solitary bone cyst, unspecified shoulder

√6ᵗʰ M85.42 Solitary bone cyst, humerus
- M85.421 Solitary bone cyst, right humerus
- M85.422 Solitary bone cyst, left humerus
- M85.429 Solitary bone cyst, unspecified humerus

√6ᵗʰ M85.43 Solitary bone cyst, ulna and radius
- M85.431 Solitary bone cyst, right ulna and radius
- M85.432 Solitary bone cyst, left ulna and radius
- M85.439 Solitary bone cyst, unspecified ulna and radius

√6ᵗʰ M85.44 Solitary bone cyst, hand
- M85.441 Solitary bone cyst, right hand
- M85.442 Solitary bone cyst, left hand
- M85.449 Solitary bone cyst, unspecified hand

√6ᵗʰ M85.45 Solitary bone cyst, pelvis
- M85.451 Solitary bone cyst, right pelvis
- M85.452 Solitary bone cyst, left pelvis
- M85.459 Solitary bone cyst, unspecified pelvis

√6ᵗʰ M85.46 Solitary bone cyst, tibia and fibula
- M85.461 Solitary bone cyst, right tibia and fibula
- M85.462 Solitary bone cyst, left tibia and fibula
- M85.469 Solitary bone cyst, unspecified tibia and fibula

√6ᵗʰ M85.47 Solitary bone cyst, ankle and foot
- M85.471 Solitary bone cyst, right ankle and foot
- M85.472 Solitary bone cyst, left ankle and foot
- M85.479 Solitary bone cyst, unspecified ankle and foot

M85.48 Solitary bone cyst, other site

√5ᵗʰ M85.5 Aneurysmal bone cyst
EXCLUDES 2 aneurysmal cyst of jaw (M27.4)

M85.50 Aneurysmal bone cyst, unspecified site

√6ᵗʰ M85.51 Aneurysmal bone cyst, shoulder
- M85.511 Aneurysmal bone cyst, right shoulder
- M85.512 Aneurysmal bone cyst, left shoulder
- M85.519 Aneurysmal bone cyst, unspecified shoulder

√6ᵗʰ M85.52 Aneurysmal bone cyst, upper arm
- M85.521 Aneurysmal bone cyst, right upper arm
- M85.522 Aneurysmal bone cyst, left upper arm
- M85.529 Aneurysmal bone cyst, unspecified upper arm

√6ᵗʰ M85.53 Aneurysmal bone cyst, forearm
- M85.531 Aneurysmal bone cyst, right forearm
- M85.532 Aneurysmal bone cyst, left forearm
- M85.539 Aneurysmal bone cyst, unspecified forearm

√6ᵗʰ M85.54 Aneurysmal bone cyst, hand
- M85.541 Aneurysmal bone cyst, right hand
- M85.542 Aneurysmal bone cyst, left hand
- M85.549 Aneurysmal bone cyst, unspecified hand

√6ᵗʰ M85.55 Aneurysmal bone cyst, thigh
- M85.551 Aneurysmal bone cyst, right thigh
- M85.552 Aneurysmal bone cyst, left thigh
- M85.559 Aneurysmal bone cyst, unspecified thigh

√6ᵗʰ M85.56 Aneurysmal bone cyst, lower leg
- M85.561 Aneurysmal bone cyst, right lower leg
- M85.562 Aneurysmal bone cyst, left lower leg
- M85.569 Aneurysmal bone cyst, unspecified lower leg

√6ᵗʰ M85.57 Aneurysmal bone cyst, ankle and foot
- M85.571 Aneurysmal bone cyst, right ankle and foot
- M85.572 Aneurysmal bone cyst, left ankle and foot
- M85.579 Aneurysmal bone cyst, unspecified ankle and foot

M85.58 **Aneurysmal bone cyst, other site**

M85.59 **Aneurysmal bone cyst, multiple sites**

✓5ᵗʰ **M85.6 Other cyst of bone**
  EXCLUDES 1 cyst of jaw NEC (M27.4)
            osteitis fibrosa cystica generalisata [von
            Recklinghausen's disease of bone] (E21.0)

M85.60 **Other cyst of bone, unspecified site**

✓6ᵗʰ M85.61 **Other cyst of bone, shoulder**
  M85.611 **Other cyst of bone, right shoulder**
  M85.612 **Other cyst of bone, left shoulder**
  M85.619 **Other cyst of bone, unspecified shoulder**

✓6ᵗʰ M85.62 **Other cyst of bone, upper arm**
  M85.621 **Other cyst of bone, right upper arm**
  M85.622 **Other cyst of bone, left upper arm**
  M85.629 **Other cyst of bone, unspecified upper arm**

✓6ᵗʰ M85.63 **Other cyst of bone, forearm**
  M85.631 **Other cyst of bone, right forearm**
  M85.632 **Other cyst of bone, left forearm**
  M85.639 **Other cyst of bone, unspecified forearm**

✓6ᵗʰ M85.64 **Other cyst of bone, hand**
  M85.641 **Other cyst of bone, right hand**
  M85.642 **Other cyst of bone, left hand**
  M85.649 **Other cyst of bone, unspecified hand**

✓6ᵗʰ M85.65 **Other cyst of bone, thigh**
  M85.651 **Other cyst of bone, right thigh**
  M85.652 **Other cyst of bone, left thigh**
  M85.659 **Other cyst of bone, unspecified thigh**

✓6ᵗʰ M85.66 **Other cyst of bone, lower leg**
  M85.661 **Other cyst of bone, right lower leg**
  M85.662 **Other cyst of bone, left lower leg**
  M85.669 **Other cyst of bone, unspecified lower leg**

✓6ᵗʰ M85.67 **Other cyst of bone, ankle and foot**
  M85.671 **Other cyst of bone, right ankle and foot**
  M85.672 **Other cyst of bone, left ankle and foot**
  M85.679 **Other cyst of bone, unspecified ankle and foot**

M85.68 **Other cyst of bone, other site**

M85.69 **Other cyst of bone, multiple sites**

✓5ᵗʰ **M85.8 Other specified disorders of bone density and structure**
  Hyperostosis of bones, except skull
  Osteosclerosis, acquired
  EXCLUDES 1 diffuse idiopathic skeletal hyperostosis [DISH] (M48.1)
            osteosclerosis congenita (Q77.4)
            osteosclerosis fragilitas (generalista) (Q78.2)
            osteosclerosis myelofibrosis (D75.81)

M85.80 **Other specified disorders of bone density and structure, unspecified site**

✓6ᵗʰ M85.81 **Other specified disorders of bone density and structure, shoulder**
  M85.811 **Other specified disorders of bone density and structure, right shoulder**
  M85.812 **Other specified disorders of bone density and structure, left shoulder**
  M85.819 **Other specified disorders of bone density and structure, unspecified shoulder**

✓6ᵗʰ M85.82 **Other specified disorders of bone density and structure, upper arm**
  M85.821 **Other specified disorders of bone density and structure, right upper arm**
  M85.822 **Other specified disorders of bone density and structure, left upper arm**
  M85.829 **Other specified disorders of bone density and structure, unspecified upper arm**

✓6ᵗʰ M85.83 **Other specified disorders of bone density and structure, forearm**
  M85.831 **Other specified disorders of bone density and structure, right forearm**
  M85.832 **Other specified disorders of bone density and structure, left forearm**
  M85.839 **Other specified disorders of bone density and structure, unspecified forearm**

✓6ᵗʰ M85.84 **Other specified disorders of bone density and structure, hand**
  M85.841 **Other specified disorders of bone density and structure, right hand**

M85.842 **Other specified disorders of bone density and structure, left hand**

M85.849 **Other specified disorders of bone density and structure, unspecified hand**

✓6ᵗʰ M85.85 **Other specified disorders of bone density and structure, thigh**
  M85.851 **Other specified disorders of bone density and structure, right thigh**
  M85.852 **Other specified disorders of bone density and structure, left thigh**
  M85.859 **Other specified disorders of bone density and structure, unspecified thigh**

✓6ᵗʰ M85.86 **Other specified disorders of bone density and structure, lower leg**
  M85.861 **Other specified disorders of bone density and structure, right lower leg**
  M85.862 **Other specified disorders of bone density and structure, left lower leg**
  M85.869 **Other specified disorders of bone density and structure, unspecified lower leg**

✓6ᵗʰ M85.87 **Other specified disorders of bone density and structure, ankle and foot**
  M85.871 **Other specified disorders of bone density and structure, right ankle and foot**
  M85.872 **Other specified disorders of bone density and structure, left ankle and foot**
  M85.879 **Other specified disorders of bone density and structure, unspecified ankle and foot**

M85.88 **Other specified disorders of bone density and structure, other site**

M85.89 **Other specified disorders of bone density and structure, multiple sites**

M85.9 Disorder of bone density and structure, unspecified

Other osteopathies (M86-M90)

  EXCLUDES 1 postprocedural osteopathies (M96.-)

✓4ᵗʰ **M86 Osteomyelitis**
  Use additional code (B95-B97) to identify infectious agent
  Use additional code to identify major osseous defect, if applicable (M89.7-)
  EXCLUDES 1 osteomyelitis due to:
            echinococcus (B67.2)
            gonococcus (A54.43)
            salmonella (A02.24)
  EXCLUDES 2 ostemyelitis of:
            orbit (H05.0-)
            petrous bone (H70.2-)
            vertebra (M46.2-)

✓5ᵗʰ **M86.0 Acute hematogenous osteomyelitis**

M86.00 **Acute hematogenous osteomyelitis, unspecified site**

✓6ᵗʰ M86.01 **Acute hematogenous osteomyelitis, shoulder**
  M86.011 **Acute hematogenous osteomyelitis, right shoulder**
  M86.012 **Acute hematogenous osteomyelitis, left shoulder**
  M86.019 **Acute hematogenous osteomyelitis, unspecified shoulder**

✓6ᵗʰ M86.02 **Acute hematogenous osteomyelitis, humerus**
  M86.021 **Acute hematogenous osteomyelitis, right humerus**
  M86.022 **Acute hematogenous osteomyelitis, left humerus**
  M86.029 **Acute hematogenous osteomyelitis, unspecified humerus**

✓6ᵗʰ M86.03 **Acute hematogenous osteomyelitis, radius and ulna**
  M86.031 **Acute hematogenous osteomyelitis, right radius and ulna**
  M86.032 **Acute hematogenous osteomyelitis, left radius and ulna**
  M86.039 **Acute hematogenous osteomyelitis, unspecified radius and ulna**

✓6ᵗʰ M86.04 **Acute hematogenous osteomyelitis, hand**
  M86.041 **Acute hematogenous osteomyelitis, right hand**
  M86.042 **Acute hematogenous osteomyelitis, left hand**

EXCLUDES 1 Not coded here   EXCLUDES 2 Not included here   N Newborn Age: 0   P Pediatric Age: 0-17   M Maternity Age: 12-55   A Adult Age: 15-124

706   ICD-10-CM 2014 (Draft)

    M86.049 **Acute hematogenous osteomyelitis, unspecified hand**

✓6ᵗʰ M86.05 Acute hematogenous osteomyelitis, femur
    M86.051 Acute hematogenous osteomyelitis, right femur
    M86.052 Acute hematogenous osteomyelitis, left femur
    M86.059 **Acute hematogenous osteomyelitis, unspecified femur**

✓6ᵗʰ M86.06 Acute hematogenous osteomyelitis, tibia and fibula
    M86.061 Acute hematogenous osteomyelitis, right tibia and fibula
    M86.062 Acute hematogenous osteomyelitis, left tibia and fibula
    M86.069 **Acute hematogenous osteomyelitis, unspecified tibia and fibula**

✓6ᵗʰ M86.07 Acute hematogenous osteomyelitis, ankle and foot
    M86.071 Acute hematogenous osteomyelitis, right ankle and foot
    M86.072 Acute hematogenous osteomyelitis, left ankle and foot
    M86.079 **Acute hematogenous osteomyelitis, unspecified ankle and foot**

    M86.08 **Acute hematogenous osteomyelitis, other sites**
    M86.09 Acute hematogenous osteomyelitis, multiple sites

✓5ᵗʰ M86.1 Other acute osteomyelitis
    M86.10 **Other acute osteomyelitis, unspecified site**

✓6ᵗʰ M86.11 Other acute osteomyelitis, shoulder
    M86.111 **Other acute osteomyelitis, right shoulder**
    M86.112 **Other acute osteomyelitis, left shoulder**
    M86.119 **Other acute osteomyelitis, unspecified shoulder**

✓6ᵗʰ M86.12 Other acute osteomyelitis, humerus
    M86.121 **Other acute osteomyelitis, right humerus**
    M86.122 **Other acute osteomyelitis, left humerus**
    M86.129 **Other acute osteomyelitis, unspecified humerus**

✓6ᵗʰ M86.13 Other acute osteomyelitis, radius and ulna
    M86.131 **Other acute osteomyelitis, right radius and ulna**
    M86.132 **Other acute osteomyelitis, left radius and ulna**
    M86.139 **Other acute osteomyelitis, unspecified radius and ulna**

✓6ᵗʰ M86.14 Other acute osteomyelitis, hand
    M86.141 **Other acute osteomyelitis, right hand**
    M86.142 **Other acute osteomyelitis, left hand**
    M86.149 **Other acute osteomyelitis, unspecified hand**

✓6ᵗʰ M86.15 Other acute osteomyelitis, femur
    M86.151 **Other acute osteomyelitis, right femur**
    M86.152 **Other acute osteomyelitis, left femur**
    M86.159 **Other acute osteomyelitis, unspecified femur**

✓6ᵗʰ M86.16 Other acute osteomyelitis, tibia and fibula
    M86.161 **Other acute osteomyelitis, right tibia and fibula**
    M86.162 **Other acute osteomyelitis, left tibia and fibula**
    M86.169 **Other acute osteomyelitis, unspecified tibia and fibula**

✓6ᵗʰ M86.17 Other acute osteomyelitis, ankle and foot
    M86.171 **Other acute osteomyelitis, right ankle and foot**
    M86.172 **Other acute osteomyelitis, left ankle and foot**
    M86.179 **Other acute osteomyelitis, unspecified ankle and foot**

    M86.18 **Other acute osteomyelitis, other site**
    M86.19 **Other acute osteomyelitis, multiple sites**

✓5ᵗʰ M86.2 Subacute osteomyelitis
    M86.20 **Subacute osteomyelitis, unspecified site**

✓6ᵗʰ M86.21 Subacute osteomyelitis, shoulder
    M86.211 Subacute osteomyelitis, right shoulder
    M86.212 Subacute osteomyelitis, left shoulder

    M86.219 **Subacute osteomyelitis, unspecified shoulder**

✓6ᵗʰ M86.22 Subacute osteomyelitis, humerus
    M86.221 Subacute osteomyelitis, right humerus
    M86.222 Subacute osteomyelitis, left humerus
    M86.229 **Subacute osteomyelitis, unspecified humerus**

✓6ᵗʰ M86.23 Subacute osteomyelitis, radius and ulna
    M86.231 Subacute osteomyelitis, right radius and ulna
    M86.232 Subacute osteomyelitis, left radius and ulna
    M86.239 **Subacute osteomyelitis, unspecified radius and ulna**

✓6ᵗʰ M86.24 Subacute osteomyelitis, hand
    M86.241 Subacute osteomyelitis, right hand
    M86.242 Subacute osteomyelitis, left hand
    M86.249 **Subacute osteomyelitis, unspecified hand**

✓6ᵗʰ M86.25 Subacute osteomyelitis, femur
    M86.251 Subacute osteomyelitis, right femur
    M86.252 Subacute osteomyelitis, left femur
    M86.259 **Subacute osteomyelitis, unspecified femur**

✓6ᵗʰ M86.26 Subacute osteomyelitis, tibia and fibula
    M86.261 Subacute osteomyelitis, right tibia and fibula
    M86.262 Subacute osteomyelitis, left tibia and fibula
    M86.269 **Subacute osteomyelitis, unspecified tibia and fibula**

✓6ᵗʰ M86.27 Subacute osteomyelitis, ankle and foot
    M86.271 Subacute osteomyelitis, right ankle and foot
    M86.272 Subacute osteomyelitis, left ankle and foot
    M86.279 **Subacute osteomyelitis, unspecified ankle and foot**

    M86.28 **Subacute osteomyelitis, other site**
    M86.29 Subacute osteomyelitis, multiple sites

✓5ᵗʰ M86.3 Chronic multifocal osteomyelitis
    M86.30 **Chronic multifocal osteomyelitis, unspecified site**

✓6ᵗʰ M86.31 Chronic multifocal osteomyelitis, shoulder
    M86.311 Chronic multifocal osteomyelitis, right shoulder
    M86.312 Chronic multifocal osteomyelitis, left shoulder
    M86.319 **Chronic multifocal osteomyelitis, unspecified shoulder**

✓6ᵗʰ M86.32 Chronic multifocal osteomyelitis, humerus
    M86.321 Chronic multifocal osteomyelitis, right humerus
    M86.322 Chronic multifocal osteomyelitis, left humerus
    M86.329 **Chronic multifocal osteomyelitis, unspecified humerus**

✓6ᵗʰ M86.33 Chronic multifocal osteomyelitis, radius and ulna
    M86.331 Chronic multifocal osteomyelitis, right radius and ulna
    M86.332 Chronic multifocal osteomyelitis, left radius and ulna
    M86.339 **Chronic multifocal osteomyelitis, unspecified radius and ulna**

✓6ᵗʰ M86.34 Chronic multifocal osteomyelitis, hand
    M86.341 Chronic multifocal osteomyelitis, right hand
    M86.342 Chronic multifocal osteomyelitis, left hand
    M86.349 **Chronic multifocal osteomyelitis, unspecified hand**

✓6ᵗʰ M86.35 Chronic multifocal osteomyelitis, femur
    M86.351 Chronic multifocal osteomyelitis, right femur
    M86.352 Chronic multifocal osteomyelitis, left femur
    M86.359 **Chronic multifocal osteomyelitis, unspecified femur**

☑ Additional Character Required   ✓7ᵗʰ Xtension Alert   Unspecified Code   Other Specified Code   Manifestation Code   ▶◀ Revised Text   ● New Code   ▲ Revised Code Title

ICD-10-CM 2014 (Draft)   **707**

√6th **M86.36** Chronic multifocal osteomyelitis, tibia and fibula

M86.361 Chronic multifocal osteomyelitis, right tibia and fibula

M86.362 Chronic multifocal osteomyelitis, left tibia and fibula

M86.369 Chronic multifocal osteomyelitis, unspecified tibia and fibula

√6th **M86.37** Chronic multifocal osteomyelitis, ankle and foot

M86.371 Chronic multifocal osteomyelitis, right ankle and foot

M86.372 Chronic multifocal osteomyelitis, left ankle and foot

M86.379 Chronic multifocal osteomyelitis, unspecified ankle and foot

M86.38 Chronic multifocal osteomyelitis, other site

M86.39 Chronic multifocal osteomyelitis, multiple sites

√5th **M86.4** Chronic osteomyelitis with draining sinus

M86.40 Chronic osteomyelitis with draining sinus, unspecified site

√6th **M86.41** Chronic osteomyelitis with draining sinus, shoulder

M86.411 Chronic osteomyelitis with draining sinus, right shoulder

M86.412 Chronic osteomyelitis with draining sinus, left shoulder

M86.419 Chronic osteomyelitis with draining sinus, unspecified shoulder

√6th **M86.42** Chronic osteomyelitis with draining sinus, humerus

M86.421 Chronic osteomyelitis with draining sinus, right humerus

M86.422 Chronic osteomyelitis with draining sinus, left humerus

M86.429 Chronic osteomyelitis with draining sinus, unspecified humerus

√6th **M86.43** Chronic osteomyelitis with draining sinus, radius and ulna

M86.431 Chronic osteomyelitis with draining sinus, right radius and ulna

M86.432 Chronic osteomyelitis with draining sinus, left radius and ulna

M86.439 Chronic osteomyelitis with draining sinus, unspecified radius and ulna

√6th **M86.44** Chronic osteomyelitis with draining sinus, hand

M86.441 Chronic osteomyelitis with draining sinus, right hand

M86.442 Chronic osteomyelitis with draining sinus, left hand

M86.449 Chronic osteomyelitis with draining sinus, unspecified hand

√6th **M86.45** Chronic osteomyelitis with draining sinus, femur

M86.451 Chronic osteomyelitis with draining sinus, right femur

M86.452 Chronic osteomyelitis with draining sinus, left femur

M86.459 Chronic osteomyelitis with draining sinus, unspecified femur

√6th **M86.46** Chronic osteomyelitis with draining sinus, tibia and fibula

M86.461 Chronic osteomyelitis with draining sinus, right tibia and fibula

M86.462 Chronic osteomyelitis with draining sinus, left tibia and fibula

M86.469 Chronic osteomyelitis with draining sinus, unspecified tibia and fibula

√6th **M86.47** Chronic osteomyelitis with draining sinus, ankle and foot

M86.471 Chronic osteomyelitis with draining sinus, right ankle and foot

M86.472 Chronic osteomyelitis with draining sinus, left ankle and foot

M86.479 Chronic osteomyelitis with draining sinus, unspecified ankle and foot

M86.48 Chronic osteomyelitis with draining sinus, other site

M86.49 Chronic osteomyelitis with draining sinus, multiple sites

√5th **M86.5** Other chronic hematogenous osteomyelitis

M86.50 Other chronic hematogenous osteomyelitis, unspecified site

√6th **M86.51** Other chronic hematogenous osteomyelitis, shoulder

M86.511 Other chronic hematogenous osteomyelitis, right shoulder

M86.512 Other chronic hematogenous osteomyelitis, left shoulder

M86.519 Other chronic hematogenous osteomyelitis, unspecified shoulder

√6th **M86.52** Other chronic hematogenous osteomyelitis, humerus

M86.521 Other chronic hematogenous osteomyelitis, right humerus

M86.522 Other chronic hematogenous osteomyelitis, left humerus

M86.529 Other chronic hematogenous osteomyelitis, unspecified humerus

√6th **M86.53** Other chronic hematogenous osteomyelitis, radius and ulna

M86.531 Other chronic hematogenous osteomyelitis, right radius and ulna

M86.532 Other chronic hematogenous osteomyelitis, left radius and ulna

M86.539 Other chronic hematogenous osteomyelitis, unspecified radius and ulna

√6th **M86.54** Other chronic hematogenous osteomyelitis, hand

M86.541 Other chronic hematogenous osteomyelitis, right hand

M86.542 Other chronic hematogenous osteomyelitis, left hand

M86.549 Other chronic hematogenous osteomyelitis, unspecified hand

√6th **M86.55** Other chronic hematogenous osteomyelitis, femur

M86.551 Other chronic hematogenous osteomyelitis, right femur

M86.552 Other chronic hematogenous osteomyelitis, left femur

M86.559 Other chronic hematogenous osteomyelitis, unspecified femur

√6th **M86.56** Other chronic hematogenous osteomyelitis, tibia and fibula

M86.561 Other chronic hematogenous osteomyelitis, right tibia and fibula

M86.562 Other chronic hematogenous osteomyelitis, left tibia and fibula

M86.569 Other chronic hematogenous osteomyelitis, unspecified tibia and fibula

√6th **M86.57** Other chronic hematogenous osteomyelitis, ankle and foot

M86.571 Other chronic hematogenous osteomyelitis, right ankle and foot

M86.572 Other chronic hematogenous osteomyelitis, left ankle and foot

M86.579 Other chronic hematogenous osteomyelitis, unspecified ankle and foot

M86.58 Other chronic hematogenous osteomyelitis, other site

M86.59 Other chronic hematogenous osteomyelitis, multiple sites

√5th **M86.6** Other chronic osteomyelitis

M86.60 Other chronic osteomyelitis, unspecified site

√6th **M86.61** Other chronic osteomyelitis, shoulder

M86.611 Other chronic osteomyelitis, right shoulder

M86.612 Other chronic osteomyelitis, left shoulder

M86.619 Other chronic osteomyelitis, unspecified shoulder

√6th **M86.62** Other chronic osteomyelitis, humerus

M86.621 Other chronic osteomyelitis, right humerus

M86.622 Other chronic osteomyelitis, left humerus

M86.629 Other chronic osteomyelitis, unspecified humerus

√6th **M86.63** Other chronic osteomyelitis, radius and ulna

M86.631 Other chronic osteomyelitis, right radius and ulna

M86.632 Other chronic osteomyelitis, left radius and ulna

EXCLUDES 1 Not coded here   EXCLUDES 2 Not included here   N Newborn Age: 0   P Pediatric Age: 0-17   M Maternity Age: 12-55   A Adult Age: 15-124

708   ICD-10-CM 2014 (Draft)

M86.639   **Other chronic osteomyelitis, unspecified radius and ulna**

✓6ᵗʰ M86.64 **Other chronic osteomyelitis, hand**
   M86.641 **Other chronic osteomyelitis, right hand**
   M86.642 **Other chronic osteomyelitis, left hand**
   M86.649 **Other chronic osteomyelitis, unspecified hand**

✓6ᵗʰ M86.65 **Other chronic osteomyelitis, thigh**
   M86.651 **Other chronic osteomyelitis, right thigh**
   M86.652 **Other chronic osteomyelitis, left thigh**
   M86.659 **Other chronic osteomyelitis, unspecified thigh**

✓6ᵗʰ M86.66 **Other chronic osteomyelitis, tibia and fibula**
   M86.661 **Other chronic osteomyelitis, right tibia and fibula**
   M86.662 **Other chronic osteomyelitis, left tibia and fibula**
   M86.669 **Other chronic osteomyelitis, unspecified tibia and fibula**

✓6ᵗʰ M86.67 **Other chronic osteomyelitis, ankle and foot**
   M86.671 **Other chronic osteomyelitis, right ankle and foot**
   M86.672 **Other chronic osteomyelitis, left ankle and foot**
   M86.679 **Other chronic osteomyelitis, unspecified ankle and foot**

   M86.68 **Other chronic osteomyelitis, other site**
   M86.69 **Other chronic osteomyelitis, multiple sites**

✓5ᵗʰ M86.8 **Other osteomyelitis**
   Brodie's abscess

✓6ᵗʰ M86.8X **Other osteomyelitis**
   M86.8X0 **Other osteomyelitis, multiple sites**
   M86.8X1 **Other osteomyelitis, shoulder**
   M86.8X2 **Other osteomyelitis, upper arm**
   M86.8X3 **Other osteomyelitis, forearm**
   M86.8X4 **Other osteomyelitis, hand**
   M86.8X5 **Other osteomyelitis, thigh**
   M86.8X6 **Other osteomyelitis, lower leg**
   M86.8X7 **Other osteomyelitis, ankle and foot**
   M86.8X8 **Other osteomyelitis, other site**
   M86.8X9 **Other osteomyelitis, unspecified sites**

M86.9 **Osteomyelitis, unspecified**
   Infection of bone NOS   Periostitis without osteomyelitis

✓4ᵗʰ **M87** **Osteonecrosis**
   INCLUDES avascular necrosis of bone
   Use additional code to identify major osseous defect, if applicable (M89.7-)
   EXCLUDES 1 *juvenile osteonecrosis (M91-M92)*
      osteochondropathies (M90-M93)

✓5ᵗʰ M87.0 **Idiopathic aseptic necrosis of bone**
   M87.00 **Idiopathic aseptic necrosis of unspecified bone**

✓6ᵗʰ M87.01 **Idiopathic aseptic necrosis of shoulder**
   Idiopathic aseptic necrosis of clavicle and scapula
   M87.011 **Idiopathic aseptic necrosis of right shoulder**
   M87.012 **Idiopathic aseptic necrosis of left shoulder**
   M87.019 **Idiopathic aseptic necrosis of unspecified shoulder**

✓6ᵗʰ M87.02 **Idiopathic aseptic necrosis of humerus**
   M87.021 **Idiopathic aseptic necrosis of right humerus**
   M87.022 **Idiopathic aseptic necrosis of left humerus**
   M87.029 **Idiopathic aseptic necrosis of unspecified humerus**

✓6ᵗʰ M87.03 **Idiopathic aseptic necrosis of radius, ulna and carpus**
   M87.031 **Idiopathic aseptic necrosis of right radius**
   M87.032 **Idiopathic aseptic necrosis of left radius**
   M87.033 **Idiopathic aseptic necrosis of unspecified radius**
   M87.034 **Idiopathic aseptic necrosis of right ulna**
   M87.035 **Idiopathic aseptic necrosis of left ulna**
   M87.036 **Idiopathic aseptic necrosis of unspecified ulna**
   M87.037 **Idiopathic aseptic necrosis of right carpus**
   M87.038 **Idiopathic aseptic necrosis of left carpus**

   M87.039 **Idiopathic aseptic necrosis of unspecified carpus**

✓6ᵗʰ M87.04 **Idiopathic aseptic necrosis of hand and fingers**
   Idiopathic aseptic necrosis of metacarpals and phalanges of hands
   M87.041 **Idiopathic aseptic necrosis of right hand**
   M87.042 **Idiopathic aseptic necrosis of left hand**
   M87.043 **Idiopathic aseptic necrosis of unspecified hand**
   M87.044 **Idiopathic aseptic necrosis of right finger(s)**
   M87.045 **Idiopathic aseptic necrosis of left finger(s)**
   M87.046 **Idiopathic aseptic necrosis of unspecified finger(s)**

✓6ᵗʰ M87.05 **Idiopathic aseptic necrosis of pelvis and femur**
   M87.050 **Idiopathic aseptic necrosis of pelvis**
   M87.051 **Idiopathic aseptic necrosis of right femur**
   M87.052 **Idiopathic aseptic necrosis of left femur**
   M87.059 **Idiopathic aseptic necrosis of unspecified femur**
      Idiopathic aseptic necrosis of hip NOS

✓6ᵗʰ M87.06 **Idiopathic aseptic necrosis of tibia and fibula**
   M87.061 **Idiopathic aseptic necrosis of right tibia**
   M87.062 **Idiopathic aseptic necrosis of left tibia**
   M87.063 **Idiopathic aseptic necrosis of unspecified tibia**
   M87.064 **Idiopathic aseptic necrosis of right fibula**
   M87.065 **Idiopathic aseptic necrosis of left fibula**
   M87.066 **Idiopathic aseptic necrosis of unspecified fibula**

✓6ᵗʰ M87.07 **Idiopathic aseptic necrosis of ankle, foot and toes**
   Idiopathic aseptic necrosis of metatarsus, tarsus, and phalanges of toes
   M87.071 **Idiopathic aseptic necrosis of right ankle**
   M87.072 **Idiopathic aseptic necrosis of left ankle**
   M87.073 **Idiopathic aseptic necrosis of unspecified ankle**
   M87.074 **Idiopathic aseptic necrosis of right foot**
   M87.075 **Idiopathic aseptic necrosis of left foot**
   M87.076 **Idiopathic aseptic necrosis of unspecified foot**
   M87.077 **Idiopathic aseptic necrosis of right toe(s)**
   M87.078 **Idiopathic aseptic necrosis of left toe(s)**
   M87.079 **Idiopathic aseptic necrosis of unspecified toe(s)**

   M87.08 **Idiopathic aseptic necrosis of bone, other site**
   M87.09 **Idiopathic aseptic necrosis of bone, multiple sites**

✓5ᵗʰ M87.1 **Osteonecrosis due to drugs**
   Use additional code for adverse effect, if applicable, to identify drug (T36-T50 with fifth or sixth character 5)
   M87.10 **Osteonecrosis due to drugs, unspecified bone**

✓6ᵗʰ M87.11 **Osteonecrosis due to drugs, shoulder**
   M87.111 **Osteonecrosis due to drugs, right shoulder**
   M87.112 **Osteonecrosis due to drugs, left shoulder**
   M87.119 **Osteonecrosis due to drugs, unspecified shoulder**

✓6ᵗʰ M87.12 **Osteonecrosis due to drugs, humerus**
   M87.121 **Osteonecrosis due to drugs, right humerus**
   M87.122 **Osteonecrosis due to drugs, left humerus**
   M87.129 **Osteonecrosis due to drugs, unspecified humerus**

✓6ᵗʰ M87.13 **Osteonecrosis due to drugs of radius, ulna and carpus**
   M87.131 **Osteonecrosis due to drugs of right radius**
   M87.132 **Osteonecrosis due to drugs of left radius**
   M87.133 **Osteonecrosis due to drugs of unspecified radius**
   M87.134 **Osteonecrosis due to drugs of right ulna**
   M87.135 **Osteonecrosis due to drugs of left ulna**
   M87.136 **Osteonecrosis due to drugs of unspecified ulna**
   M87.137 **Osteonecrosis due to drugs of right carpus**
   M87.138 **Osteonecrosis due to drugs of left carpus**
   M87.139 **Osteonecrosis due to drugs of unspecified carpus**

☑ Additional Character Required   ✓ˣ7ᵗʰ Xtension Alert   Unspecified Code   Other Specified Code   Manifestation Code   ▶◀ Revised Text   ● New Code   ▲ Revised Code Title

Diseases of the Musculoskeletal System and Connective Tissue

M87.14–M87.329

✓6ᵗʰ **M87.14** Osteonecrosis due to drugs, hand and fingers
    M87.141 Osteonecrosis due to drugs, right hand
    M87.142 Osteonecrosis due to drugs, left hand
    M87.143 Osteonecrosis due to drugs, unspecified hand
    M87.144 Osteonecrosis due to drugs, right finger(s)
    M87.145 Osteonecrosis due to drugs, left finger(s)
    M87.146 Osteonecrosis due to drugs, unspecified finger(s)

✓6ᵗʰ **M87.15** Osteonecrosis due to drugs, pelvis and femur
    M87.150 Osteonecrosis due to drugs, pelvis
    M87.151 Osteonecrosis due to drugs, right femur
    M87.152 Osteonecrosis due to drugs, left femur
    M87.159 Osteonecrosis due to drugs, unspecified femur

✓6ᵗʰ **M87.16** Osteonecrosis due to drugs, tibia and fibula
    M87.161 Osteonecrosis due to drugs, right tibia
    M87.162 Osteonecrosis due to drugs, left tibia
    M87.163 Osteonecrosis due to drugs, unspecified tibia
    M87.164 Osteonecrosis due to drugs, right fibula
    M87.165 Osteonecrosis due to drugs, left fibula
    M87.166 Osteonecrosis due to drugs, unspecified fibula

✓6ᵗʰ **M87.17** Osteonecrosis due to drugs, ankle, foot and toes
    M87.171 Osteonecrosis due to drugs, right ankle
    M87.172 Osteonecrosis due to drugs, left ankle
    M87.173 Osteonecrosis due to drugs, unspecified ankle
    M87.174 Osteonecrosis due to drugs, right foot
    M87.175 Osteonecrosis due to drugs, left foot
    M87.176 Osteonecrosis due to drugs, unspecified foot
    M87.177 Osteonecrosis due to drugs, right toe(s)
    M87.178 Osteonecrosis due to drugs, left toe(s)
    M87.179 Osteonecrosis due to drugs, unspecified toe(s)

✓6ᵗʰ **M87.18** Osteonecrosis due to drugs, other site
    M87.180 Osteonecrosis due to drugs, jaw
    M87.188 Osteonecrosis due to drugs, other site

    M87.19 Osteonecrosis due to drugs, multiple sites

✓5ᵗʰ **M87.2** Osteonecrosis due to previous trauma
    M87.20 Osteonecrosis due to previous trauma, unspecified bone

✓6ᵗʰ **M87.21** Osteonecrosis due to previous trauma, shoulder
    M87.211 Osteonecrosis due to previous trauma, right shoulder
    M87.212 Osteonecrosis due to previous trauma, left shoulder
    M87.219 Osteonecrosis due to previous trauma, unspecified shoulder

✓6ᵗʰ **M87.22** Osteonecrosis due to previous trauma, humerus
    M87.221 Osteonecrosis due to previous trauma, right humerus
    M87.222 Osteonecrosis due to previous trauma, left humerus
    M87.229 Osteonecrosis due to previous trauma, unspecified humerus

✓6ᵗʰ **M87.23** Osteonecrosis due to previous trauma of radius, ulna and carpus
    M87.231 Osteonecrosis due to previous trauma of right radius
    M87.232 Osteonecrosis due to previous trauma of left radius
    M87.233 Osteonecrosis due to previous trauma of unspecified radius
    M87.234 Osteonecrosis due to previous trauma of right ulna
    M87.235 Osteonecrosis due to previous trauma of left ulna
    M87.236 Osteonecrosis due to previous trauma of unspecified ulna
    M87.237 Osteonecrosis due to previous trauma of right carpus
    M87.238 Osteonecrosis due to previous trauma of left carpus

    M87.239 Osteonecrosis due to previous trauma of unspecified carpus

✓6ᵗʰ **M87.24** Osteonecrosis due to previous trauma, hand and fingers
    M87.241 Osteonecrosis due to previous trauma, right hand
    M87.242 Osteonecrosis due to previous trauma, left hand
    M87.243 Osteonecrosis due to previous trauma, unspecified hand
    M87.244 Osteonecrosis due to previous trauma, right finger(s)
    M87.245 Osteonecrosis due to previous trauma, left finger(s)
    M87.246 Osteonecrosis due to previous trauma, unspecified finger(s)

✓6ᵗʰ **M87.25** Osteonecrosis due to previous trauma, pelvis and femur
    M87.250 Osteonecrosis due to previous trauma, pelvis
    M87.251 Osteonecrosis due to previous trauma, right femur
    M87.252 Osteonecrosis due to previous trauma, left femur
    M87.256 Osteonecrosis due to previous trauma, unspecified femur

✓6ᵗʰ **M87.26** Osteonecrosis due to previous trauma, tibia and fibula
    M87.261 Osteonecrosis due to previous trauma, right tibia
    M87.262 Osteonecrosis due to previous trauma, left tibia
    M87.263 Osteonecrosis due to previous trauma, unspecified tibia
    M87.264 Osteonecrosis due to previous trauma, right fibula
    M87.265 Osteonecrosis due to previous trauma, left fibula
    M87.266 Osteonecrosis due to previous trauma, unspecified fibula

✓6ᵗʰ **M87.27** Osteonecrosis due to previous trauma, ankle, foot and toes
    M87.271 Osteonecrosis due to previous trauma, right ankle
    M87.272 Osteonecrosis due to previous trauma, left ankle
    M87.273 Osteonecrosis due to previous trauma, unspecified ankle
    M87.274 Osteonecrosis due to previous trauma, right foot
    M87.275 Osteonecrosis due to previous trauma, left foot
    M87.276 Osteonecrosis due to previous trauma, unspecified foot
    M87.277 Osteonecrosis due to previous trauma, right toe(s)
    M87.278 Osteonecrosis due to previous trauma, left toe(s)
    M87.279 Osteonecrosis due to previous trauma, unspecified toe(s)

    M87.28 Osteonecrosis due to previous trauma, other site
    M87.29 Osteonecrosis due to previous trauma, multiple sites

✓5ᵗʰ **M87.3** Other secondary osteonecrosis
    M87.30 Other secondary osteonecrosis, unspecified bone

✓6ᵗʰ **M87.31** Other secondary osteonecrosis, shoulder
    M87.311 Other secondary osteonecrosis, right shoulder
    M87.312 Other secondary osteonecrosis, left shoulder
    M87.319 Other secondary osteonecrosis, unspecified shoulder

✓6ᵗʰ **M87.32** Other secondary osteonecrosis, humerus
    M87.321 Other secondary osteonecrosis, right humerus
    M87.322 Other secondary osteonecrosis, left humerus
    M87.329 Other secondary osteonecrosis, unspecified humerus

---

EXCLUDES 1 Not coded here   **EXCLUDES 2** Not included here   **N** Newborn Age: 0   **P** Pediatric Age: 0-17   **M** Maternity Age: 12-55   **A** Adult Age: 15-124

✓6th **M87.33** Other secondary osteonecrosis of radius, ulna and carpus
- **M87.331** Other secondary osteonecrosis of right radius
- **M87.332** Other secondary osteonecrosis of left radius
- **M87.333** Other secondary osteonecrosis of unspecified radius
- **M87.334** Other secondary osteonecrosis of right ulna
- **M87.335** Other secondary osteonecrosis of left ulna
- **M87.336** Other secondary osteonecrosis of unspecified ulna
- **M87.337** Other secondary osteonecrosis of right carpus
- **M87.338** Other secondary osteonecrosis of left carpus
- **M87.339** Other secondary osteonecrosis of unspecified carpus

✓6th **M87.34** Other secondary osteonecrosis, hand and fingers
- **M87.341** Other secondary osteonecrosis, right hand
- **M87.342** Other secondary osteonecrosis, left hand
- **M87.343** Other secondary osteonecrosis, unspecified hand
- **M87.344** Other secondary osteonecrosis, right finger(s)
- **M87.345** Other secondary osteonecrosis, left finger(s)
- **M87.346** Other secondary osteonecrosis, unspecified finger(s)

✓6th **M87.35** Other secondary osteonecrosis, pelvis and femur
- **M87.350** Other secondary osteonecrosis, pelvis
- **M87.351** Other secondary osteonecrosis, right femur
- **M87.352** Other secondary osteonecrosis, left femur
- **M87.353** Other secondary osteonecrosis, unspecified femur

✓6th **M87.36** Other secondary osteonecrosis, tibia and fibula
- **M87.361** Other secondary osteonecrosis, right tibia
- **M87.362** Other secondary osteonecrosis, left tibia
- **M87.363** Other secondary osteonecrosis, unspecified tibia
- **M87.364** Other secondary osteonecrosis, right fibula
- **M87.365** Other secondary osteonecrosis, left fibula
- **M87.366** Other secondary osteonecrosis, unspecified fibula

✓6th **M87.37** Other secondary osteonecrosis, ankle and foot
- **M87.371** Other secondary osteonecrosis, right ankle
- **M87.372** Other secondary osteonecrosis, left ankle
- **M87.373** Other secondary osteonecrosis, unspecified ankle
- **M87.374** Other secondary osteonecrosis, right foot
- **M87.375** Other secondary osteonecrosis, left foot
- **M87.376** Other secondary osteonecrosis, unspecified foot
- **M87.377** Other secondary osteonecrosis, right toe(s)
- **M87.378** Other secondary osteonecrosis, left toe(s)
- **M87.379** Other secondary osteonecrosis, unspecified toe(s)

M87.38 Other secondary osteonecrosis, other site
M87.39 Other secondary osteonecrosis, multiple sites

✓5th **M87.8** Other osteonecrosis
M87.80 Other osteonecrosis, unspecified bone
✓6th **M87.81** Other osteonecrosis, shoulder
- **M87.811** Other osteonecrosis, right shoulder
- **M87.812** Other osteonecrosis, left shoulder
- **M87.819** Other osteonecrosis, unspecified shoulder
✓6th **M87.82** Other osteonecrosis, humerus
- **M87.821** Other osteonecrosis, right humerus
- **M87.822** Other osteonecrosis, left humerus
- **M87.829** Other osteonecrosis, unspecified humerus

✓6th **M87.83** Other osteonecrosis of radius, ulna and carpus
- **M87.831** Other osteonecrosis of right radius
- **M87.832** Other osteonecrosis of left radius
- **M87.833** Other osteonecrosis of unspecified radius
- **M87.834** Other osteonecrosis of right ulna
- **M87.835** Other osteonecrosis of left ulna
- **M87.836** Other osteonecrosis of unspecified ulna
- **M87.837** Other osteonecrosis of right carpus
- **M87.838** Other osteonecrosis of left carpus
- **M87.839** Other osteonecrosis of unspecified carpus

✓6th **M87.84** Other osteonecrosis, hand and fingers
- **M87.841** Other osteonecrosis, right hand
- **M87.842** Other osteonecrosis, left hand
- **M87.843** Other osteonecrosis, unspecified hand
- **M87.844** Other osteonecrosis, right finger(s)
- **M87.845** Other osteonecrosis, left finger(s)
- **M87.849** Other osteonecrosis, unspecified finger(s)

✓6th **M87.85** Other osteonecrosis, pelvis and femur
- **M87.850** Other osteonecrosis, pelvis
- **M87.851** Other osteonecrosis, right femur
- **M87.852** Other osteonecrosis, left femur
- **M87.859** Other osteonecrosis, unspecified femur

✓6th **M87.86** Other osteonecrosis, tibia and fibula
- **M87.861** Other osteonecrosis, right tibia
- **M87.862** Other osteonecrosis, left tibia
- **M87.863** Other osteonecrosis, unspecified tibia
- **M87.864** Other osteonecrosis, right fibula
- **M87.865** Other osteonecrosis, left fibula
- **M87.869** Other osteonecrosis, unspecified fibula

✓6th **M87.87** Other osteonecrosis, ankle, foot and toes
- **M87.871** Other osteonecrosis, right ankle
- **M87.872** Other osteonecrosis, left ankle
- **M87.873** Other osteonecrosis, unspecified ankle
- **M87.874** Other osteonecrosis, right foot
- **M87.875** Other osteonecrosis, left foot
- **M87.876** Other osteonecrosis, unspecified foot
- **M87.877** Other osteonecrosis, right toe(s)
- **M87.878** Other osteonecrosis, left toe(s)
- **M87.879** Other osteonecrosis, unspecified toe(s)

M87.88 Other osteonecrosis, other site
M87.89 Other osteonecrosis, multiple sites

M87.9 Osteonecrosis, unspecified
Necrosis of bone NOS

✓4th **M88** Osteitis deformans [Paget's disease of bone]
> EXCLUDES 1 osteitis deformans in neoplastic disease (M90.6)

M88.0 Osteitis deformans of skull
M88.1 Osteitis deformans of vertebrae
✓5th **M88.8** Osteitis deformans of other bones
✓6th **M88.81** Osteitis deformans of shoulder
- **M88.811** Osteitis deformans of right shoulder
- **M88.812** Osteitis deformans of left shoulder
- **M88.819** Osteitis deformans of unspecified shoulder
✓6th **M88.82** Osteitis deformans of upper arm
- **M88.821** Osteitis deformans of right upper arm
- **M88.822** Osteitis deformans of left upper arm
- **M88.829** Osteitis deformans of unspecified upper arm
✓6th **M88.83** Osteitis deformans of forearm
- **M88.831** Osteitis deformans of right forearm
- **M88.832** Osteitis deformans of left forearm
- **M88.839** Osteitis deformans of unspecified forearm
✓6th **M88.84** Osteitis deformans of hand
- **M88.841** Osteitis deformans of right hand
- **M88.842** Osteitis deformans of left hand
- **M88.849** Osteitis deformans of unspecified hand
✓6th **M88.85** Osteitis deformans of thigh
- **M88.851** Osteitis deformans of right thigh
- **M88.852** Osteitis deformans of left thigh
- **M88.859** Osteitis deformans of unspecified thigh

☑ Additional Character Required   ✓x7th Xtension Alert   Unspecified Code   Other Specified Code   Manifestation Code   ►◄ Revised Text   ● New Code   ▲ Revised Code Title

ICD-10-CM 2014 (Draft)   711

√6ᵗʰ **M88.86** Osteitis deformans of lower leg
- **M88.861** Osteitis deformans of right lower leg
- **M88.862** Osteitis deformans of left lower leg
- **M88.869** Osteitis deformans of unspecified lower leg

√6ᵗʰ **M88.87** Osteitis deformans of ankle and foot
- **M88.871** Osteitis deformans of right ankle and foot
- **M88.872** Osteitis deformans of left ankle and foot
- **M88.879** Osteitis deformans of unspecified ankle and foot

M88.88 Osteitis deformans of other bones
> EXCLUDES 2 osteitis deformans of skull (M88.0)
> osteitis deformans of vertebrae (M88.1)

M88.89 Osteitis deformans of multiple sites

M88.9 Osteitis deformans of unspecified bone

√4ᵗʰ **M89** Other disorders of bone

√5ᵗʰ **M89.0** Algoneurodystrophy
Shoulder-hand syndrome
Sudeck's atrophy
> EXCLUDES 1 causalgia, lower limb (G57.7-)
> causalgia, upper limb (G56.4-)
> complex regional pain syndrome II, lower limb (G57.7-)
> complex regional pain syndrome II, upper limb (G56.4-)
> reflex sympathetic dystrophy (G90.5-)

M89.00 Algoneurodystrophy, unspecified site

√6ᵗʰ **M89.01** Algoneurodystrophy, shoulder
- **M89.011** Algoneurodystrophy, right shoulder
- **M89.012** Algoneurodystrophy, left shoulder
- **M89.019** Algoneurodystrophy, unspecified shoulder

√6ᵗʰ **M89.02** Algoneurodystrophy, upper arm
- **M89.021** Algoneurodystrophy, right upper arm
- **M89.022** Algoneurodystrophy, left upper arm
- **M89.029** Algoneurodystrophy, unspecified upper arm

√6ᵗʰ **M89.03** Algoneurodystrophy, forearm
- **M89.031** Algoneurodystrophy, right forearm
- **M89.032** Algoneurodystrophy, left forearm
- **M89.039** Algoneurodystrophy, unspecified forearm

√6ᵗʰ **M89.04** Algoneurodystrophy, hand
- **M89.041** Algoneurodystrophy, right hand
- **M89.042** Algoneurodystrophy, left hand
- **M89.049** Algoneurodystrophy, unspecified hand

√6ᵗʰ **M89.05** Algoneurodystrophy, thigh
- **M89.051** Algoneurodystrophy, right thigh
- **M89.052** Algoneurodystrophy, left thigh
- **M89.059** Algoneurodystrophy, unspecified thigh

√6ᵗʰ **M89.06** Algoneurodystrophy, lower leg
- **M89.061** Algoneurodystrophy, right lower leg
- **M89.062** Algoneurodystrophy, left lower leg
- **M89.069** Algoneurodystrophy, unspecified lower leg

√6ᵗʰ **M89.07** Algoneurodystrophy, ankle and foot
- **M89.071** Algoneurodystrophy, right ankle and foot
- **M89.072** Algoneurodystrophy, left ankle and foot
- **M89.079** Algoneurodystrophy, unspecified ankle and foot

M89.08 Algoneurodystrophy, other site

M89.09 Algoneurodystrophy, multiple sites

√5ᵗʰ **M89.1** Physeal arrest
Arrest of growth plate　　　Growth plate arrest
Epiphyseal arrest

√6ᵗʰ **M89.12** Physeal arrest, humerus
- **M89.121** Complete physeal arrest, right proximal humerus
- **M89.122** Complete physeal arrest, left proximal humerus
- **M89.123** Partial physeal arrest, right proximal humerus
- **M89.124** Partial physeal arrest, left proximal humerus
- **M89.125** Complete physeal arrest, right distal humerus
- **M89.126** Complete physeal arrest, left distal humerus
- **M89.127** Partial physeal arrest, right distal humerus
- **M89.128** Partial physeal arrest, left distal humerus
- **M89.129** Physeal arrest, humerus, unspecified

√6ᵗʰ **M89.13** Physeal arrest, forearm
- **M89.131** Complete physeal arrest, right distal radius
- **M89.132** Complete physeal arrest, left distal radius
- **M89.133** Partial physeal arrest, right distal radius
- **M89.134** Partial physeal arrest, left distal radius
- **M89.138** Other physeal arrest of forearm
- **M89.139** Physeal arrest, forearm, unspecified

√6ᵗʰ **M89.15** Physeal arrest, femur
- **M89.151** Complete physeal arrest, right proximal femur
- **M89.152** Complete physeal arrest, left proximal femur
- **M89.153** Partial physeal arrest, right proximal femur
- **M89.154** Partial physeal arrest, left proximal femur
- **M89.155** Complete physeal arrest, right distal femur
- **M89.156** Complete physeal arrest, left distal femur
- **M89.157** Partial physeal arrest, right distal femur
- **M89.158** Partial physeal arrest, left distal femur
- **M89.159** Physeal arrest, femur, unspecified

√6ᵗʰ **M89.16** Physeal arrest, lower leg
- **M89.160** Complete physeal arrest, right proximal tibia
- **M89.161** Complete physeal arrest, left proximal tibia
- **M89.162** Partial physeal arrest, right proximal tibia
- **M89.163** Partial physeal arrest, left proximal tibia
- **M89.164** Complete physeal arrest, right distal tibia
- **M89.165** Complete physeal arrest, left distal tibia
- **M89.166** Partial physeal arrest, right distal tibia
- **M89.167** Partial physeal arrest, left distal tibia
- **M89.168** Other physeal arrest of lower leg
- **M89.169** Physeal arrest, lower leg, unspecified

M89.18 Physeal arrest, other site

√5ᵗʰ **M89.2** Other disorders of bone development and growth
- **M89.20** Other disorders of bone development and growth, unspecified site

√6ᵗʰ **M89.21** Other disorders of bone development and growth, shoulder
- **M89.211** Other disorders of bone development and growth, right shoulder
- **M89.212** Other disorders of bone development and growth, left shoulder
- **M89.219** Other disorders of bone development and growth, unspecified shoulder

√6ᵗʰ **M89.22** Other disorders of bone development and growth, humerus
- **M89.221** Other disorders of bone development and growth, right humerus
- **M89.222** Other disorders of bone development and growth, left humerus
- **M89.229** Other disorders of bone development and growth, unspecified humerus

√6ᵗʰ **M89.23** Other disorders of bone development and growth, ulna and radius
- **M89.231** Other disorders of bone development and growth, right ulna
- **M89.232** Other disorders of bone development and growth, left ulna
- **M89.233** Other disorders of bone development and growth, right radius
- **M89.234** Other disorders of bone development and growth, left radius
- **M89.239** Other disorders of bone development and growth, unspecified ulna and radius

EXCLUDES 1 Not coded here　　　EXCLUDES 2 Not included here　　　N Newborn Age: 0　　　P Pediatric Age: 0-17　　　M Maternity Age: 12-55　　　A Adult Age: 15-124

712　　　ICD-10-CM 2014 (Draft)

✓6th **M89.24** Other disorders of bone development and growth, hand
  M89.241 Other disorders of bone development and growth, right hand
  M89.242 Other disorders of bone development and growth, left hand
  M89.249 Other disorders of bone development and growth, unspecified hand

✓6th **M89.25** Other disorders of bone development and growth, femur
  M89.251 Other disorders of bone development and growth, right femur
  M89.252 Other disorders of bone development and growth, left femur
  M89.259 Other disorders of bone development and growth, unspecified femur

✓6th **M89.26** Other disorders of bone development and growth, tibia and fibula
  M89.261 Other disorders of bone development and growth, right tibia
  M89.262 Other disorders of bone development and growth, left tibia
  M89.263 Other disorders of bone development and growth, right fibula
  M89.264 Other disorders of bone development and growth, left fibula
  M89.269 Other disorders of bone development and growth, unspecified lower leg

✓6th **M89.27** Other disorders of bone development and growth, ankle and foot
  M89.271 Other disorders of bone development and growth, right ankle and foot
  M89.272 Other disorders of bone development and growth, left ankle and foot
  M89.279 Other disorders of bone development and growth, unspecified ankle and foot
  M89.28 Other disorders of bone development and growth, other site
  M89.29 Other disorders of bone development and growth, multiple sites

✓5th **M89.3** Hypertrophy of bone
  M89.30 Hypertrophy of bone, unspecified site
  ✓6th **M89.31** Hypertrophy of bone, shoulder
    M89.311 Hypertrophy of bone, right shoulder
    M89.312 Hypertrophy of bone, left shoulder
    M89.319 Hypertrophy of bone, unspecified shoulder
  ✓6th **M89.32** Hypertrophy of bone, humerus
    M89.321 Hypertrophy of bone, right humerus
    M89.322 Hypertrophy of bone, left humerus
    M89.329 Hypertrophy of bone, unspecified humerus
  ✓6th **M89.33** Hypertrophy of bone, ulna and radius
    M89.331 Hypertrophy of bone, right ulna
    M89.332 Hypertrophy of bone, left ulna
    M89.333 Hypertrophy of bone, right radius
    M89.334 Hypertrophy of bone, left radius
    M89.339 Hypertrophy of bone, unspecified ulna and radius
  ✓6th **M89.34** Hypertrophy of bone, hand
    M89.341 Hypertrophy of bone, right hand
    M89.342 Hypertrophy of bone, left hand
    M89.349 Hypertrophy of bone, unspecified hand
  ✓6th **M89.35** Hypertrophy of bone, femur
    M89.351 Hypertrophy of bone, right femur
    M89.352 Hypertrophy of bone, left femur
    M89.359 Hypertrophy of bone, unspecified femur
  ✓6th **M89.36** Hypertrophy of bone, tibia and fibula
    M89.361 Hypertrophy of bone, right tibia
    M89.362 Hypertrophy of bone, left tibia
    M89.363 Hypertrophy of bone, right fibula
    M89.364 Hypertrophy of bone, left fibula
    M89.369 Hypertrophy of bone, unspecified tibia and fibula

✓6th **M89.37** Hypertrophy of bone, ankle and foot
  M89.371 Hypertrophy of bone, right ankle and foot
  M89.372 Hypertrophy of bone, left ankle and foot
  M89.379 Hypertrophy of bone, unspecified ankle and foot
  M89.38 Hypertrophy of bone, other site
  M89.39 Hypertrophy of bone, multiple sites

✓5th **M89.4** Other hypertrophic osteoarthropathy
  Marie-Bamberger disease   Pachydermoperiostosis
  M89.40 Other hypertrophic osteoarthropathy, unspecified site
  ✓6th **M89.41** Other hypertrophic osteoarthropathy, shoulder
    M89.411 Other hypertrophic osteoarthropathy, right shoulder
    M89.412 Other hypertrophic osteoarthropathy, left shoulder
    M89.419 Other hypertrophic osteoarthropathy, unspecified shoulder
  ✓6th **M89.42** Other hypertrophic osteoarthropathy, upper arm
    M89.421 Other hypertrophic osteoarthropathy, right upper arm
    M89.422 Other hypertrophic osteoarthropathy, left upper arm
    M89.429 Other hypertrophic osteoarthropathy, unspecified upper arm
  ✓6th **M89.43** Other hypertrophic osteoarthropathy, forearm
    M89.431 Other hypertrophic osteoarthropathy, right forearm
    M89.432 Other hypertrophic osteoarthropathy, left forearm
    M89.439 Other hypertrophic osteoarthropathy, unspecified forearm
  ✓6th **M89.44** Other hypertrophic osteoarthropathy, hand
    M89.441 Other hypertrophic osteoarthropathy, right hand
    M89.442 Other hypertrophic osteoarthropathy, left hand
    M89.449 Other hypertrophic osteoarthropathy, unspecified hand
  ✓6th **M89.45** Other hypertrophic osteoarthropathy, thigh
    M89.451 Other hypertrophic osteoarthropathy, right thigh
    M89.452 Other hypertrophic osteoarthropathy, left thigh
    M89.459 Other hypertrophic osteoarthropathy, unspecified thigh
  ✓6th **M89.46** Other hypertrophic osteoarthropathy, lower leg
    M89.461 Other hypertrophic osteoarthropathy, right lower leg
    M89.462 Other hypertrophic osteoarthropathy, left lower leg
    M89.469 Other hypertrophic osteoarthropathy, unspecified lower leg
  ✓6th **M89.47** Other hypertrophic osteoarthropathy, ankle and foot
    M89.471 Other hypertrophic osteoarthropathy, right ankle and foot
    M89.472 Other hypertrophic osteoarthropathy, left ankle and foot
    M89.479 Other hypertrophic osteoarthropathy, unspecified ankle and foot
  M89.48 Other hypertrophic osteoarthropathy, other site
  M89.49 Other hypertrophic osteoarthropathy, multiple sites

✓5th **M89.5** Osteolysis
  Use additional code to identify major osseous defect, if applicable (M89.7-)
  EXCLUDES 2 periprosthetic osteolysis of internal prosthetic joint (T84.05-)
  M89.50 Osteolysis, unspecified site
  ✓6th **M89.51** Osteolysis, shoulder
    M89.511 Osteolysis, right shoulder
    M89.512 Osteolysis, left shoulder
    M89.519 Osteolysis, unspecified shoulder
  ✓6th **M89.52** Osteolysis, upper arm
    M89.521 Osteolysis, right upper arm
    M89.522 Osteolysis, left upper arm

M89.529 Osteolysis, unspecified upper arm

✓6ᵗʰ M89.53 Osteolysis, forearm
- M89.531 Osteolysis, right forearm
- M89.532 Osteolysis, left forearm
- M89.539 Osteolysis, unspecified forearm

✓6ᵗʰ M89.54 Osteolysis, hand
- M89.541 Osteolysis, right hand
- M89.542 Osteolysis, left hand
- M89.549 Osteolysis, unspecified hand

✓6ᵗʰ M89.55 Osteolysis, thigh
- M89.551 Osteolysis, right thigh
- M89.552 Osteolysis, left thigh
- M89.559 Osteolysis, unspecified thigh

✓6ᵗʰ M89.56 Osteolysis, lower leg
- M89.561 Osteolysis, right lower leg
- M89.562 Osteolysis, left lower leg
- M89.569 Osteolysis, unspecified lower leg

✓6ᵗʰ M89.57 Osteolysis, ankle and foot
- M89.571 Osteolysis, right ankle and foot
- M89.572 Osteolysis, left ankle and foot
- M89.579 Osteolysis, unspecified ankle and foot

M89.58 Osteolysis, other site

M89.59 Osteolysis, multiple sites

✓5ᵗʰ M89.6 Osteopathy after poliomyelitis
Use additional code (B91) to identify previous poliomyelitis
EXCLUDES 1 postpolio syndrome (G14)

M89.60 Osteopathy after poliomyelitis, unspecified site

✓6ᵗʰ M89.61 Osteopathy after poliomyelitis, shoulder
- M89.611 Osteopathy after poliomyelitis, right shoulder
- M89.612 Osteopathy after poliomyelitis, left shoulder
- M89.619 Osteopathy after poliomyelitis, unspecified shoulder

✓6ᵗʰ M89.62 Osteopathy after poliomyelitis, upper arm
- M89.621 Osteopathy after poliomyelitis, right upper arm
- M89.622 Osteopathy after poliomyelitis, left upper arm
- M89.629 Osteopathy after poliomyelitis, unspecified upper arm

✓6ᵗʰ M89.63 Osteopathy after poliomyelitis, forearm
- M89.631 Osteopathy after poliomyelitis, right forearm
- M89.632 Osteopathy after poliomyelitis, left forearm
- M89.639 Osteopathy after poliomyelitis, unspecified forearm

✓6ᵗʰ M89.64 Osteopathy after poliomyelitis, hand
- M89.641 Osteopathy after poliomyelitis, right hand
- M89.642 Osteopathy after poliomyelitis, left hand
- M89.649 Osteopathy after poliomyelitis, unspecified hand

✓6ᵗʰ M89.65 Osteopathy after poliomyelitis, thigh
- M89.651 Osteopathy after poliomyelitis, right thigh
- M89.652 Osteopathy after poliomyelitis, left thigh
- M89.659 Osteopathy after poliomyelitis, unspecified thigh

✓6ᵗʰ M89.66 Osteopathy after poliomyelitis, lower leg
- M89.661 Osteopathy after poliomyelitis, right lower leg
- M89.662 Osteopathy after poliomyelitis, left lower leg
- M89.669 Osteopathy after poliomyelitis, unspecified lower leg

✓6ᵗʰ M89.67 Osteopathy after poliomyelitis, ankle and foot
- M89.671 Osteopathy after poliomyelitis, right ankle and foot
- M89.672 Osteopathy after poliomyelitis, left ankle and foot
- M89.679 Osteopathy after poliomyelitis, unspecified ankle and foot

M89.68 Osteopathy after poliomyelitis, other site

M89.69 Osteopathy after poliomyelitis, multiple sites

✓5ᵗʰ M89.7 Major osseous defect
Code first underlying disease, if known, such as:
aseptic necrosis of bone (M87.-)
malignant neoplasm of bone (C40.-)
osteolysis (M89.5)
osteomyelitis (M86.-)
osteonecrosis (M87.-)
osteoporosis (M80.-, M81.-)
periprosthetic osteolysis (T84.05-)

M89.70 Major osseous defect, unspecified site

✓6ᵗʰ M89.71 Major osseous defect, shoulder region
Major osseous defect clavicle or scapula
- M89.711 Major osseous defect, right shoulder region
- M89.712 Major osseous defect, left shoulder region
- M89.719 Major osseous defect, unspecified shoulder region

✓6ᵗʰ M89.72 Major osseous defect, humerus
- M89.721 Major osseous defect, right humerus
- M89.722 Major osseous defect, left humerus
- M89.729 Major osseous defect, unspecified humerus

✓6ᵗʰ M89.73 Major osseous defect, forearm
Major osseous defect of radius and ulna
- M89.731 Major osseous defect, right forearm
- M89.732 Major osseous defect, left forearm
- M89.739 Major osseous defect, unspecified forearm

✓6ᵗʰ M89.74 Major osseous defect, hand
Major osseous defect of carpus, fingers, metacarpus
- M89.741 Major osseous defect, right hand
- M89.742 Major osseous defect, left hand
- M89.749 Major osseous defect, unspecified hand

✓6ᵗʰ M89.75 Major osseous defect, pelvic region and thigh
Major osseous defect of femur and pelvis
- M89.751 Major osseous defect, right pelvic region and thigh
- M89.752 Major osseous defect, left pelvic region and thigh
- M89.759 Major osseous defect, unspecified pelvic region and thigh

✓6ᵗʰ M89.76 Major osseous defect, lower leg
Major osseous defect of fibula and tibia
- M89.761 Major osseous defect, right lower leg
- M89.762 Major osseous defect, left lower leg
- M89.769 Major osseous defect, unspecified lower leg

✓6ᵗʰ M89.77 Major osseous defect, ankle and foot
Major osseous defect of metatarsus, tarsus, toes
- M89.771 Major osseous defect, right ankle and foot
- M89.772 Major osseous defect, left ankle and foot
- M89.779 Major osseous defect, unspecified ankle and foot

M89.78 Major osseous defect, other site

M89.79 Major osseous defect, multiple sites

✓5ᵗʰ M89.8 Other specified disorders of bone
Infantile cortical hyperostoses
Post-traumatic subperiosteal ossification

✓6ᵗʰ M89.8X Other specified disorders of bone
- M89.8X0 Other specified disorders of bone, multiple sites
- M89.8X1 Other specified disorders of bone, shoulder
- M89.8X2 Other specified disorders of bone, upper arm
- M89.8X3 Other specified disorders of bone, forearm
- M89.8X4 Other specified disorders of bone, hand
- M89.8X5 Other specified disorders of bone, thigh
- M89.8X6 Other specified disorders of bone, lower leg
- M89.8X7 Other specified disorders of bone, ankle and foot
- M89.8X8 Other specified disorders of bone, other site
- M89.8X9 Other specified disorders of bone, unspecified site

M89.9 Disorder of bone, unspecified

EXCLUDES 1 Not coded here   EXCLUDES 2 Not included here   N Newborn Age: 0   P Pediatric Age: 0-17   M Maternity Age: 12-55   A Adult Age: 15-124

714   ICD-10-CM 2014 (Draft)

☑️4ᵗʰ **M90 Osteopathies in diseases classified elsewhere**

> **EXCLUDES 1**   osteochondritis, osteomyelitis, and osteopathy (in):
>> cryptococcosis (B45.3)
>> diabetes mellitus (E08-E13 with .61-)
>> gonococcal (A54.43)
>> neurogenic syphilis (A52.11)
>> renal osteodystrophy (N25.0)
>> salmonellosis (A02.24)
>> secondary syphilis (A51.46)
>> syphilis (late) (A52.77)

☑️5ᵗʰ **M90.5 Osteonecrosis in diseases classified elsewhere**

> *Code first underlying disease, such as:*
>> *caisson disease (T70.3)*
>> *hemoglobinopathy (D50-D64)*

> **M90.50** *Osteonecrosis in diseases classified elsewhere, unspecified site*

> ☑️6ᵗʰ **M90.51** Osteonecrosis in diseases classified elsewhere, shoulder
>> **M90.511** *Osteonecrosis in diseases classified elsewhere, right shoulder*
>> **M90.512** *Osteonecrosis in diseases classified elsewhere, left shoulder*
>> **M90.519** *Osteonecrosis in diseases classified elsewhere, unspecified shoulder*

> ☑️6ᵗʰ **M90.52** Osteonecrosis in diseases classified elsewhere, upper arm
>> **M90.521** *Osteonecrosis in diseases classified elsewhere, right upper arm*
>> **M90.522** *Osteonecrosis in diseases classified elsewhere, left upper arm*
>> **M90.529** *Osteonecrosis in diseases classified elsewhere, unspecified upper arm*

> ☑️6ᵗʰ **M90.53** Osteonecrosis in diseases classified elsewhere, forearm
>> **M90.531** *Osteonecrosis in diseases classified elsewhere, right forearm*
>> **M90.532** *Osteonecrosis in diseases classified elsewhere, left forearm*
>> **M90.539** *Osteonecrosis in diseases classified elsewhere, unspecified forearm*

> ☑️6ᵗʰ **M90.54** Osteonecrosis in diseases classified elsewhere, hand
>> **M90.541** *Osteonecrosis in diseases classified elsewhere, right hand*
>> **M90.542** *Osteonecrosis in diseases classified elsewhere, left hand*
>> **M90.549** *Osteonecrosis in diseases classified elsewhere, unspecified hand*

> ☑️6ᵗʰ **M90.55** Osteonecrosis in diseases classified elsewhere, thigh
>> **M90.551** *Osteonecrosis in diseases classified elsewhere, right thigh*
>> **M90.552** *Osteonecrosis in diseases classified elsewhere, left thigh*
>> **M90.559** *Osteonecrosis in diseases classified elsewhere, unspecified thigh*

> ☑️6ᵗʰ **M90.56** Osteonecrosis in diseases classified elsewhere, lower leg
>> **M90.561** *Osteonecrosis in diseases classified elsewhere, right lower leg*
>> **M90.562** *Osteonecrosis in diseases classified elsewhere, left lower leg*
>> **M90.569** *Osteonecrosis in diseases classified elsewhere, unspecified lower leg*

> ☑️6ᵗʰ **M90.57** Osteonecrosis in diseases classified elsewhere, ankle and foot
>> **M90.571** *Osteonecrosis in diseases classified elsewhere, right ankle and foot*
>> **M90.572** *Osteonecrosis in diseases classified elsewhere, left ankle and foot*
>> **M90.579** *Osteonecrosis in diseases classified elsewhere, unspecified ankle and foot*

> **M90.58** *Osteonecrosis in diseases classified elsewhere, other site*

> **M90.59** *Osteonecrosis in diseases classified elsewhere, multiple sites*

☑️5ᵗʰ **M90.6 Osteitis deformans in neoplastic diseases**
> Osteitis deformans in malignant neoplasm of bone
> *Code first the neoplasm (C40-, C41-)*
> **EXCLUDES 1**   osteitis deformans [Paget's disease of bone] (M88.-)

> **M90.60** *Osteitis deformans in neoplastic diseases, unspecified site*

> ☑️6ᵗʰ **M90.61** Osteitis deformans in neoplastic diseases, shoulder
>> **M90.611** *Osteitis deformans in neoplastic diseases, right shoulder*
>> **M90.612** *Osteitis deformans in neoplastic diseases, left shoulder*
>> **M90.619** *Osteitis deformans in neoplastic diseases, unspecified shoulder*

> ☑️6ᵗʰ **M90.62** Osteitis deformans in neoplastic diseases, upper arm
>> **M90.621** *Osteitis deformans in neoplastic diseases, right upper arm*
>> **M90.622** *Osteitis deformans in neoplastic diseases, left upper arm*
>> **M90.629** *Osteitis deformans in neoplastic diseases, unspecified upper arm*

> ☑️6ᵗʰ **M90.63** Osteitis deformans in neoplastic diseases, forearm
>> **M90.631** *Osteitis deformans in neoplastic diseases, right forearm*
>> **M90.632** *Osteitis deformans in neoplastic diseases, left forearm*
>> **M90.639** *Osteitis deformans in neoplastic diseases, unspecified forearm*

> ☑️6ᵗʰ **M90.64** Osteitis deformans in neoplastic diseases, hand
>> **M90.641** *Osteitis deformans in neoplastic diseases, right hand*
>> **M90.642** *Osteitis deformans in neoplastic diseases, left hand*
>> **M90.649** *Osteitis deformans in neoplastic diseases, unspecified hand*

> ☑️6ᵗʰ **M90.65** Osteitis deformans in neoplastic diseases, thigh
>> **M90.651** *Osteitis deformans in neoplastic diseases, right thigh*
>> **M90.652** *Osteitis deformans in neoplastic diseases, left thigh*
>> **M90.659** *Osteitis deformans in neoplastic diseases, unspecified thigh*

> ☑️6ᵗʰ **M90.66** Osteitis deformans in neoplastic diseases, lower leg
>> **M90.661** *Osteitis deformans in neoplastic diseases, right lower leg*
>> **M90.662** *Osteitis deformans in neoplastic diseases, left lower leg*
>> **M90.669** *Osteitis deformans in neoplastic diseases, unspecified lower leg*

> ☑️6ᵗʰ **M90.67** Osteitis deformans in neoplastic diseases, ankle and foot
>> **M90.671** *Osteitis deformans in neoplastic diseases, right ankle and foot*
>> **M90.672** *Osteitis deformans in neoplastic diseases, left ankle and foot*
>> **M90.679** *Osteitis deformans in neoplastic diseases, unspecified ankle and foot*

> **M90.68** *Osteitis deformans in neoplastic diseases, other site*

> **M90.69** *Osteitis deformans in neoplastic diseases, multiple sites*

☑️5ᵗʰ **M90.8 Osteopathy in diseases classified elsewhere**
> *Code first underlying disease, such as:*
>> *rickets (E55.0)*
>> *vitamin-D-resistant rickets (E83.3)*

> **M90.80** *Osteopathy in diseases classified elsewhere, unspecified site*

> ☑️6ᵗʰ **M90.81** Osteopathy in diseases classified elsewhere, shoulder
>> **M90.811** *Osteopathy in diseases classified elsewhere, right shoulder*
>> **M90.812** *Osteopathy in diseases classified elsewhere, left shoulder*
>> **M90.819** *Osteopathy in diseases classified elsewhere, unspecified shoulder*

> ☑️6ᵗʰ **M90.82** Osteopathy in diseases classified elsewhere, upper arm
>> **M90.821** *Osteopathy in diseases classified elsewhere, right upper arm*
>> **M90.822** *Osteopathy in diseases classified elsewhere, left upper arm*
>> **M90.829** *Osteopathy in diseases classified elsewhere, unspecified upper arm*

☑️ Additional Character Required   ☑️x7ᵗʰ Xtension Alert   Unspecified Code   Other Specified Code   Manifestation Code   ▶◀ Revised Text   ● New Code   ▲ Revised Code Title

Diseases of the Musculoskeletal System and Connective Tissue

M90.83–M92.42

✓6ᵗʰ **M90.83 Osteopathy in diseases classified elsewhere, forearm**
- *M90.831 Osteopathy in diseases classified elsewhere, right forearm*
- *M90.832 Osteopathy in diseases classified elsewhere, left forearm*
- *M90.839 Osteopathy in diseases classified elsewhere, unspecified forearm*

✓6ᵗʰ **M90.84 Osteopathy in diseases classified elsewhere, hand**
- *M90.841 Osteopathy in diseases classified elsewhere, right hand*
- *M90.842 Osteopathy in diseases classified elsewhere, left hand*
- *M90.849 Osteopathy in diseases classified elsewhere, unspecified hand*

✓6ᵗʰ **M90.85 Osteopathy in diseases classified elsewhere, thigh**
- *M90.851 Osteopathy in diseases classified elsewhere, right thigh*
- *M90.852 Osteopathy in diseases classified elsewhere, left thigh*
- *M90.859 Osteopathy in diseases classified elsewhere, unspecified thigh*

✓6ᵗʰ **M90.86 Osteopathy in diseases classified elsewhere, lower leg**
- *M90.861 Osteopathy in diseases classified elsewhere, right lower leg*
- *M90.862 Osteopathy in diseases classified elsewhere, left lower leg*
- *M90.869 Osteopathy in diseases classified elsewhere, unspecified lower leg*

✓6ᵗʰ **M90.87 Osteopathy in diseases classified elsewhere, ankle and foot**
- *M90.871 Osteopathy in diseases classified elsewhere, right ankle and foot*
- *M90.872 Osteopathy in diseases classified elsewhere, left ankle and foot*
- *M90.879 Osteopathy in diseases classified elsewhere, unspecified ankle and foot*

M90.88 Osteopathy in diseases classified elsewhere, other site

M90.89 Osteopathy in diseases classified elsewhere, multiple sites

Chondropathies (M91-M94)

EXCLUDES1 *postprocedural chondropathies (M96.-)*

✓4ᵗʰ **M91 Juvenile osteochondrosis of hip and pelvis**
EXCLUDES1 *slipped upper femoral epiphysis (nontraumatic) (M93.0)*

M91.0 Juvenile osteochondrosis of pelvis
Osteochondrosis (juvenile) of acetabulum
Osteochondrosis (juvenile) of iliac crest [Buchanan]
Osteochondrosis (juvenile) of ischiopubic synchondrosis [van Neck]
Osteochondrosis (juvenile) of symphysis pubis [Pierson]

✓5ᵗʰ **M91.1 Juvenile osteochondrosis of head of femur [Legg-Calvé-Perthes]**
- **M91.10 Juvenile osteochondrosis of head of femur [Legg-Calvé-Perthes], unspecified leg**
- **M91.11 Juvenile osteochondrosis of head of femur [Legg-Calvé-Perthes], right leg**
- **M91.12 Juvenile osteochondrosis of head of femur [Legg-Calvé-Perthes], left leg**

✓5ᵗʰ **M91.2 Coxa plana**
Hip deformity due to previous juvenile osteochondrosis
- **M91.20 Coxa plana, unspecified hip**
- **M91.21 Coxa plana, right hip**
- **M91.22 Coxa plana, left hip**

✓5ᵗʰ **M91.3 Pseudocoxalgia**
- **M91.30 Pseudocoxalgia, unspecified hip**
- **M91.31 Pseudocoxalgia, right hip**
- **M91.32 Pseudocoxalgia, left hip**

✓5ᵗʰ **M91.4 Coxa magna**
- **M91.40 Coxa magna, unspecified hip**
- **M91.41 Coxa magna, right hip**
- **M91.42 Coxa magna, left hip**

✓5ᵗʰ **M91.8 Other juvenile osteochondrosis of hip and pelvis**
Juvenile osteochondrosis after reduction of congenital dislocation of hip
- **M91.80 Other juvenile osteochondrosis of hip and pelvis, unspecified leg**
- **M91.81 Other juvenile osteochondrosis of hip and pelvis, right leg**
- **M91.82 Other juvenile osteochondrosis of hip and pelvis, left leg**

✓5ᵗʰ **M91.9 Juvenile osteochondrosis of hip and pelvis, unspecified**
- **M91.90 Juvenile osteochondrosis of hip and pelvis, unspecified, unspecified leg**
- **M91.91 Juvenile osteochondrosis of hip and pelvis, unspecified, right leg**
- **M91.92 Juvenile osteochondrosis of hip and pelvis, unspecified, left leg**

✓4ᵗʰ **M92 Other juvenile osteochondrosis**

✓5ᵗʰ **M92.0 Juvenile osteochondrosis of humerus**
Osteochondrosis (juvenile) of capitulum of humerus [Panner]
Osteochondrosis (juvenile) of head of humerus [Haas]
- **M92.00 Juvenile osteochondrosis of humerus, unspecified arm**
- **M92.01 Juvenile osteochondrosis of humerus, right arm**
- **M92.02 Juvenile osteochondrosis of humerus, left arm**

✓5ᵗʰ **M92.1 Juvenile osteochondrosis of radius and ulna**
Osteochondrosis (juvenile) of lower ulna [Burns]
Osteochondrosis (juvenile) of radial head [Brailsford]
- **M92.10 Juvenile osteochondrosis of radius and ulna, unspecified arm**
- **M92.11 Juvenile osteochondrosis of radius and ulna, right arm**
- **M92.12 Juvenile osteochondrosis of radius and ulna, left arm**

✓5ᵗʰ **M92.2 Juvenile osteochondrosis, hand**

  ✓6ᵗʰ **M92.20 Unspecified juvenile osteochondrosis, hand**
- **M92.201 Unspecified juvenile osteochondrosis, right hand**
- **M92.202 Unspecified juvenile osteochondrosis, left hand**
- **M92.209 Unspecified juvenile osteochondrosis, unspecified hand**

  ✓6ᵗʰ **M92.21 Osteochondrosis (juvenile) of carpal lunate [Kienböck]**
- **M92.211 Osteochondrosis (juvenile) of carpal lunate [Kienböck], right hand**
- **M92.212 Osteochondrosis (juvenile) of carpal lunate [Kienböck], left hand**
- **M92.219 Osteochondrosis (juvenile) of carpal lunate [Kienböck], unspecified hand**

  ✓6ᵗʰ **M92.22 Osteochondrosis (juvenile) of metacarpal heads [Mauclaire]**
- **M92.221 Osteochondrosis (juvenile) of metacarpal heads [Mauclaire], right hand**
- **M92.222 Osteochondrosis (juvenile) of metacarpal heads [Mauclaire], left hand**
- **M92.229 Osteochondrosis (juvenile) of metacarpal heads [Mauclaire], unspecified hand**

  ✓6ᵗʰ **M92.29 Other juvenile osteochondrosis, hand**
- **M92.291 Other juvenile osteochondrosis, right hand**
- **M92.292 Other juvenile osteochondrosis, left hand**
- **M92.299 Other juvenile osteochondrosis, unspecified hand**

✓5ᵗʰ **M92.3 Other juvenile osteochondrosis, upper limb**
- **M92.30 Other juvenile osteochondrosis, unspecified upper limb**
- **M92.31 Other juvenile osteochondrosis, right upper limb**
- **M92.32 Other juvenile osteochondrosis, left upper limb**

✓5ᵗʰ **M92.4 Juvenile osteochondrosis of patella**
Osteochondrosis (juvenile) of primary patellar center [Köhler]
Osteochondrosis (juvenile) of secondary patellar centre [Sinding Larsen]
- **M92.40 Juvenile osteochondrosis of patella, unspecified knee**
- **M92.41 Juvenile osteochondrosis of patella, right knee**
- **M92.42 Juvenile osteochondrosis of patella, left knee**

EXCLUDES1 Not coded here   EXCLUDES2 Not included here   N Newborn Age: 0   P Pediatric Age: 0-17   M Maternity Age: 12-55   A Adult Age: 15-124

✓5th **M92.5 Juvenile osteochondrosis of tibia and fibula**
Osteochondrosis (juvenile) of proximal tibia [Blount]
Osteochondrosis (juvenile) of tibial tubercle [Osgood-Schlatter]
Tibia vara

M92.50 Juvenile osteochondrosis of tibia and fibula, unspecified leg

M92.51 Juvenile osteochondrosis of tibia and fibula, right leg

M92.52 Juvenile osteochondrosis of tibia and fibula, left leg

✓5th **M92.6 Juvenile osteochondrosis of tarsus**
Osteochondrosis (juvenile) of calcaneum [Sever]
Osteochondrosis (juvenile) of os tibiale externum [Haglund]
Osteochondrosis (juvenile) of talus [Diaz]
Osteochondrosis (juvenile) of tarsal navicular [Köhler]

M92.60 Juvenile osteochondrosis of tarsus, unspecified ankle

M92.61 Juvenile osteochondrosis of tarsus, right ankle

M92.62 Juvenile osteochondrosis of tarsus, left ankle

✓5th **M92.7 Juvenile osteochondrosis of metatarsus**
Osteochondrosis (juvenile) of fifth metatarsus [Iselin]
Osteochondrosis (juvenile) of second metatarsus [Freiberg]

M92.70 Juvenile osteochondrosis of metatarsus, unspecified foot

M92.71 Juvenile osteochondrosis of metatarsus, right foot

M92.72 Juvenile osteochondrosis of metatarsus, left foot

M92.8 Other specified juvenile osteochondrosis
Calcaneal apophysitis

M92.9 Juvenile osteochondrosis, unspecified
Juvenile apophysitis NOS
Juvenile epiphysitis NOS
Juvenile osteochondritis NOS
Juvenile osteochondrosis NOS

✓4th **M93 Other osteochondropathies**
EXCLUDES 2   osteochondrosis of spine (M42.-)

✓5th **M93.0 Slipped upper femoral epiphysis (nontraumatic)**
Use additional code for associated chondrolysis (M94.3)

✓6th **M93.00 Unspecified slipped upper femoral epiphysis (nontraumatic)**

M93.001 Unspecified slipped upper femoral epiphysis (nontraumatic), right hip

M93.002 Unspecified slipped upper femoral epiphysis (nontraumatic), left hip

M93.003 Unspecified slipped upper femoral epiphysis (nontraumatic), unspecified hip

✓6th **M93.01 Acute slipped upper femoral epiphysis (nontraumatic)**

M93.011 Acute slipped upper femoral epiphysis (nontraumatic), right hip

M93.012 Acute slipped upper femoral epiphysis (nontraumatic), left hip

M93.013 Acute slipped upper femoral epiphysis (nontraumatic), unspecified hip

✓6th **M93.02 Chronic slipped upper femoral epiphysis (nontraumatic)**

M93.021 Chronic slipped upper femoral epiphysis (nontraumatic), right hip

M93.022 Chronic slipped upper femoral epiphysis (nontraumatic), left hip

M93.023 Chronic slipped upper femoral epiphysis (nontraumatic), unspecified hip

✓6th **M93.03 Acute on chronic slipped upper femoral epiphysis (nontraumatic)**

M93.031 Acute on chronic slipped upper femoral epiphysis (nontraumatic), right hip

M93.032 Acute on chronic slipped upper femoral epiphysis (nontraumatic), left hip

M93.033 Acute on chronic slipped upper femoral epiphysis (nontraumatic), unspecified hip

M93.1 Kienböck's disease of adults   Ⓐ
Adult osteochondrosis of carpal lunates

✓5th **M93.2 Osteochondritis dissecans**

M93.20 Osteochondritis dissecans of unspecified site

✓6th **M93.21 Osteochondritis dissecans of shoulder**

M93.211 Osteochondritis dissecans, right shoulder

M93.212 Osteochondritis dissecans, left shoulder

M93.219 Osteochondritis dissecans, unspecified shoulder

✓6th **M93.22 Osteochondritis dissecans of elbow**

M93.221 Osteochondritis dissecans, right elbow

M93.222 Osteochondritis dissecans, left elbow

M93.229 Osteochondritis dissecans, unspecified elbow

✓6th **M93.23 Osteochondritis dissecans of wrist**

M93.231 Osteochondritis dissecans, right wrist

M93.232 Osteochondritis dissecans, left wrist

M93.239 Osteochondritis dissecans, unspecified wrist

✓6th **M93.24 Osteochondritis dissecans of joints of hand**

M93.241 Osteochondritis dissecans, joints of right hand

M93.242 Osteochondritis dissecans, joints of left hand

M93.249 Osteochondritis dissecans, joints of unspecified hand

✓6th **M93.25 Osteochondritis dissecans of hip**

M93.251 Osteochondritis dissecans, right hip

M93.252 Osteochondritis dissecans, left hip

M93.259 Osteochondritis dissecans, unspecified hip

✓6th **M93.26 Osteochondritis dissecans knee**

M93.261 Osteochondritis dissecans, right knee

M93.262 Osteochondritis dissecans, left knee

M93.269 Osteochondritis dissecans, unspecified knee

✓6th **M93.27 Osteochondritis dissecans of ankle and joints of foot**

M93.271 Osteochondritis dissecans, right ankle and joints of right foot

M93.272 Osteochondritis dissecans, left ankle and joints of left foot

M93.279 Osteochondritis dissecans, unspecified ankle and joints of foot

M93.28 Osteochondritis dissecans other site

M93.29 Osteochondritis dissecans multiple sites

✓5th **M93.8 Other specified osteochondropathies**

M93.80 Other specified osteochondropathies of unspecified site

✓6th **M93.81 Other specified osteochondropathies of shoulder**

M93.811 Other specified osteochondropathies, right shoulder

M93.812 Other specified osteochondropathies, left shoulder

M93.819 Other specified osteochondropathies, unspecified shoulder

✓6th **M93.82 Other specified osteochondropathies of upper arm**

M93.821 Other specified osteochondropathies, right upper arm

M93.822 Other specified osteochondropathies, left upper arm

M93.829 Other specified osteochondropathies, unspecified upper arm

✓6th **M93.83 Other specified osteochondropathies of forearm**

M93.831 Other specified osteochondropathies, right forearm

M93.832 Other specified osteochondropathies, left forearm

M93.839 Other specified osteochondropathies, unspecified forearm

✓6th **M93.84 Other specified osteochondropathies of hand**

M93.841 Other specified osteochondropathies, right hand

M93.842 Other specified osteochondropathies, left hand

M93.849 Other specified osteochondropathies, unspecified hand

✓6th **M93.85 Other specified osteochondropathies of thigh**

M93.851 Other specified osteochondropathies, right thigh

M93.852 Other specified osteochondropathies, left thigh

M93.859 Other specified osteochondropathies, unspecified thigh

---

✓ Additional Character Required   ✓x7th Xtension Alert   Unspecified Code   Other Specified Code   Manifestation Code   ▶◀ Revised Text   ● New Code   ▲ Revised Code Title

☑6ᵗʰ **M93.86 Other specified osteochondropathies** lower leg

     M93.861 **Other specified osteochondropathies, right lower leg**

     M93.862 **Other specified osteochondropathies, left lower leg**

     M93.869 **Other specified osteochondropathies, unspecified lower leg**

☑6ᵗʰ **M93.87 Other specified osteochondropathies of** ankle and foot

     M93.871 **Other specified osteochondropathies, right ankle and foot**

     M93.872 **Other specified osteochondropathies, left ankle and foot**

     M93.879 **Other specified osteochondropathies, unspecified ankle and foot**

     M93.88 Other specified osteochondropathies other site

     M93.89 Other specified osteochondropathies multiple sites

☑5ᵗʰ **M93.9 Osteochondropathy, unspecified**

     Apophysitis NOS   Osteochondritis NOS
     Epiphysitis NOS   Osteochondrosis NOS

     M93.90 Osteochondropathy, unspecified of unspecified site

☑6ᵗʰ **M93.91 Osteochondropathy, unspecified of** shoulder

     M93.911 **Osteochondropathy, unspecified, right shoulder**

     M93.912 **Osteochondropathy, unspecified, left shoulder**

     M93.919 **Osteochondropathy, unspecified, unspecified shoulder**

☑6ᵗʰ **M93.92 Osteochondropathy, unspecified of** upper arm

     M93.921 **Osteochondropathy, unspecified, right upper arm**

     M93.922 **Osteochondropathy, unspecified, left upper arm**

     M93.929 **Osteochondropathy, unspecified, unspecified upper arm**

☑6ᵗʰ **M93.93 Osteochondropathy, unspecified of** forearm

     M93.931 **Osteochondropathy, unspecified, right forearm**

     M93.932 **Osteochondropathy, unspecified, left forearm**

     M93.939 **Osteochondropathy, unspecified, unspecified forearm**

☑6ᵗʰ **M93.94 Osteochondropathy, unspecified of** hand

     M93.941 **Osteochondropathy, unspecified, right hand**

     M93.942 **Osteochondropathy, unspecified, left hand**

     M93.949 **Osteochondropathy, unspecified, unspecified hand**

☑6ᵗʰ **M93.95 Osteochondropathy, unspecified of** thigh

     M93.951 **Osteochondropathy, unspecified, right thigh**

     M93.952 **Osteochondropathy, unspecified, left thigh**

     M93.959 **Osteochondropathy, unspecified, unspecified thigh**

☑6ᵗʰ **M93.96 Osteochondropathy, unspecified** lower leg

     M93.961 **Osteochondropathy, unspecified, right lower leg**

     M93.962 **Osteochondropathy, unspecified, left lower leg**

     M93.969 **Osteochondropathy, unspecified, unspecified lower leg**

☑6ᵗʰ **M93.97 Osteochondropathy, unspecified of** ankle and foot

     M93.971 **Osteochondropathy, unspecified, right ankle and foot**

     M93.972 **Osteochondropathy, unspecified, left ankle and foot**

     M93.979 **Osteochondropathy, unspecified, unspecified ankle and foot**

     M93.98 Osteochondropathy, unspecified other site

     M93.99 Osteochondropathy, unspecified multiple sites

☑4ᵗʰ **M94 Other disorders of cartilage**

     M94.0 Chondrocostal junction syndrome [Tietze]
         Costochondritis

     M94.1 Relapsing polychondritis

☑5ᵗʰ **M94.2 Chondromalacia**

     EXCLUDES 1   *chondromalacia patellae (M22.4)*

     M94.20 Chondromalacia, unspecified site

☑6ᵗʰ **M94.21 Chondromalacia,** shoulder

     M94.211 **Chondromalacia,** right shoulder

     M94.212 **Chondromalacia,** left shoulder

     M94.219 **Chondromalacia, unspecified shoulder**

☑6ᵗʰ **M94.22 Chondromalacia,** elbow

     M94.221 **Chondromalacia,** right elbow

     M94.222 **Chondromalacia,** left elbow

     M94.229 **Chondromalacia, unspecified elbow**

☑6ᵗʰ **M94.23 Chondromalacia,** wrist

     M94.231 **Chondromalacia,** right wrist

     M94.232 **Chondromalacia,** left wrist

     M94.239 **Chondromalacia, unspecified wrist**

☑6ᵗʰ **M94.24 Chondromalacia,** joints of hand

     M94.241 **Chondromalacia, joints of** right hand

     M94.242 **Chondromalacia, joints of** left hand

     M94.249 **Chondromalacia, joints of unspecified hand**

☑6ᵗʰ **M94.25 Chondromalacia,** hip

     M94.251 **Chondromalacia,** right hip

     M94.252 **Chondromalacia,** left hip

     M94.259 **Chondromalacia, unspecified hip**

☑6ᵗʰ **M94.26 Chondromalacia,** knee

     M94.261 **Chondromalacia,** right knee

     M94.262 **Chondromalacia,** left knee

     M94.269 **Chondromalacia, unspecified knee**

☑6ᵗʰ **M94.27 Chondromalacia,** ankle and joints of foot

     M94.271 **Chondromalacia,** right ankle and joints of right **foot**

     M94.272 **Chondromalacia,** left ankle and joints of left **foot**

     M94.279 **Chondromalacia, unspecified ankle and joints of foot**

     M94.28 Chondromalacia, other site

     M94.29 Chondromalacia, multiple sites

☑5ᵗʰ **M94.3 Chondrolysis**

     Code first any associated slipped upper femoral epiphysis (nontraumatic) (M93.0-)

☑6ᵗʰ **M94.35 Chondrolysis, hip**

     M94.351 **Chondrolysis,** right hip

     M94.352 **Chondrolysis,** left hip

     M94.359 **Chondrolysis, unspecified hip**

☑5ᵗʰ **M94.8 Other specified disorders of cartilage**

☑6ᵗʰ **M94.8X Other specified disorders of cartilage**

     M94.8X0 **Other specified disorders of cartilage, multiple sites**

     M94.8X1 **Other specified disorders of cartilage, shoulder**

     M94.8X2 **Other specified disorders of cartilage, upper arm**

     M94.8X3 **Other specified disorders of cartilage, forearm**

     M94.8X4 **Other specified disorders of cartilage, hand**

     M94.8X5 **Other specified disorders of cartilage, thigh**

     M94.8X6 **Other specified disorders of cartilage, lower leg**

     M94.8X7 **Other specified disorders of cartilage, ankle and foot**

     M94.8X8 **Other specified disorders of cartilage, other site**

     M94.8X9 **Other specified disorders of cartilage, unspecified sites**

     M94.9 Disorder of cartilage, unspecified

EXCLUDES 1 Not coded here   EXCLUDES 2 Not included here   N Newborn Age: 0   P Pediatric Age: 0-17   M Maternity Age: 12-55   A Adult Age: 15-124

718   ICD-10-CM 2014 (Draft)

Other disorders of the musculoskeletal system and connective tissue (M95)

✓4ᵗʰ **M95 Other acquired deformities of musculoskeletal system and connective tissue**

EXCLUDES 2　*acquired absence of limbs and organs (Z89-Z90)*
acquired deformities of limbs (M20-M21)
congenital malformations and deformations of the musculoskeletal system (Q65-Q79)
deforming dorsopathies (M40-M43)
dentofacial anomalies [including malocclusion] (M26.-)
postprocedural musculoskeletal disorders (M96.-)

M95.0 Acquired deformity of nose

EXCLUDES 2　*deviated nasal septum (J34.2)*

✓5ᵗʰ **M95.1 Cauliflower ear**

EXCLUDES 2　*other acquired deformities of ear (H61.1)*

M95.10 Cauliflower ear, unspecified ear

M95.11 Cauliflower ear, right ear

M95.12 Cauliflower ear, left ear

M95.2 Other acquired deformity of head

M95.3 Acquired deformity of neck

M95.4 Acquired deformity of chest and rib

M95.5 Acquired deformity of pelvis

EXCLUDES 1　*maternal care for known or suspected disproportion (O33.-)*

M95.8 Other specified acquired deformities of musculoskeletal system

M95.9 Acquired deformity of musculoskeletal system, unspecified

Intraoperative and postprocedural complications and disorders of musculoskeletal system, not elsewhere classified (M96)

✓4ᵗʰ **M96 Intraoperative and postprocedural complications and disorders of musculoskeletal system, not elsewhere classified**

EXCLUDES 2　*arthropathy following intestinal bypass (M02.0-)*
complications of internal orthopedic prosthetic devices, implants and grafts (T84.-)
disorders associated with osteoporosis (M80)
presence of functional implants and other devices (Z96-Z97)

M96.0 Pseudarthrosis after fusion or arthrodesis

M96.1 Postlaminectomy syndrome, not elsewhere classified

M96.2 Postradiation kyphosis

M96.3 Postlaminectomy kyphosis

M96.4 Postsurgical lordosis

M96.5 Postradiation scoliosis

✓5ᵗʰ **M96.6 Fracture of bone following insertion of orthopedic implant, joint prosthesis, or bone plate**

Intraoperative fracture of bone during insertion of orthopedic implant, joint prosthesis, or bone plate

EXCLUDES 2　*complication of internal orthopedic devices, implants or grafts (T84.-)*

✓6ᵗʰ **M96.62 Fracture of humerus following insertion of orthopedic implant, joint prosthesis, or bone plate**

M96.621 Fracture of humerus following insertion of orthopedic implant, joint prosthesis, or bone plate, right arm

M96.622 Fracture of humerus following insertion of orthopedic implant, joint prosthesis, or bone plate, left arm

M96.629 Fracture of humerus following insertion of orthopedic implant, joint prosthesis, or bone plate, unspecified arm

✓6ᵗʰ **M96.63 Fracture of radius or ulna following insertion of orthopedic implant, joint prosthesis, or bone plate**

M96.631 Fracture of radius or ulna following insertion of orthopedic implant, joint prosthesis, or bone plate, right arm

M96.632 Fracture of radius or ulna following insertion of orthopedic implant, joint prosthesis, or bone plate, left arm

M96.639 Fracture of radius or ulna following insertion of orthopedic implant, joint prosthesis, or bone plate, unspecified arm

M96.65 Fracture of pelvis following insertion of orthopedic implant, joint prosthesis, or bone plate

✓6ᵗʰ **M96.66 Fracture of femur following insertion of orthopedic implant, joint prosthesis, or bone plate**

M96.661 Fracture of femur following insertion of orthopedic implant, joint prosthesis, or bone plate, right leg

M96.662 Fracture of femur following insertion of orthopedic implant, joint prosthesis, or bone plate, left leg

M96.669 Fracture of femur following insertion of orthopedic implant, joint prosthesis, or bone plate, unspecified leg

✓6ᵗʰ **M96.67 Fracture of tibia or fibula following insertion of orthopedic implant, joint prosthesis, or bone plate**

M96.671 Fracture of tibia or fibula following insertion of orthopedic implant, joint prosthesis, or bone plate, right leg

M96.672 Fracture of tibia or fibula following insertion of orthopedic implant, joint prosthesis, or bone plate, left leg

M96.679 Fracture of tibia or fibula following insertion of orthopedic implant, joint prosthesis, or bone plate, unspecified leg

M96.69 Fracture of other bone following insertion of orthopedic implant, joint prosthesis, or bone plate

✓5ᵗʰ **M96.8 Other intraoperative and postprocedural complications and disorders of musculoskeletal system, not elsewhere classified**

✓6ᵗʰ **M96.81 Intraoperative hemorrhage and hematoma of a musculoskeletal structure complicating a procedure**

EXCLUDES 1　*intraoperative hemorrhage and hematoma of a musculoskeletal structure due to accidental puncture and laceration during a procedure (M96.82-)*

M96.810 Intraoperative hemorrhage and hematoma of a musculoskeletal structure complicating a musculoskeletal system procedure

M96.811 Intraoperative hemorrhage and hematoma of a musculoskeletal structure complicating other procedure

✓6ᵗʰ **M96.82 Accidental puncture and laceration of a musculoskeletal structure during a procedure**

M96.820 Accidental puncture and laceration of a musculoskeletal structure during a musculoskeletal system procedure

M96.821 Accidental puncture and laceration of a musculoskeletal structure during other procedure

✓6ᵗʰ **M96.83 Postprocedural hemorrhage and hematoma of a musculoskeletal structure following a procedure**

M96.830 Postprocedural hemorrhage and hematoma of a musculoskeletal structure following a musculoskeletal system procedure

M96.831 Postprocedural hemorrhage and hematoma of a musculoskeletal structure following other procedure

M96.89 Other intraoperative and postprocedural complications and disorders of the musculoskeletal system

Instability of joint secondary to removal of joint prosthesis

Use additional code, if applicable, to further specify disorder

Biomechanical lesions, not elsewhere classified (M99)

✓4ᵗʰ **M99 Biomechanical lesions, not elsewhere classified**

NOTE　This category should not be used if the condition can be classified elsewhere.

✓5ᵗʰ **M99.0 Segmental and somatic dysfunction**

M99.00 Segmental and somatic dysfunction of head region

M99.01 Segmental and somatic dysfunction of cervical region

M99.02 Segmental and somatic dysfunction of thoracic region

M99.03 Segmental and somatic dysfunction of lumbar region

M99.04 Segmental and somatic dysfunction of sacral region

M99.05 Segmental and somatic dysfunction of pelvic region

M99.06 Segmental and somatic dysfunction of lower extremity

M99.07 Segmental and somatic dysfunction of upper extremity

M99.08 Segmental and somatic dysfunction of rib cage

M99.09 Segmental and somatic dysfunction of abdomen and other regions

✓5ᵗʰ **M99.1 Subluxation complex (vertebral)**

M99.10 Subluxation complex (vertebral) of head region

M99.11 Subluxation complex (vertebral) of cervical region

M99.12 Subluxation complex (vertebral) of thoracic region

M99.13 Subluxation complex (vertebral) of lumbar region

M99.14 Subluxation complex (vertebral) of sacral region

M99.15 Subluxation complex (vertebral) of pelvic region

M99.16 Subluxation complex (vertebral) of lower extremity

M99.17 Subluxation complex (vertebral) of upper extremity

M99.18 Subluxation complex (vertebral) of rib cage

M99.19 Subluxation complex (vertebral) of abdomen and other regions

✓5ᵗʰ **M99.2 Subluxation stenosis of neural canal**

M99.20 Subluxation stenosis of neural canal of head region

M99.21 Subluxation stenosis of neural canal of cervical region

M99.22 Subluxation stenosis of neural canal of thoracic region

M99.23 Subluxation stenosis of neural canal of lumbar region

M99.24 Subluxation stenosis of neural canal of sacral region

M99.25 Subluxation stenosis of neural canal of pelvic region

M99.26 Subluxation stenosis of neural canal of lower extremity

M99.27 Subluxation stenosis of neural canal of upper extremity

M99.28 Subluxation stenosis of neural canal of rib cage

M99.29 Subluxation stenosis of neural canal of abdomen and other regions

✓5ᵗʰ **M99.3 Osseous stenosis of neural canal**

M99.30 Osseous stenosis of neural canal of head region

M99.31 Osseous stenosis of neural canal of cervical region

M99.32 Osseous stenosis of neural canal of thoracic region

M99.33 Osseous stenosis of neural canal of lumbar region

M99.34 Osseous stenosis of neural canal of sacral region

M99.35 Osseous stenosis of neural canal of pelvic region

M99.36 Osseous stenosis of neural canal of lower extremity

M99.37 Osseous stenosis of neural canal of upper extremity

M99.38 Osseous stenosis of neural canal of rib cage

M99.39 Osseous stenosis of neural canal of abdomen and other regions

✓5ᵗʰ **M99.4 Connective tissue stenosis of neural canal**

M99.40 Connective tissue stenosis of neural canal of head region

M99.41 Connective tissue stenosis of neural canal of cervical region

M99.42 Connective tissue stenosis of neural canal of thoracic region

M99.43 Connective tissue stenosis of neural canal of lumbar region

M99.44 Connective tissue stenosis of neural canal of sacral region

M99.45 Connective tissue stenosis of neural canal of pelvic region

M99.46 Connective tissue stenosis of neural canal of lower extremity

M99.47 Connective tissue stenosis of neural canal of upper extremity

M99.48 Connective tissue stenosis of neural canal of rib cage

M99.49 Connective tissue stenosis of neural canal of abdomen and other regions

✓5ᵗʰ **M99.5 Intervertebral disc stenosis of neural canal**

M99.50 Intervertebral disc stenosis of neural canal of head region

M99.51 Intervertebral disc stenosis of neural canal of cervical region

M99.52 Intervertebral disc stenosis of neural canal of thoracic region

M99.53 Intervertebral disc stenosis of neural canal of lumbar region

M99.54 Intervertebral disc stenosis of neural canal of sacral region

M99.55 Intervertebral disc stenosis of neural canal of pelvic region

M99.56 Intervertebral disc stenosis of neural canal of lower extremity

M99.57 Intervertebral disc stenosis of neural canal of upper extremity

M99.58 Intervertebral disc stenosis of neural canal of rib cage

M99.59 Intervertebral disc stenosis of neural canal of abdomen and other regions

✓5ᵗʰ **M99.6 Osseous and subluxation stenosis of intervertebral foramina**

M99.60 Osseous and subluxation stenosis of intervertebral foramina of head region

M99.61 Osseous and subluxation stenosis of intervertebral foramina of cervical region

M99.62 Osseous and subluxation stenosis of intervertebral foramina of thoracic region

M99.63 Osseous and subluxation stenosis of intervertebral foramina of lumbar region

M99.64 Osseous and subluxation stenosis of intervertebral foramina of sacral region

M99.65 Osseous and subluxation stenosis of intervertebral foramina of pelvic region

M99.66 Osseous and subluxation stenosis of intervertebral foramina of lower extremity

M99.67 Osseous and subluxation stenosis of intervertebral foramina of upper extremity

M99.68 Osseous and subluxation stenosis of intervertebral foramina of rib cage

M99.69 Osseous and subluxation stenosis of intervertebral foramina of abdomen and other regions

✓5ᵗʰ **M99.7 Connective tissue and disc stenosis of intervertebral foramina**

M99.70 Connective tissue and disc stenosis of intervertebral foramina of head region

M99.71 Connective tissue and disc stenosis of intervertebral foramina of cervical region

M99.72 Connective tissue and disc stenosis of intervertebral foramina of thoracic region

M99.73 Connective tissue and disc stenosis of intervertebral foramina of lumbar region

M99.74 Connective tissue and disc stenosis of intervertebral foramina of sacral region

M99.75 Connective tissue and disc stenosis of intervertebral foramina of pelvic region

M99.76 Connective tissue and disc stenosis of intervertebral foramina of lower extremity

M99.77 Connective tissue and disc stenosis of intervertebral foramina of upper extremity

M99.78 Connective tissue and disc stenosis of intervertebral foramina of rib cage

M99.79 Connective tissue and disc stenosis of intervertebral foramina of abdomen and other regions

✓5ᵗʰ **M99.8 Other biomechanical lesions**

M99.80 Other biomechanical lesions of head region

M99.81 Other biomechanical lesions of cervical region

M99.82 Other biomechanical lesions of thoracic region

M99.83 Other biomechanical lesions of lumbar region

M99.84 Other biomechanical lesions of sacral region

M99.85 Other biomechanical lesions of pelvic region

M99.86 Other biomechanical lesions of lower extremity

M99.87 Other biomechanical lesions of upper extremity

M99.88 Other biomechanical lesions of rib cage

M99.89 Other biomechanical lesions of abdomen and other regions

M99.9 Biomechanical lesion, unspecified

EXCLUDES 1 Not coded here   **EXCLUDES 2** Not included here   **N** Newborn Age: 0   **P** Pediatric Age: 0-17   **M** Maternity Age: 12-55   **A** Adult Age: 15-124

720   ICD-10-CM 2014 (Draft)

Chapter 14. Diseases of the Genitourinary System (N00-N99)

EXCLUDES 2
*certain conditions originating in the perinatal period (P04-P96)
certain infectious and parasitic diseases (A00-B99)
complications of pregnancy, childbirth and the puerperium (O00-O9A)
congenital malformations, deformations and chromosomal abnormalities (Q00-Q99)
endocrine, nutritional and metabolic diseases (E00-E88)
injury, poisoning and certain other consequences of external causes (S00-T88)
neoplasms (C00-D49)
symptoms, signs and abnormal clinical and laboratory findings, not elsewhere classified (R00-R94)*

This chapter contains the following blocks:
- N00-N08 Glomerular diseases
- N10-N16 Renal tubulo-interstitial diseases
- N17-N19 Acute kidney failure and chronic kidney disease
- N20-N23 Urolithiasis
- N25-N29 Other disorders of kidney and ureter
- N30-N39 Other diseases of the urinary system
- N40-N53 Diseases of male genital organs
- N60-N65 Disorders of breast
- N70-N77 Inflammatory diseases of female pelvic organs
- N80-N98 Noninflammatory disorders of female genital tract
- N99 Intraoperative and postprocedural complications and disorders of genitourinary system, not elsewhere classified

Glomerular diseases (N00-N08)

Code also any associated kidney failure (N17-N19).
EXCLUDES 1 *hypertensive chronic kidney disease (I12.-)*

N00 Acute nephritic syndrome
INCLUDES acute glomerular disease
acute glomerulonephritis
acute nephritis
EXCLUDES 1 *acute tubulo-interstitial nephritis (N10)
nephritic syndrome NOS (N05.-)*

N00.0 Acute nephritic syndrome with minor glomerular abnormality
Acute nephritic syndrome with minimal change lesion

N00.1 Acute nephritic syndrome with focal and segmental glomerular lesions
Acute nephritic syndrome with focal and segmental hyalinosis
Acute nephritic syndrome with focal and segmental sclerosis
Acute nephritic syndrome with focal glomerulonephritis

N00.2 Acute nephritic syndrome with diffuse membranous glomerulonephritis

N00.3 Acute nephritic syndrome with diffuse mesangial proliferative glomerulonephritis

N00.4 Acute nephritic syndrome with diffuse endocapillary proliferative glomerulonephritis

N00.5 Acute nephritic syndrome with diffuse mesangiocapillary glomerulonephritis
Acute nephritic syndrome with membranoproliferative glomerulonephritis, types 1 and 3, or NOS

N00.6 Acute nephritic syndrome with dense deposit disease
Acute nephritic syndrome with membranoproliferative glomerulonephritis, type 2

N00.7 Acute nephritic syndrome with diffuse crescentic glomerulonephritis
Acute nephritic syndrome with extracapillary glomerulonephritis

N00.8 Acute nephritic syndrome with other morphologic changes
Acute nephritic syndrome with proliferative glomerulonephritis NOS

N00.9 Acute nephritic syndrome with unspecified morphologic changes

N01 Rapidly progressive nephritic syndrome
INCLUDES rapidly progressive glomerular disease
rapidly progressive glomerulonephritis
rapidly progressive nephritis
EXCLUDES 1 *nephritic syndrome NOS (N05.-)*

N01.0 Rapidly progressive nephritic syndrome with minor glomerular abnormality
Rapidly progressive nephritic syndrome with minimal change lesion

N01.1 Rapidly progressive nephritic syndrome with focal and segmental glomerular lesions
Rapidly progressive nephritic syndrome with focal and segmental hyalinosis
Rapidly progressive nephritic syndrome with focal and segmental sclerosis
Rapidly progressive nephritic syndrome with focal glomerulonephritis

N01.2 Rapidly progressive nephritic syndrome with diffuse membranous glomerulonephritis

N01.3 Rapidly progressive nephritic syndrome with diffuse mesangial proliferative glomerulonephritis

N01.4 Rapidly progressive nephritic syndrome with diffuse endocapillary proliferative glomerulonephritis

N01.5 Rapidly progressive nephritic syndrome with diffuse mesangiocapillary glomerulonephritis
Rapidly progressive nephritic syndrome with membranoproliferative glomerulonephritis, types 1 and 3, or NOS

N01.6 Rapidly progressive nephritic syndrome with dense deposit disease
Rapidly progressive nephritic syndrome with membranoproliferative glomerulonephritis, type 2

N01.7 Rapidly progressive nephritic syndrome with diffuse crescentic glomerulonephritis
Rapidly progressive nephritic syndrome with extracapillary glomerulonephritis

N01.8 Rapidly progressive nephritic syndrome with other morphologic changes
Rapidly progressive nephritic syndrome with proliferative glomerulonephritis NOS

N01.9 Rapidly progressive nephritic syndrome with unspecified morphologic changes

N02 Recurrent and persistent hematuria
EXCLUDES 1 *acute cystitis with hematuria (N30.01)
hematuria NOS (R31.9)
hematuria not associated with specified morphologic lesions (R31.-)*

N02.0 Recurrent and persistent hematuria with minor glomerular abnormality
Recurrent and persistent hematuria with minimal change lesion

N02.1 Recurrent and persistent hematuria with focal and segmental glomerular lesions
Recurrent and persistent hematuria with focal and segmental hyalinosis
Recurrent and persistent hematuria with focal and segmental sclerosis
Recurrent and persistent hematuria with focal glomerulonephritis

N02.2 Recurrent and persistent hematuria with diffuse membranous glomerulonephritis

N02.3 Recurrent and persistent hematuria with diffuse mesangial proliferative glomerulonephritis

N02.4 Recurrent and persistent hematuria with diffuse endocapillary proliferative glomerulonephritis

N02.5 Recurrent and persistent hematuria with diffuse mesangiocapillary glomerulonephritis
Recurrent and persistent hematuria with membranoproliferative glomerulonephritis, types 1 and 3, or NOS

N02.6 Recurrent and persistent hematuria with dense deposit disease
Recurrent and persistent hematuria with membranoproliferative glomerulonephritis, type 2

N02.7 Recurrent and persistent hematuria with diffuse crescentic glomerulonephritis
Recurrent and persistent hematuria with extracapillary glomerulonephritis

N02.8 Recurrent and persistent hematuria with other morphologic changes
Recurrent and persistent hematuria with proliferative glomerulonephritis NOS

N02.9 Recurrent and persistent hematuria with unspecified morphologic changes

Diseases of the Genitourinary System

N03–N07.3

☑4ᵗʰ **N03 Chronic nephritic syndrome**
  INCLUDES   chronic glomerular disease
  chronic glomerulonephritis
  chronic nephritis
  EXCLUDES 1   *chronic tubulo-interstitial nephritis (N11.-)*
  diffuse sclerosing glomerulonephritis (N05.8-)
  nephritic syndrome NOS (N05.-)

N03.0 Chronic nephritic syndrome with minor glomerular abnormality
  Chronic nephritic syndrome with minimal change lesion

N03.1 Chronic nephritic syndrome with focal and segmental glomerular lesions
  Chronic nephritic syndrome with focal and segmental hyalinosis
  Chronic nephritic syndrome with focal and segmental sclerosis
  Chronic nephritic syndrome with focal glomerulonephritis

N03.2 Chronic nephritic syndrome with diffuse membranous glomerulonephritis

N03.3 Chronic nephritic syndrome with diffuse mesangial proliferative glomerulonephritis

N03.4 Chronic nephritic syndrome with diffuse endocapillary proliferative glomerulonephritis

N03.5 Chronic nephritic syndrome with diffuse mesangiocapillary glomerulonephritis
  Chronic nephritic syndrome with membranoproliferative glomerulonephritis, types 1 and 3, or NOS

N03.6 Chronic nephritic syndrome with dense deposit disease
  Chronic nephritic syndrome with membranoproliferative glomerulonephritis, type 2

N03.7 Chronic nephritic syndrome with diffuse crescentic glomerulonephritis
  Chronic nephritic syndrome with extracapillary glomerulonephritis

N03.8 Chronic nephritic syndrome with other morphologic changes
  Chronic nephritic syndrome with proliferative glomerulonephritis NOS

N03.9 Chronic nephritic syndrome with unspecified morphologic changes

☑4ᵗʰ **N04 Nephrotic syndrome**
  INCLUDES   congenital nephrotic syndrome
  lipoid nephrosis

N04.0 Nephrotic syndrome with minor glomerular abnormality
  Nephrotic syndrome with minimal change lesion

N04.1 Nephrotic syndrome with focal and segmental glomerular lesions
  Nephrotic syndrome with focal and segmental hyalinosis
  Nephrotic syndrome with focal and segmental sclerosis
  Nephrotic syndrome with focal glomerulonephritis

N04.2 Nephrotic syndrome with diffuse membranous glomerulonephritis

N04.3 Nephrotic syndrome with diffuse mesangial proliferative glomerulonephritis

N04.4 Nephrotic syndrome with diffuse endocapillary proliferative glomerulonephritis

N04.5 Nephrotic syndrome with diffuse mesangiocapillary glomerulonephritis
  Nephrotic syndrome with membranoproliferative glomerulonephritis, types 1 and 3, or NOS

N04.6 Nephrotic syndrome with dense deposit disease
  Nephrotic syndrome with membranoproliferative glomerulonephritis, type 2

N04.7 Nephrotic syndrome with diffuse crescentic glomerulonephritis
  Nephrotic syndrome with extracapillary glomerulonephritis

N04.8 Nephrotic syndrome with other morphologic changes
  Nephrotic syndrome with proliferative glomerulonephritis NOS

N04.9 Nephrotic syndrome with unspecified morphologic changes

☑4ᵗʰ **N05 Unspecified nephritic syndrome**
  INCLUDES   glomerular disease NOS
  glomerulonephritis NOS
  nephritis NOS
  nephropathy NOS and renal disease NOS with morphological lesion specified in .0-.8
  EXCLUDES 1   *nephropathy NOS with no stated morphological lesion (N28.9)*
  renal disease NOS with no stated morphological lesion (N28.9)
  tubulo-interstitial nephritis NOS (N12)

N05.0 Unspecified nephritic syndrome with minor glomerular abnormality
  Unspecified nephritic syndrome with minimal change lesion

N05.1 Unspecified nephritic syndrome with focal and segmental glomerular lesions
  Unspecified nephritic syndrome with focal and segmental hyalinosis
  Unspecified nephritic syndrome with focal and segmental sclerosis
  Unspecified nephritic syndrome with focal glomerulonephritis

N05.2 Unspecified nephritic syndrome with diffuse membranous glomerulonephritis

N05.3 Unspecified nephritic syndrome with diffuse mesangial proliferative glomerulonephritis

N05.4 Unspecified nephritic syndrome with diffuse endocapillary proliferative glomerulonephritis

N05.5 Unspecified nephritic syndrome with diffuse mesangiocapillary glomerulonephritis
  Unspecified nephritic syndrome with membranoproliferative glomerulonephritis, types 1 and 3, or NOS

N05.6 Unspecified nephritic syndrome with dense deposit disease
  Unspecified nephritic syndrome with membranoproliferative glomerulonephritis, type 2

N05.7 Unspecified nephritic syndrome with diffuse crescentic glomerulonephritis
  Unspecified nephritic syndrome with extracapillary glomerulonephritis

N05.8 Unspecified nephritic syndrome with other morphologic changes
  Unspecified nephritic syndrome with proliferative glomerulonephritis NOS

N05.9 Unspecified nephritic syndrome with unspecified morphologic changes

☑4ᵗʰ **N06 Isolated proteinuria with specified morphological lesion**
  EXCLUDES 1   *proteinuria not associated with specific morphologic lesions (R80.0)*

N06.0 Isolated proteinuria with minor glomerular abnormality
  Isolated proteinuria with minimal change lesion

N06.1 Isolated proteinuria with focal and segmental glomerular lesions
  Isolated proteinuria with focal and segmental hyalinosis
  Isolated proteinuria with focal and segmental sclerosis
  Isolated proteinuria with focal glomerulonephritis

N06.2 Isolated proteinuria with diffuse membranous glomerulonephritis

N06.3 Isolated proteinuria with diffuse mesangial proliferative glomerulonephritis

N06.4 Isolated proteinuria with diffuse endocapillary proliferative glomerulonephritis

N06.5 Isolated proteinuria with diffuse mesangiocapillary glomerulonephritis
  Isolated proteinuria with membranoproliferative glomerulonephritis, types 1 and 3, or NOS

N06.6 Isolated proteinuria with dense deposit disease
  Isolated proteinuria with membranoproliferative glomerulonephritis, type 2

N06.7 Isolated proteinuria with diffuse crescentic glomerulonephritis
  Isolated proteinuria with extracapillary glomerulonephritis

N06.8 Isolated proteinuria with other morphologic lesion
  Isolated proteinuria with proliferative glomerulonephritis NOS

N06.9 Isolated proteinuria with unspecified morphologic lesion

☑4ᵗʰ **N07 Hereditary nephropathy, not elsewhere classified**
  EXCLUDES 2   *Alport's syndrome (Q87.81-)*
  hereditary amyloid nephropathy (E85.-)
  nail patella syndrome (Q87.2)
  non-neuropathic heredofamilial amyloidosis (E85.-)

N07.0 Hereditary nephropathy, not elsewhere classified with minor glomerular abnormality
  Hereditary nephropathy, not elsewhere classified with minimal change lesion

N07.1 Hereditary nephropathy, not elsewhere classified with focal and segmental glomerular lesions
  Hereditary nephropathy, not elsewhere classified with focal and segmental hyalinosis
  Hereditary nephropathy, not elsewhere classified with focal and segmental sclerosis
  Hereditary nephropathy, not elsewhere classified with focal glomerulonephritis

N07.2 Hereditary nephropathy, not elsewhere classified with diffuse membranous glomerulonephritis

N07.3 Hereditary nephropathy, not elsewhere classified with diffuse mesangial proliferative glomerulonephritis

EXCLUDES 1 Not coded here   **EXCLUDES 2** Not included here   **N** Newborn Age: 0   **P** Pediatric Age: 0-17   **M** Maternity Age: 12-55   **A** Adult Age: 15-124

722   ICD-10-CM 2014 (Draft)

N07.4 **Hereditary nephropathy, not elsewhere classified with** diffuse endocapillary proliferative glomerulonephritis

N07.5 **Hereditary nephropathy, not elsewhere classified with** diffuse mesangiocapillary glomerulonephritis
Hereditary nephropathy, not elsewhere classified with membranoproliferative glomerulonephritis, types 1 and 3, or NOS

N07.6 **Hereditary nephropathy, not elsewhere classified with** dense deposit disease
Hereditary nephropathy, not elsewhere classified with membranoproliferative glomerulonephritis, type 2

N07.7 **Hereditary nephropathy, not elsewhere classified with** diffuse crescentic glomerulonephritis
Hereditary nephropathy, not elsewhere classified with extracapillary glomerulonephritis

N07.8 **Hereditary nephropathy, not elsewhere classified with other morphologic lesions**
Hereditary nephropathy, not elsewhere classified with proliferative glomerulonephritis NOS

N07.9 **Hereditary nephropathy, not elsewhere classified with unspecified morphologic lesions**

N08 *Glomerular disorders in diseases classified elsewhere*
Glomerulonephritis
Nephritis
Nephropathy
Code first underlying disease, such as:
amyloidosis (E85.-)
congenital syphilis (A50.5)
cryoglobulinemia (D89.1)
disseminated intravascular coagulation (D65)
gout (M1A.-, M10.-)
microscopic polyangiitis (M31.7)
multiple myeloma (C90.0-)
sepsis (A40.0-A41.9)
sickle-cell disease (D57.0-D57.8)
EXCLUDES 1 *glomerulonephritis, nephritis and nephropathy (in):*
antiglomerular basement membrane disease (M31.0)
diabetes (E08-E13 with .21)
gonococcal (A54.21)
Goodpasture's syndrome (M31.0)
hemolytic-uremic syndrome (D59.3)
lupus (M32.14)
mumps (B26.83)
syphilis (A52.75)
systemic lupus erythematosus (M32.14)
Wegener's granulomatosis (M31.31)
pyelonephritis in diseases classified elsewhere (N16)
renal tubulo-interstitial disorders classified elsewhere (N16)

Renal tubulo-interstitial diseases (N10-N16)

INCLUDES pyelonephritis
EXCLUDES 1 *pyeloureteritis cystica (N28.85)*

N10 **Acute tubulo-interstitial nephritis**
Acute infectious interstitial nephritis
Acute pyelitis
Acute pyelonephritis
Hemoglobin nephrosis
Myoglobin nephrosis
Use additional code (B95-B97), to identify infectious agent

N11 **Chronic tubulo-interstitial nephritis**
INCLUDES chronic infectious interstitial nephritis
chronic pyelitis
chronic pyelonephritis
Use additional code (B95-B97), to identify infectious agent

N11.0 **Nonobstructive reflux-associated chronic pyelonephritis**
Pyelonephritis (chronic) associated with (vesicoureteral) reflux
EXCLUDES 1 *vesicoureteral reflux NOS (N13.70)*

N11.1 **Chronic obstructive pyelonephritis**
Pyelonephritis (chronic) associated with anomaly of pelviureteric junction
Pyelonephritis (chronic) associated with anomaly of pyeloureteric junction
Pyelonephritis (chronic) associated with crossing of vessel
Pyelonephritis (chronic) associated with kinking of ureter
Pyelonephritis (chronic) associated with obstruction of ureter
Pyelonephritis (chronic) associated with stricture of pelviureteric junction
Pyelonephritis (chronic) associated with stricture of ureter
EXCLUDES 1 *calculous pyelonephritis (N20.9)*
obstructive uropathy (N13.-)

N11.8 **Other chronic tubulo-interstitial nephritis**
Nonobstructive chronic pyelonephritis NOS

N11.9 **Chronic tubulo-interstitial nephritis, unspecified**
Chronic interstitial nephritis NOS
Chronic pyelitis NOS
Chronic pyelonephritis NOS

N12 **Tubulo-interstitial nephritis, not specified as acute or chronic**
Interstitial nephritis NOS
Pyelitis NOS
Pyelonephritis NOS
EXCLUDES 1 *calculous pyelonephritis (N20.9)*

N13 **Obstructive and reflux uropathy**
EXCLUDES 2 *calculus of kidney and ureter without hydronephrosis (N20.-)*
congenital obstructive defects of renal pelvis and ureter (Q62.0-Q62.3)
hydronephrosis with ureteropelvic junction obstruction (Q62.1)
obstructive pyelonephritis (N11.1)

N13.1 **Hydronephrosis with ureteral stricture, not elsewhere classified**
EXCLUDES 1 *hydronephrosis with ureteral stricture with infection (N13.6)*

N13.2 **Hydronephrosis with renal and ureteral calculous obstruction**
EXCLUDES 1 *hydronephrosis with renal and ureteral calculous obstruction with infection (N13.6)*

N13.3 **Other and unspecified hydronephrosis**
EXCLUDES 1 *hydronephrosis with infection (N13.6)*

N13.30 **Unspecified hydronephrosis**

N13.39 **Other hydronephrosis**

N13.4 **Hydroureter**
EXCLUDES 1 *congenital hydroureter (Q62.3-)*
hydroureter with infection (N13.6)
vesicoureteral-reflux with hydroureter (N13.73-)

N13.5 **Crossing vessel and stricture of ureter without hydronephrosis**
Kinking and stricture of ureter without hydronephrosis
EXCLUDES 1 *crossing vessel and stricture of ureter without hydronephrosis with infection (N13.6)*

N13.6 **Pyonephrosis**
Conditions in N13.1-N13.5 with infection
Obstructive uropathy with infection
Use additional code (B95-B97), to identify infectious agent

N13.7 **Vesicoureteral-reflux**
EXCLUDES 1 *reflux-associated pyelonephritis (N11.0)*

N13.70 **Vesicoureteral-reflux, unspecified**
Vesicoureteral-reflux NOS

N13.71 **Vesicoureteral-reflux without reflux nephropathy**

N13.72 **Vesicoureteral-reflux with reflux nephropathy without hydroureter**

N13.721 **Vesicoureteral-reflux with reflux nephropathy without hydroureter, unilateral**

N13.722 **Vesicoureteral-reflux with reflux nephropathy without hydroureter, bilateral**

N13.729 **Vesicoureteral-reflux with reflux nephropathy without hydroureter, unspecified**

N13.73 **Vesicoureteral-reflux with reflux nephropathy with hydroureter**

N13.731 **Vesicoureteral-reflux with reflux nephropathy with hydroureter, unilateral**

N13.732 **Vesicoureteral-reflux with reflux nephropathy with hydroureter, bilateral**

N13.739 **Vesicoureteral-reflux with reflux nephropathy with hydroureter, unspecified**

N13.8 **Other obstructive and reflux uropathy**
Urinary tract obstruction due to specified cause
Code first, if applicable, any causal condition, such as:
enlarged prostate (N40.1)

N13.9 **Obstructive and reflux uropathy, unspecified**
Urinary tract obstruction NOS

N14 **Drug- and heavy-metal-induced tubulo-interstitial and tubular conditions**
Code first poisoning due to drug or toxin, if applicable (T36-T65 with fifth or sixth character 1-4 or 6)
Use additional code for adverse effect, if applicable, to identify drug (T36-T50 with fifth or sixth character 5)

N14.0 **Analgesic nephropathy**

✓ Additional Character Required　　✓x7th Xtension Alert　　Unspecified Code　　Other Specified Code　　Manifestation Code　　►◄ Revised Text　　● New Code　　▲ Revised Code Title

ICD-10-CM 2014 (Draft)

723

Diseases of the Genitourinary System

N14.1–N25.1

N14.1 **Nephropathy induced by other drugs, medicaments and biological substances**

N14.2 **Nephropathy induced by unspecified drug, medicament or biological substance**

N14.3 **Nephropathy induced by heavy metals**

N14.4 **Toxic nephropathy, not elsewhere classified**

√4ᵗʰ **N15** **Other renal tubulo-interstitial diseases**

N15.0 **Balkan nephropathy**
Balkan endemic nephropathy

N15.1 **Renal and perinephric abscess**

N15.8 **Other specified renal tubulo-interstitial diseases**

N15.9 **Renal tubulo-interstitial disease, unspecified**
Infection of kidney NOS
EXCLUDES 1   *urinary tract infection NOS (N39.0)*

N16 *Renal tubulo-interstitial disorders in diseases classified elsewhere*
Pyelonephritis
Tubulo-interstitial nephritis
Code first underlying disease, such as:
   brucellosis (A23.0-A23.9)
   cryoglobulinemia (D89.1)
   glycogen storage disease (E74.0)
   leukemia (C91-C95)
   lymphoma (C81.0-C85.9, C96.0-C96.9)
   multiple myeloma (C90.0-)
   sepsis (A40.0-A41.9)
   Wilson's disease (E83.0)
EXCLUDES 1   *diphtheritic pyelonephritis and tubulo-interstitial nephritis (A36.84)*
     pyelonephritis and tubulo-interstitial nephritis in candidiasis (B37.49)
     pyelonephritis and tubulo-interstitial nephritis in cystinosis (E72.04)
     pyelonephritis and tubulo-interstitial nephritis in salmonella infection (A02.25)
     pyelonephritis and tubulo-interstitial nephritis in sarcoidosis (D86.84)
     pyelonephritis and tubulo-interstitial nephritis in sicca syndrome [Sjogren's] (M35.04)
     pyelonephritis and tubulo-interstitial nephritis in systemic lupus erythematosus (M32.15)
     pyelonephritis and tubulo-interstitial nephritis in toxoplasmosis (B58.83)
     renal tubular degeneration in diabetes (E08-E13 with .29)
     syphilitic pyelonephritis and tubulo-interstitial nephritis (A52.75)

Acute kidney failure and chronic kidney disease (N17-N19)
EXCLUDES 2   *congenital renal failure (P96.0)*
     drug- and heavy-metal-induced tubulo-interstitial and tubular conditions (N14.-)
     extrarenal uremia (R39.2)
     hemolytic-uremic syndrome (D59.3)
     hepatorenal syndrome (K76.7)
     postpartum hepatorenal syndrome (O90.4)
     posttraumatic renal failure (T79.5)
     prerenal uremia (R39.2)
     renal failure complicating abortion or ectopic or molar pregnancy (O00-O07, O08.4)
     renal failure following labor and delivery (O90.4)
     renal failure postprocedural (N99.0)

√4ᵗʰ **N17** **Acute kidney failure**
Code also associated underlying condition
EXCLUDES 1   *posttraumatic renal failure (T79.5)*

N17.0 **Acute kidney failure with tubular necrosis**
Acute tubular necrosis
Renal tubular necrosis
Tubular necrosis NOS

N17.1 **Acute kidney failure with acute cortical necrosis**
Acute cortical necrosis
Cortical necrosis NOS
Renal cortical necrosis

N17.2 **Acute kidney failure with medullary necrosis**
Medullary [papillary] necrosis NOS
Acute medullary [papillary] necrosis
Renal medullary [papillary] necrosis

N17.8 **Other acute kidney failure**

N17.9 **Acute kidney failure, unspecified**
Acute kidney injury (nontraumatic)
EXCLUDES 2   *traumatic kidney injury (S37.0-)*

√4ᵗʰ **N18** **Chronic kidney disease (CKD)**
Code first any associated:
   diabetic chronic kidney disease (E08.22, E09.22, E10.22, E11.22, E13.22)
   hypertensive chronic kidney disease (I12-, I13-)
Use additional code to identify kidney transplant status, if applicable, (Z94.0)

N18.1 **Chronic kidney disease, stage 1**

N18.2 **Chronic kidney disease, stage 2 (mild)**

N18.3 **Chronic kidney disease, stage 3 (moderate)**

N18.4 **Chronic kidney disease, stage 4 (severe)**

N18.5 **Chronic kidney disease, stage 5**
EXCLUDES 1   *chronic kidney disease, stage 5 requiring chronic dialysis (N18.6)*

N18.6 **End stage renal disease**
Chronic kidney disease requiring chronic dialysis
Use additional code to identify dialysis status (Z99.2)

N18.9 **Chronic kidney disease, unspecified**
Chronic renal disease
Chronic renal failure NOS
Chronic renal insufficiency
Chronic uremia

N19 **Unspecified kidney failure**
Uremia NOS
EXCLUDES 1   *acute kidney failure (N17.-)*
     chronic kidney disease (N18.-)
     chronic uremia (N18.9)
     extrarenal uremia (R39.2)
     prerenal uremia (R39.2)
     renal insufficiency (acute) (N28.9)
     uremia of newborn (P96.0)

Urolithiasis (N20-N23)

√4ᵗʰ **N20** **Calculus of kidney and ureter**
Calculous pyelonephritis
EXCLUDES 1   *nephrocalcinosis (E83.5)*
     that with hydronephrosis (N13.2)

N20.0 **Calculus of kidney**
Nephrolithiasis NOS
Renal calculus
Renal stone
Staghorn calculus
Stone in kidney

N20.1 **Calculus of ureter**
Ureteric stone

N20.2 **Calculus of kidney with calculus of ureter**

N20.9 **Urinary calculus, unspecified**

√4ᵗʰ **N21** **Calculus of lower urinary tract**
Calculus of lower urinary tract with cystitis and urethritis

N21.0 **Calculus in bladder**
Calculus in diverticulum of bladder
Urinary bladder stone
EXCLUDES 2   *staghorn calculus (N20.0)*

N21.1 **Calculus in urethra**
EXCLUDES 2   *calculus of prostate (N42.0)*

N21.8 **Other lower urinary tract calculus**

N21.9 **Calculus of lower urinary tract, unspecified**
EXCLUDES 1   *calculus of urinary tract NOS (N20.9)*

N22 *Calculus of urinary tract in diseases classified elsewhere*
Code first underlying disease, such as:
   gout (M1A.-, M10.-)
   schistosomiasis (B65.0-B65.9)

N23 **Unspecified renal colic**

Other disorders of kidney and ureter (N25-N29)
EXCLUDES 2   *disorders of kidney and ureter with urolithiasis (N20-N23)*

√4ᵗʰ **N25** **Disorders resulting from impaired renal tubular function**
EXCLUDES 1   *metabolic disorders classifiable to E70-E88*

N25.0 **Renal osteodystrophy**
Azotemic osteodystrophy
Phosphate-losing tubular disorders
Renal rickets
Renal short stature

N25.1 **Nephrogenic diabetes insipidus**
EXCLUDES 1   *diabetes insipidus NOS (E23.2)*

EXCLUDES 1 Not coded here   *EXCLUDES 2* Not included here   N Newborn Age: 0   P Pediatric Age: 0-17   M Maternity Age: 12-55   A Adult Age: 15-124

724   ICD-10-CM 2014 (Draft)

☑5th **N25.8 Other disorders resulting from impaired renal tubular function**

N25.81 Secondary hyperparathyroidism of renal origin

EXCLUDES 1 *secondary hyperparathyroidism, non-renal (E21.1)*

N25.89 Other disorders resulting from impaired renal tubular function

Hypokalemic nephropathy
Lightwood-Albright syndrome
Renal tubular acidosis NOS

N25.9 Disorder resulting from impaired renal tubular function, unspecified

☑4th **N26 Unspecified contracted kidney**

EXCLUDES 1 *contracted kidney due to hypertension (I12.-)*
diffuse sclerosing glomerulonephritis (N05.8-)
hypertensive nephrosclerosis (arteriolar) (arteriosclerotic) (I12.-)
small kidney of unknown cause (N27.-)

N26.1 Atrophy of kidney (terminal)

N26.2 Page kidney

N26.9 Renal sclerosis, unspecified

☑4th **N27 Small kidney of unknown cause**

INCLUDES oligonephronia

N27.0 Small kidney, unilateral

N27.1 Small kidney, bilateral

N27.9 Small kidney, unspecified

☑4th **N28 Other disorders of kidney and ureter, not elsewhere classified**

N28.0 Ischemia and infarction of kidney

Renal artery embolism   Renal artery thrombosis
Renal artery obstruction   Renal infarct
Renal artery occlusion

EXCLUDES 1 *atherosclerosis of renal artery (extrarenal part) (I70.1)*
congenital stenosis of renal artery (Q27.1)
Goldblatt's kidney (I70.1)

N28.1 Cyst of kidney, acquired

Cyst (multiple)(solitary) of kidney, acquired

EXCLUDES 1 *cystic kidney disease (congenital) (Q61.-)*

☑5th **N28.8 Other specified disorders of kidney and ureter**

EXCLUDES 1 *hydroureter (N13.4)*
ureteric stricture with hydronephrosis (N13.1)
ureteric stricture without hydronephrosis (N13.5)

N28.81 Hypertrophy of kidney

N28.82 Megaloureter

N28.83 Nephroptosis

N28.84 Pyelitis cystica

N28.85 Pyeloureteritis cystica

N28.86 Ureteritis cystica

N28.89 Other specified disorders of kidney and ureter

N28.9 Disorder of kidney and ureter, unspecified

Nephropathy NOS
Renal disease (acute) NOS
Renal insufficiency (acute)

EXCLUDES 1 *chronic renal insufficiency (N18.9)*
unspecified nephritic syndrome (N05.-)

N29 *Other disorders of kidney and ureter in diseases classified elsewhere*

Code first underlying disease, such as:
amyloidosis (E85.-)
nephrocalcinosis (E83.5)
schistosomiasis (B65.0-B65.9)

EXCLUDES 1 *disorders of kidney and ureter in:*
cystinosis (E72.0)
gonorrhea (A54.21)
syphilis (A52.75)
tuberculosis (A18.11)

Other diseases of the urinary system (N30-N39)

EXCLUDES 1 *urinary infection (complicating):*
abortion or ectopic or molar pregnancy (O00-O07, O08.8)
pregnancy, childbirth and the puerperium (O23-, O75.3, O86.2-)

☑4th **N30 Cystitis**

Use additional code to identify infectious agent (B95-B97)

EXCLUDES 1 *prostatocystitis (N41.3)*

☑5th **N30.0 Acute cystitis**

EXCLUDES 1 *irradiation cystitis (N30.4-)*
trigonitis (N30.3-)

N30.00 Acute cystitis without hematuria

N30.01 Acute cystitis with hematuria

☑5th **N30.1 Interstitial cystitis (chronic)**

N30.10 Interstitial cystitis (chronic) without hematuria

N30.11 Interstitial cystitis (chronic) with hematuria

☑5th **N30.2 Other chronic cystitis**

N30.20 Other chronic cystitis without hematuria

N30.21 Other chronic cystitis with hematuria

☑5th **N30.3 Trigonitis**

Urethrotrigonitis

N30.30 Trigonitis without hematuria

N30.31 Trigonitis with hematuria

☑5th **N30.4 Irradiation cystitis**

N30.40 Irradiation cystitis without hematuria

N30.41 Irradiation cystitis with hematuria

☑5th **N30.8 Other cystitis**

Abscess of bladder

N30.80 Other cystitis without hematuria

N30.81 Other cystitis with hematuria

☑5th **N30.9 Cystitis, unspecified**

N30.90 Cystitis, unspecified without hematuria

N30.91 Cystitis, unspecified with hematuria

☑4th **N31 Neuromuscular dysfunction of bladder, not elsewhere classified**

Use additional code to identify any associated urinary incontinence (N39.3-N39.4-)

EXCLUDES 1 *cord bladder NOS (G95.89)*
neurogenic bladder due to cauda equina syndrome (G83.4)
neuromuscular dysfunction due to spinal cord lesion (G95.89)

N31.0 Uninhibited neuropathic bladder, not elsewhere classified

N31.1 Reflex neuropathic bladder, not elsewhere classified

N31.2 Flaccid neuropathic bladder, not elsewhere classified

Atonic (motor) (sensory) neuropathic bladder
Autonomous neuropathic bladder
Nonreflex neuropathic bladder

N31.8 Other neuromuscular dysfunction of bladder

N31.9 Neuromuscular dysfunction of bladder, unspecified

Neurogenic bladder dysfunction NOS

☑4th **N32 Other disorders of bladder**

EXCLUDES 2 *calculus of bladder (N21.0)*
cystocele (N81.1-)
hernia or prolapse of bladder, female (N81.1-)

N32.0 Bladder-neck obstruction

Bladder-neck stenosis (acquired)

EXCLUDES 1 *congenital bladder-neck obstruction (Q64.3-)*

N32.1 Vesicointestinal fistula

Vesicorectal fistula

N32.2 Vesical fistula, not elsewhere classified

EXCLUDES 1 *fistula between bladder and female genital tract (N82.0-N82.1)*

N32.3 Diverticulum of bladder

EXCLUDES 1 *congenital diverticulum of bladder (Q64.6)*
diverticulitis of bladder (N30.8-)

☑5th **N32.8 Other specified disorders of bladder**

N32.81 Overactive bladder

Detrusor muscle hyperactivity

EXCLUDES 1 *frequent urination due to specified bladder condition—code to condition*

N32.89 Other specified disorders of bladder

Bladder hemorrhage
Bladder hypertrophy
Calcified bladder
Contracted bladder

N32.9 Bladder disorder, unspecified

☑ Additional Character Required   ✗x7th Xtension Alert   Unspecified Code   Other Specified Code   Manifestation Code   ◄► Revised Text   ● New Code   ▲ Revised Code Title

ICD-10-CM 2014 (Draft)

725

Diseases of the Genitourinary System

N33–N39.9

N33   Bladder disorders in diseases classified elsewhere
Code first underlying disease, such as:
schistosomiasis (B65.0-B65.9)
> EXCLUDES 1   bladder disorder in syphilis (A52.76)
> bladder disorder in tuberculosis (A18.12)
> candidal cystitis (B37.41)
> chlamydial cystitis (A56.01)
> cystitis in gonorrhea (A54.01)
> cystitis in neurogenic bladder (N31.-)
> diphtheritic cystitis (A36.85)
> neurogenic bladder (N31.-)
> syphilitic cystitis (A52.76)
> trichomonal cystitis (A59.03)

✓4th   N34   Urethritis and urethral syndrome
Use additional code (B95-B97), to identify infectious agent
> EXCLUDES 2   Reiter's disease (M02.3-)
> urethritis in diseases with a predominantly sexual mode of
> transmission (A50-A64)
> urethrotrigonitis (N30.3-)

N34.0   Urethral abscess
Abscess (of) Cowper's gland
Abscess (of) Littrés gland
Abscess (of) urethral (gland)
Periurethral abscess
> EXCLUDES 1   urethral caruncle (N36.2)

N34.1   Nonspecific urethritis
Nongonococcal urethritis
Nonvenereal urethritis

N34.2   Other urethritis
Meatitis, urethral
Postmenopausal urethritis
Ulcer of urethra (meatus)
Urethritis NOS

N34.3   Urethral syndrome, unspecified

✓4th   N35   Urethral stricture
> EXCLUDES 1   congenital urethral stricture (Q64.3-)
> postprocedural urethral stricture (N99.1-)

✓5th   N35.0   Post-traumatic urethral stricture
Urethral stricture due to injury
> EXCLUDES 1   postprocedural urethral stricture (N99.1-)

✓6th   N35.01   Post-traumatic urethral stricture, male
N35.010   Post-traumatic urethral stricture, male, meatal ♂
N35.011   Post-traumatic bulbous urethral stricture
N35.012   Post-traumatic membranous urethral stricture
N35.013   Post-traumatic anterior urethral stricture
N35.014   Post-traumatic urethral stricture, male, unspecified ♂

✓6th   N35.02   Post-traumatic urethral stricture, female
N35.021   Urethral stricture due to childbirth ♀
N35.028   Other post-traumatic urethral stricture, female ♀

✓5th   N35.1   Postinfective urethral stricture, not elsewhere classified
> EXCLUDES 1   urethral stricture associated with schistosomiasis (B65-, N29)
> gonococcal urethral stricture (A54.01)
> syphilitic urethral stricture (A52.76)

✓6th   N35.11   Postinfective urethral stricture, not elsewhere classified, male
N35.111   Postinfective urethral stricture, not elsewhere classified, male, meatal ♂
N35.112   Postinfective bulbous urethral stricture, not elsewhere classified
N35.113   Postinfective membranous urethral stricture, not elsewhere classified
N35.114   Postinfective anterior urethral stricture, not elsewhere classified
N35.119   Postinfective urethral stricture, not elsewhere classified, male, unspecified ♂

N35.12   Postinfective urethral stricture, not elsewhere classified, female ♀

N35.8   Other urethral stricture
> EXCLUDES 1   postprocedural urethral stricture (N99.1-)

N35.9   Urethral stricture, unspecified

✓4th   N36   Other disorders of urethra

N36.0   Urethral fistula
Urethroperineal fistula
Urethrorectal fistula
Urinary fistula NOS
> EXCLUDES 1   urethroscrotal fistula (N50.8)
> urethrovaginal fistula (N82.1)
> urethrovesicovaginal fistula (N82.1)

N36.1   Urethral diverticulum

N36.2   Urethral caruncle

✓5th   N36.4   Urethral functional and muscular disorders
Use additional code to identify associated urinary stress
incontinence (N39.3)

N36.41   Hypermobility of urethra

N36.42   Intrinsic sphincter deficiency (ISD)

N36.43   Combined hypermobility of urethra and intrinsic sphincter deficiency

N36.44   Muscular disorders of urethra
Bladder sphincter dyssynergy

N36.5   Urethral false passage

N36.8   Other specified disorders of urethra

N36.9   Urethral disorder, unspecified

N37   Urethral disorders in diseases classified elsewhere
Code first underlying disease
> EXCLUDES 1   urethritis (in):
> candidal infection (B37.41)
> chlamydial (A56.01)
> gonorrhea (A54.01)
> syphilis (A52.76)
> trichomonal infection (A59.03)
> tuberculosis (A18.13)

✓4th   N39   Other disorders of urinary system
> EXCLUDES 2   hematuria NOS (R31.-)
> recurrent or persistent hematuria (N02.-)
> recurrent or persistent hematuria with specified morphological lesion (N02.-)
> proteinuria NOS (R80.-)

N39.0   Urinary tract infection, site not specified
Use additional code (B95-B97), to identify infectious agent
> EXCLUDES 1   candidiasis of urinary tract (B37.4-)
> neonatal urinary tract infection (P39.3)
> urinary tract infection of specified site, such as:
> cystitis (N30.-)
> urethritis (N34.-)

AHA: 2012, Q4, 94

N39.3   Stress incontinence (female) (male)
Code also any associated overactive bladder (N32.81)
> EXCLUDES 1   mixed incontinence (N39.46)

✓5th   N39.4   Other specified urinary incontinence
Code also any associated overactive bladder (N32.81)
> EXCLUDES 1   enuresis NOS (R32)
> functional urinary incontinence (R39.81)
> urinary incontinence associated with cognitive impairment (R39.81)
> urinary incontinence NOS (R32)
> urinary incontinence of nonorganic origin (F98.0)

N39.41   Urge incontinence
> EXCLUDES 1   mixed incontinence (N39.46)

N39.42   Incontinence without sensory awareness

N39.43   Post-void dribbling

N39.44   Nocturnal enuresis

N39.45   Continuous leakage

N39.46   Mixed incontinence
Urge and stress incontinence

✓6th   N39.49   Other specified urinary incontinence
N39.490   Overflow incontinence
N39.498   Other specified urinary incontinence
Reflex incontinence
Total incontinence

N39.8   Other specified disorders of urinary system

N39.9   Disorder of urinary system, unspecified

EXCLUDES 1 Not coded here   EXCLUDES 2 Not included here   N Newborn Age: 0   P Pediatric Age: 0-17   M Maternity Age: 12-55   A Adult Age: 15-124

726   ICD-10-CM 2014 (Draft)

Diseases of male genital organs (N40-N53)

✓4th N40 Enlarged prostate
Adenofibromatous hypertrophy of prostate
Benign hypertrophy of the prostate
Benign prostatic hyperplasia
Benign prostatic hypertrophy
BPH
Nodular prostate
Polyp of prostate
EXCLUDES1 benign neoplasms of prostate (adenoma, benign)
(fibroadenoma) (fibroma) (myoma) (D29.1)
EXCLUDES2 malignant neoplasm of prostate (C61)

N40.0 Enlarged prostate without lower urinary tract symptoms A♂
Enlarged prostate NOS
Enlarged prostate without LUTS

N40.1 Enlarged prostate with lower urinary tract symptoms A♂
Enlarged prostate with LUTS
Use additional code for associated symptoms, when specified:
incomplete bladder emptying (R39.14)
nocturia (R35.1)
straining on urination (R39.16)
urinary frequency (R35.0)
urinary hesitancy (R39.11)
urinary incontinence (N39.4-)
urinary obstruction (N13.8)
urinary retention (R33.8)
urinary urgency (R39.15)
weak urinary stream (R39.12)

N40.2 Nodular prostate without lower urinary tract symptoms A♂
Nodular prostate without LUTS

N40.3 Nodular prostate with lower urinary tract symptoms A♂
Use additional code for associated symptoms, when specified:
incomplete bladder emptying (R39.14)
nocturia (R35.1)
straining on urination (R39.16)
urinary frequency (R35.0)
urinary hesitancy (R39.11)
urinary incontinence (N39.4-)
urinary obstruction (N13.8)
urinary retention (R33.8)
urinary urgency (R39.15)
weak urinary stream (R39.12)

✓4th N41 Inflammatory diseases of prostate
Use additional code (B95-B97), to identify infectious agent
N41.0 Acute prostatitis A♂
N41.1 Chronic prostatitis A♂
N41.2 Abscess of prostate A♂
N41.3 Prostatocystitis A♂
N41.4 Granulomatous prostatitis A♂
N41.8 Other inflammatory diseases of prostate A♂
N41.9 Inflammatory disease of prostate, unspecified A♂
Prostatitis NOS

✓4th N42 Other and unspecified disorders of prostate
N42.0 Calculus of prostate A♂
Prostatic stone
N42.1 Congestion and hemorrhage of prostate A♂
EXCLUDES1 enlarged prostate (N40.-)
hematuria (R31.-)
hyperplasia of prostate (N40.-)
inflammatory diseases of prostate (N41.-)
N42.3 Dysplasia of prostate ♂
Prostatic intraepithelial neoplasia I (PIN I)
Prostatic intraepithelial neoplasia II (PIN II)
EXCLUDES1 prostatic intraepithelial neoplasia III (PIN III) (D07.5)
✓5th N42.8 Other specified disorders of prostate
N42.81 Prostatodynia syndrome A♂
Painful prostate syndrome
N42.82 Prostatosis syndrome A♂
N42.83 Cyst of prostate A♂
N42.89 Other specified disorders of prostate A♂
N42.9 Disorder of prostate, unspecified A♂

✓4th N43 Hydrocele and spermatocele
INCLUDES hydrocele of spermatic cord, testis or tunica vaginalis
EXCLUDES1 congenital hydrocele (P83.5)
N43.0 Encysted hydrocele ♂
N43.1 Infected hydrocele ♂
Use additional code (B95-B97), to identify infectious agent

N43.2 Other hydrocele ♂
N43.3 Hydrocele, unspecified ♂
✓5th N43.4 Spermatocele of epididymis ♂
Spermatic cyst
N43.40 Spermatocele of epididymis, unspecified ♂
N43.41 Spermatocele of epididymis, single ♂
N43.42 Spermatocele of epididymis, multiple ♂

✓4th N44 Noninflammatory disorders of testis
✓5th N44.0 Torsion of testis
N44.00 Torsion of testis, unspecified ♂
N44.01 Extravaginal torsion of spermatic cord ♂
N44.02 Intravaginal torsion of spermatic cord ♂
Torsion of spermatic cord NOS
N44.03 Torsion of appendix testis ♂
N44.04 Torsion of appendix epididymis ♂
N44.1 Cyst of tunica albuginea testis ♂
N44.2 Benign cyst of testis ♂
N44.8 Other noninflammatory disorders of the testis ♂

✓4th N45 Orchitis and epididymitis
Use additional code (B95-B97), to identify infectious agent
N45.1 Epididymitis ♂
N45.2 Orchitis ♂
N45.3 Epididymo-orchitis ♂
N45.4 Abscess of epididymis or testis ♂

✓4th N46 Male infertility
EXCLUDES1 vasectomy status (Z98.52)
✓5th N46.0 Azoospermia
Absolute male infertility
Male infertility due to germinal (cell) aplasia
Male infertility due to spermatogenic arrest (complete)
N46.01 Organic azoospermia A♂
Azoospermia NOS
✓6th N46.02 Azoospermia due to extratesticular causes
Code also associated cause
N46.021 Azoospermia due to drug therapy A♂
N46.022 Azoospermia due to infection A♂
N46.023 Azoospermia due to obstruction of efferent ducts A♂
N46.024 Azoospermia due to radiation A♂
N46.025 Azoospermia due to systemic disease A♂
N46.029 Azoospermia due to other extratesticular causes A♂
✓5th N46.1 Oligospermia
Male infertility due to germinal cell desquamation
Male infertility due to hypospermatogenesis
Male infertility due to incomplete spermatogenic arrest
N46.11 Organic oligospermia A♂
Oligospermia NOS
✓6th N46.12 Oligospermia due to extratesticular causes
Code also associated cause
N46.121 Oligospermia due to drug therapy A♂
N46.122 Oligospermia due to infection A♂
N46.123 Oligospermia due to obstruction of efferent ducts A♂
N46.124 Oligospermia due to radiation A♂
N46.125 Oligospermia due to systemic disease A♂
N46.129 Oligospermia due to other extratesticular causes A♂
N46.8 Other male infertility A♂
N46.9 Male infertility, unspecified A♂

✓4th N47 Disorders of prepuce
N47.0 Adherent prepuce, newborn N♂
N47.1 Phimosis ♂
N47.2 Paraphimosis ♂
N47.3 Deficient foreskin ♂
N47.4 Benign cyst of prepuce ♂
N47.5 Adhesions of prepuce and glans penis ♂
N47.6 Balanoposthitis ♂
EXCLUDES1 balanitis (N48.1)
Use additional code (B95-B97), to identify infectious agent
N47.7 Other inflammatory diseases of prepuce ♂
Use additional code (B95-B97), to identify infectious agent

✔ Additional Character Required ✓x7th Xtension Alert Unspecified Code Other Specified Code Manifestation Code ►◄ Revised Text ● New Code ▲ Revised Code Title

N47.8 Other disorders of prepuce ♂

✓4ᵗʰ **N48 Other disorders of penis**

N48.0 Leukoplakia of penis ♂
Balanitis xerotica obliterans
Kraurosis of penis
Lichen sclerosus of external male genital organs
EXCLUDES 1 carcinoma in situ of penis (D07.4)

N48.1 Balanitis
EXCLUDES 1 amebic balanitis (A06.8)
balanitis xerotica obliterans (N48.0)
candidal balanitis (B37.42)
gonococcal balanitis (A54.23)
herpesviral [herpes simplex] balanitis (A60.01)
Use additional code (B95-B97), to identify infectious agent

✓5ᵗʰ **N48.2 Other inflammatory disorders of penis**
Use additional code (B95-B97), to identify infectious agent
EXCLUDES 1 balanitis (N48.1)
balanitis xerotica obliterans (N48.0)
balanoposthitis (N47.6)

N48.21 Abscess of corpus cavernosum and penis ♂
N48.22 Cellulitis of corpus cavernosum and penis ♂
N48.29 Other inflammatory disorders of penis ♂

✓5ᵗʰ **N48.3 Priapism**
Painful erection
Code first underlying cause
N48.30 Priapism, unspecified ♂
N48.31 Priapism due to trauma ♂
N48.32 Priapism due to disease classified elsewhere ♂
N48.33 Priapism, drug-induced ♂
N48.39 Other priapism ♂

N48.5 Ulcer of penis ♂

N48.6 Induration penis plastica ♂
Peyronie's disease
Plastic induration of penis

✓5ᵗʰ **N48.8 Other specified disorders of penis**
N48.81 Thrombosis of superficial vein of penis ♂
N48.82 Acquired torsion of penis ♂
Acquired torsion of penis NOS
EXCLUDES 1 congenital torsion of penis (Q55.63)
N48.83 Acquired buried penis ♂
EXCLUDES 1 congenital hidden penis (Q55.64)
N48.89 Other specified disorders of penis

N48.9 Disorder of penis, unspecified

✓4ᵗʰ **N49 Inflammatory disorders of male genital organs, not elsewhere classified**
Use additional code (B95-B97), to identify infectious agent
EXCLUDES 1 inflammation of penis (N48.1, N48.2-)
orchitis and epididymitis (N45.-)

N49.0 Inflammatory disorders of seminal vesicle ♂
Vesiculitis NOS

N49.1 Inflammatory disorders of spermatic cord, tunica vaginalis and vas deferens ♂
Vasitis

N49.2 Inflammatory disorders of scrotum ♂

N49.3 Fournier gangrene ♂

N49.8 Inflammatory disorders of other specified male genital organs ♂
Inflammation of multiple sites in male genital organs

N49.9 Inflammatory disorder of unspecified male genital organ ♂
Abscess of unspecified male genital organ
Boil of unspecified male genital organ
Carbuncle of unspecified male genital organ
Cellulitis of unspecified male genital organ

✓4ᵗʰ **N50 Other and unspecified disorders of male genital organs**
EXCLUDES 2 torsion of testis (N44.0-)

N50.0 Atrophy of testis ♂

N50.1 Vascular disorders of male genital organs ♂
Hematocele, NOS, of male genital organs
Hemorrhage of male genital organs
Thrombosis of male genital organs

N50.3 Cyst of epididymis ♂

N50.8 Other specified disorders of male genital organs ♂
Atrophy of scrotum, seminal vesicle, spermatic cord, tunica vaginalis and vas deferens
Chylocele, tunica vaginalis (nonfilarial) NOS
Edema of scrotum, seminal vesicle, spermatic cord, testis, tunica vaginalis and vas deferens
Hypertrophy of scrotum, seminal vesicle, spermatic cord, testis, tunica vaginalis and vas deferens
Stricture of spermatic cord, tunica vaginalis, and vas deferens
Ulcer of scrotum, seminal vesicle, spermatic cord, testis, tunica vaginalis and vas deferens
Urethroscrotal fistula

N50.9 Disorder of male genital organs, unspecified ♂

N51 Disorders of male genital organs in diseases classified elsewhere ♂
Code first underlying disease, such as:
filariasis (B74.0-B74.9)
EXCLUDES 1 amebic balanitis (A06.8)
candidal balanitis (B37.42)
gonococcal balanitis (A54.23)
gonococcal prostatitis (A54.22)
herpesviral [herpes simplex] balanitis (A60.01)
trichomonal prostatitis (A59.02)
tuberculous prostatitis (A18.14)

✓4ᵗʰ **N52 Male erectile dysfunction**
EXCLUDES 1 psychogenic impotence (F52.21)

✓5ᵗʰ **N52.0 Vasculogenic erectile dysfunction**
N52.01 Erectile dysfunction due to arterial insufficiency A♂
N52.02 Corporo-venous occlusive erectile dysfunction A♂
N52.03 Combined arterial insufficiency and corporo-venous occlusive erectile dysfunction A♂

N52.1 Erectile dysfunction due to diseases classified elsewhere A♂
Code first underlying disease

N52.2 Drug-induced erectile dysfunction A♂

✓5ᵗʰ **N52.3 Post-surgical erectile dysfunction**
N52.31 Erectile dysfunction following radical prostatectomy A♂
N52.32 Erectile dysfunction following radical cystectomy A♂
N52.33 Erectile dysfunction following urethral surgery A♂
N52.34 Erectile dysfunction following simple prostatectomy A♂
N52.39 Other post-surgical erectile dysfunction A♂

N52.8 Other male erectile dysfunction A♂

N52.9 Male erectile dysfunction, unspecified A♂
Impotence NOS

✓4ᵗʰ **N53 Other male sexual dysfunction**
EXCLUDES 1 psychogenic sexual dysfunction (F52.-)

✓5ᵗʰ **N53.1 Ejaculatory dysfunction**
EXCLUDES 1 premature ejaculation (F52.4)
N53.11 Retarded ejaculation ♂
N53.12 Painful ejaculation ♂
N53.13 Anejaculatory orgasm ♂
N53.14 Retrograde ejaculation ♂
N53.19 Other ejaculatory dysfunction ♂
Ejaculatory dysfunction NOS

N53.8 Other male sexual dysfunction ♂

N53.9 Unspecified male sexual dysfunction ♂

Disorders of breast (N60-N65)
EXCLUDES 1 disorders of breast associated with childbirth (O91-O92)

✓4ᵗʰ **N60 Benign mammary dysplasia**
INCLUDES fibrocystic mastopathy

✓5ᵗʰ **N60.0 Solitary cyst of breast**
Cyst of breast
N60.01 Solitary cyst of right breast
N60.02 Solitary cyst of left breast
N60.09 Solitary cyst of unspecified breast

✓5ᵗʰ **N60.1 Diffuse cystic mastopathy**
Cystic breast
Fibrocystic disease of breast
EXCLUDES 1 diffuse cystic mastopathy with epithelial proliferation (N60.3-)
N60.11 Diffuse cystic mastopathy of right breast A
N60.12 Diffuse cystic mastopathy of left breast A

EXCLUDES 1 Not coded here　　*EXCLUDES 2* Not included here　　N Newborn Age: 0　　P Pediatric Age: 0-17　　M Maternity Age: 12-55　　A Adult Age: 15-124

728　　　　　　　　　　　　　　　　　　　　　　　　　　　　　　　　　　　　ICD-10-CM 2014 (Draft)

N60.19   **Diffuse cystic mastopathy of unspecified breast** Ⓐ

✓5ᵗʰ **N60.2 Fibroadenosis of breast**
Adenofibrosis of breast
EXCLUDES 2   *fibroadenoma of breast (D24.-)*

N60.21   **Fibroadenosis of right breast**

N60.22   **Fibroadenosis of left breast**

N60.29   **Fibroadenosis of unspecified breast**

✓5ᵗʰ **N60.3 Fibrosclerosis of breast**
Cystic mastopathy with epithelial proliferation

N60.31   **Fibrosclerosis of right breast**

N60.32   **Fibrosclerosis of left breast**

N60.39   **Fibrosclerosis of unspecified breast**

✓5ᵗʰ **N60.4 Mammary duct ectasia**

N60.41   **Mammary duct ectasia of right breast**

N60.42   **Mammary duct ectasia of left breast**

N60.49   **Mammary duct ectasia of unspecified breast**

✓5ᵗʰ **N60.8 Other benign mammary dysplasias**

N60.81   **Other benign mammary dysplasias of right breast**

N60.82   **Other benign mammary dysplasias of left breast**

N60.89   **Other benign mammary dysplasias of unspecified breast**

✓5ᵗʰ **N60.9 Unspecified benign mammary dysplasia**

N60.91   **Unspecified benign mammary dysplasia of right breast**

N60.92   **Unspecified benign mammary dysplasia of left breast**

N60.99   **Unspecified benign mammary dysplasia of unspecified breast**

N61 Inflammatory disorders of breast
Abscess (acute) (chronic) (nonpuerperal) of areola
Abscess (acute) (chronic) (nonpuerperal) of breast
Carbuncle of breast
Infective mastitis (acute) (subacute) (nonpuerperal)
Mastitis (acute) (subacute) (nonpuerperal) NOS
EXCLUDES 1   *inflammatory carcinoma of breast (C50.9)*
inflammatory disorder of breast associated with childbirth (O91.-)
neonatal infective mastitis (P39.0)
thrombophlebitis of breast [Mondor's disease] (I80.8)

N62 Hypertrophy of breast
Gynecomastia
Hypertrophy of breast NOS
Massive pubertal hypertrophy of breast
EXCLUDES 1   *breast engorgement of newborn (P83.4)*
disproportion of reconstructed breast (N65.1)

N63 Unspecified lump in breast
Nodule(s) NOS in breast

✓4ᵗʰ **N64 Other disorders of breast**
EXCLUDES 2   *mechanical complication of breast prosthesis and implant (T85.4-)*

N64.0   **Fissure and fistula of nipple**

N64.1   **Fat necrosis of breast**
Fat necrosis (segmental) of breast
Code first breast necrosis due to breast graft (T85.89)

N64.2   **Atrophy of breast**

N64.3   **Galactorrhea not associated with childbirth**

N64.4   **Mastodynia**

✓5ᵗʰ N64.5   **Other signs and symptoms in breast**
EXCLUDES 2   *abnormal findings on diagnostic imaging of breast (R92.-)*

N64.51   **Induration of breast**

N64.52   **Nipple discharge**
EXCLUDES 1   *abnormal findings in nipple discharge (R89.-)*

N64.53   **Retraction of nipple**

N64.59   **Other signs and symptoms in breast**

✓5ᵗʰ N64.8   **Other specified disorders of breast**

N64.81   **Ptosis of breast** Ⓐ
EXCLUDES 1   *ptosis of native breast in relation to reconstructed breast (N65.1)*

N64.82   **Hypoplasia of breast** Ⓐ
Micromastia
EXCLUDES 1   *congenital absence of breast (Q83.0)*
hypoplasia of native breast in relation to reconstructed breast (N65.1)

N64.89   **Other specified disorders of breast**
Galactocele
Subinvolution of breast (postlactational)

N64.9   **Disorder of breast, unspecified**

✓4ᵗʰ **N65 Deformity and disproportion of reconstructed breast**

N65.0   **Deformity of reconstructed breast** Ⓐ
Contour irregularity in reconstructed breast
Excess tissue in reconstructed breast
Misshapen reconstructed breast

N65.1   **Disproportion of reconstructed breast** Ⓐ
Breast asymmetry between native breast and reconstructed breast
Disproportion between native breast and reconstructed breast

Inflammatory diseases of female pelvic organs (N70-N77)

EXCLUDES 1   *inflammatory diseases of female pelvic organs complicating:*
abortion or ectopic or molar pregnancy (O00-O07, O08.0)
pregnancy, childbirth and the puerperium (O23-, O75.3, O85, O86-)

✓4ᵗʰ **N70 Salpingitis and oophoritis**
INCLUDES   abscess (of) fallopian tube
abscess (of) ovary
pyosalpinx
salpingo-oophoritis
tubo-ovarian abscess
tubo-ovarian inflammatory disease
Use additional code (B95-B97), to identify infectious agent
EXCLUDES 1   *gonococcal infection (A54.24)*
tuberculous infection (A18.17)

✓5ᵗʰ N70.0   **Acute salpingitis and oophoritis**

N70.01   **Acute salpingitis** ♀

N70.02   **Acute oophoritis** ♀

N70.03   **Acute salpingitis and oophoritis** ♀

✓5ᵗʰ N70.1   **Chronic salpingitis and oophoritis**
Hydrosalpinx

N70.11   **Chronic salpingitis** ♀

N70.12   **Chronic oophoritis** ♀

N70.13   **Chronic salpingitis and oophoritis** ♀

✓5ᵗʰ N70.9   **Salpingitis and oophoritis, unspecified**

N70.91   **Salpingitis, unspecified** ♀

N70.92   **Oophoritis, unspecified** ♀

N70.93   **Salpingitis and oophoritis, unspecified** ♀

✓4ᵗʰ **N71 Inflammatory disease of uterus, except cervix**
Endo (myo) metritis   Pyometra
Metritis   Uterine abscess
Myometritis
Use additional code (B95-B97), to identify infectious agent
EXCLUDES 1   *hyperplastic endometritis (N85.0-)*
infection of uterus following delivery (O85, O86.-)

N71.0   **Acute inflammatory disease of uterus** ♀

N71.1   **Chronic inflammatory disease of uterus** ♀

N71.9   **Inflammatory disease of uterus, unspecified** ♀

N72 Inflammatory disease of cervix uteri ♀
Cervicitis (with or without erosion or ectropion)
Endocervicitis (with or without erosion or ectropion)
Exocervicitis (with or without erosion or ectropion)
Use additional code (B95-B97), to identify infectious agent
EXCLUDES 1   *erosion and ectropion of cervix without cervicitis (N86)*

✓4ᵗʰ **N73 Other female pelvic inflammatory diseases**
Use additional code (B95-B97), to identify infectious agent

N73.0   **Acute parametritis and pelvic cellulitis** ♀
Abscess of broad ligament
Abscess of parametrium
Pelvic cellulitis, female

N73.1   **Chronic parametritis and pelvic cellulitis** ♀
Any condition in N73.0 specified as chronic
EXCLUDES 1   *tuberculous parametritis and pelvic cellultis (A18.17)*

N73.2   **Unspecified parametritis and pelvic cellulitis** ♀
Any condition in N73.0 unspecified whether acute or chronic

N73.3   **Female acute pelvic peritonitis** ♀

N73.4   **Female chronic pelvic peritonitis** ♀
EXCLUDES 1   *tuberculous pelvic (female) peritonitis (A18.17)*

N73.5   **Female pelvic peritonitis, unspecified** ♀

N73.6   **Female pelvic peritoneal adhesions (postinfective)** ♀
EXCLUDES 2   *postprocedural pelvic peritoneal adhesions (N99.4)*

N73.8   **Other specified female pelvic inflammatory diseases** ♀

✓ Additional Character Required   ✓x7ᵗʰ Xtension Alert   Unspecified Code   Other Specified Code   Manifestation Code   ►◄ Revised Text   ● New Code   ▲ Revised Code Title

Diseases of the Genitourinary System

N73.9 Female pelvic inflammatory disease, unspecified ♀
  Female pelvic infection or inflammation NOS

N74 Female pelvic inflammatory disorders in diseases classified elsewhere ♀
  Code first underlying disease
  EXCLUDES 1 *chlamydial cervicitis (A56.02)*
  chlamydial pelvic inflammatory disease (A56.11)
  gonococcal cervicitis (A54.03)
  gonococcal pelvic inflammatory disease (A54.24)
  herpesviral [herpes simplex] cervicitis (A60.03)
  herpesviral [herpes simplex] pelvic inflammatory disease (A60.09)
  syphilitic cervicitis (A52.76)
  syphilitic pelvic inflammatory disease (A52.76)
  trichomonal cervicitis (A59.09)
  tuberculous cervicitis (A18.16)
  tuberculous pelvic inflammatory disease (A18.17)

✓4ᵗʰ N75 Diseases of Bartholin's gland
  N75.0 Cyst of Bartholin's gland ♀
  N75.1 Abscess of Bartholin's gland ♀
  N75.8 Other diseases of Bartholin's gland ♀
    Bartholinitis
  N75.9 Disease of Bartholin's gland, unspecified ♀

✓4ᵗʰ N76 Other inflammation of vagina and vulva
  Use additional code (B95-B97), to identify infectious agent
  EXCLUDES 2 *senile (atrophic) vaginitis (N95.2)*
  vulvar vestibulitis (N94.810)
  N76.0 Acute vaginitis ♀
    Acute vulvovaginitis
    Vaginitis NOS
    Vulvovaginitis NOS
  N76.1 Subacute and chronic vaginitis ♀
    Chronic vaginitis
    Subacute vulvovaginitis
  N76.2 Acute vulvitis ♀
    Vulvitis NOS
  N76.3 Subacute and chronic vulvitis ♀
  N76.4 Abscess of vulva ♀
    Furuncle of vulva
  N76.5 Ulceration of vagina ♀
  N76.6 Ulceration of vulva ♀
  ✓5ᵗʰ N76.8 Other specified inflammation of vagina and vulva
    N76.81 Mucositis (ulcerative) of vagina and vulva ♀
      Code also type of associated therapy, such as:
      antineoplastic and immunosuppressive drugs (T45.1X-)
      radiological procedure and radiotherapy (Y84.2)
      EXCLUDES 2 *gastrointestinal mucositis (ulcerative) (K92.81)*
      nasal mucositis (ulcerative) (J34.81)
      oral mucositis (ulcerative) (K12.3-)
    N76.89 Other specified inflammation of vagina and vulva ♀

✓4ᵗʰ N77 Vulvovaginal ulceration and inflammation in diseases classified elsewhere
  N77.0 Ulceration of vulva in diseases classified elsewhere ♀
    Code first underlying disease, such as:
    Behçet's disease (M35.2)
    EXCLUDES 1 *ulceration of vulva in gonococcal infection (A54.02)*
    ulceration of vulva in herpesviral [herpes simplex] infection (A60.04)
    ulceration of vulva in syphilis (A51.0)
    ulceration of vulva in tuberculosis (A18.18)
  N77.1 Vaginitis, vulvitis and vulvovaginitis in diseases classified elsewhere ♀
    Code first underlying disease, such as:
    pinworm (B80)
    EXCLUDES 1 *candidal vulvovaginitis (B37.3)*
    chlamydial vulvovaginitis (A56.02)
    gonococcal vulvovaginitis (A54.02)
    herpesviral [herpes simplex] vulvovaginitis (A60.04)
    trichomonal vulvovaginitis (A59.01)
    tuberculous vulvovaginitis (A18.18)
    vulvovaginitis in early syphilis (A51.0)
    vulvovaginitis in late syphilis (A52.76)

Noninflammatory disorders of female genital tract (N80-N98)

✓4ᵗʰ N80 Endometriosis
  N80.0 Endometriosis of uterus ♀
    Adenomyosis
    EXCLUDES 1 *stromal endometriosis (D39.0)*
  N80.1 Endometriosis of ovary ♀
  N80.2 Endometriosis of fallopian tube ♀
  N80.3 Endometriosis of pelvic peritoneum ♀
  N80.4 Endometriosis of rectovaginal septum and vagina ♀
  N80.5 Endometriosis of intestine ♀
  N80.6 Endometriosis in cutaneous scar ♀
  N80.8 Other endometriosis ♀
  N80.9 Endometriosis, unspecified ♀

✓4ᵗʰ N81 Female genital prolapse
  EXCLUDES 1 *genital prolapse complicating pregnancy, labor or delivery (O34.5-)*
  prolapse and hernia of ovary and fallopian tube (N83.4)
  prolapse of vaginal vault after hysterectomy (N99.3)
  N81.0 Urethrocele ♀
    EXCLUDES 1 *urethrocele with cystocele (N81.1-)*
    urethrocele with prolapse of uterus (N81.2-N81.4)
  ✓5ᵗʰ N81.1 Cystocele
    Cystocele with urethrocele
    Cystourethrocele
    EXCLUDES 1 *cystocele with prolapse of uterus (N81.2-N81.4)*
    N81.10 Cystocele, unspecified ♀
      Prolapse of (anterior) vaginal wall NOS
    N81.11 Cystocele, midline ♀
    N81.12 Cystocele, lateral ♀
      Paravaginal cystocele
  N81.2 Incomplete uterovaginal prolapse ♀
    First degree uterine prolapse
    Prolapse of cervix NOS
    Second degree uterine prolapse
    EXCLUDES 1 *cervical stump prolapse (N81.85)*
  N81.3 Complete uterovaginal prolapse ♀
    Procidentia (uteri) NOS
    Third degree uterine prolapse
  N81.4 Uterovaginal prolapse, unspecified ♀
    Prolapse of uterus NOS
  N81.5 Vaginal enterocele ♀
    EXCLUDES 1 *enterocele with prolapse of uterus (N81.2-N81.4)*
  N81.6 Rectocele ♀
    Prolapse of posterior vaginal wall
    Use additional code for any associated fecal incontinence, if applicable (R15.-)
    EXCLUDES 2 *perineocele (N81.81)*
    rectal prolapse (K62.3)
    rectocele with prolapse of uterus (N81.2-N81.4)
  ✓5ᵗʰ N81.8 Other female genital prolapse
    N81.81 Perineocele ♀
    N81.82 Incompetence or weakening of pubocervical tissue ♀
    N81.83 Incompetence or weakening of rectovaginal tissue ♀
    N81.84 Pelvic muscle wasting ♀
      Disuse atrophy of pelvic muscles and anal sphincter
    N81.85 Cervical stump prolapse ♀
    N81.89 Other female genital prolapse ♀
      Deficient perineum
      Old laceration of muscles of pelvic floor
  N81.9 Female genital prolapse, unspecified ♀

✓4ᵗʰ N82 Fistulae involving female genital tract
  EXCLUDES 1 *vesicointestinal fistulae (N32.1)*
  N82.0 Vesicovaginal fistula ♀
  N82.1 Other female urinary-genital tract fistulae ♀
    Cervicovesical fistula
    Ureterovaginal fistula
    Urethrovaginal fistula
    Uteroureteric fistula
    Uterovesical fistula
  N82.2 Fistula of vagina to small intestine ♀
  N82.3 Fistula of vagina to large intestine ♀
    Rectovaginal fistula

EXCLUDES 1 Not coded here   **EXCLUDES 2** Not included here   **N** Newborn Age: 0   **P** Pediatric Age: 0-17   **M** Maternity Age: 12-55   **A** Adult Age: 15-124

730   ICD-10-CM 2014 (Draft)

N82.4 Other female intestinal-genital tract fistulae ♀
Intestinouterine fistula

N82.5 Female genital tract-skin fistulae ♀
Uterus to abdominal wall fistula
Vaginoperineal fistula

N82.8 Other female genital tract fistulae ♀

N82.9 Female genital tract fistula, unspecified ♀

✓4th **N83 Noninflammatory disorders of ovary, fallopian tube and broad ligament**
EXCLUDES 2 *hydrosalpinx (N70.1-)*

N83.0 Follicular cyst of ovary ♀
Cyst of graafian follicle
Hemorrhagic follicular cyst (of ovary)

N83.1 Corpus luteum cyst ♀
Hemorrhagic corpus luteum cyst

✓5th **N83.2 Other and unspecified ovarian cysts**
EXCLUDES 1 *developmental ovarian cyst (Q50.1)*
neoplastic ovarian cyst (D27.-)
polycystic ovarian syndrome (E28.2)
Stein-Leventhal syndrome (E28.2)

    N83.20 Unspecified ovarian cysts ♀
    N83.29 Other ovarian cysts ♀
       Retention cyst of ovary
       Simple cyst of ovary

✓5th **N83.3 Acquired atrophy of ovary and fallopian tube**
    N83.31 Acquired atrophy of ovary ♀
    N83.32 Acquired atrophy of fallopian tube ♀
    N83.33 Acquired atrophy of ovary and fallopian tube ♀

N83.4 Prolapse and hernia of ovary and fallopian tube ♀

✓5th **N83.5 Torsion of ovary, ovarian pedicle and fallopian tube**
Torsion of accessory tube
    N83.51 Torsion of ovary and ovarian pedicle ♀
    N83.52 Torsion of fallopian tube ♀
       Torsion of hydatid of Morgagni
    N83.53 Torsion of ovary, ovarian pedicle and fallopian tube ♀

N83.6 Hematosalpinx
EXCLUDES 1 *hematosalpinx (with) (in):*
hematocolpos (N89.7)
hematometra (N85.7)
tubal pregnancy (O00.1)

N83.7 Hematoma of broad ligament ♀

N83.8 Other noninflammatory disorders of ovary, fallopian tube and broad ligament ♀
Broad ligament laceration syndrome [Allen-Masters]

N83.9 Noninflammatory disorder of ovary, fallopian tube and broad ligament, unspecified

✓4th **N84 Polyp of female genital tract**
EXCLUDES 1 *adenomatous polyp (D28.-)*
placental polyp (O90.89)

N84.0 Polyp of corpus uteri ♀
Polyp of endometrium
Polyp of uterus NOS
EXCLUDES 1 *polypoid endometrial hyperplasia (N85.0-)*

N84.1 Polyp of cervix uteri ♀
Mucous polyp of cervix

N84.2 Polyp of vagina ♀

N84.3 Polyp of vulva ♀
Polyp of labia

N84.8 Polyp of other parts of female genital tract ♀

N84.9 Polyp of female genital tract, unspecified ♀

✓4th **N85 Other noninflammatory disorders of uterus, except cervix**
EXCLUDES 1 *endometriosis (N80.-)*
inflammatory diseases of uterus (N71.-)
noninflammatory disorders of cervix, except malposition (N86-N88)
polyp of corpus uteri (N84.0)
uterine prolapse (N81.-)

✓5th **N85.0 Endometrial hyperplasia**
    N85.00 Endometrial hyperplasia, unspecified ♀
       Hyperplasia (adenomatous) (cystic) (glandular) of endometrium
       Hyperplastic endometritis
    N85.01 Benign endometrial hyperplasia ♀
       Endometrial hyperplasia (complex) (simple) without atypia

    N85.02 Endometrial intraepithelial neoplasia [EIN] ♀
       Endometrial hyperplasia with atypia
       EXCLUDES 1 *malignant neoplasm of endometrium (with endometrial intraepithelial neoplasia [EIN]) (C54.1)*

N85.2 Hypertrophy of uterus ♀
Bulky or enlarged uterus
EXCLUDES 1 *puerperal hypertrophy of uterus (O90.89)*

N85.3 Subinvolution of uterus ♀
EXCLUDES 1 *puerperal subinvolution of uterus (O90.89)*

N85.4 Malposition of uterus ♀
Anteversion of uterus   Retroversion of uterus
Retroflexion of uterus
EXCLUDES 1 *malposition of uterus complicating pregnancy, labor or delivery (O34.5-, O65.5)*

N85.5 Inversion of uterus ♀
EXCLUDES 1 *current obstetric trauma (O71.2)*
postpartum inversion of uterus (O71.2)

N85.6 Intrauterine synechiae ♀

N85.7 Hematometra ♀
Hematosalpinx with hematometra
EXCLUDES 1 *hematometra with hematocolpos (N89.7)*

N85.8 Other specified noninflammatory disorders of uterus ♀
Atrophy of uterus, acquired
Fibrosis of uterus NOS

N85.9 Noninflammatory disorder of uterus, unspecified ♀
Disorder of uterus NOS

N86 Erosion and ectropion of cervix uteri ♀
Decubitus (trophic) ulcer of cervix
Eversion of cervix
EXCLUDES 1 *erosion and ectropion of cervix with cervicitis (N72)*

✓4th **N87 Dysplasia of cervix uteri**
EXCLUDES 1 *abnormal results from cervical cytologic examination without histologic confirmation (R87.61-)*
carcinoma in situ of cervix uteri (D06.-)
cervical intraepithelial neoplasia III [CIN III] (D06.-)
HGSIL of cervix (R87.613)
severe dysplasia of cervix uteri (D06.-)

N87.0 Mild cervical dysplasia ♀
Cervical intraepithelial neoplasia I [CIN I]

N87.1 Moderate cervical dysplasia ♀
Cervical intraepithelial neoplasia II [CIN II]

N87.9 Dysplasia of cervix uteri, unspecified ♀
Anaplasia of cervix   Cervical dysplasia NOS
Cervical atypism

✓4th **N88 Other noninflammatory disorders of cervix uteri**
EXCLUDES 2 *inflammatory disease of cervix (N72)*
polyp of cervix (N84.1)

N88.0 Leukoplakia of cervix uteri ♀

N88.1 Old laceration of cervix uteri ♀
Adhesions of cervix
EXCLUDES 1 *current obstetric trauma (O71.3)*

N88.2 Stricture and stenosis of cervix uteri ♀
EXCLUDES 1 *stricture and stenosis of cervix uteri complicating labor (O65.5)*

N88.3 Incompetence of cervix uteri ♀
Investigation and management of (suspected) cervical incompetence in a nonpregnant woman
EXCLUDES 1 *cervical incompetence complicating pregnancy (O34.3-)*

N88.4 Hypertrophic elongation of cervix uteri ♀

N88.8 Other specified noninflammatory disorders of cervix uteri ♀
EXCLUDES 1 *current obstetric trauma (O71.3)*

N88.9 Noninflammatory disorder of cervix uteri, unspecified ♀

✓4th **N89 Other noninflammatory disorders of vagina**
EXCLUDES 1 *abnormal results from vaginal cytologic examination without histologic confirmation (R87.62-)*
carcinoma in situ of vagina (D07.2)
HGSIL of vagina (R87.623)
inflammation of vagina (N76.-)
senile (atrophic) vaginitis (N95.2)
severe dysplasia of vagina (D07.2)
trichomonal leukorrhea (A59.00)
vaginal intraepithelial neoplasia [VAIN], grade III (D07.2)

N89.0 Mild vaginal dysplasia ♀
Vaginal intraepithelial neoplasia [VAIN], grade I

✓ Additional Character Required   ✓x7th Xtension Alert   Unspecified Code   Other Specified Code   Manifestation Code   ►◄ Revised Text   ● New Code   ▲ Revised Code Title

ICD-10-CM 2014 (Draft)   731

N89.1 Moderate **vaginal dysplasia** ♀
Vaginal intraepithelial neoplasia [VAIN], grade II

N89.3 **Dysplasia of vagina, unspecified** ♀

N89.4 **Leukoplakia of vagina** ♀

N89.5 **Stricture and atresia of vagina** ♀
Vaginal adhesions
Vaginal stenosis
EXCLUDES 1   *congenital atresia or stricture (Q52.4)*
postprocedural adhesions of vagina (N99.2)

N89.6 **Tight hymenal ring** ♀
Rigid hymen
Tight introitus
EXCLUDES 1   *imperforate hymen (Q52.3)*

N89.7 **Hematocolpos** ♀
Hematocolpos with hematometra or hematosalpinx

N89.8 Other specified noninflammatory disorders of vagina ♀
Leukorrhea NOS
Old vaginal laceration
Pessary ulcer of vagina
EXCLUDES 1   *current obstetric trauma (O70-, O71.4, O71.7-O71.8)*
old laceration involving muscles of pelvic floor (N81.8)

N89.9 **Noninflammatory disorder of vagina, unspecified** ♀

✓4ᵗʰ **N90** **Other noninflammatory disorders of vulva and perineum**
EXCLUDES 1   *anogenital (venereal) warts (A63.0)*
carcinoma in situ of vulva (D07.1)
condyloma acuminatum (A63.0)
current obstetric trauma (O70-, O71.7-O71.8)
inflammation of vulva (N76.-)
severe dysplasia of vulva (D07.1)
vulvar intraepithelial neoplasm III [VIN III] (D07.1)

N90.0 Mild **vulvar dysplasia** ♀
Vulvar intraepithelial neoplasia [VIN], grade I

N90.1 Moderate **vulvar dysplasia** ♀
Vulvar intraepithelial neoplasia [VIN], grade II

N90.3 **Dysplasia of vulva, unspecified** ♀

N90.4 **Leukoplakia of vulva** ♀
Dystrophy of vulva
Kraurosis of vulva
Lichen sclerosus of external female genital organs

N90.5 **Atrophy of vulva** ♀
Stenosis of vulva

N90.6 **Hypertrophy of vulva** ♀
Hypertrophy of labia

N90.7 **Vulvar cyst** ♀

✓5ᵗʰ **N90.8** **Other specified noninflammatory disorders of vulva and perineum**

✓6ᵗʰ **N90.81** **Female genital mutilation status**
Female genital cutting status

N90.810 **Female genital mutilation status, unspecified** ♀
Female genital cutting status, unspecified
Female genital mutilation status NOS

N90.811 **Female genital mutilation Type I status** ♀
Clitorectomy status
Female genital cutting Type I status

N90.812 **Female genital mutilation Type II status** ♀
Clitorectomy with excision of labia minora status
Female genital cutting Type II status

N90.813 **Female genital mutilation Type III status** ♀
Female genital cutting Type III status
Infibulation status

N90.818 **Other female genital mutilation status** ♀
Female genital cutting Type IV status
Female genital mutilation Type IV status
Other female genital cutting status

N90.89 Other specified noninflammatory disorders of vulva and perineum ♀
Adhesions of vulva   Hypertrophy of clitoris

N90.9 **Noninflammatory disorder of vulva and perineum, unspecified** ♀

✓4ᵗʰ **N91** **Absent, scanty and rare menstruation**
EXCLUDES 1   *ovarian dysfunction (E28.-)*

N91.0 **Primary amenorrhea** ♀

N91.1 **Secondary amenorrhea** ♀

N91.2 Amenorrhea, unspecified ♀

N91.3 **Primary oligomenorrhea** ♀

N91.4 **Secondary oligomenorrhea** ♀

N91.5 **Oligomenorrhea, unspecified** ♀
Hypomenorrhea NOS

✓4ᵗʰ **N92** **Excessive, frequent and irregular menstruation**
EXCLUDES 1   *postmenopausal bleeding (N95.0)*
precocious puberty (menstruation) (E30.1)

N92.0 **Excessive and frequent menstruation** with regular cycle ♀
Heavy periods NOS
Menorrhagia NOS
Polymenorrhea

N92.1 **Excessive and frequent menstruation** with irregular cycle ♀
Irregular intermenstrual bleeding
Irregular, shortened intervals between menstrual bleeding
Menometrorrhagia
Metrorrhagia

N92.2 **Excessive menstruation at puberty** Ⓟ♀
Excessive bleeding associated with onset of menstrual periods
Pubertal menorrhagia
Puberty bleeding

N92.3 **Ovulation bleeding** ♀
Regular intermenstrual bleeding

N92.4 **Excessive bleeding in the premenopausal period** ♀
Climacteric menorrhagia or metrorrhagia
Menopausal menorrhagia or metrorrhagia
Preclimacteric menorrhagia or metrorrhagia
Premenopausal menorrhagia or metrorrhagia

N92.5 Other specified irregular menstruation ♀

N92.6 **Irregular menstruation, unspecified** ♀
Irregular bleeding NOS
Irregular periods NOS
EXCLUDES 1   *irregular menstruation with:*
lengthened intervals or scanty bleeding (N91.3-N91.5)
shortened intervals or excessive bleeding (N92.1)

✓4ᵗʰ **N93** **Other abnormal uterine and vaginal bleeding**
EXCLUDES 1   *neonatal vaginal hemorrhage (P54.6)*
precocious puberty (menstruation) (E30.1)
pseudomenses (P54.6)

N93.0 **Postcoital and contact bleeding** ♀

N93.8 Other specified abnormal uterine and vaginal bleeding ♀
Dysfunctional or functional uterine or vaginal bleeding NOS

N93.9 **Abnormal uterine and vaginal bleeding, unspecified** ♀

✓4ᵗʰ **N94** **Pain and other conditions associated with female genital organs and menstrual cycle**

N94.0 **Mittelschmerz** ♀

N94.1 **Dyspareunia** ♀
EXCLUDES 1   *psychogenic dyspareunia (F52.6)*

N94.2 **Vaginismus** ♀
EXCLUDES 1   *psychogenic vaginismus (F52.5)*

N94.3 **Premenstrual tension syndrome** ♀
Premenstrual dysphoric disorder
Code also associated menstrual migraine (G43.82-, G43.83-)

N94.4 **Primary dysmenorrhea** ♀

N94.5 **Secondary dysmenorrhea** ♀

N94.6 **Dysmenorrhea, unspecified** ♀
EXCLUDES 1   *psychogenic dysmenorrhea (F45.8)*

✓5ᵗʰ **N94.8** **Other specified conditions associated with female genital organs and menstrual cycle**

✓6ᵗʰ **N94.81** **Vulvodynia**

N94.810 **Vulvar vestibulitis** ♀

N94.818 Other vulvodynia ♀

N94.819 **Vulvodynia, unspecified** ♀
Vulvodynia NOS

N94.89 Other specified conditions associated with female genital organs and menstrual cycle ♀

N94.9 **Unspecified condition associated with female genital organs and menstrual cycle** ♀

✓4ᵗʰ **N95** **Menopausal and other perimenopausal disorders**
Menopausal and other perimenopausal disorders due to naturally occurring (age-related) menopause and perimenopause
EXCLUDES 1   *excessive bleeding in the premenopausal period (N92.4)*
menopausal and perimenopausal disorders due to artificial or premature menopause (E89.4-, E28.31-)
premature menopause (E28.31-)
EXCLUDES 2   *postmenopausal osteoporosis (M81.0-)*
postmenopausal osteoporosis with current pathological fracture (M80.0-)
postmenopausal urethritis (N34.2)

N95.0 **Postmenopausal bleeding** ♀

EXCLUDES 1 Not coded here   *EXCLUDES 2* Not included here   Ⓝ Newborn Age: 0   Ⓟ Pediatric Age: 0-17   Ⓜ Maternity Age: 12-55   Ⓐ Adult Age: 15-124

732   ICD-10-CM 2014 (Draft)

N95.1 Menopausal and female climacteric states ♀
Symptoms such as flushing, sleeplessness, headache, lack of concentration, associated with natural (age-related) menopause
Use additional code for associated symptoms
EXCLUDES 1 asymptomatic menopausal state (Z78.Ø)
symptoms associated with artificial menopause (E89.41)
symptoms associated with premature menopause (E28.31Ø)

N95.2 Postmenopausal atrophic vaginitis ♀
Senile (atrophic) vaginitis

N95.8 Other specified menopausal and perimenopausal disorders ♀

N95.9 Unspecified menopausal and perimenopausal disorder ♀

N96 Recurrent pregnancy loss ♀
Investigation or care in a nonpregnant woman with history of recurrent pregnancy loss
EXCLUDES 1 recurrent pregnancy loss with current pregnancy (O26.2-)

✓4ᵗʰ **N97 Female infertility**
INCLUDES inability to achieve a pregnancy
sterility, female NOS
EXCLUDES 1 female infertility associated with:
hypopituitarism (E23.Ø)
Stein-Leventhal syndrome (E28.2)
EXCLUDES 2 incompetence of cervix uteri (N88.3)

N97.Ø Female infertility associated with anovulation ♀

N97.1 Female infertility of tubal origin ♀
Female infertility associated with congenital anomaly of tube
Female infertility due to tubal block
Female infertility due to tubal occlusion
Female infertility due to tubal stenosis

N97.2 Female infertility of uterine origin ♀
Female infertility associated with congenital anomaly of uterus
Female infertility due to nonimplantation of ovum

N97.8 Female infertility of other origin ♀

N97.9 Female infertility, unspecified ♀

✓4ᵗʰ **N98 Complications associated with artificial fertilization**
N98.Ø Infection associated with artificial insemination ♀
N98.1 Hyperstimulation of ovaries ♀
Hyperstimulation of ovaries NOS
Hyperstimulation of ovaries associated with induced ovulation

N98.2 Complications of attempted introduction of fertilized ovum following in vitro fertilization ♀

N98.3 Complications of attempted introduction of embryo in embryo transfer ♀

N98.8 Other complications associated with artificial fertilization ♀

N98.9 Complication associated with artificial fertilization, unspecified ♀

Intraoperative and postprocedural complications and disorders of genitourinary system, not elsewhere classified (N99)

✓4ᵗʰ **N99 Intraoperative and postprocedural complications and disorders of genitourinary system, not elsewhere classified**
EXCLUDES 2 irradiation cystitis (N3Ø.4-)
postoophorectomy osteoporosis with current pathological fracture (M8Ø.8-)
postoophorectomy osteoporosis without current pathological fracture (M81.8)

N99.Ø Postprocedural (acute) (chronic) kidney failure
Use additional code to type of kidney disease

✓5ᵗʰ **N99.1 Postprocedural urethral stricture**
Postcatheterization urethral stricture

✓6ᵗʰ **N99.11 Postprocedural urethral stricture, male**
N99.11Ø Postprocedural urethral stricture, male, meatal ♂
N99.111 Postprocedural bulbous urethral stricture
N99.112 Postprocedural membranous urethral stricture
N99.113 Postprocedural anterior urethral stricture
N99.114 Postprocedural urethral stricture, male unspecified ♂
N99.12 Postprocedural urethral stricture, female ♀

N99.2 Postprocedural adhesions of vagina ♀
N99.3 Prolapse of vaginal vault after hysterectomy ♀
N99.4 Postprocedural pelvic peritoneal adhesions
EXCLUDES 2 pelvic peritoneal adhesions NOS (N73.6)
postinfective pelvic peritoneal adhesions (N73.6)

✓5ᵗʰ **N99.5 Complications of stoma of urinary tract**
EXCLUDES 2 mechanical complication of urinary (indwelling) catheter (T83.Ø-)

✓6ᵗʰ **N99.51 Complication of cystostomy**
N99.51Ø Cystostomy hemorrhage
N99.511 Cystostomy infection
N99.512 Cystostomy malfunction
N99.518 Other cystostomy complication

✓6ᵗʰ **N99.52 Complication of other external stoma of urinary tract**
N99.52Ø Hemorrhage of other external stoma of urinary tract
N99.521 Infection of other external stoma of urinary tract
N99.522 Malfunction of other external stoma of urinary tract
N99.528 Other complication of other external stoma of urinary tract

✓6ᵗʰ **N99.53 Complication of other stoma of urinary tract**
N99.53Ø Hemorrhage of other stoma of urinary tract
N99.531 Infection of other stoma of urinary tract
N99.532 Malfunction of other stoma of urinary tract
N99.538 Other complication of other stoma of urinary tract

✓5ᵗʰ **N99.6 Intraoperative hemorrhage and hematoma of a genitourinary system organ or structure complicating a procedure**
EXCLUDES 1 intraoperative hemorrhage and hematoma of a genitourinary system organ or structure due to accidental puncture or laceration during a procedure (N99.7-)

N99.61 Intraoperative hemorrhage and hematoma of a genitourinary system organ or structure complicating a genitourinary system procedure
N99.62 Intraoperative hemorrhage and hematoma of a genitourinary system organ or structure complicating other procedure

✓5ᵗʰ **N99.7 Accidental puncture and laceration of a genitourinary system organ or structure during a procedure**
N99.71 Accidental puncture and laceration of a genitourinary system organ or structure during a genitourinary system procedure
N99.72 Accidental puncture and laceration of a genitourinary system organ or structure during other procedure

✓5ᵗʰ **N99.8 Other intraoperative and postprocedural complications and disorders of genitourinary system**
N99.81 Other intraoperative complications of genitourinary system

✓6ᵗʰ **N99.82 Postprocedural hemorrhage and hematoma of a genitourinary system organ or structure following a procedure**
N99.82Ø Postprocedural hemorrhage and hematoma of a genitourinary system organ or structure following a genitourinary system procedure
N99.821 Postprocedural hemorrhage and hematoma of a genitourinary system organ or structure following other procedure

N99.83 Residual ovary syndrome ♀
N99.89 Other postprocedural complications and disorders of genitourinary system

Pregnancy, Childbirth and the Puerperium

O00–O03.31

Chapter 15. Pregnancy, Childbirth and the Puerperium (O00-O9A)

NOTE   CODES FROM THIS CHAPTER ARE FOR USE ONLY ON MATERNAL RECORDS, NEVER ON NEWBORN RECORDS.

Codes from this chapter are for use for conditions related to or aggravated by the pregnancy, childbirth, or by the puerperium (maternal causes or obstetric causes).

NOTE   Trimesters are counted from the first day of the last menstrual period. They are defined as follows:

1st trimester- less than 14 weeks 0 days
2nd trimester- 14 weeks 0 days to less than 28 weeks 0 days
3rd trimester- 28 weeks 0 days until delivery.

Use additional code from category Z3A, Weeks of gestation, to identify the specific week of the pregnancy

EXCLUDES 1   *supervision of normal pregnancy (Z34.-)*

EXCLUDES 2   *mental and behavioral disorders associated with the puerperium (F53)*
obstetrical tetanus (A34)
postpartum necrosis of pituitary gland (E23.0)
puerperal osteomalacia (M83.0)

This chapter contains the following blocks:

O00-O08   Pregnancy with abortive outcome
O09   Supervision of high risk pregnancy
O10-O16   Edema, proteinuria and hypertensive disorders in pregnancy, childbirth and the puerperium
O20-O29   Other maternal disorders predominantly related to pregnancy
O30-O48   Maternal care related to the fetus and amniotic cavity and possible delivery problems
O60-O77   Complications of labor and delivery
O80, O82   Encounter for delivery
O85-O92   Complications predominantly related to the puerperium
O94-O9A   Other obstetric conditions, not elsewhere classified

Pregnancy with abortive outcome (O00-O08)

EXCLUDES 1   *continuing pregnancy in multiple gestation after abortion of one fetus or more (O31.1-, O31.3-)*

✓4ᵗʰ O00 Ectopic pregnancy

INCLUDES   ruptured ectopic pregnancy

Use additional code from category O08 to identify any associated complication

   O00.0 Abdominal pregnancy   Ⓜ♀

     EXCLUDES 1   *maternal care for viable fetus in abdominal pregnancy (O36.7-)*

   O00.1 Tubal pregnancy   Ⓜ♀
     Fallopian pregnancy
     Rupture of (fallopian) tube due to pregnancy
     Tubal abortion

   O00.2 Ovarian pregnancy   Ⓜ♀

   O00.8 Other ectopic pregnancy   Ⓜ♀
     Cervical pregnancy
     Cornual pregnancy
     Intraligamentous pregnancy
     Mural pregnancy

   O00.9 Ectopic pregnancy, unspecified   Ⓜ♀

✓4ᵗʰ O01 Hydatidiform mole

Use additional code from category O08 to identify any associated complication

   EXCLUDES 1   *chorioadenoma (destruens) (D39.2)*
        malignant hydatidiform mole (D39.2)

   O01.0 Classical hydatidiform mole   Ⓜ♀
     Complete hydatidiform mole

   O01.1 Incomplete and partial hydatidiform mole   Ⓜ♀

   O01.9 Hydatidiform mole, unspecified   Ⓜ♀
     Trophoblastic disease NOS
     Vesicular mole NOS

✓4ᵗʰ O02 Other abnormal products of conception

Use additional code from category O08 to identify any associated complication

   EXCLUDES 1   *papyraceous fetus (O31.0-)*

   O02.0 Blighted ovum and nonhydatidiform mole   Ⓜ♀
     Carneous mole
     Fleshy mole
     Intrauterine mole NOS
     Molar pregnancy NEC
     Pathological ovum

   O02.1 Missed abortion   Ⓜ♀
     Early fetal death, before completion of 20 weeks of gestation, with retention of dead fetus

     EXCLUDES 1   *failed induced abortion (O07.-)*
        fetal death (intrauterine) (late) (O36.4)
        missed abortion with blighted ovum (O02.0)
        missed abortion with hydatidiform mole (O01.-)
        missed abortion with nonhydatidiform (O02.0)
        missed abortion with other abnormal products of conception (O02.8-)
        missed delivery (O36.4)
        stillbirth (P95)

   ✓5ᵗʰ O02.8 Other specified abnormal products of conception

     EXCLUDES 1   *abnormal products of conception with blighted ovum (O02.0)*
        abnormal products of conception with hydatidiform mole (O01.-)
        abnormal products of conception with nonhydatidiform mole (O02.0)

     O02.81 Inappropriate change in quantitative human chorionic gonadotropin (hCG) in early pregnancy   Ⓜ♀
       Biochemical pregnancy
       Chemical pregnancy
       Inappropriate level of quantitative human chorionic gonadotropin (hCG) for gestational age in early pregnancy

     O02.89 Other abnormal products of conception   Ⓜ♀

   O02.9 Abnormal product of conception, unspecified   Ⓜ♀

✓4ᵗʰ O03 Spontaneous abortion

   NOTE   Incomplete abortion includes retained products of conception following spontaneous abortion

   INCLUDES   miscarriage

   O03.0 Genital tract and pelvic infection following incomplete spontaneous abortion   Ⓜ♀
     Endometritis following incomplete spontaneous abortion
     Oophoritis following incomplete spontaneous abortion
     Parametritis following incomplete spontaneous abortion
     Pelvic peritonitis following incomplete spontaneous abortion
     Salpingitis following incomplete spontaneous abortion
     Salpingo-oophoritis following incomplete spontaneous abortion

     EXCLUDES 1   *sepsis following incomplete spontaneous abortion (O03.37)*
        urinary tract infection following incomplete spontaneous abortion (O03.38)

   O03.1 Delayed or excessive hemorrhage following incomplete spontaneous abortion   Ⓜ♀
     Afibrinogenemia following incomplete spontaneous abortion
     Defibrination syndrome following incomplete spontaneous abortion
     Hemolysis following incomplete spontaneous abortion
     Intravascular coagulation following incomplete spontaneous abortion

   O03.2 Embolism following incomplete spontaneous abortion   Ⓜ♀
     Air embolism following incomplete spontaneous abortion
     Amniotic fluid embolism following incomplete spontaneous abortion
     Blood-clot embolism following incomplete spontaneous abortion
     Embolism NOS following incomplete spontaneous abortion
     Fat embolism following incomplete spontaneous abortion
     Pulmonary embolism following incomplete spontaneous abortion
     Pyemic embolism following incomplete spontaneous abortion
     Septic or septicopyemic embolism following spontaneous abortion
     Soap embolism following incomplete spontaneous abortion

   ✓5ᵗʰ O03.3 Other and unspecified complications following incomplete spontaneous abortion

     O03.30 Unspecified complication following incomplete spontaneous abortion   Ⓜ♀

     O03.31 Shock following incomplete spontaneous abortion   Ⓜ♀
       Circulatory collapse following incomplete spontaneous abortion
       Shock (postprocedural) following incomplete spontaneous abortion

       EXCLUDES 1   *shock due to infection following incomplete spontaneous abortion (O03.37)*

EXCLUDES 1 Not coded here   **EXCLUDES 2** Not included here   Ⓝ Newborn Age: 0   Ⓟ Pediatric Age: 0-17   Ⓜ Maternity Age: 12-55   Ⓐ Adult Age: 15-124

734   ICD-10-CM 2014 (Draft)

O03.32 **Renal failure** following incomplete spontaneous ⓜ♀
abortion
Kidney failure (acute) following incomplete
spontaneous abortion
Oliguria following incomplete spontaneous abortion
Renal shutdown following incomplete spontaneous
abortion
Renal tubular necrosis following incomplete
spontaneous abortion
Uremia following incomplete spontaneous abortion

O03.33 **Metabolic disorder** following incomplete ⓜ♀
spontaneous abortion

O03.34 **Damage to pelvic organs** following incomplete ⓜ♀
spontaneous abortion
Laceration, perforation, tear or chemical damage of
bladder following incomplete spontaneous
abortion
Laceration, perforation, tear or chemical damage of
bowel following incomplete spontaneous
abortion
Laceration, perforation, tear or chemical damage of
broad ligament following incomplete
spontaneous abortion
Laceration, perforation, tear or chemical damage of
cervix following incomplete spontaneous
abortion
Laceration, perforation, tear or chemical damage of
periurethral tissue following incomplete
spontaneous abortion
Laceration, perforation, tear or chemical damage of
uterus following incomplete spontaneous
abortion
Laceration, perforation, tear or chemical damage of
vagina following incomplete spontaneous
abortion

O03.35 **Other venous complications following** ⓜ♀
incomplete spontaneous abortion

O03.36 **Cardiac arrest** following incomplete ⓜ♀
spontaneousabortion

O03.37 **Sepsis** following incomplete spontaneous ⓜ♀
abortion
Use additional code to identify infectious agent
(B95-B97)
Use additional code to identify severe sepsis, if
applicable (R65.2-)
EXCLUDES 1 *septic or septicopyemic embolism following*
incomplete spontaneous abortion
(O03.2)

O03.38 **Urinary tract infection** following incomplete ⓜ♀
spontaneous abortion
Cystitis following incomplete spontaneous abortion

O03.39 **Incomplete spontaneous abortion with other** ⓜ♀
complications

O03.4 **Incomplete** spontaneous abortion **without complication** ⓜ♀

O03.5 **Genital tract and pelvic infection following complete or** ⓜ♀
unspecified spontaneous abortion
Endometritis following complete or unspecified spontaneous
abortion
Oophoritis following complete or unspecified spontaneous
abortion
Parametritis following complete or unspecified spontaneous
abortion
Pelvic peritonitis following complete or unspecified
spontaneous abortion
Salpingitis following complete or unspecified spontaneous
abortion
Salpingo-oophoritis following complete or unspecified
spontaneous abortion
EXCLUDES 1 *sepsis following complete or unspecified spontaneous*
abortion (O03.87)
urinary tract infection following complete or
unspecified spontaneous abortion (O03.88)

O03.6 **Delayed or excessive hemorrhage following complete or** ⓜ♀
unspecified spontaneous abortion
Afibrinogenemia following complete or unspecified
spontaneous abortion
Defibrination syndrome following complete or unspecified
spontaneous abortion
Hemolysis following complete or unspecified spontaneous
abortion
Intravascular coagulation following complete or unspecified
spontaneous abortion

O03.7 **Embolism following complete or unspecified** ⓜ♀
spontaneous abortion
Air embolism following complete or unspecified spontaneous
abortion
Amniotic fluid embolism following complete or unspecified
spontaneous abortion
Blood-clot embolism following complete or unspecified
spontaneous abortion
Embolism NOS following complete or unspecified spontaneous
abortion
Fat embolism following complete or unspecified spontaneous
abortion
Pulmonary embolism following complete or unspecified
spontaneous abortion
Pyemic embolism following complete or unspecified
spontaneous abortion
Septic or septicopyemic embolism following complete or
unspecified spontaneous abortion
Soap embolism following complete or unspecified spontaneous
abortion

√5ᵗʰ **O03.8** **Other and unspecified complications following complete or**
unspecified spontaneous abortion

O03.80 **Unspecified complication following complete or** ⓜ♀
unspecified spontaneous abortion

O03.81 **Shock following complete or unspecified** ⓜ♀
spontaneous abortion
Circulatory collapse following complete or unspecified
spontaneous abortion
Shock (postprocedural) following complete or
unspecified spontaneous abortion
EXCLUDES 1 *shock due to infection following complete or*
unspecified spontaneous abortion
(O03.87)

O03.82 **Renal failure** following complete or unspecified ⓜ♀
spontaneous abortion
Kidney failure (acute) following complete or
unspecified spontaneous abortion
Oliguria following complete or unspecified
spontaneous abortion
Renal shutdown following complete or unspecified
spontaneous abortion
Renal tubular necrosis following complete or
unspecified spontaneous abortion
Uremia following complete or unspecified
spontaneous abortion

O03.83 **Metabolic disorder** following complete or ⓜ♀
unspecified spontaneous abortion

O03.84 **Damage to pelvic organs** following complete or ⓜ♀
unspecified spontaneous abortion
Laceration, perforation, tear or chemical damage of
bladder following complete or unspecified
spontaneous abortion
Laceration, perforation, tear or chemical damage of
bowel following complete or unspecified
spontaneous abortion
Laceration, perforation, tear or chemical damage of
broad ligament following complete or
unspecified spontaneous abortion
Laceration, perforation, tear or chemical damage of
cervix following complete or unspecified
spontaneous abortion
Laceration, perforation, tear or chemical damage of
periurethral tissue following complete or
unspecified spontaneous abortion
Laceration, perforation, tear or chemical damage of
uterus following complete or unspecified
spontaneous abortion
Laceration, perforation, tear or chemical damage of
vagina following complete or unspecified
spontaneous abortion

O03.85 **Other venous complications following complete** ⓜ♀
or unspecified spontaneous abortion

O03.86 **Cardiac arrest following complete or unspecified** ⓜ♀
spontaneous abortion

O03.87 **Sepsis following complete or unspecified** ⓜ♀
spontaneous abortion
Use additional code to identify infectious agent
(B95-B97)
Use additional code to identify severe sepsis, if
applicable (R65.2-)
EXCLUDES 1 *septic or septicopyemic embolism following*
complete or unspecified spontaneous
abortion (O03.7)

☑ Additional Character Required   √x7ᵗʰ Xtension Alert   **Unspecified Code**   **Other Specified Code**   Manifestation Code   ▶◀ Revised Text   ● New Code   ▲ Revised Code Title

ICD-10-CM 2014 (Draft)   **735**

O03.88   **Urinary tract infection following complete or unspecified spontaneous abortion**   Ⓜ♀
  Cystitis following complete or unspecified spontaneous abortion

O03.89   **Complete or unspecified spontaneous abortion with other complications**   Ⓜ♀

O03.9   **Complete or unspecified spontaneous abortion without complication**   Ⓜ♀
  Miscarriage NOS
  Spontaneous abortion NOS

✓4ᵗʰ **O04**   **Complications following (induced) termination of pregnancy**
  INCLUDES   complications following (induced) termination of pregnancy
  EXCLUDES 1   *encounter for elective termination of pregnancy, uncomplicated (Z33.2)*
       failed attempted termination of pregnancy (O07.-)

O04.5   **Genital tract and pelvic infection following (induced) termination of pregnancy**   Ⓜ♀
  Endometritis following (induced) termination of pregnancy
  Oophoritis following (induced) termination of pregnancy
  Parametritis following (induced) termination of pregnancy
  Pelvic peritonitis following (induced) termination of pregnancy
  Salpingitis following (induced) termination of pregnancy
  Salpingo-oophoritis following (induced) termination of pregnancy
  EXCLUDES 1   *sepsis following (induced) termination of pregnancy (O04.87)*
       urinary tract infection following (induced) termination of pregnancy (O04.88)

O04.6   **Delayed or excessive hemorrhage following (induced) termination of pregnancy**   Ⓜ♀
  Afibrinogenemia following (induced) termination of pregnancy
  Defibrination syndrome following (induced) termination of pregnancy
  Hemolysis following (induced) termination of pregnancy
  Intravascular coagulation following (induced) termination of pregnancy

O04.7   **Embolism following (induced) termination of pregnancy**   Ⓜ♀
  Air embolism following (induced) termination of pregnancy
  Amniotic fluid embolism following (induced) termination of pregnancy
  Blood-clot embolism following (induced) termination of pregnancy
  Embolism NOS following (induced) termination of pregnancy
  Fat embolism following (induced) termination of pregnancy
  Pulmonary embolism following (induced) termination of pregnancy
  Pyemic embolism following (induced) termination of pregnancy
  Septic or septicopyemic embolism following (induced) termination of pregnancy
  Soap embolism following (induced) termination of pregnancy

✓5ᵗʰ **O04.8**   **(Induced) termination of pregnancy with other and unspecified complications**

O04.80   **(Induced) termination of pregnancy with unspecified complications**   Ⓜ♀

O04.81   **Shock following (induced) termination of pregnancy**   Ⓜ♀
  Circulatory collapse following (induced) termination of pregnancy
  Shock (postprocedural) following (induced) termination of pregnancy
  EXCLUDES 1   *shock due to infection following (induced) termination of pregnancy (O04.87)*

O04.82   **Renal failure following (induced) termination of pregnancy**   Ⓜ♀
  Kidney failure (acute) following (induced) termination of pregnancy
  Oliguria following (induced) termination of pregnancy
  Renal shutdown following (induced) termination of pregnancy
  Renal tubular necrosis following (induced) termination of pregnancy
  Uremia following (induced) termination of pregnancy

O04.83   **Metabolic disorder following (induced) termination of pregnancy**   Ⓜ♀

O04.84   **Damage to pelvic organs following (induced) termination of pregnancy**   Ⓜ♀
  Laceration, perforation, tear or chemical damage of bladder following (induced) termination of pregnancy
  Laceration, perforation, tear or chemical damage of bowel following (induced) termination of pregnancy
  Laceration, perforation, tear or chemical damage of broad ligament following (induced) termination of pregnancy
  Laceration, perforation, tear or chemical damage of cervix following (induced) termination of pregnancy
  Laceration, perforation, tear or chemical damage of periurethral tissue following (induced) termination of pregnancy
  Laceration, perforation, tear or chemical damage of uterus following (induced) termination of pregnancy
  Laceration, perforation, tear or chemical damage of vagina following (induced) termination of pregnancy

O04.85   **Other venous complications following (induced) termination of pregnancy**   Ⓜ♀

O04.86   **Cardiac arrest following (induced) termination of pregnancy**   Ⓜ♀

O04.87   **Sepsis following (induced) termination of pregnancy**   Ⓜ♀
  Use additional code to identify infectious agent (B95-B97)
  Use additional code to identify severe sepsis, if applicable (R65.2-)
  EXCLUDES 1   *septic or septicopyemic embolism following (induced) termination of pregnancy (O04.7)*

O04.88   **Urinary tract infection following (induced) termination of pregnancy**   Ⓜ♀
  Cystitis following (induced) termination of pregnancy

O04.89   **(Induced) termination of pregnancy with other complications**   Ⓜ♀

✓4ᵗʰ **O07**   **Failed attempted termination of pregnancy**
  INCLUDES   failure of attempted induction of termination of pregnancy
       incomplete elective abortion
  EXCLUDES 1   *incomplete spontaneous abortion (O03.0-)*

O07.0   **Genital tract and pelvic infection following failed attempted termination of pregnancy**   Ⓜ♀
  Endometritis following failed attempted termination of pregnancy
  Oophoritis following failed attempted termination of pregnancy
  Parametritis following failed attempted termination of pregnancy
  Pelvic peritonitis following failed attempted termination of pregnancy
  Salpingitis following failed attempted termination of pregnancy
  Salpingo-oophoritis following failed attempted termination of pregnancy
  EXCLUDES 1   *sepsis following failed attempted termination of pregnancy (O07.37)*
       urinary tract infection following failed attempted termination of pregnancy (O07.38)

O07.1   **Delayed or excessive hemorrhage following failed attempted termination of pregnancy**   Ⓜ♀
  Afibrinogenemia following failed attempted termination of pregnancy
  Defibrination syndrome following failed attempted termination of pregnancy
  Hemolysis following failed attempted termination of pregnancy
  Intravascular coagulation following failed attempted termination of pregnancy

EXCLUDES 1 Not coded here   EXCLUDES 2 Not included here   Ⓝ Newborn Age: 0   Ⓟ Pediatric Age: 0-17   Ⓜ Maternity Age: 12-55   Ⓐ Adult Age: 15-124

736   ICD-10-CM 2014 (Draft)

O07.2 Embolism following failed attempted termination of pregnancy Ⓜ♀
Air embolism following failed attempted termination of pregnancy
Amniotic fluid embolism following failed attempted termination of pregnancy
Blood-clot embolism following failed attempted termination of pregnancy
Embolism NOS following failed attempted termination of pregnancy
Fat embolism following failed attempted termination of pregnancy
Pulmonary embolism following failed attempted termination of pregnancy
Pyemic embolism following failed attempted termination of pregnancy
Septic or septicopyemic embolism following failed attempted termination of pregnancy
Soap embolism following failed attempted termination of pregnancy

✓5ᵗʰ O07.3 Failed attempted termination of pregnancy with other and unspecified complications

O07.30 Failed attempted termination of pregnancy with unspecified complications Ⓜ♀

O07.31 Shock following failed attempted termination of pregnancy Ⓜ♀
Circulatory collapse following failed attempted termination of pregnancy
Shock (postprocedural) following failed attempted termination of pregnancy
EXCLUDES 1 *shock due to infection following failed attempted termination of pregnancy (O07.37)*

O07.32 Renal failure following failed attempted termination of pregnancy Ⓜ♀
Kidney failure (acute) following failed attempted termination of pregnancy
Oliguria following failed attempted termination of pregnancy
Renal shutdown following failed attempted termination of pregnancy
Renal tubular necrosis following failed attempted termination of pregnancy
Uremia following failed attempted termination of pregnancy

O07.33 Metabolic disorder following failed attempted termination of pregnancy Ⓜ♀

O07.34 Damage to pelvic organs following failed attempted termination of pregnancy Ⓜ♀
Laceration, perforation, tear or chemical damage of bladder following failed attempted termination of pregnancy
Laceration, perforation, tear or chemical damage of bowel following failed attempted termination of pregnancy
Laceration, perforation, tear or chemical damage of broad ligament following failed attempted termination of pregnancy
Laceration, perforation, tear or chemical damage of cervix following failed attempted termination of pregnancy
Laceration, perforation, tear or chemical damage of periurethral tissue following failed attempted termination of pregnancy
Laceration, perforation, tear or chemical damage of uterus following failed attempted termination of pregnancy
Laceration, perforation, tear or chemical damage of vagina following failed attempted termination of pregnancy

O07.35 Other venous complications following failed attempted termination of pregnancy Ⓜ♀

O07.36 Cardiac arrest following failed attempted termination of pregnancy Ⓜ♀

O07.37 Sepsis following failed attempted termination of pregnancy Ⓜ♀
Use additional code to identify infectious agent (B95-B97)
Use additional code to identify severe sepsis, if applicable (R65.2-)
EXCLUDES 1 *septic or septicopyemic embolism following failed attempted termination of pregnancy (O07.2)*

O07.38 Urinary tract infection following failed attempted termination of pregnancy Ⓜ♀
Cystitis following failed attempted termination of pregnancy

O07.39 Failed attempted termination of pregnancy with other complications Ⓜ♀

O07.4 Failed attempted termination of pregnancy without complication Ⓜ♀

✓4ᵗʰ O08 Complications following ectopic and molar pregnancy
This category is for use with categories O00-O02 to identify any associated complications

O08.0 Genital tract and pelvic infection following ectopic and molar pregnancy Ⓜ♀
Endometritis following ectopic and molar pregnancy
Oophoritis following ectopic and molar pregnancy
Parametritis following ectopic and molar pregnancy
Pelvic peritonitis following ectopic and molar pregnancy
Salpingitis following ectopic and molar pregnancy
Salpingo-oophoritis following ectopic and molar pregnancy
EXCLUDES 1 *sepsis following ectopic and molar pregnancy (O08.82) urinary tract infection (O08.83)*

O08.1 Delayed or excessive hemorrhage following ectopic and molar pregnancy Ⓜ♀
Afibrinogenemia following ectopic and molar pregnancy
Defibrination syndrome following ectopic and molar pregnancy
Hemolysis following ectopic and molar pregnancy
Intravascular coagulation following ectopic and molar pregnancy
EXCLUDES 1 *delayed or excessive hemorrhage due to incomplete abortion (O03.1)*

O08.2 Embolism following ectopic and molar pregnancy Ⓜ♀
Air embolism following ectopic and molar pregnancy
Amniotic fluid embolism following ectopic and molar pregnancy
Blood-clot embolism following ectopic and molar pregnancy
Embolism NOS following ectopic and molar pregnancy
Fat embolism following ectopic and molar pregnancy
Pulmonary embolism following ectopic and molar pregnancy
Pyemic embolism following ectopic and molar pregnancy
Septic or septicopyemic embolism following ectopic and molar pregnancy
Soap embolism following ectopic and molar pregnancy

O08.3 Shock following ectopic and molar pregnancy Ⓜ♀
Circulatory collapse following ectopic and molar pregnancy
Shock (postprocedural) following ectopic and molar pregnancy
EXCLUDES 1 *shock due to infection following ectopic and molar pregnancy (O08.82)*

O08.4 Renal failure following ectopic and molar pregnancy Ⓜ♀
Kidney failure (acute) following ectopic and molar pregnancy
Oliguria following ectopic and molar pregnancy
Renal shutdown following ectopic and molar pregnancy
Renal tubular necrosis following ectopic and molar pregnancy
Uremia following ectopic and molar pregnancy

O08.5 Metabolic disorders following an ectopic and molar pregnancy Ⓜ♀

O08.6 Damage to pelvic organs and tissues following an ectopic and molar pregnancy Ⓜ♀
Laceration, perforation, tear or chemical damage of bladder following an ectopic and molar pregnancy
Laceration, perforation, tear or chemical damage of bowel following an ectopic and molar pregnancy
Laceration, perforation, tear or chemical damage of broad ligament following an ectopic and molar pregnancy
Laceration, perforation, tear or chemical damage of cervix following an ectopic and molar pregnancy
Laceration, perforation, tear or chemical damage of periurethral tissue following an ectopic and molar pregnancy
Laceration, perforation, tear or chemical damage of uterus following an ectopic and molar pregnancy
Laceration, perforation, tear or chemical damage of vagina following an ectopic and molar pregnancy

O08.7 Other venous complications following an ectopic and molar pregnancy Ⓜ♀

Pregnancy, Childbirth and the Puerperium

O08.8–O09.812

√5th **O08.8** **Other complications** following an ectopic and molar pregnancy

    O08.81 **Cardiac arrest** following an ectopic and molar pregnancy   Ⓜ♀

    O08.82 **Sepsis** following ectopic and molar pregnancy   Ⓜ♀
        Use additional code to identify infectious agent (B95-B97)
        Use additional code to identify severe sepsis, if applicable (R65.2-)
        EXCLUDES 1   *septic or septicopyemic embolism following ectopic and molar pregnancy (O08.2)*

    O08.83 **Urinary tract** infection following an ectopic and molar pregnancy   Ⓜ♀
        Cystitis following an ectopic and molar pregnancy

    O08.89 Other complications following an ectopic and molar pregnancy   Ⓜ♀

√5th **O08.9** Unspecified complication following an ectopic and molar pregnancy   Ⓜ♀

Supervision of high risk pregnancy (O09)

√4th **O09** **Supervision of** high risk **pregnancy**

√5th **O09.0** **Supervision of pregnancy with** history of infertility

    O09.00 **Supervision of pregnancy with history of infertility, unspecified trimester**   Ⓜ♀

    O09.01 **Supervision of pregnancy with history of infertility, first trimester**   Ⓜ♀

    O09.02 **Supervision of pregnancy with history of infertility, second trimester**   Ⓜ♀

    O09.03 **Supervision of pregnancy with history of infertility, third trimester**   Ⓜ♀

√5th **O09.1** **Supervision of pregnancy with** history of ectopic or molar pregnancy

    O09.10 **Supervision of pregnancy with history of ectopic or molar pregnancy, unspecified trimester**   Ⓜ♀

    O09.11 **Supervision of pregnancy with history of ectopic or molar pregnancy, first trimester**   Ⓜ♀

    O09.12 **Supervision of pregnancy with history of ectopic or molar pregnancy, second trimester**   Ⓜ♀

    O09.13 **Supervision of pregnancy with history of ectopic or molar pregnancy, third trimester**   Ⓜ♀

√5th **O09.2** **Supervision of pregnancy with** other poor reproductive or obstetric history
    EXCLUDES 2   *pregnancy care for patient with history of recurrent pregnancy loss (O26.2-)*

    √6th **O09.21** **Supervision of pregnancy with** history of pre-term labor

        O09.211 **Supervision of pregnancy with history of pre-term labor, first trimester**   Ⓜ♀

        O09.212 **Supervision of pregnancy with history of pre-term labor, second trimester**   Ⓜ♀

        O09.213 **Supervision of pregnancy with history of pre-term labor, third trimester**   Ⓜ♀

        O09.219 **Supervision of pregnancy with history of pre-term labor, unspecified trimester**   Ⓜ♀

    √6th **O09.29** **Supervision of pregnancy with** other poor reproductive or obstetric history
        Supervision of pregnancy with history of neonatal death
        Supervision of pregnancy with history of stillbirth

        O09.291 **Supervision of pregnancy with other poor reproductive or obstetric history, first trimester**   Ⓜ♀

        O09.292 **Supervision of pregnancy with other poor reproductive or obstetric history, second trimester**   Ⓜ♀

        O09.293 **Supervision of pregnancy with other poor reproductive or obstetric history, third trimester**   Ⓜ♀

        O09.299 **Supervision of pregnancy with other poor reproductive or obstetric history, unspecified trimester**   Ⓜ♀

√5th **O09.3** **Supervision of pregnancy with** insufficient antenatal care
    Supervision of concealed pregnancy
    Supervision of hidden pregnancy

    O09.30 **Supervision of pregnancy with insufficient antenatal care, unspecified trimester**   Ⓜ♀

    O09.31 **Supervision of pregnancy with insufficient antenatal care, first trimester**   Ⓜ♀

    O09.32 **Supervision of pregnancy with insufficient antenatal care, second trimester**   Ⓜ♀

    O09.33 **Supervision of pregnancy with insufficient antenatal care, third trimester**   Ⓜ♀

√5th **O09.4** **Supervision of pregnancy with** grand multiparity

    O09.40 **Supervision of pregnancy with grand multiparity, unspecified trimester**   Ⓜ♀

    O09.41 **Supervision of pregnancy with grand multiparity, first trimester**   Ⓜ♀

    O09.42 **Supervision of pregnancy with grand multiparity, second trimester**   Ⓜ♀

    O09.43 **Supervision of pregnancy with grand multiparity, third trimester**   Ⓜ♀

√5th **O09.5** **Supervision of** elderly primigravida and multigravida
    Pregnancy for a female 35 years and older at expected date of delivery

    √6th **O09.51** **Supervision of** elderly primigravida

        O09.511 **Supervision of elderly primigravida, first trimester**   Ⓜ♀

        O09.512 **Supervision of elderly primigravida, second trimester**   Ⓜ♀

        O09.513 **Supervision of elderly primigravida, third trimester**   Ⓜ♀

        O09.519 **Supervision of elderly primigravida, unspecified trimester**   Ⓜ♀

    √6th **O09.52** **Supervision of** elderly multigravida

        O09.521 **Supervision of elderly multigravida, first trimester**   Ⓜ♀

        O09.522 **Supervision of elderly multigravida, second trimester**   Ⓜ♀

        O09.523 **Supervision of elderly multigravida, third trimester**   Ⓜ♀

        O09.529 **Supervision of elderly multigravida, unspecified trimester**   Ⓜ♀

√5th **O09.6** **Supervision of** young primigravida and multigravida
    Supervision of pregnancy for a female less than 16 years old at expected date of delivery

    √6th **O09.61** **Supervision of young** primigravida

        O09.611 **Supervision of young primigravida, first trimester**   Ⓜ♀

        O09.612 **Supervision of young primigravida, second trimester**   Ⓜ♀

        O09.613 **Supervision of young primigravida, third trimester**   Ⓜ♀

        O09.619 **Supervision of young primigravida, unspecified trimester**   Ⓜ♀

    √6th **O09.62** **Supervision of young** multigravida

        O09.621 **Supervision of young multigravida, first trimester**   Ⓜ♀

        O09.622 **Supervision of young multigravida, second trimester**   Ⓜ♀

        O09.623 **Supervision of young multigravida, third trimester**   Ⓜ♀

        O09.629 **Supervision of young multigravida, unspecified trimester**   Ⓜ♀

√5th **O09.7** **Supervision of high risk pregnancy due to** social problems

    O09.70 **Supervision of high risk pregnancy due to social problems, unspecified trimester**   Ⓜ♀

    O09.71 **Supervision of high risk pregnancy due to social problems, first trimester**   Ⓜ♀

    O09.72 **Supervision of high risk pregnancy due to social problems, second trimester**   Ⓜ♀

    O09.73 **Supervision of high risk pregnancy due to social problems, third trimester**   Ⓜ♀

√5th **O09.8** **Supervision of** other high risk pregnancies

    √6th **O09.81** **Supervision of pregnancy** resulting from assisted reproductive technology
        Supervision of pregnancy resulting from in-vitro fertilization

        O09.811 **Supervision of pregnancy resulting from assisted reproductive technology, first trimester**   Ⓜ♀

        O09.812 **Supervision of pregnancy resulting from assisted reproductive technology, second trimester**   Ⓜ♀

EXCLUDES 1 Not coded here   EXCLUDES 2 Not included here   Ⓝ Newborn Age: 0   Ⓟ Pediatric Age: 0-17   Ⓜ Maternity Age: 12-55   Ⓐ Adult Age: 15-124

738   ICD-10-CM 2014 (Draft)

O09.813 Supervision of pregnancy resulting from assisted reproductive technology, third trimester   Ⓜ♀

O09.819 Supervision of pregnancy resulting from assisted reproductive technology, unspecified trimester   Ⓜ♀

✓6ᵗʰ **O09.82** Supervision of pregnancy with history of in utero procedure during previous pregnancy

O09.821 Supervision of pregnancy with history of in utero procedure during previous pregnancy, first trimester   Ⓜ♀

O09.822 Supervision of pregnancy with history of in utero procedure during previous pregnancy, second trimester   Ⓜ♀

O09.823 Supervision of pregnancy with history of in utero procedure during previous pregnancy, third trimester   Ⓜ♀

O09.829 Supervision of pregnancy with history of in utero procedure during previous pregnancy, unspecified trimester   Ⓜ♀

> EXCLUDES 1   *supervision of pregnancy affected by in utero procedure during current pregnancy (O35.7)*

✓6ᵗʰ **O09.89** Supervision of other high risk pregnancies

O09.891 Supervision of other high risk pregnancies, first trimester   Ⓜ♀

O09.892 Supervision of other high risk pregnancies, second trimester   Ⓜ♀

O09.893 Supervision of other high risk pregnancies, third trimester   Ⓜ♀

O09.899 Supervision of other high risk pregnancies, unspecified trimester   Ⓜ♀

✓5ᵗʰ **O09.9** Supervision of high risk pregnancy, unspecified

O09.90 Supervision of high risk pregnancy, unspecified, unspecified trimester   Ⓜ♀

O09.91 Supervision of high risk pregnancy, unspecified, first trimester   Ⓜ♀

O09.92 Supervision of high risk pregnancy, unspecified, second trimester   Ⓜ♀

O09.93 Supervision of high risk pregnancy, unspecified, third trimester   Ⓜ♀

Edema, proteinuria and hypertensive disorders in pregnancy, childbirth and the puerperium (O10-O16)

✓4ᵗʰ **O10** Pre-existing hypertension complicating pregnancy, childbirth and the puerperium

Pre-existing hypertension with pre-existing proteinuria complicating pregnancy, childbirth and the puerperium

> EXCLUDES 2   *pre-existing hypertension with superimposed pre-eclampsia complicating pregnancy, childbirth and the puerperium (O11.-)*

✓5ᵗʰ **O10.0** Pre-existing essential hypertension complicating pregnancy, childbirth and the puerperium

Any condition in I10 specified as a reason for obstetric care during pregnancy, childbirth or the puerperium

✓6ᵗʰ **O10.01** Pre-existing essential hypertension complicating pregnancy

O10.011 Pre-existing essential hypertension complicating pregnancy, first trimester   Ⓜ♀

O10.012 Pre-existing essential hypertension complicating pregnancy, second trimester   Ⓜ♀

O10.013 Pre-existing essential hypertension complicating pregnancy, third trimester   Ⓜ♀

O10.019 Pre-existing essential hypertension complicating pregnancy, unspecified trimester   Ⓜ♀

O10.02 Pre-existing essential hypertension complicating childbirth   Ⓜ♀

O10.03 Pre-existing essential hypertension complicating the puerperium   Ⓜ♀

✓5ᵗʰ **O10.1** Pre-existing hypertensive heart disease complicating pregnancy, childbirth and the puerperium

Any condition in I11 specified as a reason for obstetric care during pregnancy, childbirth or the puerperium

Use additional code from I11 to identify the type of hypertensive heart disease

✓6ᵗʰ **O10.11** Pre-existing hypertensive heart disease complicating pregnancy

O10.111 Pre-existing hypertensive heart disease complicating pregnancy, first trimester   Ⓜ♀

O10.112 Pre-existing hypertensive heart disease complicating pregnancy, second trimester   Ⓜ♀

O10.113 Pre-existing hypertensive heart disease complicating pregnancy, third trimester   Ⓜ♀

O10.119 Pre-existing hypertensive heart disease complicating pregnancy, unspecified trimester   Ⓜ♀

O10.12 Pre-existing hypertensive heart disease complicating childbirth   Ⓜ♀

O10.13 Pre-existing hypertensive heart disease complicating the puerperium   Ⓜ♀

✓5ᵗʰ **O10.2** Pre-existing hypertensive chronic kidney disease complicating pregnancy, childbirth and the puerperium

Any condition in I12 specified as a reason for obstetric care during pregnancy, childbirth or the puerperium

Use additional code from I12 to identify the type of hypertensive chronic kidney disease

✓6ᵗʰ **O10.21** Pre-existing hypertensive chronic kidney disease complicating pregnancy

O10.211 Pre-existing hypertensive chronic kidney disease complicating pregnancy, first trimester   Ⓜ♀

O10.212 Pre-existing hypertensive chronic kidney disease complicating pregnancy, second trimester   Ⓜ♀

O10.213 Pre-existing hypertensive chronic kidney disease complicating pregnancy, third trimester   Ⓜ♀

O10.219 Pre-existing hypertensive chronic kidney disease complicating pregnancy, unspecified trimester   Ⓜ♀

O10.22 Pre-existing hypertensive chronic kidney disease complicating childbirth   Ⓜ♀

O10.23 Pre-existing hypertensive chronic kidney disease complicating the puerperium   Ⓜ♀

✓5ᵗʰ **O10.3** Pre-existing hypertensive heart and chronic kidney disease complicating pregnancy, childbirth and the puerperium

Any condition in I13 specified as a reason for obstetric care during pregnancy, childbirth or the puerperium

Use additional code from I13 to identify the type of hypertensive heart and chronic kidney disease

✓6ᵗʰ **O10.31** Pre-existing hypertensive heart and chronic kidney disease complicating pregnancy

O10.311 Pre-existing hypertensive heart and chronic kidney disease complicating pregnancy, first trimester   Ⓜ♀

O10.312 Pre-existing hypertensive heart and chronic kidney disease complicating pregnancy, second trimester   Ⓜ♀

O10.313 Pre-existing hypertensive heart and chronic kidney disease complicating pregnancy, third trimester   Ⓜ♀

O10.319 Pre-existing hypertensive heart and chronic kidney disease complicating pregnancy, unspecified trimester   Ⓜ♀

O10.32 Pre-existing hypertensive heart and chronic kidney disease complicating childbirth   Ⓜ♀

O10.33 Pre-existing hypertensive heart and chronic kidney disease complicating the puerperium   Ⓜ♀

☑ Additional Character Required   ✓×7ᵗʰ Xtension Alert   Unspecified Code   Other Specified Code   Manifestation Code   ▶◀ Revised Text   ● New Code   ▲ Revised Code Title

ICD-10-CM 2014 (Draft)   **739**

✓5ᵗʰ **O10.4 Pre-existing secondary hypertension complicating pregnancy, childbirth and the puerperium**
Any condition in I15 specified as a reason for obstetric care during pregnancy, childbirth or the puerperium
Use additional code from I15 to identify the type of secondary hypertension

    ✓6ᵗʰ **O10.41 Pre-existing secondary hypertension complicating pregnancy**

        O10.411 Pre-existing secondary hypertension complicating pregnancy, first trimester Ⓜ♀

        O10.412 Pre-existing secondary hypertension complicating pregnancy, second trimester Ⓜ♀

        O10.413 Pre-existing secondary hypertension complicating pregnancy, third trimester Ⓜ♀

        O10.419 Pre-existing secondary hypertension complicating pregnancy, unspecified trimester Ⓜ♀

    O10.42 Pre-existing secondary hypertension complicating childbirth Ⓜ♀

    O10.43 Pre-existing secondary hypertension complicating the puerperium Ⓜ♀

✓5ᵗʰ **O10.9 Unspecified pre-existing hypertension complicating pregnancy, childbirth and the puerperium**

    ✓6ᵗʰ **O10.91 Unspecified pre-existing hypertension complicating pregnancy**

        O10.911 Unspecified pre-existing hypertension complicating pregnancy, first trimester Ⓜ♀

        O10.912 Unspecified pre-existing hypertension complicating pregnancy, second trimester Ⓜ♀

        O10.913 Unspecified pre-existing hypertension complicating pregnancy, third trimester Ⓜ♀

        O10.919 Unspecified pre-existing hypertension complicating pregnancy, unspecified trimester Ⓜ♀

    O10.92 Unspecified pre-existing hypertension complicating childbirth Ⓜ♀

    O10.93 Unspecified pre-existing hypertension complicating the puerperium Ⓜ♀

✓4ᵗʰ **O11 Pre-existing hypertension with pre-eclampsia**
Conditions in O10 complicated by pre-eclampsia
Pre-eclampsia superimposed pre-existing hypertension
Use additional code from O10 to identify the type of hypertension

    O11.1 Pre-existing hypertension with pre-eclampsia, first trimester Ⓜ♀

    O11.2 Pre-existing hypertension with pre-eclampsia, second trimester Ⓜ♀

    O11.3 Pre-existing hypertension with pre-eclampsia, third trimester Ⓜ♀

    O11.9 Pre-existing hypertension with pre-eclampsia, unspecified trimester Ⓜ♀

✓4ᵗʰ **O12 Gestational [pregnancy-induced] edema and proteinuria without hypertension**

    ✓5ᵗʰ **O12.0 Gestational edema**

        O12.00 Gestational edema, unspecified trimester Ⓜ♀

        O12.01 Gestational edema, first trimester Ⓜ♀

        O12.02 Gestational edema, second trimester Ⓜ♀

        O12.03 Gestational edema, third trimester Ⓜ♀

    ✓5ᵗʰ **O12.1 Gestational proteinuria**

        O12.10 Gestational proteinuria, unspecified trimester Ⓜ♀

        O12.11 Gestational proteinuria, first trimester Ⓜ♀

        O12.12 Gestational proteinuria, second trimester Ⓜ♀

        O12.13 Gestational proteinuria, third trimester Ⓜ♀

    ✓5ᵗʰ **O12.2 Gestational edema with proteinuria**

        O12.20 Gestational edema with proteinuria, unspecified trimester Ⓜ♀

        O12.21 Gestational edema with proteinuria, first trimester Ⓜ♀

        O12.22 Gestational edema with proteinuria, second trimester Ⓜ♀

        O12.23 Gestational edema with proteinuria, third trimester Ⓜ♀

✓4ᵗʰ **O13 Gestational [pregnancy-induced] hypertension without significant proteinuria**
INCLUDES gestational hypertension NOS

    O13.1 Gestational [pregnancy-induced] hypertension without significant proteinuria, first trimester Ⓜ♀

    O13.2 Gestational [pregnancy-induced] hypertension without significant proteinuria, second trimester Ⓜ♀

    O13.3 Gestational [pregnancy-induced] hypertension without significant proteinuria, third trimester Ⓜ♀

    O13.9 Gestational [pregnancy-induced] hypertension without significant proteinuria, unspecified trimester Ⓜ♀

✓4ᵗʰ **O14 Pre-eclampsia**
EXCLUDES 1 pre-existing hypertension with pre-eclampsia (O11)

    ✓5ᵗʰ **O14.0 Mild to moderate pre-eclampsia**

        O14.00 Mild to moderate pre-eclampsia, unspecified trimester Ⓜ♀

        O14.02 Mild to moderate pre-eclampsia, second trimester Ⓜ♀

        O14.03 Mild to moderate pre-eclampsia, third trimester Ⓜ♀

    ✓5ᵗʰ **O14.1 Severe pre-eclampsia**
        EXCLUDES 1 HELLP syndrome (O14.2-)

        O14.10 Severe pre-eclampsia, unspecified trimester Ⓜ♀

        O14.12 Severe pre-eclampsia, second trimester Ⓜ♀

        O14.13 Severe pre-eclampsia, third trimester Ⓜ♀

    ✓5ᵗʰ **O14.2 HELLP syndrome**
Severe pre-eclampsia with hemolysis, elevated liver enzymes and low platelet count (HELLP)

        O14.20 HELLP syndrome (HELLP), unspecified trimester Ⓜ♀

        O14.22 HELLP syndrome (HELLP), second trimester Ⓜ♀

        O14.23 HELLP syndrome (HELLP), third trimester Ⓜ♀

    ✓5ᵗʰ **O14.9 Unspecified pre-eclampsia**

        O14.90 Unspecified pre-eclampsia, unspecified trimester Ⓜ♀

        O14.92 Unspecified pre-eclampsia, second trimester Ⓜ♀

        O14.93 Unspecified pre-eclampsia, third trimester Ⓜ♀

✓4ᵗʰ **O15 Eclampsia**
INCLUDES convulsions following conditions in O10-O14 and O16

    ✓5ᵗʰ **O15.0 Eclampsia in pregnancy**

        O15.00 Eclampsia in pregnancy, unspecified trimester Ⓜ♀

        O15.02 Eclampsia in pregnancy, second trimester Ⓜ♀

        O15.03 Eclampsia in pregnancy, third trimester Ⓜ♀

    O15.1 Eclampsia in labor Ⓜ♀

    O15.2 Eclampsia in the puerperium Ⓜ♀

    O15.9 Eclampsia, unspecified as to time period Ⓜ♀
        Eclampsia NOS

✓4ᵗʰ **O16 Unspecified maternal hypertension**

    O16.1 Unspecified maternal hypertension, first trimester Ⓜ♀

    O16.2 Unspecified maternal hypertension, second trimester Ⓜ♀

    O16.3 Unspecified maternal hypertension, third trimester Ⓜ♀

    O16.9 Unspecified maternal hypertension, unspecified trimester Ⓜ♀

Other maternal disorders predominantly related to pregnancy (O20-O29)

EXCLUDES 2 maternal care related to the fetus and amniotic cavity and possible delivery problems (O30-O48)
maternal diseases classifiable elsewhere but complicating pregnancy, labor and delivery, and the puerperium (O98-O99)

✓4ᵗʰ **O20 Hemorrhage in early pregnancy**
Hemorrhage before completion of 20 weeks gestation
EXCLUDES 1 pregnancy with abortive outcome (O00-O08)

    O20.0 Threatened abortion Ⓜ♀
        Hemorrhage specified as due to threatened abortion

    O20.8 Other hemorrhage in early pregnancy Ⓜ♀

    O20.9 Hemorrhage in early pregnancy, unspecified Ⓜ♀

✓4ᵗʰ **O21 Excessive vomiting in pregnancy**

    O21.0 Mild hyperemesis gravidarum Ⓜ♀
        Hyperemesis gravidarum, mild or unspecified, starting before the end of the 20th week of gestation

EXCLUDES 1 Not coded here   EXCLUDES 2 Not included here   Ⓝ Newborn Age: 0   Ⓟ Pediatric Age: 0-17   Ⓜ Maternity Age: 12-55   Ⓐ Adult Age: 15-124

740   ICD-10-CM 2014 (Draft)

O21.1   **Hyperemesis gravidarum with** metabolic disturbance   M♀
Hyperemesis gravidarum, starting before the end of the 20th week of gestation, with metabolic disturbance such as carbohydrate depletion
Hyperemesis gravidarum, starting before the end of the 20th week of gestation, with metabolic disturbance such as dehydration
Hyperemesis gravidarum, starting before the end of the 20th week of gestation, with metabolic disturbance such as electrolyte imbalance

O21.2   **Late** vomiting of pregnancy   M♀
Excessive vomiting starting after 20 completed weeks of gestation

O21.8   Other vomiting complicating pregnancy   M♀
Vomiting due to diseases classified elsewhere, complicating pregnancy
Use additional code, to identify cause

O21.9   **Vomiting of pregnancy, unspecified**   M♀

✓4th **O22**   **Venous complications and hemorrhoids in pregnancy**
EXCLUDES 1   venous complications of:
     abortion NOS (O03.9)
     ectopic or molar pregnancy (O08.7)
     failed attempted abortion (O07.35)
     induced abortion (O04.85)
     spontaneous abortion (O03.89)
EXCLUDES 2   obstetric pulmonary embolism (O88.-)
     venous complications and hemorrhoids of childbirth and the puerperium (O87.-)

✓5th **O22.0**   Varicose veins of lower extremity **in pregnancy**
Varicose veins NOS in pregnancy

   O22.00   **Varicose veins of lower extremity in pregnancy, unspecified trimester**   M♀

   O22.01   **Varicose veins of lower extremity in pregnancy, first trimester**   M♀

   O22.02   **Varicose veins of lower extremity in pregnancy, second trimester**   M♀

   O22.03   **Varicose veins of lower extremity in pregnancy, third trimester**   M♀

✓5th **O22.1**   Genital varices **in pregnancy**
Perineal varices in pregnancy
Vaginal varices in pregnancy
Vulval varices in pregnancy

   O22.10   **Genital varices in pregnancy, unspecified trimester**   M♀

   O22.11   **Genital varices in pregnancy,** first trimester   M♀

   O22.12   **Genital varices in pregnancy,** second trimester   M♀

   O22.13   **Genital varices in pregnancy,** third trimester   M♀

✓5th **O22.2**   Superficial thrombophlebitis **in pregnancy**
Phlebitis in pregnancy NOS
Thrombophlebitis of legs in pregnancy
Thrombosis in pregnancy NOS
Use additional code to identify the superficial thrombophlebitis (I80.0-)

   O22.20   **Superficial thrombophlebitis in pregnancy, unspecified trimester**   M♀

   O22.21   **Superficial thrombophlebitis in pregnancy, first trimester**   M♀

   O22.22   **Superficial thrombophlebitis in pregnancy, second trimester**   M♀

   O22.23   **Superficial thrombophlebitis in pregnancy, third trimester**   M♀

✓5th **O22.3**   Deep phlebothrombosis **in pregnancy**
Deep vein thrombosis, antepartum
Use additional code to identify the deep vein thrombosis (I82.4-, I82.5-, I82.62-, I82.72-)
Use additional code, if applicable, for associated long-term (current) use of anticoagulants (Z79.01)

   O22.30   **Deep phlebothrombosis in pregnancy, unspecified trimester**   M♀

   O22.31   **Deep phlebothrombosis in pregnancy, first trimester**   M♀

   O22.32   **Deep phlebothrombosis in pregnancy, second trimester**   M♀

   O22.33   **Deep phlebothrombosis in pregnancy, third trimester**   M♀

✓5th **O22.4**   Hemorrhoids **in pregnancy**

   O22.40   **Hemorrhoids in pregnancy, unspecified trimester**   M♀

   O22.41   **Hemorrhoids in pregnancy,** first trimester   M♀

   O22.42   **Hemorrhoids in pregnancy,** second trimester   M♀

   O22.43   **Hemorrhoids in pregnancy,** third trimester   M♀

✓5th **O22.5**   Cerebral venous thrombosis **in pregnancy**
Cerebrovenous sinus thrombosis in pregnancy

   O22.50   **Cerebral venous thrombosis in pregnancy, unspecified trimester**   M♀

   O22.51   **Cerebral venous thrombosis in pregnancy, first trimester**   M♀

   O22.52   **Cerebral venous thrombosis in pregnancy, second trimester**   M♀

   O22.53   **Cerebral venous thrombosis in pregnancy, third trimester**   M♀

✓5th **O22.8**   Other venous complications **in pregnancy**

   ✓6th **O22.8X**   Other venous complications in pregnancy

     O22.8X1   **Other venous complications in pregnancy,** first trimester   M♀

     O22.8X2   **Other venous complications in pregnancy,** second trimester   M♀

     O22.8X3   **Other venous complications in pregnancy,** third trimester   M♀

     O22.8X9   **Other venous complications in pregnancy, unspecified trimester**   M♀

✓5th **O22.9**   Venous complication in pregnancy, unspecified
Gestational phlebitis NOS
Gestational phlebopathy NOS
Gestational thrombosis NOS

   O22.90   **Venous complication in pregnancy, unspecified, unspecified trimester**   M♀

   O22.91   **Venous complication in pregnancy, unspecified, first trimester**   M♀

   O22.92   **Venous complication in pregnancy, unspecified, second trimester**   M♀

   O22.93   **Venous complication in pregnancy, unspecified, third trimester**   M♀

✓4th **O23**   **Infections of genitourinary tract in pregnancy**
Use additional code to identify organism (B95.-, B96.-)
EXCLUDES 2   gonococcal infections complicating pregnancy, childbirth and the puerperium (O98.2)
     infections with a predominantly sexual mode of transmission NOS complicating pregnancy, childbirth and the puerperium (O98.3)
     syphilis complicating pregnancy, childbirth and the puerperium (O98.1)
     tuberculosis of genitourinary system complicating pregnancy, childbirth and the puerperium (O98.0)
     venereal disease NOS complicating pregnancy, childbirth and the puerperium (O98.3)

✓5th **O23.0**   Infections of kidney **in pregnancy**
Pyelonephritis in pregnancy

   O23.00   **Infections of kidney in pregnancy, unspecified trimester**   M♀

   O23.01   **Infections of kidney in pregnancy,** first trimester   M♀

   O23.02   **Infections of kidney in pregnancy,** second trimester   M♀

   O23.03   **Infections of kidney in pregnancy,** third trimester   M♀

✓5th **O23.1**   Infections of bladder **in pregnancy**

   O23.10   **Infections of bladder in pregnancy, unspecified trimester**   M♀

   O23.11   **Infections of bladder in pregnancy, first trimester**   M♀

   O23.12   **Infections of bladder in pregnancy, second trimester**   M♀

   O23.13   **Infections of bladder in pregnancy, third trimester**   M♀

✓5th **O23.2**   Infections of urethra **in pregnancy**

   O23.20   **Infections of urethra in pregnancy, unspecified trimester**   M♀

   O23.21   **Infections of urethra in pregnancy, first trimester**   M♀

   O23.22   **Infections of urethra in pregnancy, second trimester**   M♀

Pregnancy, Childbirth and the Puerperium

O21.1–O23.22

☑ Additional Character Required   ✓x7th Xtension Alert   Unspecified Code   Other Specified Code   Manifestation Code   ▶◀ Revised Text   ● New Code   ▲ Revised Code Title

ICD-10-CM 2014 (Draft)   **741**

Pregnancy, Childbirth and the Puerperium

O23.23–O24.439

O23.23   **Infections of urethra in pregnancy, third trimester**   Ⓜ♀

✓5th **O23.3 Infections of other parts of urinary tract in pregnancy**

O23.30   **Infections of other parts of urinary tract in pregnancy, unspecified trimester**   Ⓜ♀

O23.31   **Infections of other parts of urinary tract in pregnancy, first trimester**   Ⓜ♀

O23.32   **Infections of other parts of urinary tract in pregnancy, second trimester**   Ⓜ♀

O23.33   **Infections of other parts of urinary tract in pregnancy, third trimester**   Ⓜ♀

✓5th **O23.4 Unspecified infection of urinary tract in pregnancy**

O23.40   **Unspecified infection of urinary tract in pregnancy, unspecified trimester**   Ⓜ♀

O23.41   **Unspecified infection of urinary tract in pregnancy, first trimester**   Ⓜ♀

O23.42   **Unspecified infection of urinary tract in pregnancy, second trimester**   Ⓜ♀

O23.43   **Unspecified infection of urinary tract in pregnancy, third trimester**   Ⓜ♀

✓5th **O23.5 Infections of the genital tract in pregnancy**

   ✓6th **O23.51 Infection of cervix in pregnancy**

     O23.511   **Infections of cervix in pregnancy, first trimester**   Ⓜ♀

     O23.512   **Infections of cervix in pregnancy, second trimester**   Ⓜ♀

     O23.513   **Infections of cervix in pregnancy, third trimester**   Ⓜ♀

     O23.519   **Infections of cervix in pregnancy, unspecified trimester**   Ⓜ♀

   ✓6th **O23.52 Salpingo-oophoritis in pregnancy**
Oophoritis in pregnancy
Salpingitis in pregnancy

     O23.521   **Salpingo-oophoritis in pregnancy, first trimester**   Ⓜ♀

     O23.522   **Salpingo-oophoritis in pregnancy, second trimester**   Ⓜ♀

     O23.523   **Salpingo-oophoritis in pregnancy, third trimester**   Ⓜ♀

     O23.529   **Salpingo-oophoritis in pregnancy, unspecified trimester**   Ⓜ♀

   ✓6th **O23.59 Infection of other part of genital tract in pregnancy**

     O23.591   **Infection of other part of genital tract in pregnancy, first trimester**   Ⓜ♀

     O23.592   **Infection of other part of genital tract in pregnancy, second trimester**   Ⓜ♀

     O23.593   **Infection of other part of genital tract in pregnancy, third trimester**   Ⓜ♀

     O23.599   **Infection of other part of genital tract in pregnancy, unspecified trimester**   Ⓜ♀

✓5th **O23.9 Unspecified genitourinary tract infection in pregnancy**
Genitourinary tract infection in pregnancy NOS

O23.90   **Unspecified genitourinary tract infection in pregnancy, unspecified trimester**   Ⓜ♀

O23.91   **Unspecified genitourinary tract infection in pregnancy, first trimester**   Ⓜ♀

O23.92   **Unspecified genitourinary tract infection in pregnancy, second trimester**   Ⓜ♀

O23.93   **Unspecified genitourinary tract infection in pregnancy, third trimester**   Ⓜ♀

✓4th **O24 Diabetes mellitus in pregnancy, childbirth, and the puerperium**

  ✓5th **O24.0 Pre-existing diabetes mellitus, type 1, in pregnancy, childbirth and the puerperium**
Juvenile onset diabetes mellitus, in pregnancy, childbirth and the puerperium
Ketosis-prone diabetes mellitus in pregnancy, childbirth and the puerperium
Use additional code from category E10 to further identify any manifestations

   ✓6th **O24.01 Pre-existing diabetes mellitus, type 1, in pregnancy**

     O24.011   **Pre-existing diabetes mellitus, type 1, in pregnancy, first trimester**   Ⓜ♀

     O24.012   **Pre-existing diabetes mellitus, type 1, in pregnancy, second trimester**   Ⓜ♀

     O24.013   **Pre-existing diabetes mellitus, type 1, in pregnancy, third trimester**   Ⓜ♀

     O24.019   **Pre-existing diabetes mellitus, type 1, in pregnancy, unspecified trimester**   Ⓜ♀

   O24.02   **Pre-existing diabetes mellitus, type 1, in childbirth**   Ⓜ♀

   O24.03   **Pre-existing diabetes mellitus, type 1, in the puerperium**   Ⓜ♀

  ✓5th **O24.1 Pre-existing diabetes mellitus, type 2, in pregnancy, childbirth and the puerperium**
Insulin-resistant diabetes mellitus in pregnancy, childbirth and the puerperium
Use additional code (for):
from category E11 to further identify any manifestations
long-term (current) use of insulin (Z79.4)

   ✓6th **O24.11 Pre-existing diabetes mellitus, type 2, in pregnancy**

     O24.111   **Pre-existing diabetes mellitus, type 2, in pregnancy, first trimester**   Ⓜ♀

     O24.112   **Pre-existing diabetes mellitus, type 2, in pregnancy, second trimester**   Ⓜ♀

     O24.113   **Pre-existing diabetes mellitus, type 2, in pregnancy, third trimester**   Ⓜ♀

     O24.119   **Pre-existing diabetes mellitus, type 2, in pregnancy, unspecified trimester**   Ⓜ♀

   O24.12   **Pre-existing diabetes mellitus, type 2, in childbirth**   Ⓜ♀

   O24.13   **Pre-existing diabetes mellitus, type 2, in the puerperium**   Ⓜ♀

  ✓5th **O24.3 Unspecified pre-existing diabetes mellitus in pregnancy, childbirth and the puerperium**
Use additional code (for):
from category E11 to further identify any manifestation
long-term (current) use of insulin (Z79.4)

   ✓6th **O24.31 Unspecified pre-existing diabetes mellitus in pregnancy**

     O24.311   **Unspecified pre-existing diabetes mellitus in pregnancy, first trimester**   Ⓜ♀

     O24.312   **Unspecified pre-existing diabetes mellitus in pregnancy, second trimester**   Ⓜ♀

     O24.313   **Unspecified pre-existing diabetes mellitus in pregnancy, third trimester**   Ⓜ♀

     O24.319   **Unspecified pre-existing diabetes mellitus in pregnancy, unspecified trimester**   Ⓜ♀

   O24.32   **Unspecified pre-existing diabetes mellitus in childbirth**   Ⓜ♀

   O24.33   **Unspecified pre-existing diabetes mellitus in the puerperium**   Ⓜ♀

  ✓5th **O24.4 Gestational diabetes mellitus**
Diabetes mellitus arising in pregnancy
Gestational diabetes mellitus NOS

   ✓6th **O24.41 Gestational diabetes mellitus in pregnancy**

     O24.410   **Gestational diabetes mellitus in pregnancy, diet controlled**   Ⓜ♀

     O24.414   **Gestational diabetes mellitus in pregnancy, insulin controlled**   Ⓜ♀

     O24.419   **Gestational diabetes mellitus in pregnancy, unspecified control**   Ⓜ♀

   ✓6th **O24.42 Gestational diabetes mellitus in childbirth**

     O24.420   **Gestational diabetes mellitus in childbirth, diet controlled**   Ⓜ♀

     O24.424   **Gestational diabetes mellitus in childbirth, insulin controlled**   Ⓜ♀

     O24.429   **Gestational diabetes mellitus in childbirth, unspecified control**   Ⓜ♀

   ✓6th **O24.43 Gestational diabetes mellitus in the puerperium**

     O24.430   **Gestational diabetes mellitus in the puerperium, diet controlled**   Ⓜ♀

     O24.434   **Gestational diabetes mellitus in the puerperium, insulin controlled**   Ⓜ♀

     O24.439   **Gestational diabetes mellitus in the puerperium, unspecified control**   Ⓜ♀

EXCLUDES 1 Not coded here   EXCLUDES 2 Not included here   Ⓝ Newborn Age: 0   Ⓟ Pediatric Age: 0-17   Ⓜ Maternity Age: 12-55   Ⓐ Adult Age: 15-124

742   ICD-10-CM 2014 (Draft)

√5ᵗʰ **O24.8** Other pre-existing **diabetes mellitus in pregnancy, childbirth, and the puerperium**
Use additional code (for):
from categories E08, E09 and E13 to further identify any manifestation
long-term (current) use of insulin (Z79.4)

√6ᵗʰ **O24.81** **Other pre-existing diabetes mellitus in** pregnancy
O24.811 **Other pre-existing diabetes mellitus in pregnancy,** first trimester Ⓜ♀
O24.812 **Other pre-existing diabetes mellitus in pregnancy,** second trimester Ⓜ♀
O24.813 **Other pre-existing diabetes mellitus in pregnancy,** third trimester Ⓜ♀
O24.819 **Other pre-existing diabetes mellitus in pregnancy, unspecified trimester** Ⓜ♀
O24.82 **Other pre-existing diabetes mellitus in** childbirth Ⓜ♀
O24.83 **Other pre-existing diabetes mellitus in the** puerperium Ⓜ♀

√5ᵗʰ **O24.9** Unspecified **diabetes mellitus in pregnancy, childbirth and the puerperium**
Use additional code for long-term (current) use of insulin (Z79.4)

√6ᵗʰ **O24.91** **Unspecified diabetes mellitus in** pregnancy
O24.911 **Unspecified diabetes mellitus in pregnancy,** first trimester Ⓜ♀
O24.912 **Unspecified diabetes mellitus in pregnancy,** second trimester Ⓜ♀
O24.913 **Unspecified diabetes mellitus in pregnancy,** third trimester Ⓜ♀
O24.919 **Unspecified diabetes mellitus in pregnancy, unspecified trimester** Ⓜ♀
O24.92 **Unspecified diabetes mellitus in** childbirth Ⓜ♀
O24.93 **Unspecified diabetes mellitus in the** puerperium Ⓜ♀

√4ᵗʰ **O25** Malnutrition **in pregnancy, childbirth and the puerperium**
√5ᵗʰ **O25.1** **Malnutrition in** pregnancy
O25.10 **Malnutrition in pregnancy, unspecified trimester** Ⓜ♀
O25.11 **Malnutrition in pregnancy,** first trimester Ⓜ♀
O25.12 **Malnutrition in pregnancy,** second trimester Ⓜ♀
O25.13 **Malnutrition in pregnancy,** third trimester Ⓜ♀
O25.2 **Malnutrition in** childbirth Ⓜ♀
O25.3 **Malnutrition in the** puerperium Ⓜ♀

√4ᵗʰ **O26** **Maternal care for other conditions predominantly related to pregnancy**
√5ᵗʰ **O26.0** **Excessive weight gain in pregnancy**
EXCLUDES 2 *gestational edema (O12.0, O12.2)*
O26.00 **Excessive weight gain in pregnancy, unspecified trimester** Ⓜ♀
O26.01 **Excessive weight gain in pregnancy,** first trimester Ⓜ♀
O26.02 **Excessive weight gain in pregnancy,** second trimester Ⓜ♀
O26.03 **Excessive weight gain in pregnancy,** third trimester Ⓜ♀

√5ᵗʰ **O26.1** **Low weight gain in pregnancy**
O26.10 **Low weight gain in pregnancy, unspecified trimester** Ⓜ♀
O26.11 **Low weight gain in pregnancy,** first trimester Ⓜ♀
O26.12 **Low weight gain in pregnancy,** second trimester Ⓜ♀
O26.13 **Low weight gain in pregnancy,** third trimester Ⓜ♀

√5ᵗʰ **O26.2** **Pregnancy care for patient with recurrent pregnancy loss**
O26.20 **Pregnancy care for patient with recurrent pregnancy loss, unspecified trimester** Ⓜ♀
O26.21 **Pregnancy care for patient with recurrent pregnancy loss,** first trimester Ⓜ♀
O26.22 **Pregnancy care for patient with recurrent pregnancy loss,** second trimester Ⓜ♀
O26.23 **Pregnancy care for patient with recurrent pregnancy loss,** third trimester Ⓜ♀

√5ᵗʰ **O26.3** **Retained intrauterine contraceptive device in pregnancy**
O26.30 **Retained intrauterine contraceptive device in pregnancy, unspecified trimester** Ⓜ♀
O26.31 **Retained intrauterine contraceptive device in pregnancy,** first trimester Ⓜ♀

O26.32 **Retained intrauterine contraceptive device in pregnancy,** second trimester Ⓜ♀
O26.33 **Retained intrauterine contraceptive device in pregnancy,** third trimester Ⓜ♀

√5ᵗʰ **O26.4** **Herpes gestationis**
O26.40 **Herpes gestationis, unspecified trimester** Ⓜ♀
O26.41 **Herpes gestationis,** first trimester Ⓜ♀
O26.42 **Herpes gestationis,** second trimester Ⓜ♀
O26.43 **Herpes gestationis,** third trimester Ⓜ♀

√5ᵗʰ **O26.5** **Maternal hypotension syndrome**
Supine hypotensive syndrome
O26.50 **Maternal hypotension syndrome, unspecified trimester** Ⓜ♀
O26.51 **Maternal hypotension syndrome,** first trimester Ⓜ♀
O26.52 **Maternal hypotension syndrome,** second trimester Ⓜ♀
O26.53 **Maternal hypotension syndrome,** third trimester Ⓜ♀

√5ᵗʰ **O26.6** **Liver and biliary tract disorders in pregnancy, childbirth and the puerperium**
Use additional code to identify the specific disorder
EXCLUDES 2 *hepatorenal syndrome following labor and delivery (O90.4)*
√6ᵗʰ **O26.61** **Liver and biliary tract disorders in** pregnancy
O26.611 **Liver and biliary tract disorders in pregnancy,** first trimester Ⓜ♀
O26.612 **Liver and biliary tract disorders in pregnancy,** second trimester Ⓜ♀
O26.613 **Liver and biliary tract disorders in pregnancy,** third trimester Ⓜ♀
O26.619 **Liver and biliary tract disorders in pregnancy, unspecified trimester** Ⓜ♀
O26.62 **Liver and biliary tract disorders in** childbirth Ⓜ♀
O26.63 **Liver and biliary tract disorders in the** puerperium Ⓜ♀

√5ᵗʰ **O26.7** **Subluxation of symphysis (pubis) in pregnancy, childbirth and the puerperium**
EXCLUDES 1 *traumatic separation of symphysis (pubis) during childbirth (O71.6)*
√6ᵗʰ **O26.71** **Subluxation of symphysis (pubis) in pregnancy**
O26.711 **Subluxation of symphysis (pubis) in pregnancy,** first trimester Ⓜ♀
O26.712 **Subluxation of symphysis (pubis) in pregnancy,** second trimester Ⓜ♀
O26.713 **Subluxation of symphysis (pubis) in pregnancy,** third trimester Ⓜ♀
O26.719 **Subluxation of symphysis (pubis) in pregnancy, unspecified trimester** Ⓜ♀
O26.72 **Subluxation of symphysis (pubis) in** childbirth Ⓜ♀
O26.73 **Subluxation of symphysis (pubis) in the** puerperium Ⓜ♀

√5ᵗʰ **O26.8** **Other specified pregnancy related conditions**
√6ᵗʰ **O26.81** **Pregnancy related exhaustion and fatigue**
O26.811 **Pregnancy related exhaustion and fatigue,** first trimester Ⓜ♀
O26.812 **Pregnancy related exhaustion and fatigue,** second trimester Ⓜ♀
O26.813 **Pregnancy related exhaustion and fatigue,** third trimester Ⓜ♀
O26.819 **Pregnancy related exhaustion and fatigue, unspecified trimester** Ⓜ♀
√6ᵗʰ **O26.82** **Pregnancy related peripheral neuritis**
O26.821 **Pregnancy related peripheral neuritis,** first trimester Ⓜ♀
O26.822 **Pregnancy related peripheral neuritis,** second trimester Ⓜ♀
O26.823 **Pregnancy related peripheral neuritis,** third trimester Ⓜ♀
O26.829 **Pregnancy related peripheral neuritis, unspecified trimester** Ⓜ♀
√6ᵗʰ **O26.83** **Pregnancy related renal disease**
Use additional code to identify the specific disorder
O26.831 **Pregnancy related renal disease,** first trimester Ⓜ♀
O26.832 **Pregnancy related renal disease,** second trimester Ⓜ♀

☑ Additional Character Required   √x7ᵗʰ Xtension Alert   Unspecified Code   Other Specified Code   Manifestation Code   ►◄ Revised Text   ● New Code   ▲ Revised Code Title

Pregnancy, Childbirth and the Puerperium

O26.833–O29.191

O26.833 **Pregnancy related renal disease,** third Ⓜ♀
trimester

O26.839 **Pregnancy related renal disease,** Ⓜ♀
unspecified trimester

✓6th O26.84 **Uterine size-date discrepancy complicating**
pregnancy
> EXCLUDES 1 *encounter for suspected problem with fetal*
> *growth ruled out (Z03.74)*

O26.841 **Uterine size-date discrepancy,** first Ⓜ♀
trimester

O26.842 **Uterine size-date discrepancy,** second Ⓜ♀
trimester

O26.843 **Uterine size-date discrepancy,** third Ⓜ♀
trimester

O26.849 **Uterine size-date discrepancy,** Ⓜ♀
unspecified trimester

✓6th O26.85 **Spotting complicating pregnancy**

O26.851 **Spotting complicating pregnancy,** Ⓜ♀
first trimester

O26.852 **Spotting complicating pregnancy,** Ⓜ♀
second trimester

O26.853 **Spotting complicating pregnancy,** Ⓜ♀
third trimester

O26.859 **Spotting complicating pregnancy,** Ⓜ♀
unspecified trimester

O26.86 **Pruritic urticarial papules and plaques of** Ⓜ♀
pregnancy (PUPPP)
Polymorphic eruption of pregnancy

✓6th O26.87 **Cervical shortening**
> EXCLUDES 1 *encounter for suspected cervical shortening*
> *ruled out (Z03.75)*

O26.872 **Cervical shortening,** second trimester Ⓜ♀
O26.873 **Cervical shortening,** third trimester Ⓜ♀
O26.879 **Cervical shortening, unspecified** Ⓜ♀
trimester

✓6th O26.89 **Other specified pregnancy related conditions**

O26.891 **Other specified pregnancy related** Ⓜ♀
conditions, first trimester

O26.892 **Other specified pregnancy related** Ⓜ♀
conditions, second trimester

O26.893 **Other specified pregnancy related** Ⓜ♀
conditions, third trimester

O26.899 **Other specified pregnancy related** Ⓜ♀
conditions, unspecified trimester

✓5th O26.9 **Pregnancy related conditions, unspecified**

O26.90 **Pregnancy related conditions, unspecified,** Ⓜ♀
unspecified trimester

O26.91 **Pregnancy related conditions, unspecified,** Ⓜ♀
first trimester

O26.92 **Pregnancy related conditions, unspecified,** Ⓜ♀
second trimester

O26.93 **Pregnancy related conditions, unspecified,** Ⓜ♀
third trimester

✓4th **O28 Abnormal findings on antenatal screening of mother**
> EXCLUDES 1 *diagnostic findings classified elsewhere—see Alphabetical*
> *Index*

O28.0 **Abnormal** hematological **finding on antenatal screening** Ⓜ♀
of mother

O28.1 **Abnormal** biochemical **finding on antenatal screening of** Ⓜ♀
mother

O28.2 **Abnormal** cytological **finding on antenatal screening** Ⓜ♀
of mother

O28.3 **Abnormal** ultrasonic **finding on antenatal screening** Ⓜ♀
of mother

O28.4 **Abnormal** radiological **finding on antenatal screening** Ⓜ♀
of mother

O28.5 **Abnormal** chromosomal and genetic **finding on antenatal** Ⓜ♀
screening of mother

O28.8 **Other abnormal findings on antenatal screening of** Ⓜ♀
mother

O28.9 **Unspecified abnormal findings on antenatal screening** Ⓜ♀
of mother

✓4th **O29 Complications of anesthesia during pregnancy**
> INCLUDES maternal complications arising from the administration of a
> general, regional or local anesthetic, analgesic or other
> sedation during pregnancy
> Use additional code, if necessary, to identify the complication
> EXCLUDES 2 *complications of anesthesia during labor and delivery (O74.-)*
> *complications of anesthesia during the puerperium (O89.-)*

✓5th O29.0 **Pulmonary complications of anesthesia during pregnancy**

✓6th O29.01 **Aspiration pneumonitis due to anesthesia during**
pregnancy
Inhalation of stomach contents or secretions NOS due
to anesthesia during pregnancy
Mendelson's syndrome due to anesthesia during
pregnancy

O29.011 **Aspiration pneumonitis due to** Ⓜ♀
anesthesia during pregnancy, first
trimester

O29.012 **Aspiration pneumonitis due to** Ⓜ♀
anesthesia during pregnancy, second
trimester

O29.013 **Aspiration pneumonitis due to** Ⓜ♀
anesthesia during pregnancy, third
trimester

O29.019 **Aspiration pneumonitis due to** Ⓜ♀
anesthesia during pregnancy,
unspecified trimester

✓6th O29.02 **Pressure collapse of lung due to anesthesia during**
pregnancy

O29.021 **Pressure collapse of lung due to** Ⓜ♀
anesthesia during pregnancy, first
trimester

O29.022 **Pressure collapse of lung due to** Ⓜ♀
anesthesia during pregnancy, second
trimester

O29.023 **Pressure collapse of lung due to** Ⓜ♀
anesthesia during pregnancy, third
trimester

O29.029 **Pressure collapse of lung due to** Ⓜ♀
anesthesia during pregnancy,
unspecified trimester

✓6th O29.09 **Other pulmonary complications of anesthesia**
during pregnancy

O29.091 **Other pulmonary complications of** Ⓜ♀
anesthesia during pregnancy, first
trimester

O29.092 **Other pulmonary complications of** Ⓜ♀
anesthesia during pregnancy, second
trimester

O29.093 **Other pulmonary complications of** Ⓜ♀
anesthesia during pregnancy, third
trimester

O29.099 **Other pulmonary complications of** Ⓜ♀
anesthesia during pregnancy,
unspecified trimester

✓5th O29.1 **Cardiac complications of anesthesia during pregnancy**

✓6th O29.11 **Cardiac arrest due to anesthesia during pregnancy**

O29.111 **Cardiac arrest due to anesthesia** Ⓜ♀
during pregnancy, first trimester

O29.112 **Cardiac arrest due to anesthesia** Ⓜ♀
during pregnancy, second trimester

O29.113 **Cardiac arrest due to anesthesia** Ⓜ♀
during pregnancy, third trimester

O29.119 **Cardiac arrest due to anesthesia** Ⓜ♀
during pregnancy, unspecified trimester

✓6th O29.12 **Cardiac failure due to anesthesia during pregnancy**

O29.121 **Cardiac failure due to anesthesia** Ⓜ♀
during pregnancy, first trimester

O29.122 **Cardiac failure due to anesthesia** Ⓜ♀
during pregnancy, second trimester

O29.123 **Cardiac failure due to anesthesia** Ⓜ♀
during pregnancy, third trimester

O29.129 **Cardiac failure due to anesthesia** Ⓜ♀
during pregnancy, unspecified trimester

✓6th O29.19 **Other cardiac complications of anesthesia during**
pregnancy

O29.191 **Other cardiac complications of** Ⓜ♀
anesthesia during pregnancy, first
trimester

EXCLUDES 1 Not coded here   EXCLUDES 2 Not included here   Ⓝ Newborn Age: 0   Ⓟ Pediatric Age: 0-17   Ⓜ Maternity Age: 12-55   Ⓐ Adult Age: 15-124

744   ICD-10-CM 2014 (Draft)

O29.192 Other cardiac complications of anesthesia during pregnancy, second trimester Ⓜ♀

O29.193 Other cardiac complications of anesthesia during pregnancy, third trimester Ⓜ♀

O29.199 Other cardiac complications of anesthesia during pregnancy, unspecified trimester Ⓜ♀

✓5ᵗʰ **O29.2** Central nervous system complications of anesthesia during pregnancy

  ✓6ᵗʰ **O29.21** Cerebral anoxia due to anesthesia during pregnancy

    O29.211 Cerebral anoxia due to anesthesia during pregnancy, first trimester Ⓜ♀

    O29.212 Cerebral anoxia due to anesthesia during pregnancy, second trimester Ⓜ♀

    O29.213 Cerebral anoxia due to anesthesia during pregnancy, third trimester Ⓜ♀

    O29.219 Cerebral anoxia due to anesthesia during pregnancy, unspecified trimester Ⓜ♀

  ✓6ᵗʰ **O29.29** Other central nervous system complications of anesthesia during pregnancy

    O29.291 Other central nervous system complications of anesthesia during pregnancy, first trimester Ⓜ♀

    O29.292 Other central nervous system complications of anesthesia during pregnancy, second trimester Ⓜ♀

    O29.293 Other central nervous system complications of anesthesia during pregnancy, third trimester Ⓜ♀

    O29.299 Other central nervous system complications of anesthesia during pregnancy, unspecified trimester Ⓜ♀

✓5ᵗʰ **O29.3** Toxic reaction to local anesthesia during pregnancy

  ✓6ᵗʰ **O29.3X** Toxic reaction to local anesthesia during pregnancy

    O29.3X1 Toxic reaction to local anesthesia during pregnancy, first trimester Ⓜ♀

    O29.3X2 Toxic reaction to local anesthesia during pregnancy, second trimester Ⓜ♀

    O29.3X3 Toxic reaction to local anesthesia during pregnancy, third trimester Ⓜ♀

    O29.3X9 Toxic reaction to local anesthesia during pregnancy, unspecified trimester Ⓜ♀

✓5ᵗʰ **O29.4** Spinal and epidural anesthesia induced headache during pregnancy

  O29.40 Spinal and epidural anesthesia induced headache during pregnancy, unspecified trimester Ⓜ♀

  O29.41 Spinal and epidural anesthesia induced headache during pregnancy, first trimester Ⓜ♀

  O29.42 Spinal and epidural anesthesia induced headache during pregnancy, second trimester Ⓜ♀

  O29.43 Spinal and epidural anesthesia induced headache during pregnancy, third trimester Ⓜ♀

✓5ᵗʰ **O29.5** Other complications of spinal and epidural anesthesia during pregnancy

  ✓6ᵗʰ **O29.5X** Other complications of spinal and epidural anesthesia during pregnancy

    O29.5X1 Other complications of spinal and epidural anesthesia during pregnancy, first trimester Ⓜ♀

    O29.5X2 Other complications of spinal and epidural anesthesia during pregnancy, second trimester Ⓜ♀

    O29.5X3 Other complications of spinal and epidural anesthesia during pregnancy, third trimester Ⓜ♀

    O29.5X9 Other complications of spinal and epidural anesthesia during pregnancy, unspecified trimester Ⓜ♀

✓5ᵗʰ **O29.6** Failed or difficult intubation for anesthesia during pregnancy

  O29.60 Failed or difficult intubation for anesthesia during pregnancy, unspecified trimester Ⓜ♀

  O29.61 Failed or difficult intubation for anesthesia during pregnancy, first trimester Ⓜ♀

  O29.62 Failed or difficult intubation for anesthesia during pregnancy, second trimester Ⓜ♀

  O29.63 Failed or difficult intubation for anesthesia during pregnancy, third trimester Ⓜ♀

✓5ᵗʰ **O29.8** Other complications of anesthesia during pregnancy

  ✓6ᵗʰ **O29.8X** Other complications of anesthesia during pregnancy

    O29.8X1 Other complications of anesthesia during pregnancy, first trimester Ⓜ♀

    O29.8X2 Other complications of anesthesia during pregnancy, second trimester Ⓜ♀

    O29.8X3 Other complications of anesthesia during pregnancy, third trimester Ⓜ♀

    O29.8X9 Other complications of anesthesia during pregnancy unspecified trimester Ⓜ♀

✓5ᵗʰ **O29.9** Unspecified complication of anesthesia during pregnancy

  O29.90 Unspecified complication of anesthesia during pregnancy, unspecified trimester Ⓜ♀

  O29.91 Unspecified complication of anesthesia during pregnancy, first trimester Ⓜ♀

  O29.92 Unspecified complication of anesthesia during pregnancy, second trimester Ⓜ♀

  O29.93 Unspecified complication of anesthesia during pregnancy, third trimester Ⓜ♀

Maternal care related to the fetus and amniotic cavity and possible delivery problems (O30-O48)

✓4ᵗʰ **O30 Multiple gestation**

Code also any complications specific to multiple gestation

✓5ᵗʰ **O30.0** Twin pregnancy

  ✓6ᵗʰ **O30.00** Twin pregnancy, unspecified number of placenta and unspecified number of amniotic sacs

    O30.001 Twin pregnancy, unspecified number of placenta and unspecified number of amniotic sacs, first trimester Ⓜ♀

    O30.002 Twin pregnancy, unspecified number of placenta and unspecified number of amniotic sacs, second trimester Ⓜ♀

    O30.003 Twin pregnancy, unspecified number of placenta and unspecified number of amniotic sacs, third trimester Ⓜ♀

    O30.009 Twin pregnancy, unspecified number of placenta and unspecified number of amniotic sacs, unspecified trimester Ⓜ♀

  ✓6ᵗʰ **O30.01** Twin pregnancy, monochorionic/monoamniotic

Twin pregnancy, one placenta, one amniotic sac

EXCLUDES 1 conjoined twins (O30.02-)

    O30.011 Twin pregnancy, monochorionic/ monoamniotic, first trimester Ⓜ♀

    O30.012 Twin pregnancy, monochorionic/ monoamniotic, second trimester Ⓜ♀

    O30.013 Twin pregnancy, monochorionic/ monoamniotic, third trimester Ⓜ♀

    O30.019 Twin pregnancy, monochorionic/ monoamniotic, unspecified trimester Ⓜ♀

  ✓6ᵗʰ **O30.02** Conjoined twin pregnancy

    O30.021 Conjoined twin pregnancy, first trimester Ⓜ♀

    O30.022 Conjoined twin pregnancy, second trimester Ⓜ♀

    O30.023 Conjoined twin pregnancy, third trimester Ⓜ♀

    O30.029 Conjoined twin pregnancy, unspecified trimester Ⓜ♀

  ✓6ᵗʰ **O30.03** Twin pregnancy, monochorionic/diamniotic

Twin pregnancy, one placenta, two amniotic sacs

    O30.031 Twin pregnancy, monochorionic/ diamniotic, first trimester Ⓜ♀

    O30.032 Twin pregnancy, monochorionic/ diamniotic, second trimester Ⓜ♀

    O30.033 Twin pregnancy, monochorionic/ diamniotic, third trimester Ⓜ♀

    O30.039 Twin pregnancy, monochorionic/ diamniotic, unspecified trimester Ⓜ♀

  ✓6ᵗʰ **O30.04** Twin pregnancy, dichorionic/diamniotic

Twin pregnancy, two placentae, two amniotic sacs

    O30.041 Twin pregnancy, dichorionic/ diamniotic, first trimester Ⓜ♀

    O30.042 Twin pregnancy, dichorionic/ diamniotic, second trimester Ⓜ♀

✓ Additional Character Required   ✓x7ᵗʰ Xtension Alert   Unspecified Code   Other Specified Code   Manifestation Code   ►◄ Revised Text   ● New Code   ▲ Revised Code Title

ICD-10-CM 2014 (Draft)   745

Pregnancy, Childbirth and the Puerperium

O30.043–O30.802

O30.043   Twin pregnancy, dichorionic/diamniotic, third trimester   Ⓜ♀

O30.049   Twin pregnancy, dichorionic/diamniotic, unspecified trimester   Ⓜ♀

√6ᵗʰ **O30.09**   Twin pregnancy, unable to determine number of placenta and number of amniotic sacs

O30.091   Twin pregnancy, unable to determine number of placenta and number of amniotic sacs, first trimester   Ⓜ♀

O30.092   Twin pregnancy, unable to determine number of placenta and number of amniotic sacs, second trimester   Ⓜ♀

O30.093   Twin pregnancy, unable to determine number of placenta and number of amniotic sacs, third trimester   Ⓜ♀

O30.099   Twin pregnancy, unable to determine number of placenta and number of amniotic sacs, unspecified trimester   Ⓜ♀

√5ᵗʰ **O30.1**   Triplet pregnancy, unspecified number of placenta and unspecified number of amniotic sacs

√6ᵗʰ **O30.10**   Triplet pregnancy, unspecified number of placenta and unspecified number of amniotic sacs

O30.101   Triplet pregnancy, unspecified number of placenta and unspecified number of amniotic sacs, first trimester   Ⓜ♀

O30.102   Triplet pregnancy, unspecified number of placenta and unspecified number of amniotic sacs, second trimester   Ⓜ♀

O30.103   Triplet pregnancy, unspecified number of placenta and unspecified number of amniotic sacs, third trimester   Ⓜ♀

O30.109   Triplet pregnancy, unspecified number of placenta and unspecified number of amniotic sacs, unspecified trimester   Ⓜ♀

√6ᵗʰ **O30.11**   Triplet pregnancy with two or more monochorionic fetuses

O30.111   Triplet pregnancy with two or more monochorionic fetuses, first trimester   Ⓜ♀

O30.112   Triplet pregnancy with two or more monochorionic fetuses, second trimester   Ⓜ♀

O30.113   Triplet pregnancy with two or more monochorionic fetuses, third trimester   Ⓜ♀

O30.119   Triplet pregnancy with two or more monochorionic fetuses, unspecified trimester   Ⓜ♀

√6ᵗʰ **O30.12**   Triplet pregnancy with two or more monoamniotic fetuses

O30.121   Triplet pregnancy with two or more monoamniotic fetuses, first trimester   Ⓜ♀

O30.122   Triplet pregnancy with two or more monoamniotic fetuses, second trimester   Ⓜ♀

O30.123   Triplet pregnancy with two or more monoamniotic fetuses, third trimester   Ⓜ♀

O30.129   Triplet pregnancy with two or more monoamniotic fetuses, unspecified trimester   Ⓜ♀

√6ᵗʰ **O30.19**   Triplet pregnancy, unable to determine number of placenta and number of amniotic sacs

O30.191   Triplet pregnancy, unable to determine number of placenta and number of amniotic sacs, first trimester   Ⓜ♀

O30.192   Triplet pregnancy, unable to determine number of placenta and number of amniotic sacs, second trimester   Ⓜ♀

O30.193   Triplet pregnancy, unable to determine number of placenta and number of amniotic sacs, third trimester   Ⓜ♀

O30.199   Triplet pregnancy, unable to determine number of placenta and number of amniotic sacs, unspecified trimester   Ⓜ♀

√6ᵗʰ **O30.2**   Quadruplet pregnancy

√6ᵗʰ **O30.20**   Quadruplet pregnancy, unspecified number of placenta and unspecified number of amniotic sacs

O30.201   Quadruplet pregnancy, unspecified number of placenta and unspecified number of amniotic sacs, first trimester   Ⓜ♀

O30.202   Quadruplet pregnancy, unspecified number of placenta and unspecified number of amniotic sacs, second trimester   Ⓜ♀

O30.203   Quadruplet pregnancy, unspecified number of placenta and unspecified number of amniotic sacs, third trimester   Ⓜ♀

O30.209   Quadruplet pregnancy, unspecified number of placenta and unspecified number of amniotic sacs, unspecified trimester   Ⓜ♀

√6ᵗʰ **O30.21**   Quadruplet pregnancy with two or more monochorionic fetuses

O30.211   Quadruplet pregnancy with two or more monochorionic fetuses, first trimester   Ⓜ♀

O30.212   Quadruplet pregnancy with two or more monochorionic fetuses, second trimester   Ⓜ♀

O30.213   Quadruplet pregnancy with two or more monochorionic fetuses, third trimester   Ⓜ♀

O30.219   Quadruplet pregnancy with two or more monochorionic fetuses, unspecified trimester   Ⓜ♀

√6ᵗʰ **O30.22**   Quadruplet pregnancy with two or more monoamniotic fetuses

O30.221   Quadruplet pregnancy with two or more monoamniotic fetuses, first trimester   Ⓜ♀

O30.222   Quadruplet pregnancy with two or more monoamniotic fetuses, second trimester   Ⓜ♀

O30.223   Quadruplet pregnancy with two or more monoamniotic fetuses, third trimester   Ⓜ♀

O30.229   Quadruplet pregnancy with two or more monoamniotic fetuses, unspecified trimester   Ⓜ♀

√6ᵗʰ **O30.29**   Quadruplet pregnancy, unable to determine number of placenta and number of amniotic sacs

O30.291   Quadruplet pregnancy, unable to determine number of placenta and number of amniotic sacs, first trimester   Ⓜ♀

O30.292   Quadruplet pregnancy, unable to determine number of placenta and number of amniotic sacs, second trimester   Ⓜ♀

O30.293   Quadruplet pregnancy, unable to determine number of placenta and number of amniotic sacs, third trimester   Ⓜ♀

O30.299   Quadruplet pregnancy, unable to determine number of placenta and number of amniotic sacs, unspecified   Ⓜ♀

√5ᵗʰ **O30.8**   Other specified multiple gestation
Multiple gestation pregnancy greater than quadruplets

√6ᵗʰ **O30.80**   Other specified multiple gestation, unspecified number of placenta and unspecified number of amniotic sacs

O30.801   Other specified multiple gestation, unspecified number of placenta and unspecified number of amniotic sacs, first trimester   Ⓜ♀

O30.802   Other specified multiple gestation, unspecified number of placenta and unspecified number of amniotic sacs, second trimester   Ⓜ♀

EXCLUDES 1 Not coded here   EXCLUDES 2 Not included here   Ⓝ Newborn Age: 0   Ⓟ Pediatric Age: 0-17   Ⓜ Maternity Age: 12-55   Ⓐ Adult Age: 15-124

746   ICD-10-CM 2014 (Draft)

O30.803 Other specified multiple gestation, unspecified number of placenta and unspecified number of amniotic sacs, third trimester Ⓜ♀

O30.809 Other specified multiple gestation, unspecified number of placenta and unspecified number of amniotic sacs, unspecified trimester Ⓜ♀

✓6th **O30.81** Other specified multiple gestation with two or more monochorionic fetuses

O30.811 Other specified multiple gestation with two or more monochorionic fetuses, first trimester Ⓜ♀

O30.812 Other specified multiple gestation with two or more monochorionic fetuses, second trimester Ⓜ♀

O30.813 Other specified multiple gestation with two or more monochorionic fetuses, third trimester Ⓜ♀

O30.819 Other specified multiple gestation with two or more monochorionic fetuses, unspecified trimester Ⓜ♀

✓6th **O30.82** Other specified multiple gestation with two or more monoamniotic fetuses

O30.821 Other specified multiple gestation with two or more monoamniotic fetuses, first trimester Ⓜ♀

O30.822 Other specified multiple gestation with two or more monoamniotic fetuses, second trimester Ⓜ♀

O30.823 Other specified multiple gestation with two or more monoamniotic fetuses, third trimester Ⓜ♀

O30.829 Other specified multiple gestation with two or more monoamniotic fetuses, unspecified trimester Ⓜ♀

✓6th **O30.89** Other specified multiple gestation, unable to determine number of placenta and number of amniotic sacs

O30.891 Other specified multiple gestation, unable to determine number of placenta and number of amniotic sacs, first trimester Ⓜ♀

O30.892 Other specified multiple gestation, unable to determine number of placenta and number of amniotic sacs, second trimester Ⓜ♀

O30.893 Other specified multiple gestation, unable to determine number of placenta and number of amniotic sacs, third trimester Ⓜ♀

O30.899 Other specified multiple gestation, unable to determine number of placenta and number of amniotic sacs, unspecified trimester Ⓜ♀

✓5th **O30.9** Multiple gestation, unspecified
Multiple pregnancy NOS

O30.90 Multiple gestation, unspecified, unspecified trimester Ⓜ♀

O30.91 Multiple gestation, unspecified, first trimester Ⓜ♀

O30.92 Multiple gestation, unspecified, second trimester Ⓜ♀

O30.93 Multiple gestation, unspecified, third trimester Ⓜ♀

✓4th **O31** Complications specific to multiple gestation
EXCLUDES 2 *delayed delivery of second twin, triplet, etc. (O63.2)*
malpresentation of one fetus or more (O32.9)
placental transfusion syndromes (O43.0-)
AHA: 2012, Q4, 107

One of the following 7th characters is to be assigned to each code under category O31. 7th character 0 is for single gestations and multiple gestations where the fetus is unspecified. 7th characters 1 through 9 are for cases of multiple gestations to identify the fetus for which the code applies. The appropriate code from category O30, Multiple gestation, must also be assigned when assigning a code from category O31 that has a 7th character of 1 through 9.
0   not applicable or unspecified   4   fetus 4
1   fetus 1   5   fetus 5
2   fetus 2   9   other fetus
3   fetus 3

✓5th **O31.0** Papyraceous fetus
Fetus compressus

✓x7th **O31.00** Papyraceous fetus, unspecified trimester Ⓜ♀

✓x7th **O31.01** Papyraceous fetus, first trimester Ⓜ♀

✓x7th **O31.02** Papyraceous fetus, second trimester Ⓜ♀

✓x7th **O31.03** Papyraceous fetus, third trimester Ⓜ♀

✓5th **O31.1** Continuing pregnancy after spontaneous abortion of one fetus or more

✓x7th **O31.10** Continuing pregnancy after spontaneous abortion of one fetus or more, unspecified trimester Ⓜ♀

✓x7th **O31.11** Continuing pregnancy after spontaneous abortion of one fetus or more, first trimester Ⓜ♀

✓x7th **O31.12** Continuing pregnancy after spontaneous abortion of one fetus or more, second trimester Ⓜ♀

✓x7th **O31.13** Continuing pregnancy after spontaneous abortion of one fetus or more, third trimester Ⓜ♀

✓5th **O31.2** Continuing pregnancy after intrauterine death of one fetus or more

✓x7th **O31.20** Continuing pregnancy after intrauterine death of one fetus or more, unspecified trimester Ⓜ♀

✓x7th **O31.21** Continuing pregnancy after intrauterine death of one fetus or more, first trimester Ⓜ♀

✓x7th **O31.22** Continuing pregnancy after intrauterine death of one fetus or more, second trimester Ⓜ♀

✓x7th **O31.23** Continuing pregnancy after intrauterine death of one fetus or more, third trimester Ⓜ♀

✓5th **O31.3** Continuing pregnancy after elective fetal reduction of one fetus or more
Continuing pregnancy after selective termination of one fetus or more

✓x7th **O31.30** Continuing pregnancy after elective fetal reduction of one fetus or more, unspecified trimester Ⓜ♀

✓x7th **O31.31** Continuing pregnancy after elective fetal reduction of one fetus or more, first trimester Ⓜ♀

✓x7th **O31.32** Continuing pregnancy after elective fetal reduction of one fetus or more, second trimester Ⓜ♀

✓x7th **O31.33** Continuing pregnancy after elective fetal reduction of one fetus or more, third trimester Ⓜ♀

✓5th **O31.8** Other complications specific to multiple gestation

✓6th **O31.8X** Other complications specific to multiple gestation

✓7th **O31.8X1** Other complications specific to multiple gestation, first trimester Ⓜ♀

✓7th **O31.8X2** Other complications specific to multiple gestation, second trimester Ⓜ♀

✓7th **O31.8X3** Other complications specific to multiple gestation, third trimester Ⓜ♀

✓7th **O31.8X9** Other complications specific to multiple gestation, unspecified trimester Ⓜ♀

Pregnancy, Childbirth and the Puerperium

O32–O34.01

✓4ᵗʰ O32 Maternal care for malpresentation of fetus

INCLUDES the listed conditions as a reason for observation, hospitalization or other obstetric care of the mother, or for cesarean delivery before onset of labor

EXCLUDES1 malpresentation of fetus with obstructed labor (O64.-)

AHA: 2012, Q4, 107

One of the following 7th characters is to be assigned to each code under category O32. 7th character Ø is for single gestations and multiple gestations where the fetus is unspecified. 7th characters 1 through 9 are for cases of multiple gestations to identify the fetus for which the code applies. The appropriate code from category O30, Multiple gestation, must also be assigned when assigning a code from category O32 that has a 7th character of 1 through 9.

Ø	not applicable or unspecified	4	fetus 4
1	fetus 1	5	fetus 5
2	fetus 2	9	other fetus
3	fetus 3		

✓x7ᵗʰ **O32.0 Maternal care for unstable lie** Ⓜ♀

✓x7ᵗʰ **O32.1 Maternal care for breech presentation** Ⓜ♀
Maternal care for buttocks presentation
Maternal care for complete breech
Maternal care for frank breech
EXCLUDES1 footling presentation (O32.8)
incomplete breech (O32.8)

✓x7ᵗʰ **O32.2 Maternal care for transverse and oblique lie** Ⓜ♀
Maternal care for oblique presentation
Maternal care for transverse presentation

✓x7ᵗʰ **O32.3 Maternal care for face, brow and chin presentation** Ⓜ♀

✓x7ᵗʰ **O32.4 Maternal care for high head at term** Ⓜ♀
Maternal care for failure of head to enter pelvic brim

✓x7ᵗʰ **O32.6 Maternal care for compound presentation** Ⓜ♀

✓x7ᵗʰ **O32.8 Maternal care for other malpresentation of fetus** Ⓜ♀
Maternal care for footling presentation
Maternal care for incomplete breech

✓x7ᵗʰ **O32.9 Maternal care for malpresentation of fetus, unspecified** Ⓜ♀

✓4ᵗʰ O33 Maternal care for disproportion

INCLUDES the listed conditions as a reason for observation, hospitalization or other obstetric care of the mother, or for cesarean delivery before onset of labor

EXCLUDES1 disproportion with obstructed labor (O65-O66)

O33.0 Maternal care for disproportion due to deformity of maternal pelvic bones Ⓜ♀
Maternal care for disproportion due to pelvic deformity causing disproportion NOS

O33.1 Maternal care for disproportion due to generally contracted pelvis Ⓜ♀
Maternal care for disproportion due to contracted pelvis NOS causing disproportion

O33.2 Maternal care for disproportion due to inlet contraction of pelvis Ⓜ♀
Maternal care for disproportion due to inlet contraction (pelvis) causing disproportion

✓x7ᵗʰ **O33.3 Maternal care for disproportion due to outlet contraction of pelvis** Ⓜ♀
Maternal care for disproportion due to mid-cavity contraction (pelvis)
Maternal care for disproportion due to outlet contraction (pelvis)

One of the following 7th characters is to be assigned to code O33.3. 7th character Ø is for single gestations and multiple gestations where the fetus is unspecified. 7th characters 1 through 9 are for cases of multiple gestations to identify the fetus for which the code applies. The appropriate code from category O30, Multiple gestation, must also be assigned when assigning code O33.3 with a 7th character of 1 through 9.

Ø	not applicable or unspecified	4	fetus 4
1	fetus 1	5	fetus 5
2	fetus 2	9	other fetus
3	fetus 3		

✓x7ᵗʰ O33.4 Maternal care for disproportion of mixed maternal and fetal origin Ⓜ♀

One of the following 7th characters is to be assigned to code O33.4. 7th character Ø is for single gestations and multiple gestations where the fetus is unspecified. 7th characters 1 through 9 are for cases of multiple gestations to identify the fetus for which the code applies. The appropriate code from category O30, Multiple gestation, must also be assigned when assigning code O33.4 with a 7th character of 1 through 9.

Ø	not applicable or unspecified	4	fetus 4
1	fetus 1	5	fetus 5
2	fetus 2	9	other fetus
3	fetus 3		

✓x7ᵗʰ O33.5 Maternal care for disproportion due to unusually large fetus Ⓜ♀

Maternal care for disproportion due to disproportion of fetal origin with normally formed fetus
Maternal care for disproportion due to fetal disproportion NOS

One of the following 7th characters is to be assigned to code O33.5. 7th character Ø is for single gestations and multiple gestations where the fetus is unspecified. 7th characters 1 through 9 are for cases of multiple gestations to identify the fetus for which the code applies. The appropriate code from category O30, Multiple gestation, must also be assigned when assigning code O33.5 with a 7th character of 1 through 9.

Ø	not applicable or unspecified	4	fetus 4
1	fetus 1	5	fetus 5
2	fetus 2	9	other fetus
3	fetus 3		

✓x7ᵗʰ O33.6 Maternal care for disproportion due to hydrocephalic fetus Ⓜ♀

One of the following 7th characters is to be assigned to code O33.6. 7th character Ø is for single gestations and multiple gestations where the fetus is unspecified. 7th characters 1 through 9 are for cases of multiple gestations to identify the fetus for which the code applies. The appropriate code from category O30, Multiple gestation, must also be assigned when assigning code O33.6 with a 7th character of 1 through 9.

Ø	not applicable or unspecified	4	fetus 4
1	fetus 1	5	fetus 5
2	fetus 2	9	other fetus
3	fetus 3		

O33.7 Maternal care for disproportion due to other fetal deformities Ⓜ♀
Maternal care for disproportion due to fetal ascites
Maternal care for disproportion due to fetal hydrops
Maternal care for disproportion due to fetal meningomyelocele
Maternal care for disproportion due to fetal sacral teratoma
Maternal care for disproportion due to fetal tumor
EXCLUDES1 obstructed labor due to other fetal deformities (O66.3)

O33.8 Maternal care for disproportion of other origin Ⓜ♀

O33.9 Maternal care for disproportion, unspecified Ⓜ♀
Maternal care for disproportion due to cephalopelvic disproportion NOS
Maternal care for disproportion due to fetopelvic disproportion NOS

✓4ᵗʰ O34 Maternal care for abnormality of pelvic organs

INCLUDES the listed conditions as a reason for hospitalization or other obstetric care of the mother, or for cesarean delivery before onset of labor

Code first any associated obstructed labor (O65.5)
Use additional code for specific condition

✓5ᵗʰ **O34.0 Maternal care for congenital malformation of uterus**

O34.00 Maternal care for unspecified congenital malformation of uterus, unspecified trimester Ⓜ♀

O34.01 Maternal care for unspecified congenital malformation of uterus, first trimester Ⓜ♀

EXCLUDES1 Not coded here   EXCLUDES2 Not included here   Ⓝ Newborn Age: 0   Ⓟ Pediatric Age: 0-17   Ⓜ Maternity Age: 12-55   Ⓐ Adult Age: 15-124

748   ICD-10-CM 2014 (Draft)

O34.02   Maternal care for unspecified congenital malformation of uterus, second trimester   Ⓜ♀

O34.03   Maternal care for unspecified congenital malformation of uterus, third trimester   Ⓜ♀

✓5ᵗʰ **O34.1**   Maternal care for benign tumor of corpus uteri

> *EXCLUDES 2*   maternal care for benign tumor of cervix (O34.4-)
> maternal care for malignant neoplasm of uterus (O9A.1-)

O34.10   Maternal care for benign tumor of corpus uteri, unspecified trimester   Ⓜ♀

O34.11   Maternal care for benign tumor of corpus uteri, first trimester   Ⓜ♀

O34.12   Maternal care for benign tumor of corpus uteri, second trimester   Ⓜ♀

O34.13   Maternal care for benign tumor of corpus uteri, third trimester   Ⓜ♀

✓5ᵗʰ **O34.2**   Maternal care due to uterine scar from previous surgery

O34.21   Maternal care for scar from previous cesarean delivery   Ⓜ♀

O34.29   Maternal care due to uterine scar from other previous surgery   Ⓜ♀

✓5ᵗʰ **O34.3**   Maternal care for cervical incompetence
> Maternal care for cerclage with or without cervical incompetence
> Maternal care for Shirodkar suture with or without cervical incompetence

O34.30   Maternal care for cervical incompetence, unspecified trimester   Ⓜ♀

O34.31   Maternal care for cervical incompetence, first trimester   Ⓜ♀

O34.32   Maternal care for cervical incompetence, second trimester   Ⓜ♀

O34.33   Maternal care for cervical incompetence, third trimester   Ⓜ♀

✓5ᵗʰ **O34.4**   Maternal care for other abnormalities of cervix

O34.40   Maternal care for other abnormalities of cervix, unspecified trimester   Ⓜ♀

O34.41   Maternal care for other abnormalities of cervix, first trimester   Ⓜ♀

O34.42   Maternal care for other abnormalities of cervix, second trimester   Ⓜ♀

O34.43   Maternal care for other abnormalities of cervix, third trimester   Ⓜ♀

✓5ᵗʰ **O34.5**   Maternal care for other abnormalities of gravid uterus

✓6ᵗʰ **O34.51**   Maternal care for incarceration of gravid uterus

O34.511   Maternal care for incarceration of gravid uterus, first trimester   Ⓜ♀

O34.512   Maternal care for incarceration of gravid uterus, second trimester   Ⓜ♀

O34.513   Maternal care for incarceration of gravid uterus, third trimester   Ⓜ♀

O34.519   Maternal care for incarceration of gravid uterus, unspecified trimester   Ⓜ♀

✓6ᵗʰ **O34.52**   Maternal care for prolapse of gravid uterus

O34.521   Maternal care for prolapse of gravid uterus, first trimester   Ⓜ♀

O34.522   Maternal care for prolapse of gravid uterus, second trimester   Ⓜ♀

O34.523   Maternal care for prolapse of gravid uterus, third trimester   Ⓜ♀

O34.529   Maternal care for prolapse of gravid uterus, unspecified trimester   Ⓜ♀

✓6ᵗʰ **O34.53**   Maternal care for retroversion of gravid uterus

O34.531   Maternal care for retroversion of gravid uterus, first trimester   Ⓜ♀

O34.532   Maternal care for retroversion of gravid uterus, second trimester   Ⓜ♀

O34.533   Maternal care for retroversion of gravid uterus, third trimester   Ⓜ♀

O34.539   Maternal care for retroversion of gravid uterus, unspecified trimester   Ⓜ♀

✓6ᵗʰ **O34.59**   Maternal care for other abnormalities of gravid uterus

O34.591   Maternal care for other abnormalities of gravid uterus, first trimester   Ⓜ♀

O34.592   Maternal care for other abnormalities of gravid uterus, second trimester   Ⓜ♀

O34.593   Maternal care for other abnormalities of gravid uterus, third trimester   Ⓜ♀

O34.599   Maternal care for other abnormalities of gravid uterus, unspecified trimester   Ⓜ♀

✓5ᵗʰ **O34.6**   Maternal care for abnormality of vagina

> *EXCLUDES 2*   maternal care for vaginal varices in pregnancy (O22.1-)

O34.60   Maternal care for abnormality of vagina, unspecified trimester   Ⓜ♀

O34.61   Maternal care for abnormality of vagina, first trimester   Ⓜ♀

O34.62   Maternal care for abnormality of vagina, second trimester   Ⓜ♀

O34.63   Maternal care for abnormality of vagina, third trimester   Ⓜ♀

✓5ᵗʰ **O34.7**   Maternal care for abnormality of vulva and perineum

> *EXCLUDES 2*   maternal care for perineal and vulval varices in pregnancy (O22.1-)

O34.70   Maternal care for abnormality of vulva and perineum, unspecified trimester   Ⓜ♀

O34.71   Maternal care for abnormality of vulva and perineum, first trimester   Ⓜ♀

O34.72   Maternal care for abnormality of vulva and perineum, second trimester   Ⓜ♀

O34.73   Maternal care for abnormality of vulva and perineum, third trimester   Ⓜ♀

✓5ᵗʰ **O34.8**   Maternal care for other abnormalities of pelvic organs

O34.80   Maternal care for other abnormalities of pelvic organs, unspecified trimester   Ⓜ♀

O34.81   Maternal care for other abnormalities of pelvic organs, first trimester   Ⓜ♀

O34.82   Maternal care for other abnormalities of pelvic organs, second trimester   Ⓜ♀

O34.83   Maternal care for other abnormalities of pelvic organs, third trimester   Ⓜ♀

✓5ᵗʰ **O34.9**   Maternal care for abnormality of pelvic organ, unspecified

O34.90   Maternal care for abnormality of pelvic organ, unspecified, unspecified trimester   Ⓜ♀

O34.91   Maternal care for abnormality of pelvic organ, unspecified, first trimester   Ⓜ♀

O34.92   Maternal care for abnormality of pelvic organ, unspecified, second trimester   Ⓜ♀

O34.93   Maternal care for abnormality of pelvic organ, unspecified, third trimester   Ⓜ♀

✓4ᵗʰ **O35**   **Maternal care for known or suspected fetal abnormality and damage**

> *INCLUDES*   the listed conditions in the fetus as a reason for hospitalization or other obstetric care to the mother, or for termination of pregnancy
>
> Code also any associated maternal condition
>
> *EXCLUDES 1*   encounter for suspected maternal and fetal conditions ruled out (Z03.7-)

> One of the following 7th characters is to be assigned to each code under category O35. 7th character 0 is for single gestations and multiple gestations where the fetus is unspecified. 7th characters 1 through 9 are for cases of multiple gestations to identify the fetus for which the code applies. The appropriate code from category O30, Multiple gestation, must also be assigned when assigning a code from category O35 that has a 7th character of 1 through 9.
> | | | | |
> |---|---|---|---|
> | 0 | not applicable or unspecified | 4 | fetus 4 |
> | 1 | fetus 1 | 5 | fetus 5 |
> | 2 | fetus 2 | 9 | other fetus |
> | 3 | fetus 3 | | |

✓x7ᵗʰ **O35.0**   Maternal care for (suspected) central nervous system malformation in fetus   Ⓜ♀
> Maternal care for fetal anencephaly
> Maternal care for fetal hydrocephalus
> Maternal care for fetal spina bifida
> *EXCLUDES 2*   chromosomal abnormality in fetus (O35.1)

✓x7ᵗʰ **O35.1**   Maternal care for (suspected) chromosomal abnormality in fetus   Ⓜ♀

✓x7ᵗʰ **O35.2**   Maternal care for (suspected) hereditary disease in fetus   Ⓜ♀
> *EXCLUDES 2*   chromosomal abnormality in fetus (O35.1)

✓x7ᵗʰ **O35.3**   Maternal care for (suspected) damage to fetus from viral disease in mother   Ⓜ♀
> Maternal care for damage to fetus from maternal cytomegalovirus infection
> Maternal care for damage to fetus from maternal rubella

☑ Additional Character Required   ✓x7ᵗʰ Xtension Alert   Unspecified Code   Other Specified Code   Manifestation Code   ▶◀ Revised Text   ● New Code   ▲ Revised Code Title

Pregnancy, Childbirth and the Puerperium

O35.4–O36.72

√x7th **O35.4 Maternal care for (suspected)** damage to fetus from alcohol   M♀

√x7th **O35.5 Maternal care for (suspected)** damage to fetus by drugs   M♀
Maternal care for damage to fetus from drug addiction

√x7th **O35.6 Maternal care for (suspected)** damage to fetus by radiation   M♀

√x7th **O35.7 Maternal care for (suspected)** damage to fetus by other medical procedures   M♀
Maternal care for damage to fetus by amniocentesis
Maternal care for damage to fetus by biopsy procedures
Maternal care for damage to fetus by hematological investigation
Maternal care for damage to fetus by intrauterine contraceptive device
Maternal care for damage to fetus by intrauterine surgery

√x7th **O35.8 Maternal care for other (suspected) fetal abnormality and damage**   M♀
Maternal care for damage to fetus from maternal listeriosis
Maternal care for damage to fetus from maternal toxoplasmosis

√x7th **O35.9 Maternal care for (suspected) fetal abnormality and damage, unspecified**   M♀

√4th **O36 Maternal care for other fetal problems**
INCLUDES the listed conditions in the fetus as a reason for hospitalization or other obstetric care of the mother, or for termination of pregnancy
EXCLUDES 1 encounter for suspected maternal and fetal conditions ruled out (Z03.7-)
placental transfusion syndromes (O43.0-)
EXCLUDES 2 labor and delivery complicated by fetal stress (O77.-)

One of the following 7th characters is to be assigned to each code under category O36. 7th character 0 is for single gestations and multiple gestations where the fetus is unspecified. 7th characters 1 through 9 are for cases of multiple gestations to identify the fetus for which the code applies. The appropriate code from category O30, Multiple gestation, must also be assigned when assigning a code from category O36 that has a 7th character of 1 through 9.
0   not applicable or unspecified   4   fetus 4
1   fetus 1   5   fetus 5
2   fetus 2   9   other fetus
3   fetus 3

√5th **O36.0 Maternal care for rhesus isoimmunization**
Maternal care for Rh incompatibility (with hydrops fetalis)

√6th **O36.01 Maternal care for** anti-D [Rh] antibodies
√7th **O36.011 Maternal care for anti-D [Rh] antibodies, first trimester**   M♀
√7th **O36.012 Maternal care for anti-D [Rh] antibodies, second trimester**   M♀
√7th **O36.013 Maternal care for anti-D [Rh] antibodies, third trimester**   M♀
√7th **O36.019 Maternal care for anti-D [Rh] antibodies, unspecified trimester**   M♀

√6th **O36.09 Maternal care for** other rhesus isoimmunization
√7th **O36.091 Maternal care for other rhesus isoimmunization, first trimester**   M♀
√7th **O36.092 Maternal care for other rhesus isoimmunization, second trimester**   M♀
√7th **O36.093 Maternal care for other rhesus isoimmunization, third trimester**   M♀
√7th **O36.099 Maternal care for other rhesus isoimmunization, unspecified trimester**   M♀

√5th **O36.1 Maternal care for other isoimmunization**
Maternal care for ABO isoimmunization

√6th **O36.11 Maternal care for** Anti-A sensitization
Maternal care for isoimmunization NOS (with hydrops fetalis)
√7th **O36.111 Maternal care for Anti-A sensitization, first trimester**   M♀
√7th **O36.112 Maternal care for Anti-A sensitization, second trimester**   M♀
√7th **O36.113 Maternal care for Anti-A sensitization, third trimester**   M♀
√7th **O36.119 Maternal care for Anti-A sensitization, unspecified trimester**   M♀

√6th **O36.19 Maternal care for** other isoimmunization
Maternal care for Anti-B sensitization
√7th **O36.191 Maternal care for other isoimmunization, first trimester**   M♀

√7th **O36.192 Maternal care for other isoimmunization, second trimester**   M♀
√7th **O36.193 Maternal care for other isoimmunization, third trimester**   M♀
√7th **O36.199 Maternal care for other isoimmunization, unspecified trimester**   M♀

√5th **O36.2 Maternal care for hydrops fetalis**
Maternal care for hydrops fetalis NOS
Maternal care for hydrops fetalis not associated with isoimmunization
EXCLUDES 1 hydrops fetalis associated with ABO isoimmunization (O36.1-)
hydrops fetalis associated with rhesus isoimmunization (O36.0-)
√x7th **O36.20 Maternal care for hydrops fetalis, unspecified trimester**   M♀
√x7th **O36.21 Maternal care for hydrops fetalis, first trimester**   M♀
√x7th **O36.22 Maternal care for hydrops fetalis, second trimester**   M♀
√x7th **O36.23 Maternal care for hydrops fetalis, third trimester**   M♀

√x7th **O36.4 Maternal care for intrauterine death**   M♀
Maternal care for intrauterine fetal death NOS
Maternal care for intrauterine fetal death after completion of 20 weeks of gestation
Maternal care for late fetal death
Maternal care for missed delivery
EXCLUDES 1 missed abortion (O02.1)
stillbirth (P95)

√5th **O36.5 Maternal care for known or suspected poor fetal growth**
√6th **O36.51 Maternal care for known or suspected placental insufficiency**
√7th **O36.511 Maternal care for known or suspected placental insufficiency, first trimester**   M♀
√7th **O36.512 Maternal care for known or suspected placental insufficiency, second trimester**   M♀
√7th **O36.513 Maternal care for known or suspected placental insufficiency, third trimester**   M♀
√7th **O36.519 Maternal care for known or suspected placental insufficiency, unspecified trimester**   M♀

√6th **O36.59 Maternal care for other known or suspected poor fetal growth**
Maternal care for known or suspected light-for-dates NOS
Maternal care for known or suspected small-for-dates NOS
√7th **O36.591 Maternal care for other known or suspected poor fetal growth, first trimester**   M♀
√7th **O36.592 Maternal care for other known or suspected poor fetal growth, second trimester**   M♀
√7th **O36.593 Maternal care for other known or suspected poor fetal growth, third trimester**   M♀
√7th **O36.599 Maternal care for other known or suspected poor fetal growth, unspecified trimester**   M♀

√5th **O36.6 Maternal care for excessive fetal growth**
Maternal care for known or suspected large-for-dates
√x7th **O36.60 Maternal care for excessive fetal growth, unspecified trimester**   M♀
√x7th **O36.61 Maternal care for excessive fetal growth, first trimester**   M♀
√x7th **O36.62 Maternal care for excessive fetal growth, second trimester**   M♀
√x7th **O36.63 Maternal care for excessive fetal growth, third trimester**   M♀

√5th **O36.7 Maternal care for viable fetus in abdominal pregnancy**
√x7th **O36.70 Maternal care for viable fetus in abdominal pregnancy, unspecified trimester**   M♀
√x7th **O36.71 Maternal care for viable fetus in abdominal pregnancy, first trimester**   M♀
√x7th **O36.72 Maternal care for viable fetus in abdominal pregnancy, second trimester**   M♀

✓x7ᵗʰ **O36.73 Maternal care for viable fetus in abdominal pregnancy, third trimester** �em♀

✓5ᵗʰ **O36.8 Maternal care for other specified fetal problems**

  ✓x7ᵗʰ **O36.80 Pregnancy with inconclusive fetal viability** �em♀
    Encounter to determine fetal viability of pregnancy

  ✓6ᵗʰ **O36.81 Decreased fetal movements**

    ✓7ᵗʰ **O36.812 Decreased fetal movements, second trimester** �em♀

    ✓7ᵗʰ **O36.813 Decreased fetal movements, third trimester** �em♀

    ✓7ᵗʰ **O36.819 Decreased fetal movements, unspecified trimester** �em♀

  ✓6ᵗʰ **O36.82 Fetal anemia and thrombocytopenia**

    ✓7ᵗʰ **O36.821 Fetal anemia and thrombocytopenia, first trimester** �em♀

    ✓7ᵗʰ **O36.822 Fetal anemia and thrombocytopenia, second trimester** �em♀

    ✓7ᵗʰ **O36.823 Fetal anemia and thrombocytopenia, third trimester** �em♀

    ✓7ᵗʰ **O36.829 Fetal anemia and thrombocytopenia, unspecified trimester** �em♀

  ✓6ᵗʰ **O36.89 Maternal care for other specified fetal problems**

    ✓7ᵗʰ **O36.891 Maternal care for other specified fetal problems, first trimester** �em♀

    ✓7ᵗʰ **O36.892 Maternal care for other specified fetal problems, second trimester** �em♀

    ✓7ᵗʰ **O36.893 Maternal care for other specified fetal problems, third trimester** �em♀

    ✓7ᵗʰ **O36.899 Maternal care for other specified fetal problems, unspecified trimester** �em♀

✓5ᵗʰ **O36.9 Maternal care for fetal problem, unspecified**

  ✓x7ᵗʰ **O36.90 Maternal care for fetal problem, unspecified, unspecified trimester** �em♀

  ✓x7ᵗʰ **O36.91 Maternal care for fetal problem, unspecified, first trimester** �em♀

  ✓x7ᵗʰ **O36.92 Maternal care for fetal problem, unspecified, second trimester** �em♀

  ✓x7ᵗʰ **O36.93 Maternal care for fetal problem, unspecified, third trimester** �em♀

✓4ᵗʰ **O40 Polyhydramnios**
Hydramnios
EXCLUDES 1 encounter for suspected maternal and fetal conditions ruled out (Z03.7-)

One of the following 7th characters is to be assigned to each code under category O40. 7th character 0 is for single gestations and multiple gestations where the fetus is unspecified. 7th characters 1 through 9 are for cases of multiple gestations to identify the fetus for which the code applies. The appropriate code from category O30, Multiple gestation, must also be assigned when assigning a code from category O40 that has a 7th character of 1 through 9.
0 not applicable or unspecified
1 fetus 1
2 fetus 2
3 fetus 3
4 fetus 4
5 fetus 5
9 other fetus

✓x7ᵗʰ **O40.1 Polyhydramnios, first trimester** �em♀

✓x7ᵗʰ **O40.2 Polyhydramnios, second trimester** �em♀

✓x7ᵗʰ **O40.3 Polyhydramnios, third trimester** �em♀

✓x7ᵗʰ **O40.9 Polyhydramnios, unspecified trimester** �em♀

✓4ᵗʰ **O41 Other disorders of amniotic fluid and membranes**
EXCLUDES 1 encounter for suspected maternal and fetal conditions ruled out (Z03.7-)

One of the following 7th characters is to be assigned to each code under category O41. 7th character 0 is for single gestations and multiple gestations where the fetus is unspecified. 7th characters 1 through 9 are for cases of multiple gestations to identify the fetus for which the code applies. The appropriate code from category O30, Multiple gestation, must also be assigned when assigning a code from category O41 that has a 7th character of 1 through 9.
0 not applicable or unspecified
1 fetus 1
2 fetus 2
3 fetus 3
4 fetus 4
5 fetus 5
9 other fetus

✓5ᵗʰ **O41.0 Oligohydramnios**
Oligohydramnios without rupture of membranes

✓x7ᵗʰ **O41.00 Oligohydramnios, unspecified trimester** �em♀

✓x7ᵗʰ **O41.01 Oligohydramnios, first trimester** �em♀

✓x7ᵗʰ **O41.02 Oligohydramnios, second trimester** �em♀

✓x7ᵗʰ **O41.03 Oligohydramnios, third trimester** �em♀

✓5ᵗʰ **O41.1 Infection of amniotic sac and membranes**

  ✓6ᵗʰ **O41.10 Infection of amniotic sac and membranes, unspecified**

    ✓7ᵗʰ **O41.101 Infection of amniotic sac and membranes, unspecified, first trimester** �em♀

    ✓7ᵗʰ **O41.102 Infection of amniotic sac and membranes, unspecified, second trimester** �em♀

    ✓7ᵗʰ **O41.103 Infection of amniotic sac and membranes, unspecified, third trimester** �em♀

    ✓7ᵗʰ **O41.109 Infection of amniotic sac and membranes, unspecified, unspecified trimester** �em♀

  ✓6ᵗʰ **O41.12 Chorioamnionitis**

    ✓7ᵗʰ **O41.121 Chorioamnionitis, first trimester** �em♀

    ✓7ᵗʰ **O41.122 Chorioamnionitis, second trimester** �em♀

    ✓7ᵗʰ **O41.123 Chorioamnionitis, third trimester** �em♀

    ✓7ᵗʰ **O41.129 Chorioamnionitis, unspecified trimester** �em♀

  ✓6ᵗʰ **O41.14 Placentitis**

    ✓7ᵗʰ **O41.141 Placentitis, first trimester** �em♀

    ✓7ᵗʰ **O41.142 Placentitis, second trimester** �em♀

    ✓7ᵗʰ **O41.143 Placentitis, third trimester** �em♀

    ✓7ᵗʰ **O41.149 Placentitis, unspecified trimester** �em♀

✓5ᵗʰ **O41.8 Other specified disorders of amniotic fluid and membranes**

  ✓6ᵗʰ **O41.8X Other specified disorders of amniotic fluid and membranes**

    ✓7ᵗʰ **O41.8X1 Other specified disorders of amniotic fluid and membranes, first trimester** �em♀

    ✓7ᵗʰ **O41.8X2 Other specified disorders of amniotic fluid and membranes, second trimester** �em♀

    ✓7ᵗʰ **O41.8X3 Other specified disorders of amniotic fluid and membranes, third trimester** �em♀

    ✓7ᵗʰ **O41.8X9 Other specified disorders of amniotic fluid and membranes, unspecified trimester** �em♀

✓5ᵗʰ **O41.9 Disorder of amniotic fluid and membranes, unspecified**

  ✓x7ᵗʰ **O41.90 Disorder of amniotic fluid and membranes, unspecified, unspecified trimester** �em♀

  ✓x7ᵗʰ **O41.91 Disorder of amniotic fluid and membranes, unspecified, first trimester** �em♀

  ✓x7ᵗʰ **O41.92 Disorder of amniotic fluid and membranes, unspecified, second trimester** �em♀

  ✓x7ᵗʰ **O41.93 Disorder of amniotic fluid and membranes, unspecified, third trimester** �em♀

✓4ᵗʰ **O42 Premature rupture of membranes**

✓5ᵗʰ **O42.0 Premature rupture of membranes, onset of labor within 24 hours of rupture**

  O42.00 Premature rupture of membranes, onset of labor within 24 hours of rupture, unspecified weeks of gestation �em♀

  ✓6ᵗʰ **O42.01 Preterm premature rupture of membranes, onset of labor within 24 hours of rupture**
    Premature rupture of membranes before 37 completed weeks of gestation

    O42.011 Preterm premature rupture of membranes, onset of labor within 24 hours of rupture, first trimester �em♀

    O42.012 Preterm premature rupture of membranes, onset of labor within 24 hours of rupture, second trimester �em♀

    O42.013 Preterm premature rupture of membranes, onset of labor within 24 hours of rupture, third trimester �em♀

    O42.019 Preterm premature rupture of membranes, onset of labor within 24 hours of rupture, unspecified trimester �em♀

O42.Ø2 Full-term premature rupture of membranes, onset of labor within 24 hours of rupture Ⓜ♀
Premature rupture of membranes after 37 completed weeks of gestation

✓5ᵗʰ **O42.1 Premature rupture of membranes,** onset of labor more than 24 hours following rupture

    O42.1Ø Premature rupture of membranes, onset of labor more than 24 hours following rupture, unspecified weeks of gestation Ⓜ♀

    ✓6ᵗʰ **O42.11 Preterm premature rupture of membranes, onset of labor more than 24 hours following rupture**
Premature rupture of membranes before 37 completed weeks of gestation

      O42.111 Preterm premature rupture of membranes, onset of labor more than 24 hours following rupture, first trimester Ⓜ♀

      O42.112 Preterm premature rupture of membranes, onset of labor more than 24 hours following rupture, second trimester Ⓜ♀

      O42.113 Preterm premature rupture of membranes, onset of labor more than 24 hours following rupture, third trimester Ⓜ♀

      O42.119 Preterm premature rupture of membranes, onset of labor more than 24 hours following rupture, unspecified trimester Ⓜ♀

    O42.12 Full-term premature rupture of membranes, onset of labor more than 24 hours following rupture Ⓜ♀
Premature rupture of membranes after 37 completed weeks of gestation

✓5ᵗʰ **O42.9 Premature rupture of membranes,** unspecified as to length of time between rupture and onset of labor

    O42.9Ø Premature rupture of membranes, unspecified as to length of time between rupture and onset of labor, unspecified weeks of gestation Ⓜ♀

    ✓6ᵗʰ **O42.91 Preterm premature rupture of membranes, unspecified as to length of time between rupture and onset of labor**
Premature rupture of membranes before 37 completed weeks of gestation

      O42.911 Preterm premature rupture of membranes, unspecified as to length of time between rupture and onset of labor, first trimester Ⓜ♀

      O42.912 Preterm premature rupture of membranes, unspecified as to length of time between rupture and onset of labor, second trimester Ⓜ♀

      O42.913 Preterm premature rupture of membranes, unspecified as to length of time between rupture and onset of labor, third trimester Ⓜ♀

      O42.919 Preterm premature rupture of membranes, unspecified as to length of time between rupture and onset of labor, unspecified trimester Ⓜ♀

    O42.92 Full-term premature rupture of membranes, unspecified as to length of time between rupture and onset of labor Ⓜ♀
Premature rupture of membranes after 37 completed weeks of gestation

✓4ᵗʰ **O43 Placental disorders**
EXCLUDES 2   maternal care for poor fetal growth due to placental insufficiency (O36.5-)
placenta previa (O44.-)
placental polyp (O9Ø.89)
placentitis (O41.14-)
premature separation of placenta [abruptio placentae] (O45.-)

✓5ᵗʰ **O43.Ø Placental transfusion syndromes**

    ✓6ᵗʰ **O43.Ø1 Fetomaternal placental transfusion syndrome**
Maternofetal placental transfusion syndrome

      O43.Ø11 Fetomaternal placental transfusion syndrome, first trimester Ⓜ♀

      O43.Ø12 Fetomaternal placental transfusion syndrome, second trimester Ⓜ♀

      O43.Ø13 Fetomaternal placental transfusion syndrome, third trimester Ⓜ♀

      O43.Ø19 Fetomaternal placental transfusion syndrome, unspecified trimester Ⓜ♀

    ✓6ᵗʰ **O43.Ø2 Fetus-to-fetus placental transfusion syndrome**

      O43.Ø21 Fetus-to-fetus placental transfusion syndrome, first trimester Ⓜ♀

      O43.Ø22 Fetus-to-fetus placental transfusion syndrome, second trimester Ⓜ♀

      O43.Ø23 Fetus-to-fetus placental transfusion syndrome, third trimester Ⓜ♀

      O43.Ø29 Fetus-to-fetus placental transfusion syndrome, unspecified trimester Ⓜ♀

✓5ᵗʰ **O43.1 Malformation of placenta**

    ✓6ᵗʰ **O43.1Ø Malformation of placenta,** unspecified
Abnormal placenta NOS

      O43.1Ø1 Malformation of placenta, unspecified, first trimester Ⓜ♀

      O43.1Ø2 Malformation of placenta, unspecified, second trimester Ⓜ♀

      O43.1Ø3 Malformation of placenta, unspecified third trimester Ⓜ♀

      O43.1Ø9 Malformation of placenta, unspecified, unspecified trimester Ⓜ♀

    ✓6ᵗʰ **O43.11 Circumvallate placenta**

      O43.111 Circumvallate placenta, first trimester Ⓜ♀

      O43.112 Circumvallate placenta, second trimester Ⓜ♀

      O43.113 Circumvallate placenta, third trimester Ⓜ♀

      O43.119 Circumvallate placenta, unspecified trimester Ⓜ♀

    ✓6ᵗʰ **O43.12 Velamentous insertion of umbilical cord**

      O43.121 Velamentous insertion of umbilical cord, first trimester Ⓜ♀

      O43.122 Velamentous insertion of umbilical cord, second trimester Ⓜ♀

      O43.123 Velamentous insertion of umbilical cord, third trimester Ⓜ♀

      O43.129 Velamentous insertion of umbilical cord, unspecified trimester Ⓜ♀

    ✓6ᵗʰ **O43.19 Other malformation of placenta**

      O43.191 Other malformation of placenta, first trimester Ⓜ♀

      O43.192 Other malformation of placenta, second trimester Ⓜ♀

      O43.193 Other malformation of placenta, third trimester Ⓜ♀

      O43.199 Other malformation of placenta, unspecified trimester Ⓜ♀

✓5ᵗʰ **O43.2 Morbidly adherent placenta**
Code also associated third stage postpartum hemorrhage, if applicable (O72.Ø)
EXCLUDES 1   retained placenta (O73.-)

    ✓6ᵗʰ **O43.21 Placenta accreta**

      O43.211 Placenta accreta, first trimester Ⓜ♀

      O43.212 Placenta accreta, second trimester Ⓜ♀

      O43.213 Placenta accreta, third trimester Ⓜ♀

      O43.219 Placenta accreta, unspecified trimester Ⓜ♀

    ✓6ᵗʰ **O43.22 Placenta increta**

      O43.221 Placenta increta, first trimester Ⓜ♀

      O43.222 Placenta increta, second trimester Ⓜ♀

      O43.223 Placenta increta, third trimester Ⓜ♀

      O43.229 Placenta increta, unspecified trimester Ⓜ♀

    ✓6ᵗʰ **O43.23 Placenta percreta**

      O43.231 Placenta percreta, first trimester Ⓜ♀

      O43.232 Placenta percreta, second trimester Ⓜ♀

      O43.233 Placenta percreta, third trimester Ⓜ♀

      O43.239 Placenta percreta, unspecified trimester Ⓜ♀

✓5ᵗʰ **O43.8 Other placental disorders**

    ✓6ᵗʰ **O43.81 Placental infarction**

      O43.811 Placental infarction, first trimester Ⓜ♀

      O43.812 Placental infarction, second trimester Ⓜ♀

      O43.813 Placental infarction, third trimester Ⓜ♀

      O43.819 Placental infarction, unspecified trimester Ⓜ♀

EXCLUDES 1 Not coded here   EXCLUDES 2 Not included here   Ⓝ Newborn Age: Ø   Ⓟ Pediatric Age: Ø-17   Ⓜ Maternity Age: 12-55   Ⓐ Adult Age: 15-124

752   ICD-1Ø-CM 2Ø14 (Draft)

√6ᵗʰ **O43.89 Other placental disorders**
Placental dysfunction

O43.891 **Other placental disorders, first trimester** ♂♀

O43.892 **Other placental disorders, second trimester** ♂♀

O43.893 **Other placental disorders, third trimester** ♂♀

O43.899 **Other placental disorders, unspecified trimester** ♂♀

√5ᵗʰ **O43.9 Unspecified placental disorder**

O43.90 **Unspecified placental disorder, unspecified trimester** ♂♀

O43.91 **Unspecified placental disorder, first trimester** ♂♀

O43.92 **Unspecified placental disorder, second trimester** ♂♀

O43.93 **Unspecified placental disorder, third trimester** ♂♀

√4ᵗʰ **O44 Placenta previa**

√5ᵗʰ **O44.0 Placenta previa specified as without hemorrhage**
Low implantation of placenta specified as without hemorrhage

O44.00 **Placenta previa specified as without hemorrhage, unspecified trimester** ♂♀

O44.01 **Placenta previa specified as without hemorrhage, first trimester** ♂♀

O44.02 **Placenta previa specified as without hemorrhage, second trimester** ♂♀

O44.03 **Placenta previa specified as without hemorrhage, third trimester** ♂♀

√5ᵗʰ **O44.1 Placenta previa with hemorrhage**
Low implantation of placenta, NOS or with hemorrhage
Marginal placenta previa, NOS or with hemorrhage
Partial placenta previa, NOS or with hemorrhage
Total placenta previa, NOS or with hemorrhage
EXCLUDES 1 *labor and delivery complicated by hemorrhage from vasa previa (O69.4)*

O44.10 **Placenta previa with hemorrhage, unspecified trimester** ♂♀

O44.11 **Placenta previa with hemorrhage, first trimester** ♂♀

O44.12 **Placenta previa with hemorrhage, second trimester** ♂♀

O44.13 **Placenta previa with hemorrhage, third trimester** ♂♀

√4ᵗʰ **O45 Premature separation of placenta [abruptio placentae]**

√5ᵗʰ **O45.0 Premature separation of placenta with coagulation defect**

√6ᵗʰ **O45.00 Premature separation of placenta with coagulation defect, unspecified**

O45.001 **Premature separation of placenta with coagulation defect, unspecified, first trimester** ♂♀

O45.002 **Premature separation of placenta with coagulation defect, unspecified, second trimester** ♂♀

O45.003 **Premature separation of placenta with coagulation defect, unspecified, third trimester** ♂♀

O45.009 **Premature separation of placenta with coagulation defect, unspecified, unspecified trimester** ♂♀

√6ᵗʰ **O45.01 Premature separation of placenta with afibrinogenemia**
Premature separation of placenta with hypofibrinogenemia

O45.011 **Premature separation of placenta with afibrinogenemia, first trimester** ♂♀

O45.012 **Premature separation of placenta with afibrinogenemia, second trimester** ♂♀

O45.013 **Premature separation of placenta with afibrinogenemia, third trimester** ♂♀

O45.019 **Premature separation of placenta with afibrinogenemia, unspecified trimester** ♂♀

√6ᵗʰ **O45.02 Premature separation of placenta with disseminated intravascular coagulation**

O45.021 **Premature separation of placenta with disseminated intravascular coagulation, first trimester** ♂♀

O45.022 **Premature separation of placenta with disseminated intravascular coagulation, second trimester** ♂♀

O45.023 **Premature separation of placenta with disseminated intravascular coagulation, third trimester** ♂♀

O45.029 **Premature separation of placenta with disseminated intravascular coagulation, unspecified trimester** ♂♀

√6ᵗʰ **O45.09 Premature separation of placenta with other coagulation defect**

O45.091 **Premature separation of placenta with other coagulation defect, first trimester** ♂♀

O45.092 **Premature separation of placenta with other coagulation defect, second trimester** ♂♀

O45.093 **Premature separation of placenta with other coagulation defect, third trimester** ♂♀

O45.099 **Premature separation of placenta with other coagulation defect, unspecified trimester** ♂♀

√5ᵗʰ **O45.8 Other premature separation of placenta**

√6ᵗʰ **O45.8X Other premature separation of placenta**

O45.8X1 **Other premature separation of placenta, first trimester** ♂♀

O45.8X2 **Other premature separation of placenta, second trimester** ♂♀

O45.8X3 **Other premature separation of placenta, third trimester** ♂♀

O45.8X9 **Other premature separation of placenta, unspecified trimester** ♂♀

√5ᵗʰ **O45.9 Premature separation of placenta, unspecified**
Abruptio placentae NOS

O45.90 **Premature separation of placenta, unspecified, unspecified trimester** ♂♀

O45.91 **Premature separation of placenta, unspecified, first trimester** ♂♀

O45.92 **Premature separation of placenta, unspecified, second trimester** ♂♀

O45.93 **Premature separation of placenta, unspecified, third trimester** ♂♀

√4ᵗʰ **O46 Antepartum hemorrhage, not elsewhere classified**
EXCLUDES 1 *hemorrhage in early pregnancy (O20.-)*
intrapartum hemorrhage NEC (O67.-)
placenta previa (O44.-)
premature separation of placenta [abruptio placentae] (O45.-)

√5ᵗʰ **O46.0 Antepartum hemorrhage with coagulation defect**

√6ᵗʰ **O46.00 Antepartum hemorrhage with coagulation defect, unspecified**

O46.001 **Antepartum hemorrhage with coagulation defect, unspecified, first trimester** ♂♀

O46.002 **Antepartum hemorrhage with coagulation defect, unspecified, second trimester** ♂♀

O46.003 **Antepartum hemorrhage with coagulation defect, unspecified, third trimester** ♂♀

O46.009 **Antepartum hemorrhage with coagulation defect, unspecified, unspecified trimester** ♂♀

√6ᵗʰ **O46.01 Antepartum hemorrhage with afibrinogenemia**
Antepartum hemorrhage with hypofibrinogenemia

O46.011 **Antepartum hemorrhage with afibrinogenemia, first trimester** ♂♀

O46.012 **Antepartum hemorrhage with afibrinogenemia, second trimester** ♂♀

O46.013 **Antepartum hemorrhage with afibrinogenemia, third trimester** ♂♀

O46.019 **Antepartum hemorrhage with afibrinogenemia, unspecified trimester** ♂♀

√6ᵗʰ **O46.02 Antepartum hemorrhage with disseminated intravascular coagulation**

O46.021 **Antepartum hemorrhage with disseminated intravascular coagulation, first trimester** ♂♀

✔ Additional Character Required   √x7ᵗʰ *Xtension Alert*   Unspecified Code   Other Specified Code   Manifestation Code   ►◄ Revised Text   ● New Code   ▲ Revised Code Title

O46.022 **Antepartum hemorrhage with disseminated intravascular coagulation, second trimester** Ⓜ♀

O46.023 **Antepartum hemorrhage with disseminated intravascular coagulation, third trimester** Ⓜ♀

O46.029 **Antepartum hemorrhage with disseminated intravascular coagulation, unspecified trimester** Ⓜ♀

✓6ᵗʰ O46.09 **Antepartum hemorrhage with** other **coagulation defect**

O46.091 **Antepartum hemorrhage with other coagulation defect,** first trimester Ⓜ♀

O46.092 **Antepartum hemorrhage with other coagulation defect,** second trimester Ⓜ♀

O46.093 **Antepartum hemorrhage with other coagulation defect,** third trimester Ⓜ♀

O46.099 **Antepartum hemorrhage with other coagulation defect, unspecified trimester** Ⓜ♀

✓5ᵗʰ O46.8 **Other antepartum hemorrhage**

✓6ᵗʰ O46.8X **Other** antepartum hemorrhage

O46.8X1 **Other antepartum hemorrhage,** first trimester Ⓜ♀

O46.8X2 **Other antepartum hemorrhage,** second trimester Ⓜ♀

O46.8X3 **Other antepartum hemorrhage,** third trimester Ⓜ♀

O46.8X9 **Other antepartum hemorrhage, unspecified trimester** Ⓜ♀

✓5ᵗʰ O46.9 **Antepartum hemorrhage,** unspecified

O46.90 **Antepartum hemorrhage, unspecified, unspecified trimester** Ⓜ♀

O46.91 **Antepartum hemorrhage, unspecified,** first trimester Ⓜ♀

O46.92 **Antepartum hemorrhage, unspecified,** second trimester Ⓜ♀

O46.93 **Antepartum hemorrhage, unspecified,** third trimester Ⓜ♀

✓4ᵗʰ **O47 False labor**
Braxton Hicks contractions
Threatened labor
EXCLUDES1 *preterm labor (O60.-)*

✓5ᵗʰ O47.0 **False labor** before 37 completed weeks of gestation

O47.00 **False labor before 37 completed weeks of gestation, unspecified trimester** Ⓜ♀

O47.02 **False labor before 37 completed weeks of gestation,** second trimester Ⓜ♀

O47.03 **False labor before 37 completed weeks of gestation,** third trimester Ⓜ♀

O47.1 **False labor** at or after 37 completed weeks of gestation Ⓜ♀

O47.9 **False labor, unspecified** Ⓜ♀

✓4ᵗʰ **O48 Late pregnancy**

O48.0 **Post-term pregnancy** Ⓜ♀
Pregnancy over 40 completed weeks to 42 completed weeks gestation

O48.1 **Prolonged pregnancy** Ⓜ♀
Pregnancy which has advanced beyond 42 completed weeks gestation

Complications of labor and delivery (O60-O77)

✓4ᵗʰ **O60 Preterm labor**
INCLUDES onset (spontaneous) of labor before 37 completed weeks of gestation
EXCLUDES1 *false labor (O47.0-)*
threatened labor NOS (O47.0-)

✓5ᵗʰ O60.0 **Preterm labor** without delivery

O60.00 **Preterm labor without delivery, unspecified trimester** Ⓜ♀

O60.02 **Preterm labor without delivery,** second trimester Ⓜ♀

O60.03 **Preterm labor without delivery,** third trimester Ⓜ♀

✓5ᵗʰ O60.1 **Preterm labor** with preterm delivery

One of the following 7th characters is to be assigned to each code under subcategory O60.1. 7th character 0 is for single gestations and multiple gestations where the fetus is unspecified. 7th characters 1 through 9 are for cases of multiple gestations to identify the fetus for which the code applies. The appropriate code from category O30, Multiple gestation, must also be assigned when assigning a code from subcategory O60.1 that has a 7th character of 1 through 9.
0	not applicable or unspecified	4	fetus 4
1	fetus 1	5	fetus 5
2	fetus 2	9	other fetus
3	fetus 3		

✓x7ᵗʰ O60.10 **Preterm labor with preterm delivery, unspecified trimester** Ⓜ♀
Preterm labor with delivery NOS

✓x7ᵗʰ O60.12 **Preterm labor** second **trimester with preterm delivery** second trimester Ⓜ♀

✓x7ᵗʰ O60.13 **Preterm labor** second **trimester with preterm delivery** third trimester Ⓜ♀

✓x7ᵗʰ O60.14 **Preterm labor** third **trimester with preterm delivery** third trimester Ⓜ♀

✓5ᵗʰ O60.2 **Term delivery with preterm labor**

One of the following 7th characters is to be assigned to each code under subcategory O60.2. 7th character 0 is for single gestations and multiple gestations where the fetus is unspecified. 7th characters 1 through 9 are for cases of multiple gestations to identify the fetus for which the code applies. The appropriate code from category O30, Multiple gestation, must also be assigned when assigning a code from subcategory O60.2 that has a 7th character of 1 through 9.
0	not applicable or unspecified	4	fetus 4
1	fetus 1	5	fetus 5
2	fetus 2	9	other fetus
3	fetus 3		

✓x7ᵗʰ O60.20 **Term delivery with preterm labor, unspecified trimester** Ⓜ♀

✓x7ᵗʰ O60.22 **Term delivery with preterm labor,** second trimester Ⓜ♀

✓x7ᵗʰ O60.23 **Term delivery with preterm labor,** third trimester Ⓜ♀

✓4ᵗʰ **O61 Failed induction of labor**

O61.0 **Failed** medical **induction of labor** Ⓜ♀
Failed induction (of labor) by oxytocin
Failed induction (of labor) by prostaglandins

O61.1 **Failed** instrumental **induction of labor** Ⓜ♀
Failed mechanical induction (of labor)
Failed surgical induction (of labor)

O61.8 **Other failed induction of labor** Ⓜ♀

O61.9 **Failed induction of labor, unspecified** Ⓜ♀

✓4ᵗʰ **O62 Abnormalities of forces of labor**

O62.0 **Primary inadequate contractions** Ⓜ♀
Failure of cervical dilatation
Primary hypotonic uterine dysfunction
Uterine inertia during latent phase of labor

O62.1 **Secondary uterine inertia** Ⓜ♀
Arrested active phase of labor
Secondary hypotonic uterine dysfunction

O62.2 **Other uterine inertia** Ⓜ♀
Atony of uterus without hemorrhage
Atony of uterus NOS
Desultory labor
Hypotonic uterine dysfunction NOS
Irregular labor
Poor contractions
Slow slope active phase of labor
Uterine inertia NOS
EXCLUDES1 *atony of uterus with hemorrhage (postpartum) (O72.1)*
postpartum atony of uterus without hemorrhage (O75.89)

O62.3 **Precipitate labor** Ⓜ♀

EXCLUDES1 Not coded here   EXCLUDES2 Not included here   Ⓝ Newborn Age: 0   Ⓟ Pediatric Age: 0-17   Ⓜ Maternity Age: 12-55   Ⓐ Adult Age: 15-124

754   ICD-10-CM 2014 (Draft)

O62.4 Hypertonic, incoordinate, and prolonged uterine contractions Ⓜ♀
Cervical spasm
Contraction ring dystocia
Dyscoordinate labor
Hour-glass contraction of uterus
Hypertonic uterine dysfunction
Incoordinate uterine action
Tetanic contractions
Uterine dystocia NOS
Uterine spasm
EXCLUDES 1 *dystocia (fetal) (maternal) NOS (O66.9)*

O62.8 Other abnormalities of forces of labor Ⓜ♀

O62.9 Abnormality of forces of labor, unspecified Ⓜ♀

✓4ᵗʰ **O63 Long labor**

O63.0 Prolonged first stage (of labor) Ⓜ♀

O63.1 Prolonged second stage (of labor) Ⓜ♀

O63.2 Delayed delivery of second twin, triplet, etc. Ⓜ♀

O63.9 Long labor, unspecified Ⓜ♀
Prolonged labor NOS

✓4ᵗʰ **O64 Obstructed labor due to malposition and malpresentation of fetus**

> One of the following 7th characters is to be assigned to each code under category O64. 7th character 0 is for single gestations and multiple gestations where the fetus is unspecified. 7th characters 1 through 9 are for cases of multiple gestations to identify the fetus for which the code applies. The appropriate code from category O30, Multiple gestation, must also be assigned when assigning a code from category O64 that has a 7th character of 1 through 9.
> 0 not applicable or unspecified 4 fetus 4
> 1 fetus 1 5 fetus 5
> 2 fetus 2 9 other fetus
> 3 fetus 3

✓x7ᵗʰ **O64.0 Obstructed labor due to incomplete rotation of fetal head** Ⓜ♀
Deep transverse arrest
Obstructed labor due to persistent occipitoiliac (position)
Obstructed labor due to persistent occipitoposterior (position)
Obstructed labor due to persistent occipitosacral (position)
Obstructed labor due to persistent occipitotransverse (position)

✓x7ᵗʰ **O64.1 Obstructed labor due to breech presentation** Ⓜ♀
Obstructed labor due to buttocks presentation
Obstructed labor due to complete breech presentation
Obstructed labor due to frank breech presentation

✓x7ᵗʰ **O64.2 Obstructed labor due to face presentation** Ⓜ♀
Obstructed labor due to chin presentation

✓x7ᵗʰ **O64.3 Obstructed labor due to brow presentation** Ⓜ♀

✓x7ᵗʰ **O64.4 Obstructed labor due to shoulder presentation** Ⓜ♀
Prolapsed arm
EXCLUDES 1 *impacted shoulders (O66.0)*
shoulder dystocia (O66.0)

✓x7ᵗʰ **O64.5 Obstructed labor due to compound presentation** Ⓜ♀

✓x7ᵗʰ **O64.8 Obstructed labor due to other malposition and malpresentation** Ⓜ♀
Obstructed labor due to footling presentation
Obstructed labor due to incomplete breech presentation

✓x7ᵗʰ **O64.9 Obstructed labor due to malposition and malpresentation, unspecified** Ⓜ♀

✓4ᵗʰ **O65 Obstructed labor due to maternal pelvic abnormality**

O65.0 Obstructed labor due to deformed pelvis Ⓜ♀

O65.1 Obstructed labor due to generally contracted pelvis Ⓜ♀

O65.2 Obstructed labor due to pelvic inlet contraction Ⓜ♀

O65.3 Obstructed labor due to pelvic outlet and mid-cavity contraction Ⓜ♀

O65.4 Obstructed labor due to fetopelvic disproportion, unspecified Ⓜ♀
EXCLUDES 1 *dystocia due to abnormality of fetus (O66.2-O66.3)*

O65.5 Obstructed labor due to abnormality of maternal pelvic organs Ⓜ♀
Obstructed labor due to conditions listed in O34-
Use additional code to identify abnormality of pelvic organs (O34.-)

O65.8 Obstructed labor due to other maternal pelvic abnormalities Ⓜ♀

O65.9 Obstructed labor due to maternal pelvic abnormality, unspecified Ⓜ♀

✓4ᵗʰ **O66 Other obstructed labor**

O66.0 Obstructed labor due to shoulder dystocia Ⓜ♀
Impacted shoulders

O66.1 Obstructed labor due to locked twins Ⓜ♀

O66.2 Obstructed labor due to unusually large fetus Ⓜ♀

O66.3 Obstructed labor due to other abnormalities of fetus Ⓜ♀
Dystocia due to fetal ascites
Dystocia due to fetal hydrops
Dystocia due to fetal meningomyelocele
Dystocia due to fetal sacral teratoma
Dystocia due to fetal tumor
Dystocia due to hydrocephalic fetus
Use additional code to identify cause of obstruction

✓5ᵗʰ **O66.4 Failed trial of labor**

O66.40 Failed trial of labor, unspecified Ⓜ♀

O66.41 Failed attempted vaginal birth after previous cesarean delivery Ⓜ♀
Code first rupture of uterus, if applicable (O71.0-, O71.1)

O66.5 Attempted application of vacuum extractor and forceps Ⓜ♀
Attempted application of vacuum or forceps, with subsequent delivery by forceps or cesarean delivery

O66.6 Obstructed labor due to other multiple fetuses Ⓜ♀

O66.8 Other specified obstructed labor Ⓜ♀
Use additional code to identify cause of obstruction

O66.9 Obstructed labor, unspecified Ⓜ♀
Dystocia NOS
Fetal dystocia NOS
Maternal dystocia NOS

✓4ᵗʰ **O67 Labor and delivery complicated by intrapartum hemorrhage, not elsewhere classified**
EXCLUDES 1 *antepartum hemorrhage NEC (O46.-)*
placenta previa (O44.-)
premature separation of placenta [abruptio placentae] (O45.-)
EXCLUDES 2 *postpartum hemorrhage (O72.-)*

O67.0 Intrapartum hemorrhage with coagulation defect Ⓜ♀
Intrapartum hemorrhage (excessive) associated with afibrinogenemia
Intrapartum hemorrhage (excessive) associated with disseminated intravascular coagulation
Intrapartum hemorrhage (excessive) associated with hyperfibrinolysis
Intrapartum hemorrhage (excessive) associated with hypofibrinogenemia

O67.8 Other intrapartum hemorrhage Ⓜ♀
Excessive intrapartum hemorrhage

O67.9 Intrapartum hemorrhage, unspecified Ⓜ♀

O68 Labor and delivery complicated by abnormality of fetal acid-base balance Ⓜ♀
Fetal acidemia complicating labor and delivery
Fetal acidosis complicating labor and delivery
Fetal alkalosis complicating labor and delivery
Fetal metabolic acidemia complicating labor and delivery
EXCLUDES 1 *fetal stress NOS (O77.9)*
labor and delivery complicated by electrocardiographic evidence of fetal stress (O77.8)
labor and delivery complicated by ultrasonic evidence of fetal stress (O77.8)
EXCLUDES 2 *abnormality in fetal heart rate or rhythm (O76)*
labor and delivery complicated by meconium in amniotic fluid (O77.0)

✓4ᵗʰ **O69 Labor and delivery complicated by umbilical cord complications**

> One of the following 7th characters is to be assigned to each code under category O69. 7th character 0 is for single gestations and multiple gestations where the fetus is unspecified. 7th characters 1 through 9 are for cases of multiple gestations to identify the fetus for which the code applies. The appropriate code from category O30, Multiple gestation, must also be assigned when assigning a code from category O69 that has a 7th character of 1 through 9.
> 0 not applicable or unspecified 3 fetus 3
>   4 fetus 4
> 1 fetus 1 5 fetus 5
> 2 fetus 2 9 other fetus

✓x7ᵗʰ **O69.0 Labor and delivery complicated by prolapse of cord** Ⓜ♀

✓x7ᵗʰ **O69.1 Labor and delivery complicated by cord around neck, with compression** Ⓜ♀
EXCLUDES 1 *labor and delivery complicated by cord around neck, without compression (O69.81)*

Pregnancy, Childbirth and the Puerperium

O69.2–O74.1

√x7ᵗʰ **O69.2 Labor and delivery complicated by other cord entanglement, with compression** Ⓜ♀
Labor and delivery complicated by compression of cord NOS
Labor and delivery complicated by entanglement of cords of twins in monoamniotic sac
Labor and delivery complicated by knot in cord
EXCLUDES 1 *labor and delivery complicated by other cord entanglement, without compression (O69.82)*

√x7ᵗʰ **O69.3 Labor and delivery complicated by short cord** Ⓜ♀

√x7ᵗʰ **O69.4 Labor and delivery complicated by vasa previa** Ⓜ♀
Labor and delivery complicated by hemorrhage from vasa previa

√x7ᵗʰ **O69.5 Labor and delivery complicated by vascular lesion of cord** Ⓜ♀
Labor and delivery complicated by cord bruising
Labor and delivery complicated by cord hematoma
Labor and delivery complicated by thrombosis of umbilical vessels

√5ᵗʰ **O69.8 Labor and delivery complicated by other cord complications**

√x7ᵗʰ **O69.81 Labor and delivery complicated by cord around neck, without compression** Ⓜ♀

√x7ᵗʰ **O69.82 Labor and delivery complicated by other cord entanglement, without compression** Ⓜ♀

√x7ᵗʰ **O69.89 Labor and delivery complicated by other cord complications** Ⓜ♀

√x7ᵗʰ **O69.9 Labor and delivery complicated by cord complication, unspecified** Ⓜ♀

√4ᵗʰ **O70 Perineal laceration during delivery**
Episiotomy extended by laceration
EXCLUDES 1 *obstetric high vaginal laceration alone (O71.4)*

O70.0 First degree perineal laceration during delivery Ⓜ♀
Perineal laceration, rupture or tear involving fourchette during delivery
Perineal laceration, rupture or tear involving labia during delivery
Perineal laceration, rupture or tear involving skin during delivery
Perineal laceration, rupture or tear involving vagina during delivery
Perineal laceration, rupture or tear involving vulva during delivery
Slight perineal laceration, rupture or tear during delivery

O70.1 Second degree perineal laceration during delivery Ⓜ♀
Perineal laceration, rupture or tear during delivery as in O70.0, also involving pelvic floor
Perineal laceration, rupture or tear during delivery as in O70.0, also involving perineal muscles
Perineal laceration, rupture or tear during delivery as in O70.0, also involving vaginal muscles
EXCLUDES 1 *perineal laceration involving anal sphincter (O70.2)*

O70.2 Third degree perineal laceration during delivery Ⓜ♀
Perineal laceration, rupture or tear during delivery as in O70.1, also involving anal sphincter
Perineal laceration, rupture or tear during delivery as in O70.1, also involving rectovaginal septum
Perineal laceration, rupture or tear during delivery as in O70.1, also involving sphincter NOS
EXCLUDES 1 *anal sphincter tear during delivery without third degree perineal laceration (O70.4)*
perineal laceration involving anal or rectal mucosa (O70.3)

O70.3 Fourth degree perineal laceration during delivery Ⓜ♀
Perineal laceration, rupture or tear during delivery as in O70.2, also involving anal mucosa
Perineal laceration, rupture or tear during delivery as in O70.2, also involving rectal mucosa

O70.4 Anal sphincter tear complicating delivery, not associated with third degree laceration Ⓜ♀
EXCLUDES 1 *anal sphincter tear with third degree perineal laceration (O70.2)*

O70.9 Perineal laceration during delivery, unspecified Ⓜ♀

√4ᵗʰ **O71 Other obstetric trauma**
Obstetric damage from instruments

√5ᵗʰ **O71.0 Rupture of uterus (spontaneous) before onset of labor**
EXCLUDES 1 *disruption of (current) cesarean delivery wound (O90.0)*
laceration of uterus, NEC (O71.81)

O71.00 Rupture of uterus before onset of labor, unspecified trimester Ⓜ♀

O71.02 Rupture of uterus before onset of labor, second trimester Ⓜ♀

O71.03 Rupture of uterus before onset of labor, third trimester Ⓜ♀

O71.1 Rupture of uterus during labor Ⓜ♀
Rupture of uterus not stated as occurring before onset of labor
EXCLUDES 1 *disruption of cesarean delivery wound (O90.0)*
laceration of uterus, NEC (O71.81)

O71.2 Postpartum inversion of uterus Ⓜ♀

O71.3 Obstetric laceration of cervix Ⓜ♀
Annular detachment of cervix

O71.4 Obstetric high vaginal laceration alone Ⓜ♀
Laceration of vaginal wall without perineal laceration
EXCLUDES 1 *obstetric high vaginal laceration with perineal laceration (O70.-)*

O71.5 Other obstetric injury to pelvic organs Ⓜ♀
Obstetric injury to bladder
Obstetric injury to urethra
EXCLUDES 2 *obstetric periurethral trauma (O71.82)*

O71.6 Obstetric damage to pelvic joints and ligaments Ⓜ♀
Obstetric avulsion of inner symphyseal cartilage
Obstetric damage to coccyx
Obstetric traumatic separation of symphysis (pubis)

O71.7 Obstetric hematoma of pelvis Ⓜ♀
Obstetric hematoma of perineum
Obstetric hematoma of vagina
Obstetric hematoma of vulva

√5ᵗʰ **O71.8 Other specified obstetric trauma**

O71.81 Laceration of uterus, not elsewhere classified Ⓜ♀

O71.82 Other specified trauma to perineum and vulva Ⓜ♀
Obstetric periurethral trauma

O71.89 Other specified obstetric trauma Ⓜ♀

O71.9 Obstetric trauma, unspecified Ⓜ♀

√4ᵗʰ **O72 Postpartum hemorrhage**
INCLUDES hemorrhage after delivery of fetus or infant

O72.0 Third-stage hemorrhage Ⓜ♀
Hemorrhage associated with retained, trapped or adherent placenta
Retained placenta NOS
Code also type of adherent placenta (O43.2-)

O72.1 Other immediate postpartum hemorrhage Ⓜ♀
Hemorrhage following delivery of placenta
Postpartum hemorrhage (atonic) NOS
Uterine atony with hemorrhage
EXCLUDES 1 *uterine atony NOS (O62.2)*
uterine atony without hemorrhage (O62.2)
postpartum atony of uterus without hemorrhage (O75.89)

O72.2 Delayed and secondary postpartum hemorrhage Ⓜ♀
Hemorrhage associated with retained portions of placenta or membranes after the first 24 hours following delivery of placenta
Retained products of conception NOS, following delivery

O72.3 Postpartum coagulation defects Ⓜ♀
Postpartum afibrinogenemia
Postpartum fibrinolysis

√4ᵗʰ **O73 Retained placenta and membranes, without hemorrhage**
EXCLUDES 1 *placenta accreta (O43.21-)*
placenta increta (O43.22-)
placenta percreta (O43.23-)

O73.0 Retained placenta without hemorrhage Ⓜ♀
Adherent placenta, without hemorrhage
Trapped placenta without hemorrhage

O73.1 Retained portions of placenta and membranes, without hemorrhage Ⓜ♀
Retained products of conception following delivery, without hemorrhage

√4ᵗʰ **O74 Complications of anesthesia during labor and delivery**
INCLUDES maternal complications arising from the administration of a general, regional or local anesthetic, analgesic or other sedation during labor and delivery
Use additional code, if applicable, to identify specific complication

O74.0 Aspiration pneumonitis due to anesthesia during labor and delivery Ⓜ♀
Inhalation of stomach contents or secretions NOS due to anesthesia during labor and delivery
Mendelson's syndrome due to anesthesia during labor and delivery

O74.1 Other pulmonary complications of anesthesia during labor and delivery Ⓜ♀

O74.2 Cardiac complications of anesthesia during labor and delivery Ⓜ♀

O74.3 Central nervous system complications of anesthesia during labor and delivery Ⓜ♀

O74.4 Toxic reaction to local anesthesia during labor and delivery Ⓜ♀

O74.5 Spinal and epidural anesthesia-induced headache during labor and delivery Ⓜ♀

O74.6 Other complications of spinal and epidural anesthesia during labor and delivery Ⓜ♀

O74.7 Failed or difficult intubation for anesthesia during labor and delivery Ⓜ♀

O74.8 Other complications of anesthesia during labor and delivery Ⓜ♀

O74.9 Complication of anesthesia during labor and delivery, unspecified Ⓜ♀

☑4ᵗʰ **O75 Other complications of labor and delivery, not elsewhere classified**
> EXCLUDES 2　*puerperal (postpartum) infection (O86.-)*
> *puerperal (postpartum) sepsis (O85)*

O75.0 Maternal distress during labor and delivery Ⓜ♀

O75.1 Shock during or following labor and delivery Ⓜ♀
> Obstetric shock following labor and delivery

O75.2 Pyrexia during labor, not elsewhere classified Ⓜ♀

O75.3 Other infection during labor Ⓜ♀
> Sepsis during labor
> Use additional code (B95-B97), to identify infectious agent

O75.4 Other complications of obstetric surgery and procedures Ⓜ♀
> Cardiac arrest following obstetric surgery or procedures
> Cardiac failure following obstetric surgery or procedures
> Cerebral anoxia following obstetric surgery or procedures
> Pulmonary edema following obstetric surgery or procedures
> Use additional code to identify specific complication
> EXCLUDES 2　*complications of anesthesia during labor and delivery (O74.-)*
> *disruption of obstetrical (surgical) wound (O90.0-O90.1)*
> *hematoma of obstetrical (surgical) wound (O90.2)*
> *infection of obstetrical (surgical) wound (O86.0)*

O75.5 Delayed delivery after artificial rupture of membranes Ⓜ♀

☑5ᵗʰ **O75.8 Other specified complications of labor and delivery**

> **O75.81 Maternal exhaustion complicating labor and delivery** Ⓜ♀

> **O75.82 Onset (spontaneous) of labor after 37 completed weeks of gestation but before 39 completed weeks gestation, with delivery by (planned) cesarean section** Ⓜ♀
> > Delivery by (planned) cesarean section occurring after 37 completed weeks of gestation but before 39 completed weeks gestation due to (spontaneous) onset of labor
> > Code first to specify reason for planned cesarean section such as:
> > cephalopelvic disproportion (normally formed fetus) (O33.9)
> > previous cesarean delivery (O34.21)

> **O75.89 Other specified complications of labor and delivery** Ⓜ♀

O75.9 Complication of labor and delivery, unspecified Ⓜ♀

O76 Abnormality in fetal heart rate and rhythm complicating labor and delivery Ⓜ♀
> Depressed fetal heart rate tones complicating labor and delivery
> Fetal bradycardia complicating labor and delivery
> Fetal heart rate decelerations complicating labor and delivery
> Fetal heart rate irregularity complicating labor and delivery
> Fetal heart rate abnormal variability complicating labor and delivery
> Fetal tachycardia complicating labor and delivery
> Non-reassuring fetal heart rate or rhythm complicating labor and delivery
> EXCLUDES 1　*fetal stress NOS (O77.9)*
> *labor and delivery complicated by electrocardiographic evidence of fetal stress (O77.8)*
> *labor and delivery complicated by ultrasonic evidence of fetal stress (O77.8)*
> EXCLUDES 2　*fetal metabolic acidemia (O68)*
> *other fetal stress (O77.0-O77.1)*

☑4ᵗʰ **O77 Other fetal stress complicating labor and delivery**

O77.0 Labor and delivery complicated by meconium in amniotic fluid Ⓜ♀

O77.1 Fetal stress in labor or delivery due to drug administration Ⓜ♀

O77.8 Labor and delivery complicated by other evidence of fetal stress Ⓜ♀
> Labor and delivery complicated by electrocardiographic evidence of fetal stress
> Labor and delivery complicated by ultrasonic evidence of fetal stress
> EXCLUDES 1　*abnormality of fetal acid-base balance (O68)*
> *abnormality in fetal heart rate or rhythm (O76)*
> *fetal metabolic acidemia (O68)*

O77.9 Labor and delivery complicated by fetal stress, unspecified
> EXCLUDES 1　*abnormality of fetal acid-base balance (O68)*
> *abnormality in fetal heart rate or rhythm (O76)*
> *fetal metabolic acidemia (O68)*

Encounter for delivery (O80, O82)

O80 Encounter for full-term uncomplicated delivery Ⓜ♀
> NOTE　Delivery requiring minimal or no assistance, with or without episiotomy, without fetal manipulation [e.g., rotation version] or instrumentation [forceps] of a spontaneous, cephalic, vaginal, full-term, single, live-born infant. This code is for use as a single diagnosis code and is not to be used with any other code from chapter 15.
> Use additional code to indicate outcome of delivery (Z37.0)

O82 Encounter for cesarean delivery without indication Ⓜ♀
> Use additional code to indicate outcome of delivery (Z37.0)

Complications predominantly related to the puerperium (O85-O92)

> EXCLUDES 2　*mental and behavioral disorders associated with the puerperium (F53)*
> *obstetrical tetanus (A34)*
> *puerperal osteomalacia (M83.0)*

O85 Puerperal sepsis Ⓜ♀
> Postpartum sepsis
> Puerperal peritonitis
> Puerperal pyemia
> Use additional code (B95-B97), to identify infectious agent
> Use additional code (R65.2-) to identify severe sepsis, if applicable
> EXCLUDES 1　*fever of unknown origin following delivery (O86.4)*
> *genital tract infection following delivery (O86.1-)*
> *obstetric pyemic and septic embolism (O88.3-)*
> *puerperal septic thrombophlebitis (O86.81)*
> *urinary tract infection following delivery (O86.2-)*
> EXCLUDES 2　*sepsis during labor (O75.3)*

☑4ᵗʰ **O86 Other puerperal infections**
> Use additional code (B95-B97), to identify infectious agent
> EXCLUDES 2　*infection during labor (O75.3)*
> *obstetrical tetanus (A34)*

O86.0 Infection of obstetric surgical wound Ⓜ♀
> Infected cesarean delivery wound following delivery
> Infected perineal repair following delivery

☑5ᵗʰ **O86.1 Other infection of genital tract following delivery**

> **O86.11 Cervicitis following delivery** Ⓜ♀

> **O86.12 Endometritis following delivery** Ⓜ♀

> **O86.13 Vaginitis following delivery** Ⓜ♀

> **O86.19 Other infection of genital tract following delivery** Ⓜ♀

☑5ᵗʰ **O86.2 Urinary tract infection following delivery**

> **O86.20 Urinary tract infection following delivery, unspecified** Ⓜ♀
> > Puerperal urinary tract infection NOS

> **O86.21 Infection of kidney following delivery** Ⓜ♀

> **O86.22 Infection of bladder following delivery**
> > Infection of urethra following delivery

> **O86.29 Other urinary tract infection following delivery** Ⓜ♀

O86.4 Pyrexia of unknown origin following delivery Ⓜ♀
> Puerperal infection NOS following delivery
> Puerperal pyrexia NOS following delivery
> EXCLUDES 1　*pyrexia during labor (O75.2)*

☑5ᵗʰ **O86.8 Other specified puerperal infections**

> **O86.81 Puerperal septic thrombophlebitis** Ⓜ♀

> **O86.89 Other specified puerperal infections** Ⓜ♀

☑ Additional Character Required　　☑7ᵗʰ Xtension Alert　　Unspecified Code　　Other Specified Code　　Manifestation Code　　►◄ Revised Text　　● New Code　　▲ Revised Code Title

Pregnancy, Childbirth and the Puerperium

O87–O90.6

✓4th **O87 Venous complications and hemorrhoids in the puerperium**
Venous complications in labor, delivery and the puerperium
EXCLUDES 2   *obstetric embolism (O88.-)*
puerperal septic thrombophlebitis (O86.81)
venous complications in pregnancy (O22.-)

O87.0 Superficial thrombophlebitis in the puerperium Ⓜ♀
Puerperal phlebitis NOS
Puerperal thrombosis NOS

O87.1 Deep phlebothrombosis in the puerperium Ⓜ♀
Deep vein thrombosis, postpartum
Pelvic thrombophlebitis, postpartum
Use additional code to identify the deep vein thrombosis (I82.4-, I82.5-, I82.62-. I82.72-)
Use additional code, if applicable, for associated long-term (current) use of anticoagulants (Z79.01)

O87.2 Hemorrhoids in the puerperium Ⓜ♀

O87.3 Cerebral venous thrombosis in the puerperium Ⓜ♀
Cerebrovenous sinus thrombosis in the puerperium

O87.4 Varicose veins of lower extremity in the puerperium Ⓜ♀

O87.8 Other venous complications in the puerperium Ⓜ♀
Genital varices in the puerperium

O87.9 Venous complication in the puerperium, unspecified Ⓜ♀
Puerperal phlebopathy NOS

✓4th **O88 Obstetric embolism**
EXCLUDES 1   *embolism complicating abortion NOS (O03.2)*
embolism complicating ectopic or molar pregnancy (O08.2)
embolism complicating failed attempted abortion (O07.2)
embolism complicating induced abortion (O04.7)
embolism complicating spontaneous abortion (O03.2, O03.7)

✓5th **O88.0 Obstetric air embolism**

✓6th **O88.01 Obstetric air embolism in pregnancy**

O88.011 Air embolism in pregnancy, first trimester Ⓜ♀

O88.012 Air embolism in pregnancy, second trimester Ⓜ♀

O88.013 Air embolism in pregnancy, third trimester Ⓜ♀

O88.019 Air embolism in pregnancy, unspecified trimester Ⓜ♀

O88.02 Air embolism in childbirth Ⓜ♀

O88.03 Air embolism in the puerperium Ⓜ♀

✓5th **O88.1 Amniotic fluid embolism**
Anaphylactoid syndrome in pregnancy

✓6th **O88.11 Amniotic fluid embolism in pregnancy**

O88.111 Amniotic fluid embolism in pregnancy, first trimester Ⓜ♀

O88.112 Amniotic fluid embolism in pregnancy, second trimester Ⓜ♀

O88.113 Amniotic fluid embolism in pregnancy, third trimester Ⓜ♀

O88.119 Amniotic fluid embolism in pregnancy, unspecified trimester Ⓜ♀

O88.12 Amniotic fluid embolism in childbirth Ⓜ♀

O88.13 Amniotic fluid embolism in the puerperium Ⓜ♀

✓5th **O88.2 Obstetric thromboembolism**

✓6th **O88.21 Thromboembolism in pregnancy**
Obstetric (pulmonary) embolism NOS

O88.211 Thromboembolism in pregnancy, first trimester Ⓜ♀

O88.212 Thromboembolism in pregnancy, second trimester Ⓜ♀

O88.213 Thromboembolism in pregnancy, third trimester Ⓜ♀

O88.219 Thromboembolism in pregnancy, unspecified trimester Ⓜ♀

O88.22 Thromboembolism in childbirth Ⓜ♀

O88.23 Thromboembolism in the puerperium Ⓜ♀
Puerperal (pulmonary) embolism NOS

✓5th **O88.3 Obstetric pyemic and septic embolism**

✓6th **O88.31 Pyemic and septic embolism in pregnancy**

O88.311 Pyemic and septic embolism in pregnancy, first trimester Ⓜ♀

O88.312 Pyemic and septic embolism in pregnancy, second trimester Ⓜ♀

O88.313 Pyemic and septic embolism in pregnancy, third trimester Ⓜ♀

O88.319 Pyemic and septic embolism in pregnancy, unspecified trimester Ⓜ♀

O88.32 Pyemic and septic embolism in childbirth Ⓜ♀

O88.33 Pyemic and septic embolism in the puerperium Ⓜ♀

✓5th **O88.8 Other obstetric embolism**
Obstetric fat embolism

✓6th **O88.81 Other embolism in pregnancy**

O88.811 Other embolism in pregnancy, first trimester Ⓜ♀

O88.812 Other embolism in pregnancy, second trimester Ⓜ♀

O88.813 Other embolism in pregnancy, third trimester Ⓜ♀

O88.819 Other embolism in pregnancy, unspecified trimester Ⓜ♀

O88.82 Other embolism in childbirth Ⓜ♀

O88.83 Other embolism in the puerperium Ⓜ♀

✓4th **O89 Complications of anesthesia during the puerperium**
INCLUDES   maternal complications arising from the administration of a general, regional or local anesthetic, analgesic or other sedation during the puerperium
Use additional code, if applicable, to identify specific complication

✓5th **O89.0 Pulmonary complications of anesthesia during the puerperium**

O89.01 Aspiration pneumonitis due to anesthesia during the puerperium Ⓜ♀
Inhalation of stomach contents or secretions NOS due to anesthesia during the puerperium
Mendelson's syndrome due to anesthesia during the puerperium

O89.09 Other pulmonary complications of anesthesia during the puerperium Ⓜ♀

O89.1 Cardiac complications of anesthesia during the puerperium Ⓜ♀

O89.2 Central nervous system complications of anesthesia during the puerperium Ⓜ♀

O89.3 Toxic reaction to local anesthesia during the puerperium Ⓜ♀

O89.4 Spinal and epidural anesthesia-induced headache during the puerperium Ⓜ♀

O89.5 Other complications of spinal and epidural anesthesia during the puerperium Ⓜ♀

O89.6 Failed or difficult intubation for anesthesia during the puerperium Ⓜ♀

O89.8 Other complications of anesthesia during the puerperium Ⓜ♀

O89.9 Complication of anesthesia during the puerperium, unspecified Ⓜ♀

✓4th **O90 Complications of the puerperium, not elsewhere classified**

O90.0 Disruption of cesarean delivery wound Ⓜ♀
Dehiscence of cesarean delivery wound
EXCLUDES 1   *rupture of uterus (spontaneous) before onset of labor (O71.0-)*
rupture of uterus during labor (O71.1)

O90.1 Disruption of perineal obstetric wound Ⓜ♀
Disruption of wound of episiotomy
Disruption of wound of perineal laceration
Secondary perineal tear

O90.2 Hematoma of obstetric wound Ⓜ♀

O90.3 Peripartum cardiomyopathy Ⓜ♀
Conditions in I42- arising during pregnancy and the puerperium
EXCLUDES 1   *pre-existing heart disease complicating pregnancy and the puerperium (O99.4-)*

O90.4 Postpartum acute kidney failure Ⓜ♀
Hepatorenal syndrome following labor and delivery

O90.5 Postpartum thyroiditis Ⓜ♀

O90.6 Postpartum mood disturbance Ⓜ♀
Postpartum blues
Postpartum dysphoria
Postpartum sadness
EXCLUDES 1   *postpartum depression (F53)*
puerperal psychosis (F53)

EXCLUDES 1 Not coded here   EXCLUDES 2 Not included here   Ⓝ Newborn Age: 0   Ⓟ Pediatric Age: 0-17   Ⓜ Maternity Age: 12-55   Ⓐ Adult Age: 15-124

O90.8 ✓5th **Other complications of the puerperium, not elsewhere classified**

    O90.81 Anemia of the puerperium Ⓜ♀
        Postpartum anemia NOS
        EXCLUDES 1   *pre-existing anemia complicating the puerperium (O99.03)*

    O90.89 Other complications of the puerperium, not elsewhere classified Ⓜ♀
        Placental polyp

O90.9 Complication of the puerperium, unspecified Ⓜ♀

O91 ✓4th **Infections of breast associated with pregnancy, the puerperium and lactation**
    Use additional code to identify infection

O91.0 ✓5th **Infection of nipple associated with pregnancy, the puerperium and lactation**

    O91.01 ✓6th **Infection of nipple associated with** pregnancy
        Gestational abscess of nipple

        O91.011 Infection of nipple associated with pregnancy, first trimester Ⓜ♀

        O91.012 Infection of nipple associated with pregnancy, second trimester Ⓜ♀

        O91.013 Infection of nipple associated with pregnancy, third trimester Ⓜ♀

        O91.019 Infection of nipple associated with pregnancy, unspecified trimester Ⓜ♀

    O91.02 Infection of nipple associated with the puerperium Ⓜ♀
        Puerperal abscess of nipple

    O91.03 Infection of nipple associated with lactation Ⓜ♀
        Abscess of nipple associated with lactation

O91.1 ✓5th **Abscess of breast associated with pregnancy, the puerperium and lactation**

    O91.11 ✓6th **Abscess of breast associated with** pregnancy
        Gestational mammary abscess
        Gestational purulent mastitis
        Gestational subareolar abscess

        O91.111 Abscess of breast associated with pregnancy, first trimester Ⓜ♀

        O91.112 Abscess of breast associated with pregnancy, second trimester Ⓜ♀

        O91.113 Abscess of breast associated with pregnancy, third trimester Ⓜ♀

        O91.119 Abscess of breast associated with pregnancy, unspecified trimester Ⓜ♀

    O91.12 Abscess of breast associated with the puerperium Ⓜ♀
        Puerperal mammary abscess
        Puerperal purulent mastitis
        Puerperal subareolar abscess

    O91.13 Abscess of breast associated with lactation Ⓜ♀
        Mammary abscess associated with lactation
        Purulent mastitis associated with lactation
        Subareolar abscess associated with lactation

O91.2 ✓5th **Nonpurulent mastitis associated with pregnancy, the puerperium and lactation**

    O91.21 ✓6th **Nonpurulent mastitis associated with** pregnancy
        Gestational interstitial mastitis
        Gestational lymphangitis of breast
        Gestational mastitis NOS
        Gestational parenchymatous mastitis

        O91.211 Nonpurulent mastitis associated with pregnancy, first trimester Ⓜ♀

        O91.212 Nonpurulent mastitis associated with pregnancy, second trimester Ⓜ♀

        O91.213 Nonpurulent mastitis associated with pregnancy, third trimester Ⓜ♀

        O91.219 Nonpurulent mastitis associated with pregnancy, unspecified trimester Ⓜ♀

    O91.22 Nonpurulent mastitis associated with the puerperium Ⓜ♀
        Puerperal interstitial mastitis
        Puerperal lymphangitis of breast
        Puerperal mastitis NOS
        Puerperal parenchymatous mastitis

    O91.23 Nonpurulent mastitis associated with lactation Ⓜ♀
        Interstitial mastitis associated with lactation
        Lymphangitis of breast associated with lactation
        Mastitis NOS associated with lactation
        Parenchymatous mastitis associated with lactation

O92 ✓4th **Other disorders of breast and disorders of lactation associated with pregnancy and the puerperium**

O92.0 ✓5th **Retracted nipple associated with pregnancy, the puerperium, and lactation**

    O92.01 ✓6th **Retracted nipple associated with** pregnancy

        O92.011 Retracted nipple associated with pregnancy, first trimester Ⓜ♀

        O92.012 Retracted nipple associated with pregnancy, second trimester Ⓜ♀

        O92.013 Retracted nipple associated with pregnancy, third trimester Ⓜ♀

        O92.019 Retracted nipple associated with pregnancy, unspecified trimester Ⓜ♀

    O92.02 Retracted nipple associated with the puerperium Ⓜ♀

    O92.03 Retracted nipple associated with lactation Ⓜ♀

O92.1 ✓5th **Cracked nipple associated with pregnancy, the puerperium, and lactation**
    Fissure of nipple, gestational or puerperal

    O92.11 ✓6th **Cracked nipple associated with** pregnancy

        O92.111 Cracked nipple associated with pregnancy, first trimester Ⓜ♀

        O92.112 Cracked nipple associated with pregnancy, second trimester Ⓜ♀

        O92.113 Cracked nipple associated with pregnancy, third trimester Ⓜ♀

        O92.119 Cracked nipple associated with pregnancy, unspecified trimester Ⓜ♀

    O92.12 Cracked nipple associated with the puerperium Ⓜ♀

    O92.13 Cracked nipple associated with lactation Ⓜ♀

O92.2 ✓5th **Other and unspecified disorders of breast associated with pregnancy and the puerperium**

    O92.20 Unspecified disorder of breast associated with pregnancy and the puerperium Ⓜ♀

    O92.29 Other disorders of breast associated with pregnancy and the puerperium Ⓜ♀

O92.3 Agalactia Ⓜ♀
    Primary agalactia
    EXCLUDES 1   *elective agalactia (O92.5)*
                secondary agalactia (O92.5)
                therapeutic agalactia (O92.5)

O92.4 Hypogalactia Ⓜ♀

O92.5 Suppressed lactation Ⓜ♀
    Elective agalactia
    Secondary agalactia
    Therapeutic agalactia
    EXCLUDES 1   *primary agalactia (O92.3)*

O92.6 Galactorrhea Ⓜ♀

O92.7 ✓5th **Other and unspecified disorders of lactation**

    O92.70 Unspecified disorders of lactation Ⓜ♀

    O92.79 Other disorders of lactation Ⓜ♀
        Puerperal galactocele

Other obstetric conditions, not elsewhere classified (O94-O9A)

O94 Sequelae of complication of pregnancy, childbirth, and the puerperium Ⓜ♀

    NOTE   This category is to be used to indicate conditions in O00-O77.-, O85-O94 and O98-O9A.- as the cause of late effects. The sequelae include conditions specified as such, or as late effects, which may occur at any time after the puerperium.

    Code first condition resulting from (sequela) of complication of pregnancy, childbirth, and the puerperium

---

☑ Additional Character Required   ✓x7th Xtension Alert   Unspecified Code   Other Specified Code   Manifestation Code   ▶◀ Revised Text   ● New Code   ▲ Revised Code Title

Pregnancy, Childbirth and the Puerperium

O98–O98.73

√4ᵗʰ **O98 Maternal infectious and parasitic diseases classifiable elsewhere but complicating pregnancy, childbirth and the puerperium**

    INCLUDES   the listed conditions when complicating the pregnant state, when aggravated by the pregnancy, or as a reason for obstetric care

    Use additional code (Chapter 1), to identify specific infectious or parasitic disease

    EXCLUDES 2   herpes gestationis (O26.4-)
                infectious carrier state (O99.82-, O99.83-)
                obstetrical tetanus (A34)
                puerperal infection (O86.-)
                puerperal sepsis (O85)
                when the reason for maternal care is that the disease is known or suspected to have affected the fetus (O35-O36)

√5ᵗʰ **O98.0 Tuberculosis complicating pregnancy, childbirth and the puerperium**
    Conditions in A15-A19

  √6ᵗʰ **O98.01 Tuberculosis complicating pregnancy**

    O98.011 Tuberculosis complicating pregnancy, first trimester ▥♀

    O98.012 Tuberculosis complicating pregnancy, second trimester ▥♀

    O98.013 Tuberculosis complicating pregnancy, third trimester ▥♀

    O98.019 Tuberculosis complicating pregnancy, unspecified trimester ▥♀

  O98.02 Tuberculosis complicating childbirth ▥♀

  O98.03 Tuberculosis complicating the puerperium ▥♀

√5ᵗʰ **O98.1 Syphilis complicating pregnancy, childbirth and the puerperium**
    Conditions in A50-A53

  √6ᵗʰ **O98.11 Syphilis complicating pregnancy**

    O98.111 Syphilis complicating pregnancy, first trimester ▥♀

    O98.112 Syphilis complicating pregnancy, second trimester ▥♀

    O98.113 Syphilis complicating pregnancy, third trimester ▥♀

    O98.119 Syphilis complicating pregnancy, unspecified trimester ▥♀

  O98.12 Syphilis complicating childbirth ▥♀

  O98.13 Syphilis complicating the puerperium ▥♀

√5ᵗʰ **O98.2 Gonorrhea complicating pregnancy, childbirth and the puerperium**
    Conditions in A54-

  √6ᵗʰ **O98.21 Gonorrhea complicating pregnancy**

    O98.211 Gonorrhea complicating pregnancy, first trimester ▥♀

    O98.212 Gonorrhea complicating pregnancy, second trimester ▥♀

    O98.213 Gonorrhea complicating pregnancy, third trimester ▥♀

    O98.219 Gonorrhea complicating pregnancy, unspecified trimester ▥♀

  O98.22 Gonorrhea complicating childbirth ▥♀

  O98.23 Gonorrhea complicating the puerperium ▥♀

√5ᵗʰ **O98.3 Other infections with a predominantly sexual mode of transmission complicating pregnancy, childbirth and the puerperium**
    Conditions in A55-A64

  √6ᵗʰ **O98.31 Other infections with a predominantly sexual mode of transmission complicating pregnancy**

    O98.311 Other infections with a predominantly sexual mode of transmission complicating pregnancy, first trimester ▥♀

    O98.312 Other infections with a predominantly sexual mode of transmission complicating pregnancy, second trimester ▥♀

    O98.313 Other infections with a predominantly sexual mode of transmission complicating pregnancy, third trimester ▥

    O98.319 Other infections with a predominantly sexual mode of transmission complicating pregnancy, unspecified trimester ▥♀

  O98.32 Other infections with a predominantly sexual mode of transmission complicating childbirth ▥♀

  O98.33 Other infections with a predominantly sexual mode of transmission complicating the puerperium ▥♀

√5ᵗʰ **O98.4 Viral hepatitis complicating pregnancy, childbirth and the puerperium**
    Conditions in B15-B19

  √6ᵗʰ **O98.41 Viral hepatitis complicating pregnancy**

    O98.411 Viral hepatitis complicating pregnancy, first trimester ▥♀

    O98.412 Viral hepatitis complicating pregnancy, second trimester ▥♀

    O98.413 Viral hepatitis complicating pregnancy, third trimester ▥♀

    O98.419 Viral hepatitis complicating pregnancy, unspecified trimester ▥♀

  O98.42 Viral hepatitis complicating childbirth ▥♀

  O98.43 Viral hepatitis complicating the puerperium ▥♀

√5ᵗʰ **O98.5 Other viral diseases complicating pregnancy, childbirth and the puerperium**
    Conditions in A80-B09, B25-B34, R87.81-, R87.82-
    EXCLUDES 1   human immunodeficiency virus [HIV] disease complicating pregnancy, childbirth and the puerperium (O98.7-)

  √6ᵗʰ **O98.51 Other viral diseases complicating pregnancy**

    O98.511 Other viral diseases complicating pregnancy, first trimester ▥♀

    O98.512 Other viral diseases complicating pregnancy, second trimester ▥♀

    O98.513 Other viral diseases complicating pregnancy, third trimester ▥♀

    O98.519 Other viral diseases complicating pregnancy, unspecified trimester ▥♀

  O98.52 Other viral diseases complicating childbirth ▥♀

  O98.53 Other viral diseases complicating the puerperium ▥♀

√5ᵗʰ **O98.6 Protozoal diseases complicating pregnancy, childbirth and the puerperium**
    Conditions in B50-B64

  √6ᵗʰ **O98.61 Protozoal diseases complicating pregnancy**

    O98.611 Protozoal diseases complicating pregnancy, first trimester ▥♀

    O98.612 Protozoal diseases complicating pregnancy, second trimester ▥♀

    O98.613 Protozoal diseases complicating pregnancy, third trimester ▥♀

    O98.619 Protozoal diseases complicating pregnancy, unspecified trimester ▥♀

  O98.62 Protozoal diseases complicating childbirth ▥♀

  O98.63 Protozoal diseases complicating the puerperium ▥♀

√5ᵗʰ **O98.7 Human immunodeficiency virus [HIV] disease complicating pregnancy, childbirth and the puerperium**

    Use additional code to identify the type of HIV disease:
        acquired immune deficiency syndrome (AIDS) (B20)
        asymptomatic HIV status (Z21)
        HIV positive NOS (Z21)
        symptomatic HIV disease (B20)

  √6ᵗʰ **O98.71 Human immunodeficiency virus [HIV] disease complicating pregnancy**

    O98.711 Human immunodeficiency virus [HIV] disease complicating pregnancy, first trimester ▥♀

    O98.712 Human immunodeficiency virus [HIV] disease complicating pregnancy, second trimester ▥♀

    O98.713 Human immunodeficiency virus [HIV] disease complicating pregnancy, third trimester ▥♀

    O98.719 Human immunodeficiency virus [HIV] disease complicating pregnancy, unspecified trimester ▥♀

  O98.72 Human immunodeficiency virus [HIV] disease complicating childbirth ▥♀

  O98.73 Human immunodeficiency virus [HIV] disease complicating the puerperium ▥♀

EXCLUDES 1 Not coded here   EXCLUDES 2 Not included here   Ⓝ Newborn Age: 0   Ⓟ Pediatric Age: 0-17   ▥ Maternity Age: 12-55   Ⓐ Adult Age: 15-124

√5th **O98.8** Other maternal infectious and parasitic diseases complicating pregnancy, childbirth and the puerperium

√6th **O98.81** Other maternal infectious and parasitic diseases complicating pregnancy

O98.811 Other maternal infectious and parasitic diseases complicating pregnancy, first trimester �♀

O98.812 Other maternal infectious and parasitic diseases complicating pregnancy, second trimester ⬜♀

O98.813 Other maternal infectious and parasitic diseases complicating pregnancy, third trimester ⬜♀

O98.819 Other maternal infectious and parasitic diseases complicating pregnancy, unspecified trimester ⬜♀

O98.82 Other maternal infectious and parasitic diseases complicating childbirth ⬜♀

O98.83 Other maternal infectious and parasitic diseases complicating the puerperium ⬜♀

√5th **O98.9** Unspecified maternal infectious and parasitic disease complicating pregnancy, childbirth and the puerperium

√6th **O98.91** Unspecified maternal infectious and parasitic disease complicating pregnancy

O98.911 Unspecified maternal infectious and parasitic disease complicating pregnancy, first trimester ⬜♀

O98.912 Unspecified maternal infectious and parasitic disease complicating pregnancy, second trimester ⬜♀

O98.913 Unspecified maternal infectious and parasitic disease complicating pregnancy, third trimester ⬜♀

O98.919 Unspecified maternal infectious and parasitic disease complicating pregnancy, unspecified trimester ⬜♀

O98.92 Unspecified maternal infectious and parasitic disease complicating childbirth ⬜♀

O98.93 Unspecified maternal infectious and parasitic disease complicating the puerperium ⬜♀

√4th **O99** Other maternal diseases classifiable elsewhere but complicating pregnancy, childbirth and the puerperium

Conditions which complicate the pregnant state, are aggravated by the pregnancy or are a main reason for obstetric care

Use additional code to identify specific condition

EXCLUDES 2 *when the reason for maternal care is that the condition is known or suspected to have affected the fetus (O35-O36)*

√5th **O99.0** Anemia complicating pregnancy, childbirth and the puerperium

Conditions in D50-D64

EXCLUDES 1 *anemia arising in the puerperium (O90.81)*
postpartum anemia NOS (O90.81)

√6th **O99.01** Anemia complicating pregnancy

O99.011 Anemia complicating pregnancy, first trimester ⬜♀

O99.012 Anemia complicating pregnancy, second trimester ⬜♀

O99.013 Anemia complicating pregnancy, third trimester ⬜♀

O99.019 Anemia complicating pregnancy, unspecified trimester ⬜♀

O99.02 Anemia complicating childbirth ⬜♀

O99.03 Anemia complicating the puerperium ⬜♀

EXCLUDES 1 *postpartum anemia not pre-existing prior to delivery (O90.81)*

√5th **O99.1** Other diseases of the blood and blood-forming organs and certain disorders involving the immune mechanism complicating pregnancy, childbirth and the puerperium

Conditions in D65-D89

EXCLUDES 2 *hemorrhage with coagulation defects (O45.-, O46.0-, O67.0, O72.3)*

√6th **O99.11** Other diseases of the blood and blood-forming organs and certain disorders involving the immune mechanism complicating pregnancy

O99.111 Other diseases of the blood and blood-forming organs and certain disorders involving the immune mechanism complicating pregnancy, first trimester ⬜♀

O99.112 Other diseases of the blood and blood-forming organs and certain disorders involving the immune mechanism complicating pregnancy, second trimester ⬜♀

O99.113 Other diseases of the blood and blood-forming organs and certain disorders involving the immune mechanism complicating pregnancy, third trimester ⬜♀

O99.119 Other diseases of the blood and blood-forming organs and certain disorders involving the immune mechanism complicating pregnancy, unspecified trimester ⬜♀

O99.12 Other diseases of the blood and blood-forming organs and certain disorders involving the immune mechanism complicating childbirth ⬜♀

O99.13 Other diseases of the blood and blood-forming organs and certain disorders involving the immune mechanism complicating the puerperium ⬜♀

√5th **O99.2** Endocrine, nutritional and metabolic diseases complicating pregnancy, childbirth and the puerperium

Conditions in E00-E88

EXCLUDES 2 *diabetes mellitus (O24.-)*
malnutrition (O25.-)
postpartum thyroiditis (O90.5)

√6th **O99.21** Obesity complicating pregnancy, childbirth, and the puerperium

Use additional code to identify the type of obesity (E66.-)

O99.210 Obesity complicating pregnancy, unspecified trimester ⬜♀

O99.211 Obesity complicating pregnancy, first trimester ⬜♀

O99.212 Obesity complicating pregnancy, second trimester ⬜♀

O99.213 Obesity complicating pregnancy, third trimester ⬜♀

O99.214 Obesity complicating childbirth ⬜♀

O99.215 Obesity complicating the puerperium ⬜♀

√6th **O99.28** Other endocrine, nutritional and metabolic diseases complicating pregnancy, childbirth and the puerperium

O99.280 Endocrine, nutritional and metabolic diseases complicating pregnancy, unspecified trimester ⬜♀

O99.281 Endocrine, nutritional and metabolic diseases complicating pregnancy, first trimester ⬜♀

O99.282 Endocrine, nutritional and metabolic diseases complicating pregnancy, second trimester ⬜♀

O99.283 Endocrine, nutritional and metabolic diseases complicating pregnancy, third trimester ⬜♀

O99.284 Endocrine, nutritional and metabolic diseases complicating childbirth ⬜♀

O99.285 Endocrine, nutritional and metabolic diseases complicating the puerperium ⬜♀

√5th **O99.3** Mental disorders and diseases of the nervous system complicating pregnancy, childbirth and the puerperium

√6th **O99.31** Alcohol use complicating pregnancy, childbirth, and the puerperium

Use additional code(s) from F10 to identify manifestations of the alcohol use

O99.310 Alcohol use complicating pregnancy, unspecified trimester ⬜♀

O99.311 Alcohol use complicating pregnancy, first trimester ⬜♀

O99.312 Alcohol use complicating pregnancy, second trimester ⬜♀

O99.313 Alcohol use complicating pregnancy, third trimester ⬜♀

O99.314 Alcohol use complicating childbirth ⬜♀

O99.315 Alcohol use complicating the puerperium ⬜♀

☑ Additional Character Required   √x7th Xtension Alert   Unspecified Code   Other Specified Code   Manifestation Code   ▶◀ Revised Text   ● New Code   ▲ Revised Code Title

√6ᵗʰ **O99.32** Drug use complicating pregnancy, childbirth, and the puerperium
     Use additional code(s) from F11-F16 and F18-F19 to identify manifestations of the drug use

O99.320 Drug use complicating pregnancy, unspecified trimester   Ⓜ♀

O99.321 Drug use complicating pregnancy, first trimester   Ⓜ♀

O99.322 Drug use complicating pregnancy, second trimester   Ⓜ♀

O99.323 Drug use complicating pregnancy, third trimester   Ⓜ♀

O99.324 Drug use complicating childbirth   Ⓜ♀

O99.325 Drug use complicating the puerperium   Ⓜ♀

√6ᵗʰ **O99.33** Smoking (tobacco) complicating pregnancy, childbirth, and the puerperium
     Use additional code from F17 to identify type of tobacco

O99.330 Smoking (tobacco) complicating pregnancy, unspecified trimester   Ⓜ♀

O99.331 Smoking (tobacco) complicating pregnancy, first trimester   Ⓜ♀

O99.332 Smoking (tobacco) complicating pregnancy, second trimester   Ⓜ♀

O99.333 Smoking (tobacco) complicating pregnancy, third trimester   Ⓜ♀

O99.334 Smoking (tobacco) complicating childbirth   Ⓜ♀

O99.335 Smoking (tobacco) complicating the puerperium   Ⓜ♀

√6ᵗʰ **O99.34** Other mental disorders complicating pregnancy, childbirth, and the puerperium
     Conditions in F01-F09 and F20-F99
     EXCLUDES 2   postpartum mood disturbance (O90.6)
                 postnatal psychosis (F53)
                 puerperal psychosis (F53)

O99.340 Other mental disorders complicating pregnancy, unspecified trimester   Ⓜ♀

O99.341 Other mental disorders complicating pregnancy, first trimester   Ⓜ♀

O99.342 Other mental disorders complicating pregnancy, second trimester   Ⓜ♀

O99.343 Other mental disorders complicating pregnancy, third trimester   Ⓜ♀

O99.344 Other mental disorders complicating childbirth   Ⓜ♀

O99.345 Other mental disorders complicating the puerperium   Ⓜ♀

√6ᵗʰ **O99.35** Diseases of the nervous system complicating pregnancy, childbirth, and the puerperium
     Conditions in G00-G99
     EXCLUDES 2   pregnancy related peripheral neuritis (O26.8-)

O99.350 Diseases of the nervous system complicating pregnancy, unspecified trimester   Ⓜ♀

O99.351 Diseases of the nervous system complicating pregnancy, first trimester   Ⓜ♀

O99.352 Diseases of the nervous system complicating pregnancy, second trimester   Ⓜ♀

O99.353 Diseases of the nervous system complicating pregnancy, third trimester   Ⓜ♀

O99.354 Diseases of the nervous system complicating childbirth   Ⓜ♀

O99.355 Diseases of the nervous system complicating the puerperium   Ⓜ♀

√5ᵗʰ **O99.4** Diseases of the circulatory system complicating pregnancy, childbirth and the puerperium
     Conditions in I00-I99
     EXCLUDES 1   peripartum cardiomyopathy (O90.3)
     EXCLUDES 2   hypertensive disorders (O10-O16)
                 obstetric embolism (O88.-)
                 venous complications and cerebrovenous sinus thrombosis in labor, childbirth and the puerperium (O87.-)
                 venous complications and cerebrovenous sinus thrombosis in pregnancy (O22.-)

√6ᵗʰ **O99.41** Diseases of the circulatory system complicating pregnancy

O99.411 Diseases of the circulatory system complicating pregnancy, first trimester   Ⓜ♀

O99.412 Diseases of the circulatory system complicating pregnancy, second trimester   Ⓜ♀

O99.413 Diseases of the circulatory system complicating pregnancy, third trimester   Ⓜ♀

O99.419 Diseases of the circulatory system complicating pregnancy, unspecified trimester   Ⓜ♀

O99.42 Diseases of the circulatory system complicating childbirth   Ⓜ♀

O99.43 Diseases of the circulatory system complicating the puerperium   Ⓜ♀

√5ᵗʰ **O99.5** Diseases of the respiratory system complicating pregnancy, childbirth and the puerperium
     Conditions in J00-J99

√6ᵗʰ **O99.51** Diseases of the respiratory system complicating pregnancy

O99.511 Diseases of the respiratory system complicating pregnancy, first trimester   Ⓜ♀

O99.512 Diseases of the respiratory system complicating pregnancy, second trimester   Ⓜ♀

O99.513 Diseases of the respiratory system complicating pregnancy, third trimester   Ⓜ♀

O99.519 Diseases of the respiratory system complicating pregnancy, unspecified trimester   Ⓜ♀

O99.52 Diseases of the respiratory system complicating childbirth   Ⓜ♀

O99.53 Diseases of the respiratory system complicating the puerperium   Ⓜ♀

√5ᵗʰ **O99.6** Diseases of the digestive system complicating pregnancy, childbirth and the puerperium
     Conditions in K00-K93
     EXCLUDES 2   liver and biliary tract disorders in pregnancy, childbirth and the puerperium (O26.6-)

√6ᵗʰ **O99.61** Diseases of the digestive system complicating pregnancy

O99.611 Diseases of the digestive system complicating pregnancy, first trimester   Ⓜ♀

O99.612 Diseases of the digestive system complicating pregnancy, second trimester   Ⓜ♀

O99.613 Diseases of the digestive system complicating pregnancy, third trimester   Ⓜ♀

O99.619 Diseases of the digestive system complicating pregnancy, unspecified trimester   Ⓜ♀

O99.62 Diseases of the digestive system complicating childbirth   Ⓜ♀

O99.63 Diseases of the digestive system complicating the puerperium   Ⓜ♀

√5ᵗʰ **O99.7** Diseases of the skin and subcutaneous tissue complicating pregnancy, childbirth and the puerperium
     Conditions in L00-L99
     EXCLUDES 2   herpes gestationis (O26.4)
                 pruritic urticarial papules and plaques of pregnancy (PUPPP) (O26.86)

√6ᵗʰ **O99.71** Diseases of the skin and subcutaneous tissue complicating pregnancy

O99.711 Diseases of the skin and subcutaneous tissue complicating pregnancy, first trimester   Ⓜ♀

O99.712 Diseases of the skin and subcutaneous tissue complicating pregnancy, second trimester   Ⓜ♀

O99.713 Diseases of the skin and subcutaneous tissue complicating pregnancy, third trimester   Ⓜ♀

EXCLUDES 1 Not coded here   EXCLUDES 2 Not included here   Ⓝ Newborn Age: 0   Ⓟ Pediatric Age: 0-17   Ⓜ Maternity Age: 12-55   Ⓐ Adult Age: 15-124

762   ICD-10-CM 2014 (Draft)

O99.719 Diseases of the skin and Ⓜ♀
subcutaneous tissue complicating
pregnancy, unspecified trimester

O99.72 Diseases of the skin and subcutaneous tissue Ⓜ♀
complicating childbirth

O99.73 Diseases of the skin and subcutaneous tissue Ⓜ♀
complicating the puerperium

✓5ᵗʰ **O99.8 Other specified diseases and conditions complicating**
pregnancy, childbirth and the puerperium
Conditions in D00-D48, H00-H95, M00-N99, and Q00-Q99
Use additional code to identify condition
EXCLUDES 2 *genitourinary infections in pregnancy (O23.-)*
infection of genitourinary tract following delivery
(O86.1-O86.3)
malignant neoplasm complicating pregnancy,
childbirth and the puerperium (O9A.1-)
maternal care for known or suspected abnormality of
maternal pelvic organs (O34.-)
postpartum acute kidney failure (O90.4)
traumatic injuries in pregnancy (O9A.2)

✓6ᵗʰ **O99.81 Abnormal glucose complicating pregnancy,**
childbirth and the puerperium
EXCLUDES 1 *gestational diabetes (O24.4-)*

O99.810 Abnormal glucose complicating Ⓜ♀
pregnancy

O99.814 Abnormal glucose complicating Ⓜ♀
childbirth

O99.815 Abnormal glucose complicating the Ⓜ♀
puerperium

✓6ᵗʰ **O99.82 Streptococcus B carrier state complicating**
pregnancy, childbirth and the puerperium

O99.820 Streptococcus B carrier state Ⓜ♀
complicating pregnancy

O99.824 Streptococcus B carrier state Ⓜ♀
complicating childbirth

O99.825 Streptococcus B carrier state Ⓜ♀
complicating the puerperium

✓6ᵗʰ **O99.83 Other infection carrier state complicating**
pregnancy, childbirth and the puerperium
Use additional code to identify the carrier state (Z22.-)

O99.830 Other infection carrier state Ⓜ♀
complicating pregnancy

O99.834 Other infection carrier state Ⓜ♀
complicating childbirth

O99.835 Other infection carrier state Ⓜ♀
complicating the puerperium

✓6ᵗʰ **O99.84 Bariatric surgery status complicating pregnancy,**
childbirth and the puerperium
Gastric banding status complicating pregnancy,
childbirth and the puerperium
Gastric bypass status for obesity complicating
pregnancy, childbirth and the puerperium
Obesity surgery status complicating pregnancy,
childbirth and the puerperium

O99.840 Bariatric surgery status complicating Ⓜ♀
pregnancy, unspecified trimester

O99.841 Bariatric surgery status complicating Ⓜ♀
pregnancy, first trimester

O99.842 Bariatric surgery status complicating Ⓜ♀
pregnancy, second trimester

O99.843 Bariatric surgery status complicating Ⓜ♀
pregnancy, third trimester

O99.844 Bariatric surgery status complicating Ⓜ♀
childbirth

O99.845 Bariatric surgery status complicating Ⓜ♀
the puerperium

O99.89 Other specified diseases and conditions Ⓜ♀
complicating pregnancy, childbirth and the
puerperium

✓4ᵗʰ **O9A Maternal malignant neoplasms, traumatic injuries and abuse**
classifiable elsewhere but complicating pregnancy, childbirth
and the puerperium

✓5ᵗʰ **O9A.1 Malignant neoplasm complicating pregnancy, childbirth and**
the puerperium
Conditions in C00-C96
Use additional code to identify neoplasm
EXCLUDES 2 *maternal care for benign tumor of corpus uteri (O34.1-)*
maternal care for benign tumor of cervix (O34.4-)

✓6ᵗʰ **O9A.11 Malignant neoplasm complicating pregnancy**

O9A.111 Malignant neoplasm complicating Ⓜ♀
pregnancy, first trimester

O9A.112 Malignant neoplasm complicating Ⓜ♀
pregnancy, second trimester

O9A.113 Malignant neoplasm complicating Ⓜ♀
pregnancy, third trimester

O9A.119 Malignant neoplasm complicating Ⓜ♀
pregnancy, unspecified trimester

O9A.12 Malignant neoplasm complicating childbirth Ⓜ♀

O9A.13 Malignant neoplasm complicating the Ⓜ♀
puerperium

✓5ᵗʰ **O9A.2 Injury, poisoning and certain other consequences of external**
causes complicating pregnancy, childbirth and the
puerperium
Conditions in S00-T88, except T74 and T76
Use additional code(s) to identify the injury or poisoning
EXCLUDES 2 *physical, sexual and psychological abuse complicating*
pregnancy, childbirth and the puerperium
(O9A.3-, O9A.4-, O9A.5-)

✓6ᵗʰ **O9A.21 Injury, poisoning and certain other consequences of**
external causes complicating pregnancy

O9A.211 Injury, poisoning and certain other Ⓜ♀
consequences of external causes
complicating pregnancy, first trimester

O9A.212 Injury, poisoning and certain other Ⓜ♀
consequences of external causes
complicating pregnancy, second trimester

O9A.213 Injury, poisoning and certain other Ⓜ♀
consequences of external causes
complicating pregnancy, third trimester

O9A.219 Injury, poisoning and certain other Ⓜ♀
consequences of external causes
complicating pregnancy, unspecified
trimester

O9A.22 Injury, poisoning and certain other Ⓜ♀
consequences of external causes complicating
childbirth

O9A.23 Injury, poisoning and certain other Ⓜ♀
consequencesof external causes complicating the
puerperium

✓5ᵗʰ **O9A.3 Physical abuse complicating pregnancy, childbirth and the**
puerperium
Conditions in T74.11 or T76.11
Use additional code (if applicable):
to identify any associated current injury due to physical abuse
to identify the perpetrator of abuse (Y07.-)
EXCLUDES 2 *sexual abuse complicating pregnancy, childbirth and*
the puerperium (O9A.4)

✓6ᵗʰ **O9A.31 Physical abuse complicating pregnancy**

O9A.311 Physical abuse complicating Ⓜ♀
pregnancy, first trimester

O9A.312 Physical abuse complicating Ⓜ♀
pregnancy,second trimester

O9A.313 Physical abuse complicating Ⓜ♀
pregnancy, third trimester

O9A.319 Physical abuse complicating Ⓜ♀
pregnancy,unspecified trimester

O9A.32 Physical abuse complicating childbirth Ⓜ♀

O9A.33 Physical abuse complicating the puerperium Ⓜ♀

✓5ᵗʰ **O9A.4** **Sexual abuse** complicating pregnancy, childbirth and the puerperium
　　Conditions in T74.21 or T76.21
　　Use additional code (if applicable):
　　　　to identify any associated current injury due to sexual abuse
　　　　to identify the perpetrator of abuse (Y07.-)

　✓6ᵗʰ **O9A.41** **Sexual abuse complicating** pregnancy
　　　　O9A.411 **Sexual abuse complicating pregnancy,** Ⓜ♀
　　　　　　　　first trimester
　　　　O9A.412 **Sexual abuse complicating pregnancy,** Ⓜ♀
　　　　　　　　second trimester
　　　　O9A.413 **Sexual abuse complicating pregnancy,** Ⓜ♀
　　　　　　　　third trimester
　　　　O9A.419 **Sexual abuse complicating** Ⓜ♀
　　　　　　　　pregnancy, unspecified trimester
　　　O9A.42 **Sexual abuse complicating** childbirth Ⓜ♀
　　　O9A.43 **Sexual abuse complicating the** puerperium Ⓜ♀

✓5ᵗʰ **O9A.5** **Psychological abuse** complicating pregnancy, childbirth and the puerperium
　　Conditions in T74.31 or T76.31
　　Use additional code to identify the perpetrator of abuse (Y07.-)

　✓6ᵗʰ **O9A.51** **Psychological abuse complicating** pregnancy
　　　　O9A.511 **Psychological abuse complicating** Ⓜ♀
　　　　　　　　pregnancy, first trimester
　　　　O9A.512 **Psychological abuse complicating** Ⓜ♀
　　　　　　　　pregnancy, second trimester
　　　　O9A.513 **Psychological abuse complicating** Ⓜ♀
　　　　　　　　pregnancy, third trimester
　　　　O9A.519 **Psychological abuse complicating** Ⓜ♀
　　　　　　　　pregnancy, unspecified trimester
　　　O9A.52 **Psychological abuse complicating** childbirth Ⓜ♀
　　　O9A.53 **Psychological abuse complicating the** Ⓜ♀
　　　　　　puerperium

Chapter 16. Certain Conditions Originating in the Perinatal Period (P00-P96)

NOTE Codes from this chapter are for use on newborn records only, never on maternal records.

INCLUDES conditions that have their origin in the fetal or perinatal period (before birth through the first 28 days after birth) even if morbidity occurs later

EXCLUDES 2 congenital malformations, deformations and chromosomal abnormalities (Q00-Q99)
endocrine, nutritional and metabolic diseases (E00-E88)
injury, poisoning and certain other consequences of external causes (S00-T88)
neoplasms (C00-D49)
tetanus neonatorum (A33)

This chapter contains the following blocks:

P00-P04	Newborn affected by maternal factors and by complications of pregnancy, labor, and delivery
P05-P08	Disorders of newborn related to length of gestation and fetal growth
P09	Abnormal findings on neonatal screening
P10-P15	Birth trauma
P19-P29	Respiratory and cardiovascular disorders specific to the perinatal period
P35-P39	Infections specific to the perinatal period
P50-P61	Hemorrhagic and hematological disorders of newborn
P70-P74	Transitory endocrine and metabolic disorders specific to newborn
P76-P78	Digestive system disorders of newborn
P80-P83	Conditions involving the integument and temperature regulation of newborn
P84	Other problems with newborn
P90-P96	Other disorders originating in the perinatal period

Newborn affected by maternal factors and by complications of pregnancy, labor, and delivery (P00-P04)

NOTE These codes are for use when the listed maternal conditions are specified as the cause of confirmed morbidity or potential morbidity which have their origin in the perinatal period (before birth through the first 28 days after birth). Codes from these categories are also for use for newborns who are suspected of having an abnormal condition resulting from exposure from the mother or the birth process, but without signs or symptoms, and, which after examination and observation, is found not to exist. These codes may be used even if treatment is begun for a suspected condition that is ruled out.

✓4ᵗʰ P00 Newborn (suspected to be) affected by maternal conditions that may be unrelated to present pregnancy

Code first any current condition in newborn

EXCLUDES 2 newborn (suspected to be) affected by maternal complications of pregnancy (P01.-)
newborn affected by maternal endocrine and metabolic disorders (P70-P74)
newborn affected by noxious substances transmitted via placenta or breast milk (P04.-)

P00.0 Newborn (suspected to be) affected by maternal hypertensive disorders N

Newborn (suspected to be) affected by maternal conditions classifiable to O10-O11, O13-O16

P00.1 Newborn (suspected to be) affected by maternal renal and urinary tract diseases N

Newborn (suspected to be) affected by maternal conditions classifiable to N00-N39

P00.2 Newborn (suspected to be) affected by maternal infectious and parasitic diseases N

Newborn (suspected to be) affected by maternal infectious disease classifiable to A00-B99, J09 and J10

EXCLUDES 1 infections specific to the perinatal period (P35-P39)
maternal genital tract or other localized infections (P00.8)

P00.3 Newborn (suspected to be) affected by other maternal circulatory and respiratory diseases N

Newborn (suspected to be) affected by maternal conditions classifiable to I00-I99, J00-J99, Q20-Q34 and not included in P00.0, P00.2

P00.4 Newborn (suspected to be) affected by maternal nutritional disorders N

Newborn (suspected to be) affected by maternal disorders classifiable to E40-E64
Maternal malnutrition NOS

P00.5 Newborn (suspected to be) affected by maternal injury N

Newborn (suspected to be) affected by maternal conditions classifiable to O9A.2-

P00.6 Newborn (suspected to be) affected by surgical procedure on mother N

Newborn (suspected to be) affected by amniocentesis

EXCLUDES 1 Cesarean delivery for present delivery (P03.4)
damage to placenta from amniocentesis, Cesarean delivery or surgical induction (P02.1)
previous surgery to uterus or pelvic organs (P03.89)

EXCLUDES 2 newborn affected by complication of (fetal) intrauterine procedure (P96.5)

P00.7 Newborn (suspected to be) affected by other medical procedures on mother, not elsewhere classified 8

Newborn (suspected to be) affected by radiation to mother

EXCLUDES 1 damage to placenta from amniocentesis, cesarean delivery or surgical induction (P02.1)
newborn affected by other complications of labor and delivery (P03.-)

✓5ᵗʰ P00.8 Newborn (suspected to be) affected by other maternal conditions

P00.81 Newborn (suspected to be) affected by periodontal disease in mother N

P00.89 Newborn (suspected to be) affected by other maternal conditions N

Newborn (suspected to be) affected by conditions classifiable to T80-T88
Newborn (suspected to be) affected by maternal genital tract or other localized infections
Newborn (suspected to be) affected by maternal systemic lupus erythematosus

P00.9 Newborn (suspected to be) affected by unspecified maternal condition N

✓4ᵗʰ P01 Newborn (suspected to be) affected by maternal complications of pregnancy

Code first any current condition in newborn

P01.0 Newborn (suspected to be) affected by incompetent cervix N

P01.1 Newborn (suspected to be) affected by premature rupture of membranes N

P01.2 Newborn (suspected to be) affected by oligohydramnios N

EXCLUDES 1 oligohydramnios due to premature rupture of membranes (P01.1)

P01.3 Newborn (suspected to be) affected by polyhydramnios N

Newborn (suspected to be) affected by hydramnios

P01.4 Newborn (suspected to be) affected by ectopic pregnancy N

Newborn (suspected to be) affected by abdominal pregnancy

P01.5 Newborn (suspected to be) affected by multiple pregnancy N

Newborn (suspected to be) affected by triplet (pregnancy)
Newborn (suspected to be) affected by twin (pregnancy)

P01.6 Newborn (suspected to be) affected by maternal death N

P01.7 Newborn (suspected to be) affected by malpresentation before labor N

Newborn (suspected to be) affected by breech presentation before labor
Newborn (suspected to be) affected by external version before labor
Newborn (suspected to be) affected by face presentation before labor
Newborn (suspected to be) affected by transverse lie before labor
Newborn (suspected to be) affected by unstable lie before labor

P01.8 Newborn (suspected to be) affected by other maternal complications of pregnancy N

P01.9 Newborn (suspected to be) affected by maternal complication of pregnancy, unspecified N

✓4ᵗʰ P02 Newborn (suspected to be) affected by complications of placenta, cord and membranes

Code first any current condition in newborn

P02.0 Newborn (suspected to be) affected by placenta previa N

P02.1 Newborn (suspected to be) affected by other forms of placental separation and hemorrhage N

Newborn (suspected to be) affected by abruptio placenta
Newborn (suspected to be) affected by accidental hemorrhage
Newborn (suspected to be) affected by antepartum hemorrhage
Newborn (suspected to be) affected by damage to placenta from amniocentesis, cesarean delivery or surgical induction
Newborn (suspected to be) affected by maternal blood loss
Newborn (suspected to be) affected by premature separation of placenta

---

☑ Additional Character Required   ✓x7ᵗʰ Xtension Alert   Unspecified Code   Other Specified Code   Manifestation Code   ►◄ Revised Text   ● New Code   ▲ Revised Code Title

√5ᵗʰ **P02.2** **Newborn (suspected to be) affected by other and unspecified morphological and functional abnormalities** of placenta

     P02.20 **Newborn (suspected to be) affected by unspecified morphological and functional abnormalities of placenta** ℕ

     P02.29 **Newborn (suspected to be) affected by other morphological and functional abnormalities of placenta** ℕ

         Newborn (suspected to be) affected by placental dysfunction

         Newborn (suspected to be) affected by placental infarction

         Newborn (suspected to be) affected by placental insufficiency

P02.3 **Newborn (suspected to be) affected by placental transfusion syndromes** ℕ

     Newborn (suspected to be) affected by placental and cord abnormalities resulting in twin-to-twin or other transplacental transfusion

P02.4 **Newborn (suspected to be) affected by prolapsed cord** ℕ

P02.5 **Newborn (suspected to be) affected by other compression of umbilical cord** ℕ

     Newborn (suspected to be) affected by umbilical cord (tightly) around neck

     Newborn (suspected to be) affected by entanglement of umbilical cord

     Newborn (suspected to be) affected by knot in umbilical cord

√5ᵗʰ **P02.6** **Newborn (suspected to be) affected by other and unspecified conditions of umbilical cord**

     P02.60 **Newborn (suspected to be) affected by unspecified conditions of umbilical cord** ℕ

     P02.69 **Newborn (suspected to be) affected by other conditions of umbilical cord** ℕ

         Newborn (suspected to be) affected by short umbilical cord

         Newborn (suspected to be) affected by vasa previa

         EXCLUDES 1   *newborn affected by single umbilical artery (Q27.0)*

P02.7 **Newborn (suspected to be) affected by chorioamnionitis** ℕ

     Newborn (suspected to be) affected by amnionitis

     Newborn (suspected to be) affected by membranitis

     Newborn (suspected to be) affected by placentitis

P02.8 **Newborn (suspected to be) affected by other abnormalities of membranes** ℕ

P02.9 **Newborn (suspected to be) affected by abnormality of membranes, unspecified** ℕ

√4ᵗʰ **P03** **Newborn (suspected to be) affected by other complications of labor and delivery**

     Code first any current condition in newborn

P03.0 **Newborn (suspected to be) affected by breech delivery and extraction** ℕ

P03.1 **Newborn (suspected to be) affected by other malpresentation, malposition and disproportion during labor and delivery** ℕ

     Newborn (suspected to be) affected by contracted pelvis

     Newborn (suspected to be) affected by conditions classifiable to O64-O66

     Newborn (suspected to be) affected by persistent occipitoposterior

     Newborn (suspected to be) affected by transverse lie

P03.2 **Newborn (suspected to be) affected by forceps delivery** ℕ

P03.3 **Newborn (suspected to be) affected by delivery by vacuum extractor [ventouse]** ℕ

P03.4 **Newborn (suspected to be) affected by Cesarean delivery** ℕ

P03.5 **Newborn (suspected to be) affected by precipitate delivery** ℕ

     Newborn (suspected to be) affected by rapid second stage

P03.6 **Newborn (suspected to be) affected by abnormal uterine contractions** ℕ

     Newborn (suspected to be) affected by conditions classifiable to O62-, except O62.3

     Newborn (suspected to be) affected by hypertonic labor

     Newborn (suspected to be) affected by uterine inertia

√5ᵗʰ **P03.8** **Newborn (suspected to be) affected by other specified complications of labor and delivery**

     √6ᵗʰ **P03.81** **Newborn (suspected to be) affected by abnormality in fetal (intrauterine) heart rate or rhythm**

         EXCLUDES 1   *neonatal cardiac dysrhythmia (P29.1-)*

         P03.810 **Newborn (suspected to be) affected by abnormality in fetal (intrauterine) heart rate or rhythm before the onset of labor** ℕ

         P03.811 **Newborn (suspected to be) affected by abnormality in fetal (intrauterine) heart rate or rhythm during labor** ℕ

         P03.819 **Newborn (suspected to be) affected by abnormality in fetal (intrauterine) heart rate or rhythm, unspecified as to time of onset** ℕ

     P03.82 **Meconium passage during delivery** ℕ

         EXCLUDES 1   *meconium aspiration (P24.00, P24.01)*

                 meconium staining (P96.83)

     P03.89 **Newborn (suspected to be) affected by other specified complications of labor and delivery** ℕ

         Newborn (suspected to be) affected by abnormality of maternal soft tissues

         Newborn (suspected to be) affected by conditions classifiable to O60-O75 and by procedures used in labor and delivery not included in P02- and P03.0-P03.6

         Newborn (suspected to be) affected by induction of labor

P03.9 **Newborn (suspected to be) affected by complication of labor and delivery, unspecified** ℕ

√4ᵗʰ **P04** **Newborn (suspected to be) affected by noxious substances transmitted via placenta or breast milk**

     INCLUDES   nonteratogenic effects of substances transmitted via placenta

     EXCLUDES 2   *congenital malformations (Q00-Q99)*

                 neonatal jaundice from excessive hemolysis due to drugs or toxins transmitted from mother (P58.4)

                 newborn in contact with and (suspected) exposures hazardous to health not transmitted via placenta or breast milk (Z77.-)

P04.0 **Newborn (suspected to be) affected by maternal anesthesia and analgesia in pregnancy, labor and delivery** ℕ

     Newborn (suspected to be) affected by reactions and intoxications from maternal opiates and tranquilizers administered during labor and delivery

P04.1 **Newborn (suspected to be) affected by other maternal medication** ℕ

     Newborn (suspected to be) affected by cancer chemotherapy

     Newborn (suspected to be) affected by cytotoxic drugs

     EXCLUDES 1   *dysmorphism due to warfarin (Q86.2)*

                 fetal hydantoin syndrome (Q86.1)

                 maternal use of drugs of addiction (P04.4-)

P04.2 **Newborn (suspected to be) affected by maternal use of tobacco** ℕ

     Newborn (suspected to be) affected by exposure in utero to tobacco smoke

     EXCLUDES 2   *newborn exposure to environmental tobacco smoke (P96.81)*

P04.3 **Newborn (suspected to be) affected by maternal use of alcohol** ℕ

     EXCLUDES 1   *fetal alcohol syndrome (Q86.0)*

√5ᵗʰ **P04.4** **Newborn (suspected to be) affected by maternal use of drugs of addiction**

     P04.41 **Newborn (suspected to be) affected by maternal use of cocaine** ℕ

         "Crack baby"

     P04.49 **Newborn (suspected to be) affected by maternal use of other drugs of addiction** ℕ

         EXCLUDES 2   *newborn (suspected to be) affected by maternal anesthesia and analgesia (P04.0)*

                 withdrawal symptoms from maternal use of drugs of addiction (P96.1)

P04.5 **Newborn (suspected to be) affected by maternal use of nutritional chemical substances** ℕ

P04.6 **Newborn (suspected to be) affected by maternal exposure to environmental chemical substances** ℕ

P04.8 **Newborn (suspected to be) affected by other maternal noxious substances** ℕ

P04.9 **Newborn (suspected to be) affected by maternal noxious substance, unspecified** ℕ

EXCLUDES 1 Not coded here   *EXCLUDES 2* Not included here   ℕ Newborn Age: 0   ℙ Pediatric Age: 0-17   ℳ Maternity Age: 12-55   🅰 Adult Age: 15-124

766   ICD-10-CM 2014 (Draft)

Disorders of newborn related to length of gestation and fetal growth (P05-P08)

✓4ᵗʰ P05　Disorders of newborn related to slow fetal growth and fetal malnutrition

✓5ᵗʰ P05.0　Newborn light for gestational age
Newborn light-for-dates

P05.00　Newborn light for gestational age, unspecified weight　N

P05.01　Newborn light for gestational age, less than 500 grams　N

P05.02　Newborn light for gestational age, 500-749 grams　N

P05.03　Newborn light for gestational age, 750-999 grams　N

P05.04　Newborn light for gestational age, 1000-1249 grams　N

P05.05　Newborn light for gestational age, 1250-1499 grams　N

P05.06　Newborn light for gestational age, 1500-1749 grams　N

P05.07　Newborn light for gestational age, 1750-1999 grams　N

P05.08　Newborn light for gestational age, 2000-2499 grams　N

✓5ᵗʰ P05.1　Newborn small for gestational age
Newborn small-and-light-for-dates
Newborn small-for-dates

P05.10　Newborn small for gestational age, unspecified weight　N

P05.11　Newborn small for gestational age, less than 500 grams　N

P05.12　Newborn small for gestational age, 500-749 grams　N

P05.13　Newborn small for gestational age, 750-999 grams　N

P05.14　Newborn small for gestational age, 1000-1249 grams　N

P05.15　Newborn small for gestational age, 1250-1499 grams　N

P05.16　Newborn small for gestational age, 1500-1749 grams　N

P05.17　Newborn small for gestational age, 1750-1999 grams　N

P05.18　Newborn small for gestational age, 2000-2499 grams　N

P05.2　Newborn affected by fetal (intrauterine) malnutrition not light or small for gestational age　N
Infant, not light or small for gestational age, showing signs of fetal malnutrition, such as dry, peeling skin and loss of subcutaneous tissue
　EXCLUDES 1　newborn affected by fetal malnutrition with light for gestational age (P05.0-)
　　newborn affected by fetal malnutrition with small for gestational age (P05.1-)

P05.9　Newborn affected by slow intrauterine growth, unspecified　N
Newborn affected by fetal growth retardation NOS

✓4ᵗʰ P07　Disorders of newborn related to short gestation and low birth weight, not elsewhere classified
　NOTE　When both birth weight and gestational age of the newborn are available, both should be coded with birth weight sequenced before gestational age
The listed conditions, without further specification, as the cause of morbidity or additional care, in newborn
　EXCLUDES 1　low birth weight due to slow fetal growth and fetal malnutrition (P05.-)

✓5ᵗʰ P07.0　Extremely low birth weight newborn
Newborn birth weight 999 g. or less

P07.00　Extremely low birth weight newborn, unspecified weight　N

P07.01　Extremely low birth weight newborn, less than 500 grams　N

P07.02　Extremely low birth weight newborn, 500-749 grams　N

P07.03　Extremely low birth weight newborn, 750-999 grams　N

✓5ᵗʰ P07.1　Other low birth weight newborn
Newborn birth weight 1000-2499 g.

P07.10　Other low birth weight newborn, unspecified weight　N

P07.14　Other low birth weight newborn, 1000-1249 grams　N

P07.15　Other low birth weight newborn, 1250-1499 grams　N

P07.16　Other low birth weight newborn, 1500-1749 grams　N

P07.17　Other low birth weight newborn, 1750-1999 grams　N

P07.18　Other low birth weight newborn, 2000-2499 grams　N

✓5ᵗʰ P07.2　Extreme immaturity of newborn
Less than 28 completed weeks (less than 196 completed days) of gestation.

P07.20　Extreme immaturity of newborn, unspecified weeks of gestation　N
Gestational age less than 28 completed weeks NOS

P07.21　Extreme immaturity of newborn, gestational age less than 23 completed weeks　N
Extreme immaturity of newborn, gestational age less than 23 weeks, 0 days

P07.22　Extreme immaturity of newborn, gestational age 23 completed weeks　N
Extreme immaturity of newborn, gestational age 23 weeks, 0 days through 23 weeks, 6 days

P07.23　Extreme immaturity of newborn, gestational age 24 completed weeks　N
Extreme immaturity of newborn, gestational age 24 weeks, 0 days through 24 weeks, 6 days

P07.24　Extreme immaturity of newborn, gestational age 25 completed weeks　N
Extreme immaturity of newborn, gestational age 25 weeks, 0 days through 25 weeks, 6 days

P07.25　Extreme immaturity of newborn, gestational age 26 completed weeks　N
Extreme immaturity of newborn, gestational age 26 weeks, 0 days through 26 weeks, 6 days

P07.26　Extreme immaturity of newborn, gestational age 27 completed weeks　N
Extreme immaturity of newborn, gestational age 27 weeks, 0 days through 27 weeks, 6 days

✓5ᵗʰ P07.3　Preterm [premature] newborn [other]
28 completed weeks or more but less than 37 completed weeks (196 completed days but less than 259 completed days) of gestation
Prematurity NOS

P07.30　Preterm newborn, unspecified weeks of gestation　N

P07.31　Preterm newborn, gestational age 28 completed weeks　N
Preterm newborn, gestational age 28 weeks, 0 days through 28 weeks, 6 days

P07.32　Preterm newborn, gestational age 29 completed weeks　N
Preterm newborn, gestational age 29 weeks, 0 days through 29 weeks, 6 days

P07.33　Preterm newborn, gestational age 30 completed weeks　N
Preterm newborn, gestational age 30 weeks, 0 days through 30 weeks, 6 days

P07.34　Preterm newborn, gestational age 31 completed weeks　N
Preterm newborn, gestational age 31 weeks, 0 days through 31 weeks, 6 days

P07.35　Preterm newborn, gestational age 32 completed weeks　N
Preterm newborn, gestational age 32 weeks, 0 days through 32 weeks, 6 days

P07.36　Preterm newborn, gestational age 33 completed weeks　N
Preterm newborn, gestational age 33 weeks, 0 days through 33 weeks, 6 days

P07.37　Preterm newborn, gestational age 34 completed weeks　N
Preterm newborn, gestational age 34 weeks, 0 days through 34 weeks, 6 days

---

✓ Additional Character Required　✓x7ᵗʰ Xtension Alert　Unspecified Code　Other Specified Code　Manifestation Code　►◄ Revised Text　● New Code　▲ Revised Code Title

Certain Conditions Originating in the Perinatal Period

P07.38–P22.9

P07.38   **Preterm newborn, gestational age 35 completed weeks**   N
Preterm newborn, gestational age 35 weeks, 0 days through 35 weeks, 6 days

P07.39   **Preterm newborn, gestational age 36 completed weeks**   N
Preterm newborn, gestational age 36 weeks, 0 days through 36 weeks, 6 days

✓4ᵗʰ **P08 Disorders of newborn related to long gestation and high birth weight**

NOTE   When both birth weight and gestational age of the newborn are available, priority of assignment should be given to birth weight

INCLUDES   the listed conditions, without further specification, as causes of morbidity or additional care, in newborn

P08.0   **Exceptionally large newborn baby**   N
Usually implies a birth weight of 4500 g. or more
EXCLUDES 1   *syndrome of infant of diabetic mother (P70.1)*
syndrome of infant of mother with gestational diabetes (P70.0)

P08.1   **Other heavy for gestational age newborn**   N
Other newborn heavy- or large-for-dates regardless of period of gestation
Usually implies a birth weight of 4000 g. to 4499 g.
EXCLUDES 1   *newborn with a birth weight of 4500 or more (P08.0)*
syndrome of infant of diabetic mother (P70.1)
syndrome of infant of mother with gestational diabetes (P70.0).

✓5ᵗʰ P08.2   **Late newborn, not heavy for gestational age**

P08.21   **Post-term newborn**   N
Newborn with gestation period over 40 completed weeks to 42 completed weeks

P08.22   **Prolonged gestation of newborn**   N
Newborn with gestation period over 42 completed weeks (294 days or more), not heavy- or large-for-dates.
Postmaturity NOS

Abnormal findings on neonatal screening (P09)

P09 Abnormal findings on neonatal screening   N
Use additional code to identify signs, symptoms and conditions associated with the screening
EXCLUDES 2   *nonspecific serologic evidence of human immunodeficiency virus [HIV] (R75)*

Birth trauma (P10-P15)

✓4ᵗʰ **P10 Intracranial laceration and hemorrhage due to birth injury**
EXCLUDES 1   *intracranial hemorrhage of newborn NOS (P52.9)*
intracranial hemorrhage of newborn due to anoxia or hypoxia (P52.-)
nontraumatic intracranial hemorrhage of newborn (P52.-)

P10.0   **Subdural hemorrhage due to birth injury**   N
Subdural hematoma (localized) due to birth injury
EXCLUDES 1   *subdural hemorrhage accompanying tentorial tear (P10.4)*

P10.1   **Cerebral hemorrhage due to birth injury**   N
P10.2   **Intraventricular hemorrhage due to birth injury**   N
P10.3   **Subarachnoid hemorrhage due to birth injury**   N
P10.4   **Tentorial tear due to birth injury**   N
P10.8   **Other intracranial lacerations and hemorrhages due to birth injury**   N
P10.9   **Unspecified intracranial laceration and hemorrhage due to birth injury**   N

✓4ᵗʰ **P11 Other birth injuries to central nervous system**
P11.0   **Cerebral edema due to birth injury**   N
P11.1   **Other specified brain damage due to birth injury**   N
P11.2   **Unspecified brain damage due to birth injury**   N
P11.3   **Birth injury to facial nerve**   N
Facial palsy due to birth injury
P11.4   **Birth injury to other cranial nerves**   N
P11.5   **Birth injury to spine and spinal cord**   N
Fracture of spine due to birth injury
P11.9   **Birth injury to central nervous system, unspecified**   N

✓4ᵗʰ **P12 Birth injury to scalp**
P12.0   **Cephalhematoma due to birth injury**   N
P12.1   **Chignon (from vacuum extraction) due to birth injury**   N
P12.2   **Epicranial subaponeurotic hemorrhage due to birth injury**   N
Subgaleal hemorrhage
P12.3   **Bruising of scalp due to birth injury**   N
P12.4   **Injury of scalp of newborn due to monitoring equipment**   N
Sampling incision of scalp of newborn
Scalp clip (electrode) injury of newborn

✓5ᵗʰ P12.8   **Other birth injuries to scalp**
P12.81   **Caput succedaneum**   N
P12.89   **Other birth injuries to scalp**   N
P12.9   **Birth injury to scalp, unspecified**   N

✓4ᵗʰ **P13 Birth injury to skeleton**
EXCLUDES 2   *birth injury to spine (P11.5)*
P13.0   **Fracture of skull due to birth injury**   N
P13.1   **Other birth injuries to skull**   N
EXCLUDES 1   *cephalhematoma (P12.0)*
P13.2   **Birth injury to femur**   N
P13.3   **Birth injury to other long bones**   N
P13.4   **Fracture of clavicle due to birth injury**   N
P13.8   **Birth injuries to other parts of skeleton**   N
P13.9   **Birth injury to skeleton, unspecified**   N

✓4ᵗʰ **P14 Birth injury to peripheral nervous system**
P14.0   **Erb's paralysis due to birth injury**   N
P14.1   **Klumpke's paralysis due to birth injury**   N
P14.2   **Phrenic nerve paralysis due to birth injury**   N
P14.3   **Other brachial plexus birth injuries**   N
P14.8   **Birth injuries to other parts of peripheral nervous system**   N
P14.9   **Birth injury to peripheral nervous system, unspecified**   N

✓4ᵗʰ **P15 Other birth injuries**
P15.0   **Birth injury to liver**   N
Rupture of liver due to birth injury
P15.1   **Birth injury to spleen**   N
Rupture of spleen due to birth injury
P15.2   **Sternomastoid injury due to birth injury**   N
P15.3   **Birth injury to eye**   N
Subconjunctival hemorrhage due to birth injury
Traumatic glaucoma due to birth injury
P15.4   **Birth injury to face**   N
Facial congestion due to birth injury
P15.5   **Birth injury to external genitalia**   N
P15.6   **Subcutaneous fat necrosis due to birth injury**   N
P15.8   **Other specified birth injuries**   N
P15.9   **Birth injury, unspecified**   N

Respiratory and cardiovascular disorders specific to the perinatal period (P19-P29)

✓4ᵗʰ **P19 Metabolic acidemia in newborn**
Metabolic acidemia in newborn
P19.0   **Metabolic acidemia in newborn first noted before onset of labor**   N
P19.1   **Metabolic acidemia in newborn first noted during labor**   N
P19.2   **Metabolic acidemia noted at birth**   N
P19.9   **Metabolic acidemia, unspecified**   N

✓4ᵗʰ **P22 Respiratory distress of newborn**
EXCLUDES 1   *respiratory arrest of newborn (P28.81)*
respiratory failure of newborn NOS (P28.5)

P22.0   **Respiratory distress syndrome of newborn**   N
Cardiorespiratory distress syndrome of newborn
Hyaline membrane disease
Idiopathic respiratory distress syndrome [IRDS or RDS] of newborn
Pulmonary hypoperfusion syndrome
Respiratory distress syndrome, type I

P22.1   **Transient tachypnea of newborn**   N
Idiopathic tachypnea of newborn
Respiratory distress syndrome, type II
Wet lung syndrome

P22.8   **Other respiratory distress of newborn**   N
P22.9   **Respiratory distress of newborn, unspecified**   N

EXCLUDES 1 Not coded here   EXCLUDES 2 Not included here   N Newborn Age: 0   P Pediatric Age: 0-17   M Maternity Age: 12-55   A Adult Age: 15-124

768   ICD-10-CM 2014 (Draft)

✓4ᵗʰ **P23** **Congenital pneumonia**
INCLUDES infective pneumonia acquired in utero or during birth
EXCLUDES1 neonatal pneumonia resulting from aspiration (P24.-)

P23.0 **Congenital pneumonia due to viral agent** N
Use additional code (B97) to identify organism
EXCLUDES1 congenital rubella pneumonitis (P35.0)

P23.1 **Congenital pneumonia due to Chlamydia** N

P23.2 **Congenital pneumonia due to staphylococcus** N

P23.3 **Congenital pneumonia due to streptococcus, group B** N

P23.4 **Congenital pneumonia due to Escherichia coli** N

P23.5 **Congenital pneumonia due to Pseudomonas** N

P23.6 **Congenital pneumonia due to other bacterial agents** N
Congenital pneumonia due to Hemophilus influenzae
Congenital pneumonia due to Klebsiella pneumoniae
Congenital pneumonia due to Mycoplasma
Congenital pneumonia due to Streptococcus, except group B
Use additional code (B95-B96) to identify organism

P23.8 **Congenital pneumonia due to other organisms** N

P23.9 **Congenital pneumonia, unspecified** N

✓4ᵗʰ **P24** **Neonatal aspiration**
INCLUDES aspiration in utero and during delivery

✓5ᵗʰ **P24.0** **Meconium aspiration**
EXCLUDES1 meconium passage (without aspiration) during delivery
(P03.82)
meconium staining (P96.83)

P24.00 **Meconium aspiration without respiratory** N
symptoms
Meconium aspiration NOS

P24.01 **Meconium aspiration with respiratory symptoms** N
Meconium aspiration pneumonia
Meconium aspiration pneumonitis
Meconium aspiration syndrome NOS
Use additional code to identify any secondary
pulmonary hypertension, if applicable (I27.2)

✓5ᵗʰ **P24.1** **Neonatal aspiration of (clear) amniotic fluid and mucus**
Neonatal aspiration of liquor (amnii)

P24.10 **Neonatal aspiration of (clear) amniotic fluid and** N
mucus without respiratory symptoms
Neonatal aspiration of amniotic fluid and mucus NOS

P24.11 **Neonatal aspiration of (clear) amniotic fluid and** N
mucus with respiratory symptoms
Neonatal aspiration of amniotic fluid and mucus with
pneumonia
Neonatal aspiration of amniotic fluid and mucus with
pneumonitis
Use additional code to identify any secondary
pulmonary hypertension, if applicable (I27.2)

✓5ᵗʰ **P24.2** **Neonatal aspiration of blood**

P24.20 **Neonatal aspiration of blood without respiratory** N
symptoms
Neonatal aspiration of blood NOS

P24.21 **Neonatal aspiration of blood with respiratory** N
symptoms
Neonatal aspiration of blood with pneumonia
Neonatal aspiration of blood with pneumonitis
Use additional code to identify any secondary
pulmonary hypertension, if applicable (I27.2)

✓5ᵗʰ **P24.3** **Neonatal aspiration of milk and regurgitated food**
Neonatal aspiration of stomach contents

P24.30 **Neonatal aspiration of milk and regurgitated** N
food without respiratory symptoms
Neonatal aspiration of milk and regurgitated food NOS

P24.31 **Neonatal aspiration of milk and regurgitated** N
food with respiratory symptoms
Neonatal aspiration of milk and regurgitated food with
pneumonia
Neonatal aspiration of milk and regurgitated food with
pneumonitis
Use additional code to identify any secondary
pulmonary hypertension, if applicable (I27.2)

✓5ᵗʰ **P24.8** **Other neonatal aspiration**

P24.80 **Other neonatal aspiration without respiratory** N
symptoms
Neonatal aspiration NEC

P24.81 **Other neonatal aspiration with respiratory** N
symptoms
Neonatal aspiration pneumonia NEC
Neonatal aspiration with pneumonitis NEC
Neonatal aspiration with pneumonia NOS
Neonatal aspiration with pneumonitis NOS
Use additional code to identify any secondary
pulmonary hypertension, if applicable (I27.2)

P24.9 **Neonatal aspiration, unspecified** N

✓4ᵗʰ **P25** **Interstitial emphysema and related conditions originating**
in the perinatal period

P25.0 **Interstitial emphysema originating in the perinatal period** N

P25.1 **Pneumothorax originating in the perinatal period** N

P25.2 **Pneumomediastinum originating in the perinatal period** N

P25.3 **Pneumopericardium originating in the perinatal period** N

P25.8 **Other conditions related to interstitial emphysema** N
originating in the perinatal period

✓4ᵗʰ **P26** **Pulmonary hemorrhage originating in the perinatal period**
EXCLUDES1 acute idiopathic hemorrhage in infants over 28 days old
(R04.81)

P26.0 **Tracheobronchial hemorrhage originating in the** N
perinatal period

P26.1 **Massive pulmonary hemorrhage originating in the** N
perinatal period

P26.8 **Other pulmonary hemorrhages originating in the** N
perinatal period

P26.9 **Unspecified pulmonary hemorrhage originating** N
in the perinatal period

✓4ᵗʰ **P27** **Chronic respiratory disease originating in the perinatal period**
EXCLUDES1 respiratory distress of newborn (P22.0-P22.9)

P27.0 **Wilson-Mikity syndrome**
Pulmonary dysmaturity

P27.1 **Bronchopulmonary dysplasia originating in the perinatal**
period

P27.8 **Other chronic respiratory diseases originating in the perinatal**
period
Congenital pulmonary fibrosis
Ventilator lung in newborn

P27.9 **Unspecified chronic respiratory disease originating in the**
perinatal period

✓4ᵗʰ **P28** **Other respiratory conditions originating in the perinatal period**
EXCLUDES1 congenital malformations of the respiratory system (Q30-Q34)

P28.0 **Primary atelectasis of newborn** N
Primary failure to expand terminal respiratory units
Pulmonary hypoplasia associated with short gestation
Pulmonary immaturity NOS

✓5ᵗʰ **P28.1** **Other and unspecified atelectasis of newborn**

P28.10 **Unspecified atelectasis of newborn** N
Atelectasis of newborn NOS

P28.11 **Resorption atelectasis without respiratory** N
distress syndrome
EXCLUDES1 resorption atelectasis with respiratory
distress syndrome (P22.0)

P28.19 **Other atelectasis of newborn** N
Partial atelectasis of newborn
Secondary atelectasis of newborn

P28.2 **Cyanotic attacks of newborn** N
EXCLUDES1 apnea of newborn (P28.3-P28.4)

P28.3 **Primary sleep apnea of newborn** N
Central sleep apnea of newborn
Obstructive sleep apnea of newborn
Sleep apnea of newborn NOS

P28.4 **Other apnea of newborn** N
Apnea of prematurity
Obstructive apnea of newborn
EXCLUDES1 obstructive sleep apnea of newborn (P28.3)

P28.5 **Respiratory failure of newborn** N
EXCLUDES1 respiratory arrest of newborn (P28.81)
respiratory distress of newborn (P22.0-)

✓5ᵗʰ **P28.8** **Other specified respiratory conditions of newborn**

P28.81 **Respiratory arrest of newborn** N

P28.89 **Other specified respiratory conditions of** N
newborn
Congenital laryngeal stridor
Sniffles in newborn
Snuffles in newborn
EXCLUDES1 early congenital syphilitic rhinitis (A50.05)

✓ Additional Character Required   ✓x7ᵗʰ Xtension Alert   Unspecified Code   Other Specified Code   Manifestation Code   ▶◀ Revised Text   ● New Code   ▲ Revised Code Title

ICD-10-CM 2014 (Draft)   **769**

P28.9 **Respiratory condition of newborn, unspecified**   N
Respiratory depression in newborn

✓4ᵗʰ **P29** **Cardiovascular disorders originating in the perinatal period**
EXCLUDES 1   congenital malformations of the circulatory system (Q20-Q28)

P29.0 **Neonatal cardiac failure**   N

✓5ᵗʰ **P29.1** **Neonatal cardiac dysrhythmia**

     P29.11 **Neonatal tachycardia**   N

     P29.12 **Neonatal bradycardia**   N

P29.2 **Neonatal hypertension**   N

P29.3 **Persistent fetal circulation**   N
Delayed closure of ductus arteriosus
(Persistent) pulmonary hypertension of newborn

P29.4 **Transient myocardial ischemia in newborn**   N

✓5ᵗʰ **P29.8** **Other cardiovascular disorders originating in the perinatal period**

     P29.81 **Cardiac arrest of newborn**   N

     P29.89 **Other cardiovascular disorders originating in the perinatal period**   N

P29.9 **Cardiovascular disorder originating in the perinatal period, unspecified**   N

Infections specific to the perinatal period (P35-P39)

Infections acquired in utero, during birth via the umbilicus, or during the first 28 days after birth

EXCLUDES 2   asymptomatic human immunodeficiency virus [HIV] infection status (Z21)
congenital gonococcal infection (A54.-)
congenital pneumonia (P23.-)
congenital syphilis (A50.-)
human immunodeficiency virus [HIV] disease (B20)
infant botulism (A48.51)
infectious diseases not specific to the perinatal period (A00-B99, J09, J10-)
intestinal infectious disease (A00-A09)
laboratory evidence of human immunodeficiency virus [HIV] (R75)
tetanus neonatorum (A33)

✓4ᵗʰ **P35** **Congenital viral diseases**
INCLUDES   infections acquired in utero or during birth

P35.0 **Congenital rubella syndrome**   N
Congenital rubella pneumonitis

P35.1 **Congenital cytomegalovirus infection**   N

P35.2 **Congenital herpesviral [herpes simplex] infection**   N

P35.3 **Congenital viral hepatitis**   N

P35.8 **Other congenital viral diseases**   N
Congenital varicella [chickenpox]

P35.9 **Congenital viral disease, unspecified**   N

✓4ᵗʰ **P36** **Bacterial sepsis of newborn**
INCLUDES   congenital sepsis
Use additional code(s), if applicable, to identify severe sepsis (R65.2-) and associated acute organ dysfunction(s)

P36.0 **Sepsis of newborn due to streptococcus, group B**   N

✓5ᵗʰ **P36.1** **Sepsis of newborn due to other and unspecified streptococci**

     P36.10 **Sepsis of newborn due to unspecified streptococci**   N

     P36.19 **Sepsis of newborn due to other streptococci**   N

P36.2 **Sepsis of newborn due to Staphylococcus aureus**   N

✓5ᵗʰ **P36.3** **Sepsis of newborn due to other and unspecified staphylococci**

     P36.30 **Sepsis of newborn due to unspecified staphylococci**   N

     P36.39 **Sepsis of newborn due to other staphylococci**   N

P36.4 **Sepsis of newborn due to Escherichia coli**   N

P36.5 **Sepsis of newborn due to anaerobes**   N

P36.8 **Other bacterial sepsis of newborn**   N
Use additional code from category B96 to identify organism

P36.9 **Bacterial sepsis of newborn, unspecified**   N

✓4ᵗʰ **P37** **Other congenital infectious and parasitic diseases**
EXCLUDES 2   congenital syphilis (A50.-)
infectious neonatal diarrhea (A00-A09)
necrotizing enterocolitis in newborn (P77.-)
noninfectious neonatal diarrhea (P78.3)
ophthalmia neonatorum due to gonococcus (A54.31)
tetanus neonatorum (A33)

P37.0 **Congenital tuberculosis**   N

P37.1 **Congenital toxoplasmosis**   N
Hydrocephalus due to congenital toxoplasmosis

P37.2 **Neonatal (disseminated) listeriosis**   N

P37.3 **Congenital falciparum malaria**   N

P37.4 **Other congenital malaria**   N

P37.5 **Neonatal candidiasis**   N

P37.8 **Other specified congenital infectious and parasitic diseases**   N

P37.9 **Congenital infectious or parasitic disease, unspecified**   N

✓4ᵗʰ **P38** **Omphalitis of newborn**
EXCLUDES 1   omphalitis not of newborn (L08.82)
tetanus omphalitis (A33)
umbilical hemorrhage of newborn (P51.-)

P38.1 **Omphalitis with mild hemorrhage**   N

P38.9 **Omphalitis without hemorrhage**   N
Omphalitis of newborn NOS

✓4ᵗʰ **P39** **Other infections specific to the perinatal period**
Use additional code to identify organism or specific infection

P39.0 **Neonatal infective mastitis**   N
EXCLUDES 1   breast engorgement of newborn (P83.4)
noninfective mastitis of newborn (P83.4)

P39.1 **Neonatal conjunctivitis and dacryocystitis**   N
Neonatal chlamydial conjunctivitis
Ophthalmia neonatorum NOS
EXCLUDES 1   gonococcal conjunctivitis (A54.31)

P39.2 **Intra-amniotic infection affecting newborn, not elsewhere classified**   N

P39.3 **Neonatal urinary tract infection**   N

P39.4 **Neonatal skin infection**   N
Neonatal pyoderma
EXCLUDES 1   pemphigus neonatorum (L00)
staphylococcal scalded skin syndrome (L00)

P39.8 **Other specified infections specific to the perinatal period**   N

P39.9 **Infection specific to the perinatal period, unspecified**   N

Hemorrhagic and hematological disorders of newborn (P50-P61)

EXCLUDES 1   congenital stenosis and stricture of bile ducts (Q44.3)
Crigler-Najjar syndrome (E80.5)
Dubin-Johnson syndrome (E80.6)
Gilbert syndrome (E80.4)
hereditary hemolytic anemias (D55-D58)

✓4ᵗʰ **P50** **Newborn affected by intrauterine (fetal) blood loss**
EXCLUDES 1   congenital anemia from intrauterine (fetal) blood loss (P61.3)

P50.0 **Newborn affected by intrauterine (fetal) blood loss from vasa previa**   N

P50.1 **Newborn affected by intrauterine (fetal) blood loss from ruptured cord**   N

P50.2 **Newborn affected by intrauterine (fetal) blood loss from placenta**   N

P50.3 **Newborn affected by hemorrhage into co-twin**   N

P50.4 **Newborn affected by hemorrhage into maternal circulation**   N

P50.5 **Newborn affected by intrauterine (fetal) blood loss from cut end of co-twin's cord**   N

P50.8 **Newborn affected by other intrauterine (fetal) blood loss**   N

P50.9 **Newborn affected by intrauterine (fetal) blood loss, unspecified**   N
Newborn affected by fetal hemorrhage NOS

✓4ᵗʰ **P51** **Umbilical hemorrhage of newborn**
EXCLUDES 1   omphalitis with mild hemorrhage (P38.1)
umbilical hemorrhage from cut end of co-twins cord (P50.5)

P51.0 **Massive umbilical hemorrhage of newborn**   N

P51.8 **Other umbilical hemorrhages of newborn**   N
Slipped umbilical ligature NOS

P51.9 **Umbilical hemorrhage of newborn, unspecified**   N

EXCLUDES 1 Not coded here   EXCLUDES 2 Not included here   N Newborn Age: 0   P Pediatric Age: 0-17   M Maternity Age: 12-55   A Adult Age: 15-124

770   ICD-10-CM 2014 (Draft)

✓4ᵗʰ **P52**   **Intracranial nontraumatic hemorrhage of newborn**
Intracranial hemorrhage due to anoxia or hypoxia
EXCLUDES 1   *intracranial hemorrhage due to birth injury (P10.-)*
intracranial hemorrhage due to other injury (S06.-)

P52.0   **Intraventricular (nontraumatic) hemorrhage, grade 1, of newborn**   N
Subependymal hemorrhage (without intraventricular extension)
Bleeding into germinal matrix

P52.1   **Intraventricular (nontraumatic) hemorrhage, grade 2, of newborn**   N
Subependymal hemorrhage with intraventricular extension
Bleeding into ventricle

✓5ᵗʰ **P52.2**   **Intraventricular (nontraumatic) hemorrhage, grade 3 and grade 4, of newborn**

    P52.21   **Intraventricular (nontraumatic) hemorrhage, grade 3, of newborn**   N
Subependymal hemorrhage with intraventricular extension with enlargement of ventricle

    P52.22   **Intraventricular (nontraumatic) hemorrhage, grade 4, of newborn**   N
Bleeding into cerebral cortex
Subependymal hemorrhage with intracerebral extension

P52.3   **Unspecified intraventricular (nontraumatic) hemorrhage of newborn**   N

P52.4   **Intracerebral (nontraumatic) hemorrhage of newborn**   N

P52.5   **Subarachnoid (nontraumatic) hemorrhage of newborn**   N

P52.6   **Cerebellar (nontraumatic) and posterior fossa hemorrhage of newborn**   N

P52.8   **Other intracranial (nontraumatic) hemorrhages of newborn**   N

P52.9   **Intracranial (nontraumatic) hemorrhage of newborn, unspecified**   N

P53   **Hemorrhagic disease of newborn**   N
Vitamin K deficiency of newborn

✓4ᵗʰ **P54**   **Other neonatal hemorrhages**
EXCLUDES 1   *newborn affected by (intrauterine) blood loss (P50.-)*
pulmonary hemorrhage originating in the perinatal period (P26.-)

P54.0   **Neonatal hematemesis**   N
EXCLUDES 1   *neonatal hematemesis due to swallowed maternal blood (P78.2)*

P54.1   **Neonatal melena**   N
EXCLUDES 1   *neonatal melena due to swallowed maternal blood (P78.2)*

P54.2   **Neonatal rectal hemorrhage**   N

P54.3   **Other neonatal gastrointestinal hemorrhage**   N

P54.4   **Neonatal adrenal hemorrhage**   N

P54.5   **Neonatal cutaneous hemorrhage**   N
Neonatal bruising
Neonatal ecchymoses
Neonatal petechiae
Neonatal superficial hematomata
EXCLUDES 2   *bruising of scalp due to birth injury (P12.3)*
cephalhematoma due to birth injury (P12.0)

P54.6   **Neonatal vaginal hemorrhage**   N♀
Neonatal pseudomenses

P54.8   **Other specified neonatal hemorrhages**   N

P54.9   **Neonatal hemorrhage, unspecified**   N

✓4ᵗʰ **P55**   **Hemolytic disease of newborn**

P55.0   **Rh isoimmunization of newborn**   N

P55.1   **ABO isoimmunization of newborn**   N

P55.8   **Other hemolytic diseases of newborn**   N

P55.9   **Hemolytic disease of newborn, unspecified**   N

✓4ᵗʰ **P56**   **Hydrops fetalis due to hemolytic disease**
EXCLUDES 1   *hydrops fetalis NOS (P83.2)*

P56.0   **Hydrops fetalis due to isoimmunization**   N

✓5ᵗʰ **P56.9**   **Hydrops fetalis due to other and unspecified hemolytic disease**

    P56.90   **Hydrops fetalis due to unspecified hemolytic disease**   N

    P56.99   **Hydrops fetalis due to other hemolytic disease**   N

✓4ᵗʰ **P57**   **Kernicterus**

P57.0   **Kernicterus due to isoimmunization**   N

P57.8   **Other specified kernicterus**   N
EXCLUDES 1   *Crigler-Najjar syndrome (E80.5)*

P57.9   **Kernicterus, unspecified**   N

✓4ᵗʰ **P58**   **Neonatal jaundice due to other excessive hemolysis**
EXCLUDES 1   *jaundice due to isoimmunization (P55-P57)*

P58.0   **Neonatal jaundice due to bruising**   N

P58.1   **Neonatal jaundice due to bleeding**   N

P58.2   **Neonatal jaundice due to infection**   N

P58.3   **Neonatal jaundice due to polycythemia**   N

✓5ᵗʰ **P58.4**   **Neonatal jaundice due to drugs or toxins transmitted from mother or given to newborn**
Code first poisoning due to drug or toxin, if applicable (T36-T65 with fifth or sixth character 1-4 or 6)
Use additional code for adverse effect, if applicable, to identify drug (T36-T50 with fifth or sixth character 5)

    P58.41   **Neonatal jaundice due to drugs or toxins transmitted from mother**   N

    P58.42   **Neonatal jaundice due to drugs or toxins given to newborn**   N

P58.5   **Neonatal jaundice due to swallowed maternal blood**   N

P58.8   **Neonatal jaundice due to other specified excessive hemolysis**   N

P58.9   **Neonatal jaundice due to excessive hemolysis, unspecified**   N

✓4ᵗʰ **P59**   **Neonatal jaundice from other and unspecified causes**
EXCLUDES 1   *jaundice due to inborn errors of metabolism (E70-E88)*
kernicterus (P57.-)

P59.0   **Neonatal jaundice associated with preterm delivery**   N
Hyperbilirubinemia of prematurity
Jaundice due to delayed conjugation associated with preterm delivery

P59.1   **Inspissated bile syndrome**   N

✓5ᵗʰ **P59.2**   **Neonatal jaundice from other and unspecified hepatocellular damage**
EXCLUDES 1   *congenital viral hepatitis (P35.3)*

    P59.20   **Neonatal jaundice from unspecified hepatocellular damage**   N

    P59.29   **Neonatal jaundice from other hepatocellular damage**   N
Neonatal giant cell hepatitis
Neonatal (idiopathic) hepatitis

P59.3   **Neonatal jaundice from breast milk inhibitor**   N

P59.8   **Neonatal jaundice from other specified causes**   N

P59.9   **Neonatal jaundice, unspecified**   N
Neonatal physiological jaundice (intense)(prolonged) NOS

P60   **Disseminated intravascular coagulation of newborn**   N
Defibrination syndrome of newborn

✓4ᵗʰ **P61**   **Other perinatal hematological disorders**
EXCLUDES 1   *transient hypogammaglobulinemia of infancy (D80.7)*

P61.0   **Transient neonatal thrombocytopenia**   N
Neonatal thrombocytopenia due to exchange transfusion
Neonatal thrombocytopenia due to idiopathic maternal thrombocytopenia
Neonatal thrombocytopenia due to isoimmunization

P61.1   **Polycythemia neonatorum**   N

P61.2   **Anemia of prematurity**   N

P61.3   **Congenital anemia from fetal blood loss**   N

P61.4   **Other congenital anemias, not elsewhere classified**   N
Congenital anemia NOS

P61.5   **Transient neonatal neutropenia**   N
EXCLUDES 1   *congenital neutropenia (nontransient) (D70.0)*

P61.6   **Other transient neonatal disorders of coagulation**   N

P61.8   **Other specified perinatal hematological disorders**   N

P61.9   **Perinatal hematological disorder, unspecified**   N

✓ Additional Character Required   ✓ˣ⁷ᵗʰ Xtension Alert   Unspecified Code   Other Specified Code   Manifestation Code   ▶◀ Revised Text   ● New Code   ▲ Revised Code Title

Transitory endocrine and metabolic disorders specific to newborn (P70-P74)

INCLUDES   transitory endocrine and metabolic disturbances caused by the infant's response to maternal endocrine and metabolic factors, or its adjustment to extrauterine environment

√4ᵗʰ **P70   Transitory disorders of carbohydrate metabolism specific to newborn**

P70.0   Syndrome of infant of mother with gestational diabetes   N
Newborn (with hypoglycemia) affected by maternal gestational diabetes
> EXCLUDES1   newborn (with hypoglycemia) affected by maternal (pre-existing) diabetes mellitus (P70.1)
> syndrome of infant of a diabetic mother (P70.1)

P70.1   Syndrome of infant of a diabetic mother   N
Newborn (with hypoglycemia) affected by maternal (pre-existing) diabetes mellitus
> EXCLUDES1   newborn (with hypoglycemia) affected by maternal gestational diabetes (P70.0)
> syndrome of infant of mother with gestational diabetes (P70.0)

P70.2   Neonatal diabetes mellitus   N

P70.3   Iatrogenic neonatal hypoglycemia   N

P70.4   Other neonatal hypoglycemia   N
Transitory neonatal hypoglycemia

P70.8   Other transitory disorders of carbohydrate metabolism of newborn   N

P70.9   Transitory disorder of carbohydrate metabolism of newborn, unspecified   N

√4ᵗʰ **P71   Transitory neonatal disorders of calcium and magnesium metabolism**

P71.0   Cow's milk hypocalcemia in newborn   N

P71.1   Other neonatal hypocalcemia   N
> EXCLUDES1   neonatal hypoparathyroidism (P71.4)

P71.2   Neonatal hypomagnesemia   N

P71.3   Neonatal tetany without calcium or magnesium deficiency   N
Neonatal tetany NOS

P71.4   Transitory neonatal hypoparathyroidism   N

P71.8   Other transitory neonatal disorders of calcium and magnesium metabolism   N

P71.9   Transitory neonatal disorder of calcium and magnesium metabolism, unspecified   N

√4ᵗʰ **P72   Other transitory neonatal endocrine disorders**
> EXCLUDES1   congenital hypothyroidism with or without goiter (E03.0-E03.1)
> dyshormogenetic goiter (E07.1)
> Pendred's syndrome (E07.1)

P72.0   Neonatal goiter, not elsewhere classified   N
Transitory congenital goiter with normal functioning

P72.1   Transitory neonatal hyperthyroidism   N
Neonatal thyrotoxicosis

P72.2   Other transitory neonatal disorders of thyroid function, not elsewhere classified   N
Transitory neonatal hypothyroidism

P72.8   Other specified transitory neonatal endocrine disorders   N

P72.9   Transitory neonatal endocrine disorder, unspecified   N

√4ᵗʰ **P74   Other transitory neonatal electrolyte and metabolic disturbances**

P74.0   Late metabolic acidosis of newborn   N
> EXCLUDES1   (fetal) metabolic acidosis of newborn (P19)

P74.1   Dehydration of newborn   N

P74.2   Disturbances of sodium balance of newborn   N

P74.3   Disturbances of potassium balance of newborn   N

P74.4   Other transitory electrolyte disturbances of newborn   N

P74.5   Transitory tyrosinemia of newborn   N

P74.6   Transitory hyperammonemia of newborn   N

P74.8   Other transitory metabolic disturbances of newborn   N
Amino-acid metabolic disorders described as transitory

P74.9   Transitory metabolic disturbance of newborn, unspecified   N

Digestive system disorders of newborn (P76-P78)

√4ᵗʰ **P76   Other intestinal obstruction of newborn**

P76.0   Meconium plug syndrome   N
Meconium ileus NOS
> EXCLUDES1   meconium ileus in cystic fibrosis (E84.11)

P76.1   Transitory ileus of newborn   N
> EXCLUDES1   Hirschsprung's disease (Q43.1)

P76.2   Intestinal obstruction due to inspissated milk   N

P76.8   Other specified intestinal obstruction of newborn   N
> EXCLUDES1   intestinal obstruction classifiable to K56-

P76.9   Intestinal obstruction of newborn, unspecified   N

√4ᵗʰ **P77   Necrotizing enterocolitis of newborn**

P77.1   Stage 1 necrotizing enterocolitis in newborn   N
Necrotizing enterocolitis without pneumatosis, without perforation

P77.2   Stage 2 necrotizing enterocolitis in newborn   N
Necrotizing enterocolitis with pneumatosis, without perforation

P77.3   Stage 3 necrotizing enterocolitis in newborn   N
Necrotizing enterocolitis with perforation
Necrotizing enterocolitis with pneumatosis and perforation

P77.9   Necrotizing enterocolitis in newborn, unspecified   N
Necrotizing enterocolitis in newborn, NOS

√4ᵗʰ **P78   Other perinatal digestive system disorders**
> EXCLUDES1   cystic fibrosis (E84.0-E84.9)
> neonatal gastrointestinal hemorrhages (P54.0-P54.3)

P78.0   Perinatal intestinal perforation   N
Meconium peritonitis

P78.1   Other neonatal peritonitis   N
Neonatal peritonitis NOS

P78.2   Neonatal hematemesis and melena due to swallowed maternal blood   N

P78.3   Noninfective neonatal diarrhea   N
Neonatal diarrhea NOS

√5ᵗʰ **P78.8   Other specified perinatal digestive system disorders**

P78.81   Congenital cirrhosis (of liver)   N

P78.82   Peptic ulcer of newborn   N

P78.83   Newborn esophageal reflux   N
Neonatal esophageal reflux

P78.89   Other specified perinatal digestive system disorders   N

P78.9   Perinatal digestive system disorder, unspecified   N

Conditions involving the integument and temperature regulation of newborn (P80-P83)

√4ᵗʰ **P80   Hypothermia of newborn**

P80.0   Cold injury syndrome   N
Severe and usually chronic hypothermia associated with a pink flushed appearance, edema and neurological and biochemical abnormalities.
> EXCLUDES1   mild hypothermia of newborn (P80.8)

P80.8   Other hypothermia of newborn   N
Mild hypothermia of newborn

P80.9   Hypothermia of newborn, unspecified   N

√4ᵗʰ **P81   Other disturbances of temperature regulation of newborn**

P81.0   Environmental hyperthermia of newborn   N

P81.8   Other specified disturbances of temperature regulation of newborn   N

P81.9   Disturbance of temperature regulation of newborn, unspecified   N
Fever of newborn NOS

√4ᵗʰ **P83   Other conditions of integument specific to newborn**
> EXCLUDES1   congenital malformations of skin and integument (Q80-Q84)
> hydrops fetalis due to hemolytic disease (P56.-)
> neonatal skin infection (P39.4)
> staphylococcal scalded skin syndrome (L00)
> EXCLUDES2   cradle cap (L21.0)
> diaper [napkin] dermatitis (L22)

P83.0   Sclerema neonatorum   N

P83.1   Neonatal erythema toxicum   N

P83.2   Hydrops fetalis not due to hemolytic disease   N
Hydrops fetalis NOS

√5ᵗʰ **P83.3   Other and unspecified edema specific to newborn**

P83.30   Unspecified edema specific to newborn   N

P83.39   Other edema specific to newborn   N

P83.4   Breast engorgement of newborn   N
Noninfective mastitis of newborn

P83.5   Congenital hydrocele   ♂

P83.6   Umbilical polyp of newborn   N

EXCLUDES1 Not coded here   EXCLUDES2 Not included here   N Newborn Age: 0   P Pediatric Age: 0-17   M Maternity Age: 12-55   A Adult Age: 15-124

772   ICD-10-CM 2014 (Draft)

P83.8 Other specified conditions of integument specific to newborn   N
Bronze baby syndrome
Neonatal scleroderma
Urticaria neonatorum

P83.9 Condition of the integument specific to newborn, unspecified   N

Other problems with newborn (P84)

P84 Other problems with newborn   N
Acidemia of newborn
Acidosis of newborn
Anoxia of newborn NOS
Asphyxia of newborn NOS
Hypercapnia of newborn
Hypoxemia of newborn
Hypoxia of newborn NOS
Mixed metabolic and respiratory acidosis of newborn
EXCLUDES 1   intracranial hemorrhage due to anoxia or hypoxia (P52.-)
hypoxic ischemic encephalopathy [HIE] (P91.6-)
late metabolic acidosis of newborn (P74.0)

Other disorders originating in the perinatal period (P90-P96)

P90 Convulsions of newborn   N
EXCLUDES 1   benign myoclonic epilepsy in infancy (G40.3-)
benign neonatal convulsions (familial) (G40.3-)

✓4th **P91 Other disturbances of cerebral status of newborn**
P91.0 Neonatal cerebral ischemia   N
P91.1 Acquired periventricular cysts of newborn   N
P91.2 Neonatal cerebral leukomalacia   N
Periventricular leukomalacia
P91.3 Neonatal cerebral irritability   N
P91.4 Neonatal cerebral depression   N
P91.5 Neonatal coma   N
✓5th **P91.6 Hypoxic ischemic encephalopathy [HIE]**
P91.60 Hypoxic ischemic encephalopathy [HIE], unspecified   N
P91.61 Mild hypoxic ischemic encephalopathy [HIE]   N
P91.62 Moderate hypoxic ischemic encephalopathy [HIE]   N
P91.63 Severe hypoxic ischemic encephalopathy [HIE]   N
P91.8 Other specified disturbances of cerebral status of newborn   N
P91.9 Disturbance of cerebral status of newborn, unspecified   N

✓4th **P92 Feeding problems of newborn**
EXCLUDES 1   feeding problems in child over 28 days old (R63.3)
✓5th **P92.0 Vomiting of newborn**
EXCLUDES 1   vomiting of child over 28 days old (R11.-)
P92.01 Bilious vomiting of newborn   N
EXCLUDES 1   bilious vomiting in child over 28 days old (R11.14)
P92.09 Other vomiting of newborn   N
EXCLUDES 1   regurgitation of food in newborn (P92.1)
P92.1 Regurgitation and rumination of newborn   N
P92.2 Slow feeding of newborn   N
P92.3 Underfeeding of newborn   N
P92.4 Overfeeding of newborn   N
P92.5 Neonatal difficulty in feeding at breast   N
P92.6 Failure to thrive in newborn   N
EXCLUDES 1   failure to thrive in child over 28 days old (R62.51)
P92.8 Other feeding problems of newborn   N
P92.9 Feeding problem of newborn, unspecified   N

✓4th **P93 Reactions and intoxications due to drugs administered to newborn**
INCLUDES   reactions and intoxications due to drugs administered to fetus affecting newborn
EXCLUDES 1   jaundice due to drugs or toxins transmitted from mother or given to newborn (P58.4-)
reactions and intoxications from maternal opiates, tranquilizers and other medication (P04.0-P04.1, P04.4)
withdrawal symptoms from maternal use of drugs of addiction (P96.1)
withdrawal symptoms from therapeutic use of drugs in newborn (P96.2)
P93.0 Grey baby syndrome   N
Grey syndrome from chloramphenicol administration in newborn
P93.8 Other reactions and intoxications due to drugs administered to newborn   N
Use additional code for adverse effect, if applicable, to identify drug (T36-T50 with fifth or sixth character 5)

✓4th **P94 Disorders of muscle tone of newborn**
P94.0 Transient neonatal myasthenia gravis   N
EXCLUDES 1   myasthenia gravis (G70.0)
P94.1 Congenital hypertonia   N
P94.2 Congenital hypotonia   N
Floppy baby syndrome, unspecified
P94.8 Other disorders of muscle tone of newborn   N
P94.9 Disorder of muscle tone of newborn, unspecified   N

P95 Stillbirth   N
Deadborn fetus NOS
Fetal death of unspecified cause
Stillbirth NOS
EXCLUDES 1   maternal care for intrauterine death (O36.4)
missed abortion (O02.1)
outcome of delivery, stillbirth (Z37.1, Z37.3, Z37.4, Z37.7)

✓4th **P96 Other conditions originating in the perinatal period**
P96.0 Congenital renal failure   N
Uremia of newborn
P96.1 Neonatal withdrawal symptoms from maternal use of drugs of addiction   N
Drug withdrawal syndrome in infant of dependent mother
Neonatal abstinence syndrome
EXCLUDES 1   reactions and intoxications from maternal opiates and tranquilizers administered during labor and delivery (P04.0)
P96.2 Withdrawal symptoms from therapeutic use of drugs in newborn   N
P96.3 Wide cranial sutures of newborn   N
Neonatal craniotabes
P96.5 Complication to newborn due to (fetal) intrauterine procedure   N
EXCLUDES 2   newborn (suspected to be) affected by amniocentesis (P00.6)
✓5th **P96.8 Other specified conditions originating in the perinatal period**
P96.81 Exposure to (parental) (environmental) tobacco smoke in the perinatal period
EXCLUDES 2   newborn affected by in utero exposure to tobacco (P04.2)
exposure to environmental tobacco smoke after the perinatal period (Z77.22)
P96.82 Delayed separation of umbilical cord   N
P96.83 Meconium staining   N
EXCLUDES 1   meconium aspiration (P24.00, P24.01)
meconium passage during delivery (P03.82)
P96.89 Other specified conditions originating in the perinatal period
Use additional code to specify condition
P96.9 Condition originating in the perinatal period, unspecified   N
Congenital debility NOS

Congenital Malformations, Deformations and Chromosomal Abnormalities

Q00–Q07.00

Chapter 17. Congenital Malformations, Deformations and Chromosomal Abnormalities(Q00-Q99)

NOTE   Codes from this chapter are not for use on maternal or fetal records.

EXCLUDES 2   *inborn errors of metabolism (E70-E88)*

This chapter contains the following blocks:

Q00-Q07   Congenital malformations of the nervous system
Q10-Q18   Congenital malformations of eye, ear, face and neck
Q20-Q28   Congenital malformations of the circulatory system
Q30-Q34   Congenital malformations of the respiratory system
Q35-Q37   Cleft lip and cleft palate
Q38-Q45   Other congenital malformations of the digestive system
Q50-Q56   Congenital malformations of genital organs
Q60-Q64   Congenital malformations of the urinary system
Q65-Q79   Congenital malformations and deformations of the musculoskeletal system
Q80-Q89   Other congenital malformations
Q90-Q99   Chromosomal abnormalities, not elsewhere classified

Congenital malformations of the nervous system (Q00-Q07)

✓4ᵗʰ Q00 Anencephaly and similar malformations

   Q00.0 Anencephaly
     Acephaly
     Acrania
     Amyelencephaly
     Hemianencephaly
     Hemicephaly

   Q00.1 Craniorachischisis

   Q00.2 Iniencephaly

✓4ᵗʰ Q01 Encephalocele

   INCLUDES   Arnold-Chiari syndrome, type III
     encephalocystocele
     encephalomyelocele
     hydroencephalocele
     hydromeningocele, cranial
     meningocele, cerebral
     meningoencephalocele

   EXCLUDES 1   *Meckel-Gruber syndrome (Q61.9)*

   Q01.0 Frontal encephalocele

   Q01.1 Nasofrontal encephalocele

   Q01.2 Occipital encephalocele

   Q01.8 Encephalocele of other sites

   Q01.9 Encephalocele, unspecified

Q02 Microcephaly

   INCLUDES   hydromicrocephaly
     micrencephalon

   EXCLUDES 1   *Meckel-Gruber syndrome (Q61.9)*

✓4ᵗʰ Q03 Congenital hydrocephalus

   INCLUDES   hydrocephalus in newborn

   EXCLUDES 1   *Arnold-Chiari syndrome, type II (Q07.0-)*
     acquired hydrocephalus (G91.-)
     hydrocephalus due to congenital toxoplasmosis (P37.1)
     hydrocephalus with spina bifida (Q05.0-Q05.4)

   Q03.0 Malformations of aqueduct of Sylvius
     Anomaly of aqueduct of Sylvius
     Obstruction of aqueduct of Sylvius, congenital
     Stenosis of aqueduct of Sylvius

   Q03.1 Atresia of foramina of Magendie and Luschka
     Dandy-Walker syndrome

   Q03.8 Other congenital hydrocephalus

   Q03.9 Congenital hydrocephalus, unspecified

✓4ᵗʰ Q04 Other congenital malformations of brain

   EXCLUDES 1   *cyclopia (Q87.0)*
     macrocephaly (Q75.3)

   Q04.0 Congenital malformations of corpus callosum
     Agenesis of corpus callosum

   Q04.1 Arhinencephaly

   Q04.2 Holoprosencephaly

   Q04.3 Other reduction deformities of brain
     Absence of part of brain
     Agenesis of part of brain
     Agyria
     Aplasia of part of brain
     Hydranencephaly
     Hypoplasia of part of brain
     Lissencephaly
     Microgyria
     Pachygyria

     EXCLUDES 1   *congenital malformations of corpus callosum (Q04.0)*

   Q04.4 Septo-optic dysplasia of brain

   Q04.5 Megalencephaly

   Q04.6 Congenital cerebral cysts
     Porencephaly
     Schizencephaly

     EXCLUDES 1   *acquired porencephalic cyst (G93.0)*

   Q04.8 Other specified congenital malformations of brain
     Arnold-Chiari syndrome, type IV
     Macrogyria

   Q04.9 Congenital malformation of brain, unspecified
     Congenital anomaly NOS of brain
     Congenital deformity NOS of brain
     Congenital disease or lesion NOS of brain
     Multiple anomalies NOS of brain, congenital

✓4ᵗʰ Q05 Spina bifida

   Hydromeningocele (spinal)
   Meningocele (spinal)
   Meningomyelocele
   Myelocele
   Myelomeningocele
   Rachischisis
   Spina bifida (aperta)(cystica)
   Syringomyelocele

   Use additional code for any associated paraplegia (paraparesis) (G82.2-)

   EXCLUDES 1   *Arnold-Chiari syndrome, type II (Q07.0-)*
     spina bifida occulta (Q76.0)

   Q05.0 Cervical spina bifida with hydrocephalus

   Q05.1 Thoracic spina bifida with hydrocephalus
     Dorsal spina bifida with hydrocephalus
     Thoracolumbar spina bifida with hydrocephalus

   Q05.2 Lumbar spina bifida with hydrocephalus
     Lumbosacral spina bifida with hydrocephalus

   Q05.3 Sacral spina bifida with hydrocephalus

   Q05.4 Unspecified spina bifida with hydrocephalus

   Q05.5 Cervical spina bifida without hydrocephalus

   Q05.6 Thoracic spina bifida without hydrocephalus
     Dorsal spina bifida NOS
     Thoracolumbar spina bifida NOS

   Q05.7 Lumbar spina bifida without hydrocephalus
     Lumbosacral spina bifida NOS

   Q05.8 Sacral spina bifida without hydrocephalus

   Q05.9 Spina bifida, unspecified

✓4ᵗʰ Q06 Other congenital malformations of spinal cord

   Q06.0 Amyelia

   Q06.1 Hypoplasia and dysplasia of spinal cord
     Atelomyelia
     Myelatelia
     Myelodysplasia of spinal cord

   Q06.2 Diastematomyelia

   Q06.3 Other congenital cauda equina malformations

   Q06.4 Hydromyelia
     Hydrorachis

   Q06.8 Other specified congenital malformations of spinal cord

   Q06.9 Congenital malformation of spinal cord, unspecified
     Congenital anomaly NOS of spinal cord
     Congenital deformity NOS of spinal cord
     Congenital disease or lesion NOS of spinal cord

✓4ᵗʰ Q07 Other congenital malformations of nervous system

   EXCLUDES 2   *congenital central alveolar hypoventilation syndrome (G47.35)*
     familial dysautonomia [Riley-Day] (G90.1)
     neurofibromatosis (nonmalignant) (Q85.0-)

   ✓5ᵗʰ Q07.0 Arnold-Chiari syndrome
     Arnold-Chiari syndrome, type II

     EXCLUDES 1   *Arnold-Chiari syndrome, type III (Q01.-)*
      Arnold-Chiari syndrome, type IV (Q04.8)

     Q07.00 Arnold-Chiari syndrome without spina bifida or hydrocephalus

---

EXCLUDES 1 Not coded here   **EXCLUDES 2** Not included here   **N** Newborn Age: 0   **P** Pediatric Age: 0-17   **M** Maternity Age: 12-55   **A** Adult Age: 15-124

Q07.01 **Arnold-Chiari syndrome** with spina bifida

Q07.02 **Arnold-Chiari syndrome** with hydrocephalus

Q07.03 **Arnold-Chiari syndrome** with spina bifida and hydrocephalus

Q07.8 **Other specified congenital malformations of nervous system**
Agenesis of nerve
Displacement of brachial plexus
Jaw-winking syndrome
Marcus Gunn's syndrome

Q07.9 **Congenital malformation of nervous system, unspecified**
Congenital anomaly NOS of nervous system
Congenital deformity NOS of nervous system
Congenital disease or lesion NOS of nervous system

Congenital malformations of eye, ear, face and neck (Q10-Q18)

EXCLUDES 2 cleft lip and cleft palate (Q35-Q37)
congenital malformation of cervical spine (Q05.0, Q05.5, Q67.5, Q76.0-Q76.4)
congenital malformation of larynx (Q31.-)
congenital malformation of lip NEC (Q38.0)
congenital malformation of nose (Q30.-)
congenital malformation of parathyroid gland (Q89.2)
congenital malformation of thyroid gland (Q89.2)

✓4ᵗʰ **Q10 Congenital malformations of eyelid, lacrimal apparatus and orbit**

EXCLUDES 1 cryptophthalmos NOS (Q11.2)
cryptophthalmos syndrome (Q87.0)

Q10.0 **Congenital ptosis**

Q10.1 **Congenital ectropion**

Q10.2 **Congenital entropion**

Q10.3 **Other congenital malformations of eyelid**
Ablepharon
Blepharophimosis, congenital
Coloboma of eyelid
Congenital absence or agenesis of cilia
Congenital absence or agenesis of eyelid
Congenital accessory eyelid
Congenital accessory eye muscle
Congenital malformation of eyelid NOS

Q10.4 **Absence and agenesis of lacrimal apparatus**
Congenital absence of punctum lacrimale

Q10.5 **Congenital stenosis and stricture of lacrimal duct**

Q10.6 **Other congenital malformations of lacrimal apparatus**
Congenital malformation of lacrimal apparatus NOS

Q10.7 **Congenital malformation of orbit**

✓4ᵗʰ **Q11 Anophthalmos, microphthalmos and macrophthalmos**

Q11.0 **Cystic eyeball**

Q11.1 **Other anophthalmos**
Anophthalmos NOS
Agenesis of eye
Aplasia of eye

Q11.2 **Microphthalmos**
Cryptophthalmos NOS
Dysplasia of eye
Hypoplasia of eye
Rudimentary eye
EXCLUDES 1 cryptophthalmos syndrome (Q87.0)

Q11.3 **Macrophthalmos**
EXCLUDES 1 macrophthalmos in congenital glaucoma (Q15.0)

✓4ᵗʰ **Q12 Congenital lens malformations**

Q12.0 **Congenital cataract**

Q12.1 **Congenital displaced lens**

Q12.2 **Coloboma of lens**

Q12.3 **Congenital aphakia**

Q12.4 **Spherophakia**

Q12.8 **Other congenital lens malformations**
Microphakia

Q12.9 **Congenital lens malformation, unspecified**

✓4ᵗʰ **Q13 Congenital malformations of anterior segment of eye**

Q13.0 **Coloboma of iris**
Coloboma NOS

Q13.1 **Absence of iris**
Aniridia
Use additional code for associated glaucoma (H42)

Q13.2 **Other congenital malformations of iris**
Anisocoria, congenital
Atresia of pupil
Congenital malformation of iris NOS
Corectopia

Q13.3 **Congenital corneal opacity**

Q13.4 **Other congenital corneal malformations**
Congenital malformation of cornea NOS
Microcornea
Peter's anomaly

Q13.5 **Blue sclera**

✓5ᵗʰ Q13.8 **Other congenital malformations of anterior segment of eye**

Q13.81 **Rieger's anomaly**
Use additional code for associated glaucoma (H42)

Q13.89 **Other congenital malformations of anterior segment of eye**

Q13.9 **Congenital malformation of anterior segment of eye, unspecified**

✓4ᵗʰ **Q14 Congenital malformations of posterior segment of eye**
EXCLUDES 2 optic nerve hypoplasia (H47.03-)

Q14.0 **Congenital malformation of vitreous humor**
Congenital vitreous opacity

Q14.1 **Congenital malformation of retina**
Congenital retinal aneurysm

Q14.2 **Congenital malformation of optic disc**
Coloboma of optic disc

Q14.3 **Congenital malformation of choroid**

Q14.8 **Other congenital malformations of posterior segment of eye**
Coloboma of the fundus

Q14.9 **Congenital malformation of posterior segment of eye, unspecified**

✓4ᵗʰ **Q15 Other congenital malformations of eye**
EXCLUDES 1 congenital nystagmus (H55.01)
ocular albinism (E70.31-)
optic nerve hypoplasia (H47.03-)
retinitis pigmentosa (H35.52)

Q15.0 **Congenital glaucoma**
Axenfeld's anomaly
Buphthalmos
Glaucoma of childhood
Glaucoma of newborn
Hydrophthalmos
Keratoglobus, congenital, with glaucoma
Macrocornea with glaucoma
Macrophthalmos in congenital glaucoma
Megalocornea with glaucoma

Q15.8 **Other specified congenital malformations of eye**

Q15.9 **Congenital malformation of eye, unspecified**
Congenital anomaly of eye
Congenital deformity of eye

✓4ᵗʰ **Q16 Congenital malformations of ear causing impairment of hearing**
EXCLUDES 1 congenital deafness (H90.-)

Q16.0 **Congenital absence of (ear) auricle**

Q16.1 **Congenital absence, atresia and stricture of auditory canal (external)**
Congenital atresia or stricture of osseous meatus

Q16.2 **Absence of eustachian tube**

Q16.3 **Congenital malformation of ear ossicles**
Congenital fusion of ear ossicles

Q16.4 **Other congenital malformations of middle ear**
Congenital malformation of middle ear NOS

Q16.5 **Congenital malformation of inner ear**
Congenital anomaly of membranous labyrinth
Congenital anomaly of organ of Corti

Q16.9 **Congenital malformation of ear causing impairment of hearing, unspecified**
Congenital absence of ear NOS

✓4ᵗʰ **Q17 Other congenital malformations of ear**
EXCLUDES 1 congenital malformations of ear with impairment of hearing (Q16.0- Q16.9)
preauricular sinus (Q18.1)

Q17.0 **Accessory auricle**
Accessory tragus
Polyotia
Preauricular appendage or tag
Supernumerary ear
Supernumerary lobule

Q17.1 **Macrotia**

Q17.2 Microtia

Q17.3 Other misshapen ear
Pointed ear

Q17.4 Misplaced ear
Low-set ears
EXCLUDES 1 *cervical auricle (Q18.2)*

Q17.5 Prominent ear
Bat ear

Q17.8 Other specified congenital malformations of ear
Congenital absence of lobe of ear

Q17.9 Congenital malformation of ear, unspecified
Congenital anomaly of ear NOS

✓4ᵗʰ **Q18 Other congenital malformations of face and neck**
EXCLUDES 1 *cleft lip and cleft palate (Q35-Q37)*
conditions classified to Q67.0-Q67.4
congenital malformations of skull and face bones (Q75.-)
cyclopia (Q87.0)
dentofacial anomalies [including malocclusion] (M26.-)
malformation syndromes affecting facial appearance (Q87.0)
persistent thyroglossal duct (Q89.2)

Q18.0 Sinus, fistula and cyst of branchial cleft
Branchial vestige

Q18.1 Preauricular sinus and cyst
Fistula of auricle, congenital
Cervicoaural fistula

Q18.2 Other branchial cleft malformations
Branchial cleft malformation NOS
Cervical auricle
Otocephaly

Q18.3 Webbing of neck
Pterygium colli

Q18.4 Macrostomia

Q18.5 Microstomia

Q18.6 Macrocheilia
Hypertrophy of lip, congenital

Q18.7 Microcheilia

Q18.8 Other specified congenital malformations of face and neck
Medial cyst of face and neck
Medial fistula of face and neck
Medial sinus of face and neck

Q18.9 Congenital malformation of face and neck, unspecified
Congenital anomaly NOS of face and neck

Congenital malformations of the circulatory system (Q20-Q28)

✓4ᵗʰ **Q20 Congenital malformations of cardiac chambers and connections**
EXCLUDES 1 *dextrocardia with situs inversus (Q89.3)*
mirror-image atrial arrangement with situs inversus (Q89.3)

Q20.0 Common arterial trunk
Persistent truncus arteriosus
EXCLUDES 1 *aortic septal defect (Q21.4)*

Q20.1 Double outlet right ventricle
Taussig-Bing syndrome

Q20.2 Double outlet left ventricle

Q20.3 Discordant ventriculoarterial connection
Dextrotransposition of aorta
Transposition of great vessels (complete)

Q20.4 Double inlet ventricle
Common ventricle
Cor triloculare biatriatum
Single ventricle

Q20.5 Discordant atrioventricular connection
Corrected transposition
Levotransposition
Ventricular inversion

Q20.6 Isomerism of atrial appendages
Isomerism of atrial appendages with asplenia or polysplenia

Q20.8 Other congenital malformations of cardiac chambers and connections
Cor binoculare

Q20.9 Congenital malformation of cardiac chambers and connections, unspecified

✓4ᵗʰ **Q21 Congenital malformations of cardiac septa**
EXCLUDES 1 *acquired cardiac septal defect (I51.0)*

Q21.0 Ventricular septal defect
Roger's disease

Q21.1 Atrial septal defect
Coronary sinus defect
Patent or persistent foramen ovale
Patent or persistent ostium secundum defect (type II)
Patent or persistent sinus venosus defect

Q21.2 Atrioventricular septal defect
Common atrioventricular canal
Endocardial cushion defect
Ostium primum atrial septal defect (type I)

Q21.3 Tetralogy of Fallot
Ventricular septal defect with pulmonary stenosis or atresia, dextroposition of aorta and hypertrophy of right ventricle.

Q21.4 Aortopulmonary septal defect
Aortic septal defect
Aortopulmonary window

Q21.8 Other congenital malformations of cardiac septa
Eisenmenger's defect
Pentalogy of Fallot
EXCLUDES 1 *Eisenmenger's complex (I27.8)*
Eisenmenger's syndrome (I27.8)

Q21.9 Congenital malformation of cardiac septum, unspecified
Septal (heart) defect NOS

✓4ᵗʰ **Q22 Congenital malformations of pulmonary and tricuspid valves**

Q22.0 Pulmonary valve atresia

Q22.1 Congenital pulmonary valve stenosis

Q22.2 Congenital pulmonary valve insufficiency
Congenital pulmonary valve regurgitation

Q22.3 Other congenital malformations of pulmonary valve
Congenital malformation of pulmonary valve NOS
Supernumerary cusps of pulmonary valve

Q22.4 Congenital tricuspid stenosis
Congenital tricuspid atresia

Q22.5 Ebstein's anomaly

Q22.6 Hypoplastic right heart syndrome

Q22.8 Other congenital malformations of tricuspid valve

Q22.9 Congenital malformation of tricuspid valve, unspecified

✓4ᵗʰ **Q23 Congenital malformations of aortic and mitral valves**

Q23.0 Congenital stenosis of aortic valve
Congenital aortic atresia
Congenital aortic stenosis NOS
EXCLUDES 1 *congenital stenosis of aortic valve in hypoplastic left heart syndrome (Q23.4)*
congenital subaortic stenosis (Q24.4)
supravalvular aortic stenosis (congenital) (Q25.3)

Q23.1 Congenital insufficiency of aortic valve
Bicuspid aortic valve
Congenital aortic insufficiency

Q23.2 Congenital mitral stenosis
Congenital mitral atresia

Q23.3 Congenital mitral insufficiency

Q23.4 Hypoplastic left heart syndrome

Q23.8 Other congenital malformations of aortic and mitral valves

Q23.9 Congenital malformation of aortic and mitral valves, unspecified

✓4ᵗʰ **Q24 Other congenital malformations of heart**
EXCLUDES 1 *endocardial fibroelastosis (I42.4)*

Q24.0 Dextrocardia
EXCLUDES 1 *dextrocardia with situs inversus (Q89.3)*
isomerism of atrial appendages (with asplenia or polysplenia) (Q20.6)
mirror-image atrial arrangement with situs inversus (Q89.3)

Q24.1 Levocardia

Q24.2 Cor triatriatum

Q24.3 Pulmonary infundibular stenosis
Subvalvular pulmonic stenosis

Q24.4 Congenital subaortic stenosis

Q24.5 Malformation of coronary vessels
Congenital coronary (artery) aneurysm

Q24.6 Congenital heart block

Q24.8 Other specified congenital malformations of heart
Congenital diverticulum of left ventricle
Congenital malformation of myocardium
Congenital malformation of pericardium
Malposition of heart
Uhl's disease

EXCLUDES 1 Not coded here   **EXCLUDES 2** Not included here   **N** Newborn Age: 0   **P** Pediatric Age: 0-17   **M** Maternity Age: 12-55   **A** Adult Age: 15-124

776   ICD-10-CM 2014 (Draft)

Q24.9 Congenital malformation of heart, unspecified
Congenital anomaly of heart
Congenital disease of heart

✓4ᵗʰ **Q25 Congenital malformations of great arteries**

Q25.0 Patent ductus arteriosus
Patent ductus Botallo
Persistent ductus arteriosus

Q25.1 Coarctation of aorta
Coarctation of aorta (preductal) (postductal)

Q25.2 Atresia of aorta

Q25.3 Supravalvular aortic stenosis
EXCLUDES 1 congenital aortic stenosis NOS (Q23.0)
congenital stenosis of aortic valve (Q23.0)

Q25.4 Other congenital malformations of aorta
Absence of aorta
Aneurysm of sinus of Valsalva (ruptured)
Aplasia of aorta
Congenital aneurysm of aorta
Congenital malformations of aorta
Congenital dilatation of aorta
Double aortic arch [vascular ring of aorta]
Hypoplasia of aorta
Persistent convolutions of aortic arch
Persistent right aortic arch
EXCLUDES 1 hypoplasia of aorta in hypoplastic left heart syndrome (Q23.4)

Q25.5 Atresia of pulmonary artery

Q25.6 Stenosis of pulmonary artery
Supravalvular pulmonary stenosis

✓5ᵗʰ **Q25.7 Other congenital malformations of pulmonary artery**

Q25.71 Coarctation of pulmonary artery

Q25.72 Congenital pulmonary arteriovenous malformation
Congenital pulmonary arteriovenous aneurysm

Q25.79 Other congenital malformations of pulmonary artery
Aberrant pulmonary artery
Agenesis of pulmonary artery
Congenital aneurysm of pulmonary artery
Congenital anomaly of pulmonary artery
Hypoplasia of pulmonary artery

Q25.8 Other congenital malformations of other great arteries

Q25.9 Congenital malformation of great arteries, unspecified

✓4ᵗʰ **Q26 Congenital malformations of great veins**

Q26.0 Congenital stenosis of vena cava
Congenital stenosis of vena cava (inferior)(superior)

Q26.1 Persistent left superior vena cava

Q26.2 Total anomalous pulmonary venous connection
Total anomalous pulmonary venous return [TAPVR], subdiaphragmatic
Total anomalous pulmonary venous return [TAPVR], supradiaphragmatic

Q26.3 Partial anomalous pulmonary venous connection
Partial anomalous pulmonary venous return

Q26.4 Anomalous pulmonary venous connection, unspecified

Q26.5 Anomalous portal venous connection

Q26.6 Portal vein-hepatic artery fistula

Q26.8 Other congenital malformations of great veins
Absence of vena cava (inferior) (superior)
Azygos continuation of inferior vena cava
Persistent left posterior cardinal vein
Scimitar syndrome

Q26.9 Congenital malformation of great vein, unspecified
Congenital anomaly of vena cava (inferior) (superior) NOS

✓4ᵗʰ **Q27 Other congenital malformations of peripheral vascular system**
EXCLUDES 2 anomalies of cerebral and precerebral vessels (Q28.0-Q28.3)
anomalies of coronary vessels (Q24.5)
anomalies of pulmonary artery (Q25.5-Q25.7)
congenital retinal aneurysm (Q14.1)
hemangioma and lymphangioma (D18.-)

Q27.0 Congenital absence and hypoplasia of umbilical artery
Single umbilical artery

Q27.1 Congenital renal artery stenosis

Q27.2 Other congenital malformations of renal artery
Congenital malformation of renal artery NOS
Multiple renal arteries

✓5ᵗʰ **Q27.3 Arteriovenous malformation (peripheral)**
Arteriovenous aneurysm
EXCLUDES 1 acquired arteriovenous aneurysm (I77.0)
EXCLUDES 2 arteriovenous malformation of cerebral vessels (Q28.2)
arteriovenous malformation of precerebral vessels (Q28.0)

Q27.30 Arteriovenous malformation, site unspecified

Q27.31 Arteriovenous malformation of vessel of upper limb

Q27.32 Arteriovenous malformation of vessel of lower limb

Q27.33 Arteriovenous malformation of digestive system vessel

Q27.34 Arteriovenous malformation of renal vessel

Q27.39 Arteriovenous malformation, other site

Q27.4 Congenital phlebectasia

Q27.8 Other specified congenital malformations of peripheral vascular system
Absence of peripheral vascular system
Atresia of peripheral vascular system
Congenital aneurysm (peripheral)
Congenital stricture, artery
Congenital varix
EXCLUDES 1 arteriovenous malformation (Q27.3-)

Q27.9 Congenital malformation of peripheral vascular system, unspecified
Anomaly of artery or vein NOS

✓4ᵗʰ **Q28 Other congenital malformations of circulatory system**
EXCLUDES 1 congenital aneurysm NOS (Q27.8)
congenital coronary aneurysm (Q24.5)
ruptured cerebral arteriovenous malformation (I60.8)
ruptured malformation of precerebral vessels (I72.0)
EXCLUDES 2 congenital peripheral aneurysm (Q27.8)
congenital pulmonary aneurysm (Q25.79)
congenital retinal aneurysm (Q14.1)

Q28.0 Arteriovenous malformation of precerebral vessels
Congenital arteriovenous precerebral aneurysm (nonruptured)

Q28.1 Other malformations of precerebral vessels
Congenital malformation of precerebral vessels NOS
Congenital precerebral aneurysm (nonruptured)

Q28.2 Arteriovenous malformation of cerebral vessels
Arteriovenous malformation of brain NOS
Congenital arteriovenous cerebral aneurysm (nonruptured)

Q28.3 Other malformations of cerebral vessels
Congenital cerebral aneurysm (nonruptured)
Congenital malformation of cerebral vessels NOS
Developmental venous anomaly

Q28.8 Other specified congenital malformations of circulatory system
Congenital aneurysm, specified site NEC
Spinal vessel anomaly

Q28.9 Congenital malformation of circulatory system, unspecified

Congenital malformations of the respiratory system (Q30-Q34)

✓4ᵗʰ **Q30 Congenital malformations of nose**
EXCLUDES 1 congenital deviation of nasal septum (Q67.4)

Q30.0 Choanal atresia
Atresia of nares (anterior) (posterior)
Congenital stenosis of nares (anterior) (posterior)

Q30.1 Agenesis and underdevelopment of nose
Congenital absent of nose

Q30.2 Fissured, notched and cleft nose

Q30.3 Congenital perforated nasal septum

Q30.8 Other congenital malformations of nose
Accessory nose
Congenital anomaly of nasal sinus wall

Q30.9 Congenital malformation of nose, unspecified

✓4ᵗʰ **Q31 Congenital malformations of larynx**
EXCLUDES 1 congenital laryngeal stridor NOS (P28.89)

Q31.0 Web of larynx
Glottic web of larynx
Subglottic web of larynx
Web of larynx NOS

Q31.1 Congenital subglottic stenosis

Q31.2 Laryngeal hypoplasia

Q31.3 Laryngocele

Q31.5 Congenital laryngomalacia

☑ Additional Character Required   ✓x7ᵗʰ Xtension Alert   Unspecified Code   Other Specified Code   Manifestation Code   ►◄ Revised Text   ● New Code   ▲ Revised Code Title

ICD-10-CM 2014 (Draft)   777

Q31.8 Other congenital malformations of larynx
Absence of larynx
Agenesis of larynx
Atresia of larynx
Congenital cleft thyroid cartilage
Congenital fissure of epiglottis
Congenital stenosis of larynx NEC
Posterior cleft of cricoid cartilage

Q31.9 Congenital malformation of larynx, unspecified

✓4ᵗʰ **Q32 Congenital malformations of trachea and bronchus**
EXCLUDES 1 congenital bronchiectasis (Q33.4)

Q32.0 Congenital tracheomalacia

Q32.1 Other congenital malformations of trachea
Atresia of trachea
Congenital anomaly of tracheal cartilage
Congenital dilatation of trachea
Congenital malformation of trachea
Congenital stenosis of trachea
Congenital tracheocele

Q32.2 Congenital bronchomalacia

Q32.3 Congenital stenosis of bronchus

Q32.4 Other congenital malformations of bronchus
Absence of bronchus
Agenesis of bronchus
Atresia of bronchus
Congenital diverticulum of bronchus
Congenital malformation of bronchus NOS

✓4ᵗʰ **Q33 Congenital malformations of lung**

Q33.0 Congenital cystic lung
Congenital cystic lung disease
Congenital honeycomb lung
Congenital polycystic lung disease
EXCLUDES 1 cystic fibrosis (E84.0)
cystic lung disease, acquired or unspecified (J98.4)

Q33.1 Accessory lobe of lung
Azygos lobe (fissured), lung

Q33.2 Sequestration of lung

Q33.3 Agenesis of lung
Congenital absence of lung (lobe)

Q33.4 Congenital bronchiectasis

Q33.5 Ectopic tissue in lung

Q33.6 Congenital hypoplasia and dysplasia of lung
EXCLUDES 1 pulmonary hypoplasia associated with short gestation (P28.0)

Q33.8 Other congenital malformations of lung

Q33.9 Congenital malformation of lung, unspecified

✓4ᵗʰ **Q34 Other congenital malformations of respiratory system**
EXCLUDES 2 congenital central alveolar hypoventilation syndrome (G47.35)

Q34.0 Anomaly of pleura

Q34.1 Congenital cyst of mediastinum

Q34.8 Other specified congenital malformations of respiratory system
Atresia of nasopharynx

Q34.9 Congenital malformation of respiratory system, unspecified
Congenital absence of respiratory system
Congenital anomaly of respiratory system NOS

Cleft lip and cleft palate (Q35-Q37)

Use additional code to identify associated malformation of the nose (Q30.2)
EXCLUDES 1 Robin syndrome (Q87.0)

✓4ᵗʰ **Q35 Cleft palate**
INCLUDES fissure of palate
palatoschisis
EXCLUDES 1 cleft palate with cleft lip (Q37.-)

Q35.1 Cleft hard palate

Q35.3 Cleft soft palate

Q35.5 Cleft hard palate with cleft soft palate

Q35.7 Cleft uvula

Q35.9 Cleft palate, unspecified
Cleft palate NOS

✓4ᵗʰ **Q36 Cleft lip**
Cheiloschisis
Congenital fissure of lip
Harelip
Labium leporinum
EXCLUDES 1 cleft lip with cleft palate (Q37.-)

Q36.0 Cleft lip, bilateral

Q36.1 Cleft lip, median

Q36.9 Cleft lip, unilateral
Cleft lip NOS

✓4ᵗʰ **Q37 Cleft palate with cleft lip**
Cheilopalatoschisis

Q37.0 Cleft hard palate with bilateral cleft lip

Q37.1 Cleft hard palate with unilateral cleft lip
Cleft hard palate with cleft lip NOS

Q37.2 Cleft soft palate with bilateral cleft lip

Q37.3 Cleft soft palate with unilateral cleft lip
Cleft soft palate with cleft lip NOS

Q37.4 Cleft hard and soft palate with bilateral cleft lip

Q37.5 Cleft hard and soft palate with unilateral cleft lip
Cleft hard and soft palate with cleft lip NOS

Q37.8 Unspecified cleft palate with bilateral cleft lip

Q37.9 Unspecified cleft palate with unilateral cleft lip
Cleft palate with cleft lip NOS

Other congenital malformations of the digestive system (Q38-Q45)

✓4ᵗʰ **Q38 Other congenital malformations of tongue, mouth and pharynx**
EXCLUDES 1 dentofacial anomalies (M26.-)
macrostomia (Q18.4)
microstomia (Q18.5)

Q38.0 Congenital malformations of lips, not elsewhere classified
Congenital fistula of lip
Congenital malformation of lip NOS
Van der Woude's syndrome
EXCLUDES 1 cleft lip (Q36.-)
cleft lip with cleft palate (Q37.-)
macrocheilia (Q18.6)
microcheilia (Q18.7)

Q38.1 Ankyloglossia
Tongue tie

Q38.2 Macroglossia
Congenital hypertrophy of tongue

Q38.3 Other congenital malformations of tongue
Aglossia
Bifid tongue
Congenital adhesion of tongue
Congenital fissure of tongue
Congenital malformation of tongue NOS
Double tongue
Hypoglossia
Hypoplasia of tongue
Microglossia

Q38.4 Congenital malformations of salivary glands and ducts
Atresia of salivary glands and ducts
Congenital absence of salivary glands and ducts
Congenital accessory salivary glands and ducts
Congenital fistula of salivary gland

Q38.5 Congenital malformations of palate, not elsewhere classified
Congenital absence of uvula
Congenital malformation of palate NOS
Congenital high arched palate
EXCLUDES 1 cleft palate (Q35.-)
cleft palate with cleft lip (Q37.-)

Q38.6 Other congenital malformations of mouth
Congenital malformation of mouth NOS

Q38.7 Congenital pharyngeal pouch
Congenital diverticulum of pharynx
EXCLUDES 1 pharyngeal pouch syndrome (D82.1)

Q38.8 Other congenital malformations of pharynx
Congenital malformation of pharynx NOS
Imperforate pharynx

✓4ᵗʰ **Q39 Congenital malformations of esophagus**

Q39.0 Atresia of esophagus without fistula
Atresia of esophagus NOS

Q39.1 Atresia of esophagus with tracheo-esophageal fistula
Atresia of esophagus with broncho-esophageal fistula

EXCLUDES 1 Not coded here   EXCLUDES 2 Not included here   N Newborn Age: 0   P Pediatric Age: 0-17   M Maternity Age: 12-55   A Adult Age: 15-124

778   ICD-10-CM 2014 (Draft)

Q39.2 Congenital tracheo-esophageal fistula without atresia
Congenital tracheo-esophageal fistula NOS

Q39.3 Congenital stenosis and stricture of esophagus

Q39.4 Esophageal web

Q39.5 Congenital dilatation of esophagus
Congenital cardiospasm

Q39.6 Congenital diverticulum of esophagus
Congenital esophageal pouch

Q39.8 Other congenital malformations of esophagus
Congenital absence of esophagus
Congenital displacement of esophagus
Congenital duplication of esophagus

Q39.9 Congenital malformation of esophagus, unspecified

✓4ᵗʰ **Q40 Other congenital malformations of upper alimentary tract**

Q40.0 Congenital hypertrophic pyloric stenosis
Congenital or infantile constriction
Congenital or infantile hypertrophy
Congenital or infantile spasm
Congenital or infantile stenosis
Congenital or infantile stricture

Q40.1 Congenital hiatus hernia
Congenital displacement of cardia through esophageal hiatus
EXCLUDES 1 *congenital diaphragmatic hernia (Q79.0)*

Q40.2 Other specified congenital malformations of stomach
Congenital displacement of stomach
Congenital diverticulum of stomach
Congenital hourglass stomach
Congenital duplication of stomach
Megalogastria
Microgastria

Q40.3 Congenital malformation of stomach, unspecified

Q40.8 Other specified congenital malformations of upper alimentary tract

Q40.9 Congenital malformation of upper alimentary tract, unspecified
Congenital anomaly of upper alimentary tract
Congenital deformity of upper alimentary tract

✓4ᵗʰ **Q41 Congenital absence, atresia and stenosis of small intestine**
Congenital obstruction, occlusion or stricture of small intestine or intestine NOS
EXCLUDES 1 *cystic fibrosis with intestinal manifestation (E84.11)*
meconium ileus NOS (without cystic fibrosis) (P76.0)

Q41.0 Congenital absence, atresia and stenosis of duodenum

Q41.1 Congenital absence, atresia and stenosis of jejunum
Apple peel syndrome
Imperforate jejunum

Q41.2 Congenital absence, atresia and stenosis of ileum

Q41.8 Congenital absence, atresia and stenosis of other specified parts of small intestine

Q41.9 Congenital absence, atresia and stenosis of small intestine, part unspecified
Congenital absence, atresia and stenosis of intestine NOS

✓4ᵗʰ **Q42 Congenital absence, atresia and stenosis of large intestine**
Congenital obstruction, occlusion and stricture of large intestine

Q42.0 Congenital absence, atresia and stenosis of rectum with fistula

Q42.1 Congenital absence, atresia and stenosis of rectum without fistula
Imperforate rectum

Q42.2 Congenital absence, atresia and stenosis of anus with fistula

Q42.3 Congenital absence, atresia and stenosis of anus without fistula
Imperforate anus

Q42.8 Congenital absence, atresia and stenosis of other parts of large intestine

Q42.9 Congenital absence, atresia and stenosis of large intestine, part unspecified

✓4ᵗʰ **Q43 Other congenital malformations of intestine**

Q43.0 Meckel's diverticulum (displaced) (hypertrophic)
Persistent omphalomesenteric duct
Persistent vitelline duct

Q43.1 Hirschsprung's disease
Aganglionosis
Congenital (aganglionic) megacolon

Q43.2 Other congenital functional disorders of colon
Congenital dilatation of colon

Q43.3 Congenital malformations of intestinal fixation
Congenital omental, anomalous adhesions [bands]
Congenital peritoneal adhesions [bands]
Incomplete rotation of cecum and colon
Insufficient rotation of cecum and colon
Jackson's membrane
Malrotation of colon
Rotation failure of cecum and colon
Universal mesentery

Q43.4 Duplication of intestine

Q43.5 Ectopic anus

Q43.6 Congenital fistula of rectum and anus
EXCLUDES 1 *congenital fistula of anus with absence, atresia and stenosis (Q42.2)*
congenital fistula of rectum with absence, atresia and stenosis (Q42.0)
congenital rectovaginal fistula (Q52.2)
congenital urethrorectal fistula (Q64.73)
pilonidal fistula or sinus (L05.-)

Q43.7 Persistent cloaca
Cloaca NOS

Q43.8 Other specified congenital malformations of intestine
Congenital blind loop syndrome
Congenital diverticulitis, colon
Congenital diverticulum, intestine
Dolichocolon
Megaloappendix
Megaloduodenum
Microcolon
Transposition of appendix
Transposition of colon
Transposition of intestine

Q43.9 Congenital malformation of intestine, unspecified

✓4ᵗʰ **Q44 Congenital malformations of gallbladder, bile ducts and liver**

Q44.0 Agenesis, aplasia and hypoplasia of gallbladder
Congenital absence of gallbladder

Q44.1 Other congenital malformations of gallbladder
Congenital malformation of gallbladder NOS
Intrahepatic gallbladder

Q44.2 Atresia of bile ducts

Q44.3 Congenital stenosis and stricture of bile ducts

Q44.4 Choledochal cyst

Q44.5 Other congenital malformations of bile ducts
Accessory hepatic duct
Biliary duct duplication
Congenital malformation of bile duct NOS
Cystic duct duplication

Q44.6 Cystic disease of liver
Fibrocystic disease of liver

Q44.7 Other congenital malformations of liver
Accessory liver
Alagille's syndrome
Congenital absence of liver
Congenital hepatomegaly
Congenital malformation of liver NOS

✓4ᵗʰ **Q45 Other congenital malformations of digestive system**
EXCLUDES 2 *congenital diaphragmatic hernia (Q79.0)*
congenital hiatus hernia (Q40.1)

Q45.0 Agenesis, aplasia and hypoplasia of pancreas
Congenital absence of pancreas

Q45.1 Annular pancreas

Q45.2 Congenital pancreatic cyst

Q45.3 Other congenital malformations of pancreas and pancreatic duct
Accessory pancreas
Congenital malformation of pancreas or pancreatic duct NOS
EXCLUDES 1 *congenital diabetes mellitus (E10.-)*
cystic fibrosis (E84.0-E84.9)
fibrocystic disease of pancreas (E84.-)
neonatal diabetes mellitus (P70.2)

Q45.8 Other specified congenital malformations of digestive system
Absence (complete) (partial) of alimentary tract NOS
Duplication of digestive system
Malposition, congenital of digestive system

Q45.9 Congenital malformation of digestive system, unspecified
Congenital anomaly of digestive system
Congenital deformity of digestive system

✓ Additional Character Required   ✓x7ᵗʰ Xtension Alert   Unspecified Code   Other Specified Code   Manifestation Code   ▶◀ Revised Text   ● New Code   ▲ Revised Code Title

Congenital malformations of genital organs (Q50-Q56)

EXCLUDES 1 androgen insensitivity syndrome (E34.5-)
syndromes associated with anomalies in the number and form of chromosomes (Q90-Q99)

☑4th **Q50 Congenital malformations of ovaries, fallopian tubes and broad ligaments**

☑5th **Q50.0 Congenital absence of ovary**
   EXCLUDES 1 Turner's syndrome (Q96.-)

   Q50.01 Congenital absence of ovary, unilateral ♀
   Q50.02 Congenital absence of ovary, bilateral ♀

Q50.1 Developmental ovarian cyst ♀

Q50.2 Congenital torsion of ovary ♀

☑5th **Q50.3 Other congenital malformations of ovary**

   Q50.31 Accessory ovary ♀
   Q50.32 Ovarian streak ♀
     46, XX with streak gonads
   Q50.39 Other congenital malformation of ovary ♀
     Congenital malformation of ovary NOS

Q50.4 Embryonic cyst of fallopian tube ♀
   Fimbrial cyst

Q50.5 Embryonic cyst of broad ligament ♀
   Epoophoron cyst
   Parovarian cyst

Q50.6 Other congenital malformations of fallopian tube and broad ligament ♀
   Absence of fallopian tube and broad ligament
   Accessory fallopian tube and broad ligament
   Atresia of fallopian tube and broad ligament
   Congenital malformation of fallopian tube or broad ligament NOS

☑4th **Q51 Congenital malformations of uterus and cervix**

Q51.0 Agenesis and aplasia of uterus ♀
   Congenital absence of uterus

☑5th **Q51.1 Doubling of uterus with doubling of cervix and vagina**

   Q51.10 Doubling of uterus with doubling of cervix and vagina without obstruction ♀
     Doubling of uterus with doubling of cervix and vagina NOS
   Q51.11 Doubling of uterus with doubling of cervix and vagina with obstruction ♀

Q51.2 Other doubling of uterus ♀
   Doubling of uterus NOS
   Septate uterus, complete or partial

Q51.3 Bicornate uterus ♀
   Bicornate uterus, complete or partial

Q51.4 Unicornate uterus ♀
   Unicornate uterus with or without a separate uterine horn
   Uterus with only one functioning horn

Q51.5 Agenesis and aplasia of cervix ♀
   Congenital absence of cervix

Q51.6 Embryonic cyst of cervix ♀

Q51.7 Congenital fistulae between uterus and digestive and urinary tracts ♀

☑5th **Q51.8 Other congenital malformations of uterus and cervix**

  ☑6th **Q51.81 Other congenital malformations of uterus**
     Q51.810 Arcuate uterus ♀
       Arcuatus uterus
     Q51.811 Hypoplasia of uterus ♀
     Q51.818 Other congenital malformations of uterus ♀
       Müllerian anomaly of uterus NEC

  ☑6th **Q51.82 Other congenital malformations of cervix**
     Q51.820 Cervical duplication ♀
     Q51.821 Hypoplasia of cervix ♀
     Q51.828 Other congenital malformations of cervix ♀

Q51.9 Congenital malformation of uterus and cervix, unspecified ♀

☑4th **Q52 Other congenital malformations of female genitalia**

Q52.0 Congenital absence of vagina ♀
   Vaginal agenesis, total or partial

☑5th **Q52.1 Doubling of vagina**
   EXCLUDES 1 doubling of vagina with doubling of uterus and cervix (Q51.1-)

   Q52.10 Doubling of vagina, unspecified ♀
     Septate vagina NOS

   Q52.11 Transverse vaginal septum ♀
   Q52.12 Longitudinal vaginal septum ♀
     Longitudinal vaginal septum with or without obstruction

Q52.2 Congenital rectovaginal fistula ♀
   EXCLUDES 1 cloaca (Q43.7)

Q52.3 Imperforate hymen ♀

Q52.4 Other congenital malformations of vagina ♀
   Canal of Nuck cyst, congenital
   Congenital malformation of vagina NOS
   Embryonic vaginal cyst
   Gartner's duct cyst

Q52.5 Fusion of labia ♀

Q52.6 Congenital malformation of clitoris ♀

☑5th **Q52.7 Other and unspecified congenital malformations of vulva**
   Q52.70 Unspecified congenital malformations of vulva ♀
     Congenital malformation of vulva NOS
   Q52.71 Congenital absence of vulva ♀
   Q52.79 Other congenital malformations of vulva ♀
     Congenital cyst of vulva

Q52.8 Other specified congenital malformations of female genitalia ♀

Q52.9 Congenital malformation of female genitalia, unspecified ♀

☑4th **Q53 Undescended and ectopic testicle**

☑5th **Q53.0 Ectopic testis**
   Q53.00 Ectopic testis, unspecified ♂
   Q53.01 Ectopic testis, unilateral ♂
   Q53.02 Ectopic testes, bilateral ♂

☑5th **Q53.1 Undescended testicle, unilateral**
   Q53.10 Unspecified undescended testicle, unilateral ♂
   Q53.11 Abdominal testis, unilateral ♂
   Q53.12 Ectopic perineal testis, unilateral ♂

☑5th **Q53.2 Undescended testicle, bilateral**
   Q53.20 Undescended testicle, unspecified, bilateral ♂
   Q53.21 Abdominal testis, bilateral ♂
   Q53.22 Ectopic perineal testis, bilateral ♂

Q53.9 Undescended testicle, unspecified ♂
   Cryptorchism NOS

☑4th **Q54 Hypospadias**
   EXCLUDES 1 epispadias (Q64.0)

Q54.0 Hypospadias, balanic ♂
   Hypospadias, coronal
   Hypospadias, glandular

Q54.1 Hypospadias, penile ♂

Q54.2 Hypospadias, penoscrotal ♂

Q54.3 Hypospadias, perineal ♂

Q54.4 Congenital chordee ♂
   Chordee without hypospadias

Q54.8 Other hypospadias ♂
   Hypospadias with intersex state

Q54.9 Hypospadias, unspecified ♂

☑4th **Q55 Other congenital malformations of male genital organs**
   EXCLUDES 1 congenital hydrocele (P83.5)
     hypospadias (Q54.-)

Q55.0 Absence and aplasia of testis ♂
   Monorchism

Q55.1 Hypoplasia of testis and scrotum ♂
   Fusion of testes

☑5th **Q55.2 Other and unspecified congenital malformations of testis and scrotum**
   Q55.20 Unspecified congenital malformations of testis and scrotum ♂
     Congenital malformation of testis or scrotum NOS
   Q55.21 Polyorchism ♂
   Q55.22 Retractile testis ♂
   Q55.23 Scrotal transposition ♂
   Q55.29 Other congenital malformations of testis and scrotum ♂

Q55.3 Atresia of vas deferens ♂
   Code first any associated cystic fibrosis (E84.-)

EXCLUDES 1 Not coded here   **EXCLUDES 2** Not included here   N Newborn Age: 0   P Pediatric Age: 0-17   M Maternity Age: 12-55   A Adult Age: 15-124

780   ICD-10-CM 2014 (Draft)

Q55.4 **Other congenital malformations of vas deferens, epididymis, seminal vesicles and prostate**   ♂
    Absence or aplasia of prostate
    Absence or aplasia of spermatic cord
    Congenital malformation of vas deferens, epididymis, seminal vesicles or prostate NOS

Q55.5 **Congenital absence and aplasia of penis**   ♂

✓5ᵗʰ **Q55.6** **Other congenital malformations of penis**

    Q55.61 **Curvature of penis (lateral)**   ♂

    Q55.62 **Hypoplasia of penis**   ♂
        Micropenis

    Q55.63 **Congenital torsion of penis**   ♂
        EXCLUDES 1 *acquired torsion of penis (N48.82)*

    Q55.64 **Hidden penis**   ♂
        Buried penis
        Concealed penis
        EXCLUDES 1 *acquired buried penis (N48.83)*

    Q55.69 **Other congenital malformation of penis**   ♂
        Congenital malformation of penis NOS

Q55.7 **Congenital vasocutaneous fistula**   ♂

Q55.8 **Other specified congenital malformations of male genital organs**   ♂

Q55.9 **Congenital malformation of male genital organ, unspecified**   ♂
    Congenital anomaly of male genital organ
    Congenital deformity of male genital organ

✓4ᵗʰ **Q56** **Indeterminate sex and pseudohermaphroditism**
    EXCLUDES 1 *46, XX true hermaphrodite (Q99.1)*
        androgen insensitivity syndrome (E34.5-)
        chimera 46, XX/46, XY true hermaphrodite (Q99.0)
        female pseudohermaphroditism with adrenocortical disorder (E25.-)
        pseudohermaphroditism with specified chromosomal anomaly (Q96-Q99)
        pure gonadal dysgenesis (Q99.1)

    Q56.0 **Hermaphroditism, not elsewhere classified**
        Ovotestis

    Q56.1 **Male pseudohermaphroditism, not elsewhere classified**   ♂
        46, XY with streak gonads
        Male pseudohermaphroditism NOS

    Q56.2 **Female pseudohermaphroditism, not elsewhere classified**   ♀
        Female pseudohermaphroditism NOS

    Q56.3 **Pseudohermaphroditism, unspecified**

    Q56.4 **Indeterminate sex, unspecified**
        Ambiguous genitalia

Congenital malformations of the urinary system (Q60-Q64)

✓4ᵗʰ **Q60** **Renal agenesis and other reduction defects of kidney**
    Congenital absence of kidney
    Congenital atrophy of kidney
    Infantile atrophy of kidney

    Q60.0 **Renal agenesis, unilateral**

    Q60.1 **Renal agenesis, bilateral**

    Q60.2 **Renal agenesis, unspecified**

    Q60.3 **Renal hypoplasia, unilateral**

    Q60.4 **Renal hypoplasia, bilateral**

    Q60.5 **Renal hypoplasia, unspecified**

    Q60.6 **Potter's syndrome**

✓4ᵗʰ **Q61** **Cystic kidney disease**
    EXCLUDES 1 *acquired cyst of kidney (N28.1)*
        Potter's syndrome (Q60.6)

✓5ᵗʰ **Q61.0** **Congenital renal cyst**

    Q61.00 **Congenital renal cyst, unspecified**
        Cyst of kidney NOS (congenital)

    Q61.01 **Congenital single renal cyst**

    Q61.02 **Congenital multiple renal cysts**

✓5ᵗʰ **Q61.1** **Polycystic kidney, infantile type**
    Polycystic kidney, autosomal recessive

    Q61.11 **Cystic dilatation of collecting ducts**

    Q61.19 **Other polycystic kidney, infantile type**

    Q61.2 **Polycystic kidney, adult type**
        Polycystic kidney, autosomal dominant

    Q61.3 **Polycystic kidney, unspecified**

Q61.4 **Renal dysplasia**
    Multicystic dysplastic kidney
    Multicystic kidney (development)
    Multicystic kidney disease
    Multicystic renal dysplasia
    EXCLUDES 1 *polycystic kidney disease (Q61.11-Q61.3)*

Q61.5 **Medullary cystic kidney**
    Nephronopthisis
    Sponge kidney NOS

Q61.8 **Other cystic kidney diseases**
    Fibrocystic kidney
    Fibrocystic renal degeneration or disease

Q61.9 **Cystic kidney disease, unspecified**
    Meckel-Gruber syndrome

✓4ᵗʰ **Q62** **Congenital obstructive defects of renal pelvis and congenital malformations of ureter**

    Q62.0 **Congenital hydronephrosis**

✓5ᵗʰ **Q62.1** **Congenital occlusion of ureter**
    Atresia and stenosis of ureter

    Q62.10 **Congenital occlusion of ureter, unspecified**

    Q62.11 **Congenital occlusion of ureteropelvic junction**

    Q62.12 **Congenital occlusion of ureterovesical orifice**

    Q62.2 **Congenital megaureter**
        Congenital dilatation of ureter

✓5ᵗʰ **Q62.3** **Other obstructive defects of renal pelvis and ureter**

    Q62.31 **Congenital ureterocele, orthotopic**

    Q62.32 **Cecoureterocele**
        Ectopic ureterocele

    Q62.39 **Other obstructive defects of renal pelvis and ureter**
        Ureteropelvic junction obstruction NOS

    Q62.4 **Agenesis of ureter**
        Congenital absence ureter

    Q62.5 **Duplication of ureter**
        Accessory ureter
        Double ureter

✓5ᵗʰ **Q62.6** **Malposition of ureter**

    Q62.60 **Malposition of ureter, unspecified**

    Q62.61 **Deviation of ureter**

    Q62.62 **Displacement of ureter**

    Q62.63 **Anomalous implantation of ureter**
        Ectopia of ureter
        Ectopic ureter

    Q62.69 **Other malposition of ureter**

    Q62.7 **Congenital vesico-uretero-renal reflux**

    Q62.8 **Other congenital malformations of ureter**
        Anomaly of ureter NOS

✓4ᵗʰ **Q63** **Other congenital malformations of kidney**
    EXCLUDES 1 *congenital nephrotic syndrome (N04.-)*

    Q63.0 **Accessory kidney**

    Q63.1 **Lobulated, fused and horseshoe kidney**

    Q63.2 **Ectopic kidney**
        Congenital displaced kidney
        Malrotation of kidney

    Q63.3 **Hyperplastic and giant kidney**
        Compensatory hypertrophy of kidney

    Q63.8 **Other specified congenital malformations of kidney**
        Congenital renal calculi

    Q63.9 **Congenital malformation of kidney, unspecified**

✓4ᵗʰ **Q64** **Other congenital malformations of urinary system**

    Q64.0 **Epispadias**   ♂
        EXCLUDES 1 *hypospadias (Q54.-)*

✓5ᵗʰ **Q64.1** **Exstrophy of urinary bladder**

    Q64.10 **Exstrophy of urinary bladder, unspecified**
        Ectopia vesicae

    Q64.11 **Supravesical fissure of urinary bladder**

    Q64.12 **Cloacal extrophy of urinary bladder**

    Q64.19 **Other exstrophy of urinary bladder**
        Extroversion of bladder

    Q64.2 **Congenital posterior urethral valves**

✓5ᵗʰ **Q64.3** **Other atresia and stenosis of urethra and bladder neck**

    Q64.31 **Congenital bladder neck obstruction**
        Congenital obstruction of vesicourethral orifice

    Q64.32 **Congenital stricture of urethra**

    Q64.33 **Congenital stricture of urinary meatus**

✓ Additional Character Required   ✓x7ᵗʰ Xtension Alert   Unspecified Code   Other Specified Code   Manifestation Code   ▶◀ Revised Text   ● New Code   ▲ Revised Code Title

Q64.39   **Other atresia and stenosis of urethra and bladder neck**
Atresia and stenosis of urethra and bladder neck NOS

Q64.4   **Malformation of urachus**
Cyst of urachus
Patent urachus
Prolapse of urachus

Q64.5   **Congenital absence of bladder and urethra**

Q64.6   **Congenital diverticulum of bladder**

✓5ᵗʰ **Q64.7**   **Other and unspecified congenital malformations of bladder and urethra**
> EXCLUDES 1   *congenital prolapse of bladder (mucosa) (Q79.4)*

     Q64.70   **Unspecified congenital malformation of bladder and urethra**
Malformation of bladder or urethra NOS

     Q64.71   **Congenital prolapse of urethra**

     Q64.72   **Congenital prolapse of urinary meatus**

     Q64.73   **Congenital urethrorectal fistula**

     Q64.74   **Double urethra**

     Q64.75   **Double urinary meatus**

     Q64.79   **Other congenital malformations of bladder and urethra**

Q64.8   **Other specified congenital malformations of urinary system**

Q64.9   **Congenital malformation of urinary system, unspecified**
Congenital anomaly NOS of urinary system
Congenital deformity NOS of urinary system

Congenital malformations and deformations of the musculoskeletal system (Q65-Q79)

✓4ᵗʰ **Q65**   **Congenital deformities of hip**
> EXCLUDES 1   *clicking hip (R29.4)*

✓5ᵗʰ **Q65.0**   **Congenital dislocation of hip, unilateral**

     Q65.00   **Congenital dislocation of unspecified hip, unilateral**

     Q65.01   **Congenital dislocation of right hip, unilateral**

     Q65.02   **Congenital dislocation of left hip, unilateral**

Q65.1   **Congenital dislocation of hip, bilateral**

Q65.2   **Congenital dislocation of hip, unspecified**

✓5ᵗʰ **Q65.3**   **Congenital partial dislocation of hip, unilateral**

     Q65.30   **Congenital partial dislocation of unspecified hip, unilateral**

     Q65.31   **Congenital partial dislocation of right hip, unilateral**

     Q65.32   **Congenital partial dislocation of left hip, unilateral**

Q65.4   **Congenital partial dislocation of hip, bilateral**

Q65.5   **Congenital partial dislocation of hip, unspecified**

Q65.6   **Congenital unstable hip**
Congenital dislocatable hip

✓5ᵗʰ **Q65.8**   **Other congenital deformities of hip**

     Q65.81   **Congenital coxa valga**

     Q65.82   **Congenital coxa vara**

     Q65.89   **Other specified congenital deformities of hip**
Anteversion of femoral neck
Congenital acetabular dysplasia

Q65.9   **Congenital deformity of hip, unspecified**

✓4ᵗʰ **Q66**   **Congenital deformities of feet**
> EXCLUDES 1   *reduction defects of feet (Q72.-)*
> *valgus deformities (acquired) (M21.0-)*
> *varus deformities (acquired) (M21.1-)*

Q66.0   **Congenital talipes equinovarus**

Q66.1   **Congenital talipes calcaneovarus**

Q66.2   **Congenital metatarsus (primus) varus**

Q66.3   **Other congenital varus deformities of feet**
Hallux varus, congenital

Q66.4   **Congenital talipes calcaneovalgus**

✓5ᵗʰ **Q66.5**   **Congenital pes planus**
Congenital flat foot
Congenital rigid flat foot
Congenital spastic (everted) flat foot
> EXCLUDES 1   *pes planus, acquired (M21.4)*

     Q66.50   **Congenital pes planus, unspecified foot**

     Q66.51   **Congenital pes planus, right foot**

     Q66.52   **Congenital pes planus, left foot**

Q66.6   **Other congenital valgus deformities of feet**
Congenital metatarsus valgus

Q66.7   **Congenital pes cavus**

✓5ᵗʰ **Q66.8**   **Other congenital deformities of feet**

     Q66.80   **Congenital vertical talus deformity, unspecified foot**

     Q66.81   **Congenital vertical talus deformity, right foot**

     Q66.82   **Congenital vertical talus deformity, left foot**

     Q66.89   **Other specified congenital deformities of feet**
Congenital asymmetric talipes
Congenital clubfoot NOS
Congenital talipes NOS
Congenital tarsal coalition
Hammer toe, congenital

Q66.9   **Congenital deformity of feet, unspecified**

✓4ᵗʰ **Q67**   **Congenital musculoskeletal deformities of head, face, spine and chest**
> EXCLUDES 1   *congenital malformation syndromes classified to Q87-Potter's syndrome (Q60.6)*

Q67.0   **Congenital facial asymmetry**

Q67.1   **Congenital compression facies**

Q67.2   **Dolichocephaly**

Q67.3   **Plagiocephaly**

Q67.4   **Other congenital deformities of skull, face and jaw**
Congenital depressions in skull
Congenital hemifacial atrophy or hypertrophy
Deviation of nasal septum, congenital
Squashed or bent nose, congenital
> EXCLUDES 1   *dentofacial anomalies [including malocclusion] (M26.-)*
> *syphilitic saddle nose (A50.5)*

Q67.5   **Congenital deformity of spine**
Congenital postural scoliosis
Congenital scoliosis NOS
> EXCLUDES 1   *infantile idiopathic scoliosis (M41.0)*
> *scoliosis due to congenital bony malformation (Q76.3)*

Q67.6   **Pectus excavatum**
Congenital funnel chest

Q67.7   **Pectus carinatum**
Congenital pigeon chest

Q67.8   **Other congenital deformities of chest**
Congenital deformity of chest wall NOS

✓4ᵗʰ **Q68**   **Other congenital musculoskeletal deformities**
> EXCLUDES 1   *reduction defects of limb(s) (Q71-Q73)*
> EXCLUDES 2   *congenital myotonic chondrodystrophy (G71.13)*

Q68.0   **Congenital deformity of sternocleidomastoid muscle**
Congenital contracture of sternocleidomastoid (muscle)
Congenital (sternomastoid) torticollis
Sternomastoid tumor (congenital)

Q68.1   **Congenital deformity of finger(s) and hand**
Congenital clubfinger
Spade-like hand (congenital)

Q68.2   **Congenital deformity of knee**
Congenital dislocation of knee
Congenital genu recurvatum

Q68.3   **Congenital bowing of femur**
> EXCLUDES 1   *anteversion of femur (neck) (Q65.89)*

Q68.4   **Congenital bowing of tibia and fibula**

Q68.5   **Congenital bowing of long bones of leg, unspecified**

Q68.6   **Discoid meniscus**

Q68.8   **Other specified congenital musculoskeletal deformities**
Congenital deformity of clavicle
Congenital deformity of elbow
Congenital deformity of forearm
Congenital deformity of scapula
Congenital deformity of wrist
Congenital dislocation of elbow
Congenital dislocation of shoulder
Congenital dislocation of wrist

✓4ᵗʰ **Q69**   **Polydactyly**

Q69.0   **Accessory finger(s)**

Q69.1   **Accessory thumb(s)**

Q69.2   **Accessory toe(s)**
Accessory hallux

Q69.9   **Polydactyly, unspecified**
Supernumerary digit(s) NOS

EXCLUDES 1 Not coded here   EXCLUDES 2 Not included here   N Newborn Age: 0   P Pediatric Age: 0-17   M Maternity Age: 12-55   A Adult Age: 15-124

782   ICD-10-CM 2014 (Draft)

✓4th **Q70　Syndactyly**

✓5th **Q70.0　Fused fingers**
　　　　Complex syndactyly of fingers with synostosis
　　Q70.00　Fused fingers, unspecified hand
　　Q70.01　Fused fingers, right hand
　　Q70.02　Fused fingers, left hand
　　Q70.03　Fused fingers, bilateral

✓5th **Q70.1　Webbed fingers**
　　　　Simple syndactyly of fingers without synostosis
　　Q70.10　Webbed fingers, unspecified hand
　　Q70.11　Webbed fingers, right hand
　　Q70.12　Webbed fingers, left hand
　　Q70.13　Webbed fingers, bilateral

✓5th **Q70.2　Fused toes**
　　　　Complex syndactyly of toes with synostosis
　　Q70.20　Fused toes, unspecified foot
　　Q70.21　Fused toes, right foot
　　Q70.22　Fused toes, left foot
　　Q70.23　Fused toes, bilateral

✓5th **Q70.3　Webbed toes**
　　　　Simple syndactyly of toes without synostosis
　　Q70.30　Webbed toes, unspecified foot
　　Q70.31　Webbed toes, right foot
　　Q70.32　Webbed toes, left foot
　　Q70.33　Webbed toes, bilateral

Q70.4　Polysyndactyly, unspecified
　　EXCLUDES 1 *specified syndactyly of hand and feet—code to specified conditions (Q70.0-Q70.3-)*

Q70.9　Syndactyly, unspecified
　　　　Symphalangy NOS

✓4th **Q71　Reduction defects of upper limb**

✓5th **Q71.0　Congenital complete absence of upper limb**
　　Q71.00　Congenital complete absence of unspecified upper limb
　　Q71.01　Congenital complete absence of right upper limb
　　Q71.02　Congenital complete absence of left upper limb
　　Q71.03　Congenital complete absence of upper limb, bilateral

✓5th **Q71.1　Congenital absence of upper arm and forearm with hand present**
　　Q71.10　Congenital absence of unspecified upper arm and forearm with hand present
　　Q71.11　Congenital absence of right upper arm and forearm with hand present
　　Q71.12　Congenital absence of left upper arm and forearm with hand present
　　Q71.13　Congenital absence of upper arm and forearm with hand present, bilateral

✓5th **Q71.2　Congenital absence of both forearm and hand**
　　Q71.20　Congenital absence of both forearm and hand, unspecified upper limb
　　Q71.21　Congenital absence of both forearm and hand, right upper limb
　　Q71.22　Congenital absence of both forearm and hand, left upper limb
　　Q71.23　Congenital absence of both forearm and hand, bilateral

✓5th **Q71.3　Congenital absence of hand and finger**
　　Q71.30　Congenital absence of unspecified hand and finger
　　Q71.31　Congenital absence of right hand and finger
　　Q71.32　Congenital absence of left hand and finger
　　Q71.33　Congenital absence of hand and finger, bilateral

✓5th **Q71.4　Longitudinal reduction defect of radius**
　　　　Clubhand (congenital)
　　　　Radial clubhand
　　Q71.40　Longitudinal reduction defect of unspecified radius
　　Q71.41　Longitudinal reduction defect of right radius
　　Q71.42　Longitudinal reduction defect of left radius
　　Q71.43　Longitudinal reduction defect of radius, bilateral

✓5th **Q71.5　Longitudinal reduction defect of ulna**
　　Q71.50　Longitudinal reduction defect of unspecified ulna
　　Q71.51　Longitudinal reduction defect of right ulna

Q71.52　Longitudinal reduction defect of left ulna
Q71.53　Longitudinal reduction defect of ulna, bilateral

✓5th **Q71.6　Lobster-claw hand**
　　Q71.60　Lobster-claw hand, unspecified hand
　　Q71.61　Lobster-claw right hand
　　Q71.62　Lobster-claw left hand
　　Q71.63　Lobster-claw hand, bilateral

✓5th **Q71.8　Other reduction defects of upper limb**
　✓6th **Q71.81　Congenital shortening of upper limb**
　　　Q71.811　Congenital shortening of right upper limb
　　　Q71.812　Congenital shortening of left upper limb
　　　Q71.813　Congenital shortening of upper limb, bilateral
　　　Q71.819　Congenital shortening of unspecified upper limb
　✓6th **Q71.89　Other reduction defects of upper limb**
　　　Q71.891　Other reduction defects of right upper limb
　　　Q71.892　Other reduction defects of left upper limb
　　　Q71.893　Other reduction defects of upper limb, bilateral
　　　Q71.899　Other reduction defects of unspecified upper limb

✓5th **Q71.9　Unspecified reduction defect of upper limb**
　　Q71.90　Unspecified reduction defect of unspecified upper limb
　　Q71.91　Unspecified reduction defect of right upper limb
　　Q71.92　Unspecified reduction defect of left upper limb
　　Q71.93　Unspecified reduction defect of upper limb, bilateral

✓4th **Q72　Reduction defects of lower limb**

✓5th **Q72.0　Congenital complete absence of lower limb**
　　Q72.00　Congenital complete absence of unspecified lower limb
　　Q72.01　Congenital complete absence of right lower limb
　　Q72.02　Congenital complete absence of left lower limb
　　Q72.03　Congenital complete absence of lower limb, bilateral

✓5th **Q72.1　Congenital absence of thigh and lower leg with foot present**
　　Q72.10　Congenital absence of unspecified thigh and lower leg with foot present
　　Q72.11　Congenital absence of right thigh and lower leg with foot present
　　Q72.12　Congenital absence of left thigh and lower leg with foot present
　　Q72.13　Congenital absence of thigh and lower leg with foot present, bilateral

✓5th **Q72.2　Congenital absence of both lower leg and foot**
　　Q72.20　Congenital absence of both lower leg and foot, unspecified lower limb
　　Q72.21　Congenital absence of both lower leg and foot, right lower limb
　　Q72.22　Congenital absence of both lower leg and foot, left lower limb
　　Q72.23　Congenital absence of both lower leg and foot, bilateral

✓5th **Q72.3　Congenital absence of foot and toe(s)**
　　Q72.30　Congenital absence of unspecified foot and toe(s)
　　Q72.31　Congenital absence of right foot and toe(s)
　　Q72.32　Congenital absence of left foot and toe(s)
　　Q72.33　Congenital absence of foot and toe(s), bilateral

✓5th **Q72.4　Longitudinal reduction defect of femur**
　　　　Proximal femoral focal deficiency
　　Q72.40　Longitudinal reduction defect of unspecified femur
　　Q72.41　Longitudinal reduction defect of right femur
　　Q72.42　Longitudinal reduction defect of left femur
　　Q72.43　Longitudinal reduction defect of femur, bilateral

✓5th **Q72.5　Longitudinal reduction defect of tibia**
　　Q72.50　Longitudinal reduction defect of unspecified tibia
　　Q72.51　Longitudinal reduction defect of right tibia
　　Q72.52　Longitudinal reduction defect of left tibia
　　Q72.53　Longitudinal reduction defect of tibia, bilateral

✓5th **Q72.6　Longitudinal reduction defect of fibula**
　　Q72.60　Longitudinal reduction defect of unspecified fibula

☑ Additional Character Required　　✓x7th *Xtension* Alert　　Unspecified Code　　Other Specified Code　　Manifestation Code　　▶◀ Revised Text　　● New Code　　▲ Revised Code Title

Q72.61   Longitudinal reduction defect of right fibula
Q72.62   Longitudinal reduction defect of left fibula
Q72.63   Longitudinal reduction defect of fibula, bilateral

Q72.7 Split foot
Q72.70   Split foot, unspecified lower limb
Q72.71   Split foot, right lower limb
Q72.72   Split foot, left lower limb
Q72.73   Split foot, bilateral

Q72.8 Other reduction defects of lower limb
Q72.81   Congenital shortening of lower limb
Q72.811   Congenital shortening of right lower limb
Q72.812   Congenital shortening of left lower limb
Q72.813   Congenital shortening of lower limb, bilateral
Q72.819   Congenital shortening of unspecified lower limb
Q72.89   Other reduction defects of lower limb
Q72.891   Other reduction defects of right lower limb
Q72.892   Other reduction defects of left lower limb
Q72.893   Other reduction defects of lower limb, bilateral
Q72.899   Other reduction defects of unspecified lower limb

Q72.9 Unspecified reduction defect of lower limb
Q72.90   Unspecified reduction defect of unspecified lower limb
Q72.91   Unspecified reduction defect of right lower limb
Q72.92   Unspecified reduction defect of left lower limb
Q72.93   Unspecified reduction defect of lower limb, bilateral

Q73 Reduction defects of unspecified limb
Q73.0   Congenital absence of unspecified limb(s)
Amelia NOS
Q73.1   Phocomelia, unspecified limb(s)
Phocomelia NOS
Q73.8   Other reduction defects of unspecified limb(s)
Longitudinal reduction deformity of unspecified limb(s)
Ectromelia of limb NOS
Hemimelia of limb NOS
Reduction defect of limb NOS

Q74 Other congenital malformations of limb(s)
EXCLUDES1   polydactyly (Q69.-)
reduction defect of limb (Q71-Q73)
syndactyly (Q70.-)
Q74.0   Other congenital malformations of upper limb(s), including shoulder girdle
Accessory carpal bones
Cleidocranial dysostosis
Congenital pseudarthrosis of clavicle
Macrodactylia (fingers)
Madelung's deformity
Radioulnar synostosis
Sprengel's deformity
Triphalangeal thumb
Q74.1   Congenital malformation of knee
Congenital absence of patella
Congenital dislocation of patella
Congenital genu valgum
Congenital genu varum
Rudimentary patella
EXCLUDES1   congenital dislocation of knee (Q68.2)
congenital genu recurvatum (Q68.2)
nail patella syndrome (Q87.2)
Q74.2   Other congenital malformations of lower limb(s), including pelvic girdle
Congenital fusion of sacroiliac joint
Congenital malformation of ankle joint
Congenital malformation of sacroiliac joint
EXCLUDES1   anteversion of femur (neck) (Q65.89)
Q74.3   Arthrogryposis multiplex congenita
Q74.8   Other specified congenital malformations of limb(s)
Q74.9   Unspecified congenital malformation of limb(s)
Congenital anomaly of limb(s) NOS

Q75 Other congenital malformations of skull and face bones
EXCLUDES1   congenital malformation of face NOS (Q18.-)
congenital malformation syndromes classified to Q87.-
dentofacial anomalies [including malocclusion] (M26.-)
musculoskeletal deformities of head and face (Q67.0-Q67.4)
skull defects associated with congenital anomalies of brain such as:
anencephaly (Q00.0)
encephalocele (Q01.-)
hydrocephalus (Q03.-)
microcephaly (Q02)
Q75.0   Craniosynostosis
Acrocephaly
Imperfect fusion of skull
Oxycephaly
Trigonocephaly
Q75.1   Craniofacial dysostosis
Crouzon's disease
Q75.2   Hypertelorism
Q75.3   Macrocephaly
Q75.4   Mandibulofacial dysostosis
Franceschetti syndrome
Treacher Collins syndrome
Q75.5   Oculomandibular dysostosis
Q75.8   Other specified congenital malformations of skull and face bones
Absence of skull bone, congenital
Congenital deformity of forehead
Platybasia
Q75.9   Congenital malformation of skull and face bones, unspecified
Congenital anomaly of face bones NOS
Congenital anomaly of skull NOS

Q76 Congenital malformations of spine and bony thorax
EXCLUDES1   congenital musculoskeletal deformities of spine and chest (Q67.5-Q67.8)
Q76.0   Spina bifida occulta
EXCLUDES1   meningocele (spinal) (Q05.-)
spina bifida (aperta) (cystica) (Q05.-)
Q76.1   Klippel-Feil syndrome
Cervical fusion syndrome
Q76.2   Congenital spondylolisthesis
Congenital spondylolysis
EXCLUDES1   spondylolisthesis (acquired) (M43.1-)
spondylolysis (acquired) (M43.0-)
Q76.3   Congenital scoliosis due to congenital bony malformation
Hemivertebra fusion or failure of segmentation with scoliosis
Q76.4   Other congenital malformations of spine, not associated with scoliosis
Q76.41   Congenital kyphosis
Q76.411   Congenital kyphosis, occipito-atlanto-axial region
Q76.412   Congenital kyphosis, cervical region
Q76.413   Congenital kyphosis, cervicothoracic region
Q76.414   Congenital kyphosis, thoracic region
Q76.415   Congenital kyphosis, thoracolumbar region
Q76.419   Congenital kyphosis, unspecified region
Q76.42   Congenital lordosis
Q76.425   Congenital lordosis, thoracolumbar region
Q76.426   Congenital lordosis, lumbar region
Q76.427   Congenital lordosis, lumbosacral region
Q76.428   Congenital lordosis, sacral and sacrococcygeal region
Q76.429   Congenital lordosis, unspecified region
Q76.49   Other congenital malformations of spine, not associated with scoliosis
Congenital absence of vertebra NOS
Congenital fusion of spine NOS
Congenital malformation of lumbosacral (joint) (region) NOS
Congenital malformation of spine NOS
Hemivertebra NOS
Malformation of spine NOS
Platyspondylisis NOS
Supernumerary vertebra NOS
Q76.5   Cervical rib
Supernumerary rib in cervical region

Q76.6 **Other congenital malformations of** ribs
- Accessory rib
- Congenital absence of rib
- Congenital fusion of ribs
- Congenital malformation of ribs NOS
  - **EXCLUDES 1**   short rib syndrome (Q77.2)

Q76.7 **Congenital malformation of** sternum
- Congenital absence of sternum
- Sternum bifidum

Q76.8 **Other congenital malformations of bony thorax**

Q76.9 **Congenital malformation of bony thorax, unspecified**

✓4th **Q77** **Osteochondrodysplasia with defects of growth of tubular bones and spine**
- **EXCLUDES 1**   mucopolysaccharidosis (E76.0-E76.3)
- **EXCLUDES 2**   congenital myotonic chondrodystrophy (G71.13)

Q77.0 **Achondrogenesis**
- Hypochondrogenesis

Q77.1 **Thanatophoric short stature**

Q77.2 **Short rib syndrome**
- Asphyxiating thoracic dysplasia [Jeune]

Q77.3 **Chondrodysplasia punctata**
- **EXCLUDES 1**   Rhizomelic chondrodysplasia punctata (E71.43)

Q77.4 **Achondroplasia**
- Hypochondroplasia
- Osteosclerosis congenita

Q77.5 **Diastrophic dysplasia**

Q77.6 **Chondroectodermal dysplasia**
- Ellis-van Creveld syndrome

Q77.7 **Spondyloepiphyseal dysplasia**

Q77.8 **Other osteochondrodysplasia with defects of growth of tubular bones and spine**

Q77.9 **Osteochondrodysplasia with defects of growth of tubular bones and spine, unspecified**

✓4th **Q78** **Other osteochondrodysplasias**
- **EXCLUDES 2**   congenital myotonic chondrodystrophy (G71.13)

Q78.0 **Osteogenesis imperfecta**
- Fragilitas ossium
- Osteopsathyrosis

Q78.1 **Polyostotic fibrous dysplasia**
- Albright(-McCune)(-Sternberg) syndrome

Q78.2 **Osteopetrosis**
- Albers-Schönberg syndrome
- Osteosclerosis NOS

Q78.3 **Progressive diaphyseal dysplasia**
- Camurati-Engelmann syndrome

Q78.4 **Enchondromatosis**
- Maffucci's syndrome
- Ollier's disease

Q78.5 **Metaphyseal dysplasia**
- Pyle's syndrome

Q78.6 **Multiple congenital exostoses**
- Diaphyseal aclasis

Q78.8 **Other specified osteochondrodysplasias**
- Osteopoikilosis

Q78.9 **Osteochondrodysplasia, unspecified**
- Chondrodystrophy NOS
- Osteodystrophy NOS

✓4th **Q79** **Congenital malformations of musculoskeletal system, not elsewhere classified**
- **EXCLUDES 2**   congenital (sternomastoid) torticollis (Q68.0)

Q79.0 **Congenital diaphragmatic hernia**
- **EXCLUDES 1**   congenital hiatus hernia (Q40.1)

Q79.1 **Other congenital malformations of diaphragm**
- Absence of diaphragm
- Congenital malformation of diaphragm NOS
- Eventration of diaphragm

Q79.2 **Exomphalos**
- Omphalocele
- **EXCLUDES 1**   umbilical hernia (K42.-)

Q79.3 **Gastroschisis**

Q79.4 **Prune belly syndrome**
- Congenital prolapse of bladder mucosa
- Eagle-Barrett syndrome

✓5th **Q79.5** **Other congenital malformations of abdominal wall**
- **EXCLUDES 1**   umbilical hernia (K42.-)

Q79.51 **Congenital hernia of bladder**

Q79.59 **Other congenital malformations of** abdominal wall

Q79.6 **Ehlers-Danlos syndrome**

Q79.8 **Other congenital malformations of musculoskeletal system**
- Absence of muscle
- Absence of tendon
- Accessory muscle
- Amyotrophia congenita
- Congenital constricting bands
- Congenital shortening of tendon
- Poland syndrome

Q79.9 **Congenital malformation of musculoskeletal system, unspecified**
- Congenital anomaly of musculoskeletal system NOS
- Congenital deformity of musculoskeletal system NOS

Other congenital malformations (Q80-Q89)

✓4th **Q80** **Congenital ichthyosis**
- **EXCLUDES 1**   Refsum's disease (G60.1)

Q80.0 **Ichthyosis** vulgaris

Q80.1 **X-linked** ichthyosis

Q80.2 **Lamellar** ichthyosis
- Collodion baby

Q80.3 **Congenital** bullous **ichthyosiform erythroderma**

Q80.4 **Harlequin fetus**

Q80.8 **Other congenital ichthyosis**

Q80.9 **Congenital ichthyosis, unspecified**

✓4th **Q81** **Epidermolysis bullosa**

Q81.0 **Epidermolysis bullosa** simplex
- **EXCLUDES 1**   Cockayne's syndrome (Q87.1)

Q81.1 **Epidermolysis bullosa** letalis
- Herlitz' syndrome

Q81.2 **Epidermolysis bullosa** dystrophica

Q81.8 **Other epidermolysis bullosa**

Q81.9 **Epidermolysis bullosa, unspecified**

✓4th **Q82** **Other congenital malformations of skin**
- **EXCLUDES 1**   acrodermatitis enteropathica (E83.2)
  - congenital erythropoietic porphyria (E80.0)
  - pilonidal cyst or sinus (L05.-)
  - Sturge-Weber (-Dimitri) syndrome (Q85.8)

Q82.0 **Hereditary lymphedema**

Q82.1 **Xeroderma pigmentosum**

Q82.2 **Mastocytosis**
- Urticaria pigmentosa
- **EXCLUDES 1**   malignant mastocytosis (C96.2)

Q82.3 **Incontinentia pigmenti**

Q82.4 **Ectodermal dysplasia (anhidrotic)**
- **EXCLUDES 1**   Ellis-van Creveld syndrome (Q77.6)

Q82.5 **Congenital non-neoplastic nevus**

Birthmark NOS	Strawberry Nevus
Flammeus Nevus	Vascular Nevus NOS
Portwine Nevus	Verrucous Nevus
Sanguineous Nevus	

- **EXCLUDES 2**   araneus nevus (I78.1)
  - café au lait spots (L81.3)
  - lentigo (L81.4)
  - melanocytic nevus (D22.-)
  - nevus NOS (D22.-)
  - pigmented nevus (D22.-)
  - spider nevus (I78.1)
  - stellar nevus (I78.1)

Q82.8 **Other specified congenital malformations of skin**
- Abnormal palmar creases
- Accessory skin tags
- Benign familial pemphigus [Hailey-Hailey]
- Congenital poikiloderma
- Cutis laxa (hyperelastica)
- Dermatoglyphic anomalies
- Inherited keratosis palmaris et plantaris
- Keratosis follicularis [Darier-White]
  - **EXCLUDES 1**   Ehlers-Danlos syndrome (Q79.6)

Q82.9 **Congenital malformation of skin, unspecified**

✓4th **Q83** **Congenital malformations of** breast
- **EXCLUDES 2**   absence of pectoral muscle (Q79.8)
  - hypoplasia of breast (N64.82)
  - micromastia (N64.82)

Q83.0 **Congenital** absence of breast **with** absent nipple

☑ Additional Character Required   ✓x7th Xtension Alert   Unspecified Code   Other Specified Code   Manifestation Code   ▶◀ Revised Text   ● New Code   ▲ Revised Code Title

ICD-10-CM 2014 (Draft)   **785**

Q83.1 Accessory breast
Supernumerary breast

Q83.2 Absent nipple

Q83.3 Accessory nipple
Supernumerary nipple

Q83.8 Other congenital malformations of breast

Q83.9 Congenital malformation of breast, unspecified

✓4ᵗʰ **Q84** Other congenital malformations of integument

Q84.0 Congenital alopecia
Congenital atrichosis

Q84.1 Congenital morphological disturbances of hair, not elsewhere classified
Beaded hair   Pili annulati
Monilethrix
EXCLUDES 1 *Menkes' kinky hair syndrome (E83.0)*

Q84.2 Other congenital malformations of hair
Congenital hypertrichosis
Congenital malformation of hair NOS
Persistent lanugo

Q84.3 Anonychia
EXCLUDES 1 *nail patella syndrome (Q87.2)*

Q84.4 Congenital leukonychia

Q84.5 Enlarged and hypertrophic nails
Congenital onychauxis   Pachyonychia

Q84.6 Other congenital malformations of nails
Congenital clubnail
Congenital koilonychia
Congenital malformation of nail NOS

Q84.8 Other specified congenital malformations of integument
Aplasia cutis congenita

Q84.9 Congenital malformation of integument, unspecified
Congenital anomaly of integument NOS
Congenital deformity of integument NOS

✓4ᵗʰ **Q85** Phakomatoses, not elsewhere classified
EXCLUDES 1 *ataxia telangiectasia [Louis-Bar] (G11.3)*
familial dysautonomia [Riley-Day] (G90.1)

✓5ᵗʰ **Q85.0** Neurofibromatosis (nonmalignant)

Q85.00 Neurofibromatosis, unspecified

Q85.01 Neurofibromatosis, type 1
Von Recklinghausen disease

Q85.02 Neurofibromatosis, type 2
Acoustic neurofibromatosis

Q85.03 Schwannomatosis

Q85.09 Other neurofibromatosis

Q85.1 Tuberous sclerosis
Bourneville's disease
Epiloia

Q85.8 Other phakomatoses, not elsewhere classified
Peutz-Jeghers Syndrome
Sturge-Weber(-Dimitri) syndrome
von Hippel-Lindau syndrome
EXCLUDES 1 *Meckel-Gruber syndrome (Q61.9)*

Q85.9 Phakomatosis, unspecified
Hamartosis NOS

✓4ᵗʰ **Q86** Congenital malformation syndromes due to known exogenous causes, not elsewhere classified
EXCLUDES 2 *iodine-deficiency-related hypothyroidism (E00-E02)*
nonteratogenic effects of substances transmitted via placenta or breast milk (P04.-)

Q86.0 Fetal alcohol syndrome (dysmorphic)

Q86.1 Fetal hydantoin syndrome   N
Meadow's syndrome

Q86.2 Dysmorphism due to warfarin

Q86.8 Other congenital malformation syndromes due to known exogenous causes

✓4ᵗʰ **Q87** Other specified congenital malformation syndromes affecting multiple systems
Use additional code(s) to identify all associated manifestations

Q87.0 Congenital malformation syndromes predominantly affecting facial appearance
Acrocephalopolysyndactyly   Robin syndrome
Acrocephalosyndactyly [Apert]   Whistling face
Cryptophthalmos syndrome
Cyclopia
Goldenhar syndrome
Moebius syndrome
Oro-facial-digital syndrome

Q87.1 Congenital malformation syndromes predominantly associated with short stature
Aarskog syndrome   Robinow-Silverman-Smith
Cockayne syndrome   syndrome
De Lange syndrome   Russell-Silver syndrome
Dubowitz syndrome   Seckel syndrome
Noonan syndrome
Prader-Willi syndrome
EXCLUDES 1 *Ellis-van Creveld syndrome (Q77.6)*
Smith-Lemli-Opitz syndrome (E78.72)

Q87.2 Congenital malformation syndromes predominantly involving limbs
Holt-Oram syndrome
Klippel-Trenaunay-Weber syndrome
Nail patella syndrome
Rubinstein-Taybi syndrome
Sirenomelia syndrome
Thrombocytopenia with absent radius [TAR] syndrome
VATER syndrome

Q87.3 Congenital malformation syndromes involving early overgrowth
Beckwith-Wiedemann syndrome   Weaver syndrome
Sotos syndrome

✓5ᵗʰ **Q87.4** Marfan's syndrome

Q87.40 Marfan's syndrome, unspecified

✓6ᵗʰ **Q87.41** Marfan's syndrome with cardiovascular manifestations

Q87.410 Marfan's syndrome with aortic dilation

Q87.418 Marfan's syndrome with other cardiovascular manifestations

Q87.42 Marfan's syndrome with ocular manifestations

Q87.43 Marfan's syndrome with skeletal manifestation

Q87.5 Other congenital malformation syndromes with other skeletal changes

✓5ᵗʰ **Q87.8** Other specified congenital malformation syndromes, not elsewhere classified
EXCLUDES 1 *Zellweger syndrome (E71.510)*

Q87.81 Alport syndrome
Use additional code to identify stage of chronic kidney disease (N18.1-N18.6)

Q87.89 Other specified congenital malformation syndromes, not elsewhere classified
Laurence-Moon (-Bardet)-Biedl syndrome

✓4ᵗʰ **Q89** Other congenital malformations, not elsewhere classified

✓5ᵗʰ **Q89.0** Congenital absence and malformations of spleen
EXCLUDES 1 *isomerism of atrial appendages (with asplenia or polysplenia) (Q20.6)*

Q89.01 Asplenia (congenital)

Q89.09 Congenital malformations of spleen
Congenital splenomegaly

Q89.1 Congenital malformations of adrenal gland
EXCLUDES 1 *adrenogenital disorders (E25.-)*
congenital adrenal hyperplasia (E25.0)

Q89.2 Congenital malformations of other endocrine glands
Congenital malformation of parathyroid or thyroid gland
Persistent thyroglossal duct
Thyroglossal cyst
EXCLUDES 1 *congenital goiter (E03.0)*
congenital hypothyroidism (E03.1)

Q89.3 Situs inversus
Dextrocardia with situs inversus
Mirror-image atrial arrangement with situs inversus
Situs inversus or transversus abdominalis
Situs inversus or transversus thoracis
Transposition of abdominal viscera
Transposition of thoracic viscera
EXCLUDES 1 *dextrocardia NOS (Q24.0)*

Q89.4 Conjoined twins
Craniopagus   Pygopagus
Dicephaly   Thoracopagus

Q89.7 Multiple congenital malformations, not elsewhere classified
Multiple congenital anomalies NOS
Multiple congenital deformities NOS
EXCLUDES 1 *congenital malformation syndromes affecting multiple systems (Q87.-)*

Q89.8 Other specified congenital malformations
Use additional code(s) to identify all associated manifestations

Q89.9 Congenital malformation, unspecified
Congenital anomaly NOS   Congenital deformity NOS

EXCLUDES 1 Not coded here   EXCLUDES 2 Not included here   N Newborn Age: 0   P Pediatric Age: 0-17   M Maternity Age: 12-55   A Adult Age: 15-124

Chromosomal abnormalities, not elsewhere classified (Q90-Q99)

EXCLUDES 2 *mitochondrial metabolic disorders (E88.4-)*

√4th **Q90 Down syndrome**
Use additional code(s) to identify any associated physical conditions and degree of intellectual disabilities (F70-F79)

Q90.0 Trisomy 21, nonmosaicism (meiotic nondisjunction)

Q90.1 Trisomy 21, mosaicism (mitotic nondisjunction)

Q90.2 Trisomy 21, translocation

Q90.9 Down syndrome, unspecified
Trisomy 21 NOS

√4th **Q91 Trisomy 18 and Trisomy 13**

Q91.0 Trisomy 18, nonmosaicism (meiotic nondisjunction)

Q91.1 Trisomy 18, mosaicism (mitotic nondisjunction)

Q91.2 Trisomy 18, translocation

Q91.3 Trisomy 18, unspecified

Q91.4 Trisomy 13, nonmosaicism (meiotic nondisjunction)

Q91.5 Trisomy 13, mosaicism (mitotic nondisjunction)

Q91.6 Trisomy 13, translocation

Q91.7 Trisomy 13, unspecified

√4th **Q92 Other trisomies and partial trisomies of the autosomes, not elsewhere classified**
INCLUDES unbalanced translocations and insertions
EXCLUDES 1 *trisomies of chromosomes 13, 18, 21 (Q90-Q91)*

Q92.0 Whole chromosome trisomy, nonmosaicism (meiotic nondisjunction)

Q92.1 Whole chromosome trisomy, mosaicism (mitotic nondisjunction)

Q92.2 Partial trisomy
Less than whole arm duplicated
Whole arm or more duplicated
EXCLUDES 1 *partial trisomy due to unbalanced translocation (Q92.5)*

Q92.5 Duplications with other complex rearrangements
Partial trisomy due to unbalanced translocations
Code also any associated deletions due to unbalanced translocations, inversions and insertions (Q93.7)

√5th **Q92.6 Marker chromosomes**
Trisomies due to dicentrics
Trisomies due to extra rings
Trisomies due to isochromosomes
Individual with marker heterochromatin

Q92.61 Marker chromosomes in normal individual

Q92.62 Marker chromosomes in abnormal individual

Q92.7 Triploidy and polyploidy

Q92.8 Other specified trisomies and partial trisomies of autosomes
Duplications identified by fluorescence in situ hybridization (FISH)
Duplications identified by in situ hybridization (ISH)
Duplications seen only at prometaphase

Q92.9 Trisomy and partial trisomy of autosomes, unspecified

√4th **Q93 Monosomies and deletions from the autosomes, not elsewhere classified**

Q93.0 Whole chromosome monosomy, nonmosaicism (meiotic nondisjunction)

Q93.1 Whole chromosome monosomy, mosaicism (mitotic nondisjunction)

Q93.2 Chromosome replaced with ring, dicentric or isochromosome

Q93.3 Deletion of short arm of chromosome 4
Wolff-Hirschorn syndrome

Q93.4 Deletion of short arm of chromosome 5
Cri-du-chat syndrome

Q93.5 Other deletions of part of a chromosome
Angelman syndrome

Q93.7 Deletions with other complex rearrangements
Deletions due to unbalanced translocations, inversions and insertions
Code also any associated duplications due to unbalanced translocations, inversions and insertions (Q92.5)

√5th **Q93.8 Other deletions from the autosomes**

Q93.81 Velo-cardio-facial syndrome
Deletion 22q11.2

Q93.88 Other microdeletions
Miller-Dieker syndrome
Smith-Magenis syndrome

Q93.89 Other deletions from the autosomes
Deletions identified by fluorescence in situ hybridization (FISH)
Deletions identified by in situ hybridization (ISH)
Deletions seen only at prometaphase

Q93.9 Deletion from autosomes, unspecified

√4th **Q95 Balanced rearrangements and structural markers, not elsewhere classified**
INCLUDES Robertsonian and balanced reciprocal translocations and insertions

Q95.0 Balanced translocation and insertion in normal individual

Q95.1 Chromosome inversion in normal individual

Q95.2 Balanced autosomal rearrangement in abnormal individual

Q95.3 Balanced sex/autosomal rearrangement in abnormal individual

Q95.5 Individual with autosomal fragile site

Q95.8 Other balanced rearrangements and structural markers

Q95.9 Balanced rearrangement and structural marker, unspecified

√4th **Q96 Turner's syndrome**
EXCLUDES 1 *Noonan syndrome (Q87.1)*

Q96.0 Karyotype 45, X ♀

Q96.1 Karyotype 46, X iso (Xq) ♀
Karyotype 46, isochromosome Xq

Q96.2 Karyotype 46, X with abnormal sex chromosome, except iso (Xq) ♀
Karyotype 46, X with abnormal sex chromosome, except isochromosome Xq

Q96.3 Mosaicism, 45, X/46, XX or XY ♀

Q96.4 Mosaicism, 45, X/other cell line(s) with abnormal sex chromosome ♀

Q96.8 Other variants of Turner's syndrome ♀

Q96.9 Turner's syndrome, unspecified ♀

√4th **Q97 Other sex chromosome abnormalities, female phenotype, not elsewhere classified**
EXCLUDES 1 *Turner's syndrome (Q96.-)*

Q97.0 Karyotype 47, XXX ♀

Q97.1 Female with more than three X chromosomes ♀

Q97.2 Mosaicism, lines with various numbers of X chromosomes ♀

Q97.3 Female with 46, XY karyotype ♀

Q97.8 Other specified sex chromosome abnormalities, female phenotype ♀

Q97.9 Sex chromosome abnormality, female phenotype, unspecified ♀

√4th **Q98 Other sex chromosome abnormalities, male phenotype, not elsewhere classified**

Q98.0 Klinefelter syndrome karyotype 47, XXY ♂

Q98.1 Klinefelter syndrome, male with more than two X chromosomes ♂

Q98.3 Other male with 46, XX karyotype ♂

Q98.4 Klinefelter syndrome, unspecified ♂

Q98.5 Karyotype 47, XYY ♂

Q98.6 Male with structurally abnormal sex chromosome ♂

Q98.7 Male with sex chromosome mosaicism ♂

Q98.8 Other specified sex chromosome abnormalities, male phenotype ♂

Q98.9 Sex chromosome abnormality, male phenotype, unspecified ♂

√4th **Q99 Other chromosome abnormalities, not elsewhere classified**

Q99.0 Chimera 46, XX/46, XY
Chimera 46, XX/46, XY true hermaphrodite

Q99.1 46, XX true hermaphrodite
46, XX with streak gonads   Pure gonadal dysgenesis
46, XY with streak gonads

Q99.2 Fragile X chromosome
Fragile X syndrome

Q99.8 Other specified chromosome abnormalities

Q99.9 Chromosomal abnormality, unspecified

Chapter 18. Symptoms, Signs and Abnormal Clinical and Laboratory Findings, Not Elsewhere Classified (R00-R99)

This chapter includes symptoms, signs, abnormal results of clinical or other investigative procedures, and ill-defined conditions regarding which no diagnosis classifiable elsewhere is recorded.

Signs and symptoms that point rather definitely to a given diagnosis have been assigned to a category in other chapters of the classification. In general, categories in this chapter include the less well-defined conditions and symptoms that, without the necessary study of the case to establish a final diagnosis, point perhaps equally to two or more diseases or to two or more systems of the body. Practically all categories in the chapter could be designated "not otherwise specified", "unknown etiology" or "transient". The Alphabetical Index should be consulted to determine which symptoms and signs are to be allocated here and which to other chapters. The residual subcategories, numbered .8, are generally provided for other relevant symptoms that cannot be allocated elsewhere in the classification.

The conditions and signs or symptoms included in categories R00-R94 consist of:

(a) cases for which no more specific diagnosis can be made even after all the facts bearing on the case have been investigated;

(b) signs or symptoms existing at the time of initial encounter that proved to be transient and whose causes could not be determined;

(c) provisional diagnosis in a patient who failed to return for further investigation or care;

(d) cases referred elsewhere for investigation or treatment before the diagnosis was made;

(e) cases in which a more precise diagnosis was not available for any other reason;

(f) certain symptoms, for which supplementary information is provided, that represent important problems in medical care in their own right.

EXCLUDES 2 abnormal findings on antenatal screening of mother (O28.-)
certain conditions originating in the perinatal period (P04-P96)
signs and symptoms classified in the body system chapters
signs and symptoms of breast (N63, N64.5)

This chapter contains the following blocks:

R00-R09 Symptoms and signs involving the circulatory and respiratory systems
R10-R19 Symptoms and signs involving the digestive system and abdomen
R20-R23 Symptoms and signs involving the skin and subcutaneous tissue
R25-R29 Symptoms and signs involving the nervous and musculoskeletal systems
R30-R39 Symptoms and signs involving the genitourinary system
R40-R46 Symptoms and signs involving cognition, perception, emotional state and behavior
R47-R49 Symptoms and signs involving speech and voice
R50-R69 General symptoms and signs
R70-R79 Abnormal findings on examination of blood, without diagnosis
R80-R82 Abnormal findings on examination of urine, without diagnosis
R83-R89 Abnormal findings on examination of other body fluids, substances and tissues, without diagnosis
R90-R94 Abnormal findings on diagnostic imaging and in function studies, without diagnosis
R97 Abnormal tumor markers
R99 Ill-defined and unknown cause of mortality

Symptoms and signs involving the circulatory and respiratory systems (R00-R09)

☑4ᵗʰ **R00 Abnormalities of heart beat**
EXCLUDES 1 abnormalities originating in the perinatal period (P29.1-)
specified arrhythmias (I47-I49)

R00.0 Tachycardia, unspecified
Rapid heart beat
Sinoauricular tachycardia NOS
Sinus [sinusal] tachycardia NOS
EXCLUDES 1 neonatal tachycardia (P29.11)
paroxysmal tachycardia (I47.-)

R00.1 Bradycardia, unspecified
Sinoatrial bradycardia
Sinus bradycardia
Slow heart beat
Vagal bradycardia
Use additional code for adverse effect, if applicable, to identify drug (T36-T50 with fifth or sixth character 5)
EXCLUDES 1 neonatal bradycardia (P29.12)

R00.2 Palpitations
Awareness of heart beat

R00.8 Other abnormalities of heart beat

R00.9 Unspecified abnormalities of heart beat

☑4ᵗʰ **R01 Cardiac murmurs and other cardiac sounds**
EXCLUDES 1 cardiac murmurs and sounds originating in the perinatal period (P29.8)

R01.0 Benign and innocent cardiac murmurs
Functional cardiac murmur

R01.1 Cardiac murmur, unspecified
Cardiac bruit NOS
Heart murmur NOS

R01.2 Other cardiac sounds
Cardiac dullness, increased or decreased
Precordial friction

☑4ᵗʰ **R03 Abnormal blood-pressure reading, without diagnosis**

R03.0 Elevated blood-pressure reading, without diagnosis of hypertension
NOTE This category is to be used to record an episode of elevated blood pressure in a patient in whom no formal diagnosis of hypertension has been made, or as an isolated incidental finding.

R03.1 Nonspecific low blood-pressure reading
EXCLUDES 1 hypotension (I95.-)
maternal hypotension syndrome (O26.5-)
neurogenic orthostatic hypotension (G90.3)

☑4ᵗʰ **R04 Hemorrhage from respiratory passages**

R04.0 Epistaxis
Hemorrhage from nose
Nosebleed

R04.1 Hemorrhage from throat
EXCLUDES 2 hemoptysis (R04.2)

R04.2 Hemoptysis
Blood-stained sputum
Cough with hemorrhage

☑5ᵗʰ **R04.8 Hemorrhage from other sites in respiratory passages**

R04.81 Acute idiopathic pulmonary hemorrhage in infants P
AIPHI
Acute idiopathic hemorrhage in infants over 28 days old
EXCLUDES 1 perinatal pulmonary hemorrhage (P26.-)
von Willebrand's disease (D68.0)

R04.89 Hemorrhage from other sites in respiratory passages
Pulmonary hemorrhage NOS

R04.9 Hemorrhage from respiratory passages, unspecified

R05 Cough
EXCLUDES 1 cough with hemorrhage (R04.2)
smoker's cough (J41.0)

☑4ᵗʰ **R06 Abnormalities of breathing**
EXCLUDES 1 acute respiratory distress syndrome (J80)
respiratory arrest (R09.2)
respiratory arrest of newborn (P28.81)
respiratory distress syndrome of newborn (P22.-)
respiratory failure (J96.-)
respiratory failure of newborn (P28.5)

☑5ᵗʰ **R06.0 Dyspnea**
EXCLUDES 1 tachypnea NOS (R06.82)
transient tachypnea of newborn (P22.1)

R06.00 Dyspnea, unspecified

R06.01 Orthopnea

R06.02 Shortness of breath

R06.09 Other forms of dyspnea

R06.1 Stridor
EXCLUDES 1 congenital laryngeal stridor (P28.89)
laryngismus (stridulus) (J38.5)

R06.2 Wheezing
EXCLUDES 1 asthma (J45.-)

R06.3 Periodic breathing
Cheyne-Stokes breathing

R06.4 Hyperventilation
EXCLUDES 1 psychogenic hyperventilation (F45.8)

R06.5 Mouth breathing
EXCLUDES 2 dry mouth NOS (R68.2)

R06.6 Hiccough
EXCLUDES 1 psychogenic hiccough (F45.8)

R06.7 Sneezing

Symptoms, Signs and Abnormal Clinical and Laboratory Findings

R06.8–R10.827

✓5ᵗʰ **R06.8** **Other abnormalities of breathing**

R06.81 **Apnea, not elsewhere classified**
Apnea NOS
EXCLUDES 1 *apnea (of) newborn (P28.4)*
sleep apnea (G47.3-)
sleep apnea of newborn (primary) (P28.3)

R06.82 **Tachypnea, not elsewhere classified**
Tachypnea NOS
EXCLUDES 1 *transitory tachypnea of newborn (P22.1)*

R06.83 Snoring

R06.89 Other abnormalities of breathing
Breath-holding (spells)
Sighing

R06.9 **Unspecified abnormalities of breathing**

✓4ᵗʰ **R07** **Pain in throat and chest**
EXCLUDES 1 *epidemic myalgia (B33.0)*
EXCLUDES 2 *jaw pain (R68.84)*
pain in breast (N64.4)

R07.0 **Pain in throat**
EXCLUDES 1 *chronic sore throat (J31.2)*
sore throat (acute) NOS (J02.9)
EXCLUDES 2 *dysphagia (R13.1-)*
pain in neck (M54.2)

R07.1 **Chest pain on breathing**
Painful respiration

R07.2 **Precordial pain**

✓5ᵗʰ **R07.8** **Other chest pain**

R07.81 **Pleurodynia**
Pleurodynia NOS
EXCLUDES 1 *epidemic pleurodynia (B33.0)*

R07.82 **Intercostal pain**

R07.89 **Other chest pain**
Anterior chest-wall pain NOS

R07.9 **Chest pain, unspecified**

✓4ᵗʰ **R09** **Other symptoms and signs involving the circulatory and respiratory system**
EXCLUDES 1 *acute respiratory distress syndrome (J80)*
respiratory arrest of newborn (P28.81)
respiratory distress syndrome of newborn (P22.0)
respiratory failure (J96.-)
respiratory failure of newborn (P28.5)

✓5ᵗʰ **R09.0** **Asphyxia and hypoxemia**
EXCLUDES 1 *asphyxia due to carbon monoxide (T58.-)*
asphyxia due to foreign body in respiratory tract (T17.-)
birth (intrauterine) asphyxia (P84)
hypercapnia (R06.4)
hyperventilation (R06.4)
traumatic asphyxia (T71.-)

R09.01 **Asphyxia**

R09.02 **Hypoxemia**

R09.1 **Pleurisy**
EXCLUDES 1 *pleurisy with effusion (J90)*

R09.2 **Respiratory arrest**
Cardiorespiratory failure
EXCLUDES 1 *cardiac arrest (I46.-)*
respiratory arrest of newborn (P28.81)
respiratory distress of newborn (P22.0)
respiratory failure (J96.-)
respiratory failure of newborn (P28.5)
respiratory insufficiency (R06.89)
respiratory insufficiency of newborn (P28.5)

R09.3 **Abnormal sputum**
Abnormal amount of sputum
Abnormal color of sputum
Abnormal odor of sputum
Excessive sputum
EXCLUDES 1 *blood-stained sputum (R04.2)*

✓5ᵗʰ **R09.8** **Other specified symptoms and signs involving the circulatory and respiratory systems**

R09.81 **Nasal congestion**

R09.82 **Postnasal drip**

R09.89 **Other specified symptoms and signs involving the circulatory and respiratory systems**
Abnormal chest percussion
Bruit (arterial)
Chest tympany
Choking sensation
Feeling of foreign body in throat
Friction sounds in chest
Rales
Weak pulse
EXCLUDES 2 *foreign body in throat (T17.2-)*
wheezing (R06.2)

Symptoms and signs involving the digestive system and abdomen (R10-R19)

EXCLUDES 1 *congenital or infantile pylorospasm (Q40.0)*
gastrointestinal hemorrhage (K92.0-K92.2)
intestinal obstruction (K56.-)
newborn gastrointestinal hemorrhage (P54.0-P54.3)
newborn intestinal obstruction (P76.-)
pylorospasm (K31.3)
signs and symptoms involving the urinary system (R30-R39)
symptoms referable to female genital organs (N94.-)
symptoms referable to male genital organs male (N48-N50)

✓4ᵗʰ **R10** **Abdominal and pelvic pain**
EXCLUDES 1 *renal colic (N23)*
EXCLUDES 2 *dorsalgia (M54.-)*
flatulence and related conditions (R14.-)

R10.0 **Acute abdomen**
Severe abdominal pain (generalized) (with abdominal rigidity)
EXCLUDES 1 *abdominal rigidity NOS (R19.3)*
generalized abdominal pain NOS (R10.84)
localized abdominal pain (R10.1-R10.3-)

✓5ᵗʰ **R10.1** **Pain localized to upper abdomen**

R10.10 **Upper abdominal pain, unspecified**

R10.11 **Right upper quadrant pain**

R10.12 **Left upper quadrant pain**

R10.13 **Epigastric pain**
Dyspepsia
EXCLUDES 1 *functional dyspepsia (K30)*

R10.2 **Pelvic and perineal pain**
EXCLUDES 1 *vulvodynia (N94.81)*

✓5ᵗʰ **R10.3** **Pain localized to other parts of lower abdomen**

R10.30 **Lower abdominal pain, unspecified**

R10.31 **Right lower quadrant pain**

R10.32 **Left lower quadrant pain**

R10.33 **Periumbilical pain**

✓5ᵗʰ **R10.8** **Other abdominal pain**

✓6ᵗʰ **R10.81** **Abdominal tenderness**
Abdominal tenderness NOS

R10.811 **Right upper quadrant abdominal tenderness**

R10.812 **Left upper quadrant abdominal tenderness**

R10.813 **Right lower quadrant abdominal tenderness**

R10.814 **Left lower quadrant abdominal tenderness**

R10.815 **Periumbilic abdominal tenderness**

R10.816 **Epigastric abdominal tenderness**

R10.817 **Generalized abdominal tenderness**

R10.819 **Abdominal tenderness, unspecified site**

✓6ᵗʰ **R10.82** **Rebound abdominal tenderness**

R10.821 **Right upper quadrant rebound abdominal tenderness**

R10.822 **Left upper quadrant rebound abdominal tenderness**

R10.823 **Right lower quadrant rebound abdominal tenderness**

R10.824 **Left lower quadrant rebound abdominal tenderness**

R10.825 **Periumbilic rebound abdominal tenderness**

R10.826 **Epigastric rebound abdominal tenderness**

R10.827 **Generalized rebound abdominal tenderness**

EXCLUDES 1 Not coded here　　　EXCLUDES 2 Not included here　　　N Newborn Age: 0　　　P Pediatric Age: 0-17　　　M Maternity Age: 12-55　　　A Adult Age: 15-124

790　　　　　　　　　　　　　　　　　　　　　　　　　　　　　　　　　　ICD-10-CM 2014 (Draft)

R10.829 **Rebound** abdominal tenderness, unspecified site

R10.83 Colic   🄿
Colic NOS
Infantile colic
EXCLUDES 1   colic in adult and child over 12 months old (R10.84)

R10.84 **Generalized** abdominal pain
EXCLUDES 1   generalized abdominal pain associated with acute abdomen (R10.0)

R10.9 **Unspecified** abdominal pain

✓4ᵗʰ R11 Nausea and vomiting
EXCLUDES 1   cyclical vomiting associated with migraine (G43.A-)
excessive vomiting in pregnancy (O21.-)
hematemesis (K92.0)
neonatal hematemesis (P54.0)
newborn vomiting (P92.0-)
psychogenic vomiting (F50.8)
vomiting associated with bulimia nervosa (F50.2)
vomiting following gastrointestinal surgery (K91.0)

R11.0 **Nausea**
Nausea NOS
Nausea without vomiting

✓5ᵗʰ R11.1 **Vomiting**
R11.10 **Vomiting,** unspecified
Vomiting NOS
R11.11 **Vomiting** without nausea
R11.12 **Projectile** vomiting
R11.13 **Vomiting** of fecal matter
R11.14 **Bilious** vomiting
Bilious emesis

R11.2 **Nausea** with vomiting, unspecified
Persistent nausea with vomiting NOS

R12 Heartburn
EXCLUDES 1   dyspepsia NOS (R10.13)
functional dyspepsia (K30)

✓4ᵗʰ R13 Aphagia and dysphagia
R13.0 **Aphagia**
Inability to swallow
EXCLUDES 1   psychogenic aphagia (F50.9)

✓5ᵗʰ R13.1 **Dysphagia**
Code first, if applicable, dysphagia following cerebrovascular disease (I69. with final characters -91)
EXCLUDES 1   psychogenic dysphagia (F45.8)
R13.10 **Dysphagia,** unspecified
Difficulty in swallowing NOS
R13.11 **Dysphagia,** oral phase
R13.12 **Dysphagia,** oropharyngeal phase
R13.13 **Dysphagia,** pharyngeal phase
R13.14 **Dysphagia,** pharyngoesophageal phase
R13.19 **Other dysphagia**
Cervical dysphagia
Neurogenic dysphagia

✓4ᵗʰ R14 Flatulence and related conditions
EXCLUDES 1   psychogenic aerophagy (F45.8)
R14.0 **Abdominal distension (gaseous)**
Bloating
Tympanites (abdominal) (intestinal)
R14.1 **Gas pain**
R14.2 **Eructation**
R14.3 **Flatulence**

✓4ᵗʰ R15 Fecal incontinence
Encopresis NOS
EXCLUDES 1   fecal incontinence of nonorganic origin (F98.1)
R15.0 **Incomplete defecation**
EXCLUDES 1   constipation (K59.0-)
fecal impaction (K56.41)
R15.1 **Fecal smearing**
Fecal soiling
R15.2 **Fecal urgency**
R15.9 **Full incontinence of feces**
Fecal incontinence NOS

✓4ᵗʰ R16 Hepatomegaly and splenomegaly, not elsewhere classified
R16.0 **Hepatomegaly, not elsewhere classified**
Hepatomegaly NOS

R16.1 **Splenomegaly, not elsewhere classified**
Splenomegaly NOS
R16.2 **Hepatomegaly with splenomegaly, not elsewhere classified**
Hepatosplenomegaly NOS

R17 Unspecified jaundice
EXCLUDES 1   neonatal jaundice (P55, P57-P59)

✓4ᵗʰ R18 Ascites
INCLUDES   fluid in peritoneal cavity
EXCLUDES 1   ascites in alcoholic cirrhosis (K70.31)
ascites in alcoholic hepatitis (K70.11)
ascites in toxic liver disease with chronic active hepatitis (K71.51)

R18.0 **Malignant** ascites
Code first malignancy, such as:
malignant neoplasm of ovary (C56.-)
secondary malignant neoplasm of retroperitoneum and peritoneum (C78.6)
R18.8 **Other ascites**
Ascites NOS
Peritoneal effusion (chronic)

✓4ᵗʰ R19 Other symptoms and signs involving the digestive system and abdomen
EXCLUDES 1   acute abdomen (R10.0)

✓5ᵗʰ R19.0 **Intra-abdominal and pelvic swelling, mass and lump**
EXCLUDES 1   abdominal distension (gaseous) (R14.-)
ascites (R18.-)
R19.00 **Intra-abdominal and pelvic swelling, mass and lump, unspecified site**
R19.01 **Right upper quadrant** abdominal swelling, mass and lump
R19.02 **Left upper quadrant** abdominal swelling, mass and lump
R19.03 **Right lower quadrant** abdominal swelling, mass and lump
R19.04 **Left lower quadrant** abdominal swelling, mass and lump
R19.05 **Periumbilic** swelling, mass or lump
Diffuse or generalized umbilical swelling or mass
R19.06 **Epigastric** swelling, mass or lump
R19.07 **Generalized** intra-abdominal and pelvic swelling, mass and lump
Diffuse or generalized intra-abdominal swelling or mass NOS
Diffuse or generalized pelvic swelling or mass NOS
R19.09 **Other intra-abdominal and pelvic swelling, mass and lump**

✓5ᵗʰ R19.1 **Abnormal bowel sounds**
R19.11 **Absent** bowel sounds
R19.12 **Hyperactive** bowel sounds
R19.15 **Other abnormal bowel sounds**
Abnormal bowel sounds NOS

R19.2 **Visible peristalsis**
Hyperperistalsis

✓5ᵗʰ R19.3 **Abdominal rigidity**
EXCLUDES 1   abdominal rigidity with severe abdominal pain (R10.0)
R19.30 **Abdominal rigidity, unspecified site**
R19.31 **Right upper quadrant** abdominal rigidity
R19.32 **Left upper quadrant** abdominal rigidity
R19.33 **Right lower quadrant** abdominal rigidity
R19.34 **Left lower quadrant** abdominal rigidity
R19.35 **Periumbilic** abdominal rigidity
R19.36 **Epigastric** abdominal rigidity
R19.37 **Generalized** abdominal rigidity

R19.4 **Change in bowel habit**
EXCLUDES 1   constipation (K59.0-)
functional diarrhea (K59.1)

R19.5 **Other fecal abnormalities**
Abnormal stool color
Bulky stools
Mucus in stools
Occult blood in feces
Occult blood in stools
EXCLUDES 1   melena (K92.1)
neonatal melena (P54.1)

R19.6 **Halitosis**

Symptoms, Signs and Abnormal Clinical and Laboratory Findings

R19.7–R29.5

R19.7 Diarrhea, unspecified
Diarrhea NOS
EXCLUDES 1   *functional diarrhea (K59.1)*
neonatal diarrhea (P78.3)
psychogenic diarrhea (F45.8)

R19.8 Other specified symptoms and signs involving the digestive system and abdomen

Symptoms and signs involving the skin and subcutaneous tissue (R2Ø-R23)

EXCLUDES 2   *symptoms relating to breast (N64.4-N64.5)*

✓4ᵗʰ **R2Ø Disturbances of skin sensation**
EXCLUDES 1   *dissociative anesthesia and sensory loss (F44.6)*
psychogenic disturbances (F45.8)

R2Ø.Ø Anesthesia of skin

R2Ø.1 Hypoesthesia of skin

R2Ø.2 Paresthesia of skin
Formication
Pins and needles
Tingling skin
EXCLUDES 1   *acroparesthesia (I73.8)*

R2Ø.3 Hyperesthesia

R2Ø.8 Other disturbances of skin sensation

R2Ø.9 Unspecified disturbances of skin sensation

R21 Rash and other nonspecific skin eruption
Rash NOS
EXCLUDES 1   *specified type of rash—code to condition*
vesicular eruption (R23.8)

✓4ᵗʰ **R22 Localized swelling, mass and lump of skin and subcutaneous tissue**
Subcutaneous nodules (localized)(superficial)
EXCLUDES 1   *abnormal findings on diagnostic imaging (R9Ø-R93)*
edema (R6Ø.-)
enlarged lymph nodes (R59.-)
localized adiposity (E65)
swelling of joint (M25.4-)

R22.Ø Localized swelling, mass and lump, head

R22.1 Localized swelling, mass and lump, neck

R22.2 Localized swelling, mass and lump, trunk
EXCLUDES 1   *intra-abdominal or pelvic mass and lump (R19.Ø-)*
intra-abdominal or pelvic swelling (R19.Ø-)
EXCLUDES 2   *breast mass and lump (N63)*

✓5ᵗʰ **R22.3 Localized swelling, mass and lump, upper limb**

    R22.3Ø Localized swelling, mass and lump, unspecified upper limb

    R22.31 Localized swelling, mass and lump, right upper limb

    R22.32 Localized swelling, mass and lump, left upper limb

    R22.33 Localized swelling, mass and lump, upper limb, bilateral

✓5ᵗʰ **R22.4 Localized swelling, mass and lump, lower limb**

    R22.4Ø Localized swelling, mass and lump, unspecified lower limb

    R22.41 Localized swelling, mass and lump, right lower limb

    R22.42 Localized swelling, mass and lump, left lower limb

    R22.43 Localized swelling, mass and lump, lower limb, bilateral

R22.9 Localized swelling, mass and lump, unspecified

✓4ᵗʰ **R23 Other skin changes**

R23.Ø Cyanosis
EXCLUDES 1   *acrocyanosis (I73.8)*
cyanotic attacks of newborn (P28.2)

R23.1 Pallor
Clammy skin

R23.2 Flushing
Excessive blushing
Code first, if applicable, menopausal and female climacteric states (N95.1)

R23.3 Spontaneous ecchymoses
Petechiae
EXCLUDES 1   *ecchymoses of newborn (P54.5)*
purpura (D69.-)

R23.4 Changes in skin texture
Desquamation of skin
Induration of skin
Scaling of skin
EXCLUDES 1   *epidermal thickening NOS (L85.9)*

R23.8 Other skin changes

R23.9 Unspecified skin changes

Symptoms and signs involving the nervous and musculoskeletal systems (R25-R29)

✓4ᵗʰ **R25 Abnormal involuntary movements**
EXCLUDES 1   *specific movement disorders (G2Ø-G26)*
stereotyped movement disorders (F98.4)
tic disorders (F95.-)

R25.Ø Abnormal head movements

R25.1 Tremor, unspecified
EXCLUDES 1   *chorea NOS (G25.5)*
essential tremor (G25.Ø)
hysterical tremor (F44.4)
intention tremor (G25.2)

R25.2 Cramp and spasm
EXCLUDES 2   *carpopedal spasm (R29.Ø)*
charley-horse (M62.831)
infantile spasms (G4Ø.4-)
muscle spasm of back (M62.83Ø)
muscle spasm of calf (M62.831)

R25.3 Fasciculation
Twitching NOS

R25.8 Other abnormal involuntary movements

R25.9 Unspecified abnormal involuntary movements

✓4ᵗʰ **R26 Abnormalities of gait and mobility**
EXCLUDES 1   *ataxia NOS (R27.Ø)*
hereditary ataxia (G11.-)
locomotor (syphilitic) ataxia (A52.11)
immobility syndrome (paraplegic) (M62.3)

R26.Ø Ataxic gait
Staggering gait

R26.1 Paralytic gait
Spastic gait

R26.2 Difficulty in walking, not elsewhere classified
EXCLUDES 1   *falling (R29.6)*
unsteadiness on feet (R26.81)

✓5ᵗʰ **R26.8 Other abnormalities of gait and mobility**

    R26.81 Unsteadiness on feet

    R26.89 Other abnormalities of gait and mobility

R26.9 Unspecified abnormalities of gait and mobility

✓4ᵗʰ **R27 Other lack of coordination**
EXCLUDES 1   *ataxic gait (R26.Ø)*
hereditary ataxia (G11.-)
vertigo NOS (R42)

R27.Ø Ataxia, unspecified
EXCLUDES 1   *ataxia following cerebrovascular disease (I69. with final characters -93)*

R27.8 Other lack of coordination

R27.9 Unspecified lack of coordination

✓4ᵗʰ **R29 Other symptoms and signs involving the nervous and musculoskeletal systems**

R29.Ø Tetany
Carpopedal spasm
EXCLUDES 1   *hysterical tetany (F44.5)*
neonatal tetany (P71.3)
parathyroid tetany (E2Ø.9)
post-thyroidectomy tetany (E89.2)

R29.1 Meningismus

R29.2 Abnormal reflex
EXCLUDES 2   *abnormal pupillary reflex (H57.Ø)*
hyperactive gag reflex (J39.2)
vasovagal reaction or syncope (R55)

R29.3 Abnormal posture

R29.4 Clicking hip
EXCLUDES 1   *congenital deformities of hip (Q65.-)*

R29.5 Transient paralysis
Code first any associated spinal cord injury (S14.Ø, S14.1-, S24.Ø, S24.1-, S34.Ø-, S34.1-)
EXCLUDES 1   *transient ischemic attack (G45.9)*

EXCLUDES 1 Not coded here   *EXCLUDES 2* Not included here   **N** Newborn Age: Ø   **P** Pediatric Age: Ø-17   **M** Maternity Age: 12-55   **A** Adult Age: 15-124

792   ICD-1Ø-CM 2Ø14 (Draft)

R29.6 Repeated falls
Falling
Tendency to fall
EXCLUDES 2   at risk for falling (Z91.81)
              history of falling (Z91.81)

R29.8 Other symptoms and signs involving the nervous and musculoskeletal systems

R29.81 Other symptoms and signs involving the nervous system

R29.810 Facial weakness
Facial droop
EXCLUDES 1   Bell's palsy (G51.0)
          facial weakness following cerebrovascular disease (I69. with final characters -92)

R29.818 Other symptoms and signs involving the nervous system

R29.89 Other symptoms and signs involving the musculoskeletal system
EXCLUDES 2   pain in limb (M79.6-)

R29.890 Loss of height
EXCLUDES 1   osteoporosis (M80-M81)

R29.891 Ocular torticollis
EXCLUDES 1   congenital (sternomastoid) torticollis Q68.0
          psychogenic torticollis (F45.8)
          spasmodic torticollis (G24.3)
          torticollis due to birth injury (P15.8)
          torticollis NOS M43.6

R29.898 Other symptoms and signs involving the musculoskeletal system

R29.9 Unspecified symptoms and signs involving the nervous and musculoskeletal systems

R29.90 Unspecified symptoms and signs involving the nervous system

R29.91 Unspecified symptoms and signs involving the musculoskeletal system

Symptoms and signs involving the genitourinary system (R30-R39)

R30 Pain associated with micturition
EXCLUDES 1   psychogenic pain associated with micturition (F45.8)

R30.0 Dysuria
Strangury

R30.1 Vesical tenesmus

R30.9 Painful micturition, unspecified
Painful urination NOS

R31 Hematuria
EXCLUDES 1   hematuria included with underlying conditions, such as:
          acute cystitis with hematuria (N30.01)
          recurrent and persistent hematuria in glomerular diseases (N02.-)

R31.0 Gross hematuria

R31.1 Benign essential microscopic hematuria

R31.2 Other microscopic hematuria

R31.9 Hematuria, unspecified

R32 Unspecified urinary incontinence
Enuresis NOS
EXCLUDES 1   functional urinary incontinence (R39.81)
          nonorganic enuresis (F98.0)
          stress incontinence and other specified urinary incontinence (N39.3-N39.4-)
          urinary incontinence associated with cognitive impairment (R39.81)

R33 Retention of urine
EXCLUDES 1   psychogenic retention of urine (F45.8)

R33.0 Drug induced retention of urine
Use additional code for adverse effect, if applicable, to identify drug (T36-T50 with fifth or sixth character 5)

R33.8 Other retention of urine
Code first, if applicable, any causal condition, such as:
enlarged prostate (N40.1)

R33.9 Retention of urine, unspecified

R34 Anuria and oliguria
EXCLUDES 1   anuria and oliguria complicating abortion or ectopic or molar pregnancy (O00-O07, O08.4)
          anuria and oliguria complicating pregnancy (O26.83-)
          anuria and oliguria complicating the puerperium (O90.4)

R35 Polyuria
Code first, if applicable, any causal condition, such as:
enlarged prostate (N40.1)
EXCLUDES 1   psychogenic polyuria (F45.8)

R35.0 Frequency of micturition

R35.1 Nocturia

R35.8 Other polyuria
Polyuria NOS

R36 Urethral discharge

R36.0 Urethral discharge without blood

R36.1 Hematospermia

R36.9 Urethral discharge, unspecified
Penile discharge NOS
Urethrorrhea

R37 Sexual dysfunction, unspecified

R39 Other and unspecified symptoms and signs involving the genitourinary system

R39.0 Extravasation of urine

R39.1 Other difficulties with micturition
Code first, if applicable, any causal condition, such as:
enlarged prostate (N40.1)

R39.11 Hesitancy of micturition

R39.12 Poor urinary stream
Weak urinary steam

R39.13 Splitting of urinary stream

R39.14 Feeling of incomplete bladder emptying

R39.15 Urgency of urination
EXCLUDES 1   urge incontinence (N39.41, N39.46)

R39.16 Straining to void

R39.19 Other difficulties with micturition

R39.2 Extrarenal uremia
Prerenal uremia
EXCLUDES 1   uremia NOS (N19)

R39.8 Other symptoms and signs involving the genitourinary system

R39.81 Functional urinary incontinence
Urinary incontinence due to cognitive impairment, or severe physical disability or immobility
EXCLUDES 1   stress incontinence and other specified urinary incontinence (N39.3-N39.4-)
          urinary incontinence NOS (R32)

R39.89 Other symptoms and signs involving the genitourinary system

R39.9 Unspecified symptoms and signs involving the genitourinary system

Symptoms and signs involving cognition, perception, emotional state and behavior (R40-R46)

EXCLUDES 1   symptoms and signs constituting part of a pattern of mental disorder (F01-F99)

R40 Somnolence, stupor and coma
EXCLUDES 1   neonatal coma (P91.5)
          somnolence, stupor and coma in diabetes (E08-E13)
          somnolence, stupor and coma in hepatic failure (K72.-)
          somnolence, stupor and coma in hypoglycemia (nondiabetic) (E15)

R40.0 Somnolence
Drowsiness
EXCLUDES 1   coma (R40.2-)

R40.1 Stupor
Catatonic stupor
Semicoma
EXCLUDES 1   catatonic schizophrenia (F20.2)
          coma (R40.2-)
          depressive stupor (F31-F33)
          dissociative stupor (F44.2)
          manic stupor (F30.2)

Additional Character Required   Xtension Alert   Unspecified Code   Other Specified Code   Manifestation Code   ►◄ Revised Text   ● New Code   ▲ Revised Code Title

✓5ᵗʰ R40.2 Coma
  Code first any associated:
    fracture of skull (S02.-)
    intracranial injury (S06.-)
  NOTE One code from subcategories R40.21-R40.23 is required to complete the coma scale

  R40.20 Unspecified coma
    Coma NOS
    Unconsciousness NOS

  ✓6ᵗʰ R40.21 Coma scale, eyes open

    The following appropriate 7th character is to be added to subcategory R40.21-.
    0   unspecified time
    1   in the field [EMT or ambulance]
    2   at arrival to emergency department
    3   at hospital admission
    4   24 hours or more after hospital admission

    ✓7ᵗʰ R40.211 Coma scale, eyes open, never
    ✓7ᵗʰ R40.212 Coma scale, eyes open, to pain
    ✓7ᵗʰ R40.213 Coma scale, eyes open, to sound
    ✓7ᵗʰ R40.214 Coma scale, eyes open, spontaneous

  ✓6ᵗʰ R40.22 Coma scale, best verbal response

    The following appropriate 7th character is to be added to subcategory R40.22-.
    0   unspecified time
    1   in the field [EMT or ambulance]
    2   at arrival to emergency department
    3   at hospital admission
    4   24 hours or more after hospital admission

    ✓7ᵗʰ R40.221 Coma scale, best verbal response, none
    ✓7ᵗʰ R40.222 Coma scale, best verbal response, incomprehensible words
    ✓7ᵗʰ R40.223 Coma scale, best verbal response, inappropriate words
    ✓7ᵗʰ R40.224 Coma scale, best verbal response, confused conversation
    ✓7ᵗʰ R40.225 Coma scale, best verbal response, oriented

  ✓6ᵗʰ R40.23 Coma scale, best motor response

    The following appropriate 7th character is to be added to subcategory R40.23-.
    0   unspecified time
    1   in the field [EMT or ambulance]
    2   at arrival to emergency department
    3   at hospital admission
    4   24 hours or more after hospital admission

    ✓7ᵗʰ R40.231 Coma scale, best motor response, none
    ✓7ᵗʰ R40.232 Coma scale, best motor response, extension
    ✓7ᵗʰ R40.233 Coma scale, best motor response, abnormal
    ✓7ᵗʰ R40.234 Coma scale, best motor response, flexion withdrawal
    ✓7ᵗʰ R40.235 Coma scale, best motor response, localizes pain
    ✓7ᵗʰ R40.236 Coma scale, best motor response, obeys commands

  ✓6ᵗʰ R40.24 Glasgow coma scale, total score
    Use codes R40.21- through R40.23- only when the individual score(s) are documented
    R40.241 Glasgow coma scale score 13-15
    R40.242 Glasgow coma scale score 9-12
    R40.243 Glasgow coma scale score 3-8
    R40.244 Other coma, without documented Glasgow coma scale score, or with partial score reported

  R40.3 Persistent vegetative state
  R40.4 Transient alteration of awareness

✓4ᵗʰ R41 Other symptoms and signs involving cognitive functions and awareness
  EXCLUDES 1 *dissociative [conversion] disorders (F44.-)*
    mild cognitive impairment, so stated (G31.84)

  R41.0 Disorientation, unspecified
    Confusion NOS
    Delirium NOS

  R41.1 Anterograde amnesia
  R41.2 Retrograde amnesia
  R41.3 Other amnesia
    Amnesia NOS
    Memory loss NOS
    EXCLUDES 1 *amnestic disorder due to known physiologic condition (F04)*
      amnestic syndrome due to psychoactive substance use (F10-F19 with 5th character .6)
      mild memory disturbance due to known physiological condition (F06.8)
      transient global amnesia (G45.4)

  R41.4 Neurologic neglect syndrome
    Asomatognosia
    Hemi-akinesia
    Hemi-inattention
    Hemispatial neglect
    Left-sided neglect
    Sensory neglect
    Visuospatial neglect
    EXCLUDES 1 *visuospatial deficit (R41.842)*

  ✓5ᵗʰ R41.8 Other symptoms and signs involving cognitive functions and awareness
    R41.81 Age-related cognitive decline　　🅰
      Senility NOS
    R41.82 Altered mental status, unspecified
      Change in mental status NOS
      EXCLUDES 1 *altered level of consciousness (R40.-)*
        altered mental status due to known condition—code to condition
        delirium NOS (R41.0)
      AHA: 2012, Q4, 97
    R41.83 Borderline intellectual functioning
      IQ level 71 to 84
      EXCLUDES 1 *intellectual disabilities (F70-F79)*
    ✓6ᵗʰ R41.84 Other specified cognitive deficit
      R41.840 Attention and concentration deficit
        EXCLUDES 1 *attention-deficit hyperactivity disorders (F90.-)*
      R41.841 Cognitive communication deficit
      R41.842 Visuospatial deficit
      R41.843 Psychomotor deficit
      R41.844 Frontal lobe and executive function deficit
    R41.89 Other symptoms and signs involving cognitive functions and awareness
      Anosognosia

  R41.9 Unspecified symptoms and signs involving cognitive functions and awareness

R42 Dizziness and giddiness
  Light-headedness
  Vertigo NOS
  EXCLUDES 1 *vertiginous syndromes (H81.-)*
    vertigo from infrasound (T75.23)

✓4ᵗʰ R43 Disturbances of smell and taste
  R43.0 Anosmia
  R43.1 Parosmia
  R43.2 Parageusia
  R43.8 Other disturbances of smell and taste
    Mixed disturbance of smell and taste
  R43.9 Unspecified disturbances of smell and taste

✓4ᵗʰ R44 Other symptoms and signs involving general sensations and perceptions
  EXCLUDES 1 *alcoholic hallucinations (F1.5)*
    hallucinations in drug psychosis (F11-F19 with .5)
    hallucinations in mood disorders with psychotic symptoms (F30.2, F31.5, F32.3, F33.3)
    hallucinations in schizophrenia, schizotypal and delusional disorders (F20-F29)
  EXCLUDES 2 *disturbances of skin sensation (R20.-)*
  R44.0 Auditory hallucinations
  R44.1 Visual hallucinations

EXCLUDES 1 Not coded here　　　*EXCLUDES 2* Not included here　　　Ⓝ Newborn Age: 0　　　Ⓟ Pediatric Age: 0-17　　　Ⓜ Maternity Age: 12-55　　　🅰 Adult Age: 15-124

R44.2   **Other hallucinations**

R44.3   **Hallucinations, unspecified**

R44.8   **Other symptoms and signs involving general sensations and perceptions**

R44.9   **Unspecified symptoms and signs involving general sensations and perceptions**

✓4ᵗʰ **R45   Symptoms and signs involving emotional state**

R45.0   **Nervousness**
Nervous tension

R45.1   **Restlessness and agitation**

R45.2   **Unhappiness**

R45.3   **Demoralization and apathy**
EXCLUDES 1   *anhedonia (R45.84)*

R45.4   **Irritability and anger**

R45.5   **Hostility**

R45.6   **Violent behavior**

R45.7   **State of emotional shock and stress, unspecified**

✓5ᵗʰ R45.8   **Other symptoms and signs involving emotional state**

R45.81   **Low self-esteem**

R45.82   **Worries**

R45.83   **Excessive crying of child, adolescent or adult**
EXCLUDES 1   *excessive crying of infant (baby) R68.11*

R45.84   **Anhedonia**

✓6ᵗʰ R45.85   **Homicidal and suicidal ideations**
EXCLUDES 1   *suicide attempt (T14.91)*

R45.850   **Homicidal ideations**

R45.851   **Suicidal ideations**

R45.86   **Emotional lability**

R45.87   **Impulsiveness**

R45.89   **Other symptoms and signs involving emotional state**

✓4ᵗʰ **R46   Symptoms and signs involving appearance and behavior**
EXCLUDES 1   *appearance and behavior in schizophrenia, schizotypal and delusional disorders (F20-F29)*
mental and behavioral disorders (F01-F99)

R46.0   **Very low level of personal hygiene**

R46.1   **Bizarre personal appearance**

R46.2   **Strange and inexplicable behavior**

R46.3   **Overactivity**

R46.4   **Slowness and poor responsiveness**
EXCLUDES 1   *stupor (R40.1)*

R46.5   **Suspiciousness and marked evasiveness**

R46.6   **Undue concern and preoccupation with stressful events**

R46.7   **Verbosity and circumstantial detail obscuring reason for contact**

✓5ᵗʰ R46.8   **Other symptoms and signs involving appearance and behavior**

R46.81   **Obsessive-compulsive behavior**
EXCLUDES 1   *obsessive-compulsive disorder (F42)*

R46.89   **Other symptoms and signs involving appearance and behavior**

Symptoms and signs involving speech and voice (R47-R49)

✓4ᵗʰ **R47   Speech disturbances, not elsewhere classified**
EXCLUDES 1   *autism (F84.0)*
cluttering (F80.81)
specific developmental disorders of speech and language (F80.-)
stuttering (F80.81)

✓5ᵗʰ R47.0   **Dysphasia and aphasia**

R47.01   **Aphasia**
EXCLUDES 1   *aphasia following cerebrovascular disease (I69. with final characters -20)*
progressive isolated aphasia (G31.01)

R47.02   **Dysphasia**
EXCLUDES 1   *dysphasia following cerebrovascular disease (I69. with final characters -21)*

R47.1   **Dysarthria and anarthria**
EXCLUDES 1   *dysarthria following cerebrovascular disease (I69. with final characters -22)*

✓5ᵗʰ R47.8   **Other speech disturbances**
EXCLUDES 1   *dysarthria following cerebrovascular disease (I69. with final characters -28)*

R47.81   **Slurred speech**

R47.82   ***Fluency disorder in conditions classified elsewhere***
Stuttering in conditions classified elsewhere
Code first underlying disease or condition, such as:
Parkinson's disease (G20)
EXCLUDES 1   *adult onset fluency disorder (F98.5)*
childhood onset fluency disorder (F80.81)
fluency disorder (stuttering) following cerebrovascular disease (I69. with final characters-23)

R47.89   **Other speech disturbances**

R47.9   **Unspecified speech disturbances**

✓4ᵗʰ **R48   Dyslexia and other symbolic dysfunctions, not elsewhere classified**
EXCLUDES 1   *specific developmental disorders of scholastic skills (F81.-)*

R48.0   **Dyslexia and alexia**

R48.1   **Agnosia**
Astereognosia (astereognosis)
Autotopagnosia
EXCLUDES 1   *visual object agnosia (R48.3)*

R48.2   **Apraxia**
EXCLUDES 1   *apraxia following cerebrovascular disease (I69. with final characters -90)*

R48.3   **Visual agnosia**
Prosopagnosia
Simultanagnosia (asimultagnosia)

R48.8   **Other symbolic dysfunctions**
Acalculia
Agraphia

R48.9   **Unspecified symbolic dysfunctions**

✓4ᵗʰ **R49   Voice and resonance disorders**
EXCLUDES 1   *psychogenic voice and resonance disorders (F44.4)*

R49.0   **Dysphonia**
Hoarseness

R49.1   **Aphonia**
Loss of voice

✓5ᵗʰ R49.2   **Hypernasality and hyponasality**

R49.21   **Hypernasality**

R49.22   **Hyponasality**

R49.8   **Other voice and resonance disorders**

R49.9   **Unspecified voice and resonance disorder**
Change in voice NOS
Resonance disorder NOS

General symptoms and signs (R50-R69)

✓4ᵗʰ **R50   Fever of other and unknown origin**
EXCLUDES 1   *chills without fever (R68.83)*
febrile convulsions (R56.0-)
fever of unknown origin during labor (O75.2)
fever of unknown origin in newborn (P81.9)
hypothermia due to illness (R68.0)
malignant hyperthermia due to anesthesia (T88.3)
puerperal pyrexia NOS (O86.4)

R50.2   **Drug induced fever**
Use additional code for adverse effect, if applicable, to identify drug (T36-T50 with fifth or sixth character 5)
EXCLUDES 1   *postvaccination (postimmunization) fever (R50.83)*

✓5ᵗʰ R50.8   **Other specified fever**

R50.81   ***Fever presenting with conditions classified elsewhere***
Code first underlying condition when associated fever is present, such as with:
leukemia (C91-C95)
neutropenia (D70.-)
sickle-cell disease (D57.-)

R50.82   **Postprocedural fever**
EXCLUDES 1   *postprocedural infection (T81.4)*
posttransfusion fever (R50.84)
postvaccination (postimmunization) fever (R50.83)

R50.83   **Postvaccination fever**
Postimmunization fever

R50.84   **Febrile nonhemolytic transfusion reaction**
FNHTR
Posttransfusion fever

☑ Additional Character Required   ✓7ᵗʰ Xtension Alert   Unspecified Code   Other Specified Code   Manifestation Code   ▶◀ Revised Text   ● New Code   ▲ Revised Code Title

R50.9 Fever, unspecified
Fever NOS
Fever of unknown origin [FUO]
Fever with chills
Fever with rigors
Hyperpyrexia NOS
Persistent fever
Pyrexia NOS

R51 Headache
Facial pain NOS
EXCLUDES 1   atypical face pain (G50.1)
migraine and other headache syndromes (G43-G44)
trigeminal neuralgia (G50.0)

R52 Pain, unspecified
Acute pain NOS
Generalized pain NOS
Pain NOS
EXCLUDES 1   acute and chronic pain, not elsewhere classified (G89.-)
localized pain, unspecified type—code to pain by site, such as:
abdomen pain (R10.-)
back pain (M54.9)
breast pain (N64.4)
chest pain (R07.1-R07.9)
ear pain (H92.0-)
eye pain (H57.1)
headache (R51)
joint pain (M25.5-)
limb pain (M79.6-)
lumbar region pain (M54.5)
pelvic and perineal pain (R10.2)
shoulder pain (M25.51-)
spine pain (M54.-)
throat pain (R07.0)
tongue pain (K14.6)
tooth pain (K08.8)
renal colic (N23)
pain disorders exclusively related to psychological factors (F45.41)

√4th R53 Malaise and fatigue

R53.0 Neoplastic (malignant) related fatigue
Code first associated neoplasm

R53.1 Weakness
Asthenia NOS
EXCLUDES 1   age-related weakness (R54)
muscle weakness (M62.8-)
senile asthenia (R54)

R53.2 Functional quadriplegia
Complete immobility due to severe physical disability or frailty
EXCLUDES 1   frailty NOS (R54)
hysterical paralysis (F44.4)
immobility syndrome (M62.3)
neurologic quadriplegia (G82.5-)
quadriplegia (G82.50)

√5th R53.8 Other malaise and fatigue
EXCLUDES 1   combat exhaustion and fatigue (F43.0)
congenital debility (P96.9)
exhaustion and fatigue due to depressive episode (F32.-)
exhaustion and fatigue due to excessive exertion (T73.3)
exhaustion and fatigue due to exposure (T73.2)
exhaustion and fatigue due to heat (T67.-)
exhaustion and fatigue due to pregnancy (O26.8-)
exhaustion and fatigue due to recurrent depressive episode (F33)
exhaustion and fatigue due to senile debility (R54)

R53.81 Other malaise
Chronic debility
Debility NOS
General physical deterioration
Malaise NOS
Nervous debility
EXCLUDES 1   age-related physical debility (R54)

R53.82 Chronic fatigue, unspecified
Chronic fatigue syndrome NOS
EXCLUDES 1   postviral fatigue syndrome (G93.3)

R53.83 Other fatigue
Fatigue NOS
Lack of energy
Lethargy
Tiredness

R54 Age-related physical debility   Ⓐ
Frailty
Old age
Senescence
Senile asthenia
Senile debility
EXCLUDES 1   age-related cognitive decline (R41.81)
senile psychosis (F03)
senility NOS (R41.81)

R55 Syncope and collapse
Blackout
Fainting
Vasovagal attack
EXCLUDES 1   cardiogenic shock (R57.0)
carotid sinus syncope (G90.01)
heat syncope (T67.1)
neurocirculatory asthenia (F45.8)
neurogenic orthostatic hypotension (G90.3)
orthostatic hypotension (I95.1)
postprocedural shock (T81.1-)
psychogenic syncope (F48.8)
shock NOS (R57.9)
shock complicating or following abortion or ectopic or molar pregnancy (O00-O07, O08.3)
shock complicating or following labor and delivery (O75.1)
Stokes-Adams attack (I45.9)
unconsciousness NOS (R40.2-)

√4th R56 Convulsions, not elsewhere classified
EXCLUDES 1   dissociative convulsions and seizures (F44.5)
epileptic convulsions and seizures (G40.-)
newborn convulsions and seizures (P90)

√5th R56.0 Febrile convulsions

R56.00 Simple febrile convulsions
Febrile convulsion NOS
Febrile seizure NOS

R56.01 Complex febrile convulsions
Atypical febrile seizure
Complex febrile seizure
Complicated febrile seizure
EXCLUDES 1   status epilepticus (G40.901)

R56.1 Post traumatic seizures
EXCLUDES 1   post traumatic epilepsy (G40.-)

R56.9 Unspecified convulsions
Convulsion disorder
Fit NOS
Recurrent convulsions
Seizure(s) (convulsive) NOS

√4th R57 Shock, not elsewhere classified
EXCLUDES 1   anaphylactic shock NOS (T78.2)
anaphylactic reaction or shock due to adverse food reaction (T78.0-)
anaphylactic shock due to adverse effect of correct drug or medicament properly administered (T88.6)
anaphylactic shock due to serum (T80.5-)
anesthetic shock (T88.3)
electric shock (T75.4)
obstetric shock (O75.1)
postprocedural shock (T81.1-)
psychic shock (F43.0)
septic shock (R65.21)
shock complicating or following ectopic or molar pregnancy (O00-O07, O08.3)
shock due to lightning (T75.01)
traumatic shock (T79.4)
toxic shock syndrome (A48.3)

R57.0 Cardiogenic shock

R57.1 Hypovolemic shock

R57.8 Other shock

R57.9 Shock, unspecified
Failure of peripheral circulation NOS

R58 Hemorrhage, not elsewhere classified
Hemorrhage NOS
EXCLUDES 1   hemorrhage included with underlying conditions, such as:
acute duodenal ulcer with hemorrhage (K26.0)
acute gastritis with bleeding (K29.01)
ulcerative enterocolitis with rectal bleeding (K51.01)

EXCLUDES 1 Not coded here   *EXCLUDES 2* Not included here   Ⓝ Newborn Age: 0   Ⓟ Pediatric Age: 0-17   Ⓜ Maternity Age: 12-55   Ⓐ Adult Age: 15-124

796   ICD-10-CM 2014 (Draft)

☑4ᵗʰ **R59 Enlarged lymph nodes**

     INCLUDES   swollen glands

     EXCLUDES 1   *acute lymphadenitis (L04.-)*
                chronic lymphadenitis (I88.1)
                lymphadenitis NOS (I88.9)
                mesenteric (acute) (chronic) lymphadenitis (I88.0)

     R59.0 Localized enlarged lymph nodes

     R59.1 Generalized enlarged lymph nodes
            Lymphadenopathy NOS

     R59.9 Enlarged lymph nodes, unspecified

☑4ᵗʰ **R60 Edema, not elsewhere classified**

     EXCLUDES 1   *angioneurotic edema (T78.3)*
                ascites (R18.-)
                cerebral edema (G93.6)
                cerebral edema due to birth injury (P11.0)
                edema of larynx (J38.4)
                edema of nasopharynx (J39.2)
                edema of pharynx (J39.2)
                gestational edema (O12.0-)
                hereditary edema (Q82.0)
                hydrops fetalis NOS (P83.2)
                hydrothorax (J94.8)
                nutritional edema (E40-E46)
                hydrops fetalis NOS (P83.2)
                newborn edema (P83.3)
                pulmonary edema (J81.-)

     R60.0 Localized edema

     R60.1 Generalized edema

     R60.9 Edema, unspecified
            Fluid retention NOS

R61 Generalized hyperhidrosis

     Excessive sweating
     Night sweats
     Secondary hyperhidrosis
     Code first, if applicable, menopausal and female climacteric states
            (N95.1)

     EXCLUDES 1   *focal (primary) (secondary) hyperhidrosis (L74.5-)*
                Frey's syndrome (L74.52)
                localized (primary) (secondary) hyperhidrosis (L74.5-)

☑4ᵗʰ **R62 Lack of expected normal physiological development in childhood and adults**

     EXCLUDES 1   *delayed puberty (E30.0)*
                gonadal dysgenesis (Q99.1)
                hypopituitarism (E23.0)

     R62.0 Delayed milestone in childhood   P
            Delayed attainment of expected physiological developmental
                stage
            Late talker
            Late walker

     ☑5ᵗʰ **R62.5 Other and unspecified lack of expected normal physiological development in childhood**

            EXCLUDES 1   *HIV disease resulting in failure to thrive (B20)*
                        physical retardation due to malnutrition (E45)

            R62.50 Unspecified lack of expected normal physiological development in childhood   P
                   Infantilism NOS

            R62.51 Failure to thrive (child)   P
                   Failure to gain weight
                   EXCLUDES 1   *failure to thrive in child under 28 days old*
                              (P92.6)

            R62.52 Short stature (child)   P
                   Lack of growth
                   Physical retardation
                   Short stature NOS
                   EXCLUDES 1   *short stature due to endocrine disorder*
                              (E34.3)

            R62.59 Other lack of expected normal physiological development in childhood   P

     R62.7 Adult failure to thrive   A

☑4ᵗʰ **R63 Symptoms and signs concerning food and fluid intake**

     EXCLUDES 1   *bulimia NOS (F50.2)*
                eating disorders of nonorganic origin (F50.-)
                 malnutrition (E40-E46)

     R63.0 Anorexia
            Loss of appetite
            EXCLUDES 1   *anorexia nervosa (F50.0-)*
                        loss of appetite of nonorganic origin (F50.8)

     R63.1 Polydipsia
            Excessive thirst

     R63.2 Polyphagia
            Excessive eating
            Hyperalimentation NOS

     R63.3 Feeding difficulties
            Feeding problem (elderly) (infant) NOS
            EXCLUDES 1   *feeding problems of newborn (P92.-)*
                        infant feeding disorder of nonorganic origin (F98.2-)

     R63.4 Abnormal weight loss

     R63.5 Abnormal weight gain
            EXCLUDES 1   *excessive weight gain in pregnancy (O26.0-)*
                        obesity (E66.-)

     R63.6 Underweight
            Use additional code to identify body mass index (BMI), if known
                (Z68.-)
            EXCLUDES 1   *abnormal weight loss (R63.4)*
                        anorexia nervosa (F50.0-)
                        malnutrition (E40-E46)

     R63.8 Other symptoms and signs concerning food and fluid intake

R64 Cachexia

     Wasting syndrome
     Code first underlying condition, if known
     EXCLUDES 1   *abnormal weight loss (R63.4)*
                nutritional marasmus (E41)

☑4ᵗʰ **R65 Symptoms and signs specifically associated with systemic inflammation and infection**

     ☑5ᵗʰ **R65.1 Systemic inflammatory response syndrome [SIRS] of non-infectious origin**
            Code first underlying condition, such as:
                heatstroke (T67.0)
                injury and trauma (S00-T88)
            EXCLUDES 1   *sepsis—code to infection*
                        severe sepsis (R65.2)

            R65.10 Systemic inflammatory response syndrome [SIRS] of non-infectious origin without acute organ dysfunction
                   Systemic inflammatory response syndrome (SIRS) NOS

            R65.11 Systemic inflammatory response syndrome [SIRS] of non-infectious origin with acute organ dysfunction
                   Use additional code to identify specific acute organ
                      dysfunction, such as:
                   acute kidney failure (N17.-)
                   acute respiratory failure (J96.0-)
                   critical illness myopathy (G72.81)
                   critical illness polyneuropathy (G62.81)
                   disseminated intravascular coagulopathy [DIC]
                      (D65)
                   encephalopathy (metabolic) (septic) (G93.41)
                   hepatic failure (K72.0-)

     ☑5ᵗʰ **R65.2 Severe sepsis**
            Infection with associated acute organ dysfunction
            Sepsis with acute organ dysfunction
            Sepsis with multiple organ dysfunction
            Systemic inflammatory response syndrome due to infectious
                process with acute organ dysfunction
            Code first underlying infection, such as:
                infection following a procedure (T81.4)
                infections following infusion, transfusion and therapeutic
                   injection (T80.2-)
                puerperal sepsis (O85)
                sepsis following complete or unspecified spontaneous
                   abortion (O03.87)
                sepsis following ectopic and molar pregnancy (O08.82)
                sepsis following incomplete spontaneous abortion (O03.37)
                sepsis following (induced) termination of pregnancy (O04.87)
                sepsis NOS (A41.9)
            Use additional code to identify specific acute organ dysfunction,
                such as:
                acute kidney failure (N17.-)
                acute respiratory failure (J96.0-)
                critical illness myopathy (G72.81)
                critical illness polyneuropathy (G62.81)
                disseminated intravascular coagulopathy [DIC] (D65)
                encephalopathy (metabolic) (septic) (G93.41)
                hepatic failure (K72.0-)

            R65.20 Severe sepsis without septic shock
                   Severe sepsis NOS

            R65.21 Severe sepsis with septic shock

☑ Additional Character Required   ✕x7ᵗʰ Xtension Alert   **Unspecified Code**   **Other Specified Code**   **Manifestation Code**   ►◄ Revised Text   ● New Code   ▲ Revised Code Title

ICD-10-CM 2014 (Draft)   **797**

Symptoms, Signs and Abnormal Clinical and Laboratory Findings

R68 Other general symptoms and signs

R68.0 Hypothermia, not associated with low environmental temperature
EXCLUDES1 hypothermia NOS (accidental) (T68)
hypothermia due to anesthesia (T88.51)
hypothermia due to low environmental temperature (T68)
newborn hypothermia (P80.-)

R68.1 Nonspecific symptoms peculiar to infancy
EXCLUDES1 colic, infantile (R10.83)
neonatal cerebral irritability (P91.3)
teething syndrome (K00.7)

R68.11 Excessive crying of infant (baby) P
EXCLUDES1 excessive crying of child, adolescent, or adult (R45.83)

R68.12 Fussy infant (baby) P
Irritable infant

R68.13 Apparent life threatening event in infant [ALTE] P
Apparent life threatening event in newborn
Code first confirmed diagnosis, if known
Use additional code(s) for associated signs and symptoms if no confirmed diagnosis established, or if signs and symptoms are not associated routinely with confirmed diagnosis, or provide additional information for cause of ALTE

R68.19 Other nonspecific symptoms peculiar to infancy P

R68.2 Dry mouth, unspecified
EXCLUDES1 dry mouth due to dehydration (E86.0)
dry mouth due to sicca syndrome [Sjögren] (M35.0-)
salivary gland hyposecretion (K11.7)

R68.3 Clubbing of fingers
Clubbing of nails
EXCLUDES1 congenital clubfinger (Q68.1)

R68.8 Other general symptoms and signs

R68.81 Early satiety

R68.82 Decreased libido A
Decreased sexual desire

R68.83 Chills (without fever)
Chills NOS
EXCLUDES1 chills with fever (R50.9)

R68.84 Jaw pain
Mandibular pain
Maxilla pain
EXCLUDES1 temporomandibular joint arthralgia (M26.62)

R68.89 Other general symptoms and signs

R69 Illness, unspecified
Unknown and unspecified cases of morbidity

Abnormal findings on examination of blood, without diagnosis (R70-R79)

EXCLUDES1 abnormalities (of)(on):
abnormal findings on antenatal screening of mother (O28.-)
coagulation hemorrhagic disorders (D65-D68)
lipids (E78.-)
platelets and thrombocytes (D69.-)
white blood cells classified elsewhere (D70-D72)
diagnostic abnormal findings classified elsewhere—see Alphabetical Index
hemorrhagic and hematological disorders of newborn (P50-P61)

R70 Elevated erythrocyte sedimentation rate and abnormality of plasma viscosity

R70.0 Elevated erythrocyte sedimentation rate

R70.1 Abnormal plasma viscosity

R71 Abnormality of red blood cells
EXCLUDES1 anemias (D50-D64)
anemia of premature infant (P61.2)
benign (familial) polycythemia (D75.0)
congenital anemias (P61.2-P61.4)
newborn anemia due to isoimmunization (P55.-)
polycythemia neonatorum (P61.1)
polycythemia NOS (D75.1)
polycythemia vera (D45)
secondary polycythemia (D75.1)

R71.0 Precipitous drop in hematocrit
Drop (precipitous) in hemoglobin
Drop in hematocrit

R71.8 Other abnormality of red blood cells
Abnormal red-cell morphology NOS
Abnormal red-cell volume NOS
Anisocytosis
Poikilocytosis

R73 Elevated blood glucose level
EXCLUDES1 diabetes mellitus (E08-E13)
diabetes mellitus in pregnancy, childbirth and the puerperium (O24.-)
neonatal disorders (P70.0-P70.2)
postsurgical hypoinsulinemia (E89.1)

R73.0 Abnormal glucose
EXCLUDES1 abnormal glucose in pregnancy (O99.81-)
diabetes mellitus (E08-E13)
dysmetabolic syndrome X (E88.81)
gestational diabetes (O24.4-)
glycosuria (R81)
hypoglycemia (E16.2)

R73.01 Impaired fasting glucose
Elevated fasting glucose

R73.02 Impaired glucose tolerance (oral)
Elevated glucose tolerance

R73.09 Other abnormal glucose
Abnormal glucose NOS
Abnormal non-fasting glucose tolerance
Latent diabetes
Prediabetes

R73.9 Hyperglycemia, unspecified

R74 Abnormal serum enzyme levels

R74.0 Nonspecific elevation of levels of transaminase and lactic acid dehydrogenase [LDH]

R74.8 Abnormal levels of other serum enzymes
Abnormal level of acid phosphatase
Abnormal level of alkaline phosphatase
Abnormal level of amylase
Abnormal level of lipase [triacylglycerol lipase]

R74.9 Abnormal serum enzyme level, unspecified

R75 Inconclusive laboratory evidence of human immunodeficiency virus [HIV]
Nonconclusive HIV-test finding in infants
EXCLUDES1 asymptomatic human immunodeficiency virus [HIV] infection status (Z21)
human immunodeficiency virus [HIV] disease (B20)

R76 Other abnormal immunological findings in serum

R76.0 Raised antibody titer
EXCLUDES1 isoimmunization in pregnancy (O36.0-O36.1)
isoimmunization affecting newborn (P55.-)

R76.1 Nonspecific reaction to test for tuberculosis

R76.11 Nonspecific reaction to tuberculin skin test without active tuberculosis
Abnormal result of Mantoux test
PPD positive
Tuberculin (skin test) positive
Tuberculin (skin test) reactor
EXCLUDES1 nonspecific reaction to cell mediated immunity measurement of gamma interferon antigen response without active tuberculosis (R76.12)

R76.12 Nonspecific reaction to cell mediated immunity measurement of gamma interferon antigen response without active tuberculosis
Nonspecific reaction to QuantiFERON-TB test (QFT) without active tuberculosis
EXCLUDES1 nonspecific reaction to tuberculin skin test without active tuberculosis (R76.11)
positive tuberculin skin test (R76.11)

R76.8 Other specified abnormal immunological findings in serum
Raised level of immunoglobulins NOS

R76.9 Abnormal immunological finding in serum, unspecified

R77 Other abnormalities of plasma proteins
EXCLUDES1 disorders of plasma-protein metabolism (E88.0)

R77.0 Abnormality of albumin

R77.1 Abnormality of globulin
Hyperglobulinemia NOS

R77.2 Abnormality of alphafetoprotein

R77.8 Other specified abnormalities of plasma proteins

R77.9 Abnormality of plasma protein, unspecified

☑4ᵗʰ **R78**   **Findings of drugs and other substances, not normally found in blood**

Use additional code to identify any retained foreign body, if applicable (Z18.-)

EXCLUDES 1   *mental or behavioral disorders due to psychoactive substance use (F10-F19)*

R78.0   **Finding of alcohol in blood**

Use additional external cause code (Y90.-), for detail regarding alcohol level

R78.1   **Finding of opiate drug in blood**

R78.2   **Finding of cocaine in blood**

R78.3   **Finding of hallucinogen in blood**

R78.4   **Finding of other drugs of addictive potential in blood**

R78.5   **Finding of other psychotropic drug in blood**

R78.6   **Finding of steroid agent in blood**

☑5ᵗʰ **R78.7**   **Finding of abnormal level of heavy metals in blood**

     R78.71   **Abnormal lead level in blood**

         EXCLUDES 1   *lead poisoning (T56.0-)*

     R78.79   **Finding of abnormal level of heavy metals in blood**

☑5ᵗʰ **R78.8**   **Finding of other specified substances, not normally found in blood**

     R78.81   **Bacteremia**

         EXCLUDES 1   *sepsis—code to specified infection (A00-B99)*

     R78.89   **Finding of other specified substances, not normally found in blood**

         Finding of abnormal level of lithium in blood

R78.9   **Finding of unspecified substance, not normally found in blood**

☑4ᵗʰ **R79**   **Other abnormal findings of blood chemistry**

Use additional code to identify any retained foreign body, if applicable (Z18.-)

EXCLUDES 1   *abnormality of fluid, electrolyte or acid-base balance (E86-E87)*
asymptomatic hyperuricemia (E79.0)
hyperglycemia NOS (R73.9)
hypoglycemia NOS (E16.2)
neonatal hypoglycemia (P70.3-P70.4)
specific findings indicating disorder of amino-acid metabolism (E70-E72)
specific findings indicating disorder of carbohydrate metabolism (E73-E74)
specific findings indicating disorder of lipid metabolism (E75.-)

R79.0   **Abnormal level of blood mineral**

Abnormal blood level of cobalt
Abnormal blood level of copper
Abnormal blood level of iron
Abnormal blood level of magnesium
Abnormal blood level of mineral NEC
Abnormal blood level of zinc

EXCLUDES 1   *abnormal level of lithium (R78.89)*
disorders of mineral metabolism (E83.-)
neonatal hypomagnesemia (P71.2)
nutritional mineral deficiency (E58-E61)

R79.1   **Abnormal coagulation profile**

Abnormal or prolonged bleeding time
Abnormal or prolonged coagulation time
Abnormal or prolonged partial thromboplastin time [PTT]
Abnormal or prolonged prothrombin time [PT]

EXCLUDES 1   *coagulation defects (D68.-)*

☑5ᵗʰ **R79.8**   **Other specified abnormal findings of blood chemistry**

     R79.81   **Abnormal blood-gas level**

     R79.82   **Elevated C-reactive protein [CRP]**

     R79.89   **Other specified abnormal findings of blood chemistry**

R79.9   **Abnormal finding of blood chemistry, unspecified**

Abnormal findings on examination of urine, without diagnosis (R80-R82)

EXCLUDES 1   *abnormal findings on antenatal screening of mother (O28.-)*
diagnostic abnormal findings classified elsewhere—see Alphabetical Index
specific findings indicating disorder of amino-acid metabolism (E70-E72)
specific findings indicating disorder of carbohydrate metabolism (E73-E74)

☑4ᵗʰ **R80**   **Proteinuria**

EXCLUDES 1   *gestational proteinuria (O12.1-)*

R80.0   **Isolated proteinuria**

Idiopathic proteinuria

EXCLUDES 1   *isolated proteinuria with specific morphological lesion (N06.-)*

R80.1   **Persistent proteinuria, unspecified**

R80.2   **Orthostatic proteinuria, unspecified**

Postural proteinuria

R80.3   **Bence Jones proteinuria**

R80.8   **Other proteinuria**

R80.9   **Proteinuria, unspecified**

Albuminuria NOS

R81   **Glycosuria**

EXCLUDES 1   *renal glycosuria (E74.8)*

☑4ᵗʰ **R82**   **Other and unspecified abnormal findings in urine**

Chromoabnormalities in urine

Use additional code to identify any retained foreign body, if applicable (Z18.-)

EXCLUDES 2   *hematuria (R31.-)*

R82.0   **Chyluria**

EXCLUDES 1   *filarial chyluria (B74.-)*

R82.1   **Myoglobinuria**

R82.2   **Biliuria**

R82.3   **Hemoglobinuria**

EXCLUDES 1   *hemoglobinuria due to hemolysis from external causes NEC (D59.6)*
hemoglobinuria due to paroxysmal nocturnal [Marchiafava-Micheli] (D59.5)

R82.4   **Acetonuria**

Ketonuria

R82.5   **Elevated urine levels of drugs, medicaments and biological substances**

Elevated urine levels of catecholamines
Elevated urine levels of indoleacetic acid
Elevated urine levels of 17-ketosteroids
Elevated urine levels of steroids

R82.6   **Abnormal urine levels of substances chiefly nonmedicinal as to source**

Abnormal urine level of heavy metals

R82.7   **Abnormal findings on microbiological examination of urine**

Positive culture findings of urine

EXCLUDES 1   *colonization status (Z22.-)*

R82.8   **Abnormal findings on cytological and histological examination of urine**

☑5ᵗʰ **R82.9**   **Other and unspecified abnormal findings in urine**

     R82.90   **Unspecified abnormal findings in urine**

     R82.91   **Other chromoabnormalities of urine**

         Chromoconversion (dipstick)
         Idiopathic dipstick converts positive for blood with no cellular forms in sediment

         EXCLUDES 1   *hemoglobinuria (R82.3)*
                   myoglobinuria (R82.1)

     R82.99   **Other abnormal findings in urine**

         Cells and casts in urine
         Crystalluria
         Melanuria

☑ Additional Character Required   ✗7ᵗʰ Xtension Alert   Unspecified Code   Other Specified Code   Manifestation Code   ▶◀ Revised Text   ● New Code   ▲ Revised Code Title

ICD-10-CM 2014 (Draft)   **799**

Symptoms, Signs and Abnormal Clinical and Laboratory Findings

R83–R86.1

Abnormal findings on examination of other body fluids, substances and tissues, without diagnosis (R83-R89)

> EXCLUDES 1   *abnormal findings on antenatal screening of mother (O28.-)*
> *diagnostic abnormal findings classified elsewhere—see Alphabetical Index*

> EXCLUDES 2   *abnormal findings on examination of blood, without diagnosis (R70-R79)*
> *abnormal findings on examination of urine, without diagnosis (R80-R82)*
> *abnormal tumor markers (R97.-)*

✓4ᵗʰ **R83**   **Abnormal findings in cerebrospinal fluid**

     R83.0   **Abnormal level of enzymes in cerebrospinal fluid**

     R83.1   **Abnormal level of hormones in cerebrospinal fluid**

     R83.2   **Abnormal level of other drugs, medicaments and biological substances in cerebrospinal fluid**

     R83.3   **Abnormal level of substances chiefly nonmedicinal as to source in cerebrospinal fluid**

     R83.4   **Abnormal immunological findings in cerebrospinal fluid**

     R83.5   **Abnormal microbiological findings in cerebrospinal fluid**
         Positive culture findings in cerebrospinal fluid
         EXCLUDES 1   *colonization status (Z22.-)*

     R83.6   **Abnormal cytological findings in cerebrospinal fluid**

     R83.8   **Other abnormal findings in cerebrospinal fluid**
         Abnormal chromosomal findings in cerebrospinal fluid

     R83.9   **Unspecified abnormal finding in cerebrospinal fluid**

✓4ᵗʰ **R84**   **Abnormal findings in specimens from respiratory organs and thorax**
         Abnormal findings in bronchial washings
         Abnormal findings in nasal secretions
         Abnormal findings in pleural fluid
         Abnormal findings in sputum
         Abnormal findings in throat scrapings
         EXCLUDES 1   *blood-stained sputum (R04.2)*

     R84.0   **Abnormal level of enzymes in specimens from respiratory organs and thorax**

     R84.1   **Abnormal level of hormones in specimens from respiratory organs and thorax**

     R84.2   **Abnormal level of other drugs, medicaments and biological substances in specimens from respiratory organs and thorax**

     R84.3   **Abnormal level of substances chiefly nonmedicinal as to source in specimens from respiratory organs and thorax**

     R84.4   **Abnormal immunological findings in specimens from respiratory organs and thorax**

     R84.5   **Abnormal microbiological findings in specimens from respiratory organs and thorax**
         Positive culture findings in specimens from respiratory organs and thorax
         EXCLUDES 1   *colonization status (Z22.-)*

     R84.6   **Abnormal cytological findings in specimens from respiratory organs and thorax**

     R84.7   **Abnormal histological findings in specimens from respiratory organs and thorax**

     R84.8   **Other abnormal findings in specimens from respiratory organs and thorax**
         Abnormal chromosomal findings in specimens from respiratory organs and thorax

     R84.9   **Unspecified abnormal finding in specimens from respiratory organs and thorax**

✓4ᵗʰ **R85**   **Abnormal findings in specimens from digestive organs and abdominal cavity**
         INCLUDES   abnormal findings in peritoneal fluid
            abnormal findings in saliva
         EXCLUDES 1   *cloudy peritoneal dialysis effluent (R88.0)*
                     fecal abnormalities (R19.5)

     R85.0   **Abnormal level of enzymes in specimens from digestive organs and abdominal cavity**

     R85.1   **Abnormal level of hormones in specimens from digestive organs and abdominal cavity**

     R85.2   **Abnormal level of other drugs, medicaments and biological substances in specimens from digestive organs and abdominal cavity**

     R85.3   **Abnormal level of substances chiefly nonmedicinal as to source in specimens from digestive organs and abdominal cavity**

     R85.4   **Abnormal immunological findings in specimens from digestive organs and abdominal cavity**

     R85.5   **Abnormal microbiological findings in specimens from digestive organs and abdominal cavity**
         Positive culture findings in specimens from digestive organs and abdominal cavity
         EXCLUDES 1   *colonization status (Z22.-)*

✓5ᵗʰ   **R85.6**   **Abnormal cytological findings in specimens from digestive organs and abdominal cavity**

     ✓6ᵗʰ   **R85.61**   **Abnormal cytologic smear of anus**
         EXCLUDES 1   *abnormal cytological findings in specimens from other digestive organs and abdominal cavity (R85.69)*
                    carcinoma in situ of anus (histologically confirmed) (D01.3)
                    anal intraepithelial neoplasia I [AIN I] (K62.82)
                    anal intraepithelial neoplasia II [AIN II] (K62.82)
                    anal intraepithelial neoplasia III [AIN III] (D01.3)
                    dysplasia (mild) (moderate) of anus (histologically confirmed) (K62.82)
                    severe dysplasia of anus (histologically confirmed) (D01.3)
         EXCLUDES 2   *anal high risk human papillomavirus (HPV) DNA test positive (R85.81)*
                    anal low risk human papillomavirus (HPV) DNA test positive (R85.82)

         R85.610   **Atypical squamous cells of undetermined significance on cytologic smear of anus [ASC-US]**

         R85.611   **Atypical squamous cells cannot exclude high grade squamous intraepithelial lesion on cytologic smear of anus [ASC-H]**

         R85.612   **Low grade squamous intraepithelial lesion on cytologic smear of anus [LGSIL]**

         R85.613   **High grade squamous intraepithelial lesion on cytologic smear of anus [HGSIL]**

         R85.614   **Cytologic evidence of malignancy on smear of anus**

         R85.615   **Unsatisfactory cytologic smear of anus**
            Inadequate sample of cytologic smear of anus

         R85.616   **Satisfactory anal smear but lacking transformation zone**

         R85.618   **Other abnormal cytological findings on specimens from anus**

         R85.619   **Unspecified abnormal cytological findings in specimens from anus**
            Abnormal anal cytology NOS
            Atypical glandular cells of anus NOS

     R85.69   **Abnormal cytological findings in specimens from other digestive organs and abdominal cavity**

     R85.7   **Abnormal histological findings in specimens from digestive organs and abdominal cavity**

✓5ᵗʰ   **R85.8**   **Other abnormal findings in specimens from digestive organs and abdominal cavity**

     R85.81   **Anal high risk human papillomavirus [HPV] DNA test positive**
         EXCLUDES 1   *anogenital warts due to human papillomavirus (HPV) (A63.0)*
                    condyloma acuminatum (A63.0)

     R85.82   **Anal low risk human papillomavirus [HPV] DNA test positive**
         Use additional code for associated human papillomavirus (B97.7)

     R85.89   **Other abnormal findings in specimens from digestive organs and abdominal cavity**
         Abnormal chromosomal findings in specimens from digestive organs and abdominal cavity

     R85.9   **Unspecified abnormal finding in specimens from digestive organs and abdominal cavity**

✓4ᵗʰ **R86**   **Abnormal findings in specimens from male genital organs**
         INCLUDES   abnormal findings in prostatic secretions
            abnormal findings in semen, seminal fluid
            abnormal spermatozoa
         EXCLUDES 1   *azoospermia (N46.0-)*
                    oligospermia (N46.1-)

     R86.0   **Abnormal level of enzymes in specimens from male genital organs** ♂

     R86.1   **Abnormal level of hormones in specimens from male genital organs** ♂

EXCLUDES 1 Not coded here   EXCLUDES 2 Not included here   N Newborn Age: 0   P Pediatric Age: 0-17   M Maternity Age: 12-55   A Adult Age: 15-124

800   ICD-10-CM 2014 (Draft)

R86.2 Abnormal level of other drugs, medicaments and biological substances in specimens from male genital organs ♂

R86.3 Abnormal level of substances chiefly nonmedicinal as to source in specimens from male genital organs ♂

R86.4 Abnormal immunological findings in specimens from male genital organs ♂

R86.5 Abnormal microbiological findings in specimens from male genital organs ♂
    Positive culture findings in specimens from male genital organs
    EXCLUDES 1   colonization status (Z22.-)

R86.6 Abnormal cytological findings in specimens from male genital organs ♂

R86.7 Abnormal histological findings in specimens from male genital organs ♂

R86.8 Other abnormal findings in specimens from male genital organs ♂
    Abnormal chromosomal findings in specimens from male genital organs

R86.9 Unspecified abnormal finding in specimens from male genital organs ♂

√4ᵗʰ **R87** Abnormal findings in specimens from female genital organs
    Abnormal findings in secretion and smears from cervix uteri
    Abnormal findings in secretion and smears from vagina
    Abnormal findings in secretion and smears from vulva

R87.0 Abnormal level of enzymes in specimens from female genital organs ♀

R87.1 Abnormal level of hormones in specimens from female genital organs ♀

R87.2 Abnormal level of other drugs, medicaments and biological substances in specimens from female genital organs ♀

R87.3 Abnormal level of substances chiefly nonmedicinal as to source in specimens from female genital organs ♀

R87.4 Abnormal immunological findings in specimens from female genital organs ♀

R87.5 Abnormal microbiological findings in specimens from female genital organs ♀
    Positive culture findings in specimens from female genital organs
    EXCLUDES 1   colonization status (Z22.-)

√5ᵗʰ **R87.6** Abnormal cytological findings in specimens from female genital organs

√6ᵗʰ **R87.61** Abnormal cytological findings in specimens from cervix uteri
    EXCLUDES 1   abnormal cytological findings in specimens from other female genital organs (R87.69)
        abnormal cytological findings in specimens from vagina (R87.62-)
        carcinoma in situ of cervix uteri (histologically confirmed) (D06.-)
        cervical intraepithelial neoplasia I [CIN I] (N87.0)
        cervical intraepithelial neoplasia II [CIN II] (N87.1)
        cervical intraepithelial neoplasia III [CIN III] (D06.-)
        dysplasia (mild) (moderate) of cervix uteri (histologically confirmed) (N87.-)
        severe dysplasia of cervix uteri (histologically confirmed) (D06.-)
    EXCLUDES 2   cervical high risk human papillomavirus (HPV) DNA test positive (R87.810)
        cervical low risk human papillomavirus (HPV) DNA test positive (R87.820)

R87.610 Atypical squamous cells of undetermined significance on cytologic smear of cervix [ASC-US] ♀

R87.611 Atypical squamous cells cannot exclude high grade squamous intraepithelial lesion on cytologic smear of cervix [ASC-H] ♀

R87.612 Low grade squamous intraepithelial lesion on cytologic smear of cervix [LGSIL] ♀

R87.613 High grade squamous intraepithelial lesion on cytologic smear of cervix [HGSIL] ♀

R87.614 Cytologic evidence of malignancy on smear of cervix ♀

R87.615 Unsatisfactory cytologic smear of cervix ♀
    Inadequate sample of cytologic smear of cervix

R87.616 Satisfactory cervical smear but lacking transformation zone ♀

R87.618 Other abnormal cytological findings on specimens from cervix uteri ♀

R87.619 Unspecified abnormal cytological findings in specimens from cervix uteri ♀
    Abnormal cervical cytology NOS
    Abnormal Papanicolaou smear of cervix NOS
    Abnormal thin preparation smear of cervix NOS
    Atypical endocervical cells of cervix NOS
    Atypical endometrial cells of cervix NOS
    Atypical glandular cells of cervix NOS

√6ᵗʰ **R87.62** Abnormal cytological findings in specimens from vagina
    Use additional code to identify acquired absence of uterus and cervix, if applicable (Z90.71-)
    EXCLUDES 1   abnormal cytological findings in specimens from cervix uteri (R87.61-)
        abnormal cytological findings in specimens from other female genital organs (R87.69)
        carcinoma in situ of vagina (histologically confirmed) (D07.2)
        dysplasia (mild) (moderate) of vagina (histologically confirmed) (N89.-)
        severe dysplasia of vagina (histologically confirmed) (D07.2)
        vaginal intraepithelial neoplasia I [VAIN I] (N89.0)
        vaginal intraepithelial neoplasia II [VAIN II] (N89.1)
        vaginal intraepithelial neoplasia III [VAIN III] (D07.2)
    EXCLUDES 2   vaginal high risk human papillomavirus (HPV) DNA test positive (R87.811)
        vaginal low risk human papillomavirus (HPV) DNA test positive (R87.821)

R87.620 Atypical squamous cells of undetermined significance on cytologic smear of vagina [ASC-US] ♀

R87.621 Atypical squamous cells cannot exclude high grade squamous intraepithelial lesion on cytologic smear of vagina [ASC-H] ♀

R87.622 Low grade squamous intraepithelial lesion on cytologic smear of vagina [LGSIL] ♀

R87.623 High grade squamous intraepithelial lesion on cytologic smear of vagina [HGSIL] ♀

R87.624 Cytologic evidence of malignancy on smear of vagina ♀

R87.625 Unsatisfactory cytologic smear of vagina ♀
    Inadequate sample of cytologic smear of vagina

R87.628 Other abnormal cytological findings on specimens from vagina ♀

R87.629 Unspecified abnormal cytological findings in specimens from vagina ♀
    Abnormal Papanicolaou smear of vagina NOS
    Abnormal thin preparation smear of vagina NOS
    Abnormal vaginal cytology NOS
    Atypical endocervical cells of vagina NOS
    Atypical endometrial cells of vagina NOS
    Atypical glandular cells of vagina NOS

R87.69 Abnormal cytological findings in specimens from other female genital organs ♀
    Abnormal cytological findings in specimens from female genital organs NOS
    EXCLUDES 1   dysplasia of vulva (histologically confirmed) (N90.0-N90.3)

√ Additional Character Required   √×7ᵗʰ Xtension Alert   Unspecified Code   Other Specified Code   Manifestation Code   ►◄ Revised Text   ● New Code   ▲ Revised Code Title

R87.7 **Abnormal histological findings in specimens from female genital organs** ♀
  EXCLUDES 1 *carcinoma in situ (histologically confirmed) of female genital organs (D06-D07.3)*
  cervical intraepithelial neoplasia I [CIN I] (N87.0)
  cervical intraepithelial neoplasia II [CIN II] (N87.1)
  cervical intraepithelial neoplasia III [CIN III] (D06.-)
  dysplasia (mild) (moderate) of cervix uteri (histologically confirmed) (N87.-)
  dysplasia (mild) (moderate) of vagina (histologically confirmed) (N89.-)
  severe dysplasia of cervix uteri (histologically confirmed) (D06.-)
  severe dysplasia of vagina (histologically confirmed) (D07.2)
  vaginal intraepithelial neoplasia I [VAIN I] (N89.0)
  vaginal intraepithelial neoplasia II [VAIN II] (N89.1)
  vaginal intraepithelial neoplasia III [VAIN III] (D07.2)

✓5ᵗʰ **R87.8** **Other abnormal findings in specimens from female genital organs**

  ✓6ᵗʰ **R87.81** **High risk human papillomavirus [HPV] DNA test positive from female genital organs**
    EXCLUDES 1 *anogenital warts due to human papillomavirus (HPV) (A63.0)*
    condyloma acuminatum (A63.0)

    R87.810 **Cervical high risk human papillomavirus [HPV] DNA test positive** ♀
    R87.811 **Vaginal high risk human papillomavirus [HPV] DNA test positive** ♀

  ✓6ᵗʰ **R87.82** **Low risk human papillomavirus [HPV] DNA test positive from female genital organs**
    Use additional code for associated human papillomavirus (B97.7)

    R87.820 **Cervical low risk human papillomavirus [HPV] DNA test positive** ♀
    R87.821 **Vaginal low risk human papillomavirus [HPV] DNA test positive** ♀

  R87.89 **Other abnormal findings in specimens from female genital organs** ♀
    Abnormal chromosomal findings in specimens from female genital organs

  R87.9 **Unspecified abnormal finding in specimens from female genital organs** ♀

✓4ᵗʰ **R88** **Abnormal findings in other body fluids and substances**
  R88.0 **Cloudy (hemodialysis) (peritoneal) dialysis effluent**
  R88.8 **Abnormal findings in other body fluids and substances**

✓4ᵗʰ **R89** **Abnormal findings in specimens from other organs, systems and tissues**
  INCLUDES abnormal findings in nipple discharge
    abnormal findings in synovial fluid
    abnormal findings in wound secretions
  R89.0 **Abnormal level of enzymes in specimens from other organs, systems and tissues**
  R89.1 **Abnormal level of hormones in specimens from other organs, systems and tissues**
  R89.2 **Abnormal level of other drugs, medicaments and biological substances in specimens from other organs, systems and tissues**
  R89.3 **Abnormal level of substances chiefly nonmedicinal as to source in specimens from other organs, systems and tissues**
  R89.4 **Abnormal immunological findings in specimens from other organs, systems and tissues**
  R89.5 **Abnormal microbiological findings in specimens from other organs, systems and tissues**
    Positive culture findings in specimens from other organs, systems and tissues
    EXCLUDES 1 *colonization status (Z22.-)*
  R89.6 **Abnormal cytological findings in specimens from other organs, systems and tissues**
  R89.7 **Abnormal histological findings in specimens from other organs, systems and tissues**
  R89.8 **Other abnormal findings in specimens from other organs, systems and tissues**
    Abnormal chromosomal findings in specimens from other organs, systems and tissues
  R89.9 **Unspecified abnormal finding in specimens from other organs, systems and tissues**

Abnormal findings on diagnostic imaging and in function studies, without diagnosis (R90-R94)
  INCLUDES nonspecific abnormal findings on diagnostic imaging by computerized axial tomography [CAT scan]
    nonspecific abnormal findings on diagnostic imaging by magnetic resonance imaging [MRI][NMR]
    nonspecific abnormal findings on diagnostic imaging by positron emission tomography [PET scan]
    nonspecific abnormal findings on diagnostic imaging by thermography
    nonspecific abnormal findings on diagnostic imaging by ultrasound [echogram]
    nonspecific abnormal findings on diagnostic imaging by X-ray examination
  EXCLUDES 1 *abnormal findings on antenatal screening of mother (O28.-)*
    diagnostic abnormal findings classified elsewhere—see Alphabetical Index

✓4ᵗʰ **R90** **Abnormal findings on diagnostic imaging of central nervous system**
  R90.0 **Intracranial space-occupying lesion found on diagnostic imaging of central nervous system**
  ✓5ᵗʰ **R90.8** **Other abnormal findings on diagnostic imaging of central nervous system**
    R90.81 **Abnormal echoencephalogram**
    R90.82 **White matter disease, unspecified**
    R90.89 **Other abnormal findings on diagnostic imaging of central nervous system**
      Other cerebrovascular abnormality found on diagnostic imaging of central nervous system

✓4ᵗʰ **R91** **Abnormal findings on diagnostic imaging of lung**
  R91.1 **Solitary pulmonary nodule**
    Coin lesion lung
    Solitary pulmonary nodule, subsegmental branch of the bronchial tree
  R91.8 **Other nonspecific abnormal finding of lung field**
    Lung mass NOS found on diagnostic imaging of lung
    Pulmonary infiltrate NOS
    Shadow, lung

✓4ᵗʰ **R92** **Abnormal and inconclusive findings on diagnostic imaging of breast**
  R92.0 **Mammographic microcalcification found on diagnostic imaging of breast**
    EXCLUDES 2 *mammographic calcification (calculus) found on diagnostic imaging of breast (R92.1)*
  R92.1 **Mammographic calcification found on diagnostic imaging of breast**
    Mammographic calculus found on diagnostic imaging of breast
  R92.2 **Inconclusive mammogram**
    Dense breasts NOS
    Inconclusive mammogram NEC
    Inconclusive mammography due to dense breasts
    Inconclusive mammography NEC
  R92.8 **Other abnormal and inconclusive findings on diagnostic imaging of breast**

✓4ᵗʰ **R93** **Abnormal findings on diagnostic imaging of other body structures**
  R93.0 **Abnormal findings on diagnostic imaging of skull and head, not elsewhere classified**
    EXCLUDES 1 *intracranial space-occupying lesion found on diagnostic imaging (R90.0)*
  R93.1 **Abnormal findings on diagnostic imaging of heart and coronary circulation**
    Abnormal echocardiogram NOS
    Abnormal heart shadow
  R93.2 **Abnormal findings on diagnostic imaging of liver and biliary tract**
    Nonvisualization of gallbladder
  R93.3 **Abnormal findings on diagnostic imaging of other parts of digestive tract**
  R93.4 **Abnormal findings on diagnostic imaging of urinary organs**
    Filling defect of bladder found on diagnostic imaging
    Filling defect of kidney found on diagnostic imaging
    Filling defect of ureter found on diagnostic imaging
    EXCLUDES 1 *hypertrophy of kidney (N28.81)*
  R93.5 **Abnormal findings on diagnostic imaging of other abdominal regions, including retroperitoneum**

R93.6 **Abnormal findings on diagnostic imaging of** limbs
> EXCLUDES 2 *abnormal finding in skin and subcutaneous tissue (R93.8)*

R93.7 **Abnormal findings on diagnostic imaging of** other parts of musculoskeletal system
> EXCLUDES 2 *abnormal findings on diagnostic imaging of skull (R93.0)*

R93.8 **Abnormal findings on diagnostic imaging of other specified body structures**
Abnormal finding by radioisotope localization of placenta
Abnormal radiological finding in skin and subcutaneous tissue
Mediastinal shift

R93.9 **Diagnostic imaging inconclusive due to** excess body fat of patient

☑4ᵗʰ **R94 Abnormal results of function studies**
> INCLUDES abnormal results of radionuclide [radioisotope] uptake studies
> abnormal results of scintigraphy

☑5ᵗʰ R94.0 **Abnormal results of function studies of** central nervous system

R94.01 **Abnormal** electroencephalogram [EEG]

R94.02 **Abnormal** brain scan

R94.09 **Abnormal results of other function studies of central nervous system**

☑5ᵗʰ R94.1 **Abnormal results of function studies of** peripheral nervous system and special senses

☑6ᵗʰ R94.11 **Abnormal results of function studies of** eye

R94.110 **Abnormal** electro-oculogram [EOG]

R94.111 **Abnormal** electroretinogram [ERG]
Abnormal retinal function study

R94.112 **Abnormal** visually evoked potential [VEP]

R94.113 **Abnormal** oculomotor study

R94.118 **Abnormal results of other function studies of eye**

☑6ᵗʰ R94.12 **Abnormal results of function studies of** ear and other special senses

R94.120 **Abnormal** auditory function study

R94.121 **Abnormal** vestibular function study

R94.128 **Abnormal results of other function studies of ear and other special senses**

☑6ᵗʰ R94.13 **Abnormal results of function studies of** peripheral nervous system

R94.130 **Abnormal response to nerve stimulation, unspecified**

R94.131 **Abnormal** electromyogram [EMG]
> EXCLUDES 1 *electromyogram of eye (R94.113)*

R94.138 **Abnormal results of other function studies of peripheral nervous system**

R94.2 **Abnormal results of** pulmonary function studies
Reduced ventilatory capacity
Reduced vital capacity

☑5ᵗʰ R94.3 **Abnormal results of** cardiovascular function studies

R94.30 **Abnormal result of cardiovascular function study, unspecified**

R94.31 **Abnormal** electrocardiogram [ECG] [EKG]
> EXCLUDES 1 *long QT syndrome (I45.81)*

R94.39 **Abnormal result of other cardiovascular function study**
Abnormal electrophysiological intracardiac studies
Abnormal phonocardiogram
Abnormal vectorcardiogram

R94.4 **Abnormal results of** kidney function studies
Abnormal renal function test

R94.5 **Abnormal results of** liver function studies

R94.6 **Abnormal results of** thyroid function studies

R94.7 **Abnormal results of other endocrine function studies**
> EXCLUDES 2 *abnormal glucose (R73.0-)*

R94.8 **Abnormal results of function studies of** other organs and systems
Abnormal basal metabolic rate [BMR]
Abnormal bladder function test
Abnormal splenic function test

Abnormal tumor markers (R97)

☑4ᵗʰ **R97 Abnormal tumor markers**
Elevated tumor associated antigens [TAA]
Elevated tumor specific antigens [TSA]

R97.0 **Elevated carcinoembryonic antigen [CEA]**

R97.1 **Elevated cancer antigen 125 [CA 125]**   ♀

R97.2 **Elevated prostate specific antigen [PSA]**   A♂

R97.8 **Other abnormal tumor markers**

Ill-defined and unknown cause of mortality (R99)

R99 **Ill-defined and unknown cause of mortality**
Death (unexplained) NOS
Unspecified cause of mortality

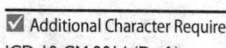

Chapter 19. Injury, Poisoning and Certain Other Consequences of External Causes (S00-T88)

NOTE   Use secondary code(s) from Chapter 20, External causes of morbidity, to indicate cause of injury. Codes within the T section that include the external cause do not require an additional external cause code.

Use additional code to identify any retained foreign body, if applicable (Z18.-)

EXCLUDES 1   birth trauma (P10-P15)
         obstetric trauma (O70-O71)

This chapter contains the following blocks:

S00-S09	Injuries to the head
S10-S19	Injuries to the neck
S20-S29	Injuries to the thorax
S30-S39	Injuries to the abdomen, lower back, lumbar spine, pelvis and external genitals
S40-S49	Injuries to the shoulder and upper arm
S50-S59	Injuries to the elbow and forearm
S60-S69	Injuries to the wrist, hand and fingers
S70-S79	Injuries to the hip and thigh
S80-S89	Injuries to the knee and lower leg
S90-S99	Injuries to the ankle and foot
T07	Injuries involving multiple body regions
T14	Injury of unspecified body region
T15-T19	Effects of foreign body entering through natural orifice
T20-T25	Burns and corrosions of external body surface, specified by site
T26-T28	Burns and corrosions confined to eye and internal organs
T30-T32	Burns and corrosions of multiple and unspecified body regions
T33-T34	Frostbite
T36-T50	Poisoning by, adverse effect of and underdosing of drugs, medicaments and biological substances
T51-T65	Toxic effects of substances chiefly nonmedicinal as to source
T66-T78	Other and unspecified effects of external causes
T79	Certain early complications of trauma
T80-T88	Complications of surgical and medical care, not elsewhere classified

The chapter uses the S-section for coding different types of injuries related to single body regions and the T-section to cover injuries to unspecified body regions as well as poisoning and certain other consequences of external causes.

Injuries to the head (S00-S09)

INCLUDES   injuries of ear
         injuries of eye
         injuries of face [any part]
         injuries of gum
         injuries of jaw
         injuries of oral cavity
         injuries of palate
         injuries of periocular area
         injuries of scalp
         injuries of temporomandibular joint area
         injuries of tongue
         injuries of tooth

Code also for any associated infection

EXCLUDES 2   burns and corrosions (T20-T32)
         effects of foreign body in ear (T16)
         effects of foreign body in larynx (T17.3)
         effects of foreign body in mouth NOS (T18.0)
         effects of foreign body in nose (T17.0-T17.1)
         effects of foreign body in pharynx (T17.2)
         effects of foreign body on external eye (T15.-)
         frostbite (T33-T34)
         insect bite or sting, venomous (T63.4)

☑4ᵗʰ S00   **Superficial injury of head**

     EXCLUDES 1   diffuse cerebral contusion (S06.2-)
                 focal cerebral contusion (S06.3-)
                 injury of eye and orbit (S05.-)
                 open wound of head (S01.-)

> The appropriate 7th character is to be added to each code from category S00.
> A   initial encounter
> D   subsequent encounter
> S   sequela

   ☑5ᵗʰ S00.0   **Superficial injury of scalp**

     ☑x7ᵗʰ S00.00   **Unspecified superficial injury of scalp**

     ☑x7ᵗʰ S00.01   **Abrasion of scalp**

     ☑x7ᵗʰ S00.02   **Blister (nonthermal) of scalp**

     ☑x7ᵗʰ S00.03   **Contusion of scalp**
                   Bruise of scalp
                   Hematoma of scalp

     ☑x7ᵗʰ S00.04   **External constriction of part of scalp**

     ☑x7ᵗʰ S00.05   **Superficial foreign body of scalp**
                   Splinter in the scalp

     ☑x7ᵗʰ S00.06   **Insect bite (nonvenomous) of scalp**

     ☑x7ᵗʰ S00.07   **Other superficial bite of scalp**
         EXCLUDES 1   open bite of scalp (S01.05)

   ☑5ᵗʰ S00.1   **Contusion of eyelid and periocular area**
         Black eye
     EXCLUDES 2   contusion of eyeball and orbital tissues (S05.1)

     ☑x7ᵗʰ S00.10   **Contusion of unspecified eyelid and periocular area**

     ☑x7ᵗʰ S00.11   **Contusion of right eyelid and periocular area**

     ☑x7ᵗʰ S00.12   **Contusion of left eyelid and periocular area**

   ☑5ᵗʰ S00.2   **Other and unspecified superficial injuries of eyelid and periocular area**
     EXCLUDES 2   superficial injury of conjunctiva and cornea (S05.0-)

     ☑6ᵗʰ S00.20   **Unspecified superficial injury of eyelid and periocular area**

       ☑7ᵗʰ S00.201   **Unspecified superficial injury of right eyelid and periocular area**

       ☑7ᵗʰ S00.202   **Unspecified superficial injury of left eyelid and periocular area**

       ☑7ᵗʰ S00.209   **Unspecified superficial injury of unspecified eyelid and periocular area**

     ☑6ᵗʰ S00.21   **Abrasion of eyelid and periocular area**

       ☑7ᵗʰ S00.211   **Abrasion of right eyelid and periocular area**

       ☑7ᵗʰ S00.212   **Abrasion of left eyelid and periocular area**

       ☑7ᵗʰ S00.219   **Abrasion of unspecified eyelid and periocular area**

     ☑6ᵗʰ S00.22   **Blister (nonthermal) of eyelid and periocular area**

       ☑7ᵗʰ S00.221   **Blister (nonthermal) of right eyelid and periocular area**

       ☑7ᵗʰ S00.222   **Blister (nonthermal) of left eyelid and periocular area**

       ☑7ᵗʰ S00.229   **Blister (nonthermal) of unspecified eyelid and periocular area**

     ☑6ᵗʰ S00.24   **External constriction of eyelid and periocular area**

       ☑7ᵗʰ S00.241   **External constriction of right eyelid and periocular area**

       ☑7ᵗʰ S00.242   **External constriction of left eyelid and periocular area**

       ☑7ᵗʰ S00.249   **External constriction of unspecified eyelid and periocular area**

     ☑6ᵗʰ S00.25   **Superficial foreign body of eyelid and periocular area**
         Splinter of eyelid and periocular area
       EXCLUDES 2   retained foreign body in eyelid (H02.81-)

       ☑7ᵗʰ S00.251   **Superficial foreign body of right eyelid and periocular area**

       ☑7ᵗʰ S00.252   **Superficial foreign body of left eyelid and periocular area**

       ☑7ᵗʰ S00.259   **Superficial foreign body of unspecified eyelid and periocular area**

     ☑6ᵗʰ S00.26   **Insect bite (nonvenomous) of eyelid and periocular area**

       ☑7ᵗʰ S00.261   **Insect bite (nonvenomous) of right eyelid and periocular area**

       ☑7ᵗʰ S00.262   **Insect bite (nonvenomous) of left eyelid and periocular area**

       ☑7ᵗʰ S00.269   **Insect bite (nonvenomous) of unspecified eyelid and periocular area**

     ☑6ᵗʰ S00.27   **Other superficial bite of eyelid and periocular area**
       EXCLUDES 1   open bite of eyelid and periocular area (S01.15)

       ☑7ᵗʰ S00.271   **Other superficial bite of right eyelid and periocular area**

       ☑7ᵗʰ S00.272   **Other superficial bite of left eyelid and periocular area**

       ☑7ᵗʰ S00.279   **Other superficial bite of unspecified eyelid and periocular area**

   ☑5ᵗʰ S00.3   **Superficial injury of nose**

     ☑x7ᵗʰ S00.30   **Unspecified superficial injury of nose**

     ☑x7ᵗʰ S00.31   **Abrasion of nose**

     ☑x7ᵗʰ S00.32   **Blister (nonthermal) of nose**

EXCLUDES 1 Not coded here   **EXCLUDES 2** Not included here   **N** Newborn Age: 0   **P** Pediatric Age: 0-17   **M** Maternity Age: 12-55   **A** Adult Age: 15-124

804   ICD-10-CM 2014 (Draft)

√x7ᵗʰ **S00.33** **Contusion of nose**
Bruise of nose
Hematoma of nose

√x7ᵗʰ **S00.34** **External constriction of nose**

√x7ᵗʰ **S00.35** **Superficial foreign body of nose**
Splinter in the nose

√x7ᵗʰ **S00.36** **Insect bite (nonvenomous) of nose**

√x7ᵗʰ **S00.37** **Other superficial bite of nose**
EXCLUDES 1 open bite of nose (S01.25)

√5ᵗʰ **S00.4** **Superficial injury of ear**

√6ᵗʰ **S00.40** **Unspecified superficial injury of ear**

√7ᵗʰ **S00.401** **Unspecified superficial injury of right ear**

√7ᵗʰ **S00.402** **Unspecified superficial injury of left ear**

√7ᵗʰ **S00.409** **Unspecified superficial injury of unspecified ear**

√6ᵗʰ **S00.41** **Abrasion of ear**

√7ᵗʰ **S00.411** **Abrasion of right ear**

√7ᵗʰ **S00.412** **Abrasion of left ear**

√7ᵗʰ **S00.419** **Abrasion of unspecified ear**

√6ᵗʰ **S00.42** **Blister (nonthermal) of ear**

√7ᵗʰ **S00.421** **Blister (nonthermal) of right ear**

√7ᵗʰ **S00.422** **Blister (nonthermal) of left ear**

√7ᵗʰ **S00.429** **Blister (nonthermal) of unspecified ear**

√6ᵗʰ **S00.43** **Contusion of ear**
Bruise of ear
Hematoma of ear

√7ᵗʰ **S00.431** **Contusion of right ear**

√7ᵗʰ **S00.432** **Contusion of left ear**

√7ᵗʰ **S00.439** **Contusion of unspecified ear**

√6ᵗʰ **S00.44** **External constriction of ear**

√7ᵗʰ **S00.441** **External constriction of right ear**

√7ᵗʰ **S00.442** **External constriction of left ear**

√7ᵗʰ **S00.449** **External constriction of unspecified ear**

√6ᵗʰ **S00.45** **Superficial foreign body of ear**
Splinter in the ear

√7ᵗʰ **S00.451** **Superficial foreign body of right ear**

√7ᵗʰ **S00.452** **Superficial foreign body of left ear**

√7ᵗʰ **S00.459** **Superficial foreign body of unspecified ear**

√6ᵗʰ **S00.46** **Insect bite (nonvenomous) of ear**

√7ᵗʰ **S00.461** **Insect bite (nonvenomous) of right ear**

√7ᵗʰ **S00.462** **Insect bite (nonvenomous) of left ear**

√7ᵗʰ **S00.469** **Insect bite (nonvenomous) of unspecified ear**

√6ᵗʰ **S00.47** **Other superficial bite of ear**
EXCLUDES 1 open bite of ear (S01.35)

√7ᵗʰ **S00.471** **Other superficial bite of right ear**

√7ᵗʰ **S00.472** **Other superficial bite of left ear**

√7ᵗʰ **S00.479** **Other superficial bite of unspecified ear**

√5ᵗʰ **S00.5** **Superficial injury of lip and oral cavity**

√6ᵗʰ **S00.50** **Unspecified superficial injury of lip and oral cavity**

√7ᵗʰ **S00.501** **Unspecified superficial injury of lip**

√7ᵗʰ **S00.502** **Unspecified superficial injury of oral cavity**

√6ᵗʰ **S00.51** **Abrasion of lip and oral cavity**

√7ᵗʰ **S00.511** **Abrasion of lip**

√7ᵗʰ **S00.512** **Abrasion of oral cavity**

√6ᵗʰ **S00.52** **Blister (nonthermal) of lip and oral cavity**

√7ᵗʰ **S00.521** **Blister (nonthermal) of lip**

√7ᵗʰ **S00.522** **Blister (nonthermal) of oral cavity**

√6ᵗʰ **S00.53** **Contusion of lip and oral cavity**

√7ᵗʰ **S00.531** **Contusion of lip**
Bruise of lip
Hematoma of oral cavity

√7ᵗʰ **S00.532** **Contusion of oral cavity**
Bruise of lip
Hematoma of oral cavity

√6ᵗʰ **S00.54** **External constriction of lip and oral cavity**

√7ᵗʰ **S00.541** **External constriction of lip**

√7ᵗʰ **S00.542** **External constriction of oral cavity**

√6ᵗʰ **S00.55** **Superficial foreign body of lip and oral cavity**

√7ᵗʰ **S00.551** **Superficial foreign body of lip**
Splinter of lip and oral cavity

√7ᵗʰ **S00.552** **Superficial foreign body of oral cavity**
Splinter of lip and oral cavity

√6ᵗʰ **S00.56** **Insect bite (nonvenomous) of lip and oral cavity**

√7ᵗʰ **S00.561** **Insect bite (nonvenomous) of lip**

√7ᵗʰ **S00.562** **Insect bite (nonvenomous) of oral cavity**

√6ᵗʰ **S00.57** **Other superficial bite of lip and oral cavity**

√7ᵗʰ **S00.571** **Other superficial bite of lip**
EXCLUDES 1 open bite of lip (S01.551)

√7ᵗʰ **S00.572** **Other superficial bite of oral cavity**
EXCLUDES 1 open bite of oral cavity (S01.552)

√5ᵗʰ **S00.8** **Superficial injury of other parts of head**

√x7ᵗʰ **S00.80** **Unspecified superficial injury of other part of head**

√x7ᵗʰ **S00.81** **Abrasion of other part of head**

√x7ᵗʰ **S00.82** **Blister (nonthermal) of other part of head**

√x7ᵗʰ **S00.83** **Contusion of other part of head**
Bruise of other part of head
Hematoma of other part of head

√x7ᵗʰ **S00.84** **External constriction of other part of head**

√x7ᵗʰ **S00.85** **Superficial foreign body of other part of head**
Splinter in other part of head

√x7ᵗʰ **S00.86** **Insect bite (nonvenomous) of other part of head**

√x7ᵗʰ **S00.87** **Other superficial bite of other part of head**
EXCLUDES 1 open bite of other part of head (S01.85)

√5ᵗʰ **S00.9** **Superficial injury of unspecified part of head**

√x7ᵗʰ **S00.90** **Unspecified superficial injury of unspecified part of head**

√x7ᵗʰ **S00.91** **Abrasion of unspecified part of head**

√x7ᵗʰ **S00.92** **Blister (nonthermal) of unspecified part of head**

√x7ᵗʰ **S00.93** **Contusion of unspecified part of head**
Bruise of head
Hematoma of head

√x7ᵗʰ **S00.94** **External constriction of unspecified part of head**

√x7ᵗʰ **S00.95** **Superficial foreign body of unspecified part of head**
Splinter of head

√x7ᵗʰ **S00.96** **Insect bite (nonvenomous) of unspecified part of head**

√x7ᵗʰ **S00.97** **Other superficial bite of unspecified part of head**
EXCLUDES 1 open bite of head (S01.95)

√4ᵗʰ **S01** **Open wound of head**
Code also any associated:
injury of cranial nerve (S04.-)
injury of muscle and tendon of head (S09.1-)
intracranial injury (S06.-)
wound infection
EXCLUDES 1 open skull fracture (S02- with 7th character B)
EXCLUDES 2 injury of eye and orbit (S05.-)
traumatic amputation of part of head (S08.-)

The appropriate 7th character is to be added to each code from category S01.
A initial encounter
D subsequent encounter
S sequela

√5ᵗʰ **S01.0** **Open wound of scalp**
EXCLUDES 1 avulsion of scalp (S08.0)

√x7ᵗʰ **S01.00** **Unspecified open wound of scalp**

√x7ᵗʰ **S01.01** **Laceration without foreign body of scalp**

√x7ᵗʰ **S01.02** **Laceration with foreign body of scalp**

√x7ᵗʰ **S01.03** **Puncture wound without foreign body of scalp**

√x7ᵗʰ **S01.04** **Puncture wound with foreign body of scalp**

√x7ᵗʰ **S01.05** **Open bite of scalp**
Bite of scalp NOS
EXCLUDES 1 superficial bite of scalp (S00.06, S00.07-)

√5ᵗʰ **S01.1** **Open wound of eyelid and periocular area**
Open wound of eyelid and periocular area with or without involvement of lacrimal passages

√6ᵗʰ **S01.10** **Unspecified open wound of eyelid and periocular area**

√7ᵗʰ **S01.101** **Unspecified open wound of right eyelid and periocular area**

√7ᵗʰ **S01.102 Unspecified open wound of** left **eyelid and periocular area**

√7ᵗʰ **S01.109 Unspecified open wound of unspecified eyelid and periocular area**

√6ᵗʰ **S01.11 Laceration without foreign body of eyelid and periocular area**

√7ᵗʰ **S01.111 Laceration without foreign body of** right **eyelid and periocular area**

√7ᵗʰ **S01.112 Laceration without foreign body of** left **eyelid and periocular area**

√7ᵗʰ **S01.119 Laceration without foreign body of unspecified eyelid and periocular area**

√6ᵗʰ **S01.12 Laceration with foreign body of eyelid and periocular area**

√7ᵗʰ **S01.121 Laceration with foreign body of** right **eyelid and periocular area**

√7ᵗʰ **S01.122 Laceration with foreign body of** left **eyelid and periocular area**

√7ᵗʰ **S01.129 Laceration with foreign body of unspecified eyelid and periocular area**

√6ᵗʰ **S01.13 Puncture wound without foreign body of eyelid and periocular area**

√7ᵗʰ **S01.131 Puncture wound without foreign body of** right **eyelid and periocular area**

√7ᵗʰ **S01.132 Puncture wound without foreign body of** left **eyelid and periocular area**

√7ᵗʰ **S01.139 Puncture wound without foreign body of unspecified eyelid and periocular area**

√6ᵗʰ **S01.14 Puncture wound with foreign body of eyelid and periocular area**

√7ᵗʰ **S01.141 Puncture wound with foreign body of** right **eyelid and periocular area**

√7ᵗʰ **S01.142 Puncture wound with foreign body of** left **eyelid and periocular area**

√7ᵗʰ **S01.149 Puncture wound with foreign body of unspecified eyelid and periocular area**

√6ᵗʰ **S01.15 Open bite of eyelid and periocular area**
Bite of eyelid and periocular area NOS

EXCLUDES 1 superficial bite of eyelid and periocular area (S00.26, S00.27)

√7ᵗʰ **S01.151 Open bite of** right **eyelid and periocular area**

√7ᵗʰ **S01.152 Open bite of** left **eyelid and periocular area**

√7ᵗʰ **S01.159 Open bite of unspecified eyelid and periocular area**

√5ᵗʰ **S01.2 Open wound of** nose

√x7ᵗʰ **S01.20 Unspecified open wound of nose**

√x7ᵗʰ **S01.21 Laceration without foreign body of nose**

√x7ᵗʰ **S01.22 Laceration with foreign body of nose**

√x7ᵗʰ **S01.23 Puncture wound without foreign body of nose**

√x7ᵗʰ **S01.24 Puncture wound with foreign body of nose**

√x7ᵗʰ **S01.25 Open bite of nose**
Bite of nose NOS

EXCLUDES 1 superficial bite of nose (S00.36, S00.37)

√5ᵗʰ **S01.3 Open wound of** ear

√6ᵗʰ **S01.30 Unspecified open wound of ear**

√7ᵗʰ **S01.301 Unspecified open wound of** right **ear**

√7ᵗʰ **S01.302 Unspecified open wound of** left **ear**

√7ᵗʰ **S01.309 Unspecified open wound of unspecified ear**

√6ᵗʰ **S01.31 Laceration without foreign body of ear**

√7ᵗʰ **S01.311 Laceration without foreign body of** right **ear**

√7ᵗʰ **S01.312 Laceration without foreign body of** left **ear**

√7ᵗʰ **S01.319 Laceration without foreign body of unspecified ear**

√6ᵗʰ **S01.32 Laceration with foreign body of ear**

√7ᵗʰ **S01.321 Laceration with foreign body of** right **ear**

√7ᵗʰ **S01.322 Laceration with foreign body of** left **ear**

√7ᵗʰ **S01.329 Laceration with foreign body of unspecified ear**

√6ᵗʰ **S01.33 Puncture wound without foreign body of ear**

√7ᵗʰ **S01.331 Puncture wound without foreign body of** right **ear**

√7ᵗʰ **S01.332 Puncture wound without foreign body of** left **ear**

√7ᵗʰ **S01.339 Puncture wound without foreign body of unspecified ear**

√6ᵗʰ **S01.34 Puncture wound with foreign body of ear**

√7ᵗʰ **S01.341 Puncture wound with foreign body of** right **ear**

√7ᵗʰ **S01.342 Puncture wound with foreign body of** left **ear**

√7ᵗʰ **S01.349 Puncture wound with foreign body of unspecified ear**

√6ᵗʰ **S01.35 Open bite of ear**
Bite of ear NOS

EXCLUDES 1 superficial bite of ear (S00.46, S00.47)

√7ᵗʰ **S01.351 Open bite of** right **ear**

√7ᵗʰ **S01.352 Open bite of** left **ear**

√7ᵗʰ **S01.359 Open bite of unspecified ear**

√5ᵗʰ **S01.4 Open wound of** cheek and temporomandibular area

√6ᵗʰ **S01.40 Unspecified open wound of cheek and temporomandibular area**

√7ᵗʰ **S01.401 Unspecified open wound of** right **cheek and temporomandibular area**

√7ᵗʰ **S01.402 Unspecified open wound of** left **cheek and temporomandibular area**

√7ᵗʰ **S01.409 Unspecified open wound of unspecified cheek and temporomandibular area**

√6ᵗʰ **S01.41 Laceration without foreign body of cheek and temporomandibular area**

√7ᵗʰ **S01.411 Laceration without foreign body of** right **cheek and temporomandibular area**

√7ᵗʰ **S01.412 Laceration without foreign body of** left **cheek and temporomandibular area**

√7ᵗʰ **S01.419 Laceration without foreign body of unspecified cheek and temporomandibular area**

√6ᵗʰ **S01.42 Laceration with foreign body of cheek and temporomandibular area**

√7ᵗʰ **S01.421 Laceration with foreign body of** right **cheek and temporomandibular area**

√7ᵗʰ **S01.422 Laceration with foreign body of** left **cheek and temporomandibular area**

√7ᵗʰ **S01.429 Laceration with foreign body of unspecified cheek and temporomandibular area**

√6ᵗʰ **S01.43 Puncture wound without foreign body of cheek and temporomandibular area**

√7ᵗʰ **S01.431 Puncture wound without foreign body of** right **cheek and temporomandibular area**

√7ᵗʰ **S01.432 Puncture wound without foreign body of** left **cheek and temporomandibular area**

√7ᵗʰ **S01.439 Puncture wound without foreign body of unspecified cheek and temporomandibular area**

√6ᵗʰ **S01.44 Puncture wound with foreign body of cheek and temporomandibular area**

√7ᵗʰ **S01.441 Puncture wound with foreign body of** right **cheek and temporomandibular area**

√7ᵗʰ **S01.442 Puncture wound with foreign body of** left **cheek and temporomandibular area**

√7ᵗʰ **S01.449 Puncture wound with foreign body of unspecified cheek and temporomandibular area**

√6ᵗʰ **S01.45 Open bite of cheek and temporomandibular area**
Bite of cheek and temporomandibular area NOS

EXCLUDES 2 superficial bite of cheek and temporomandibular area (S00.86, S00.87)

√7ᵗʰ **S01.451 Open bite of** right **cheek and temporomandibular area**

√7ᵗʰ **S01.452 Open bite of** left **cheek and temporomandibular area**

√7ᵗʰ **S01.459 Open bite of unspecified cheek and temporomandibular area**

EXCLUDES 1 Not coded here   *EXCLUDES 2* Not included here   N Newborn Age: 0   P Pediatric Age: 0-17   M Maternity Age: 12-55   A Adult Age: 15-124

806   ICD-10-CM 2014 (Draft)

√5th S01.5 Open wound of lip and oral cavity
> EXCLUDES 2   tooth dislocation (S03.2)
> tooth fracture (S02.5)

   √6th S01.50 Unspecified open wound of lip and oral cavity
     √7th S01.501 Unspecified open wound of lip
     √7th S01.502 Unspecified open wound of oral cavity

   √6th S01.51 Laceration of lip and oral cavity without foreign body
     √7th S01.511 Laceration without foreign body of lip
     √7th S01.512 Laceration without foreign body of oral cavity

   √6th S01.52 Laceration of lip and oral cavity with foreign body
     √7th S01.521 Laceration with foreign body of lip
     √7th S01.522 Laceration with foreign body of oral cavity

   √6th S01.53 Puncture wound of lip and oral cavity without foreign body
     √7th S01.531 Puncture wound without foreign body of lip
     √7th S01.532 Puncture wound without foreign body of oral cavity

   √6th S01.54 Puncture wound of lip and oral cavity with foreign body
     √7th S01.541 Puncture wound with foreign body of lip
     √7th S01.542 Puncture wound with foreign body of oral cavity

   √6th S01.55 Open bite of lip and oral cavity
     √7th S01.551 Open bite of lip
       Bite of lip NOS
       EXCLUDES 1   superficial bite of lip (S00.571)
     √7th S01.552 Open bite of oral cavity
       Bite of oral cavity NOS
       EXCLUDES 1   superficial bite of oral cavity (S00.572)

√5th S01.8 Open wound of other parts of head
   √x7th S01.80 Unspecified open wound of other part of head
   √x7th S01.81 Laceration without foreign body of other part of head
   √x7th S01.82 Laceration with foreign body of other part of head
   √x7th S01.83 Puncture wound without foreign body of other part of head
   √x7th S01.84 Puncture wound with foreign body of other part of head
   √x7th S01.85 Open bite of other part of head
     Bite of other part of head NOS
     EXCLUDES 1   superficial bite of other part of head (S00.85)

√5th S01.9 Open wound of unspecified part of head
   √x7th S01.90 Unspecified open wound of unspecified part of head
   √x7th S01.91 Laceration without foreign body of unspecified part of head
   √x7th S01.92 Laceration with foreign body of unspecified part of head
   √x7th S01.93 Puncture wound without foreign body of unspecified part of head
   √x7th S01.94 Puncture wound with foreign body of unspecified part of head
   √x7th S01.95 Open bite of unspecified part of head
     Bite of head NOS
     EXCLUDES 1   superficial bite of head NOS (S00.97)

√4th S02 Fracture of skull and facial bones
> NOTE   A fracture not indicated as open or closed should be coded to closed.
> Code also any associated intracranial injury (S06.-).

The appropriate 7th character is to be added to each code from category S02.
A   initial encounter for closed fracture
B   initial encounter for open fracture
D   subsequent encounter for fracture with routine healing
G   subsequent encounter for fracture with delayed healing
K   subsequent encounter for fracture with nonunion
S   sequela

√x7th S02.0 Fracture of vault of skull
   Fracture of frontal bone
   Fracture of parietal bone

√5th S02.1 Fracture of base of skull
> EXCLUDES 1   orbit NOS (S02.8)
> EXCLUDES 2   orbital floor (S02.3-)

   √x7th S02.10 Unspecified fracture of base of skull
   √6th S02.11 Fracture of occiput
     √7th S02.110 Type I occipital condyle fracture
     √7th S02.111 Type II occipital condyle fracture
     √7th S02.112 Type III occipital condyle fracture
     √7th S02.113 Unspecified occipital condyle fracture
     √7th S02.118 Other fracture of occiput
     √7th S02.119 Unspecified fracture of occiput

   √x7th S02.19 Other fracture of base of skull
     Fracture of anterior fossa of base of skull
     Fracture of ethmoid sinus
     Fracture of frontal sinus
     Fracture of middle fossa of base of skull
     Fracture of orbital roof
     Fracture of posterior fossa of base of skull
     Fracture of sphenoid
     Fracture of temporal bone

√x7th S02.2 Fracture of nasal bones

√x7th S02.3 Fracture of orbital floor
> EXCLUDES 1   orbit NOS (S02.8)
> EXCLUDES 2   orbital roof (S02.1-)

√5th S02.4 Fracture of malar, maxillary and zygoma bones
   Fracture of superior maxilla
   Fracture of upper jaw (bone)
   Fracture of zygomatic process of temporal bone

   √6th S02.40 Fracture of malar, maxillary and zygoma bones, unspecified
     √7th S02.400 Malar fracture unspecified
     √7th S02.401 Maxillary fracture, unspecified
     √7th S02.402 Zygomatic fracture, unspecified
   √6th S02.41 LeFort fracture
     √7th S02.411 LeFort I fracture
     √7th S02.412 LeFort II fracture
     √7th S02.413 LeFort III fracture
   √x7th S02.42 Fracture of alveolus of maxilla

√x7th S02.5 Fracture of tooth (traumatic)
   Broken tooth
> EXCLUDES 1   cracked tooth (nontraumatic) (K03.81)

√5th S02.6 Fracture of mandible
   Fracture of lower jaw (bone)
   √6th S02.60 Fracture of mandible, unspecified
     √7th S02.600 Fracture of unspecified part of body of mandible
     √7th S02.609 Fracture of mandible, unspecified
   √x7th S02.61 Fracture of condylar process of mandible
   √x7th S02.62 Fracture of subcondylar process of mandible
   √x7th S02.63 Fracture of coronoid process of mandible
   √x7th S02.64 Fracture of ramus of mandible
   √x7th S02.65 Fracture of angle of mandible
   √x7th S02.66 Fracture of symphysis of mandible
   √x7th S02.67 Fracture of alveolus of mandible
   √x7th S02.69 Fracture of mandible of other specified site

√x7th S02.8 Fractures of other specified skull and facial bones
   Fracture of orbit NOS
   Fracture of palate
> EXCLUDES 1   fracture of orbital floor (S02.3-)
> fracture of orbital roof (S02.1-)

√5th S02.9 Fracture of unspecified skull and facial bones
   √x7th S02.91 Unspecified fracture of skull
   √x7th S02.92 Unspecified fracture of facial bones

☑4ᵗʰ **S03   Dislocation and sprain of joints and ligaments of head**
> INCLUDES   avulsion of joint (capsule) or ligament of head
> laceration of cartilage, joint (capsule) or ligament of head
> sprain of cartilage, joint (capsule) or ligament of head
> traumatic hemarthrosis of joint or ligament of head
> traumatic rupture of joint or ligament of head
> traumatic subluxation of joint or ligament of head
> traumatic tear of joint or ligament of head

> Code also any associated open wound
> EXCLUDES 2   strain of muscle or tendon of head (S09.1)

> The appropriate 7th character is to be added to each code from category S03.
> A   initial encounter
> D   subsequent encounter
> S   sequela

☑x7ᵗʰ **S03.0   Dislocation of jaw**
> Dislocation of jaw (cartilage) (meniscus)
> Dislocation of mandible
> Dislocation of temporomandibular (joint)

☑x7ᵗʰ **S03.1   Dislocation of septal cartilage of nose**

☑x7ᵗʰ **S03.2   Dislocation of tooth**

☑x7ᵗʰ **S03.4   Sprain of jaw**
> Sprain of temporomandibular (joint) (ligament)

☑x7ᵗʰ **S03.8   Sprain of joints and ligaments of other parts of head**

☑x7ᵗʰ **S03.9   Sprain of joints and ligaments of unspecified parts of head**

☑4ᵗʰ **S04   Injury of cranial nerve**
> The selection of side should be based on the side of the body being affected
> Codes first any associated intracranial injury (S06.-)
> Code also any associated:
>   open wound of head (S01.-)
>   skull fracture (S02.-)

> The appropriate 7th character is to be added to each code from category S04.
> A   initial encounter
> D   subsequent encounter
> S   sequela

☑5ᵗʰ **S04.0   Injury of optic nerve and pathways**
> Use additional code to identify any visual field defect or blindness (H53.4-, H54)

☑6ᵗʰ **S04.01   Injury of optic nerve**
> Injury of 2nd cranial nerve

> ☑7ᵗʰ **S04.011   Injury of optic nerve, right eye**
> ☑7ᵗʰ **S04.012   Injury of optic nerve, left eye**
> ☑7ᵗʰ **S04.019   Injury of optic nerve, unspecified eye**
>   Injury of optic nerve NOS

☑x7ᵗʰ **S04.02   Injury of optic chiasm**

☑6ᵗʰ **S04.03   Injury of optic tract and pathways**
> Injury of optic radiation

> ☑7ᵗʰ **S04.031   Injury of optic tract and pathways, right eye**
> ☑7ᵗʰ **S04.032   Injury of optic tract and pathways, left eye**
> ☑7ᵗʰ **S04.039   Injury of optic tract and pathways, unspecified eye**
>   Injury of optic tract and pathways NOS

☑6ᵗʰ **S04.04   Injury of visual cortex**
> ☑7ᵗʰ **S04.041   Injury of visual cortex, right eye**
> ☑7ᵗʰ **S04.042   Injury of visual cortex, left eye**
> ☑7ᵗʰ **S04.049   Injury of visual cortex, unspecified eye**
>   Injury of visual cortex NOS

☑5ᵗʰ **S04.1   Injury of oculomotor nerve**
> Injury of 3rd cranial nerve

> ☑x7ᵗʰ **S04.10   Injury of oculomotor nerve, unspecified side**
> ☑x7ᵗʰ **S04.11   Injury of oculomotor nerve, right side**
> ☑x7ᵗʰ **S04.12   Injury of oculomotor nerve, left side**

☑5ᵗʰ **S04.2   Injury of trochlear nerve**
> Injury of 4th cranial nerve

> ☑x7ᵗʰ **S04.20   Injury of trochlear nerve, unspecified side**
> ☑x7ᵗʰ **S04.21   Injury of trochlear nerve, right side**
> ☑x7ᵗʰ **S04.22   Injury of trochlear nerve, left side**

☑5ᵗʰ **S04.3   Injury of trigeminal nerve**
> Injury of 5th cranial nerve

> ☑x7ᵗʰ **S04.30   Injury of trigeminal nerve, unspecified side**

> ☑x7ᵗʰ **S04.31   Injury of trigeminal nerve, right side**
> ☑x7ᵗʰ **S04.32   Injury of trigeminal nerve, left side**

☑5ᵗʰ **S04.4   Injury of abducent nerve**
> Injury of 6th cranial nerve

> ☑x7ᵗʰ **S04.40   Injury of abducent nerve, unspecified side**
> ☑x7ᵗʰ **S04.41   Injury of abducent nerve, right side**
> ☑x7ᵗʰ **S04.42   Injury of abducent nerve, left side**

☑5ᵗʰ **S04.5   Injury of facial nerve**
> Injury of 7th cranial nerve

> ☑x7ᵗʰ **S04.50   Injury of facial nerve, unspecified side**
> ☑x7ᵗʰ **S04.51   Injury of facial nerve, right side**
> ☑x7ᵗʰ **S04.52   Injury of facial nerve, left side**

☑5ᵗʰ **S04.6   Injury of acoustic nerve**
> Injury of auditory nerve
> Injury of 8th cranial nerve

> ☑x7ᵗʰ **S04.60   Injury of acoustic nerve, unspecified side**
> ☑x7ᵗʰ **S04.61   Injury of acoustic nerve, right side**
> ☑x7ᵗʰ **S04.62   Injury of acoustic nerve, left side**

☑5ᵗʰ **S04.7   Injury of accessory nerve**
> Injury of 11th cranial nerve

> ☑x7ᵗʰ **S04.70   Injury of accessory nerve, unspecified side**
> ☑x7ᵗʰ **S04.71   Injury of accessory nerve, right side**
> ☑x7ᵗʰ **S04.72   Injury of accessory nerve, left side**

☑5ᵗʰ **S04.8   Injury of other cranial nerves**
> ☑6ᵗʰ **S04.81   Injury of olfactory [1st] nerve**
> > ☑7ᵗʰ **S04.811   Injury of olfactory [1st] nerve, right side**
> > ☑7ᵗʰ **S04.812   Injury of olfactory [1st] nerve, left side**
> > ☑7ᵗʰ **S04.819   Injury of olfactory [1st] nerve, unspecified side**

> ☑6ᵗʰ **S04.89   Injury of other cranial nerves**
> > Injury of vagus [10th] nerve
> > ☑7ᵗʰ **S04.891   Injury of other cranial nerves, right side**
> > ☑7ᵗʰ **S04.892   Injury of other cranial nerves, left side**
> > ☑7ᵗʰ **S04.899   Injury of other cranial nerves, unspecified side**

S04.9   Injury of unspecified cranial nerve

☑4ᵗʰ **S05   Injury of eye and orbit**
> Open wound of eye and orbit
> EXCLUDES 2   2nd cranial [optic] nerve injury (S04.0-)
>   3rd cranial [oculomotor] nerve injury (S04.1-)
>   open wound of eyelid and periocular area (S01.1-)
>   orbital bone fracture (S02.1-, S02.3-, S02.8-)
>   superficial injury of eyelid (S00.1-S00.2)

> The appropriate 7th character is to be added to each code from category S05.
> A   initial encounter
> D   subsequent encounter
> S   sequela

☑5ᵗʰ **S05.0   Injury of conjunctiva and corneal abrasion without foreign body**
> EXCLUDES 1   foreign body in conjunctival sac (T15.1)
>   foreign body in cornea (T15.0)

> ☑x7ᵗʰ **S05.00   Injury of conjunctiva and corneal abrasion without foreign body, unspecified eye**
> ☑x7ᵗʰ **S05.01   Injury of conjunctiva and corneal abrasion without foreign body, right eye**
> ☑x7ᵗʰ **S05.02   Injury of conjunctiva and corneal abrasion without foreign body, left eye**

☑5ᵗʰ **S05.1   Contusion of eyeball and orbital tissues**
> Traumatic hyphema
> EXCLUDES 2   black eye NOS (S00.1)
>   contusion of eyelid and periocular area (S00.1)

> ☑x7ᵗʰ **S05.10   Contusion of eyeball and orbital tissues, unspecified eye**
> ☑x7ᵗʰ **S05.11   Contusion of eyeball and orbital tissues, right eye**
> ☑x7ᵗʰ **S05.12   Contusion of eyeball and orbital tissues, left eye**

☑5ᵗʰ **S05.2   Ocular laceration and rupture with prolapse or loss of intraocular tissue**
> ☑x7ᵗʰ **S05.20   Ocular laceration and rupture with prolapse or loss of intraocular tissue, unspecified eye**
> ☑x7ᵗʰ **S05.21   Ocular laceration and rupture with prolapse or loss of intraocular tissue, right eye**

EXCLUDES 1 Not coded here   EXCLUDES 2 Not included here   N Newborn Age: 0   P Pediatric Age: 0-17   M Maternity Age: 12-55   A Adult Age: 15-124

808   ICD-10-CM 2014 (Draft)

✓x 7ᵗʰ **S05.22** **Ocular laceration and rupture with prolapse or loss of intraocular tissue, left eye**

✓5ᵗʰ **S05.3** **Ocular laceration** without prolapse or loss of intraocular tissue
Laceration of eye NOS

✓x 7ᵗʰ **S05.30** **Ocular laceration without prolapse or loss of intraocular tissue, unspecified eye**

✓x 7ᵗʰ **S05.31** **Ocular laceration without prolapse or loss of intraocular tissue, right eye**

✓x 7ᵗʰ **S05.32** **Ocular laceration without prolapse or loss of intraocular tissue, left eye**

✓5ᵗʰ **S05.4** **Penetrating wound** of orbit with or without foreign body
EXCLUDES 2 *retained (old) foreign body following penetrating wound in orbit (H05.5-)*

✓x 7ᵗʰ **S05.40** **Penetrating wound of orbit with or without foreign body, unspecified eye**

✓x 7ᵗʰ **S05.41** **Penetrating wound of orbit with or without foreign body, right eye**

✓x 7ᵗʰ **S05.42** **Penetrating wound of orbit with or without foreign body, left eye**

✓5ᵗʰ **S05.5** **Penetrating wound with foreign body** of eyeball
EXCLUDES 2 *retained (old) intraocular foreign body (H44.6-, H44.7)*

✓x 7ᵗʰ **S05.50** **Penetrating wound with foreign body of unspecified eyeball**

✓x 7ᵗʰ **S05.51** **Penetrating wound with foreign body of right eyeball**

✓x 7ᵗʰ **S05.52** **Penetrating wound with foreign body of left eyeball**

✓5ᵗʰ **S05.6** **Penetrating wound without foreign body** of eyeball
Ocular penetration NOS

✓x 7ᵗʰ **S05.60** **Penetrating wound without foreign body of unspecified eyeball**

✓x 7ᵗʰ **S05.61** **Penetrating wound without foreign body of right eyeball**

✓x 7ᵗʰ **S05.62** **Penetrating wound without foreign body of left eyeball**

✓5ᵗʰ **S05.7** **Avulsion of eye**
Traumatic enucleation

✓x 7ᵗʰ **S05.70** **Avulsion of unspecified eye**

✓x 7ᵗʰ **S05.71** **Avulsion of right eye**

✓x 7ᵗʰ **S05.72** **Avulsion of left eye**

✓5ᵗʰ **S05.8** **Other injuries of eye and orbit**
Lacrimal duct injury

✓6ᵗʰ **S05.8X** **Other injuries of eye and orbit**

✓7ᵗʰ **S05.8X1** **Other injuries of right eye and orbit**

✓7ᵗʰ **S05.8X2** **Other injuries of left eye and orbit**

✓7ᵗʰ **S05.8X9** **Other injuries of unspecified eye and orbit**

✓5ᵗʰ **S05.9** **Unspecified injury of eye and orbit**
Injury of eye NOS

✓x 7ᵗʰ **S05.90** **Unspecified injury of unspecified eye and orbit**

✓x 7ᵗʰ **S05.91** **Unspecified injury of right eye and orbit**

✓x 7ᵗʰ **S05.92** **Unspecified injury of left eye and orbit**

✓4ᵗʰ **S06** **Intracranial injury**
Traumatic brain injury
Code also any associated:
open wound of head (S01.-)
skull fracture (S02.-)
EXCLUDES 1 *head injury NOS (S09.90)*

The appropriate 7th character is to be added to each code from category S06.
A   initial encounter
D   subsequent encounter
S   sequela

✓5ᵗʰ **S06.0** **Concussion**
Commotio cerebri
EXCLUDES 1 *concussion with other intracranial injuries classified in category S06—code to specified intracranial injury*

✓6ᵗʰ **S06.0X** **Concussion**

✓7ᵗʰ **S06.0X0** **Concussion** without loss of consciousness

✓7ᵗʰ **S06.0X1** **Concussion with loss of consciousness of 30 minutes or less**

✓7ᵗʰ **S06.0X2** **Concussion with loss of consciousness of 31 minutes to 59 minutes**

✓7ᵗʰ **S06.0X3** **Concussion with loss of consciousness of 1 hour to 5 hours 59 minutes**

✓7ᵗʰ **S06.0X4** **Concussion with loss of consciousness of 6 hours to 24 hours**

✓7ᵗʰ **S06.0X5** **Concussion with loss of consciousness** greater than 24 hours with return to pre-existing conscious level

✓7ᵗʰ **S06.0X6** **Concussion with loss of consciousness** greater than 24 hours without return to pre-existing conscious level with patient surviving

✓7ᵗʰ **S06.0X7** **Concussion with loss of consciousness of** any duration with death due to brain injury prior to regaining consciousness

✓7ᵗʰ **S06.0X8** **Concussion with loss of consciousness of any duration with death due to other cause prior to regaining consciousness**

✓7ᵗʰ **S06.0X9** **Concussion with loss of consciousness of unspecified duration**
Concussion NOS

✓5ᵗʰ **S06.1** **Traumatic cerebral edema**
Diffuse traumatic cerebral edema
Focal traumatic cerebral edema

✓6ᵗʰ **S06.1X** **Traumatic** cerebral edema

✓7ᵗʰ **S06.1X0** **Traumatic cerebral edema** without loss of consciousness

✓7ᵗʰ **S06.1X1** **Traumatic cerebral edema with loss of consciousness of 30 minutes or less**

✓7ᵗʰ **S06.1X2** **Traumatic cerebral edema with loss of consciousness of 31 minutes to 59 minutes**

✓7ᵗʰ **S06.1X3** **Traumatic cerebral edema with loss of consciousness of 1 hour to 5 hours 59 minutes**

✓7ᵗʰ **S06.1X4** **Traumatic cerebral edema with loss of consciousness of 6 hours to 24 hours**

✓7ᵗʰ **S06.1X5** **Traumatic cerebral edema with loss of consciousness** greater than 24 hours with return to pre-existing conscious level

✓7ᵗʰ **S06.1X6** **Traumatic cerebral edema with loss of consciousness** greater than 24 hours without return to pre-existing conscious level with patient surviving

✓7ᵗʰ **S06.1X7** **Traumatic cerebral edema with loss of consciousness of** any duration with death due to brain injury prior to regaining consciousness

✓7ᵗʰ **S06.1X8** **Traumatic cerebral edema with loss of consciousness of** any duration with death due to other cause prior to regaining consciousness

✓7ᵗʰ **S06.1X9** **Traumatic cerebral edema with loss of consciousness of unspecified duration**
Traumatic cerebral edema NOS

✓5ᵗʰ **S06.2** **Diffuse traumatic brain injury**
Diffuse axonal brain injury
EXCLUDES 1 *traumatic diffuse cerebral edema (S06.1X-)*

✓6ᵗʰ **S06.2X** **Diffuse traumatic brain injury**

✓7ᵗʰ **S06.2X0** **Diffuse traumatic brain injury** without loss of consciousness

✓7ᵗʰ **S06.2X1** **Diffuse traumatic brain injury with loss of consciousness of 30 minutes or less**

✓7ᵗʰ **S06.2X2** **Diffuse traumatic brain injury with loss of consciousness of 31 minutes to 59 minutes**

✓7ᵗʰ **S06.2X3** **Diffuse traumatic brain injury with loss of consciousness of 1 hour to 5 hours 59 minutes**

✓7ᵗʰ **S06.2X4** **Diffuse traumatic brain injury with loss of consciousness of 6 hours to 24 hours**

✓7ᵗʰ **S06.2X5** **Diffuse traumatic brain injury with loss of consciousness** greater than 24 hours with return to pre-existing conscious levels

✓7ᵗʰ **S06.2X6** **Diffuse traumatic brain injury with loss of consciousness** greater than 24 hours without return to pre-existing conscious level with patient surviving

✓ Additional Character Required   ✓x 7ᵗʰ Xtension Alert   Unspecified Code   Other Specified Code   Manifestation Code   ▶◀ Revised Text   ● New Code   ▲ Revised Code Title

ICD-10-CM 2014 (Draft)   **809**

✓7ᵗʰ **S06.2X7** **Diffuse traumatic brain injury with loss of consciousness of** any duration with death due to brain injury prior to regaining consciousness

✓7ᵗʰ **S06.2X8** **Diffuse traumatic brain injury with loss of consciousness of** any duration with death due to **other** cause prior to regaining consciousness

✓7ᵗʰ **S06.2X9** **Diffuse traumatic brain injury with loss of consciousness of unspecified duration**
Diffuse traumatic brain injury NOS

✓5ᵗʰ **S06.3** **Focal traumatic brain injury**
EXCLUDES 1   any condition classifiable to S06.4-S06.6
focal cerebral edema (S06.1)

✓6ᵗʰ **S06.30** **Unspecified focal traumatic brain injury**

✓7ᵗʰ **S06.300** **Unspecified focal traumatic brain injury** without loss of consciousness

✓7ᵗʰ **S06.301** **Unspecified focal traumatic brain injury with loss of consciousness of** 30 minutes or less

✓7ᵗʰ **S06.302** **Unspecified focal traumatic brain injury with loss of consciousness of** 31 minutes to 59 minutes

✓7ᵗʰ **S06.303** **Unspecified focal traumatic brain injury with loss of consciousness of** 1 hour to 5 hours 59 minutes

✓7ᵗʰ **S06.304** **Unspecified focal traumatic brain injury with loss of consciousness of** 6 hours to 24 hours

✓7ᵗʰ **S06.305** **Unspecified focal traumatic brain injury with loss of consciousness** greater than 24 hours with return to pre-existing conscious level

✓7ᵗʰ **S06.306** **Unspecified focal traumatic brain injury with loss of consciousness** greater than 24 hours without return to pre-existing conscious level with patient surviving

✓7ᵗʰ **S06.307** **Unspecified focal traumatic brain injury with loss of consciousness of** any duration with death due to brain injury prior to regaining consciousness

✓7ᵗʰ **S06.308** **Unspecified focal traumatic brain injury with loss of** any duration with death due to **other** cause prior to regaining consciousness

✓7ᵗʰ **S06.309** **Unspecified focal traumatic brain injury with loss of consciousness of unspecified duration**
Unspecified focal traumatic brain injury NOS

✓6ᵗʰ **S06.31** **Contusion and laceration of** right cerebrum

✓7ᵗʰ **S06.310** **Contusion and laceration of right cerebrum** without loss of consciousness

✓7ᵗʰ **S06.311** **Contusion and laceration of right cerebrum with loss of consciousness of** 30 minutes or less

✓7ᵗʰ **S06.312** **Contusion and laceration of right cerebrum with loss of consciousness of** 31 minutes to 59 minutes

✓7ᵗʰ **S06.313** **Contusion and laceration of right cerebrum with loss of consciousness of** 1 hour to 5 hours 59 minutes

✓7ᵗʰ **S06.314** **Contusion and laceration of right cerebrum with loss of consciousness of** 6 hours to 24 hours

✓7ᵗʰ **S06.315** **Contusion and laceration of right cerebrum with loss of consciousness** greater than 24 hours with return to pre-existing conscious level

✓7ᵗʰ **S06.316** **Contusion and laceration of right cerebrum with loss of consciousness** greater than 24 hours without return to pre-existing conscious level with patient surviving

✓7ᵗʰ **S06.317** **Contusion and laceration of right cerebrum with loss of consciousness of** any duration with death due to brain injury prior to regaining consciousness

✓7ᵗʰ **S06.318** **Contusion and laceration of right cerebrum with loss of consciousness of** any duration with death due to **other** cause prior to regaining consciousness

✓7ᵗʰ **S06.319** **Contusion and laceration of right cerebrum with loss of consciousness of unspecified duration**
Contusion and laceration of right cerebrum NOS

✓6ᵗʰ **S06.32** **Contusion and laceration of** left cerebrum

✓7ᵗʰ **S06.320** **Contusion and laceration of left cerebrum** without loss of consciousness

✓7ᵗʰ **S06.321** **Contusion and laceration of left cerebrum with loss of consciousness of** 30 minutes or less

✓7ᵗʰ **S06.322** **Contusion and laceration of left cerebrum with loss of consciousness of** 31 minutes to 59 minutes

✓7ᵗʰ **S06.323** **Contusion and laceration of left cerebrum with loss of consciousness of** 1 hour to 5 hours 59 minutes

✓7ᵗʰ **S06.324** **Contusion and laceration of left cerebrum with loss of consciousness of** 6 hours to 24 hours

✓7ᵗʰ **S06.325** **Contusion and laceration of left cerebrum with loss of consciousness** greater than 24 hours with return to pre-existing conscious level

✓7ᵗʰ **S06.326** **Contusion and laceration of left cerebrum with loss of consciousness** greater than 24 hours with return to pre-existing conscious level with patient surviving

✓7ᵗʰ **S06.327** **Contusion and laceration of left cerebrum with loss of consciousness of** any duration with death due to brain injury prior to regaining consciousness

✓7ᵗʰ **S06.328** **Contusion and laceration of left cerebrum with loss of consciousness of** any duration with death due to other cause prior to regaining consciousness

✓7ᵗʰ **S06.329** **Contusion and laceration of left cerebrum with loss of consciousness of unspecified duration**
Contusion and laceration of left cerebrum NOS

✓6ᵗʰ **S06.33** **Contusion and laceration of** cerebrum, unspecified

✓7ᵗʰ **S06.330** **Contusion and laceration of cerebrum, unspecified,** without loss of consciousness

✓7ᵗʰ **S06.331** **Contusion and laceration of cerebrum, unspecified, with loss of consciousness of** 30 minutes or less

✓7ᵗʰ **S06.332** **Contusion and laceration of cerebrum, unspecified, with loss of consciousness of** 31 minutes to 59 minutes

✓7ᵗʰ **S06.333** **Contusion and laceration of cerebrum, unspecified, with loss of consciousness of** 1 hour to 5 hours 59 minutes

✓7ᵗʰ **S06.334** **Contusion and laceration of cerebrum, unspecified, with loss of consciousness of** 6 hours to 24 hours

✓7ᵗʰ **S06.335** **Contusion and laceration of cerebrum, unspecified, with loss of consciousness** greater than 24 hours with return to pre-existing conscious level

✓7ᵗʰ **S06.336** **Contusion and laceration of cerebrum, unspecified, with loss of consciousness** greater than 24 hours without return to pre-existing conscious level with patient surviving

✓7ᵗʰ **S06.337** **Contusion and laceration of cerebrum, unspecified, with loss of consciousness of** any duration with death due to brain injury prior to regaining consciousness

✓7ᵗʰ **S06.338** **Contusion and laceration of cerebrum, unspecified, with loss of consciousness of** any duration with death due to other cause prior to regaining consciousness

☑7ᵗʰ **S06.339 Contusion and laceration of cerebrum, unspecified, with loss of consciousness of unspecified duration**
Contusion and laceration of cerebrum NOS

☑6ᵗʰ **S06.34 Traumatic hemorrhage of** right cerebrum
Traumatic intracerebral hemorrhage and hematoma of right cerebrum

☑7ᵗʰ **S06.340 Traumatic hemorrhage of right cerebrum** without loss of consciousness

☑7ᵗʰ **S06.341 Traumatic hemorrhage of right cerebrum with loss of consciousness of** 30 minutes or less

☑7ᵗʰ **S06.342 Traumatic hemorrhage of right cerebrum with loss of consciousness of** 31 minutes to 59 minutes

☑7ᵗʰ **S06.343 Traumatic hemorrhage of right cerebrum with loss of consciousness of** 1 hours to 5 hours 59 minutes

☑7ᵗʰ **S06.344 Traumatic hemorrhage of right cerebrum with loss of consciousness of** 6 hours to 24 hours

☑7ᵗʰ **S06.345 Traumatic hemorrhage of right cerebrum with loss of consciousness** greater than 24 hours with return to pre-existing conscious level

☑7ᵗʰ **S06.346 Traumatic hemorrhage of right cerebrum with loss of consciousness** greater than 24 hours without return to pre-existing conscious level with patient surviving

☑7ᵗʰ **S06.347 Traumatic hemorrhage of right cerebrum with loss of consciousness of** any duration with death due to brain injury prior to regaining consciousness

☑7ᵗʰ **S06.348 Traumatic hemorrhage of right cerebrum with loss of consciousness of** any duration with death due to **other** cause prior to regaining consciousness

☑7ᵗʰ **S06.349 Traumatic hemorrhage of right cerebrum with loss of consciousness of unspecified duration**
Traumatic hemorrhage of right cerebrum NOS

☑6ᵗʰ **S06.35 Traumatic hemorrhage of** left cerebrum
Traumatic intracerebral hemorrhage and hematoma of left cerebrum

☑7ᵗʰ **S06.350 Traumatic hemorrhage of left cerebrum** without loss of consciousness

☑7ᵗʰ **S06.351 Traumatic hemorrhage of left cerebrum with loss of consciousness of** 30 minutes or less

☑7ᵗʰ **S06.352 Traumatic hemorrhage of left cerebrum with loss of consciousness of** 31 minutes to 59 minutes

☑7ᵗʰ **S06.353 Traumatic hemorrhage of left cerebrum with loss of consciousness of** 1 hours to 5 hours 59 minutes

☑7ᵗʰ **S06.354 Traumatic hemorrhage of left cerebrum with loss of consciousness of** 6 hours to 24 hours

☑7ᵗʰ **S06.355 Traumatic hemorrhage of left cerebrum with loss of consciousness** greater than 24 hours with return to pre-existing conscious level

☑7ᵗʰ **S06.356 Traumatic hemorrhage of left cerebrum with loss of consciousness** greater than 24 hours without return to pre-existing conscious level with patient surviving

☑7ᵗʰ **S06.357 Traumatic hemorrhage of left cerebrum with loss of consciousness of** any duration with death due to brain injury prior to regaining consciousness

☑7ᵗʰ **S06.358 Traumatic hemorrhage of left cerebrum with loss of consciousness of** any duration with death due to **other** cause prior to regaining consciousness

☑7ᵗʰ **S06.359 Traumatic hemorrhage of left cerebrum with loss of consciousness of unspecified duration**
Traumatic hemorrhage of left cerebrum NOS

☑6ᵗʰ **S06.36 Traumatic hemorrhage of** cerebrum, unspecified
Traumatic intracerebral hemorrhage and hematoma, unspecified

☑7ᵗʰ **S06.360 Traumatic hemorrhage of cerebrum, unspecified,** without loss of consciousness

☑7ᵗʰ **S06.361 Traumatic hemorrhage of cerebrum, unspecified, with loss of consciousness of** 30 minutes or less

☑7ᵗʰ **S06.362 Traumatic hemorrhage of cerebrum, unspecified, with loss of consciousness of** 31 minutes to 59 minutes

☑7ᵗʰ **S06.363 Traumatic hemorrhage of cerebrum, unspecified, with loss of consciousness of** 1 hours to 5 hours 59 minutes

☑7ᵗʰ **S06.364 Traumatic hemorrhage of cerebrum, unspecified, with loss of consciousness of** 6 hours to 24 hours

☑7ᵗʰ **S06.365 Traumatic hemorrhage of cerebrum, unspecified, with loss of consciousness** greater than 24 hours with return to pre-existing conscious level

☑7ᵗʰ **S06.366 Traumatic hemorrhage of cerebrum, unspecified, with loss of consciousness** greater than 24 hours without return to pre-existing conscious level with patient surviving

☑7ᵗʰ **S06.367 Traumatic hemorrhage of cerebrum, unspecified, with loss of consciousness of** any duration with death due to brain injury prior to regaining consciousness

☑7ᵗʰ **S06.368 Traumatic hemorrhage of cerebrum, unspecified, with loss of consciousness of** any duration with death due to **other** cause prior to regaining consciousness

☑7ᵗʰ **S06.369 Traumatic hemorrhage of cerebrum, unspecified, with loss of consciousness of unspecified duration**
Traumatic hemorrhage of cerebrum NOS

☑6ᵗʰ **S06.37 Contusion, laceration, and hemorrhage of cerebellum**

☑7ᵗʰ **S06.370 Contusion, laceration, and hemorrhage of cerebellum** without loss of consciousness

☑7ᵗʰ **S06.371 Contusion, laceration, and hemorrhage of cerebellum with loss of consciousness of** 30 minutes or less

☑7ᵗʰ **S06.372 Contusion, laceration, and hemorrhage of cerebellum with loss of consciousness of** 31 minutes to 59 minutes

☑7ᵗʰ **S06.373 Contusion, laceration, and hemorrhage of cerebellum with loss of consciousness of** 1 hour to 5 hours 59 minutes

☑7ᵗʰ **S06.374 Contusion, laceration, and hemorrhage of cerebellum with loss of consciousness of** 6 hours to 24 hours

☑7ᵗʰ **S06.375 Contusion, laceration, and hemorrhage of cerebellum with loss of consciousness** greater than 24 hours with return to pre-existing conscious level

☑7ᵗʰ **S06.376 Contusion, laceration, and hemorrhage of cerebellum with loss of consciousness** greater than 24 hours without return to pre-existing conscious level with patient surviving

☑7ᵗʰ **S06.377 Contusion, laceration, and hemorrhage of cerebellum with loss of consciousness of** any duration with death due to brain injury prior to regaining consciousness

☑7ᵗʰ **S06.378 Contusion, laceration, and hemorrhage of cerebellum with loss of consciousness of** any duration with death due to **other** cause prior to regaining consciousness

☑7ᵗʰ **S06.379 Contusion, laceration, and hemorrhage of cerebellum with loss of consciousness of unspecified duration**
Contusion, laceration, and hemorrhage of cerebellum NOS

☑6ᵗʰ **S06.38 Contusion, laceration, and hemorrhage of** brainstem

☑7ᵗʰ **S06.380 Contusion, laceration, and hemorrhage of brainstem** without loss of consciousness

---

☑ Additional Character Required   ✓ₓ7ᵗʰ Xtension Alert   Unspecified Code   Other Specified Code   Manifestation Code   ►◄ Revised Text   ● New Code   ▲ Revised Code Title

√7ᵗʰ **S06.381** Contusion, laceration, and hemorrhage of brainstem with loss of consciousness of 30 minutes or less

√7ᵗʰ **S06.382** Contusion, laceration, and hemorrhage of brainstem with loss of consciousness of 31 minutes to 59 minutes

√7ᵗʰ **S06.383** Contusion, laceration, and hemorrhage of brainstem with loss of consciousness of 1 hour to 5 hours 59 minutes

√7ᵗʰ **S06.384** Contusion, laceration, and hemorrhage of brainstem with loss of consciousness of 6 hours to 24 hours

√7ᵗʰ **S06.385** Contusion, laceration, and hemorrhage of brainstem with loss of consciousness greater than 24 hours with return to pre-existing conscious level

√7ᵗʰ **S06.386** Contusion, laceration, and hemorrhage of brainstem with loss of consciousness greater than 24 hours without return to pre-existing conscious level with patient surviving

√7ᵗʰ **S06.387** Contusion, laceration, and hemorrhage of brainstem with loss of consciousness of any duration with death due to brain injury prior to regaining consciousness

√7ᵗʰ **S06.388** Contusion, laceration, and hemorrhage of brainstem with loss of consciousness of any duration with death due to other cause prior to regaining consciousness

√7ᵗʰ **S06.389** Contusion, laceration, and hemorrhage of brainstem with loss of consciousness of unspecified duration
    Contusion, laceration, and hemorrhage of brainstem NOS

√5ᵗʰ **S06.4** Epidural hemorrhage
    Extradural hemorrhage NOS
    Extradural hemorrhage (traumatic)

√6ᵗʰ **S06.4X** Epidural hemorrhage

√7ᵗʰ **S06.4X0** Epidural hemorrhage without loss of consciousness

√7ᵗʰ **S06.4X1** Epidural hemorrhage with loss of consciousness of 30 minutes or less

√7ᵗʰ **S06.4X2** Epidural hemorrhage with loss of consciousness of 31 minutes to 59 minutes

√7ᵗʰ **S06.4X3** Epidural hemorrhage with loss of consciousness of 1 hour to 5 hours 59 minutes

√7ᵗʰ **S06.4X4** Epidural hemorrhage with loss of consciousness of 6 hours to 24 hours

√7ᵗʰ **S06.4X5** Epidural hemorrhage with loss of consciousness greater than 24 hours with return to pre-existing conscious level

√7ᵗʰ **S06.4X6** Epidural hemorrhage with loss of consciousness greater than 24 hours without return to pre-existing conscious level with patient surviving

√7ᵗʰ **S06.4X7** Epidural hemorrhage with loss of consciousness of any duration with death due to brain injury prior to regaining consciousness

√7ᵗʰ **S06.4X8** Epidural hemorrhage with loss of consciousness of any duration with death due to other causes prior to regaining consciousness

√7ᵗʰ **S06.4X9** Epidural hemorrhage with loss of consciousness of unspecified duration
    Epidural hemorrhage NOS

√5ᵗʰ **S06.5** Traumatic subdural hemorrhage

√6ᵗʰ **S06.5X** Traumatic subdural hemorrhage

√7ᵗʰ **S06.5X0** Traumatic subdural hemorrhage without loss of consciousness

√7ᵗʰ **S06.5X1** Traumatic subdural hemorrhage with loss of consciousness of 30 minutes or less

√7ᵗʰ **S06.5X2** Traumatic subdural hemorrhage with loss of consciousness of 31 minutes to 59 minutes

√7ᵗʰ **S06.5X3** Traumatic subdural hemorrhage with loss of consciousness of 1 hour to 5 hours 59 minutes

√7ᵗʰ **S06.5X4** Traumatic subdural hemorrhage with loss of consciousness of 6 hours to 24 hours

√7ᵗʰ **S06.5X5** Traumatic subdural hemorrhage with loss of consciousness greater than 24 hours with return to pre-existing conscious level

√7ᵗʰ **S06.5X6** Traumatic subdural hemorrhage with loss of consciousness greater than 24 hours without return to pre-existing conscious level with patient surviving

√7ᵗʰ **S06.5X7** Traumatic subdural hemorrhage with loss of consciousness of any duration with death due to brain injury before regaining consciousness

√7ᵗʰ **S06.5X8** Traumatic subdural hemorrhage with loss of consciousness of any duration with death due to other cause before regaining consciousness

√7ᵗʰ **S06.5X9** Traumatic subdural hemorrhage with loss of consciousness of unspecified duration
    Traumatic subdural hemorrhage NOS

√5ᵗʰ **S06.6** Traumatic subarachnoid hemorrhage

√6ᵗʰ **S06.6X** Traumatic subarachnoid hemorrhage

√7ᵗʰ **S06.6X0** Traumatic subarachnoid hemorrhage without loss of consciousness

√7ᵗʰ **S06.6X1** Traumatic subarachnoid hemorrhage with loss of consciousness of 30 minutes or less

√7ᵗʰ **S06.6X2** Traumatic subarachnoid hemorrhage with loss of consciousness of 31 minutes to 59 minutes

√7ᵗʰ **S06.6X3** Traumatic subarachnoid hemorrhage with loss of consciousness of 1 hour to 5 hours 59 minutes

√7ᵗʰ **S06.6X4** Traumatic subarachnoid hemorrhage with loss of consciousness of 6 hours to 24 hours

√7ᵗʰ **S06.6X5** Traumatic subarachnoid hemorrhage with loss of consciousness greater than 24 hours with return to pre-existing conscious level

√7ᵗʰ **S06.6X6** Traumatic subarachnoid hemorrhage with loss of consciousness greater than 24 hours without return to pre-existing conscious level with patient surviving

√7ᵗʰ **S06.6X7** Traumatic subarachnoid hemorrhage with loss of consciousness of any duration with death due to brain injury prior to regaining consciousness

√7ᵗʰ **S06.6X8** Traumatic subarachnoid hemorrhage with loss of consciousness of any duration with death due to other cause prior to regaining consciousness

√7ᵗʰ **S06.6X9** Traumatic subarachnoid hemorrhage with loss of consciousness of unspecified duration
    Traumatic subarachnoid hemorrhage NOS

√5ᵗʰ **S06.8** Other specified intracranial injuries

√6ᵗʰ **S06.81** Injury of right internal carotid artery, intracranial portion, not elsewhere classified

√7ᵗʰ **S06.810** Injury of right internal carotid artery, intracranial portion, not elsewhere classified without loss of consciousness

√7ᵗʰ **S06.811** Injury of right internal carotid artery, intracranial portion, not elsewhere classified with loss of consciousness of 30 minutes or less

√7ᵗʰ **S06.812** Injury of right internal carotid artery, intracranial portion, not elsewhere classified with loss of consciousness of 31 minutes to 59 minutes

√7ᵗʰ **S06.813** Injury of right internal carotid artery, intracranial portion, not elsewhere classified with loss of consciousness of 1 hour to 5 hours 59 minutes

√7ᵗʰ **S06.814** Injury of right internal carotid artery, intracranial portion, not elsewhere classified with loss of consciousness of 6 hours to 24 hours

---

EXCLUDES1 Not coded here   **EXCLUDES2** Not included here   **N** Newborn Age: 0   **P** Pediatric Age: 0-17   **M** Maternity Age: 12-55   **A** Adult Age: 15-124

✓7ᵗʰ **S06.815** **Injury of right internal carotid artery, intracranial portion, not elsewhere classified with loss of consciousness** greater than 24 hours with return to pre-existing conscious level

✓7ᵗʰ **S06.816** **Injury of right internal carotid artery, intracranial portion, not elsewhere classified with loss of consciousness** greater than 24 hours without return to pre-existing conscious level with patient surviving

✓7ᵗʰ **S06.817** **Injury of right internal carotid artery, intracranial portion, not elsewhere classified with loss of consciousness of** any duration with death due to brain injury prior to regaining consciousness

✓7ᵗʰ **S06.818** **Injury of right internal carotid artery, intracranial portion, not elsewhere classified with loss of consciousness of** any duration with death due to **other** cause prior to regaining consciousness

✓7ᵗʰ **S06.819** **Injury of right internal carotid artery, intracranial portion, not elsewhere classified with loss of consciousness of unspecified duration**
Injury of right internal carotid artery, intracranial portion, not elsewhere classified NOS

✓6ᵗʰ **S06.82** **Injury of** left internal carotid artery, **intracranial portion, not elsewhere classified**

✓7ᵗʰ **S06.820** **Injury of left internal carotid artery, intracranial portion, not elsewhere classified** without loss of consciousness

✓7ᵗʰ **S06.821** **Injury of left internal carotid artery, intracranial portion, not elsewhere classified with loss of consciousness of** 30 minutes or less

✓7ᵗʰ **S06.822** **Injury of left internal carotid artery, intracranial portion, not elsewhere classified with loss of consciousness of** 31 minutes to 59 minutes

✓7ᵗʰ **S06.823** **Injury of left internal carotid artery, intracranial portion, not elsewhere classified with loss of consciousness of** 1 hour to 5 hours 59 minutes

✓7ᵗʰ **S06.824** **Injury of left internal carotid artery, intracranial portion, not elsewhere classified with loss of consciousness of** 6 hours to 24 hours

✓7ᵗʰ **S06.825** **Injury of left internal carotid artery, intracranial portion, not elsewhere classified with loss of consciousness** greater than 24 hours with return to pre-existing conscious level

✓7ᵗʰ **S06.826** **Injury of left internal carotid artery, intracranial portion, not elsewhere classified with loss of consciousness** greater than 24 hours without return to pre-existing conscious level with patient surviving

✓7ᵗʰ **S06.827** **Injury of left internal carotid artery, intracranial portion, not elsewhere classified with loss of consciousness of** any duration with death due to brain injury prior to regaining consciousness

✓7ᵗʰ **S06.828** **Injury of left internal carotid artery, intracranial portion, not elsewhere classified with loss of consciousness of** any duration with death due to other cause prior to regaining consciousness

✓7ᵗʰ **S06.829** **Injury of left internal carotid artery, intracranial portion, not elsewhere classified with loss of consciousness of unspecified duration**
Injury of left internal carotid artery, intracranial portion, not elsewhere classified NOS

✓6ᵗʰ **S06.89** **Other** specified intracranial injury

✓7ᵗʰ **S06.890** **Other specified intracranial injury** without loss of consciousness

✓7ᵗʰ **S06.891** **Other specified intracranial injury with loss of consciousness of** 30 minutes or less

✓7ᵗʰ **S06.892** **Other specified intracranial injury with loss of consciousness of** 31 minutes to 59 minutes

✓7ᵗʰ **S06.893** **Other specified intracranial injury with loss of consciousness of** 1 hour to 5 hours 59 minutes

✓7ᵗʰ **S06.894** **Other specified intracranial injury with loss of consciousness of** 6 hours to 24 hours

✓7ᵗʰ **S06.895** **Other specified intracranial injury with loss of consciousness** greater than 24 hours with return to pre-existing conscious level

✓7ᵗʰ **S06.896** **Other specified intracranial injury with loss of consciousness** greater than 24 hours without return to pre-existing conscious level with patient surviving

✓7ᵗʰ **S06.897** **Other specified intracranial injury with loss of consciousness of** any duration with death due to brain injury prior to regaining consciousness

✓7ᵗʰ **S06.898** **Other specified intracranial injury with loss of consciousness of** any duration with death due to other cause prior to regaining consciousness

✓7ᵗʰ **S06.899** **Other specified intracranial injury with loss of consciousness of unspecified duration**

✓5ᵗʰ **S06.9** **Unspecified intracranial injury**
Brain injury NOS
Head injury NOS with loss of consciousness
EXCLUDES 1 head injury NOS (S09.90)

✓6ᵗʰ **S06.9X** **Unspecified** intracranial injury

✓7ᵗʰ **S06.9X0** **Unspecified intracranial injury** without loss of consciousness

✓7ᵗʰ **S06.9X1** **Unspecified intracranial injury with loss of consciousness of** 30 minutes or less

✓7ᵗʰ **S06.9X2** **Unspecified intracranial injury with loss of consciousness of** 31 minutes to 59 minutes

✓7ᵗʰ **S06.9X3** **Unspecified intracranial injury with loss of consciousness of** 1 hour to 5 hours 59 minutes

✓7ᵗʰ **S06.9X4** **Unspecified intracranial injury with loss of consciousness of** 6 hours to 24 hours

✓7ᵗʰ **S06.9X5** **Unspecified intracranial injury with loss of consciousness** greater than 24 hours with return to pre-existing conscious level

✓7ᵗʰ **S06.9X6** **Unspecified intracranial injury with loss of consciousness** greater than 24 hours without return to pre-existing conscious level with patient surviving

✓7ᵗʰ **S06.9X7** **Unspecified intracranial injury with loss of consciousness of** any duration with death due to brain injury prior to regaining consciousness

✓7ᵗʰ **S06.9X8** **Unspecified intracranial injury with loss of consciousness of** any duration with death due to **other** cause prior to regaining consciousness

✓7ᵗʰ **S06.9X9** **Unspecified intracranial injury with loss of consciousness of unspecified duration**

✓4ᵗʰ **S07** **Crushing injury of head**
Use additional code for all associated injuries, such as:
intracranial injuries (S06.-)
skull fractures (S02.-)

The appropriate 7th character is to be added to each code from category S07.
A   initial encounter
D   subsequent encounter
S   sequela

✓x7ᵗʰ **S07.0** **Crushing injury of** face

✓x7ᵗʰ **S07.1** **Crushing injury of** skull

✓x7ᵗʰ **S07.8** **Crushing injury of** other parts of head

✓x7ᵗʰ **S07.9** **Crushing injury of** head, part unspecified

Injury, Poisoning and Certain Other Consequences of External Causes   S06.815–S07.9

√4ᵗʰ **S08 Avulsion and traumatic amputation of part of head**

> **NOTE** An amputation not identified as partial or complete should be coded to complete

> The appropriate 7th character is to be added to each code from category S08.
> A   initial encounter
> D   subsequent encounter
> S   sequela

√x7ᵗʰ **S08.0 Avulsion of** scalp

√5ᵗʰ **S08.1 Traumatic amputation of ear**

> √6ᵗʰ **S08.11 Complete traumatic amputation of ear**
> > √7ᵗʰ **S08.111 Complete traumatic amputation of** right ear
> > √7ᵗʰ **S08.112 Complete traumatic amputation of** left ear
> > √7ᵗʰ **S08.119 Complete traumatic amputation of unspecified ear**

> √6ᵗʰ **S08.12 Partial traumatic amputation of ear**
> > √7ᵗʰ **S08.121 Partial traumatic amputation of** right ear
> > √7ᵗʰ **S08.122 Partial traumatic amputation of** left ear
> > √7ᵗʰ **S08.129 Partial traumatic amputation of unspecified ear**

√5ᵗʰ **S08.8 Traumatic amputation of** other parts of head

> √6ᵗʰ **S08.81 Traumatic amputation of** nose
> > √7ᵗʰ **S08.811 Complete traumatic amputation of nose**
> > √7ᵗʰ **S08.812 Partial traumatic amputation of nose**

> √x7ᵗʰ **S08.89 Traumatic amputation of other parts of head**

√4ᵗʰ **S09 Other and unspecified injuries of head**

> The appropriate 7th character is to be added to each code from category S09.
> A   initial encounter
> D   subsequent encounter
> S   sequela

√x7ᵗʰ **S09.0 Injury of** blood vessels **of head, not elsewhere classified**
> **EXCLUDES 1** injury of cerebral blood vessels (S06.-)
> injury of precerebral blood vessels (S15.-)

√5ᵗʰ **S09.1 Injury of** muscle and tendon **of head**
> Code also any associated open wound (S01.-)
> **EXCLUDES 2** sprain to joints and ligament of head (S03.9)

> √x7ᵗʰ **S09.10 Unspecified injury of muscle and tendon of head**
> Injury of muscle and tendon of head NOS
> √x7ᵗʰ **S09.11 Strain of muscle and tendon of head**
> √x7ᵗʰ **S09.12 Laceration of muscle and tendon of head**
> √x7ᵗʰ **S09.19 Other specified injury of muscle and tendon of head**

√5ᵗʰ **S09.2 Traumatic rupture of** ear drum
> **EXCLUDES 1** traumatic rupture of ear drum due to blast injury (S09.31-)

> √x7ᵗʰ **S09.20 Traumatic rupture of unspecified ear drum**
> √x7ᵗʰ **S09.21 Traumatic rupture of** right **ear drum**
> √x7ᵗʰ **S09.22 Traumatic rupture of** left **ear drum**

√5ᵗʰ **S09.3 Other specified and unspecified injury of middle and inner ear**
> **EXCLUDES 1** injury to ear NOS (S09.91-)
> **EXCLUDES 2** injury to external ear (S00.4-, S01.3-, S08.1-)

> √6ᵗʰ **S09.30 Unspecified injury of** middle and inner ear
> > √7ᵗʰ **S09.301 Unspecified injury of** right **middle and inner ear**
> > √7ᵗʰ **S09.302 Unspecified injury of** left **middle and inner ear**
> > √7ᵗʰ **S09.309 Unspecified injury of unspecified middle and inner ear**

> √6ᵗʰ **S09.31 Primary** blast injury **of ear**
> Blast injury of ear NOS
> > √7ᵗʰ **S09.311 Primary blast injury of** right **ear**
> > √7ᵗʰ **S09.312 Primary blast injury of** left **ear**
> > √7ᵗʰ **S09.313 Primary blast injury of ear,** bilateral
> > √7ᵗʰ **S09.319 Primary blast injury of unspecified ear**

> √6ᵗʰ **S09.39 Other** specified injury of middle and inner ear
> Secondary blast injury to ear
> > √7ᵗʰ **S09.391 Other specified injury of** right **middle and inner ear**

> > √7ᵗʰ **S09.392 Other specified injury of** left **middle and inner ear**
> > √7ᵗʰ **S09.399 Other specified injury of unspecified middle and inner ear**

√x7ᵗʰ **S09.8 Other specified injuries of head**

√5ᵗʰ **S09.9 Unspecified injury of face and head**

> √x7ᵗʰ **S09.90 Unspecified injury of** head
> Head injury NOS
> **EXCLUDES 1** brain injury NOS (S06.9-)
> head injury NOS with loss of consciousness (S06.9-)
> intracranial injury NOS (S06.9-)

> √x7ᵗʰ **S09.91 Unspecified injury of** ear
> Injury of ear NOS

> √x7ᵗʰ **S09.92 Unspecified injury of** nose
> Injury of nose NOS

> √x7ᵗʰ **S09.93 Unspecified injury of** face
> Injury of face NOS

Injuries to the neck (S10-S19)

INCLUDES injuries of nape
injuries of supraclavicular region
injuries of throat

EXCLUDES 2 burns and corrosions (T20-T32)
effects of foreign body in esophagus (T18.1)
effects of foreign body in larynx (T17.3)
effects of foreign body in pharynx (T17.2)
effects of foreign body in trachea (T17.4)
frostbite (T33-T34)
insect bite or sting, venomous (T63.4)

√4ᵗʰ **S10 Superficial injury of neck**

> The appropriate 7th character is to be added to each code from category S10.
> A   initial encounter
> D   subsequent encounter
> S   sequela

√x7ᵗʰ **S10.0 Contusion of throat**
> Contusion of cervical esophagus
> Contusion of larynx
> Contusion of pharynx
> Contusion of trachea

√5ᵗʰ **S10.1 Other and unspecified superficial injuries of throat**

> √x7ᵗʰ **S10.10 Unspecified superficial injuries of throat**
> √x7ᵗʰ **S10.11 Abrasion of throat**
> √x7ᵗʰ **S10.12 Blister (nonthermal) of throat**
> √x7ᵗʰ **S10.14 External constriction of part of throat**
> √x7ᵗʰ **S10.15 Superficial foreign body of throat**
> Splinter in the throat
> √x7ᵗʰ **S10.16 Insect bite (nonvenomous) of throat**
> √x7ᵗʰ **S10.17 Other superficial** bite **of throat**
> **EXCLUDES 1** open bite of throat (S11.85)

√5ᵗʰ **S10.8 Superficial injury of** other specified parts of neck

> √x7ᵗʰ **S10.80 Unspecified superficial injury of other specified part of neck**
> √x7ᵗʰ **S10.81 Abrasion of other specified part of neck**
> √x7ᵗʰ **S10.82 Blister (nonthermal) of other specified part of neck**
> √x7ᵗʰ **S10.83 Contusion of other specified part of neck**
> √x7ᵗʰ **S10.84 External constriction of other specified part of neck**
> √x7ᵗʰ **S10.85 Superficial** foreign body **of other specified part of neck**
> Splinter in other specified part of neck
> √x7ᵗʰ **S10.86 Insect bite of other specified part of neck**
> √x7ᵗʰ **S10.87 Other superficial** bite **of other specified part of neck**
> **EXCLUDES 1** open bite of other specified parts of neck (S11.85)

√5ᵗʰ **S10.9 Superficial injury of** unspecified part of neck

> √x7ᵗʰ **S10.90 Unspecified superficial injury of unspecified part of neck**
> √x7ᵗʰ **S10.91 Abrasion of unspecified part of neck**
> √x7ᵗʰ **S10.92 Blister (nonthermal) of unspecified part of neck**
> √x7ᵗʰ **S10.93 Contusion of unspecified part of neck**
> √x7ᵗʰ **S10.94 External constriction of unspecified part of neck**
> √x7ᵗʰ **S10.95 Superficial** foreign body **of unspecified part of neck**

EXCLUDES 1 Not coded here   **EXCLUDES 2** Not included here   N Newborn Age: 0   P Pediatric Age: 0-17   M Maternity Age: 12-55   A Adult Age: 15-124

814   ICD-10-CM 2014 (Draft)

☑x7ᵗʰ **S10.96** Insect bite of unspecified part of neck

☑x7ᵗʰ **S10.97** Other superficial bite of unspecified part of neck

☑4ᵗʰ **S11 Open wound of neck**

Code also any associated:
    spinal cord injury (S14.0, S14.1-)
    wound infection

EXCLUDES 2   *open fracture of vertebra (S12- with 7th character B)*

The appropriate 7th character is to be added to each code from category S11.
    A   initial encounter
    D   subsequent encounter
    S   sequela

☑5ᵗʰ **S11.0 Open wound of larynx and trachea**

   ☑6ᵗʰ **S11.01 Open wound of** larynx

     EXCLUDES 2   *open wound of vocal cord (S11.03)*

    ☑7ᵗʰ **S11.011 Laceration without foreign body of larynx**

    ☑7ᵗʰ **S11.012 Laceration with foreign body of larynx**

    ☑7ᵗʰ **S11.013 Puncture wound without foreign body of larynx**

    ☑7ᵗʰ **S11.014 Puncture wound with foreign body of larynx**

    ☑7ᵗʰ **S11.015** Open bite of larynx
       Bite of larynx NOS

    ☑7ᵗʰ **S11.019 Unspecified open wound of larynx**

   ☑6ᵗʰ **S11.02 Open wound of** trachea
     Open wound of cervical trachea
     Open wound of trachea NOS
     EXCLUDES 2   *open wound of thoracic trachea (S27.5-)*

    ☑7ᵗʰ **S11.021 Laceration without foreign body of trachea**

    ☑7ᵗʰ **S11.022 Laceration with foreign body of trachea**

    ☑7ᵗʰ **S11.023 Puncture wound without foreign body of trachea**

    ☑7ᵗʰ **S11.024 Puncture wound with foreign body of trachea**

    ☑7ᵗʰ **S11.025** Open bite of trachea
       Bite of trachea NOS

    ☑7ᵗʰ **S11.029 Unspecified open wound of trachea**

   ☑6ᵗʰ **S11.03 Open wound of** vocal cord

    ☑7ᵗʰ **S11.031 Laceration without foreign body of vocal cord**

    ☑7ᵗʰ **S11.032 Laceration with foreign body of vocal cord**

    ☑7ᵗʰ **S11.033 Puncture wound without foreign body of vocal cord**

    ☑7ᵗʰ **S11.034 Puncture wound with foreign body of vocal cord**

    ☑7ᵗʰ **S11.035** Open bite of vocal cord
       Bite of vocal cord NOS

    ☑7ᵗʰ **S11.039 Unspecified open wound of vocal cord**

☑5ᵗʰ **S11.1 Open wound of** thyroid gland

   ☑x7ᵗʰ **S11.10 Unspecified open wound of thyroid gland**

   ☑x7ᵗʰ **S11.11** Laceration without foreign body of thyroid gland

   ☑x7ᵗʰ **S11.12** Laceration with foreign body of thyroid gland

   ☑x7ᵗʰ **S11.13** Puncture wound without foreign body of thyroid gland

   ☑x7ᵗʰ **S11.14** Puncture wound with foreign body of thyroid gland

   ☑x7ᵗʰ **S11.15** Open bite of thyroid gland
      Bite of thyroid gland NOS

☑5ᵗʰ **S11.2 Open wound of** pharynx and cervical esophagus

    EXCLUDES 1   *open wound of esophagus NOS (S27.8-)*

   ☑x7ᵗʰ **S11.20 Unspecified open wound of pharynx and cervical esophagus**

   ☑x7ᵗʰ **S11.21** Laceration without foreign body of pharynx and cervical esophagus

   ☑x7ᵗʰ **S11.22** Laceration with foreign body of pharynx and cervical esophagus

   ☑x7ᵗʰ **S11.23** Puncture wound without foreign body of pharynx and cervical esophagus

   ☑x7ᵗʰ **S11.24** Puncture wound with foreign body of pharynx and cervical esophagus

   ☑x7ᵗʰ **S11.25** Open bite of pharynx and cervical esophagus
      Bite of pharynx and cervical esophagus NOS

☑5ᵗʰ **S11.8 Open wound of** other specified parts of neck

   ☑x7ᵗʰ **S11.80 Unspecified open wound of other specified part of neck**

   ☑x7ᵗʰ **S11.81** Laceration without foreign body of other specified part of neck

   ☑x7ᵗʰ **S11.82** Laceration with foreign body of other specified part of neck

   ☑x7ᵗʰ **S11.83** Puncture wound without foreign body of other specified part of neck

   ☑x7ᵗʰ **S11.84** Puncture wound with foreign body of other specified part of neck

   ☑x7ᵗʰ **S11.85** Open bite of other specified part of neck
      Bite of other specified part of neck NOS
      EXCLUDES 1   *superficial bite of other specified part of neck (S10.87)*

   ☑x7ᵗʰ **S11.89** Other open wound of other specified part of neck

☑5ᵗʰ **S11.9 Open wound of** unspecified part of neck

   ☑x7ᵗʰ **S11.90 Unspecified open wound of unspecified part of neck**

   ☑x7ᵗʰ **S11.91** Laceration without foreign body of unspecified part of neck

   ☑x7ᵗʰ **S11.92** Laceration with foreign body of unspecified part of neck

   ☑x7ᵗʰ **S11.93** Puncture wound without foreign body of unspecified part of neck

   ☑x7ᵗʰ **S11.94** Puncture wound with foreign body of unspecified part of neck

   ☑x7ᵗʰ **S11.95** Open bite of unspecified part of neck
      Bite of neck NOS
      EXCLUDES 1   *superficial bite of neck (S10.97)*

☑4ᵗʰ **S12 Fracture of cervical vertebra and other parts of neck**

   NOTE   A fracture not indicated as nondisplaced or displaced should be classified to displaced.
      A fracture not indicated as open or closed should be coded to closed.

   INCLUDES   fracture of cervical neural arch
      fracture of cervical spine
      fracture of cervical spinous process
      fracture of cervical transverse process
      fracture of cervical vertebral arch
      fracture of neck

Code first any associated cervical spinal cord injury (S14.0, S14.1-)

The appropriate 7th character is to be added to all codes from subcategories S12.0-S12.6.
   A   initial encounter for closed fracture
   B   initial encounter for open fracture
   D   subsequent encounter for fracture with routine healing
   G   subsequent encounter for fracture with delayed healing
   K   subsequent encounter for fracture with nonunion
   S   sequela

☑5ᵗʰ **S12.0 Fracture of first cervical vertebra**
    Atlas

   ☑6ᵗʰ **S12.00 Unspecified fracture of first cervical vertebra**

    ☑7ᵗʰ **S12.000 Unspecified displaced fracture of first cervical vertebra**

    ☑7ᵗʰ **S12.001 Unspecified nondisplaced fracture of first cervical vertebra**

   ☑x7ᵗʰ **S12.01** Stable burst fracture of first cervical vertebra

   ☑x7ᵗʰ **S12.02** Unstable burst fracture of first cervical vertebra

   ☑6ᵗʰ **S12.03** Posterior arch fracture of first cervical vertebra

    ☑7ᵗʰ **S12.030** Displaced posterior arch fracture of first cervical vertebra

    ☑7ᵗʰ **S12.031** Nondisplaced posterior arch fracture of first cervical vertebra

   ☑6ᵗʰ **S12.04** Lateral mass fracture of first cervical vertebra

    ☑7ᵗʰ **S12.040** Displaced lateral mass fracture of first cervical vertebra

    ☑7ᵗʰ **S12.041** Nondisplaced lateral mass fracture of first cervical vertebra

   ☑x7ᵗʰ **S12.09** Other fracture of first cervical vertebra

    ☑7ᵗʰ **S12.090** Other displaced fracture of first cervical vertebra

    ☑7ᵗʰ **S12.091** Other nondisplaced fracture of first cervical vertebra

☑ Additional Character Required   ☑x7ᵗʰ Xtension Alert   Unspecified Code   Other Specified Code   Manifestation Code   ▶◀ Revised Text   ● New Code   ▲ Revised Code Title

ICD-10-CM 2014 (Draft)   **815**

Injury, Poisoning and Certain Other Consequences of External Causes

S12.1–S12.590

√5ᵗʰ **S12.1** Fracture of second cervical vertebra
Axis

  √6ᵗʰ **S12.10** Unspecified fracture of second cervical vertebra

    √7ᵗʰ **S12.100** Unspecified displaced fracture of second cervical vertebra

    √7ᵗʰ **S12.101** Unspecified nondisplaced fracture of second cervical vertebra

  √6ᵗʰ **S12.11** Type II dens fracture

    √7ᵗʰ **S12.110** Anterior displaced Type II dens fracture

    √7ᵗʰ **S12.111** Posterior displaced Type II dens fracture

    √7ᵗʰ **S12.112** Nondisplaced Type II dens fracture

  √6ᵗʰ **S12.12** Other dens fracture

    √7ᵗʰ **S12.120** Other displaced dens fracture

    √7ᵗʰ **S12.121** Other nondisplaced dens fracture

  √6ᵗʰ **S12.13** Unspecified traumatic spondylolisthesis of second cervical vertebra

    √7ᵗʰ **S12.130** Unspecified traumatic displaced spondylolisthesis of second cervical vertebra

    √7ᵗʰ **S12.131** Unspecified traumatic nondisplaced spondylolisthesis of second cervical vertebra

  √x7ᵗʰ **S12.14** Type III traumatic spondylolisthesis of second cervical vertebra

  √6ᵗʰ **S12.15** Other traumatic spondylolisthesis of second cervical vertebra

    √7ᵗʰ **S12.150** Other traumatic displaced spondylolisthesis of second cervical vertebra

    √7ᵗʰ **S12.151** Other traumatic nondisplaced spondylolisthesis of second cervical vertebra

  √6ᵗʰ **S12.19** Other fracture of second cervical vertebra

    √7ᵗʰ **S12.190** Other displaced fracture of second cervical vertebra

    √7ᵗʰ **S12.191** Other nondisplaced fracture of second cervical vertebra

√5ᵗʰ **S12.2** Fracture of third cervical vertebra

  √6ᵗʰ **S12.20** Unspecified fracture of third cervical vertebra

    √7ᵗʰ **S12.200** Unspecified displaced fracture of third cervical vertebra

    √7ᵗʰ **S12.201** Unspecified nondisplaced fracture of third cervical vertebra

  √6ᵗʰ **S12.23** Unspecified traumatic spondylolisthesis of third cervical vertebra

    √7ᵗʰ **S12.230** Unspecified traumatic displaced spondylolisthesis of third cervical vertebra

    √7ᵗʰ **S12.231** Unspecified traumatic nondisplaced spondylolisthesis of third cervical vertebra

  √x7ᵗʰ **S12.24** Type III traumatic spondylolisthesis of third cervical vertebra

  √6ᵗʰ **S12.25** Other traumatic spondylolisthesis of third cervical vertebra

    √7ᵗʰ **S12.250** Other traumatic displaced spondylolisthesis of third cervical vertebra

    √7ᵗʰ **S12.251** Other traumatic nondisplaced spondylolisthesis of third cervical vertebra

  √6ᵗʰ **S12.29** Other fracture of third cervical vertebra

    √7ᵗʰ **S12.290** Other displaced fracture of third cervical vertebra

    √7ᵗʰ **S12.291** Other nondisplaced fracture of third cervical vertebra

√5ᵗʰ **S12.3** Fracture of fourth cervical vertebra

  √6ᵗʰ **S12.30** Unspecified fracture of fourth cervical vertebra

    √7ᵗʰ **S12.300** Unspecified displaced fracture of fourth cervical vertebra

    √7ᵗʰ **S12.301** Unspecified nondisplaced fracture of fourth cervical vertebra

  √6ᵗʰ **S12.33** Unspecified traumatic spondylolisthesis of fourth cervical vertebra

    √7ᵗʰ **S12.330** Unspecified traumatic displaced spondylolisthesis of fourth cervical vertebra

    √7ᵗʰ **S12.331** Unspecified traumatic nondisplaced spondylolisthesis of fourth cervical vertebra

  √x7ᵗʰ **S12.34** Type III traumatic spondylolisthesis of fourth cervical vertebra

  √6ᵗʰ **S12.35** Other traumatic spondylolisthesis of fourth cervical vertebra

    √7ᵗʰ **S12.350** Other traumatic displaced spondylolisthesis of fourth cervical vertebra

    √7ᵗʰ **S12.351** Other traumatic nondisplaced spondylolisthesis of fourth cervical vertebra

  √6ᵗʰ **S12.39** Other fracture of fourth cervical vertebra

    √7ᵗʰ **S12.390** Other displaced fracture of fourth cervical vertebra

    √7ᵗʰ **S12.391** Other nondisplaced fracture of fourth cervical vertebra

√5ᵗʰ **S12.4** Fracture of fifth cervical vertebra

  √6ᵗʰ **S12.40** Unspecified fracture of fifth cervical vertebra

    √7ᵗʰ **S12.400** Unspecified displaced fracture of fifth cervical vertebra

    √7ᵗʰ **S12.401** Unspecified nondisplaced fracture of fifth cervical vertebra

  √6ᵗʰ **S12.43** Unspecified traumatic spondylolisthesis of fifth cervical vertebra

    √7ᵗʰ **S12.430** Unspecified traumatic displaced spondylolisthesis of fifth cervical vertebra

    √7ᵗʰ **S12.431** Unspecified traumatic nondisplaced spondylolisthesis of fifth cervical vertebra

  √x7ᵗʰ **S12.44** Type III traumatic spondylolisthesis of fifth cervical vertebra

  √6ᵗʰ **S12.45** Other traumatic spondylolisthesis of fifth cervical vertebra

    √7ᵗʰ **S12.450** Other traumatic displaced spondylolisthesis of fifth cervical vertebra

    √7ᵗʰ **S12.451** Other traumatic nondisplaced spondylolisthesis of fifth cervical vertebra

  √6ᵗʰ **S12.49** Other fracture of fifth cervical vertebra

    √7ᵗʰ **S12.490** Other displaced fracture of fifth cervical vertebra

    √7ᵗʰ **S12.491** Other nondisplaced fracture of fifth cervical vertebra

√5ᵗʰ **S12.5** Fracture of sixth cervical vertebra

  √6ᵗʰ **S12.50** Unspecified fracture of sixth cervical vertebra

    √7ᵗʰ **S12.500** Unspecified displaced fracture of sixth cervical vertebra

    √7ᵗʰ **S12.501** Unspecified nondisplaced fracture of sixth cervical vertebra

  √6ᵗʰ **S12.53** Unspecified traumatic spondylolisthesis of sixth cervical vertebra

    √7ᵗʰ **S12.530** Unspecified traumatic displaced spondylolisthesis of sixth cervical vertebra

    √7ᵗʰ **S12.531** Unspecified traumatic nondisplaced spondylolisthesis of sixth cervical vertebra

  √x7ᵗʰ **S12.54** Type III traumatic spondylolisthesis of sixth cervical vertebra

  √6ᵗʰ **S12.55** Other traumatic spondylolisthesis of sixth cervical vertebra

    √7ᵗʰ **S12.550** Other traumatic displaced spondylolisthesis of sixth cervical vertebra

    √7ᵗʰ **S12.551** Other traumatic nondisplaced spondylolisthesis of sixth cervical vertebra

  √6ᵗʰ **S12.59** Other fracture of sixth cervical vertebra

    √7ᵗʰ **S12.590** Other displaced fracture of sixth cervical vertebra

EXCLUDES 1 Not coded here   EXCLUDES 2 Not included here   N Newborn Age: 0   P Pediatric Age: 0-17   M Maternity Age: 12-55   A Adult Age: 15-124

816   ICD-10-CM 2014 (Draft)

√7ᵗʰ **S12.591** **Other nondisplaced fracture of sixth cervical vertebra**

√6ᵗʰ **S12.6 Fracture of seventh cervical vertebra**

√6ᵗʰ **S12.60** **Unspecified fracture of seventh cervical vertebra**

√7ᵗʰ **S12.600** **Unspecified displaced fracture of seventh cervical vertebra**

√7ᵗʰ **S12.601** **Unspecified nondisplaced fracture of seventh cervical vertebra**

√6ᵗʰ **S12.63** **Unspecified traumatic spondylolisthesis of seventh cervical vertebra**

√7ᵗʰ **S12.630** **Unspecified traumatic displaced spondylolisthesis of seventh cervical vertebra**

√7ᵗʰ **S12.631** **Unspecified traumatic nondisplaced spondylolisthesis of seventh cervical vertebra**

√x7ᵗʰ **S12.64** **Type III traumatic spondylolisthesis of seventh cervical vertebra**

√6ᵗʰ **S12.65** **Other traumatic spondylolisthesis of seventh cervical vertebra**

√7ᵗʰ **S12.650** **Other traumatic displaced spondylolisthesis of seventh cervical vertebra**

√7ᵗʰ **S12.651** **Other traumatic nondisplaced spondylolisthesis of seventh cervical vertebra**

√6ᵗʰ **S12.69** **Other fracture of seventh cervical vertebra**

√7ᵗʰ **S12.690** **Other displaced fracture of seventh cervical vertebra**

√7ᵗʰ **S12.691** **Other nondisplaced fracture of seventh cervical vertebra**

√x7ᵗʰ **S12.8 Fracture of other parts of neck**

The appropriate 7th character is to be added to code S12.8.
A   initial encounter
D   subsequent encounter
S   sequela

Hyoid bone
Larynx
Thyroid cartilage
Trachea

√x7ᵗʰ **S12.9 Fracture of neck, unspecified**

The appropriate 7th character is to be added to code S12.9.
A   initial encounter
D   subsequent encounter
S   sequela

Fracture of cervical spine NOS
Fracture of cervical vertebra NOS
Fracture of neck NOS

√4ᵗʰ **S13 Dislocation and sprain of joints and ligaments at neck level**

INCLUDES   avulsion of joint or ligament at neck level
laceration of cartilage, joint or ligament at neck level
sprain of cartilage, joint or ligament at neck level
traumatic hemarthrosis of joint or ligament at neck level
traumatic rupture of joint or ligament at neck level
traumatic subluxation of joint or ligament at neck level
traumatic tear of joint or ligament at neck level

Code also: any associated open wound
EXCLUDES 2   *strain of muscle or tendon at neck level (S16.1)*

The appropriate 7th character is to be added to each code from
category S13.
A   initial encounter
D   subsequent encounter
S   sequela

√x7ᵗʰ **S13.0 Traumatic rupture of cervical intervertebral disc**

EXCLUDES 1   *rupture or displacement (nontraumatic) of cervical intervertebral disc NOS (M50.-)*

√5ᵗʰ **S13.1 Subluxation and dislocation of cervical vertebrae**

Code also any associated:
open wound of neck (S11.-)
spinal cord injury (S14.1-)
EXCLUDES 2   *fracture of cervical vertebrae (S12.0--S12.3-)*

√6ᵗʰ **S13.10** **Subluxation and dislocation of unspecified cervical vertebrae**

√7ᵗʰ **S13.100** **Subluxation of unspecified cervical vertebra**

√7ᵗʰ **S13.101** **Dislocation of unspecified cervical vertebrae**

√6ᵗʰ **S13.11** **Subluxation and dislocation of C0/C1 cervical vertebrae**

Subluxation and dislocation of atlantooccipital joint
Subluxation and dislocation of atloidooccipital joint
Subluxation and dislocation of occipitoatloid joint

√7ᵗʰ **S13.110** **Subluxation of C0/C1 cervical vertebrae**

√7ᵗʰ **S13.111** **Dislocation of C0/C1 cervical vertebrae**

√6ᵗʰ **S13.12** **Subluxation and dislocation of C1/C2 cervical vertebrae**

Subluxation and dislocation of atlantoaxial joint

√7ᵗʰ **S13.120** **Subluxation of C1/C2 cervical vertebrae**

√7ᵗʰ **S13.121** **Dislocation of C1/C2 cervical vertebrae**

√6ᵗʰ **S13.13** **Subluxation and dislocation of C2/C3 cervical vertebrae**

√7ᵗʰ **S13.130** **Subluxation of C2/C3 cervical vertebrae**

√7ᵗʰ **S13.131** **Dislocation of C2/C3 cervical vertebrae**

√6ᵗʰ **S13.14** **Subluxation and dislocation of C3/C4 cervical vertebrae**

√7ᵗʰ **S13.140** **Subluxation of C3/C4 cervical vertebrae**

√7ᵗʰ **S13.141** **Dislocation of C3/C4 cervical vertebrae**

√6ᵗʰ **S13.15** **Subluxation and dislocation of C4/C5 cervical vertebrae**

√7ᵗʰ **S13.150** **Subluxation of C4/C5 cervical vertebrae**

√7ᵗʰ **S13.151** **Dislocation of C4/C5 cervical vertebrae**

√6ᵗʰ **S13.16** **Subluxation and dislocation of C5/C6 cervical vertebrae**

√7ᵗʰ **S13.160** **Subluxation of C5/C6 cervical vertebrae**

√7ᵗʰ **S13.161** **Dislocation of C5/C6 cervical vertebrae**

√6ᵗʰ **S13.17** **Subluxation and dislocation of C6/C7 cervical vertebrae**

√7ᵗʰ **S13.170** **Subluxation of C6/C7 cervical vertebrae**

√7ᵗʰ **S13.171** **Dislocation of C6/C7 cervical vertebrae**

√6ᵗʰ **S13.18** **Subluxation and dislocation of C7/T1 cervical vertebrae**

√7ᵗʰ **S13.180** **Subluxation of C7/T1 cervical vertebrae**

√7ᵗʰ **S13.181** **Dislocation of C7/T1 cervical vertebrae**

√5ᵗʰ **S13.2 Dislocation of other and unspecified parts of neck**

√x7ᵗʰ **S13.20** **Dislocation of unspecified parts of neck**

√x7ᵗʰ **S13.29** **Dislocation of other parts of neck**

√x7ᵗʰ **S13.4 Sprain of ligaments of cervical spine**

Sprain of anterior longitudinal (ligament), cervical
Sprain of atlanto-axial (joints)
Sprain of atlanto-occipital (joints)
Whiplash injury of cervical spine

√x7ᵗʰ **S13.5 Sprain of thyroid region**

Sprain of cricoarytenoid (joint) (ligament)
Sprain of cricothyroid (joint) (ligament)
Sprain of thyroid cartilage

√x7ᵗʰ **S13.8 Sprain of joints and ligaments of other parts of neck**

√x7ᵗʰ **S13.9 Sprain of joints and ligaments of unspecified parts of neck**

√4ᵗʰ **S14 Injury of nerves and spinal cord at neck level**

NOTE   Code to highest level of cervical cord injury.

Code also any associated:
fracture of cervical vertebra (S12.0--S12.6-)
open wound of neck (S11.-)
transient paralysis (R29.5)

The appropriate 7th character is to be added to each code from
category S14.
A   initial encounter
D   subsequent encounter
S   sequela

√x7ᵗʰ **S14.0 Concussion and edema of cervical spinal cord**

√5ᵗʰ **S14.1 Other and unspecified injuries of cervical spinal cord**

√6ᵗʰ **S14.10** **Unspecified injury of cervical spinal cord**

√7ᵗʰ **S14.101** **Unspecified injury at C1 level of cervical spinal cord**

√7ᵗʰ **S14.102** **Unspecified injury at C2 level of cervical spinal cord**

√7ᵗʰ **S14.103** **Unspecified injury at C3 level of cervical spinal cord**

☑ Additional Character Required   √x7ᵗʰ Xtension Alert   Unspecified Code   Other Specified Code   Manifestation Code   ▶◀ Revised Text   ● New Code   ▲ Revised Code Title

Injury, Poisoning and Certain Other Consequences of External Causes

S14.104–S15.029

√7th **S14.104** **Unspecified injury at** C4 level **of cervical spinal cord**

√7th **S14.105** **Unspecified injury at** C5 level **of cervical spinal cord**

√7th **S14.106** **Unspecified injury at** C6 level **of cervical spinal cord**

√7th **S14.107** **Unspecified injury at** C7 level **of cervical spinal cord**

√7th **S14.108** **Unspecified injury at** C8 level **of cervical spinal cord**

√7th **S14.109** **Unspecified injury at unspecified level of cervical spinal cord**
   Injury of cervical spinal cord NOS

√6th **S14.11** Complete lesion **of cervical spinal cord**

√7th **S14.111** **Complete lesion at** C1 level **of cervical spinal cord**

√7th **S14.112** **Complete lesion at** C2 level **of cervical spinal cord**

√7th **S14.113** **Complete lesion at** C3 level **of cervical spinal cord**

√7th **S14.114** **Complete lesion at** C4 level **of cervical spinal cord**

√7th **S14.115** **Complete lesion at** C5 level **of cervical spinal cord**

√7th **S14.116** **Complete lesion at** C6 level **of cervical spinal cord**

√7th **S14.117** **Complete lesion at** C7 level **of cervical spinal cord**

√7th **S14.118** **Complete lesion at** C8 level **of cervical spinal cord**

√7th **S14.119** **Complete lesion at unspecified level of cervical spinal cord**

√6th **S14.12** Central cord syndrome **of cervical spinal cord**

√7th **S14.121** **Central cord syndrome at** C1 level **of cervical spinal cord**

√7th **S14.122** **Central cord syndrome at** C2 level **of cervical spinal cord**

√7th **S14.123** **Central cord syndrome at** C3 level **of cervical spinal cord**

√7th **S14.124** **Central cord syndrome at** C4 level **of cervical spinal cord**

√7th **S14.125** **Central cord syndrome at** C5 level **of cervical spinal cord**

√7th **S14.126** **Central cord syndrome at** C6 level **of cervical spinal cord**

√7th **S14.127** **Central cord syndrome at** C7 level **of cervical spinal cord**

√7th **S14.128** **Central cord syndrome at** C8 level **of cervical spinal cord**

√7th **S14.129** **Central cord syndrome at unspecified level of cervical spinal cord**

√6th **S14.13** Anterior cord syndrome **of cervical spinal cord**

√7th **S14.131** **Anterior cord syndrome at** C1 level **of cervical spinal cord**

√7th **S14.132** **Anterior cord syndrome at** C2 level **of cervical spinal cord**

√7th **S14.133** **Anterior cord syndrome at** C3 level **of cervical spinal cord**

√7th **S14.134** **Anterior cord syndrome at** C4 level **of cervical spinal cord**

√7th **S14.135** **Anterior cord syndrome at** C5 level **of cervical spinal cord**

√7th **S14.136** **Anterior cord syndrome at** C6 level **of cervical spinal cord**

√7th **S14.137** **Anterior cord syndrome at** C7 level **of cervical spinal cord**

√7th **S14.138** **Anterior cord syndrome at** C8 level **of cervical spinal cord**

√7th **S14.139** **Anterior cord syndrome at unspecified level of cervical spinal cord**

√6th **S14.14** Brown-Séquard syndrome **of cervical spinal cord**

√7th **S14.141** **Brown-Séquard syndrome at** C1 level **of cervical spinal cord**

√7th **S14.142** **Brown-Séquard syndrome at** C2 level **of cervical spinal cord**

√7th **S14.143** **Brown-Séquard syndrome at** C3 level **of cervical spinal cord**

√7th **S14.144** **Brown-Séquard syndrome at** C4 level **of cervical spinal cord**

√7th **S14.145** **Brown-Séquard syndrome at** C5 level **of cervical spinal cord**

√7th **S14.146** **Brown-Séquard syndrome at** C6 level **of cervical spinal cord**

√7th **S14.147** **Brown-Séquard syndrome at** C7 level **of cervical spinal cord**

√7th **S14.148** **Brown-Séquard syndrome at** C8 level **of cervical spinal cord**

√7th **S14.149** **Brown-Séquard syndrome at unspecified level of cervical spinal cord**

√6th **S14.15** Other incomplete lesions **of cervical spinal cord**
   Incomplete lesion of cervical spinal cord NOS
   Posterior cord syndrome of cervical spinal cord

√7th **S14.151** **Other incomplete lesion at** C1 level **of cervical spinal cord**

√7th **S14.152** **Other incomplete lesion at** C2 level **of cervical spinal cord**

√7th **S14.153** **Other incomplete lesion at** C3 level **of cervical spinal cord**

√7th **S14.154** **Other incomplete lesion at** C4 level **of cervical spinal cord**

√7th **S14.155** **Other incomplete lesion at** C5 level **of cervical spinal cord**

√7th **S14.156** **Other incomplete lesion at** C6 level **of cervical spinal cord**

√7th **S14.157** **Other incomplete lesion at** C7 level **of cervical spinal cord**

√7th **S14.158** **Other incomplete lesion at** C8 level **of cervical spinal cord**

√7th **S14.159** **Other incomplete lesion at unspecified level of cervical spinal cord**

√x7th **S14.2** **Injury of** nerve root of cervical spine

√x7th **S14.3** **Injury of** brachial plexus

√x7th **S14.4** **Injury of** peripheral nerves of neck

√x7th **S14.5** **Injury of** cervical sympathetic nerves

√x7th **S14.8** **Injury of other specified nerves of neck**

√x7th **S14.9** **Injury of unspecified nerves of neck**

√4th **S15** **Injury of blood vessels at neck level**
   Code also any associated open wound (S11.-)

> The appropriate 7th character is to be added to each code from category S15.
> A   initial encounter
> D   subsequent encounter
> S   sequela

√5th **S15.0** **Injury of** carotid artery **of neck**
   Injury of carotid artery (common) (external) (internal, extracranial portion)
   Injury of carotid artery NOS
   EXCLUDES 1 injury of internal carotid artery, intracranial portion (S06.8)

√6th **S15.00** Unspecified **injury of carotid artery**

√7th **S15.001** **Unspecified injury of** right **carotid artery**

√7th **S15.002** **Unspecified injury of** left **carotid artery**

√7th **S15.009** **Unspecified injury of unspecified carotid artery**

√6th **S15.01** Minor laceration **of carotid artery**
   Incomplete transection of carotid artery
   Laceration of carotid artery NOS
   Superficial laceration of carotid artery

√7th **S15.011** **Minor laceration of** right **carotid artery**

√7th **S15.012** **Minor laceration of** left **carotid artery**

√7th **S15.019** **Minor laceration of unspecified carotid artery**

√6th **S15.02** Major laceration **of carotid artery**
   Complete transection of carotid artery
   Traumatic rupture of carotid artery

√7th **S15.021** **Major laceration of** right **carotid artery**

√7th **S15.022** **Major laceration of** left **carotid artery**

√7th **S15.029** **Major laceration of unspecified carotid artery**

EXCLUDES 1 Not coded here   **EXCLUDES 2** Not included here   **N** Newborn Age: 0   **P** Pediatric Age: 0-17   **M** Maternity Age: 12-55   **A** Adult Age: 15-124

818   ICD-10-CM 2014 (Draft)

√6ᵗʰ **S15.09** Other **specified injury of carotid artery**

  √7ᵗʰ **S15.091** **Other specified injury of** right **carotid artery**

  √7ᵗʰ **S15.092** **Other specified injury of** left **carotid artery**

  √7ᵗʰ **S15.099** **Other specified injury of unspecified carotid artery**

√5ᵗʰ **S15.1** Injury of vertebral artery

√6ᵗʰ **S15.10** Unspecified **injury of vertebral artery**

  √7ᵗʰ **S15.101** **Unspecified injury of** right **vertebral artery**

  √7ᵗʰ **S15.102** **Unspecified injury of** left **vertebral artery**

  √7ᵗʰ **S15.109** **Unspecified injury of unspecified vertebral artery**

√6ᵗʰ **S15.11** Minor laceration **of vertebral artery**

  Incomplete transection of vertebral artery
  Laceration of vertebral artery NOS
  Superficial laceration of vertebral artery

  √7ᵗʰ **S15.111** **Minor laceration of** right **vertebral artery**

  √7ᵗʰ **S15.112** **Minor laceration of** left **vertebral artery**

  √7ᵗʰ **S15.119** **Minor laceration of unspecified vertebral artery**

√6ᵗʰ **S15.12** Major laceration **of vertebral artery**

  Complete transection of vertebral artery
  Traumatic rupture of vertebral artery

  √7ᵗʰ **S15.121** **Major laceration of** right **vertebral artery**

  √7ᵗʰ **S15.122** **Major laceration of** left **vertebral artery**

  √7ᵗʰ **S15.129** **Major laceration of unspecified vertebral artery**

√6ᵗʰ **S15.19** Other **specified injury of vertebral artery**

  √7ᵗʰ **S15.191** **Other specified injury of** right **vertebral artery**

  √7ᵗʰ **S15.192** **Other specified injury of** left **vertebral artery**

  √7ᵗʰ **S15.199** **Other specified injury of unspecified vertebral artery**

√5ᵗʰ **S15.2** Injury of external jugular vein

√6ᵗʰ **S15.20** Unspecified **injury of external jugular vein**

  √7ᵗʰ **S15.201** **Unspecified injury of** right **external jugular vein**

  √7ᵗʰ **S15.202** **Unspecified injury of** left **external jugular vein**

  √7ᵗʰ **S15.209** **Unspecified injury of unspecified external jugular vein**

√6ᵗʰ **S15.21** Minor laceration **of external jugular vein**

  Incomplete transection of external jugular vein
  Laceration of external jugular vein NOS
  Superficial laceration of external jugular vein

  √7ᵗʰ **S15.211** **Minor laceration of** right **external jugular vein**

  √7ᵗʰ **S15.212** **Minor laceration of** left **external jugular vein**

  √7ᵗʰ **S15.219** **Minor laceration of unspecified external jugular vein**

√6ᵗʰ **S15.22** Major laceration **of external jugular vein**

  Complete transection of external jugular vein
  Traumatic rupture of external jugular vein

  √7ᵗʰ **S15.221** **Major laceration of** right **external jugular vein**

  √7ᵗʰ **S15.222** **Major laceration of** left **external jugular vein**

  √7ᵗʰ **S15.229** **Major laceration of unspecified external jugular vein**

√6ᵗʰ **S15.29** Other **specified injury of external jugular vein**

  √7ᵗʰ **S15.291** **Other specified injury of** right **external jugular vein**

  √7ᵗʰ **S15.292** **Other specified injury of** left **external jugular vein**

  √7ᵗʰ **S15.299** **Other specified injury of unspecified external jugular vein**

√5ᵗʰ **S15.3** Injury of internal jugular vein

√6ᵗʰ **S15.30** Unspecified **injury of internal jugular vein**

  √7ᵗʰ **S15.301** **Unspecified injury of** right **internal jugular vein**

  √7ᵗʰ **S15.302** **Unspecified injury of** left **internal jugular vein**

  √7ᵗʰ **S15.309** **Unspecified injury of unspecified internal jugular vein**

√6ᵗʰ **S15.31** Minor laceration **of internal jugular vein**

  Incomplete transection of internal jugular vein
  Laceration of internal jugular vein NOS
  Superficial laceration of internal jugular vein

  √7ᵗʰ **S15.311** **Minor laceration of** right **internal jugular vein**

  √7ᵗʰ **S15.312** **Minor laceration of** left **internal jugular vein**

  √7ᵗʰ **S15.319** **Minor laceration of unspecified internal jugular vein**

√6ᵗʰ **S15.32** Major laceration **of internal jugular vein**

  Complete transection of internal jugular vein
  Traumatic rupture of internal jugular vein

  √7ᵗʰ **S15.321** **Major laceration of** right **internal jugular vein**

  √7ᵗʰ **S15.322** **Major laceration of** left **internal jugular vein**

  √7ᵗʰ **S15.329** **Major laceration of unspecified internal jugular vein**

√6ᵗʰ **S15.39** Other **specified injury of internal jugular vein**

  √7ᵗʰ **S15.391** **Other specified injury of** right **internal jugular vein**

  √7ᵗʰ **S15.392** **Other specified injury of** left **internal jugular vein**

  √7ᵗʰ **S15.399** **Other specified injury of unspecified internal jugular vein**

√x7ᵗʰ **S15.8** **Injury of other specified blood vessels at neck level**

√x7ᵗʰ **S15.9** **Injury of unspecified blood vessel at neck level**

√4ᵗʰ **S16** **Injury of muscle, fascia and tendon at neck level**

  Code also any associated open wound (S11.-)
  EXCLUDES 2 sprain of joint or ligament at neck level (S13.9)

  The appropriate 7th character is to be added to each code from category S16.
  A   initial encounter
  D   subsequent encounter
  S   sequela

√x7ᵗʰ **S16.1** **Strain of muscle, fascia and tendon at neck level**

√x7ᵗʰ **S16.2** **Laceration of muscle, fascia and tendon at neck level**

√x7ᵗʰ **S16.8** **Other specified injury of muscle, fascia and tendon at neck level**

√x7ᵗʰ **S16.9** **Unspecified injury of muscle, fascia and tendon at neck level**

√4ᵗʰ **S17** **Crushing injury of neck**

  Use additional code for all associated injuries, such as:
    injury of blood vessels (S15.-)
    open wound of neck (S11.-)
    spinal cord injury (S14.0, S14.1-)
    vertebral fracture (S12.0--S12.3-)

  The appropriate 7th character is to be added to each code from category S17.
  A   initial encounter
  D   subsequent encounter
  S   sequela

√x7ᵗʰ **S17.0** **Crushing injury of larynx and trachea**

√x7ᵗʰ **S17.8** **Crushing injury of other specified parts of neck**

√x7ᵗʰ **S17.9** **Crushing injury of neck, part unspecified**

√4ᵗʰ **S19** **Other specified and unspecified injuries of neck**

  The appropriate 7th character is to be added to each code from category S19.
  A   initial encounter
  D   subsequent encounter
  S   sequela

√5ᵗʰ **S19.8** Other specified injuries of neck

√x7ᵗʰ **S19.80** **Other specified injuries of unspecified part of neck**

√x7ᵗʰ **S19.81** **Other specified injuries of** larynx

√x7ᵗʰ **S19.82** **Other specified injuries of cervical** trachea

  EXCLUDES 2 other specified injury of thoracic trachea (S27.5-)

√x7ᵗʰ **S19.83** **Other specified injuries of** vocal cord

√x7ᵗʰ **S19.84** **Other specified injuries of** thyroid gland

---

☑ Additional Character Required √x7ᵗʰ Xtension Alert Unspecified Code Other Specified Code Manifestation Code ►◄ Revised Text ● New Code ▲ Revised Code Title

√x7ᵗʰ **S19.85** **Other specified injuries of** pharynx and cervical esophagus

√x7ᵗʰ **S19.89** **Other specified injuries of other specified part of neck**

√x7ᵗʰ **S19.9** **Unspecified injury of neck**

Injuries to the thorax (S20-S29)

INCLUDES   injuries of breast
      injuries of chest (wall)
      injuries of interscapular area

EXCLUDES 2   burns and corrosions (T20-T32)
      effects of foreign body in bronchus (T17.5)
      effects of foreign body in esophagus (T18.1)
      effects of foreign body in lung (T17.8)
      effects of foreign body in trachea (T17.4)
      frostbite (T33-T34)
      injuries of axilla
      injuries of clavicle
      injuries of scapular region
      injuries of shoulder
      insect bite or sting, venomous (T63.4)

√4ᵗʰ **S20** **Superficial injury of thorax**

> The appropriate 7th character is to be added to each code from category S20.
> A   initial encounter
> D   subsequent encounter
> S   sequela

√5ᵗʰ **S20.0** **Contusion** of breast

√x7ᵗʰ **S20.00** **Contusion of breast, unspecified breast**

√x7ᵗʰ **S20.01** **Contusion of** right **breast**

√x7ᵗʰ **S20.02** **Contusion of** left **breast**

√5ᵗʰ **S20.1** **Other and unspecified superficial injuries of breast**

√6ᵗʰ **S20.10** **Unspecified superficial injuries of breast**

√7ᵗʰ **S20.101** **Unspecified superficial injuries of breast, right breast**

√7ᵗʰ **S20.102** **Unspecified superficial injuries of breast, left breast**

√7ᵗʰ **S20.109** **Unspecified superficial injuries of breast, unspecified breast**

√6ᵗʰ **S20.11** **Abrasion** of breast

√7ᵗʰ **S20.111** **Abrasion of breast,** right **breast**

√7ᵗʰ **S20.112** **Abrasion of breast,** left **breast**

√7ᵗʰ **S20.119** **Abrasion of breast, unspecified breast**

√6ᵗʰ **S20.12** **Blister** (nonthermal) of breast

√7ᵗʰ **S20.121** **Blister (nonthermal) of breast,** right **breast**

√7ᵗʰ **S20.122** **Blister (nonthermal) of breast,** left **breast**

√7ᵗʰ **S20.129** **Blister (nonthermal) of breast, unspecified breast**

√6ᵗʰ **S20.14** **External constriction** of part of breast

√7ᵗʰ **S20.141** **External constriction of part of breast, right breast**

√7ᵗʰ **S20.142** **External constriction of part of breast,** left **breast**

√7ᵗʰ **S20.149** **External constriction of part of breast, unspecified breast**

√6ᵗʰ **S20.15** **Superficial** foreign body **of breast**
      Splinter in the breast

√7ᵗʰ **S20.151** **Superficial foreign body of breast, right breast**

√7ᵗʰ **S20.152** **Superficial foreign body of breast,** left **breast**

√7ᵗʰ **S20.159** **Superficial foreign body of breast, unspecified breast**

√6ᵗʰ **S20.16** **Insect bite** (nonvenomous) of breast

√7ᵗʰ **S20.161** **Insect bite (nonvenomous) of breast, right breast**

√7ᵗʰ **S20.162** **Insect bite (nonvenomous) of breast, left breast**

√7ᵗʰ **S20.169** **Insect bite (nonvenomous) of breast, unspecified breast**

√6ᵗʰ **S20.17** **Other** superficial bite **of breast**
      EXCLUDES 1   open bite of breast (S21.05-)

√7ᵗʰ **S20.171** **Other superficial bite of breast, right breast**

√7ᵗʰ **S20.172** **Other superficial bite of breast,** left **breast**

√7ᵗʰ **S20.179** **Other superficial bite of breast, unspecified breast**

√5ᵗʰ **S20.2** **Contusion of thorax**

√x7ᵗʰ **S20.20** **Contusion of thorax, unspecified**

√6ᵗʰ **S20.21** **Contusion of** front wall **of thorax**

√7ᵗʰ **S20.211** **Contusion of** right **front wall of thorax**

√7ᵗʰ **S20.212** **Contusion of** left **front wall of thorax**

√7ᵗʰ **S20.219** **Contusion of unspecified front wall of thorax**

√6ᵗʰ **S20.22** **Contusion of** back wall **of thorax**

√7ᵗʰ **S20.221** **Contusion of** right **back wall of thorax**

√7ᵗʰ **S20.222** **Contusion of** left **back wall of thorax**

√7ᵗʰ **S20.229** **Contusion of unspecified back wall of thorax**

√5ᵗʰ **S20.3** **Other and unspecified superficial injuries of** front wall **of thorax**

√6ᵗʰ **S20.30** **Unspecified superficial injuries of front wall of thorax**

√7ᵗʰ **S20.301** **Unspecified superficial injuries of** right **front wall of thorax**

√7ᵗʰ **S20.302** **Unspecified superficial injuries of** left **front wall of thorax**

√7ᵗʰ **S20.309** **Unspecified superficial injuries of unspecified front wall of thorax**

√6ᵗʰ **S20.31** **Abrasion** of front wall of thorax

√7ᵗʰ **S20.311** **Abrasion of** right **front wall of thorax**

√7ᵗʰ **S20.312** **Abrasion of** left **front wall of thorax**

√7ᵗʰ **S20.319** **Abrasion of unspecified front wall of thorax**

√6ᵗʰ **S20.32** **Blister** (nonthermal) of front wall of thorax

√7ᵗʰ **S20.321** **Blister (nonthermal) of** right **front wall of thorax**

√7ᵗʰ **S20.322** **Blister (nonthermal) of** left **front wall of thorax**

√7ᵗʰ **S20.329** **Blister (nonthermal) of unspecified front wall of thorax**

√6ᵗʰ **S20.34** **External constriction** of front wall of thorax

√7ᵗʰ **S20.341** **External constriction of** right **front wall of thorax**

√7ᵗʰ **S20.342** **External constriction of** left **front wall of thorax**

√7ᵗʰ **S20.349** **External constriction of unspecified front wall of thorax**

√6ᵗʰ **S20.35** **Superficial** foreign body **of front wall of thorax**
      Splinter in front wall of thorax

√7ᵗʰ **S20.351** **Superficial foreign body of** right **front wall of thorax**

√7ᵗʰ **S20.352** **Superficial foreign body of** left **front wall of thorax**

√7ᵗʰ **S20.359** **Superficial foreign body of unspecified front wall of thorax**

√6ᵗʰ **S20.36** **Insect bite** (nonvenomous) of front wall of thorax

√7ᵗʰ **S20.361** **Insect bite (nonvenomous) of** right **front wall of thorax**

√7ᵗʰ **S20.362** **Insect bite (nonvenomous) of** left **front wall of thorax**

√7ᵗʰ **S20.369** **Insect bite (nonvenomous) of unspecified front wall of thorax**

√6ᵗʰ **S20.37** **Other** superficial bite **of front wall of thorax**
      EXCLUDES 1   open bite of front wall of thorax (S21.15)

√7ᵗʰ **S20.371** **Other superficial bite of** right **front wall of thorax**

√7ᵗʰ **S20.372** **Other superficial bite of** left **front wall of thorax**

√7ᵗʰ **S20.379** **Other superficial bite of unspecified front wall of thorax**

√5ᵗʰ **S20.4** **Other and unspecified superficial injuries of** back wall **of thorax**

√6ᵗʰ **S20.40** **Unspecified superficial injuries of back wall of thorax**

√7ᵗʰ **S20.401** **Unspecified superficial injuries of** right **back wall of thorax**

EXCLUDES 1 Not coded here   EXCLUDES 2 Not included here   N Newborn Age: 0   P Pediatric Age: 0-17   M Maternity Age: 12-55   A Adult Age: 15-124

820   ICD-10-CM 2014 (Draft)

√7ᵗʰ **S20.402** Unspecified superficial injuries of left back wall of thorax

√7ᵗʰ **S20.409** Unspecified superficial injuries of unspecified back wall of thorax

√6ᵗʰ **S20.41** Abrasion of back wall of thorax

√7ᵗʰ **S20.411** Abrasion of right back wall of thorax

√7ᵗʰ **S20.412** Abrasion of left back wall of thorax

√7ᵗʰ **S20.419** Abrasion of unspecified back wall of thorax

√6ᵗʰ **S20.42** Blister (nonthermal) of back wall of thorax

√7ᵗʰ **S20.421** Blister (nonthermal) of right back wall of thorax

√7ᵗʰ **S20.422** Blister (nonthermal) of left back wall of thorax

√7ᵗʰ **S20.429** Blister (nonthermal) of unspecified back wall of thorax

√6ᵗʰ **S20.44** External constriction of back wall of thorax

√7ᵗʰ **SS20.441** External constriction of right back wall of thorax

√7ᵗʰ **S20.442** External constriction of left back wall of thorax

√7ᵗʰ **S20.449** External constriction of unspecified back wall of thorax

√6ᵗʰ **S20.45** Superficial foreign body of back wall of thorax
  Splinter of back wall of thorax

√7ᵗʰ **S20.451** Superficial foreign body of right back wall of thorax

√7ᵗʰ **S20.452** Superficial foreign body of left back wall of thorax

√7ᵗʰ **S20.459** Superficial foreign body of unspecified back wall of thorax

√6ᵗʰ **S20.46** Insect bite (nonvenomous) of back wall of thorax

√7ᵗʰ **S20.461** Insect bite (nonvenomous) of right back wall of thorax

√7ᵗʰ **S20.462** Insect bite (nonvenomous) of left back wall of thorax

√7ᵗʰ **S20.469** Insect bite (nonvenomous) of unspecified back wall of thorax

√6ᵗʰ **S20.47** Other superficial bite of back wall of thorax
  EXCLUDES 1 *open bite of back wall of thorax (S21.25)*

√7ᵗʰ **S20.471** Other superficial bite of right back wall of thorax

√7ᵗʰ **S20.472** Other superficial bite of left back wall of thorax

√7ᵗʰ **S20.479** Other superficial bite of unspecified back wall of thorax

√5ᵗʰ **S20.9** Superficial injury of unspecified parts of thorax
  EXCLUDES 1 *contusion of thorax NOS (S20.20)*

√x7ᵗʰ **S20.90** Unspecified superficial injury of unspecified parts of thorax
  Superficial injury of thoracic wall NOS

√x7ᵗʰ **S20.91** Abrasion of unspecified parts of thorax

√x7ᵗʰ **S20.92** Blister (nonthermal) of unspecified parts of thorax

√x7ᵗʰ **S20.94** External constriction of unspecified parts of thorax

√x7ᵗʰ **S20.95** Superficial foreign body of unspecified parts of thorax
  Splinter in thorax NOS

√x7ᵗʰ **S20.96** Insect bite (nonvenomous) of unspecified parts of thorax

√x7ᵗʰ **S20.97** Other superficial bite of unspecified parts of thorax
  EXCLUDES 1 *open bite of thorax NOS (S21.95)*

√4ᵗʰ **S21** **Open wound of thorax**
  Code also any associated injury such as:
    injury of heart (S26.-)
    injury of intrathoracic organs (S27.-)
    rib fracture (S22.3-, S22.4-)
    spinal cord injury (S24.0-, S24.1-)
    traumatic hemothorax (S27.1)
    traumatic hemopneumothorax (S27.3)
    traumatic pneumothorax (S27.0)
    wound infection
  EXCLUDES 1 *traumatic amputation (partial) of thorax (S28.1)*

  The appropriate 7th character is to be added to each code from category S21.
  A   initial encounter
  D   subsequent encounter
  S   sequela

√5ᵗʰ **S21.0** Open wound of breast

√6ᵗʰ **S21.00** Unspecified open wound of breast

√7ᵗʰ **S21.001** Unspecified open wound of right breast

√7ᵗʰ **S21.002** Unspecified open wound of left breast

√7ᵗʰ **S21.009** Unspecified open wound of unspecified breast

√6ᵗʰ **S21.01** Laceration without foreign body of breast

√7ᵗʰ **S21.011** Laceration without foreign body of right breast

√7ᵗʰ **S21.012** Laceration without foreign body of left breast

√7ᵗʰ **S21.019** Laceration without foreign body of unspecified breast

√6ᵗʰ **S21.02** Laceration with foreign body of breast

√7ᵗʰ **S21.021** Laceration with foreign body of right breast

√7ᵗʰ **S21.022** Laceration with foreign body of left breast

√7ᵗʰ **S21.029** Laceration with foreign body of unspecified breast

√6ᵗʰ **S21.03** Puncture wound without foreign body of breast

√7ᵗʰ **S21.031** Puncture wound without foreign body of right breast

√7ᵗʰ **S21.032** Puncture wound without foreign body of left breast

√7ᵗʰ **S21.039** Puncture wound without foreign body of unspecified breast

√6ᵗʰ **S21.04** Puncture wound with foreign body of breast

√7ᵗʰ **S21.041** Puncture wound with foreign body of right breast

√7ᵗʰ **S21.042** Puncture wound with foreign body of left breast

√7ᵗʰ **S21.049** Puncture wound with foreign body of unspecified breast

√6ᵗʰ **S21.05** Open bite of breast
  Bite of breast NOS
  EXCLUDES 1 *superficial bite of breast (S20.17)*

√7ᵗʰ **S21.051** Open bite of right breast

√7ᵗʰ **S21.052** Open bite of left breast

√7ᵗʰ **S21.059** Open bite of unspecified breast

√5ᵗʰ **S21.1** Open wound of front wall of thorax without penetration into thoracic cavity
  Open wound of chest without penetration into thoracic cavity

√6ᵗʰ **S21.10** Unspecified open wound of front wall of thorax without penetration into thoracic cavity

√7ᵗʰ **S21.101** Unspecified open wound of right front wall of thorax without penetration into thoracic cavity

√7ᵗʰ **S21.102** Unspecified open wound of left front wall of thorax without penetration into thoracic cavity

√7ᵗʰ **S21.109** Unspecified open wound of unspecified front wall of thorax without penetration into thoracic cavity

√6ᵗʰ **S21.11** Laceration without foreign body of front wall of thorax without penetration into thoracic cavity

√7ᵗʰ **S21.111** Laceration without foreign body of right front wall of thorax without penetration into thoracic cavity

☑ Additional Character Required   √x7ᵗʰ Xtension Alert   Unspecified Code   Other Specified Code   Manifestation Code   ►◄ Revised Text   ● New Code   ▲ Revised Code Title

ICD-10-CM 2014 (Draft)

821

√7ᵗʰ **S21.112** Laceration without foreign body of left front wall of thorax without penetration into thoracic cavity

√7ᵗʰ **S21.119** Laceration without foreign body of unspecified front wall of thorax without penetration into thoracic cavity

√6ᵗʰ **S21.12** Laceration with foreign body of front wall of thorax without penetration into thoracic cavity

√7ᵗʰ **S21.121** Laceration with foreign body of right front wall of thorax without penetration into thoracic cavity

√7ᵗʰ **S21.122** Laceration with foreign body of left front wall of thorax without penetration into thoracic cavity

√7ᵗʰ **S21.129** Laceration with foreign body of unspecified front wall of thorax without penetration into thoracic cavity

√6ᵗʰ **S21.13** Puncture wound without foreign body of front wall of thorax without penetration into thoracic cavity

√7ᵗʰ **S21.131** Puncture wound without foreign body of right front wall of thorax without penetration into thoracic cavity

√7ᵗʰ **S21.132** Puncture wound without foreign body of left front wall of thorax without penetration into thoracic cavity

√7ᵗʰ **S21.139** Puncture wound without foreign body of unspecified front wall of thorax without penetration into thoracic cavity

√6ᵗʰ **S21.14** Puncture wound with foreign body of front wall of thorax without penetration into thoracic cavity

√7ᵗʰ **S21.141** Puncture wound with foreign body of right front wall of thorax without penetration into thoracic cavity

√7ᵗʰ **S21.142** Puncture wound with foreign body of left front wall of thorax without penetration into thoracic cavity

√7ᵗʰ **S21.149** Puncture wound with foreign body of unspecified front wall of thorax without penetration into thoracic cavity

√6ᵗʰ **S21.15** Open bite of front wall of thorax without penetration into thoracic cavity
Bite of front wall of thorax NOS
EXCLUDES 1 superficial bite of front wall of thorax (S20.37)

√7ᵗʰ **S21.151** Open bite of right front wall of thorax without penetration into thoracic cavity

√7ᵗʰ **S21.152** Open bite of left front wall of thorax without penetration into thoracic cavity

√7ᵗʰ **S21.159** Open bite of unspecified front wall of thorax without penetration into thoracic cavity

√5ᵗʰ **S21.2** Open wound of back wall of thorax without penetration into thoracic cavity

√6ᵗʰ **S21.20** Unspecified open wound of back wall of thorax without penetration into thoracic cavity

√7ᵗʰ **S21.201** Unspecified open wound of right back wall of thorax without penetration into thoracic cavity

√7ᵗʰ **S21.202** Unspecified open wound of left back wall of thorax without penetration into thoracic cavity

√7ᵗʰ **S21.209** Unspecified open wound of unspecified back wall of thorax without penetration into thoracic cavity

√6ᵗʰ **S21.21** Laceration without foreign body of back wall of thorax without penetration into thoracic cavity

√7ᵗʰ **S21.211** Laceration without foreign body of right back wall of thorax without penetration into thoracic cavity

√7ᵗʰ **S21.212** Laceration without foreign body of left back wall of thorax without penetration into thoracic cavity

√7ᵗʰ **S21.219** Laceration without foreign body of unspecified back wall of thorax without penetration into thoracic cavity

√6ᵗʰ **S21.22** Laceration with foreign body of back wall of thorax without penetration into thoracic cavity

√7ᵗʰ **S21.221** Laceration with foreign body of right back wall of thorax without penetration into thoracic cavity

√7ᵗʰ **S21.222** Laceration with foreign body of left back wall of thorax without penetration into thoracic cavity

√7ᵗʰ **S21.229** Laceration with foreign body of unspecified back wall of thorax without penetration into thoracic cavity

√6ᵗʰ **S21.23** Puncture wound without foreign body of back wall of thorax without penetration into thoracic cavity

√7ᵗʰ **S21.231** Puncture wound without foreign body of right back wall of thorax without penetration into thoracic cavity

√7ᵗʰ **S21.232** Puncture wound without foreign body of left back wall of thorax without penetration into thoracic cavity

√7ᵗʰ **S21.239** Puncture wound without foreign body of unspecified back wall of thorax without penetration into thoracic cavity

√6ᵗʰ **S21.24** Puncture wound with foreign body of back wall of thorax without penetration into thoracic cavity

√7ᵗʰ **S21.241** Puncture wound with foreign body of right back wall of thorax without penetration into thoracic cavity

√7ᵗʰ **S21.242** Puncture wound with foreign body of left back wall of thorax without penetration into thoracic cavity

√7ᵗʰ **S21.249** Puncture wound with foreign body of unspecified back wall of thorax without penetration into thoracic cavity

√6ᵗʰ **S21.25** Open bite of back wall of thorax without penetration into thoracic cavity
Bite of back wall of thorax NOS
EXCLUDES 1 superficial bite of back wall of thorax (S20.47)

√7ᵗʰ **S21.251** Open bite of right back wall of thorax without penetration into thoracic cavity

√7ᵗʰ **S21.252** Open bite of left back wall of thorax without penetration into thoracic cavity

√7ᵗʰ **S21.259** Open bite of unspecified back wall of thorax without penetration into thoracic cavity

√5ᵗʰ **S21.3** Open wound of front wall of thorax with penetration into thoracic cavity
Open wound of chest with penetration into thoracic cavity

√6ᵗʰ **S21.30** Unspecified open wound of front wall of thorax with penetration into thoracic cavity

√7ᵗʰ **S21.301** Unspecified open wound of right front wall of thorax with penetration into thoracic cavity

√7ᵗʰ **S21.302** Unspecified open wound of left front wall of thorax with penetration into thoracic cavity

√7ᵗʰ **S21.309** Unspecified open wound of unspecified front wall of thorax with penetration into thoracic cavity

√6ᵗʰ **S21.31** Laceration without foreign body of front wall of thorax with penetration into thoracic cavity

√7ᵗʰ **S21.311** Laceration without foreign body of right front wall of thorax with penetration into thoracic cavity

√7ᵗʰ **S21.312** Laceration without foreign body of left front wall of thorax with penetration into thoracic cavity

√7ᵗʰ **S21.319** Laceration without foreign body of unspecified front wall of thorax with penetration into thoracic cavity

√6ᵗʰ **S21.32** Laceration with foreign body of front wall of thorax with penetration into thoracic cavity

√7ᵗʰ **S21.321** Laceration with foreign body of right front wall of thorax with penetration into thoracic cavity

√7ᵗʰ **S21.322** Laceration with foreign body of left front wall of thorax with penetration into thoracic cavity

---

EXCLUDES 1 Not coded here   *EXCLUDES 2* Not included here   N Newborn Age: 0   P Pediatric Age: 0-17   M Maternity Age: 12-55   A Adult Age: 15-124

822   ICD-10-CM 2014 (Draft)

√7th **S21.329** Laceration with foreign body of unspecified front wall of thorax with penetration into thoracic cavity

√6th **S21.33** Puncture wound without foreign body of front wall of thorax with penetration into thoracic cavity

√7th **S21.331** Puncture wound without foreign body of right front wall of thorax with penetration into thoracic cavity

√7th **S21.332** Puncture wound without foreign body of left front wall of thorax with penetration into thoracic cavity

√7th **S21.339** Puncture wound without foreign body of unspecified front wall of thorax with penetration into thoracic cavity

√6th **S21.34** Puncture wound with foreign body of front wall of thorax with penetration into thoracic cavity

√7th **S21.341** Puncture wound with foreign body of right front wall of thorax with penetration into thoracic cavity

√7th **S21.342** Puncture wound with foreign body of left front wall of thorax with penetration into thoracic cavity

√7th **S21.349** Puncture wound with foreign body of unspecified front wall of thorax with penetration into thoracic cavity

√6th **S21.35** Open bite of front wall of thorax with penetration into thoracic cavity
> EXCLUDES 1   superficial bite of front wall of thorax (S20.37)

√7th **S21.351** Open bite of right front wall of thorax with penetration into thoracic cavity

√7th **S21.352** Open bite of left front wall of thorax with penetration into thoracic cavity

√7th **S21.359** Open bite of unspecified front wall of thorax with penetration into thoracic cavity

√5th **S21.4** Open wound of back wall of thorax with penetration into thoracic cavity

√6th **S21.40** Unspecified open wound of back wall of thorax with penetration into thoracic cavity

√7th **S21.401** Unspecified open wound of right back wall of thorax with penetration into thoracic cavity

√7th **S21.402** Unspecified open wound of left back wall of thorax with penetration into thoracic cavity

√7th **S21.409** Unspecified open wound of unspecified back wall of thorax with penetration into thoracic cavity

√6th **S21.41** Laceration without foreign body of back wall of thorax with penetration into thoracic cavity

√7th **S21.411** Laceration without foreign body of right back wall of thorax with penetration into thoracic cavity

√7th **S21.412** Laceration without foreign body of left back wall of thorax with penetration into thoracic cavity

√7th **S21.419** Laceration without foreign body of unspecified back wall of thorax with penetration into thoracic cavity

√6th **S21.42** Laceration with foreign body of back wall of thorax with penetration into thoracic cavity

√7th **S21.421** Laceration with foreign body of right back wall of thorax with penetration into thoracic cavity

√7th **S21.422** Laceration with foreign body of left back wall of thorax with penetration into thoracic cavity

√7th **S21.429** Laceration with foreign body of unspecified back wall of thorax with penetration into thoracic cavity

√6th **S21.43** Puncture wound without foreign body of back wall of thorax with penetration into thoracic cavity

√7th **S21.431** Puncture wound without foreign body of right back wall of thorax with penetration into thoracic cavity

√7th **S21.432** Puncture wound without foreign body of left back wall of thorax with penetration into thoracic cavity

√7th **S21.439** Puncture wound without foreign body of unspecified back wall of thorax with penetration into thoracic cavity

√6th **S21.44** Puncture wound with foreign body of back wall of thorax with penetration into thoracic cavity

√7th **S21.441** Puncture wound with foreign body of right back wall of thorax with penetration into thoracic cavity

√7th **S21.442** Puncture wound with foreign body of left back wall of thorax with penetration into thoracic cavity

√7th **S21.449** Puncture wound with foreign body of unspecified back wall of thorax with penetration into thoracic cavity

√6th **S21.45** Open bite of back wall of thorax with penetration into thoracic cavity
> Bite of back wall of thorax NOS
> EXCLUDES 1   superficial bite of back wall of thorax (S20.47)

√7th **S21.451** Open bite of right back wall of thorax with penetration into thoracic cavity

√7th **S21.452** Open bite of left back wall of thorax with penetration into thoracic cavity

√7th **S21.459** Open bite of unspecified back wall of thorax with penetration into thoracic cavity

√5th **S21.9** Open wound of unspecified part of thorax
> Open wound of thoracic wall NOS

√x7th **S21.90** Unspecified open wound of unspecified part of thorax

√x7th **S21.91** Laceration without foreign body of unspecified part of thorax

√x7th **S21.92** Laceration with foreign body of unspecified part of thorax

√x7th **S21.93** Puncture wound without foreign body of unspecified part of thorax

√x7th **S21.94** Puncture wound with foreign body of unspecified part of thorax

√x7th **S21.95** Open bite of unspecified part of thorax
> EXCLUDES 1   superficial bite of thorax (S20.97)

√4th **S22** Fracture of rib(s), sternum and thoracic spine
> NOTE   A fracture not indicated as nondisplaced or displaced should be classified to displaced.
> A fracture not indicated as open or closed should be coded to closed.
> Fracture of thoracic neural arch
> Fracture of thoracic spinous process
> Fracture of thoracic transverse process
> Fracture of thoracic vertebra
> Fracture of thoracic vertebral arch
> Codes first any associated:
>   injury of intrathoracic organ (S27.-)
>   spinal cord injury (S24.0-, S24.1-)
> EXCLUDES 1   transection of thorax (S28.1)
> EXCLUDES 2   fracture of clavicle (S42.0-)
>   fracture of scapula (S42.1-)

> The appropriate 7th character is to be added to each code from category S22.
> A   initial encounter for closed fracture
> B   initial encounter for open fracture
> D   subsequent encounter for fracture with routine healing
> G   subsequent encounter for fracture with delayed healing
> K   subsequent encounter for fracture with nonunion
> S   sequela

√5th **S22.0** Fracture of thoracic vertebra

√6th **S22.00** Fracture of unspecified thoracic vertebra

√7th **S22.000** Wedge compression fracture of unspecified thoracic vertebra

√7th **S22.001** Stable burst fracture of unspecified thoracic vertebra

√7th **S22.002** Unstable burst fracture of unspecified thoracic vertebra

√7th **S22.008** Other fracture of unspecified thoracic vertebra

√7th **S22.009** Unspecified fracture of unspecified thoracic vertebra

√6ᵗʰ **S22.01** Fracture of first thoracic vertebra
- √7ᵗʰ **S22.010** Wedge compression fracture of first thoracic vertebra
- √7ᵗʰ **S22.011** Stable burst fracture of first thoracic vertebra
- √7ᵗʰ **S22.012** Unstable burst fracture of first thoracic vertebra
- √7ᵗʰ **S22.018** Other fracture of first thoracic vertebra
- √7ᵗʰ **S22.019** Unspecified fracture of first thoracic vertebra

√6ᵗʰ **S22.02** Fracture of second thoracic vertebra
- √7ᵗʰ **S22.020** Wedge compression fracture of second thoracic vertebra
- √7ᵗʰ **S22.021** Stable burst fracture of second thoracic vertebra
- √7ᵗʰ **S22.022** Unstable burst fracture of second thoracic vertebra
- √7ᵗʰ **S22.028** Other fracture of second thoracic vertebra
- √7ᵗʰ **S22.029** Unspecified fracture of second thoracic vertebra

√6ᵗʰ **S22.03** Fracture of third thoracic vertebra
- √7ᵗʰ **S22.030** Wedge compression fracture of third thoracic vertebra
- √7ᵗʰ **S22.031** Stable burst fracture of third thoracic vertebra
- √7ᵗʰ **S22.032** Unstable burst fracture of third thoracic vertebra
- √7ᵗʰ **S22.038** Other fracture of third thoracic vertebra
- √7ᵗʰ **S22.039** Unspecified fracture of third thoracic vertebra

√6ᵗʰ **S22.04** Fracture of fourth thoracic vertebra
- √7ᵗʰ **S22.040** Wedge compression fracture of fourth thoracic vertebra
- √7ᵗʰ **S22.041** Stable burst fracture of fourth thoracic vertebra
- √7ᵗʰ **S22.042** Unstable burst fracture of fourth thoracic vertebra
- √7ᵗʰ **S22.048** Other fracture of fourth thoracic vertebra
- √7ᵗʰ **S22.049** Unspecified fracture of fourth thoracic vertebra

√6ᵗʰ **S22.05** Fracture of T5-T6 vertebra
- √7ᵗʰ **S22.050** Wedge compression fracture of T5-T6 vertebra
- √7ᵗʰ **S22.051** Stable burst fracture of T5-T6 vertebra
- √7ᵗʰ **S22.052** Unstable burst fracture of T5-T6 vertebra
- √7ᵗʰ **S22.058** Other fracture of T5-T6 vertebra
- √7ᵗʰ **S22.059** Unspecified fracture of T5-T6 vertebra

√6ᵗʰ **S22.06** Fracture of T7-T8 vertebra
- √7ᵗʰ **S22.060** Wedge compression fracture of T7-T8 vertebra
- √7ᵗʰ **S22.061** Stable burst fracture of T7-T8 vertebra
- √7ᵗʰ **S22.062** Unstable burst fracture of T7-T8 vertebra
- √7ᵗʰ **S22.068** Other fracture of T7-T8 thoracic vertebra
- √7ᵗʰ **S22.069** Unspecified fracture of T7-T8 vertebra

√6ᵗʰ **S22.07** Fracture of T9-T10 vertebra
- √7ᵗʰ **S22.070** Wedge compression fracture of T9-T10 vertebra
- √7ᵗʰ **S22.071** Stable burst fracture of T9-T10 vertebra
- √7ᵗʰ **S22.072** Unstable burst fracture of T9-T10 vertebra
- √7ᵗʰ **S22.078** Other fracture of T9-T10 vertebra
- √7ᵗʰ **S22.079** Unspecified fracture of T9-T10 vertebra

√6ᵗʰ **S22.08** Fracture of T11-T12 vertebra
- √7ᵗʰ **S22.080** Wedge compression fracture of T11-T12 vertebra
- √7ᵗʰ **S22.081** Stable burst fracture of T11-T12 vertebra
- √7ᵗʰ **S22.082** Unstable burst fracture of T11-T12 vertebra
- √7ᵗʰ **S22.088** Other fracture of T11-T12 vertebra
- √7ᵗʰ **S22.089** Unspecified fracture of T11-T12 vertebra

√5ᵗʰ **S22.2** Fracture of sternum
- √x7ᵗʰ **S22.20** Unspecified fracture of sternum

√x7ᵗʰ **S22.21** Fracture of manubrium
√x7ᵗʰ **S22.22** Fracture of body of sternum
√x7ᵗʰ **S22.23** Sternal manubrial dissociation
√x7ᵗʰ **S22.24** Fracture of xiphoid process

√5ᵗʰ **S22.3** Fracture of one rib
- √x7ᵗʰ **S22.31** Fracture of one rib, right side
- √x7ᵗʰ **S22.32** Fracture of one rib, left side
- √x7ᵗʰ **S22.39** Fracture of one rib, unspecified side

√5ᵗʰ **S22.4** Multiple fractures of ribs
Fractures of two or more ribs
> **EXCLUDES 1**   flail chest (S22.5-)
- √x7ᵗʰ **S22.41** Multiple fractures of ribs, right side
- √x7ᵗʰ **S22.42** Multiple fractures of ribs, left side
- √x7ᵗʰ **S22.43** Multiple fractures of ribs, bilateral
- √x7ᵗʰ **S22.49** Multiple fractures of ribs, unspecified side

√x7ᵗʰ **S22.5** Flail chest
√x7ᵗʰ **S22.9** Fracture of bony thorax, part unspecified

√4ᵗʰ **S23** Dislocation and sprain of joints and ligaments of thorax
> **INCLUDES**   avulsion of joint or ligament of thorax
> laceration of cartilage, joint or ligament of thorax
> sprain of cartilage, joint or ligament of thorax
> traumatic hemarthrosis of joint or ligament of thorax
> traumatic rupture of joint or ligament of thorax
> traumatic subluxation of joint or ligament of thorax
> traumatic tear of joint or ligament of thorax

Code also any associated open wound
> **EXCLUDES 2**   dislocation, sprain of sternoclavicular joint (S43.2, S43.6)
> strain of muscle or tendon of thorax (S29.01-)

The appropriate 7th character is to be added to each code from category S23.
A   initial encounter
D   subsequent encounter
S   sequela

√x7ᵗʰ **S23.0** Traumatic rupture of thoracic intervertebral disc
> **EXCLUDES 1**   rupture or displacement (nontraumatic) of thoracic intervertebral disc NOS (M51- with fifth character 4)

√5ᵗʰ **S23.1** Subluxation and dislocation of thoracic vertebra
Code also any associated
open wound of thorax (S21.-)
spinal cord injury (S24.0-, S24.1-)
> **EXCLUDES 2**   fracture of thoracic vertebrae (S22.0-)

√6ᵗʰ **S23.10** Subluxation and dislocation of unspecified thoracic vertebra
- √7ᵗʰ **S23.100** Subluxation of unspecified thoracic vertebra
- √7ᵗʰ **S23.101** Dislocation of unspecified thoracic vertebra

√6ᵗʰ **S23.11** Subluxation and dislocation of T1/T2 thoracic vertebra
- √7ᵗʰ **S23.110** Subluxation of T1/T2 thoracic vertebra
- √7ᵗʰ **S23.111** Dislocation of T1/T2 thoracic vertebra

√6ᵗʰ **S23.12** Subluxation and dislocation of T2/T3-T3/T4 thoracic vertebra
- √7ᵗʰ **S23.120** Subluxation of T2/T3 thoracic vertebra
- √7ᵗʰ **S23.121** Dislocation of T2/T3 thoracic vertebra
- √7ᵗʰ **S23.122** Subluxation of T3/T4 thoracic vertebra
- √7ᵗʰ **S23.123** Dislocation of T3/T4 thoracic vertebra

√6ᵗʰ **S23.13** Subluxation and dislocation of T4/T5-T5/T6 thoracic vertebra
- √7ᵗʰ **S23.130** Subluxation of T4/T5 thoracic vertebra
- √7ᵗʰ **S23.131** Dislocation of T4/T5 thoracic vertebra
- √7ᵗʰ **S23.132** Subluxation of T5/T6 thoracic vertebra
- √7ᵗʰ **S23.133** Dislocation of T5/T6 thoracic vertebra

√6ᵗʰ **S23.14** Subluxation and dislocation of T6/T7-T7/T8 thoracic vertebra
- √7ᵗʰ **S23.140** Subluxation of T6/T7 thoracic vertebra
- √7ᵗʰ **S23.141** Dislocation of T6/T7 thoracic vertebra
- √7ᵗʰ **S23.142** Subluxation of T7/T8 thoracic vertebra
- √7ᵗʰ **S23.143** Dislocation of T7/T8 thoracic vertebra

EXCLUDES 1 Not coded here   **EXCLUDES 2** Not included here   **N** Newborn Age: 0   **P** Pediatric Age: 0-17   **M** Maternity Age: 12-55   **A** Adult Age: 15-124

824   ICD-10-CM 2014 (Draft)

✓6th **S23.15** **Subluxation and dislocation of** T8/T9-T9/T10 **thoracic vertebra**

   ✓7th **S23.150** **Subluxation of** T8/T9 **thoracic vertebra**

   ✓7th **S23.151** **Dislocation of** T8/T9 **thoracic vertebra**

   ✓7th **S23.152** **Subluxation of** T9/T10 **thoracic vertebra**

   ✓7th **S23.153** **Dislocation of** T9/T10 **thoracic vertebra**

✓6th **S23.16** **Subluxation and dislocation of** T10/T11-T11/T12 **thoracic vertebra**

   ✓7th **S23.160** **Subluxation of** T10/T11 **thoracic vertebra**

   ✓7th **S23.161** **Dislocation of** T10/T11 **thoracic vertebra**

   ✓7th **S23.162** **Subluxation of** T11/T12 **thoracic vertebra**

   ✓7th **S23.163** **Dislocation of** T11/T12 **thoracic vertebra**

✓6th **S23.17** **Subluxation and dislocation of** T12/L1 **thoracic vertebra**

   ✓7th **S23.170** **Subluxation of** T12/L1 **thoracic vertebra**

   ✓7th **S23.171** **Dislocation of** T12/L1 **thoracic vertebra**

✓5th **S23.2** **Dislocation of other and unspecified parts of thorax**

   ✓x7th **S23.20** **Dislocation of unspecified part of thorax**

   ✓x7th **S23.29** **Dislocation of other parts of thorax**

✓x7th **S23.3** **Sprain of ligaments of thoracic spine**

✓5th **S23.4** **Sprain of ribs and sternum**

   ✓x7th **S23.41** **Sprain of ribs**

   ✓6th **S23.42** **Sprain of sternum**

      ✓7th **S23.420** **Sprain of sternoclavicular (joint) (ligament)**

      ✓7th **S23.421** **Sprain of chondrosternal joint**

      ✓7th **S23.428** **Other sprain of sternum**

      ✓7th **S23.429** **Unspecified sprain of sternum**

✓x7th **S23.8** **Sprain of other specified parts of thorax**

✓x7th **S23.9** **Sprain of unspecified parts of thorax**

✓4th **S24** **Injury of nerves and spinal cord at thorax level**

> NOTE   Code to highest level of thoracic spinal cord injury.
> Injuries to the spinal cord (S24.0 and S24.1) refer to the cord level and not bone level injury, and can affect nerve roots at and below the level given.

Code also any associated:
   fracture of thoracic vertebra (S22.0-)
   open wound of thorax (S21.-)
   transient paralysis (R29.5)

EXCLUDES 2   injury of brachial plexus (S14.3)

The appropriate 7th character is to be added to each code from category S24.
A   initial encounter
D   subsequent encounter
S   sequela

✓x7th **S24.0** **Concussion and edema of thoracic spinal cord**

✓5th **S24.1** **Other and unspecified injuries of thoracic spinal cord**

   ✓6th **S24.10** **Unspecified injury of thoracic spinal cord**

      ✓7th **S24.101** **Unspecified injury at** T1 **level of thoracic spinal cord**

      ✓7th **S24.102** **Unspecified injury at** T2-T6 **level of thoracic spinal cord**

      ✓7th **S24.103** **Unspecified injury at** T7-T10 **level of thoracic spinal cord**

      ✓7th **S24.104** **Unspecified injury at** T11-T12 **level of thoracic spinal cord**

      ✓7th **S24.109** **Unspecified injury at unspecified level of thoracic spinal cord**
        Injury of thoracic spinal cord NOS

   ✓6th **S24.11** **Complete lesion of thoracic spinal cord**

      ✓7th **S24.111** **Complete lesion at** T1 **level of thoracic spinal cord**

      ✓7th **S24.112** **Complete lesion at** T2-T6 **level of thoracic spinal cord**

      ✓7th **S24.113** **Complete lesion at** T7-T10 **level of thoracic spinal cord**

      ✓7th **S24.114** **Complete lesion at** T11-T12 **level of thoracic spinal cord**

      ✓7th **S24.119** **Complete lesion at unspecified level of thoracic spinal cord**

✓6th **S24.13** **Anterior cord syndrome of thoracic spinal cord**

   ✓7th **S24.131** **Anterior cord syndrome at** T1 **level of thoracic spinal cord**

   ✓7th **S24.132** **Anterior cord syndrome at** T2-T6 **level of thoracic spinal cord**

   ✓7th **S24.133** **Anterior cord syndrome at** T7-T10 **level of thoracic spinal cord**

   ✓7th **S24.134** **Anterior cord syndrome at** T11-T12 **level of thoracic spinal cord**

   ✓7th **S24.139** **Anterior cord syndrome at unspecified level of thoracic spinal cord**

✓6th **S24.14** **Brown-Séquard syndrome of thoracic spinal cord**

   ✓7th **S24.141** **Brown-Séquard syndrome at** T1 **level of thoracic spinal cord**

   ✓7th **S24.142** **Brown-Séquard syndrome at** T2-T6 **level of thoracic spinal cord**

   ✓7th **S24.143** **Brown-Séquard syndrome at** T7-T10 **level of thoracic spinal cord**

   ✓7th **S24.144** **Brown-Séquard syndrome at** T11-T12 **level of thoracic spinal cord**

   ✓7th **S24.149** **Brown-Séquard syndrome at unspecified level of thoracic spinal cord**

✓6th **S24.15** **Other incomplete lesions of thoracic spinal cord**
    Incomplete lesion of thoracic spinal cord NOS
    Posterior cord syndrome of thoracic spinal cord

   ✓7th **S24.151** **Other incomplete lesion at** T1 **level of thoracic spinal cord**

   ✓7th **S24.152** **Other incomplete lesion at** T2-T6 **level of thoracic spinal cord**

   ✓7th **S24.153** **Other incomplete lesion at** T7-T10 **level of thoracic spinal cord**

   ✓7th **S24.154** **Other incomplete lesion at** T11-T12 **level of thoracic spinal cord**

   ✓7th **S24.159** **Other incomplete lesion at unspecified level of thoracic spinal cord**

✓x7th **S24.2** **Injury of nerve root of thoracic spine**

✓x7th **S24.3** **Injury of peripheral nerves of thorax**

✓x7th **S24.4** **Injury of thoracic sympathetic nervous system**
    Injury of cardiac plexus
    Injury of esophageal plexus
    Injury of pulmonary plexus
    Injury of stellate ganglion
    Injury of thoracic sympathetic ganglion

✓x7th **S24.8** **Injury of other specified nerves of thorax**

✓x7th **S24.9** **Injury of unspecified nerve of thorax**

✓4th **S25** **Injury of blood vessels of thorax**
   Code also any associated open wound (S21.-)

The appropriate 7th character is to be added to each code from category S25.
A   initial encounter
D   subsequent encounter
S   sequela

✓5th **S25.0** **Injury of thoracic aorta**
   Injury of aorta NOS

   ✓x7th **S25.00** **Unspecified injury of thoracic aorta**

   ✓x7th **S25.01** **Minor laceration of thoracic aorta**
      Incomplete transection of thoracic aorta
      Laceration of thoracic aorta NOS
      Superficial laceration of thoracic aorta

   ✓x7th **S25.02** **Major laceration of thoracic aorta**
      Complete transection of thoracic aorta
      Traumatic rupture of thoracic aorta

   ✓x7th **S25.09** **Other specified injury of thoracic aorta**

✓5th **S25.1** **Injury of innominate or subclavian artery**

   ✓6th **S25.10** **Unspecified injury of innominate or subclavian artery**

      ✓7th **S25.101** **Unspecified injury of right innominate or subclavian artery**

      ✓7th **S25.102** **Unspecified injury of left innominate or subclavian artery**

      ✓7th **S25.109** **Unspecified injury of unspecified innominate or subclavian artery**

✓ Additional Character Required   ✓x7th Xtension Alert   Unspecified Code   Other Specified Code   Manifestation Code   ►◄ Revised Text   ● New Code   ▲ Revised Code Title

ICD-10-CM 2014 (Draft)   825

√6ᵗʰ **S25.11** Minor laceration of innominate or subclavian artery
Incomplete transection of innominate or subclavian artery
Laceration of innominate or subclavian artery NOS
Superficial laceration of innominate or subclavian artery

√7ᵗʰ **S25.111** Minor laceration of right innominate or subclavian artery

√7ᵗʰ **S25.112** Minor laceration of left innominate or subclavian artery

√7ᵗʰ **S25.119** Minor laceration of unspecified innominate or subclavian artery

√6ᵗʰ **S25.12** Major laceration of innominate or subclavian artery
Complete transection of innominate or subclavian artery
Traumatic rupture of innominate or subclavian artery

√7ᵗʰ **S25.121** Major laceration of right innominate or subclavian artery

√7ᵗʰ **S25.122** Major laceration of left innominate or subclavian artery

√7ᵗʰ **S25.129** Major laceration of unspecified innominate or subclavian artery

√6ᵗʰ **S25.19** Other specified injury of innominate or subclavian artery

√7ᵗʰ **S25.191** Other specified injury of right innominate or subclavian artery

√7ᵗʰ **S25.192** Other specified injury of left innominate or subclavian artery

√7ᵗʰ **S25.199** Other specified injury of unspecified innominate or subclavian artery

√5ᵗʰ **S25.2** Injury of superior vena cava
Injury of vena cava NOS

√x7ᵗʰ **S25.20** Unspecified injury of superior vena cava

√x7ᵗʰ **S25.21** Minor laceration of superior vena cava
Incomplete transection of superior vena cava
Laceration of superior vena cava NOS
Superficial laceration of superior vena cava

√x7ᵗʰ **S25.22** Major laceration of superior vena cava
Complete transection of superior vena cava
Traumatic rupture of superior vena cava

√x7ᵗʰ **S25.29** Other specified injury of superior vena cava

√5ᵗʰ **S25.3** Injury of innominate or subclavian vein

√6ᵗʰ **S25.30** Unspecified injury of innominate or subclavian vein

√7ᵗʰ **S25.301** Unspecified injury of right innominate or subclavian vein

√7ᵗʰ **S25.302** Unspecified injury of left innominate or subclavian vein

√7ᵗʰ **S25.309** Unspecified injury of unspecified innominate or subclavian vein

√6ᵗʰ **S25.31** Minor laceration of innominate or subclavian vein
Incomplete transection of innominate or subclavian vein
Laceration of innominate or subclavian vein NOS
Superficial laceration of innominate or subclavian vein

√7ᵗʰ **S25.311** Minor laceration of right innominate or subclavian vein

√7ᵗʰ **S25.312** Minor laceration of left innominate or subclavian vein

√7ᵗʰ **S25.319** Minor laceration of unspecified innominate or subclavian vein

√6ᵗʰ **S25.32** Major laceration of innominate or subclavian vein
Complete transection of innominate or subclavian vein
Traumatic rupture of innominate or subclavian vein

√7ᵗʰ **S25.321** Major laceration of right innominate or subclavian vein

√7ᵗʰ **S25.322** Major laceration of left innominate or subclavian vein

√7ᵗʰ **S25.329** Major laceration of unspecified innominate or subclavian vein

√6ᵗʰ **S25.39** Other specified injury of innominate or subclavian vein

√7ᵗʰ **S25.391** Other specified injury of right innominate or subclavian vein

√7ᵗʰ **S25.392** Other specified injury of left innominate or subclavian vein

√7ᵗʰ **S25.399** Other specified injury of unspecified innominate or subclavian vein

√5ᵗʰ **S25.4** Injury of pulmonary blood vessels

√6ᵗʰ **S25.40** Unspecified injury of pulmonary blood vessels

√7ᵗʰ **S25.401** Unspecified injury of right pulmonary blood vessels

√7ᵗʰ **S25.402** Unspecified injury of left pulmonary blood vessels

√7ᵗʰ **S25.409** Unspecified injury of unspecified pulmonary blood vessels

√6ᵗʰ **S25.41** Minor laceration of pulmonary blood vessels
Incomplete transection of pulmonary blood vessels
Laceration of pulmonary blood vessels NOS
Superficial laceration of pulmonary blood vessels

√7ᵗʰ **S25.411** Minor laceration of right pulmonary blood vessels

√7ᵗʰ **S25.412** Minor laceration of left pulmonary blood vessels

√7ᵗʰ **S25.419** Minor laceration of unspecified pulmonary blood vessels

√6ᵗʰ **S25.42** Major laceration of pulmonary blood vessels
Complete transection of pulmonary blood vessels
Traumatic rupture of pulmonary blood vessels

√7ᵗʰ **S25.421** Major laceration of right pulmonary blood vessels

√7ᵗʰ **S25.422** Major laceration of left pulmonary blood vessels

√7ᵗʰ **S25.429** Major laceration of unspecified pulmonary blood vessels

√6ᵗʰ **S25.49** Other specified injury of pulmonary blood vessels

√7ᵗʰ **S25.491** Other specified injury of right pulmonary blood vessels

√7ᵗʰ **S25.492** Other specified injury of left pulmonary blood vessels

√7ᵗʰ **S25.499** Other specified injury of unspecified pulmonary blood vessels

√5ᵗʰ **S25.5** Injury of intercostal blood vessels

√6ᵗʰ **S25.50** Unspecified injury of intercostal blood vessels

√7ᵗʰ **S25.501** Unspecified injury of intercostal blood vessels, right side

√7ᵗʰ **S25.502** Unspecified injury of intercostal blood vessels, left side

√7ᵗʰ **S25.509** Unspecified injury of intercostal blood vessels, unspecified side

√6ᵗʰ **S25.51** Laceration of intercostal blood vessels

√7ᵗʰ **S25.511** Laceration of intercostal blood vessels, right side

√7ᵗʰ **S25.512** Laceration of intercostal blood vessels, left side

√7ᵗʰ **S25.519** Laceration of intercostal blood vessels, unspecified side

√6ᵗʰ **S25.59** Other specified injury of intercostal blood vessels

√7ᵗʰ **S25.591** Other specified injury of intercostal blood vessels, right side

√7ᵗʰ **S25.592** Other specified injury of intercostal blood vessels, left side

√7ᵗʰ **S25.599** Other specified injury of intercostal blood vessels, unspecified side

√5ᵗʰ **S25.8** Injury of other blood vessels of thorax
Injury of azygos vein   Injury of mammary artery or vein

√6ᵗʰ **S25.80** Unspecified injury of other blood vessels of thorax

√7ᵗʰ **S25.801** Unspecified injury of other blood vessels of thorax, right side

√7ᵗʰ **S25.802** Unspecified injury of other blood vessels of thorax, left side

√7ᵗʰ **S25.809** Unspecified injury of other blood vessels of thorax, unspecified side

√6ᵗʰ **S25.81** Laceration of other blood vessels of thorax

√7ᵗʰ **S25.811** Laceration of other blood vessels of thorax, right side

√7ᵗʰ **S25.812** Laceration of other blood vessels of thorax, left side

√7ᵗʰ **S25.819** Laceration of other blood vessels of thorax, unspecified side

EXCLUDES 1 Not coded here   **EXCLUDES 2** Not included here   **N** Newborn Age: 0   **P** Pediatric Age: 0-17   **M** Maternity Age: 12-55   **A** Adult Age: 15-124

826   ICD-10-CM 2014 (Draft)

☑6th **S25.89** Other specified injury of other blood vessels of thorax

  ☑7th **S25.891** Other specified injury of other blood vessels of thorax, right side

  ☑7th **S25.892** Other specified injury of other blood vessels of thorax, left side

  ☑7th **S25.899** Other specified injury of other blood vessels of thorax, unspecified side

☑5th **S25.9** Injury of unspecified blood vessel of thorax

  ☑x7th **S25.90** Unspecified injury of unspecified blood vessel of thorax

  ☑x7th **S25.91** Laceration of unspecified blood vessel of thorax

  ☑x7th **S25.99** Other specified injury of unspecified blood vessel of thorax

☑4th **S26** **Injury of heart**

  Code also any associated:
    open wound of thorax (S21.-)
    traumatic hemopneumothorax (S27.2)
    traumatic hemothorax (S27.1)
    traumatic pneumothorax (S27.0)

  The appropriate 7th character is to be added to each code from category S26.
  A   initial encounter
  D   subsequent encounter
  S   sequela

  ☑5th **S26.0** Injury of heart with hemopericardium

    ☑x7th **S26.00** Unspecified injury of heart with hemopericardium

    ☑x7th **S26.01** Contusion of heart with hemopericardium

    ☑6th **S26.02** Laceration of heart with hemopericardium

      ☑7th **S26.020** Mild laceration of heart with hemopericardium
        Laceration of heart without penetration of heart chamber

      ☑7th **S26.021** Moderate laceration of heart with hemopericardium
        Laceration of heart with penetration of heart chamber

      ☑7th **S26.022** Major laceration of heart with hemopericardium
        Laceration of heart with penetration of multiple heart chambers

    ☑x7th **S26.09** Other injury of heart with hemopericardium

  ☑5th **S26.1** Injury of heart without hemopericardium

    ☑x7th **S26.10** Unspecified injury of heart without hemopericardium

    ☑x7th **S26.11** Contusion of heart without hemopericardium

    ☑x7th **S26.12** Laceration of heart without hemopericardium

    ☑x7th **S26.19** Other injury of heart without hemopericardium

  ☑5th **S26.9** Injury of heart, unspecified with or without hemopericardium

    ☑x7th **S26.90** Unspecified injury of heart, unspecified with or without hemopericardium

    ☑x7th **S26.91** Contusion of heart, unspecified with or without hemopericardium

    ☑x7th **S26.92** Laceration of heart, unspecified with or without hemopericardium
      Laceration of heart NOS

    ☑x7th **S26.99** Other injury of heart, unspecified with or without hemopericardium

☑4th **S27** **Injury of other and unspecified intrathoracic organs**

  Code also any associated open wound of thorax (S21.-)

  EXCLUDES 2 injury of cervical esophagus (S10-S19)
            injury of trachea (cervical) (S10-S19)

  The appropriate 7th character is to be added to each code from category S27.
  A   initial encounter
  D   subsequent encounter
  S   sequela

  ☑x7th **S27.0** Traumatic pneumothorax

    EXCLUDES 1 spontaneous pneumothorax (J93.-)

  ☑x7th **S27.1** Traumatic hemothorax

  ☑x7th **S27.2** Traumatic hemopneumothorax

  ☑5th **S27.3** Other and unspecified injuries of lung

    ☑6th **S27.30** Unspecified injury of lung

      ☑7th **S27.301** Unspecified injury of lung, unilateral

      ☑7th **S27.302** Unspecified injury of lung, bilateral

      ☑7th **S27.309** Unspecified injury of lung, unspecified

    ☑6th **S27.31** Primary blast injury of lung
      Blast injury of lung NOS

      ☑7th **S27.311** Primary blast injury of lung, unilateral

      ☑7th **S27.312** Primary blast injury of lung, bilateral

      ☑7th **S27.319** Primary blast injury of lung, unspecified

    ☑6th **S27.32** Contusion of lung

      ☑7th **S27.321** Contusion of lung, unilateral

      ☑7th **S27.322** Contusion of lung, bilateral

      ☑7th **S27.329** Contusion of lung, unspecified

    ☑6th **S27.33** Laceration of lung

      ☑7th **S27.331** Laceration of lung, unilateral

      ☑7th **S27.332** Laceration of lung, bilateral

      ☑7th **S27.339** Laceration of lung, unspecified

    ☑6th **S27.39** Other injuries of lung
      Secondary blast injury of lung

      ☑7th **S27.391** Other injuries of lung, unilateral

      ☑7th **S27.392** Other injuries of lung, bilateral

      ☑7th **S27.399** Other injuries of lung, unspecified

  ☑5th **S27.4** Injury of bronchus

    ☑6th **S27.40** Unspecified injury of bronchus

      ☑7th **S27.401** Unspecified injury of bronchus, unilateral

      ☑7th **S27.402** Unspecified injury of bronchus, bilateral

      ☑7th **S27.409** Unspecified injury of bronchus, unspecified

    ☑6th **S27.41** Primary blast injury of bronchus
      Blast injury of bronchus NOS

      ☑7th **S27.411** Primary blast injury of bronchus, unilateral

      ☑7th **S27.412** Primary blast injury of bronchus, bilateral

      ☑7th **S27.419** Primary blast injury of bronchus, unspecified

    ☑6th **S27.42** Contusion of bronchus

      ☑7th **S27.421** Contusion of bronchus, unilateral

      ☑7th **S27.422** Contusion of bronchus, bilateral

      ☑7th **S27.429** Contusion of bronchus, unspecified

    ☑6th **S27.43** Laceration of bronchus

      ☑7th **S27.431** Laceration of bronchus, unilateral

      ☑7th **S27.432** Laceration of bronchus, bilateral

      ☑7th **S27.439** Laceration of bronchus, unspecified

    ☑6th **S27.49** Other injury of bronchus
      Secondary blast injury of bronchus

      ☑7th **S27.491** Other injury of bronchus, unilateral

      ☑7th **S27.492** Other injury of bronchus, bilateral

      ☑7th **S27.499** Other injury of bronchus, unspecified

  ☑5th **S27.5** Injury of thoracic trachea

    ☑x7th **S27.50** Unspecified injury of thoracic trachea

    ☑x7th **S27.51** Primary blast injury of thoracic trachea
      Blast injury of thoracic trachea NOS

    ☑x7th **S27.52** Contusion of thoracic trachea

    ☑x7th **S27.53** Laceration of thoracic trachea

    ☑x7th **S27.59** Other injury of thoracic trachea
      Secondary blast injury of thoracic trachea

  ☑5th **S27.6** Injury of pleura

    ☑x7th **S27.60** Unspecified injury of pleura

    ☑x7th **S27.63** Laceration of pleura

    ☑x7th **S27.69** Other injury of pleura

  ☑5th **S27.8** Injury of other specified intrathoracic organs

    ☑6th **S27.80** Injury of diaphragm

      ☑7th **S27.802** Contusion of diaphragm

      ☑7th **S27.803** Laceration of diaphragm

      ☑7th **S27.808** Other injury of diaphragm

      ☑7th **S27.809** Unspecified injury of diaphragm

    ☑6th **S27.81** Injury of esophagus (thoracic part)

      ☑7th **S27.812** Contusion of esophagus (thoracic part)

      ☑7th **S27.813** Laceration of esophagus (thoracic part)

☑ Additional Character Required   ☑x7th Xtension Alert   Unspecified Code   Other Specified Code   Manifestation Code   ►◄ Revised Text   ● New Code   ▲ Revised Code Title

ICD-10-CM 2014 (Draft)

827

✓7ᵗʰ **S27.818** Other injury of esophagus (thoracic part)

✓7ᵗʰ **S27.819** Unspecified injury of esophagus (thoracic part)

✓6ᵗʰ **S27.89** Injury of other specified intrathoracic organs
Injury of lymphatic thoracic duct
Injury of thymus gland

    ✓7ᵗʰ **S27.892** Contusion of other specified intrathoracic organs

    ✓7ᵗʰ **S27.893** Laceration of other specified intrathoracic organs

    ✓7ᵗʰ **S27.898** Other injury of other specified intrathoracic organs

    ✓7ᵗʰ **S27.899** Unspecified injury of other specified intrathoracic organs

✓ₓ7ᵗʰ **S27.9** Injury of unspecified intrathoracic organ

✓4ᵗʰ **S28** Crushing injury of thorax, and traumatic amputation of part of thorax

> The appropriate 7th character is to be added to each code from category S28.
> A   initial encounter
> D   subsequent encounter
> S   sequela

✓ₓ7ᵗʰ **S28.0** Crushed chest
Use additional code for all associated injuries
EXCLUDES 1   flail chest (S22.5)

✓ₓ7ᵗʰ **S28.1** Traumatic amputation (partial) of part of thorax, except breast

✓5ᵗʰ **S28.2** Traumatic amputation of breast

    ✓6ᵗʰ **S28.21** Complete traumatic amputation of breast
Traumatic amputation of breast NOS

       ✓7ᵗʰ **S28.211** Complete traumatic amputation of right breast

       ✓7ᵗʰ **S28.212** Complete traumatic amputation of left breast

       ✓7ᵗʰ **S28.219** Complete traumatic amputation of unspecified breast

    ✓6ᵗʰ **S28.22** Partial traumatic amputation of breast

       ✓7ᵗʰ **S28.221** Partial traumatic amputation of right breast

       ✓7ᵗʰ **S28.222** Partial traumatic amputation of left breast

       ✓7ᵗʰ **S28.229** Partial traumatic amputation of unspecified breast

✓4ᵗʰ **S29** Other and unspecified injuries of thorax
Code also any associated open wound (S21.-)

> The appropriate 7th character is to be added to each code from category S29.
> A   initial encounter
> D   subsequent encounter
> S   sequela

✓5ᵗʰ **S29.0** Injury of muscle and tendon at thorax level

    ✓6ᵗʰ **S29.00** Unspecified injury of muscle and tendon of thorax

       ✓7ᵗʰ **S29.001** Unspecified injury of muscle and tendon of front wall of thorax

       ✓7ᵗʰ **S29.002** Unspecified injury of muscle and tendon of back wall of thorax

       ✓7ᵗʰ **S29.009** Unspecified injury of muscle and tendon of unspecified wall of thorax

    ✓6ᵗʰ **S29.01** Strain of muscle and tendon of thorax

       ✓7ᵗʰ **S29.011** Strain of muscle and tendon of front wall of thorax

       ✓7ᵗʰ **S29.012** Strain of muscle and tendon of back wall of thorax

       ✓7ᵗʰ **S29.019** Strain of muscle and tendon of unspecified wall of thorax

    ✓6ᵗʰ **S29.02** Laceration of muscle and tendon of thorax

       ✓7ᵗʰ **S29.021** Laceration of muscle and tendon of front wall of thorax

       ✓7ᵗʰ **S29.022** Laceration of muscle and tendon of back wall of thorax

       ✓7ᵗʰ **S29.029** Laceration of muscle and tendon of unspecified wall of thorax

    ✓6ᵗʰ **S29.09** Other injury of muscle and tendon of thorax

       ✓7ᵗʰ **S29.091** Other injury of muscle and tendon of front wall of thorax

       ✓7ᵗʰ **S29.092** Other injury of muscle and tendon of back wall of thorax

       ✓7ᵗʰ **S29.099** Other injury of muscle and tendon of unspecified wall of thorax

✓ₓ7ᵗʰ **S29.8** Other specified injuries of thorax

✓ₓ7ᵗʰ **S29.9** Unspecified injury of thorax

Injuries to the abdomen, lower back, lumbar spine, pelvis and external genitals (S30-S39)

INCLUDES   injuries to the abdominal wall
injuries to the anus
injuries to the buttock
injuries to the external genitalia
injuries to the flank
injuries to the groin

EXCLUDES 2   burns and corrosions (T20-T32)
effects of foreign body in anus and rectum (T18.5)
effects of foreign body in genitourinary tract (T19.-)
effects of foreign body in stomach, small intestine and colon (T18.2-T18.4)
frostbite (T33-T34)
insect bite or sting, venomous (T63.4)

✓4ᵗʰ **S30** Superficial injury of abdomen, lower back, pelvis and external genitals
EXCLUDES 2   superficial injury of hip (S70.-)

> The appropriate 7th character is to be added to each code from category S30.
> A   initial encounter
> D   subsequent encounter
> S   sequela

✓ₓ7ᵗʰ **S30.0** Contusion of lower back and pelvis
Contusion of buttock

✓ₓ7ᵗʰ **S30.1** Contusion of abdominal wall
Contusion of flank   Contusion of groin

✓5ᵗʰ **S30.2** Contusion of external genital organs

    ✓6ᵗʰ **S30.20** Contusion of unspecified external genital organ

       ✓7ᵗʰ **S30.201** Contusion of unspecified external genital organ, male   ♂

       ✓7ᵗʰ **S30.202** Contusion of unspecified external genital organ, female   ♀

    ✓ₓ7ᵗʰ **S30.21** Contusion of penis   ♂

    ✓ₓ7ᵗʰ **S30.22** Contusion of scrotum and testes   ♂

    ✓ₓ7ᵗʰ **S30.23** Contusion of vagina and vulva   ♀

✓ₓ7ᵗʰ **S30.3** Contusion of anus

✓5ᵗʰ **S30.8** Other superficial injuries of abdomen, lower back, pelvis and external genitals

    ✓6ᵗʰ **S30.81** Abrasion of abdomen, lower back, pelvis and external genitals

       ✓7ᵗʰ **S30.810** Abrasion of lower back and pelvis

       ✓7ᵗʰ **S30.811** Abrasion of abdominal wall

       ✓7ᵗʰ **S30.812** Abrasion of penis   ♂

       ✓7ᵗʰ **S30.813** Abrasion of scrotum and testes   ♂

       ✓7ᵗʰ **S30.814** Abrasion of vagina and vulva   ♀

       ✓7ᵗʰ **S30.815** Abrasion of unspecified external genital organs, male   ♂

       ✓7ᵗʰ **S30.816** Abrasion of unspecified external genital organs, female   ♀

       ✓7ᵗʰ **S30.817** Abrasion of anus

    ✓6ᵗʰ **S30.82** Blister (nonthermal) of abdomen, lower back, pelvis and external genitals

       ✓7ᵗʰ **S30.820** Blister (nonthermal) of lower back and pelvis

       ✓7ᵗʰ **S30.821** Blister (nonthermal) of abdominal wall

       ✓7ᵗʰ **S30.822** Blister (nonthermal) of penis   ♂

       ✓7ᵗʰ **S30.823** Blister (nonthermal) of scrotum and testes   ♂

       ✓7ᵗʰ **S30.824** Blister (nonthermal) of vagina and vulva   ♀

       ✓7ᵗʰ **S30.825** Blister (nonthermal) of unspecified external genital organs, male   ♂

EXCLUDES 1 Not coded here   EXCLUDES 2 Not included here   N Newborn Age: 0   P Pediatric Age: 0-17   M Maternity Age: 12-55   A Adult Age: 15-124

828   ICD-10-CM 2014 (Draft)

✓7th **S30.826** **Blister (nonthermal) of** unspecified external genital organs, female ♀

✓7th **S30.827** **Blister (nonthermal) of** anus

✓6th **S30.84** **External constriction of abdomen, lower back, pelvis and external genitals**

✓7th **S30.840** **External constriction of** lower back and pelvis

✓7th **S30.841** **External constriction of** abdominal wall

✓7th **S30.842** **External constriction of** penis ♂
Hair tourniquet syndrome of penis
Use additional cause code to identify the constricting item (W49.0-)

✓7th **S30.843** **External constriction of** scrotum and testes ♂

✓7th **S30.844** **External constriction of** vagina and vulva ♀

✓7th **S30.845** **External constriction of unspecified** external genital organs, male ♂

✓7th **S30.846** **External constriction of unspecified** external genital organs, female ♀

✓6th **S30.85** **Superficial** foreign body **of abdomen, lower back, pelvis and external genitals**
Splinter in the abdomen, lower back, pelvis and external genitals

✓7th **S30.850** **Superficial foreign body of** lower back and pelvis

✓7th **S30.851** **Superficial foreign body of** abdominal wall

✓7th **S30.852** **Superficial foreign body of** penis ♂

✓7th **S30.853** **Superficial foreign body of** scrotum and testes ♂

✓7th **S30.854** **Superficial foreign body of** vagina and vulva ♀

✓7th **S30.855** **Superficial foreign body of unspecified** external genital organs, male ♂

✓7th **S30.856** **Superficial foreign body of unspecified** external genital organs, female ♀

✓7th **S30.857** **Superficial foreign body of** anus

✓6th **S30.86** **Insect bite (nonvenomous) of abdomen, lower back, pelvis and external genitals**

✓7th **S30.860** **Insect bite (nonvenomous) of** lower back and pelvis

✓7th **S30.861** **Insect bite (nonvenomous) of** abdominal wall

✓7th **S30.862** **Insect bite (nonvenomous) of** penis ♂

✓7th **S30.863** **Insect bite (nonvenomous) of** scrotum and testes ♂

✓7th **S30.864** **Insect bite (nonvenomous) of** vagina and vulva ♀

✓7th **S30.865** **Insect bite (nonvenomous) of unspecified** external genital organs, male ♂

✓7th **S30.866** **Insect bite (nonvenomous) of unspecified** external genital organs, female ♀

✓7th **S30.867** **Insect bite (nonvenomous) of** anus

✓6th **S30.87** **Other** superficial bite **of abdomen, lower back, pelvis and external genitals**
EXCLUDES 1 open bite of abdomen, lower back, pelvis and external genitals (S31.05, S31.15, S31.25, S31.35, S31.45, S31.55)

✓7th **S30.870** **Other superficial bite of** lower back and pelvis

✓7th **S30.871** **Other superficial bite of** abdominal wall

✓7th **S30.872** **Other superficial bite of** penis ♂

✓7th **S30.873** **Other superficial bite of** scrotum and testes ♂

✓7th **S30.874** **Other superficial bite of** vagina and vulva ♀

✓7th **S30.875** **Other superficial bite of unspecified** external genital organs, male ♂

✓7th **S30.876** **Other superficial bite of unspecified** external genital organs, female ♀

✓7th **S30.877** **Other superficial bite of** anus

✓5th **S30.9** Unspecified **superficial injury of abdomen, lower back, pelvis and external genitals**

✓x7th **S30.91** **Unspecified superficial injury of** lower back and pelvis

✓x7th **S30.92** **Unspecified superficial injury of** abdominal wall

✓x7th **S30.93** **Unspecified superficial injury of** penis ♂

✓x7th **S30.94** **Unspecified superficial injury of** scrotum and testes ♂

✓x7th **S30.95** **Unspecified superficial injury of** vagina and vulva ♀

✓x7th **S30.96** **Unspecified superficial injury of unspecified** external genital organs, male ♂

✓x7th **S30.97** **Unspecified superficial injury of unspecified** external genital organs, female ♀

✓x7th **S30.98** **Unspecified superficial injury of** anus

✓4th **S31** **Open wound of abdomen, lower back, pelvis and external genitals**
Code also any associated:
spinal cord injury (S24.0, S24.1-, S34.0-, S34.1-)
wound infection
EXCLUDES 1 traumatic amputation of part of abdomen, lower back and pelvis (S38.2-, S38.3)
EXCLUDES 2 open wound of hip (S71.00-S71.02)
open fracture of pelvis (S32.1--S32.9 with 7th character B)

The appropriate 7th character is to be added to each code from category S31.
A   initial encounter
D   subsequent encounter
S   sequela

✓5th **S31.0** **Open wound of** lower back and pelvis

✓6th **S31.00** Unspecified **open wound of lower back and pelvis**

✓7th **S31.000** **Unspecified open wound of lower back and pelvis** without penetration into retroperitoneum
Unspecified open wound of lower back and pelvis NOS

✓7th **S31.001** **Unspecified open wound of lower back and pelvis** with penetration into retroperitoneum

✓6th **S31.01** Laceration without foreign body **of lower back and pelvis**

✓7th **S31.010** **Laceration without foreign body of lower back and pelvis** without penetration into retroperitoneum
Laceration without foreign body of lower back and pelvis NOS

✓7th **S31.011** **Laceration without foreign body of lower back and pelvis** with penetration into retroperitoneum

✓6th **S31.02** Laceration with foreign body **of lower back and pelvis**

✓7th **S31.020** **Laceration with foreign body of lower back and pelvis** without penetration into retroperitoneum
Laceration with foreign body of lower back and pelvis NOS

✓7th **S31.021** **Laceration with foreign body of lower back and pelvis** with penetration into retroperitoneum

✓6th **S31.03** Puncture wound without foreign body **of lower back and pelvis**

✓7th **S31.030** **Puncture wound without foreign body of lower back and pelvis** without penetration into retroperitoneum
Puncture wound without foreign body of lower back and pelvis NOS

✓7th **S31.031** **Puncture wound without foreign body of lower back and pelvis** with penetration into retroperitoneum

✓6th **S31.04** Puncture wound with foreign body **of lower back and pelvis**

✓7th **S31.040** **Puncture wound with foreign body of lower back and pelvis** without penetration into retroperitoneum
Puncture wound with foreign body of lower back and pelvis NOS

✓ Additional Character Required   ✓x7th Xtension Alert   Unspecified Code   Other Specified Code   Manifestation Code   ▶◀ Revised Text   ● New Code   ▲ Revised Code Title
ICD-10-CM 2014 (Draft)

829

√7ᵗʰ **S31.041** **Puncture wound with foreign body of lower back and pelvis** with penetration into retroperitoneum

√6ᵗʰ **S31.05** **Open bite** of lower back and pelvis
Bite of lower back and pelvis NOS
EXCLUDES 1 *superficial bite of lower back and pelvis (S30.860, S30.870)*

√7ᵗʰ **S31.050** **Open bite of lower back and pelvis** without penetration into retroperitoneum
Open bite of lower back and pelvis NOS

√7ᵗʰ **S31.051** **Open bite of lower back and pelvis** with penetration into retroperitoneum

√5ᵗʰ **S31.1** **Open wound of** abdominal wall without penetration into peritoneal cavity
Open wound of abdominal wall NOS
EXCLUDES 2 *open wound of abdominal wall with penetration into peritoneal cavity (S31.6-)*

√6ᵗʰ **S31.10** **Unspecified** open wound of abdominal wall without penetration into peritoneal cavity

√7ᵗʰ **S31.100** **Unspecified open wound of abdominal wall,** right upper quadrant **without penetration into peritoneal cavity**

√7ᵗʰ **S31.101** **Unspecified open wound of abdominal wall,** left upper quadrant **without penetration into peritoneal cavity**

√7ᵗʰ **S31.102** **Unspecified open wound of abdominal wall,** epigastric region **without penetration into peritoneal cavity**

√7ᵗʰ **S31.103** **Unspecified open wound of abdominal wall,** right lower quadrant **without penetration into peritoneal cavity**

√7ᵗʰ **S31.104** **Unspecified open wound of abdominal wall,** left lower quadrant **without penetration into peritoneal cavity**

√7ᵗʰ **S31.105** **Unspecified open wound of abdominal wall,** periumbilic region **without penetration into peritoneal cavity**

√7ᵗʰ **S31.109** **Unspecified open wound of abdominal wall, unspecified quadrant without penetration into peritoneal cavity**
Unspecified open wound of abdominal wall NOS

√6ᵗʰ **S31.11** **Laceration without foreign body** of abdominal wall without penetration into peritoneal cavity

√7ᵗʰ **S31.110** **Laceration without foreign body of abdominal wall,** right upper quadrant **without penetration into peritoneal cavity**

√7ᵗʰ **S31.111** **Laceration without foreign body of abdominal wall,** left upper quadrant **without penetration into peritoneal cavity**

√7ᵗʰ **S31.112** **Laceration without foreign body of abdominal wall,** epigastric region **without penetration into peritoneal cavity**

√7ᵗʰ **S31.113** **Laceration without foreign body of abdominal wall,** right lower quadrant **without penetration into peritoneal cavity**

√7ᵗʰ **S31.114** **Laceration without foreign body of abdominal wall,** left lower quadrant **without penetration into peritoneal cavity**

√7ᵗʰ **S31.115** **Laceration without foreign body of abdominal wall,** periumbilic region **without penetration into peritoneal cavity**

√7ᵗʰ **S31.119** **Laceration without foreign body of abdominal wall, unspecified quadrant without penetration into peritoneal cavity**

√6ᵗʰ **S31.12** **Laceration with foreign body** of abdominal wall without penetration into peritoneal cavity

√7ᵗʰ **S31.120** **Laceration of abdominal wall with foreign body,** right upper quadrant **without penetration into peritoneal cavity**

√7ᵗʰ **S31.121** **Laceration of abdominal wall with foreign body,** left upper quadrant **without penetration into peritoneal cavity**

√7ᵗʰ **S31.122** **Laceration of abdominal wall with foreign body,** epigastric region **without penetration into peritoneal cavity**

√7ᵗʰ **S31.123** **Laceration of abdominal wall with foreign body,** right lower quadrant **without penetration into peritoneal cavity**

√7ᵗʰ **S31.124** **Laceration of abdominal wall with foreign body,** left lower quadrant **without penetration into peritoneal cavity**

√7ᵗʰ **S31.125** **Laceration of abdominal wall with foreign body,** periumbilic region **without penetration into peritoneal cavity**

√7ᵗʰ **S31.129** **Laceration of abdominal wall with foreign body, unspecified quadrant without penetration into peritoneal cavity**

√6ᵗʰ **S31.13** **Puncture wound** of abdominal wall without foreign body without penetration into peritoneal cavity

√7ᵗʰ **S31.130** **Puncture wound of abdominal wall without foreign body,** right upper quadrant **without penetration into peritoneal cavity**

√7ᵗʰ **S31.131** **Puncture wound of abdominal wall without foreign body,** left upper quadrant **without penetration into peritoneal cavity**

√7ᵗʰ **S31.132** **Puncture wound of abdominal wall without foreign body,** epigastric region **without penetration into peritoneal cavity**

√7ᵗʰ **S31.133** **Puncture wound of abdominal wall without foreign body,** right lower quadrant **without penetration into peritoneal cavity**

√7ᵗʰ **S31.134** **Puncture wound of abdominal wall without foreign body,** left lower quadrant **without penetration into peritoneal cavity**

√7ᵗʰ **S31.135** **Puncture wound of abdominal wall without foreign body,** periumbilic region **without penetration into peritoneal cavity**

√7ᵗʰ **S31.139** **Puncture wound of abdominal wall without foreign body, unspecified quadrant without penetration into peritoneal cavity**

√6ᵗʰ **S31.14** **Puncture wound** of abdominal wall with foreign body without penetration into peritoneal cavity

√7ᵗʰ **S31.140** **Puncture wound of abdominal wall with foreign body,** right upper quadrant **without penetration into peritoneal cavity**

√7ᵗʰ **S31.141** **Puncture wound of abdominal wall with foreign body,** left upper quadrant **without penetration into peritoneal cavity**

√7ᵗʰ **S31.142** **Puncture wound of abdominal wall with foreign body,** epigastric region **without penetration into peritoneal cavity**

√7ᵗʰ **S31.143** **Puncture wound of abdominal wall with foreign body,** right lower quadrant **without penetration into peritoneal cavity**

√7ᵗʰ **S31.144** **Puncture wound of abdominal wall with foreign body,** left lower quadrant **without penetration into peritoneal cavity**

√7ᵗʰ **S31.145** **Puncture wound of abdominal wall with foreign body,** periumbilic region **without penetration into peritoneal cavity**

√7ᵗʰ **S31.149** **Puncture wound of abdominal wall with foreign body, unspecified quadrant without penetration into peritoneal cavity**

√6ᵗʰ **S31.15** **Open bite** of abdominal wall without penetration into peritoneal cavity
Bite of abdominal wall NOS
EXCLUDES 1 *superficial bite of abdominal wall (S30.871)*

√7ᵗʰ **S31.150** **Open bite of abdominal wall,** right upper quadrant **without penetration into peritoneal cavity**

√7ᵗʰ **S31.151** **Open bite of abdominal wall,** left upper quadrant **without penetration into peritoneal cavity**

√7ᵗʰ **S31.152** **Open bite of abdominal wall,** epigastric region **without penetration into peritoneal cavity**

√7ᵗʰ **S31.153** **Open bite of abdominal wall,** right lower quadrant **without penetration into peritoneal cavity**

√7ᵗʰ **S31.154** **Open bite of abdominal wall,** left lower quadrant **without penetration into peritoneal cavity**

EXCLUDES 1 Not coded here   **EXCLUDES 2** Not included here   Ⓝ Newborn Age: 0   Ⓟ Pediatric Age: 0-17   Ⓜ Maternity Age: 12-55   Ⓐ Adult Age: 15-124

830   ICD-10-CM 2014 (Draft)

√7ᵗʰ **S31.155 Open bite of abdominal wall,** periumbilic region **without penetration into peritoneal cavity**

√7ᵗʰ **S31.159 Open bite of abdominal wall, unspecified quadrant without penetration into peritoneal cavity**

√5ᵗʰ **S31.2 Open wound of** penis

√x7ᵗʰ **S31.20 Unspecified open wound of penis** ♂

√x7ᵗʰ **S31.21** Laceration without foreign body **of penis** ♂

√x7ᵗʰ **S31.22** Laceration with foreign body **of penis** ♂

√x7ᵗʰ **S31.23** Puncture wound without foreign body **of penis** ♂

√x7ᵗʰ **S31.24** Puncture wound with foreign body **of penis** ♂

√x7ᵗʰ **S31.25** Open bite **of penis** ♂
    Bite of penis NOS
    EXCLUDES 1   *superficial bite of penis (S30.862, S30.872)*

√5ᵗʰ **S31.3 Open wound of** scrotum and testes

√x7ᵗʰ **S31.30 Unspecified open wound of scrotum and testes** ♂

√x7ᵗʰ **S31.31** Laceration without foreign body **of scrotum and testes** ♂

√x7ᵗʰ **S31.32** Laceration with foreign body **of scrotum and testes** ♂

√x7ᵗʰ **S31.33** Puncture wound without foreign body **of scrotum and testes** ♂

√x7ᵗʰ **S31.34** Puncture wound with foreign body **of scrotum and testes** ♂

√x7ᵗʰ **S31.35** Open bite **of scrotum and testes** ♂
    Bite of scrotum and testes NOS
    EXCLUDES 1   *superficial bite of scrotum and testes (S30.863, S30.873)*

√5ᵗʰ **S31.4 Open wound of** vagina and vulva
    EXCLUDES 1   *injury to vagina and vulva during delivery (O70-, O71.4)*

√x7ᵗʰ **S31.40 Unspecified open wound of vagina and vulva** ♀

√x7ᵗʰ **S31.41** Laceration without foreign body **of vagina and vulva** ♀

√x7ᵗʰ **S31.42** Laceration with foreign body **of vagina and vulva** ♀

√x7ᵗʰ **S31.43** Puncture wound without foreign body **of vagina and vulva** ♀

√x7ᵗʰ **S31.44** Puncture wound with foreign body **of vagina and vulva** ♀

√x7ᵗʰ **S31.45** Open bite **of vagina and vulva** ♀
    Bite of vagina and vulva NOS
    EXCLUDES 1   *superficial bite of vagina and vulva (S30.864, S30.874)*

√5ᵗʰ **S31.5 Open wound of** unspecified external genital organs
    EXCLUDES 1   *traumatic amputation of external genital organs (S38.21, S38.22)*

√6ᵗʰ **S31.50 Unspecified open wound of unspecified external genital organs**

√7ᵗʰ **S31.501 Unspecified open wound of unspecified external genital organs,** male ♂

√7ᵗʰ **S31.502 Unspecified open wound of unspecified external genital organs,** female ♀

√6ᵗʰ **S31.51** Laceration without foreign body **of unspecified external genital organs**

√7ᵗʰ **S31.511 Laceration without foreign body of unspecified external genital organs,** male ♂

√7ᵗʰ **S31.512 Laceration without foreign body of unspecified external genital organs,** female ♀

√6ᵗʰ **S31.52** Laceration with foreign body **of unspecified external genital organs**

√7ᵗʰ **S31.521 Laceration with foreign body of unspecified external genital organs,** male ♂

√7ᵗʰ **S31.522 Laceration with foreign body of unspecified external genital organs,** female ♀

√6ᵗʰ **S31.53** Puncture wound without foreign body **of unspecified external genital organs**

√7ᵗʰ **S31.531 Puncture wound without foreign body of unspecified external genital organs,** male ♂

√7ᵗʰ **S31.532 Puncture wound without foreign body of unspecified external genital organs,** female ♀

√6ᵗʰ **S31.54** Puncture wound with foreign body **of unspecified external genital organs**

√7ᵗʰ **S31.541 Puncture wound with foreign body of unspecified external genital organs,** male ♂

√7ᵗʰ **S31.542 Puncture wound with foreign body of unspecified external genital organs,** female ♀

√6ᵗʰ **S31.55** Open bite **of unspecified external genital organs**
    Bite of unspecified external genital organs NOS
    EXCLUDES 1   *superficial bite of unspecified external genital organs (S30.865, S30.866, S30.875, S30.876)*

√7ᵗʰ **S31.551 Open bite of unspecified external genital organs,** male ♂

√7ᵗʰ **S31.552 Open bite of unspecified external genital organs,** female ♀

√5ᵗʰ **S31.6 Open wound of** abdominal wall with penetration into peritoneal cavity

√6ᵗʰ **S31.60 Unspecified** open wound of abdominal wall with penetration into peritoneal cavity

√7ᵗʰ **S31.600 Unspecified open wound of abdominal wall,** right upper quadrant **with penetration into peritoneal cavity**

√7ᵗʰ **S31.601 Unspecified open wound of abdominal wall,** left upper quadrant **with penetration into peritoneal cavity**

√7ᵗʰ **S31.602 Unspecified open wound of abdominal wall,** epigastric region **with penetration into peritoneal cavity**

√7ᵗʰ **S31.603 Unspecified open wound of abdominal wall,** right lower quadrant **with penetration into peritoneal cavity**

√7ᵗʰ **S31.604 Unspecified open wound of abdominal wall,** left lower quadrant **with penetration into peritoneal cavity**

√7ᵗʰ **S31.605 Unspecified open wound of abdominal wall,** periumbilic region **with penetration into peritoneal cavity**

√7ᵗʰ **S31.609 Unspecified open wound of abdominal wall, unspecified quadrant with penetration into peritoneal cavity**

√6ᵗʰ **S31.61** Laceration without foreign body **of abdominal wall with penetration into peritoneal cavity**

√7ᵗʰ **S31.610 Laceration without foreign body of abdominal wall,** right upper quadrant **with penetration into peritoneal cavity**

√7ᵗʰ **S31.611 Laceration without foreign body of abdominal wall,** left upper quadrant **with penetration into peritoneal cavity**

√7ᵗʰ **S31.612 Laceration without foreign body of abdominal wall,** epigastric region **with penetration into peritoneal cavity**

√7ᵗʰ **S31.613 Laceration without foreign body of abdominal wall,** right lower quadrant **with penetration into peritoneal cavity**

√7ᵗʰ **S31.614 Laceration without foreign body of abdominal wall,** left lower quadrant **with penetration into peritoneal cavity**

√7ᵗʰ **S31.615 Laceration without foreign body of abdominal wall,** periumbilic region **with penetration into peritoneal cavity**

√7ᵗʰ **S31.619 Laceration without foreign body of abdominal wall, unspecified quadrant with penetration into peritoneal cavity**

√6ᵗʰ **S31.62** Laceration with foreign body **of abdominal wall with penetration into peritoneal cavity**

√7ᵗʰ **S31.620 Laceration with foreign body of abdominal wall,** right upper quadrant **with penetration into peritoneal cavity**

√7ᵗʰ **S31.621 Laceration with foreign body of abdominal wall,** left upper quadrant **with penetration into peritoneal cavity**

√7ᵗʰ **S31.622** Laceration with foreign body of abdominal wall, epigastric region with penetration into peritoneal cavity

√7ᵗʰ **S31.623** Laceration with foreign body of abdominal wall, right lower quadrant with penetration into peritoneal cavity

√7ᵗʰ **S31.624** Laceration with foreign body of abdominal wall, left lower quadrant with penetration into peritoneal cavity

√7ᵗʰ **S31.625** Laceration with foreign body of abdominal wall, periumbilic region with penetration into peritoneal cavity

√7ᵗʰ **S31.629** Laceration with foreign body of abdominal wall, unspecified quadrant with penetration into peritoneal cavity

√6ᵗʰ **S31.63** Puncture wound without foreign body of abdominal wall with penetration into peritoneal cavity

√7ᵗʰ **S31.630** Puncture wound without foreign body of abdominal wall, right upper quadrant with penetration into peritoneal cavity

√7ᵗʰ **S31.631** Puncture wound without foreign body of abdominal wall, left upper quadrant with penetration into peritoneal cavity

√7ᵗʰ **S31.632** Puncture wound without foreign body of abdominal wall, epigastric region with penetration into peritoneal cavity

√7ᵗʰ **S31.633** Puncture wound without foreign body of abdominal wall, right lower quadrant with penetration into peritoneal cavity

√7ᵗʰ **S31.634** Puncture wound without foreign body of abdominal wall, left lower quadrant with penetration into peritoneal cavity

√7ᵗʰ **S31.635** Puncture wound without foreign body of abdominal wall, periumbilic region with penetration into peritoneal cavity

√7ᵗʰ **S31.639** Puncture wound without foreign body of abdominal wall, unspecified quadrant with penetration into peritoneal cavity

√6ᵗʰ **S31.64** Puncture wound with foreign body of abdominal wall with penetration into peritoneal cavity

√7ᵗʰ **S31.640** Puncture wound with foreign body of abdominal wall, right upper quadrant with penetration into peritoneal cavity

√7ᵗʰ **S31.641** Puncture wound with foreign body of abdominal wall, left upper quadrant with penetration into peritoneal cavity

√7ᵗʰ **S31.642** Puncture wound with foreign body of abdominal wall, epigastric region with penetration into peritoneal cavity

√7ᵗʰ **S31.643** Puncture wound with foreign body of abdominal wall, right lower quadrant with penetration into peritoneal cavity

√7ᵗʰ **S31.644** Puncture wound with foreign body of abdominal wall, left lower quadrant with penetration into peritoneal cavity

√7ᵗʰ **S31.645** Puncture wound with foreign body of abdominal wall, periumbilic region with penetration into peritoneal cavity

√7ᵗʰ **S31.649** Puncture wound with foreign body of abdominal wall, unspecified quadrant with penetration into peritoneal cavity

√6ᵗʰ **S31.65** Open bite of abdominal wall with penetration into peritoneal cavity

     EXCLUDES 1   superficial bite of abdominal wall (S30.861, S30.871)

√7ᵗʰ **S31.650** Open bite of abdominal wall, right upper quadrant with penetration into peritoneal cavity

√7ᵗʰ **S31.651** Open bite of abdominal wall, left upper quadrant with penetration into peritoneal cavity

√7ᵗʰ **S31.652** Open bite of abdominal wall, epigastric region with penetration into peritoneal cavity

√7ᵗʰ **S31.653** Open bite of abdominal wall, right lower quadrant with penetration into peritoneal cavity

√7ᵗʰ **S31.654** Open bite of abdominal wall, left lower quadrant with penetration into peritoneal cavity

√7ᵗʰ **S31.655** Open bite of abdominal wall, periumbilic region with penetration into peritoneal cavity

√7ᵗʰ **S31.659** Open bite of abdominal wall, unspecified quadrant with penetration into peritoneal cavity

√5ᵗʰ **S31.8** **Open wound of other parts of abdomen, lower back and pelvis**

√6ᵗʰ **S31.80** Open wound of unspecified buttock

√7ᵗʰ **S31.801** Laceration without foreign body of unspecified buttock

√7ᵗʰ **S31.802** Laceration with foreign body of unspecified buttock

√7ᵗʰ **S31.803** Puncture wound without foreign body of unspecified buttock

√7ᵗʰ **S31.804** Puncture wound with foreign body of unspecified buttock

√7ᵗʰ **S31.805** Open bite of unspecified buttock

     Bite of buttock NOS

     EXCLUDES 1   superficial bite of buttock (S30.870)

√7ᵗʰ **S31.809** Unspecified open wound of unspecified buttock

√6ᵗʰ **S31.81** Open wound of right buttock

√7ᵗʰ **S31.811** Laceration without foreign body of right buttock

√7ᵗʰ **S31.812** Laceration with foreign body of right buttock

√7ᵗʰ **S31.813** Puncture wound without foreign body of right buttock

√7ᵗʰ **S31.814** Puncture wound with foreign body of right buttock

√7ᵗʰ **S31.815** Open bite of right buttock

     Bite of right buttock NOS

     EXCLUDES 1   superficial bite of buttock (S30.870)

√7ᵗʰ **S31.819** Unspecified open wound of right buttock

√6ᵗʰ **S31.82** Open wound of left buttock

√7ᵗʰ **S31.821** Laceration without foreign body of left buttock

√7ᵗʰ **S31.822** Laceration with foreign body of left buttock

√7ᵗʰ **S31.823** Puncture wound without foreign body of left buttock

√7ᵗʰ **S31.824** Puncture wound with foreign body of left buttock

√7ᵗʰ **S31.825** Open bite of left buttock

     Bite of left buttock NOS

     EXCLUDES 1   superficial bite of buttock (S30.870)

√7ᵗʰ **S31.829** Unspecified open wound of left buttock

√6ᵗʰ **S31.83** Open wound of anus

√7ᵗʰ **S31.831** Laceration without foreign body of anus

√7ᵗʰ **S31.832** Laceration with foreign body of anus

√7ᵗʰ **S31.833** Puncture wound without foreign body of anus

√7ᵗʰ **S31.834** Puncture wound with foreign body of anus

√7ᵗʰ **S31.835** Open bite of anus

     Bite of anus NOS

     EXCLUDES 1   superficial bite of anus (S30.877)

√7ᵗʰ **S31.839** Unspecified open wound of anus

EXCLUDES 1 Not coded here   EXCLUDES 2 Not included here   N Newborn Age: 0   P Pediatric Age: 0–17   M Maternity Age: 12–55   A Adult Age: 15–124

832   ICD-10-CM 2014 (Draft)

✓4th **S32 Fracture of lumbar spine and pelvis**

> **NOTE** A fracture not indicated as displaced or nondisplaced should be coded to displaced.
> A fracture not indicated as opened or closed should be coded to closed.
> **INCLUDES** fracture of lumbosacral neural arch
> fracture of lumbosacral spinous process
> fracture of lumbosacral transverse process
> fracture of lumbosacral vertebra
> fracture of lumbosacral vertebral arch

Codes first any associated spinal cord and spinal nerve injury (S34.-)

EXCLUDES 1 transection of abdomen (S38.3)
EXCLUDES 2 fracture of hip NOS (S72.0-)

> The appropriate 7th character is to be added to each code from category S32.
> A   initial encounter for closed fracture
> B   initial encounter for open fracture
> D   subsequent encounter for fracture with routine healing
> G   subsequent encounter for fracture with delayed healing
> K   subsequent encounter for fracture with nonunion
> S   sequela

✓5th **S32.0 Fracture of lumbar vertebra**
Fracture of lumbar spine NOS

✓6th **S32.00 Fracture of unspecified lumbar vertebra**

✓7th **S32.000 Wedge compression fracture of unspecified lumbar vertebra**

✓7th **S32.001 Stable burst fracture of unspecified lumbar vertebra**

✓7th **S32.002 Unstable burst fracture of unspecified lumbar vertebra**

✓7th **S32.008 Other fracture of unspecified lumbar vertebra**

✓7th **S32.009 Unspecified fracture of unspecified lumbar vertebra**

✓6th **S32.01 Fracture of first lumbar vertebra**

✓7th **S32.010 Wedge compression fracture of first lumbar vertebra**

✓7th **S32.011 Stable burst fracture of first lumbar vertebra**

✓7th **S32.012 Unstable burst fracture of first lumbar vertebra**

✓7th **S32.018 Other fracture of first lumbar vertebra**

✓7th **S32.019 Unspecified fracture of first lumbar vertebra**

✓6th **S32.02 Fracture of second lumbar vertebra**

✓7th **S32.020 Wedge compression fracture of second lumbar vertebra**

✓7th **S32.021 Stable burst fracture of second lumbar vertebra**

✓7th **S32.022 Unstable burst fracture of second lumbar vertebra**

✓7th **S32.028 Other fracture of second lumbar vertebra**

✓7th **S32.029 Unspecified fracture of second lumbar vertebra**

✓6th **S32.03 Fracture of third lumbar vertebra**

✓7th **S32.030 Wedge compression fracture of third lumbar vertebra**

✓7th **S32.031 Stable burst fracture of third lumbar vertebra**

✓7th **S32.032 Unstable burst fracture of third lumbar vertebra**

✓7th **S32.038 Other fracture of third lumbar vertebra**

✓7th **S32.039 Unspecified fracture of third lumbar vertebra**

✓6th **S32.04 Fracture of fourth lumbar vertebra**

✓7th **S32.040 Wedge compression fracture of fourth lumbar vertebra**

✓7th **S32.041 Stable burst fracture of fourth lumbar vertebra**

✓7th **S32.042 Unstable burst fracture of fourth lumbar vertebra**

✓7th **S32.048 Other fracture of fourth lumbar vertebra**

✓7th **S32.049 Unspecified fracture of fourth lumbar vertebra**

✓6th **S32.05 Fracture of fifth lumbar vertebra**

✓7th **S32.050 Wedge compression fracture of fifth lumbar vertebra**

✓7th **S32.051 Stable burst fracture of fifth lumbar vertebra**

✓7th **S32.052 Unstable burst fracture of fifth lumbar vertebra**

✓7th **S32.058 Other fracture of fifth lumbar vertebra**

✓7th **S32.059 Unspecified fracture of fifth lumbar vertebra**

✓5th **S32.1 Fracture of sacrum**

> **NOTE** For vertical fractures, code to most medial fracture extension.
> Use two codes if both a vertical and transverse fracture are present.

Code also any associated fracture of pelvic ring (S32.8-)

✓x7th **S32.10 Unspecified fracture of sacrum**

✓6th **S32.11 Zone I fracture of sacrum**
Vertical sacral ala fracture of sacrum

✓7th **S32.110 Nondisplaced Zone I fracture of sacrum**

✓7th **S32.111 Minimally displaced Zone I fracture of sacrum**

✓7th **S32.112 Severely displaced Zone I fracture of sacrum**

✓7th **S32.119 Unspecified Zone I fracture of sacrum**

✓6th **S32.12 Zone II fracture of sacrum**
Vertical foraminal region fracture of sacrum

✓7th **S32.120 Nondisplaced Zone II fracture of sacrum**

✓7th **S32.121 Minimally displaced Zone II fracture of sacrum**

✓7th **S32.122 Severely displaced Zone II fracture of sacrum**

✓7th **S32.129 Unspecified Zone II fracture of sacrum**

✓6th **S32.13 Zone III fracture of sacrum**
Vertical fracture into spinal canal region of sacrum

✓7th **S32.130 Nondisplaced Zone III fracture of sacrum**

✓7th **S32.131 Minimally displaced Zone III fracture of sacrum**

✓7th **S32.132 Severely displaced Zone III fracture of sacrum**

✓7th **S32.139 Unspecified Zone III fracture of sacrum**

✓x7th **S32.14 Type 1 fracture of sacrum**
Transverse flexion fracture of sacrum without displacement

✓x7th **S32.15 Type 2 fracture of sacrum**
Transverse flexion fracture of sacrum with posterior displacement

✓x7th **S32.16 Type 3 fracture of sacrum**
Transverse extension fracture of sacrum with anterior displacement

✓x7th **S32.17 Type 4 fracture of sacrum**
Transverse segmental comminution of upper sacrum

✓x7th **S32.19 Other fracture of sacrum**

✓x7th **S32.2 Fracture of coccyx**

✓5th **S32.3 Fracture of ilium**

> **EXCLUDES 1** fracture of ilium with associated disruption of pelvic ring (S32.8-)

✓6th **S32.30 Unspecified fracture of ilium**

✓7th **S32.301 Unspecified fracture of right ilium**

✓7th **S32.302 Unspecified fracture of left ilium**

✓7th **S32.309 Unspecified fracture of unspecified ilium**

✓6th **S32.31 Avulsion fracture of ilium**

✓7th **S32.311 Displaced avulsion fracture of right ilium**

✓7th **S32.312 Displaced avulsion fracture of left ilium**

✓7th **S32.313 Displaced avulsion fracture of unspecified ilium**

✓7th **S32.314 Nondisplaced avulsion fracture of right ilium**

✓7th **S32.315 Nondisplaced avulsion fracture of left ilium**

✓7th **S32.316 Nondisplaced avulsion fracture of unspecified ilium**

✓6ᵗʰ **S32.39** Other fracture of ilium
    ✓7ᵗʰ **S32.391** Other fracture of right ilium
    ✓7ᵗʰ **S32.392** Other fracture of left ilium
    ✓7ᵗʰ **S32.399** Other fracture of unspecified ilium

✓5ᵗʰ **S32.4** Fracture of acetabulum
    Code also any associated fracture of pelvic ring (S32.8-)

    ✓6ᵗʰ **S32.40** Unspecified fracture of acetabulum
      ✓7ᵗʰ **S32.401** Unspecified fracture of right acetabulum
      ✓7ᵗʰ **S32.402** Unspecified fracture of left acetabulum
      ✓7ᵗʰ **S32.409** Unspecified fracture of unspecified acetabulum

    ✓6ᵗʰ **S32.41** Fracture of anterior wall of acetabulum
      ✓7ᵗʰ **S32.411** Displaced fracture of anterior wall of right acetabulum
      ✓7ᵗʰ **S32.412** Displaced fracture of anterior wall of left acetabulum
      ✓7ᵗʰ **S32.413** Displaced fracture of anterior wall of unspecified acetabulum
      ✓7ᵗʰ **S32.414** Nondisplaced fracture of anterior wall of right acetabulum
      ✓7ᵗʰ **S32.415** Nondisplaced fracture of anterior wall of left acetabulum
      ✓7ᵗʰ **S32.416** Nondisplaced fracture of anterior wall of unspecified acetabulum

    ✓6ᵗʰ **S32.42** Fracture of posterior wall of acetabulum
      ✓7ᵗʰ **S32.421** Displaced fracture of posterior wall of right acetabulum
      ✓7ᵗʰ **S32.422** Displaced fracture of posterior wall of left acetabulum
      ✓7ᵗʰ **S32.423** Displaced fracture of posterior wall of unspecified acetabulum
      ✓7ᵗʰ **S32.424** Nondisplaced fracture of posterior wall of right acetabulum
      ✓7ᵗʰ **S32.425** Nondisplaced fracture of posterior wall of left acetabulum
      ✓7ᵗʰ **S32.426** Nondisplaced fracture of posterior wall of unspecified acetabulum

    ✓6ᵗʰ **S32.43** Fracture of anterior column [iliopubic] of acetabulum
      ✓7ᵗʰ **S32.431** Displaced fracture of anterior column [iliopubic] of right acetabulum
      ✓7ᵗʰ **S32.432** Displaced fracture of anterior column [iliopubic] of left acetabulum
      ✓7ᵗʰ **S32.433** Displaced fracture of anterior column [iliopubic] of unspecified acetabulum
      ✓7ᵗʰ **S32.434** Nondisplaced fracture of anterior column [iliopubic] of right acetabulum
      ✓7ᵗʰ **S32.435** Nondisplaced fracture of anterior column [iliopubic] of left acetabulum
      ✓7ᵗʰ **S32.436** Nondisplaced fracture of anterior column [iliopubic] of unspecified acetabulum

    ✓6ᵗʰ **S32.44** Fracture of posterior column [ilioischial] of acetabulum
      ✓7ᵗʰ **S32.441** Displaced fracture of posterior column [ilioischial] of right acetabulum
      ✓7ᵗʰ **S32.442** Displaced fracture of posterior column [ilioischial] of left acetabulum
      ✓7ᵗʰ **S32.443** Displaced fracture of posterior column [ilioischial] of unspecified acetabulum
      ✓7ᵗʰ **S32.444** Nondisplaced fracture of posterior column [ilioischial] of right acetabulum
      ✓7ᵗʰ **S32.445** Nondisplaced fracture of posterior column [ilioischial] of left acetabulum
      ✓7ᵗʰ **S32.446** Nondisplaced fracture of posterior column [ilioischial] of unspecified acetabulum

    ✓6ᵗʰ **S32.45** Transverse fracture of acetabulum
      ✓7ᵗʰ **S32.451** Displaced transverse fracture of right acetabulum
      ✓7ᵗʰ **S32.452** Displaced transverse fracture of left acetabulum
      ✓7ᵗʰ **S32.453** Displaced transverse fracture of unspecified acetabulum
      ✓7ᵗʰ **S32.454** Nondisplaced transverse fracture of right acetabulum
      ✓7ᵗʰ **S32.455** Nondisplaced transverse fracture of left acetabulum
      ✓7ᵗʰ **S32.456** Nondisplaced transverse fracture of unspecified acetabulum

    ✓6ᵗʰ **S32.46** Associated transverse-posterior fracture of acetabulum
      ✓7ᵗʰ **S32.461** Displaced associated transverse-posterior fracture of right acetabulum
      ✓7ᵗʰ **S32.462** Displaced associated transverse-posterior fracture of left acetabulum
      ✓7ᵗʰ **S32.463** Displaced associated transverse-posterior fracture of unspecified acetabulum
      ✓7ᵗʰ **S32.464** Nondisplaced associated transverse-posterior fracture of right acetabulum
      ✓7ᵗʰ **S32.465** Nondisplaced associated transverse-posterior fracture of left acetabulum
      ✓7ᵗʰ **S32.466** Nondisplaced associated transverse-posterior fracture of unspecified acetabulum

    ✓6ᵗʰ **S32.47** Fracture of medial wall of acetabulum
      ✓7ᵗʰ **S32.471** Displaced fracture of medial wall of right acetabulum
      ✓7ᵗʰ **S32.472** Displaced fracture of medial wall of left acetabulum
      ✓7ᵗʰ **S32.473** Displaced fracture of medial wall of unspecified acetabulum
      ✓7ᵗʰ **S32.474** Nondisplaced fracture of medial wall of right acetabulum
      ✓7ᵗʰ **S32.475** Nondisplaced fracture of medial wall of left acetabulum
      ✓7ᵗʰ **S32.476** Nondisplaced fracture of medial wall of unspecified acetabulum

    ✓6ᵗʰ **S32.48** Dome fracture of acetabulum
      ✓7ᵗʰ **S32.481** Displaced dome fracture of right acetabulum
      ✓7ᵗʰ **S32.482** Displaced dome fracture of left acetabulum
      ✓7ᵗʰ **S32.483** Displaced dome fracture of unspecified acetabulum
      ✓7ᵗʰ **S32.484** Nondisplaced dome fracture of right acetabulum
      ✓7ᵗʰ **S32.485** Nondisplaced dome fracture of left acetabulum
      ✓7ᵗʰ **S32.486** Nondisplaced dome fracture of unspecified acetabulum

    ✓6ᵗʰ **S32.49** Other specified fracture of acetabulum
      ✓7ᵗʰ **S32.491** Other specified fracture of right acetabulum
      ✓7ᵗʰ **S32.492** Other specified fracture of left acetabulum
      ✓7ᵗʰ **S32.499** Other specified fracture of unspecified acetabulum

✓5ᵗʰ **S32.5** Fracture of pubis
    EXCLUDES 1 fracture of pubis with associated disruption of pelvic ring (S32.8-)

    ✓6ᵗʰ **S32.50** Unspecified fracture of pubis
      ✓7ᵗʰ **S32.501** Unspecified fracture of right pubis
      ✓7ᵗʰ **S32.502** Unspecified fracture of left pubis
      ✓7ᵗʰ **S32.509** Unspecified fracture of unspecified pubis

    ✓6ᵗʰ **S32.51** Fracture of superior rim of pubis
      ✓7ᵗʰ **S32.511** Fracture of superior rim of right pubis
      ✓7ᵗʰ **S32.512** Fracture of superior rim of left pubis
      ✓7ᵗʰ **S32.519** Fracture of superior rim of unspecified pubis

    ✓6ᵗʰ **S32.59** Other specified fracture of pubis
      ✓7ᵗʰ **S32.591** Other specified fracture of right pubis
      ✓7ᵗʰ **S32.592** Other specified fracture of left pubis
      ✓7ᵗʰ **S32.599** Other specified fracture of unspecified pubis

EXCLUDES 1 Not coded here   **EXCLUDES 2** Not included here   **N** Newborn Age: 0   **P** Pediatric Age: 0-17   **M** Maternity Age: 12-55   **A** Adult Age: 15-124

834   ICD-10-CM 2014 (Draft)

√5th **S32.6　Fracture of ischium**

> EXCLUDES 1　*fracture of ischium with associated disruption of pelvic ring (S32.8-)*

√6th **S32.60　Unspecified fracture of ischium**

√7th　S32.601　**Unspecified fracture of right ischium**

√7th　S32.602　**Unspecified fracture of left ischium**

√7th　S32.609　**Unspecified fracture of unspecified ischium**

√6th **S32.61　Avulsion fracture of ischium**

√7th　S32.611　**Displaced avulsion fracture of right ischium**

√7th　S32.612　**Displaced avulsion fracture of left ischium**

√7th　S32.613　**Displaced avulsion fracture of unspecified ischium**

√7th　S32.614　**Nondisplaced avulsion fracture of right ischium**

√7th　S32.615　**Nondisplaced avulsion fracture of left ischium**

√7th　S32.616　**Nondisplaced avulsion fracture of unspecified ischium**

√6th **S32.69　Other specified fracture of ischium**

√7th　S32.691　**Other specified fracture of right ischium**

√7th　S32.692　**Other specified fracture of left ischium**

√7th　S32.699　**Other specified fracture of unspecified ischium**

√5th **S32.8　Fracture of other parts of pelvis**

> Code also any associated:
> fracture of acetabulum (S32.4-)
> sacral fracture (S32.1-)

√6th **S32.81　Multiple fractures of pelvis with disruption of pelvic ring**

> Multiple pelvic fractures with disruption of pelvic circle

√7th　S32.810　**Multiple fractures of pelvis with stable disruption of pelvic ring**

√7th　S32.811　**Multiple fractures of pelvis with unstable disruption of pelvic ring**

√6th **S32.82　Multiple fractures of pelvis without disruption of pelvic ring**

> Multiple pelvic fractures without disruption of pelvic circle

√x7th　S32.89　**Fracture of other parts of pelvis**

√x7th **S32.9　Fracture of unspecified parts of lumbosacral spine and pelvis**

> Fracture of lumbosacral spine NOS
> Fracture of pelvis NOS
> **AHA:** 2012, Q4, 93

√4th **S33　Dislocation and sprain of joints and ligaments of lumbar spine and pelvis**

> INCLUDES　avulsion of joint or ligament of lumbar spine and pelvis
> laceration of cartilage, joint or ligament of lumbar spine and pelvis
> sprain of cartilage, joint or ligament of lumbar spine and pelvis
> traumatic hemarthrosis of joint or ligament of lumbar spine and pelvis
> traumatic rupture of joint or ligament of lumbar spine and pelvis
> traumatic subluxation of joint or ligament of lumbar spine and pelvis
> traumatic tear of joint or ligament of lumbar spine and pelvis
>
> Code also any associated open wound
>
> EXCLUDES 1　*nontraumatic rupture or displacement of lumbar intervertebral disc NOS (M51.-)*
> *obstetric damage to pelvic joints and ligaments (O71.6)*
>
> EXCLUDES 2　*dislocation and sprain of joints and ligaments of hip (S73.-)*
> *strain of muscle of lower back and pelvis (S39.01-)*

> The appropriate 7th character is to be added to each code from category S33.
> A　initial encounter
> D　subsequent encounter
> S　sequela

√x7th **S33.0　Traumatic rupture of lumbar intervertebral disc**

> EXCLUDES 1　*rupture or displacement (nontraumatic) of lumbar inter- vertebral disc NOS (M51- with fifth character 6)*

√5th **S33.1　Subluxation and dislocation of lumbar vertebra**

> Code also any associated:
> open wound of abdomen, lower back and pelvis (S31)
> spinal cord injury (S24.0, S24.1-, S34.0-, S34.1-)
> EXCLUDES 2　*fracture of lumbar vertebrae (S32.0-)*

√6th **S33.10　Subluxation and dislocation of unspecified lumbar vertebra**

√7th　S33.100　**Subluxation of unspecified lumbar vertebra**

√7th　S33.101　**Dislocation of unspecified lumbar vertebra**

√6th **S33.11　Subluxation and dislocation of L1/L2 lumbar vertebra**

√7th　S33.110　**Subluxation of L1/L2 lumbar vertebra**

√7th　S33.111　**Dislocation of L1/L2 lumbar vertebra**

√6th **S33.12　Subluxation and dislocation of L2/L3 lumbar vertebra**

√7th　S33.120　**Subluxation of L2/L3 lumbar vertebra**

√7th　S33.121　**Dislocation of L2/L3 lumbar vertebra**

√6th **S33.13　Subluxation and dislocation of L3/L4 lumbar vertebra**

√7th　S33.130　**Subluxation of L3/L4 lumbar vertebra**

√7th　S33.131　**Dislocation of L3/L4 lumbar vertebra**

√6th **S33.14　Subluxation and dislocation of L4/L5 lumbar vertebra**

√7th　S33.140　**Subluxation of L4/L5 lumbar vertebra**

√7th　S33.141　**Dislocation of L4/L5 lumbar vertebra**

√x7th **S33.2　Dislocation of sacroiliac and sacrococcygeal joint**

√5th **S33.3　Dislocation of other and unspecified parts of lumbar spine and pelvis**

√x7th　S33.30　**Dislocation of unspecified parts of lumbar spine and pelvis**

√x7th　S33.39　**Dislocation of other parts of lumbar spine and pelvis**

√x7th **S33.4　Traumatic rupture of symphysis pubis**

√x7th **S33.5　Sprain of ligaments of lumbar spine**

√x7th **S33.6　Sprain of sacroiliac joint**

√x7th **S33.8　Sprain of other parts of lumbar spine and pelvis**

√x7th **S33.9　Sprain of unspecified parts of lumbar spine and pelvis**

√4th **S34　Injury of lumbar and sacral spinal cord and nerves at abdomen, lower back and pelvis level**

> NOTE　Code to highest level of lumbar cord injury.
> Injuries to the spinal cord (S34.0 and S34.1) refer to the cord level and not bone level injury, and can affect nerve roots at and below the level given.
>
> Code also any associated:
> fracture of vertebra (S22.0-, S32.0-)
> open wound of abdomen, lower back and pelvis (S31.-)
> transient paralysis (R29.5)

> The appropriate 7th character is to be added to each code from category S34.
> A　initial encounter
> D　subsequent encounter
> S　sequela

√5th **S34.0　Concussion and edema of lumbar and sacral spinal cord**

√x7th　S34.01　**Concussion and edema of lumbar spinal cord**

√x7th　S34.02　**Concussion and edema of sacral spinal cord**

> Concussion and edema of conus medullaris

√5th **S34.1　Other and unspecified injury of lumbar and sacral spinal cord**

√6th **S34.10　Unspecified injury to lumbar spinal cord**

√7th　S34.101　**Unspecified injury to L1 level of lumbar spinal cord**

√7th　S34.102　**Unspecified injury to L2 level of lumbar spinal cord**

√7th　S34.103　**Unspecified injury to L3 level of lumbar spinal cord**

√7th　S34.104　**Unspecified injury to L4 level of lumbar spinal cord**

√7th　S34.105　**Unspecified injury to L5 level of lumbar spinal cord**

√7th　S34.109　**Unspecified injury to unspecified level of lumbar spinal cord**

☑ Additional Character Required　　√x7th Xtension Alert　　Unspecified Code　　Other Specified Code　　Manifestation Code　　►◄ Revised Text　　● New Code　　▲ Revised Code Title

√6ᵗʰ **S34.11** Complete lesion of lumbar spinal cord

     √7ᵗʰ **S34.111** Complete lesion of L1 level of lumbar spinal cord

     √7ᵗʰ **S34.112** Complete lesion of L2 level of lumbar spinal cord

     √7ᵗʰ **S34.113** Complete lesion of L3 level of lumbar spinal cord

     √7ᵗʰ **S34.114** Complete lesion of L4 level of lumbar spinal cord

     √7ᵗʰ **S34.115** Complete lesion of L5 level of lumbar spinal cord

     √7ᵗʰ **S34.119** Complete lesion of unspecified level of lumbar spinal cord

√6ᵗʰ **S34.12** Incomplete lesion of lumbar spinal cord

     √7ᵗʰ **S34.121** Incomplete lesion of L1 level of lumbar spinal cord

     √7ᵗʰ **S34.122** Incomplete lesion of L2 level of lumbar spinal cord

     √7ᵗʰ **S34.123** Incomplete lesion of L3 level of lumbar spinal cord

     √7ᵗʰ **S34.124** Incomplete lesion of L4 level of lumbar spinal cord

     √7ᵗʰ **S34.125** Incomplete lesion of L5 level of lumbar spinal cord

     √7ᵗʰ **S34.129** Incomplete lesion of unspecified level of lumbar spinal cord

√6ᵗʰ **S34.13** Other and unspecified injury to sacral spinal cord
     Other injury to conus medullaris

     √7ᵗʰ **S34.131** Complete lesion of sacral spinal cord
        Complete lesion of conus medullaris

     √7ᵗʰ **S34.132** Incomplete lesion of sacral spinal cord
        Incomplete lesion of conus medullaris

     √7ᵗʰ **S34.139** Unspecified injury to sacral spinal cord
        Unspecified injury of conus medullaris

√5ᵗʰ **S34.2** Injury of nerve root of lumbar and sacral spine

     √x7ᵗʰ **S34.21** Injury of nerve root of lumbar spine

     √x7ᵗʰ **S34.22** Injury of nerve root of sacral spine

√x7ᵗʰ **S34.3** Injury of cauda equina

√x7ᵗʰ **S34.4** Injury of lumbosacral plexus

√x7ᵗʰ **S34.5** Injury of lumbar, sacral and pelvic sympathetic nerves
     Injury of celiac ganglion or plexus
     Injury of hypogastric plexus
     Injury of mesenteric plexus (inferior) (superior)
     Injury of splanchnic nerve

√x7ᵗʰ **S34.6** Injury of peripheral nerve(s) at abdomen, lower back and pelvis level

√x7ᵗʰ **S34.8** Injury of other nerves at abdomen, lower back and pelvis level

√x7ᵗʰ **S34.9** Injury of unspecified nerves at abdomen, lower back and pelvis level

√4ᵗʰ **S35** Injury of blood vessels at abdomen, lower back and pelvis level
     Code also any associated open wound (S31.-)

     The appropriate 7th character is to be added to each code from category S35.
     A   initial encounter
     D   subsequent encounter
     S   sequela

√5ᵗʰ **S35.0** Injury of abdominal aorta
     EXCLUDES 1 injury of aorta NOS (S25.0)

     √x7ᵗʰ **S35.00** Unspecified injury of abdominal aorta

     √x7ᵗʰ **S35.01** Minor laceration of abdominal aorta
        Incomplete transection of abdominal aorta
        Laceration of abdominal aorta NOS
        Superficial laceration of abdominal aorta

     √x7ᵗʰ **S35.02** Major laceration of abdominal aorta
        Complete transection of abdominal aorta
        Traumatic rupture of abdominal aorta

     √x7ᵗʰ **S35.09** Other injury of abdominal aorta

√5ᵗʰ **S35.1** Injury of inferior vena cava
     Injury of hepatic vein
     EXCLUDES 1 injury of vena cava NOS (S25.2)

     √x7ᵗʰ **S35.10** Unspecified injury of inferior vena cava

√x7ᵗʰ **S35.11** Minor laceration of inferior vena cava
     Incomplete transection of inferior vena cava
     Laceration of inferior vena cava NOS
     Superficial laceration of inferior vena cava

√x7ᵗʰ **S35.12** Major laceration of inferior vena cava
     Complete transection of inferior vena cava
     Traumatic rupture of inferior vena cava

√x7ᵗʰ **S35.19** Other injury of inferior vena cava

√5ᵗʰ **S35.2** Injury of celiac or mesenteric artery and branches

     √6ᵗʰ **S35.21** Injury of celiac artery

        √7ᵗʰ **S35.211** Minor laceration of celiac artery
           Incomplete transection of celiac artery
           Laceration of celiac artery NOS
           Superficial laceration of celiac artery

        √7ᵗʰ **S35.212** Major laceration of celiac artery
           Complete transection of celiac artery
           Traumatic rupture of celiac artery

        √7ᵗʰ **S35.218** Other injury of celiac artery

        √7ᵗʰ **S35.219** Unspecified injury of celiac artery

     √6ᵗʰ **S35.22** Injury of superior mesenteric artery

        √7ᵗʰ **S35.221** Minor laceration of superior mesenteric artery
           Incomplete transection of superior mesenteric artery
           Laceration of superior mesenteric artery NOS
           Superficial laceration of superior mesenteric artery

        √7ᵗʰ **S35.222** Major laceration of superior mesenteric artery
           Complete transection of superior mesenteric artery
           Traumatic rupture of superior mesenteric artery

        √7ᵗʰ **S35.228** Other injury of superior mesenteric artery

        √7ᵗʰ **S35.229** Unspecified injury of superior mesenteric artery

     √6ᵗʰ **S35.23** Injury of inferior mesenteric artery

        √7ᵗʰ **S35.231** Minor laceration of inferior mesenteric artery
           Incomplete transection of inferior mesenteric artery
           Laceration of inferior mesenteric artery NOS
           Superficial laceration of inferior mesenteric artery

        √7ᵗʰ **S35.232** Major laceration of inferior mesenteric artery
           Complete transection of inferior mesenteric artery
           Traumatic rupture of inferior mesenteric artery

        √7ᵗʰ **S35.238** Other injury of inferior mesenteric artery

        √7ᵗʰ **S35.239** Unspecified injury of inferior mesenteric artery

     √6ᵗʰ **S35.29** Injury of branches of celiac and mesenteric artery
        Injury of gastric artery
        Injury of gastroduodenal artery
        Injury of hepatic artery
        Injury of splenic artery

        √7ᵗʰ **S35.291** Minor laceration of branches of celiac and mesenteric artery
           Incomplete transection of branches of celiac and mesenteric artery
           Laceration of branches of celiac and mesenteric artery NOS
           Superficial laceration of branches of celiac and mesenteric artery

        √7ᵗʰ **S35.292** Major laceration of branches of celiac and mesenteric artery
           Complete transection of branches of celiac and mesenteric artery
           Traumatic rupture of branches of celiac and mesenteric artery

        √7ᵗʰ **S35.298** Other injury of branches of celiac and mesenteric artery

        √7ᵗʰ **S35.299** Unspecified injury of branches of celiac and mesenteric artery

---

EXCLUDES 1 Not coded here   **EXCLUDES 2** Not included here   N Newborn Age: 0   P Pediatric Age: 0-17   M Maternity Age: 12-55   A Adult Age: 15-124

836   ICD-10-CM 2014 (Draft)

✓5ᵗʰ **S35.3** Injury of portal or splenic vein and branches

  ✓6ᵗʰ **S35.31** Injury of portal vein

    ✓7ᵗʰ **S35.311** Laceration of portal vein

    ✓7ᵗʰ **S35.318** Other specified injury of portal vein

    ✓7ᵗʰ **S35.319** Unspecified injury of portal vein

  ✓6ᵗʰ **S35.32** Injury of splenic vein

    ✓7ᵗʰ **S35.321** Laceration of splenic vein

    ✓7ᵗʰ **S35.328** Other specified injury of splenic vein

    ✓7ᵗʰ **S35.329** Unspecified injury of splenic vein

  ✓6ᵗʰ **S35.33** Injury of superior mesenteric vein

    ✓7ᵗʰ **S35.331** Laceration of superior mesenteric vein

    ✓7ᵗʰ **S35.338** Other specified injury of superior mesenteric vein

    ✓7ᵗʰ **S35.339** Unspecified injury of superior mesenteric vein

  ✓6ᵗʰ **S35.34** Injury of inferior mesenteric vein

    ✓7ᵗʰ **S35.341** Laceration of inferior mesenteric vein

    ✓7ᵗʰ **S35.348** Other specified injury of inferior mesenteric vein

    ✓7ᵗʰ **S35.349** Unspecified injury of inferior mesenteric vein

✓5ᵗʰ **S35.4** Injury of renal blood vessels

  ✓6ᵗʰ **S35.40** Unspecified injury of renal blood vessel

    ✓7ᵗʰ **S35.401** Unspecified injury of right renal artery

    ✓7ᵗʰ **S35.402** Unspecified injury of left renal artery

    ✓7ᵗʰ **S35.403** Unspecified injury of unspecified renal artery

    ✓7ᵗʰ **S35.404** Unspecified injury of right renal vein

    ✓7ᵗʰ **S35.405** Unspecified injury of left renal vein

    ✓7ᵗʰ **S35.406** Unspecified injury of unspecified renal vein

  ✓6ᵗʰ **S35.41** Laceration of renal blood vessel

    ✓7ᵗʰ **S35.411** Laceration of right renal artery

    ✓7ᵗʰ **S35.412** Laceration of left renal artery

    ✓7ᵗʰ **S35.413** Laceration of unspecified renal artery

    ✓7ᵗʰ **S35.414** Laceration of right renal vein

    ✓7ᵗʰ **S35.415** Laceration of left renal vein

    ✓7ᵗʰ **S35.416** Laceration of unspecified renal vein

  ✓6ᵗʰ **S35.49** Other specified injury of renal blood vessel

    ✓7ᵗʰ **S35.491** Other specified injury of right renal artery

    ✓7ᵗʰ **S35.492** Other specified injury of left renal artery

    ✓7ᵗʰ **S35.493** Other specified injury of unspecified renal artery

    ✓7ᵗʰ **S35.494** Other specified injury of right renal vein

    ✓7ᵗʰ **S35.495** Other specified injury of left renal vein

    ✓7ᵗʰ **S35.496** Other specified injury of unspecified renal vein

✓5ᵗʰ **S35.5** Injury of iliac blood vessels

  ✓x7ᵗʰ **S35.50** Injury of unspecified iliac blood vessel(s)

  ✓6ᵗʰ **S35.51** Injury of iliac artery or vein

    Injury of hypogastric artery or vein

    ✓7ᵗʰ **S35.511** Injury of right iliac artery

    ✓7ᵗʰ **S35.512** Injury of left iliac artery

    ✓7ᵗʰ **S35.513** Injury of unspecified iliac artery

    ✓7ᵗʰ **S35.514** Injury of right iliac vein

    ✓7ᵗʰ **S35.515** Injury of left iliac vein

    ✓7ᵗʰ **S35.516** Injury of unspecified iliac vein

  ✓6ᵗʰ **S35.53** Injury of uterine artery or vein

    ✓7ᵗʰ **S35.531** Injury of right uterine artery ♀

    ✓7ᵗʰ **S35.532** Injury of left uterine artery ♀

    ✓7ᵗʰ **S35.533** Injury of unspecified uterine artery ♀

    ✓7ᵗʰ **S35.534** Injury of right uterine vein ♀

    ✓7ᵗʰ **S35.535** Injury of left uterine vein ♀

    ✓7ᵗʰ **S35.536** Injury of unspecified uterine vein ♀

  ✓x7ᵗʰ **S35.59** Injury of other iliac blood vessels

✓5ᵗʰ **S35.8** Injury of other blood vessels at abdomen, lower back and pelvis level

    Injury of ovarian artery or vein

  ✓6ᵗʰ **S35.8X** Injury of other blood vessels at abdomen, lower back and pelvis level

    ✓7ᵗʰ **S35.8X1** Laceration of other blood vessels at abdomen, lower back and pelvis level ♀

    ✓7ᵗʰ **S35.8X8** Other specified injury of other blood vessels at abdomen, lower back and pelvis level ♀

    ✓7ᵗʰ **S35.8X9** Unspecified injury of other blood vessels at abdomen, lower back and pelvis level

✓5ᵗʰ **S35.9** Injury of unspecified blood vessel at abdomen, lower back and pelvis level

  ✓x7ᵗʰ **S35.90** Unspecified injury of unspecified blood vessel at abdomen, lower back and pelvis level

  ✓x7ᵗʰ **S35.91** Laceration of unspecified blood vessel at abdomen, lower back and pelvis level

  ✓x7ᵗʰ **S35.99** Other specified injury of unspecified blood vessel at abdomen, lower back and pelvis level

✓4ᵗʰ **S36** Injury of intra-abdominal organs

  Code also any associated open wound (S31.-)

> The appropriate 7th character is to be added to each code from category S36.
> A   initial encounter
> D   subsequent encounter
> S   sequela

✓5ᵗʰ **S36.0** Injury of spleen

  ✓x7ᵗʰ **S36.00** Unspecified injury of spleen

  ✓6ᵗʰ **S36.02** Contusion of spleen

    ✓7ᵗʰ **S36.020** Minor contusion of spleen
      Contusion of spleen less than 2 cm

    ✓7ᵗʰ **S36.021** Major contusion of spleen
      Contusion of spleen greater than 2 cm

    ✓7ᵗʰ **S36.029** Unspecified contusion of spleen

  ✓6ᵗʰ **S36.03** Laceration of spleen

    ✓7ᵗʰ **S36.030** Superficial (capsular) laceration of spleen
      Laceration of spleen less than 1cm
      Minor laceration of spleen

    ✓7ᵗʰ **S36.031** Moderate laceration of spleen
      Laceration of spleen 1 to 3 cm

    ✓7ᵗʰ **S36.032** Major laceration of spleen
      Avulsion of spleen
      Laceration of spleen greater than 3 cm
      Massive laceration of spleen
      Multiple moderate lacerations of spleen
      Stellate laceration of spleen

    ✓7ᵗʰ **S36.039** Unspecified laceration of spleen

  ✓x7ᵗʰ **S36.09** Other injury of spleen

✓5ᵗʰ **S36.1** Injury of liver and gallbladder and bile duct

  ✓6ᵗʰ **S36.11** Injury of liver

    ✓7ᵗʰ **S36.112** Contusion of liver

    ✓7ᵗʰ **S36.113** Laceration of liver, unspecified degree

    ✓7ᵗʰ **S36.114** Minor laceration of liver
      Laceration involving capsule only, or, without significant involvement of hepatic parenchyma [i.e., less than 1cm deep]

    ✓7ᵗʰ **S36.115** Moderate laceration of liver
      Laceration involving parenchyma but without major disruption of parenchyma [i.e., less than 10 cm long and less than 3 cm deep]

    ✓7ᵗʰ **S36.116** Major laceration of liver
      Laceration with significant disruption of hepatic parenchyma [i.e., greater than 10 cm long and 3 cm deep]
      Multiple moderate lacerations, with or without hematoma
      Stellate laceration of liver

    ✓7ᵗʰ **S36.118** Other injury of liver

    ✓7ᵗʰ **S36.119** Unspecified injury of liver

  ✓6ᵗʰ **S36.12** Injury of gallbladder

    ✓7ᵗʰ **S36.122** Contusion of gallbladder

    ✓7ᵗʰ **S36.123** Laceration of gallbladder

✓ Additional Character Required   ✓x7ᵗʰ Xtension Alert   Unspecified Code   Other Specified Code   Manifestation Code   ►◄ Revised Text   ● New Code   ▲ Revised Code Title

ICD-10-CM 2014 (Draft)   837

√7th **S36.128 Other injury of gallbladder**
√7th **S36.129 Unspecified injury of gallbladder**
√x7th **S36.13 Injury of** bile duct
√5th **S36.2 Injury of** pancreas
√6th **S36.20 Unspecified injury of pancreas**
√7th **S36.200 Unspecified injury of** head **of pancreas**
√7th **S36.201 Unspecified injury of** body **of pancreas**
√7th **S36.202 Unspecified injury of** tail **of pancreas**
√7th **S36.209 Unspecified injury of unspecified part of pancreas**
√6th **S36.22 Contusion of pancreas**
√7th **S36.220 Contusion of** head **of pancreas**
√7th **S36.221 Contusion of** body **of pancreas**
√7th **S36.222 Contusion of** tail **of pancreas**
√7th **S36.229 Contusion of unspecified part of pancreas**
√6th **S36.23 Laceration of pancreas, unspecified degree**
√7th **S36.230 Laceration of** head **of pancreas, unspecified degree**
√7th **S36.231 Laceration of** body **of pancreas, unspecified degree**
√7th **S36.232 Laceration of** tail **of pancreas, unspecified degree**
√7th **S36.239 Laceration of unspecified part of pancreas, unspecified degree**
√6th **S36.24 Minor laceration of pancreas**
√7th **S36.240 Minor laceration of** head **of pancreas**
√7th **S36.241 Minor laceration of** body **of pancreas**
√7th **S36.242 Minor laceration of** tail **of pancreas**
√7th **S36.249 Minor laceration of unspecified part of pancreas**
√6th **S36.25 Moderate laceration of pancreas**
√7th **S36.250 Moderate laceration of** head **of pancreas**
√7th **S36.251 Moderate laceration of** body **of pancreas**
√7th **S36.252 Moderate laceration of** tail **of pancreas**
√7th **S36.259 Moderate laceration of unspecified part of pancreas**
√6th **S36.26 Major laceration of pancreas**
√7th **S36.260 Major laceration of** head **of pancreas**
√7th **S36.261 Major laceration of** body **of pancreas**
√7th **S36.262 Major laceration of** tail **of pancreas**
√7th **S36.269 Major laceration of unspecified part of pancreas**
√6th **S36.29 Other injury of pancreas**
√7th **S36.290 Other injury of** head **of pancreas**
√7th **S36.291 Other injury of** body **of pancreas**
√7th **S36.292 Other injury of** tail **of pancreas**
√7th **S36.299 Other injury of unspecified part of pancreas**
√5th **S36.3 Injury of** stomach
√x7th **S36.30 Unspecified injury of stomach**
√x7th **S36.32 Contusion of stomach**
√x7th **S36.33 Laceration of stomach**
√x7th **S36.39 Other injury of stomach**
√5th **S36.4 Injury of** small intestine
√6th **S36.40 Unspecified injury of small intestine**
√7th **S36.400 Unspecified injury of** duodenum
√7th **S36.408 Unspecified injury of other part of small intestine**
√7th **S36.409 Unspecified injury of unspecified part of small intestine**
√6th **S36.41 Primary blast injury of small intestine**
Blast injury of small intestine NOS
√7th **S36.410 Primary blast injury of** duodenum
√7th **S36.418 Primary blast injury of other part of small intestine**
√7th **S36.419 Primary blast injury of unspecified part of small intestine**
√6th **S36.42 Contusion of small intestine**
√7th **S36.420 Contusion of** duodenum
√7th **S36.428 Contusion of other part of small intestine**

√7th **S36.429 Contusion of unspecified part of small intestine**
√6th **S36.43 Laceration of small intestine**
√7th **S36.430 Laceration of** duodenum
√7th **S36.438 Laceration of other part of small intestine**
√7th **S36.439 Laceration of unspecified part of small intestine**
√6th **S36.49 Other injury of small intestine**
√7th **S36.490 Other injury of** duodenum
√7th **S36.498 Other injury of other part of small intestine**
√7th **S36.499 Other injury of unspecified part of small intestine**
√5th **S36.5 Injury of** colon
EXCLUDES 2 injury of rectum (S36.6-)
√6th **S36.50 Unspecified injury of colon**
√7th **S36.500 Unspecified injury of** ascending [right] **colon**
√7th **S36.501 Unspecified injury of** transverse **colon**
√7th **S36.502 Unspecified injury of** descending [left] **colon**
√7th **S36.503 Unspecified injury of** sigmoid **colon**
√7th **S36.508 Unspecified injury of other part of colon**
√7th **S36.509 Unspecified injury of unspecified part of colon**
√6th **S36.51 Primary blast injury of colon**
Blast injury of colon NOS
√7th **S36.510 Primary blast injury of** ascending [right] **colon**
√7th **S36.511 Primary blast injury of** transverse **colon**
√7th **S36.512 Primary blast injury of** descending [left] **colon**
√7th **S36.513 Primary blast injury of** sigmoid **colon**
√7th **S36.518 Primary blast injury of other part of colon**
√7th **S36.519 Primary blast injury of unspecified part of colon**
√6th **S36.52 Contusion of colon**
√7th **S36.520 Contusion of** ascending [right] **colon**
√7th **S36.521 Contusion of** transverse **colon**
√7th **S36.522 Contusion of** descending [left] **colon**
√7th **S36.523 Contusion of** sigmoid **colon**
√7th **S36.528 Contusion of other part of colon**
√7th **S36.529 Contusion of unspecified part of colon**
√6th **S36.53 Laceration of colon**
√7th **S36.530 Laceration of** ascending [right] **colon**
√7th **S36.531 Laceration of** transverse **colon**
√7th **S36.532 Laceration of** descending [left] **colon**
√7th **S36.533 Laceration of** sigmoid **colon**
√7th **S36.538 Laceration of other part of colon**
√7th **S36.539 Laceration of unspecified part of colon**
√6th **S36.59 Other injury of colon**
Secondary blast injury of colon
√7th **S36.590 Other injury of** ascending [right] **colon**
√7th **S36.591 Other injury of** transverse **colon**
√7th **S36.592 Other injury of** descending [left] **colon**
√7th **S36.593 Other injury of** sigmoid **colon**
√7th **S36.598 Other injury of other part of colon**
√7th **S36.599 Other injury of unspecified part of colon**
√5th **S36.6 Injury of** rectum
√x7th **S36.60 Unspecified injury of rectum**
√x7th **S36.61 Primary blast injury of rectum**
Blast injury of rectum NOS
√x7th **S36.62 Contusion of rectum**
√x7th **S36.63 Laceration of rectum**
√x7th **S36.69 Other injury of rectum**
Secondary blast injury of rectum
√5th **S36.8 Injury of other intra-abdominal organs**
√x7th **S36.81 Injury of** peritoneum
√6th **S36.89 Injury of** other **intra-abdominal organs**
Injury of retroperitoneum

EXCLUDES 1 Not coded here   EXCLUDES 2 Not included here   N Newborn Age: 0   P Pediatric Age: 0-17   M Maternity Age: 12-55   A Adult Age: 15-124

838   ICD-10-CM 2014 (Draft)

√7ᵗʰ **S36.892** Contusion of other intra-abdominal organs

√7ᵗʰ **S36.893** Laceration of other intra-abdominal organs

√7ᵗʰ **S36.898** Other injury of other intra-abdominal organs

√7ᵗʰ **S36.899** Unspecified injury of other intra-abdominal organs

√5ᵗʰ **S36.9** Injury of unspecified intra-abdominal organ

√x7ᵗʰ **S36.90** Unspecified injury of unspecified intra-abdominal organ

√x7ᵗʰ **S36.92** Contusion of unspecified intra-abdominal organ

√x7ᵗʰ **S36.93** Laceration of unspecified intra-abdominal organ

√x7ᵗʰ **S36.99** Other injury of unspecified intra-abdominal organ

√4ᵗʰ **S37** **Injury of urinary and pelvic organs**

Code also any associated open wound (S31.-)

EXCLUDES 1 obstetric trauma to pelvic organs (O71.-)

EXCLUDES 2 injury of peritoneum (S36.81)
injury of retroperitoneum (S36.89-)

The appropriate 7th character is to be added to each code from category S37.
A   initial encounter
D   subsequent encounter
S   sequela

√5ᵗʰ **S37.0** **Injury of kidney**

EXCLUDES 2 acute kidney injury (nontraumatic) (N17.9)

√6ᵗʰ **S37.00** Unspecified injury of kidney

√7ᵗʰ **S37.001** Unspecified injury of right kidney

√7ᵗʰ **S37.002** Unspecified injury of left kidney

√7ᵗʰ **S37.009** Unspecified injury of unspecified kidney

√6ᵗʰ **S37.01** Minor contusion of kidney
Contusion of kidney less than 2 cm
Contusion of kidney NOS

√7ᵗʰ **S37.011** Minor contusion of right kidney

√7ᵗʰ **S37.012** Minor contusion of left kidney

√7ᵗʰ **S37.019** Minor contusion of unspecified kidney

√6ᵗʰ **S37.02** Major contusion of kidney
Contusion of kidney greater than 2 cm

√7ᵗʰ **S37.021** Major contusion of right kidney

√7ᵗʰ **S37.022** Major contusion of left kidney

√7ᵗʰ **S37.029** Major contusion of unspecified kidney

√6ᵗʰ **S37.03** Laceration of kidney, unspecified degree

√7ᵗʰ **S37.031** Laceration of right kidney, unspecified degree

√7ᵗʰ **S37.032** Laceration of left kidney, unspecified degree

√7ᵗʰ **S37.039** Laceration of unspecified kidney, unspecified degree

√6ᵗʰ **S37.04** Minor laceration of kidney
Laceration of kidney less than 1 cm

√7ᵗʰ **S37.041** Minor laceration of right kidney

√7ᵗʰ **S37.042** Minor laceration of left kidney

√7ᵗʰ **S37.049** Minor laceration of unspecified kidney

√6ᵗʰ **S37.05** Moderate laceration of kidney
Laceration of kidney 1 to 3 cm

√7ᵗʰ **S37.051** Moderate laceration of right kidney

√7ᵗʰ **S37.052** Moderate laceration of left kidney

√7ᵗʰ **S37.059** Moderate laceration of unspecified kidney

√6ᵗʰ **S37.06** Major laceration of kidney
Avulsion of kidney
Laceration of kidney greater than 3 cm
Massive laceration of kidney
Multiple moderate lacerations of kidney
Stellate laceration of kidney

√7ᵗʰ **S37.061** Major laceration of right kidney

√7ᵗʰ **S37.062** Major laceration of left kidney

√7ᵗʰ **S37.069** Major laceration of unspecified kidney

√6ᵗʰ **S37.09** Other injury of kidney

√7ᵗʰ **S37.091** Other injury of right kidney

√7ᵗʰ **S37.092** Other injury of left kidney

√7ᵗʰ **S37.099** Other injury of unspecified kidney

√5ᵗʰ **S37.1** Injury of ureter

√x7ᵗʰ **S37.10** Unspecified injury of ureter

√x7ᵗʰ **S37.12** Contusion of ureter

√x7ᵗʰ **S37.13** Laceration of ureter

√x7ᵗʰ **S37.19** Other injury of ureter

√5ᵗʰ **S37.2** Injury of bladder

√x7ᵗʰ **S37.20** Unspecified injury of bladder

√x7ᵗʰ **S37.22** Contusion of bladder

√x7ᵗʰ **S37.23** Laceration of bladder

√x7ᵗʰ **S37.29** Other injury of bladder

√5ᵗʰ **S37.3** Injury of urethra

√x7ᵗʰ **S37.30** Unspecified injury of urethra

√x7ᵗʰ **S37.32** Contusion of urethra

√x7ᵗʰ **S37.33** Laceration of urethra

√x7ᵗʰ **S37.39** Other injury of urethra

√5ᵗʰ **S37.4** Injury of ovary

√6ᵗʰ **S37.40** Unspecified injury of ovary

√7ᵗʰ **S37.401** Unspecified injury of ovary, unilateral ♀

√7ᵗʰ **S37.402** Unspecified injury of ovary, bilateral ♀

√7ᵗʰ **S37.409** Unspecified injury of ovary, unspecified ♀

√6ᵗʰ **S37.42** Contusion of ovary

√7ᵗʰ **S37.421** Contusion of ovary, unilateral ♀

√7ᵗʰ **S37.422** Contusion of ovary, bilateral ♀

√7ᵗʰ **S37.429** Contusion of ovary, unspecified ♀

√6ᵗʰ **S37.43** Laceration of ovary

√7ᵗʰ **S37.431** Laceration of ovary, unilateral ♀

√7ᵗʰ **S37.432** Laceration of ovary, bilateral ♀

√7ᵗʰ **S37.439** Laceration of ovary, unspecified ♀

√6ᵗʰ **S37.49** Other injury of ovary

√7ᵗʰ **S37.491** Other injury of ovary, unilateral ♀

√7ᵗʰ **S37.492** Other injury of ovary, bilateral ♀

√7ᵗʰ **S37.499** Other injury of ovary, unspecified ♀

√5ᵗʰ **S37.5** Injury of fallopian tube

S37.50 Unspecified injury of fallopian tube

√7ᵗʰ **S37.501** Unspecified injury of fallopian tube, unilateral ♀

√7ᵗʰ **S37.502** Unspecified injury of fallopian tube, bilateral ♀

√7ᵗʰ **S37.509** Unspecified injury of fallopian tube, unspecified ♀

√6ᵗʰ **S37.51** Primary blast injury of fallopian tube
Blast injury of fallopian tube NOS

√7ᵗʰ **S37.511** Primary blast injury of fallopian tube, unilateral ♀

√7ᵗʰ **S37.512** Primary blast injury of fallopian tube, bilateral ♀

√7ᵗʰ **S37.519** Primary blast injury of fallopian tube, unspecified ♀

√6ᵗʰ **S37.52** Contusion of fallopian tube

√7ᵗʰ **S37.521** Contusion of fallopian tube, unilateral ♀

√7ᵗʰ **S37.522** Contusion of fallopian tube, bilateral ♀

√7ᵗʰ **S37.529** Contusion of fallopian tube, unspecified ♀

√6ᵗʰ **S37.53** Laceration of fallopian tube

√7ᵗʰ **S37.531** Laceration of fallopian tube, unilateral ♀

√7ᵗʰ **S37.532** Laceration of fallopian tube, bilateral ♀

√7ᵗʰ **S37.539** Laceration of fallopian tube, unspecified ♀

√6ᵗʰ **S37.59** Other injury of fallopian tube
Secondary blast injury of fallopian tube

√7ᵗʰ **S37.591** Other injury of fallopian tube, unilateral ♀

√7ᵗʰ **S37.592** Other injury of fallopian tube, bilateral ♀

√7ᵗʰ **S37.599** Other injury of fallopian tube, unspecified ♀

√5ᵗʰ **S37.6** Injury of uterus

EXCLUDES 1 injury to gravid uterus (O9A.2-)
injury to uterus during delivery (O71.-)

√x7ᵗʰ **S37.60** Unspecified injury of uterus ♀

√x7ᵗʰ **S37.62** Contusion of uterus ♀

√x7ᵗʰ **S37.63** Laceration of uterus ♀

✔ Additional Character Required   √x7ᵗʰ Xtension Alert   Unspecified Code   Other Specified Code   Manifestation Code   ►◄ Revised Text   ● New Code   ▲ Revised Code Title

ICD-10-CM 2014 (Draft)

839

S37.69–S39.94

Injury, Poisoning and Certain Other Consequences of External Causes

√x7ᵗʰ **S37.69** Other injury of uterus ♀

√5ᵗʰ **S37.8** Injury of other urinary and pelvic organs
- √6ᵗʰ **S37.81** Injury of adrenal gland
  - √7ᵗʰ **S37.812** Contusion of adrenal gland
  - √7ᵗʰ **S37.813** Laceration of adrenal gland
  - √7ᵗʰ **S37.818** Other injury of adrenal gland
  - √7ᵗʰ **S37.819** Unspecified injury of adrenal gland
- √6ᵗʰ **S37.82** Injury of prostate
  - √7ᵗʰ **S37.822** Contusion of prostate ♂
  - √7ᵗʰ **S37.823** Laceration of prostate ♂
  - √7ᵗʰ **S37.828** Other injury of prostate ♂
  - √7ᵗʰ **S37.829** Unspecified injury of prostate ♂
- √6ᵗʰ **S37.89** Injury of other urinary and pelvic organ
  - √7ᵗʰ **S37.892** Contusion of other urinary and pelvic organ
  - √7ᵗʰ **S37.893** Laceration of other urinary and pelvic organ
  - √7ᵗʰ **S37.898** Other injury of other urinary and pelvic organ
  - √7ᵗʰ **S37.899** Unspecified injury of other urinary and pelvic organ

√5ᵗʰ **S37.9** Injury of unspecified urinary and pelvic organ
- √x7ᵗʰ **S37.90** Unspecified injury of unspecified urinary and pelvic organ
- √x7ᵗʰ **S37.92** Contusion of unspecified urinary and pelvic organ
- √x7ᵗʰ **S37.93** Laceration of unspecified urinary and pelvic organ
- √x7ᵗʰ **S37.99** Other injury of unspecified urinary and pelvic organ

√4ᵗʰ **S38** Crushing injury and traumatic amputation of abdomen, lower back, pelvis and external genitals

NOTE An amputation not identified as partial or complete should be coded to complete.

The appropriate 7th character is to be added to each code from category S38.
- A initial encounter
- D subsequent encounter
- S sequela

√5ᵗʰ **S38.0** Crushing injury of external genital organs
Use additional code for any associated injuries
- √6ᵗʰ **S38.00** Crushing injury of unspecified external genital organs
  - √7ᵗʰ **S38.001** Crushing injury of unspecified external genital organs, male ♂
  - √7ᵗʰ **S38.002** Crushing injury of unspecified external genital organs, female ♀
- √x7ᵗʰ **S38.01** Crushing injury of penis ♂
- √x7ᵗʰ **S38.02** Crushing injury of scrotum and testis ♂
- √x7ᵗʰ **S38.03** Crushing injury of vulva ♀

√x7ᵗʰ **S38.1** Crushing injury of abdomen, lower back, and pelvis
Use additional code for all associated injuries, such as:
fracture of thoracic or lumbar spine and pelvis (S22.0-, S32-)
injury to intra-abdominal organs (S36.-)
injury to urinary and pelvic organs (S37.-)
open wound of abdominal wall (S31.-)
spinal cord injury (S34.0, S34.1-)
EXCLUDES 2 crushing injury of external genital organs (S38.0-)

√5ᵗʰ **S38.2** Traumatic amputation of external genital organs
- √6ᵗʰ **S38.21** Traumatic amputation of female external genital organs
  Traumatic amputation of clitoris
  Traumatic amputation of labium (majus) (minus)
  Traumatic amputation of vulva
  - √7ᵗʰ **S38.211** Complete traumatic amputation of female external genital organs ♀
  - √7ᵗʰ **S38.212** Partial traumatic amputation of female external genital organs ♀
- √6ᵗʰ **S38.22** Traumatic amputation of penis
  - √7ᵗʰ **S38.221** Complete traumatic amputation of penis ♂
  - √7ᵗʰ **S38.222** Partial traumatic amputation of penis ♂
- √6ᵗʰ **S38.23** Traumatic amputation of scrotum and testis
  - √7ᵗʰ **S38.231** Complete traumatic amputation of scrotum and testis ♂

  - √7ᵗʰ **S38.232** Partial traumatic amputation of scrotum and testis ♂

√x7ᵗʰ **S38.3** Transection (partial) of abdomen

√4ᵗʰ **S39** Other and unspecified injuries of abdomen, lower back, pelvis and external genitals
Code also any associated open wound (S31.-)
EXCLUDES 2 sprain of joints and ligaments of lumbar spine and pelvis (S33.-)

The appropriate 7th character is to be added to each code from category S39.
- A initial encounter
- D subsequent encounter
- S sequela

√5ᵗʰ **S39.0** Injury of muscle, fascia and tendon of abdomen, lower back and pelvis
- √6ᵗʰ **S39.00** Unspecified injury of muscle, fascia and tendon of abdomen, lower back and pelvis
  - √7ᵗʰ **S39.001** Unspecified injury of muscle, fascia and tendon of abdomen
  - √7ᵗʰ **S39.002** Unspecified injury of muscle, fascia and tendon of lower back
  - √7ᵗʰ **S39.003** Unspecified injury of muscle, fascia and tendon of pelvis
- √6ᵗʰ **S39.01** Strain of muscle, fascia and tendon of abdomen, lower back and pelvis
  - √7ᵗʰ **S39.011** Strain of muscle, fascia and tendon of abdomen
  - √7ᵗʰ **S39.012** Strain of muscle, fascia and tendon of lower back
  - √7ᵗʰ **S39.013** Strain of muscle, fascia and tendon of pelvis
- √6ᵗʰ **S39.02** Laceration of muscle, fascia and tendon of abdomen, lower back and pelvis
  - √7ᵗʰ **S39.021** Laceration of muscle, fascia and tendon of abdomen
  - √7ᵗʰ **S39.022** Laceration of muscle, fascia and tendon of lower back
  - √7ᵗʰ **S39.023** Laceration of muscle, fascia and tendon of pelvis
- √6ᵗʰ **S39.09** Other injury of muscle, fascia and tendon of abdomen, lower back and pelvis
  - √7ᵗʰ **S39.091** Other injury of muscle, fascia and tendon of abdomen
  - √7ᵗʰ **S39.092** Other injury of muscle, fascia and tendon of lower back
  - √7ᵗʰ **S39.093** Other injury of muscle, fascia and tendon of pelvis

√5ᵗʰ **S39.8** Other specified injuries of abdomen, lower back, pelvis and external genitals
- √x7ᵗʰ **S39.81** Other specified injuries of abdomen
- √x7ᵗʰ **S39.82** Other specified injuries of lower back
- √x7ᵗʰ **S39.83** Other specified injuries of pelvis
- √6ᵗʰ **S39.84** Other specified injuries of external genitals
  - √7ᵗʰ **S39.840** Fracture of corpus cavernosum penis ♂
  - √7ᵗʰ **S39.848** Other specified injuries of external genitals

√5ᵗʰ **S39.9** Unspecified injury of abdomen, lower back, pelvis and external genitals
- √x7ᵗʰ **S39.91** Unspecified injury of abdomen
- √x7ᵗʰ **S39.92** Unspecified injury of lower back
- √x7ᵗʰ **S39.93** Unspecified injury of pelvis
- √x7ᵗʰ **S39.94** Unspecified injury of external genitals

EXCLUDES 1 Not coded here **EXCLUDES 2** Not included here N Newborn Age: 0 P Pediatric Age: 0-17 M Maternity Age: 12-55 A Adult Age: 15-124

840 ICD-10-CM 2014 (Draft)

Injuries to the shoulder and upper arm (S40-S49)

INCLUDES injuries of axilla
injuries of scapular region

EXCLUDES 2 *burns and corrosions (T20-T32)*
frostbite (T33-T34)
injuries of elbow (S50-S59)
insect bite or sting, venomous (T63.4)

✓4th **S40   Superficial injury of shoulder and upper arm**

The appropriate 7th character is to be added to each code from category S40.
A   initial encounter
D   subsequent encounter
S   sequela

✓5th **S40.0   Contusion of shoulder and upper arm**

✓6th **S40.01   Contusion of shoulder**

✓7th S40.011   Contusion of right shoulder

✓7th S40.012   Contusion of left shoulder

✓7th S40.019   Contusion of unspecified shoulder

✓6th **S40.02   Contusion of upper arm**

✓7th S40.021   Contusion of right upper arm

✓7th S40.022   Contusion of left upper arm

✓7th S40.029   Contusion of unspecified upper arm

✓5th **S40.2   Other superficial injuries of shoulder**

✓6th **S40.21   Abrasion of shoulder**

✓7th S40.211   Abrasion of right shoulder

✓7th S40.212   Abrasion of left shoulder

✓7th S40.219   Abrasion of unspecified shoulder

✓6th **S40.22   Blister (nonthermal) of shoulder**

✓7th S40.221   Blister (nonthermal) of right shoulder

✓7th S40.222   Blister (nonthermal) of left shoulder

✓7th S40.229   Blister (nonthermal) of unspecified shoulder

✓6th **S40.24   External constriction of shoulder**

✓7th S40.241   External constriction of right shoulder

✓7th S40.242   External constriction of left shoulder

✓7th S40.249   External constriction of unspecified shoulder

✓6th **S40.25   Superficial foreign body of shoulder**
Splinter in the shoulder

✓7th S40.251   Superficial foreign body of right shoulder

✓7th S40.252   Superficial foreign body of left shoulder

✓7th S40.259   Superficial foreign body of unspecified shoulder

✓6th **S40.26   Insect bite (nonvenomous) of shoulder**

✓7th S40.261   Insect bite (nonvenomous) of right shoulder

✓7th S40.262   Insect bite (nonvenomous) of left shoulder

✓7th S40.269   Insect bite (nonvenomous) of unspecified shoulder

✓6th **S40.27   Other superficial bite of shoulder**
EXCLUDES 1 *open bite of shoulder (S41.05)*

✓7th S40.271   Other superficial bite of right shoulder

✓7th S40.272   Other superficial bite of left shoulder

✓7th S40.279   Other superficial bite of unspecified shoulder

✓5th **S40.8   Other superficial injuries of upper arm**

✓6th **S40.81   Abrasion of upper arm**

✓7th S40.811   Abrasion of right upper arm

✓7th S40.812   Abrasion of left upper arm

✓7th S40.819   Abrasion of unspecified upper arm

✓6th **S40.82   Blister (nonthermal) of upper arm**

✓7th S40.821   Blister (nonthermal) of right upper arm

✓7th S40.822   Blister (nonthermal) of left upper arm

✓7th S40.829   Blister (nonthermal) of unspecified upper arm

✓6th **S40.84   External constriction of upper arm**

✓7th S40.841   External constriction of right upper arm

✓7th S40.842   External constriction of left upper arm

✓7th S40.849   External constriction of unspecified upper arm

✓6th **S40.85   Superficial foreign body of upper arm**
Splinter in the upper arm

✓7th S40.851   Superficial foreign body of right upper arm

✓7th S40.852   Superficial foreign body of left upper arm

✓7th S40.859   Superficial foreign body of unspecified upper arm

✓6th **S40.86   Insect bite (nonvenomous) of upper arm**

✓7th S40.861   Insect bite (nonvenomous) of right upper arm

✓7th S40.862   Insect bite (nonvenomous) of left upper arm

✓7th S40.869   Insect bite (nonvenomous) of unspecified upper arm

✓6th **S40.87   Other superficial bite of upper arm**
EXCLUDES 1 *open bite of upper arm (S41.14)*
EXCLUDES 2 *other superficial bite of shoulder (S40.27-)*

✓7th S40.871   Other superficial bite of right upper arm

✓7th S40.872   Other superficial bite of left upper arm

✓7th S40.879   Other superficial bite of unspecified upper arm

✓5th **S40.9   Unspecified superficial injury of shoulder and upper arm**

✓6th **S40.91   Unspecified superficial injury of shoulder**

✓7th S40.911   Unspecified superficial injury of right shoulder

✓7th S40.912   Unspecified superficial injury of left shoulder

✓7th S40.919   Unspecified superficial injury of unspecified shoulder

✓6th **S40.92   Unspecified superficial injury of upper arm**

✓7th S40.921   Unspecified superficial injury of right upper arm

✓7th S40.922   Unspecified superficial injury of left upper arm

✓7th S40.929   Unspecified superficial injury of unspecified upper arm

✓4th **S41   Open wound of shoulder and upper arm**
Code also any associated wound infection
EXCLUDES 1 *traumatic amputation of shoulder and upper arm (S48.-)*
EXCLUDES 2 *open fracture of shoulder and upper arm (S42.- with 7th character B)*

The appropriate 7th character is to be added to each code from category S41.
A   initial encounter
D   subsequent encounter
S   sequela

✓5th **S41.0   Open wound of shoulder**

✓6th **S41.00   Unspecified open wound of shoulder**

✓7th S41.001   Unspecified open wound of right shoulder

✓7th S41.002   Unspecified open wound of left shoulder

✓7th S41.009   Unspecified open wound of unspecified shoulder

✓6th **S41.01   Laceration without foreign body of shoulder**

✓7th S41.011   Laceration without foreign body of right shoulder

✓7th S41.012   Laceration without foreign body of left shoulder

✓7th S41.019   Laceration without foreign body of unspecified shoulder

✓6th **S41.02   Laceration with foreign body of shoulder**

✓7th S41.021   Laceration with foreign body of right shoulder

✓7th S41.022   Laceration with foreign body of left shoulder

✓7th S41.029   Laceration with foreign body of unspecified shoulder

✓6th **S41.03   Puncture wound without foreign body of shoulder**

✓7th S41.031   Puncture wound without foreign body of right shoulder

✓7th S41.032   Puncture wound without foreign body of left shoulder

✓7th S41.039   Puncture wound without foreign body of unspecified shoulder

☑ Additional Character Required   ✓x7th Xtension Alert   Unspecified Code   Other Specified Code   Manifestation Code   ►◄ Revised Text   ● New Code   ▲ Revised Code Title

ICD-10-CM 2014 (Draft)   841

Injury, Poisoning and Certain Other Consequences of External Causes

S41.04–S42.122

✓6th **S41.04 Puncture wound with foreign body** of shoulder

✓7th **S41.041 Puncture wound with foreign body of right shoulder**

✓7th **S41.042 Puncture wound with foreign body of left shoulder**

✓7th **S41.049 Puncture wound with foreign body of unspecified shoulder**

✓6th **S41.05 Open bite** of shoulder
Bite of shoulder NOS
EXCLUDES 1 superficial bite of shoulder (S40.27)

✓7th **S41.051 Open bite of right shoulder**

✓7th **S41.052 Open bite of left shoulder**

✓7th **S41.059 Open bite of unspecified shoulder**

✓5th **S41.1 Open wound of** upper arm

✓6th **S41.10 Unspecified open wound of upper arm**

✓7th **S41.101 Unspecified open wound of right upper arm**

✓7th **S41.102 Unspecified open wound of left upper arm**

✓7th **S41.109 Unspecified open wound of unspecified upper arm**

✓6th **S41.11 Laceration without foreign body** of upper arm

✓7th **S41.111 Laceration without foreign body of right upper arm**

✓7th **S41.112 Laceration without foreign body of left upper arm**

✓7th **S41.119 Laceration without foreign body of unspecified upper arm**

✓6th **S41.12 Laceration with foreign body** of upper arm

✓7th **S41.121 Laceration with foreign body of right upper arm**

✓7th **S41.122 Laceration with foreign body of left upper arm**

✓7th **S41.129 Laceration with foreign body of unspecified upper arm**

✓6th **S41.13 Puncture wound without foreign body** of upper arm

✓7th **S41.131 Puncture wound without foreign body of right upper arm**

✓7th **S41.132 Puncture wound without foreign body of left upper arm**

✓7th **S41.139 Puncture wound without foreign body of unspecified upper arm**

✓6th **S41.14 Puncture wound with foreign body** of upper arm

✓7th **S41.141 Puncture wound with foreign body of right upper arm**

✓7th **S41.142 Puncture wound with foreign body of left upper arm**

✓7th **S41.149 Puncture wound with foreign body of unspecified upper arm**

✓6th **S41.15 Open bite** of upper arm
Bite of upper arm NOS
EXCLUDES 1 superficial bite of upper arm (S40.87)

✓7th **S41.151 Open bite of right upper arm**

✓7th **S41.152 Open bite of left upper arm**

✓7th **S41.159 Open bite of unspecified upper arm**

✓4th **S42 Fracture of shoulder and upper arm**

NOTE A fracture not indicated as displaced or nondisplaced should be coded to displaced.
A fracture not indicated as open or closed should be coded to closed.

EXCLUDES 1 traumatic amputation of shoulder and upper arm (S48.-)

The appropriate 7th character is to be added to all codes from category S42 [unless otherwise indicated].
A initial encounter for closed fracture
B initial encounter for open fracture
D subsequent encounter for fracture with routine healing
G subsequent encounter for fracture with delayed healing
K subsequent encounter for fracture with nonunion
P subsequent encounter for fracture with malunion
S sequela

✓5th **S42.0 Fracture of** clavicle

✓6th **S42.00 Fracture of** unspecified part of clavicle

✓7th **S42.001 Fracture of unspecified part of right clavicle**

✓7th **S42.002 Fracture of unspecified part of left clavicle**

✓7th **S42.009 Fracture of unspecified part of unspecified clavicle**
AHA: 2012, Q4, 93

✓6th **S42.01 Fracture of** sternal end of clavicle

✓7th **S42.011 Anterior displaced fracture of sternal end of right clavicle**

✓7th **S42.012 Anterior displaced fracture of sternal end of left clavicle**

✓7th **S42.013 Anterior displaced fracture of sternal end of unspecified clavicle**
Displaced fracture of sternal end of clavicle NOS

✓7th **S42.014 Posterior displaced fracture of sternal end of right clavicle**

✓7th **S42.015 Posterior displaced fracture of sternal end of left clavicle**

✓7th **S42.016 Posterior displaced fracture of sternal end of unspecified clavicle**

✓7th **S42.017 Nondisplaced fracture of sternal end of right clavicle**

✓7th **S42.018 Nondisplaced fracture of sternal end of left clavicle**

✓7th **S42.019 Nondisplaced fracture of sternal end of unspecified clavicle**

✓6th **S42.02 Fracture of** shaft of clavicle

✓7th **S42.021 Displaced fracture of shaft of right clavicle**

✓7th **S42.022 Displaced fracture of shaft of left clavicle**

✓7th **S42.023 Displaced fracture of shaft of unspecified clavicle**

✓7th **S42.024 Nondisplaced fracture of shaft of right clavicle**

✓7th **S42.025 Nondisplaced fracture of shaft of left clavicle**

✓7th **S42.026 Nondisplaced fracture of shaft of unspecified clavicle**

✓6th **S42.03 Fracture of** lateral end of clavicle
Fracture of acromial end of clavicle

✓7th **S42.031 Displaced fracture of lateral end of right clavicle**

✓7th **S42.032 Displaced fracture of lateral end of left clavicle**

✓7th **S42.033 Displaced fracture of lateral end of unspecified clavicle**

✓7th **S42.034 Nondisplaced fracture of lateral end of right clavicle**

✓7th **S42.035 Nondisplaced fracture of lateral end of left clavicle**

✓7th **S42.036 Nondisplaced fracture of lateral end of unspecified clavicle**

✓5th **S42.1 Fracture of** scapula

✓6th **S42.10 Fracture of** unspecified part of scapula

✓7th **S42.101 Fracture of unspecified part of scapula, right shoulder**

✓7th **S42.102 Fracture of unspecified part of scapula, left shoulder**

✓7th **S42.109 Fracture of unspecified part of scapula, unspecified shoulder**

✓6th **S42.11 Fracture of** body of scapula

✓7th **S42.111 Displaced fracture of body of scapula, right shoulder**

✓7th **S42.112 Displaced fracture of body of scapula, left shoulder**

✓7th **S42.113 Displaced fracture of body of scapula, unspecified shoulder**

✓7th **S42.114 Nondisplaced fracture of body of scapula, right shoulder**

✓7th **S42.115 Nondisplaced fracture of body of scapula, left shoulder**

✓7th **S42.116 Nondisplaced fracture of body of scapula, unspecified shoulder**

✓6th **S42.12 Fracture of** acromial process

✓7th **S42.121 Displaced fracture of acromial process, right shoulder**

✓7th **S42.122 Displaced fracture of acromial process, left shoulder**

EXCLUDES 1 Not coded here   *EXCLUDES 2* Not included here   N Newborn Age: 0   P Pediatric Age: 0-17   M Maternity Age: 12-55   A Adult Age: 15-124

842   ICD-10-CM 2014 (Draft)

√7ᵗʰ **S42.123** Displaced **fracture of acromial process, unspecified shoulder**

√7ᵗʰ **S42.124** Nondisplaced **fracture of acromial process, right shoulder**

√7ᵗʰ **S42.125** Nondisplaced **fracture of acromial process, left shoulder**

√7ᵗʰ **S42.126** Nondisplaced **fracture of acromial process, unspecified shoulder**

√6ᵗʰ **S42.13** Fracture of coracoid process

√7ᵗʰ **S42.131** Displaced **fracture of coracoid process, right shoulder**

√7ᵗʰ **S42.132** Displaced **fracture of coracoid process, left shoulder**

√7ᵗʰ **S42.133** Displaced **fracture of coracoid process, unspecified shoulder**

√7ᵗʰ **S42.134** Nondisplaced **fracture of coracoid process, right shoulder**

√7ᵗʰ **S42.135** Nondisplaced **fracture of coracoid process, left shoulder**

√7ᵗʰ **S42.136** Nondisplaced **fracture of coracoid process, unspecified shoulder**

√6ᵗʰ **S42.14** Fracture of glenoid cavity of scapula

√7ᵗʰ **S42.141** Displaced **fracture of glenoid cavity of scapula, right shoulder**

√7ᵗʰ **S42.142** Displaced **fracture of glenoid cavity of scapula, left shoulder**

√7ᵗʰ **S42.143** Displaced **fracture of glenoid cavity of scapula, unspecified shoulder**

√7ᵗʰ **S42.144** Nondisplaced **fracture of glenoid cavity of scapula, right shoulder**

√7ᵗʰ **S42.145** Nondisplaced **fracture of glenoid cavity of scapula, left shoulder**

√7ᵗʰ **S42.146** Nondisplaced **fracture of glenoid cavity of scapula, unspecified shoulder**

√6ᵗʰ **S42.15** Fracture of neck of scapula

√7ᵗʰ **S42.151** Displaced **fracture of neck of scapula, right shoulder**

√7ᵗʰ **S42.152** Displaced **fracture of neck of scapula, left shoulder**

√7ᵗʰ **S42.153** Displaced **fracture of neck of scapula, unspecified shoulder**

√7ᵗʰ **S42.154** Nondisplaced **fracture of neck of scapula, right shoulder**

√7ᵗʰ **S42.155** Nondisplaced **fracture of neck of scapula, left shoulder**

√7ᵗʰ **S42.156** Nondisplaced **fracture of neck of scapula, unspecified shoulder**

√6ᵗʰ **S42.19** Fracture of other part of scapula

√7ᵗʰ **S42.191** Fracture of other part of scapula, right shoulder

√7ᵗʰ **S42.192** Fracture of other part of scapula, left shoulder

√7ᵗʰ **S42.199** Fracture of other part of scapula, unspecified shoulder

√5ᵗʰ **S42.2** Fracture of upper end of humerus
Fracture of proximal end of humerus
EXCLUDES 2   *fracture of shaft of humerus (S42.3-)*
physeal fracture of upper end of humerus (S49.0-)

√6ᵗʰ **S42.20** Unspecified **fracture of upper end of humerus**

√7ᵗʰ **S42.201** Unspecified **fracture of upper end of right humerus**

√7ᵗʰ **S42.202** Unspecified **fracture of upper end of left humerus**

√7ᵗʰ **S42.209** Unspecified **fracture of upper end of unspecified humerus**

√6ᵗʰ **S42.21** Unspecified **fracture of surgical neck of humerus**
Fracture of neck of humerus NOS

√7ᵗʰ **S42.211** Unspecified displaced **fracture of surgical neck of right humerus**

√7ᵗʰ **S42.212** Unspecified displaced **fracture of surgical neck of left humerus**

√7ᵗʰ **S42.213** Unspecified displaced **fracture of surgical neck of unspecified humerus**

√7ᵗʰ **S42.214** Unspecified nondisplaced **fracture of surgical neck of right humerus**

√7ᵗʰ **S42.215** Unspecified nondisplaced **fracture of surgical neck of left humerus**

√7ᵗʰ **S42.216** Unspecified nondisplaced **fracture of surgical neck of unspecified humerus**

√6ᵗʰ **S42.22** 2-part **fracture of surgical neck of humerus**

√7ᵗʰ **S42.221** 2-part displaced **fracture of surgical neck of right humerus**

√7ᵗʰ **S42.222** 2-part displaced **fracture of surgical neck of left humerus**

√7ᵗʰ **S42.223** 2-part displaced **fracture of surgical neck of unspecified humerus**

√7ᵗʰ **S42.224** 2-part nondisplaced **fracture of surgical neck of right humerus**

√7ᵗʰ **S42.225** 2-part nondisplaced **fracture of surgical neck of left humerus**

√7ᵗʰ **S42.226** 2-part nondisplaced **fracture of surgical neck of unspecified humerus**

√6ᵗʰ **S42.23** 3-part **fracture of surgical neck of humerus**

√7ᵗʰ **S42.231** 3-part fracture of surgical neck of right humerus

√7ᵗʰ **S42.232** 3-part fracture of surgical neck of left humerus

√7ᵗʰ **S42.239** 3-part fracture of surgical neck of unspecified humerus

√6ᵗʰ **S42.24** 4-part **fracture of surgical neck of humerus**

√7ᵗʰ **S42.241** 4-part fracture of surgical neck of right humerus

√7ᵗʰ **S42.242** 4-part fracture of surgical neck of left humerus

√7ᵗʰ **S42.249** 4-part fracture of surgical neck of unspecified humerus

√6ᵗʰ **S42.25** Fracture of greater tuberosity of humerus

√7ᵗʰ **S42.251** Displaced **fracture of greater tuberosity of right humerus**

√7ᵗʰ **S42.252** Displaced **fracture of greater tuberosity of left humerus**

√7ᵗʰ **S42.253** Displaced **fracture of greater tuberosity of unspecified humerus**

√7ᵗʰ **S42.254** Nondisplaced **fracture of greater tuberosity of right humerus**

√7ᵗʰ **S42.255** Nondisplaced **fracture of greater tuberosity of left humerus**

√7ᵗʰ **S42.256** Nondisplaced **fracture of greater tuberosity of unspecified humerus**

√6ᵗʰ **S42.26** Fracture of lesser tuberosity of humerus

√7ᵗʰ **S42.261** Displaced **fracture of lesser tuberosity of right humerus**

√7ᵗʰ **S42.262** Displaced **fracture of lesser tuberosity of left humerus**

√7ᵗʰ **S42.263** Displaced **fracture of lesser tuberosity of unspecified humerus**

√7ᵗʰ **S42.264** Nondisplaced **fracture of lesser tuberosity of right humerus**

√7ᵗʰ **S42.265** Nondisplaced **fracture of lesser tuberosity of left humerus**

√7ᵗʰ **S42.266** Nondisplaced **fracture of lesser tuberosity of unspecified humerus**

√6ᵗʰ **S42.27** Torus **fracture of upper end of humerus**

The appropriate 7th character is to be added to all codes in subcategory S42.27.
A   initial encounter for closed fracture
D   subsequent encounter for fracture with routine healing
G   subsequent encounter for fracture with delayed healing
K   subsequent encounter for fracture with nonunion
P   subsequent encounter for fracture with malunion
S   sequela

√7ᵗʰ **S42.271** Torus **fracture of upper end of right humerus**

√7ᵗʰ **S42.272** Torus **fracture of upper end of left humerus**

√7ᵗʰ **S42.279** **Torus fracture of upper end of unspecified humerus**

√6ᵗʰ **S42.29** **Other fracture of upper end of humerus**
Fracture of anatomical neck of humerus
Fracture of articular head of humerus

√7ᵗʰ **S42.291** **Other displaced fracture of upper end of right humerus**

√7ᵗʰ **S42.292** **Other displaced fracture of upper end of left humerus**

√7ᵗʰ **S42.293** **Other displaced fracture of upper end of unspecified humerus**

√7ᵗʰ **S42.294** **Other nondisplaced fracture of upper end of right humerus**

√7ᵗʰ **S42.295** **Other nondisplaced fracture of upper end of left humerus**

√7ᵗʰ **S42.296** **Other nondisplaced fracture of upper end of unspecified humerus**

√5ᵗʰ **S42.3** **Fracture of shaft of humerus**
Fracture of humerus NOS
Fracture of upper arm NOS
EXCLUDES 2   physeal fractures of upper end of humerus (S49.0-)
physeal fractures of lower end of humerus (S49.1-)

√6ᵗʰ **S42.30** **Unspecified fracture of shaft of humerus**

√7ᵗʰ **S42.301** **Unspecified fracture of shaft of humerus, right arm**

√7ᵗʰ **S42.302** **Unspecified fracture of shaft of humerus, left arm**

√7ᵗʰ **S42.309** **Unspecified fracture of shaft of humerus, unspecified arm**

√6ᵗʰ **S42.31** **Greenstick fracture of shaft of humerus**

The appropriate 7th character is to be added to all codes in subcategory S42.31.
A   initial encounter for closed fracture
D   subsequent encounter for fracture with routine healing
G   subsequent encounter for fracture with delayed healing
K   subsequent encounter for fracture with nonunion
P   subsequent encounter for fracture with malunion
S   sequela

√7ᵗʰ **S42.311** **Greenstick fracture of shaft of humerus, right arm**

√7ᵗʰ **S42.312** **Greenstick fracture of shaft of humerus, left arm**

√7ᵗʰ **S42.319** **Greenstick fracture of shaft of humerus, unspecified arm**

√6ᵗʰ **S42.32** **Transverse fracture of shaft of humerus**

√7ᵗʰ **S42.321** **Displaced transverse fracture of shaft of humerus, right arm**

√7ᵗʰ **S42.322** **Displaced transverse fracture of shaft of humerus, left arm**

√7ᵗʰ **S42.323** **Displaced transverse fracture of shaft of humerus, unspecified arm**

√7ᵗʰ **S42.324** **Nondisplaced transverse fracture of shaft of humerus, right arm**

√7ᵗʰ **S42.325** **Nondisplaced transverse fracture of shaft of humerus, left arm**

√7ᵗʰ **S42.326** **Nondisplaced transverse fracture of shaft of humerus, unspecified arm**

√6ᵗʰ **S42.33** **Oblique fracture of shaft of humerus**

√7ᵗʰ **S42.331** **Displaced oblique fracture of shaft of humerus, right arm**

√7ᵗʰ **S42.332** **Displaced oblique fracture of shaft of humerus, left arm**

√7ᵗʰ **S42.333** **Displaced oblique fracture of shaft of humerus, unspecified arm**

√7ᵗʰ **S42.334** **Nondisplaced oblique fracture of shaft of humerus, right arm**

√7ᵗʰ **S42.335** **Nondisplaced oblique fracture of shaft of humerus, left arm**

√7ᵗʰ **S42.336** **Nondisplaced oblique fracture of shaft of humerus, unspecified arm**

√6ᵗʰ **S42.34** **Spiral fracture of shaft of humerus**

√7ᵗʰ **S42.341** **Displaced spiral fracture of shaft of humerus, right arm**

√7ᵗʰ **S42.342** **Displaced spiral fracture of shaft of humerus, left arm**

√7ᵗʰ **S42.343** **Displaced spiral fracture of shaft of humerus, unspecified arm**

√7ᵗʰ **S42.344** **Nondisplaced spiral fracture of shaft of humerus, right arm**

√7ᵗʰ **S42.345** **Nondisplaced spiral fracture of shaft of humerus, left arm**

√7ᵗʰ **S42.346** **Nondisplaced spiral fracture of shaft of humerus, unspecified arm**

√6ᵗʰ **S42.35** **Comminuted fracture of shaft of humerus**

√7ᵗʰ **S42.351** **Displaced comminuted fracture of shaft of humerus, right arm**

√7ᵗʰ **S42.352** **Displaced comminuted fracture of shaft of humerus, left arm**

√7ᵗʰ **S42.353** **Displaced comminuted fracture of shaft of humerus, unspecified arm**

√7ᵗʰ **S42.354** **Nondisplaced comminuted fracture of shaft of humerus, right arm**

√7ᵗʰ **S42.355** **Nondisplaced comminuted fracture of shaft of humerus, left arm**

√7ᵗʰ **S42.356** **Nondisplaced comminuted fracture of shaft of humerus, unspecified arm**

√6ᵗʰ **S42.36** **Segmental fracture of shaft of humerus**

√7ᵗʰ **S42.361** **Displaced segmental fracture of shaft of humerus, right arm**

√7ᵗʰ **S42.362** **Displaced segmental fracture of shaft of humerus, left arm**

√7ᵗʰ **S42.363** **Displaced segmental fracture of shaft of humerus, unspecified arm**

√7ᵗʰ **S42.364** **Nondisplaced segmental fracture of shaft of humerus, right arm**

√7ᵗʰ **S42.365** **Nondisplaced segmental fracture of shaft of humerus, left arm**

√7ᵗʰ **S42.366** **Nondisplaced segmental fracture of shaft of humerus, unspecified arm**

√6ᵗʰ **S42.39** **Other fracture of shaft of humerus**

√7ᵗʰ **S42.391** **Other fracture of shaft of right humerus**

√7ᵗʰ **S42.392** **Other fracture of shaft of left humerus**

√7ᵗʰ **S42.399** **Other fracture of shaft of unspecified humerus**

√5ᵗʰ **S42.4** **Fracture of lower end of humerus**
Fracture of distal end of humerus
EXCLUDES 2   fracture of shaft of humerus (S42.3-)
physeal fracture of lower end of humerus (S49.1-)

√6ᵗʰ **S42.40** **Unspecified fracture of lower end of humerus**
Fracture of elbow NOS

√7ᵗʰ **S42.401** **Unspecified fracture of lower end of right humerus**

√7ᵗʰ **S42.402** **Unspecified fracture of lower end of left humerus**

√7ᵗʰ **S42.409** **Unspecified fracture of lower end of unspecified humerus**

√6ᵗʰ **S42.41** **Simple supracondylar fracture without intercondylar fracture of humerus**

√7ᵗʰ **S42.411** **Displaced simple supracondylar fracture without intercondylar fracture of right humerus**

√7ᵗʰ **S42.412** **Displaced simple supracondylar fracture without intercondylar fracture of left humerus**

√7ᵗʰ **S42.413** **Displaced simple supracondylar fracture without intercondylar fracture of unspecified humerus**

√7ᵗʰ **S42.414** **Nondisplaced simple supracondylar fracture without intercondylar fracture of right humerus**

√7ᵗʰ **S42.415** **Nondisplaced simple supracondylar fracture without intercondylar fracture of left humerus**

√7ᵗʰ **S42.416** **Nondisplaced simple supracondylar fracture without intercondylar fracture of unspecified humerus**

EXCLUDES 1 Not coded here   EXCLUDES 2 Not included here   N Newborn Age: 0   P Pediatric Age: 0-17   M Maternity Age: 12-55   A Adult Age: 15-124

844   ICD-10-CM 2014 (Draft)

√6ᵗʰ **S42.42** Comminuted supracondylar **fracture** without intercondylar **fracture of humerus**

√7ᵗʰ **S42.421** Displaced **comminuted supracondylar fracture** without **intercondylar fracture of right humerus**

√7ᵗʰ **S42.422** Displaced **comminuted supracondylar fracture** without **intercondylar fracture of left humerus**

√7ᵗʰ **S42.423** Displaced **comminuted supracondylar fracture** without **intercondylar fracture of unspecified humerus**

√7ᵗʰ **S42.424** Nondisplaced **comminuted supracondylar fracture** without **intercondylar fracture of right humerus**

√7ᵗʰ **S42.425** Nondisplaced **comminuted supracondylar fracture** without **intercondylar fracture of left humerus**

√7ᵗʰ **S42.426** Nondisplaced **comminuted supracondylar fracture** without **intercondylar fracture of unspecified humerus**

√6ᵗʰ **S42.43** Fracture (avulsion) of lateral epicondyle of humerus

√7ᵗʰ **S42.431** Displaced **fracture (avulsion) of lateral epicondyle of right humerus**

√7ᵗʰ **S42.432** Displaced **fracture (avulsion) of lateral epicondyle of left humerus**

√7ᵗʰ **S42.433** Displaced **fracture (avulsion) of lateral epicondyle of unspecified humerus**

√7ᵗʰ **S42.434** Nondisplaced **fracture (avulsion) of lateral epicondyle of right humerus**

√7ᵗʰ **S42.435** Nondisplaced **fracture (avulsion) of lateral epicondyle of left humerus**

√7ᵗʰ **S42.436** Nondisplaced **fracture (avulsion) of lateral epicondyle of unspecified humerus**

√6ᵗʰ **S42.44** Fracture (avulsion) of medial epicondyle of humerus

S42.441 Displaced **fracture (avulsion) of medial epicondyle of right humerus**

√7ᵗʰ **S42.442** Displaced **fracture (avulsion) of medial epicondyle of left humerus**

√7ᵗʰ **S42.443** Displaced **fracture (avulsion) of medial epicondyle of unspecified humerus**

√7ᵗʰ **S42.444** Nondisplaced **fracture (avulsion) of medial epicondyle of right humerus**

√7ᵗʰ **S42.445** Nondisplaced **fracture (avulsion) of medial epicondyle of left humerus**

√7ᵗʰ **S42.446** Nondisplaced **fracture (avulsion) of medial epicondyle of unspecified humerus**

√7ᵗʰ **S42.447** Incarcerated **fracture (avulsion) of medial epicondyle of right humerus**

√7ᵗʰ **S42.448** Incarcerated **fracture (avulsion) of medial epicondyle of left humerus**

√7ᵗʰ **S42.449** Incarcerated **fracture (avulsion) of medial epicondyle of unspecified humerus**

√6ᵗʰ **S42.45** Fracture of lateral condyle of humerus
Fracture of capitellum of humerus

√7ᵗʰ **S42.451** Displaced **fracture of lateral condyle of right humerus**

√7ᵗʰ **S42.452** Displaced **fracture of lateral condyle of left humerus**

√7ᵗʰ **S42.453** Displaced **fracture of lateral condyle of unspecified humerus**

√7ᵗʰ **S42.454** Nondisplaced **fracture of lateral condyle of right humerus**

√7ᵗʰ **S42.455** Nondisplaced **fracture of lateral condyle of left humerus**

√7ᵗʰ **S42.456** Nondisplaced **fracture of lateral condyle of unspecified humerus**

√6ᵗʰ **S42.46** Fracture of medial condyle of humerus
Trochlea fracture of humerus

√7ᵗʰ **S42.461** Displaced **fracture of medial condyle of right humerus**

√7ᵗʰ **S42.462** Displaced **fracture of medial condyle of left humerus**

√7ᵗʰ **S42.463** Displaced **fracture of medial condyle of unspecified humerus**

√7ᵗʰ **S42.464** Nondisplaced **fracture of medial condyle of right humerus**

√7ᵗʰ **S42.465** Nondisplaced **fracture of medial condyle of left humerus**

√7ᵗʰ **S42.466** Nondisplaced **fracture of medial condyle of unspecified humerus**

√6ᵗʰ **S42.47** Transcondylar **fracture of humerus**

√7ᵗʰ **S42.471** Displaced **transcondylar fracture of right humerus**

√7ᵗʰ **S42.472** Displaced **transcondylar fracture of left humerus**

√7ᵗʰ **S42.473** Displaced **transcondylar fracture of unspecified humerus**

√7ᵗʰ **S42.474** Nondisplaced **transcondylar fracture of right humerus**

√7ᵗʰ **S42.475** Nondisplaced **transcondylar fracture of left humerus**

√7ᵗʰ **S42.476** Nondisplaced **transcondylar fracture of unspecified humerus**

√6ᵗʰ **S42.48** Torus fracture of lower end of humerus

The appropriate 7th character is to be added to all codes in subcategory S42.48.
A   initial encounter for closed fracture
D   subsequent encounter for fracture with routine healing
G   subsequent encounter for fracture with delayed healing
K   subsequent encounter for fracture with nonunion
P   subsequent encounter for fracture with malunion
S   sequela

√7ᵗʰ **S42.481** Torus fracture of lower end of right **humerus**

√7ᵗʰ **S42.482** Torus fracture of lower end of left **humerus**

√7ᵗʰ **S42.489** Torus fracture of lower end of unspecified **humerus**

√6ᵗʰ **S42.49** Other fracture of lower end of humerus

√7ᵗʰ **S42.491** Other displaced **fracture of lower end of right humerus**

√7ᵗʰ **S42.492** Other displaced **fracture of lower end of left humerus**

√7ᵗʰ **S42.493** Other displaced **fracture of lower end of unspecified humerus**

√7ᵗʰ **S42.494** Other nondisplaced **fracture of lower end of right humerus**

√7ᵗʰ **S42.495** Other nondisplaced **fracture of lower end of left humerus**

√7ᵗʰ **S42.496** Other nondisplaced **fracture of lower end of unspecified humerus**

√5ᵗʰ **S42.9** Fracture of shoulder girdle, part unspecified
Fracture of shoulder NOS

√x7ᵗʰ **S42.90** Fracture of unspecified shoulder girdle, part unspecified

√x7ᵗʰ **S42.91** Fracture of right shoulder girdle, part unspecified

√x7ᵗʰ **S42.92** Fracture of left shoulder girdle, part unspecified

✓4ᵗʰ S43 Dislocation and sprain of joints and ligaments of shoulder girdle

INCLUDES   avulsion of joint or ligament of shoulder girdle
laceration of cartilage, joint or ligament of shoulder girdle
sprain of cartilage, joint or ligament of shoulder girdle
traumatic hemarthrosis of joint or ligament of shoulder girdle
traumatic rupture of joint or ligament of shoulder girdle
traumatic subluxation of joint or ligament of shoulder girdle
traumatic tear of joint or ligament of shoulder girdle

Code also any associated open wound

EXCLUDES 2   strain of muscle, fascia and tendon of shoulder and upper arm (S46.-)

The appropriate 7th character is to be added to each code from category S43.
A   initial encounter
D   subsequent encounter
S   sequela

✓5ᵗʰ S43.0 Subluxation and dislocation of shoulder joint
Dislocation of glenohumeral joint
Subluxation of glenohumeral joint

✓6ᵗʰ S43.00 Unspecified subluxation and dislocation of shoulder joint
Dislocation of humerus NOS
Subluxation of humerus NOS

✓7ᵗʰ S43.001 Unspecified subluxation of right shoulder joint

✓7ᵗʰ S43.002 Unspecified subluxation of left shoulder joint

✓7ᵗʰ S43.003 Unspecified subluxation of unspecified shoulder joint

✓7ᵗʰ S43.004 Unspecified dislocation of right shoulder joint

✓7ᵗʰ S43.005 Unspecified dislocation of left shoulder joint

✓7ᵗʰ S43.006 Unspecified dislocation of unspecified shoulder joint

✓6ᵗʰ S43.01 Anterior subluxation and dislocation of humerus

✓7ᵗʰ S43.011 Anterior subluxation of right humerus

✓7ᵗʰ S43.012 Anterior subluxation of left humerus

✓7ᵗʰ S43.013 Anterior subluxation of unspecified humerus

✓7ᵗʰ S43.014 Anterior dislocation of right humerus

✓7ᵗʰ S43.015 Anterior dislocation of left humerus

✓7ᵗʰ S43.016 Anterior dislocation of unspecified humerus

✓6ᵗʰ S43.02 Posterior subluxation and dislocation of humerus

✓7ᵗʰ S43.021 Posterior subluxation of right humerus

✓7ᵗʰ S43.022 Posterior subluxation of left humerus

✓7ᵗʰ S43.023 Posterior subluxation of unspecified humerus

✓7ᵗʰ S43.024 Posterior dislocation of right humerus

✓7ᵗʰ S43.025 Posterior dislocation of left humerus

✓7ᵗʰ S43.026 Posterior dislocation of unspecified humerus

✓6ᵗʰ S43.03 Inferior subluxation and dislocation of humerus

✓7ᵗʰ S43.031 Inferior subluxation of right humerus

✓7ᵗʰ S43.032 Inferior subluxation of left humerus

✓7ᵗʰ S43.033 Inferior subluxation of unspecified humerus

✓7ᵗʰ S43.034 Inferior dislocation of right humerus

✓7ᵗʰ S43.035 Inferior dislocation of left humerus

✓7ᵗʰ S43.036 Inferior dislocation of unspecified humerus

✓6ᵗʰ S43.08 Other subluxation and dislocation of shoulder joint

✓7ᵗʰ S43.081 Other subluxation of right shoulder joint

✓7ᵗʰ S43.082 Other subluxation of left shoulder joint

✓7ᵗʰ S43.083 Other subluxation of unspecified shoulder joint

✓7ᵗʰ S43.084 Other dislocation of right shoulder joint

✓7ᵗʰ S43.085 Other dislocation of left shoulder joint

✓7ᵗʰ S43.086 Other dislocation of unspecified shoulder joint

✓5ᵗʰ S43.1 Subluxation and dislocation of acromioclavicular joint

✓6ᵗʰ S43.10 Unspecified dislocation of acromioclavicular joint

✓7ᵗʰ S43.101 Unspecified dislocation of right acromioclavicular joint

✓7ᵗʰ S43.102 Unspecified dislocation of left acromioclavicular joint

✓7ᵗʰ S43.109 Unspecified dislocation of unspecified acromioclavicular joint

✓6ᵗʰ S43.11 Subluxation of acromioclavicular joint

✓7ᵗʰ S43.111 Subluxation of right acromioclavicular joint

✓7ᵗʰ S43.112 Subluxation of left acromioclavicular joint

✓7ᵗʰ S43.119 Subluxation of unspecified acromioclavicular joint

✓6ᵗʰ S43.12 Dislocation of acromioclavicular joint, 100%-200% displacement

✓7ᵗʰ S43.121 Dislocation of right acromioclavicular joint, 100%-200% displacement

✓7ᵗʰ S43.122 Dislocation of left acromioclavicular joint, 100%-200% displacement

✓7ᵗʰ S43.129 Dislocation of unspecified acromioclavicular joint, 100%-200% displacement

✓6ᵗʰ S43.13 Dislocation of acromioclavicular joint, greater than 200% displacement

✓7ᵗʰ S43.131 Dislocation of right acromioclavicular joint, greater than 200% displacement

✓7ᵗʰ S43.132 Dislocation of left acromioclavicular joint, greater than 200% displacement

✓7ᵗʰ S43.139 Dislocation of unspecified acromioclavicular joint, greater than 200% displacement

✓6ᵗʰ S43.14 Inferior dislocation of acromioclavicular joint

✓7ᵗʰ S43.141 Inferior dislocation of right acromioclavicular joint

✓7ᵗʰ S43.142 Inferior dislocation of left acromioclavicular joint

✓7ᵗʰ S43.149 Inferior dislocation of unspecified acromioclavicular joint

✓6ᵗʰ S43.15 Posterior dislocation of acromioclavicular joint

✓7ᵗʰ S43.151 Posterior dislocation of right acromioclavicular joint

✓7ᵗʰ S43.152 Posterior dislocation of left acromioclavicular joint

✓7ᵗʰ S43.159 Posterior dislocation of unspecified acromioclavicular joint

✓5ᵗʰ S43.2 Subluxation and dislocation of sternoclavicular joint

✓6ᵗʰ S43.20 Unspecified subluxation and dislocation of sternoclavicular joint

✓7ᵗʰ S43.201 Unspecified subluxation of right sternoclavicular joint

✓7ᵗʰ S43.202 Unspecified subluxation of left sternoclavicular joint

✓7ᵗʰ S43.203 Unspecified subluxation of unspecified sternoclavicular joint

✓7ᵗʰ S43.204 Unspecified dislocation of right sternoclavicular joint

✓7ᵗʰ S43.205 Unspecified dislocation of left sternoclavicular joint

✓7ᵗʰ S43.206 Unspecified dislocation of unspecified sternoclavicular joint

✓6ᵗʰ S43.21 Anterior subluxation and dislocation of sternoclavicular joint

✓7ᵗʰ S43.211 Anterior subluxation of right sternoclavicular joint

✓7ᵗʰ S43.212 Anterior subluxation of left sternoclavicular joint

✓7ᵗʰ S43.213 Anterior subluxation of unspecified sternoclavicular joint

✓7ᵗʰ S43.214 Anterior dislocation of right sternoclavicular joint

✓7ᵗʰ S43.215 Anterior dislocation of left sternoclavicular joint

✓7ᵗʰ S43.216 Anterior dislocation of unspecified sternoclavicular joint

EXCLUDES 1 Not coded here   EXCLUDES 2 Not included here   N Newborn Age: 0   P Pediatric Age: 0-17   M Maternity Age: 12-55   A Adult Age: 15-124

846   ICD-10-CM 2014 (Draft)

√6ᵗʰ **S43.22** Posterior subluxation and dislocation of sternoclavicular joint

√7ᵗʰ **S43.221** Posterior subluxation of right sternoclavicular joint

√7ᵗʰ **S43.222** Posterior subluxation of left sternoclavicular joint

√7ᵗʰ **S43.223** Posterior subluxation of unspecified sternoclavicular joint

√7ᵗʰ **S43.224** Posterior dislocation of right sternoclavicular joint

√7ᵗʰ **S43.225** Posterior dislocation of left sternoclavicular joint

√7ᵗʰ **S43.226** Posterior dislocation of unspecified sternoclavicular joint

√5ᵗʰ **S43.3** Subluxation and dislocation of other and unspecified parts of shoulder girdle

√6ᵗʰ **S43.30** Subluxation and dislocation of unspecified parts of shoulder girdle

Dislocation of shoulder girdle NOS
Subluxation of shoulder girdle NOS

√7ᵗʰ **S43.301** Subluxation of unspecified parts of right shoulder girdle

√7ᵗʰ **S43.302** Subluxation of unspecified parts of left shoulder girdle

√7ᵗʰ **S43.303** Subluxation of unspecified parts of unspecified shoulder girdle

√7ᵗʰ **S43.304** Dislocation of unspecified parts of right shoulder girdle

√7ᵗʰ **S43.305** Dislocation of unspecified parts of left shoulder girdle

√7ᵗʰ **S43.306** Dislocation of unspecified parts of unspecified shoulder girdle

√6ᵗʰ **S43.31** Subluxation and dislocation of scapula

√7ᵗʰ **S43.311** Subluxation of right scapula

√7ᵗʰ **S43.312** Subluxation of left scapula

√7ᵗʰ **S43.313** Subluxation of unspecified scapula

√7ᵗʰ **S43.314** Dislocation of right scapula

√7ᵗʰ **S43.315** Dislocation of left scapula

√7ᵗʰ **S43.316** Dislocation of unspecified scapula

√6ᵗʰ **S43.39** Subluxation and dislocation of other parts of shoulder girdle

√7ᵗʰ **S43.391** Subluxation of other parts of right shoulder girdle

√7ᵗʰ **S43.392** Subluxation of other parts of left shoulder girdle

√7ᵗʰ **S43.393** Subluxation of other parts of unspecified shoulder girdle

√7ᵗʰ **S43.394** Dislocation of other parts of right shoulder girdle

√7ᵗʰ **S43.395** Dislocation of other parts of left shoulder girdle

√7ᵗʰ **S43.396** Dislocation of other parts of unspecified shoulder girdle

√5ᵗʰ **S43.4** Sprain of shoulder joint

√6ᵗʰ **S43.40** Unspecified sprain of shoulder joint

√7ᵗʰ **S43.401** Unspecified sprain of right shoulder joint

√7ᵗʰ **S43.402** Unspecified sprain of left shoulder joint

√7ᵗʰ **S43.409** Unspecified sprain of unspecified shoulder joint

√6ᵗʰ **S43.41** Sprain of coracohumeral (ligament)

√7ᵗʰ **S43.411** Sprain of right coracohumeral (ligament)

√7ᵗʰ **S43.412** Sprain of left coracohumeral (ligament)

√7ᵗʰ **S43.419** Sprain of unspecified coracohumeral (ligament)

√6ᵗʰ **S43.42** Sprain of rotator cuff capsule

EXCLUDES 1 *rotator cuff syndrome (complete) (incomplete), not specified as traumatic (M75.1-)*

EXCLUDES 2 *injury of tendon of rotator cuff (S46.0-)*

√7ᵗʰ **S43.421** Sprain of right rotator cuff capsule

√7ᵗʰ **S43.422** Sprain of left rotator cuff capsule

√7ᵗʰ **S43.429** Sprain of unspecified rotator cuff capsule

√6ᵗʰ **S43.43** Superior glenoid labrum lesion

SLAP lesion

√7ᵗʰ **S43.431** Superior glenoid labrum lesion of right shoulder

√7ᵗʰ **S43.432** Superior glenoid labrum lesion of left shoulder

√7ᵗʰ **S43.439** Superior glenoid labrum lesion of unspecified shoulder

√6ᵗʰ **S43.49** Other sprain of shoulder joint

√7ᵗʰ **S43.491** Other sprain of right shoulder joint

√7ᵗʰ **S43.492** Other sprain of left shoulder joint

√7ᵗʰ **S43.499** Other sprain of unspecified shoulder joint

√5ᵗʰ **S43.5** Sprain of acromioclavicular joint

Sprain of acromioclavicular ligament

√x7ᵗʰ **S43.50** Sprain of unspecified acromioclavicular joint

√x7ᵗʰ **S43.51** Sprain of right acromioclavicular joint

√x7ᵗʰ **S43.52** Sprain of left acromioclavicular joint

√5ᵗʰ **S43.6** Sprain of sternoclavicular joint

√x7ᵗʰ **S43.60** Sprain of unspecified sternoclavicular joint

√x7ᵗʰ **S43.61** Sprain of right sternoclavicular joint

√x7ᵗʰ **S43.62** Sprain of left sternoclavicular joint

√5ᵗʰ **S43.8** Sprain of other specified parts of shoulder girdle

√x7ᵗʰ **S43.80** Sprain of other specified parts of unspecified shoulder girdle

√x7ᵗʰ **S43.81** Sprain of other specified parts of right shoulder girdle

√x7ᵗʰ **S43.82** Sprain of other specified parts of left shoulder girdle

√5ᵗʰ **S43.9** Sprain of unspecified parts of shoulder girdle

√x7ᵗʰ **S43.90** Sprain of unspecified parts of unspecified shoulder girdle

Sprain of shoulder girdle NOS

√x7ᵗʰ **S43.91** Sprain of unspecified parts of right shoulder girdle

√x7ᵗʰ **S43.92** Sprain of unspecified parts of left shoulder girdle

√4ᵗʰ **S44** **Injury of nerves at shoulder and upper arm level**

Code also any associated open wound (S41.-)

EXCLUDES 2 *injury of brachial plexus (S14.3-)*

The appropriate 7th character is to be added to each code from category S44.
A   initial encounter
D   subsequent encounter
S   sequela

√5ᵗʰ **S44.0** Injury of ulnar nerve at upper arm level

EXCLUDES 1 *ulnar nerve NOS (S54.0)*

√x7ᵗʰ **S44.00** Injury of ulnar nerve at upper arm level, unspecified arm

√x7ᵗʰ **S44.01** Injury of ulnar nerve at upper arm level, right arm

√x7ᵗʰ **S44.02** Injury of ulnar nerve at upper arm level, left arm

√5ᵗʰ **S44.1** Injury of median nerve at upper arm level

EXCLUDES 1 *median nerve NOS (S54.1)*

√x7ᵗʰ **S44.10** Injury of median nerve at upper arm level, unspecified arm

√x7ᵗʰ **S44.11** Injury of median nerve at upper arm level, right arm

√x7ᵗʰ **S44.12** Injury of median nerve at upper arm level, left arm

√5ᵗʰ **S44.2** Injury of radial nerve at upper arm level

EXCLUDES 1 *radial nerve NOS (S54.2)*

√x7ᵗʰ **S44.20** Injury of radial nerve at upper arm level, unspecified arm

√x7ᵗʰ **S44.21** Injury of radial nerve at upper arm level, right arm

√x7ᵗʰ **S44.22** Injury of radial nerve at upper arm level, left arm

√5ᵗʰ **S44.3** Injury of axillary nerve

√x7ᵗʰ **S44.30** Injury of axillary nerve, unspecified arm

√x7ᵗʰ **S44.31** Injury of axillary nerve, right arm

√x7ᵗʰ **S44.32** Injury of axillary nerve, left arm

√5ᵗʰ **S44.4** Injury of musculocutaneous nerve

√x7ᵗʰ **S44.40** Injury of musculocutaneous nerve, unspecified arm

√x7ᵗʰ **S44.41** Injury of musculocutaneous nerve, right arm

√x7ᵗʰ **S44.42** Injury of musculocutaneous nerve, left arm

✅ Additional Character Required   √x7ᵗʰ Xtension Alert   Unspecified Code   Other Specified Code   Manifestation Code   ►◄ Revised Text   ● New Code   ▲ Revised Code Title

Injury, Poisoning and Certain Other Consequences of External Causes

S44.5–S45.891

✓5ᵗʰ S44.5 Injury of cutaneous sensory nerve **at shoulder and upper arm level**

     ✓x7ᵗʰ **S44.50 Injury of cutaneous sensory nerve at shoulder and upper arm level, unspecified arm**

     ✓x7ᵗʰ **S44.51 Injury of cutaneous sensory nerve at shoulder and upper arm level, right arm**

     ✓x7ᵗʰ **S44.52 Injury of cutaneous sensory nerve at shoulder and upper arm level, left arm**

✓5ᵗʰ S44.8 Injury of other nerves at shoulder and upper arm level

     ✓6ᵗʰ **S44.8X Injury of** other nerves **at shoulder and upper arm level**

         ✓7ᵗʰ **S44.8X1 Injury of other nerves at shoulder and upper arm level, right arm**

         ✓7ᵗʰ **S44.8X2 Injury of other nerves at shoulder and upper arm level, left arm**

         ✓7ᵗʰ **S44.8X9 Injury of other nerves at shoulder and upper arm level, unspecified arm**

✓5ᵗʰ S44.9 Injury of unspecified nerve **at shoulder and upper arm level**

     ✓x7ᵗʰ **S44.90 Injury of unspecified nerve at shoulder and upper arm level, unspecified arm**

     ✓x7ᵗʰ **S44.91 Injury of unspecified nerve at shoulder and upper arm level, right arm**

     ✓x7ᵗʰ **S44.92 Injury of unspecified nerve at shoulder and upper arm level, left arm**

✓4ᵗʰ S45 Injury of blood vessels at shoulder and upper arm level

     Code also any associated open wound (S41.-)

     EXCLUDES 2 *injury of subclavian artery (S25.1)*
                    injury of subclavian vein (S25.3)

     The appropriate 7th character is to be added to each code from category S45.
     A   initial encounter
     D   subsequent encounter
     S   sequela

✓5ᵗʰ S45.0 Injury of axillary artery

     ✓6ᵗʰ **S45.00 Unspecified injury of axillary artery**

         ✓7ᵗʰ **S45.001 Unspecified injury of axillary artery, right side**

         ✓7ᵗʰ **S45.002 Unspecified injury of axillary artery, left side**

         ✓7ᵗʰ **S45.009 Unspecified injury of axillary artery, unspecified side**

     ✓6ᵗʰ **S45.01 Laceration of axillary artery**

         ✓7ᵗʰ **S45.011 Laceration of axillary artery, right side**

         ✓7ᵗʰ **S45.012 Laceration of axillary artery, left side**

         ✓7ᵗʰ **S45.019 Laceration of axillary artery, unspecified side**

     ✓6ᵗʰ **S45.09 Other specified injury of axillary artery**

         ✓7ᵗʰ **S45.091 Other specified injury of axillary artery, right side**

         ✓7ᵗʰ **S45.092 Other specified injury of axillary artery, left side**

         ✓7ᵗʰ **S45.099 Other specified injury of axillary artery, unspecified side**

✓5ᵗʰ S45.1 Injury of brachial artery

     ✓6ᵗʰ **S45.10 Unspecified injury of brachial artery**

         ✓7ᵗʰ **S45.101 Unspecified injury of brachial artery, right side**

         ✓7ᵗʰ **S45.102 Unspecified injury of brachial artery, left side**

         ✓7ᵗʰ **S45.109 Unspecified injury of brachial artery, unspecified side**

     ✓6ᵗʰ **S45.11 Laceration of brachial artery**

         ✓7ᵗʰ **S45.111 Laceration of brachial artery, right side**

         ✓7ᵗʰ **S45.112 Laceration of brachial artery, left side**

         ✓7ᵗʰ **S45.119 Laceration of brachial artery, unspecified side**

     ✓6ᵗʰ **S45.19 Other specified injury of brachial artery**

         ✓7ᵗʰ **S45.191 Other specified injury of brachial artery, right side**

         ✓7ᵗʰ **S45.192 Other specified injury of brachial artery, left side**

         ✓7ᵗʰ **S45.199 Other specified injury of brachial artery, unspecified side**

✓5ᵗʰ S45.2 Injury of axillary or brachial vein

     ✓6ᵗʰ **S45.20 Unspecified injury of axillary or brachial vein**

         ✓7ᵗʰ **S45.201 Unspecified injury of axillary or brachial vein, right side**

         ✓7ᵗʰ **S45.202 Unspecified injury of axillary or brachial vein, left side**

         ✓7ᵗʰ **S45.209 Unspecified injury of axillary or brachial vein, unspecified side**

     ✓6ᵗʰ **S45.21 Laceration of axillary or brachial vein**

         ✓7ᵗʰ **S45.211 Laceration of axillary or brachial vein, right side**

         ✓7ᵗʰ **S45.212 Laceration of axillary or brachial vein, left side**

         ✓7ᵗʰ **S45.219 Laceration of axillary or brachial vein, unspecified side**

     ✓6ᵗʰ **S45.29 Other** specified injury of axillary or brachial vein

         ✓7ᵗʰ **S45.291 Other specified injury of axillary or brachial vein, right side**

         ✓7ᵗʰ **S45.292 Other specified injury of axillary or brachial vein, left side**

         ✓7ᵗʰ **S45.299 Other specified injury of axillary or brachial vein, unspecified side**

✓5ᵗʰ S45.3 Injury of superficial vein **at shoulder and upper arm level**

     ✓6ᵗʰ **S45.30 Unspecified injury of superficial vein at shoulder and upper arm level**

         ✓7ᵗʰ **S45.301 Unspecified injury of superficial vein at shoulder and upper arm level, right arm**

         ✓7ᵗʰ **S45.302 Unspecified injury of superficial vein at shoulder and upper arm level, left arm**

         ✓7ᵗʰ **S45.309 Unspecified injury of superficial vein at shoulder and upper arm level, unspecified arm**

     ✓6ᵗʰ **S45.31 Laceration of superficial vein at shoulder and upper arm level**

         ✓7ᵗʰ **S45.311 Laceration of superficial vein at shoulder and upper arm level, right arm**

         ✓7ᵗʰ **S45.312 Laceration of superficial vein at shoulder and upper arm level, left arm**

         ✓7ᵗʰ **S45.319 Laceration of superficial vein at shoulder and upper arm level, unspecified arm**

     ✓6ᵗʰ **S45.39 Other** specified injury of superficial vein at shoulder and upper arm level

         ✓7ᵗʰ **S45.391 Other specified injury of superficial vein at shoulder and upper arm level, right arm**

         ✓7ᵗʰ **S45.392 Other specified injury of superficial vein at shoulder and upper arm level, left arm**

         ✓7ᵗʰ **S45.399 Other specified injury of superficial vein at shoulder and upper arm level, unspecified arm**

✓5ᵗʰ S45.8 Injury of other specified blood vessels **at shoulder and upper arm level**

     ✓6ᵗʰ **S45.80 Unspecified injury of other specified blood vessels at shoulder and upper arm level**

         ✓7ᵗʰ **S45.801 Unspecified injury of other specified blood vessels at shoulder and upper arm level, right arm**

         ✓7ᵗʰ **S45.802 Unspecified injury of other specified blood vessels at shoulder and upper arm level, left arm**

         ✓7ᵗʰ **S45.809 Unspecified injury of other specified blood vessels at shoulder and upper arm level, unspecified arm**

     ✓6ᵗʰ **S45.81 Laceration of other specified blood vessels at shoulder and upper arm level**

         ✓7ᵗʰ **S45.811 Laceration of other specified blood vessels at shoulder and upper arm level, right arm**

         ✓7ᵗʰ **S45.812 Laceration of other specified blood vessels at shoulder and upper arm level, left arm**

         ✓7ᵗʰ **S45.819 Laceration of other specified blood vessels at shoulder and upper arm level, unspecified arm**

     ✓6ᵗʰ **S45.89 Other** specified injury of other specified blood vessels at shoulder and upper arm level

         ✓7ᵗʰ **S45.891 Other specified injury of other specified blood vessels at shoulder and upper arm level, right arm**

EXCLUDES 1 Not coded here   **EXCLUDES 2** Not included here   **N** Newborn Age: 0   **P** Pediatric Age: 0-17   **M** Maternity Age: 12-55   **A** Adult Age: 15-124

848   ICD-10-CM 2014 (Draft)

√7ᵗʰ **S45.892** Other specified injury of other specified blood vessels at shoulder and upper arm level, left arm

√7ᵗʰ **S45.899** Other specified injury of other specified blood vessels at shoulder and upper arm level, unspecified arm

√5ᵗʰ **S45.9** Injury of unspecified blood vessel at shoulder and upper arm level

√6ᵗʰ **S45.90** Unspecified injury of unspecified blood vessel at shoulder and upper arm level

√7ᵗʰ **S45.901** Unspecified injury of unspecified blood vessel at shoulder and upper arm level, right arm

√7ᵗʰ **S45.902** Unspecified injury of unspecified blood vessel at shoulder and upper arm level, left arm

√7ᵗʰ **S45.909** Unspecified injury of unspecified blood vessel at shoulder and upper arm level, unspecified arm

√6ᵗʰ **S45.91** Laceration of unspecified blood vessel at shoulder and upper arm level

√7ᵗʰ **S45.911** Laceration of unspecified blood vessel at shoulder and upper arm level, right arm

√7ᵗʰ **S45.912** Laceration of unspecified blood vessel at shoulder and upper arm level, left arm

√7ᵗʰ **S45.919** Laceration of unspecified blood vessel at shoulder and upper arm level, unspecified arm

√6ᵗʰ **S45.99** Other specified injury of unspecified blood vessel at shoulder and upper arm level

√7ᵗʰ **S45.991** Other specified injury of unspecified blood vessel at shoulder and upper arm level, right arm

√7ᵗʰ **S45.992** Other specified injury of unspecified blood vessel at shoulder and upper arm level, left arm

√7ᵗʰ **S45.999** Other specified injury of unspecified blood vessel at shoulder and upper arm level, unspecified arm

√4ᵗʰ **S46** Injury of muscle, fascia and tendon at shoulder and upper arm level

Code also any associated open wound (S41.-)

EXCLUDES 2 injury of muscle, fascia and tendon at elbow (S56.-)
sprain of joints and ligaments of shoulder girdle (S43.9)

The appropriate 7th character is to be added to each code from category S46.
A   initial encounter
D   subsequent encounter
S   sequela

√5ᵗʰ **S46.0** Injury of muscle(s) and tendon(s) of the rotator cuff of shoulder

√6ᵗʰ **S46.00** Unspecified injury of muscle(s) and tendon(s) of the rotator cuff of shoulder

√7ᵗʰ **S46.001** Unspecified injury of muscle(s) and tendon(s) of the rotator cuff of right shoulder

√7ᵗʰ **S46.002** Unspecified injury of muscle(s) and tendon(s) of the rotator cuff of left shoulder

√7ᵗʰ **S46.009** Unspecified injury of muscle(s) and tendon(s) of the rotator cuff of unspecified shoulder

√6ᵗʰ **S46.01** Strain of muscle(s) and tendon(s) of the rotator cuff of shoulder

√7ᵗʰ **S46.011** Strain of muscle(s) and tendon(s) of the rotator cuff of right shoulder

√7ᵗʰ **S46.012** Strain of muscle(s) and tendon(s) of the rotator cuff of left shoulder

√7ᵗʰ **S46.019** Strain of muscle(s) and tendon(s) of the rotator cuff of unspecified shoulder

√6ᵗʰ **S46.02** Laceration of muscle(s) and tendon(s) of the rotator cuff of shoulder

√7ᵗʰ **S46.021** Laceration of muscle(s) and tendon(s) of the rotator cuff of right shoulder

√7ᵗʰ **S46.022** Laceration of muscle(s) and tendon(s) of the rotator cuff of left shoulder

√7ᵗʰ **S46.029** Laceration of muscle(s) and tendon(s) of the rotator cuff of unspecified shoulder

√6ᵗʰ **S46.09** Other injury of muscle(s) and tendon(s) of the rotator cuff of shoulder

√7ᵗʰ **S46.091** Other injury of muscle(s) and tendon(s) of the rotator cuff of right shoulder

√7ᵗʰ **S46.092** Other injury of muscle(s) and tendon(s) of the rotator cuff of left shoulder

√7ᵗʰ **S46.099** Other injury of muscle(s) and tendon(s) of the rotator cuff of unspecified shoulder

√5ᵗʰ **S46.1** Injury of muscle, fascia and tendon of long head of biceps

√6ᵗʰ **S46.10** Unspecified injury of muscle, fascia and tendon of long head of biceps

√7ᵗʰ **S46.101** Unspecified injury of muscle, fascia and tendon of long head of biceps, right arm

√7ᵗʰ **S46.102** Unspecified injury of muscle, fascia and tendon of long head of biceps, left arm

√7ᵗʰ **S46.109** Unspecified injury of muscle, fascia and tendon of long head of biceps, unspecified arm

√6ᵗʰ **S46.11** Strain of muscle, fascia and tendon of long head of biceps

√7ᵗʰ **S46.111** Strain of muscle, fascia and tendon of long head of biceps, right arm

√7ᵗʰ **S46.112** Strain of muscle, fascia and tendon of long head of biceps, left arm

√7ᵗʰ **S46.119** Strain of muscle, fascia and tendon of long head of biceps, unspecified arm

√6ᵗʰ **S46.12** Laceration of muscle, fascia and tendon of long head of biceps

√7ᵗʰ **S46.121** Laceration of muscle, fascia and tendon of long head of biceps, right arm

√7ᵗʰ **S46.122** Laceration of muscle, fascia and tendon of long head of biceps, left arm

√7ᵗʰ **S46.129** Laceration of muscle, fascia and tendon of long head of biceps, unspecified arm

√6ᵗʰ **S46.19** Other injury of muscle, fascia and tendon of long head of biceps

√7ᵗʰ **S46.191** Other injury of muscle, fascia and tendon of long head of biceps, right arm

√7ᵗʰ **S46.192** Other injury of muscle, fascia and tendon of long head of biceps, left arm

√7ᵗʰ **S46.199** Other injury of muscle, fascia and tendon of long head of biceps, unspecified arm

√5ᵗʰ **S46.2** Injury of muscle, fascia and tendon of other parts of biceps

√6ᵗʰ **S46.20** Unspecified injury of muscle, fascia and tendon of other parts of biceps

√7ᵗʰ **S46.201** Unspecified injury of muscle, fascia and tendon of other parts of biceps, right arm

√7ᵗʰ **S46.202** Unspecified injury of muscle, fascia and tendon of other parts of biceps, left arm

√7ᵗʰ **S46.209** Unspecified injury of muscle, fascia and tendon of other parts of biceps, unspecified arm

√6ᵗʰ **S46.21** Strain of muscle, fascia and tendon of other parts of biceps

√7ᵗʰ **S46.211** Strain of muscle, fascia and tendon of other parts of biceps, right arm

√7ᵗʰ **S46.212** Strain of muscle, fascia and tendon of other parts of biceps, left arm

√7ᵗʰ **S46.219** Strain of muscle, fascia and tendon of other parts of biceps, unspecified arm

√6ᵗʰ **S46.22** Laceration of muscle, fascia and tendon of other parts of biceps

√7ᵗʰ **S46.221** Laceration of muscle, fascia and tendon of other parts of biceps, right arm

√7ᵗʰ **S46.222** Laceration of muscle, fascia and tendon of other parts of biceps, left arm

√7ᵗʰ **S46.229** Laceration of muscle, fascia and tendon of other parts of biceps, unspecified arm

√6ᵗʰ **S46.29** Other injury of muscle, fascia and tendon of other parts of biceps

√7ᵗʰ **S46.291** Other injury of muscle, fascia and tendon of other parts of biceps, right arm

√7ᵗʰ **S46.292** Other injury of muscle, fascia and tendon of other parts of biceps, left arm

√7ᵗʰ **S46.299** Other injury of muscle, fascia and tendon of other parts of biceps, unspecified arm

√5ᵗʰ **S46.3** Injury of muscle, fascia and tendon of triceps

√6ᵗʰ **S46.30** Unspecified injury of muscle, fascia and tendon of triceps

√7ᵗʰ **S46.301** Unspecified injury of muscle, fascia and tendon of triceps, right arm

√7ᵗʰ **S46.302** Unspecified injury of muscle, fascia and tendon of triceps, left arm

√7ᵗʰ **S46.309** Unspecified injury of muscle, fascia and tendon of triceps, unspecified arm

√6ᵗʰ **S46.31** Strain of muscle, fascia and tendon of triceps

√7ᵗʰ **S46.311** Strain of muscle, fascia and tendon of triceps, right arm

√7ᵗʰ **S46.312** Strain of muscle, fascia and tendon of triceps, left arm

√7ᵗʰ **S46.319** Strain of muscle, fascia and tendon of triceps, unspecified arm

√6ᵗʰ **S46.32** Laceration of muscle, fascia and tendon of triceps

√7ᵗʰ **S46.321** Laceration of muscle, fascia and tendon of triceps, right arm

√7ᵗʰ **S46.322** Laceration of muscle, fascia and tendon of triceps, left arm

√7ᵗʰ **S46.329** Laceration of muscle, fascia and tendon of triceps, unspecified arm

√6ᵗʰ **S46.39** Other injury of muscle, fascia and tendon of triceps

√7ᵗʰ **S46.391** Other injury of muscle, fascia and tendon of triceps, right arm

√7ᵗʰ **S46.392** Other injury of muscle, fascia and tendon of triceps, left arm

√7ᵗʰ **S46.399** Other injury of muscle, fascia and tendon of triceps, unspecified arm

√5ᵗʰ **S46.8** Injury of other muscles, fascia and tendons at shoulder and upper arm level

√6ᵗʰ **S46.80** Unspecified injury of other muscles, fascia and tendons at shoulder and upper arm level

√7ᵗʰ **S46.801** Unspecified injury of other muscles, fascia and tendons at shoulder and upper arm level, right arm

√7ᵗʰ **S46.802** Unspecified injury of other muscles, fascia and tendons at shoulder and upper arm level, left arm

√7ᵗʰ **S46.809** Unspecified injury of other muscles, fascia and tendons at shoulder and upper arm level, unspecified arm

√6ᵗʰ **S46.81** Strain of other muscles, fascia and tendons at shoulder and upper arm level

√7ᵗʰ **S46.811** Strain of other muscles, fascia and tendons at shoulder and upper arm level, right arm

√7ᵗʰ **S46.812** Strain of other muscles, fascia and tendons at shoulder and upper arm level, left arm

√7ᵗʰ **S46.819** Strain of other muscles, fascia and tendons at shoulder and upper arm level, unspecified arm

√6ᵗʰ **S46.82** Laceration of other muscles, fascia and tendons at shoulder and upper arm level

√7ᵗʰ **S46.821** Laceration of other muscles, fascia and tendons at shoulder and upper arm level, right arm

√7ᵗʰ **S46.822** Laceration of other muscles, fascia and tendons at shoulder and upper arm level, left arm

√7ᵗʰ **S46.829** Laceration of other muscles, fascia and tendons at shoulder and upper arm level, unspecified arm

√6ᵗʰ **S46.89** Other injury of other muscles, fascia and tendons at shoulder and upper arm level

√7ᵗʰ **S46.891** Other injury of other muscles, fascia and tendons at shoulder and upper arm level, right arm

√7ᵗʰ **S46.892** Other injury of other muscles, fascia and tendons at shoulder and upper arm level, left arm

√7ᵗʰ **S46.899** Other injury of other muscles, fascia and tendons at shoulder and upper arm level, unspecified arm

√5ᵗʰ **S46.9** Injury of unspecified muscle, fascia and tendon at shoulder and upper arm level

√6ᵗʰ **S46.90** Unspecified injury of unspecified muscle, fascia and tendon at shoulder and upper arm level

√7ᵗʰ **S46.901** Unspecified injury of unspecified muscle, fascia and tendon at shoulder and upper arm level, right arm

√7ᵗʰ **S46.902** Unspecified injury of unspecified muscle, fascia and tendon at shoulder and upper arm level, left arm

√7ᵗʰ **S46.909** Unspecified injury of unspecified muscle, fascia and tendon at shoulder and upper arm level, unspecified arm

√6ᵗʰ **S46.91** Strain of unspecified muscle, fascia and tendon at shoulder and upper arm level

√7ᵗʰ **S46.911** Strain of unspecified muscle, fascia and tendon at shoulder and upper arm level, right arm

√7ᵗʰ **S46.912** Strain of unspecified muscle, fascia and tendon at shoulder and upper arm level, left arm

√7ᵗʰ **S46.919** Strain of unspecified muscle, fascia and tendon at shoulder and upper arm level, unspecified arm

√6ᵗʰ **S46.92** Laceration of unspecified muscle, fascia and tendon at shoulder and upper arm level

√7ᵗʰ **S46.921** Laceration of unspecified muscle, fascia and tendon at shoulder and upper arm level, right arm

√7ᵗʰ **S46.922** Laceration of unspecified muscle, fascia and tendon at shoulder and upper arm level, left arm

√7ᵗʰ **S46.929** Laceration of unspecified muscle, fascia and tendon at shoulder and upper arm level, unspecified arm

√6ᵗʰ **S46.99** Other injury of unspecified muscle, fascia and tendon at shoulder and upper arm level

√7ᵗʰ **S46.991** Other injury of unspecified muscle, fascia and tendon at shoulder and upper arm level, right arm

√7ᵗʰ **S46.992** Other injury of unspecified muscle, fascia and tendon at shoulder and upper arm level, left arm

√7ᵗʰ **S46.999** Other injury of unspecified muscle, fascia and tendon at shoulder and upper arm level, unspecified arm

√4ᵗʰ **S47** Crushing injury of shoulder and upper arm

Use additional code for all associated injuries

EXCLUDES 2 crushing injury of elbow (S57.0-)

The appropriate 7th character is to be added to each code from category S47.
A initial encounter
D subsequent encounter
S sequela

√x7ᵗʰ **S47.1** Crushing injury of right shoulder and upper arm

√x7ᵗʰ **S47.2** Crushing injury of left shoulder and upper arm

√x7ᵗʰ **S47.9** Crushing injury of shoulder and upper arm, unspecified arm

√4ᵗʰ **S48** Traumatic amputation of shoulder and upper arm

NOTE An amputation not identified as partial or complete should be coded to complete.

EXCLUDES 1 traumatic amputation at elbow level (S58.0)

The appropriate 7th character is to be added to each code from category S48.
A initial encounter
D subsequent encounter
S sequela

√5ᵗʰ **S48.0** Traumatic amputation at shoulder joint

√6ᵗʰ **S48.01** Complete traumatic amputation at shoulder joint

√7ᵗʰ **S48.011** Complete traumatic amputation at right shoulder joint

EXCLUDES 1 Not coded here   EXCLUDES 2 Not included here   N Newborn Age: 0   P Pediatric Age: 0-17   M Maternity Age: 12-55   A Adult Age: 15-124

850   ICD-10-CM 2014 (Draft)

S48.012 Complete traumatic amputation at left shoulder joint

S48.019 Complete traumatic amputation at unspecified shoulder joint

S48.02 Partial traumatic amputation at shoulder joint

S48.021 Partial traumatic amputation at right shoulder joint

S48.022 Partial traumatic amputation at left shoulder joint

S48.029 Partial traumatic amputation at unspecified shoulder joint

S48.1 Traumatic amputation at level between shoulder and elbow

S48.11 Complete traumatic amputation at level between shoulder and elbow

S48.111 Complete traumatic amputation at level between right shoulder and elbow

S48.112 Complete traumatic amputation at level between left shoulder and elbow

S48.119 Complete traumatic amputation at level between unspecified shoulder and elbow

S48.12 Partial traumatic amputation at level between shoulder and elbow

S48.121 Partial traumatic amputation at level between right shoulder and elbow

S48.122 Partial traumatic amputation at level between left shoulder and elbow

S48.129 Partial traumatic amputation at level between unspecified shoulder and elbow

S48.9 Traumatic amputation of shoulder and upper arm, level unspecified

S48.91 Complete traumatic amputation of shoulder and upper arm, level unspecified

S48.911 Complete traumatic amputation of right shoulder and upper arm, level unspecified

S48.912 Complete traumatic amputation of left shoulder and upper arm, level unspecified

S48.919 Complete traumatic amputation of unspecified shoulder and upper arm, level unspecified

S48.92 Partial traumatic amputation of shoulder and upper arm, level unspecified

S48.921 Partial traumatic amputation of right shoulder and upper arm, level unspecified

S48.922 Partial traumatic amputation of left shoulder and upper arm, level unspecified

S48.929 Partial traumatic amputation of unspecified shoulder and upper arm, level unspecified

S49 Other and unspecified injuries of shoulder and upper arm

The appropriate 7th character is to be added to each code from subcategories S49.0 and S49.1.
A   initial encounter for closed fracture
D   subsequent encounter for fracture with routine healing
G   subsequent encounter for fracture with delayed healing
K   subsequent encounter for fracture with nonunion
P   subsequent encounter for fracture with malunion
S   sequela

S49.0 Physeal fracture of upper end of humerus

S49.00 Unspecified physeal fracture of upper end of humerus

S49.001 Unspecified physeal fracture of upper end of humerus, right arm

S49.002 Unspecified physeal fracture of upper end of humerus, left arm

S49.009 Unspecified physeal fracture of upper end of humerus, unspecified arm

S49.01 Salter-Harris Type I physeal fracture of upper end of humerus

S49.011 Salter-Harris Type I physeal fracture of upper end of humerus, right arm

S49.012 Salter-Harris Type I physeal fracture of upper end of humerus, left arm

S49.019 Salter-Harris Type I physeal fracture of upper end of humerus, unspecified arm

S49.02 Salter-Harris Type II physeal fracture of upper end of humerus

S49.021 Salter-Harris Type II physeal fracture of upper end of humerus, right arm

S49.022 Salter-Harris Type II physeal fracture of upper end of humerus, left arm

S49.029 Salter-Harris Type II physeal fracture of upper end of humerus, unspecified arm

S49.03 Salter-Harris Type III physeal fracture of upper end of humerus

S49.031 Salter Harris Type III physeal fracture of upper end of humerus, right arm

S49.032 Salter-Harris Type III physeal fracture of upper end of humerus, left arm

S49.039 Salter-Harris Type III physeal fracture of upper end of humerus, unspecified arm

S49.04 Salter-Harris Type IV physeal fracture of upper end of humerus

S49.041 Salter-Harris Type IV physeal fracture of upper end of humerus, right arm

S49.042 Salter-Harris Type IV physeal fracture of upper end of humerus, left arm

S49.049 Salter-Harris Type IV physeal fracture of upper end of humerus, unspecified arm

S49.09 Other physeal fracture of upper end of humerus

S49.091 Other physeal fracture of upper end of humerus, right arm

S49.092 Other physeal fracture of upper end of humerus, left arm

S49.099 Other physeal fracture of upper end of humerus, unspecified arm

S49.1 Physeal fracture of lower end of humerus

S49.10 Unspecified physeal fracture of lower end of humerus

S49.101 Unspecified physeal fracture of lower end of humerus, right arm

S49.102 Unspecified physeal fracture of lower end of humerus, left arm

S49.109 Unspecified physeal fracture of lower end of humerus, unspecified arm

S49.11 Salter-Harris Type I physeal fracture of lower end of humerus

S49.111 Salter-Harris Type I physeal fracture of lower end of humerus, right arm

S49.112 Salter-Harris Type I physeal fracture of lower end of humerus, left arm

S49.119 Salter-Harris Type I physeal fracture of lower end of humerus, unspecified arm

S49.12 Salter-Harris Type II physeal fracture of lower end of humerus

S49.121 Salter-Harris Type II physeal fracture of lower end of humerus, right arm

S49.122 Salter-Harris Type II physeal fracture of lower end of humerus, left arm

S49.129 Salter-Harris Type II physeal fracture of lower end of humerus, unspecified arm

S49.13 Salter Harris Type III physeal fracture of lower end of humerus

S49.131 Salter Harris Type III physeal fracture of lower end of humerus, right arm

S49.132 Salter Harris Type III physeal fracture of lower end of humerus, left arm

S49.139 Salter Harris Type III physeal fracture of lower end of humerus, unspecified arm

S49.14 Salter-Harris Type IV physeal fracture of lower end of humerus

S49.141 Salter-Harris Type IV physeal fracture of lower end of humerus, right arm

S49.142 Salter-Harris Type IV physeal fracture of lower end of humerus, left arm

S49.149 Salter-Harris Type IV physeal fracture of lower end of humerus, unspecified arm

S49.19 Other physeal fracture of lower end of humerus

S49.191 Other physeal fracture of lower end of humerus, right arm

Injury, Poisoning and Certain Other Consequences of External Causes

S49.192–S51.002

√7ᵗʰ **S49.192** **Other physeal fracture of lower end of humerus, left arm**

√7ᵗʰ **S49.199** **Other physeal fracture of lower end of humerus, unspecified arm**

√5ᵗʰ **S49.8** **Other specified injuries of shoulder and upper arm**

The appropriate 7th character is to be added to each code in subcategory S49.8.
- A   initial encounter
- D   subsequent encounter
- S   sequela

√x7ᵗʰ **S49.80** **Other specified injuries of shoulder and upper arm, unspecified arm**

√x7ᵗʰ **S49.81** **Other specified injuries of right shoulder and upper arm**

√x7ᵗʰ **S49.82** **Other specified injuries of left shoulder and upper arm**

√5ᵗʰ **S49.9** **Unspecified injury of shoulder and upper arm**

The appropriate 7th character is to be added to each code in subcategory S49.9.
- A   initial encounter
- D   subsequent encounter
- S   sequela

√x7ᵗʰ **S49.90** **Unspecified injury of shoulder and upper arm, unspecified arm**

√x7ᵗʰ **S49.91** **Unspecified injury of right shoulder and upper arm**

√x7ᵗʰ **S49.92** **Unspecified injury of left shoulder and upper arm**

Injuries to the elbow and forearm (S50-S59)

EXCLUDES 2   burns and corrosions (T20-T32)
frostbite (T33-T34)
injuries of wrist and hand (S60-S69)
insect bite or sting, venomous (T63.4)

√4ᵗʰ **S50** **Superficial injury of elbow and forearm**

EXCLUDES 2   superficial injury of wrist and hand (S60.-)

The appropriate 7th character is to be added to each code from category S50.
- A   initial encounter
- D   subsequent encounter
- S   sequela

√5ᵗʰ **S50.0** **Contusion of elbow**

√x7ᵗʰ **S50.00** **Contusion of unspecified elbow**

√x7ᵗʰ **S50.01** **Contusion of right elbow**

√x7ᵗʰ **S50.02** **Contusion of left elbow**

√5ᵗʰ **S50.1** **Contusion of forearm**

√x7ᵗʰ **S50.10** **Contusion of unspecified forearm**

√x7ᵗʰ **S50.11** **Contusion of right forearm**

√x7ᵗʰ **S50.12** **Contusion of left forearm**

√5ᵗʰ **S50.3** **Other superficial injuries of elbow**

√6ᵗʰ **S50.31** **Abrasion of elbow**

√7ᵗʰ **S50.311** **Abrasion of right elbow**

√7ᵗʰ **S50.312** **Abrasion of left elbow**

√7ᵗʰ **S50.319** **Abrasion of unspecified elbow**

√6ᵗʰ **S50.32** **Blister (nonthermal) of elbow**

√7ᵗʰ **S50.321** **Blister (nonthermal) of right elbow**

√7ᵗʰ **S50.322** **Blister (nonthermal) of left elbow**

√7ᵗʰ **S50.329** **Blister (nonthermal) of unspecified elbow**

√6ᵗʰ **S50.34** **External constriction of elbow**

√7ᵗʰ **S50.341** **External constriction of right elbow**

√7ᵗʰ **S50.342** **External constriction of left elbow**

√7ᵗʰ **S50.349** **External constriction of unspecified elbow**

√6ᵗʰ **S50.35** **Superficial foreign body of elbow**
Splinter in the elbow

√7ᵗʰ **S50.351** **Superficial foreign body of right elbow**

√7ᵗʰ **S50.352** **Superficial foreign body of left elbow**

√7ᵗʰ **S50.359** **Superficial foreign body of unspecified elbow**

√6ᵗʰ **S50.36** **Insect bite (nonvenomous) of elbow**

√7ᵗʰ **S50.361** **Insect bite (nonvenomous) of right elbow**

√7ᵗʰ **S50.362** **Insect bite (nonvenomous) of left elbow**

√7ᵗʰ **S50.369** **Insect bite (nonvenomous) of unspecified elbow**

√6ᵗʰ **S50.37** **Other superficial bite of elbow**
EXCLUDES 1   open bite of elbow (S51.05)

√7ᵗʰ **S50.371** **Other superficial bite of right elbow**

√7ᵗʰ **S50.372** **Other superficial bite of left elbow**

√7ᵗʰ **S50.379** **Other superficial bite of unspecified elbow**

√5ᵗʰ **S50.8** **Other superficial injuries of forearm**

√6ᵗʰ **S50.81** **Abrasion of forearm**

√7ᵗʰ **S50.811** **Abrasion of right forearm**

√7ᵗʰ **S50.812** **Abrasion of left forearm**

√7ᵗʰ **S50.819** **Abrasion of unspecified forearm**

√6ᵗʰ **S50.82** **Blister (nonthermal) of forearm**

√7ᵗʰ **S50.821** **Blister (nonthermal) of right forearm**

√7ᵗʰ **S50.822** **Blister (nonthermal) of left forearm**

√7ᵗʰ **S50.829** **Blister (nonthermal) of unspecified forearm**

√6ᵗʰ **S50.84** **External constriction of forearm**

√7ᵗʰ **S50.841** **External constriction of right forearm**

√7ᵗʰ **S50.842** **External constriction of left forearm**

√7ᵗʰ **S50.849** **External constriction of unspecified forearm**

√6ᵗʰ **S50.85** **Superficial foreign body of forearm**
Splinter in the forearm

√7ᵗʰ **S50.851** **Superficial foreign body of right forearm**

√7ᵗʰ **S50.852** **Superficial foreign body of left forearm**

√7ᵗʰ **S50.859** **Superficial foreign body of unspecified forearm**

√6ᵗʰ **S50.86** **Insect bite (nonvenomous) of forearm**

√7ᵗʰ **S50.861** **Insect bite (nonvenomous) of right forearm**

√7ᵗʰ **S50.862** **Insect bite (nonvenomous) of left forearm**

√7ᵗʰ **S50.869** **Insect bite (nonvenomous) of unspecified forearm**

√6ᵗʰ **S50.87** **Other superficial bite of forearm**
EXCLUDES 1   open bite of forearm (S51.85)

√7ᵗʰ **S50.871** **Other superficial bite of right forearm**

√7ᵗʰ **S50.872** **Other superficial bite of left forearm**

√7ᵗʰ **S50.879** **Other superficial bite of unspecified forearm**

√5ᵗʰ **S50.9** **Unspecified superficial injury of elbow and forearm**

√6ᵗʰ **S50.90** **Unspecified superficial injury of elbow**

√7ᵗʰ **S50.901** **Unspecified superficial injury of right elbow**

√7ᵗʰ **S50.902** **Unspecified superficial injury of left elbow**

√7ᵗʰ **S50.909** **Unspecified superficial injury of unspecified elbow**

√6ᵗʰ **S50.91** **Unspecified superficial injury of forearm**

√7ᵗʰ **S50.911** **Unspecified superficial injury of right forearm**

√7ᵗʰ **S50.912** **Unspecified superficial injury of left forearm**

√7ᵗʰ **S50.919** **Unspecified superficial injury of unspecified forearm**

√4ᵗʰ **S51** **Open wound of elbow and forearm**

Code also any associated wound infection

EXCLUDES 1   open fracture of elbow and forearm (S52- with open fracture 7th character)
traumatic amputation of elbow and forearm (S58.-)

EXCLUDES 2   open wound of wrist and hand (S61.-)

The appropriate 7th character is to be added to each code from category S51.
- A   initial encounter
- D   subsequent encounter
- S   sequela

√5ᵗʰ **S51.0** **Open wound of elbow**

√6ᵗʰ **S51.00** **Unspecified open wound of elbow**

√7ᵗʰ **S51.001** **Unspecified open wound of right elbow**
AHA: 2012, Q4, 108

√7ᵗʰ **S51.002** **Unspecified open wound of left elbow**

EXCLUDES 1 Not coded here   EXCLUDES 2 Not included here   N Newborn Age: 0   P Pediatric Age: 0-17   M Maternity Age: 12-55   A Adult Age: 15-124

852   ICD-10-CM 2014 (Draft)

✓7ᵗʰ **S51.009** **Unspecified open wound of unspecified elbow**
Open wound of elbow NOS

✓6ᵗʰ **S51.01** Laceration without foreign body of elbow

✓7ᵗʰ **S51.011** **Laceration without foreign body of** right **elbow**

✓7ᵗʰ **S51.012** **Laceration without foreign body of** left **elbow**

✓7ᵗʰ **S51.019** **Laceration without foreign body of unspecified elbow**

✓6ᵗʰ **S51.02** Laceration with foreign body of elbow

✓7ᵗʰ **S51.021** **Laceration with foreign body of** right **elbow**

✓7ᵗʰ **S51.022** **Laceration with foreign body of** left **elbow**

✓7ᵗʰ **S51.029** **Laceration with foreign body of unspecified elbow**

✓6ᵗʰ **S51.03** Puncture wound without foreign body of elbow

✓7ᵗʰ **S51.031** **Puncture wound without foreign body of** right **elbow**

✓7ᵗʰ **S51.032** **Puncture wound without foreign body of** left **elbow**

✓7ᵗʰ **S51.039** **Puncture wound without foreign body of unspecified elbow**

✓6ᵗʰ **S51.04** Puncture wound with foreign body of elbow

✓7ᵗʰ **S51.041** **Puncture wound with foreign body of** right **elbow**

✓7ᵗʰ **S51.042** **Puncture wound with foreign body of** left **elbow**

✓7ᵗʰ **S51.049** **Puncture wound with foreign body of unspecified elbow**

✓6ᵗʰ **S51.05** Open bite of elbow
Bite of elbow NOS
EXCLUDES 1 *superficial bite of elbow (S50.36, S50.37)*

✓7ᵗʰ **S51.051** **Open bite,** right **elbow**

✓7ᵗʰ **S51.052** **Open bite,** left **elbow**

✓7ᵗʰ **S51.059** **Open bite, unspecified elbow**

✓5ᵗʰ **S51.8** **Open wound of forearm**
EXCLUDES 2 *open wound of elbow (S51.0-)*

✓6ᵗʰ **S51.80** **Unspecified open wound of forearm**

✓7ᵗʰ **S51.801** **Unspecified open wound of** right **forearm**

✓7ᵗʰ **S51.802** **Unspecified open wound of** left **forearm**

✓7ᵗʰ **S51.809** **Unspecified open wound of unspecified forearm**
Open wound of forearm NOS

✓6ᵗʰ **S51.81** Laceration without foreign body of forearm

✓7ᵗʰ **S51.811** **Laceration without foreign body of** right **forearm**

✓7ᵗʰ **S51.812** **Laceration without foreign body of** left **forearm**

✓7ᵗʰ **S51.819** **Laceration without foreign body of unspecified forearm**

✓6ᵗʰ **S51.82** Laceration with foreign body of forearm

✓7ᵗʰ **S51.821** **Laceration with foreign body of** right **forearm**

✓7ᵗʰ **S51.822** **Laceration with foreign body of** left **forearm**

✓7ᵗʰ **S51.829** **Laceration with foreign body of unspecified forearm**

✓6ᵗʰ **S51.83** Puncture wound without foreign body of forearm

✓7ᵗʰ **S51.831** **Puncture wound without foreign body of** right **forearm**

✓7ᵗʰ **S51.832** **Puncture wound without foreign body of** left **forearm**

✓7ᵗʰ **S51.839** **Puncture wound without foreign body of unspecified forearm**

✓6ᵗʰ **S51.84** Puncture wound with foreign body of forearm

✓7ᵗʰ **S51.841** **Puncture wound with foreign body of** right **forearm**

✓7ᵗʰ **S51.842** **Puncture wound with foreign body of** left **forearm**

✓7ᵗʰ **S51.849** **Puncture wound with foreign body of unspecified forearm**

✓6ᵗʰ **S51.85** Open bite of forearm
Bite of forearm NOS
EXCLUDES 1 *superficial bite of forearm (S50.86, S50.87)*

✓7ᵗʰ **S51.851** **Open bite of** right **forearm**

✓7ᵗʰ **S51.852** **Open bite of** left **forearm**

✓7ᵗʰ **S51.859** **Open bite of unspecified forearm**

✓4ᵗʰ **S52** **Fracture of forearm**

NOTE   A fracture not indicated as displaced or nondisplaced should be coded to displaced.
A fracture not indicated as open or closed should be coded to closed.
The open fracture designations are based on the Gustilo open fracture classification.
EXCLUDES 1 *traumatic amputation of forearm (S58.-)*
EXCLUDES 2 *fracture at wrist and hand level (S62.-)*

The appropriate 7th character is to be added to all codes from category S52 [unless otherwise indicated].
A   initial encounter for closed fracture
B   initial encounter for open fracture type I or II
initial encounter for open fracture NOS
C   initial encounter for open fracture type IIIA, IIIB, or IIIC
D   subsequent encounter for closed fracture with routine healing
E   subsequent encounter for open fracture type I or II with routine healing
F   subsequent encounter for open fracture type IIIA, IIIB, or IIIC with routine healing
G   subsequent encounter for closed fracture with delayed healing
H   subsequent encounter for open fracture type I or II with delayed healing
J   subsequent encounter for open fracture type IIIA, IIIB, or IIIC with delayed healing
K   subsequent encounter for closed fracture with nonunion
M   subsequent encounter for open fracture type I or II with nonunion
N   subsequent encounter for open fracture type IIIA, IIIB, or IIIC with nonunion
P   subsequent encounter for closed fracture with malunion
Q   subsequent encounter for open fracture type I or II with malunion
R   subsequent encounter for open fracture type IIIA, IIIB, or IIIC with malunion
S   sequela

✓5ᵗʰ **S52.0** **Fracture of upper end of ulna**
Fracture of proximal end of ulna
EXCLUDES 2 *fracture of elbow NOS (S42.40-)*
fractures of shaft of ulna (S52.2-)

✓6ᵗʰ **S52.00** **Unspecified fracture of upper end of ulna**

✓7ᵗʰ **S52.001** **Unspecified fracture of upper end of** right **ulna**

✓7ᵗʰ **S52.002** **Unspecified fracture of upper end of** left **ulna**

✓7ᵗʰ **S52.009** **Unspecified fracture of upper end of unspecified ulna**

✓6ᵗʰ **S52.01** **Torus fracture of upper end of ulna**

The appropriate 7th character is to be added to all codes in subcategory S52.01.
A   initial encounter for closed fracture
D   subsequent encounter for fracture with routine healing
G   subsequent encounter for fracture with delayed healing
K   subsequent encounter for fracture with nonunion
P   subsequent encounter for fracture with malunion
S   sequela

✓7ᵗʰ **S52.011** **Torus fracture of upper end of** right **ulna**

✓7ᵗʰ **S52.012** **Torus fracture of upper end of** left **ulna**

✓7ᵗʰ **S52.019** **Torus fracture of upper end of unspecified ulna**

✓6ᵗʰ **S52.02** **Fracture of** olecranon process without intraarticular extension **of ulna**

✓7ᵗʰ **S52.021** **Displaced fracture of olecranon process without intraarticular extension of** right **ulna**

✓ Additional Character Required   ✓7ᵗʰ Xtension Alert   Unspecified Code   Other Specified Code   Manifestation Code   ►◄ Revised Text   ● New Code   ▲ Revised Code Title

ICD-10-CM 2014 (Draft)

853

Injury, Poisoning and Certain Other Consequences of External Causes

S52.022–S52.232

✓7ᵗʰ **S52.022** Displaced fracture of olecranon process without intraarticular extension of left ulna

✓7ᵗʰ **S52.023** Displaced fracture of olecranon process without intraarticular extension of unspecified ulna

✓7ᵗʰ **S52.024** Nondisplaced fracture of olecranon process without intraarticular extension of right ulna

✓7ᵗʰ **S52.025** Nondisplaced fracture of olecranon process without intraarticular extension of left ulna

✓7ᵗʰ **S52.026** Nondisplaced fracture of olecranon process without intraarticular extension of unspecified ulna

✓6ᵗʰ **S52.03** Fracture of olecranon process with intraarticular extension of ulna

✓7ᵗʰ **S52.031** Displaced fracture of olecranon process with intraarticular extension of right ulna

✓7ᵗʰ **S52.032** Displaced fracture of olecranon process with intraarticular extension of left ulna

✓7ᵗʰ **S52.033** Displaced fracture of olecranon process with intraarticular extension of unspecified ulna

✓7ᵗʰ **S52.034** Nondisplaced fracture of olecranon process with intraarticular extension of right ulna

✓7ᵗʰ **S52.035** Nondisplaced fracture of olecranon process with intraarticular extension of left ulna

✓7ᵗʰ **S52.036** Nondisplaced fracture of olecranon process with intraarticular extension of unspecified ulna

✓6ᵗʰ **S52.04** Fracture of coronoid process of ulna

✓7ᵗʰ **S52.041** Displaced fracture of coronoid process of right ulna

✓7ᵗʰ **S52.042** Displaced fracture of coronoid process of left ulna

✓7ᵗʰ **S52.043** Displaced fracture of coronoid process of unspecified ulna

✓7ᵗʰ **S52.044** Nondisplaced fracture of coronoid process of right ulna

✓7ᵗʰ **S52.045** Nondisplaced fracture of coronoid process of left ulna

✓7ᵗʰ **S52.046** Nondisplaced fracture of coronoid process of unspecified ulna

✓6ᵗʰ **S52.09** Other fracture of upper end of ulna

✓7ᵗʰ **S52.091** Other fracture of upper end of right ulna

✓7ᵗʰ **S52.092** Other fracture of upper end of left ulna

✓7ᵗʰ **S52.099** Other fracture of upper end of unspecified ulna

✓5ᵗʰ **S52.1** **Fracture of upper end of radius**
Fracture of proximal end of radius

EXCLUDES 2   physeal fractures of upper end of radius (S59.2-)
fracture of shaft of radius (S52.3-)

✓6ᵗʰ **S52.10** Unspecified fracture of upper end of radius

✓7ᵗʰ **S52.101** Unspecified fracture of upper end of right radius

✓7ᵗʰ **S52.102** Unspecified fracture of upper end of left radius

✓7ᵗʰ **S52.109** Unspecified fracture of upper end of unspecified radius

✓6ᵗʰ **S52.11** Torus fracture of upper end of radius

The appropriate 7th character is to be added to all codes in subcategory S52.11.
A   initial encounter for closed fracture
D   subsequent encounter for fracture with routine healing
G   subsequent encounter for fracture with delayed healing
K   subsequent encounter for fracture with nonunion
P   subsequent encounter for fracture with malunion
S   sequela

✓7ᵗʰ **S52.111** Torus fracture of upper end of right radius

✓7ᵗʰ **S52.112** Torus fracture of upper end of left radius

✓7ᵗʰ **S52.119** Torus fracture of upper end of unspecified radius

✓6ᵗʰ **S52.12** Fracture of head of radius

✓7ᵗʰ **S52.121** Displaced fracture of head of right radius

✓7ᵗʰ **S52.122** Displaced fracture of head of left radius

✓7ᵗʰ **S52.123** Displaced fracture of head of unspecified radius

✓7ᵗʰ **S52.124** Nondisplaced fracture of head of right radius

✓7ᵗʰ **S52.125** Nondisplaced fracture of head of left radius

✓7ᵗʰ **S52.126** Nondisplaced fracture of head of unspecified radius

✓6ᵗʰ **S52.13** Fracture of neck of radius

✓7ᵗʰ **S52.131** Displaced fracture of neck of right radius

✓7ᵗʰ **S52.132** Displaced fracture of neck of left radius

✓7ᵗʰ **S52.133** Displaced fracture of neck of unspecified radius

✓7ᵗʰ **S52.134** Nondisplaced fracture of neck of right radius

✓7ᵗʰ **S52.135** Nondisplaced fracture of neck of left radius

✓7ᵗʰ **S52.136** Nondisplaced fracture of neck of unspecified radius

✓6ᵗʰ **S52.18** Other fracture of upper end of radius

✓7ᵗʰ **S52.181** Other fracture of upper end of right radius

✓7ᵗʰ **S52.182** Other fracture of upper end of left radius

✓7ᵗʰ **S52.189** Other fracture of upper end of unspecified radius

✓5ᵗʰ **S52.2** **Fracture of shaft of ulna**

✓6ᵗʰ **S52.20** Unspecified fracture of shaft of ulna
Fracture of ulna NOS

✓7ᵗʰ **S52.201** Unspecified fracture of shaft of right ulna

✓7ᵗʰ **S52.202** Unspecified fracture of shaft of left ulna

✓7ᵗʰ **S52.209** Unspecified fracture of shaft of unspecified ulna

✓6ᵗʰ **S52.21** Greenstick fracture of shaft of ulna

The appropriate 7th character is to be added to all codes in subcategory S52.21.
A   initial encounter for closed fracture
D   subsequent encounter for fracture with routine healing
G   subsequent encounter for fracture with delayed healing
K   subsequent encounter for fracture with nonunion
P   subsequent encounter for fracture with malunion
S   sequela

✓7ᵗʰ **S52.211** Greenstick fracture of shaft of right ulna

✓7ᵗʰ **S52.212** Greenstick fracture of shaft of left ulna

✓7ᵗʰ **S52.219** Greenstick fracture of shaft of unspecified ulna

✓6ᵗʰ **S52.22** Transverse fracture of shaft of ulna

✓7ᵗʰ **S52.221** Displaced transverse fracture of shaft of right ulna

✓7ᵗʰ **S52.222** Displaced transverse fracture of shaft of left ulna

✓7ᵗʰ **S52.223** Displaced transverse fracture of shaft of unspecified ulna

✓7ᵗʰ **S52.224** Nondisplaced transverse fracture of shaft of right ulna

✓7ᵗʰ **S52.225** Nondisplaced transverse fracture of shaft of left ulna

✓7ᵗʰ **S52.226** Nondisplaced transverse fracture of shaft of unspecified ulna

✓6ᵗʰ **S52.23** Oblique fracture of shaft of ulna

✓7ᵗʰ **S52.231** Displaced oblique fracture of shaft of right ulna

✓7ᵗʰ **S52.232** Displaced oblique fracture of shaft of left ulna

EXCLUDES 1 Not coded here   EXCLUDES 2 Not included here   N Newborn Age: 0   P Pediatric Age: 0-17   M Maternity Age: 12-55   A Adult Age: 15-124

854   ICD-10-CM 2014 (Draft)

√7th **S52.233** Displaced oblique fracture of shaft of unspecified ulna

√7th **S52.234** Nondisplaced oblique fracture of shaft of right ulna

√7th **S52.235** Nondisplaced oblique fracture of shaft of left ulna

√7th **S52.236** Nondisplaced oblique fracture of shaft of unspecified ulna

√6th **S52.24** Spiral fracture of shaft of ulna

√7th **S52.241** Displaced spiral fracture of shaft of ulna, right arm

√7th **S52.242** Displaced spiral fracture of shaft of ulna, left arm

√7th **S52.243** Displaced spiral fracture of shaft of ulna, unspecified arm

√7th **S52.244** Nondisplaced spiral fracture of shaft of ulna, right arm

√7th **S52.245** Nondisplaced spiral fracture of shaft of ulna, left arm

√7th **S52.246** Nondisplaced spiral fracture of shaft of ulna, unspecified arm

√6th **S52.25** Comminuted fracture of shaft of ulna

√7th **S52.251** Displaced comminuted fracture of shaft of ulna, right arm

√7th **S52.252** Displaced comminuted fracture of shaft of ulna, left arm

√7th **S52.253** Displaced comminuted fracture of shaft of ulna, unspecified arm

√7th **S52.254** Nondisplaced comminuted fracture of shaft of ulna, right arm

√7th **S52.255** Nondisplaced comminuted fracture of shaft of ulna, left arm

√7th **S52.256** Nondisplaced comminuted fracture of shaft of ulna, unspecified arm

√6th **S52.26** Segmental fracture of shaft of ulna

√7th **S52.261** Displaced segmental fracture of shaft of ulna, right arm

√7th **S52.262** Displaced segmental fracture of shaft of ulna, left arm

√7th **S52.263** Displaced segmental fracture of shaft of ulna, unspecified arm

√7th **S52.264** Nondisplaced segmental fracture of shaft of ulna, right arm

√7th **S52.265** Nondisplaced segmental fracture of shaft of ulna, left arm

√7th **S52.266** Nondisplaced segmental fracture of shaft of ulna, unspecified arm

√6th **S52.27** Monteggia's fracture of ulna
Fracture of upper shaft of ulna with dislocation of radial head

√7th **S52.271** Monteggia's fracture of right ulna

√7th **S52.272** Monteggia's fracture of left ulna

√7th **S52.279** Monteggia's fracture of unspecified ulna

√6th **S52.28** Bent bone of ulna

√7th **S52.281** Bent bone of right ulna

√7th **S52.282** Bent bone of left ulna

√7th **S52.283** Bent bone of unspecified ulna

√6th **S52.29** Other fracture of shaft of ulna

√7th **S52.291** Other fracture of shaft of right ulna

√7th **S52.292** Other fracture of shaft of left ulna

√7th **S52.299** Other fracture of shaft of unspecified ulna

√5th **S52.3** Fracture of shaft of radius

√6th **S52.30** Unspecified fracture of shaft of radius

√7th **S52.301** Unspecified fracture of shaft of right radius

√7th **S52.302** Unspecified fracture of shaft of left radius

√7th **S52.309** Unspecified fracture of shaft of unspecified radius

√6th **S52.31** Greenstick fracture of shaft of radius

> The appropriate 7th character is to be added to all codes in subcategory S52.31.
> A initial encounter for closed fracture
> D subsequent encounter for fracture with routine healing
> G subsequent encounter for fracture with delayed healing
> K subsequent encounter for fracture with nonunion
> P subsequent encounter for fracture with malunion
> S sequela

√7th **S52.311** Greenstick fracture of shaft of radius, right arm

√7th **S52.312** Greenstick fracture of shaft of radius, left arm

√7th **S52.319** Greenstick fracture of shaft of radius, unspecified arm

√6th **S52.32** Transverse fracture of shaft of radius

√7th **S52.321** Displaced transverse fracture of shaft of right radius

√7th **S52.322** Displaced transverse fracture of shaft of left radius

√7th **S52.323** Displaced transverse fracture of shaft of unspecified radius

√7th **S52.324** Nondisplaced transverse fracture of shaft of right radius

√7th **S52.325** Nondisplaced transverse fracture of shaft of left radius

√7th **S52.326** Nondisplaced transverse fracture of shaft of unspecified radius

√6th **S52.33** Oblique fracture of shaft of radius

√7th **S52.331** Displaced oblique fracture of shaft of right radius

√7th **S52.332** Displaced oblique fracture of shaft of left radius

√7th **S52.333** Displaced oblique fracture of shaft of unspecified radius

√7th **S52.334** Nondisplaced oblique fracture of shaft of right radius

√7th **S52.335** Nondisplaced oblique fracture of shaft of left radius

√7th **S52.336** Nondisplaced oblique fracture of shaft of unspecified radius

√6th **S52.34** Spiral fracture of shaft of radius

√7th **S52.341** Displaced spiral fracture of shaft of radius, right arm

√7th **S52.342** Displaced spiral fracture of shaft of radius, left arm

√7th **S52.343** Displaced spiral fracture of shaft of radius, unspecified arm

√7th **S52.344** Nondisplaced spiral fracture of shaft of radius, right arm

√7th **S52.345** Nondisplaced spiral fracture of shaft of radius, left arm

√7th **S52.346** Nondisplaced spiral fracture of shaft of radius, unspecified arm

√6th **S52.35** Comminuted fracture of shaft of radius

√7th **S52.351** Displaced comminuted fracture of shaft of radius, right arm

√7th **S52.352** Displaced comminuted fracture of shaft of radius, left arm

√7th **S52.353** Displaced comminuted fracture of shaft of radius, unspecified arm

√7th **S52.354** Nondisplaced comminuted fracture of shaft of radius, right arm

√7th **S52.355** Nondisplaced comminuted fracture of shaft of radius, left arm

√7th **S52.356** Nondisplaced comminuted fracture of shaft of radius, unspecified arm

√6th **S52.36** Segmental fracture of shaft of radius

√7th **S52.361** Displaced segmental fracture of shaft of radius, right arm

Injury, Poisoning and Certain Other Consequences of External Causes   **S52.362–S52.92**

    ✓7ᵗʰ **S52.362** Displaced segmental fracture of shaft of radius, left arm

    ✓7ᵗʰ **S52.363** Displaced segmental fracture of shaft of radius, unspecified arm

    ✓7ᵗʰ **S52.364** Nondisplaced segmental fracture of shaft of radius, right arm

    ✓7ᵗʰ **S52.365** Nondisplaced segmental fracture of shaft of radius, left arm

    ✓7ᵗʰ **S52.366** Nondisplaced segmental fracture of shaft of radius, unspecified arm

 ✓6ᵗʰ **S52.37** Galeazzi's fracture

     Fracture of lower shaft of radius with radioulnar joint dislocation

    ✓7ᵗʰ **S52.371** Galeazzi's fracture of right radius

    ✓7ᵗʰ **S52.372** Galeazzi's fracture of left radius

    ✓7ᵗʰ **S52.379** Galeazzi's fracture of unspecified radius

 ✓6ᵗʰ **S52.38** Bent bone of radius

    ✓7ᵗʰ **S52.381** Bent bone of right radius

    ✓7ᵗʰ **S52.382** Bent bone of left radius

    ✓7ᵗʰ **S52.389** Bent bone of unspecified radius

 ✓6ᵗʰ **S52.39** Other fracture of shaft of radius

    ✓7ᵗʰ **S52.391** Other fracture of shaft of radius, right arm

    ✓7ᵗʰ **S52.392** Other fracture of shaft of radius, left arm

    ✓7ᵗʰ **S52.399** Other fracture of shaft of radius, unspecified arm

✓5ᵗʰ **S52.5** Fracture of lower end of radius

    Fracture of distal end of radius

    EXCLUDES 2   *physeal fractures of lower end of radius (S59.2-)*

 ✓6ᵗʰ **S52.5Ø** Unspecified fracture of the lower end of radius

    ✓7ᵗʰ **S52.5Ø1** Unspecified fracture of the lower end of right radius

    ✓7ᵗʰ **S52.5Ø2** Unspecified fracture of the lower end of left radius

    ✓7ᵗʰ **S52.5Ø9** Unspecified fracture of the lower end of unspecified radius

 ✓6ᵗʰ **S52.51** Fracture of radial styloid process

    ✓7ᵗʰ **S52.511** Displaced fracture of right radial styloid process

    ✓7ᵗʰ **S52.512** Displaced fracture of left radial styloid process

    ✓7ᵗʰ **S52.513** Displaced fracture of unspecified radial styloid process

    ✓7ᵗʰ **S52.514** Nondisplaced fracture of right radial styloid process

    ✓7ᵗʰ **S52.515** Nondisplaced fracture of left radial styloid process

    ✓7ᵗʰ **S52.516** Nondisplaced fracture of unspecified radial styloid process

 ✓6ᵗʰ **S52.52** Torus fracture of lower end of radius

> The appropriate 7th character is to be added to all codes in subcategory S52.52.
> A   initial encounter for closed fracture
> D   subsequent encounter for fracture with routine healing
> G   subsequent encounter for fracture with delayed healing
> K   subsequent encounter for fracture with nonunion
> P   subsequent encounter for fracture with malunion
> S   sequela

    ✓7ᵗʰ **S52.521** Torus fracture of lower end of right radius

    ✓7ᵗʰ **S52.522** Torus fracture of lower end of left radius

    ✓7ᵗʰ **S52.529** Torus fracture of lower end of unspecified radius

 ✓6ᵗʰ **S52.53** Colles' fracture

    ✓7ᵗʰ **S52.531** Colles' fracture of right radius

    ✓7ᵗʰ **S52.532** Colles' fracture of left radius

    ✓7ᵗʰ **S52.539** Colles' fracture of unspecified radius

 ✓6ᵗʰ **S52.54** Smith's fracture

    ✓7ᵗʰ **S52.541** Smith's fracture of right radius

    ✓7ᵗʰ **S52.542** Smith's fracture of left radius

    ✓7ᵗʰ **S52.549** Smith's fracture of unspecified radius

 ✓6ᵗʰ **S52.55** Other extraarticular fracture of lower end of radius

    ✓7ᵗʰ **S52.551** Other extraarticular fracture of lower end of right radius

    ✓7ᵗʰ **S52.552** Other extraarticular fracture of lower end of left radius

    ✓7ᵗʰ **S52.559** Other extraarticular fracture of lower end of unspecified radius

 ✓6ᵗʰ **S52.56** Barton's fracture

    ✓7ᵗʰ **S52.561** Barton's fracture of right radius

    ✓7ᵗʰ **S52.562** Barton's fracture of left radius

    ✓7ᵗʰ **S52.569** Barton's fracture of unspecified radius

 ✓6ᵗʰ **S52.57** Other intraarticular fracture of lower end of radius

    ✓7ᵗʰ **S52.571** Other intraarticular fracture of lower end of right radius

    ✓7ᵗʰ **S52.572** Other intraarticular fracture of lower end of left radius

    ✓7ᵗʰ **S52.579** Other intraarticular fracture of lower end of unspecified radius

 ✓6ᵗʰ **S52.59** Other fractures of lower end of radius

    ✓7ᵗʰ **S52.591** Other fractures of lower end of right radius

    ✓7ᵗʰ **S52.592** Other fractures of lower end of left radius

    ✓7ᵗʰ **S52.599** Other fractures of lower end of unspecified radius

✓5ᵗʰ **S52.6** Fracture of lower end of ulna

 ✓6ᵗʰ **S52.6Ø** Unspecified fracture of lower end of ulna

    ✓7ᵗʰ **S52.6Ø1** Unspecified fracture of lower end of right ulna

    ✓7ᵗʰ **S52.6Ø2** Unspecified fracture of lower end of left ulna

    ✓7ᵗʰ **S52.6Ø9** Unspecified fracture of lower end of unspecified ulna

 ✓6ᵗʰ **S52.61** Fracture of ulna styloid process

    ✓7ᵗʰ **S52.611** Displaced fracture of right ulna styloid process

    ✓7ᵗʰ **S52.612** Displaced fracture of left ulna styloid process

    ✓7ᵗʰ **S52.613** Displaced fracture of unspecified ulna styloid process

    ✓7ᵗʰ **S52.614** Nondisplaced fracture of right ulna styloid process

    ✓7ᵗʰ **S52.615** Nondisplaced fracture of left ulna styloid process

    ✓7ᵗʰ **S52.616** Nondisplaced fracture of unspecified ulna styloid process

 ✓6ᵗʰ **S52.62** Torus fracture of lower end of ulna

> The appropriate 7th character is to be added to all codes in subcategory S52.62.
> A   initial encounter for closed fracture
> D   subsequent encounter for fracture with routine healing
> G   subsequent encounter for fracture with delayed healing
> K   subsequent encounter for fracture with nonunion
> P   subsequent encounter for fracture with malunion
> S   sequela

    ✓7ᵗʰ **S52.621** Torus fracture of lower end of right ulna

    ✓7ᵗʰ **S52.622** Torus fracture of lower end of left ulna

    ✓7ᵗʰ **S52.629** Torus fracture of lower end of unspecified ulna

 ✓6ᵗʰ **S52.69** Other fracture of lower end of ulna

    ✓7ᵗʰ **S52.691** Other fracture of lower end of right ulna

    ✓7ᵗʰ **S52.692** Other fracture of lower end of left ulna

    ✓7ᵗʰ **S52.699** Other fracture of lower end of unspecified ulna

✓5ᵗʰ **S52.9** Unspecified fracture of forearm

 ✓x7ᵗʰ **S52.9Ø** Unspecified fracture of unspecified forearm

 ✓x7ᵗʰ **S52.91** Unspecified fracture of right forearm

 ✓x7ᵗʰ **S52.92** Unspecified fracture of left forearm

EXCLUDES 1 Not coded here   *EXCLUDES 2* Not included here   **N** Newborn Age: Ø   **P** Pediatric Age: Ø-17   **M** Maternity Age: 12-55   **A** Adult Age: 15-124

856   ICD-1Ø-CM 2Ø14 (Draft)

√4th **S53** **Dilocation and sprain of joints and ligaments of elbow**

INCLUDES   avulsion of joint or ligament of elbow
laceration of cartilage, joint or ligament of elbow
sprain of cartilage, joint or ligament of elbow
traumatic hemarthrosis of joint or ligament of elbow
traumatic rupture of joint or ligament of elbow
traumatic subluxation of joint or ligament of elbow
traumatic tear of joint or ligament of elbow

Code also any associated open wound

EXCLUDES 2   strain of muscle, fascia and tendon at forearm level (S56.-)

The appropriate 7th character is to be added to each code from category S53.
A   initial encounter
D   subsequent encounter
S   sequela

√5th **S53.0** **Subluxation and dislocation of** radial head

Dislocation of radiohumeral joint
Subluxation of radiohumeral joint

EXCLUDES 1   Monteggia's fracture-dislocation (S52.27-)

√6th   **S53.00**   **Unspecified** subluxation and dislocation of radial head

√7th   **S53.001**   **Unspecified** subluxation of right **radial head**

√7th   **S53.002**   **Unspecified** subluxation of left **radial head**

√7th   **S53.003**   **Unspecified** subluxation of unspecified **radial head**

√7th   **S53.004**   **Unspecified** dislocation of right **radial head**

√7th   **S53.005**   **Unspecified** dislocation of left **radial head**

√7th   **S53.006**   **Unspecified** dislocation of unspecified **radial head**

√6th   **S53.01**   **Anterior** subluxation and dislocation of radial head

Anteriomedial subluxation and dislocation of radial head

√7th   **S53.011**   **Anterior** subluxation of right **radial head**

√7th   **S53.012**   **Anterior** subluxation of left **radial head**

√7th   **S53.013**   **Anterior** subluxation of unspecified **radial head**

√7th   **S53.014**   **Anterior** dislocation of right **radial head**

√7th   **S53.015**   **Anterior** dislocation of left **radial head**

√7th   **S53.016**   **Anterior** dislocation of unspecified **radial head**

√6th   **S53.02**   **Posterior** subluxation and dislocation of radial head

Posteriolateral subluxation and dislocation of radial head

√7th   **S53.021**   **Posterior** subluxation of right **radial head**

√7th   **S53.022**   **Posterior** subluxation of left **radial head**

√7th   **S53.023**   **Posterior** subluxation of unspecified **radial head**

√7th   **S53.024**   **Posterior** dislocation of right **radial head**

√7th   **S53.025**   **Posterior** dislocation of left **radial head**

√7th   **S53.026**   **Posterior** dislocation of unspecified radial head

√6th   **S53.03**   **Nursemaid's elbow**

√7th   **S53.031**   **Nursemaid's elbow,** right **elbow**

√7th   **S53.032**   **Nursemaid's elbow,** left **elbow**

√7th   **S53.033**   **Nursemaid's elbow, unspecified elbow**

√6th   **S53.09**   **Other** subluxation and dislocation of radial head

√7th   **S53.091**   **Other** subluxation of right **radial head**

√7th   **S53.092**   **Other** subluxation of left **radial head**

√7th   **S53.093**   **Other** subluxation of unspecified radial head

√7th   **S53.094**   **Other** dislocation of right **radial head**

√7th   **S53.095**   **Other** dislocation of left **radial head**

√7th   **S53.096**   **Other** dislocation of unspecified radial head

√5th **S53.1** **Subluxation and dislocation of** ulnohumeral joint

Subluxation and dislocation of elbow NOS

EXCLUDES 1   dislocation of radial head alone (S53.0-)

√6th   **S53.10**   **Unspecified** subluxation and dislocation of ulnohumeral joint

√7th   **S53.101**   **Unspecified** subluxation of right ulnohumeral joint

√7th   **S53.102**   **Unspecified** subluxation of left ulnohumeral joint

√7th   **S53.103**   **Unspecified** subluxation of unspecified ulnohumeral joint

√7th   **S53.104**   **Unspecified** dislocation of right ulnohumeral joint

√7th   **S53.105**   **Unspecified** dislocation of left ulnohumeral joint

√7th   **S53.106**   **Unspecified** dislocation of unspecified ulnohumeral joint

√6th   **S53.11**   **Anterior** subluxation and dislocation of ulnohumeral joint

√7th   **S53.111**   **Anterior** subluxation of right ulnohumeral joint

√7th   **S53.112**   **Anterior** subluxation of left **ulnohumeral joint**

√7th   **S53.113**   **Anterior** subluxation of unspecified ulnohumeral joint

√7th   **S53.114**   **Anterior** dislocation of right ulnohumeral joint

AHA: 2012, Q4, 108

√7th   **S53.115**   **Anterior** dislocation of left ulnohumeral joint

√7th   **S53.116**   **Anterior** dislocation of unspecified ulnohumeral joint

√6th   **S53.12**   **Posterior** subluxation and dislocation of ulnohumeral joint

√7th   **S53.121**   **Posterior** subluxation of right ulnohumeral joint

√7th   **S53.122**   **Posterior** subluxation of left ulnohumeral joint

√7th   **S53.123**   **Posterior** subluxation of unspecified ulnohumeral joint

√7th   **S53.124**   **Posterior** dislocation of right ulnohumeral joint

√7th   **S53.125**   **Posterior** dislocation of left ulnohumeral joint

√7th   **S53.126**   **Posterior** dislocation of unspecified ulnohumeral joint

√6th   **S53.13**   **Medial** subluxation and dislocation of ulnohumeral joint

√7th   **S53.131**   **Medial** subluxation of right ulnohumeral joint

√7th   **S53.132**   **Medial** subluxation of left ulnohumeral joint

√7th   **S53.133**   **Medial** subluxation of unspecified ulnohumeral joint

√7th   **S53.134**   **Medial** dislocation of right ulnohumeral joint

√7th   **S53.135**   **Medial** dislocation of left ulnohumeral joint

√7th   **S53.136**   **Medial** dislocation of unspecified ulnohumeral joint

√6th   **S53.14**   **Lateral** subluxation and dislocation of ulnohumeral joint

√7th   **S53.141**   **Lateral** subluxation of right ulnohumeral joint

√7th   **S53.142**   **Lateral** subluxation of left ulnohumeral joint

√7th   **S53.143**   **Lateral** subluxation of unspecified ulnohumeral joint

√7th   **S53.144**   **Lateral** dislocation of right ulnohumeral joint

√7th   **S53.145**   **Lateral** dislocation of left ulnohumeral joint

√7th   **S53.146**   **Lateral** dislocation of unspecified ulnohumeral joint

√6th   **S53.19**   **Other** subluxation and dislocation of ulnohumeral joint

√7th   **S53.191**   **Other** subluxation of right ulnohumeral joint

√7th   **S53.192**   **Other** subluxation of left ulnohumeral joint

√7th   **S53.193**   **Other** subluxation of unspecified ulnohumeral joint

√ Additional Character Required   √7th Xtension Alert   Unspecified Code   Other Specified Code   Manifestation Code   ►◄ Revised Text   ● New Code   ▲ Revised Code Title

ICD-10-CM 2014 (Draft)   **857**

Injury, Poisoning and Certain Other Consequences of External Causes

S53.194–S55.111

√7ᵗʰ **S53.194** Other dislocation of right ulnohumeral joint

√7ᵗʰ **S53.195** Other dislocation of left ulnohumeral joint

√7ᵗʰ **S53.196** Other dislocation of unspecified ulnohumeral joint

√5ᵗʰ **S53.2** Traumatic rupture of radial collateral ligament
     EXCLUDES 1   sprain of radial collateral ligament NOS (S53.43-)

√x7ᵗʰ **S53.20** Traumatic rupture of unspecified radial collateral ligament

√x7ᵗʰ **S53.21** Traumatic rupture of right radial collateral ligament

√x7ᵗʰ **S53.22** Traumatic rupture of left radial collateral ligament

√5ᵗʰ **S53.3** Traumatic rupture of ulnar collateral ligament
     EXCLUDES 1   sprain of ulnar collateral ligament (S53.44-)

√x7ᵗʰ **S53.30** Traumatic rupture of unspecified ulnar collateral ligament

√x7ᵗʰ **S53.31** Traumatic rupture of right ulnar collateral ligament

√x7ᵗʰ **S53.32** Traumatic rupture of left ulnar collateral ligament

√5ᵗʰ **S53.4** Sprain of elbow
     EXCLUDES 2   traumatic rupture of radial collateral ligament (S53.2-)
                 traumatic rupture of ulnar collateral ligament (S53.3-)

√6ᵗʰ **S53.40** Unspecified sprain of elbow

√7ᵗʰ **S53.401** Unspecified sprain of right elbow

√7ᵗʰ **S53.402** Unspecified sprain of left elbow

√7ᵗʰ **S53.409** Unspecified sprain of unspecified elbow
         Sprain of elbow NOS

√6ᵗʰ **S53.41** Radiohumeral (joint) sprain

√7ᵗʰ **S53.411** Radiohumeral (joint) sprain of right elbow

√7ᵗʰ **S53.412** Radiohumeral (joint) sprain of left elbow

√7ᵗʰ **S53.419** Radiohumeral (joint) sprain of unspecified elbow

√6ᵗʰ **S53.42** Ulnohumeral (joint) sprain

√7ᵗʰ **S53.421** Ulnohumeral (joint) sprain of right elbow

√7ᵗʰ **S53.422** Ulnohumeral (joint) sprain of left elbow

√7ᵗʰ **S53.429** Ulnohumeral (joint) sprain of unspecified elbow

√6ᵗʰ **S53.43** Radial collateral ligament sprain

√7ᵗʰ **S53.431** Radial collateral ligament sprain of right elbow

√7ᵗʰ **S53.432** Radial collateral ligament sprain of left elbow

√7ᵗʰ **S53.439** Radial collateral ligament sprain of unspecified elbow

√6ᵗʰ **S53.44** Ulnar collateral ligament sprain

√7ᵗʰ **S53.441** Ulnar collateral ligament sprain of right elbow

√7ᵗʰ **S53.442** Ulnar collateral ligament sprain of left elbow

√7ᵗʰ **S53.449** Ulnar collateral ligament sprain of unspecified elbow

√6ᵗʰ **S53.49** Other sprain of elbow

√7ᵗʰ **S53.491** Other sprain of right elbow

√7ᵗʰ **S53.492** Other sprain of left elbow

√7ᵗʰ **S53.499** Other sprain of unspecified elbow

√4ᵗʰ **S54** Injury of nerves at forearm level
     Code also any associated open wound (S51.-)
     EXCLUDES 2   injury of nerves at wrist and hand level (S64.-)

     The appropriate 7th character is to be added to each code from category S54.
     A   initial encounter
     D   subsequent encounter
     S   sequela

√5ᵗʰ **S54.0** Injury of ulnar nerve at forearm level
     Injury of ulnar nerve NOS

√x7ᵗʰ **S54.00** Injury of ulnar nerve at forearm level, unspecified arm

√x7ᵗʰ **S54.01** Injury of ulnar nerve at forearm level, right arm

√x7ᵗʰ **S54.02** Injury of ulnar nerve at forearm level, left arm

√5ᵗʰ **S54.1** Injury of median nerve at forearm level
     Injury of median nerve NOS

√x7ᵗʰ **S54.10** Injury of median nerve at forearm level, unspecified arm

√x7ᵗʰ **S54.11** Injury of median nerve at forearm level, right arm

√x7ᵗʰ **S54.12** Injury of median nerve at forearm level, left arm

√5ᵗʰ **S54.2** Injury of radial nerve at forearm level
     Injury of radial nerve NOS

√x7ᵗʰ **S54.20** Injury of radial nerve at forearm level, unspecified arm

√x7ᵗʰ **S54.21** Injury of radial nerve at forearm level, right arm

√x7ᵗʰ **S54.22** Injury of radial nerve at forearm level, left arm

√5ᵗʰ **S54.3** Injury of cutaneous sensory nerve at forearm level

√x7ᵗʰ **S54.30** Injury of cutaneous sensory nerve at forearm level, unspecified arm

√x7ᵗʰ **S54.31** Injury of cutaneous sensory nerve at forearm level, right arm

√x7ᵗʰ **S54.32** Injury of cutaneous sensory nerve at forearm level, left arm

√5ᵗʰ **S54.8** Injury of other nerves at forearm level

√6ᵗʰ **S54.8X** Unspecified injury of other nerves at forearm level

√7ᵗʰ **S54.8X1** Unspecified injury of other nerves at forearm level, right arm

√7ᵗʰ **S54.8X2** Unspecified injury of other nerves at forearm level, left arm

√7ᵗʰ **S54.8X9** Unspecified injury of other nerves at forearm level, unspecified arm

√5ᵗʰ **S54.9** Injury of unspecified nerve at forearm level

√x7ᵗʰ **S54.90** Injury of unspecified nerve at forearm level, unspecified arm

√x7ᵗʰ **S54.91** Injury of unspecified nerve at forearm level, right arm

√x7ᵗʰ **S54.92** Injury of unspecified nerve at forearm level, left arm

√4ᵗʰ **S55** Injury of blood vessels at forearm level
     Code also any associated open wound (S51.-)
     EXCLUDES 2   injury of blood vessels at wrist and hand level (S65.-)
                 injury of brachial vessels (S45.1-S45.2)

     The appropriate 7th character is to be added to each code from category S55.
     A   initial encounter
     D   subsequent encounter
     S   sequela

√5ᵗʰ **S55.0** Injury of ulnar artery at forearm level

√6ᵗʰ **S55.00** Unspecified injury of ulnar artery at forearm level

√7ᵗʰ **S55.001** Unspecified injury of ulnar artery at forearm level, right arm

√7ᵗʰ **S55.002** Unspecified injury of ulnar artery at forearm level, left arm

√7ᵗʰ **S55.009** Unspecified injury of ulnar artery at forearm level, unspecified arm

√6ᵗʰ **S55.01** Laceration of ulnar artery at forearm level

√7ᵗʰ **S55.011** Laceration of ulnar artery at forearm level, right arm

√7ᵗʰ **S55.012** Laceration of ulnar artery at forearm level, left arm

√7ᵗʰ **S55.019** Laceration of ulnar artery at forearm level, unspecified arm

√6ᵗʰ **S55.09** Other specified injury of ulnar artery at forearm level

√7ᵗʰ **S55.091** Other specified injury of ulnar artery at forearm level, right arm

√7ᵗʰ **S55.092** Other specified injury of ulnar artery at forearm level, left arm

√7ᵗʰ **S55.099** Other specified injury of ulnar artery at forearm level, unspecified arm

√5ᵗʰ **S55.1** Injury of radial artery at forearm level

√6ᵗʰ **S55.10** Unspecified injury of radial artery at forearm level

√7ᵗʰ **S55.101** Unspecified injury of radial artery at forearm level, right arm

√7ᵗʰ **S55.102** Unspecified injury of radial artery at forearm level, left arm

√7ᵗʰ **S55.109** Unspecified injury of radial artery at forearm level, unspecified arm

√6ᵗʰ **S55.11** Laceration of radial artery at forearm level

√7ᵗʰ **S55.111** Laceration of radial artery at forearm level, right arm

---

EXCLUDES 1 Not coded here   EXCLUDES 2 Not included here   N Newborn Age: 0   P Pediatric Age: 0-17   M Maternity Age: 12-55   A Adult Age: 15-124

858   ICD-10-CM 2014 (Draft)

√7ᵗʰ **S55.112** Laceration of radial artery at forearm level, **left** arm

√7ᵗʰ **S55.119** Laceration of radial artery at forearm level, unspecified arm

√6ᵗʰ **S55.19** **Other** specified injury of radial artery at forearm level

√7ᵗʰ **S55.191** Other specified injury of radial artery at forearm level, **right** arm

√7ᵗʰ **S55.192** Other specified injury of radial artery at forearm level, **left** arm

√7ᵗʰ **S55.199** Other specified injury of radial artery at forearm level, unspecified arm

√5ᵗʰ **S55.2** Injury of **vein** at forearm level

√6ᵗʰ **S55.2Ø** **Unspecified** injury of vein at forearm level

√7ᵗʰ **S55.2Ø1** Unspecified injury of vein at forearm level, **right** arm

√7ᵗʰ **S55.2Ø2** Unspecified injury of vein at forearm level, **left** arm

√7ᵗʰ **S55.2Ø9** Unspecified injury of vein at forearm level, unspecified arm

√6ᵗʰ **S55.21** **Laceration** of vein at forearm level

√7ᵗʰ **S55.211** Laceration of vein at forearm level, **right** arm

√7ᵗʰ **S55.212** Laceration of vein at forearm level, **left** arm

√7ᵗʰ **S55.219** Laceration of vein at forearm level, unspecified arm

√6ᵗʰ **S55.29** Other specified injury of vein at forearm level

√7ᵗʰ **S55.291** Other specified injury of vein at forearm level, **right** arm

√7ᵗʰ **S55.292** Other specified injury of vein at forearm level, **left** arm

√7ᵗʰ **S55.299** Other specified injury of vein at forearm level, unspecified arm

√5ᵗʰ **S55.8** Injury of **other blood vessels** at forearm level

√6ᵗʰ **S55.8Ø** **Unspecified** injury of other blood vessels at forearm level

√7ᵗʰ **S55.8Ø1** Unspecified injury of other blood vessels at forearm level, **right** arm

√7ᵗʰ **S55.8Ø2** Unspecified injury of other blood vessels at forearm level, **left** arm

√7ᵗʰ **S55.8Ø9** Unspecified injury of other blood vessels at forearm level, unspecified arm

√6ᵗʰ **S55.81** **Laceration** of other blood vessels at forearm level

√7ᵗʰ **S55.811** Laceration of other blood vessels at forearm level, **right** arm

√7ᵗʰ **S55.812** Laceration of other blood vessels at forearm level, **left** arm

√7ᵗʰ **S55.819** Laceration of other blood vessels at forearm level, unspecified arm

√6ᵗʰ **S55.89** **Other** specified injury of other blood vessels at forearm level

√7ᵗʰ **S55.891** Other specified injury of other blood vessels at forearm level, **right** arm

√7ᵗʰ **S55.892** Other specified injury of other blood vessels at forearm level, **left** arm

√7ᵗʰ **S55.899** Other specified injury of other blood vessels at forearm level, unspecified arm

√5ᵗʰ **S55.9** Injury of **unspecified blood vessel** at forearm level

√6ᵗʰ **S55.9Ø** **Unspecified** injury of unspecified blood vessel at forearm level

√7ᵗʰ **S55.9Ø1** Unspecified injury of unspecified blood vessel at forearm level, **right** arm

√7ᵗʰ **S55.9Ø2** Unspecified injury of unspecified blood vessel at forearm level, **left** arm

√7ᵗʰ **S55.9Ø9** Unspecified injury of unspecified blood vessel at forearm level, unspecified arm

√6ᵗʰ **S55.91** **Laceration** of unspecified blood vessel at forearm level

√7ᵗʰ **S55.911** Laceration of unspecified blood vessel at forearm level, **right** arm

√7ᵗʰ **S55.912** Laceration of unspecified blood vessel at forearm level, **left** arm

√7ᵗʰ **S55.919** Laceration of unspecified blood vessel at forearm level, unspecified arm

√6ᵗʰ **S55.99** **Other** specified injury of unspecified blood vessel at forearm level

√7ᵗʰ **S55.991** Other specified injury of unspecified blood vessel at forearm level, **right** arm

√7ᵗʰ **S55.992** Other specified injury of unspecified blood vessel at forearm level, **left** arm

√7ᵗʰ **S55.999** Other specified injury of unspecified blood vessel at forearm level, unspecified arm

√4ᵗʰ **S56** **Injury of muscle, fascia and tendon at forearm level**

Code also any associated open wound (S51.-)

EXCLUDES 2   injury of muscle, fascia and tendon at or below wrist (S66.-)
     sprain of joints and ligaments of elbow (S53.4-)

The appropriate 7th character is to be added to each code from category S56.
A   initial encounter
D   subsequent encounter
S   sequela

√5ᵗʰ **S56.Ø** Injury of **flexor** muscle, fascia and tendon of **thumb** at forearm level

√6ᵗʰ **S56.ØØ** **Unspecified** injury of flexor muscle, fascia and tendon of thumb at forearm level

√7ᵗʰ **S56.ØØ1** Unspecified injury of flexor muscle, fascia and tendon of **right thumb** at forearm level

√7ᵗʰ **S56.ØØ2** Unspecified injury of flexor muscle, fascia and tendon of **left thumb** at forearm level

√7ᵗʰ **S56.ØØ9** Unspecified injury of flexor muscle, fascia and tendon of unspecified thumb at forearm level

√6ᵗʰ **S56.Ø1** **Strain** of flexor muscle, fascia and tendon of thumb at forearm level

√7ᵗʰ **S56.Ø11** Strain of flexor muscle, fascia and tendon of **right thumb** at forearm level

√7ᵗʰ **S56.Ø12** Strain of flexor muscle, fascia and tendon of **left thumb** at forearm level

√7ᵗʰ **S56.Ø19** Strain of flexor muscle, fascia and tendon of unspecified thumb at forearm level

√6ᵗʰ **S56.Ø2** **Laceration** of flexor muscle, fascia and tendon of thumb at forearm level

√7ᵗʰ **S56.Ø21** Laceration of flexor muscle, fascia and tendon of **right thumb** at forearm level

√7ᵗʰ **S56.Ø22** Laceration of flexor muscle, fascia and tendon of **left thumb** at forearm level

√7ᵗʰ **S56.Ø29** Laceration of flexor muscle, fascia and tendon of unspecified thumb at forearm level

√6ᵗʰ **S56.Ø9** **Other** injury of flexor muscle, fascia and tendon of thumb at forearm level

√7ᵗʰ **S56.Ø91** Other injury of flexor muscle, fascia and tendon of **right thumb** at forearm level

√7ᵗʰ **S56.Ø92** Other injury of flexor muscle, fascia and tendon of **left thumb** at forearm level

√7ᵗʰ **S56.Ø99** Other injury of flexor muscle, fascia and tendon of unspecified thumb at forearm level

√5ᵗʰ **S56.1** Injury of **flexor** muscle, fascia and tendon of other and unspecified **finger** at forearm level

√6ᵗʰ **S56.1Ø** **Unspecified** injury of flexor muscle, fascia and tendon of other and unspecified finger at forearm level

√7ᵗʰ **S56.1Ø1** Unspecified injury of flexor muscle, fascia and tendon of **right index finger** at forearm level

√7ᵗʰ **S56.1Ø2** Unspecified injury of flexor muscle, fascia and tendon of **left index finger** at forearm level

√7ᵗʰ **S56.1Ø3** Unspecified injury of flexor muscle, fascia and tendon of **right middle finger** at forearm level

√7ᵗʰ **S56.1Ø4** Unspecified injury of flexor muscle, fascia and tendon of **left middle finger** at forearm level

---

☑ Additional Character Required   √ₓ7ᵗʰ Xtension Alert   Unspecified Code   Other Specified Code   Manifestation Code   ▶◀ Revised Text   ● New Code   ▲ Revised Code Title

ICD-1Ø-CM 2Ø14 (Draft)   859

Injury, Poisoning and Certain Other Consequences of External Causes

S56.105–S56.32

√7ᵗʰ **S56.105** Unspecified injury of flexor muscle, fascia and tendon of right ring finger at forearm level

√7ᵗʰ **S56.106** Unspecified injury of flexor muscle, fascia and tendon of left ring finger at forearm level

√7ᵗʰ **S56.107** Unspecified injury of flexor muscle, fascia and tendon of right little finger at forearm level

√7ᵗʰ **S56.108** Unspecified injury of flexor muscle, fascia and tendon of left little finger at forearm level

√7ᵗʰ **S56.109** Unspecified injury of flexor muscle, fascia and tendon of unspecified finger at forearm level

√6ᵗʰ **S56.11** Strain of flexor muscle, fascia and tendon of other and unspecified finger at forearm level

√7ᵗʰ **S56.111** Strain of flexor muscle, fascia and tendon of right index finger at forearm level

√7ᵗʰ **S56.112** Strain of flexor muscle, fascia and tendon of left index finger at forearm level

√7ᵗʰ **S56.113** Strain of flexor muscle, fascia and tendon of right middle finger at forearm level

√7ᵗʰ **S56.114** Strain of flexor muscle, fascia and tendon of left middle finger at forearm level

√7ᵗʰ **S56.115** Strain of flexor muscle, fascia and tendon of right ring finger at forearm level

√7ᵗʰ **S56.116** Strain of flexor muscle, fascia and tendon of left ring finger at forearm level

√7ᵗʰ **S56.117** Strain of flexor muscle, fascia and tendon of right little finger at forearm level

√7ᵗʰ **S56.118** Strain of flexor muscle, fascia and tendon of left little finger at forearm level

√7ᵗʰ **S56.119** Strain of flexor muscle, fascia and tendon of finger of unspecified finger at forearm level

√6ᵗʰ **S56.12** Laceration of flexor muscle, fascia and tendon of other and unspecified finger at forearm level

√7ᵗʰ **S56.121** Laceration of flexor muscle, fascia and tendon of right index finger at forearm level

√7ᵗʰ **S56.122** Laceration of flexor muscle, fascia and tendon of left index finger at forearm level

√7ᵗʰ **S56.123** Laceration of flexor muscle, fascia and tendon of right middle finger at forearm level

√7ᵗʰ **S56.124** Laceration of flexor muscle, fascia and tendon of left middle finger at forearm level

√7ᵗʰ **S56.125** Laceration of flexor muscle, fascia and tendon of right ring finger at forearm level

√7ᵗʰ **S56.126** Laceration of flexor muscle, fascia and tendon of left ring finger at forearm level

√7ᵗʰ **S56.127** Laceration of flexor muscle, fascia and tendon of right little finger at forearm level

√7ᵗʰ **S56.128** Laceration of flexor muscle, fascia and tendon of left little finger at forearm level

√7ᵗʰ **S56.129** Laceration of flexor muscle, fascia and tendon of unspecified finger at forearm level

√6ᵗʰ **S56.19** Other injury of flexor muscle, fascia and tendon of other and unspecified finger at forearm level

√7ᵗʰ **S56.191** Other injury of flexor muscle, fascia and tendon of right index finger at forearm level

√7ᵗʰ **S56.192** Other injury of flexor muscle, fascia and tendon of left index finger at forearm level

√7ᵗʰ **S56.193** Other injury of flexor muscle, fascia and tendon of right middle finger at forearm level

√7ᵗʰ **S56.194** Other injury of flexor muscle, fascia and tendon of left middle finger at forearm level

√7ᵗʰ **S56.195** Other injury of flexor muscle, fascia and tendon of right ring finger at forearm level

√7ᵗʰ **S56.196** Other injury of flexor muscle, fascia and tendon of left ring finger at forearm level

√7ᵗʰ **S56.197** Other injury of flexor muscle, fascia and tendon of right little finger at forearm level

√7ᵗʰ **S56.198** Other injury of flexor muscle, fascia and tendon of left little finger at forearm level

√7ᵗʰ **S56.199** Other injury of flexor muscle, fascia and tendon of unspecified finger at forearm level

√5ᵗʰ **S56.2** Injury of other flexor muscle, fascia and tendon at forearm level

√6ᵗʰ **S56.20** Unspecified injury of other flexor muscle, fascia and tendon at forearm level

√7ᵗʰ **S56.201** Unspecified injury of other flexor muscle, fascia and tendon at forearm level, right arm

√7ᵗʰ **S56.202** Unspecified injury of other flexor muscle, fascia and tendon at forearm level, left arm

√7ᵗʰ **S56.209** Unspecified injury of other flexor muscle, fascia and tendon at forearm level, unspecified arm

√6ᵗʰ **S56.21** Strain of other flexor muscle, fascia and tendon at forearm level

√7ᵗʰ **S56.211** Strain of other flexor muscle, fascia and tendon at forearm level, right arm

√7ᵗʰ **S56.212** Strain of other flexor muscle, fascia and tendon at forearm level, left arm

√7ᵗʰ **S56.219** Strain of other flexor muscle, fascia and tendon at forearm level, unspecified arm

√6ᵗʰ **S56.22** Laceration of other flexor muscle, fascia and tendon at forearm level

√7ᵗʰ **S56.221** Laceration of other flexor muscle, fascia and tendon at forearm level, right arm

√7ᵗʰ **S56.222** Laceration of other flexor muscle, fascia and tendon at forearm level, left arm

√7ᵗʰ **S56.229** Laceration of other flexor muscle, fascia and tendon at forearm level, unspecified arm

√6ᵗʰ **S56.29** Other injury of other flexor muscle, fascia and tendon at forearm level

√7ᵗʰ **S56.291** Other injury of other flexor muscle, fascia and tendon at forearm level, right arm

√7ᵗʰ **S56.292** Other injury of other flexor muscle, fascia and tendon at forearm level, left arm

√7ᵗʰ **S56.299** Other injury of other flexor muscle, fascia and tendon at forearm level, unspecified arm

√5ᵗʰ **S56.3** Injury of extensor or abductor muscles, fascia and tendons of thumb at forearm level

√6ᵗʰ **S56.30** Unspecified injury of extensor or abductor muscles, fascia and tendons of thumb at forearm level

√7ᵗʰ **S56.301** Unspecified injury of extensor or abductor muscles, fascia and tendons of right thumb at forearm level

√7ᵗʰ **S56.302** Unspecified injury of extensor or abductor muscles, fascia and tendons of left thumb at forearm level

√7ᵗʰ **S56.309** Unspecified injury of extensor or abductor muscles, fascia and tendons of unspecified thumb at forearm level

√6ᵗʰ **S56.31** Strain of extensor or abductor muscles, fascia and tendons of thumb at forearm level

√7ᵗʰ **S56.311** Strain of extensor or abductor muscles, fascia and tendons of right thumb at forearm level

√7ᵗʰ **S56.312** Strain of extensor or abductor muscles, fascia and tendons of left thumb at forearm level

√7ᵗʰ **S56.319** Strain of extensor or abductor muscles, fascia and tendons of unspecified thumb at forearm level

√6ᵗʰ **S56.32** Laceration of extensor or abductor muscles, fascia and tendons of thumb at forearm level

EXCLUDES 1 Not coded here   **EXCLUDES 2** Not included here   **N** Newborn Age: 0   **P** Pediatric Age: 0-17   **M** Maternity Age: 12-55   **A** Adult Age: 15-124

860   ICD-10-CM 2014 (Draft)

√7ᵗʰ **S56.321** Laceration of extensor or abductor muscles, fascia and tendons of right thumb at forearm level

√7ᵗʰ **S56.322** Laceration of extensor or abductor muscles, fascia and tendons of left thumb at forearm level

√7ᵗʰ **S56.329** Laceration of extensor or abductor muscles, fascia and tendons of unspecified thumb at forearm level

√6ᵗʰ **S56.39** Other injury of extensor or abductor muscles, fascia and tendons of thumb at forearm level

√7ᵗʰ **S56.391** Other injury of extensor or abductor muscles, fascia and tendons of right thumb at forearm level

√7ᵗʰ **S56.392** Other injury of extensor or abductor muscles, fascia and tendons of left thumb at forearm level

√7ᵗʰ **S56.399** Other injury of extensor or abductor muscles, fascia and tendons of unspecified thumb at forearm level

√5ᵗʰ **S56.4** Injury of extensor muscle, fascia and tendon of other and unspecified finger at forearm level

√6ᵗʰ **S56.40** Unspecified injury of extensor muscle, fascia and tendon of other and unspecified finger at forearm level

√7ᵗʰ **S56.401** Unspecified injury of extensor muscle, fascia and tendon of right index finger at forearm level

√7ᵗʰ **S56.402** Unspecified injury of extensor muscle, fascia and tendon of left index finger at forearm level

√7ᵗʰ **S56.403** Unspecified injury of extensor muscle, fascia and tendon of right middle finger at forearm level

√7ᵗʰ **S56.404** Unspecified injury of extensor muscle, fascia and tendon of left middle finger at forearm level

√7ᵗʰ **S56.405** Unspecified injury of extensor muscle, fascia and tendon of right ring finger at forearm level

√7ᵗʰ **S56.406** Unspecified injury of extensor muscle, fascia and tendon of left ring finger at forearm level

√7ᵗʰ **S56.407** Unspecified injury of extensor muscle, fascia and tendon of right little finger at forearm level

√7ᵗʰ **S56.408** Unspecified injury of extensor muscle, fascia and tendon of left little finger at forearm level

√7ᵗʰ **S56.409** Unspecified injury of extensor muscle, fascia and tendon of unspecified finger at forearm level

√6ᵗʰ **S56.41** Strain of extensor muscle, fascia and tendon of other and unspecified finger at forearm level

S56.411 Strain of extensor muscle, fascia and tendon of right index finger at forearm level

√7ᵗʰ **S56.412** Strain of extensor muscle, fascia and tendon of left index finger at forearm level

√7ᵗʰ **S56.413** Strain of extensor muscle, fascia and tendon of right middle finger at forearm level

√7ᵗʰ **S56.414** Strain of extensor muscle, fascia and tendon of left middle finger at forearm level

√7ᵗʰ **S56.415** Strain of extensor muscle, fascia and tendon of right ring finger at forearm level

√7ᵗʰ **S56.416** Strain of extensor muscle, fascia and tendon of left ring finger at forearm level

√7ᵗʰ **S56.417** Strain of extensor muscle, fascia and tendon of right little finger at forearm level

√7ᵗʰ **S56.418** Strain of extensor muscle, fascia and tendon of left little finger at forearm level

√7ᵗʰ **S56.419** Strain of extensor muscle, fascia and tendon of finger, unspecified finger at forearm level

√6ᵗʰ **S56.42** Laceration of extensor muscle, fascia and tendon of other and unspecified finger at forearm level

S56.421 Laceration of extensor muscle, fascia and tendon of right index finger at forearm level

√7ᵗʰ **S56.422** Laceration of extensor muscle, fascia and tendon of left index finger at forearm level

√7ᵗʰ **S56.423** Laceration of extensor muscle, fascia and tendon of right middle finger at forearm level

√7ᵗʰ **S56.424** Laceration of extensor muscle, fascia and tendon of left middle finger at forearm level

√7ᵗʰ **S56.425** Laceration of extensor muscle, fascia and tendon of right ring finger at forearm level

√7ᵗʰ **S56.426** Laceration of extensor muscle, fascia and tendon of left ring finger at forearm level

√7ᵗʰ **S56.427** Laceration of extensor muscle, fascia and tendon of right little finger at forearm level

√7ᵗʰ **S56.428** Laceration of extensor muscle, fascia and tendon of left little finger at forearm level

√7ᵗʰ **S56.429** Laceration of extensor muscle, fascia and tendon of unspecified finger at forearm level

√6ᵗʰ **S56.49** Other injury of extensor muscle, fascia and tendon of other and unspecified finger at forearm level

√7ᵗʰ **S56.491** Other injury of extensor muscle, fascia and tendon of right index finger at forearm level

√7ᵗʰ **S56.492** Other injury of extensor muscle, fascia and tendon of left index finger at forearm level

√7ᵗʰ **S56.493** Other injury of extensor muscle, fascia and tendon of right middle finger at forearm level

√7ᵗʰ **S56.494** Other injury of extensor muscle, fascia and tendon of left middle finger at forearm level

√7ᵗʰ **S56.495** Other injury of extensor muscle, fascia and tendon of right ring finger at forearm level

√7ᵗʰ **S56.496** Other injury of extensor muscle, fascia and tendon of left ring finger at forearm level

√7ᵗʰ **S56.497** Other injury of extensor muscle, fascia and tendon of right little finger at forearm level

√7ᵗʰ **S56.498** Other injury of extensor muscle, fascia and tendon of left little finger at forearm level

√7ᵗʰ **S56.499** Other injury of extensor muscle, fascia and tendon of unspecified finger at forearm level

√5ᵗʰ **S56.5** Injury of other extensor muscle, fascia and tendon at forearm level

√6ᵗʰ **S56.50** Unspecified injury of other extensor muscle, fascia and tendon at forearm level

√7ᵗʰ **S56.501** Unspecified injury of other extensor muscle, fascia and tendon at forearm level, right arm

√7ᵗʰ **S56.502** Unspecified injury of other extensor muscle, fascia and tendon at forearm level, left arm

√7ᵗʰ **S56.509** Unspecified injury of other extensor muscle, fascia and tendon at forearm level, unspecified arm

√6ᵗʰ **S56.51** Strain of other extensor muscle, fascia and tendon at forearm level

√7ᵗʰ **S56.511** Strain of other extensor muscle, fascia and tendon at forearm level, right arm

√7ᵗʰ **S56.512** Strain of other extensor muscle, fascia and tendon at forearm level, left arm

√7ᵗʰ **S56.519** Strain of other extensor muscle, fascia and tendon at forearm level, unspecified arm

√6ᵗʰ **S56.52** Laceration of other extensor muscle, fascia and tendon at forearm level

√7ᵗʰ **S56.521** Laceration of other extensor muscle, fascia and tendon at forearm level, right arm

☑ Additional Character Required   √x7ᵗʰ Xtension Alert   Unspecified Code   Other Specified Code   Manifestation Code   ►◄ Revised Text   ● New Code   ▲ Revised Code Title

ICD-10-CM 2014 (Draft)   861

√7ᵗʰ **S56.522** **Laceration of other extensor muscle, fascia and tendon at forearm level, left arm**

√7ᵗʰ **S56.529** **Laceration of other extensor muscle, fascia and tendon at forearm level, unspecified arm**

√6ᵗʰ **S56.59** Other injury of other extensor muscle, fascia and tendon at forearm level

√7ᵗʰ **S56.591** **Other injury of other extensor muscle, fascia and tendon at forearm level, right arm**

√7ᵗʰ **S56.592** **Other injury of other extensor muscle, fascia and tendon at forearm level, left arm**

√7ᵗʰ **S56.599** **Other injury of other extensor muscle, fascia and tendon at forearm level, unspecified arm**

√5ᵗʰ **S56.8** Injury of other muscles, fascia and tendons at forearm level

√6ᵗʰ **S56.80** Unspecified injury of other muscles, fascia and tendons at forearm level

√7ᵗʰ **S56.801** **Unspecified injury of other muscles, fascia and tendons at forearm level, right arm**

√7ᵗʰ **S56.802** **Unspecified injury of other muscles, fascia and tendons at forearm level, left arm**

√7ᵗʰ **S56.809** **Unspecified injury of other muscles, fascia and tendons at forearm level, unspecified arm**

√6ᵗʰ **S56.81** Strain of other muscles, fascia and tendons at forearm level

√7ᵗʰ **S56.811** **Strain of other muscles, fascia and tendons at forearm level, right arm**

√7ᵗʰ **S56.812** **Strain of other muscles, fascia and tendons at forearm level, left arm**

√7ᵗʰ **S56.819** **Strain of other muscles, fascia and tendons at forearm level, unspecified arm**

√6ᵗʰ **S56.82** Laceration of other muscles, fascia and tendons at forearm level

√7ᵗʰ **S56.821** **Laceration of other muscles, fascia and tendons at forearm level, right arm**

√7ᵗʰ **S56.822** **Laceration of other muscles, fascia and tendons at forearm level, left arm**

√7ᵗʰ **S56.829** **Laceration of other muscles, fascia and tendons at forearm level, unspecified arm**

√6ᵗʰ **S56.89** Other injury of other muscles, fascia and tendons at forearm level

√7ᵗʰ **S56.891** **Other injury of other muscles, fascia and tendons at forearm level, right arm**

√7ᵗʰ **S56.892** **Other injury of other muscles, fascia and tendons at forearm level, left arm**

√7ᵗʰ **S56.899** **Other injury of other muscles, fascia and tendons at forearm level, unspecified arm**

√5ᵗʰ **S56.9** Injury of unspecified muscles, fascia and tendons at forearm level

√6ᵗʰ **S56.90** Unspecified injury of unspecified muscles, fascia and tendons at forearm level

√7ᵗʰ **S56.901** **Unspecified injury of unspecified muscles, fascia and tendons at forearm level, right arm**

√7ᵗʰ **S56.902** **Unspecified injury of unspecified muscles, fascia and tendons at forearm level, left arm**

√7ᵗʰ **S56.909** **Unspecified injury of unspecified muscles, fascia and tendons at forearm level, unspecified arm**

√6ᵗʰ **S56.91** Strain of unspecified muscles, fascia and tendons at forearm level

√7ᵗʰ **S56.911** **Strain of unspecified muscles, fascia and tendons at forearm level, right arm**

√7ᵗʰ **S56.912** **Strain of unspecified muscles, fascia and tendons at forearm level, left arm**

√7ᵗʰ **S56.919** **Strain of unspecified muscles, fascia and tendons at forearm level, unspecified arm**

√6ᵗʰ **S56.92** Laceration of unspecified muscles, fascia and tendons at forearm level

√7ᵗʰ **S56.921** **Laceration of unspecified muscles, fascia and tendons at forearm level, right arm**

√7ᵗʰ **S56.922** **Laceration of unspecified muscles, fascia and tendons at forearm level, left arm**

√7ᵗʰ **S56.929** **Laceration of unspecified muscles, fascia and tendons at forearm level, unspecified arm**

√6ᵗʰ **S56.99** Other injury of unspecified muscles, fascia and tendons at forearm level

√7ᵗʰ **S56.991** **Other injury of unspecified muscles, fascia and tendons at forearm level, right arm**

√7ᵗʰ **S56.992** **Other injury of unspecified muscles, fascia and tendons at forearm level, left arm**

√7ᵗʰ **S56.999** **Other injury of unspecified muscles, fascia and tendons at forearm level, unspecified arm**

√4ᵗʰ **S57** **Crushing injury of elbow and forearm**
Use additional code(s) for all associated injuries
EXCLUDES 2　crushing injury of wrist and hand (S67.-)

The appropriate 7th character is to be added to each code from category S57.
A　initial encounter
D　subsequent encounter
S　sequela

√5ᵗʰ **S57.0** Crushing injury of elbow

√x7ᵗʰ **S57.00** **Crushing injury of unspecified elbow**

√x7ᵗʰ **S57.01** **Crushing injury of right elbow**

√x7ᵗʰ **S57.02** **Crushing injury of left elbow**

√5ᵗʰ **S57.8** Crushing injury of forearm

√x7ᵗʰ **S57.80** **Crushing injury of unspecified forearm**

√x7ᵗʰ **S57.81** **Crushing injury of right forearm**

√x7ᵗʰ **S57.82** **Crushing injury of left forearm**

√4ᵗʰ **S58** **Traumatic amputation of elbow and forearm**
NOTE　An amputation not identified as partial or complete should be coded to complete.
EXCLUDES 1　traumatic amputation of wrist and hand (S68.-)

The appropriate 7th character is to be added to each code from category S58.
A　initial encounter
D　subsequent encounter
S　sequela

√5ᵗʰ **S58.0** Traumatic amputation at elbow level

√6ᵗʰ **S58.01** Complete traumatic amputation at elbow level

√7ᵗʰ **S58.011** **Complete traumatic amputation at elbow level, right arm**

√7ᵗʰ **S58.012** **Complete traumatic amputation at elbow level, left arm**

√7ᵗʰ **S58.019** **Complete traumatic amputation at elbow level, unspecified arm**

√6ᵗʰ **S58.02** Partial traumatic amputation at elbow level

√7ᵗʰ **S58.021** **Partial traumatic amputation at elbow level, right arm**

√7ᵗʰ **S58.022** **Partial traumatic amputation at elbow level, left arm**

√7ᵗʰ **S58.029** **Partial traumatic amputation at elbow level, unspecified arm**

√5ᵗʰ **S58.1** Traumatic amputation at level between elbow and wrist

√6ᵗʰ **S58.11** Complete traumatic amputation at level between elbow and wrist

√7ᵗʰ **S58.111** **Complete traumatic amputation at level between elbow and wrist, right arm**

√7ᵗʰ **S58.112** **Complete traumatic amputation at level between elbow and wrist, left arm**

√7ᵗʰ **S58.119** **Complete traumatic amputation at level between elbow and wrist, unspecified arm**

√6ᵗʰ **S58.12** Partial traumatic amputation at level between elbow and wrist

√7ᵗʰ **S58.121** **Partial traumatic amputation at level between elbow and wrist, right arm**

√7ᵗʰ **S58.122** **Partial traumatic amputation at level between elbow and wrist, left arm**

EXCLUDES 1 Not coded here　　**EXCLUDES 2** Not included here　　N Newborn Age: 0　　P Pediatric Age: 0-17　　M Maternity Age: 12-55　　A Adult Age: 15-124

862　　ICD-10-CM 2014 (Draft)

☑7th **S58.129** Partial traumatic amputation at level between elbow and wrist, unspecified arm

☑5th **S58.9** Traumatic amputation of forearm, level unspecified
EXCLUDES 1 *traumatic amputation of wrist (S68.-)*

☑6th **S58.91** Complete traumatic amputation of forearm, level unspecified

☑7th **S58.911** Complete traumatic amputation of right forearm, level unspecified

☑7th **S58.912** Complete traumatic amputation of left forearm, level unspecified

☑7th **S58.919** Complete traumatic amputation of unspecified forearm, level unspecified

☑6th **S58.92** Partial traumatic amputation of forearm, level unspecified

☑7th **S58.921** Partial traumatic amputation of right forearm, level unspecified

☑7th **S58.922** Partial traumatic amputation of left forearm, level unspecified

☑7th **S58.929** Partial traumatic amputation of unspecified forearm, level unspecified

☑4th **S59** Other and unspecified injuries of elbow and forearm
EXCLUDES 2 *other and unspecified injuries of wrist and hand (S69.-)*

The appropriate 7th character is to be added to each code from subcategories S59.0, S59.1, and S59.2.
A initial encounter for closed fracture
D subsequent encounter for fracture with routine healing
G subsequent encounter for fracture with delayed healing
K subsequent encounter for fracture with nonunion
P subsequent encounter for fracture with malunion
S sequela

☑5th **S59.0** Physeal fracture of lower end of ulna

☑6th **S59.00** Unspecified physeal fracture of lower end of ulna

☑7th **S59.001** Unspecified physeal fracture of lower end of ulna, right arm

☑7th **S59.002** Unspecified physeal fracture of lower end of ulna, left arm

☑7th **S59.009** Unspecified physeal fracture of lower end of ulna, unspecified arm

☑6th **S59.01** Salter-Harris Type I physeal fracture of lower end of ulna

☑7th **S59.011** Salter-Harris Type I physeal fracture of lower end of ulna, right arm

☑7th **S59.012** Salter-Harris Type I physeal fracture of lower end of ulna, left arm

☑7th **S59.019** Salter-Harris Type I physeal fracture of lower end of ulna, unspecified arm

☑6th **S59.02** Salter-Harris Type II physeal fracture of lower end of ulna

☑7th **S59.021** Salter-Harris Type II physeal fracture of lower end of ulna, right arm

☑7th **S59.022** Salter-Harris Type II physeal fracture of lower end of ulna, left arm

☑7th **S59.029** Salter-Harris Type II physeal fracture of lower end of ulna, unspecified arm

☑6th **S59.03** Salter-Harris Type III physeal fracture of lower end of ulna

☑7th **S59.031** Salter-Harris Type III physeal fracture of lower end of ulna, right arm

☑7th **S59.032** Salter-Harris Type III physeal fracture of lower end of ulna, left arm

☑7th **S59.039** Salter-Harris Type III physeal fracture of lower end of ulna, unspecified arm

☑6th **S59.04** Salter-Harris Type IV physeal fracture of lower end of ulna

☑7th **S59.041** Salter-Harris Type IV physeal fracture of lower end of ulna, right arm

☑7th **S59.042** Salter-Harris Type IV physeal fracture of lower end of ulna, left arm

☑7th **S59.049** Salter-Harris Type IV physeal fracture of lower end of ulna, unspecified arm

☑6th **S59.09** Other physeal fracture of lower end of ulna

☑7th **S59.091** Other physeal fracture of lower end of ulna, right arm

☑7th **S59.092** Other physeal fracture of lower end of ulna, left arm

☑7th **S59.099** Other physeal fracture of lower end of ulna, unspecified arm

☑5th **S59.1** Physeal fracture of upper end of radius

☑6th **S59.10** Unspecified physeal fracture of upper end of radius

☑7th **S59.101** Unspecified physeal fracture of upper end of radius, right arm

☑7th **S59.102** Unspecified physeal fracture of upper end of radius, left arm

☑7th **S59.109** Unspecified physeal fracture of upper end of radius, unspecified arm

☑6th **S59.11** Salter-Harris Type I physeal fracture of upper end of radius

☑7th **S59.111** Salter-Harris Type I physeal fracture of upper end of radius, right arm

☑7th **S59.112** Salter-Harris Type I physeal fracture of upper end of radius, left arm

☑7th **S59.119** Salter-Harris Type I physeal fracture of upper end of radius, unspecified arm

☑6th **S59.12** Salter-Harris Type II physeal fracture of upper end of radius

☑7th **S59.121** Salter-Harris Type II physeal fracture of upper end of radius, right arm

☑7th **S59.122** Salter-Harris Type II physeal fracture of upper end of radius, left arm

☑7th **S59.129** Salter-Harris Type II physeal fracture of upper end of radius, unspecified arm

☑6th **S59.13** Salter-Harris Type III physeal fracture of upper end of radius

☑7th **S59.131** Salter-Harris Type III physeal fracture of upper end of radius, right arm

☑7th **S59.132** Salter-Harris Type III physeal fracture of upper end of radius, left arm

☑7th **S59.139** Salter-Harris Type III physeal fracture of upper end of radius, unspecified arm

☑6th **S59.14** Salter-Harris Type IV physeal fracture of upper end of radius

☑7th **S59.141** Salter-Harris Type IV physeal fracture of upper end of radius, right arm

☑7th **S59.142** Salter-Harris Type IV physeal fracture of upper end of radius, left arm

☑7th **S59.149** Salter-Harris Type IV physeal fracture of upper end of radius, unspecified arm

☑6th **S59.19** Other physeal fracture of upper end of radius

☑7th **S59.191** Other physeal fracture of upper end of radius, right arm

☑7th **S59.192** Other physeal fracture of upper end of radius, left arm

☑7th **S59.199** Other physeal fracture of upper end of radius, unspecified arm

☑5th **S59.2** Physeal fracture of lower end of radius

☑6th **S59.20** Unspecified physeal fracture of lower end of radius

☑7th **S59.201** Unspecified physeal fracture of lower end of radius, right arm

☑7th **S59.202** Unspecified physeal fracture of lower end of radius, left arm

☑7th **S59.209** Unspecified physeal fracture of lower end of radius, unspecified arm

☑6th **S59.21** Salter-Harris Type I physeal fracture of lower end of radius

☑7th **S59.211** Salter-Harris Type I physeal fracture of lower end of radius, right arm

☑7th **S59.212** Salter-Harris Type I physeal fracture of lower end of radius, left arm

☑7th **S59.219** Salter-Harris Type I physeal fracture of lower end of radius, unspecified arm

☑6th **S59.22** Salter-Harris Type II physeal fracture of lower end of radius

☑7th **S59.221** Salter-Harris Type II physeal fracture of lower end of radius, right arm

☑7th **S59.222** Salter-Harris Type II physeal fracture of lower end of radius, left arm

☑7th **S59.229** Salter-Harris Type II physeal fracture of lower end of radius, unspecified arm

Injury, Poisoning and Certain Other Consequences of External Causes   S59.23–S60.211

✓6ᵗʰ **S59.23** Salter-Harris Type III physeal fracture of lower end of radius

   ✓7ᵗʰ **S59.231** Salter-Harris Type III physeal fracture of lower end of radius, right arm

   ✓7ᵗʰ **S59.232** Salter-Harris Type III physeal fracture of lower end of radius, left arm

   ✓7ᵗʰ **S59.239** Salter-Harris Type III physeal fracture of lower end of radius, unspecified arm

✓6ᵗʰ **S59.24** Salter-Harris Type IV physeal fracture of lower end of radius

   ✓7ᵗʰ **S59.241** Salter-Harris Type IV physeal fracture of lower end of radius, right arm

   ✓7ᵗʰ **S59.242** Salter-Harris Type IV physeal fracture of lower end of radius, left arm

   ✓7ᵗʰ **S59.249** Salter-Harris Type IV physeal fracture of lower end of radius, unspecified arm

✓6ᵗʰ **S59.29** Other physeal fracture of lower end of radius

   ✓7ᵗʰ **S59.291** Other physeal fracture of lower end of radius, right arm

   ✓7ᵗʰ **S59.292** Other physeal fracture of lower end of radius, left arm

   ✓7ᵗʰ **S59.299** Other physeal fracture of lower end of radius, unspecified arm

✓5ᵗʰ **S59.8** Other specified injuries of elbow and forearm

> The appropriate 7th character is to be added to each code in subcategory S59.8.
> A   initial encounter
> D   subsequent encounter
> S   sequela

✓6ᵗʰ **S59.80** Other specified injuries of elbow

   ✓7ᵗʰ **S59.801** Other specified injuries of right elbow

   ✓7ᵗʰ **S59.802** Other specified injuries of left elbow

   ✓7ᵗʰ **S59.809** Other specified injuries of unspecified elbow

✓6ᵗʰ **S59.81** Other specified injuries of forearm

   ✓7ᵗʰ **S59.811** Other specified injuries right forearm

   ✓7ᵗʰ **S59.812** Other specified injuries left forearm

   ✓7ᵗʰ **S59.819** Other specified injuries unspecified forearm

✓5ᵗʰ **S59.9** Unspecified injury of elbow and forearm

> The appropriate 7th character is to be added to each code in subcategory S59.9.
> A   initial encounter
> D   subsequent encounter
> S   sequela

✓6ᵗʰ **S59.90** Unspecified injury of elbow

   ✓7ᵗʰ **S59.901** Unspecified injury of right elbow

   ✓7ᵗʰ **S59.902** Unspecified injury of left elbow

   ✓7ᵗʰ **S59.909** Unspecified injury of unspecified elbow

✓6ᵗʰ **S59.91** Unspecified injury of forearm

   ✓7ᵗʰ **S59.911** Unspecified injury of right forearm

   ✓7ᵗʰ **S59.912** Unspecified injury of left forearm

   ✓7ᵗʰ **S59.919** Unspecified injury of unspecified forearm

Injuries to the wrist, hand and fingers (S60-S69)

EXCLUDES 2   burns and corrosions (T20-T32)
frostbite (T33-T34)
insect bite or sting, venomous (T63.4)

✓4ᵗʰ **S60** Superficial injury of wrist, hand and fingers

> The appropriate 7th character is to be added to each code from category S60.
> A   initial encounter
> D   subsequent encounter
> S   sequela

✓5ᵗʰ **S60.0** Contusion of finger without damage to nail

   EXCLUDES 1   contusion involving nail (matrix) (S60.1)

✓x7ᵗʰ **S60.00** Contusion of unspecified finger without damage to nail

   Contusion of finger(s) NOS

✓6ᵗʰ **S60.01** Contusion of thumb without damage to nail

   ✓7ᵗʰ **S60.011** Contusion of right thumb without damage to nail

   ✓7ᵗʰ **S60.012** Contusion of left thumb without damage to nail

   ✓7ᵗʰ **S60.019** Contusion of unspecified thumb without damage to nail

✓6ᵗʰ **S60.02** Contusion of index finger without damage to nail

   ✓7ᵗʰ **S60.021** Contusion of right index finger without damage to nail

   ✓7ᵗʰ **S60.022** Contusion of left index finger without damage to nail

   ✓7ᵗʰ **S60.029** Contusion of unspecified index finger without damage to nail

✓6ᵗʰ **S60.03** Contusion of middle finger without damage to nail

   ✓7ᵗʰ **S60.031** Contusion of right middle finger without damage to nail

   ✓7ᵗʰ **S60.032** Contusion of left middle finger without damage to nail

   ✓7ᵗʰ **S60.039** Contusion of unspecified middle finger without damage to nail

✓6ᵗʰ **S60.04** Contusion of ring finger without damage to nail

   ✓7ᵗʰ **S60.041** Contusion of right ring finger without damage to nail

   ✓7ᵗʰ **S60.042** Contusion of left ring finger without damage to nail

   ✓7ᵗʰ **S60.049** Contusion of unspecified ring finger without damage to nail

✓6ᵗʰ **S60.05** Contusion of little finger without damage to nail

   ✓7ᵗʰ **S60.051** Contusion of right little finger without damage to nail

   ✓7ᵗʰ **S60.052** Contusion of left little finger without damage to nail

   ✓7ᵗʰ **S60.059** Contusion of unspecified little finger without damage to nail

✓5ᵗʰ **S60.1** Contusion of finger with damage to nail

✓x7ᵗʰ **S60.10** Contusion of unspecified finger with damage to nail

✓6ᵗʰ **S60.11** Contusion of thumb with damage to nail

   ✓7ᵗʰ **S60.111** Contusion of right thumb with damage to nail

   ✓7ᵗʰ **S60.112** Contusion of left thumb with damage to nail

   ✓7ᵗʰ **S60.119** Contusion of unspecified thumb with damage to nail

✓6ᵗʰ **S60.12** Contusion of index finger with damage to nail

   ✓7ᵗʰ **S60.121** Contusion of right index finger with damage to nail

   ✓7ᵗʰ **S60.122** Contusion of left index finger with damage to nail

   ✓7ᵗʰ **S60.129** Contusion of unspecified index finger with damage to nail

✓6ᵗʰ **S60.13** Contusion of middle finger with damage to nail

   ✓7ᵗʰ **S60.131** Contusion of right middle finger with damage to nail

   ✓7ᵗʰ **S60.132** Contusion of left middle finger with damage to nail

   ✓7ᵗʰ **S60.139** Contusion of unspecified middle finger with damage to nail

✓6ᵗʰ **S60.14** Contusion of ring finger with damage to nail

   ✓7ᵗʰ **S60.141** Contusion of right ring finger with damage to nail

   ✓7ᵗʰ **S60.142** Contusion of left ring finger with damage to nail

   ✓7ᵗʰ **S60.149** Contusion of unspecified ring finger with damage to nail

✓6ᵗʰ **S60.15** Contusion of little finger with damage to nail

   ✓7ᵗʰ **S60.151** Contusion of right little finger with damage to nail

   ✓7ᵗʰ **S60.152** Contusion of left little finger with damage to nail

   ✓7ᵗʰ **S60.159** Contusion of unspecified little finger with damage to nail

✓5ᵗʰ **S60.2** Contusion of wrist and hand

   EXCLUDES 2   contusion of fingers (S60.0-, S60.1-)

✓6ᵗʰ **S60.21** Contusion of wrist

   ✓7ᵗʰ **S60.211** Contusion of right wrist

EXCLUDES 1 Not coded here   EXCLUDES 2 Not included here   N Newborn Age: 0   P Pediatric Age: 0-17   M Maternity Age: 12-55   A Adult Age: 15-124

864   ICD-10-CM 2014 (Draft)

√7ᵗʰ **S60.212** Contusion of left wrist

√7ᵗʰ **S60.219** Contusion of unspecified wrist

√6ᵗʰ **S60.22** Contusion of hand

√7ᵗʰ **S60.221** Contusion of right hand

√7ᵗʰ **S60.222** Contusion of left hand

√7ᵗʰ **S60.229** Contusion of unspecified hand

√5ᵗʰ **S60.3** Other superficial injuries of thumb

√6ᵗʰ **S60.31** Abrasion of thumb

√7ᵗʰ **S60.311** Abrasion of right thumb

√7ᵗʰ **S60.312** Abrasion of left thumb

√7ᵗʰ **S60.319** Abrasion of unspecified thumb

√6ᵗʰ **S60.32** Blister (nonthermal) of thumb

√7ᵗʰ **S60.321** Blister (nonthermal) of right thumb

√7ᵗʰ **S60.322** Blister (nonthermal) of left thumb

√7ᵗʰ **S60.329** Blister (nonthermal) of unspecified thumb

√6ᵗʰ **S60.34** External constriction of thumb

Hair tourniquet syndrome of thumb

Use additional cause code to identify the constricting item (W49.0-)

√7ᵗʰ **S60.341** External constriction of right thumb

√7ᵗʰ **S60.342** External constriction of left thumb

√7ᵗʰ **S60.349** External constriction of unspecified thumb

√6ᵗʰ **S60.35** Superficial foreign body of thumb

Splinter in the thumb

√7ᵗʰ **S60.351** Superficial foreign body of right thumb

√7ᵗʰ **S60.352** Superficial foreign body of left thumb

√7ᵗʰ **S60.359** Superficial foreign body of unspecified thumb

√6ᵗʰ **S60.36** Insect bite (nonvenomous) of thumb

√7ᵗʰ **S60.361** Insect bite (nonvenomous) of right thumb

√7ᵗʰ **S60.362** Insect bite (nonvenomous) of left thumb

√7ᵗʰ **S60.369** Insect bite (nonvenomous) of unspecified thumb

√6ᵗʰ **S60.37** Other superficial bite of thumb

EXCLUDES 1 *open bite of thumb (S61.05-, S61.15-)*

√7ᵗʰ **S60.371** Other superficial bite of right thumb

√7ᵗʰ **S60.372** Other superficial bite of left thumb

√7ᵗʰ **S60.379** Other superficial bite of unspecified thumb

√6ᵗʰ **S60.39** Other superficial injuries of thumb

√7ᵗʰ **S60.391** Other superficial injuries of right thumb

√7ᵗʰ **S60.392** Other superficial injuries of left thumb

√7ᵗʰ **S60.399** Other superficial injuries of unspecified thumb

√5ᵗʰ **S60.4** Other superficial injuries of other fingers

√6ᵗʰ **S60.41** Abrasion of fingers

√7ᵗʰ **S60.410** Abrasion of right index finger

√7ᵗʰ **S60.411** Abrasion of left index finger

√7ᵗʰ **S60.412** Abrasion of right middle finger

√7ᵗʰ **S60.413** Abrasion of left middle finger

√7ᵗʰ **S60.414** Abrasion of right ring finger

√7ᵗʰ **S60.415** Abrasion of left ring finger

√7ᵗʰ **S60.416** Abrasion of right little finger

√7ᵗʰ **S60.417** Abrasion of left little finger

√7ᵗʰ **S60.418** Abrasion of other finger

Abrasion of specified finger with unspecified laterality

√7ᵗʰ **S60.419** Abrasion of unspecified finger

√6ᵗʰ **S60.42** Blister (nonthermal) of fingers

√7ᵗʰ **S60.420** Blister (nonthermal) of right index finger

√7ᵗʰ **S60.421** Blister (nonthermal) of left index finger

√7ᵗʰ **S60.422** Blister (nonthermal) of right middle finger

√7ᵗʰ **S60.423** Blister (nonthermal) of left middle finger

√7ᵗʰ **S60.424** Blister (nonthermal) of right ring finger

√7ᵗʰ **S60.425** Blister (nonthermal) of left ring finger

√7ᵗʰ **S60.426** Blister (nonthermal) of right little finger

√7ᵗʰ **S60.427** Blister (nonthermal) of left little finger

√7ᵗʰ **S60.428** Blister (nonthermal) of other finger

Blister (nonthermal) of specified finger with unspecified laterality

√7ᵗʰ **S60.429** Blister (nonthermal) of unspecified finger

√6ᵗʰ **S60.44** External constriction of fingers

Hair tourniquet syndrome of finger

Use additional cause code to identify the constricting item (W49.0-)

√7ᵗʰ **S60.440** External constriction of right index finger

√7ᵗʰ **S60.441** External constriction of left index finger

√7ᵗʰ **S60.442** External constriction of right middle finger

√7ᵗʰ **S60.443** External constriction of left middle finger

√7ᵗʰ **S60.444** External constriction of right ring finger

√7ᵗʰ **S60.445** External constriction of left ring finger

√7ᵗʰ **S60.446** External constriction of right little finger

√7ᵗʰ **S60.447** External constriction of left little finger

√7ᵗʰ **S60.448** External constriction of other finger

External constriction of specified finger with unspecified laterality

√7ᵗʰ **S60.449** External constriction of unspecified finger

√6ᵗʰ **S60.45** Superficial foreign body of fingers

Splinter in the finger(s)

√7ᵗʰ **S60.450** Superficial foreign body of right index finger

√7ᵗʰ **S60.451** Superficial foreign body of left index finger

√7ᵗʰ **S60.452** Superficial foreign body of right middle finger

√7ᵗʰ **S60.453** Superficial foreign body of left middle finger

√7ᵗʰ **S60.454** Superficial foreign body of right ring finger

√7ᵗʰ **S60.455** Superficial foreign body of left ring finger

√7ᵗʰ **S60.456** Superficial foreign body of right little finger

√7ᵗʰ **S60.457** Superficial foreign body of left little finger

√7ᵗʰ **S60.458** Superficial foreign body of other finger

Superficial foreign body of specified finger with unspecified laterality

√7ᵗʰ **S60.459** Superficial foreign body of unspecified finger

√6ᵗʰ **S60.46** Insect bite (nonvenomous) of fingers

√7ᵗʰ **S60.460** Insect bite (nonvenomous) of right index finger

√7ᵗʰ **S60.461** Insect bite (nonvenomous) of left index finger

√7ᵗʰ **S60.462** Insect bite (nonvenomous) of right middle finger

√7ᵗʰ **S60.463** Insect bite (nonvenomous) of left middle finger

√7ᵗʰ **S60.464** Insect bite (nonvenomous) of right ring finger

√7ᵗʰ **S60.465** Insect bite (nonvenomous) of left ring finger

√7ᵗʰ **S60.466** Insect bite (nonvenomous) of right little finger

√7ᵗʰ **S60.467** Insect bite (nonvenomous) of left little finger

√7ᵗʰ **S60.468** Insect bite (nonvenomous) of other finger

Insect bite (nonvenomous) of specified finger with unspecified laterality

√7ᵗʰ **S60.469** Insect bite (nonvenomous) of unspecified finger

√6ᵗʰ **S60.47** Other superficial bite of fingers

EXCLUDES 1 *open bite of fingers (S61.25-, S61.35-)*

√7ᵗʰ **S60.470** Other superficial bite of right index finger

√7ᵗʰ **S60.471** Other superficial bite of left index finger

√7ᵗʰ **S60.472** Other superficial bite of right middle finger

√7ᵗʰ **S60.473** Other superficial bite of left middle finger

√7ᵗʰ **S60.474** Other superficial bite of right ring finger

√7ᵗʰ **S60.475** Other superficial bite of left ring finger

√7ᵗʰ **S60.476** Other superficial bite of right little finger

✓ Additional Character Required   √x7ᵗʰ Xtension Alert   Unspecified Code   Other Specified Code   Manifestation Code   ►◄ Revised Text   ● New Code   ▲ Revised Code Title

ICD-10-CM 2014 (Draft)   865

Injury, Poisoning and Certain Other Consequences of External Causes   S60.477–S61.021

✓7ᵗʰ   **S60.477**   **Other superficial bite of** left little **finger**

✓7ᵗʰ   **S60.478**   **Other superficial bite of other finger**
       Other superficial bite of specified finger with xc vunspecified laterality

✓7ᵗʰ   **S60.479**   **Other superficial bite of unspecified finger**

✓5ᵗʰ   **S60.5**   **Other superficial injuries of** hand
     EXCLUDES 2   *superficial injuries of fingers (S60.3-, S60.4-)*

   ✓6ᵗʰ   **S60.51**   **Abrasion** of hand
     ✓7ᵗʰ   **S60.511**   **Abrasion of** right **hand**
     ✓7ᵗʰ   **S60.512**   **Abrasion of** left **hand**
     ✓7ᵗʰ   **S60.519**   **Abrasion of unspecified hand**

   ✓6ᵗʰ   **S60.52**   **Blister (nonthermal)** of hand
     ✓7ᵗʰ   **S60.521**   **Blister (nonthermal) of** right **hand**
     ✓7ᵗʰ   **S60.522**   **Blister (nonthermal) of** left **hand**
     ✓7ᵗʰ   **S60.529**   **Blister (nonthermal) of unspecified hand**

   ✓6ᵗʰ   **S60.54**   **External constriction** of hand
     ✓7ᵗʰ   **S60.541**   **External constriction of** right **hand**
     ✓7ᵗʰ   **S60.542**   **External constriction of** left **hand**
     ✓7ᵗʰ   **S60.549**   **External constriction of unspecified hand**

   ✓6ᵗʰ   **S60.55**   **Superficial** foreign body **of hand**
       Splinter in the hand
     ✓7ᵗʰ   **S60.551**   **Superficial foreign body of** right **hand**
     ✓7ᵗʰ   **S60.552**   **Superficial foreign body of** left **hand**
     ✓7ᵗʰ   **S60.559**   **Superficial foreign body of unspecified hand**

   ✓6ᵗʰ   **S60.56**   **Insect bite (nonvenomous)** of hand
     ✓7ᵗʰ   **S60.561**   **Insect bite (nonvenomous) of** right **hand**
     ✓7ᵗʰ   **S60.562**   **Insect bite (nonvenomous) of** left **hand**
     ✓7ᵗʰ   **S60.569**   **Insect bite (nonvenomous) of unspecified hand**

   ✓6ᵗʰ   **S60.57**   **Other** superficial bite **of hand**
     EXCLUDES 1   *open bite of hand (S61.45-)*
     ✓7ᵗʰ   **S60.571**   **Other superficial bite of hand of** right **hand**
     ✓7ᵗʰ   **S60.572**   **Other superficial bite of hand of** left **hand**
     ✓7ᵗʰ   **S60.579**   **Other superficial bite of hand of unspecified hand**

✓5ᵗʰ   **S60.8**   **Other superficial injuries of** wrist

   ✓6ᵗʰ   **S60.81**   **Abrasion** of wrist
     ✓7ᵗʰ   **S60.811**   **Abrasion of** right **wrist**
     ✓7ᵗʰ   **S60.812**   **Abrasion of** left **wrist**
     ✓7ᵗʰ   **S60.819**   **Abrasion of unspecified wrist**

   ✓6ᵗʰ   **S60.82**   **Blister (nonthermal)** of wrist
     ✓7ᵗʰ   **S60.821**   **Blister (nonthermal) of** right **wrist**
     ✓7ᵗʰ   **S60.822**   **Blister (nonthermal) of** left **wrist**
     ✓7ᵗʰ   **S60.829**   **Blister (nonthermal) of unspecified wrist**

   ✓6ᵗʰ   **S60.84**   **External constriction** of wrist
     ✓7ᵗʰ   **S60.841**   **External constriction of** right **wrist**
     ✓7ᵗʰ   **S60.842**   **External constriction of** left **wrist**
     ✓7ᵗʰ   **S60.849**   **External constriction of unspecified wrist**

   ✓6ᵗʰ   **S60.85**   **Superficial** foreign body **of wrist**
       Splinter in the wrist
     ✓7ᵗʰ   **S60.851**   **Superficial foreign body of** right **wrist**
     ✓7ᵗʰ   **S60.852**   **Superficial foreign body of** left **wrist**
     ✓7ᵗʰ   **S60.859**   **Superficial foreign body of unspecified wrist**

   ✓6ᵗʰ   **S60.86**   **Insect bite (nonvenomous)** of wrist
     ✓7ᵗʰ   **S60.861**   **Insect bite (nonvenomous) of** right **wrist**
     ✓7ᵗʰ   **S60.862**   **Insect bite (nonvenomous) of** left **wrist**
     ✓7ᵗʰ   **S60.869**   **Insect bite (nonvenomous) of unspecified wrist**

   ✓6ᵗʰ   **S60.87**   **Other** superficial bite **of wrist**
     EXCLUDES 1   *open bite of wrist (S61.55)*
     ✓7ᵗʰ   **S60.871**   **Other superficial bite of** right **wrist**
     ✓7ᵗʰ   **S60.872**   **Other superficial bite of** left **wrist**
     ✓7ᵗʰ   **S60.879**   **Other superficial bite of unspecified wrist**

✓5ᵗʰ   **S60.9**   **Unspecified** superficial injury of wrist, hand and fingers

   ✓6ᵗʰ   **S60.91**   **Unspecified superficial injury of** wrist

---

     ✓7ᵗʰ   **S60.911**   **Unspecified superficial injury of** right **wrist**
     ✓7ᵗʰ   **S60.912**   **Unspecified superficial injury of** left **wrist**
     ✓7ᵗʰ   **S60.919**   **Unspecified superficial injury of unspecified wrist**

   ✓6ᵗʰ   **S60.92**   **Unspecified superficial injury of** hand
     ✓7ᵗʰ   **S60.921**   **Unspecified superficial injury of** right **hand**
     ✓7ᵗʰ   **S60.922**   **Unspecified superficial injury of** left **hand**
     ✓7ᵗʰ   **S60.929**   **Unspecified superficial injury of unspecified hand**

   ✓6ᵗʰ   **S60.93**   **Unspecified superficial injury of** thumb
     ✓7ᵗʰ   **S60.931**   **Unspecified superficial injury of** right **thumb**
     ✓7ᵗʰ   **S60.932**   **Unspecified superficial injury of** left **thumb**
     ✓7ᵗʰ   **S60.939**   **Unspecified superficial injury of unspecified thumb**

   ✓6ᵗʰ   **S60.94**   **Unspecified superficial injury of other** fingers
     ✓7ᵗʰ   **S60.940**   **Unspecified superficial injury of** right index **finger**
     ✓7ᵗʰ   **S60.941**   **Unspecified superficial injury of** left index **finger**
     ✓7ᵗʰ   **S60.942**   **Unspecified superficial injury of** right middle **finger**
     ✓7ᵗʰ   **S60.943**   **Unspecified superficial injury of** left middle **finger**
     ✓7ᵗʰ   **S60.944**   **Unspecified superficial injury of** right ring **finger**
     ✓7ᵗʰ   **S60.945**   **Unspecified superficial injury of** left ring **finger**
     ✓7ᵗʰ   **S60.946**   **Unspecified superficial injury of** right little **finger**
     ✓7ᵗʰ   **S60.947**   **Unspecified superficial injury of** left little **finger**
     ✓7ᵗʰ   **S60.948**   **Unspecified superficial injury of other finger**
       Unspecified superficial injury of specified finger with unspecified laterality
     ✓7ᵗʰ   **S60.949**   **Unspecified superficial injury of unspecified finger**

✓4ᵗʰ   **S61**   **Open wound of wrist, hand and fingers**
   Code also any associated wound infection
     EXCLUDES 1   *open fracture of wrist, hand and finger (S62- with 7th character B)*
           traumatic amputation of wrist and hand (S68.-)

> The appropriate 7th character is to be added to each code from category S61.
> A   initial encounter
> D   subsequent encounter
> S   sequela

✓5ᵗʰ   **S61.0**   **Open wound of** thumb without damage to nail
     EXCLUDES 1   *open wound of thumb with damage to nail (S61.1-)*

   ✓6ᵗʰ   **S61.00**   **Unspecified open wound of thumb without damage to nail**
     ✓7ᵗʰ   **S61.001**   **Unspecified open wound of** right **thumb without damage to nail**
     ✓7ᵗʰ   **S61.002**   **Unspecified open wound of** left **thumb without damage to nail**
     ✓7ᵗʰ   **S61.009**   **Unspecified open wound of unspecified thumb without damage to nail**

   ✓6ᵗʰ   **S61.01**   **Laceration without foreign body of thumb without damage to nail**
     ✓7ᵗʰ   **S61.011**   **Laceration without foreign body of** right **thumb without damage to nail**
     ✓7ᵗʰ   **S61.012**   **Laceration without foreign body of** left **thumb without damage to nail**
     ✓7ᵗʰ   **S61.019**   **Laceration without foreign body of unspecified thumb without damage to nail**

   ✓6ᵗʰ   **S61.02**   **Laceration with foreign body of thumb without damage to nail**
     ✓7ᵗʰ   **S61.021**   **Laceration with foreign body of** right **thumb without damage to nail**

EXCLUDES 1 Not coded here   EXCLUDES 2 Not included here   N Newborn Age: 0   P Pediatric Age: 0–17   M Maternity Age: 12–55   A Adult Age: 15–124

866   ICD-10-CM 2014 (Draft)

√7th **S61.022** Laceration with foreign body of left thumb without damage to nail

√7th **S61.029** Laceration with foreign body of unspecified thumb without damage to nail

√6th **S61.03** Puncture wound without foreign body of thumb without damage to nail

√7th **S61.031** Puncture wound without foreign body of right thumb without damage to nail

√7th **S61.032** Puncture wound without foreign body of left thumb without damage to nail

√7th **S61.039** Puncture wound without foreign body of unspecified thumb without damage to nail

√6th **S61.04** Puncture wound with foreign body of thumb without damage to nail

√7th **S61.041** Puncture wound with foreign body of right thumb without damage to nail

√7th **S61.042** Puncture wound with foreign body of left thumb without damage to nail

√7th **S61.049** Puncture wound with foreign body of unspecified thumb without damage to nail

√6th **S61.05** Open bite of thumb without damage to nail
Bite of thumb NOS
EXCLUDES 1 superficial bite of thumb (S60.36-, S60.37-)

√7th **S61.051** Open bite of right thumb without damage to nail

√7th **S61.052** Open bite of left thumb without damage to nail

√7th **S61.059** Open bite of unspecified thumb without damage to nail

√5th **S61.1** Open wound of thumb with damage to nail

√6th **S61.10** Unspecified open wound of thumb with damage to nail

√7th **S61.101** Unspecified open wound of right thumb with damage to nail

√7th **S61.102** Unspecified open wound of left thumb with damage to nail

√7th **S61.109** Unspecified open wound of unspecified thumb with damage to nail

√6th **S61.11** Laceration without foreign body of thumb with damage to nail

√7th **S61.111** Laceration without foreign body of right thumb with damage to nail

√7th **S61.112** Laceration without foreign body of left thumb with damage to nail

√7th **S61.119** Laceration without foreign body of unspecified thumb with damage to nail

√6th **S61.12** Laceration with foreign body of thumb with damage to nail

√7th **S61.121** Laceration with foreign body of right thumb with damage to nail

√7th **S61.122** Laceration with foreign body of left thumb with damage to nail

√7th **S61.129** Laceration with foreign body of unspecified thumb with damage to nail

√6th **S61.13** Puncture wound without foreign body of thumb with damage to nail

√7th **S61.131** Puncture wound without foreign body of right thumb with damage to nail

√7th **S61.132** Puncture wound without foreign body of left thumb with damage to nail

√7th **S61.139** Puncture wound without foreign body of unspecified thumb with damage to nail

√6th **S61.14** Puncture wound with foreign body of thumb with damage to nail

√7th **S61.141** Puncture wound with foreign body of right thumb with damage to nail

√7th **S61.142** Puncture wound with foreign body of left thumb with damage to nail

√7th **S61.149** Puncture wound with foreign body of unspecified thumb with damage to nail

√6th **S61.15** Open bite of thumb with damage to nail
Bite of thumb with damage to nail NOS
EXCLUDES 1 superficial bite of thumb (S60.36-, S60.37-)

√7th **S61.151** Open bite of right thumb with damage to nail

√7th **S61.152** Open bite of left thumb with damage to nail

√7th **S61.159** Open bite of unspecified thumb with damage to nail

√5th **S61.2** Open wound of other finger without damage to nail
EXCLUDES 1 open wound of finger involving nail (matrix) (S61.3-)
EXCLUDES 2 open wound of thumb without damage to nail (S61.0-)

√6th **S61.20** Unspecified open wound of other finger without damage to nail

√7th **S61.200** Unspecified open wound of right index finger without damage to nail

√7th **S61.201** Unspecified open wound of left index finger without damage to nail

√7th **S61.202** Unspecified open wound of right middle finger without damage to nail

√7th **S61.203** Unspecified open wound of left middle finger without damage to nail

√7th **S61.204** Unspecified open wound of right ring finger without damage to nail

√7th **S61.205** Unspecified open wound of left ring finger without damage to nail

√7th **S61.206** Unspecified open wound of right little finger without damage to nail

√7th **S61.207** Unspecified open wound of left little finger without damage to nail

√7th **S61.208** Unspecified open wound of other finger without damage to nail
Unspecified open wound of specified finger with unspecified laterality without damage to nail

√7th **S61.209** Unspecified open wound of unspecified finger without damage to nail

√6th **S61.21** Laceration without foreign body of finger without damage to nail

√7th **S61.210** Laceration without foreign body of right index finger without damage to nail

√7th **S61.211** Laceration without foreign body of left index finger without damage to nail

√7th **S61.212** Laceration without foreign body of right middle finger without damage to nail

√7th **S61.213** Laceration without foreign body of left middle finger without damage to nail

√7th **S61.214** Laceration without foreign body of right ring finger without damage to nail

√7th **S61.215** Laceration without foreign body of left ring finger without damage to nail

√7th **S61.216** Laceration without foreign body of right little finger without damage to nail

√7th **S61.217** Laceration without foreign body of left little finger without damage to nail

√7th **S61.218** Laceration without foreign body of other finger without damage to nail
Laceration without foreign body of specified finger with unspecified laterality without damage to nail

√7th **S61.219** Laceration without foreign body of unspecified finger without damage to nail

√6th **S61.22** Laceration with foreign body of finger without damage to nail

√7th **S61.220** Laceration with foreign body of right index finger without damage to nail

√7th **S61.221** Laceration with foreign body of left index finger without damage to nail

√7th **S61.222** Laceration with foreign body of right middle finger without damage to nail

√7th **S61.223** Laceration with foreign body of left middle finger without damage to nail

√7th **S61.224** Laceration with foreign body of right ring finger without damage to nail

√7th **S61.225** Laceration with foreign body of left ring finger without damage to nail

√7th **S61.226** Laceration with foreign body of right little finger without damage to nail

✓7ᵗʰ **S61.227** **Laceration with foreign body of** left little finger **without damage to nail**

✓7ᵗʰ **S61.228** **Laceration with foreign body of other finger without damage to nail**
Laceration with foreign body of specified finger with unspecified laterality without damage to nail

✓7ᵗʰ **S61.229** **Laceration with foreign body of unspecified finger without damage to nail**

✓6ᵗʰ **S61.23** Puncture wound without foreign body **of finger without damage to nail**

✓7ᵗʰ **S61.230** **Puncture wound without foreign body of** right index **finger without damage to nail**

✓7ᵗʰ **S61.231** **Puncture wound without foreign body of** left index **finger without damage to nail**

✓7ᵗʰ **S61.232** **Puncture wound without foreign body of** right middle **finger without damage to nail**

✓7ᵗʰ **S61.233** **Puncture wound without foreign body of** left middle **finger without damage to nail**

✓7ᵗʰ **S61.234** **Puncture wound without foreign body of** right ring **finger without damage to nail**

✓7ᵗʰ **S61.235** **Puncture wound without foreign body of** left ring **finger without damage to nail**

✓7ᵗʰ **S61.236** **Puncture wound without foreign body of** right little **finger without damage to nail**

✓7ᵗʰ **S61.237** **Puncture wound without foreign body of** left little **finger without damage to nail**

✓7ᵗʰ **S61.238** **Puncture wound without foreign body of other finger without damage to nail**
Puncture wound without foreign body of specified finger with unspecified laterality without damage to nail

✓7ᵗʰ **S61.239** **Puncture wound without foreign body of unspecified finger without damage to nail**

✓6ᵗʰ **S61.24** Puncture wound with foreign body **of finger without damage to nail**

✓7ᵗʰ **S61.240** **Puncture wound with foreign body of** right index **finger without damage to nail**

✓7ᵗʰ **S61.241** **Puncture wound with foreign body of** left index **finger without damage to nail**

✓7ᵗʰ **S61.242** **Puncture wound with foreign body of** right middle **finger without damage to nail**

✓7ᵗʰ **S61.243** **Puncture wound with foreign body of** left middle **finger without damage to nail**

✓7ᵗʰ **S61.244** **Puncture wound with foreign body of** right ring **finger without damage to nail**

✓7ᵗʰ **S61.245** **Puncture wound with foreign body of** left ring **finger without damage to nail**

✓7ᵗʰ **S61.246** **Puncture wound with foreign body of** right little **finger without damage to nail**

✓7ᵗʰ **S61.247** **Puncture wound with foreign body of** left little **finger without damage to nail**

✓7ᵗʰ **S61.248** **Puncture wound with foreign body of other finger without damage to nail**
Puncture wound with foreign body of specified finger with unspecified laterality without damage to nail

✓7ᵗʰ **S61.249** **Puncture wound with foreign body of unspecified finger without damage to nail**

✓6ᵗʰ **S61.25** Open bite **of finger without damage to nail**
Bite of finger without damage to nail NOS
EXCLUDES 1 *superficial bite of finger (S60.46-, S60.47-)*

✓7ᵗʰ **S61.250** **Open bite of** right index **finger without damage to nail**

✓7ᵗʰ **S61.251** **Open bite of** left index **finger without damage to nail**

✓7ᵗʰ **S61.252** **Open bite of** right middle **finger without damage to nail**

✓7ᵗʰ **S61.253** **Open bite of** left middle **finger without damage to nail**

✓7ᵗʰ **S61.254** **Open bite of** right ring **finger without damage to nail**

✓7ᵗʰ **S61.255** **Open bite of** left ring **finger without damage to nail**

✓7ᵗʰ **S61.256** **Open bite of** right little **finger without damage to nail**

✓7ᵗʰ **S61.257** **Open bite of** left little **finger without damage to nail**

✓7ᵗʰ **S61.258** **Open bite of other finger without damage to nail**
Open bite of specified finger with unspecified laterality without damage to nail

✓7ᵗʰ **S61.259** **Open bite of unspecified finger without damage to nail**

✓5ᵗʰ **S61.3** Open wound of other finger with damage to nail

✓6ᵗʰ **S61.30** Unspecified **open wound of finger with damage to nail**

✓7ᵗʰ **S61.300** **Unspecified open wound of** right index **finger with damage to nail**

✓7ᵗʰ **S61.301** **Unspecified open wound of** left index **finger with damage to nail**

✓7ᵗʰ **S61.302** **Unspecified open wound of** right middle **finger with damage to nail**

✓7ᵗʰ **S61.303** **Unspecified open wound of** left middle **finger with damage to nail**

✓7ᵗʰ **S61.304** **Unspecified open wound of** right ring **finger with damage to nail**

✓7ᵗʰ **S61.305** **Unspecified open wound of** left ring **finger with damage to nail**

✓7ᵗʰ **S61.306** **Unspecified open wound of** right little **finger with damage to nail**

✓7ᵗʰ **S61.307** **Unspecified open wound of** left little **finger with damage to nail**

✓7ᵗʰ **S61.308** **Unspecified open wound of other finger with damage to nail**
Unspecified open wound of specified finger with unspecified laterality with damage to nail

✓7ᵗʰ **S61.309** **Unspecified open wound of unspecified finger with damage to nail**

✓6ᵗʰ **S61.31** Laceration without foreign body **of finger with damage to nail**

✓7ᵗʰ **S61.310** **Laceration without foreign body of** right index **finger with damage to nail**

✓7ᵗʰ **S61.311** **Laceration without foreign body of** left index **finger with damage to nail**

✓7ᵗʰ **S61.312** **Laceration without foreign body of** right middle **finger with damage to nail**

✓7ᵗʰ **S61.313** **Laceration without foreign body of** left middle **finger with damage to nail**

✓7ᵗʰ **S61.314** **Laceration without foreign body of** right ring **finger with damage to nail**

✓7ᵗʰ **S61.315** **Laceration without foreign body of** left ring **finger with damage to nail**

✓7ᵗʰ **S61.316** **Laceration without foreign body of** right little **finger with damage to nail**

✓7ᵗʰ **S61.317** **Laceration without foreign body of** left little **finger with damage to nail**

✓7ᵗʰ **S61.318** **Laceration without foreign body of other finger with damage to nail**
Laceration without foreign body of specified finger with unspecified laterality with damage to nail

✓7ᵗʰ **S61.319** **Laceration without foreign body of unspecified finger with damage to nail**

✓6ᵗʰ **S61.32** Laceration with foreign body **of finger with damage to nail**

✓7ᵗʰ **S61.320** **Laceration with foreign body of** right index **finger with damage to nail**

✓7ᵗʰ **S61.321** **Laceration with foreign body of** left index **finger with damage to nail**

✓7ᵗʰ **S61.322** **Laceration with foreign body of** right middle **finger with damage to nail**

✓7ᵗʰ **S61.323** **Laceration with foreign body of** left middle **finger with damage to nail**

✓7ᵗʰ **S61.324** **Laceration with foreign body of** right ring **finger with damage to nail**

✓7ᵗʰ **S61.325** **Laceration with foreign body of** left ring **finger with damage to nail**

EXCLUDES 1 Not coded here   EXCLUDES 2 Not included here   N Newborn Age: 0   P Pediatric Age: 0-17   M Maternity Age: 12-55   A Adult Age: 15-124

868   ICD-10-CM 2014 (Draft)

√7th **S61.326** Laceration with foreign body of right little finger with damage to nail

√7th **S61.327** Laceration with foreign body of left little finger with damage to nail

√7th **S61.328** Laceration with foreign body of other finger with damage to nail
Laceration with foreign body of specified finger with unspecified laterality with damage to nail

√7th **S61.329** Laceration with foreign body of unspecified finger with damage to nail

√6th **S61.33** Puncture wound without foreign body of finger with damage to nail

√7th **S61.330** Puncture wound without foreign body of right index finger with damage to nail

√7th **S61.331** Puncture wound without foreign body of left index finger with damage to nail

√7th **S61.332** Puncture wound without foreign body of right middle finger with damage to nail

√7th **S61.333** Puncture wound without foreign body of left middle finger with damage to nail

√7th **S61.334** Puncture wound without foreign body of right ring finger with damage to nail

√7th **S61.335** Puncture wound without foreign body of left ring finger with damage to nail

√7th **S61.336** Puncture wound without foreign body of right little finger with damage to nail

√7th **S61.337** Puncture wound without foreign body of left little finger with damage to nail

√7th **S61.338** Puncture wound without foreign body of other finger with damage to nail
Puncture wound without foreign body of specified finger with unspecified laterality with damage to nail

√7th **S61.339** Puncture wound without foreign body of unspecified finger with damage to nail

√6th **S61.34** Puncture wound with foreign body of finger with damage to nail

√7th **S61.340** Puncture wound with foreign body of right index finger with damage to nail

√7th **S61.341** Puncture wound with foreign body of left index finger with damage to nail

√7th **S61.342** Puncture wound with foreign body of right middle finger with damage to nail

√7th **S61.343** Puncture wound with foreign body of left middle finger with damage to nail

√7th **S61.344** Puncture wound with foreign body of right ring finger with damage to nail

√7th **S61.345** Puncture wound with foreign body of left ring finger with damage to nail

√7th **S61.346** Puncture wound with foreign body of right little finger with damage to nail

√7th **S61.347** Puncture wound with foreign body of left little finger with damage to nail

√7th **S61.348** Puncture wound with foreign body of other finger with damage to nail
Puncture wound with foreign body of specified finger with unspecified laterality with damage to nail

√7th **S61.349** Puncture wound with foreign body of unspecified finger with damage to nail

√6th **S61.35** Open bite of finger with damage to nail
Bite of finger with damage to nail NOS
EXCLUDES 1 superficial bite of finger (S60.46-, S60.47-)

√7th **S61.350** Open bite of right index finger with damage to nail

√7th **S61.351** Open bite of left index finger with damage to nail

√7th **S61.352** Open bite of right middle finger with damage to nail

√7th **S61.353** Open bite of left middle finger with damage to nail

√7th **S61.354** Open bite of right ring finger with damage to nail

√7th **S61.355** Open bite of left ring finger with damage to nail

√7th **S61.356** Open bite of right little finger with damage to nail

√7th **S61.357** Open bite of left little finger with damage to nail

√7th **S61.358** Open bite of other finger with damage to nail
Open bite of specified finger with unspecified laterality with damage to nail

√7th **S61.359** Open bite of unspecified finger with damage to nail

√5th **S61.4** Open wound of hand

√6th **S61.40** Unspecified open wound of hand

√7th **S61.401** Unspecified open wound of right hand

√7th **S61.402** Unspecified open wound of left hand

√7th **S61.409** Unspecified open wound of unspecified hand

√6th **S61.41** Laceration without foreign body of hand

√7th **S61.411** Laceration without foreign body of right hand

√7th **S61.412** Laceration without foreign body of left hand

√7th **S61.419** Laceration without foreign body of unspecified hand

√6th **S61.42** Laceration with foreign body of hand

√7th **S61.421** Laceration with foreign body of right hand

√7th **S61.422** Laceration with foreign body of left hand

√7th **S61.429** Laceration with foreign body of unspecified hand

√6th **S61.43** Puncture wound without foreign body of hand

√7th **S61.431** Puncture wound without foreign body of right hand

√7th **S61.432** Puncture wound without foreign body of left hand

√7th **S61.439** Puncture wound without foreign body of unspecified hand

√6th **S61.44** Puncture wound with foreign body of hand

√7th **S61.441** Puncture wound with foreign body of right hand

√7th **S61.442** Puncture wound with foreign body of left hand

√7th **S61.449** Puncture wound with foreign body of unspecified hand

√6th **S61.45** Open bite of hand
Bite of hand NOS
EXCLUDES 1 superficial bite of hand (S60.56-, S60.57-)

√7th **S61.451** Open bite of right hand

√7th **S61.452** Open bite of left hand

√7th **S61.459** Open bite of unspecified hand

√5th **S61.5** Open wound of wrist

√6th **S61.50** Unspecified open wound of wrist

√7th **S61.501** Unspecified open wound of right wrist

√7th **S61.502** Unspecified open wound of left wrist

√7th **S61.509** Unspecified open wound of unspecified wrist

√6th **S61.51** Laceration without foreign body of wrist

√7th **S61.511** Laceration without foreign body of right wrist

√7th **S61.512** Laceration without foreign body of left wrist

√7th **S61.519** Laceration without foreign body of unspecified wrist

√6th **S61.52** Laceration with foreign body of wrist

√7th **S61.521** Laceration with foreign body of right wrist

√7th **S61.522** Laceration with foreign body of left wrist

√7th **S61.529** Laceration with foreign body of unspecified wrist

√6th **S61.53** Puncture wound without foreign body of wrist

√7th **S61.531** Puncture wound without foreign body of right wrist

√7th **S61.532** Puncture wound without foreign body of left wrist

☑ Additional Character Required   √x7th Xtension Alert   Unspecified Code   Other Specified Code   Manifestation Code   ▶◀ Revised Text   ● New Code   ▲ Revised Code Title

ICD-10-CM 2014 (Draft)   **869**

Injury, Poisoning and Certain Other Consequences of External Causes

✓7th **S61.539** **Puncture wound without foreign body of unspecified wrist**

✓6th **S61.54** Puncture wound with foreign body of wrist

    ✓7th **S61.541** **Puncture wound with foreign body of right wrist**

    ✓7th **S61.542** **Puncture wound with foreign body of left wrist**

    ✓7th **S61.549** **Puncture wound with foreign body of unspecified wrist**

✓6th **S61.55** Open bite of wrist
    Bite of wrist NOS
    EXCLUDES 1   superficial bite of wrist (S60.86-, S60.87-)

    ✓7th **S61.551** **Open bite of right wrist**

    ✓7th **S61.552** **Open bite of left wrist**

    ✓7th **S61.559** **Open bite of unspecified wrist**

✓4th **S62** **Fracture at wrist and hand level**

    NOTE   A fracture not indicated as displaced or nondisplaced should be coded to displaced.
    A fracture not indicated as open or closed should be coded to closed.

    EXCLUDES 1   traumatic amputation of wrist and hand (S68.-)
    EXCLUDES 2   fracture of distal parts of ulna and radius (S52.-)

The appropriate 7th character is to be added to each code from category S62.
A   initial encounter for closed fracture
B   initial encounter for open fracture
D   subsequent encounter for fracture with routine healing
G   subsequent encounter for fracture with delayed healing
K   subsequent encounter for fracture with nonunion
P   subsequent encounter for fracture with malunion
S   sequela

✓5th **S62.0** Fracture of navicular [scaphoid] bone of wrist

    ✓6th **S62.00** Unspecified fracture of navicular [scaphoid] bone of wrist

        ✓7th **S62.001** **Unspecified fracture of navicular [scaphoid] bone of right wrist**

        ✓7th **S62.002** **Unspecified fracture of navicular [scaphoid] bone of left wrist**
            AHA: 2012, Q4, 106

        ✓7th **S62.009** **Unspecified fracture of navicular [scaphoid] bone of unspecified wrist**

    ✓6th **S62.01** Fracture of distal pole of navicular [scaphoid] bone of wrist
        Fracture of volar tuberosity of navicular [scaphoid] bone of wrist

        ✓7th **S62.011** Displaced **fracture of distal pole of navicular [scaphoid] bone of right wrist**

        ✓7th **S62.012** Displaced **fracture of distal pole of navicular [scaphoid] bone of left wrist**

        ✓7th **S62.013** Displaced **fracture of distal pole of navicular [scaphoid] bone of unspecified wrist**

        ✓7th **S62.014** Nondisplaced **fracture of distal pole of navicular [scaphoid] bone of right wrist**

        ✓7th **S62.015** Nondisplaced **fracture of distal pole of navicular [scaphoid] bone of left wrist**

        ✓7th **S62.016** Nondisplaced **fracture of distal pole of navicular [scaphoid] bone of unspecified wrist**

    ✓6th **S62.02** Fracture of middle third of navicular [scaphoid] bone of wrist

        ✓7th **S62.021** Displaced **fracture of middle third of navicular [scaphoid] bone of right wrist**

        ✓7th **S62.022** Displaced **fracture of middle third of navicular [scaphoid] bone of left wrist**

        ✓7th **S62.023** Displaced **fracture of middle third of navicular [scaphoid] bone of unspecified wrist**

        ✓7th **S62.024** Nondisplaced **fracture of middle third of navicular [scaphoid] bone of right wrist**

        ✓7th **S62.025** Nondisplaced **fracture of middle third of navicular [scaphoid] bone of left wrist**

        ✓7th **S62.026** Nondisplaced **fracture of middle third of navicular [scaphoid] bone of unspecified wrist**

✓6th **S62.03** Fracture of proximal third of navicular [scaphoid] bone of wrist

    ✓7th **S62.031** Displaced **fracture of proximal third of navicular [scaphoid] bone of right wrist**

    ✓7th **S62.032** Displaced **fracture of proximal third of navicular [scaphoid] bone of left wrist**

    ✓7th **S62.033** Displaced **fracture of proximal third of navicular [scaphoid] bone of unspecified wrist**

    ✓7th **S62.034** Nondisplaced **fracture of proximal third of navicular [scaphoid] bone of right wrist**

    ✓7th **S62.035** Nondisplaced **fracture of proximal third of navicular [scaphoid] bone of left wrist**

    ✓7th **S62.036** Nondisplaced **fracture of proximal third of navicular [scaphoid] bone of unspecified wrist**

✓5th **S62.1** Fracture of other and unspecified carpal bone(s)
    EXCLUDES 2   fracture of scaphoid of wrist (S62.0-)

    ✓6th **S62.10** Fracture of unspecified carpal bone
        Fracture of wrist NOS

        ✓7th **S62.101** **Fracture of unspecified carpal bone, right wrist**

        ✓7th **S62.102** **Fracture of unspecified carpal bone, left wrist**
            AHA: 2012, Q4, 95

        ✓7th **S62.109** **Fracture of unspecified carpal bone, unspecified wrist**

    ✓6th **S62.11** Fracture of triquetrum [cuneiform] bone of wrist

        ✓7th **S62.111** Displaced **fracture of triquetrum [cuneiform] bone, right wrist**

        ✓7th **S62.112** Displaced **fracture of triquetrum [cuneiform] bone, left wrist**

        ✓7th **S62.113** Displaced **fracture of triquetrum [cuneiform] bone, unspecified wrist**

        ✓7th **S62.114** Nondisplaced **fracture of triquetrum [cuneiform] bone, right wrist**

        ✓7th **S62.115** Nondisplaced **fracture of triquetrum [cuneiform] bone, left wrist**

        ✓7th **S62.116** Nondisplaced **fracture of triquetrum [cuneiform] bone, unspecified wrist**

    ✓6th **S62.12** Fracture of lunate [semilunar]

        ✓7th **S62.121** Displaced **fracture of lunate [semilunar], right wrist**

        ✓7th **S62.122** Displaced **fracture of lunate [semilunar], left wrist**

        ✓7th **S62.123** Displaced **fracture of lunate [semilunar], unspecified wrist**

        ✓7th **S62.124** Nondisplaced **fracture of lunate [semilunar], right wrist**

        ✓7th **S62.125** Nondisplaced **fracture of lunate [semilunar], left wrist**

        ✓7th **S62.126** Nondisplaced **fracture of lunate [semilunar], unspecified wrist**

    ✓6th **S62.13** Fracture of capitate [os magnum] bone

        ✓7th **S62.131** Displaced **fracture of capitate [os magnum] bone, right wrist**

        ✓7th **S62.132** Displaced **fracture of capitate [os magnum] bone, left wrist**

        ✓7th **S62.133** Displaced **fracture of capitate [os magnum] bone, unspecified wrist**

        ✓7th **S62.134** Nondisplaced **fracture of capitate [os magnum] bone, right wrist**

        ✓7th **S62.135** Nondisplaced **fracture of capitate [os magnum] bone, left wrist**

        ✓7th **S62.136** Nondisplaced **fracture of capitate [os magnum] bone, unspecified wrist**

    ✓6th **S62.14** Fracture of body of hamate [unciform] bone
        Fracture of hamate [unciform] bone NOS

        ✓7th **S62.141** Displaced **fracture of body of hamate [unciform] bone, right wrist**

        ✓7th **S62.142** Displaced **fracture of body of hamate [unciform] bone, left wrist**

        ✓7th **S62.143** Displaced **fracture of body of hamate [unciform] bone, unspecified wrist**

EXCLUDES 1 Not coded here   *EXCLUDES 2* Not included here   **N** Newborn Age: 0   **P** Pediatric Age: 0-17   **M** Maternity Age: 12-55   **A** Adult Age: 15-124

870   ICD-10-CM 2014 (Draft)

√7ᵗʰ **S62.144** Nondisplaced **fracture of body of hamate [unciform] bone**, **right wrist**

√7ᵗʰ **S62.145** Nondisplaced **fracture of body of hamate [unciform] bone, left wrist**

√7ᵗʰ **S62.146** Nondisplaced **fracture of body of hamate [unciform] bone, unspecified wrist**

√6ᵗʰ **S62.15** Fracture of hook process of hamate [unciform] bone
Fracture of unciform process of hamate [unciform] bone

√7ᵗʰ **S62.151** Displaced **fracture of hook process of hamate [unciform] bone, right wrist**

√7ᵗʰ **S62.152** Displaced **fracture of hook process of hamate [unciform] bone, left wrist**

√7ᵗʰ **S62.153** Displaced **fracture of hook process of hamate [unciform] bone, unspecified wrist**

√7ᵗʰ **S62.154** Nondisplaced **fracture of hook process of hamate [unciform] bone, right wrist**

√7ᵗʰ **S62.155** Nondisplaced **fracture of hook process of hamate [unciform] bone, left wrist**

√7ᵗʰ **S62.156** Nondisplaced **fracture of hook process of hamate [unciform] bone, unspecified wrist**

√6ᵗʰ **S62.16** Fracture of pisiform

√7ᵗʰ **S62.161** Displaced **fracture of pisiform, right wrist**

√7ᵗʰ **S62.162** Displaced **fracture of pisiform, left wrist**

√7ᵗʰ **S62.163** Displaced **fracture of pisiform, unspecified wrist**

√7ᵗʰ **S62.164** Nondisplaced **fracture of pisiform, right wrist**

√7ᵗʰ **S62.165** Nondisplaced **fracture of pisiform, left wrist**

√7ᵗʰ **S62.166** Nondisplaced **fracture of pisiform, unspecified wrist**

√6ᵗʰ **S62.17** Fracture of trapezium [larger multangular]

√7ᵗʰ **S62.171** Displaced **fracture of trapezium [larger multangular], right wrist**

√7ᵗʰ **S62.172** Displaced **fracture of trapezium [larger multangular], left wrist**

√7ᵗʰ **S62.173** Displaced **fracture of trapezium [larger multangular], unspecified wrist**

√7ᵗʰ **S62.174** Nondisplaced **fracture of trapezium [larger multangular], right wrist**

√7ᵗʰ **S62.175** Nondisplaced **fracture of trapezium [larger multangular], left wrist**

√7ᵗʰ **S62.176** Nondisplaced **fracture of trapezium [larger multangular], unspecified wrist**

√6ᵗʰ **S62.18** Fracture of trapezoid [smaller multangular]

√7ᵗʰ **S62.181** Displaced **fracture of trapezoid [smaller multangular], right wrist**

√7ᵗʰ **S62.182** Displaced **fracture of trapezoid [smaller multangular], left wrist**

√7ᵗʰ **S62.183** Displaced **fracture of trapezoid [smaller multangular], unspecified wrist**

√7ᵗʰ **S62.184** Nondisplaced **fracture of trapezoid [smaller multangular], right wrist**

√7ᵗʰ **S62.185** Nondisplaced **fracture of trapezoid [smaller multangular], left wrist**

√7ᵗʰ **S62.186** Nondisplaced **fracture of trapezoid [smaller multangular], unspecified wrist**

√5ᵗʰ **S62.2** Fracture of first metacarpal bone

√6ᵗʰ **S62.20** Unspecified fracture of first metacarpal bone

√7ᵗʰ **S62.201** Unspecified **fracture of first metacarpal bone, right hand**

√7ᵗʰ **S62.202** Unspecified **fracture of first metacarpal bone, left hand**

√7ᵗʰ **S62.209** Unspecified **fracture of first metacarpal bone, unspecified hand**

√6ᵗʰ **S62.21** Bennett's fracture

√7ᵗʰ **S62.211** Bennett's **fracture, right hand**

√7ᵗʰ **S62.212** Bennett's **fracture, left hand**

√7ᵗʰ **S62.213** Bennett's **fracture, unspecified hand**

√6ᵗʰ **S62.22** Rolando's fracture

√7ᵗʰ **S62.221** Displaced **Rolando's fracture, right hand**

√7ᵗʰ **S62.222** Displaced **Rolando's fracture, left hand**

√7ᵗʰ **S62.223** Displaced **Rolando's fracture, unspecified hand**

√7ᵗʰ **S62.224** Nondisplaced **Rolando's fracture, right hand**

√7ᵗʰ **S62.225** Nondisplaced **Rolando's fracture, left hand**

√7ᵗʰ **S62.226** Nondisplaced **Rolando's fracture, unspecified hand**

√6ᵗʰ **S62.23** Other fracture of base of first metacarpal bone

√7ᵗʰ **S62.231** Other displaced **fracture of base of first metacarpal bone, right hand**

√7ᵗʰ **S62.232** Other displaced **fracture of base of first metacarpal bone, left hand**

√7ᵗʰ **S62.233** Other displaced **fracture of base of first metacarpal bone, unspecified hand**

√7ᵗʰ **S62.234** Other nondisplaced **fracture of base of first metacarpal bone, right hand**

√7ᵗʰ **S62.235** Other nondisplaced **fracture of base of first metacarpal bone, left hand**

√7ᵗʰ **S62.236** Other nondisplaced **fracture of base of first metacarpal bone, unspecified hand**

√6ᵗʰ **S62.24** Fracture of shaft of first metacarpal bone

√7ᵗʰ **S62.241** Displaced **fracture of shaft of first metacarpal bone, right hand**

√7ᵗʰ **S62.242** Displaced **fracture of shaft of first metacarpal bone, left hand**

√7ᵗʰ **S62.243** Displaced **fracture of shaft of first metacarpal bone, unspecified hand**

√7ᵗʰ **S62.244** Nondisplaced **fracture of shaft of first metacarpal bone, right hand**

√7ᵗʰ **S62.245** Nondisplaced **fracture of shaft of first metacarpal bone, left hand**

√7ᵗʰ **S62.246** Nondisplaced **fracture of shaft of first metacarpal bone, unspecified hand**

√6ᵗʰ **S62.25** Fracture of neck of first metacarpal bone

√7ᵗʰ **S62.251** Displaced **fracture of neck of first metacarpal bone, right hand**

√7ᵗʰ **S62.252** Displaced **fracture of neck of first metacarpal bone, left hand**

√7ᵗʰ **S62.253** Displaced **fracture of neck of first metacarpal bone, unspecified hand**

√7ᵗʰ **S62.254** Nondisplaced **fracture of neck of first metacarpal bone, right hand**

√7ᵗʰ **S62.255** Nondisplaced **fracture of neck of first metacarpal bone, left hand**

√7ᵗʰ **S62.256** Nondisplaced **fracture of neck of first metacarpal bone, unspecified hand**

√6ᵗʰ **S62.29** Other fracture of first metacarpal bone

√7ᵗʰ **S62.291** Other **fracture of first metacarpal bone, right hand**

√7ᵗʰ **S62.292** Other **fracture of first metacarpal bone, left hand**

√7ᵗʰ **S62.299** Other **fracture of first metacarpal bone, unspecified hand**

√5ᵗʰ **S62.3** Fracture of other and unspecified metacarpal bone
EXCLUDES 2 *fracture of first metacarpal bone (S62.2-)*

√6ᵗʰ **S62.30** Unspecified fracture of other metacarpal bone

√7ᵗʰ **S62.300** Unspecified **fracture of second metacarpal bone, right hand**

√7ᵗʰ **S62.301** Unspecified **fracture of second metacarpal bone, left hand**

√7ᵗʰ **S62.302** Unspecified **fracture of third metacarpal bone, right hand**

√7ᵗʰ **S62.303** Unspecified **fracture of third metacarpal bone, left hand**

√7ᵗʰ **S62.304** Unspecified **fracture of fourth metacarpal bone, right hand**

√7ᵗʰ **S62.305** Unspecified **fracture of fourth metacarpal bone, left hand**

√7ᵗʰ **S62.306** Unspecified **fracture of fifth metacarpal bone, right hand**

√7ᵗʰ **S62.307** Unspecified **fracture of fifth metacarpal bone, left hand**

☑ Additional Character Required　√x7ᵗʰ Xtension Alert　Unspecified Code　Other Specified Code　Manifestation Code　▶◀ Revised Text　● New Code　▲ Revised Code Title

ICD-10-CM 2014 (Draft)

871

Injury, Poisoning and Certain Other Consequences of External Causes

S62.308–S62.367

√7ᵗʰ **S62.308** **Unspecified fracture of other metacarpal bone**
Unspecified fracture of specified metacarpal bone with unspecified laterality

√7ᵗʰ **S62.309** **Unspecified fracture of unspecified metacarpal bone**

√6ᵗʰ **S62.31** Displaced fracture of base of other metacarpal bone

√7ᵗʰ **S62.310** **Displaced fracture of base of second metacarpal bone, right hand**

√7ᵗʰ **S62.311** **Displaced fracture of base of second metacarpal bone. left hand**

√7ᵗʰ **S62.312** **Displaced fracture of base of third metacarpal bone, right hand**

√7ᵗʰ **S62.313** **Displaced fracture of base of third metacarpal bone, left hand**

√7ᵗʰ **S62.314** **Displaced fracture of base of fourth metacarpal bone, right hand**

√7ᵗʰ **S62.315** **Displaced fracture of base of fourth metacarpal bone, left hand**

√7ᵗʰ **S62.316** **Displaced fracture of base of fifth metacarpal bone, right hand**

√7ᵗʰ **S62.317** **Displaced fracture of base of fifth metacarpal bone, left hand**

√7ᵗʰ **S62.318** **Displaced fracture of base of other metacarpal bone**
Displaced fracture of base of specified metacarpal bone with unspecified laterality

√7ᵗʰ **S62.319** **Displaced fracture of base of unspecified metacarpal bone**

√6ᵗʰ **S62.32** Displaced fracture of shaft of other metacarpal bone

√7ᵗʰ **S62.320** **Displaced fracture of shaft of second metacarpal bone, right hand**

√7ᵗʰ **S62.321** **Displaced fracture of shaft of second metacarpal bone, left hand**

√7ᵗʰ **S62.322** **Displaced fracture of shaft of third metacarpal bone, right hand**

√7ᵗʰ **S62.323** **Displaced fracture of shaft of third metacarpal bone, left hand**

√7ᵗʰ **S62.324** **Displaced fracture of shaft of fourth metacarpal bone, right hand**

√7ᵗʰ **S62.325** **Displaced fracture of shaft of fourth metacarpal bone, left hand**

√7ᵗʰ **S62.326** **Displaced fracture of shaft of fifth metacarpal bone, right hand**

√7ᵗʰ **S62.327** **Displaced fracture of shaft of fifth metacarpal bone, left hand**

√7ᵗʰ **S62.328** **Displaced fracture of shaft of other metacarpal bone**
Displaced fracture of shaft of specified metacarpal bone with unspecified laterality

√7ᵗʰ **S62.329** **Displaced fracture of shaft of unspecified metacarpal bone**

√6ᵗʰ **S62.33** Displaced fracture of neck of other metacarpal bone

√7ᵗʰ **S62.330** **Displaced fracture of neck of second metacarpal bone, right hand**

√7ᵗʰ **S62.331** **Displaced fracture of neck of second metacarpal bone, left hand**

√7ᵗʰ **S62.332** **Displaced fracture of neck of third metacarpal bone, right hand**

√7ᵗʰ **S62.333** **Displaced fracture of neck of third metacarpal bone, left hand**

√7ᵗʰ **S62.334** **Displaced fracture of neck of fourth metacarpal bone, right hand**

√7ᵗʰ **S62.335** **Displaced fracture of neck of fourth metacarpal bone, left hand**

√7ᵗʰ **S62.336** **Displaced fracture of neck of fifth metacarpal bone, right hand**

√7ᵗʰ **S62.337** **Displaced fracture of neck of fifth metacarpal bone, left hand**

√7ᵗʰ **S62.338** **Displaced fracture of neck of other metacarpal bone**
Displaced fracture of neck of specified metacarpal bone with unspecified laterality

√7ᵗʰ **S62.339** **Displaced fracture of neck of unspecified metacarpal bone**

√6ᵗʰ **S62.34** Nondisplaced fracture of base of other metacarpal bone

√7ᵗʰ **S62.340** **Nondisplaced fracture of base of second metacarpal bone, right hand**

√7ᵗʰ **S62.341** **Nondisplaced fracture of base of second metacarpal bone. left hand**

√7ᵗʰ **S62.342** **Nondisplaced fracture of base of third metacarpal bone, right hand**

√7ᵗʰ **S62.343** **Nondisplaced fracture of base of third metacarpal bone, left hand**

√7ᵗʰ **S62.344** **Nondisplaced fracture of base of fourth metacarpal bone, right hand**

√7ᵗʰ **S62.345** **Nondisplaced fracture of base of fourth metacarpal bone, left hand**

√7ᵗʰ **S62.346** **Nondisplaced fracture of base of fifth metacarpal bone, right hand**

√7ᵗʰ **S62.347** **Nondisplaced fracture of base of fifth metacarpal bone, left hand**

√7ᵗʰ **S62.348** **Nondisplaced fracture of base of other metacarpal bone**
Nondisplaced fracture of base of specified metacarpal bone with unspecified laterality

√7ᵗʰ **S62.349** **Nondisplaced fracture of base of unspecified metacarpal bone**

√6ᵗʰ **S62.35** Nondisplaced fracture of shaft of other metacarpal bone

√7ᵗʰ **S62.350** **Nondisplaced fracture of shaft of second metacarpal bone, right hand**

√7ᵗʰ **S62.351** **Nondisplaced fracture of shaft of second metacarpal bone, left hand**

√7ᵗʰ **S62.352** **Nondisplaced fracture of shaft of third metacarpal bone, right hand**

√7ᵗʰ **S62.353** **Nondisplaced fracture of shaft of third metacarpal bone, left hand**

√7ᵗʰ **S62.354** **Nondisplaced fracture of shaft of fourth metacarpal bone, right hand**

√7ᵗʰ **S62.355** **Nondisplaced fracture of shaft of fourth metacarpal bone, left hand**

√7ᵗʰ **S62.356** **Nondisplaced fracture of shaft of fifth metacarpal bone, right hand**

√7ᵗʰ **S62.357** **Nondisplaced fracture of shaft of fifth metacarpal bone, left hand**

√7ᵗʰ **S62.358** **Nondisplaced fracture of shaft of other metacarpal bone**
Nondisplaced fracture of shaft of specified metacarpal bone with unspecified laterality

√7ᵗʰ **S62.359** **Nondisplaced fracture of shaft of unspecified metacarpal bone**

√6ᵗʰ **S62.36** Nondisplaced fracture of neck of other metacarpal bone

√7ᵗʰ **S62.360** **Nondisplaced fracture of neck of second metacarpal bone, right hand**

√7ᵗʰ **S62.361** **Nondisplaced fracture of neck of second metacarpal bone, left hand**

√7ᵗʰ **S62.362** **Nondisplaced fracture of neck of third metacarpal bone, right hand**

√7ᵗʰ **S62.363** **Nondisplaced fracture of neck of third metacarpal bone, left hand**

√7ᵗʰ **S62.364** **Nondisplaced fracture of neck of fourth metacarpal bone, right hand**

√7ᵗʰ **S62.365** **Nondisplaced fracture of neck of fourth metacarpal bone, left hand**

√7ᵗʰ **S62.366** **Nondisplaced fracture of neck of fifth metacarpal bone, right hand**

√7ᵗʰ **S62.367** **Nondisplaced fracture of neck of fifth metacarpal bone, left hand**

EXCLUDES 1 Not coded here   **EXCLUDES 2** Not included here   N Newborn Age: 0   P Pediatric Age: 0-17   M Maternity Age: 12-55   A Adult Age: 15-124

872   ICD-10-CM 2014 (Draft)

✓7th **S62.368 Nondisplaced fracture of neck of other metacarpal bone**
     Nondisplaced fracture of neck of specified metacarpal bone with unspecified laterality

✓7th **S62.369 Nondisplaced fracture of neck of unspecified metacarpal bone**

✓6th **S62.39 Other fracture of other metacarpal bone**

✓7th **S62.390 Other fracture of second metacarpal bone, right hand**

✓7th **S62.391 Other fracture of second metacarpal bone, left hand**

✓7th **S62.392 Other fracture of third metacarpal bone, right hand**

✓7th **S62.393 Other fracture of third metacarpal bone, left hand**

✓7th **S62.394 Other fracture of fourth metacarpal bone, right hand**

✓7th **S62.395 Other fracture of fourth metacarpal bone, left hand**

✓7th **S62.396 Other fracture of fifth metacarpal bone, right hand**

✓7th **S62.397 Other fracture of fifth metacarpal bone, left hand**

✓7th **S62.398 Other fracture of other metacarpal bone**
     Other fracture of specified metacarpal bone with unspecified laterality

✓7th **S62.399 Other fracture of unspecified metacarpal bone**

✓5th **S62.5 Fracture of thumb**

✓6th **S62.50 Fracture of unspecified phalanx of thumb**

✓7th **S62.501 Fracture of unspecified phalanx of right thumb**

✓7th **S62.502 Fracture of unspecified phalanx of left thumb**

✓7th **S62.509 Fracture of unspecified phalanx of unspecified thumb**

✓6th **S62.51 Fracture of proximal phalanx of thumb**

✓7th **S62.511 Displaced fracture of proximal phalanx of right thumb**

✓7th **S62.512 Displaced fracture of proximal phalanx of left thumb**

✓7th **S62.513 Displaced fracture of proximal phalanx of unspecified thumb**

✓7th **S62.514 Nondisplaced fracture of proximal phalanx of right thumb**

✓7th **S62.515 Nondisplaced fracture of proximal phalanx of left thumb**

✓7th **S62.516 Nondisplaced fracture of proximal phalanx of unspecified thumb**

✓6th **S62.52 Fracture of distal phalanx of thumb**

✓7th **S62.521 Displaced fracture of distal phalanx of right thumb**

✓7th **S62.522 Displaced fracture of distal phalanx of left thumb**

✓7th **S62.523 Displaced fracture of distal phalanx of unspecified thumb**

✓7th **S62.524 Nondisplaced fracture of distal phalanx of right thumb**

✓7th **S62.525 Nondisplaced fracture of distal phalanx of left thumb**

✓7th **S62.526 Nondisplaced fracture of distal phalanx of unspecified thumb**

✓5th **S62.6 Fracture of other and unspecified finger(s)**
     EXCLUDES 2   fracture of thumb (S62.5-)

✓6th **S62.60 Fracture of unspecified phalanx of finger**

✓7th **S62.600 Fracture of unspecified phalanx of right index finger**

✓7th **S62.601 Fracture of unspecified phalanx of left index finger**

✓7th **S62.602 Fracture of unspecified phalanx of right middle finger**

✓7th **S62.603 Fracture of unspecified phalanx of left middle finger**

✓7th **S62.604 Fracture of unspecified phalanx of right ring finger**

✓7th **S62.605 Fracture of unspecified phalanx of left ring finger**

✓7th **S62.606 Fracture of unspecified phalanx of right little finger**

✓7th **S62.607 Fracture of unspecified phalanx of left little finger**

✓7th **S62.608 Fracture of unspecified phalanx of other finger**
     Fracture of unspecified phalanx of specified finger with unspecified laterality

✓7th **S62.609 Fracture of unspecified phalanx of unspecified finger**

✓6th **S62.61 Displaced fracture of proximal phalanx of finger**

✓7th **S62.610 Displaced fracture of proximal phalanx of right index finger**

✓7th **S62.611 Displaced fracture of proximal phalanx of left index finger**

✓7th **S62.612 Displaced fracture of proximal phalanx of right middle finger**

✓7th **S62.613 Displaced fracture of proximal phalanx of left middle finger**

✓7th **S62.614 Displaced fracture of proximal phalanx of right ring finger**

✓7th **S62.615 Displaced fracture of proximal phalanx of left ring finger**

✓7th **S62.616 Displaced fracture of proximal phalanx of right little finger**

✓7th **S62.617 Displaced fracture of proximal phalanx of left little finger**

✓7th **S62.618 Displaced fracture of proximal phalanx of other finger**
     Displaced fracture of proximal phalanx of specified finger with unspecified laterality

✓7th **S62.619 Displaced fracture of proximal phalanx of unspecified finger**

✓6th **S62.62 Displaced fracture of medial phalanx of finger**

✓7th **S62.620 Displaced fracture of medial phalanx of right index finger**

✓7th **S62.621 Displaced fracture of medial phalanx of left index finger**

✓7th **S62.622 Displaced fracture of medial phalanx of right middle finger**

✓7th **S62.623 Displaced fracture of medial phalanx of left middle finger**

✓7th **S62.624 Displaced fracture of medial phalanx of right ring finger**

✓7th **S62.625 Displaced fracture of medial phalanx of left ring finger**

✓7th **S62.626 Displaced fracture of medial phalanx of right little finger**

✓7th **S62.627 Displaced fracture of medial phalanx of left little finger**

✓7th **S62.628 Displaced fracture of medial phalanx of other finger**
     Displaced fracture of medial phalanx of specified finger with unspecified laterality

✓7th **S62.629 Displaced fracture of medial phalanx of unspecified finger**

✓6th **S62.63 Displaced fracture of distal phalanx of finger**

✓7th **S62.630 Displaced fracture of distal phalanx of right index finger**

✓7th **S62.631 Displaced fracture of distal phalanx of left index finger**

✓7th **S62.632 Displaced fracture of distal phalanx of right middle finger**

✓7th **S62.633 Displaced fracture of distal phalanx of left middle finger**

✓7th **S62.634 Displaced fracture of distal phalanx of right ring finger**

✓7th **S62.635 Displaced fracture of distal phalanx of left ring finger**

✓ Additional Character Required   ✓x7th Xtension Alert   Unspecified Code   Other Specified Code   Manifestation Code   ►◄ Revised Text   ● New Code   ▲ Revised Code Title

ICD-10-CM 2014 (Draft)   **873**

✓7th **S62.636 Displaced fracture of distal phalanx of right little finger**

✓7th **S62.637 Displaced fracture of distal phalanx of left little finger**

✓7th **S62.638 Displaced fracture of distal phalanx of other finger**
Displaced fracture of distal phalanx of specified finger with unspecified laterality

✓7th **S62.639 Displaced fracture of distal phalanx of unspecified finger**

✓6th **S62.64 Nondisplaced fracture of proximal phalanx of finger**

✓7th **S62.640 Nondisplaced fracture of proximal phalanx of right index finger**

✓7th **S62.641 Nondisplaced fracture of proximal phalanx of left index finger**

✓7th **S62.642 Nondisplaced fracture of proximal phalanx of right middle finger**

✓7th **S62.643 Nondisplaced fracture of proximal phalanx of left middle finger**

✓7th **S62.644 Nondisplaced fracture of proximal phalanx of right ring finger**

✓7th **S62.645 Nondisplaced fracture of proximal phalanx of left ring finger**

✓7th **S62.646 Nondisplaced fracture of proximal phalanx of right little finger**

✓7th **S62.647 Nondisplaced fracture of proximal phalanx of left little finger**

✓7th **S62.648 Nondisplaced fracture of proximal phalanx of other finger**
Nondisplaced fracture of proximal phalanx of specified finger with unspecified laterality

✓7th **S62.649 Nondisplaced fracture of proximal phalanx of unspecified finger**

✓6th **S62.65 Nondisplaced fracture of medial phalanx of finger**

✓7th **S62.650 Nondisplaced fracture of medial phalanx of right index finger**

✓7th **S62.651 Nondisplaced fracture of medial phalanx of left index finger**

✓7th **S62.652 Nondisplaced fracture of medial phalanx of right middle finger**

✓7th **S62.653 Nondisplaced fracture of medial phalanx of left middle finger**

✓7th **S62.654 Nondisplaced fracture of medial phalanx of right ring finger**

✓7th **S62.655 Nondisplaced fracture of medial phalanx of left ring finger**

✓7th **S62.656 Nondisplaced fracture of medial phalanx of right little finger**

✓7th **S62.657 Nondisplaced fracture of medial phalanx of left little finger**

✓7th **S62.658 Nondisplaced fracture of medial phalanx of other finger**
Nondisplaced fracture of medial phalanx of specified finger with unspecified laterality

✓7th **S62.659 Nondisplaced fracture of medial phalanx of unspecified finger**

✓6th **S62.66 Nondisplaced fracture of distal phalanx of finger**

✓7th **S62.660 Nondisplaced fracture of distal phalanx of right index finger**

✓7th **S62.661 Nondisplaced fracture of distal phalanx of left index finger**

✓7th **S62.662 Nondisplaced fracture of distal phalanx of right middle finger**

✓7th **S62.663 Nondisplaced fracture of distal phalanx of left middle finger**

✓7th **S62.664 Nondisplaced fracture of distal phalanx of right ring finger**

✓7th **S62.665 Nondisplaced fracture of distal phalanx of left ring finger**

✓7th **S62.666 Nondisplaced fracture of distal phalanx of right little finger**

✓7th **S62.667 Nondisplaced fracture of distal phalanx of left little finger**

✓7th **S62.668 Nondisplaced fracture of distal phalanx of other finger**
Nondisplaced fracture of distal phalanx of specified finger with unspecified laterality

✓7th **S62.669 Nondisplaced fracture of distal phalanx of unspecified finger**

✓5th **S62.9 Unspecified fracture of wrist and hand**

✓x7th **S62.90 Unspecified fracture of unspecified wrist and hand**

✓x7th **S62.91 Unspecified fracture of right wrist and hand**

✓x7th **S62.92 Unspecified fracture of left wrist and hand**

✓4th **S63 Dislocation and sprain of joints and ligaments at wrist and hand level**

INCLUDES   avulsion of joint or ligament at wrist and hand level
laceration of cartilage, joint or ligament at wrist and hand level
sprain of cartilage, joint or ligament at wrist and hand level
traumatic hemarthrosis of joint or ligament at wrist and hand level
traumatic rupture of joint or ligament at wrist and hand level
traumatic subluxation of joint or ligament at wrist and hand level
traumatic tear of joint or ligament at wrist and hand level

Code also any associated open wound

EXCLUDES 2   strain of muscle, fascia and tendon of wrist and hand (S66.-)

The appropriate 7th character is to be added to each code from category S63.
A   initial encounter
D   subsequent encounter
S   sequela

✓5th **S63.0 Subluxation and dislocation of wrist and hand joints**

✓6th **S63.00 Unspecified subluxation and dislocation of wrist and hand**
Dislocation of carpal bone NOS
Dislocation of distal end of radius NOS
Subluxation of carpal bone NOS
Subluxation of distal end of radius NOS

✓7th **S63.001 Unspecified subluxation of right wrist and hand**

✓7th **S63.002 Unspecified subluxation of left wrist and hand**

✓7th **S63.003 Unspecified subluxation of unspecified wrist and hand**

✓7th **S63.004 Unspecified dislocation of right wrist and hand**

✓7th **S63.005 Unspecified dislocation of left wrist and hand**

✓7th **S63.006 Unspecified dislocation of unspecified wrist and hand**

✓6th **S63.01 Subluxation and dislocation of distal radioulnar joint**

✓7th **S63.011 Subluxation of distal radioulnar joint of right wrist**

✓7th **S63.012 Subluxation of distal radioulnar joint of left wrist**

✓7th **S63.013 Subluxation of distal radioulnar joint of unspecified wrist**

✓7th **S63.014 Dislocation of distal radioulnar joint of right wrist**

✓7th **S63.015 Dislocation of distal radioulnar joint of left wrist**

✓7th **S63.016 Dislocation of distal radioulnar joint of unspecified wrist**

✓6th **S63.02 Subluxation and dislocation of radiocarpal joint**

✓7th **S63.021 Subluxation of radiocarpal joint of right wrist**

✓7th **S63.022 Subluxation of radiocarpal joint of left wrist**

✓7th **S63.023 Subluxation of radiocarpal joint of unspecified wrist**

✓7th **S63.024 Dislocation of radiocarpal joint of right wrist**

✓7th **S63.025 Dislocation of radiocarpal joint of left wrist**

EXCLUDES 1 Not coded here   EXCLUDES 2 Not included here   N Newborn Age: 0   P Pediatric Age: 0-17   M Maternity Age: 12-55   A Adult Age: 15-124

874   ICD-10-CM 2014 (Draft)

√7ᵗʰ **S63.026** Dislocation of radiocarpal joint of unspecified wrist

√6ᵗʰ **S63.03** Subluxation and dislocation of midcarpal joint

√7ᵗʰ **S63.031** Subluxation of midcarpal joint of right wrist

√7ᵗʰ **S63.032** Subluxation of midcarpal joint of left wrist

√7ᵗʰ **S63.033** Subluxation of midcarpal joint of unspecified wrist

√7ᵗʰ **S63.034** Dislocation of midcarpal joint of right wrist

√7ᵗʰ **S63.035** Dislocation of midcarpal joint of left wrist

√7ᵗʰ **S63.036** Dislocation of midcarpal joint of unspecified wrist

√6ᵗʰ **S63.04** Subluxation and dislocation of carpometacarpal joint of thumb

EXCLUDES 2 interphalangeal subluxation and dislocation of thumb (S63.1-)

√7ᵗʰ **S63.041** Subluxation of carpometacarpal joint of right thumb

√7ᵗʰ **S63.042** Subluxation of carpometacarpal joint of left thumb

√7ᵗʰ **S63.043** Subluxation of carpometacarpal joint of unspecified thumb

√7ᵗʰ **S63.044** Dislocation of carpometacarpal joint of right thumb

√7ᵗʰ **S63.045** Dislocation of carpometacarpal joint of left thumb

√7ᵗʰ **S63.046** Dislocation of carpometacarpal joint of unspecified thumb

√6ᵗʰ **S63.05** Subluxation and dislocation of other carpometacarpal joint

EXCLUDES 2 subluxation and dislocation of carpometacarpal joint of thumb (S63.04-)

√7ᵗʰ **S63.051** Subluxation of other carpometacarpal joint of right hand

√7ᵗʰ **S63.052** Subluxation of other carpometacarpal joint of left hand

√7ᵗʰ **S63.053** Subluxation of other carpometacarpal joint of unspecified hand

√7ᵗʰ **S63.054** Dislocation of other carpometacarpal joint of right hand

√7ᵗʰ **S63.055** Dislocation of other carpometacarpal joint of left hand

√7ᵗʰ **S63.056** Dislocation of other carpometacarpal joint of unspecified hand

√6ᵗʰ **S63.06** Subluxation and dislocation of metacarpal (bone), proximal end

√7ᵗʰ **S63.061** Subluxation of metacarpal (bone), proximal end of right hand

√7ᵗʰ **S63.062** Subluxation of metacarpal (bone), proximal end of left hand

√7ᵗʰ **S63.063** Subluxation of metacarpal (bone), proximal end of unspecified hand

√7ᵗʰ **S63.064** Dislocation of metacarpal (bone), proximal end of right hand

√7ᵗʰ **S63.065** Dislocation of metacarpal (bone), proximal end of left hand

√7ᵗʰ **S63.066** Dislocation of metacarpal (bone), proximal end of unspecified hand

√6ᵗʰ **S63.07** Subluxation and dislocation of distal end of ulna

√7ᵗʰ **S63.071** Subluxation of distal end of right ulna

√7ᵗʰ **S63.072** Subluxation of distal end of left ulna

√7ᵗʰ **S63.073** Subluxation of distal end of unspecified ulna

√7ᵗʰ **S63.074** Dislocation of distal end of right ulna

√7ᵗʰ **S63.075** Dislocation of distal end of left ulna

√7ᵗʰ **S63.076** Dislocation of distal end of unspecified ulna

√6ᵗʰ **S63.09** Other subluxation and dislocation of wrist and hand

√7ᵗʰ **S63.091** Other subluxation of right wrist and hand

√7ᵗʰ **S63.092** Other subluxation of left wrist and hand

√7ᵗʰ **S63.093** Other subluxation of unspecified wrist and hand

√7ᵗʰ **S63.094** Other dislocation of right wrist and hand

√7ᵗʰ **S63.095** Other dislocation of left wrist and hand

√7ᵗʰ **S63.096** Other dislocation of unspecified wrist and hand

√5ᵗʰ **S63.1** Subluxation and dislocation of thumb

√6ᵗʰ **S63.10** Unspecified subluxation and dislocation of thumb

√7ᵗʰ **S63.101** Unspecified subluxation of right thumb

√7ᵗʰ **S63.102** Unspecified subluxation of left thumb

√7ᵗʰ **S63.103** Unspecified subluxation of unspecified thumb

√7ᵗʰ **S63.104** Unspecified dislocation of right thumb

√7ᵗʰ **S63.105** Unspecified dislocation of left thumb

√7ᵗʰ **S63.106** Unspecified dislocation of unspecified thumb

√6ᵗʰ **S63.11** Subluxation and dislocation of metacarpophalangeal joint of thumb

√7ᵗʰ **S63.111** Subluxation of metacarpophalangeal joint of right thumb

√7ᵗʰ **S63.112** Subluxation of metacarpophalangeal joint of left thumb

√7ᵗʰ **S63.113** Subluxation of metacarpophalangeal joint of unspecified thumb

√7ᵗʰ **S63.114** Dislocation of metacarpophalangeal joint of right thumb

√7ᵗʰ **S63.115** Dislocation of metacarpophalangeal joint of left thumb

√7ᵗʰ **S63.116** Dislocation of metacarpophalangeal joint of unspecified thumb

√6ᵗʰ **S63.12** Subluxation and dislocation of unspecified interphalangeal joint of thumb

√7ᵗʰ **S63.121** Subluxation of unspecified interphalangeal joint of right thumb

√7ᵗʰ **S63.122** Subluxation of unspecified interphalangeal joint of left thumb

√7ᵗʰ **S63.123** Subluxation of unspecified interphalangeal joint of unspecified thumb

√7ᵗʰ **S63.124** Dislocation of unspecified interphalangeal joint of right thumb

√7ᵗʰ **S63.125** Dislocation of unspecified interphalangeal joint of left thumb

√7ᵗʰ **S63.126** Dislocation of unspecified interphalangeal joint of unspecified thumb

√6ᵗʰ **S63.13** Subluxation and dislocation of proximal interphalangeal joint of thumb

√7ᵗʰ **S63.131** Subluxation of proximal interphalangeal joint of right thumb

√7ᵗʰ **S63.132** Subluxation of proximal interphalangeal joint of left thumb

√7ᵗʰ **S63.133** Subluxation of proximal interphalangeal joint of unspecified thumb

√7ᵗʰ **S63.134** Dislocation of proximal interphalangeal joint of right thumb

√7ᵗʰ **S63.135** Dislocation of proximal interphalangeal joint of left thumb

√7ᵗʰ **S63.136** Dislocation of proximal interphalangeal joint of unspecified thumb

√6ᵗʰ **S63.14** Subluxation and dislocation of distal interphalangeal joint of thumb

√7ᵗʰ **S63.141** Subluxation of distal interphalangeal joint of right thumb

√7ᵗʰ **S63.142** Subluxation of distal interphalangeal joint of left thumb

√7ᵗʰ **S63.143** Subluxation of distal interphalangeal joint of unspecified thumb

√7ᵗʰ **S63.144** Dislocation of distal interphalangeal joint of right thumb

√7ᵗʰ **S63.145** Dislocation of distal interphalangeal joint of left thumb

√7ᵗʰ **S63.146** Dislocation of distal interphalangeal joint of unspecified thumb

√5ᵗʰ **S63.2** Subluxation and dislocation of other finger(s)

EXCLUDES 2 subluxation and dislocation of thumb (S63.1-)

√6ᵗʰ **S63.20** Unspecified subluxation of other finger

☑ Additional Character Required   √ₓ7ᵗʰ Xtension Alert   Unspecified Code   Other Specified Code   Manifestation Code   ▶◀ Revised Text   ● New Code   ▲ Revised Code Title

ICD-10-CM 2014 (Draft)

875

√7th **S63.200** **Unspecified subluxation of** right index finger

√7th **S63.201** **Unspecified subluxation of** left index finger

√7th **S63.202** **Unspecified subluxation of** right middle finger

√7th **S63.203** **Unspecified subluxation of** left middle finger

√7th **S63.204** **Unspecified subluxation of** right ring finger

√7th **S63.205** **Unspecified subluxation of** left ring finger

√7th **S63.206** **Unspecified subluxation of** right little finger

√7th **S63.207** **Unspecified subluxation of** left little finger

√7th **S63.208** **Unspecified subluxation of other finger**
Unspecified subluxation of specified finger with unspecified laterality

√7th **S63.209** **Unspecified subluxation of unspecified finger**

√6th **S63.21** Subluxation of metacarpophalangeal joint of finger

√7th **S63.210** **Subluxation of metacarpophalangeal joint of** right index finger

√7th **S63.211** **Subluxation of metacarpophalangeal joint of** left index finger

√7th **S63.212** **Subluxation of metacarpophalangeal joint of** right middle finger

√7th **S63.213** **Subluxation of metacarpophalangeal joint of** left middle finger

√7th **S63.214** **Subluxation of metacarpophalangeal joint of** right ring finger

√7th **S63.215** **Subluxation of metacarpophalangeal joint of** left ring finger

√7th **S63.216** **Subluxation of metacarpophalangeal joint of** right little finger

√7th **S63.217** **Subluxation of metacarpophalangeal joint of** left little finger

√7th **S63.218** **Subluxation of metacarpophalangeal joint of other finger**
Subluxation of metacarpophalangeal joint of specified finger with unspecified laterality

√7th **S63.219** **Subluxation of metacarpophalangeal joint of unspecified finger**

√6th **S63.22** Subluxation of unspecified interphalangeal joint of finger

√7th **S63.220** **Subluxation of unspecified interphalangeal joint of** right index finger

√7th **S63.221** **Subluxation of unspecified interphalangeal joint of** left index finger

√7th **S63.222** **Subluxation of unspecified interphalangeal joint of** right middle finger

√7th **S63.223** **Subluxation of unspecified interphalangeal joint of** left middle finger

√7th **S63.224** **Subluxation of unspecified interphalangeal joint of** right ring finger

√7th **S63.225** **Subluxation of unspecified interphalangeal joint of** left ring finger

√7th **S63.226** **Subluxation of unspecified interphalangeal joint of** right little finger

√7th **S63.227** **Subluxation of unspecified interphalangeal joint of** left little finger

√7th **S63.228** **Subluxation of unspecified interphalangeal joint of other finger**
Subluxation of unspecified interphalangeal joint of specified finger with unspecified laterality

√7th **S63.229** **Subluxation of unspecified interphalangeal joint of unspecified finger**

√6th **S63.23** Subluxation of proximal interphalangeal joint of finger

√7th **S63.230** **Subluxation of proximal interphalangeal joint of** right index finger

√7th **S63.231** **Subluxation of proximal interphalangeal joint of** left index finger

√7th **S63.232** **Subluxation of proximal interphalangeal joint of** right middle finger

√7th **S63.233** **Subluxation of proximal interphalangeal joint of** left middle finger

√7th **S63.234** **Subluxation of proximal interphalangeal joint of** right ring finger

√7th **S63.235** **Subluxation of proximal interphalangeal joint of** left ring finger

√7th **S63.236** **Subluxation of proximal interphalangeal joint of** right little finger

√7th **S63.237** **Subluxation of proximal interphalangeal joint of** left little finger

√7th **S63.238** **Subluxation of proximal interphalangeal joint of other finger**
Subluxation of proximal interphalangeal joint of specified finger with unspecified laterality

√7th **S63.239** **Subluxation of proximal interphalangeal joint of unspecified finger**

√6th **S63.24** Subluxation of distal interphalangeal joint of finger

√7th **S63.240** **Subluxation of distal interphalangeal joint of** right index finger

√7th **S63.241** **Subluxation of distal interphalangeal joint of** left index finger

√7th **S63.242** **Subluxation of distal interphalangeal joint of** right middle finger

√7th **S63.243** **Subluxation of distal interphalangeal joint of** left middle finger

√7th **S63.244** **Subluxation of distal interphalangeal joint of** right ring finger

√7th **S63.245** **Subluxation of distal interphalangeal joint of** left ring finger

√7th **S63.246** **Subluxation of distal interphalangeal joint of** right little finger

√7th **S63.247** **Subluxation of distal interphalangeal joint of** left little finger

√7th **S63.248** **Subluxation of distal interphalangeal joint of other finger**
Subluxation of distal interphalangeal joint of specified finger with unspecified laterality

√7th **S63.249** **Subluxation of distal interphalangeal joint of unspecified finger**

√6th **S63.25** Unspecified dislocation of other finger

√7th **S63.250** **Unspecified dislocation of** right index finger

√7th **S63.251** **Unspecified dislocation of** left index finger

√7th **S63.252** **Unspecified dislocation of** right middle finger

√7th **S63.253** **Unspecified dislocation of** left middle finger

√7th **S63.254** **Unspecified dislocation of** right ring finger

√7th **S63.255** **Unspecified dislocation of** left ring finger

√7th **S63.256** **Unspecified dislocation of** right little finger

√7th **S63.257** **Unspecified dislocation of** left little finger

√7th **S63.258** **Unspecified dislocation of other finger**
Unspecified dislocation of specified finger with unspecified laterality

√7th **S63.259** **Unspecified dislocation of unspecified finger**
Unspecified dislocation of specified finger with unspecified laterality

√6th **S63.26** Dislocation of metacarpophalangeal joint of finger

√7th **S63.260** **Dislocation of metacarpophalangeal joint of** right index finger

√7th **S63.261** **Dislocation of metacarpophalangeal joint of** left index finger

√7th **S63.262** **Dislocation of metacarpophalangeal joint of** right middle finger

√7th **S63.263** **Dislocation of metacarpophalangeal joint of** left middle finger

√7th **S63.264** **Dislocation of metacarpophalangeal joint of** right ring finger

√7th **S63.265** **Dislocation of metacarpophalangeal joint of** left ring finger

EXCLUDES 1 Not coded here | EXCLUDES 2 Not included here | N Newborn Age: 0 | P Pediatric Age: 0-17 | M Maternity Age: 12-55 | A Adult Age: 15-124

876 | ICD-10-CM 2014 (Draft)

☑7ᵗʰ **S63.266 Dislocation of metacarpophalangeal joint of right little finger**

☑7ᵗʰ **S63.267 Dislocation of metacarpophalangeal joint of left little finger**

☑7ᵗʰ **S63.268 Dislocation of metacarpophalangeal joint of other finger**
Dislocation of metacarpophalangeal joint of specified finger with unspecified laterality

☑7ᵗʰ **S63.269 Dislocation of metacarpophalangeal joint of unspecified finger**

☑6ᵗʰ **S63.27 Dislocation of unspecified interphalangeal joint of finger**

☑7ᵗʰ **S63.270 Dislocation of unspecified interphalangeal joint of right index finger**

☑7ᵗʰ **S63.271 Dislocation of unspecified interphalangeal joint of left index finger**

☑7ᵗʰ **S63.272 Dislocation of unspecified interphalangeal joint of right middle finger**

☑7ᵗʰ **S63.273 Dislocation of unspecified interphalangeal joint of left middle finger**

☑7ᵗʰ **S63.274 Dislocation of unspecified interphalangeal joint of right ring finger**

☑7ᵗʰ **S63.275 Dislocation of unspecified interphalangeal joint of left ring finger**

☑7ᵗʰ **S63.276 Dislocation of unspecified interphalangeal joint of right little finger**

☑7ᵗʰ **S63.277 Dislocation of unspecified interphalangeal joint of left little finger**

☑7ᵗʰ **S63.278 Dislocation of unspecified interphalangeal joint of other finger**
Dislocation of unspecified interphalangeal joint of specified finger with unspecified laterality

☑7ᵗʰ **S63.279 Dislocation of unspecified interphalangeal joint of unspecified finger**
Dislocation of unspecified interphalangeal joint of specified finger without specified laterality

☑6ᵗʰ **S63.28 Dislocation of proximal interphalangeal joint of finger**

☑7ᵗʰ **S63.280 Dislocation of proximal interphalangeal joint of right index finger**

☑7ᵗʰ **S63.281 Dislocation of proximal interphalangeal joint of left index finger**

☑7ᵗʰ **S63.282 Dislocation of proximal interphalangeal joint of right middle finger**

☑7ᵗʰ **S63.283 Dislocation of proximal interphalangeal joint of left middle finger**

☑7ᵗʰ **S63.284 Dislocation of proximal interphalangeal joint of right ring finger**

☑7ᵗʰ **S63.285 Dislocation of proximal interphalangeal joint of left ring finger**

☑7ᵗʰ **S63.286 Dislocation of proximal interphalangeal joint of right little finger**

☑7ᵗʰ **S63.287 Dislocation of proximal interphalangeal joint of left little finger**

☑7ᵗʰ **S63.288 Dislocation of proximal interphalangeal joint of other finger**
Dislocation of proximal interphalangeal joint of specified finger with unspecified laterality

☑7ᵗʰ **S63.289 Dislocation of proximal interphalangeal joint of unspecified finger**

☑6ᵗʰ **S63.29 Dislocation of distal interphalangeal joint of finger**

☑7ᵗʰ **S63.290 Dislocation of distal interphalangeal joint of right index finger**

☑7ᵗʰ **S63.291 Dislocation of distal interphalangeal joint of left index finger**

☑7ᵗʰ **S63.292 Dislocation of distal interphalangeal joint of right middle finger**

☑7ᵗʰ **S63.293 Dislocation of distal interphalangeal joint of left middle finger**

☑7ᵗʰ **S63.294 Dislocation of distal interphalangeal joint of right ring finger**

☑7ᵗʰ **S63.295 Dislocation of distal interphalangeal joint of left ring finger**

☑7ᵗʰ **S63.296 Dislocation of distal interphalangeal joint of right little finger**

☑7ᵗʰ **S63.297 Dislocation of distal interphalangeal joint of left little finger**

☑7ᵗʰ **S63.298 Dislocation of distal interphalangeal joint of other finger**
Dislocation of distal interphalangeal joint of specified finger with unspecified laterality

☑7ᵗʰ **S63.299 Dislocation of distal interphalangeal joint of unspecified finger**

☑5ᵗʰ **S63.3 Traumatic rupture of ligament of wrist**

☑6ᵗʰ **S63.30 Traumatic rupture of unspecified ligament of wrist**

☑7ᵗʰ **S63.301 Traumatic rupture of unspecified ligament of right wrist**

☑7ᵗʰ **S63.302 Traumatic rupture of unspecified ligament of left wrist**

☑7ᵗʰ **S63.309 Traumatic rupture of unspecified ligament of unspecified wrist**

☑6ᵗʰ **S63.31 Traumatic rupture of collateral ligament of wrist**

☑7ᵗʰ **S63.311 Traumatic rupture of collateral ligament of right wrist**

☑7ᵗʰ **S63.312 Traumatic rupture of collateral ligament of left wrist**

☑7ᵗʰ **S63.319 Traumatic rupture of collateral ligament of unspecified wrist**

☑6ᵗʰ **S63.32 Traumatic rupture of radiocarpal ligament**

☑7ᵗʰ **S63.321 Traumatic rupture of right radiocarpal ligament**

☑7ᵗʰ **S63.322 Traumatic rupture of left radiocarpal ligament**

☑7ᵗʰ **S63.329 Traumatic rupture of unspecified radiocarpal ligament**

☑6ᵗʰ **S63.33 Traumatic rupture of ulnocarpal (palmar) ligament**

☑7ᵗʰ **S63.331 Traumatic rupture of right ulnocarpal (palmar) ligament**

☑7ᵗʰ **S63.332 Traumatic rupture of left ulnocarpal (palmar) ligament**

☑7ᵗʰ **S63.339 Traumatic rupture of unspecified ulnocarpal (palmar) ligament**

☑6ᵗʰ **S63.39 Traumatic rupture of other ligament of wrist**

☑7ᵗʰ **S63.391 Traumatic rupture of other ligament of right wrist**

☑7ᵗʰ **S63.392 Traumatic rupture of other ligament of left wrist**

☑7ᵗʰ **S63.399 Traumatic rupture of other ligament of unspecified wrist**

☑5ᵗʰ **S63.4 Traumatic rupture of ligament of finger at metacarpophalangeal and interphalangeal joint(s)**

☑6ᵗʰ **S63.40 Traumatic rupture of unspecified ligament of finger at metacarpophalangeal and interphalangeal joint**

☑7ᵗʰ **S63.400 Traumatic rupture of unspecified ligament of right index finger at metacarpophalangeal and interphalangeal joint**

☑7ᵗʰ **S63.401 Traumatic rupture of unspecified ligament of left index finger at metacarpophalangeal and interphalangeal joint**

☑7ᵗʰ **S63.402 Traumatic rupture of unspecified ligament of right middle finger at metacarpophalangeal and interphalangeal joint**

☑7ᵗʰ **S63.403 Traumatic rupture of unspecified ligament of left middle finger at metacarpophalangeal and interphalangeal joint**

☑7ᵗʰ **S63.404 Traumatic rupture of unspecified ligament of right ring finger at metacarpophalangeal and interphalangeal joint**

☑7ᵗʰ **S63.405 Traumatic rupture of unspecified ligament of left ring finger at metacarpophalangeal and interphalangeal joint**

☑7ᵗʰ **S63.406 Traumatic rupture of unspecified ligament of right little finger at metacarpophalangeal and interphalangeal joint**

☑ Additional Character Required   ☑7ᵗʰ Xtension Alert   Unspecified Code   Other Specified Code   Manifestation Code   ▶◀ Revised Text   ● New Code   ▲ Revised Code Title

ICD-10-CM 2014 (Draft)   877

✓7th **S63.407** **Traumatic rupture of unspecified ligament of left little finger at metacarpophalangeal and interphalangeal joint**

✓7th **S63.408** **Traumatic rupture of unspecified ligament of other finger at metacarpophalangeal and interphalangeal joint**
Traumatic rupture of unspecified ligament of specified finger with unspecified laterality at metacarpophalangeal and interphalangeal joint

✓7th **S63.409** **Traumatic rupture of unspecified ligament of unspecified finger at metacarpophalangeal and interphalangeal joint**

✓6th **S63.41** **Traumatic rupture of collateral ligament of finger at metacarpophalangeal and interphalangeal joint**

✓7th **S63.410** **Traumatic rupture of collateral ligament of right index finger at metacarpophalangeal and interphalangeal joint**

✓7th **S63.411** **Traumatic rupture of collateral ligament of left index finger at metacarpophalangeal and interphalangeal joint**

✓7th **S63.412** **Traumatic rupture of collateral ligament of right middle finger at metacarpophalangeal and interphalangeal joint**

✓7th **S63.413** **Traumatic rupture of collateral ligament of left middle finger at metacarpophalangeal and interphalangeal joint**

✓7th **S63.414** **Traumatic rupture of collateral ligament of right ring finger at metacarpophalangeal and interphalangeal joint**

✓7th **S63.415** **Traumatic rupture of collateral ligament of left ring finger at metacarpophalangeal and interphalangeal joint**

✓7th **S63.416** **Traumatic rupture of collateral ligament of right little finger at metacarpophalangeal and interphalangeal joint**

✓7th **S63.417** **Traumatic rupture of collateral ligament of left little finger at metacarpophalangeal and interphalangeal joint**

✓7th **S63.418** **Traumatic rupture of collateral ligament of other finger at metacarpophalangeal and interphalangeal joint**
Traumatic rupture of collateral ligament of specified finger with unspecified laterality at metacarpophalangeal and interphalangeal joint

✓7th **S63.419** **Traumatic rupture of collateral ligament of unspecified finger at metacarpophalangeal and interphalangeal joint**

✓6th **S63.42** **Traumatic rupture of palmar ligament of finger at metacarpophalangeal and interphalangeal joint**

✓7th **S63.420** **Traumatic rupture of palmar ligament of right index finger at metacarpophalangeal and interphalangeal joint**

✓7th **S63.421** **Traumatic rupture of palmar ligament of left index finger at metacarpophalangeal and interphalangeal joint**

✓7th **S63.422** **Traumatic rupture of palmar ligament of right middle finger at metacarpophalangeal and interphalangeal joint**

✓7th **S63.423** **Traumatic rupture of palmar ligament of left middle finger at metacarpophalangeal and interphalangeal joint**

✓7th **S63.424** **Traumatic rupture of palmar ligament of right ring finger at metacarpophalangeal and interphalangeal joint**

✓7th **S63.425** **Traumatic rupture of palmar ligament of left ring finger at metacarpophalangeal and interphalangeal joint**

✓7th **S63.426** **Traumatic rupture of palmar ligament of right little finger at metacarpophalangeal and interphalangeal joint**

✓7th **S63.427** **Traumatic rupture of palmar ligament of left little finger at metacarpophalangeal and interphalangeal joint**

✓7th **S63.428** **Traumatic rupture of palmar ligament of other finger at metacarpophalangeal and interphalangeal joint**
Traumatic rupture of palmar ligament of specified finger with unspecified laterality at metacarpophalangeal and interphalangeal joint

✓7th **S63.429** **Traumatic rupture of palmar ligament of unspecified finger at metacarpophalangeal and interphalangeal joint**

✓6th **S63.43** **Traumatic rupture of volar plate of finger at metacarpophalangeal and interphalangeal joint**

✓7th **S63.430** **Traumatic rupture of volar plate of right index finger at metacarpophalangeal and interphalangeal joint**

✓7th **S63.431** **Traumatic rupture of volar plate of left index finger at metacarpophalangeal and interphalangeal joint**

✓7th **S63.432** **Traumatic rupture of volar plate of right middle finger at metacarpophalangeal and interphalangeal joint**

✓7th **S63.433** **Traumatic rupture of volar plate of left middle finger at metacarpophalangeal and interphalangeal joint**

✓7th **S63.434** **Traumatic rupture of volar plate of right ring finger at metacarpophalangeal and interphalangeal joint**

✓7th **S63.435** **Traumatic rupture of volar plate of left ring finger at metacarpophalangeal and interphalangeal joint**

✓7th **S63.436** **Traumatic rupture of volar plate of right little finger at metacarpophalangeal and interphalangeal joint**

✓7th **S63.437** **Traumatic rupture of volar plate of left little finger at metacarpophalangeal and interphalangeal joint**

✓7th **S63.438** **Traumatic rupture of volar plate of other finger at metacarpophalangeal and interphalangeal joint**
Traumatic rupture of volar plate of specified finger with unspecified laterality at metacarpophalangeal and interphalangeal joint

✓7th **S63.439** **Traumatic rupture of volar plate of unspecified finger at metacarpophalangeal and interphalangeal joint**

✓6th **S63.49** **Traumatic rupture of other ligament of finger at metacarpophalangeal and interphalangeal joint**

✓7th **S63.490** **Traumatic rupture of other ligament of right index finger at metacarpophalangeal and interphalangeal joint**

✓7th **S63.491** **Traumatic rupture of other ligament of left index finger at metacarpophalangeal and interphalangeal joint**

✓7th **S63.492** **Traumatic rupture of other ligament of right middle finger at metacarpophalangeal and interphalangeal joint**

✓7th **S63.493** **Traumatic rupture of other ligament of left middle finger at metacarpophalangeal and interphalangeal joint**

✓7th **S63.494** **Traumatic rupture of other ligament of right ring finger at metacarpophalangeal and interphalangeal joint**

✓7th **S63.495** **Traumatic rupture of other ligament of left ring finger at metacarpophalangeal and interphalangeal joint**

✓7th **S63.496** **Traumatic rupture of other ligament of right little finger at metacarpophalangeal and interphalangeal joint**

✓7th **S63.497** **Traumatic rupture of other ligament of left little finger at metacarpophalangeal and interphalangeal joint**

✓7th **S63.498** **Traumatic rupture of other ligament of other finger at metacarpophalangeal and interphalangeal joint**
Traumatic rupture of ligament of specified finger with unspecified laterality at metacarpophalangeal and interphalangeal joint

---

EXCLUDES 1 Not coded here   **EXCLUDES 2** Not included here   **N** Newborn Age: 0   **P** Pediatric Age: 0-17   **M** Maternity Age: 12-55   **A** Adult Age: 15-124

878   ICD-10-CM 2014 (Draft)

√7ᵗʰ **S63.499 Traumatic rupture of other ligament of unspecified finger at metacarpophalangeal and interphalangeal joint**

√5ᵗʰ **S63.5 Other and unspecified** sprain of wrist

√6ᵗʰ **S63.50** Unspecified **sprain of wrist**

√7ᵗʰ **S63.501 Unspecified sprain of** right **wrist**

√7ᵗʰ **S63.502 Unspecified sprain of** left **wrist**

√7ᵗʰ **S63.509 Unspecified sprain of unspecified wrist**

√6ᵗʰ **S63.51 Sprain of** carpal (joint)

√7ᵗʰ **S63.511 Sprain of carpal joint of** right **wrist**

√7ᵗʰ **S63.512 Sprain of carpal joint of** left **wrist**

√7ᵗʰ **S63.519 Sprain of carpal joint of unspecified wrist**

√6ᵗʰ **S63.52 Sprain of** radiocarpal **joint**

EXCLUDES 1   *traumatic rupture of radiocarpal ligament (S63.32-)*

√7ᵗʰ **S63.521 Sprain of radiocarpal joint of** right **wrist**

√7ᵗʰ **S63.522 Sprain of radiocarpal joint of** left **wrist**

√7ᵗʰ **S63.529 Sprain of radiocarpal joint of unspecified wrist**

√6ᵗʰ **S63.59** Other **specified sprain of wrist**

√7ᵗʰ **S63.591 Other specified sprain of** right **wrist**

√7ᵗʰ **S63.592 Other specified sprain of** left **wrist**

√7ᵗʰ **S63.599 Other specified sprain of unspecified wrist**

√5ᵗʰ **S63.6 Other and unspecified sprain of finger(s)**

EXCLUDES 1   *traumatic rupture of ligament of finger at metacarpophalangeal and interphalangeal joint(s) (S63.4-)*

√6ᵗʰ **S63.60** Unspecified **sprain of** thumb

√7ᵗʰ **S63.601 Unspecified sprain of** right **thumb**

√7ᵗʰ **S63.602 Unspecified sprain of** left **thumb**

√7ᵗʰ **S63.609 Unspecified sprain of unspecified thumb**

√6ᵗʰ **S63.61** Unspecified **sprain of** other and unspecified finger(s)

√7ᵗʰ **S63.610 Unspecified sprain of** right index **finger**

√7ᵗʰ **S63.611 Unspecified sprain of** left index **finger**

√7ᵗʰ **S63.612 Unspecified sprain of** right middle **finger**

√7ᵗʰ **S63.613 Unspecified sprain of** left middle **finger**

√7ᵗʰ **S63.614 Unspecified sprain of** right ring **finger**

√7ᵗʰ **S63.615 Unspecified sprain of** left ring **finger**

√7ᵗʰ **S63.616 Unspecified sprain of** right little **finger**

√7ᵗʰ **S63.617 Unspecified sprain of** left little **finger**

√7ᵗʰ **S63.618 Unspecified sprain of other finger**

Unspecified sprain of specified finger with unspecified laterality

√7ᵗʰ **S63.619 Unspecified sprain of unspecified finger**

√6ᵗʰ **S63.62 Sprain of** interphalangeal joint of thumb

√7ᵗʰ **S63.621 Sprain of interphalangeal joint of** right **thumb**

√7ᵗʰ **S63.622 Sprain of interphalangeal joint of** left **thumb**

√7ᵗʰ **S63.629 Sprain of interphalangeal joint of unspecified thumb**

√6ᵗʰ **S63.63 Sprain of** interphalangeal joint of other and unspecified finger(s)

√7ᵗʰ **S63.630 Sprain of interphalangeal joint of** right index **finger**

√7ᵗʰ **S63.631 Sprain of interphalangeal joint of** left index **finger**

√7ᵗʰ **S63.632 Sprain of interphalangeal joint of** right middle **finger**

√7ᵗʰ **S63.633 Sprain of interphalangeal joint of** left middle **finger**

√7ᵗʰ **S63.634 Sprain of interphalangeal joint of** right ring **finger**

√7ᵗʰ **S63.635 Sprain of interphalangeal joint of** left ring **finger**

√7ᵗʰ **S63.636 Sprain of interphalangeal joint of** right little **finger**

√7ᵗʰ **S63.637 Sprain of interphalangeal joint of** left little **finger**

√7ᵗʰ **S63.638 Sprain of interphalangeal joint of other finger**

√7ᵗʰ **S63.639 Sprain of interphalangeal joint of unspecified finger**

√6ᵗʰ **S63.64 Sprain of** metacarpophalangeal joint of thumb

√7ᵗʰ **S63.641 Sprain of metacarpophalangeal joint of** right **thumb**

√7ᵗʰ **S63.642 Sprain of metacarpophalangeal joint of** left **thumb**

√7ᵗʰ **S63.649 Sprain of metacarpophalangeal joint of unspecified thumb**

√6ᵗʰ **S63.65 Sprain of** metacarpophalangeal joint of other and unspecified finger(s)

√7ᵗʰ **S63.650 Sprain of metacarpophalangeal joint of** right index **finger**

√7ᵗʰ **S63.651 Sprain of metacarpophalangeal joint of** left index **finger**

√7ᵗʰ **S63.652 Sprain of metacarpophalangeal joint of** right middle **finger**

√7ᵗʰ **S63.653 Sprain of metacarpophalangeal joint of** left middle **finger**

√7ᵗʰ **S63.654 Sprain of metacarpophalangeal joint of** right ring **finger**

√7ᵗʰ **S63.655 Sprain of metacarpophalangeal joint of** left ring **finger**

√7ᵗʰ **S63.656 Sprain of metacarpophalangeal joint of** right little **finger**

√7ᵗʰ **S63.657 Sprain of metacarpophalangeal joint of** left little **finger**

√7ᵗʰ **S63.658 Sprain of metacarpophalangeal joint of other finger**

Sprain of metacarpophalangeal joint of specified finger with unspecified laterality

√7ᵗʰ **S63.659 Sprain of metacarpophalangeal joint of unspecified finger**

√6ᵗʰ **S63.68 Other sprain of** thumb

√7ᵗʰ **S63.681 Other sprain of** right **thumb**

√7ᵗʰ **S63.682 Other sprain of** left **thumb**

√7ᵗʰ **S63.689 Other sprain of unspecified thumb**

√6ᵗʰ **S63.69 Other sprain of** other and unspecified finger(s)

√7ᵗʰ **S63.690 Other sprain of** right index **finger**

√7ᵗʰ **S63.691 Other sprain of** left index **finger**

√7ᵗʰ **S63.692 Other sprain of** right middle **finger**

√7ᵗʰ **S63.693 Other sprain of** left middle **finger**

√7ᵗʰ **S63.694 Other sprain of** right ring **finger**

√7ᵗʰ **S63.695 Other sprain of** left ring **finger**

√7ᵗʰ **S63.696 Other sprain of** right little **finger**

√7ᵗʰ **S63.697 Other sprain of** left little **finger**

√7ᵗʰ **S63.698 Other sprain of other finger**

Other sprain of specified finger with unspecified laterality

√7ᵗʰ **S63.699 Other sprain of unspecified finger**

√5ᵗʰ **S63.8 Sprain of other part of wrist and hand**

√6ᵗʰ **S63.8X Sprain of other part of wrist and hand**

√7ᵗʰ **S63.8X1 Sprain of other part of** right **wrist and hand**

√7ᵗʰ **S63.8X2 Sprain of other part of** left **wrist and hand**

√7ᵗʰ **S63.8X9 Sprain of other part of unspecified wrist and hand**

√5ᵗʰ **S63.9 Sprain of unspecified part of wrist and hand**

√x7ᵗʰ **S63.90 Sprain of unspecified part of unspecified wrist and hand**

√x7ᵗʰ **S63.91 Sprain of unspecified part of** right **wrist and hand**

√x7ᵗʰ **S63.92 Sprain of unspecified part of** left **wrist and hand**

√4ᵗʰ **S64 Injury of nerves at wrist and hand level**

Code also any associated open wound (S61.-)

The appropriate 7th character is to be added to each code from category S64.
A   initial encounter
D   subsequent encounter
S   sequela

√5ᵗʰ **S64.0 Injury of** ulnar **nerve at wrist and hand level**

✓ Additional Character Required   √x7ᵗʰ *X*tension Alert   Unspecified Code   Other Specified Code   Manifestation Code   ►◄ Revised Text   ● New Code   ▲ Revised Code Title

√x7ᵗʰ **S64.00** Injury of ulnar nerve at wrist and hand level of unspecified arm

√x7ᵗʰ **S64.01** Injury of ulnar nerve at wrist and hand level of right arm

√x7ᵗʰ **S64.02** Injury of ulnar nerve at wrist and hand level of left arm

√5ᵗʰ **S64.1** Injury of median nerve at wrist and hand level

√x7ᵗʰ **S64.10** Injury of median nerve at wrist and hand level of unspecified arm

√x7ᵗʰ **S64.11** Injury of median nerve at wrist and hand level of right arm

√x7ᵗʰ **S64.12** Injury of median nerve at wrist and hand level of left arm

√5ᵗʰ **S64.2** Injury of radial nerve at wrist and hand level

√x7ᵗʰ **S64.20** Injury of radial nerve at wrist and hand level of unspecified arm

√x7ᵗʰ **S64.21** Injury of radial nerve at wrist and hand level of right arm

√x7ᵗʰ **S64.22** Injury of radial nerve at wrist and hand level of left arm

√5ᵗʰ **S64.3** Injury of digital nerve of thumb

√x7ᵗʰ **S64.30** Injury of digital nerve of unspecified thumb

√x7ᵗʰ **S64.31** Injury of digital nerve of right thumb

√x7ᵗʰ **S64.32** Injury of digital nerve of left thumb

√5ᵗʰ **S64.4** Injury of digital nerve of other and unspecified finger

√x7ᵗʰ **S64.40** Injury of digital nerve of unspecified finger

√6ᵗʰ **S64.49** Injury of digital nerve of other finger

√7ᵗʰ **S64.490** Injury of digital nerve of right index finger

√7ᵗʰ **S64.491** Injury of digital nerve of left index finger

√7ᵗʰ **S64.492** Injury of digital nerve of right middle finger

√7ᵗʰ **S64.493** Injury of digital nerve of left middle finger

√7ᵗʰ **S64.494** Injury of digital nerve of right ring finger

√7ᵗʰ **S64.495** Injury of digital nerve of left ring finger

√7ᵗʰ **S64.496** Injury of digital nerve of right little finger

√7ᵗʰ **S64.497** Injury of digital nerve of left little finger

√7ᵗʰ **S64.498** Injury of digital nerve of other finger
Injury of digital nerve of specified finger with unspecified laterality

√5ᵗʰ **S64.8** Injury of other nerves at wrist and hand level

√6ᵗʰ **S64.8X** Injury of other nerves at wrist and hand level

√7ᵗʰ **S64.8X1** Injury of other nerves at wrist and hand level of right arm

√7ᵗʰ **S64.8X2** Injury of other nerves at wrist and hand level of left arm

√7ᵗʰ **S64.8X9** Injury of other nerves at wrist and hand level of unspecified arm

√5ᵗʰ **S64.9** Injury of unspecified nerve at wrist and hand level

√x7ᵗʰ **S64.90** Injury of unspecified nerve at wrist and hand level of unspecified arm

√x7ᵗʰ **S64.91** Injury of unspecified nerve at wrist and hand level of right arm

√x7ᵗʰ **S64.92** Injury of unspecified nerve at wrist and hand level of left arm

√4ᵗʰ **S65** **Injury of blood vessels at wrist and hand level**
Code also any associated open wound (S61.-)

The appropriate 7th character is to be added to each code from category S65.
A   initial encounter
D   subsequent encounter
S   sequela

√5ᵗʰ **S65.0** Injury of ulnar artery at wrist and hand level

√6ᵗʰ **S65.00** Unspecified injury of ulnar artery at wrist and hand level

√7ᵗʰ **S65.001** Unspecified injury of ulnar artery at wrist and hand level of right arm

√7ᵗʰ **S65.002** Unspecified injury of ulnar artery at wrist and hand level of left arm

√7ᵗʰ **S65.009** Unspecified injury of ulnar artery at wrist and hand level of unspecified arm

√6ᵗʰ **S65.01** Laceration of ulnar artery at wrist and hand level

√7ᵗʰ **S65.011** Laceration of ulnar artery at wrist and hand level of right arm

√7ᵗʰ **S65.012** Laceration of ulnar artery at wrist and hand level of left arm

√7ᵗʰ **S65.019** Laceration of ulnar artery at wrist and hand level of unspecified arm

√6ᵗʰ **S65.09** Other specified injury of ulnar artery at wrist and hand level

√7ᵗʰ **S65.091** Other specified injury of ulnar artery at wrist and hand level of right arm

√7ᵗʰ **S65.092** Other specified injury of ulnar artery at wrist and hand level of left arm

√7ᵗʰ **S65.099** Other specified injury of ulnar artery at wrist and hand level of unspecified arm

√5ᵗʰ **S65.1** Injury of radial artery at wrist and hand level

√6ᵗʰ **S65.10** Unspecified injury of radial artery at wrist and hand level

√7ᵗʰ **S65.101** Unspecified injury of radial artery at wrist and hand level of right arm

√7ᵗʰ **S65.102** Unspecified injury of radial artery at wrist and hand level of left arm

√7ᵗʰ **S65.109** Unspecified injury of radial artery at wrist and hand level of unspecified arm

√6ᵗʰ **S65.11** Laceration of radial artery at wrist and hand level

√7ᵗʰ **S65.111** Laceration of radial artery at wrist and hand level of right arm

√7ᵗʰ **S65.112** Laceration of radial artery at wrist and hand level of left arm

√7ᵗʰ **S65.119** Laceration of radial artery at wrist and hand level of unspecified arm

√6ᵗʰ **S65.19** Other specified injury of radial artery at wrist and hand level

√7ᵗʰ **S65.191** Other specified injury of radial artery at wrist and hand level of right arm

√7ᵗʰ **S65.192** Other specified injury of radial artery at wrist and hand level of left arm

√7ᵗʰ **S65.199** Other specified injury of radial artery at wrist and hand level of unspecified arm

√5ᵗʰ **S65.2** Injury of superficial palmar arch

√6ᵗʰ **S65.20** Unspecified injury of superficial palmar arch

√7ᵗʰ **S65.201** Unspecified injury of superficial palmar arch of right hand

√7ᵗʰ **S65.202** Unspecified injury of superficial palmar arch of left hand

√7ᵗʰ **S65.209** Unspecified injury of superficial palmar arch of unspecified hand

√6ᵗʰ **S65.21** Laceration of superficial palmar arch

√7ᵗʰ **S65.211** Laceration of superficial palmar arch of right hand

√7ᵗʰ **S65.212** Laceration of superficial palmar arch of left hand

√7ᵗʰ **S65.219** Laceration of superficial palmar arch of unspecified hand

√6ᵗʰ **S65.29** Other specified injury of superficial palmar arch

√7ᵗʰ **S65.291** Other specified injury of superficial palmar arch of right hand

√7ᵗʰ **S65.292** Other specified injury of superficial palmar arch of left hand

√7ᵗʰ **S65.299** Other specified injury of superficial palmar arch of unspecified hand

√5ᵗʰ **S65.3** Injury of deep palmar arch

√6ᵗʰ **S65.30** Unspecified injury of deep palmar arch

√7ᵗʰ **S65.301** Unspecified injury of deep palmar arch of right hand

√7ᵗʰ **S65.302** Unspecified injury of deep palmar arch of left hand

√7ᵗʰ **S65.309** Unspecified injury of deep palmar arch of unspecified hand

√6ᵗʰ **S65.31** Laceration of deep palmar arch

√7ᵗʰ **S65.311** Laceration of deep palmar arch of right hand

√7ᵗʰ **S65.312** Laceration of deep palmar arch of left hand

EXCLUDES 1 Not coded here   EXCLUDES 2 Not included here   N Newborn Age: 0   P Pediatric Age: 0-17   M Maternity Age: 12-55   A Adult Age: 15-124

880

ICD-10-CM 2014 (Draft)

√7ᵗʰ **S65.319 Laceration of deep palmar arch of unspecified hand**

√6ᵗʰ **S65.39** Other specified injury of deep palmar arch

√7ᵗʰ **S65.391 Other specified injury of deep palmar arch of right hand**

√7ᵗʰ **S65.392 Other specified injury of deep palmar arch of left hand**

√7ᵗʰ **S65.399 Other specified injury of deep palmar arch of unspecified hand**

√5ᵗʰ **S65.4** Injury of blood vessel of thumb

√6ᵗʰ **S65.40** Unspecified injury of blood vessel of thumb

√7ᵗʰ **S65.401 Unspecified injury of blood vessel of right thumb**

√7ᵗʰ **S65.402 Unspecified injury of blood vessel of left thumb**

√7ᵗʰ **S65.409 Unspecified injury of blood vessel of unspecified thumb**

√6ᵗʰ **S65.41** Laceration of blood vessel of thumb

√7ᵗʰ **S65.411 Laceration of blood vessel of right thumb**

√7ᵗʰ **S65.412 Laceration of blood vessel of left thumb**

√7ᵗʰ **S65.419 Laceration of blood vessel of unspecified thumb**

√6ᵗʰ **S65.49** Other specified injury of blood vessel of thumb

√7ᵗʰ **S65.491 Other specified injury of blood vessel of right thumb**

√7ᵗʰ **S65.492 Other specified injury of blood vessel of left thumb**

√7ᵗʰ **S65.499 Other specified injury of blood vessel of unspecified thumb**

√5ᵗʰ **S65.5** Injury of blood vessel of other and unspecified finger

√6ᵗʰ **S65.50** Unspecified injury of blood vessel of other and unspecified finger

√7ᵗʰ **S65.500 Unspecified injury of blood vessel of right index finger**

√7ᵗʰ **S65.501 Unspecified injury of blood vessel of left index finger**

√7ᵗʰ **S65.502 Unspecified injury of blood vessel of right middle finger**

√7ᵗʰ **S65.503 Unspecified injury of blood vessel of left middle finger**

√7ᵗʰ **S65.504 Unspecified injury of blood vessel of right ring finger**

√7ᵗʰ **S65.505 Unspecified injury of blood vessel of left ring finger**

√7ᵗʰ **S65.506 Unspecified injury of blood vessel of right little finger**

√7ᵗʰ **S65.507 Unspecified injury of blood vessel of left little finger**

√7ᵗʰ **S65.508 Unspecified injury of blood vessel of other finger**
Unspecified injury of blood vessel of specified finger with unspecified laterality

√7ᵗʰ **S65.509 Unspecified injury of blood vessel of unspecified finger**

√6ᵗʰ **S65.51** Laceration of blood vessel of other and unspecified finger

√7ᵗʰ **S65.510 Laceration of blood vessel of right index finger**

√7ᵗʰ **S65.511 Laceration of blood vessel of left index finger**

√7ᵗʰ **S65.512 Laceration of blood vessel of right middle finger**

√7ᵗʰ **S65.513 Laceration of blood vessel of left middle finger**

√7ᵗʰ **S65.514 Laceration of blood vessel of right ring finger**

√7ᵗʰ **S65.515 Laceration of blood vessel of left ring finger**

√7ᵗʰ **S65.516 Laceration of blood vessel of right little finger**

√7ᵗʰ **S65.517 Laceration of blood vessel of left little finger**

√7ᵗʰ **S65.518 Laceration of blood vessel of other finger**
Laceration of blood vessel of specified finger with unspecified laterality

√7ᵗʰ **S65.519 Laceration of blood vessel of unspecified finger**

√6ᵗʰ **S65.59** Other specified injury of blood vessel of other and unspecified finger

√7ᵗʰ **S65.590 Other specified injury of blood vessel of right index finger**

√7ᵗʰ **S65.591 Other specified injury of blood vessel of left index finger**

√7ᵗʰ **S65.592 Other specified injury of blood vessel of right middle finger**

√7ᵗʰ **S65.593 Other specified injury of blood vessel of left middle finger**

√7ᵗʰ **S65.594 Other specified injury of blood vessel of right ring finger**

√7ᵗʰ **S65.595 Other specified injury of blood vessel of left ring finger**

√7ᵗʰ **S65.596 Other specified injury of blood vessel of right little finger**

√7ᵗʰ **S65.597 Other specified injury of blood vessel of left little finger**

√7ᵗʰ **S65.598 Other specified injury of blood vessel of other finger**
Other specified injury of blood vessel of specified finger with unspecified laterality

√7ᵗʰ **S65.599 Other specified injury of blood vessel of unspecified finger**

√5ᵗʰ **S65.8** Injury of other blood vessels at wrist and hand level

√6ᵗʰ **S65.80** Unspecified injury of other blood vessels at wrist and hand level

√7ᵗʰ **S65.801 Unspecified injury of other blood vessels at wrist and hand level of right arm**

√7ᵗʰ **S65.802 Unspecified injury of other blood vessels at wrist and hand level of left arm**

√7ᵗʰ **S65.809 Unspecified injury of other blood vessels at wrist and hand level of unspecified arm**

√6ᵗʰ **S65.81** Laceration of other blood vessels at wrist and hand level

√7ᵗʰ **S65.811 Laceration of other blood vessels at wrist and hand level of right arm**

√7ᵗʰ **S65.812 Laceration of other blood vessels at wrist and hand level of left arm**

√7ᵗʰ **S65.819 Laceration of other blood vessels at wrist and hand level of unspecified arm**

√6ᵗʰ **S65.89** Other specified injury of other blood vessels at wrist and hand level

√7ᵗʰ **S65.891 Other specified injury of other blood vessels at wrist and hand level of right arm**

√7ᵗʰ **S65.892 Other specified injury of other blood vessels at wrist and hand level of left arm**

√7ᵗʰ **S65.899 Other specified injury of other blood vessels at wrist and hand level of unspecified arm**

√5ᵗʰ **S65.9** Injury of unspecified blood vessel at wrist and hand level

√6ᵗʰ **S65.90** Unspecified injury of unspecified blood vessel at wrist and hand level

√7ᵗʰ **S65.901 Unspecified injury of unspecified blood vessel at wrist and hand level of right arm**

√7ᵗʰ **S65.902 Unspecified injury of unspecified blood vessel at wrist and hand level of left arm**

√7ᵗʰ **S65.909 Unspecified injury of unspecified blood vessel at wrist and hand level of unspecified arm**

√6ᵗʰ **S65.91** Laceration of unspecified blood vessel at wrist and hand level

√7ᵗʰ **S65.911 Laceration of unspecified blood vessel at wrist and hand level of right arm**

√7ᵗʰ **S65.912 Laceration of unspecified blood vessel at wrist and hand level of left arm**

√7ᵗʰ **S65.919 Laceration of unspecified blood vessel at wrist and hand level of unspecified arm**

√6ᵗʰ **S65.99** Other specified injury of unspecified blood vessel at wrist and hand level

  √7ᵗʰ **S65.991** Other specified injury of unspecified blood vessel at wrist and hand of right arm

  √7ᵗʰ **S65.992** Other specified injury of unspecified blood vessel at wrist and hand of left arm

  √7ᵗʰ **S65.999** Other specified injury of unspecified blood vessel at wrist and hand of unspecified arm

√4ᵗʰ **S66** **Injury of muscle, fascia and tendon at wrist and hand level**

Code also any associated open wound (S61.-)

EXCLUDES 2 *sprain of joints and ligaments of wrist and hand (S63.-)*

The appropriate 7th character is to be added to each code from category S66.
A   initial encounter
D   subsequent encounter
S   sequela

√5ᵗʰ **S66.0** **Injury of long flexor muscle, fascia and tendon of thumb at wrist and hand level**

  √6ᵗʰ **S66.00** Unspecified injury of long flexor muscle, fascia and tendon of thumb at wrist and hand level

    √7ᵗʰ **S66.001** Unspecified injury of long flexor muscle, fascia and tendon of right thumb at wrist and hand level

    √7ᵗʰ **S66.002** Unspecified injury of long flexor muscle, fascia and tendon of left thumb at wrist and hand level

    √7ᵗʰ **S66.009** Unspecified injury of long flexor muscle, fascia and tendon of unspecified thumb at wrist and hand level

  √6ᵗʰ **S66.01** Strain of long flexor muscle, fascia and tendon of thumb at wrist and hand level

    √7ᵗʰ **S66.011** Strain of long flexor muscle, fascia and tendon of right thumb at wrist and hand level

    √7ᵗʰ **S66.012** Strain of long flexor muscle, fascia and tendon of left thumb at wrist and hand level

    √7ᵗʰ **S66.019** Strain of long flexor muscle, fascia and tendon of unspecified thumb at wrist and hand level

  √6ᵗʰ **S66.02** Laceration of long flexor muscle, fascia and tendon of thumb at wrist and hand level

    √7ᵗʰ **S66.021** Laceration of long flexor muscle, fascia and tendon of right thumb at wrist and hand level

    √7ᵗʰ **S66.022** Laceration of long flexor muscle, fascia and tendon of left thumb at wrist and hand level

    √7ᵗʰ **S66.029** Laceration of long flexor muscle, fascia and tendon of unspecified thumb at wrist and hand level

  √6ᵗʰ **S66.09** Other specified injury of long flexor muscle, fascia and tendon of thumb at wrist and hand level

    √7ᵗʰ **S66.091** Other specified injury of long flexor muscle, fascia and tendon of right thumb at wrist and hand level

    √7ᵗʰ **S66.092** Other specified injury of long flexor muscle, fascia and tendon of left thumb at wrist and hand level

    √7ᵗʰ **S66.099** Other specified injury of long flexor muscle, fascia and tendon of unspecified thumb at wrist and hand level

√5ᵗʰ **S66.1** **Injury of flexor muscle, fascia and tendon of other and unspecified finger at wrist and hand level**

EXCLUDES 2 *Injury of long flexor muscle, fascia and tendon of thumb at wrist and hand level (S66.0-)*

  √6ᵗʰ **S66.10** Unspecified injury of flexor muscle, fascia and tendon of other and unspecified finger at wrist and hand level

    √7ᵗʰ **S66.100** Unspecified injury of flexor muscle, fascia and tendon of right index finger at wrist and hand level

    √7ᵗʰ **S66.101** Unspecified injury of flexor muscle, fascia and tendon of left index finger at wrist and hand level

    √7ᵗʰ **S66.102** Unspecified injury of flexor muscle, fascia and tendon of right middle finger at wrist and hand level

    √7ᵗʰ **S66.103** Unspecified injury of flexor muscle, fascia and tendon of left middle finger at wrist and hand level

    √7ᵗʰ **S66.104** Unspecified injury of flexor muscle, fascia and tendon of right ring finger at wrist and hand level

    √7ᵗʰ **S66.105** Unspecified injury of flexor muscle, fascia and tendon of left ring finger at wrist and hand level

    √7ᵗʰ **S66.106** Unspecified injury of flexor muscle, fascia and tendon of right little finger at wrist and hand level

    √7ᵗʰ **S66.107** Unspecified injury of flexor muscle, fascia and tendon of left little finger at wrist and hand level

    √7ᵗʰ **S66.108** Unspecified injury of flexor muscle, fascia and tendon of other finger at wrist and hand level

Unspecified injury of flexor muscle, fascia and tendon of specified finger with unspecified laterality at wrist and hand level

    √7ᵗʰ **S66.109** Unspecified injury of flexor muscle, fascia and tendon of unspecified finger at wrist and hand level

  √6ᵗʰ **S66.11** Strain of flexor muscle, fascia and tendon of other and unspecified finger at wrist and hand level

    √7ᵗʰ **S66.110** Strain of flexor muscle, fascia and tendon of right index finger at wrist and hand level

    √7ᵗʰ **S66.111** Strain of flexor muscle, fascia and tendon of left index finger at wrist and hand level

    √7ᵗʰ **S66.112** Strain of flexor muscle, fascia and tendon of right middle finger at wrist and hand level

    √7ᵗʰ **S66.113** Strain of flexor muscle, fascia and tendon of left middle finger at wrist and hand level

    √7ᵗʰ **S66.114** Strain of flexor muscle, fascia and tendon of right ring finger at wrist and hand level

    √7ᵗʰ **S66.115** Strain of flexor muscle, fascia and tendon of left ring finger at wrist and hand level

    √7ᵗʰ **S66.116** Strain of flexor muscle, fascia and tendon of right little finger at wrist and hand level

    √7ᵗʰ **S66.117** Strain of flexor muscle, fascia and tendon of left little finger at wrist and hand level

    √7ᵗʰ **S66.118** Strain of flexor muscle, fascia and tendon of other finger at wrist and hand level

Strain of flexor muscle, fascia and tendon of specified finger with unspecified laterality at wrist and hand level

    √7ᵗʰ **S66.119** Strain of flexor muscle, fascia and tendon of unspecified finger at wrist and hand level

  √6ᵗʰ **S66.12** Laceration of flexor muscle, fascia and tendon of other and unspecified finger at wrist and hand level

    √7ᵗʰ **S66.120** Laceration of flexor muscle, fascia and tendon of right index finger at wrist and hand level

    √7ᵗʰ **S66.121** Laceration of flexor muscle, fascia and tendon of left index finger at wrist and hand level

    √7ᵗʰ **S66.122** Laceration of flexor muscle, fascia and tendon of right middle finger at wrist and hand level

    √7ᵗʰ **S66.123** Laceration of flexor muscle, fascia and tendon of left middle finger at wrist and hand level

    √7ᵗʰ **S66.124** Laceration of flexor muscle, fascia and tendon of right ring finger at wrist and hand level

    √7ᵗʰ **S66.125** Laceration of flexor muscle, fascia and tendon of left ring finger at wrist and hand level

EXCLUDES 1 Not coded here   EXCLUDES 2 Not included here   N Newborn Age: 0   P Pediatric Age: 0-17   M Maternity Age: 12-55   A Adult Age: 15-124

882   ICD-10-CM 2014 (Draft)

√7ᵗʰ **S66.126 Laceration of flexor muscle, fascia and tendon of right little finger at wrist and hand level**

√7ᵗʰ **S66.127 Laceration of flexor muscle, fascia and tendon of left little finger at wrist and hand level**

√7ᵗʰ **S66.128 Laceration of flexor muscle, fascia and tendon of other finger at wrist and hand level**

    Laceration of flexor muscle, fascia and tendon of specified finger with unspecified laterality at wrist and hand level

√7ᵗʰ **S66.129 Laceration of flexor muscle, fascia and tendon of unspecified finger at wrist and hand level**

√6ᵗʰ **S66.19 Other injury of flexor muscle, fascia and tendon of other and unspecified finger at wrist and hand level**

√7ᵗʰ **S66.190 Other injury of flexor muscle, fascia and tendon of right index finger at wrist and hand level**

√7ᵗʰ **S66.191 Other injury of flexor muscle, fascia and tendon of left index finger at wrist and hand level**

√7ᵗʰ **S66.192 Other injury of flexor muscle, fascia and tendon of right middle finger at wrist and hand level**

√7ᵗʰ **S66.193 Other injury of flexor muscle, fascia and tendon of left middle finger at wrist and hand level**

√7ᵗʰ **S66.194 Other injury of flexor muscle, fascia and tendon of right ring finger at wrist and hand level**

√7ᵗʰ **S66.195 Other injury of flexor muscle, fascia and tendon of left ring finger at wrist and hand level**

√7ᵗʰ **S66.196 Other injury of flexor muscle, fascia and tendon of right little finger at wrist and hand level**

√7ᵗʰ **S66.197 Other injury of flexor muscle, fascia and tendon of left little finger at wrist and hand level**

√7ᵗʰ **S66.198 Other injury of flexor muscle, fascia and tendon of other finger at wrist and hand level**

    Other injury of flexor muscle, fascia and tendon of specified finger with unspecified laterality at wrist and hand level

√7ᵗʰ **S66.199 Other injury of flexor muscle, fascia and tendon of unspecified finger at wrist and hand level**

√5ᵗʰ **S66.2 Injury of extensor muscle, fascia and tendon of thumb at wrist and hand level**

√6ᵗʰ **S66.20 Unspecified injury of extensor muscle, fascia and tendon of thumb at wrist and hand level**

√7ᵗʰ **S66.201 Unspecified injury of extensor muscle, fascia and tendon of right thumb at wrist and hand level**

√7ᵗʰ **S66.202 Unspecified injury of extensor muscle, fascia and tendon of left thumb at wrist and hand level**

√7ᵗʰ **S66.209 Unspecified injury of extensor muscle, fascia and tendon of unspecified thumb at wrist and hand level**

√6ᵗʰ **S66.21 Strain of extensor muscle, fascia and tendon of thumb at wrist and hand level**

√7ᵗʰ **S66.211 Strain of extensor muscle, fascia and tendon of right thumb at wrist and hand level**

√7ᵗʰ **S66.212 Strain of extensor muscle, fascia and tendon of left thumb at wrist and hand level**

√7ᵗʰ **S66.219 Strain of extensor muscle, fascia and tendon of unspecified thumb at wrist and hand level**

√6ᵗʰ **S66.22 Laceration of extensor muscle, fascia and tendon of thumb at wrist and hand level**

√7ᵗʰ **S66.221 Laceration of extensor muscle, fascia and tendon of right thumb at wrist and hand level**

√7ᵗʰ **S66.222 Laceration of extensor muscle, fascia and tendon of left thumb at wrist and hand level**

√7ᵗʰ **S66.229 Laceration of extensor muscle, fascia and tendon of unspecified thumb at wrist and hand level**

√6ᵗʰ **S66.29 Other specified injury of extensor muscle, fascia and tendon of thumb at wrist and hand level**

√7ᵗʰ **S66.291 Other specified injury of extensor muscle, fascia and tendon of right thumb at wrist and hand level**

√7ᵗʰ **S66.292 Other specified injury of extensor muscle, fascia and tendon of left thumb at wrist and hand level**

√7ᵗʰ **S66.299 Other specified injury of extensor muscle, fascia and tendon of unspecified thumb at wrist and hand level**

√5ᵗʰ **S66.3 Injury of extensor muscle, fascia and tendon of other and unspecified finger at wrist and hand level**

    EXCLUDES 2 *Injury of extensor muscle, fascia and tendon of thumb at wrist and hand level (S66.2-)*

√6ᵗʰ **S66.30 Unspecified injury of extensor muscle, fascia and tendon of other and unspecified finger at wrist and hand level**

√7ᵗʰ **S66.300 Unspecified injury of extensor muscle, fascia and tendon of right index finger at wrist and hand level**

√7ᵗʰ **S66.301 Unspecified injury of extensor muscle, fascia and tendon of left index finger at wrist and hand level**

√7ᵗʰ **S66.302 Unspecified injury of extensor muscle, fascia and tendon of right middle finger at wrist and hand level**

√7ᵗʰ **S66.303 Unspecified injury of extensor muscle, fascia and tendon of left middle finger at wrist and hand level**

√7ᵗʰ **S66.304 Unspecified injury of extensor muscle, fascia and tendon of right ring finger at wrist and hand level**

√7ᵗʰ **S66.305 Unspecified injury of extensor muscle, fascia and tendon of left ring finger at wrist and hand level**

√7ᵗʰ **S66.306 Unspecified injury of extensor muscle, fascia and tendon of right little finger at wrist and hand level**

√7ᵗʰ **S66.307 Unspecified injury of extensor muscle, fascia and tendon of left little finger at wrist and hand level**

√7ᵗʰ **S66.308 Unspecified injury of extensor muscle, fascia and tendon of other finger at wrist and hand level**

    Unspecified injury of extensor muscle, fascia and tendon of specified finger with unspecified laterality at wrist and hand level

√7ᵗʰ **S66.309 Unspecified injury of extensor muscle, fascia and tendon of unspecified finger at wrist and hand level**

√6ᵗʰ **S66.31 Strain of extensor muscle, fascia and tendon of other and unspecified finger at wrist and hand level**

√7ᵗʰ **S66.310 Strain of extensor muscle, fascia and tendon of right index finger at wrist and hand level**

√7ᵗʰ **S66.311 Strain of extensor muscle, fascia and tendon of left index finger at wrist and hand level**

√7ᵗʰ **S66.312 Strain of extensor muscle, fascia and tendon of right middle finger at wrist and hand level**

√7ᵗʰ **S66.313 Strain of extensor muscle, fascia and tendon of left middle finger at wrist and hand level**

√7ᵗʰ **S66.314 Strain of extensor muscle, fascia and tendon of right ring finger at wrist and hand level**

√ Additional Character Required   √x7ᵗʰ *X*tension Alert   Unspecified Code   Other Specified Code   Manifestation Code   ►◄ Revised Text   ● New Code   ▲ Revised Code Title

✓7ᵗʰ **S66.315** Strain of extensor muscle, fascia and tendon of left ring finger at wrist and hand level

✓7ᵗʰ **S66.316** Strain of extensor muscle, fascia and tendon of right little finger at wrist and hand level

✓7ᵗʰ **S66.317** Strain of extensor muscle, fascia and tendon of left little finger at wrist and hand level

✓7ᵗʰ **S66.318** Strain of extensor muscle, fascia and tendon of other finger at wrist and hand level

Strain of extensor muscle, fascia and tendon of specified finger with unspecified laterality at wrist and hand level

✓7ᵗʰ **S66.319** Strain of extensor muscle, fascia and tendon of unspecified finger at wrist and hand level

✓6ᵗʰ **S66.32** Laceration of extensor muscle, fascia and tendon of other and unspecified finger at wrist and hand level

✓7ᵗʰ **S66.320** Laceration of extensor muscle, fascia and tendon of right index finger at wrist and hand level

✓7ᵗʰ **S66.321** Laceration of extensor muscle, fascia and tendon of left index finger at wrist and hand level

✓7ᵗʰ **S66.322** Laceration of extensor muscle, fascia and tendon of right middle finger at wrist and hand level

✓7ᵗʰ **S66.323** Laceration of extensor muscle, fascia and tendon of left middle finger at wrist and hand level

✓7ᵗʰ **S66.324** Laceration of extensor muscle, fascia and tendon of right ring finger at wrist and hand level

✓7ᵗʰ **S66.325** Laceration of extensor muscle, fascia and tendon of left ring finger at wrist and hand level

✓7ᵗʰ **S66.326** Laceration of extensor muscle, fascia and tendon of right little finger at wrist and hand level

✓7ᵗʰ **S66.327** Laceration of extensor muscle, fascia and tendon of left little finger at wrist and hand level

✓7ᵗʰ **S66.328** Laceration of extensor muscle, fascia and tendon of other finger at wrist and hand level

Laceration of extensor muscle, fascia and tendon of specified finger with unspecified laterality at wrist and hand level

✓7ᵗʰ **S66.329** Laceration of extensor muscle, fascia and tendon of unspecified finger at wrist and hand level

✓6ᵗʰ **S66.39** Other injury of extensor muscle, fascia and tendon of other and unspecified finger at wrist and hand level

✓7ᵗʰ **S66.390** Other injury of extensor muscle, fascia and tendon of right index finger at wrist and hand level

✓7ᵗʰ **S66.391** Other injury of extensor muscle, fascia and tendon of left index finger at wrist and hand level

✓7ᵗʰ **S66.392** Other injury of extensor muscle, fascia and tendon of right middle finger at wrist and hand level

✓7ᵗʰ **S66.393** Other injury of extensor muscle, fascia and tendon of left middle finger at wrist and hand level

✓7ᵗʰ **S66.394** Other injury of extensor muscle, fascia and tendon of right ring finger at wrist and hand level

✓7ᵗʰ **S66.395** Other injury of extensor muscle, fascia and tendon of left ring finger at wrist and hand level

✓7ᵗʰ **S66.396** Other injury of extensor muscle, fascia and tendon of right little finger at wrist and hand level

✓7ᵗʰ **S66.397** Other injury of extensor muscle, fascia and tendon of left little finger at wrist and hand level

✓7ᵗʰ **S66.398** Other injury of extensor muscle, fascia and tendon of other finger at wrist and hand level

Other injury of extensor muscle, fascia and tendon of specified finger with unspecified laterality at wrist and hand level

✓7ᵗʰ **S66.399** Other injury of extensor muscle, fascia and tendon of unspecified finger at wrist and hand level

✓5ᵗʰ **S66.4** Injury of intrinsic muscle, fascia and tendon of thumb at wrist and hand level

✓6ᵗʰ **S66.40** Unspecified injury of intrinsic muscle, fascia and tendon of thumb at wrist and hand level

✓7ᵗʰ **S66.401** Unspecified injury of intrinsic muscle, fascia and tendon of right thumb at wrist and hand level

✓7ᵗʰ **S66.402** Unspecified injury of intrinsic muscle, fascia and tendon of left thumb at wrist and hand level

✓7ᵗʰ **S66.409** Unspecified injury of intrinsic muscle, fascia and tendon of unspecified thumb at wrist and hand level

✓6ᵗʰ **S66.41** Strain of intrinsic muscle, fascia and tendon of thumb at wrist and hand level

✓7ᵗʰ **S66.411** Strain of intrinsic muscle, fascia and tendon of right thumb at wrist and hand level

✓7ᵗʰ **S66.412** Strain of intrinsic muscle, fascia and tendon of left thumb at wrist and hand level

✓7ᵗʰ **S66.419** Strain of intrinsic muscle, fascia and tendon of unspecified thumb at wrist and hand level

✓6ᵗʰ **S66.42** Laceration of intrinsic muscle, fascia and tendon of thumb at wrist and hand level

✓7ᵗʰ **S66.421** Laceration of intrinsic muscle, fascia and tendon of right thumb at wrist and hand level

✓7ᵗʰ **S66.422** Laceration of intrinsic muscle, fascia and tendon of left thumb at wrist and hand

✓7ᵗʰ **S66.429** Laceration of intrinsic muscle, fascia and tendon of unspecified thumb at wrist and hand level of side

✓6ᵗʰ **S66.49** Other specified injury of intrinsic muscle, fascia and tendon of thumb at wrist and hand level

✓7ᵗʰ **S66.491** Other specified injury of intrinsic muscle, fascia and tendon of right thumb at wrist and hand level

✓7ᵗʰ **S66.492** Other specified injury of intrinsic muscle, fascia and tendon of left thumb at wrist and hand level

✓7ᵗʰ **S66.499** Other specified injury of intrinsic muscle, fascia and tendon of unspecified thumb at wrist and hand level

✓5ᵗʰ **S66.5** Injury of intrinsic muscle, fascia and tendon of other and unspecified finger at wrist and hand level

EXCLUDES 2   injury of intrinsic muscle, fascia and tendon of thumb at wrist and hand level (S66.4-)

✓6ᵗʰ **S66.50** Unspecified injury of intrinsic muscle, fascia and tendon of other and unspecified finger at wrist and hand level

✓7ᵗʰ **S66.500** Unspecified injury of intrinsic muscle, fascia and tendon of right index finger at wrist and hand level

✓7ᵗʰ **S66.501** Unspecified injury of intrinsic muscle, fascia and tendon of left index finger at wrist and hand level

✓7ᵗʰ **S66.502** Unspecified injury of intrinsic muscle, fascia and tendon of right middle finger at wrist and hand level

✓7ᵗʰ **S66.503** Unspecified injury of intrinsic muscle, fascia and tendon of left middle finger at wrist and hand level

EXCLUDES 1 Not coded here   EXCLUDES 2 Not included here   N Newborn Age: 0   P Pediatric Age: 0-17   M Maternity Age: 12-55   A Adult Age: 15-124

884   ICD-10-CM 2014 (Draft)

√7ᵗʰ **S66.504** **Unspecified injury of intrinsic muscle, fascia and tendon of right ring finger at wrist and hand level**

√7ᵗʰ **S66.505** **Unspecified injury of intrinsic muscle, fascia and tendon of left ring finger at wrist and hand level**

√7ᵗʰ **S66.506** **Unspecified injury of intrinsic muscle, fascia and tendon of right little finger at wrist and hand level**

√7ᵗʰ **S66.507** **Unspecified injury of intrinsic muscle, fascia and tendon of left little finger at wrist and hand level**

√7ᵗʰ **S66.508** **Unspecified injury of intrinsic muscle, fascia and tendon of other finger at wrist and hand level**

Unspecified injury of intrinsic muscle, fascia and tendon of specified finger with unspecified laterality at wrist and hand level

√7ᵗʰ **S66.509** **Unspecified injury of intrinsic muscle, fascia and tendon of unspecified finger at wrist and hand level**

√6ᵗʰ **S66.51** Strain of intrinsic muscle, fascia and tendon of other and unspecified finger at wrist and hand level

√7ᵗʰ **S66.510** **Strain of intrinsic muscle, fascia and tendon of right index finger at wrist and hand level**

√7ᵗʰ **S66.511** **Strain of intrinsic muscle, fascia and tendon of left index finger at wrist and hand level**

√7ᵗʰ **S66.512** **Strain of intrinsic muscle, fascia and tendon of right middle finger at wrist and hand level**

√7ᵗʰ **S66.513** **Strain of intrinsic muscle, fascia and tendon of left middle finger at wrist and hand level**

√7ᵗʰ **S66.514** **Strain of intrinsic muscle, fascia and tendon of right ring finger at wrist and hand level**

√7ᵗʰ **S66.515** **Strain of intrinsic muscle, fascia and tendon of left ring finger at wrist and hand level**

√7ᵗʰ **S66.516** **Strain of intrinsic muscle, fascia and tendon of right little finger at wrist and hand level**

√7ᵗʰ **S66.517** **Strain of intrinsic muscle, fascia and tendon of left little finger at wrist and hand level**

√7ᵗʰ **S66.518** **Strain of intrinsic muscle, fascia and tendon of other finger at wrist and hand level**

Strain of intrinsic muscle, fascia and tendon of specified finger with unspecified laterality at wrist and hand level

√7ᵗʰ **S66.519** **Strain of intrinsic muscle, fascia and tendon of unspecified finger at wrist and hand level**

√6ᵗʰ **S66.52** Laceration of intrinsic muscle, fascia and tendon of other and unspecified finger at wrist and hand level

√7ᵗʰ **S66.520** **Laceration of intrinsic muscle, fascia and tendon of right index finger at wrist and hand level**

√7ᵗʰ **S66.521** **Laceration of intrinsic muscle, fascia and tendon of left index finger at wrist and hand level**

√7ᵗʰ **S66.522** **Laceration of intrinsic muscle, fascia and tendon of right middle finger at wrist and hand level**

√7ᵗʰ **S66.523** **Laceration of intrinsic muscle, fascia and tendon of left middle finger at wrist and hand level**

√7ᵗʰ **S66.524** **Laceration of intrinsic muscle, fascia and tendon of right ring finger at wrist and hand level**

√7ᵗʰ **S66.525** **Laceration of intrinsic muscle, fascia and tendon of left ring finger at wrist and hand level**

√7ᵗʰ **S66.526** **Laceration of intrinsic muscle, fascia and tendon of right little finger at wrist and hand level**

√7ᵗʰ **S66.527** **Laceration of intrinsic muscle, fascia and tendon of left little finger at wrist and hand level**

√7ᵗʰ **S66.528** **Laceration of intrinsic muscle, fascia and tendon of other finger at wrist and hand level**

Laceration of intrinsic muscle, fascia and tendon of specified finger with unspecified laterality at wrist and hand level

√7ᵗʰ **S66.529** **Laceration of intrinsic muscle, fascia and tendon of unspecified finger at wrist and hand level**

√6ᵗʰ **S66.59** Other injury of intrinsic muscle, fascia and tendon of other and unspecified finger at wrist and hand level

√7ᵗʰ **S66.590** **Other injury of intrinsic muscle, fascia and tendon of right index finger at wrist and hand level**

√7ᵗʰ **S66.591** **Other injury of intrinsic muscle, fascia and tendon of left index finger at wrist and hand level**

√7ᵗʰ **S66.592** **Other injury of intrinsic muscle, fascia and tendon of right middle finger at wrist and hand level**

√7ᵗʰ **S66.593** **Other injury of intrinsic muscle, fascia and tendon of left middle finger at wrist and hand level**

√7ᵗʰ **S66.594** **Other injury of intrinsic muscle, fascia and tendon of right ring finger at wrist and hand level**

√7ᵗʰ **S66.595** **Other injury of intrinsic muscle, fascia and tendon of left ring finger at wrist and hand level**

√7ᵗʰ **S66.596** **Other injury of intrinsic muscle, fascia and tendon of right little finger at wrist and hand level**

√7ᵗʰ **S66.597** **Other injury of intrinsic muscle, fascia and tendon of left little finger at wrist and hand level**

√7ᵗʰ **S66.598** **Other injury of intrinsic muscle, fascia and tendon of other finger at wrist and hand level**

Other injury of intrinsic muscle, fascia and tendon of specified finger with unspecified laterality at wrist and hand level

√7ᵗʰ **S66.599** **Other injury of intrinsic muscle, fascia and tendon of unspecified finger at wrist and hand level**

√5ᵗʰ **S66.8** Injury of other specified muscles, fascia and tendons at wrist and hand level

√6ᵗʰ **S66.80** Unspecified injury of other specified muscles, fascia and tendons at wrist and hand level

√7ᵗʰ **S66.801** **Unspecified injury of other specified muscles, fascia and tendons at wrist and hand level, right hand**

√7ᵗʰ **S66.802** **Unspecified injury of other specified muscles, fascia and tendons at wrist and hand level, left hand**

√7ᵗʰ **S66.809** **Unspecified injury of other specified muscles, fascia and tendons at wrist and hand level, unspecified hand**

√6ᵗʰ **S66.81** Strain of other specified muscles, fascia and tendons at wrist and hand level

√7ᵗʰ **S66.811** **Strain of other specified muscles, fascia and tendons at wrist and hand level, right hand**

√7ᵗʰ **S66.812** **Strain of other specified muscles, fascia and tendons at wrist and hand level, left hand**

√7ᵗʰ **S66.819** **Strain of other specified muscles, fascia and tendons at wrist and hand level, unspecified hand**

√6ᵗʰ **S66.82** Laceration of other specified muscles, fascia and tendons at wrist and hand level

√7ᵗʰ **S66.821** **Laceration of other specifed muscles, fascia and tendons at wrist and hand level, right hand**

☑ Additional Character Required   √x7ᵗʰ Xtension Alert   Unspecified Code   Other Specified Code   Manifestation Code   ▶◀ Revised Text   ● New Code   ▲ Revised Code Title

ICD-10-CM 2014 (Draft)   885

S66.822–S68.029

Injury, Poisoning and Certain Other Consequences of External Causes

√7ᵗʰ **S66.822 Laceration** of other specified muscles, fascia and tendons at wrist and hand level, left hand

√7ᵗʰ **S66.829 Laceration** of other specified muscles, fascia and tendons at wrist and hand level, unspecified hand

√6ᵗʰ **S66.89 Other** injury of other specified muscles, fascia and tendons at wrist and hand level

√7ᵗʰ **S66.891 Other** injury of other specified muscles, fascia and tendons at wrist and hand level, right hand

√7ᵗʰ **S66.892 Other** injury of other specified muscles, fascia and tendons at wrist and hand level, left hand

√7ᵗʰ **S66.899 Other** injury of other specified muscles, fascia and tendons at wrist and hand level, unspecified hand

√5ᵗʰ **S66.9 Injury** of unspecified muscle, fascia and tendon at wrist and hand level

√6ᵗʰ **S66.90 Unspecified** injury of unspecified muscle, fascia and tendon at wrist and hand level

√7ᵗʰ **S66.901 Unspecified** injury of unspecified muscle, fascia and tendon at wrist and hand level, right hand

√7ᵗʰ **S66.902 Unspecified** injury of unspecified muscle, fascia and tendon at wrist and hand level, left hand

√7ᵗʰ **S66.909 Unspecified** injury of unspecified muscle, fascia and tendon at wrist and hand level, unspecified hand

√6ᵗʰ **S66.91 Strain** of unspecified muscle, fascia and tendon at wrist and hand level

√7ᵗʰ **S66.911 Strain** of unspecified muscle, fascia and tendon at wrist and hand level, right hand

√7ᵗʰ **S66.912 Strain** of unspecified muscle, fascia and tendon at wrist and hand level, left hand

√7ᵗʰ **S66.919 Strain** of unspecified muscle, fascia and tendon at wrist and hand level, unspecified hand

√6ᵗʰ **S66.92 Laceration** of unspecified muscle, fascia and tendon at wrist and hand level

√7ᵗʰ **S66.921 Laceration** of unspecified muscle, fascia and tendon at wrist and hand level, right hand

√7ᵗʰ **S66.922 Laceration** of unspecified muscle, fascia and tendon at wrist and hand level, left hand

√7ᵗʰ **S66.929 Laceration** of unspecified muscle, fascia and tendon at wrist and hand level, unspecified hand

√6ᵗʰ **S66.99 Other** injury of unspecified muscle, fascia and tendon at wrist and hand level

√7ᵗʰ **S66.991 Other** injury of unspecified muscle, fascia and tendon at wrist and hand level, right hand

√7ᵗʰ **S66.992 Other** injury of unspecified muscle, fascia and tendon at wrist and hand level, left hand

√7ᵗʰ **S66.999 Other** injury of unspecified muscle, fascia and tendon at wrist and hand level, unspecified hand

√4ᵗʰ **S67 Crushing injury of wrist, hand and fingers**

Use additional code for all associated injuries, such as:
    fracture of wrist and hand (S62.-)
    open wound of wrist and hand (S61.-)

The appropriate 7th character is to be added to each code from category S67.
   A   initial encounter
   D   subsequent encounter
   S   sequela

√5ᵗʰ **S67.0 Crushing injury of thumb**

√x7ᵗʰ **S67.00 Crushing injury of unspecified thumb**

√x7ᵗʰ **S67.01 Crushing injury of right thumb**

√x7ᵗʰ **S67.02 Crushing injury of left thumb**

√5ᵗʰ **S67.1 Crushing injury of other and unspecified finger(s)**

EXCLUDES 2   crushing injury of thumb (S67.0-)

√x7ᵗʰ **S67.10 Crushing injury of unspecified finger(s)**

√6ᵗʰ **S67.19 Crushing injury of other finger(s)**

√7ᵗʰ **S67.190 Crushing injury of right index finger**

√7ᵗʰ **S67.191 Crushing injury of left index finger**

√7ᵗʰ **S67.192 Crushing injury of right middle finger**

√7ᵗʰ **S67.193 Crushing injury of left middle finger**

√7ᵗʰ **S67.194 Crushing injury of right ring finger**

√7ᵗʰ **S67.195 Crushing injury of left ring finger**

√7ᵗʰ **S67.196 Crushing injury of right little finger**

√7ᵗʰ **S67.197 Crushing injury of left little finger**

√7ᵗʰ **S67.198 Crushing injury of other finger**
Crushing injury of specified finger with unspecified laterality

√5ᵗʰ **S67.2 Crushing injury of hand**

EXCLUDES 2   crushing injury of fingers (S67.1-)
              crushing injury of thumb (S67.0-)

√x7ᵗʰ **S67.20 Crushing injury of unspecified hand**

√x7ᵗʰ **S67.21 Crushing injury of right hand**

√x7ᵗʰ **S67.22 Crushing injury of left hand**

√5ᵗʰ **S67.3 Crushing injury of wrist**

√x7ᵗʰ **S67.30 Crushing injury of unspecified wrist**

√x7ᵗʰ **S67.31 Crushing injury of right wrist**

√x7ᵗʰ **S67.32 Crushing injury of left wrist**

√5ᵗʰ **S67.4 Crushing injury of wrist and hand**

EXCLUDES 1   crushing injury of hand alone (S67.2-)
              crushing injury of wrist alone (S67.3-)

EXCLUDES 2   crushing injury of fingers (S67.1-)
              crushing injury of thumb (S67.0-)

√x7ᵗʰ **S67.40 Crushing injury of unspecified wrist and hand**

√x7ᵗʰ **S67.41 Crushing injury of right wrist and hand**

√x7ᵗʰ **S67.42 Crushing injury of left wrist and hand**

√5ᵗʰ **S67.9 Crushing injury of unspecified part(s) of wrist, hand and fingers**

√x7ᵗʰ **S67.90 Crushing injury of unspecified part(s) of unspecified wrist, hand and fingers**

√x7ᵗʰ **S67.91 Crushing injury of unspecified part(s) of right wrist, hand and fingers**

√x7ᵗʰ **S67.92 Crushing injury of unspecified part(s) of left wrist, hand and fingers**

√4ᵗʰ **S68 Traumatic amputation of wrist, hand and fingers**

NOTE   An amputation not identified as partial or complete should be coded to complete.

The appropriate 7th character is to be added to each code from category S68.
   A   initial encounter
   D   subsequent encounter
   S   sequela

√5ᵗʰ **S68.0 Traumatic metacarpophalangeal amputation of thumb**
Traumatic amputation of thumb NOS

√6ᵗʰ **S68.01 Complete traumatic metacarpophalangeal amputation of thumb**

√7ᵗʰ **S68.011 Complete traumatic metacarpophalangeal amputation of right thumb**

√7ᵗʰ **S68.012 Complete traumatic metacarpophalangeal amputation of left thumb**

√7ᵗʰ **S68.019 Complete traumatic metacarpophalangeal amputation of unspecified thumb**

√6ᵗʰ **S68.02 Partial traumatic metacarpophalangeal amputation of thumb**

√7ᵗʰ **S68.021 Partial traumatic metacarpophalangeal amputation of right thumb**

√7ᵗʰ **S68.022 Partial traumatic metacarpophalangeal amputation of left thumb**

√7ᵗʰ **S68.029 Partial traumatic metacarpophalangeal amputation of unspecified thumb**

EXCLUDES 1 Not coded here   EXCLUDES 2 Not included here   N Newborn Age: 0   P Pediatric Age: 0-17   M Maternity Age: 12-55   A Adult Age: 15-124

886   ICD-10-CM 2014 (Draft)

√5ᵗʰ **S68.1** Traumatic metacarpophalangeal amputation of other and unspecified finger

Traumatic amputation of finger NOS

EXCLUDES 2 *traumatic metacarpophalangeal amputation of thumb (S68.0-)*

√6ᵗʰ **S68.11** Complete traumatic metacarpophalangeal amputation of other and unspecified finger

√7ᵗʰ **S68.110** Complete traumatic metacarpophalangeal amputation of right index finger

√7ᵗʰ **S68.111** Complete traumatic metacarpophalangeal amputation of left index finger

√7ᵗʰ **S68.112** Complete traumatic metacarpophalangeal amputation of right middle finger

√7ᵗʰ **S68.113** Complete traumatic metacarpophalangeal amputation of left middle finger

√7ᵗʰ **S68.114** Complete traumatic metacarpophalangeal amputation of right ring finger

√7ᵗʰ **S68.115** Complete traumatic metacarpophalangeal amputation of left ring finger

√7ᵗʰ **S68.116** Complete traumatic metacarpophalangeal amputation of right little finger

√7ᵗʰ **S68.117** Complete traumatic metacarpophalangeal amputation of left little finger

√7ᵗʰ **S68.118** Complete traumatic metacarpophalangeal amputation of other finger

Complete traumatic metacarpophalangeal amputation of specified finger with unspecified laterality

√7ᵗʰ **S68.119** Complete traumatic metacarpophalangeal amputation of unspecified finger

√6ᵗʰ **S68.12** Partial traumatic metacarpophalangeal amputation of other and unspecified finger

√7ᵗʰ **S68.120** Partial traumatic metacarpophalangeal amputation of right index finger

√7ᵗʰ **S68.121** Partial traumatic metacarpophalangeal amputation of left index finger

√7ᵗʰ **S68.122** Partial traumatic metacarpophalangeal amputation of right middle finger

√7ᵗʰ **S68.123** Partial traumatic metacarpophalangeal amputation of left middle finger

√7ᵗʰ **S68.124** Partial traumatic metacarpophalangeal amputation of right ring finger

√7ᵗʰ **S68.125** Partial traumatic metacarpophalangeal amputation of left ring finger

√7ᵗʰ **S68.126** Partial traumatic metacarpophalangeal amputation of right little finger

√7ᵗʰ **S68.127** Partial traumatic metacarpophalangeal amputation of left little finger

√7ᵗʰ **S68.128** Partial traumatic metacarpophalangeal amputation of other finger

Partial traumatic metacarpophalangeal amputation of specified finger with unspecified laterality

√7ᵗʰ **S68.129** Partial traumatic metacarpophalangeal amputation of unspecified finger

√5ᵗʰ **S68.4** Traumatic amputation of hand at wrist level

Traumatic amputation of hand NOS

Traumatic amputation of wrist

√6ᵗʰ **S68.41** Complete traumatic amputation of hand at wrist level

√7ᵗʰ **S68.411** Complete traumatic amputation of right hand at wrist level

√7ᵗʰ **S68.412** Complete traumatic amputation of left hand at wrist level

√7ᵗʰ **S68.419** Complete traumatic amputation of unspecified hand at wrist level

√6ᵗʰ **S68.42** Partial traumatic amputation of hand at wrist level

√7ᵗʰ **S68.421** Partial traumatic amputation of right hand at wrist level

√7ᵗʰ **S68.422** Partial traumatic amputation of left hand at wrist level

√7ᵗʰ **S68.429** Partial traumatic amputation of unspecified hand at wrist level

√5ᵗʰ **S68.5** Traumatic transphalangeal amputation of thumb

Traumatic interphalangeal joint amputation of thumb

√6ᵗʰ **S68.51** Complete traumatic transphalangeal amputation of thumb

√7ᵗʰ **S68.511** Complete traumatic transphalangeal amputation of right thumb

√7ᵗʰ **S68.512** Complete traumatic transphalangeal amputation of left thumb

√7ᵗʰ **S68.519** Complete traumatic transphalangeal amputation of unspecified thumb

√6ᵗʰ **S68.52** Partial traumatic transphalangeal amputation of thumb

√7ᵗʰ **S68.521** Partial traumatic transphalangeal amputation of right thumb

√7ᵗʰ **S68.522** Partial traumatic transphalangeal amputation of left thumb

√7ᵗʰ **S68.529** Partial traumatic transphalangeal amputation of unspecified thumb

√5ᵗʰ **S68.6** Traumatic transphalangeal amputation of other and unspecified finger

√6ᵗʰ **S68.61** Complete traumatic transphalangeal amputation of other and unspecified finger(s)

√7ᵗʰ **S68.610** Complete traumatic transphalangeal amputation of right index finger

√7ᵗʰ **S68.611** Complete traumatic transphalangeal amputation of left index finger

√7ᵗʰ **S68.612** Complete traumatic transphalangeal amputation of right middle finger

√7ᵗʰ **S68.613** Complete traumatic transphalangeal amputation of left middle finger

√7ᵗʰ **S68.614** Complete traumatic transphalangeal amputation of right ring finger

√7ᵗʰ **S68.615** Complete traumatic transphalangeal amputation of left ring finger

√7ᵗʰ **S68.616** Complete traumatic transphalangeal amputation of right little finger

√7ᵗʰ **S68.617** Complete traumatic transphalangeal amputation of left little finger

√7ᵗʰ **S68.618** Complete traumatic transphalangeal amputation of other finger

Complete traumatic transphalangeal amputation of specified finger with unspecified laterality

√7ᵗʰ **S68.619** Complete traumatic transphalangeal amputation of unspecified finger

√6ᵗʰ **S68.62** Partial traumatic transphalangeal amputation of other and unspecified finger

√7ᵗʰ **S68.620** Partial traumatic transphalangeal amputation of right index finger

√7ᵗʰ **S68.621** Partial traumatic transphalangeal amputation of left index finger

√7ᵗʰ **S68.622** Partial traumatic transphalangeal amputation of right middle finger

√7ᵗʰ **S68.623** Partial traumatic transphalangeal amputation of left middle finger

√7ᵗʰ **S68.624** Partial traumatic transphalangeal amputation of right ring finger

√7ᵗʰ **S68.625** Partial traumatic transphalangeal amputation of left ring finger

√7ᵗʰ **S68.626** Partial traumatic transphalangeal amputation of right little finger

√7ᵗʰ **S68.627** Partial traumatic transphalangeal amputation of left little finger

√7ᵗʰ **S68.628** Partial traumatic transphalangeal amputation of other finger

Partial traumatic transphalangeal amputation of specified finger with unspecified laterality

√7ᵗʰ **S68.629** Partial traumatic transphalangeal amputation of unspecified finger

√5ᵗʰ **S68.7** Traumatic transmetacarpal amputation of hand

√6ᵗʰ **S68.71** Complete traumatic transmetacarpal amputation of hand

☑ Additional Character Required   √x7ᵗʰ Xtension Alert   Unspecified Code   Other Specified Code   Manifestation Code   ▶◀ Revised Text   ● New Code   ▲ Revised Code Title

Injury, Poisoning and Certain Other Consequences of External Causes

S68.711–S71.002

- √7th **S68.711** Complete traumatic transmetacarpal amputation of right hand
- √7th **S68.712** Complete traumatic transmetacarpal amputation of left hand
- √7th **S68.719** Complete traumatic transmetacarpal amputation of unspecified hand

- √6th **S68.72** Partial traumatic transmetacarpal amputation of hand
  - √7th **S68.721** Partial traumatic transmetacarpal amputation of right hand
  - √7th **S68.722** Partial traumatic transmetacarpal amputation of left hand
  - √7th **S68.729** Partial traumatic transmetacarpal amputation of unspecified hand

√4th **S69** Other and unspecified injuries of wrist, hand and finger(s)

The appropriate 7th character is to be added to each code from category S69.
- A   initial encounter
- D   subsequent encounter
- S   sequela

- √5th **S69.8** Other specified injuries of wrist, hand and finger(s)
  - √x7th **S69.80** Other specified injuries of unspecified wrist, hand and finger(s)
  - √x7th **S69.81** Other specified injuries of right wrist, hand and finger(s)
  - √x7th **S69.82** Other specified injuries of left wrist, hand and finger(s)
- √5th **S69.9** Unspecified injury of wrist, hand and finger(s)
  - √x7th **S69.90** Unspecified injury of unspecified wrist, hand and finger(s)
  - √x7th **S69.91** Unspecified injury of right wrist, hand and finger(s)
  - √x7th **S69.92** Unspecified injury of left wrist, hand and finger(s)

Injuries to the hip and thigh (S70-S79)

EXCLUDES 2   burns and corrosions (T20-T32)
frostbite (T33-T34)
snake bite (T63.0-)
venomous insect bite or sting (T63.4-)

√4th **S70** Superficial injury of hip and thigh

The appropriate 7th character is to be added to each code from category S70.
- A   initial encounter
- D   subsequent encounter
- S   sequela

- √5th **S70.0** Contusion of hip
  - √x7th **S70.00** Contusion of unspecified hip
  - √x7th **S70.01** Contusion of right hip
  - √x7th **S70.02** Contusion of left hip
- √5th **S70.1** Contusion of thigh
  - √x7th **S70.10** Contusion of unspecified thigh
  - √x7th **S70.11** Contusion of right thigh
  - √x7th **S70.12** Contusion of left thigh
- √5th **S70.2** Other superficial injuries of hip
  - √6th **S70.21** Abrasion of hip
    - √7th **S70.211** Abrasion, right hip
    - √7th **S70.212** Abrasion, left hip
    - √7th **S70.219** Abrasion, unspecified hip
  - √6th **S70.22** Blister (nonthermal) of hip
    - √7th **S70.221** Blister (nonthermal), right hip
    - √7th **S70.222** Blister (nonthermal), left hip
    - √7th **S70.229** Blister (nonthermal), unspecified hip
  - √6th **S70.24** External constriction of hip
    - √7th **S70.241** External constriction, right hip
    - √7th **S70.242** External constriction, left hip
    - √7th **S70.249** External constriction, unspecified hip
  - √6th **S70.25** Superficial foreign body of hip
    Splinter in the hip
    - √7th **S70.251** Superficial foreign body, right hip

- √7th **S70.252** Superficial foreign body, left hip
- √7th **S70.259** Superficial foreign body, unspecified hip
- √6th **S70.26** Insect bite (nonvenomous) of hip
  - √7th **S70.261** Insect bite (nonvenomous), right hip
  - √7th **S70.262** Insect bite (nonvenomous), left hip
  - √7th **S70.269** Insect bite (nonvenomous), unspecified hip
- √6th **S70.27** Other superficial bite of hip
  EXCLUDES 1   open bite of hip (S71.05-)
  - √7th **S70.271** Other superficial bite of hip, right hip
  - √7th **S70.272** Other superficial bite of hip, left hip
  - √7th **S70.279** Other superficial bite of hip, unspecified hip
- √5th **S70.3** Other superficial injuries of thigh
  - √6th **S70.31** Abrasion of thigh
    - √7th **S70.311** Abrasion, right thigh
    - √7th **S70.312** Abrasion, left thigh
    - √7th **S70.319** Abrasion, unspecified thigh
  - √6th **S70.32** Blister (nonthermal) of thigh
    - √7th **S70.321** Blister (nonthermal), right thigh
    - √7th **S70.322** Blister (nonthermal), left thigh
    - √7th **S70.329** Blister (nonthermal), unspecified thigh
  - √6th **S70.34** External constriction of thigh
    - √7th **S70.341** External constriction, right thigh
    - √7th **S70.342** External constriction, left thigh
    - √7th **S70.349** External constriction, unspecified thigh
  - √6th **S70.35** Superficial foreign body of thigh
    Splinter in the thigh
    - √7th **S70.351** Superficial foreign body, right thigh
    - √7th **S70.352** Superficial foreign body, left thigh
    - √7th **S70.359** Superficial foreign body, unspecified thigh
  - √6th **S70.36** Insect bite (nonvenomous) of thigh
    - √7th **S70.361** Insect bite (nonvenomous), right thigh
    - √7th **S70.362** Insect bite (nonvenomous), left thigh
    - √7th **S70.369** Insect bite (nonvenomous), unspecified thigh
  - √6th **S70.37** Other superficial bite of thigh
    EXCLUDES 1   open bite of thigh (S71.15)
    - √7th **S70.371** Other superficial bite of right thigh
    - √7th **S70.372** Other superficial bite of left thigh
    - √7th **S70.379** Other superficial bite of unspecified thigh
- √5th **S70.9** Unspecified superficial injury of hip and thigh
  - √6th **S70.91** Unspecified superficial injury of hip
    - √7th **S70.911** Unspecified superficial injury of right hip
    - √7th **S70.912** Unspecified superficial injury of left hip
    - √7th **S70.919** Unspecified superficial injury of unspecified hip
  - √6th **S70.92** Unspecified superficial injury of thigh
    - √7th **S70.921** Unspecified superficial injury of right thigh
    - √7th **S70.922** Unspecified superficial injury of left thigh
    - √7th **S70.929** Unspecified superficial injury of unspecified thigh

√4th **S71** Open wound of hip and thigh
Code also any associated wound infection
EXCLUDES 1   open fracture of hip and thigh (S72.-)
traumatic amputation of hip and thigh (S78.-)
EXCLUDES 2   bite of venomous animal (T63.-)
open wound of ankle, foot and toes (S91.-)
open wound of knee and lower leg (S81.-)

The appropriate 7th character is to be added to each code from category S71.
- A   initial encounter
- D   subsequent encounter
- S   sequela

- √5th **S71.0** Open wound of hip
  - √6th **S71.00** Unspecified open wound of hip
    - √7th **S71.001** Unspecified open wound, right hip
    - √7th **S71.002** Unspecified open wound, left hip

EXCLUDES 1 Not coded here   EXCLUDES 2 Not included here   N Newborn Age: 0   P Pediatric Age: 0-17   M Maternity Age: 12-55   A Adult Age: 15-124

888   ICD-10-CM 2014 (Draft)

☑7ᵗʰ **S71.009** **Unspecified open wound, unspecified hip**

☑6ᵗʰ **S71.01** Laceration without foreign body of hip

  ☑7ᵗʰ **S71.011** **Laceration without foreign body, right hip**

  ☑7ᵗʰ **S71.012** **Laceration without foreign body, left hip**

  ☑7ᵗʰ **S71.019** **Laceration without foreign body, unspecified hip**

☑6ᵗʰ **S71.02** Laceration with foreign body of hip

  ☑7ᵗʰ **S71.021** **Laceration with foreign body, right hip**

  ☑7ᵗʰ **S71.022** **Laceration with foreign body, left hip**

  ☑7ᵗʰ **S71.029** **Laceration with foreign body, unspecified hip**

☑6ᵗʰ **S71.03** Puncture wound without foreign body of hip

  ☑7ᵗʰ **S71.031** **Puncture wound without foreign body, right hip**

  ☑7ᵗʰ **S71.032** **Puncture wound without foreign body, left hip**

  ☑7ᵗʰ **S71.039** **Puncture wound without foreign body, unspecified hip**

☑6ᵗʰ **S71.04** Puncture wound with foreign body of hip

  ☑7ᵗʰ **S71.041** **Puncture wound with foreign body, right hip**

  ☑7ᵗʰ **S71.042** **Puncture wound with foreign body, left hip**

  ☑7ᵗʰ **S71.049** **Puncture wound with foreign body, unspecified hip**

☑6ᵗʰ **S71.05** Open bite of hip
    Bite of hip NOS
    EXCLUDES 1   superficial bite of hip (S70.26, S70.27)

  ☑7ᵗʰ **S71.051** **Open bite, right hip**

  ☑7ᵗʰ **S71.052** **Open bite, left hip**

  ☑7ᵗʰ **S71.059** **Open bite, unspecified hip**

☑5ᵗʰ **S71.1** **Open wound of thigh**

☑6ᵗʰ **S71.10** Unspecified open wound of thigh

  ☑7ᵗʰ **S71.101** **Unspecified open wound, right thigh**

  ☑7ᵗʰ **S71.102** **Unspecified open wound, left thigh**

  ☑7ᵗʰ **S71.109** **Unspecified open wound, unspecified thigh**

☑6ᵗʰ **S71.11** Laceration without foreign body of thigh

  ☑7ᵗʰ **S71.111** **Laceration without foreign body, right thigh**

  ☑7ᵗʰ **S71.112** **Laceration without foreign body, left thigh**

  ☑7ᵗʰ **S71.119** **Laceration without foreign body, unspecified thigh**

☑6ᵗʰ **S71.12** Laceration with foreign body of thigh

  ☑7ᵗʰ **S71.121** **Laceration with foreign body, right thigh**

  ☑7ᵗʰ **S71.122** **Laceration with foreign body, left thigh**

  ☑7ᵗʰ **S71.129** **Laceration with foreign body, unspecified thigh**

☑6ᵗʰ **S71.13** Puncture wound without foreign body of thigh

  ☑7ᵗʰ **S71.131** **Puncture wound without foreign body, right thigh**

  ☑7ᵗʰ **S71.132** **Puncture wound without foreign body, left thigh**

  ☑7ᵗʰ **S71.139** **Puncture wound without foreign body, unspecified thigh**

☑6ᵗʰ **S71.14** Puncture wound with foreign body of thigh

  ☑7ᵗʰ **S71.141** **Puncture wound with foreign body, right thigh**

  ☑7ᵗʰ **S71.142** **Puncture wound with foreign body, left thigh**

  ☑7ᵗʰ **S71.149** **Puncture wound with foreign body, unspecified thigh**

☑6ᵗʰ **S71.15** Open bite of thigh
    Bite of thigh NOS
    EXCLUDES 1   superficial bite of thigh (S70.37-)

  ☑7ᵗʰ **S71.151** **Open bite, right thigh**

  ☑7ᵗʰ **S71.152** **Open bite, left thigh**

  ☑7ᵗʰ **S71.159** **Open bite, unspecified thigh**

☑4ᵗʰ **S72** **Fracture of femur**
    NOTE   A fracture not indicated as displaced or nondisplaced should be coded to displaced.
          The open fracture designations are based on the Gustilo open fracture classification.
          A fracture not indicated as open or closed should be coded to closed.
    EXCLUDES 1   traumatic amputation of hip and thigh (S78.-)
    EXCLUDES 2   fracture of lower leg and ankle (S82.-)
          fracture of foot (S92.-)
          periprosthetic fracture of prosthetic implant of hip (T84.040, T84.041)

The appropriate 7th character is to be added to all codes from category S72 [unless otherwise indicated].

A	initial encounter for closed fracture
B	initial encounter for open fracture type I or II
	initial encounter for open fracture NOS
C	initial encounter for open fracture type IIIA, IIIB, or IIIC
D	subsequent encounter for closed fracture with routine healing
E	subsequent encounter for open fracture type I or II with routine healing
F	subsequent encounter for open fracture type IIIA, IIIB, or IIIC with routine healing
G	subsequent encounter for closed fracture with delayed healing
H	subsequent encounter for open fracture type I or II with delayed healing
J	subsequent encounter for open fracture type IIIA, IIIB, or IIIC with delayed healing
K	subsequent encounter for closed fracture with nonunion
M	subsequent encounter for open fracture type I or I with nonunion
N	subsequent encounter for open fracture type IIIA, IIIB, or IIIC with nonunion
P	subsequent encounter for closed fracture with malunion
Q	subsequent encounter for open fracture type I or II with malunion
R	subsequent encounter for open fracture type IIIA, IIIB, or IIIC with malunion
S	sequela

☑5ᵗʰ **S72.0** **Fracture of head and neck of femur**
    EXCLUDES 2   physeal fracture of upper end of femur (S79.0-)

☑6ᵗʰ **S72.00** Fracture of unspecified part of neck of femur
    Fracture of hip NOS   Fracture of neck of femur NOS

  ☑7ᵗʰ **S72.001** **Fracture of unspecified part of neck of right femur**

  ☑7ᵗʰ **S72.002** **Fracture of unspecified part of neck of left femur**

  ☑7ᵗʰ **S72.009** **Fracture of unspecified part of neck of unspecified femur**

☑6ᵗʰ **S72.01** Unspecified intracapsular fracture of femur
    Subcapital fracture of femur

  ☑7ᵗʰ **S72.011** **Unspecified intracapsular fracture of right femur**

  ☑7ᵗʰ **S72.012** **Unspecified intracapsular fracture of left femur**

  ☑7ᵗʰ **S72.019** **Unspecified intracapsular fracture of unspecified femur**

☑6ᵗʰ **S72.02** Fracture of epiphysis (separation) (upper) of femur
    Transepiphyseal fracture of femur
    EXCLUDES 1   capital femoral epiphyseal fracture (pediatric) of femur (S79.01-)
          Salter-Harris Type I physeal fracture of upper end of femur (S79.01-)

  ☑7ᵗʰ **S72.021** **Displaced fracture of epiphysis (separation) (upper) of right femur**

  ☑7ᵗʰ **S72.022** **Displaced fracture of epiphysis (separation) (upper) of left femur**

  ☑7ᵗʰ **S72.023** **Displaced fracture of epiphysis (separation) (upper) of unspecified femur**

  ☑7ᵗʰ **S72.024** **Nondisplaced fracture of epiphysis (separation) (upper) of right femur**

  ☑7ᵗʰ **S72.025** **Nondisplaced fracture of epiphysis (separation) (upper) of left femur**

  ☑7ᵗʰ **S72.026** **Nondisplaced fracture of epiphysis (separation) (upper) of unspecified femur**

☑6ᵗʰ **S72.03** Midcervical fracture of femur
    Transcervical fracture of femur NOS

  ☑7ᵗʰ **S72.031** **Displaced midcervical fracture of right femur**

☑ Additional Character Required   ☑x7ᵗʰ *X*tension Alert   Unspecified Code   Other Specified Code   Manifestation Code   ►◄ Revised Text   ● New Code   ▲ Revised Code Title

ICD-10-CM 2014 (Draft)

889

√7ᵗʰ **S72.032** Displaced midcervical fracture of left femur

√7ᵗʰ **S72.033** Displaced midcervical fracture of unspecified femur

√7ᵗʰ **S72.034** Nondisplaced midcervical fracture of right femur

√7ᵗʰ **S72.035** Nondisplaced midcervical fracture of left femur

√7ᵗʰ **S72.036** Nondisplaced midcervical fracture of unspecified femur

√6ᵗʰ **S72.04** Fracture of base of neck of femur
Cervicotrochanteric fracture of femur

√7ᵗʰ **S72.041** Displaced fracture of base of neck of right femur

√7ᵗʰ **S72.042** Displaced fracture of base of neck of left femur

√7ᵗʰ **S72.043** Displaced fracture of base of neck of unspecified femur

√7ᵗʰ **S72.044** Nondisplaced fracture of base of neck of right femur

√7ᵗʰ **S72.045** Nondisplaced fracture of base of neck of left femur

√7ᵗʰ **S72.046** Nondisplaced fracture of base of neck of unspecified femur

√6ᵗʰ **S72.05** Unspecified fracture of head of femur
Fracture of head of femur NOS

√7ᵗʰ **S72.051** Unspecified fracture of head of right femur

√7ᵗʰ **S72.052** Unspecified fracture of head of left femur

√7ᵗʰ **S72.059** Unspecified fracture of head of unspecified femur

√6ᵗʰ **S72.06** Articular fracture of head of femur

√7ᵗʰ **S72.061** Displaced articular fracture of head of right femur

√7ᵗʰ **S72.062** Displaced articular fracture of head of left femur

√7ᵗʰ **S72.063** Displaced articular fracture of head of unspecified femur

√7ᵗʰ **S72.064** Nondisplaced articular fracture of head of right femur

√7ᵗʰ **S72.065** Nondisplaced articular fracture of head of left femur

√7ᵗʰ **S72.066** Nondisplaced articular fracture of head of unspecified femur

√6ᵗʰ **S72.09** Other fracture of head and neck of femur

√7ᵗʰ **S72.091** Other fracture of head and neck of right femur

√7ᵗʰ **S72.092** Other fracture of head and neck of left femur

√7ᵗʰ **S72.099** Other fracture of head and neck of unspecified femur

√5ᵗʰ **S72.1** Pertrochanteric fracture

√6ᵗʰ **S72.10** Unspecified trochanteric fracture of femur
Fracture of trochanter NOS

√7ᵗʰ **S72.101** Unspecified trochanteric fracture of right femur

√7ᵗʰ **S72.102** Unspecified trochanteric fracture of left femur

√7ᵗʰ **S72.109** Unspecified trochanteric fracture of unspecified femur

√6ᵗʰ **S72.11** Fracture of greater trochanter of femur

√7ᵗʰ **S72.111** Displaced fracture of greater trochanter of right femur

√7ᵗʰ **S72.112** Displaced fracture of greater trochanter of left femur

√7ᵗʰ **S72.113** Displaced fracture of greater trochanter of unspecified femur

√7ᵗʰ **S72.114** Nondisplaced fracture of greater trochanter of right femur

√7ᵗʰ **S72.115** Nondisplaced fracture of greater trochanter of left femur

√7ᵗʰ **S72.116** Nondisplaced fracture of greater trochanter of unspecified femur

√6ᵗʰ **S72.12** Fracture of lesser trochanter of femur

√7ᵗʰ **S72.121** Displaced fracture of lesser trochanter of right femur

√7ᵗʰ **S72.122** Displaced fracture of lesser trochanter of left femur

√7ᵗʰ **S72.123** Displaced fracture of lesser trochanter of unspecified femur

√7ᵗʰ **S72.124** Nondisplaced fracture of lesser trochanter of right femur

√7ᵗʰ **S72.125** Nondisplaced fracture of lesser trochanter of left femur

√7ᵗʰ **S72.126** Nondisplaced fracture of lesser trochanter of unspecified femur

√6ᵗʰ **S72.13** Apophyseal fracture of femur
EXCLUDES 1   chronic (nontraumatic) slipped upper femoral epiphysis (M93.0-)

√7ᵗʰ **S72.131** Displaced apophyseal fracture of right femur

√7ᵗʰ **S72.132** Displaced apophyseal fracture of left femur

√7ᵗʰ **S72.133** Displaced apophyseal fracture of unspecified femur

√7ᵗʰ **S72.134** Nondisplaced apophyseal fracture of right femur

√7ᵗʰ **S72.135** Nondisplaced apophyseal fracture of left femur

√7ᵗʰ **S72.136** Nondisplaced apophyseal fracture of unspecified femur

√6ᵗʰ **S72.14** Intertrochanteric fracture of femur

√7ᵗʰ **S72.141** Displaced intertrochanteric fracture of right femur

√7ᵗʰ **S72.142** Displaced intertrochanteric fracture of left femur

√7ᵗʰ **S72.143** Displaced intertrochanteric fracture of unspecified femur

√7ᵗʰ **S72.144** Nondisplaced intertrochanteric fracture of right femur

√7ᵗʰ **S72.145** Nondisplaced intertrochanteric fracture of left femur

√7ᵗʰ **S72.146** Nondisplaced intertrochanteric fracture of unspecified femur

√5ᵗʰ **S72.2** Subtrochanteric fracture of femur

√x7ᵗʰ **S72.21** Displaced subtrochanteric fracture of right femur

√x7ᵗʰ **S72.22** Displaced subtrochanteric fracture of left femur

√x7ᵗʰ **S72.23** Displaced subtrochanteric fracture of unspecified femur

√x7ᵗʰ **S72.24** Nondisplaced subtrochanteric fracture of right femur

√x7ᵗʰ **S72.25** Nondisplaced subtrochanteric fracture of left femur

√x7ᵗʰ **S72.26** Nondisplaced subtrochanteric fracture of unspecified femur

√5ᵗʰ **S72.3** Fracture of shaft of femur

√6ᵗʰ **S72.30** Unspecified fracture of shaft of femur

√7ᵗʰ **S72.301** Unspecified fracture of shaft of right femur

√7ᵗʰ **S72.302** Unspecified fracture of shaft of left femur

√7ᵗʰ **S72.309** Unspecified fracture of shaft of unspecified femur

√6ᵗʰ **S72.32** Transverse fracture of shaft of femur

√7ᵗʰ **S72.321** Displaced transverse fracture of shaft of right femur

√7ᵗʰ **S72.322** Displaced transverse fracture of shaft of left femur

√7ᵗʰ **S72.323** Displaced transverse fracture of shaft of unspecified femur

√7ᵗʰ **S72.324** Nondisplaced transverse fracture of shaft of right femur

√7ᵗʰ **S72.325** Nondisplaced transverse fracture of shaft of left femur

√7ᵗʰ **S72.326** Nondisplaced transverse fracture of shaft of unspecified femur

√6ᵗʰ **S72.33** Oblique fracture of shaft of femur

√7ᵗʰ **S72.331** Displaced oblique fracture of shaft of right femur

---

EXCLUDES 1 Not coded here   EXCLUDES 2 Not included here   N Newborn Age: 0   P Pediatric Age: 0-17   M Maternity Age: 12-55   A Adult Age: 15-124

890   ICD-10-CM 2014 (Draft)

√7ᵗʰ **S72.332** Displaced **oblique fracture of shaft of** left **femur**

√7ᵗʰ **S72.333** Displaced **oblique fracture of shaft of unspecified femur**

√7ᵗʰ **S72.334** Nondisplaced **oblique fracture of shaft of** right **femur**

√7ᵗʰ **S72.335** Nondisplaced **oblique fracture of shaft of** left **femur**

√7ᵗʰ **S72.336** Nondisplaced **oblique fracture of shaft of unspecified femur**

√6ᵗʰ **S72.34** Spiral **fracture of shaft of femur**

√7ᵗʰ **S72.341** Displaced **spiral fracture of shaft of** right **femur**

√7ᵗʰ **S72.342** Displaced **spiral fracture of shaft of** left **femur**

√7ᵗʰ **S72.343** Displaced **spiral fracture of shaft of unspecified femur**

√7ᵗʰ **S72.344** Nondisplaced **spiral fracture of shaft of** right **femur**

√7ᵗʰ **S72.345** Nondisplaced **spiral fracture of shaft of** left **femur**

√7ᵗʰ **S72.346** Nondisplaced **spiral fracture of shaft of unspecified femur**

√6ᵗʰ **S72.35** Comminuted **fracture of shaft of femur**

√7ᵗʰ **S72.351** Displaced **comminuted fracture of shaft of** right **femur**

√7ᵗʰ **S72.352** Displaced **comminuted fracture of shaft of** left **femur**

√7ᵗʰ **S72.353** Displaced **comminuted fracture of shaft of unspecified femur**

√7ᵗʰ **S72.354** Nondisplaced **comminuted fracture of shaft of** right **femur**

√7ᵗʰ **S72.355** Nondisplaced **comminuted fracture of shaft of** left **femur**

√7ᵗʰ **S72.356** Nondisplaced **comminuted fracture of shaft of unspecified femur**

√6ᵗʰ **S72.36** Segmental **fracture of shaft of femur**

√7ᵗʰ **S72.361** Displaced **segmental fracture of shaft of** right **femur**

√7ᵗʰ **S72.362** Displaced **segmental fracture of shaft of** left **femur**

√7ᵗʰ **S72.363** Displaced **segmental fracture of shaft of unspecified femur**

√7ᵗʰ **S72.364** Nondisplaced **segmental fracture of shaft of** right **femur**

√7ᵗʰ **S72.365** Nondisplaced **segmental fracture of shaft of** left **femur**

√7ᵗʰ **S72.366** Nondisplaced **segmental fracture of shaft of unspecified femur**

√6ᵗʰ **S72.39** Other **fracture of shaft of femur**

√7ᵗʰ **S72.391** Other **fracture of shaft of** right **femur**

√7ᵗʰ **S72.392** Other **fracture of shaft of** left **femur**

√7ᵗʰ **S72.399** Other **fracture of shaft of unspecified femur**

√5ᵗʰ **S72.4** Fracture of lower end **of femur**
Fracture of distal end of femur
EXCLUDES 2   fracture of shaft of femur (S72.3-)
physeal fracture of lower end of femur (S79.1-)

√6ᵗʰ **S72.40** Unspecified **fracture of lower end of femur**

√7ᵗʰ **S72.401** Unspecified **fracture of lower end of** right **femur**

√7ᵗʰ **S72.402** Unspecified **fracture of lower end of** left **femur**

√7ᵗʰ **S72.409** Unspecified **fracture of lower end of unspecified femur**

√6ᵗʰ **S72.41** Unspecified condyle **fracture of lower end of femur**
Condyle fracture of femur NOS

√7ᵗʰ **S72.411** Displaced **unspecified condyle fracture of lower end of** right **femur**

√7ᵗʰ **S72.412** Displaced **unspecified condyle fracture of lower end of** left **femur**

√7ᵗʰ **S72.413** Displaced **unspecified condyle fracture of lower end of unspecified femur**

√7ᵗʰ **S72.414** Nondisplaced **unspecified condyle fracture of lower end of** right **femur**

√7ᵗʰ **S72.415** Nondisplaced **unspecified condyle fracture of lower end of** left **femur**

√7ᵗʰ **S72.416** Nondisplaced **unspecified condyle fracture of lower end of unspecified femur**

√6ᵗʰ **S72.42** Fracture of lateral condyle **of femur**

√7ᵗʰ **S72.421** Displaced **fracture of lateral condyle of** right **femur**

√7ᵗʰ **S72.422** Displaced **fracture of lateral condyle of** left **femur**

√7ᵗʰ **S72.423** Displaced **fracture of lateral condyle of unspecified femur**

√7ᵗʰ **S72.424** Nondisplaced **fracture of lateral condyle of** right **femur**

√7ᵗʰ **S72.425** Nondisplaced **fracture of lateral condyle of** left **femur**

√7ᵗʰ **S72.426** Nondisplaced **fracture of lateral condyle of unspecified femur**

√6ᵗʰ **S72.43** Fracture of medial condyle **of femur**

√7ᵗʰ **S72.431** Displaced **fracture of medial condyle of** right **femur**

√7ᵗʰ **S72.432** Displaced **fracture of medial condyle of** left **femur**

√7ᵗʰ **S72.433** Displaced **fracture of medial condyle of unspecified femur**

√7ᵗʰ **S72.434** Nondisplaced **fracture of medial condyle of** right **femur**

√7ᵗʰ **S72.435** Nondisplaced **fracture of medial condyle of** left **femur**

√7ᵗʰ **S72.436** Nondisplaced **fracture of medial condyle of unspecified femur**

√6ᵗʰ **S72.44** Fracture of lower epiphysis (separation) **of femur**
EXCLUDES 1   Salter-Harris Type I physeal fracture of lower end of femur (S79.11-)

√7ᵗʰ **S72.441** Displaced **fracture of lower epiphysis (separation) of** right **femur**

√7ᵗʰ **S72.442** Displaced **fracture of lower epiphysis (separation) of** left **femur**

√7ᵗʰ **S72.443** Displaced **fracture of lower epiphysis (separation) of unspecified femur**

√7ᵗʰ **S72.444** Nondisplaced **fracture of lower epiphysis (separation) of** right **femur**

√7ᵗʰ **S72.445** Nondisplaced **fracture of lower epiphysis (separation) of** left **femur**

√7ᵗʰ **S72.446** Nondisplaced **fracture of lower epiphysis (separation) of unspecified femur**

√6ᵗʰ **S72.45** Supracondylar **fracture without intracondylar extension of lower end of femur**
Supracondylar fracture of lower end of femur NOS
EXCLUDES 1   supracondylar fracture with intracondylar extension of lower end of femur (S72.46-)

√7ᵗʰ **S72.451** Displaced **supracondylar fracture without intracondylar extension of lower end of** right **femur**

√7ᵗʰ **S72.452** Displaced **supracondylar fracture without intracondylar extension of lower end of** left **femur**

√7ᵗʰ **S72.453** Displaced **supracondylar fracture without intracondylar extension of lower end of unspecified femur**

√7ᵗʰ **S72.454** Nondisplaced **supracondylar fracture without intracondylar extension of lower end of** right **femur**

√7ᵗʰ **S72.455** Nondisplaced **supracondylar fracture without intracondylar extension of lower end of** left **femur**

√7ᵗʰ **S72.456** Nondisplaced **supracondylar fracture without intracondylar extension of lower end of unspecified femur**

√6ᵗʰ **S72.46** Supracondylar **fracture with intracondylar extension of lower end of femur**
EXCLUDES 1   supracondylar fracture without intracondylar extension of lower end of femur (S72.45-)

√7ᵗʰ **S72.461** Displaced **supracondylar fracture with intracondylar extension of lower end of** right **femur**

☑ Additional Character Required   √x7ᵗʰ Xtension Alert   Unspecified Code   Other Specified Code   Manifestation Code   ►◄ Revised Text   ● New Code   ▲ Revised Code Title

√7ᵗʰ **S72.462** Displaced **supracondylar fracture with intracondylar extension of lower end of left** femur

√7ᵗʰ **S72.463** Displaced **supracondylar fracture with intracondylar extension of lower end of unspecified** femur

√7ᵗʰ **S72.464** Nondisplaced **supracondylar fracture with intracondylar extension of lower end of right** femur

√7ᵗʰ **S72.465** Nondisplaced **supracondylar fracture with intracondylar extension of lower end of left** femur

√7ᵗʰ **S72.466** Nondisplaced **supracondylar fracture with intracondylar extension of lower end of unspecified** femur

√6ᵗʰ **S72.47** Torus **fracture of lower end of femur**

> The appropriate 7th character is to be added to all codes in subcategory S72.47.
> A   initial encounter for closed fracture
> D   subsequent encounter for fracture with routine healing
> G   subsequent encounter for fracture with delayed healing
> K   subsequent encounter for fracture with nonunion
> P   subsequent encounter for fracture with malunion
> S   sequela

√7ᵗʰ **S72.471** Torus **fracture of lower end of right femur**

√7ᵗʰ **S72.472** Torus **fracture of lower end of left femur**

√7ᵗʰ **S72.479** Torus **fracture of lower end of unspecified femur**

√6ᵗʰ **S72.49** Other **fracture of lower end of femur**

√7ᵗʰ **S72.491** Other **fracture of lower end of right femur**

√7ᵗʰ **S72.492** Other **fracture of lower end of left femur**

√7ᵗʰ **S72.499** Other **fracture of lower end of unspecified femur**

√5ᵗʰ **S72.8** Other **fracture of femur**

√6ᵗʰ **S72.8X** Other **fracture of femur**

√7ᵗʰ **S72.8X1** Other **fracture of right femur**

√7ᵗʰ **S72.8X2** Other **fracture of left femur**

√7ᵗʰ **S72.8X9** Other **fracture of unspecified femur**

√5ᵗʰ **S72.9** Unspecified **fracture of femur**
Fracture of thigh NOS
Fracture of upper leg NOS
> EXCLUDES 1   fracture of hip NOS (S72.00-, S72.01-)

√x7ᵗʰ **S72.90** Unspecified **fracture of unspecified femur**
AHA: 2012, Q4, 93

√x7ᵗʰ **S72.91** Unspecified **fracture of right femur**

√x7ᵗʰ **S72.92** Unspecified **fracture of left femur**

√4ᵗʰ **S73** **Dislocation and sprain of joint and ligaments of hip**
> INCLUDES   avulsion of joint or ligament of hip
> laceration of cartilage, joint or ligament of hip
> sprain of cartilage, joint or ligament of hip
> traumatic hemarthrosis of joint or ligament of hip
> traumatic rupture of joint or ligament of hip
> traumatic subluxation of joint or ligament of hip
> traumatic tear of joint or ligament of hip

Code also any associated open wound
> EXCLUDES 2   strain of muscle, fascia and tendon of hip and thigh (S76.-)

> The appropriate 7th character is to be added to each code from category S73.
> A   initial encounter
> D   subsequent encounter
> S   sequela

√5ᵗʰ **S73.0** Subluxation and dislocation of **hip**
> EXCLUDES 2   dislocation and subluxation of hip prosthesis (T84.020, T84.021)

√6ᵗʰ **S73.00** Unspecified **subluxation and dislocation of hip**
Dislocation of hip NOS
Subluxation of hip NOS

√7ᵗʰ **S73.001** Unspecified **subluxation of right hip**

√7ᵗʰ **S73.002** Unspecified **subluxation of left hip**

√7ᵗʰ **S73.003** Unspecified **subluxation of unspecified hip**

√7ᵗʰ **S73.004** Unspecified **dislocation of right hip**

√7ᵗʰ **S73.005** Unspecified **dislocation of left hip**

√7ᵗʰ **S73.006** Unspecified **dislocation of unspecified hip**

√6ᵗʰ **S73.01** Posterior **subluxation and dislocation of hip**

√7ᵗʰ **S73.011** Posterior **subluxation of right hip**

√7ᵗʰ **S73.012** Posterior **subluxation of left hip**

√7ᵗʰ **S73.013** Posterior **subluxation of unspecified hip**

√7ᵗʰ **S73.014** Posterior **dislocation of right hip**

√7ᵗʰ **S73.015** Posterior **dislocation of left hip**

√7ᵗʰ **S73.016** Posterior **dislocation of unspecified hip**

√6ᵗʰ **S73.02** Obturator **subluxation and dislocation of hip**

√7ᵗʰ **S73.021** Obturator **subluxation of right hip**

√7ᵗʰ **S73.022** Obturator **subluxation of left hip**

√7ᵗʰ **S73.023** Obturator **subluxation of unspecified hip**

√7ᵗʰ **S73.024** Obturator **dislocation of right hip**

√7ᵗʰ **S73.025** Obturator **dislocation of left hip**

√7ᵗʰ **S73.026** Obturator **dislocation of unspecified hip**

√6ᵗʰ **S73.03** Other anterior **dislocation of hip**

√7ᵗʰ **S73.031** Other anterior **subluxation of right hip**

√7ᵗʰ **S73.032** Other anterior **subluxation of left hip**

√7ᵗʰ **S73.033** Other anterior **subluxation of unspecified hip**

√7ᵗʰ **S73.034** Other anterior **dislocation of right hip**

√7ᵗʰ **S73.035** Other anterior **dislocation of left hip**

√7ᵗʰ **S73.036** Other anterior **dislocation of unspecified hip**

√6ᵗʰ **S73.04** Central **dislocation of hip**

√7ᵗʰ **S73.041** Central **subluxation of right hip**

√7ᵗʰ **S73.042** Central **subluxation of left hip**

√7ᵗʰ **S73.043** Central **subluxation of unspecified hip**

√7ᵗʰ **S73.044** Central **dislocation of right hip**

√7ᵗʰ **S73.045** Central **dislocation of left hip**

√7ᵗʰ **S73.046** Central **dislocation of unspecified hip**

√5ᵗʰ **S73.1** Sprain of **hip**

√6ᵗʰ **S73.10** Unspecified **sprain of hip**

√7ᵗʰ **S73.101** Unspecified **sprain of right hip**

√7ᵗʰ **S73.102** Unspecified **sprain of left hip**

√7ᵗʰ **S73.109** Unspecified **sprain of unspecified hip**

√6ᵗʰ **S73.11** Iliofemoral ligament **sprain of hip**

√7ᵗʰ **S73.111** Iliofemoral ligament **sprain of right hip**

√7ᵗʰ **S73.112** Iliofemoral ligament **sprain of left hip**

√7ᵗʰ **S73.119** Iliofemoral ligament **sprain of unspecified hip**

√6ᵗʰ **S73.12** Ischiocapsular (ligament) **sprain of hip**

√7ᵗʰ **S73.121** Ischiocapsular ligament **sprain of right hip**

√7ᵗʰ **S73.122** Ischiocapsular ligament **sprain of left hip**

√7ᵗʰ **S73.129** Ischiocapsular ligament **sprain of unspecified hip**

√6ᵗʰ **S73.19** Other **sprain of hip**

√7ᵗʰ **S73.191** Other **sprain of right hip**

√7ᵗʰ **S73.192** Other **sprain of left hip**

√7ᵗʰ **S73.199** Other **sprain of unspecified hip**

√4ᵗʰ **S74** **Injury of nerves at hip and thigh level**
Code also any associated open wound (S71.-)
> EXCLUDES 2   injury of nerves at ankle and foot level (S94.-)
> injury of nerves at lower leg level (S84.-)

> The appropriate 7th character is to be added to each code from category S74.
> A   initial encounter
> D   subsequent encounter
> S   sequela

√5ᵗʰ **S74.0** Injury of **sciatic nerve at hip and thigh level**

√x7ᵗʰ **S74.00** Injury of sciatic nerve at hip and thigh level, unspecified leg

√x7ᵗʰ **S74.01** Injury of sciatic nerve at hip and thigh level, right leg

√x7ᵗʰ **S74.02** Injury of sciatic nerve at hip and thigh level, left leg

---

EXCLUDES 1 Not coded here   EXCLUDES 2 Not included here   N Newborn Age: 0   P Pediatric Age: 0-17   M Maternity Age: 12-55   A Adult Age: 15-124

892   ICD-10-CM 2014 (Draft)

√5ᵗʰ **S74.1** Injury of femoral nerve at hip and thigh level

    √x7ᵗʰ **S74.10** **Injury of femoral nerve at hip and thigh level, unspecified leg**

    √x7ᵗʰ **S74.11** Injury of femoral nerve at hip and thigh level, right leg

    √x7ᵗʰ **S74.12** Injury of femoral nerve at hip and thigh level, left leg

√5ᵗʰ **S74.2** Injury of cutaneous sensory nerve at hip and thigh level

    √x7ᵗʰ **S74.20** **Injury of cutaneous sensory nerve at hip and thigh level, unspecified leg**

    √x7ᵗʰ **S74.21** Injury of cutaneous sensory nerve at hip and high level, right leg

    √x7ᵗʰ **S74.22** Injury of cutaneous sensory nerve at hip and thigh level, left leg

√5ᵗʰ **S74.8** Injury of other nerves at hip and thigh level

    √6ᵗʰ **S74.8X** Injury of other nerves at hip and thigh level

        √7ᵗʰ **S74.8X1** **Injury of other nerves at hip and thigh level, right leg**

        √7ᵗʰ **S74.8X2** **Injury of other nerves at hip and thigh level, left leg**

        √7ᵗʰ **S74.8X9** **Injury of other nerves at hip and thigh level, unspecified leg**

√5ᵗʰ **S74.9** Injury of unspecified nerve at hip and thigh level

    √x7ᵗʰ **S74.90** **Injury of unspecified nerve at hip and thigh level, unspecified leg**

    √x7ᵗʰ **S74.91** **Injury of unspecified nerve at hip and thigh level, right leg**

    √x7ᵗʰ **S74.92** **Injury of unspecified nerve at hip and thigh level, left leg**

√4ᵗʰ **S75** **Injury of blood vessels at hip and thigh level**

Code also any associated open wound (S71.-)

EXCLUDES 2   injury of blood vessels at lower leg level (S85.-)
                injury of popliteal artery (S85.0)

The appropriate 7th character is to be added to each code from category S75.
A   initial encounter
D   subsequent encounter
S   sequela

√5ᵗʰ **S75.0** Injury of femoral artery

    √6ᵗʰ **S75.00** Unspecified injury of femoral artery

        √7ᵗʰ **S75.001** **Unspecified injury of femoral artery, right leg**

        √7ᵗʰ **S75.002** **Unspecified injury of femoral artery, left leg**

        √7ᵗʰ **S75.009** **Unspecified injury of femoral artery, unspecified leg**

    √6ᵗʰ **S75.01** Minor laceration of femoral artery
        Incomplete transection of femoral artery
        Laceration of femoral artery NOS
        Superficial laceration of femoral artery

        √7ᵗʰ **S75.011** **Minor laceration of femoral artery, right leg**

        √7ᵗʰ **S75.012** **Minor laceration of femoral artery, left leg**

        √7ᵗʰ **S75.019** **Minor laceration of femoral artery, unspecified leg**

    √6ᵗʰ **S75.02** Major laceration of femoral artery
        Complete transection of femoral artery
        Traumatic rupture of femoral artery

        √7ᵗʰ **S75.021** **Major laceration of femoral artery, right leg**

        √7ᵗʰ **S75.022** **Major laceration of femoral artery, left leg**

        √7ᵗʰ **S75.029** **Major laceration of femoral artery, unspecified leg**

    √6ᵗʰ **S75.09** Other specified injury of femoral artery

        √7ᵗʰ **S75.091** **Other specified injury of femoral artery, right leg**

        √7ᵗʰ **S75.092** **Other specified injury of femoral artery, left leg**

        √7ᵗʰ **S75.099** **Other specified injury of femoral artery, unspecified leg**

√5ᵗʰ **S75.1** Injury of femoral vein at hip and thigh level

    √6ᵗʰ **S75.10** Unspecified injury of femoral vein at hip and thigh level

        √7ᵗʰ **S75.101** **Unspecified injury of femoral vein at hip and thigh level, right leg**

        √7ᵗʰ **S75.102** **Unspecified injury of femoral vein at hip and thigh level, left leg**

        √7ᵗʰ **S75.109** **Unspecified injury of femoral vein at hip and thigh level, unspecified leg**

    √6ᵗʰ **S75.11** Minor laceration of femoral vein at hip and thigh level
        Incomplete transection of femoral vein at hip and thigh level
        Laceration of femoral vein at hip and thigh level NOS
        Superficial laceration of femoral vein at hip and thigh level

        √7ᵗʰ **S75.111** **Minor laceration of femoral vein at hip and thigh level, right leg**

        √7ᵗʰ **S75.112** **Minor laceration of femoral vein at hip and thigh level, left leg**

        √7ᵗʰ **S75.119** **Minor laceration of femoral vein at hip and thigh level, unspecified leg**

    √6ᵗʰ **S75.12** Major laceration of femoral vein at hip and thigh level
        Complete transection of femoral vein at hip and thigh level
        Traumatic rupture of femoral vein at hip and thigh level

        √7ᵗʰ **S75.121** **Major laceration of femoral vein at hip and thigh level, right leg**

        √7ᵗʰ **S75.122** **Major laceration of femoral vein at hip and thigh level, left leg**

        √7ᵗʰ **S75.129** **Major laceration of femoral vein at hip and thigh level, unspecified leg**

    √6ᵗʰ **S75.19** Other specified injury of femoral vein at hip and thigh level

        √7ᵗʰ **S75.191** **Other specified injury of femoral vein at hip and thigh level, right leg**

        √7ᵗʰ **S75.192** **Other specified injury of femoral vein at hip and thigh level, left leg**

        √7ᵗʰ **S75.199** **Other specified injury of femoral vein at hip and thigh level, unspecified leg**

√5ᵗʰ **S75.2** Injury of greater saphenous vein at hip and thigh level

    EXCLUDES 1   greater saphenous vein NOS (S85.3)

    √6ᵗʰ **S75.20** Unspecified injury of greater saphenous vein at hip and thigh level

        √7ᵗʰ **S75.201** **Unspecified injury of greater saphenous vein at hip and thigh level, right leg**

        √7ᵗʰ **S75.202** **Unspecified injury of greater saphenous vein at hip and thigh level, left leg**

        √7ᵗʰ **S75.209** **Unspecified injury of greater saphenous vein at hip and thigh level, unspecified leg**

    √6ᵗʰ **S75.21** Minor laceration of greater saphenous vein at hip and thigh level
        Incomplete transection of greater saphenous vein at hip and thigh level
        Laceration of greater saphenous vein at hip and thigh level NOS
        Superficial laceration of greater saphenous vein at hip and thigh level

        √7ᵗʰ **S75.211** **Minor laceration of greater saphenous vein at hip and thigh level, right leg**

        √7ᵗʰ **S75.212** **Minor laceration of greater saphenous vein at hip and thigh level, left leg**

        √7ᵗʰ **S75.219** **Minor laceration of greater saphenous vein at hip and thigh level, unspecified leg**

    √6ᵗʰ **S75.22** Major laceration of greater saphenous vein at hip and thigh level
        Complete transection of greater saphenous vein at hip and thigh level
        Traumatic rupture of greater saphenous vein at hip and thigh level

        √7ᵗʰ **S75.221** **Major laceration of greater saphenous vein at hip and thigh level, right leg**

        √7ᵗʰ **S75.222** **Major laceration of greater saphenous vein at hip and thigh level, left leg**

        √7ᵗʰ **S75.229** **Major laceration of greater saphenous vein at hip and thigh level, unspecified leg**

✔ Additional Character Required   √x7ᵗʰ Xtension Alert   Unspecified Code   Other Specified Code   Manifestation Code   ►◄ Revised Text   ● New Code   ▲ Revised Code Title

√6ᵗʰ **S75.29** Other specified injury of greater saphenous vein at hip and thigh level

   √7ᵗʰ **S75.291** **Other specified injury of greater saphenous vein at hip and thigh level, right leg**

   √7ᵗʰ **S75.292** **Other specified injury of greater saphenous vein at hip and thigh level, left leg**

   √7ᵗʰ **S75.299** **Other specified injury of greater saphenous vein at hip and thigh level, unspecified leg**

√5ᵗʰ **S75.8** Injury of other blood vessels at hip and thigh level

  √6ᵗʰ **S75.80** Unspecified injury of other blood vessels at hip and thigh level

   √7ᵗʰ **S75.801** **Unspecified injury of other blood vessels at hip and thigh level, right leg**

   √7ᵗʰ **S75.802** **Unspecified injury of other blood vessels at hip and thigh level, left leg**

   √7ᵗʰ **S75.809** **Unspecified injury of other blood vessels at hip and thigh level, unspecified leg**

  √6ᵗʰ **S75.81** Laceration of other blood vessels at hip and thigh level

   √7ᵗʰ **S75.811** **Laceration of other blood vessels at hip and thigh level, right leg**

   √7ᵗʰ **S75.812** **Laceration of other blood vessels at hip and thigh level, left leg**

   √7ᵗʰ **S75.819** **Laceration of other blood vessels at hip and thigh level, unspecified leg**

  √6ᵗʰ **S75.89** Other specified injury of other blood vessels at hip and thigh level

   √7ᵗʰ **S75.891** **Other specified injury of other blood vessels at hip and thigh level, right leg**

   √7ᵗʰ **S75.892** **Other specified injury of other blood vessels at hip and thigh level, left leg**

   √7ᵗʰ **S75.899** **Other specified injury of other blood vessels at hip and thigh level, unspecified leg**

√5ᵗʰ **S75.9** Injury of unspecified blood vessel at hip and thigh level

  √6ᵗʰ **S75.90** Unspecified injury of unspecified blood vessel at hip and thigh level

   √7ᵗʰ **S75.901** **Unspecified injury of unspecified blood vessel at hip and thigh level, right leg**

   √7ᵗʰ **S75.902** **Unspecified injury of unspecified blood vessel at hip and thigh level, left leg**

   √7ᵗʰ **S75.909** **Unspecified injury of unspecified blood vessel at hip and thigh level, unspecified leg**

  √6ᵗʰ **S75.91** Laceration of unspecified blood vessel at hip and thigh level

   √7ᵗʰ **S75.911** **Laceration of unspecified blood vessel at hip and thigh level, right leg**

   √7ᵗʰ **S75.912** **Laceration of unspecified blood vessel at hip and thigh level, left leg**

   √7ᵗʰ **S75.919** **Laceration of unspecified blood vessel at hip and thigh level, unspecified leg**

  √6ᵗʰ **S75.99** Other specified injury of unspecified blood vessel at hip and thigh level

   √7ᵗʰ **S75.991** **Other specified injury of unspecified blood vessel at hip and thigh level, right leg**

   √7ᵗʰ **S75.992** **Other specified injury of unspecified blood vessel at hip and thigh level, left leg**

   √7ᵗʰ **S75.999** **Other specified injury of unspecified blood vessel at hip and thigh level, unspecified leg**

√4ᵗʰ **S76** Injury of muscle, fascia and tendon at hip and thigh level

  Code also any associated open wound (S71.-)

  EXCLUDES 2   *injury of muscle, fascia and tendon at lower leg level (S86)*
        sprain of joint and ligament of hip (S73.1)

  The appropriate 7th character is to be added to each code from category S76.
  A   initial encounter
  D   subsequent encounter
  S   sequela

√5ᵗʰ **S76.0** Injury of muscle, fascia and tendon of hip

  √6ᵗʰ **S76.00** Unspecified injury of muscle, fascia and tendon of hip

   √7ᵗʰ **S76.001** **Unspecified injury of muscle, fascia and tendon of right hip**

   √7ᵗʰ **S76.002** **Unspecified injury of muscle, fascia and tendon of left hip**

   √7ᵗʰ **S76.009** **Unspecified injury of muscle, fascia and tendon of unspecified hip**

  √6ᵗʰ **S76.01** Strain of muscle, fascia and tendon of hip

   √7ᵗʰ **S76.011** **Strain of muscle, fascia and tendon of right hip**

   √7ᵗʰ **S76.012** **Strain of muscle, fascia and tendon of left hip**

   √7ᵗʰ **S76.019** **Strain of muscle, fascia and tendon of unspecified hip**

  √6ᵗʰ **S76.02** Laceration of muscle, fascia and tendon of hip

   √7ᵗʰ **S76.021** **Laceration of muscle, fascia and tendon of right hip**

   √7ᵗʰ **S76.022** **Laceration of muscle, fascia and tendon of left hip**

   √7ᵗʰ **S76.029** **Laceration of muscle, fascia and tendon of unspecified hip**

  √6ᵗʰ **S76.09** Other specified injury of muscle, fascia and tendon of hip

   √7ᵗʰ **S76.091** **Other specified injury of muscle, fascia and tendon of right hip**

   √7ᵗʰ **S76.092** **Other specified injury of muscle, fascia and tendon of left hip**

   √7ᵗʰ **S76.099** **Other specified injury of muscle, fascia and tendon of unspecified hip**

√5ᵗʰ **S76.1** Injury of quadriceps muscle, fascia and tendon
  Injury of patellar ligament (tendon)

  √6ᵗʰ **S76.10** Unspecified injury of quadriceps muscle, fascia and tendon

   √7ᵗʰ **S76.101** **Unspecified injury of right quadriceps muscle, fascia and tendon**

   √7ᵗʰ **S76.102** **Unspecified injury of left quadriceps muscle, fascia and tendon**

   √7ᵗʰ **S76.109** **Unspecified injury of unspecified quadriceps muscle, fascia and tendon**

  √6ᵗʰ **S76.11** Strain of quadriceps muscle, fascia and tendon

   √7ᵗʰ **S76.111** **Strain of right quadriceps muscle, fascia and tendon**

   √7ᵗʰ **S76.112** **Strain of left quadriceps muscle, fascia and tendon**

   √7ᵗʰ **S76.119** **Strain of unspecified quadriceps muscle, fascia and tendon**

  √6ᵗʰ **S76.12** Laceration of quadriceps muscle, fascia and tendon

   √7ᵗʰ **S76.121** **Laceration of right quadriceps muscle, fascia and tendon**

   √7ᵗʰ **S76.122** **Laceration of left quadriceps muscle, fascia and tendon**

   √7ᵗʰ **S76.129** **Laceration of unspecified quadriceps muscle, fascia and tendon**

  √6ᵗʰ **S76.19** Other specified injury of quadriceps muscle, fascia and tendon

   √7ᵗʰ **S76.191** **Other specified injury of right quadriceps muscle, fascia and tendon**

   √7ᵗʰ **S76.192** **Other specified injury of left quadriceps muscle, fascia and tendon**

   √7ᵗʰ **S76.199** **Other specified injury of unspecified quadriceps muscle, fascia and tendon**

EXCLUDES 1 Not coded here   EXCLUDES 2 Not included here   N Newborn Age: 0   P Pediatric Age: 0-17   M Maternity Age: 12-55   A Adult Age: 15-124

894   ICD-10-CM 2014 (Draft)

√5th **S76.2** Injury of adductor muscle, fascia and tendon of thigh

√6th **S76.20** Unspecified injury of adductor muscle, fascia and tendon of thigh

√7th **S76.201** Unspecified injury of adductor muscle, fascia and tendon of right thigh

√7th **S76.202** Unspecified injury of adductor muscle, fascia and tendon of left thigh

√7th **S76.209** Unspecified injury of adductor muscle, fascia and tendon of unspecified thigh

√6th **S76.21** Strain of adductor muscle, fascia and tendon of thigh

√7th **S76.211** Strain of adductor muscle, fascia and tendon of right thigh

√7th **S76.212** Strain of adductor muscle, fascia and tendon of left thigh

√7th **S76.219** Strain of adductor muscle, fascia and tendon of unspecified thigh

√6th **S76.22** Laceration of adductor muscle, fascia and tendon of thigh

√7th **S76.221** Laceration of adductor muscle, fascia and tendon of right thigh

√7th **S76.222** Laceration of adductor muscle, fascia and tendon of left thigh

√7th **S76.229** Laceration of adductor muscle, fascia and tendon of unspecified thigh

√6th **S76.29** Other injury of adductor muscle, fascia and tendon of thigh

√7th **S76.291** Other injury of adductor muscle, fascia and tendon of right thigh

√7th **S76.292** Other injury of adductor muscle, fascia and tendon of left thigh

√7th **S76.299** Other injury of adductor muscle, fascia and tendon of unspecified thigh

√5th **S76.3** Injury of muscle, fascia and tendon of the posterior muscle group at thigh level

√6th **S76.30** Unspecified injury of muscle, fascia and tendon of the posterior muscle group at thigh level

√7th **S76.301** Unspecified injury of muscle, fascia and tendon of the posterior muscle group at thigh level, right thigh

√7th **S76.302** Unspecified injury of muscle, fascia and tendon of the posterior muscle group at thigh level, left thigh

√7th **S76.309** Unspecified injury of muscle, fascia and tendon of the posterior muscle group at thigh level, unspecified thigh

√6th **S76.31** Strain of muscle, fascia and tendon of the posterior muscle group at thigh level

√7th **S76.311** Strain of muscle, fascia and tendon of the posterior muscle group at thigh level, right thigh

√7th **S76.312** Strain of muscle, fascia and tendon of the posterior muscle group at thigh level, left thigh

√7th **S76.319** Strain of muscle, fascia and tendon of the posterior muscle group at thigh level, unspecified thigh

√6th **S76.32** Laceration of muscle, fascia and tendon of the posterior muscle group at thigh level

√7th **S76.321** Laceration of muscle, fascia and tendon of the posterior muscle group at thigh level, right thigh

√7th **S76.322** Laceration of muscle, fascia and tendon of the posterior muscle group at thigh level, left thigh

√7th **S76.329** Laceration of muscle, fascia and tendon of the posterior muscle group at thigh level, unspecified thigh

√6th **S76.39** Other specified injury of muscle, fascia and tendon of the posterior muscle group at thigh level

√7th **S76.391** Other specified injury of muscle, fascia and tendon of the posterior muscle group at thigh level, right thigh

√7th **S76.392** Other specified injury of muscle, fascia and tendon of the posterior muscle group at thigh level, left thigh

√7th **S76.399** Other specified injury of muscle, fascia and tendon of the posterior muscle group at thigh level, unspecified thigh

√5th **S76.8** Injury of other specified muscles, fascia and tendons at thigh level

√6th **S76.80** Unspecified injury of other specified muscles, fascia and tendons at thigh level

√7th **S76.801** Unspecified injury of other specified muscles, fascia and tendons at thigh level, right thigh

√7th **S76.802** Unspecified injury of other specified muscles, fascia and tendons at thigh level, left thigh

√7th **S76.809** Unspecified injury of other specified muscles, fascia and tendons at thigh level, unspecified thigh

√6th **S76.81** Strain of other specified muscles, fascia and tendons at thigh level

√7th **S76.811** Strain of other specified muscles, fascia and tendons at thigh level, right thigh

√7th **S76.812** Strain of other specified muscles, fascia and tendons at thigh level, left thigh

√7th **S76.819** Strain of other specified muscles, fascia and tendons at thigh level, unspecified thigh

√6th **S76.82** Laceration of other specified muscles, fascia and tendons at thigh level

√7th **S76.821** Laceration of other specified muscles, fascia and tendons at thigh level, right thigh

√7th **S76.822** Laceration of other specified muscles, fascia and tendons at thigh level, left thigh

√7th **S76.829** Laceration of other specified muscles, fascia and tendons at thigh level, unspecified thigh

√6th **S76.89** Other injury of other specified muscles, fascia and tendons at thigh level

√7th **S76.891** Other injury of other specified muscles, fascia and tendons at thigh level, right thigh

√7th **S76.892** Other injury of other specified muscles, fascia and tendons at thigh level, left thigh

√7th **S76.899** Other injury of other specified muscles, fascia and tendons at thigh level, unspecified thigh

√5th **S76.9** Injury of unspecified muscles, fascia and tendons at thigh level

√6th **S76.90** Unspecified injury of unspecified muscles, fascia and tendons at thigh level

√7th **S76.901** Unspecified injury of unspecified muscles, fascia and tendons at thigh level, right thigh

√7th **S76.902** Unspecified injury of unspecified muscles, fascia and tendons at thigh level, left thigh

√7th **S76.909** Unspecified injury of unspecified muscles, fascia and tendons at thigh level, unspecified thigh

√6th **S76.91** Strain of unspecified muscles, fascia and tendons at thigh level

√7th **S76.911** Strain of unspecified muscles, fascia and tendons at thigh level, right thigh

√7th **S76.912** Strain of unspecified muscles, fascia and tendons at thigh level, left thigh

√7th **S76.919** Strain of unspecified muscles, fascia and tendons at thigh level, unspecified thigh

√6th **S76.92** Laceration of unspecified muscles, fascia and tendons at thigh level

√7th **S76.921** Laceration of unspecified muscles, fascia and tendons at thigh level, right thigh

√7th **S76.922** Laceration of unspecified muscles, fascia and tendons at thigh level, left thigh

√7th **S76.929** Laceration of unspecified muscles, fascia and tendons at thigh level, unspecified thigh

---

☑ Additional Character Required √x7th *X*tension Alert   Unspecified Code   Other Specified Code   Manifestation Code   ►◄ Revised Text   ● New Code   ▲ Revised Code Title

Injury, Poisoning and Certain Other Consequences of External Causes

✓6ᵗʰ **S76.99** Other specified injury of unspecified muscles, fascia and tendons at thigh level

   ✓7ᵗʰ **S76.991** Other specified injury of unspecified muscles, fascia and tendons at thigh level, right thigh

   ✓7ᵗʰ **S76.992** Other specified injury of unspecified muscles, fascia and tendons at thigh level, left thigh

   ✓7ᵗʰ **S76.999** Other specified injury of unspecified muscles, fascia and tendons at thigh level, unspecified thigh

✓4ᵗʰ **S77 Crushing injury of hip and thigh**

Use additional code(s) for all associated injuries

EXCLUDES 2   crushing injury of ankle and foot (S97.-)
crushing injury of lower leg (S87.-)

The appropriate 7th character is to be added to each code from category S77.
A   initial encounter
D   subsequent encounter
S   sequela

✓5ᵗʰ **S77.0 Crushing injury of hip**

  ✓x7ᵗʰ **S77.00 Crushing injury of unspecified hip**
  ✓x7ᵗʰ **S77.01 Crushing injury of right hip**
  ✓x7ᵗʰ **S77.02 Crushing injury of left hip**

✓5ᵗʰ **S77.1 Crushing injury of thigh**

  ✓x7ᵗʰ **S77.10 Crushing injury of unspecified thigh**
  ✓x7ᵗʰ **S77.11 Crushing injury of right thigh**
  ✓x7ᵗʰ **S77.12 Crushing injury of left thigh**

✓5ᵗʰ **S77.2 Crushing injury of hip with thigh**

  ✓x7ᵗʰ **S77.20 Crushing injury of unspecified hip with thigh**
  ✓x7ᵗʰ **S77.21 Crushing injury of right hip with thigh**
  ✓x7ᵗʰ **S77.22 Crushing injury of left hip with thigh**

✓4ᵗʰ **S78 Traumatic amputation of hip and thigh**

NOTE   An amputation not identified as partial or complete should be coded to complete.

EXCLUDES 1   traumatic amputation of knee (S88.0-)

The appropriate 7th character is to be added to each code from category S78.
A   initial encounter
D   subsequent encounter
S   sequela

✓5ᵗʰ **S78.0 Traumatic amputation at hip joint**

 ✓6ᵗʰ **S78.01 Complete traumatic amputation at hip joint**

  ✓7ᵗʰ **S78.011 Complete traumatic amputation at right hip joint**
  ✓7ᵗʰ **S78.012 Complete traumatic amputation at left hip joint**
  ✓7ᵗʰ **S78.019 Complete traumatic amputation at unspecified hip joint**

 ✓6ᵗʰ **S78.02 Partial traumatic amputation at hip joint**

  ✓7ᵗʰ **S78.021 Partial traumatic amputation at right hip joint**
  ✓7ᵗʰ **S78.022 Partial traumatic amputation at left hip joint**
  ✓7ᵗʰ **S78.029 Partial traumatic amputation at unspecified hip joint**

✓5ᵗʰ **S78.1 Traumatic amputation at level between hip and knee**

EXCLUDES 1   traumatic amputation of knee (S88.0-)

 ✓6ᵗʰ **S78.11 Complete traumatic amputation at level between hip and knee**

  ✓7ᵗʰ **S78.111 Complete traumatic amputation at level between right hip and knee**
  ✓7ᵗʰ **S78.112 Complete traumatic amputation at level between left hip and knee**
  ✓7ᵗʰ **S78.119 Complete traumatic amputation at level between unspecified hip and knee**

 ✓6ᵗʰ **S78.12 Partial traumatic amputation at level between hip and knee**

  ✓7ᵗʰ **S78.121 Partial traumatic amputation at level between right hip and knee**
  ✓7ᵗʰ **S78.122 Partial traumatic amputation at level between left hip and knee**

  ✓7ᵗʰ **S78.129 Partial traumatic amputation at level between unspecified hip and knee**

✓5ᵗʰ **S78.9 Traumatic amputation of hip and thigh, level unspecified**

 ✓6ᵗʰ **S78.91 Complete traumatic amputation of hip and thigh, level unspecified**

  ✓7ᵗʰ **S78.911 Complete traumatic amputation of right hip and thigh, level unspecified**
  ✓7ᵗʰ **S78.912 Complete traumatic amputation of left hip and thigh, level unspecified**
  ✓7ᵗʰ **S78.919 Complete traumatic amputation of unspecified hip and thigh, level unspecified**

 ✓6ᵗʰ **S78.92 Partial traumatic amputation of hip and thigh, level unspecified**

  ✓7ᵗʰ **S78.921 Partial traumatic amputation of right hip and thigh, level unspecified**
  ✓7ᵗʰ **S78.922 Partial traumatic amputation of left hip and thigh, level unspecified**
  ✓7ᵗʰ **S78.929 Partial traumatic amputation of unspecified hip and thigh, level unspecified**

✓4ᵗʰ **S79 Other and unspecified injuries of hip and thigh**

✓5ᵗʰ **S79.0 Physeal fracture of upper end of femur**

NOTE   A fracture not indicated as open or closed should be coded to closed.

EXCLUDES 1   apophyseal fracture of upper end of femur (S72.13-)
nontraumatic slipped upper femoral epiphysis (M93.0-)

The appropriate 7th character is to be added to each code from subcategory S79.0.
A   initial encounter for closed fracture
D   subsequent encounter for fracture with routine healing
G   subsequent encounter for fracture with delayed healing
K   subsequent encounter for fracture with nonunion
P   subsequent encounter for fracture with malunion
S   sequela

 ✓6ᵗʰ **S79.00 Unspecified physeal fracture of upper end of femur**

  ✓7ᵗʰ **S79.001 Unspecified physeal fracture of upper end of right femur**
  ✓7ᵗʰ **S79.002 Unspecified physeal fracture of upper end of left femur**
  ✓7ᵗʰ **S79.009 Unspecified physeal fracture of upper end of unspecified femur**

 ✓6ᵗʰ **S79.01 Salter-Harris Type I physeal fracture of upper end of femur**

Acute on chronic slipped capital femoral epiphysis (traumatic)
Acute slipped capital femoral epiphysis (traumatic)
Capital femoral epiphyseal fracture

EXCLUDES 1   chronic slipped upper femoral epiphysis (nontraumatic) (M93.02-)

  ✓7ᵗʰ **S79.011 Salter-Harris Type I physeal fracture of upper end of right femur**
  ✓7ᵗʰ **S79.012 Salter-Harris Type I physeal fracture of upper end of left femur**
  ✓7ᵗʰ **S79.019 Salter-Harris Type I physeal fracture of upper end of unspecified femur**

 ✓6ᵗʰ **S79.09 Other physeal fracture of upper end of femur**

  ✓7ᵗʰ **S79.091 Other physeal fracture of upper end of right femur**
  ✓7ᵗʰ **S79.092 Other physeal fracture of upper end of left femur**
  ✓7ᵗʰ **S79.099 Other physeal fracture of upper end of unspecified femur**

EXCLUDES 1 Not coded here   EXCLUDES 2 Not included here   N Newborn Age: 0   P Pediatric Age: 0-17   M Maternity Age: 12-55   A Adult Age: 15-124

896   ICD-10-CM 2014 (Draft)

√5ᵗʰ **S79.1** Physeal **fracture of** lower end of femur

> **NOTE** A fracture not indicated as open or closed should be coded to closed.

> The appropriate 7th character is to be added to each code from subcategory S79.1.
> A initial encounter for closed fracture
> D subsequent encounter for fracture with routine healing
> G subsequent encounter for fracture with delayed healing
> K subsequent encounter for fracture with nonunion
> P subsequent encounter for fracture with malunion
> S sequela

√6ᵗʰ **S79.10** Unspecified physeal fracture of lower end of femur

√7ᵗʰ **S79.101** Unspecified physeal fracture of lower end of right femur

√7ᵗʰ **S79.102** Unspecified physeal fracture of lower end of left femur

√7ᵗʰ **S79.109** Unspecified physeal fracture of lower end of unspecified femur

√6ᵗʰ **S79.11** Salter-Harris Type I physeal fracture of lower end of femur

√7ᵗʰ **S79.111** Salter-Harris Type I physeal fracture of lower end of right femur

√7ᵗʰ **S79.112** Salter-Harris Type I physeal fracture of lower end of left femur

√7ᵗʰ **S79.119** Salter-Harris Type I physeal fracture of lower end of unspecified femur

√6ᵗʰ **S79.12** Salter-Harris Type II physeal fracture of lower end of femur

√7ᵗʰ **S79.121** Salter-Harris Type II physeal fracture of lower end of right femur

√7ᵗʰ **S79.122** Salter-Harris Type II physeal fracture of lower end of left femur

√7ᵗʰ **S79.129** Salter-Harris Type II physeal fracture of lower end of unspecified femur

√6ᵗʰ **S79.13** Salter-Harris Type III physeal fracture of lower end of femur

√7ᵗʰ **S79.131** Salter-Harris Type III physeal fracture of lower end of right femur

√7ᵗʰ **S79.132** Salter-Harris Type III physeal fracture of lower end of left femur

√7ᵗʰ **S79.139** Salter-Harris Type III physeal fracture of lower end of unspecified femur

√6ᵗʰ **S79.14** Salter-Harris Type IV physeal fracture of lower end of femur

√7ᵗʰ **S79.141** Salter-Harris Type IV physeal fracture of lower end of right femur

√7ᵗʰ **S79.142** Salter-Harris Type IV physeal fracture of lower end of left femur

√7ᵗʰ **S79.149** Salter-Harris Type IV physeal fracture of lower end of unspecified femur

√6ᵗʰ **S79.19** Other physeal fracture of lower end of femur

√7ᵗʰ **S79.191** Other physeal fracture of lower end of right femur

√7ᵗʰ **S79.192** Other physeal fracture of lower end of left femur

√7ᵗʰ **S79.199** Other physeal fracture of lower end of unspecified femur

√5ᵗʰ **S79.8** Other specified injuries of hip and thigh

> The appropriate 7th character is to be added to each code in subcategory S79.8.
> A initial encounter
> D subsequent encounter
> S sequela

√6ᵗʰ **S79.81** Other specified injuries of hip

√7ᵗʰ **S79.811** Other specified injuries of right hip

√7ᵗʰ **S79.812** Other specified injuries of left hip

√7ᵗʰ **S79.819** Other specified injuries of unspecified hip

√6ᵗʰ **S79.82** Other specified injuries of thigh

√7ᵗʰ **S79.821** Other specified injuries of right thigh

√7ᵗʰ **S79.822** Other specified injuries of left thigh

√7ᵗʰ **S79.829** Other specified injuries of unspecified thigh

√5ᵗʰ **S79.9** Unspecified injury of hip and thigh

> The appropriate 7th character is to be added to each code in subcategory S79.9.
> A initial encounter
> D subsequent encounter
> S sequela

√6ᵗʰ **S79.91** Unspecified injury of hip

√7ᵗʰ **S79.911** Unspecified injury of right hip

√7ᵗʰ **S79.912** Unspecified injury of left hip

√7ᵗʰ **S79.919** Unspecified injury of unspecified hip

√6ᵗʰ **S79.92** Unspecified injury of thigh

√7ᵗʰ **S79.921** Unspecified injury of right thigh

√7ᵗʰ **S79.922** Unspecified injury of left thigh

√7ᵗʰ **S79.929** Unspecified injury of unspecified thigh

Injuries to the knee and lower leg (S80-S89)

EXCLUDES 2 burns and corrosions (T20-T32)
frostbite (T33-T34)
injuries of ankle and foot, except fracture of ankle and malleolus (S90-S99)
insect bite or sting, venomous (T63.4)

√4ᵗʰ **S80** Superficial injury of knee and lower leg

> **EXCLUDES 2** superficial injury of ankle and foot (S90.-)

> The appropriate 7th character is to be added to each code from category S80.
> A initial encounter
> D subsequent encounter
> S sequela

√5ᵗʰ **S80.0** Contusion of knee

√x7ᵗʰ **S80.00** Contusion of unspecified knee

√x7ᵗʰ **S80.01** Contusion of right knee

√x7ᵗʰ **S80.02** Contusion of left knee

√5ᵗʰ **S80.1** Contusion of lower leg

√x7ᵗʰ **S80.10** Contusion of unspecified lower leg

√x7ᵗʰ **S80.11** Contusion of right lower leg

√x7ᵗʰ **S80.12** Contusion of left lower leg

√5ᵗʰ **S80.2** Other superficial injuries of knee

√6ᵗʰ **S80.21** Abrasion of knee

√7ᵗʰ **S80.211** Abrasion, right knee

√7ᵗʰ **S80.212** Abrasion, left knee

√7ᵗʰ **S80.219** Abrasion, unspecified knee

√6ᵗʰ **S80.22** Blister (nonthermal) of knee

√7ᵗʰ **S80.221** Blister (nonthermal), right knee

√7ᵗʰ **S80.222** Blister (nonthermal), left knee

√7ᵗʰ **S80.229** Blister (nonthermal), unspecified knee

√6ᵗʰ **S80.24** External constriction of knee

√7ᵗʰ **S80.241** External constriction, right knee

√7ᵗʰ **S80.242** External constriction, left knee

√7ᵗʰ **S80.249** External constriction, unspecified knee

√6ᵗʰ **S80.25** Superficial foreign body of knee
Splinter in the knee

√7ᵗʰ **S80.251** Superficial foreign body, right knee

√7ᵗʰ **S80.252** Superficial foreign body, left knee

√7ᵗʰ **S80.259** Superficial foreign body, unspecified knee

√6ᵗʰ **S80.26** Insect bite (nonvenomous) of knee

√7ᵗʰ **S80.261** Insect bite (nonvenomous), right knee

√7ᵗʰ **S80.262** Insect bite (nonvenomous), left knee

√7ᵗʰ **S80.269** Insect bite (nonvenomous), unspecified knee

√6ᵗʰ **S80.27** Other superficial bite of knee

> **EXCLUDES 1** open bite of knee (S81.05-)

√7ᵗʰ **S80.271** Other superficial bite of right knee

√7ᵗʰ **S80.272** Other superficial bite of left knee

√7ᵗʰ **S80.279** Other superficial bite of unspecified knee

√5ᵗʰ **S80.8** Other superficial injuries of lower leg

√6ᵗʰ **S80.81** Abrasion of lower leg

√7ᵗʰ **S80.811** Abrasion, right lower leg

√7ᵗʰ **S80.812** Abrasion, left lower leg

√7ᵗʰ **S80.819** Abrasion, unspecified lower leg

✓6th **S80.82 Blister (nonthermal) of lower leg**
- ✓7th **S80.821** Blister (nonthermal), right lower leg
- ✓7th **S80.822** Blister (nonthermal), left lower leg
- ✓7th **S80.829** Blister (nonthermal), unspecified lower leg

✓6th **S80.84 External constriction of lower leg**
- ✓7th **S80.841** External constriction, right lower leg
- ✓7th **S80.842** External constriction, left lower leg
- ✓7th **S80.849** External constriction, unspecified lower leg

✓6th **S80.85 Superficial foreign body of lower leg**
Splinter in the lower leg
- ✓7th **S80.851** Superficial foreign body, right lower leg
- ✓7th **S80.852** Superficial foreign body, left lower leg
- ✓7th **S80.859** Superficial foreign body, unspecified lower leg

✓6th **S80.86 Insect bite (nonvenomous) of lower leg**
- ✓7th **S80.861** Insect bite (nonvenomous), right lower leg
- ✓7th **S80.862** Insect bite (nonvenomous), left lower leg
- ✓7th **S80.869** Insect bite (nonvenomous), unspecified lower leg

✓6th **S80.87 Other superficial bite of lower leg**
EXCLUDES1 open bite of lower leg (S81.85-)
- ✓7th **S80.871** Other superficial bite, right lower leg
- ✓7th **S80.872** Other superficial bite, left lower leg
- ✓7th **S80.879** Other superficial bite, unspecified lower leg

✓5th **S80.9 Unspecified superficial injury of knee and lower leg**
✓6th **S80.91 Unspecified superficial injury of knee**
- ✓7th **S80.911** Unspecified superficial injury of right knee
- ✓7th **S80.912** Unspecified superficial injury of left knee
- ✓7th **S80.919** Unspecified superficial injury of unspecified knee

✓6th **S80.92 Unspecified superficial injury of lower leg**
- ✓7th **S80.921** Unspecified superficial injury of right lower leg
- ✓7th **S80.922** Unspecified superficial injury of left lower leg
- ✓7th **S80.929** Unspecified superficial injury of unspecified lower leg

✓4th **S81 Open wound of knee and lower leg**
Code also any associated wound infection
EXCLUDES1 open fracture of knee and lower leg (S82.-)
   traumatic amputation of lower leg (S88.-)
EXCLUDES2 open wound of ankle and foot (S91.-)

The appropriate 7th character is to be added to each code from category S81.
A   initial encounter
D   subsequent encounter
S   sequela

✓5th **S81.0 Open wound of knee**
✓6th **S81.00 Unspecified open wound of knee**
- ✓7th **S81.001** Unspecified open wound, right knee
- ✓7th **S81.002** Unspecified open wound, left knee
- ✓7th **S81.009** Unspecified open wound, unspecified knee

✓6th **S81.01 Laceration without foreign body of knee**
- ✓7th **S81.011** Laceration without foreign body, right knee
- ✓7th **S81.012** Laceration without foreign body, left knee
- ✓7th **S81.019** Laceration without foreign body, unspecified knee

✓6th **S81.02 Laceration with foreign body of knee**
- ✓7th **S81.021** Laceration with foreign body, right knee
- ✓7th **S81.022** Laceration with foreign body, left knee
- ✓7th **S81.029** Laceration with foreign body, unspecified knee

✓6th **S81.03 Puncture wound without foreign body of knee**
- ✓7th **S81.031** Puncture wound without foreign body, right knee

- ✓7th **S81.032** Puncture wound without foreign body, left knee
- ✓7th **S81.039** Puncture wound without foreign body, unspecified knee

✓6th **S81.04 Puncture wound with foreign body of knee**
- ✓7th **S81.041** Puncture wound with foreign body, right knee
- ✓7th **S81.042** Puncture wound with foreign body, left knee
- ✓7th **S81.049** Puncture wound with foreign body, unspecified knee

✓6th **S81.05 Open bite of knee**
Bite of knee NOS
EXCLUDES1 superficial bite of knee (S80.27-)
- ✓7th **S81.051** Open bite, right knee
- ✓7th **S81.052** Open bite, left knee
- ✓7th **S81.059** Open bite, unspecified knee

✓5th **S81.8 Open wound of lower leg**
✓6th **S81.80 Unspecified open wound of lower leg**
- ✓7th **S81.801** Unspecified open wound, right lower leg
- ✓7th **S81.802** Unspecified open wound, left lower leg
- ✓7th **S81.809** Unspecified open wound, unspecified lower leg

✓6th **S81.81 Laceration without foreign body of lower leg**
- ✓7th **S81.811** Laceration without foreign body, right lower leg
- ✓7th **S81.812** Laceration without foreign body, left lower leg
- ✓7th **S81.819** Laceration without foreign body, unspecified lower leg

✓6th **S81.82 Laceration with foreign body of lower leg**
- ✓7th **S81.821** Laceration with foreign body, right lower leg
- ✓7th **S81.822** Laceration with foreign body, left lower leg
- ✓7th **S81.829** Laceration with foreign body, unspecified lower leg

✓6th **S81.83 Puncture wound without foreign body of lower leg**
- ✓7th **S81.831** Puncture wound without foreign body, right lower leg
- ✓7th **S81.832** Puncture wound without foreign body, left lower leg
- ✓7th **S81.839** Puncture wound without foreign body, unspecified lower leg

✓6th **S81.84 Puncture wound with foreign body of lower leg**
- ✓7th **S81.841** Puncture wound with foreign body, right lower leg
- ✓7th **S81.842** Puncture wound with foreign body, left lower leg
- ✓7th **S81.849** Puncture wound with foreign body, unspecified lower leg

✓6th **S81.85 Open bite of lower leg**
Bite of lower leg NOS
EXCLUDES1 superficial bite of lower leg (S80.86-, S80.87-)
- ✓7th **S81.851** Open bite, right lower leg
- ✓7th **S81.852** Open bite, left lower leg
- ✓7th **S81.859** Open bite, unspecified lower leg

☑4ᵗʰ **S82 Fracture of lower leg, including ankle**

> NOTE   A fracture not indicated as displaced or nondisplaced should be coded to displaced.
> A fracture not designated as open or closed should be coded to closed.
> The open fracture designations are based on the Gustilo open fracture classification.
>
> INCLUDES   fracture of malleolus
> EXCLUDES 1 *traumatic amputation of lower leg (S88.-)*
> EXCLUDES 2 *fracture of foot, except ankle (S92.-)*
> *periprosthetic fracture of prosthetic implant of knee (T84.042, T84.043)*

> The appropriate 7th character is to be added to all codes from category S82 [unless otherwise indicated].
> A   initial encounter for closed fracture
> B   initial encounter for open fracture type I or II
>   initial encounter for open fracture NOS
> C   initial encounter for open fracture type IIIA, IIIB, or IIIC
> D   subsequent encounter for closed fracture with routine healing
> E   subsequent encounter for open fracture type I or II with routine healing
> F   subsequent encounter for open fracture type IIIA, IIIB, or IIIC with routine healing
> G   subsequent encounter for closed fracture with delayed healing
> H   subsequent encounter for open fracture type I or II with delayed healing
> J   subsequent encounter for open fracture type IIIA, IIIB or IIIC with delayed healing
> K   subsequent encounter for closed fracture with nonunion
> M   subsequent encounter for open fracture type I or II with nonunion
> N   subsequent encounter for open fracture type IIIA, IIIB or IIIC with nonunion
> P   subsequent encounter for closed fracture with malunion
> Q   subsequent encounter for open fracture type I or II with malunion
> R   subsequent encounter for open fracture type IIIA, IIIB or IIIC with malunion
> S   sequela

☑5ᵗʰ **S82.0 Fracture of patella**
Knee cap

 ☑6ᵗʰ **S82.00 Unspecified fracture of patella**
  ☑7ᵗʰ S82.001 **Unspecified fracture of right patella**
  ☑7ᵗʰ S82.002 **Unspecified fracture of left patella**
  ☑7ᵗʰ S82.009 **Unspecified fracture of unspecified patella**

 ☑6ᵗʰ **S82.01 Osteochondral fracture of patella**
  ☑7ᵗʰ S82.011 **Displaced osteochondral fracture of right patella**
  ☑7ᵗʰ S82.012 **Displaced osteochondral fracture of left patella**
  ☑7ᵗʰ S82.013 **Displaced osteochondral fracture of unspecified patella**
  ☑7ᵗʰ S82.014 **Nondisplaced osteochondral fracture of right patella**
  ☑7ᵗʰ S82.015 **Nondisplaced osteochondral fracture of left patella**
  ☑7ᵗʰ S82.016 **Nondisplaced osteochondral fracture of unspecified patella**

 ☑6ᵗʰ **S82.02 Longitudinal fracture of patella**
  ☑7ᵗʰ S82.021 **Displaced longitudinal fracture of right patella**
  ☑7ᵗʰ S82.022 **Displaced longitudinal fracture of left patella**
  ☑7ᵗʰ S82.023 **Displaced longitudinal fracture of unspecified patella**
  ☑7ᵗʰ S82.024 **Nondisplaced longitudinal fracture of right patella**
  ☑7ᵗʰ S82.025 **Nondisplaced longitudinal fracture of left patella**
  ☑7ᵗʰ S82.026 **Nondisplaced longitudinal fracture of unspecified patella**

 ☑6ᵗʰ **S82.03 Transverse fracture of patella**
  ☑7ᵗʰ S82.031 **Displaced transverse fracture of right patella**
  ☑7ᵗʰ S82.032 **Displaced transverse fracture of left patella**

☑7ᵗʰ S82.033 **Displaced transverse fracture of unspecified patella**
☑7ᵗʰ S82.034 **Nondisplaced transverse fracture of right patella**
☑7ᵗʰ S82.035 **Nondisplaced transverse fracture of left patella**
☑7ᵗʰ S82.036 **Nondisplaced transverse fracture of unspecified patella**

 ☑6ᵗʰ **S82.04 Comminuted fracture of patella**
  ☑7ᵗʰ S82.041 **Displaced comminuted fracture of right patella**
  ☑7ᵗʰ S82.042 **Displaced comminuted fracture of left patella**
  ☑7ᵗʰ S82.043 **Displaced comminuted fracture of unspecified patella**
  ☑7ᵗʰ S82.044 **Nondisplaced comminuted fracture of right patella**
  ☑7ᵗʰ S82.045 **Nondisplaced comminuted fracture of left patella**
  ☑7ᵗʰ S82.046 **Nondisplaced comminuted fracture of unspecified patella**

 ☑6ᵗʰ **S82.09 Other fracture of patella**
  ☑7ᵗʰ S82.091 **Other fracture of right patella**
  ☑7ᵗʰ S82.092 **Other fracture of left patella**
  ☑7ᵗʰ S82.099 **Other fracture of unspecified patella**

☑5ᵗʰ **S82.1 Fracture of upper end of tibia**
Fracture of proximal end of tibia
> EXCLUDES 2 *fracture of shaft of tibia (S82.2-)*
> *physeal fracture of upper end of tibia (S89.0-)*

 ☑6ᵗʰ **S82.10 Unspecified fracture of upper end of tibia**
  ☑7ᵗʰ S82.101 **Unspecified fracture of upper end of right tibia**
  ☑7ᵗʰ S82.102 **Unspecified fracture of upper end of left tibia**
  ☑7ᵗʰ S82.109 **Unspecified fracture of upper end of unspecified tibia**

 ☑6ᵗʰ **S82.11 Fracture of tibial spine**
  ☑7ᵗʰ S82.111 **Displaced fracture of right tibial spine**
  ☑7ᵗʰ S82.112 **Displaced fracture of left tibial spine**
  ☑7ᵗʰ S82.113 **Displaced fracture of unspecified tibial spine**
  ☑7ᵗʰ S82.114 **Nondisplaced fracture of right tibial spine**
  ☑7ᵗʰ S82.115 **Nondisplaced fracture of left tibial spine**
  ☑7ᵗʰ S82.116 **Nondisplaced fracture of unspecified tibial spine**

 ☑6ᵗʰ **S82.12 Fracture of lateral condyle of tibia**
  ☑7ᵗʰ S82.121 **Displaced fracture of lateral condyle of right tibia**
  ☑7ᵗʰ S82.122 **Displaced fracture of lateral condyle of left tibia**
  ☑7ᵗʰ S82.123 **Displaced fracture of lateral condyle of unspecified tibia**
  ☑7ᵗʰ S82.124 **Nondisplaced fracture of lateral condyle of right tibia**
  ☑7ᵗʰ S82.125 **Nondisplaced fracture of lateral condyle of left tibia**
  ☑7ᵗʰ S82.126 **Nondisplaced fracture of lateral condyle of unspecified tibia**

 ☑6ᵗʰ **S82.13 Fracture of medial condyle of tibia**
  ☑7ᵗʰ S82.131 **Displaced fracture of medial condyle of right tibia**
  ☑7ᵗʰ S82.132 **Displaced fracture of medial condyle of left tibia**
  ☑7ᵗʰ S82.133 **Displaced fracture of medial condyle of unspecified tibia**
  ☑7ᵗʰ S82.134 **Nondisplaced fracture of medial condyle of right tibia**
  ☑7ᵗʰ S82.135 **Nondisplaced fracture of medial condyle of left tibia**
  ☑7ᵗʰ S82.136 **Nondisplaced fracture of medial condyle of unspecified tibia**

 ☑6ᵗʰ **S82.14 Bicondylar fracture of tibia**
Fracture of tibial plateau NOS
  ☑7ᵗʰ S82.141 **Displaced bicondylar fracture of right tibia**

√7ᵗʰ **S82.142** Displaced **bicondylar fracture of** left **tibia**

√7ᵗʰ **S82.143** Displaced **bicondylar fracture of unspecified tibia**

√7ᵗʰ **S82.144** Nondisplaced **bicondylar fracture of** right **tibia**

√7ᵗʰ **S82.145** Nondisplaced **bicondylar fracture of** left **tibia**

√7ᵗʰ **S82.146** Nondisplaced **bicondylar fracture of unspecified tibia**

√6ᵗʰ **S82.15** Fracture of tibial tuberosity

√7ᵗʰ **S82.151** Displaced **fracture of** right **tibial tuberosity**

√7ᵗʰ **S82.152** Displaced **fracture of** left **tibial tuberosity**

√7ᵗʰ **S82.153** Displaced **fracture of unspecified tibial tuberosity**

√7ᵗʰ **S82.154** Nondisplaced **fracture of** right **tibial tuberosity**

√7ᵗʰ **S82.155** Nondisplaced **fracture of** left **tibial tuberosity**

√7ᵗʰ **S82.156** Nondisplaced **fracture of unspecified tibial tuberosity**

√6ᵗʰ **S82.16** Torus **fracture of upper end of tibia**

> The appropriate 7th character is to be added to all codes in subcategory S82.16.
> A   initial encounter for closed fracture
> D   subsequent encounter for fracture with routine healing
> G   subsequent encounter for fracture with delayed healing
> K   subsequent encounter for fracture with nonunion
> P   subsequent encounter for fracture with malunion
> S   sequela

√7ᵗʰ **S82.161** Torus **fracture of upper end of** right **tibia**

√7ᵗʰ **S82.162** Torus **fracture of upper end of** left **tibia**

√7ᵗʰ **S82.169** Torus **fracture of upper end of unspecified tibia**

√6ᵗʰ **S82.19** Other **fracture of upper end of tibia**

√7ᵗʰ **S82.191** Other **fracture of upper end of** right **tibia**

√7ᵗʰ **S82.192** Other **fracture of upper end of** left **tibia**

√7ᵗʰ **S82.199** Other **fracture of upper end of unspecified tibia**

√5ᵗʰ **S82.2** Fracture of shaft of tibia

√6ᵗʰ **S82.20** Unspecified **fracture of shaft of tibia**
Fracture of tibia NOS

√7ᵗʰ **S82.201** Unspecified **fracture of shaft of** right **tibia**

√7ᵗʰ **S82.202** Unspecified **fracture of shaft of** left **tibia**

√7ᵗʰ **S82.209** Unspecified **fracture of shaft of unspecified tibia**

√6ᵗʰ **S82.22** Transverse **fracture of shaft of tibia**

√7ᵗʰ **S82.221** Displaced **transverse fracture of shaft of** right **tibia**

√7ᵗʰ **S82.222** Displaced **transverse fracture of shaft of** left **tibia**

√7ᵗʰ **S82.223** Displaced **transverse fracture of shaft of unspecified tibia**

√7ᵗʰ **S82.224** Nondisplaced **transverse fracture of shaft of** right **tibia**

√7ᵗʰ **S82.225** Nondisplaced **transverse fracture of shaft of** left **tibia**

√7ᵗʰ **S82.226** Nondisplaced **transverse fracture of shaft of unspecified tibia**

√6ᵗʰ **S82.23** Oblique **fracture of shaft of tibia**

√7ᵗʰ **S82.231** Displaced **oblique fracture of shaft of** right **tibia**

√7ᵗʰ **S82.232** Displaced **oblique fracture of shaft of** left **tibia**

√7ᵗʰ **S82.233** Displaced **oblique fracture of shaft of unspecified tibia**

√7ᵗʰ **S82.234** Nondisplaced **oblique fracture of shaft of** right **tibia**

√7ᵗʰ **S82.235** Nondisplaced **oblique fracture of shaft of** left **tibia**

√7ᵗʰ **S82.236** Nondisplaced **oblique fracture of shaft of unspecified tibia**

√6ᵗʰ **S82.24** Spiral **fracture of shaft of tibia**
Toddler fracture

√7ᵗʰ **S82.241** Displaced **spiral fracture of shaft of** right **tibia**

√7ᵗʰ **S82.242** Displaced **spiral fracture of shaft of** left **tibia**

√7ᵗʰ **S82.243** Displaced **spiral fracture of shaft of unspecified tibia**

√7ᵗʰ **S82.244** Nondisplaced **spiral fracture of shaft of** right **tibia**

√7ᵗʰ **S82.245** Nondisplaced **spiral fracture of shaft of** left **tibia**

√7ᵗʰ **S82.246** Nondisplaced **spiral fracture of shaft of unspecified tibia**

√6ᵗʰ **S82.25** Comminuted **fracture of shaft of tibia**

√7ᵗʰ **S82.251** Displaced **comminuted fracture of shaft of** right **tibia**

√7ᵗʰ **S82.252** Displaced **comminuted fracture of shaft of** left **tibia**

√7ᵗʰ **S82.253** Displaced **comminuted fracture of shaft of unspecified tibia**

√7ᵗʰ **S82.254** Nondisplaced **comminuted fracture of shaft of** right **tibia**

√7ᵗʰ **S82.255** Nondisplaced **comminuted fracture of shaft of** left **tibia**

√7ᵗʰ **S82.256** Nondisplaced **comminuted fracture of shaft of unspecified tibia**

√6ᵗʰ **S82.26** Segmental **fracture of shaft of tibia**

√7ᵗʰ **S82.261** Displaced **segmental fracture of shaft of** right **tibia**

√7ᵗʰ **S82.262** Displaced **segmental fracture of shaft of** left **tibia**

√7ᵗʰ **S82.263** Displaced **segmental fracture of shaft of unspecified tibia**

√7ᵗʰ **S82.264** Nondisplaced **segmental fracture of shaft of** right **tibia**

√7ᵗʰ **S82.265** Nondisplaced **segmental fracture of shaft of** left **tibia**

√7ᵗʰ **S82.266** Nondisplaced **segmental fracture of shaft of unspecified tibia**

√6ᵗʰ **S82.29** Other **fracture of shaft of tibia**

√7ᵗʰ **S82.291** Other **fracture of shaft of** right **tibia**

√7ᵗʰ **S82.292** Other **fracture of shaft of** left **tibia**

√7ᵗʰ **S82.299** Other **fracture of shaft of unspecified tibia**

√5ᵗʰ **S82.3** Fracture of lower end of tibia

EXCLUDES 1   bimalleolar fracture of lower leg (S82.84-)
fracture of medial malleolus alone (S82.5-)
Maisonneuve's fracture (S82.86-)
pilon fracture of distal tibia (S82.87-)
trimalleolar fractures of lower leg (S82.85-)

√6ᵗʰ **S82.30** Unspecified **fracture of lower end of tibia**

√7ᵗʰ **S82.301** Unspecified **fracture of lower end of** right **tibia**

√7ᵗʰ **S82.302** Unspecified **fracture of lower end of** left **tibia**

√7ᵗʰ **S82.309** Unspecified **fracture of lower end of unspecified tibia**

√6ᵗʰ **S82.31** Torus **fracture of lower end of tibia**

> The appropriate 7th character is to be added to all codes in subcategory S82.31.
> A   initial encounter for closed fracture
> D   subsequent encounter for fracture with routine healing
> G   subsequent encounter for fracture with delayed healing
> K   subsequent encounter for fracture with nonunion
> P   subsequent encounter for fracture with malunion
> S   sequela

√7ᵗʰ **S82.311** Torus **fracture of lower end of** right **tibia**

√7ᵗʰ **S82.312** Torus **fracture of lower end of** left **tibia**

EXCLUDES 1 Not coded here   **EXCLUDES 2** Not included here   **N** Newborn Age: 0   **P** Pediatric Age: 0-17   **M** Maternity Age: 12-55   **A** Adult Age: 15-124

900   ICD-10-CM 2014 (Draft)

√7ᵗʰ **S82.319** Torus fracture of lower end of unspecified tibia

√6ᵗʰ **S82.39** Other fracture of lower end of tibia

  √7ᵗʰ **S82.391** Other fracture of lower end of right tibia

  √7ᵗʰ **S82.392** Other fracture of lower end of left tibia

  √7ᵗʰ **S82.399** Other fracture of lower end of unspecified tibia

√5ᵗʰ **S82.4** Fracture of shaft of fibula

  EXCLUDES 2   *fracture of lateral malleolus alone (S82.6-)*

√6ᵗʰ **S82.40** Unspecified fracture of shaft of fibula

  √7ᵗʰ **S82.401** Unspecified fracture of shaft of right fibula

  √7ᵗʰ **S82.402** Unspecified fracture of shaft of left fibula

  √7ᵗʰ **S82.409** Unspecified fracture of shaft of unspecified fibula

√6ᵗʰ **S82.42** Transverse fracture of shaft of fibula

  √7ᵗʰ **S82.421** Displaced transverse fracture of shaft of right fibula

  √7ᵗʰ **S82.422** Displaced transverse fracture of shaft of left fibula

  √7ᵗʰ **S82.423** Displaced transverse fracture of shaft of unspecified fibula

  √7ᵗʰ **S82.424** Nondisplaced transverse fracture of shaft of right fibula

  √7ᵗʰ **S82.425** Nondisplaced transverse fracture of shaft of left fibula

  √7ᵗʰ **S82.426** Nondisplaced transverse fracture of shaft of unspecified fibula

√6ᵗʰ **S82.43** Oblique fracture of shaft of fibula

  √7ᵗʰ **S82.431** Displaced oblique fracture of shaft of right fibula

  √7ᵗʰ **S82.432** Displaced oblique fracture of shaft of left fibula

  √7ᵗʰ **S82.433** Displaced oblique fracture of shaft of unspecified fibula

  √7ᵗʰ **S82.434** Nondisplaced oblique fracture of shaft of right fibula

  √7ᵗʰ **S82.435** Nondisplaced oblique fracture of shaft of left fibula

  √7ᵗʰ **S82.436** Nondisplaced oblique fracture of shaft of unspecified fibula

√6ᵗʰ **S82.44** Spiral fracture of shaft of fibula

  √7ᵗʰ **S82.441** Displaced spiral fracture of shaft of right fibula

  √7ᵗʰ **S82.442** Displaced spiral fracture of shaft of left fibula

  √7ᵗʰ **S82.443** Displaced spiral fracture of shaft of unspecified fibula

  √7ᵗʰ **S82.444** Nondisplaced spiral fracture of shaft of right fibula

  √7ᵗʰ **S82.445** Nondisplaced spiral fracture of shaft of left fibula

  √7ᵗʰ **S82.446** Nondisplaced spiral fracture of shaft of unspecified fibula

√6ᵗʰ **S82.45** Comminuted fracture of shaft of fibula

  √7ᵗʰ **S82.451** Displaced comminuted fracture of shaft of right fibula

  √7ᵗʰ **S82.452** Displaced comminuted fracture of shaft of left fibula

  √7ᵗʰ **S82.453** Displaced comminuted fracture of shaft of unspecified fibula

  √7ᵗʰ **S82.454** Nondisplaced comminuted fracture of shaft of right fibula

  √7ᵗʰ **S82.455** Nondisplaced comminuted fracture of shaft of left fibula

  √7ᵗʰ **S82.456** Nondisplaced comminuted fracture of shaft of unspecified fibula

√6ᵗʰ **S82.46** Segmental fracture of shaft of fibula

  √7ᵗʰ **S82.461** Displaced segmental fracture of shaft of right fibula

  √7ᵗʰ **S82.462** Displaced segmental fracture of shaft of left fibula

  √7ᵗʰ **S82.463** Displaced segmental fracture of shaft of unspecified fibula

  √7ᵗʰ **S82.464** Nondisplaced segmental fracture of shaft of right fibula

  √7ᵗʰ **S82.465** Nondisplaced segmental fracture of shaft of left fibula

  √7ᵗʰ **S82.466** Nondisplaced segmental fracture of shaft of unspecified fibula

√6ᵗʰ **S82.49** Other fracture of shaft of fibula

  √7ᵗʰ **S82.491** Other fracture of shaft of right fibula

  √7ᵗʰ **S82.492** Other fracture of shaft of left fibula

  √7ᵗʰ **S82.499** Other fracture of shaft of unspecified fibula

√5ᵗʰ **S82.5** Fracture of medial malleolus

  EXCLUDES 1   *pilon fracture of distal tibia (S82.87-)*
                    Salter-Harris type III of lower end of tibia (S89.13-)
                    Salter-Harris type IV of lower end of tibia (S89.14-)

√×7ᵗʰ **S82.51** Displaced fracture of medial malleolus of right tibia

√×7ᵗʰ **S82.52** Displaced fracture of medial malleolus of left tibia

√×7ᵗʰ **S82.53** Displaced fracture of medial malleolus of unspecified tibia

√×7ᵗʰ **S82.54** Nondisplaced fracture of medial malleolus of right tibia

√×7ᵗʰ **S82.55** Nondisplaced fracture of medial malleolus of left tibia

√×7ᵗʰ **S82.56** Nondisplaced fracture of medial malleolus of unspecified tibia

√5ᵗʰ **S82.6** Fracture of lateral malleolus

  EXCLUDES 1   *pilon fracture of distal tibia (S82.87-)*

√×7ᵗʰ **S82.61** Displaced fracture of lateral malleolus of right fibula

√×7ᵗʰ **S82.62** Displaced fracture of lateral malleolus of left fibula

√×7ᵗʰ **S82.63** Displaced fracture of lateral malleolus of unspecified fibula

√×7ᵗʰ **S82.64** Nondisplaced fracture of lateral malleolus of right fibula

√×7ᵗʰ **S82.65** Nondisplaced fracture of lateral malleolus of left fibula

√×7ᵗʰ **S82.66** Nondisplaced fracture of lateral malleolus of unspecified fibula

√5ᵗʰ **S82.8** Other fractures of lower leg

√6ᵗʰ **S82.81** Torus fracture of upper end of fibula

The appropriate 7th character is to be added to all codes in subcategory S82.81.	
A	initial encounter for closed fracture
D	subsequent encounter for fracture with routine healing
G	subsequent encounter for fracture with delayed healing
K	subsequent encounter for fracture with nonunion
P	subsequent encounter for fracture with malunion
S	sequela

  √7ᵗʰ **S82.811** Torus fracture of upper end of right fibula

  √7ᵗʰ **S82.812** Torus fracture of upper end of left fibula

  √7ᵗʰ **S82.819** Torus fracture of upper end of unspecified fibula

√6ᵗʰ **S82.82** Torus fracture of lower end of fibula

The appropriate 7th character is to be added to all codes in subcategory S82.82.	
A	initial encounter for closed fracture
D	subsequent encounter for fracture with routine healing
G	subsequent encounter for fracture with delayed healing
K	subsequent encounter for fracture with nonunion
P	subsequent encounter for fracture with malunion
S	sequela

  √7ᵗʰ **S82.821** Torus fracture of lower end of right fibula

  √7ᵗʰ **S82.822** Torus fracture of lower end of left fibula

  √7ᵗʰ **S82.829** Torus fracture of lower end of unspecified fibula

---

☑ Additional Character Required   √×7ᵗʰ Xtension Alert   Unspecified Code   Other Specified Code   Manifestation Code   ▶◀ Revised Text   ● New Code   ▲ Revised Code Title

√6ᵗʰ **S82.83** Other fracture of upper and lower end of fibula

     √7ᵗʰ **S82.831** Other fracture of upper and lower end of right fibula

     √7ᵗʰ **S82.832** Other fracture of upper and lower end of left fibula

     √7ᵗʰ **S82.839** Other fracture of upper and lower end of unspecified fibula

√6ᵗʰ **S82.84** Bimalleolar fracture of lower leg

     √7ᵗʰ **S82.841** Displaced bimalleolar fracture of right lower leg

     √7ᵗʰ **S82.842** Displaced bimalleolar fracture of left lower leg

     √7ᵗʰ **S82.843** Displaced bimalleolar fracture of unspecified lower leg

     √7ᵗʰ **S82.844** Nondisplaced bimalleolar fracture of right lower leg

     √7ᵗʰ **S82.845** Nondisplaced bimalleolar fracture of left lower leg

     √7ᵗʰ **S82.846** Nondisplaced bimalleolar fracture of unspecified lower leg

√6ᵗʰ **S82.85** Trimalleolar fracture of lower leg

     √7ᵗʰ **S82.851** Displaced trimalleolar fracture of right lower leg

     √7ᵗʰ **S82.852** Displaced trimalleolar fracture of left lower leg

     √7ᵗʰ **S82.853** Displaced trimalleolar fracture of unspecified lower leg

     √7ᵗʰ **S82.854** Nondisplaced trimalleolar fracture of right lower leg

     √7ᵗʰ **S82.855** Nondisplaced trimalleolar fracture of left lower leg

     √7ᵗʰ **S82.856** Nondisplaced trimalleolar fracture of unspecified lower leg

√6ᵗʰ **S82.86** Maisonneuve's fracture

     √7ᵗʰ **S82.861** Displaced Maisonneuve's fracture of right leg

     √7ᵗʰ **S82.862** Displaced Maisonneuve's fracture of left leg

     √7ᵗʰ **S82.863** Displaced Maisonneuve's fracture of unspecified leg

     √7ᵗʰ **S82.864** Nondisplaced Maisonneuve's fracture of right leg

     √7ᵗʰ **S82.865** Nondisplaced Maisonneuve's fracture of left leg

     √7ᵗʰ **S82.866** Nondisplaced Maisonneuve's fracture of unspecified leg

√6ᵗʰ **S82.87** Pilon fracture of tibia

     √7ᵗʰ **S82.871** Displaced pilon fracture of right tibia

     √7ᵗʰ **S82.872** Displaced pilon fracture of left tibia

     √7ᵗʰ **S82.873** Displaced pilon fracture of unspecified tibia

     √7ᵗʰ **S82.874** Nondisplaced pilon fracture of right tibia

     √7ᵗʰ **S82.875** Nondisplaced pilon fracture of left tibia

     √7ᵗʰ **S82.876** Nondisplaced pilon fracture of unspecified tibia

√6ᵗʰ **S82.89** Other fractures of lower leg

     Fracture of ankle NOS

     √7ᵗʰ **S82.891** Other fracture of right lower leg

     √7ᵗʰ **S82.892** Other fracture of left lower leg

     √7ᵗʰ **S82.899** Other fracture of unspecified lower leg

√5ᵗʰ **S82.9** Unspecified fracture of lower leg

     √x7ᵗʰ **S82.9Ø** Unspecified fracture of unspecified lower leg

     √x7ᵗʰ **S82.91** Unspecified fracture of right lower leg

     √x7ᵗʰ **S82.92** Unspecified fracture of left lower leg

√4ᵗʰ **S83** Dislocation and sprain of joints and ligaments of knee

     INCLUDES   avulsion of joint or ligament of knee
         laceration of cartilage, joint or ligament of knee
         sprain of cartilage, joint or ligament of knee
         traumatic hemarthrosis of joint or ligament of knee
         traumatic rupture of joint or ligament of knee
         traumatic subluxation of joint or ligament of knee
         traumatic tear of joint or ligament of knee

     Code also any associated open wound

     EXCLUDES 1   *derangement of patella (M22.Ø-M22.3)*
         injury of patellar ligament (tendon) (S76.1-)
         internal derangement of knee (M23.-)
         old dislocation of knee (M23.8X-)
         pathological dislocation of knee (M24.36)
         recurrent dislocation of knee (M22.Ø)

     EXCLUDES 2   *strain of muscle, fascia and tendon of lower leg (S86.-)*

     The appropriate 7th character is to be added to each code from category S83.
     A   initial encounter
     D   subsequent encounter
     S   sequela

√5ᵗʰ **S83.Ø** Subluxation and dislocation of patella

     √6ᵗʰ **S83.ØØ** Unspecified subluxation and dislocation of patella

         √7ᵗʰ **S83.ØØ1** Unspecified subluxation of right patella

         √7ᵗʰ **S83.ØØ2** Unspecified subluxation of left patella

         √7ᵗʰ **S83.ØØ3** Unspecified subluxation of unspecified patella

         √7ᵗʰ **S83.ØØ4** Unspecified dislocation of right patella

         √7ᵗʰ **S83.ØØ5** Unspecified dislocation of left patella

         √7ᵗʰ **S83.ØØ6** Unspecified dislocation of unspecified patella

     √6ᵗʰ **S83.Ø1** Lateral subluxation and dislocation of patella

         √7ᵗʰ **S83.Ø11** Lateral subluxation of right patella

         √7ᵗʰ **S83.Ø12** Lateral subluxation of left patella

         √7ᵗʰ **S83.Ø13** Lateral subluxation of unspecified patella

         √7ᵗʰ **S83.Ø14** Lateral dislocation of right patella

         √7ᵗʰ **S83.Ø15** Lateral dislocation of left patella

         √7ᵗʰ **S83.Ø16** Lateral dislocation of unspecified patella

     √6ᵗʰ **S83.Ø9** Other subluxation and dislocation of patella

         √7ᵗʰ **S83.Ø91** Other subluxation of right patella

         √7ᵗʰ **S83.Ø92** Other subluxation of left patella

         √7ᵗʰ **S83.Ø93** Other subluxation of unspecified patella

         √7ᵗʰ **S83.Ø94** Other dislocation of right patella

         √7ᵗʰ **S83.Ø95** Other dislocation of left patella

         √7ᵗʰ **S83.Ø96** Other dislocation of unspecified patella

√5ᵗʰ **S83.1** Subluxation and dislocation of knee

     EXCLUDES 2   *instability of knee prosthesis (T84.Ø22, T84.Ø23)*

     √6ᵗʰ **S83.1Ø** Unspecified subluxation and dislocation of knee

         √7ᵗʰ **S83.1Ø1** Unspecified subluxation of right knee

         √7ᵗʰ **S83.1Ø2** Unspecified subluxation of left knee

         √7ᵗʰ **S83.1Ø3** Unspecified subluxation of unspecified knee

         √7ᵗʰ **S83.1Ø4** Unspecified dislocation of right knee

         √7ᵗʰ **S83.1Ø5** Unspecified dislocation of left knee

         √7ᵗʰ **S83.1Ø6** Unspecified dislocation of unspecified knee

     √6ᵗʰ **S83.11** Anterior subluxation and dislocation of proximal end of tibia

         Posterior subluxation and dislocation of distal end of femur

         √7ᵗʰ **S83.111** Anterior subluxation of proximal end of tibia, right knee

         √7ᵗʰ **S83.112** Anterior subluxation of proximal end of tibia, left knee

         √7ᵗʰ **S83.113** Anterior subluxation of proximal end of tibia, unspecified knee

         √7ᵗʰ **S83.114** Anterior dislocation of proximal end of tibia, right knee

         √7ᵗʰ **S83.115** Anterior dislocation of proximal end of tibia, left knee

         √7ᵗʰ **S83.116** Anterior dislocation of proximal end of tibia, unspecified knee

EXCLUDES 1 Not coded here   EXCLUDES 2 Not included here   N Newborn Age: Ø   P Pediatric Age: Ø-17   M Maternity Age: 12-55   A Adult Age: 15-124

902   ICD-1Ø-CM 2Ø14 (Draft)

√6ᵗʰ **S83.12** Posterior subluxation and dislocation of proximal end of tibia
　　　Anterior dislocation of distal end of femur

√7ᵗʰ **S83.121** Posterior subluxation of proximal end of tibia, right knee

√7ᵗʰ **S83.122** Posterior subluxation of proximal end of tibia, left knee

√7ᵗʰ **S83.123** Posterior subluxation of proximal end of tibia, unspecified knee

√7ᵗʰ **S83.124** Posterior dislocation of proximal end of tibia, right knee

√7ᵗʰ **S83.125** Posterior dislocation of proximal end of tibia, left knee

√7ᵗʰ **S83.126** Posterior dislocation of proximal end of tibia, unspecified knee

√6ᵗʰ **S83.13** Medial subluxation and dislocation of proximal end of tibia

√7ᵗʰ **S83.131** Medial subluxation of proximal end of tibia, right knee

√7ᵗʰ **S83.132** Medial subluxation of proximal end of tibia, left knee

√7ᵗʰ **S83.133** Medial subluxation of proximal end of tibia, unspecified knee

√7ᵗʰ **S83.134** Medial dislocation of proximal end of tibia, right knee

√7ᵗʰ **S83.135** Medial dislocation of proximal end of tibia, left knee

√7ᵗʰ **S83.136** Medial dislocation of proximal end of tibia, unspecified knee

√6ᵗʰ **S83.14** Lateral subluxation and dislocation of proximal end of tibia

√7ᵗʰ **S83.141** Lateral subluxation of proximal end of tibia, right knee

√7ᵗʰ **S83.142** Lateral subluxation of proximal end of tibia, left knee

√7ᵗʰ **S83.143** Lateral subluxation of proximal end of tibia, unspecified knee

√7ᵗʰ **S83.144** Lateral dislocation of proximal end of tibia, right knee

√7ᵗʰ **S83.145** Lateral dislocation of proximal end of tibia, left knee

√7ᵗʰ **S83.146** Lateral dislocation of proximal end of tibia, unspecified knee

√6ᵗʰ **S83.19** Other subluxation and dislocation of knee

√7ᵗʰ **S83.191** Other subluxation of right knee

√7ᵗʰ **S83.192** Other subluxation of left knee

√7ᵗʰ **S83.193** Other subluxation of unspecified knee

√7ᵗʰ **S83.194** Other dislocation of right knee

√7ᵗʰ **S83.195** Other dislocation of left knee

√7ᵗʰ **S83.196** Other dislocation of unspecified knee

√5ᵗʰ **S83.2** Tear of meniscus, current injury
　　EXCLUDES 1　old bucket-handle tear (M23.2)

√6ᵗʰ **S83.20** Tear of unspecified meniscus, current injury
　　　Tear of meniscus of knee NOS

√7ᵗʰ **S83.200** Bucket-handle tear of unspecified meniscus, current injury, right knee

√7ᵗʰ **S83.201** Bucket-handle tear of unspecified meniscus, current injury, left knee

√7ᵗʰ **S83.202** Bucket-handle tear of unspecified meniscus, current injury, unspecified knee

√7ᵗʰ **S83.203** Other tear of unspecified meniscus, current injury, right knee

√7ᵗʰ **S83.204** Other tear of unspecified meniscus, current injury, left knee

√7ᵗʰ **S83.205** Other tear of unspecified meniscus, current injury, unspecified knee

√7ᵗʰ **S83.206** Unspecified tear of unspecified meniscus, current injury, right knee

√7ᵗʰ **S83.207** Unspecified tear of unspecified meniscus, current injury, left knee

√7ᵗʰ **S83.209** Unspecified tear of unspecified meniscus, current injury, unspecified knee

√6ᵗʰ **S83.21** Bucket-handle tear of medial meniscus, current injury

√7ᵗʰ **S83.211** Bucket-handle tear of medial meniscus, current injury, right knee

√7ᵗʰ **S83.212** Bucket-handle tear of medial meniscus, current injury, left knee

√7ᵗʰ **S83.219** Bucket-handle tear of medial meniscus, current injury, unspecified knee

√6ᵗʰ **S83.22** Peripheral tear of medial meniscus, current injury

√7ᵗʰ **S83.221** Peripheral tear of medial meniscus, current injury, right knee

√7ᵗʰ **S83.222** Peripheral tear of medial meniscus, current injury, left knee

√7ᵗʰ **S83.229** Peripheral tear of medial meniscus, current injury, unspecified knee

√6ᵗʰ **S83.23** Complex tear of medial meniscus, current injury

√7ᵗʰ **S83.231** Complex tear of medial meniscus, current injury, right knee

√7ᵗʰ **S83.232** Complex tear of medial meniscus, current injury, left knee

√7ᵗʰ **S83.239** Complex tear of medial meniscus, current injury, unspecified knee

√6ᵗʰ **S83.24** Other tear of medial meniscus, current injury

√7ᵗʰ **S83.241** Other tear of medial meniscus, current injury, right knee

√7ᵗʰ **S83.242** Other tear of medial meniscus, current injury, left knee

√7ᵗʰ **S83.249** Other tear of medial meniscus, current injury, unspecified knee

√6ᵗʰ **S83.25** Bucket-handle tear of lateral meniscus, current injury

√7ᵗʰ **S83.251** Bucket-handle tear of lateral meniscus, current injury, right knee

√7ᵗʰ **S83.252** Bucket-handle tear of lateral meniscus, current injury, left knee

√7ᵗʰ **S83.259** Bucket-handle tear of lateral meniscus, current injury, unspecified knee

√6ᵗʰ **S83.26** Peripheral tear of lateral meniscus, current injury

√7ᵗʰ **S83.261** Peripheral tear of lateral meniscus, current injury, right knee

√7ᵗʰ **S83.262** Peripheral tear of lateral meniscus, current injury, left knee

√7ᵗʰ **S83.269** Peripheral tear of lateral meniscus, current injury, unspecified knee

√6ᵗʰ **S83.27** Complex tear of lateral meniscus, current injury

√7ᵗʰ **S83.271** Complex tear of lateral meniscus, current injury, right knee

√7ᵗʰ **S83.272** Complex tear of lateral meniscus, current injury, left knee

√7ᵗʰ **S83.279** Complex tear of lateral meniscus, current injury, unspecified knee

√6ᵗʰ **S83.28** Other tear of lateral meniscus, current injury

√7ᵗʰ **S83.281** Other tear of lateral meniscus, current injury, right knee

√7ᵗʰ **S83.282** Other tear of lateral meniscus, current injury, left knee

√7ᵗʰ **S83.289** Other tear of lateral meniscus, current injury, unspecified knee

√5ᵗʰ **S83.3** Tear of articular cartilage of knee, current

√x7ᵗʰ **S83.30** Tear of articular cartilage of unspecified knee, current

√x7ᵗʰ **S83.31** Tear of articular cartilage of right knee, current

√x7ᵗʰ **S83.32** Tear of articular cartilage of left knee, current

√5ᵗʰ **S83.4** Sprain of collateral ligament of knee

√6ᵗʰ **S83.40** Sprain of unspecified collateral ligament of knee

√7ᵗʰ **S83.401** Sprain of unspecified collateral ligament of right knee

√7ᵗʰ **S83.402** Sprain of unspecified collateral ligament of left knee

√7ᵗʰ **S83.409** Sprain of unspecified collateral ligament of unspecified knee

---

Injury, Poisoning and Certain Other Consequences of External Causes

S83.41–S85.122

√6ᵗʰ **S83.41** Sprain of medial collateral ligament of knee
Sprain of tibial collateral ligament

  √7ᵗʰ **S83.411** Sprain of medial collateral ligament of right knee

  √7ᵗʰ **S83.412** Sprain of medial collateral ligament of left knee

  √7ᵗʰ **S83.419** Sprain of medial collateral ligament of unspecified knee

√6ᵗʰ **S83.42** Sprain of lateral collateral ligament of knee
Sprain of fibular collateral ligament

  √7ᵗʰ **S83.421** Sprain of lateral collateral ligament of right knee

  √7ᵗʰ **S83.422** Sprain of lateral collateral ligament of left knee

  √7ᵗʰ **S83.429** Sprain of lateral collateral ligament of unspecified knee

√5ᵗʰ **S83.5** Sprain of cruciate ligament of knee

  √6ᵗʰ **S83.50** Sprain of unspecified cruciate ligament of knee

    √7ᵗʰ **S83.501** Sprain of unspecified cruciate ligament of right knee

    √7ᵗʰ **S83.502** Sprain of unspecified cruciate ligament of left knee

    √7ᵗʰ **S83.509** Sprain of unspecified cruciate ligament of unspecified knee

  √6ᵗʰ **S83.51** Sprain of anterior cruciate ligament of knee

    √7ᵗʰ **S83.511** Sprain of anterior cruciate ligament of right knee

    √7ᵗʰ **S83.512** Sprain of anterior cruciate ligament of left knee

    √7ᵗʰ **S83.519** Sprain of anterior cruciate ligament of unspecified knee

  √6ᵗʰ **S83.52** Sprain of posterior cruciate ligament of knee

    √7ᵗʰ **S83.521** Sprain of posterior cruciate ligament of right knee

    √7ᵗʰ **S83.522** Sprain of posterior cruciate ligament of left knee

    √7ᵗʰ **S83.529** Sprain of posterior cruciate ligament of unspecified knee

√5ᵗʰ **S83.6** Sprain of the superior tibiofibular joint and ligament

  √x7ᵗʰ **S83.60** Sprain of the superior tibiofibular joint and ligament, unspecified knee

  √x7ᵗʰ **S83.61** Sprain of the superior tibiofibular joint and ligament, right knee

  √x7ᵗʰ **S83.62** Sprain of the superior tibiofibular joint and ligament, left knee

√5ᵗʰ **S83.8** Sprain of other specified parts of knee

  √6ᵗʰ **S83.8X** Sprain of other specified parts of knee

    √7ᵗʰ **S83.8X1** Sprain of other specified parts of right knee

    √7ᵗʰ **S83.8X2** Sprain of other specified parts of left knee

    √7ᵗʰ **S83.8X9** Sprain of other specified parts of unspecified knee

√5ᵗʰ **S83.9** Sprain of unspecified site of knee

  √x7ᵗʰ **S83.90** Sprain of unspecified site of unspecified knee

  √x7ᵗʰ **S83.91** Sprain of unspecified site of right knee

  √x7ᵗʰ **S83.92** Sprain of unspecified site of left knee

√4ᵗʰ **S84** Injury of nerves at lower leg level
Code also any associated open wound (S81.-)
EXCLUDES 2   injury of nerves at ankle and foot level (S94.-)

The appropriate 7th character is to be added to each code from category S84.
A   initial encounter
D   subsequent encounter
S   sequela

√5ᵗʰ **S84.0** Injury of tibial nerve at lower leg level

  √x7ᵗʰ **S84.00** Injury of tibial nerve at lower leg level, unspecified leg

  √x7ᵗʰ **S84.01** Injury of tibial nerve at lower leg level, right leg

  √x7ᵗʰ **S84.02** Injury of tibial nerve at lower leg level, left leg

√5ᵗʰ **S84.1** Injury of peroneal nerve at lower leg level

  √x7ᵗʰ **S84.10** Injury of peroneal nerve at lower leg level, unspecified leg

  √x7ᵗʰ **S84.11** Injury of peroneal nerve at lower leg level, right leg

  √x7ᵗʰ **S84.12** Injury of peroneal nerve at lower leg level, left leg

√5ᵗʰ **S84.2** Injury of cutaneous sensory nerve at lower leg level

  √x7ᵗʰ **S84.20** Injury of cutaneous sensory nerve at lower leg level, unspecified leg

  √x7ᵗʰ **S84.21** Injury of cutaneous sensory nerve at lower leg level, right leg

  √x7ᵗʰ **S84.22** Injury of cutaneous sensory nerve at lower leg level, left leg

√5ᵗʰ **S84.8** Injury of other nerves at lower leg level

  √6ᵗʰ **S84.80** Injury of other nerves at lower leg level

    √7ᵗʰ **S84.801** Injury of other nerves at lower leg level, right leg

    √7ᵗʰ **S84.802** Injury of other nerves at lower leg level, left leg

    √7ᵗʰ **S84.809** Injury of other nerves at lower leg level, unspecified leg

√5ᵗʰ **S84.9** Injury of unspecified nerve at lower leg level

  √x7ᵗʰ **S84.90** Injury of unspecified nerve at lower leg level, unspecified leg

  √x7ᵗʰ **S84.91** Injury of unspecified nerve at lower leg level, right leg

  √x7ᵗʰ **S84.92** Injury of unspecified nerve at lower leg level, left leg

√4ᵗʰ **S85** Injury of blood vessels at lower leg level
Code also any associated open wound (S81.-)
EXCLUDES 2   injury of blood vessels at ankle and foot level (S95.-)

The appropriate 7th character is to be added to each code from category S85.
A   initial encounter
D   subsequent encounter
S   sequela

√5ᵗʰ **S85.0** Injury of popliteal artery

  √6ᵗʰ **S85.00** Unspecified injury of popliteal artery

    √7ᵗʰ **S85.001** Unspecified injury of popliteal artery, right leg

    √7ᵗʰ **S85.002** Unspecified injury of popliteal artery, left leg

    √7ᵗʰ **S85.009** Unspecified injury of popliteal artery, unspecified leg

  √6ᵗʰ **S85.01** Laceration of popliteal artery

    √7ᵗʰ **S85.011** Laceration of popliteal artery, right leg

    √7ᵗʰ **S85.012** Laceration of popliteal artery, left leg

    √7ᵗʰ **S85.019** Laceration of popliteal artery, unspecified leg

  √6ᵗʰ **S85.09** Other specified injury of popliteal artery

    √7ᵗʰ **S85.091** Other specified injury of popliteal artery, right leg

    √7ᵗʰ **S85.092** Other specified injury of popliteal artery, left leg

    √7ᵗʰ **S85.099** Other specified injury of popliteal artery, unspecified leg

√5ᵗʰ **S85.1** Injury of tibial artery

  √6ᵗʰ **S85.10** Unspecified injury of unspecified tibial artery
Injury of tibial artery NOS

    √7ᵗʰ **S85.101** Unspecified injury of unspecified tibial artery, right leg

    √7ᵗʰ **S85.102** Unspecified injury of unspecified tibial artery, left leg

    √7ᵗʰ **S85.109** Unspecified injury of unspecified tibial artery, unspecified leg

  √6ᵗʰ **S85.11** Laceration of unspecified tibial artery

    √7ᵗʰ **S85.111** Laceration of unspecified tibial artery, right leg

    √7ᵗʰ **S85.112** Laceration of unspecified tibial artery, left leg

    √7ᵗʰ **S85.119** Laceration of unspecified tibial artery, unspecified leg

  √6ᵗʰ **S85.12** Other specified injury of unspecified tibial artery

    √7ᵗʰ **S85.121** Other specified injury of unspecified tibial artery, right leg

    √7ᵗʰ **S85.122** Other specified injury of unspecified tibial artery, left leg

EXCLUDES 1 Not coded here   EXCLUDES 2 Not included here   N Newborn Age: 0   P Pediatric Age: 0-17   M Maternity Age: 12-55   A Adult Age: 15-124

904   ICD-10-CM 2014 (Draft)

√7ᵗʰ **S85.129** Other specified injury of unspecified tibial artery, unspecified leg

√6ᵗʰ **S85.13** Unspecified injury of anterior tibial artery
√7ᵗʰ **S85.131** Unspecified injury of anterior tibial artery, right leg
√7ᵗʰ **S85.132** Unspecified injury of anterior tibial artery, left leg
√7ᵗʰ **S85.139** Unspecified injury of anterior tibial artery, unspecified leg

√6ᵗʰ **S85.14** Laceration of anterior tibial artery
√7ᵗʰ **S85.141** Laceration of anterior tibial artery, right leg
√7ᵗʰ **S85.142** Laceration of anterior tibial artery, left leg
√7ᵗʰ **S85.149** Laceration of anterior tibial artery, unspecified leg

√6ᵗʰ **S85.15** Other specified injury of anterior tibial artery
√7ᵗʰ **S85.151** Other specified injury of anterior tibial artery, right leg
√7ᵗʰ **S85.152** Other specified injury of anterior tibial artery, left leg
√7ᵗʰ **S85.159** Other specified injury of anterior tibial artery, unspecified leg

√6ᵗʰ **S85.16** Unspecified injury of posterior tibial artery
√7ᵗʰ **S85.161** Unspecified injury of posterior tibial artery, right leg
√7ᵗʰ **S85.162** Unspecified injury of posterior tibial artery, left leg
√7ᵗʰ **S85.169** Unspecified injury of posterior tibial artery, unspecified leg

√6ᵗʰ **S85.17** Laceration of posterior tibial artery
√7ᵗʰ **S85.171** Laceration of posterior tibial artery, right leg
√7ᵗʰ **S85.172** Laceration of posterior tibial artery, left leg
√7ᵗʰ **S85.179** Laceration of posterior tibial artery, unspecified leg

√6ᵗʰ **S85.18** Other specified injury of posterior tibial artery
√7ᵗʰ **S85.181** Other specified injury of posterior tibial artery, right leg
√7ᵗʰ **S85.182** Other specified injury of posterior tibial artery, left leg
√7ᵗʰ **S85.189** Other specified injury of posterior tibial artery, unspecified leg

√5ᵗʰ **S85.2** Injury of peroneal artery
√6ᵗʰ **S85.20** Unspecified injury of peroneal artery
√7ᵗʰ **S85.201** Unspecified injury of peroneal artery, right leg
√7ᵗʰ **S85.202** Unspecified injury of peroneal artery, left leg
√7ᵗʰ **S85.209** Unspecified injury of peroneal artery, unspecified leg

√6ᵗʰ **S85.21** Laceration of peroneal artery
√7ᵗʰ **S85.211** Laceration of peroneal artery, right leg
√7ᵗʰ **S85.212** Laceration of peroneal artery, left leg
√7ᵗʰ **S85.219** Laceration of peroneal artery, unspecified leg

√6ᵗʰ **S85.29** Other specified injury of peroneal artery
√7ᵗʰ **S85.291** Other specified injury of peroneal artery, right leg
√7ᵗʰ **S85.292** Other specified injury of peroneal artery, left leg
√7ᵗʰ **S85.299** Other specified injury of peroneal artery, unspecified leg

√5ᵗʰ **S85.3** Injury of greater saphenous vein at lower leg level
Injury of greater saphenous vein NOS
Injury of saphenous vein NOS
√6ᵗʰ **S85.30** Unspecified injury of greater saphenous vein at lower leg level
√7ᵗʰ **S85.301** Unspecified injury of greater saphenous vein at lower leg level, right leg
√7ᵗʰ **S85.302** Unspecified injury of greater saphenous vein at lower leg level, left leg
√7ᵗʰ **S85.309** Unspecified injury of greater saphenous vein at lower leg level, unspecified leg

√6ᵗʰ **S85.31** Laceration of greater saphenous vein at lower leg level
√7ᵗʰ **S85.311** Laceration of greater saphenous vein at lower leg level, right leg
√7ᵗʰ **S85.312** Laceration of greater saphenous vein at lower leg level, left leg
√7ᵗʰ **S85.319** Laceration of greater saphenous vein at lower leg level, unspecified leg

√6ᵗʰ **S85.39** Other specified injury of greater saphenous vein at lower leg level
√7ᵗʰ **S85.391** Other specified injury of greater saphenous vein at lower leg level, right leg
√7ᵗʰ **S85.392** Other specified injury of greater saphenous vein at lower leg level, left leg
√7ᵗʰ **S85.399** Other specified injury of greater saphenous vein at lower leg level, unspecified leg

√5ᵗʰ **S85.4** Injury of lesser saphenous vein at lower leg level
√6ᵗʰ **S85.40** Unspecified injury of lesser saphenous vein at lower leg level
√7ᵗʰ **S85.401** Unspecified injury of lesser saphenous vein at lower leg level, right leg
√7ᵗʰ **S85.402** Unspecified injury of lesser saphenous vein at lower leg level, left leg
√7ᵗʰ **S85.409** Unspecified injury of lesser saphenous vein at lower leg level, unspecified leg

√6ᵗʰ **S85.41** Laceration of lesser saphenous vein at lower leg level
√7ᵗʰ **S85.411** Laceration of lesser saphenous vein at lower leg level, right leg
√7ᵗʰ **S85.412** Laceration of lesser saphenous vein at lower leg level, left leg
√7ᵗʰ **S85.419** Laceration of lesser saphenous vein at lower leg level, unspecified leg

√6ᵗʰ **S85.49** Other specified injury of lesser saphenous vein at lower leg level
√7ᵗʰ **S85.491** Other specified injury of lesser saphenous vein at lower leg level, right leg
√7ᵗʰ **S85.492** Other specified injury of lesser saphenous vein at lower leg level, left leg
√7ᵗʰ **S85.499** Other specified injury of lesser saphenous vein at lower leg level, unspecified leg

√5ᵗʰ **S85.5** Injury of popliteal vein
√6ᵗʰ **S85.50** Unspecified injury of popliteal vein
√7ᵗʰ **S85.501** Unspecified injury of popliteal vein, right leg
√7ᵗʰ **S85.502** Unspecified injury of popliteal vein, left leg
√7ᵗʰ **S85.509** Unspecified injury of popliteal vein, unspecified leg

√6ᵗʰ **S85.51** Laceration of popliteal vein
√7ᵗʰ **S85.511** Laceration of popliteal vein, right leg
√7ᵗʰ **S85.512** Laceration of popliteal vein, left leg
√7ᵗʰ **S85.519** Laceration of popliteal vein, unspecified leg

√6ᵗʰ **S85.59** Other specified injury of popliteal vein
√7ᵗʰ **S85.591** Other specified injury of popliteal vein, right leg
√7ᵗʰ **S85.592** Other specified injury of popliteal vein, left leg
√7ᵗʰ **S85.599** Other specified injury of popliteal vein, unspecified leg

√5ᵗʰ **S85.8** Injury of other blood vessels at lower leg level
√6ᵗʰ **S85.80** Unspecified injury of other blood vessels at lower leg level
√7ᵗʰ **S85.801** Unspecified injury of other blood vessels at lower leg level, right leg
√7ᵗʰ **S85.802** Unspecified injury of other blood vessels at lower leg level, left leg
√7ᵗʰ **S85.809** Unspecified injury of other blood vessels at lower leg level, unspecified leg

---

☑ Additional Character Required   √x7ᵗʰ Xtension Alert   Unspecified Code   Other Specified Code   Manifestation Code   ►◄ Revised Text   ● New Code   ▲ Revised Code Title

✓6ᵗʰ **S85.81** Laceration of other blood vessels at lower leg level

    ✓7ᵗʰ **S85.811** Laceration of other blood vessels at lower leg level, right leg

    ✓7ᵗʰ **S85.812** Laceration of other blood vessels at lower leg level, left leg

    ✓7ᵗʰ **S85.819** Laceration of other blood vessels at lower leg level, unspecified leg

✓6ᵗʰ **S85.89** Other specified injury of other blood vessels at lower leg level

    ✓7ᵗʰ **S85.891** Other specified injury of other blood vessels at lower leg level, right leg

    ✓7ᵗʰ **S85.892** Other specified injury of other blood vessels at lower leg level, left leg

    ✓7ᵗʰ **S85.899** Other specified injury of other blood vessels at lower leg level, unspecified leg

✓5ᵗʰ **S85.9** Injury of unspecified blood vessel at lower leg level

  ✓6ᵗʰ **S85.90** Unspecified injury of unspecified blood vessel at lower leg level

    ✓7ᵗʰ **S85.901** Unspecified injury of unspecified blood vessel at lower leg level, right leg

    ✓7ᵗʰ **S85.902** Unspecified injury of unspecified blood vessel at lower leg level, left leg

    ✓7ᵗʰ **S85.909** Unspecified injury of unspecified blood vessel at lower leg level, unspecified leg

  ✓6ᵗʰ **S85.91** Laceration of unspecified blood vessel at lower leg level

    ✓7ᵗʰ **S85.911** Laceration of unspecified blood vessel at lower leg level, right leg

    ✓7ᵗʰ **S85.912** Laceration of unspecified blood vessel at lower leg level, left leg

    ✓7ᵗʰ **S85.919** Laceration of unspecified blood vessel at lower leg level, unspecified leg

  ✓6ᵗʰ **S85.99** Other specified injury of unspecified blood vessel at lower leg level

    ✓7ᵗʰ **S85.991** Other specified injury of unspecified blood vessel at lower leg level, right leg

    ✓7ᵗʰ **S85.992** Other specified injury of unspecified blood vessel at lower leg level, left leg

    ✓7ᵗʰ **S85.999** Other specified injury of unspecified blood vessel at lower leg level, unspecified leg

✓4ᵗʰ **S86** **Injury of muscle, fascia and tendon at lower leg level**

Code also any associated open wound (S81.-)

EXCLUDES 2   *injury of muscle, fascia and tendon at ankle (S96.-)*
injury of patellar ligament (tendon) (S76.1-)
sprain of joints and ligaments of knee (S83.-)

The appropriate 7th character is to be added to each code from category S86.
A   initial encounter
D   subsequent encounter
S   sequela

✓5ᵗʰ **S86.0** Injury of Achilles tendon

  ✓6ᵗʰ **S86.00** Unspecified injury of Achilles tendon

    ✓7ᵗʰ **S86.001** Unspecified injury of right Achilles tendon

    ✓7ᵗʰ **S86.002** Unspecified injury of left Achilles tendon

    ✓7ᵗʰ **S86.009** Unspecified injury of unspecified Achilles tendon

  ✓6ᵗʰ **S86.01** Strain of Achilles tendon

    ✓7ᵗʰ **S86.011** Strain of right Achilles tendon

    ✓7ᵗʰ **S86.012** Strain of left Achilles tendon

    ✓7ᵗʰ **S86.019** Strain of unspecified Achilles tendon

  ✓6ᵗʰ **S86.02** Laceration of Achilles tendon

    ✓7ᵗʰ **S86.021** Laceration of right Achilles tendon

    ✓7ᵗʰ **S86.022** Laceration of left Achilles tendon

    ✓7ᵗʰ **S86.029** Laceration of unspecified Achilles tendon

  ✓6ᵗʰ **S86.09** Other specified injury of Achilles tendon

    ✓7ᵗʰ **S86.091** Other specified injury of right Achilles tendon

    ✓7ᵗʰ **S86.092** Other specified injury of left Achilles tendon

    ✓7ᵗʰ **S86.099** Other specified injury of unspecified Achilles tendon

✓5ᵗʰ **S86.1** Injury of other muscle(s) and tendon(s) of posterior muscle group at lower leg level

  ✓6ᵗʰ **S86.10** Unspecified injury of other muscle(s) and tendon(s) of posterior muscle group at lower leg level

    ✓7ᵗʰ **S86.101** Unspecified injury of other muscle(s) and tendon(s) of posterior muscle group at lower leg level, right leg

    ✓7ᵗʰ **S86.102** Unspecified injury of other muscle(s) and tendon(s) of posterior muscle group at lower leg level, left leg

    ✓7ᵗʰ **S86.109** Unspecified injury of other muscle(s) and tendon(s) of posterior muscle group at lower leg level, unspecified leg

  ✓6ᵗʰ **S86.11** Strain of other muscle(s) and tendon(s) of posterior muscle group at lower leg level

    ✓7ᵗʰ **S86.111** Strain of other muscle(s) and tendon(s) of posterior muscle group at lower leg level, right leg

    ✓7ᵗʰ **S86.112** Strain of other muscle(s) and tendon(s) of posterior muscle group at lower leg level, left leg

    ✓7ᵗʰ **S86.119** Strain of other muscle(s) and tendon(s) of posterior muscle group at lower leg level, unspecified leg

  ✓6ᵗʰ **S86.12** Laceration of other muscle(s) and tendon(s) of posterior muscle group at lower leg level

    ✓7ᵗʰ **S86.121** Laceration of other muscle(s) and tendon(s) of posterior muscle group at lower leg level, right leg

    ✓7ᵗʰ **S86.122** Laceration of other muscle(s) and tendon(s) of posterior muscle group at lower leg level, left leg

    ✓7ᵗʰ **S86.129** Laceration of other muscle(s) and tendon(s) of posterior muscle group at lower leg level, unspecified leg

  ✓6ᵗʰ **S86.19** Other injury of other muscle(s) and tendon(s) of posterior muscle group at lower leg level

    ✓7ᵗʰ **S86.191** Other injury of other muscle(s) and tendon(s) of posterior muscle group at lower leg level, right leg

    ✓7ᵗʰ **S86.192** Other injury of other muscle(s) and tendon(s) of posterior muscle group at lower leg level, left leg

    ✓7ᵗʰ **S86.199** Other injury of other muscle(s) and tendon(s) of posterior muscle group at lower leg level, unspecified leg

✓5ᵗʰ **S86.2** Injury of muscle(s) and tendon(s) of anterior muscle group at lower leg level

  ✓6ᵗʰ **S86.20** Unspecified injury of muscle(s) and tendon(s) of anterior muscle group at lower leg level

    ✓7ᵗʰ **S86.201** Unspecified injury of muscle(s) and tendon(s) of anterior muscle group at lower leg level, right leg

    ✓7ᵗʰ **S86.202** Unspecified injury of muscle(s) and tendon(s) of anterior muscle group at lower leg level, left leg

    ✓7ᵗʰ **S86.209** Unspecified injury of muscle(s) and tendon(s) of anterior muscle group at lower leg level, unspecified leg

  ✓6ᵗʰ **S86.21** Strain of muscle(s) and tendon(s) of anterior muscle group at lower leg level

    ✓7ᵗʰ **S86.211** Strain of muscle(s) and tendon(s) of anterior muscle group at lower leg level, right leg

    ✓7ᵗʰ **S86.212** Strain of muscle(s) and tendon(s) of anterior muscle group at lower leg level, left leg

    ✓7ᵗʰ **S86.219** Strain of muscle(s) and tendon(s) of anterior muscle group at lower leg level, unspecified leg

  ✓6ᵗʰ **S86.22** Laceration of muscle(s) and tendon(s) of anterior muscle group at lower leg level

    ✓7ᵗʰ **S86.221** Laceration of muscle(s) and tendon(s) of anterior muscle group at lower leg level, right leg

    ✓7ᵗʰ **S86.222** Laceration of muscle(s) and tendon(s) of anterior muscle group at lower leg level, left leg

EXCLUDES 1 Not coded here   EXCLUDES 2 Not included here   N Newborn Age: 0   P Pediatric Age: 0-17   M Maternity Age: 12-55   A Adult Age: 15-124

906   ICD-10-CM 2014 (Draft)

✅7th **S86.229** Laceration of muscle(s) and tendon(s) of anterior muscle group at lower leg level, unspecified leg

✅6th **S86.29** Other injury of muscle(s) and tendon(s) of anterior muscle group at lower leg level

  ✅7th **S86.291** Other injury of muscle(s) and tendon(s) of anterior muscle group at lower leg level, right leg

  ✅7th **S86.292** Other injury of muscle(s) and tendon(s) of anterior muscle group at lower leg level, left leg

  ✅7th **S86.299** Other injury of muscle(s) and tendon(s) of anterior muscle group at lower leg level, unspecified leg

✅5th **S86.3** Injury of muscle(s) and tendon(s) of peroneal muscle group at lower leg level

  ✅6th **S86.30** Unspecified injury of muscle(s) and tendon(s) of peroneal muscle group at lower leg level

    ✅7th **S86.301** Unspecified injury of muscle(s) and tendon(s) of peroneal muscle group at lower leg level, right leg

    ✅7th **S86.302** Unspecified injury of muscle(s) and tendon(s) of peroneal muscle group at lower leg level, left leg

    ✅7th **S86.309** Unspecified injury of muscle(s) and tendon(s) of peroneal muscle group at lower leg level, unspecified leg

  ✅6th **S86.31** Strain of muscle(s) and tendon(s) of peroneal muscle group at lower leg level

    ✅7th **S86.311** Strain of muscle(s) and tendon(s) of peroneal muscle group at lower leg level, right leg

    ✅7th **S86.312** Strain of muscle(s) and tendon(s) of peroneal muscle group at lower leg level, left leg

    ✅7th **S86.319** Strain of muscle(s) and tendon(s) of peroneal muscle group at lower leg level, unspecified leg

  ✅6th **S86.32** Laceration of muscle(s) and tendon(s) of peroneal muscle group at lower leg level

    ✅7th **S86.321** Laceration of muscle(s) and tendon(s) of peroneal muscle group at lower leg level, right leg

    ✅7th **S86.322** Laceration of muscle(s) and tendon(s) of peroneal muscle group at lower leg level, left leg

    ✅7th **S86.329** Laceration of muscle(s) and tendon(s) of peroneal muscle group at lower leg level, unspecified leg

  ✅6th **S86.39** Other injury of muscle(s) and tendon(s) of peroneal muscle group at lower leg level

    ✅7th **S86.391** Other injury of muscle(s) and tendon(s) of peroneal muscle group at lower leg level, right leg

    ✅7th **S86.392** Other injury of muscle(s) and tendon(s) of peroneal muscle group at lower leg level, left leg

    ✅7th **S86.399** Other injury of muscle(s) and tendon(s) of peroneal muscle group at lower leg level, unspecified leg

✅5th **S86.8** Injury of other muscles and tendons at lower leg level

  ✅6th **S86.80** Unspecified injury of other muscles and tendons at lower leg level

    ✅7th **S86.801** Unspecified injury of other muscle(s) and tendon(s) at lower leg level, right leg

    ✅7th **S86.802** Unspecified injury of other muscle(s) and tendon(s) at lower leg level, left leg

    ✅7th **S86.809** Unspecified injury of other muscle(s) and tendon(s) at lower leg level, unspecified leg

  ✅6th **S86.81** Strain of other muscles and tendons at lower leg level

    ✅7th **S86.811** Strain of other muscle(s) and tendon(s) at lower leg level, right leg

    ✅7th **S86.812** Strain of other muscle(s) and tendon(s) at lower leg level, left leg

✅7th **S86.819** Strain of other muscle(s) and tendon(s) at lower leg level, unspecified leg

✅6th **S86.82** Laceration of other muscles and tendons at lower leg level

  ✅7th **S86.821** Laceration of other muscle(s) and tendon(s) at lower leg level, right leg

  ✅7th **S86.822** Laceration of other muscle(s) and tendon(s) at lower leg level, left leg

  ✅7th **S86.829** Laceration of other muscle(s) and tendon(s) at lower leg level, unspecified leg

✅6th **S86.89** Other injury of other muscles and tendons at lower leg level

  ✅7th **S86.891** Other injury of other muscle(s) and tendon(s) at lower leg level, right leg

  ✅7th **S86.892** Other injury of other muscle(s) and tendon(s) at lower leg level, left leg

  ✅7th **S86.899** Other injury of other muscle(s) and tendon(s) at lower leg level, unspecified leg

✅5th **S86.9** Injury of unspecified muscle and tendon at lower leg level

  ✅6th **S86.90** Unspecified injury of unspecified muscle and tendon at lower leg level

    ✅7th **S86.901** Unspecified injury of unspecified muscle(s) and tendon(s) at lower leg level, right leg

    ✅7th **S86.902** Unspecified injury of unspecified muscle(s) and tendon(s) at lower leg level, left leg

    ✅7th **S86.909** Unspecified injury of unspecified muscle(s) and tendon(s) at lower leg level, unspecified leg

  ✅6th **S86.91** Strain of unspecified muscle and tendon at lower leg level

    ✅7th **S86.911** Strain of unspecified muscle(s) and tendon(s) at lower leg level, right leg

    ✅7th **S86.912** Strain of unspecified muscle(s) and tendon(s) at lower leg level, left leg

    ✅7th **S86.919** Strain of unspecified muscle(s) and tendon(s) at lower leg level, unspecified leg

  ✅6th **S86.92** Laceration of unspecified muscle and tendon at lower leg level

    ✅7th **S86.921** Laceration of unspecified muscle(s) and tendon(s) at lower leg level, right leg

    ✅7th **S86.922** Laceration of unspecified muscle(s) and tendon(s) at lower leg level, left leg

    ✅7th **S86.929** Laceration of unspecified muscle(s) and tendon(s) at lower leg level, unspecified leg

  ✅6th **S86.99** Other injury of unspecified muscle and tendon at lower leg level

    ✅7th **S86.991** Other injury of unspecified muscle(s) and tendon(s) at lower leg level, right leg

    ✅7th **S86.992** Other injury of unspecified muscle(s) and tendon(s) at lower leg level, left leg

    ✅7th **S86.999** Other injury of unspecified muscle(s) and tendon(s) at lower leg level, unspecified leg

✅4th **S87** Crushing injury of lower leg

Use additional code(s) for all associated injuries

EXCLUDES 2 *crushing injury of ankle and foot (S97.-)*

The appropriate 7th character is to be added to each code from category S87.
A   initial encounter
D   subsequent encounter
S   sequela

✅5th **S87.0** Crushing injury of knee

  ✅x7th **S87.00** Crushing injury of unspecified knee

  ✅x7th **S87.01** Crushing injury of right knee

  ✅x7th **S87.02** Crushing injury of left knee

✅5th **S87.8** Crushing injury of lower leg

  ✅x7th **S87.80** Crushing injury of unspecified lower leg

  ✅x7th **S87.81** Crushing injury of right lower leg

✅ Additional Character Required   ✅x7th Xtension Alert   Unspecified Code   Other Specified Code   Manifestation Code   ►◄ Revised Text   ● New Code   ▲ Revised Code Title

√x7ᵗʰ S87.82 Crushing injury of left lower leg

√4ᵗʰ S88 **Traumatic amputation of lower leg**

> **NOTE** An amputation not identified as partial or complete should be coded to complete.
>
> **EXCLUDES1** traumatic amputation of ankle and foot (S98.-)

> The appropriate 7th character is to be added to each code from category S88.
> A   initial encounter
> D   subsequent encounter
> S   sequela

√5ᵗʰ S88.0 **Traumatic amputation at knee level**

    √6ᵗʰ S88.01 **Complete** traumatic amputation at knee level

       √7ᵗʰ S88.011 Complete traumatic amputation at knee level, right lower leg

       √7ᵗʰ S88.012 Complete traumatic amputation at knee level, left lower leg

       √7ᵗʰ S88.019 Complete traumatic amputation at knee level, unspecified lower leg

    √6ᵗʰ S88.02 **Partial** traumatic amputation at knee level

       √7ᵗʰ S88.021 Partial traumatic amputation at knee level, right lower leg

       √7ᵗʰ S88.022 Partial traumatic amputation at knee level, left lower leg

       √7ᵗʰ S88.029 Partial traumatic amputation at knee level, unspecified lower leg

√5ᵗʰ S88.1 **Traumatic amputation at level** between knee and ankle

    √6ᵗʰ S88.11 **Complete** traumatic amputation at level between knee and ankle

       √7ᵗʰ S88.111 Complete traumatic amputation at level between knee and ankle, right lower leg

       √7ᵗʰ S88.112 Complete traumatic amputation at level between knee and ankle, left lower leg

       √7ᵗʰ S88.119 Complete traumatic amputation at level between knee and ankle, unspecified lower leg

    √6ᵗʰ S88.12 **Partial** traumatic amputation at level between knee and ankle

       √7ᵗʰ S88.121 Partial traumatic amputation at level between knee and ankle, right lower leg

       √7ᵗʰ S88.122 Partial traumatic amputation at level between knee and ankle, left lower leg

       √7ᵗʰ S88.129 Partial traumatic amputation at level between knee and ankle, unspecified lower leg

√5ᵗʰ S88.9 **Traumatic amputation of lower leg,** level unspecified

    √6ᵗʰ S88.91 **Complete** traumatic amputation of lower leg, level unspecified

       √7ᵗʰ S88.911 Complete traumatic amputation of right lower leg, level unspecified

       √7ᵗʰ S88.912 Complete traumatic amputation of left lower leg, level unspecified

       √7ᵗʰ S88.919 Complete traumatic amputation of unspecified lower leg, level unspecified

    √6ᵗʰ S88.92 **Partial** traumatic amputation of lower leg, level unspecified

       √7ᵗʰ S88.921 Partial traumatic amputation of right lower leg, level unspecified

       √7ᵗʰ S88.922 Partial traumatic amputation of left lower leg, level unspecified

       √7ᵗʰ S88.929 Partial traumatic amputation of unspecified lower leg, level unspecified

√4ᵗʰ S89 **Other and unspecified injuries of lower leg**

> **NOTE** A fracture not indicated as open or closed should be coded to closed.
>
> **EXCLUDES2** other and unspecified injuries of ankle and foot (S99.-)

> The appropriate 7th character is to be added to each code from subcategories S89.0, S89.1, S89.2, and S89.3.
> A   initial encounter for closed fracture
> D   subsequent encounter for fracture with routine healing
> G   subsequent encounter for fracture with delayed healing
> K   subsequent encounter for fracture with nonunion
> P   subsequent encounter for fracture with malunion
> S   sequela

√5ᵗʰ S89.0 **Physeal fracture of** upper end of tibia

    √6ᵗʰ S89.00 **Unspecified** physeal fracture of upper end of tibia

       √7ᵗʰ S89.001 Unspecified physeal fracture of upper end of right tibia

       √7ᵗʰ S89.002 Unspecified physeal fracture of upper end of left tibia

       √7ᵗʰ S89.009 Unspecified physeal fracture of upper end of unspecified tibia

    √6ᵗʰ S89.01 **Salter-Harris Type I** physeal fracture of upper end of tibia

       √7ᵗʰ S89.011 Salter-Harris Type I physeal fracture of upper end of right tibia

       √7ᵗʰ S89.012 Salter-Harris Type I physeal fracture of upper end of left tibia

       √7ᵗʰ S89.019 Salter-Harris Type I physeal fracture of upper end of unspecified tibia

    √6ᵗʰ S89.02 **Salter-Harris Type II** physeal fracture of upper end of tibia

       √7ᵗʰ S89.021 Salter-Harris Type II physeal fracture of upper end of right tibia

       √7ᵗʰ S89.022 Salter-Harris Type II physeal fracture of upper end of left tibia

       √7ᵗʰ S89.029 Salter-Harris Type II physeal fracture of upper end of unspecified tibia

    √6ᵗʰ S89.03 **Salter-Harris Type III** physeal fracture of upper end of tibia

       √7ᵗʰ S89.031 Salter-Harris Type III physeal fracture of upper end of right tibia

       √7ᵗʰ S89.032 Salter-Harris Type III physeal fracture of upper end of left tibia

       √7ᵗʰ S89.039 Salter-Harris Type III physeal fracture of upper end of unspecified tibia

    √6ᵗʰ S89.04 **Salter-Harris Type IV** physeal fracture of upper end of tibia

       √7ᵗʰ S89.041 Salter-Harris Type IV physeal fracture of upper end of right tibia

       √7ᵗʰ S89.042 Salter-Harris Type IV physeal fracture of upper end of left tibia

       √7ᵗʰ S89.049 Salter-Harris Type IV physeal fracture of upper end of unspecified tibia

    √6ᵗʰ S89.09 **Other** physeal fracture of upper end of tibia

       √7ᵗʰ S89.091 Other physeal fracture of upper end of right tibia

       √7ᵗʰ S89.092 Other physeal fracture of upper end of left tibia

       √7ᵗʰ S89.099 Other physeal fracture of upper end of unspecified tibia

√5ᵗʰ S89.1 **Physeal fracture of** lower end of tibia

    √6ᵗʰ S89.10 **Unspecified** physeal fracture of lower end of tibia

       √7ᵗʰ S89.101 Unspecified physeal fracture of lower end of right tibia

       √7ᵗʰ S89.102 Unspecified physeal fracture of lower end of left tibia

       √7ᵗʰ S89.109 Unspecified physeal fracture of lower end of unspecified tibia

    √6ᵗʰ S89.11 **Salter-Harris Type I** lphyseal fracture of ower end of tibia

       √7ᵗʰ S89.111 Salter-Harris Type I physeal fracture of lower end of right tibia

       √7ᵗʰ S89.112 Salter-Harris Type I physeal fracture of lower end of left tibia

       √7ᵗʰ S89.119 Salter-Harris Type I physeal fracture of lower end of unspecified tibia

    √6ᵗʰ S89.12 **Salter-Harris Type II** physeal fracture of lower end of tibia

       √7ᵗʰ S89.121 Salter-Harris Type II physeal fracture of lower end of right tibia

       √7ᵗʰ S89.122 Salter-Harris Type II physeal fracture of lower end of left tibia

       √7ᵗʰ S89.129 Salter-Harris Type II physeal fracture of lower end of unspecified tibia

---

EXCLUDES1 Not coded here   **EXCLUDES2** Not included here   **N** Newborn Age: 0   **P** Pediatric Age: 0-17   **M** Maternity Age: 12-55   **A** Adult Age: 15-124

908   ICD-10-CM 2014 (Draft)

√6ᵗʰ **S89.13** Salter-Harris Type III physeal fracture of lower end of tibia

EXCLUDES 1 *fracture of medial malleolus (adult) (S82.5-)*

√7ᵗʰ **S89.131** Salter-Harris Type III physeal fracture of lower end of right tibia

√7ᵗʰ **S89.132** Salter-Harris Type III physeal fracture of lower end of left tibia

√7ᵗʰ **S89.139** Salter-Harris Type III physeal fracture of lower end of unspecified tibia

√6ᵗʰ **S89.14** Salter-Harris Type IV physeal fracture of lower end of tibia

EXCLUDES 1 *fracture of medial malleolus (adult) (S82.5-)*

√7ᵗʰ **S89.141** Salter-Harris Type IV physeal fracture of lower end of right tibia

√7ᵗʰ **S89.142** Salter-Harris Type IV physeal fracture of lower end of left tibia

√7ᵗʰ **S89.149** Salter-Harris Type IV physeal fracture of lower end of unspecified tibia

√6ᵗʰ **S89.19** Other physeal fracture of lower end of tibia

√7ᵗʰ **S89.191** Other physeal fracture of lower end of right tibia

√7ᵗʰ **S89.192** Other physeal fracture of lower end of left tibia

√7ᵗʰ **S89.199** Other physeal fracture of lower end of unspecified tibia

√5ᵗʰ **S89.2** Physeal fracture of upper end of fibula

√6ᵗʰ **S89.20** Unspecified physeal fracture of upper end of fibula

√7ᵗʰ **S89.201** Unspecified physeal fracture of upper end of right fibula

√7ᵗʰ **S89.202** Unspecified physeal fracture of upper end of left fibula

√7ᵗʰ **S89.209** Unspecified physeal fracture of upper end of unspecified fibula

√6ᵗʰ **S89.21** Salter-Harris Type I physeal fracture of upper end of fibula

√7ᵗʰ **S89.211** Salter-Harris Type I physeal fracture of upper end of right fibula

√7ᵗʰ **S89.212** Salter-Harris Type I physeal fracture of upper end of left fibula

√7ᵗʰ **S89.219** Salter-Harris Type I physeal fracture of upper end of unspecified fibula

√6ᵗʰ **S89.22** Salter-Harris Type II physeal fracture of upper end of fibula

√7ᵗʰ **S89.221** Salter-Harris Type II physeal fracture of upper end of right fibula

√7ᵗʰ **S89.222** Salter-Harris Type II physeal fracture of upper end of left fibula

√7ᵗʰ **S89.229** Salter-Harris Type II physeal fracture of upper end of unspecified fibula

√6ᵗʰ **S89.29** Other physeal fracture of upper end of fibula

√7ᵗʰ **S89.291** Other physeal fracture of upper end of right fibula

√7ᵗʰ **S89.292** Other physeal fracture of upper end of left fibula

√7ᵗʰ **S89.299** Other physeal fracture of upper end of unspecified fibula

√5ᵗʰ **S89.3** Physeal fracture of lower end of fibula

√6ᵗʰ **S89.30** Unspecified physeal fracture of lower end of fibula

√7ᵗʰ **S89.301** Unspecified physeal fracture of lower end of right fibula

√7ᵗʰ **S89.302** Unspecified physeal fracture of lower end of left fibula

√7ᵗʰ **S89.309** Unspecified physeal fracture of lower end of unspecified fibula

√6ᵗʰ **S89.31** Salter-Harris Type I physeal fracture of lower end of fibula

√7ᵗʰ **S89.311** Salter-Harris Type I physeal fracture of lower end of right fibula

√7ᵗʰ **S89.312** Salter-Harris Type I physeal fracture of lower end of left fibula

√7ᵗʰ **S89.319** Salter-Harris Type I physeal fracture of lower end of unspecified fibula

√6ᵗʰ **S89.32** Salter-Harris Type II physeal fracture of lower end of fibula

√7ᵗʰ **S89.321** Salter-Harris Type II physeal fracture of lower end of right fibula

√7ᵗʰ **S89.322** Salter-Harris Type II physeal fracture of lower end of left fibula

√7ᵗʰ **S89.329** Salter-Harris Type II physeal fracture of lower end of unspecified fibula

√6ᵗʰ **S89.39** Other physeal fracture of lower end of fibula

√7ᵗʰ **S89.391** Other physeal fracture of lower end of right fibula

√7ᵗʰ **S89.392** Other physeal fracture of lower end of left fibula

√7ᵗʰ **S89.399** Other physeal fracture of lower end of unspecified fibula

√5ᵗʰ **S89.8** Other specified injuries of lower leg

The appropriate 7th character is to be added to each code in subcategory S89.8.
A   initial encounter
D   subsequent encounter
S   sequela

√x7ᵗʰ **S89.80** Other specified injuries of unspecified lower leg

√x7ᵗʰ **S89.81** Other specified injuries of right lower leg

√x7ᵗʰ **S89.82** Other specified injuries of left lower leg

√5ᵗʰ **S89.9** Unspecified injury of lower leg

The appropriate 7th character is to be added to each code in subcategory S89.9.
A   initial encounter
D   subsequent encounter
S   sequela

√x7ᵗʰ **S89.90** Unspecified injury of unspecified lower leg

√x7ᵗʰ **S89.91** Unspecified injury of right lower leg

√x7ᵗʰ **S89.92** Unspecified injury of left lower leg

Injuries to the ankle and foot (S90-S99)

EXCLUDES 2 *burns and corrosions (T20-T32)*
fracture of ankle and malleolus (S82.-)
frostbite (T33-T34)
insect bite or sting, venomous (T63.4)

√4ᵗʰ **S90** **Superficial injury of ankle, foot and toes**

The appropriate 7th character is to be added to each code from category S90.
A   initial encounter
D   subsequent encounter
S   sequela

√5ᵗʰ **S90.0** Contusion of ankle

√x7ᵗʰ **S90.00** Contusion of unspecified ankle

√x7ᵗʰ **S90.01** Contusion of right ankle

√x7ᵗʰ **S90.02** Contusion of left ankle

√5ᵗʰ **S90.1** Contusion of toe without damage to nail

√6ᵗʰ **S90.11** Contusion of great toe without damage to nail

√7ᵗʰ **S90.111** Contusion of right great toe without damage to nail

√7ᵗʰ **S90.112** Contusion of left great toe without damage to nail

√7ᵗʰ **S90.119** Contusion of unspecified great toe without damage to nail

√6ᵗʰ **S90.12** Contusion of lesser toe without damage to nail

√7ᵗʰ **S90.121** Contusion of right lesser toe(s) without damage to nail

√7ᵗʰ **S90.122** Contusion of left lesser toe(s) without damage to nail

√7ᵗʰ **S90.129** Contusion of unspecified lesser toe(s) without damage to nail
Contusion of toe NOS

√5ᵗʰ **S90.2** Contusion of toe with damage to nail

√6ᵗʰ **S90.21** Contusion of great toe with damage to nail

√7ᵗʰ **S90.211** Contusion of right great toe with damage to nail

√7ᵗʰ **S90.212** Contusion of left great toe with damage to nail

---

Injury, Poisoning and Certain Other Consequences of External Causes   S90.219–S90.921

✓7ᵗʰ **S90.219** **Contusion of unspecified great toe with damage to nail**

✓6ᵗʰ **S90.22** **Contusion of lesser toe with damage to nail**

     ✓7ᵗʰ **S90.221** **Contusion of right lesser toe(s) with damage to nail**

     ✓7ᵗʰ **S90.222** **Contusion of left lesser toe(s) with damage to nail**

     ✓7ᵗʰ **S90.229** **Contusion of unspecified lesser toe(s) with damage to nail**

✓5ᵗʰ **S90.3** **Contusion of foot**

     EXCLUDES 2   contusion of toes (S90.1-, S90.2-)

     ✓x7ᵗʰ **S90.30** **Contusion of unspecified foot**
         Contusion of foot NOS

     ✓x7ᵗʰ **S90.31** **Contusion of right foot**

     ✓x7ᵗʰ **S90.32** **Contusion of left foot**

✓5ᵗʰ **S90.4** **Other superficial injuries of toe**

     ✓6ᵗʰ **S90.41** **Abrasion of toe**

         ✓7ᵗʰ **S90.411** **Abrasion, right great toe**

         ✓7ᵗʰ **S90.412** **Abrasion, left great toe**

         ✓7ᵗʰ **S90.413** **Abrasion, unspecified great toe**

         ✓7ᵗʰ **S90.414** **Abrasion, right lesser toe(s)**

         ✓7ᵗʰ **S90.415** **Abrasion, left lesser toe(s)**

         ✓7ᵗʰ **S90.416** **Abrasion, unspecified lesser toe(s)**

     ✓6ᵗʰ **S90.42** **Blister (nonthermal) of toe**

         ✓7ᵗʰ **S90.421** **Blister (nonthermal), right great toe**

         ✓7ᵗʰ **S90.422** **Blister (nonthermal), left great toe**

         ✓7ᵗʰ **S90.423** **Blister (nonthermal), unspecified great toe**

         ✓7ᵗʰ **S90.424** **Blister (nonthermal), right lesser toe(s)**

         ✓7ᵗʰ **S90.425** **Blister (nonthermal), left lesser toe(s)**

         ✓7ᵗʰ **S90.426** **Blister (nonthermal), unspecified lesser toe(s)**

     ✓6ᵗʰ **S90.44** **External constriction of toe**
         Hair tourniquet syndrome of toe

         ✓7ᵗʰ **S90.441** **External constriction, right great toe**

         ✓7ᵗʰ **S90.442** **External constriction, left great toe**

         ✓7ᵗʰ **S90.443** **External constriction, unspecified great toe**

         ✓7ᵗʰ **S90.444** **External constriction, right lesser toe(s)**

         ✓7ᵗʰ **S90.445** **External constriction, left lesser toe(s)**

         ✓7ᵗʰ **S90.446** **External constriction, unspecified lesser toe(s)**

     ✓6ᵗʰ **S90.45** **Superficial foreign body of toe**
         Splinter in the toe

         ✓7ᵗʰ **S90.451** **Superficial foreign body, right great toe**

         ✓7ᵗʰ **S90.452** **Superficial foreign body, left great toe**

         ✓7ᵗʰ **S90.453** **Superficial foreign body, unspecified great toe**

         ✓7ᵗʰ **S90.454** **Superficial foreign body, right lesser toe(s)**

         ✓7ᵗʰ **S90.455** **Superficial foreign body, left lesser toe(s)**

         ✓7ᵗʰ **S90.456** **Superficial foreign body, unspecified lesser toe(s)**

     ✓6ᵗʰ **S90.46** **Insect bite (nonvenomous) of toe**

         ✓7ᵗʰ **S90.461** **Insect bite (nonvenomous), right great toe**

         ✓7ᵗʰ **S90.462** **Insect bite (nonvenomous), left great toe**

         ✓7ᵗʰ **S90.463** **Insect bite (nonvenomous), unspecified great toe**

         ✓7ᵗʰ **S90.464** **Insect bite (nonvenomous), right lesser toe(s)**

         ✓7ᵗʰ **S90.465** **Insect bite (nonvenomous), left lesser toe(s)**

         ✓7ᵗʰ **S90.466** **Insect bite (nonvenomous), unspecified lesser toe(s)**

     ✓6ᵗʰ **S90.47** **Other superficial bite of toe**
         EXCLUDES 1   open bite of toe (S91.15-, S91.25-)

         ✓7ᵗʰ **S90.471** **Other superficial bite of right great toe**

         ✓7ᵗʰ **S90.472** **Other superficial bite of left great toe**

         ✓7ᵗʰ **S90.473** **Other superficial bite of unspecified great toe**

         ✓7ᵗʰ **S90.474** **Other superficial bite of right lesser toe(s)**

         ✓7ᵗʰ **S90.475** **Other superficial bite of left lesser toe(s)**

         ✓7ᵗʰ **S90.476** **Other superficial bite of unspecified lesser toe(s)**

✓5ᵗʰ **S90.5** **Other superficial injuries of ankle**

     ✓6ᵗʰ **S90.51** **Abrasion of ankle**

         ✓7ᵗʰ **S90.511** **Abrasion, right ankle**

         ✓7ᵗʰ **S90.512** **Abrasion, left ankle**

         ✓7ᵗʰ **S90.519** **Abrasion, unspecified ankle**

     ✓6ᵗʰ **S90.52** **Blister (nonthermal) of ankle**

         ✓7ᵗʰ **S90.521** **Blister (nonthermal), right ankle**

         ✓7ᵗʰ **S90.522** **Blister (nonthermal), left ankle**

         ✓7ᵗʰ **S90.529** **Blister (nonthermal), unspecified ankle**

     ✓6ᵗʰ **S90.54** **External constriction of ankle**

         ✓7ᵗʰ **S90.541** **External constriction, right ankle**

         ✓7ᵗʰ **S90.542** **External constriction, left ankle**

         ✓7ᵗʰ **S90.549** **External constriction, unspecified ankle**

     ✓6ᵗʰ **S90.55** **Superficial foreign body of ankle**
         Splinter in the ankle

         ✓7ᵗʰ **S90.551** **Superficial foreign body, right ankle**

         ✓7ᵗʰ **S90.552** **Superficial foreign body, left ankle**

         ✓7ᵗʰ **S90.559** **Superficial foreign body, unspecified ankle**

     ✓6ᵗʰ **S90.56** **Insect bite (nonvenomous) of ankle**

         ✓7ᵗʰ **S90.561** **Insect bite (nonvenomous), right ankle**

         ✓7ᵗʰ **S90.562** **Insect bite (nonvenomous), left ankle**

         ✓7ᵗʰ **S90.569** **Insect bite (nonvenomous), unspecified ankle**

     ✓6ᵗʰ **S90.57** **Other superficial bite of ankle**
         EXCLUDES 1   open bite of ankle (S91.05-)

         ✓7ᵗʰ **S90.571** **Other superficial bite of ankle, right ankle**

         ✓7ᵗʰ **S90.572** **Other superficial bite of ankle, left ankle**

         ✓7ᵗʰ **S90.579** **Other superficial bite of ankle, unspecified ankle**

✓5ᵗʰ **S90.8** **Other superficial injuries of foot**

     ✓6ᵗʰ **S90.81** **Abrasion of foot**

         ✓7ᵗʰ **S90.811** **Abrasion, right foot**

         ✓7ᵗʰ **S90.812** **Abrasion, left foot**

         ✓7ᵗʰ **S90.819** **Abrasion, unspecified foot**

     ✓6ᵗʰ **S90.82** **Blister (nonthermal) of foot**

         ✓7ᵗʰ **S90.821** **Blister (nonthermal), right foot**

         ✓7ᵗʰ **S90.822** **Blister (nonthermal), left foot**

         ✓7ᵗʰ **S90.829** **Blister (nonthermal), unspecified foot**

     ✓6ᵗʰ **S90.84** **External constriction of foot**

         ✓7ᵗʰ **S90.841** **External constriction, right foot**

         ✓7ᵗʰ **S90.842** **External constriction, left foot**

         ✓7ᵗʰ **S90.849** **External constriction, unspecified foot**

     ✓6ᵗʰ **S90.85** **Superficial foreign body of foot**
         Splinter in the foot

         ✓7ᵗʰ **S90.851** **Superficial foreign body, right foot**

         ✓7ᵗʰ **S90.852** **Superficial foreign body, left foot**

         ✓7ᵗʰ **S90.859** **Superficial foreign body, unspecified foot**

     ✓6ᵗʰ **S90.86** **Insect bite (nonvenomous) of foot**

         ✓7ᵗʰ **S90.861** **Insect bite (nonvenomous), right foot**

         ✓7ᵗʰ **S90.862** **Insect bite (nonvenomous), left foot**

         ✓7ᵗʰ **S90.869** **Insect bite (nonvenomous), unspecified foot**

     ✓6ᵗʰ **S90.87** **Other superficial bite of foot**
         EXCLUDES 1   open bite of foot (S91.35-)

         ✓7ᵗʰ **S90.871** **Other superficial bite of right foot**

         ✓7ᵗʰ **S90.872** **Other superficial bite of left foot**

         ✓7ᵗʰ **S90.879** **Other superficial bite of unspecified foot**

✓5ᵗʰ **S90.9** **Unspecified superficial injury of ankle, foot and toe**

     ✓6ᵗʰ **S90.91** **Unspecified superficial injury of ankle**

         ✓7ᵗʰ **S90.911** **Unspecified superficial injury of right ankle**

         ✓7ᵗʰ **S90.912** **Unspecified superficial injury of left ankle**

         ✓7ᵗʰ **S90.919** **Unspecified superficial injury of unspecified ankle**

     ✓6ᵗʰ **S90.92** **Unspecified superficial injury of foot**

         ✓7ᵗʰ **S90.921** **Unspecified superficial injury of right foot**

EXCLUDES 1 Not coded here   **EXCLUDES 2** Not included here   N Newborn Age: 0   P Pediatric Age: 0-17   M Maternity Age: 12-55   A Adult Age: 15-124

910   ICD-10-CM 2014 (Draft)

| ✓7th | S90.922 | Unspecified superficial injury of left foot |
| ✓7th | S90.929 | Unspecified superficial injury of unspecified foot |

✓6th **S90.93** Unspecified superficial injury of toes

✓7th	S90.931	Unspecified superficial injury of right great toe
✓7th	S90.932	Unspecified superficial injury of left great toe
✓7th	S90.933	Unspecified superficial injury of unspecified great toe
✓7th	S90.934	Unspecified superficial injury of right lesser toe(s)
✓7th	S90.935	Unspecified superficial injury of left lesser toe(s)
✓7th	S90.936	Unspecified superficial injury of unspecified lesser toe(s)

✓4th **S91 Open wound of ankle, foot and toes**

Code also any associated wound infection

EXCLUDES 1 open fracture of ankle, foot and toes (S92-with 7th character B)
traumatic amputation of ankle and foot (S98.-)

The appropriate 7th character is to be added to each code from category S91.
A initial encounter
D subsequent encounter
S sequela

✓5th **S91.0 Open wound of ankle**

✓6th **S91.00** Unspecified open wound of ankle

✓7th	S91.001	Unspecified open wound, right ankle
✓7th	S91.002	Unspecified open wound, left ankle
✓7th	S91.009	Unspecified open wound, unspecified ankle

✓6th **S91.01** Laceration without foreign body of ankle

✓7th	S91.011	Laceration without foreign body, right ankle
✓7th	S91.012	Laceration without foreign body, left ankle
✓7th	S91.019	Laceration without foreign body, unspecified ankle

✓6th **S91.02** Laceration with foreign body of ankle

✓7th	S91.021	Laceration with foreign body, right ankle
✓7th	S91.022	Laceration with foreign body, left ankle
✓7th	S91.029	Laceration with foreign body, unspecified ankle

✓6th **S91.03** Puncture wound without foreign body of ankle

✓7th	S91.031	Puncture wound without foreign body, right ankle
✓7th	S91.032	Puncture wound without foreign body, left ankle
✓7th	S91.039	Puncture wound without foreign body, unspecified ankle

✓6th **S91.04** Puncture wound with foreign body of ankle

✓7th	S91.041	Puncture wound with foreign body, right ankle
✓7th	S91.042	Puncture wound with foreign body, left ankle
✓7th	S91.049	Puncture wound with foreign body, unspecified ankle

✓6th **S91.05** Open bite of ankle

EXCLUDES 1 superficial bite of ankle (S90.56-, S90.57-)

✓7th	S91.051	Open bite, right ankle
✓7th	S91.052	Open bite, left ankle
✓7th	S91.059	Open bite, unspecified ankle

✓5th **S91.1 Open wound of toe without damage to nail**

✓6th **S91.10** Unspecified open wound of toe without damage to nail

✓7th	S91.101	Unspecified open wound of right great toe without damage to nail
✓7th	S91.102	Unspecified open wound of left great toe without damage to nail
✓7th	S91.103	Unspecified open wound of unspecified great toe without damage to nail
✓7th	S91.104	Unspecified open wound of right lesser toe(s) without damage to nail

✓7th	S91.105	Unspecified open wound of left lesser toe(s) without damage to nail
✓7th	S91.106	Unspecified open wound of unspecified lesser toe(s) without damage to nail
✓7th	S91.109	Unspecified open wound of unspecified toe(s) without damage to nail

✓6th **S91.11** Laceration without foreign body of toe without damage to nail

✓7th	S91.111	Laceration without foreign body of right great toe without damage to nail
✓7th	S91.112	Laceration without foreign body of left great toe without damage to nail
✓7th	S91.113	Laceration without foreign body of unspecified great toe without damage to nail
✓7th	S91.114	Laceration without foreign body of right lesser toe(s) without damage to nail
✓7th	S91.115	Laceration without foreign body of left lesser toe(s) without damage to nail
✓7th	S91.116	Laceration without foreign body of unspecified lesser toe(s) without damage to nail
✓7th	S91.119	Laceration without foreign body of unspecified toe without damage to nail

✓6th **S91.12** Laceration with foreign body of toe without damage to nail

✓7th	S91.121	Laceration with foreign body of right great toe without damage to nail
✓7th	S91.122	Laceration with foreign body of left great toe without damage to nail
✓7th	S91.123	Laceration with foreign body of unspecified great toe without damage to nail
✓7th	S91.124	Laceration with foreign body of right lesser toe(s) without damage to nail
✓7th	S91.125	Laceration with foreign body of left lesser toe(s) without damage to nail
✓7th	S91.126	Laceration with foreign body of unspecified lesser toe(s) without damage to nail
✓7th	S91.129	Laceration with foreign body of unspecified toe(s) without damage to nail

✓6th **S91.13** Puncture wound without foreign body of toe without damage to nail

✓7th	S91.131	Puncture wound without foreign body of right great toe without damage to nail
✓7th	S91.132	Puncture wound without foreign body of left great toe without damage to nail
✓7th	S91.133	Puncture wound without foreign body of unspecified great toe without damage to nail
✓7th	S91.134	Puncture wound without foreign body of right lesser toe(s) without damage to nail
✓7th	S91.135	Puncture wound without foreign body of left lesser toe(s) without damage to nail
✓7th	S91.136	Puncture wound without foreign body of unspecified lesser toe(s) without damage to nail
✓7th	S91.139	Puncture wound without foreign body of unspecified toe(s) without damage to nail

✓6th **S91.14** Puncture wound with foreign body of toe without damage to nail

✓7th	S91.141	Puncture wound with foreign body of right great toe without damage to nail
✓7th	S91.142	Puncture wound with foreign body of left great toe without damage to nail
✓7th	S91.143	Puncture wound with foreign body of unspecified great toe without damage to nail
✓7th	S91.144	Puncture wound with foreign body of right lesser toe(s) without damage to nail
✓7th	S91.145	Puncture wound with foreign body of left lesser toe(s) without damage to nail
✓7th	S91.146	Puncture wound with foreign body of unspecified lesser toe(s) without damage to nail

✓ Additional Character Required   ✓x7th Xtension Alert   Unspecified Code   Other Specified Code   Manifestation Code   ►◄ Revised Text   ● New Code   ▲ Revised Code Title

☑7ᵗʰ **S91.149**   **Puncture wound with foreign body of unspecified toe(s) without damage to nail**

☑6ᵗʰ **S91.15**   **Open bite** of toe without damage to nail
Bite of toe NOS
EXCLUDES 1   *superficial bite of toe (S90.46-, S90.47-)*

☑7ᵗʰ **S91.151**   **Open bite of** right great **toe without damage to nail**

☑7ᵗʰ **S91.152**   **Open bite of** left great **toe without damage to nail**

☑7ᵗʰ **S91.153**   **Open bite of unspecified great toe without damage to nail**

☑7ᵗʰ **S91.154**   **Open bite of** right lesser **toe(s) without damage to nail**

☑7ᵗʰ **S91.155**   **Open bite of** left lesser **toe(s) without damage to nail**

☑7ᵗʰ **S91.156**   **Open bite of unspecified lesser toe(s) without damage to nail**

☑7ᵗʰ **S91.159**   **Open bite of unspecified toe(s) without damage to nail**

☑5ᵗʰ **S91.2**   **Open wound** of toe with damage to nail

☑6ᵗʰ **S91.20**   Unspecified **open wound of toe with damage to nail**

☑7ᵗʰ **S91.201**   **Unspecified open wound of** right great **toe with damage to nail**

☑7ᵗʰ **S91.202**   **Unspecified open wound of** left great **toe with damage to nail**

☑7ᵗʰ **S91.203**   **Unspecified open wound of unspecified great toe with damage to nail**

☑7ᵗʰ **S91.204**   **Unspecified open wound of** right lesser **toe(s) with damage to nail**

☑7ᵗʰ **S91.205**   **Unspecified open wound of** left lesser **toe(s) with damage to nail**

☑7ᵗʰ **S91.206**   **Unspecified open wound of unspecified lesser toe(s) with damage to nail**

☑7ᵗʰ **S91.209**   **Unspecified open wound of unspecified toe(s) with damage to nail**

☑6ᵗʰ **S91.21**   **Laceration** without foreign body **of toe with damage to nail**

☑7ᵗʰ **S91.211**   **Laceration without foreign body of** right great **toe with damage to nail**

☑7ᵗʰ **S91.212**   **Laceration without foreign body of** left great **toe with damage to nail**

☑7ᵗʰ **S91.213**   **Laceration without foreign body of unspecified great toe with damage to nail**

☑7ᵗʰ **S91.214**   **Laceration without foreign body of** right lesser **toe(s) with damage to nail**

☑7ᵗʰ **S91.215**   **Laceration without foreign body of** left lesser **toe(s) with damage to nail**

☑7ᵗʰ **S91.216**   **Laceration without foreign body of unspecified lesser toe(s) with damage to nail**

☑7ᵗʰ **S91.219**   **Laceration without foreign body of unspecified toe(s) with damage to nail**

☑6ᵗʰ **S91.22**   **Laceration** with foreign body **of toe with damage to nail**

☑7ᵗʰ **S91.221**   **Laceration with foreign body of** right great **toe with damage to nail**

☑7ᵗʰ **S91.222**   **Laceration with foreign body of** left great **toe with damage to nail**

☑7ᵗʰ **S91.223**   **Laceration with foreign body of unspecified great toe with damage to nail**

☑7ᵗʰ **S91.224**   **Laceration with foreign body of** right lesser **toe(s) with damage to nail**

☑7ᵗʰ **S91.225**   **Laceration with foreign body of** left lesser **toe(s) with damage to nail**

☑7ᵗʰ **S91.226**   **Laceration with foreign body of unspecified lesser toe(s) with damage to nail**

☑7ᵗʰ **S91.229**   **Laceration with foreign body of unspecified toe(s) with damage to nail**

☑6ᵗʰ **S91.23**   **Puncture wound** without foreign body **of toe with damage to nail**

☑7ᵗʰ **S91.231**   **Puncture wound without foreign body of** right great **toe with damage to nail**

☑7ᵗʰ **S91.232**   **Puncture wound without foreign body of** left great **toe with damage to nail**

☑7ᵗʰ **S91.233**   **Puncture wound without foreign body of unspecified great toe with damage to nail**

☑7ᵗʰ **S91.234**   **Puncture wound without foreign body of** right lesser **toe(s) with damage to nail**

☑7ᵗʰ **S91.235**   **Puncture wound without foreign body of** left lesser **toe(s) with damage to nail**

☑7ᵗʰ **S91.236**   **Puncture wound without foreign body of unspecified lesser toe(s) with damage to nail**

☑7ᵗʰ **S91.239**   **Puncture wound without foreign body of unspecified toe(s) with damage to nail**

☑6ᵗʰ **S91.24**   **Puncture wound** with foreign body **of toe with damage to nail**

☑7ᵗʰ **S91.241**   **Puncture wound with foreign body of** right great **toe with damage to nail**

☑7ᵗʰ **S91.242**   **Puncture wound with foreign body of** left great **toe with damage to nail**

☑7ᵗʰ **S91.243**   **Puncture wound with foreign body of unspecified great toe with damage to nail**

☑7ᵗʰ **S91.244**   **Puncture wound with foreign body of** right lesser **toe(s) with damage to nail**

☑7ᵗʰ **S91.245**   **Puncture wound with foreign body of** left lesser **toe(s) with damage to nail**

☑7ᵗʰ **S91.246**   **Puncture wound with foreign body of unspecified lesser toe(s) with damage to nail**

☑7ᵗʰ **S91.249**   **Puncture wound with foreign body of unspecified toe(s) with damage to nail**

☑6ᵗʰ **S91.25**   **Open bite** of toe with damage to nail
Bite of toe with damage to nail NOS
EXCLUDES 1   *superficial bite of toe (S90.46-, S90.47-)*

☑7ᵗʰ **S91.251**   **Open bite of** right great **toe with damage to nail**

☑7ᵗʰ **S91.252**   **Open bite of** left great **toe with damage to nail**

☑7ᵗʰ **S91.253**   **Open bite of unspecified great toe with damage to nail**

☑7ᵗʰ **S91.254**   **Open bite of** right lesser **toe(s) with damage to nail**

☑7ᵗʰ **S91.255**   **Open bite of** left lesser **toe(s) with damage to nail**

☑7ᵗʰ **S91.256**   **Open bite of unspecified lesser toe(s) with damage to nail**

☑7ᵗʰ **S91.259**   **Open bite of unspecified toe(s) with damage to nail**

☑5ᵗʰ **S91.3**   **Open wound** of foot

☑6ᵗʰ **S91.30**   Unspecified **open wound of foot**

☑7ᵗʰ **S91.301**   **Unspecified open wound,** right **foot**

☑7ᵗʰ **S91.302**   **Unspecified open wound,** left **foot**

☑7ᵗʰ **S91.309**   **Unspecified open wound, unspecified foot**

☑6ᵗʰ **S91.31**   **Laceration** without foreign body **of foot**

☑7ᵗʰ **S91.311**   **Laceration without foreign body,** right **foot**

☑7ᵗʰ **S91.312**   **Laceration without foreign body,** left **foot**

☑7ᵗʰ **S91.319**   **Laceration without foreign body, unspecified foot**

☑6ᵗʰ **S91.32**   **Laceration** with foreign body **of foot**

☑7ᵗʰ **S91.321**   **Laceration with foreign body,** right **foot**

☑7ᵗʰ **S91.322**   **Laceration with foreign body,** left **foot**

☑7ᵗʰ **S91.329**   **Laceration with foreign body, unspecified foot**

☑6ᵗʰ **S91.33**   **Puncture wound** without foreign body **of foot**

☑7ᵗʰ **S91.331**   **Puncture wound without foreign body,** right **foot**

☑7ᵗʰ **S91.332**   **Puncture wound without foreign body,** left **foot**

☑7ᵗʰ **S91.339**   **Puncture wound without foreign body, unspecified foot**

☑6ᵗʰ **S91.34**   **Puncture wound** with foreign body **of foot**

☑7ᵗʰ **S91.341**   **Puncture wound with foreign body,** right **foot**

☑7ᵗʰ **S91.342**   **Puncture wound with foreign body,** left **foot**

EXCLUDES 1 Not coded here   EXCLUDES 2 Not included here   N Newborn Age: 0   P Pediatric Age: 0-17   M Maternity Age: 12-55   A Adult Age: 15-124

912   ICD-10-CM 2014 (Draft)

☑7ᵗʰ **S91.349** **Puncture wound with foreign body, unspecified foot**

☑6ᵗʰ **S91.35** Open bite of foot
> EXCLUDES 1 *superficial bite of foot (S90.86-, S90.87-)*

☑7ᵗʰ **S91.351** **Open bite, right foot**

☑7ᵗʰ **S91.352** **Open bite, left foot**

☑7ᵗʰ **S91.359** **Open bite, unspecified foot**

☑4ᵗʰ **S92** **Fracture of foot and toe, except ankle**
> NOTE A fracture not indicated as displaced or nondisplaced should be coded to displaced.
> A fracture not indicated as open or closed should be coded to closed.
> EXCLUDES 1 *traumatic amputation of ankle and foot (S98.-)*
> EXCLUDES 2 *fracture of ankle (S82.-)*
> *fracture of malleolus (S82.-)*

> The appropriate 7th character is to be added to each code from category S92.
> A initial encounter for closed fracture
> B initial encounter for open fracture
> D subsequent encounter for fracture with routine healing
> G subsequent encounter for fracture with delayed healing
> K subsequent encounter for fracture with nonunion
> P subsequent encounter for fracture with malunion
> S sequela

☑5ᵗʰ **S92.0** **Fracture of** calcaneus
> Heel bone
> Os calcis

☑6ᵗʰ **S92.00** Unspecified fracture of calcaneus

☑7ᵗʰ **S92.001** **Unspecified fracture of right calcaneus**

☑7ᵗʰ **S92.002** **Unspecified fracture of left calcaneus**

☑7ᵗʰ **S92.009** **Unspecified fracture of unspecified calcaneus**

☑6ᵗʰ **S92.01** Fracture of body of calcaneus

☑7ᵗʰ **S92.011** **Displaced fracture of body of right calcaneus**

☑7ᵗʰ **S92.012** **Displaced fracture of body of left calcaneus**

☑7ᵗʰ **S92.013** **Displaced fracture of body of unspecified calcaneus**

☑7ᵗʰ **S92.014** **Nondisplaced fracture of body of right calcaneus**

☑7ᵗʰ **S92.015** **Nondisplaced fracture of body of left calcaneus**

☑7ᵗʰ **S92.016** **Nondisplaced fracture of body of unspecified calcaneus**

☑6ᵗʰ **S92.02** Fracture of anterior process of calcaneus

☑7ᵗʰ **S92.021** **Displaced fracture of anterior process of right calcaneus**

☑7ᵗʰ **S92.022** **Displaced fracture of anterior process of left calcaneus**

☑7ᵗʰ **S92.023** **Displaced fracture of anterior process of unspecified calcaneus**

☑7ᵗʰ **S92.024** **Nondisplaced fracture of anterior process of right calcaneus**

☑7ᵗʰ **S92.025** **Nondisplaced fracture of anterior process of left calcaneus**

☑7ᵗʰ **S92.026** **Nondisplaced fracture of anterior process of unspecified calcaneus**

☑6ᵗʰ **S92.03** Avulsion fracture of tuberosity of calcaneus

☑7ᵗʰ **S92.031** **Displaced avulsion fracture of tuberosity of right calcaneus**

☑7ᵗʰ **S92.032** **Displaced avulsion fracture of tuberosity of left calcaneus**

☑7ᵗʰ **S92.033** **Displaced avulsion fracture of tuberosity of unspecified calcaneus**

☑7ᵗʰ **S92.034** **Nondisplaced avulsion fracture of tuberosity of right calcaneus**

☑7ᵗʰ **S92.035** **Nondisplaced avulsion fracture of tuberosity of left calcaneus**

☑7ᵗʰ **S92.036** **Nondisplaced avulsion fracture of tuberosity of unspecified calcaneus**

☑6ᵗʰ **S92.04** Other fracture of tuberosity of calcaneus

☑7ᵗʰ **S92.041** **Displaced other fracture of tuberosity of right calcaneus**

☑7ᵗʰ **S92.042** **Displaced other fracture of tuberosity of left calcaneus**

☑7ᵗʰ **S92.043** **Displaced other fracture of tuberosity of unspecified calcaneus**

☑7ᵗʰ **S92.044** **Nondisplaced other fracture of tuberosity of right calcaneus**

☑7ᵗʰ **S92.045** **Nondisplaced other fracture of tuberosity of left calcaneus**

☑7ᵗʰ **S92.046** **Nondisplaced other fracture of tuberosity of unspecified calcaneus**

☑6ᵗʰ **S92.05** Other extraarticular fracture of calcaneus

☑7ᵗʰ **S92.051** **Displaced other extraarticular fracture of right calcaneus**

☑7ᵗʰ **S92.052** **Displaced other extraarticular fracture of left calcaneus**

☑7ᵗʰ **S92.053** **Displaced other extraarticular fracture of unspecified calcaneus**

☑7ᵗʰ **S92.054** **Nondisplaced other extraarticular fracture of right calcaneus**

☑7ᵗʰ **S92.055** **Nondisplaced other extraarticular fracture of left calcaneus**

☑7ᵗʰ **S92.056** **Nondisplaced other extraarticular fracture of unspecified calcaneus**

☑6ᵗʰ **S92.06** Intraarticular fracture of calcaneus

☑7ᵗʰ **S92.061** **Displaced intraarticular fracture of right calcaneus**

☑7ᵗʰ **S92.062** **Displaced intraarticular fracture of left calcaneus**

☑7ᵗʰ **S92.063** **Displaced intraarticular fracture of unspecified calcaneus**

☑7ᵗʰ **S92.064** **Nondisplaced intraarticular fracture of right calcaneus**

☑7ᵗʰ **S92.065** **Nondisplaced intraarticular fracture of left calcaneus**

☑7ᵗʰ **S92.066** **Nondisplaced intraarticular fracture of unspecified calcaneus**

☑5ᵗʰ **S92.1** **Fracture of** talus
> Astragalus

☑6ᵗʰ **S92.10** Unspecified fracture of talus

☑7ᵗʰ **S92.101** **Unspecified fracture of right talus**

☑7ᵗʰ **S92.102** **Unspecified fracture of left talus**

☑7ᵗʰ **S92.109** **Unspecified fracture of unspecified talus**

☑6ᵗʰ **S92.11** Fracture of neck of talus

☑7ᵗʰ **S92.111** **Displaced fracture of neck of right talus**

☑7ᵗʰ **S92.112** **Displaced fracture of neck of left talus**

☑7ᵗʰ **S92.113** **Displaced fracture of neck of unspecified talus**

☑7ᵗʰ **S92.114** **Nondisplaced fracture of neck of right talus**

☑7ᵗʰ **S92.115** **Nondisplaced fracture of neck of left talus**

☑7ᵗʰ **S92.116** **Nondisplaced fracture of neck of unspecified talus**

☑6ᵗʰ **S92.12** Fracture of body of talus

☑7ᵗʰ **S92.121** **Displaced fracture of body of right talus**

☑7ᵗʰ **S92.122** **Displaced fracture of body of left talus**

☑7ᵗʰ **S92.123** **Displaced fracture of body of unspecified talus**

☑7ᵗʰ **S92.124** **Nondisplaced fracture of body of right talus**

☑7ᵗʰ **S92.125** **Nondisplaced fracture of body of left talus**

☑7ᵗʰ **S92.126** **Nondisplaced fracture of body of unspecified talus**

☑6ᵗʰ **S92.13** Fracture of posterior process of talus

☑7ᵗʰ **S92.131** **Displaced fracture of posterior process of right talus**

☑7ᵗʰ **S92.132** **Displaced fracture of posterior process of left talus**

☑7ᵗʰ **S92.133** **Displaced fracture of posterior process of unspecified talus**

☑7ᵗʰ **S92.134** **Nondisplaced fracture of posterior process of right talus**

☑7ᵗʰ **S92.135** **Nondisplaced fracture of posterior process of left talus**

☑ Additional Character Required ☑x7ᵗʰ Xtension Alert Unspecified Code Other Specified Code Manifestation Code ►◄ Revised Text ● New Code ▲ Revised Code Title

ICD-10-CM 2014 (Draft) 913

√7th **S92.136** Nondisplaced **fracture of posterior process of unspecified talus**

√6th **S92.14** Dome **fracture of talus**
     EXCLUDES 1   osteochondritis dissecans (M93.2)
√7th **S92.141** Displaced **dome fracture of** right **talus**
√7th **S92.142** Displaced **dome fracture of** left **talus**
√7th **S92.143** Displaced **dome fracture of unspecified talus**
√7th **S92.144** Nondisplaced **dome fracture of** right **talus**
√7th **S92.145** Nondisplaced **dome fracture of** left **talus**
√7th **S92.146** Nondisplaced **dome fracture of unspecified talus**

√6th **S92.15** Avulsion **fracture (chip fracture) of talus**
√7th **S92.151** Displaced **avulsion fracture (chip fracture) of** right **talus**
√7th **S92.152** Displaced **avulsion fracture (chip fracture) of** left **talus**
√7th **S92.153** Displaced **avulsion fracture (chip fracture) of unspecified talus**
√7th **S92.154** Nondisplaced **avulsion fracture (chip fracture) of** right **talus**
√7th **S92.155** Nondisplaced **avulsion fracture (chip fracture) of** left **talus**
√7th **S92.156** Nondisplaced **avulsion fracture (chip fracture) of unspecified talus**

√6th **S92.19** Other **fracture of talus**
√7th **S92.191** Other **fracture of** right **talus**
√7th **S92.192** Other **fracture of** left **talus**
√7th **S92.199** Other **fracture of unspecified talus**

√5th **S92.2** Fracture of other and unspecified tarsal bone(s)
√6th **S92.20** Fracture of unspecified tarsal bone(s)
√7th **S92.201** Fracture of unspecified tarsal bone(s) of right foot
√7th **S92.202** Fracture of unspecified tarsal bone(s) of left foot
√7th **S92.209** Fracture of unspecified tarsal bone(s) of unspecified foot

√6th **S92.21** Fracture of cuboid bone
√7th **S92.211** Displaced **fracture of cuboid bone of** right **foot**
√7th **S92.212** Displaced **fracture of cuboid bone of** left **foot**
√7th **S92.213** Displaced **fracture of cuboid bone of unspecified foot**
√7th **S92.214** Nondisplaced **fracture of cuboid bone of** right **foot**
√7th **S92.215** Nondisplaced **fracture of cuboid bone of** left **foot**
√7th **S92.216** Nondisplaced **fracture of cuboid bone of unspecified foot**

√6th **S92.22** Fracture of lateral cuneiform
√7th **S92.221** Displaced **fracture of lateral cuneiform of** right **foot**
√7th **S92.222** Displaced **fracture of lateral cuneiform of** left **foot**
√7th **S92.223** Displaced **fracture of lateral cuneiform of unspecified foot**
√7th **S92.224** Nondisplaced **fracture of lateral cuneiform of** right **foot**
√7th **S92.225** Nondisplaced **fracture of lateral cuneiform of** left **foot**
√7th **S92.226** Nondisplaced **fracture of lateral cuneiform of unspecified foot**

√6th **S92.23** Fracture of intermediate cuneiform
√7th **S92.231** Displaced **fracture of intermediate cuneiform of** right **foot**
√7th **S92.232** Displaced **fracture of intermediate cuneiform of** left **foot**
√7th **S92.233** Displaced **fracture of intermediate cuneiform of unspecified foot**
√7th **S92.234** Nondisplaced **fracture of intermediate cuneiform of** right **foot**
√7th **S92.235** Nondisplaced **fracture of intermediate cuneiform of** left **foot**

√7th **S92.236** Nondisplaced **fracture of intermediate cuneiform of unspecified foot**

√6th **S92.24** Fracture of medial cuneiform
√7th **S92.241** Displaced **fracture of medial cuneiform of** right **foot**
√7th **S92.242** Displaced **fracture of medial cuneiform of** left **foot**
√7th **S92.243** Displaced **fracture of medial cuneiform of unspecified foot**
√7th **S92.244** Nondisplaced **fracture of medial cuneiform of** right **foot**
√7th **S92.245** Nondisplaced **fracture of medial cuneiform of** left **foot**
√7th **S92.246** Nondisplaced **fracture of medial cuneiform of unspecified foot**

√6th **S92.25** Fracture of navicular [scaphoid] of foot
√7th **S92.251** Displaced **fracture of navicular [scaphoid] of** right **foot**
√7th **S92.252** Displaced **fracture of navicular [scaphoid] of** left **foot**
√7th **S92.253** Displaced **fracture of navicular [scaphoid] of unspecified foot**
√7th **S92.254** Nondisplaced **fracture of navicular [scaphoid] of** right **foot**
√7th **S92.255** Nondisplaced **fracture of navicular [scaphoid] of** left **foot**
√7th **S92.256** Nondisplaced **fracture of navicular [scaphoid] of unspecified foot**

√5th **S92.3** Fracture of metatarsal bone(s)
√6th **S92.30** Fracture of unspecified metatarsal bone(s)
√7th **S92.301** Fracture of unspecified metatarsal bone(s), right foot
√7th **S92.302** Fracture of unspecified metatarsal bone(s), left foot
√7th **S92.309** Fracture of unspecified metatarsal bone(s), unspecified foot

√6th **S92.31** Fracture of first metatarsal bone
√7th **S92.311** Displaced **fracture of first metatarsal bone,** right **foot**
√7th **S92.312** Displaced **fracture of first metatarsal bone,** left **foot**
√7th **S92.313** Displaced **fracture of first metatarsal bone, unspecified foot**
√7th **S92.314** Nondisplaced **fracture of first metatarsal bone,** right **foot**
√7th **S92.315** Nondisplaced **fracture of first metatarsal bone,** left **foot**
√7th **S92.316** Nondisplaced **fracture of first metatarsal bone, unspecified foot**

√6th **S92.32** Fracture of second metatarsal bone
√7th **S92.321** Displaced **fracture of second metatarsal bone,** right **foot**
√7th **S92.322** Displaced **fracture of second metatarsal bone,** left **foot**
√7th **S92.323** Displaced **fracture of second metatarsal bone, unspecified foot**
√7th **S92.324** Nondisplaced **fracture of second metatarsal bone,** right **foot**
√7th **S92.325** Nondisplaced **fracture of second metatarsal bone,** left **foot**
√7th **S92.326** Nondisplaced **fracture of second metatarsal bone, unspecified foot**

√6th **S92.33** Fracture of third metatarsal bone
√7th **S92.331** Displaced **fracture of third metatarsal bone,** right **foot**
√7th **S92.332** Displaced **fracture of third metatarsal bone,** left **foot**
√7th **S92.333** Displaced **fracture of third metatarsal bone, unspecified foot**
√7th **S92.334** Nondisplaced **fracture of third metatarsal bone,** right **foot**
√7th **S92.335** Nondisplaced **fracture of third metatarsal bone,** left **foot**
√7th **S92.336** Nondisplaced **fracture of third metatarsal bone, unspecified foot**

EXCLUDES 1 Not coded here   *EXCLUDES 2* Not included here   N Newborn Age: 0   P Pediatric Age: 0-17   M Maternity Age: 12-55   A Adult Age: 15-124

914   ICD-10-CM 2014 (Draft)

✓6ᵗʰ **S92.34** Fracture of fourth metatarsal bone

    ✓7ᵗʰ **S92.341** Displaced fracture of fourth metatarsal bone, right foot

    ✓7ᵗʰ **S92.342** Displaced fracture of fourth metatarsal bone, left foot

    ✓7ᵗʰ **S92.343** Displaced fracture of fourth metatarsal bone, unspecified foot

    ✓7ᵗʰ **S92.344** Nondisplaced fracture of fourth metatarsal bone, right foot

    ✓7ᵗʰ **S92.345** Nondisplaced fracture of fourth metatarsal bone, left foot

    ✓7ᵗʰ **S92.346** Nondisplaced fracture of fourth metatarsal bone, unspecified foot

✓6ᵗʰ **S92.35** Fracture of fifth metatarsal bone

    ✓7ᵗʰ **S92.351** Displaced fracture of fifth metatarsal bone, right foot

    ✓7ᵗʰ **S92.352** Displaced fracture of fifth metatarsal bone, left foot

    ✓7ᵗʰ **S92.353** Displaced fracture of fifth metatarsal bone, unspecified foot

    ✓7ᵗʰ **S92.354** Nondisplaced fracture of fifth metatarsal bone, right foot

    ✓7ᵗʰ **S92.355** Nondisplaced fracture of fifth metatarsal bone, left foot

    ✓7ᵗʰ **S92.356** Nondisplaced fracture of fifth metatarsal bone, unspecified foot

✓5ᵗʰ **S92.4** Fracture of great toe

   ✓6ᵗʰ **S92.40** Unspecified fracture of great toe

    ✓7ᵗʰ **S92.401** Displaced unspecified fracture of right great toe

    ✓7ᵗʰ **S92.402** Displaced unspecified fracture of left great toe

    ✓7ᵗʰ **S92.403** Displaced unspecified fracture of unspecified great toe

    ✓7ᵗʰ **S92.404** Nondisplaced unspecified fracture of right great toe

    ✓7ᵗʰ **S92.405** Nondisplaced unspecified fracture of left great toe

    ✓7ᵗʰ **S92.406** Nondisplaced unspecified fracture of unspecified great toe

   ✓6ᵗʰ **S92.41** Fracture of proximal phalanx of great toe

    ✓7ᵗʰ **S92.411** Displaced fracture of proximal phalanx of right great toe

    ✓7ᵗʰ **S92.412** Displaced fracture of proximal phalanx of left great toe

    ✓7ᵗʰ **S92.413** Displaced fracture of proximal phalanx of unspecified great toe

    ✓7ᵗʰ **S92.414** Nondisplaced fracture of proximal phalanx of right great toe

    ✓7ᵗʰ **S92.415** Nondisplaced fracture of proximal phalanx of left great toe

    ✓7ᵗʰ **S92.416** Nondisplaced fracture of proximal phalanx of unspecified great toe

   ✓6ᵗʰ **S92.42** Fracture of distal phalanx of great toe

    ✓7ᵗʰ **S92.421** Displaced fracture of distal phalanx of right great toe

    ✓7ᵗʰ **S92.422** Displaced fracture of distal phalanx of left great toe

    ✓7ᵗʰ **S92.423** Displaced fracture of distal phalanx of unspecified great toe

    ✓7ᵗʰ **S92.424** Nondisplaced fracture of distal phalanx of right great toe

    ✓7ᵗʰ **S92.425** Nondisplaced fracture of distal phalanx of left great toe

    ✓7ᵗʰ **S92.426** Nondisplaced fracture of distal phalanx of unspecified great toe

   ✓6ᵗʰ **S92.49** Other fracture of great toe

    ✓7ᵗʰ **S92.491** Other fracture of right great toe

    ✓7ᵗʰ **S92.492** Other fracture of left great toe

    ✓7ᵗʰ **S92.499** Other fracture of unspecified great toe

✓5ᵗʰ **S92.5** Fracture of lesser toe(s)

   ✓6ᵗʰ **S92.50** Unspecified fracture of lesser toe(s)

    ✓7ᵗʰ **S92.501** Displaced unspecified fracture of right lesser toe(s)

    ✓7ᵗʰ **S92.502** Displaced unspecified fracture of left lesser toe(s)

    ✓7ᵗʰ **S92.503** Displaced unspecified fracture of unspecified lesser toe(s)

    ✓7ᵗʰ **S92.504** Nondisplaced unspecified fracture of right lesser toe(s)

    ✓7ᵗʰ **S92.505** Nondisplaced unspecified fracture of left lesser toe(s)

    ✓7ᵗʰ **S92.506** Nondisplaced unspecified fracture of unspecified lesser toe(s)

   ✓6ᵗʰ **S92.51** Fracture of proximal phalanx of lesser toe(s)

    ✓7ᵗʰ **S92.511** Displaced fracture of proximal phalanx of right lesser toe(s)

    ✓7ᵗʰ **S92.512** Displaced fracture of proximal phalanx of left lesser toe(s)

    ✓7ᵗʰ **S92.513** Displaced fracture of proximal phalanx of unspecified lesser toe(s)

    ✓7ᵗʰ **S92.514** Nondisplaced fracture of proximal phalanx of right lesser toe(s)

    ✓7ᵗʰ **S92.515** Nondisplaced fracture of proximal phalanx of left lesser toe(s)

    ✓7ᵗʰ **S92.516** Nondisplaced fracture of proximal phalanx of unspecified lesser toe(s)

   ✓6ᵗʰ **S92.52** Fracture of medial phalanx of lesser toe(s)

    ✓7ᵗʰ **S92.521** Displaced fracture of medial phalanx of right lesser toe(s)

    ✓7ᵗʰ **S92.522** Displaced fracture of medial phalanx of left lesser toe(s)

    ✓7ᵗʰ **S92.523** Displaced fracture of medial phalanx of unspecified lesser toe(s)

    ✓7ᵗʰ **S92.524** Nondisplaced fracture of medial phalanx of right lesser toe(s)

    ✓7ᵗʰ **S92.525** Nondisplaced fracture of medial phalanx of left lesser toe(s)

    ✓7ᵗʰ **S92.526** Nondisplaced fracture of medial phalanx of unspecified lesser toe(s)

   ✓6ᵗʰ **S92.53** Fracture of distal phalanx of lesser toe(s)

    ✓7ᵗʰ **S92.531** Displaced fracture of distal phalanx of right lesser toe(s)

    ✓7ᵗʰ **S92.532** Displaced fracture of distal phalanx of left lesser toe(s)

    ✓7ᵗʰ **S92.533** Displaced fracture of distal phalanx of unspecified lesser toe(s)

    ✓7ᵗʰ **S92.534** Nondisplaced fracture of distal phalanx of right lesser toe(s)

    ✓7ᵗʰ **S92.535** Nondisplaced fracture of distal phalanx of left lesser toe(s)

    ✓7ᵗʰ **S92.536** Nondisplaced fracture of distal phalanx of unspecified lesser toe(s)

   ✓6ᵗʰ **S92.59** Other fracture of lesser toe(s)

    ✓7ᵗʰ **S92.591** Other fracture of right lesser toe(s)

    ✓7ᵗʰ **S92.592** Other fracture of left lesser toe(s)

    ✓7ᵗʰ **S92.599** Other fracture of unspecified lesser toe(s)

✓5ᵗʰ **S92.9** Unspecified fracture of foot and toe

   ✓6ᵗʰ **S92.90** Unspecified fracture of foot

    ✓7ᵗʰ **S92.901** Unspecified fracture of right foot

    ✓7ᵗʰ **S92.902** Unspecified fracture of left foot

    ✓7ᵗʰ **S92.909** Unspecified fracture of unspecified foot

   ✓6ᵗʰ **S92.91** Unspecified fracture of toe

    ✓7ᵗʰ **S92.911** Unspecified fracture of right toe(s)

    ✓7ᵗʰ **S92.912** Unspecified fracture of left toe(s)

    ✓7ᵗʰ **S92.919** Unspecified fracture of unspecified toe(s)

✓ Additional Character Required   ✓x7ᵗʰ Xtension Alert   Unspecified Code   Other Specified Code   Manifestation Code   ►◄ Revised Text   ● New Code   ▲ Revised Code Title

ICD-10-CM 2014 (Draft)   **915**

✓4ᵗʰ **S93 Dislocation and sprain of joints and ligaments at ankle, foot and toe level**

     INCLUDES   avulsion of joint or ligament of ankle, foot and toe
                 laceration of cartilage, joint or ligament of ankle, foot and toe
                 sprain of cartilage, joint or ligament of ankle, foot and toe
                 traumatic hemarthrosis of joint or ligament of ankle, foot and toe
                 traumatic rupture of joint or ligament of ankle, foot and toe
                 traumatic subluxation of joint or ligament of ankle, foot and toe
                 traumatic tear of joint or ligament of ankle, foot and toe

     Code also any associated open wound

     EXCLUDES 2   *strain of muscle and tendon of ankle and foot (S96.-)*

> The appropriate 7th character is to be added to each code from category S93.
> A   initial encounter
> D   subsequent encounter
> S   sequela

✓5ᵗʰ **S93.0 Subluxation and dislocation of** ankle joint
     Subluxation and dislocation of astragalus
     Subluxation and dislocation of fibula, lower end
     Subluxation and dislocation of talus
     Subluxation and dislocation of tibia, lower end

     ✓x7ᵗʰ **S93.01 Subluxation** of right ankle joint
     ✓x7ᵗʰ **S93.02 Subluxation** of left ankle joint
     ✓x7ᵗʰ **S93.03 Subluxation of unspecified ankle joint**
     ✓x7ᵗʰ **S93.04 Dislocation** of right ankle joint
     ✓x7ᵗʰ **S93.05 Dislocation** of left ankle joint
     ✓x7ᵗʰ **S93.06 Dislocation of unspecified ankle joint**

✓5ᵗʰ **S93.1 Subluxation and dislocation of** toe
     ✓6ᵗʰ **S93.10 Unspecified subluxation and dislocation of toe**
         Dislocation of toe NOS
         Subluxation of toe NOS

         ✓7ᵗʰ **S93.101 Unspecified** subluxation of right toe(s)
         ✓7ᵗʰ **S93.102 Unspecified** subluxation of left toe(s)
         ✓7ᵗʰ **S93.103 Unspecified** subluxation of unspecified toe(s)
         ✓7ᵗʰ **S93.104 Unspecified** dislocation of right toe(s)
         ✓7ᵗʰ **S93.105 Unspecified** dislocation of left toe(s)
         ✓7ᵗʰ **S93.106 Unspecified** dislocation of unspecified toe(s)

     ✓6ᵗʰ **S93.11 Dislocation of** interphalangeal joint
         ✓7ᵗʰ **S93.111 Dislocation of interphalangeal joint of** right great toe
         ✓7ᵗʰ **S93.112 Dislocation of interphalangeal joint of** left great toe
         ✓7ᵗʰ **S93.113 Dislocation of interphalangeal joint of unspecified great toe**
         ✓7ᵗʰ **S93.114 Dislocation of interphalangeal joint of right lesser** toe(s)
         ✓7ᵗʰ **S93.115 Dislocation of interphalangeal joint of** left lesser toe(s)
         ✓7ᵗʰ **S93.116 Dislocation of interphalangeal joint of unspecified lesser toe(s)**
         ✓7ᵗʰ **S93.119 Dislocation of interphalangeal joint of unspecified toe(s)**

     ✓6ᵗʰ **S93.12 Dislocation of** metatarsophalangeal joint
         ✓7ᵗʰ **S93.121 Dislocation of metatarsophalangeal joint of right great toe**
         ✓7ᵗʰ **S93.122 Dislocation of metatarsophalangeal joint of left great toe**
         ✓7ᵗʰ **S93.123 Dislocation of metatarsophalangeal joint of unspecified great toe**
         ✓7ᵗʰ **S93.124 Dislocation of metatarsophalangeal joint of right lesser toe(s)**
         ✓7ᵗʰ **S93.125 Dislocation of metatarsophalangeal joint of left lesser toe(s)**
         ✓7ᵗʰ **S93.126 Dislocation of metatarsophalangeal joint of unspecified lesser toe(s)**
         ✓7ᵗʰ **S93.129 Dislocation of metatarsophalangeal joint of unspecified toe(s)**

✓6ᵗʰ **S93.13 Subluxation of** interphalangeal joint
     ✓7ᵗʰ **S93.131 Subluxation of interphalangeal joint of right great toe**
     ✓7ᵗʰ **S93.132 Subluxation of interphalangeal joint of left great toe**
     ✓7ᵗʰ **S93.133 Subluxation of interphalangeal joint of unspecified great toe**
     ✓7ᵗʰ **S93.134 Subluxation of interphalangeal joint of right lesser toe(s)**
     ✓7ᵗʰ **S93.135 Subluxation of interphalangeal joint of left lesser toe(s)**
     ✓7ᵗʰ **S93.136 Subluxation of interphalangeal joint of unspecified lesser toe(s)**
     ✓7ᵗʰ **S93.139 Subluxation of interphalangeal joint of unspecified toe(s)**

✓6ᵗʰ **S93.14 Subluxation of** metatarsophalangeal joint
     ✓7ᵗʰ **S93.141 Subluxation of metatarsophalangeal joint of right great toe**
     ✓7ᵗʰ **S93.142 Subluxation of metatarsophalangeal joint of left great toe**
     ✓7ᵗʰ **S93.143 Subluxation of metatarsophalangeal joint of unspecified great toe**
     ✓7ᵗʰ **S93.144 Subluxation of metatarsophalangeal joint of right lesser toe(s)**
     ✓7ᵗʰ **S93.145 Subluxation of metatarsophalangeal joint of left lesser toe(s)**
     ✓7ᵗʰ **S93.146 Subluxation of metatarsophalangeal joint of unspecified lesser toe(s)**
     ✓7ᵗʰ **S93.149 Subluxation of metatarsophalangeal joint of unspecified toe(s)**

✓5ᵗʰ **S93.3 Subluxation and dislocation of** foot
     EXCLUDES 2   *dislocation of toe (S93.1-)*

     ✓6ᵗʰ **S93.30 Unspecified subluxation and dislocation of foot**
         Dislocation of foot NOS
         Subluxation of foot NOS

         ✓7ᵗʰ **S93.301 Unspecified** subluxation of right foot
         ✓7ᵗʰ **S93.302 Unspecified** subluxation of left foot
         ✓7ᵗʰ **S93.303 Unspecified** subluxation of unspecified foot
         ✓7ᵗʰ **S93.304 Unspecified** dislocation of right foot
         ✓7ᵗʰ **S93.305 Unspecified** dislocation of left foot
         ✓7ᵗʰ **S93.306 Unspecified** dislocation of unspecified foot

     ✓6ᵗʰ **S93.31 Subluxation and dislocation of** tarsal joint
         ✓7ᵗʰ **S93.311 Subluxation of tarsal joint of** right foot
         ✓7ᵗʰ **S93.312 Subluxation of tarsal joint of** left foot
         ✓7ᵗʰ **S93.313 Subluxation of tarsal joint of unspecified foot**
         ✓7ᵗʰ **S93.314 Dislocation** of tarsal joint of right foot
         ✓7ᵗʰ **S93.315 Dislocation** of tarsal joint of left foot
         ✓7ᵗʰ **S93.316 Dislocation of tarsal joint of unspecified foot**

     ✓6ᵗʰ **S93.32 Subluxation and dislocation of** tarsometatarsal joint
         ✓7ᵗʰ **S93.321 Subluxation of tarsometatarsal joint of right foot**
         ✓7ᵗʰ **S93.322 Subluxation of tarsometatarsal joint of left foot**
         ✓7ᵗʰ **S93.323 Subluxation of tarsometatarsal joint of unspecified foot**
         ✓7ᵗʰ **S93.324 Dislocation of tarsometatarsal joint of right foot**
         ✓7ᵗʰ **S93.325 Dislocation of tarsometatarsal joint of** left foot
         ✓7ᵗʰ **S93.326 Dislocation of tarsometatarsal joint of unspecified foot**

     ✓6ᵗʰ **S93.33 Other subluxation and dislocation of foot**
         ✓7ᵗʰ **S93.331 Other** subluxation of right foot
         ✓7ᵗʰ **S93.332 Other** subluxation of left foot
         ✓7ᵗʰ **S93.333 Other** subluxation of unspecified foot
         ✓7ᵗʰ **S93.334 Other** dislocation of right foot
         ✓7ᵗʰ **S93.335 Other** dislocation of left foot
         ✓7ᵗʰ **S93.336 Other** dislocation of unspecified foot

EXCLUDES 1 Not coded here   EXCLUDES 2 Not included here   N Newborn Age: 0   P Pediatric Age: 0-17   M Maternity Age: 12-55   A Adult Age: 15-124

916   ICD-10-CM 2014 (Draft)

√5ᵗʰ **S93.4 Sprain of** ankle
  EXCLUDES 2 *injury of Achilles tendon (S86.0-)*

√6ᵗʰ **S93.40 Sprain of** unspecified **ligament of ankle**
    Sprain of ankle NOS
    Sprained ankle NOS

√7ᵗʰ **S93.401 Sprain of unspecified ligament of** right **ankle**

√7ᵗʰ **S93.402 Sprain of unspecified ligament of** left **ankle**

√7ᵗʰ **S93.409 Sprain of unspecified ligament of unspecified ankle**

√6ᵗʰ **S93.41 Sprain of** calcaneofibular **ligament**

√7ᵗʰ **S93.411 Sprain of calcaneofibular ligament of** right **ankle**

√7ᵗʰ **S93.412 Sprain of calcaneofibular ligament of** left **ankle**

√7ᵗʰ **S93.419 Sprain of calcaneofibular ligament of unspecified ankle**

√6ᵗʰ **S93.42 Sprain of** deltoid **ligament**

√7ᵗʰ **S93.421 Sprain of deltoid ligament of** right **ankle**

√7ᵗʰ **S93.422 Sprain of deltoid ligament of** left **ankle**

√7ᵗʰ **S93.429 Sprain of deltoid ligament of unspecified ankle**

√6ᵗʰ **S93.43 Sprain of** tibiofibular **ligament**

√7ᵗʰ **S93.431 Sprain of tibiofibular ligament of** right **ankle**

√7ᵗʰ **S93.432 Sprain of tibiofibular ligament of** left **ankle**

√7ᵗʰ **S93.439 Sprain of tibiofibular ligament of unspecified ankle**

√6ᵗʰ **S93.49 Sprain of** other **ligament of ankle**
    Sprain of internal collateral ligament
    Sprain of talofibular ligament

√7ᵗʰ **S93.491 Sprain of other ligament of** right **ankle**

√7ᵗʰ **S93.492 Sprain of other ligament of** left **ankle**

√7ᵗʰ **S93.499 Sprain of other ligament of unspecified ankle**

√5ᵗʰ **S93.5 Sprain of** toe

√6ᵗʰ **S93.50 Unspecified sprain of toe**

√7ᵗʰ **S93.501 Unspecified sprain of** right great **toe**

√7ᵗʰ **S93.502 Unspecified sprain of** left great **toe**

√7ᵗʰ **S93.503 Unspecified sprain of unspecified great toe**

√7ᵗʰ **S93.504 Unspecified sprain of** right lesser **toe(s)**

√7ᵗʰ **S93.505 Unspecified sprain of** left lesser **toe(s)**

√7ᵗʰ **S93.506 Unspecified sprain of unspecified lesser toe(s)**

√7ᵗʰ **S93.509 Unspecified sprain of unspecified toe(s)**

√6ᵗʰ **S93.51 Sprain of** interphalangeal joint **of toe**

√7ᵗʰ **S93.511 Sprain of interphalangeal joint of** right great **toe**

√7ᵗʰ **S93.512 Sprain of interphalangeal joint of** left great **toe**

√7ᵗʰ **S93.513 Sprain of interphalangeal joint of unspecified great toe**

√7ᵗʰ **S93.514 Sprain of interphalangeal joint of** right lesser **toe(s)**

√7ᵗʰ **S93.515 Sprain of interphalangeal joint of** left lesser **toe(s)**

√7ᵗʰ **S93.516 Sprain of interphalangeal joint of unspecified lesser toe(s)**

√7ᵗʰ **S93.519 Sprain of interphalangeal joint of unspecified toe(s)**

√6ᵗʰ **S93.52 Sprain of** metatarsophalangeal joint **of toe**

√7ᵗʰ **S93.521 Sprain of metatarsophalangeal joint of right great toe**

√7ᵗʰ **S93.522 Sprain of metatarsophalangeal joint of left great toe**

√7ᵗʰ **S93.523 Sprain of metatarsophalangeal joint of unspecified great toe**

√7ᵗʰ **S93.524 Sprain of metatarsophalangeal joint of right lesser toe(s)**

√7ᵗʰ **S93.525 Sprain of metatarsophalangeal joint of left lesser toe(s)**

√7ᵗʰ **S93.526 Sprain of metatarsophalangeal joint of unspecified lesser toe(s)**

√7ᵗʰ **S93.529 Sprain of metatarsophalangeal joint of unspecified toe(s)**

√5ᵗʰ **S93.6 Sprain of** foot
  EXCLUDES 2 *sprain of metatarsophalangeal joint of toe (S93.52-)*
    sprain of toe (S93.5-)

√6ᵗʰ **S93.60 Unspecified sprain of foot**

√7ᵗʰ **S93.601 Unspecified sprain of** right **foot**

√7ᵗʰ **S93.602 Unspecified sprain of** left **foot**

√7ᵗʰ **S93.609 Unspecified sprain of unspecified foot**

√6ᵗʰ **S93.61 Sprain of** tarsal ligament **of foot**

√7ᵗʰ **S93.611 Sprain of tarsal ligament of** right **foot**

√7ᵗʰ **S93.612 Sprain of tarsal ligament of** left **foot**

√7ᵗʰ **S93.619 Sprain of tarsal ligament of unspecified foot**

√6ᵗʰ **S93.62 Sprain of** tarsometatarsal ligament **of foot**

√7ᵗʰ **S93.621 Sprain of tarsometatarsal ligament of** right **foot**

√7ᵗʰ **S93.622 Sprain of tarsometatarsal ligament of** left **foot**

√7ᵗʰ **S93.629 Sprain of tarsometatarsal ligament of unspecified foot**

√6ᵗʰ **S93.69 Other sprain of foot**

√7ᵗʰ **S93.691 Other sprain of** right **foot**

√7ᵗʰ **S93.692 Other sprain of** left **foot**

√7ᵗʰ **S93.699 Other sprain of unspecified foot**

√4ᵗʰ **S94 Injury of nerves at ankle and foot level**
  Code also any associated open wound (S91.-)

  The appropriate 7th character is to be added to each code from category S94.
  A   initial encounter
  D   subsequent encounter
  S   sequela

√5ᵗʰ **S94.0 Injury of** lateral plantar **nerve**

√x7ᵗʰ **S94.00 Injury of lateral plantar nerve, unspecified leg**

√x7ᵗʰ **S94.01 Injury of lateral plantar nerve,** right **leg**

√x7ᵗʰ **S94.02 Injury of lateral plantar nerve,** left **leg**

√5ᵗʰ **S94.1 Injury of** medial plantar **nerve**

√x7ᵗʰ **S94.10 Injury of medial plantar nerve, unspecified leg**

√x7ᵗʰ **S94.11 Injury of medial plantar nerve,** right **leg**

√x7ᵗʰ **S94.12 Injury of medial plantar nerve,** left **leg**

√5ᵗʰ **S94.2 Injury of** deep peroneal **nerve at ankle and foot level**
    Injury of terminal, lateral branch of deep peroneal nerve

√x7ᵗʰ **S94.20 Injury of deep peroneal nerve at ankle and foot level, unspecified leg**

√x7ᵗʰ **S94.21 Injury of deep peroneal nerve at ankle and foot level,** right **leg**

√x7ᵗʰ **S94.22 Injury of deep peroneal nerve at ankle and foot level,** left **leg**

√5ᵗʰ **S94.3 Injury of** cutaneous sensory **nerve at ankle and foot level**

√x7ᵗʰ **S94.30 Injury of cutaneous sensory nerve at ankle and foot level, unspecified leg**

√x7ᵗʰ **S94.31 Injury of cutaneous sensory nerve at ankle and foot level,** right **leg**

√x7ᵗʰ **S94.32 Injury of cutaneous sensory nerve at ankle and foot level,** left **leg**

√5ᵗʰ **S94.8 Injury of** other **nerves at ankle and foot level**

√6ᵗʰ **S94.8X Injury of other nerves at ankle and foot level**

√7ᵗʰ **S94.8X1 Injury of other nerves at ankle and foot level,** right **leg**

√7ᵗʰ **S94.8X2 Injury of other nerves at ankle and foot level,** left **leg**

√7ᵗʰ **S94.8X9 Injury of other nerves at ankle and foot level, unspecified leg**

√5ᵗʰ **S94.9 Injury of** unspecified **nerve at ankle and foot level**

✓Additional Character Required   √x7ᵗʰ Xtension Alert   Unspecified Code   Other Specified Code   Manifestation Code   ►◄ Revised Text   ● New Code   ▲ Revised Code Title

ICD-10-CM 2014 (Draft)   917

S94.90 Injury of unspecified nerve at ankle and foot level, unspecified leg

S94.91 Injury of unspecified nerve at ankle and foot level, right leg

S94.92 Injury of unspecified nerve at ankle and foot level, left leg

S95   Injury of blood vessels at ankle and foot level

Code also any associated open wound (S91.-)

EXCLUDES 2   injury of posterior tibial artery and vein (S85.1-, S85.8-)

The appropriate 7th character is to be added to each code from category S95.
A   initial encounter
D   subsequent encounter
S   sequela

S95.0   Injury of dorsal artery of foot

   S95.00   Unspecified injury of dorsal artery of foot

     S95.001   Unspecified injury of dorsal artery of right foot

     S95.002   Unspecified injury of dorsal artery of left foot

     S95.009   Unspecified injury of dorsal artery of unspecified foot

   S95.01   Laceration of dorsal artery of foot

     S95.011   Laceration of dorsal artery of right foot

     S95.012   Laceration of dorsal artery of left foot

     S95.019   Laceration of dorsal artery of unspecified foot

   S95.09   Other specified injury of dorsal artery of foot

     S95.091   Other specified injury of dorsal artery of right foot

     S95.092   Other specified injury of dorsal artery of left foot

     S95.099   Other specified injury of dorsal artery of unspecified foot

S95.1   Injury of plantar artery of foot

   S95.10   Unspecified injury of plantar artery of foot

     S95.101   Unspecified injury of plantar artery of right foot

     S95.102   Unspecified injury of plantar artery of left foot

     S95.109   Unspecified injury of plantar artery of unspecified foot

   S95.11   Laceration of plantar artery of foot

     S95.111   Laceration of plantar artery of right foot

     S95.112   Laceration of plantar artery of left foot

     S95.119   Laceration of plantar artery of unspecified foot

   S95.19   Other specified injury of plantar artery of foot

     S95.191   Other specified injury of plantar artery of right foot

     S95.192   Other specified injury of plantar artery of left foot

     S95.199   Other specified injury of plantar artery of unspecified foot

S95.2   Injury of dorsal vein of foot

   S95.20   Unspecified injury of dorsal vein of foot

     S95.201   Unspecified injury of dorsal vein of right foot

     S95.202   Unspecified injury of dorsal vein of left foot

     S95.209   Unspecified injury of dorsal vein of unspecified foot

   S95.21   Laceration of dorsal vein of foot

     S95.211   Laceration of dorsal vein of right foot

     S95.212   Laceration of dorsal vein of left foot

     S95.219   Laceration of dorsal vein of unspecified foot

   S95.29   Other specified injury of dorsal vein of foot

     S95.291   Other specified injury of dorsal vein of right foot

     S95.292   Other specified injury of dorsal vein of left foot

     S95.299   Other specified injury of dorsal vein of unspecified foot

S95.8   Injury of other blood vessels at ankle and foot level

   S95.80   Unspecified injury of other blood vessels at ankle and foot level

     S95.801   Unspecified injury of other blood vessels at ankle and foot level, right leg

     S95.802   Unspecified injury of other blood vessels at ankle and foot level, left leg

     S95.809   Unspecified injury of other blood vessels at ankle and foot level, unspecified leg

   S95.81   Laceration of other blood vessels at ankle and foot level

     S95.811   Laceration of other blood vessels at ankle and foot level, right leg

     S95.812   Laceration of other blood vessels at ankle and foot level, left leg

     S95.819   Laceration of other blood vessels at ankle and foot level, unspecified leg

   S95.89   Other specified injury of other blood vessels at ankle and foot level

     S95.891   Other specified injury of other blood vessels at ankle and foot level, right leg

     S95.892   Other specified injury of other blood vessels at ankle and foot level, left leg

     S95.899   Other specified injury of other blood vessels at ankle and foot level, unspecified leg

S95.9   Injury of unspecified blood vessel at ankle and foot level

   S95.90   Unspecified injury of unspecified blood vessel at ankle and foot level

     S95.901   Unspecified injury of unspecified blood vessel at ankle and foot level, right leg

     S95.902   Unspecified injury of unspecified blood vessel at ankle and foot level, left leg

     S95.909   Unspecified injury of unspecified blood vessel at ankle and foot level, unspecified leg

   S95.91   Laceration of unspecified blood vessel at ankle and foot level

     S95.911   Laceration of unspecified blood vessel at ankle and foot level, right leg

     S95.912   Laceration of unspecified blood vessel at ankle and foot level, left leg

     S95.919   Laceration of unspecified blood vessel at ankle and foot level, unspecified leg

   S95.99   Other specified injury of unspecified blood vessel at ankle and foot level

     S95.991   Other specified injury of unspecified blood vessel at ankle and foot level, right leg

     S95.992   Other specified injury of unspecified blood vessel at ankle and foot level, left leg

     S95.999   Other specified injury of unspecified blood vessel at ankle and foot level, unspecified leg

S96   Injury of muscle and tendon at ankle and foot level

Code also any associated open wound (S91.-)

EXCLUDES 2   injury of Achilles tendon (S86.0-)
                sprain of joints and ligaments of ankle and foot (S93.-)

The appropriate 7th character is to be added to each code from category S96.
A   initial encounter
D   subsequent encounter
S   sequela

S96.0   Injury of muscle and tendon of long flexor muscle of toe at ankle and foot level

   S96.00   Unspecified injury of muscle and tendon of long flexor muscle of toe at ankle and foot level

     S96.001   Unspecified injury of muscle and tendon of long flexor muscle of toe at ankle and foot level, right foot

     S96.002   Unspecified injury of muscle and tendon of long flexor muscle of toe at ankle and foot level, left foot

EXCLUDES 1 Not coded here   EXCLUDES 2 Not included here   N Newborn Age: 0   P Pediatric Age: 0-17   M Maternity Age: 12-55   A Adult Age: 15-124

918   ICD-10-CM 2014 (Draft)

√7ᵗʰ **S96.009** Unspecified injury of muscle and tendon of long flexor muscle of toe at ankle and foot level, unspecified foot

√6ᵗʰ **S96.01** Strain of muscle and tendon of long flexor muscle of toe at ankle and foot level

√7ᵗʰ **S96.011** Strain of muscle and tendon of long flexor muscle of toe at ankle and foot level, right foot

√7ᵗʰ **S96.012** Strain of muscle and tendon of long flexor muscle of toe at ankle and foot level, left foot

√7ᵗʰ **S96.019** Strain of muscle and tendon of long flexor muscle of toe at ankle and foot level, unspecified foot

√6ᵗʰ **S96.02** Laceration of muscle and tendon of long flexor muscle of toe at ankle and foot level

√7ᵗʰ **S96.021** Laceration of muscle and tendon of long flexor muscle of toe at ankle and foot level, right foot

√7ᵗʰ **S96.022** Laceration of muscle and tendon of long flexor muscle of toe at ankle and foot level, left foot

√7ᵗʰ **S96.029** Laceration of muscle and tendon of long flexor muscle of toe at ankle and foot level, unspecified foot

√6ᵗʰ **S96.09** Other injury of muscle and tendon of long flexor muscle of toe at ankle and foot level

√7ᵗʰ **S96.091** Other injury of muscle and tendon of long flexor muscle of toe at ankle and foot level, right foot

√7ᵗʰ **S96.092** Other injury of muscle and tendon of long flexor muscle of toe at ankle and foot level, left foot

√7ᵗʰ **S96.099** Other injury of muscle and tendon of long flexor muscle of toe at ankle and foot level, unspecified foot

√5ᵗʰ **S96.1** Injury of muscle and tendon of long extensor muscle of toe at ankle and foot level

√6ᵗʰ **S96.10** Unspecified injury of muscle and tendon of long extensor muscle of toe at ankle and foot level

√7ᵗʰ **S96.101** Unspecified injury of muscle and tendon of long extensor muscle of toe at ankle and foot level, right foot

√7ᵗʰ **S96.102** Unspecified injury of muscle and tendon of long extensor muscle of toe at ankle and foot level, left foot

√7ᵗʰ **S96.109** Unspecified injury of muscle and tendon of long extensor muscle of toe at ankle and foot level, unspecified foot

√6ᵗʰ **S96.11** Strain of muscle and tendon of long extensor muscle of toe at ankle and foot level

√7ᵗʰ **S96.111** Strain of muscle and tendon of long extensor muscle of toe at ankle and foot level, right foot

√7ᵗʰ **S96.112** Strain of muscle and tendon of long extensor muscle of toe at ankle and foot level, left foot

√7ᵗʰ **S96.119** Strain of muscle and tendon of long extensor muscle of toe at ankle and foot level, unspecified foot

√6ᵗʰ **S96.12** Laceration of muscle and tendon of long extensor muscle of toe at ankle and foot level

√7ᵗʰ **S96.121** Laceration of muscle and tendon of long extensor muscle of toe at ankle and foot level, right foot

√7ᵗʰ **S96.122** Laceration of muscle and tendon of long extensor muscle of toe at ankle and foot level, left foot

√7ᵗʰ **S96.129** Laceration of muscle and tendon of long extensor muscle of toe at ankle and foot level, unspecified foot

√6ᵗʰ **S96.19** Other specified injury of muscle and tendon of long extensor muscle of toe at ankle and foot level

√7ᵗʰ **S96.191** Other specified injury of muscle and tendon of long extensor muscle of toe at ankle and foot level, right foot

√7ᵗʰ **S96.192** Other specified injury of muscle and tendon of long extensor muscle of toe at ankle and foot level, left foot

√7ᵗʰ **S96.199** Other specified injury of muscle and tendon of long extensor muscle of toe at ankle and foot level, unspecified foot

√5ᵗʰ **S96.2** Injury of intrinsic muscle and tendon at ankle and foot level

√6ᵗʰ **S96.20** Unspecified injury of intrinsic muscle and tendon at ankle and foot level

√7ᵗʰ **S96.201** Unspecified injury of intrinsic muscle and tendon at ankle and foot level, right foot

√7ᵗʰ **S96.202** Unspecified injury of intrinsic muscle and tendon at ankle and foot level, left foot

√7ᵗʰ **S96.209** Unspecified injury of intrinsic muscle and tendon at ankle and foot level, unspecified foot

√6ᵗʰ **S96.21** Strain of intrinsic muscle and tendon at ankle and foot level

√7ᵗʰ **S96.211** Strain of intrinsic muscle and tendon at ankle and foot level, right foot

√7ᵗʰ **S96.212** Strain of intrinsic muscle and tendon at ankle and foot level, left foot

√7ᵗʰ **S96.219** Strain of intrinsic muscle and tendon at ankle and foot level, unspecified foot

√6ᵗʰ **S96.22** Laceration of intrinsic muscle and tendon at ankle and foot level

√7ᵗʰ **S96.221** Laceration of intrinsic muscle and tendon at ankle and foot level, right foot

√7ᵗʰ **S96.222** Laceration of intrinsic muscle and tendon at ankle and foot level, left foot

√7ᵗʰ **S96.229** Laceration of intrinsic muscle and tendon at ankle and foot level, unspecified foot

√6ᵗʰ **S96.29** Other specified injury of intrinsic muscle and tendon at ankle and foot level

√7ᵗʰ **S96.291** Other specified injury of intrinsic muscle and tendon at ankle and foot level, right foot

√7ᵗʰ **S96.292** Other specified injury of intrinsic muscle and tendon at ankle and foot level, left foot

√7ᵗʰ **S96.299** Other specified injury of intrinsic muscle and tendon at ankle and foot level, unspecified foot

√5ᵗʰ **S96.8** Injury of other specified muscles and tendons at ankle and foot level

√6ᵗʰ **S96.80** Unspecified injury of other specified muscles and tendons at ankle and foot level

√7ᵗʰ **S96.801** Unspecified injury of other specified muscles and tendons at ankle and foot level, right foot

√7ᵗʰ **S96.802** Unspecified injury of other specified muscles and tendons at ankle and foot level, left foot

√7ᵗʰ **S96.809** Unspecified injury of other specified muscles and tendons at ankle and foot level, unspecified foot

√6ᵗʰ **S96.81** Strain of other specified muscles and tendons at ankle and foot level

√7ᵗʰ **S96.811** Strain of other specified muscles and tendons at ankle and foot level, right foot

√7ᵗʰ **S96.812** Strain of other specified muscles and tendons at ankle and foot level, left foot

√7ᵗʰ **S96.819** Strain of other specified muscles and tendons at ankle and foot level, unspecified foot

√6ᵗʰ **S96.82** Laceration of other specified muscles and tendons at ankle and foot level

√7ᵗʰ **S96.821** Laceration of other specified muscles and tendons at ankle and foot level, right foot

√7ᵗʰ **S96.822** Laceration of other specified muscles and tendons at ankle and foot level, left foot

√7ᵗʰ **S96.829** Laceration of other specified muscles and tendons at ankle and foot level, unspecified foot

☑ Additional Character Required   √7ᵗʰ Xtension Alert   Unspecified Code   Other Specified Code   Manifestation Code   ►◄ Revised Text   ● New Code   ▲ Revised Code Title

ICD-10-CM 2014 (Draft)   919

✓6ᵗʰ **S96.89** Other specified injury of other specified muscles and tendons at ankle and foot level

   ✓7ᵗʰ **S96.891** Other specified injury of other specified muscles and tendons at ankle and foot level, right foot

   ✓7ᵗʰ **S96.892** Other specified injury of other specified muscles and tendons at ankle and foot level, left foot

   ✓7ᵗʰ **S96.899** Other specified injury of other specified muscles and tendons at ankle and foot level, unspecified foot

✓5ᵗʰ **S96.9** Injury of unspecified muscle and tendon at ankle and foot level

   ✓6ᵗʰ **S96.90** Unspecified injury of unspecified muscle and tendon at ankle and foot level

     ✓7ᵗʰ **S96.901** Unspecified injury of unspecified muscle and tendon at ankle and foot level, right foot

     ✓7ᵗʰ **S96.902** Unspecified injury of unspecified muscle and tendon at ankle and foot level, left foot

     ✓7ᵗʰ **S96.909** Unspecified injury of unspecified muscle and tendon at ankle and foot level, unspecified foot

   ✓6ᵗʰ **S96.91** Strain of unspecified muscle and tendon at ankle and foot level

     ✓7ᵗʰ **S96.911** Strain of unspecified muscle and tendon at ankle and foot level, right foot

     ✓7ᵗʰ **S96.912** Strain of unspecified muscle and tendon at ankle and foot level, left foot

     ✓7ᵗʰ **S96.919** Strain of unspecified muscle and tendon at ankle and foot level, unspecified foot

   ✓6ᵗʰ **S96.92** Laceration of unspecified muscle and tendon at ankle and foot level

     ✓7ᵗʰ **S96.921** Laceration of unspecified muscle and tendon at ankle and foot level, right foot

     ✓7ᵗʰ **S96.922** Laceration of unspecified muscle and tendon at ankle and foot level, left foot

     ✓7ᵗʰ **S96.929** Laceration of unspecified muscle and tendon at ankle and foot level, unspecified foot

   ✓6ᵗʰ **S96.99** Other specified injury of unspecified muscle and tendon at ankle and foot level

     ✓7ᵗʰ **S96.991** Other specified injury of unspecified muscle and tendon at ankle and foot level, right foot

     ✓7ᵗʰ **S96.992** Other specified injury of unspecified muscle and tendon at ankle and foot level, left foot

     ✓7ᵗʰ **S96.999** Other specified injury of unspecified muscle and tendon at ankle and foot level, unspecified foot

✓4ᵗʰ **S97** **Crushing injury of ankle and foot**

Use additional code(s) for all associated injuries

The appropriate 7th character is to be added to each code from category S97.
A   initial encounter
D   subsequent encounter
S   sequela

✓5ᵗʰ **S97.0** **Crushing injury of** ankle

   ✓×7ᵗʰ **S97.00** Crushing injury of unspecified ankle

   ✓×7ᵗʰ **S97.01** Crushing injury of right ankle

   ✓×7ᵗʰ **S97.02** Crushing injury of left ankle

✓5ᵗʰ **S97.1** **Crushing injury of** toe

   ✓6ᵗʰ **S97.10** Crushing injury of unspecified toe(s)

     ✓7ᵗʰ **S97.101** Crushing injury of unspecified right toe(s)

     ✓7ᵗʰ **S97.102** Crushing injury of unspecified left toe(s)

     ✓7ᵗʰ **S97.109** Crushing injury of unspecified toe(s)
       Crushing injury of toe NOS

   ✓6ᵗʰ **S97.11** Crushing injury of great toe

     ✓7ᵗʰ **S97.111** Crushing injury of right great toe

     ✓7ᵗʰ **S97.112** Crushing injury of left great toe

     ✓7ᵗʰ **S97.119** Crushing injury of unspecified great toe

   ✓6ᵗʰ **S97.12** Crushing injury of lesser toe(s)

     ✓7ᵗʰ **S97.121** Crushing injury of right lesser toe(s)

     ✓7ᵗʰ **S97.122** Crushing injury of left lesser toe(s)

     ✓7ᵗʰ **S97.129** Crushing injury of unspecified lesser toe(s)

✓5ᵗʰ **S97.8** **Crushing injury of** foot

   ✓×7ᵗʰ **S97.80** Crushing injury of unspecified foot
     Crushing injury of foot NOS

   ✓×7ᵗʰ **S97.81** Crushing injury of right foot

   ✓×7ᵗʰ **S97.82** Crushing injury of left foot

✓4ᵗʰ **S98** **Traumatic amputation of ankle and foot**

An amputation not identified as partial or complete should be coded to complete

The appropriate 7th character is to be added to each code from category S98.
A   initial encounter
D   subsequent encounter
S   sequela

✓5ᵗʰ **S98.0** **Traumatic amputation of** foot at ankle level

   ✓6ᵗʰ **S98.01** Complete traumatic amputation of foot at ankle level

     ✓7ᵗʰ **S98.011** Complete traumatic amputation of right foot at ankle level

     ✓7ᵗʰ **S98.012** Complete traumatic amputation of left foot at ankle level

     ✓7ᵗʰ **S98.019** Complete traumatic amputation of unspecified foot at ankle level

   ✓6ᵗʰ **S98.02** Partial traumatic amputation of foot at ankle level

     ✓7ᵗʰ **S98.021** Partial traumatic amputation of right foot at ankle level

     ✓7ᵗʰ **S98.022** Partial traumatic amputation of left foot at ankle level

     ✓7ᵗʰ **S98.029** Partial traumatic amputation of unspecified foot at ankle level

✓5ᵗʰ **S98.1** **Traumatic amputation of** one toe

   ✓6ᵗʰ **S98.11** Complete traumatic amputation of great toe

     ✓7ᵗʰ **S98.111** Complete traumatic amputation of right great toe

     ✓7ᵗʰ **S98.112** Complete traumatic amputation of left great toe

     ✓7ᵗʰ **S98.119** Complete traumatic amputation of unspecified great toe

   ✓6ᵗʰ **S98.12** Partial traumatic amputation of great toe

     ✓7ᵗʰ **S98.121** Partial traumatic amputation of right great toe

     ✓7ᵗʰ **S98.122** Partial traumatic amputation of left great toe

     ✓7ᵗʰ **S98.129** Partial traumatic amputation of unspecified great toe

   ✓6ᵗʰ **S98.13** Complete traumatic amputation of one lesser toe
     Traumatic amputation of toe NOS

     ✓7ᵗʰ **S98.131** Complete traumatic amputation of one right lesser toe

     ✓7ᵗʰ **S98.132** Complete traumatic amputation of one left lesser toe

     ✓7ᵗʰ **S98.139** Complete traumatic amputation of one unspecified lesser toe

   ✓6ᵗʰ **S98.14** Partial traumatic amputation of one lesser toe

     ✓7ᵗʰ **S98.141** Partial traumatic amputation of one right lesser toe

     ✓7ᵗʰ **S98.142** Partial traumatic amputation of one left lesser toe

     ✓7ᵗʰ **S98.149** Partial traumatic amputation of one unspecified lesser toe

✓5ᵗʰ **S98.2** **Traumatic amputation of** two or more lesser toes

   ✓6ᵗʰ **S98.21** Complete traumatic amputation of two or more lesser toes

     ✓7ᵗʰ **S98.211** Complete traumatic amputation of two or more right lesser toes

     ✓7ᵗʰ **S98.212** Complete traumatic amputation of two or more left lesser toes

     ✓7ᵗʰ **S98.219** Complete traumatic amputation of two or more unspecified lesser toes

EXCLUDES 1 Not coded here   **EXCLUDES 2** Not included here   **N** Newborn Age: 0   **P** Pediatric Age: 0-17   **M** Maternity Age: 12-55   **A** Adult Age: 15-124

920   ICD-10-CM 2014 (Draft)

✓6ᵗʰ **S98.22 Partial** traumatic amputation of two or more lesser toes

✓7ᵗʰ **S98.221 Partial** traumatic amputation of two or more **right** lesser toes

✓7ᵗʰ **S98.222 Partial** traumatic amputation of two or more **left** lesser toes

✓7ᵗʰ **S98.229 Partial traumatic amputation of two or more unspecified lesser toes**

✓5ᵗʰ **S98.3 Traumatic amputation of** midfoot

✓6ᵗʰ **S98.31 Complete** traumatic amputation of midfoot

✓7ᵗʰ **S98.311 Complete** traumatic amputation of **right** midfoot

✓7ᵗʰ **S98.312 Complete** traumatic amputation of **left** midfoot

✓7ᵗʰ **S98.319 Complete traumatic amputation of unspecified midfoot**

✓6ᵗʰ **S98.32 Partial** traumatic amputation of midfoot

✓7ᵗʰ **S98.321 Partial** traumatic amputation of **right** midfoot

✓7ᵗʰ **S98.322 Partial** traumatic amputation of **left** midfoot

✓7ᵗʰ **S98.329 Partial traumatic amputation of unspecified midfoot**

✓5ᵗʰ **S98.9 Traumatic amputation of** foot, level unspecified

✓6ᵗʰ **S98.91 Complete** traumatic amputation of foot, level unspecified

✓7ᵗʰ **S98.911 Complete traumatic amputation of** right **foot, level unspecified**

✓7ᵗʰ **S98.912 Complete traumatic amputation of** left **foot, level unspecified**

✓7ᵗʰ **S98.919 Complete traumatic amputation of unspecified foot, level unspecified**

✓6ᵗʰ **S98.92 Partial** traumatic amputation of foot, level unspecified

✓7ᵗʰ **S98.921 Partial traumatic amputation of** right**foot, level unspecified**

✓7ᵗʰ **S98.922 Partial traumatic amputation of** left**foot, level unspecified**

✓7ᵗʰ **S98.929 Partial traumatic amputation of unspecified foot, level unspecified**

✓4ᵗʰ **S99 Other and unspecified injuries of ankle and foot**

The appropriate 7th character is to be added to each code from category S99.
A   initial encounter
D   subsequent encounter
S   sequela

✓5ᵗʰ **S99.8 Other** specified injuries of ankle and foot

✓6ᵗʰ **S99.81 Other specified injuries of** ankle

✓7ᵗʰ **S99.811 Other specified injuries of** right **ankle**

✓7ᵗʰ **S99.812 Other specified injuries of** left **ankle**

✓7ᵗʰ **S99.819 Other specified injuries of unspecified ankle**

✓6ᵗʰ **S99.82 Other specified injuries of** foot

✓7ᵗʰ **S99.821 Other specified injuries of** right**foot**

✓7ᵗʰ **S99.822 Other specified injuries of** left**foot**

✓7ᵗʰ **S99.829 Other specified injuries of unspecified foot**

✓5ᵗʰ **S99.9 Unspecified** injury of ankle and foot

✓6ᵗʰ **S99.91 Unspecified injury of** ankle

✓7ᵗʰ **S99.911 Unspecified injury of** right **ankle**

✓7ᵗʰ **S99.912 Unspecified injury of** left **ankle**

✓7ᵗʰ **S99.919 Unspecified injury of unspecified ankle**

✓6ᵗʰ **S99.92 Unspecified injury of** foot

✓7ᵗʰ **S99.921 Unspecified injury of** right**foot**

✓7ᵗʰ **S99.922 Unspecified injury of** left**foot**

✓7ᵗʰ **S99.929 Unspecified injury of unspecified foot**

Injury, Poisoning And Other Consequences Of External Causes (T07-T88)

Injuries involving multiple body regions (T07)

EXCLUDES 1   *burns and corrosions (T20-T32)*
frostbite (T33-T34)
insect bite or sting, venomous (T63.4)
sunburn (L55.-)

T07 Unspecified multiple injuries

EXCLUDES 1   *injury NOS (T14)*

Injury of unspecified body region (T14)

✓4ᵗʰ **T14 Injury of unspecified body region**

EXCLUDES 1   *multiple unspecified injuries (T07)*

T14.8 Other injury of unspecified body region
Abrasion NOS
Contusion NOS
Crush injury NOS
Fracture NOS
Skin injury NOS
Vascular injury NOS

✓5ᵗʰ **T14.9 Unspecified injury**

T14.90 Injury, unspecified
Injury NOS

T14.91 Suicide attempt
Attempted suicide NOS

Effects of foreign body entering through natural orifice (T15-T19)

EXCLUDES 2   *foreign body accidentally left in operation wound (T81.5-)*
foreign body in penetrating wound—See open wound by body region
residual foreign body in soft tissue (M79.5)
splinter, without open wound—See superficial injury by body region

✓4ᵗʰ **T15 Foreign body on external eye**

EXCLUDES 2   *foreign body in penetrating wound of orbit and eye ball (S05.4-, S05.5-)*
open wound of eyelid and periocular area (S01.1-)
retained foreign body in eyelid (H02.8-)
retained (old) foreign body in penetrating wound of orbit and eye ball (H05.5-, H44.6-, H44.7-)
superficial foreign body of eyelid and periocular area (S00.25-)

The appropriate 7th character is to be added to each code from category T15.
A   initial encounter
D   subsequent encounter
S   sequela

✓5ᵗʰ **T15.0 Foreign body in** cornea

✓x7ᵗʰ **T15.00 Foreign body in cornea, unspecified eye**

✓x7ᵗʰ **T15.01 Foreign body in cornea,** right **eye**

✓x7ᵗʰ **T15.02 Foreign body in cornea,** left **eye**

✓5ᵗʰ **T15.1 Foreign body in** conjunctival sac

✓x7ᵗʰ **T15.10 Foreign body in conjunctival sac, unspecified eye**

✓x7ᵗʰ **T15.11 Foreign body in conjunctival sac,** right **eye**

✓x7ᵗʰ **T15.12 Foreign body in conjunctival sac,** left **eye**

✓5ᵗʰ **T15.8 Foreign body in other and** multiple parts **of external eye**
Foreign body in lacrimal punctum

✓x7ᵗʰ **T15.80 Foreign body in other and multiple parts of external eye, unspecified eye**

✓x7ᵗʰ **T15.81 Foreign body in other and multiple parts of external eye,** right**eye**

✓x7ᵗʰ **T15.82 Foreign body in other and multiple parts of external eye,** left**eye**

✓5ᵗʰ **T15.9 Foreign body on external eye,** part unspecified

✓x7ᵗʰ **T15.90 Foreign body on external eye, part unspecified, unspecified eye**

✓x7ᵗʰ **T15.91 Foreign body on external eye, part unspecified,** right **eye**

✓x7ᵗʰ **T15.92 Foreign body on external eye, part unspecified,** left**eye**

Injury, Poisoning and Certain Other Consequences of External Causes

T16–T17.900

☑4ᵗʰ **T16 Foreign body in ear**
Foreign body in auditory canal

> The appropriate 7th character is to be added to each code from category T16.
> A   initial encounter
> D   subsequent encounter
> S   sequela

☑x7ᵗʰ **T16.1 Foreign body in right ear**
☑x7ᵗʰ **T16.2 Foreign body in left ear**
☑x7ᵗʰ **T16.9 Foreign body in ear, unspecified ear**

☑4ᵗʰ **T17 Foreign body in respiratory tract**

> The appropriate 7th character is to be added to each code from category T17.
> A   initial encounter
> D   subsequent encounter
> S   sequela

☑x7ᵗʰ **T17.0 Foreign body in nasal sinus**
☑x7ᵗʰ **T17.1 Foreign body in nostril**
Foreign body in nose NOS

☑5ᵗʰ **T17.2 Foreign body in pharynx**
Foreign body in nasopharynx
Foreign body in throat NOS

    ☑6ᵗʰ **T17.20 Unspecified foreign body in pharynx**
        ☑7ᵗʰ **T17.200 Unspecified foreign body in pharynx causing asphyxiation**
        ☑7ᵗʰ **T17.208 Unspecified foreign body in pharynx causing other injury**

    ☑6ᵗʰ **T17.21 Gastric contents in pharynx**
Aspiration of gastric contents into pharynx
Vomitus in pharynx
        ☑7ᵗʰ **T17.210 Gastric contents in pharynx causing asphyxiation**
        ☑7ᵗʰ **T17.218 Gastric contents in pharynx causing other injury**

    ☑6ᵗʰ **T17.22 Food in pharynx**
Bones in pharynx
Seeds in pharynx
        ☑7ᵗʰ **T17.220 Food in pharynx causing asphyxiation**
        ☑7ᵗʰ **T17.228 Food in pharynx causing other injury**

    ☑6ᵗʰ **T17.29 Other foreign object in pharynx**
        ☑7ᵗʰ **T17.290 Other foreign object in pharynx causing asphyxiation**
        ☑7ᵗʰ **T17.298 Other foreign object in pharynx causing other injury**

☑5ᵗʰ **T17.3 Foreign body in larynx**

    ☑6ᵗʰ **T17.30 Unspecified foreign body in larynx**
        ☑7ᵗʰ **T17.300 Unspecified foreign body in larynx causing asphyxiation**
        ☑7ᵗʰ **T17.308 Unspecified foreign body in larynx causing other injury**

    ☑6ᵗʰ **T17.31 Gastric contents in larynx**
Aspiration of gastric contents into larynx
Vomitus in larynx
        ☑7ᵗʰ **T17.310 Gastric contents in larynx causing asphyxiation**
        ☑7ᵗʰ **T17.318 Gastric contents in larynx causing other injury**

    ☑6ᵗʰ **T17.32 Food in larynx**
Bones in larynx
Seeds in larynx
        ☑7ᵗʰ **T17.320 Food in larynx causing asphyxiation**
        ☑7ᵗʰ **T17.328 Food in larynx causing other injury**

    ☑6ᵗʰ **T17.39 Other foreign object in larynx**
        ☑7ᵗʰ **T17.390 Other foreign object in larynx causing asphyxiation**
        ☑7ᵗʰ **T17.398 Other foreign object in larynx causing other injury**

☑5ᵗʰ **T17.4 Foreign body in trachea**

    ☑6ᵗʰ **T17.40 Unspecified foreign body in trachea**
        ☑7ᵗʰ **T17.400 Unspecified foreign body in trachea causing asphyxiation**
        ☑7ᵗʰ **T17.408 Unspecified foreign body in trachea causing other injury**

    ☑6ᵗʰ **T17.41 Gastric contents in trachea**
Aspiration of gastric contents into trachea
Vomitus in trachea
        ☑7ᵗʰ **T17.410 Gastric contents in trachea causing asphyxiation**
        ☑7ᵗʰ **T17.418 Gastric contents in trachea causing other injury**

    ☑6ᵗʰ **T17.42 Food in trachea**
Bones in trachea
Seeds in trachea
        ☑7ᵗʰ **T17.420 Food in trachea causing asphyxiation**
        ☑7ᵗʰ **T17.428 Food in trachea causing other injury**

    ☑6ᵗʰ **T17.49 Other foreign object in trachea**
        ☑7ᵗʰ **T17.490 Other foreign object in trachea causing asphyxiation**
        ☑7ᵗʰ **T17.498 Other foreign object in trachea causing other injury**

☑5ᵗʰ **T17.5 Foreign body in bronchus**

    ☑6ᵗʰ **T17.50 Unspecified foreign body in bronchus**
        ☑7ᵗʰ **T17.500 Unspecified foreign body in bronchus causing asphyxiation**
        ☑7ᵗʰ **T17.508 Unspecified foreign body in bronchus causing other injury**

    ☑6ᵗʰ **T17.51 Gastric contents in bronchus**
Aspiration of gastric contents into bronchus
Vomitus in bronchus
        ☑7ᵗʰ **T17.510 Gastric contents in bronchus causing asphyxiation**
        ☑7ᵗʰ **T17.518 Gastric contents in bronchus causing other injury**

    ☑6ᵗʰ **T17.52 Food in bronchus**
Bones in bronchus   Seeds in bronchus
        ☑7ᵗʰ **T17.520 Food in bronchus causing asphyxiation**
        ☑7ᵗʰ **T17.528 Food in bronchus causing other injury**

    ☑6ᵗʰ **T17.59 Other foreign object in bronchus**
        ☑7ᵗʰ **T17.590 Other foreign object in bronchus causing asphyxiation**
        ☑7ᵗʰ **T17.598 Other foreign object in bronchus causing other injury**

☑5ᵗʰ **T17.8 Foreign body in other parts of respiratory tract**
Foreign body in bronchioles
Foreign body in lung

    ☑6ᵗʰ **T17.80 Unspecified foreign body in other parts of respiratory tract**
        ☑7ᵗʰ **T17.800 Unspecified foreign body in other parts of respiratory tract causing asphyxiation**
        ☑7ᵗʰ **T17.808 Unspecified foreign body in other parts of respiratory tract causing other injury**

    ☑6ᵗʰ **T17.81 Gastric contents in other parts of respiratory tract**
Aspiration of gastric contents into other parts of respiratory tract
Vomitus in other parts of respiratory tract
        ☑7ᵗʰ **T17.810 Gastric contents in other parts of respiratory tract causing asphyxiation**
        ☑7ᵗʰ **T17.818 Gastric contents in other parts of respiratory tract causing other injury**

    ☑6ᵗʰ **T17.82 Food in other parts of respiratory tract**
Bones in other parts of respiratory tract
Seeds in other parts of respiratory tract
        ☑7ᵗʰ **T17.820 Food in other parts of respiratory tract causing asphyxiation**
        ☑7ᵗʰ **T17.828 Food in other parts of respiratory tract causing other injury**

    ☑6ᵗʰ **T17.89 Other foreign object in other parts of respiratory tract**
        ☑7ᵗʰ **T17.890 Other foreign object in other parts of respiratory tract causing asphyxiation**
        ☑7ᵗʰ **T17.898 Other foreign object in other parts of respiratory tract causing other injury**

☑5ᵗʰ **T17.9 Foreign body in respiratory tract, part unspecified**

    ☑6ᵗʰ **T17.90 Unspecified foreign body in respiratory tract, part unspecified**
        ☑7ᵗʰ **T17.900 Unspecified foreign body in respiratory tract, part unspecified causing asphyxiation**

EXCLUDES 1 Not coded here   **EXCLUDES 2** Not included here   N Newborn Age: 0   P Pediatric Age: 0-17   M Maternity Age: 12-55   A Adult Age: 15-124

922   ICD-10-CM 2014 (Draft)

✓7th **T17.908** **Unspecified foreign body in respiratory tract, part unspecified causing other injury**

✓6th **T17.91** **Gastric contents in respiratory tract, part unspecified**
Aspiration of gastric contents into respiratory tract, part unspecified
Vomitus in trachea respiratory tract, part unspecified

✓7th **T17.910** **Gastric contents in respiratory tract, part unspecified causing asphyxiation**

✓7th **T17.918** **Gastric contents in respiratory tract, part unspecified causing other injury**

✓6th **T17.92** **Food in respiratory tract, part unspecified**
Bones in respiratory tract, part unspecified
Seeds in respiratory tract, part unspecified

✓7th **T17.920** **Food in respiratory tract, part unspecified causing asphyxiation**

✓7th **T17.928** **Food in respiratory tract, part unspecified causing other injury**

✓6th **T17.99** **Other foreign object in respiratory tract, part unspecified**

✓7th **T17.990** **Other foreign object in respiratory tract, part unspecified in causing asphyxiation**

✓7th **T17.998** **Other foreign object in respiratory tract, part unspecified causing other injury**

✓4th **T18** **Foreign body in alimentary tract**
EXCLUDES 2 *foreign body in pharynx (T17.2-)*

The appropriate 7th character is to be added to each code from category T18.
A   initial encounter
D   subsequent encounter
S   sequela

✓x7th **T18.0** **Foreign body in mouth**

✓5th **T18.1** **Foreign body in esophagus**
EXCLUDES 2 *foreign body in respiratory tract (T17.-)*

✓6th **T18.10** **Unspecified foreign body in esophagus**

✓7th **T18.100** **Unspecified foreign body in esophagus causing compression of trachea**
Unspecified foreign body in esophagus causing obstruction of respiration

✓7th **T18.108** **Unspecified foreign body in esophagus causing other injury**

✓6th **T18.11** **Gastric contents in esophagus**
Vomitus in esophagus

✓7th **T18.110** **Gastric contents in esophagus causing compression of trachea**
Gastric contents in esophagus causing obstruction of respiration

✓7th **T18.118** **Gastric contents in esophagus causing other injury**

✓6th **T18.12** **Food in esophagus**
Bones in esophagus
Seeds in esophagus

✓7th **T18.120** **Food in esophagus causing compression of trachea**
Food in esophagus causing obstruction of respiration

✓7th **T18.128** **Food in esophagus causing other injury**

✓6th **T18.19** **Other foreign object in esophagus**

✓7th **T18.190** **Other foreign object in esophagus causing compression of trachea**
Other foreign body in esophagus causing obstruction of respiration

✓7th **T18.198** **Other foreign object in esophagus causing other injury**

✓x7th **T18.2** **Foreign body in stomach**

✓x7th **T18.3** **Foreign body in small intestine**

✓x7th **T18.4** **Foreign body in colon**

✓x7th **T18.5** **Foreign body in anus and rectum**
Foreign body in rectosigmoid (junction)

✓x7th **T18.8** **Foreign body in other parts of alimentary tract**

✓x7th **T18.9** **Foreign body of alimentary tract, part unspecified**
Foreign body in digestive system NOS
Swallowed foreign body NOS

✓4th **T19** **Foreign body in genitourinary tract**
EXCLUDES 2 *complications due to implanted mesh (T83.7-)*
mechanical complications of contraceptive device (intrauterine) (vaginal) (T83.3-)
presence of contraceptive device (intrauterine) (vaginal) (Z97.5)

The appropriate 7th character is to be added to each code from category T19.
A   initial encounter
D   subsequent encounter
S   sequela

✓x7th **T19.0** **Foreign body in urethra**

✓x7th **T19.1** **Foreign body in bladder**

✓x7th **T19.2** **Foreign body in vulva and vagina**   ♀

✓x7th **T19.3** **Foreign body in uterus**   ♀

✓x7th **T19.4** **Foreign body in penis**   ♂

✓x7th **T19.8** **Foreign body in other parts of genitourinary tract**

✓x7th **T19.9** **Foreign body in genitourinary tract, part unspecified**

Burns and corrosions (T20-T32)

INCLUDES   burns (thermal) from electrical heating appliances
burns (thermal) from electricity
burns (thermal) from flame
burns (thermal) from friction
burns (thermal) from hot air and hot gases
burns (thermal) from hot objects
burns (thermal) from lightning
burns (thermal) from radiation
chemical burn [corrosion] (external) (internal)
scalds
EXCLUDES 2 *erythema [dermatitis] ab igne (L59.0)*
radiation-related disorders of the skin and subcutaneous tissue (L55-L59)
sunburn (L55.-)

Burns and corrosions of external body surface, specified by site (T20-T25)

INCLUDES   burns and corrosions of first degree [erythema]
burns and corrosions of second degree [blisters] [epidermal loss]
burns and corrosions of third degree [deep necrosis of underlying tissue] [full-thickness skin loss]
Use additional code from category T31 or T32 to identify extent of body surface involved

✓4th **T20** **Burn and corrosion of head, face, and neck**
EXCLUDES 2 *burn and corrosion of ear drum (T28.41, T28.91)*
burn and corrosion of eye and adnexa (T26.-)
burn and corrosion of mouth and pharynx (T28.0)

The appropriate 7th character is to be added to each code from category T20.
A   initial encounter
D   subsequent encounter
S   sequela

✓5th **T20.0** **Burn of unspecified degree of head, face, and neck**
Use additional external cause code to identify the source, place and intent of the burn (X00-X19, X75-X77, X96-X98, Y92)

✓x7th **T20.00** **Burn of unspecified degree of head, face, and neck, unspecified site**

✓6th **T20.01** **Burn of unspecified degree of ear [any part, except ear drum]**
EXCLUDES 2 *burn of ear drum (T28.41-)*

✓7th **T20.011** **Burn of unspecified degree of right ear [any part, except ear drum]**

✓7th **T20.012** **Burn of unspecified degree of left ear [any part, except ear drum]**

✓7th **T20.019** **Burn of unspecified degree of unspecified ear [any part, except ear drum]**

✓x7th **T20.02** **Burn of unspecified degree of lip(s)**

✓x7th **T20.03** **Burn of unspecified degree of chin**

✓x7th **T20.04** **Burn of unspecified degree of nose (septum)**

✓x7th **T20.05** **Burn of unspecified degree of scalp [any part]**

✓x7th **T20.06** **Burn of unspecified degree of forehead and cheek**

✓x7th **T20.07** **Burn of unspecified degree of neck**

✓x7th **T20.09** **Burn of unspecified degree of multiple sites of head, face, and neck**

✓5th **T20.1** Burn of first degree of head, face, and neck
Use additional external cause code to identify the source, place and intent of the burn (X00-X19, X75-X77, X96-X98, Y92)

✓x7th **T20.10** **Burn of first degree of head, face, and neck, unspecified site**

✓6th **T20.11** **Burn of first degree of ear [any part, except ear drum]**
EXCLUDES 2 *burn of ear drum (T28.41-)*

✓7th **T20.111** **Burn of first degree of right ear [any part, except ear drum]**

✓7th **T20.112** **Burn of first degree of left ear [any part, except ear drum]**

✓7th **T20.119** **Burn of first degree of unspecified ear [any part, except ear drum]**

✓x7th **T20.12** **Burn of first degree of lip(s)**

✓x7th **T20.13** **Burn of first degree of chin**

✓x7th **T20.14** **Burn of first degree of nose (septum)**

✓x7th **T20.15** **Burn of first degree of scalp [any part]**

✓x7th **T20.16** **Burn of first degree of forehead and cheek**

✓x7th **T20.17** **Burn of first degree of neck**

✓x7th **T20.19** **Burn of first degree of multiple sites of head, face, and neck**

✓5th **T20.2** Burn of second degree of head, face, and neck
Use additional external cause code to identify the source, place and intent of the burn (X00-X19, X75-X77, X96-X98, Y92)

✓x7th **T20.20** **Burn of second degree of head, face, and neck, unspecified site**

✓6th **T20.21** **Burn of second degree of ear [any part, except ear drum]**
EXCLUDES 2 *burn of ear drum (T28.41-)*

✓7th **T20.211** **Burn of second degree of right ear [any part, except ear drum]**

✓7th **T20.212** **Burn of second degree of left ear [any part, except ear drum]**

✓7th **T20.219** **Burn of second degree of unspecified ear [any part, except ear drum]**

✓x7th **T20.22** **Burn of second degree of lip(s)**

✓x7th **T20.23** **Burn of second degree of chin**

✓x7th **T20.24** **Burn of second degree of nose (septum)**

✓x7th **T20.25** **Burn of second degree of scalp [any part]**

✓x7th **T20.26** **Burn of second degree of forehead and cheek**

✓x7th **T20.27** **Burn of second degree of neck**

✓x7th **T20.29** **Burn of second degree of multiple sites of head, face, and neck**

✓5th **T20.3** Burn of third degree of head, face, and neck
Use additional external cause code to identify the source, place and intent of the burn (X00-X19, X75-X77, X96-X98, Y92)

✓x7th **T20.30** **Burn of third degree of head, face, and neck, unspecified site**

✓6th **T20.31** **Burn of third degree of ear [any part, except ear drum]**
EXCLUDES 2 *burn of ear drum (T28.41-)*

✓7th **T20.311** **Burn of third degree of right ear [any part, except ear drum]**

✓7th **T20.312** **Burn of third degree of left ear [any part, except ear drum]**

✓7th **T20.319** **Burn of third degree of unspecified ear [any part, except ear drum]**

✓x7th **T20.32** **Burn of third degree of lip(s)**

✓x7th **T20.33** **Burn of third degree of chin**

✓x7th **T20.34** **Burn of third degree of nose (septum)**

✓x7th **T20.35** **Burn of third degree of scalp [any part]**

✓x7th **T20.36** **Burn of third degree of forehead and cheek**

✓x7th **T20.37** **Burn of third degree of neck**

✓x7th **T20.39** **Burn of third degree of multiple sites of head, face, and neck**

✓5th **T20.4** Corrosion of unspecified degree of head, face, and neck
Code first (T51-T65) to identify chemical and intent
Use additional external cause code to identify place (Y92)

✓x7th **T20.40** **Corrosion of unspecified degree of head, face, and neck, unspecified site**

✓6th **T20.41** **Corrosion of unspecified degree of ear [any part, except ear drum]**
EXCLUDES 2 *corrosion of ear drum (T28.91-)*

✓7th **T20.411** **Corrosion of unspecified degree of right ear [any part, except ear drum]**

✓7th **T20.412** **Corrosion of unspecified degree of left ear [any part, except ear drum]**

✓7th **T20.419** **Corrosion of unspecified degree of unspecified ear [any part, except ear drum]**

✓x7th **T20.42** **Corrosion of unspecified degree of lip(s)**

✓x7th **T20.43** **Corrosion of unspecified degree of chin**

✓x7th **T20.44** **Corrosion of unspecified degree of nose (septum)**

✓x7th **T20.45** **Corrosion of unspecified degree of scalp [any part]**

✓x7th **T20.46** **Corrosion of unspecified degree of forehead and cheek**

✓x7th **T20.47** **Corrosion of unspecified degree of neck**

✓x7th **T20.49** **Corrosion of unspecified degree of multiple sites of head, face, and neck**

✓5th **T20.5** Corrosion of first degree of head, face, and neck
Code first (T51-T65) to identify chemical and intent
Use additional external cause code to identify place (Y92)

✓x7th **T20.50** **Corrosion of first degree of head, face, and neck, unspecified site**

✓6th **T20.51** **Corrosion of first degree of ear [any part, except ear drum]**
EXCLUDES 2 *corrosion of ear drum (T28.91-)*

✓7th **T20.511** **Corrosion of first degree of right ear [any part, except ear drum]**

✓7th **T20.512** **Corrosion of first degree of left ear [any part, except ear drum]**

✓7th **T20.519** **Corrosion of first degree of unspecified ear [any part, except ear drum]**

✓x7th **T20.52** **Corrosion of first degree of lip(s)**

✓x7th **T20.53** **Corrosion of first degree of chin**

✓x7th **T20.54** **Corrosion of first degree of nose (septum)**

✓x7th **T20.55** **Corrosion of first degree of scalp [any part]**

✓x7th **T20.56** **Corrosion of first degree of forehead and cheek**

✓x7th **T20.57** **Corrosion of first degree of neck**

✓x7th **T20.59** **Corrosion of first degree of multiple sites of head, face, and neck**

✓5th **T20.6** Corrosion of second degree of head, face, and neck
Code first (T51-T65) to identify chemical and intent
Use additional external cause code to identify place (Y92)

✓x7th **T20.60** **Corrosion of second degree of head, face, and neck, unspecified site**

✓6th **T20.61** **Corrosion of second degree of ear [any part, except ear drum]**
EXCLUDES 2 *corrosion of ear drum (T28.91-)*

✓7th **T20.611** **Corrosion of second degree of right ear [any part, except ear drum]**

✓7th **T20.612** **Corrosion of second degree of left ear [any part, except ear drum]**

✓7th **T20.619** **Corrosion of second degree of unspecified ear [any part, except ear drum]**

✓x7th **T20.62** **Corrosion of second degree of lip(s)**

✓x7th **T20.63** **Corrosion of second degree of chin**

✓x7th **T20.64** **Corrosion of second degree of nose (septum)**

✓x7th **T20.65** **Corrosion of second degree of scalp [any part]**

✓x7th **T20.66** **Corrosion of second degree of forehead and cheek**

✓x7th **T20.67** **Corrosion of second degree of neck**

✓x7th **T20.69** **Corrosion of second degree of multiple sites of head, face, and neck**

✓5th **T20.7** Corrosion of third degree of head, face, and neck
Code first (T51-T65) to identify chemical and intent
Use additional external cause code to identify place (Y92)

✓x7th **T20.70** **Corrosion of third degree of head, face, and neck, unspecified site**

EXCLUDES 1 Not coded here   EXCLUDES 2 Not included here   N Newborn Age: 0   P Pediatric Age: 0-17   M Maternity Age: 12-55   A Adult Age: 15-124

924   ICD-10-CM 2014 (Draft)

√6ᵗʰ **T20.71** **Corrosion of third degree of** ear [any part, except ear drum]
> *EXCLUDES 2* corrosion of ear drum (T28.91-)

√7ᵗʰ **T20.711** **Corrosion of third degree of** right ear [any part, except ear drum]

√7ᵗʰ **T20.712** **Corrosion of third degree of** left ear [any part, except ear drum]

√7ᵗʰ **T20.719** **Corrosion of third degree of unspecified ear [any part, except ear drum]**

√x7ᵗʰ **T20.72** **Corrosion of third degree of** lip(s)

√x7ᵗʰ **T20.73** **Corrosion of third degree of** chin

√x7ᵗʰ **T20.74** **Corrosion of third degree of** nose (septum)

√x7ᵗʰ **T20.75** **Corrosion of third degree of** scalp [any part]

√x7ᵗʰ **T20.76** **Corrosion of third degree of** forehead and cheek

√x7ᵗʰ **T20.77** **Corrosion of third degree of** neck

√x7ᵗʰ **T20.79** **Corrosion of third degree of** multiple sites of head, face, and neck

√4ᵗʰ **T21** **Burn and corrosion of trunk**
Burns and corrosion of hip region
> *EXCLUDES 2* burns and corrosion of axilla (T22.- with fifth character 4)
> burns and corrosion of scapular region (T22.- with fifth character 6)
> burns and corrosion of shoulder (T22.- with fifth character 5)

> The appropriate 7th character is to be added to each code from category T21.
> A   initial encounter
> D   subsequent encounter
> S   sequela

√5ᵗʰ **T21.0** **Burn of** unspecified degree of trunk
> Use additional external cause code to identify the source, place and intent of the burn (X00-X19, X75-X77, X96-X98, Y92)

√x7ᵗʰ **T21.00** **Burn of unspecified degree of trunk, unspecified site**

√x7ᵗʰ **T21.01** **Burn of unspecified degree of** chest wall
Burn of of unspecified degree of breast

√x7ᵗʰ **T21.02** **Burn of unspecified degree of** abdominal wall
Burn of unspecified degree of flank
Burn of unspecified degree of groin

√x7ᵗʰ **T21.03** **Burn of unspecified degree of** upper back
Burn of unspecified degree of interscapular region

√x7ᵗʰ **T21.04** **Burn of unspecified degree of** lower back

√x7ᵗʰ **T21.05** **Burn of unspecified degree of** buttock
Burn of unspecified degree of anus

√x7ᵗʰ **T21.06** **Burn of unspecified degree of** male genital region ♂
Burn of unspecified degree of penis
Burn of unspecified degree of scrotum
Burn of unspecified degree of testis

√x7ᵗʰ **T21.07** **Burn of unspecified degree of** female genital region ♀
Burn of unspecified degree of labium (majus) (minus)
Burn of unspecified degree of perineum
Burn of unspecified degree of vulva
> *EXCLUDES 2* burn of vagina (T28.3)

√x7ᵗʰ **T21.09** **Burn of unspecified degree of other site of trunk**

√5ᵗʰ **T21.1** **Burn of** first degree of trunk
> Use additional external cause code to identify the source, place and intent of the burn (X00-X19, X75-X77, X96-X98, Y92)

√x7ᵗʰ **T21.10** **Burn of first degree of trunk, unspecified site**

√x7ᵗʰ **T21.11** **Burn of first degree of** chest wall
Burn of first degree of breast

√x7ᵗʰ **T21.12** **Burn of first degree of** abdominal wall
Burn of first degree of flank
Burn of first degree of groin

√x7ᵗʰ **T21.13** **Burn of first degree of** upper back
Burn of first degree of interscapular region

√x7ᵗʰ **T21.14** **Burn of first degree of** lower back

√x7ᵗʰ **T21.15** **Burn of first degree of** buttock
Burn of first degree of anus

√x7ᵗʰ **T21.16** **Burn of first degree of** male genital region ♂
Burn of first degree of penis
Burn of first degree of scrotum
Burn of first degree of testis

√x7ᵗʰ **T21.17** **Burn of first degree of** female genital region ♀
Burn of first degree of labium (majus) (minus)
Burn of first degree of perineum
Burn of first degree of vulva
> *EXCLUDES 2* burn of vagina (T28.3)

√x7ᵗʰ **T21.19** **Burn of first degree of other site of trunk**

√5ᵗʰ **T21.2** **Burn of** second degree of trunk
> Use additional external cause code to identify the source, place and intent of the burn (X00-X19, X75-X77, X96-X98, Y92)

√x7ᵗʰ **T21.20** **Burn of second degree of trunk, unspecified site**

√x7ᵗʰ **T21.21** **Burn of second degree of** chest wall
Burn of second degree of breast

√x7ᵗʰ **T21.22** **Burn of second degree of** abdominal wall
Burn of second degree of flank
Burn of second degree of groin

√x7ᵗʰ **T21.23** **Burn of second degree of** upper back
Burn of second degree of interscapular region

√x7ᵗʰ **T21.24** **Burn of second degree of** lower back

√x7ᵗʰ **T21.25** **Burn of second degree of** buttock
Burn of second degree of anus

√x7ᵗʰ **T21.26** **Burn of second degree of** male genital region ♂
Burn of second degree of penis
Burn of second degree of scrotum
Burn of second degree of testis

√x7ᵗʰ **T21.27** **Burn of second degree of** female genital region ♀
Burn of second degree of labium (majus) (minus)
Burn of second degree of perineum
Burn of second degree of vulva
> *EXCLUDES 2* burn of vagina (T28.3)

√x7ᵗʰ **T21.29** **Burn of second degree of other site of trunk**

√5ᵗʰ **T21.3** **Burn of** third degree of trunk
> Use additional external cause code to identify the source, place and intent of the burn (X00-X19, X75-X77, X96-X98, Y92)

√x7ᵗʰ **T21.30** **Burn of third degree of trunk, unspecified site**

√x7ᵗʰ **T21.31** **Burn of third degree of** chest wall
Burn of third degree of breast

√x7ᵗʰ **T21.32** **Burn of third degree of** abdominal wall
Burn of third degree of flank
Burn of third degree of groin

√x7ᵗʰ **T21.33** **Burn of third degree of** upper back
Burn of third degree of interscapular region

√x7ᵗʰ **T21.34** **Burn of third degree of** lower back

√x7ᵗʰ **T21.35** **Burn of third degree of** buttock
Burn of third degree of anus

√x7ᵗʰ **T21.36** **Burn of third degree of** male genital region ♂
Burn of third degree of penis
Burn of third degree of scrotum
Burn of third degree of testis

√x7ᵗʰ **T21.37** **Burn of third degree of** female genital region ♀
Burn of third degree of labium (majus) (minus)
Burn of third degree of perineum
Burn of third degree of vulva
> *EXCLUDES 2* burn of vagina (T28.3)

√x7ᵗʰ **T21.39** **Burn of third degree of other site of trunk**

√5ᵗʰ **T21.4** **Corrosion of** unspecified degree of trunk
> Code first (T51-T65) to identify chemical and intent
> Use additional external cause code to identify place (Y92)

√x7ᵗʰ **T21.40** **Corrosion of unspecified degree of trunk, unspecified site**

√x7ᵗʰ **T21.41** **Corrosion of unspecified degree of** chest wall
Corrosion of unspecified degree of breast

√x7ᵗʰ **T21.42** **Corrosion of unspecified degree of** abdominal wall
Corrosion of unspecified degree of flank
Corrosion of unspecified degree of groin

√x7ᵗʰ **T21.43** **Corrosion of unspecified degree of** upper back
Corrosion of unspecified degree of interscapular region

√x7ᵗʰ **T21.44** **Corrosion of unspecified degree of** lower back

√x7ᵗʰ **T21.45** **Corrosion of unspecified degree of** buttock
Corrosion of unspecified degree of anus

√x7ᵗʰ **T21.46** **Corrosion of unspecified degree of** male genital region ♂
Corrosion of unspecified degree of penis
Corrosion of unspecified degree of scrotum
Corrosion of unspecified degree of testis

Injury, Poisoning and Certain Other Consequences of External Causes

T21.47–T22.099

√x7th **T21.47** **Corrosion of unspecified degree of** female genital ♀
region
Corrosion of unspecified degree of labium (majus)
(minus)
Corrosion of unspecified degree of perineum
Corrosion of unspecified degree of vulva
EXCLUDES 2   *corrosion of vagina (T28.8)*

√x7th **T21.49** **Corrosion of unspecified degree of other site of**
trunk

√5th **T21.5** **Corrosion of** first degree **of trunk**
Code first (T51-T65) to identify chemical and intent
Use additional external cause code to identify place (Y92)

√x7th **T21.50** **Corrosion of first degree of trunk, unspecified site**

√x7th **T21.51** **Corrosion of first degree of** chest wall
Corrosion of first degree of breast

√x7th **T21.52** **Corrosion of first degree of** abdominal wall
Corrosion of first degree of flank
Corrosion of first degree of groin

√x7th **T21.53** **Corrosion of first degree of** upper back
Corrosion of first degree of interscapular region

√x7th **T21.54** **Corrosion of first degree of** lower back

√x7th **T21.55** **Corrosion of first degree of** buttock
Corrosion of first degree of anus

√x7th **T21.56** **Corrosion of first degree of** male genital region ♂
Corrosion of first degree of penis
Corrosion of first degree of scrotum
Corrosion of first degree of testis

√x7th **T21.57** **Corrosion of first degree of** female genital region ♀
Corrosion of first degree of labium (majus) (minus)
Corrosion of first degree of perineum
Corrosion of first degree of vulva
EXCLUDES 2   *corrosion of vagina (T28.8)*

√x7th **T21.59** **Corrosion of first degree of other site of trunk**

√5th **T21.6** **Corrosion of** second degree **of trunk**
Code first (T51-T65) to identify chemical and intent
Use additional external cause code to identify place (Y92)

√x7th **T21.60** **Corrosion of second degree of trunk, unspecified site**

√x7th **T21.61** **Corrosion of second degree of** chest wall
Corrosion of second degree of breast

√x7th **T21.62** **Corrosion of second degree of** abdominal wall
Corrosion of second degree of flank
Corrosion of second degree of groin

√x7th **T21.63** **Corrosion of second degree of** upper back
Corrosion of second degree of interscapular region

√x7th **T21.64** **Corrosion of second degree of** lower back

√x7th **T21.65** **Corrosion of second degree of** buttock
Corrosion of second degree of anus

√x7th **T21.66** **Corrosion of second degree of** male genital region ♂
Corrosion of second degree of penis
Corrosion of second degree of scrotum
Corrosion of second degree of testis

√x7th **T21.67** **Corrosion of second degree of** female genital ♀
region
Corrosion of second degree of labium (majus) (minus)
Corrosion of second degree of perineum
Corrosion of second degree of vulva
EXCLUDES 2   *corrosion of vagina (T28.8)*

√x7th **T21.69** **Corrosion of second degree of other site of trunk**

√5th **T21.7** **Corrosion of** third degree **of trunk**
Code first (T51-T65) to identify chemical and intent
Use additional external cause code to identify place (Y92)

√x7th **T21.70** **Corrosion of third degree of trunk, unspecified site**

√x7th **T21.71** **Corrosion of third degree of** chest wall
Corrosion of third degree of breast

√x7th **T21.72** **Corrosion of third degree of** abdominal wall
Corrosion of third degree of flank
Corrosion of third degree of groin

√x7th **T21.73** **Corrosion of third degree of** upper back
Corrosion of third degree of interscapular region

√x7th **T21.74** **Corrosion of third degree of** lower back

√x7th **T21.75** **Corrosion of third degree of** buttock
Corrosion of third degree of anus

√x7th **T21.76** **Corrosion of third degree of** male genital region ♂
Corrosion of third degree of penis
Corrosion of third degree of scrotum
Corrosion of third degree of testis

√x7th **T21.77** **Corrosion of third degree of** female genital region ♀
Corrosion of third degree of labium (majus) (minus)
Corrosion of third degree of perineum
Corrosion of third degree of vulva
EXCLUDES 2   *corrosion of vagina (T28.8)*

√x7th **T21.79** **Corrosion of third degree of other site of trunk**

√4th **T22** **Burn and corrosion of shoulder and upper limb, except wrist and**
hand
EXCLUDES 2   *burn and corrosion of interscapular region (T21.-)*
burn and corrosion of wrist and hand (T23.-)

The appropriate 7th character is to be added to each code from
category T22.
A   initial encounter
D   subsequent encounter
S   sequela

√5th **T22.0** **Burn of** unspecified degree **of shoulder and upper limb,**
except wrist and hand
Use additional external cause code to identify the source, place
and intent of the burn (X00-X19, X75-X77, X96-X98, Y92)

√x7th **T22.00** **Burn of unspecified degree of shoulder and upper**
limb, except wrist and hand, unspecified site

√6th **T22.01** **Burn of unspecified degree of** forearm

   √7th **T22.011** **Burn of unspecified degree of** right
forearm

   √7th **T22.012** **Burn of unspecified degree of** left forearm

   √7th **T22.019** **Burn of unspecified degree of** unspecified
forearm

√6th **T22.02** **Burn of unspecified degree of** elbow

   √7th **T22.021** **Burn of unspecified degree of** right elbow

   √7th **T22.022** **Burn of unspecified degree of** left elbow

   √7th **T22.029** **Burn of unspecified degree of** unspecified
elbow

√6th **T22.03** **Burn of unspecified degree of** upper arm

   √7th **T22.031** **Burn of unspecified degree of** right upper
arm

   √7th **T22.032** **Burn of unspecified degree of** left upper
arm

   √7th **T22.039** **Burn of unspecified degree of** unspecified
upper arm

√6th **T22.04** **Burn of unspecified degree of** axilla

   √7th **T22.041** **Burn of unspecified degree of** right axilla

   √7th **T22.042** **Burn of unspecified degree of** left axilla

   √7th **T22.049** **Burn of unspecified degree of** unspecified
axilla

√6th **T22.05** **Burn of unspecified degree of** shoulder

   √7th **T22.051** **Burn of unspecified degree of** right
shoulder

   √7th **T22.052** **Burn of unspecified degree of** left
shoulder

   √7th **T22.059** **Burn of unspecified degree of** unspecified
shoulder

√6th **T22.06** **Burn of unspecified degree of** scapular region

   √7th **T22.061** **Burn of unspecified degree of** right
scapular region

   √7th **T22.062** **Burn of unspecified degree of** left scapular
region

   √7th **T22.069** **Burn of unspecified degree of** unspecified
scapular region

√6th **T22.09** **Burn of unspecified degree of** multiple sites **of**
shoulder and upper limb, except wrist and hand

   √7th **T22.091** **Burn of unspecified degree of multiple**
sites of right shoulder and upper limb,
except wrist and hand

   √7th **T22.092** **Burn of unspecified degree of multiple**
sites of left shoulder and upper limb,
except wrist and hand

   √7th **T22.099** **Burn of unspecified degree of multiple**
sites of unspecified shoulder and upper
limb, except wrist and hand

EXCLUDES 1 Not coded here   EXCLUDES 2 Not included here   N Newborn Age: 0   P Pediatric Age: 0-17   M Maternity Age: 12-55   A Adult Age: 15-124

926   ICD-10-CM 2014 (Draft)

☑5ᵗʰ **T22.1** Burn of first degree of shoulder and upper limb, except wrist and hand
    Use additional external cause code to identify the source, place and intent of the burn (X00-X19, X75-X77, X96-X98, Y92)

☑x7ᵗʰ **T22.10** **Burn of first degree of shoulder and upper limb, except wrist and hand, unspecified site**

☑6ᵗʰ **T22.11** **Burn of first degree of forearm**

☑7ᵗʰ **T22.111** **Burn of first degree of right forearm**

☑7ᵗʰ **T22.112** **Burn of first degree of left forearm**

☑7ᵗʰ **T22.119** **Burn of first degree of unspecified forearm**

☑6ᵗʰ **T22.12** **Burn of first degree of elbow**

☑7ᵗʰ **T22.121** **Burn of first degree of right elbow**

☑7ᵗʰ **T22.122** **Burn of first degree of left elbow**

☑7ᵗʰ **T22.129** **Burn of first degree of unspecified elbow**

☑6ᵗʰ **T22.13** **Burn of first degree of upper arm**

☑7ᵗʰ **T22.131** **Burn of first degree of right upper arm**

☑7ᵗʰ **T22.132** **Burn of first degree of left upper arm**

☑7ᵗʰ **T22.139** **Burn of first degree of unspecified upper arm**

☑6ᵗʰ **T22.14** **Burn of first degree of axilla**

☑7ᵗʰ **T22.141** **Burn of first degree of right axilla**

☑7ᵗʰ **T22.142** **Burn of first degree of left axilla**

☑7ᵗʰ **T22.149** **Burn of first degree of unspecified axilla**

☑6ᵗʰ **T22.15** **Burn of first degree of shoulder**

☑7ᵗʰ **T22.151** **Burn of first degree of right shoulder**

☑7ᵗʰ **T22.152** **Burn of first degree of left shoulder**

☑7ᵗʰ **T22.159** **Burn of first degree of unspecified shoulder**

☑6ᵗʰ **T22.16** **Burn of first degree of scapular region**

☑7ᵗʰ **T22.161** **Burn of first degree of right scapular region**

☑7ᵗʰ **T22.162** **Burn of first degree of left scapular region**

☑7ᵗʰ **T22.169** **Burn of first degree of unspecified scapular region**

☑6ᵗʰ **T22.19** **Burn of first degree of multiple sites of shoulder and upper limb, except wrist and hand**

☑7ᵗʰ **T22.191** **Burn of first degree of multiple sites of right shoulder and upper limb, except wrist and hand**

☑7ᵗʰ **T22.192** **Burn of first degree of multiple sites of left shoulder and upper limb, except wrist and hand**

☑7ᵗʰ **T22.199** **Burn of first degree of multiple sites of unspecified shoulder and upper limb, except wrist and hand**

☑5ᵗʰ **T22.2** Burn of second degree of shoulder and upper limb, except wrist and hand
    Use additional external cause code to identify the source, place and intent of the burn (X00-X19, X75-X77, X96-X98, Y92)

☑x7ᵗʰ **T22.20** **Burn of second degree of shoulder and upper limb, except wrist and hand, unspecified site**

☑6ᵗʰ **T22.21** **Burn of second degree of forearm**

☑7ᵗʰ **T22.211** **Burn of second degree of right forearm**

☑7ᵗʰ **T22.212** **Burn of second degree of left forearm**

☑7ᵗʰ **T22.219** **Burn of second degree of unspecified forearm**

☑6ᵗʰ **T22.22** **Burn of second degree of elbow**

☑7ᵗʰ **T22.221** **Burn of second degree of right elbow**

☑7ᵗʰ **T22.222** **Burn of second degree of left elbow**

☑7ᵗʰ **T22.229** **Burn of second degree of unspecified elbow**

☑6ᵗʰ **T22.23** **Burn of second degree of upper arm**

☑7ᵗʰ **T22.231** **Burn of second degree of right upper arm**

☑7ᵗʰ **T22.232** **Burn of second degree of left upper arm**

☑7ᵗʰ **T22.239** **Burn of second degree of unspecified upper arm**

☑6ᵗʰ **T22.24** **Burn of second degree of axilla**

☑7ᵗʰ **T22.241** **Burn of second degree of right axilla**

☑7ᵗʰ **T22.242** **Burn of second degree of left axilla**

☑7ᵗʰ **T22.249** **Burn of second degree of unspecified axilla**

☑6ᵗʰ **T22.25** **Burn of second degree of shoulder**

☑7ᵗʰ **T22.251** **Burn of second degree of right shoulder**

☑7ᵗʰ **T22.252** **Burn of second degree of left shoulder**

☑7ᵗʰ **T22.259** **Burn of second degree of unspecified shoulder**

☑6ᵗʰ **T22.26** **Burn of second degree of scapular region**

☑7ᵗʰ **T22.261** **Burn of second degree of right scapular region**

☑7ᵗʰ **T22.262** **Burn of second degree of left scapular region**

☑7ᵗʰ **T22.269** **Burn of second degree of unspecified scapular region**

☑6ᵗʰ **T22.29** **Burn of second degree of multiple sites of shoulder and upper limb, except wrist and hand**

☑7ᵗʰ **T22.291** **Burn of second degree of multiple sites of right shoulder and upper limb, except wrist and hand**

☑7ᵗʰ **T22.292** **Burn of second degree of multiple sites of left shoulder and upper limb, except wrist and hand**

☑7ᵗʰ **T22.299** **Burn of second degree of multiple sites of unspecified shoulder and upper limb, except wrist and hand**

☑5ᵗʰ **T22.3** Burn of third degree of shoulder and upper limb, except wrist and hand
    Use additional external cause code to identify the source, place and intent of the burn (X00-X19, X75-X77, X96-X98, Y92)

☑x7ᵗʰ **T22.30** **Burn of third degree of shoulder and upper limb, except wrist and hand, unspecified site**

☑6ᵗʰ **T22.31** **Burn of third degree of forearm**

☑7ᵗʰ **T22.311** **Burn of third degree of right forearm**

☑7ᵗʰ **T22.312** **Burn of third degree of left forearm**

☑7ᵗʰ **T22.319** **Burn of third degree of unspecified forearm**

☑6ᵗʰ **T22.32** **Burn of third degree of elbow**

☑7ᵗʰ **T22.321** **Burn of third degree of right elbow**

☑7ᵗʰ **T22.322** **Burn of third degree of left elbow**

☑7ᵗʰ **T22.329** **Burn of third degree of unspecified elbow**

☑6ᵗʰ **T22.33** **Burn of third degree of upper arm**

☑7ᵗʰ **T22.331** **Burn of third degree of right upper arm**

☑7ᵗʰ **T22.332** **Burn of third degree of left upper arm**

☑7ᵗʰ **T22.339** **Burn of third degree of unspecified upper arm**

☑6ᵗʰ **T22.34** **Burn of third degree of axilla**

☑7ᵗʰ **T22.341** **Burn of third degree of right axilla**

☑7ᵗʰ **T22.342** **Burn of third degree of left axilla**

☑7ᵗʰ **T22.349** **Burn of third degree of unspecified axilla**

☑6ᵗʰ **T22.35** **Burn of third degree of shoulder**

☑7ᵗʰ **T22.351** **Burn of third degree of right shoulder**

☑7ᵗʰ **T22.352** **Burn of third degree of left shoulder**

☑7ᵗʰ **T22.359** **Burn of third degree of unspecified shoulder**

☑6ᵗʰ **T22.36** **Burn of third degree of scapular region**

☑7ᵗʰ **T22.361** **Burn of third degree of right scapular region**

☑7ᵗʰ **T22.362** **Burn of third degree of left scapular region**

☑7ᵗʰ **T22.369** **Burn of third degree of unspecified scapular region**

☑6ᵗʰ **T22.39** **Burn of third degree of multiple sites of shoulder and upper limb, except wrist and hand**

☑7ᵗʰ **T22.391** **Burn of third degree of multiple sites of right shoulder and upper limb, except wrist and hand**

☑7ᵗʰ **T22.392** **Burn of third degree of multiple sites of left shoulder and upper limb, except wrist and hand**

☑7ᵗʰ **T22.399** **Burn of third degree of multiple sites of unspecified shoulder and upper limb, except wrist and hand**

☑ Additional Character Required   ☑x7ᵗʰ Xtension Alert   Unspecified Code   Other Specified Code   Manifestation Code   ▶◀ Revised Text   ● New Code   ▲ Revised Code Title

ICD-10-CM 2014 (Draft)   **927**

Injury, Poisoning and Certain Other Consequences of External Causes

T22.4–T22.659

✓5th **T22.4** **Corrosion of** unspecified degree **of shoulder and upper limb, except wrist and hand**

    Code first (T51-T65) to identify chemical and intent
    Use additional external cause code to identify place (Y92)

  ✓x7th **T22.40** **Corrosion of unspecified degree of shoulder and upper limb, except wrist and hand, unspecified site**

  ✓6th **T22.41** **Corrosion of unspecified degree of** forearm

    ✓7th **T22.411** **Corrosion of unspecified degree of** right **forearm**

    ✓7th **T22.412** **Corrosion of unspecified degree of** left **forearm**

    ✓7th **T22.419** **Corrosion of unspecified degree of unspecified forearm**

  ✓6th **T22.42** **Corrosion of unspecified degree of** elbow

    ✓7th **T22.421** **Corrosion of unspecified degree of** right **elbow**

    ✓7th **T22.422** **Corrosion of unspecified degree of** left **elbow**

    ✓7th **T22.429** **Corrosion of unspecified degree of unspecified elbow**

  ✓6th **T22.43** **Corrosion of unspecified degree of** upper arm

    ✓7th **T22.431** **Corrosion of unspecified degree of** right **upper arm**

    ✓7th **T22.432** **Corrosion of unspecified degree of** left **upper arm**

    ✓7th **T22.439** **Corrosion of unspecified degree of unspecified upper arm**

  ✓6th **T22.44** **Corrosion of unspecified degree of** axilla

    ✓7th **T22.441** **Corrosion of unspecified degree of** right **axilla**

    ✓7th **T22.442** **Corrosion of unspecified degree of** left **axilla**

    ✓7th **T22.449** **Corrosion of unspecified degree of unspecified axilla**

  ✓6th **T22.45** **Corrosion of unspecified degree of** shoulder

    ✓7th **T22.451** **Corrosion of unspecified degree of** right **shoulder**

    ✓7th **T22.452** **Corrosion of unspecified degree of** left **shoulder**

    ✓7th **T22.459** **Corrosion of unspecified degree of unspecified shoulder**

  ✓6th **T22.46** **Corrosion of unspecified degree of** scapular region

    ✓7th **T22.461** **Corrosion of unspecified degree of** right **scapular region**

    ✓7th **T22.462** **Corrosion of unspecified degree of** left **scapular region**

    ✓7th **T22.469** **Corrosion of unspecified degree of unspecified scapular region**

  ✓6th **T22.49** **Corrosion of unspecified degree of** multiple sites **of shoulder and upper limb, except wrist and hand**

    ✓7th **T22.491** **Corrosion of unspecified degree of multiple sites of** right **shoulder and upper limb, except wrist and hand**

    ✓7th **T22.492** **Corrosion of unspecified degree of multiple sites of** left **shoulder and upper limb, except wrist and hand**

    ✓7th **T22.499** **Corrosion of unspecified degree of multiple sites of unspecified shoulder and upper limb, except wrist and hand**

✓5th **T22.5** **Corrosion of** first degree **of shoulder and upper limb, except wrist and hand**

    Code first (T51-T65) to identify chemical and intent
    Use additional external cause code to identify place (Y92)

  ✓x7th **T22.50** **Corrosion of first degree of shoulder and upper limb, except wrist and hand unspecified site**

  ✓6th **T22.51** **Corrosion of first degree of** forearm

    ✓7th **T22.511** **Corrosion of first degree of** right **forearm**

    ✓7th **T22.512** **Corrosion of first degree of** left **forearm**

    ✓7th **T22.519** **Corrosion of first degree of unspecified forearm**

  ✓6th **T22.52** **Corrosion of first degree of** elbow

    ✓7th **T22.521** **Corrosion of first degree of** right **elbow**

    ✓7th **T22.522** **Corrosion of first degree of** left **elbow**

  ✓7th **T22.529** **Corrosion of first degree of unspecified elbow**

  ✓6th **T22.53** **Corrosion of first degree of** upper arm

    ✓7th **T22.531** **Corrosion of first degree of** right **upper arm**

    ✓7th **T22.532** **Corrosion of first degree of** left **upper arm**

    ✓7th **T22.539** **Corrosion of first degree of unspecified upper arm**

  ✓6th **T22.54** **Corrosion of first degree of** axilla

    ✓7th **T22.541** **Corrosion of first degree of** right **axilla**

    ✓7th **T22.542** **Corrosion of first degree of** left **axilla**

    ✓7th **T22.549** **Corrosion of first degree of unspecified axilla**

  ✓6th **T22.55** **Corrosion of first degree of** shoulder

    ✓7th **T22.551** **Corrosion of first degree of** right **shoulder**

    ✓7th **T22.552** **Corrosion of first degree of** left **shoulder**

    ✓7th **T22.559** **Corrosion of first degree of unspecified shoulder**

  ✓6th **T22.56** **Corrosion of first degree of** scapular region

    ✓7th **T22.561** **Corrosion of first degree of** right **scapular region**

    ✓7th **T22.562** **Corrosion of first degree of** left **scapular region**

    ✓7th **T22.569** **Corrosion of first degree of unspecified scapular region**

  ✓6th **T22.59** **Corrosion of first degree of** multiple sites **of shoulder and upper limb, except wrist and hand**

    ✓7th **T22.591** **Corrosion of first degree of multiple sites of** right **shoulder and upper limb, except wrist and hand**

    ✓7th **T22.592** **Corrosion of first degree of multiple sites of** left **shoulder and upper limb, except wrist and hand**

    ✓7th **T22.599** **Corrosion of first degree of multiple sites of unspecified shoulder and upper limb, except wrist and hand**

✓5th **T22.6** **Corrosion of** second degree **of shoulder and upper limb, except wrist and hand**

    Code first (T51-T65) to identify chemical and intent
    Use additional external cause code to identify place (Y92)

  ✓x7th **T22.60** **Corrosion of second degree of shoulder and upper limb, except wrist and hand, unspecified site**

  ✓6th **T22.61** **Corrosion of second degree of** forearm

    ✓7th **T22.611** **Corrosion of second degree of** right **forearm**

    ✓7th **T22.612** **Corrosion of second degree of** left **forearm**

    ✓7th **T22.619** **Corrosion of second degree of unspecified forearm**

  ✓6th **T22.62** **Corrosion of second degree of** elbow

    ✓7th **T22.621** **Corrosion of second degree of** right **elbow**

    ✓7th **T22.622** **Corrosion of second degree of** left **elbow**

    ✓7th **T22.629** **Corrosion of second degree of unspecified elbow**

  ✓6th **T22.63** **Corrosion of second degree of** upper arm

    ✓7th **T22.631** **Corrosion of second degree of** right **upper arm**

    ✓7th **T22.632** **Corrosion of second degree of** left **upper arm**

    ✓7th **T22.639** **Corrosion of second degree of unspecified upper arm**

  ✓6th **T22.64** **Corrosion of second degree of** axilla

    ✓7th **T22.641** **Corrosion of second degree of** right **axilla**

    ✓7th **T22.642** **Corrosion of second degree of** left **axilla**

    ✓7th **T22.649** **Corrosion of second degree of unspecified axilla**

  ✓6th **T22.65** **Corrosion of second degree of** shoulder

    ✓7th **T22.651** **Corrosion of second degree of** right **shoulder**

    ✓7th **T22.652** **Corrosion of second degree of** left **shoulder**

    ✓7th **T22.659** **Corrosion of second degree of unspecified shoulder**

EXCLUDES 1 Not coded here   EXCLUDES 2 Not included here   N Newborn Age: 0   P Pediatric Age: 0-17   M Maternity Age: 12-55   A Adult Age: 15-124

928   ICD-10-CM 2014 (Draft)

✓6th **T22.66** Corrosion of second degree of scapular region

  ✓7th **T22.661** Corrosion of second degree of right scapular region

  ✓7th **T22.662** Corrosion of second degree of left scapular region

  ✓7th **T22.669 Corrosion of second degree of unspecified scapular region**

✓6th **T22.69** Corrosion of second degree of multiple sites of shoulder and upper limb, except wrist and hand

  ✓7th **T22.691 Corrosion of second degree of multiple sites of right shoulder and upper limb, except wrist and hand**

  ✓7th **T22.692 Corrosion of second degree of multiple sites of left shoulder and upper limb, except wrist and hand**

  ✓7th **T22.699 Corrosion of second degree of multiple sites of unspecified shoulder and upper limb, except wrist and hand**

✓5th **T22.7** Corrosion of third degree of shoulder and upper limb, except wrist and hand

  Code first (T51-T65) to identify chemical and intent

  Use additional external cause code to identify place (Y92)

  ✓x7th **T22.70 Corrosion of third degree of shoulder and upper limb, except wrist and hand, unspecified site**

✓6th **T22.71** Corrosion of third degree of forearm

  ✓7th **T22.711** Corrosion of third degree of right forearm

  ✓7th **T22.712** Corrosion of third degree of left forearm

  ✓7th **T22.719 Corrosion of third degree of unspecified forearm**

✓6th **T22.72** Corrosion of third degree of elbow

  ✓7th **T22.721** Corrosion of third degree of right elbow

  ✓7th **T22.722** Corrosion of third degree of left elbow

  ✓7th **T22.729 Corrosion of third degree of unspecified elbow**

✓6th **T22.73** Corrosion of third degree of upper arm

  ✓7th **T22.731** Corrosion of third degree of right upper arm

  ✓7th **T22.732** Corrosion of third degree of left upper arm

  ✓7th **T22.739 Corrosion of third degree of unspecified upper arm**

✓6th **T22.74** Corrosion of third degree of axilla

  ✓7th **T22.741** Corrosion of third degree of right axilla

  ✓7th **T22.742** Corrosion of third degree of left axilla

  ✓7th **T22.749 Corrosion of third degree of unspecified axilla**

✓6th **T22.75** Corrosion of third degree of shoulder

  ✓7th **T22.751** Corrosion of third degree of right shoulder

  ✓7th **T22.752** Corrosion of third degree of left shoulder

  ✓7th **T22.759 Corrosion of third degree of unspecified shoulder**

✓6th **T22.76** Corrosion of third degree of scapular region

  ✓7th **T22.761 Corrosion of third degree of right scapular region**

  ✓7th **T22.762 Corrosion of third degree of left scapular region**

  ✓7th **T22.769 Corrosion of third degree of unspecified scapular region**

✓6th **T22.79** Corrosion of third degree of multiple sites of shoulder and upper limb, except wrist and hand

  ✓7th **T22.791 Corrosion of third degree of multiple sites of right shoulder and upper limb, except wrist and hand**

  ✓7th **T22.792 Corrosion of third degree of multiple sites of left shoulder and upper limb, except wrist and hand**

  ✓7th **T22.799 Corrosion of third degree of multiple sites of unspecified shoulder and upper limb, except wrist and hand**

✓4th **T23** Burn and corrosion of wrist and hand

The appropriate 7th character is to be added to each code from category T23.
A   initial encounter
D   subsequent encounter
S   sequela

✓5th **T23.0** Burn of unspecified degree of wrist and hand

  Use additional external cause code to identify the source, place and intent of the burn (X00-X19, X75-X77, X96-X98, Y92)

✓6th **T23.00** Burn of unspecified degree of hand, unspecified site

  ✓7th **T23.001 Burn of unspecified degree of right hand, unspecified site**

  ✓7th **T23.002 Burn of unspecified degree of left hand, unspecified site**

  ✓7th **T23.009 Burn of unspecified degree of unspecified hand, unspecified site**

✓6th **T23.01** Burn of unspecified degree of thumb (nail)

  ✓7th **T23.011 Burn of unspecified degree of right thumb (nail)**

  ✓7th **T23.012 Burn of unspecified degree of left thumb (nail)**

  ✓7th **T23.019 Burn of unspecified degree of unspecified thumb (nail)**

✓6th **T23.02** Burn of unspecified degree of single finger (nail) except thumb

  ✓7th **T23.021 Burn of unspecified degree of single right finger (nail) except thumb**

  ✓7th **T23.022 Burn of unspecified degree of single left finger (nail) except thumb**

  ✓7th **T23.029 Burn of unspecified degree of unspecified single finger (nail) except thumb**

✓6th **T23.03** Burn of unspecified degree of multiple fingers (nail), not including thumb

  ✓7th **T23.031 Burn of unspecified degree of multiple right fingers (nail), not including thumb**

  ✓7th **T23.032 Burn of unspecified degree of multiple left fingers (nail), not including thumb**

  ✓7th **T23.039 Burn of unspecified degree of unspecified multiple fingers (nail), not including thumb**

✓6th **T23.04** Burn of unspecified degree of multiple fingers (nail), including thumb

  ✓7th **T23.041 Burn of unspecified degree of multiple right fingers (nail), including thumb**

  ✓7th **T23.042 Burn of unspecified degree of multiple left fingers (nail), including thumb**

  ✓7th **T23.049 Burn of unspecified degree of unspecified multiple fingers (nail), including thumb**

✓6th **T23.05** Burn of unspecified degree of palm

  ✓7th **T23.051** Burn of unspecified degree of right palm

  ✓7th **T23.052** Burn of unspecified degree of left palm

  ✓7th **T23.059 Burn of unspecified degree of unspecified palm**

✓6th **T23.06** Burn of unspecified degree of back of hand

  ✓7th **T23.061 Burn of unspecified degree of back of right hand**

  ✓7th **T23.062 Burn of unspecified degree of back of left hand**

  ✓7th **T23.069 Burn of unspecified degree of back of unspecified hand**

✓6th **T23.07** Burn of unspecified degree of wrist

  ✓7th **T23.071** Burn of unspecified degree of right wrist

  ✓7th **T23.072** Burn of unspecified degree of left wrist

  ✓7th **T23.079 Burn of unspecified degree of unspecified wrist**

✓6th **T23.09** Burn of unspecified degree of multiple sites of wrist and hand

  ✓7th **T23.091 Burn of unspecified degree of multiple sites of right wrist and hand**

  ✓7th **T23.092 Burn of unspecified degree of multiple sites of left wrist and hand**

  ✓7th **T23.099 Burn of unspecified degree of multiple sites of unspecified wrist and hand**

✓ Additional Character Required   ✓x7th Xtension Alert   Unspecified Code   Other Specified Code   Manifestation Code   ▶◀ Revised Text   ● New Code   ▲ Revised Code Title

ICD-10-CM 2014 (Draft)   **929**

✓5ᵗʰ **T23.1** Burn of first degree of wrist and hand

Use additional external cause code to identify the source, place and intent of the burn (X00-X19, X75-X77, X96-X98, Y92)

✓6ᵗʰ **T23.10** Burn of first degree of hand, unspecified site

✓7ᵗʰ **T23.101** Burn of first degree of right hand, unspecified site

✓7ᵗʰ **T23.102** Burn of first degree of left hand, unspecified site

✓7ᵗʰ **T23.109** Burn of first degree of unspecified hand, unspecified site

✓6ᵗʰ **T23.11** Burn of first degree of thumb (nail)

✓7ᵗʰ **T23.111** Burn of first degree of right thumb (nail)

✓7ᵗʰ **T23.112** Burn of first degree of left thumb (nail)

✓7ᵗʰ **T23.119** Burn of first degree of unspecified thumb (nail)

✓6ᵗʰ **T23.12** Burn of first degree of single finger (nail) except thumb

✓7ᵗʰ **T23.121** Burn of first degree of single right finger (nail) except thumb

✓7ᵗʰ **T23.122** Burn of first degree of single left finger (nail) except thumb

✓7ᵗʰ **T23.129** Burn of first degree of unspecified single finger (nail) except thumb

✓6ᵗʰ **T23.13** Burn of first degree of multiple fingers (nail), not including thumb

✓7ᵗʰ **T23.131** Burn of first degree of multiple right fingers (nail), not including thumb

✓7ᵗʰ **T23.132** Burn of first degree of multiple left fingers (nail), not including thumb

✓7ᵗʰ **T23.139** Burn of first degree of unspecified multiple fingers (nail), not including thumb

✓6ᵗʰ **T23.14** Burn of first degree of multiple fingers (nail), including thumb

✓7ᵗʰ **T23.141** Burn of first degree of multiple right fingers (nail), including thumb

✓7ᵗʰ **T23.142** Burn of first degree of multiple left fingers (nail), including thumb

✓7ᵗʰ **T23.149** Burn of first degree of unspecified multiple fingers (nail), including thumb

✓6ᵗʰ **T23.15** Burn of first degree of palm

✓7ᵗʰ **T23.151** Burn of first degree of right palm

✓7ᵗʰ **T23.152** Burn of first degree of left palm

✓7ᵗʰ **T23.159** Burn of first degree of unspecified palm

✓6ᵗʰ **T23.16** Burn of first degree of back of hand

✓7ᵗʰ **T23.161** Burn of first degree of back of right hand

✓7ᵗʰ **T23.162** Burn of first degree of back of left hand

✓7ᵗʰ **T23.169** Burn of first degree of back of unspecified hand

✓6ᵗʰ **T23.17** Burn of first degree of wrist

✓7ᵗʰ **T23.171** Burn of first degree of right wrist

✓7ᵗʰ **T23.172** Burn of first degree of left wrist

✓7ᵗʰ **T23.179** Burn of first degree of unspecified wrist

✓6ᵗʰ **T23.19** Burn of first degree of multiple sites of wrist and hand

✓7ᵗʰ **T23.191** Burn of first degree of multiple sites of right wrist and hand

✓7ᵗʰ **T23.192** Burn of first degree of multiple sites of left wrist and hand

✓7ᵗʰ **T23.199** Burn of first degree of multiple sites of unspecified wrist and hand

✓5ᵗʰ **T23.2** Burn of second degree of wrist and hand

Use additional external cause code to identify the source, place and intent of the burn (X00-X19, X75-X77, X96-X98, Y92)

✓6ᵗʰ **T23.20** Burn of second degree of hand, unspecified site

✓7ᵗʰ **T23.201** Burn of second degree of right hand, unspecified site

✓7ᵗʰ **T23.202** Burn of second degree of left hand, unspecified site

✓7ᵗʰ **T23.209** Burn of second degree of unspecified hand, unspecified site

✓6ᵗʰ **T23.21** Burn of second degree of thumb (nail)

✓7ᵗʰ **T23.211** Burn of second degree of right thumb (nail)

✓7ᵗʰ **T23.212** Burn of second degree of left thumb (nail)

✓7ᵗʰ **T23.219** Burn of second degree of unspecified thumb (nail)

✓6ᵗʰ **T23.22** Burn of second degree of single finger (nail) except thumb

✓7ᵗʰ **T23.221** Burn of second degree of single right finger (nail) except thumb

✓7ᵗʰ **T23.222** Burn of second degree of single left finger (nail) except thumb

✓7ᵗʰ **T23.229** Burn of second degree of unspecified single finger (nail) except thumb

✓6ᵗʰ **T23.23** Burn of second degree of multiple fingers (nail), not including thumb

✓7ᵗʰ **T23.231** Burn of second degree of multiple right fingers (nail), not including thumb

✓7ᵗʰ **T23.232** Burn of second degree of multiple left fingers (nail), not including thumb

✓7ᵗʰ **T23.239** Burn of second degree of unspecified multiple fingers (nail), not including thumb

✓6ᵗʰ **T23.24** Burn of second degree of multiple fingers (nail), including thumb

✓7ᵗʰ **T23.241** Burn of second degree of multiple right fingers (nail), including thumb

✓7ᵗʰ **T23.242** Burn of second degree of multiple left fingers (nail), including thumb

✓7ᵗʰ **T23.249** Burn of second degree of unspecified multiple fingers (nail), including thumb

✓6ᵗʰ **T23.25** Burn of second degree of palm

✓7ᵗʰ **T23.251** Burn of second degree of right palm

✓7ᵗʰ **T23.252** Burn of second degree of left palm

✓7ᵗʰ **T23.259** Burn of second degree of unspecified palm

✓6ᵗʰ **T23.26** Burn of second degree of back of hand

✓7ᵗʰ **T23.261** Burn of second degree of back of right hand

✓7ᵗʰ **T23.262** Burn of second degree of back of left hand

✓7ᵗʰ **T23.269** Burn of second degree of back of unspecified hand

✓6ᵗʰ **T23.27** Burn of second degree of wrist

✓7ᵗʰ **T23.271** Burn of second degree of right wrist

✓7ᵗʰ **T23.272** Burn of second degree of left wrist

✓7ᵗʰ **T23.279** Burn of second degree of unspecified wrist

✓6ᵗʰ **T23.29** Burn of second degree of multiple sites of wrist and hand

✓7ᵗʰ **T23.291** Burn of second degree of multiple sites of right wrist and hand

✓7ᵗʰ **T23.292** Burn of second degree of multiple sites of left wrist and hand

✓7ᵗʰ **T23.299** Burn of second degree of multiple sites of unspecified wrist and hand

✓5ᵗʰ **T23.3** Burn of third degree of wrist and hand

Use additional external cause code to identify the source, place and intent of the burn (X00-X19, X75-X77, X96-X98, Y92)

✓6ᵗʰ **T23.30** Burn of third degree of hand, unspecified site

✓7ᵗʰ **T23.301** Burn of third degree of right hand, unspecified site

✓7ᵗʰ **T23.302** Burn of third degree of left hand, unspecified site

✓7ᵗʰ **T23.309** Burn of third degree of unspecified hand, unspecified site

✓6ᵗʰ **T23.31** Burn of third degree of thumb (nail)

✓7ᵗʰ **T23.311** Burn of third degree of right thumb (nail)

✓7ᵗʰ **T23.312** Burn of third degree of left thumb (nail)

✓7ᵗʰ **T23.319** Burn of third degree of unspecified thumb (nail)

✓6ᵗʰ **T23.32** Burn of third degree of single finger (nail) except thumb

✓7ᵗʰ **T23.321** Burn of third degree of single right finger (nail) except thumb

EXCLUDES 1 Not coded here   EXCLUDES 2 Not included here   N Newborn Age: 0   P Pediatric Age: 0-17   M Maternity Age: 12-55   A Adult Age: 15-124

930   ICD-10-CM 2014 (Draft)

✓7th **T23.322** Burn of third degree of single left finger (nail) except thumb

✓7th **T23.329** **Burn of third degree of unspecified single finger (nail) except thumb**

✓6th **T23.33** Burn of third degree of multiple fingers (nail), not including thumb

✓7th **T23.331** Burn of third degree of multiple right fingers (nail), not including thumb

✓7th **T23.332** Burn of third degree of multiple left fingers (nail), not including thumb

✓7th **T23.339** **Burn of third degree of unspecified multiple fingers (nail), not including thumb**

✓6th **T23.34** Burn of third degree of multiple fingers (nail), including thumb

✓7th **T23.341** Burn of third degree of multiple right fingers (nail), including thumb

✓7th **T23.342** Burn of third degree of multiple left fingers (nail), including thumb

✓7th **T23.349** **Burn of third degree of unspecified multiple fingers (nail), including thumb**

✓6th **T23.35** Burn of third degree of palm

✓7th **T23.351** Burn of third degree of right palm

✓7th **T23.352** Burn of third degree of left palm

✓7th **T23.359** **Burn of third degree of unspecified palm**

✓6th **T23.36** Burn of third degree of back of hand

✓7th **T23.361** Burn of third degree of back of right hand

✓7th **T23.362** Burn of third degree of back of left hand

✓7th **T23.369** **Burn of third degree of back of unspecified hand**

✓6th **T23.37** Burn of third degree of wrist

✓7th **T23.371** Burn of third degree of right wrist

✓7th **T23.372** Burn of third degree of left wrist

✓7th **T23.379** **Burn of third degree of unspecified wrist**

✓6th **T23.39** Burn of third degree of multiple sites of wrist and hand

✓7th **T23.391** Burn of third degree of multiple sites of right wrist and hand

✓7th **T23.392** Burn of third degree of multiple sites of left wrist and hand

✓7th **T23.399** **Burn of third degree of multiple sites of unspecified wrist and hand**

✓5th **T23.4** Corrosion of unspecified degree of wrist and hand
   Code first (T51-T65) to identify chemical and intent
   Use additional external cause code to identify place (Y92)

✓6th **T23.40** **Corrosion of unspecified degree of hand, unspecified site**

✓7th **T23.401** **Corrosion of unspecified degree of right hand, unspecified site**

✓7th **T23.402** **Corrosion of uealtnspecified degree of left hand, unspecified site**

✓7th **T23.409** **Corrosion of unspecified degree of unspecified hand, unspecified site**

✓6th **T23.41** Corrosion of unspecified degree of thumb (nail)

✓7th **T23.411** **Corrosion of unspecified degree of right thumb (nail)**

✓7th **T23.412** **Corrosion of unspecified degree of left thumb (nail)**

✓7th **T23.419** **Corrosion of unspecified degree of unspecified thumb (nail)**

✓6th **T23.42** Corrosion of unspecified degree of single finger (nail) except thumb

✓7th **T23.421** **Corrosion of unspecified degree of single right finger (nail) except thumb**

✓7th **T23.422** **Corrosion of unspecified degree of single left finger (nail) except thumb**

✓7th **T23.429** **Corrosion of unspecified degree of unspecified single finger (nail) except thumb**

✓6th **T23.43** Corrosion of unspecified degree of multiple fingers (nail), not including thumb

✓7th **T23.431** **Corrosion of unspecified degree of multiple right fingers (nail), not including thumb**

✓7th **T23.432** **Corrosion of unspecified degree of multiple left fingers (nail), not including thumb**

✓7th **T23.439** **Corrosion of unspecified degree of unspecified multiple fingers (nail), not including thumb**

✓6th **T23.44** Corrosion of unspecified degree of multiple fingers (nail), including thumb

✓7th **T23.441** **Corrosion of unspecified degree of multiple right fingers (nail), including thumb**

✓7th **T23.442** **Corrosion of unspecified degree of multiple left fingers (nail), including thumb**

✓7th **T23.449** **Corrosion of unspecified degree of unspecified multiple fingers (nail), including thumb**

✓6th **T23.45** Corrosion of unspecified degree of palm

✓7th **T23.451** **Corrosion of unspecified degree of right palm**

✓7th **T23.452** **Corrosion of unspecified degree of left palm**

✓7th **T23.459** **Corrosion of unspecified degree of unspecified palm**

✓6th **T23.46** Corrosion of unspecified degree of back of hand

✓7th **T23.461** **Corrosion of unspecified degree of back of right hand**

✓7th **T23.462** **Corrosion of unspecified degree of back of left hand**

✓7th **T23.469** **Corrosion of unspecified degree of back of unspecified hand**

✓6th **T23.47** Corrosion of unspecified degree of wrist

✓7th **T23.471** **Corrosion of unspecified degree of right wrist**

✓7th **T23.472** **Corrosion of unspecified degree of left wrist**

✓7th **T23.479** **Corrosion of unspecified degree of unspecified wrist**

✓6th **T23.49** Corrosion of unspecified degree of multiple sites of wrist and hand

✓7th **T23.491** **Corrosion of unspecified degree of multiple sites of right wrist and hand**

✓7th **T23.492** **Corrosion of unspecified degree of multiple sites of left wrist and hand**

✓7th **T23.499** **Corrosion of unspecified degree of multiple sites of unspecified wrist and hand**

✓5th **T23.5** Corrosion of first degree of wrist and hand
   Code first (T51-T65) to identify chemical and intent
   Use additional external cause code to identify place (Y92)

✓6th **T23.50** Corrosion of first degree of hand, unspecified site

✓7th **T23.501** **Corrosion of first degree of right hand, unspecified site**

✓7th **T23.502** **Corrosion of first degree of left hand, unspecified site**

✓7th **T23.509** **Corrosion of first degree of unspecified hand, unspecified site**

✓6th **T23.51** Corrosion of first degree of thumb (nail)

✓7th **T23.511** Corrosion of first degree of right thumb (nail)

✓7th **T23.512** Corrosion of first degree of left thumb (nail)

✓7th **T23.519** **Corrosion of first degree of unspecified thumb (nail)**

✓6th **T23.52** Corrosion of first degree of single finger (nail) except thumb

✓7th **T23.521** Corrosion of first degree of single right finger (nail) except thumb

✓7th **T23.522** Corrosion of first degree of single left finger (nail) except thumb

✓7th **T23.529** **Corrosion of first degree of unspecified single finger (nail) except thumb**

☑ Additional Character Required   ✓x7th Xtension Alert   Unspecified Code   Other Specified Code   Manifestation Code   ►◄ Revised Text   ● New Code   ▲ Revised Code Title

ICD-10-CM 2014 (Draft)   931

Injury, Poisoning and Certain Other Consequences of External Causes

T23.53–T23.741

✓6ᵗʰ **T23.53** Corrosion of first degree of multiple fingers (nail), not including thumb
  ✓7ᵗʰ **T23.531** Corrosion of first degree of multiple right fingers (nail), not including thumb
  ✓7ᵗʰ **T23.532** Corrosion of first degree of multiple left fingers (nail), not including thumb
  ✓7ᵗʰ **T23.539** Corrosion of first degree of unspecified multiple fingers (nail), not including thumb

✓6ᵗʰ **T23.54** Corrosion of first degree of multiple fingers (nail), including thumb
  ✓7ᵗʰ **T23.541** Corrosion of first degree of multiple right fingers (nail), including thumb
  ✓7ᵗʰ **T23.542** Corrosion of first degree of multiple left fingers (nail), including thumb
  ✓7ᵗʰ **T23.549** Corrosion of first degree of unspecified multiple fingers (nail), including thumb

✓6ᵗʰ **T23.55** Corrosion of first degree of palm
  ✓7ᵗʰ **T23.551** Corrosion of first degree of right palm
  ✓7ᵗʰ **T23.552** Corrosion of first degree of left palm
  ✓7ᵗʰ **T23.559** Corrosion of first degree of unspecified palm

✓6ᵗʰ **T23.56** Corrosion of first degree of back of hand
  ✓7ᵗʰ **T23.561** Corrosion of first degree of back of right hand
  ✓7ᵗʰ **T23.562** Corrosion of first degree of back of left hand
  ✓7ᵗʰ **T23.569** Corrosion of first degree of back of unspecified hand

✓6ᵗʰ **T23.57** Corrosion of first degree of wrist
  ✓7ᵗʰ **T23.571** Corrosion of first degree of right wrist
  ✓7ᵗʰ **T23.572** Corrosion of first degree of left wrist
  ✓7ᵗʰ **T23.579** Corrosion of first degree of unspecified wrist

✓6ᵗʰ **T23.59** Corrosion of first degree of multiple sites of wrist and hand
  ✓7ᵗʰ **T23.591** Corrosion of first degree of multiple sites of right wrist and hand
  ✓7ᵗʰ **T23.592** Corrosion of first degree of multiple sites of left wrist and hand
  ✓7ᵗʰ **T23.599** Corrosion of first degree of multiple sites of unspecified wrist and hand

✓5ᵗʰ **T23.6** Corrosion of second degree of wrist and hand
Code first (T51-T65) to identify chemical and intent
Use additional external cause code to identify place (Y92)

✓6ᵗʰ **T23.60** Corrosion of second degree of hand, unspecified site
  ✓7ᵗʰ **T23.601** Corrosion of second degree of right hand, unspecified site
  ✓7ᵗʰ **T23.602** Corrosion of second degree of left hand, unspecified site
  ✓7ᵗʰ **T23.609** Corrosion of first degree of unspecified hand, unspecified site

✓6ᵗʰ **T23.61** Corrosion of second degree of thumb (nail)
  ✓7ᵗʰ **T23.611** Corrosion of second degree of right thumb (nail)
  ✓7ᵗʰ **T23.612** Corrosion of second degree of left thumb (nail)
  ✓7ᵗʰ **T23.619** Corrosion of second degree of unspecified thumb (nail)

✓6ᵗʰ **T23.62** Corrosion of second degree of single finger (nail) except thumb
  ✓7ᵗʰ **T23.621** Corrosion of second degree of single right finger (nail) except thumb
  ✓7ᵗʰ **T23.622** Corrosion of second degree of single left finger (nail) except thumb
  ✓7ᵗʰ **T23.629** Corrosion of second degree of unspecified single finger (nail) except thumb

✓6ᵗʰ **T23.63** Corrosion of second degree of multiple fingers (nail), not including thumb
  ✓7ᵗʰ **T23.631** Corrosion of second degree of multiple right fingers (nail), not including thumb
  ✓7ᵗʰ **T23.632** Corrosion of second degree of multiple left fingers (nail), not including thumb

✓7ᵗʰ **T23.639** Corrosion of second degree of unspecified multiple fingers (nail), not including thumb

✓6ᵗʰ **T23.64** Corrosion of second degree of multiple fingers (nail), including thumb
  ✓7ᵗʰ **T23.641** Corrosion of second degree of multiple right fingers (nail), including thumb
  ✓7ᵗʰ **T23.642** Corrosion of second degree of multiple left fingers (nail), including thumb
  ✓7ᵗʰ **T23.649** Corrosion of second degree of unspecified multiple fingers (nail), including thumb

✓6ᵗʰ **T23.65** Corrosion of second degree of palm
  ✓7ᵗʰ **T23.651** Corrosion of second degree of right palm
  ✓7ᵗʰ **T23.652** Corrosion of second degree of left palm
  ✓7ᵗʰ **T23.659** Corrosion of second degree of unspecified palm

✓6ᵗʰ **T23.66** Corrosion of second degree of back of hand
  ✓7ᵗʰ **T23.661** Corrosion of second degree back of right hand
  ✓7ᵗʰ **T23.662** Corrosion of second degree back of left hand
  ✓7ᵗʰ **T23.669** Corrosion of second degree back of unspecified hand

✓6ᵗʰ **T23.67** Corrosion of second degree of wrist
  ✓7ᵗʰ **T23.671** Corrosion of second degree of right wrist
  ✓7ᵗʰ **T23.672** Corrosion of second degree of left wrist
  ✓7ᵗʰ **T23.679** Corrosion of second degree of unspecified wrist

✓6ᵗʰ **T23.69** Corrosion of second degree of multiple sites of wrist and hand
  ✓7ᵗʰ **T23.691** Corrosion of second degree of multiple sites of right wrist and hand
  ✓7ᵗʰ **T23.692** Corrosion of second degree of multiple sites of left wrist and hand
  ✓7ᵗʰ **T23.699** Corrosion of second degree of multiple sites of unspecified wrist and hand

✓5ᵗʰ **T23.7** Corrosion of third degree of wrist and hand
Code first (T51-T65) to identify chemical and intent
Use additional external cause code to identify place (Y92)

✓6ᵗʰ **T23.70** Corrosion of third degree of hand, unspecified site
  ✓7ᵗʰ **T23.701** Corrosion of third degree of right hand, unspecified site
  ✓7ᵗʰ **T23.702** Corrosion of third degree of left hand, unspecified site
  ✓7ᵗʰ **T23.709** Corrosion of third degree of unspecified hand, unspecified site

✓6ᵗʰ **T23.71** Corrosion of third degree of thumb (nail)
  ✓7ᵗʰ **T23.711** Corrosion of third degree of right thumb (nail)
  ✓7ᵗʰ **T23.712** Corrosion of third degree of left thumb (nail)
  ✓7ᵗʰ **T23.719** Corrosion of third degree of unspecified thumb (nail)

✓6ᵗʰ **T23.72** Corrosion of third degree of single finger (nail) except thumb
  ✓7ᵗʰ **T23.721** Corrosion of third degree of single right finger (nail) except thumb
  ✓7ᵗʰ **T23.722** Corrosion of third degree of single left finger (nail) except thumb
  ✓7ᵗʰ **T23.729** Corrosion of third degree of unspecified single finger (nail) except thumb

✓6ᵗʰ **T23.73** Corrosion of third degree of multiple fingers (nail), not including thumb
  ✓7ᵗʰ **T23.731** Corrosion of third degree of multiple right fingers (nail), not including thumb
  ✓7ᵗʰ **T23.732** Corrosion of third degree of multiple left fingers (nail), not including thumb
  ✓7ᵗʰ **T23.739** Corrosion of third degree of unspecified multiple fingers (nail), not including thumb

✓6ᵗʰ **T23.74** Corrosion of third degree of multiple fingers (nail), including thumb
  ✓7ᵗʰ **T23.741** Corrosion of third degree of multiple right fingers (nail), including thumb

---

EXCLUDES1 Not coded here   EXCLUDES2 Not included here   N Newborn Age: 0   P Pediatric Age: 0-17   M Maternity Age: 12-55   A Adult Age: 15-124

932   ICD-10-CM 2014 (Draft)

√7ᵗʰ **T23.742** Corrosion of third degree of multiple left fingers (nail), including thumb

√7ᵗʰ **T23.749** Corrosion of third degree of unspecified multiple fingers (nail), including thumb

√6ᵗʰ **T23.75** Corrosion of third degree of palm

√7ᵗʰ **T23.751** Corrosion of third degree of right palm

√7ᵗʰ **T23.752** Corrosion of third degree of left palm

√7ᵗʰ **T23.759** Corrosion of third degree of unspecified palm

√6ᵗʰ **T23.76** Corrosion of third degree of back of hand

√7ᵗʰ **T23.761** Corrosion of third degree of back of right hand

√7ᵗʰ **T23.762** Corrosion of third degree of back of left hand

√7ᵗʰ **T23.769** Corrosion of third degree back of unspecified hand

√6ᵗʰ **T23.77** Corrosion of third degree of wrist

√7ᵗʰ **T23.771** Corrosion of third degree of right wrist

√7ᵗʰ **T23.772** Corrosion of third degree of left wrist

√7ᵗʰ **T23.779** Corrosion of third degree of unspecified wrist

√6ᵗʰ **T23.79** Corrosion of third degree of multiple sites of wrist and hand

√7ᵗʰ **T23.791** Corrosion of third degree of multiple sites of right wrist and hand

√7ᵗʰ **T23.792** Corrosion of third degree of multiple sites of left wrist and hand

√7ᵗʰ **T23.799** Corrosion of third degree of multiple sites of unspecified wrist and hand

√4ᵗʰ **T24** Burn and corrosion of lower limb, except ankle and foot

EXCLUDES 2 burn and corrosion of ankle and foot (T25.-)
burn and corrosion of hip region (T21.-)

The appropriate 7th character is to be added to each code from category T24.
A   initial encounter
D   subsequent encounter
S   sequela

√5ᵗʰ **T24.0** Burn of unspecified degree of lower limb, except ankle and foot

Use additional external cause code to identify the source, place and intent of the burn (X00-X19, X75-X77, X96-X98, Y92)

√6ᵗʰ **T24.00** Burn of unspecified degree of unspecified site of lower limb, except ankle and foot

√7ᵗʰ **T24.001** Burn of unspecified degree of unspecified site of right lower limb, except ankle and foot

√7ᵗʰ **T24.002** Burn of unspecified degree of unspecified site of left lower limb, except ankle and foot

√7ᵗʰ **T24.009** Burn of unspecified degree of unspecified site of unspecified lower limb, except ankle and foot

√6ᵗʰ **T24.01** Burn of unspecified degree of thigh

√7ᵗʰ **T24.011** Burn of unspecified degree of right thigh

√7ᵗʰ **T24.012** Burn of unspecified degree of left thigh

√7ᵗʰ **T24.019** Burn of unspecified degree of unspecified thigh

√6ᵗʰ **T24.02** Burn of unspecified degree of knee

√7ᵗʰ **T24.021** Burn of unspecified degree of right knee

√7ᵗʰ **T24.022** Burn of unspecified degree of left knee

√7ᵗʰ **T24.029** Burn of unspecified degree of unspecified knee

√6ᵗʰ **T24.03** Burn of unspecified degree of lower leg

√7ᵗʰ **T24.031** Burn of unspecified degree of right lower leg

√7ᵗʰ **T24.032** Burn of unspecified degree of left lower leg

√7ᵗʰ **T24.039** Burn of unspecified degree of unspecified lower leg

√6ᵗʰ **T24.09** Burn of unspecified degree of multiple sites of lower limb, except ankle and foot

√7ᵗʰ **T24.091** Burn of unspecified degree of multiple sites of right lower limb, except ankle and foot

√7ᵗʰ **T24.092** Burn of unspecified degree of multiple sites of left lower limb, except ankle and foot

√7ᵗʰ **T24.099** Burn of unspecified degree of multiple sites of unspecified lower limb, except ankle and foot

√5ᵗʰ **T24.1** Burn of first degree of lower limb, except ankle and foot

Use additional external cause code to identify the source, place and intent of the burn (X00-X19, X75-X77, X96-X98, Y92)

√6ᵗʰ **T24.10** Burn of first degree of unspecified site of lower limb, except ankle and foot

√7ᵗʰ **T24.101** Burn of first degree of unspecified site of right lower limb, except ankle and foot

√7ᵗʰ **T24.102** Burn of first degree of unspecified site of left lower limb, except ankle and foot

√7ᵗʰ **T24.109** Burn of first degree of unspecified site of unspecified lower limb, except ankle and foot

√6ᵗʰ **T24.11** Burn of first degree of thigh

√7ᵗʰ **T24.111** Burn of first degree of right thigh

√7ᵗʰ **T24.112** Burn of first degree of left thigh

√7ᵗʰ **T24.119** Burn of first degree of unspecified thigh

√6ᵗʰ **T24.12** Burn of first degree of knee

√7ᵗʰ **T24.121** Burn of first degree of right knee

√7ᵗʰ **T24.122** Burn of first degree of left knee

√7ᵗʰ **T24.129** Burn of first degree of unspecified knee

√6ᵗʰ **T24.13** Burn of first degree of lower leg

√7ᵗʰ **T24.131** Burn of first degree of right lower leg

√7ᵗʰ **T24.132** Burn of first degree of left lower leg

√7ᵗʰ **T24.139** Burn of first degree of unspecified lower leg

√6ᵗʰ **T24.19** Burn of first degree of multiple sites of lower limb, except ankle and foot

√7ᵗʰ **T24.191** Burn of first degree of multiple sites of right lower limb, except ankle and foot

√7ᵗʰ **T24.192** Burn of first degree of multiple sites of left lower limb, except ankle and foot

√7ᵗʰ **T24.199** Burn of first degree of multiple sites of unspecified lower limb, except ankle and foot

√5ᵗʰ **T24.2** Burn of second degree of lower limb, except ankle and foot

Use additional external cause code to identify the source, place and intent of the burn (X00-X19, X75-X77, X96-X98, Y92)

√6ᵗʰ **T24.20** Burn of second degree of unspecified site of lower limb, except ankle and foot

√7ᵗʰ **T24.201** Burn of second degree of unspecified site of right lower limb, except ankle and foot

√7ᵗʰ **T24.202** Burn of second degree of unspecified site of left lower limb, except ankle and foot

√7ᵗʰ **T24.209** Burn of second degree of unspecified site of unspecified lower limb, except ankle and foot

√6ᵗʰ **T24.21** Burn of second degree of thigh

√7ᵗʰ **T24.211** Burn of second degree of right thigh

√7ᵗʰ **T24.212** Burn of second degree of left thigh

√7ᵗʰ **T24.219** Burn of second degree of unspecified thigh

√6ᵗʰ **T24.22** Burn of second degree of knee

√7ᵗʰ **T24.221** Burn of second degree of right knee

√7ᵗʰ **T24.222** Burn of second degree of left knee

√7ᵗʰ **T24.229** Burn of second degree of unspecified knee

√6ᵗʰ **T24.23** Burn of second degree of lower leg

√7ᵗʰ **T24.231** Burn of second degree of right lower leg

√7ᵗʰ **T24.232** Burn of second degree of left lower leg

√7ᵗʰ **T24.239** Burn of second degree of unspecified lower leg

√6ᵗʰ **T24.29** Burn of second degree of multiple sites of lower limb, except ankle and foot

√7ᵗʰ **T24.291** Burn of second degree of multiple sites of right lower limb, except ankle and foot

√7ᵗʰ **T24.292** Burn of second degree of multiple sites of left lower limb, except ankle and foot

√7ᵗʰ **T24.299** Burn of second degree of multiple sites of unspecified lower limb, except ankle and foot

√5ᵗʰ **T24.3** Burn of third degree of lower limb, except ankle and foot
Use additional external cause code to identify the source, place and intent of the burn (X00-X19, X75-X77, X96-X98, Y92)

√6ᵗʰ **T24.30** Burn of third degree of unspecified site of lower limb, except ankle and foot

√7ᵗʰ **T24.301** Burn of third degree of unspecified site of right lower limb, except ankle and foot

√7ᵗʰ **T24.302** Burn of third degree of unspecified site of left lower limb, except ankle and foot

√7ᵗʰ **T24.309** Burn of third degree of unspecified site of unspecified lower limb, except ankle and foot

√6ᵗʰ **T24.31** Burn of third degree of thigh

√7ᵗʰ **T24.311** Burn of third degree of right thigh

√7ᵗʰ **T24.312** Burn of third degree of left thigh

√7ᵗʰ **T24.319** Burn of third degree of unspecified thigh

√6ᵗʰ **T24.32** Burn of third degree of knee

√7ᵗʰ **T24.321** Burn of third degree of right knee

√7ᵗʰ **T24.322** Burn of third degree of left knee

√7ᵗʰ **T24.329** Burn of third degree of unspecified knee

√6ᵗʰ **T24.33** Burn of third degree of lower leg

√7ᵗʰ **T24.331** Burn of third degree of right lower leg

√7ᵗʰ **T24.332** Burn of third degree of left lower leg

√7ᵗʰ **T24.339** Burn of third degree of unspecified lower leg

√6ᵗʰ **T24.39** Burn of third degree of multiple sites of lower limb, except ankle and foot

√7ᵗʰ **T24.391** Burn of third degree of multiple sites of right lower limb, except ankle and foot

√7ᵗʰ **T24.392** Burn of third degree of multiple sites of left lower limb, except ankle and foot

√7ᵗʰ **T24.399** Burn of third degree of multiple sites of unspecified lower limb, except ankle and foot

√5ᵗʰ **T24.4** Corrosion of unspecified degree of lower limb, except ankle and foot
Code first (T51-T65) to identify chemical and intent
Use additional external cause code to identify place (Y92)

√6ᵗʰ **T24.40** Corrosion of unspecified degree of unspecified site of lower limb, except ankle and foot

√7ᵗʰ **T24.401** Corrosion of unspecified degree of unspecified site of right lower limb, except ankle and foot

√7ᵗʰ **T24.402** Corrosion of unspecified degree of unspecified site of left lower limb, except ankle and foot

√7ᵗʰ **T24.409** Corrosion of unspecified degree of unspecified site of unspecified lower limb, except ankle and foot

√6ᵗʰ **T24.41** Corrosion of unspecified degree of thigh

√7ᵗʰ **T24.411** Corrosion of unspecified degree of right thigh

√7ᵗʰ **T24.412** Corrosion of unspecified degree of left thigh

√7ᵗʰ **T24.419** Corrosion of unspecified degree of unspecified thigh

√6ᵗʰ **T24.42** Corrosion of unspecified degree of knee

√7ᵗʰ **T24.421** Corrosion of unspecified degree of right knee

√7ᵗʰ **T24.422** Corrosion of unspecified degree of left knee

√7ᵗʰ **T24.429** Corrosion of unspecified degree of unspecified knee

√6ᵗʰ **T24.43** Corrosion of unspecified degree of lower leg

√7ᵗʰ **T24.431** Corrosion of unspecified degree of right lower leg

√7ᵗʰ **T24.432** Corrosion of unspecified degree of left lower leg

√7ᵗʰ **T24.439** Corrosion of unspecified degree of unspecified lower leg

√6ᵗʰ **T24.49** Corrosion of unspecified degree of multiple sites of lower limb, except ankle and foot

√7ᵗʰ **T24.491** Corrosion of unspecified degree of multiple sites of right lower limb, except ankle and foot

√7ᵗʰ **T24.492** Corrosion of unspecified degree of multiple sites of left lower limb, except ankle and foot

√7ᵗʰ **T24.499** Corrosion of unspecified degree of multiple sites of unspecified lower limb, except ankle and foot

√5ᵗʰ **T24.5** Corrosion of first degree of lower limb, except ankle and foot
Code first (T51-T65) to identify chemical and intent
Use additional external cause code to identify place (Y92)

√6ᵗʰ **T24.50** Corrosion of first degree of unspecified site of lower limb, except ankle and foot

√7ᵗʰ **T24.501** Corrosion of first degree of unspecified site of right lower limb, except ankle and foot

√7ᵗʰ **T24.502** Corrosion of first degree of unspecified site of left lower limb, except ankle and foot

√7ᵗʰ **T24.509** Corrosion of first degree of unspecified site of unspecified lower limb, except ankle and foot

√6ᵗʰ **T24.51** Corrosion of first degree of thigh

√7ᵗʰ **T24.511** Corrosion of first degree of right thigh

√7ᵗʰ **T24.512** Corrosion of first degree of left thigh

√7ᵗʰ **T24.519** Corrosion of first degree of unspecified thigh

√6ᵗʰ **T24.52** Corrosion of first degree of knee

√7ᵗʰ **T24.521** Corrosion of first degree of right knee

√7ᵗʰ **T24.522** Corrosion of first degree of left knee

√7ᵗʰ **T24.529** Corrosion of first degree of unspecified knee

√6ᵗʰ **T24.53** Corrosion of first degree of lower leg

√7ᵗʰ **T24.531** Corrosion of first degree of right lower leg

√7ᵗʰ **T24.532** Corrosion of first degree of left lower leg

√7ᵗʰ **T24.539** Corrosion of first degree of unspecified lower leg

√6ᵗʰ **T24.59** Corrosion of first degree of multiple sites of lower limb, except ankle and foot

√7ᵗʰ **T24.591** Corrosion of first degree of multiple sites of right lower limb, except ankle and foot

√7ᵗʰ **T24.592** Corrosion of first degree of multiple sites of left lower limb, except ankle and foot

√7ᵗʰ **T24.599** Corrosion of first degree of multiple sites of unspecified lower limb, except ankle and foot

√5ᵗʰ **T24.6** Corrosion of second degree of lower limb, except ankle and foot
Code first (T51-T65) to identify chemical and intent
Use additional external cause code to identify place (Y92)

√6ᵗʰ **T24.60** Corrosion of second degree of unspecified site of lower limb, except ankle and foot

√7ᵗʰ **T24.601** Corrosion of second degree of unspecified site of right lower limb, except ankle and foot

√7ᵗʰ **T24.602** Corrosion of second degree of unspecified site of left lower limb, except ankle and foot

√7ᵗʰ **T24.609** Corrosion of second degree of unspecified site of unspecified lower limb, except ankle and foot

√6ᵗʰ **T24.61** Corrosion of second degree of thigh

√7ᵗʰ **T24.611** Corrosion of second degree of right thigh

√7ᵗʰ **T24.612** Corrosion of second degree of left thigh

√7ᵗʰ **T24.619** Corrosion of second degree of unspecified thigh

√6ᵗʰ **T24.62** Corrosion of second degree of knee

√7ᵗʰ **T24.621** Corrosion of second degree of right knee

√7ᵗʰ **T24.622** Corrosion of second degree of left knee

√7ᵗʰ **T24.629** Corrosion of second degree of unspecified knee

---

EXCLUDES 1 Not coded here   **EXCLUDES 2** Not included here   Ⓝ Newborn Age: 0   Ⓟ Pediatric Age: 0-17   Ⓜ Maternity Age: 12-55   Ⓐ Adult Age: 15-124

✓6ᵗʰ **T24.63** Corrosion of second degree of lower leg

     ✓7ᵗʰ **T24.631** Corrosion of second degree of right lower leg

     ✓7ᵗʰ **T24.632** Corrosion of second degree of left lower leg

     ✓7ᵗʰ **T24.639** Corrosion of second degree of unspecified lower leg

✓6ᵗʰ **T24.69** Corrosion of second degree of multiple sites of lower limb, except ankle and foot

     ✓7ᵗʰ **T24.691** Corrosion of second degree of multiple sites of right lower limb, except ankle and foot

     ✓7ᵗʰ **T24.692** Corrosion of second degree of multiple sites of left lower limb, except ankle and foot

     ✓7ᵗʰ **T24.699** Corrosion of second degree of multiple sites of unspecified lower limb, except ankle and foot

✓5ᵗʰ **T24.7** Corrosion of third degree of lower limb, except ankle and foot

     Code first (T51-T65) to identify chemical and intent
     Use additional external cause code to identify place (Y92)

✓6ᵗʰ **T24.70** Corrosion of third degree of unspecified site of lower limb, except ankle and foot

     ✓7ᵗʰ **T24.701** Corrosion of third degree of unspecified site of right lower limb, except ankle and foot

     ✓7ᵗʰ **T24.702** Corrosion of third degree of unspecified site of left lower limb, except ankle and foot

     ✓7ᵗʰ **T24.709** Corrosion of third degree of unspecified site of unspecified lower limb, except ankle and foot

✓6ᵗʰ **T24.71** Corrosion of third degree of thigh

     ✓7ᵗʰ **T24.711** Corrosion of third degree of right thigh

     ✓7ᵗʰ **T24.712** Corrosion of third degree of left thigh

     ✓7ᵗʰ **T24.719** Corrosion of third degree of unspecified thigh

✓6ᵗʰ **T24.72** Corrosion of third degree of knee

     ✓7ᵗʰ **T24.721** Corrosion of third degree of right knee

     ✓7ᵗʰ **T24.722** Corrosion of third degree of left knee

     ✓7ᵗʰ **T24.729** Corrosion of third degree of unspecified knee

✓6ᵗʰ **T24.73** Corrosion of third degree of lower leg

     ✓7ᵗʰ **T24.731** Corrosion of third degree of right lower leg

     ✓7ᵗʰ **T24.732** Corrosion of third degree of left lower leg

     ✓7ᵗʰ **T24.739** Corrosion of third degree of unspecified lower leg

✓6ᵗʰ **T24.79** Corrosion of third degree of multiple sites of lower limb, except ankle and foot

     ✓7ᵗʰ **T24.791** Corrosion of third degree of multiple sites of right lower limb, except ankle and foot

     ✓7ᵗʰ **T24.792** Corrosion of third degree of multiple sites of left lower limb, except ankle and foot

     ✓7ᵗʰ **T24.799** Corrosion of third degree of multiple sites of unspecified lower limb, except ankle and foot

✓4ᵗʰ **T25** **Burn and corrosion of ankle and foot**

     The appropriate 7th character is to be added to each code from category T25.
     A   initial encounter
     D   subsequent encounter
     S   sequela

✓5ᵗʰ **T25.0** Burn of unspecified degree of ankle and foot

     Use additional external cause code to identify the source, place and intent of the burn (X00-X19, X75-X77, X96-X98, Y92)

✓6ᵗʰ **T25.01** Burn of unspecified degree of ankle

     ✓7ᵗʰ **T25.011** Burn of unspecified degree of right ankle

     ✓7ᵗʰ **T25.012** Burn of unspecified degree of left ankle

     ✓7ᵗʰ **T25.019** Burn of unspecified degree of unspecified ankle

✓6ᵗʰ **T25.02** Burn of unspecified degree of foot

     EXCLUDES 2   burn of unspecified degree of toe(s) (nail) (T25.03-)

     ✓7ᵗʰ **T25.021** Burn of unspecified degree of right foot

     ✓7ᵗʰ **T25.022** Burn of unspecified degree of left foot

     ✓7ᵗʰ **T25.029** Burn of unspecified degree of unspecified foot

✓6ᵗʰ **T25.03** Burn of unspecified degree of toe(s) (nail)

     ✓7ᵗʰ **T25.031** Burn of unspecified degree of right toe(s) (nail)

     ✓7ᵗʰ **T25.032** Burn of unspecified degree of left toe(s) (nail)

     ✓7ᵗʰ **T25.039** Burn of unspecified degree of unspecified toe(s) (nail)

✓6ᵗʰ **T25.09** Burn of unspecified degree of multiple sites of ankle and foot

     ✓7ᵗʰ **T25.091** Burn of unspecified degree of multiple sites of right ankle and foot

     ✓7ᵗʰ **T25.092** Burn of unspecified degree of multiple sites of left ankle and foot

     ✓7ᵗʰ **T25.099** Burn of unspecified degree of multiple sites of unspecified ankle and foot

✓5ᵗʰ **T25.1** Burn of first degree of ankle and foot

     Use additional external cause code to identify the source, place and intent of the burn (X00-X19, X75-X77, X96-X98, Y92)

✓6ᵗʰ **T25.11** Burn of first degree of ankle

     ✓7ᵗʰ **T25.111** Burn of first degree of right ankle

     ✓7ᵗʰ **T25.112** Burn of first degree of left ankle

     ✓7ᵗʰ **T25.119** Burn of first degree of unspecified ankle

✓6ᵗʰ **T25.12** Burn of first degree of foot

     EXCLUDES 2   burn of first degree of toe(s) (nail) (T25.13-)

     ✓7ᵗʰ **T25.121** Burn of first degree of right foot

     ✓7ᵗʰ **T25.122** Burn of first degree of left foot

     ✓7ᵗʰ **T25.129** Burn of first degree of unspecified foot

✓6ᵗʰ **T25.13** Burn of first degree of toe(s) (nail)

     ✓7ᵗʰ **T25.131** Burn of first degree of right toe(s) (nail)

     ✓7ᵗʰ **T25.132** Burn of first degree of left toe(s) (nail)

     ✓7ᵗʰ **T25.139** Burn of first degree of unspecified toe(s) (nail)

✓6ᵗʰ **T25.19** Burn of first degree of multiple sites of ankle and foot

     ✓7ᵗʰ **T25.191** Burn of first degree of multiple sites of right ankle and foot

     ✓7ᵗʰ **T25.192** Burn of first degree of multiple sites of left ankle and foot

     ✓7ᵗʰ **T25.199** Burn of first degree of multiple sites of unspecified ankle and foot

✓5ᵗʰ **T25.2** Burn of second degree of ankle and foot

     Use additional external cause code to identify the source, place and intent of the burn (X00-X19, X75-X77, X96-X98, Y92)

✓6ᵗʰ **T25.21** Burn of second degree of ankle

     ✓7ᵗʰ **T25.211** Burn of second degree of right ankle

     ✓7ᵗʰ **T25.212** Burn of second degree of left ankle

     ✓7ᵗʰ **T25.219** Burn of second degree of unspecified ankle

✓6ᵗʰ **T25.22** Burn of second degree of foot

     EXCLUDES 2   burn of second degree of toe(s) (nail) (T25.23-)

     ✓7ᵗʰ **T25.221** Burn of second degree of right foot

     ✓7ᵗʰ **T25.222** Burn of second degree of left foot

     ✓7ᵗʰ **T25.229** Burn of second degree of unspecified foot

✓6ᵗʰ **T25.23** Burn of second degree of toe(s) (nail)

     ✓7ᵗʰ **T25.231** Burn of second degree of right toe(s) (nail)

     ✓7ᵗʰ **T25.232** Burn of second degree of left toe(s) (nail)

     ✓7ᵗʰ **T25.239** Burn of second degree of unspecified toe(s) (nail)

✓6ᵗʰ **T25.29** Burn of second degree of multiple sites of ankle and foot

     ✓7ᵗʰ **T25.291** Burn of second degree of multiple sites of right ankle and foot

     ✓7ᵗʰ **T25.292** Burn of second degree of multiple sites of left ankle and foot

     ✓7ᵗʰ **T25.299** Burn of second degree of multiple sites of unspecified ankle and foot

✓ Additional Character Required   ✓7ᵗʰ Xtension Alert   Unspecified Code   Other Specified Code   Manifestation Code   ▶◀ Revised Text   ● New Code   ▲ Revised Code Title

ICD-10-CM 2014 (Draft)   **935**

Injury, Poisoning and Certain Other Consequences of External Causes

T25.3–T25.792

✓5ᵗʰ **T25.3 Burn of third degree of ankle and foot**
Use additional external cause code to identify the source, place and intent of the burn (X00-X19, X75-X77, X96-X98, Y92)

   ✓6ᵗʰ **T25.31 Burn of third degree of ankle**
      ✓7ᵗʰ **T25.311 Burn of third degree of right ankle**
      ✓7ᵗʰ **T25.312 Burn of third degree of left ankle**
      ✓7ᵗʰ **T25.319 Burn of third degree of unspecified ankle**

   ✓6ᵗʰ **T25.32 Burn of third degree of foot**
      EXCLUDES 2   *burn of third degree of toe(s) (nail) (T25.33-)*
      ✓7ᵗʰ **T25.321 Burn of third degree of right foot**
      ✓7ᵗʰ **T25.322 Burn of third degree of left foot**
      ✓7ᵗʰ **T25.329 Burn of third degree of unspecified foot**

   ✓6ᵗʰ **T25.33 Burn of third degree of toe(s) (nail)**
      ✓7ᵗʰ **T25.331 Burn of third degree of right toe(s) (nail)**
      ✓7ᵗʰ **T25.332 Burn of third degree of left toe(s) (nail)**
      ✓7ᵗʰ **T25.339 Burn of third degree of unspecified toe(s) (nail)**

   ✓6ᵗʰ **T25.39 Burn of third degree of multiple sites of ankle and foot**
      ✓7ᵗʰ **T25.391 Burn of third degree of multiple sites of right ankle and foot**
      ✓7ᵗʰ **T25.392 Burn of third degree of multiple sites of left ankle and foot**
      ✓7ᵗʰ **T25.399 Burn of third degree of multiple sites of unspecified ankle and foot**

✓5ᵗʰ **T25.4 Corrosion of unspecified degree of ankle and foot**
Code first (T51-T65) to identify chemical and intent
Use additional external cause code to identify place (Y92)

   ✓6ᵗʰ **T25.41 Corrosion of unspecified degree of ankle**
      ✓7ᵗʰ **T25.411 Corrosion of unspecified degree of right ankle**
      ✓7ᵗʰ **T25.412 Corrosion of unspecified degree of left ankle**
      ✓7ᵗʰ **T25.419 Corrosion of unspecified degree of unspecified ankle**

   ✓6ᵗʰ **T25.42 Corrosion of unspecified degree of foot**
      EXCLUDES 2   *corrosion of unspecified degree of toe(s) (nail) (T25.43-)*
      ✓7ᵗʰ **T25.421 Corrosion of unspecified degree of right foot**
      ✓7ᵗʰ **T25.422 Corrosion of unspecified degree of left foot**
      ✓7ᵗʰ **T25.429 Corrosion of unspecified degree of unspecified foot**

   ✓6ᵗʰ **T25.43 Corrosion of unspecified degree of toe(s) (nail)**
      ✓7ᵗʰ **T25.431 Corrosion of unspecified degree of right toe(s) (nail)**
      ✓7ᵗʰ **T25.432 Corrosion of unspecified degree of left toe(s) (nail)**
      ✓7ᵗʰ **T25.439 Corrosion of unspecified degree of unspecified toe(s) (nail)**

   ✓6ᵗʰ **T25.49 Corrosion of unspecified degree of multiple sites of ankle and foot**
      ✓7ᵗʰ **T25.491 Corrosion of unspecified degree of multiple sites of right ankle and foot**
      ✓7ᵗʰ **T25.492 Corrosion of unspecified degree of multiple sites of left ankle and foot**
      ✓7ᵗʰ **T25.499 Corrosion of unspecified degree of multiple sites of unspecified ankle and foot**

✓5ᵗʰ **T25.5 Corrosion of first degree of ankle and foot**
Code first (T51-T65) to identify chemical and intent
Use additional external cause code to identify place (Y92)

   ✓6ᵗʰ **T25.51 Corrosion of first degree of ankle**
      ✓7ᵗʰ **T25.511 Corrosion of first degree of right ankle**
      ✓7ᵗʰ **T25.512 Corrosion of first degree of left ankle**
      ✓7ᵗʰ **T25.519 Corrosion of first degree of unspecified ankle**

   ✓6ᵗʰ **T25.52 Corrosion of first degree of foot**
      EXCLUDES 2   *corrosion of first degree of toe(s) (nail) (T25.53-)*
      ✓7ᵗʰ **T25.521 Corrosion of first degree of right foot**
      ✓7ᵗʰ **T25.522 Corrosion of first degree of left foot**

      ✓7ᵗʰ **T25.529 Corrosion of first degree of unspecified foot**

   ✓6ᵗʰ **T25.53 Corrosion of first degree of toe(s) (nail)**
      ✓7ᵗʰ **T25.531 Corrosion of first degree of right toe(s) (nail)**
      ✓7ᵗʰ **T25.532 Corrosion of first degree of left toe(s) (nail)**
      ✓7ᵗʰ **T25.539 Corrosion of first degree of unspecified toe(s) (nail)**

   ✓6ᵗʰ **T25.59 Corrosion of first degree of multiple sites of ankle and foot**
      ✓7ᵗʰ **T25.591 Corrosion of first degree of multiple sites of right ankle and foot**
      ✓7ᵗʰ **T25.592 Corrosion of first degree of multiple sites of left ankle and foot**
      ✓7ᵗʰ **T25.599 Corrosion of first degree of multiple sites of unspecified ankle and foot**

✓5ᵗʰ **T25.6 Corrosion of second degree of ankle and foot**
Code first (T51-T65) to identify chemical and intent
Use additional external cause code to identify place (Y92)

   ✓6ᵗʰ **T25.61 Corrosion of second degree of ankle**
      ✓7ᵗʰ **T25.611 Corrosion of second degree of right ankle**
      ✓7ᵗʰ **T25.612 Corrosion of second degree of left ankle**
      ✓7ᵗʰ **T25.619 Corrosion of second degree of unspecified ankle**

   ✓6ᵗʰ **T25.62 Corrosion of second degree of foot**
      EXCLUDES 2   *corrosion of second degree of toe(s) (nail) (T25.63-)*
      ✓7ᵗʰ **T25.621 Corrosion of second degree of right foot**
      ✓7ᵗʰ **T25.622 Corrosion of second degree of left foot**
      ✓7ᵗʰ **T25.629 Corrosion of second degree of unspecified foot**

   ✓6ᵗʰ **T25.63 Corrosion of second degree of toe(s) (nail)**
      ✓7ᵗʰ **T25.631 Corrosion of second degree of right toe(s) (nail)**
      ✓7ᵗʰ **T25.632 Corrosion of second degree of left toe(s) (nail)**
      ✓7ᵗʰ **T25.639 Corrosion of second degree of unspecified toe(s) (nail)**

   ✓6ᵗʰ **T25.69 Corrosion of second degree of multiple sites of ankle and foot**
      ✓7ᵗʰ **T25.691 Corrosion of second degree of right ankle and foot**
      ✓7ᵗʰ **T25.692 Corrosion of second degree of left ankle and foot**
      ✓7ᵗʰ **T25.699 Corrosion of second degree of unspecified ankle and foot**

✓5ᵗʰ **T25.7 Corrosion of third degree of ankle and foot**
Code first (T51-T65) to identify chemical and intent
Use additional external cause code to identify place (Y92)

   ✓6ᵗʰ **T25.71 Corrosion of third degree of ankle**
      ✓7ᵗʰ **T25.711 Corrosion of third degree of right ankle**
      ✓7ᵗʰ **T25.712 Corrosion of third degree of left ankle**
      ✓7ᵗʰ **T25.719 Corrosion of third degree of unspecified ankle**

   ✓6ᵗʰ **T25.72 Corrosion of third degree of foot**
      EXCLUDES 2   *corrosion of third degree of toe(s) (nail) (T25.73-)*
      ✓7ᵗʰ **T25.721 Corrosion of third degree of right foot**
      ✓7ᵗʰ **T25.722 Corrosion of third degree of left foot**
      ✓7ᵗʰ **T25.729 Corrosion of third degree of unspecified foot**

   ✓6ᵗʰ **T25.73 Corrosion of third degree of toe(s) (nail)**
      ✓7ᵗʰ **T25.731 Corrosion of third degree of right toe(s) (nail)**
      ✓7ᵗʰ **T25.732 Corrosion of third degree of left toe(s) (nail)**
      ✓7ᵗʰ **T25.739 Corrosion of third degree of unspecified toe(s) (nail)**

   ✓6ᵗʰ **T25.79 Corrosion of third degree of multiple sites of ankle and foot**
      ✓7ᵗʰ **T25.791 Corrosion of third degree of multiple sites of right ankle and foot**
      ✓7ᵗʰ **T25.792 Corrosion of third degree of multiple sites of left ankle and foot**

EXCLUDES 1 Not coded here   EXCLUDES 2 Not included here   N Newborn Age: 0   P Pediatric Age: 0-17   M Maternity Age: 12-55   A Adult Age: 15-124

936   ICD-10-CM 2014 (Draft)

√7ᵗʰ **T25.799**   **Corrosion of third degree of multiple sites of unspecified ankle and foot**

Burns and corrosions confined to eye and internal organs (T26-T28)

√4ᵗʰ **T26**   **Burn and corrosion confined to eye and adnexa**

> The appropriate 7th character is to be added to each code from category T26.
> A   initial encounter
> D   subsequent encounter
> S   sequela

√5ᵗʰ **T26.0**   **Burn of** eyelid and periocular area
> Use additional external cause code to identify the source, place and intent of the burn (X00-X19, X75-X77, X96-X98, Y92)

√x7ᵗʰ **T26.00**   **Burn of unspecified eyelid and periocular area**
√x7ᵗʰ **T26.01**   **Burn of** right **eyelid and periocular area**
√x7ᵗʰ **T26.02**   **Burn of** left **eyelid and periocular area**

√5ᵗʰ **T26.1**   **Burn of** cornea and conjunctival sac
> Use additional external cause code to identify the source, place and intent of the burn (X00-X19, X75-X77, X96-X98, Y92)

√x7ᵗʰ **T26.10**   **Burn of cornea and conjunctival sac, unspecified eye**
√x7ᵗʰ **T26.11**   **Burn of cornea and conjunctival sac,** right **eye**
√x7ᵗʰ **T26.12**   **Burn of cornea and conjunctival sac,** left **eye**

√5ᵗʰ **T26.2**   **Burn with resulting** rupture and destruction of eyeball
> Use additional external cause code to identify the source, place and intent of the burn (X00-X19, X75-X77, X96-X98, Y92)

√x7ᵗʰ **T26.20**   **Burn with resulting rupture and destruction of unspecified eyeball**
√x7ᵗʰ **T26.21**   **Burn with resulting rupture and destruction of** right **eyeball**
√x7ᵗʰ **T26.22**   **Burn with resulting rupture and destruction of** left **eyeball**

√5ᵗʰ **T26.3**   **Burns of** other specified parts of eye and adnexa
> Use additional external cause code to identify the source, place and intent of the burn (X00-X19, X75-X77, X96-X98, Y92)

√x7ᵗʰ **T26.30**   **Burns of other specified parts of unspecified eye and adnexa**
√x7ᵗʰ **T26.31**   **Burns of other specified parts of** right **eye and adnexa**
√x7ᵗʰ **T26.32**   **Burns of other specified parts of** left **eye and adnexa**

√5ᵗʰ **T26.4**   **Burn of eye and adnexa,** part unspecified
> Use additional external cause code to identify the source, place and intent of the burn (X00-X19, X75-X77, X96-X98, Y92)

√x7ᵗʰ **T26.40**   **Burn of unspecified eye and adnexa, part unspecified**
√x7ᵗʰ **T26.41**   **Burn of** right **eye and adnexa, part unspecified**
√x7ᵗʰ **T26.42**   **Burn of** left **eye and adnexa, part unspecified**

√5ᵗʰ **T26.5**   **Corrosion of** eyelid and periocular area
> Code first (T51-T65) to identify chemical and intent
> Use additional external cause code to identify place (Y92)

√x7ᵗʰ **T26.50**   **Corrosion of unspecified eyelid and periocular area**
√x7ᵗʰ **T26.51**   **Corrosion of** right **eyelid and periocular area**
√x7ᵗʰ **T26.52**   **Corrosion of** left **eyelid and periocular area**

√5ᵗʰ **T26.6**   **Corrosion of** cornea and conjunctival sac
> Code first (T51-T65) to identify chemical and intent
> Use additional external cause code to identify place (Y92)

√x7ᵗʰ **T26.60**   **Corrosion of cornea and conjunctival sac, unspecified eye**
√x7ᵗʰ **T26.61**   **Corrosion of cornea and conjunctival sac,** right **eye**
√x7ᵗʰ **T26.62**   **Corrosion of cornea and conjunctival sac,** left **eye**

√5ᵗʰ **T26.7**   **Corrosion with resulting** rupture and destruction of eyeball
> Code first (T51-T65) to identify chemical and intent
> Use additional external cause code to identify place (Y92)

√x7ᵗʰ **T26.70**   **Corrosion with resulting rupture and destruction of unspecified eyeball**
√x7ᵗʰ **T26.71**   **Corrosion with resulting rupture and destruction of** right **eyeball**
√x7ᵗʰ **T26.72**   **Corrosion with resulting rupture and destruction of** left **eyeball**

√5ᵗʰ **T26.8**   **Corrosions of** other specified parts of eye and adnexa
> Code first (T51-T65) to identify chemical and intent
> Use additional external cause code to identify place (Y92)

√x7ᵗʰ **T26.80**   **Corrosions of other specified parts of unspecified eye and adnexa**
√x7ᵗʰ **T26.81**   **Corrosions of other specified parts of** right **eye and adnexa**
√x7ᵗʰ **T26.82**   **Corrosions of other specified parts of** left **eye and adnexa**

√5ᵗʰ **T26.9**   **Corrosion of eye and adnexa,** part unspecified
> Code first (T51-T65) to identify chemical and intent
> Use additional external cause code to identify place (Y92)

√x7ᵗʰ **T26.90**   **Corrosion of unspecified eye and adnexa, part unspecified**
√x7ᵗʰ **T26.91**   **Corrosion of** right **eye and adnexa, part unspecified**
√x7ᵗʰ **T26.92**   **Corrosion of** left **eye and adnexa, part unspecified**

√4ᵗʰ **T27**   **Burn and corrosion of respiratory tract**
> Use additional external cause code to identify the source and intent of the burn (X00-X19, X75-X77, X96-X98)
> Use additional external cause code to identify place (Y92)

> The appropriate 7th character is to be added to each code from category T27.
> A   initial encounter
> D   subsequent encounter
> S   sequela

√x7ᵗʰ **T27.0**   **Burn of** larynx and trachea
√x7ᵗʰ **T27.1**   **Burn involving** larynx and trachea with lung
√x7ᵗʰ **T27.2**   **Burn of other** parts of respiratory tract
> Burn of thoracic cavity
√x7ᵗʰ **T27.3**   **Burn of respiratory tract, part unspecified**
> Code first (T51-T65) to identify chemical and intent for codes T27.4-T27.7
√x7ᵗʰ **T27.4**   **Corrosion of** larynx and trachea
√x7ᵗʰ **T27.5**   **Corrosion involving** larynx and trachea with lung
√x7ᵗʰ **T27.6**   **Corrosion of other** parts of respiratory tract
√x7ᵗʰ **T27.7**   **Corrosion of respiratory tract, part unspecified**

√4ᵗʰ **T28**   **Burn and corrosion of other internal organs**
> Use additional external cause code to identify the source and intent of the burn (X00- X19, X75-X77, X96-X98)
> Use additional external cause code to identify place (Y92)

> The appropriate 7th character is to be added to each code from category T28.
> A   initial encounter
> D   subsequent encounter
> S   sequela

√x7ᵗʰ **T28.0**   **Burn of** mouth and pharynx
√x7ᵗʰ **T28.1**   **Burn of** esophagus
√x7ᵗʰ **T28.2**   **Burn of other parts of** alimentary tract
√x7ᵗʰ **T28.3**   **Burn of** internal genitourinary organs   ♀
√5ᵗʰ **T28.4**   **Burns of other and unspecified internal organs**

√x7ᵗʰ **T28.40**   **Burn of unspecified internal organ**
√6ᵗʰ **T28.41**   **Burn of** ear drum
> √7ᵗʰ **T28.411**   **Burn of** right **ear drum**
> √7ᵗʰ **T28.412**   **Burn of** left **ear drum**
> √7ᵗʰ **T28.419**   **Burn of unspecified ear drum**
√x7ᵗʰ **T28.49**   **Burn of other internal organ**
> Code first (T51-T65) to identify chemical and intent for T28.5-T28.9-

√x7ᵗʰ **T28.5**   **Corrosion of** mouth and pharynx
√x7ᵗʰ **T28.6**   **Corrosion of** esophagus
√x7ᵗʰ **T28.7**   **Corrosion of other parts of** alimentary tract
√x7ᵗʰ **T28.8**   **Corrosion of internal** genitourinary organs   ♀
√x7ᵗʰ **T28.9**   **Corrosions of other and unspecified internal organs**

√x7ᵗʰ **T28.90**   **Corrosions of unspecified internal organs**
√6ᵗʰ **T28.91**   **Corrosions of** ear drum
> √7ᵗʰ **T28.911**   **Corrosions of** right **ear drum**
> √7ᵗʰ **T28.912**   **Corrosions of** left **ear drum**
> √7ᵗʰ **T28.919**   **Corrosions of unspecified ear drum**
√x7ᵗʰ **T28.99**   **Corrosions of other internal organs**

☑ Additional Character Required   √x7ᵗʰ Xtension Alert   Unspecified Code   Other Specified Code   Manifestation Code   ▶◀ Revised Text   ● New Code   ▲ Revised Code Title

ICD-10-CM 2014 (Draft)   937

Injury, Poisoning and Certain Other Consequences of External Causes

T30–T32.0

Burns and corrosions of multiple and unspecified body regions (T30-T32)

☑4ᵗʰ **T30** **Burn and corrosion, body region unspecified**

    T30.0 **Burn of unspecified body region, unspecified degree**
       NOTE   This code is not for inpatient use. Code to specified site and degree of burns.
       Burn NOS
       Multiple burns NOS

    T30.4 **Corrosion of unspecified body region, unspecified degree**
       NOTE   This code is not for inpatient use. Code to specified site and degree of corrosion.
       Corrosion NOS
       Multiple corrosion NOS

☑4ᵗʰ **T31** **Burns classified according to extent of body surface involved**
       NOTE   This category is to be used as the primary code only when the site of the burn is unspecified. It should be used as a supplementary code with categories T20-T25 when the site is specified.

    T31.0 **Burns involving less than 10% of body surface**

    ☑5ᵗʰ **T31.1** **Burns involving 10-19% of body surface**
       T31.10 **Burns involving 10-19% of body surface with 0% to 9% third degree burns**
          Burns involving 10-19% of body surface NOS
       T31.11 **Burns involving 10-19% of body surface with 10-19% third degree burns**

    ☑5ᵗʰ **T31.2** **Burns involving 20-29% of body surface**
       T31.20 **Burns involving 20-29% of body surface with 0% to 9% third degree burns**
          Burns involving 20-29% of body surface NOS
       T31.21 **Burns involving 20-29% of body surface with 10-19% third degree burns**
       T31.22 **Burns involving 20-29% of body surface with 20-29% third degree burns**

    ☑5ᵗʰ **T31.3** **Burns involving 30-39% of body surface**
       T31.30 **Burns involving 30-39% of body surface with 0% to 9% third degree burns**
          Burns involving 30-39% of body surface NOS
       T31.31 **Burns involving 30-39% of body surface with 10-19% third degree burns**
       T31.32 **Burns involving 30-39% of body surface with 20-29% third degree burns**
       T31.33 **Burns involving 30-39% of body surface with 30-39% third degree burns**

    ☑5ᵗʰ **T31.4** **Burns involving 40-49% of body surface**
       T31.40 **Burns involving 40-49% of body surface with 0% to 9% third degree burns**
          Burns involving 40-49% of body surface NOS
       T31.41 **Burns involving 40-49% of body surface with 10-19% third degree burns**
       T31.42 **Burns involving 40-49% of body surface with 20-29% third degree burns**
       T31.43 **Burns involving 40-49% of body surface with 30-39% third degree burns**
       T31.44 **Burns involving 40-49% of body surface with 40-49% third degree burns**

    ☑5ᵗʰ **T31.5** **Burns involving 50-59% of body surface**
       T31.50 **Burns involving 50-59% of body surface with 0% to 9% third degree burns**
          Burns involving 50-59% of body surface NOS
       T31.51 **Burns involving 50-59% of body surface with 10-19% third degree burns**
       T31.52 **Burns involving 50-59% of body surface with 20-29% third degree burns**
       T31.53 **Burns involving 50-59% of body surface with 30-39% third degree burns**
       T31.54 **Burns involving 50-59% of body surface with 40-49% third degree burns**
       T31.55 **Burns involving 50-59% of body surface with 50-59% third degree burns**

    ☑5ᵗʰ **T31.6** **Burns involving 60-69% of body surface**
       T31.60 **Burns involving 60-69% of body surface with 0% to 9% third degree burns**
          Burns involving 60-69% of body surface NOS
       T31.61 **Burns involving 60-69% of body surface with 10-19% third degree burns**

       T31.62 **Burns involving 60-69% of body surface with 20-29% third degree burns**
       T31.63 **Burns involving 60-69% of body surface with 30-39% third degree burns**
       T31.64 **Burns involving 60-69% of body surface with 40-49% third degree burns**
       T31.65 **Burns involving 60-69% of body surface with 50-59% third degree burns**
       T31.66 **Burns involving 60-69% of body surface with 60-69% third degree burns**

    ☑5ᵗʰ **T31.7** **Burns involving 70-79% of body surface**
       T31.70 **Burns involving 70-79% of body surface with 0% to 9% third degree burns**
          Burns involving 70-79% of body surface NOS
       T31.71 **Burns involving 70-79% of body surface with 10-19% third degree burns**
       T31.72 **Burns involving 70-79% of body surface with 20-29% third degree burns**
       T31.73 **Burns involving 70-79% of body surface with 30-39% third degree burns**
       T31.74 **Burns involving 70-79% of body surface with 40-49% third degree burns**
       T31.75 **Burns involving 70-79% of body surface with 50-59% third degree burns**
       T31.76 **Burns involving 70-79% of body surface with 60-69% third degree burns**
       T31.77 **Burns involving 70-79% of body surface with 70-79% third degree burns**

    ☑5ᵗʰ **T31.8** **Burns involving 80-89% of body surface**
       T31.80 **Burns involving 80-89% of body surface with 0% to 9% third degree burns**
          Burns involving 80-89% of body surface NOS
       T31.81 **Burns involving 80-89% of body surface with 10-19% third degree burns**
       T31.82 **Burns involving 80-89% of body surface with 20-29% third degree burns**
       T31.83 **Burns involving 80-89% of body surface with 30-39% third degree burns**
       T31.84 **Burns involving 80-89% of body surface with 40-49% third degree burns**
       T31.85 **Burns involving 80-89% of body surface with 50-59% third degree burns**
       T31.86 **Burns involving 80-89% of body surface with 60-69% third degree burns**
       T31.87 **Burns involving 80-89% of body surface with 70-79% third degree burns**
       T31.88 **Burns involving 80-89% of body surface with 80-89% third degree burns**

    ☑5ᵗʰ **T31.9** **Burns involving 90% or more of body surface**
       T31.90 **Burns involving 90% or more of body surface with 0% to 9% third degree burns**
          Burns involving 90% or more of body surface NOS
       T31.91 **Burns involving 90% or more of body surface with 10-19% third degree burns**
       T31.92 **Burns involving 90% or more of body surface with 20-29% third degree burns**
       T31.93 **Burns involving 90% or more of body surface with 30-39% third degree burns**
       T31.94 **Burns involving 90% or more of body surface with 40-49% third degree burns**
       T31.95 **Burns involving 90% or more of body surface with 50-59% third degree burns**
       T31.96 **Burns involving 90% or more of body surface with 60-69% third degree burns**
       T31.97 **Burns involving 90% or more of body surface with 70-79% third degree burns**
       T31.98 **Burns involving 90% or more of body surface with 80-89% third degree burns**
       T31.99 **Burns involving 90% or more of body surface with 90% or more third degree burns**

☑4ᵗʰ **T32** **Corrosions classified according to extent of body surface involved**
       NOTE   This category is to be used as the primary code only when the site of the corrosion is unspecified. It may be used as a supplementary code with categories T20-T25 when the site is specified.

    T32.0 **Corrosions involving less than 10% of body surface**

EXCLUDES 1 Not coded here   **EXCLUDES 2** Not included here   **N** Newborn Age: 0   **P** Pediatric Age: 0-17   **M** Maternity Age: 12-55   **A** Adult Age: 15-124

938   ICD-10-CM 2014 (Draft)

✓5ᵗʰ **T32.1** **Corrosions involving 10-19% of body surface**

  T32.10 **Corrosions involving 10-19% of body surface with 0% to 9% third degree corrosion**
    Corrosions involving 10-19% of body surface NOS

  T32.11 **Corrosions involving 10-19% of body surface with 10-19% third degree corrosion**

✓5ᵗʰ **T32.2** **Corrosions involving 20-29% of body surface**

  T32.20 **Corrosions involving 20-29% of body surface with 0% to 9% third degree corrosion**

  T32.21 **Corrosions involving 20-29% of body surface with 10-19% third degree corrosion**

  T32.22 **Corrosions involving 20-29% of body surface with 20-29% third degree corrosion**

✓5ᵗʰ **T32.3** **Corrosions involving 30-39% of body surface**

  T32.30 **Corrosions involving 30-39% of body surface with 0% to 9% third degree corrosion**

  T32.31 **Corrosions involving 30-39% of body surface with 10-19% third degree corrosion**

  T32.32 **Corrosions involving 30-39% of body surface with 20-29% third degree corrosion**

  T32.33 **Corrosions involving 30-39% of body surface with 30-39% third degree corrosion**

✓5ᵗʰ **T32.4** **Corrosions involving 40-49% of body surface**

  T32.40 **Corrosions involving 40-49% of body surface with 0% to 9% third degree corrosion**

  T32.41 **Corrosions involving 40-49% of body surface with 10-19% third degree corrosion**

  T32.42 **Corrosions involving 40-49% of body surface with 20-29% third degree corrosion**

  T32.43 **Corrosions involving 40-49% of body surface with 30-39% third degree corrosion**

  T32.44 **Corrosions involving 40-49% of body surface with 40-49% third degree corrosion**

✓5ᵗʰ **T32.5** **Corrosions involving 50-59% of body surface**

  T32.50 **Corrosions involving 50-59% of body surface with 0% to 9% third degree corrosion**

  T32.51 **Corrosions involving 50-59% of body surface with 10-19% third degree corrosion**

  T32.52 **Corrosions involving 50-59% of body surface with 20-29% third degree corrosion**

  T32.53 **Corrosions involving 50-59% of body surface with 30-39% third degree corrosion**

  T32.54 **Corrosions involving 50-59% of body surface with 40-49% third degree corrosion**

  T32.55 **Corrosions involving 50-59% of body surface with 50-59% third degree corrosion**

✓5ᵗʰ **T32.6** **Corrosions involving 60-69% of body surface**

  T32.60 **Corrosions involving 60-69% of body surface with 0% to 9% third degree corrosion**

  T32.61 **Corrosions involving 60-69% of body surface with 10-19% third degree corrosion**

  T32.62 **Corrosions involving 60-69% of body surface with 20-29% third degree corrosion**

  T32.63 **Corrosions involving 60-69% of body surface with 30-39% third degree corrosion**

  T32.64 **Corrosions involving 60-69% of body surface with 40-49% third degree corrosion**

  T32.65 **Corrosions involving 60-69% of body surface with 50-59% third degree corrosion**

  T32.66 **Corrosions involving 60-69% of body surface with 60-69% third degree corrosion**

✓5ᵗʰ **T32.7** **Corrosions involving 70-79% of body surface**

  T32.70 **Corrosions involving 70-79% of body surface with 0% to 9% third degree corrosion**

  T32.71 **Corrosions involving 70-79% of body surface with 10-19% third degree corrosion**

  T32.72 **Corrosions involving 70-79% of body surface with 20-29% third degree corrosion**

  T32.73 **Corrosions involving 70-79% of body surface with 30-39% third degree corrosion**

  T32.74 **Corrosions involving 70-79% of body surface with 40-49% third degree corrosion**

  T32.75 **Corrosions involving 70-79% of body surface with 50-59% third degree corrosion**

  T32.76 **Corrosions involving 70-79% of body surface with 60-69% third degree corrosion**

  T32.77 **Corrosions involving 70-79% of body surface with 70-79% third degree corrosion**

✓5ᵗʰ **T32.8** **Corrosions involving 80-89% of body surface**

  T32.80 **Corrosions involving 80-89% of body surface with 0% to 9% third degree corrosion**

  T32.81 **Corrosions involving 80-89% of body surface with 10-19% third degree corrosion**

  T32.82 **Corrosions involving 80-89% of body surface with 20-29% third degree corrosion**

  T32.83 **Corrosions involving 80-89% of body surface with 30-39% third degree corrosion**

  T32.84 **Corrosions involving 80-89% of body surface with 40-49% third degree corrosion**

  T32.85 **Corrosions involving 80-89% of body surface with 50-59% third degree corrosion**

  T32.86 **Corrosions involving 80-89% of body surface with 60-69% third degree corrosion**

  T32.87 **Corrosions involving 80-89% of body surface with 70-79% third degree corrosion**

  T32.88 **Corrosions involving 80-89% of body surface with 80-89% third degree corrosion**

✓5ᵗʰ **T32.9** **Corrosions involving 90% or more of body surface**

  T32.90 **Corrosions involving 90% or more of body surface with 0% to 9% third degree corrosion**

  T32.91 **Corrosions involving 90% or more of body surface with 10-19% third degree corrosion**

  T32.92 **Corrosions involving 90% or more of body surface with 20-29% third degree corrosion**

  T32.93 **Corrosions involving 90% or more of body surface with 30-39% third degree corrosion**

  T32.94 **Corrosions involving 90% or more of body surface with 40-49% third degree corrosion**

  T32.95 **Corrosions involving 90% or more of body surface with 50-59% third degree corrosion**

  T32.96 **Corrosions involving 90% or more of body surface with 60-69% third degree corrosion**

  T32.97 **Corrosions involving 90% or more of body surface with 70-79% third degree corrosion**

  T32.98 **Corrosions involving 90% or more of body surface with 80-89% third degree corrosion**

  T32.99 **Corrosions involving 90% or more of body surface with 90% or more third degree corrosion**

Frostbite (T33-T34)

EXCLUDES 2 *hypothermia and other effects of reduced temperature (T68, T69-)*

✓4ᵗʰ **T33** **Superficial frostbite**
  INCLUDES frostbite with partial thickness skin loss

  The appropriate 7th character is to be added to each code from category T33.
  A   initial encounter
  D   subsequent encounter
  S   sequela

✓5ᵗʰ **T33.0** **Superficial frostbite of head**

  ✓6ᵗʰ **T33.01** **Superficial frostbite of ear**

    ✓7ᵗʰ **T33.011** **Superficial frostbite of right ear**

    ✓7ᵗʰ **T33.012** **Superficial frostbite of left ear**

    ✓7ᵗʰ **T33.019** **Superficial frostbite of unspecified ear**

  ✓x7ᵗʰ **T33.02** **Superficial frostbite of nose**

  ✓x7ᵗʰ **T33.09** **Superficial frostbite of other part of head**

✓x7ᵗʰ **T33.1** **Superficial frostbite of neck**

✓x7ᵗʰ **T33.2** **Superficial frostbite of thorax**

✓x7ᵗʰ **T33.3** **Superficial frostbite of abdominal wall, lower back and pelvis**

✓5ᵗʰ **T33.4** **Superficial frostbite of arm**
  EXCLUDES 2 *superficial frostbite of wrist and hand (T33.5-)*

  ✓x7ᵗʰ **T33.40** **Superficial frostbite of unspecified arm**

  ✓x7ᵗʰ **T33.41** **Superficial frostbite of right arm**

  ✓x7ᵗʰ **T33.42** **Superficial frostbite of left arm**

✓5ᵗʰ **T33.5** **Superficial frostbite of wrist, hand, and fingers**

  ✓6ᵗʰ **T33.51** **Superficial frostbite of wrist**

    ✓7ᵗʰ **T33.511** **Superficial frostbite of right wrist**

    ✓7ᵗʰ **T33.512** **Superficial frostbite of left wrist**

✓ Additional Character Required   ✓x7ᵗʰ Xtension Alert   Unspecified Code   Other Specified Code   Manifestation Code   ▶◀ Revised Text   ● New Code   ▲ Revised Code Title

Injury, Poisoning and Certain Other Consequences of External Causes   T33.519–T34.99

✓7ᵗʰ   **T33.519**   **Superficial frostbite of unspecified wrist**

✓6ᵗʰ   **T33.52**   **Superficial frostbite of hand**
- EXCLUDES 2   *superficial frostbite of fingers (T33.53-)*

   ✓7ᵗʰ   **T33.521**   **Superficial frostbite of right hand**

   ✓7ᵗʰ   **T33.522**   **Superficial frostbite of left hand**

   ✓7ᵗʰ   **T33.529**   **Superficial frostbite of unspecified hand**

✓6ᵗʰ   **T33.53**   **Superficial frostbite of finger(s)**

   ✓7ᵗʰ   **T33.531**   **Superficial frostbite of right finger(s)**

   ✓7ᵗʰ   **T33.532**   **Superficial frostbite of left finger(s)**

   ✓7ᵗʰ   **T33.539**   **Superficial frostbite of unspecified finger(s)**

✓5ᵗʰ   **T33.6**   **Superficial frostbite of hip and thigh**

   ✓x7ᵗʰ   **T33.60**   **Superficial frostbite of unspecified hip and thigh**

   ✓x7ᵗʰ   **T33.61**   **Superficial frostbite of right hip and thigh**

   ✓x7ᵗʰ   **T33.62**   **Superficial frostbite of left hip and thigh**

✓5ᵗʰ   **T33.7**   **Superficial frostbite of knee and lower leg**
- EXCLUDES 2   *superficial frostbite of ankle and foot (T33.8-)*

   ✓x7ᵗʰ   **T33.70**   **Superficial frostbite of unspecified knee and lower leg**

   ✓x7ᵗʰ   **T33.71**   **Superficial frostbite of right knee and lower leg**

   ✓x7ᵗʰ   **T33.72**   **Superficial frostbite of left knee and lower leg**

✓5ᵗʰ   **T33.8**   **Superficial frostbite of ankle, foot, and toe(s)**

   ✓6ᵗʰ   **T33.81**   **Superficial frostbite of ankle**

     ✓7ᵗʰ   **T33.811**   **Superficial frostbite of right ankle**

     ✓7ᵗʰ   **T33.812**   **Superficial frostbite of left ankle**

     ✓7ᵗʰ   **T33.819**   **Superficial frostbite of unspecified ankle**

   ✓6ᵗʰ   **T33.82**   **Superficial frostbite of foot**

     ✓7ᵗʰ   **T33.821**   **Superficial frostbite of right foot**

     ✓7ᵗʰ   **T33.822**   **Superficial frostbite of left foot**

     ✓7ᵗʰ   **T33.829**   **Superficial frostbite of unspecified foot**

   ✓6ᵗʰ   **T33.83**   **Superficial frostbite of toe(s)**

     ✓7ᵗʰ   **T33.831**   **Superficial frostbite of right toe(s)**

     ✓7ᵗʰ   **T33.832**   **Superficial frostbite of left toe(s)**

     ✓7ᵗʰ   **T33.839**   **Superficial frostbite of unspecified toe(s)**

✓5ᵗʰ   **T33.9**   **Superficial frostbite of other and unspecified sites**

   ✓x7ᵗʰ   **T33.90**   **Superficial frostbite of unspecified sites**
Superficial frostbite NOS

   ✓x7ᵗʰ   **T33.99**   **Superficial frostbite of other sites**
Superficial frostbite of leg NOS
Superficial frostbite of trunk NOS

✓4ᵗʰ   **T34**   **Frostbite with tissue necrosis**

The appropriate 7th character is to be added to each code from category T34.
A   initial encounter
D   subsequent encounter
S   sequela

✓5ᵗʰ   **T34.0**   **Frostbite with tissue necrosis of head**

   ✓6ᵗʰ   **T34.01**   **Frostbite with tissue necrosis of ear**

     ✓7ᵗʰ   **T34.011**   **Frostbite with tissue necrosis of right ear**

     ✓7ᵗʰ   **T34.012**   **Frostbite with tissue necrosis of left ear**

     ✓7ᵗʰ   **T34.019**   **Frostbite with tissue necrosis of unspecified ear**

   ✓x7ᵗʰ   **T34.02**   **Frostbite with tissue necrosis of nose**

   ✓x7ᵗʰ   **T34.09**   **Frostbite with tissue necrosis of other part of head**

✓x7ᵗʰ   **T34.1**   **Frostbite with tissue necrosis of neck**

✓x7ᵗʰ   **T34.2**   **Frostbite with tissue necrosis of thorax**

✓x7ᵗʰ   **T34.3**   **Frostbite with tissue necrosis of abdominal wall, lower back and pelvis**

✓5ᵗʰ   **T34.4**   **Frostbite with tissue necrosis of arm**
- EXCLUDES 2   *frostbite with tissue necrosis of wrist and hand (T34.5-)*

   ✓x7ᵗʰ   **T34.40**   **Frostbite with tissue necrosis of unspecified arm**

   ✓x7ᵗʰ   **T34.41**   **Frostbite with tissue necrosis of right arm**

   ✓x7ᵗʰ   **T34.42**   **Frostbite with tissue necrosis of left arm**

✓5ᵗʰ   **T34.5**   **Frostbite with tissue necrosis of wrist, hand, and finger(s)**

   ✓6ᵗʰ   **T34.51**   **Frostbite with tissue necrosis of wrist**

     ✓7ᵗʰ   **T34.511**   **Frostbite with tissue necrosis of right wrist**

     ✓7ᵗʰ   **T34.512**   **Frostbite with tissue necrosis of left wrist**

   ✓7ᵗʰ   **T34.519**   **Frostbite with tissue necrosis of unspecified wrist**

✓6ᵗʰ   **T34.52**   **Frostbite with tissue necrosis of hand**
- EXCLUDES 2   *frostbite with tissue necrosis of finger(s) (T34.53-)*

   ✓7ᵗʰ   **T34.521**   **Frostbite with tissue necrosis of right hand**

   ✓7ᵗʰ   **T34.522**   **Frostbite with tissue necrosis of left hand**

   ✓7ᵗʰ   **T34.529**   **Frostbite with tissue necrosis of unspecified hand**

✓6ᵗʰ   **T34.53**   **Frostbite with tissue necrosis of finger(s)**

   ✓7ᵗʰ   **T34.531**   **Frostbite with tissue necrosis of right finger(s)**

   ✓7ᵗʰ   **T34.532**   **Frostbite with tissue necrosis of left finger(s)**

   ✓7ᵗʰ   **T34.539**   **Frostbite with tissue necrosis of unspecified finger(s)**

✓5ᵗʰ   **T34.6**   **Frostbite with tissue necrosis of hip and thigh**

   ✓x7ᵗʰ   **T34.60**   **Frostbite with tissue necrosis of unspecified hip and thigh**

   ✓x7ᵗʰ   **T34.61**   **Frostbite with tissue necrosis of right hip and thigh**

   ✓x7ᵗʰ   **T34.62**   **Frostbite with tissue necrosis of left hip and thigh**

✓5ᵗʰ   **T34.7**   **Frostbite with tissue necrosis of knee and lower leg**
- EXCLUDES 2   *frostbite with tissue necrosis of ankle and foot (T34.8-)*

   ✓x7ᵗʰ   **T34.70**   **Frostbite with tissue necrosis of unspecified knee and lower leg**

   ✓x7ᵗʰ   **T34.71**   **Frostbite with tissue necrosis of right knee and lower leg**

   ✓x7ᵗʰ   **T34.72**   **Frostbite with tissue necrosis of left knee and lower leg**

✓5ᵗʰ   **T34.8**   **Frostbite with tissue necrosis of ankle, foot, and toe(s)**

   ✓7ᵗʰ   **T34.81**   **Frostbite with tissue necrosis of ankle**

     ✓7ᵗʰ   **T34.811**   **Frostbite with tissue necrosis of right ankle**

     ✓7ᵗʰ   **T34.812**   **Frostbite with tissue necrosis of left ankle**

     ✓7ᵗʰ   **T34.819**   **Frostbite with tissue necrosis of unspecified ankle**

   ✓6ᵗʰ   **T34.82**   **Frostbite with tissue necrosis of foot**

     ✓7ᵗʰ   **T34.821**   **Frostbite with tissue necrosis of right foot**

     ✓7ᵗʰ   **T34.822**   **Frostbite with tissue necrosis of left foot**

     ✓7ᵗʰ   **T34.829**   **Frostbite with tissue necrosis of unspecified foot**

   ✓6ᵗʰ   **T34.83**   **Frostbite with tissue necrosis of toe(s)**

     ✓7ᵗʰ   **T34.831**   **Frostbite with tissue necrosis of right toe(s)**

     ✓7ᵗʰ   **T34.832**   **Frostbite with tissue necrosis of left toe(s)**

     ✓7ᵗʰ   **T34.839**   **Frostbite with tissue necrosis of unspecified toe(s)**

✓5ᵗʰ   **T34.9**   **Frostbite with tissue necrosis of other and unspecified sites**

   ✓x7ᵗʰ   **T34.90**   **Frostbite with tissue necrosis of unspecified sites**
Frostbite with tissue necrosis NOS

   ✓x7ᵗʰ   **T34.99**   **Frostbite with tissue necrosis of other sites**
Frostbite with tissue necrosis of leg NOS
Frostbite with tissue necrosis of trunk NOS

EXCLUDES 1 Not coded here   EXCLUDES 2 Not included here   N Newborn Age: 0   P Pediatric Age: 0-17   M Maternity Age: 12-55   A Adult Age: 15-124

940   ICD-10-CM 2014 (Draft)

Poisoning by, adverse effects of and underdosing of drugs, medicaments and biological substances (T36-T50)

INCLUDES adverse effect of correct substance properly administered
poisoning by overdose of substance
poisoning by wrong substance given or taken in error
underdosing by (inadvertently) (deliberately) taking less substance than prescribed or instructed

Code first, for adverse effects, the nature of the adverse effect, such as:
adverse effect NOS (T88.7)
aspirin gastritis (K29.-)
blood disorders (D56-D76)
contact dermatitis (L23-L25)
dermatitis due to substances taken internally (L27.-)
nephropathy (N14.0-N14.2)

NOTE The drug giving rise to the adverse effect should be identified by use of codes from categories T36-T50 with fifth or sixth character 5.

Use additional code(s) to specify:
manifestations of poisoning
underdosing or failure in dosage during medical and surgical care (Y63.6, Y63.8-Y63.9)
underdosing of medication regimen (Z91.12-, Z91.13-)

EXCLUDES 1 toxic reaction to local anesthesia in pregnancy (O29.3-)
EXCLUDES 2 abuse and dependence of psychoactive substances (F10-F19)
abuse of non-dependence-producing substances (F55.-)
drug reaction and poisoning affecting newborn (P00-P96)
pathological drug intoxication (inebriation) (F10-F19)

☑4ᵗʰ **T36** **Poisoning by, adverse effect of and underdosing of systemic antibiotics**

EXCLUDES 1 antineoplastic antibiotics (T45.1-)
locally applied antibiotic NEC (T49.0)
topically used antibiotic for ear, nose and throat (T49.6)
topically used antibiotic for eye (T49.5)

The appropriate 7th character is to be added to each code from category T36.
A   initial encounter
D   subsequent encounter
S   sequela

☑5ᵗʰ **T36.0** **Poisoning by, adverse effect of and underdosing of penicillins**

☑6ᵗʰ **T36.0X** **Poisoning by, adverse effect of and underdosing of penicillins**

☑7ᵗʰ **T36.0X1** **Poisoning by penicillins, accidental (unintentional)**
Poisoning by penicillins NOS

☑7ᵗʰ **T36.0X2** **Poisoning by penicillins, intentional self-harm**

☑7ᵗʰ **T36.0X3** **Poisoning by penicillins, assault**

☑7ᵗʰ **T36.0X4** **Poisoning by penicillins, undetermined**

☑7ᵗʰ **T36.0X5** **Adverse effect of penicillins**

☑7ᵗʰ **T36.0X6** **Underdosing of penicillins**

☑5ᵗʰ **T36.1** **Poisoning by, adverse effect of and underdosing of cephalosporins and other beta-lactam antibiotics**

☑6ᵗʰ **T36.1X** **Poisoning by, adverse effect of and underdosing of cephalosporins and other beta-lactam antibiotics**

☑7ᵗʰ **T36.1X1** **Poisoning by cephalosporins and other beta-lactam antibiotics, accidental (unintentional)**
Poisoning by cephalosporins and other beta-lactam antibiotics NOS

☑7ᵗʰ **T36.1X2** **Poisoning by cephalosporins and other beta-lactam antibiotics, intentional self-harm**

☑7ᵗʰ **T36.1X3** **Poisoning by cephalosporins and other beta-lactam antibiotics, assault**

☑7ᵗʰ **T36.1X4** **Poisoning by cephalosporins and other beta-lactam antibiotics, undetermined**

☑7ᵗʰ **T36.1X5** **Adverse effect of cephalosporins and other beta-lactam antibiotics**

☑7ᵗʰ **T36.1X6** **Underdosing of cephalosporins and other beta-lactam antibiotics**

☑5ᵗʰ **T36.2** **Poisoning by, adverse effect of and underdosing of chloramphenicol group**

☑6ᵗʰ **T36.2X** **Poisoning by, adverse effect of and underdosing of chloramphenicol group**

☑7ᵗʰ **T36.2X1** **Poisoning by chloramphenicol group, accidental (unintentional)**
Poisoning by chloramphenicol group NOS

☑7ᵗʰ **T36.2X2** **Poisoning by chloramphenicol group, intentional self-harm**

☑7ᵗʰ **T36.2X3** **Poisoning by chloramphenicol group, assault**

☑7ᵗʰ **T36.2X4** **Poisoning by chloramphenicol group, undetermined**

☑7ᵗʰ **T36.2X5** **Adverse effect of chloramphenicol group**

☑7ᵗʰ **T36.2X6** **Underdosing of chloramphenicol group**

☑5ᵗʰ **T36.3** **Poisoning by, adverse effect of and underdosing of macrolides**

☑6ᵗʰ **T36.3X** **Poisoning by, adverse effect of and underdosing of macrolides**

☑7ᵗʰ **T36.3X1** **Poisoning by macrolides, accidental (unintentional)**
Poisoning by macrolides NOS

☑7ᵗʰ **T36.3X2** **Poisoning by macrolides, intentional self-harm**

☑7ᵗʰ **T36.3X3** **Poisoning by macrolides, assault**

☑7ᵗʰ **T36.3X4** **Poisoning by macrolides, undetermined**

☑7ᵗʰ **T36.3X5** **Adverse effect of macrolides**

☑7ᵗʰ **T36.3X6** **Underdosing of macrolides**

☑5ᵗʰ **T36.4** **Poisoning by, adverse effect of and underdosing of tetracyclines**

☑6ᵗʰ **T36.4X** **Poisoning by, adverse effect of and underdosing of tetracyclines**

☑7ᵗʰ **T36.4X1** **Poisoning by tetracyclines, accidental (unintentional)**
Poisoning by tetracyclines NOS

☑7ᵗʰ **T36.4X2** **Poisoning by tetracyclines, intentional self-harm**

☑7ᵗʰ **T36.4X3** **Poisoning by tetracyclines, assault**

☑7ᵗʰ **T36.4X4** **Poisoning by tetracyclines, undetermined**

☑7ᵗʰ **T36.4X5** **Adverse effect of tetracyclines**

☑7ᵗʰ **T36.4X6** **Underdosing of tetracyclines**

☑5ᵗʰ **T36.5** **Poisoning by, adverse effect of and underdosing of aminoglycosides**
Poisoning by, adverse effect of and underdosing of streptomycin

☑6ᵗʰ **T36.5X** **Poisoning by, adverse effect of and underdosing of aminoglycosides**

☑7ᵗʰ **T36.5X1** **Poisoning by aminoglycosides, accidental (unintentional)**
Poisoning by aminoglycosides NOS

☑7ᵗʰ **T36.5X2** **Poisoning by aminoglycosides, intentional self-harm**

☑7ᵗʰ **T36.5X3** **Poisoning by aminoglycosides, assault**

☑7ᵗʰ **T36.5X4** **Poisoning by aminoglycosides, undetermined**

☑7ᵗʰ **T36.5X5** **Adverse effect of aminoglycosides**

☑7ᵗʰ **T36.5X6** **Underdosing of aminoglycosides**

☑5ᵗʰ **T36.6** **Poisoning by, adverse effect of and underdosing of rifampicins**

☑6ᵗʰ **T36.6X** **Poisoning by, adverse effect of and underdosing of rifampicins**

☑7ᵗʰ **T36.6X1** **Poisoning by rifampicins, accidental (unintentional)**
Poisoning by rifampicins NOS

☑7ᵗʰ **T36.6X2** **Poisoning by rifampicins, intentional self-harm**

☑7ᵗʰ **T36.6X3** **Poisoning by rifampicins, assault**

☑7ᵗʰ **T36.6X4** **Poisoning by rifampicins, undetermined**

☑7ᵗʰ **T36.6X5** **Adverse effect of rifampicins**

☑7ᵗʰ **T36.6X6** **Underdosing of rifampicins**

☑5ᵗʰ **T36.7** **Poisoning by, adverse effect of and underdosing of antifungal antibiotics, systemically used**

☑6ᵗʰ **T36.7X** **Poisoning by, adverse effect of and underdosing of antifungal antibiotics, systemically used**

☑7ᵗʰ **T36.7X1** **Poisoning by antifungal antibiotics, systemically used, accidental (unintentional)**
Poisoning by antifungal antibiotics, systemically used NOS

☑7ᵗʰ **T36.7X2** **Poisoning by antifungal antibiotics, systemically used, intentional self-harm**

☑ Additional Character Required   ✓ₓ7ᵗʰ *X*tension Alert   Unspecified Code   Other Specified Code   Manifestation Code   ►◄ Revised Text   ● New Code   ▲ Revised Code Title

ICD-10-CM 2014 (Draft)   **941**

✓7th **T36.7X3** **Poisoning by antifungal antibiotics, systemically used,** assault

✓7th **T36.7X4** **Poisoning by antifungal antibiotics, systemically used,** undetermined

✓7th **T36.7X5** Adverse effect of antifungal antibiotics, systemically used

✓7th **T36.7X6** Underdosing of antifungal antibiotics, systemically used

✓5th **T36.8** **Poisoning by, adverse effect of and underdosing of other systemic antibiotics**

✓6th **T36.8X** **Poisoning by, adverse effect of and underdosing of other systemic antibiotics**

✓7th **T36.8X1** **Poisoning by other systemic antibiotics, accidental (unintentional)**
Poisoning by other systemic antibiotics NOS

✓7th **T36.8X2** **Poisoning by other systemic antibiotics, intentional self-harm**

✓7th **T36.8X3** **Poisoning by other systemic antibiotics, assault**

✓7th **T36.8X4** **Poisoning by other systemic antibiotics, undetermined**

✓7th **T36.8X5** Adverse effect of other systemic antibiotics

✓7th **T36.8X6** Underdosing of other systemic antibiotics

✓5th **T36.9** **Poisoning by, adverse effect of and underdosing of unspecified systemic antibiotic**

✓x7th **T36.91** **Poisoning by unspecified systemic antibiotic, accidental (unintentional)**
Poisoning by systemic antibiotic NOS

✓x7th **T36.92** **Poisoning by unspecified systemic antibiotic, intentional self-harm**

✓x7th **T36.93** **Poisoning by unspecified systemic antibiotic, assault**

✓x7th **T36.94** **Poisoning by unspecified systemic antibiotic, undetermined**

✓x7th **T36.95** Adverse effect of unspecified systemic antibiotic

✓x7th **T36.96** Underdosing of unspecified systemic antibiotic

✓4th **T37** **Poisoning by, adverse effect of and underdosing of other systemic anti- infectives and antiparasitics**

EXCLUDES 1 anti-infectives topically used for ear, nose and throat (T49.6-)
anti-infectives topically used for eye (T49.5-)
locally applied anti-infectives NEC (T49.0-)

The appropriate 7th character is to be added to each code from category T37.
A   initial encounter
D   subsequent encounter
S   sequela

✓5th **T37.0** **Poisoning by, adverse effect of and underdosing of sulfonamides**

✓6th **T37.0X** **Poisoning by, adverse effect of and underdosing of sulfonamides**

✓7th **T37.0X1** **Poisoning by sulfonamides, accidental (unintentional)**
Poisoning by sulfonamides NOS

✓7th **T37.0X2** **Poisoning by sulfonamides, intentional self-harm**

✓7th **T37.0X3** **Poisoning by sulfonamides, assault**

✓7th **T37.0X4** **Poisoning by sulfonamides, undetermined**

✓7th **T37.0X5** Adverse effect of sulfonamides

✓7th **T37.0X6** Underdosing of sulfonamides

✓5th **T37.1** **Poisoning by, adverse effect of and underdosing of antimycobacterial drugs**

EXCLUDES 1 rifampicins (T36.6-)
streptomycin (T36.5-)

✓6th **T37.1X** **Poisoning by, adverse effect of and underdosing of antimycobacterial drugs**

✓7th **T37.1X1** **Poisoning by antimycobacterial drugs, accidental (unintentional)**
Poisoning by antimycobacterial drugs NOS

✓7th **T37.1X2** **Poisoning by antimycobacterial drugs, intentional self-harm**

✓7th **T37.1X3** **Poisoning by antimycobacterial drugs, assault**

✓7th **T37.1X4** **Poisoning by antimycobacterial drugs, undetermined**

✓7th **T37.1X5** Adverse effect of antimycobacterial drugs

✓7th **T37.1X6** Underdosing of antimycobacterial drugs

✓5th **T37.2** **Poisoning by, adverse effect of and underdosing of antimalarials and drugs acting on other blood protozoa**

EXCLUDES 1 hydroxyquinoline derivatives (T37.8-)

✓6th **T37.2X** **Poisoning by, adverse effect of and underdosing of antimalarials and drugs acting on other blood protozoa**

✓7th **T37.2X1** **Poisoning by antimalarials and drugs acting on other blood protozoa, accidental (unintentional)**
Poisoning by antimalarials and drugs acting on other blood protozoa NOS

✓7th **T37.2X2** **Poisoning by antimalarials and drugs acting on other blood protozoa, intentional self-harm**

✓7th **T37.2X3** **Poisoning by antimalarials and drugs acting on other blood protozoa, assault**

✓7th **T37.2X4** **Poisoning by antimalarials and drugs acting on other blood protozoa, undetermined**

✓7th **T37.2X5** Adverse effect of antimalarials and drugs acting on other blood protozoa

✓7th **T37.2X6** Underdosing of antimalarials and drugs acting on other blood protozoa

✓5th **T37.3** **Poisoning by, adverse effect of and underdosing of other antiprotozoal drugs**

✓6th **T37.3X** **Poisoning by, adverse effect of and underdosing of other antiprotozoal drugs**

✓7th **T37.3X1** **Poisoning by other antiprotozoal drugs, accidental (unintentional)**
Poisoning by other antiprotozoal drugs NOS

✓7th **T37.3X2** **Poisoning by other antiprotozoal drugs, intentional self-harm**

✓7th **T37.3X3** **Poisoning by other antiprotozoal drugs, assault**

✓7th **T37.3X4** **Poisoning by other antiprotozoal drugs, undetermined**

✓7th **T37.3X5** Adverse effect of other antiprotozoal drugs

✓7th **T37.3X6** Underdosing of other antiprotozoal drugs

✓5th **T37.4** **Poisoning by, adverse effect of and underdosing of anthelminthics**

✓6th **T37.4X** **Poisoning by, adverse effect of and underdosing of anthelminthics**

✓7th **T37.4X1** **Poisoning by anthelminthics, accidental (unintentional)**
Poisoning by anthelminthics NOS

✓7th **T37.4X2** **Poisoning by anthelminthics, intentional self-harm**

✓7th **T37.4X3** **Poisoning by anthelminthics, assault**

✓7th **T37.4X4** **Poisoning by anthelminthics, undetermined**

✓7th **T37.4X5** Adverse effect of anthelminthics

✓7th **T37.4X6** Underdosing of anthelminthics

✓5th **T37.5** **Poisoning by, adverse effect of and underdosing of antiviral drugs**

EXCLUDES 1 amantadine (T42.8-)
cytarabine (T45.1-)

✓6th **T37.5X** **Poisoning by, adverse effect of and underdosing of antiviral drugs**

✓7th **T37.5X1** **Poisoning by antiviral drugs, accidental (unintentional)**
Poisoning by antiviral drugs NOS

✓7th **T37.5X2** **Poisoning by antiviral drugs, intentional self-harm**

✓7th **T37.5X3** **Poisoning by antiviral drugs, assault**

✓7th **T37.5X4** **Poisoning by antiviral drugs, undetermined**

✓7th **T37.5X5** Adverse effect of antiviral drugs

✓7th **T37.5X6** Underdosing of antiviral drugs

EXCLUDES 1 Not coded here   EXCLUDES 2 Not included here   N Newborn Age: 0   P Pediatric Age: 0-17   M Maternity Age: 12-55   A Adult Age: 15-124

942   ICD-10-CM 2014 (Draft)

√5th **T37.8 Poisoning by, adverse effect of and underdosing of other specified systemic anti-infectives and antiparasitics**
Poisoning by, adverse effect of and underdosing of hydroxyquinoline derivatives
EXCLUDES 1 *antimalarial drugs (T37.2-)*

√6th **T37.8X Poisoning by, adverse effect of and underdosing of other specified systemic anti-infectives and antiparasitics**

√7th **T37.8X1 Poisoning by other specified systemic anti-infectives and antiparasitics, accidental (unintentional)**
Poisoning by other specified systemic anti-infectives and antiparasitics NOS

√7th **T37.8X2 Poisoning by other specified systemic anti-infectives and antiparasitics, intentional self-harm**

√7th **T37.8X3 Poisoning by other specified systemic anti-infectives and antiparasitics, assault**

√7th **T37.8X4 Poisoning by other specified systemic anti-infectives and antiparasitics, undetermined**

√7th **T37.8X5 Adverse effect of other specified systemic anti-infectives and antiparasitics**

√7th **T37.8X6 Underdosing of other specified systemic anti-infectives and antiparasitics**

√5th **T37.9 Poisoning by, adverse effect of and underdosing of unspecified systemic anti-infective and antiparasitics**

√x7th **T37.91 Poisoning by unspecified systemic anti-infective and antiparasitics, accidental (unintentional)**
Poisoning by, adverse effect of and underdosing of systemic anti-infective and antiparasitics NOS

√x7th **T37.92 Poisoning by unspecified systemic anti-infective and antiparasitics, intentional self-harm**

√x7th **T37.93 Poisoning by unspecified systemic anti-infective and antiparasitics, assault**

√x7th **T37.94 Poisoning by unspecified systemic anti-infective and antiparasitics, undetermined**

√x7th **T37.95 Adverse effect of unspecified systemic anti-infective and antiparasitic**

√x7th **T37.96 Underdosing of unspecified systemic anti-infectives and antiparasitics**

√4th **T38 Poisoning by, adverse effect of and underdosing of hormones and their synthetic substitutes and antagonists, not elsewhere classified**
EXCLUDES 1 *mineralocorticoids and their antagonists (T5Ø.Ø-)*
oxytocic hormones (T48.Ø-)
parathyroid hormones and derivatives (T5Ø.9-)

The appropriate 7th character is to be added to each code from category T38.
A   initial encounter
D   subsequent encounter
S   sequela

√5th **T38.Ø Poisoning by, adverse effect of and underdosing of glucocorticoids and synthetic analogues**
EXCLUDES 1 *glucocorticoids, topically used (T49.-)*

√6th **T38.ØX Poisoning by, adverse effect of and underdosing of glucocorticoids and synthetic analogues**

√7th **T38.ØX1 Poisoning by glucocorticoids and synthetic analogues, accidental (unintentional)**
Poisoning by glucocorticoids and synthetic analogues NOS

√7th **T38.ØX2 Poisoning by glucocorticoids and synthetic analogues, intentional self-harm**

√7th **T38.ØX3 Poisoning by glucocorticoids and synthetic analogues, assault**

√7th **T38.ØX4 Poisoning by glucocorticoids and synthetic analogues, undetermined**

√7th **T38.ØX5 Adverse effect of glucocorticoids and synthetic analogues**

√7th **T38.ØX6 Underdosing of glucocorticoids and synthetic analogues**

√5th **T38.1 Poisoning by, adverse effect of and underdosing of thyroid hormones and substitutes**

√6th **T38.1X Poisoning by, adverse effect of and underdosing of thyroid hormones and substitutes**

√7th **T38.1X1 Poisoning by thyroid hormones and substitutes, accidental (unintentional)**
Poisoning by thyroid hormones and substitutes NOS

√7th **T38.1X2 Poisoning by thyroid hormones and substitutes, intentional self-harm**

√7th **T38.1X3 Poisoning by thyroid hormones and substitutes, assault**

√7th **T38.1X4 Poisoning by thyroid hormones and substitutes, undetermined**

√7th **T38.1X5 Adverse effect of thyroid hormones and substitutes**

√7th **T38.1X6 Underdosing of thyroid hormones and substitutes**

√5th **T38.2 Poisoning by, adverse effect of and underdosing of antithyroid drugs**

√6th **T38.2X Poisoning by, adverse effect of and underdosing of antithyroid drugs**

√7th **T38.2X1 Poisoning by antithyroid drugs, accidental (unintentional)**
Poisoning by antithyroid drugs NOS

√7th **T38.2X2 Poisoning by antithyroid drugs, intentional self-harm**

√7th **T38.2X3 Poisoning by antithyroid drugs, assault**

√7th **T38.2X4 Poisoning by antithyroid drugs, undetermined**

√7th **T38.2X5 Adverse effect of antithyroid drugs**

√7th **T38.2X6 Underdosing of antithyroid drugs**

√5th **T38.3 Poisoning by, adverse effect of and underdosing of insulin and oral hypoglycemic [antidiabetic] drugs**

√6th **T38.3X Poisoning by, adverse effect of and underdosing of insulin and oral hypoglycemic [antidiabetic] drugs**

√7th **T38.3X1 Poisoning by insulin and oral hypoglycemic [antidiabetic] drugs, accidental (unintentional)**
Poisoning by insulin and oral hypoglycemic [antidiabetic] drugs NOS

√7th **T38.3X2 Poisoning by insulin and oral hypoglycemic [antidiabetic] drugs, intentional self-harm**

√7th **T38.3X3 Poisoning by insulin and oral hypoglycemic [antidiabetic] drugs, assault**

√7th **T38.3X4 Poisoning by insulin and oral hypoglycemic [antidiabetic] drugs, undetermined**

√7th **T38.3X5 Adverse effect of insulin and oral hypoglycemic [antidiabetic] drugs**

√7th **T38.3X6 Underdosing of insulin and oral hypoglycemic [antidiabetic] drugs**

√5th **T38.4 Poisoning by, adverse effect of and underdosing of oral contraceptives**
Poisoning by, adverse effect of and underdosing of multiple- and single-ingredient oral contraceptive preparations

√6th **T38.4X Poisoning by, adverse effect of and underdosing of oral contraceptives**

√7th **T38.4X1 Poisoning by oral contraceptives, accidental (unintentional)**
Poisoning by oral contraceptives NOS

√7th **T38.4X2 Poisoning by oral contraceptives, intentional self-harm**

√7th **T38.4X3 Poisoning by oral contraceptives, assault**

√7th **T38.4X4 Poisoning by oral contraceptives, undetermined**

√7th **T38.4X5 Adverse effect of oral contraceptives**

√7th **T38.4X6 Underdosing of oral contraceptives**

☑ Additional Character Required   √x7th Xtension Alert   Unspecified Code   Other Specified Code   Manifestation Code   ▶◀ Revised Text   ● New Code   ▲ Revised Code Title

✓5th **T38.5** **Poisoning by, adverse effect of and underdosing of other estrogens and progestogens**
Poisoning by, adverse effect of and underdosing of estrogens and progestogens mixtures and substitutes

✓6th **T38.5X** **Poisoning by, adverse effect of and underdosing of other estrogens and progestogens**

✓7th **T38.5X1** **Poisoning by other estrogens and progestogens, accidental (unintentional)**
Poisoning by other estrogens and progestogens NOS

✓7th **T38.5X2** **Poisoning by other estrogens and progestogens, intentional self-harm**

✓7th **T38.5X3** **Poisoning by other estrogens and progestogens, assault**

✓7th **T38.5X4** **Poisoning by other estrogens and progestogens, undetermined**

✓7th **T38.5X5** **Adverse effect of other estrogens and progestogens**

✓7th **T38.5X6** **Underdosing of other estrogens and progestogens**

✓5th **T38.6** **Poisoning by, adverse effect of and underdosing of antigonadotrophins, antiestrogens, antiandrogens, not elsewhere classified**
Poisoning by, adverse effect of and underdosing of tamoxifen

✓6th **T38.6X** **Poisoning by, adverse effect of and underdosing of antigonadotrophins, antiestrogens, antiandrogens, not elsewhere classified**

✓7th **T38.6X1** **Poisoning by antigonadotrophins, antiestrogens, antiandrogens, not elsewhere classified, accidental (unintentional)**
Poisoning by antigonadotrophins, antiestrogens, antiandrogens, not elsewhere classified NOS

✓7th **T38.6X2** **Poisoning by antigonadotrophins, antiestrogens, antiandrogens, not elsewhere classified, intentional self-harm**

✓7th **T38.6X3** **Poisoning by antigonadotrophins, antiestrogens, antiandrogens, not elsewhere classified, assault**

✓7th **T38.6X4** **Poisoning by antigonadotrophins, antiestrogens, antiandrogens, not elsewhere classified, undetermined**

✓7th **T38.6X5** **Adverse effect of antigonadotrophins, antiestrogens, antiandrogens, not elsewhere classified**

✓7th **T38.6X6** **Underdosing of antigonadotrophins, antiestrogens, antiandrogens, not elsewhere classified**

✓5th **T38.7** **Poisoning by, adverse effect of and underdosing of androgens and anabolic congeners**

✓6th **T38.7X** **Poisoning by, adverse effect of and underdosing of androgens and anabolic congeners**

✓7th **T38.7X1** **Poisoning by androgens and anabolic congeners, accidental (unintentional)**
Poisoning by androgens and anabolic congeners NOS

✓7th **T38.7X2** **Poisoning by androgens and anabolic congeners, intentional self-harm**

✓7th **T38.7X3** **Poisoning by androgens and anabolic congeners, assault**

✓7th **T38.7X4** **Poisoning by androgens and anabolic congeners, undetermined**

✓7th **T38.7X5** **Adverse effect of androgens and anabolic congeners**

✓7th **T38.7X6** **Underdosing of androgens and anabolic congeners**

✓5th **T38.8** **Poisoning by, adverse effect of and underdosing of other and unspecified hormones and synthetic substitutes**

✓6th **T38.80** **Poisoning by, adverse effect of and underdosing of unspecified hormones and synthetic substitutes**

✓7th **T38.801** **Poisoning by unspecified hormones and synthetic substitutes, accidental (unintentional)**
Poisoning by unspecified hormones and synthetic substitutes NOS

✓7th **T38.802** **Poisoning by unspecified hormones and synthetic substitutes, intentional self-harm**

✓7th **T38.803** **Poisoning by unspecified hormones and synthetic substitutes, assault**

✓7th **T38.804** **Poisoning by unspecified hormones and synthetic substitutes, undetermined**

✓7th **T38.805** **Adverse effect of unspecified hormones and synthetic substitutes**

✓7th **T38.806** **Underdosing of unspecified hormones and synthetic substitutes**

✓6th **T38.81** **Poisoning by, adverse effect of and underdosing of anterior pituitary [adenohypophyseal] hormones**

✓7th **T38.811** **Poisoning by anterior pituitary [adenohypophyseal] hormones, accidental (unintentional)**
Poisoning by anterior pituitary [adenohypophyseal] hormones NOS

✓7th **T38.812** **Poisoning by anterior pituitary [adenohypophyseal] hormones, intentional self-harm**

✓7th **T38.813** **Poisoning by anterior pituitary [adenohypophyseal] hormones, assault**

✓7th **T38.814** **Poisoning by anterior pituitary [adenohypophyseal] hormones, undetermined**

✓7th **T38.815** **Adverse effect of anterior pituitary [adenohypophyseal] hormones**

✓7th **T38.816** **Underdosing of anterior pituitary [adenohypophyseal] hormones**

✓6th **T38.89** **Poisoning by, adverse effect of and underdosing of other hormones and synthetic substitutes**

✓7th **T38.891** **Poisoning by other hormones and synthetic substitutes, accidental (unintentional)**
Poisoning by other hormones and synthetic substitutes NOS

✓7th **T38.892** **Poisoning by other hormones and synthetic substitutes, intentional self-harm**

✓7th **T38.893** **Poisoning by other hormones and synthetic substitutes, assault**

✓7th **T38.894** **Poisoning by other hormones and synthetic substitutes, undetermined**

✓7th **T38.895** **Adverse effect of other hormones and synthetic substitutes**

✓7th **T38.896** **Underdosing of other hormones and synthetic substitutes**

✓5th **T38.9** **Poisoning by, adverse effect of and underdosing of other and unspecified hormone antagonists**

✓6th **T38.90** **Poisoning by, adverse effect of and underdosing of unspecified hormone antagonists**

✓7th **T38.901** **Poisoning by unspecified hormone antagonists, accidental (unintentional)**
Poisoning by unspecified hormone antagonists NOS

✓7th **T38.902** **Poisoning by unspecified hormone antagonists, intentional self-harm**

✓7th **T38.903** **Poisoning by unspecified hormone antagonists, assault**

✓7th **T38.904** **Poisoning by unspecified hormone antagonists, undetermined**

✓7th **T38.905** **Adverse effect of unspecified hormone antagonists**

✓7th **T38.906** **Underdosing of unspecified hormone antagonists**

✓6th **T38.99** **Poisoning by, adverse effect of and underdosing of other hormone antagonists**

✓7th **T38.991** **Poisoning by other hormone antagonists, accidental (unintentional)**
Poisoning by other hormone antagonists NOS

✓7th **T38.992** **Poisoning by other hormone antagonists, intentional self-harm**

✓7th **T38.993** **Poisoning by other hormone antagonists, assault**

EXCLUDES 1 Not coded here   **EXCLUDES 2** Not included here   N Newborn Age: 0   P Pediatric Age: 0-17   M Maternity Age: 12-55   A Adult Age: 15-124

944   ICD-10-CM 2014 (Draft)

√7ʰ **T38.994** Poisoning by other hormone antagonists, undetermined

√7ʰ **T38.995** Adverse effect of other hormone antagonists

√7ʰ **T38.996** Underdosing of other hormone antagonists

√4ʰ **T39** **Poisoning by, adverse effect of and underdosing of nonopioid analgesics, antipyretics and antirheumatics**

> The appropriate 7th character is to be added to each code from category T39.
> A   initial encounter
> D   subsequent encounter
> S   sequela

√5ʰ **T39.0** **Poisoning by, adverse effect of and underdosing of salicylates**

√6ʰ **T39.01** Poisoning by, adverse effect of and underdosing of aspirin

> Poisoning by, adverse effect of and underdosing of acetylsalicylic acid

√7ʰ **T39.011** Poisoning by aspirin, accidental (unintentional)

√7ʰ **T39.012** Poisoning by aspirin, intentional self-harm

√7ʰ **T39.013** Poisoning by aspirin, assault

√7ʰ **T39.014** Poisoning by aspirin, undetermined

√7ʰ **T39.015** Adverse effect of aspirin

√7ʰ **T39.016** Underdosing of aspirin

√6ʰ **T39.09** Poisoning by, adverse effect of and underdosing of other salicylates

√7ʰ **T39.091** Poisoning by salicylates, accidental (unintentional)

> Poisoning by salicylates NOS

√7ʰ **T39.092** Poisoning by salicylates, intentional self-harm

√7ʰ **T39.093** Poisoning by salicylates, assault

√7ʰ **T39.094** Poisoning by salicylates, undetermined

√7ʰ **T39.095** Adverse effect of salicylates

√7ʰ **T39.096** Underdosing of salicylates

√5ʰ **T39.1** Poisoning by, adverse effect of and underdosing of 4-Aminophenol derivatives

√6ʰ **T39.1X** Poisoning by, adverse effect of and underdosing of 4-Aminophenol derivatives

√7ʰ **T39.1X1** Poisoning by 4-Aminophenol derivatives, accidental (unintentional)

> Poisoning by 4-Aminophenol derivatives NOS

√7ʰ **T39.1X2** Poisoning by 4-Aminophenol derivatives, intentional self-harm

√7ʰ **T39.1X3** Poisoning by 4-Aminophenol derivatives, assault

√7ʰ **T39.1X4** Poisoning by 4-Aminophenol derivatives, undetermined

√7ʰ **T39.1X5** Adverse effect of 4-Aminophenol derivatives

√7ʰ **T39.1X6** Underdosing of 4-Aminophenol derivatives

√5ʰ **T39.2** Poisoning by, adverse effect of and underdosing of pyrazolone derivatives

√6ʰ **T39.2X** Poisoning by, adverse effect of and underdosing of pyrazolone derivatives

√7ʰ **T39.2X1** Poisoning by pyrazolone derivatives, accidental (unintentional)

> Poisoning by pyrazolone derivatives NOS

√7ʰ **T39.2X2** Poisoning by pyrazolone derivatives, intentional self-harm

√7ʰ **T39.2X3** Poisoning by pyrazolone derivatives, assault

√7ʰ **T39.2X4** Poisoning by pyrazolone derivatives, undetermined

√7ʰ **T39.2X5** Adverse effect of pyrazolone derivatives

√7ʰ **T39.2X6** Underdosing of pyrazolone derivatives

√5ʰ **T39.3** Poisoning by, adverse effect of and underdosing of other nonsteroidal anti-inflammatory drugs [NSAID]

√6ʰ **T39.31** Poisoning by, adverse effect of and underdosing of propionic acid derivatives

> Poisoning by, adverse effect of and underdosing of fenoprofen
> Poisoning by, adverse effect of and underdosing of flurbiprofen
> Poisoning by, adverse effect of and underdosing of ibuprofen
> Poisoning by, adverse effect of and underdosing of ketoprofen
> Poisoning by, adverse effect of and underdosing of naproxen
> Poisoning by, adverse effect of and underdosing of oxaprozin

√7ʰ **T39.311** Poisoning by propionic acid derivatives, accidental (unintentional)

√7ʰ **T39.312** Poisoning by propionic acid derivatives, intentional self-harm

√7ʰ **T39.313** Poisoning by propionic acid derivatives, assault

√7ʰ **T39.314** Poisoning by propionic acid derivatives, undetermined

√7ʰ **T39.315** Adverse effect of propionic acid derivatives

√7ʰ **T39.316** Underdosing of propionic acid derivatives

√6ʰ **T39.39** Poisoning by, adverse effect of and underdosing of other nonsteroidal anti-inflammatory drugs [NSAID]

√7ʰ **T39.391** Poisoning by other nonsteroidal anti-inflammatory drugs [NSAID], accidental (unintentional)

> Poisoning by other nonsteroidal anti-inflammatory drugs NOS

√7ʰ **T39.392** Poisoning by other nonsteroidal anti-inflammatory drugs [NSAID], intentional self-harm

√7ʰ **T39.393** Poisoning by other nonsteroidal anti-inflammatory drugs [NSAID], assault

√7ʰ **T39.394** Poisoning by other nonsteroidal anti-inflammatory drugs [NSAID], undetermined

√7ʰ **T39.395** Adverse effect of other nonsteroidal anti-inflammatory drugs [NSAID]

√7ʰ **T39.396** Underdosing of other nonsteroidal anti-inflammatory drugs [NSAID]

√5ʰ **T39.4** Poisoning by, adverse effect of and underdosing of antirheumatics, not elsewhere classified

> **EXCLUDES 1** *poisoning by, adverse effect of and underdosing of glucocorticoids (T38.0-)*
> *poisoning by, adverse effect of and underdosing of salicylates (T39.0-)*

√6ʰ **T39.4X** Poisoning by, adverse effect of and underdosing of antirheumatics, not elsewhere classified

√7ʰ **T39.4X1** Poisoning by antirheumatics, not elsewhere classified, accidental (unintentional)

> Poisoning by antirheumatics, not elsewhere classified NOS

√7ʰ **T39.4X2** Poisoning by antirheumatics, not elsewhere classified, intentional self-harm

√7ʰ **T39.4X3** Poisoning by antirheumatics, not elsewhere classified, assault

√7ʰ **T39.4X4** Poisoning by antirheumatics, not elsewhere classified, undetermined

√7ʰ **T39.4X5** Adverse effect of antirheumatics, not elsewhere classified

√7ʰ **T39.4X6** Underdosing of antirheumatics, not elsewhere classified

Injury, Poisoning and Certain Other Consequences of External Causes

T39.8–T40.691

✓5ᵗʰ **T39.8** Poisoning by, adverse effect of and underdosing of other nonopioid analgesics and antipyretics, not elsewhere classified

    ✓6ᵗʰ **T39.8X** Poisoning by, adverse effect of and underdosing of other nonopioid analgesics and antipyretics, not elsewhere classified

       ✓7ᵗʰ **T39.8X1** Poisoning by other nonopioid analgesics and antipyretics, not elsewhere classified, accidental (unintentional)

          Poisoning by other nonopioid analgesics and antipyretics, not elsewhere classified NOS

       ✓7ᵗʰ **T39.8X2** Poisoning by other nonopioid analgesics and antipyretics, not elsewhere classified, intentional self-harm

       ✓7ᵗʰ **T39.8X3** Poisoning by other nonopioid analgesics and antipyretics, not elsewhere classified, assault

       ✓7ᵗʰ **T39.8X4** Poisoning by other nonopioid analgesics and antipyretics, not elsewhere classified, undetermined

       ✓7ᵗʰ **T39.8X5** Adverse effect of other nonopioid analgesics and antipyretics, not elsewhere classified

       ✓7ᵗʰ **T39.8X6** Underdosing of other nonopioid analgesics and antipyretics, not elsewhere classified

✓5ᵗʰ **T39.9** Poisoning by, adverse effect of and underdosing of unspecified nonopioid analgesic, antipyretic and antirheumatic

    ✓x7ᵗʰ **T39.91** Poisoning by unspecified nonopioid analgesic, antipyretic and antirheumatic, accidental (unintentional)

       Poisoning by nonopioid analgesic, antipyretic and antirheumatic NOS

    ✓x7ᵗʰ **T39.92** Poisoning by unspecified nonopioid analgesic, antipyretic and antirheumatic, intentional self-harm

    ✓x7ᵗʰ **T39.93** Poisoning by unspecified nonopioid analgesic, antipyretic and antirheumatic, assault

    ✓x7ᵗʰ **T39.94** Poisoning by unspecified nonopioid analgesic, antipyretic and antirheumatic, undetermined

    ✓x7ᵗʰ **T39.95** Adverse effect of unspecified nonopioid analgesic and antirheumatic

    ✓x7ᵗʰ **T39.96** Underdosing of unspecified nonopioid analgesic, antipyretic and antirheumatic

✓4ᵗʰ **T40** Poisoning by, adverse effect of and underdosing of narcotics and psychodysleptics [hallucinogens]

    EXCLUDES 2   *drug dependence and related mental and behavioral disorders due to psychoactive substance use (F10-F19-)*

    The appropriate 7th character is to be added to each code from category T40.
    A   initial encounter
    D   subsequent encounter
    S   sequela

✓5ᵗʰ **T40.0** Poisoning by, adverse effect of and underdosing of opium

    ✓6ᵗʰ **T40.0X** Poisoning by, adverse effect of and underdosing of opium

       ✓7ᵗʰ **T40.0X1** Poisoning by opium, accidental (unintentional)
          Poisoning by opium NOS

       ✓7ᵗʰ **T40.0X2** Poisoning by opium, intentional self-harm

       ✓7ᵗʰ **T40.0X3** Poisoning by opium, assault

       ✓7ᵗʰ **T40.0X4** Poisoning by opium, undetermined

       ✓7ᵗʰ **T40.0X5** Adverse effect of opium

       ✓7ᵗʰ **T40.0X6** Underdosing of opium

✓5ᵗʰ **T40.1** Poisoning by and adverse effect of heroin

    ✓6ᵗʰ **T40.1X** Poisoning by and adverse effect of heroin

       ✓7ᵗʰ **T40.1X1** Poisoning by heroin, accidental (unintentional)
          Poisoning by heroin NOS

       ✓7ᵗʰ **T40.1X2** Poisoning by heroin, intentional self-harm

       ✓7ᵗʰ **T40.1X3** Poisoning by heroin, assault

       ✓7ᵗʰ **T40.1X4** Poisoning by heroin, undetermined

✓5ᵗʰ **T40.2** Poisoning by, adverse effect of and underdosing of other opioids

    ✓6ᵗʰ **T40.2X** Poisoning by, adverse effect of and underdosing of other opioids

       ✓7ᵗʰ **T40.2X1** Poisoning by other opioids, accidental (unintentional)
          Poisoning by other opioids NOS

       ✓7ᵗʰ **T40.2X2** Poisoning by other opioids, intentional self-harm

       ✓7ᵗʰ **T40.2X3** Poisoning by other opioids, assault

       ✓7ᵗʰ **T40.2X4** Poisoning by other opioids, undetermined

       ✓7ᵗʰ **T40.2X5** Adverse effect of other opioids

       ✓7ᵗʰ **T40.2X6** Underdosing of other opioids

✓5ᵗʰ **T40.3** Poisoning by, adverse effect of and underdosing of methadone

    ✓6ᵗʰ **T40.3X** Poisoning by, adverse effect of and underdosing of methadone

       ✓7ᵗʰ **T40.3X1** Poisoning by methadone, accidental (unintentional)
          Poisoning by methadone NOS

       ✓7ᵗʰ **T40.3X2** Poisoning by methadone, intentional self-harm

       ✓7ᵗʰ **T40.3X3** Poisoning by methadone, assault

       ✓7ᵗʰ **T40.3X4** Poisoning by methadone, undetermined

       ✓7ᵗʰ **T40.3X5** Adverse effect of methadone

       ✓7ᵗʰ **T40.3X6** Underdosing of methadone

✓5ᵗʰ **T40.4** Poisoning by, adverse effect of and underdosing of other synthetic narcotics

    ✓6ᵗʰ **T40.4X** Poisoning by, adverse effect of and underdosing of other synthetic narcotics

       ✓7ᵗʰ **T40.4X1** Poisoning by other synthetic narcotics, accidental (unintentional)
          Poisoning by other synthetic narcotics NOS

       ✓7ᵗʰ **T40.4X2** Poisoning by other synthetic narcotics, intentional self-harm

       ✓7ᵗʰ **T40.4X3** Poisoning by other synthetic narcotics, assault

       ✓7ᵗʰ **T40.4X4** Poisoning by other synthetic narcotics, undetermined

       ✓7ᵗʰ **T40.4X5** Adverse effect of other synthetic narcotics

       ✓7ᵗʰ **T40.4X6** Underdosing of other synthetic narcotics

✓5ᵗʰ **T40.5** Poisoning by, adverse effect of and underdosing of cocaine

    ✓6ᵗʰ **T40.5X** Poisoning by, adverse effect of and underdosing of cocaine

       ✓7ᵗʰ **T40.5X1** Poisoning by cocaine, accidental (unintentional)
          Poisoning by cocaine NOS

       ✓7ᵗʰ **T40.5X2** Poisoning by cocaine, intentional self-harm

       ✓7ᵗʰ **T40.5X3** Poisoning by cocaine, assault

       ✓7ᵗʰ **T40.5X4** Poisoning by cocaine, undetermined

       ✓7ᵗʰ **T40.5X5** Adverse effect of cocaine

       ✓7ᵗʰ **T40.5X6** Underdosing of cocaine

✓5ᵗʰ **T40.6** Poisoning by, adverse effect of and underdosing of other and unspecified narcotics

    ✓6ᵗʰ **T40.60** Poisoning by, adverse effect of and underdosing of unspecified narcotics

       ✓7ᵗʰ **T40.601** Poisoning by unspecified narcotics, accidental (unintentional)
          Poisoning by narcotics NOS

       ✓7ᵗʰ **T40.602** Poisoning by unspecified narcotics, intentional self-harm

       ✓7ᵗʰ **T40.603** Poisoning by unspecified narcotics, assault

       ✓7ᵗʰ **T40.604** Poisoning by unspecified narcotics, undetermined

       ✓7ᵗʰ **T40.605** Adverse effect of unspecified narcotics

       ✓7ᵗʰ **T40.606** Underdosing of unspecified narcotics

    ✓6ᵗʰ **T40.69** Poisoning by, adverse effect of and underdosing of other narcotics

       ✓7ᵗʰ **T40.691** Poisoning by other narcotics, accidental (unintentional)
          Poisoning by other narcotics NOS

EXCLUDES 1 Not coded here   EXCLUDES 2 Not included here   N Newborn Age: 0   P Pediatric Age: 0-17   M Maternity Age: 12-55   A Adult Age: 15-124

946   ICD-10-CM 2014 (Draft)

✓7ᵗʰ **T40.692** Poisoning by other narcotics, intentional self-harm

✓7ᵗʰ **T40.693** Poisoning by other narcotics, assault

✓7ᵗʰ **T40.694** Poisoning by other narcotics, undetermined

✓7ᵗʰ **T40.695** Adverse effect of other narcotics

✓7ᵗʰ **T40.696** Underdosing of other narcotics

✓5ᵗʰ **T40.7** Poisoning by, adverse effect of and underdosing of cannabis (derivatives)

✓6ᵗʰ **T40.7X** Poisoning by, adverse effect of and underdosing of cannabis (derivatives)

✓7ᵗʰ **T40.7X1** Poisoning by cannabis (derivatives), accidental (unintentional)
Poisoning by cannabis NOS

✓7ᵗʰ **T40.7X2** Poisoning by cannabis (derivatives), intentional self-harm

✓7ᵗʰ **T40.7X3** Poisoning by cannabis (derivatives), assault

✓7ᵗʰ **T40.7X4** Poisoning by cannabis (derivatives), undetermined

✓7ᵗʰ **T40.7X5** Adverse effect of cannabis (derivatives)

✓7ᵗʰ **T40.7X6** Underdosing of cannabis (derivatives)

✓5ᵗʰ **T40.8** Poisoning by and adverse effect of lysergide [LSD]

✓6ᵗʰ **T40.8X** Poisoning by and adverse effect of lysergide [LSD]

✓7ᵗʰ **T40.8X1** Poisoning by lysergide [LSD], accidental (unintentional)
Poisoning by lysergide [LSD]NOS

✓7ᵗʰ **T40.8X2** Poisoning by lysergide [LSD], intentional self-harm

✓7ᵗʰ **T40.8X3** Poisoning by lysergide [LSD], assault

✓7ᵗʰ **T40.8X4** Poisoning by lysergide [LSD], undetermined

✓5ᵗʰ **T40.9** Poisoning by, adverse effect of and underdosing of other and unspecified psychodysleptics [hallucinogens]

✓6ᵗʰ **T40.90** Poisoning by, adverse effect of and underdosing of unspecified psychodysleptics [hallucinogens]

✓7ᵗʰ **T40.901** Poisoning by unspecified psychodysleptics [hallucinogens], accidental (unintentional)

✓7ᵗʰ **T40.902** Poisoning by unspecified psychodysleptics [hallucinogens], intentional self-harm

✓7ᵗʰ **T40.903** Poisoning by unspecified psychodysleptics [hallucinogens], assault

✓7ᵗʰ **T40.904** Poisoning by unspecified psychodysleptics [hallucinogens], undetermined

✓7ᵗʰ **T40.905** Adverse effect of unspecified psychodysleptics [hallucinogens]

✓7ᵗʰ **T40.906** Underdosing of unspecified psychodysleptics

✓6ᵗʰ **T40.99** Poisoning by, adverse effect of and underdosing of other psychodysleptics [hallucinogens]

✓7ᵗʰ **T40.991** Poisoning by other psychodysleptics [hallucinogens], accidental (unintentional)
Poisoning by other psychodysleptics [hallucinogens] NOS

✓7ᵗʰ **T40.992** Poisoning by other psychodysleptics [hallucinogens], intentional self-harm

✓7ᵗʰ **T40.993** Poisoning by other psychodysleptics [hallucinogens], assault

✓7ᵗʰ **T40.994** Poisoning by other psychodysleptics [hallucinogens], undetermined

✓7ᵗʰ **T40.995** Adverse effect of other psychodysleptics [hallucinogens]

✓7ᵗʰ **T40.996** Underdosing of other psychodysleptics

✓4ᵗʰ **T41** **Poisoning by, adverse effect of and underdosing of anesthetics and therapeutic gases**

EXCLUDES 1 benzodiazepines (T42.4-)
cocaine (T40.5-)
complications of anesthesia during pregnancy (O29.-)
complications of anesthesia during labor and delivery (O74.-)
complications of anesthesia during the puerperium (O89.-)
opioids (T40.0-T40.2-)

The appropriate 7th character is to be added to each code from category T41.
A   initial encounter
D   subsequent encounter
S   sequela

✓5ᵗʰ **T41.0** Poisoning by, adverse effect of and underdosing of inhaled anesthetics

EXCLUDES 1 oxygen (T41.5-)

✓6ᵗʰ **T41.0X** Poisoning by, adverse effect of and underdosing of inhaled anesthetics

✓7ᵗʰ **T41.0X1** Poisoning by inhaled anesthetics, accidental (unintentional)
Poisoning by inhaled anesthetics NOS

✓7ᵗʰ **T41.0X2** Poisoning by inhaled anesthetics, intentional self-harm

✓7ᵗʰ **T41.0X3** Poisoning by inhaled anesthetics, assault

✓7ᵗʰ **T41.0X4** Poisoning by inhaled anesthetics, undetermined

✓7ᵗʰ **T41.0X5** Adverse effect of inhaled anesthetics

✓7ᵗʰ **T41.0X6** Underdosing of inhaled anesthetics

✓5ᵗʰ **T41.1** Poisoning by, adverse effect of and underdosing of intravenous anesthetics
Poisoning by, adverse effect of and underdosing of thiobarbiturates

✓6ᵗʰ **T41.1X** Poisoning by, adverse effect of and underdosing of intravenous anesthetics

✓7ᵗʰ **T41.1X1** Poisoning by intravenous anesthetics, accidental (unintentional)
Poisoning by intravenous anesthetics NOS

✓7ᵗʰ **T41.1X2** Poisoning by intravenous anesthetics, intentional self-harm

✓7ᵗʰ **T41.1X3** Poisoning by intravenous anesthetics, assault

✓7ᵗʰ **T41.1X4** Poisoning by intravenous anesthetics, undetermined

✓7ᵗʰ **T41.1X5** Adverse effect of intravenous anesthetics

✓7ᵗʰ **T41.1X6** Underdosing of intravenous anesthetics

✓5ᵗʰ **T41.2** Poisoning by, adverse effect of and underdosing of other and unspecified general anesthetics

✓6ᵗʰ **T41.20** Poisoning by, adverse effect of and underdosing of unspecified general anesthetics

✓7ᵗʰ **T41.201** Poisoning by unspecified general anesthetics, accidental (unintentional)
Poisoning by general anesthetics NOS

✓7ᵗʰ **T41.202** Poisoning by unspecified general anesthetics, intentional self-harm

✓7ᵗʰ **T41.203** Poisoning by unspecified general anesthetics, assault

✓7ᵗʰ **T41.204** Poisoning by unspecified general anesthetics, undetermined

✓7ᵗʰ **T41.205** Adverse effect of unspecified general anesthetics

✓7ᵗʰ **T41.206** Underdosing of unspecified general anesthetics

✓6ᵗʰ **T41.29** Poisoning by, adverse effect of and underdosing of other general anesthetics

✓7ᵗʰ **T41.291** Poisoning by other general anesthetics, accidental (unintentional)
Poisoning by other general anesthetics NOS

✓7ᵗʰ **T41.292** Poisoning by other general anesthetics, intentional self-harm

✓7ᵗʰ **T41.293** Poisoning by other general anesthetics, assault

✓7ᵗʰ **T41.294** Poisoning by other general anesthetics, undetermined

✓7ᵗʰ **T41.295** Adverse effect of other general anesthetics

✓ Additional Character Required   ✓x7ᵗʰ Xtension Alert   Unspecified Code   Other Specified Code   Manifestation Code   ►◄ Revised Text   ● New Code   ▲ Revised Code Title

ICD-10-CM 2014 (Draft)   **947**

✓7ᵗʰ **T41.296** Underdosing of other general anesthetics

✓5ᵗʰ **T41.3** **Poisoning by, adverse effect of and underdosing of local anesthetics**
Cocaine (topical)
EXCLUDES 2 *poisoning by cocaine used as a central nervous system stimulant (T40.5X1-T40.5X4)*

  ✓6ᵗʰ **T41.3X** **Poisoning by, adverse effect of and underdosing of local anesthetics**

    ✓7ᵗʰ **T41.3X1** **Poisoning by local anesthetics, accidental (unintentional)**
Poisoning by local anesthetics NOS

    ✓7ᵗʰ **T41.3X2** **Poisoning by local anesthetics, intentional self-harm**

    ✓7ᵗʰ **T41.3X3** **Poisoning by local anesthetics, assault**

    ✓7ᵗʰ **T41.3X4** **Poisoning by local anesthetics, undetermined**

    ✓7ᵗʰ **T41.3X5** **Adverse effect of local anesthetics**

    ✓7ᵗʰ **T41.3X6** Underdosing of local anesthetics

✓5ᵗʰ **T41.4** **Poisoning by, adverse effect of and underdosing of unspecified anesthetic**

  ✓x7ᵗʰ **T41.41** **Poisoning by unspecified anesthetic, accidental (unintentional)**
Poisoning by anesthetic NOS

  ✓x7ᵗʰ **T41.42** **Poisoning by unspecified anesthetic, intentional self-harm**

  ✓x7ᵗʰ **T41.43** **Poisoning by unspecified anesthetic, assault**

  ✓x7ᵗʰ **T41.44** **Poisoning by unspecified anesthetic, undetermined**

  ✓x7ᵗʰ **T41.45** Adverse effect of unspecified anesthetic

  ✓x7ᵗʰ **T41.46** Underdosing of unspecified anesthetics

✓5ᵗʰ **T41.5** **Poisoning by, adverse effect of and underdosing of therapeutic gases**

  ✓6ᵗʰ **T41.5X** **Poisoning by, adverse effect of and underdosing of therapeutic gases**

    ✓7ᵗʰ **T41.5X1** **Poisoning by therapeutic gases, accidental (unintentional)**
Poisoning by therapeutic gases NOS

    ✓7ᵗʰ **T41.5X2** **Poisoning by therapeutic gases, intentional self-harm**

    ✓7ᵗʰ **T41.5X3** **Poisoning by therapeutic gases, assault**

    ✓7ᵗʰ **T41.5X4** **Poisoning by therapeutic gases, undetermined**

    ✓7ᵗʰ **T41.5X5** **Adverse effect of therapeutic gases**

    ✓7ᵗʰ **T41.5X6** Underdosing of therapeutic gases

✓4ᵗʰ **T42** **Poisoning by, adverse effect of and underdosing of antiepileptic, sedative- hypnotic and antiparkinsonism drugs**
EXCLUDES 2 *drug dependence and related mental and behavioral disorders due to psychoactive substance use (F10--F19-)*

The appropriate 7th character is to be added to each code from category T42.
A   initial encounter
D   subsequent encounter
S   sequela

✓5ᵗʰ **T42.0** **Poisoning by, adverse effect of and underdosing of hydantoin derivatives**

  ✓6ᵗʰ **T42.0X** **Poisoning by, adverse effect of and underdosing of hydantoin derivatives**

    ✓7ᵗʰ **T42.0X1** **Poisoning by hydantoin derivatives, accidental (unintentional)**
Poisoning by hydantoin derivatives NOS

    ✓7ᵗʰ **T42.0X2** **Poisoning by hydantoin derivatives, intentional self-harm**

    ✓7ᵗʰ **T42.0X3** **Poisoning by hydantoin derivatives, assault**

    ✓7ᵗʰ **T42.0X4** **Poisoning by hydantoin derivatives, undetermined**

    ✓7ᵗʰ **T42.0X5** **Adverse effect of hydantoin derivatives**

    ✓7ᵗʰ **T42.0X6** Underdosing of hydantoin derivatives

✓5ᵗʰ **T42.1** **Poisoning by, adverse effect of and underdosing of iminostilbenes**
Poisoning by, adverse effect of and underdosing of carbamazepine

  ✓6ᵗʰ **T42.1X** **Poisoning by, adverse effect of and underdosing of iminostilbenes**

    ✓7ᵗʰ **T42.1X1** **Poisoning by iminostilbenes, accidental (unintentional)**
Poisoning by iminostilbenes NOS

    ✓7ᵗʰ **T42.1X2** **Poisoning by iminostilbenes, intentional self-harm**

    ✓7ᵗʰ **T42.1X3** **Poisoning by iminostilbenes, assault**

    ✓7ᵗʰ **T42.1X4** **Poisoning by iminostilbenes, undetermined**

    ✓7ᵗʰ **T42.1X5** **Adverse effect of iminostilbenes**

    ✓7ᵗʰ **T42.1X6** Underdosing of iminostilbenes

✓5ᵗʰ **T42.2** **Poisoning by, adverse effect of and underdosing of succinimides and oxazolidinediones**

  ✓6ᵗʰ **T42.2X** **Poisoning by, adverse effect of and underdosing of succinimides and oxazolidinediones**

    ✓7ᵗʰ **T42.2X1** **Poisoning by succinimides and oxazolidinediones, accidental (unintentional)**
Poisoning by succinimides and oxazolidinediones NOS

    ✓7ᵗʰ **T42.2X2** **Poisoning by succinimides and oxazolidinediones, intentional self-harm**

    ✓7ᵗʰ **T42.2X3** **Poisoning by succinimides and oxazolidinediones, assault**

    ✓7ᵗʰ **T42.2X4** **Poisoning by succinimides and oxazolidinediones, undetermined**

    ✓7ᵗʰ **T42.2X5** **Adverse effect of succinimides and oxazolidinediones**

    ✓7ᵗʰ **T42.2X6** Underdosing of succinimides and oxazolidinediones

✓5ᵗʰ **T42.3** **Poisoning by, adverse effect of and underdosing of barbiturates**
EXCLUDES 1 *poisoning by, adverse effect of and underdosing of thiobarbiturates (T41.1-)*

  ✓6ᵗʰ **T42.3X** **Poisoning by, adverse effect of and underdosing of barbiturates**

    ✓7ᵗʰ **T42.3X1** **Poisoning by barbiturates, accidental (unintentional)**
Poisoning by barbiturates NOS

    ✓7ᵗʰ **T42.3X2** **Poisoning by barbiturates, intentional self-harm**

    ✓7ᵗʰ **T42.3X3** **Poisoning by barbiturates, assault**

    ✓7ᵗʰ **T42.3X4** **Poisoning by barbiturates, undetermined**

    ✓7ᵗʰ **T42.3X5** **Adverse effect of barbiturates**

    ✓7ᵗʰ **T42.3X6** Underdosing of barbiturates

✓5ᵗʰ **T42.4** **Poisoning by, adverse effect of and underdosing of benzodiazepines**

  ✓6ᵗʰ **T42.4X** **Poisoning by, adverse effect of and underdosing of benzodiazepines**

    ✓7ᵗʰ **T42.4X1** **Poisoning by benzodiazepines, accidental (unintentional)**
Poisoning by benzodiazepines NOS

    ✓7ᵗʰ **T42.4X2** **Poisoning by benzodiazepines, intentional self-harm**

    ✓7ᵗʰ **T42.4X3** **Poisoning by benzodiazepines, assault**

    ✓7ᵗʰ **T42.4X4** **Poisoning by benzodiazepines, undetermined**

    ✓7ᵗʰ **T42.4X5** **Adverse effect of benzodiazepines**

    ✓7ᵗʰ **T42.4X6** Underdosing of benzodiazepines

✓5ᵗʰ **T42.5** **Poisoning by, adverse effect of and underdosing of mixed antiepileptics**

  ✓6ᵗʰ **T42.5X** **Poisoning by, adverse effect of and underdosing of antiepileptics**

    ✓7ᵗʰ **T42.5X1** **Poisoning by mixed antiepileptics, accidental (unintentional)**
Poisoning by mixed antiepileptics NOS

    ✓7ᵗʰ **T42.5X2** **Poisoning by mixed antiepileptics, intentional self-harm**

    ✓7ᵗʰ **T42.5X3** **Poisoning by mixed antiepileptics, assault**

EXCLUDES 1 Not coded here   **EXCLUDES 2** Not included here   **N** Newborn Age: 0   **P** Pediatric Age: 0-17   **M** Maternity Age: 12-55   **A** Adult Age: 15-124

948   ICD-10-CM 2014 (Draft)

✓7th **T42.5X4 Poisoning by mixed antiepileptics, undetermined**

✓7th **T42.5X5** Adverse effect of mixed antiepileptics

✓7th **T42.5X6** Underdosing of mixed antiepileptics

✓5th **T42.6 Poisoning by, adverse effect of and underdosing of other antiepileptic and sedative-hypnotic drugs**
Poisoning by, adverse effect of and underdosing of methaqualone
Poisoning by, adverse effect of and underdosing of valproic acid
EXCLUDES 1   *poisoning by, adverse effect of and underdosing of carbamazepine (T42.1-)*

✓6th **T42.6X Poisoning by, adverse effect of and underdosing of other antiepileptic and sedative-hypnotic drugs**

✓7th **T42.6X1 Poisoning by other antiepileptic and sedative-hypnotic drugs, accidental (unintentional)**
Poisoning by other antiepileptic and sedative-hypnotic drugs NOS

✓7th **T42.6X2 Poisoning by other antiepileptic and sedative-hypnotic drugs, intentional self-harm**

✓7th **T42.6X3 Poisoning by other antiepileptic and sedative-hypnotic drugs, assault**

✓7th **T42.6X4 Poisoning by other antiepileptic and sedative-hypnotic drugs, undetermined**

✓7th **T42.6X5** Adverse effect of other antiepileptic and sedative-hypnotic drugs

✓7th **T42.6X6** Underdosing of other antiepileptic and sedative-hypnotic drugs

✓5th **T42.7 Poisoning by, adverse effect of and underdosing of unspecified antiepileptic and sedative-hypnotic drugs**

✓x7th **T42.71 Poisoning by unspecified antiepileptic and sedative-hypnotic drugs, accidental (unintentional)**
Poisoning by antiepileptic and sedative-hypnotic drugs NOS

✓x7th **T42.72 Poisoning by unspecified antiepileptic and sedative-hypnotic drugs, intentional self-harm**

✓x7th **T42.73 Poisoning by unspecified antiepileptic and sedative-hypnotic drugs, assault**

✓x7th **T42.74 Poisoning by unspecified antiepileptic and sedative-hypnotic drugs, undetermined**

✓x7th **T42.75** Adverse effect of unspecified antiepileptic and sedative-hypnotic drugs

✓x7th **T42.76** Underdosing of unspecified antiepileptic and sedative-hypnotic drugs

✓5th **T42.8 Poisoning by, adverse effect of and underdosing of antiparkinsonism drugs and other central muscle-tone depressants**
Poisoning by, adverse effect of and underdosing of amantadine

✓6th **T42.8X Poisoning by, adverse effect of and underdosing of antiparkinsonism drugs and other central muscle-tone depressants**

✓7th **T42.8X1 Poisoning by antiparkinsonism drugs and other central muscle-tone depressants, accidental (unintentional)**
Poisoning by antiparkinsonism drugs and other central muscle-tone depressants NOS

✓7th **T42.8X2 Poisoning by antiparkinsonism drugs and other central muscle-tone depressants, intentional self-harm**

✓7th **T42.8X3 Poisoning by antiparkinsonism drugs and other central muscle-tone depressants, assault**

✓7th **T42.8X4 Poisoning by antiparkinsonism drugs and other central muscle-tone depressants, undetermined**

✓7th **T42.8X5** Adverse effect of antiparkinsonism drugs and other central muscle-tone depressants

✓7th **T42.8X6** Underdosing of antiparkinsonism drugs and other central muscle-tone depressants

✓4th **T43 Poisoning by, adverse effect of and underdosing of psychotropic drugs, not elsewhere classified**
EXCLUDES 1   *appetite depressants (T50.5-)*
barbiturates (T42.3-)
benzodiazepines (T42.4-)
methaqualone (T42.6-)
psychodysleptics [hallucinogens] (T40.7-T40.9-)
EXCLUDES 2   *drug dependence and related mental and behavioral disorders due to psychoactive substance use (F10--F19-)*

The appropriate 7th character is to be added to each code from category T43.
A   initial encounter
D   subsequent encounter
S   sequela

✓5th **T43.0 Poisoning by, adverse effect of and underdosing of tricyclic and tetracyclic antidepressants**

✓6th **T43.01 Poisoning by, adverse effect of and underdosing of tricyclic antidepressants**

✓7th **T43.011 Poisoning by tricyclic antidepressants, accidental (unintentional)**
Poisoning by tricyclic antidepressants NOS

✓7th **T43.012 Poisoning by tricyclic antidepressants, intentional self-harm**

✓7th **T43.013 Poisoning by tricyclic antidepressants, assault**

✓7th **T43.014 Poisoning by tricyclic antidepressants, undetermined**

✓7th **T43.015** Adverse effect of tricyclic antidepressants

✓7th **T43.016** Underdosing of tricyclic antidepressants

✓6th **T43.02 Poisoning by, adverse effect of and underdosing of tetracyclic antidepressants**

✓7th **T43.021 Poisoning by tetracyclic antidepressants, accidental (unintentional)**
Poisoning by tetracyclic antidepressants NOS

✓7th **T43.022 Poisoning by tetracyclic antidepressants, intentional self-harm**

✓7th **T43.023 Poisoning by tetracyclic antidepressants, assault**

✓7th **T43.024 Poisoning by tetracyclic antidepressants, undetermined**

✓7th **T43.025** Adverse effect of tetracyclic antidepressants

✓7th **T43.026** Underdosing of tetracyclic antidepressants

✓5th **T43.1 Poisoning by, adverse effect of and underdosing of monoamine-oxidase-inhibitor antidepressants**

✓6th **T43.1X Poisoning by, adverse effect of and underdosing of monoamine-oxidase-inhibitor antidepressants**

✓7th **T43.1X1 Poisoning by monoamine-oxidase-inhibitor antidepressants, accidental (unintentional)**
Poisoning by monoamine-oxidase-inhibitor antidepressants NOS

✓7th **T43.1X2 Poisoning by monoamine-oxidase-inhibitor antidepressants, intentional self-harm**

✓7th **T43.1X3 Poisoning by monoamine-oxidase-inhibitor antidepressants, assault**

✓7th **T43.1X4 Poisoning by monoamine-oxidase-inhibitor antidepressants, undetermined**

✓7th **T43.1X5** Adverse effect of monoamine-oxidase-inhibitor antidepressants

✓7th **T43.1X6** Underdosing of monoamine-oxidase-inhibitor antidepressants

✓5th **T43.2 Poisoning by, adverse effect of and underdosing of other and unspecified antidepressants**

✓6th **T43.20 Poisoning by, adverse effect of and underdosing of unspecified antidepressants**

✓7th **T43.201 Poisoning by unspecified antidepressants, accidental (unintentional)**
Poisoning by antidepressants NOS

✓7th **T43.202 Poisoning by unspecified antidepressants, intentional self-harm**

✓7th **T43.203 Poisoning by unspecified antidepressants, assault**

√7ᵗʰ **T43.204** Poisoning by unspecified antidepressants, undetermined

√7ᵗʰ **T43.205** Adverse effect of unspecified antidepressants

√7ᵗʰ **T43.206** Underdosing of unspecified antidepressants

√6ᵗʰ **T43.21** Poisoning by, adverse effect of and underdosing of selective serotonin and norepinephrine reuptake inhibitors
  Poisoning by, adverse effect of and underdosing of SSNRI antidepressants

√7ᵗʰ **T43.211** Poisoning by selective serotonin and norepinephrine reuptake inhibitors, accidental (unintentional)

√7ᵗʰ **T43.212** Poisoning by selective serotonin and norepinephrine reuptake inhibitors, intentional self-harm

√7ᵗʰ **T43.213** Poisoning by selective serotonin and norepinephrine reuptake inhibitors, assault

√7ᵗʰ **T43.214** Poisoning by selective serotonin and norepinephrine reuptake inhibitors, undetermined

√7ᵗʰ **T43.215** Adverse effect of selective serotonin and norepinephrine reuptake inhibitors

√7ᵗʰ **T43.216** Underdosing of selective serotonin and norepinephrine reuptake inhibitors

√6ᵗʰ **T43.22** Poisoning by, adverse effect of and underdosing of selective serotonin reuptake inhibitors
  Poisoning by, adverse effect of and underdosing of SSRI antidepressants

√7ᵗʰ **T43.221** Poisoning by selective serotonin reuptake inhibitors, accidental (unintentional)

√7ᵗʰ **T43.222** Poisoning by selective serotonin reuptake inhibitors, intentional self-harm

√7ᵗʰ **T43.223** Poisoning by selective serotonin reuptake inhibitors, assault

√7ᵗʰ **T43.224** Poisoning by selective serotonin reuptake inhibitors, undetermined

√7ᵗʰ **T43.225** Adverse effect of selective serotonin reuptake inhibitors

√7ᵗʰ **T43.226** Underdosing of selective serotonin reuptake inhibitors

√6ᵗʰ **T43.29** Poisoning by, adverse effect of and underdosing of other antidepressants

√7ᵗʰ **T43.291** Poisoning by other antidepressants, accidental (unintentional)
  Poisoning by other antidepressants NOS

√7ᵗʰ **T43.292** Poisoning by other antidepressants, intentional self-harm

√7ᵗʰ **T43.293** Poisoning by other antidepressants, assault

√7ᵗʰ **T43.294** Poisoning by other antidepressants, undetermined

√7ᵗʰ **T43.295** Adverse effect of other antidepressants

√7ᵗʰ **T43.296** Underdosing of other antidepressants

√5ᵗʰ **T43.3** Poisoning by, adverse effect of and underdosing of phenothiazine antipsychotics and neuroleptics

√6ᵗʰ **T43.3X** Poisoning by, adverse effect of and underdosing of phenothiazine antipsychotics and neuroleptics

√7ᵗʰ **T43.3X1** Poisoning by phenothiazine antipsychotics and neuroleptics, accidental (unintentional)
  Poisoning by phenothiazine antipsychotics and neuroleptics NOS

√7ᵗʰ **T43.3X2** Poisoning by phenothiazine antipsychotics and neuroleptics, intentional self-harm

√7ᵗʰ **T43.3X3** Poisoning by phenothiazine antipsychotics and neuroleptics, assault

√7ᵗʰ **T43.3X4** Poisoning by phenothiazine antipsychotics and neuroleptics, undetermined

√7ᵗʰ **T43.3X5** Adverse effect of phenothiazine antipsychotics and neuroleptics

√7ᵗʰ **T43.3X6** Underdosing of phenothiazine antipsychotics and neuroleptics

√5ᵗʰ **T43.4** Poisoning by, adverse effect of and underdosing of butyrophenone and thiothixene neuroleptics

√6ᵗʰ **T43.4X** Poisoning by, adverse effect of and underdosing of butyrophenone and thiothixene neuroleptics

√7ᵗʰ **T43.4X1** Poisoning by butyrophenone and thiothixene neuroleptics, accidental (unintentional)
  Poisoning by butyrophenone and thiothixene neuroleptics NOS

√7ᵗʰ **T43.4X2** Poisoning by butyrophenone and thiothixene neuroleptics, intentional self-harm

√7ᵗʰ **T43.4X3** Poisoning by butyrophenone and thiothixene neuroleptics, assault

√7ᵗʰ **T43.4X4** Poisoning by butyrophenone and thiothixene neuroleptics, undetermined

√7ᵗʰ **T43.4X5** Adverse effect of butyrophenone and thiothixene neuroleptics

√7ᵗʰ **T43.4X6** Underdosing of butyrophenone and thiothixene neuroleptics

√5ᵗʰ **T43.5** Poisoning by, adverse effect of and underdosing of other and unspecified antipsychotics and neuroleptics
  EXCLUDES 1 poisoning by, adverse effect of and underdosing of rauwolfia (T46.5-)

√6ᵗʰ **T43.50** Poisoning by, adverse effect of and underdosing of unspecified antipsychotics and neuroleptics

√7ᵗʰ **T43.501** Poisoning by unspecified antipsychotics and neuroleptics, accidental (unintentional)
  Poisoning by antipsychotics and neuroleptics NOS

√7ᵗʰ **T43.502** Poisoning by unspecified antipsychotics and neuroleptics, intentional self-harm

√7ᵗʰ **T43.503** Poisoning by unspecified antipsychotics and neuroleptics, assault

√7ᵗʰ **T43.504** Poisoning by unspecified antipsychotics and neuroleptics, undetermined

√7ᵗʰ **T43.505** Adverse effect of unspecified antipsychotics and neuroleptics

√7ᵗʰ **T43.506** Underdosing of unspecified antipsychotics and neuroleptics

√6ᵗʰ **T43.59** Poisoning by, adverse effect of and underdosing of other antipsychotics and neuroleptics

√7ᵗʰ **T43.591** Poisoning by other antipsychotics and neuroleptics, accidental (unintentional)
  Poisoning by other antipsychotics and neuroleptics NOS

√7ᵗʰ **T43.592** Poisoning by other antipsychotics and neuroleptics, intentional self-harm

√7ᵗʰ **T43.593** Poisoning by other antipsychotics and neuroleptics, assault

√7ᵗʰ **T43.594** Poisoning by other antipsychotics and neuroleptics, undetermined

√7ᵗʰ **T43.595** Adverse effect of other antipsychotics and neuroleptics

√7ᵗʰ **T43.596** Underdosing of other antipsychotics and neuroleptics

√5ᵗʰ **T43.6** Poisoning by, adverse effect of and underdosing of psychostimulants
  EXCLUDES 1 poisoning by, adverse effect of and underdosing of cocaine (T40.5-)

√6ᵗʰ **T43.60** Poisoning by, adverse effect of and underdosing of unspecified psychostimulant

√7ᵗʰ **T43.601** Poisoning by unspecified psychostimulants, accidental (unintentional)
  Poisoning by psychostimulants NOS

√7ᵗʰ **T43.602** Poisoning by unspecified psychostimulants, intentional self-harm

√7ᵗʰ **T43.603** Poisoning by unspecified psychostimulants, assault

√7ᵗʰ **T43.604** Poisoning by unspecified psychostimulants, undetermined

√7ᵗʰ **T43.605** Adverse effect of unspecified psychostimulants

√7ᵗʰ **T43.606** Underdosing of unspecified psychostimulants

EXCLUDES 1 Not coded here   EXCLUDES 2 Not included here   N Newborn Age: 0   P Pediatric Age: 0-17   M Maternity Age: 12-55   A Adult Age: 15-124

950   ICD-10-CM 2014 (Draft)

√6ᵗʰ **T43.61** **Poisoning by, adverse effect of and underdosing of** caffeine

     √7ᵗʰ **T43.611** **Poisoning by caffeine,** accidental (unintentional)
         Poisoning by caffeine NOS

     √7ᵗʰ **T43.612** **Poisoning by caffeine,** intentional self-harm

     √7ᵗʰ **T43.613** **Poisoning by caffeine,** assault

     √7ᵗʰ **T43.614** **Poisoning by caffeine,** undetermined

     √7ᵗʰ **T43.615** Adverse effect **of caffeine**

     √7ᵗʰ **T43.616** Underdosing **of caffeine**

√6ᵗʰ **T43.62** **Poisoning by, adverse effect of and underdosing of** amphetamines
     Poisoning by, adverse effect of and underdosing of methamphetamines

     √7ᵗʰ **T43.621** **Poisoning by amphetamines,** accidental (unintentional)
         Poisoning by amphetamines NOS

     √7ᵗʰ **T43.622** **Poisoning by amphetamines,** intentional self-harm

     √7ᵗʰ **T43.623** **Poisoning by amphetamines,** assault

     √7ᵗʰ **T43.624** **Poisoning by amphetamines, undetermined**

     √7ᵗʰ **T43.625** Adverse effect **of amphetamines**

     √7ᵗʰ **T43.626** Underdosing **of amphetamines**

√6ᵗʰ **T43.63** **Poisoning by, adverse effect of and underdosing of** methylphenidate

     √7ᵗʰ **T43.631** **Poisoning by methylphenidate,** accidental (unintentional)
         Poisoning by methylphenidate NOS

     √7ᵗʰ **T43.632** **Poisoning by methylphenidate, intentional self-harm**

     √7ᵗʰ **T43.633** **Poisoning by methylphenidate,** assault

     √7ᵗʰ **T43.634** **Poisoning by methylphenidate, undetermined**

     √7ᵗʰ **T43.635** Adverse effect **of methylphenidate**

     √7ᵗʰ **T43.636** Underdosing **of methylphenidate**

√6ᵗʰ **T43.69** **Poisoning by, adverse effect of and underdosing of** other psychostimulants

     √7ᵗʰ **T43.691** **Poisoning by other psychostimulants, accidental (unintentional)**
         Poisoning by other psychostimulants NOS

     √7ᵗʰ **T43.692** **Poisoning by other psychostimulants, intentional self-harm**

     √7ᵗʰ **T43.693** **Poisoning by other psychostimulants, assault**

     √7ᵗʰ **T43.694** **Poisoning by other psychostimulants, undetermined**

     √7ᵗʰ **T43.695** Adverse effect **of other psychostimulants**

     √7ᵗʰ **T43.696** Underdosing **of other psychostimulants**

√5ᵗʰ **T43.8** **Poisoning by, adverse effect of and underdosing of other psychotropic drugs**

 √6ᵗʰ **T43.8X** **Poisoning by, adverse effect of and underdosing of** other psychotropic **drugs**

     √7ᵗʰ **T43.8X1** **Poisoning by other psychotropic drugs, accidental (unintentional)**
         Poisoning by other psychotropic drugs NOS

     √7ᵗʰ **T43.8X2** **Poisoning by other psychotropic drugs, intentional self-harm**

     √7ᵗʰ **T43.8X3** **Poisoning by other psychotropic drugs, assault**

     √7ᵗʰ **T43.8X4** **Poisoning by other psychotropic drugs, undetermined**

     √7ᵗʰ **T43.8X5** Adverse effect **of other psychotropic drugs**

     √7ᵗʰ **T43.8X6** Underdosing **of other psychotropic drugs**

√5ᵗʰ **T43.9** **Poisoning by, adverse effect of and underdosing of** unspecified psychotropic **drug**

 √x7ᵗʰ **T43.91** **Poisoning by unspecified psychotropic drug, accidental (unintentional)**
     Poisoning by psychotropic drug NOS

 √x7ᵗʰ **T43.92** **Poisoning by unspecified psychotropic drug, intentional self-harm**

 √x7ᵗʰ **T43.93** **Poisoning by unspecified psychotropic drug,** assault

 √x7ᵗʰ **T43.94** **Poisoning by unspecified psychotropic drug, undetermined**

 √x7ᵗʰ **T43.95** Adverse effect **of unspecified psychotropic drug**

 √x7ᵗʰ **T43.96** Underdosing **of unspecified psychotropic drug**

√4ᵗʰ **T44** **Poisoning by, adverse effect of and underdosing of drugs primarily affecting the autonomic nervous system**

> The appropriate 7th character is to be added to each code from category T44.
> A   initial encounter
> D   subsequent encounter
> S   sequela

√5ᵗʰ **T44.0** **Poisoning by, adverse effect of and underdosing of** anticholinesterase agents

 √6ᵗʰ **T44.0X** **Poisoning by, adverse effect of and underdosing of** anticholinesterase agents

     √7ᵗʰ **T44.0X1** **Poisoning by anticholinesterase agents,** accidental (unintentional)
         Poisoning by anticholinesterase agents NOS

     √7ᵗʰ **T44.0X2** **Poisoning by anticholinesterase agents,** intentional self-harm

     √7ᵗʰ **T44.0X3** **Poisoning by anticholinesterase agents,** assault

     √7ᵗʰ **T44.0X4** **Poisoning by anticholinesterase agents, undetermined**

     √7ᵗʰ **T44.0X5** Adverse effect **of anticholinesterase agents**

     √7ᵗʰ **T44.0X6** Underdosing **of anticholinesterase agents**

√5ᵗʰ **T44.1** **Poisoning by, adverse effect of and underdosing of other parasympathomimetics [cholinergics]**

 √6ᵗʰ **T44.1X** **Poisoning by, adverse effect of and underdosing of other** parasympathomimetics **[cholinergics]**

     √7ᵗʰ **T44.1X1** **Poisoning by other parasympathomimetics [cholinergics], accidental (unintentional)**
         Poisoning by other parasympathomimetics [cholinergics] NOS

     √7ᵗʰ **T44.1X2** **Poisoning by other parasympathomimetics [cholinergics], intentional self-harm**

     √7ᵗʰ **T44.1X3** **Poisoning by other parasympathomimetics [cholinergics], assault**

     √7ᵗʰ **T44.1X4** **Poisoning by other parasympathomimetics [cholinergics], undetermined**

     √7ᵗʰ **T44.1X5** Adverse effect **of other parasympathomimetics [cholinergics]**

     √7ᵗʰ **T44.1X6** Underdosing **of other parasympathomimetics**

√5ᵗʰ **T44.2** **Poisoning by, adverse effect of and underdosing of ganglionic blocking drugs**

 √6ᵗʰ **T44.2X** **Poisoning by, adverse effect of and underdosing of** ganglionic blocking drugs

     √7ᵗʰ **T44.2X1** **Poisoning by ganglionic blocking drugs, accidental (unintentional)**
         Poisoning by ganglionic blocking drugs NOS

     √7ᵗʰ **T44.2X2** **Poisoning by ganglionic blocking drugs, intentional self-harm**

     √7ᵗʰ **T44.2X3** **Poisoning by ganglionic blocking drugs, assault**

     √7ᵗʰ **T44.2X4** **Poisoning by ganglionic blocking drugs, undetermined**

     √7ᵗʰ **T44.2X5** Adverse effect **of ganglionic blocking drugs**

     √7ᵗʰ **T44.2X6** Underdosing **of ganglionic blocking drugs**

☑ Additional Character Required   √x7ᵗʰ Xtension Alert   Unspecified Code   Other Specified Code   Manifestation Code   ►◄ Revised Text   ● New Code   ▲ Revised Code Title

ICD-10-CM 2014 (Draft)   951

Injury, Poisoning and Certain Other Consequences of External Causes

T44.3–T44.8X6

✓5th **T44.3** Poisoning by, adverse effect of and underdosing of other parasympatholytics [anticholinergics and antimuscarinics] and spasmolytics
Poisoning by, adverse effect of and underdosing of papaverine

✓6th **T44.3X** Poisoning by, adverse effect of and underdosing of other parasympatholytics [anticholinergics and antimuscarinics] and spasmolytics

✓7th **T44.3X1** Poisoning by other parasympatholytics [anticholinergics and antimuscarinics] and spasmolytics, accidental (unintentional)
Poisoning by other parasympatholytics [anticholinergics and antimuscarinics] and spasmolytics NOS

✓7th **T44.3X2** Poisoning by other parasympatholytics [anticholinergics and antimuscarinics] and spasmolytics, intentional self-harm

✓7th **T44.3X3** Poisoning by other parasympatholytics [anticholinergics and antimuscarinics] and spasmolytics, assault

✓7th **T44.3X4** Poisoning by other parasympatholytics [anticholinergics and antimuscarinics] and spasmolytics, undetermined

✓7th **T44.3X5** Adverse effect of other parasympatholytics [anticholinergics and antimuscarinics] and spasmolytics

✓7th **T44.3X6** Underdosing of other parasympatholytics [anticholinergics and antimuscarinics] and spasmolytics

✓5th **T44.4** Poisoning by, adverse effect of and underdosing of predominantly alpha-adrenoreceptor agonists
Poisoning by, adverse effect of and underdosing of metaraminol

✓6th **T44.4X** Poisoning by, adverse effect of and underdosing of predominantly alpha-adrenoreceptor agonists

✓7th **T44.4X1** Poisoning by predominantly alpha-adrenoreceptor agonists, accidental (unintentional)
Poisoning by predominantly alpha-adrenoreceptor agonists NOS

✓7th **T44.4X2** Poisoning by predominantly alpha-adrenoreceptor agonists, intentional self-harm

✓7th **T44.4X3** Poisoning by predominantly alpha-adrenoreceptor agonists, assault

✓7th **T44.4X4** Poisoning by predominantly alpha-adrenoreceptor agonists, undetermined

✓7th **T44.4X5** Adverse effect of predominantly alpha-adrenoreceptor agonists

✓7th **T44.4X6** Underdosing of predominantly alpha-adrenoreceptor agonists

✓5th **T44.5** Poisoning by, adverse effect of and underdosing of predominantly beta-adrenoreceptor agonists
EXCLUDES 1 poisoning by, adverse effect of and underdosing of beta-adrenoreceptor agonists used in asthma therapy (T48.6-)

✓6th **T44.5X** Poisoning by, adverse effect of and underdosing of predominantly beta-adrenoreceptor agonists

✓7th **T44.5X1** Poisoning by predominantly beta-adrenoreceptor agonists, accidental (unintentional)
Poisoning by predominantly beta-adrenoreceptor agonists NOS

✓7th **T44.5X2** Poisoning by predominantly beta-adrenoreceptor agonists, intentional self-harm

✓7th **T44.5X3** Poisoning by predominantly beta-adrenoreceptor agonists, assault

✓7th **T44.5X4** Poisoning by predominantly beta-adrenoreceptor agonists, undetermined

✓7th **T44.5X5** Adverse effect of predominantly beta-adrenoreceptor agonists

✓7th **T44.5X6** Underdosing of predominantly beta-adrenoreceptor agonists

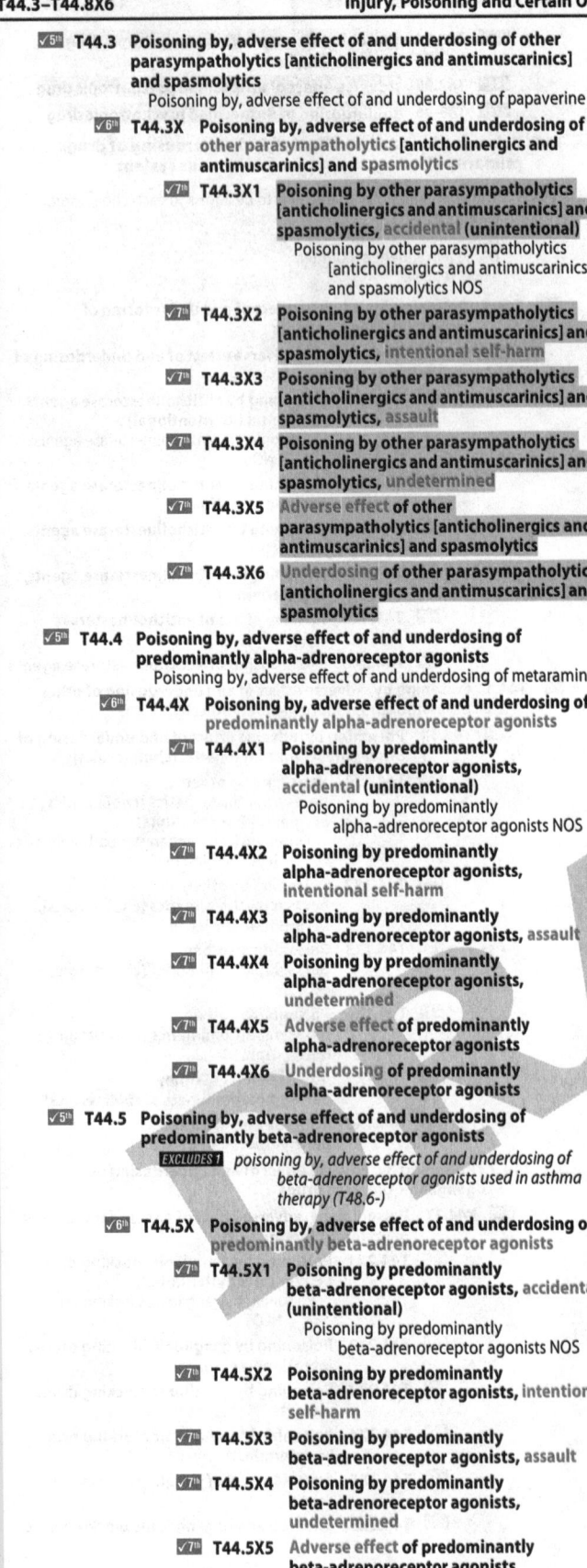

✓5th **T44.6** Poisoning by, adverse effect of and underdosing of alpha-adrenoreceptor antagonists
EXCLUDES 1 poisoning by, adverse effect of and underdosing of ergot alkaloids (T48.0)

✓6th **T44.6X** Poisoning by, adverse effect of and underdosing of alpha-adrenoreceptor antagonists

✓7th **T44.6X1** Poisoning by alpha-adrenoreceptor antagonists, accidental (unintentional)
Poisoning by alpha-adrenoreceptor antagonists NOS

✓7th **T44.6X2** Poisoning by alpha-adrenoreceptor antagonists, intentional self-harm

✓7th **T44.6X3** Poisoning by alpha-adrenoreceptor antagonists, assault

✓7th **T44.6X4** Poisoning by alpha-adrenoreceptor antagonists, undetermined

✓7th **T44.6X5** Adverse effect of alpha-adrenoreceptor antagonists

✓7th **T44.6X6** Underdosing of alpha-adrenoreceptor antagonists

✓5th **T44.7** Poisoning by, adverse effect of and underdosing of beta-adrenoreceptor antagonists

✓6th **T44.7X** Poisoning by, adverse effect of and underdosing of beta-adrenoreceptor antagonists

✓7th **T44.7X1** Poisoning by beta-adrenoreceptor antagonists, accidental (unintentional)
Poisoning by beta-adrenoreceptor antagonists NOS

✓7th **T44.7X2** Poisoning by beta-adrenoreceptor antagonists, intentional self-harm

✓7th **T44.7X3** Poisoning by beta-adrenoreceptor antagonists, assault

✓7th **T44.7X4** Poisoning by beta-adrenoreceptor antagonists, undetermined

✓7th **T44.7X5** Adverse effect of beta-adrenoreceptor antagonists

✓7th **T44.7X6** Underdosing of beta-adrenoreceptor antagonists

✓5th **T44.8** Poisoning by, adverse effect of and underdosing of centrally-acting and adrenergic-neuron- blocking agents
EXCLUDES 1 poisoning by, adverse effect of and underdosing of clonidine (T46.5)
poisoning by, adverse effect of and underdosing of guanethidine (T46.5)

✓6th **T44.8X** Poisoning by, adverse effect of and underdosing of centrally-acting and adrenergic- neuron-blocking agents

✓7th **T44.8X1** Poisoning by centrally-acting and adrenergic-neuron-blocking agents, accidental (unintentional)
Poisoning by centrally-acting and adrenergic-neuron-blocking agents NOS

✓7th **T44.8X2** Poisoning by centrally-acting and adrenergic-neuron-blocking agents, intentional self-harm

✓7th **T44.8X3** Poisoning by centrally-acting and adrenergic-neuron-blocking agents, assault

✓7th **T44.8X4** Poisoning by centrally-acting and adrenergic-neuron-blocking agents, undetermined

✓7th **T44.8X5** Adverse effect of centrally-acting and adrenergic-neuron-blocking agents

✓7th **T44.8X6** Underdosing of centrally-acting and adrenergic-neuron-blocking agents

EXCLUDES 1 Not coded here   EXCLUDES 2 Not included here   N Newborn Age: 0   P Pediatric Age: 0-17   M Maternity Age: 12-55   A Adult Age: 15-124

952   ICD-10-CM 2014 (Draft)

Injury, Poisoning and Certain Other Consequences of External Causes   T44.9–T45.511

√5th **T44.9 Poisoning by, adverse effect of and underdosing of other and unspecified drugs** *primarily affecting the autonomic nervous system*

Poisoning by, adverse effect of and underdosing of drug stimulating both alpha and beta-adrenoreceptors

√6th **T44.90 Poisoning by, adverse effect of and underdosing of unspecified drugs primarily affecting the autonomic nervous system**

√7th **T44.901 Poisoning by unspecified drugs primarily affecting the autonomic nervous system, accidental (unintentional)**

Poisoning by unspecified drugs primarily affecting the autonomic nervous system NOS

√7th **T44.902 Poisoning by unspecified drugs primarily affecting the autonomic nervous system, intentional self-harm**

√7th **T44.903 Poisoning by unspecified drugs primarily affecting the autonomic nervous system, assault**

√7th **T44.904 Poisoning by unspecified drugs primarily affecting the autonomic nervous system, undetermined**

√7th **T44.905 Adverse effect of unspecified drugs primarily affecting the autonomic nervous system**

√7th **T44.906 Underdosing of unspecified drugs primarily affecting the autonomic nervous system**

√6th **T44.99 Poisoning by, adverse effect of and underdosing of other drugs primarily affecting the autonomic nervous system**

√7th **T44.991 Poisoning by other drug primarily affecting the autonomic nervous system, accidental (unintentional)**

Poisoning by other drugs primarily affecting the autonomic nervous system NOS

√7th **T44.992 Poisoning by other drug primarily affecting the autonomic nervous system, intentional self-harm**

√7th **T44.993 Poisoning by other drug primarily affecting the autonomic nervous system, assault**

√7th **T44.994 Poisoning by other drug primarily affecting the autonomic nervous system, undetermined**

√7th **T44.995 Adverse effect of other drug primarily affecting the autonomic nervous system**

√7th **T44.996 Underdosing of other drug primarily affecting the autonomic nervous system**

√4th **T45 Poisoning by, adverse effect of and underdosing of primarily systemic and hematological agents, not elsewhere classified**

The appropriate 7th character is to be added to each code from category T45.
A   initial encounter
D   subsequent encounter
S   sequela

√5th **T45.0 Poisoning by, adverse effect of and underdosing of antiallergic and antiemetic drugs**

EXCLUDES 1   poisoning by, adverse effect of and underdosing of phenothiazine-based neuroleptics (T43.3)

√6th **T45.0X Poisoning by, adverse effect of and underdosing of antiallergic and antiemetic drugs**

√7th **T45.0X1 Poisoning by antiallergic and antiemetic drugs, accidental (unintentional)**

Poisoning by antiallergic and antiemetic drugs NOS

√7th **T45.0X2 Poisoning by antiallergic and antiemetic drugs, intentional self-harm**

√7th **T45.0X3 Poisoning by antiallergic and antiemetic drugs, assault**

√7th **T45.0X4 Poisoning by antiallergic and antiemetic drugs, undetermined**

√7th **T45.0X5 Adverse effect of antiallergic and antiemetic drugs**

√7th **T45.0X6 Underdosing of antiallergic and antiemetic drugs**

√5th **T45.1 Poisoning by, adverse effect of and underdosing of antineoplastic and immunosuppressive drugs**

EXCLUDES 1   poisoning by, adverse effect of and underdosing of tamoxifen (T38.6)

√6th **T45.1X Poisoning by, adverse effect of and underdosing of antineoplastic and immunosuppressive drugs**

√7th **T45.1X1 Poisoning by antineoplastic and immunosuppressive drugs, accidental (unintentional)**

Poisoning by antineoplastic and immunosuppressive drugs NOS

√7th **T45.1X2 Poisoning by antineoplastic and immunosuppressive drugs, intentional self-harm**

√7th **T45.1X3 Poisoning by antineoplastic and immunosuppressive drugs, assault**

√7th **T45.1X4 Poisoning by antineoplastic and immunosuppressive drugs, undetermined**

√7th **T45.1X5 Adverse effect of antineoplastic and immunosuppressive drugs**

√7th **T45.1X6 Underdosing of antineoplastic and immunosuppressive drugs**

√5th **T45.2 Poisoning by, adverse effect of and underdosing of vitamins**

EXCLUDES 2   poisoning by, adverse effect of and underdosing of nicotinic acid (derivatives) (T46.7)
poisoning by, adverse effect of and underdosing of iron (T45.4)
poisoning by, adverse effect of and underdosing of vitamin K (T45.7)

√6th **T45.2X Poisoning by, adverse effect of and underdosing of vitamins**

√7th **T45.2X1 Poisoning by vitamins, accidental (unintentional)**

Poisoning by vitamins NOS

√7th **T45.2X2 Poisoning by vitamins, intentional self-harm**

√7th **T45.2X3 Poisoning by vitamins, assault**

√7th **T45.2X4 Poisoning by vitamins, undetermined**

√7th **T45.2X5 Adverse effect of vitamins**

√7th **T45.2X6 Underdosing of vitamins**
EXCLUDES 1   vitamin deficiencies (E50-E56)

√5th **T45.3 Poisoning by, adverse effect of and underdosing of enzymes**

√6th **T45.3X Poisoning by, adverse effect of and underdosing of enzymes**

√7th **T45.3X1 Poisoning by enzymes, accidental (unintentional)**

Poisoning by enzymes NOS

√7th **T45.3X2 Poisoning by enzymes, intentional self-harm**

√7th **T45.3X3 Poisoning by enzymes, assault**

√7th **T45.3X4 Poisoning by enzymes, undetermined**

√7th **T45.3X5 Adverse effect of enzymes**

√7th **T45.3X6 Underdosing of enzymes**

√5th **T45.4 Poisoning by, adverse effect of and underdosing of iron and its compounds**

√6th **T45.4X Poisoning by, adverse effect of and underdosing of iron and its compounds**

T45.4X1 Poisoning by iron and its compounds, accidental (unintentional)

Poisoning by iron and its compounds NOS

√7th **T45.4X2 Poisoning by iron and its compounds, intentional self-harm**

√7th **T45.4X3 Poisoning by iron and its compounds, assault**

√7th **T45.4X4 Poisoning by iron and its compounds, undetermined**

√7th **T45.4X5 Adverse effect of iron and its compounds**

√7th **T45.4X6 Underdosing of iron and its compounds**
EXCLUDES 1   iron deficiency (E61.1)

√5th **T45.5 Poisoning by, adverse effect of and underdosing of anticoagulants and antithrombotic drugs**

√6th **T45.51 Poisoning by, adverse effect of and underdosing of anticoagulants**

√7th **T45.511 Poisoning by anticoagulants, accidental (unintentional)**

Poisoning by anticoagulants NOS

√7ᵗʰ **T45.512** **Poisoning by anticoagulants, intentional self-harm**

√7ᵗʰ **T45.513** **Poisoning by anticoagulants, assault**

√7ᵗʰ **T45.514** **Poisoning by anticoagulants, undetermined**

√7ᵗʰ **T45.515** **Adverse effect of anticoagulants**

√7ᵗʰ **T45.516** **Underdosing of anticoagulants**

√6ᵗʰ **T45.52** **Poisoning by, adverse effect of and underdosing of antithrombotic drugs**
Poisoning by, adverse effect of and underdosing of antiplatelet drugs
EXCLUDES 2 *poisoning by, adverse effect of and underdosing of aspirin (T39.01-)*
poisoning by, adverse effect of and underdosing of acetylsalicylic acid (T39.01-)

√7ᵗʰ **T45.521** **Poisoning by antithrombotic drugs, accidental (unintentional)**
Poisoning by antithrombotic drug NOS

√7ᵗʰ **T45.522** **Poisoning by antithrombotic drugs, intentional self-harm**

√7ᵗʰ **T45.523** **Poisoning by antithrombotic drugs, assault**

√7ᵗʰ **T45.524** **Poisoning by antithrombotic drugs, undetermined**

√7ᵗʰ **T45.525** **Adverse effect of antithrombotic drugs**

√7ᵗʰ **T45.526** **Underdosing of antithrombotic drugs**

√5ᵗʰ **T45.6** **Poisoning by, adverse effect of and underdosing of fibrinolysis-affecting drugs**

√6ᵗʰ **T45.60** **Poisoning by, adverse effect of and underdosing of unspecified fibrinolysis-affecting drugs**

√7ᵗʰ **T45.601** **Poisoning by unspecified fibrinolysis-affecting drugs, accidental (unintentional)**
Poisoning by fibrinolysis-affecting drug NOS

√7ᵗʰ **T45.602** **Poisoning by unspecified fibrinolysis-affecting drugs, intentional self-harm**

√7ᵗʰ **T45.603** **Poisoning by unspecified fibrinolysis-affecting drugs, assault**

√7ᵗʰ **T45.604** **Poisoning by unspecified fibrinolysis-affecting drugs, undetermined**

√7ᵗʰ **T45.605** **Adverse effect of unspecified fibrinolysis-affecting drugs**

√7ᵗʰ **T45.606** **Underdosing of unspecified fibrinolysis-affecting drugs**

√6ᵗʰ **T45.61** **Poisoning by, adverse effect of and underdosing of thrombolytic drugs**

√7ᵗʰ **T45.611** **Poisoning by thrombolytic drug, accidental (unintentional)**
Poisoning by thrombolytic drug NOS

√7ᵗʰ **T45.612** **Poisoning by thrombolytic drug, intentional self-harm**

√7ᵗʰ **T45.613** **Poisoning by thrombolytic drug, assault**

√7ᵗʰ **T45.614** **Poisoning by thrombolytic drug, undetermined**

√7ᵗʰ **T45.615** **Adverse effect of thrombolytic drugs**

√7ᵗʰ **T45.616** **Underdosing of thrombolytic drugs**

√6ᵗʰ **T45.62** **Poisoning by, adverse effect of and underdosing of hemostatic drugs**

√7ᵗʰ **T45.621** **Poisoning by hemostatic drug, accidental (unintentional)**
Poisoning by hemostatic drug NOS

√7ᵗʰ **T45.622** **Poisoning by hemostatic drug, intentional self-harm**

√7ᵗʰ **T45.623** **Poisoning by hemostatic drug, assault**

√7ᵗʰ **T45.624** **Poisoning by hemostatic drug, undetermined**

√7ᵗʰ **T45.625** **Adverse effect of hemostatic drug**

√7ᵗʰ **T45.626** **Underdosing of hemostatic drugs**

√6ᵗʰ **T45.69** **Poisoning by, adverse effect of and underdosing of other fibrinolysis-affecting drugs**

√7ᵗʰ **T45.691** **Poisoning by other fibrinolysis-affecting drugs, accidental (unintentional)**
Poisoning by other fibrinolysis-affecting drug NOS

√7ᵗʰ **T45.692** **Poisoning by other fibrinolysis-affecting drugs, intentional self-harm**

√7ᵗʰ **T45.693** **Poisoning by other fibrinolysis-affecting drugs, assault**

√7ᵗʰ **T45.694** **Poisoning by other fibrinolysis-affecting drugs, undetermined**

√7ᵗʰ **T45.695** **Adverse effect of other fibrinolysis-affecting drugs**

√7ᵗʰ **T45.696** **Underdosing of other fibrinolysis-affecting drugs**

√5ᵗʰ **T45.7** **Poisoning by, adverse effect of and underdosing of anticoagulant antagonists, vitamin K and other coagulants**

√6ᵗʰ **T45.7X** **Poisoning by, adverse effect of and underdosing of anticoagulant antagonists, vitamin K and other coagulants**

√7ᵗʰ **T45.7X1** **Poisoning by anticoagulant antagonists, vitamin K and other coagulants, accidental (unintentional)**
Poisoning by anticoagulant antagonists, vitamin K and other coagulants NOS

√7ᵗʰ **T45.7X2** **Poisoning by anticoagulant antagonists, vitamin K and other coagulants, intentional self-harm**

√7ᵗʰ **T45.7X3** **Poisoning by anticoagulant antagonists, vitamin K and other coagulants, assault**

√7ᵗʰ **T45.7X4** **Poisoning by anticoagulant antagonists, vitamin K and other coagulants, undetermined**

√7ᵗʰ **T45.7X5** **Adverse effect of anticoagulant antagonists, vitamin K and other coagulants**

√7ᵗʰ **T45.7X6** **Underdosing of anticoagulant antagonist, vitamin K and other coagulants**
EXCLUDES 1 *vitamin K deficiency (E56.1)*

√5ᵗʰ **T45.8** **Poisoning by, adverse effect of and underdosing of other primarily systemic and hematological agents**
Poisoning by, adverse effect of and underdosing of liver preparations and other antianemic agents
Poisoning by, adverse effect of and underdosing of natural blood and blood products
Poisoning by, adverse effect of and underdosing of plasma substitute
EXCLUDES 2 *poisoning by, adverse effect of and underdosing of immunoglobulin (T50.Z1)*
poisoning by, adverse effect of and underdosing of iron (T45.4)
transfusion reactions (T80.-)

√6ᵗʰ **T45.8X** **Poisoning by, adverse effect of and underdosing of other primarily systemic and hematological agents**

√7ᵗʰ **T45.8X1** **Poisoning by other primarily systemic and hematological agents, accidental (unintentional)**
Poisoning by other primarily systemic and hematological agents NOS

√7ᵗʰ **T45.8X2** **Poisoning by other primarily systemic and hematological agents, intentional self-harm**

√7ᵗʰ **T45.8X3** **Poisoning by other primarily systemic and hematological agents, assault**

√7ᵗʰ **T45.8X4** **Poisoning by other primarily systemic and hematological agents, undetermined**

√7ᵗʰ **T45.8X5** **Adverse effect of other primarily systemic and hematological agents**

√7ᵗʰ **T45.8X6** **Underdosing of other primarily systemic and hematological agents**

√5ᵗʰ **T45.9** **Poisoning by, adverse effect of and underdosing of unspecified primarily systemic and hematological agent**

√x7ᵗʰ **T45.91** **Poisoning by unspecified primarily systemic and hematological agent, accidental (unintentional)**
Poisoning by primarily systemic and hematological agent NOS

√x7ᵗʰ **T45.92** **Poisoning by unspecified primarily systemic and hematological agent, intentional self-harm**

√x7ᵗʰ **T45.93** **Poisoning by unspecified primarily systemic and hematological agent, assault**

√x7ᵗʰ **T45.94** **Poisoning by unspecified primarily systemic and hematological agent, undetermined**

EXCLUDES 1 Not coded here   *EXCLUDES 2* Not included here   **N** Newborn Age: 0   **P** Pediatric Age: 0-17   **M** Maternity Age: 12-55   **A** Adult Age: 15-124

954 ICD-10-CM 2014 (Draft)

√x7ᵗʰ **T45.95** Adverse effect of unspecified primarily systemic and hematological agent

√x7ᵗʰ **T45.96** Underdosing of unspecified primarily systemic and hematological agent

√4ᵗʰ **T46** **Poisoning by, adverse effect of and underdosing of agents primarily affecting the cardiovascular system**

EXCLUDES 1 *poisoning by, adverse effect of and underdosing of metaraminol (T44.4)*

The appropriate 7th character is to be added to each code from category T46.
A initial encounter
D subsequent encounter
S sequela

√5ᵗʰ **T46.0** **Poisoning by, adverse effect of and underdosing of cardiac-stimulant glycosides and drugs of similar action**

√6ᵗʰ **T46.0X** Poisoning by, adverse effect of and underdosing of cardiac-stimulant glycosides and drugs of similar action

√7ᵗʰ **T46.0X1** Poisoning by cardiac-stimulant glycosides and drugs of similar action, accidental (unintentional)
Poisoning by cardiac-stimulant glycosides and drugs of similar action NOS

√7ᵗʰ **T46.0X2** Poisoning by cardiac-stimulant glycosides and drugs of similar action, intentional self-harm

√7ᵗʰ **T46.0X3** Poisoning by cardiac-stimulant glycosides and drugs of similar action, assault

√7ᵗʰ **T46.0X4** Poisoning by cardiac-stimulant glycosides and drugs of similar action, undetermined

√7ᵗʰ **T46.0X5** Adverse effect of cardiac-stimulant glycosides and drugs of similar action

√7ᵗʰ **T46.0X6** Underdosing of cardiac-stimulant glycosides and drugs of similar action

√5ᵗʰ **T46.1** **Poisoning by, adverse effect of and underdosing of calcium-channel blockers**

√6ᵗʰ **T46.1X** Poisoning by, adverse effect of and underdosing of calcium-channel blockers

√7ᵗʰ **T46.1X1** Poisoning by calcium-channel blockers, accidental (unintentional)
Poisoning by calcium-channel blockers NOS

√7ᵗʰ **T46.1X2** Poisoning by calcium-channel blockers, intentional self-harm

√7ᵗʰ **T46.1X3** Poisoning by calcium-channel blockers, assault

√7ᵗʰ **T46.1X4** Poisoning by calcium-channel blockers, undetermined

√7ᵗʰ **T46.1X5** Adverse effect of calcium-channel blockers

√7ᵗʰ **T46.1X6** Underdosing of calcium-channel blockers

√5ᵗʰ **T46.2** **Poisoning by, adverse effect of and underdosing of other antidysrhythmic drugs, not elsewhere classified**

EXCLUDES 1 *poisoning by, adverse effect of and underdosing of beta-adrenoreceptor antagonists (T44.7-)*

√6ᵗʰ **T46.2X** Poisoning by, adverse effect of and underdosing of other antidysrhythmic drugs

√7ᵗʰ **T46.2X1** Poisoning by other antidysrhythmic drugs, accidental (unintentional)
Poisoning by other antidysrhythmic drugs NOS

√7ᵗʰ **T46.2X2** Poisoning by other antidysrhythmic drugs, intentional self-harm

√7ᵗʰ **T46.2X3** Poisoning by other antidysrhythmic drugs, assault

√7ᵗʰ **T46.2X4** Poisoning by other antidysrhythmic drugs, undetermined

√7ᵗʰ **T46.2X5** Adverse effect of other antidysrhythmic drugs

√7ᵗʰ **T46.2X6** Underdosing of other antidysrhythmic drugs

√5ᵗʰ **T46.3** **Poisoning by, adverse effect of and underdosing of coronary vasodilators**
Poisoning by, adverse effect of and underdosing of dipyridamole

EXCLUDES 1 *poisoning by, adverse effect of and underdosing of calcium-channel blockers (T46.1)*

√6ᵗʰ **T46.3X** Poisoning by, adverse effect of and underdosing of coronary vasodilators

√7ᵗʰ **T46.3X1** Poisoning by coronary vasodilators, accidental (unintentional)
Poisoning by coronary vasodilators NOS

√7ᵗʰ **T46.3X2** Poisoning by coronary vasodilators, intentional self-harm

√7ᵗʰ **T46.3X3** Poisoning by coronary vasodilators, assault

√7ᵗʰ **T46.3X4** Poisoning by coronary vasodilators, undetermined

√7ᵗʰ **T46.3X5** Adverse effect of coronary vasodilators

√7ᵗʰ **T46.3X6** Underdosing of coronary vasodilators

√5ᵗʰ **T46.4** **Poisoning by, adverse effect of and underdosing of angiotensin-converting-enzyme inhibitors**

√6ᵗʰ **T46.4X** Poisoning by, adverse effect of and underdosing of angiotensin-converting-enzyme inhibitors

√7ᵗʰ **T46.4X1** Poisoning by angiotensin-converting-enzyme inhibitors, accidental (unintentional)
Poisoning by angiotensin-converting-enzyme inhibitors NOS

√7ᵗʰ **T46.4X2** Poisoning by angiotensin-converting-enzyme inhibitors, intentional self-harm

√7ᵗʰ **T46.4X3** Poisoning by angiotensin-converting-enzyme inhibitors, assault

√7ᵗʰ **T46.4X4** Poisoning by angiotensin-converting-enzyme inhibitors, undetermined

√7ᵗʰ **T46.4X5** Adverse effect of angiotensin-converting-enzyme inhibitors

√7ᵗʰ **T46.4X6** Underdosing of angiotensin-converting-enzyme inhibitors

√5ᵗʰ **T46.5** **Poisoning by, adverse effect of and underdosing of other antihypertensive drugs**

EXCLUDES 2 *poisoning by, adverse effect of and underdosing of beta-adrenoreceptor antagonists (T44.7)*
poisoning by, adverse effect of and underdosing of calcium-channel blockers (T46.1)
poisoning by, adverse effect of and underdosing of diuretics (T50.0-T50.2)

√6ᵗʰ **T46.5X** Poisoning by, adverse effect of and underdosing of other antihypertensive drugs

√7ᵗʰ **T46.5X1** Poisoning by other antihypertensive drugs, accidental (unintentional)
Poisoning by other antihypertensive drugs NOS

√7ᵗʰ **T46.5X2** Poisoning by other antihypertensive drugs, intentional self-harm

√7ᵗʰ **T46.5X3** Poisoning by other antihypertensive drugs, assault

√7ᵗʰ **T46.5X4** Poisoning by other antihypertensive drugs, undetermined

√7ᵗʰ **T46.5X5** Adverse effect of other antihypertensive drugs

√7ᵗʰ **T46.5X6** Underdosing of other antihypertensive drugs

√5ᵗʰ **T46.6** **Poisoning by, adverse effect of and underdosing of antihyperlipidemic and antiarteriosclerotic drugs**

√6ᵗʰ **T46.6X** Poisoning by, adverse effect of and underdosing of antihyperlipidemic and antiarteriosclerotic drugs

√7ᵗʰ **T46.6X1** Poisoning by antihyperlipidemic and antiarteriosclerotic drugs, accidental (unintentional)
Poisoning by antihyperlipidemic and antiarteriosclerotic drugs NOS

√7ᵗʰ **T46.6X2** Poisoning by antihyperlipidemic and antiarteriosclerotic drugs, intentional self-harm

√7ᵗʰ **T46.6X3** Poisoning by antihyperlipidemic and antiarteriosclerotic drugs, assault

√7ᵗʰ **T46.6X4** Poisoning by antihyperlipidemic and antiarteriosclerotic drugs, undetermined

√7ᵗʰ **T46.6X5** Adverse effect of antihyperlipidemic and antiarteriosclerotic drugs

√7ᵗʰ **T46.6X6** Underdosing of antihyperlipidemic and antiarteriosclerotic drugs

√5ᵗʰ **T46.7** Poisoning by, adverse effect of and underdosing of peripheral vasodilators
Poisoning by, adverse effect of and underdosing of nicotinic acid (derivatives)
EXCLUDES 1 poisoning by, adverse effect of and underdosing of papaverine (T44.3)

√6ᵗʰ **T46.7X** Poisoning by, adverse effect of and underdosing of peripheral vasodilators

√7ᵗʰ **T46.7X1** Poisoning by peripheral vasodilators, accidental (unintentional)
Poisoning by peripheral vasodilators NOS

√7ᵗʰ **T46.7X2** Poisoning by peripheral vasodilators, intentional self-harm

√7ᵗʰ **T46.7X3** Poisoning by peripheral vasodilators, assault

√7ᵗʰ **T46.7X4** Poisoning by peripheral vasodilators, undetermined

√7ᵗʰ **T46.7X5** Adverse effect of peripheral vasodilators

√7ᵗʰ **T46.7X6** Underdosing of peripheral vasodilators

√5ᵗʰ **T46.8** Poisoning by, adverse effect of and underdosing of antivaricose drugs, including sclerosing agents

√6ᵗʰ **T46.8X** Poisoning by, adverse effect of and underdosing of antivaricose drugs, including sclerosing agents

√7ᵗʰ **T46.8X1** Poisoning by antivaricose drugs, including sclerosing agents, accidental (unintentional)
Poisoning by antivaricose drugs, including sclerosing agents NOS

√7ᵗʰ **T46.8X2** Poisoning by antivaricose drugs, including sclerosing agents, intentional self-harm

√7ᵗʰ **T46.8X3** Poisoning by antivaricose drugs, including sclerosing agents, assault

√7ᵗʰ **T46.8X4** Poisoning by antivaricose drugs, including sclerosing agents, undetermined

√7ᵗʰ **T46.8X5** Adverse effect of antivaricose drugs, including sclerosing agents

√7ᵗʰ **T46.8X6** Underdosing of antivaricose drugs, including sclerosing agents

√5ᵗʰ **T46.9** Poisoning by, adverse effect of and underdosing of other and unspecified agents primarily affecting the cardiovascular system

√6ᵗʰ **T46.90** Poisoning by, adverse effect of and underdosing of unspecified agents primarily affecting the cardiovascular system

√7ᵗʰ **T46.901** Poisoning by unspecified agents primarily affecting the cardiovascular system, accidental (unintentional)

√7ᵗʰ **T46.902** Poisoning by unspecified agents primarily affecting the cardiovascular system, intentional self-harm

√7ᵗʰ **T46.903** Poisoning by unspecified agents primarily affecting the cardiovascular system, assault

√7ᵗʰ **T46.904** Poisoning by unspecified agents primarily affecting the cardiovascular system, undetermined

√7ᵗʰ **T46.905** Adverse effect of unspecified agents primarily affecting the cardiovascular system

√7ᵗʰ **T46.906** Underdosing of unspecified agents primarily affecting the cardiovascular system

√6ᵗʰ **T46.99** Poisoning by, adverse effect of and underdosing of other agents primarily affecting the cardiovascular system

√7ᵗʰ **T46.991** Poisoning by other agents primarily affecting the cardiovascular system, accidental (unintentional)

√7ᵗʰ **T46.992** Poisoning by other agents primarily affecting the cardiovascular system, intentional self-harm

√7ᵗʰ **T46.993** Poisoning by other agents primarily affecting the cardiovascular system, assault

√7ᵗʰ **T46.994** Poisoning by other agents primarily affecting the cardiovascular system, undetermined

√7ᵗʰ **T46.995** Adverse effect of other agents primarily affecting the cardiovascular system

√7ᵗʰ **T46.996** Underdosing of other agents primarily affecting the cardiovascular system

√4ᵗʰ **T47** Poisoning by, adverse effect of and underdosing of agents primarily affecting the gastrointestinal system

The appropriate 7th character is to be added to each code from category T47.
A initial encounter
D subsequent encounter
S sequela

√5ᵗʰ **T47.0** Poisoning by, adverse effect of and underdosing of histamine H2-receptor blockers

√6ᵗʰ **T47.0X** Poisoning by, adverse effect of and underdosing of histamine H2-receptor blockers

√7ᵗʰ **T47.0X1** Poisoning by histamine H2-receptor blockers, accidental (unintentional)
Poisoning by histamine H2-receptor blockers NOS

√7ᵗʰ **T47.0X2** Poisoning by histamine H2-receptor blockers, intentional self-harm

√7ᵗʰ **T47.0X3** Poisoning by histamine H2-receptor blockers, assault

√7ᵗʰ **T47.0X4** Poisoning by histamine H2-receptor blockers, undetermined

√7ᵗʰ **T47.0X5** Adverse effect of histamine H2-receptor blockers

√7ᵗʰ **T47.0X6** Underdosing of histamine H2-receptor blockers

√5ᵗʰ **T47.1** Poisoning by, adverse effect of and underdosing of other antacids and anti-gastric-secretion drugs

√6ᵗʰ **T47.1X** Poisoning by, adverse effect of and underdosing of other antacids and anti-gastric-secretion drugs

√7ᵗʰ **T47.1X1** Poisoning by other antacids and anti-gastric-secretion drugs, accidental (unintentional)
Poisoning by other antacids and anti-gastric-secretion drugs NOS

√7ᵗʰ **T47.1X2** Poisoning by other antacids and anti-gastric-secretion drugs, intentional self-harm

√7ᵗʰ **T47.1X3** Poisoning by other antacids and anti-gastric-secretion drugs, assault

√7ᵗʰ **T47.1X4** Poisoning by other antacids and anti-gastric-secretion drugs, undetermined

√7ᵗʰ **T47.1X5** Adverse effect of other antacids and anti-gastric-secretion drugs

√7ᵗʰ **T47.1X6** Underdosing of other antacids and anti-gastric-secretion drugs

√5ᵗʰ **T47.2** Poisoning by, adverse effect of and underdosing of stimulant laxatives

√6ᵗʰ **T47.2X** Poisoning by, adverse effect of and underdosing of stimulant laxatives

√7ᵗʰ **T47.2X1** Poisoning by stimulant laxatives, accidental (unintentional)
Poisoning by stimulant laxatives NOS

√7ᵗʰ **T47.2X2** Poisoning by stimulant laxatives, intentional self-harm

√7ᵗʰ **T47.2X3** Poisoning by stimulant laxatives, assault

√7ᵗʰ **T47.2X4** Poisoning by stimulant laxatives, undetermined

√7ᵗʰ **T47.2X5** Adverse effect of stimulant laxatives

√7ᵗʰ **T47.2X6** Underdosing of stimulant laxatives

EXCLUDES 1 Not coded here   EXCLUDES 2 Not included here   N Newborn Age: 0   P Pediatric Age: 0-17   M Maternity Age: 12-55   A Adult Age: 15-124

956   ICD-10-CM 2014 (Draft)

☑5ᵗʰ **T47.3 Poisoning by, adverse effect of and underdosing of saline and osmotic laxatives**

  ☑6ᵗʰ **T47.3X Poisoning by and adverse effect of** saline and osmotic laxatives

    ☑7ᵗʰ **T47.3X1 Poisoning by saline and osmotic laxatives, accidental (unintentional)**
    Poisoning by saline and osmotic laxatives NOS

    ☑7ᵗʰ **T47.3X2 Poisoning by saline and osmotic laxatives, intentional self-harm**

    ☑7ᵗʰ **T47.3X3 Poisoning by saline and osmotic laxatives, assault**

    ☑7ᵗʰ **T47.3X4 Poisoning by saline and osmotic laxatives, undetermined**

    ☑7ᵗʰ **T47.3X5 Adverse effect of saline and osmotic laxatives**

    ☑7ᵗʰ **T47.3X6 Underdosing of saline and osmotic laxatives**

☑5ᵗʰ **T47.4 Poisoning by, adverse effect of and underdosing of other laxatives**

  ☑6ᵗʰ **T47.4X Poisoning by, adverse effect of and underdosing of other laxatives**

    ☑7ᵗʰ **T47.4X1 Poisoning by other laxatives, accidental (unintentional)**
    Poisoning by other laxatives NOS

    ☑7ᵗʰ **T47.4X2 Poisoning by other laxatives, intentional self-harm**

    ☑7ᵗʰ **T47.4X3 Poisoning by other laxatives, assault**

    ☑7ᵗʰ **T47.4X4 Poisoning by other laxatives, undetermined**

    ☑7ᵗʰ **T47.4X5 Adverse effect of other laxatives**

    ☑7ᵗʰ **T47.4X6 Underdosing of other laxatives**

☑5ᵗʰ **T47.5 Poisoning by, adverse effect of and underdosing of digestants**

  ☑6ᵗʰ **T47.5X Poisoning by, adverse effect of and underdosing of digestants**

    ☑7ᵗʰ **T47.5X1 Poisoning by digestants, accidental (unintentional)**
    Poisoning by digestants NOS

    ☑7ᵗʰ **T47.5X2 Poisoning by digestants, intentional self-harm**

    ☑7ᵗʰ **T47.5X3 Poisoning by digestants, assault**

    ☑7ᵗʰ **T47.5X4 Poisoning by digestants, undetermined**

    ☑7ᵗʰ **T47.5X5 Adverse effect of digestants**

    ☑7ᵗʰ **T47.5X6 Underdosing of digestants**

☑5ᵗʰ **T47.6 Poisoning by, adverse effect of and underdosing of antidiarrheal drugs**

    EXCLUDES 2 *poisoning by, adverse effect of and underdosing of systemic antibiotics and other anti-infectives (T36-T37)*

  ☑6ᵗʰ **T47.6X Poisoning by, adverse effect of and underdosing of antidiarrheal drugs**

    ☑7ᵗʰ **T47.6X1 Poisoning by antidiarrheal drugs, accidental (unintentional)**
    Poisoning by antidiarrheal drugs NOS

    ☑7ᵗʰ **T47.6X2 Poisoning by antidiarrheal drugs, intentional self-harm**

    ☑7ᵗʰ **T47.6X3 Poisoning by antidiarrheal drugs, assault**

    ☑7ᵗʰ **T47.6X4 Poisoning by antidiarrheal drugs, undetermined**

    ☑7ᵗʰ **T47.6X5 Adverse effect of antidiarrheal drugs**

    ☑7ᵗʰ **T47.6X6 Underdosing of antidiarrheal drugs**

☑5ᵗʰ **T47.7 Poisoning by, adverse effect of and underdosing of emetics**

  ☑6ᵗʰ **T47.7X Poisoning by, adverse effect of and underdosing of emetics**

    ☑7ᵗʰ **T47.7X1 Poisoning by emetics, accidental (unintentional)**
    Poisoning by emetics NOS

    ☑7ᵗʰ **T47.7X2 Poisoning by emetics, intentional self-harm**

    ☑7ᵗʰ **T47.7X3 Poisoning by emetics, assault**

    ☑7ᵗʰ **T47.7X4 Poisoning by emetics, undetermined**

    ☑7ᵗʰ **T47.7X5 Adverse effect of emetics**

    ☑7ᵗʰ **T47.7X6 Underdosing of emetics**

☑5ᵗʰ **T47.8 Poisoning by, adverse effect of and underdosing of other agents primarily affecting gastrointestinal system**

  ☑6ᵗʰ **T47.8X Poisoning by, adverse effect of and underdosing of other agents primarily affecting gastrointestinal system**

    ☑7ᵗʰ **T47.8X1 Poisoning by other agents primarily affecting gastrointestinal system, accidental (unintentional)**
    Poisoning by other agents primarily affecting gastrointestinal system NOS

    ☑7ᵗʰ **T47.8X2 Poisoning by other agents primarily affecting gastrointestinal system, intentional self-harm**

    ☑7ᵗʰ **T47.8X3 Poisoning by other agents primarily affecting gastrointestinal system, assault**

    ☑7ᵗʰ **T47.8X4 Poisoning by other agents primarily affecting gastrointestinal system, undetermined**

    ☑7ᵗʰ **T47.8X5 Adverse effect of other agents primarily affecting gastrointestinal system**

    ☑7ᵗʰ **T47.8X6 Underdosing of other agents primarily affecting gastrointestinal system**

☑5ᵗʰ **T47.9 Poisoning by, adverse effect of and underdosing of unspecified agents primarily affecting the gastrointestinal system**

    ☑x7ᵗʰ **T47.91 Poisoning by unspecified agents primarily affecting the gastrointestinal system, accidental (unintentional)**
    Poisoning by agents primarily affecting the gastrointestinal system NOS

    ☑x7ᵗʰ **T47.92 Poisoning by unspecified agents primarily affecting the gastrointestinal system, intentional self-harm**

    ☑x7ᵗʰ **T47.93 Poisoning by unspecified agents primarily affecting the gastrointestinal system, assault**

    ☑x7ᵗʰ **T47.94 Poisoning by unspecified agents primarily affecting the gastrointestinal system, undetermined**

    ☑x7ᵗʰ **T47.95 Adverse effect of unspecified agents primarily affecting the gastrointestinal system**

    ☑x7ᵗʰ **T47.96 Underdosing of unspecified agents primarily affecting the gastrointestinal system**

☑4ᵗʰ **T48 Poisoning by, adverse effect of and underdosing of agents primarily acting on smooth and skeletal muscles and the respiratory system**

The appropriate 7th character is to be added to each code from category T48.
A   initial encounter
D   subsequent encounter
S   sequela

☑5ᵗʰ **T48.0 Poisoning by, adverse effect of and underdosing of oxytocic drugs**

    EXCLUDES 1 *poisoning by, adverse effect of and underdosing of estrogens, progestogens and antagonists (T38.4-T38.6)*

  ☑6ᵗʰ **T48.0X Poisoning by, adverse effect of and underdosing of oxytocic drugs**

    ☑7ᵗʰ **T48.0X1 Poisoning by oxytocic drugs, accidental (unintentional)**
    Poisoning by oxytocic drugs NOS

    ☑7ᵗʰ **T48.0X2 Poisoning by oxytocic drugs, intentional self-harm**

    ☑7ᵗʰ **T48.0X3 Poisoning by oxytocic drugs, assault**

    ☑7ᵗʰ **T48.0X4 Poisoning by oxytocic drugs, undetermined**

    ☑7ᵗʰ **T48.0X5 Adverse effect of oxytocic drugs**

    ☑7ᵗʰ **T48.0X6 Underdosing of oxytocic drugs**

☑5ᵗʰ **T48.1 Poisoning by, adverse effect of and underdosing of skeletal muscle relaxants [neuromuscular blocking agents]**

  ☑6ᵗʰ **T48.1X Poisoning by, adverse effect of and underdosing of skeletal muscle relaxants [neuromuscular blocking agents]**

    ☑7ᵗʰ **T48.1X1 Poisoning by skeletal muscle relaxants [neuromuscular blocking agents], accidental (unintentional)**
    Poisoning by skeletal muscle relaxants [neuromuscular blocking agents] NOS

✓7th **T48.1X2** **Poisoning by skeletal muscle relaxants [neuromuscular blocking agents], intentional self-harm**

✓7th **T48.1X3** **Poisoning by skeletal muscle relaxants [neuromuscular blocking agents], assault**

✓7th **T48.1X4** **Poisoning by skeletal muscle relaxants [neuromuscular blocking agents], undetermined**

✓7th **T48.1X5** **Adverse effect of skeletal muscle relaxants [neuromuscular blocking agents]**

✓7th **T48.1X6** **Underdosing of skeletal muscle relaxants [neuromuscular blocking agents]**

✓5th **T48.2** **Poisoning by, adverse effect of and underdosing of other and unspecified drugs acting on muscles**

✓6th **T48.20** **Poisoning by, adverse effect of and underdosing of unspecified drugs acting on muscles**

✓7th **T48.201** **Poisoning by unspecified drugs acting on muscles, accidental (unintentional)**
Poisoning by unspecified drugs acting on muscles NOS

✓7th **T48.202** **Poisoning by unspecified drugs acting on muscles, intentional self-harm**

✓7th **T48.203** **Poisoning by unspecified drugs acting on muscles, assault**

✓7th **T48.204** **Poisoning by unspecified drugs acting on muscles, undetermined**

✓7th **T48.205** **Adverse effect of unspecified drugs acting on muscles**

✓7th **T48.206** **Underdosing of unspecified drugs acting on muscles**

✓6th **T48.29** **Poisoning by, adverse effect of and underdosing of other drugs acting on muscles**

✓7th **T48.291** **Poisoning by other drugs acting on muscles, accidental (unintentional)**
Poisoning by other drugs acting on muscles NOS

✓7th **T48.292** **Poisoning by other drugs acting on muscles, intentional self-harm**

✓7th **T48.293** **Poisoning by other drugs acting on muscles, assault**

✓7th **T48.294** **Poisoning by other drugs acting on muscles, undetermined**

✓7th **T48.295** **Adverse effect of other drugs acting on muscles**

✓7th **T48.296** **Underdosing of other drugs acting on muscles**

✓5th **T48.3** **Poisoning by, adverse effect of and underdosing of antitussives**

✓6th **T48.3X** **Poisoning by, adverse effect of and underdosing of antitussives**

✓7th **T48.3X1** **Poisoning by antitussives, accidental (unintentional)**
Poisoning by antitussives NOS

✓7th **T48.3X2** **Poisoning by antitussives, intentional self-harm**

✓7th **T48.3X3** **Poisoning by antitussives, assault**

✓7th **T48.3X4** **Poisoning by antitussives, undetermined**

✓7th **T48.3X5** **Adverse effect of antitussives**

✓7th **T48.3X6** **Underdosing of antitussives**

✓5th **T48.4** **Poisoning by, adverse effect of and underdosing of expectorants**

✓6th **T48.4X** **Poisoning by, adverse effect of and underdosing of expectorants**

✓7th **T48.4X1** **Poisoning by expectorants, accidental (unintentional)**
Poisoning by expectorants NOS

✓7th **T48.4X2** **Poisoning by expectorants, intentional self-harm**

✓7th **T48.4X3** **Poisoning by expectorants, assault**

✓7th **T48.4X4** **Poisoning by expectorants, undetermined**

✓7th **T48.4X5** **Adverse effect of expectorants**

✓7th **T48.4X6** **Underdosing of expectorants**

✓5th **T48.5** **Poisoning by, adverse effect of and underdosing of other anti-common-cold drugs**
Poisoning by, adverse effect of and underdosing of decongestants

EXCLUDES 2   poisoning by, adverse effect of and underdosing of antipyretics, NEC (T39.9-)
poisoning by, adverse effect of and underdosing of non-steroidal antiinflammatory drugs (T39.3-)
poisoning by, adverse effect of and underdosing of salicylates (T39.0-)

✓6th **T48.5X** **Poisoning by, adverse effect of and underdosing of other anti-common-cold drugs**

✓7th **T48.5X1** **Poisoning by other anti-common-cold drugs, accidental (unintentional)**
Poisoning by other anti-common-cold drugs NOS

✓7th **T48.5X2** **Poisoning by other anti-common-cold drugs, intentional self-harm**

✓7th **T48.5X3** **Poisoning by other anti-common-cold drugs, assault**

✓7th **T48.5X4** **Poisoning by other anti-common-cold drugs, undetermined**

✓7th **T48.5X5** **Adverse effect of other anti-common-cold drugs**

✓7th **T48.5X6** **Underdosing of other anti-common-cold drugs**

✓5th **T48.6** **Poisoning by, adverse effect of and underdosing of antiasthmatics, not elsewhere classified**
Poisoning by, adverse effect of and underdosing of beta-adrenoreceptor agonists used in asthma therapy

EXCLUDES 1   poisoning by, adverse effect of and underdosing of beta-adrenoreceptor agonists not used in asthma therapy (T44.5)
poisoning by, adverse effect of and underdosing of anterior pituitary [adenohypophyseal] hormones (T38.8)

✓6th **T48.6X** **Poisoning by, adverse effect of and underdosing of antiasthmatics**

✓7th **T48.6X1** **Poisoning by antiasthmatics, accidental (unintentional)**
Poisoning by antiasthmatics NOS

✓7th **T48.6X2** **Poisoning by antiasthmatics, intentional self-harm**

✓7th **T48.6X3** **Poisoning by antiasthmatics, assault**

✓7th **T48.6X4** **Poisoning by antiasthmatics, undetermined**

✓7th **T48.6X5** **Adverse effect of antiasthmatics**

✓7th **T48.6X6** **Underdosing of antiasthmatics**

✓5th **T48.9** **Poisoning by, adverse effect of and underdosing of other and unspecified agents primarily acting on the respiratory system**

✓6th **T48.90** **Poisoning by, adverse effect of and underdosing of unspecified agents primarily acting on the respiratory system**

✓7th **T48.901** **Poisoning by unspecified agents primarily acting on the respiratory system, accidental (unintentional)**

✓7th **T48.902** **Poisoning by unspecified agents primarily acting on the respiratory system, intentional self-harm**

✓7th **T48.903** **Poisoning by unspecified agents primarily acting on the respiratory system, assault**

✓7th **T48.904** **Poisoning by unspecified agents primarily acting on the respiratory system, undetermined**

✓7th **T48.905** **Adverse effect of unspecified agents primarily acting on the respiratory system**

✓7th **T48.906** **Underdosing of unspecified agents primarily acting on the respiratory system**

✓6th **T48.99** **Poisoning by, adverse effect of and underdosing of other agents primarily acting on the respiratory system**

✓7th **T48.991** **Poisoning by other agents primarily acting on the respiratory system, accidental (unintentional)**

✓7th **T48.992** **Poisoning by other agents primarily acting on the respiratory system, intentional self-harm**

EXCLUDES 1 Not coded here   *EXCLUDES 2* Not included here   Ⓝ Newborn Age: 0   Ⓟ Pediatric Age: 0-17   Ⓜ Maternity Age: 12-55   Ⓐ Adult Age: 15-124

958   ICD-10-CM 2014 (Draft)

✓7th **T48.993** Poisoning by other agents primarily acting on the respiratory system, assault

✓7th **T48.994** Poisoning by other agents primarily acting on the respiratory system, undetermined

✓7th **T48.995** Adverse effect of other agents primarily acting on the respiratory system

✓7th **T48.996** Underdosing of other agents primarily acting on the respiratory system

✓4th **T49** Poisoning by, adverse effect of and underdosing of topical agents primarily affecting skin and mucous membrane and by ophthalmological, otorhinolaryngological and dental drugs
Poisoning by, adverse effect of and underdosing of glucocorticoids, topically used

The appropriate 7th character is to be added to each code from category T49.
A   initial encounter
D   subsequent encounter
S   sequela

✓5th **T49.0** Poisoning by, adverse effect of and underdosing of local antifungal, anti-infective and anti-inflammatory drugs

✓6th **T49.0X** Poisoning by, adverse effect of and underdosing of local antifungal, anti-infective and anti-inflammatory drugs

✓7th **T49.0X1** Poisoning by local antifungal, anti-infective and anti-inflammatory drugs, accidental (unintentional)
Poisoning by local antifungal, anti-infective and anti-inflammatory drugs NOS

✓7th **T49.0X2** Poisoning by local antifungal, anti-infective and anti-inflammatory drugs, intentional self-harm

✓7th **T49.0X3** Poisoning by local antifungal, anti-infective and anti-inflammatory drugs, assault

✓7th **T49.0X4** Poisoning by local antifungal, anti-infective and anti-inflammatory drugs, undetermined

✓7th **T49.0X5** Adverse effect of local antifungal, anti-infective and anti-inflammatory drugs

✓7th **T49.0X6** Underdosing of local antifungal, anti-infective and anti-inflammatory drugs

✓5th **T49.1** Poisoning by, adverse effect of and underdosing of antipruritics

✓6th **T49.1X** Poisoning by, adverse effect of and underdosing of antipruritics

✓7th **T49.1X1** Poisoning by antipruritics, accidental (unintentional)
Poisoning by antipruritics NOS

✓7th **T49.1X2** Poisoning by antipruritics, intentional self-harm

✓7th **T49.1X3** Poisoning by antipruritics, assault

✓7th **T49.1X4** Poisoning by antipruritics, undetermined

✓7th **T49.1X5** Adverse effect of antipruritics

✓7th **T49.1X6** Underdosing of antipruritics

✓5th **T49.2** Poisoning by, adverse effect of and underdosing of local astringents and local detergents

✓6th **T49.2X** Poisoning by, adverse effect of and underdosing of local astringents and local detergents

✓7th **T49.2X1** Poisoning by local astringents and local detergents, accidental (unintentional)
Poisoning by local astringents and local detergents NOS

✓7th **T49.2X2** Poisoning by local astringents and local detergents, intentional self-harm

✓7th **T49.2X3** Poisoning by local astringents and local detergents, assault

✓7th **T49.2X4** Poisoning by local astringents and local detergents, undetermined

✓7th **T49.2X5** Adverse effect of local astringents and local detergents

✓7th **T49.2X6** Underdosing of local astringents and local detergents

✓5th **T49.3** Poisoning by, adverse effect of and underdosing of emollients, demulcents and protectants

✓6th **T49.3X** Poisoning by, adverse effect of and underdosing of emollients, demulcents and protectants

✓7th **T49.3X1** Poisoning by emollients, demulcents and protectants, accidental (unintentional)
Poisoning by emollients, demulcents and protectants NOS

✓7th **T49.3X2** Poisoning by emollients, demulcents and protectants, intentional self-harm

✓7th **T49.3X3** Poisoning by emollients, demulcents and protectants, assault

✓7th **T49.3X4** Poisoning by emollients, demulcents and protectants, undetermined

✓7th **T49.3X5** Adverse effect of emollients, demulcents and protectants

✓7th **T49.3X6** Underdosing of emollients, demulcents and protectants

✓5th **T49.4** Poisoning by, adverse effect of and underdosing of keratolytics, keratoplastics, and other hair treatment drugs and preparations

✓6th **T49.4X** Poisoning by, adverse effect of and underdosing of keratolytics, keratoplastics, and other hair treatment drugs and preparations

✓7th **T49.4X1** Poisoning by keratolytics, keratoplastics, and other hair treatment drugs and preparations, accidental (unintentional)
Poisoning by keratolytics, keratoplastics, and other hair treatment drugs and preparations NOS

✓7th **T49.4X2** Poisoning by keratolytics, keratoplastics, and other hair treatment drugs and preparations, intentional self-harm

✓7th **T49.4X3** Poisoning by keratolytics, keratoplastics, and other hair treatment drugs and preparations, assault

✓7th **T49.4X4** Poisoning by keratolytics, keratoplastics, and other hair treatment drugs and preparations, undetermined

✓7th **T49.4X5** Adverse effect of keratolytics, keratoplastics, and other hair treatment drugs and preparations

✓7th **T49.4X6** Underdosing of keratolytics, keratoplastics, and other hair treatment drugs and preparations

✓5th **T49.5** Poisoning by, adverse effect of and underdosing of ophthalmological drugs and preparations

✓6th **T49.5X** Poisoning by, adverse effect of and underdosing of ophthalmological drugs and preparations

✓7th **T49.5X1** Poisoning by ophthalmological drugs and preparations, accidental (unintentional)
Poisoning by ophthalmological drugs and preparations NOS

✓7th **T49.5X2** Poisoning by ophthalmological drugs and preparations, intentional self-harm

✓7th **T49.5X3** Poisoning by ophthalmological drugs and preparations, assault

✓7th **T49.5X4** Poisoning by ophthalmological drugs and preparations, undetermined

✓7th **T49.5X5** Adverse effect of ophthalmological drugs and preparations

✓7th **T49.5X6** Underdosing of ophthalmological drugs and preparations

✓5th **T49.6** Poisoning by, adverse effect of and underdosing of otorhinolaryngological drugs and preparations

✓6th **T49.6X** Poisoning by, adverse effect of and underdosing of otorhinolaryngological drugs and preparations

✓7th **T49.6X1** Poisoning by otorhinolaryngological drugs and preparations, accidental (unintentional)
Poisoning by otorhinolaryngological drugs and preparations NOS

✓7th **T49.6X2** Poisoning by otorhinolaryngological drugs and preparations, intentional self-harm

✓7th **T49.6X3** Poisoning by otorhinolaryngological drugs and preparations, assault

☑ Additional Character Required   ✓x7th Xtension Alert   Unspecified Code   Other Specified Code   Manifestation Code   ▶◀ Revised Text   ● New Code   ▲ Revised Code Title

ICD-10-CM 2014 (Draft)   959

Injury, Poisoning and Certain Other Consequences of External Causes

T49.6X4–T50.3X6

√7ᵗʰ **T49.6X4** Poisoning by otorhinolaryngological drugs and preparations, undetermined

√7ᵗʰ **T49.6X5** Adverse effect of otorhinolaryngological drugs and preparations

√7ᵗʰ **T49.6X6** Underdosing of otorhinolaryngological drugs and preparations

√5ᵗʰ **T49.7** Poisoning by, adverse effect of and underdosing of dental drugs, topically applied

√6ᵗʰ **T49.7X** Poisoning by, adverse effect of and underdosing of dental drugs, topically applied

√7ᵗʰ **T49.7X1** Poisoning by dental drugs, topically applied, accidental (unintentional)
Poisoning by dental drugs, topically applied NOS

√7ᵗʰ **T49.7X2** Poisoning by dental drugs, topically applied, intentional self-harm

√7ᵗʰ **T49.7X3** Poisoning by dental drugs, topically applied, assault

√7ᵗʰ **T49.7X4** Poisoning by dental drugs, topically applied, undetermined

√7ᵗʰ **T49.7X5** Adverse effect of dental drugs, topically applied

√7ᵗʰ **T49.7X6** Underdosing of dental drugs, topically applied

√5ᵗʰ **T49.8** Poisoning by, adverse effect of and underdosing of other topical agents
Poisoning by, adverse effect of and underdosing of spermicides

√6ᵗʰ **T49.8X** Poisoning by, adverse effect of and underdosing of other topical agents

√7ᵗʰ **T49.8X1** Poisoning by other topical agents, accidental (unintentional)
Poisoning by other topical agents NOS

√7ᵗʰ **T49.8X2** Poisoning by other topical agents, intentional self-harm

√7ᵗʰ **T49.8X3** Poisoning by other topical agents, assault

√7ᵗʰ **T49.8X4** Poisoning by other topical agents, undetermined

√7ᵗʰ **T49.8X5** Adverse effect of other topical agents

√7ᵗʰ **T49.8X6** Underdosing of other topical agents

√5ᵗʰ **T49.9** Poisoning by, adverse effect of and underdosing of unspecified topical agent

√x7ᵗʰ **T49.91** Poisoning by unspecified topical agent, accidental (unintentional)

√x7ᵗʰ **T49.92** Poisoning by unspecified topical agent, intentional self-harm

√x7ᵗʰ **T49.93** Poisoning by unspecified topical agent, assault

√x7ᵗʰ **T49.94** Poisoning by unspecified topical agent, undetermined

√x7ᵗʰ **T49.95** Adverse effect of unspecified topical agent

√x7ᵗʰ **T49.96** Underdosing of unspecified topical agent

√4ᵗʰ **T50** Poisoning by, adverse effect of and underdosing of diuretics and other and unspecified drugs, medicaments and biological substances

The appropriate 7th character is to be added to each code from category T50.
A   initial encounter
D   subsequent encounter
S   sequela

√5ᵗʰ **T50.0** Poisoning by, adverse effect of and underdosing of mineralocorticoids and their antagonists

√6ᵗʰ **T50.0X** Poisoning by, adverse effect of and underdosing of mineralocorticoids and their antagonists

√7ᵗʰ **T50.0X1** Poisoning by mineralocorticoids and their antagonists, accidental (unintentional)
Poisoning by mineralocorticoids and their antagonists NOS

√7ᵗʰ **T50.0X2** Poisoning by mineralocorticoids and their antagonists, intentional self-harm

√7ᵗʰ **T50.0X3** Poisoning by mineralocorticoids and their antagonists, assault

√7ᵗʰ **T50.0X4** Poisoning by mineralocorticoids and their antagonists, undetermined

√7ᵗʰ **T50.0X5** Adverse effect of mineralocorticoids and their antagonists

√7ᵗʰ **T50.0X6** Underdosing of mineralocorticoids and their antagonists

√5ᵗʰ **T50.1** Poisoning by, adverse effect of and underdosing of loop [high-ceiling] diuretics

√6ᵗʰ **T50.1X** Poisoning by, adverse effect of and underdosing of loop [high-ceiling] diuretics

√7ᵗʰ **T50.1X1** Poisoning by loop [high-ceiling] diuretics, accidental (unintentional)
Poisoning by loop [high-ceiling] diuretics NOS

√7ᵗʰ **T50.1X2** Poisoning by loop [high-ceiling] diuretics, intentional self-harm

√7ᵗʰ **T50.1X3** Poisoning by loop [high-ceiling] diuretics, assault

√7ᵗʰ **T50.1X4** Poisoning by loop [high-ceiling] diuretics, undetermined

√7ᵗʰ **T50.1X5** Adverse effect of loop [high-ceiling] diuretics

√7ᵗʰ **T50.1X6** Underdosing of loop [high-ceiling] diuretics

√5ᵗʰ **T50.2** Poisoning by, adverse effect of and underdosing of carbonic-anhydrase inhibitors, benzothiadiazides and other diuretics
Poisoning by, adverse effect of and underdosing of acetazolamide

√6ᵗʰ **T50.2X** Poisoning by, adverse effect of and underdosing of carbonic-anhydrase inhibitors, benzothiadiazides and other diuretics

√7ᵗʰ **T50.2X1** Poisoning by carbonic-anhydrase inhibitors, benzothiadiazides and other diuretics, accidental (unintentional)
Poisoning by carbonic-anhydrase inhibitors, benzothiadiazides and other diuretics NOS

√7ᵗʰ **T50.2X2** Poisoning by carbonic-anhydrase inhibitors, benzothiadiazides and other diuretics, intentional self-harm

√7ᵗʰ **T50.2X3** Poisoning by carbonic-anhydrase inhibitors, benzothiadiazides and other diuretics, assault

√7ᵗʰ **T50.2X4** Poisoning by carbonic-anhydrase inhibitors, benzothiadiazides and other diuretics, undetermined

√7ᵗʰ **T50.2X5** Adverse effect of carbonic-anhydrase inhibitors, benzothiadiazides and other diuretics

√7ᵗʰ **T50.2X6** Underdosing of carbonic-anhydrase inhibitors, benzothiadiazides and other diuretics

√5ᵗʰ **T50.3** Poisoning by, adverse effect of and underdosing of electrolytic, caloric and water-balance agents
Poisoning by, adverse effect of and underdosing of oral rehydration salts

√6ᵗʰ **T50.3X** Poisoning by, adverse effect of and underdosing of electrolytic, caloric and water-balance agents

√7ᵗʰ **T50.3X1** Poisoning by electrolytic, caloric and water-balance agents, accidental (unintentional)
Poisoning by electrolytic, caloric and water-balance agents NOS

√7ᵗʰ **T50.3X2** Poisoning by electrolytic, caloric and water-balance agents, intentional self-harm

√7ᵗʰ **T50.3X3** Poisoning by electrolytic, caloric and water-balance agents, assault

√7ᵗʰ **T50.3X4** Poisoning by electrolytic, caloric and water-balance agents, undetermined

√7ᵗʰ **T50.3X5** Adverse effect of electrolytic, caloric and water-balance agents

√7ᵗʰ **T50.3X6** Underdosing of electrolytic, caloric and water-balance agents

EXCLUDES 1 Not coded here   EXCLUDES 2 Not included here   N Newborn Age: 0   P Pediatric Age: 0-17   M Maternity Age: 12-55   A Adult Age: 15-124

960   ICD-10-CM 2014 (Draft)

✓5th **T50.4** Poisoning by, adverse effect of and underdosing of drugs affecting uric acid metabolism

  ✓6th **T50.4X** Poisoning by, adverse effect of and underdosing of drugs affecting uric acid metabolism

    ✓7th **T50.4X1** Poisoning by drugs affecting uric acid metabolism, accidental (unintentional)
      Poisoning by drugs affecting uric acid metabolism NOS

    ✓7th **T50.4X2** Poisoning by drugs affecting uric acid metabolism, intentional self-harm

    ✓7th **T50.4X3** Poisoning by drugs affecting uric acid metabolism, assault

    ✓7th **T50.4X4** Poisoning by drugs affecting uric acid metabolism, undetermined

    ✓7th **T50.4X5** Adverse effect of drugs affecting uric acid metabolism

    ✓7th **T50.4X6** Underdosing of drugs affecting uric acid metabolism

✓5th **T50.5** Poisoning by, adverse effect of and underdosing of appetite depressants

  ✓6th **T50.5X** Poisoning by, adverse effect of and underdosing of appetite depressants

    ✓7th **T50.5X1** Poisoning by appetite depressants, accidental (unintentional)
      Poisoning by appetite depressants NOS

    ✓7th **T50.5X2** Poisoning by appetite depressants, intentional self-harm

    ✓7th **T50.5X3** Poisoning by appetite depressants, assault

    ✓7th **T50.5X4** Poisoning by appetite depressants, undetermined

    ✓7th **T50.5X5** Adverse effect of appetite depressants

    ✓7th **T50.5X6** Underdosing of appetite depressants

✓5th **T50.6** Poisoning by, adverse effect of and underdosing of antidotes and chelating agents
  Poisoning by, adverse effect of and underdosing of alcohol deterrents

  ✓6th **T50.6X** Poisoning by, adverse effect of and underdosing of antidotes and chelating agents

    ✓7th **T50.6X1** Poisoning by antidotes and chelating agents, accidental (unintentional)
      Poisoning by antidotes and chelating agents NOS

    ✓7th **T50.6X2** Poisoning by antidotes and chelating agents, intentional self-harm

    ✓7th **T50.6X3** Poisoning by antidotes and chelating agents, assault

    ✓7th **T50.6X4** Poisoning by antidotes and chelating agents, undetermined

    ✓7th **T50.6X5** Adverse effect of antidotes and chelating agents

    ✓7th **T50.6X6** Underdosing of antidotes and chelating agents

✓5th **T50.7** Poisoning by, adverse effect of and underdosing of analeptics and opioid receptor antagonists

  ✓6th **T50.7X** Poisoning by, adverse effect of and underdosing of analeptics and opioid receptor antagonists

    ✓7th **T50.7X1** Poisoning by analeptics and opioid receptor antagonists, accidental (unintentional)
      Poisoning by analeptics and opioid receptor antagonists NOS

    ✓7th **T50.7X2** Poisoning by analeptics and opioid receptor antagonists, intentional self-harm

    ✓7th **T50.7X3** Poisoning by analeptics and opioid receptor antagonists, assault

    ✓7th **T50.7X4** Poisoning by analeptics and opioid receptor antagonists, undetermined

    ✓7th **T50.7X5** Adverse effect of analeptics and opioid receptor antagonists

    ✓7th **T50.7X6** Underdosing of analeptics and opioid receptor antagonists

✓5th **T50.8** Poisoning by, adverse effect of and underdosing of diagnostic agents

  ✓6th **T50.8X** Poisoning by, adverse effect of and underdosing of diagnostic agents

    ✓7th **T50.8X1** Poisoning by diagnostic agents, accidental (unintentional)
      Poisoning by diagnostic agents NOS

    ✓7th **T50.8X2** Poisoning by diagnostic agents, intentional self-harm

    ✓7th **T50.8X3** Poisoning by diagnostic agents, assault

    ✓7th **T50.8X4** Poisoning by diagnostic agents, undetermined

    ✓7th **T50.8X5** Adverse effect of diagnostic agents

    ✓7th **T50.8X6** Underdosing of diagnostic agents

✓5th **T50.A** Poisoning by, adverse effect of and underdosing of bacterial vaccines

  ✓6th **T50.A1** Poisoning by, adverse effect of and underdosing of pertussis vaccine, including combinations with a pertussis component

    ✓7th **T50.A11** Poisoning by pertussis vaccine, including combinations with a pertussis component, accidental (unintentional)

    ✓7th **T50.A12** Poisoning by pertussis vaccine, including combinations with a pertussis component, intentional self-harm

    ✓7th **T50.A13** Poisoning by pertussis vaccine, including combinations with a pertussis component, assault

    ✓7th **T50.A14** Poisoning by pertussis vaccine, including combinations with a pertussis component, undetermined

    ✓7th **T50.A15** Adverse effect of pertussis vaccine, including combinations with a pertussis component

    ✓7th **T50.A16** Underdosing of pertussis vaccine, including combinations with a pertussis component

  ✓6th **T50.A2** Poisoning by, adverse effect of and underdosing of mixed bacterial vaccines without a pertussis component

    ✓7th **T50.A21** Poisoning by mixed bacterial vaccines without a pertussis component, accidental (unintentional)

    ✓7th **T50.A22** Poisoning by mixed bacterial vaccines without a pertussis component, intentional self-harm

    ✓7th **T50.A23** Poisoning by mixed bacterial vaccines without a pertussis component, assault

    ✓7th **T50.A24** Poisoning by mixed bacterial vaccines without a pertussis component, undetermined

    ✓7th **T50.A25** Adverse effect of mixed bacterial vaccines without a pertussis component

    ✓7th **T50.A26** Underdosing of mixed bacterial vaccines without a pertussis component

  ✓6th **T50.A9** Poisoning by, adverse effect of and underdosing of other bacterial vaccines

    ✓7th **T50.A91** Poisoning by other bacterial vaccines, accidental (unintentional)

    ✓7th **T50.A92** Poisoning by other bacterial vaccines, intentional self-harm

    ✓7th **T50.A93** Poisoning by other bacterial vaccines, assault

    ✓7th **T50.A94** Poisoning by other bacterial vaccines, undetermined

    ✓7th **T50.A95** Adverse effect of other bacterial vaccines

    ✓7th **T50.A96** Underdosing of other bacterial vaccines

✓5th **T50.B** Poisoning by, adverse effect of and underdosing of viral vaccines

  ✓6th **T50.B1** Poisoning by, adverse effect of and underdosing of smallpox vaccines

    ✓7th **T50.B11** Poisoning by smallpox vaccines, accidental (unintentional)

    ✓7th **T50.B12** Poisoning by smallpox vaccines, intentional self-harm

    ✓7th **T50.B13** Poisoning by smallpox vaccines, assault

☑ Additional Character Required   ✓7th Xtension Alert   **Unspecified Code**   Other Specified Code   Manifestation Code   ►◄ Revised Text   ● New Code   ▲ Revised Code Title

ICD-10-CM 2014 (Draft)   **961**

√7ᵗʰ **T50.B14** Poisoning by smallpox vaccines, undetermined

√7ᵗʰ **T50.B15** Adverse effect of smallpox vaccines

√7ᵗʰ **T50.B16** Underdosing of smallpox vaccines

√6ᵗʰ **T50.B9** Poisoning by, adverse effect of and underdosing of other viral vaccines

    √7ᵗʰ **T50.B91** Poisoning by other viral vaccines, accidental (unintentional)

    √7ᵗʰ **T50.B92** Poisoning by other viral vaccines, intentional self-harm

    √7ᵗʰ **T50.B93** Poisoning by other viral vaccines, assault

    √7ᵗʰ **T50.B94** Poisoning by other viral vaccines, undetermined

    √7ᵗʰ **T50.B95** Adverse effect of other viral vaccines

    √7ᵗʰ **T50.B96** Underdosing of other viral vaccines

√5ᵗʰ **T50.Z** Poisoning by, adverse effect of and underdosing of other vaccines and biological substances

    √6ᵗʰ **T50.Z1** Poisoning by, adverse effect of and underdosing of immunoglobulin

       √7ᵗʰ **T50.Z11** Poisoning by immunoglobulin, accidental (unintentional)

       √7ᵗʰ **T50.Z12** Poisoning by immunoglobulin, intentional self-harm

       √7ᵗʰ **T50.Z13** Poisoning by immunoglobulin, assault

       √7ᵗʰ **T50.Z14** Poisoning by immunoglobulin, undetermined

       √7ᵗʰ **T50.Z15** Adverse effect of immunoglobulin

       √7ᵗʰ **T50.Z16** Underdosing of immunoglobulin

    √6ᵗʰ **T50.Z9** Poisoning by, adverse effect of and underdosing of other vaccines and biological substances

       √7ᵗʰ **T50.Z91** Poisoning by other vaccines and biological substances, accidental (unintentional)

       √7ᵗʰ **T50.Z92** Poisoning by other vaccines and biological substances, intentional self-harm

       √7ᵗʰ **T50.Z93** Poisoning by other vaccines and biological substances, assault

       √7ᵗʰ **T50.Z94** Poisoning by other vaccines and biological substances, undetermined

       √7ᵗʰ **T50.Z95** Adverse effect of other vaccines and biological substances

       √7ᵗʰ **T50.Z96** Underdosing of other vaccines and biological substances

√5ᵗʰ **T50.9** Poisoning by, adverse effect of and underdosing of other and unspecified drugs, medicaments and biological substances

    √6ᵗʰ **T50.90** Poisoning by, adverse effect of and underdosing of unspecified drugs, medicaments and biological substances

       √7ᵗʰ **T50.901** Poisoning by unspecified drugs, medicaments and biological substances, accidental (unintentional)

       √7ᵗʰ **T50.902** Poisoning by unspecified drugs, medicaments and biological substances, intentional self-harm

       √7ᵗʰ **T50.903** Poisoning by unspecified drugs, medicaments and biological substances, assault

       √7ᵗʰ **T50.904** Poisoning by unspecified drugs, medicaments and biological substances, undetermined

       √7ᵗʰ **T50.905** Adverse effect of unspecified drugs, medicaments and biological substances

       √7ᵗʰ **T50.906** Underdosing of unspecified drugs, medicaments and biological substances

    √6ᵗʰ **T50.99** Poisoning by, adverse effect of and underdosing of other drugs, medicaments and biological substances

       √7ᵗʰ **T50.991** Poisoning by other drugs, medicaments and biological substances, accidental (unintentional)

       √7ᵗʰ **T50.992** Poisoning by other drugs, medicaments and biological substances, intentional self-harm

       √7ᵗʰ **T50.993** Poisoning by other drugs, medicaments and biological substances, assault

       √7ᵗʰ **T50.994** Poisoning by other drugs, medicaments and biological substances, undetermined

√7ᵗʰ **T50.995** Adverse effect of other drugs, medicaments and biological substances

√7ᵗʰ **T50.996** Underdosing of other drugs, medicaments and biological substances

Toxic effects of substances chiefly nonmedicinal as to source (T51-T65)

Use additional code(s) for all associated manifestations of toxic effect, such as:
personal history of foreign body fully removed (Z87.821)
respiratory conditions due to external agents (J60-J70)
to identify any retained foreign body, if applicable (Z18.-)

NOTE When no intent is indicated code to accidental. Undetermined intent is only for use when there is specific documentation in the record that the intent of the toxic effect cannot be determined.

EXCLUDES 1 contact with and (suspected) exposure to toxic substances (Z77.-)

√4ᵗʰ **T51** Toxic effect of alcohol

The appropriate 7th character is to be added to each code from category T51.
A   initial encounter
D   subsequent encounter
S   sequela

√5ᵗʰ **T51.0** Toxic effect of ethanol
Toxic effect of ethyl alcohol
EXCLUDES 2 acute alcohol intoxication or 'hangover' effects (F10.129, F10.229, F10.929)
drunkenness (F10.129, F10.229, F10.929)
pathological alcohol intoxication (F10.129, F10.229, F10.929)

    √6ᵗʰ **T51.0X** Toxic effect of ethanol

       √7ᵗʰ **T51.0X1** Toxic effect of ethanol, accidental (unintentional)
Toxic effect of ethanol NOS

       √7ᵗʰ **T51.0X2** Toxic effect of ethanol, intentional self-harm

       √7ᵗʰ **T51.0X3** Toxic effect of ethanol, assault

       √7ᵗʰ **T51.0X4** Toxic effect of ethanol, undetermined

√5ᵗʰ **T51.1** Toxic effect of methanol
Toxic effect of methyl alcohol

    √6ᵗʰ **T51.1X** Toxic effect of methanol

       √7ᵗʰ **T51.1X1** Toxic effect of methanol, accidental (unintentional)
Toxic effect of methanol NOS

       √7ᵗʰ **T51.1X2** Toxic effect of methanol, intentional self-harm

       √7ᵗʰ **T51.1X3** Toxic effect of methanol, assault

       √7ᵗʰ **T51.1X4** Toxic effect of methanol, undetermined

√5ᵗʰ **T51.2** Toxic effect of 2-Propanol
Toxic effect of isopropyl alcohol

    √6ᵗʰ **T51.2X** Toxic effect of 2-Propanol

       √7ᵗʰ **T51.2X1** Toxic effect of 2-Propanol, accidental (unintentional)
Toxic effect of 2-Propanol NOS

       √7ᵗʰ **T51.2X2** Toxic effect of 2-Propanol, intentional self-harm

       √7ᵗʰ **T51.2X3** Toxic effect of 2-Propanol, assault

       √7ᵗʰ **T51.2X4** Toxic effect of 2-Propanol, undetermined

√5ᵗʰ **T51.3** Toxic effect of fusel oil
Toxic effect of amyl alcohol
Toxic effect of butyl [1-butanol] alcohol
Toxic effect of propyl [1-propanol] alcohol

    √6ᵗʰ **T51.3X** Toxic effect of fusel oil

       √7ᵗʰ **T51.3X1** Toxic effect of fusel oil, accidental (unintentional)
Toxic effect of fusel oil NOS

       √7ᵗʰ **T51.3X2** Toxic effect of fusel oil, intentional self-harm

       √7ᵗʰ **T51.3X3** Toxic effect of fusel oil, assault

       √7ᵗʰ **T51.3X4** Toxic effect of fusel oil, undetermined

√5ᵗʰ **T51.8** Toxic effect of other alcohols

    √6ᵗʰ **T51.8X** Toxic effect of other alcohols

       √7ᵗʰ **T51.8X1** Toxic effect of other alcohols, accidental (unintentional)
Toxic effect of other alcohols NOS

EXCLUDES 1 Not coded here   **EXCLUDES 2** Not included here   **N** Newborn Age: 0   **P** Pediatric Age: 0-17   **M** Maternity Age: 12-55   **A** Adult Age: 15-124

962   ICD-10-CM 2014 (Draft)

√7th T51.8X2 **Toxic effect of other alcohols,** intentional self-harm

√7th T51.8X3 **Toxic effect of other alcohols,** assault

√7th T51.8X4 **Toxic effect of other alcohols,** undetermined

√5th **T51.9 Toxic effect of** unspecified **alcohol**

√x7th T51.91 **Toxic effect of unspecified alcohol,** accidental **(unintentional)**

√x7th T51.92 **Toxic effect of unspecified alcohol,** intentional self-harm

√x7th T51.93 **Toxic effect of unspecified alcohol,** assault

√x7th T51.94 **Toxic effect of unspecified alcohol,** undetermined

√4th **T52 Toxic effect of organic solvents**

> EXCLUDES 1 *halogen derivatives of aliphatic and aromatic hydrocarbons (T53.-)*

> The appropriate 7th character is to be added to each code from category T52.
> A initial encounter
> D subsequent encounter
> S sequela

√5th **T52.0 Toxic effects of petroleum products**
Toxic effects of gasoline [petrol]
Toxic effects of kerosene [paraffin oil]
Toxic effects of paraffin wax
Toxic effects of ether petroleum
Toxic effects of naphtha petroleum
Toxic effects of spirit petroleum

√6th **T52.0X Toxic effects of** petroleum products

√7th T52.0X1 **Toxic effect of petroleum products,** accidental **(unintentional)**
Toxic effects of petroleum products NOS

√7th T52.0X2 **Toxic effect of petroleum products,** intentional self-harm

√7th T52.0X3 **Toxic effect of petroleum products,** assault

√7th T52.0X4 **Toxic effect of petroleum products,** undetermined

√5th **T52.1 Toxic effects of benzene**

> EXCLUDES 1 *homologues of benzene (T52.2)*
> *nitroderivatives and aminoderivatives of benzene and its homologues (T65.3)*

√6th **T52.1X Toxic effects of** benzene

√7th T52.1X1 **Toxic effect of benzene,** accidental **(unintentional)**
Toxic effects of benzene NOS

√7th T52.1X2 **Toxic effect of benzene,** intentional self-harm

√7th T52.1X3 **Toxic effect of benzene,** assault

√7th T52.1X4 **Toxic effect of benzene,** undetermined

√5th **T52.2 Toxic effects of homologues of benzene**
Toxic effects of toluene [methylbenzene]
Toxic effects of xylene [dimethylbenzene]

√6th **T52.2X Toxic effects of** homologues of benzene

√7th T52.2X1 **Toxic effect of homologues of benzene,** accidental **(unintentional)**
Toxic effects of homologues of benzene NOS

√7th T52.2X2 **Toxic effect of homologues of benzene,** intentional self-harm

√7th T52.2X3 **Toxic effect of homologues of benzene,** assault

√7th T52.2X4 **Toxic effect of homologues of benzene,** undetermined

√5th **T52.3 Toxic effects of glycols**

√6th **T52.3X Toxic effects of** glycols

√7th T52.3X1 **Toxic effect of glycols,** accidental **(unintentional)**
Toxic effects of glycols NOS

√7th T52.3X2 **Toxic effect of glycols,** intentional self-harm

√7th T52.3X3 **Toxic effect of glycols,** assault

√7th T52.3X4 **Toxic effect of glycols,** undetermined

√5th **T52.4 Toxic effects of ketones**

√6th **T52.4X Toxic effects of** ketones

√7th T52.4X1 **Toxic effect of ketones,** accidental **(unintentional)**
Toxic effects of ketones NOS

√7th T52.4X2 **Toxic effect of ketones,** intentional self-harm

√7th T52.4X3 **Toxic effect of ketones,** assault

√7th T52.4X4 **Toxic effect of ketones,** undetermined

√5th **T52.8 Toxic effects of other organic solvents**

√6th **T52.8X Toxic effects of** other organic solvents

√7th T52.8X1 **Toxic effect of other organic solvents,** accidental **(unintentional)**
Toxic effects of other organic solvents NOS

√7th T52.8X2 **Toxic effect of other organic solvents,** intentional self-harm

√7th T52.8X3 **Toxic effect of other organic solvents,** assault

√7th T52.8X4 **Toxic effect of other organic solvents,** undetermined

√5th **T52.9 Toxic effects of** unspecified **organic solvent**

√x7th T52.91 **Toxic effect of unspecified organic solvent,** accidental **(unintentional)**

√x7th T52.92 **Toxic effect of unspecified organic solvent,** intentional self-harm

√x7th T52.93 **Toxic effect of unspecified organic solvent,** assault

√x7th T52.94 **Toxic effect of unspecified organic solvent,** undetermined

√4th **T53 Toxic effect of halogen derivatives of aliphatic and aromatic hydrocarbons**

> The appropriate 7th character is to be added to each code from category T53.
> A initial encounter
> D subsequent encounter
> S sequela

√5th **T53.0 Toxic effects of carbon tetrachloride**
Toxic effects of tetrachloromethane

√6th **T53.0X Toxic effects of** carbon tetrachloride

√7th T53.0X1 **Toxic effect of carbon tetrachloride,** accidental **(unintentional)**
Toxic effects of carbon tetrachloride NOS

√7th T53.0X2 **Toxic effect of carbon tetrachloride,** intentional self-harm

√7th T53.0X3 **Toxic effect of carbon tetrachloride,** assault

√7th T53.0X4 **Toxic effect of carbon tetrachloride,** undetermined

√5th **T53.1 Toxic effects of chloroform**
Toxic effects of trichloromethane

√6th **T53.1X Toxic effects of** chloroform

√7th T53.1X1 **Toxic effect of chloroform,** accidental **(unintentional)**
Toxic effects of chloroform NOS

√7th T53.1X2 **Toxic effect of chloroform,** intentional self-harm

√7th T53.1X3 **Toxic effect of chloroform,** assault

√7th T53.1X4 **Toxic effect of chloroform,** undetermined

√5th **T53.2 Toxic effects of trichloroethylene**
Toxic effects of trichloroethene

√6th **T53.2X Toxic effects of** trichloroethylene

√7th T53.2X1 **Toxic effect of trichloroethylene,** accidental **(unintentional)**
Toxic effects of trichloroethylene NOS

√7th T53.2X2 **Toxic effect of trichloroethylene,** intentional self-harm

√7th T53.2X3 **Toxic effect of trichloroethylene,** assault

√7th T53.2X4 **Toxic effect of trichloroethylene,** undetermined

☑ Additional Character Required   √x7th Xtension Alert   Unspecified Code   Other Specified Code   Manifestation Code   ►◄ Revised Text   ● New Code   ▲ Revised Code Title

ICD-10-CM 2014 (Draft)

963

√5ᵗʰ **T53.3 Toxic effects of tetrachloroethylene**
Toxic effects of perchloroethylene
Toxic effect of tetrachloroethene

  √6ᵗʰ **T53.3X Toxic effects of** tetrachloroethylene

    √7ᵗʰ **T53.3X1 Toxic effect of tetrachloroethylene, accidental (unintentional)**
Toxic effects of tetrachloroethylene NOS

    √7ᵗʰ **T53.3X2 Toxic effect of tetrachloroethylene, intentional self-harm**

    √7ᵗʰ **T53.3X3 Toxic effect of tetrachloroethylene, assault**

    √7ᵗʰ **T53.3X4 Toxic effect of tetrachloroethylene, undetermined**

√5ᵗʰ **T53.4 Toxic effects of dichloromethane**
Toxic effects of methylene chloride

  √6ᵗʰ **T53.4X Toxic effects of** dichloromethane

    √7ᵗʰ **T53.4X1 Toxic effect of dichloromethane, accidental (unintentional)**
Toxic effects of dichloromethane NOS

    √7ᵗʰ **T53.4X2 Toxic effect of dichloromethane, intentional self-harm**

    √7ᵗʰ **T53.4X3 Toxic effect of dichloromethane, assault**

    √7ᵗʰ **T53.4X4 Toxic effect of dichloromethane, undetermined**

√5ᵗʰ **T53.5 Toxic effects of chlorofluorocarbons**

  √6ᵗʰ **T53.5X Toxic effects of** chlorofluorocarbons

    √7ᵗʰ **T53.5X1 Toxic effect of chlorofluorocarbons, accidental (unintentional)**
Toxic effects of chlorofluorocarbons NOS

    √7ᵗʰ **T53.5X2 Toxic effect of chlorofluorocarbons, intentional self-harm**

    √7ᵗʰ **T53.5X3 Toxic effect of chlorofluorocarbons, assault**

    √7ᵗʰ **T53.5X4 Toxic effect of chlorofluorocarbons, undetermined**

√5ᵗʰ **T53.6 Toxic effects of other halogen derivatives of aliphatic hydrocarbons**

  √6ᵗʰ **T53.6X Toxic effects of other** halogen derivatives of aliphatic hydrocarbons

    √7ᵗʰ **T53.6X1 Toxic effect of other halogen derivatives of aliphatic hydrocarbons, accidental (unintentional)**
Toxic effects of other halogen derivatives of aliphatic hydrocarbons NOS

    √7ᵗʰ **T53.6X2 Toxic effect of other halogen derivatives of aliphatic hydrocarbons, intentional self-harm**

    √7ᵗʰ **T53.6X3 Toxic effect of other halogen derivatives of aliphatic hydrocarbons, assault**

    √7ᵗʰ **T53.6X4 Toxic effect of other halogen derivatives of aliphatic hydrocarbons, undetermined**

√5ᵗʰ **T53.7 Toxic effects of other halogen derivatives of aromatic hydrocarbons**

  √6ᵗʰ **T53.7X Toxic effects of other** halogen derivatives of aromatic hydrocarbons

    √7ᵗʰ **T53.7X1 Toxic effect of other halogen derivatives of aromatic hydrocarbons, accidental (unintentional)**
Toxic effects of other halogen derivatives of aromatic hydrocarbons NOS

    √7ᵗʰ **T53.7X2 Toxic effect of other halogen derivatives of aromatic hydrocarbons, intentional self-harm**

    √7ᵗʰ **T53.7X3 Toxic effect of other halogen derivatives of aromatic hydrocarbons, assault**

    √7ᵗʰ **T53.7X4 Toxic effect of other halogen derivatives of aromatic hydrocarbons, undetermined**

√5ᵗʰ **T53.9 Toxic effects of unspecified halogen derivatives of aliphatic and aromatic hydrocarbons**

  √x7ᵗʰ **T53.91 Toxic effect of unspecified halogen derivatives of aliphatic and aromatic hydrocarbons, accidental (unintentional)**

  √7ᵗʰ **T53.92 Toxic effect of unspecified halogen derivatives of aliphatic and aromatic hydrocarbons, intentional self-harm**

  √x7ᵗʰ **T53.93 Toxic effect of unspecified halogen derivatives of aliphatic and aromatic hydrocarbons, assault**

  √x7ᵗʰ **T53.94 Toxic effect of unspecified halogen derivatives of aliphatic and aromatic hydrocarbons, undetermined**

√4ᵗʰ **T54 Toxic effect of corrosive substances**

> The appropriate 7th character is to be added to each code from category T54.
> A   initial encounter
> D   subsequent encounter
> S   sequela

√5ᵗʰ **T54.0 Toxic effects of phenol and phenol homologues**

  √6ᵗʰ **T54.0X Toxic effects of** phenol and phenol homologues

    √7ᵗʰ **T54.0X1 Toxic effect of phenol and phenol homologues, accidental (unintentional)**
Toxic effects of phenol and phenol homologues NOS

    √7ᵗʰ **T54.0X2 Toxic effect of phenol and phenol homologues, intentional self-harm**

    √7ᵗʰ **T54.0X3 Toxic effect of phenol and phenol homologues, assault**

    √7ᵗʰ **T54.0X4 Toxic effect of phenol and phenol homologues, undetermined**

√5ᵗʰ **T54.1 Toxic effects of other corrosive organic compounds**

  √6ᵗʰ **T54.1X Toxic effects of** other corrosive organic compounds

    √7ᵗʰ **T54.1X1 Toxic effect of other corrosive organic compounds, accidental (unintentional)**
Toxic effects of other corrosive organic compounds NOS

    √7ᵗʰ **T54.1X2 Toxic effect of other corrosive organic compounds, intentional self-harm**

    √7ᵗʰ **T54.1X3 Toxic effect of other corrosive organic compounds, assault**

    √7ᵗʰ **T54.1X4 Toxic effect of other corrosive organic compounds, undetermined**

√5ᵗʰ **T54.2 Toxic effects of corrosive acids and acid-like substances**
Toxic effects of hydrochloric acid
Toxic effects of sulfuric acid

  √6ᵗʰ **T54.2X Toxic effects of corrosive** acids and acid-like substances

    √7ᵗʰ **T54.2X1 Toxic effect of corrosive acids and acid-like substances, accidental (unintentional)**
Toxic effects of corrosive acids and acid-like substances NOS

    √7ᵗʰ **T54.2X2 Toxic effect of corrosive acids and acid-like substances, intentional self-harm**

    √7ᵗʰ **T54.2X3 Toxic effect of corrosive acids and acid-like substances, assault**

    √7ᵗʰ **T54.2X4 Toxic effect of corrosive acids and acid-like substances, undetermined**

√5ᵗʰ **T54.3 Toxic effects of corrosive alkalis and alkali-like substances**
Toxic effects of potassium hydroxide
Toxic effects of sodium hydroxide

  √6ᵗʰ **T54.3X Toxic effects of corrosive** alkalis and alkali-like substances

    √7ᵗʰ **T54.3X1 Toxic effect of corrosive alkalis and alkali-like substances, accidental (unintentional)**
Toxic effects of corrosive alkalis and alkali-like substances NOS

    √7ᵗʰ **T54.3X2 Toxic effect of corrosive alkalis and alkali-like substances, intentional self-harm**

    √7ᵗʰ **T54.3X3 Toxic effect of corrosive alkalis and alkali-like substances, assault**

    √7ᵗʰ **T54.3X4 Toxic effect of corrosive alkalis and alkali-like substances, undetermined**

√5ᵗʰ **T54.9 Toxic effects of unspecified corrosive substance**

  √x7ᵗʰ **T54.91 Toxic effect of unspecified corrosive substance, accidental (unintentional)**

  √x7ᵗʰ **T54.92 Toxic effect of unspecified corrosive substance, intentional self-harm**

  √x7ᵗʰ **T54.93 Toxic effect of unspecified corrosive substance, assault**

  √x7ᵗʰ **T54.94 Toxic effect of unspecified corrosive substance, undetermined**

EXCLUDES1 Not coded here   EXCLUDES2 Not included here   N Newborn Age: 0   P Pediatric Age: 0-17   M Maternity Age: 12-55   A Adult Age: 15-124

964   ICD-10-CM 2014 (Draft)

☑4ᵗʰ **T55 Toxic effect of soaps and detergents**

> The appropriate 7th character is to be added to each code from category T55.
> A   initial encounter
> D   subsequent encounter
> S   sequela

☑5ᵗʰ **T55.0 Toxic effect of soaps**

    ☑6ᵗʰ **T55.0X Toxic effect of** soaps

       ☑7ᵗʰ **T55.0X1 Toxic effect of soaps,** accidental **(unintentional)**
          Toxic effect of soaps NOS

       ☑7ᵗʰ **T55.0X2 Toxic effect of soaps,** intentional self-harm

       ☑7ᵗʰ **T55.0X3 Toxic effect of soaps,** assault

       ☑7ᵗʰ **T55.0X4 Toxic effect of soaps,** undetermined

☑5ᵗʰ **T55.1 Toxic effect of detergents**

    ☑6ᵗʰ **T55.1X Toxic effect of** detergents

       ☑7ᵗʰ **T55.1X1 Toxic effect of detergents,** accidental **(unintentional)**
          Toxic effect of detergents NOS

       ☑7ᵗʰ **T55.1X2 Toxic effect of detergents,** intentional self-harm

       ☑7ᵗʰ **T55.1X3 Toxic effect of detergents,** assault

       ☑7ᵗʰ **T55.1X4 Toxic effect of detergents,** undetermined

☑4ᵗʰ **T56 Toxic effect of metals**

> **INCLUDES**   toxic effects of fumes and vapors of metals
>   toxic effects of metals from all sources, except medicinal substances
> Use additional code to identify any retained metal foreign body, if applicable (Z18.0-, T18.1-)
> **EXCLUDES 1**   *arsenic and its compounds (T57.0)*
>   *manganese and its compounds (T57.2)*

> The appropriate 7th character is to be added to each code from category T56.
> A   initial encounter
> D   subsequent encounter
> S   sequela

☑5ᵗʰ **T56.0 Toxic effects of lead and its compounds**

    ☑6ᵗʰ **T56.0X Toxic effects of** lead **and its compounds**

       ☑7ᵗʰ **T56.0X1 Toxic effect of lead and its compounds,** accidental **(unintentional)**
          Toxic effects of lead and its compounds NOS

       ☑7ᵗʰ **T56.0X2 Toxic effect of lead and its compounds,** intentional self-harm

       ☑7ᵗʰ **T56.0X3 Toxic effect of lead and its compounds,** assault

       ☑7ᵗʰ **T56.0X4 Toxic effect of lead and its compounds,** undetermined

☑5ᵗʰ **T56.1 Toxic effects of mercury and its compounds**

    ☑6ᵗʰ **T56.1X Toxic effects of** mercury **and its compounds**

       ☑7ᵗʰ **T56.1X1 Toxic effect of mercury and its compounds,** accidental **(unintentional)**
          Toxic effects of mercury and its compounds NOS

       ☑7ᵗʰ **T56.1X2 Toxic effect of mercury and its compounds,** intentional self-harm

       ☑7ᵗʰ **T56.1X3 Toxic effect of mercury and its compounds,** assault

       ☑7ᵗʰ **T56.1X4 Toxic effect of mercury and its compounds,** undetermined

☑5ᵗʰ **T56.2 Toxic effects of chromium and its compounds**

    ☑6ᵗʰ **T56.2X Toxic effects of** chromium **and its compounds**

       ☑7ᵗʰ **T56.2X1 Toxic effect of chromium and its compounds,** accidental **(unintentional)**
          Toxic effects of chromium and its compounds NOS

       ☑7ᵗʰ **T56.2X2 Toxic effect of chromium and its compounds,** intentional self-harm

       ☑7ᵗʰ **T56.2X3 Toxic effect of chromium and its compounds,** assault

       ☑7ᵗʰ **T56.2X4 Toxic effect of chromium and its compounds,** undetermined

☑5ᵗʰ **T56.3 Toxic effects of** cadmium **and its compounds**

    ☑6ᵗʰ **T56.3X Toxic effects of cadmium and its compounds**

       ☑7ᵗʰ **T56.3X1 Toxic effect of cadmium and its compounds,** accidental **(unintentional)**
          Toxic effects of cadmium and its compounds NOS

       ☑7ᵗʰ **T56.3X2 Toxic effect of cadmium and its compounds,** intentional self-harm

       ☑7ᵗʰ **T56.3X3 Toxic effect of cadmium and its compounds,** assault

       ☑7ᵗʰ **T56.3X4 Toxic effect of cadmium and its compounds,** undetermined

☑5ᵗʰ **T56.4 Toxic effects of copper and its compounds**

    ☑6ᵗʰ **T56.4X Toxic effects of** copper **and its compounds**

       ☑7ᵗʰ **T56.4X1 Toxic effect of copper and its compounds,** accidental **(unintentional)**
          Toxic effects of copper and its compounds NOS

       ☑7ᵗʰ **T56.4X2 Toxic effect of copper and its compounds,** intentional self-harm

       ☑7ᵗʰ **T56.4X3 Toxic effect of copper and its compounds,** assault

       ☑7ᵗʰ **T56.4X4 Toxic effect of copper and its compounds,** undetermined

☑5ᵗʰ **T56.5 Toxic effects of zinc and its compounds**

    ☑6ᵗʰ **T56.5X Toxic effects of** zinc **and its compounds**

       ☑7ᵗʰ **T56.5X1 Toxic effect of zinc and its compounds,** accidental **(unintentional)**
          Toxic effects of zinc and its compounds NOS

       ☑7ᵗʰ **T56.5X2 Toxic effect of zinc and its compounds,** intentional self-harm

       ☑7ᵗʰ **T56.5X3 Toxic effect of zinc and its compounds,** assault

       ☑7ᵗʰ **T56.5X4 Toxic effect of zinc and its compounds,** undetermined

☑5ᵗʰ **T56.6 Toxic effects of tin and its compounds**

    ☑6ᵗʰ **T56.6X Toxic effects of** tin **and its compounds**

       ☑7ᵗʰ **T56.6X1 Toxic effect of tin and its compounds,** accidental **(unintentional)**
          Toxic effects of tin and its compounds NOS

       ☑7ᵗʰ **T56.6X2 Toxic effect of tin and its compounds,** intentional self-harm

       ☑7ᵗʰ **T56.6X3 Toxic effect of tin and its compounds,** assault

       ☑7ᵗʰ **T56.6X4 Toxic effect of tin and its compounds,** undetermined

☑5ᵗʰ **T56.7 Toxic effects of beryllium and its compounds**

    ☑6ᵗʰ **T56.7X Toxic effects of** beryllium **and its compounds**

       ☑7ᵗʰ **T56.7X1 Toxic effect of beryllium and its compounds,** accidental **(unintentional)**
          Toxic effects of beryllium and its compounds NOS

       ☑7ᵗʰ **T56.7X2 Toxic effect of beryllium and its compounds,** intentional self-harm

       ☑7ᵗʰ **T56.7X3 Toxic effect of beryllium and its compounds,** assault

       ☑7ᵗʰ **T56.7X4 Toxic effect of beryllium and its compounds,** undetermined

☑5ᵗʰ **T56.8 Toxic effects of** other metals

    ☑6ᵗʰ **T56.81 Toxic effect of** thallium

       ☑7ᵗʰ **T56.811 Toxic effect of thallium,** accidental **(unintentional)**
          Toxic effect of thallium NOS

       ☑7ᵗʰ **T56.812 Toxic effect of thallium,** intentional self-harm

       ☑7ᵗʰ **T56.813 Toxic effect of thallium,** assault

       ☑7ᵗʰ **T56.814 Toxic effect of thallium,** undetermined

    ☑6ᵗʰ **T56.89 Toxic effects of** other metals

       ☑7ᵗʰ **T56.891 Toxic effect of other metals,** accidental **(unintentional)**
          Toxic effects of other metals NOS

       ☑7ᵗʰ **T56.892 Toxic effect of other metals,** intentional self-harm

       ☑7ᵗʰ **T56.893 Toxic effect of other metals,** assault

---

☑ Additional Character Required   ✔x7ᵗʰ Xtension Alert   Unspecified Code   Other Specified Code   Manifestation Code   ►◄ Revised Text   ● New Code   ▲ Revised Code Title

Injury, Poisoning and Certain Other Consequences of External Causes

T56.894–T58.91

√7ᵗʰ **T56.894** **Toxic effect of other metals, undetermined**

√5ᵗʰ **T56.9** **Toxic effects of unspecified metal**

√x7ᵗʰ **T56.91** **Toxic effect of unspecified metal, accidental (unintentional)**

√x7ᵗʰ **T56.92** **Toxic effect of unspecified metal, intentional self-harm**

√x7ᵗʰ **T56.93** **Toxic effect of unspecified metal, assault**

√x7ᵗʰ **T56.94** **Toxic effect of unspecified metal, undetermined**

√4ᵗʰ **T57** **Toxic effect of other inorganic substances**

> The appropriate 7th character is to be added to each code from category T57.
> A   initial encounter
> D   subsequent encounter
> S   sequela

√5ᵗʰ **T57.0** **Toxic effect of arsenic and its compounds**

√6ᵗʰ **T57.0X** **Toxic effect of arsenic and its compounds**

√7ᵗʰ **T57.0X1** **Toxic effect of arsenic and its compounds, accidental (unintentional)**
Toxic effect of arsenic and its compounds NOS

√7ᵗʰ **T57.0X2** **Toxic effect of arsenic and its compounds, intentional self-harm**

√7ᵗʰ **T57.0X3** **Toxic effect of arsenic and its compounds, assault**

√7ᵗʰ **T57.0X4** **Toxic effect of arsenic and its compounds, undetermined**

√5ᵗʰ **T57.1** **Toxic effect of phosphorus and its compounds**
EXCLUDES 1   *organophosphate insecticides (T60.0)*

√6ᵗʰ **T57.1X** **Toxic effect of phosphorus and its compounds**

√7ᵗʰ **T57.1X1** **Toxic effect of phosphorus and its compounds, accidental (unintentional)**
Toxic effect of phosphorus and its compounds NOS

√7ᵗʰ **T57.1X2** **Toxic effect of phosphorus and its compounds, intentional self-harm**

√7ᵗʰ **T57.1X3** **Toxic effect of phosphorus and its compounds, assault**

√7ᵗʰ **T57.1X4** **Toxic effect of phosphorus and its compounds, undetermined**

√5ᵗʰ **T57.2** **Toxic effect of manganese and its compounds**

√6ᵗʰ **T57.2X** **Toxic effect of manganese and its compounds**

√7ᵗʰ **T57.2X1** **Toxic effect of manganese and its compounds, accidental (unintentional)**
Toxic effect of manganese and its compounds NOS

√7ᵗʰ **T57.2X2** **Toxic effect of manganese and its compounds, intentional self-harm**

√7ᵗʰ **T57.2X3** **Toxic effect of manganese and its compounds, assault**

√7ᵗʰ **T57.2X4** **Toxic effect of manganese and its compounds, undetermined**

√5ᵗʰ **T57.3** **Toxic effect of hydrogen cyanide**

√6ᵗʰ **T57.3X** **Toxic effect of hydrogen cyanide**

√7ᵗʰ **T57.3X1** **Toxic effect of hydrogen cyanide, accidental (unintentional)**
Toxic effect of hydrogen cyanide NOS

√7ᵗʰ **T57.3X2** **Toxic effect of hydrogen cyanide, intentional self-harm**

√7ᵗʰ **T57.3X3** **Toxic effect of hydrogen cyanide, assault**

√7ᵗʰ **T57.3X4** **Toxic effect of hydrogen cyanide, undetermined**

√5ᵗʰ **T57.8** **Toxic effect of other specified inorganic substances**

√6ᵗʰ **T57.8X** **Toxic effect of other specified inorganic substances**

√7ᵗʰ **T57.8X1** **Toxic effect of other specified inorganic substances, accidental (unintentional)**
Toxic effect of other specified inorganic substances NOS

√7ᵗʰ **T57.8X2** **Toxic effect of other specified inorganic substances, intentional self-harm**

√7ᵗʰ **T57.8X3** **Toxic effect of other specified inorganic substances, assault**

√7ᵗʰ **T57.8X4** **Toxic effect of other specified inorganic substances, undetermined**

√5ᵗʰ **T57.9** **Toxic effect of unspecified inorganic substance**

√x7ᵗʰ **T57.91** **Toxic effect of unspecified inorganic substance, accidental (unintentional)**

√x7ᵗʰ **T57.92** **Toxic effect of unspecified inorganic substance, intentional self-harm**

√x7ᵗʰ **T57.93** **Toxic effect of unspecified inorganic substance, assault**

√x7ᵗʰ **T57.94** **Toxic effect of unspecified inorganic substance, undetermined**

√4ᵗʰ **T58** **Toxic effect of carbon monoxide**
INCLUDES   asphyxiation from carbon monoxide
toxic effect of carbon monoxide from all sources

> The appropriate 7th character is to be added to each code from category T58.
> A   initial encounter
> D   subsequent encounter
> S   sequela

√5ᵗʰ **T58.0** **Toxic effect of carbon monoxide from motor vehicle exhaust**
Toxic effect of exhaust gas from gas engine
Toxic effect of exhaust gas from motor pump

√x7ᵗʰ **T58.01** **Toxic effect of carbon monoxide from motor vehicle exhaust, accidental (unintentional)**

√x7ᵗʰ **T58.02** **Toxic effect of carbon monoxide from motor vehicle exhaust, intentional self-harm**

√x7ᵗʰ **T58.03** **Toxic effect of carbon monoxide from motor vehicle exhaust, assault**

√x7ᵗʰ **T58.04** **Toxic effect of carbon monoxide from motor vehicle exhaust, undetermined**

√5ᵗʰ **T58.1** **Toxic effect of carbon monoxide from utility gas**
Toxic effect of acetylene
Toxic effect of gas NOS used for lighting, heating, cooking
Toxic effect of water gas

√x7ᵗʰ **T58.11** **Toxic effect of carbon monoxide from utility gas, accidental (unintentional)**

√x7ᵗʰ **T58.12** **Toxic effect of carbon monoxide from utility gas, intentional self-harm**

√x7ᵗʰ **T58.13** **Toxic effect of carbon monoxide from utility gas, assault**

√x7ᵗʰ **T58.14** **Toxic effect of carbon monoxide from utility gas, undetermined**

√5ᵗʰ **T58.2** **Toxic effect of carbon monoxide from incomplete combustion of other domestic fuels**
Toxic effect of carbon monoxide from incomplete combustion of coal, coke, kerosene, wood

√6ᵗʰ **T58.2X** **Toxic effect of carbon monoxide from incomplete combustion of other domestic fuels**

√7ᵗʰ **T58.2X1** **Toxic effect of carbon monoxide from incomplete combustion of other domestic fuels, accidental (unintentional)**

√7ᵗʰ **T58.2X2** **Toxic effect of carbon monoxide from incomplete combustion of other domestic fuels, intentional self-harm**

√7ᵗʰ **T58.2X3** **Toxic effect of carbon monoxide from incomplete combustion of other domestic fuels, assault**

√7ᵗʰ **T58.2X4** **Toxic effect of carbon monoxide from incomplete combustion of other domestic fuels, undetermined**

√5ᵗʰ **T58.8** **Toxic effect of carbon monoxide from other source**
Toxic effect of carbon monoxide from blast furnace gas
Toxic effect of carbon monoxide from fuels in industrial use
Toxic effect of carbon monoxide from kiln vapor

√6ᵗʰ **T58.8X** **Toxic effect of carbon monoxide from other source**

√7ᵗʰ **T58.8X1** **Toxic effect of carbon monoxide from other source, accidental (unintentional)**

√7ᵗʰ **T58.8X2** **Toxic effect of carbon monoxide from other source, intentional self-harm**

√7ᵗʰ **T58.8X3** **Toxic effect of carbon monoxide from other source, assault**

√7ᵗʰ **T58.8X4** **Toxic effect of carbon monoxide from other source, undetermined**

√5ᵗʰ **T58.9** **Toxic effect of carbon monoxide from unspecified source**

√x7ᵗʰ **T58.91** **Toxic effect of carbon monoxide from unspecified source, accidental (unintentional)**

EXCLUDES 1 Not coded here   EXCLUDES 2 Not included here   N Newborn Age: 0   P Pediatric Age: 0-17   M Maternity Age: 12-55   A Adult Age: 15-124

√x7ᵗʰ **T58.92** **Toxic effect of carbon monoxide from unspecified source, intentional self-harm**

√x7ᵗʰ **T58.93** **Toxic effect of carbon monoxide from unspecified source, assault**

√x7ᵗʰ **T58.94** **Toxic effect of carbon monoxide from unspecified source, undetermined**

√4ᵗʰ **T59** **Toxic effect of other gases, fumes and vapors**
> INCLUDES   aerosol propellants
> EXCLUDES 1   *chlorofluorocarbons (T53.5)*

> The appropriate 7th character is to be added to each code from category T59.
> A   initial encounter
> D   subsequent encounter
> S   sequela

√5ᵗʰ **T59.0** **Toxic effect of nitrogen oxides**

√6ᵗʰ **T59.0X** **Toxic effect of nitrogen oxides**

√7ᵗʰ **T59.0X1** **Toxic effect of nitrogen oxides, accidental (unintentional)**
Toxic effect of nitrogen oxides NOS

√7ᵗʰ **T59.0X2** **Toxic effect of nitrogen oxides, intentional self-harm**

√7ᵗʰ **T59.0X3** **Toxic effect of nitrogen oxides, assault**

√7ᵗʰ **T59.0X4** **Toxic effect of nitrogen oxides, undetermined**

√5ᵗʰ **T59.1** **Toxic effect of sulfur dioxide**

√6ᵗʰ **T59.1X** **Toxic effect of sulfur dioxide**

√7ᵗʰ **T59.1X1** **Toxic effect of sulfur dioxide, accidental (unintentional)**
Toxic effect of sulfur dioxide NOS

√7ᵗʰ **T59.1X2** **Toxic effect of sulfur dioxide, intentional self-harm**

√7ᵗʰ **T59.1X3** **Toxic effect of sulfur dioxide, assault**

√7ᵗʰ **T59.1X4** **Toxic effect of sulfur dioxide, undetermined**

√5ᵗʰ **T59.2** **Toxic effect of formaldehyde**

√6ᵗʰ **T59.2X** **Toxic effect of formaldehyde**

√7ᵗʰ **T59.2X1** **Toxic effect of formaldehyde, accidental (unintentional)**
Toxic effect of formaldehyde NOS

√7ᵗʰ **T59.2X2** **Toxic effect of formaldehyde, intentional self-harm**

√7ᵗʰ **T59.2X3** **Toxic effect of formaldehyde, assault**

√7ᵗʰ **T59.2X4** **Toxic effect of formaldehyde, undetermined**

√5ᵗʰ **T59.3** **Toxic effect of lacrimogenic gas**
Toxic effect of tear gas

√6ᵗʰ **T59.3X** **Toxic effect of lacrimogenic gas**

√7ᵗʰ **T59.3X1** **Toxic effect of lacrimogenic gas, accidental (unintentional)**
Toxic effect of lacrimogenic gas NOS

√7ᵗʰ **T59.3X2** **Toxic effect of lacrimogenic gas, intentional self-harm**

√7ᵗʰ **T59.3X3** **Toxic effect of lacrimogenic gas, assault**

√7ᵗʰ **T59.3X4** **Toxic effect of lacrimogenic gas, undetermined**

√5ᵗʰ **T59.4** **Toxic effect of chlorine gas**

√6ᵗʰ **T59.4X** **Toxic effect of chlorine gas**

√7ᵗʰ **T59.4X1** **Toxic effect of chlorine gas, accidental (unintentional)**
Toxic effect of chlorine gas NOS

√7ᵗʰ **T59.4X2** **Toxic effect of chlorine gas, intentional self-harm**

√7ᵗʰ **T59.4X3** **Toxic effect of chlorine gas, assault**

√7ᵗʰ **T59.4X4** **Toxic effect of chlorine gas, undetermined**

√5ᵗʰ **T59.5** **Toxic effect of fluorine gas and hydrogen fluoride**

√6ᵗʰ **T59.5X** **Toxic effect of fluorine gas and hydrogen fluoride**

√7ᵗʰ **T59.5X1** **Toxic effect of fluorine gas and hydrogen fluoride, accidental (unintentional)**
Toxic effect of fluorine gas and hydrogen fluoride NOS

√7ᵗʰ **T59.5X2** **Toxic effect of fluorine gas and hydrogen fluoride, intentional self-harm**

√7ᵗʰ **T59.5X3** **Toxic effect of fluorine gas and hydrogen fluoride, assault**

√7ᵗʰ **T59.5X4** **Toxic effect of fluorine gas and hydrogen fluoride, undetermined**

√5ᵗʰ **T59.6** **Toxic effect of hydrogen sulfide**

√6ᵗʰ **T59.6X** **Toxic effect of hydrogen sulfide**

√7ᵗʰ **T59.6X1** **Toxic effect of hydrogen sulfide, accidental (unintentional)**
Toxic effect of hydrogen sulfide NOS

√7ᵗʰ **T59.6X2** **Toxic effect of hydrogen sulfide, intentional self-harm**

√7ᵗʰ **T59.6X3** **Toxic effect of hydrogen sulfide, assault**

√7ᵗʰ **T59.6X4** **Toxic effect of hydrogen sulfide, undetermined**

√5ᵗʰ **T59.7** **Toxic effect of carbon dioxide**

√6ᵗʰ **T59.7X** **Toxic effect of carbon dioxide**

√7ᵗʰ **T59.7X1** **Toxic effect of carbon dioxide, accidental (unintentional)**
Toxic effect of carbon dioxide NOS

√7ᵗʰ **T59.7X2** **Toxic effect of carbon dioxide, intentional self-harm**

√7ᵗʰ **T59.7X3** **Toxic effect of carbon dioxide, assault**

√7ᵗʰ **T59.7X4** **Toxic effect of carbon dioxide, undetermined**

√5ᵗʰ **T59.8** **Toxic effect of other specified gases, fumes and vapors**

√6ᵗʰ **T59.81** **Toxic effect of smoke**
Smoke inhalation
> EXCLUDES 2   *toxic effect of cigarette (tobacco) smoke (T65.22-)*

√7ᵗʰ **T59.811** **Toxic effect of smoke, accidental (unintentional)**
Toxic effect of smoke NOS

√7ᵗʰ **T59.812** **Toxic effect of smoke, intentional self-harm**

√7ᵗʰ **T59.813** **Toxic effect of smoke, assault**

√7ᵗʰ **T59.814** **Toxic effect of smoke, undetermined**

√6ᵗʰ **T59.89** **Toxic effect of other specified gases, fumes and vapors**

√7ᵗʰ **T59.891** **Toxic effect of other specified gases, fumes and vapors, accidental (unintentional)**

√7ᵗʰ **T59.892** **Toxic effect of other specified gases, fumes and vapors, intentional self-harm**

√7ᵗʰ **T59.893** **Toxic effect of other specified gases, fumes and vapors, assault**

√7ᵗʰ **T59.894** **Toxic effect of other specified gases, fumes and vapors, undetermined**

√5ᵗʰ **T59.9** **Toxic effect of unspecified gases, fumes and vapors**

√x7ᵗʰ **T59.91** **Toxic effect of unspecified gases, fumes and vapors, accidental (unintentional)**

√x7ᵗʰ **T59.92** **Toxic effect of unspecified gases, fumes and vapors, intentional self-harm**

√x7ᵗʰ **T59.93** **Toxic effect of unspecified gases, fumes and vapors, assault**

√x7ᵗʰ **T59.94** **Toxic effect of unspecified gases, fumes and vapors, undetermined**

√4ᵗʰ **T60** **Toxic effect of pesticides**
> INCLUDES   toxic effect of wood preservatives

> The appropriate 7th character is to be added to each code from category T60.
> A   initial encounter
> D   subsequent encounter
> S   sequela

√5ᵗʰ **T60.0** **Toxic effect of organophosphate and carbamate insecticides**

√6ᵗʰ **T60.0X** **Toxic effect of organophosphate and carbamate insecticides**

√7ᵗʰ **T60.0X1** **Toxic effect of organophosphate and carbamate insecticides, accidental (unintentional)**
Toxic effect of organophosphate and carbamate insecticides NOS

√7ᵗʰ **T60.0X2** **Toxic effect of organophosphate and carbamate insecticides, intentional self-harm**

☑ Additional Character Required   √x7ᵗʰ Xtension Alert   Unspecified Code   Other Specified Code   Manifestation Code   ►◄ Revised Text   ● New Code   ▲ Revised Code Title

ICD-10-CM 2014 (Draft)

967

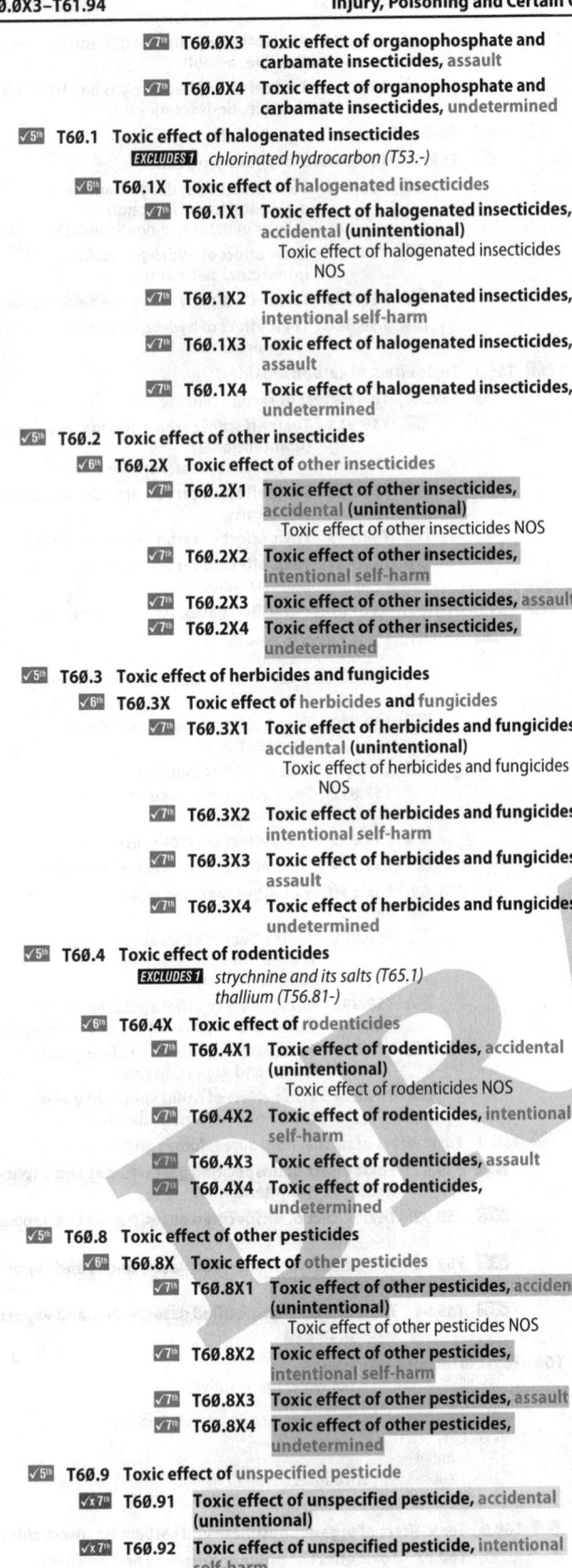

   ☑7ᵗʰ **T60.0X3** **Toxic effect of organophosphate and carbamate insecticides,** assault

   ☑7ᵗʰ **T60.0X4** **Toxic effect of organophosphate and carbamate insecticides,** undetermined

☑5ᵗʰ **T60.1** **Toxic effect of halogenated insecticides**
EXCLUDES 1   chlorinated hydrocarbon (T53.-)

   ☑6ᵗʰ **T60.1X** **Toxic effect of** halogenated insecticides

      ☑7ᵗʰ **T60.1X1** **Toxic effect of halogenated insecticides,** accidental (unintentional)
          Toxic effect of halogenated insecticides NOS

      ☑7ᵗʰ **T60.1X2** **Toxic effect of halogenated insecticides,** intentional self-harm

      ☑7ᵗʰ **T60.1X3** **Toxic effect of halogenated insecticides,** assault

      ☑7ᵗʰ **T60.1X4** **Toxic effect of halogenated insecticides,** undetermined

☑5ᵗʰ **T60.2** **Toxic effect of other insecticides**

   ☑6ᵗʰ **T60.2X** **Toxic effect of** other insecticides

      ☑7ᵗʰ **T60.2X1** **Toxic effect of other insecticides, accidental (unintentional)**
          Toxic effect of other insecticides NOS

      ☑7ᵗʰ **T60.2X2** **Toxic effect of other insecticides, intentional self-harm**

      ☑7ᵗʰ **T60.2X3** **Toxic effect of other insecticides,** assault

      ☑7ᵗʰ **T60.2X4** **Toxic effect of other insecticides, undetermined**

☑5ᵗʰ **T60.3** **Toxic effect of herbicides and fungicides**

   ☑6ᵗʰ **T60.3X** **Toxic effect of** herbicides and fungicides

      ☑7ᵗʰ **T60.3X1** **Toxic effect of herbicides and fungicides,** accidental (unintentional)
          Toxic effect of herbicides and fungicides NOS

      ☑7ᵗʰ **T60.3X2** **Toxic effect of herbicides and fungicides,** intentional self-harm

      ☑7ᵗʰ **T60.3X3** **Toxic effect of herbicides and fungicides,** assault

      ☑7ᵗʰ **T60.3X4** **Toxic effect of herbicides and fungicides,** undetermined

☑5ᵗʰ **T60.4** **Toxic effect of rodenticides**
EXCLUDES 1   strychnine and its salts (T65.1)
         thallium (T56.81-)

   ☑6ᵗʰ **T60.4X** **Toxic effect of** rodenticides

      ☑7ᵗʰ **T60.4X1** **Toxic effect of rodenticides,** accidental (unintentional)
          Toxic effect of rodenticides NOS

      ☑7ᵗʰ **T60.4X2** **Toxic effect of rodenticides,** intentional self-harm

      ☑7ᵗʰ **T60.4X3** **Toxic effect of rodenticides,** assault

      ☑7ᵗʰ **T60.4X4** **Toxic effect of rodenticides,** undetermined

☑5ᵗʰ **T60.8** **Toxic effect of other pesticides**

   ☑6ᵗʰ **T60.8X** **Toxic effect of** other pesticides

      ☑7ᵗʰ **T60.8X1** **Toxic effect of other pesticides,** accidental (unintentional)
          Toxic effect of other pesticides NOS

      ☑7ᵗʰ **T60.8X2** **Toxic effect of other pesticides, intentional self-harm**

      ☑7ᵗʰ **T60.8X3** **Toxic effect of other pesticides,** assault

      ☑7ᵗʰ **T60.8X4** **Toxic effect of other pesticides, undetermined**

☑5ᵗʰ **T60.9** **Toxic effect of** unspecified pesticide

   ☑x7ᵗʰ **T60.91** **Toxic effect of unspecified pesticide,** accidental (unintentional)

   ☑x7ᵗʰ **T60.92** **Toxic effect of unspecified pesticide, intentional self-harm**

   ☑x7ᵗʰ **T60.93** **Toxic effect of unspecified pesticide,** assault

   ☑x7ᵗʰ **T60.94** **Toxic effect of unspecified pesticide,** undetermined

---

☑4ᵗʰ **T61** **Toxic effect of noxious substances eaten as seafood**
EXCLUDES 1   *allergic reaction to food, such as:*
      anaphylactic reaction or shock due to adverse food reaction (T78.0-)
      dermatitis (L23.6, L25.4, L27.2)
      gastroenteritis (noninfective) (K52.2)
    bacterial foodborne intoxications (A05.-)
    toxic effect of aflatoxin and other mycotoxins (T64)
    toxic effect of cyanides (T65.0-)
    toxic effect of harmful algae bloom (T65.82-)
    toxic effect of hydrogen cyanide (T57.3-)
    toxic effect of mercury (T56.1-)
    toxic effect of red tide (T65.82-)

The appropriate 7th character is to be added to each code from category T61.
A   initial encounter
D   subsequent encounter
S   sequela

☑5ᵗʰ **T61.0** **Ciguatera fish poisoning**

   ☑x7ᵗʰ **T61.01** **Ciguatera fish poisoning,** accidental (unintentional)

   ☑x7ᵗʰ **T61.02** **Ciguatera fish poisoning,** intentional self-harm

   ☑x7ᵗʰ **T61.03** **Ciguatera fish poisoning,** assault

   ☑x7ᵗʰ **T61.04** **Ciguatera fish poisoning,** undetermined

☑5ᵗʰ **T61.1** **Scombroid fish poisoning**
      Histamine-like syndrome

   ☑x7ᵗʰ **T61.11** **Scombroid fish poisoning,** accidental (unintentional)

   ☑x7ᵗʰ **T61.12** **Scombroid fish poisoning,** intentional self-harm

   ☑x7ᵗʰ **T61.13** **Scombroid fish poisoning,** assault

   ☑x7ᵗʰ **T61.14** **Scombroid fish poisoning,** undetermined

☑5ᵗʰ **T61.7** **Other fish and shellfish poisoning**

   ☑6ᵗʰ **T61.77** **Other** fish **poisoning**

      ☑7ᵗʰ **T61.771** **Other fish poisoning,** accidental (unintentional)

      ☑7ᵗʰ **T61.772** **Other fish poisoning,** intentional self-harm

      ☑7ᵗʰ **T61.773** **Other fish poisoning,** assault

      ☑7ᵗʰ **T61.774** **Other fish poisoning,** undetermined

   ☑6ᵗʰ **T61.78** **Other** shellfish **poisoning**

      ☑7ᵗʰ **T61.781** **Other shellfish poisoning,** accidental (unintentional)

      ☑7ᵗʰ **T61.782** **Other shellfish poisoning,** intentional self-harm

      ☑7ᵗʰ **T61.783** **Other shellfish poisoning,** assault

      ☑7ᵗʰ **T61.784** **Other shellfish poisoning,** undetermined

☑5ᵗʰ **T61.8** **Toxic effect of other seafood**

   ☑6ᵗʰ **T61.8X** **Toxic effect of** other seafood

      ☑7ᵗʰ **T61.8X1** **Toxic effect of other seafood,** accidental (unintentional)

      ☑7ᵗʰ **T61.8X2** **Toxic effect of other seafood,** intentional self-harm

      ☑7ᵗʰ **T61.8X3** **Toxic effect of other seafood,** assault

      ☑7ᵗʰ **T61.8X4** **Toxic effect of other seafood,** undetermined

☑5ᵗʰ **T61.9** **Toxic effect of** unspecified seafood

   ☑x7ᵗʰ **T61.91** **Toxic effect of unspecified seafood,** accidental (unintentional)

   ☑x7ᵗʰ **T61.92** **Toxic effect of unspecified seafood,** intentional self-harm

   ☑x7ᵗʰ **T61.93** **Toxic effect of unspecified seafood,** assault

   ☑x7ᵗʰ **T61.94** **Toxic effect of unspecified seafood,** undetermined

---

EXCLUDES 1 Not coded here   EXCLUDES 2 Not included here   N Newborn Age: 0   P Pediatric Age: 0-17   M Maternity Age: 12-55   A Adult Age: 15-124

                                                          ICD-10-CM 2014 (Draft)

☑4ᵗʰ T62 Toxic effect of other noxious substances eaten as food

EXCLUDES 1 allergic reaction to food, such as:
anaphylactic shock (reaction) due to adverse food reaction (T78.0-)
dermatitis (L23.6, L25.4, L27.2)
gastroenteritis (noninfective) (K52.2)
bacterial food borne intoxications (A05.-)
toxic effect of aflatoxin and other mycotoxins (T64)
toxic effect of cyanides (T65.0-)
toxic effect of hydrogen cyanide (T57.3-)
toxic effect of mercury (T56.1-)

The appropriate 7th character is to be added to each code from category T62.
A initial encounter
D subsequent encounter
S sequela

☑5ᵗʰ T62.0 Toxic effect of ingested mushrooms

☑6ᵗʰ T62.0X Toxic effect of ingested mushrooms

☑7ᵗʰ T62.0X1 Toxic effect of ingested mushrooms, accidental (unintentional)
Toxic effect of ingested mushrooms NOS

☑7ᵗʰ T62.0X2 Toxic effect of ingested mushrooms, intentional self-harm

☑7ᵗʰ T62.0X3 Toxic effect of ingested mushrooms, assault

☑7ᵗʰ T62.0X4 Toxic effect of ingested mushrooms, undetermined

☑5ᵗʰ T62.1 Toxic effect of ingested berries

☑6ᵗʰ T62.1X Toxic effect of ingested berries

☑7ᵗʰ T62.1X1 Toxic effect of ingested berries, accidental (unintentional)
Toxic effect of ingested berries NOS

☑7ᵗʰ T62.1X2 Toxic effect of ingested berries, intentional self-harm

☑7ᵗʰ T62.1X3 Toxic effect of ingested berries, assault

☑7ᵗʰ T62.1X4 Toxic effect of ingested berries, undetermined

☑5ᵗʰ T62.2 Toxic effect of other ingested (parts of) plant(s)

☑6ᵗʰ T62.2X Toxic effect of other ingested (parts of) plant(s)

☑7ᵗʰ T62.2X1 Toxic effect of other ingested (parts of) plant(s), accidental (unintentional)
Toxic effect of other ingested (parts of) plant(s) NOS

☑7ᵗʰ T62.2X2 Toxic effect of other ingested (parts of) plant(s), intentional self-harm

☑7ᵗʰ T62.2X3 Toxic effect of other ingested (parts of) plant(s), assault

☑7ᵗʰ T62.2X4 Toxic effect of other ingested (parts of) plant(s), undetermined

☑5ᵗʰ T62.8 Toxic effect of other specified noxious substances eaten as food

☑6ᵗʰ T62.8X Toxic effect of other specified noxious substances eaten as food

☑7ᵗʰ T62.8X1 Toxic effect of other specified noxious substances eaten as food, accidental (unintentional)
Toxic effect of other specified noxious substances eaten as food NOS

☑7ᵗʰ T62.8X2 Toxic effect of other specified noxious substances eaten as food, intentional self-harm

☑7ᵗʰ T62.8X3 Toxic effect of other specified noxious substances eaten as food, assault

☑7ᵗʰ T62.8X4 Toxic effect of other specified noxious substances eaten as food, undetermined

☑5ᵗʰ T62.9 Toxic effect of unspecified noxious substance eaten as food

☑x7ᵗʰ T62.91 Toxic effect of unspecified noxious substance eaten as food, accidental (unintentional)
Toxic effect of unspecified noxious substance eaten as food NOS

☑x7ᵗʰ T62.92 Toxic effect of unspecified noxious substance eaten as food, intentional self-harm

☑x7ᵗʰ T62.93 Toxic effect of unspecified noxious substance eaten as food, assault

☑x7ᵗʰ T62.94 Toxic effect of unspecified noxious substance eaten as food, undetermined

☑4ᵗʰ T63 Toxic effect of contact with venomous animals and plants

INCLUDES bite or touch of venomous animal
pricked or stuck by thorn or leaf
EXCLUDES 2 ingestion of toxic animal or plant (T61-, T62-))

The appropriate 7th character is to be added to each code from category T63.
A initial encounter
D subsequent encounter
S sequela

☑5ᵗʰ T63.0 Toxic effect of snake venom

☑6ᵗʰ T63.00 Toxic effect of unspecified snake venom

☑7ᵗʰ T63.001 Toxic effect of unspecified snake venom, accidental (unintentional)
Toxic effect of unspecified snake venom NOS

☑7ᵗʰ T63.002 Toxic effect of unspecified snake venom, intentional self-harm

☑7ᵗʰ T63.003 Toxic effect of unspecified snake venom, assault

☑7ᵗʰ T63.004 Toxic effect of unspecified snake venom, undetermined

☑6ᵗʰ T63.01 Toxic effect of rattlesnake venom

☑7ᵗʰ T63.011 Toxic effect of rattlesnake venom, accidental (unintentional)
Toxic effect of rattlesnake venom NOS

☑7ᵗʰ T63.012 Toxic effect of rattlesnake venom, intentional self-harm

☑7ᵗʰ T63.013 Toxic effect of rattlesnake venom, assault

☑7ᵗʰ T63.014 Toxic effect of rattlesnake venom, undetermined

☑6ᵗʰ T63.02 Toxic effect of coral snake venom

☑7ᵗʰ T63.021 Toxic effect of coral snake venom, accidental (unintentional)
Toxic effect of coral snake venom NOS

☑7ᵗʰ T63.022 Toxic effect of coral snake venom, intentional self-harm

☑7ᵗʰ T63.023 Toxic effect of coral snake venom, assault

☑7ᵗʰ T63.024 Toxic effect of coral snake venom, undetermined

☑6ᵗʰ T63.03 Toxic effect of taipan venom

☑7ᵗʰ T63.031 Toxic effect of taipan venom, accidental (unintentional)
Toxic effect of taipan venom NOS

☑7ᵗʰ T63.032 Toxic effect of taipan venom, intentional self-harm

☑7ᵗʰ T63.033 Toxic effect of taipan venom, assault

☑7ᵗʰ T63.034 Toxic effect of taipan venom, undetermined

☑6ᵗʰ T63.04 Toxic effect of cobra venom

☑7ᵗʰ T63.041 Toxic effect of cobra venom, accidental (unintentional)
Toxic effect of cobra venom NOS

☑7ᵗʰ T63.042 Toxic effect of cobra venom, intentional self-harm

☑7ᵗʰ T63.043 Toxic effect of cobra venom, assault

☑7ᵗʰ T63.044 Toxic effect of cobra venom, undetermined

☑6ᵗʰ T63.06 Toxic effect of venom of other North and South American snake

☑7ᵗʰ T63.061 Toxic effect of venom of other North and South American snake, accidental (unintentional)
Toxic effect of venom of other North and South American snake NOS

☑7ᵗʰ T63.062 Toxic effect of venom of other North and South American snake, intentional self-harm

☑7ᵗʰ T63.063 Toxic effect of venom of other North and South American snake, assault

☑7ᵗʰ T63.064 Toxic effect of venom of other North and South American snake, undetermined

☑ Additional Character Required ☑x7ᵗʰ Xtension Alert Unspecified Code Other Specified Code Manifestation Code ►◄ Revised Text ● New Code ▲ Revised Code Title

T63.07 Toxic effect of venom of other Australian snake

- **T63.071** Toxic effect of venom of other Australian snake, accidental (unintentional)
  Toxic effect of venom of other Australian snake NOS
- **T63.072** Toxic effect of venom of other Australian snake, intentional self-harm
- **T63.073** Toxic effect of venom of other Australian snake, assault
- **T63.074** Toxic effect of venom of other Australian snake, undetermined

T63.08 Toxic effect of venom of other African and Asian snake

- **T63.081** Toxic effect of venom of other African and Asian snake, accidental (unintentional)
  Toxic effect of venom of other African and Asian snake NOS
- **T63.082** Toxic effect of venom of other African and Asian snake, intentional self-harm
- **T63.083** Toxic effect of venom of other African and Asian snake, assault
- **T63.084** Toxic effect of venom of other African and Asian snake, undetermined

T63.09 Toxic effect of venom of other snake

- **T63.091** Toxic effect of venom of other snake, accidental (unintentional)
  Toxic effect of venom of other snake NOS
- **T63.092** Toxic effect of venom of other snake, intentional self-harm
- **T63.093** Toxic effect of venom of other snake, assault
- **T63.094** Toxic effect of venom of other snake, undetermined

T63.1 Toxic effect of venom of other reptiles

T63.11 Toxic effect of venom of gila monster

- **T63.111** Toxic effect of venom of gila monster, accidental (unintentional)
  Toxic effect of venom of gila monster NOS
- **T63.112** Toxic effect of venom of gila monster, intentional self-harm
- **T63.113** Toxic effect of venom of gila monster, assault
- **T63.114** Toxic effect of venom of gila monster, undetermined

T63.12 Toxic effect of venom of other venomous lizard

- **T63.121** Toxic effect of venom of other venomous lizard, accidental (unintentional)
  Toxic effect of venom of other venomous lizard NOS
- **T63.122** Toxic effect of venom of other venomous lizard, intentional self-harm
- **T63.123** Toxic effect of venom of other venomous lizard, assault
- **T63.124** Toxic effect of venom of other venomous lizard, undetermined

T63.19 Toxic effect of venom of other reptiles

- **T63.191** Toxic effect of venom of other reptiles, accidental (unintentional)
  Toxic effect of venom of other reptiles NOS
- **T63.192** Toxic effect of venom of other reptiles, intentional self-harm
- **T63.193** Toxic effect of venom of other reptiles, assault
- **T63.194** Toxic effect of venom of other reptiles, undetermined

T63.2 Toxic effect of venom of scorpion

T63.2X Toxic effect of venom of scorpion

- **T63.2X1** Toxic effect of venom of scorpion, accidental (unintentional)
  Toxic effect of venom of scorpion NOS
- **T63.2X2** Toxic effect of venom of scorpion, intentional self-harm
- **T63.2X3** Toxic effect of venom of scorpion, assault
- **T63.2X4** Toxic effect of venom of scorpion, undetermined

T63.3 Toxic effect of venom of spider

T63.30 Toxic effect of unspecified spider venom

- **T63.301** Toxic effect of unspecified spider venom, accidental (unintentional)
- **T63.302** Toxic effect of unspecified spider venom, intentional self-harm
- **T63.303** Toxic effect of unspecified spider venom, assault
- **T63.304** Toxic effect of unspecified spider venom, undetermined

T63.31 Toxic effect of venom of black widow spider

- **T63.311** Toxic effect of venom of black widow spider, accidental (unintentional)
- **T63.312** Toxic effect of venom of black widow spider, intentional self-harm
- **T63.313** Toxic effect of venom of black widow spider, assault
- **T63.314** Toxic effect of venom of black widow spider, undetermined

T63.32 Toxic effect of venom of tarantula

- **T63.321** Toxic effect of venom of tarantula, accidental (unintentional)
- **T63.322** Toxic effect of venom of tarantula, intentional self-harm
- **T63.323** Toxic effect of venom of tarantula, assault
- **T63.324** Toxic effect of venom of tarantula, undetermined

T63.33 Toxic effect of venom of brown recluse spider

- **T63.331** Toxic effect of venom of brown recluse spider, accidental (unintentional)
- **T63.332** Toxic effect of venom of brown recluse spider, intentional self-harm
- **T63.333** Toxic effect of venom of brown recluse spider, assault
- **T63.334** Toxic effect of venom of brown recluse spider, undetermined

T63.39 Toxic effect of venom of other spider

- **T63.391** Toxic effect of venom of other spider, accidental (unintentional)
- **T63.392** Toxic effect of venom of other spider, intentional self-harm
- **T63.393** Toxic effect of venom of other spider, assault
- **T63.394** Toxic effect of venom of other spider, undetermined

T63.4 Toxic effect of venom of other arthropods

T63.41 Toxic effect of venom of centipedes and venomous millipedes

- **T63.411** Toxic effect of venom of centipedes and venomous millipedes, accidental (unintentional)
- **T63.412** Toxic effect of venom of centipedes and venomous millipedes, intentional self-harm
- **T63.413** Toxic effect of venom of centipedes and venomous millipedes, assault
- **T63.414** Toxic effect of venom of centipedes and venomous millipedes, undetermined

T63.42 Toxic effect of venom of ants

- **T63.421** Toxic effect of venom of ants, accidental (unintentional)
- **T63.422** Toxic effect of venom of ants, intentional self-harm
- **T63.423** Toxic effect of venom of ants, assault
- **T63.424** Toxic effect of venom of ants, undetermined

T63.43 Toxic effect of venom of caterpillars

- **T63.431** Toxic effect of venom of caterpillars, accidental (unintentional)
- **T63.432** Toxic effect of venom of caterpillars, intentional self-harm
- **T63.433** Toxic effect of venom of caterpillars, assault

EXCLUDES 1 Not coded here   EXCLUDES 2 Not included here   N Newborn Age: 0   P Pediatric Age: 0-17   M Maternity Age: 12-55   A Adult Age: 15-124

970   ICD-10-CM 2014 (Draft)

✓7th **T63.434 Toxic effect of venom of caterpillars, undetermined**

✓6th **T63.44 Toxic effect of venom of bees**

✓7th **T63.441 Toxic effect of venom of bees, accidental (unintentional)**

✓7th **T63.442 Toxic effect of venom of bees, intentional self-harm**

✓7th **T63.443 Toxic effect of venom of bees, assault**

✓7th **T63.444 Toxic effect of venom of bees, undetermined**

✓6th **T63.45 Toxic effect of venom of hornets**

✓7th **T63.451 Toxic effect of venom of hornets, accidental (unintentional)**

✓7th **T63.452 Toxic effect of venom of hornets, intentional self-harm**

✓7th **T63.453 Toxic effect of venom of hornets, assault**

✓7th **T63.454 Toxic effect of venom of hornets, undetermined**

✓6th **T63.46 Toxic effect of venom of wasps**
Toxic effect of yellow jacket

✓7th **T63.461 Toxic effect of venom of wasps, accidental (unintentional)**

✓7th **T63.462 Toxic effect of venom of wasps, intentional self-harm**

✓7th **T63.463 Toxic effect of venom of wasps, assault**

✓7th **T63.464 Toxic effect of venom of wasps, undetermined**

✓6th **T63.48 Toxic effect of venom of other arthropod**

✓7th **T63.481 Toxic effect of venom of other arthropod, accidental (unintentional)**

✓7th **T63.482 Toxic effect of venom of other arthropod, intentional self-harm**

✓7th **T63.483 Toxic effect of venom of other arthropod, assault**

✓7th **T63.484 Toxic effect of venom of other arthropod, undetermined**

✓5th **T63.5 Toxic effect of contact with venomous fish**
EXCLUDES 2   poisoning by ingestion of fish (T61.-)

✓6th **T63.51 Toxic effect of contact with stingray**

✓7th **T63.511 Toxic effect of contact with stingray, accidental (unintentional)**

✓7th **T63.512 Toxic effect of contact with stingray, intentional self-harm**

✓7th **T63.513 Toxic effect of contact with stingray, assault**

✓7th **T63.514 Toxic effect of contact with stingray, undetermined**

✓6th **T63.59 Toxic effect of contact with other venomous fish**

✓7th **T63.591 Toxic effect of contact with other venomous fish, accidental (unintentional)**

✓7th **T63.592 Toxic effect of contact with other venomous fish, intentional self-harm**

✓7th **T63.593 Toxic effect of contact with other venomous fish, assault**

✓7th **T63.594 Toxic effect of contact with other venomous fish, undetermined**

✓5th **T63.6 Toxic effect of contact with other venomous marine animals**
EXCLUDES 1   sea-snake venom (T63.09)
EXCLUDES 2   poisoning by ingestion of shellfish (T61.78-)

✓6th **T63.61 Toxic effect of contact with Portugese Man-o-war**
Toxic effect of contact with bluebottle

✓7th **T63.611 Toxic effect of contact with Portugese Man-o-war, accidental (unintentional)**

✓7th **T63.612 Toxic effect of contact with Portugese Man-o-war, intentional self-harm**

✓7th **T63.613 Toxic effect of contact with Portugese Man-o-war, assault**

✓7th **T63.614 Toxic effect of contact with Portugese Man-o-war, undetermined**

✓6th **T63.62 Toxic effect of contact with other jellyfish**

✓7th **T63.621 Toxic effect of contact with other jellyfish, accidental (unintentional)**

✓7th **T63.622 Toxic effect of contact with other jellyfish, intentional self-harm**

✓7th **T63.623 Toxic effect of contact with other jellyfish, assault**

✓7th **T63.624 Toxic effect of contact with other jellyfish, undetermined**

✓6th **T63.63 Toxic effect of contact with sea anemone**

✓7th **T63.631 Toxic effect of contact with sea anemone, accidental (unintentional)**

✓7th **T63.632 Toxic effect of contact with sea anemone, intentional self-harm**

✓7th **T63.633 Toxic effect of contact with sea anemone, assault**

✓7th **T63.634 Toxic effect of contact with sea anemone, undetermined**

✓6th **T63.69 Toxic effect of contact with other venomous marine animals**

✓7th **T63.691 Toxic effect of contact with other venomous marine animals, accidental (unintentional)**

✓7th **T63.692 Toxic effect of contact with other venomous marine animals, intentional self-harm**

✓7th **T63.693 Toxic effect of contact with other venomous marine animals, assault**

✓7th **T63.694 Toxic effect of contact with other venomous marine animals, undetermined**

✓5th **T63.7 Toxic effect of contact with venomous plant**

✓6th **T63.71 Toxic effect of contact with venomous marine plant**

✓7th **T63.711 Toxic effect of contact with venomous marine plant, accidental (unintentional)**

✓7th **T63.712 Toxic effect of contact with venomous marine plant, intentional self-harm**

✓7th **T63.713 Toxic effect of contact with venomous marine plant, assault**

✓7th **T63.714 Toxic effect of contact with venomous marine plant, undetermined**

✓6th **T63.79 Toxic effect of contact with other venomous plant**

✓7th **T63.791 Toxic effect of contact with other venomous plant, accidental (unintentional)**

✓7th **T63.792 Toxic effect of contact with other venomous plant, intentional self-harm**

✓7th **T63.793 Toxic effect of contact with other venomous plant, assault**

✓7th **T63.794 Toxic effect of contact with other venomous plant, undetermined**

✓5th **T63.8 Toxic effect of contact with other venomous animals**

✓6th **T63.81 Toxic effect of contact with venomous frog**
EXCLUDES 1   contact with nonvenomous frog (W62.0)

✓7th **T63.811 Toxic effect of contact with venomous frog, accidental (unintentional)**

✓7th **T63.812 Toxic effect of contact with venomous frog, intentional self-harm**

✓7th **T63.813 Toxic effect of contact with venomous frog, assault**

✓7th **T63.814 Toxic effect of contact with venomous frog, undetermined**

✓6th **T63.82 Toxic effect of contact with venomous toad**
EXCLUDES 1   contact with nonvenomous toad (W62.1)

✓7th **T63.821 Toxic effect of contact with venomous toad, accidental (unintentional)**

✓7th **T63.822 Toxic effect of contact with venomous toad, intentional self-harm**

✓7th **T63.823 Toxic effect of contact with venomous toad, assault**

✓7th **T63.824 Toxic effect of contact with venomous toad, undetermined**

✓6th **T63.83 Toxic effect of contact with other venomous amphibian**
EXCLUDES 1   contact with nonvenomous amphibian (W62.9)

✓7th **T63.831 Toxic effect of contact with other venomous amphibian, accidental (unintentional)**

✓7th **T63.832 Toxic effect of contact with other venomous amphibian, intentional self-harm**

✓7th **T63.833 Toxic effect of contact with other venomous amphibian, assault**

✓7th **T63.834 Toxic effect of contact with other venomous amphibian, undetermined**

✓6th **T63.89 Toxic effect of contact with other venomous animals**

✓7th **T63.891 Toxic effect of contact with other venomous animals, accidental (unintentional)**

✓7th **T63.892 Toxic effect of contact with other venomous animals, intentional self-harm**

✓7th **T63.893 Toxic effect of contact with other venomous animals, assault**

✓7th **T63.894 Toxic effect of contact with other venomous animals, undetermined**

✓5th **T63.9 Toxic effect of contact with unspecified venomous animal**

✓x7th **T63.91 Toxic effect of contact with unspecified venomous animal, accidental (unintentional)**

✓x7th **T63.92 Toxic effect of contact with unspecified venomous animal, intentional self-harm**

✓x7th **T63.93 Toxic effect of contact with unspecified venomous animal, assault**

✓x7th **T63.94 Toxic effect of contact with unspecified venomous animal, undetermined**

✓4th **T64 Toxic effect of aflatoxin and other mycotoxin food contaminants**

> The appropriate 7th character is to be added to each code from category T64.
> A   initial encounter
> D   subsequent encounter
> S   sequela

✓5th **T64.0 Toxic effect of aflatoxin**

✓x7th **T64.01 Toxic effect of aflatoxin, accidental (unintentional)**

✓x7th **T64.02 Toxic effect of aflatoxin, intentional self-harm**

✓x7th **T64.03 Toxic effect of aflatoxin, assault**

✓x7th **T64.04 Toxic effect of aflatoxin, undetermined**

✓5th **T64.8 Toxic effect of other mycotoxin food contaminants**

✓x7th **T64.81 Toxic effect of other mycotoxin food contaminants, accidental (unintentional)**

✓x7th **T64.82 Toxic effect of other mycotoxin food contaminants, intentional self-harm**

✓x7th **T64.83 Toxic effect of other mycotoxin food contaminants, assault**

✓x7th **T64.84 Toxic effect of other mycotoxin food contaminants, undetermined**

✓4th **T65 Toxic effect of other and unspecified substances**

> The appropriate 7th character is to be added to each code from category T65.
> A   initial encounter
> D   subsequent encounter
> S   sequela

✓5th **T65.0 Toxic effect of cyanides**
EXCLUDES 1 *hydrogen cyanide (T57.3-)*

✓6th **T65.0X Toxic effect of cyanides**

✓7th **T65.0X1 Toxic effect of cyanides, accidental (unintentional)**
Toxic effect of cyanides NOS

✓7th **T65.0X2 Toxic effect of cyanides, intentional self-harm**

✓7th **T65.0X3 Toxic effect of cyanides, assault**

✓7th **T65.0X4 Toxic effect of cyanides, undetermined**

✓5th **T65.1 Toxic effect of strychnine and its salts**

✓6th **T65.1X Toxic effect of strychnine and its salts**

✓7th **T65.1X1 Toxic effect of strychnine and its salts, accidental (unintentional)**
Toxic effect of strychnine and its salts NOS

✓7th **T65.1X2 Toxic effect of strychnine and its salts, intentional self-harm**

✓7th **T65.1X3 Toxic effect of strychnine and its salts, assault**

✓7th **T65.1X4 Toxic effect of strychnine and its salts, undetermined**

✓5th **T65.2 Toxic effect of tobacco and nicotine**
EXCLUDES 2 *nicotine dependence (F17.-)*

✓6th **T65.21 Toxic effect of chewing tobacco**

✓7th **T65.211 Toxic effect of chewing tobacco, accidental (unintentional)**
Toxic effect of chewing tobacco NOS

✓7th **T65.212 Toxic effect of chewing tobacco, intentional self-harm**

✓7th **T65.213 Toxic effect of chewing tobacco, assault**

✓7th **T65.214 Toxic effect of chewing tobacco, undetermined**

✓6th **T65.22 Toxic effect of tobacco cigarettes**
Toxic effect of tobacco smoke
Use additional code for exposure to second hand tobacco smoke (Z57.31, Z77.22)

✓7th **T65.221 Toxic effect of tobacco cigarettes, accidental (unintentional)**
Toxic effect of tobacco cigarettes NOS

✓7th **T65.222 Toxic effect of tobacco cigarettes, intentional self-harm**

✓7th **T65.223 Toxic effect of tobacco cigarettes, assault**

✓7th **T65.224 Toxic effect of tobacco cigarettes, undetermined**

✓6th **T65.29 Toxic effect of other tobacco and nicotine**

✓7th **T65.291 Toxic effect of other tobacco and nicotine, accidental (unintentional)**
Toxic effect of other tobacco and nicotine NOS

✓7th **T65.292 Toxic effect of other tobacco and nicotine, intentional self-harm**

✓7th **T65.293 Toxic effect of other tobacco and nicotine, assault**

✓7th **T65.294 Toxic effect of other tobacco and nicotine, undetermined**

✓5th **T65.3 Toxic effect of nitroderivatives and aminoderivatives of benzene and its homologues**
Toxic effect of anilin [benzenamine]
Toxic effect of nitrobenzene
Toxic effect of trinitrotoluene

✓6th **T65.3X Toxic effect of nitroderivatives and aminoderivatives of benzene and its homologues**

✓7th **T65.3X1 Toxic effect of nitroderivatives and aminoderivatives of benzene and its homologues, accidental (unintentional)**
Toxic effect of nitroderivatives and aminoderivatives of benzene and its homologues NOS

✓7th **T65.3X2 Toxic effect of nitroderivatives and aminoderivatives of benzene and its homologues, intentional self-harm**

✓7th **T65.3X3 Toxic effect of nitroderivatives and aminoderivatives of benzene and its homologues, assault**

✓7th **T65.3X4 Toxic effect of nitroderivatives and aminoderivatives of benzene and its homologues, undetermined**

✓5th **T65.4 Toxic effect of carbon disulfide**

✓6th **T65.4X Toxic effect of carbon disulfide**

✓7th **T65.4X1 Toxic effect of carbon disulfide, accidental (unintentional)**
Toxic effect of carbon disulfide NOS

✓7th **T65.4X2 Toxic effect of carbon disulfide, intentional self-harm**

✓7th **T65.4X3 Toxic effect of carbon disulfide, assault**

✓7th **T65.4X4 Toxic effect of carbon disulfide, undetermined**

✓5th **T65.5 Toxic effect of nitroglycerin and other nitric acids and esters**
Toxic effect of 1,2,3-Propanetriol trinitrate

✓6th **T65.5X Toxic effect of nitroglycerin and other nitric acids and esters**

✓7th **T65.5X1 Toxic effect of nitroglycerin and other nitric acids and esters, accidental (unintentional)**
Toxic effect of nitroglycerin and other nitric acids and esters NOS

EXCLUDES 1 Not coded here   EXCLUDES 2 Not included here   N Newborn Age: 0   P Pediatric Age: 0-17   M Maternity Age: 12-55   A Adult Age: 15-124

972   ICD-10-CM 2014 (Draft)

✓7ᵗʰ **T65.5X2** **Toxic effect of nitroglycerin and other nitric acids and esters, intentional self-harm**

✓7ᵗʰ **T65.5X3** **Toxic effect of nitroglycerin and other nitric acids and esters, assault**

✓7ᵗʰ **T65.5X4** **Toxic effect of nitroglycerin and other nitric acids and esters, undetermined**

✓5ᵗʰ **T65.6** **Toxic effect of paints and dyes, not elsewhere classified**

✓6ᵗʰ **T65.6X** **Toxic effect of paints and dyes, not elsewhere classified**

✓7ᵗʰ **T65.6X1** **Toxic effect of paints and dyes, not elsewhere classified, accidental (unintentional)**
Toxic effect of paints and dyes NOS

✓7ᵗʰ **T65.6X2** **Toxic effect of paints and dyes, not elsewhere classified, intentional self-harm**

✓7ᵗʰ **T65.6X3** **Toxic effect of paints and dyes, not elsewhere classified, assault**

✓7ᵗʰ **T65.6X4** **Toxic effect of paints and dyes, not elsewhere classified, undetermined**

✓5ᵗʰ **T65.8** **Toxic effect of other specified substances**

✓6ᵗʰ **T65.81** **Toxic effect of latex**

✓7ᵗʰ **T65.811** **Toxic effect of latex, accidental (unintentional)**
Toxic effect of latex NOS

✓7ᵗʰ **T65.812** **Toxic effect of latex, intentional self-harm**

✓7ᵗʰ **T65.813** **Toxic effect of latex, assault**

✓7ᵗʰ **T65.814** **Toxic effect of latex, undetermined**

✓6ᵗʰ **T65.82** **Toxic effect of harmful algae and algae toxins**
Toxic effect of (harmful) algae bloom NOS
Toxic effect of blue-green algae bloom
Toxic effect of brown tide
Toxic effect of cyanobacteria bloom
Toxic effect of Florida red tide
Toxic effect of pfiesteria piscicida
Toxic effect of red tide

✓7ᵗʰ **T65.821** **Toxic effect of harmful algae and algae toxins, accidental (unintentional)**
Toxic effect of harmful algae and algae toxins NOS

✓7ᵗʰ **T65.822** **Toxic effect of harmful algae and algae toxins, intentional self-harm**

✓7ᵗʰ **T65.823** **Toxic effect of harmful algae and algae toxins, assault**

✓7ᵗʰ **T65.824** **Toxic effect of harmful algae and algae toxins, undetermined**

✓6ᵗʰ **T65.83** **Toxic effect of fiberglass**

✓7ᵗʰ **T65.831** **Toxic effect of fiberglass, accidental (unintentional)**
Toxic effect of fiberglass NOS

✓7ᵗʰ **T65.832** **Toxic effect of fiberglass, intentional self-harm**

✓7ᵗʰ **T65.833** **Toxic effect of fiberglass, assault**

✓7ᵗʰ **T65.834** **Toxic effect of fiberglass, undetermined**

✓6ᵗʰ **T65.89** **Toxic effect of other specified substances**

✓7ᵗʰ **T65.891** **Toxic effect of other specified substances, accidental (unintentional)**
Toxic effect of other specified substances NOS

✓7ᵗʰ **T65.892** **Toxic effect of other specified substances, intentional self-harm**

✓7ᵗʰ **T65.893** **Toxic effect of other specified substances, assault**

✓7ᵗʰ **T65.894** **Toxic effect of other specified substances, undetermined**

✓5ᵗʰ **T65.9** **Toxic effect of unspecified substance**

✓x7ᵗʰ **T65.91** **Toxic effect of unspecified substance, accidental (unintentional)**
Poisoning NOS

✓x7ᵗʰ **T65.92** **Toxic effect of unspecified substance, intentional self-harm**

✓x7ᵗʰ **T65.93** **Toxic effect of unspecified substance, assault**

✓x7ᵗʰ **T65.94** **Toxic effect of unspecified substance, undetermined**

Other and unspecified effects of external causes (T66-T78)

✓x7ᵗʰ **T66** **Radiation sickness, unspecified**
EXCLUDES 1 specified adverse effects of radiation, such as:
    burns (T20-T31)
    leukemia (C91-C95)
    radiation gastroenteritis and colitis (K52.0)
    radiation pneumonitis (J70.0)
    radiation related disorders of the skin and subcutaneous tissue (L55-L59)
    radiation sunburn (L55.-)

The appropriate 7th character is to be added to code T66.
A   initial encounter
D   subsequent encounter
S   sequela

✓4ᵗʰ **T67** **Effects of heat and light**
EXCLUDES 1 erythema [dermatitis] ab igne (L59.0)
    malignant hyperpyrexia due to anesthesia (T88.3)
    radiation-related disorders of the skin and subcutaneous tissue (L55-L59)
EXCLUDES 2 burns (T20-T31)
    sunburn (L55.-)
    sweat disorder due to heat (L74-L75))

The appropriate 7th character is to be added to each code from category T67.
A   initial encounter
D   subsequent encounter
S   sequela

✓x7ᵗʰ **T67.0** **Heatstroke and sunstroke**
Heat apoplexy   Siriasis
Heat pyrexia   Thermoplegia
Use additional code(s) to identify any associated complications of heatstroke, such as:
    coma and stupor (R40.-)
    systemic inflammatory response syndrome (R65.1-)

✓x7ᵗʰ **T67.1** **Heat syncope**
Heat collapse

✓x7ᵗʰ **T67.2** **Heat cramp**

✓x7ᵗʰ **T67.3** **Heat exhaustion, anhydrotic**
Heat prostration due to water depletion
EXCLUDES 1 heat exhaustion due to salt depletion (T67.4)

✓x7ᵗʰ **T67.4** **Heat exhaustion due to salt depletion**
Heat prostration due to salt (and water) depletion

✓x7ᵗʰ **T67.5** **Heat exhaustion, unspecified**
Heat prostration NOS

✓x7ᵗʰ **T67.6** **Heat fatigue, transient**

✓x7ᵗʰ **T67.7** **Heat edema**

✓x7ᵗʰ **T67.8** **Other effects of heat and light**

✓x7ᵗʰ **T67.9** **Effect of heat and light, unspecified**

✓x7ᵗʰ **T68** **Hypothermia**
Accidental hypothermia   Hypothermia NOS
EXCLUDES 1 hypothermia following anesthesia (T88.51)
    hypothermia not associated with low environmental temperature (R68.0)
    hypothermia of newborn (P80.-)
EXCLUDES 2 frostbite (T33-T34)
Use additional code to identify source of exposure:
    exposure to excessive cold of man-made origin (W93)
    exposure to excessive cold of natural origin (X31)

The appropriate 7th character is to be added to code T68.
A   initial encounter
D   subsequent encounter
S   sequela

✓4ᵗʰ **T69** **Other effects of reduced temperature**
EXCLUDES 2 frostbite (T33-T34)
Use additional code to identify source of exposure:
    exposure to excessive cold of man-made origin (W93)
    exposure to excessive cold of natural origin (X31)

The appropriate 7th character is to be added to each code from category T69.
A   initial encounter
D   subsequent encounter
S   sequela

✓5ᵗʰ **T69.0** **Immersion hand and foot**

✓6ᵗʰ **T69.01** **Immersion hand**

✓7ᵗʰ **T69.011** **Immersion hand, right hand**

Injury, Poisoning and Certain Other Consequences of External Causes   **T69.012–T71.221**

√7ᵗʰ **T69.012** Immersion hand, left hand

√7ᵗʰ **T69.019** Immersion hand, unspecified hand

√6ᵗʰ **T69.02** Immersion foot
     Trench foot

√7ᵗʰ **T69.021** Immersion foot, right foot

√7ᵗʰ **T69.022** Immersion foot, left foot

√7ᵗʰ **T69.029** Immersion foot, unspecified foot

√x7ᵗʰ **T69.1** Chilblains

√x7ᵗʰ **T69.8** Other specified effects of reduced temperature

√x7ᵗʰ **T69.9** Effect of reduced temperature, unspecified

√4ᵗʰ **T70** Effects of air pressure and water pressure

> The appropriate 7th character is to be added to each code from category T70.
> A   initial encounter
> D   subsequent encounter
> S   sequela

√x7ᵗʰ **T70.0** Otitic barotrauma
     Aero-otitis media
     Effects of change in ambient atmospheric pressure or water pressure on ears

√x7ᵗʰ **T70.1** Sinus barotrauma
     Aerosinusitis
     Effects of change in ambient atmospheric pressure on sinuses

√5ᵗʰ **T70.2** Other and unspecified effects of high altitude
     EXCLUDES 2 *polycythemia due to high altitude (D75.1)*

√x7ᵗʰ **T70.20** Unspecified effects of high altitude

√x7ᵗʰ **T70.29** Other effects of high altitude
     Alpine sickness
     Anoxia due to high altitude
     Barotrauma NOS
     Hypobaropathy
     Mountain sickness

√x7ᵗʰ **T70.3** Caisson disease [decompression sickness]
     Compressed-air disease
     Diver's palsy or paralysis

√x7ᵗʰ **T70.4** Effects of high-pressure fluids
     Hydraulic jet injection (industrial)
     Pneumatic jet injection (industrial)
     Traumatic jet injection (industrial)

√x7ᵗʰ **T70.8** Other effects of air pressure and water pressure

√x7ᵗʰ **T70.9** Effect of air pressure and water pressure, unspecified

√4ᵗʰ **T71** Asphyxiation
     Mechanical suffocation
     Traumatic suffocation
     EXCLUDES 1 *acute respiratory distress (syndrome) (J80)*
     anoxia due to high altitude (T70.2)
     asphyxia NOS (R09.01)
     asphyxia from carbon monoxide (T58.-)
     asphyxia from inhalation of food or foreign body (T17.-)
     asphyxia from other gases, fumes and vapors (T59.-)
     respiratory distress (syndrome) in newborn (P22.-)

> The appropriate 7th character is to be added to each code from category T71.
> A   initial encounter
> D   subsequent encounter
> S   sequela

√5ᵗʰ **T71.1** Asphyxiation due to mechanical threat to breathing
     Suffocation due to mechanical threat to breathing

√6ᵗʰ **T71.11** Asphyxiation due to smothering under pillow

√7ᵗʰ **T71.111** Asphyxiation due to smothering under pillow, accidental
     Asphyxiation due to smothering under pillow NOS

√7ᵗʰ **T71.112** Asphyxiation due to smothering under pillow, intentional self-harm

√7ᵗʰ **T71.113** Asphyxiation due to smothering under pillow, assault

√7ᵗʰ **T71.114** Asphyxiation due to smothering under pillow, undetermined

√6ᵗʰ **T71.12** Asphyxiation due to plastic bag

√7ᵗʰ **T71.121** Asphyxiation due to plastic bag, accidental
     Asphyxiation due to plastic bag NOS

√7ᵗʰ **T71.122** Asphyxiation due to plastic bag, intentional self-harm

√7ᵗʰ **T71.123** Asphyxiation due to plastic bag, assault

√7ᵗʰ **T71.124** Asphyxiation due to plastic bag, undetermined

√6ᵗʰ **T71.13** Asphyxiation due to being trapped in bed linens

√7ᵗʰ **T71.131** Asphyxiation due to being trapped in bed linens, accidental
     Asphyxiation due to being trapped in bed linens NOS

√7ᵗʰ **T71.132** Asphyxiation due to being trapped in bed linens, intentional self-harm

√7ᵗʰ **T71.133** Asphyxiation due to being trapped in bed linens, assault

√7ᵗʰ **T71.134** Asphyxiation due to being trapped in bed linens, undetermined

√6ᵗʰ **T71.14** Asphyxiation due to smothering under another person's body (in bed)

√7ᵗʰ **T71.141** Asphyxiation due to smothering under another person's body (in bed), accidental
     Asphyxiation due to smothering under another person's body (in bed) NOS

√7ᵗʰ **T71.143** Asphyxiation due to smothering under another person's body (in bed), assault

√7ᵗʰ **T71.144** Asphyxiation due to smothering under another person's body (in bed), undetermined

√6ᵗʰ **T71.15** Asphyxiation due to smothering in furniture

√7ᵗʰ **T71.151** Asphyxiation due to smothering in furniture, accidental
     Asphyxiation due to smothering in furniture NOS

√7ᵗʰ **T71.152** Asphyxiation due to smothering in furniture, intentional self-harm

√7ᵗʰ **T71.153** Asphyxiation due to smothering in furniture, assault

√7ᵗʰ **T71.154** Asphyxiation due to smothering in furniture, undetermined

√6ᵗʰ **T71.16** Asphyxiation due to hanging
     Hanging by window shade cord
     Use additional code for any associated injuries, such as:
     crushing injury of neck (S17.-)
     fracture of cervical vertebrae (S12.0-S12.2-)
     open wound of neck (S11.-)

√7ᵗʰ **T71.161** Asphyxiation due to hanging, accidental
     Asphyxiation due to hanging NOS
     Hanging NOS

√7ᵗʰ **T71.162** Asphyxiation due to hanging, intentional self-harm

√7ᵗʰ **T71.163** Asphyxiation due to hanging, assault

√7ᵗʰ **T71.164** Asphyxiation due to hanging, undetermined

√6ᵗʰ **T71.19** Asphyxiation due to mechanical threat to breathing due to other causes

√7ᵗʰ **T71.191** Asphyxiation due to mechanical threat to breathing due to other causes, accidental
     Asphyxiation due to other causes NOS

√7ᵗʰ **T71.192** Asphyxiation due to mechanical threat to breathing due to other causes, intentional self-harm

√7ᵗʰ **T71.193** Asphyxiation due to mechanical threat to breathing due to other causes, assault

√7ᵗʰ **T71.194** Asphyxiation due to mechanical threat to breathing due to other causes, undetermined

√5ᵗʰ **T71.2** Asphyxiation due to systemic oxygen deficiency due to low oxygen content in ambient air
     Suffocation due to systemic oxygen deficiency due to low oxygen content in ambient air

√x7ᵗʰ **T71.20** Asphyxiation due to systemic oxygen deficiency due to low oxygen content in ambient air due to unspecified cause

√x7ᵗʰ **T71.21** Asphyxiation due to cave-in or falling earth
     Use additional code for any associated cataclysm (X34-X38)

√6ᵗʰ **T71.22** Asphyxiation due to being trapped in a car trunk

√7ᵗʰ **T71.221** Asphyxiation due to being trapped in a car trunk, accidental

---

EXCLUDES 1 Not coded here   EXCLUDES 2 Not included here   N Newborn Age: 0   P Pediatric Age: 0-17   M Maternity Age: 12-55   A Adult Age: 15-124

974   ICD-10-CM 2014 (Draft)

√7ᵗʰ **T71.222** Asphyxiation due to being trapped in a car trunk, intentional self-harm

√7ᵗʰ **T71.223** Asphyxiation due to being trapped in a car trunk, assault

√7ᵗʰ **T71.224** Asphyxiation due to being trapped in a car trunk, undetermined

√6ᵗʰ **T71.23** Asphyxiation due to being trapped in a (discarded) refrigerator

√7ᵗʰ **T71.231** Asphyxiation due to being trapped in a (discarded) refrigerator, accidental

√7ᵗʰ **T71.232** Asphyxiation due to being trapped in a (discarded) refrigerator, intentional self-harm

√7ᵗʰ **T71.233** Asphyxiation due to being trapped in a (discarded) refrigerator, assault

√7ᵗʰ **T71.234** Asphyxiation due to being trapped in a (discarded) refrigerator, undetermined

√x7ᵗʰ **T71.29** Asphyxiation due to being trapped in other low oxygen environment

√x7ᵗʰ **T71.9** Asphyxiation due to unspecified cause
Suffocation (by strangulation) due to unspecified cause
Suffocation NOS
Systemic oxygen deficiency due to low oxygen content in ambient air due to unspecified cause
Systemic oxygen deficiency due to mechanical threat to breathing due to unspecified cause
Traumatic asphyxia NOS

√4ᵗʰ **T73** **Effects of other deprivation**

The appropriate 7th character is to be added to each code from category T73.
A   initial encounter
D   subsequent encounter
S   sequela

√x7ᵗʰ **T73.0** Starvation
Deprivation of food

√x7ᵗʰ **T73.1** Deprivation of water

√x7ᵗʰ **T73.2** Exhaustion due to exposure

√x7ᵗʰ **T73.3** Exhaustion due to excessive exertion
Exhaustion due to overexertion

√x7ᵗʰ **T73.8** Other effects of deprivation

√x7ᵗʰ **T73.9** Effect of deprivation, unspecified

√4ᵗʰ **T74** **Adult and child abuse, neglect and other maltreatment, confirmed**
EXCLUDES 1 abuse and maltreatment in pregnancy (O9A.3-, O9A.4-, O9A.5-)
adult and child maltreatment, suspected (T76.-)
Use additional code, if applicable, to identify any associated current injury
Use additional external cause code to identify perpetrator, if known (Y07.-)

The appropriate 7th character is to be added to each code from category T74.
A   initial encounter
D   subsequent encounter
S   sequela

√5ᵗʰ **T74.0** Neglect or abandonment, confirmed

√x7ᵗʰ **T74.01** Adult neglect or abandonment, confirmed 🄰

√x7ᵗʰ **T74.02** Child neglect or abandonment, confirmed 🄿

√5ᵗʰ **T74.1** Physical abuse, confirmed
EXCLUDES 2 sexual abuse (T74.2-)

√x7ᵗʰ **T74.11** Adult physical abuse, confirmed 🄰

√x7ᵗʰ **T74.12** Child physical abuse, confirmed 🄿
EXCLUDES 2 shaken infant syndrome (T74.4)

√5ᵗʰ **T74.2** Sexual abuse, confirmed
Rape, confirmed
Sexual assault, confirmed

√x7ᵗʰ **T74.21** Adult sexual abuse, confirmed 🄰

√x7ᵗʰ **T74.22** Child sexual abuse, confirmed 🄿

√5ᵗʰ **T74.3** Psychological abuse, confirmed

√x7ᵗʰ **T74.31** Adult psychological abuse, confirmed 🄰

√x7ᵗʰ **T74.32** Child psychological abuse, confirmed 🄿

√x7ᵗʰ **T74.4** Shaken infant syndrome

√5ᵗʰ **T74.9** Unspecified maltreatment, confirmed

√x7ᵗʰ **T74.91** Unspecified adult maltreatment, confirmed 🄰

√x7ᵗʰ **T74.92** Unspecified child maltreatment, confirmed 🄿

√4ᵗʰ **T75** **Other and unspecified effects of other external causes**
EXCLUDES 1 adverse effects NEC (T78.-)
EXCLUDES 2 burns (electric) (T20-T31)

The appropriate 7th character is to be added to each code from category T75.
A   initial encounter
D   subsequent encounter
S   sequela

√5ᵗʰ **T75.0** Effects of lightning
Struck by lightning

√x7ᵗʰ **T75.00** Unspecified effects of lightning
Struck by lightning NOS

√x7ᵗʰ **T75.01** Shock due to being struck by lightning

√x7ᵗʰ **T75.09** Other effects of lightning
Use additional code for other effects of lightning

√x7ᵗʰ **T75.1** Unspecified effects of drowning and nonfatal submersion
Immersion
EXCLUDES 1 specified effects of drowning—code to effects

√5ᵗʰ **T75.2** Effects of vibration

√x7ᵗʰ **T75.20** Unspecified effects of vibration

√x7ᵗʰ **T75.21** Pneumatic hammer syndrome

√x7ᵗʰ **T75.22** Traumatic vasospastic syndrome

√x7ᵗʰ **T75.23** Vertigo from infrasound
EXCLUDES 1 vertigo NOS (R42)

√x7ᵗʰ **T75.29** Other effects of vibration

√x7ᵗʰ **T75.3** Motion sickness
Airsickness
Seasickness
Travel sickness
Use additional external cause code to identify vehicle or type of motion (Y92.81-, Y93.5-)

√x7ᵗʰ **T75.4** Electrocution
Shock from electric current
Shock from electroshock gun (taser)

√5ᵗʰ **T75.8** Other specified effects of external causes

√x7ᵗʰ **T75.81** Effects of abnormal gravitation [G] forces

√x7ᵗʰ **T75.82** Effects of weightlessness

√x7ᵗʰ **T75.89** Other specified effects of external causes

√4ᵗʰ **T76** **Adult and child abuse, neglect and other maltreatment, suspected**
EXCLUDES 1 adult and child maltreatment, confirmed (T74.-)
suspected abuse and maltreatment in pregnancy (O9A.3-, O9A.4-, O9A.5-)
suspected adult physical abuse, ruled out (Z04.71)
suspected adult sexual abuse, ruled out (Z04.41)
suspected child physical abuse, ruled out (Z04.72)
suspected child sexual abuse, ruled out (Z04.42)
Use additional code, if applicable, to identify any associated current injury

The appropriate 7th character is to be added to each code from category T76.
A   initial encounter
D   subsequent encounter
S   sequela

√5ᵗʰ **T76.0** Neglect or abandonment, suspected

√x7ᵗʰ **T76.01** Adult neglect or abandonment, suspected 🄰

√x7ᵗʰ **T76.02** Child neglect or abandonment, suspected 🄿

√5ᵗʰ **T76.1** Physical abuse, suspected

√x7ᵗʰ **T76.11** Adult physical abuse, suspected 🄰

√x7ᵗʰ **T76.12** Child physical abuse, suspected 🄿

√5ᵗʰ **T76.2** Sexual abuse, suspected
Rape, suspected
Sexual abuse, suspected
EXCLUDES 1 alleged abuse, ruled out (Z04.7)

√x7ᵗʰ **T76.21** Adult sexual abuse, suspected 🄰

√x7ᵗʰ **T76.22** Child sexual abuse, suspected 🄿

√5ᵗʰ **T76.3** Psychological abuse, suspected

√x7ᵗʰ **T76.31** Adult psychological abuse, suspected 🄰

√x7ᵗʰ **T76.32** Child psychological abuse, suspected 🄿

Injury, Poisoning and Certain Other Consequences of External Causes

T71.222–T76.32

T76.9 Unspecified maltreatment, suspected

   √x7ᵗʰ **T76.91** **Unspecified adult maltreatment, suspected**   A

   √x7ᵗʰ **T76.92** **Unspecified child maltreatment, suspected**   P

√4ᵗʰ **T78** **Adverse effects, not elsewhere classified**

   EXCLUDES 2   complications of surgical and medical care NEC (T80-T88)

> The appropriate 7th character is to be added to each code from category T78.
> A   initial encounter
> D   subsequent encounter
> S   sequela

√5ᵗʰ **T78.0** **Anaphylactic reaction due to food**
     Anaphylactic reaction due to adverse food reaction
     Anaphylactic shock or reaction due to nonpoisonous foods
     Anaphylactoid reaction due to food

   √x7ᵗʰ **T78.00** **Anaphylactic reaction due to unspecified food**

   √x7ᵗʰ **T78.01** **Anaphylactic reaction due to peanuts**

   √x7ᵗʰ **T78.02** **Anaphylactic reaction due to shellfish (crustaceans)**

   √x7ᵗʰ **T78.03** **Anaphylactic reaction due to other fish**

   √x7ᵗʰ **T78.04** **Anaphylactic reaction due to fruits and vegetables**

   √x7ᵗʰ **T78.05** **Anaphylactic reaction due to tree nuts and seeds**
       EXCLUDES 1   anaphylactic reaction due to peanuts (T78.01)

   √x7ᵗʰ **T78.06** **Anaphylactic reaction due to food additives**

   √x7ᵗʰ **T78.07** **Anaphylactic reaction due to milk and dairy products**

   √x7ᵗʰ **T78.08** **Anaphylactic reaction due to eggs**

   √x7ᵗʰ **T78.09** **Anaphylactic reaction due to other food products**

√x7ᵗʰ **T78.1** **Other adverse food reactions, not elsewhere classified**
     Use additional code to identify the type of reaction
     EXCLUDES 1   anaphylactic reaction or shock due to adverse food reaction (T78.0-)
       anaphylactic reaction due to food (T78.0-)
       bacterial food borne intoxications (A05.-)
     EXCLUDES 2   allergic and dietetic gastroenteritis and colitis (K52.2)
       allergic rhinitis due to food (J30.5)
       dermatitis due to food in contact with skin (L23.6, L24.6, L25.4)
       dermatitis due to ingested food (L27.2)

√x7ᵗʰ **T78.2** **Anaphylactic shock, unspecified**
     Allergic shock
     Anaphylactic reaction
     Anaphylaxis
     EXCLUDES 1   anaphylactic reaction or shock due to adverse effect of correct medicinal substance properly administered (T88.6)
       anaphylactic reaction or shock due to adverse food reaction (T78.0-)
       anaphylactic reaction or shock due to serum (T80.5-)

√x7ᵗʰ **T78.3** **Angioneurotic edema**
     Allergic angioedema
     Giant urticaria
     Quincke's edema
     EXCLUDES 1   serum urticaria (T80.6-)
       urticaria (L50.-)

√5ᵗʰ **T78.4** **Other and unspecified allergy**
     EXCLUDES 1   specified types of allergic reaction such as:
       allergic diarrhea (K52.2)
       allergic gastroenteritis and colitis (K52.2)
       dermatitis (L23-L25, L27-)
       hay fever (J30.1)

   √x7ᵗʰ **T78.40** **Allergy, unspecified**
       Allergic reaction NOS
       Hypersensitivity NOS

   √x7ᵗʰ **T78.41** **Arthus phenomenon**
       Arthus reaction

   √x7ᵗʰ **T78.49** **Other allergy**

√x7ᵗʰ **T78.8** **Other adverse effects, not elsewhere classified**

Certain early complications of trauma (T79)

√4ᵗʰ **T79** **Certain early complications of trauma, not elsewhere classified**

   EXCLUDES 2   acute respiratory distress syndrome (J80)
       complications occurring during or following medical procedures (T80-T88)
       complications of surgical and medical care NEC (T80-T88)
       newborn respiratory distress syndrome (P22.0)

> The appropriate 7th character is to be added to each code from category T79.
> A   initial encounter
> D   subsequent encounter
> S   sequela

√x7ᵗʰ **T79.0** **Air embolism (traumatic)**
     EXCLUDES 1   air embolism complicating abortion or ectopic or molar pregnancy (O00-O07, O08.2)
       air embolism complicating pregnancy, childbirth and the puerperium (O88.0)
       air embolism following infusion, transfusion, and therapeutic injection (T80.0)
       air embolism following procedure NEC (T81.7-)

√x7ᵗʰ **T79.1** **Fat embolism (traumatic)**
     EXCLUDES 1   fat embolism complicating:
       abortion or ectopic or molar pregnancy (O00-O07, O08.2)
       pregnancy, childbirth and the puerperium (O88.8)

√x7ᵗʰ **T79.2** **Traumatic secondary and recurrent hemorrhage and seroma**

√x7ᵗʰ **T79.4** **Traumatic shock**
     Shock (immediate) (delayed) following injury
     EXCLUDES 1   anaphylactic shock due to adverse food reaction (T78.0-)
       anaphylactic shock due to correct medicinal substance properly administered (T88.6)
       anaphylactic shock due to serum (T80.5-)
       anaphylactic shock NOS (T78.2)
       anesthetic shock (T88.2)
       electric shock (T75.4)
       nontraumatic shock NEC (R57.-)
       obstetric shock (O75.1)
       postprocedural shock (T81.1-)
       septic shock (R65.21)
       shock complicating abortion or ectopic or molar pregnancy (O00-O07, O08.3)
       shock due to lightning (T75.01)
       shock NOS (R57.9)

√x7ᵗʰ **T79.5** **Traumatic anuria**
     Crush syndrome
     Renal failure following crushing

√x7ᵗʰ **T79.6** **Traumatic ischemia of muscle**
     Traumatic rhabdomyolysis
     Volkmann's ischemic contracture
     EXCLUDES 2   anterior tibial syndrome (M76.8)
       compartment syndrome (traumatic) (T79.A-)
       nontraumatic ischemia of muscle (M62.2-)

√x7ᵗʰ **T79.7** **Traumatic subcutaneous emphysema**
     EXCLUDES 1   emphysema NOS (J43)
       emphysema (subcutaneous) resulting from a procedure (T81.82)

√5ᵗʰ **T79.A** **Traumatic compartment syndrome**
     EXCLUDES 1   fibromyalgia (M79.7)
       nontraumatic compartment syndrome (M79.A-)
       traumatic ischemic infarction of muscle (T79.6)

   √x7ᵗʰ **T79.A0** **Compartment syndrome, unspecified**
       Compartment syndrome NOS

   √6ᵗʰ **T79.A1** **Traumatic compartment syndrome of upper extremity**
       Traumatic compartment syndrome of shoulder, arm, forearm, wrist, hand, and fingers

     √7ᵗʰ **T79.A11** **Traumatic compartment syndrome of right upper extremity**

     √7ᵗʰ **T79.A12** **Traumatic compartment syndrome of left upper extremity**

     √7ᵗʰ **T79.A19** **Traumatic compartment syndrome of unspecified upper extremity**

EXCLUDES 1 Not coded here   EXCLUDES 2 Not included here   N Newborn Age: 0   P Pediatric Age: 0-17   M Maternity Age: 12-55   A Adult Age: 15-124

976   ICD-10-CM 2014 (Draft)

√6ᵗʰ **T79.A2 Traumatic compartment syndrome of** lower
extremity
Traumatic compartment syndrome of hip, buttock,
thigh, leg, foot, and toes

√7ᵗʰ **T79.A21 Traumatic compartment syndrome of**
right **lower extremity**

√7ᵗʰ **T79.A22 Traumatic compartment syndrome of** left
lower extremity

√7ᵗʰ **T79.A29 Traumatic compartment syndrome of**
unspecified lower extremity

√x7ᵗʰ **T79.A3 Traumatic compartment syndrome of** abdomen

√x7ᵗʰ **T79.A9 Traumatic compartment syndrome of other sites**

√x7ᵗʰ **T79.8 Other early complications of trauma**

√x7ᵗʰ **T79.9 Unspecified early complication of trauma**

Complications of surgical and medical care, not elsewhere classified (T80-T88)

Use additional code for adverse effect, if applicable, to identify drug (T36-T50
with fifth or sixth character 5)

Use additional code(s) to identify the specified condition resulting from the
complication

Use additional code to identify devices involved and details of circumstances
(Y62-Y82)

EXCLUDES 2 *any encounters with medical care for postprocedural conditions in
which no complications are present, such as:*
artificial opening status (Z93.-)
closure of external stoma (Z43.-)
fitting and adjustment of external prosthetic device (Z44.-)
burns and corrosions from local applications and irradiation (T20-T32)
*complications of surgical procedures during pregnancy, childbirth and
the puerperium (O00-O9A)*
disorders of fluid and electrolyte imbalance (E86-E87)
mechanical complication of respirator [ventilator] (J95.850)
ostomy complications (J95.0-, K94.-, N99.5-)
*poisoning and toxic effects of drugs and chemicals (T36-T65 with fifth
or sixth character 1-4 or 6)*
postprocedural fever (R50.82)
specified complications classified elsewhere, such as:
cerebrospinal fluid leak from spinal puncture (G97.0)
colostomy malfunction (K94.0-)
disorders of fluid and electrolyte imbalance (E86-E87)
functional disturbances following cardiac surgery (I97.0-I97.1)
*intraoperative and postprocedural complications of specified body
systems (D78-, E36-, E89-, G97.3-, G97.4, H59.3-, H59-,
H95.2-, H95.3, I97.4-, I97.5, J95.6-, J95.7, K91.6-, L76-, M96-,
N99-)*
ostomy complications (J95.0-, K94-, N99.5-)
postgastric surgery syndromes (K91.1)
postlaminectomy syndrome NEC (M96.1)
postmastectomy lymphedema syndrome (I97.2)
postsurgical blind-loop syndrome (K91.2)
ventilator associated pneumonia (J95.851)

√4ᵗʰ **T80 Complications following infusion, transfusion and therapeutic**
injection

INCLUDES *complications following perfusion*

EXCLUDES 2 *bone marrow transplant rejection (T86.01)*
febrile nonhemolytic transfusion reaction (R50.84)
fluid overload due to transfusion (E87.71)
posttransfusion purpura (D69.51)
transfusion associated circulatory overload (TACO) (E87.71)
*transfusion (red blood cell) associated hemochromatosis
(E83.111)*
transfusion related acute lung injury (TRALI) (J95.84)

The appropriate 7th character is to be added to each code from
category T80.
A   initial encounter
D   subsequent encounter
S   sequela

√x7ᵗʰ **T80.0 Air embolism following infusion, transfusion and therapeutic**
injection

√x7ᵗʰ **T80.1 Vascular complications following infusion, transfusion and**
therapeutic injection

Use additional code to identify the vascular complication

EXCLUDES 2 *extravasation of vesicant agent (T80.81-)*
infiltration of vesicant agent (T80.81-)
*vascular complications specified as due to prosthetic
devices, implants and grafts (T82.8-, T83.8,
T84.8-, T85.8)*
postprocedural vascular complications (T81.7-)

√5ᵗʰ **T80.2 Infections following infusion, transfusion and therapeutic**
injection

Use additional code to identify the specific infection, such as:
sepsis (A41.9)

Use additional code (R65.2-) to identify severe sepsis, if
applicable

EXCLUDES 2 *infections specified as due to prosthetic devices,
implants and grafts (T82.6-T82.7, T83.5-T83.6,
T84.5-T84.7, T85.7)*
postprocedural infections (T81.4)

√6ᵗʰ **T80.21 Infection** due to central venous catheter

√7ᵗʰ **T80.211 Bloodstream infection** due to central
venous catheter
Catheter-related bloodstream infection
(CRBSI) NOS
Central line-associated bloodstream
infection (CLABSI)
Bloodstream infection due to Hickman
catheter
Bloodstream infection due to peripherally
inserted central catheter (PICC)
Bloodstream infection due to portacath
(port-a-cath)
Bloodstream infection due to triple lumen
catheter
Bloodstream infection due to umbilical
venous catheter

√7ᵗʰ **T80.212 Local infection** due to central venous
catheter
Exit or insertion site infection
Local infection due to Hickman catheter
Local infection due to peripherally inserted
central catheter (PICC)
Local infection due to portacath
(port-a-cath)
Local infection due to triple lumen catheter
Local infection due to umbilical venous
catheter
Port or reservoir infection
Tunnel infection

√7ᵗʰ **T80.218 Other infection due to central venous**
catheter
Other central line-associated infection
Other infection due to Hickman catheter
Other infection due to peripherally inserted
central catheter (PICC)
Other infection due to portacath
(port-a-cath)
Other infection due to triple lumen
catheter
Other infection due to umbilical venous
catheter

√7ᵗʰ **T80.219 Unspecified infection due to central**
venous catheter
Central line-associated infection NOS
Unspecified infection due to Hickman
catheter
Unspecified infection due to peripherally
inserted central catheter (PICC)
Unspecified infection due to portacath
(port-a-cath)
Unspecified infection due to triple lumen
catheter
Unspecified infection due to umbilical
venous catheter

√x7ᵗʰ **T80.22 Acute infection following transfusion, infusion, or**
injection of blood and blood products

√x7ᵗʰ **T80.29 Infection following other infusion, transfusion and**
therapeutic injection

✓ Additional Character Required   √x7ᵗʰ Xtension Alert   Unspecified Code   Other Specified Code   Manifestation Code   ►◄ Revised Text   ● New Code   ▲ Revised Code Title

ICD-10-CM 2014 (Draft)   977

T80.3 ABO incompatibility reaction due to transfusion of blood or blood products

> *EXCLUDES 1*   minor blood group antigens reactions (Duffy) (E) (K(ell)) (Kidd) (Lewis) (M) (N) (P) (S) (T80.A)

✓x7th **T80.30** **ABO incompatibility reaction due to transfusion of blood or blood products, unspecified**
> ABO incompatibility blood transfusion NOS
> Reaction to ABO incompatibility from transfusion NOS

✓6th **T80.31** **ABO incompatibility with hemolytic transfusion reaction**

> ✓7th **T80.310** **ABO incompatibility with acute hemolytic transfusion reaction**
> > ABO incompatibility with hemolytic transfusion reaction less than 24 hours after transfusion
> > Acute hemolytic transfusion reaction (AHTR) due to ABO incompatibility

> ✓7th **T80.311** **ABO incompatibility with delayed hemolytic transfusion reaction**
> > ABO incompatibility with hemolytic transfusion reaction 24 hours or more after transfusion
> > Delayed hemolytic transfusion reaction (DHTR) due to ABO incompatibility

> ✓7th **T80.319** **ABO incompatibility with hemolytic transfusion reaction, unspecified**
> > ABO incompatibility with hemolytic transfusion reaction at unspecified time after transfusion
> > Hemolytic transfusion reaction (HTR) due to ABO incompatibility NOS

✓x7th **T80.39** **Other ABO incompatibility reaction due to transfusion of blood or blood products**
> Delayed serologic transfusion reaction (DSTR) from ABO incompatibility
> Other ABO incompatible blood transfusion
> Other reaction to ABO incompatible blood transfusion

✓x7th **T80.4** Rh incompatibility reaction due to transfusion of blood or blood products
> Reaction due to incompatibility of Rh antigens (C) (c) (D) (E) (e)

✓x7th **T80.40** **Rh incompatibility reaction due to transfusion of blood or blood products, unspecified**
> Reaction due to Rh factor in transfusion NOS
> Rh incompatible blood transfusion NOS

✓6th **T80.41** **Rh incompatibility with hemolytic transfusion reaction**

> ✓7th **T80.410** **Rh incompatibility with acute hemolytic transfusion reaction**
> > Acute hemolytic transfusion reaction (AHTR) due to Rh incompatibility
> > Rh incompatibility with hemolytic transfusion reaction less than 24 hours after transfusion

> ✓7th **T80.411** **Rh incompatibility with delayed hemolytic transfusion reaction**
> > Delayed hemolytic transfusion reaction (DHTR) due to Rh incompatibility
> > Rh incompatibility with hemolytic transfusion reaction 24 hours or more after transfusion

> ✓7th **T80.419** **Rh incompatibility with hemolytic transfusion reaction, unspecified**
> > Hemolytic transfusion reaction (HTR) due to Rh incompatibility NOS
> > Rh incompatibility with hemolytic transfusion reaction at unspecified time after transfusion

✓x7th **T80.49** **Other Rh incompatibility reaction due to transfusion of blood or blood products**
> Delayed serologic transfusion reaction (DSTR) from Rh incompatibility
> Other reaction to Rh incompatible blood transfusion

✓5th **T80.A** Non-ABO incompatibility reaction due to transfusion of blood or blood products
> Reaction due to incompatibility of minor antigens (Duffy) (Kell) (Kidd) (Lewis) (M) (N) (P) (S)

✓x7th **T80.A0** **Non-ABO incompatibility reaction due to transfusion of blood or blood products, unspecified**
> Non-ABO antigen incompatibility reaction from transfusion NOS

✓6th **T80.A1** **Non-ABO incompatibility with hemolytic transfusion reaction**

> ✓7th **T80.A10** **Non-ABO incompatibility with acute hemolytic transfusion reaction**
> > Acute hemolytic transfusion reaction (AHTR) due to non-ABO incompatibility
> > Non-ABO incompatibility with hemolytic transfusion reaction less than 24 hours after transfusion

> ✓7th **T80.A11** **Non-ABO incompatibility with delayed hemolytic transfusion reaction**
> > Delayed hemolytic transfusion reaction (DHTR) due to non-ABO incompatibility
> > Non-ABO incompatibility with hemolytic transfusion reaction 24 or more hours after transfusion

> ✓7th **T80.A19** **Non-ABO incompatibility with hemolytic transfusion reaction, unspecified**
> > Hemolytic transfusion reaction (HTR) due to non-ABO incompatibility NOS
> > Non-ABO incompatibility with hemolytic transfusion reaction at unspecified time after transfusion

✓x7th **T80.A9** **Other non-ABO incompatibility reaction due to transfusion of blood or blood products**
> Delayed serologic transfusion reaction (DSTR) from non-ABO incompatibility
> Other reaction to non-ABO incompatible blood transfusion

✓5th **T80.5** Anaphylactic reaction due to serum
> Allergic shock due to serum
> Anaphylactic shock due to serum
> Anaphylactoid reaction due to serum
> Anaphylaxis due to serum

> *EXCLUDES 1*   ABO incompatibility reaction due to transfusion of blood or blood products (T80.3-)
> allergic reaction or shock NOS (T78.2)
> anaphylactic reaction or shock NOS (T78.2)
> anaphylactic reaction or shock due to adverse effect of correct medicinal substance properly administered (T88.6)
> other serum reaction (T80.6-)

✓x7th **T80.51** **Anaphylactic reaction due to administration of blood and blood products**

✓x7th **T80.52** **Anaphylactic reaction due to vaccination**

✓x7th **T80.59** **Anaphylactic reaction due to other serum**

✓5th **T80.6** Other serum reactions
> Intoxication by serum
> Protein sickness
> Serum rash
> Serum sickness
> Serum urticaria

> *EXCLUDES 2*   serum hepatitis (B16.-)

✓x7th **T80.61** **Other serum reaction due to administration of blood and blood products**

✓x7th **T80.62** **Other serum reaction due to vaccination**

✓x7th **T80.69** **Other serum reaction due to other serum**

✓5th **T80.8** Other complications following infusion, transfusion and therapeutic injection

✓6th **T80.81** **Extravasation of vesicant agent**
> Infiltration of vesicant agent

> ✓7th **T80.810** **Extravasation of vesicant antineoplastic chemotherapy**
> > Infiltration of vesicant antineoplastic chemotherapy

> ✓7th **T80.818** **Extravasation of other vesicant agent**
> > Infiltration of other vesicant agent

✓x7th **T80.89** **Other complications following infusion, transfusion and therapeutic injection**
> Delayed serologic transfusion reaction (DSTR), unspecified incompatibility
> Use additional code to identify graft-versus-host reaction, if applicable, (D89.81-)

✓5th **T80.9** Unspecified complication following infusion, transfusion and therapeutic injection

✓x7th **T80.90** **Unspecified complication following infusion and therapeutic injection**

EXCLUDES 1 Not coded here   *EXCLUDES 2* Not included here   N Newborn Age: 0   P Pediatric Age: 0-17   M Maternity Age: 12-55   A Adult Age: 15-124

✓6ᵗʰ **T80.91 Hemolytic transfusion reaction**, unspecified incompatibility

> EXCLUDES 1   *ABO incompatibility with hemolytic transfusion reaction (T80.31-)*
> *Non-ABO incompatibility with hemolytic transfusion reaction (T80.A1-)*
> *Rh incompatibility with hemolytic transfusion reaction (T80.41-)*

✓7ᵗʰ **T80.910 Acute hemolytic transfusion reaction, unspecified incompatibility**

✓7ᵗʰ **T80.911 Delayed hemolytic transfusion reaction, unspecified incompatibility**

✓7ᵗʰ **T80.919 Hemolytic transfusion reaction, unspecified incompatibility, unspecified as acute or delayed**
> Hemolytic transfusion reaction NOS

✓x7ᵗʰ **T80.92 Unspecified transfusion reaction**
> Transfusion reaction NOS

✓4ᵗʰ **T81 Complications of procedures, not elsewhere classified**
> Use additional code for adverse effect, if applicable, to identify drug (T36-T50 with fifth or sixth character 5)
> EXCLUDES 2   *complications following immunization (T88.0-T88.1)*
> *complications following infusion, transfusion and therapeutic injection (T80.-)*
> *complications of transplanted organs and tissue (T86.-)*
> *intraoperative and postprocedural complications of specific body system (D78.-, E36.-, E89.-, G97.3-, G97.4, H59.3-, H59.-, H95.2-, H95.3, I97.4-, I97.5, J95, K91.-, L76.-, M96.-, N99.-)*
> *specified complications classified elsewhere, such as:*
>   *complication of prosthetic devices, implants and grafts (T82-T85)*
>   *dermatitis due to drugs and medicaments (L23.3, L24.4, L25.1, L27.0-L27.1)*
>   *endosseous dental implant failure (M27.6-)*
>   *floppy iris syndrome (IFIS) (intraoperative) H21.81*
>   *intraoperative and postprocedural complications of specific body system (D78-, E36- E89-, G97.3-, G97.4, H59.3-, H59-, H95.2-, H95.3, I97.4-, I97.5, J95, K91-, L76-, M96-, N99-)*
>   *ostomy complications (J95.0-, K94-, N99.5-)*
>   *plateau iris syndrome (post-iridectomy) (postprocedural) H21.82*
>   *poisoning and toxic effects of drugs and chemicals (T36-T65 with fifth or sixth character 1-4 or 6)*

The appropriate 7th character is to be added to each code from category T81.
A   initial encounter
D   subsequent encounter
S   sequela

✓5ᵗʰ **T81.1 Postprocedural shock**
> Shock during or resulting from a procedure, not elsewhere classified
> EXCLUDES 1   *anaphylactic shock NOS (T78.2)*
> *anaphylactic shock due to correct substance properly administered (T88.6)*
> *anaphylactic shock due to serum (T80.5-)*
> *anesthetic shock (T88.2)*
> *electric shock (T75.4)*
> *obstetric shock (O75.1)*
> *septic shock (R65.21)*
> *shock following abortion or ectopic or molar pregnancy (O00-O07, O08.3)*
> *traumatic shock (T79.4)*

✓x7ᵗʰ **T81.10 Postprocedural shock unspecified**
> Collapse NOS during or resulting from a procedure, not elsewhere classified
> Postprocedural failure of peripheral circulation
> Postprocedural shock NOS

✓x7ᵗʰ **T81.11 Postprocedural cardiogenic shock**

✓x7ᵗʰ **T81.12 Postprocedural septic shock**
> Postprocedural endotoxic shock during or resulting from a procedure, not elsewhere classified
> Postprocedural gram-negative shock during or resulting from a procedure, not elsewhere classified
> Code first underlying infection
> Use additional code, to identify any associated acute organ dysfunction, if applicable

✓x7ᵗʰ **T81.19 Other postprocedural shock**
> Postprocedural hypovolemic shock

✓5ᵗʰ **T81.3 Disruption of wound, not elsewhere classified**
> Disruption of any suture materials or other closure methods
> EXCLUDES 1   *breakdown (mechanical) of permanent sutures (T85.612)*
> *displacement of permanent sutures (T85.622)*
> *disruption of cesarean delivery wound (O90.0)*
> *disruption of perineal obstetric wound (O90.1)*
> *mechanical complication of permanent sutures NEC (T85.692)*

✓x7ᵗʰ **T81.30 Disruption of wound, unspecified**
> Disruption of wound NOS

✓x7ᵗʰ **T81.31 Disruption of external operation (surgical) wound, not elsewhere classified**
> Dehiscence of operation wound NOS
> Disruption of operation wound NOS
> Disruption or dehiscence of closure of cornea
> Disruption or dehiscence of closure of mucosa
> Disruption or dehiscence of closure of skin and subcutaneous tissue
> Full-thickness skin disruption or dehiscence
> Superficial disruption or dehiscence of operation wound
> EXCLUDES 1   *dehiscence of amputation stump (T87.81)*

✓x7ᵗʰ **T81.32 Disruption of internal operation (surgical) wound, not elsewhere classified**
> Deep disruption or dehiscence of operation wound NOS
> Disruption or dehiscence of closure of internal organ or other internal tissue
> Disruption or dehiscence of closure of muscle or muscle flap
> Disruption or dehiscence of closure of ribs or rib cage
> Disruption or dehiscence of closure of skull or craniotomy
> Disruption or dehiscence of closure of sternum or sternotomy
> Disruption or dehiscence of closure of tendon or ligament
> Disruption or dehiscence of closure of superficial or muscular fascia

✓x7ᵗʰ **T81.33 Disruption of traumatic injury wound repair**
> Disruption or dehiscence of closure of traumatic laceration (external) (internal)

✓x7ᵗʰ **T81.4 Infection following a procedure**
> Intra-abdominal abscess following a procedure
> Postprocedural infection, not elsewhere classified
> Sepsis following a procedure
> Stitch abscess following a procedure
> Subphrenic abscess following a procedure
> Wound abscess following a procedure
> Use additional code to identify infection
> Use additional code (R65.2-) to identify severe sepsis, if applicable
> EXCLUDES 1   *obstetric surgical wound infection (O86.0)*
> *postprocedural fever NOS (R50.82)*
> *postprocedural retroperitoneal abscess (K68.11)*
> EXCLUDES 2   *bleb associated endophthalmitis (H59.4-)*
> *infection due to infusion, transfusion and therapeutic injection (T80.2-)*
> *infection due to prosthetic devices, implants and grafts (T82.6-T82.7, T83.5-T83.6, T84.5-T84.7, T85.7)*

✓5ᵗʰ **T81.5 Complications of foreign body accidentally left in body following procedure**

✓6ᵗʰ **T81.50 Unspecified complication of foreign body accidentally left in body following procedure**

✓7ᵗʰ **T81.500 Unspecified complication of foreign body accidentally left in body following surgical operation**

✓7ᵗʰ **T81.501 Unspecified complication of foreign body accidentally left in body following infusion or transfusion**

✓7ᵗʰ **T81.502 Unspecified complication of foreign body accidentally left in body following kidney dialysis**

✓7ᵗʰ **T81.503 Unspecified complication of foreign body accidentally left in body following injection or immunization**

✓7ᵗʰ **T81.504 Unspecified complication of foreign body accidentally left in body following endoscopic examination**

☑ Additional Character Required   ✓x7ᵗʰ Xtension Alert   Unspecified Code   Other Specified Code   Manifestation Code   ▶◀ Revised Text   ● New Code   ▲ Revised Code Title

ICD-10-CM 2014 (Draft)   979

√7th **T81.505** **Unspecified complication of foreign body accidentally left in body following heart catheterization**

√7th **T81.506** **Unspecified complication of foreign body accidentally left in body following aspiration, puncture or other catheterization**

√7th **T81.507** **Unspecified complication of foreign body accidentally left in body following removal of catheter or packing**

√7th **T81.508** **Unspecified complication of foreign body accidentally left in body following other procedure**

√7th **T81.509** **Unspecified complication of foreign body accidentally left in body following unspecified procedure**

√6th **T81.51** Adhesions **due to foreign body accidentally left in body following procedure**

√7th **T81.510** **Adhesions due to foreign body accidentally left in body following surgical operation**

√7th **T81.511** **Adhesions due to foreign body accidentally left in body following infusion or transfusion**

√7th **T81.512** **Adhesions due to foreign body accidentally left in body following kidney dialysis**

√7th **T81.513** **Adhesions due to foreign body accidentally left in body following injection or immunization**

√7th **T81.514** **Adhesions due to foreign body accidentally left in body following endoscopic examination**

√7th **T81.515** **Adhesions due to foreign body accidentally left in body following heart catheterization**

√7th **T81.516** **Adhesions due to foreign body accidentally left in body following aspiration, puncture or other catheterization**

√7th **T81.517** **Adhesions due to foreign body accidentally left in body following removal of catheter or packing**

√7th **T81.518** **Adhesions due to foreign body accidentally left in body following other procedure**

√7th **T81.519** **Adhesions due to foreign body accidentally left in body following unspecified procedure**

√6th **T81.52** Obstruction **due to foreign body accidentally left in body following procedure**

√7th **T81.520** **Obstruction due to foreign body accidentally left in body following surgical operation**

√7th **T81.521** **Obstruction due to foreign body accidentally left in body following infusion or transfusion**

√7th **T81.522** **Obstruction due to foreign body accidentally left in body following kidney dialysis**

√7th **T81.523** **Obstruction due to foreign body accidentally left in body following injection or immunization**

√7th **T81.524** **Obstruction due to foreign body accidentally left in body following endoscopic examination**

√7th **T81.525** **Obstruction due to foreign body accidentally left in body following heart catheterization**

√7th **T81.526** **Obstruction due to foreign body accidentally left in body following aspiration, puncture or other catheterization**

√7th **T81.527** **Obstruction due to foreign body accidentally left in body following removal of catheter or packing**

√7th **T81.528** **Obstruction due to foreign body accidentally left in body following other procedure**

√7th **T81.529** **Obstruction due to foreign body accidentally left in body following unspecified procedure**

√6th **T81.53** Perforation **due to foreign body accidentally left in body following procedure**

√7th **T81.530** **Perforation due to foreign body accidentally left in body following surgical operation**

√7th **T81.531** **Perforation due to foreign body accidentally left in body following infusion or transfusion**

√7th **T81.532** **Perforation due to foreign body accidentally left in body following kidney dialysis**

√7th **T81.533** **Perforation due to foreign body accidentally left in body following injection or immunization**

√7th **T81.534** **Perforation due to foreign body accidentally left in body following endoscopic examination**

√7th **T81.535** **Perforation due to foreign body accidentally left in body following heart catheterization**

√7th **T81.536** **Perforation due to foreign body accidentally left in body following aspiration, puncture or other catheterization**

√7th **T81.537** **Perforation due to foreign body accidentally left in body following removal of catheter or packing**

√7th **T81.538** **Perforation due to foreign body accidentally left in body following other procedure**

√7th **T81.539** **Perforation due to foreign body accidentally left in body following unspecified procedure**

√6th **T81.59** Other **complications of foreign body accidentally left in body following procedure**

EXCLUDES 2   *obstruction or perforation due to prosthetic devices and implants intentionally left in body (T82.0-T82.5, T83.0-T83.4, T83.7, T84.0-T84.4, T85.0-T85.6)*

√7th **T81.590** **Other complications of foreign body accidentally left in body following surgical operation**

√7th **T81.591** **Other complications of foreign body accidentally left in body following infusion or transfusion**

√7th **T81.592** **Other complications of foreign body accidentally left in body following kidney dialysis**

√7th **T81.593** **Other complications of foreign body accidentally left in body following injection or immunization**

√7th **T81.594** **Other complications of foreign body accidentally left in body following endoscopic examination**

√7th **T81.595** **Other complications of foreign body accidentally left in body following heart catheterization**

√7th **T81.596** **Other complications of foreign body accidentally left in body following aspiration, puncture or other catheterization**

√7th **T81.597** **Other complications of foreign body accidentally left in body following removal of catheter or packing**

√7th **T81.598** **Other complications of foreign body accidentally left in body following other procedure**

√7th **T81.599** **Other complications of foreign body accidentally left in body following unspecified procedure**

EXCLUDES 1 Not coded here   EXCLUDES 2 Not included here   N Newborn Age: 0   P Pediatric Age: 0-17   M Maternity Age: 12-55   A Adult Age: 15-124

980   ICD-10-CM 2014 (Draft)

✓5th **T81.6 Acute reaction to foreign substance accidentally left during a procedure**

> EXCLUDES 2   *complications of foreign body accidentally left in body cavity or operation wound following procedure (T81.5-)*

  ✓x7th **T81.60 Unspecified acute reaction to foreign substance accidentally left during a procedure**

  ✓x7th **T81.61 Aseptic peritonitis due to foreign substance accidentally left during a procedure**
Chemical peritonitis

  ✓x7th **T81.69 Other acute reaction to foreign substance accidentally left during a procedure**

✓5th **T81.7 Vascular complications following a procedure, not elsewhere classified**
Air embolism following procedure NEC
Phlebitis or thrombophlebitis resulting from a procedure

> EXCLUDES 1   *embolism complicating abortion or ectopic or molar pregnancy (O00–O07, O08.2)*
> *embolism complicating pregnancy, childbirth and the puerperium (O88.-)*
> *traumatic embolism (T79.0)*

> EXCLUDES 2   *embolism due to prosthetic devices, implants and grafts (T82.8-, T83.8, T84.8-, T85.8)*
> *embolism following infusion, transfusion and therapeutic injection (T80.0)*

  ✓6th **T81.71 Complication of artery following a procedure, not elsewhere classified**

    ✓7th **T81.710 Complication of mesenteric artery following a procedure, not elsewhere classified**

    ✓7th **T81.711 Complication of renal artery following a procedure, not elsewhere classified**

    ✓7th **T81.718 Complication of other artery following a procedure, not elsewhere classified**

    ✓7th **T81.719 Complication of unspecified artery following a procedure, not elsewhere classified**

  ✓x7th **T81.72 Complication of vein following a procedure, not elsewhere classified**

✓5th **T81.8 Other complications of procedures, not elsewhere classified**

> EXCLUDES 2   *hypothermia following anesthesia (T88.51)*
> *malignant hyperpyrexia due to anesthesia (T88.3)*

  ✓x7th **T81.81 Complication of inhalation therapy**

  ✓x7th **T81.82 Emphysema (subcutaneous) resulting from a procedure**

  ✓x7th **T81.83 Persistent postprocedural fistula**

  ✓x7th **T81.89 Other complications of procedures, not elsewhere classified**
Use additional code to specify complication, such as: postprocedural delirium (F05)

✓x7th **T81.9 Unspecified complication of procedure**

✓4th **T82 Complications of cardiac and vascular prosthetic devices, implants and grafts**

> EXCLUDES 2   *failure and rejection of transplanted organs and tissue (T86.-)*

The appropriate 7th character is to be added to each code from category T82.
A   initial encounter
D   subsequent encounter
S   sequela

✓5th **T82.0 Mechanical complication of heart valve prosthesis**
Mechanical complication of artificial heart valve

> EXCLUDES 1   *mechanical complication of biological heart valve graft (T82.22-)*

  ✓x7th **T82.01 Breakdown (mechanical) of heart valve prosthesis**

  ✓x7th **T82.02 Displacement of heart valve prosthesis**
Malposition of heart valve prosthesis

  ✓x7th **T82.03 Leakage of heart valve prosthesis**

  ✓x7th **T82.09 Other mechanical complication of heart valve prosthesis**
Obstruction (mechanical) of heart valve prosthesis
Perforation of heart valve prosthesis
Protrusion of heart valve prosthesis

✓5th **T82.1 Mechanical complication of cardiac electronic device**

  ✓6th **T82.11 Breakdown (mechanical) of cardiac electronic device**

    ✓7th **T82.110 Breakdown (mechanical) of cardiac electrode**

    ✓7th **T82.111 Breakdown (mechanical) of cardiac pulse generator (battery)**

    ✓7th **T82.118 Breakdown (mechanical) of other cardiac electronic device**

    ✓7th **T82.119 Breakdown (mechanical) of unspecified cardiac electronic device**

  ✓6th **T82.12 Displacement of cardiac electronic device**
Malposition of cardiac electronic device

    ✓7th **T82.120 Displacement of cardiac electrode**

    ✓7th **T82.121 Displacement of cardiac pulse generator (battery)**

    ✓7th **T82.128 Displacement of other cardiac electronic device**

    ✓7th **T82.129 Displacement of unspecified cardiac electronic device**

  ✓6th **T82.19 Other mechanical complication of cardiac electronic device**
Leakage of cardiac electronic device
Obstruction of cardiac electronic device
Perforation of cardiac electronic device
Protrusion of cardiac electronic device

    ✓7th **T82.190 Other mechanical complication of cardiac electrode**

    ✓7th **T82.191 Other mechanical complication of cardiac pulse generator (battery)**

    ✓7th **T82.198 Other mechanical complication of other cardiac electronic device**

    ✓7th **T82.199 Other mechanical complication of unspecified cardiac device**

✓5th **T82.2 Mechanical complication of coronary artery bypass graft and biological heart valve graft**

> EXCLUDES 1   *mechanical complication of artificial heart valve prosthesis (T82.0-)*

  ✓6th **T82.21 Mechanical complication of coronary artery bypass graft**

    ✓7th **T82.211 Breakdown (mechanical) of coronary artery bypass graft**

    ✓7th **T82.212 Displacement of coronary artery bypass graft**
Malposition of coronary artery bypass graft

    ✓7th **T82.213 Leakage of coronary artery bypass graft**

    ✓7th **T82.218 Other mechanical complication of coronary artery bypass graft**
Obstruction, mechanical of coronary artery bypass graft
Perforation of coronary artery bypass graft
Protrusion of coronary artery bypass graft

  ✓6th **T82.22 Mechanical complication of biological heart valve graft**

    ✓7th **T82.221 Breakdown (mechanical) of biological heart valve graft**

    ✓7th **T82.222 Displacement of biological heart valve graft**
Malposition of biological heart valve graft

    ✓7th **T82.223 Leakage of biological heart valve graft**

    ✓7th **T82.228 Other mechanical complication of biological heart valve graft**
Obstruction of biological heart valve graft
Perforation of biological heart valve graft
Protrusion of biological heart valve graft

✓5th **T82.3 Mechanical complication of other vascular grafts**

  ✓6th **T82.31 Breakdown (mechanical) of other vascular grafts**

    ✓7th **T82.310 Breakdown (mechanical) of aortic (bifurcation) graft (replacement)**

    ✓7th **T82.311 Breakdown (mechanical) of carotid arterial graft (bypass)**

    ✓7th **T82.312 Breakdown (mechanical) of femoral arterial graft (bypass)**

    ✓7th **T82.318 Breakdown (mechanical) of other vascular grafts**

    ✓7th **T82.319 Breakdown (mechanical) of unspecified vascular grafts**

  ✓6th **T82.32 Displacement of other vascular grafts**
Malposition of other vascular grafts

    ✓7th **T82.320 Displacement of aortic (bifurcation) graft (replacement)**

Injury, Poisoning and Certain Other Consequences of External

T82.321–T82.847

√7th **T82.321** **Displacement** of carotid arterial graft (bypass)

√7th **T82.322** **Displacement** of femoral arterial graft (bypass)

√7th **T82.328** **Displacement of other vascular grafts**

√7th **T82.329** **Displacement of unspecified vascular grafts**

√6th **T82.33** Leakage of other vascular grafts

     √7th **T82.330** **Leakage of** aortic (bifurcation) graft (replacement)

     √7th **T82.331** **Leakage of** carotid arterial graft (bypass)

     √7th **T82.332** **Leakage of** femoral arterial graft (bypass)

     √7th **T82.338** **Leakage of other vascular grafts**

     √7th **T82.339** **Leakage of unspecified vascular graft**

√6th **T82.39** Other mechanical complication of other vascular grafts
> Obstruction (mechanical) of other vascular grafts
> Perforation of other vascular grafts
> Protrusion of other vascular grafts

     √7th **T82.390** **Other mechanical complication of** aortic (bifurcation) graft (replacement)

     √7th **T82.391** **Other mechanical complication of** carotid arterial graft (bypass)

     √7th **T82.392** **Other mechanical complication of** femoral arterial graft (bypass)

     √7th **T82.398** **Other mechanical complication of other vascular grafts**

     √7th **T82.399** **Other mechanical complication of unspecified vascular grafts**

√5th **T82.4** **Mechanical complication of** vascular dialysis catheter
Mechanical complication of hemodialysis catheter
> **EXCLUDES 1** mechanical complication of intraperitoneal dialysis catheter (T85.62)

√x7th **T82.41** **Breakdown (mechanical) of** vascular dialysis catheter

√x7th **T82.42** **Displacement** of vascular dialysis catheter
Malposition of vascular dialysis catheter

√x7th **T82.43** **Leakage** of vascular dialysis catheter

√x7th **T82.49** **Other complication of** vascular dialysis catheter
> Obstruction (mechanical) of vascular dialysis catheter
> Perforation of vascular dialysis catheter
> Protrusion of vascular dialysis catheter

√5th **T82.5** **Mechanical complication of** other cardiac and vascular devices and implants
> **EXCLUDES 2** mechanical complication of epidural and subdural infusion catheter (T85.61)

√6th **T82.51** Breakdown (mechanical) of other cardiac and vascular devices and implants

     √7th **T82.510** **Breakdown (mechanical) of** surgically created arteriovenous fistula

     √7th **T82.511** **Breakdown (mechanical) of** surgically created arteriovenous shunt

     √7th **T82.512** **Breakdown (mechanical) of** artificial heart

     √7th **T82.513** **Breakdown (mechanical) of** balloon (counterpulsation) device

     √7th **T82.514** **Breakdown (mechanical) of** infusion catheter

     √7th **T82.515** **Breakdown (mechanical) of** umbrella device

     √7th **T82.518** **Breakdown (mechanical) of other cardiac and vascular devices and implants**

     √7th **T82.519** **Breakdown (mechanical) of unspecified cardiac and vascular devices and implants**

√6th **T82.52** Displacement of other cardiac and vascular devices and implants
> Malposition of other cardiac and vascular devices and implants

     √7th **T82.520** **Displacement of** surgically created arteriovenous fistula

     √7th **T82.521** **Displacement of** surgically created arteriovenous shunt

     √7th **T82.522** **Displacement of** artificial heart

     √7th **T82.523** **Displacement of** balloon (counterpulsation) device

     √7th **T82.524** **Displacement of** infusion catheter

√7th **T82.525** **Displacement of** umbrella device

√7th **T82.528** **Displacement of other cardiac and vascular devices and implants**

√7th **T82.529** **Displacement of unspecified cardiac and vascular devices and implants**

√6th **T82.53** Leakage of other cardiac and vascular devices and implants

     √7th **T82.530** **Leakage of** surgically created arteriovenous fistula

     √7th **T82.531** **Leakage of** surgically created arteriovenous shunt

     √7th **T82.532** **Leakage of** artificial heart

     √7th **T82.533** **Leakage of** balloon (counterpulsation) device

     √7th **T82.534** **Leakage of** infusion catheter

     √7th **T82.535** **Leakage of** umbrella device

     √7th **T82.538** **Leakage of other cardiac and vascular devices and implants**

     √7th **T82.539** **Leakage of unspecified cardiac and vascular devices and implants**

√6th **T82.59** Other mechanical complication of other cardiac and vascular devices and implants
> Obstruction (mechanical) of other cardiac and vascular devices and implants
> Perforation of other cardiac and vascular devices and implants
> Protrusion of other cardiac and vascular devices and implants

     √7th **T82.590** **Other mechanical complication of** surgically created arteriovenous fistula

     √7th **T82.591** **Other mechanical complication of** surgically created arteriovenous shunt

     √7th **T82.592** **Other mechanical complication of** artificial heart

     √7th **T82.593** **Other mechanical complication of** balloon (counterpulsation) device

     √7th **T82.594** **Other mechanical complication of** infusion catheter

     √7th **T82.595** **Other mechanical complication of** umbrella device

     √7th **T82.598** **Other mechanical complication of other cardiac and vascular devices and implants**

     √7th **T82.599** **Other mechanical complication of unspecified cardiac and vascular devices and implants**

√x7th **T82.6** **Infection and inflammatory reaction due to** cardiac valve prosthesis
Use additional code to identify infection

√x7th **T82.7** **Infection and inflammatory reaction due to** other cardiac and vascular devices, implants and grafts
Use additional code to identify infection

√5th **T82.8** Other specified complications of cardiac and vascular prosthetic devices, implants and grafts

√6th **T82.81** Embolism of cardiac and vascular prosthetic devices, implants and grafts

     √7th **T82.817** **Embolism of** cardiac prosthetic devices, implants and grafts

     √7th **T82.818** **Embolism of** vascular prosthetic devices, implants and grafts

√6th **T82.82** Fibrosis of cardiac and vascular prosthetic devices, implants and grafts

     √7th **T82.827** **Fibrosis of** cardiac prosthetic devices, implants and grafts

     √7th **T82.828** **Fibrosis of** vascular prosthetic devices, implants and grafts

√6th **T82.83** Hemorrhage of cardiac and vascular prosthetic devices, implants and grafts

     √7th **T82.837** **Hemorrhage of** cardiac prosthetic devices, implants and grafts

     √7th **T82.838** **Hemorrhage of** vascular prosthetic devices, implants and grafts

√6th **T82.84** Pain from cardiac and vascular prosthetic devices, implants and grafts

     √7th **T82.847** **Pain from** cardiac prosthetic devices, implants and grafts

---

EXCLUDES 1 Not coded here   **EXCLUDES 2** Not included here   **N** Newborn Age: 0   **P** Pediatric Age: 0-17   **M** Maternity Age: 12-55   **A** Adult Age: 15-124

982   ICD-10-CM 2014 (Draft)

√7th **T82.848** **Pain from** vascular **prosthetic devices, implants and grafts**

√6th **T82.85** Stenosis **of cardiac and vascular prosthetic devices, implants and grafts**

√7th **T82.857** **Stenosis of** cardiac **prosthetic devices, implants and grafts**

√7th **T82.858** **Stenosis of** vascular **prosthetic devices, implants and grafts**

√6th **T82.86** Thrombosis **of cardiac and vascular prosthetic devices, implants and grafts**

√7th **T82.867** **Thrombosis of** cardiac **prosthetic devices, implants and grafts**

√7th **T82.868** **Thrombosis of** vascular **prosthetic devices, implants and grafts**

√6th **T82.89** Other **specified complication of cardiac and vascular prosthetic devices, implants and grafts**

√7th **T82.897** **Other specified complication of** cardiac **prosthetic devices, implants and grafts**

√7th **T82.898** **Other specified complication of** vascular **prosthetic devices, implants and grafts**

√x7th **T82.9** **Unspecified complication of cardiac and vascular prosthetic device, implant and graft**

√4th **T83** **Complications of genitourinary prosthetic devices, implants and grafts**

> EXCLUDES 2 *failure and rejection of transplanted organs and tissue (T86.-)*

> The appropriate 7th character is to be added to each code from category T83.
> A   initial encounter
> D   subsequent encounter
> S   sequela

√5th **T83.0** **Mechanical complication of** urinary (indwelling) **catheter**

> EXCLUDES 2 *complications of stoma of urinary tract (N99.5-)*

√6th **T83.01** Breakdown (mechanical) **of urinary (indwelling) catheter**

√7th **T83.010** **Breakdown (mechanical) of** cystostomy **catheter**

√7th **T83.018** **Breakdown (mechanical) of other indwelling** urethral **catheter**

√6th **T83.02** Displacement **of urinary (indwelling) catheter**
Malposition of urinary (indwelling) catheter

√7th **T83.020** **Displacement of** cystostomy **catheter**

√7th **T83.028** **Displacement of other indwelling** urethral **catheter**

√6th **T83.03** Leakage **of urinary (indwelling) catheter**

√7th **T83.030** **Leakage of** cystostomy **catheter**

√7th **T83.038** **Leakage of other indwelling** urethral **catheter**

√6th **T83.09** Other **mechanical complication of urinary (indwelling) catheter**
Obstruction (mechanical) of urinary (indwelling) catheter
Perforation of urinary (indwelling) catheter
Protrusion of urinary (indwelling) catheter

√7th **T83.090** **Other mechanical complication of** cystostomy **catheter**

√7th **T83.098** **Other mechanical complication of other indwelling** urethral **catheter**

√5th **T83.1** **Mechanical complication of** other urinary devices and implants

√6th **T83.11** Breakdown (mechanical) **of other urinary devices and implants**

√7th **T83.110** **Breakdown (mechanical) of urinary** electronic stimulator device

√7th **T83.111** **Breakdown (mechanical) of urinary** sphincter implant

√7th **T83.112** **Breakdown (mechanical) of urinary** stent

√7th **T83.118** **Breakdown (mechanical) of other urinary devices and implants**

√6th **T83.12** Displacement **of other urinary devices and implants**
Malposition of other urinary devices and implants

√7th **T83.120** **Displacement of urinary** electronic stimulator device

√7th **T83.121** **Displacement of urinary** sphincter implant

√7th **T83.122** **Displacement of urinary** stent

√7th **T83.128** **Displacement of other urinary devices and implants**

√6th **T83.19** Other **mechanical complication of other urinary devices and implants**
Leakage of other urinary devices and implants
Obstruction (mechanical) of other urinary devices and implants
Perforation of other urinary devices and implants
Protrusion of other urinary devices and implants

√7th **T83.190** **Other mechanical complication of urinary** electronic stimulator device

√7th **T83.191** **Other mechanical complication of urinary** sphincter implant

√7th **T83.192** **Other mechanical complication of urinary** stent

√7th **T83.198** **Other mechanical complication of other urinary devices and implants**

√5th **T83.2** **Mechanical complication of** graft of urinary organ

√x7th **T83.21** Breakdown (mechanical) **of graft of urinary organ**

√x7th **T83.22** Displacement **of graft of urinary organ**
Malposition of graft of urinary organ

√x7th **T83.23** Leakage **of graft of urinary organ**

√x7th **T83.29** Other **mechanical complication of graft of urinary organ**
Obstruction (mechanical) of graft of urinary organ
Perforation of graft of urinary organ
Protrusion of graft of urinary organ

√5th **T83.3** **Mechanical complication of** intrauterine contraceptive device

√x7th **T83.31** Breakdown (mechanical) **of intrauterine contraceptive device** ♀

√x7th **T83.32** Displacement **of intrauterine contraceptive device** ♀
Malposition of intrauterine contraceptive device

√x7th **T83.39** Other **mechanical complication of intrauterine contraceptive device** ♀
Leakage of intrauterine contraceptive device
Obstruction (mechanical) of intrauterine contraceptive device
Perforation of intrauterine contraceptive device
Protrusion of intrauterine contraceptive device

√5th **T83.4** **Mechanical complication of** other prosthetic devices, implants and grafts of genital tract

√6th **T83.41** Breakdown (mechanical) **of other prosthetic devices, implants and grafts of genital tract**

√7th **T83.410** **Breakdown (mechanical) of** penile (implanted) prosthesis ♂

√7th **T83.418** **Breakdown (mechanical) of other prosthetic devices, implants and grafts of genital tract**

√6th **T83.42** Displacement **of other prosthetic devices, implants and grafts of genital tract**
Malposition of other prosthetic devices, implants and grafts of genital tract

√7th **T83.420** **Displacement of** penile (implanted) prosthesis ♂

√7th **T83.428** **Displacement of other prosthetic devices, implants and grafts of genital tract**

√6th **T83.49** Other **mechanical complication of other prosthetic devices, implants and grafts of genital tract**
Leakage of other prosthetic devices, implants and grafts of genital tract
Obstruction, mechanical of other prosthetic devices, implants and grafts of genital tract
Perforation of other prosthetic devices, implants and grafts of genital tract
Protrusion of other prosthetic devices, implants and grafts of genital tract

√7th **T83.490** **Other mechanical complication of** penile (implanted) prosthesis ♂

√7th **T83.498** **Other mechanical complication of other prosthetic devices, implants and grafts of genital tract**

√5th **T83.5** **Infection and inflammatory reaction due to prosthetic device, implant and graft in** urinary system
Use additional code to identify infection

√x7th **T83.51** **Infection and inflammatory reaction due to indwelling urinary catheter**

> EXCLUDES 2 *complications of stoma of urinary tract (N99.5-)*

✓x7ᵗʰ **T83.59 Infection and inflammatory reaction due to** prosthetic device, implant and graft in urinary system

✓x7ᵗʰ **T83.6 Infection and inflammatory reaction due to prosthetic device, implant and graft in** genital tract
Use additional code to identify infection

✓5ᵗʰ **T83.7 Complications due to** implanted mesh and other prosthetic materials

✓6ᵗʰ **T83.71 Erosion** of implanted mesh and other prosthetic materials to surrounding organ or tissue

✓7ᵗʰ **T83.711 Erosion of implanted** vaginal **mesh and other prosthetic materials to surrounding organ or tissue** ♀
Erosion of implanted vaginal mesh and other prosthetic materials into pelvic floor muscles

✓7ᵗʰ **T83.718 Erosion of other implanted mesh and other prosthetic materials to surrounding organ or tissue**

✓6ᵗʰ **T83.72 Exposure** of implanted mesh and other prosthetic materials into surrounding organ or tissue

✓7ᵗʰ **T83.721 Exposure of implanted** vaginal **mesh and other prosthetic materials into vagina** ♀
Exposure of implanted vaginal mesh and other prosthetic materials through vaginal wall

✓7ᵗʰ **T83.728 Exposure of** other **implanted mesh and other prosthetic materials to surrounding organ or tissue**

✓5ᵗʰ **T83.8 Other specified complications of** genitourinary prosthetic devices, implants and grafts

✓x7ᵗʰ **T83.81 Embolism** of genitourinary prosthetic devices, implants and grafts

✓x7ᵗʰ **T83.82 Fibrosis** of genitourinary prosthetic devices, implants and grafts

✓x7ᵗʰ **T83.83 Hemorrhage** of genitourinary prosthetic devices, implants and grafts

✓x7ᵗʰ **T83.84 Pain from** genitourinary prosthetic devices, implants and grafts

✓x7ᵗʰ **T83.85 Stenosis** of genitourinary prosthetic devices, implants and grafts

✓x7ᵗʰ **T83.86 Thrombosis** of genitourinary prosthetic devices, implants and grafts

✓x7ᵗʰ **T83.89 Other specified complication of genitourinary prosthetic devices, implants and grafts**

✓x7ᵗʰ **T83.9 Unspecified complication of genitourinary prosthetic device, implant and graft**

✓4ᵗʰ **T84 Complications of internal orthopedic prosthetic devices, implants and grafts**
EXCLUDES 2 *failure and rejection of transplanted organs and tissues (T86.-)*
fracture of bone following insertion of orthopedic implant, joint prosthesis or bone plate (M96.6)

The appropriate 7th character is to be added to each code from category T84.
A   initial encounter
D   subsequent encounter
S   sequela

✓5ᵗʰ **T84.0 Mechanical complication of** internal joint prosthesis

✓6ᵗʰ **T84.01 Broken** internal joint prosthesis
Breakage (fracture) of prosthetic joint
Broken prosthetic joint implant
EXCLUDES 1 *periprosthetic joint implant fracture (T84.04)*

✓7ᵗʰ **T84.010 Broken internal** right hip **prosthesis**

✓7ᵗʰ **T84.011 Broken internal** left hip **prosthesis**

✓7ᵗʰ **T84.012 Broken internal** right knee **prosthesis**

✓7ᵗʰ **T84.013 Broken internal** left knee **prosthesis**

✓7ᵗʰ **T84.018 Broken internal joint prosthesis, other site**
Use additional code to identify the joint (Z96.6-)

✓7ᵗʰ **T84.019 Broken internal joint prosthesis, unspecified site**

✓6ᵗʰ **T84.02 Dislocation** of internal joint prosthesis
Instability of internal joint prosthesis
Subluxation of internal joint prosthesis

✓7ᵗʰ **T84.020 Dislocation of internal** right hip **prosthesis**

✓7ᵗʰ **T84.021 Dislocation of internal** left hip **prosthesis**

✓7ᵗʰ **T84.022 Instability of internal** right knee **prosthesis**

✓7ᵗʰ **T84.023 Instability of internal** left knee **prosthesis**

✓7ᵗʰ **T84.028 Dislocation of other internal joint prosthesis**
Use additional code to identify the joint (Z96.6-)

✓7ᵗʰ **T84.029 Dislocation of unspecified internal joint prosthesis**

✓6ᵗʰ **T84.03 Mechanical loosening** of internal prosthetic joint
Aseptic loosening of prosthetic joint

✓7ᵗʰ **T84.030 Mechanical loosening of internal** right hip **prosthetic joint**

✓7ᵗʰ **T84.031 Mechanical loosening of internal** left hip **prosthetic joint**

✓7ᵗʰ **T84.032 Mechanical loosening of internal** right knee **prosthetic joint**

✓7ᵗʰ **T84.033 Mechanical loosening of internal** left knee **prosthetic joint**

✓7ᵗʰ **T84.038 Mechanical loosening of other internal prosthetic joint**
Use additional code to identify the joint (Z96.6-)

✓7ᵗʰ **T84.039 Mechanical loosening of unspecified internal prosthetic joint**

✓6ᵗʰ **T84.04 Periprosthetic fracture around internal prosthetic joint**
EXCLUDES 2 *breakage (fracture) of prosthetic joint (T84.01)*

✓7ᵗʰ **T84.040 Periprosthetic fracture around internal prosthetic** right hip **joint**

✓7ᵗʰ **T84.041 Periprosthetic fracture around internal prosthetic** left hip **joint**

✓7ᵗʰ **T84.042 Periprosthetic fracture around internal prosthetic** right knee **joint**

✓7ᵗʰ **T84.043 Periprosthetic fracture around internal prosthetic** left knee **joint**

✓7ᵗʰ **T84.048 Periprosthetic fracture around other internal prosthetic joint**
Use additional code to identify the joint (Z96.6-)

✓7ᵗʰ **T84.049 Periprosthetic fracture around unspecified internal prosthetic joint**

✓6ᵗʰ **T84.05 Periprosthetic osteolysis of internal prosthetic joint**
Use additional code to identify major osseous defect, if applicable (M89.7-)

✓7ᵗʰ **T84.050 Periprosthetic osteolysis of internal prosthetic** right hip **joint**

✓7ᵗʰ **T84.051 Periprosthetic osteolysis of internal prosthetic** left hip **joint**

✓7ᵗʰ **T84.052 Periprosthetic osteolysis of internal prosthetic** right knee **joint**

✓7ᵗʰ **T84.053 Periprosthetic osteolysis of internal prosthetic** left knee **joint**

✓7ᵗʰ **T84.058 Periprosthetic osteolysis of other internal prosthetic joint**
Use additional code to identify the joint (Z96.6-)

✓7ᵗʰ **T84.059 Periprosthetic osteolysis of unspecified internal prosthetic joint**

✓6ᵗʰ **T84.06 Wear of articular bearing surface of internal prosthetic joint**

✓7ᵗʰ **T84.060 Wear of articular bearing surface of internal prosthetic** right hip **joint**

✓7ᵗʰ **T84.061 Wear of articular bearing surface of internal prosthetic** left hip **joint**

✓7ᵗʰ **T84.062 Wear of articular bearing surface of internal prosthetic** right knee **joint**

✓7ᵗʰ **T84.063 Wear of articular bearing surface of internal prosthetic** left knee **joint**

✓7ᵗʰ **T84.068 Wear of articular bearing surface of other internal prosthetic joint**
Use additional code to identify the joint (Z96.6-)

✓7ᵗʰ **T84.069 Wear of articular bearing surface of unspecified internal prosthetic joint**

EXCLUDES 1 Not coded here   EXCLUDES 2 Not included here   N Newborn Age: 0   P Pediatric Age: 0-17   M Maternity Age: 12-55   A Adult Age: 15-124

984   ICD-10-CM 2014 (Draft)

√6ᵗʰ **T84.09** Other mechanical complication of internal joint prosthesis

     Prosthetic joint implant failure NOS

√7ᵗʰ **T84.090** Other mechanical complication of internal right hip prosthesis

√7ᵗʰ **T84.091** Other mechanical complication of internal left hip prosthesis

√7ᵗʰ **T84.092** Other mechanical complication of internal right knee prosthesis

√7ᵗʰ **T84.093** Other mechanical complication of internal left knee prosthesis

√7ᵗʰ **T84.098** Other mechanical complication of other internal joint prosthesis

     Use additional code to identify the joint (Z96.6-)

√7ᵗʰ **T84.099** Other mechanical complication of unspecified internal joint prosthesis

√5ᵗʰ **T84.1** Mechanical complication of internal fixation device of bones of limb

     EXCLUDES 2   mechanical complication of internal fixation device of bones of feet (T84.2-)

         mechanical complication of internal fixation device of bones of fingers (T84.2-)

         mechanical complication of internal fixation device of bones of hands (T84.2-)

         mechanical complication of internal fixation device of bones of toes (T84.2-)

√6ᵗʰ **T84.11** Breakdown (mechanical) of internal fixation device of bones of limb

√7ᵗʰ **T84.110** Breakdown (mechanical) of internal fixation device of right humerus

√7ᵗʰ **T84.111** Breakdown (mechanical) of internal fixation device of left humerus

√7ᵗʰ **T84.112** Breakdown (mechanical) of internal fixation device of bone of right forearm

√7ᵗʰ **T84.113** Breakdown (mechanical) of internal fixation device of bone of left forearm

√7ᵗʰ **T84.114** Breakdown (mechanical) of internal fixation device of right femur

√7ᵗʰ **T84.115** Breakdown (mechanical) of internal fixation device of left femur

√7ᵗʰ **T84.116** Breakdown (mechanical) of internal fixation device of bone of right lower leg

√7ᵗʰ **T84.117** Breakdown (mechanical) of internal fixation device of bone of left lower leg

√7ᵗʰ **T84.119** Breakdown (mechanical) of internal fixation device of unspecified bone of limb

√6ᵗʰ **T84.12** Displacement of internal fixation device of bones of limb

     Malposition of internal fixation device of bones of limb

√7ᵗʰ **T84.120** Displacement of internal fixation device of right humerus

√7ᵗʰ **T84.121** Displacement of internal fixation device of left humerus

√7ᵗʰ **T84.122** Displacement of internal fixation device of bone of right forearm

√7ᵗʰ **T84.123** Displacement of internal fixation device of bone of left forearm

√7ᵗʰ **T84.124** Displacement of internal fixation device of right femur

√7ᵗʰ **T84.125** Displacement of internal fixation device of left femur

√7ᵗʰ **T84.126** Displacement of internal fixation device of bone of right lower leg

√7ᵗʰ **T84.127** Displacement of internal fixation device of bone of left lower leg

√7ᵗʰ **T84.129** Displacement of internal fixation device of unspecified bone of limb

√6ᵗʰ **T84.19** Other mechanical complication of internal fixation device of bones of limb

     Obstruction (mechanical) of internal fixation device of bones of limb

     Perforation of internal fixation device of bones of limb

     Protrusion of internal fixation device of bones of limb

√7ᵗʰ **T84.190** Other mechanical complication of internal fixation device of right humerus

√7ᵗʰ **T84.191** Other mechanical complication of internal fixation device of left humerus

√7ᵗʰ **T84.192** Other mechanical complication of internal fixation device of bone of right forearm

√7ᵗʰ **T84.193** Other mechanical complication of internal fixation device of bone of left forearm

√7ᵗʰ **T84.194** Other mechanical complication of internal fixation device of right femur

√7ᵗʰ **T84.195** Other mechanical complication of internal fixation device of left femur

√7ᵗʰ **T84.196** Other mechanical complication of internal fixation device of bone of right lower leg

√7ᵗʰ **T84.197** Other mechanical complication of internal fixation device of bone of left lower leg

√7ᵗʰ **T84.199** Other mechanical complication of internal fixation device of unspecified bone of limb

√5ᵗʰ **T84.2** Mechanical complication of internal fixation device of other bones

√6ᵗʰ **T84.21** Breakdown (mechanical) of internal fixation device of other bones

√7ᵗʰ **T84.210** Breakdown (mechanical) of internal fixation device of bones of hand and fingers

√7ᵗʰ **T84.213** Breakdown (mechanical) of internal fixation device of bones of foot and toes

√7ᵗʰ **T84.216** Breakdown (mechanical) of internal fixation device of vertebrae

√7ᵗʰ **T84.218** Breakdown (mechanical) of internal fixation device of other bones

√6ᵗʰ **T84.22** Displacement of internal fixation device of other bones

     Malposition of internal fixation device of other bones

√7ᵗʰ **T84.220** Displacement of internal fixation device of bones of hand and fingers

√7ᵗʰ **T84.223** Displacement of internal fixation device of bones of foot and toes

√7ᵗʰ **T84.226** Displacement of internal fixation device of vertebrae

√7ᵗʰ **T84.228** Displacement of internal fixation device of other bones

√6ᵗʰ **T84.29** Other mechanical complication of internal fixation device of other bones

     Obstruction (mechanical) of internal fixation device of other bones

     Perforation of internal fixation device of other bones

     Protrusion of internal fixation device of other bones

√7ᵗʰ **T84.290** Other mechanical complication of internal fixation device of bones of hand and fingers

√7ᵗʰ **T84.293** Other mechanical complication of internal fixation device of bones of foot and toes

√7ᵗʰ **T84.296** Other mechanical complication of internal fixation device of vertebrae

√7ᵗʰ **T84.298** Other mechanical complication of internal fixation device of other bones

√5ᵗʰ **T84.3** Mechanical complication of other bone devices, implants and grafts

     EXCLUDES 2   other complications of bone graft (T86.83-)

√6ᵗʰ **T84.31** Breakdown (mechanical) of other bone devices, implants and grafts

√7ᵗʰ **T84.310** Breakdown (mechanical) of electronic bone stimulator

√7ᵗʰ **T84.318** Breakdown (mechanical) of other bone devices, implants and grafts

√6ᵗʰ **T84.32** Displacement of other bone devices, implants and grafts

     Malposition of other bone devices, implants and grafts

√7ᵗʰ **T84.320** Displacement of electronic bone stimulator

√7ᵗʰ **T84.328** Displacement of other bone devices, implants and grafts

√6ᵗʰ **T84.39** Other mechanical complication of other bone devices, implants and grafts

     Obstruction (mechanical) of other bone devices, implants and grafts

     Perforation of other bone devices, implants and grafts

     Protrusion of other bone devices, implants and grafts

√7ᵗʰ **T84.390** Other mechanical complication of electronic bone stimulator

---

✓ Additional Character Required   √x7ᵗʰ Xtension Alert   Unspecified Code   Other Specified Code   Manifestation Code   ▶◀ Revised Text   ● New Code   ▲ Revised Code Title

ICD-10-CM 2014 (Draft)   **985**

✓7ᵗʰ **T84.398** **Other mechanical complication of other bone devices, implants and grafts**

✓5ᵗʰ **T84.4** **Mechanical complication of** other internal orthopedic devices, implants and grafts

✓6ᵗʰ **T84.41** Breakdown (mechanical) of other internal orthopedic devices, implants and grafts

✓7ᵗʰ **T84.410** **Breakdown (mechanical) of** muscle and tendon graft

✓7ᵗʰ **T84.418** **Breakdown (mechanical) of other** internal orthopedic devices, implants and grafts

✓6ᵗʰ **T84.42** Displacement of other internal orthopedic devices, implants and grafts

Malposition of other internal orthopedic devices, implants and grafts

✓7ᵗʰ **T84.420** **Displacement of** muscle and tendon graft

✓7ᵗʰ **T84.428** **Displacement of other internal orthopedic devices, implants and grafts**

✓6ᵗʰ **T84.49** Other mechanical complication of other internal orthopedic devices, implants and grafts

Mechanical complication of other internal orthopedic devices, implants and grafts NOS

Obstruction (mechanical) of other internal orthopedic devices, implants and grafts

Perforation of other internal orthopedic devices, implants and grafts

Protrusion of other internal orthopedic devices, implants and grafts

✓7ᵗʰ **T84.490** **Other mechanical complication of** muscle and tendon graft

✓7ᵗʰ **T84.498** **Other mechanical complication of other** internal orthopedic devices, implants and grafts

✓5ᵗʰ **T84.5** **Infection and inflammatory reaction due to** internal joint prosthesis

Use additional code to identify infection

✓x7ᵗʰ **T84.50** **Infection and inflammatory reaction due to unspecified internal joint prosthesis**

✓x7ᵗʰ **T84.51** **Infection and inflammatory reaction due to internal** right hip **prosthesis**

✓x7ᵗʰ **T84.52** **Infection and inflammatory reaction due to internal** left hip **prosthesis**

✓x7ᵗʰ **T84.53** **Infection and inflammatory reaction due to internal** right knee **prosthesis**

✓x7ᵗʰ **T84.54** **Infection and inflammatory reaction due to internal** left knee **prosthesis**

✓x7ᵗʰ **T84.59** **Infection and inflammatory reaction due to other internal joint prosthesis**

✓5ᵗʰ **T84.6** **Infection and inflammatory reaction due to** internal fixation device

Use additional code to identify infection

✓x7ᵗʰ **T84.60** **Infection and inflammatory reaction due to internal fixation device of unspecified site**

✓6ᵗʰ **T84.61** Infection and inflammatory reaction due to internal fixation device of arm

✓7ᵗʰ **T84.610** **Infection and inflammatory reaction due to internal fixation device of** right humerus

✓7ᵗʰ **T84.611** **Infection and inflammatory reaction due to internal fixation device of** left humerus

✓7ᵗʰ **T84.612** **Infection and inflammatory reaction due to internal fixation device of** right radius

✓7ᵗʰ **T84.613** **Infection and inflammatory reaction due to internal fixation device of** left radius

✓7ᵗʰ **T84.614** **Infection and inflammatory reaction due to internal fixation device of** right ulna

✓7ᵗʰ **T84.615** **Infection and inflammatory reaction due to internal fixation device of** left ulna

✓7ᵗʰ **T84.619** **Infection and inflammatory reaction due to internal fixation device of unspecified bone of arm**

✓6ᵗʰ **T84.62** Infection and inflammatory reaction due to internal fixation device of leg

✓7ᵗʰ **T84.620** **Infection and inflammatory reaction due to internal fixation device of** right femur

✓7ᵗʰ **T84.621** **Infection and inflammatory reaction due to internal fixation device of** left femur

✓7ᵗʰ **T84.622** **Infection and inflammatory reaction due to internal fixation device of** right tibia

✓7ᵗʰ **T84.623** **Infection and inflammatory reaction due to internal fixation device of** left tibia

✓7ᵗʰ **T84.624** **Infection and inflammatory reaction due to internal fixation device of** right fibula

✓7ᵗʰ **T84.625** **Infection and inflammatory reaction due to internal fixation device of** left fibula

✓7ᵗʰ **T84.629** **Infection and inflammatory reaction due to internal fixation device of unspecified bone of leg**

✓x7ᵗʰ **T84.63** Infection and inflammatory reaction due to internal fixation device of spine

✓x7ᵗʰ **T84.69** **Infection and inflammatory reaction due to internal fixation device of other site**

✓x7ᵗʰ **T84.7** **Infection and inflammatory reaction due to other internal orthopedic prosthetic devices, implants and grafts**

Use additional code to identify infection

✓5ᵗʰ **T84.8** **Other specified complications of internal orthopedic prosthetic devices, implants and grafts**

✓x7ᵗʰ **T84.81** Embolism due to internal orthopedic prosthetic devices, implants and grafts

✓x7ᵗʰ **T84.82** Fibrosis due to internal orthopedic prosthetic devices, implants and grafts

✓x7ᵗʰ **T84.83** Hemorrhage due to internal orthopedic prosthetic devices, implants and grafts

✓x7ᵗʰ **T84.84** Pain due to internal orthopedic prosthetic devices, implants and grafts

✓x7ᵗʰ **T84.85** Stenosis due to internal orthopedic prosthetic devices, implants and grafts

✓x7ᵗʰ **T84.86** Thrombosis due to internal orthopedic prosthetic devices, implants and grafts

✓x7ᵗʰ **T84.89** **Other specified complication of internal orthopedic prosthetic devices, implants and grafts**

✓x7ᵗʰ **T84.9** **Unspecified complication of internal orthopedic prosthetic device, implant and graft**

✓4ᵗʰ **T85** **Complications of other internal prosthetic devices, implants and grafts**

EXCLUDES 2   failure and rejection of transplanted organs and tissue (T86.-)

The appropriate 7th character is to be added to each code from category T85.
A   initial encounter
D   subsequent encounter
S   sequela

✓5ᵗʰ **T85.0** **Mechanical complication of** ventricular intracranial (communicating) shunt

✓x7ᵗʰ **T85.01** Breakdown (mechanical) of ventricular intracranial (communicating) shunt

✓x7ᵗʰ **T85.02** Displacement of ventricular intracranial (communicating) shunt

Malposition of ventricular intracranial (communicating) shunt

✓x7ᵗʰ **T85.03** Leakage of ventricular intracranial (communicating) shunt

✓x7ᵗʰ **T85.09** Other mechanical complication of ventricular intracranial (communicating) shunt

Obstruction (mechanical) of ventricular intracranial (communicating) shunt

Perforation of ventricular intracranial (communicating) shunt

Protrusion of ventricular intracranial (communicating) shunt

✓5ᵗʰ **T85.1** **Mechanical complication of** implanted electronic stimulator of nervous system

✓6ᵗʰ **T85.11** Breakdown (mechanical) of implanted electronic stimulator of nervous system

✓7ᵗʰ **T85.110** Breakdown (mechanical) of implanted electronic neurostimulator (electrode) of brain

✓7ᵗʰ **T85.111** Breakdown (mechanical) of implanted electronic neurostimulator (electrode) of peripheral nerve

✓7ᵗʰ **T85.112** Breakdown (mechanical) of implanted electronic neurostimulator (electrode) of spinal cord

EXCLUDES 1 Not coded here   EXCLUDES 2 Not included here   N Newborn Age: 0   P Pediatric Age: 0-17   M Maternity Age: 12-55   A Adult Age: 15-124

986   ICD-10-CM 2014 (Draft)

√7ᵗʰ **T85.118 Breakdown (mechanical) of other implanted electronic stimulator of nervous system**

√6ᵗʰ **T85.12** Displacement of implanted electronic stimulator of nervous system
Malposition of implanted electronic stimulator of nervous system

√7ᵗʰ **T85.120 Displacement of implanted electronic neurostimulator (electrode) of brain**

√7ᵗʰ **T85.121 Displacement of implanted electronic neurostimulator (electrode) of peripheral nerve**

√7ᵗʰ **T85.122 Displacement of implanted electronic neurostimulator (electrode) of spinal cord**

√7ᵗʰ **T85.128 Displacement of other implanted electronic stimulator of nervous system**

√6ᵗʰ **T85.19** Other mechanical complication of implanted electronic stimulator of nervous system
Leakage of implanted electronic stimulator of nervous system
Obstruction (mechanical) of implanted electronic stimulator of nervous system
Perforation of implanted electronic stimulator of nervous system
Protrusion of implanted electronic stimulator of nervous system

√7ᵗʰ **T85.190 Other mechanical complication of implanted electronic neurostimulator (electrode) of brain**

√7ᵗʰ **T85.191 Other mechanical complication of implanted electronic neurostimulator (electrode) of peripheral nerve**

√7ᵗʰ **T85.192 Other mechanical complication of implanted electronic neurostimulator (electrode) of spinal cord**

√7ᵗʰ **T85.199 Other mechanical complication of other implanted electronic stimulator of nervous system**

√5ᵗʰ **T85.2** Mechanical complication of intraocular lens

√x7ᵗʰ **T85.21** Breakdown (mechanical) of intraocular lens

√x7ᵗʰ **T85.22** Displacement of intraocular lens
Malposition of intraocular lens

√x7ᵗʰ **T85.29** Other mechanical complication of intraocular lens
Obstruction (mechanical) of intraocular lens
Perforation of intraocular lens
Protrusion of intraocular lens

√5ᵗʰ **T85.3** Mechanical complication of other ocular prosthetic devices, implants and grafts
EXCLUDES 2 other complications of corneal graft (T86.84-)

√6ᵗʰ **T85.31** Breakdown (mechanical) of other ocular prosthetic devices, implants and grafts

√7ᵗʰ **T85.310 Breakdown (mechanical) of prosthetic orbit of right eye**

√7ᵗʰ **T85.311 Breakdown (mechanical) of prosthetic orbit of left eye**

√7ᵗʰ **T85.318 Breakdown (mechanical) of other ocular prosthetic devices, implants and grafts**

√6ᵗʰ **T85.32** Displacement of other ocular prosthetic devices, implants and grafts
Malposition of other ocular prosthetic devices, implants and grafts

√7ᵗʰ **T85.320 Displacement of prosthetic orbit of right eye**

√7ᵗʰ **T85.321 Displacement of prosthetic orbit of left eye**

√7ᵗʰ **T85.328 Displacement of other ocular prosthetic devices, implants and grafts**

√6ᵗʰ **T85.39** Other mechanical complication of other ocular prosthetic devices, implants and grafts
Obstruction (mechanical) of other ocular prosthetic devices, implants and grafts
Perforation of other ocular prosthetic devices, implants and grafts
Protrusion of other ocular prosthetic devices, implants and grafts

√7ᵗʰ **T85.390 Other mechanical complication of prosthetic orbit of right eye**

√7ᵗʰ **T85.391 Other mechanical complication of prosthetic orbit of left eye**

√7ᵗʰ **T85.398 Other mechanical complication of other ocular prosthetic devices, implants and grafts**

√5ᵗʰ **T85.4** Mechanical complication of breast prosthesis and implant

√x7ᵗʰ **T85.41** Breakdown (mechanical) of breast prosthesis and implant

√x7ᵗʰ **T85.42** Displacement of breast prosthesis and implant
Malposition of breast prosthesis and implant

√x7ᵗʰ **T85.43** Leakage of breast prosthesis and implant

√x7ᵗʰ **T85.44** Capsular contracture of breast implant

√x7ᵗʰ **T85.49** Other mechanical complication of breast prosthesis and implant
Obstruction (mechanical) of breast prosthesis and implant
Perforation of breast prosthesis and implant
Protrusion of breast prosthesis and implant

√5ᵗʰ **T85.5** Mechanical complication of gastrointestinal prosthetic devices, implants and grafts

√6ᵗʰ **T85.51** Breakdown (mechanical) of gastrointestinal prosthetic devices, implants and grafts

√7ᵗʰ **T85.510 Breakdown (mechanical) of bile duct prosthesis**

√7ᵗʰ **T85.511 Breakdown (mechanical) of esophageal anti-reflux device**

√7ᵗʰ **T85.518 Breakdown (mechanical) of other gastrointestinal prosthetic devices, implants and grafts**

√6ᵗʰ **T85.52** Displacement of gastrointestinal prosthetic devices, implants and grafts
Malposition of gastrointestinal prosthetic devices, implants and grafts

√7ᵗʰ **T85.520 Displacement of bile duct prosthesis**

√7ᵗʰ **T85.521 Displacement of esophageal anti-reflux device**

√7ᵗʰ **T85.528 Displacement of other gastrointestinal prosthetic devices, implants and grafts**

√6ᵗʰ **T85.59** Other mechanical complication of gastrointestinal prosthetic devices, implants and
Obstruction, mechanical of gastrointestinal prosthetic devices, implants and grafts
Perforation of gastrointestinal prosthetic devices, implants and grafts
Protrusion of gastrointestinal prosthetic devices, implants and grafts

√7ᵗʰ **T85.590 Other mechanical complication of bile duct prosthesis**

√7ᵗʰ **T85.591 Other mechanical complication of esophageal anti-reflux device**

√7ᵗʰ **T85.598 Other mechanical complication of other gastrointestinal prosthetic devices, implants and grafts**

√5ᵗʰ **T85.6** Mechanical complication of other specified internal and external prosthetic devices, implants and grafts

√6ᵗʰ **T85.61** Breakdown (mechanical) of other specified internal prosthetic devices, implants and grafts

√7ᵗʰ **T85.610 Breakdown (mechanical) of epidural and subdural infusion catheter**

√7ᵗʰ **T85.611 Breakdown (mechanical) of intraperitoneal dialysis catheter**
EXCLUDES 1 mechanical complication of vascular dialysis catheter (T82.4-)

√7ᵗʰ **T85.612 Breakdown (mechanical) of permanent sutures**
EXCLUDES 1 mechanical complication of permanent (wire) suture used in bone repair (T84.1-T84.2)

Injury, Poisoning and Certain Other Consequences of External Causes

T85.613–T86.32

√7ᵗʰ **T85.613 Breakdown (mechanical) of** artificial skin graft and decellularized allodermis
  Failure of artificial skin graft and decellularized allodermis
  Non-adherence of artificial skin graft and decellularized allodermis
  Poor incorporation of artificial skin graft and decellularized allodermis
  Shearing of artificial skin graft and decellularized allodermis

√7ᵗʰ **T85.614 Breakdown (mechanical) of** insulin pump

√7ᵗʰ **T85.618 Breakdown (mechanical) of other specified internal prosthetic devices, implants and grafts**

√6ᵗʰ **T85.62 Displacement of other specified internal prosthetic devices, implants and grafts**
  Malposition of other specified internal prosthetic devices, implants and grafts

√7ᵗʰ **T85.620 Displacement of** epidural and subdural infusion catheter

√7ᵗʰ **T85.621 Displacement of** intraperitoneal dialysis catheter
  EXCLUDES 1   mechanical complication of vascular dialysis catheter (T82.4-)

√7ᵗʰ **T85.622 Displacement of** permanent sutures
  EXCLUDES 1   mechanical complication of permanent (wire) suture used in bone repair (T84.1-T84.2)

√7ᵗʰ **T85.623 Displacement of** artificial skin graft and decellularized allodermis
  Dislodgement of artificial skin graft and decellularized allodermis
  Displacement of artificial skin graft and decellularized allodermis

√7ᵗʰ **T85.624 Displacement of** insulin pump

√7ᵗʰ **T85.628 Displacement of other specified internal prosthetic devices, implants and grafts**

√6ᵗʰ **T85.63 Leakage of other specified internal prosthetic devices, implants and grafts**

√7ᵗʰ **T85.630 Leakage of** epidural and subdural infusion catheter

√7ᵗʰ **T85.631 Leakage of** intraperitoneal dialysis catheter
  EXCLUDES 1   mechanical complication of vascular dialysis catheter (T82.4)

√7ᵗʰ **T85.633 Leakage of** insulin pump

√7ᵗʰ **T85.638 Leakage of other specified internal prosthetic devices, implants and grafts**

√6ᵗʰ **T85.69 Other** mechanical complication of other specified internal prosthetic devices, implants and grafts
  Obstruction, mechanical of other specified internal prosthetic devices, implants and grafts
  Perforation of other specified internal prosthetic devices, implants and grafts
  Protrusion of other specified internal prosthetic devices, implants and grafts

√7ᵗʰ **T85.690 Other mechanical complication of epidural and subdural infusion catheter**

√7ᵗʰ **T85.691 Other mechanical complication of intraperitoneal dialysis catheter**
  EXCLUDES 1   mechanical complication of vascular dialysis catheter (T82.4)

√7ᵗʰ **T85.692 Other mechanical complication of permanent sutures**
  EXCLUDES 1   mechanical complication of permanent (wire) suture used in bone repair (T84.1-T84.2)

√7ᵗʰ **T85.693 Other mechanical complication of** artificial skin graft and decellularized allodermis

√7ᵗʰ **T85.694 Other mechanical complication of** insulin pump

√7ᵗʰ **T85.698 Other mechanical complication of other specified internal prosthetic devices, implants and grafts**
  Mechanical complication of nonabsorbable surgical material NOS

√5ᵗʰ **T85.7 Infection and inflammatory reaction due to other internal prosthetic devices, implants and grafts**
  Use additional code to identify infection

√x7ᵗʰ **T85.71 Infection and inflammatory reaction due to** peritoneal dialysis catheter

√x7ᵗʰ **T85.72 Infection and inflammatory reaction due to** insulin pump

√x7ᵗʰ **T85.79 Infection and inflammatory reaction due to other internal prosthetic devices, implants and grafts**

√5ᵗʰ **T85.8 Other specified complications of internal prosthetic devices, implants and grafts, not elsewhere classified**

√x7ᵗʰ **T85.81 Embolism due to internal prosthetic devices, implants and grafts, not elsewhere classified**

√x7ᵗʰ **T85.82 Fibrosis due to internal prosthetic devices, implants and grafts, not elsewhere classified**

√x7ᵗʰ **T85.83 Hemorrhage due to internal prosthetic devices, implants and grafts, not elsewhere classified**

√x7ᵗʰ **T85.84 Pain due to internal prosthetic devices, implants and grafts, not elsewhere classified**

√x7ᵗʰ **T85.85 Stenosis due to internal prosthetic devices, implants and grafts, not elsewhere classified**

√x7ᵗʰ **T85.86 Thrombosis due to internal prosthetic devices, implants and grafts, not elsewhere classified**

√x7ᵗʰ **T85.89 Other specified complication of internal prosthetic devices, implants and grafts, not elsewhere classified**

√x7ᵗʰ **T85.9 Unspecified complication of internal prosthetic device, implant and graft**
  Complication of internal prosthetic device, implant and graft NOS

√4ᵗʰ **T86 Complications of transplanted organs and tissue**
  Use additional code to identify other transplant complications, such as:
  graft-versus-host disease (D89.81-)
  malignancy associated with organ transplant (C80.2)
  post-transplant lymphoproliferative disorders (PTLD) (D47.Z1)

√5ᵗʰ **T86.0 Complications of** bone marrow transplant

T86.00 Unspecified complication of bone marrow transplant

T86.01 Bone marrow transplant rejection

T86.02 Bone marrow transplant failure

T86.03 Bone marrow transplant infection

T86.09 Other complications of bone marrow transplant

√5ᵗʰ **T86.1 Complications of** kidney transplant

T86.10 Unspecified complication of kidney transplant

T86.11 Kidney transplant rejection

T86.12 Kidney transplant failure

T86.13 Kidney transplant infection
  Use additional code to specify infection

T86.19 Other complication of kidney transplant

√5ᵗʰ **T86.2 Complications of** heart transplant
  EXCLUDES 1   complication of:
  artificial heart device (T82.5)
  heart-lung transplant (T86.3)

T86.20 Unspecified complication of heart transplant

T86.21 Heart transplant rejection

T86.22 Heart transplant failure

T86.23 Heart transplant infection
  Use additional code to specify infection

√6ᵗʰ **T86.29 Other complications of heart transplant**

T86.290 Cardiac allograft vasculopathy
  EXCLUDES 1   atherosclerosis of coronary arteries (I25.75-, I25.76-, I25.81-)

T86.298 Other complications of heart transplant

√5ᵗʰ **T86.3 Complications of** heart-lung transplant

T86.30 Unspecified complication of heart-lung transplant

T86.31 Heart-lung transplant rejection

T86.32 Heart-lung transplant failure

EXCLUDES 1 Not coded here   *EXCLUDES 2* Not included here   N Newborn Age: 0   P Pediatric Age: 0-17   M Maternity Age: 12-55   A Adult Age: 15-124

988   ICD-10-CM 2014 (Draft)

T86.33   **Heart-lung transplant** infection
Use additional code to specify infection

T86.39   **Other complications of heart-lung transplant**

√5ᵗʰ **T86.4   Complications of** liver **transplant**

T86.40   **Unspecified complication of liver transplant**

T86.41   **Liver transplant** rejection

T86.42   **Liver transplant** failure

T86.43   **Liver transplant** infection
Use additional code to identify infection, such as:
cytomegalovirus (CMV) infection (B25.-)

T86.49   **Other complications of liver transplant**

T86.5   Complications of stem cell **transplant**
Complications from stem cells from peripheral blood
Complications from stem cells from umbilical cord

√5ᵗʰ **T86.8   Complications of** other **transplanted organs and tissues**

√6ᵗʰ **T86.81   Complications of** lung **transplant**
EXCLUDES 1   complication of heart-lung transplant (T86.3-)

T86.810   **Lung transplant** rejection

T86.811   **Lung transplant** failure

T86.812   **Lung transplant** infection
Use additional code to specify infection

T86.818   **Other complications of lung transplant**

T86.819   **Unspecified complication of lung transplant**

√6ᵗʰ **T86.82   Complications of** skin graft (allograft) (autograft)
EXCLUDES 2   complication of artificial skin graft (T85.693)

T86.820   **Skin graft (allograft)** rejection

T86.821   **Skin graft (allograft) (autograft)** failure

T86.822   **Skin graft (allograft) (autograft)** infection
Use additional code to specify infection

T86.828   **Other complications of skin graft (allograft) (autograft)**

T86.829   **Unspecified complication of skin graft (allograft) (autograft)**

√6ᵗʰ **T86.83   Complications of** bone graft
EXCLUDES 2   mechanical complications of bone graft (T84.3-)

T86.830   **Bone graft** rejection

T86.831   **Bone graft** failure

T86.832   **Bone graft** infection
Use additional code to specify infection

T86.838   **Other complications of bone graft**

T86.839   **Unspecified complication of bone graft**

√6ᵗʰ **T86.84   Complications of** corneal **transplant**
EXCLUDES 2   mechanical complications of corneal graft (T85.3-)

T86.840   **Corneal transplant** rejection

T86.841   **Corneal transplant** failure

T86.842   **Corneal transplant** infection
Use additional code to specify infection

T86.848   **Other complications of corneal transplant**

T86.849   **Unspecified complication of corneal transplant**

√6ᵗʰ **T86.85   Complication of** intestine **transplant**

T86.850   **Intestine transplant** rejection

T86.851   **Intestine transplant** failure

T86.852   **Intestine transplant** infection
Use additional code to specify infection

T86.858   **Other complications of intestine transplant**

T86.859   **Unspecified complication of intestine transplant**

√6ᵗʰ **T86.89   Complications of** other **transplanted tissue**
Transplant failure or rejection of pancreas

T86.890   **Other transplanted tissue** rejection

T86.891   **Other transplanted tissue** failure

T86.892   **Other transplanted tissue** infection
Use additional code to specify infection

T86.898   **Other complications of other transplanted tissue**

T86.899   **Unspecified complication of other transplanted tissue**

√5ᵗʰ **T86.9   Complication of** unspecified **transplanted** organ and tissue

T86.90   **Unspecified complication of unspecified transplanted organ and tissue**

T86.91   **Unspecified transplanted organ and tissue** rejection

T86.92   **Unspecified transplanted organ and tissue** failure

T86.93   **Unspecified transplanted organ and tissue** infection
Use additional code to specify infection

T86.99   **Other complications of unspecified transplanted organ and tissue**

√4ᵗʰ **T87   Complications peculiar to reattachment and amputation**

√5ᵗʰ **T87.0   Complications of reattached (part of)** upper extremity

√6ᵗʰ **T87.0X   Complications of reattached (part of) upper extremity**

T87.0X1   **Complications of reattached (part of)** right **upper extremity**

T87.0X2   **Complications of reattached (part of)** left **upper extremity**

T87.0X9   **Complications of reattached (part of) unspecified upper extremity**

√5ᵗʰ **T87.1   Complications of reattached (part of)** lower extremity

√6ᵗʰ **T87.1X   Complications of reattached (part of) lower extremity**

T87.1X1   **Complications of reattached (part of)** right **lower extremity**

T87.1X2   **Complications of reattached (part of)** left **lower extremity**

T87.1X9   **Complications of reattached (part of) unspecified lower extremity**

T87.2   Complications of other reattached body part

√5ᵗʰ **T87.3   Neuroma** of amputation stump

T87.30   **Neuroma of amputation stump, unspecified extremity**

T87.31   **Neuroma of amputation stump,** right upper extremity

T87.32   **Neuroma of amputation stump,** left upper **extremity**

T87.33   **Neuroma of amputation stump,** right lower extremity

T87.34   **Neuroma of amputation stump,** left lower **extremity**

√5ᵗʰ **T87.4   Infection** of amputation stump

T87.40   **Infection of amputation stump, unspecified extremity**

T87.41   **Infection of amputation stump,** right upper extremity

T87.42   **Infection of amputation stump,** left upper **extremity**

T87.43   **Infection of amputation stump,** right lower extremity

T87.44   **Infection of amputation stump,** left lower **extremity**

√5ᵗʰ **T87.5   Necrosis** of amputation stump

T87.50   **Necrosis of amputation stump, unspecified extremity**

T87.51   **Necrosis of amputation stump,** right upper extremity

T87.52   **Necrosis of amputation stump,** left upper **extremity**

T87.53   **Necrosis of amputation stump,** right lower **extremity**

T87.54   **Necrosis of amputation stump,** left lower **extremity**

√5ᵗʰ **T87.8   Other** complications of amputation stump

T87.81   **Dehiscence** of amputation stump

T87.89   **Other complications of amputation stump**
Amputation stump contracture
Amputation stump contracture of next proximal joint
Amputation stump flexion
Amputation stump edema
Amputation stump hematoma
EXCLUDES 2   phantom limb syndrome (G54.6-G54.7)

T87.9   **Unspecified complications of amputation stump**

☑ Additional Character Required   √x7ᵗʰ Xtension Alert   Unspecified Code   Other Specified Code   Manifestation Code   ►◄ Revised Text   ● New Code   ▲ Revised Code Title

ICD-10-CM 2014 (Draft)

989

Injury, Poisoning and Certain Other Consequences of External Causes

T88–T88.9

✓4th **T88** **Other complications of surgical and medical care, not elsewhere classified**

    EXCLUDES 2   *complication following infusion, transfusion and therapeutic injection (T80.-)*
      complication following procedure NEC (T81.-)
      complications of anesthesia in labor and delivery (O74.-)
      complications of anesthesia in pregnancy (O29.-)
      complications of anesthesia in puerperium (O89.-)
      complications of devices, implants and grafts (T82-T85)
      complications of obstetric surgery and procedure (O75.4)
      dermatitis due to drugs and medicaments (L23.3, L24.4, L25.1, L27.0-L27.1)
      poisoning and toxic effects of drugs and chemicals (T36-T65 with fifth or sixth character 1-4 or 6)
      specified complications classified elsewhere

The appropriate 7th character is to be added to each code from category T88.
A   initial encounter
D   subsequent encounter
S   sequela

✓x7th **T88.0** **Infection following immunization**
    Sepsis following immunization

✓x7th **T88.1** **Other complications following immunization, not elsewhere classified**
    Generalized vaccinia
    Rash following immunization
    EXCLUDES 1   *vaccinia not from vaccine (B08.011)*
    EXCLUDES 2   *anaphylactic shock due to serum (T80.5-)*
      other serum reactions (T80.6-)
      postimmunization arthropathy (M02.2)
      postimmunization encephalitis (G04.02)
      postimmunization fever (R50.83)

✓x7th **T88.2** **Shock due to anesthesia**
    Use additional code for adverse effect, if applicable, to identify drug (T41.- with fifth or sixth character 5)
    EXCLUDES 1   *complications of anesthesia (in):*
      labor and delivery (O74.-)
      pregnancy (O29.-)
      puerperium (O89.-)
      postprocedural shock NOS (T81.1-)

✓x7th **T88.3** **Malignant hyperthermia due to anesthesia**
    Use additional code for adverse effect, if applicable, to identify drug (T41.- with fifth or sixth character 5)

✓x7th **T88.4** **Failed or difficult intubation**

✓5th **T88.5** **Other complications of anesthesia**
    Use additional code for adverse effect, if applicable, to identify drug (T41.- with fifth or sixth character 5)

    ✓x7th **T88.51** **Hypothermia following anesthesia**

    ✓x7th **T88.52** **Failed moderate sedation during procedure**
      Failed conscious sedation during procedure
      EXCLUDES 2   *personal history of failed moderate sedation (Z92.83)*

    ✓x7th **T88.59** **Other complications of anesthesia**

✓x7th **T88.6** **Anaphylactic reaction due to adverse effect of correct drug or medicament properly administered**
    Anaphylactic shock due to adverse effect of correct drug or medicament properly administered
    Anaphylactoid reaction NOS
    Use additional code for adverse effect, if applicable, to identify drug (T36-T50 with fifth or sixth character 5)
    EXCLUDES 1   *anaphylactic reaction due to serum (T80.5-)*
      anaphylactic shock or reaction due to adverse food reaction (T78.0-)

✓x7th **T88.7** **Unspecified adverse effect of drug or medicament**
    Use additional code for adverse effect, if applicable, to identify drug (T36-T50 with fifth or sixth character 5)
    Drug hypersensitivity NOS
    Drug reaction NOS
    EXCLUDES 1   *specified adverse effects of drugs and medicaments (A00-R94 and T80-T88.6, T88.8)*

✓x7th **T88.8** **Other specified complications of surgical and medical care, not elsewhere classified**
    Use additional code to identify the complication

✓x7th **T88.9** **Complication of surgical and medical care, unspecified**

Chapter 20. External Causes of Morbidity (V00-Y99)

NOTE This chapter permits the classification of environmental events and circumstances as the cause of injury, and other adverse effects. Where a code from this section is applicable, it is intended that it shall be used secondary to a code from another chapter of the Classification indicating the nature of the condition. Most often, the condition will be classifiable to Chapter 19, Injury, poisoning and certain other consequences of external causes (S00-T88). Other conditions that may be stated to be due to external causes are classified in Chapters I to XVIII. For these conditions, codes from Chapter 20 should be used to provide additional information as to the cause of the condition.

This chapter contains the following blocks:

V00-V09	Pedestrian injured in transport accident
V10-V19	Pedal cycle rider injured in transport accident
V20-V29	Motorcycle rider injured in transport accident
V30-V39	Occupant of three-wheeled motor vehicle injured in transport accident
V40-V49	Car occupant injured in transport accident
V50-V59	Occupant of pick-up truck or van injured in transport accident
V60-V69	Occupant of heavy transport vehicle injured in transport accident
V70-V79	Bus occupant injured in transport accident
V80-V89	Other land transport accidents
V90-V94	Water transport accidents
V95-V97	Air and space transport accidents
V98-V99	Other and unspecified transport accidents
W00-X58	Other external causes of accidental injury
W00-W19	Slipping, tripping, stumbling and falls
W20-W49	Exposure to inanimate mechanical forces
W50-W64	Exposure to animate mechanical forces
W65-W74	Accidental non-transport drowning and submersion
W85-W99	Exposure to electric current, radiation and extreme ambient air temperature and pressure
X00-X08	Exposure to smoke, fire and flames
X10-X19	Contact with heat and hot substances
X30-X39	Exposure to forces of nature
X52, X58	Accidental exposure to other specified factors
X71-X83	Intentional self-harm
X92-Y08	Assault
Y21-Y33	Event of undetermined intent
Y35-Y38	Legal intervention, operations of war, military operations, and terrorism
Y62-Y84	Complications of medical and surgical care
Y62-Y69	Misadventures to patients during surgical and medical care
Y70-Y82	Medical devices associated with adverse incidents in diagnostic and therapeutic use
Y83-Y84	Surgical and other medical procedures as the cause of abnormal reaction of the patient, or of later complication, without mention of misadventure at the time of the procedure
Y90-Y99	Supplementary factors related to causes of morbidity classified elsewhere

Transport accidents (V00-V99)

NOTE This section is structured in 12 groups. Those relating to land transport accidents (V01-V89) reflect the victim's mode of transport and are subdivided to identify the victim's 'counterpart' or the type of event. The vehicle of which the injured person is an occupant is identified in the first two characters since it is seen as the most important factor to identify for prevention purposes. A transport accident is one in which the vehicle involved must be moving or running or in use for transport purposes at the time of the accident.

Use additional code to identify:
airbag injury (W22.1)
type of street or road (Y92.4-)
use of cellular telephone and other electronic equipment at the time of the transport accident (Y93.C-)

EXCLUDES 1 agricultural vehicles in stationary use or maintenance (W31.-)
assault by crashing of motor vehicle (Y03.-)
automobile or motor cycle in stationary use or maintenance—code to type of accident
crashing of motor vehicle, undetermined intent (Y32)
intentional self-harm by crashing of motor vehicle (X82)

EXCLUDES 2 transport accidents due to cataclysm (X34-X38)

NOTE This section is structured in 12 groups. Those relating to land transport accidents (V01-V89) reflect the victim's mode of transport and are subdivided to identify the victim's 'counterpart' or the type of event. The vehicle of which the injured person is an occupant is identified in the first two characters since it is seen as the most important factor to identify for prevention purposes. A transport accident is one in which the vehicle involved must be moving or running or in use for transport purposes at the time of the accident.

Definitions of transport vehicles:

(a) A transport accident is any accident involving a device designed primarily for, or used at the time primarily for, conveying persons or good from one place to another.

(b) A public highway [trafficway] or street is the entire width between property lines (or other boundary lines) of land open to the public as a matter of right or custom for purposes of moving persons or property from one place to another. A roadway is that part of the public highway designed, improved and customarily used for vehicular traffic.

(c) A traffic accident is any vehicle accident occurring on the public highway [i.e. originating on, terminating on, or involving a vehicle partially on the highway]. A vehicle accident is assumed to have occurred on the public highway unless another place is specified, except in the case of accidents involving only off-road motor vehicles, which are classified as nontraffic accidents unless the contrary is stated.

(d) A nontraffic accident is any vehicle accident that occurs entirely in any place other than a public highway.

(e) A pedestrian is any person involved in an accident who was not at the time of the accident riding in or on a motor vehicle, railway train, streetcar or animal-drawn or other vehicle, or on a pedal cycle or animal. This includes, a person changing a tire or working on a parked car. It also includes, the use of a pedestrian conveyance such as a baby carriage, ice-skates, roller skates, a skateboard, nonmotorized or motorized wheelchair, motorized mobility scooter, or nonmotorized scooter.

(f) A driver is an occupant of a transport vehicle who is operating or intending to operate it.

(g) A passenger is any occupant of a transport vehicle other than the driver, except a person traveling on the outside of the vehicle.

(h) A person on the outside of a vehicle is any person being transported by a vehicle but not occupying the space normally reserved for the driver or passengers, or the space intended for the transport of property. This includes the body, bumper, fender, roof, running board or step of a vehicle.

(i) A pedal cycle is any land transport vehicle operated solely by nonmotorized pedals including a bicycle or tricycle.

(j) A pedal cyclist is any person riding a pedal cycle or in a sidecar or trailer attached to a pedal cycle.

(k) A motorcycle is a two-wheeled motor vehicle with one or two riding saddles and sometimes with a third wheel for the support of a sidecar. The sidecar is considered part of the motorcycle.

(l) A motorcycle rider is any person riding a motorcycle or in a sidecar or trailer attached to the motorcycle.

(m) A three-wheeled motor vehicle is a motorized tricycle designed primarily for on-road use. This includes a motor-driven tricycle, a motorized rickshaw, or a three-wheeled motor car.

(n) A car [automobile] is a four-wheeled motor vehicle designed primarily for carrying up to 7 persons. A trailer being towed by the car is considered part of the car.

(o) A pick-up truck or van is a four or six-wheeled motor vehicle designed for carrying passengers as well as property or cargo weighing less than the local limit for classification as a heavy goods vehicle, and not requiring a special driver's license. This includes a minivan and a sport-utility vehicle (SUV).

(p) A heavy transport vehicle is a motor vehicle designed primarily for carrying property, meeting local criteria for classification as a heavy goods vehicle in terms of weight and requiring a special driver's license.

(q) A bus (coach) is a motor vehicle designed or adapted primarily for carrying more than 10 passengers, and requiring a special driver's license.

(r) A railway train or railway vehicle is any device, with or without freight or passenger cars couple to it, designed for traffic on a railway track. This includes subterranean (subways) or elevated trains.

(s) A streetcar, is a device designed and used primarily for transporting passengers within a municipality, running on rails, usually subject to normal traffic control signals, and operated principally on a right-of-way that forms part of the roadway. This includes a tram or trolley that runs on rails. A trailer being towed by a streetcar is considered part of the streetcar.

(t) A special vehicle mainly used on industrial premises is a motor vehicle designed primarily for use within the buildings and premises of industrial or commercial establishments. This includes battery-powered trucks, forklifts, coal-cars in a coal mine, logging cars and trucks used in mines or quarries.

(u) A special vehicle mainly used in agriculture is a motor vehicle designed specifically for use in farming and agriculture (horticulture), to work the land, tend and harvest crops and transport materials on the farm. This includes harvesters, farm machinery and tractor and trailers.

(v) A special construction vehicle is a motor vehicle designed specifically for use on construction and demolition sites. This includes bulldozers, diggers, earth levelers, dump trucks. backhoes, front-end loaders, pavers, and mechanical shovels.

(w) A special all-terrain vehicle is a motor vehicle of special design to enable it to negotiate over rough or soft terrain, snow or sand. This includes snow mobiles, All-terrain vehicles (ATV), and dune buggies. It does not include passenger vehicle designated as Sport Utility Vehicles (SUV).

☑ Additional Character Required   ✓x7th Xtension Alert   **Unspecified Code**   Other Specified Code   Manifestation Code   ►◄ Revised Text   ● New Code   ▲ Revised Code Title

ICD-10-CM 2014 (Draft)   **991**

(x) A watercraft is any device designed for transporting passengers or goods on water. This includes motor or sailboats, ships, and hovercraft.

(y) An aircraft is any device for transporting passengers or goods in the air. This includes hot-air balloons, gliders, helicopters and airplanes.

(z) A military vehicle is any motorized vehicle operating on a public roadway owned by the military and being operated by a member of the military.

Pedestrian injured in transport accident (V00-V09)

INCLUDES   person changing tire on transport vehicle
person examining engine of vehicle broken down in (on side of) road

EXCLUDES1   fall due to non-transport collision with other person (W03)
pedestrian on foot falling (slipping) on ice and snow (W00.-)
struck or bumped by another person (W51)

✓4ᵗʰ **V00 Pedestrian conveyance accident**

Use additional place of occurrence and activity external cause codes, if known (Y92-, Y93-)

EXCLUDES1   collision with another person without fall (W51)
fall due to person on foot colliding with another person on foot (W03)
fall from non-moving wheelchair, nonmotorized scooter and motorized mobility scooter without collision (W05.-)
pedestrian (conveyance) collision with other land transport vehicle (V01-V09)
pedestrian on foot falling (slipping) on ice and snow (W00.-)

The appropriate 7th character is to be added to each code from category V00.
A   initial encounter
D   subsequent encounter
S   sequela

✓5ᵗʰ **V00.0 Pedestrian on foot injured in collision with pedestrian conveyance**

✓x7ᵗʰ **V00.01 Pedestrian on foot injured in collision with roller-skater**

✓x7ᵗʰ **V00.02 Pedestrian on foot injured in collision with skateboarder**

✓x7ᵗʰ **V00.09 Pedestrian on foot injured in collision with other pedestrian conveyance**

✓5ᵗʰ **V00.1 Rolling-type pedestrian conveyance accident**

EXCLUDES1   accident with babystroller (V00.82-)
accident with motorized mobility scooter (V00.83-)
accident with wheelchair (powered) (V00.81-)

✓6ᵗʰ **V00.11 In-line roller-skate accident**

✓7ᵗʰ **V00.111 Fall from in-line roller-skates**

✓7ᵗʰ **V00.112 In-line roller-skater colliding with stationary object**

✓7ᵗʰ **V00.118 Other in-line roller-skate accident**
EXCLUDES1   roller-skater collision with other land transport vehicle (V01-V09 with 5th character 1)

✓6ᵗʰ **V00.12 Non-in-line roller-skate accident**

✓7ᵗʰ **V00.121 Fall from non-in-line roller-skates**

✓7ᵗʰ **V00.122 Non-in-line roller-skater colliding with stationary object**

✓7ᵗʰ **V00.128 Other non-in-line roller-skating accident**
EXCLUDES1   roller-skater collision with other land transport vehicle (V01-V09 with 5th character 1)

✓6ᵗʰ **V00.13 Skateboard accident**

✓7ᵗʰ **V00.131 Fall from skateboard**

✓7ᵗʰ **V00.132 Skateboarder colliding with stationary object**

✓7ᵗʰ **V00.138 Other skateboard accident**
EXCLUDES1   skateboarder collision with other land transport vehicle (V01-V09 with 5th character 2)

✓6ᵗʰ **V00.14 Scooter (nonmotorized) accident**
EXCLUDES1   motorscooter accident (V20-V29)

✓7ᵗʰ **V00.141 Fall from scooter (nonmotorized)**

✓7ᵗʰ **V00.142 Scooter (nonmotorized) colliding with stationary object**

✓7ᵗʰ **V00.148 Other scooter (nonmotorized) accident**
EXCLUDES1   scooter (nonmotorized) collision with other land transport vehicle (V01-V09 with fifth character 9)

✓6ᵗʰ **V00.15 Heelies accident**
Rolling shoe
Wheeled shoe
Wheelies accident

✓7ᵗʰ **V00.151 Fall from heelies**

✓7ᵗʰ **V00.152 Heelies colliding with stationary object**

✓7ᵗʰ **V00.158 Other heelies accident**

✓6ᵗʰ **V00.18 Accident on other rolling-type pedestrian conveyance**

✓7ᵗʰ **V00.181 Fall from other rolling-type pedestrian conveyance**

✓7ᵗʰ **V00.182 Pedestrian on other rolling-type pedestrian conveyance colliding with stationary object**

✓7ᵗʰ **V00.188 Other accident on other rolling-type pedestrian conveyance**

✓5ᵗʰ **V00.2 Gliding-type pedestrian conveyance accident**

✓6ᵗʰ **V00.21 Ice-skates accident**

✓7ᵗʰ **V00.211 Fall from ice-skates**

✓7ᵗʰ **V00.212 Ice-skater colliding with stationary object**

✓7ᵗʰ **V00.218 Other ice-skates accident**
EXCLUDES1   ice-skater collision with other land transport vehicle (V01-V09 with 5th digit 9)

✓6ᵗʰ **V00.22 Sled accident**

✓7ᵗʰ **V00.221 Fall from sled**

✓7ᵗʰ **V00.222 Sledder colliding with stationary object**

✓7ᵗʰ **V00.228 Other sled accident**
EXCLUDES1   sled collision with other land transport vehicle (V01-V09 with 5th digit 9)

✓6ᵗʰ **V00.28 Other gliding-type pedestrian conveyance accident**

✓7ᵗʰ **V00.281 Fall from other gliding-type pedestrian conveyance**

✓7ᵗʰ **V00.282 Pedestrian on other gliding-type pedestrian conveyance colliding with stationary object**

✓7ᵗʰ **V00.288 Other accident on other gliding-type pedestrian conveyance**
EXCLUDES1   gliding-type pedestrian conveyance collision with other land transport vehicle (V01-V09 with 5th digit 9)

✓5ᵗʰ **V00.3 Flat-bottomed pedestrian conveyance accident**

✓6ᵗʰ **V00.31 Snowboard accident**

✓7ᵗʰ **V00.311 Fall from snowboard**

✓7ᵗʰ **V00.312 Snowboarder colliding with stationary object**

✓7ᵗʰ **V00.318 Other snowboard accident**
EXCLUDES1   snowboarder collision with other land transport vehicle (V01-V09 with 5th digit 9)

✓6ᵗʰ **V00.32 Snow-ski accident**

✓7ᵗʰ **V00.321 Fall from snow-skis**

✓7ᵗʰ **V00.322 Snow-skier colliding with stationary object**

✓7ᵗʰ **V00.328 Other snow-ski accident**
EXCLUDES1   snow-skier collision with other land transport vehicle (V01-V09 with 5th digit 9)

✓6ᵗʰ **V00.38 Other flat-bottomed pedestrian conveyance accident**

✓7ᵗʰ **V00.381 Fall from other flat-bottomed pedestrian conveyance**

✓7ᵗʰ **V00.382 Pedestrian on other flat-bottomed pedestrian conveyance colliding with stationary object**

✓7ᵗʰ **V00.388 Other accident on other flat-bottomed pedestrian conveyance**

✓5ᵗʰ **V00.8 Accident on other pedestrian conveyance**

✓6ᵗʰ **V00.81 Accident with wheelchair (powered)**

✓7ᵗʰ **V00.811 Fall from moving wheelchair (powered)**
EXCLUDES1   fall from non-moving wheelchair (W05.0)

EXCLUDES1 Not coded here   EXCLUDES2 Not included here   N Newborn Age: 0   P Pediatric Age: 0-17   M Maternity Age: 12-55   A Adult Age: 15-124

☑7th **V00.812** Wheelchair (powered) colliding with stationary object

☑7th **V00.818** Other accident with wheelchair (powered)

☑6th **V00.82** **Accident with** babystroller

☑7th **V00.821** Fall from **babystroller**

☑7th **V00.822** **Babystroller** colliding with stationary object

☑7th **V00.828** Other accident with babystroller

☑6th **V00.83** **Accident with motorized** mobility scooter

V00.831 Fall from **motorized mobility scooter**

EXCLUDES 1 *fall from non-moving motorized mobility scooter (W05.2)*

V00.832 Motorized mobility scooter **colliding with stationary object**

V00.838 Other accident with motorized mobility scooter

☑6th **V00.89** **Accident on** other pedestrian **conveyance**

☑7th **V00.891** Fall from **other pedestrian conveyance**

☑7th **V00.892** **Pedestrian on other pedestrian conveyance** colliding with stationary object

☑7th **V00.898** Other accident on other pedestrian conveyance

EXCLUDES 1 *other pedestrian (conveyance) collision with other land transport vehicle (V01-V09 with 5th digit 9)*

☑4th **V01** **Pedestrian injured in collision with pedal cycle**

The appropriate 7th character is to be added to each code from category V01.
A   initial encounter
D   subsequent encounter
S   sequela

☑5th **V01.0** **Pedestrian injured in collision with pedal cycle in** nontraffic accident

☑x 7th **V01.00** Pedestrian on foot **injured in collision with pedal cycle in nontraffic accident**

Pedestrian NOS injured in collision with pedal cycle in nontraffic accident

☑x 7th **V01.01** **Pedestrian** on roller-skates **injured in collision with pedal cycle in nontraffic accident**

☑x 7th **V01.02** **Pedestrian** on skateboard **injured in collision with pedal cycle in nontraffic accident**

☑x 7th **V01.09** **Pedestrian with other** conveyance **injured in collision with pedal cycle in nontraffic accident**

Pedestrian with babystroller injured in collision with pedal cycle in nontraffic accident

Pedestrian on ice-skates injured in collision with pedal cycle in nontraffic accident

Pedestrian on nonmotorized scooter injured in collision with pedal cycle in nontraffic accident

Pedestrian on sled injured in collision with pedal cycle in nontraffic accident

Pedestrian on snowboard injured in collision with pedal cycle in nontraffic accident

Pedestrian on snow-skis injured in collision with pedal cycle in nontraffic accident

Pedestrian in wheelchair (powered) injured in collision with pedal cycle in nontraffic accident

Pedestrian in motorized mobility scooter injured in collision with pedal cycle in nontraffic accident

☑5th **V01.1** **Pedestrian injured in collision with pedal cycle in** traffic accident

☑x 7th **V01.10** **Pedestrian** on foot **injured in collision with pedal cycle in traffic accident**

Pedestrian NOS injured in collision with pedal cycle in traffic accident

☑x 7th **V01.11** **Pedestrian** on roller-skates **injured in collision with pedal cycle in traffic accident**

☑x 7th **V01.12** **Pedestrian** on skateboard **injured in collision with pedal cycle in traffic accident**

☑x 7th **V01.19** **Pedestrian with other** conveyance **injured in collision with pedal cycle in traffic accident**

Pedestrian with babystroller injured in collision with pedal cycle in traffic accident

Pedestrian on ice-skates injured in collision with pedal cycle in traffic accident

Pedestrian on nonmotorized scooter injured in collision with pedal cycle in traffic accident

Pedestrian on sled injured in collision with pedal cycle in traffic accident

Pedestrian on snowboard injured in collision with pedal cycle in traffic accident

Pedestrian on snow-skis injured in collision with pedal cycle in traffic accident

Pedestrian in wheelchair (powered) injured in collision with pedal cycle in traffic accident

Pedestrian in motorized mobility scooter injured in collision with pedal cycle in traffic accident

☑5th **V01.9** **Pedestrian injured in collision with pedal cycle,** unspecified whether traffic or nontraffic accident

☑x 7th **V01.90** **Pedestrian** on foot **injured in collision with pedal cycle, unspecified whether traffic or nontraffic accident**

Pedestrian NOS injured in collision with pedal cycle, unspecified whether traffic or nontraffic accident

☑x 7th **V01.91** **Pedestrian** on roller-skates **injured in collision with pedal cycle, unspecified whether traffic or nontraffic accident**

☑x 7th **V01.92** **Pedestrian** on skateboard **injured in collision with pedal cycle, unspecified whether traffic or nontraffic accident**

☑x 7th **V01.99** **Pedestrian with other** conveyance **injured in collision with pedal cycle, unspecified whether traffic or nontraffic accident**

Pedestrian with babystroller injured in collision with pedal cycle, unspecified whether traffic or nontraffic accident

Pedestrian on ice-skates injured in collision with pedal cycle unspecified, whether traffic or nontraffic accident

Pedestrian on nonmotorized scooter injured in collision with pedal cycle, unspecified whether traffic or nontraffic accident

Pedestrian on sled injured in collision with pedal cycle unspecified, whether traffic or nontraffic accident

Pedestrian on snowboard injured in collision with pedal cycle, unspecified whether traffic or nontraffic accident

Pedestrian on snow-skis injured in collision with pedal cycle, unspecified whether traffic or nontraffic accident

Pedestrian in wheelchair (powered) injured in collision with pedal cycle, unspecified whether traffic or nontraffic accident

Pedestrian in motorized mobility scooter injured in collision with pedal cycle, unspecified whether traffic or nontraffic accident

☑4th **V02** **Pedestrian injured in collision with two- or three-wheeled motor vehicle**

The appropriate 7th character is to be added to each code from category V02.
A   initial encounter
D   subsequent encounter
S   sequela

☑5th **V02.0** **Pedestrian injured in collision with two- or three-wheeled motor vehicle in** nontraffic accident

☑x 7th **V02.00** **Pedestrian** on foot **injured in collision with two- or three-wheeled motor vehicle in nontraffic accident**

Pedestrian NOS injured in collision with two- or three-wheeled motor vehicle in nontraffic accident

☑x 7th **V02.01** **Pedestrian** on roller-skates **injured in collision with two- or three-wheeled motor vehicle in nontraffic accident**

☑x 7th **V02.02** **Pedestrian** on skateboard **injured in collision with two- or three-wheeled motor vehicle in nontraffic accident**

☑ Additional Character Required   ☑x7th Xtension Alert   Unspecified Code   Other Specified Code   Manifestation Code   ▶◀ Revised Text   ● New Code   ▲ Revised Code Title

ICD-10-CM 2014 (Draft)   993

✓x7th V02.09 Pedestrian with other conveyance injured in collision with two- or three-wheeled motor vehicle in nontraffic accident

Pedestrian with babystroller injured in collision with two- or three-wheeled motor vehicle in nontraffic accident

Pedestrian on ice-skates injured in collision with two- or three-wheeled motor vehicle in nontraffic accident

Pedestrian on nonmotorized scooter injured in collision with two- or three-wheeled motor vehicle in nontraffic accident

Pedestrian on sled injured in collision with two- or three-wheeled motor vehicle in nontraffic accident

Pedestrian on snowboard injured in collision with two- or three-wheeled motor vehicle in nontraffic accident

Pedestrian on snow-skis injured in collision with two- or three-wheeled motor vehicle in nontraffic accident

Pedestrian in wheelchair (powered) injured in collision with two- or three-wheeled motor vehicle in nontraffic accident

Pedestrian in motorized mobility scooter injured in collision with two- or three-wheeled motor vehicle in nontraffic accident

✓5th V02.1 Pedestrian injured in collision with two- or three-wheeled motor vehicle in traffic accident

✓x7th V02.10 Pedestrian on foot injured in collision with two- or three-wheeled motor vehicle in traffic accident

Pedestrian NOS injured in collision with two- or three-wheeled motor vehicle in traffic accident

✓x7th V02.11 Pedestrian on roller-skates injured in collision with two- or three-wheeled motor vehicle in traffic accident

✓x7th V02.12 Pedestrian on skateboard injured in collision with two- or three-wheeled motor vehicle in traffic accident

✓x7th V02.19 Pedestrian with other conveyance injured in collision with two- or three-wheeled motor vehicle in traffic accident

Pedestrian with babystroller injured in collision with two- or three-wheeled motor vehicle in traffic accident

Pedestrian on ice-skates injured in collision with two- or three-wheeled motor vehicle in traffic accident

Pedestrian on nonmotorized scooter injured in collision with two- or three-wheeled motor vehicle in traffic accident

Pedestrian on sled injured in collision with two- or three-wheeled motor vehicle in traffic accident

Pedestrian on snowboard injured in collision with two- or three-wheeled motor vehicle in traffic accident

Pedestrian on snow-skis injured in collision with two- or three-wheeled motor vehicle in traffic accident

Pedestrian in wheelchair (powered) injured in collision with two- or three-wheeled motor vehicle in traffic accident

Pedestrian in motorized mobility scooter injured in collision with two- or three-wheeled motor vehicle in traffic accident

✓5th V02.9 Pedestrian injured in collision with two- or three-wheeled motor vehicle, unspecified whether traffic or nontraffic accident

✓x7th V02.90 Pedestrian on foot injured in collision with two- or three-wheeled motor vehicle, unspecified whether traffic or nontraffic accident

Pedestrian NOS injured in collision with two- or three-wheeled motor vehicle, unspecified whether traffic or nontraffic accident

✓x7th V02.91 Pedestrian on roller-skates injured in collision with two- or three-wheeled motor vehicle, unspecified whether traffic or nontraffic accident

✓x7th V02.92 Pedestrian on skateboard injured in collision with two- or three-wheeled motor vehicle, unspecified whether traffic or nontraffic accident

✓x7th V02.99 Pedestrian with other conveyance injured in collision with two- or three-wheeled motor vehicle, unspecified whether traffic or nontraffic accident

Pedestrian with babystroller injured in collision with two- or three-wheeled motor vehicle, unspecified whether traffic or nontraffic accident

Pedestrian on ice-skates injured in collision with two- or three-wheeled motor vehicle, unspecified whether traffic or nontraffic accident

Pedestrian on nonmotorized scooter injured in collision with two- or three-wheeled motor vehicle, unspecified whether traffic or nontraffic accident

Pedestrian on sled injured in collision with two- or three-wheeled motor vehicle, unspecified whether traffic or nontraffic accident

Pedestrian on snowboard injured in collision with two- or three-wheeled motor vehicle, unspecified whether traffic or nontraffic accident

Pedestrian on snow-skis injured in collision with two- or three-wheeled motor vehicle, unspecified whether traffic or nontraffic accident

Pedestrian in wheelchair (powered) injured in collision with two- or three-wheeled motor vehicle, unspecified whether traffic or nontraffic accident

Pedestrian in motorized mobility scooter injured in collision with two- or three-wheeled motor vehicle, unspecified whether traffic or nontraffic accident

✓4th V03 Pedestrian injured in collision with car, pick-up truck or van

The appropriate 7th character is to be added to each code from category V03.
A   initial encounter
D   subsequent encounter
S   sequela

✓5th V03.0 Pedestrian injured in collision with car, pick-up truck or van in nontraffic accident

✓x7th V03.00 Pedestrian on foot injured in collision with car, pick-up truck or van in nontraffic accident

Pedestrian NOS injured in collision with car, pick-up truck or van in nontraffic accident

✓x7th V03.01 Pedestrian on roller-skates injured in collision with car, pick-up truck or van in nontraffic accident

✓x7th V03.02 Pedestrian on skateboard injured in collision with car, pick-up truck or van in nontraffic accident

✓x7th V03.09 Pedestrian with other conveyance injured in collision with car, pick-up truck or van in nontraffic accident

Pedestrian with babystroller injured in collision with car, pick-up truck or van in nontraffic accident

Pedestrian on ice-skates injured in collision with car, pick-up truck or van in nontraffic accident

Pedestrian on nonmotorized scooter injured in collision with car, pick-up truck or van in nontraffic accident

Pedestrian on sled injured in collision with car, pick-up truck or van in nontraffic accident

Pedestrian on snowboard injured in collision with car, pick-up truck or van in nontraffic accident

Pedestrian on snow-skis injured in collision with car, pick-up truck or van in nontraffic accident

Pedestrian in wheelchair (powered) injured in collision with car, pick-up truck or van in nontraffic accident

Pedestrian in motorized mobility scooter injured in collision with car, pick-up truck or van in nontraffic accident

✓5th V03.1 Pedestrian injured in collision with car, pick-up truck or van in traffic accident

✓x7th V03.10 Pedestrian on foot injured in collision with car, pick-up truck or van in traffic accident

Pedestrian NOS injured in collision with car, pick-up truck or van in traffic accident

✓x7th V03.11 Pedestrian on roller-skates injured in collision with car, pick-up truck or van in traffic accident

✓x7th V03.12 Pedestrian on skateboard injured in collision with car, pick-up truck or van in traffic accident

EXCLUDES 1 Not coded here   EXCLUDES 2 Not included here   N Newborn Age: 0   P Pediatric Age: 0-17   M Maternity Age: 12-55   A Adult Age: 15-124

994   ICD-10-CM 2014 (Draft)

√x7th **V03.19 Pedestrian with other conveyance injured in collision with car, pick-up truck or van in traffic accident**

> Pedestrian with babystroller injured in collision with car, pick-up truck or van in traffic accident
> Pedestrian on ice-skates injured in collision with car, pick-up truck or van in traffic accident
> Pedestrian on nonmotorized scooter injured in collision with car, pick-up truck or van in traffic accident
> Pedestrian on sled injured in collision with car, pick-up truck or van in traffic accident
> Pedestrian on snowboard injured in collision with car, pick-up truck or van in traffic accident
> Pedestrian on snow-skis injured in collision with car, pick-up truck or van in traffic accident
> Pedestrian in wheelchair (powered) injured in collision with car, pick-up truck or van in traffic accident
> Pedestrian in motorized mobility scooter injured in collision with car, pick-up truck or van in traffic accident

√5th **V03.9 Pedestrian injured in collision with car, pick-up truck or van, unspecified whether traffic or nontraffic accident**

√x7th **V03.90 Pedestrian on foot injured in collision with car, pick-up truck or van, unspecified whether traffic or nontraffic accident**

> Pedestrian NOS injured in collision with car, pick-up truck or van, unspecified whether traffic or nontraffic accident

√x7th **V03.91 Pedestrian on roller-skates injured in collision with car, pick-up truck or van, unspecified whether traffic or nontraffic accident**

√x7th **V03.92 Pedestrian on skateboard injured in collision with car, pick-up truck or van, unspecified whether traffic or nontraffic accident**

√x7th **V03.99 Pedestrian with other conveyance injured in collision with car, pick-up truck or van, unspecified whether traffic or nontraffic accident**

> Pedestrian with babystroller injured in collision with car, pick-up truck or van, unspecified whether traffic or nontraffic accident
> Pedestrian on ice-skates injured in collision with car, pick-up truck or van, unspecified whether traffic or nontraffic accident
> Pedestrian on nonmotorized scooter injured in collision with car, pick-up truck or van, unspecified whether traffic or nontraffic accident
> Pedestrian on sled injured in collision with car, pick-up truck or van in nontraffic accident
> Pedestrian on snowboard injured in collision with car, pick-up truck or van, unspecified whether traffic or nontraffic accident
> Pedestrian on snow-skis injured in collision with car, pick-up truck or van, unspecified whether traffic or nontraffic accident
> Pedestrian in wheelchair (powered) injured in collision with car, pick-up truck or van, unspecified whether traffic or nontraffic accident
> Pedestrian in motorized mobility scooter injured in collision with car, pick-up truck or van, unspecified whether traffic or nontraffic accident

√4th **V04 Pedestrian injured in collision with heavy transport vehicle or bus**

> EXCLUDES 1   *pedestrian injured in collision with military vehicle (V09.01, V09.21)*

> The appropriate 7th character is to be added to each code from category V04.
> A   initial encounter
> D   subsequent encounter
> S   sequela

√5th **V04.0 Pedestrian injured in collision with heavy transport vehicle or bus in nontraffic accident**

√x7th **V04.00 Pedestrian on foot injured in collision with heavy transport vehicle or bus in nontraffic accident**

> Pedestrian NOS injured in collision with heavy transport vehicle or bus in nontraffic accident

√x7th **V04.01 Pedestrian on roller-skates injured in collision with heavy transport vehicle or bus in nontraffic accident**

√x7th **V04.02 Pedestrian on skateboard injured in collision with heavy transport vehicle or bus in nontraffic accident**

√x7th **V04.09 Pedestrian with other conveyance injured in collision with heavy transport vehicle or bus in nontraffic accident**

> Pedestrian with babystroller injured in collision with heavy transport vehicle or bus in nontraffic accident
> Pedestrian on ice-skates injured in collision with heavy transport vehicle or bus in nontraffic accident
> Pedestrian on nonmotorized scooter injured in collision with heavy transport vehicle or bus in nontraffic accident
> Pedestrian on sled injured in collision with heavy transport vehicle or bus in nontraffic accident
> Pedestrian on snowboard injured in collision with heavy transport vehicle or bus in nontraffic accident
> Pedestrian on snow-skis injured in collision with heavy transport vehicle or bus in nontraffic accident
> Pedestrian in wheelchair (powered) injured in collision with heavy transport vehicle or bus in nontraffic accident
> Pedestrian in motorized mobility scooter injured in collision with heavy transport vehicle or bus in nontraffic accident

√5th **V04.1 Pedestrian injured in collision with heavy transport vehicle or bus in traffic accident**

√x7th **V04.10 Pedestrian on foot injured in collision with heavy transport vehicle or bus in traffic accident**

> Pedestrian NOS injured in collision with heavy transport vehicle or bus in traffic accident

√x7th **V04.11 Pedestrian on roller-skates injured in collision with heavy transport vehicle or bus in traffic accident**

√x7th **V04.12 Pedestrian on skateboard injured in collision with heavy transport vehicle or bus in traffic accident**

√x7th **V04.19 Pedestrian with other conveyance injured in collision with heavy transport vehicle or bus in traffic accident**

> Pedestrian with babystroller injured in collision with heavy transport vehicle or bus in traffic accident
> Pedestrian on ice-skates injured in collision with heavy transport vehicle or bus in traffic accident
> Pedestrian on nonmotorized scooter injured in collision with heavy transport vehicle or bus in traffic accident
> Pedestrian on sled injured in collision with heavy transport vehicle or bus in traffic accident
> Pedestrian on snowboard injured in collision with heavy transport vehicle or bus in traffic accident
> Pedestrian on snow-skis injured in collision with heavy transport vehicle or bus in traffic accident
> Pedestrian in wheelchair (powered) injured in collision with heavy transport vehicle or bus in traffic accident
> Pedestrian in motorized mobility scooter injured in collision with heavy transport vehicle or bus in traffic accident

√5th **V04.9 Pedestrian injured in collision with heavy transport vehicle or bus, unspecified whether traffic or nontraffic accident**

√x7th **V04.90 Pedestrian on foot injured in collision with heavy transport vehicle or bus, unspecified whether traffic or nontraffic accident**

> Pedestrian NOS injured in collision with heavy transport vehicle or bus, unspecified whether traffic or nontraffic accident

√x7th **V04.91 Pedestrian on roller-skates injured in collision with heavy transport vehicle or bus, unspecified whether traffic or nontraffic accident**

√x7th **V04.92 Pedestrian on skateboard injured in collision with heavy transport vehicle or bus, unspecified whether traffic or nontraffic accident**

✓ Additional Character Required   √x7th *X*tension Alert   Unspecified Code   Other Specified Code   Manifestation Code   ►◄ Revised Text   ● New Code   ▲ Revised Code Title

ICD-10-CM 2014 (Draft)   995

☑x7th **V04.99** **Pedestrian with other conveyance injured in collision with heavy transport vehicle or bus, unspecified whether traffic or nontraffic accident**
> Pedestrian with babystroller injured in collision with heavy transport vehicle or bus, unspecified whether traffic or nontraffic accident
> Pedestrian on ice-skates injured in collision with heavy transport vehicle or bus, unspecified whether traffic or nontraffic accident
> Pedestrian on nonmotorized scooter injured in collision with heavy transport vehicle or bus, unspecified whether traffic or nontraffic accident
> Pedestrian on sled injured in collision with heavy transport vehicle or bus, unspecified whether traffic or nontraffic accident
> Pedestrian on snowboard injured in collision with heavy transport vehicle or bus, unspecified whether traffic or nontraffic accident
> Pedestrian on snow-skis injured in collision with heavy transport vehicle or bus, unspecified whether traffic or nontraffic accident
> Pedestrian in wheelchair (powered) injured in collision with heavy transport vehicle or bus, unspecified whether traffic or nontraffic accident
> Pedestrian in motorized mobility scooter injured in collision with heavy transport vehicle or bus, unspecified whether traffic or nontraffic accident

☑4th **V05** **Pedestrian injured in collision with railway train or railway vehicle**

> The appropriate 7th character is to be added to each code from category V05.
> A   initial encounter
> D   subsequent encounter
> S   sequela

☑5th **V05.0** **Pedestrian injured in collision with railway train or railway vehicle in nontraffic accident**

☑x7th **V05.00** **Pedestrian on foot injured in collision with railway train or railway vehicle in nontraffic accident**
> Pedestrian NOS injured in collision with railway train or railway vehicle in nontraffic accident

☑x7th **V05.01** **Pedestrian on roller-skates injured in collision with railway train or railway vehicle in nontraffic accident**

☑x7th **V05.02** **Pedestrian on skateboard injured in collision with railway train or railway vehicle in nontraffic accident**

☑x7th **V05.09** **Pedestrian with other conveyance injured in collision with railway train or railway vehicle in nontraffic accident**
> Pedestrian with babystroller injured in collision with railway train or railway vehicle in nontraffic accident
> Pedestrian on ice-skates injured in collision with railway train or railway vehicle in nontraffic accident
> Pedestrian on nonmotorized scooter injured in collision with railway train or railway vehicle in nontraffic accident
> Pedestrian on sled injured in collision with railway train or railway vehicle in nontraffic accident
> Pedestrian on snowboard injured in collision with railway train or railway vehicle in nontraffic accident
> Pedestrian on snow-skis injured in collision with railway train or railway vehicle in nontraffic accident
> Pedestrian in wheelchair (powered) injured in collision with railway train or railway vehicle in nontraffic accident
> Pedestrian in motorized mobility scooter injured in collision with railway train or railway vehicle in nontraffic accident

☑5th **V05.1** **Pedestrian injured in collision with railway train or railway vehicle in traffic accident**

☑x7th **V05.10** **Pedestrian on foot injured in collision with railway train or railway vehicle in traffic accident**
> Pedestrian NOS injured in collision with railway train or railway vehicle in traffic accident

☑x7th **V05.11** **Pedestrian on roller-skates injured in collision with railway train or railway vehicle in traffic accident**

☑x7th **V05.12** **Pedestrian on skateboard injured in collision with railway train or railway vehicle in traffic accident**

☑x7th **V05.19** **Pedestrian with other conveyance injured in collision with railway train or railway vehicle in traffic accident**
> Pedestrian with babystroller injured in collision with railway train or railway vehicle in traffic accident
> Pedestrian on ice-skates injured in collision with railway train or railway vehicle in traffic accident
> Pedestrian on nonmotorized scooter injured in collision with railway train or railway vehicle in traffic accident
> Pedestrian on sled injured in collision with railway train or railway vehicle in traffic accident
> Pedestrian on snowboard injured in collision with railway train or railway vehicle in traffic accident
> Pedestrian on snow-skis injured in collision with railway train or railway vehicle in traffic accident
> Pedestrian in wheelchair (powered) injured in collision with railway train or railway vehicle in traffic accident
> Pedestrian in motorized mobility scooter injured in collision with railway train or railway vehicle in traffic accident

☑5th **V05.9** **Pedestrian injured in collision with railway train or railway vehicle, unspecified whether traffic or nontraffic accident**

☑x7th **V05.90** **Pedestrian on foot injured in collision with railway train or railway vehicle, unspecified whether traffic or nontraffic accident**
> Pedestrian NOS injured in collision with railway train or railway vehicle, unspecified whether traffic or nontraffic accident

☑x7th **V05.91** **Pedestrian on roller-skates injured in collision with railway train or railway vehicle, unspecified whether traffic or nontraffic accident**

☑x7th **V05.92** **Pedestrian on skateboard injured in collision with railway train or railway vehicle, unspecified whether traffic or nontraffic accident**

☑x7th **V05.99** **Pedestrian with other conveyance injured in collision with railway train or railway vehicle, unspecified whether traffic or nontraffic accident**
> Pedestrian with babystroller injured in collision with railway train or railway vehicle, unspecified whether traffic or nontraffic
> Pedestrian on ice-skates injured in collision with railway train or railway vehicle, unspecified whether traffic or nontraffic
> Pedestrian on nonmotorized scooter injured in collision with railway train or railway vehicle, unspecified whether traffic or nontraffic
> Pedestrian on sled injured in collision with railway train or railway vehicle, unspecified whether traffic or nontraffic
> Pedestrian on snowboard injured in collision with railway train or railway vehicle, unspecified whether traffic or nontraffic
> Pedestrian on snow-skis injured in collision with railway train or railway vehicle, unspecified whether traffic or nontraffic
> Pedestrian in wheelchair (powered) injured in collision with railway train or railway vehicle, unspecified whether traffic or nontraffic
> Pedestrian in motorized mobility scooter injured in collision with railway train or railway vehicle, unspecified whether traffic or nontraffic

☑4th **V06** **Pedestrian injured in collision with other nonmotor vehicle**
> INCLUDES   collision with animal-drawn vehicle, animal being ridden, nonpowered streetcar
> EXCLUDES 1   pedestrian injured in collision with pedestrian conveyance (V00.0-)

> The appropriate 7th character is to be added to each code from category V06.
> A   initial encounter
> D   subsequent encounter
> S   sequela

☑5th **V06.0** **Pedestrian injured in collision with other nonmotor vehicle in nontraffic accident**

☑x7th **V06.00** **Pedestrian on foot injured in collision with other nonmotor vehicle in nontraffic accident**
> Pedestrian NOS injured in collision with other nonmotor vehicle in nontraffic accident

☑x7th **V06.01** **Pedestrian on roller-skates injured in collision with other nonmotor vehicle in nontraffic accident**

EXCLUDES 1 Not coded here   EXCLUDES 2 Not included here   N Newborn Age: 0   P Pediatric Age: 0-17   M Maternity Age: 12-55   A Adult Age: 15-124

996   ICD-10-CM 2014 (Draft)

√x7ᵗʰ **V06.02 Pedestrian** on skateboard **injured in collision with other nonmotor vehicle in nontraffic accident**

√x7ᵗʰ **V06.09 Pedestrian with other** conveyance **injured in collision with other nonmotor vehicle in nontraffic accident**
     Pedestrian with babystroller injured in collision with other nonmotor vehicle in nontraffic accident
     Pedestrian on ice-skates injured in collision with other nonmotor vehicle in nontraffic accident
     Pedestrian on nonmotorized scooter injured in collision with other nonmotor vehicle in nontraffic accident
     Pedestrian on sled injured in collision with other nonmotor vehicle in nontraffic accident
     Pedestrian on snowboard injured in collision with other nonmotor vehicle in nontraffic accident
     Pedestrian on snow-skis injured in collision with other nonmotor vehicle in nontraffic accident
     Pedestrian in wheelchair (powered) injured in collision with other nonmotor vehicle in nontraffic accident
     Pedestrian in motorized mobility scooter injured in collision with other nonmotor vehicle in nontraffic accident

√5ᵗʰ **V06.1 Pedestrian injured in collision with other nonmotor vehicle** in traffic accident

√x7ᵗʰ **V06.10 Pedestrian** on foot **injured in collision with other nonmotor vehicle in traffic accident**
     Pedestrian NOS injured in collision with other nonmotor vehicle in traffic accident

√x7ᵗʰ **V06.11 Pedestrian** on roller-skates **injured in collision with other nonmotor vehicle in traffic accident**

√x7ᵗʰ **V06.12 Pedestrian** on skateboard **injured in collision with other nonmotor vehicle in traffic accident**

√x7ᵗʰ **V06.19 Pedestrian with other** conveyance **injured in collision with other nonmotor vehicle in traffic accident**
     Pedestrian with babystroller injured in collision with other nonmotor vehicle in nontraffic accident
     Pedestrian on ice-skates injured in collision with other nonmotor vehicle in traffic accident
     Pedestrian on nonmotorized scooter injured in collision with other nonmotor vehicle in traffic accident
     Pedestrian on sled injured in collision with other nonmotor vehicle in traffic accident
     Pedestrian on snowboard injured in collision with other nonmotor vehicle in traffic accident
     Pedestrian on snow-skis injured in collision with other nonmotor vehicle in traffic accident
     Pedestrian in wheelchair (powered) injured in collision with other nonmotor vehicle in traffic accident
     Pedestrian in motorized mobility scooter injured in collision with other nonmotor vehicle in traffic accident

√5ᵗʰ **V06.9 Pedestrian injured in collision with other nonmotor vehicle, unspecified whether traffic or nontraffic accident**

√x7ᵗʰ **V06.90 Pedestrian** on foot **injured in collision with other nonmotor vehicle, unspecified whether traffic or nontraffic accident**
     Pedestrian NOS injured in collision with other nonmotor vehicle, unspecified whether traffic or nontraffic accident

√x7ᵗʰ **V06.91 Pedestrian** on roller-skates **injured in collision with other nonmotor vehicle, unspecified whether traffic or nontraffic accident**

√x7ᵗʰ **V06.92 Pedestrian** on skateboard **injured in collision with other nonmotor vehicle, unspecified whether traffic or nontraffic accident**

√x7ᵗʰ **V06.99 Pedestrian with other** conveyance **injured in collision with other nonmotor vehicle, unspecified whether traffic or nontraffic accident**
     Pedestrian with babystroller injured in collision with other nonmotor vehicle, unspecified whether traffic or nontraffic accident
     Pedestrian on ice-skates injured in collision with other nonmotor vehicle, unspecified whether traffic or nontraffic accident
     Pedestrian on nonmotorized scooter injured in collision with other nonmotor vehicle, unspecified whether traffic or nontraffic accident
     Pedestrian on sled injured in collision with other nonmotor vehicle, unspecified whether traffic or nontraffic accident
     Pedestrian on snowboard injured in collision with other nonmotor vehicle, unspecified whether traffic or nontraffic accident
     Pedestrian on snow-skis injured in collision with other nonmotor vehicle, unspecified whether traffic or nontraffic accident
     Pedestrian in wheelchair (powered) injured in collision with other nonmotor vehicle, unspecified whether traffic or nontraffic accident
     Pedestrian in motorized mobility scooter injured in collision with other nonmotor vehicle, unspecified whether traffic or nontraffic accident

√4ᵗʰ **V09 Pedestrian injured in other and unspecified transport accidents**

> The appropriate 7th character is to be added to each code from category V09.
> A   initial encounter
> D   subsequent encounter
> S   sequela

√5ᵗʰ **V09.0 Pedestrian injured in** nontraffic **accident involving** other **and unspecified motor vehicles**

√x7ᵗʰ **V09.00 Pedestrian injured in nontraffic accident involving unspecified motor vehicles**

√x7ᵗʰ **V09.01 Pedestrian injured in nontraffic accident involving** military **vehicle**

√x7ᵗʰ **V09.09 Pedestrian injured in nontraffic accident involving other motor vehicles**
     Pedestrian injured in nontraffic accident by special vehicle

√x7ᵗʰ **V09.1 Pedestrian injured in unspecified** nontraffic **accident**

√5ᵗʰ **V09.2 Pedestrian injured in** traffic accident **involving other and unspecified motor vehicles**

√x7ᵗʰ **V09.20 Pedestrian injured in traffic accident involving unspecified motor vehicles**

√x7ᵗʰ **V09.21 Pedestrian injured in traffic accident involving** military vehicle

√x7ᵗʰ **V09.29 Pedestrian injured in traffic accident involving other motor vehicles**

√x7ᵗʰ **V09.3 Pedestrian injured in unspecified** traffic **accident**

√x7ᵗʰ **V09.9 Pedestrian injured in unspecified** transport **accident**

Pedal cycle rider injured in transport accident (V10-V19)

INCLUDES   any non-motorized vehicle, excluding an animal-drawn vehicle, or a sidecar or trailer attached to the pedal cycle
EXCLUDES 2   *rupture of pedal cycle tire (W37.0)*

√4ᵗʰ **V10 Pedal cycle rider injured in collision with pedestrian or animal**
     EXCLUDES 1   *pedal cycle rider collision with animal-drawn vehicle or animal being ridden (V16.-)*

> The appropriate 7th character is to be added to each code from category V10.
> A   initial encounter
> D   subsequent encounter
> S   sequela

√x7ᵗʰ **V10.0 Pedal cycle** driver **injured in collision with pedestrian or animal** in nontraffic accident

√x7ᵗʰ **V10.1 Pedal cycle** passenger **injured in collision with pedestrian or animal** in nontraffic accident

√x7ᵗʰ **V10.2 Unspecified pedal cyclist injured in collision with pedestrian or animal** in nontraffic accident

√x7ᵗʰ **V10.3 Person boarding or alighting a pedal cycle injured in collision with pedestrian or animal**

√x7ᵗʰ **V10.4 Pedal cycle** driver **injured in collision with pedestrian or animal** in traffic accident

External Causes of Morbidity

V10.5–V16.9

√x7ᵗʰ **V10.5**   **Pedal cycle** passenger **injured in collision with pedestrian or animal** in traffic accident

√x7ᵗʰ **V10.9**   **Unspecified pedal cyclist injured in collision with pedestrian or animal** in traffic accident

√4ᵗʰ **V11**   **Pedal cycle rider injured in collision with other pedal cycle**

> The appropriate 7th character is to be added to each code from category V11.
> A   initial encounter
> D   subsequent encounter
> S   sequela

√x7ᵗʰ **V11.0**   **Pedal cycle** driver **injured in collision with other pedal cycle** in nontraffic accident

√x7ᵗʰ **V11.1**   **Pedal cycle** passenger **injured in collision with other pedal cycle** in nontraffic accident

√x7ᵗʰ **V11.2**   **Unspecified pedal cyclist injured in collision with other pedal cycle** in nontraffic accident

√x7ᵗʰ **V11.3**   Person boarding or alighting **a pedal cycle injured in collision with other pedal cycle**

√x7ᵗʰ **V11.4**   **Pedal cycle** driver **injured in collision with other pedal cycle** in traffic accident

√x7ᵗʰ **V11.5**   **Pedal cycle** passenger **injured in collision with other pedal cycle** in traffic accident

√x7ᵗʰ **V11.9**   **Unspecified pedal cyclist injured in collision with other pedal cycle** in traffic accident

√4ᵗʰ **V12**   **Pedal cycle rider injured in collision with two- or three-wheeled motor vehicle**

> The appropriate 7th character is to be added to each code from category V12.
> A   initial encounter
> D   subsequent encounter
> S   sequela

√x7ᵗʰ **V12.0**   **Pedal cycle** driver **injured in collision with two- or three-wheeled motor vehicle** in nontraffic accident

√x7ᵗʰ **V12.1**   **Pedal cycle** passenger **injured in collision with two- or three-wheeled motor vehicle** in nontraffic accident

√x7ᵗʰ **V12.2**   **Unspecified pedal cyclist injured in collision with two- or three-wheeled motor vehicle** in nontraffic accident

√x7ᵗʰ **V12.3**   Person boarding or alighting **a pedal cycle injured in collision with two- or three-wheeled motor vehicle**

√x7ᵗʰ **V12.4**   **Pedal cycle** driver **injured in collision with two- or three-wheeled motor vehicle** in traffic accident

√x7ᵗʰ **V12.5**   **Pedal cycle** passenger **injured in collision with two- or three-wheeled motor vehicle** in traffic accident

√x7ᵗʰ **V12.9**   **Unspecified pedal cyclist injured in collision with two- or three-wheeled motor vehicle** in traffic accident

√4ᵗʰ **V13**   **Pedal cycle rider injured in collision with car, pick-up truck or van**

> The appropriate 7th character is to be added to each code from category V13.
> A   initial encounter
> D   subsequent encounter
> S   sequela

√x7ᵗʰ **V13.0**   **Pedal cycle** driver **injured in collision with car, pick-up truck or van** in nontraffic accident

√x7ᵗʰ **V13.1**   **Pedal cycle** passenger **injured in collision with car, pick-up truck or van** in nontraffic accident

√x7ᵗʰ **V13.2**   **Unspecified pedal cyclist injured in collision with car, pick-up truck or van** in nontraffic accident

√x7ᵗʰ **V13.3**   Person boarding or alighting **a pedal cycle injured in collision with car, pick-up truck or van**

√x7ᵗʰ **V13.4**   **Pedal cycle** driver **injured in collision with car, pick-up truck or van** in traffic accident

√x7ᵗʰ **V13.5**   **Pedal cycle** passenger **injured in collision with car, pick-up truck or van** in traffic accident

√x7ᵗʰ **V13.9**   **Unspecified pedal cyclist injured in collision with car, pick-up truck or van** in traffic accident

√4ᵗʰ **V14**   **Pedal cycle rider injured in collision with heavy transport vehicle or bus**

> **EXCLUDES 1**   pedal cycle rider injured in collision with military vehicle (V19.81)

> The appropriate 7th character is to be added to each code from category V14.
> A   initial encounter
> D   subsequent encounter
> S   sequela

√x7ᵗʰ **V14.0**   **Pedal cycle** driver **injured in collision with heavy transport vehicle or bus** in nontraffic accident

√x7ᵗʰ **V14.1**   **Pedal cycle** passenger **injured in collision with heavy transport vehicle or bus** in nontraffic accident

√x7ᵗʰ **V14.2**   **Unspecified pedal cyclist injured in collision with heavy transport vehicle or bus** in nontraffic accident

√x7ᵗʰ **V14.3**   Person boarding or alighting **a pedal cycle injured in collision with heavy transport vehicle or bus**

√x7ᵗʰ **V14.4**   **Pedal cycle** driver **injured in collision with heavy transport vehicle or bus** in traffic accident

√x7ᵗʰ **V14.5**   **Pedal cycle** passenger **injured in collision with heavy transport vehicle or bus** in traffic accident

√x7ᵗʰ **V14.9**   **Unspecified pedal cyclist injured in collision with heavy transport vehicle or bus** in traffic accident

√4ᵗʰ **V15**   **Pedal cycle rider injured in collision with railway train or railway vehicle**

> The appropriate 7th character is to be added to each code from category V15.
> A   initial encounter
> D   subsequent encounter
> S   sequela

√x7ᵗʰ **V15.0**   **Pedal cycle** driver **injured in collision with railway train or railway vehicle** in nontraffic accident

√x7ᵗʰ **V15.1**   **Pedal cycle** passenger **injured in collision with railway train or railway vehicle** in nontraffic accident

√x7ᵗʰ **V15.2**   **Unspecified pedal cyclist injured in collision with railway train or railway vehicle** in nontraffic accident

√x7ᵗʰ **V15.3**   Person boarding or alighting **a pedal cycle injured in collision with railway train or railway vehicle**

√x7ᵗʰ **V15.4**   **Pedal cycle** driver **injured in collision with railway train or railway vehicle** in traffic accident

√x7ᵗʰ **V15.5**   **Pedal cycle** passenger **injured in collision with railway train or railway vehicle** in traffic accident

√x7ᵗʰ **V15.9**   **Unspecified pedal cyclist injured in collision with railway train or railway vehicle** in traffic accident

√4ᵗʰ **V16**   **Pedal cycle rider injured in collision with other nonmotor vehicle**

> **INCLUDES**   collision with animal-drawn vehicle, animal being ridden, streetcar

> The appropriate 7th character is to be added to each code from category V16.
> A   initial encounter
> D   subsequent encounter
> S   sequela

√x7ᵗʰ **V16.0**   **Pedal cycle** driver **injured in collision with other nonmotor vehicle** in nontraffic accident

√x7ᵗʰ **V16.1**   **Pedal cycle** passenger **injured in collision with other nonmotor vehicle** in nontraffic accident

√x7ᵗʰ **V16.2**   **Unspecified pedal cyclist injured in collision with other nonmotor vehicle** in nontraffic accident

√x7ᵗʰ **V16.3**   Person boarding or alighting **a pedal cycle injured in collision with other nonmotor vehicle** in nontraffic accident

√x7ᵗʰ **V16.4**   **Pedal cycle** driver **injured in collision with other nonmotor vehicle** in traffic accident

√x7ᵗʰ **V16.5**   **Pedal cycle** passenger **injured in collision with other nonmotor vehicle** in traffic accident

√x7ᵗʰ **V16.9**   **Unspecified pedal cyclist injured in collision with other nonmotor vehicle** in traffic accident

EXCLUDES 1 Not coded here   **EXCLUDES 2** Not included here   **N** Newborn Age: 0   **P** Pediatric Age: 0-17   **M** Maternity Age: 12-55   **A** Adult Age: 15-124

998   ICD-10-CM 2014 (Draft)

✓4th **V17 Pedal cycle rider injured in collision with fixed or stationary object**

The appropriate 7th character is to be added to each code from category V17.
A   initial encounter
D   subsequent encounter
S   sequela

✓x7th **V17.0 Pedal cycle** driver **injured in collision with fixed or stationary object** in nontraffic accident

✓x7th **V17.1 Pedal cycle** passenger **injured in collision with fixed or stationary object** in nontraffic accident

✓x7th **V17.2 Unspecified pedal cyclist injured in collision with fixed or stationary object** in nontraffic accident

✓x7th **V17.3** Person boarding or alighting **a pedal cycle injured in collision with fixed or stationary object**

✓x7th **V17.4 Pedal cycle** driver **injured in collision with fixed or stationary object** in traffic accident

✓x7th **V17.5 Pedal cycle** passenger **injured in collision with fixed or stationary object** in traffic accident

✓x7th **V17.9 Unspecified pedal cyclist injured in collision with fixed or stationary object** in traffic accident

✓4th **V18 Pedal cycle rider injured in noncollision transport accident**

   INCLUDES   fall or thrown from pedal cycle (without antecedent collision)
            overturning pedal cycle NOS
            overturning pedal cycle without collision

The appropriate 7th character is to be added to each code from category V18.
A   initial encounter
D   subsequent encounter
S   sequela

✓x7th **V18.0 Pedal cycle** driver **injured in noncollision transport accident** in nontraffic accident

✓x7th **V18.1 Pedal cycle** passenger **injured in noncollision transport accident** in nontraffic accident

✓x7th **V18.2 Unspecified pedal cyclist injured in noncollision transport accident** in nontraffic accident

✓x7th **V18.3** Person boarding or alighting **a pedal cycle injured in noncollision transport accident**

✓x7th **V18.4 Pedal cycle** driver **injured in noncollision transport accident** in traffic accident

✓x7th **V18.5 Pedal cycle** passenger **injured in noncollision transport accident** in traffic accident

✓x7th **V18.9 Unspecified pedal cyclist injured in noncollision transport accident** in traffic accident

✓4th **V19 Pedal cycle rider injured in other and unspecified transport accidents**

The appropriate 7th character is to be added to each code from category V19.
A   initial encounter
D   subsequent encounter
S   sequela

✓5th **V19.0 Pedal cycle** driver **injured in collision with other and unspecified motor vehicles in nontraffic accident**

   ✓x7th **V19.00 Pedal cycle driver injured in collision with unspecified motor vehicles in nontraffic accident**

   ✓x7th **V19.09 Pedal cycle driver injured in collision with other motor vehicles in nontraffic accident**

✓5th **V19.1 Pedal cycle** passenger **injured in collision with other and unspecified motor vehicles in nontraffic accident**

   ✓x7th **V19.10 Pedal cycle passenger injured in collision with unspecified motor vehicles in nontraffic accident**

   ✓x7th **V19.19 Pedal cycle passenger injured in collision with other motor vehicles in nontraffic accident**

✓5th **V19.2 Unspecified pedal cyclist injured in collision with** other and unspecified motor vehicles in nontraffic accident

   ✓x7th **V19.20 Unspecified pedal cyclist injured in collision with unspecified motor vehicles in nontraffic accident**
         Pedal cycle collision NOS, nontraffic

   ✓x7th **V19.29 Unspecified pedal cyclist injured in collision with other motor vehicles in nontraffic accident**

✓x7th **V19.3 Pedal cyclist (driver) (passenger) injured in unspecified nontraffic accident**
     Pedal cycle accident NOS, nontraffic
     Pedal cyclist injured in nontraffic accident NOS

✓5th **V19.4 Pedal cycle** driver **injured in collision with other and unspecified motor vehicles in traffic accident**

   ✓x7th **V19.40 Pedal cycle driver injured in collision with unspecified motor vehicles in traffic accident**

   ✓x7th **V19.49 Pedal cycle driver injured in collision with other motor vehicles in traffic accident**

✓5th **V19.5 Pedal cycle** passenger **injured in collision with other and unspecified motor vehicles in traffic accident**

   ✓x7th **V19.50 Pedal cycle passenger injured in collision with unspecified motor vehicles in traffic accident**

   ✓x7th **V19.59 Pedal cycle passenger injured in collision with other motor vehicles in traffic accident**

✓5th **V19.6** Unspecified **pedal cyclist injured in collision with** other and unspecified motor vehicles in traffic accident

   ✓x7th **V19.60 Unspecified pedal cyclist injured in collision with unspecified motor vehicles in traffic accident**
         Pedal cycle collision NOS (traffic)

   ✓x7th **V19.69 Unspecified pedal cyclist injured in collision with other motor vehicles in traffic accident**

✓5th **V19.8 Pedal cyclist (driver) (passenger) injured in** other specified transport accidents

   ✓x7th **V19.81 Pedal cyclist (driver) (passenger) injured in transport accident with** military vehicle

   ✓x7th **V19.88 Pedal cyclist (driver) (passenger) injured in other specified transport accidents**

✓x7th **V19.9 Pedal cyclist (driver) (passenger) injured in unspecified traffic accident**
     Pedal cycle accident NOS

Motorcycle rider injured in transport accident (V20-V29)

   INCLUDES   moped
            motorcycle with sidecar
            motorized bicycle
            motor scooter
   EXCLUDES 1   three-wheeled motor vehicle (V30-V39)

✓4th **V20 Motorcycle rider injured in collision with pedestrian or animal**

   EXCLUDES 1   motorcycle rider collision with animal-drawn vehicle or animal being ridden (V26.-)

The appropriate 7th character is to be added to each code from category V20.
A   initial encounter
D   subsequent encounter
S   sequela

✓x7th **V20.0 Motorcycle** driver **injured in collision with pedestrian or animal** in nontraffic accident

✓x7th **V20.1 Motorcycle** passenger **injured in collision with pedestrian or animal** in nontraffic accident

✓x7th **V20.2 Unspecified motorcycle rider injured in collision with pedestrian or animal** in nontraffic accident

✓x7th **V20.3** Person boarding or alighting **a motorcycle injured in collision with pedestrian or animal**

✓x7th **V20.4 Motorcycle** driver **injured in collision with pedestrian or animal** in traffic accident

✓x7th **V20.5 Motorcycle** passenger **injured in collision with pedestrian or animal** in traffic accident

✓x7th **V20.9 Unspecified motorcycle rider injured in collision with pedestrian or animal** in traffic accident

✓4th **V21 Motorcycle rider injured in collision with pedal cycle**

The appropriate 7th character is to be added to each code from category V21.
A   initial encounter
D   subsequent encounter
S   sequela

✓x7th **V21.0 Motorcycle** driver **injured in collision with pedal cycle** in nontraffic accident

✓x7th **V21.1 Motorcycle** passenger **injured in collision with pedal cycle** in nontraffic accident

✓x7th **V21.2 Unspecified motorcycle rider injured in collision with pedal cycle** in nontraffic accident

---

✓ Additional Character Required   ✓x7th Xtension Alert   Unspecified Code   Other Specified Code   Manifestation Code   ►◄ Revised Text   ● New Code   ▲ Revised Code Title

ICD-10-CM 2014 (Draft)   999

External Causes of Morbidity

V21.3–V27.9

√x7th **V21.3** Person boarding or alighting a motorcycle injured in collision with pedal cycle

√x7th **V21.4** Motorcycle driver injured in collision with pedal cycle in traffic accident

√x7th **V21.5** Motorcycle passenger injured in collision with pedal cycle in traffic accident

√x7th **V21.9** Unspecified motorcycle rider injured in collision with pedal cycle in traffic accident

√4th **V22** Motorcycle rider injured in collision with two- or three-wheeled motor vehicle

The appropriate 7th character is to be added to each code from category V22.
A   initial encounter
D   subsequent encounter
S   sequela

√x7th **V22.0** Motorcycle driver injured in collision with two- or three-wheeled motor vehicle in nontraffic accident

√x7th **V22.1** Motorcycle passenger injured in collision with two- or three-wheeled motor vehicle in nontraffic accident

√x7th **V22.2** Unspecified motorcycle rider injured in collision with two- or three-wheeled motor vehicle in nontraffic accident

√x7th **V22.3** Person boarding or alighting a motorcycle injured in collision with two- or three-wheeled motor vehicle

√x7th **V22.4** Motorcycle driver injured in collision with two- or three-wheeled motor vehicle in traffic accident

√x7th **V22.5** Motorcycle passenger injured in collision with two- or three-wheeled motor vehicle in traffic accident

√x7th **V22.9** Unspecified motorcycle rider injured in collision with two- or three-wheeled motor vehicle in traffic accident

√4th **V23** Motorcycle rider injured in collision with car, pick-up truck or van

The appropriate 7th character is to be added to each code from category V23.
A   initial encounter
D   subsequent encounter
S   sequela

√x7th **V23.0** Motorcycle driver injured in collision with car, pick-up truck or van in nontraffic accident

√x7th **V23.1** Motorcycle passenger injured in collision with car, pick-up truck or van in nontraffic accident

√x7th **V23.2** Unspecified motorcycle rider injured in collision with car, pick-up truck or van in nontraffic accident

√x7th **V23.3** Person boarding or alighting a motorcycle injured in collision with car, pick-up truck or van

√x7th **V23.4** Motorcycle driver injured in collision with car, pick-up truck or van in traffic accident

√x7th **V23.5** Motorcycle passenger injured in collision with car, pick-up truck or van in traffic accident

√x7th **V23.9** Unspecified motorcycle rider injured in collision with car, pick-up truck or van in traffic accident

√4th **V24** Motorcycle rider injured in collision with heavy transport vehicle or bus

EXCLUDES 1   motorcycle rider injured in collision with military vehicle (V29.81)

The appropriate 7th character is to be added to each code from category V24.
A   initial encounter
D   subsequent encounter
S   sequela

√x7th **V24.0** Motorcycle driver injured in collision with heavy transport vehicle or bus in nontraffic accident

√x7th **V24.1** Motorcycle passenger injured in collision with heavy transport vehicle or bus in nontraffic accident

√x7th **V24.2** Unspecified motorcycle rider injured in collision with heavy transport vehicle or bus in nontraffic accident

√x7th **V24.3** Person boarding or alighting a motorcycle injured in collision with heavy transport vehicle or bus

√x7th **V24.4** Motorcycle driver injured in collision with heavy transport vehicle or bus in traffic accident

√x7th **V24.5** Motorcycle passenger injured in collision with heavy transport vehicle or bus in traffic accident

√x7th **V24.9** Unspecified motorcycle rider injured in collision with heavy transport vehicle or bus in traffic accident

√4th **V25** Motorcycle rider injured in collision with railway train or railway vehicle

The appropriate 7th character is to be added to each code from category V25.
A   initial encounter
D   subsequent encounter
S   sequela

√x7th **V25.0** Motorcycle driver injured in collision with railway train or railway vehicle in nontraffic accident

√x7th **V25.1** Motorcycle passenger injured in collision with railway train or railway vehicle in nontraffic accident

√x7th **V25.2** Unspecified motorcycle rider injured in collision with railway train or railway vehicle in nontraffic accident

√x7th **V25.3** Person boarding or alighting a motorcycle injured in collision with railway train or railway vehicle

√x7th **V25.4** Motorcycle driver injured in collision with railway train or railway vehicle in traffic accident

√x7th **V25.5** Motorcycle passenger injured in collision with railway train or railway vehicle in traffic accident

√x7th **V25.9** Unspecified motorcycle rider injured in collision with railway train or railway vehicle in traffic accident

√4th **V26** Motorcycle rider injured in collision with other nonmotor vehicle

INCLUDES   collision with animal-drawn vehicle, animal being ridden, streetcar

The appropriate 7th character is to be added to each code from category V26.
A   initial encounter
D   subsequent encounter
S   sequela

√x7th **V26.0** Motorcycle driver injured in collision with other nonmotor vehicle in nontraffic accident

√x7th **V26.1** Motorcycle passenger injured in collision with other nonmotor vehicle in nontraffic accident

√x7th **V26.2** Unspecified motorcycle rider injured in collision with other nonmotor vehicle in nontraffic accident

√x7th **V26.3** Person boarding or alighting a motorcycle injured in collision with other nonmotor vehicle

√x7th **V26.4** Motorcycle driver injured in collision with other nonmotor vehicle in traffic accident

√x7th **V26.5** Motorcycle passenger injured in collision with other nonmotor vehicle in traffic accident

√x7th **V26.9** Unspecified motorcycle rider injured in collision with other nonmotor vehicle in traffic accident

√4th **V27** Motorcycle rider injured in collision with fixed or stationary object

The appropriate 7th character is to be added to each code from category V27.
A   initial encounter
D   subsequent encounter
S   sequela

√x7th **V27.0** Motorcycle driver injured in collision with fixed or stationary object in nontraffic accident

√x7th **V27.1** Motorcycle passenger injured in collision with fixed or stationary object in nontraffic accident

√x7th **V27.2** Unspecified motorcycle rider injured in collision with fixed or stationary object in nontraffic accident

√x7th **V27.3** Person boarding or alighting a motorcycle injured in collision with fixed or stationary object

√x7th **V27.4** Motorcycle driver injured in collision with fixed or stationary object in traffic accident

√x7th **V27.5** Motorcycle passenger injured in collision with fixed or stationary object in traffic accident

√x7th **V27.9** Unspecified motorcycle rider injured in collision with fixed or stationary object in traffic accident

EXCLUDES 1 Not coded here   EXCLUDES 2 Not included here   N Newborn Age: 0   P Pediatric Age: 0-17   M Maternity Age: 12-55   A Adult Age: 15-124

1000   ICD-10-CM 2014 (Draft)

☑4ᵗʰ **V28 Motorcycle rider injured in noncollision transport accident**

INCLUDES fall or thrown from motorcycle (without antecedent collision)
overturning motorcycle NOS
overturning motorcycle without collision

The appropriate 7th character is to be added to each code from
category V28.
A   initial encounter
D   subsequent encounter
S   sequela

√x7ᵗʰ **V28.0 Motorcycle driver injured in noncollision transport accident in nontraffic accident**

√x7ᵗʰ **V28.1 Motorcycle passenger injured in noncollision transport accident in nontraffic accident**

√x7ᵗʰ **V28.2 Unspecified motorcycle rider injured in noncollision transport accident in nontraffic accident**

√x7ᵗʰ **V28.3 Person boarding or alighting a motorcycle injured in noncollision transport accident**

√x7ᵗʰ **V28.4 Motorcycle driver injured in noncollision transport accident in traffic accident**

√x7ᵗʰ **V28.5 Motorcycle passenger injured in noncollision transport accident in traffic accident**

√x7ᵗʰ **V28.9 Unspecified motorcycle rider injured in noncollision transport accident in traffic accident**

☑4ᵗʰ **V29 Motorcycle rider injured in other and unspecified transport accidents**

The appropriate 7th character is to be added to each code from
category V29.
A   initial encounter
D   subsequent encounter
S   sequela

√5ᵗʰ **V29.0 Motorcycle driver injured in collision with other and unspecified motor vehicles in nontraffic accident**

√x7ᵗʰ **V29.00 Motorcycle driver injured in collision with unspecified motor vehicles in nontraffic accident**

√x7ᵗʰ **V29.09 Motorcycle driver injured in collision with other motor vehicles in nontraffic accident**

√5ᵗʰ **V29.1 Motorcycle passenger injured in collision with other and unspecified motor vehicles in nontraffic accident**

√x7ᵗʰ **V29.10 Motorcycle passenger injured in collision with unspecified motor vehicles in nontraffic accident**

√x7ᵗʰ **V29.19 Motorcycle passenger injured in collision with other motor vehicles in nontraffic accident**

√5ᵗʰ **V29.2 Unspecified motorcycle rider injured in collision with other and unspecified motor vehicles in nontraffic accident**

√x7ᵗʰ **V29.20 Unspecified motorcycle rider injured in collision with unspecified motor vehicles in nontraffic accident**
Motorcycle collision NOS, nontraffic

√x7ᵗʰ **V29.29 Unspecified motorcycle rider injured in collision with other motor vehicles in nontraffic accident**

√x7ᵗʰ **V29.3 Motorcycle rider (driver) (passenger) injured in unspecified nontraffic accident**
Motorcycle accident NOS, nontraffic
Motorcycle rider injured in nontraffic accident NOS

√5ᵗʰ **V29.4 Motorcycle driver injured in collision with other and unspecified motor vehicles in traffic accident**

√x7ᵗʰ **V29.40 Motorcycle driver injured in collision with unspecified motor vehicles in traffic accident**

√x7ᵗʰ **V29.49 Motorcycle driver injured in collision with other motor vehicles in traffic accident**

√5ᵗʰ **V29.5 Motorcycle passenger injured in collision with other and unspecified motor vehicles in traffic accident**

√x7ᵗʰ **V29.50 Motorcycle passenger injured in collision with unspecified motor vehicles in traffic accident**

√x7ᵗʰ **V29.59 Motorcycle passenger injured in collision with other motor vehicles in traffic accident**

√5ᵗʰ **V29.6 Unspecified motorcycle rider injured in collision with other and unspecified motor vehicles in traffic accident**

√x7ᵗʰ **V29.60 Unspecified motorcycle rider injured in collision with unspecified motor vehicles in traffic accident**
Motorcycle collision NOS (traffic)

√x7ᵗʰ **V29.69 Unspecified motorcycle rider injured in collision with other motor vehicles in traffic accident**

√5ᵗʰ **V29.8 Motorcycle rider (driver) (passenger) injured in other specified transport accidents**

√x7ᵗʰ **V29.81 Motorcycle rider (driver) (passenger) injured in transport accident with military vehicle**

√x7ᵗʰ **V29.88 Motorcycle rider (driver) (passenger) injured in other specified transport accidents**

√x7ᵗʰ **V29.9 Motorcycle rider (driver) (passenger) injured in unspecified traffic accident**
Motorcycle accident NOS

Occupant of three-wheeled motor vehicle injured in transport accident (V30-V39)

INCLUDES motorized tricycle
motorized rickshaw
three-wheeled motor car
EXCLUDES 1 all-terrain vehicles (V86.-)
motorcycle with sidecar (V20-V29)
vehicle designed primarily for off-road use (V86.-)

☑4ᵗʰ **V30 Occupant of three-wheeled motor vehicle injured in collision with pedestrian or animal**

EXCLUDES 1 three-wheeled motor vehicle collision with animal-drawn vehicle or animal being ridden (V36.-)

The appropriate 7th character is to be added to each code from
category V30.
A   initial encounter
D   subsequent encounter
S   sequela

√x7ᵗʰ **V30.0 Driver of three-wheeled motor vehicle injured in collision with pedestrian or animal in nontraffic accident**

√x7ᵗʰ **V30.1 Passenger in three-wheeled motor vehicle injured in collision with pedestrian or animal in nontraffic accident**

√x7ᵗʰ **V30.2 Person on outside of three-wheeled motor vehicle injured in collision with pedestrian or animal in nontraffic accident**

√x7ᵗʰ **V30.3 Unspecified occupant of three-wheeled motor vehicle injured in collision with pedestrian or animal in nontraffic accident**

√x7ᵗʰ **V30.4 Person boarding or alighting a three-wheeled motor vehicle injured in collision with pedestrian or animal**

√x7ᵗʰ **V30.5 Driver of three-wheeled motor vehicle injured in collision with pedestrian or animal in traffic accident**

√x7ᵗʰ **V30.6 Passenger in three-wheeled motor vehicle injured in collision with pedestrian or animal in traffic accident**

√x7ᵗʰ **V30.7 Person on outside of three-wheeled motor vehicle injured in collision with pedestrian or animal in traffic accident**

√x7ᵗʰ **V30.9 Unspecified occupant of three-wheeled motor vehicle injured in collision with pedestrian or animal in traffic accident**

☑4ᵗʰ **V31 Occupant of three-wheeled motor vehicle injured in collision with pedal cycle**

The appropriate 7th character is to be added to each code from
category V31.
A   initial encounter
D   subsequent encounter
S   sequela

√x7ᵗʰ **V31.0 Driver of three-wheeled motor vehicle injured in collision with pedal cycle in nontraffic accident**

√x7ᵗʰ **V31.1 Passenger in three-wheeled motor vehicle injured in collision with pedal cycle in nontraffic accident**

√x7ᵗʰ **V31.2 Person on outside of three-wheeled motor vehicle injured in collision with pedal cycle in nontraffic accident**

√x7ᵗʰ **V31.3 Unspecified occupant of three-wheeled motor vehicle injured in collision with pedal cycle in nontraffic accident**

√x7ᵗʰ **V31.4 Person boarding or alighting a three-wheeled motor vehicle injured in collision with pedal cycle**

√x7ᵗʰ **V31.5 Driver of three-wheeled motor vehicle injured in collision with pedal cycle in traffic accident**

√x7ᵗʰ **V31.6 Passenger in three-wheeled motor vehicle injured in collision with pedal cycle in traffic accident**

√x7ᵗʰ **V31.7 Person on outside of three-wheeled motor vehicle injured in collision with pedal cycle in traffic accident**

√x7ᵗʰ **V31.9 Unspecified occupant of three-wheeled motor vehicle injured in collision with pedal cycle in traffic accident**

☑ Additional Character Required   √x7ᵗʰ Xtension Alert   Unspecified Code   Other Specified Code   Manifestation Code   ▶◀ Revised Text   ● New Code   ▲ Revised Code Title

ICD-10-CM 2014 (Draft)   1001

External Causes of Morbidity

V32–V36.9

☑4ᵗʰ **V32 Occupant of three-wheeled motor vehicle injured in collision with two- or three-wheeled motor vehicle**

> The appropriate 7th character is to be added to each code from category V32.
> A   initial encounter
> D   subsequent encounter
> S   sequela

√x7ᵗʰ **V32.0** Driver of three-wheeled motor vehicle injured in collision with two- or three-wheeled motor vehicle in nontraffic accident

√x7ᵗʰ **V32.1** Passenger in three-wheeled motor vehicle injured in collision with two- or three-wheeled motor vehicle in nontraffic accident

√x7ᵗʰ **V32.2** Person on outside of three-wheeled motor vehicle injured in collision with two- or three-wheeled motor vehicle in nontraffic accident

√x7ᵗʰ **V32.3** Unspecified occupant of three-wheeled motor vehicle injured in collision with two- or three-wheeled motor vehicle in nontraffic accident

√x7ᵗʰ **V32.4** Person boarding or alighting a three-wheeled motor vehicle injured in collision with two- or three-wheeled motor vehicle

√x7ᵗʰ **V32.5** Driver of three-wheeled motor vehicle injured in collision with two- or three-wheeled motor vehicle in traffic accident

√x7ᵗʰ **V32.6** Passenger in three-wheeled motor vehicle injured in collision with two- or three-wheeled motor vehicle in traffic accident

√x7ᵗʰ **V32.7** Person on outside of three-wheeled motor vehicle injured in collision with two- or three-wheeled motor vehicle in traffic accident

√x7ᵗʰ **V32.9** Unspecified occupant of three-wheeled motor vehicle injured in collision with two- or three-wheeled motor vehicle in traffic accident

☑4ᵗʰ **V33 Occupant of three-wheeled motor vehicle injured in collision with car, pick-up truck or van**

> The appropriate 7th character is to be added to each code from category V33.
> A   initial encounter
> D   subsequent encounter
> S   sequela

√x7ᵗʰ **V33.0** Driver of three-wheeled motor vehicle injured in collision with car, pick-up truck or van in nontraffic accident

√x7ᵗʰ **V33.1** Passenger in three-wheeled motor vehicle injured in collision with car, pick-up truck or van in nontraffic accident

√x7ᵗʰ **V33.2** Person on outside of three-wheeled motor vehicle injured in collision with car, pick-up truck or van in nontraffic accident

√x7ᵗʰ **V33.3** Unspecified occupant of three-wheeled motor vehicle injured in collision with car, pick-up truck or van in nontraffic accident

√x7ᵗʰ **V33.4** Person boarding or alighting a three-wheeled motor vehicle injured in collision with car, pick-up truck or van

√x7ᵗʰ **V33.5** Driver of three-wheeled motor vehicle injured in collision with car, pick-up truck or van in traffic accident

√x7ᵗʰ **V33.6** Passenger in three-wheeled motor vehicle injured in collision with car, pick-up truck or van in traffic accident

√x7ᵗʰ **V33.7** Person on outside of three-wheeled motor vehicle injured in collision with car, pick-up truck or van in traffic accident

√x7ᵗʰ **V33.9** Unspecified occupant of three-wheeled motor vehicle injured in collision with car, pick-up truck or van in traffic accident

☑4ᵗʰ **V34 Occupant of three-wheeled motor vehicle injured in collision with heavy transport vehicle or bus**

> EXCLUDES 1   occupant of three-wheeled motor vehicle injured in collision with military vehicle (V39.81)

> The appropriate 7th character is to be added to each code from category V34.
> A   initial encounter
> D   subsequent encounter
> S   sequela

√x7ᵗʰ **V34.0** Driver of three-wheeled motor vehicle injured in collision with heavy transport vehicle or bus in nontraffic accident

√x7ᵗʰ **V34.1** Passenger in three-wheeled motor vehicle injured in collision with heavy transport vehicle or bus in nontraffic accident

√x7ᵗʰ **V34.2** Person on outside of three-wheeled motor vehicle injured in collision with heavy transport vehicle or bus in nontraffic accident

√x7ᵗʰ **V34.3** Unspecified occupant of three-wheeled motor vehicle injured in collision with heavy transport vehicle or bus in nontraffic accident

√x7ᵗʰ **V34.4** Person boarding or alighting a three-wheeled motor vehicle injured in collision with heavy transport vehicle or bus

√x7ᵗʰ **V34.5** Driver of three-wheeled motor vehicle injured in collision with heavy transport vehicle or bus in traffic accident

√x7ᵗʰ **V34.6** Passenger in three-wheeled motor vehicle injured in collision with heavy transport vehicle or bus in traffic accident

√x7ᵗʰ **V34.7** Person on outside of three-wheeled motor vehicle injured in collision with heavy transport vehicle or bus in traffic accident

√x7ᵗʰ **V34.9** Unspecified occupant of three-wheeled motor vehicle injured in collision with heavy transport vehicle or bus in traffic accident

☑4ᵗʰ **V35 Occupant of three-wheeled motor vehicle injured in collision with railway train or railway vehicle**

> The appropriate 7th character is to be added to each code from category V35.
> A   initial encounter
> D   subsequent encounter
> S   sequela

√x7ᵗʰ **V35.0** Driver of three-wheeled motor vehicle injured in collision with railway train or railway vehicle in nontraffic accident

√x7ᵗʰ **V35.1** Passenger in three-wheeled motor vehicle injured in collision with railway train or railway vehicle in nontraffic accident

√x7ᵗʰ **V35.2** Person on outside of three-wheeled motor vehicle injured in collision with railway train or railway vehicle in nontraffic accident

√x7ᵗʰ **V35.3** Unspecified occupant of three-wheeled motor vehicle injured in collision with railway train or railway vehicle in nontraffic accident

√x7ᵗʰ **V35.4** Person boarding or alighting a three-wheeled motor vehicle injured in collision with railway train or railway vehicle

√x7ᵗʰ **V35.5** Driver of three-wheeled motor vehicle injured in collision with railway train or railway vehicle in traffic accident

√x7ᵗʰ **V35.6** Passenger in three-wheeled motor vehicle injured in collision with railway train or railway vehicle in traffic accident

√x7ᵗʰ **V35.7** Person on outside of three-wheeled motor vehicle injured in collision with railway train or railway vehicle in traffic accident

√x7ᵗʰ **V35.9** Unspecified occupant of three-wheeled motor vehicle injured in collision with railway train or railway vehicle in traffic accident

☑4ᵗʰ **V36 Occupant of three-wheeled motor vehicle injured in collision with other nonmotor vehicle**

> INCLUDES   collision with animal-drawn vehicle, animal being ridden, streetcar

> The appropriate 7th character is to be added to each code from category V36.
> A   initial encounter
> D   subsequent encounter
> S   sequela

√x7ᵗʰ **V36.0** Driver of three-wheeled motor vehicle injured in collision with other nonmotor vehicle in nontraffic accident

√x7ᵗʰ **V36.1** Passenger in three-wheeled motor vehicle injured in collision with other nonmotor vehicle in nontraffic accident

√x7ᵗʰ **V36.2** Person on outside of three-wheeled motor vehicle injured in collision with other nonmotor vehicle in nontraffic accident

√x7ᵗʰ **V36.3** Unspecified occupant of three-wheeled motor vehicle injured in collision with other nonmotor vehicle in nontraffic accident

√x7ᵗʰ **V36.4** Person boarding or alighting a three-wheeled motor vehicle injured in collision with other nonmotor vehicle

√x7ᵗʰ **V36.5** Driver of three-wheeled motor vehicle injured in collision with other nonmotor vehicle in traffic accident

√x7ᵗʰ **V36.6** Passenger in three-wheeled motor vehicle injured in collision with other nonmotor vehicle in traffic accident

√x7ᵗʰ **V36.7** Person on outside of three-wheeled motor vehicle injured in collision with other nonmotor vehicle in traffic accident

√x7ᵗʰ **V36.9** Unspecified occupant of three-wheeled motor vehicle injured in collision with other nonmotor vehicle in traffic accident

EXCLUDES 1 Not coded here   EXCLUDES 2 Not included here   N Newborn Age: 0   P Pediatric Age: 0–17   M Maternity Age: 12–55   A Adult Age: 15–124

1002   ICD-10-CM 2014 (Draft)

☑4ᵗʰ V37　Occupant of three-wheeled motor vehicle injured in collision with fixed or stationary object

> The appropriate 7th character is to be added to each code from category V37.
> A　initial encounter
> D　subsequent encounter
> S　sequela

☑x7ᵗʰ **V37.0　Driver** of three-wheeled motor vehicle injured in collision with fixed or stationary object **in nontraffic accident**

☑x7ᵗʰ **V37.1　Passenger** in three-wheeled motor vehicle injured in collision with fixed or stationary object **in nontraffic accident**

☑x7ᵗʰ **V37.2　Person on outside** of three-wheeled motor vehicle injured in collision with fixed or stationary object **in nontraffic accident**

☑x7ᵗʰ **V37.3　Unspecified occupant** of three-wheeled motor vehicle injured in collision with other nonmotor vehicle **in traffic accident**

☑x7ᵗʰ **V37.4　Person boarding or alighting** a three-wheeled motor vehicle injured in collision with fixed or stationary object

☑x7ᵗʰ **V37.5　Driver** of three-wheeled motor vehicle injured in collision with fixed or stationary object **in traffic accident**

☑x7ᵗʰ **V37.6　Passenger** in three-wheeled motor vehicle injured in collision with fixed or stationary object **in traffic accident**

☑x7ᵗʰ **V37.7　Person on outside** of three-wheeled motor vehicle injured in collision with fixed or stationary object **in traffic accident**

☑x7ᵗʰ **V37.9　Unspecified occupant** of three-wheeled motor vehicle injured in collision with fixed or stationary object **in traffic accident**

V38　Occupant of three-wheeled motor vehicle injured in noncollision transport accident

> **INCLUDES**　fall or thrown from three-wheeled motor vehicle
> overturning of three-wheeled motor vehicle NOS
> overturning of three-wheeled motor vehicle without collision

> The appropriate 7th character is to be added to each code from category V38.
> A　initial encounter
> D　subsequent encounter
> S　sequela

☑x7ᵗʰ **V38.0　Driver** of three-wheeled motor vehicle injured in noncollision transport accident **in nontraffic accident**

☑x7ᵗʰ **V38.1　Passenger** in three-wheeled motor vehicle injured in noncollision transport accident **in nontraffic accident**

☑x7ᵗʰ **V38.2　Person on outside** of three-wheeled motor vehicle injured in noncollision transport accident **in nontraffic accident**

☑x7ᵗʰ **V38.3　Unspecified occupant** of three-wheeled motor vehicle injured in noncollision transport accident **in nontraffic accident**

☑x7ᵗʰ **V38.4　Person boarding or alighting** a three-wheeled motor vehicle injured in noncollision transport accident

☑x7ᵗʰ **V38.5　Driver** of three-wheeled motor vehicle injured in noncollision transport accident **in traffic accident**

☑x7ᵗʰ **V38.6　Passenger** in three-wheeled motor vehicle injured in noncollision transport accident **in traffic accident**

☑x7ᵗʰ **V38.7　Person on outside** of three-wheeled motor vehicle injured in noncollision transport accident **in traffic accident**

☑x7ᵗʰ **V38.9　Unspecified occupant** of three-wheeled motor vehicle injured in noncollision transport accident **in traffic accident**

☑4ᵗʰ V39　Occupant of three-wheeled motor vehicle injured in other and unspecified transport accidents

> The appropriate 7th character is to be added to each code from category V39.
> A　initial encounter
> D　subsequent encounter
> S　sequela

☑5ᵗʰ **V39.0　Driver** of three-wheeled motor vehicle injured in collision with other and unspecified motor vehicles **in nontraffic accident**

☑x7ᵗʰ **V39.00　Driver** of three-wheeled motor vehicle injured in collision with unspecified motor vehicles in nontraffic accident

☑x7ᵗʰ **V39.09　Driver** of three-wheeled motor vehicle injured in collision with other motor vehicles in nontraffic accident

☑5ᵗʰ **V39.1　Passenger** in three-wheeled motor vehicle injured in collision with other and unspecified motor vehicles **in nontraffic accident**

☑x7ᵗʰ **V39.10　Passenger** in three-wheeled motor vehicle injured in collision with unspecified motor vehicles in nontraffic accident

☑x7ᵗʰ **V39.19　Passenger** in three-wheeled motor vehicle injured in collision with other motor vehicles in nontraffic accident

☑5ᵗʰ **V39.2　Unspecified** occupant of three-wheeled motor vehicle injured in collision with other and unspecified motor vehicles **in nontraffic accident**

☑x7ᵗʰ **V39.20　Unspecified** occupant of three-wheeled motor vehicle injured in collision with unspecified motor vehicles in nontraffic accident
> Collision NOS involving three-wheeled motor vehicle, nontraffic

☑x7ᵗʰ **V39.29　Unspecified** occupant of three-wheeled motor vehicle injured in collision with other motor vehicles in nontraffic accident

☑x7ᵗʰ **V39.3　Occupant (driver) (passenger)** of three-wheeled motor vehicle injured in unspecified **nontraffic accident**
> Accident NOS involving three-wheeled motor vehicle, nontraffic
> Occupant of three-wheeled motor vehicle injured in nontraffic accident NOS

☑5ᵗʰ **V39.4　Driver** of three-wheeled motor vehicle injured in collision with other and unspecified motor vehicles **in traffic accident**

☑x7ᵗʰ **V39.40　Driver** of three-wheeled motor vehicle injured in collision with unspecified motor vehicles in traffic accident

☑x7ᵗʰ **V39.49　Driver** of three-wheeled motor vehicle injured in collision with other motor vehicles in traffic accident

☑5ᵗʰ **V39.5　Passenger** in three-wheeled motor vehicle injured in collision with other and unspecified motor vehicles **in traffic accident**

☑x7ᵗʰ **V39.50　Passenger** in three-wheeled motor vehicle injured in collision with unspecified motor vehicles in traffic accident

☑x7ᵗʰ **V39.59　Passenger** in three-wheeled motor vehicle injured in collision with other motor vehicles in traffic accident

☑5ᵗʰ **V39.6　Unspecified** occupant of three-wheeled motor vehicle injured in collision with other and unspecified motor vehicles in **traffic accident**

☑x7ᵗʰ **V39.60　Unspecified** occupant of three-wheeled motor vehicle injured in collision with unspecified motor vehicles in traffic accident
> Collision NOS involving three-wheeled motor vehicle (traffic)

☑x7ᵗʰ **V39.69　Unspecified** occupant of three-wheeled motor vehicle injured in collision with other motor vehicles in traffic accident

☑5ᵗʰ **V39.8　Occupant (driver) (passenger)** of three-wheeled motor vehicle injured in **other specified transport accidents**

☑x7ᵗʰ **V39.81　Occupant (driver) (passenger)** of three-wheeled motor vehicle injured in transport accident with **military vehicle**

☑x7ᵗʰ **V39.89　Occupant (driver) (passenger)** of three-wheeled motor vehicle injured in other **specified** transport accidents

☑x7ᵗʰ **V39.9　Occupant (driver) (passenger)** of three-wheeled motor vehicle injured in unspecified **traffic accident**
> Accident NOS involving three-wheeled motor vehicle

☑ Additional Character Required　☑x7ᵗʰ *X*tension Alert　Unspecified Code　Other Specified Code　Manifestation Code　►◄ Revised Text　● New Code　▲ Revised Code Title

ICD-10-CM 2014 (Draft)　　　　　1003

occupant injured in transport accident (V40-V49)

INCLUDES   a four-wheeled motor vehicle designed primarily for carrying passengers
automobile (pulling a trailer or camper)

EXCLUDES1   bus (V50-V59)
minibus (V50-V59)
minivan (V50-V59)
motorcoach (V70-V79)
pick-up truck (V50-V59)
sport utility vehicle (SUV) (V50-V59)

✓4th **V40 Car occupant injured in collision with pedestrian or animal**

EXCLUDES1   car collision with animal-drawn vehicle or animal being ridden (V46.-)

The appropriate 7th character is to be added to each code from category V40.
A   initial encounter
D   subsequent encounter
S   sequela

✓x7th **V40.0** Car driver injured in collision with pedestrian or animal in nontraffic accident

✓x7th **V40.1** Car passenger injured in collision with pedestrian or animal in nontraffic accident

✓x7th **V40.2** Person on outside of car injured in collision with pedestrian or animal in nontraffic accident

✓x7th **V40.3** Unspecified car occupant injured in collision with pedestrian or animal in nontraffic accident

✓x7th **V40.4** Person boarding or alighting a car injured in collision with pedestrian or animal

✓x7th **V40.5** Car driver injured in collision with pedestrian or animal in traffic accident

✓x7th **V40.6** Car passenger injured in collision with pedestrian or animal in traffic accident

✓x7th **V40.7** Person on outside of car injured in collision with pedestrian or animal in traffic accident

✓x7th **V40.9** Unspecified car occupant injured in collision with pedestrian or animal in traffic accident

✓4th **V41 Car occupant injured in collision with pedal cycle**

The appropriate 7th character is to be added to each code from category V41.
A   initial encounter
D   subsequent encounter
S   sequela

✓x7th **V41.0** Car driver injured in collision with pedal cycle in nontraffic accident

✓x7th **V41.1** Car passenger injured in collision with pedal cycle in nontraffic accident

✓x7th **V41.2** Person on outside of car injured in collision with pedal cycle in nontraffic accident

✓x7th **V41.3** Unspecified car occupant injured in collision with pedal cycle in nontraffic accident

✓x7th **V41.4** Person boarding or alighting a car injured in collision with pedal cycle

✓x7th **V41.5** Car driver injured in collision with pedal cycle in traffic accident

✓x7th **V41.6** Car passenger injured in collision with pedal cycle in traffic accident

✓x7th **V41.7** Person on outside of car injured in collision with pedal cycle in traffic accident

✓x7th **V41.9** Unspecified car occupant injured in collision with pedal cycle in traffic accident

✓4th **V42 Car occupant injured in collision with two- or three-wheeled motor vehicle**

The appropriate 7th character is to be added to each code from category V42.
A   initial encounter
D   subsequent encounter
S   sequela

✓x7th **V42.0** Car driver injured in collision with two- or three-wheeled motor vehicle in nontraffic accident

✓x7th **V42.1** Car passenger injured in collision with two- or three-wheeled motor vehicle in nontraffic accident

✓x7th **V42.2** Person on outside of car injured in collision with two- or three-wheeled motor vehicle in nontraffic accident

✓x7th **V42.3** Unspecified car occupant injured in collision with two- or three-wheeled motor vehicle in nontraffic accident

✓x7th **V42.4** Person boarding or alighting a car injured in collision with two- or three-wheeled motor vehicle

✓x7th **V42.5** Car driver injured in collision with two- or three-wheeled motor vehicle in traffic accident

✓x7th **V42.6** Car passenger injured in collision with two- or three-wheeled motor vehicle in traffic accident

✓x7th **V42.7** Person on outside of car injured in collision with two- or three-wheeled motor vehicle in traffic accident

✓x7th **V42.9** Unspecified car occupant injured in collision with two- or three-wheeled motor vehicle in traffic accident

✓4th **V43 Car occupant injured in collision with car, pick-up truck or van**

The appropriate 7th character is to be added to each code from category V43.
A   initial encounter
D   subsequent encounter
S   sequela

✓5th **V43.0** Car driver injured in collision with car, pick-up truck or van in nontraffic accident

    ✓x7th **V43.01** Car driver injured in collision with sport utility vehicle in nontraffic accident

    ✓x7th **V43.02** Car driver injured in collision with other type car in nontraffic accident

    ✓x7th **V43.03** Car driver injured in collision with pick-up truck in nontraffic accident

    ✓x7th **V43.04** Car driver injured in collision with van in nontraffic accident

✓5th **V43.1** Car passenger injured in collision with car, pick-up truck or van in nontraffic accident

    ✓x7th **V43.11** Car passenger injured in collision with sport utility vehicle in nontraffic accident

    ✓x7th **V43.12** Car passenger injured in collision with other type car in nontraffic accident

    ✓x7th **V43.13** Car passenger injured in collision with pick-up in nontraffic accident

    ✓x7th **V43.14** Car passenger injured in collision with van in nontraffic accident

✓5th **V43.2** Person on outside of car injured in collision with car, pick-up truck or van in nontraffic accident

    ✓x7th **V43.21** Person on outside of car injured in collision with sport utility vehicle in nontraffic accident

    ✓x7th **V43.22** Person on outside of car injured in collision with other type car in nontraffic accident

    ✓x7th **V43.23** Person on outside of car injured in collision with pick-up truck in nontraffic accident

    ✓x7th **V43.24** Person on outside of car injured in collision with van in nontraffic accident

✓5th **V43.3** Unspecified car occupant injured in collision with car, pick-up truck or van in nontraffic accident

    ✓x7th **V43.31** Unspecified car occupant injured in collision with sport utility vehicle in nontraffic accident

    ✓x7th **V43.32** Unspecified car occupant injured in collision with other type car in nontraffic accident

    ✓x7th **V43.33** Unspecified car occupant injured in collision with pick-up truck in nontraffic accident

    ✓x7th **V43.34** Unspecified car occupant injured in collision with van in nontraffic accident

✓5th **V43.4** Person boarding or alighting a car injured in collision with car, pick-up truck or van

    ✓x7th **V43.41** Person boarding or alighting a car injured in collision with sport utility vehicle

    ✓x7th **V43.42** Person boarding or alighting a car injured in collision with other type car

    ✓x7th **V43.43** Person boarding or alighting a car injured in collision with pick-up truck

    ✓x7th **V43.44** Person boarding or alighting a car injured in collision with van

✓5th **V43.5** Car driver injured in collision with car, pick-up truck or van in traffic accident

    ✓x7th **V43.51** Car driver injured in collision with sport utility vehicle in traffic accident

EXCLUDES1 Not coded here   EXCLUDES2 Not included here   N Newborn Age: 0   P Pediatric Age: 0-17   M Maternity Age: 12-55   A Adult Age: 15-124

1004   ICD-10-CM 2014 (Draft)

V40-V43.51 (side tab)

√x7ᵗʰ **V43.52** Car driver injured in collision with other type car in traffic accident

√x7ᵗʰ **V43.53** Car driver injured in collision with pick-up truck in traffic accident

√x7ᵗʰ **V43.54** Car driver injured in collision with van in traffic accident

√5ᵗʰ **V43.6** Car passenger injured in collision with car, pick-up truck or van in traffic accident

√x7ᵗʰ **V43.61** Car passenger injured in collision with sport utility vehicle in traffic accident

√x7ᵗʰ **V43.62** Car passenger injured in collision with other type car in traffic accident

√x7ᵗʰ **V43.63** Car passenger injured in collision with pick-up truck in traffic accident

√x7ᵗʰ **V43.64** Car passenger injured in collision with van in traffic accident

√5ᵗʰ **V43.7** Person on outside of car injured in collision with car, pick-up truck or van in traffic accident

√x7ᵗʰ **V43.71** Person on outside of car injured in collision with sport utility vehicle in traffic accident

√x7ᵗʰ **V43.72** Person on outside of car injured in collision with other type car in traffic accident

√x7ᵗʰ **V43.73** Person on outside of car injured in collision with pick-up truck in traffic accident

√x7ᵗʰ **V43.74** Person on outside of car injured in collision with van in traffic accident

√5ᵗʰ **V43.9** Unspecified car occupant injured in collision with car, pick-up truck or van in traffic accident

√x7ᵗʰ **V43.91** Unspecified car occupant injured in collision with sport utility vehicle in traffic accident

√x7ᵗʰ **V43.92** Unspecified car occupant injured in collision with other type car in traffic accident

√x7ᵗʰ **V43.93** Unspecified car occupant injured in collision with pick-up truck in traffic accident

√x7ᵗʰ **V43.94** Unspecified car occupant injured in collision with van in traffic accident

√4ᵗʰ **V44** Car occupant injured in collision with heavy transport vehicle or bus

> EXCLUDES 1   car occupant injured in collision with military vehicle (V49.81)

> The appropriate 7th character is to be added to each code from category V44.
> A   initial encounter
> D   subsequent encounter
> S   sequela

√x7ᵗʰ **V44.0** Car driver injured in collision with heavy transport vehicle or bus in nontraffic accident

√x7ᵗʰ **V44.1** Car passenger injured in collision with heavy transport vehicle or bus in nontraffic accident

√x7ᵗʰ **V44.2** Person on outside of car injured in collision with heavy transport vehicle or bus in nontraffic accident

√x7ᵗʰ **V44.3** Unspecified car occupant injured in collision with heavy transport vehicle or bus in nontraffic accident

√x7ᵗʰ **V44.4** Person boarding or alighting a car injured in collision with heavy transport vehicle or bus

√x7ᵗʰ **V44.5** Car driver injured in collision with heavy transport vehicle or bus in traffic accident

√x7ᵗʰ **V44.6** Car passenger injured in collision with heavy transport vehicle or bus in traffic accident

√x7ᵗʰ **V44.7** Person on outside of car injured in collision with heavy transport vehicle or bus in traffic accident

√x7ᵗʰ **V44.9** Unspecified car occupant injured in collision with heavy transport vehicle or bus in traffic accident

√4ᵗʰ **V45** Car occupant injured in collision with railway train or railway vehicle

> The appropriate 7th character is to be added to each code from category V45.
> A   initial encounter
> D   subsequent encounter
> S   sequela

√x7ᵗʰ **V45.0** Car driver injured in collision with railway train or railway vehicle in nontraffic accident

√x7ᵗʰ **V45.1** Car passenger injured in collision with railway train or railway vehicle in nontraffic accident

√x7ᵗʰ **V45.2** Person on outside of car injured in collision with railway train or railway vehicle in nontraffic accident

√x7ᵗʰ **V45.3** Unspecified car occupant injured in collision with railway train or railway vehicle in nontraffic accident

√x7ᵗʰ **V45.4** Person boarding or alighting a car injured in collision with railway train or railway vehicle

√x7ᵗʰ **V45.5** Car driver injured in collision with railway train or railway vehicle in traffic accident

√x7ᵗʰ **V45.6** Car passenger injured in collision with railway train or railway vehicle in traffic accident

√x7ᵗʰ **V45.7** Person on outside of car injured in collision with railway train or railway vehicle in traffic accident

√x7ᵗʰ **V45.9** Unspecified car occupant injured in collision with railway train or railway vehicle in traffic accident

√4ᵗʰ **V46** Car occupant injured in collision with other nonmotor vehicle

> INCLUDES   collision with animal-drawn vehicle, animal being ridden, streetcar

> The appropriate 7th character is to be added to each code from category V46.
> A   initial encounter
> D   subsequent encounter
> S   sequela

√x7ᵗʰ **V46.0** Car driver injured in collision with other nonmotor vehicle in nontraffic accident

√x7ᵗʰ **V46.1** Car passenger injured in collision with other nonmotor vehicle in nontraffic accident

√x7ᵗʰ **V46.2** Person on outside of car injured in collision with other nonmotor vehicle in nontraffic accident

√x7ᵗʰ **V46.3** Unspecified car occupant injured in collision with other nonmotor vehicle in nontraffic accident

√x7ᵗʰ **V46.4** Person boarding or alighting a car injured in collision with other nonmotor vehicle

√x7ᵗʰ **V46.5** Car driver injured in collision with other nonmotor vehicle in traffic accident

√x7ᵗʰ **V46.6** Car passenger injured in collision with other nonmotor vehicle in traffic accident

√x7ᵗʰ **V46.7** Person on outside of car injured in collision with other nonmotor vehicle in traffic accident

√x7ᵗʰ **V46.9** Unspecified car occupant injured in collision with other nonmotor vehicle in traffic accident

√4ᵗʰ **V47** Car occupant injured in collision with fixed or stationary object

> The appropriate 7th character is to be added to each code from category V47.
> A   initial encounter
> D   subsequent encounter
> S   sequela

√5ᵗʰ **V47.0** Car driver injured in collision with fixed or stationary object in nontraffic accident

√x7ᵗʰ **V47.01** Driver of sport utility vehicle injured in collision with fixed or stationary object in nontraffic accident

√x7ᵗʰ **V47.02** Driver of other type car injured in collision with fixed or stationary object in nontraffic accident

√5ᵗʰ **V47.1** Car passenger injured in collision with fixed or stationary object in nontraffic accident

√x7ᵗʰ **V47.11** Passenger of sport utility vehicle injured in collision with fixed or stationary object in nontraffic accident

√x7ᵗʰ **V47.12** Passenger of other type car injured in collision with fixed or stationary object in nontraffic accident

√x7ᵗʰ **V47.2** Person on outside of car injured in collision with fixed or stationary object in nontraffic accident

√5ᵗʰ **V47.3** Unspecified car occupant injured in collision with fixed or stationary object in nontraffic accident

√x7ᵗʰ **V47.31** Unspecified occupant of sport utility vehicle injured in collision with fixed or stationary object in nontraffic accident

√x7ᵗʰ **V47.32** Unspecified occupant of other type car injured in collision with fixed or stationary object in nontraffic accident

√x7ᵗʰ **V47.4** Person boarding or alighting a car injured in collision with fixed or stationary object

√5ᵗʰ **V47.5** Car driver injured in collision with fixed or stationary object in traffic accident

√x7ᵗʰ **V47.51** Driver of sport utility vehicle injured in collision with fixed or stationary object in traffic accident

---

☑ Additional Character Required   √x7ᵗʰ Xtension Alert   Unspecified Code   Other Specified Code   Manifestation Code   ►◄ Revised Text   ● New Code   ▲ Revised Code Title

External Causes of Morbidity

V47.52–V50.9

✓7ᵗʰ **V47.52 Driver of other type car injured in collision with fixed or stationary object in traffic accident**

✓5ᵗʰ **V47.6 Car** passenger **injured in collision with fixed or stationary object in traffic accident**

✓7ᵗʰ **V47.61 Passenger of** sport utility vehicle **injured in collision with fixed or stationary object in traffic accident**

✓7ᵗʰ **V47.62 Passenger of other type car injured in collision with fixed or stationary object in traffic accident**

✓7ᵗʰ **V47.7 Person on outside of car injured in collision with fixed or stationary object** in traffic accident

✓5ᵗʰ **V47.9 Unspecified car occupant injured in collision with fixed or stationary object** in traffic accident

✓7ᵗʰ **V47.91 Unspecified occupant of** sport utility vehicle **injured in collision with fixed or stationary object in traffic accident**

✓7ᵗʰ **V47.92 Unspecified occupant of other type car injured in collision with fixed or stationary object in traffic accident**

✓4ᵗʰ **V48 Car occupant injured in noncollision transport accident**

INCLUDES   overturning car NOS
overturning car without collision

The appropriate 7th character is to be added to each code from category V48.
A   initial encounter
D   subsequent encounter
S   sequela

✓7ᵗʰ **V48.0 Car** driver **injured in noncollision transport accident in** nontraffic accident

✓7ᵗʰ **V48.1 Car** passenger **injured in noncollision transport accident in** nontraffic accident

✓7ᵗʰ **V48.2 Person on outside of car injured in noncollision transport accident in** nontraffic accident

✓7ᵗʰ **V48.3 Unspecified car occupant injured in noncollision transport accident in** nontraffic accident

✓7ᵗʰ **V48.4 Person boarding or alighting a car injured in noncollision transport accident**

✓7ᵗʰ **V48.5 Car** driver **injured in noncollision transport accident in** traffic accident

✓7ᵗʰ **V48.6 Car** passenger **injured in noncollision transport accident in** traffic accident

✓7ᵗʰ **V48.7 Person on outside of car injured in noncollision transport accident in** traffic accident

✓7ᵗʰ **V48.9 Unspecified car occupant injured in noncollision transport accident in** traffic accident

✓4ᵗʰ **V49 Car occupant injured in other and unspecified transport accidents**

The appropriate 7th character is to be added to each code from category V49.
A   initial encounter
D   subsequent encounter
S   sequela

✓5ᵗʰ **V49.0 Driver injured in collision with other and unspecified motor vehicles in** nontraffic accident

✓7ᵗʰ **V49.00 Driver injured in collision with unspecified motor vehicles in nontraffic accident**

✓7ᵗʰ **V49.09 Driver injured in collision with other motor vehicles in nontraffic accident**

✓5ᵗʰ **V49.1 Passenger injured in collision with other and unspecified motor vehicles in** nontraffic accident

✓7ᵗʰ **V49.10 Passenger injured in collision with unspecified motor vehicles in nontraffic accident**

✓7ᵗʰ **V49.19 Passenger injured in collision with other motor vehicles in nontraffic accident**

✓5ᵗʰ **V49.2 Unspecified car occupant injured in collision with other and** unspecified motor vehicles in nontraffic accident

✓7ᵗʰ **V49.20 Unspecified car occupant injured in collision with unspecified motor vehicles in nontraffic accident**
Car collision NOS, nontraffic

✓7ᵗʰ **V49.29 Unspecified car occupant injured in collision with other motor vehicles in nontraffic accident**

✓7ᵗʰ **V49.3 Car occupant (driver) (passenger) injured in unspecified** nontraffic accident
Car accident NOS, nontraffic
Car occupant injured in nontraffic accident NOS

✓5ᵗʰ **V49.4 Driver injured in collision with other and unspecified motor vehicles in** traffic accident

✓7ᵗʰ **V49.40 Driver injured in collision with unspecified motor vehicles in traffic accident**

✓7ᵗʰ **V49.49 Driver injured in collision with other motor vehicles in traffic accident**

✓5ᵗʰ **V49.5 Passenger injured in collision with other and unspecified motor vehicles in** traffic accident

✓7ᵗʰ **V49.50 Passenger injured in collision with unspecified motor vehicles in traffic accident**

✓7ᵗʰ **V49.59 Passenger injured in collision with other motor vehicles in traffic accident**

✓5ᵗʰ **V49.6 Unspecified car occupant injured in collision with other and unspecified motor vehicles in** traffic accident

✓7ᵗʰ **V49.60 Unspecified car occupant injured in collision with unspecified motor vehicles in traffic accident**
Car collision NOS (traffic)

✓7ᵗʰ **V49.69 Unspecified car occupant injured in collision with other motor vehicles in traffic accident**

✓5ᵗʰ **V49.8 Car** occupant (driver) (passenger) **injured in other specified transport accidents**

✓7ᵗʰ **V49.81 Car occupant (driver) (passenger) injured in transport accident** with military vehicle

✓7ᵗʰ **V49.88 Car occupant (driver) (passenger) injured in other** specified **transport accidents**

✓7ᵗʰ **V49.9 Car occupant (driver) (passenger) injured in unspecified** traffic accident
Car accident NOS

Occupant of pick-up truck or van injured in transport accident (V50-V59)

INCLUDES   a four or six wheel motor vehicle designed primarily for carrying passengers and property but weighing less than the local limit for classification as a heavy goods vehicle
minibus
minivan
sport utility vehicle (SUV)
truck
van

EXCLUDES 1   heavy transport vehicle (V60-V69)

✓4ᵗʰ **V50 Occupant of pick-up truck or van injured in collision with pedestrian or animal**

EXCLUDES 1   pick-up truck or van collision with animal-drawn vehicle or animal being ridden (V56.-)

The appropriate 7th character is to be added to each code from category V50.
A   initial encounter
D   subsequent encounter
S   sequela

✓7ᵗʰ **V50.0 Driver of pick-up truck or van injured in collision with pedestrian or animal** in nontraffic accident

✓7ᵗʰ **V50.1 Passenger in pick-up truck or van injured in collision with pedestrian or animal** in nontraffic accident

✓7ᵗʰ **V50.2 Person on outside of pick-up truck or van injured in collision with pedestrian or animal** in nontraffic accident

✓7ᵗʰ **V50.3 Unspecified occupant of pick-up truck or van injured in collision with pedestrian or animal** in nontraffic accident

✓7ᵗʰ **V50.4 Person boarding or alighting a pick-up truck or van injured in collision with pedestrian or animal**

✓7ᵗʰ **V50.5 Driver of pick-up truck or van injured in collision with pedestrian or animal** in traffic accident

✓7ᵗʰ **V50.6 Passenger in pick-up truck or van injured in collision with pedestrian or animal** in traffic accident

✓7ᵗʰ **V50.7 Person on outside of pick-up truck or van injured in collision with pedestrian or animal** in traffic accident

✓7ᵗʰ **V50.9 Unspecified occupant of pick-up truck or van injured in collision with pedestrian or animal** in traffic accident

EXCLUDES 1 Not coded here   EXCLUDES 2 Not included here   N Newborn Age: 0   P Pediatric Age: 0-17   M Maternity Age: 12-55   A Adult Age: 15-124

1006   ICD-10-CM 2014 (Draft)

✓4ᵗʰ **V51** **Occupant of pick-up truck or van injured in collision with pedal cycle**

The appropriate 7th character is to be added to each code from category V51.
- A   initial encounter
- D   subsequent encounter
- S   sequela

✓x7ᵗʰ **V51.0** Driver of pick-up truck or van injured in collision with pedal cycle in nontraffic accident

✓x7ᵗʰ **V51.1** Passenger in pick-up truck or van injured in collision with pedal cycle in nontraffic accident

✓x7ᵗʰ **V51.2** Person on outside of pick-up truck or van injured in collision with pedal cycle in nontraffic accident

✓x7ᵗʰ **V51.3** **Unspecified occupant of pick-up truck or van injured in collision with pedal cycle in nontraffic accident**

✓x7ᵗʰ **V51.4** Person boarding or alighting a pick-up truck or van injured in collision with pedal cycle

✓x7ᵗʰ **V51.5** Driver of pick-up truck or van injured in collision with pedal cycle in traffic accident

✓x7ᵗʰ **V51.6** Passenger in pick-up truck or van injured in collision with pedal cycle in traffic accident

✓x7ᵗʰ **V51.7** Person on outside of pick-up truck or van injured in collision with pedal cycle in traffic accident

✓x7ᵗʰ **V51.9** **Unspecified occupant of pick-up truck or van injured in collision with pedal cycle in traffic accident**

✓4ᵗʰ **V52** **Occupant of pick-up truck or van injured in collision with two- or three-wheeled motor vehicle**

The appropriate 7th character is to be added to each code from category V52.
- A   initial encounter
- D   subsequent encounter
- S   sequela

✓x7ᵗʰ **V52.0** Driver of pick-up truck or van injured in collision with two- or three-wheeled motor vehicle in nontraffic accident

✓x7ᵗʰ **V52.1** Passenger in pick-up truck or van injured in collision with two- or three-wheeled motor vehicle in nontraffic accident

✓x7ᵗʰ **V52.2** Person on outside of pick-up truck or van injured in collision with two- or three-wheeled motor vehicle in nontraffic accident

✓x7ᵗʰ **V52.3** **Unspecified occupant of pick-up truck or van injured in collision with two- or three-wheeled motor vehicle in nontraffic accident**

✓x7ᵗʰ **V52.4** Person boarding or alighting a pick-up truck or van injured in collision with two- or three-wheeled motor vehicle

✓x7ᵗʰ **V52.5** Driver of pick-up truck or van injured in collision with two- or three-wheeled motor vehicle in traffic accident

✓x7ᵗʰ **V52.6** Passenger in pick-up truck or van injured in collision with two- or three-wheeled motor vehicle in traffic accident

✓x7ᵗʰ **V52.7** Person on outside of pick-up truck or van injured in collision with two- or three-wheeled motor vehicle in traffic accident

✓x7ᵗʰ **V52.9** **Unspecified occupant of pick-up truck or van injured in collision with two- or three-wheeled motor vehicle in traffic accident**

✓4ᵗʰ **V53** **Occupant of pick-up truck or van injured in collision with car, pick-up truck or van**

The appropriate 7th character is to be added to each code from category V53.
- A   initial encounter
- D   subsequent encounter
- S   sequela

✓x7ᵗʰ **V53.0** Driver of pick-up truck or van injured in collision with car, pick-up truck or van in nontraffic accident

✓x7ᵗʰ **V53.1** Passenger in pick-up truck or van injured in collision with car, pick-up truck or van in nontraffic accident

✓x7ᵗʰ **V53.2** Person on outside of pick-up truck or van injured in collision with car, pick-up truck or van in nontraffic accident

✓x7ᵗʰ **V53.3** **Unspecified occupant of pick-up truck or van injured in collision with car, pick-up truck or van in nontraffic accident**

✓x7ᵗʰ **V53.4** Person boarding or alighting a pick-up truck or van injured in collision with car, pick-up truck or van

✓x7ᵗʰ **V53.5** Driver of pick-up truck or van injured in collision with car, pick-up truck or van in traffic accident

✓x7ᵗʰ **V53.6** Passenger in pick-up truck or van injured in collision with car, pick-up truck or van in traffic accident

✓x7ᵗʰ **V53.7** Person on outside of pick-up truck or van injured in collision with car, pick-up truck or van in traffic accident

✓x7ᵗʰ **V53.9** **Unspecified occupant of pick-up truck or van injured in collision with car, pick-up truck or van in traffic accident**

✓4ᵗʰ **V54** **Occupant of pick-up truck or van injured in collision with heavy transport vehicle or bus**

EXCLUDES 1   occupant of pick-up truck or van injured in collision with military vehicle (V59.81)

The appropriate 7th character is to be added to each code from category V54.
- A   initial encounter
- D   subsequent encounter
- S   sequela

✓x7ᵗʰ **V54.0** Driver of pick-up truck or van injured in collision with heavy transport vehicle or bus in nontraffic accident

✓x7ᵗʰ **V54.1** Passenger in pick-up truck or van injured in collision with heavy transport vehicle or bus in nontraffic accident

✓x7ᵗʰ **V54.2** Person on outside of pick-up truck or van injured in collision with heavy transport vehicle or bus in nontraffic accident

✓x7ᵗʰ **V54.3** **Unspecified occupant of pick-up truck or van injured in collision with heavy transport vehicle or bus in nontraffic accident**

✓x7ᵗʰ **V54.4** Person boarding or alighting a pick-up truck or van injured in collision with heavy transport vehicle or bus

✓x7ᵗʰ **V54.5** Driver of pick-up truck or van injured in collision with heavy transport vehicle or bus in traffic accident

✓x7ᵗʰ **V54.6** Passenger in pick-up truck or van injured in collision with heavy transport vehicle or bus in traffic accident

✓x7ᵗʰ **V54.7** Person on outside of pick-up truck or van injured in collision with heavy transport vehicle or bus in traffic accident

✓x7ᵗʰ **V54.9** **Unspecified occupant of pick-up truck or van injured in collision with heavy transport vehicle or bus in traffic accident**

✓4ᵗʰ **V55** **Occupant of pick-up truck or van injured in collision with railway train or railway vehicle**

The appropriate 7th character is to be added to each code from category V55.
- A   initial encounter
- D   subsequent encounter
- S   sequela

✓x7ᵗʰ **V55.0** Driver of pick-up truck or van injured in collision with railway train or railway vehicle in nontraffic accident

✓x7ᵗʰ **V55.1** Passenger in pick-up truck or van injured in collision with railway train or railway vehicle in nontraffic accident

✓x7ᵗʰ **V55.2** Person on outside of pick-up truck or van injured in collision with railway train or railway vehicle in nontraffic accident

✓x7ᵗʰ **V55.3** **Unspecified occupant of pick-up truck or van injured in collision with railway train or railway vehicle in nontraffic accident**

✓x7ᵗʰ **V55.4** Person boarding or alighting a pick-up truck or van injured in collision with railway train or railway vehicle

✓x7ᵗʰ **V55.5** Driver of pick-up truck or van injured in collision with railway train or railway vehicle in traffic accident

✓x7ᵗʰ **V55.6** Passenger in pick-up truck or van injured in collision with railway train or railway vehicle in traffic accident

✓x7ᵗʰ **V55.7** Person on outside of pick-up truck or van injured in collision with railway train or railway vehicle in traffic accident

✓x7ᵗʰ **V55.9** **Unspecified occupant of pick-up truck or van injured in collision with railway train or railway vehicle in nontraffic accident**

✓4ᵗʰ **V56** **Occupant of pick-up truck or van injured in collision with other nonmotor vehicle**

INCLUDES   collision with animal-drawn vehicle, animal being ridden, streetcar

The appropriate 7th character is to be added to each code from category V56.
- A   initial encounter
- D   subsequent encounter
- S   sequela

✓x7ᵗʰ **V56.0** Driver of pick-up truck or van injured in collision with other nonmotor vehicle in nontraffic accident

✓x7ᵗʰ **V56.1** Passenger in pick-up truck or van injured in collision with other nonmotor vehicle in nontraffic accident

---

☑ Additional Character Required   ✓x7ᵗʰ Xtension Alert   Unspecified Code   Other Specified Code   Manifestation Code   ▶◀ Revised Text   ● New Code   ▲ Revised Code Title

✓x7ᵗʰ **V56.2 Person on outside** of pick-up truck or van injured in collision with other nonmotor vehicle **in nontraffic accident**

✓x7ᵗʰ **V56.3 Unspecified occupant** of pick-up truck or van injured in collision with other nonmotor vehicle **in nontraffic accident**

✓x7ᵗʰ **V56.4 Person boarding or alighting** a pick-up truck or van injured in collision with other nonmotor vehicle

✓x7ᵗʰ **V56.5 Driver of** pick-up truck or van injured in collision with other nonmotor vehicle **in traffic accident**

✓x7ᵗʰ **V56.6 Passenger in** pick-up truck or van injured in collision with other nonmotor vehicle **in traffic accident**

✓x7ᵗʰ **V56.7 Person on outside** of pick-up truck or van injured in collision with other nonmotor vehicle **in traffic accident**

✓x7ᵗʰ **V56.9 Unspecified occupant** of pick-up truck or van injured in collision with fixed or stationary object **in traffic accident**

✓4ᵗʰ **V57 Occupant of pick-up truck or van injured in collision with fixed or stationary object**

The appropriate 7th character is to be added to each code from category V57.
A   initial encounter
D   subsequent encounter
S   sequela

✓x7ᵗʰ **V57.0 Driver** of pick-up truck or van injured in collision with fixed or stationary object **in nontraffic accident**

✓x7ᵗʰ **V57.1 Passenger in** pick-up truck or van injured in collision with fixed or stationary object **in nontraffic accident**

✓x7ᵗʰ **V57.2 Person on outside** of pick-up truck or van injured in collision with fixed or stationary object **in nontraffic accident**

✓x7ᵗʰ **V57.3 Unspecified occupant** of pick-up truck or van injured in collision with other nonmotor vehicle **in nontraffic accident**

✓x7ᵗʰ **V57.4 Person boarding or alighting** a pick-up truck or van injured in collision with fixed or stationary object

✓x7ᵗʰ **V57.5 Driver of** pick-up truck or van injured in collision with fixed or stationary object **in traffic accident**

✓x7ᵗʰ **V57.6 Passenger in** pick-up truck or van injured in collision with fixed or stationary object **in traffic accident**

✓x7ᵗʰ **V57.7 Person on outside** of pick-up truck or van injured in collision with fixed or stationary object **in traffic accident**

✓x7ᵗʰ **V57.9 Unspecified occupant** of pick-up truck or van injured in collision with other nonmotor vehicle **in nontraffic accident**

✓4ᵗʰ **V58 Occupant of pick-up truck or van injured in noncollision transport accident**
   INCLUDES   overturning pick-up truck or van NOS
                overturning pick-up truck or van without collision

The appropriate 7th character is to be added to each code from category V58.
A   initial encounter
D   subsequent encounter
S   sequela

✓x7ᵗʰ **V58.0 Driver** of pick-up truck or van injured in noncollision transport accident **in nontraffic accident**

✓x7ᵗʰ **V58.1 Passenger in** pick-up truck or van injured in noncollision transport accident **in nontraffic accident**

✓x7ᵗʰ **V58.2 Person on outside** of pick-up truck or van injured in noncollision transport accident **in nontraffic accident**

✓x7ᵗʰ **V58.3 Unspecified occupant** of pick-up truck or van injured in collision with other nonmotor vehicle **in nontraffic accident**

✓x7ᵗʰ **V58.4 Person boarding or alighting** a pick-up truck or van injured in noncollision transport accident

✓x7ᵗʰ **V58.5 Driver** of pick-up truck or van injured in noncollision transport accident **in traffic accident**

✓x7ᵗʰ **V58.6 Passenger in** pick-up truck or van injured in noncollision transport accident **in traffic accident**

✓x7ᵗʰ **V58.7 Person on outside** of pick-up truck or van injured in noncollision transport accident **in traffic accident**

✓x7ᵗʰ **V58.9 Unspecified occupant** of pick-up truck or van injured in collision with other nonmotor vehicle **in nontraffic accident**

✓4ᵗʰ **V59 Occupant of pick-up truck or van injured in other and unspecified transport accidents**

The appropriate 7th character is to be added to each code from category V59.
A   initial encounter
D   subsequent encounter
S   sequela

✓5ᵗʰ **V59.0 Driver** of pick-up truck or van injured in collision with other and unspecified motor vehicles **in nontraffic accident**

     ✓x7ᵗʰ **V59.00 Driver of** pick-up truck or van injured in collision with unspecified motor vehicles in nontraffic accident

     ✓x7ᵗʰ **V59.09 Driver of** pick-up truck or van injured in collision with other motor vehicles in nontraffic accident

✓5ᵗʰ **V59.1 Passenger in** pick-up truck or van injured in collision with other and unspecified motor vehicles **in nontraffic accident**

     ✓x7ᵗʰ **V59.10 Passenger in** pick-up truck or van injured in collision with unspecified motor vehicles in nontraffic accident

     ✓x7ᵗʰ **V59.19 Passenger in** pick-up truck or van injured in collision with other motor vehicles in nontraffic accident

✓5ᵗʰ **V59.2 Unspecified occupant** of pick-up truck or van injured in collision with other and unspecified motor vehicles **in nontraffic accident**

     ✓x7ᵗʰ **V59.20 Unspecified occupant** of pick-up truck or van injured in collision with unspecified motor vehicles in nontraffic accident
         Collision NOS involving pick-up truck or van, nontraffic

     ✓x7ᵗʰ **V59.29 Unspecified occupant** of pick-up truck or van injured in collision with other motor vehicles in nontraffic accident

✓x7ᵗʰ **V59.3 Occupant (driver) (passenger)** of pick-up truck or van injured in unspecified nontraffic accident
         Accident NOS involving pick-up truck or van, nontraffic
         Occupant of pick-up truck or van injured in nontraffic accident NOS

✓5ᵗʰ **V59.4 Driver** of pick-up truck or van injured in collision with other and unspecified motor vehicles **in traffic accident**

     ✓x7ᵗʰ **V59.40 Driver of** pick-up truck or van injured in collision with unspecified motor vehicles in traffic accident

     ✓x7ᵗʰ **V59.49 Driver of** pick-up truck or van injured in collision with other motor vehicles in traffic accident

✓5ᵗʰ **V59.5 Passenger in** pick-up truck or van injured in collision with other and unspecified motor vehicles **in traffic accident**

     ✓x7ᵗʰ **V59.50 Passenger in** pick-up truck or van injured in collision with unspecified motor vehicles in traffic accident

     ✓x7ᵗʰ **V59.59 Passenger in** pick-up truck or van injured in collision with other motor vehicles in traffic accident

✓5ᵗʰ **V59.6 Unspecified occupant** of pick-up truck or van injured in collision with other and unspecified motor vehicles **in traffic accident**

     ✓x7ᵗʰ **V59.60 Unspecified occupant** of pick-up truck or van injured in collision with unspecified motor vehicles in traffic accident
         Collision NOS involving pick-up truck or van (traffic)

     ✓x7ᵗʰ **V59.69 Unspecified occupant** of pick-up truck or van injured in collision with other motor vehicles in traffic accident

✓5ᵗʰ **V59.8 Occupant (driver) (passenger)** of pick-up truck or van injured in other specified transport accidents

     ✓x7ᵗʰ **V59.81 Occupant (driver) (passenger)** of pick-up truck or van injured in transport accident with military vehicle

     ✓x7ᵗʰ **V59.88 Occupant (driver) (passenger)** of pick-up truck or van injured in other specified transport accidents

✓x7ᵗʰ **V59.9 Occupant (driver) (passenger)** of pick-up truck or van injured in unspecified traffic accident
         Accident NOS involving pick-up truck or van

EXCLUDES 1 Not coded here   EXCLUDES 2 Not included here   N Newborn Age: 0   P Pediatric Age: 0-17   M Maternity Age: 12-55   A Adult Age: 15-124

1008   ICD-10-CM 2014 (Draft)

Occupant of heavy transport vehicle injured in transport accident (V60-V69)

INCLUDES	18 wheeler
	armored car
	panel truck
EXCLUDES 1	bus
	motorcoach

☑4ᵗʰ **V60   Occupant of heavy transport vehicle injured in collision with pedestrian or animal**

> EXCLUDES 1   *heavy transport vehicle collision with animal-drawn vehicle or animal being ridden (V66.-)*

> The appropriate 7th character is to be added to each code from category V60.
> A   initial encounter
> D   subsequent encounter
> S   sequela

√x7ᵗʰ **V60.0   Driver** of heavy transport vehicle injured in collision with pedestrian or animal in nontraffic accident

√x7ᵗʰ **V60.1   Passenger** in heavy transport vehicle injured in collision with pedestrian or animal in nontraffic accident

√x7ᵗʰ **V60.2   Person on outside** of heavy transport vehicle injured in collision with pedestrian or animal in nontraffic accident

√x7ᵗʰ **V60.3   Unspecified occupant** of heavy transport vehicle injured in collision with pedestrian or animal in nontraffic accident

√x7ᵗʰ **V60.4   Person boarding or alighting** a heavy transport vehicle injured in collision with pedestrian or animal

√x7ᵗʰ **V60.5   Driver** of heavy transport vehicle injured in collision with pedestrian or animal in traffic accident

√x7ᵗʰ **V60.6   Passenger** in heavy transport vehicle injured in collision with pedestrian or animal in traffic accident

√x7ᵗʰ **V60.7   Person on outside** of heavy transport vehicle injured in collision with pedestrian or animal in traffic accident

√x7ᵗʰ **V60.9   Unspecified occupant** of heavy transport vehicle injured in collision with pedestrian or animal in traffic accident

☑4ᵗʰ **V61   Occupant of heavy transport vehicle injured in collision with pedal cycle**

> The appropriate 7th character is to be added to each code from category V61.
> A   initial encounter
> D   subsequent encounter
> S   sequela

√x7ᵗʰ **V61.0   Driver** of heavy transport vehicle injured in collision with pedal cycle in nontraffic accident

√x7ᵗʰ **V61.1   Passenger** in heavy transport vehicle injured in collision with pedal cycle in nontraffic accident

√x7ᵗʰ **V61.2   Person on outside** of heavy transport vehicle injured in collision with pedal cycle in nontraffic accident

√x7ᵗʰ **V61.3   Unspecified occupant** of heavy transport vehicle injured in collision with pedal cycle in nontraffic accident

√x7ᵗʰ **V61.4   Person boarding or alighting** a heavy transport vehicle injured in collision with pedal cycle while boarding or alighting

√x7ᵗʰ **V61.5   Driver** of heavy transport vehicle injured in collision with pedal cycle in traffic accident

√x7ᵗʰ **V61.6   Passenger** in heavy transport vehicle injured in collision with pedal cycle in traffic accident

√x7ᵗʰ **V61.7   Person on outside** of heavy transport vehicle injured in collision with pedal cycle in traffic accident

√x7ᵗʰ **V61.9   Unspecified occupant** of heavy transport vehicle injured in collision with pedal cycle in traffic accident

☑4ᵗʰ **V62   Occupant of heavy transport vehicle injured in collision with two- or three-wheeled motor vehicle**

> The appropriate 7th character is to be added to each code from category V62.
> A   initial encounter
> D   subsequent encounter
> S   sequela

√x7ᵗʰ **V62.0   Driver** of heavy transport vehicle injured in collision with two- or three-wheeled motor vehicle in nontraffic accident

√x7ᵗʰ **V62.1   Passenger** in heavy transport vehicle injured in collision with two- or three-wheeled motor vehicle in nontraffic accident

√x7ᵗʰ **V62.2   Person on outside** of heavy transport vehicle injured in collision with two- or three-wheeled motor vehicle in nontraffic accident

√x7ᵗʰ **V62.3   Unspecified occupant** of heavy transport vehicle injured in collision with two- or three-wheeled motor vehicle in nontraffic accident

√x7ᵗʰ **V62.4   Person boarding or alighting** a heavy transport vehicle injured in collision with two- or three-wheeled motor vehicle

√x7ᵗʰ **V62.5   Driver** of heavy transport vehicle injured in collision with two- or three-wheeled motor vehicle in traffic accident

√x7ᵗʰ **V62.6   Passenger** in heavy transport vehicle injured in collision with two- or three-wheeled motor vehicle in traffic accident

√x7ᵗʰ **V62.7   Person on outside** of heavy transport vehicle injured in collision with two- or three-wheeled motor vehicle in traffic accident

√x7ᵗʰ **V62.9   Unspecified occupant** of heavy transport vehicle injured in collision with two- or three-wheeled motor vehicle in traffic accident

☑4ᵗʰ **V63   Occupant of heavy transport vehicle injured in collision with car, pick-up truck or van**

> The appropriate 7th character is to be added to each code from category V63.
> A   initial encounter
> D   subsequent encounter
> S   sequela

√x7ᵗʰ **V63.0   Driver** of heavy transport vehicle injured in collision with car, pick-up truck or van in nontraffic accident

√x7ᵗʰ **V63.1   Passenger** in heavy transport vehicle injured in collision with car, pick-up truck or van in nontraffic accident

√x7ᵗʰ **V63.2   Person on outside** of heavy transport vehicle injured in collision with car, pick-up truck or van in nontraffic accident

√x7ᵗʰ **V63.3   Unspecified occupant** of heavy transport vehicle injured in collision with car, pick-up truck or van in nontraffic accident

√x7ᵗʰ **V63.4   Person boarding or alighting** a heavy transport vehicle injured in collision with car, pick-up truck or van

√x7ᵗʰ **V63.5   Driver** of heavy transport vehicle injured in collision with car, pick-up truck or van in traffic accident

√x7ᵗʰ **V63.6   Passenger** in heavy transport vehicle injured in collision with car, pick-up truck or van in traffic accident

√x7ᵗʰ **V63.7   Person on outside** of heavy transport vehicle injured in collision with car, pick-up truck or van in traffic accident

√x7ᵗʰ **V63.9   Unspecified occupant** of heavy transport vehicle injured in collision with car, pick-up truck or van in traffic accident

☑4ᵗʰ **V64   Occupant of heavy transport vehicle injured in collision with heavy transport vehicle or bus**

> EXCLUDES 1   *occupant of heavy transport vehicle injured in collision with military vehicle (V69.81)*

> The appropriate 7th character is to be added to each code from category V64.
> A   initial encounter
> D   subsequent encounter
> S   sequela

√x7ᵗʰ **V64.0   Driver** of heavy transport vehicle injured in collision with heavy transport vehicle or bus in nontraffic accident

√x7ᵗʰ **V64.1   Passenger** in heavy transport vehicle injured in collision with heavy transport vehicle or bus in nontraffic accident

√x7ᵗʰ **V64.2   Person on outside** of heavy transport vehicle injured in collision with heavy transport vehicle or bus in nontraffic accident

√x7ᵗʰ **V64.3   Unspecified occupant** of heavy transport vehicle injured in collision with heavy transport vehicle or bus in nontraffic accident

√x7ᵗʰ **V64.4   Person boarding or alighting** a heavy transport vehicle injured in collision with heavy transport vehicle or bus while boarding or alighting

√x7ᵗʰ **V64.5   Driver** of heavy transport vehicle injured in collision with heavy transport vehicle or bus in traffic accident

√x7ᵗʰ **V64.6   Passenger** in heavy transport vehicle injured in collision with heavy transport vehicle or bus in traffic accident

√x7ᵗʰ **V64.7   Person on outside** of heavy transport vehicle injured in collision with heavy transport vehicle or bus in traffic accident

√x7ᵗʰ **V64.9   Unspecified occupant** of heavy transport vehicle injured in collision with heavy transport vehicle or bus in traffic accident

---

☑ Additional Character Required   √x7ᵗʰ Xtension Alert   Unspecified Code   Other Specified Code   Manifestation Code   ▶◀ Revised Text   ● New Code   ▲ Revised Code Title

External Causes of Morbidity

V65–V69.3

√4th **V65 Occupant of heavy transport vehicle injured in collision with railway train or railway vehicle**

> The appropriate 7th character is to be added to each code from category V65.
> A   initial encounter
> D   subsequent encounter
> S   sequela

√x7th **V65.0 Driver** of heavy transport vehicle injured in collision with railway train or railway vehicle **in nontraffic accident**

√x7th **V65.1 Passenger** in heavy transport vehicle injured in collision with railway train or railway vehicle **in nontraffic accident**

√x7th **V65.2 Person on outside** of heavy transport vehicle injured in collision with railway train or railway vehicle **in nontraffic accident**

√x7th **V65.3 Unspecified occupant** of heavy transport vehicle injured in collision with railway train or railway vehicle **in nontraffic accident**

√x7th **V65.4 Person boarding or alighting** a heavy transport vehicle injured in collision with railway train or railway vehicle

√x7th **V65.5 Driver** of heavy transport vehicle injured in collision with railway train or railway vehicle **in traffic accident**

√x7th **V65.6 Passenger** in heavy transport vehicle injured in collision with railway train or railway vehicle **in traffic accident**

√x7th **V65.7 Person on outside** of heavy transport vehicle injured in collision with railway train or railway vehicle **in traffic accident**

√x7th **V65.9 Unspecified occupant** of heavy transport vehicle injured in collision with railway train or railway vehicle **in traffic accident**

√4th **V66 Occupant of heavy transport vehicle injured in collision with other nonmotor vehicle**

> **INCLUDES** collision with animal-drawn vehicle, animal being ridden, streetcar

> The appropriate 7th character is to be added to each code from category V66.
> A   initial encounter
> D   subsequent encounter
> S   sequela

√x7th **V66.0 Driver** of heavy transport vehicle injured in collision with other nonmotor vehicle **in nontraffic accident**

√x7th **V66.1 Passenger** in heavy transport vehicle injured in collision with other nonmotor vehicle **in nontraffic accident**

√x7th **V66.2 Person on outside** of heavy transport vehicle injured in collision with other nonmotor vehicle **in nontraffic accident**

√x7th **V66.3 Unspecified occupant** of heavy transport vehicle injured in collision with other nonmotor vehicle **in nontraffic accident**

√x7th **V66.4 Person boarding or alighting** a heavy transport vehicle injured in collision with other nonmotor vehicle

√x7th **V66.5 Driver** of heavy transport vehicle injured in collision with other nonmotor vehicle **in traffic accident**

√x7th **V66.6 Passenger** in heavy transport vehicle injured in collision with other nonmotor vehicle **in traffic accident**

√x7th **V66.7 Person on outside** of heavy transport vehicle injured in collision with other nonmotor vehicle **in traffic accident**

√x7th **V66.9 Unspecified occupant** of heavy transport vehicle injured in collision with other nonmotor vehicle **in traffic accident**

√4th **V67 Occupant of heavy transport vehicle injured in collision with fixed or stationary object**

> The appropriate 7th character is to be added to each code from category V67.
> A   initial encounter
> D   subsequent encounter
> S   sequela

√x7th **V67.0 Driver** of heavy transport vehicle injured in collision with fixed or stationary object **in nontraffic accident**

√x7th **V67.1 Passenger** in heavy transport vehicle injured in collision with fixed or stationary object **in nontraffic accident**

√x7th **V67.2 Person on outside** of heavy transport vehicle injured in collision with fixed or stationary object **in nontraffic accident**

√x7th **V67.3 Unspecified occupant** of heavy transport vehicle injured in collision with fixed or stationary object **in nontraffic accident**

√x7th **V67.4 Person boarding or alighting** a heavy transport vehicle injured in collision with fixed or stationary object

√x7th **V67.5 Driver** of heavy transport vehicle injured in collision with fixed or stationary object **in traffic accident**

√x7th **V67.6 Passenger** in heavy transport vehicle injured in collision with fixed or stationary object **in traffic accident**

√x7th **V67.7 Person on outside** of heavy transport vehicle injured in collision with fixed or stationary object **in traffic accident**

√x7th **V67.9 Unspecified occupant** of heavy transport vehicle injured in collision with fixed or stationary object **in traffic accident**

√4th **V68 Occupant of heavy transport vehicle injured in noncollision transport accident**

> **INCLUDES** overturning heavy transport vehicle NOS
> overturning heavy transport vehicle without collision

> The appropriate 7th character is to be added to each code from category V68.
> A   initial encounter
> D   subsequent encounter
> S   sequela

√x7th **V68.0 Driver** of heavy transport vehicle injured in noncollision transport accident **in nontraffic accident**

√x7th **V68.1 Passenger** in heavy transport vehicle injured in noncollision transport accident **in nontraffic accident**

√x7th **V68.2 Person on outside** of heavy transport vehicle injured in noncollision transport accident **in nontraffic accident**

√x7th **V68.3 Unspecified occupant** of heavy transport vehicle injured in noncollision transport accident **in nontraffic accident**

√x7th **V68.4 Person boarding or alighting** a heavy transport vehicle injured in noncollision transport accident

√x7th **V68.5 Driver** of heavy transport vehicle injured in noncollision transport accident **in traffic accident**

√x7th **V68.6 Passenger** in heavy transport vehicle injured in noncollision transport accident **in traffic accident**

√x7th **V68.7 Person on outside** of heavy transport vehicle injured in noncollision transport accident **in traffic accident**

√x7th **V68.9 Unspecified occupant** of heavy transport vehicle injured in noncollision transport accident **in traffic accident**

√4th **V69 Occupant of heavy transport vehicle injured in other and unspecified transport accidents**

> The appropriate 7th character is to be added to each code from category V69.
> A   initial encounter
> D   subsequent encounter
> S   sequela

√5th **V69.0 Driver** of heavy transport vehicle injured in collision with other and unspecified motor vehicles **in nontraffic accident**

√x7th **V69.00 Driver** of heavy transport vehicle injured in collision with unspecified **motor vehicles in nontraffic accident**

√x7th **V69.09 Driver** of heavy transport vehicle injured in collision with other **motor vehicles in nontraffic accident**

√5th **V69.1 Passenger** in heavy transport vehicle injured in collision with other and unspecified motor vehicles **in nontraffic accident**

√x7th **V69.10 Passenger** in heavy transport vehicle injured in collision with unspecified **motor vehicles** in nontraffic accident

√x7th **V69.19 Passenger** in heavy transport vehicle injured in collision with other **motor vehicles** in nontraffic accident

√5th **V69.2 Unspecified** occupant of heavy transport vehicle injured in collision with other and unspecified motor vehicles **in nontraffic accident**

√x7th **V69.20 Unspecified occupant** of heavy transport vehicle injured in collision with unspecified **motor vehicles in nontraffic accident**

> Collision NOS involving heavy transport vehicle, nontraffic

√x7th **V69.29 Unspecified occupant** of heavy transport vehicle injured in collision with other **motor vehicles in nontraffic accident**

√x7th **V69.3 Occupant (driver) (passenger)** of heavy transport vehicle injured in unspecified **nontraffic accident**

> Accident NOS involving heavy transport vehicle, nontraffic
> Occupant of heavy transport vehicle injured in nontraffic accident NOS

EXCLUDES 1 Not coded here   **EXCLUDES 2** Not included here   N Newborn Age: 0   P Pediatric Age: 0-17   M Maternity Age: 12-55   A Adult Age: 15-124

1010   ICD-10-CM 2014 (Draft)

✓5th **V69.4** Driver of heavy transport vehicle injured in collision with other and unspecified motor vehicles in traffic accident

✓x7th **V69.40** Driver of heavy transport vehicle injured in collision with unspecified motor vehicles in traffic accident

✓x7th **V69.49** Driver of heavy transport vehicle injured in collision with other motor vehicles in traffic accident

✓5th **V69.5** Passenger in heavy transport vehicle injured in collision with other and unspecified motor vehicles in traffic accident

✓x7th **V69.50** Passenger in heavy transport vehicle injured in collision with unspecified motor vehicles in traffic accident

✓x7th **V69.59** Passenger in heavy transport vehicle injured in collision with other motor vehicles in traffic accident

✓5th **V69.6** Unspecified occupant of heavy transport vehicle injured in collision with other and unspecified motor vehicles in traffic accident

✓x7th **V69.60** Unspecified occupant of heavy transport vehicle injured in collision with unspecified motor vehicles in traffic accident
Collision NOS involving heavy transport vehicle (traffic)

✓x7th **V69.69** Unspecified occupant of heavy transport vehicle injured in collision with other motor vehicles in traffic accident

✓5th **V69.8** Occupant (driver) (passenger) of heavy transport vehicle injured in other specified transport accidents

✓x7th **V69.81** Occupant (driver) (passenger) of heavy transport vehicle injured in transport accidents with military vehicle

✓x7th **V69.88** Occupant (driver) (passenger) of heavy transport vehicle injured in other specified transport accidents

✓x7th **V69.9** Occupant (driver) (passenger) of heavy transport vehicle injured in unspecified traffic accident
Accident NOS involving heavy transport vehicle

Bus occupant injured in transport accident (V70-V79)

INCLUDES motorcoach

EXCLUDES 1 minibus (V50-V59)

✓4th **V70** Bus occupant injured in collision with pedestrian or animal

The appropriate 7th character is to be added to each code from category V70.
A   initial encounter
D   subsequent encounter
S   sequela

EXCLUDES 1 bus collision with animal-drawn vehicle or animal being ridden (V76.-)

✓x7th **V70.0** Driver of bus injured in collision with pedestrian or animal in nontraffic accident

✓x7th **V70.1** Passenger on bus injured in collision with pedestrian or animal in nontraffic accident

✓x7th **V70.2** Person on outside of bus injured in collision with pedestrian or animal in nontraffic accident

✓x7th **V70.3** Unspecified occupant of bus injured in collision with pedestrian or animal in nontraffic accident

✓x7th **V70.4** Person boarding or alighting from bus injured in collision with pedestrian or animal

✓x7th **V70.5** Driver of bus injured in collision with pedestrian or animal in traffic accident

✓x7th **V70.6** Passenger on bus injured in collision with pedestrian or animal in traffic accident

✓x7th **V70.7** Person on outside of bus injured in collision with pedestrian or animal in traffic accident

✓x7th **V70.9** Unspecified occupant of bus injured in collision with pedestrian or animal in traffic accident

✓4th **V71** Bus occupant injured in collision with pedal cycle

The appropriate 7th character is to be added to each code from category V71.
A   initial encounter
D   subsequent encounter
S   sequela

✓x7th **V71.0** Driver of bus injured in collision with pedal cycle in nontraffic accident

✓x7th **V71.1** Passenger on bus injured in collision with pedal cycle in nontraffic accident

✓x7th **V71.2** Person on outside of bus injured in collision with pedal cycle in nontraffic accident

✓x7th **V71.3** Unspecified occupant of bus injured in collision with pedal cycle in nontraffic accident

✓x7th **V71.4** Person boarding or alighting from bus injured in collision with pedal cycle

✓x7th **V71.5** Driver of bus injured in collision with pedal cycle in traffic accident

✓x7th **V71.6** Passenger on bus injured in collision with pedal cycle in traffic accident

✓x7th **V71.7** Person on outside of bus injured in collision with pedal cycle in traffic accident

✓x7th **V71.9** Unspecified occupant of bus injured in collision with pedal cycle in traffic accident

✓4th **V72** Bus occupant injured in collision with two- or three-wheeled motor vehicle

The appropriate 7th character is to be added to each code from category V72.
A   initial encounter
D   subsequent encounter
S   sequela

✓x7th **V72.0** Driver of bus injured in collision with two- or three-wheeled motor vehicle in nontraffic accident

✓x7th **V72.1** Passenger on bus injured in collision with two- or three-wheeled motor vehicle in nontraffic accident

✓x7th **V72.2** Person on outside of bus injured in collision with two- or three-wheeled motor vehicle in nontraffic accident

✓x7th **V72.3** Unspecified occupant of bus injured in collision with two- or three-wheeled motor vehicle in nontraffic accident

✓x7th **V72.4** Person boarding or alighting from bus injured in collision with two- or three-wheeled motor vehicle

✓x7th **V72.5** Driver of bus injured in collision with two- or three-wheeled motor vehicle in traffic accident

✓x7th **V72.6** Passenger on bus injured in collision with two- or three-wheeled motor vehicle in traffic accident

✓x7th **V72.7** Person on outside of bus injured in collision with two- or three-wheeled motor vehicle in traffic accident

✓x7th **V72.9** Unspecified occupant of bus injured in collision with two- or three-wheeled motor vehicle in traffic accident

✓4th **V73** Bus occupant injured in collision with car, pick-up truck or van

The appropriate 7th character is to be added to each code from category V73.
A   initial encounter
D   subsequent encounter
S   sequela

✓x7th **V73.0** Driver of bus injured in collision with car, pick-up truck or van in nontraffic accident

✓x7th **V73.1** Passenger on bus injured in collision with car, pick-up truck or van in nontraffic accident

✓x7th **V73.2** Person on outside of bus injured in collision with car, pick-up truck or van in nontraffic accident

✓x7th **V73.3** Unspecified occupant of bus injured in collision with car, pick-up truck or van in nontraffic accident

✓x7th **V73.4** Person boarding or alighting from bus injured in collision with car, pick-up truck or van

✓x7th **V73.5** Driver of bus injured in collision with car, pick-up truck or van in traffic accident

✓x7th **V73.6** Passenger on bus injured in collision with car, pick-up truck or van in traffic accident

✓x7th **V73.7** Person on outside of bus injured in collision with car, pick-up truck or van in traffic accident

✓x7th **V73.9** Unspecified occupant of bus injured in collision with car, pick-up truck or van in traffic accident

✓4th **V74** Bus occupant injured in collision with heavy transport vehicle or bus

EXCLUDES 1 bus occupant injured in collision with military vehicle (V79.81)

The appropriate 7th character is to be added to each code from category V74.
A   initial encounter
D   subsequent encounter
S   sequela

✓x7th **V74.0** Driver of bus injured in collision with heavy transport vehicle or bus in nontraffic accident

---

☑ Additional Character Required   ✓x7th Xtension Alert   Unspecified Code   Other Specified Code   Manifestation Code   ▶◀ Revised Text   ● New Code   ▲ Revised Code Title

ICD-10-CM 2014 (Draft)   1011

External Causes of Morbidity

V74.1–V79.19

√x7th **V74.1** Passenger on bus injured in collision with heavy transport vehicle or bus in nontraffic accident

√x7th **V74.2** Person on outside of bus injured in collision with heavy transport vehicle or bus in nontraffic accident

√x7th **V74.3** Unspecified occupant of bus injured in collision with heavy transport vehicle or bus in nontraffic accident

√x7th **V74.4** Person boarding or alighting from bus injured in collision with heavy transport vehicle or bus

√x7th **V74.5** Driver of bus injured in collision with heavy transport vehicle or bus in traffic accident

√x7th **V74.6** Passenger on bus injured in collision with heavy transport vehicle or bus in traffic accident

√x7th **V74.7** Person on outside of bus injured in collision with heavy transport vehicle or bus in traffic accident

√x7th **V74.9** Unspecified occupant of bus injured in collision with heavy transport vehicle or bus in traffic accident

√4th **V75 Bus occupant injured in collision with railway train or railway vehicle**

The appropriate 7th character is to be added to each code from category V75.
A   initial encounter
D   subsequent encounter
S   sequela

√x7th **V75.0** Driver of bus injured in collision with railway train or railway vehicle in nontraffic accident

√x7th **V75.1** Passenger on bus injured in collision with railway train or railway vehicle in nontraffic accident

√x7th **V75.2** Person on outside of bus injured in collision with railway train or railway vehicle in nontraffic accident

√x7th **V75.3** Unspecified occupant of bus injured in collision with railway train or railway vehicle in nontraffic accident

√x7th **V75.4** Person boarding or alighting from bus injured in collision with railway train or railway vehicle

√x7th **V75.5** Driver of bus injured in collision with railway train or railway vehicle in traffic accident

√x7th **V75.6** Passenger on bus injured in collision with railway train or railway vehicle in traffic accident

√x7th **V75.7** Person on outside of bus injured in collision with railway train or railway vehicle in traffic accident

√x7th **V75.9** Unspecified occupant of bus injured in collision with railway train or railway vehicle in traffic accident

√4th **V76 Bus occupant injured in collision with other nonmotor vehicle**
INCLUDES   collision with animal-drawn vehicle, animal being ridden, streetcar

The appropriate 7th character is to be added to each code from category V76.
A   initial encounter
D   subsequent encounter
S   sequela

√x7th **V76.0** Driver of bus injured in collision with other nonmotor vehicle in nontraffic accident

√x7th **V76.1** Passenger on bus injured in collision with other nonmotor vehicle in nontraffic accident

√x7th **V76.2** Person on outside of bus injured in collision with other nonmotor vehicle in nontraffic accident

√x7th **V76.3** Unspecified occupant of bus injured in collision with other nonmotor vehicle in nontraffic accident

√x7th **V76.4** Person boarding or alighting from bus injured in collision with other nonmotor vehicle

√x7th **V76.5** Driver of bus injured in collision with other nonmotor vehicle in traffic accident

√x7th **V76.6** Passenger on bus injured in collision with other nonmotor vehicle in traffic accident

√x7th **V76.7** Person on outside of bus injured in collision with other nonmotor vehicle in traffic accident

√x7th **V76.9** Unspecified occupant of bus injured in collision with other nonmotor vehicle in traffic accident

√4th **V77 Bus occupant injured in collision with fixed or stationary object**

The appropriate 7th character is to be added to each code from category V77.
A   initial encounter
D   subsequent encounter
S   sequela

√x7th **V77.0** Driver of bus injured in collision with fixed or stationary object in nontraffic accident

√x7th **V77.1** Passenger on bus injured in collision with fixed or stationary object in nontraffic accident

√x7th **V77.2** Person on outside of bus injured in collision with fixed or stationary object in nontraffic accident

√x7th **V77.3** Unspecified occupant of bus injured in collision with fixed or stationary object in nontraffic accident

√x7th **V77.4** Person boarding or alighting from bus injured in collision with fixed or stationary object

√x7th **V77.5** Driver of bus injured in collision with fixed or stationary object in traffic accident

√x7th **V77.6** Passenger on bus injured in collision with fixed or stationary object in traffic accident

√x7th **V77.7** Person on outside of bus injured in collision with fixed or stationary object in traffic accident

√x7th **V77.9** Unspecified occupant of bus injured in collision with fixed or stationary object in traffic accident

√4th **V78 Bus occupant injured in noncollision transport accident**
INCLUDES   overturning bus NOS
      overturning bus without collision

The appropriate 7th character is to be added to each code from category V78.
A   initial encounter
D   subsequent encounter
S   sequela

√x7th **V78.0** Driver of bus injured in noncollision transport accident in nontraffic accident

√x7th **V78.1** Passenger on bus injured in noncollision transport accident in nontraffic accident

√x7th **V78.2** Person on outside of bus injured in noncollision transport accident in nontraffic accident

√x7th **V78.3** Unspecified occupant of bus injured in noncollision transport accident in nontraffic accident

√x7th **V78.4** Person boarding or alighting from bus injured in noncollision transport accident

√x7th **V78.5** Driver of bus injured in noncollision transport accident in traffic accident

√x7th **V78.6** Passenger on bus injured in noncollision transport accident in traffic accident

√x7th **V78.7** Person on outside of bus injured in noncollision transport accident in traffic accident

√x7th **V78.9** Unspecified occupant of bus injured in noncollision transport accident in traffic accident

√4th **V79 Bus occupant injured in other and unspecified transport accidents**

The appropriate 7th character is to be added to each code from category V79.
A   initial encounter
D   subsequent encounter
S   sequela

√5th **V79.0** Driver of bus injured in collision with other and unspecified motor vehicles in nontraffic accident

√x7th **V79.00** Driver of bus injured in collision with unspecified motor vehicles in nontraffic accident

√x7th **V79.09** Driver of bus injured in collision with other motor vehicles in nontraffic accident

√5th **V79.1** Passenger on bus injured in collision with other and unspecified motor vehicles in nontraffic accident

√x7th **V79.10** Passenger on bus injured in collision with unspecified motor vehicles in nontraffic accident

√x7th **V79.19** Passenger on bus injured in collision with other motor vehicles in nontraffic accident

EXCLUDES 1 Not coded here   EXCLUDES 2 Not included here   N Newborn Age: 0   P Pediatric Age: 0-17   M Maternity Age: 12-55   A Adult Age: 15-124

1012   ICD-10-CM 2014 (Draft)

☑5th V79.2 Unspecified **bus** occupant injured in collision with other and unspecified motor vehicles in nontraffic accident

　　✓x7th V79.20 Unspecified bus occupant injured in collision with unspecified motor vehicles in nontraffic accident
　　　　Bus collision NOS, nontraffic

　　✓x7th V79.29 Unspecified bus occupant injured in collision with other motor vehicles in nontraffic accident

✓x7th V79.3 Bus occupant (driver) (passenger) injured in unspecified nontraffic accident
　　Bus accident NOS, nontraffic
　　Bus occupant injured in nontraffic accident NOS

☑5th V79.4 Driver of bus injured in collision with other and unspecified motor vehicles in traffic accident

　　✓x7th V79.40 Driver of bus injured in collision with unspecified motor vehicles in traffic accident

　　✓x7th V79.49 Driver of bus injured in collision with other motor vehicles in traffic accident

☑5th V79.5 Passenger on bus injured in collision with other and unspecified motor vehicles in traffic accident

　　✓x7th V79.50 Passenger on bus injured in collision with unspecified motor vehicles in traffic accident

　　✓x7th V79.59 Passenger on bus injured in collision with other motor vehicles in traffic accident

☑5th V79.6 Unspecified **bus** occupant injured in collision with other and unspecified motor vehicles in traffic accident

　　✓x7th V79.60 Unspecified bus occupant injured in collision with unspecified motor vehicles in traffic accident
　　　　Bus collision NOS (traffic)

　　✓x7th V79.69 Unspecified bus occupant injured in collision with other motor vehicles in traffic accident

☑5th V79.8 Bus occupant (driver) (passenger) injured in other specified transport accidents

　　✓x7th V79.81 Bus occupant (driver) (passenger) injured in transport accidents with military vehicle

　　✓x7th V79.88 Bus occupant (driver) (passenger) injured in other specified transport accidents

✓x7th V79.9 Bus occupant (driver) (passenger) injured in unspecified traffic accident
　　Bus accident NOS

Other land transport accidents (V80-V89)

☑4th V80 Animal-rider or occupant of animal-drawn vehicle injured in transport accident

　　The appropriate 7th character is to be added to each code from category V80.
　　A　initial encounter
　　D　subsequent encounter
　　S　sequela

☑5th V80.0 Animal-rider or occupant of animal drawn vehicle injured by fall from or being thrown from animal or animal-drawn vehicle in noncollision accident

　　☑6th V80.01 Animal-rider injured by fall from or being thrown from animal in noncollision accident

　　　　✓7th V80.010 Animal-rider injured by fall from or being thrown from horse in noncollision accident

　　　　✓7th V80.018 Animal-rider injured by fall from or being thrown from other animal in noncollision accident

　　✓x7th V80.02 Occupant of animal-drawn vehicle injured by fall from or being thrown from animal-drawn vehicle in noncollision accident
　　　　Overturning animal-drawn vehicle NOS
　　　　Overturning animal-drawn vehicle without collision

☑5th V80.1 Animal-rider or occupant of animal-drawn vehicle injured in collision with pedestrian or animal

　　EXCLUDES 1 *animal-rider or animal-drawn vehicle collision with animal-drawn vehicle or animal being ridden (V80.7)*

　　✓x7th V80.11 Animal-rider injured in collision with pedestrian or animal

　　✓x7th V80.12 Occupant of animal-drawn vehicle injured in collision with pedestrian or animal

☑5th V80.2 Animal-rider or occupant of animal-drawn vehicle injured in collision with pedal cycle

　　✓x7th V80.21 Animal-rider injured in collision with pedal cycle

　　✓x7th V80.22 Occupant of animal-drawn vehicle injured in collision with pedal cycle

☑5th V80.3 Animal-rider or occupant of animal-drawn vehicle injured in collision with two- or three-wheeled motor vehicle

　　✓x7th V80.31 Animal-rider injured in collision with two- or three-wheeled motor vehicle

　　✓x7th V80.32 Occupant of animal-drawn vehicle injured in collision with two- or three-wheeled motor vehicle

☑5th V80.4 Animal-rider or occupant of animal-drawn vehicle injured in collision with car, pick-up truck, van, heavy transport vehicle or bus

　　EXCLUDES 1 *animal-rider injured in collision with military vehicle (V80.910)*
　　　　occupant of animal-drawn vehicle injured in collision with military vehicle (V80.920)

　　✓x7th V80.41 Animal-rider injured in collision with car, pick-up truck, van, heavy transport vehicle or bus

　　✓x7th V80.42 Occupant of animal-drawn vehicle injured in collision with car, pick-up truck, van, heavy transport vehicle or bus

☑5th V80.5 Animal-rider or occupant of animal-drawn vehicle injured in collision with other specified motor vehicle

　　✓x7th V80.51 Animal-rider injured in collision with other specified motor vehicle

　　✓x7th V80.52 Occupant of animal-drawn vehicle injured in collision with other specified motor vehicle

☑5th V80.6 Animal-rider or occupant of animal-drawn vehicle injured in collision with railway train or railway vehicle

　　✓x7th V80.61 Animal-rider injured in collision with railway train or railway vehicle

　　✓x7th V80.62 Occupant of animal-drawn vehicle injured in collision with railway train or railway vehicle

☑5th V80.7 Animal-rider or occupant of animal-drawn vehicle injured in collision with other nonmotor vehicles

　　☑6th V80.71 Animal-rider or occupant of animal-drawn vehicle injured in collision with animal being ridden

　　　　✓7th V80.710 Animal-rider injured in collision with other animal being ridden

　　　　✓7th V80.711 Occupant of animal-drawn vehicle injured in collision with animal being ridden

　　☑6th V80.72 Animal-rider or occupant of animal-drawn vehicle injured in collision with other animal-drawn vehicle

　　　　✓7th V80.720 Animal-rider injured in collision with animal-drawn vehicle

　　　　✓7th V80.721 Occupant of animal-drawn vehicle injured in collision with other animal-drawn vehicle

　　☑6th V80.73 Animal-rider or occupant of animal-drawn vehicle injured in collision with streetcar

　　　　✓7th V80.730 Animal-rider injured in collision with streetcar

　　　　✓7th V80.731 Occupant of animal-drawn vehicle injured in collision with streetcar

　　☑6th V80.79 Animal-rider or occupant of animal-drawn vehicle injured in collision with other nonmotor vehicles

　　　　✓7th V80.790 Animal-rider injured in collision with other nonmotor vehicles

　　　　✓7th V80.791 Occupant of animal-drawn vehicle injured in collision with other nonmotor vehicles

☑5th V80.8 Animal-rider or occupant of animal-drawn vehicle injured in collision with fixed or stationary object

　　✓x7th V80.81 Animal-rider injured in collision with fixed or stationary object

　　✓x7th V80.82 Occupant of animal-drawn vehicle injured in collision with fixed or stationary object

☑5th V80.9 Animal-rider or occupant of animal-drawn vehicle injured in other and unspecified transport accidents

　　☑6th V80.91 Animal-rider injured in other and unspecified transport accidents

　　　　✓7th V80.910 Animal-rider injured in transport accident with military vehicle

☑ Additional Character Required　✓x7th Xtension Alert　Unspecified Code　Other Specified Code　Manifestation Code　►◄ Revised Text　● New Code　▲ Revised Code Title

ICD-10-CM 2014 (Draft)

1013

External Causes of Morbidity

V80.918–V83.7

√7th **V80.918 Animal-rider injured in other transport accident**

√7th **V80.919 Animal-rider injured in unspecified transport accident**
Animal rider accident NOS

√6th **V80.92 Occupant of animal-drawn vehicle injured in other and unspecified transport accidents**

√7th **V80.920 Occupant of animal-drawn vehicle injured in transport accident with military vehicle**

√7th **V80.928 Occupant of animal-drawn vehicle injured in other transport accident**

√7th **V80.929 Occupant of animal-drawn vehicle injured in unspecified transport accident**
Animal-drawn vehicle accident NOS

√4th **V81 Occupant of railway train or railway vehicle injured in transport accident**
INCLUDES derailment of railway train or railway vehicle
person on outside of train
EXCLUDES 1 *streetcar (V82.-)*

The appropriate 7th character is to be added to each code from category V81.
A   initial encounter
D   subsequent encounter
S   sequela

√x7th **V81.0 Occupant of railway train or railway vehicle injured in collision with motor vehicle in nontraffic accident**
EXCLUDES 1 *occupant of railway train or railway vehicle injured due to collision with military vehicle (V81.83)*

√x7th **V81.1 Occupant of railway train or railway vehicle injured in collision with motor vehicle in traffic accident**
EXCLUDES 1 *occupant of railway train or railway vehicle injured due to collision with military vehicle (V81.83)*

√x7th **V81.2 Occupant of railway train or railway vehicle injured in collision with or hit by rolling stock**

√x7th **V81.3 Occupant of railway train or railway vehicle injured in collision with other object**
Railway collision NOS

√x7th **V81.4 Person injured while boarding or alighting from railway train or railway vehicle**

√x7th **V81.5 Occupant of railway train or railway vehicle injured by fall in railway train or railway vehicle**

√x7th **V81.6 Occupant of railway train or railway vehicle injured by fall from railway train or railway vehicle**

√x7th **V81.7 Occupant of railway train or railway vehicle injured in derailment without antecedent collision**

√5th **V81.8 Occupant of railway train or railway vehicle injured in other specified railway accidents**

√x7th **V81.81 Occupant of railway train or railway vehicle injured due to explosion or fire on train**

√x7th **V81.82 Occupant of railway train or railway vehicle injured due to object falling onto train**
Occupant of railway train or railway vehicle injured due to falling earth onto train
Occupant of railway train or railway vehicle injured due to falling rocks onto train
Occupant of railway train or railway vehicle injured due to falling snow onto train
Occupant of railway train or railway vehicle injured due to falling trees onto train

√x7th **V81.83 Occupant of railway train or railway vehicle injured due to collision with military vehicle**

√x7th **V81.89 Occupant of railway train or railway vehicle injured due to other specified railway accident**

√x7th **V81.9 Occupant of railway train or railway vehicle injured in unspecified railway accident**
Railway accident NOS

√4th **V82 Occupant of powered streetcar injured in transport accident**
INCLUDES interurban electric car
person on outside of streetcar
tram (car)
trolley (car)
EXCLUDES 1 *bus (V70-V79)*
motorcoach (V70-V79)
nonpowered streetcar (V76.-)
train (V81.-)

The appropriate 7th character is to be added to each code from category V82.
A   initial encounter
D   subsequent encounter
S   sequela

√x7th **V82.0 Occupant of streetcar injured in collision with motor vehicle in nontraffic accident**

√x7th **V82.1 Occupant of streetcar injured in collision with motor vehicle in traffic accident**

√x7th **V82.2 Occupant of streetcar injured in collision with or hit by rolling stock**

√x7th **V82.3 Occupant of streetcar injured in collision with other object**
EXCLUDES 1 *collision with animal-drawn vehicle or animal being ridden (V82.8)*

√x7th **V82.4 Person injured while boarding or alighting from streetcar**

√x7th **V82.5 Occupant of streetcar injured by fall in streetcar**
EXCLUDES 1 *fall in streetcar:*
while boarding or alighting (V82.4)
with antecedent collision (V82.0-V82.3)

√x7th **V82.6 Occupant of streetcar injured by fall from streetcar**
EXCLUDES 1 *fall from streetcar:*
while boarding or alighting (V82.4)
with antecedent collision (V82.0-V82.3)

√x7th **V82.7 Occupant of streetcar injured in derailment without antecedent collision**
EXCLUDES 1 *occupant of streetcar injured in derailment with antecedent collision (V82.0-V82.3)*

√x7th **V82.8 Occupant of streetcar injured in other specified transport accidents**
Streetcar collision with military vehicle
Streetcar collision with train or nonmotor vehicles

√x7th **V82.9 Occupant of streetcar injured in unspecified traffic accident**
Streetcar accident NOS

√4th **V83 Occupant of special vehicle mainly used on industrial premises injured in transport accident**
INCLUDES battery-powered airport passenger vehicle
battery-powered truck (baggage) (mail)
coal-car in mine
forklift (truck)
logging car
self-propelled industrial truck
station baggage truck (powered)
tram, truck, or tub (powered) in mine or quarry
EXCLUDES 1 *special construction vehicles (V85.-)*
special industrial vehicle in stationary use or maintenance (W31.-)

The appropriate 7th character is to be added to each code from category V83.
A   initial encounter
D   subsequent encounter
S   sequela

√x7th **V83.0 Driver of special industrial vehicle injured in traffic accident**

√x7th **V83.1 Passenger of special industrial vehicle injured in traffic accident**

√x7th **V83.2 Person on outside of special industrial vehicle injured in traffic accident**

√x7th **V83.3 Unspecified occupant of special industrial vehicle injured in traffic accident**

√x7th **V83.4 Person injured while boarding or alighting from special industrial vehicle**

√x7th **V83.5 Driver of special industrial vehicle injured in nontraffic accident**

√x7th **V83.6 Passenger of special industrial vehicle injured in nontraffic accident**

√x7th **V83.7 Person on outside of special industrial vehicle injured in nontraffic accident**

EXCLUDES 1 Not coded here   EXCLUDES 2 Not included here   N Newborn Age: 0   P Pediatric Age: 0-17   M Maternity Age: 12-55   A Adult Age: 15-124

1014   ICD-10-CM 2014 (Draft)

✓x7th **V83.9** **Unspecified occupant of special industrial vehicle injured in nontraffic accident**
　　　Special-industrial-vehicle accident NOS

✓4th **V84** **Occupant of special vehicle mainly used in agriculture injured in transport accident**
　　INCLUDES　self-propelled farm machinery
　　　　　　tractor (and trailer)
　　EXCLUDES 1　animal-powered farm machinery accident (W30.8-)
　　　　　　contact with combine harvester (W30.0)
　　　　　　special agricultural vehicle in stationary use or maintenance (W30.-)

The appropriate 7th character is to be added to each code from category V84.
A　initial encounter
D　subsequent encounter
S　sequela

✓x7th **V84.0** **Driver** of special agricultural vehicle injured in traffic accident

✓x7th **V84.1** **Passenger** of special agricultural vehicle injured in traffic accident

✓x7th **V84.2** **Person on outside** of special agricultural vehicle injured in traffic accident

✓x7th **V84.3** **Unspecified occupant of special agricultural vehicle injured in traffic accident**

✓x7th **V84.4** **Person injured while** boarding or alighting **from special agricultural vehicle**

✓x7th **V84.5** **Driver** of special agricultural vehicle injured in nontraffic accident

✓x7th **V84.6** **Passenger** of special agricultural vehicle injured in nontraffic accident

✓x7th **V84.7** **Person on outside** of special agricultural vehicle injured in nontraffic accident

✓x7th **V84.9** **Unspecified occupant of special agricultural vehicle injured in nontraffic accident**
　　　Special-agricultural vehicle accident NOS

✓4th **V85** **Occupant of special construction vehicle injured in transport accident**
　　INCLUDES　bulldozer
　　　　　　digger
　　　　　　dump truck
　　　　　　earth-leveller
　　　　　　mechanical shovel
　　　　　　road-roller
　　EXCLUDES 1　special industrial vehicle (V83.-)
　　　　　　special construction vehicle in stationary use or maintenance (W31.-)

The appropriate 7th character is to be added to each code from category V85.
A　initial encounter
D　subsequent encounter
S　sequela

✓x7th **V85.0** **Driver** of special construction vehicle injured in traffic accident

✓x7th **V85.1** **Passenger** of special construction vehicle injured in traffic accident

✓x7th **V85.2** **Person on outside** of special construction vehicle injured in traffic accident

✓x7th **V85.3** **Unspecified occupant of special construction vehicle injured in traffic accident**

✓x7th **V85.4** **Person injured while** boarding or alighting **from special construction vehicle**

✓x7th **V85.5** **Driver** of special construction vehicle injured in nontraffic accident

✓x7th **V85.6** **Passenger** of special construction vehicle injured in nontraffic accident

✓x7th **V85.7** **Person on outside** of special construction vehicle injured in nontraffic accident

✓x7th **V85.9** **Unspecified occupant of special construction vehicle injured in nontraffic accident**
　　　Special-construction-vehicle accident NOS

✓4th **V86** **Occupant of special all-terrain or other off-road motor vehicle, injured in transport accident**
　　EXCLUDES 1　special all-terrain vehicle in stationary use or maintenance (W31.-)
　　　　　　sport-utility vehicle (V50-V59)
　　　　　　three-wheeled motor vehicle designed for on-road use (V30-V39)

The appropriate 7th character is to be added to each code from category V86.
A　initial encounter
D　subsequent encounter
S　sequela

✓5th **V86.0** **Driver** of special all-terrain or other off-road motor vehicle injured in traffic accident

　✓x7th **V86.01** **Driver of** ambulance or fire engine **injured in traffic accident**

　✓x7th **V86.02** **Driver of** snowmobile **injured in traffic accident**

　✓x7th **V86.03** **Driver of** dune buggy **injured in traffic accident**

　✓x7th **V86.04** **Driver of** military vehicle **injured in traffic accident**

　✓x7th **V86.09** **Driver of other special all-terrain or other off-road motor vehicle injured in traffic accident**
　　　Driver of dirt bike injured in traffic accident
　　　Driver of go cart injured in traffic accident
　　　Driver of golf cart injured in traffic accident

✓5th **V86.1** **Passenger** of special all-terrain or other off-road motor vehicle injured in traffic accident

　✓x7th **V86.11** **Passenger of** ambulance or fire engine **injured in traffic accident**

　✓x7th **V86.12** **Passenger of** snowmobile **injured in traffic accident**

　✓x7th **V86.13** **Passenger of** dune buggy **injured in traffic accident**

　✓x7th **V86.14** **Passenger of** military vehicle **injured in traffic accident**

　✓x7th **V86.19** **Passenger of other special all-terrain or other off-road motor vehicle injured in traffic accident**
　　　Passenger of dirt bike injured in traffic accident
　　　Passenger of go cart injured in traffic accident
　　　Passenger of golf cart injured in traffic accident

✓5th **V86.2** **Person on outside** of special all-terrain or other off-road motor vehicle injured in traffic accident

　✓x7th **V86.21** **Person on outside of** ambulance or fire engine **injured in traffic accident**

　✓x7th **V86.22** **Person on outside of** snowmobile **injured in traffic accident**

　✓x7th **V86.23** **Person on outside of** dune buggy **injured in traffic accident**

　✓x7th **V86.24** **Person on outside of** military vehicle **injured in traffic accident**

　✓x7th **V86.29** **Person on outside of other special all-terrain or other off-road motor vehicle injured in traffic accident**
　　　Person on outside of dirt bike injured in traffic accident
　　　Person on outside of go cart in traffic accident
　　　Person on outside of golf cart injured in traffic accident

✓5th **V86.3** **Unspecified occupant** of special all-terrain or other off-road motor vehicle injured in traffic accident

　✓x7th **V86.31** **Unspecified occupant of** ambulance or fire engine **injured in traffic accident**

　✓x7th **V86.32** **Unspecified occupant of** snowmobile **injured in traffic accident**

　✓x7th **V86.33** **Unspecified occupant of** dune buggy **injured in traffic accident**

　✓x7th **V86.34** **Unspecified occupant of** military vehicle **injured in traffic accident**

　✓x7th **V86.39** **Unspecified occupant of other special all-terrain or other off-road motor vehicle injured in traffic accident**
　　　Unspecified occupant of dirt bike injured in traffic accident
　　　Unspecified occupant of go cart injured in traffic accident
　　　Unspecified occupant of golf cart injured in traffic accident

✓5th **V86.4** **Person injured while** boarding or alighting **from special all-terrain or other off-road motor vehicle**

　✓x7th **V86.41** **Person injured while boarding or alighting from** ambulance or fire engine

√x7th **V86.42** Person injured while boarding or alighting from snowmobile

√x7th **V86.43** Person injured while boarding or alighting from dune buggy

√x7th **V86.44** Person injured while boarding or alighting from military vehicle

√x7th **V86.49** Person injured while boarding or alighting from other special all-terrain or other off-road motor vehicle

Person injured while boarding or alighting from dirt bike

Person injured while boarding or alighting from go cart

Person injured while boarding or alighting from golf cart

√5th **V86.5** Driver of special all-terrain or other off-road motor vehicle injured in nontraffic accident

√x7th **V86.51** Driver of ambulance or fire engine injured in nontraffic accident

√x7th **V86.52** Driver of snowmobile injured in nontraffic accident

√x7th **V86.53** Driver of dune buggy injured in nontraffic accident

√x7th **V86.54** Driver of military vehicle injured in nontraffic accident

√x7th **V86.59** Driver of other special all-terrain or other off-road motor vehicle injured in nontraffic accident

Driver of dirt bike injured in nontraffic accident

Driver of go cart injured in nontraffic accident

Driver of golf cart injured in nontraffic accident

√5th **V86.6** Passenger of special all-terrain or other off-road motor vehicle injured in nontraffic accident

√x7th **V86.61** Passenger of ambulance or fire engine injured in nontraffic accident

√x7th **V86.62** Passenger of snowmobile injured in nontraffic accident

√x7th **V86.63** Passenger of dune buggy injured in nontraffic accident

√x7th **V86.64** Passenger of military vehicle injured in nontraffic accident

√x7th **V86.69** Passenger of other special all-terrain or other off-road motor vehicle injured in nontraffic accident

Passenger of dirt bike injured in nontraffic accident

Passenger of go cart injured in nontraffic accident

Passenger of golf cart injured in nontraffic accident

√5th **V86.7** Person on outside of special all-terrain or other off-road motor vehicle injured in nontraffic accident

√x7th **V86.71** Person on outside of ambulance or fire engine injured in nontraffic accident

√x7th **V86.72** Person on outside of snowmobile injured in nontraffic accident

√x7th **V86.73** Person on outside of dune buggy injured in nontraffic accident

√x7th **V86.74** Person on outside of military vehicle injured in nontraffic accident

√x7th **V86.79** Person on outside of other special all-terrain or other off-road motor vehicles injured in nontraffic accident

Person on outside of dirt bike injured in nontraffic accident

Person on outside of go cart injured in nontraffic accident

Person on outside of golf cart injured in nontraffic accident

√5th **V86.9** Unspecified occupant of special all-terrain or other off-road motor vehicle injured in nontraffic accident

√x7th **V86.91** Unspecified occupant of ambulance or fire engine injured in nontraffic accident

√x7th **V86.92** Unspecified occupant of snowmobile injured in nontraffic accident

√x7th **V86.93** Unspecified occupant of dune buggy injured in nontraffic accident

√x7th **V86.94** Unspecified occupant of military vehicle injured in nontraffic accident

√x7th **V86.99** Unspecified occupant of other special all-terrain or other off-road motor vehicle injured in nontraffic accident

All-terrain motor-vehicle accident NOS

Off-road motor-vehicle accident NOS

Other motor-vehicle accident NOS

Unspecified occupant of dirt bike injured in nontraffic accident

Unspecified occupant of go cart injured in nontraffic accident

Unspecified occupant of golf cart injured in nontraffic accident

√4th **V87** Traffic accident of specified type but victim's mode of transport unknown

EXCLUDES 1 collision involving:
pedal cycle (V10-V19)
pedestrian (V01-V09)

The appropriate 7th character is to be added to each code from category V87.
A initial encounter
D subsequent encounter
S sequela

√x7th **V87.0** Person injured in collision between car and two- or three-wheeled powered vehicle (traffic)

√x7th **V87.1** Person injured in collision between other motor vehicle and two- or three-wheeled motor vehicle (traffic)

√x7th **V87.2** Person injured in collision between car and pick-up truck or van (traffic)

√x7th **V87.3** Person injured in collision between car and bus (traffic)

√x7th **V87.4** Person injured in collision between car and heavy transport vehicle (traffic)

√x7th **V87.5** Person injured in collision between heavy transport vehicle and bus (traffic)

√x7th **V87.6** Person injured in collision between railway train or railway vehicle and car (traffic)

√x7th **V87.7** Person injured in collision between other specified motor vehicles (traffic)

√x7th **V87.8** Person injured in other specified noncollision transport accidents involving motor vehicle (traffic)

√x7th **V87.9** Person injured in other specified (collision)(noncollision) transport accidents involving nonmotor vehicle (traffic)

√4th **V88** Nontraffic accident of specified type but victim's mode of transport unknown

EXCLUDES 1 collision involving:
pedal cycle (V10-V19)
pedestrian (V01-V09)

The appropriate 7th character is to be added to each code from category V88.
A initial encounter
D subsequent encounter
S sequela

√x7th **V88.0** Person injured in collision between car and two- or three-wheeled motor vehicle, nontraffic

√x7th **V88.1** Person injured in collision between other motor vehicle and two- or three-wheeled motor vehicle, nontraffic

√x7th **V88.2** Person injured in collision between car and pick-up truck or van, nontraffic

√x7th **V88.3** Person injured in collision between car and bus, nontraffic

√x7th **V88.4** Person injured in collision between car and heavy transport vehicle, nontraffic

√x7th **V88.5** Person injured in collision between heavy transport vehicle and bus, nontraffic

√x7th **V88.6** Person injured in collision between railway train or railway vehicle and car, nontraffic

√x7th **V88.7** Person injured in collision between other specified motor vehicle, nontraffic

√x7th **V88.8** Person injured in other specified noncollision transport accidents involving motor vehicle, nontraffic

√x7th **V88.9** Person injured in other specified (collision)(noncollision) transport accidents involving nonmotor vehicle, nontraffic

EXCLUDES 1 Not coded here   EXCLUDES 2 Not included here   N Newborn Age: 0   P Pediatric Age: 0-17   M Maternity Age: 12-55   A Adult Age: 15-124

1016   ICD-10-CM 2014 (Draft)

✓4ᵗʰ **V89   Motor- or nonmotor-vehicle accident, type of vehicle unspecified**

> The appropriate 7th character is to be added to each code from category V89.
> A   initial encounter
> D   subsequent encounter
> S   sequela

✓x7ᵗʰ **V89.0   Person injured in unspecified motor-vehicle accident, nontraffic**
> Motor-vehicle accident NOS, nontraffic

✓x7ᵗʰ **V89.1   Person injured in unspecified nonmotor-vehicle accident, nontraffic**
> Nonmotor-vehicle accident NOS (nontraffic)

✓x7ᵗʰ **V89.2   Person injured in unspecified motor-vehicle accident, traffic**
> Motor-vehicle accident [MVA] NOS
> Road (traffic) accident [RTA] NOS

✓x7ᵗʰ **V89.3   Person injured in unspecified nonmotor-vehicle accident, traffic**
> Nonmotor-vehicle traffic accident NOS

✓x7ᵗʰ **V89.9   Person injured in unspecified vehicle accident**
> Collision NOS

Water transport accidents (V90-V94)

✓4ᵗʰ **V90   Drowning and submersion due to accident to watercraft**

> EXCLUDES 1   civilian water transport accident involving military watercraft (V94.81-)
> fall into water not from watercraft (W16.-)
> military watercraft accident in military or war operations (Y36.0-, Y37.0-)
> water-transport-related drowning or submersion without accident to watercraft (V92.-)

> The appropriate 7th character is to be added to each code from category V90.
> A   initial encounter
> D   subsequent encounter
> S   sequela

✓5ᵗʰ **V90.0   Drowning and submersion due to watercraft overturning**

✓x7ᵗʰ **V90.00   Drowning and submersion due to merchant ship overturning**

✓x7ᵗʰ **V90.01   Drowning and submersion due to passenger ship overturning**
> Drowning and submersion due to Ferry-boat overturning
> Drowning and submersion due to Liner overturning

✓x7ᵗʰ **V90.02   Drowning and submersion due to fishing boat overturning**

✓x7ᵗʰ **V90.03   Drowning and submersion due to other powered watercraft overturning**
> Drowning and submersion due to Hovercraft (on open water) overturning
> Drowning and submersion due to Jet ski overturning

✓x7ᵗʰ **V90.04   Drowning and submersion due to sailboat overturning**

✓x7ᵗʰ **V90.05   Drowning and submersion due to canoe or kayak overturning**

✓x7ᵗʰ **V90.06   Drowning and submersion due to (nonpowered) inflatable craft overturning**

✓x7ᵗʰ **V90.08   Drowning and submersion due to other unpowered watercraft overturning**
> Drowning and submersion due to windsurfer overturning

✓x7ᵗʰ **V90.09   Drowning and submersion due to unspecified watercraft overturning**
> Drowning and submersion due to boat NOS overturning
> Drowning and submersion due to ship NOS overturning
> Drowning and submersion due to watercraft NOS overturning

✓5ᵗʰ **V90.1   Drowning and submersion due to watercraft sinking**

✓x7ᵗʰ **V90.10   Drowning and submersion due to merchant ship sinking**

✓x7ᵗʰ **V90.11   Drowning and submersion due to passenger ship sinking**
> Drowning and submersion due to Ferry-boat sinking
> Drowning and submersion due to Liner sinking

✓x7ᵗʰ **V90.12   Drowning and submersion due to fishing boat sinking**

✓x7ᵗʰ **V90.13   Drowning and submersion due to other powered watercraft sinking**
> Drowning and submersion due to Hovercraft (on open water) sinking
> Drowning and submersion due to Jet ski sinking

✓x7ᵗʰ **V90.14   Drowning and submersion due to sailboat sinking**

✓x7ᵗʰ **V90.15   Drowning and submersion due to canoe or kayak sinking**

✓x7ᵗʰ **V90.16   Drowning and submersion due to (nonpowered) inflatable craft sinking**

✓x7ᵗʰ **V90.18   Drowning and submersion due to other unpowered watercraft sinking**

✓x7ᵗʰ **V90.19   Drowning and submersion due to unspecified watercraft sinking**
> Drowning and submersion due to boat NOS sinking
> Drowning and submersion due to ship NOS sinking
> Drowning and submersion due to watercraft NOS sinking

✓5ᵗʰ **V90.2   Drowning and submersion due to falling or jumping from burning watercraft**

✓x7ᵗʰ **V90.20   Drowning and submersion due to falling or jumping from burning merchant ship**

✓x7ᵗʰ **V90.21   Drowning and submersion due to falling or jumping from burning passenger ship**
> Drowning and submersion due to falling or jumping from burning Ferry-boat
> Drowning and submersion due to falling or jumping from burning Liner

✓x7ᵗʰ **V90.22   Drowning and submersion due to falling or jumping from burning fishing boat**

✓x7ᵗʰ **V90.23   Drowning and submersion due to falling or jumping from other burning powered watercraft**
> Drowning and submersion due to falling and jumping from burning Hovercraft (on open water)
> Drowning and submersion due to falling and jumping from burning Jet ski

✓x7ᵗʰ **V90.24   Drowning and submersion due to falling or jumping from burning sailboat**

✓x7ᵗʰ **V90.25   Drowning and submersion due to falling or jumping from burning canoe or kayak**

✓x7ᵗʰ **V90.26   Drowning and submersion due to falling or jumping from burning (nonpowered) inflatable craft**

✓x7ᵗʰ **V90.27   Drowning and submersion due to falling or jumping from burning water-skis**

✓x7ᵗʰ **V90.28   Drowning and submersion due to falling or jumping from other burning unpowered watercraft**
> Drowning and submersion due to falling and jumping from burning surf-board
> Drowning and submersion due to falling and jumping from burning windsurfer

✓x7ᵗʰ **V90.29   Drowning and submersion due to falling or jumping from unspecified burning watercraft**
> Drowning and submersion due to falling or jumping from burning boat NOS
> Drowning and submersion due to falling or jumping from burning ship NOS
> Drowning and submersion due to falling or jumping from burning watercraft NOS

✓5ᵗʰ **V90.3   Drowning and submersion due to falling or jumping from crushed watercraft**

✓x7ᵗʰ **V90.30   Drowning and submersion due to falling or jumping from crushed merchant ship**

✓x7ᵗʰ **V90.31   Drowning and submersion due to falling or jumping from crushed passenger ship**
> Drowning and submersion due to falling and jumping from crushed Ferry boat
> Drowning and submersion due to falling and jumping from crushed Liner

✓x7ᵗʰ **V90.32   Drowning and submersion due to falling or jumping from crushed fishing boat**

✓x7ᵗʰ **V90.33   Drowning and submersion due to falling or jumping from other crushed powered watercraft**
> Drowning and submersion due to falling and jumping from crushed Hovercraft
> Drowning and submersion due to falling and jumping from crushed Jet ski

✓x7ᵗʰ **V90.34   Drowning and submersion due to falling or jumping from crushed sailboat**

☑ Additional Character Required   ✓x7ᵗʰ Xtension Alert   Unspecified Code   Other Specified Code   Manifestation Code   ►◄ Revised Text   ● New Code   ▲ Revised Code Title

ICD-10-CM 2014 (Draft)   1017

√x7th **V90.35** Drowning and submersion due to falling or jumping from crushed canoe or kayak

√x7th **V90.36** Drowning and submersion due to falling or jumping from crushed (nonpowered) inflatable craft

√x7th **V90.37** Drowning and submersion due to falling or jumping from crushed water-skis

√x7th **V90.38** Drowning and submersion due to falling or jumping from other crushed unpowered watercraft
Drowning and submersion due to falling and jumping from crushed surf-board
Drowning and submersion due to falling and jumping from crushed windsurfer

√x7th **V90.39** Drowning and submersion due to falling or jumping from crushed unspecified watercraft
Drowning and submersion due to falling and jumping from crushed boat NOS
Drowning and submersion due to falling and jumping from crushed ship NOS
Drowning and submersion due to falling and jumping from crushed watercraft NOS

√5th **V90.8** Drowning and submersion due to other accident to watercraft

√x7th **V90.80** Drowning and submersion due to other accident to merchant ship

√x7th **V90.81** Drowning and submersion due to other accident to passenger ship
Drowning and submersion due to other accident to Ferry-boat
Drowning and submersion due to other accident to Liner

√x7th **V90.82** Drowning and submersion due to other accident to fishing boat

√x7th **V90.83** Drowning and submersion due to other accident to other powered watercraft
Drowning and submersion due to other accident to Hovercraft (on open water)
Drowning and submersion due to other accident to Jet ski

√x7th **V90.84** Drowning and submersion due to other accident to sailboat

√x7th **V90.85** Drowning and submersion due to other accident to canoe or kayak

√x7th **V90.86** Drowning and submersion due to other accident to (nonpowered) inflatable craft

√x7th **V90.87** Drowning and submersion due to other accident to water-skis

√x7th **V90.88** Drowning and submersion due to other accident to other unpowered watercraft
Drowning and submersion due to other accident to surf-board
Drowning and submersion due to other accident to windsurfer

√x7th **V90.89** Drowning and submersion due to other accident to unspecified watercraft
Drowning and submersion due to other accident to boat NOS
Drowning and submersion due to other accident to ship NOS
Drowning and submersion due to other accident to watercraft NOS

√4th **V91** Other injury due to accident to watercraft
INCLUDES any injury except drowning and submersion as a result of an accident to watercraft
EXCLUDES 1 civilian water transport accident involving military watercraft (V94.81-)
military watercraft accident in military or war operations (Y36, Y37.-)
EXCLUDES 2 drowning and submersion due to accident to watercraft (V90.-)

The appropriate 7th character is to be added to each code from category V91.
A initial encounter
D subsequent encounter
S sequela

√5th **V91.0** Burn due to watercraft on fire
EXCLUDES 1 burn from localized fire or explosion on board ship without accident to watercraft (V93.-)

√x7th **V91.00** Burn due to merchant ship on fire

√x7th **V91.01** Burn due to passenger ship on fire
Burn due to Ferry-boat on fire
Burn due to Liner on fire

√x7th **V91.02** Burn due to fishing boat on fire

√x7th **V91.03** Burn due to other powered watercraft on fire
Burn due to Hovercraft (on open water) on fire
Burn due to Jet ski on fire

√x7th **V91.04** Burn due to sailboat on fire

√x7th **V91.05** Burn due to canoe or kayak on fire

√x7th **V91.06** Burn due to (nonpowered) inflatable craft on fire

√x7th **V91.07** Burn due to water-skis on fire

√x7th **V91.08** Burn due to other unpowered watercraft on fire

√x7th **V91.09** Burn due to unspecified watercraft on fire
Burn due to boat NOS on fire
Burn due to ship NOS on fire
Burn due to watercraft NOS on fire

√5th **V91.1** Crushed between watercraft and other watercraft or other object due to collision
Crushed by lifeboat after abandoning ship in a collision
NOTE select the specified type of watercraft that the victim was on at the time of the collision

√x7th **V91.10** Crushed between merchant ship and other watercraft or other object due to collision

√x7th **V91.11** Crushed between passenger ship and other watercraft or other object due to collision
Crushed between Ferry-boat and other watercraft or other object due to collision
Crushed between Liner and other watercraft or other object due to collision

√x7th **V91.12** Crushed between fishing boat and other watercraft or other object due to collision

√x7th **V91.13** Crushed between other powered watercraft and other watercraft or other object due to collision
Crushed between Hovercraft (on open water) and other watercraft or other object due to collision
Crushed between Jet ski and other watercraft or other object due to collision

√x7th **V91.14** Crushed between sailboat and other watercraft or other object due to collision

√x7th **V91.15** Crushed between canoe or kayak and other watercraft or other object due to collision

√x7th **V91.16** Crushed between (nonpowered) inflatable craft and other watercraft or other object due to collision

√x7th **V91.18** Crushed between other unpowered watercraft and other watercraft or other object due to collision
Crushed between surfboard and other watercraft or other object due to collision
Crushed between windsurfer and other watercraft or other object due to collision

√x7th **V91.19** Crushed between unspecified watercraft and other watercraft or other object due to collision
Crushed between boat NOS and other watercraft or other object due to collision
Crushed between ship NOS and other watercraft or other object due to collision
Crushed between watercraft NOS and other watercraft or other object due to collision

√5th **V91.2** Fall due to collision between watercraft and other watercraft or other object
Fall while remaining on watercraft after collision
NOTE Select the specified type of watercraft that the victim was on at the time of the collision.
EXCLUDES 1 crushed between watercraft and other watercraft and other object due to collision (V91.1-)
drowning and submersion due to falling from crushed watercraft (V90.3-)

√x7th **V91.20** Fall due to collision between merchant ship and other watercraft or other object

√x7th **V91.21** Fall due to collision between passenger ship and other watercraft or other object
Fall due to collision between Ferry-boat and other watercraft or other object
Fall due to collision between Liner and other watercraft or other object

√x7th **V91.22** Fall due to collision between fishing boat and other watercraft or other object

√x7th **V91.23 Fall due to collision between other** powered **watercraft and other watercraft or other object**
 Fall due to collision between Hovercraft (on open water) and other watercraft or other object
 Fall due to collision between Jet ski and other watercraft or other object

√x7th **V91.24 Fall due to collision between** sailboat **and other watercraft or other object**

√x7th **V91.25 Fall due to collision between** canoe or kayak **and other watercraft or other object**

√x7th **V91.26 Fall due to collision between** (nonpowered) inflatable craft **and other watercraft or other object**

√x7th **V91.29 Fall due to collision between unspecified watercraft and other watercraft or other object**
 Fall due to collision between boat NOS and other watercraft or other object
 Fall due to collision between ship NOS and other watercraft or other object
 Fall due to collision between watercraft NOS and other watercraft or other object

√5th **V91.3 Hit or struck by falling object due to accident to watercraft**
 Hit or struck by falling object (part of damaged watercraft or other object) after falling or jumping from damaged watercraft
 EXCLUDES 2 *drowning or submersion due to fall or jumping from damaged watercraft (V90.2-, V90.3-)*

√x7th **V91.30 Hit or struck by falling object due to accident to** merchant ship

√x7th **V91.31 Hit or struck by falling object due to accident to** passenger ship
 Hit or struck by falling object due to accident to Ferry-boat
 Hit or struck by falling object due to accident to Liner

√x7th **V91.32 Hit or struck by falling object due to accident to** fishing boat

√x7th **V91.33 Hit or struck by falling object due to accident to other** powered **watercraft**
 Hit or struck by falling object due to accident to Hovercraft (on open water)
 Hit or struck by falling object due to accident to Jet ski

√x7th **V91.34 Hit or struck by falling object due to accident to** sailboat

√x7th **V91.35 Hit or struck by falling object due to accident to** canoe or kayak

√x7th **V91.36 Hit or struck by falling object due to accident to** (nonpowered) inflatable craft

√x7th **V91.37 Hit or struck by falling object due to accident to** water-skis
 Hit by water-skis after jumping off of waterskis

√x7th **V91.38 Hit or struck by falling object due to accident to other** unpowered **watercraft**
 Hit or struck by surf-board after falling off damaged surf-board
 Hit or struck by object after falling off damaged windsurfer

√x7th **V91.39 Hit or struck by falling object due to accident to unspecified watercraft**
 Hit or struck by falling object due to accident to boat NOS
 Hit or struck by falling object due to accident to ship NOS
 Hit or struck by falling object due to accident to watercraft NOS

√5th **V91.8 Other injury due to other accident to watercraft**

√x7th **V91.80 Other injury due to other accident to** merchant ship

√x7th **V91.81 Other injury due to other accident to** passenger ship
 Other injury due to other accident to Ferry-boat
 Other injury due to other accident to Liner

√x7th **V91.82 Other injury due to other accident to** fishing boat

√x7th **V91.83 Other injury due to other accident to other** powered **watercraft**
 Other injury due to other accident to Hovercraft (on open water)
 Other injury due to other accident to Jet ski

√x7th **V91.84 Other injury due to other accident to** sailboat

√x7th **V91.85 Other injury due to other accident to** canoe or kayak

√x7th **V91.86 Other injury due to other accident to (nonpowered)** inflatable craft

√x7th **V91.87 Other injury due to other accident to** water-skis

√x7th **V91.88 Other injury due to other accident to other** unpowered **watercraft**
 Other injury due to other accident to surf-board
 Other injury due to other accident to windsurfer

√x7th **V91.89 Other injury due to other accident to unspecified watercraft**
 Other injury due to other accident to boat NOS
 Other injury due to other accident to ship NOS
 Other injury due to other accident to watercraft NOS

√4th **V92 Drowning and submersion due to accident on board watercraft, without accident to watercraft**
 EXCLUDES 1 *civilian water transport accident involving military watercraft (V94.81-)*
  drowning or submersion due to accident to watercraft (V90-V91)
  drowning or submersion of diver who voluntarily jumps from boat not involved in an accident (W16.711, W16.721)
  fall into water without watercraft (W16.-)
  military watercraft accident in military or war operations (Y36, Y37)

The appropriate 7th character is to be added to each code from category V92.
A initial encounter
D subsequent encounter
S sequela

√5th **V92.0 Drowning and submersion due to** fall off **watercraft**
 Drowning and submersion due to fall from gangplank of watercraft
 Drowning and submersion due to fall overboard watercraft
 EXCLUDES 2 *hitting head on object or bottom of body of water due to fall from watercraft (V94.0-)*

√x7th **V92.00 Drowning and submersion due to fall off** merchant ship

√x7th **V92.01 Drowning and submersion due to fall off** passenger ship
 Drowning and submersion due to fall off Ferry-boat
 Drowning and submersion due to fall off Liner

√x7th **V92.02 Drowning and submersion due to fall off** fishing boat

√x7th **V92.03 Drowning and submersion due to fall off other** powered **watercraft**
 Drowning and submersion due to fall off Hovercraft (on open water)
 Drowning and submersion due to fall off Jet ski

√x7th **V92.04 Drowning and submersion due to fall off** sailboat

√x7th **V92.05 Drowning and submersion due to fall off** canoe or kayak

√x7th **V92.06 Drowning and submersion due to fall off** (nonpowered) inflatable craft

√x7th **V92.07 Drowning and submersion due to fall off** water-skis
 EXCLUDES 1 *drowning and submersion due to falling off burning water-skis (V90.27)*
  drowning and submersion due to falling off crushed water-skis (V90.37)
  hit by boat while water-skiing NOS (V94.X)

√x7th **V92.08 Drowning and submersion due to fall off other** unpowered **watercraft**
 Drowning and submersion due to fall off surf-board
 Drowning and submersion due to fall off windsurfer
 EXCLUDES 1 *drowning and submersion due to fall off burning unpowered watercraft (V90.28)*
  drowning and submersion due to fall off crushed unpowered watercraft (V90.38)
  drowning and submersion due to fall off damaged unpowered watercraft (V90.88)
  drowning and submersion due to rider of nonpowered watercraft being hit by other watercraft (V94.-)
  other injury due to rider of nonpowered watercraft being hit by other watercraft (V94.-)

√x7th **V92.09 Drowning and submersion due to fall off unspecified watercraft**
 Drowning and submersion due to fall off boat NOS
 Drowning and submersion due to fall off ship
 Drowning and submersion due to fall off watercraft NOS

External Causes of Morbidity

V92.1–V93.32

√5ᵗʰ **V92.1 Drowning and submersion due to being thrown overboard by motion of watercraft**

> EXCLUDES 1   *drowning and submersion due to fall off surf-board (V92.08)*
> *drowning and submersion due to fall off water-skis (V92.07)*
> *drowning and submersion due to fall off windsurfer (V92.08)*

√x7ᵗʰ **V92.10 Drowning and submersion due to being thrown overboard by motion of merchant ship**

√x7ᵗʰ **V92.11 Drowning and submersion due to being thrown overboard by motion of passenger ship**
> Drowning and submersion due to being thrown overboard by motion of Ferry-boat
> Drowning and submersion due to being thrown overboard by motion of Liner

√x7ᵗʰ **V92.12 Drowning and submersion due to being thrown overboard by motion of fishing boat**

√x7ᵗʰ **V92.13 Drowning and submersion due to being thrown overboard by motion of other powered watercraft**
> Drowning and submersion due to being thrown overboard by motion of Hovercraft

√x7ᵗʰ **V92.14 Drowning and submersion due to being thrown overboard by motion of sailboat**

√x7ᵗʰ **V92.15 Drowning and submersion due to being thrown overboard by motion of canoe or kayak**

√x7ᵗʰ **V92.16 Drowning and submersion due to being thrown overboard by motion of (nonpowered) inflatable craft**

√x7ᵗʰ **V92.19 Drowning and submersion due to being thrown overboard by motion of unspecified watercraft**
> Drowning and submersion due to being thrown overboard by motion of boat NOS
> Drowning and submersion due to being thrown overboard by motion of ship NOS
> Drowning and submersion due to being thrown overboard by motion of watercraft NOS

√5ᵗʰ **V92.2 Drowning and submersion due to being washed overboard from watercraft**

> Code first any associated cataclysm (X37.0-)

√x7ᵗʰ **V92.20 Drowning and submersion due to being washed overboard from merchant ship**

√x7ᵗʰ **V92.21 Drowning and submersion due to being washed overboard from passenger ship**
> Drowning and submersion due to being washed overboard from Ferry-boat
> Drowning and submersion due to being washed overboard from Liner

√x7ᵗʰ **V92.22 Drowning and submersion due to being washed overboard from fishing boat**

√x7ᵗʰ **V92.23 Drowning and submersion due to being washed overboard from other powered watercraft**
> Drowning and submersion due to being washed overboard from Hovercraft (on open water)
> Drowning and submersion due to being washed overboard from Jet ski

√x7ᵗʰ **V92.24 Drowning and submersion due to being washed overboard from sailboat**

√x7ᵗʰ **V92.25 Drowning and submersion due to being washed overboard from canoe or kayak**

√x7ᵗʰ **V92.26 Drowning and submersion due to being washed overboard from (nonpowered) inflatable craft**

√x7ᵗʰ **V92.27 Drowning and submersion due to being washed overboard from water-skis**
> EXCLUDES 1   *drowning and submersion due to fall off water-skis (V92.07)*

√x7ᵗʰ **V92.28 Drowning and submersion due to being washed overboard from other unpowered watercraft**
> Drowning and submersion due to being washed overboard from surf-board
> Drowning and submersion due to being washed overboard from windsurfer

√x7ᵗʰ **V92.29 Drowning and submersion due to being washed overboard from unspecified watercraft**
> Drowning and submersion due to being washed overboard from boat NOS
> Drowning and submersion due to being washed overboard from ship NOS
> Drowning and submersion due to being washed overboard from watercraft NOS

√4ᵗʰ **V93 Other injury due to accident on board watercraft, without accident to watercraft**

> EXCLUDES 1   *civilian water transport accident involving military watercraft (V94.81-)*
> *other injury due to accident to watercraft (V91.-)*
> *military watercraft accident in military or war operations (Y36, Y37.-)*
> EXCLUDES 2   *drowning and submersion due to accident on board watercraft, without accident to watercraft (V92.-)*

> The appropriate 7th character is to be added to each code from category V93.
> A   initial encounter
> D   subsequent encounter
> S   sequela

√5ᵗʰ **V93.0 Burn due to localized fire on board watercraft**
> EXCLUDES 1   *burn due to watercraft on fire (V91.0-)*

√x7ᵗʰ **V93.00 Burn due to localized fire on board merchant vessel**

√x7ᵗʰ **V93.01 Burn due to localized fire on board passenger vessel**
> Burn due to localized fire on board Ferry-boat
> Burn due to localized fire on board Liner

√x7ᵗʰ **V93.02 Burn due to localized fire on board fishing boat**

√x7ᵗʰ **V93.03 Burn due to localized fire on board other powered watercraft**
> Burn due to localized fire on board Hovercraft
> Burn due to localized fire on board Jet ski

√x7ᵗʰ **V93.04 Burn due to localized fire on board sailboat**

√x7ᵗʰ **V93.09 Burn due to localized fire on board unspecified watercraft**
> Burn due to localized fire on board boat NOS
> Burn due to localized fire on board ship NOS
> Burn due to localized fire on board watercraft NOS

√5ᵗʰ **V93.1 Other burn on board watercraft**
> Burn due to source other than fire on board watercraft
> EXCLUDES 1   *burn due to watercraft on fire (V91.0-)*

√x7ᵗʰ **V93.10 Other burn on board merchant vessel**

√x7ᵗʰ **V93.11 Other burn on board passenger vessel**
> Other burn on board Ferry-boat
> Other burn on board Liner

√x7ᵗʰ **V93.12 Other burn on board fishing boat**

√x7ᵗʰ **V93.13 Other burn on board other powered watercraft**
> Other burn on board Hovercraft
> Other burn on board Jet ski

√x7ᵗʰ **V93.14 Other burn on board sailboat**

√x7ᵗʰ **V93.19 Other burn on board unspecified watercraft**
> Other burn on board boat NOS
> Other burn on board ship NOS
> Other burn on board watercraft NOS

√5ᵗʰ **V93.2 Heat exposure on board watercraft**
> EXCLUDES 1   *exposure to man-made heat not aboard watercraft (W92)*
> *exposure to natural heat while on board watercraft (X30)*
> *exposure to sunlight while on board watercraft (X32)*
> EXCLUDES 2   *burn due to fire on board watercraft (V93.0-)*

√x7ᵗʰ **V93.20 Heat exposure on board merchant ship**

√x7ᵗʰ **V93.21 Heat exposure on board passenger ship**
> Heat exposure on board Ferry-boat
> Heat exposure on board Liner

√x7ᵗʰ **V93.22 Heat exposure on board fishing boat**

√x7ᵗʰ **V93.23 Heat exposure on board other powered watercraft**
> Heat exposure on board hovercraft

√x7ᵗʰ **V93.24 Heat exposure on board sailboat**

√x7ᵗʰ **V93.29 Heat exposure on board unspecified watercraft**
> Heat exposure on board boat NOS
> Heat exposure on board ship NOS
> Heat exposure on board watercraft NOS

√5ᵗʰ **V93.3 Fall on board watercraft**
> EXCLUDES 1   *fall due to collision of watercraft (V91.2-)*

√x7ᵗʰ **V93.30 Fall on board merchant ship**

√x7ᵗʰ **V93.31 Fall on board passenger ship**
> Fall on board Ferry-boat
> Fall on board Liner

√x7ᵗʰ **V93.32 Fall on board fishing boat**

EXCLUDES 1 Not coded here   EXCLUDES 2 Not included here   N Newborn Age: 0   P Pediatric Age: 0-17   M Maternity Age: 12-55   A Adult Age: 15-124

1020   ICD-10-CM 2014 (Draft)

✓x7th **V93.33** **Fall on board other** powered **watercraft**
Fall on board Hovercraft (on open water)
Fall on board Jet ski

✓x7th **V93.34** **Fall on board** sailboat

✓x7th **V93.35** **Fall on board** canoe or kayak

✓x7th **V93.36** **Fall on board (nonpowered)** inflatable craft

✓x7th **V93.38** **Fall on board other** unpowered **watercraft**

✓x7th **V93.39** **Fall on board unspecified watercraft**
Fall on board boat NOS
Fall on board ship NOS
Fall on board watercraft NOS

✓5th **V93.4** **Struck by falling object on board watercraft**
Hit by falling object on board watercraft
EXCLUDES 1 *struck by falling object due to accident to watercraft (V91.3)*

✓x7th **V93.40** **Struck by falling object on** merchant ship

✓x7th **V93.41** **Struck by falling object on** passenger ship
Struck by falling object on Ferry-boat
Struck by falling object on Liner

✓x7th **V93.42** **Struck by falling object on** fishing boat

✓x7th **V93.43** **Struck by falling object on other** powered **watercraft**
Struck by falling object on Hovercraft

✓x7th **V93.44** **Struck by falling object on** sailboat

✓x7th **V93.48** **Struck by falling object on other** unpowered **watercraft**

✓x7th **V93.49** **Struck by falling object on unspecified watercraft**

✓5th **V93.5** **Explosion on board watercraft**
Boiler explosion on steamship
EXCLUDES 2 *fire on board watercraft (V93.0-)*

✓x7th **V93.50** **Explosion on board** merchant ship

✓x7th **V93.51** **Explosion on board** passenger ship
Explosion on board Ferry-boat
Explosion on board Liner

✓x7th **V93.52** **Explosion on board** fishing boat

✓x7th **V93.53** **Explosion on board other** powered **watercraft**
Explosion on board Hovercraft
Explosion on board Jet ski

✓x7th **V93.54** **Explosion on board** sailboat

✓x7th **V93.59** **Explosion on board unspecified watercraft**
Explosion on board boat NOS
Explosion on board ship NOS
Explosion on board watercraft NOS

✓5th **V93.6** **Machinery accident on board watercraft**
EXCLUDES 1 *machinery explosion on board watercraft (V93.4-)*
machinery fire on board watercraft (V93.0-)

✓x7th **V93.60** **Machinery accident on board** merchant ship

✓x7th **V93.61** **Machinery accident on board** passenger ship
Machinery accident on board Ferry-boat
Machinery accident on board Liner

✓x7th **V93.62** **Machinery accident on board** fishing boat

✓x7th **V93.63** **Machinery accident on board other** powered **watercraft**
Machinery accident on board Hovercraft

✓x7th **V93.64** **Machinery accident on board** sailboat

✓x7th **V93.69** **Machinery accident on board unspecified watercraft**
Machinery accident on board boat NOS
Machinery accident on board ship NOS
Machinery accident on board watercraft NOS

✓5th **V93.8** **Other injury due to other accident on board watercraft**
Accidental poisoning by gases or fumes on watercraft

✓x7th **V93.80** **Other injury due to other accident on board** merchant ship

✓x7th **V93.81** **Other injury due to other accident on board** passenger ship
Other injury due to other accident on board Ferry-boat
Other injury due to other accident on board Liner

✓x7th **V93.82** **Other injury due to other accident on board** fishing boat

✓x7th **V93.83** **Other injury due to other accident on board other** powered **watercraft**
Other injury due to other accident on board Hovercraft
Other injury due to other accident on board Jet ski

✓x7th **V93.84** **Other injury due to other accident on board** sailboat

✓x7th **V93.85** **Other injury due to other accident on board** canoe or kayak

✓x7th **V93.86** **Other injury due to other accident on board (nonpowered)** inflatable craft

✓x7th **V93.87** **Other injury due to other accident on board** water-skis
Hit or struck by object while waterskiing

✓x7th **V93.88** **Other injury due to other accident on board other** unpowered **watercraft**
Hit or struck by object while surfing
Hit or struck by object while on board windsurfer

✓x7th **V93.89** **Other injury due to other accident on board unspecified watercraft**
Other injury due to other accident on board boat NOS
Other injury due to other accident on board ship NOS
Other injury due to other accident on board watercraft NOS

✓4th **V94** **Other and unspecified water transport accidents**
EXCLUDES 1 *military watercraft accidents in military or war operations (Y36, Y37)*

The appropriate 7th character is to be added to each code from category V94.
A   initial encounter
D   subsequent encounter
S   sequela

✓x7th **V94.0** **Hitting object or bottom of body of water due to fall from watercraft**
EXCLUDES 2 *drowning and submersion due to fall from watercraft (V92.0-)*

✓5th **V94.1** **Bather struck by watercraft**
Swimmer hit by watercraft

✓x7th **V94.11** **Bather struck by** powered **watercraft**

✓x7th **V94.12** **Bather struck by** nonpowered **watercraft**

✓5th **V94.2** **Rider of nonpowered watercraft struck by other watercraft**

✓x7th **V94.21** **Rider of nonpowered watercraft struck by other** nonpowered **watercraft**
Canoer hit by other nonpowered watercraft
Surfer hit by other nonpowered watercraft
Windsurfer hit by other nonpowered watercraft

✓x7th **V94.22** **Rider of nonpowered watercraft struck by** powered **watercraft**
Canoer hit by motorboat
Surfer hit by motorboat
Windsurfer hit by motorboat

✓5th **V94.3** **Injury to rider of (inflatable) watercraft being pulled behind other watercraft**

✓x7th **V94.31** **Injury to rider of (inflatable)** recreational **watercraft being pulled behind other watercraft**
Injury to rider of inner-tube pulled behind motor boat

✓x7th **V94.32** **Injury to rider of** non-recreational **watercraft being pulled behind other watercraft**
Injury to occupant of dingy being pulled behind boat or ship
Injury to occupant of life-raft being pulled behind boat or ship

✓x7th **V94.4** **Injury to barefoot water-skier**
Injury to person being pulled behind boat or ship

✓5th **V94.8** **Other water transport accident**

✓6th **V94.81** **Water transport accident involving military watercraft**

✓7th **V94.810** **Civilian watercraft involved in water transport accident with military watercraft**
Passenger on civilian watercraft injured due to accident with military watercraft

✓7th **V94.811** **Civilian in water injured by military watercraft**

✓7th **V94.818** **Other water transport accident involving military watercraft**

✓x7th **V94.89** **Other water transport accident**

✓x7th **V94.9** **Unspecified water transport accident**
Water transport accident NOS

✓ Additional Character Required   ✓x7th Xtension Alert   Unspecified Code   Other Specified Code   Manifestation Code   ►◄ Revised Text   ● New Code   ▲ Revised Code Title

ICD-10-CM 2014 (Draft)   1021

External Causes of Morbidity

V95–V97.22

Air and space transport accidents (V95-V97)

EXCLUDES 1   *military aircraft accidents in military or war operations (Y36, Y37)*

☑4ᵗʰ V95   Accident to powered aircraft causing injury to occupant

> The appropriate 7th character is to be added to each code from category V95.
> A   initial encounter
> D   subsequent encounter
> S   sequela

☑5ᵗʰ V95.0   Helicopter accident injuring occupant

    ✓x7ᵗʰ **V95.00   Unspecified helicopter accident injuring occupant**

    ✓x7ᵗʰ **V95.01   Helicopter crash injuring occupant**

    ✓x7ᵗʰ **V95.02   Forced landing of helicopter injuring occupant**

    ✓x7ᵗʰ **V95.03   Helicopter collision injuring occupant**
       Helicopter collision with any object, fixed, movable or moving

    ✓x7ᵗʰ **V95.04   Helicopter fire injuring occupant**

    ✓x7ᵗʰ **V95.05   Helicopter explosion injuring occupant**

    ✓x7ᵗʰ **V95.09   Other helicopter accident injuring occupant**

☑5ᵗʰ V95.1   Ultralight, microlight or powered-glider accident injuring occupant

    ✓x7ᵗʰ **V95.10   Unspecified ultralight, microlight or powered-glider accident injuring occupant**

    ✓x7ᵗʰ **V95.11   Ultralight, microlight or powered-glider crash injuring occupant**

    ✓x7ᵗʰ **V95.12   Forced landing of ultralight, microlight or powered-glider injuring occupant**

    ✓x7ᵗʰ **V95.13   Ultralight, microlight or powered-glider collision injuring occupant**
       Ultralight, microlight or powered-glider collision with any object, fixed, movable or moving

    ✓x7ᵗʰ **V95.14   Ultralight, microlight or powered-glider fire injuring occupant**

    ✓x7ᵗʰ **V95.15   Ultralight, microlight or powered-glider explosion injuring occupant**

    ✓x7ᵗʰ **V95.19   Other ultralight, microlight or powered-glider accident injuring occupant**

☑5ᵗʰ V95.2   Other private fixed-wing aircraft accident injuring occupant

    ✓x7ᵗʰ **V95.20   Unspecified accident to other private fixed-wing aircraft, injuring occupant**

    ✓x7ᵗʰ **V95.21   Other private fixed-wing aircraft crash injuring occupant**

    ✓x7ᵗʰ **V95.22   Forced landing of other private fixed-wing aircraft injuring occupant**

    ✓x7ᵗʰ **V95.23   Other private fixed-wing aircraft collision injuring occupant**
       Other private fixed-wing aircraft collision with any object, fixed, movable or moving

    ✓x7ᵗʰ **V95.24   Other private fixed-wing aircraft fire injuring occupant**

    ✓x7ᵗʰ **V95.25   Other private fixed-wing aircraft explosion injuring occupant**

    ✓x7ᵗʰ **V95.29   Other accident to other private fixed-wing aircraft injuring occupant**

☑5ᵗʰ V95.3   Commercial fixed-wing aircraft accident injuring occupant

    ✓x7ᵗʰ **V95.30   Unspecified accident to commercial fixed-wing aircraft injuring occupant**

    ✓x7ᵗʰ **V95.31   Commercial fixed-wing aircraft crash injuring occupant**

    ✓x7ᵗʰ **V95.32   Forced landing of commercial fixed-wing aircraft injuring occupant**

    ✓x7ᵗʰ **V95.33   Commercial fixed-wing aircraft collision injuring occupant**
       Commercial fixed-wing aircraft collision with any object, fixed, movable or moving

    ✓x7ᵗʰ **V95.34   Commercial fixed-wing aircraft fire injuring occupant**

    ✓x7ᵗʰ **V95.35   Commercial fixed-wing aircraft explosion injuring occupant**

    ✓x7ᵗʰ **V95.39   Other accident to commercial fixed-wing aircraft injuring occupant**

☑5ᵗʰ V95.4   Spacecraft accident injuring occupant

    ✓x7ᵗʰ **V95.40   Unspecified spacecraft accident injuring occupant**

    ✓x7ᵗʰ **V95.41   Spacecraft crash injuring occupant**

    ✓x7ᵗʰ **V95.42   Forced landing of spacecraft injuring occupant**

    ✓x7ᵗʰ **V95.43   Spacecraft collision injuring occupant**
       Spacecraft collision with any object, fixed, moveable or moving

    ✓x7ᵗʰ **V95.44   Spacecraft fire injuring occupant**

    ✓x7ᵗʰ **V95.45   Spacecraft explosion injuring occupant**

    ✓x7ᵗʰ **V95.49   Other spacecraft accident injuring occupant**

    ✓x7ᵗʰ **V95.8   Other powered aircraft accidents injuring occupant**

    ✓x7ᵗʰ **V95.9   Unspecified aircraft accident injuring occupant**
       Aircraft accident NOS
       Air transport accident NOS

☑4ᵗʰ V96   Accident to nonpowered aircraft causing injury to occupant

> The appropriate 7th character is to be added to each code from category V96.
> A   initial encounter
> D   subsequent encounter
> S   sequela

☑5ᵗʰ V96.0   Balloon accident injuring occupant

    ✓x7ᵗʰ **V96.00   Unspecified balloon accident injuring occupant**

    ✓x7ᵗʰ **V96.01   Balloon crash injuring occupant**

    ✓x7ᵗʰ **V96.02   Forced landing of balloon injuring occupant**

    ✓x7ᵗʰ **V96.03   Balloon collision injuring occupant**
       Balloon collision with any object, fixed, moveable or moving

    ✓x7ᵗʰ **V96.04   Balloon fire injuring occupant**

    ✓x7ᵗʰ **V96.05   Balloon explosion injuring occupant**

    ✓x7ᵗʰ **V96.09   Other balloon accident injuring occupant**

☑5ᵗʰ V96.1   Hang-glider accident injuring occupant

    ✓x7ᵗʰ **V96.10   Unspecified hang-glider accident injuring occupant**

    ✓x7ᵗʰ **V96.11   Hang-glider crash injuring occupant**

    ✓x7ᵗʰ **V96.12   Forced landing of hang-glider injuring occupant**

    ✓x7ᵗʰ **V96.13   Hang-glider collision injuring occupant**
       Hang-glider collision with any object, fixed, moveable or moving

    ✓x7ᵗʰ **V96.14   Hang-glider fire injuring occupant**

    ✓x7ᵗʰ **V96.15   Hang-glider explosion injuring occupant**

    ✓x7ᵗʰ **V96.19   Other hang-glider accident injuring occupant**

☑5ᵗʰ V96.2   Glider (nonpowered) accident injuring occupant

    ✓x7ᵗʰ **V96.20   Unspecified glider (nonpowered) accident injuring occupant**

    ✓x7ᵗʰ **V96.21   Glider (nonpowered) crash injuring occupant**

    ✓x7ᵗʰ **V96.22   Forced landing of glider (nonpowered) injuring occupant**

    ✓x7ᵗʰ **V96.23   Glider (nonpowered) collision injuring occupant**
       Glider (nonpowered) collision with any object, fixed, moveable or moving

    ✓x7ᵗʰ **V96.24   Glider (nonpowered) fire injuring occupant**

    ✓x7ᵗʰ **V96.25   Glider (nonpowered) explosion injuring occupant**

    ✓x7ᵗʰ **V96.29   Other glider (nonpowered) accident injuring occupant**

    ✓x7ᵗʰ **V96.8   Other nonpowered-aircraft accidents injuring occupant**
       Kite carrying a person accident injuring occupant

    ✓x7ᵗʰ **V96.9   Unspecified nonpowered-aircraft accident injuring occupant**
       Nonpowered-aircraft accident NOS

☑4ᵗʰ V97   Other specified air transport accidents

> The appropriate 7th character is to be added to each code from category V97.
> A   initial encounter
> D   subsequent encounter
> S   sequela

    ✓x7ᵗʰ **V97.0   Occupant of aircraft injured in other specified air transport accidents**
       Fall in, on or from aircraft in air transport accident
       EXCLUDES 1   *accident while boarding or alighting aircraft (V97.1)*

    ✓x7ᵗʰ **V97.1   Person injured while boarding or alighting from aircraft**

☑5ᵗʰ V97.2   Parachutist accident

    ✓x7ᵗʰ **V97.21   Parachutist entangled in object**
       Parachutist landing in tree

    ✓x7ᵗʰ **V97.22   Parachutist injured on landing**

EXCLUDES 1 Not coded here   **EXCLUDES 2** Not included here   N Newborn Age: 0   P Pediatric Age: 0-17   M Maternity Age: 12-55   A Adult Age: 15-124

1022   ICD-10-CM 2014 (Draft)

√x7ᵗʰ **V97.29 Other parachutist accident**

√5ᵗʰ **V97.3 Person on ground injured in air transport accident**

√x7ᵗʰ **V97.31 Hit by object falling from aircraft**
Hit by crashing aircraft
Injured by aircraft hitting house
Injured by aircraft hitting car

√x7ᵗʰ **V97.32 Injured by rotating propeller**

√x7ᵗʰ **V97.33 Sucked into jet engine**

√x7ᵗʰ **V97.39 Other injury to person on ground due to air transport accident**

√5ᵗʰ **V97.8 Other air transport accidents, not elsewhere classified**
EXCLUDES1 aircraft accident NOS (V95.9)
exposure to changes in air pressure during ascent or descent (W94.-)

√6ᵗʰ **V97.81 Air transport accident involving military aircraft**

7ᵗʰ **V97.810 Civilian aircraft involved in air transport accident with military aircraft**
Passenger in civilian aircraft injured due to accident with military aircraft

7ᵗʰ **V97.811 Civilian injured by military aircraft**

7ᵗʰ **V97.818 Other air transport accident involving military aircraft**

√x7ᵗʰ **V97.89 Other air transport accidents, not elsewhere classified**
Injury from machinery on aircraft

Other and unspecified transport accidents (V98-V99)
EXCLUDES1 vehicle accident, type of vehicle unspecified (V89.-)

√4ᵗʰ **V98 Other specified transport accidents**

The appropriate 7th character is to be added to each code from category V98.
A   initial encounter
D   subsequent encounter
S   sequela

√x7ᵗʰ **V98.0 Accident to, on or involving cable-car, not on rails**
Caught or dragged by cable-car, not on rails
Fall or jump from cable-car, not on rails
Object thrown from or in cable-car, not on rails

√x7ᵗʰ **V98.1 Accident to, on or involving land-yacht**

√x7ᵗʰ **V98.2 Accident to, on or involving ice yacht**

√x7ᵗʰ **V98.3 Accident to, on or involving ski lift**
Accident to, on or involving ski chair-lift
Accident to, on or involving ski-lift with gondola

√x7ᵗʰ **V98.8 Other specified transport accidents**

√x7ᵗʰ **V99 Unspecified transport accident**

The appropriate 7th character is to be added to code V99.
A   initial encounter
D   subsequent encounter
S   sequela

OTHER EXTERNAL CAUSES OF ACCIDENTAL INJURY (W00-X58)

Slipping, tripping, stumbling and falls (W00-W19)
EXCLUDES1 assault involving a fall (Y01-Y02)
fall from animal (V80.-)
fall (in) (from) machinery (in operation) (W28-W31)
fall (in) (from) transport vehicle (V01-V99)
intentional self-harm involving a fall (X80-X81)
EXCLUDES2 at risk for fall (history of fall) (Z91.81)
fall (in) (from) burning building (X00.-)
fall into fire (X00-X04, X08-X09)

√4ᵗʰ **W00 Fall due to ice and snow**
INCLUDES pedestrian on foot falling (slipping) on ice and snow
EXCLUDES1 fall on (from) ice and snow involving pedestrian conveyance (V00.-)
fall from stairs and steps not due to ice and snow (W10.-)

The appropriate 7th character is to be added to each code from category W00.
A   initial encounter
D   subsequent encounter
S   sequela

√x7ᵗʰ **W00.0 Fall on same level due to ice and snow**

√x7ᵗʰ **W00.1 Fall from stairs and steps due to ice and snow**

√x7ᵗʰ **W00.2 Other fall from one level to another due to ice and snow**

√x7ᵗʰ **W00.9 Unspecified fall due to ice and snow**

√4ᵗʰ **W01 Fall on same level from slipping, tripping and stumbling**
INCLUDES fall on moving sidewalk
EXCLUDES1 fall due to bumping (striking) against object (W18.0-)
fall in shower or bathtub (W18.2-)
fall on same level NOS (W18.30)
fall on same level from slipping, tripping and stumbling due to ice or snow (W00.0)
fall off or from toilet (W18.1-)
slipping, tripping and stumbling NOS (W18.40)
slipping, tripping and stumbling without falling (W18.4-)

The appropriate 7th character is to be added to each code from category W01.
A   initial encounter
D   subsequent encounter
S   sequela

√x7ᵗʰ **W01.0 Fall on same level from slipping, tripping and stumbling without subsequent striking against object**
Falling over animal

√5ᵗʰ **W01.1 Fall on same level from slipping, tripping and stumbling with subsequent striking against object**

√x7ᵗʰ **W01.10 Fall on same level from slipping, tripping and stumbling with subsequent striking against unspecified object**

√6ᵗʰ **W01.11 Fall on same level from slipping, tripping and stumbling with subsequent striking against sharp object**

7ᵗʰ **W01.110 Fall on same level from slipping, tripping and stumbling with subsequent striking against sharp glass**

7ᵗʰ **W01.111 Fall on same level from slipping, tripping and stumbling with subsequent striking against power tool or machine**

7ᵗʰ **W01.118 Fall on same level from slipping, tripping and stumbling with subsequent striking against other sharp object**

7ᵗʰ **W01.119 Fall on same level from slipping, tripping and stumbling with subsequent striking against unspecified sharp object**

√6ᵗʰ **W01.19 Fall on same level from slipping, tripping and stumbling with subsequent striking against other object**

7ᵗʰ **W01.190 Fall on same level from slipping, tripping and stumbling with subsequent striking against furniture**

7ᵗʰ **W01.198 Fall on same level from slipping, tripping and stumbling with subsequent striking against other object**

√x7ᵗʰ **W03 Other fall on same level due to collision with another person**
Fall due to non-transport collision with other person
EXCLUDES1 collision with another person without fall (W51)
crushed or pushed by a crowd or human stampede (W52)
fall involving pedestrian conveyance (V00-V09)
fall due to ice or snow (W00)
fall on same level NOS (W18.30)

The appropriate 7th character is to be added to code W03.
A   initial encounter
D   subsequent encounter
S   sequela

√x7ᵗʰ **W04 Fall while being carried or supported by other persons**
Accidentally dropped while being carried

The appropriate 7th character is to be added to code W04.
A   initial encounter
D   subsequent encounter
S   sequela

☑ Additional Character Required   √x7ᵗʰ Xtension Alert   Unspecified Code   Other Specified Code   Manifestation Code   ▶◀ Revised Text   ● New Code   ▲ Revised Code Title

W05 Fall from non-moving wheelchair, nonmotorized scooter and motorized mobility scooter
EXCLUDES 1 fall from moving wheelchair (powered) (V00.811)
fall from moving motorized mobility scooter (V00.831)
fall from nonmotorized scooter (V00.141)

The appropriate 7th character is to be added to each code from category W05.
A initial encounter
D subsequent encounter
S sequela

W05.0 Fall from non-moving wheelchair

W05.1 Fall from non-moving nonmotorized scooter

W05.2 Fall from non-moving motorized mobility scooter

W06 Fall from bed

The appropriate 7th character is to be added to code W06.
A initial encounter
D subsequent encounter
S sequela

W07 Fall from chair

The appropriate 7th character is to be added to code W07.
A initial encounter
D subsequent encounter
S sequela

W08 Fall from other furniture

The appropriate 7th character is to be added to code W08.
A initial encounter
D subsequent encounter
S sequela

W09 Fall on and from playground equipment
EXCLUDES 1 fall involving recreational machinery (W31)

The appropriate 7th character is to be added to each code from category W09.
A initial encounter
D subsequent encounter
S sequela

W09.0 Fall on or from playground slide

W09.1 Fall from playground swing

W09.2 Fall on or from jungle gym

W09.8 Fall on or from other playground equipment

W10 Fall on and from stairs and steps
EXCLUDES 1 Fall from stairs and steps due to ice and snow (W00.1)

The appropriate 7th character is to be added to each code from category W10.
A initial encounter
D subsequent encounter
S sequela

W10.0 Fall (on)(from) escalator

W10.1 Fall (on)(from) sidewalk curb

W10.2 Fall (on)(from) incline
Fall (on) (from) ramp

W10.8 Fall (on) (from) other stairs and steps

W10.9 Fall (on) (from) unspecified stairs and steps

W11 Fall on and from ladder

The appropriate 7th character is to be added to code W11.
A initial encounter
D subsequent encounter
S sequela

W12 Fall on and from scaffolding

The appropriate 7th character is to be added to code W12.
A initial encounter
D subsequent encounter
S sequela

W13 Fall from, out of or through building or structure

The appropriate 7th character is to be added to each code from category W13.
A initial encounter
D subsequent encounter
S sequela

W13.0 Fall from, out of or through balcony
Fall from, out of or through railing

W13.1 Fall from, out of or through bridge

W13.2 Fall from, out of or through roof

W13.3 Fall through floor

W13.4 Fall from, out of or through window
EXCLUDES 2 fall with subsequent striking against sharp glass (W01.110)

W13.8 Fall from, out of or through other building or structure
Fall from, out of or through viaduct
Fall from, out of or through wall
Fall from, out of or through flag-pole

W13.9 Fall from, out of or through building, not otherwise specified
EXCLUDES 1 collapse of a building or structure (W20.-)
fall or jump from burning building or structure (X00.-)

W14 Fall from tree

The appropriate 7th character is to be added to code W14.
A initial encounter
D subsequent encounter
S sequela

W15 Fall from cliff

The appropriate 7th character is to be added to code W15.
A initial encounter
D subsequent encounter
S sequela

W16 Fall, jump or diving into water
EXCLUDES 1 accidental non-watercraft drowning and submersion not involving fall (W65-W74)
effects of air pressure from diving (W94.-)
fall into water from watercraft (V90-V94)
hitting an object or against bottom when falling from watercraft (V94.0)
EXCLUDES 2 striking or hitting diving board (W21.4)

The appropriate 7th character is to be added to each code from category W16.
A initial encounter
D subsequent encounter
S sequela

W16.0 Fall into swimming pool
Fall into swimming pool NOS
EXCLUDES 1 fall into empty swimming pool (W17.3)

W16.01 Fall into swimming pool striking water surface

W16.011 Fall into swimming pool striking water surface causing drowning and submersion
EXCLUDES 1 drowning and submersion while in swimming pool without fall (W67)

W16.012 Fall into swimming pool striking water surface causing other injury

W16.02 Fall into swimming pool striking bottom

W16.021 Fall into swimming pool striking bottom causing drowning and submersion
EXCLUDES 1 drowning and submersion while in swimming pool without fall (W67)

W16.022 Fall into swimming pool striking bottom causing other injury

W16.03 Fall into swimming pool striking wall

W16.031 Fall into swimming pool striking wall causing drowning and submersion
EXCLUDES 1 drowning and submersion while in swimming pool without fall (W67)

W16.032 Fall into swimming pool striking wall causing other injury

EXCLUDES 1 Not coded here   EXCLUDES 2 Not included here   N Newborn Age: 0   P Pediatric Age: 0-17   M Maternity Age: 12-55   A Adult Age: 15-124

1024   ICD-10-CM 2014 (Draft)

✓5ᵗʰ **W16.1 Fall into natural body of water**
Fall into lake
Fall into open sea
Fall into river
Fall into stream

✓6ᵗʰ **W16.11 Fall into natural body of water** striking water surface

✓7ᵗʰ **W16.111 Fall into natural body of water striking water surface causing** drowning **and submersion**
EXCLUDES 1 *drowning and submersion while in natural body of water without fall (W69)*

✓7ᵗʰ **W16.112 Fall into natural body of water striking water surface causing other injury**

✓6ᵗʰ **W16.12 Fall into natural body of water** striking bottom

✓7ᵗʰ **W16.121 Fall into natural body of water striking bottom causing** drowning **and submersion**
EXCLUDES 1 *drowning and submersion while in natural body of water without fall (W69)*

✓7ᵗʰ **W16.122 Fall into natural body of water striking bottom causing other injury**

✓6ᵗʰ **W16.13 Fall into natural body of water** striking side

✓7ᵗʰ **W16.131 Fall into natural body of water striking side causing** drowning **and submersion**
EXCLUDES 1 *drowning and submersion while in natural body of water without fall (W69)*

✓7ᵗʰ **W16.132 Fall into natural body of water striking side causing other injury**

✓5ᵗʰ **W16.2 Fall in (into) filled bathtub or bucket of water**

✓6ᵗʰ **W16.21 Fall in (into)** filled bathtub
EXCLUDES 1 *fall into empty bathtub (W18.2)*

✓7ᵗʰ **W16.211 Fall in (into) filled bathtub causing** drowning **and submersion**
EXCLUDES 1 *drowning and submersion while in filled bathtub without fall (W65)*

✓7ᵗʰ **W16.212 Fall in (into) filled bathtub causing other injury**

✓6ᵗʰ **W16.22 Fall in (into)** bucket of water

✓7ᵗʰ **W16.221 Fall in (into) bucket of water causing** drowning **and submersion**

✓7ᵗʰ **W16.222 Fall in (into) bucket of water causing other injury**

✓5ᵗʰ **W16.3 Fall into other water**
Fall into fountain
Fall into reservoir

✓6ᵗʰ **W16.31 Fall into other water** striking water surface

✓7ᵗʰ **W16.311 Fall into other water striking water surface causing** drowning **and submersion**
EXCLUDES 1 *drowning and submersion while in other water without fall (W73)*

✓7ᵗʰ **W16.312 Fall into other water striking water surface causing other injury**

✓6ᵗʰ **W16.32 Fall into other water** striking bottom

✓7ᵗʰ **W16.321 Fall into other water striking bottom causing** drowning **and submersion**
EXCLUDES 1 *drowning and submersion while in other water without fall (W73)*

✓7ᵗʰ **W16.322 Fall into other water striking bottom causing other injury**

✓6ᵗʰ **W16.33 Fall into other water** striking wall

✓7ᵗʰ **W16.331 Fall into other water striking wall causing** drowning **and submersion**
EXCLUDES 1 *drowning and submersion while in other water without fall (W73)*

✓7ᵗʰ **W16.332 Fall into other water striking wall causing other injury**

✓5ᵗʰ **W16.4 Fall into unspecified water**

✓x7ᵗʰ **W16.41 Fall into unspecified water causing drowning and submersion**

✓x7ᵗʰ **W16.42 Fall into unspecified water causing other injury**

✓5ᵗʰ **W16.5 Jumping or diving into swimming pool**

✓6ᵗʰ **W16.51 Jumping or diving into swimming pool** striking water surface

✓7ᵗʰ **W16.511 Jumping or diving into swimming pool striking water surface causing** drowning **and submersion**
EXCLUDES 1 *drowning and submersion while in swimming pool without jumping or diving (W67)*

✓7ᵗʰ **W16.512 Jumping or diving into swimming pool striking water surface causing other injury**

✓6ᵗʰ **W16.52 Jumping or diving into swimming pool** striking bottom

✓7ᵗʰ **W16.521 Jumping or diving into swimming pool striking bottom causing** drowning **and submersion**
EXCLUDES 1 *drowning and submersion while in swimming pool without jumping or diving (W67)*

✓7ᵗʰ **W16.522 Jumping or diving into swimming pool striking bottom causing other injury**

✓6ᵗʰ **W16.53 Jumping or diving into swimming pool** striking wall

✓7ᵗʰ **W16.531 Jumping or diving into swimming pool striking wall causing** drowning **and submersion**
EXCLUDES 1 *drowning and submersion while in swimming pool without jumping or diving (W67)*

✓7ᵗʰ **W16.532 Jumping or diving into swimming pool striking wall causing other injury**

✓5ᵗʰ **W16.6 Jumping or diving into** natural body of water
Jumping or diving into lake
Jumping or diving into open sea
Jumping or diving into river
Jumping or diving into stream

✓6ᵗʰ **W16.61 Jumping or diving into natural body of water** striking water surface

✓7ᵗʰ **W16.611 Jumping or diving into natural body of water striking water surface causing** drowning **and submersion**
EXCLUDES 1 *drowning and submersion while in natural body of water without jumping or diving (W69)*

✓7ᵗʰ **W16.612 Jumping or diving into natural body of water striking water surface causing other injury**

✓6ᵗʰ **W16.62 Jumping or diving into natural body of water** striking bottom

✓7ᵗʰ **W16.621 Jumping or diving into natural body of water striking bottom causing** drowning **and submersion**
EXCLUDES 1 *drowning and submersion while in natural body of water without jumping or diving (W69)*

✓7ᵗʰ **W16.622 Jumping or diving into natural body of water striking bottom causing other injury**

✓5ᵗʰ **W16.7 Jumping or diving** from boat
EXCLUDES 1 *Fall from boat into water—see watercraft accident (V90-V94)*

✓6ᵗʰ **W16.71 Jumping or diving from boat** striking water surface

✓7ᵗʰ **W16.711 Jumping or diving from boat striking water surface causing** drowning **and submersion**

✓7ᵗʰ **W16.712 Jumping or diving from boat striking water surface causing other injury**

✓6ᵗʰ **W16.72 Jumping or diving from boat** striking bottom

✓7ᵗʰ **W16.721 Jumping or diving from boat striking bottom causing** drowning **and submersion**

✓7ᵗʰ **W16.722 Jumping or diving from boat striking bottom causing other injury**

External Causes of Morbidity

W16.1–W16.722

External Causes of Morbidity

W16.8–W20.8

✓5ᵗʰ **W16.8 Jumping or diving into other water**
Jumping or diving into fountain
Jumping or diving into reservoir

✓6ᵗʰ **W16.81 Jumping or diving into other water striking water surface**

✓7ᵗʰ **W16.811 Jumping or diving into other water striking water surface causing drowning and submersion**
EXCLUDES 1   drowning and submersion while in other water without jumping or diving (W73)

✓7ᵗʰ **W16.812 Jumping or diving into other water striking water surface causing other injury**

✓6ᵗʰ **W16.82 Jumping or diving into other water striking bottom**

✓7ᵗʰ **W16.821 Jumping or diving into other water striking bottom causing drowning and submersion**
EXCLUDES 1   drowning and submersion while in other water without jumping or diving (W73)

✓7ᵗʰ **W16.822 Jumping or diving into other water striking bottom causing other injury**

✓6ᵗʰ **W16.83 Jumping or diving into other water striking wall**

✓7ᵗʰ **W16.831 Jumping or diving into other water striking wall causing drowning and submersion**
EXCLUDES 1   drowning and submersion while in other water without jumping or diving (W73)

✓7ᵗʰ **W16.832 Jumping or diving into other water striking wall causing other injury**

✓5ᵗʰ **W16.9 Jumping or diving into unspecified water**

✓x7ᵗʰ **W16.91 Jumping or diving into unspecified water causing drowning and submersion**

✓x7ᵗʰ **W16.92 Jumping or diving into unspecified water causing other injury**

✓4ᵗʰ **W17 Other fall from one level to another**

The appropriate 7th character is to be added to each code from category W17.
A   initial encounter
D   subsequent encounter
S   sequela

✓x7ᵗʰ **W17.0 Fall into well**

✓x7ᵗʰ **W17.1 Fall into storm drain or manhole**

✓x7ᵗʰ **W17.2 Fall into hole**
Fall into pit

✓x7ᵗʰ **W17.3 Fall into empty swimming pool**
EXCLUDES 1   fall into filled swimming pool (W16.0-)

✓x7ᵗʰ **W17.4 Fall from dock**

✓5ᵗʰ **W17.8 Other fall from one level to another**

✓x7ᵗʰ **W17.81 Fall down embankment (hill)**

✓x7ᵗʰ **W17.82 Fall from (out of) grocery cart**
Fall due to grocery cart tipping over

✓x7ᵗʰ **W17.89 Other fall from one level to another**
Fall from cherry picker
Fall from lifting device
Fall from mobile elevated work platform [MEWP]
Fall from sky lift

✓4ᵗʰ **W18 Other slipping, tripping and stumbling and falls**

The appropriate 7th character is to be added to each code from category W18.
A   initial encounter
D   subsequent encounter
S   sequela

✓5ᵗʰ **W18.0 Fall due to bumping against object**
Striking against object with subsequent fall
EXCLUDES 1   fall on same level due to slipping, tripping, or stumbling with subsequent striking against object (W01.1-)

✓x7ᵗʰ **W18.00 Striking against unspecified object with subsequent fall**

✓x7ᵗʰ **W18.01 Striking against sports equipment with subsequent fall**

✓x7ᵗʰ **W18.02 Striking against glass with subsequent fall**

✓x7ᵗʰ **W18.09 Striking against other object with subsequent fall**

✓5ᵗʰ **W18.1 Fall from or off toilet**

✓x7ᵗʰ **W18.11 Fall from or off toilet without subsequent striking against object**
Fall from (off) toilet NOS

✓x7ᵗʰ **W18.12 Fall from or off toilet with subsequent striking against object**

✓x7ᵗʰ **W18.2 Fall in (into) shower or empty bathtub**
EXCLUDES 1   fall in full bathtub causing drowning or submersion (W16.21-)

✓5ᵗʰ **W18.3 Other and unspecified fall on same level**

✓x7ᵗʰ **W18.30 Fall on same level, unspecified**

✓x7ᵗʰ **W18.31 Fall on same level due to stepping on an object**
Fall on same level due to stepping on an animal
EXCLUDES 1   slipping, tripping and stumbling without fall due to stepping on animal (W18.41)

✓x7ᵗʰ **W18.39 Other fall on same level**

✓5ᵗʰ **W18.4 Slipping, tripping and stumbling without falling**
EXCLUDES 1   collision with another person without fall (W51)

✓x7ᵗʰ **W18.40 Slipping, tripping and stumbling without falling, unspecified**

✓x7ᵗʰ **W18.41 Slipping, tripping and stumbling without falling due to stepping on object**
Slipping, tripping and stumbling without falling due to stepping on animal
EXCLUDES 1   slipping, tripping and stumbling with fall due to stepping on animal (W18.31)

✓x7ᵗʰ **W18.42 Slipping, tripping and stumbling without falling due to stepping into hole or opening**

✓x7ᵗʰ **W18.43 Slipping, tripping and stumbling without falling due to stepping from one level to another**

✓x7ᵗʰ **W18.49 Other slipping, tripping and stumbling without falling**

✓x7ᵗʰ **W19 Unspecified fall**
Accidental fall NOS

The appropriate 7th character is to be added to code W19.
A   initial encounter
D   subsequent encounter
S   sequela

Exposure to inanimate mechanical forces (W20-W49)

EXCLUDES 1   assault (X92-Y08)
contact or collision with animals or persons (W50-W64)
exposure to inanimate mechanical forces involving military or war operations (Y36-, Y37-)
intentional self-harm (X71-X83)

✓4ᵗʰ **W20 Struck by thrown, projected or falling object**
Code first any associated:
cataclysm (X34-X39)
lightning strike (T75.00)
EXCLUDES 1   falling object in machinery accident (W24, W28-W31)
falling object in transport accident (V01-V99)
object set in motion by explosion (W35-W40)
object set in motion by firearm (W32-W34)

The appropriate 7th character is to be added to each code from category W20.
A   initial encounter
D   subsequent encounter
S   sequela

✓x7ᵗʰ **W20.0 Struck by falling object in cave-in**
EXCLUDES 2   asphyxiation due to cave-in (T71.21)

✓x7ᵗʰ **W20.1 Struck by object due to collapse of building**
EXCLUDES 1   struck by object due to collapse of burning building (X00.2, X02.2)

✓x7ᵗʰ **W20.8 Other cause of strike by thrown, projected or falling object**
EXCLUDES 1   struck by thrown sports equipment (W21.-)

EXCLUDES 1 Not coded here   EXCLUDES 2 Not included here   N Newborn Age: 0   P Pediatric Age: 0-17   M Maternity Age: 12-55   A Adult Age: 15-124

1026   ICD-10-CM 2014 (Draft)

☑4ᵗʰ **W21 Striking against or struck by sports equipment**
     EXCLUDES 1   *assault with sports equipment (Y08.0-)*
                striking against or struck by sports equipment with subsequent fall (W18.01)

The appropriate 7th character is to be added to each code from category W21.
A   initial encounter
D   subsequent encounter
S   sequela

☑5ᵗʰ **W21.0 Struck by hit or thrown ball**
     ✓x7ᵗʰ **W21.00 Struck by hit or thrown ball, unspecified type**
     ✓x7ᵗʰ **W21.01 Struck by football**
     ✓x7ᵗʰ **W21.02 Struck by soccer ball**
     ✓x7ᵗʰ **W21.03 Struck by baseball**
     ✓x7ᵗʰ **W21.04 Struck by golf ball**
     ✓x7ᵗʰ **W21.05 Struck by basketball**
     ✓x7ᵗʰ **W21.06 Struck by volleyball**
     ✓x7ᵗʰ **W21.07 Struck by softball**
     ✓x7ᵗʰ **W21.09 Struck by other hit or thrown ball**

☑5ᵗʰ **W21.1 Struck by bat, racquet or club**
     ✓x7ᵗʰ **W21.11 Struck by baseball bat**
     ✓x7ᵗʰ **W21.12 Struck by tennis racquet**
     ✓x7ᵗʰ **W21.13 Struck by golf club**
     ✓x7ᵗʰ **W21.19 Struck by other bat, racquet or club**

☑5ᵗʰ **W21.2 Struck by hockey stick or puck**
     ✓6ᵗʰ **W21.21 Struck by hockey stick**
         ✓7ᵗʰ **W21.210 Struck by ice hockey stick**
         ✓7ᵗʰ **W21.211 Struck by field hockey stick**
     ✓6ᵗʰ **W21.22 Struck by hockey puck**
         ✓7ᵗʰ **W21.220 Struck by ice hockey puck**
         ✓7ᵗʰ **W21.221 Struck by field hockey puck**

☑5ᵗʰ **W21.3 Struck by sports foot wear**
     ✓x7ᵗʰ **W21.31 Struck by shoe cleats**
            Stepped on by shoe cleats
     ✓x7ᵗʰ **W21.32 Struck by skate blades**
            Skated over by skate blades
     ✓x7ᵗʰ **W21.39 Struck by other sports foot wear**

✓x7ᵗʰ **W21.4 Striking against diving board**
     Use additional code for subsequent falling into water, if applicable (W16.-)

☑5ᵗʰ **W21.8 Striking against or struck by other sports equipment**
     ✓x7ᵗʰ **W21.81 Striking against or struck by football helmet**
     ✓x7ᵗʰ **W21.89 Striking against or struck by other sports equipment**

✓x7ᵗʰ **W21.9 Striking against or struck by unspecified sports equipment**

☑4ᵗʰ **W22 Striking against or struck by other objects**
     EXCLUDES 1   *striking against or struck by object with subsequent fall (W18.09)*

The appropriate 7th character is to be added to each code from category W22.
A   initial encounter
D   subsequent encounter
S   sequela

☑5ᵗʰ **W22.0 Striking against stationary object**
     EXCLUDES 1   *striking against stationary sports equipment (W21.8)*
     ✓x7ᵗʰ **W22.01 Walked into wall**
     ✓x7ᵗʰ **W22.02 Walked into lamppost**
     ✓x7ᵗʰ **W22.03 Walked into furniture**
     ✓6ᵗʰ **W22.04 Striking against wall of swimming pool**
         ✓7ᵗʰ **W22.041 Striking against wall of swimming pool causing drowning and submersion**
             EXCLUDES 1   *drowning and submersion while swimming without striking against wall (W67)*
         ✓7ᵗʰ **W22.042 Striking against wall of swimming pool causing other injury**
     ✓x7ᵗʰ **W22.09 Striking against other stationary object**

☑5ᵗʰ **W22.1 Striking against or struck by automobile airbag**
     ✓x7ᵗʰ **W22.10 Striking against or struck by unspecified automobile airbag**

     ✓x7ᵗʰ **W22.11 Striking against or struck by driver side automobile airbag**
     ✓x7ᵗʰ **W22.12 Striking against or struck by front passenger side automobile airbag**
     ✓x7ᵗʰ **W22.19 Striking against or struck by other automobile airbag**

☑x7ᵗʰ **W22.8 Striking against or struck by other objects**
     Striking against or struck by object NOS
     EXCLUDES 1   *struck by thrown, projected or falling object (W20.-)*

☑4ᵗʰ **W23 Caught, crushed, jammed or pinched in or between objects**
     EXCLUDES 1   *injury caused by cutting or piercing instruments (W25-W27)*
                injury caused by firearms malfunction (W32.1, W33.1-, W34.1-)
                injury caused by lifting and transmission devices (W24.-)
                injury caused by machinery (W28-W31)
                injury caused by nonpowered hand tools (W27.-)
                injury caused by transport vehicle being used as a means of transportation (V01-V99)
                injury caused by struck by thrown, projected or falling object (W20.-)

The appropriate 7th character is to be added to each code from category W23.
A   initial encounter
D   subsequent encounter
S   sequela

✓x7ᵗʰ **W23.0 Caught, crushed, jammed, or pinched between moving objects**

✓x7ᵗʰ **W23.1 Caught, crushed, jammed, or pinched between stationary objects**

☑4ᵗʰ **W24 Contact with lifting and transmission devices, not elsewhere classified**
     EXCLUDES 1   *transport accidents (V01-V99)*

The appropriate 7th character is to be added to each code from category W24.
A   initial encounter
D   subsequent encounter
S   sequela

✓x7ᵗʰ **W24.0 Contact with lifting devices, not elsewhere classified**
     Contact with chain hoist
     Contact with drive belt
     Contact with pulley (block)

✓x7ᵗʰ **W24.1 Contact with transmission devices, not elsewhere classified**
     Contact with transmission belt or cable

✓x7ᵗʰ **W25 Contact with sharp glass**
     Code first any associated:
       injury due to flying glass from explosion or firearm discharge (W32-W40)
       transport accident (V00-V99)
     EXCLUDES 1   *fall on same level due to slipping, tripping and stumbling with subsequent striking against sharp glass (W01.10)*
                striking against sharp glass with subsequent fall (W18.02)

The appropriate 7th character is to be added to code W25.
A   initial encounter
D   subsequent encounter
S   sequela

☑4ᵗʰ **W26 Contact with knife, sword or dagger**

The appropriate 7th character is to be added to each code from category W26.
A   initial encounter
D   subsequent encounter
S   sequela

✓x7ᵗʰ **W26.0 Contact with knife**
     EXCLUDES 1   *contact with electric knife (W29.1)*

✓x7ᵗʰ **W26.1 Contact with sword or dagger**

☑4ᵗʰ **W27 Contact with nonpowered hand tool**

The appropriate 7th character is to be added to each code from category W27.
A   initial encounter
D   subsequent encounter
S   sequela

✓x7ᵗʰ **W27.0 Contact with workbench tool**
     Contact with auger
     Contact with axe
     Contact with chisel
     Contact with handsaw
     Contact with screwdriver

External Causes of Morbidity

W27.1–W31.9

✓x7th **W27.1 Contact with garden tool**
 Contact with hoe
 Contact with nonpowered lawn mower
 Contact with pitchfork
 Contact with rake

✓x7th **W27.2 Contact with scissors**

✓x7th **W27.3 Contact with needle (sewing)**
 EXCLUDES 1 *contact with hypodermic needle (W46.-)*

✓x7th **W27.4 Contact with kitchen utensil**
 Contact with fork
 Contact with ice-pick
 Contact with can-opener NOS

✓x7th **W27.5 Contact with paper-cutter**

✓x7th **W27.8 Contact with other nonpowered hand tool**
 Contact with nonpowered sewing machine
 Contact with shovel

✓x7th **W28 Contact with powered lawn mower**
 Powered lawn mower (commercial) (residential)
 EXCLUDES 1 *contact with nonpowered lawn mower (W27.1)*
 EXCLUDES 2 *exposure to electric current (W86.-)*

 The appropriate 7th character is to be added to code W28.
 A initial encounter
 D subsequent encounter
 S sequela

✓4th **W29 Contact with other powered hand tools and household machinery**
 EXCLUDES 1 *contact with commercial machinery (W31.82)*
 contact with hot household appliance (X15)
 contact with nonpowered hand tool (W27.-)
 exposure to electric current (W86)

 The appropriate 7th character is to be added to each code from category W29.
 A initial encounter
 D subsequent encounter
 S sequela

✓x7th **W29.0 Contact with powered kitchen appliance**
 Contact with blender
 Contact with can-opener
 Contact with garbage disposal
 Contact with mixer

✓x7th **W29.1 Contact with electric knife**

✓x7th **W29.2 Contact with other powered household machinery**
 Contact with electric fan
 Contact with powered dryer (clothes) (powered) (spin)
 Contact with washing-machine
 Contact with sewing machine

✓x7th **W29.3 Contact with powered garden and outdoor hand tools and machinery**
 Contact with chainsaw
 Contact with edger
 Contact with garden cultivator (tiller)
 Contact with hedge trimmer
 Contact with other powered garden tool
 EXCLUDES 1 *contact with powered lawn mower (W28)*

✓x7th **W29.4 Contact with nail gun**

✓x7th **W29.8 Contact with other powered hand tools and household machinery**
 Contact with do-it-yourself tool NOS

✓4th **W30 Contact with agricultural machinery**
 INCLUDES animal-powered farm machine
 EXCLUDES 1 *agricultural transport vehicle accident (V01-V99)*
 explosion of grain store (W40.8)
 exposure to electric current (W86.-)

 The appropriate 7th character is to be added to each code from category W30.
 A initial encounter
 D subsequent encounter
 S sequela

✓x7th **W30.0 Contact with combine harvester**
 Contact with reaper
 Contact with thresher

✓x7th **W30.1 Contact with power take-off devices (PTO)**

✓x7th **W30.2 Contact with hay derrick**

✓x7th **W30.3 Contact with grain storage elevator**
 EXCLUDES 1 *explosion of grain store (W40.8)*

✓5th **W30.8 Contact with other specified agricultural machinery**

✓x7th **W30.81 Contact with agricultural transport vehicle in stationary use**
 Contact with agricultural transport vehicle under repair, not on public roadway
 EXCLUDES 1 *agricultural transport vehicle accident (V01-V99)*

✓x7th **W30.89 Contact with other specified agricultural machinery**

✓x7th **W30.9 Contact with unspecified agricultural machinery**
 Contact with farm machinery NOS

✓4th **W31 Contact with other and unspecified machinery**
 EXCLUDES 1 *contact with agricultural machinery (W30.-)*
 contact with machinery in transport under own power or being towed by a vehicle (V01-V99)
 exposure to electric current (W86)

 The appropriate 7th character is to be added to each code from category W31.
 A initial encounter
 D subsequent encounter
 S sequela

✓x7th **W31.0 Contact with mining and earth-drilling machinery**
 Contact with bore or drill (land) (seabed)
 Contact with shaft hoist
 Contact with shaft lift
 Contact with undercutter

✓x7th **W31.1 Contact with metalworking machines**
 Contact with abrasive wheel
 Contact with forging machine
 Contact with lathe
 Contact with mechanical shears
 Contact with metal drilling machine
 Contact with milling machine
 Contact with power press
 Contact with rolling-mill
 Contact with metal sawing machine

✓x7th **W31.2 Contact with powered woodworking and forming machines**
 Contact with band saw
 Contact with bench saw
 Contact with circular saw
 Contact with molding machine
 Contact with overhead plane
 Contact with powered saw
 Contact with radial saw
 Contact with sander
 EXCLUDES 1 *nonpowered woodworking tools (W27.0)*

✓x7th **W31.3 Contact with prime movers**
 Contact with gas turbine
 Contact with internal combustion engine
 Contact with steam engine
 Contact with water driven turbine

✓5th **W31.8 Contact with other specified machinery**

✓x7th **W31.81 Contact with recreational machinery**
 Contact with roller coaster

✓x7th **W31.82 Contact with other commercial machinery**
 Contact with commercial electric fan
 Contact with commercial kitchen appliances
 Contact with commercial powered dryer (clothes) (powered) (spin)
 Contact with commercial washing-machine
 Contact with commercial sewing machine
 EXCLUDES 1 *contact with household machinery (W29.-)*
 contact with powered lawn mower (W28)

✓x7th **W31.83 Contact with special construction vehicle in stationary use**
 Contact with special construction vehicle under repair, not on public roadway
 EXCLUDES 1 *special construction vehicle accident (V01-V99)*

✓x7th **W31.89 Contact with other specified machinery**

✓x7th **W31.9 Contact with unspecified machinery**
 Contact with machinery NOS

☑4ᵗʰ **W32 Accidental handgun discharge and malfunction**

     INCLUDES   Accidental discharge and malfunction of gun for single hand use

         Accidental discharge and malfunction of pistol

         Accidental discharge and malfunction of revolver

         Handgun discharge and malfunction NOS

     EXCLUDES 1   *accidental airgun discharge and malfunction (W34.010, W34.110)*

         accidental BB gun discharge and malfunction (W34.010, W34.110)

         accidental pellet gun discharge and malfunction (W34.010, W34.110)

         accidental shotgun discharge and malfunction (W33.01, W33.11)

         assault by handgun discharge (X93)

         handgun discharge involving legal intervention (Y35.0-)

         handgun discharge involving military or war operations (Y36.4-)

         intentional self-harm by handgun discharge (X72)

         Very pistol discharge and malfunction (W34.09, W34.19)

     The appropriate 7th character is to be added to each code from category W32.

     A   initial encounter

     D   subsequent encounter

     S   sequela

√x7ᵗʰ **W32.0 Accidental handgun discharge**

√x7ᵗʰ **W32.1 Accidental handgun malfunction**

     Injury due to explosion of handgun (parts)

     Injury due to malfunction of mechanism or component of handgun

     Injury due to recoil of handgun

     Powder burn from handgun

☑4ᵗʰ **W33 Accidental rifle, shotgun and larger firearm discharge and malfunction**

     INCLUDES   rifle, shotgun and larger firearm discharge and malfunction NOS

     EXCLUDES 1   *accidental airgun discharge and malfunction (W34.010, W34.110)*

         accidental BB gun discharge and malfunction (W34.010, W34.110)

         accidental handgun discharge and malfunction (W32.-)

         accidental pellet gun discharge and malfunction (W34.010, W34.110)

         assault by rifle, shotgun and larger firearm discharge (X94)

         firearm discharge involving legal intervention (Y35.0-)

         firearm discharge involving military or war operations (Y36.4-)

         intentional self-harm by rifle, shotgun and larger firearm discharge (X73)

     The appropriate 7th character is to be added to each code from category W33.

     A   initial encounter

     D   subsequent encounter

     S   sequela

☑5ᵗʰ **W33.0 Accidental rifle, shotgun and larger firearm discharge**

√x7ᵗʰ **W33.00 Accidental discharge of unspecified larger firearm**

     Discharge of unspecified larger firearm NOS

√x7ᵗʰ **W33.01 Accidental discharge of shotgun**

     Discharge of shotgun NOS

√x7ᵗʰ **W33.02 Accidental discharge of hunting rifle**

     Discharge of hunting rifle NOS

√x7ᵗʰ **W33.03 Accidental discharge of machine gun**

     Discharge of machine gun NOS

√x7ᵗʰ **W33.09 Accidental discharge of other larger firearm**

     Discharge of other larger firearm NOS

☑5ᵗʰ **W33.1 Accidental rifle, shotgun and larger firearm malfunction**

     Injury due to explosion of rifle, shotgun and larger firearm (parts)

     Injury due to malfunction of mechanism or component of rifle, shotgun and larger firearm

     Injury due to piercing, cutting, crushing or pinching due to (by) slide trigger mechanism, scope or other gun part

     Injury due to recoil of rifle, shotgun and larger firearm

     Powder burn from rifle, shotgun and larger firearm

√x7ᵗʰ **W33.10 Accidental malfunction of unspecified larger firearm**

     Malfunction of unspecified larger firearm NOS

√x7ᵗʰ **W33.11 Accidental malfunction of shotgun**

     Malfunction of shotgun NOS

√x7ᵗʰ **W33.12 Accidental malfunction of hunting rifle**

     Malfunction of hunting rifle NOS

√x7ᵗʰ **W33.13 Accidental malfunction of machine gun**

     Malfunction of machine gun NOS

√x7ᵗʰ **W33.19 Accidental malfunction of other larger firearm**

     Malfunction of other larger firearm NOS

☑4ᵗʰ **W34 Accidental discharge and malfunction from other and unspecified firearms and guns**

     The appropriate 7th character is to be added to each code from category W34.

     A   initial encounter

     D   subsequent encounter

     S   sequela

☑5ᵗʰ **W34.0 Accidental discharge from other and unspecified firearms and guns**

√x7ᵗʰ **W34.00 Accidental discharge from unspecified firearms or gun**

     Discharge from firearm NOS

     Gunshot wound NOS

     Shot NOS

☑6ᵗʰ **W34.01 Accidental discharge of gas, air or spring-operated guns**

√7ᵗʰ **W34.010 Accidental discharge of airgun**

     Accidental discharge of BB gun

     Accidental discharge of pellet gun

√7ᵗʰ **W34.011 Accidental discharge of paintball gun**

     Accidental injury due to paintball discharge

√7ᵗʰ **W34.018 Accidental discharge of other gas, air or spring-operated gun**

√x7ᵗʰ **W34.09 Accidental discharge from other specified firearms**

     Accidental discharge from Very pistol [flare]

☑5ᵗʰ **W34.1 Accidental malfunction from other and unspecified firearms and guns**

√x7ᵗʰ **W34.10 Accidental malfunction from unspecified firearms or gun**

     Firearm malfunction NOS

☑6ᵗʰ **W34.11 Accidental malfunction of gas, air or spring-operated guns**

√7ᵗʰ **W34.110 Accidental malfunction of airgun**

     Accidental malfunction of BB gun

     Accidental malfunction of pellet gun

√7ᵗʰ **W34.111 Accidental malfunction of paintball gun**

     Accidental injury due to paintball gun malfunction

√7ᵗʰ **W34.118 Accidental malfunction of other gas, air or spring-operated gun**

√x7ᵗʰ **W34.19 Accidental malfunction from other specified firearms**

     Accidental malfunction from Very pistol [flare]

√x7ᵗʰ **W35 Explosion and rupture of boiler**

     EXCLUDES 1   *explosion and rupture of boiler on watercraft (V93.4)*

     The appropriate 7th character is to be added to code W35.

     A   initial encounter

     D   subsequent encounter

     S   sequela

☑4ᵗʰ **W36 Explosion and rupture of gas cylinder**

     The appropriate 7th character is to be added to each code from category W36.

     A   initial encounter

     D   subsequent encounter

     S   sequela

√x7ᵗʰ **W36.1 Explosion and rupture of aerosol can**

√x7ᵗʰ **W36.2 Explosion and rupture of air tank**

√x7ᵗʰ **W36.3 Explosion and rupture of pressurized-gas tank**

√x7ᵗʰ **W36.8 Explosion and rupture of other gas cylinder**

√x7ᵗʰ **W36.9 Explosion and rupture of unspecified gas cylinder**

☑4ᵗʰ **W37 Explosion and rupture of pressurized tire, pipe or hose**

     The appropriate 7th character is to be added to each code from category W37.

     A   initial encounter

     D   subsequent encounter

     S   sequela

√x7ᵗʰ **W37.0 Explosion of bicycle tire**

√x7ᵗʰ **W37.8 Explosion and rupture of other pressurized tire, pipe or hose**

☑ Additional Character Required   √x7ᵗʰ Xtension Alert   Unspecified Code   Other Specified Code   Manifestation Code   ►◄ Revised Text   ● New Code   ▲ Revised Code Title

External Causes of Morbidity

W38–W52

✓x7th W38 Explosion and rupture of other specified pressurized devices

> The appropriate 7th character is to be added to code W38.
> A   initial encounter
> D   subsequent encounter
> S   sequela

✓x7th W39 Discharge of firework

> The appropriate 7th character is to be added to code W39.
> A   initial encounter
> D   subsequent encounter
> S   sequela

✓4th W40 Explosion of other materials

> EXCLUDES1   assault by explosive material (X96)
> explosion involving legal intervention (Y35.1-)
> explosion involving military or war operations (Y36.0-, Y36.2-)
> intentional self-harm by explosive material (X75)

> The appropriate 7th character is to be added to each code from category W40.
> A   initial encounter
> D   subsequent encounter
> S   sequela

✓x7th W40.0 Explosion of blasting material
> Explosion of blasting cap
> Explosion of detonator
> Explosion of dynamite
> Explosion of explosive (any) used in blasting operations

✓x7th W40.1 Explosion of explosive gases
> Explosion of acetylene
> Explosion of butane
> Explosion of coal gas
> Explosion in mine NOS
> Explosion of explosive gas
> Explosion of fire damp
> Explosion of gasoline fumes
> Explosion of methane
> Explosion of propane

✓x7th W40.8 Explosion of other specified explosive materials
> Explosion in dump NOS
> Explosion in factory NOS
> Explosion in grain store
> Explosion in munitions
> EXCLUDES1   explosion involving legal intervention (Y35.1-)
> explosion involving military or war operations (Y36.0-, Y36.2-)

✓x7th W40.9 Explosion of unspecified explosive materials
> Explosion NOS

✓4th W42 Exposure to noise

> The appropriate 7th character is to be added to each code from category W42.
> A   initial encounter
> D   subsequent encounter
> S   sequela

✓x7th W42.0 Exposure to supersonic waves
✓x7th W42.9 Exposure to other noise
> Exposure to sound waves NOS

✓4th W45 Foreign body or object entering through skin

> EXCLUDES2   contact with hand tools (nonpowered) (powered) (W27-W29)
> contact with knife, sword or dagger (W26.-)
> contact with sharp glass (W25.-)
> struck by objects (W20-W22)

> The appropriate 7th character is to be added to each code from category W45.
> A   initial encounter
> D   subsequent encounter
> S   sequela

✓x7th W45.0 Nail entering through skin
✓x7th W45.1 Paper entering through skin
> Paper cut
✓x7th W45.2 Lid of can entering through skin
✓x7th W45.8 Other foreign body or object entering through skin
> Splinter in skin NOS

✓4th W46 Contact with hypodermic needle

> The appropriate 7th character is to be added to each code from category W46.
> A   initial encounter
> D   subsequent encounter
> S   sequela

✓x7th W46.0 Contact with hypodermic needle
> Hypodermic needle stick NOS
✓x7th W46.1 Contact with contaminated hypodermic needle

✓4th W49 Exposure to other inanimate mechanical forces
> INCLUDES   exposure to abnormal gravitational [G] forces
> exposure to inanimate mechanical forces NEC
> EXCLUDES1   exposure to inanimate mechanical forces involving military or war operations (Y36-, Y37-)

> The appropriate 7th character is to be added to each code from category W49.
> A   initial encounter
> D   subsequent encounter
> S   sequela

✓5th W49.0 Item causing external constriction
✓x7th W49.01 Hair causing external constriction
✓x7th W49.02 String or thread causing external constriction
✓x7th W49.03 Rubber band causing external constriction
✓x7th W49.04 Ring or other jewelry causing external constriction
✓x7th W49.09 Other specified item causing external constriction
✓x7th W49.9 Exposure to other inanimate mechanical forces

Exposure to animate mechanical forces (W50-W64)
> EXCLUDES1   Toxic effect of contact with venomous animals and plants (T63.-)

✓4th W50 Accidental hit, strike, kick, twist, bite or scratch by another person
> Hit, strike, kick, twist, bite, or scratch by another person NOS
> EXCLUDES1   assault by bodily force (Y04)
> struck by objects (W20-W22)

> The appropriate 7th character is to be added to each code from category W50.
> A   initial encounter
> D   subsequent encounter
> S   sequela

✓x7th W50.0 Accidental hit or strike by another person
> Hit or strike by another person NOS
✓x7th W50.1 Accidental kick by another person
> Kick by another person NOS
✓x7th W50.2 Accidental twist by another person
> Twist by another person NOS
✓x7th W50.3 Accidental bite by another person
> Human bite
> Bite by another person NOS
✓x7th W50.4 Accidental scratch by another person
> Scratch by another person NOS

✓x7th W51 Accidental striking against or bumped into by another person
> EXCLUDES1   assault by striking against or bumping into by another person (Y04.2)
> fall due to collision with another person (W03)

> The appropriate 7th character is to be added to code W51.
> A   initial encounter
> D   subsequent encounter
> S   sequela

✓x7th W52 Crushed, pushed or stepped on by crowd or human stampede
> Crushed, pushed or stepped on by crowd or human stampede with or without fall

> The appropriate 7th character is to be added to code W52.
> A   initial encounter
> D   subsequent encounter
> S   sequela

✓4ᵗʰ W53 Contact with rodent
Contact with saliva, feces or urine of rodent

The appropriate 7th character is to be added to each code from category W53.
A   initial encounter
D   subsequent encounter
S   sequela

✓5ᵗʰ W53.0 Contact with mouse
 ✓x7ᵗʰ W53.01 Bitten by mouse
 ✓x7ᵗʰ W53.09 Other contact with mouse

✓5ᵗʰ W53.1 Contact with rat
 ✓x7ᵗʰ W53.11 Bitten by rat
 ✓x7ᵗʰ W53.19 Other contact with rat

✓5ᵗʰ W53.2 Contact with squirrel
 ✓x7ᵗʰ W53.21 Bitten by squirrel
 ✓x7ᵗʰ W53.29 Other contact with squirrel

✓5ᵗʰ W53.8 Contact with other rodent
 ✓x7ᵗʰ W53.81 Bitten by other rodent
 ✓x7ᵗʰ W53.89 Other contact with other rodent

✓4ᵗʰ W54 Contact with dog
Contact with saliva, feces or urine of dog

The appropriate 7th character is to be added to each code from category W54.
A   initial encounter
D   subsequent encounter
S   sequela

 ✓x7ᵗʰ W54.0 Bitten by dog
 ✓x7ᵗʰ W54.1 Struck by dog
Knocked over by dog
 ✓x7ᵗʰ W54.8 Other contact with dog

✓4ᵗʰ W55 Contact with other mammals
Contact with saliva, feces or urine of mammal
EXCLUDES1 animal being ridden—see transport accidents
bitten or struck by dog (W54)
bitten or struck by rodent (W53.-)
contact with marine mammals (W56.-)

The appropriate 7th character is to be added to each code from category W55.
A   initial encounter
D   subsequent encounter
S   sequela

✓5ᵗʰ W55.0 Contact with cat
 ✓x7ᵗʰ W55.01 Bitten by cat
 ✓x7ᵗʰ W55.03 Scratched by cat
 ✓x7ᵗʰ W55.09 Other contact with cat

✓5ᵗʰ W55.1 Contact with horse
 ✓x7ᵗʰ W55.11 Bitten by horse
 ✓x7ᵗʰ W55.12 Struck by horse
 ✓x7ᵗʰ W55.19 Other contact with horse

✓5ᵗʰ W55.2 Contact with cow
Contact with bull
 ✓x7ᵗʰ W55.21 Bitten by cow
 ✓x7ᵗʰ W55.22 Struck by cow
Gored by bull
 ✓x7ᵗʰ W55.29 Other contact with cow

✓5ᵗʰ W55.3 Contact with other hoof stock
Contact with goats
Contact with sheep
 ✓x7ᵗʰ W55.31 Bitten by other hoof stock
 ✓x7ᵗʰ W55.32 Struck by other hoof stock
Gored by goat
Gored by ram
 ✓x7ᵗʰ W55.39 Other contact with other hoof stock

✓5ᵗʰ W55.4 Contact with pig
 ✓x7ᵗʰ W55.41 Bitten by pig
 ✓x7ᵗʰ W55.42 Struck by pig
 ✓x7ᵗʰ W55.49 Other contact with pig

✓5ᵗʰ W55.5 Contact with raccoon
 ✓x7ᵗʰ W55.51 Bitten by raccoon

 ✓x7ᵗʰ W55.52 Struck by raccoon
 ✓x7ᵗʰ W55.59 Other contact with raccoon

✓5ᵗʰ W55.8 Contact with other mammals
 ✓x7ᵗʰ W55.81 Bitten by other mammals
 ✓x7ᵗʰ W55.82 Struck by other mammals
 ✓x7ᵗʰ W55.89 Other contact with other mammals

✓4ᵗʰ W56 Contact with nonvenomous marine animal
EXCLUDES1 contact with venomous marine animal (T63.-)

The appropriate 7th character is to be added to each code from category W56.
A   initial encounter
D   subsequent encounter
S   sequela

✓5ᵗʰ W56.0 Contact with dolphin
 ✓x7ᵗʰ W56.01 Bitten by dolphin
 ✓x7ᵗʰ W56.02 Struck by dolphin
 ✓x7ᵗʰ W56.09 Other contact with dolphin

✓5ᵗʰ W56.1 Contact with sea lion
 ✓x7ᵗʰ W56.11 Bitten by sea lion
 ✓x7ᵗʰ W56.12 Struck by sea lion
 ✓x7ᵗʰ W56.19 Other contact with sea lion

✓5ᵗʰ W56.2 Contact with orca
Contact with killer whale
 ✓x7ᵗʰ W56.21 Bitten by orca
 ✓x7ᵗʰ W56.22 Struck by orca
 ✓x7ᵗʰ W56.29 Other contact with orca

✓5ᵗʰ W56.3 Contact with other marine mammals
 ✓x7ᵗʰ W56.31 Bitten by other marine mammals
 ✓x7ᵗʰ W56.32 Struck by other marine mammals
 ✓x7ᵗʰ W56.39 Other contact with other marine mammals

✓5ᵗʰ W56.4 Contact with shark
 ✓x7ᵗʰ W56.41 Bitten by shark
 ✓x7ᵗʰ W56.42 Struck by shark
 ✓x7ᵗʰ W56.49 Other contact with shark

✓5ᵗʰ W56.5 Contact with other fish
 ✓x7ᵗʰ W56.51 Bitten by other fish
 ✓x7ᵗʰ W56.52 Struck by other fish
 ✓x7ᵗʰ W56.59 Other contact with other fish

✓5ᵗʰ W56.8 Contact with other nonvenomous marine animals
 ✓x7ᵗʰ W56.81 Bitten by other nonvenomous marine animals
 ✓x7ᵗʰ W56.82 Struck by other nonvenomous marine animals
 ✓x7ᵗʰ W56.89 Other contact with other nonvenomous marine animals

✓x7ᵗʰ W57 Bitten or stung by nonvenomous insect and other nonvenomous arthropods
EXCLUDES1 contact with venomous insects and arthropods (T63.2-, T63.3-, T63.4-)

The appropriate 7th character is to be added to code W57.
A   initial encounter
D   subsequent encounter
S   sequela

✓4ᵗʰ W58 Contact with crocodile or alligator

The appropriate 7th character is to be added to each code from category W58.
A   initial encounter
D   subsequent encounter
S   sequela

✓5ᵗʰ W58.0 Contact with alligator
 ✓x7ᵗʰ W58.01 Bitten by alligator
 ✓x7ᵗʰ W58.02 Struck by alligator
 ✓x7ᵗʰ W58.03 Crushed by alligator
 ✓x7ᵗʰ W58.09 Other contact with alligator

✓5ᵗʰ W58.1 Contact with crocodile
 ✓x7ᵗʰ W58.11 Bitten by crocodile
 ✓x7ᵗʰ W58.12 Struck by crocodile
 ✓x7ᵗʰ W58.13 Crushed by crocodile
 ✓x7ᵗʰ W58.19 Other contact with crocodile

✓ Additional Character Required   ✓x7ᵗʰ Xtension Alert   Unspecified Code   Other Specified Code   Manifestation Code   ▶◀ Revised Text   ● New Code   ▲ Revised Code Title

√4ᵗʰ **W59 Contact with other nonvenomous reptiles**
    EXCLUDES 1   contact with venomous reptile (T63.0-, T63.1-)

    The appropriate 7th character is to be added to each code from category W59.
    A   initial encounter
    D   subsequent encounter
    S   sequela

√5ᵗʰ **W59.0 Contact with nonvenomous lizards**
   √x7ᵗʰ **W59.01 Bitten by nonvenomous lizards**
   √x7ᵗʰ **W59.02 Struck by nonvenomous lizards**
   √x7ᵗʰ **W59.09 Other contact with nonvenomous lizards**
       Exposure to nonvenomous lizards

√5ᵗʰ **W59.1 Contact with nonvenomous snakes**
   √x7ᵗʰ **W59.11 Bitten by nonvenomous snake**
   √x7ᵗʰ **W59.12 Struck by nonvenomous snake**
   √x7ᵗʰ **W59.13 Crushed by nonvenomous snake**
   √x7ᵗʰ **W59.19 Other contact with nonvenomous snake**

√5ᵗʰ **W59.2 Contact with turtles**
     EXCLUDES 1   contact with tortoises (W59.8-)
   √x7ᵗʰ **W59.21 Bitten by turtle**
   √x7ᵗʰ **W59.22 Struck by turtle**
   √x7ᵗʰ **W59.29 Other contact with turtle**
       Exposure to turtles

√5ᵗʰ **W59.8 Contact with other nonvenomous reptiles**
   √x7ᵗʰ **W59.81 Bitten by other nonvenomous reptiles**
   √x7ᵗʰ **W59.82 Struck by other nonvenomous reptiles**
   √x7ᵗʰ **W59.83 Crushed by other nonvenomous reptiles**
   √x7ᵗʰ **W59.89 Other contact with other nonvenomous reptiles**

√x7ᵗʰ **W60 Contact with nonvenomous plant thorns and spines and sharp leaves**
    EXCLUDES 1   contact with venomous plants (T63.7-)

    The appropriate 7th character is to be added to code W60.
    A   initial encounter
    D   subsequent encounter
    S   sequela

√4ᵗʰ **W61 Contact with birds (domestic) (wild)**
    Contact with excreta of birds

    The appropriate 7th character is to be added to each code from category W61.
    A   initial encounter
    D   subsequent encounter
    S   sequela

√5ᵗʰ **W61.0 Contact with parrot**
   √x7ᵗʰ **W61.01 Bitten by parrot**
   √x7ᵗʰ **W61.02 Struck by parrot**
   √x7ᵗʰ **W61.09 Other contact with parrot**
       Exposure to parrots

√5ᵗʰ **W61.1 Contact with macaw**
   √x7ᵗʰ **W61.11 Bitten by macaw**
   √x7ᵗʰ **W61.12 Struck by macaw**
   √x7ᵗʰ **W61.19 Other contact with macaw**
       Exposure to macaws

√5ᵗʰ **W61.2 Contact with other psittacines**
   √x7ᵗʰ **W61.21 Bitten by other psittacines**
   √x7ᵗʰ **W61.22 Struck by other psittacines**
   √x7ᵗʰ **W61.29 Other contact with other psittacines**
       Exposure to other psittacines

√5ᵗʰ **W61.3 Contact with chicken**
   √x7ᵗʰ **W61.32 Struck by chicken**
   √x7ᵗʰ **W61.33 Pecked by chicken**
   √x7ᵗʰ **W61.39 Other contact with chicken**
       Exposure to chickens

√5ᵗʰ **W61.4 Contact with turkey**
   √x7ᵗʰ **W61.42 Struck by turkey**
   √x7ᵗʰ **W61.43 Pecked by turkey**
   √x7ᵗʰ **W61.49 Other contact with turkey**

√5ᵗʰ **W61.5 Contact with goose**
   √x7ᵗʰ **W61.51 Bitten by goose**

√x7ᵗʰ **W61.52 Struck by goose**
√x7ᵗʰ **W61.59 Other contact with goose**
√5ᵗʰ **W61.6 Contact with duck**
   √x7ᵗʰ **W61.61 Bitten by duck**
   √x7ᵗʰ **W61.62 Struck by duck**
   √x7ᵗʰ **W61.69 Other contact with duck**
√5ᵗʰ **W61.9 Contact with other birds**
   √x7ᵗʰ **W61.91 Bitten by other birds**
   √x7ᵗʰ **W61.92 Struck by other birds**
   √x7ᵗʰ **W61.99 Other contact with other birds**
       Contact with bird NOS

√4ᵗʰ **W62 Contact with nonvenomous amphibians**
    EXCLUDES 1   contact with venomous amphibians (T63.81-R63.83)

    The appropriate 7th character is to be added to each code from category W62.
    A   initial encounter
    D   subsequent encounter
    S   sequela

√x7ᵗʰ **W62.0 Contact with nonvenomous frogs**
√x7ᵗʰ **W62.1 Contact with nonvenomous toads**
√x7ᵗʰ **W62.9 Contact with other nonvenomous amphibians**

√x7ᵗʰ **W64 Exposure to other animate mechanical forces**
    Exposure to nonvenomous animal NOS
    EXCLUDES 1   contact with venomous animal (T63.-)

    The appropriate 7th character is to be added to code W64.
    A   initial encounter
    D   subsequent encounter
    S   sequela

Accidental non-transport drowning and submersion (W65-W74)

   EXCLUDES 1   accidental drowning and submersion due to fall into water (W16.-)
              accidental drowning and submersion due to water transport accident (V90-, V92-)
   EXCLUDES 2   accidental drowning and submersion due to cataclysm (X34-X39)

√x7ᵗʰ **W65 Accidental drowning and submersion while in bath-tub**
    EXCLUDES 1   accidental drowning and submersion due to fall in (into) bathtub (W16.211)

    The appropriate 7th character is to be added to code W65.
    A   initial encounter
    D   subsequent encounter
    S   sequela

√x7ᵗʰ **W67 Accidental drowning and submersion while in swimming-pool**
    EXCLUDES 1   accidental drowning and submersion due to fall into swimming pool (W16.011, W16.021, W16.031)
              accidental drowning and submersion due to striking into wall of swimming pool (W22.041)

    The appropriate 7th character is to be added to code W67.
    A   initial encounter
    D   subsequent encounter
    S   sequela

√x7ᵗʰ **W69 Accidental drowning and submersion while in natural water**
    Accidental drowning and submersion while in lake
    Accidental drowning and submersion while in open sea
    Accidental drowning and submersion while in river
    Accidental drowning and submersion while in stream
    EXCLUDES 1   accidental drowning and submersion due to fall into natural body of water (W16.111, W16.121, W16.131)

    The appropriate 7th character is to be added to code W69.
    A   initial encounter
    D   subsequent encounter
    S   sequela

√x7ᵗʰ **W73 Other specified cause of accidental non-transport drowning and submersion**
    Accidental drowning and submersion while in quenching tank
    Accidental drowning and submersion while in reservoir
    EXCLUDES 1   accidental drowning and submersion due to fall into other water (W16.311, W16.321, W16.331)

    The appropriate 7th character is to be added to code W73.
    A   initial encounter
    D   subsequent encounter
    S   sequela

EXCLUDES 1 Not coded here   *EXCLUDES 2* Not included here   N Newborn Age: 0   P Pediatric Age: 0-17   M Maternity Age: 12-55   A Adult Age: 15-124

1032   ICD-10-CM 2014 (Draft)

✓x7th **W74 Unspecified cause of accidental drowning and submersion**
Drowning NOS

The appropriate 7th character is to be added to code W74.
A   initial encounter
D   subsequent encounter
S   sequela

Exposure to electric current, radiation and extreme ambient air temperature and pressure (W85-W99)

EXCLUDES 1   exposure to:
   failure in dosage of radiation or temperature during surgical and medical care (Y63.2-Y63.5)
   lightning (T75.0-)
   natural cold (X31)
   natural heat (X30)
   natural radiation NOS (X39)
   radiological procedure and radiotherapy (Y84.2)
   sunlight (X32)

✓x7th **W85 Exposure to electric transmission lines**
Broken power line

The appropriate 7th character is to be added to code W85.
A   initial encounter
D   subsequent encounter
S   sequela

✓4th **W86 Exposure to other specified electric current**

The appropriate 7th character is to be added to each code from category W86.
A   initial encounter
D   subsequent encounter
S   sequela

✓x7th **W86.0 Exposure to domestic wiring and appliances**

✓x7th **W86.1 Exposure to industrial wiring, appliances and electrical machinery**
Exposure to conductors
Exposure to control apparatus
Exposure to electrical equipment and machinery
Exposure to transformers

✓x7th **W86.8 Exposure to other electric current**
Exposure to wiring and appliances in or on farm (not farmhouse)
Exposure to wiring and appliances outdoors
Exposure to wiring and appliances in or on public building
Exposure to wiring and appliances in or on residential institutions
Exposure to wiring and appliances in or on schools

✓4th **W88 Exposure to ionizing radiation**
EXCLUDES 1   exposure to sunlight (X32)

The appropriate 7th character is to be added to each code from category W88.
A   initial encounter
D   subsequent encounter
S   sequela

✓x7th **W88.0 Exposure to X-rays**
✓x7th **W88.1 Exposure to radioactive isotopes**
✓x7th **W88.8 Exposure to other ionizing radiation**

✓4th **W89 Exposure to man-made visible and ultraviolet light**
Exposure to welding light (arc)
EXCLUDES 2   exposure to sunlight (X32)

The appropriate 7th character is to be added to each code from category W89.
A   initial encounter
D   subsequent encounter
S   sequela

✓x7th **W89.0 Exposure to welding light (arc)**
✓x7th **W89.1 Exposure to tanning bed**
✓x7th **W89.8 Exposure to other man-made visible and ultraviolet light**
✓x7th **W89.9 Exposure to unspecified man-made visible and ultraviolet light**

✓4th **W90 Exposure to other nonionizing radiation**
EXCLUDES 1   exposure to sunlight (X32)

The appropriate 7th character is to be added to each code from category W90.
A   initial encounter
D   subsequent encounter
S   sequela

✓x7th **W90.0 Exposure to radiofrequency**
✓x7th **W90.1 Exposure to infrared radiation**
✓x7th **W90.2 Exposure to laser radiation**
✓x7th **W90.8 Exposure to other nonionizing radiation**

✓x7th **W92 Exposure to excessive heat of man-made origin**

The appropriate 7th character is to be added to code W92.
A   initial encounter
D   subsequent encounter
S   sequela

✓4th **W93 Exposure to excessive cold of man-made origin**

The appropriate 7th character is to be added to each code from category W93.
A   initial encounter
D   subsequent encounter
S   sequela

✓5th **W93.0 Contact with or inhalation of dry ice**
  ✓x7th **W93.01 Contact with dry ice**
  ✓x7th **W93.02 Inhalation of dry ice**
✓5th **W93.1 Contact with or inhalation of liquid air**
  ✓x7th **W93.11 Contact with liquid air**
    Contact with liquid hydrogen
    Contact with liquid nitrogen
  ✓x7th **W93.12 Inhalation of liquid air**
    Inhalation of liquid hydrogen
    Inhalation of liquid nitrogen
✓x7th **W93.2 Prolonged exposure in deep freeze unit or refrigerator**
✓x7th **W93.8 Exposure to other excessive cold of man-made origin**

✓4th **W94 Exposure to high and low air pressure and changes in air pressure**

The appropriate 7th character is to be added to each code from category W94.
A   initial encounter
D   subsequent encounter
S   sequela

✓x7th **W94.0 Exposure to prolonged high air pressure**
✓5th **W94.1 Exposure to prolonged low air pressure**
  ✓x7th **W94.11 Exposure to residence or prolonged visit at high altitude**
  ✓x7th **W94.12 Exposure to other prolonged low air pressure**
✓5th **W94.2 Exposure to rapid changes in air pressure during ascent**
  ✓x7th **W94.21 Exposure to reduction in atmospheric pressure while surfacing from deep-water diving**
  ✓x7th **W94.22 Exposure to reduction in atmospheric pressure while surfacing from underground**
  ✓x7th **W94.23 Exposure to sudden change in air pressure in aircraft during ascent**
  ✓x7th **W94.29 Exposure to other rapid changes in air pressure during ascent**
✓5th **W94.3 Exposure to rapid changes in air pressure during descent**
  ✓x7th **W94.31 Exposure to sudden change in air pressure in aircraft during descent**
  ✓x7th **W94.32 Exposure to high air pressure from rapid descent in water**
  ✓x7th **W94.39 Exposure to other rapid changes in air pressure during descent**

✓x7th **W99 Exposure to other man-made environmental factors**

The appropriate 7th character is to be added to code W99.
A   initial encounter
D   subsequent encounter
S   sequela

Exposure to smoke, fire and flames (X00-X08)

EXCLUDES 1 arson (X97)
EXCLUDES 2 explosions (W35-W40)
lightning (T75.0-)
transport accident (V01-V99)

√4ᵗʰ **X00 Exposure to uncontrolled fire in building or structure**
Conflagration in building or structure
Code first any associated cataclysm
EXCLUDES 2 exposure to ignition or melting of nightwear (X05)
exposure to ignition or melting of other clothing and apparel (X06.-)
exposure to other specified smoke, fire and flames (X08.-)

The appropriate 7th character is to be added to each code from category X00.
A initial encounter
D subsequent encounter
S sequela

√x7ᵗʰ **X00.0 Exposure to flames in uncontrolled fire in building or structure**

√x7ᵗʰ **X00.1 Exposure to smoke in uncontrolled fire in building or structure**

√x7ᵗʰ **X00.2 Injury due to collapse of burning building or structure in uncontrolled fire**
EXCLUDES 1 injury due to collapse of building not on fire (W20.1)

√x7ᵗʰ **X00.3 Fall from burning building or structure in uncontrolled fire**

√x7ᵗʰ **X00.4 Hit by object from burning building or structure in uncontrolled fire**

√x7ᵗʰ **X00.5 Jump from burning building or structure in uncontrolled fire**

√x7ᵗʰ **X00.8 Other exposure to uncontrolled fire in building or structure**

√4ᵗʰ **X01 Exposure to uncontrolled fire, not in building or structure**
Exposure to forest fire

The appropriate 7th character is to be added to each code from category X01.
A initial encounter
D subsequent encounter
S sequela

√x7ᵗʰ **X01.0 Exposure to flames in uncontrolled fire, not in building or structure**

√x7ᵗʰ **X01.1 Exposure to smoke in uncontrolled fire, not in building or structure**

√x7ᵗʰ **X01.3 Fall due to uncontrolled fire, not in building or structure**

√x7ᵗʰ **X01.4 Hit by object due to uncontrolled fire, not in building or structure**

√x7ᵗʰ **X01.8 Other exposure to uncontrolled fire, not in building or structure**

√4ᵗʰ **X02 Exposure to controlled fire in building or structure**
Exposure to fire in fireplace
Exposure to fire in stove

The appropriate 7th character is to be added to each code from category X02.
A initial encounter
D subsequent encounter
S sequela

√x7ᵗʰ **X02.0 Exposure to flames in controlled fire in building or structure**

√x7ᵗʰ **X02.1 Exposure to smoke in controlled fire in building or structure**

√x7ᵗʰ **X02.2 Injury due to collapse of burning building or structure in controlled fire**
EXCLUDES 1 injury due to collapse of building not on fire (W20.1)

√x7ᵗʰ **X02.3 Fall from burning building or structure in controlled fire**

√x7ᵗʰ **X02.4 Hit by object from burning building or structure in controlled fire**

√x7ᵗʰ **X02.5 Jump from burning building or structure in controlled fire**

√x7ᵗʰ **X02.8 Other exposure to controlled fire in building or structure**

√4ᵗʰ **X03 Exposure to controlled fire, not in building or structure**
Exposure to bon fire
Exposure to camp-fire
Exposure to trash fire

The appropriate 7th character is to be added to each code from category X03.
A initial encounter
D subsequent encounter
S sequela

√x7ᵗʰ **X03.0 Exposure to flames in controlled fire, not in building or structure**

√x7ᵗʰ **X03.1 Exposure to smoke in controlled fire, not in building or structure**

√x7ᵗʰ **X03.3 Fall due to controlled fire, not in building or structure**

√x7ᵗʰ **X03.4 Hit by object due to controlled fire, not in building or structure**

√x7ᵗʰ **X03.8 Other exposure to controlled fire, not in building or structure**

√x7ᵗʰ **X04 Exposure to ignition of highly flammable material**
Exposure to ignition of gasoline
Exposure to ignition of kerosene
Exposure to ignition of petrol
EXCLUDES 2 exposure to ignition or melting of nightwear (X05)
exposure to ignition or melting of other clothing and apparel (X06)

The appropriate 7th character is to be added to code X04.
A initial encounter
D subsequent encounter
S sequela

√x7ᵗʰ **X05 Exposure to ignition or melting of nightwear**
EXCLUDES 2 exposure to uncontrolled fire in building or structure (X00.-)
exposure to uncontrolled fire, not in building or structure (X01.-)
exposure to controlled fire in building or structure (X02.-)
exposure to controlled fire, not in building or structure (X03.-)
exposure to ignition of highly flammable materials (X04.-)

The appropriate 7th character is to be added to code X05.
A initial encounter
D subsequent encounter
S sequela

√4ᵗʰ **X06 Exposure to ignition or melting of other clothing and apparel**
EXCLUDES 2 exposure to uncontrolled fire in building or structure (X00.-)
exposure to uncontrolled fire, not in building or structure (X01.-)
exposure to controlled fire in building or structure (X02.-)
exposure to controlled fire, not in building or structure (X03.-)
exposure to ignition of highly flammable materials (X04.-)

The appropriate 7th character is to be added to each code from category X06.
A initial encounter
D subsequent encounter
S sequela

√x7ᵗʰ **X06.0 Exposure to ignition of plastic jewelry**
√x7ᵗʰ **X06.1 Exposure to melting of plastic jewelry**
√x7ᵗʰ **X06.2 Exposure to ignition of other clothing and apparel**
√x7ᵗʰ **X06.3 Exposure to melting of other clothing and apparel**

√4ᵗʰ **X08 Exposure to other specified smoke, fire and flames**

The appropriate 7th character is to be added to each code from category X08.
A initial encounter
D subsequent encounter
S sequela

√5ᵗʰ **X08.0 Exposure to bed fire**
Exposure to mattress fire
√x7ᵗʰ **X08.00 Exposure to bed fire due to unspecified burning material**
√x7ᵗʰ **X08.01 Exposure to bed fire due to burning cigarette**
√x7ᵗʰ **X08.09 Exposure to bed fire due to other burning material**

√5ᵗʰ **X08.1 Exposure to sofa fire**
√x7ᵗʰ **X08.10 Exposure to sofa fire due to unspecified burning material**
√x7ᵗʰ **X08.11 Exposure to sofa fire due to burning cigarette**
√x7ᵗʰ **X08.19 Exposure to sofa fire due to other burning material**

√5ᵗʰ **X08.2 Exposure to other furniture fire**
√x7ᵗʰ **X08.20 Exposure to other furniture fire due to unspecified burning material**

√x7th **X08.21 Exposure to other furniture fire due to** burning cigarette

√x7th **X08.29 Exposure to other furniture fire due to other burning material**

√x7th **X08.8 Exposure to other specified smoke, fire and flames**

Contact with heat and hot substances (X10-X19)

EXCLUDES 1   *exposure to excessive natural heat (X30)*
              exposure to fire and flames (X00-X09)

✓4th **X10 Contact with hot drinks, food, fats and cooking oils**

> The appropriate 7th character is to be added to each code from category X10.
> A   initial encounter
> D   subsequent encounter
> S   sequela

√x7th **X10.0 Contact with hot** drinks

√x7th **X10.1 Contact with hot** food

√x7th **X10.2 Contact with** fats and cooking oils

✓4th **X11 Contact with hot tap-water**
Contact with boiling tap-water
Contact with boiling water NOS
EXCLUDES 1   *contact with water heated on stove (X12)*

> The appropriate 7th character is to be added to each code from category X11.
> A   initial encounter
> D   subsequent encounter
> S   sequela

√x7th **X11.0 Contact with hot water** in bath or tub
    EXCLUDES 1   *contact with running hot water in bath or tub (X11.1)*

√x7th **X11.1 Contact with** running **hot water**
Contact with hot water running out of hose
Contact with hot water running out of tap

√x7th **X11.8 Contact with other hot tap-water**
Contact with hot water in bucket
Contact with hot tap-water NOS

√x7th **X12 Contact with other hot fluids**
Contact with water heated on stove
EXCLUDES 1   *hot (liquid) metals (X18)*

> The appropriate 7th character is to be added to code X12.
> A   initial encounter
> D   subsequent encounter
> S   sequela

✓4th **X13 Contact with steam and other hot vapors**

> The appropriate 7th character is to be added to each code from category X13.
> A   initial encounter
> D   subsequent encounter
> S   sequela

√x7th **X13.0 Inhalation of steam and other hot vapors**

√x7th **X13.1 Other contact with steam and other hot vapors**

✓4th **X14 Contact with hot air and other hot gases**

> The appropriate 7th character is to be added to each code from category X14.
> A   initial encounter
> D   subsequent encounter
> S   sequela

√x7th **X14.0 Inhalation of hot air and gases**

√x7th **X14.1 Other contact with hot air and other hot gases**

✓4th **X15 Contact with hot household appliances**
EXCLUDES 1   *contact with heating appliances (X16)*
          contact with powered household appliances (W29.-)
          exposure to controlled fire in building or structure due to household appliance (X02.8)
          exposure to household appliances electrical current (W86.0)

> The appropriate 7th character is to be added to each code from category X15.
> A   initial encounter
> D   subsequent encounter
> S   sequela

√x7th **X15.0 Contact with hot** stove (kitchen)

√x7th **X15.1 Contact with hot** toaster

√x7th **X15.2 Contact with** hotplate

√x7th **X15.3 Contact with hot** saucepan or skillet

√x7th **X15.8 Contact with other hot household appliances**
Contact with cooker   Contact with light bulbs
Contact with kettle

√x7th **X16 Contact with hot heating appliances, radiators and pipes**
EXCLUDES 1   *contact with powered appliances (W29.-)*
          exposure to controlled fire in building or structure due to appliance (X02.8)
          exposure to industrial appliances electrical current (W86.1)

> The appropriate 7th character is to be added to code X16.
> A   initial encounter
> D   subsequent encounter
> S   sequela

√x7th **X17 Contact with hot engines, machinery and tools**
EXCLUDES 1   *contact with hot heating appliances, radiators and pipes (X16)*
          contact with hot household appliances (X15)

> The appropriate 7th character is to be added to code X17.
> A   initial encounter
> D   subsequent encounter
> S   sequela

√x7th **X18 Contact with other hot metals**
Contact with liquid metal

> The appropriate 7th character is to be added to code X18.
> A   initial encounter
> D   subsequent encounter
> S   sequela

√x7th **X19 Contact with other heat and hot substances**
EXCLUDES 1   *objects that are not normally hot, e.g., an object made hot by a house fire (X00-X09)*

> The appropriate 7th character is to be added to code X19.
> A   initial encounter
> D   subsequent encounter
> S   sequela

Exposure to forces of nature (X30-X39)

√x7th **X30 Exposure to excessive** natural heat
Exposure to excessive heat as the cause of sunstroke
Exposure to heat NOS
EXCLUDES 1   *excessive heat of man-made origin (W92)*
          exposure to man-made radiation (W89)
          exposure to sunlight (X32)
          exposure to tanning bed (W89)

> The appropriate 7th character is to be added to code X30.
> A   initial encounter
> D   subsequent encounter
> S   sequela

√x7th **X31 Exposure to excessive** natural cold
Excessive cold as the cause of chilblains NOS
Excessive cold as the cause of immersion foot or hand
Exposure to cold NOS
Exposure to weather conditions
EXCLUDES 1   *cold of man-made origin (W93.-)*
          contact with or inhalation of dry ice (W93.-)
          contact with or inhalation of liquefied gas (W93.-)

> The appropriate 7th character is to be added to code X31.
> A   initial encounter
> D   subsequent encounter
> S   sequela

√x7th **X32 Exposure to sunlight**
EXCLUDES 1   *radiation-related disorders of the skin and subcutaneous tissue (L55-L59)*
          man-made radiation (tanning bed) (W89)

> The appropriate 7th character is to be added to code X32.
> A   initial encounter
> D   subsequent encounter
> S   sequela

√x7th **X34 Earthquake**
EXCLUDES 2   *tidal wave (tsunami) due to earthquake (X37.41)*

> The appropriate 7th character is to be added to code X34.
> A   initial encounter
> D   subsequent encounter
> S   sequela

✓ Additional Character Required   √x7th Xtension Alert   Unspecified Code   Other Specified Code   Manifestation Code   ►◄ Revised Text   ● New Code   ▲ Revised Code Title

External Causes of Morbidity

X35–X74.09

√x7th **X35 Volcanic eruption**

EXCLUDES 2   *tidal wave (tsunami) due to volcanic eruption (X37.41)*

The appropriate 7th character is to be added to code X35.
A   initial encounter
D   subsequent encounter
S   sequela

√4th **X36 Avalanche, landslide and other earth movements**

INCLUDES   victim of mudslide of cataclysmic nature
EXCLUDES 1   *earthquake (X34)*
EXCLUDES 2   *transport accident involving collision with avalanche or landslide not in motion (V01-V99)*

The appropriate 7th character is to be added to each code from category X36.
A   initial encounter
D   subsequent encounter
S   sequela

√x7th **X36.0 Collapse of dam or man-made structure causing earth movement**

√x7th **X36.1 Avalanche, landslide, or mudslide**

√4th **X37 Cataclysmic storm**

The appropriate 7th character is to be added to each code from category X37.
A   initial encounter
D   subsequent encounter
S   sequela

√x7th **X37.0 Hurricane**
Storm surge
Typhoon

√x7th **X37.1 Tornado**
Cyclone
Twister

√x7th **X37.2 Blizzard (snow)(ice)**

√x7th **X37.3 Dust storm**

√5th **X37.4 Tidalwave**

√x7th **X37.41 Tidal wave due to earthquake or volcanic eruption**
Tidal wave NOS
Tsunami

√x7th **X37.42 Tidal wave due to storm**

√x7th **X37.43 Tidal wave due to landslide**

√x7th **X37.8 Other cataclysmic storms**
Cloudburst
Torrential rain
EXCLUDES 2   *flood (X38)*

√x7th **X37.9 Unspecified cataclysmic storm**
Storm NOS
EXCLUDES 1   *collapse of dam or man-made structure causing earth movement (X36.0)*

√x7th **X38 Flood**
Flood arising from remote storm
Flood of cataclysmic nature arising from melting snow
Flood resulting directly from storm
EXCLUDES 1   *collapse of dam or man-made structure causing earth movement (X36.0)*
tidal wave NOS (X37.41)
tidal wave caused by storm (X37.42)

The appropriate 7th character is to be added to code X38.
A   initial encounter
D   subsequent encounter
S   sequela

√4th **X39 Exposure to other forces of nature**

The appropriate 7th character is to be added to each code from category X39.
A   initial encounter
D   subsequent encounter
S   sequela

√5th **X39.0 Exposure to natural radiation**
EXCLUDES 1   *contact with and (suspected) exposure to radon and other naturally occuring radiation (Z77.123)*
exposure to man-made radiation (W88-W90)
exposure to sunlight (X32)

√x7th **X39.01 Exposure to radon**

√x7th **X39.08 Exposure to other natural radiation**

√x7th **X39.8 Other exposure to forces of nature**

Accidental exposure to other specified factors (X52, X58)

√x7th **X52 Prolonged stay in weightless environment**
Weightlessness in spacecraft (simulator)

The appropriate 7th character is to be added to code X52.
A   initial encounter
D   subsequent encounter
S   sequela

√x7th **X58 Exposure to other specified factors**
Accident NOS
Exposure NOS

The appropriate 7th character is to be added to code X58.
A   initial encounter
D   subsequent encounter
S   sequela

Intentional self-harm (X71-X83)

Purposely self-inflicted injury
Suicide (attempted)

√4th **X71 Intentional self-harm by drowning and submersion**

The appropriate 7th character is to be added to each code from category X71.
A   initial encounter
D   subsequent encounter
S   sequela

√x7th **X71.0 Intentional self-harm by drowning and submersion while in bathtub**

√x7th **X71.1 Intentional self-harm by drowning and submersion while in swimming pool**

√x7th **X71.2 Intentional self-harm by drowning and submersion after jump into swimming pool**

√x7th **X71.3 Intentional self-harm by drowning and submersion in natural water**

√x7th **X71.8 Other intentional self-harm by drowning and submersion**

√x7th **X71.9 Intentional self-harm by drowning and submersion, unspecified**

√x7th **X72 Intentional self-harm by handgun discharge**
Intentional self-harm by gun for single hand use
Intentional self-harm by pistol
Intentional self-harm by revolver
EXCLUDES 1   *Very pistol (X74.8)*

The appropriate 7th character is to be added to code X72.
A   initial encounter
D   subsequent encounter
S   sequela

√4th **X73 Intentional self-harm by rifle, shotgun and larger firearm discharge**
EXCLUDES 1   *airgun (X74.01)*

The appropriate 7th character is to be added to each code from category X73.
A   initial encounter
D   subsequent encounter
S   sequela

√x7th **X73.0 Intentional self-harm by shotgun discharge**

√x7th **X73.1 Intentional self-harm by hunting rifle discharge**

√x7th **X73.2 Intentional self-harm by machine gun discharge**

√x7th **X73.8 Intentional self-harm by other larger firearm discharge**

√x7th **X73.9 Intentional self-harm by unspecified larger firearm discharge**

√4th **X74 Intentional self-harm by other and unspecified firearm and gun discharge**

The appropriate 7th character is to be added to each code from category X74.
A   initial encounter
D   subsequent encounter
S   sequela

√5th **X74.0 Intentional self-harm by gas, air or spring-operated guns**

√x7th **X74.01 Intentional self-harm by airgun**
Intentional self-harm by BB gun discharge
Intentional self-harm by pellet gun discharge

√x7th **X74.02 Intentional self-harm by paintball gun**

√x7th **X74.09 Intentional self-harm by other gas, air or spring-operated gun**

EXCLUDES 1 Not coded here   EXCLUDES 2 Not included here   N Newborn Age: 0   P Pediatric Age: 0-17   M Maternity Age: 12-55   A Adult Age: 15-124

√x7ᵗʰ **X74.8** **Intentional self-harm by other firearm discharge**
      Intentional self-harm by Very pistol [flare] discharge

√x7ᵗʰ **X74.9** **Intentional self-harm by unspecified firearm discharge**

√x7ᵗʰ **X75** **Intentional self-harm by explosive material**

> The appropriate 7th character is to be added to code X75.
> A   initial encounter
> D   subsequent encounter
> S   sequela

√x7ᵗʰ **X76** **Intentional self-harm by smoke, fire and flames**

> The appropriate 7th character is to be added to code X76.
> A   initial encounter
> D   subsequent encounter
> S   sequela

√4ᵗʰ **X77** **Intentional self-harm by steam, hot vapors and hot objects**

> The appropriate 7th character is to be added to each code from category X77.
> A   initial encounter
> D   subsequent encounter
> S   sequela

√x7ᵗʰ **X77.0** **Intentional self-harm by steam or hot vapors**

√x7ᵗʰ **X77.1** **Intentional self-harm by hot tap water**

√x7ᵗʰ **X77.2** **Intentional self-harm by other hot fluids**

√x7ᵗʰ **X77.3** **Intentional self-harm by hot household appliances**

√x7ᵗʰ **X77.8** **Intentional self-harm by other hot objects**

√x7ᵗʰ **X77.9** **Intentional self-harm by unspecified hot objects**

√4ᵗʰ **X78** **Intentional self-harm by sharp object**

> The appropriate 7th character is to be added to each code from category X78.
> A   initial encounter
> D   subsequent encounter
> S   sequela

√x7ᵗʰ **X78.0** **Intentional self-harm by sharp glass**

√x7ᵗʰ **X78.1** **Intentional self-harm by knife**

√x7ᵗʰ **X78.2** **Intentional self-harm by sword or dagger**

√x7ᵗʰ **X78.8** **Intentional self-harm by other sharp object**

√x7ᵗʰ **X78.9** **Intentional self-harm by unspecified sharp object**

√x7ᵗʰ **X79** **Intentional self-harm by blunt object**

> The appropriate 7th character is to be added to code X79.
> A   initial encounter
> D   subsequent encounter
> S   sequela

√x7ᵗʰ **X80** **Intentional self-harm by jumping from a high place**
      Intentional fall from one level to another

> The appropriate 7th character is to be added to code X80.
> A   initial encounter
> D   subsequent encounter
> S   sequela

√4ᵗʰ **X81** **Intentional self-harm by jumping or lying in front of moving object**

> The appropriate 7th character is to be added to each code from category X81.
> A   initial encounter
> D   subsequent encounter
> S   sequela

√x7ᵗʰ **X81.0** **Intentional self-harm by jumping or lying in front of motor vehicle**

√x7ᵗʰ **X81.1** **Intentional self-harm by jumping or lying in front of (subway) train**

√x7ᵗʰ **X81.8** **Intentional self-harm by jumping or lying in front of other moving object**

√4ᵗʰ **X82** **Intentional self-harm by crashing of motor vehicle**

> The appropriate 7th character is to be added to each code from category X82.
> A   initial encounter
> D   subsequent encounter
> S   sequela

√x7ᵗʰ **X82.0** **Intentional collision of motor vehicle with other motor vehicle**

√x7ᵗʰ **X82.1** **Intentional collision of motor vehicle with train**

√x7ᵗʰ **X82.2** **Intentional collision of motor vehicle with tree**

√x7ᵗʰ **X82.8** **Other intentional self-harm by crashing of motor vehicle**

√4ᵗʰ **X83** **Intentional self-harm by other specified means**
      EXCLUDES 1 *intentional self-harm by poisoning or contact with toxic substance—see Table of Drugs and Chemicals*

> The appropriate 7th character is to be added to each code from category X83.
> A   initial encounter
> D   subsequent encounter
> S   sequela

√x7ᵗʰ **X83.0** **Intentional self-harm by crashing of aircraft**

√x7ᵗʰ **X83.1** **Intentional self-harm by electrocution**

√x7ᵗʰ **X83.2** **Intentional self-harm by exposure to extremes of cold**

√x7ᵗʰ **X83.8** **Intentional self-harm by other specified means**

Assault (X92-Y08)

INCLUDES   homicide
          injuries inflicted by another person with intent to injure or kill, by any means

EXCLUDES 1 *injuries due to legal intervention (Y35.-)*
          injuries due to operations of war (Y36.-)
          injuries due to terrorism (Y38.-)

√4ᵗʰ **X92** **Assault by drowning and submersion**

> The appropriate 7th character is to be added to each code from category X92.
> A   initial encounter
> D   subsequent encounter
> S   sequela

√x7ᵗʰ **X92.0** **Assault by drowning and submersion while in bathtub**

√x7ᵗʰ **X92.1** **Assault by drowning and submersion while in swimming pool**

√x7ᵗʰ **X92.2** **Assault by drowning and submersion after push into swimming pool**

√x7ᵗʰ **X92.3** **Assault by drowning and submersion in natural water**

√x7ᵗʰ **X92.8** **Other assault by drowning and submersion**

√x7ᵗʰ **X92.9** **Assault by drowning and submersion, unspecified**

√x7ᵗʰ **X93** **Assault by handgun discharge**
      Assault by discharge of gun for single hand use
      Assault by discharge of pistol
      Assault by discharge of revolver
      EXCLUDES 1 *Very pistol (X95.8)*

> The appropriate 7th character is to be added to code X93.
> A   initial encounter
> D   subsequent encounter
> S   sequela

√4ᵗʰ **X94** **Assault by rifle, shotgun and larger firearm discharge**
      EXCLUDES 1 *airgun (X95.01)*

> The appropriate 7th character is to be added to each code from category X94.
> A   initial encounter
> D   subsequent encounter
> S   sequela

√x7ᵗʰ **X94.0** **Assault by shotgun**

√x7ᵗʰ **X94.1** **Assault by hunting rifle**

√x7ᵗʰ **X94.2** **Assault by machine gun**

√x7ᵗʰ **X94.8** **Assault by other larger firearm discharge**

√x7ᵗʰ **X94.9** **Assault by unspecified larger firearm discharge**

√4ᵗʰ **X95** **Assault by other and unspecified firearm and gun discharge**

> The appropriate 7th character is to be added to each code from category X95.
> A   initial encounter
> D   subsequent encounter
> S   sequela

√5ᵗʰ **X95.0** **Assault by gas, air or spring-operated guns**

√x7ᵗʰ **X95.01** **Assault by airgun discharge**
       Assault by BB gun discharge
       Assault by pellet gun discharge

√x7ᵗʰ **X95.02** **Assault by paintball gun discharge**

√x7ᵗʰ **X95.09** **Assault by other gas, air or spring-operated gun**

√x7ᵗʰ **X95.8** **Assault by other firearm discharge**
       Assault by Very pistol [flare] discharge

☑ Additional Character Required   √x7ᵗʰ Xtension Alert   Unspecified Code   Other Specified Code   Manifestation Code   ▶◀ Revised Text   ● New Code   ▲ Revised Code Title

ICD-10-CM 2014 (Draft)   1037

☑7ᵗʰ X95.9 Assault by unspecified firearm discharge

☑4ᵗʰ X96 Assault by explosive material
> **EXCLUDES 1**   *incendiary device (X97)*
> *terrorism involving explosive material (Y38.2-)*

> The appropriate 7th character is to be added to each code from category X96.
> A   initial encounter
> D   subsequent encounter
> S   sequela

☑7ᵗʰ X96.0 Assault by antipersonnel bomb
> **EXCLUDES 1**   *antipersonnel bomb use in military or war (Y36.2-)*

☑7ᵗʰ X96.1 Assault by gasoline bomb

☑7ᵗʰ X96.2 Assault by letter bomb

☑7ᵗʰ X96.3 Assault by fertilizer bomb

☑7ᵗʰ X96.4 Assault by pipe bomb

☑7ᵗʰ X96.8 Assault by other specified explosive

☑7ᵗʰ X96.9 Assault by unspecified explosive

☑x7ᵗʰ X97 Assault by smoke, fire and flames
> Assault by arson
> Assault by cigarettes
> Assault by incendiary device

> The appropriate 7th character is to be added to code X97.
> A   initial encounter
> D   subsequent encounter
> S   sequela

☑4ᵗʰ X98 Assault by steam, hot vapors and hot objects

> The appropriate 7th character is to be added to each code from category X98.
> A   initial encounter
> D   subsequent encounter
> S   sequela

☑x7ᵗʰ X98.0 Assault by steam or hot vapors

☑x7ᵗʰ X98.1 Assault by hot tap water

☑x7ᵗʰ X98.2 Assault by hot fluids

☑x7ᵗʰ X98.3 Assault by hot household appliances

☑x7ᵗʰ X98.8 Assault by other hot objects

☑x7ᵗʰ X98.9 Assault by unspecified hot objects

☑4ᵗʰ X99 Assault by sharp object
> **EXCLUDES 1**   *assault by strike by sports equipment (Y08.0-)*

> The appropriate 7th character is to be added to each code from category X99.
> A   initial encounter
> D   subsequent encounter
> S   sequela

☑x7ᵗʰ X99.0 Assault by sharp glass

☑x7ᵗʰ X99.1 Assault by knife

☑x7ᵗʰ X99.2 Assault by sword or dagger

☑x7ᵗʰ X99.8 Assault by other sharp object

☑x7ᵗʰ X99.9 Assault by unspecified sharp object
> Assault by stabbing NOS

☑x7ᵗʰ Y00 Assault by blunt object
> **EXCLUDES 1**   *assault by strike by sports equipment (Y08.0-)*

> The appropriate 7th character is to be added to code Y00.
> A   initial encounter
> D   subsequent encounter
> S   sequela

☑x7ᵗʰ Y01 Assault by pushing from high place

> The appropriate 7th character is to be added to code Y01.
> A   initial encounter
> D   subsequent encounter
> S   sequela

☑4ᵗʰ Y02 Assault by pushing or placing victim in front of moving object

> The appropriate 7th character is to be added to each code from category Y02.
> A   initial encounter
> D   subsequent encounter
> S   sequela

☑x7ᵗʰ Y02.0 Assault by pushing or placing victim in front of motor vehicle

☑x7ᵗʰ Y02.1 Assault by pushing or placing victim in front of (subway) train

☑x7ᵗʰ Y02.8 Assault by pushing or placing victim in front of other moving object

☑4ᵗʰ Y03 Assault by crashing of motor vehicle

> The appropriate 7th character is to be added to each code from category Y03.
> A   initial encounter
> D   subsequent encounter
> S   sequela

☑x7ᵗʰ Y03.0 Assault by being hit or run over by motor vehicle

☑x7ᵗʰ Y03.8 Other assault by crashing of motor vehicle

☑4ᵗʰ Y04 Assault by bodily force
> **EXCLUDES 1**   *assault by:*
> *submersion (X92.-)*
> *use of weapon (X93-X95, X99, Y00)*

> The appropriate 7th character is to be added to each code from category Y04.
> A   initial encounter
> D   subsequent encounter
> S   sequela

☑x7ᵗʰ Y04.0 Assault by unarmed brawl or fight

☑x7ᵗʰ Y04.1 Assault by human bite

☑x7ᵗʰ Y04.2 Assault by strike against or bumped into by another person

☑x7ᵗʰ Y04.8 Assault by other bodily force
> Assault by bodily force NOS

☑4ᵗʰ Y07 Perpetrator of assault, maltreatment and neglect
> **NOTE**   Codes from this category are for use only in cases of confirmed abuse (T74.-)
> Selection of the correct perpetrator code is based on the relationship between the perpetrator and the victim
> **INCLUDES**   perpetrator of abandonment
> perpetrator of emotional neglect
> perpetrator of mental cruelty
> perpetrator of physical abuse
> perpetrator of physical neglect
> perpetrator of sexual abuse
> perpetrator of torture

☑5ᵗʰ Y07.0 Spouse or partner, perpetrator of maltreatment and neglect
> **NOTE**   Spouse or partner, perpetrator of maltreatment and neglect against spouse or partner

> **Y07.01 Husband, perpetrator of maltreatment and neglect**

> **Y07.02 Wife, perpetrator of maltreatment and neglect**

> **Y07.03 Male partner, perpetrator of maltreatment and neglect**

> **Y07.04 Female partner, perpetrator of maltreatment and neglect**

☑5ᵗʰ Y07.1 Parent (adoptive) (biological), perpetrator of maltreatment and neglect

> **Y07.11 Biological father, perpetrator of maltreatment and neglect**

> **Y07.12 Biological mother, perpetrator of maltreatment and neglect**

> **Y07.13 Adoptive father, perpetrator of maltreatment and neglect**

> **Y07.14 Adoptive mother, perpetrator of maltreatment and neglect**

☑5ᵗʰ Y07.4 Other family member, perpetrator of maltreatment and neglect

> **☑6ᵗʰ Y07.41 Sibling, perpetrator of maltreatment and neglect**
> > **EXCLUDES 1**   *stepsibling, perpetrator of maltreatment and neglect (Y07.435, Y07.436)*

> > **Y07.410 Brother, perpetrator of maltreatment and neglect**

> > **Y07.411 Sister, perpetrator of maltreatment and neglect**

> **☑6ᵗʰ Y07.42 Foster parent, perpetrator of maltreatment and neglect**

> > **Y07.420 Foster father, perpetrator of maltreatment and neglect**

> > **Y07.421 Foster mother, perpetrator of maltreatment and neglect**

> **☑6ᵗʰ Y07.43 Stepparent or stepsibling, perpetrator of maltreatment and neglect**

> > **Y07.430 Stepfather, perpetrator of maltreatment and neglect**

EXCLUDES 1 Not coded here   **EXCLUDES 2** Not included here   **N** Newborn Age: 0   **P** Pediatric Age: 0-17   **M** Maternity Age: 12-55   **A** Adult Age: 15-124

1038   ICD-10-CM 2014 (Draft)

Y07.432 **Male friend of parent (co-residing in household), perpetrator of maltreatment and neglect**

Y07.433 **Stepmother**, perpetrator of maltreatment and neglect

Y07.434 **Female friend of parent (co-residing in household), perpetrator of maltreatment and neglect**

Y07.435 **Stepbrother, perpetrator or maltreatment and neglect**

Y07.436 **Stepsister**, perpetrator of maltreatment and neglect

✓6ᵗʰ Y07.49 Other **family member, perpetrator of maltreatment and neglect**

Y07.490 **Male cousin, perpetrator of maltreatment and neglect**

Y07.491 **Female cousin, perpetrator of maltreatment and neglect**

Y07.499 **Other family member, perpetrator of maltreatment and neglect**

✓5ᵗʰ Y07.5 Non-family member, perpetrator of maltreatment and neglect

Y07.50 **Unspecified non-family member, perpetrator of maltreatment and neglect**

✓6ᵗʰ Y07.51 **Daycare provider, perpetrator of maltreatment and neglect**

Y07.510 **At-home childcare provider, perpetrator of maltreatment and neglect**

Y07.511 **Daycare center childcare provider, perpetrator of maltreatment and neglect**

Y07.512 **At-home adultcare provider, perpetrator of maltreatment and neglect**

Y07.513 **Adultcare center provider, perpetrator of maltreatment and neglect**

Y07.519 **Unspecified daycare provider, perpetrator of maltreatment and neglect**

✓6ᵗʰ Y07.52 **Healthcare provider, perpetrator of maltreatment and neglect**

Y07.521 **Mental health provider, perpetrator of maltreatment and neglect**

Y07.528 **Other therapist or healthcare provider, perpetrator of maltreatment and neglect**

Nurse, perpetrator of maltreatment and neglect

Occupational therapist, perpetrator of maltreatment and neglect

Physical therapist, perpetrator of maltreatment and neglect

Speech therapist, perpetrator of maltreatment and neglect

Y07.529 **Unspecified healthcare provider, perpetrator of maltreatment and neglect**

Y07.53 **Teacher or instructor, perpetrator of maltreatment and neglect**

Coach, perpetrator of maltreatment and neglect

Y07.59 **Other non-family member, perpetrator of maltreatment and neglect**

Y07.9 Unspecified perpetrator of maltreatment and neglect

✓4ᵗʰ **Y08 Assault by other specified means**

The appropriate 7th character is to be added to each code from category Y08.
A   initial encounter
D   subsequent encounter
S   sequela

✓5ᵗʰ **Y08.0 Assault by strike by sport equipment**

✓7ᵗʰ Y08.01 **Assault by strike by hockey stick**

✓7ᵗʰ Y08.02 **Assault by strike by baseball bat**

✓7ᵗʰ Y08.09 **Assault by strike by other specified type of sport equipment**

✓5ᵗʰ **Y08.8 Assault by other specified means**

✓7ᵗʰ Y08.81 **Assault by crashing of aircraft**

✓7ᵗʰ Y08.89 **Assault by other specified means**

Y09 Assault by unspecified means
Assassination (attempted) NOS
Homicide (attempted) NOS
Manslaughter (attempted) NOS
Murder (attempted) NOS

Event of undetermined intent (Y21-Y33)

Undetermined intent is only for use when there is specific documentation in the record that the intent of the injury cannot be determined. If no such documentation is present, code to accidental (unintentional)

✓4ᵗʰ **Y21 Drowning and submersion, undetermined intent**

The appropriate 7th character is to be added to each code from category Y21.
A   initial encounter
D   subsequent encounter
S   sequela

✓x7ᵗʰ Y21.0 **Drowning and submersion while in bathtub, undetermined intent**

✓x7ᵗʰ Y21.1 **Drowning and submersion after fall into bathtub, undetermined intent**

✓x7ᵗʰ Y21.2 **Drowning and submersion while in swimming pool, undetermined intent**

✓x7ᵗʰ Y21.3 **Drowning and submersion after fall into swimming pool, undetermined intent**

✓x7ᵗʰ Y21.4 **Drowning and submersion in natural water, undetermined intent**

✓x7ᵗʰ Y21.8 **Other drowning and submersion, undetermined intent**

✓x7ᵗʰ Y21.9 **Unspecified drowning and submersion, undetermined intent**

✓x7ᵗʰ **Y22 Handgun discharge, undetermined intent**
Discharge of gun for single hand use, undetermined intent
Discharge of pistol, undetermined intent
Discharge of revolver, undetermined intent
EXCLUDES 2   *Very pistol (Y24.8)*

The appropriate 7th character is to be added to code Y22.
A   initial encounter
D   subsequent encounter
S   sequela

✓4ᵗʰ **Y23 Rifle, shotgun and larger firearm discharge, undetermined intent**
EXCLUDES 2   *airgun (Y24.0)*

The appropriate 7th character is to be added to each code from category Y23.
A   initial encounter
D   subsequent encounter
S   sequela

✓x7ᵗʰ Y23.0 **Shotgun discharge, undetermined intent**

✓x7ᵗʰ Y23.1 **Hunting rifle discharge, undetermined intent**

✓x7ᵗʰ Y23.2 **Military firearm discharge, undetermined intent**

✓x7ᵗʰ Y23.3 **Machine gun discharge, undetermined intent**

✓x7ᵗʰ Y23.8 **Other larger firearm discharge, undetermined intent**

✓x7ᵗʰ Y23.9 **Unspecified larger firearm discharge, undetermined intent**

✓4ᵗʰ **Y24 Other and unspecified firearm discharge, undetermined intent**

The appropriate 7th character is to be added to each code from category Y24.
A   initial encounter
D   subsequent encounter
S   sequela

✓x7ᵗʰ Y24.0 **Airgun discharge, undetermined intent**
BB gun discharge, undetermined intent
Pellet gun discharge, undetermined intent

✓x7ᵗʰ Y24.8 **Other firearm discharge, undetermined intent**
Paintball gun discharge, undetermined intent
Very pistol [flare] discharge, undetermined intent

✓x7ᵗʰ Y24.9 **Unspecified firearm discharge, undetermined intent**

✓x7ᵗʰ **Y25 Contact with explosive material, undetermined intent**

The appropriate 7th character is to be added to code Y25.
A   initial encounter
D   subsequent encounter
S   sequela

External Causes of Morbidity

Y26–Y35.103

√x7th **Y26 Exposure to smoke, fire and flames, undetermined intent**

> The appropriate 7th character is to be added to code Y26.
> A   initial encounter
> D   subsequent encounter
> S   sequela

√4th **Y27 Contact with steam, hot vapors and hot objects, undetermined intent**

> The appropriate 7th character is to be added to each code from category Y27.
> A   initial encounter
> D   subsequent encounter
> S   sequela

√x7th **Y27.0 Contact with steam and hot vapors, undetermined intent**

√x7th **Y27.1 Contact with hot tap water, undetermined intent**

√x7th **Y27.2 Contact with hot fluids, undetermined intent**

√x7th **Y27.3 Contact with hot household appliance, undetermined intent**

√x7th **Y27.8 Contact with other hot objects, undetermined intent**

√x7th **Y27.9 Contact with unspecified hot objects, undetermined intent**

√4th **Y28 Contact with sharp object, undetermined intent**

> The appropriate 7th character is to be added to each code from category Y28.
> A   initial encounter
> D   subsequent encounter
> S   sequela

√x7th **Y28.0 Contact with sharp glass, undetermined intent**

√x7th **Y28.1 Contact with knife, undetermined intent**

√x7th **Y28.2 Contact with sword or dagger, undetermined intent**

√x7th **Y28.8 Contact with other sharp object, undetermined intent**

√x7th **Y28.9 Contact with unspecified hot objects, undetermined intent**

√x7th **Y29 Contact with blunt object, undetermined intent**

> The appropriate 7th character is to be added to code Y29.
> A   initial encounter
> D   subsequent encounter
> S   sequela

√x7th **Y30 Falling, jumping or pushed from a high place, undetermined intent**

> Victim falling from one level to another, undetermined intent

> The appropriate 7th character is to be added to code Y30.
> A   initial encounter
> D   subsequent encounter
> S   sequela

√x7th **Y31 Falling, lying or running before or into moving object, undetermined intent**

> The appropriate 7th character is to be added to code Y31.
> A   initial encounter
> D   subsequent encounter
> S   sequela

√x7th **Y32 Crashing of motor vehicle, undetermined intent**

> The appropriate 7th character is to be added to code Y32.
> A   initial encounter
> D   subsequent encounter
> S   sequela

√x7th **Y33 Other specified events, undetermined intent**

> The appropriate 7th character is to be added to code Y33.
> A   initial encounter
> D   subsequent encounter
> S   sequela

Legal intervention, operations of war, military operations, and terrorism (Y35-Y38)

√4th **Y35 Legal intervention**

> INCLUDES   any injury sustained as a result of an encounter with any law enforcement official, serving in any capacity at the time of the encounter, whether on-duty or off-duty. Includes: injury to law enforcement official, suspect and bystander

√5th **Y35.0 Legal intervention involving firearm discharge**

√6th **Y35.00 Legal intervention involving unspecified firearm discharge**

> Legal intervention involving gunshot wound
> Legal intervention involving shot NOS

√7th **Y35.001 Legal intervention involving unspecified firearm discharge, law enforcement official injured**

√7th **Y35.002 Legal intervention involving unspecified firearm discharge, bystander injured**

√7th **Y35.003 Legal intervention involving unspecified firearm discharge, suspect injured**

√6th **Y35.01 Legal intervention involving injury by machine gun**

√7th **Y35.011 Legal intervention involving injury by machine gun, law enforcement official injured**

√7th **Y35.012 Legal intervention involving injury by machine gun, bystander injured**

√7th **Y35.013 Legal intervention involving injury by machine gun, suspect injured**

√6th **Y35.02 Legal intervention involving injury by handgun**

√7th **Y35.021 Legal intervention involving injury by handgun, law enforcement official injured**

√7th **Y35.022 Legal intervention involving injury by handgun, bystander injured**

√7th **Y35.023 Legal intervention involving injury by handgun, suspect injured**

√6th **Y35.03 Legal intervention involving injury by rifle pellet**

√7th **Y35.031 Legal intervention involving injury by rifle pellet, law enforcement official injured**

√7th **Y35.032 Legal intervention involving injury by rifle pellet, bystander injured**

√7th **Y35.033 Legal intervention involving injury by rifle pellet, suspect injured**

√6th **Y35.04 Legal intervention involving injury by rubber bullet**

√7th **Y35.041 Legal intervention involving injury by rubber bullet, law enforcement official injured**

√7th **Y35.042 Legal intervention involving injury by rubber bullet, bystander injured**

√7th **Y35.043 Legal intervention involving injury by rubber bullet, suspect injured**

√6th **Y35.09 Legal intervention involving other firearm discharge**

√7th **Y35.091 Legal intervention involving other firearm discharge, law enforcement official injured**

√7th **Y35.092 Legal intervention involving other firearm discharge, bystander injured**

√7th **Y35.093 Legal intervention involving other firearm discharge, suspect injured**

√5th **Y35.1 Legal intervention involving explosives**

√6th **Y35.10 Legal intervention involving unspecified explosives**

√7th **Y35.101 Legal intervention involving unspecified explosives, law enforcement official injured**

√7th **Y35.102 Legal intervention involving unspecified explosives, bystander injured**

√7th **Y35.103 Legal intervention involving unspecified explosives, suspect injured**

EXCLUDES 1 Not coded here   EXCLUDES 2 Not included here   N Newborn Age: 0   P Pediatric Age: 0-17   M Maternity Age: 12-55   A Adult Age: 15-124

1040   ICD-10-CM 2014 (Draft)

√6ᵗʰ **Y35.11** Legal intervention involving injury by dynamite

    √7ᵗʰ **Y35.111** Legal intervention involving injury by dynamite, law enforcement official injured

    √7ᵗʰ **Y35.112** Legal intervention involving injury by dynamite, bystander injured

    √7ᵗʰ **Y35.113** Legal intervention involving injury by dynamite, suspect injured

√6ᵗʰ **Y35.12** Legal intervention involving injury by explosive shell

    √7ᵗʰ **Y35.121** Legal intervention involving injury by explosive shell, law enforcement official injured

    √7ᵗʰ **Y35.122** Legal intervention involving injury by explosive shell, bystander injured

    √7ᵗʰ **Y35.123** Legal intervention involving injury by explosive shell, suspect injured

√6ᵗʰ **Y35.19** Legal intervention involving other explosives
Legal intervention involving injury by grenade
Legal intervention involving injury by mortar bomb

    √7ᵗʰ **Y35.191** Legal intervention involving other explosives, law enforcement official injured

    √7ᵗʰ **Y35.192** Legal intervention involving other explosives, bystander injured

    √7ᵗʰ **Y35.193** Legal intervention involving other explosives, suspect injured

√5ᵗʰ **Y35.2** Legal intervention involving gas
Legal intervention involving asphyxiation by gas
Legal intervention involving poisoning by gas

√6ᵗʰ **Y35.20** Legal intervention involving unspecified gas

    √7ᵗʰ **Y35.201** Legal intervention involving unspecified gas, law enforcement official injured

    √7ᵗʰ **Y35.202** Legal intervention involving unspecified gas, bystander injured

    √7ᵗʰ **Y35.203** Legal intervention involving unspecified gas, suspect injured

√6ᵗʰ **Y35.21** Legal intervention involving injury by tear gas

    √7ᵗʰ **Y35.211** Legal intervention involving injury by tear gas, law enforcement official injured

    √7ᵗʰ **Y35.212** Legal intervention involving injury by tear gas, bystander injured

    √7ᵗʰ **Y35.213** Legal intervention involving injury by tear gas, suspect injured

√6ᵗʰ **Y35.29** Legal intervention involving other gas

    √7ᵗʰ **Y35.291** Legal intervention involving other gas, law enforcement official injured

    √7ᵗʰ **Y35.292** Legal intervention involving other gas, bystander injured

    √7ᵗʰ **Y35.293** Legal intervention involving other gas, suspect injured

√5ᵗʰ **Y35.3** Legal intervention involving blunt objects
Legal intervention involving being hit or struck by blunt object

√6ᵗʰ **Y35.30** Legal intervention involving unspecified blunt objects

    √7ᵗʰ **Y35.301** Legal intervention involving unspecified blunt objects, law enforcement official injured

    √7ᵗʰ **Y35.302** Legal intervention involving unspecified blunt objects, bystander injured

    √7ᵗʰ **Y35.303** Legal intervention involving unspecified blunt objects, suspect injured

√6ᵗʰ **Y35.31** Legal intervention involving baton

    √7ᵗʰ **Y35.311** Legal intervention involving baton, law enforcement official injured

    √7ᵗʰ **Y35.312** Legal intervention involving baton, bystander injured

    √7ᵗʰ **Y35.313** Legal intervention involving baton, suspect injured

√6ᵗʰ **Y35.39** Legal intervention involving other blunt objects

    √7ᵗʰ **Y35.391** Legal intervention involving other blunt objects, law enforcement official injured

    √7ᵗʰ **Y35.392** Legal intervention involving other blunt objects, bystander injured

    √7ᵗʰ **Y35.393** Legal intervention involving other blunt objects, suspect injured

√5ᵗʰ **Y35.4** Legal intervention involving sharp objects
Legal intervention involving being cut by sharp objects
Legal intervention involving being stabbed by sharp objects

√6ᵗʰ **Y35.40** Legal intervention involving unspecified sharp objects

    √7ᵗʰ **Y35.401** Legal intervention involving unspecified sharp objects, law enforcement official injured

    √7ᵗʰ **Y35.402** Legal intervention involving unspecified sharp objects, bystander injured

    √7ᵗʰ **Y35.403** Legal intervention involving unspecified sharp objects, suspect injured

√6ᵗʰ **Y35.41** Legal intervention involving bayonet

    √7ᵗʰ **Y35.411** Legal intervention involving bayonet, law enforcement official injured

    √7ᵗʰ **Y35.412** Legal intervention involving bayonet, bystander injured

    √7ᵗʰ **Y35.413** Legal intervention involving bayonet, suspect injured

√6ᵗʰ **Y35.49** Legal intervention involving other sharp objects

    √7ᵗʰ **Y35.491** Legal intervention involving other sharp objects, law enforcement official injured

    √7ᵗʰ **Y35.492** Legal intervention involving other sharp objects, bystander injured

    √7ᵗʰ **Y35.493** Legal intervention involving other sharp objects, suspect injured

√5ᵗʰ **Y35.8** Legal intervention involving other specified means

√6ᵗʰ **Y35.81** Legal intervention involving manhandling

    √7ᵗʰ **Y35.811** Legal intervention involving manhandling, law enforcement official injured

    √7ᵗʰ **Y35.812** Legal intervention involving manhandling, bystander injured

    √7ᵗʰ **Y35.813** Legal intervention involving manhandling, suspect injured

√6ᵗʰ **Y35.89** Legal intervention involving other specified means

    √7ᵗʰ **Y35.891** Legal intervention involving other specified means, law enforcement official injured

    √7ᵗʰ **Y35.892** Legal intervention involving other specified means, bystander injured

    √7ᵗʰ **Y35.893** Legal intervention involving other specified means, suspect injured

√5ᵗʰ **Y35.9** Legal intervention, means unspecified

    √x7ᵗʰ **Y35.91** Legal intervention, means unspecified, law enforcement official injured

    √x7ᵗʰ **Y35.92** Legal intervention, means unspecified, bystander injured

    √x7ᵗʰ **Y35.93** Legal intervention, means unspecified, suspect injured

√4ᵗʰ **Y36 Operations of war**

    INCLUDES   injuries to military personnel and civilians caused by war, civil insurrection, and peacekeeping missions

    EXCLUDES 1   *injury to military personnel occurring during peacetime military operations (Y37.-)*
military vehicles involved in transport accidents with non-military vehicle during peacetime (V09.01, V09.21, V19.81, V29.81, V39.81, V49.81, V59.81, V69.81, V79.81)

The appropriate 7th character is to be added to each code from category Y36.
A   initial encounter
D   subsequent encounter
S   sequela

√5ᵗʰ **Y36.0** War operations involving explosion of marine weapons

√6ᵗʰ **Y36.00** War operations involving explosion of unspecified marine weapon
War operations involving underwater blast NOS

    √7ᵗʰ **Y36.000** War operations involving explosion of unspecified marine weapon, military personnel

    √7ᵗʰ **Y36.001** War operations involving explosion of unspecified marine weapon, civilian

---

☑ Additional Character Required   √x7ᵗʰ Xtension Alert   Unspecified Code   Other Specified Code   Manifestation Code   ▶◀ Revised Text   ● New Code   ▲ Revised Code Title

ICD-10-CM 2014 (Draft)   1041

✓6th **Y36.01** War operations involving explosion of depth-charge

    ✓7th **Y36.010** War operations involving explosion of depth-charge, military personnel

    ✓7th **Y36.011** War operations involving explosion of depth-charge, civilian

✓6th **Y36.02** War operations involving explosion of marine mine
    War operations involving explosion of marine mine, at sea or in harbor

    ✓7th **Y36.020** War operations involving explosion of marine mine, military personnel

    ✓7th **Y36.021** War operations involving explosion of marine mine, civilian

✓6th **Y36.03** War operations involving explosion of sea-based artillery shell

    ✓7th **Y36.030** War operations involving explosion of sea-based artillery shell, military personnel

    ✓7th **Y36.031** War operations involving explosion of sea-based artillery shell, civilian

✓6th **Y36.04** War operations involving explosion of torpedo

    ✓7th **Y36.040** War operations involving explosion of torpedo, military personnel

    ✓7th **Y36.041** War operations involving explosion of torpedo, civilian

✓6th **Y36.05** War operations involving accidental detonation of onboard marine weapons

    ✓7th **Y36.050** War operations involving accidental detonation of onboard marine weapons, military personnel

    ✓7th **Y36.051** War operations involving accidental detonation of onboard marine weapons, civilian

✓6th **Y36.09** War operations involving explosion of other marine weapons

    ✓7th **Y36.090** War operations involving explosion of other marine weapons, military personnel

    ✓7th **Y36.091** War operations involving explosion of other marine weapons, civilian

✓5th **Y36.1** War operations involving destruction of aircraft

✓6th **Y36.10** War operations involving unspecified destruction of aircraft

    ✓7th **Y36.100** War operations involving unspecified destruction of aircraft, military personnel

    ✓7th **Y36.101** War operations involving unspecified destruction of aircraft, civilian

✓6th **Y36.11** War operations involving destruction of aircraft due to enemy fire or explosives
    War operations involving destruction of aircraft due to air to air missile
    War operations involving destruction of aircraft due to explosive placed on aircraft
    War operations involving destruction of aircraft due to rocket propelled grenade [RPG]
    War operations involving destruction of aircraft due to small arms fire
    War operations involving destruction of aircraft due to surface to air missile

    ✓7th **Y36.110** War operations involving destruction of aircraft due to enemy fire or explosives, military personnel

    ✓7th **Y36.111** War operations involving destruction of aircraft due to enemy fire or explosives, civilian

✓6th **Y36.12** War operations involving destruction of aircraft due to collision with other aircraft

    ✓7th **Y36.120** War operations involving destruction of aircraft due to collision with other aircraft, military personnel

    ✓7th **Y36.121** War operations involving destruction of aircraft due to collision with other aircraft, civilian

✓6th **Y36.13** War operations involving destruction of aircraft due to onboard fire

    ✓7th **Y36.130** War operations involving destruction of aircraft due to onboard fire, military personnel

    ✓7th **Y36.131** War operations involving destruction of aircraft due to onboard fire, civilian

✓6th **Y36.14** War operations involving destruction of aircraft due to accidental detonation of onboard munitions and explosives

    ✓7th **Y36.140** War operations involving destruction of aircraft due to accidental detonation of onboard munitions and explosives, military personnel

    ✓7th **Y36.141** War operations involving destruction of aircraft due to accidental detonation of onboard munitions and explosives, civilian

✓6th **Y36.19** War operations involving other destruction of aircraft

    ✓7th **Y36.190** War operations involving other destruction of aircraft, military personnel

    ✓7th **Y36.191** War operations involving other destruction of aircraft, civilian

✓5th **Y36.2** War operations involving other explosions and fragments

    EXCLUDES 1 war operations involving explosion of aircraft (Y36.1-)
        war operations involving explosion of marine weapons (Y36.0-)
        war operations involving explosion of nuclear weapons (Y36.5-)
        war operations involving explosion occurring after cessation of hostilities (Y36.8-)

✓6th **Y36.20** War operations involving unspecified explosion and fragments
    War operations involving air blast NOS
    War operations involving blast NOS
    War operations involving blast fragments NOS
    War operations involving blast wave NOS
    War operations involving blast wind NOS
    War operations involving explosion NOS
    War operations involving explosion of bomb NOS

    ✓7th **Y36.200** War operations involving unspecified explosion and fragments, military personnel

    ✓7th **Y36.201** War operations involving unspecified explosion and fragments, civilian

✓6th **Y36.21** War operations involving explosion of aerial bomb

    ✓7th **Y36.210** War operations involving explosion of aerial bomb, military personnel

    ✓7th **Y36.211** War operations involving explosion of aerial bomb, civilian

✓6th **Y36.22** War operations involving explosion of guided missile

    ✓7th **Y36.220** War operations involving explosion of guided missile, military personnel

    ✓7th **Y36.221** War operations involving explosion of guided missile, civilian

✓6th **Y36.23** War operations involving explosion of improvised explosive device [IED]
    War operations involving explosion of person-borne improvised explosive device [IED]
    War operations involving explosion of vehicle-borne improvised explosive device [IED]
    War operations involving explosion of roadside improvised explosive device [IED]

    ✓7th **Y36.230** War operations involving explosion of improvised explosive device [IED], military personnel

    ✓7th **Y36.231** War operations involving explosion of improvised explosive device [IED], civilian

✓6th **Y36.24** War operations involving explosion due to accidental detonation and discharge of own munitions or munitions launch device

    ✓7th **Y36.240** War operations involving explosion due to accidental detonation and discharge of own munitions or munitions launch device, military personnel

    ✓7th **Y36.241** War operations involving explosion due to accidental detonation and discharge of own munitions or munitions launch device, civilian

✓6th **Y36.25** War operations involving fragments from munitions

    ✓7th **Y36.250** War operations involving fragments from munitions, military personnel

EXCLUDES 1 Not coded here   **EXCLUDES 2** Not included here   **N** Newborn Age: 0   **P** Pediatric Age: 0-17   **M** Maternity Age: 12-55   **A** Adult Age: 15-124

1042   ICD-10-CM 2014 (Draft)

✓7ᵗʰ Y36.251 War operations involving fragments from munitions, civilian

✓6ᵗʰ Y36.26 War operations involving fragments of improvised explosive device [IED]
War operations involving fragments of person-borne improvised explosive device [IED]
War operations involving fragments of vehicle-borne improvised explosive device [IED]
War operations involving fragments of roadside improvised explosive device [IED]

     ✓7ᵗʰ Y36.260 War operations involving fragments of improvised explosive device [IED], military personnel

     ✓7ᵗʰ Y36.261 War operations involving fragments of improvised explosive device [IED], civilian

✓6ᵗʰ Y36.27 War operations involving fragments from weapons

     ✓7ᵗʰ Y36.270 War operations involving fragments from weapons, military personnel

     ✓7ᵗʰ Y36.271 War operations involving fragments from weapons, civilian

✓6ᵗʰ Y36.29 War operations involving other explosions and fragments
War operations involving explosion of grenade
War operations involving explosions of land mine
War operations involving shrapnel NOS

     ✓7ᵗʰ Y36.290 War operations involving other explosions and fragments, military personnel

     ✓7ᵗʰ Y36.291 War operations involving other explosions and fragments, civilian

✓5ᵗʰ Y36.3 War operations involving fires, conflagrations and hot substances
War operations involving smoke, fumes, and heat from fires, conflagrations and hot substances

> **EXCLUDES 1** *war operations involving fires and conflagrations aboard military aircraft (Y36.1-)*
> *war operations involving fires and conflagrations aboard military watercraft (Y36.0-)*
> *war operations involving fires and conflagrations caused indirectly by conventional weapons (Y36.2-)*
> *war operations involving fires and thermal effects of nuclear weapons (Y36.53-)*

✓6ᵗʰ Y36.30 War operations involving unspecified fire, conflagration and hot substance

     ✓7ᵗʰ Y36.300 War operations involving unspecified fire, conflagration and hot substance, military personnel

     ✓7ᵗʰ Y36.301 War operations involving unspecified fire, conflagration and hot substance, civilian

✓6ᵗʰ Y36.31 War operations involving gasoline bomb
War operations involving incendiary bomb
War operations involving petrol bomb

     ✓7ᵗʰ Y36.310 War operations involving gasoline bomb, military personnel

     ✓7ᵗʰ Y36.311 War operations involving gasoline bomb, civilian

✓6ᵗʰ Y36.32 War operations involving incendiary bullet

     ✓7ᵗʰ Y36.320 War operations involving incendiary bullet, military personnel

     ✓7ᵗʰ Y36.321 War operations involving incendiary bullet, civilian

✓6ᵗʰ Y36.33 War operations involving flamethrower

     ✓7ᵗʰ Y36.330 War operations involving flamethrower, military personnel

     ✓7ᵗʰ Y36.331 War operations involving flamethrower, civilian

✓6ᵗʰ Y36.39 War operations involving other fires, conflagrations and hot substances

     ✓7ᵗʰ Y36.390 War operations involving other fires, conflagrations and hot substances, military personnel

     ✓7ᵗʰ Y36.391 War operations involving other fires, conflagrations and hot substances, civilian

✓5ᵗʰ Y36.4 War operations involving firearm discharge and other forms of conventional warfare

✓6ᵗʰ Y36.41 War operations involving rubber bullets

     ✓7ᵗʰ Y36.410 War operations involving rubber bullets, military personnel

     ✓7ᵗʰ Y36.411 War operations involving rubber bullets, civilian

✓6ᵗʰ Y36.42 War operations involving firearms pellets

     ✓7ᵗʰ Y36.420 War operations involving firearms pellets, military personnel

     ✓7ᵗʰ Y36.421 War operations involving firearms pellets, civilian

✓6ᵗʰ Y36.43 War operations involving other firearms discharge
War operations involving bullets NOS

> **EXCLUDES 1** *war operations involving munitions fragments (Y36.25-)*
> *war operations involving incendiary bullets (Y36.32-)*

     ✓7ᵗʰ Y36.430 War operations involving other firearms discharge, military personnel

     ✓7ᵗʰ Y36.431 War operations involving other firearms discharge, civilian

✓6ᵗʰ Y36.44 War operations involving unarmed hand to hand combat

> **EXCLUDES 1** *war operations involving combat using blunt or piercing object (Y36.45-)*
> *war operations involving intentional restriction of air and airway (Y36.46-)*
> *war operations involving unintentional restriction of air and airway (Y36.47-)*

     ✓7ᵗʰ Y36.440 War operations involving unarmed hand to hand combat, military personnel

     ✓7ᵗʰ Y36.441 War operations involving unarmed hand to hand combat, civilian

✓6ᵗʰ Y36.45 War operations involving combat using blunt or piercing object

     ✓7ᵗʰ Y36.450 War operations involving combat using blunt or piercing object, military personnel

     ✓7ᵗʰ Y36.451 War operations involving combat using blunt or piercing object, civilian

✓6ᵗʰ Y36.46 War operations involving intentional restriction of air and airway

     ✓7ᵗʰ Y36.460 War operations involving intentional restriction of air and airway, military personnel

     ✓7ᵗʰ Y36.461 War operations involving intentional restriction of air and airway, civilian

✓6ᵗʰ Y36.47 War operations involving unintentional restriction of air and airway

     ✓7ᵗʰ Y36.470 War operations involving unintentional restriction of air and airway, military personnel

     ✓7ᵗʰ Y36.471 War operations involving unintentional restriction of air and airway, civilian

✓6ᵗʰ Y36.49 War operations involving other forms of conventional warfare

     ✓7ᵗʰ Y36.490 War operations involving other forms of conventional warfare, military personnel

     ✓7ᵗʰ Y36.491 War operations involving other forms of conventional warfare, civilian

✓5ᵗʰ Y36.5 War operations involving nuclear weapons
War operations involving dirty bomb NOS

✓6ᵗʰ Y36.50 War operations involving unspecified effect of nuclear weapon

     ✓7ᵗʰ Y36.500 War operations involving unspecified effect of nuclear weapon, military personnel

     ✓7ᵗʰ Y36.501 War operations involving unspecified effect of nuclear weapon, civilian

✓6ᵗʰ Y36.51 War operations involving direct blast effect of nuclear weapon
War operations involving blast pressure of nuclear weapon

     ✓7ᵗʰ Y36.510 War operations involving direct blast effect of nuclear weapon, military personnel

✓ Additional Character Required   ✓7ᵗʰ Xtension Alert   Unspecified Code   Other Specified Code   Manifestation Code   ▶◀ Revised Text   ● New Code   ▲ Revised Code Title

ICD-10-CM 2014 (Draft)

1043

√7ᵗʰ **Y36.511** War operations involving direct blast effect of nuclear weapon, civilian

√6ᵗʰ **Y36.52** War operations involving indirect blast effect of nuclear weapon
War operations involving being thrown by blast of nuclear weapon
War operations involving being struck or crushed by blast debris of nuclear weapon

√7ᵗʰ **Y36.520** War operations involving indirect blast effect of nuclear weapon, military personnel

√7ᵗʰ **Y36.521** War operations involving indirect blast effect of nuclear weapon, civilian

√6ᵗʰ **Y36.53** War operations involving thermal radiation effect of nuclear weapon
War operations involving direct heat from nuclear weapon
War operation involving fireball effects from nuclear weapon

√7ᵗʰ **Y36.530** War operations involving thermal radiation effect of nuclear weapon, military personnel

√7ᵗʰ **Y36.531** War operations involving thermal radiation effect of nuclear weapon, civilian

√6ᵗʰ **Y36.54** War operation involving nuclear radiation effects of nuclear weapon
War operation involving acute radiation exposure from nuclear weapon
War operation involving exposure to immediate ionizing radiation from nuclear weapon
War operation involving fallout exposure from nuclear weapon
War operation involving secondary effects of nuclear weapons

√7ᵗʰ **Y36.540** War operation involving nuclear radiation effects of nuclear weapon, military personnel

√7ᵗʰ **Y36.541** War operation involving nuclear radiation effects of nuclear weapon, civilian

√6ᵗʰ **Y36.59** War operation involving other effects of nuclear weapons

√7ᵗʰ **Y36.590** War operation involving other effects of nuclear weapons, military personnel

√7ᵗʰ **Y36.591** War operation involving other effects of nuclear weapons, civilian

√5ᵗʰ **Y36.6** War operations involving biological weapons

√6ᵗʰ **Y36.6X** War operations involving biological weapons

√7ᵗʰ **Y36.6X0** War operations involving biological weapons, military personnel

√7ᵗʰ **Y36.6X1** War operations involving biological weapons, civilian

√5ᵗʰ **Y36.7** War operations involving chemical weapons and other forms of unconventional warfare

EXCLUDES 1   war operations involving incendiary devices (Y36.3-, Y36.5-)

√6ᵗʰ **Y36.7X** War operations involving chemical weapons and other forms of unconventional warfare

√7ᵗʰ **Y36.7X0** War operations involving chemical weapons and other forms of unconventional warfare, military personnel

√7ᵗʰ **Y36.7X1** War operations involving chemical weapons and other forms of unconventional warfare, civilian

√5ᵗʰ **Y36.8** War operations occurring after cessation of hostilities
War operations classifiable to categories Y36.0-Y36.8 but occurring after cessation of hostilities

√6ᵗʰ **Y36.81** Explosion of mine placed during war operations but exploding after cessation of hostilities

√7ᵗʰ **Y36.810** Explosion of mine placed during war operations but exploding after cessation of hostilities, military personnel

√7ᵗʰ **Y36.811** Explosion of mine placed during war operations but exploding after cessation of hostilities, civilian

√6ᵗʰ **Y36.82** Explosion of bomb placed during war operations but exploding after cessation of hostilities

√7ᵗʰ **Y36.820** Explosion of bomb placed during war operations but exploding after cessation of hostilities, military personnel

√7ᵗʰ **Y36.821** Explosion of bomb placed during war operations but exploding after cessation of hostilities, civilian

√6ᵗʰ **Y36.88** Other war operations occurring after cessation of hostilities

√7ᵗʰ **Y36.880** Other war operations occurring after cessation of hostilities, military personnel

√7ᵗʰ **Y36.881** Other war operations occurring after cessation of hostilities, civilian

√6ᵗʰ **Y36.89** Unspecified war operations occurring after cessation of hostilities

√7ᵗʰ **Y36.890** Unspecified war operations occurring after cessation of hostilities, military personnel

√7ᵗʰ **Y36.891** Unspecified war operations occurring after cessation of hostilities, civilian

√5ᵗʰ **Y36.9** Other and unspecified war operations

√x7ᵗʰ **Y36.90** War operations, unspecified

√x7ᵗʰ **Y36.91** War operations involving unspecified weapon of mass destruction [WMD]

√x7ᵗʰ **Y36.92** War operations involving friendly fire

√4ᵗʰ **Y37** **Military operations**

INCLUDES   injuries to military personnel and civilians occurring during peacetime on military property and during routine military exercises and operations

EXCLUDES 1   military aircraft involved in aircraft accident with civilian aircraft (V97.81-)
military vehicles involved in transport accident with civilian vehicle (V09.01, V09.21, V19.81, V29.81, V39.81, V49.81, V59.81, V69.81, V79.81)
military watercraft involved in water transport accident with civilian watercraft (V94.81-)
war operations (Y36.-)

The appropriate 7th character is to be added to each code from category Y37.
A   initial encounter
D   subsequent encounter
S   sequela

√5ᵗʰ **Y37.0** Military operations involving explosion of marine weapons

√6ᵗʰ **Y37.00** Military operations involving explosion of unspecified marine weapon
Military operations involving underwater blast NOS

√7ᵗʰ **Y37.000** Military operations involving explosion of unspecified marine weapon, military personnel

√7ᵗʰ **Y37.001** Military operations involving explosion of unspecified marine weapon, civilian

√6ᵗʰ **Y37.01** Military operations involving explosion of depth-charge

√7ᵗʰ **Y37.010** Military operations involving explosion of depth-charge, military personnel

√7ᵗʰ **Y37.011** Military operations involving explosion of depth-charge, civilian

√6ᵗʰ **Y37.02** Military operations involving explosion of marine mine
Military operations involving explosion of marine mine, at sea or in harbor

√7ᵗʰ **Y37.020** Military operations involving explosion of marine mine, military personnel

√7ᵗʰ **Y37.021** Military operations involving explosion of marine mine, civilian

√6ᵗʰ **Y37.03** Military operations involving explosion of sea-based artillery shell

√7ᵗʰ **Y37.030** Military operations involving explosion of sea-based artillery shell, military personnel

√7ᵗʰ **Y37.031** Military operations involving explosion of sea-based artillery shell, civilian

√6ᵗʰ **Y37.04** Military operations involving explosion of torpedo

√7ᵗʰ **Y37.040** Military operations involving explosion of torpedo, military personnel

EXCLUDES 1 Not coded here   EXCLUDES 2 Not included here   N Newborn Age: 0   P Pediatric Age: 0-17   M Maternity Age: 12-55   A Adult Age: 15-124

1044   ICD-10-CM 2014 (Draft)

√7th **Y37.041** **Military operations involving explosion of torpedo, civilian**

√6th **Y37.05** **Military operations involving accidental detonation of onboard marine weapons**

√7th **Y37.050** **Military operations involving accidental detonation of onboard marine weapons, military personnel**

√7th **Y37.051** **Military operations involving accidental detonation of onboard marine weapons, civilian**

√6th **Y37.09** **Military operations involving explosion of other marine weapons**

√7th **Y37.090** **Military operations involving explosion of other marine weapons, military personnel**

√7th **Y37.091** **Military operations involving explosion of other marine weapons, civilian**

√5th **Y37.1** **Military operations involving destruction of aircraft**

√6th **Y37.10** **Military operations involving unspecified destruction of aircraft**

√7th **Y37.100** **Military operations involving unspecified destruction of aircraft, military personnel**

√7th **Y37.101** **Military operations involving unspecified destruction of aircraft, civilian**

√6th **Y37.11** **Military operations involving destruction of aircraft due to enemy fire or explosives**

Military operations involving destruction of aircraft due to air to air missile
Military operations involving destruction of aircraft due to explosive placed on aircraft
Military operations involving destruction of aircraft due to rocket propelled grenade [RPG]
Military operations involving destruction of aircraft due to small arms fire
Military operations involving destruction of aircraft due to surface to air missile

√7th **Y37.110** **Military operations involving destruction of aircraft due to enemy fire or explosives, military personnel**

√7th **Y37.111** **Military operations involving destruction of aircraft due to enemy fire or explosives, civilian**

√6th **Y37.12** **Military operations involving destruction of aircraft due to collision with other aircraft**

√7th **Y37.120** **Military operations involving destruction of aircraft due to collision with other aircraft, military personnel**

√7th **Y37.121** **Military operations involving destruction of aircraft due to collision with other aircraft, civilian**

√6th **Y37.13** **Military operations involving destruction of aircraft due to onboard fire**

√7th **Y37.130** **Military operations involving destruction of aircraft due to onboard fire, military personnel**

√7th **Y37.131** **Military operations involving destruction of aircraft due to onboard fire, civilian**

√6th **Y37.14** **Military operations involving destruction of aircraft due to accidental detonation of onboard munitions and explosives**

√7th **Y37.140** **Military operations involving destruction of aircraft due to accidental detonation of onboard munitions and explosives, military personnel**

√7th **Y37.141** **Military operations involving destruction of aircraft due to accidental detonation of onboard munitions and explosives, civilian**

√6th **Y37.19** **Military operations involving other destruction of aircraft**

√7th **Y37.190** **Military operations involving other destruction of aircraft, military personnel**

√7th **Y37.191** **Military operations involving other destruction of aircraft, civilian**

√5th **Y37.2** **Military operations involving other explosions and fragments**

EXCLUDES 1   *military operations involving explosion of aircraft (Y37.1-)*
military operations involving explosion of marine weapons (Y37.0-)
military operations involving explosion of nuclear weapons (Y37.5-)

√6th **Y37.20** **Military operations involving unspecified explosion and fragments**

Military operations involving air blast NOS
Military operations involving blast NOS
Military operations involving blast fragments NOS
Military operations involving blast wave NOS
Military operations involving blast wind NOS
Military operations involving explosion NOS
Military operations involving explosion of bomb NOS

√7th **Y37.200** **Military operations involving unspecified explosion and fragments, military personnel**

√7th **Y37.201** **Military operations involving unspecified explosion and fragments, civilian**

√6th **Y37.21** **Military operations involving explosion of aerial bomb**

√7th **Y37.210** **Military operations involving explosion of aerial bomb, military personnel**

√7th **Y37.211** **Military operations involving explosion of aerial bomb, civilian**

√6th **Y37.22** **Military operations involving explosion of guided missile**

√7th **Y37.220** **Military operations involving explosion of guided missile, military personnel**

√7th **Y37.221** **Military operations involving explosion of guided missile, civilian**

√6th **Y37.23** **Military operations involving explosion of improvised explosive device [IED]**

Military operations involving explosion of person-borne improvised explosive device [IED]
Military operations involving explosion of vehicle-borne improvised explosive device [IED]
Military operations involving explosion of roadside improvised explosive device [IED]

√7th **Y37.230** **Military operations involving explosion of improvised explosive device [IED], military personnel**

√7th **Y37.231** **Military operations involving explosion of improvised explosive device [IED], civilian**

√6th **Y37.24** **Military operations involving explosion due to accidental detonation and discharge of own munitions or munitions launch device**

√7th **Y37.240** **Military operations involving explosion due to accidental detonation and discharge of own munitions or munitions launch device, military personnel**

√7th **Y37.241** **Military operations involving explosion due to accidental detonation and discharge of own munitions or munitions launch device, civilian**

√6th **Y37.25** **Military operations involving fragments from munitions**

√7th **Y37.250** **Military operations involving fragments from munitions, military personnel**

√7th **Y37.251** **Military operations involving fragments from munitions, civilian**

√6th **Y37.26** **Military operations involving fragments of improvised explosive device [IED]**

Military operations involving fragments of person-borne improvised explosive device [IED]
Military operations involving fragments of vehicle-borne improvised explosive device [IED]
Military operations involving fragments of roadside improvised explosive device [IED]

√7th **Y37.260** **Military operations involving fragments of improvised explosive device [IED], military personnel**

√7th **Y37.261** **Military operations involving fragments of improvised explosive device [IED], civilian**

✓6ᵗʰ **Y37.27 Military operations involving fragments from weapons**

✓7ᵗʰ **Y37.270 Military operations involving fragments from weapons, military personnel**

✓7ᵗʰ **Y37.271 Military operations involving fragments from weapons, civilian**

✓6ᵗʰ **Y37.29 Military operations involving other explosions and fragments**
Military operations involving explosion of grenade
Military operations involving explosions of land mine
Military operations involving shrapnel NOS

✓7ᵗʰ **Y37.290 Military operations involving other explosions and fragments, military personnel**

✓7ᵗʰ **Y37.291 Military operations involving other explosions and fragments, civilian**

✓5ᵗʰ **Y37.3 Military operations involving fires, conflagrations and hot substances**
Military operations involving smoke, fumes, and heat from fires, conflagrations and hot substances

EXCLUDES 1 *military operations involving fires and conflagrations aboard military aircraft (Y37.1-)*
military operations involving fires and conflagrations aboard military watercraft (Y37.0-)
military operations involving fires and conflagrations caused indirectly by conventional weapons (Y37.2-)
military operations involving fires and thermal effects of nuclear weapons (Y36.53-)

✓6ᵗʰ **Y37.30 Military operations involving unspecified fire, conflagration and hot substance**

✓7ᵗʰ **Y37.300 Military operations involving unspecified fire, conflagration and hot substance, military personnel**

✓7ᵗʰ **Y37.301 Military operations involving unspecified fire, conflagration and hot substance, civilian**

✓6ᵗʰ **Y37.31 Military operations involving gasoline bomb**
Military operations involving incendiary bomb
Military operations involving petrol bomb

✓7ᵗʰ **Y37.310 Military operations involving gasoline bomb, military personnel**

✓7ᵗʰ **Y37.311 Military operations involving gasoline bomb, civilian**

✓6ᵗʰ **Y37.32 Military operations involving incendiary bullet**

✓7ᵗʰ **Y37.320 Military operations involving incendiary bullet, military personnel**

✓7ᵗʰ **Y37.321 Military operations involving incendiary bullet, civilian**

✓6ᵗʰ **Y37.33 Military operations involving flamethrower**

✓7ᵗʰ **Y37.330 Military operations involving flamethrower, military personnel**

✓7ᵗʰ **Y37.331 Military operations involving flamethrower, civilian**

✓6ᵗʰ **Y37.39 Military operations involving other fires, conflagrations and hot substances**

✓7ᵗʰ **Y37.390 Military operations involving other fires, conflagrations and hot substances, military personnel**

✓7ᵗʰ **Y37.391 Military operations involving other fires, conflagrations and hot substances, civilian**

✓5ᵗʰ **Y37.4 Military operations involving firearm discharge and other forms of conventional warfare**

✓6ᵗʰ **Y37.41 Military operations involving rubber bullets**

✓7ᵗʰ **Y37.410 Military operations involving rubber bullets, military personnel**

✓7ᵗʰ **Y37.411 Military operations involving rubber bullets, civilian**

✓6ᵗʰ **Y37.42 Military operations involving firearms pellets**

✓7ᵗʰ **Y37.420 Military operations involving firearms pellets, military personnel**

✓7ᵗʰ **Y37.421 Military operations involving firearms pellets, civilian**

✓6ᵗʰ **Y37.43 Military operations involving other firearms discharge**
Military operations involving bullets NOS

EXCLUDES 1 *military operations involving munitions fragments (Y37.25-)*
military operations involving incendiary bullets (Y37.32-)

✓7ᵗʰ **Y37.430 Military operations involving other firearms discharge, military personnel**

✓7ᵗʰ **Y37.431 Military operations involving other firearms discharge, civilian**

✓6ᵗʰ **Y37.44 Military operations involving unarmed hand to hand combat**

EXCLUDES 1 *military operations involving combat using blunt or piercing object (Y37.45-)*
military operations involving intentional restriction of air and airway (Y37.46-)
military operations involving unintentional restriction of air and airway (Y37.47-)

✓7ᵗʰ **Y37.440 Military operations involving unarmed hand to hand combat, military personnel**

✓7ᵗʰ **Y37.441 Military operations involving unarmed hand to hand combat, civilian**

✓6ᵗʰ **Y37.45 Military operations involving combat using blunt or piercing object**

✓7ᵗʰ **Y37.450 Military operations involving combat using blunt or piercing object, military personnel**

✓7ᵗʰ **Y37.451 Military operations involving combat using blunt or piercing object, civilian**

✓6ᵗʰ **Y37.46 Military operations involving intentional restriction of air and airway**

✓7ᵗʰ **Y37.460 Military operations involving intentional restriction of air and airway, military personnel**

✓7ᵗʰ **Y37.461 Military operations involving intentional restriction of air and airway, civilian**

✓6ᵗʰ **Y37.47 Military operations involving unintentional restriction of air and airway**

✓7ᵗʰ **Y37.470 Military operations involving unintentional restriction of air and airway, military personnel**

✓7ᵗʰ **Y37.471 Military operations involving unintentional restriction of air and airway, civilian**

✓6ᵗʰ **Y37.49 Military operations involving other forms of conventional warfare**

✓7ᵗʰ **Y37.490 Military operations involving other forms of conventional warfare, military personnel**

✓7ᵗʰ **Y37.491 Military operations involving other forms of conventional warfare, civilian**

✓5ᵗʰ **Y37.5 Military operations involving nuclear weapons**
Military operation involving dirty bomb NOS

✓6ᵗʰ **Y37.50 Military operations involving unspecified effect of nuclear weapon**

✓7ᵗʰ **Y37.500 Military operations involving unspecified effect of nuclear weapon, military personnel**

✓7ᵗʰ **Y37.501 Military operations involving unspecified effect of nuclear weapon, civilian**

✓6ᵗʰ **Y37.51 Military operations involving direct blast effect of nuclear weapon**
Military operations involving blast pressure of nuclear weapon

✓7ᵗʰ **Y37.510 Military operations involving direct blast effect of nuclear weapon, military personnel**

✓7ᵗʰ **Y37.511 Military operations involving direct blast effect of nuclear weapon, civilian**

EXCLUDES 1 Not coded here   EXCLUDES 2 Not included here   N Newborn Age: 0   P Pediatric Age: 0-17   M Maternity Age: 12-55   A Adult Age: 15-124

1046   ICD-10-CM 2014 (Draft)

√6ᵗʰ **Y37.52** **Military operations involving** indirect blast effect of nuclear weapon
Military operations involving being thrown by blast of nuclear weapon
Military operations involving being struck or crushed by blast debris of nuclear weapon

√7ᵗʰ **Y37.520** **Military operations involving indirect blast effect of nuclear weapon,** military personnel

√7ᵗʰ **Y37.521** **Military operations involving indirect blast effect of nuclear weapon,** civilian

√6ᵗʰ **Y37.53** **Military operations involving** thermal radiation effect of nuclear weapon
Military operations involving direct heat from nuclear weapon
Military operation involving fireball effects from nuclear weapon

√7ᵗʰ **Y37.530** **Military operations involving thermal radiation effect of nuclear weapon,** military personnel

√7ᵗʰ **Y37.531** **Military operations involving thermal radiation effect of nuclear weapon,** civilian

√6ᵗʰ **Y37.54** **Military operation involving** nuclear radiation effects of nuclear weapon
Military operation involving acute radiation exposure from nuclear weapon
Military operation involving exposure to immediate ionizing radiation from nuclear weapon
Military operation involving fallout exposure from nuclear weapon
Military operation involving secondary effects of nuclear weapons

√7ᵗʰ **Y37.540** **Military operation involving nuclear radiation effects of nuclear weapon,** military personnel

√7ᵗʰ **Y37.541** **Military operation involving nuclear radiation effects of nuclear weapon,** civilian

√6ᵗʰ **Y37.59** **Military operation involving** other effects of nuclear weapons

√7ᵗʰ **Y37.590** **Military operation involving other effects of nuclear weapons,** military personnel

√7ᵗʰ **Y37.591** **Military operation involving other effects of nuclear weapons,** civilian

√5ᵗʰ **Y37.6** **Military operations involving** biological weapons

√6ᵗʰ **Y37.6X** **Military operations involving** biological weapons

√7ᵗʰ **Y37.6X0** **Military operations involving biological weapons,** military personnel

√7ᵗʰ **Y37.6X1** **Military operations involving biological weapons,** civilian

√5ᵗʰ **Y37.7** **Military operations involving chemical weapons and other forms of unconventional warfare**
EXCLUDES 1 *military operations involving incendiary devices (Y36.3-, Y36.5-)*

√6ᵗʰ **Y37.7X** **Military operations involving** chemical weapons and other forms of unconventional warfare

√7ᵗʰ **Y37.7X0** **Military operations involving chemical weapons and other forms of unconventional warfare,** military personnel

√7ᵗʰ **Y37.7X1** **Military operations involving chemical weapons and other forms of unconventional warfare,** civilian

√5ᵗʰ **Y37.9** **Other and unspecified military operations**

√x7ᵗʰ **Y37.90** **Military operations, unspecified**

√x7ᵗʰ **Y37.91** **Military operations involving unspecified** weapon of mass destruction **[WMD]**

√x7ᵗʰ **Y37.92** **Military operations** involving friendly fire

√4ᵗʰ **Y38** **Terrorism**
NOTE These codes are for use to identify injuries resulting from the unlawful use of force or violence against persons or property to intimidate or coerce a Government, the civilian population, or any segment thereof, in furtherance of political or social objective.
Use additional code for place of occurrence (Y92.-)

The appropriate 7th character is to be added to each code from category Y38.
A initial encounter
D subsequent encounter
S sequela

√5ᵗʰ **Y38.0** **Terrorism involving explosion of marine weapons**
Terrorism involving depth-charge
Terrorism involving marine mine
Terrorism involving mine NOS, at sea or in harbor
Terrorism involving sea-based artillery shell
Terrorism involving torpedo
Terrorism involving underwater blast

√6ᵗʰ **Y38.0X** **Terrorism involving explosion of** marine weapons

√7ᵗʰ **Y38.0X1** **Terrorism involving explosion of marine weapons,** public safety official injured

√7ᵗʰ **Y38.0X2** **Terrorism involving explosion of marine weapons,** civilian injured

√7ᵗʰ **Y38.0X3** **Terrorism involving explosion of marine weapons,** terrorist injured

√5ᵗʰ **Y38.1** **Terrorism involving destruction of aircraft**
Terrorism involving aircraft burned
Terrorism involving aircraft exploded
Terrorism involving aircraft being shot down
Terrorism involving aircraft used as a weapon

√6ᵗʰ **Y38.1X** **Terrorism involving** destruction of aircraft

√7ᵗʰ **Y38.1X1** **Terrorism involving destruction of aircraft,** public safety official injured

√7ᵗʰ **Y38.1X2** **Terrorism involving destruction of aircraft,** civilian injured

√7ᵗʰ **Y38.1X3** **Terrorism involving destruction of aircraft,** terrorist injured

√5ᵗʰ **Y38.2** **Terrorism involving other explosions and fragments**
Terrorism involving antipersonnel (fragments) bomb
Terrorism involving blast NOS
Terrorism involving explosion NOS
Terrorism involving explosion of breech block
Terrorism involving explosion of cannon block
Terrorism involving explosion (fragments) of artillery shell
Terrorism involving explosion (fragments) of bomb
Terrorism involving explosion (fragments) of grenade
Terrorism involving explosion (fragments) of guided missile
Terrorism involving explosion (fragments) of land mine
Terrorism involving explosion of mortar bomb
Terrorism involving explosion of munitions
Terrorism involving explosion (fragments) of rocket
Terrorism involving explosion (fragments) of shell
Terrorism involving shrapnel
Terrorism involving mine NOS, on land
EXCLUDES 1 *terrorism involving explosion of nuclear weapon (Y38.5)*
terrorism involving suicide bomber (Y38.81)

√6ᵗʰ **Y38.2X** **Terrorism involving** other explosions and fragments

√7ᵗʰ **Y38.2X1** **Terrorism involving other explosions and fragments,** public safety official injured

√7ᵗʰ **Y38.2X2** **Terrorism involving other explosions and fragments,** civilian injured

√7ᵗʰ **Y38.2X3** **Terrorism involving other explosions and fragments,** terrorist injured

√5ᵗʰ **Y38.3** **Terrorism involving fires, conflagration and hot substances**
Terrorism involving conflagration NOS
Terrorism involving fire NOS
Terrorism involving petrol bomb
EXCLUDES 1 *terrorism involving fire or heat of nuclear weapon (Y38.5)*

√6ᵗʰ **Y38.3X** **Terrorism involving** fires, conflagration and hot substances

√7ᵗʰ **Y38.3X1** **Terrorism involving fires, conflagration and hot substances,** public safety official injured

√7ᵗʰ **Y38.3X2** **Terrorism involving fires, conflagration and hot substances,** civilian injured

External Causes of Morbidity

Y38.3X3–Y65.51

   ✓7th **Y38.3X3** **Terrorism involving fires, conflagration and hot substances,** terrorist **injured**

✓5th **Y38.4 Terrorism involving firearms**
Terrorism involving carbine bullet
Terrorism involving machine gun bullet
Terrorism involving pellets (shotgun)
Terrorism involving pistol bullet
Terrorism involving rifle bullet
Terrorism involving rubber (rifle) bullet

  ✓6th **Y38.4X Terrorism involving** firearms

    ✓7th **Y38.4X1 Terrorism involving firearms,** public safety official **injured**

    ✓7th **Y38.4X2 Terrorism involving firearms,** civilian **injured**

    ✓7th **Y38.4X3 Terrorism involving firearms,** terrorist **injured**

✓5th **Y38.5 Terrorism involving nuclear weapons**
Terrorism involving blast effects of nuclear weapon
Terrorism involving exposure to ionizing radiation from nuclear weapon
Terrorism involving fireball effect of nuclear weapon
Terrorism involving heat from nuclear weapon

  ✓6th **Y38.5X Terrorism involving** nuclear weapons

    ✓7th **Y38.5X1 Terrorism involving nuclear weapons,** public safety official **injured**

    ✓7th **Y38.5X2 Terrorism involving nuclear weapons,** civilian **injured**

    ✓7th **Y38.5X3 Terrorism involving nuclear weapons,** terrorist **injured**

✓5th **Y38.6 Terrorism involving biological weapons**
Terrorism involving anthrax
Terrorism involving cholera
Terrorism involving smallpox

  ✓6th **Y38.6X Terrorism involving** biological weapons

    ✓7th **Y38.6X1 Terrorism involving biological weapons,** public safety official **injured**

    ✓7th **Y38.6X2 Terrorism involving biological weapons,** civilian **injured**

    ✓7th **Y38.6X3 Terrorism involving biological weapons,** terrorist **injured**

✓5th **Y38.7 Terrorism involving chemical weapons**
Terrorism involving gases, fumes, chemicals
Terrorism involving hydrogen cyanide
Terrorism involving phosgene
Terrorism involving sarin

  ✓6th **Y38.7X Terrorism involving** chemical weapons

    ✓7th **Y38.7X1 Terrorism involving chemical weapons,** public safety official **injured**

    ✓7th **Y38.7X2 Terrorism involving chemical weapons,** civilian **injured**

    ✓7th **Y38.7X3 Terrorism involving chemical weapons,** terrorist **injured**

✓5th **Y38.8 Terrorism involving other and unspecified means**

  Y38.80 Terrorism involving unspecified means
Terrorism NOS

  ✓6th **Y38.81 Terrorism involving** suicide bomber

    ✓7th **Y38.811 Terrorism involving suicide bomber,** public safety official **injured**

    ✓7th **Y38.812 Terrorism involving suicide bomber,** civilian **injured**

  ✓6th **Y38.89 Terrorism involving** other **means**
Terrorism involving drowning and submersion
Terrorism involving lasers
Terrorism involving piercing or stabbing instruments

    ✓7th **Y38.891 Terrorism involving other means,** public safety official **injured**

    ✓7th **Y38.892 Terrorism involving other means,** civilian **injured**

    ✓7th **Y38.893 Terrorism involving other means,** terrorist **injured**

✓5th **Y38.9 Terrorism, secondary effects**
  NOTE This code is for use to identify injuries occurring subsequent to a terrorist attack, not those that are due to the initial terrorist attack.

  ✓6th **Y38.9X Terrorism,** secondary effects

    ✓7th **Y38.9X1 Terrorism, secondary effects,** public safety official **injured**

    ✓7th **Y38.9X2 Terrorism, secondary effects,** civilian **injured**

Complications of medical and surgical care (Y62-Y84)

INCLUDES complications of medical devices
surgical and medical procedures as the cause of abnormal reaction of the patient, or of later complication, without mention of misadventure at the time of the procedure

Misadventures to patients during surgical and medical care (Y62-Y69)

EXCLUDES 2 breakdown or malfunctioning of medical device (during procedure) (after implantation) (ongoing use) (Y70-Y82)
surgical and medical procedures as the cause of abnormal reaction of the patient, without mention of misadventure at the time of the procedure (Y83-Y84)

✓4th **Y62 Failure of** sterile precautions **during surgical and medical care**

  Y62.0 Failure of sterile precautions during surgical operation

  Y62.1 Failure of sterile precautions during infusion or transfusion

  Y62.2 Failure of sterile precautions during kidney dialysis and other perfusion

  Y62.3 Failure of sterile precautions during injection or immunization

  Y62.4 Failure of sterile precautions during endoscopic examination

  Y62.5 Failure of sterile precautions during heart catheterization

  Y62.6 Failure of sterile precautions during aspiration, puncture and other catheterization

  Y62.8 Failure of sterile precautions during other surgical and medical care

  Y62.9 Failure of sterile precautions during unspecified surgical and medical care

✓4th **Y63 Failure in** dosage **during surgical and medical care**
  EXCLUDES 2 accidental overdose of drug or wrong drug given in error (T36-T50)

  Y63.0 Excessive amount of blood or other fluid given during transfusion or infusion

  Y63.1 Incorrect dilution of fluid used during infusion

  Y63.2 Overdose of radiation given during therapy

  Y63.3 Inadvertent exposure of patient to radiation during medical care

  Y63.4 Failure in dosage in electroshock or insulin-shock therapy

  Y63.5 Inappropriate temperature in local application and packing

  Y63.6 Underdosing and nonadministration of necessary drug, medicament or biological substance

  Y63.8 Failure in dosage during other surgical and medical care

  Y63.9 Failure in dosage during unspecified surgical and medical care

✓4th **Y64 Contaminated medical or biological substances**

  Y64.0 Contaminated medical or biological substance, transfused or infused

  Y64.1 Contaminated medical or biological substance, injected or used for immunization

  Y64.8 Contaminated medical or biological substance administered by other means

  Y64.9 Contaminated medical or biological substance administered by unspecified means
Administered contaminated medical or biological substance NOS

✓4th **Y65 Other misadventures during surgical and medical care**

  Y65.0 Mismatched blood in transfusion

  Y65.1 Wrong fluid used in infusion

  Y65.2 Failure in suture or ligature during surgical operation

  Y65.3 Endotracheal tube wrongly placed during anesthetic procedure

  Y65.4 Failure to introduce or to remove other tube or instrument

  ✓5th **Y65.5 Performance of** wrong procedure (operation)

    Y65.51 Performance of wrong procedure (operation) on correct patient
Wrong device implanted into correct surgical site
    EXCLUDES 1 performance of correct procedure (operation) on wrong side or body part (Y65.53)

EXCLUDES 1 Not coded here   **EXCLUDES 2** Not included here   N Newborn Age: 0   P Pediatric Age: 0-17   M Maternity Age: 12-55   A Adult Age: 15-124

1048   ICD-10-CM 2014 (Draft)

Y65.52   **Performance of procedure (operation) on patient not scheduled for surgery**
Performance of procedure (operation) intended for another patient
Performance of procedure (operation) on wrong patient

Y65.53   **Performance of correct procedure (operation) on wrong side or body part**
Performance of correct procedure (operation) on wrong side
Performance of correct procedure (operation) on wrong site

Y65.8   **Other specified misadventures during surgical and medical care**

Y66   **Nonadministration of surgical and medical care**
Premature cessation of surgical and medical care
EXCLUDES 1   *DNR status (Z66)*
palliative care (Z51.5)

Y69   **Unspecified misadventure during surgical and medical care**

Medical devices associated with adverse incidents in diagnostic and therapeutic use (Y70-Y82)

INCLUDES   breakdown or malfunction of medical devices (during use) (after implantation) (ongoing use)

EXCLUDES 1   *misadventure to patients during surgical and medical care, classifiable to (Y62-Y69)*
later complications following use of medical devices without breakdown or malfunctioning of device (Y83-Y84)

✓4ᵗʰ **Y70**   **Anesthesiology devices associated with adverse incidents**

Y70.0   Diagnostic and monitoring anesthesiology devices associated with adverse incidents

Y70.1   Therapeutic (nonsurgical) and rehabilitative anesthesiology devices associated with adverse incidents

Y70.2   Prosthetic and other implants, materials and accessory anesthesiology devices associated with adverse incidents

Y70.3   Surgical instruments, materials and anesthesiology devices (including sutures) associated with adverse incidents

Y70.8   Miscellaneous anesthesiology devices associated with adverse incidents, not elsewhere classified

✓4ᵗʰ **Y71**   **Cardiovascular devices associated with adverse incidents**

Y71.0   Diagnostic and monitoring cardiovascular devices associated with adverse incidents

Y71.1   Therapeutic (nonsurgical) and rehabilitative cardiovascular devices associated with adverse incidents

Y71.2   Prosthetic and other implants, materials and accessory cardiovascular devices associated with adverse incidents

Y71.3   Surgical instruments, materials and cardiovascular devices (including sutures) associated with adverse incidents

Y71.8   Miscellaneous cardiovascular devices associated with adverse incidents, not elsewhere classified

✓4ᵗʰ **Y72**   **Otorhinolaryngological devices associated with adverse incidents**

Y72.0   Diagnostic and monitoring otorhinolaryngological devices associated with adverse incidents

Y72.1   Therapeutic (nonsurgical) and rehabilitative otorhinolaryngological devices associated with adverse incidents

Y72.2   Prosthetic and other implants, materials and accessory otorhinolaryngological devices associated with adverse incidents

Y72.3   Surgical instruments, materials and otorhinolaryngological devices (including sutures) associated with adverse incidents

Y72.8   Miscellaneous otorhinolaryngological devices associated with adverse incidents, not elsewhere classified

✓4ᵗʰ **Y73**   **Gastroenterology and urology devices associated with adverse incidents**

Y73.0   Diagnostic and monitoring gastroenterology and urology devices associated with adverse incidents

Y73.1   Therapeutic (nonsurgical) and rehabilitative gastroenterology and urology devices associated with adverse incidents

Y73.2   Prosthetic and other implants, materials and accessory gastroenterology and urology devices associated with adverse incidents

Y73.3   Surgical instruments, materials and gastroenterology and urology devices (including sutures) associated with adverse incidents

Y73.8   Miscellaneous gastroenterology and urology devices associated with adverse incidents, not elsewhere classified

✓4ᵗʰ **Y74**   **General hospital and personal-use devices associated with adverse incidents**

Y74.0   Diagnostic and monitoring general hospital and personal-use devices associated with adverse incidents

Y74.1   Therapeutic (nonsurgical) and rehabilitative general hospital and personal-use devices associated with adverse incidents

Y74.2   Prosthetic and other implants, materials and accessory general hospital and personal-use devices associated with adverse incidents

Y74.3   Surgical instruments, materials and general hospital and personal-use devices (including sutures) associated with adverse incidents

Y74.8   Miscellaneous general hospital and personal-use devices associated with adverse incidents, not elsewhere classified

✓4ᵗʰ **Y75**   **Neurological devices associated with adverse incidents**

Y75.0   Diagnostic and monitoring neurological devices associated with adverse incidents

Y75.1   Therapeutic (nonsurgical) and rehabilitative neurological devices associated with adverse incidents

Y75.2   Prosthetic and other implants, materials and neurological devices associated with adverse incidents

Y75.3   Surgical instruments, materials and neurological devices (including sutures) associated with adverse incidents

Y75.8   Miscellaneous neurological devices associated with adverse incidents, not elsewhere classified

✓4ᵗʰ **Y76**   **Obstetric and gynecological devices associated with adverse incidents**

Y76.0   Diagnostic and monitoring obstetric and gynecological devices associated with adverse incidents   ♀

Y76.1   Therapeutic (nonsurgical) and rehabilitative obstetric and gynecological devices associated with adverse incidents   ♀

Y76.2   Prosthetic and other implants, materials and accessory obstetric and gynecological devices associated with adverse incidents   ♀

Y76.3   Surgical instruments, materials and obstetric and gynecological devices (including sutures) associated with adverse incidents   ♀

Y76.8   Miscellaneous obstetric and gynecological devices associated with adverse incidents, not elsewhere classified   ♀

✓4ᵗʰ **Y77**   **Ophthalmic devices associated with adverse incidents**

Y77.0   Diagnostic and monitoring ophthalmic devices associated with adverse incidents

Y77.1   Therapeutic (nonsurgical) and rehabilitative ophthalmic devices associated with adverse incidents

Y77.2   Prosthetic and other implants, materials and accessory ophthalmic devices associated with adverse incidents

Y77.3   Surgical instruments, materials and ophthalmic devices (including sutures) associated with adverse incidents

Y77.8   Miscellaneous ophthalmic devices associated with adverse incidents, not elsewhere classified

✓4ᵗʰ **Y78**   **Radiological devices associated with adverse incidents**

Y78.0   Diagnostic and monitoring radiological devices associated with adverse incidents

Y78.1   Therapeutic (nonsurgical) and rehabilitative radiological devices associated with adverse incidents

Y78.2   Prosthetic and other implants, materials and accessory radiological devices associated with adverse incidents

Y78.3   Surgical instruments, materials and radiological devices (including sutures) associated with adverse incidents

Y78.8   Miscellaneous radiological devices associated with adverse incidents, not elsewhere classified

✓4ᵗʰ **Y79**   **Orthopedic devices associated with adverse incidents**

Y79.0   Diagnostic and monitoring orthopedic devices associated with adverse incidents

Y79.1   Therapeutic (nonsurgical) and rehabilitative orthopedic devices associated with adverse incidents

Y79.2   Prosthetic and other implants, materials and accessory orthopedic devices associated with adverse incidents

Y79.3   Surgical instruments, materials and orthopedic devices (including sutures) associated with adverse incidents

Y79.8   Miscellaneous orthopedic devices associated with adverse incidents, not elsewhere classified

✓ Additional Character Required   ✓7ᵗʰ Xtension Alert   Unspecified Code   Other Specified Code   Manifestation Code   ►◄ Revised Text   ● New Code   ▲ Revised Code Title

ICD-10-CM 2014 (Draft)

1049

Y65.52–Y79.8

✓4ᵗʰ Y80 Physical medicine devices associated with adverse incidents

Y80.0 Diagnostic and monitoring physical medicine devices associated with adverse incidents

Y80.1 Therapeutic (nonsurgical) and rehabilitative physical medicine devices associated with adverse incidents

Y80.2 Prosthetic and other implants, materials and accessory physical medicine devices associated with adverse incidents

Y80.3 Surgical instruments, materials and physical medicine devices (including sutures) associated with adverse incidents

Y80.8 Miscellaneous physical medicine devices associated with adverse incidents, not elsewhere classified

✓4ᵗʰ Y81 General- and plastic-surgery devices associated with adverse incidents

Y81.0 Diagnostic and monitoring general- and plastic-surgery devices associated with adverse incidents

Y81.1 Therapeutic (nonsurgical) and rehabilitative general- and plastic-surgery devices associated with adverse incidents

Y81.2 Prosthetic and other implants, materials and accessory general- and plastic-surgery devices associated with adverse incidents

Y81.3 Surgical instruments, materials and general- and plastic-surgery devices (including sutures) associated with adverse incidents

Y81.8 Miscellaneous general- and plastic-surgery devices associated with adverse incidents, not elsewhere classified

✓4ᵗʰ Y82 Other and unspecified medical devices associated with adverse incidents

Y82.8 Other medical devices associated with adverse incidents

Y82.9 Unspecified medical devices associated with adverse incidents

Surgical and other medical procedures as the cause of abnormal reaction of the patient, or of later complication, without mention of misadventure at the time of the procedure (Y83-Y84)

EXCLUDES 1 misadventures to patients during surgical and medical care, classifiable to (Y62-Y69)

✓4ᵗʰ Y83 Surgical operation and other surgical procedures as the cause of abnormal reaction of the patient, or of later complication, without mention of misadventure at the time of the procedure

Y83.0 Surgical operation with transplant of whole organ as the cause of abnormal reaction of the patient, or of later complication, without mention of misadventure at the time of the procedure

Y83.1 Surgical operation with implant of artificial internal device as the cause of abnormal reaction of the patient, or of later complication, without mention of misadventure at the time of the procedure

Y83.2 Surgical operation with anastomosis, bypass or graft as the cause of abnormal reaction of the patient, or of later complication, without mention of misadventure at the time of the procedure

Y83.3 Surgical operation with formation of external stoma as the cause of abnormal reaction of the patient, or of later complication, without mention of misadventure at the time of the procedure

Y83.4 Other reconstructive surgery as the cause of abnormal reaction of the patient, or of later complication, without mention of misadventure at the time of the procedure

Y83.5 Amputation of limb(s) as the cause of abnormal reaction of the patient, or of later complication, without mention of misadventure at the time of the procedure

Y83.6 Removal of other organ (partial) (total) as the cause of abnormal reaction of the patient, or of later complication, without mention of misadventure at the time of the procedure

Y83.8 Other surgical procedures as the cause of abnormal reaction of the patient, or of later complication, without mention of misadventure at the time of the procedure

Y83.9 Surgical procedure, unspecified as the cause of abnormal reaction of the patient, or of later complication, without mention of misadventure at the time of the procedure

✓4ᵗʰ Y84 Other medical procedures as the cause of abnormal reaction of the patient, or of later complication, without mention of misadventure at the time of the procedure

Y84.0 Cardiac catheterization as the cause of abnormal reaction of the patient, or of later complication, without mention of misadventure at the time of the procedure

Y84.1 Kidney dialysis as the cause of abnormal reaction of the patient, or of later complication, without mention of misadventure at the time of the procedure

Y84.2 Radiological procedure and radiotherapy as the cause of abnormal reaction of the patient, or of later complication, without mention of misadventure at the time of the procedure

Y84.3 Shock therapy as the cause of abnormal reaction of the patient, or of later complication, without mention of misadventure at the time of the procedure

Y84.4 Aspiration of fluid as the cause of abnormal reaction of the patient, or of later complication, without mention of misadventure at the time of the procedure

Y84.5 Insertion of gastric or duodenal sound as the cause of abnormal reaction of the patient, or of later complication, without mention of misadventure at the time of the procedure

Y84.6 Urinary catheterization as the cause of abnormal reaction of the patient, or of later complication, without mention of misadventure at the time of the procedure

Y84.7 Blood-sampling as the cause of abnormal reaction of the patient, or of later complication, without mention of misadventure at the time of the procedure

Y84.8 Other medical procedures as the cause of abnormal reaction of the patient, or of later complication, without mention of misadventure at the time of the procedure

Y84.9 Medical procedure, unspecified as the cause of abnormal reaction of the patient, or of later complication, without mention of misadventure at the time of the procedure

Supplementary factors related to causes of morbidity classified elsewhere (Y90-Y99)

NOTE These categories may be used to provide supplementary information concerning causes of morbidity. They are not to be used for single-condition coding.

✓4ᵗʰ Y90 Evidence of alcohol involvement determined by blood alcohol level

Code first any associated alcohol related disorders (F10)

Y90.0 Blood alcohol level of less than 20 mg/100 ml

Y90.1 Blood alcohol level of 20-39 mg/100 ml

Y90.2 Blood alcohol level of 40-59 mg/100 ml

Y90.3 Blood alcohol level of 60-79 mg/100 ml

Y90.4 Blood alcohol level of 80-99 mg/100 ml

Y90.5 Blood alcohol level of 100-119 mg/100 ml

Y90.6 Blood alcohol level of 120-199 mg/100 ml

Y90.7 Blood alcohol level of 200-239 mg/100 ml

Y90.8 Blood alcohol level of 240 mg/100 ml or more

Y90.9 Presence of alcohol in blood, level not specified

✓4ᵗʰ Y92 Place of occurrence of the external cause

The following category is for use, when relevant, to identify the place of occurrence of the external cause. Use in conjunction with an activity code.

Place of occurrence should be recorded only at the initial encounter for treatment

✓5ᵗʰ Y92.0 Non-institutional (private) residence as the place of occurrence of the external cause

EXCLUDES 1 abandoned or derelict house (Y92.89)
home under construction but not yet occupied (Y92.6-)
institutional place of residence (Y92.1-)

✓6ᵗʰ Y92.00 Unspecified non-institutional (private) residence as the place of occurrence of the external cause

Y92.000 Kitchen of unspecified non-institutional (private) residence as the place of occurrence of the external cause

Y92.001 Dining room of unspecified non-institutional (private) residence as the place of occurrence of the external cause

Y92.002 Bathroom of unspecified non-institutional (private) residence single-family (private) house as the place of occurrence of the external cause

Y92.003 Bedroom of unspecified non-institutional (private) residence as the place of occurrence of the external cause

Y92.007 Garden or yard of unspecified non-institutional (private) residence as the place of occurrence of the external cause

Y92.008 Other place in unspecified non-institutional (private) residence as the place of occurrence of the external cause

Y92.009 Unspecified place in unspecified non-institutional (private) residence as the place of occurrence of the external cause
Home (NOS) as the place of occurrence of the external cause

✓6ᵗʰ **Y92.01** Single-family non-institutional (private) house as the place of occurrence of the external cause
Farmhouse as the place of occurrence of the external cause
EXCLUDES 1 barn (Y92.71)
chicken coop or hen house (Y92.72)
farm field (Y92.73)
orchard (Y92.74)
single family mobile home or trailer (Y92.02-)
slaughter house (Y92.86)

Y92.010 Kitchen of single-family (private) house as the place of occurrence of the external cause

Y92.011 Dining room of single-family (private) house as the place of occurrence of the external cause

Y92.012 Bathroom of single-family (private) house as the place of occurrence of the external cause

Y92.013 Bedroom of single-family (private) house as the place of occurrence of the external cause

Y92.014 Private driveway to single-family (private) house as the place of occurrence of the external cause

Y92.015 Private garage of single-family (private) house as the place of occurrence of the external cause

Y92.016 Swimming-pool in single-family (private) house or garden as the place of occurrence of the external cause

Y92.017 Garden or yard in single-family (private) house as the place of occurrence of the external cause

Y92.018 Other place in single-family (private) house as the place of occurrence of the external cause

Y92.019 Unspecified place in single-family (private) house as the place of occurrence of the external cause

✓6ᵗʰ **Y92.02** Mobile home as the place of occurrence of the external cause

Y92.020 Kitchen in mobile home as the place of occurrence of the external cause

Y92.021 Dining room in mobile home as the place of occurrence of the external cause

Y92.022 Bathroom in mobile home as the place of occurrence of the external cause

Y92.023 Bedroom in mobile home as the place of occurrence of the external cause

Y92.024 Driveway of mobile home as the place of occurrence of the external cause

Y92.025 Garage of mobile home as the place of occurrence of the external cause

Y92.026 Swimming-pool of mobile home as the place of occurrence of the external cause

Y92.027 Garden or yard of mobile home as the place of occurrence of the external cause

Y92.028 Other place in mobile home as the place of occurrence of the external cause

Y92.029 Unspecified place in mobile home as the place of occurrence of the external cause

✓6ᵗʰ **Y92.03** Apartment as the place of occurrence of the external cause
Condominium as the place of occurrence of the external cause
Co-op apartment as the place of occurrence of the external cause

Y92.030 Kitchen in apartment as the place of occurrence of the external cause

Y92.031 Bathroom in apartment as the place of occurrence of the external cause

Y92.032 Bedroom in apartment as the place of occurrence of the external cause

Y92.038 Other place in apartment as the place of occurrence of the external cause

Y92.039 Unspecified place in apartment as the place of occurrence of the external cause

✓6ᵗʰ **Y92.04** Boarding-house as the place of occurrence of the external cause

Y92.040 Kitchen in boarding-house as the place of occurrence of the external cause

Y92.041 Bathroom in boarding-house as the place of occurrence of the external cause

Y92.042 Bedroom in boarding-house as the place of occurrence of the external cause

Y92.043 Driveway of boarding-house as the place of occurrence of the external cause

Y92.044 Garage of boarding-house as the place of occurrence of the external cause

Y92.045 Swimming-pool of boarding-house as the place of occurrence of the external cause

Y92.046 Garden or yard of boarding-house as the place of occurrence of the external cause

Y92.048 Other place in boarding-house as the place of occurrence of the external cause

Y92.049 Unspecified place in boarding-house as the place of occurrence of the external cause

✓6ᵗʰ **Y92.09** Other non-institutional residence as the place of occurrence of the external cause

Y92.090 Kitchen in other non-institutional residence as the place of occurrence of the external cause

Y92.091 Bathroom in other non-institutional residence as the place of occurrence of the external cause

Y92.092 Bedroom in other non-institutional residence as the place of occurrence of the external cause

Y92.093 Driveway of other non-institutional residence as the place of occurrence of the external cause

Y92.094 Garage of other non-institutional residence as the place of occurrence of the external cause

Y92.095 Swimming-pool of other non-institutional residence as the place of occurrence of the external cause

Y92.096 Garden or yard of other non-institutional residence as the place of occurrence of the external cause

Y92.098 Other place in other non-institutional residence as the place of occurrence of the external cause

Y92.099 Unspecified place in other non-institutional residence as the place of occurrence of the external cause

✓5ᵗʰ **Y92.1** Institutional (nonprivate) residence as the place of occurrence of the external cause

Y92.10 Unspecified residential institution as the place of occurrence of the external cause

✓6ᵗʰ **Y92.11** Children's home and orphanage as the place of occurrence of the external cause

Y92.110 Kitchen in children's home and orphanage as the place of occurrence of the external cause

Y92.111 Bathroom in children's home and orphanage as the place of occurrence of the external cause

Y92.112 Bedroom in children's home and orphanage as the place of occurrence of the external cause

Y92.113 Driveway of children's home and orphanage as the place of occurrence of the external cause

Y92.114 Garage of children's home and orphanage as the place of occurrence of the external cause

Y92.115 Swimming-pool of children's home and orphanage as the place of occurrence of the external cause

✔ Additional Character Required ✔x7ᵗʰ Xtension Alert Unspecified Code Other Specified Code Manifestation Code ▶◀ Revised Text ● New Code ▲ Revised Code Title

ICD-10-CM 2014 (Draft) 1051

Y92.116 Garden or yard of children's home and orphanage as the place of occurrence of the external cause

Y92.118 Other place in children's home and orphanage as the place of occurrence of the external cause

Y92.119 Unspecified place in children's home and orphanage as the place of occurrence of the external cause

✓6ᵗʰ **Y92.12** Nursing home as the place of occurrence of the external cause

Home for the sick as the place of occurrence of the external cause

Hospice as the place of occurrence of the external cause

Y92.120 Kitchen in nursing home as the place of occurrence of the external cause

Y92.121 Bathroom in nursing home as the place of occurrence of the external cause

Y92.122 Bedroom in nursing home as the place of occurrence of the external cause

Y92.123 Driveway of nursing home as the place of occurrence of the external cause

Y92.124 Garage of nursing home as the place of occurrence of the external cause

Y92.125 Swimming-pool of nursing home as the place of occurrence of the external cause

Y92.126 Garden or yard of nursing home as the place of occurrence of the external cause

Y92.128 Other place in nursing home as the place of occurrence of the external cause

Y92.129 Unspecified place in nursing home as the place of occurrence of the external cause

✓6ᵗʰ **Y92.13** Military base as the place of occurrence of the external cause

EXCLUDES 1　military training grounds (Y92.84)

Y92.130 Kitchen on military base as the place of occurrence of the external cause

Y92.131 Mess hall on military base as the place of occurrence of the external cause

Y92.133 Barracks on military base as the place of occurrence of the external cause

Y92.135 Garage on military base as the place of occurrence of the external cause

Y92.136 Swimming-pool on military base as the place of occurrence of the external cause

Y92.137 Garden or yard on military base as the place of occurrence of the external cause

Y92.138 Other place on military base as the place of occurrence of the external cause

Y92.139 Unspecified place military base as the place of occurrence of the external cause

✓6ᵗʰ **Y92.14** Prison as the place of occurrence of the external cause

Y92.140 Kitchen in prison as the place of occurrence of the external cause

Y92.141 Dining room in prison as the place of occurrence of the external cause

Y92.142 Bathroom in prison as the place of occurrence of the external cause

Y92.143 Cell of prison as the place of occurrence of the external cause

Y92.146 Swimming-pool of prison as the place of occurrence of the external cause

Y92.147 Courtyard of prison as the place of occurrence of the external cause

Y92.148 Other place in prison as the place of occurrence of the external cause

Y92.149 Unspecified place in prison as the place of occurrence of the external cause

✓6ᵗʰ **Y92.15** Reform school as the place of occurrence of the external cause

Y92.150 Kitchen in reform school as the place of occurrence of the external cause

Y92.151 Dining room in reform school as the place of occurrence of the external cause

Y92.152 Bathroom in reform school as the place of occurrence of the external cause

Y92.153 Bedroom in reform school as the place of occurrence of the external cause

Y92.154 Driveway of reform school as the place of occurrence of the external cause

Y92.155 Garage of reform school as the place of occurrence of the external cause

Y92.156 Swimming-pool of reform school as the place of occurrence of the external cause

Y92.157 Garden or yard of reform school as the place of occurrence of the external cause

Y92.158 Other place in reform school as the place of occurrence of the external cause

Y92.159 Unspecified place in reform school as the place of occurrence of the external cause

✓6ᵗʰ **Y92.16** School dormitory as the place of occurrence of the external cause

EXCLUDES 1　reform school as the place of occurrence of the external cause (Y92.15-)
school buildings and grounds as the place of occurrence of the external cause (Y92.2-)
school sports and athletic areas as the place of occurrence of the external cause (Y92.3-)

Y92.160 Kitchen in school dormitory as the place of occurrence of the external cause

Y92.161 Dining room in school dormitory as the place of occurrence of the external cause

Y92.162 Bathroom in school dormitory as the place of occurrence of the external cause

Y92.163 Bedroom in school dormitory as the place of occurrence of the external cause

Y92.168 Other place in school dormitory as the place of occurrence of the external cause

Y92.169 Unspecified place in school dormitory as the place of occurrence of the external cause

✓6ᵗʰ **Y92.19** Other specified residential institution as the place of occurrence of the external cause

Y92.190 Kitchen in other specified residential institution as the place of occurrence of the external cause

Y92.191 Dining room in other specified residential institution as the place of occurrence of the external cause

Y92.192 Bathroom in other specified residential institution as the place of occurrence of the external cause

Y92.193 Bedroom in other specified residential institution as the place of occurrence of the external cause

Y92.194 Driveway of other specified residential institution as the place of occurrence of the external cause

Y92.195 Garage of other specified residential institution as the place of occurrence of the external cause

Y92.196 Pool of other specified residential institution as the place of occurrence of the external cause

Y92.197 Garden or yard of other specified residential institution as the place of occurrence of the external cause

Y92.198 Other place in other specified residential institution as the place of occurrence of the external cause

Y92.199 Unspecified place in other specified residential institution as the place of occurrence of the external cause

EXCLUDES 1 Not coded here　　EXCLUDES 2 Not included here　　N Newborn Age: 0　　P Pediatric Age: 0-17　　M Maternity Age: 12-55　　A Adult Age: 15-124

1052　　ICD-10-CM 2014 (Draft)

√6th **Y92.2** **School, other institution and public administrative area as the place of occurrence of the external cause**
　　Building and adjacent grounds used by the general public or by a particular group of the public
　　　EXCLUDES 1 *building under construction as the place of occurrence of the external cause (Y92.6)*
　　　　　residential institution as the place of occurrence of the external cause (Y92.1)
　　　　　school dormitory as the place of occurrence of the external cause (Y92.16-)
　　　　　sports and athletics area of schools as the place of occurrence of the external cause (Y92.3-)

√6th **Y92.21** **School (private) (public) (state) as the place of occurrence of the external cause**
　　Y92.210 **Daycare center as the place of occurrence of the external cause**
　　Y92.211 **Elementary school as the place of occurrence of the external cause**
　　　　Kindergarten as the place of occurrence of the external cause
　　Y92.212 **Middle school as the place of occurrence of the external cause**
　　Y92.213 **High school as the place of occurrence of the external cause**
　　　　AHA: 2012, Q4, 108
　　Y92.214 **College as the place of occurrence of the external cause**
　　　　University as the place of occurrence of the external cause
　　Y92.215 **Trade school as the place of occurrence of the external cause**
　　Y92.218 **Other school as the place of occurrence of the external cause**
　　Y92.219 **Unspecified school as the place of occurrence of the external cause**

Y92.22 **Religious institution as the place of occurrence of the external cause**
　　Church as the place of occurrence of the external cause
　　Mosque as the place of occurrence of the external cause
　　Synagogue as the place of occurrence of the external cause

√6th **Y92.23** **Hospital as the place of occurrence of the external cause**
　　　EXCLUDES 1 *ambulatory (outpatient) health services establishments (Y92.53-)*
　　　　　home for the sick as the place of occurrence of the external cause (Y92.12-)
　　　　　hospice as the place of occurrence of the external cause (Y92.12-)
　　　　　nursing home as the place of occurrence of the external cause (Y92.12-)
　　Y92.230 **Patient room in hospital as the place of occurrence of the external cause**
　　Y92.231 **Patient bathroom in hospital as the place of occurrence of the external cause**
　　Y92.232 **Corridor of hospital as the place of occurrence of the external cause**
　　Y92.233 **Cafeteria of hospital as the place of occurrence of the external cause**
　　Y92.234 **Operating room of hospital as the place of occurrence of the external cause**
　　Y92.238 **Other place in hospital as the place of occurrence of the external cause**
　　Y92.239 **Unspecified place in hospital as the place of occurrence of the external cause**

√6th **Y92.24** **Public administrative building as the place of occurrence of the external cause**
　　Y92.240 **Courthouse as the place of occurrence of the external cause**
　　Y92.241 **Library as the place of occurrence of the external cause**
　　Y92.242 **Post office as the place of occurrence of the external cause**
　　Y92.243 **City hall as the place of occurrence of the external cause**
　　Y92.248 **Other public administrative building as the place of occurrence of the external cause**

√6th **Y92.25** **Cultural building as the place of occurrence of the external cause**
　　Y92.250 **Art Gallery as the place of occurrence of the external cause**
　　Y92.251 **Museum as the place of occurrence of the external cause**
　　Y92.252 **Music hall as the place of occurrence of the external cause**
　　Y92.253 **Opera house as the place of occurrence of the external cause**
　　Y92.254 **Theater (live) as the place of occurrence of the external cause**
　　Y92.258 **Other cultural public building as the place of occurrence of the external cause**

Y92.26 **Movie house or cinema as the place of occurrence of the external cause**

Y92.29 **Other specified public building as the place of occurrence of the external cause**
　　Assembly hall as the place of occurrence of the external cause
　　Clubhouse as the place of occurrence of the external cause

√5th **Y92.3** **Sports and athletics area as the place of occurrence of the external cause**

√6th **Y92.31** **Athletic court as the place of occurrence of the external cause**
　　　EXCLUDES 1 *tennis court in private home or garden (Y92.09)*
　　Y92.310 **Basketball court as the place of occurrence of the external cause**
　　Y92.311 **Squash court as the place of occurrence of the external cause**
　　Y92.312 **Tennis court as the place of occurrence of the external cause**
　　Y92.318 **Other athletic court as the place of occurrence of the external cause**

√6th **Y92.32** **Athletic field as the place of occurrence of the external cause**
　　Y92.320 **Baseball field as the place of occurrence of the external cause**
　　Y92.321 **Football field as the place of occurrence of the external cause**
　　Y92.322 **Soccer field as the place of occurrence of the external cause**
　　Y92.328 **Other athletic field as the place of occurrence of the external cause**
　　　　Cricket field as the place of occurrence of the external cause
　　　　Hockey field as the place of occurrence of the external cause

√6th **Y92.33** **Skating rink as the place of occurrence of the external cause**
　　Y92.330 **Ice skating rink (indoor) (outdoor) as the place of occurrence of the external cause**
　　Y92.331 **Roller skating rink as the place of occurrence of the external cause**

Y92.34 **Swimming pool (public) as the place of occurrence of the external cause**
　　　EXCLUDES 1 *swimming pool in private home or garden (Y92.016)*

Y92.39 **Other specified sports and athletic area as the place of occurrence of the external cause**
　　Golf-course as the place of occurrence of the external cause
　　Gymnasium as the place of occurrence of the external cause
　　Riding-school as the place of occurrence of the external cause
　　Stadium as the place of occurrence of the external cause

√5th **Y92.4** **Street, highway and other paved roadways as the place of occurrence of the external cause**
　　　EXCLUDES 1 *private driveway of residence (Y92.014, Y92.024, Y92.043, Y92.093, Y92.113, Y92.123, Y92.154, Y92.194)*

☑ Additional Character Required　　√x7th Xtension Alert　　Unspecified Code　　Other Specified Code　　Manifestation Code　　►◄ Revised Text　　● New Code　　▲ Revised Code Title

ICD-10-CM 2014 (Draft)　　　　　　　　　　　　　　　　　　　　　　　　　　　　　　　　　1053

External Causes of Morbidity

Y92.41–Y92.813

✓6th **Y92.41** Street and highway as the place of occurrence of the external cause

     Y92.410 Unspecified street and highway as the place of occurrence of the external cause
         Road NOS as the place of occurrence of the external cause

     Y92.411 Interstate highway as the place of occurrence of the external cause
         Freeway as the place of occurrence of the external cause
         Motorway as the place of occurrence of the external cause

     Y92.412 Parkway as the place of occurrence of the external cause

     Y92.413 State road as the place of occurrence of the external cause

     Y92.414 Local residential or business street as the place of occurrence of the external cause

     Y92.415 Exit ramp or entrance ramp of street or highway as the place of occurrence of the external cause

✓6th **Y92.48** Other paved roadways as the place of occurrence of the external cause

     Y92.480 Sidewalk as the place of occurrence of the external cause

     Y92.481 Parking lot as the place of occurrence of the external cause

     Y92.482 Bike path as the place of occurrence of the external cause

     Y92.488 Other paved roadways as the place of occurrence of the external cause

✓5th **Y92.5** Trade and service area as the place of occurrence of the external cause
     EXCLUDES 1   garage in private home (Y92.015)
            schools and other public administration buildings (Y92.2-)

✓6th **Y92.51** Private commercial establishments as the place of occurrence of the external cause

     Y92.510 Bank as the place of occurrence of the external cause

     Y92.511 Restaurant or café as the place of occurrence of the external cause

     Y92.512 Supermarket, store or market as the place of occurrence of the external cause

     Y92.513 Shop (commercial) as the place of occurrence of the external cause

✓6th **Y92.52** Service areas as the place of occurrence of the external cause

     Y92.520 Airport as the place of occurrence of the external cause

     Y92.521 Bus station as the place of occurrence of the external cause

     Y92.522 Railway station as the place of occurrence of the external cause

     Y92.523 Highway rest stop as the place of occurrence of the external cause

     Y92.524 Gas station as the place of occurrence of the external cause
         Petroleum station as the place of occurrence of the external cause
         Service station as the place of occurrence of the external cause

✓6th **Y92.53** Ambulatory health services establishments as the place of occurrence of the external cause

     Y92.530 Ambulatory surgery center as the place of occurrence of the external cause
         Outpatient surgery center, including that connected with a hospital as the place of occurrence of the external cause
         Same day surgery center, including that connected with a hospital as the place of occurrence of the external cause

     Y92.531 Health care provider office as the place of occurrence of the external cause
         Physician office as the place of occurrence of the external cause

     Y92.532 Urgent care center as the place of occurrence of the external cause

     Y92.538 Other ambulatory health services establishments as the place of occurrence of the external cause

     Y92.59 Other trade areas as the place of occurrence of the external cause
         Office building as the place of occurrence of the external cause
         Casino as the place of occurrence of the external cause
         Garage (commercial) as the place of occurrence of the external cause
         Hotel as the place of occurrence of the external cause
         Radio or television station as the place of occurrence of the external cause
         Shopping mall as the place of occurrence of the external cause
         Warehouse as the place of occurrence of the external cause

✓5th **Y92.6** Industrial and construction area as the place of occurrence of the external cause

     Y92.61 Building [any] under construction as the place of occurrence of the external cause

     Y92.62 Dock or shipyard as the place of occurrence of the external cause
         Dockyard as the place of occurrence of the external cause
         Dry dock as the place of occurrence of the external cause
         Shipyard as the place of occurrence of the external cause

     Y92.63 Factory as the place of occurrence of the external cause
         Factory building as the place of occurrence of the external cause
         Factory premises as the place of occurrence of the external cause
         Industrial yard as the place of occurrence of the external cause

     Y92.64 Mine or pit as the place of occurrence of the external cause
         Mine as the place of occurrence of the external cause

     Y92.65 Oil rig as the place of occurrence of the external cause
         Pit (coal) (gravel) (sand) as the place of occurrence of the external cause

     Y92.69 Other specified industrial and construction area as the place of occurrence of the external cause
         Gasworks as the place of occurrence of the external cause
         Power-station (coal) (nuclear) (oil) as the place of occurrence of the external cause
         Tunnel under construction as the place of occurrence of the external cause
         Workshop as the place of occurrence of the external cause

✓5th **Y92.7** Farm as the place of occurrence of the external cause
     Ranch as the place of occurrence of the external cause
     EXCLUDES 1   farmhouse and home premises of farm (Y92.01-)

     Y92.71 Barn as the place of occurrence of the external cause

     Y92.72 Chicken coop as the place of occurrence of the external cause
         Hen house as the place of occurrence of the external cause

     Y92.73 Farm field as the place of occurrence of the external cause

     Y92.74 Orchard as the place of occurrence of the external cause

     Y92.79 Other farm location as the place of occurrence of the external cause

✓5th **Y92.8** Other places as the place of occurrence of the external cause

     ✓6th **Y92.81** Transport vehicle as the place of occurrence of the external cause
         EXCLUDES 1   transport accidents (V00-V99)

     Y92.810 Car as the place of occurrence of the external cause

     Y92.811 Bus as the place of occurrence of the external cause

     Y92.812 Truck as the place of occurrence of the external cause

     Y92.813 Airplane as the place of occurrence of the external cause

---

EXCLUDES 1 Not coded here   *EXCLUDES 2* Not included here   N Newborn Age: 0   P Pediatric Age: 0-17   M Maternity Age: 12-55   A Adult Age: 15-124

Y92.814 Boat as the place of occurrence of the external cause

Y92.815 Train as the place of occurrence of the external cause

Y92.816 Subway car as the place of occurrence of the external cause

Y92.818 Other transport vehicle as the place of occurrence of the external cause

✓6ᵗʰ **Y92.82** Wilderness area

Y92.820 Desert as the place of occurrence of the external cause

Y92.821 Forest as the place of occurrence of the external cause

Y92.828 Other wilderness area as the place of occurrence of the external cause
Swamp as the place of occurrence of the external cause
Mountain as the place of occurrence of the external cause
Marsh as the place of occurrence of the external cause
Prairie as the place of occurrence of the external cause

✓6ᵗʰ **Y92.83** Recreation area as the place of occurrence of the external cause

Y92.830 Public park as the place of occurrence of the external cause

Y92.831 Amusement park as the place of occurrence of the external cause

Y92.832 Beach as the place of occurrence of the external cause
Seashore as the place of occurrence of the external cause

Y92.833 Campsite as the place of occurrence of the external cause

Y92.834 Zoological garden (Zoo) as the place of occurrence of the external cause

Y92.838 Other recreation area as the place of occurrence of the external cause

Y92.84 Military training ground as the place of occurrence of the external cause

Y92.85 Railroad track as the place of occurrence of the external cause

Y92.86 Slaughter house as the place of occurrence of the external cause

Y92.89 Other specified places as the place of occurrence of the external cause
Derelict house as the place of occurrence of the external cause

Y92.9 Unspecified place or not applicable

✓4ᵗʰ **Y93** Activity codes

NOTE   Category Y93 is provided for use to indicate the activity of the person seeking healthcare for an injury or health condition, such as a heart attack while shoveling snow, which resulted from, or was contributed to, by the activity. These codes are appropriate for use for both acute injuries, such as those from chapter 19, and conditions that are due to the long-term, cumulative effects of an activity, such as those from chapter 13. They are also appropriate for use with external cause codes for cause and intent if identifying the activity provides additional information on the event. These codes should be used in conjunction with codes for external cause status (Y99) and place of occurrence (Y92).

This section contains the following broad activity categories:

Y93.0   Activities involving walking and running
Y93.1   Activities involving water and water craft
Y93.2   Activities involving ice and snow
Y93.3   Activities involving climbing, rappelling, and jumping off
Y93.4   Activities involving dancing and other rhythmic movement
Y93.5   Activities involving other sports and athletics played individually
Y93.6   Activities involving other sports and athletics played as a team or group
Y93.7   Activities involving other specified sports and athletics
Y93.A   Activities involving other cardiorespiratory exercise
Y93.B   Activities involving other muscle strengthening exercises
Y93.C   Activities involving computer technology and electronic devices
Y93.D   Activities involving arts and handcrafts
Y93.E   Activities involving personal hygiene and interior property and clothing maintenance
Y93.F   Activities involving caregiving
Y93.G   Activities involving food preparation, cooking and grilling
Y93.H   Activities involving exterior property and land maintenance, building and construction
Y93.I   Activities involving roller coasters and other types of external motion
Y93.J   Activities involving playing musical instrument
Y93.K   Activities involving animal care
Y93.8   Activities, other specified
Y93.9   Activity, unspecified

✓5ᵗʰ **Y93.0** Activities involving walking and running
EXCLUDES 1   activity, walking an animal (Y93.K1)
activity, walking or running on a treadmill (Y93.A1)

Y93.01 Activity, walking, marching and hiking
Activity, walking, marching and hiking on level or elevated terrain
EXCLUDES 1   activity, mountain climbing (Y93.31)

Y93.02 Activity, running

✓5ᵗʰ **Y93.1** Activities involving water and water craft
EXCLUDES 1   activities involving ice (Y93.2-)

Y93.11 Activity, swimming

Y93.12 Activity, springboard and platform diving

Y93.13 Activity, water polo

Y93.14 Activity, water aerobics and water exercise

Y93.15 Activity, underwater diving and snorkeling
Activity, SCUBA diving

Y93.16 Activity, rowing, canoeing, kayaking, rafting and tubing
Activity, canoeing, kayaking, rafting and tubing in calm and turbulent water

Y93.17 Activity, water skiing and wake boarding

Y93.18 Activity, surfing, windsurfing and boogie boarding
Activity, water sliding

Y93.19 Activity, other activity involving water and watercraft
Activity involving water NOS
Activity, parasailing
Activity, water survival training and testing

✓5ᵗʰ **Y93.2** Activities involving ice and snow
EXCLUDES 1   activity, shoveling ice and snow (Y93.H1)

Y93.21 Activity, ice skating
Activity, figure skating (singles) (pairs)
Activity, ice dancing
EXCLUDES 1   activity, ice hockey (Y93.22)

Y93.22 Activity, ice hockey

Y93.23   **Activity, snow (alpine) (downhill) skiing, snow boarding, sledding, tobogganing and snow tubing**
> EXCLUDES 1   *activity, cross country skiing (Y93.24)*

Y93.24   **Activity, cross country skiing**
Activity, nordic skiing

Y93.29   **Activity, other involving ice and snow**
Activity involving ice and snow NOS

✓5ᵗʰ **Y93.3**   **Activities involving climbing, rappelling and jumping off**
> EXCLUDES 1   *activity, hiking on level or elevated terrain (Y93.01)*
> *activity, jumping rope (Y93.56)*
> *activity, trampoline jumping (Y93.44)*

Y93.31   **Activity, mountain climbing, rock climbing and wall climbing**

Y93.32   **Activity, rappelling**

Y93.33   **Activity, BASE jumping**
Activity, Building, Antenna, Span, Earth jumping

Y93.34   **Activity, bungee jumping**

Y93.35   **Activity, hang gliding**

Y93.39   **Activity, other involving climbing, rappelling and jumping off**

✓5ᵗʰ **Y93.4**   **Activities involving dancing and other rhythmic movement**
> EXCLUDES 1   *activity, martial arts (Y93.75)*

Y93.41   **Activity, dancing**
AHA: 2012, Q4, 108

Y93.42   **Activity, yoga**

Y93.43   **Activity, gymnastics**
Activity, rhythmic gymnastics
> EXCLUDES 1   *activity, trampolining (Y93.44)*

Y93.44   **Activity, trampolining**

Y93.45   **Activity, cheerleading**

Y93.49   **Activity, other involving dancing and other rhythmic movements**

✓5ᵗʰ **Y93.5**   **Activities involving other sports and athletics played individually**
> EXCLUDES 1   *activity, dancing (Y93.41)*
> *activity, gymnastic (Y93.43)*
> *activity, trampolining (Y93.44)*
> *activity, yoga (Y93.42)*

Y93.51   **Activity, roller skating (inline) and skateboarding**

Y93.52   **Activity, horseback riding**

Y93.53   **Activity, golf**

Y93.54   **Activity, bowling**

Y93.55   **Activity, bike riding**

Y93.56   **Activity, jumping rope**

Y93.57   **Activity, non-running track and field events**
> EXCLUDES 1   *activity, running (any form) (Y93.02)*

Y93.59   **Activity, other involving other sports and athletics played individually**
> EXCLUDES 1   *activities involving climbing, rappelling, and jumping (Y93.3-)*
> *activities involving ice and snow (Y93.2-)*
> *activities involving walking and running (Y93.0-)*
> *activities involving water and watercraft (Y93.1-)*

✓5ᵗʰ **Y93.6**   **Activities involving other sports and athletics played as a team or group**
> EXCLUDES 1   *activity, ice hockey (Y93.22)*
> *activity, water polo (Y93.13)*

Y93.61   **Activity, American tackle football**
Activity, football NOS

Y93.62   **Activity, American flag or touch football**

Y93.63   **Activity, rugby**

Y93.64   **Activity, baseball**
Activity, softball

Y93.65   **Activity, lacrosse and field hockey**

Y93.66   **Activity, soccer**

Y93.67   **Activity, basketball**

Y93.68   **Activity, volleyball (beach) (court)**

Y93.6A   **Activity, physical games generally associated with school recess, summer camp and children**   P
Activity, capture the flag
Activity, dodge ball
Activity, four square
Activity, kickball

Y93.69   **Activity, other involving other sports and athletics played as a team or group**
Activity, cricket

✓5ᵗʰ **Y93.7**   **Activities involving other specified sports and athletics**

Y93.71   **Activity, boxing**

Y93.72   **Activity, wrestling**

Y93.73   **Activity, racquet and hand sports**
Activity, handball
Activity, racquetball
Activity, squash
Activity, tennis

Y93.74   **Activity, frisbee**
Activity, ultimate frisbee

Y93.75   **Activity, martial arts**
Activity, combatives

Y93.79   **Activity, other specified sports and athletics**
> EXCLUDES 1   *sports and athletics activities specified in categories Y93.0-Y93.6*

✓5ᵗʰ **Y93.A**   **Activities involving other cardiorespiratory exercise**
Activities involving physical training

Y93.A1   **Activity, exercise machines primarily for cardiorespiratory conditioning**
Activity, elliptical and stepper machines
Activity, stationary bike
Activity, treadmill

Y93.A2   **Activity, calisthenics**
Activity, jumping jacks
Activity, warm up and cool down

Y93.A3   **Activity, aerobic and step exercise**

Y93.A4   **Activity, circuit training**

Y93.A5   **Activity, obstacle course**
Activity, challenge course
Activity, confidence course

Y93.A6   **Activity, grass drills**
Activity, guerilla drills

Y93.A9   **Activity, other involving other cardiorespiratory exercise**
> EXCLUDES 1   *activities involving cardiorespiratory exercise specified in categories Y93.0-Y93.7*

✓5ᵗʰ **Y93.B**   **Activities involving other muscle strengthening exercises**

Y93.B1   **Activity, exercise machines primarily for muscle strengthening**

Y93.B2   **Activity, push-ups, pull-ups, sit-ups**

Y93.B3   **Activity, free weights**
Activity, barbells
Activity, dumbbells

Y93.B4   **Activity, pilates**

Y93.B9   **Activity, other involving other muscle strengthening exercises**
> EXCLUDES 1   *activities involving muscle strengthening specified in categories Y93.0-Y93.A*

✓5ᵗʰ **Y93.C**   **Activities involving computer technology and electronic devices**
> EXCLUDES 1   *activity, electronic musical keyboard or instruments (Y93.J-)*

Y93.C1   **Activity, computer keyboarding**
Activity, electronic game playing using keyboard or other stationary device

Y93.C2   **Activity, hand held interactive electronic device**
Activity, cellular telephone and communication device
Activity, electronic game playing using interactive device
> EXCLUDES 1   *activity, electronic game playing using keyboard or other stationary device (Y93.C1)*

Y93.C9   **Activity, other involving computer technology and electronic devices**

✓5ᵗʰ **Y93.D**   **Activities involving arts and handcrafts**
> EXCLUDES 1   *activities involving playing musical instrument (Y93.J-)*

Y93.D1   **Activity, knitting and crocheting**

Y93.D2   **Activity, sewing**

Y93.D3   **Activity, furniture building and finishing**
Activity, furniture repair

Y93.D9   **Activity, involving other arts and handcrafts**

EXCLUDES 1 Not coded here   EXCLUDES 2 Not included here   N Newborn Age: 0   P Pediatric Age: 0-17   M Maternity Age: 12-55   A Adult Age: 15-124

1056   ICD-10-CM 2014 (Draft)

✓5ᵗʰ **Y93.E Activities involving personal hygiene and interior property and clothing maintenance**

> **EXCLUDES 1** *activities involving cooking and grilling (Y93.G-)*
> *activities involving exterior property and land maintenance, building and construction (Y93.H-)*
> *activities involving caregiving (Y93.F-)*
> *activity, dishwashing (Y93.G1)*
> *activity, food preparation (Y93.G1)*
> *activity, gardening (Y93.H2)*

Y93.E1 Activity, personal bathing and showering

Y93.E2 Activity, laundry

Y93.E3 Activity, vacuuming

Y93.E4 Activity, ironing

Y93.E5 Activity, floor mopping and cleaning

Y93.E6 Activity, residential relocation
Activity, packing up and unpacking involved in moving to a new residence

Y93.E8 Activity, other personal hygiene

Y93.E9 Activity, other interior property and clothing maintenance

✓5ᵗʰ **Y93.F Activities involving caregiving**
Activity involving the provider of caregiving

Y93.F1 Activity, caregiving, bathing

Y93.F2 Activity, caregiving, lifting

Y93.F9 Activity, other caregiving

✓5ᵗʰ **Y93.G Activities involving food preparation, cooking and grilling**

Y93.G1 Activity, food preparation and clean up
Activity, dishwashing

Y93.G2 Activity, grilling and smoking food

Y93.G3 Activity, cooking and baking
Activity, use of stove, oven and microwave oven

Y93.G9 Activity, other involving cooking and grilling

✓5ᵗʰ **Y93.H Activities involving exterior property and land maintenance, building and construction**

Y93.H1 Activity, digging, shoveling and raking
Activity, dirt digging
Activity, raking leaves
Activity, snow shoveling

Y93.H2 Activity, gardening and landscaping
Activity, pruning, trimming shrubs, weeding

Y93.H3 Activity, building and construction

Y93.H9 Activity, other involving exterior property and land maintenance, building and construction

✓5ᵗʰ **Y93.I Activities involving roller coasters and other types of external motion**

Y93.I1 Activity, rollercoaster riding

Y93.I9 Activity, other involving external motion

✓5ᵗʰ **Y93.J Activities involving playing musical instrument**
Activity involving playing electric musical instrument

Y93.J1 Activity, piano playing
Activity, musical keyboard (electronic) playing

Y93.J2 Activity, drum and other percussion instrument playing

Y93.J3 Activity, string instrument playing

Y93.J4 Activity, winds and brass instrument playing

✓5ᵗʰ **Y93.K Activities involving animal care**

> **EXCLUDES 1** *activity, horseback riding (Y93.52)*

Y93.K1 Activity, walking an animal

Y93.K2 Activity, milking an animal

Y93.K3 Activity, grooming and shearing an animal

Y93.K9 Activity, other involving animal care

✓5ᵗʰ **Y93.8 Activities, other specified**

Y93.81 Activity, refereeing a sports activity

Y93.82 Activity, spectator at an event

Y93.83 Activity, rough housing and horseplay

Y93.84 Activity, sleeping

Y93.89 Activity, other specified

Y93.9 Activity, unspecified

Y95 Nosocomial condition

✓4ᵗʰ **Y99 External cause status**

> **NOTE** A single code from category Y99 should be used in conjunction with the external cause code(s) assigned to a record to indicate the status of the person at the time the event occurred.

Y99.0 Civilian activity done for income or pay
Civilian activity done for financial or other compensation

> **EXCLUDES 1** *military activity (Y99.1)*
> *volunteer activity (Y99.2)*

Y99.1 Military activity

> **EXCLUDES 1** *activity of off duty military personnel (Y99.8)*

Y99.2 Volunteer activity

> **EXCLUDES 1** *activity of child or other family member assisting in compensated work of other family member (Y99.8)*

Y99.8 Other external cause status
Activity NEC
Activity of child or other family member assisting in compensated work of other family member
Hobby not done for income
Leisure activity
Off-duty activity of military personnel
Recreation or sport not for income or while a student
Student activity

> **EXCLUDES 1** *civilian activity done for income or compensation (Y99.0)*
> *military activity (Y99.1)*

AHA: 2012, Q4, 108

Y99.9 Unspecified external cause status

✓ Additional Character Required   ✓x7ᵗʰ Xtension Alert   Unspecified Code   Other Specified Code   Manifestation Code   ▶◀ Revised Text   ● New Code   ▲ Revised Code Title

ICD-10-CM 2014 (Draft)   1057

Chapter 21. Factors Influencing Health Status and Contact With Health Services (Z00-Z99)

NOTE   Z codes represent reasons for encounters. A corresponding procedure code must accompany a Z code if a procedure is performed. Categories Z00-Z99 are provided for occasions when circumstances other than a disease, injury or external cause classifiable to categories A00-Y89 are recorded as "diagnoses" or "problems". This can arise in two main ways:

(a) When a person who may or may not be sick encounters the health services for some specific purpose, such as to receive limited care or service for a current condition, to donate an organ or tissue, to receive prophylactic vaccination (immunization), or to discuss a problem which is in itself not a disease or injury.

(b) When some circumstance or problem is present which influences the person's health status but is not in itself a current illness or injury.

This chapter contains the following blocks:

Z00-Z13	Persons encountering health services for examinations
Z14-Z15	Genetic carrier and genetic susceptibility to disease
Z16	Resistance to antimicrobial drugs
Z17	Estrogen receptor status
Z18	Retained foreign body fragments
Z20-Z28	Persons with potential health hazards related to communicable diseases
Z30-Z39	Persons encountering health services in circumstances related to reproduction
Z40-Z53	Encounters for other specific health care
Z55-Z65	Persons with potential health hazards related to socioeconomic and psychosocial circumstances
Z66	Do not resuscitate status
Z67	Blood type
Z68	Body mass index (BMI)
Z69-Z76	Persons encountering health services in other circumstances
Z77-Z99	Persons with potential health hazards related to family and personal history and certain conditions influencing health status

Persons encountering health services for examinations (Z00-Z13)

NOTE   Nonspecific abnormal findings disclosed at the time of these examinations are classified to categories R70-R94.

EXCLUDES 1   *examinations related to pregnancy and reproduction (Z30-Z36, Z39-)*

✓4ᵗʰ **Z00**   **Encounter for general examination without complaint, suspected or reported diagnosis**

EXCLUDES 1   *encounter for examination for administrative purposes (Z02.-)*

EXCLUDES 2   *encounter for pre-procedural examinations (Z01.81-)*
special screening examinations (Z11-Z13)

✓5ᵗʰ **Z00.0**   **Encounter for general adult medical examination**
Encounter for adult periodic examination (annual) (physical) and any associated laboratory and radiologic examinations

EXCLUDES 1   *encounter for examination of sign or symptom—code to sign or symptom*
general health check-up of infant or child (Z00.12-)

    Z00.00   **Encounter for general adult medical examination without abnormal findings**   **A PDx**
Encounter for adult health check-up NOS

    Z00.01   **Encounter for general adult medical examination with abnormal findings**   **A PDx**
Use additional code to identify abnormal findings

✓5ᵗʰ **Z00.1**   **Encounter for newborn, infant and child health examinations**

   ✓6ᵗʰ **Z00.11**   **Newborn health examination**
Health check for child under 29 days old
Use additional code to identify any abnormal findings

EXCLUDES 1   *health check for child over 28 days old (Z00.12-)*

    Z00.110   **Health examination for newborn under 8 days old**   **N PDx**
Health check for newborn under 8 days old

    Z00.111   **Health examination for newborn 8 to 28 days old**   **N PDx**
Health check for newborn 8 to 28 days old
Newborn weight check

   ✓6ᵗʰ **Z00.12**   **Encounter for routine child health examination**
Encounter for development testing of infant or child
Health check (routine) for child over 28 days old

EXCLUDES 1   *health check for child under 29 days old (Z00.11-)*
health supervision of foundling or other healthy infant or child (Z76.1-Z76.2)
newborn health examination (Z00.11-)

    Z00.121   **Encounter for routine child health examination with abnormal findings**   **P PDx**
Use additional code to identify abnormal findings

    Z00.129   **Encounter for routine child health examination without abnormal findings**   **P PDx**
Encounter for routine child health examination NOS

Z00.2   **Encounter for examination for period of rapid growth in childhood**   **P PDx**

Z00.3   **Encounter for examination for adolescent development state**   **P PDx**
Encounter for puberty development state

Z00.5   **Encounter for examination of potential donor of organ and tissue**   **PDx**

Z00.6   **Encounter for examination for normal comparison and control in clinical research program**   **PDx**
Examination of participant or control in clinical research program

✓5ᵗʰ **Z00.7**   **Encounter for examination for period of delayed growth in childhood**

    Z00.70   **Encounter for examination for period of delayed growth in childhood without abnormal findings**   **P PDx**

    Z00.71   **Encounter for examination for period of delayed growth in childhood with abnormal findings**   **P PDx**
Use additional code to identify abnormal findings

Z00.8   **Encounter for other general examination**
Encounter for health examination in population surveys

✓4ᵗʰ **Z01**   **Encounter for other special examination without complaint, suspected or reported diagnosis**

INCLUDES   routine examination of specific system

NOTE   Codes from category Z01 represent the reason for the encounter. A separate procedure code is required to identify any examinations or procedures performed.

EXCLUDES 1   *encounter for examination for administrative purposes (Z02.-)*
encounter for examination for suspected conditions, proven not to exist (Z03.-)
encounter for laboratory and radiologic examinations as a component of general medical examinations (Z00.0-)
encounter for laboratory, radiologic and imaging examinations for sign(s) and symptom(s)—code to the sign(s) or symptom(s)

EXCLUDES 2   *screening examinations (Z11-Z13)*

✓5ᵗʰ **Z01.0**   **Encounter for examination of eyes and vision**

EXCLUDES 1   *examination for driving license (Z02.4)*

    Z01.00   **Encounter for examination of eyes and vision without abnormal findings**   **PDx**
Encounter for examination of eyes and vision NOS

    Z01.01   **Encounter for examination of eyes and vision with abnormal findings**   **PDx**
Use additional code to identify abnormal findings

✓5ᵗʰ **Z01.1**   **Encounter for examination of ears and hearing**

    Z01.10   **Encounter for examination of ears and hearing without abnormal findings**   **PDx**
Encounter for examination of ears and hearing NOS

   ✓6ᵗʰ **Z01.11**   **Encounter for examination of ears and hearing with abnormal findings**

    Z01.110   **Encounter for hearing examination following failed hearing screening**   **PDx**

    Z01.118   **Encounter for examination of ears and hearing with other abnormal findings**   **PDx**
Use additional code to identify abnormal findings

    Z01.12   **Encounter for hearing conservation and treatment**

✓5ᵗʰ **Z01.2**   **Encounter for dental examination and cleaning**

    Z01.20   **Encounter for dental examination and cleaning without abnormal findings**   **PDx**
Encounter for dental examination and cleaning NOS

    Z01.21   **Encounter for dental examination and cleaning with abnormal findings**   **PDx**
Use additional code to identify abnormal findings

EXCLUDES 1 Not coded here   **EXCLUDES 2** Not included here   **PDx** Primary Diagnosis Only   **N** Newborn Age: 0   **P** Pediatric Age: 0-17   **M** Maternity Age: 12-55   **A** Adult Age: 15-124

1058   ICD-10-CM 2014 (Draft)

√5ᵗʰ **Z01.3** **Encounter for examination of** blood pressure

Z01.30 **Encounter for examination of blood pressure without abnormal findings** `PDx`
Encounter for examination of blood pressure NOS

Z01.31 **Encounter for examination of blood pressure with abnormal findings** `PDx`
Use additional code to identify abnormal findings

√5ᵗʰ **Z01.4** **Encounter for** gynecological **examination**
EXCLUDES 2 *pregnancy examination or test (Z32.0-)*
routine examination for contraceptive maintenance (Z30.4-)

√6ᵗʰ **Z01.41** **Encounter for** routine gynecological **examination**
Encounter for general gynecological examination with or without cervical smear
Encounter for gynecological examination (general) (routine) NOS
Encounter for pelvic examination (annual) (periodic)
Use additional code:
for screening for human papillomavirus, if applicable, (Z11.51)
for screening vaginal pap smear, if applicable (Z12.72)
to identify acquired absence of uterus, if applicable (Z90.71-)
EXCLUDES 1 *gynecologic examination status-post hysterectomy for malignant condition (Z08)*
screening cervical pap smear not a part of a routine gynecological examination (Z12.4)

Z01.411 **Encounter for gynecological examination (general) (routine) with abnormal findings** ♀ `PDx`
Use additional code to identify abnormal findings

Z01.419 **Encounter for gynecological examination (general) (routine) without abnormal findings** ♀ `PDx`

Z01.42 **Encounter for** cervical smear to confirm findings **of recent normal smear following initial abnormal smear** ♀ `PDx`

√5ᵗʰ **Z01.8** **Encounter for** other specified special **examinations**

√6ᵗʰ **Z01.81** **Encounter for** preprocedural **examinations**
Encounter for preoperative examinations
Encounter for radiological and imaging examinations as part of preprocedural examination

Z01.810 **Encounter for preprocedural** cardiovascular **examination** `PDx`

Z01.811 **Encounter for preprocedural** respiratory **examination** `PDx`

Z01.812 **Encounter for preprocedural** laboratory **examination** `PDx`
Blood and urine tests prior to treatment or procedure

Z01.818 **Encounter for other preprocedural examination** `PDx`
Encounter for preprocedural examination NOS
Encounter for examinations prior to antineoplastic chemotherapy

Z01.82 **Encounter for** allergy testing `PDx`
EXCLUDES 1 *encounter for antibody response examination (Z01.84)*

Z01.83 **Encounter for** blood typing `PDx`
Encounter for Rh typing

Z01.84 **Encounter for** antibody response examination `PDx`
Encounter for immunity status testing
EXCLUDES 1 *encounter for allergy testing (Z01.82)*

Z01.89 **Encounter for other specified special examinations** `PDx`

√4ᵗʰ **Z02** **Encounter for** administrative **examination**

Z02.0 **Encounter for examination for** admission to educational institution
Encounter for examination for admission to preschool (education)
Encounter for examination for re-admission to school following illness or medical treatment

Z02.1 **Encounter for** pre-employment **examination** `PDx`

Z02.2 **Encounter for examination for** admission to residential institution `PDx`
EXCLUDES 1 *examination for admission to prison (Z02.89)*

Z02.3 **Encounter for examination for** recruitment to armed forces `PDx`

Z02.4 **Encounter for examination for** driving license `PDx`

Z02.5 **Encounter for examination for** participation in sport `PDx`
EXCLUDES 1 *blood-alcohol and blood-drug test (Z02.83)*

Z02.6 **Encounter for examination for** insurance purposes `PDx`

√5ᵗʰ **Z02.7** **Encounter for** issue of medical certificate
EXCLUDES 1 *encounter for general medical examination (Z00-Z01, Z02.0-Z02.6, Z02.8-Z02.9)*

Z02.71 **Encounter for** disability determination `PDx`
Encounter for issue of medical certificate of incapacity
Encounter for issue of medical certificate of invalidity

Z02.79 **Encounter for issue of other medical certificate** `PDx`

√5ᵗʰ **Z02.8** **Encounter for** other administrative examinations

Z02.81 **Encounter for** paternity testing `PDx`

Z02.82 **Encounter for** adoption services `PDx`

Z02.83 **Encounter for** blood-alcohol and blood-drug test `PDx`
Use additional code for findings of alcohol or drugs in blood (R78.-)

Z02.89 **Encounter for other administrative examinations** `PDx`
Encounter for examination for admission to prison
Encounter for examination for admission to summer camp
Encounter for immigration examination
Encounter for naturalization examination
Encounter for premarital examination
EXCLUDES 1 *health supervision of foundling or other healthy infant or child (Z76.1-Z76.2)*

Z02.9 **Encounter for administrative examinations, unspecified** `PDx`

√4ᵗʰ **Z03** **Encounter for** medical observation **for suspected diseases and conditions ruled out**
NOTE This category is to be used when a person without a diagnosis is suspected of having an abnormal condition, without signs or symptoms, which requires study, but after examination and observation, is ruled out. This category is also for use for administrative and legal observation status.
EXCLUDES 1 *contact with and (suspected) exposures hazardous to health (Z77.-)*
newborn observation for suspected condition, ruled out (P00-P04)
person with feared complaint in whom no diagnosis is made (Z71.1)
signs or symptoms under study—code to signs or symptoms

Z03.6 **Encounter for observation for suspected** toxic effect from ingested substance **ruled out** `PDx`
Encounter for observation for suspected adverse effect from drug
Encounter for observation for suspected poisoning

√5ᵗʰ **Z03.7** **Encounter for suspected** maternal and fetal conditions **ruled out**
Encounter for suspected maternal and fetal conditions not found
EXCLUDES 1 *known or suspected fetal anomalies affecting management of mother, not ruled out (O26-, O35-, O36-, O40-, O41-)*

Z03.71 **Encounter for suspected problem with amniotic cavity and membrane ruled out** Ⓜ ♀ `PDx`
Encounter for suspected oligohydramnios ruled out
Encounter for suspected polyhydramnios ruled out

Z03.72 **Encounter for suspected** placental problem **ruled out** Ⓜ ♀ `PDx`

Z03.73 **Encounter for suspected** fetal anomaly **ruled out** Ⓜ ♀ `PDx`

Z03.74 **Encounter for suspected** problem with fetal growth **ruled out** Ⓜ ♀ `PDx`

Z03.75 **Encounter for suspected** cervical shortening **ruled out** Ⓜ ♀ `PDx`

Z03.79 **Encounter for other suspected maternal and fetal conditions ruled out** Ⓜ ♀ `PDx`

✓5ᵗʰ **Z03.8 Encounter for observation for other suspected diseases and conditions ruled out**

   ✓6ᵗʰ **Z03.81 Encounter for observation for suspected exposure to biological agents ruled out**

   Z03.810 Encounter for observation for suspected exposure to anthrax ruled out   PDx

   Z03.818 Encounter for observation for suspected exposure to other biological agents ruled out   PDx

   Z03.89 Encounter for observation for other suspected diseases and conditions ruled out   PDx

✓4ᵗʰ **Z04 Encounter for examination and observation for other reasons**

   INCLUDES encounter for examination for medicolegal reasons

   NOTE This category is to be used when a person without a diagnosis is suspected of having an abnormal condition, without signs or symptoms, which requires study, but after examination and observation, is ruled-out. This category is also for use for administrative and legal observation status.

   Z04.1 Encounter for examination and observation following transport accident   PDx

   EXCLUDES 1 encounter for examination and observation following work accident (Z04.2)

   Z04.2 Encounter for examination and observation following work accident   PDx

   Z04.3 Encounter for examination and observation following other accident   PDx

   ✓5ᵗʰ **Z04.4 Encounter for examination and observation following alleged rape**

   Encounter for examination and observation of victim following alleged rape
   Encounter for examination and observation of victim following alleged sexual abuse

   Z04.41 Encounter for examination and observation following alleged adult rape   A PDx
   Suspected adult rape, ruled out
   Suspected adult sexual abuse, ruled out

   Z04.42 Encounter for examination and observation following alleged child rape   P PDx
   Suspected child rape, ruled out
   Suspected child sexual abuse, ruled out

   Z04.6 Encounter for general psychiatric examination, requested by authority   PDx

   ✓5ᵗʰ **Z04.7 Encounter for examination and observation following alleged physical abuse**

   Z04.71 Encounter for examination and observation following alleged adult physical abuse   A PDx
   Suspected adult physical abuse, ruled out
   EXCLUDES 1 confirmed case of adult physical abuse (T74.-)
   encounter for examination and observation following alleged adult sexual abuse (Z04.41)
   suspected case of adult physical abuse, not ruled out (T76.-)

   Z04.72 Encounter for examination and observation following alleged child physical abuse   P PDx
   Suspected child physical abuse, ruled out
   EXCLUDES 1 confirmed case of child physical abuse (T74.-)
   encounter for examination and observation following alleged child sexual abuse (Z04.42)
   suspected case of child physical abuse, not ruled out (T76.-)

   Z04.8 Encounter for examination and observation for other specified reasons   PDx
   Encounter for examination and observation for request for expert evidence

   Z04.9 Encounter for examination and observation for unspecified reason   PDx
   Encounter for observation NOS

Z08 Encounter for follow-up examination after completed treatment for malignant neoplasm
   Medical surveillance following completed treatment
   Use additional code to identify any acquired absence of organs (Z90.-)
   Use additional code to identify the personal history of malignant neoplasm (Z85.-)
   EXCLUDES 1 aftercare following medical care (Z43-Z49, Z51)

Z09 Encounter for follow-up examination after completed treatment for conditions other than malignant neoplasm
   Medical surveillance following completed treatment
   Use additional code to identify any applicable history of disease code (Z86-. Z87-)
   EXCLUDES 1 aftercare following medical care (Z43-Z49, Z51)
   surveillance of contraception (Z30.4-)
   surveillance of prosthetic and other medical devices (Z44-Z46)

✓4ᵗʰ **Z11 Encounter for screening for infectious and parasitic diseases**
   NOTE Screening is the testing for disease or disease precursors in asymptomatic individuals so that early detection and treatment can be provided for those who test positive for the disease.
   EXCLUDES 1 encounter for diagnostic examination—code to sign or symptom

   Z11.0 Encounter for screening for intestinal infectious diseases

   Z11.1 Encounter for screening for respiratory tuberculosis

   Z11.2 Encounter for screening for other bacterial diseases

   Z11.3 Encounter for screening for infections with a predominantly sexual mode of transmission
   EXCLUDES 2 encounter for screening for human immunodeficiency virus [HIV] (Z11.4)
   encounter for screening for human papillomavirus (Z11.51)

   Z11.4 Encounter for screening for human immunodeficiency virus [HIV]

   ✓5ᵗʰ **Z11.5 Encounter for screening for other viral diseases**
   EXCLUDES 2 encounter for screening for viral intestinal disease (Z11.0)

   Z11.51 Encounter for screening for human papillomavirus (HPV)

   Z11.59 Encounter for screening for other viral diseases

   Z11.6 Encounter for screening for other protozoal diseases and helminthiases
   EXCLUDES 2 encounter for screening for protozoal intestinal disease (Z11.0)

   Z11.8 Encounter for screening for other infectious and parasitic diseases
   Encounter for screening for chlamydia
   Encounter for screening for rickettsial
   Encounter for screening for spirochetal
   Encounter for screening for mycoses

   Z11.9 Encounter for screening for infectious and parasitic diseases, unspecified

✓4ᵗʰ **Z12 Encounter for screening for malignant neoplasms**
   NOTE Screening is the testing for disease or disease precursors in asymptomatic individuals so that early detection and treatment can be provided for those who test positive for the disease.
   Use additional code to identify any family history of malignant neoplasm (Z80.-)
   EXCLUDES 1 encounter for diagnostic examination—code to sign or symptom

   Z12.0 Encounter for screening for malignant neoplasm of stomach

   ✓5ᵗʰ **Z12.1 Encounter for screening for malignant neoplasm of intestinal tract**

   Z12.10 Encounter for screening for malignant neoplasm of intestinal tract, unspecified

   Z12.11 Encounter for screening for malignant neoplasm of colon
   Encounter for screening colonoscopy NOS

   Z12.12 Encounter for screening for malignant neoplasm of rectum

   Z12.13 Encounter for screening for malignant neoplasm of small intestine

   Z12.2 Encounter for screening for malignant neoplasm of respiratory organs

   ✓5ᵗʰ **Z12.3 Encounter for screening for malignant neoplasm of breast**

   Z12.31 Encounter for screening mammogram for malignant neoplasm of breast
   EXCLUDES 1 inconclusive mammogram (R92.2)

   Z12.39 Encounter for other screening for malignant neoplasm of breast

---

EXCLUDES 1 Not coded here   EXCLUDES 2 Not included here   PDx Primary Diagnosis Only   N Newborn Age: 0   P Pediatric Age: 0-17   M Maternity Age: 12-55   A Adult Age: 15-124

1060   ICD-10-CM 2014 (Draft)

Z12.4 **Encounter for screening for malignant neoplasm of** cervix ♀
Encounter for screening pap smear for malignant neoplasm of cervix
EXCLUDES 1 *encounter for screening for human papillomavirus (Z11.51)*
when screening is part of general gynecological examination (Z01.4-)

Z12.5 **Encounter for screening for malignant neoplasm of** prostate ♂

Z12.6 **Encounter for screening for malignant neoplasm of** bladder

√5th **Z12.7** **Encounter for screening for malignant neoplasm of** other genitourinary organs

    Z12.71 **Encounter for screening for malignant neoplasm of** testis ♂

    Z12.72 **Encounter for screening for malignant neoplasm of** vagina ♀
Vaginal pap smear status-post hysterectomy for non-malignant condition
Use additional code to identify acquired absence of uterus (Z90.71-)
EXCLUDES 1 *vaginal pap smear status-post hysterectomy for malignant conditions (Z08)*

    Z12.73 **Encounter for screening for malignant neoplasm of** ovary ♀

    Z12.79 **Encounter for screening for malignant neoplasm of other genitourinary organs**

√5th **Z12.8** **Encounter for screening for malignant neoplasm of** other sites

    Z12.81 **Encounter for screening for malignant neoplasm of** oral cavity

    Z12.82 **Encounter for screening for malignant neoplasm of** nervous system

    Z12.83 **Encounter for screening for malignant neoplasm of** skin

    Z12.89 **Encounter for screening for malignant neoplasm of other sites**

Z12.9 **Encounter for screening for malignant neoplasm, site unspecified**

√4th **Z13** **Encounter for screening for** other diseases and disorders
NOTE Screening is the testing for disease or disease precursors in asymptomatic individuals so that early detection and treatment can be provided for those who test positive for the disease.
EXCLUDES 1 *encounter for diagnostic examination—code to sign or symptom*

Z13.0 **Encounter for screening for diseases of the** blood and blood-forming organs **and certain disorders involving the immune mechanism**

Z13.1 **Encounter for screening for** diabetes mellitus

√5th **Z13.2** **Encounter for screening for nutritional, metabolic and other endocrine disorders**

    Z13.21 **Encounter for screening for** nutritional disorder

    √6th **Z13.22** **Encounter for screening for** metabolic disorder

        Z13.220 **Encounter for screening for** lipoid disorders
Encounter for screening for cholesterol level
Encounter for screening for hypercholesterolemia
Encounter for screening for hyperlipidemia

        Z13.228 **Encounter for screening for other metabolic disorders**

    Z13.29 **Encounter for screening for other suspected endocrine disorder**
EXCLUDES 1 *encounter for screening for diabetes mellitus (Z13.1)*

Z13.4 **Encounter for screening for certain** developmental disorders in childhood ℗
Encounter for screening for developmental handicaps in early childhood
EXCLUDES 1 *routine development testing of infant or child (Z00.1-)*

Z13.5 **Encounter for screening for** eye and ear disorders
EXCLUDES 2 *encounter for general hearing examination (Z01.1-)*
encounter for general vision examination (Z01.0-)

Z13.6 **Encounter for screening for** cardiovascular disorders

√5th **Z13.7** **Encounter for screening for** genetic and chromosomal anomalies
EXCLUDES 1 *genetic testing for procreative management (Z31.4-)*

    Z13.71 **Encounter for nonprocreative screening for genetic disease carrier status**

    Z13.79 **Encounter for other screening for genetic and chromosomal anomalies**

√5th **Z13.8** **Encounter for screening for** other specified diseases and disorders
EXCLUDES 2 *screening for malignant neoplasms (Z12.-)*

    √6th **Z13.81** **Encounter for screening for** digestive system disorders

        Z13.810 **Encounter for screening for** upper gastrointestinal disorder

        Z13.811 **Encounter for screening for** lower gastrointestinal disorder
EXCLUDES 1 *encounter for screening for intestinal infectious disease (Z11.0)*

        Z13.818 **Encounter for screening for other digestive system disorders**

    √6th **Z13.82** **Encounter for screening for** musculoskeletal disorder

        Z13.820 **Encounter for screening for** osteoporosis

        Z13.828 **Encounter for screening for other musculoskeletal disorder**

    Z13.83 **Encounter for screening for** respiratory disorder NEC
EXCLUDES 1 *encounter for screening for respiratory tuberculosis (Z11.1)*

    Z13.84 **Encounter for screening for** dental disorders

    √6th **Z13.85** **Encounter for screening for** nervous system disorders

        Z13.850 **Encounter for screening for** traumatic brain injury

        Z13.858 **Encounter for screening for other nervous system disorders**

    Z13.88 **Encounter for screening for disorder** due to exposure to contaminants
EXCLUDES 1 *those exposed to contaminants without suspected disorders (Z57-Z77-)*

    Z13.89 **Encounter for screening for other disorder**
Encounter for screening for genitourinary disorders

Z13.9 **Encounter for screening, unspecified**

Genetic carrier and genetic susceptibility to disease (Z14-Z15)

√4th **Z14** **Genetic carrier**

√5th **Z14.0** Hemophilia A carrier

    Z14.01 **Asymptomatic** hemophilia A carrier

    Z14.02 **Symptomatic** hemophilia A carrier

Z14.1 Cystic fibrosis carrier

Z14.8 **Genetic carrier of other disease**

√4th **Z15** **Genetic susceptibility** to disease
Confirmed abnormal gene
Use additional code, if applicable, for any associated family history of the disease (Z80-Z84)
EXCLUDES 1 *chromosomal anomalies (Q90-Q99)*

√5th **Z15.0** **Genetic susceptibility to** malignant neoplasm
Code first, if applicable, any current malignant neoplasm (C00-C75, C81-C96)
Use additional code, if applicable, for any personal history of malignant neoplasm (Z85.-)

    Z15.01 **Genetic susceptibility to malignant neoplasm of** breast

    Z15.02 **Genetic susceptibility to malignant neoplasm of** ovary ♀

    Z15.03 **Genetic susceptibility to malignant neoplasm of** prostate ♂

    Z15.04 **Genetic susceptibility to malignant neoplasm of** endometrium ♀

    Z15.09 **Genetic susceptibility to other malignant neoplasm**

√5th **Z15.8** **Genetic susceptibility to other disease**

    Z15.81 **Genetic susceptibility to** multiple endocrine neoplasia [MEN]
EXCLUDES 1 *multiple endocrine neoplasia [MEN] syndromes (E31.2-)*

    Z15.89 **Genetic susceptibility to other disease**

✓ Additional Character Required   √x7th Xtension Alert   Unspecified Code   Other Specified Code   Manifestation Code   ►◄ Revised Text   ● New Code   ▲ Revised Code Title

ICD-10-CM 2014 (Draft)   1061

Resistance to antimicrobial drugs (Z16)

☑4ᵗʰ **Z16 Resistance to antimicrobial drugs**

NOTE The codes in this category are provided for use as additional codes to identify the resistance and non-responsiveness of a condition to antimicrobial drugs.

Code first the infection

EXCLUDES 1 *Methicillin resistant Staphylococcus aureus infection (A49.02)*
Methicillin resistant Staphylococcus aureus infection in diseases classified elsewhere (B95.62)
Methicillin resistant Staphylococcus aureus pneumonia (J15.212)
Sepsis due to Methicillin resistant Staphylococcus aureus (A41.02)

☑5ᵗʰ **Z16.1 Resistance to beta lactam antibiotics**

Z16.10 Resistance to unspecified beta lactam antibiotics

Z16.11 Resistance to penicillins
Resistance to amoxicillin   Resistance to ampicillin

Z16.12 Extended spectrum beta lactamase (ESBL) resistance

Z16.19 Resistance to other specified beta lactam antibiotics
Resistance to cephalosporins

☑5ᵗʰ **Z16.2 Resistance to other antibiotics**

Z16.20 Resistance to unspecified antibiotic
Resistance to antibiotics NOS

Z16.21 Resistance to vancomycin

Z16.22 Resistance to vancomycin related antibiotics

Z16.23 Resistance to quinolones and fluoroquinolones

Z16.24 Resistance to multiple antibiotics

Z16.29 Resistance to other single specified antibiotic
Resistance to aminoglycosides
Resistance to macrolides
Resistance to sulfonamides
Resistance to tetracyclines

☑5ᵗʰ **Z16.3 Resistance to other antimicrobial drugs**
EXCLUDES 1 *resistance to antibiotics (Z16.1-, Z16.2-)*

Z16.30 Resistance to unspecified antimicrobial drugs
Drug resistance NOS

Z16.31 Resistance to antiparasitic drug(s)
Resistance to quinine and related compounds

Z16.32 Resistance to antifungal drug(s)

Z16.33 Resistance to antiviral drug(s)

☑6ᵗʰ **Z16.34 Resistance to antimycobacterial drug(s)**
Resistance to tuberculostatics

Z16.341 Resistance to single antimycobacterial drug
Resistance to antimycobacterial drug NOS

Z16.342 Resistance to multiple antimycobacterial drugs

Z16.35 Resistance to multiple antimicrobial drugs
EXCLUDES 1 *Resistance to multiple antibiotics only (Z16.24)*

Z16.39 Resistance to other specified antimicrobial drug

Estrogen receptor status (Z17)

☑4ᵗʰ **Z17 Estrogen receptor status**
Code first malignant neoplasm of breast (C50.-)

Z17.0 Estrogen receptor positive status [ER+]

Z17.1 Estrogen receptor negative status [ER-]

Retained foreign body fragment (Z18)

☑4ᵗʰ **Z18 Retained foreign body fragments**
Embedded fragment (status)
Embedded splinter (status)
Retained foreign body status
EXCLUDES 1 *artificial joint prosthesis status (Z96.6-)*
foreign body accidentally left during a procedure (T81.5-)
foreign body entering through orifice (T15-T19)
in situ cardiac device (Z95.-)
organ or tissue replaced by means other than transplant (Z96.-, Z97.-)
organ or tissue replaced by transplant (Z94.-)
personal history of retained foreign body fully removed (Z87.821)
superficial foreign body (non-embedded splinter)—code to superficial foreign body, by site

☑5ᵗʰ **Z18.0 Retained radioactive fragments**

Z18.01 Retained depleted uranium fragments

Z18.09 Other retained radioactive fragments
Other retained depleted isotope fragments
Retained nontherapeutic radioactive fragments

☑5ᵗʰ **Z18.1 Retained metal fragments**
EXCLUDES 1 *retained radioactive metal fragments (Z18.01-Z18.09)*

Z18.10 Retained metal fragments, unspecified
Retained metal fragment NOS

Z18.11 Retained magnetic metal fragments

Z18.12 Retained nonmagnetic metal fragments

Z18.2 Retained plastic fragments
Acrylics fragments
Diethylhexylphthalates fragments
Isocyanate fragments

☑5ᵗʰ **Z18.3 Retained organic fragments**

Z18.31 Retained animal quills or spines

Z18.32 Retained tooth

Z18.33 Retained wood fragments

Z18.39 Other retained organic fragments

☑5ᵗʰ **Z18.8 Other specified retained foreign body**

Z18.81 Retained glass fragments

Z18.83 Retained stone or crystalline fragments
Retained concrete or cement fragments

Z18.89 Other specified retained foreign body fragments

Z18.9 Retained foreign body fragments, unspecified material

Persons with potential health hazards related to communicable diseases (Z20-Z28)

☑4ᵗʰ **Z20 Contact with and (suspected) exposure to communicable diseases**
EXCLUDES 1 *carrier of infectious disease (Z22.-)*
diagnosed current infectious or parasitic disease—see Alphabetic Index
EXCLUDES 2 *personal history of infectious and parasitic diseases (Z86.1-)*

☑5ᵗʰ **Z20.0 Contact with and (suspected) exposure to intestinal infectious diseases**

Z20.01 Contact with and (suspected) exposure to intestinal infectious diseases due to Escherichia coli (E. coli)

Z20.09 Contact with and (suspected) exposure to other intestinal infectious diseases

Z20.1 Contact with and (suspected) exposure to tuberculosis

Z20.2 Contact with and (suspected) exposure to infections with a predominantly sexual mode of transmission

Z20.3 Contact with and (suspected) exposure to rabies

Z20.4 Contact with and (suspected) exposure to rubella

Z20.5 Contact with and (suspected) exposure to viral hepatitis

Z20.6 Contact with and (suspected) exposure to human immunodeficiency virus [HIV]
EXCLUDES 1 *asymptomatic human immunodeficiency virus [HIV] HIV infection status (Z21)*

Z20.7 Contact with and (suspected) exposure to pediculosis, acariasis and other infestations

☑5ᵗʰ **Z20.8 Contact with and (suspected) exposure to other communicable diseases**

☑6ᵗʰ **Z20.81 Contact with and (suspected) exposure to other bacterial communicable diseases**

Z20.810 Contact with and (suspected) exposure to anthrax

Z20.811 Contact with and (suspected) exposure to meningococcus

Z20.818 Contact with and (suspected) exposure to other bacterial communicable diseases

☑6ᵗʰ **Z20.82 Contact with and (suspected) exposure to other viral communicable diseases**

Z20.820 Contact with and (suspected) exposure to varicella

Z20.828 Contact with and (suspected) exposure to other viral communicable diseases

Z20.89 Contact with and (suspected) exposure to other communicable diseases

Z20.9 Contact with and (suspected) exposure to unspecified communicable disease

EXCLUDES 1 Not coded here   **EXCLUDES 2** Not included here   **PDX** Primary Diagnosis Only   **N** Newborn Age: 0   **P** Pediatric Age: 0-17   **M** Maternity Age: 12-55   **A** Adult Age: 15-124

1062   ICD-10-CM 2014 (Draft)

Z21   Asymptomatic human immunodeficiency virus [HIV] infection status

HIV positive NOS

Code first human immunodeficiency virus [HIV] disease complicating pregnancy, childbirth and the puerperium, if applicable (O98.7-)

EXCLUDES 1   *acquired immunodeficiency syndrome (B20)*
contact with human immunodeficiency virus [HIV] (Z20.6)
exposure to human immunodeficiency virus [HIV] (Z20.6)
human immunodeficiency virus [HIV] disease (B20)
inconclusive laboratory evidence of human immunodeficiency virus [HIV] (R75)

✓4th **Z22   Carrier of infectious disease**

Colonization status
Suspected carrier

Z22.0   Carrier of typhoid

Z22.1   Carrier of other intestinal infectious diseases

Z22.2   Carrier of diphtheria

✓5th **Z22.3   Carrier of other specified bacterial diseases**

Z22.31   Carrier of bacterial disease due to meningococci

✓6th **Z22.32   Carrier of bacterial disease due to staphylococci**

Z22.321   Carrier or suspected carrier of Methicillin susceptible Staphylococcus aureus
MSSA colonization

Z22.322   Carrier or suspected carrier of Methicillin resistant Staphylococcus aureus
MRSA colonization

✓6th **Z22.33   Carrier of bacterial disease due to streptococci**

Z22.330   Carrier of Group B streptococcus

Z22.338   Carrier of other streptococcus

Z22.39   Carrier of other specified bacterial diseases

Z22.4   Carrier of infections with a predominantly sexual mode of transmission

✓5th **Z22.5   Carrier of viral hepatitis**

Z22.50   Carrier of unspecified viral hepatitis

Z22.51   Carrier of viral hepatitis B
Hepatitis B surface antigen [HBsAg] carrier

Z22.52   Carrier of viral hepatitis C

Z22.59   Carrier of other viral hepatitis

Z22.6   Carrier of human T-lymphotropic virus type-1 [HTLV-1] infection

Z22.8   Carrier of other infectious diseases

Z22.9   Carrier of infectious disease, unspecified

Z23   Encounter for immunization

Code first any routine childhood examination

NOTE   Procedure codes are required to identify the types of immunizations given

✓4th **Z28   Immunization not carried out and underimmunization status**

Vaccination not carried out

✓5th **Z28.0   Immunization not carried out because of contraindication**

Z28.01   Immunization not carried out because of acute illness of patient

Z28.02   Immunization not carried out because of chronic illness or condition of patient

Z28.03   Immunization not carried out because of immune compromised state of patient

Z28.04   Immunization not carried out because of patient allergy to vaccine or component

Z28.09   Immunization not carried out because of other contraindication

Z28.1   Immunization not carried out because of patient decision for reasons of belief or group pressure
Immunization not carried out because of religious belief

✓5th **Z28.2   Immunization not carried out because of patient decision for other and unspecified reason**

Z28.20   Immunization not carried out because of patient decision for unspecified reason

Z28.21   Immunization not carried out because of patient refusal

Z28.29   Immunization not carried out because of patient decision for other reason

Z28.3   Underimmunization status
Delinquent immunization status
Lapsed immunization schedule status

✓5th **Z28.8   Immunization not carried out for other reason**

Z28.81   Immunization not carried out due to patient having had the disease

Z28.82   Immunization not carried out because of caregiver refusal
Immunization not carried out because of guardian refusal
Immunization not carried out because of parent refusal

EXCLUDES 1   *immunization not carried out because of caregiver refusal because of religious belief (Z28.1)*

Z28.89   Immunization not carried out for other reason

Z28.9   Immunization not carried out for unspecified reason

Persons encountering health services in circumstances related to reproduction (Z30-Z39)

✓4th **Z30   Encounter for contraceptive management**

✓5th **Z30.0   Encounter for general counseling and advice on contraception**

✓6th **Z30.01   Encounter for initial prescription of contraceptives**

EXCLUDES 1   *encounter for surveillance of contraceptives (Z30.4-)*

Z30.011   Encounter for initial prescription of contraceptive pills   ♀

Z30.012   Encounter for prescription of emergency contraception   ♀
Encounter for postcoital contraception

Z30.013   Encounter for initial prescription of injectable contraceptive   ♀

Z30.014   Encounter for initial prescription of intrauterine contraceptive device   ♀

EXCLUDES 1   *encounter for insertion of intrauterine contraceptive device (Z30.430, Z30.432)*

Z30.018   Encounter for initial prescription of other contraceptives

Z30.019   Encounter for initial prescription of contraceptives, unspecified   ♀

Z30.02   Counseling and instruction in natural family planning to avoid pregnancy

Z30.09   Encounter for other general counseling and advice on contraception
Encounter for family planning advice NOS

Z30.2   Encounter for sterilization

✓5th **Z30.4   Encounter for surveillance of contraceptives**

Z30.40   Encounter for surveillance of contraceptives, unspecified

Z30.41   Encounter for surveillance of contraceptive pills   ♀
Encounter for repeat prescription for contraceptive pill

Z30.42   Encounter for surveillance of injectable contraceptive   ♀

✓6th **Z30.43   Encounter for surveillance of intrauterine contraceptive device**

Z30.430   Encounter for insertion of intrauterine contraceptive device   ♀

Z30.431   Encounter for routine checking of intrauterine contraceptive device   ♀

Z30.432   Encounter for removal of intrauterine contraceptive device   ♀

Z30.433   Encounter for removal and reinsertion of intrauterine contraceptive device   ♀
Encounter for replacement of intrauterine contraceptive device

Z30.49   Encounter for surveillance of other contraceptives   ♀

Z30.8   Encounter for other contraceptive management   ♀
Encounter for postvasectomy sperm count
Encounter for routine examination for contraceptive maintenance

EXCLUDES 1   *sperm count following sterilization reversal (Z31.42)*
sperm count for fertility testing (Z31.41)

Z30.9   Encounter for contraceptive management, unspecified

✓4th **Z31   Encounter for procreative management**

EXCLUDES 1   *complications associated with artificial fertilization (N98.-)*
female infertility (N97.-)
male infertility (N46.-)

Z31.0   Encounter for reversal of previous sterilization

☑ Additional Character Required   ✓x7th Xtension Alert   Unspecified Code   Other Specified Code   Manifestation Code   ▶◀ Revised Text   ● New Code   ▲ Revised Code Title

✓5ᵗʰ **Z31.4 Encounter for** procreative investigation and testing
    EXCLUDES 1 *postvasectomy sperm count (Z30.8)*
- **Z31.41 Encounter for** fertility testing
  - Encounter for fallopian tube patency testing
  - Encounter for sperm count for fertility testing
- **Z31.42 Aftercare following** sterilization reversal
  - Sperm count following sterilization reversal

✓6ᵗʰ **Z31.43 Encounter for genetic testing of** female **for procreative management**
    Use additional code for recurrent pregnancy loss, if applicable (N96, O26.2-)
    EXCLUDES 1 *nonprocreative genetic testing (Z13.7-)*
- **Z31.430 Encounter of female for testing for genetic** disease carrier status **for procreative management** ♀
- **Z31.438 Encounter for other genetic testing of female for procreative management** ♀

✓6ᵗʰ **Z31.44 Encounter for genetic testing of** male **for procreative management**
    EXCLUDES 1 *nonprocreative genetic testing (Z13.7-)*
- **Z31.440 Encounter of male for testing for genetic** disease carrier status **for procreative management** ♂
- **Z31.441 Encounter for testing of male partner patient with** recurrent pregnancy loss Ⓐ♂
- **Z31.448 Encounter for other genetic testing of male for procreative management** Ⓐ♂
- **Z31.49 Encounter for other procreative investigation and testing**

Z31.5 Encounter for genetic counseling

✓5ᵗʰ **Z31.6 Encounter for general counseling and advice on procreation**
- **Z31.61 Procreative counseling and advice using** natural family planning
- **Z31.62 Encounter for** fertility preservation **counseling**
  - Encounter for fertility preservation counseling prior to cancer therapy
  - Encounter for fertility preservation counseling prior to surgical removal of gonads
- **Z31.69 Encounter for other general counseling and advice on procreation**

✓5ᵗʰ **Z31.8 Encounter for** other procreative management
- **Z31.81 Encounter for** male factor **infertility in female patient** ♀ PDx
- **Z31.82 Encounter for** Rh incompatibility **status** ♀ PDx
- **Z31.83 Encounter for** assisted reproductive fertility procedure cycle ♀ PDx
  - Patient undergoing in vitro fertilization cycle
  - Use additional code to identify the type of infertility
  - EXCLUDES 1 *pre-cycle diagnosis and testing—code to reason for encounter*
- **Z31.84 Encounter for** fertility preservation **procedure** PDx
  - Encounter for fertility preservation procedure prior to cancer therapy
  - Encounter for fertility preservation procedure prior to surgical removal of gonads
- **Z31.89 Encounter for other procreative management**

Z31.9 Encounter for procreative management, unspecified

✓4ᵗʰ **Z32 Encounter for pregnancy test and childbirth and childcare instruction**

✓5ᵗʰ **Z32.0 Encounter for** pregnancy test
- **Z32.00 Encounter for pregnancy test,** result unknown ♀
  - Encounter for pregnancy test NOS
- **Z32.01 Encounter for pregnancy test,** result positive Ⓜ♀
- **Z32.02 Encounter for pregnancy test,** result negative ♀
- **Z32.2 Encounter for** childbirth instruction
- **Z32.3 Encounter for** childcare instruction
  - Encounter for prenatal or postpartum childcare instruction

✓4ᵗʰ **Z33 Pregnant state**
- **Z33.1 Pregnant state,** incidental Ⓜ♀
  - Pregnant state NOS
  - EXCLUDES 1 *complications of pregnancy (O00-O9A)*
- **Z33.2 Encounter for** elective termination of pregnancy Ⓜ♀ PDx
  - EXCLUDES 1 *early fetal death with retention of dead fetus (O02.1)*
    late fetal death (O36.4)
    spontaneous abortion (O03)

✓4ᵗʰ **Z34 Encounter for supervision of normal pregnancy**
    EXCLUDES 1 *any complication of pregnancy (O00-O9A)*
    encounter for pregnancy test (Z32.0-)
    encounter for supervision of high risk pregnancy (O09.-)

✓5ᵗʰ **Z34.0 Encounter for supervision of normal** first **pregnancy**
- **Z34.00 Encounter for supervision of normal first pregnancy, unspecified trimester** Ⓜ♀ PDx
- **Z34.01 Encounter for supervision of normal first pregnancy,** first **trimester** Ⓜ♀ PDx
- **Z34.02 Encounter for supervision of normal first pregnancy,** second **trimester** Ⓜ♀ PDx
- **Z34.03 Encounter for supervision of normal first pregnancy,** third **trimester** Ⓜ♀ PDx

✓5ᵗʰ **Z34.8 Encounter for supervision of** other **normal pregnancy**
- **Z34.80 Encounter for supervision of other normal pregnancy, unspecified trimester** Ⓜ♀ PDx
- **Z34.81 Encounter for supervision of other normal pregnancy,** first **trimester** Ⓜ♀ PDx
- **Z34.82 Encounter for supervision of other normal pregnancy,** second **trimester** Ⓜ♀ PDx
- **Z34.83 Encounter for supervision of other normal pregnancy,** third **trimester** Ⓜ♀ PDx

✓5ᵗʰ **Z34.9 Encounter for supervision of normal pregnancy,** unspecified
- **Z34.90 Encounter for supervision of normal pregnancy, unspecified, unspecified trimester** Ⓜ♀ PDx
- **Z34.91 Encounter for supervision of normal pregnancy, unspecified,** first **trimester** Ⓜ♀ PDx
- **Z34.92 Encounter for supervision of normal pregnancy, unspecified,** second **trimester** Ⓜ♀ PDx
- **Z34.93 Encounter for supervision of normal pregnancy, unspecified,** third **trimester** Ⓜ♀ PDx

Z36 Encounter for antenatal screening of mother Ⓜ♀
    EXCLUDES 1 *abnormal findings on antenatal screening of mother (O28.-)*
    diagnostic examination—code to sign or symptom
    encounter for suspected maternal and fetal conditions ruled out (Z03.7-)
    suspected fetal condition affecting management of pregnancy—code to condition in Chapter 15
    EXCLUDES 2 *genetic counseling and testing (Z31.43-, Z31.5)*
    routine prenatal care (Z34)

✓4ᵗʰ **Z3A Weeks of gestation**
    NOTE Codes from category Z3A are for use, only on the maternal record, to indicate the weeks of gestation of the pregnancy.
    Code first complications of pregnancy, childbirth and the puerperium (O00-O9A)

✓5ᵗʰ **Z3A.0 Weeks of gestation of pregnancy,** unspecified or less than 10 weeks
- **Z3A.00 Weeks of gestation of pregnancy** not specified Ⓜ♀
- **Z3A.01 Less than 8 weeks gestation of pregnancy** Ⓜ♀
- **Z3A.08 8 weeks gestation of pregnancy** Ⓜ♀
- **Z3A.09 9 weeks gestation of pregnancy** Ⓜ♀

✓5ᵗʰ **Z3A.1 Weeks of gestation of pregnancy, weeks** 10-19
- **Z3A.10 10 weeks gestation of pregnancy** Ⓜ♀
- **Z3A.11 11 weeks gestation of pregnancy** Ⓜ♀
- **Z3A.12 12 weeks gestation of pregnancy** Ⓜ♀
- **Z3A.13 13 weeks gestation of pregnancy** Ⓜ♀
- **Z3A.14 14 weeks gestation of pregnancy** Ⓜ♀
- **Z3A.15 15 weeks gestation of pregnancy** Ⓜ♀
- **Z3A.16 16 weeks gestation of pregnancy** Ⓜ♀
- **Z3A.17 17 weeks gestation of pregnancy** Ⓜ♀
- **Z3A.18 18 weeks gestation of pregnancy** Ⓜ♀
- **Z3A.19 19 weeks gestation of pregnancy** Ⓜ♀

✓5ᵗʰ **Z3A.2 Weeks of gestation of pregnancy, weeks** 20-29
- **Z3A.20 20 weeks gestation of pregnancy** Ⓜ♀
- **Z3A.21 21 weeks gestation of pregnancy** Ⓜ♀
- **Z3A.22 22 weeks gestation of pregnancy** Ⓜ♀
- **Z3A.23 23 weeks gestation of pregnancy** Ⓜ♀
- **Z3A.24 24 weeks gestation of pregnancy** Ⓜ♀
- **Z3A.25 25 weeks gestation of pregnancy** Ⓜ♀
- **Z3A.26 26 weeks gestation of pregnancy** Ⓜ♀
- **Z3A.27 27 weeks gestation of pregnancy** Ⓜ♀
- **Z3A.28 28 weeks gestation of pregnancy** Ⓜ♀
- **Z3A.29 29 weeks gestation of pregnancy** Ⓜ♀

EXCLUDES 1 Not coded here EXCLUDES 2 Not included here PDx Primary Diagnosis Only Ⓝ Newborn Age: 0 Ⓟ Pediatric Age: 0-17 Ⓜ Maternity Age: 12-55 Ⓐ Adult Age: 15-124

1064   ICD-10-CM 2014 (Draft)

✓5th **Z3A.3 Weeks of gestation of pregnancy, weeks 30-39**
- Z3A.30 30 weeks gestation of pregnancy   M♀
- Z3A.31 31 weeks gestation of pregnancy   M♀
- Z3A.32 32 weeks gestation of pregnancy   M♀
- Z3A.33 33 weeks gestation of pregnancy   M♀
- Z3A.34 34 weeks gestation of pregnancy   M♀
- Z3A.35 35 weeks gestation of pregnancy   M♀
- Z3A.36 36 weeks gestation of pregnancy   M♀
- Z3A.37 37 weeks gestation of pregnancy   M♀
- Z3A.38 38 weeks gestation of pregnancy   M♀
- Z3A.39 39 weeks gestation of pregnancy   M♀

✓5th **Z3A.4 Weeks of gestation of pregnancy, weeks 40 or greater**
- Z3A.40 40 weeks gestation of pregnancy   M♀
- Z3A.41 41 weeks gestation of pregnancy   M♀
- Z3A.42 42 weeks gestation of pregnancy   M♀
- Z3A.49 Greater than 42 weeks gestation of pregnancy   M♀

✓4th **Z37 Outcome of delivery**
> NOTE: This category is intended for use as an additional code to identify the outcome of delivery on the mother's record. It is not for use on the newborn record.
> EXCLUDES 1: stillbirth (P95)

- Z37.0 Single live birth   M♀
- Z37.1 Single stillbirth   M♀
- Z37.2 Twins, both liveborn   M♀
- Z37.3 Twins, one liveborn and one stillborn   M♀
- Z37.4 Twins, both stillborn   M♀

✓5th **Z37.5 Other multiple births, all liveborn**
- Z37.50 Multiple births, unspecified, all liveborn   M♀
- Z37.51 Triplets, all liveborn   M♀
- Z37.52 Quadruplets, all liveborn   M♀
- Z37.53 Quintuplets, all liveborn   M♀
- Z37.54 Sextuplets, all liveborn   M♀
- Z37.59 Other multiple births, all liveborn   M♀

✓5th **Z37.6 Other multiple births, some liveborn**
- Z37.60 Multiple births, unspecified, some liveborn   M♀
- Z37.61 Triplets, some liveborn   M♀
- Z37.62 Quadruplets, some liveborn   M♀
- Z37.63 Quintuplets, some liveborn   M♀
- Z37.64 Sextuplets, some liveborn   M♀
- Z37.69 Other multiple births, some liveborn

- Z37.7 Other multiple births, all stillborn   M♀
- Z37.9 Outcome of delivery, unspecified   M♀
  - Multiple birth NOS
  - Single birth NOS

✓4th **Z38 Liveborn infants according to place of birth and type of delivery**
> NOTE: This category is for use as the principal code on the initial record of a newborn baby. It is to be used for the initial birth record only. It is not to be used on the mother's record.

✓5th **Z38.0 Single liveborn infant, born in hospital**
> Single liveborn infant, born in birthing center or other health care facility
- Z38.00 Single liveborn infant, delivered vaginally   N PDx
- Z38.01 Single liveborn infant, delivered by cesarean   N PDx
- Z38.1 Single liveborn infant, born outside hospital   N PDx
- Z38.2 Single liveborn infant, unspecified as to place of birth   N PDx
  - Single liveborn infant NOS

✓5th **Z38.3 Twin liveborn infant, born in hospital**
- Z38.30 Twin liveborn infant, delivered vaginally   N PDx
- Z38.31 Twin liveborn infant, delivered by cesarean   N PDx
- Z38.4 Twin liveborn infant, born outside hospital   N PDx
- Z38.5 Twin liveborn infant, unspecified as to place of birth   N PDx

✓5th **Z38.6 Other multiple liveborn infant, born in hospital**
- Z38.61 Triplet liveborn infant, delivered vaginally   N PDx
- Z38.62 Triplet liveborn infant, delivered by cesarean   N PDx
- Z38.63 Quadruplet liveborn infant, delivered vaginally   N PDx
- Z38.64 Quadruplet liveborn infant, delivered by cesarean   N PDx
- Z38.65 Quintuplet liveborn infant, delivered vaginally   N PDx

- Z38.66 Quintuplet liveborn infant, delivered by cesarean   N PDx
- Z38.68 Other multiple liveborn infant, delivered vaginally   N PDx
- Z38.69 Other multiple liveborn infant, delivered by cesarean   N PDx
- Z38.7 Other multiple liveborn infant, born outside hospital   N PDx
- Z38.8 Other multiple liveborn infant, unspecified as to place of birth   N PDx

✓4th **Z39 Encounter for maternal postpartum care and examination**
- Z39.0 Encounter for care and examination of mother immediately after delivery   M♀ PDx
  > Care and observation in uncomplicated cases when the delivery occurs outside a healthcare facility
  > EXCLUDES 1: care for postpartum complication—see Alphabetic index
- Z39.1 Encounter for care and examination of lactating mother   M♀ PDx
  > Encounter for supervision of lactation
  > EXCLUDES 1: disorders of lactation (O92.-)
- Z39.2 Encounter for routine postpartum follow-up   M♀ PDx

Encounters for other specific health care (Z40-Z53)

> NOTE: Categories Z40-Z53 are intended for use to indicate a reason for care. They may be used for patients who have already been treated for a disease or injury, but who are receiving aftercare or prophylactic care, or care to consolidate the treatment, or to deal with a residual state.
> EXCLUDES 2: follow-up examination for medical surveillance after treatment (Z08-Z09)

✓4th **Z40 Encounter for prophylactic surgery**
> EXCLUDES 1: organ donations (Z52.-)
> therapeutic organ removal—code to condition

✓5th **Z40.0 Encounter for prophylactic surgery for risk factors related to malignant neoplasms**
> Admission for prophylactic organ removal
> Use additional code to identify risk factor
- Z40.00 Encounter for prophylactic removal of unspecified organ
- Z40.01 Encounter for prophylactic removal of breast
- Z40.02 Encounter for prophylactic removal of ovary   ♀
- Z40.09 Encounter for prophylactic removal of other organ
- Z40.8 Encounter for other prophylactic surgery
- Z40.9 Encounter for prophylactic surgery, unspecified

✓4th **Z41 Encounter for procedures for purposes other than remedying health state**
- Z41.1 Encounter for cosmetic surgery
  > Encounter for cosmetic breast implant
  > Encounter for cosmetic procedure
  > EXCLUDES 1: encounter for plastic and reconstructive surgery following medical procedure or healed injury (Z42.-)
  > encounter for post-mastectomy breast implantation (Z42.1)
- Z41.2 Encounter for routine and ritual male circumcision   ♂
- Z41.3 Encounter for ear piercing
- Z41.8 Encounter for other procedures for purposes other than remedying health state
- Z41.9 Encounter for procedure for purposes other than remedying health state, unspecified

✓4th **Z42 Encounter for plastic and reconstructive surgery following medical procedure or healed injury**
> EXCLUDES 1: encounter for cosmetic plastic surgery (Z41.1)
> encounter for plastic surgery for treatment of current injury—code to relevent injury
- Z42.1 Encounter for breast reconstruction following mastectomy   A PDx
  > EXCLUDES 1: deformity and disproportion of reconstructed breast (N65.1-)
- Z42.8 Encounter for other plastic and reconstructive surgery following medical procedure or healed injury   PDx

✓4th **Z43 Encounter for attention to artificial openings**

INCLUDES closure of artificial openings
passage of sounds or bougies through artificial openings
reforming artificial openings
removal of catheter from artificial openings
toilet or cleansing of artificial openings

EXCLUDES 1 artificial opening status only, without need for care (Z93.-)
complications of external stoma (J95.0-, K94.-, N99.5-)

EXCLUDES 2 fitting and adjustment of prosthetic and other devices (Z44-Z46)

Z43.0 Encounter for attention to tracheostomy

Z43.1 Encounter for attention to gastrostomy

Z43.2 Encounter for attention to ileostomy

Z43.3 Encounter for attention to colostomy

Z43.4 Encounter for attention to other artificial openings of digestive tract

Z43.5 Encounter for attention to cystostomy

Z43.6 Encounter for attention to other artificial openings of urinary tract
Encounter for attention to nephrostomy
Encounter for attention to ureterostomy
Encounter for attention to urethrostomy

Z43.7 Encounter for attention to artificial vagina

Z43.8 Encounter for attention to other artificial openings

Z43.9 Encounter for attention to unspecified artificial opening

✓4th **Z44 Encounter for fitting and adjustment of external prosthetic device**

INCLUDES removal or replacement of external prosthetic device

EXCLUDES 1 malfunction or other complications of device—see Alphabetical Index
presence of prosthetic device (Z97.-)

✓5th **Z44.0 Encounter for fitting and adjustment of** artificial arm

✓6th **Z44.00 Encounter for fitting and adjustment of** unspecified artificial arm

Z44.001 Encounter for fitting and adjustment of unspecified right **artificial arm**

Z44.002 Encounter for fitting and adjustment of unspecified left **artificial arm**

Z44.009 Encounter for fitting and adjustment of unspecified artificial arm, unspecified arm

✓6th **Z44.01 Encounter for fitting and adjustment of** complete **artificial arm**

Z44.011 Encounter for fitting and adjustment of complete right **artificial arm**

Z44.012 Encounter for fitting and adjustment of complete left **artificial arm**

Z44.019 Encounter for fitting and adjustment of complete artificial arm, unspecified arm

✓6th **Z44.02 Encounter for fitting and adjustment of** partial **artificial arm**

Z44.021 Encounter for fitting and adjustment of partial artificial right **arm**

Z44.022 Encounter for fitting and adjustment of partial artificial left **arm**

Z44.029 Encounter for fitting and adjustment of partial artificial arm, unspecified arm

✓5th **Z44.1 Encounter for fitting and adjustment of** artificial leg

✓6th **Z44.10 Encounter for fitting and adjustment of** unspecified **artificial leg**

Z44.101 Encounter for fitting and adjustment of unspecified right **artificial leg**

Z44.102 Encounter for fitting and adjustment of unspecified left **artificial leg**

Z44.109 Encounter for fitting and adjustment of unspecified artificial leg, unspecified leg

✓6th **Z44.11 Encounter for fitting and adjustment of** complete **artificial leg**

Z44.111 Encounter for fitting and adjustment of complete right **artificial leg**

Z44.112 Encounter for fitting and adjustment of complete left **artificial leg**

Z44.119 Encounter for fitting and adjustment of complete artificial leg, unspecified leg

✓6th **Z44.12 Encounter for fitting and adjustment of** partial **artificial leg**

Z44.121 Encounter for fitting and adjustment of partial artificial right **leg**

Z44.122 Encounter for fitting and adjustment of partial artificial left **leg**

Z44.129 Encounter for fitting and adjustment of partial artificial leg, unspecified leg

✓5th **Z44.2 Encounter for fitting and adjustment of** artificial eye

EXCLUDES 1 mechanical complication of ocular prosthesis (T85.3)

Z44.20 Encounter for fitting and adjustment of artificial eye, unspecified

Z44.21 Encounter for fitting and adjustment of artificial right **eye**

Z44.22 Encounter for fitting and adjustment of artificial left **eye**

✓5th **Z44.3 Encounter for fitting and adjustment of** external breast prosthesis

EXCLUDES 1 complications of breast implant (T85.4-)
encounter for adjustment or removal of breast implant (Z45.81-)
encounter for initial breast implant insertion for cosmetic breast augmentation (Z41.1)
encounter for breast reconstruction following mastectomy (Z42.1)

Z44.30 Encounter for fitting and adjustment of external breast prosthesis, unspecified breast ♀

Z44.31 Encounter for fitting and adjustment of external right **breast prosthesis** ♀

Z44.32 Encounter for fitting and adjustment of external left **breast prosthesis** ♀

Z44.8 Encounter for fitting and adjustment of other external prosthetic devices

Z44.9 Encounter for fitting and adjustment of unspecified external prosthetic device

✓4th **Z45 Encounter for adjustment and management of implanted device**

INCLUDES removal or replacement of implanted device

EXCLUDES 1 malfunction or other complications of device—see Alphabetical Index
presence of prosthetic and other devices (Z95-Z97)

EXCLUDES 2 encounter for fitting and adjustment of non-implanted device (Z46.-)

✓5th **Z45.0 Encounter for adjustment and management of** cardiac device

✓6th **Z45.01 Encounter for adjustment and management of** cardiac pacemaker

EXCLUDES 1 encounter for adjustment and management of automatic implantable cardiac defibrillator with synchronous cardiac pacemaker (Z45.02)

Z45.010 Encounter for checking and testing of cardiac pacemaker pulse generator **[battery]**
Encounter for replacing cardiac pacemaker pulse generator [battery]

Z45.018 Encounter for adjustment and management of other part of cardiac pacemaker

Z45.02 Encounter for adjustment and management of automatic implantable cardiac defibrillator
Encounter for adjustment and management of automatic implantable cardiac defibrillator with synchronous cardiac pacemaker

Z45.09 Encounter for adjustment and management of other cardiac device

Z45.1 Encounter for adjustment and management of infusion pump

Z45.2 Encounter for adjustment and management of vascular access device
Encounter for adjustment and management of vascular catheters

EXCLUDES 1 encounter for adjustment and management of renal dialysis catheter (Z49.01)

✓5th **Z45.3 Encounter for adjustment and management of implanted** devices of the special senses

Z45.31 Encounter for adjustment and management of implanted visual **substitution device**

✓6th **Z45.32 Encounter for adjustment and management of implanted** hearing **device**

EXCLUDES 1 Encounter for fitting and adjustment of hearing aide (Z46.1)

Z45.320 Encounter for adjustment and management of bone conduction **device**

Z45.321 Encounter for adjustment and management of cochlear **device**

EXCLUDES 1 Not coded here   EXCLUDES 2 Not included here   PDx Primary Diagnosis Only   N Newborn Age: 0   P Pediatric Age: 0-17   M Maternity Age: 12-55   A Adult Age: 15-124

1066   ICD-10-CM 2014 (Draft)

      Z45.328 **Encounter for adjustment and management of other implanted hearing device**

✓5ᵗʰ **Z45.4** **Encounter for adjustment and management of implanted nervous system device**

   Z45.41 **Encounter for adjustment and management of cerebrospinal fluid drainage device**
Encounter for adjustment and management of cerebral ventricular (communicating) shunt

   Z45.42 **Encounter for adjustment and management of neuropacemaker (brain) (peripheral nerve) (spinal cord)**

   Z45.49 **Encounter for adjustment and management of other implanted nervous system device**

✓5ᵗʰ **Z45.8** **Encounter for adjustment and management of other implanted devices**

   ✓6ᵗʰ **Z45.81** **Encounter for adjustment or removal of breast implant**
Encounter for elective implant exchange (different material) (different size)
Encounter removal of tissue expander without synchronous insertion of permanent implant
    EXCLUDES 1 *complications of breast implant (T85.4-)*
encounter for initial breast implant insertion for cosmetic breast augmentation (Z41.1)
encounter for breast reconstruction following mastectomy (Z42.1)

    Z45.811 **Encounter for adjustment or removal of ♀ right breast implant**
    Z45.812 **Encounter for adjustment or removal of ♀ left breast implant**
    Z45.819 **Encounter for adjustment or removal of ♀ unspecified breast implant**

   Z45.82 **Encounter for adjustment or removal of myringotomy device (stent) (tube)**

   Z45.89 **Encounter for adjustment and management of other implanted devices**

Z45.9 **Encounter for adjustment and management of unspecified implanted device**

✓4ᵗʰ **Z46** **Encounter for fitting and adjustment of other devices**
INCLUDES removal or replacement of other device
EXCLUDES 1 *malfunction or other complications of device—see Alphabetical Index*
EXCLUDES 2 *encounter for fitting and management of implanted devices (Z45.-)*
issue of repeat prescription only (Z76.0)
presence of prosthetic and other devices (Z95-Z97)

Z46.0 **Encounter for fitting and adjustment of spectacles and contact lenses**

Z46.1 **Encounter for fitting and adjustment of hearing aid**
EXCLUDES 1 *encounter for adjustment and management of implanted hearing device (Z45.32-)*

Z46.2 **Encounter for fitting and adjustment of other devices related to nervous system and special senses**
EXCLUDES 2 *encounter for adjustment and management of implanted nervous system device (Z45.4-)*
encounter for adjustment and management of implanted visual substitution device (Z45.31)

Z46.3 **Encounter for fitting and adjustment of dental prosthetic device**
Encounter for fitting and adjustment of dentures

Z46.4 **Encounter for fitting and adjustment of orthodontic device**

✓5ᵗʰ **Z46.5** **Encounter for fitting and adjustment of other gastrointestinal appliance and device**
EXCLUDES 1 *encounter for attention to artificial openings of digestive tract (Z43.1-Z43.4)*

   Z46.51 **Encounter for fitting and adjustment of gastric lap band**

   Z46.59 **Encounter for fitting and adjustment of other gastrointestinal appliance and device**

Z46.6 **Encounter for fitting and adjustment of urinary device**
EXCLUDES 2 *attention to artificial openings of urinary tract (Z43.5, Z43.6)*

✓5ᵗʰ **Z46.8** **Encounter for fitting and adjustment of other specified devices**

   Z46.81 **Encounter for fitting and adjustment of insulin pump**
Encounter for insulin pump titration
Encounter for insulin pump instruction and training

   Z46.82 **Encounter for fitting and adjustment of non-vascular catheter**

   Z46.89 **Encounter for fitting and adjustment of other specified devices**
Encounter for fitting and adjustment of wheelchair

Z46.9 **Encounter for fitting and adjustment of unspecified device**

✓4ᵗʰ **Z47** **Orthopedic aftercare**
EXCLUDES 1 *aftercare for healing fracture—code to fracture with 7th character D*

Z47.1 **Aftercare following joint replacement surgery**
Use additional code to identify the joint (Z96.6-)

Z47.2 **Encounter for removal of internal fixation device**
EXCLUDES 1 *encounter for adjustment of internal fixation device for fracture treatment—code to fracture with appropriate 7th character*
encounter for removal of external fixation device—code to fracture with 7th character D
infection or inflammatory reaction to internal fixation device (T84.6-)
mechanical complication of internal fixation device (T84.1-)

✓5ᵗʰ **Z47.3** **Aftercare following explanation of joint prosthesis**
Aftercare following explanation of joint prosthesis, staged procedure
Encounter for joint prosthesis insertion following prior explanation of joint prosthesis

   Z47.31 **Aftercare following explanation of shoulder joint prosthesis**
EXCLUDES 1 *acquired absence of shoulder joint following prior explanation of shoulder joint prosthesis (Z89.23-)*
shoulder joint prosthesis explanation status (Z89.23-)

   Z47.32 **Aftercare following explanation of hip joint prosthesis**
EXCLUDES 1 *acquired absence of hip joint following prior explanation of hip joint prosthesis (Z89.62-)*
hip joint prosthesis explanation status (Z89.62-)

   Z47.33 **Aftercare following explanation of knee joint prosthesis**
EXCLUDES 1 *acquired absence of knee joint following prior explanation of knee prosthesis (Z89.52-)*
knee joint prosthesis explanation status (Z89.52-)

✓5ᵗʰ **Z47.8** **Encounter for other orthopedic aftercare**

   Z47.81 **Encounter for orthopedic aftercare following surgical amputation**
Use additional code to identify the limb amputated (Z89.-)

   Z47.82 **Encounter for orthopedic aftercare following scoliosis surgery**

   Z47.89 **Encounter for other orthopedic aftercare**

✓4ᵗʰ **Z48** **Encounter for other postprocedural aftercare**
EXCLUDES 1 *encounter for follow-up examination after completed treatment (Z08-Z09)*
EXCLUDES 2 *encounter for attention to artificial openings (Z43.-)*
encounter for fitting and adjustment of prosthetic and other devices (Z44-Z46)

✓5ᵗʰ **Z48.0** **Encounter for attention to dressings, sutures and drains**
EXCLUDES 1 *encounter for planned postprocedural wound closure (Z48.1)*

   Z48.00 **Encounter for change or removal of nonsurgical wound dressing**
Encounter for change or removal of wound dressing NOS

   Z48.01 **Encounter for change or removal of surgical wound dressing**

   Z48.02 **Encounter for removal of sutures**
Encounter for removal of staples

   Z48.03 **Encounter for change or removal of drains**

Z48.1   **Encounter for planned postprocedural wound closure**
> *EXCLUDES 1*   *encounter for attention to dressings and sutures (Z48.0-)*

✓5ᵗʰ **Z48.2**   **Encounter for aftercare following organ transplant**

     Z48.21   **Encounter for aftercare following heart transplant**

     Z48.22   **Encounter for aftercare following kidney transplant**

     Z48.23   **Encounter for aftercare following liver transplant**

     Z48.24   **Encounter for aftercare following lung transplant**

     ✓6ᵗʰ **Z48.28**   **Encounter for aftercare following multiple organ transplant**

         Z48.280   **Encounter for aftercare following heart-lung transplant**

         Z48.288   **Encounter for aftercare following multiple organ transplant**

     ✓6ᵗʰ **Z48.29**   **Encounter for aftercare following other organ transplant**

         Z48.290   **Encounter for aftercare following bone marrow transplant**

         Z48.298   **Encounter for aftercare following other organ transplant**

Z48.3   **Aftercare following surgery for neoplasm**
> Use additional code to identify the neoplasm

✓5ᵗʰ **Z48.8**   **Encounter for other specified postprocedural aftercare**

     ✓6ᵗʰ **Z48.81**   **Encounter for surgical aftercare following surgery on specified body systems**
> **NOTE**   These codes identify the body system requiring aftercare. They are for use in conjunction with other aftercare codes to fully explain the aftercare encounter. The condition treated should also be coded if still present.
>
> *EXCLUDES 1*   *aftercare for injury—code the injury with 7th character D*
> *aftercare following surgery for neoplasm (Z48.3)*
> *EXCLUDES 2*   *aftercare following organ transplant (Z48.2-)*
> *orthopedic aftercare (Z47.-)*

         Z48.810   **Encounter for surgical aftercare following surgery on the sense organs**

         Z48.811   **Encounter for surgical aftercare following surgery on the nervous system**
> *EXCLUDES 2*   *encounter for surgical aftercare following surgery on the sense organs (Z48.810)*

         Z48.812   **Encounter for surgical aftercare following surgery on the circulatory system**
> AHA: 2012, Q4, 96

         Z48.813   **Encounter for surgical aftercare following surgery on the respiratory system**

         Z48.814   **Encounter for surgical aftercare following surgery on the teeth or oral cavity**

         Z48.815   **Encounter for surgical aftercare following surgery on the digestive system**

         Z48.816   **Encounter for surgical aftercare following surgery on the genitourinary system**
> *EXCLUDES 1*   *encounter for aftercare following sterilization reversal (Z31.42)*

         Z48.817   **Encounter for surgical aftercare following surgery on the skin and subcutaneous tissue**

     Z48.89   **Encounter for other specified surgical aftercare**

✓4ᵗʰ **Z49**   **Encounter for care involving renal dialysis**
> Code also associated end stage renal disease (N18.6)

     ✓5ᵗʰ **Z49.0**   **Preparatory care for renal dialysis**
> Encounter for dialysis instruction and training

     Z49.01   **Encounter for fitting and adjustment of extracorporeal dialysis catheter**
> Removal or replacement of renal dialysis catheter
> Toilet or cleansing of renal dialysis catheter

     Z49.02   **Encounter for fitting and adjustment of peritoneal dialysis catheter**

     ✓5ᵗʰ **Z49.3**   **Encounter for adequacy testing for dialysis**

     Z49.31   **Encounter for adequacy testing for hemodialysis**

     Z49.32   **Encounter for adequacy testing for peritoneal dialysis**
> Encounter for peritoneal equilibration test

✓4ᵗʰ **Z51**   **Encounter for other aftercare**
> Code also condition requiring care
> *EXCLUDES 1*   *follow-up examination after treatment (Z08-Z09)*

     Z51.0   **Encounter for antineoplastic radiation therapy**   PDx

     ✓5ᵗʰ **Z51.1**   **Encounter for antineoplastic chemotherapy and immunotherapy**
> *EXCLUDES 2*   *encounter for chemotherapy and immunotherapy for nonneoplastic condition—code to condition*

     Z51.11   **Encounter for antineoplastic chemotherapy**   PDx

     Z51.12   **Encounter for antineoplastic immunotherapy**   PDx

     Z51.5   **Encounter for palliative care**

     ✓5ᵗʰ **Z51.8**   **Encounter for other specified aftercare**
> *EXCLUDES 1*   *holiday relief care (Z75.5)*

     Z51.81   **Encounter for therapeutic drug level monitoring**
> Code also any long-term (current) drug therapy (Z79.-)
> *EXCLUDES 1*   *encounter for blood-drug test for administrative or medicolegal reasons (Z02.83)*

     Z51.89   **Encounter for other specified aftercare**
> AHA: 2012, Q4, 95-97

✓4ᵗʰ **Z52**   **Donors of organs and tissues**
> *INCLUDES*   autologous and other living donors
> *EXCLUDES 1*   *cadaveric donor—omit code*
> *examination of potential donor (Z00.5)*
> AHA: 2012, Q4, 99

     ✓5ᵗʰ **Z52.0**   **Blood donor**

     ✓6ᵗʰ **Z52.00**   **Unspecified blood donor**

         Z52.000   **Unspecified donor, whole blood**   PDx

         Z52.001   **Unspecified donor, stem cells**   PDx

         Z52.008   **Unspecified donor, other blood**   PDx

     ✓6ᵗʰ **Z52.01**   **Autologous blood donor**

         Z52.010   **Autologous donor, whole blood**   PDx

         Z52.011   **Autologous donor, stem cells**   PDx

         Z52.018   **Autologous donor, other blood**   PDx

     ✓6ᵗʰ **Z52.09**   **Other blood donor**
> Volunteer donor

         Z52.090   **Other blood donor, whole blood**   PDx

         Z52.091   **Other blood donor, stem cells**   PDx

         Z52.098   **Other blood donor, other blood**   PDx

     ✓5ᵗʰ **Z52.1**   **Skin donor**

     Z52.10   **Skin donor, unspecified**   PDx

     Z52.11   **Skin donor, autologous**   PDx

     Z52.19   **Skin donor, other**   PDx

     ✓5ᵗʰ **Z52.2**   **Bone donor**

     Z52.20   **Bone donor, unspecified**   PDx

     Z52.21   **Bone donor, autologous**   PDx

     Z52.29   **Bone donor, other**   PDx

     Z52.3   **Bone marrow donor**   PDx

     Z52.4   **Kidney donor**   PDx

     Z52.5   **Cornea donor**   PDx

     Z52.6   **Liver donor**   PDx

     ✓5ᵗʰ **Z52.8**   **Donor of other specified organs or tissues**

     ✓6ᵗʰ **Z52.81**   **Egg (Oocyte) donor**

         Z52.810   **Egg (Oocyte) donor under age 35, anonymous recipient**   ♀ PDx
> Egg donor under age 35 NOS

         Z52.811   **Egg (Oocyte) donor under age 35, designated recipient**   ♀ PDx

         Z52.812   **Egg (Oocyte) donor age 35 and over, anonymous recipient**   ♀ PDx
> Egg donor age 35 and over NOS

         Z52.813   **Egg (Oocyte) donor age 35 and over, designated recipient**   ♀ PDx

         Z52.819   **Egg (Oocyte) donor, unspecified**   ♀ PDx

     Z52.89   **Donor of other specified organs or tissues**   PDx

     Z52.9   **Donor of unspecified organ or tissue**   PDx
> Donor NOS

✓4ᵗʰ **Z53**   **Persons encountering health services for specific procedures and treatment, not carried out**

     ✓5ᵗʰ **Z53.0**   **Procedure and treatment not carried out because of contraindication**

     Z53.01   **Procedure and treatment not carried out due to patient smoking**

EXCLUDES 1 Not coded here   *EXCLUDES 2* Not included here   PDx Primary Diagnosis Only   N Newborn Age: 0   P Pediatric Age: 0-17   M Maternity Age: 12-55   A Adult Age: 15-124

1068   ICD-10-CM 2014 (Draft)

Z53.09 Procedure and treatment not carried out because of other contraindication

Z53.1 Procedure and treatment not carried out because of patient's decision for reasons of belief and group pressure

☑5ᵗʰ **Z53.2** Procedure and treatment not carried out because of patient's decision for other and unspecified reasons

　　Z53.20 Procedure and treatment not carried out because of patient's decision for unspecified reasons

　　Z53.21 Procedure and treatment not carried out due to patient leaving prior to being seen by health care provider

　　Z53.29 Procedure and treatment not carried out because of patient's decision for other reasons

Z53.8 Procedure and treatment not carried out for other reasons

Z53.9 Procedure and treatment not carried out, unspecified reason

Persons with potential health hazards related to socioeconomic and psychosocial circumstances (Z55-Z65)

☑4ᵗʰ **Z55** Problems related to education and literacy
EXCLUDES1 disorders of psychological development (F80-F89)

Z55.0 Illiteracy and low-level literacy

Z55.1 Schooling unavailable and unattainable

Z55.2 Failed school examinations

Z55.3 Underachievement in school

Z55.4 Educational maladjustment and discord with teachers and classmates

Z55.8 Other problems related to education and literacy
Problems related to inadequate teaching

Z55.9 Problems related to education and literacy, unspecified
Academic problems NOS

☑4ᵗʰ **Z56** Problems related to employment and unemployment
EXCLUDES2 occupational exposure to risk factors (Z57.-)
problems related to housing and economic circumstances (Z59.-)

Z56.0 Unemployment, unspecified

Z56.1 Change of job

Z56.2 Threat of job loss

Z56.3 Stressful work schedule

Z56.4 Discord with boss and workmates

Z56.5 Uncongenial work environment
Difficult conditions at work

Z56.6 Other physical and mental strain related to work

☑5ᵗʰ **Z56.8** Other problems related to employment

　　Z56.81 Sexual harassment on the job

　　Z56.82 Military deployment status
Individual (civilian or military) currently deployed in theater or in support of military war, peacekeeping and humanitarian operations

　　Z56.89 Other problems related to employment

Z56.9 Unspecified problems related to employment
Occupational problems NOS

☑4ᵗʰ **Z57** Occupational exposure to risk factors

Z57.0 Occupational exposure to noise

Z57.1 Occupational exposure to radiation

Z57.2 Occupational exposure to dust

☑5ᵗʰ **Z57.3** Occupational exposure to other air contaminants

　　Z57.31 Occupational exposure to environmental tobacco smoke
EXCLUDES2 exposure to environmental tobacco smoke (Z77.22)

　　Z57.39 Occupational exposure to other air contaminants

Z57.4 Occupational exposure to toxic agents in agriculture
Occupational exposure to solids, liquids, gases or vapors in agriculture

Z57.5 Occupational exposure to toxic agents in other industries
Occupational exposure to solids, liquids, gases or vapors in other industries

Z57.6 Occupational exposure to extreme temperature

Z57.7 Occupational exposure to vibration

Z57.8 Occupational exposure to other risk factors

Z57.9 Occupational exposure to unspecified risk factor

☑4ᵗʰ **Z59** Problems related to housing and economic circumstances
EXCLUDES2 problems related to upbringing (Z62.-)

Z59.0 Homelessness

Z59.1 Inadequate housing
Lack of heating
Restriction of space
Technical defects in home preventing adequate care
Unsatisfactory surroundings
EXCLUDES1 problems related to the natural and physical environment (Z77.1-)

Z59.2 Discord with neighbors, lodgers and landlord

Z59.3 Problems related to living in residential institution
Boarding-school resident
EXCLUDES1 institutional upbringing (Z62.2)

Z59.4 Lack of adequate food and safe drinking water
Inadequate drinking water supply
EXCLUDES1 effects of hunger (T73.0)
inappropriate diet or eating habits (Z72.4)
malnutrition (E40-E46)

Z59.5 Extreme poverty

Z59.6 Low income

Z59.7 Insufficient social insurance and welfare support

Z59.8 Other problems related to housing and economic circumstances
Foreclosure on loan
Isolated dwelling
Problems with creditors

Z59.9 Problem related to housing and economic circumstances, unspecified

☑4ᵗʰ **Z60** Problems related to social environment

Z60.0 Problems of adjustment to life-cycle transitions
Empty nest syndrome
Phase of life problem
Problem with adjustment to retirement [pension]

Z60.2 Problems related to living alone

Z60.3 Acculturation difficulty
Problem with migration
Problem with social transplantation

Z60.4 Social exclusion and rejection
Exclusion and rejection on the basis of personal characteristics, such as unusual physical appearance, illness or behavior.
EXCLUDES1 target of adverse discrimination such as for racial or religious reasons (Z60.5)

Z60.5 Target of (perceived) adverse discrimination and persecution
EXCLUDES1 social exclusion and rejection (Z60.4)

Z60.8 Other problems related to social environment

Z60.9 Problem related to social environment, unspecified

☑4ᵗʰ **Z62** Problems related to upbringing
Current and past negative life events in childhood
Current and past problems of a child related to upbringing
EXCLUDES2 maltreatment syndrome (T74.-)
problems related to housing and economic circumstances (Z59.-)

Z62.0 Inadequate parental supervision and control

Z62.1 Parental overprotection

☑5ᵗʰ **Z62.2** Upbringing away from parents
EXCLUDES1 problems with boarding school (Z59.3)

　　Z62.21 Child in welfare custody　　P
Child in care of non-parental family member
Child in foster care
EXCLUDES2 problem for parent due to child in welfare custody (Z63.5)

　　Z62.22 Institutional upbringing
Child living in orphanage or group home

　　Z62.29 Other upbringing away from parents

Z62.3 Hostility towards and scapegoating of child　　P

Z62.6 Inappropriate (excessive) parental pressure

☑5ᵗʰ **Z62.8** Other specified problems related to upbringing

☑6ᵗʰ　**Z62.81** Personal history of abuse in childhood

　　　Z62.810 Personal history of physical and sexual abuse in childhood
EXCLUDES1 current child physical abuse (T74.12, T76.12)
current child sexual abuse (T74.22, T76.22)

　　　Z62.811 Personal history of psychological abuse in childhood
EXCLUDES1 current child psychological abuse (T74.32, T76.32)

☑ Additional Character Required　　✗x7ᵗʰ Xtension Alert　　Unspecified Code　　Other Specified Code　　Manifestation Code　　▶◀ Revised Text　　● New Code　　▲ Revised Code Title

         Z62.812 **Personal history of neglect in childhood**
              EXCLUDES 1 *current child neglect (T74.02, T76.02)*

         Z62.819 **Personal history of unspecified abuse in childhood**
              EXCLUDES 1 *current child abuse NOS (T74.92, T76.92)*

    ✓6th **Z62.82** **Parent-child conflict**
         Z62.820 **Parent-biological child conflict**
              Parent-child problem NOS
         Z62.821 **Parent-adopted child conflict**
         Z62.822 **Parent-foster child conflict**

    ✓6th **Z62.89** **Other specified problems related to upbringing**
         Z62.890 **Parent-child estrangement NEC**
         Z62.891 **Sibling rivalry**
         Z62.898 **Other specified problems related to upbringing**

   Z62.9 **Problem related to upbringing, unspecified**

✓4th **Z63** **Other problems related to primary support group, including family circumstances**
    EXCLUDES 2 *maltreatment syndrome (T74-, T76)*
          parent-child problems (Z62.-)
          problems related to negative life events in childhood (Z62.-)
          problems related to upbringing (Z62.-)

   Z63.0 **Problems in relationship with spouse or partner**
       EXCLUDES 1 *counseling for spousal or partner abuse problems (Z69.1)*
           counseling related to sexual attitude, behavior, and orientation (Z70.-)

   Z63.1 **Problems in relationship with in-laws**

    ✓5th **Z63.3** **Absence of family member**
       EXCLUDES 1 *absence of family member due to disappearance and death (Z63.4)*
           absence of family member due to separation and divorce (Z63.5)

      Z63.31 **Absence of family member due to military deployment**
          Individual or family affected by other family member being on military deployment
         EXCLUDES 1 *family disruption due to return of family member from military deployment (Z63.71)*

      Z63.32 **Other absence of family member**

   Z63.4 **Disappearance and death of family member**
          Assumed death of family member
          Bereavement

   Z63.5 **Disruption of family by separation and divorce**
          Marital estrangement

   Z63.6 **Dependent relative needing care at home**

    ✓5th **Z63.7** **Other stressful life events affecting family and household**
      Z63.71 **Stress on family due to return of family member from military deployment**
          Individual or family affected by family member having returned from military deployment (current or past conflict)
      Z63.72 **Alcoholism and drug addiction in family**
      Z63.79 **Other stressful life events affecting family and household**
          Anxiety (normal) about sick person in family
          Health problems within family
          Ill or disturbed family member
          Isolated family

   Z63.8 **Other specified problems related to primary support group**
          Family discord NOS
          Family estrangement NOS
          High expressed emotional level within family
          Inadequate family support NOS
          Inadequate or distorted communication within family

   Z63.9 **Problem related to primary support group, unspecified**
          Relationship disorder NOS

✓4th **Z64** **Problems related to certain psychosocial circumstances**
   Z64.0 **Problems related to unwanted pregnancy**   M ♀
   Z64.1 **Problems related to multiparity**   ♀
   Z64.4 **Discord with counselors**
          Discord with probation officer
          Discord with social worker

✓4th **Z65** **Problems related to other psychosocial circumstances**
   Z65.0 **Conviction in civil and criminal proceedings without imprisonment**
   Z65.1 **Imprisonment and other incarceration**
   Z65.2 **Problems related to release from prison**
   Z65.3 **Problems related to other legal circumstances**
          Arrest
          Child custody or support proceedings
          Litigation
          Prosecution
   Z65.4 **Victim of crime and terrorism**
          Victim of torture
   Z65.5 **Exposure to disaster, war and other hostilities**   A
       EXCLUDES 1 *target of perceived discrimination or persecution (Z60.5)*
   Z65.8 **Other specified problems related to psychosocial circumstances**
   Z65.9 **Problem related to unspecified psychosocial circumstances**

Do not resuscitate status (Z66)

Z66 **Do not resuscitate**
       DNR status

Blood type (Z67)

✓4th **Z67** **Blood type**
    ✓5th **Z67.1** **Type A blood**
      Z67.10 **Type A blood, Rh positive**
      Z67.11 **Type A blood, Rh negative**
    ✓5th **Z67.2** **Type B blood**
      Z67.20 **Type B blood, Rh positive**
      Z67.21 **Type B blood, Rh negative**
    ✓5th **Z67.3** **Type AB blood**
      Z67.30 **Type AB blood, Rh positive**
      Z67.31 **Type AB blood, Rh negative**
    ✓5th **Z67.4** **Type O blood**
      Z67.40 **Type O blood, Rh positive**
      Z67.41 **Type O blood, Rh negative**
    ✓5th **Z67.9** **Unspecified blood type**
      Z67.90 **Unspecified blood type, Rh positive**
      Z67.91 **Unspecified blood type, Rh negative**

Body mass index [BMI] (Z68)

✓4th **Z68** **Body mass index [BMI]**
       Kilograms per meters squared
       NOTE BMI adult codes are for use for persons 21 years of age or older.
          BMI pediatric codes are for use for persons 2-20 years of age. These percentiles are based on the growth charts published by the Centers for Disease Control and Prevention (CDC).
   Z68.1 **Body mass index [BMI] 19 or less, adult**   A
    ✓5th **Z68.2** **Body mass index [BMI] 20-29, adult**
      Z68.20 **Body mass index [BMI] 20.0-20.9, adult**   A
      Z68.21 **Body mass index [BMI] 21.0-21.9, adult**   A
      Z68.22 **Body mass index [BMI] 22.0-22.9, adult**   A
      Z68.23 **Body mass index [BMI] 23.0-23.9, adult**   A
      Z68.24 **Body mass index [BMI] 24.0-24.9, adult**   A
      Z68.25 **Body mass index [BMI] 25.0-25.9, adult**   A
      Z68.26 **Body mass index [BMI] 26.0-26.9, adult**   A
      Z68.27 **Body mass index [BMI] 27.0-27.9, adult**   A
      Z68.28 **Body mass index [BMI] 28.0-28.9, adult**   A
      Z68.29 **Body mass index [BMI] 29.0-29.9, adult**   A
    ✓5th **Z68.3** **Body mass index [BMI] 30-39, adult**
      Z68.30 **Body mass index [BMI] 30.0-30.9, adult**   A
      Z68.31 **Body mass index [BMI] 31.0-31.9, adult**   A
      Z68.32 **Body mass index [BMI] 32.0-32.9, adult**   A
      Z68.33 **Body mass index [BMI] 33.0-33.9, adult**   A
      Z68.34 **Body mass index [BMI] 34.0-34.9, adult**   A
      Z68.35 **Body mass index [BMI] 35.0-35.9, adult**   A
      Z68.36 **Body mass index [BMI] 36.0-36.9, adult**   A
      Z68.37 **Body mass index [BMI] 37.0-37.9, adult**   A
      Z68.38 **Body mass index [BMI] 38.0-38.9, adult**   A

EXCLUDES 1 Not coded here   EXCLUDES 2 Not included here   PDx Primary Diagnosis Only   N Newborn Age: 0   P Pediatric Age: 0-17   M Maternity Age: 12-55   A Adult Age: 15-124

1070   ICD-10-CM 2014 (Draft)

Z68.39 Body mass index [BMI] 39.0-39.9, adult A

√5ᵗʰ **Z68.4 Body mass index [BMI] 40 or greater, adult**
Z68.41 Body mass index [BMI] 40.0-44.9, adult A
Z68.42 Body mass index [BMI] 45.0-49.9, adult A
Z68.43 Body mass index [BMI] 50-59.9, adult A
Z68.44 Body mass index [BMI] 60.0-69.9, adult A
Z68.45 Body mass index [BMI] 70 or greater, adult A

√5ᵗʰ **Z68.5 Body mass index [BMI] pediatric**
Z68.51 Body mass index [BMI] pediatric, less than 5th P
percentile for age
Z68.52 Body mass index [BMI] pediatric, 5th percentile P
to less than 85th percentile for age
Z68.53 Body mass index [BMI] pediatric, 85th percentile P
to less than 95th percentile for age
Z68.54 Body mass index [BMI] pediatric, greater than or P
equal to 95th percentile for age

Persons encountering health services in other circumstances (Z69-Z76)

√4ᵗʰ **Z69 Encounter for mental health services for victim and perpetrator of abuse**
Counseling for victims and perpetrators of abuse

√5ᵗʰ **Z69.0 Encounter for mental health services for child abuse problems**

√6ᵗʰ **Z69.01 Encounter for mental health services for parental child abuse**
Z69.010 Encounter for mental health services P
for victim of parental child abuse
Z69.011 Encounter for mental health services for
perpetrator of parental child abuse
EXCLUDES 1 *encounter for mental health
services for non-parental
child abuse (Z69.02-)*

√6ᵗʰ **Z69.02 Encounter for mental health services for non-parental child abuse**
Z69.020 Encounter for mental health services P
for victim of non-parental child abuse
Z69.021 Encounter for mental health services for
perpetrator of non-parental child abuse

√5ᵗʰ **Z69.1 Encounter for mental health services for spousal or partner abuse problems**
Z69.11 Encounter for mental health services for victim of
spousal or partner abuse
Z69.12 Encounter for mental health services for perpetrator
of spousal or partner abuse

√5ᵗʰ **Z69.8 Encounter for mental health services for victim or perpetrator of other abuse**
Z69.81 Encounter for mental health services for victim of
other abuse
Encounter for rape victim counseling
Z69.82 Encounter for mental health services for perpetrator
of other abuse

√4ᵗʰ **Z70 Counseling related to sexual attitude, behavior and orientation**
Encounter for mental health services for sexual attitude, behavior and
orientation
EXCLUDES 2 *contraceptive or procreative counseling (Z30-Z31)*
Z70.0 Counseling related to sexual attitude
Z70.1 Counseling related to patient's sexual behavior and
orientation
Patient concerned regarding impotence
Patient concerned regarding non-responsiveness
Patient concerned regarding promiscuity
Patient concerned regarding sexual orientation
Z70.2 Counseling related to sexual behavior and orientation of
third party
Advice sought regarding sexual behavior and orientation of
child
Advice sought regarding sexual behavior and orientation of
partner
Advice sought regarding sexual behavior and orientation of
spouse
Z70.3 Counseling related to combined concerns regarding sexual
attitude, behavior and orientation
Z70.8 Other sex counseling
Encounter for sex education
Z70.9 Sex counseling, unspecified

√4ᵗʰ **Z71 Persons encountering health services for other counseling and medical advice, not elsewhere classified**
EXCLUDES 2 *contraceptive or procreation counseling (Z30-Z31)*
sex counseling (Z70.-)
Z71.0 Person encountering health services to consult on behalf of
another person
Person encountering health services to seek advice or treatment
for non-attending third party
EXCLUDES 2 *anxiety (normal) about sick person in family (Z63.7)*
*expectant (adoptive) parent(s) pre-birth pediatrician
visit (Z76.81)*
Z71.1 Person with feared health complaint in whom no diagnosis is
made
Person encountering health services with feared condition
which was not demonstrated
Person encountering health services in which problem was
normal state
"Worried well"
EXCLUDES 1 *medical observation for suspected diseases and
conditions proven not to exist (Z03.-)*
Z71.2 Person consulting for explanation of examination or test
findings
Z71.3 Dietary counseling and surveillance
Use additional code for any associated underlying medical
condition
Use additional code to identify body mass index (BMI), if known
(Z68.-)
√5ᵗʰ **Z71.4 Alcohol abuse counseling and surveillance**
Use additional code for alcohol abuse or dependence (F10.-)
Z71.41 Alcohol abuse counseling and surveillance of
alcoholic
Z71.42 Counseling for family member of alcoholic
Counseling for significant other, partner, or friend of
alcoholic
√5ᵗʰ **Z71.5 Drug abuse counseling and surveillance**
Use additional code for drug abuse or dependence (F11-F16,
F18-F19)
Z71.51 Drug abuse counseling and surveillance of drug
abuser
Z71.52 Counseling for family member of drug abuser
Counseling for significant other, partner, or friend of
drug abuser
Z71.6 Tobacco abuse counseling
Use additional code for nicotine dependence (F17.-)
Z71.7 Human immunodeficiency virus [HIV] counseling
√5ᵗʰ **Z71.8 Other specified counseling**
EXCLUDES 2 *counseling for contraception (Z30.0-)*
counseling for genetics (Z31.5)
counseling for procreative management (Z31.6-)
Z71.81 Spiritual or religious counseling
Z71.89 Other specified counseling
Z71.9 Counseling, unspecified
Encounter for medical advice NOS

√4ᵗʰ **Z72 Problems related to lifestyle**
EXCLUDES 2 *problems related to life-management difficulty (Z73.-)*
*problems related to socioeconomic and psychosocial
circumstances (Z55-Z65)*
Z72.0 Tobacco use
Tobacco use NOS
EXCLUDES 1 *history of tobacco dependence (Z87.891)*
nicotine dependence (F17.2-)
tobacco dependence (F17.2-)
tobacco use during pregnancy (O99.33-)
Z72.3 Lack of physical exercise
Z72.4 Inappropriate diet and eating habits
EXCLUDES 1 *behavioral eating disorders of infancy or childhood
(F98.2- F98.3)*
eating disorders (F50.-)
lack of adequate food (Z59.4)
*malnutrition and other nutritional deficiencies
(E40-E64)*
√5ᵗʰ **Z72.5 High risk sexual behavior**
Promiscuity
EXCLUDES 1 *paraphilias (F65)*
Z72.51 High risk heterosexual behavior
Z72.52 High risk homosexual behavior
Z72.53 High risk bisexual behavior

☑ Additional Character Required √x7ᵗʰ Xtension Alert Unspecified Code Other Specified Code Manifestation Code ►◄ Revised Text ● New Code ▲ Revised Code Title

Z72.6   **Gambling and betting**
     EXCLUDES 1   *compulsive or pathological gambling (F63.0)*

☑5ᵗʰ **Z72.8**   **Other problems related to lifestyle**

   ☑6ᵗʰ **Z72.81**   **Antisocial behavior**
       EXCLUDES 1   *conduct disorders (F91.-)*

       Z72.810   **Child and adolescent antisocial**   **P**
               behavior
               Antisocial behavior (child) (adolescent)
                     without manifest psychiatric disorder
               Delinquency NOS
               Group delinquency
               Offenses in the context of gang
                     membership
               Stealing in company with others
               Truancy from school

       Z72.811   **Adult antisocial behavior**   **A**
               Adult antisocial behavior without manifest
                     psychiatric disorder

   ☑6ᵗʰ **Z72.82**   **Problems related to sleep**

       Z72.820   **Sleep deprivation**
               Lack of adequate sleep
               EXCLUDES 1   *insomnia (G47.0-)*

       Z72.821   **Inadequate sleep hygiene**
               Bad sleep habits
               Irregular sleep habits
               Unhealthy sleep wake schedule
               EXCLUDES 1   *insomnia (F51.0-, G47.0-)*

     Z72.89   **Other problems related to lifestyle**
            Self-damaging behavior

Z72.9   **Problem related to lifestyle, unspecified**

☑4ᵗʰ **Z73**   **Problems related to life management difficulty**
     EXCLUDES 2   *problems related to socioeconomic and psychosocial*
                    circumstances (Z55-Z65)

   Z73.0   **Burn-out**

   Z73.1   **Type A behavior pattern**

   Z73.2   **Lack of relaxation and leisure**

   Z73.3   **Stress, not elsewhere classified**
           Physical and mental strain NOS
       EXCLUDES 1   *stress related to employment or unemployment (Z56.-)*

   Z73.4   **Inadequate social skills, not elsewhere classified**

   Z73.5   **Social role conflict, not elsewhere classified**

   Z73.6   **Limitation of activities due to disability**
       EXCLUDES 1   *care-provider dependency (Z74.-)*

   ☑5ᵗʰ **Z73.8**   **Other problems related to life management difficulty**

     ☑6ᵗʰ **Z73.81**   **Behavioral insomnia of childhood**

       Z73.810   **Behavioral insomnia of childhood,**   **P**
               sleep-onset association type

       Z73.811   **Behavioral insomnia of childhood, limit**   **P**
               setting type

       Z73.812   **Behavioral insomnia of childhood,**   **P**
               combined type

       Z73.819   **Behavioral insomnia of childhood,**   **P**
               unspecified type

     Z73.82   **Dual sensory impairment**

     Z73.89   **Other problems related to life management difficulty**

   Z73.9   **Problem related to life management difficulty, unspecified**

☑4ᵗʰ **Z74**   **Problems related to care provider dependency**
     EXCLUDES 2   *dependence on enabling machines or devices NEC (Z99.-)*

   ☑5ᵗʰ **Z74.0**   **Reduced mobility**

     Z74.01   **Bed confinement status**
           Bedridden

     Z74.09   **Other reduced mobility**
           Chair ridden
           Reduced mobility NOS
       EXCLUDES 2   *wheelchair dependence (Z99.3)*

   Z74.1   **Need for assistance with personal care**

   Z74.2   **Need for assistance at home and no other household member able to render care**

   Z74.3   **Need for continuous supervision**

   Z74.8   **Other problems related to care provider dependency**

   Z74.9   **Problem related to care provider dependency, unspecified**

☑4ᵗʰ **Z75**   **Problems related to medical facilities and other health care**

   Z75.0   **Medical services not available in home**
       EXCLUDES 1   *no other household member able to render care (Z74.2)*

Z75.1   **Person awaiting admission to adequate facility elsewhere**

Z75.2   **Other waiting period for investigation and treatment**

Z75.3   **Unavailability and inaccessibility of health-care facilities**
     EXCLUDES 1   *bed unavailable (Z75.1)*

Z75.4   **Unavailability and inaccessibility of other helping agencies**

Z75.5   **Holiday relief care**

Z75.8   **Other problems related to medical facilities and other health care**

Z75.9   **Unspecified problem related to medical facilities and other health care**

☑4ᵗʰ **Z76**   **Persons encountering health services in other circumstances**

   Z76.0   **Encounter for issue of repeat prescription**
          Encounter for issue of repeat prescription for appliance
          Encounter for issue of repeat prescription for medicaments
          Encounter for issue of repeat prescription for spectacles
       EXCLUDES 2   *issue of medical certificate (Z02.7)*
                     repeat prescription for contraceptive (Z30.4-)

   Z76.1   **Encounter for health supervision and care of foundling**   **PDx**

   Z76.2   **Encounter for health supervision and care of other**   **P** **PDx**
          healthy infant and child
          Encounter for medical or nursing care or supervision of healthy
               infant under circumstances such as adverse socioeconomic
               conditions at home
          Encounter for medical or nursing care or supervision of healthy
               infant under circumstances such as awaiting foster or
               adoptive placement
          Encounter for medical or nursing care or supervision of healthy
               infant under circumstances such as maternal illness
          Encounter for medical or nursing care or supervision of healthy
               infant under circumstances such as number of children at
               home preventing or interfering with normal care

   Z76.3   **Healthy person accompanying sick person**

   Z76.4   **Other boarder to healthcare facility**
       EXCLUDES 1   *homelessness (Z59.0)*

   Z76.5   **Malingerer [conscious simulation]**
          Person feigning illness (with obvious motivation)
       EXCLUDES 1   *factitious disorder (F68.1-)*
                     peregrinating patient (F68.1-)

   ☑5ᵗʰ **Z76.8**   **Persons encountering health services in other specified circumstances**

     Z76.81   **Expectant parent(s) prebirth pediatrician visit**
           Pre-adoption pediatrician visit for adoptive parent(s)

     Z76.82   **Awaiting organ transplant status**
           Patient waiting for organ availability

     Z76.89   **Persons encountering health services in other specified circumstances**
           Persons encountering health services NOS

Persons with potential health hazards related to family and personal history and certain conditions influencing health status (Z77-Z99)

Code also any follow-up examination (Z08-Z09)

☑4ᵗʰ **Z77**   **Other contact with and (suspected) exposures hazardous to health**
     INCLUDES   contact with and (suspected) exposures to potential hazards
                 to health
     EXCLUDES 2   *contact with and (suspected) exposure to communicable*
                 diseases (Z20.-)
               exposure to (parental) (environmental) tobacco smoke in the
                 perinatal period (P96.81)
               newborn (suspected to be) affected by noxious substances
                 transmitted via placenta or breast milk (P04.-)
               occupational exposure to risk factors (Z57.-)
               retained foreign body (Z18.-)
               retained foreign body fully removed (Z87.821)
               toxic effects of substances chiefly nonmedicinal as to source
                 (T51-T65)

   ☑5ᵗʰ **Z77.0**   **Contact with and (suspected) exposure to hazardous, chiefly nonmedicinal, chemicals**

     ☑6ᵗʰ **Z77.01**   **Contact with and (suspected) exposure to hazardous metals**

       Z77.010   **Contact with and (suspected) exposure to arsenic**

       Z77.011   **Contact with and (suspected) exposure to lead**

EXCLUDES 1 Not coded here   EXCLUDES 2 Not included here   PDx Primary Diagnosis Only   N Newborn Age: 0   P Pediatric Age: 0-17   M Maternity Age: 12-55   A Adult Age: 15-124

1072   ICD-10-CM 2014 (Draft)

Z77.012   **Contact with and (suspected) exposure to uranium**
    EXCLUDES 1   *retained depleted uranium fragments (Z18.01)*

Z77.018   **Contact with and (suspected) exposure to other hazardous metals**
    Contact with and (suspected) exposure to chromium compounds
    Contact with and (suspected) exposure to nickel dust

✓6ᵗʰ **Z77.02**   **Contact with and (suspected) exposure to hazardous aromatic compounds**

    Z77.020   **Contact with and (suspected) exposure to aromatic amines**

    Z77.021   **Contact with and (suspected) exposure to benzene**

    Z77.028   **Contact with and (suspected) exposure to other hazardous aromatic compounds**
      Aromatic dyes NOS
      Polycyclic aromatic hydrocarbons

✓6ᵗʰ **Z77.09**   **Contact with and (suspected) exposure to other hazardous, chiefly nonmedicinal, chemicals**

    Z77.090   **Contact with and (suspected) exposure to asbestos**

    Z77.098   **Contact with and (suspected) exposure to other hazardous, chiefly nonmedicinal, chemicals**
      Dyes NOS

✓5ᵗʰ **Z77.1**   **Contact with and (suspected) exposure to environmental pollution and hazards in the physical environment**

   ✓6ᵗʰ **Z77.11**   **Contact with and (suspected) exposure to environmental pollution**

    Z77.110   **Contact with and (suspected) exposure to air pollution**

    Z77.111   **Contact with and (suspected) exposure to water pollution**

    Z77.112   **Contact with and (suspected) exposure to soil pollution**

    Z77.118   **Contact with and (suspected) exposure to other environmental pollution**

   ✓6ᵗʰ **Z77.12**   **Contact with and (suspected) exposure to hazards in the physical environment**

    Z77.120   **Contact with and (suspected) exposure to mold (toxic)**

    Z77.121   **Contact with and (suspected) exposure to harmful algae and algae toxins**
      Contact with and (suspected) exposure to (harmful) algae bloom NOS
      Contact with and (suspected) exposure to blue-green algae bloom
      Contact with and (suspected) exposure to brown tide
      Contact with and (suspected) exposure to cyanobacteria bloom
      Contact with and (suspected) exposure to Florida red tide
      Contact with and (suspected) exposure to pfiesteria piscicida
      Contact with and (suspected) exposure to red tide

    Z77.122   **Contact with and (suspected) exposure to noise**

    Z77.123   **Contact with and (suspected) exposure to radon and other naturally occuring radiation**
      EXCLUDES 2   *radiation exposure as the cause of a confirmed condition (W88-W90, X39.0-)*
        radiation sickness NOS (T66)

    Z77.128   **Contact with and (suspected) exposure to other hazards in the physical environment**

✓5ᵗʰ **Z77.2**   **Contact with and (suspected) exposure to other hazardous substances**

    Z77.21   **Contact with and (suspected) exposure to potentially hazardous body fluids**

Z77.22   **Contact with and (suspected) exposure to environmental tobacco smoke (acute) (chronic)**
    Exposure to second hand tobacco smoke (acute) (chronic)
    Passive smoking (acute) (chronic)
    EXCLUDES 1   *nicotine dependence (F17.-)*
       tobacco use (Z72.0)
    EXCLUDES 2   *occupational exposure to environmental tobacco smoke (Z57.31)*

Z77.29   **Contact with and (suspected) exposure to other hazardous substances**

Z77.9   **Other contact with and (suspected) exposures hazardous to health**

✓4ᵗʰ **Z78**   **Other specified health status**
    EXCLUDES 2   *asymptomatic human immunodeficiency virus [HIV] infection status (Z21)*
       postprocedural status (Z93- Z99)
       sex reassignment status (Z87.890)

Z78.0   **Asymptomatic menopausal state**   Ⓐ♀
    Menopausal state NOS
    Postmenopausal status NOS
    EXCLUDES 2   *symptomatic menopausal state (N95.1)*

Z78.1   **Physical restraint status**
    EXCLUDES 1   *physical restraint due to a procedure - omit code*

Z78.9   **Other specified health status**

✓4ᵗʰ **Z79**   **Long term (current) drug therapy**
    INCLUDES   long term (current) drug use for prophylactic purposes
    Code also any therapeutic drug level monitoring (Z51.81)
    EXCLUDES 2   *drug abuse and dependence (F11-F19)*
       drug use complicating pregnancy, childbirth, and the puerperium (O99.32-)

   ✓5ᵗʰ **Z79.0**   **Long term (current) use of anticoagulants and antithrombotics/antiplatelets**
    EXCLUDES 2   *long term (current) use of aspirin (Z79.82)*

    Z79.01   **Long term (current) use of anticoagulants**

    Z79.02   **Long term (current) use of antithrombotics/antiplatelets**

Z79.1   **Long term (current) use of non-steroidal anti-inflammatories (NSAID)**
    EXCLUDES 2   *long term (current) use of aspirin (Z79.82)*

Z79.2   **Long term (current) use of antibiotics**

Z79.3   **Long term (current) use of hormonal contraceptives**
    Long term (current) use of birth control pill or patch

Z79.4   **Long term (current) use of insulin**

   ✓5ᵗʰ **Z79.5**   **Long term (current) use of steroids**

    Z79.51   **Long term (current) use of inhaled steroids**

    Z79.52   **Long term (current) use of systemic steroids**

   ✓5ᵗʰ **Z79.8**   **Other long term (current) drug therapy**

   ✓6ᵗʰ **Z79.81**   **Long term (current) use of agents affecting estrogen receptors and estrogen levels**
    Code first, if applicable:
      malignant neoplasm of breast (C50.-)
      malignant neoplasm of prostate (C61)
    Use additional code, if applicable, to identify:
      estrogen receptor positive status (Z17.0)
      family history of breast cancer (Z80.3)
      genetic susceptibility to malignant neoplasm (cancer) (Z15.0-)
      personal history of breast cancer (Z85.3)
      personal history of prostate cancer (Z85.46)
      postmenopausal status (Z78.0)
    EXCLUDES 1   *hormone replacement therapy (postmenopausal) (Z79.890)*

    Z79.810   **Long term (current) use of selective estrogen receptor modulators (SERMs)**
      Long term (current) use of raloxifene (Evista)
      Long term (current) use of tamoxifen (Nolvadex)
      Long term (current) use of toremifene (Fareston)

    Z79.811   **Long term (current) use of aromatase inhibitors**
      Long term (current) use of anastrozole (Arimidex)
      Long term (current) use of exemestane (Aromasin)
      Long term (current) use of letrozole (Femara)

☑ Additional Character Required   ✓x7ᵗʰ Xtension Alert   Unspecified Code   Other Specified Code   Manifestation Code   ▶◀ Revised Text   ● New Code   ▲ Revised Code Title

ICD-10-CM 2014 (Draft)   1073

Factors Influencing Health Status and Contact With Health Services

Z79.818–Z83.6

Z79.818   **Long term (current) use of other agents affecting estrogen receptors and estrogen levels**

Long term (current) use of estrogen receptor downregulators

Long term (current) use of fulvestrant (Faslodex)

Long term (current) use of gonadotropin-releasing hormone (GnRH) agonist

Long term (current) use of goserelin acetate (Zoladex)

Long term (current) use of leuprolide acetate (leuprorelin) (Lupron)

Long term (current) use of megestrol acetate (Megace)

Z79.82   **Long term (current) use of aspirin**

Z79.83   **Long term (current) use of bisphosphonates**

✓6ᵗʰ **Z79.89**   **Other long term (current) drug therapy**

Z79.890   **Hormone replacement therapy (postmenopausal)** ♀

Z79.891   **Long term (current) use of opiate analgesic**

Long term (current) use of methadone for pain management

EXCLUDES 1   methodone use NOS (F11.2-)

use of methodone for treatment of heroin addiction (F11.2-)

Z79.899   **Other long term (current) drug therapy**

✓4ᵗʰ **Z80**   **Family history of primary malignant neoplasm**

Z80.0   **Family history of malignant neoplasm of digestive organs**

Conditions classifiable to C15-C26

Z80.1   **Family history of malignant neoplasm of trachea, bronchus and lung**

Conditions classifiable to C33-C34

Z80.2   **Family history of malignant neoplasm of other respiratory and intrathoracic organs**

Conditions classifiable to C30-C32, C37-C39

Z80.3   **Family history of malignant neoplasm of breast**

Conditions classifiable to C50-

✓5ᵗʰ **Z80.4**   **Family history of malignant neoplasm of genital organs**

Conditions classifiable to C51-C63

Z80.41   **Family history of malignant neoplasm of ovary** ♀

Z80.42   **Family history of malignant neoplasm of prostate** ♂

Z80.43   **Family history of malignant neoplasm of testis** ♂

Z80.49   **Family history of malignant neoplasm of other genital organs**

✓5ᵗʰ **Z80.5**   **Family history of malignant neoplasm of urinary tract**

Conditions classifiable to C64-C68

Z80.51   **Family history of malignant neoplasm of kidney**

Z80.52   **Family history of malignant neoplasm of bladder**

Z80.59   **Family history of malignant neoplasm of other urinary tract organ**

Z80.6   **Family history of leukemia**

Conditions classifiable to C91-C95

Z80.7   **Family history of other malignant neoplasms of lymphoid, hematopoietic and related tissues**

Conditions classifiable to C81-C90, C96-

Z80.8   **Family history of malignant neoplasm of other organs or systems**

Conditions classifiable to C00-C14, C40-C49, C69-C79

Z80.9   **Family history of malignant neoplasm, unspecified**

Conditions classifiable to C80.1

✓4ᵗʰ **Z81**   **Family history of mental and behavioral disorders**

Z81.0   **Family history of intellectual disabilities**

Conditions classifiable to F70-F79

Z81.1   **Family history of alcohol abuse and dependence**

Conditions classifiable to F10-

Z81.2   **Family history of tobacco abuse and dependence**

Conditions classifiable to F17-

Z81.3   **Family history of other psychoactive substance abuse and dependence**

Conditions classifiable to F11-F16, F18-F19

Z81.4   **Family history of other substance abuse and dependence**

Conditions classifiable to F55

Z81.8   **Family history of other mental and behavioral disorders**

Conditions classifiable elsewhere in F01-F99

✓4ᵗʰ **Z82**   **Family history of certain disabilities and chronic diseases (leading to disablement)**

Z82.0   **Family history of epilepsy and other diseases of the nervous system**

Conditions classifiable to G00-G99

Z82.1   **Family history of blindness and visual loss**

Conditions classifiable to H54-

Z82.2   **Family history of deafness and hearing loss**

Conditions classifiable to H90-H91

Z82.3   **Family history of stroke**

Conditions classifiable to I60-I64

✓5ᵗʰ **Z82.4**   **Family history of ischemic heart disease and other diseases of the circulatory system**

Conditions classifiable to I00-I52, I65-I99

Z82.41   **Family history of sudden cardiac death**

Z82.49   **Family history of ischemic heart disease and other diseases of the circulatory system**

Z82.5   **Family history of asthma and other chronic lower respiratory diseases**

Conditions classifiable to J40-J47

EXCLUDES 2   family history of other diseases of the respiratory system (Z83.6)

✓5ᵗʰ **Z82.6**   **Family history of arthritis and other diseases of the musculoskeletal system and connective tissue**

Conditions classifiable to M00-M99

Z82.61   **Family history of arthritis**

Z82.62   **Family history of osteoporosis**

Z82.69   **Family history of other diseases of the musculoskeletal system and connective tissue**

✓5ᵗʰ **Z82.7**   **Family history of congenital malformations, deformations and chromosomal abnormalities**

Conditions classifiable to Q00-Q99

Z82.71   **Family history of polycystic kidney**

Z82.79   **Family history of other congenital malformations, deformations and chromosomal abnormalities**

Z82.8   **Family history of other disabilities and chronic diseases leading to disablement, not elsewhere classified**

✓4ᵗʰ **Z83**   **Family history of other specific disorders**

EXCLUDES 2   contact with and (suspected) exposure to communicable disease in the family (Z20.-)

Z83.0   **Family history of human immunodeficiency virus [HIV] disease**

Conditions classifiable to B20

Z83.1   **Family history of other infectious and parasitic diseases**

Conditions classifiable to A00-B19, B25-B94, B99

Z83.2   **Family history of diseases of the blood and blood-forming organs and certain disorders involving the immune mechanism**

Conditions classifiable to D50-D89

Z83.3   **Family history of diabetes mellitus**

Conditions classifiable to E08-E13

✓5ᵗʰ **Z83.4**   **Family history of other endocrine, nutritional and metabolic diseases**

Conditions classifiable to E00-E07, E15-E88

Z83.41   **Family history of multiple endocrine neoplasia [MEN] syndrome**

Z83.49   **Family history of other endocrine, nutritional and metabolic diseases**

✓5ᵗʰ **Z83.5**   **Family history of eye and ear disorders**

✓6ᵗʰ **Z83.51**   **Family history of eye disorders**

Conditions classifiable to H00-H53, H55-H59

EXCLUDES 2   family history of blindness and visual loss (Z82.1)

Z83.511   **Family history of glaucoma**

Z83.518   **Family history of other specified eye disorder**

Z83.52   **Family history of ear disorders**

Conditions classifiable to H60-H83, H92-H95

EXCLUDES 2   family history of deafness and hearing loss (Z82.2)

Z83.6   **Family history of other diseases of the respiratory system**

Conditions classifiable to J00-J39, J60-J99

EXCLUDES 2   family history of asthma and other chronic lower respiratory diseases (Z82.5)

EXCLUDES 1 Not coded here   EXCLUDES 2 Not included here   PDx Primary Diagnosis Only   N Newborn Age: 0   P Pediatric Age: 0-17   M Maternity Age: 12-55   A Adult Age: 15-124

1074   ICD-10-CM 2014 (Draft)

√5ᵗʰ **Z83.7 Family history of diseases of the digestive system**
Conditions classifiable to K00-K93

    Z83.71 Family history of colonic polyps
        EXCLUDES 1 *family history of malignant neoplasm of digestive organs (Z80.0)*

    Z83.79 Family history of other diseases of the digestive system

√4ᵗʰ **Z84 Family history of other conditions**

    Z84.0 Family history of diseases of the skin and subcutaneous tissue
      Conditions classifiable to L00-L99

    Z84.1 Family history of disorders of kidney and ureter
      Conditions classifiable to N00-N29

    Z84.2 Family history of other diseases of the genitourinary system
      Conditions classifiable to N30-N99

    Z84.3 Family history of consanguinity

√5ᵗʰ **Z84.8 Family history of other specified conditions**

    Z84.81 Family history of carrier of genetic disease
    Z84.89 Family history of other specified conditions

√4ᵗʰ **Z85 Personal history of malignant neoplasm**
Code first any follow-up examination after treatment of malignant neoplasm (Z08)
Use additional code to identify:
  alcohol use and dependence (F10.-)
  exposure to environmental tobacco smoke (Z77.22)
  history of tobacco use (Z87.891)
  occupational exposure to environmental tobacco smoke (Z57.31)
  tobacco dependence (F17.-)
  tobacco use (Z72.0)
  EXCLUDES 2 *personal history of benign neoplasm (Z86.01-)*
        personal history of carcinoma-in-situ (Z86.00-)

√5ᵗʰ **Z85.0 Personal history of malignant neoplasm of digestive organs**

    Z85.00 Personal history of malignant neoplasm of unspecified digestive organ

    Z85.01 Personal history of malignant neoplasm of esophagus
      Conditions classifiable to C15

    √6ᵗʰ **Z85.02 Personal history of malignant neoplasm of stomach**

      Z85.020 Personal history of malignant carcinoid tumor of stomach
        Conditions classifiable to C7A.092

      Z85.028 Personal history of other malignant neoplasm of stomach
        Conditions classifiable to C16

    √6ᵗʰ **Z85.03 Personal history of malignant neoplasm of large intestine**

      Z85.030 Personal history of malignant carcinoid tumor of large intestine
        Conditions classifiable to C7A.022-C7A.025, C7A.029

      Z85.038 Personal history of other malignant neoplasm of large intestine
        Conditions classifiable to C18

    √6ᵗʰ **Z85.04 Personal history of malignant neoplasm of rectum, rectosigmoid junction, and anus**

      Z85.040 Personal history of malignant carcinoid tumor of rectum
        Conditions classifiable to C7A.026

      Z85.048 Personal history of other malignant neoplasm of rectum, rectosigmoid junction, and anus
        Conditions classifiable to C19-C21

    Z85.05 Personal history of malignant neoplasm of liver
      Conditions classifiable to C22

    √6ᵗʰ **Z85.06 Personal history of malignant neoplasm of small intestine**

      Z85.060 Personal history of malignant carcinoid tumor of small intestine
        Conditions classifiable to C7A.01-

      Z85.068 Personal history of other malignant neoplasm of small intestine
        Conditions classifiable to C17

    Z85.07 Personal history of malignant neoplasm of pancreas
      Conditions classifiable to C25

    Z85.09 Personal history of malignant neoplasm of other digestive organs

√5ᵗʰ **Z85.1 Personal history of malignant neoplasm of trachea, bronchus and lung**

    √6ᵗʰ **Z85.11 Personal history of malignant neoplasm of bronchus and lung**

      Z85.110 Personal history of malignant carcinoid tumor of bronchus and lung
        Conditions classifiable to C7A.090

      Z85.118 Personal history of other malignant neoplasm of bronchus and lung
        Conditions classifiable to C34

    Z85.12 Personal history of malignant neoplasm of trachea
      Conditions classifiable to C33

√5ᵗʰ **Z85.2 Personal history of malignant neoplasm of other respiratory and intrathoracic organs**

    Z85.20 Personal history of malignant neoplasm of unspecified respiratory organ

    Z85.21 Personal history of malignant neoplasm of larynx
      Conditions classifiable to C32

    Z85.22 Personal history of malignant neoplasm of nasal cavities, middle ear, and accessory sinuses
      Conditions classifiable to C30-C31

    √6ᵗʰ **Z85.23 Personal history of malignant neoplasm of thymus**

      Z85.230 Personal history of malignant carcinoid tumor of thymus
        Conditions classifiable to C7A.091

      Z85.238 Personal history of other malignant neoplasm of thymus
        Conditions classifiable to C37

    Z85.29 Personal history of malignant neoplasm of other respiratory and intrathoracic organs

    Z85.3 Personal history of malignant neoplasm of breast
      Conditions classifiable to C50-

√5ᵗʰ **Z85.4 Personal history of malignant neoplasm of genital organs**
Conditions classifiable to C51-C63

    Z85.40 Personal history of malignant neoplasm of unspecified female genital organ ♀

    Z85.41 Personal history of malignant neoplasm of cervix uteri ♀

    Z85.42 Personal history of malignant neoplasm of other parts of uterus ♀

    Z85.43 Personal history of malignant neoplasm of ovary ♀

    Z85.44 Personal history of malignant neoplasm of other female genital organs ♀

    Z85.45 Personal history of malignant neoplasm of unspecified male genital organ ♂

    Z85.46 Personal history of malignant neoplasm of prostate ♂

    Z85.47 Personal history of malignant neoplasm of testis ♂

    Z85.48 Personal history of malignant neoplasm of epididymis

    Z85.49 Personal history of malignant neoplasm of other male genital organs ♂

√5ᵗʰ **Z85.5 Personal history of malignant neoplasm of urinary tract**
Conditions classifiable to C64-C68

    Z85.50 Personal history of malignant neoplasm of unspecified urinary tract organ

    Z85.51 Personal history of malignant neoplasm of bladder

    √6ᵗʰ **Z85.52 Personal history of malignant neoplasm of kidney**
      EXCLUDES 1 *personal history of malignant neoplasm of renal pelvis (Z85.53)*

      Z85.520 Personal history of malignant carcinoid tumor of kidney
        Conditions classifiable to C7A.093

      Z85.528 Personal history of other malignant neoplasm of kidney
        Conditions classifiable to C64

    Z85.53 Personal history of malignant neoplasm of renal pelvis

    Z85.54 Personal history of malignant neoplasm of ureter

    Z85.59 Personal history of malignant neoplasm of other urinary tract organ

    Z85.6 Personal history of leukemia
      Conditions classifiable to C91-C95
      EXCLUDES 1 *leukemia in remission C91.0-C95.9 with 5th character 1*

☑ Additional Character Required   **√x7ᵗʰ** Xtension Alert   Unspecified Code   Other Specified Code   Manifestation Code   ►◄ Revised Text   ● New Code   ▲ Revised Code Title

ICD-10-CM 2014 (Draft)   1075

✓5ᵗʰ **Z85.7** **Personal history of other malignant neoplasms of lymphoid, hematopoietic and related tissues**

Z85.71 **Personal history of** Hodgkin lymphoma
Conditions classifiable to C81

Z85.72 **Personal history of** non-Hodgkin lymphomas
Conditions classifiable to C82-C85

Z85.79 **Personal history of other malignant neoplasms of lymphoid, hematopoietic and related tissues**
Conditions classifiable to C88-C90, C96
EXCLUDES 1 multiple myeloma in remission (C90.01)
plasma cell leukemia in remission (C90.11)
plasmacytoma in remission (C90.21)

✓5ᵗʰ **Z85.8** **Personal history of malignant neoplasms of other organs and systems**
Conditions classifiable to C00-C14, C40-C49, C69-C79, C7A.098

✓6ᵗʰ **Z85.81** **Personal history of malignant neoplasm of** lip, oral cavity, and pharynx

Z85.810 **Personal history of malignant neoplasm of** tongue

Z85.818 **Personal history of malignant neoplasm of** other sites of lip, oral cavity, and pharynx

Z85.819 **Personal history of malignant neoplasm of** unspecified site of lip, oral cavity, and pharynx

✓6ᵗʰ **Z85.82** **Personal history of malignant neoplasm of** skin

Z85.820 **Personal history of malignant** melanoma of skin
Conditions classifiable to C43

Z85.821 **Personal history of** Merkel cell carcinoma
Conditions classifiable to C4A

Z85.828 **Personal history of other malignant neoplasm of skin**
Conditions classifiable to C44

✓6ᵗʰ **Z85.83** **Personal history of malignant neoplasm of** bone and soft tissue

Z85.830 **Personal history of malignant neoplasm of** bone

Z85.831 **Personal history of malignant neoplasm of** soft tissue
EXCLUDES 2 personal history of malignant neoplasm of skin (Z85.82-)

✓6ᵗʰ **Z85.84** **Personal history of malignant neoplasm of** eye and nervous tissue

Z85.840 **Personal history of malignant neoplasm of** eye

Z85.841 **Personal history of malignant neoplasm of** brain

Z85.848 **Personal history of malignant neoplasm of** other parts of nervous tissue

✓6ᵗʰ **Z85.85** **Personal history of malignant neoplasm of** endocrine glands

Z85.850 **Personal history of malignant neoplasm of** thyroid

Z85.858 **Personal history of malignant neoplasm of** other endocrine glands

Z85.89 **Personal history of malignant neoplasm of other organs and systems**

Z85.9 **Personal history of malignant neoplasm, unspecified**
Conditions classifiable to C7A.00, C80.1

✓4ᵗʰ **Z86** **Personal history of certain other diseases**
Code first any follow-up examination after treatment (Z09)

✓5ᵗʰ **Z86.0** **Personal history of in-situ and benign neoplasms and neoplasms of uncertain behavior**
EXCLUDES 2 personal history of malignant neoplasms (Z85.-)

✓6ᵗʰ **Z86.00** **Personal history of** in-situ neoplasm

Z86.000 **Personal history of in-situ neoplasm of** breast

Z86.001 **Personal history of in-situ neoplasm of** cervix uteri ♀

Z86.008 **Personal history of in-situ neoplasm of** other site

✓6ᵗʰ **Z86.01** **Personal history of** benign neoplasm

Z86.010 **Personal history of** colonic polyps

Z86.011 **Personal history of benign neoplasm of** the brain

Z86.012 **Personal history of benign** carcinoid tumor

Z86.018 **Personal history of other benign neoplasm**

Z86.03 **Personal history of** neoplasm of uncertain behavior

✓5ᵗʰ **Z86.1** **Personal history of** infectious and parasitic diseases
Conditions classifiable to A00-B89, B99
EXCLUDES 1 personal history of infectious diseases specific to a body system
sequelae of infectious and parasitic diseases (B90-B94)

Z86.11 **Personal history of** tuberculosis

Z86.12 **Personal history of** poliomyelitis

Z86.13 **Personal history of** malaria

Z86.14 **Personal history of** Methicillin resistant Staphylococcus aureus infection
Personal history of MRSA infection

Z86.19 **Personal history of other infectious and parasitic diseases**

Z86.2 **Personal history of diseases of the** blood and blood-forming organs and certain disorders involving the immune mechanism
Conditions classifiable to D50-D89

✓5ᵗʰ **Z86.3** **Personal history of** endocrine, nutritional and metabolic diseases
Conditions classifiable to E00-E88

Z86.31 **Personal history of** diabetic foot ulcer
EXCLUDES 2 current diabetic foot ulcer (E08.621, E09.621, E10.621, E11.621, E13.621)

Z86.32 **Personal history of** gestational diabetes ♀
Personal history of conditions classifiable to O24.4-
EXCLUDES 1 gestational diabetes mellitus in current pregnancy (O24.4-)

Z86.39 **Personal history of other endocrine, nutritional and metabolic disease**

✓5ᵗʰ **Z86.5** **Personal history of** mental and behavioral disorders
Conditions classifiable to F40-F59

Z86.51 **Personal history of** combat and operational stress reaction 🅰

Z86.59 **Personal history of other mental and behavioral disorders**

✓5ᵗʰ **Z86.6** **Personal history of diseases of the** nervous system and sense organs
Conditions classifiable to G00-G99, H00-H95
EXCLUDES 2 personal history of anaphylactic shock (Z87.892)

Z86.61 **Personal history of** infections of the central nervous system
Personal history of encephalitis
Personal history of meningitis

Z86.69 **Personal history of other diseases of the nervous system and sense organs**

✓5ᵗʰ **Z86.7** **Personal history of diseases of the** circulatory system
Conditions classifiable to I00-I99
EXCLUDES 2 old myocardial infarction (I25.2)
personal history of anaphylactic shock (Z87.892)
postmyocardial infarction syndrome (I24.1)

✓6ᵗʰ **Z86.71** **Personal history of** venous thrombosis and embolism

Z86.711 **Personal history of** pulmonary embolism

Z86.718 **Personal history of other venous thrombosis and embolism**

Z86.72 **Personal history of** thrombophlebitis

Z86.73 **Personal history of** transient ischemic attack (TIA), and cerebral infarction without residual deficits
Personal history of prolonged reversible ischemic neurological deficit (PRIND)
Personal history of stroke NOS without residual deficits
EXCLUDES 1 personal history of traumatic brain injury (Z87.820)
sequelae of cerebrovascular disease (I69.-)
AHA: 2012, Q4, 92

Z86.74 **Personal history of** sudden cardiac arrest
Personal history of sudden cardiac death successfully resuscitated

Z86.79 **Personal history of other diseases of the circulatory system**

✓4ᵗʰ **Z87** **Personal history of other diseases and conditions**
Code first any follow-up examination after treatment (Z09)

✓5ᵗʰ **Z87.0** **Personal history of diseases of the** respiratory system
Conditions classifiable to J00-J99

EXCLUDES 1 Not coded here *EXCLUDES 2* Not included here **PDx** Primary Diagnosis Only **N** Newborn Age: 0 **P** Pediatric Age: 0-17 **M** Maternity Age: 12-55 **🅰** Adult Age: 15-124
ICD-10-CM 2014 (Draft)

Z87.01 Personal history of pneumonia (recurrent)

Z87.09 Personal history of other diseases of the circulatory system

☑5ᵗʰ **Z87.1** Personal history of diseases of the digestive system
Conditions classifiable to K00-K93

Z87.11 Personal history of peptic ulcer disease

Z87.19 Personal history of other diseases of the digestive system

Z87.2 Personal history of diseases of the skin and subcutaneous tissue
Conditions classifiable to L00-L99
EXCLUDES 2 personal history of diabetic foot ulcer (Z86.31)

☑5ᵗʰ **Z87.3** Personal history of diseases of the musculoskeletal system and connective tissue
Conditions classifiable to M00-M99
EXCLUDES 2 personal history of (healed) traumatic fracture (Z87.81)

☑6ᵗʰ **Z87.31** Personal history of (healed) nontraumatic fracture

Z87.310 Personal history of (healed) osteoporosis fracture
Personal history of (healed) fragility fracture
Personal history of (healed) collapsed vertebra due to osteoporosis

Z87.311 Personal history of (healed) other pathological fracture
Personal history of (healed) collapsed vertebra NOS
EXCLUDES 2 personal history of osteoporosis fracture (Z87.310)

Z87.312 Personal history of (healed) stress fracture
Personal history of (healed) fatigue fracture

Z87.39 Personal history of other diseases of the musculoskeletal system and connective tissue

☑5ᵗʰ **Z87.4** Personal history of diseases of the genitourinary system
Conditions classifiable to N00-N99

☑6ᵗʰ **Z87.41** Personal history of dysplasia of the female genital tract
EXCLUDES 1 personal history of malignant neoplasm of female genital tract (Z85.40-Z85.44)

Z87.410 Personal history of cervical dysplasia ♀
Z87.411 Personal history of vaginal dysplasia ♀
Z87.412 Personal history of vulvar dysplasia ♀

Z87.42 Personal history of other diseases of the female genital tract ♀

☑6ᵗʰ **Z87.43** Personal history of diseases of the male genital organs

Z87.430 Personal history of prostatic dysplasia
EXCLUDES 1 personal history of malignant neoplasm of prostate (Z85.46)

Z87.438 Personal history of other diseases of male genital organs

☑6ᵗʰ **Z87.44** Personal history of diseases of the urinary system
EXCLUDES 1 personal history of malignant neoplasm of cervix uteri (Z85.41)

Z87.440 Personal history of urinary (tract) infections

Z87.441 Personal history of nephrotic syndrome

Z87.442 Personal history of urinary calculi
Personal history of kidney stones

Z87.448 Personal history of other diseases of urinary system

☑5ᵗʰ **Z87.5** Personal history of complications of pregnancy, childbirth and the puerperium
Conditions classifiable to O00-O9A
EXCLUDES 2 recurrent pregnancy loss (N96)

Z87.51 Personal history of pre-term labor ♀
EXCLUDES 1 current pregnancy with history of pre-term labor (O09.21-)

Z87.59 Personal history of other complications of pregnancy, childbirth and the puerperium ♀
Personal history of trophoblastic disease

☑5ᵗʰ **Z87.7** Personal history of (corrected) congenital malformations
Conditions classifiable to Q00-Q89 that have been repaired or corrected
EXCLUDES 1 congenital malformations that have been partially corrected or repaired but which still require medical treatment—code to condition
EXCLUDES 2 other postprocedural states (Z98.-)
personal history of medical treatment (Z92.-)
presence of cardiac and vascular implants and grafts (Z95.-)
presence of other devices (Z97.-)
presence of other functional implants (Z96.-)
transplanted organ and tissue status (Z94.-)

☑6ᵗʰ **Z87.71** Personal history of (corrected) congenital malformations of genitourinary system

Z87.710 Personal history of (corrected) hypospadias ♂

Z87.718 Personal history of other specified (corrected) congenital malformations of genitourinary system

☑6ᵗʰ **Z87.72** Personal history of (corrected) congenital malformations of nervous system and sense organs

Z87.720 Personal history of (corrected) congenital malformations of eye

Z87.721 Personal history of (corrected) congenital malformations of ear

Z87.728 Personal history of other specified (corrected) congenital malformations of nervous system and sense organs

☑6ᵗʰ **Z87.73** Personal history of (corrected) congenital malformations of digestive system

Z87.730 Personal history of (corrected) cleft lip and palate

Z87.738 Personal history of other specified (corrected) congenital malformations of digestive system

Z87.74 Personal history of (corrected) congenital malformations of heart and circulatory system

Z87.75 Personal history of (corrected) congenital malformations of respiratory system

Z87.76 Personal history of (corrected) congenital malformations of integument, limbs and musculoskeletal system

☑6ᵗʰ **Z87.79** Personal history of other (corrected) congenital malformations

Z87.790 Personal history of (corrected) congenital malformations of face and neck

Z87.798 Personal history of other (corrected) congenital malformations

☑5ᵗʰ **Z87.8** Personal history of other specified conditions
EXCLUDES 2 personal history of self harm (Z91.5)

Z87.81 Personal history of (healed) traumatic fracture
EXCLUDES 2 personal history of (healed) nontraumatic fracture (Z87.31-)

☑6ᵗʰ **Z87.82** Personal history of other (healed) physical injury and trauma
Conditions classifiable to S00-T88, except traumatic fractures

Z87.820 Personal history of traumatic brain injury
EXCLUDES 1 personal history of transient ischemic attack (TIA), and cerebral infarction without residual deficits (Z86.73)

Z87.821 Personal history of retained foreign body fully removed

Z87.828 Personal history of other (healed) physical injury and trauma

☑6ᵗʰ **Z87.89** Personal history of other specified conditions

Z87.890 Personal history of sex reassignment

Z87.891 Personal history of nicotine dependence
EXCLUDES 1 current nicotine dependence (F17.2-)

Z87.892 Personal history of anaphylaxis
Code also allergy status such as:
allergy status to drugs, medicaments and biological substances (Z88.-)
allergy status, other than to drugs and biological substances (Z91.0-)

Z87.898 Personal history of other specified conditions

Z88   Allergy status to drugs, medicaments and biological substances
> EXCLUDES 2   *allergy status, other than to drugs and biological substances (Z91.0-)*

   Z88.0   Allergy status to penicillin

   Z88.1   Allergy status to other antibiotic agents status

   Z88.2   Allergy status to sulfonamides status

   Z88.3   Allergy status to other anti-infective agents status

   Z88.4   Allergy status to anesthetic agent status

   Z88.5   Allergy status to narcotic agent status

   Z88.6   Allergy status to analgesic agent status

   Z88.7   Allergy status to serum and vaccine status

   Z88.8   Allergy status to other drugs, medicaments and biological substances status

   Z88.9   Allergy status to unspecified drugs, medicaments and biological substances status

√4th **Z89   Acquired absence of limb**
> INCLUDES   amputation status
> postprocedural loss of limb
> post-traumatic loss of limb
> EXCLUDES 1   *acquired deformities of limbs (M20-M21)*
> *congenital absence of limbs (Q71-Q73)*

   √5th **Z89.0   Acquired absence of thumb and other finger(s)**

     √6th **Z89.01   Acquired absence of thumb**

       Z89.011   Acquired absence of right thumb

       Z89.012   Acquired absence of left thumb

       Z89.019   Acquired absence of unspecified thumb

     √6th **Z89.02   Acquired absence of other finger(s)**
>   EXCLUDES 2   *acquired absence of thumb (Z89.01-)*

       Z89.021   Acquired absence of right finger(s)

       Z89.022   Acquired absence of left finger(s)

       Z89.029   Acquired absence of unspecified finger(s)

   √5th **Z89.1   Acquired absence of hand and wrist**

     √6th **Z89.11   Acquired absence of hand**

       Z89.111   Acquired absence of right hand

       Z89.112   Acquired absence of left hand

       Z89.119   Acquired absence of unspecified hand

     √6th **Z89.12   Acquired absence of wrist**
> Disarticulation at wrist

       Z89.121   Acquired absence of right wrist

       Z89.122   Acquired absence of left wrist

       Z89.129   Acquired absence of unspecified wrist

   √5th **Z89.2   Acquired absence of upper limb above wrist**

     √6th **Z89.20   Acquired absence of upper limb, unspecified level**

       Z89.201   Acquired absence of right upper limb, unspecified level

       Z89.202   Acquired absence of left upper limb, unspecified level

       Z89.209   Acquired absence of unspecified upper limb, unspecified level
> Acquired absence of arm NOS

     √6th **Z89.21   Acquired absence of upper limb below elbow**

       Z89.211   Acquired absence of right upper limb below elbow

       Z89.212   Acquired absence of left upper limb below elbow

       Z89.219   Acquired absence of unspecified upper limb below elbow

     √6th **Z89.22   Acquired absence of upper limb above elbow**
> Disarticulation at elbow

       Z89.221   Acquired absence of right upper limb above elbow

       Z89.222   Acquired absence of left upper limb above elbow

       Z89.229   Acquired absence of unspecified upper limb above elbow

     √6th **Z89.23   Acquired absence of shoulder**
> Acquired absence of shoulder joint following explantation of shoulder joint prosthesis, with or without presence of antibiotic-impregnated cement spacer

       Z89.231   Acquired absence of right shoulder

       Z89.232   Acquired absence of left shoulder

       Z89.239   Acquired absence of unspecified shoulder

   √5th **Z89.4   Acquired absence of toe(s), foot, and ankle**

     √6th **Z89.41   Acquired absence of great toe**

       Z89.411   Acquired absence of right great toe

       Z89.412   Acquired absence of left great toe

       Z89.419   Acquired absence of unspecified great toe

     √6th **Z89.42   Acquired absence of other toe(s)**
>   EXCLUDES 2   *acquired absence of great toe (Z89.41-)*

       Z89.421   Acquired absence of other right toe(s)

       Z89.422   Acquired absence of other left toe(s)

       Z89.429   Acquired absence of other toe(s), unspecified side

     √6th **Z89.43   Acquired absence of foot**

       Z89.431   Acquired absence of right foot

       Z89.432   Acquired absence of left foot

       Z89.439   Acquired absence of unspecified foot

     √6th **Z89.44   Acquired absence of ankle**
> Disarticulation of ankle

       Z89.441   Acquired absence of right ankle

       Z89.442   Acquired absence of left ankle

       Z89.449   Acquired absence of unspecified ankle

   √5th **Z89.5   Acquired absence of leg below knee**

     √6th **Z89.51   Acquired absence of leg below knee**

       Z89.511   Acquired absence of right leg below knee

       Z89.512   Acquired absence of left leg below knee

       Z89.519   Acquired absence of unspecified leg below knee

     √6th **Z89.52   Acquired absence of knee**
> Acquired absence of knee joint following explantation of knee joint prosthesis, with or without presence of antibiotic-impregnated cement spacer

       Z89.521   Acquired absence of right knee

       Z89.522   Acquired absence of left knee

       Z89.529   Acquired absence of unspecified knee

   √5th **Z89.6   Acquired absence of leg above knee**

     √6th **Z89.61   Acquired absence of leg above knee**
> Acquired absence of leg NOS
> Disarticulation at knee

       Z89.611   Acquired absence of right leg above knee

       Z89.612   Acquired absence of left leg above knee

       Z89.619   Acquired absence of unspecified leg above knee

     √6th **Z89.62   Acquired absence of hip**
> Acquired absence of hip joint following explantation of hip joint prosthesis, with or without presence of antibiotic-impregnated cement spacer
> Disarticulation at hip

       Z89.621   Acquired absence of right hip joint

       Z89.622   Acquired absence of left hip joint

       Z89.629   Acquired absence of unspecified hip joint

   Z89.9   Acquired absence of limb, unspecified

√4th **Z90   Acquired absence of organs, not elsewhere classified**
> INCLUDES   postprocedural or post-traumatic loss of body part NEC
> EXCLUDES 1   *congenital absence—see Alphabetical Index*
> EXCLUDES 2   *postprocedural absence of endocrine glands (E89.-)*

   √5th **Z90.0   Acquired absence of part of head and neck**

     Z90.01   Acquired absence of eye

     Z90.02   Acquired absence of larynx

     Z90.09   Acquired absence of other part of head and neck
> Acquired absence of nose
> EXCLUDES 2   *teeth (K08.1)*

   √5th **Z90.1   Acquired absence of breast and nipple**

     Z90.10   Acquired absence of unspecified breast and nipple

     Z90.11   Acquired absence of right breast and nipple

     Z90.12   Acquired absence of left breast and nipple

     Z90.13   Acquired absence of bilateral breasts and nipples

   Z90.2   Acquired absence of lung [part of]

   Z90.3   Acquired absence of stomach [part of]

EXCLUDES 1 Not coded here   EXCLUDES 2 Not included here   PDx Primary Diagnosis Only   N Newborn Age: 0   P Pediatric Age: 0-17   M Maternity Age: 12-55   A Adult Age: 15-124

ICD-10-CM 2014 (Draft)

1078

✓5ᵗʰ Z90.4 Acquired absence of other specified parts of digestive tract

  ✓6ᵗʰ Z90.41 Acquired absence of pancreas
    Use additional code to identify any associated:
    insulin use (Z79.4)
    diabetes mellitus, postpancreatectomy (E13.-)

    Z90.410 Acquired total absence of pancreas
      Acquired absence of pancreas NOS

    Z90.411 Acquired partial absence of pancreas

  Z90.49 Acquired absence of other specified parts of digestive tract

Z90.5 Acquired absence of kidney

Z90.6 Acquired absence of other parts of urinary tract
  Acquired absence of bladder

✓5ᵗʰ Z90.7 Acquired absence of genital organ(s)
  EXCLUDES 1 personal history of sex reassignment (Z87.890)
  EXCLUDES 2 female genital mutilation status (N90.81-)

  ✓6ᵗʰ Z90.71 Acquired absence of cervix and uterus

    Z90.710 Acquired absence of both cervix and uterus ♀
      Acquired absence of uterus NOS
      Status post total hysterectomy

    Z90.711 Acquired absence of uterus with remaining cervical stump ♀
      Status post partial hysterectomy with remaining cervical stump

    Z90.712 Acquired absence of cervix with remaining uterus ♀

  ✓6ᵗʰ Z90.72 Acquired absence of ovaries
    Z90.721 Acquired absence of ovaries, unilateral ♀
    Z90.722 Acquired absence of ovaries, bilateral ♀

  Z90.79 Acquired absence of other genital organ(s)

✓5ᵗʰ Z90.8 Acquired absence of other organs
  Z90.81 Acquired absence of spleen
  Z90.89 Acquired absence of other organs

✓4ᵗʰ Z91 Personal risk factors, not elsewhere classified
  EXCLUDES 2 contact with and (suspected) exposures hazardous to health (Z77.-)
  exposure to pollution and other problems related to physical environment (Z77.1-)
  personal history of physical injury and trauma (Z87.81, Z87.82-)
  occupational exposure to risk factors (Z57.-)

  ✓5ᵗʰ Z91.0 Allergy status, other than to drugs and biological substances
    EXCLUDES 2 allergy status to drugs, medicaments, and biological substances (Z88.-)

    ✓6ᵗʰ Z91.01 Food allergy status
      EXCLUDES 2 food additives allergy status (Z91.02)

      Z91.010 Allergy to peanuts
      Z91.011 Allergy to milk products
        EXCLUDES 1 lactose intolerance (E73.-)

      Z91.012 Allergy to eggs
      Z91.013 Allergy to seafood
        Allergy to shellfish
        Allergy to octopus or squid ink

      Z91.018 Allergy to other foods
        Allergy to nuts other than peanuts

    Z91.02 Food additives allergy status

    ✓6ᵗʰ Z91.03 Insect allergy status
      Z91.030 Bee allergy status
      Z91.038 Other insect allergy status

    ✓6ᵗʰ Z91.04 Nonmedicinal substance allergy status
      Z91.040 Latex allergy status
        Latex sensitivity status

      Z91.041 Radiographic dye allergy status
        Allergy status to contrast media used for diagnostic X-ray procedure

      Z91.048 Other nonmedicinal substance allergy status

    Z91.09 Other allergy status, other than to drugs and biological substances

  ✓5ᵗʰ Z91.1 Patient's noncompliance with medical treatment and regimen

    Z91.11 Patient's noncompliance with dietary regimen

    ✓6ᵗʰ Z91.12 Patient's intentional underdosing of medication regimen
      Code first underdosing of medication (T36-T50) with fifth or sixth character 6
      EXCLUDES 1 adverse effect of prescribed drug taken as directed—code to adverse effect
      poisoning (overdose)—code to poisoning

      Z91.120 Patient's intentional underdosing of medication regimen due to financial hardship

      Z91.128 Patient's intentional underdosing of medication regimen for other reason

    ✓6ᵗʰ Z91.13 Patient's unintentional underdosing of medication regimen
      Code first underdosing of medication (T36-T50) with fifth or sixth character 6
      EXCLUDES 1 adverse effect of prescribed drug taken as directed—code to adverse effect
      poisoning (overdose)—code to poisoning

      Z91.130 Patient's unintentional underdosing of medication regimen due to age-related debility

      Z91.138 Patient's unintentional underdosing of medication regimen for other reason

    Z91.14 Patient's other noncompliance with medication regimen
      Patient's underdosing of medication NOS

    Z91.15 Patient's noncompliance with renal dialysis

    Z91.19 Patient's noncompliance with other medical treatment and regimen

  ✓5ᵗʰ Z91.4 Personal history of psychological trauma, not elsewhere classified

    ✓6ᵗʰ Z91.41 Personal history of adult abuse
      EXCLUDES 2 personal history of abuse in childhood (Z62.81-)

      Z91.410 Personal history of adult physical and sexual abuse Ⓐ
        EXCLUDES 1 current adult physical abuse (T74.11, T76.11)
        current adult sexual abuse (T74.21, T76.11)

      Z91.411 Personal history of adult psychological abuse Ⓐ

      Z91.412 Personal history of adult neglect Ⓐ
        EXCLUDES 1 current adult neglect (T74.01, T76.01)

      Z91.419 Personal history of unspecified adult abuse Ⓐ

    Z91.49 Other personal history of psychological trauma, not elsewhere classified

  Z91.5 Personal history of self-harm
    Personal history of parasuicide
    Personal history of self-poisoning
    Personal history of suicide attempt

  ✓5ᵗʰ Z91.8 Other specified personal risk factors, not elsewhere classified

    Z91.81 History of falling
      At risk for falling

    Z91.82 Personal history of military deployment
      Individual (civilian or military) with past history of military war, peacekeeping and humanitarian deployment (current or past conflict)
      Returned from military deployment

    Z91.83 *Wandering in diseases classified elsewhere*
      Code first underlying disorder such as:
      Alzheimer's disease (G30.-)
      autism or pervasive developmental disorder (F84.-)
      intellectual disabilities (F70-F79)
      unspecified dementia with behavioral disturbance (F03.9-)

    Z91.89 Other specified personal risk factors, not elsewhere classified

✓4ᵗʰ Z92 Personal history of medical treatment
  EXCLUDES 2 postprocedural states (Z98.-)

  Z92.0 Personal history of contraception
    EXCLUDES 1 counseling or management of current contraceptive practices (Z30.-)
    long term (current) use of contraception (Z79.3)
    presence of (intrauterine) contraceptive device (Z97.5)

✓ Additional Character Required   ✓7ᵗʰ Xtension Alert   Unspecified Code   Other Specified Code   Manifestation Code   ►◄ Revised Text   ● New Code   ▲ Revised Code Title

✓5ᵗʰ **Z92.2　Personal history of** drug therapy
　　　EXCLUDES 2　long term (current) drug therapy (Z79.-)

　　Z92.21　Personal history of antineoplastic chemotherapy

　　Z92.22　Personal history of monoclonal drug therapy

　　Z92.23　Personal history of estrogen therapy

✓6ᵗʰ **Z92.24　Personal history of** steroid therapy

　　　　Z92.240　Personal history of inhaled steroid therapy

　　　　Z92.241　Personal history of systemic steroid therapy
　　　　　　　Personal history of steroid therapy NOS

　　Z92.25　Personal history of immunosupression therapy
　　　　EXCLUDES 2　personal history of steroid therapy (Z92.24)

　　Z92.29　Personal history of other drug therapy

Z92.3　Personal history of irradiation
　　　Personal history of exposure to therapeutic radiation
　　　EXCLUDES 1　exposure to radiation in the physical environment (Z77.12)
　　　　occupational exposure to radiation (Z57.1)

✓5ᵗʰ **Z92.8　Personal history of other medical treatment**

　　Z92.81　Personal history of extracorporeal membrane oxygenation (ECMO)

　　Z92.82　Status post administration of tPA (rtPA) in a different facility within the last 24 hours prior to admission to current facility
　　　　Code first condition requiring tPA administration, such as:
　　　　　acute cerebral infarction (I63.-)
　　　　　acute myocardial infarction (I21-, I22-)

　　Z92.83　Personal history of failed moderate sedation
　　　　Personal history of failed conscious sedation
　　　　EXCLUDES 2　failed moderate sedation during procedure (T88.52)

　　Z92.89　Personal history of other medical treatment

✓4ᵗʰ **Z93　Artificial opening status**
　　　EXCLUDES 1　artificial openings requiring attention or management (Z43.-)
　　　　complications of external stoma (J95.0-, K94.-, N99.5-)

Z93.0　Tracheostomy status

Z93.1　Gastrostomy status

Z93.2　Ileostomy status

Z93.3　Colostomy status

Z93.4　Other artificial openings of gastrointestinal tract status

✓5ᵗʰ **Z93.5　Cystostomy status**

　　Z93.50　Unspecified cystostomy status

　　Z93.51　Cutaneous-vesicostomy status

　　Z93.52　Appendico-vesicostomy status

　　Z93.59　Other cystostomy status

Z93.6　Other artificial openings of urinary tract **status**
　　　Nephrostomy status
　　　Ureterostomy status
　　　Urethrostomy status

Z93.8　Other artificial opening status

Z93.9　Artificial opening status, unspecified

✓4ᵗʰ **Z94　Transplanted organ and tissue status**
　　　INCLUDES　organ or tissue replaced by heterogenous or homogenous transplant
　　　EXCLUDES 1　complications of transplanted organ or tissue—see Alphabetical Index
　　　EXCLUDES 2　presence of vascular grafts (Z95.-)

Z94.0　Kidney transplant status

Z94.1　Heart transplant status
　　　EXCLUDES 1　artificial heart status (Z95.812)
　　　　heart-valve replacement status (Z95.2-Z95.4)

Z94.2　Lung transplant status

Z94.3　Heart and lungs transplant status

Z94.4　Liver transplant status

Z94.5　Skin transplant status
　　　Autogenous skin transplant status

Z94.6　Bone transplant status

Z94.7　Corneal transplant status

✓5ᵗʰ **Z94.8　Other transplanted organ and tissue status**

　　Z94.81　Bone marrow transplant status

　　Z94.82　Intestine transplant status

　　Z94.83　Pancreas transplant status

　　Z94.84　Stem cells transplant status

　　Z94.89　Other transplanted organ and tissue status

Z94.9　Transplanted organ and tissue status, unspecified

✓4ᵗʰ **Z95　Presence of cardiac and vascular implants and grafts**
　　　EXCLUDES 1　complications of cardiac and vascular devices, implants and grafts (T82.-)

Z95.0　Presence of cardiac pacemaker
　　　EXCLUDES 1　adjustment or management of cardiac pacemaker (Z45.0)
　　　　presence of automatic (implantable) cardiac defibrillator with synchronous cardiac pacemaker (Z95.810)

Z95.1　Presence of aortocoronary bypass graft

Z95.2　Presence of prosthetic heart valve
　　　Presence of heart valve NOS

Z95.3　Presence of xenogenic heart valve

Z95.4　Presence of other heart-valve **replacement**

Z95.5　Presence of coronary angioplasty **implant and graft**
　　　EXCLUDES 1　coronary angioplasty status without implant and graft (Z98.61)

✓5ᵗʰ **Z95.8　Presence of other cardiac and vascular implants and grafts**

✓6ᵗʰ **Z95.81　Presence of** other cardiac implants and grafts

　　　　Z95.810　Presence of automatic (implantable) cardiac defibrillator
　　　　　　　Presence of automatic (implantable) cardiac defibrillator with synchronous cardiac pacemaker

　　　　Z95.811　Presence of heart assist device

　　　　Z95.812　Presence of fully implantable artificial heart

　　　　Z95.818　Presence of other cardiac implants and grafts

✓6ᵗʰ **Z95.82　Presence of other vascular implants and grafts**

　　　　Z95.820　Peripheral vascular angioplasty status **with implants and grafts**
　　　　　　　EXCLUDES 1　peripheral vascular angioplasty without implant and graft (Z98.62)

　　　　Z95.828　Presence of other vascular implants and grafts
　　　　　　　Presence of intravascular prosthesis NEC

Z95.9　Presence of cardiac and vascular implant and graft, unspecified

✓4ᵗʰ **Z96　Presence of other functional implants**
　　　EXCLUDES 2　complications of internal prosthetic devices, implants and grafts (T82-T85)
　　　　fitting and adjustment of prosthetic and other devices (Z44-Z46)

Z96.0　Presence of urogenital **implants**

Z96.1　Presence of intraocular lens
　　　Presence of pseudophakia

✓5ᵗʰ **Z96.2　Presence of** otological and audiological **implants**

　　Z96.20　Presence of otological and audiological implant, unspecified

　　Z96.21　Cochlear implant status

　　Z96.22　Myringotomy tube(s) status

　　Z96.29　Presence of other otological and audiological implants
　　　　Presence of bone-conduction hearing device
　　　　Presence of eustachian tube stent
　　　　Stapes replacement

Z96.3　Presence of artificial larynx

✓5ᵗʰ **Z96.4　Presence of** endocrine **implants**

　　Z96.41　Presence of insulin pump (external) (internal)

　　Z96.49　Presence of other endocrine implants

Z96.5　Presence of tooth-root and mandibular **implants**

✓5ᵗʰ **Z96.6　Presence of** orthopedic joint **implants**

　　Z96.60　Presence of unspecified orthopedic joint implant

✓6ᵗʰ **Z96.61　Presence of** artificial shoulder joint

　　　　Z96.611　Presence of right artificial shoulder joint

　　　　Z96.612　Presence of left artificial shoulder joint

　　　　Z96.619　Presence of unspecified artificial shoulder joint

✓6ᵗʰ **Z96.62　Presence of** artificial elbow joint

　　　　Z96.621　Presence of right artificial elbow joint

　　　　Z96.622　Presence of left artificial elbow joint

EXCLUDES 1 Not coded here　　EXCLUDES 2 Not included here　　PDx Primary Diagnosis Only　　N Newborn Age: 0　　P Pediatric Age: 0-17　　M Maternity Age: 12-55　　A Adult Age: 15-124

1080　　　　　　　　　　　　　　　　　　　　　　　　　　　　　　　　　　　　ICD-10-CM 2014 (Draft)

Z96.629   **Presence of unspecified artificial elbow joint**

✓6ᵗʰ **Z96.63**   Presence of artificial wrist joint

Z96.631   **Presence of right artificial wrist joint**

Z96.632   **Presence of left artificial wrist joint**

Z96.639   **Presence of unspecified artificial wrist joint**

✓6ᵗʰ **Z96.64**   Presence of artificial hip joint
     Hip-joint replacement (partial) (total)

Z96.641   **Presence of right artificial hip joint**

Z96.642   **Presence of left artificial hip joint**

Z96.643   **Presence of artificial hip joint, bilateral**

Z96.649   **Presence of unspecified artificial hip joint**

✓6ᵗʰ **Z96.65**   Presence of artificial knee joint

Z96.651   **Presence of right artificial knee joint**

Z96.652   **Presence of left artificial knee joint**

Z96.653   **Presence of artificial knee joint, bilateral**

Z96.659   **Presence of unspecified artificial knee joint**

✓6ᵗʰ **Z96.66**   Presence of artificial ankle joint

Z96.661   **Presence of right artificial ankle joint**

Z96.662   **Presence of left artificial ankle joint**

Z96.669   **Presence of unspecified artificial ankle joint**

✓6ᵗʰ **Z96.69**   Presence of other orthopedic joint implants

Z96.691   **Finger-joint replacement of right hand**

Z96.692   **Finger-joint replacement of left hand**

Z96.693   **Finger-joint replacement, bilateral**

Z96.698   **Presence of other orthopedic joint implants**

Z96.7   **Presence of other bone and tendon implants**
     Presence of skull plate

✓5ᵗʰ **Z96.8**   Presence of other specified functional implants

Z96.81   **Presence of artificial skin**

Z96.89   **Presence of other specified functional implants**

Z96.9   **Presence of functional implant, unspecified**

✓4ᵗʰ **Z97**   **Presence of other devices**

EXCLUDES 1   *complications of internal prosthetic devices, implants and grafts (T82-T85)*
     fitting and adjustment of prosthetic and other devices (Z44-Z46)

EXCLUDES 2   *presence of cerebrospinal fluid drainage device (Z98.2)*

Z97.0   **Presence of artificial eye**

✓5ᵗʰ **Z97.1**   Presence of artificial limb (complete) (partial)

Z97.10   **Presence of artificial limb (complete) (partial), unspecified**

Z97.11   **Presence of artificial right arm (complete) (partial)**

Z97.12   **Presence of artificial left arm (complete) (partial)**

Z97.13   **Presence of artificial right leg (complete) (partial)**

Z97.14   **Presence of artificial left leg (complete) (partial)**

Z97.15   **Presence of artificial arms, bilateral (complete) (partial)**

Z97.16   **Presence of artificial legs, bilateral (complete) (partial)**

Z97.2   **Presence of dental prosthetic device (complete) (partial)**
     Presence of dentures (complete) (partial)

Z97.3   **Presence of spectacles and contact lenses**

Z97.4   **Presence of external hearing-aid**

Z97.5   **Presence of (intrauterine) contraceptive device**   ♀

EXCLUDES 1   *checking, reinsertion or removal of contraceptive device (Z30.43)*

Z97.8   **Presence of other specified devices**

✓4ᵗʰ **Z98**   **Other postprocedural states**

EXCLUDES 2   *aftercare (Z43-Z49, Z51)*
     follow-up medical care (Z08- Z09)
     postprocedural complication—see Alphabetical Index

Z98.0   **Intestinal bypass and anastomosis status**

EXCLUDES 2   *bariatric surgery status (Z98.84)*
     gastric bypass status (Z98.84)
     obesity surgery status (Z98.84)

Z98.1   **Arthrodesis status**

Z98.2   **Presence of cerebrospinal fluid drainage device**
     Presence of CSF shunt

Z98.3   **Post therapeutic collapse of lung status**
     Code first underlying disease

✓5ᵗʰ **Z98.4**   Cataract extraction status
     Use additional code to identify intraocular lens implant status (Z96.1)

EXCLUDES 1   *aphakia (H27.0)*

Z98.41   **Cataract extraction status, right eye**

Z98.42   **Cataract extraction status, left eye**

Z98.49   **Cataract extraction status, unspecified eye**

✓5ᵗʰ **Z98.5**   Sterilization status

EXCLUDES 1   *female infertility (N97.-)*
     male infertility (N46.-)

Z98.51   **Tubal ligation status**   ♀

Z98.52   **Vasectomy status**   Ⓐ♂

✓5ᵗʰ **Z98.6**   Angioplasty status

Z98.61   **Coronary angioplasty status**

EXCLUDES 1   *coronary angioplasty status with implant and graft (Z95.5)*

Z98.62   **Peripheral vascular angioplasty status**

EXCLUDES 1   *peripheral vascular angioplasty status with implant and graft (Z95.820)*

✓5ᵗʰ **Z98.8**   Other specified postprocedural states

✓6ᵗʰ **Z98.81**   Dental procedure status

Z98.810   **Dental sealant status**

Z98.811   **Dental restoration status**
     Dental crown status
     Dental fillings status

Z98.818   **Other dental procedure status**

Z98.82   **Breast implant status**

EXCLUDES 1   *breast implant removal status (Z98.86)*

Z98.83   **Filtering (vitreous) bleb after glaucoma surgery status**

EXCLUDES 1   *inflammation (infection) of postprocedural bleb (H59.4-)*

Z98.84   **Bariatric surgery status**
     Gastric banding status
     Gastric bypass status for obesity
     Obesity surgery status

EXCLUDES 1   *bariatric surgery status complicating pregnancy, childbirth, or the puerperium (O99.84)*

EXCLUDES 2   *intestinal bypass and anastomosis status (Z98.0)*

Z98.85   **Transplanted organ removal status**
     Transplanted organ previously removed due to complication, failure, rejection or infection

EXCLUDES 1   *encounter for removal of transplanted organ—code to complication of transplanted organ (T86.-)*

Z98.86   **Personal history of breast implant removal**

✓6ᵗʰ **Z98.87**   Personal history of in utero procedure

Z98.870   **Personal history of in utero procedure during pregnancy**   ♀

EXCLUDES 2   *complications from in utero procedure for current pregnancy (O35.7)*
     supervision of current pregnancy with history of in utero procedure during previous pregnancy (O09.82-)

Z98.871   **Personal history of in utero procedure while a fetus**

Z98.89   **Other specified postprocedural states**
     Personal history of surgery, not elsewhere classified

✓4ᵗʰ **Z99**   **Dependence on enabling machines and devices, not elsewhere classified**

EXCLUDES 1   *cardiac pacemaker status (Z95.0)*

Z99.0   **Dependence on aspirator**

✓5ᵗʰ **Z99.1**   Dependence on respirator
     Dependence on ventilator

Z99.11   **Dependence on respirator [ventilator] status**

Z99.12   **Encounter for respirator [ventilator] dependence during power failure**   PDx

EXCLUDES 1   *mechanical complication of respirator [ventilator] (J95.850)*

✓ Additional Character Required   ✗⁷ᵗʰ Xtension Alert   Unspecified Code   Other Specified Code   Manifestation Code   ▶◀ Revised Text   ● New Code   ▲ Revised Code Title

Factors Influencing Health Status and Contact With Health Service.

Z99.2–Z99.89

Z99.2   **Dependence on** renal dialysis
       Hemodialysis status
       Peritoneal dialysis status
       Presence of arteriovenous shunt for dialysis
       Renal dialysis status NOS
       EXCLUDES 1   *encounter for fitting and adjustment of dialysis catheter (Z49.0-)*
                     noncompliance with renal dialysis (Z91.15)

Z99.3   **Dependence on** wheelchair
       Wheelchair confinement status
       Code first cause of dependence, such as:
          muscular dystrophy (G71.0)
          obesity (E66.-)

√5th   **Z99.8**   **Dependence on other enabling machines and devices**

       Z99.81   **Dependence on** supplemental oxygen
                 Dependence on long-term oxygen

       Z99.89   **Dependence on other enabling machines and devices**
                 Dependence on machine or device NOS

EXCLUDES 1 Not coded here   **EXCLUDES 2** Not included here   **PDx** Primary Diagnosis Only   **N** Newborn Age: 0   **P** Pediatric Age: 0-17   **M** Maternity Age: 12-55   **A** Adult Age: 15-124

1082   ICD-10-CM 2014 (Draft)

Illustrations

Peripheral Nervous System

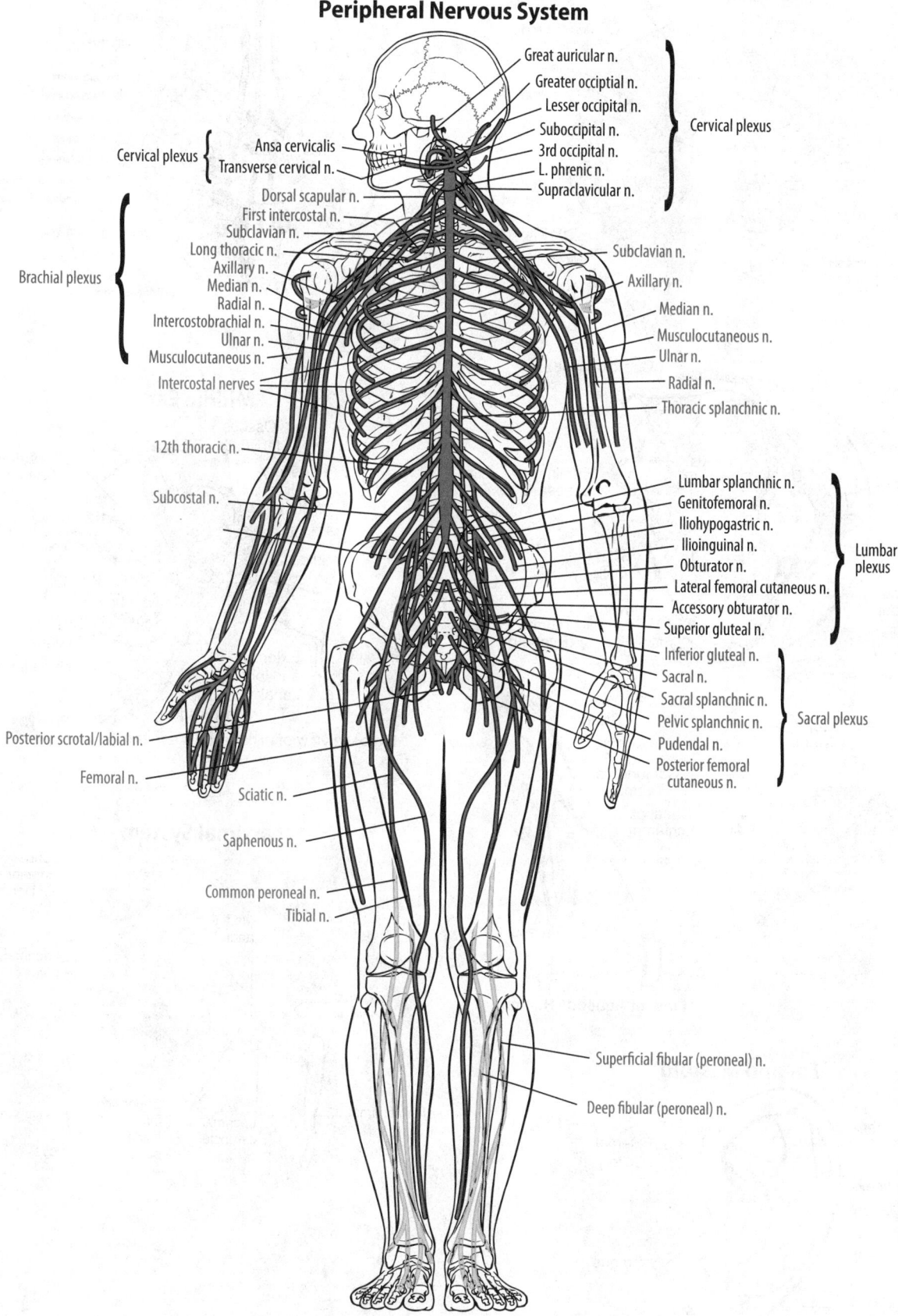

Great auricular n.
Greater occiptial n.
Lesser occipital n.
Suboccipital n.
3rd occipital n.
L. phrenic n.
Supraclavicular n.

Cervical plexus

Ansa cervicalis
Transverse cervical n.

Cervical plexus

Dorsal scapular n.
First intercostal n.
Subclavian n.
Long thoracic n.
Axillary n.
Median n.
Radial n.
Intercostobrachial n.
Ulnar n.
Musculocutaneous n.
Intercostal nerves

Brachial plexus

Subclavian n.
Axillary n.
Median n.
Musculocutaneous n.
Ulnar n.
Radial n.
Thoracic splanchnic n.

12th thoracic n.

Subcostal n.

Lumbar splanchnic n.
Genitofemoral n.
Iliohypogastric n.
Ilioinguinal n.
Obturator n.
Lateral femoral cutaneous n.
Accessory obturator n.
Superior gluteal n.

Lumbar plexus

Inferior gluteal n.
Sacral n.
Sacral splanchnic n.
Pelvic splanchnic n.
Pudendal n.
Posterior femoral cutaneous n.

Sacral plexus

Posterior scrotal/labial n.

Femoral n.

Sciatic n.

Saphenous n.

Common peroneal n.
Tibial n.

Superficial fibular (peroneal) n.

Deep fibular (peroneal) n.

Brain

Cranial Nerves

Eye

Globe (Eyeball)

Middle Ear

Exposed view of middle and inner ear

Posterior Pole of Globe

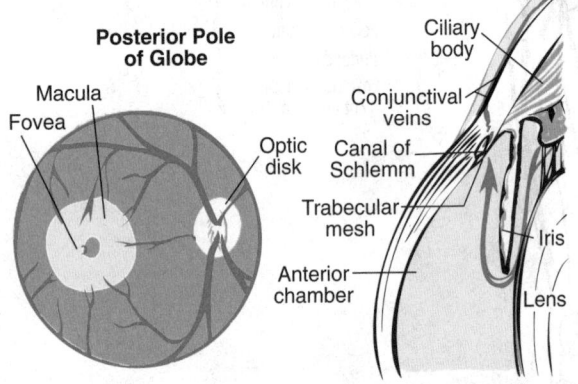

Flow of Aqueous Humor

Lacrimal System

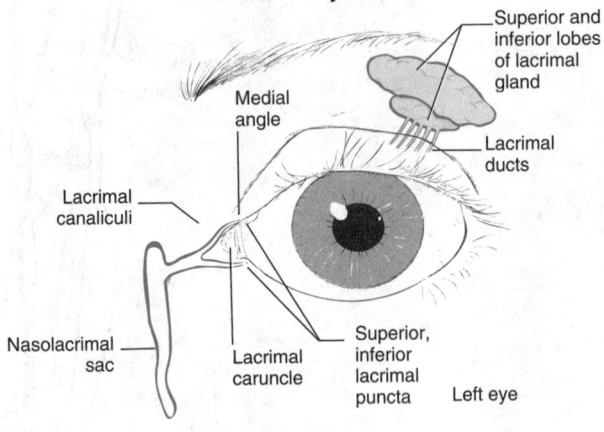

Left eye

Ear and Mastoid

Arteries

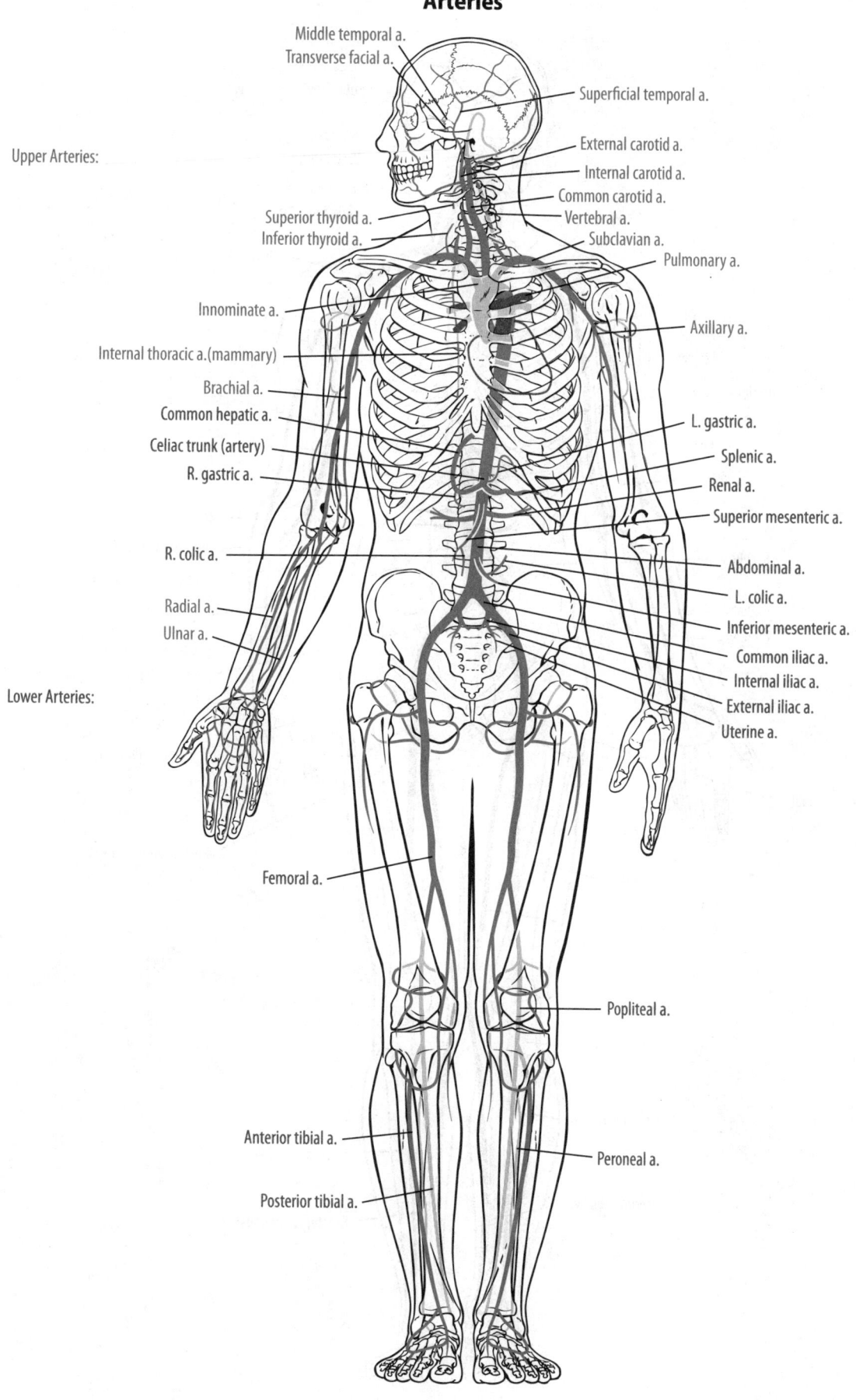

Upper Arteries:

Lower Arteries:

Middle temporal a.
Transverse facial a.
Superficial temporal a.
External carotid a.
Internal carotid a.
Common carotid a.
Superior thyroid a.
Inferior thyroid a.
Vertebral a.
Subclavian a.
Pulmonary a.
Innominate a.
Axillary a.
Internal thoracic a.(mammary)
Brachial a.
Common hepatic a.
L. gastric a.
Celiac trunk (artery)
Splenic a.
R. gastric a.
Renal a.
Superior mesenteric a.
R. colic a.
Abdominal a.
Radial a.
L. colic a.
Ulnar a.
Inferior mesenteric a.
Common iliac a.
Internal iliac a.
External iliac a.
Uterine a.
Femoral a.
Popliteal a.
Anterior tibial a.
Peroneal a.
Posterior tibial a.

Veins

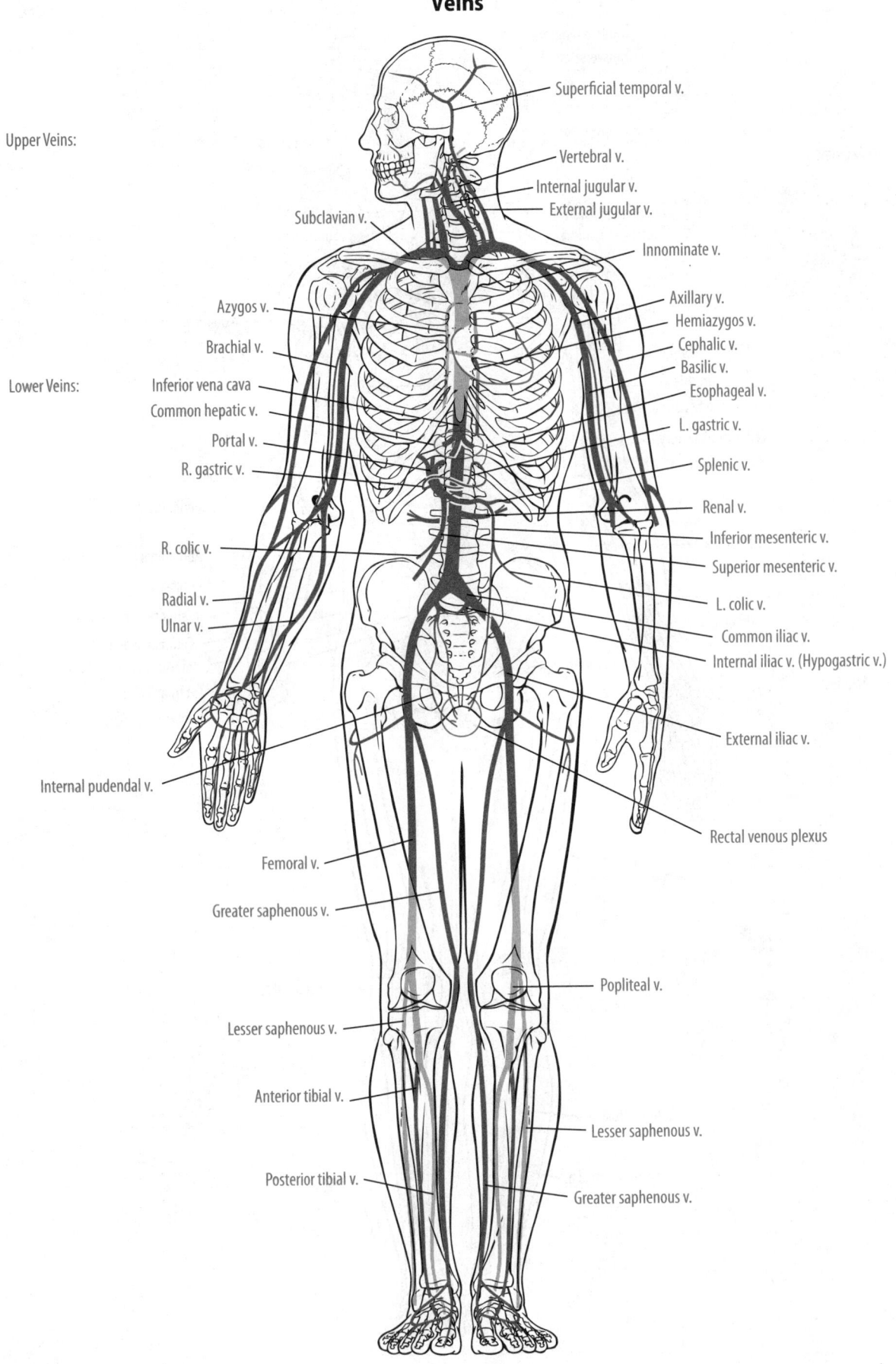

Upper Veins:

Lower Veins:

Superficial temporal v.

Vertebral v.

Internal jugular v.

External jugular v.

Subclavian v.

Innominate v.

Azygos v.

Axillary v.

Brachial v.

Hemiazygos v.

Cephalic v.

Inferior vena cava

Basilic v.

Common hepatic v.

Esophageal v.

Portal v.

L. gastric v.

R. gastric v.

Splenic v.

Renal v.

R. colic v.

Inferior mesenteric v.

Superior mesenteric v.

Radial v.

L. colic v.

Ulnar v.

Common iliac v.

Internal iliac v. (Hypogastric v.)

External iliac v.

Internal pudendal v.

Rectal venous plexus

Femoral v.

Greater saphenous v.

Popliteal v.

Lesser saphenous v.

Anterior tibial v.

Lesser saphenous v.

Posterior tibial v.

Greater saphenous v.

Anatomy of Heart

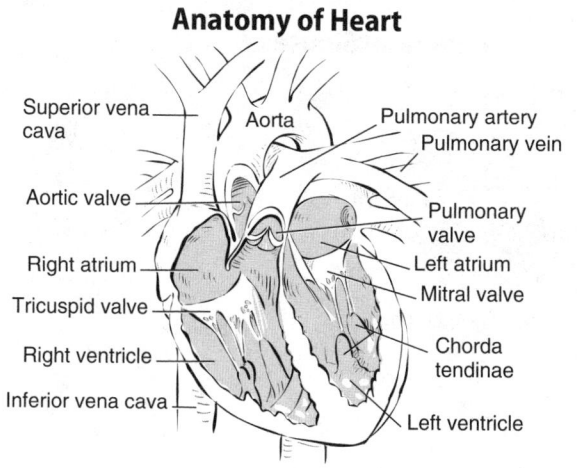

- Superior vena cava
- Aorta
- Pulmonary artery
- Pulmonary vein
- Aortic valve
- Pulmonary valve
- Right atrium
- Left atrium
- Mitral valve
- Tricuspid valve
- Right ventricle
- Chorda tendinae
- Inferior vena cava
- Left ventricle

Arteries of Heart

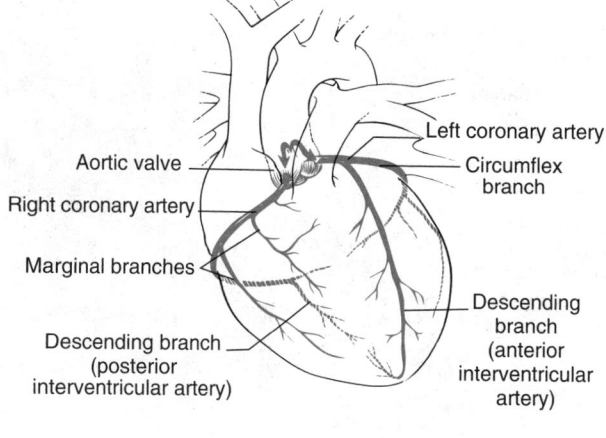

- Aortic valve
- Left coronary artery
- Circumflex branch
- Right coronary artery
- Marginal branches
- Descending branch (posterior interventricular artery)
- Descending branch (anterior interventricular artery)

Cerebrovascular Arteries

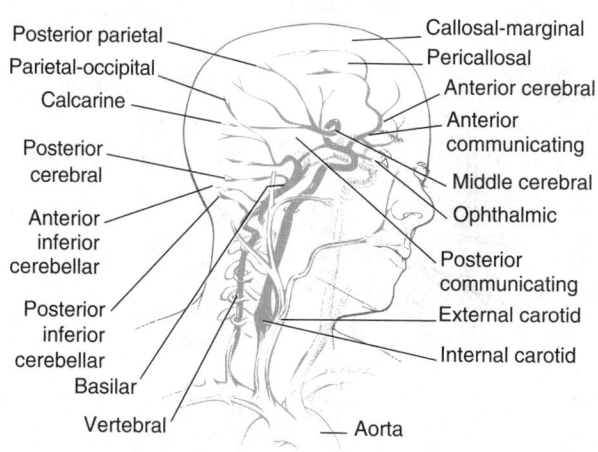

- Posterior parietal
- Callosal-marginal
- Parietal-occipital
- Pericallosal
- Calcarine
- Anterior cerebral
- Posterior cerebral
- Anterior communicating
- Middle cerebral
- Ophthalmic
- Anterior inferior cerebellar
- Posterior communicating
- Posterior inferior cerebellar
- External carotid
- Basilar
- Internal carotid
- Vertebral
- Aorta

Veins of Head and Neck

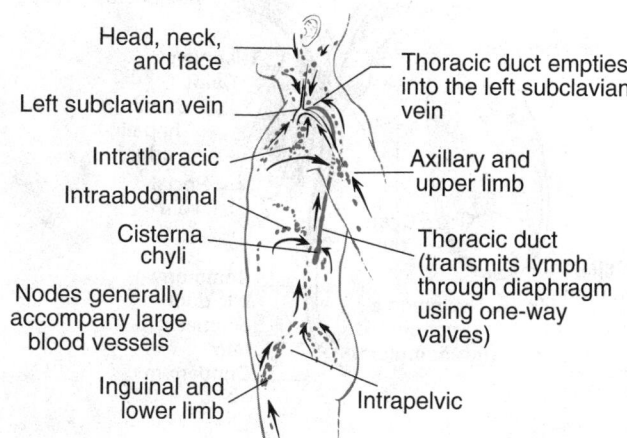

- Superficial temporal vein
- Superior sagittal sinus
- Inferior sagittal sinus
- Superior ophthalmic vein
- Straight sinus
- Retro-mandibular vein
- Transverse sinus
- Facial vein
- Occipital sinus
- Lingual vein
- Posterior auricular vein
- Thyroid veins
- Deep cervical vein
- Anterior jugular
- External jugular vein
- External jugular vein
- Bracheocephalic vein
- Vertebral vein
- Subclavian vein

Lymphatic System of Head and Neck

- Afferent vessels (in)
- Blood vessels
- Hilum
- Efferent vessel (out)

Schematic of lymph node

- Jugulodigastric
- Superficial parotid
- Submental
- Occipital
- Submandibular
- Jugulomyohyoid
- Anterior cervical

Lymphatic drainage of the head, neck, and face

Lymph Nodes

- Head, neck, and face
- Thoracic duct empties into the left subclavian vein
- Left subclavian vein
- Intrathoracic
- Axillary and upper limb
- Intraabdominal
- Cisterna chyli
- Thoracic duct (transmits lymph through diaphragm using one-way valves)
- Nodes generally accompany large blood vessels
- Inguinal and lower limb
- Intrapelvic

Respiratory System

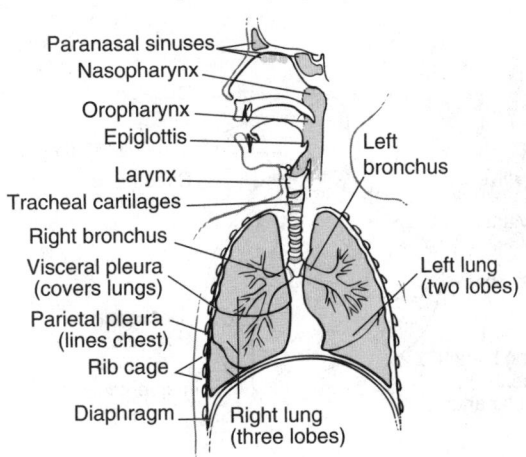

Paranasal sinuses
Nasopharynx
Oropharynx
Epiglottis
Larynx
Tracheal cartilages
Right bronchus
Visceral pleura (covers lungs)
Parietal pleura (lines chest)
Rib cage
Diaphragm
Left bronchus
Left lung (two lobes)
Right lung (three lobes)

Paranasal Sinuses

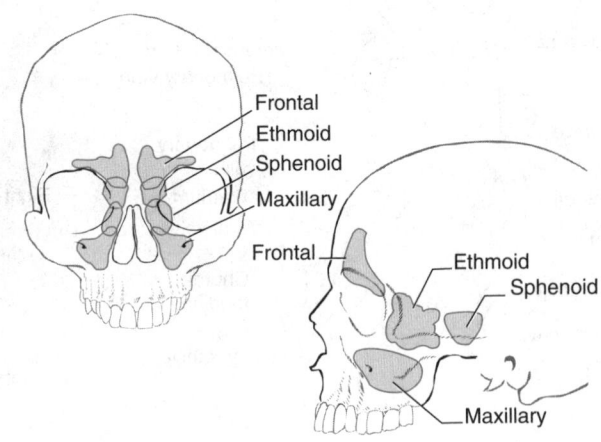

Frontal
Ethmoid
Sphenoid
Maxillary
Frontal
Ethmoid
Sphenoid
Maxillary

Oral Cavity

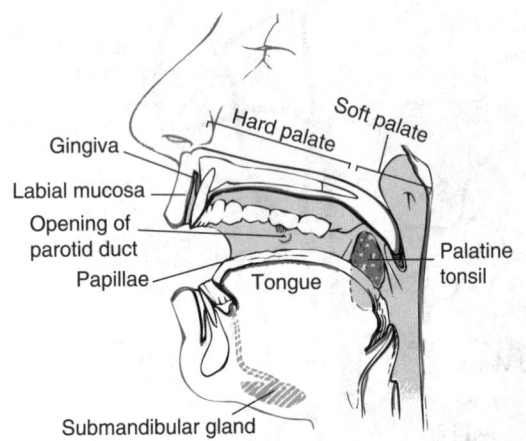

Gingiva
Labial mucosa
Opening of parotid duct
Papillae
Submandibular gland
Hard palate
Soft palate
Tongue
Palatine tonsil

Pancreas

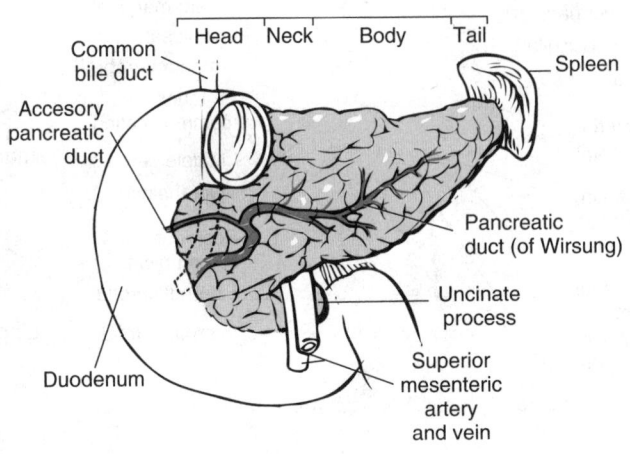

Head   Neck   Body   Tail
Common bile duct
Accesory pancreatic duct
Duodenum
Spleen
Pancreatic duct (of Wirsung)
Uncinate process
Superior mesenteric artery and vein

Gallbladder and Bile Ducts

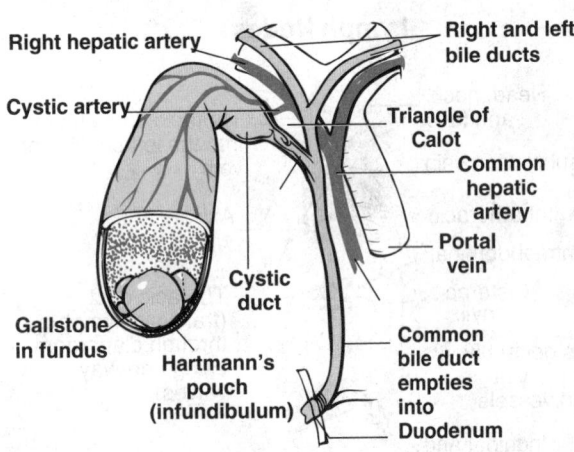

Right hepatic artery
Cystic artery
Gallstone in fundus
Hartmann's pouch (infundibulum)
Cystic duct
Right and left bile ducts
Triangle of Calot
Common hepatic artery
Portal vein
Common bile duct empties into Duodenum

Liver

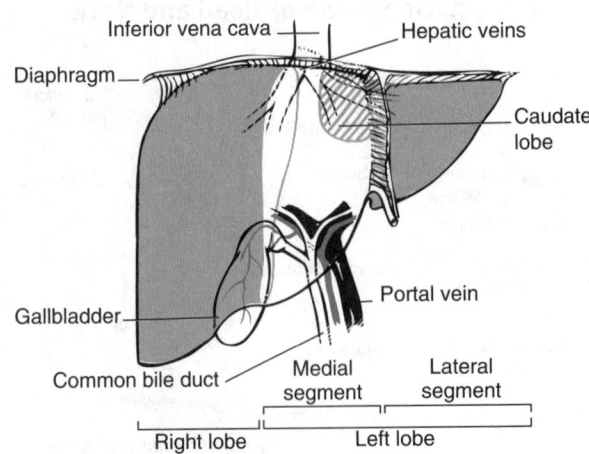

Inferior vena cava
Diaphragm
Gallbladder
Common bile duct
Hepatic veins
Caudate lobe
Portal vein
Medial segment
Lateral segment
Right lobe
Left lobe

Gastrointestinal System

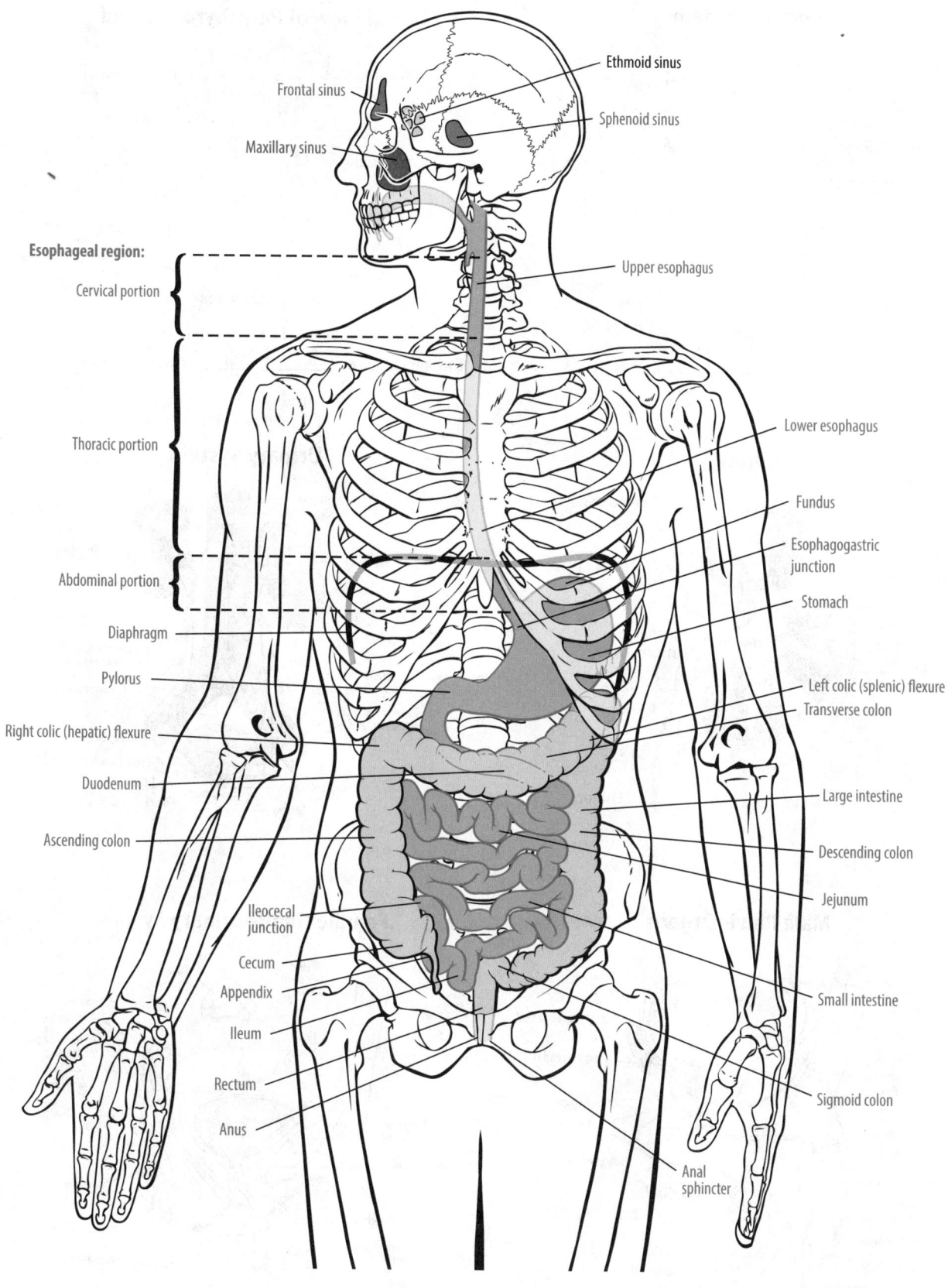

Ethmoid sinus

Frontal sinus

Sphenoid sinus

Maxillary sinus

Esophageal region:

Cervical portion

Thoracic portion

Abdominal portion

Diaphragm

Pylorus

Right colic (hepatic) flexure

Duodenum

Ascending colon

Ileocecal junction

Cecum

Appendix

Ileum

Rectum

Anus

Upper esophagus

Lower esophagus

Fundus

Esophagogastric junction

Stomach

Left colic (splenic) flexure

Transverse colon

Large intestine

Descending colon

Jejunum

Small intestine

Sigmoid colon

Anal sphincter

Endocrine System

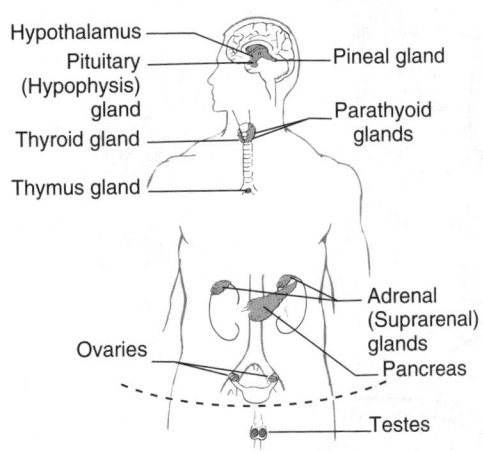

Hypothalamus
Pituitary (Hypophysis) gland
Thyroid gland
Thymus gland
Ovaries
Pineal gland
Parathyroid glands
Adrenal (Suprarenal) glands
Pancreas
Testes

Dorsal View of Parathyroid Gland

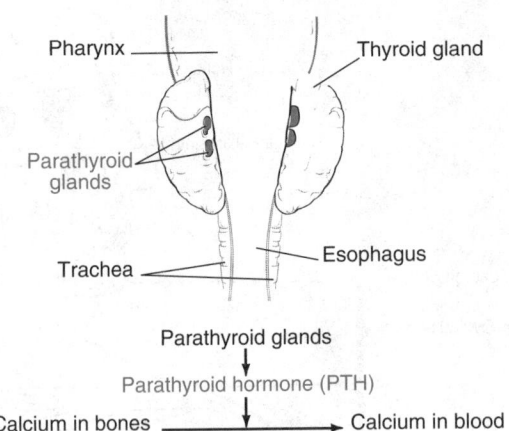

Pharynx
Parathyroid glands
Trachea
Thyroid gland
Esophagus

Parathyroid glands
↓
Parathyroid hormone (PTH)
↓
Calcium in bones ——→ Calcium in blood

Kidney

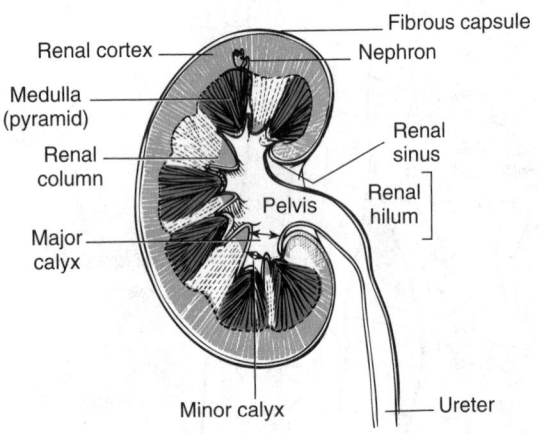

Renal cortex
Medulla (pyramid)
Renal column
Major calyx
Fibrous capsule
Nephron
Renal sinus
Renal hilum
Pelvis
Minor calyx
Ureter

Urinary System

Inferior vena cava
Aorta
Right kidney
Left kidney
Ureter
Ovarian or testicular artery and vein
Anterior division of Internal iliac artery
Superior and inferior vesicular arteries
Fundus of bladder
Urinary bladder
Ureteral orifice
Trigone
Uvula of bladder
Urogenital diaphragm
Urethra

Male Pelvic Organs

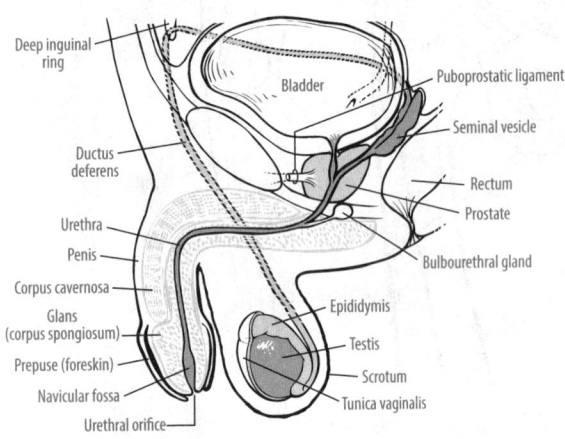

Deep inguinal ring
Ductus deferens
Urethra
Penis
Corpus cavernosa
Glans (corpus spongiosum)
Prepuse (foreskin)
Navicular fossa
Urethral orifice
Bladder
Puboprostatic ligament
Seminal vesicle
Rectum
Prostate
Bulbourethral gland
Epididymis
Testis
Scrotum
Tunica vaginalis

Female Genitourinary System

Uterine (fallopian) tube
Ovary
Uterus (fundus)
Symphysis pubis
Arcuate pubic ligament
Clitoris
Urogenital diaphragm
Urethral orifice (meatus)
Labia minora
Labia majora
Bladder
Posterior fornix
Rectouterine pouch (of Douglas)
Cervix
Rectum
Anus
Vaginal canal

Joints

Shoulder (Anterior View)

Shoulder (Posterior View)

Elbow (Anterior View)

Elbow (Posterior View)

Hand

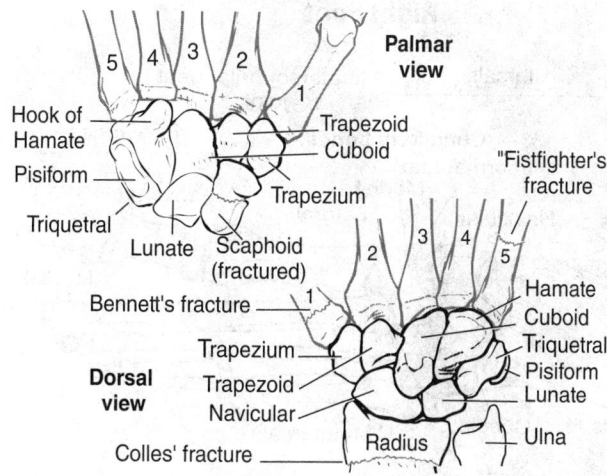

Joints

Hip (Anterior View)

Hip (Posterior View)

Knee (Anterior View)

Knee (Posterior View)

Right Foot

Bones/Joints

Muscles

Temporalis m.

Frontalis m.

Orbicularis oculi m.

Orbicularis oris m.

Depressor labii inferioris m.

Mentalis m.

Masseter m.

Zygomaticus major m.

Splenius m.

Omohyoid m.

Sternocleidomastoid m. (Clavicular head)

Sternocleidomastoid m. (Sternal head)

Levator scapulae m.

Platysma m.

Deltoid m.

Pectoralis major m.

Latissimus dorsi m.

Coracobrachialis m.

Biceps brachii m. (short head)

Biceps brachii m. (long head)

Serratus anterior m.

Biceps brachii m.

Linea alba

Triceps m.

Brachialis m.

Rectus abdominis m.

Brachioradialis m.

Extensor carpi radialis longus m.

Bicipital aponeurosis

External oblique m.

Flexor carpi radialis m.

Palmaris longus m.

Flexor carpi ulnaris m.

Flexor digitorum superficialis m.

Brachioradialis m.

Pronator teres m.

Flexor carpi radialis m.

Extensor carpi radialis longus m.

Extensor carpi radialis brevis m.

Extensor digitorum m.

Extensor retinaculum

Anterior
Superior
Iliac Spine

Extensor digiti minimi m.

Extensor retinaculum

Iliopsoas m.

Pectineus m.

Adductor longus m.

Sartorius m.

Pudendal n.

Pubic
tubercle

Gracilis m.

Tensor fascia latae m.

Vastus lateralis m.

Vastus medialis m.

Rectus femoris m.

Tensor fascia latae m.

Patella

Gastrocnemius m.

Tibialis anterior m.

Peroneus longus m.

Extensor digitorum longus m.

Tibia

Soleus m.

Superior extensor retinaculum

Medial maleolus

Lateral maleolus